Te Linde's
Operative
Gynecology

NINTH EDITION

John A. Rock, MD
Chancellor
Louisiana State University Health Sciences Center
Professor
Department of Gynecology and Obstetrics
Louisiana State University School of Medicine
New Orleans, Louisiana

Howard W. Jones III, MD
Director
Department of Gynecology and Obstetrics
Vanderbilt University Medical Center
Nashville, Tennessee

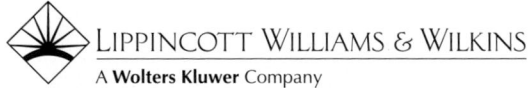
LIPPINCOTT WILLIAMS & WILKINS
A **Wolters Kluwer** Company

Acquisitions Editor: *Lisa McAllister*
Developmental Editor: *Tanya Lazar*
Production Editor: *Patrick Carr*
Manufacturing Manager: *Benjamin Rivera*
Cover Designer: *Marsha Cohen*
Indexer: *Ann Blum*
Compositor: *Graphic World*
Printer: *Quebecor-World*

9 8 7 6 5 4 3 2 1

Library of Congress Cataloging-in-Publication Data
te Lind's operative gynecology.--9th ed. / [edited by] John A. Rock, Howard W. Jones III.
    p. ; cm.
  Includes bibliographical references and index.
  ISBN 0-7817-2859-2
    1. Generative organs, Female—Surgery. I. Title: Operative gynecology. II. Te Linde.
Richard W. (Richard Wesley), 1894– III. Rock, John A. IV. Jones, Howard W. (Howard
Wilbur), 1942–
  [DNLM: 1. Gynecologic Surgical Procedures. WP 660 T2721 2003]
RG104.T4 2003
618.1′45—dc21

                                                            2003045803

Care has been taken to confirm the accuracy of the information presented and to describe generally accepted practices. However, the authors, editors, and publisher are not responsible for errors or omissions or for any consequences from application of the information in this book and make no warranty, expressed or implied, with respect to the contents of the publication.

The authors, editors, and publisher have exerted every effort to ensure that drug selection and dosage set forth in this text are in accordance with current recommendations and practice at the time of publication. However, in view of ongoing research, changes in government regulations, and the constant flow of information relating to drug therapy and drug reactions, the reader is urged to check the package insert for each drug for any change in indications and dosage and for added warnings and precautions. This is particularly important when the recommended agent is a new or infrequently employed drug.

Some drugs and medical devices presented in this publication have Food and Drug Administration (FDA) clearance for limited use in restricted research settings. It is the responsibility of the health care provider to ascertain the FDA status of each drug or device planned for use in their clinical practice.

Leon Schlossberg was an illustrator in the Department of Surgery and an educator in the Department of Art as Applied to Medicine at Johns Hopkins University until his death in 1999. During his career, which spanned over sixty years, Mr. Schlossberg inspired countless surgeons, clinicians, and students throughout the world with his elegant portrayals of surgical techniques. His illustrations are respected for their anatomical accuracy, ability to educate, and creativity.

Mr. Schlossberg has been a contributor to *Operative Gynecology* ever since Dr. Richard W. Te Linde published the first edition in 1946. He studied the work of Max Brödel, his mentor at the Johns Hopkins University Department of Art as Applied to Medicine. Leon's intricate, detailed illustrations of anatomy in surgical procedures are reflective of his passion for living, functional anatomy. Just as many of Max Brödel's original illustrations are still included in the ninth edition of *TeLinde's Operative Gynecology*, Leon Schlossberg has over 45 illustrations in this edition, in addition to those of his students.

As was noted by Gary Lees, Chair of the Department of Art as Applied to Medicine at Johns Hopkins University, "he and his work are respected for their anatomical accuracy and artistic creativity." He has been recognized as "the dean of medical illustrators because of his wide range of knowledge and tenure in depicting surgery and anatomy."

In appreciation, the ninth edition of *TeLinde's Operative Gynecology* is respectfully dedicated to Leon Schlossberg.

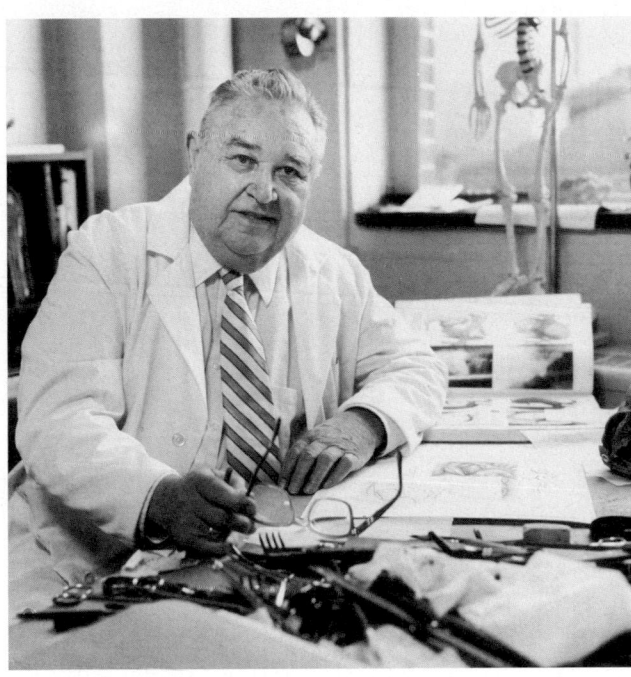

A scholarship fund has been established in the Department of Art as Applied to Medicine to honor Leon Schlossberg's legacy to medical science, medical education, and medical illustration. Contributions can be made to:

The Leon Schlossberg Scholarship Fund
C/o The Fund for Johns Hopkins Medicine
One Charles Center
100 North Charles Street, Suite 200
Baltimore, Maryland 21201

More information about the Fund or the Department of Art as Applied to Medicine can be obtained at (410) 955-3213.

Contents

Contributors

Nadeem R. Abu-Rustum, MD
Director of Minimally Invasive Surgery
Department of Surgery
Memorial Sloan-Kettering Cancer Center
New York, New York

Rony A. Adam, MD
Assistant Professor
Department of Gynecology and Obstetrics
Emory University
Director, Division of Gynecology and Section of
Urogynecology and Pelvic Reconstructive
Surgery
Department of Gynecology and Obstetrics
Emory University Hospital
Atlanta, Georgia
Grady Memorial Hospital
Atlanta, Georgia

Mark D. Adelson, MD
Clinical Professor
Department of Obstetrics and Gynecology
State University of New York—Upstate Medical
Center
Syracuse, New York
Director
Comprehensive Gynecology, PC
Syracuse, New York

Kaled M. Alektiar, MD
Memorial Sloan Kettering Cancer Center
Department of Radiation Oncology
New York, New York

Michael P. Aronson, MD
Associate Professor
Department of Obstetrics and Gynecology
University of Massachusetts Medical School
Worcester, Massachusetts
Director, Women's Health Services
Department of Obstetrics and Gynecology
University of Massachusetts Medical Center
Worcester, Massachusetts

Michael S. Baggish, MD
Chairman
Department of Obstetrics and Gynecology
Good Samaritan Hospital
Director, Residency Education
Department of Obstetrics and Gynecology
TriHealth Medical System (Good Samaritan
Hospital, Bethesda Hospital)
Professor
Obstetrics and Gynecology
University of Cincinnati College of Medicine
Cincinnati, Ohio

Jack B. Basil, MD
Assistant Professor
Department of Gynecology and Obstetrics
Emory University School of Medicine
Emory University Hospital
Atlanta, Georgia

Lesley L. Breech, MD
Assistant Professor
Department of Gynecology and Obstetrics
Emory University School of Medicine
Attending Physician
Department of Gynecology and Obstetrics
Emory University Hospital
Atlanta, Georgia

Gert H. Brieger, MD, PHD
Distinguished Service Professor
Johns Hopkins University School of Medicine
Baltimore, Maryland

Joseph B. Bruner, MD
Associate Professor
Department of Obstetrics and Gynecology
Vanderbilt University School of Medicine
Nashville, Tennessee

James Joseph Burke II, MD
Assistant Professor
Department of Obstetrics and Gynecology
Mercer University School of Medicine
Savannah, Georgia
Staff
Department of Obstetrics and Gynecology
Memorial Health University Medical Center
Savannah, Georgia

Thomas W. Burke, MD
Professor
Department of Gynecologic Oncology
The University of Texas M.D. Anderson Cancer
    Center
Houston, Texas

Joseph Buscema, MD
Assistant Professor
Department of Obstetrics and Gynecology
The Johns Hopkins University Medical
    Institutions
The Johns Hopkins Hospital
Lutherville, Maryland
Director of Gynecology and Obstetrics
The Cancer Center at St. Agnes Healthcare
Baltimore, Maryland

William J. Butler, MD
Professor
Department of Obstetrics and Gynecology
Mercer University School of Medicine
Macon, Georgia
Director
Central Georgia Fertility Institute
Medical Center of Central Georgia
Macon, Georgia

Dennis S. Chi, MD
Director, Fellowship Program, Gynecology Service
Co-Director, Pelvic Reconstructive Surgery,
    Department of Surgery
Memorial Sloan-Kettering Cancer Center
New York, New York

William T. Creasman, MD
J. Marion Sims Professor
Department of Obstetrics and Gynecology
Medical University of South Carolina
Charleston, South Carolina

Mark A. Damario, MD
Associate Professor
Department of Obstetrics, Gynecology, and
    Women's Health
University of Minnesota
Minneapolis, Minnesota
Medical Director
Reproductive Medicine Center
Minneapolis, Minnesota

John O. L. DeLancey, MD
Norman F. Miller Professor of Gynecology
Department of Obstetrics and Gynecology
University of Michigan Health System
Ann Arbor, Michigan

Celia E. Dominguez, MD
Assistant Professor
Department of Gynecology and Obstetrics
Emory University
Atlanta, Georgia
Grady Memorial Hospital
Department of Gynecology and Obstetrics
Atlanta, Georgia

James H. Dorsey, MD
Assistant Professor and Chair
Greater Baltimore Medical Center
Baltimore, Maryland

Donald George Gallup, MD
Professor
Department of Obstetrics and Gynecology
Mercer University School of Medicine
Savannah, Georgia
Chairman
Department of Obstetrics and Gynecology
Memorial Health University Medical Center
Savannah, Georgia

David M. Gershenson, MD
Professor and Chairman
Department of Gynecologic Oncology
University of Texas M.D. Anderson Cancer
    Center
Houston, Texas

Victor Gomel, MD
Professor and Head
Department of Obstetrics and Gynecology
University of British Columbia
Vancouver, British Columbia
Canada

Victoria L. Green, MD, MHSA, MBA, JD
Associate Professor
Department of Gynecology and Obstetrics
Emory University
Atlanta, Georgia

David A. Grimes, MD
Clinical Professor
Department of Obstetrics and Gynecology
University of North Carolina
Chapel Hill, North Carolina
Attending Physician
Department of Obstetrics and Gynecology
University of North Carolina Hospitals
Chapel Hill, North Carolina

Marvin H. Terry Grody, MD
Professor
Department of Obstetrics and Gynecology
Robert Wood Johnson School of Medicine
University of Medicine and Dentistry of New Jersey
Camden, New Jersey
Senior Attending Consultant
Division of Female Pelvic Medicine and
    Reconstructive Surgery
Department of Obstetrics and Gynecology
Cooper Hospital Health System
Camden, New Jersey

W. David Hager, MD, FACOG
Professor
Department of Obstetrics and Gynecology
University of Kentucky, Chandler Medical Center
Lexington, Kentucky
Director
University of Kentucky Affiliated Residency
    Training Program
Department of Obstetrics and Gynecology
Central Baptist Hospital
Lexington, Kentucky

John S. Hesla, MD
Medical Director
Portland Center for Reproductive Medicine
Clinical Assistant Professor
Oregon Health and Sciences University School of
    Medicine
Portland, Oregon

Mitchel Scott Hoffman, MD
Professor and Director
Division of Gynecologic Oncology
Department of Obstetrics and Gynecology
University of South Florida College of Medicine
Tampa, Florida
Medical Doctor and Professor
Department of Obstetrics and Gynecology
Tampa General Hospital
Tampa, Florida

Ira R. Horowitz, MD
Professor
Department of Gynecology and Obstetrics
Emory University School of Medicine
Atlanta, Georgia

William J. Hoskins, MD
Professor
Department of Obstetrics and Gynecology
Mercer University School of Medicine
Savannah, Georgia
Director and Senior Vice-President
The Curtis and Elizabeth Anderson Cancer
    Institute
Memorial Health University Medical Center
Savannah, Georgia

Barry K. Jarnagin, MD
Assistant Professor
Department of Obstetrics and Gynocology
Vanderbilt University Medical Center
Vanderbilt Hospital
Nashville, Tennessee

Howard W. Jones, Jr., MD
Professor Emeritus
Department of Obstetrics and Gynecology
Eastern Virginia Medical School
Norfolk, Virginia

Howard W. Jones III, MD
Department of Gynecology and Obstetrics
Vanderbilt University Medical Center
Nashville, Tennessee

Mickey Karram, MD
Professor
Department of Obstetrics and Gynecology
University of Cincinnati
Director of Urogynecology
Department of Obstetrics and Gynecology
Good Samaritan Hospital
Cincinnati, Ohio

Steven D. Kleeman, MD
Clinical Assistant Professor
Department of Obstetrics and Gynecology
Wright State University
Dayton, Ohio
Clinical Instructor
Department of Obstetrics and Gynecology
Good Samaritan Hospital
Cincinnati, Ohio

Raymond A. Lee, MD
Professor
Department of Obstetrics and Gynecology
Division of Gynecologic Surgery
Mayo Clinic
Rochester, Minnesota

Frank W. Ling, MD
Professor and Chairman
Department of Obstetrics and Gynecology
University of Tennessee
Memphis, Tennessee

Gary H. Lipscomb, MD
Professor
Department of Obstetrics and Gynecology
University of Tennessee
Memphis, Tennessee
Chief
Division of Gynecology
Department of Obstetrics and Gynecology
Regional Medical Center
Memphis, Tennessee

Bhagirath Majmudar, MD
Professor
Department of Pathology
Associate Professor
Department of Obstetrics and Gynecology
Emory University
Atlanta, Georgia
Pathologist
Department of Pathology
Grady Health System
Atlanta, Georgia

Sanford M. Markham, MD
Associate Professor
Department of Obstetrics and Gynecology
University of Iowa Hospitals and Clinics
Iowa City, Iowa
Department of Obstetrics and Gynecology
Roy J. and Lucille A. Carver College of Medicine
Iowa City, Iowa

Mark G. Martens, MD
Professor
Department of Obstetrics and Gynecology
University of Oklahoma
Tulsa, Oklahoma
Vice Chairman for Research
Director, Division of
    Obstetrics/Gynecology/Infectious Disease
Hillcrest Medical Center
Tulsa, Oklahoma

G. Rodney Meeks, MD
Professor
Department of Obstetrics and Gynecology
University of Mississippi Medical Center
Jackson, Mississippi

Luis E. Mendez, MD
Assistant Professor
Department of Obstetrics and Gynecology
Division of Gynecologic Oncology
University of Miami/Sylvester Cancer Center
Miami, Florida
Department of Obstetrics and Gynecology
Division of Gynecologic Oncology
Jackson Memorial Medical Center
Miami, Florida

Kelly L. Molpus, MD
Associate Professor and Director
Department of Gynecologic Oncology
Vice-President
Department of Obstetrics and Gynecology
University of Nebraska Medical Center
Omaha, Nebraska

Frederick J. Montz, MD
Professor and Director
The Kelly Gynecologic Oncology Service
Johns Hopkins University School of Medicine
Baltimore, Maryland
Professor
Department of Gynecology and Obstetrics
Johns Hopkins Hospital and Medical Institution
Baltimore, Maryland

Ana Alvarez Murphy, MD
Anne Winship Bates Leach Professor
Department of Gynecology and Obstetrics
Emory University School of Medicine
Atlanta, Georgia

Anne Brawner Namnoum, MD
Assistant Professor
Division of Reproductive Endocrinology
Department of Obstetrics and Gynecology
Emory University/Crawford Long Hospital
Atlanta, Georgia

Lynn P. Parker, MD
Assistant Professor
Department of Obstetrics and Gynecology
Division of Gynecologic Oncology
Vanderbilt University Medical Center
Nashville, Tennessee

Manuel Penalver, MD
Professor and Chairman
Department of Obstetrics and Gynecology
University of Miami School of Medicine
Miami, Florida
Chairman and Chief of Service
Department of Obstetrics and Gynecology
Jackson Memorial Hospital
Miami, Florida

Herbert B. Peterson, MD
Reproductive Health and Research
World Health Organization
Geneva, Switzerland

Amy E. Pollack, MD, MPH
Adjunct Assistant Professor
Mailman School of Public Health
Columbia University
New York, New York
President
Endgenderhealth
New York, New York

John Aubrey Rock, MD
Professor and Chancellor
Department of Gynecology and Obstetrics
Louisiana State University Health Sciences Center
New Orleans, Louisiana

Robert M. Rogers, Jr., MD
Attending Gynecologist
Department of Obstetrics and Gynecology
The Reading Hospital and Medical Center
West Reading, Pennsylvania

Audrey A. Romero, MD
Assistant Professor
Department of Obstetrics and Gynecology
University of New Mexico School of Medicine
Albuquerque, New Mexico

Kenneth J. Ryan, MD
Professor and Chairman Emeritus
Department of Obstetrics and Gynecology and
    Reproductive Biology
Harvard Medical Center
Boston, Massachusetts
Chief Emeritus
Department of Obstetrics and Gynecology
Brigham & Women's Hospital
Boston, Massachusetts

Joseph S. Sanfilippo, MD
Professor
Department of Obstetrics and Gynecology
MCP Hahnemann School of Medicine
Philadelphia, Pennsylvania
Chairman
Department of Obstetrics and Gynecology
Allegheny General Hospital
Pittsburgh, Pennsylvania

Kenneth W. Sharp, MD
Professor and Division Chief, General Surgery
Department of Surgery
Vanderbilt University Medical Center
Nashville, Tennessee

Bob L. Shull, MD
Professor
Department of Obstetrics and Gynecology
Texas A&M Health Sciences Center
Temple, Texas
Professor
Department of Obstetrics and Gynecology
Scott & White Clinic and Hospital
Temple, Texas

Harriet O. Smith, MD
Professor
Department of Obstetrics and Gynecology
Director
Division of Gynecologic Oncology
University of New Mexico Health Sciences Center
Albuquerque, New Mexico

Richard Mathew Soderstrom, MD
Clinical Professor
Department of Obstetrics and Gynecology
University of Washington School of Medicine
Seattle, Washington
Emeritus Staff
Department of Obstetrics and Gynecology
Swedish Medical Center
Seattle, Washington

Betty Ruth Speir, MD
Clinical Associate Professor
Department of Obstetrics and Gynecology
Clinical Professor
General Surgery
University of South Alabama School of Medicine
Mobile, Alabama

John F. Steege, MD
Professor and Chief
Division of Advanced Laparoscopy and
    Gynecological Surgery
Department of Obstetrics and Gynecology
University of North Carolina
Chapel Hill, North Carolina

L. Lewis Wall, MD, D. PHIL
Department of Obstetrics and Gynecology
Cedars-Sinai Medical Center
Los Angeles, California

Charles J. Ward, MD, FACOG, FACS
Associate Professor
Department of Obstetrics and Gynecology
Emory University
Atlanta, Georgia

Jeffrey S. Warshaw, MD
Assistant Professor and Director of
    Urogynecology
Department of Obstetrics and Gynecology
University of Minnesota School of Medicine
Hennepin County Medical Center
Minneapolis, Minnesota

Carl Zimmerman, MD
Clinical Professor
Department of Obstetrics and Gynecology
Vanderbilt University Medical Center
Nashville, Tennessee

Preface

Over the past decade the field of gynecologic surgery has rapidly advanced. Advances in suture material, adhesion prevention, instrumentation, and video technology have resulted in more efficient and successful surgical procedures. Cutting edge robotics may forecast a time where the gynecologic surgeon operates with safety and accuracy "away" from the patient. Nevertheless, new vistas will certainly challenge the surgeon to rethink his or her surgical approach.

The ninth edition of *Te Linde's Operative Gynecology* presents a synthesis of current gynecologic surgical practice. This edition was undertaken in recognition of the rapid changes encountered in the practice of gynecology. With the introduction of new procedures, there is a need to address their efficacy and critically evaluate their place in the surgical armamentarium. The contributors to *Te Linde's Operative Gynecology* look at previous experience in light of advances to try to clarify what is "state of the art" in gynecologic surgery.

This edition of *Te Linde's Operative Gynecology* reflects not only the basic, sound principles for established gynecologic surgical techniques, but also what is new and controversial in the sometimes slow and steady advance of knowledge in the field. Also considered is the often surprisingly quick-changing landscape of operative gynecology: reproductive technologies that allow the creation of life, and the surgical techniques that relieve suffering, correct anatomical defects, and save lives. Major topics have been addressed, building on past editions, with twenty-four new authors who have updated or totally rewritten chapters. There are new illustrations and figures in the chapters on Leiomyoma Uteri and Myomectomy, Breast Diseases, and Surgical Conditions of the Vagina and Urethra, among many others.

A new chapter, Training the Gynecologic Surgeon, by Robert M. Rogers, Jr. is a valuable addition to this text. Dr. Rogers addresses the issues of how to train surgeons in newer surgical modalities such as laparoscopic and hysteroscopic techniques, and the pressures faced in training a new generation of gynecologists facing reimbursement and financial crises. The chapter on pelvic support has also been extensively revised to reflect the latest concepts of pelvic anatomy and new concepts concerning correction of pelvic support defects. Featured in this edition is the study tool of an Appendix of questions and answers for each chapter. We thank Nathaniel Zoneraich, MD, and Ellen Hayes, MD, Reproductive Fellows at Emory University School of Medicine, and residents in Obstetrics and Gynecology at Vanderbilt University for their efforts in writing the questions for many chapters.

The editors thank all of the contributing authors and gratefully acknowledge the assistance of Claire Hackworth, Glenda Walker, Lynne Black, and Patsy Shepherd, and the editorial team of Lippincott Williams & Wilkins: Lisa McAllister, Tanya Lazar, Patrick Carr, and designer Marsha Cohen, for their attention to details and hard work in the preparation of this book. As always, we are deeply indebted to those authors and editors who have labored to write the previous editions of this text; the current edition would not exist without their dedication. We owe a sincere debt of gratitude to Drs. Richard W. Te Linde, Richard Mattingly, and John D. Thompson.

TE LINDE'S
Operative Gynecology
NINTH EDITION

GENERAL TOPICS AFFECTING GYNECOLOGIC SURGERY PRACTICE

Te Linde's Operative Gynecology, ninth edition, edited by John A. Rock and Howard W. Jones, III. Lippincott Williams & Wilkins, Philadelphia, © 2003.

CHAPTER

1

▼

A Brief History of Operative Gynecology

GERT H. BRIEGER

Gynecology, spelled gynaecology, is defined by the *Oxford English Dictionary* as "That department of medical science which treats of the functions and diseases peculiar to women." The word was first used as such in the middle of the 19th century. In 1867, gynecology represented the physiology and pathology of the nonpregnant state. Although most histories of gynecology trace its roots back to antiquity, the field of medicine we call by that name today really has had a fairly recent origin. The successful removal of an ovarian tumor by Ephraim McDowell in 1809 was as rare an event as it was a spectacular one. In the preceding centuries, the history of gynecologic surgery was closely tied to the history of general surgery, and the obstacles that had to be overcome were the same. Infection, hemorrhage and shock, and pain were all effective barriers to any but emergency surgical procedures in the days before anesthesia.

"The history of gynecology," Howard Kelly wrote in 1912, "seems to me more full of dramatic interest than the evolution of any other medical or surgical specialty." Himself an accomplished historian of medicine, among his many other skills, Kelly noted that, "It was, notably, anesthesia which robbed surgery of its horrors, asepsis which robbed it of its dangers, and cellular pathology which came as a godsend to enable the operator to discriminate between malignant and non-malignant growths." Here, in a nutshell, we have the landmarks of much of the history of gynecology of the last 150 years.

There are many ways to approach the history of a medical and surgical specialty such as gynecology. The usual practice in textbooks that make an attempt to include some history is to tell the story in terms of who discovered what and who did which operation first. These facts are of interest but hardly constitute the history of the field. Besides the surgical operations of gynecology, the techniques devised, and the instruments to carry them out, there is much to be learned from the changing picture of diseases and their diagnoses; from the professionalization of the field, including the societies, journals, and textbooks that have been created; and from the education required to master the science and practice of operative gynecology. It is in these terms, rather than in tracing simply the great ideas and their creators, that this historical introduction proceeds.

Any major medical textbook can itself serve as a convenient window through which we can see history unfold. Robert Hahn has vividly described the changing world view of obstetrics by examining the succeeding editions of Williams' *Obstetrics* since its first edition in 1903. Likewise, the 50 years that have elapsed since the first edition of Richard Wesley Te Linde's *Operative Gynecology* provide an equal opportunity to describe the major developments in the companion field of gynecology.

BARRIERS TO SURGICAL PROGRESS

In ancient times, the lack of real anatomic knowledge was a barrier to the development of surgery. It is sometimes said that because the ancient Egyptians had effective techniques for the evisceration of bodies for mummification, they must have had a good knowledge of the body. However, removal of the internal organs during the embalming process was performed by technicians who did not concern themselves with the structure of the bodies they were preparing.

Anatomy was pursued in Alexandria during the Hellenistic period, but it had few, if any, practical applications until a later time. By the end of the 13th century, anatomic dissection again became more common, but often it was limited to one or two public dissections a year or the study of animals. Surgeons were responsible for the few autopsies that were performed to determine the cause of death. This was especially important if a crime was suspected or drowning had to be established.

Soranus, the Roman physician and writer who practiced in the reign of the Emperors Trajan (98–117) and Hadrian (117–138), is perhaps best known for his text entitled, *Gynecology*. This book is somewhat mistitled because it is mostly devoted to what we would call obstetrics. Soranus wrote about prenatal and postnatal problems, as well as those associated with delivery itself. This ancient text has been translated and has an excellent introduction by Owsei Temkin. Recently, it has been reissued in a paperback edition.

Although Soranus' *Gynecology* still makes interesting reading, it hardly qualifies as an early text on the subject of operative gynecology. However, like other physicians of his time, Soranus clearly noted that the best midwife was one who was trained in all branches of therapy, ". . . for some cases must be treated by diet, others by surgery, while still others must be cured by drugs."

Although there were instances of human anatomy in earlier times, we generally begin the story with the work of Andreas Vesalius and the publication of his *De humani corporis fabrica* in 1543. Before this time, anatomic knowledge was not tied to the teaching and practice of medicine. The tradition of the surgeon-anatomists, of whom Vesalius was a stellar example, culminated in the late 18th century with the work of the English surgical teacher John Hunter (1728–1793) and his older brother William (1718–1783). It was William's classic book about the gravid uterus with its detailed engravings that shed new light on the structures of the female pelvis.

In the 19th century, for all types of surgery, the problems of pain, hemorrhage, and infection had to be solved before operations could be undertaken safely. The problems of surgical dressings and postoperative infections were generally a matter of trial and error. The Scottish surgeon and gynecologist Sir James Simpson (1811–1870) urged his surgical colleagues to perform their operations on the kitchen tables of their patients to avoid the dangers of hospital infections, or "hospitalism" as it came to be called.

In the 1840s, the Hungarian obstetrician Ignaz Semmelweis (1818–1865) showed clearly that puerperal fever could be prevented by disinfecting the hands of doctors before they examined their patients during the course of delivery. Despite good statistical evidence, his method of washing hands in chlorinated lime solution was not widely adopted. In fact, it met with outright resistance from most physicians. In this country, the Harvard anatomist and writer Oliver Wendell Holmes (1809–1894) met similar disbelief and resistance when he suggested in 1842 that it was the physicians themselves who were carrying the dreaded puerperal infections to their patients.

In the middle 1860s, Joseph Lister (1827–1912), while working in Glasgow, began experiments using carbolic acid, a phenol derivative, to clean the instruments, sutures, and dressings he was using in his operations. He based his work on an understanding of the germ theory of disease, which was then just in its infancy as a major theory of disease causation. Lister believed it was important to prevent the germs present in the air or on instruments and sutures from entering the wound, which would prevent the formation of the heretofore much desired laudable pus. Lister, too, met much opposition to his method of antisepsis. Partly because of the frequent changes in the system he was developing, which made it difficult for others to follow him, and because of the inadequate understanding of the germ theory by most surgeons, it took nearly two decades for antiseptic surgery to become routine. In Lister's case, as was also true for Holmes and Semmelweis, some of the resistance undoubtedly stemmed from the fact that doctors never like being told that what they are doing is actually causing harm to their patients.

Lister encountered a great deal of opposition, particularly in his own country. Lawson Tait (1845–1899), an active and polemical gynecologist who settled in Birmingham, was staunchly opposed to Lister's system of antisepsis. Tait paid much attention to general cleanliness when he was operating, and he actually achieved quite good results. However, his older colleague, Spencer Wells (1818–1897) of London, was a devoted follower of the antiseptic system in his many ovarian operations, perhaps because he had a clear grasp of the role of microbes. In 1864, the year before Lister began using carbolic acid in Glasgow and 3 years before he published his first results, Wells published a paper in the *British Medical Journal* entitled "Some Causes of Excessive Mortality After Surgical Operations." Wells clearly described the recent work on germs by Louis Pasteur (1822–1895) in France. There is no definite proof that Lister was aware of the paper, but it is hard to imagine that he did not know what was appearing in the national medical journal. Thus, gynecologists probably had a much greater hand in the development of safe surgery in the last century than is usually acknowledged.

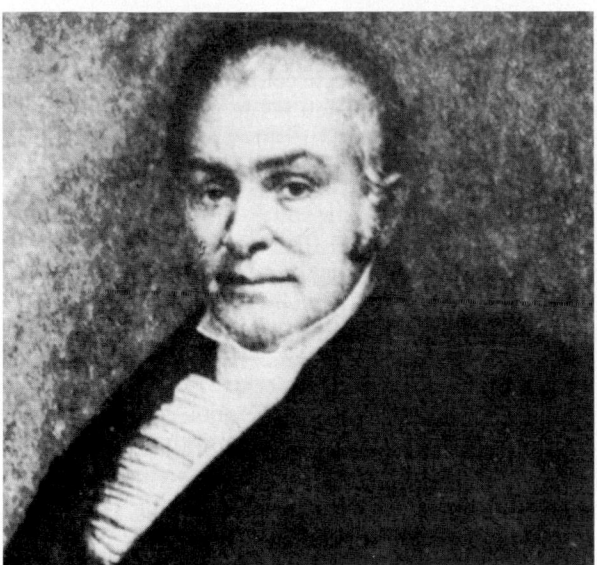

FIGURE 1.1. Ephraim McDowell (1771–1830). One of the earliest abdominal surgeons.

BEGINNINGS OF GYNECOLOGIC SURGERY IN 19TH-CENTURY AMERICA

Opening the abdominal cavity to remove extrauterine pregnancies was successfully accomplished several times in the later 18th century but did not become routine until the advent of anesthesia and antisepsis/asepsis. Ephraim McDowell (1771–1830) (Fig. 1.1) made surgical history with his successful removal of a large ovarian cyst in his patient Jane Todd Crawford, who in 1809 rode 60 miles to her doctor's house in Danville, Kentucky, to undergo an untried operation without any assurance of cure and without the benefit of anesthesia. Although McDowell is often referred to as a backwoods physician, he was in fact a well-trained surgeon. His Edinburgh training probably gave him confidence in his diagnosis and courage to attempt a surgical cure rather than have his patient face certain death from her relentlessly growing tumor. During his study tour in Scotland, he probably heard that in the previous century the popular surgical teacher John Hunter had suggested such an operation, believing that "women could bear spaying just as well as did animals."

The drama of McDowell's case is best described in the words of the surgeon himself:

> In December, 1809, I was called to see a Mrs. Crawford, who had for several months thought herself pregnant. She was affected with pains similar to labor pains, from which she could find no relief. So strong was the presumption of her being in the last stage of pregnancy, that two physicians, who were consulted on her case, requested my aid in delivering her. The abdomen was considerably enlarged, and had the appearance of pregnancy, though the inclination of the tumor was to one side, admitting of an easy removal to the other. Upon examination, per vaginum, I found
> nothing in the uterus; which induced the conclusion that it must be an enlarged ovarium. Having never seen so large a substance extracted, nor heard of an attempt, or success attending any operation, such as this required, I gave to the unhappy woman information of her dangerous situation. She appeared willing to undergo an experiment, which I promised to perform if she would come to Danville. . . . With the assistance of my nephew and colleague, James McDowell, M.D., I commenced the operation, which was concluded as follows: Having placed her on a table of the ordinary height, on her back, and removed all her dressing which might in any way impede the operation, I made an incision about three inches from the musculus rectus abdominis, on the left side, continuing the same nine inches in length, parallel with the fibers of the above named muscle, extending into the cavity of the abdomen, the parietes of which were a good deal contused, which we ascribed to the resting of the tumor on the horn of the saddle during her journey. The tumor then appeared in full view, but was so large that we could not take it away entire. We put a strong ligature around the fallopian tube near to the uterus; we then cut open the tumor, which was the ovarium and fibrinous part of the fallopian tube very much enlarged. We took out fifteen pounds of a dirty, gelatinous looking substance. After which we cut through the fallopian tube, and extracted the sack, which weighed seven pounds and one half. As soon as the external opening was made, the intestines rushed out upon the table; and so completely was the abdomen filled by the tumor, that they could not be replaced during the operation, which was terminated in about twenty-five minutes. We then turned her upon her left side, so as to permit the blood to escape; after which, we closed the external opening with the interrupted suture, leaving out, at the lower end of the incision, the ligature which surrounded the fallopian tube. Between every two stitches we put a strip of adhesive plaster, which, by keeping the parts in contact, hastened the healing of the incision. We then applied the usual dressing, put her to bed, and prescribed a strict observance of the antiphlogistic regimen. In five days I visited her, and much to my astonishment found her engaged in making up her bed. I gave her particular caution for the future; and in twenty five days, she returned home as she came, in good health, which she continues to enjoy.

McDowell's patient long outlived her surgeon. He did not publish his feat until 1816, by which time he had performed several more oophorectomies. McDowell is sometimes cited as a pioneer of early ambulation, unwitting as it was in his case. If his sturdy patient had not recovered so well, her failure would surely have been blamed on rising too early from her bed after such extensive surgery. McDowell also did not mention the intense drama of this Christmas Day operation. When the townsfolk of Danville heard about his plan, they were incensed. They gathered in a tense group outside his house, with a rope slung over a tree, ready to lynch the surgeon if his "experiment" proved a failure. McDowell certainly had the nature of a true pioneer.

T.G. Thomas, in his 1876 centennial review of obstetrics and gynecology, reported that Alexander Dunlap of Springfield, Ohio claimed he did his first ovarian operation in 1843. Dunlap said he sent the report of this case to a medical journal, which sent it back to him saying that they "could not publish the case of such an unjustifiable operation."

By 1876, Thomas wrote, "It is to estimate the amount of good this operation has bestowed upon humanity. Practised today in every civilized country in the world, yielding the statistics of seventy to seventy-five per cent of recoveries, and daily being improved in its various steps, it may well be regarded as one of the greatest surgical triumphs of the century."

In the middle decades of the 19th century, another American surgeon working in the South helped to popularize gynecologic surgery by another set of pioneering feats. James Marion Sims (1813–1883) told the dramatic tale of his development of a successful technique to repair vesicovaginal fistulas in his widely read autobiography *The Story of My Life,* which was published the year after his death (Fig. 1.2). He described his repeated attempts to achieve a permanent closure of these fistulas in a few of his young slave-women patients. Sims began his experiments in 1845 and continued them for 4 years. In these preanesthesia and preantiseptic days, Sims produced remarkable results. He had had no experience in pelvic surgery, and in fact claimed that he disliked it. It was his custom to turn away patients with pelvic disorders, referring them to other doctors in his Alabama neighborhood. Many of his planter friends owned slaves, some of whom suffered from vesicovaginal fistulas as a result of traumatic births. These wounds were considered incurable and made the young women unacceptable for household work. After several entreaties to help one of his planter friends who had such a slave, Sims began with a small group of women, operating on some of them repeatedly over the course of 4 years.

Sims' many failures only increased his determination to succeed. The colleagues who at first assisted him at the

operations abandoned him, and his friends, he claimed, begged him to give up what was considered to be a hopeless effort. He trained other young slave patients to assist him, and on his 29th operation on one of the patients, he finally succeeded. In reviewing his work in 1852, Sims did cite several successful cases by other American surgeons between 1839 and 1849. He claimed originality for:

> 1st. for the discovery of a method by which the vagina can be thoroughly explored, and the operation easily performed [the Sims, or lateral, position]. 2nd. For the introduction of a new suture apparatus, which lies imbedded in the tissues for an indefinite period without danger of cutting its way out, as do silk ligatures. And 3rd. For the invention of a self-retaining catheter, which can be worn with the greatest comfort by the patient during the whole process of treatment.

The new "suture apparatus" used silver wire. This provided the breakthrough needed for the successful repair of vesico-vaginal fistulae. Sims used silver in many of his other operations. In a tenth anniversary lecture at the New York Academy of Medicine in 1858, Sims somewhat immodestly told his august audience that the use of silver suture was one of the great achievements of 19th-century surgery.

On the 21st of June in 1849, Sims proclaimed, "After nearly four years of fruitless labor, silver wire was fortunately substituted, for silk as a suture, and lo! a new era dawns upon surgery."

Sims soon left the South, and after a stay in Europe during the Civil War, he settled in New York, where a newly founded Woman's Hospital allowed him to develop gynecologic surgery with great success. With the advent of anesthesia and the use of antiseptic techniques, such surgery became increasingly routine. The repair of vesicovaginal fistulas and the removal of ovaries for a wide variety of indications were the beginning of the field of operative gynecology as it is known today. The story is, of course, not purely an American one. The English, French, and German contributions were important and can be found in any general history of medicine or of obstetrics and gynecology. In 1876 Sims became President of the American Medical Association, and in the same year he and others founded the American Gynecological Association.

Even with the advent of effective and relatively safe anesthesia after 1846, it was several decades before surgeons were ready to increase the number of their operations. At mid-century and during the Civil War in the 1860s, surgery was generally confined to amputations after accidents; hernia repair when the intestine became incarcerated in the hernia sac, thus threatening life; an occasional ligation of a major vessel for aneurysm; and cystotomy for bladder stones. Therefore, Sims, operating in the 1840s, was truly a pioneer.

Also pioneers in the field of gynecologic surgery by mid-century were the Atlee brothers of Lancaster, Pennsylvania. They rediscovered oophorectomy, which was also being done in England by the 1860s, and were among the early leaders who performed myomectomy for fibroid tumors of the uterus.

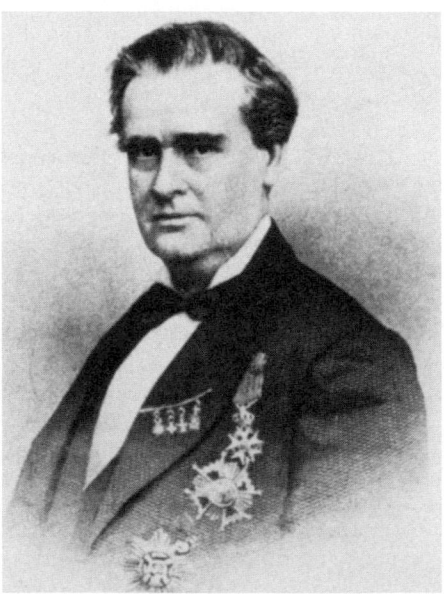

FIGURE 1.2. James Marion Sims (1813–1883).

Of semantic interest is the changing terminology for ovarian surgery. Ovariotomy, often used imprecisely to refer to removal of the ovary, actually was first used in that way in the 1850s by James Simpson and other British gynecologists. Ovariotomy means to cut into the ovary for removal of a cyst or tumor. In the 1870s, gynecologists such as Edmund Peaslee of New York, in his book on ovarian tumors, stated that oophorectomy was a more precise and distinctive term for removal of the ovary.

John Light Atlee (1799–1885) actively practiced medicine for 65 years, during which time he performed over 2,000 operations and attended 3,200 births. John Atlee performed 78 ovarian operations between 1843 and 1883, with 64 recoveries and only 14 deaths. Thus, he validated McDowell's work of the early part of the 19th century. Atlee's younger brother, Washington Lemuel Atlee (1808–1878) (Fig. 1.3), also was involved in some of the ovarian cases, but deserves separate credit for being one of the first to successfully treat the problem of uterine leiomyomata.

The Atlee brothers were relatively conservative gynecologic surgeons. It was their careful approach coupled with their obvious successes that gave other surgeons increasing confidence to operate. Thus, they played an important role in the early stages of operative gynecology as it developed into the specialty it would become in the next generation. Ovariotomy, the most controversial of gynecologic procedures, was also the key to making it a surgical specialty. Indeed, some gynecologists claimed that operating for ovarian cysts and tumors laid the groundwork for all abdominal surgery in the last decades of the 19th century.

By the 1880s, the specialty of gynecology, or the science of women, as some historians have called it, was well on its way to being established as one of the subdivisions of medical labor. Ornella Moscucci, in her perceptive history of gynecology in Britain, quotes the eminent surgeon from Birmingham, Lawson Tait, in his aptly titled book of 1889, *Diseases of Women and Abdominal Surgery:*

> The great function of woman's life has for years made her the subject of specialists, male and female, the obstetricians. The subsidiary relations of her special organs and the special requirements of her physique, based upon these, have necessitated the establishment of another class of specialist, the gynecologist.

WOMEN AS PATIENTS IN THE 19TH CENTURY

The growth of interest in women's diseases began long before the 19th century. In the Renaissance, for instance, the publication of a large, encyclopedic work entitled *Gynaecia,* by Caspar Wolf (1532–1601), and later similar collections, represented what had been written since antiquity. The mere existence of such texts, however, does not mean that much attention was given to the treatment of women, except as it related to childbirth.

Any discussion of the treatment of women's diseases since the latter half of the 19th century must take into account a variety of interpretations of women's role in society and both professional and lay views of women's health. Historical assessments in our own time have contributed to the furthering of interest in the issues of women's health. Today's discussions are best understood in the light of their historical roots.

Historians of the family and the role of women in the 19th century have written much about the separate spheres for women and the cult of domesticity in which there was a rigid distinction between the home, where it was thought women belonged, and the economic world outside. Thus, the "cult of true womanhood," as historians have called it, made sharp distinctions between women's place in the family and the working world of men. As the social role of women was increasingly defined, they were, in a sense, held hostage in the home. Women were judged by the male world and themselves according to four cardinal virtues: piety, purity, submissiveness, and domesticity.

To these social distinctions between men and women were added the biologic differences. The biologic notions of women in the 19th century ranged widely, but they included the idea that women were not only physically weaker than men (although morally superior), but inherently diseased or pathologic. Their cyclical physiology was believed to make women unsuitable for sustained work or learning. Feminist historians of recent times have taken doctors of an earlier era to task for cast-

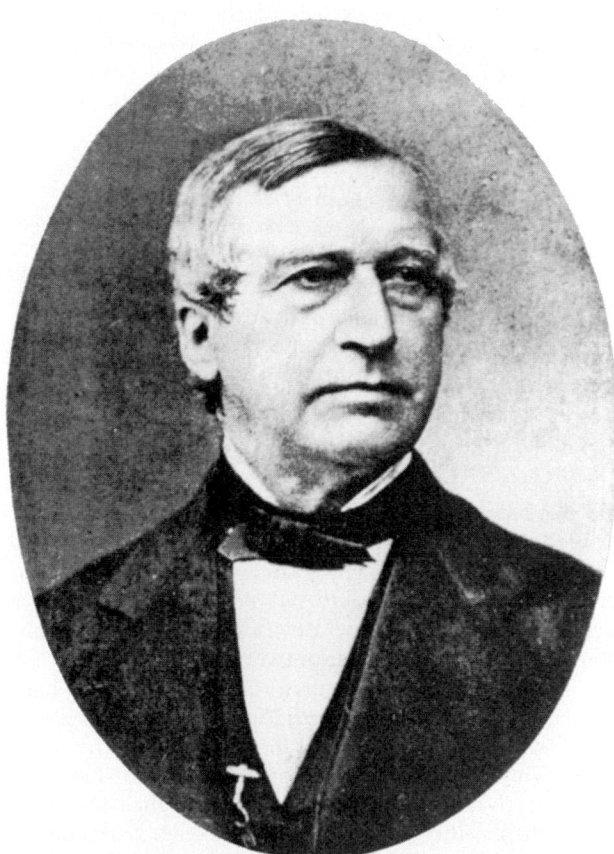

FIGURE 1.3. Washington Lemuel Atlee (1808–1878).

ing women as frail creatures entirely dependent on their biology, destined to be kept from the male world of education, politics, the professions, and any but domestic work. As Ornella Moscucci points out, however, the medical ideas about the social destiny of women were far more complex than has been assumed.

On both sides of the Atlantic, the view of Victorian women was influenced by the writings of eminent physicians. In Boston, a Harvard Medical School professor, Edward H. Clarke (1820–1877), wrote a book in 1873 entitled *Sex in Education; or, A Fair Chance for the Girls.* This book was widely reviewed and discussed. Similarly, Henry Maudsley (1835–1918) in England, an influential psychiatrist and medical teacher, also wrote about the supposed harm of higher education on the physiologic development of postpubescent girls. Clarke's book, which has become known as a uterine manifesto, clearly set the brain and the uterus in opposition. Higher education, Clarke claimed, might be good for developing the intellect, but that occurred at the expense of the reproductive organs, thus dooming the woman to a state of stunted womanhood and lifelong invalidism.

Sex in Education went through 17 printings and editions in the space of a few years. Because of its popularity and notoriety, it is worth citing one of Clarke's case reports:

> Miss D—went to college in good physical condition. During the four years of her college life, her parents and the college faculty required her to get what is popularly called an education. Nature required her, during the same period, to build and put in working order a large and complicated reproductive mechanism a matter that is popularly ignored—shoved out of sight like a disgrace. She naturally obeyed the requirements of the faculty, which she could see, rather than the requirements of the mechanism within her, that she could not see. Subjected to the college regimen, she worked four years in getting a liberal education. Her way of work was sustained and continuous, and out of harmony with the rhythmical periodicity of the female organization. The stream of vital and constructive force evolved within her was turned steadily to the brain, and away from the ovaries and their accessories. The result of this sort of education was, that these last-mentioned organs, deprived of sufficient opportunity and nutriment, first began to perform their functions with pain, a warning of error that was unheeded; then, to cease to grow; . . . And so Miss D—spent the few years next succeeding her graduation in conflict with dysmenorrhea, headache, neuralgia, and hysteria.

Many writings in the 1870s and 1880s attempted to refute the medical notions of physicians such as Clarke and Maudsley. In this country, Mary Putnam Jacobi (1842–1906), a physician and future champion of women in higher education and the professions, submitted a prize-winning essay that refuted Clarke's contentions that work by the brain interfered with uterine function and the menses. In Britain, the pioneer woman-physician Elizabeth Garrett Anderson (1836–1917) claimed that it was boredom that caused the medical complaints of middle-class women, not higher education.

By the middle of the 19th century, even the use of the speculum as a diagnostic instrument stirred controversy. The speculum was known to the ancients, but it fell into disuse by the early modern period. Early in the 19th century, Joseph Recamier (1774–1852) reintroduced it in Paris, and soon the speculum was routinely used in treating inflammatory disease. It was also used in the routine examination of prostitutes in France and England.

In the Victorian climate of concern about women and their diseases, as well as their moral sensibilities, vaginal examinations were not routine. When they were performed, great efforts were made to preserve the patient's privacy and dignity, as the accompanying illustrations show (Figs. 1.4 and 1.5). A battle over the morality of the use of the speculum also ensued. The speculum, opponents of its use believed, could lead to sexual stimulation and sexual excesses. The term "speculum rape" was used in the debates over the Contagious Disease Acts in England in the 1860s.

Meanwhile, the surgeons went about debating the advisability of oophorectomy. One of the most prominent proponents of ovarian surgery for symptoms not just associated with demonstrable ovarian disease was an American surgeon named Robert Battey (1828–1895), of Georgia. In 1872, he removed the ovaries of a 32-year-old woman who had claimed invalidism for 16 years. Battey reported that his patient was cured after the bilateral oophorectomy. (Cured of what remains the intriguing question.) In succeeding years, the Battey operation became popular with some surgeons. Battey himself tried a vaginal approach to the ovaries but soon reverted to abdominal section. He advocated bilateral removal of the ovaries, whether or not they revealed any sign of disease, to ameliorate menstrual difficulties or psychological symptoms.

With historical examples such as the Battey operation, it is no surprise that feminist historians today level charges of male physicians' exploitation of their female patients. One of the most drastic charges claimed that most of the gynecologic surgery of the late 19th century was a calculated plot against women, a tacit conspiracy between insecure husbands and anxious gynecologists.

Ann Douglas, a literary historian and feminist, was one of the earliest to invoke the notion of a conspiracy of male physicians to subject their female patients to mutilating, harmful, and unnecessary surgery. She simply dismissed 19th-century doctors as ignorant because they did not receive the kind of medical training we have now come to take for granted. However, because the physician of 1870 did not yet have the understanding of physiology or pathophysiology enjoyed by his colleagues a century later, calling most earlier doctors ignorant, callous, or worse was not warranted.

Those with a less conspiratorial view of history have shown that other views of both husbands and male physicians existed in the late part of the last century. The economist Thorstein Veblen, for instance, believed that non-working wives served as status symbols for their husbands rather than as threats or temptations to eager surgeons.

Women learned and taught surgery, including gynecologic procedures, at The Women's Medical College of

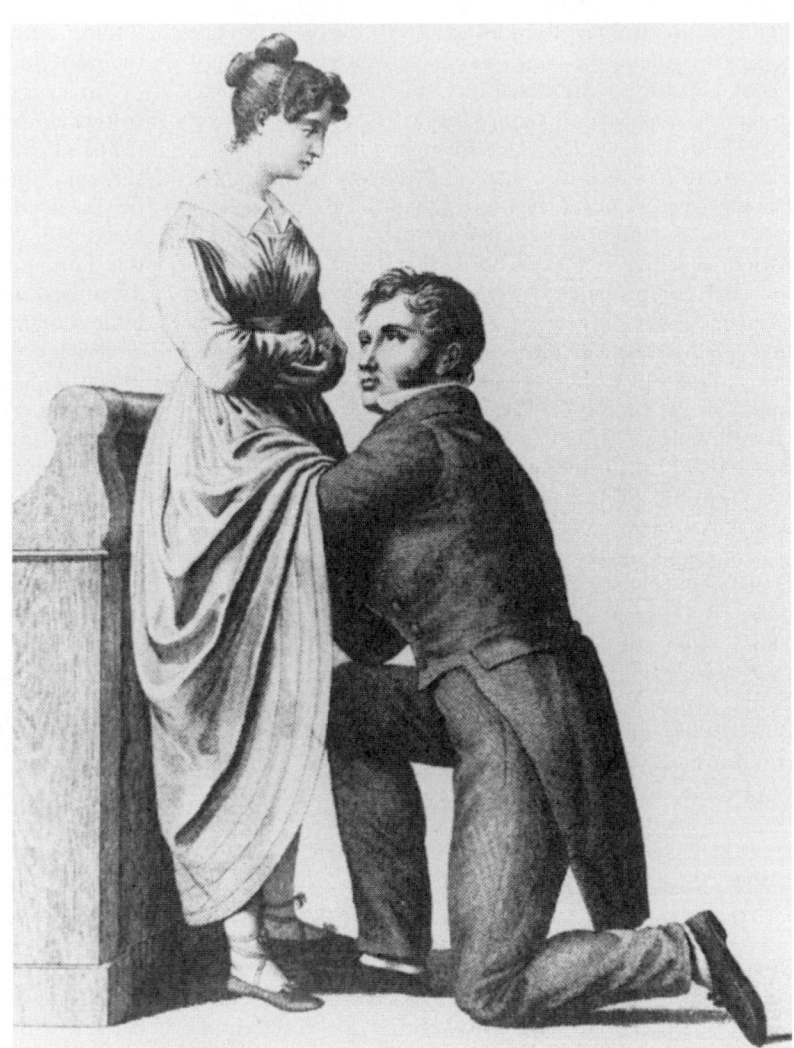

FIGURE 1.4. This famous illustration of "the touch" in a gynecologic examination is from a 19th-century French text frequently used in America. Note the avoidance of eye contact between doctor and patient and the dress shielding the woman's body from view. (From: Wertz RW, Wertz DC. *Lying-in: a history of childbirth in America,* expanded edition. New Haven, CT: Yale University Press, 1989:78, with permission.)

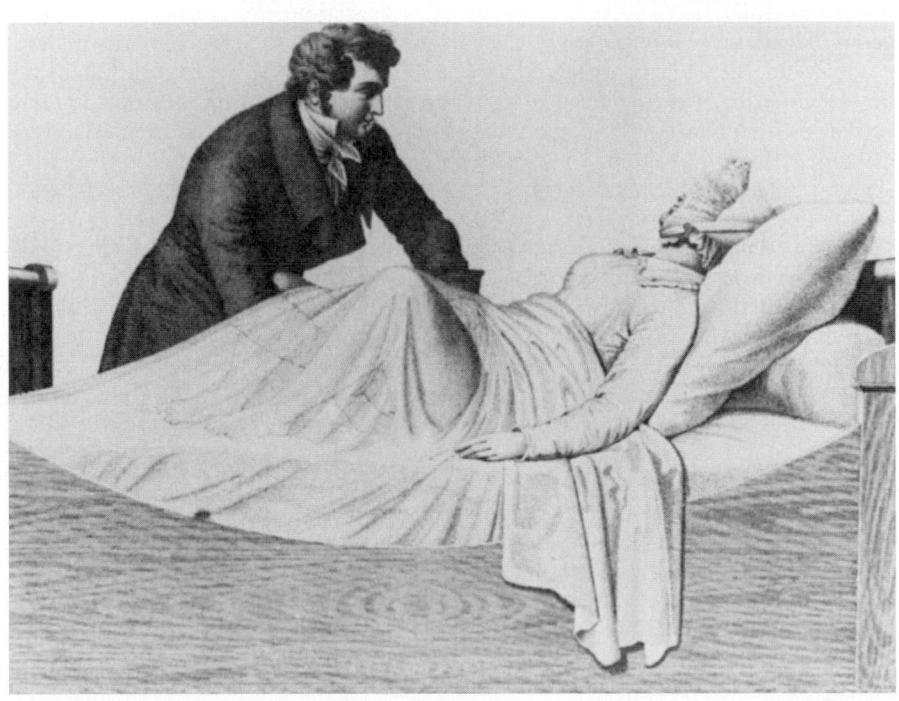

FIGURE 1.5. This 19th-century drawing illustrates another technique for preserving the patient's modesty: the doctor conducting a gynecologic examination looks directly into the woman's eyes to assure her that her private parts are safe from his gaze. (From: Wertz RW, Wertz DC. *Lying-in: a history of childbirth in America,* expanded edition. New Haven, CT: Yale University Press, 1989:84, with permission.)

Pennsylvania from its founding in 1850. But it is also fair to say that there were few women actively practicing gynecologic surgery until well into this century. A notable exception was Mary Dixon Jones of Brooklyn, who by the 1890s had won respect from her male colleagues. Her story has recently been told by Regina Morantz-Sanchez, whose observations of Dixon Jones' career help us to understand how a woman made it in a man's world. Morantz-Sanchez, in her book about the libel trial of Dixon-Jones in the early 1890s, charts the development of gynecologic surgery as a specialty. Dixon-Jones was unusual because she was a successful woman-surgeon, but also because she was on the cusp of the developments in gynecology and its evolution from a field that viewed women in their social as well as their biological roles, to a 20th-century surgical specialty that concentrated on the pathology of diseased organs and the most appropriate and effective surgical techniques.

Morantz-Sanchez nicely illustrates this evolution of gynecology by framing the developments by the textbooks of Thomas Addis Emmet and J.C. Skene of the 1880s, still using the language of women as "other" than men, with the 1909 text of Howard Kelly and Charles Noble, *Gynecology and Abdominal Surgery,* in which there is no discussion of women's social roles because the focus is on surgical technique. Thus, the language of medicine can be used to trace the changes in medicine itself.

THE RELATION BETWEEN SURGERY AND GYNECOLOGY

The complex relation between general surgery and gynecology played a continuing role in the professional definition of gynecology as a 20th-century specialty. Moreover, several important contributions to surgery, such as chloroform anesthesia, rubber gloves, and early ambulation, were influenced by gynecologists as well as surgeons. The latter two items are discussed subsequently.

By 1905, the Chicago gynecologist Franklin H. Martin (1857–1935) was convinced that the three closely allied fields—surgery, gynecology, and obstetrics—were making sufficient progress to warrant a new journal. There was a shared feeling, Martin wrote in the opening editorial of *Surgery, Gynecology, and Obstetrics,* ". . . that the field of the three allied specialties represented by its title is not over-cultivated, and that there is already a place for a creditable magazine representing in one publication these three divisions of surgery."

Another of the founding editors of the journal, the gynecologist J. Clarence Webster, wrote a provocative editorial in the first issue on "The Future of Gynecology." Webster firmly laid to rest an idea that had gained some acceptance by 1905—that gynecology was doomed to extinction, to be gradually merged with the practice of the general surgeon. Webster assured his readers that contrary to what some had claimed, much advance had occurred in the preceding decades, and, moreover, ". . . it is very evident that almost all the important advances have resulted from the work of men who have given their entire energies to the specialty. At the present day the leading authorities everywhere are those who still limit their attention to this sphere of work."

In a programmatic statement to the American Gynecological Society in 1920, Robert L. Dickinson (1861–1950) contended that gynecologists promote surgery. "But if we be just surgeons, by surgeons we may be displaced." In this presidential address to the Society, Dickinson claimed that gynecologic procedures constituted one fourth of all surgery, but this hardly accounted for the extent of the field, ". . . since operation is needed by less than one-tenth of the patients that come to the doctor for ailments peculiar to women (childbearing not included)." It was true, of course, that for much of the preceding century, gynecology was a medical rather than a surgical discipline, often taught in medical schools as part of the course on diseases of women and children.

In the early decades of the 20th century, the professional battles between the general surgeons (who increasingly dominated the field of abdominal surgery) and the gynecologists (who wished to lay claim to the same territory) waxed and waned. Dr. Howard Longyear of Detroit noted in 1917 that general surgeons tended to scorn the area of the pelvis, while this area was being increasingly perfected by gynecologists. These surgeons wanted to move upward in the body from surgery of the female genitalia and the pelvis to the abdomen. Longyear also noted that the Sims operation for vesicovaginal fistula did more to establish operative gynecology as a specialty than did any other single procedure or development.

The complex relations between surgery and gynecology also can be traced by following the name changes in the American Medical Association specialty section. In 1903, at its founding, it was called Section on Obstetrics and Gynecology. From 1912 until 1936, it was called Section on Obstetrics, Gynecology, and Abdominal Surgery. Then the name was changed once again and dropped the abdominal surgery component.

One area of joint progress forged by surgeons and gynecologists was the introduction of the use of rubber gloves, which helped to expand the work of all surgeons. The idea of using some form of protective covering for the surgeon's hands occasionally appeared in the medical literature in the early decades of the 19th century, but it was not until the end of the century that some of the associates of Dr. William S. Halsted (1852–1922) at the Johns Hopkins Hospital in Baltimore began to use gloves routinely. About two decades after their introduction, Dr. Halsted recalled the story:

> In the winter of 1889 and 1890—I cannot recall the month—the nurse in charge of my operating room complained that the solutions of mercuric chloride produced a dermatitis of her arms and hands. As she was an unusually efficient woman, I gave the matter my consideration and one day in New York requested the Goodyear Rubber Company to make as an experiment two pair of thin rubber gloves with gauntlets. On trial these proved to be so satisfactory that additional gloves were ordered. In the autumn, on my return to town, the assistant who passed the instruments and threaded the needles was also provided with rubber gloves to wear at the operations. At first the operator wore them

only when exploratory incisions into joints were made. After a time the assistants became so accustomed to working in gloves that they also wore them as operators and would remark that they seemed to be less expert with the bare hands than with the gloved hands.

I think it was Dr. Bloodgood, my house surgeon, who first made this comment and that he was the first to wear them invariably, when operating. . . . Dr. Hunter Robb in 1894, in his book on aseptic technic recommended that the operator wear rubber gloves. Dr. Robb was, at that time, resident gynecologist of the Johns Hopkins Hospital and had frequent opportunities to observe the technic of the surgical clinic.

Gynecologists were also closely involved in the form of postoperative care we have now come to take for granted—early ambulation after surgery. With the change from 2 or 3 weeks of enforced bed rest after surgery to active ambulation within a few hours of the operation, we have improved recovery, shortened hospital stays, and reduced costs as well as postoperative complications. But like all new techniques or practices, early rising after surgery did not win rapid acceptance.

Ephraim McDowell's patient in 1809 not only was ambulant early, but also engaged in physical tasks such as making her own bed. Her surgeon clearly was not pleased with her activity, which was not in keeping with customary and usual practices of the day.

What we call early ambulation was not found again in the medical literature until the very last year of the 19th century, when Emil Ries, a professor of gynecology in Chicago, published a landmark paper, which soon disappeared from view. It was rediscovered four decades later. Ries noted in his 1899 paper that he wanted to change treatment radically by freeing patients from ". . . many irksome and disagreeable features of convalescence following vaginal and abdominal surgery." Ries found that his patients could be fed and allowed out of bed much sooner than was the usual custom. "Very soon I found," he wrote, "that the period for which it was advisable to confine such cases to bed could be counted by hours instead of days, so that of late I have allowed my patients to get up within twenty-four to forty-eight hours and to leave the hospital four to six days after their vaginal celiotomy." These patients, Ries also noted, did not have the listlessness or muscular weakness that was usually seen after 2 or 3 weeks in bed.

In the preoperative preparation of his patients, Ries also went against the usual custom of completely emptying the bowel. Most textbooks, he said, claimed that early action of the bowels helped to prevent peritonitis. However, in most patients with an empty intestinal tract, regular movements did not resume until after they were eating a regular diet. Ries maintained that cause and effect were confused because it was not movement of the bowels that prevented peritonitis, but freedom from inflammation that allowed the bowels to move.

At the meeting of the Southern Surgical and Gynecological Society in Baltimore in 1906, H.J. Boldt described 384 cases of early ambulation that he had accumulated since 1890. All recovered well. Ironically, Boldt reported, the most serious objection raised by his colleagues was that early ambulation increased the risk of thrombosis. This was clearly wrong, he said, from both a theoretic and an empirical point of view, because his patients had a better circulation from exercising.

Early ambulation was discussed repeatedly in the succeeding decade, but it received far from universal acceptance. Even Howard Kelly, the country's leading teacher of gynecology, noted in 1911 that great progress was made as a result of Boldt's and Ries' work, but that it was far from standard practice. Early ambulation really became a routine practice with the exigencies of World War II (which resulted in a shortage of hospital personnel) and with the work of Daniel J. Leithauser, a general surgeon from Detroit who rediscovered Boldt and Ries. Although doctors may not have prescribed early ambulation, as in the case of McDowell, patients probably were up and about far more often than we realize. Dr. Bert Dunphy of San Francisco told me that when he had a hernia repair while he was a house officer at the Peter Bent Brigham Hospital in 1938, his surgeon prescribed strict bed rest after the operation. Dunphy was up on the first day and thereafter and felt perfectly well, if a bit guilty.

GYNECOLOGY IN THE 20TH CENTURY AND DR. TE LINDE'S BOOK

In the 1890s, when Thomas Cullen (1868–1953) was a medical student in Toronto, he recalled that ". . . there were anteversions, anteflexions, retroversions, and retroflexions and that some of the displacements might be relieved by appropriate pessaries." Abdominal gynecologic operations, Cullen continued, ". . . were limited almost entirely to the removal of large ovarian cysts. An occasional myomatous uterus was removed, but the fatality in this class of cases was so high that the operation was rarely attempted." Cullen also said that he did hear of cancers of the uterus in his student days, but only cauterization or curettage was performed. Entire removal of the uterus was not yet being done.

By the turn of the 20th century, the leadership of gynecology in this country had clearly moved to the new Johns Hopkins Hospital, where Howard A. Kelly (1858–1943) (Fig. 1.6) began to train a series of young men who put gynecology on a strong academic footing in the next two generations. Kelly received both his bachelor's and medical degrees from the University of Pennsylvania. After his medical graduation in 1882, Kelly spent some time in Germany learning the latest surgical and pathologic techniques. Back in Philadelphia at Kensington Hospital, he soon acquired a reputation as a brilliant operator. When his fellow Philadelphian William Osler became Chief of Medicine at the opening of the Johns Hopkins Hospital in 1889, he urged the trustees to hire Kelly as Chief of Obstetrics and Gynecology.

At age 31, the youthful-appearing Kelly, who many patients thought was still a student or resident, initiated a residency program in gynecology with a strong link to the pathology department. Even more than half a century later, the leading texts in the field—Eastman's

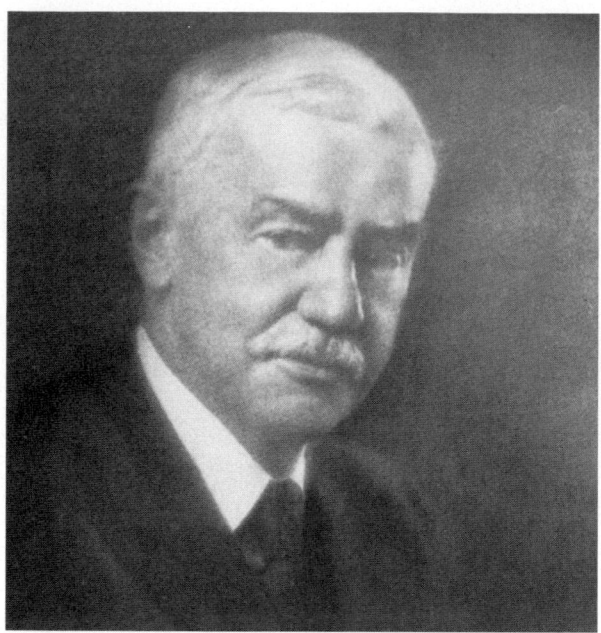

FIGURE 1.6. Howard A. Kelly (1858–1943). (From: Davis AW. *Dr. Kelly of Hopkins*. Baltimore: The Johns Hopkins Press, 1959, with permission.)

(Williams') *Obstetrics*, Te Linde's *Operative Gynecology*, and Novak's *Gynecologic and Obstetric Pathology*—were written by professors in Baltimore who had received their training at Hopkins with Kelly and his assistants.

Kelly soon found that his interests and skills were in gynecologic surgery; therefore, he turned the obstetric service over to J. Whitridge Williams (1866–1931), who became a leader in that field and the author of the most

widely used textbook of the time. Kelly had a great interest in the female urinary system, realizing that the symptomatology of urinary tract disease is often intertwined with that of the reproductive organs. He invented the air cystoscope and devised ureteral catheters. He was the first to plicate the vesical sphincter for stress incontinence of urine. Physicians from all over the world came to Baltimore to watch him operate (Figs. 1.7 and 1.8).

Kelly's legendary operative skill was well described by Cullen, who later became one of Kelly's outstanding residents and successors to the chair at Hopkins. Kelly and Hunter Robb, his earlier resident, went to the Toronto General Hospital not long after Kelly became Chief at Hopkins. Cullen was an intern in Toronto at the time and handled the instruments during an operation that Kelly and Robb had agreed to perform. Cullen's description speaks for itself:

> I turned around to thread a needle and when I turned back found to my amazement that the operator had the abdomen open. Operators in the General often took ten minutes to get that far. After cutting through the skin, fat and fascia they were apt to get lost in the muscles. Kelly and Robb working together used dissecting forceps as I had never seen them used. One man pulling each way, the cleavage between the muscles was seen at once and the opening in the abdomen could be completed without difficulty. I watched, fascinated, while Kelly went ahead and finished that operation and did the second, working with clock-like precision and at a speed I had not imagined possible. By the time he had finished, the course of my professional life was decided. Up to that afternoon I had intended to be a physician. From that afternoon I knew I had to be a surgeon.

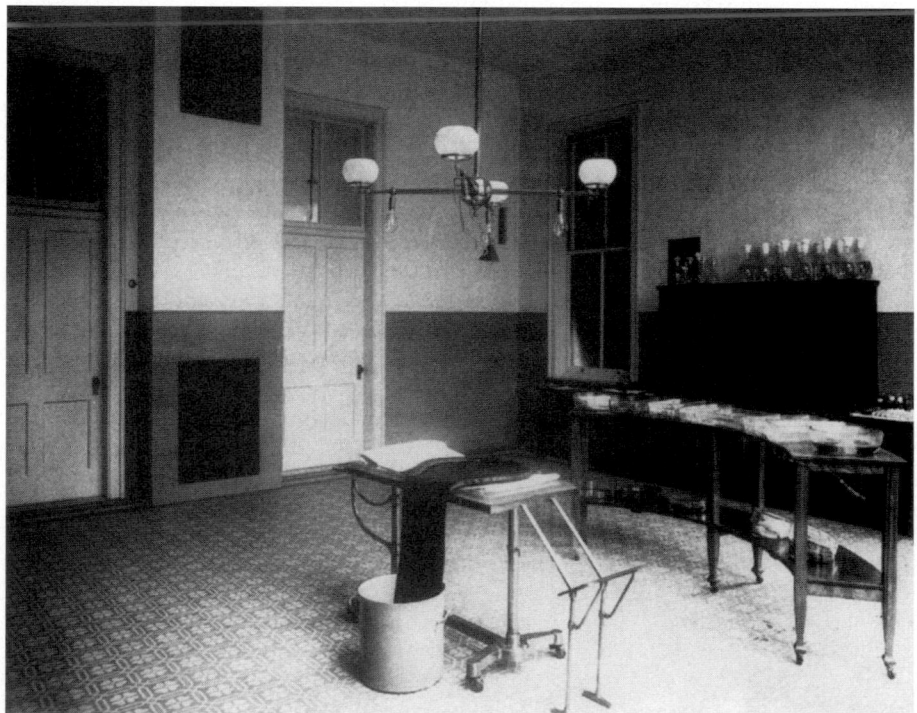

FIGURE 1.7. Dr. Howard A. Kelly's operating room at the Johns Hopkins Hospital. To the left is the door to the corridor. In the center is the door to the ether room. The rubber pad was used for drainage during irrigation of the abdomen. A similar pad was developed by Dr. Kelly for drainage of blood and amniotic fluid during and after a vaginal delivery.

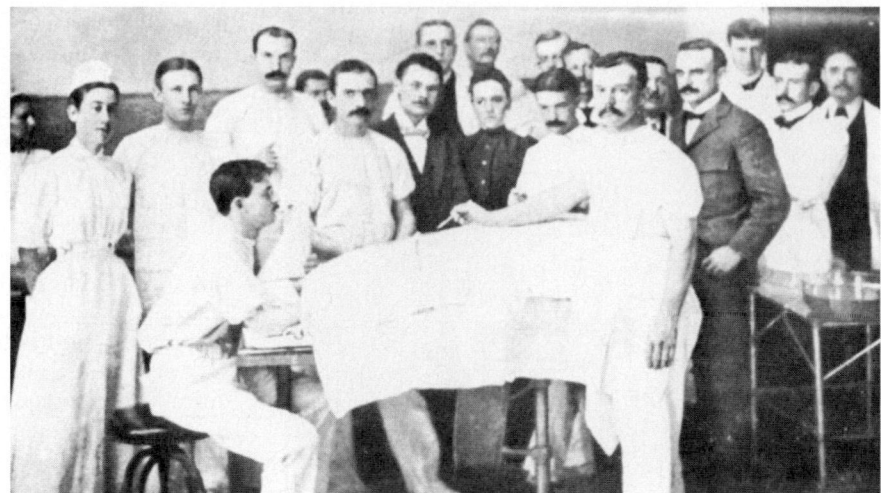

FIGURE 1.8. Howard Kelly operates. Grouped about the operating table, left to right, are: Emma Beckwith, head nurse; Jay Durkee *(seated);* Thomas S. Cullen; Max Brödel *(center);* Elisabeth Hurdon; J.E. Stokes; and John G. Clark. (From: Davis AW. *Dr. Kelly of Hopkins.* Baltimore: The Johns Hopkins Press, 1959, with permission.)

Chance often determines the course of one's life, so it was fortunate for Cullen that he had to wait 6 months for his residency with Kelly to start. He used this time to begin the study of pathology with William H. Welch at Hopkins, and it was the close alliance of gynecology and pathology, begun by Kelly and continued by Cullen, that shaped the careers of many future gynecologists at Hopkins and elsewhere and determined the course of the field itself.

In 1898, Kelly published a two-volume textbook called *Operative Gynecology,* certainly the direct ancestor of the volume you have in your hands. Kelly wrote in the preface, "My aim in writing this book has been to place in the hands of the many friends who have from time to time visited me and followed my work, a convenient summary of the various gynecological operations I have found best in my own practice."

Although gynecology at the end of the last century was still a very young science, in Kelly's words, change was at hand: "Although I have spent several years in the preparation of my book, so rapid have been the changes in the gynecological field that I have found it necessary to rewrite some of the chapters two and even three times." A little more than a dozen years later, in the preface to his text entitled *Medical Gynecology,* Kelly reiterated the pace of the changes: "What a transformation two generations have witnessed in the field of gynecology! From modest beginnings, as a sort of minor specialty coupled with diseases of children and often professed by general practitioners with no special training, it has grown to the dignity of a major surgical specialty, so extensive that many gynecologists of today [1912] claim the entire field of abdominal surgery as their proper domain by right of discovery and conquest." This was also a time when radical or complete removal of tumors and repair of hernias became increasingly common. Kelly and his residents were pioneers in radical hysterectomy when Hugh Young of Hopkins introduced radical prostatectomy.

What imparted even greater value to all of Kelly's texts were the illustrations of Max Brödel, a German medical illustrator brought to Hopkins by Kelly (Fig.

1.9). Brödel's contributions to operative gynecology, including Te Linde's text 50 years after Kelly's, were portrayals of operative techniques, pelvic anatomy, and pathologic conditions. He set a standard for medical illustration never attained before or surpassed since.

As long ago as 1900, in his classic text, *Cancer of the Uterus,* Thomas Cullen, student of and successor to Kelly (Fig. 1.10), wrote that, "The number of cases of cancer of the genital tract coming too late for operation is so appalling that the surgeon is ever seeking to devise ways and means by which the dread malady may be more generally detected at the earliest possible moment—at a time when complete removal of the malignant tissue is still possible. . . . But since it is the general practitioner who, as a rule, is the first consulted, upon him largely falls the responsibility of arriving at a timely diagnosis."

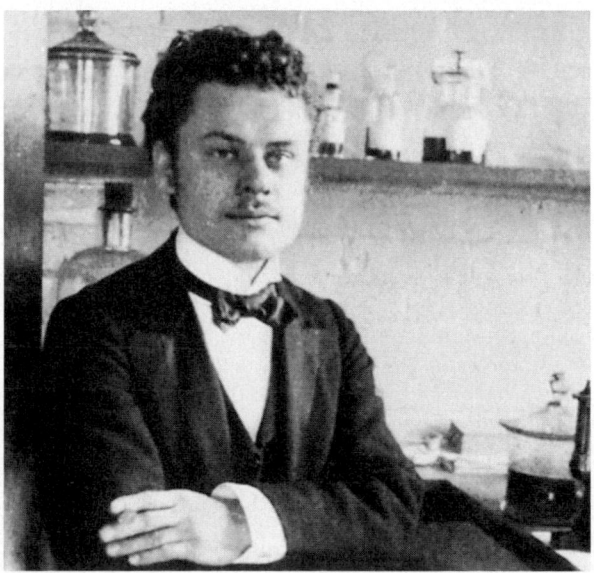

FIGURE 1.9. Max Brödel. (From: Robinson J. *Tom Cullen of Baltimore.* New York: Oxford University Press, 1949, with permission.)

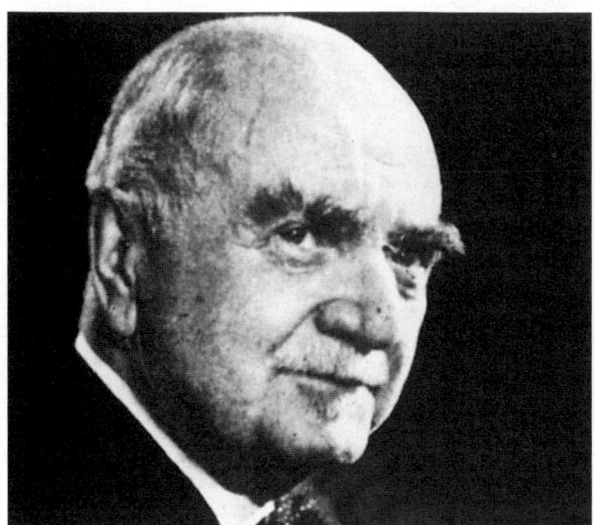

FIGURE 1.10. Thomas S. Cullen (1868–1953). (From: Robinson J. *Tom Cullen of Baltimore.* New York: Oxford University Press, 1949, with permission.)

One of the greatest advances in gynecology in this century has been the improvement in the early detection and cure rate of cancer of the uterine cervix that has resulted from the development of cytology and the recognition of carcinoma *in situ.* In 1943, George N. Papanicolaou (1883–1962) and Herbert Traut (1894–1963) published their seminal monograph entitled *Diagnosis of Uterine Cancer by the Vaginal Smear.* Papanicolaou had worked on this technique since the 1920s, but, like many other innovations in medicine, it took years to find widespread acceptance. Further publications by Papanicolaou and others, notably Ruth Graham, demonstrated beyond a doubt that cytologic studies could almost infallibly detect cervical cancer.

Cancer *in situ* was recognized early in the century by Cullen and in 1912 by J. Schottlander and F. Kermauner, but its relation to invasive cancer was not well understood. This relation was more clearly described in 1944 by G.A. Galvin and Te Linde in several reports. Since then, the relation has been amply confirmed, and early cervical cancer has become a detectable and curable disease. Since its inception by Hans Hinselmann in Germany in the 1920s, colposcopy has given a new dimension to the assessment of cervical carcinoma, making blind, random cervical biopsies unnecessary and providing more accuracy in finding and treating localized lesions.

By the early 1970s, the editor of a new journal, *Gynecologic Oncology,* pointed out that ". . . the scientific importance of gynecologic oncology may be gained from the observation that the tumors that we study and treat are prototypes for cancer in other areas of the body, for the histogenesis of the two principal uterine cancers is probably understood better than that of any other tumor in the body."

Another diagnostic and therapeutic procedure that has been a milestone in the history of pelvic surgery is the use of the laparoscope. The idea of viewing the in-traabdominal organs was explained in 1911 by Bertram Bernheim, a surgical resident at Hopkins. He described two cases in which a proctoscope was passed through a small abdominal incision. He observed the organs in the abdomen by using a reflected light. Others soon tried the technique, and by the late 1920s, H. Kalk, a German surgeon, was avidly promoting peritoneoscopy. The method gained credibility through his many examinations and publications. Diagnostic possibilities were further increased in the late 1940s with the introduction of fiberoptics.

Culdoscopy has been replaced by laparoscopy now. In recent years, many operative and diagnostic procedures formerly requiring a major pelvic operation have been performed successfully through the laparoscope. Among these are tubal sterilization, lysis of pelvic adhesions, evaluation of chronic pelvic pain and infertility, evaluation of treated pelvic malignancies, and, more recently, use of the carbon dioxide laser for vaporization of endometriosis implants throughout the pelvis.

The immediate post–World War II years were a period of truly astounding medical developments and saw the explosive growth of medical research funding and new hospital construction. After 1945, penicillin became available for civilian use, and this was soon followed by other antibiotics. Hormone replacement became increasingly possible, and in 1946, the year that Richard Te Linde published the first edition of this textbook, Congress passed the Hill-Burton Act, making federal funds available to localities for the construction of new hospitals. These and other developments of the time greatly changed and expanded the work of medicine.

OPERATIVE GYNECOLOGY, FIRST EDITION, 1946

Richard Wesley Te Linde was born in Wisconsin in 1894, and except for the years he attended a small liberal arts college in Holland, Michigan, he spent all his formative years in Wisconsin. When he was ready to go to medical school, he went to Madison, but in 1916 the University of Wisconsin had only a 2-year school. Te Linde completed the 2 preclinical years and then transferred to Johns Hopkins for the final 2 years. He graduated with the class of 1920 and spent the rest of his professional career associated with Hopkins, where he became chief of the gynecology division of the Department of Surgery and then chair of the separate Department of Gynecology in 1939. He held that post until his retirement in 1960, when the newly reunified Department of Obstetrics and Gynecology was reestablished.

Just as his teacher Howard Kelly had felt the need to compile a textbook of operative gynecology half a century earlier, Te Linde believed that the many-sided specialty that gynecology had become by World War II required a new text. With Kelly's earlier text as a model, Te Linde wished to incorporate the vast changes that had occurred in the period separating the two books. During this 50-year span, there were changes in our knowledge of the hormones, new surgical techniques, and the ability to visualize the abdominal and pelvic organs.

Te Linde chose the same simple title for his own text. Although Kelly's had been published by Appleton in New York, Te Linde chose Lippincott in Philadelphia. Gynecology, Te Linde wrote in the preface in 1946, was no longer to be considered simply a branch of general surgery. The gynecologist, he stressed, must still be a good surgeon but must also master the pathology of gynecologic disorders and the newly burgeoning field of endocrinology. New books were appearing in all these fields except gynecologic surgery, and it was this void that Te Linde wished to fill.

Te Linde wrote his text with the ". . . primary purpose of describing the technic of the usual and some of the rarer operative procedures. It also includes indications for and against operations as well as pre- and postoperative care of patients." Gynecologic pathology, Te Linde stressed in the Hopkins tradition, is the bedrock of good gynecologic surgery. "Without an understanding of it, surgery becomes merely a mechanical job, and errors in surgical judgment are inevitable." In the organization of his text and in the subsequent editions over the succeeding half century to the present edition, one can readily see important landmarks in the history of operative gynecology. Some of these were discussed in the preceding.

The 751-page first edition of 1946, all of it written by Te Linde, had a first printing of 5,000 copies, which quickly sold out. A second printing was equally successful. The reviews have always been laudatory. Of the sixth edition of 1985, edited by Richard Mattingly and John Thompson, the *Journal of the American Medical Association* reviewer ended by saying, "I cannot imagine any gynecologist who performs surgery doing without it, first as a primer and then as a reminder." By 1962, when the third edition appeared and Te Linde had retired from the chairmanship of his department, he decided that, like all the other major medical textbooks of the time, his book needed a group of authors to bring out new revisions. In the preface to that edition, he states that his book has never been simply a manual of surgical technique—that surgical philosophy is equally important. "What does it profit a woman if the operation is technically perfect and the procedure unnecessary or even harmful?" One reason unnecessary procedures still prevailed, Te Linde noted, was the lack of knowledge of gynecologic pathology, still the "bedrock upon which good surgery is done." Therefore, Te Linde justified including a considerable amount of pathology in his text. Pathology is what has differentiated gynecologic surgery from general surgery since Howard Kelly's years at the turn of the century. Surgical texts, and by implication their surgical readers, have generally not devoted nearly as much attention to pathology as have gynecologists, some of whose leaders have actually been very well versed in pathology.

The fact that Te Linde could produce three editions, each larger than the first, is a testament to his broad knowledge of his field, his ability as a writer, and his stamina for hard work. He died in Baltimore in 1989 at the age of 95.

In the decades since the third edition of 1962, the world of medicine and the society in which it is practiced have seen much change. By the mid-1960s, when significant advances in the treatment of infections, malignancies, and hormonal disorders had become evident, these successes had an impact on gynecology just as they did in other areas of medicine. The reduction in mastoid infections, for instance, has changed the practice of the otolaryngologist considerably. In gynecology, the reduction in major pelvic inflammatory disease forced gynecologists to focus more of their attention on other disorders. Also affecting gynecologic surgery by the middle of this century were significant improvements in obstetric practices, which sharply reduced injuries to the bladder and rectum. Hysterectomies and suspensory operations were not performed for vague complaints of illness as often as they had been.

We have also lived through social revolutions that have changed the way our society carries on its business and dispenses its social prerogatives. Especially prominent in the 1960s, a civil rights movement, greater concern for our environment, a resurgence of consumer rights, and a revitalized women's movement profoundly affected our social institutions, including medicine. Within medicine, no specialty has been more touched by these trends than obstetrics and gynecology.

The new feminism viewed abortion, childbirth, contraception, and gynecologic surgery as a means of social control of female patients by doctors, most of whom were male. The feminist movement challenged not only the domination of doctors but also the supposed benevolence of their knowledge and practices.

As the world has changed, so have our expectations. In the decades after the first edition of Te Linde's book appeared, when wonder drugs were touted as curing previously untreatable illnesses, the public began to expect much from its doctors, and we were not shy in claiming that ever-greater investments in medical research would lead to more cures. It is hardly surprising, then, that in these last few decades, as we began to spend increasing amounts of our gross national product for health, those who paid the bill became increasingly interested in seeing just what their money was actually buying. Like most other social institutions, medicine lost much of the autonomy it had for so long taken for granted. Although as a profession we did not always get all we wanted, we were for decades amazingly adept at preventing those things we did not want. Now that, too, has changed, as has the practice of medicine.

The division of labor in all areas of medicine grew as the 20th century progressed. In the last decades of the century, what used to be called general practice became the specialty of family practice. In the Anglo-American world of the late 20th century, both obstetrics and gynecology were caught in the middle of the battles between specialists and generalists. Likewise, they became involved in the tensions among primary, secondary, and tertiary medical care. Similar strife occurred in earlier centuries among those vying for a place and for status among physicians caring for women in childbirth and in disease. If one looks at the Table of Contents of this edition and compares it to a simpler period of half a century or a century ago, one will see what great breadth the field of operative gynecology continues to enjoy.

BIBLIOGRAPHY

Anderson EG. Sex in mind and education: a reply. *Fortnightly Review* 1874;15:582.

Beacham WD. The American Academy of Obstetrics and Gynecology: first presidential address. *Obstet Gynecol* 1953;1:115.

Boldt HJ. The management of laparotomy patients and their modified after-treatment. *NY Med J* 1907;85:145.

Brieger GH. The development of surgery: historical aspects important in the origin and development of modern surgical science. In: Sabiston, DC, ed. *Christopher's textbook of surgery,* 14th ed. Philadelphia: WB Saunders, 1991:1.

Brieger GH. Early ambulation: a study in the history of surgery. *Ann Surg* 1983;197:443.

Brunschwig A. Whither gynecology? *Am J Obstet Gynecol* 1968;100:122.

Cullen TS. *Cancer of the uterus: its pathology, symptomatology, diagnosis, and treatment.* New York: Appleton, 1900.

Cullen TS. The evolution of gynecology. *Ohio State Med J* 1924;20:484.

Cullen TS. The relation of obstetrics, gynecology and abdominal surgery to the public welfare. *JAMA* 1916;66:239.

Davis A. *Dr. Kelly of Hopkins.* Baltimore: The Johns Hopkins Press, 1959.

Dickinson RL. Original communications: a program for American Gynecology Society presidential address. *Am J Obstet Gynecol* 1920,1921;1:2.

Ehrenreich B, English D. *For her own good: 150 years of the experts' advice to women.* Garden City, NY: Anchor Press/Doubleday, 1978.

Gusberg SB. An introduction to volume 1. *Gynecol Oncol* 1972;1:i.

Hahn R. *Sickness and health: an anthropological perspective.* New Haven, CT: Yale University Press, 1995:209.

Halsted WS. The employment of fine silk in preference to catgut and the advantages of transfixing tissues and vessels in controlling haemorrhage. *JAMA* 1913;60:1119.

Harris S. *Woman's surgeon: the life story of J. Marion Sims.* New York: Macmillan, 1950.

Jacobi MP. *A question of rest for women during menstruation.* London: Smith & Elder, 1878.

Jones HW Jr, Jones GS, Ticknor WE. *Richard Wesley TeLinde.* Baltimore: Williams & Wilkins, 1986.

Kelly HA. *History of gynecology in America. A Cyclopedia of American Medical Biography,* 2 vols. Philadelphia: WB Saunders, 1912: xxxix–xl.

Kelly HA. Getting up early after grave surgical operations. *Surg Gynecol Obstet* 1911;13:78.

Kelly HA. *Medical gynecology.* New York: Appleton, 1912.

Kelly HA. *Operative gynecology.* New York: Appleton, 1898.

Longo LD. The rise and fall of Battey's operation: a fashion in surgery. *Bull Hist Med* 1979;53:244.

Longyear HW. The relations of gynecology to general surgery, past and present. *JAMA* 1917;69:501.

Martin FH. Surgery, gynecology, and obstetrics. *Surg Gynecol Obstet* 1905;1:62.

Maudsley H. Sex in mind and on education. *Fortnightly Review* 1874;15:466.

McDowell E. Extirpation of diseased ovaria. *Eclectic Repertory* 1817;7:742. Reprinted in Brieger GH, ed. *Medical America in the nineteenth century.* Baltimore: The Johns Hopkins Press, 1972.

Meigs JV. *Progress in gynecology. Fifty years of surgical progress, 1905–1955.* Chicago: The Franklin H. Martin Memorial Foundation, 1955. Reprinted from Davis L, ed. *Surgery: gynecology and obstetrics with international abstracts of surgery.*

Morantz R. The lady and her physician. In: Hartman M, Banner L, eds. *Clio's consciousness raised: new perspectives on the history of women.* New York: Harper & Row, 1974:38.

Morantz-Sanchez R. Making it in a man's world: the late nineteenth-century surgical career of Mary Amanda Dixon Jones. *Bull Hist Med* 1995;69:542.

Morantz-Sanchez R. *Conduct unbecoming a woman: medicine on trial in turn of-the-century.* New York: Oxford University Press, 1999.

Moscucci O. *The science of woman: gynaecology and gender in England 1800–1929.* Cambridge: Cambridge University Press, 1990:30.

O'Dowd MJ, Philipp EE. *The history of obstetrics and gynecology.* New York: Parthenon Publishing Group, 1994.

Ricci JV. *The development of gynaecological surgery and instruments.* Philadelphia: Blakiston, 1949.

Ries E. Some radical changes in the after-treatment of celiotomy cases. *JAMA* 1899;33:454.

Robinson J. *Tom Cullen of Baltimore.* London: Oxford University Press, 1949.

Rock JA, Johnson TRB, Woodruff JD, eds. *The first 100 years: Department of Gynecology and Obstetrics of The Johns Hopkins Hospital.* Baltimore: The Johns Hopkins University Press, 1991.

Sims JM. On the treatment of vesico-vaginal fistula. *Am J Med Sci* 1852;23:59.

Sims JM. *Silver sutures in surgery. The anniversary discourse, the New York Academy of Medicine.* New York: S&W Wood, 1858.

Sims JM. *The story of my life.* New York: Appleton, 1884. Reprinted by Dacapo Press, 1968.

Simpson JY. *Hospitalism: its effects on the results of surgical operations.* Edinburgh: Oliver Boyd, 1869.

Speert H. *Obstetrics and gynecology in America.* Chicago: American College of Obstetrics and Gynecology, 1980.

Temkin O, trans. *Soranus' gynecology.* Baltimore: The Johns Hopkins Press, 1956.

Thomas TG. A century of American medicine, 1776–1876: obstetrics and gynecology. *Am J Med Sci* 1876;72:138.

Webster JC. The future of gynecology. *Surg Gynecol Obstet* 1905;1:63.

Wells TS. Some causes of excessive mortality after surgical operations. *Br Med J* 1864;2:384. See also Brieger G. American surgery and the germ theory of disease. *Bull Hist Med* 1966;40:135.

Wood AD. The fashionable diseases: women's complaints and their treatment in nineteenth century America. *J Interdisc Hist* 1973;4:25. Reprinted in Hartman M, Banner L, eds. *Clio's consciousness raised: new perspectives on the history of women.* New York: Harper & Row, 1974:1.

Te Linde's Operative Gynecology, ninth edition, edited by John A. Rock and Howard W. Jones, III. Lippincott Williams & Wilkins, Philadelphia, © 2003.

CHAPTER

2

▼

The Ethics of Pelvic Surgery

KENNETH J. RYAN

THEORY AND PRACTICE IN MEDICAL ETHICS

Ethics is concerned with the right and wrong, the good and bad of human behavior as it materially affects other human beings and some would say even all other sentient beings. In medicine, ethics has been embodied in the venerable Hippocratic oath and aphorisms that have provided a guide over the centuries on how physicians should deal with their patients. The major goals of medicine have been to provide relief from pain and suffering, to try to treat disease, and at least minimize harm in the process. Over the years, medical ethics has also been influenced by religious traditions of charity and the Good Samaritan and by the evolution of medicine into a profession with formal licensure and societal obligations. For all its good works, medicine also has had morally problematic traditions of being paternalistic and autocratic. These traditions were severely criticized during the social upheavals of the 1960s concerned with civil rights, women's issues, and the celebration of individual autonomy. It was this social unrest in the 1960s and 1970s, as well as the revolutionary changes in medical technology such as organ transplantation, artificial organs, mechanical life support systems, genetic engineering, and assisted reproductive technologies that gave birth to a broader field of bioethics and generated the public discussions and need for formal teaching of ethics in medical schools and residency training.

Physicians have learned a new vocabulary as well as the theoretical basics of applied and normative ethics, have participated in public debates, and have communicated with moral philosophers, lawyers, and social scientists, who have been attracted to the problems in this field and often participate on hospital ethics committees. Hospital ethics committees are now reviewed by the Joint Commission for the Accreditation of Hospitals when evaluating a hospital's protection of patients' rights in matters such as terminal care and informed consent. In a 1962 edition of this text, Dr. Te Linde wrote a short piece on the moral issues of induced abortion at a time when it seemed to everyone that abortion was the only moral problem the gynecologist faced. This narrow view of ethics was common in most medical texts and medical schools. The teaching of specific courses in medical ethics began in earnest only in the past 20 years or so. This chapter recognizes the more explicit role that ethics now plays in the practice of the discipline and acknowledges the profound changes in ethical concerns brought about by advances in medical technology and surgery.

During the course of the events described in the preceding, the concept of medical ethics changed from the paternalistic Hippocratic ideal, which emphasized physician concern for the patient's well-being, to a principle- and rights-based ethic in which physicians' obligations were more clearly defined. In 1973, the American Hospital Association issued "A Patient's Bill of Rights," which emphasized institutional responsibility and the new dimension in the traditional physician–patient relationship when care is provided in the hospital. The disclosure by the physician to the patient would now include not only information on choices in diagnosis and treatment, but also how residents and students participate in patient care and procedures, whether any research is involved, and any financial relationship to laboratories or diagnostic facilities that might pose conflicts of interest for the doctor.

In 1978, the Belmont Report was issued by the National Commission for the Protection of Human Subjects of Biomedical and Behavioral Research. This report responded to the query by the US Congress concerning the ethical principles that should underlie the conduct of research and medical practice when funded by the US government. The report emphasized the following principles.

- *Respect for persons.* Treating research subjects and patients as autonomous individuals and obtaining informed consent for all research and medical treatments proposed. This principle was derived with Emanuel Kant's practical imperative in mind: to treat others as an end and never simply as a means.
- *Beneficence.* Doing a risk-benefit analysis and favoring procedures and treatments that protect or benefit subjects and patients and avoid unnecessary harm. This principle was derived with the classic Hippocratic admonition: to help and at least not harm.
- *Justice.* Being fair in the process of selecting subjects or patients and fair in the risks borne and the benefits received by them.

This final principle was derived with John Rawls' elaborate "Theory of Justice" in mind (Table 2.1).

These principles are guidelines for considering ethical issues in research and practice, but they provide less assistance when there is conflict in applying them to specific cases. In general, precedence in the law and most ethical teaching is that the patient's autonomy and right to respect require that a physician must not do anything even to benefit the patient without the patient's express permission, unless in an emergency when such permission cannot be obtained readily. Individuals of diminished autonomy, such as small children and those with mental handicaps, are protected by a requirement that physicians seek informed consent from the next of kin or a designated proxy.

There are many other approaches to ethical analysis. Some have advocated a case-based method, working from analogy or the pragmatic approach, which is to consider in the broadest terms what difference there would be in taking one or another course of action. There is much to medical ethics not covered by this discussion that still requires wisdom and judgment by the practicing physician for resolution and, when needed, the assistance of colleagues and the hospital ethics committee.

ETHICAL ISSUES IN SURGICAL TRAINING

Most surgeons trained before World War II attended medical schools and participated in residency programs affiliated with large, inner-city hospitals, where patients without adequate resources or health insurance received care. It was accepted that these patients would receive treatment and even surgery by students, interns, and residents, preferably under the watchful eyes of skilled volunteers or paid clinical faculty and only when the trainee had reached the necessary level of competence. The trade-off was free care for helping to train the doctors of the future. The care was not as luxurious as in the private pavilions or hospitals, but the quality of care was usually as good and sometimes better than private care because of the openness of the process and the enthusiasm and dedication of the young doctors-in-training and their supervisors.

When health care became an entitlement under Medicare and Medicaid government funding and health insurance became more prevalent, many patients sought the services of private physicians. The so-called free care or resident services were often unable to recruit sufficient patients to provide adequate training for new surgeons. This was particularly true in pelvic surgery; given the choice, these patients sought refuge from the clinic, where privacy and dignity were hard to maintain, and fled in large numbers to private doctors' offices. Surgical teaching thereafter often involved the private patient, with the resident ultimately doing complete procedures under the watchful eye and assistance of the patient's private doctor. The problem with this arrangement was that patients were poorly informed or uninformed about the role played by physicians-in-training, and this often became apparent only when complications arose or the medical records were reviewed in malpractice cases. There was even an expose of this on national television when an investigative reporter informed a deceived patient on camera that it was the resident and not the professor who had actually done his complex surgery. We recall that the patient said he did not believe it.

Patients are typically better informed now, and it is ethically necessary to inform the patient about teaching or training in each case so that objections can be dealt with or other arrangements made. Most surgeons involved in teaching programs tell their patients that modern surgery involves a team effort and that residents may be involved in assisting or operating with them, but that, as the private surgeons of record, they not only will be present but also will be in charge and responsible for all that takes place. Teaching should not take place in the operating room

---

TABLE 2.1.
Ethical Principles for Medical Research and Practice

Show *respect* for patients and research subjects by obtaining voluntary informed consent.

Demonstrate *beneficence* toward patients and research subjects by seeking their well-being and avoiding harm.

Provide *justice* to patients and research subjects by treating them fairly in the distribution of benefits and burdens.

without such a disclosure and the patient's informed consent. The resident's role, status, and experience should be clear to the patient. We are long past introducing medical students to patients as doctors rather than revealing their true status. Another troubling aspect of modern surgical care is the disappearance of preoperative admission time so that surgery is scheduled on the day of arrival. This further diminishes the opportunity for contact preoperatively of the resident-in-training with the patient and compromises care and education even further.

ETHICAL ISSUES IN RESEARCH ON HUMAN SUBJECTS

Although the Nuremberg medical war crimes trials of Nazi doctors and the ensuing Nuremberg Code in 1949 represent a landmark in bioethics on human subject research, they made little impact on research practices in the United States. Biomedical research expanded exponentially after World War II without much in the way of regulations or oversight. The Nuremberg Code established the need for the "voluntary consent of the human subject." It covers such other matters as the need to justify a study in terms of expected beneficial results and risks, avoiding harm and injury to subjects, freedom for the subject to withdraw, and obligation of the investigator to stop a study if continuation would likely cause injury, disability, or death. This had to do with Nazi Germany, however, and did not seem applicable to democratic countries like the United States. Much of the US medical community lost sight of the fact that the German doctors involved were distinguished professors and academicians and that they were breaking their own laws regarding the protection of vulnerable populations. In the war crimes trials, these doctors used familiar excuses to justify their research, such as that the end (more knowledge) justified the means they employed.

In 1966, the US Public Health Service introduced the requirement that all human subject research funded by the government must be peer reviewed by a local institutional review board. The objective was to protect the rights of the individuals involved, and review the quality of the informed consent and the risks and benefits of the study. This regulation was the result of a growing awareness that these kinds of safeguards often were not followed even in the best academic institutions in the United States.

In 1966, Dr. Henry K. Beecher, professor of anesthesia at Harvard University, published an article in the *New England Journal of Medicine* describing ethically troubling studies published in good journals from prestigious institutions. One example involved surgeons who performed thymectomies to check the survival of skin homografts in children from 3½ months to 18 years of age as an add-on to cardiac surgery. Another publication described transplantation of a malignant melanoma from a terminally ill daughter to her consenting mother to look for tumor antibodies. The mother died of diffuse melanoma a little more than 1 year later.

The most notorious nonsurgical studies that reached the attention of the public included the following.

1. In the Jewish Chronic Disease Hospital, cancer cells were injected into patients in 1963 without their knowledge or consent to see if they would reject them. This study originated at the Memorial Sloan-Kettering Cancer Institute.
2. The Tuskegee study, which ran from 1932 to 1972, was organized by the US Public Health Service to follow the natural history of syphilis in a cohort of 400 rural black men without providing any treatment and without any real informed consent.
3. In the Willowbrook study, new residents on admission to an institution for the retarded were infected with hepatitis virus to study the course of the disease and search for a vaccine.

When news of such studies reached the public, the US Congress in 1974 formed the National Commission for the Protection of Human Subjects of Biomedical and Behavioral Research (see the preceding) to craft suitable federal regulations on the ethical conduct of research and develop the Belmont Report to establish the ethical standards that should prevail. Although the regulations apply to research funded by the government, they should cover all research involving human subjects, regardless of the source of funding. Surgeons continually try to innovate and improve their skills and the procedures used, but they must be mindful of the possible need of antecedent work in basic science and the animal laboratory and the need for informed consent of the patient and peer review when significant deviation from standard practice is contemplated. In most instances, new surgical procedures should be developed in appropriately controlled research trials with all the safeguards needed for the protection of human subjects.

INFORMED CONSENT AND THE OPERATIVE PERMIT

It is difficult now to operate on a patient without first having a signed consent form in the medical record. Strange as this may seem to the surgeon today, this has not always been the case. The practice of requiring a signed operative permit or consent gained momentum in the 1970s and has followed the change in attitudes about patient rights and medical ethics. It has also followed successful court cases in which the patient—suffering a complication of surgery not caused by negligence—could prove that the physician failed to inform him or her adequately of the gravity or frequency of a risk or failed to mention the risk altogether. Physicians have sometimes withheld complete disclosure of risks to avoid frightening the patient or ensure that the patient would not refuse surgery. The courts have held that the physician has a duty to disclose all the information a reasonable person would require to make an informed decision. According to the courts, the patient has a right to the in-

TABLE 2.2.
Elements and Content of Informed Consent

Disclosure: Advise patients of their diagnoses and suggest surgical therapy, alternatives, and risks and benefits of all options, including no therapy, in sufficient detail to satisfy the needs of a reasonable person to make an informed choice.

Comprehension: Use language and descriptive materials appropriate to the patient's level of comprehension, and determine that the patient understands by asking for a summary in the patient's own words.

Voluntariness: Be certain the patient is free of coercion or constraints on his or her ability to choose freely.

Competence: Determine that the patient has no evidence of limitation in ability to understand and act independently on the information disclosed.

Validation: Obtain the written consent.

---

formation even if it results in a decision to forgo a life-saving procedure.

Before 1960, there seldom was a requirement for a written document; the transfer of information and patient consent, if they occurred, were private transactions between patients and their doctors. The demand for informed consent started in research (see the preceding) and then spread to the practice of medicine, fostered by more openness in medicine, a greater interest in patient autonomy, and court decisions requiring disclosure. Today, informed consent is required for all operative procedures and has at least five elements (Table 2.2).

In practice, this involves informing the patient of the diagnosis, including the degree of certainty of the diagnosis; the recommended surgery; and possible alternatives with their expected outcomes, risks, and benefits, including those of no therapy. Determining the correct content to disclose to the patient still requires some judgment because it is impossible to disclose every contingency. The shared experience of colleagues and an institutional record of previous operative complications are helpful, as are preprinted consent forms that have been prepared for various procedures based on a collective experience. The consent should be obtained by the operative surgeon well in advance of surgery in a comfortable setting with adequate time for the patient to ask questions and make an informed decision. It is important to remember that risks have two dimensions—incidence and severity—and that sometimes a rare occurrence needs mentioning if it is of a sufficiently severe nature. Although an important obligation of the physician is to benefit the patient, there are few instances in which withholding important information can be justified on this basis.

SURGICAL COMPETENCE AS A MORAL COMMITMENT

Competence of the surgeon is a moral commitment to the patient, especially before undertaking a new procedure. It is essential that adequate preparation in the basic and clinical sciences and training in surgical techniques be accomplished before any new surgical procedure is introduced into clinical medicine. An illustrative example of an overenthusiastic rush into a procedure was the sudden popularity of cardiac transplantation in the 1960s. The preparatory laboratory work in cardiac transplantation started in 1905, but the first successful replacement of the heart in a dog took place in 1960. Immune suppression, which is crucial to the procedure, was introduced in 1958, and long-time survival of grafts occurred by 1965. A chimpanzee heart transplanted into a human in 1964 functioned for only a brief time. Christian Barnard reported the first successful human heart transplantation in December 1967 in South Africa. By the end of 1968, 101 human heart transplantations had been performed by 64 surgical groups in 22 countries. Most patients improved briefly and then died of rejection of the transplant or infection. In 2 years, the procedure was largely discredited, and it took more than 10 additional years to reestablish wide acceptance of the operation. This experience illustrates the need to limit difficult and complex procedures to specialized centers that have the resources and adequately trained surgeons to perform them.

This is equally true for complex pelvic surgery. The move to the subspecialty boards in gynecologic oncology and reproductive biology and the creation of programs in advanced gynecologic surgery have helped to emphasize the need for specialized training in surgical techniques for pelvic surgeons. The rapid expansion of the use of laparoscopic surgery, which started in a disorganized manner with many accompanying complications, is another example of a rush into routine practice. The use of this procedure is now better organized, with the establishment of guidelines for training, and preceptorships, before a surgeon is qualified. It is likely that standards will be developed for the number and type of operative cases that must be performed each year by a pelvic surgeon in order to maintain competence. This will further ensure the qualifications needed to maintain operative privileges.

MORAL AND LEGAL ISSUES OF ABORTION

The moral controversy in the United States has been bitter and divisive since the Supreme Court's *Roe v. Wade* decision of 1973, which legalized abortion throughout the country. In keeping with the Puritan and other religious traditions during our first 200 years of development as a nation, abortion had always been considered by some to be morally wrong, but it was covered legally under the common law and generally dealt with leniently until the mid-19th century. During this period, abortion before quickening typically was not considered criminal. The American Medical Association was founded in 1847 and became the framework for an organized effort to change public policy on abortion. A physician-led crusade against abortion started in the 1850s and continued well into the 20th century with the objective of making abortion a crime. The expressed objectives were not only to establish a moral standard, but also to protect women from being harmed by the procedure and to drive "abortionists," who were usually nonphysicians, out of business. This set the standard for state laws until the Supreme Court action in 1973, which established a national standard.

Abortion in the pre–*Roe v. Wade* era usually was performed illegally by poorly trained individuals and often was performed under life- or health-threatening conditions. By the 1950s, fatal illegal abortion had become the number one cause of maternal death in New York City. Some abortions were carried out safely by physicians in hospitals to protect the mother's life from medical or pregnancy complications, but a new ploy was introduced. Psychiatric consultants recommended abortions under the justification of the threat of suicide by the pregnant woman, and this became a popular way to get around the laws and perform an abortion safely in a hospital. However, this latter mechanism for obtaining a safe abortion was demeaning to women and was available mainly to private patients and the wealthy. Because many countries other than the United States had more liberal abortion laws, the wealthy could also simply travel abroad to seek abortions.

After World War II, attitudes toward abortion softened in the United States. In 1959, the American Law Institute, reflecting the popular mood, introduced model legislation to allow abortion for so-called hard reasons: if the woman's life or health is endangered, if the infant will have a severe birth defect, or if the pregnancy was the result of rape or incest. This was not enacted until some states, such as New York and California, liberalized their laws in the early 1970s. In the 1960s, there was a widespread and severe rubella epidemic, during which many women of all walks of life sought and received abortions to avoid having children with severe congenital anomalies. These abortions were performed using the deception of a psychiatric indication under threat of suicide (noted in the preceding). In many instances, however, the demand for abortion by pregnant women with rubella was so great and widespread that the laws were simply ignored. Also, amniocentesis and prenatal diagnosis were just beginning to be used, and this new technology further changed public attitudes.

The *Roe v. Wade* decision was more liberal than the American Law Institute's model in that it made abortion a privacy right and, at least in the first trimester of pregnancy, allowed for abortion without restrictions. In the second trimester, restrictions on where and how abortions were performed could be set by law if necessary to protect the woman's health. In the third trimester, the state can have a legitimate interest in protecting fetal life and can restrict abortion, but not if it adversely affects the pregnant woman's life or health. Some have claimed that the animus and intensity of the antiabortion movement is based on the too-liberal nature of the law. Since the time of the Supreme Court decision, much has been written about both the validity of the logic of the Court's majority legal opinion and the moral arguments for and against abortion itself. The moral arguments are deceptively simple in the extremes. One argument is based on the moral status of the fetus, and the other argument is based on the rights of the pregnant woman versus those of the fetus when their interests conflict.

In the first argument, abortion is morally wrong because the fetus is an innocent human life; it is wrong to harm the fetus from conception on, or deprive it of life, just as it is wrong to harm any human living creature. The counter argument is that abortion is not morally wrong because the developing life in the uterus—a zygote (fertilized egg), preembryo, embryo, or the early fetus—although technically living and human, is still developing from a microscopic single cell into a complex organism. At no stage before viability does it constitute the status of a freely living human person, and at these early stages of development it does not require the absolute respect for life that is afforded the late fetus or a born child.

In the second argument, abortion is morally right because a woman should not be forced to use her body to bear a child against her will. The universal moral justification would be that no one should be forced to use his or her body for the benefit of someone else. The counter argument is that abortion is not morally right because the woman has an obligation to the fetus (even one resulting from rape) and should not harm or destroy it, regardless of her preferences or needs about the use of her body.

One can embellish or modify these two arguments, but they constitute the core of the rationales generally offered for and against abortion. One can even see the possibilities of accommodation between the two positions based on the gestational age of the pregnancy (early), the specification of certain justifiable circumstances (e.g., rape and incest), or the use of the American Law Institute's model code mentioned in the preceding. In fact, there has been little willingness to give any ground on either side of the argument. We believe both sides have merit depending on one's beliefs, religious or otherwise, about the moral status of the fetus and about a woman's rights. There is no single morally correct answer for everyone in our diverse society, but even this position of seeing merit in the opposing arguments is attacked by extremists on both sides. The major challenge is not to convince one or the other side that they are wrong, but rather to try to convince the two entrenched opposing sides that they have to learn to live together in a democratic society without the intense rhetoric and deadly violence that has occurred. It is important for the gynecologist to determine how he or she feels about these issues and to deal fairly and honestly with patients who ask for advice about abortion or request abortion services. It is generally accepted that physicians should be free to follow their own beliefs and not be forced to engage in practices that are in their own minds morally wrong, but it is difficult as a practicing gynecologist to stay completely neutral on this issue. In the year 2000, the Food and Drug Administration approved the use of the oral abortion drug RU 486 (mifepristone), which has done little to change the dynamic of the controversy.

TERMINAL ILLNESS, ADVANCE DIRECTIVES, AND EUTHANASIA

The moral agenda on issues regarding death and dying has been set largely by the courts as doctors, patients, patients' families, and hospital administrators have sought to have the intractable controversies that arise among them resolved before a judge. Problems with managing terminal illness and persistent coma typically stem from the introduction of technology, such as the respirator, that can keep the human body functioning biologically and either delay or prolong dying without the prospect of a return to even a diminished level of normalcy. The problem with treatment of terminal cancer is often the willingness of the surgeon or patient to try extreme courses of chemotherapy and surgery beyond reasonable bounds of hope for even limited prolongation of a meaningful life. When patients, their families, and their health care teams all agree on one of these courses of action, there is usually no overt problem, except the question of the prudent use of scarce resources. When there is agreement among all parties, there is seldom a need to go to court, and courts discourage bringing these cases before them. When there is disagreement and the patient, the patient's family, or both want therapy and life support stopped and the doctors want it continued, or when the family and patient insist on so-called futile or nonindicated therapy or life support and the doctors believe otherwise, the stage is set for conflict that often ends up in court. The courts have provided guidance in each of these types of cases. The cases followed one another over the years and influenced public attitudes. Although not every case and its outcome are comparable, the general consensus is that the patient's autonomous choices are binding and that the ultimate goal of medicine is not to preserve life at any cost, but to relieve pain and suffering in keeping with the patient's wishes.

Karen Ann Quinlan was a 21-year-old woman who had been in a prolonged coma after an overdose of alcohol and drugs at a birthday party. She had been put on a respirator when she developed pneumonia, and it was expected she would die if the respirator were withdrawn. When the likelihood of recovery disappeared, her family requested removal of the respirator. The hospital went to court because of the uncertainty about liability. Although the lower courts denied the parents' request, the New Jersey Supreme Court overturned these decisions and allowed removal of the respirator. Ironically, Karen lived another 10 years in the persistent vegetative state before dying. It was in this decision that the court suggested the use of a hospital ethics committee to help in prognosis. This case, as well as the subsequent need for ethics committees for treatment decisions in the newborn nursery, prompted the development of hospital ethics committees nationwide.

In the case of *Brophy v. New England Sinai Hospital,* the patient was a 49-year-old firefighter from Boston who was in a persistent vegetative state from which he would not recover because of a massive brain hemorrhage. He had previously indicated to his family that he would not want to be kept alive under such circumstances, and his family requested the withdrawal of his feeding tube. There was much public discussion and debate in the press, including objections by religious leaders, but the Massachusetts Supreme Court in 1986 granted the family's wish, and the patient was allowed to die peacefully at home. It took essentially 10 years between these two cases to go from withdrawing a respirator to withdrawing food and fluid, and the moral arguments changed. Allowing someone to die under such circumstances became not only permissible, but also desirable, when this is what they would have wanted. Maintaining life without cognition was no longer an obligation.

In the case of Nancy Cruzan of Missouri, which reached the US Supreme Court and was decided in 1990, the issue was similar to the Brophy case. Nancy Cruzan was in a prolonged coma, and her parents wanted to withdraw food and fluid. There was no record of her prior stated wishes, and Missouri has a state law forbidding withdrawal without such evidence. The US Supreme Court found the Missouri statute constitutional; therefore, the parents did not have immediate relief. In the course of handing down this decision, the US Supreme Court established the right of competent patients to refuse any kind of treatment, even life-sustaining treatment, and that no distinction was necessary between artificial feeding and other forms of therapy. Finally, evidence was found of Nancy Cruzan's prior wishes that she would not want to be kept alive in a permanent coma, and she was allowed to die after treatment was withdrawn.

In a diametrically opposite type of case, Helen Wanglie was an 86-year-old woman in a persistent vegetative state. Her family wanted everything done to maintain her, whereas the doctors objected because there was no hope for recovery and the cost was enormous. The case went to court. In this case, the family maintained that this is what the patient would want because she felt life should be preserved at all costs. The court found for the family and treatment continued. This is nonetheless consistent with most of the other court decisions that make the patient's prior wishes a determining factor in the determination whether or not to continue therapy.

Many of these cases did not deal directly with the issue of withholding or withdrawing therapy from patients with a terminal illness, but they provided the moral and legal environment in which such requests can more readily be honored by the physician. There had been sufficient consensus on this issue that in 1990, the Patient Self Determination Act was passed by Congress, requiring hospitals to promote the use of advance directives by their patients to qualify for federal funds for Medicare and Medicaid. Practically every state in the country has enacted laws that allow health care proxies, durable power of attorney, living wills, or advance directives for withholding or withdrawing care and protecting the rights of the terminally ill. Pelvic surgeons should familiarize themselves with applicable laws and discuss these issues with their patients and their families, preferably before such decisions are actually needed for implementation. The advanced directive provides physicians with essential guidance on the need for do-not-resuscitate (DNR) orders and the type of care and treatment to be provided for patients with terminal or fatal diseases when discharge from the hospital or recovery is not expected. A problem arises when a patient with DNR orders must go to surgery and either the anesthetist or surgeon objects to having restrictions on resuscitation during a surgical procedure. Often the surgery is for a problem incidental to the long-term illness. Institutional policy should be developed for such cases; the tendency has been to allow patients to keep their DNR orders and still be allowed surgery.

Although there is widespread acceptance of foregoing therapy in terminal illness or a permanent coma, also known as *passive euthanasia,* there is still dissension about whether active euthanasia or physician-assisted suicide should be allowed or encouraged. The argument has been advanced that there is no real moral difference between passive and active euthanasia because the objective is to relieve pain or suffering by death in both cases. This argument misses the emotional significance for physicians and patients of the conceptual difference between allowing death and killing. It also misses the concerns about possible abuse, "brutalization" of the physician, and an erosion of trust between the public and the medical profession. Physician-assisted suicide is a halfway measure that at least ensures patient participation. There is much public interest in active euthanasia and physician-assisted suicide, and one or the other issue has been on several state ballots for popular vote. So far, these have all been defeated with close margins, except for the passage of a law in Oregon permitting physician-assisted suicide under restricted conditions. In the first year of the Oregon law in 1998, 15 patients availed themselves of assisted suicide, most with terminal cancer.

Unless controls are stringent, there are concerns that patients with undetected depression might request assisted suicide or that patients might seek this solely for economic reasons. Holland has had many years of experience dealing with a permissive policy on euthanasia, and based on interpretations of this experience, arguments have been advanced to support or condemn the practice, depending on the observer's bias. In the year 2000, the Dutch Parliament finally legalized Euthanasia and Assisted Suicide. Actually the first legalization of euthanasia occurred in the Northern Territory of Australia in 1996.

As a profession, we do a poor job in providing adequate medication for pain relief, especially with cancer. The Agency for Health Care Policy and Research of the Department of Health and Human Services issued new practice guidelines in 1994 to improve performance in this area. It is possible that more attention to pain relief and wider availability of hospice care may relieve some of the pressure for euthanasia. Although many physicians and their medical societies are against changing the laws about euthanasia at this time, the public may be moving in this direction faster than the profession. The shift in attitude and more lenient enforcement of laws on use of morphinelike drugs allow physicians more latitude. Physicians have reported a greater willingness to use doses of drugs for pain relief that may in the end hasten the patient's death.

BIBLIOGRAPHY

Beecher HK. Ethics and clinical research. *N Engl J Med* 1966;274:1354.

Faden RR, Beauchamp TL. *A history and theory of informed consent.* New York: Oxford University Press, 1986.

Jacox A, Carr DB, Payne R. New clinical-practice guidelines for the management of pain in patients with cancer. *N Engl J Med* 1994;330:651.

Jonsen AR. *The birth of bioethics.* New York: Oxford University Press, 1998.

King NMP. *Making sense of advance directives.* Dordrecht, The Netherlands: Kluwer Academic Publishers, 1993.

LaFollette H, ed. *Ethics in practice, an anthology.* Cambridge: Blackwell, 1997.

Rothman DJ. *Strangers at the bedside.* New York: Basic Books, 1991.

Ryan KJ. Abortion or motherhood, madness and suicide. *Am J Obstet Gynecol* 1992;160:1415.

Veatch RM. *Medical ethics.* Boston: Jones & Bartlett, 1989.

Te Linde's Operative Gynecology, ninth edition, edited by John A. Rock and Howard W. Jones, III. Lippincott Williams & Wilkins, Philadelphia, © 2003.

CHAPTER

3

▼

Psychological Aspects of Pelvic Surgery

BETTY RUTH SPEIR

PSYCHOLOGICAL ASPECTS OF PELVIC SURGERY

The technological revolution has presented today's surgeon with a vast array of sophisticated equipment. In capable hands, miraculous surgical feats can be performed on a woman's body, but at what cost to her psychological self?

The removal or reconstruction of diseased or dysfunctional anatomy sets off a chain reaction of parallel events in a woman's psyche.

For a surgeon, the gynecologic operation is an ordinary event of usually simple dimension. For the patient, each procedure is a unique experience. Her sense of well-being and health are threatened. She will definitely lose control over her body for some indefinite period of time. She may perceive the planned procedure as temporarily or even permanently affecting her sexual identity.

As even complicated procedures become routine, the surgeon risks losing perspective about the impact of surgery on the life of the individual woman. The patient who experiences ablative genital (or breast) surgery is strongly influenced by her emotions. These vary in degree but are usually cumulative. As the patient passes through the presurgical, surgical, and postsurgical experiences, she is stressed and may be inundated beyond her capacity to compensate. If help is not available to facilitate emotional healing and rehabilitation, permanent psychological damage might result.

The majority of women do heal and take up their lives, raise their children, work at their jobs, and relate well to their husbands or lovers. For them, the healing interval is relatively quick, and the stress is modest. Do not underestimate what can be learned from this segment of psychologically healthy women patients. In the 1940s, Abraham Maslow studied people with exceptional mental health to develop his hierarchy of needs theory. He discovered that these people's potential had never been weakened by negative thinking, destructive outlook, or destructive self-image. "The rest of us," he declared, "fixate at a lower level because someone or thing has implanted notions of limitations."

Once you become cognizant of the success statistics in your own patient population, you may discover why most women recover after gynecologic surgery to zestfully re-embrace life, whereas others begin to slowly turn away from its possibilities.

It will never be enough for a surgeon to be a trained mechanic, able only to diagnose and repair. He or she must also be prepared to predict, recognize, and begin treatment of the psychological consequences of gynecologic disorders. This chapter is designed to help surgeons and other physicians better understand the female perspective and to use that knowledge to facilitate multidimensional healing.

ANKH

The ansate cross, Egyptian emblem of generation, symbol for life and soul and eternity, is a mark universally designated to depict femaleness (Fig. 3.1). By using this hieroglyph, modern scientists continue an ancient tradition of respect and reverence for women. Within the inner sanctum of every woman's mind lie symbols that are powerful and personal. These feminine identity markers are guarded and guided by her instincts, and no surgeon can successfully maneuver in this labyrinth of psychological and psychosexual emotion and cause no harm unless the female patient acts as a guide.

Egyptian writings from 2,000 years ago in the Kahan Papyrus depict the uterus as having an important and powerful effect on mental life, and current research tends to agree with the ancient scribes. The uterus has great symbolic value for many modern women, too. Beginning with the rite of passage called menstruation, a strong invisible bond is formed between a woman and her body. Her biological clock has been set. For the next 40 years or so, she will be reminded each month that she is a woman, and menstruation is regarded by many as palpable proof of their femininity.

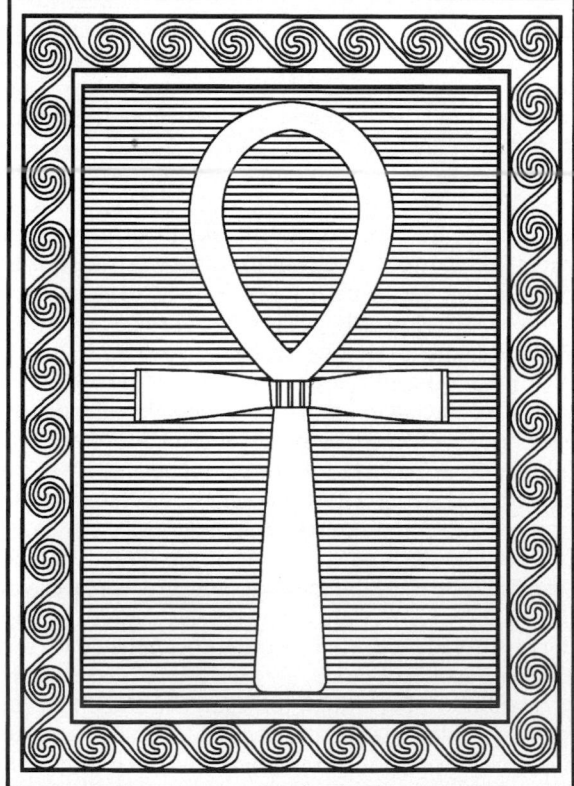

FIGURE 3.1. The ansate cross, or ankh amulet, is an ancient Egyptian symbol of life and sexuality.

Others believe that menstruation is part of a natural cleansing cycle that purges the body of poisons that accumulate during the month. They know from experience that the premenstrual symptoms of edema, bloating, headaches, and emotional tension will be washed away in the tide of their monthly flow.

For some, the rhythm of the menstrual cycle is used as a way to time and order their lives. Like the phases of the moon, this cycle bestows a sense of routine, regularity, and predictability that has emotional significance. With the onset of menstruation, a woman is forever changed. Surgical removal of any of the reproductive organs will change her again, but how?

The fact that many medical conditions are affected by a woman's menstrual cycle is well documented. Medical suppression of ovulation is commonly used as a way to evaluate and treat such chronic conditions as migraine headache, epilepsy, asthma, rheumatoid arthritis, irritable bowel syndrome, and diabetes.

Current research is trying to determine if removal of malignant breast tumors during specific times of the menstrual cycle might affect long-term survival rates. Other scientists are investigating the circulating levels of sex hormones to determine whether or not the fluctuations produce a direct effect on the immune system and consequently, the disease processes. Hormones secreted during a woman's menstrual cycle certainly affect her mood. Could the decline of these hormones during the natural aging process contribute to dementia? The future is alive with fascinating possibilities of eventual elucidation, but today's woman is backlit by the present. Her concerns about her body and the way it will work after surgery are immediate and quite often, heart-wrenching.

A woman about to undergo a hysterectomy might wonder if her lover will be able to detect the absence of her uterus? After the surgery, will she be thought of as less of a woman? Will her partner abandon her for someone who is still complete, either in the sense of being able to offer the possibility of a child or complete in the sense of having experienced no unnatural surgical transformations?

Will orgasm be as pleasurable for her after the surgery? For many women, the uterus has symbolic significance as a sexual organ. The uterus contracts during orgasm. Some women perceive this as most pleasurable. If the patient believes the uterus is essential to sexual response, then, in fact, it often becomes so, and women with this mindset may become sexually dysfunctional when it is removed.

Once the procedure is accomplished, will she still look and sound like a woman, or will she become noticeably more masculine? For others, the uterus is closely tied to feelings of attractiveness and sexual desirability. To a few women, removal of the uterus or ovaries or both constitutes a desexing, a permanent destruction of female identity and function. Sadly, certain members of the medical community as well as the feminist community perpetuate this notion and increase the attendant fear when they refer to women who must have their ovaries removed as castrates.

Some women become distressed when they learn they must deal with the certainty of absolute sterility. For those who choose motherhood, the personality, uterus, ovaries, breasts, and vagina work in harmony to attract a necessary mate and get down to the business of creating new life. These organs become vital coconspirators in the sexual and reproductive aspects of a woman's life. Impending loss of these physical structures because of disease or dysfunction sometimes creates deep angst that must be resolved before surgery is attempted. Many women who have all the children they want and who do not wish to get pregnant again are still sometimes disturbed by the finality of the decision. The gynecologist should assure these maternal women that, although they will no longer be able to conceive a child, the powerful urge to create will never leave them. In time, they will learn to direct this primal energy into other areas of their lives and be immensely satisfied with the results.

Today's modern woman, for the most part, is an avid information seeker. She surfs the net, buys the latest books, reads magazine articles, and conducts in-depth interviews with peers who have experienced similar gynecologic problems. A certain proportion of the harvested material is useful to her and perhaps even illuminating for the physician, but unfortunately, some of the sources are inherently flawed, prejudicial, illogical, or without scientific basis in medical reality. It is the physician's responsibility to separate the grains of truth from the chaff. All the information she has gathered represents her attempt to prepare herself psychologically for the ordeal ahead, and she must never be condemned or made to feel small for trying to protect herself.

For the gynecologist, it is not necessary to change a patient's basic attitude or feelings. It is, however, vital to acknowledge them. The right information, reassurance, and support usually quickly modify many negative factors and lead to a healthier attitude and understanding of the surgical process. It is crucial that the patient be allowed to vent her anxiety and speak of her fears.

COMMUNICATION

Patients in General

Diplomats the world over understand the significance of effective communication. Indeed, the possibility of world peace depends on their ability to interact efficiently. A female patient's psychological bearing before, during, and after the gynecologic procedure can depend on the communication techniques employed by her physician. Once you establish rapport, begin to speak of the real and present danger to her health and then, elaborate on your plans to protect her.

Whenever possible, provide pleasant surroundings where you and your patient can comfortably hold a private conversation. Push all other thoughts out of your mind. These few minutes belong exclusively to her, and the quality of the time you spend actively communicating will pay healthy dividends for you both.

Whether explaining the simplicity of a needle-directed breast biopsy or the intricacies of hysterectomy, you must be able to highlight the technical details of the procedure and its postsurgical realities in a nonthreatening but utterly truthful manner. Begin the presentation using simple but thorough explanations and examples of the procedures. Your patient will let you know how much information she can or wishes to process by the questions she asks.

Besides technical competence, the patient needs two assurances from her surgeon during the presurgical consultation. One, is to know that she has your complete attention, that her problem is being taken seriously, and two, that you are qualified to competently help her cope with all of the ramifications of this new experience.

Dealing with the patient's feelings usually is not difficult if the surgeon accepts the viewpoint that many of the patient's emotions are part of the gynecologic situation. To the physician, the presurgical tension is predictable, familiar, transient, and simply comes with the territory, but to each new patient, it represents a dramatic and life-altering experience.

To interpret the patient's true feelings, simply listen to her. Listening well is both an art and a skill, and the surgeon who cares about the patient's physical and mental health as well as her quick recovery works diligently to hone a sharp edge on this valuable tool. Listen and you will hear the woman give a name to her most profound doubts and fears. Repeat her words so that you are absolutely certain you understand what she said, and she is absolutely assured that you are listening to her.

Begin the communication process by finding out what the patient perceives will be done to her body and why the procedure is necessary. Find out what she believes the consequences of the surgery will be. How does she think the surgery will impact her life? As she discusses the implications of her decision, her knowledge, fears, and biases emerge. At this point, you should be able to supplement the patient's perspective with appropriate explanations about anatomy, physiology, and pathology. After this, it is time to describe in detail the usual preoperative, operative, and postoperative routines. Address the patient's questions and fears in as many ways as it takes for her to become confident that she understands what is about to happen to her.

Carefully explain what you are going to do to help her. If she wants to know, or needs to know, describe the common physical sensations, bandages, incisions, catheters, tubing, and medications that are associated with her particular procedure. Define the patient's role in her own convalescence and recovery. Give her a general timetable for how long she will feel discomfort, have to use pain medication, when she will be ambulatory, and finally, when she will be discharged from the hospital or outpatient center.

Relate the most common complications that might occur as the result of the pelvic surgery. Injuries that might affect the quality of her life, even temporarily, should never come as a postsurgical surprise, nor should they be glossed over during the signing of the consent forms.

Iatrogenic injury remains the most common cause of lower urinary tract trauma. An understanding of the prevention, recognition, and treatment of urologic complications is important for every surgeon performing major pelvic surgery. Injury to a woman's genitourinary system may take 10 to 20 years to develop full-blown symptoms, about the same time line as from multiple childbirths, but it remains a possibility. Physicians, however, disagree on whether or not to tell the patient that urinary incontinence after hysterectomy because of damage to the pelvic nerves or pelvic supportive structures could be a long-term adverse effect because only 4% of the hysterectomies performed are for relief from symptoms of incontinence.

Complications such as the formation of adhesions may occur in as many as 55% to 100% of patients after gynecologic surgery. These adhesions can become a critical issue from a standpoint of reproductive potential, and their presence is also strongly associated with pelvic pain, abnormal bowel function, and small bowel obstruction.

The mentally competent patient has a moral, legal, and ethical right to make an intelligent informed decision and can only do it if she is privy to all of the available facts concerning her situation. It is essential that you involve her in the decision-making processes, because the more committed she is to the proposed treatment, the more involved she will become in her own preparation and rehabilitation.

The art of touching, the therapeutic laying on of the hands, is important. Being lonely, frightened, and sick is a reason for the patient to be touched by her physician, especially if she seems particularly overwhelmed by her situation. To hold the patient's hand while talking to her or touch her shoulder is therapeutic. Even a comforting hug is appropriate if it fits the circumstances and the patient reaches out to you. Before fetal monitoring, quality of labor was evaluated by sitting at the patient's bedside with the physician's hand on her abdomen to feel uterine contractions. Often, the presence of the physician and a warm hand on her abdomen made the patient relax, rest, and become calmer during active labor. Cancer patients, especially, on hearing bad news, need immediate human-to-human contact to stay grounded enough to face that terrible moment. The professional boundaries of roles, time, place and space, gifts and services, chaperoned examinations, physical contact, money and formal language, were never intended to be an impermeable membrane separating a doctor's ability to administer human kindness from the patient's need to receive it. A healer's touch can often comfort a distressed patient when words are inadequate.

A patient's family is a vital part of her support system, too, and can be a potent ally, or not, to the health care team. If your patient requests that family members be present during her consultation, allow it, but speak directly to her whenever possible.

Once the initial presurgical discussions are complete, your patient may need some time to digest all the new information she has received. After assimilation, expect her to contact you for clarification or to ask more questions. You should be available to her. Too often, office personnel believe their role is to shield the physician from patients rather than to facilitate meaningful contact.

Multicultural Patients

Multicultural patients abound in the United States and their numbers are increasing dramatically. The populations are sometimes situated in dense clusters in specific regions and physicians in these areas are often multilingual or have assistants who are able to act as interpreters. No matter where your practice is located, chances are that at some point during your career as a physician, an individual from another culture will need your help.

Mull makes the following suggestions for communicating effectively with a person whose language you do not speak and whose culture is foreign to you: Make sure that your office staff are courteous and respectful. Show the genuine concern you feel. Be friendly and helpful to build rapport and develop a repertoire of knowledge. Familiarize yourself with the general principles of their traditional medicine. Learn a few key phrases from their language, and use these for initial greeting and during examinations. Include, at least in discussion, any family members your patient considers influential. Always ask what they have done to treat themselves. Have they consulted an influential family member? A healer? Have they used home or herbal remedies?

Physicians should be aware of common themes that exist in cross-cultural medicine, including the following.

Fear of blood loss
Fear of cold
Tradition of male dominance
Conservatism in sexual matters relative to teenage girls
Poorly developed concept of preventive medicine
Intolerance of side effects from medication
Expectation of expeditious wellness
Reluctance to discuss emotions with people who are not family members

Diaz-Gilbert cautions health care professionals to check their prejudices at the door and not to assume that a non–English speaking person is uneducated. The following are some guidelines for effective communication with multicultural patients.

Allot extra time for the multicultural patient.
Address every patient initially in English.
Ask if the patient carries a bilingual dictionary.
Gesture or write down simple words or phrases.
Use visual cues, such as insurance forms, calendars, medication bottles, or anatomic sketches. If necessary, draw a picture to convey what you mean.

If the patient needs to perform a specific task, such as disrobing, carefully pantomime each step. Remain aware that direct eye contact, certain hand or finger gestures,

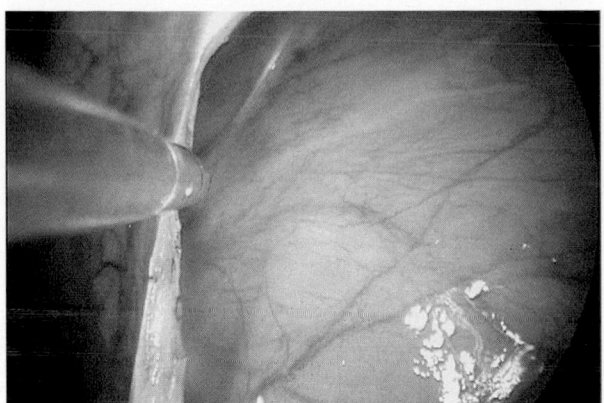

COLOR FIGURE 15.9.

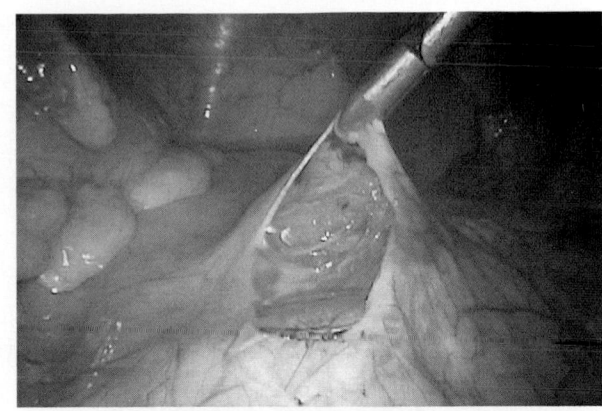

COLOR FIGURE 15.10.

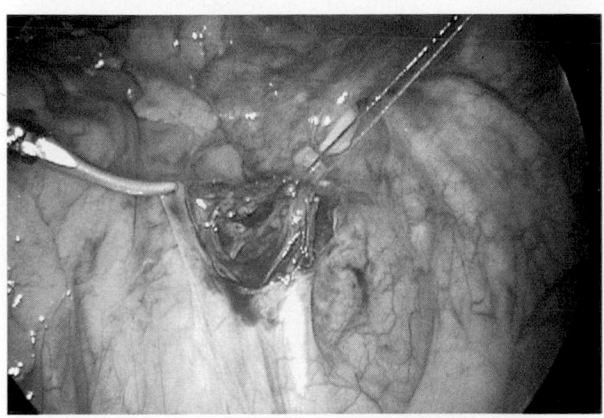

COLOR FIGURE 15.11.

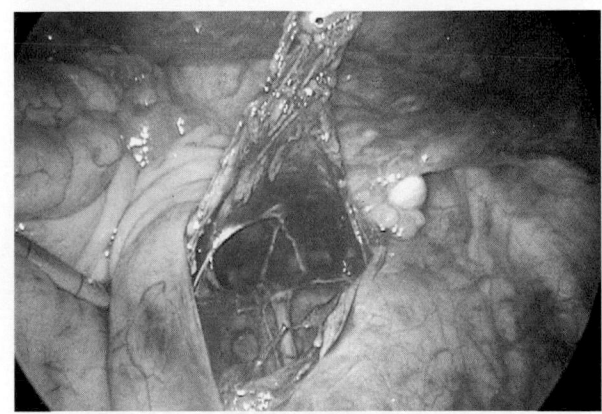

COLOR FIGURE 15.12.

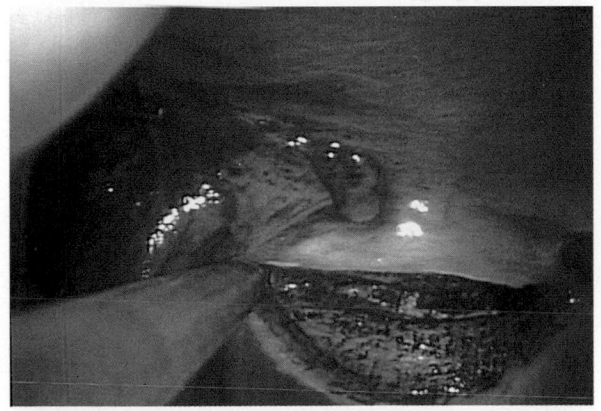

COLOR FIGURE 15.13.

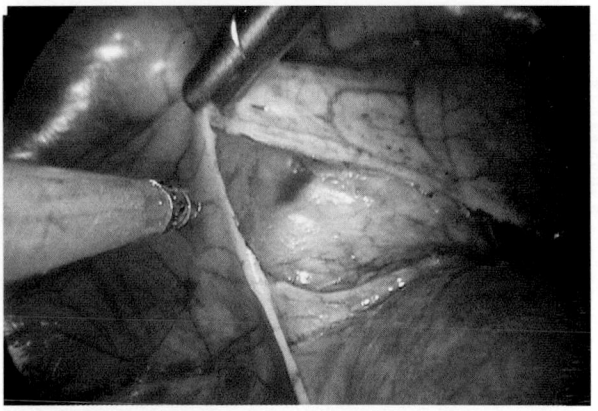

COLOR FIGURE 15.14.

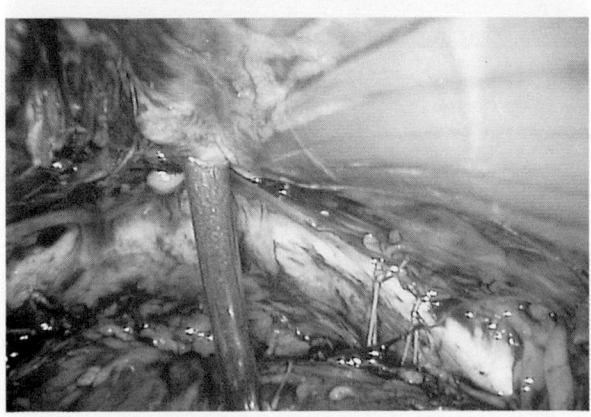

COLOR FIGURE 15.15.

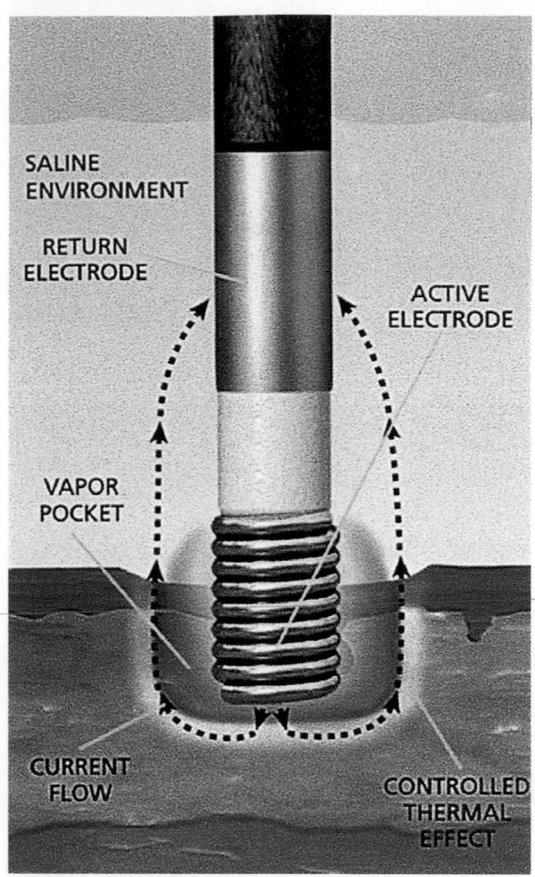

COLOR FIGURE 17.9.

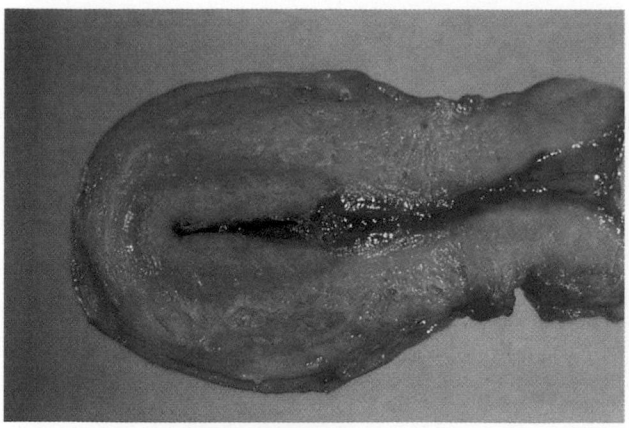

COLOR FIGURE 17.34.

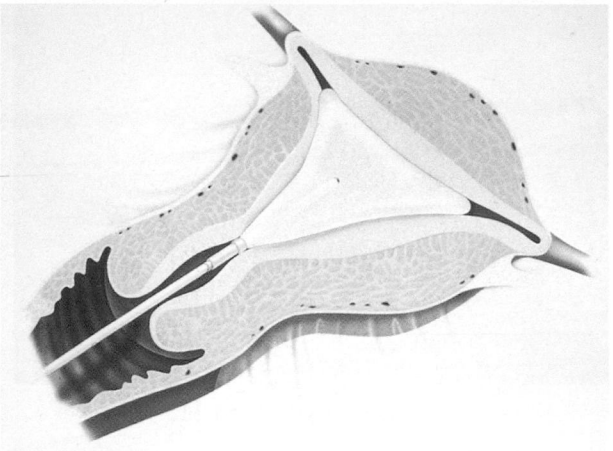

COLOR FIGURE 17.36.

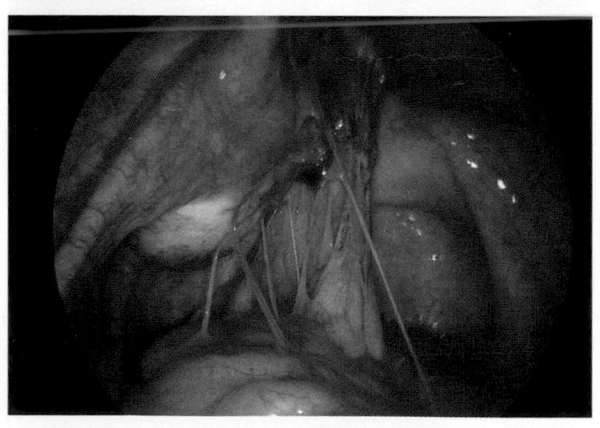

COLOR FIGURE 24.9.

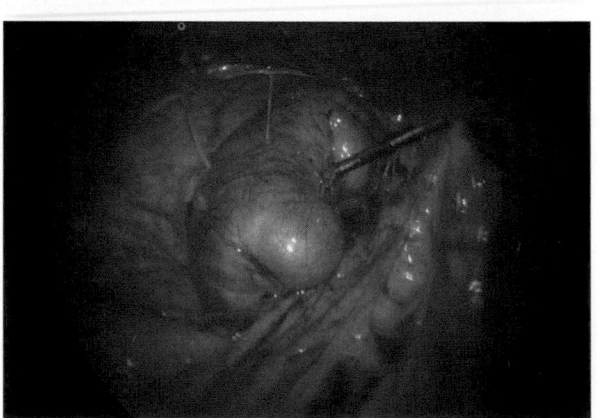

COLOR FIGURE 24.10.

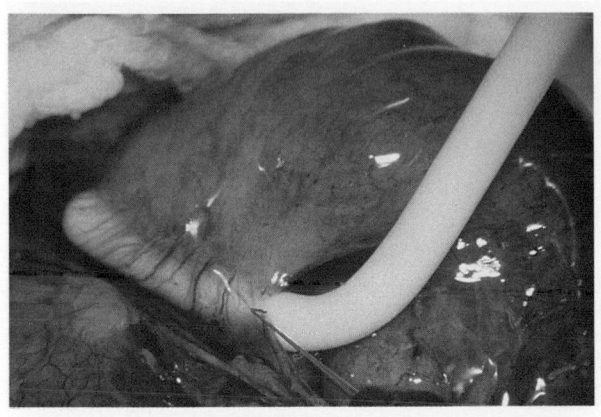

COLOR FIGURE 24.13.

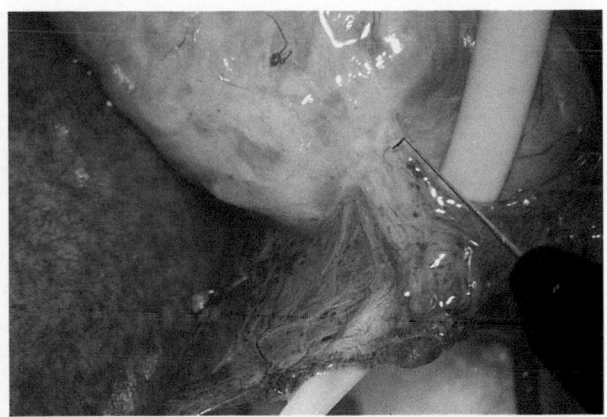

COLOR FIGURE 24.14.

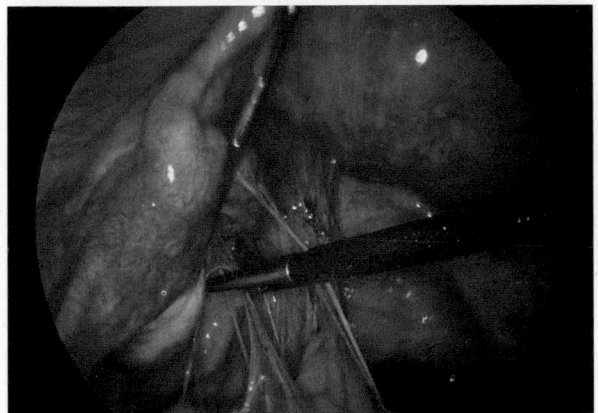

COLOR FIGURE 24.15.

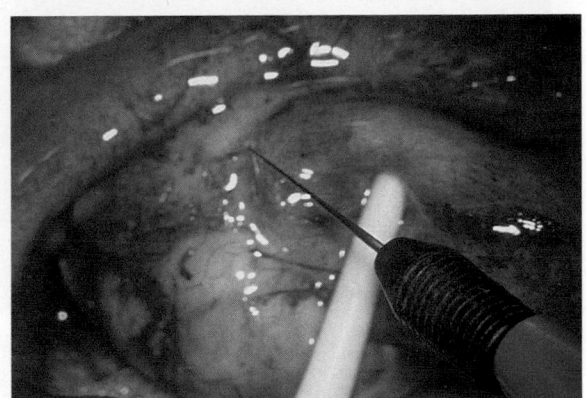

COLOR FIGURE 24.19.

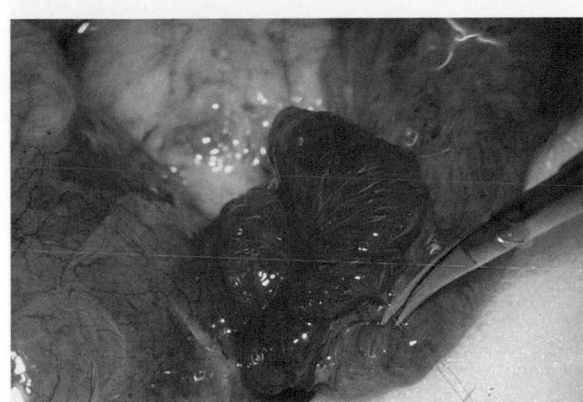

COLOR FIGURE 24.21.

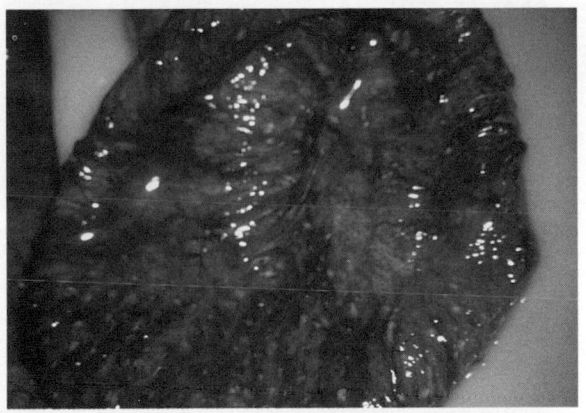

COLOR FIGURE 24.22.

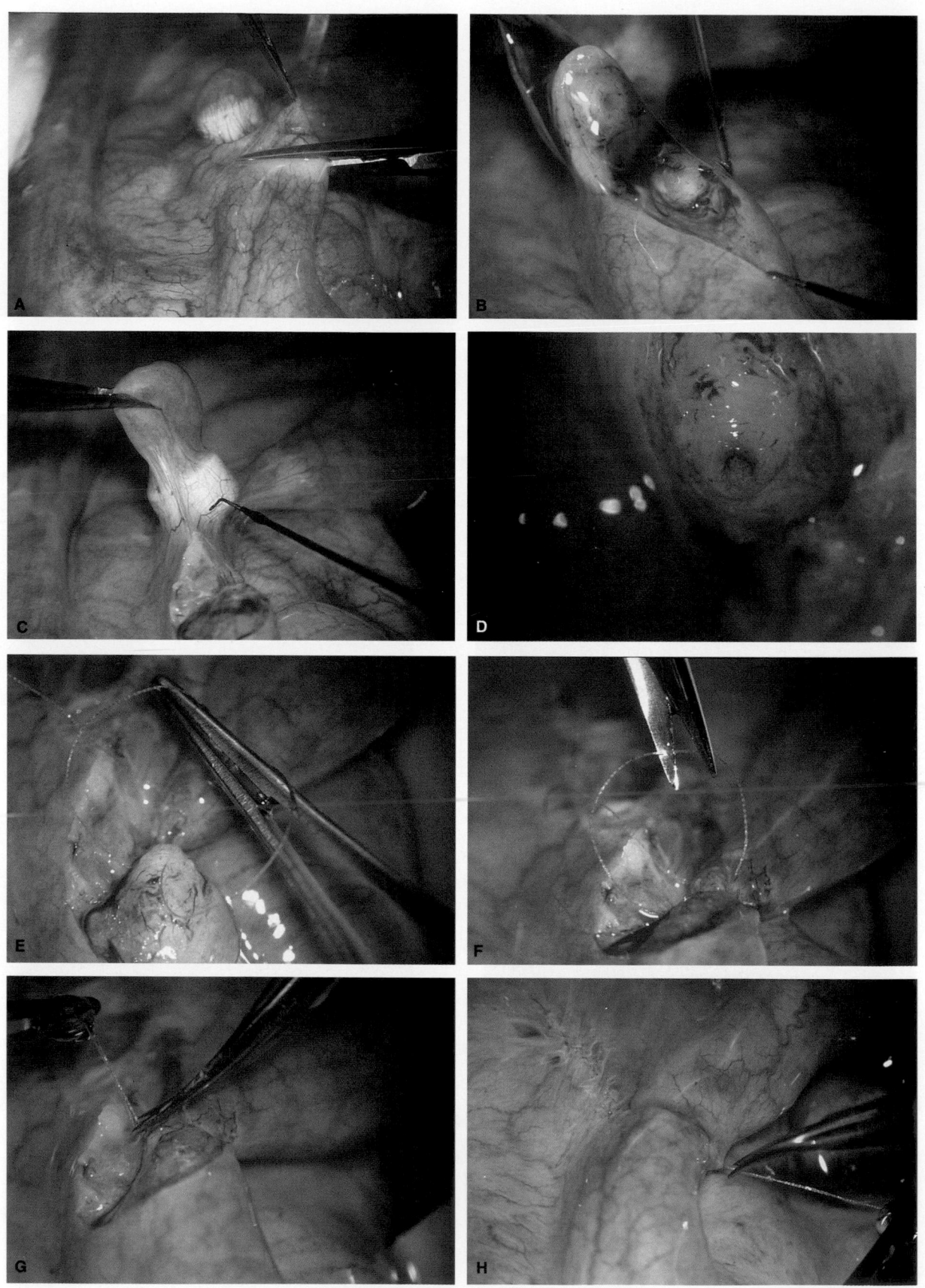

COLOR FIGURE 24.23.

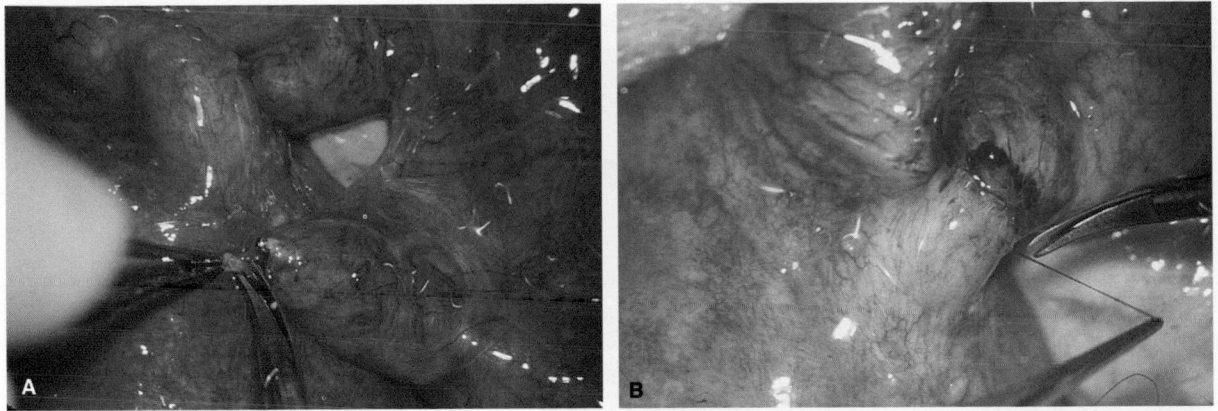

COLOR FIGURE 24.25.

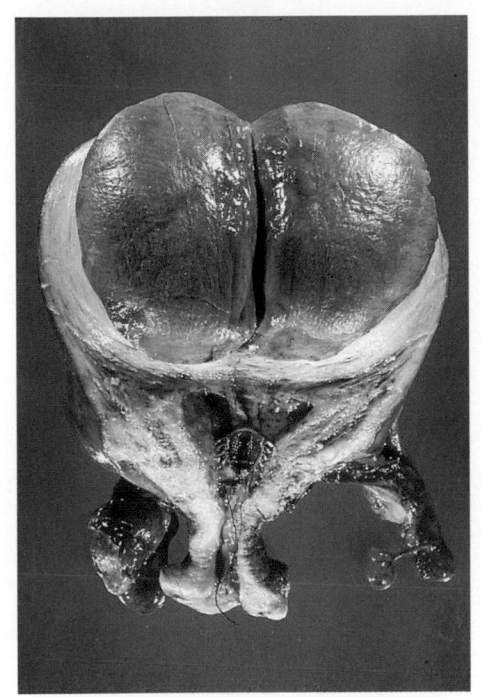

COLOR FIGURE 30.7.

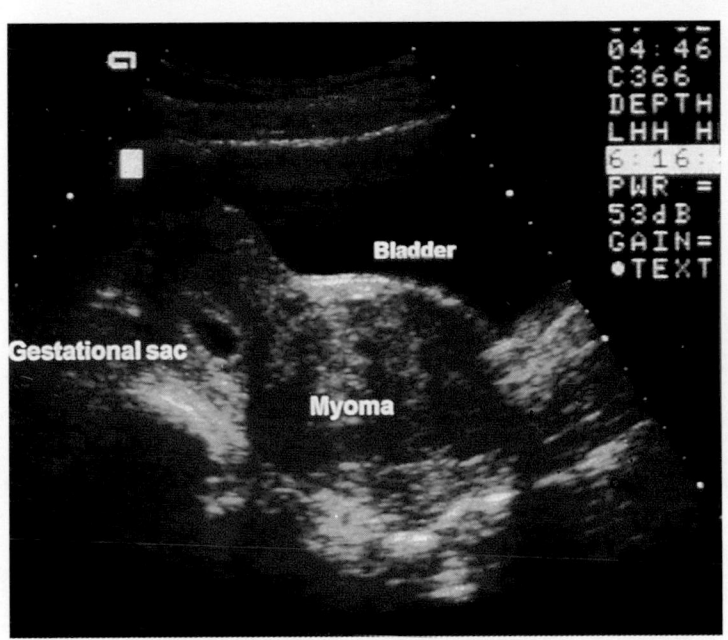

COLOR FIGURE 30.14.

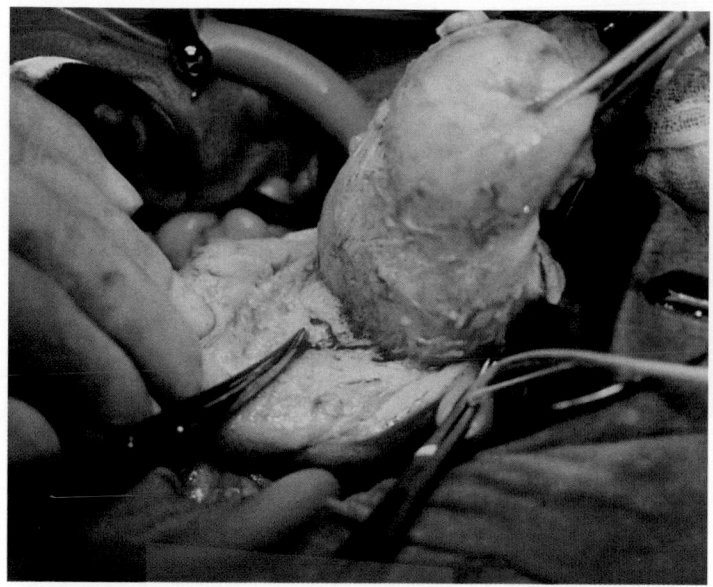

COLOR FIGURE 30.24.

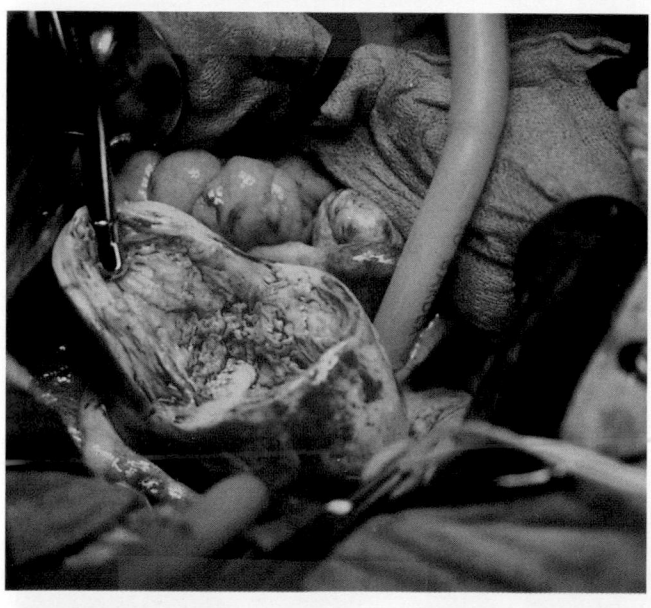

COLOR FIGURE 30.25.

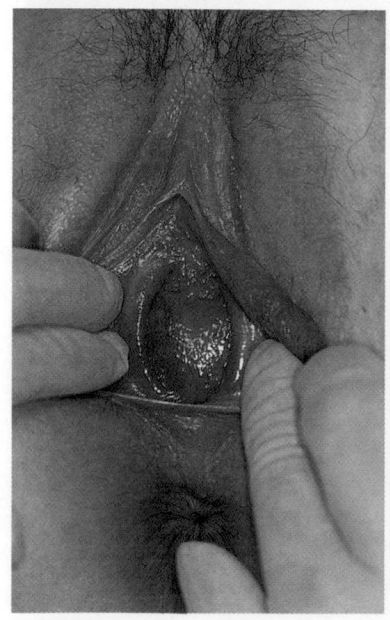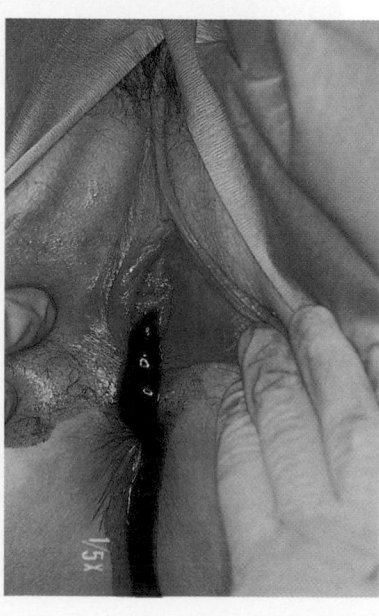

COLOR FIGURE 34.1.

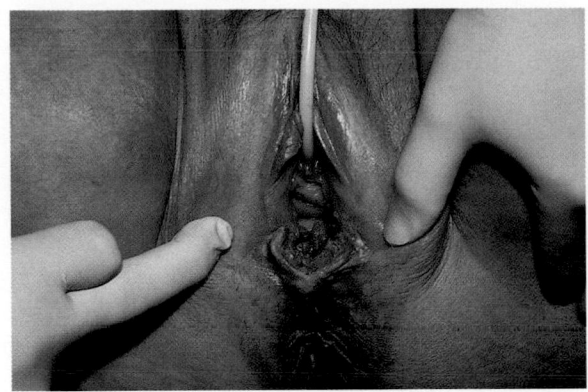

COLOR FIGURE 44.11.

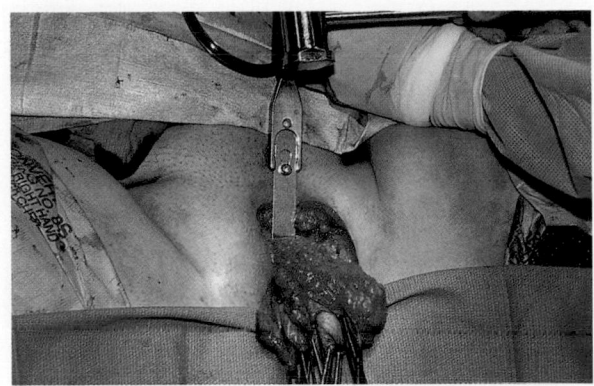

COLOR FIGURE 44.13.

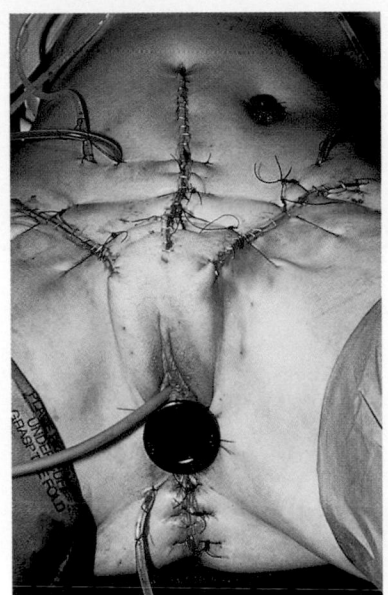

COLOR FIGURE 44.14.

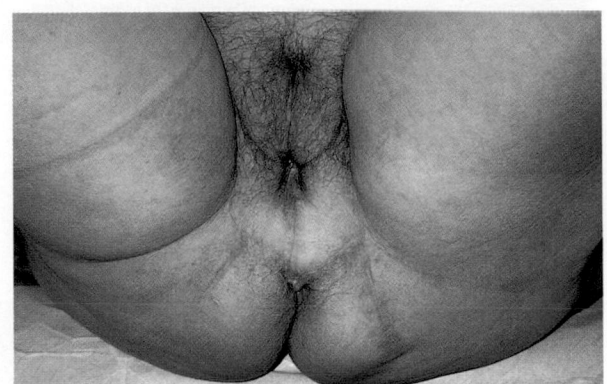

COLOR FIGURE 44.47.

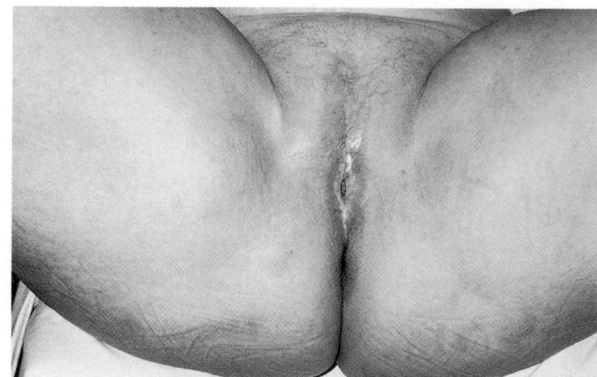

COLOR FIGURE 44.49.

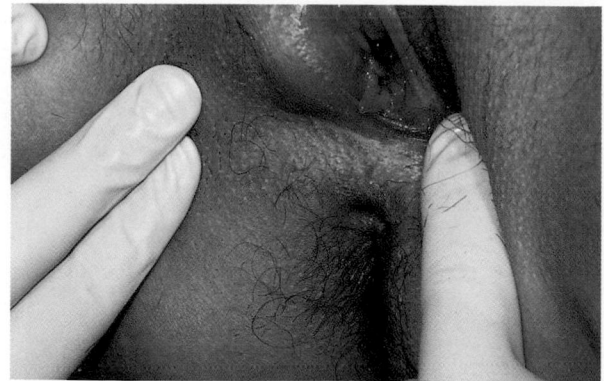

COLOR FIGURE 44.52.

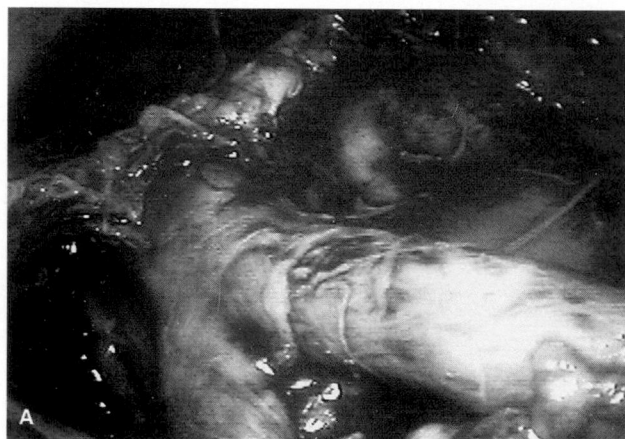
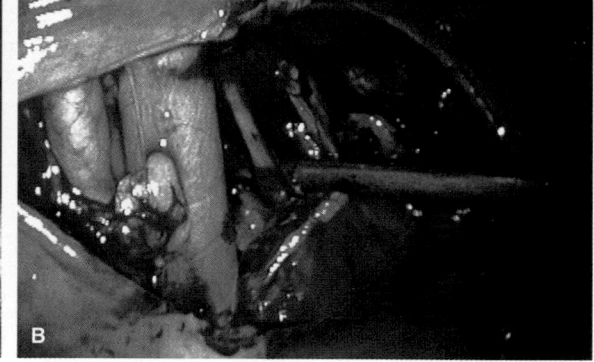

COLOR FIGURE 47.3.

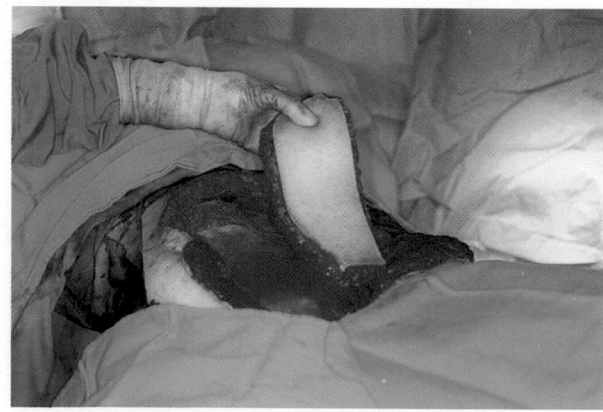

COLOR FIGURE 50.11.

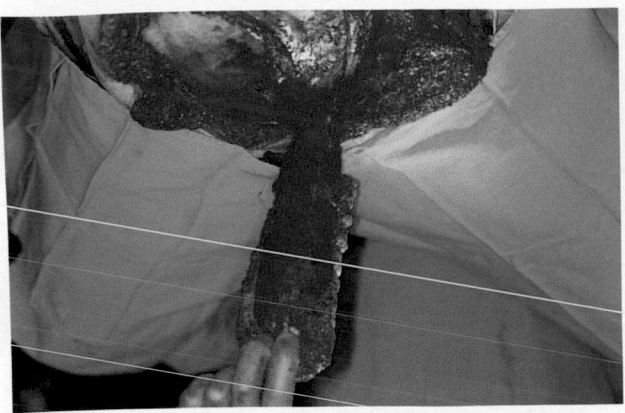

COLOR FIGURE 50.12.

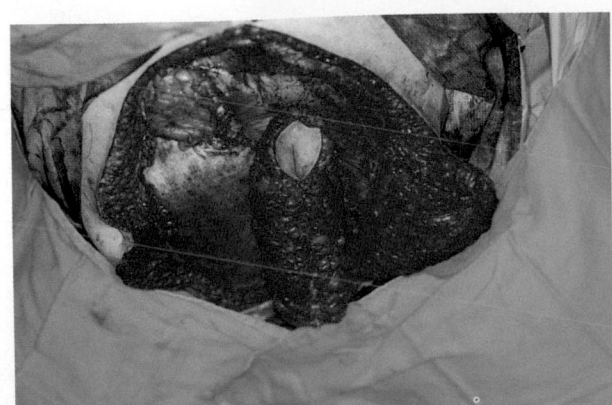 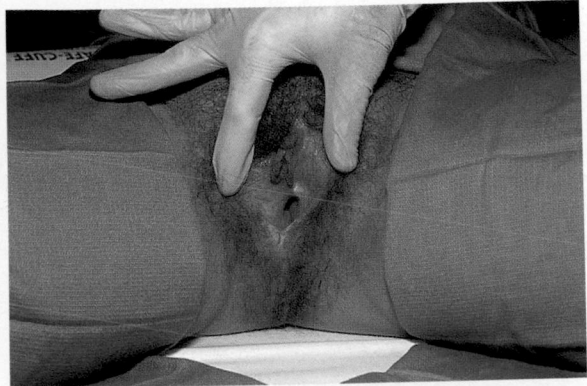

COLOR FIGURE 50.13.

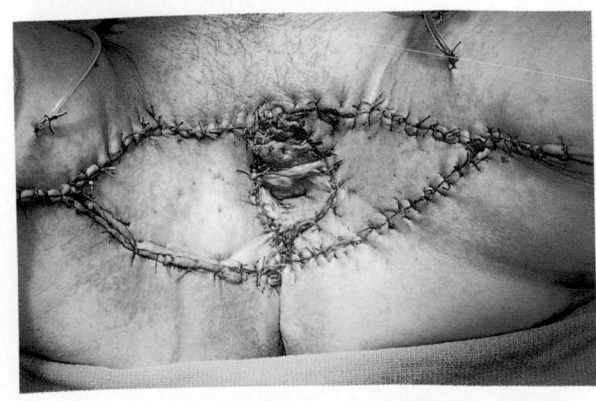 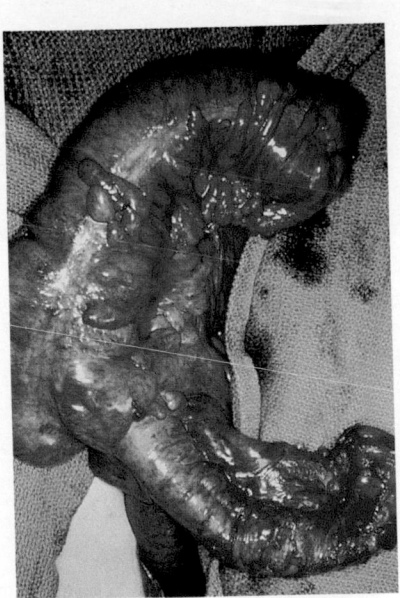

COLOR FIGURE 50.17.   COLOR FIGURE 50.21.

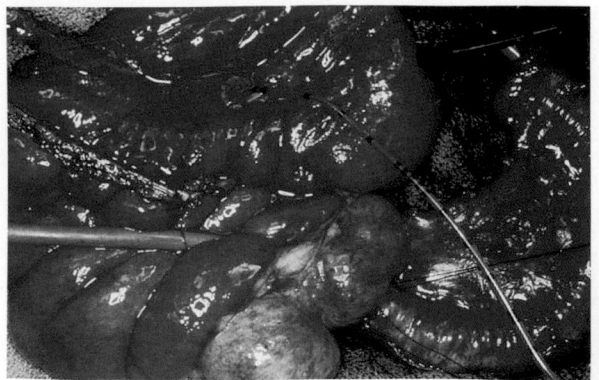

COLOR FIGURE 50.23.

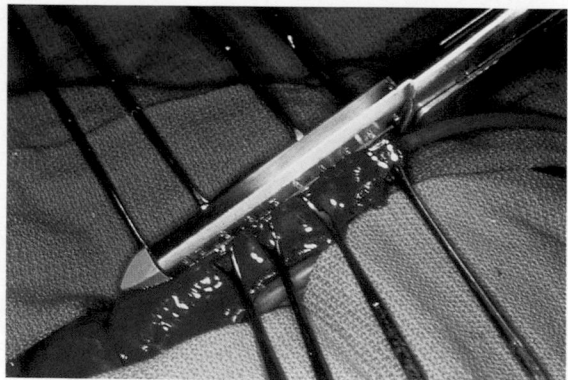

COLOR FIGURE 50.24.

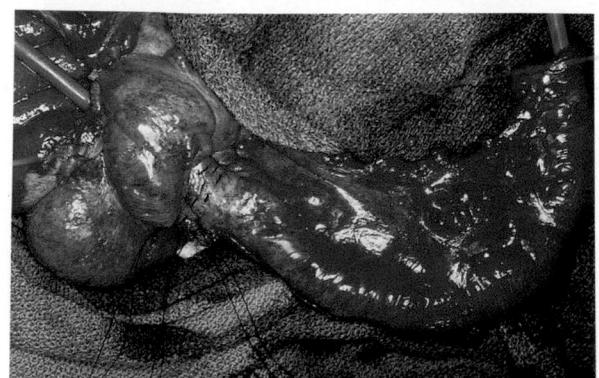

COLOR FIGURE 50.25.

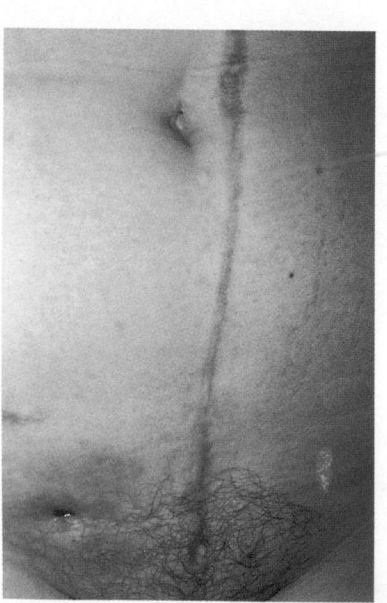

COLOR FIGURE 50.26.

and physical touch are offensive, disrespectful, or can be construed as sexually suggestive in certain cultures.

When a cultural language barrier exists, reliance on body language becomes crucially important. Work at learning to read it. These patients experience the same emotional responses to surgery and need the same education and reassurances. Having to use the services of a foreign doctor in an alien land makes the surgical process even more frightening for them.

PSYCHOLOGICAL PREPARATION FOR SURGERY

Massler and Devansan said there is an emotional response to any physical assault on the body. The magnitude of the response is expected to be proportional to the degree of emotional investment one has in the part of the body under siege. Among women, anatomic entities most vulnerable to this emotional reaction are the face, hair, breasts, genitalia, and abdominal wall.

After Caesarian birth, hysterectomy is the most frequently performed major surgical procedure done on reproductive-aged women. Over 600,000 women a year have a hysterectomy in the United States. The majority recover quickly from the procedure and enjoy the new freedom that comes to an individual when a chronic health problem has been solved. Indeed, studies show that hysterectomy is not associated with severe depression in older women and bilateral oophorectomy is associated with only slight increases in depression scores. Your patients, however, are not always older, wiser women and they do not always recover quickly. If you know the signs to look for, you will be able to help that patient who is having a harder time adjusting to pelvic surgery, especially if it was a radical, life-threatening, or unexpected event.

In his book, *Matters of Life and Death,* Daniel Bruns writes, "Even the strongest person can be shaken by the horrors of some medical cures. Beyond this, life anxiety is even more common in persons with pre-existing emotional difficulties or characterological disorders. These persons may go through life like eggshells, intact and functioning, but with psychological fragility. When faced with an extreme life stressor, such a person may simply shatter." How will you, as the physician, recognize the vulnerable?

Roeske researched 13 factors related to poor prognosis for excellent mental health after hysterectomy. These factors begin to define for you the patient who might react negatively to genital surgical stress.

1. Gender identity
2. Previous adverse reactions to stress
3. Previous depressive episodes
4. Family history of mental illness
5. History of multiple physical complaints, especially lower back pain
6. Numerous hospitalizations or surgeries
7. Age less than 35 years at time of hysterectomy
8. Desire for a child or more children
9. Fear of loss of libido
10. Significant other's negative attitude toward procedure
11. Marital dissatisfaction or instability
12. Cultural or religious disapproval
13. Lack of vocation or hobbies

Barnes and Tinkham's research also indicates that patients tend to react to current stress in much the same way as they reacted to past crises and personal losses. Well-established patterns of behavior repeat themselves. By taking a patient's history, the surgeon can be forewarned about which patients are likely to have the most difficult time handling the emotional aspects of gynecologic surgery. Equipped with this information, the surgeon can prepare to offer extra support in the form of reassurance, educational information, and, if indicated or requested, the names of psychotherapists who are trained to deal with women's health issues.

COMMON EMOTIONAL RESPONSES TO SURGERY

Insecurity

Feelings of insecurity and vulnerability are often a realistic appraisal of the patient's situation. Giving up control of one's body, even temporarily, is uncomfortable for all of us, but it is terrifying for people who feel generally insecure. One of the most common defense mechanisms against feelings of insecurity is to institute rigid controls over all aspects of life. These patients had no control over getting sick. They will have little control, if any, during the surgical procedures. Postsurgical setting will be a hospital room where the staff tells the patient when to awake, take medicine, eat, bathe, walk, have visitors, and get blood drawn. The health care workers will probe such personal matters as urination, defecation, and passage of flatus. Anxiety, anger, and feelings of being assaulted combine with insecurity to produce an unhappy, fearful, and sometimes raging patient.

These feelings are greatly diminished when the patient believes the surgery will improve the quality of her life. There will eventually be relief of pain, removal of cancer, an end to heavy bleeding, restoration of fertility, or some other positive result. She will be better than she was before the surgery. The transition to becoming this healthier person is made easier when she trusts and believes in her physician.

Anxiety or Fear

Anxiety or fear associated with surgery is essentially universal. Most common is fear of the unknown or of what the patient imagines she will be forced to endure during hospitalization. Factual information about the surgical and recovery process and competent care by a compassionate hospital staff help to diminish this fear. Surgeons are responsible for the behavior of the hospital staff toward their particular patients. When a patient complains of ill treatment by any of the health care providers, the physician should personally deal with the situation, because this will decrease the probability of a future recurrence of the offensive or thoughtless behavior.

Patients also fear the loss of economic competence. A woman who has worked hard every day for many years is afraid she will be partially or totally disabled for some variable length of time. The loss of this familiar role, even temporarily, jeopardizes her sense of usefulness. Whether she is a major or minor financial player, the contribution she makes to her family's economic stability is important to her. Many women create an identity for themselves based on their job description. Any threat to the survival of the career also menaces a woman's self-esteem.

Fear of anesthesia is often a thinly disguised fear of dying as well as a fear of loss of control. It may be appropriate to confront the fear of dying directly so that the patient has the opportunity to express why she is afraid. Is the fear general or specific? Did a close relative suffer from the same affliction and die during or shortly after surgery? Does the patient have a strong intuitive feeling that something will go wrong? If so, ask her what you can do to modify the surgical situation. Determine whether the scheduled date of surgery or the particular hospital is significant. The fact that you consider her feelings an important issue and a normal part of the gynecologic disease process may be enough to calm her fears.

Regression and Dependency

In most people who are ill or who undergo surgery, regression to a more dependent state is fairly common. Dealing with a woman who is no longer self-sufficient or emotionally stable is difficult for the patient's family and friends. These members of her supporting cast are accustomed to her presurgical roles as wage earner, wife, mother, friend, cook, advisor, shopper, housekeeper, taxi driver, entertainer, and more. When she becomes ill and can no longer function to make their lives easier, family members and friends often become frustrated and angry. They may apply overt or subtle pressure to try to force the woman to exert herself and fulfill her usual roles. A change in roles is difficult, but often the illness teaches family and friends why this particular woman is valuable to them. Those who temporarily assume her normal duties or help her cope with the surgical experience will have the opportunity to learn that taking care of another human being somehow makes us stronger than we ever were before.

When the disease and prospect of surgery are new, all these factors, as well as a feeling of non-health, contribute to an emotional fragility that yields extremely labile emotions, including feelings of sadness, despondency, tearfulness, and irritability. The usual defense mechanisms are often temporarily weakened or destroyed. The woman is vulnerable to attack on all personal and professional fronts. She needs time with people she cares about, and she needs time alone to sort out her thoughts.

Grief

Grief is a normal, natural reaction to illness or loss of any kind, and is essential to emotional healing. Recognizing the various stages of grief allows the surgeon to help the female patient understand what is happening to her.

Denial is the first and most primitive emotional response to loss and can take many forms. The patient may demonstrate denial by not going to the doctor when she finds a lump in her breast or when she notices abnormal bleeding. She may pretend the symptoms do not exist or are a temporary nuisance. Not remembering instructions the physician gave her could be a manifestation of denial. She may forget important facts or deny the seriousness of the problem. Denial allows people to function for a little while in a make-believe world. With this primitive mechanism, they survive emotional stresses they might otherwise be unable to handle.

Bargaining with a higher power is the second stage of grief. Patients feel they have carte blanche to bargain when they are experiencing a loss. "Make this bad thing that has happened to me go away, and I swear, I will become a better person."

Guilt can surface before or after a loss. Most guilty feelings are completely inappropriate, in that the guilty act rarely is directly related to the cause of the loss. When sick, many people feel that they are being punished for not being perfect. Explain to your guilt-ridden patients that their feelings are normal for the circumstances. Although guilt can sometimes deliver devastating, incapacitating blows, the good news is that it is usually transitory.

Depression comes in varying degrees to most people experiencing grief and is characterized by feelings of helplessness, hopelessness, and worthlessness. Other symptoms include middle-of-the-night insomnia, nightmares, loss of appetite or excessive eating, lethargy, difficulty making decisions, psychosomatic symptoms, and fatigue unexplained by activity.

Ask the patient if she has any of these symptoms. Postsurgical depression is common. Depressed patients usually admit that the sad feelings are routine and occur daily. When prolonged, they indicate the patient has been unable to work through the grief process. Something emotional has yet to be resolved.

Rage turned inward often manifests as depression. When the patient is able to identify what she is angry about, to ventilate the rage, the depression usually begins to lift. When she takes charge of her life again and makes decisions, even small ones, she begins to feel better, and feelings of helplessness, hopelessness, and worthlessness abate. However, when the depressed patient becomes suicidal, stringent intervention must occur. The suicidal patient presents serious challenges and so is discussed in specific detail later in this chapter.

The stage at which the patient ventilates her anger can be difficult for those providing care, but it should be accepted as healthy. The patient may go to extremes, writing letters to the newspaper or speaking of suing her physician. She may complain bitterly about the nursing staff and her hospital bill. Such actions are a form of protest at the stress that has been dealt to her body and mind. In most instances, this behavior means that the depression is lifting and the patient is beginning to move toward the resolution of her grief. The depressed patient should be encouraged to ventilate by talking, establish an enjoyable form of physical exercise, and begin to take charge of her own life.

Resolution and integration eventually occur. The stressful experience of loss finally becomes an accepted part of her life. The memory causes sadness and regret, but no longer the devastating immobilization found in the earlier stages of grief. Integration does not mean the experience is forgotten, only that it has less trauma associated with it. After integration, certain stimuli can provoke flashback grief. The painful emotional tapes begin to play again, but the patient learns that the bad time is a rerun and will not last long.

The stages of grief do not always occur in order. The patient may feel fragments of several of them at the same time. If a female patient's behavior seems bizarre, excessive, or out of the realm of what would usually be anticipated during her particular surgical experience, look for the role grief might be playing in her life.

PSYCHODYNAMICS SPECIFIC TO DIAGNOSIS AND SURGERY

Patient–Physician Bonding

Neither scalpel nor laser can divide the psyche and soma. As technical skills have improved and multiplied, comprehensive care of the gynecologic patient has declined. Increased emphasis on scientific and procedural care usually means less time in the consultation room and more time in the examining or procedure rooms. This is unfortunate for all concerned, because it takes *time* to explore the concepts, fears, and psychological well-being of the individual patient both before and after surgery.

It takes time to at least scan the books and magazines women read, to search the same Internet sites, to listen to the voices of their advocates, and essentially, evaluate, critique, and learn from their sources of information. It is important to make the effort. Otherwise, you run the risk of appearing out of touch, or worse still, arrogant and condescending. Women in general have a sixth sense about these attitudes, and women about to undergo surgery or those recovering from surgical trauma to their bodies are hypersensitive to all manner of psychological stimuli.

The medicolegal climate has also potentiated perioperative anxiety. When you inform your patient, as she prepares for surgery, that she can bleed to death, be subjected to blood transfusions, have an adverse reaction to anesthesia, or sustain bowel or urinary tract injuries, you augment her innate fear of surgery. With strong emphasis from the women's rights groups on the patient to seek and maintain a controlling role in her life, over her destiny, and over the surgeon, it is more necessary than ever before that the pelvic surgeon take the time to explore the patient's psyche in the preoperative and post-operative periods to avoid undesirable psychological sequelae.

It is a good thing to have personable, competent health care workers in your office who assist in preparing your patient for surgery. Anatomic charts have become works of art and they, as well as video movie tapes and other teaching aids, are useful in explaining the technical details; however, despite all the educational tools and patient assistance, the most important person remains you, the doctor. Unless you sit and answer questions on a one-to-one basis, you are neglecting your responsibility to her.

Much of the time, the questions will deal with information the patient has gleaned from literature, popular talk shows, and the Internet. Some of the opinions she reads or hears will frighten her or make her suspicious, and a few patients may initially come to your office thinking of you as a potential enemy. A staunch feminist may express the belief that you are just another insistently prosurgical doctor out to highjack her womb and add it to your trophy collection.

Popular literature today often stresses sexism, ageism, and greed on the part of doctors. *The Silent Passage* and *Our Bodies, Ourselves* were among the first widely read books on which patients depended for their gynecologic information. In these, they read that "for well over a century in the United States, women's uteri and ovaries have been subject to routine medical abuse," and "one should not be railroaded into hysterectomy nor onto hormones." Hysterectomy is described as "devastating" surgery, and for some women, it certainly can be. These books found a wide audience and led to the publication of other books, which took an even more radical approach, all in the name of protecting women from castrating medical experts who might use their position of authority to hurt, not help, them.

The Ultimate Rape: What Every Woman Should Know About Hysterectomies and Ovarian Removal was inspired after the author underwent a hysterectomy. She suffered extreme physical and emotional trauma following the surgery, but when she complained to her physicians, they advised her to go see a psychiatrist, because all her symptoms were in her head. The book's title is evidence of the rage she felt at their pronouncement. Now her voice is joined by others who believe every woman has the right to be thoroughly informed about procedures and consequences before consenting to gynecologic modifications. And certainly, a woman should.

In *No More Hysterectomies,* touted as the first living textbook on the web, the reader learns how the male-dominated medical profession and the insurance industry have sanctioned millions of unwarranted hysterectomies. One testimonial to the ideas presented in the book describes the current medical environment as a "woman's hormonal holocaust."

The enlightening news is that interest generated by these sources and their legions of followers has had a positive and direct effect on women's health research. Global studies are numerous and are concentrating on traditional as well as alternative methods of treatment for menopause, hysterectomy, hormone replacement therapy, cancer, endometriosis, fibroids, and dementia. For the first time in the history of medical science, ethnic research is being conducted on a large scale to determine how women in various cultures and with variances in their physiology react to menopause, gynecologic surgery, hormone therapy, and sexual function. Future generations of women will reap the benefits from this research, but the overwhelming aura that prevails in today's gynecologic patient is one of confusion.

After reading just a sampling of the lay literature, some women feel that surgical removal of their female organs and commencement of hormonal therapy constitutes an unnatural, chemotherapy-like assault on their physical bodies. It is the task of the physician to admit into evidence the medical facts necessary to correct any gross misconceptions that could affect patient care. Sometimes, it may seem as if the patient, armed with advice about natural remedies for her severe pelvic pain, heavy bleeding, or hot flashes, wants to drag you with her back into the Dark Ages. Be patient and also prepared, if necessary, to explain the medically sound benefits of life lived outside the cave.

Be compassionate. No matter how routine the job becomes, compassion is a vital requisite to becoming an exceptional communicator and healer. Empathy often follows experience, and those times when you are able to make a noticeably positive difference in your patient's life are inspirational. To try the one new thing that might help many patients in the future, it is necessary to earn the trust of a single patient in the present.

The days are gone when a doctor was considered omnipotent, when he, and rarely, she, received a hock of ham for the birth of a child, or had to tell a woman that she would have to live with the eventual hump on her back because it was a natural process of aging. Patients know about osteoporosis and heart disease and reproductive technology and brain neurotransmitters. The media have turned every living room into a medical school. Some patients present videos and clippings detailing current research and experimental treatments relative to their specific diagnoses. They know a little, and they want to know more. Many patients want to participate in their health care and absolutely should be encouraged to do so. Unlike the doctors of old, who, for the most part, had to contend with an uneducated populace, the modern physician must form a partnership with the modern patient. Mutual responsibility, respect, and trust eventually strengthen this bond. The cornerstone of the initial work is truth.

Use good judgment about when to tell all the facts, particularly those that point to a devastating diagnosis, but never lie. In 1961, 90% of physicians surveyed in a single large urban hospital stated that they withheld the diagnosis of cancer from their patients. By 1977, the position had been totally reversed, with 97% reporting that they did reveal the true diagnosis of cancer.

Doctors, however, are not the only members of the team with ethical considerations. Patients also have the responsibility to tell the physician the truth relative to their symptoms, medications, allergies, past medical his-

tories, and to relate any significant traumas or family history that could bear on their current situations.

Question your patient specifically about stressful life events. Did she respond to these in a positive or negative way? Of all inquiries, this is the most important indicator of how the patient will respond to any current stress. Once the physician knows the answer, psychological preparation for diagnosis or surgery can begin in earnest.

Researchers in the United Kingdom have compiled data from multiple trial studies confirming that psychological preparation for surgery is effective. The general hypothesis was that communication and counseling are important determinants of numerous factors, including the following.

Accuracy of the diagnosis
Effectiveness of disease management
Disease or problem prevention
Patient satisfaction
Adherence to treatment
Psychological well-being
Patient understanding of procedures
Professional satisfaction and levels of stress

Information about each of these parameters was compiled, and considerable evidence existed to support all the hypotheses. In review, Davis and Johnston reported that psychological preparation is effective in reducing negative effect, pain, medication, length of hospital stay, and in improving behavioral recovery and physiologic functioning.

Surgical Whispers

The surgeon should make it a point to be with the patient while anesthesia is administered. Knowing that you are there with her from the beginning will help her feel safe.

At the end of each surgical procedure, whisper into your patient's ear, "You're going to be well very soon." You may be surprised to find she needs less pain medication and recovers quicker than patients without the benefit of this positive prophecy, because the mind itself is a powerful force.

Youngs and colleagues believe the surgeon or a familiar associate also should be present immediately after surgery to reassure the patient, orient her to her surroundings, and make certain she has adequate pain relief. Even if the patient appears unresponsive during the immediate postoperative phase, a familiar voice and reassuring word can be immensely beneficial.

Immediate Postoperative Care

Hospital stays are much shorter than in the past, and outpatient hysterectomy is performed in some areas. This has a positive psychological effect on the patient. She knows that she is getting well when she no longer requires needles and is able to ambulate and urinate without assistance. It has long been known that early ambulation significantly reduces morbidity as well as the incidence of phlebitis and pneumonia. As long as intravenous therapy and urethral catheterization are maintained, the patient remains immobile and consequently at higher risk for venous stasis, ileus, and pulmonary complications. The incidence of pulmonary embolus in the postoperative hysterectomy patient has decreased in the past decades with shortened stay and early ambulation.

Crisis Intervention

It is important to recognize a patient who is overwhelmed by stress. This event can occur during any phase between diagnosis and recuperation. A *crisis* has been described as an obstacle to important life goals that becomes insurmountable when the individual employs customary methods of problem solving. Kaplan highlighted the following four phases of crisis.

1. Arousal occurs and attempts are made at problem solving.
2. Increased tension leads to distress and disorganization because arousal *hinders* rather than promotes coping behavior. Insomnia and fatigue frequently result.
3. Internal and external emergency resources are mobilized. Novel methods of coping are tried.
4. A state of progressive deterioration, exhaustion, and decompensation ensues as the problems drag on and on without resolution.

Dennerstein and van Hall report that the types of problems dealt with in crisis therapy include loss, change in status or role, interpersonal problems, and problems of choice between two or more alternatives. As an advocate, encourage your patient to communicate her feelings, to understand the problem enough to identify and define it, and then, help her rehearse alternative ways of coping.

One of the best concepts to apply during any stressful situation is to give the assurance that this particular moment, no matter how painful, is temporary. The surgical procedure and all the stages of mending that follow will have a beginning, middle, and an end.

PSYCHOSEXUAL REHABILITATION

The goal of psychosexual rehabilitation after gynecologic or breast surgery is to restore sexual function, sexual identity, body image, and self-esteem. Most of the work must be done by the patient herself, but she may need assistance from her doctor and other health care providers because the experience is new to her. She has no gauge to measure what is normal for her particular situation and what is aberrant. You do.

She may expect too much too soon from herself or she may head off in the opposite direction and begin to assume the role of invalid, but in most cases, she will be caught somewhere in-between these two extremes. Once she begins to exhibit her normal patterns of relating to others, you will know she has officially begun the process of genuine healing.

You will be able to tell when she enters the healing phase because she will become less dependent on you, the nurses, and even her family members. As her strength increases, she will want to resume her usual activities.

The inevitable, normal, uncomfortable grief process will commence. Encourage the patient to talk about her feelings rather than repress them and begin to brood, because worry and rumination are forms of repetitive thought that are concomitant and predictive of negative mood. Dreary thoughts fuel a depressed mood and turn it into something ugly and dangerous that has the potential to burn the thinker beyond recognition.

The patient has the power within to effect change in herself. Family members and friends should be cautioned, at this point, to allow verbal ventilation. It's a form of healthy discontent that frequently provides the impetus to hurry and lose the sick image and begin to see herself well and strong again.

Cosmetics, dress, and grooming are important parts of the rehabilitation process. When a postoperative patient combs her hair, puts on lipstick, and demands her own nightgown instead of hospital garb, she has begun to heal. When a patient feels that the surgery was disfiguring, she needs to compensate by learning new ways to dress or groom. She needs to feel whole and complete and responsible again as quickly as possible.

The surgical patient begins to see herself as a sexual person when her sexual identity is validated by her sexual partner, friends, family, and even admiring strangers she passes on the street. The woman who has had a mastectomy or other body-altering surgery needs to know her partner still finds her attractive and desirable. Without this affirmation, she may have a great deal of trouble seeing herself as a sexual being. Some sexual partners cannot accept an incomplete person. This is another potential problem.

Some surgical procedures result in loss of vulva, clitoris, or vagina. Radical pelvic surgery can leave a woman with a colostomy or urinary diversion. A severely altered body image concurrent with loss of health and vigor poses a serious threat to a woman's self-esteem. The woman who has lost her sexual identity feels damaged beyond repair. Some complain of continuing pelvic pain without obvious structural cause. Interest in sex vanishes, and the patient may actually leave her sexual partner or force the partner to abandon her. As she terminates her sexual identity, she feels old before her time and begins to draw in the edges of her life. These women need intense psychosexual therapy if they are ever to heal emotionally. Table 3.1 outlines the major factors that occur with psychosexual dysfunction.

Most of the time, the mate or lover of the woman is good to her. There is genuine concern for her health, hope for a quick recovery, and the willingness to assume many aspects of her role until she is well. Often there is a deepening of affection between the couple as gifts of love and concern are given and received. That special someone is in the waiting room during the surgical ordeal and by the patient's bedside when she awakes. There are flowers and gifts and promises made and kept. There is an abundance of reciprocal love. Adjustment to new roles is relatively smooth, causing new bonds to form and old ones to strengthen.

In other cases, the woman's partner becomes a bigger problem than her physical disability. It is possible her sig-

TABLE 3.1.
Major Factors in Psychosexual Dysfunction

Symptomatic

Interpersonal (discord with significant other)
Organic (disease, malnutrition, malfunction of body organs)
Psychiatric (anxiety, depression, schizophrenia)
Alcohol or drug abuse
Iatrogenic (suggestions, medication, surgery)

Learned

Family (childhood negative sexual associations, experiences)
Religion (imposed prohibitions internalized)
Early unpleasant sexual experiences
Gynecologic disorders (damaged genitalia, loss of breasts, uterus)

Intrapsychic conflict

Failure to develop psychosexually
Restrictive childrearing
Religious influences

nificant other constructed a fragile emotional bond with body parts rather than with the actual woman. If she had or has cancer, the partner may irrationally feel that the cancer is contagious. If she is receiving radiation treatment, he may feel that if he resumes sexual relations with her, he, too, might absorb radiation from her body and be burned. The couple may be accustomed to frequent sex and any change in the woman's availability stresses the relationship. The fear of causing pain also has an inhibiting effect. Emotional isolation and loss of nurturing occur in both partners when the woman experiences physical disability. As surgeon to the postoperative patient, you are her first line of psychosexual defense and yours will not be an easy job.

Depending on the study cited, sexual dysfunction exists in 23% to 43% of women and 31% of the men surveyed in the *general* population. One third of the women lacked sexual interest, one fourth were unable to experience orgasm in the menopause, one fifth reported lubrication difficulties, and another one fifth said they did not find sex pleasurable.

These figures come from members of the population willing to discuss sexual dysfunction. Many women and their physicians, who sometimes fear they are not qualified to help, are reluctant to speak of personal problems such as libido, arousal, coital pain, or past traumatic sexual events. Much of this reluctance can be overcome if the gynecologist knows what questions to ask when taking a sexual history, preferably during an initial or annual examination prior to any body-altering surgery.

Sexual Cycle Primer

Davis suggests that the physician ask the following open-ended questions to obtain a sexual history: Are you sexually active? Are you or your partner having any sexual difficulties at this time? Has there been any change in your sexual activity? Have you ever experienced any unwanted or harmful sexual activity? Another good question is: What sort of sexual problems do you have?

Even if the patient is initially reluctant to discuss such personal issues, she will have learned that you are willing to discuss them should the need arise. Davis also believes that a physician's confidence in dealing with sexual issues increase when the cycles of sexual response (desire, arousal, plateau, orgasm, and resolution) are learned and factors that affect them (psychological, environmental, and physiologic) understood.

Davis, in a sexual and sexual dysfunction tutorial describes the following stages.

Desire is the motivation and inclination to be sexual. It is dependent on internal (fantasies) and external sexual cues and also on adequate neuroendocrine functioning.

Arousal is characterized by erotic feelings and vaginal lubrication as blood flow increases to the vagina. In addition to feelings of sexual tension, the sexually excited woman may experience tachycardia, rapid breathing, elevated blood pressure, breast engorgement, muscle tension, nipple erection, and other physical signs of arousal such as a flush. This is the stage where the vagina lengthens, distends, and dilates, and the uterus elevates partially out of the pelvis.

During the plateau phase, sexual tension, erotic feelings, and vasocongestion reach maximum intensity. The labia become more swollen and turn dark red, the lower third of the vagina swells and thickens to form the orgasmic platform. The clitoris becomes more swollen and elevated, and the uterus elevates fully out of the pelvis. Eventually, women reach the threshold point of orgasmic inevitability. Orgasm is a myotonic response mediated by the sympathetic nervous system and is experienced as a sudden release of the tension built up during previous phases. Women, unlike men, experience no refractory period but can experience multiple orgasms during a single cycle. They can also experience orgasms before, during, and after intercourse provided they receive enough clitoral stimulation.

The last phase is called the resolution phase. Women experience a feeling of relaxation and well-being. The body returns to a resting state. Complete uterine descent, detumescence of the clitoris and orgasmic platform, and decongestion of the vagina and labia take about 5 to 10 minutes.

Sexual adjustment is often significantly impaired in women after pelvic exenteration and gracilis myocutaneous vaginal reconstruction. Eighty-four percent of the patients in one of the few studies that exist resumed sexual activity within the first year after surgery. A modified version of the Sexual Adjustment Questionnaire was used and the responses outlined the most common problems patients face after the surgery: self-consciousness about a urostomy or colostomy, being seen in the nude by their partner, vaginal dryness, and vaginal discharge. It is hoped that future modifications in surgical technique, more realistic patient counseling, and aggressive postoperative support will minimize these problems in the future. Less serious matters can cause self-esteem and body image problems, too, if their aftermath includes or leads to bowel incontinence, urinary incontinence, vaginal vault prolapse, and scarring.

Bowel incontinence is rarely discussed even with a woman's physician because it is so embarrassing. Whether from obstetric injuries, injury to the anal muscles, infections, or diminished muscle strength from aging, once the cause and severity are determined, treatments can begin that include dietary changes, constipating medications, muscle strengthening exercises, biofeedback techniques, and sometimes, surgical repair of the muscle. Some or all of these remedies help the woman control the discharge of embarrassing gas or stool. It is most important to discuss possible remedies because many women feel there is nothing that can be done for them but the frightening colostomy, when in actual fact, colostomy is a procedure that is rarely required.

As many as 50% of all women experience occasional urinary incontinence. In an attempt to lessen the blow to a woman's ego and make the event more socially acceptable, manufacturers hire movie stars to make commercials about the effectiveness of diapers for grown women. Diapers do treat the symptoms and allow for more freedom of movement, but not in an intimate setting. For many years, gynecologists have instructed patients about Kegel exercises to tighten the muscles of the pelvic floor, but this may not be enough to stop the embarrassing leakage of urine. The patient needs to know that there are tests that can determine the exact cause of the problem, and treatment using bladder retaining therapy, medications, and surgery. Urinary incontinence may be more socially acceptable today, but it is never normal, no matter what the woman's age.

Both bowel and urinary incontinence can be caused by vaginal vault prolapse and this condition must be ruled out because it drastically affects sexual functioning. The presence of a mass can cause painful intercourse, difficulty accepting penetration, and a great deal of psychological anxiety when the tissue can be seen in the vaginal opening. This condition, if left untreated, only worsens with time, but techniques that correct female organ–supporting defects in the pelvis can restore sexual functioning and with it, a woman's sense of vitality and feminine allure.

Patients who talk about their sex lives frequently describe four pleasures associated with sexuality. These universal elements are touching, genital caressing, orgasm, and gratifying a partner. When a patient is recovering from surgery or has experienced surgical loss of coital function, genital caressing as a receiver or giver can be satisfying. Once a woman learns early in life how to be orgasmic, she can often learn to be so again despite major genital loss, including her clitoris. When the ability to experience orgasm by one favorite means is destroyed by disease, the patient can be encouraged to experiment with alternative methods that do not conflict with her value system. Women who will never experience vaginal intercourse again can discover they are able, with education and imagination, to fulfill their feminine role as givers of pleasure if they choose to do so.

When a patient's psychosexual rehabilitation after surgery seems to be impaired and she fails to make steady progress toward resumption of her usual role, with appropriate self-esteem, energy, identity, and ability to handle stress, she should be offered help. Help should be offered as soon as she mentions the problem. Early intervention is often easy and brief. The surgeon should be the first person to help the patient, with counseling and, if necessary, suitable medications.

Hormonal Therapy

A 16-year study that involved 60,000 postmenopausal female nurses found that those who took hormone replacement therapy for 10 years reduced their risk of dying from all causes by 37%, with the most dramatic reduction being death from cardiac disease. After 10 years, the reduced risk for all causes was 16% because of the increased risk of dying from breast cancer. That risk rose to 43% but the women who contracted breast cancer during the first 10 years had a lower death rate from the disease than women who had never taken hormones, probably because of early detection. Chances of early detection of breast cancer are probably better for hormone users because they receive regular check-ups.

Before starting therapy, patients need to be aware of their risk factors for cardiovascular disease, osteoporosis, and breast cancer in order to make informed choices. The screening process that provides such information may include a thorough history and physical and an accurate measurement of body weight and height, blood pressure, cholesterol level, and, for some women, bone density. In an extensive review of current literature on the subject, dubbed "the New Science of Estrogen," Hammond provides an overview of the risks and benefits of hormone replacement therapy and also includes information on therapeutic alternatives.

Current theories indicate that estrogen has extraordinarily complex biological effects that translate into a variety of actions in diverse tissues. There is growing scientific evidence that estrogen exerts its beneficial actions on tissues of the skeletal, urogenital, digestive, cardiovascular, ocular, and nervous systems. However, many women are afraid to use it because the media repeatedly tell them that estrogen greatly increases their risk for breast cancer.

Statistics show overwhelmingly that cardiovascular disease (CVD)—*not* cancer—is the leading cause of mortality for postmenopausal women. In fact, one in two women will eventually die of heart disease or stroke, whereas only one in 25 women die of breast cancer. Although the incidence of heart disease, including coronary artery disease and stroke, is low in premenopausal women, heart disease is the most frequent cause of death in women over the age of 50. Since 1984, the death rate from CVD in men has decreased, whereas the death rate for women has increased. Numerous epidemiologic studies support the long-term benefit of estrogen in preventing CVD. Observational studies, such as the Postmenopausal Estrogen/Progestin Intervention Study (PEPI) sponsored by the National Institutes of Health, revealed that hormone replacement therapy (HRT) can increase high-density lipoprotein cholesterol and decrease low-density lipoprotein cholesterol. The Nurses' Health Study demonstrated a reduction in the risk of CVD of up to 50% among current HRT users. Women who use estrogen have significantly less coronary artery stenosis than women who do not use it. Moreover, patients with the most advanced coronary artery disease experience the most benefit from estrogen replacement therapy (ERT), but only 35% of women surveyed were aware of the connection between heart disease and menopause.

ERT/HRT is also first-line therapy for osteoporosis for most women, and treatment should begin as soon as possible after the menopause. Discontinuation of therapy is followed by bone loss, which could result in a subsequent increase in the occurrence of fractures. Preliminary data suggest that even the elderly respond to estrogen replacement. However, there are therapeutic alternatives and lifestyle modifications (diet and routine exercise) that perimenopausal women must be counseled about to create a comprehensive preventive program. Such an effort can have a significant impact on long-term morbidity and mortality associated with osteoporosis.

Women have phenomenal memories because one of their jobs is to find every needle that gets lost in the proverbial haystacks of their homes. When they become less adept at remembering where they and other people put their things, they fear the worst—that they are losing their minds, and this fear is not illogical. Women comprise 72% of the population over the age of 85 years, and roughly half of this group has Alzheimer disease (AD). Not only do women constitute a greater proportion of this older population, but AD is expressed earlier in women than men. This may be related to the estrogen loss that occurs with menopause. Hammond cites a study that found women who took estrogen for more than 1 year experienced a dramatic delay in AD onset. But even the group of women who averaged only 4 months of estrogen therapy and most likely took the medication to control symptoms such as hot flushes experienced a delay in AD onset. It has been speculated that a brief exposure to estrogen influenced AD expression *20 to 30 years later* by preventing an irreversible loss of neurons associated with the occurrence of hot flushes. Research is ongoing but one study found that estrogen replacement therapy in postmenopausal women is associated with a 50% reduction in the risk of developing AD because it slows the decline of visual memory.

Colon cancer occurs more often in women than men and is a leading cause of cancer incidence and cancer deaths in women. Even though mortality rates for colon cancer have decreased 25% among women in the last 20 years, it remains the third leading cause of cancer deaths in this group. The concept that postmenopausal ERT may decrease the risk of colorectal cancer has received considerable attention, even though the hormone has no indication for this use. Some 20 epidemiologic studies have been published that examined this relationship. The majority of these suggest an inverse, protective effect for estrogen, particularly with current use. Although the precise mechanism by which estrogen reduces colon cancer risk is unknown, it has been hypothesized that it affects bile acid metabolism or promotes tumor suppressor activity. The inclusion of estrogen as a measure to prevent colon cancer should be part of the discussions between menopausal women and their physicians. Counseling should include the American Cancer Society recommendations for annual digital rectal examination and fecal occult blood testing as well as a flexible sigmoidoscopy every 5 years or colonoscopy every 10 years.

Age-related macular degeneration (AMD) may be reduced by estrogen administration. This disease is the leading cause of legal blindness in the United States, accounting for as many as 60% of all new cases. There is no medical treatment, and surgical management in the form of photocoagulation is effective in only a small percentage of patients with the wet type of the disease. In the Rotterdam study, women who experienced menopause at an earlier age had a 90% increased risk of exhibiting signs of late AMD compared with those who experienced menopause at a later age. These data suggest that HRT reduces the risk of developing AMD.

Counseling women about replacement therapy must be combined with discussions about the importance of lifestyle changes, including the following.

- Normalization of weight
- Dietary intervention
- Smoking cessation
- Regular exercise
- Control of hypertension
- Control of diabetes
- Control of alcohol consumption
- Control of lipid elevations

Routinely, ERT/HRT counseling should go beyond simple symptom control to include both short- and long-term benefits, contraindications, common patient concerns, and misconceptions.

The contraindications to estrogen replacement, which have been established by the Food and Drug Administration (FDA) include: known or suspected pregnancy or breast cancer, estrogen-dependent neoplasia, undiagnosed abnormal genital bleeding, and active thromboembolic disorders. However, ongoing research suggests that some of these contraindications may not be absolute. In the meantime, all of the relative contraindications must be carefully discussed and weighed against the risk of not prescribing ERT/HRT. This is also a good time to discuss the common concerns and misconceptions that women have about estrogen, even if patients do not raise them. For example, many women are concerned that estrogen may bring on the return of monthly bleeding, restore fertility, or produce weight gain.

For perimenopausal women who choose HRT, there are two common regimens: continuous estrogen and progestin or cyclic (continuous estrogen plus progestin for only 10 to 14 days per month). In ERT, unopposed estrogen is administered without interruption to women without a uterus. For the perimenopausal woman, counseling must go beyond symptom control to include prevention of heart disease and osteoporosis, control of body weight, restrictions on alcohol and tobacco consumption, encouragement of regular exercise, maintenance of mental health (including sexuality), and cancer screening.

When bilateral oophorectomy is anticipated in a premenopausal patient, hormonal replacement therapy should be discussed before surgery because one of the greatest fears of younger women is surgery-induced menopause. Patients should be told that estrogen therapy can be started immediately after surgery and that hot flashes and other menopausal symptoms can be avoided. The natural conjugated estrogens do not cause hypercoagulability and are safe during the immediate convalescent period.

The long-term benefits of estrogen replacement therapy in preventing osteoporosis, cardiovascular disease, and colon cancer are well established. The health of the vagina and lower urinary tract is maintained. The vagina lubricates more easily with sexual arousal, and intercourse is more comfortable with an estrogenic vaginal mucosa. Many women report an increased interest in and enjoyment of sex.

For women who do experience a loss of libido, even while taking estrogenic hormones, the new androgen therapies look promising as a way to improve sexual function and psychological well-being. Testosterone delivered via transdermal patches or gel bypasses the liver and has no negative effect on cholesterol. The skin serves as a constant reservoir; therefore, blood levels show fewer fluctuations.

However, there are physicians who believe hormonal balances induced by prescription medications should only be offered for relief of extreme menopausal symptoms and only for a short while. The author of *Dr. Susan Love's Hormone Book* and *Dr. Susan Love's Breast Book,* is one such physician. She is a staunch supporter of eating soybean products and using herbal remedies such as black cohosh to maintain estrogen levels, the use of acupuncture and paced-respiration for hot flashes, exercise, and using vitamin and calcium supplements. But even she, admitted in an interview, "If my symptoms [for menopause] worsen, I may feel that I want to take some kind of drug. I certainly would be open to that."

SPECIAL CASES

Every patient is special, of course, but some women in tumultuous life situations require a great deal of compassion and sensitivity from a surgeon. These women can present the greatest challenges to the surgeon's ability to handle patients in emotional turmoil.

The Teenager

Bluestein and Starling report that one million teenagers a year conceive. Of these million pregnancies, 400,000 end in abortion and 100,000 in miscarriage. Childbearing teenagers face a 60% excess in maternal mortality compared with adults and are most likely to suffer toxemia, anemia, hemorrhage, cervical trauma, cephalopelvic disproportion, excessive weight gain, and premature labor. These complications are due more to social and behavioral correlates than inherent adolescent aspects. Correlates include inadequate prenatal care, poor nutrition, substance abuse, and emotional distress.

One to two teenagers per 1,000 who have first-trimester abortions experience fever, hemorrhage, and emergency abdominal surgical procedures. These numbers are lower than for older women, but the rate for cervical injury, which could affect future childbearing, is 5.5 per 1,000 teenagers, notably higher than the 1.7 to 3.1 per 1,000 for adults. Bluestein and Starling recommend the following communication techniques for the teenage patient: Guarantee confidentiality to build trust. Conduct the initial interview alone. Teenage girls may want to relate private information to the physician but not in the presence of a parent. Be patient. Gear communication to the patient's emotional and intellectual development. Be nonjudgmental. Gently explore the teenager's family and social environments. Will family members and friends support or harm your patient? Discuss the teenager's long-term plans. Be aware of ethnic differences in health-related matters.

Female patients who belong to local or national gangs come into the health care system with a unique set of problems and values. It is imperative that the surgeon not add to the patient's stress more than is absolutely necessary. Sometimes, the simple act of being treated like a human being worthy of consideration is a novel and humbling experience.

The Senior Woman

It is easy to imagine a grandmother baking cookies or rocking a new baby in the family. Our culture makes it a little more difficult to imagine this same woman flushed and happy from an energetic romp in the sack with her favorite beau. Sex after 60 is a reality for many women and men. These people enjoyed sex when they were young, they perfected it as the years flowed by, and the thought of doing without expression of the natural urges, even temporarily, is discomforting.

When an older woman faces gynecologic surgery, do not assume she is asexual. She may simply view her sex life as her private business and be loath to discuss it. Do not antagonize or humiliate the senior patient by assuming her sexuality is a thing of the past.

If the surgical procedure will affect her sexually, explain the consequences. Assure her that the surgery will leave her as whole and as functional as possible. Give this woman the opportunity to express her anxieties and to ask questions. If her mate or lover is present, include this person in the discussion. In the senior woman who has a large cystocele, rectocele, or uterine or vault prolapse, every effort should be made to avoid colpocleisis. Sacrospinous colpopexies and vaginal reconstructive surgery are indicated. The fact that a woman is older and sexually inactive at the time of surgery does not mean that she will never be active again. Much preparation and explanation must be given to evaluate and prepare her for the closing off of her vagina or its subsequent reconstruction should that become necessary.

Butler and colleagues advise that, when taking a sexual history, ask if the symptoms started after a period of sexual activity. Excretory urogram and cystoscopy sometimes can be avoided with a diagnosis of postcoital cystitis and subsequent antibiotic treatment. A history of traumatic intercourse in the presence of an atrophic vagina can lead to estrogen therapy and lubricants rather than dilation and curettage. Butler and colleagues, also, caution physicians not to assume an older woman is sexually inactive. They advise checking for sexually transmitted diseases in older women as you would in younger ones.

When surgery is indicated, perform it as if the senior woman was still young and had many years of sexuality ahead of her, because she probably does. If the surgery occurs in the genital area, do not shave her pubic hair. The procedure is archaic and microbiologically unnecessary if competent sterilization procedures are followed. As men age, they sometimes lose hair on the head. As women age, the pubic hair sometimes thins and once shaved, may never grow back.

Many older women have had to curb their sexual appetites to compensate for physiologic changes that have occurred in a mate. Removal of excessive vaginal mucosa during pelvic surgery compromises the vagina, which is already losing elasticity. This inhibits penetration during coitus and can cause painful intercourse. Be understanding and helpful if solutions are possible. If the dysfunction resulting from the surgery will be permanent, encourage the couple to experiment with various ways to please each other or seek the advice of a sex therapist that is knowledgeable about creative sexual play.

Butler instructs physicians to educate themselves about the effects of medications on sexuality. More than 200 medications have sexual dysfunction as a side effect. Many are effective in lower doses that do not harm the libido or the patient's physical ability.

The positive benefits of a healthy sex life are multiple. Emotional intimacy and the ability to connect physically with another human being brings great joy and satisfaction. This need to connect intensifies rather than diminishes with age.

The Sexually Assaulted Patient

Reported rape and sexual assault in the United States, at the rate of 34.4 victims per 100,000 people showed no evidence in the late 1990s of being on the decline. It is estimated that only about 16% of the rapes that occur are ever reported. One in three sexually assaulted victims is under the age of 12. Convicted rape and sexual assault offenders testify that two thirds of their victims are younger than 18. Two thirds of the victims older than 18 knew their attacker prior to the rape. A sad fact is that almost one fifth of the women who are raped before the age of 18 are raped again after the age of 18. Many require medical attention, up to 22% suffer genital trauma, up to 40% incur sexually transmitted disease, and 1% to 5% become pregnant as a result of the rape. Rape survivors are 13 times more likely than the general population to attempt suicide.

Most hospital emergency rooms have strict protocols to follow when treating sexually assaulted patients. The proper collection of evidence and initial treatment of injuries is a priority. The surgeon who repairs the gynecologic damage done to these female patients should be aware of the general characteristics of psychological trauma associated with rape.

The symptoms of rape trauma syndrome compiled by Blair and Warner can be found in Table 3.2.

Many of these symptoms are the same as seen in posttraumatic stress disorder. These authors also outlined the following necessary skills that any caregivers attempting to help a sexually assaulted victim should possess the following.

Understand rape and sexual assault
Assess how the patient perceives the act
Identify and reinforce patient's ability to cope
Assist significant others
Coordinate care and help if victim needs assistance
Mobilize community resources

The female gynecologic patient, from the youngest child to the oldest adult, has survived the attack on her physical body. Most gynecologists are familiar with the legacy of these attacks (up to 75% of patients seen with chronic pelvic pain were physically or emotionally abused). The assaulted patient now needs reassurance from her surgeon and other health care workers that she will also survive the damage done to her psyche.

The Cancer Patient

Bloch cautions physicians that the manner in which the diagnosis of cancer is disclosed to the patient can determine whether the patient lives or dies. It is impera-

---

TABLE 3.2.
Symptoms of Rape Trauma Syndrome

Recurrent, painful recollections or dreams of the event
Suddenly acting or feeling as if the event were recurring
Demonstrations of fear, anger, or anxiety
Crying, restlessness, or tenseness
Controlled feelings masked by a false demeanor of calmness, composure, or subdued attitude
Matter-of-fact answering of questions
Inappropriate smiles or laughter
Inability to remember parts of the event because re-exposure to stimuli present during the traumatic moment reinvokes the associated pain
Decreased interest in important activities
Lack of future plans
Limited range of affect
Detachment toward others
Sleep disorders
Difficulty concentrating
Hypervigilance
Irritability
Angry outbursts

tive to instill hope and the desire to fight the disease. A diagnosis of cancer by telephone can be devastating and is viewed by many physicians and patients as a form of cruelty.

The cancer patient shares the same fears common to all surgical patients. She may be psychologically attached to the body part that must be removed. She may fear anesthesia, disfigurement, the unknown, the hospital experience and staff, debility, loss of economic competence, and sexual function.

In addition to the normal realm of anxiety associated with surgery, a diagnosis of cancer brings special stresses to a woman's life. Schain describes universal concerns experienced by people diagnosed with cancer no matter where in the body the cancer is located. These people fear death, postoperative adjuvant treatment, and recurrence.

The cancer patient is concerned about dying or being injured during the operation. Preoperative anxiety can manifest as anorexia, insomnia, tachycardia, fear, and panic. Acute depression is not uncommon and can lead to suicidal tendencies.

The patient is afraid of becoming unable to take care of her family members. Will she be sick for long? Who will raise her children if she dies? Who will care for her parents? Will her loved ones be supportive, or will they begin to back away from her? If the woman is alone, without mate or family, she fears becoming unable to care for herself.

The treating surgeon can ease some of the cancer patient's fear by free and open communication. Educate the patient about exactly what to expect, and offer reassurance if possible. Explain the procedure she is about to undergo and the positive benefits that you both hope will result.

Surgery and cancer in the urogenital region can be consciously or unconsciously interpreted as mutilation. The possibility of some degree of postoperative sexual dysfunction can create a fear of abandonment by the sexual partner. Assure both the patient and her partner that they will continue to be able to bring joy, pleasure, and comfort to each other.

The psychological effect of cancer on a woman is largely determined by whether the malignancy is primary, recurrent, or terminal. The surgeon is usually the patient's first big gun aimed at the cancer and the patient's greatest hope for a complete cure. The surgeon most likely is the first physician to learn the stage of growth of the cancer, and the family will be waiting to hear the results of the surgical experience. How advanced is the cancer? What is the prognosis? What happens next?

If the news is good, the patient recovers and has routine checkups to monitor her health for the rest of her life. If the news is not good, the results should be revealed with as much sensitivity and hope as possible. No patient should ever be given an absolute death sentence.

Ethically and morally, the surgeon must wrestle with personal internal conflicts when the surgery for the cancer patient is palliative. Should procedures be performed that extend death and not life? If she is able, the patient herself must make the choice.

If the cancer patient elects to have the procedure, the surgeon's job is primarily over once she has recovered from her operation. If the cancer has spread, radiologists, chemotherapists, and others who specialize in cancer treatment will assume the lead roles in trying to get the patient well or at least enhance the quality of the remainder of her life. Meaningful psychosocial support should be based on established concepts of crisis intervention because cancer is a major life crisis. Counseling should be designed to support adaptive behaviors and feelings that reduce the psychological stress, restore and consolidate the patient's self-image, and normalize sexual functioning as quickly as possible. It is the surgeon's job to foster courage, not hope, in the terminal patient.

The Suicidal Patient

Approximately 30,000 people commit suicide each year in the United States. Cooper, Rosa, and Daniel studied over 6,000 individuals and found that *hopelessness* ranked the highest of all symptoms associated with suicidal ideation in psychiatric patients and adolescents.

A surgeon probably will not know if a patient is contemplating suicide unless the patient admits to thinking about ending her life or unless a family member voices concern. Subtle warning signs include a chronic state of depression, lethargy, an inability to relate to others, weight loss or gain, lack of interest in life in general or the surgical procedure in question, a change in personal appearance, abnormal sleep patterns, or any strange behavior uncharacteristic of the particular patient. Many of these symptoms are normal for the presurgical and postsurgical patient, so it is easy to see how suicidal tendencies could hide within the maze.

To determine a patient's suicide potential, ask: Have you been troubled with thoughts of hurting yourself? Barbee advises physicians to ask directly: Have you ever thought of taking your own life? Do you feel like taking your life now? If the patient answers yes, the physician should find out if the patient has a simple, straightforward suicide plan that is likely to succeed.

A patient with low to moderate suicide potential is noticeably depressed but can identify some support system. There may be suicidal thoughts but no specific plan.

A patient with a high suicide potential feels profoundly helpless. Little or no support system seems to exist. Thoughts of suicide are frequent, and a plan exists that is likely to succeed.

The surgeon may be the first person to realize the patient is in emotional trouble and could be the only support system available if the patient has significantly withdrawn from others. Crisis therapy for the suicidal patient begins when the patient requests help or when someone recognizes her potential for self-destruction. By showing interest in her feelings and concern for her welfare, the surgeon initiates crisis intervention.

Medcast News Networks reported an interesting study that was presented at the 152nd American Psychiatric Association. Antti Tanskanen and colleagues followed approximately 40,000 Finnish men and women for 15 years. Observing their health habits and causes of death, they found that those individuals with high cholesterol (309.4 mg/dL) were more than twice as likely to commit violent suicide compared with those whose blood lipids were in the normal range (193.3 mg/dL). This is a simple thing to check and one that might make a life-or-death difference for a patient.

DEALING WITH DEATH

Death is a taboo subject for most physicians. Many doctors go to great lengths to avoid discussing the eventuality, and most are uncomfortable dealing with the emotional consequences of the death of a patient. To many physicians, death is viewed as a personal failure. Regardless of any internal attitudes, the surgeon is responsible for communicating the facts of the death to the family and for being the first person to help them cope with the loss of their loved one.

When a patient dies, explain to the family, to the best of your ability, exactly what happened. Assure them that everything medically possible was done. Ufema suggests the following guidelines to make the death experience as bearable as possible for all concerned.

> Ask about donations for transplantation.
> Provide an area where the family members can say goodbye.
> If it is true, tell the family members how the patient affected you personally.
> Transfer your protective feelings for the patient to the family members.
> Begin the grief process by saying, "Jane's body is ready for the morgue now. Would you like to say a final goodbye?"
> If family members want a lock of hair, allow them to take it.
> Give family members the patient's belongings.
> Provide an escort for any family member who is alone.
> Help the hospital staff cope with the loss.

Remember that it is permissible for the physician to show emotion with the family if the emotion is genuine. Someone is gone and will never see tomorrow.

FUTURE TRENDS

The new millennium was heralded with great joy and celebration. Its predominant theme was one of hope, and nowhere is this more evident than in the field of medicine, specifically, for women's health issues. The hand that rocks the cradle now rules important aspects of the research world. During the next 20 years, 45 million women will enter menopause and live one third to one half of their lives postmenopausally. Research into improving the quality of their lives and subsequently, all those they touch, has never been more important or timely.

As a multitude of women move through the life stages of maiden, mother, and crone, the health care they receive during one stage will be reflected in all those that follow. Boomer women, born between 1946 and 1964, will continue their legacy of reform by participating in medical clinical studies concerning endocrinology, gynecology, neurology, oncology, genetics, and finally, geriatrics. The daughters and sons they presented to the world will advance reproductive technology in all its genetic and social ramifications.

Virtual surgery is a recent gift of the technological world. Medical students will soon be able to perfect their surgical techniques using cyberscalpels, simulated lifelike patient bodies, three-dimensional models, and long distance mentors. The space industry has also yielded a smart surgical probe that will be used for breast biopsies. The small disposable needle with multiple sensors will be able to distinguish normal tissue from tumor tissue and greatly reduce the 18,000 breast biopsies per week now performed on women with suspicious lesions. Originally conceived as a robotic tool to aid astronaut/physicians during long-duration space flights, it has found a medical application on Earth in neurosurgery.

Voice-activated language programs will make it possible to effectively communicate with multicultural patients and international colleagues. Advances in documentation techniques will make keeping accurate records less of a burden. More ethics classes will emerge to better prepare the medical student for the real-world challenges such as end-of-life issues, fiduciary responsibilities, confidentiality, informed consent, and religious or philosophical conflicts.

As surgeons, it will be your duty and privilege to witness, record, and practice the new knowledge and incorporate it with what is already known so that you can make a positive difference in the lives of women now living as well as those yet to be born.

CONCLUSION

Technology will never change the fact that women are emotional creatures by nature, even when they have the choice to menstruate or not. Few experiences give women more satisfaction than sexuality and conception. Surgery on or near her reproductive tract is potentially fraught with emotional sequelae. The gynecologic surgeon's responsibility transcends a stunning performance in the surgical arena. Making appropriate decisions about the surgical procedure and considerately managing the patient's return to physical and psychological health will be the hallmarks of an accomplished surgeon in this millennium and the next.

BIBLIOGRAPHY

Abel G. *How to avoid being accused of sexual harassment.* The American Association of Sex Educators, Counselors, and Therapists (AASECT), 2000 Annual Conference. May 10–14.

Bowel incontinence (patient brochure). Arlington Heights, IL: American Society of Colon and Rectal Surgeons (ASCRS). *ascrs@fascrs.org*

Andersen BL, Hacker NF. Psychosexual adjustment following pelvic exenteration. *Obstet Gynecol* 1983;61:331.

Andersen BL, Hacker NF. Psychosexual adjustment of gynecologic oncology patients: a proposed model for future investigation. *Gynecol Oncol* 1983;15:214.

Andersen BL, Hacker NF. Psychosexual adjustment after vulva surgery. *Obstet Gynecol* 1983;67:477.

Andersen BL, Turnquist D, La Polla J, et al. Sexual functioning after treatment of in situ vulvar cancer: preliminary report. *Obstet Gynecol* 1988;71:15.

Barbee MA. Recognizing suicide. *Nursing* 1993;(Oct):32N.

Barnes AB, Tinkham CG. Surgical gynecology. In: Notman MT Nadelson CC, eds. *The woman patient: medical and psychological interfaces.* New York: Plenum Press, 1978.

Bernal EW. Hysterectomy and autonomy. *Theor Med* 1988;9:73.

Blair TMH, Warner CG. Sexual assault. *Topics Emerg Med* 1992;(Dec):58.

Bloch R. Disclosing cancer diagnosis to a patient. *JNCI* 1994;86:38.

Bluestein D, Starling E. Helping pregnant teenagers. *West J Med* 1994;161:140.

Brinton LA, Schairer C. Postmenopausal hormone-replacement therapy—time for a reappraisal? *N Engl J Med* 1997;336:1821–1822

Brown J, Seeley D, et al. Correspondence re: Urinary incontinence after hysterectomy. *Lancet* 2000;356:2012.

Bruns D. *Matters of life and death.* Greeley, CO: Health Psychology Associates.

Butler RN, Hoffman E, Whitehead DE, et al. Love and sex after sixty: how physical changes affect intimate expression. *Geriatrics* 1994;49:20.

Campion MJ, Brown JR, McCance DJ, et al. A psychosexual trauma of an abnormal cervical smear. *Br J Obstet Gynecol* 1988;95:175.

Case AM, Reid RL. Effects of the menstrual cycle on medical disorders. *Arch Intern Med* 1998;158:1405–1412.

Chang S, Hulka BS, et al. Breast cancer survival and the timing of tumor removal during the menstrual cycle. *Cancer Epidemiol Biomarkers Prev* 1997;6:881–886.

Cutler WB, Garcia CR. *The medical management of menopause and premenopause.* Philadelphia: JB Lippincott, 1984.

Daly MJ, Sadock BJ, Kaplan HI, et al. Psychological impact of surgical procedures on women. In: Sadock BJ, Kaplan HI, Freedman AM, eds. *The sexual experience.* Baltimore: Williams & Wilkins, 1976:308.

Davis H, Johnston M. The effects of communication/counselling in medical practice: an evaluation. *J R Soc Med* 1994;87:429.

Dennerstein AO, Franz CP. *Conference report: third annual female sexual function forum: new perspectives in the management of female sexual dysfunction.* U.S. National Health and Social Life Survey and Kinsey Institute for Research on Sex, Gender, and Reproduction, Indiana University. Boston: October 26–29, 2000.

Dennerstein L, Wood C, Burrows G. Hormone therapy: effects and side effects. In: Dennerstein L, ed. *Hysterectomy.* Melbourne: Oxford University Press, 1982:107.

Dennerstein L, van Hall E. Etiology of sexual dysfunction. In: *Psychosomatic gynecology.* Lancaster, UK: Parthenon, 1986.

Derogatis LR. Breast and gynecologic cancers: their unique impact on body image and sexual identity in women. In: Vaeth JM, Blomberg RC, Adler L, eds. *Body image, self-esteem, and sexuality in cancer patients.* New York: Karger, 1980.

Diaz-Gilbert M. Culturally diverse patients. *Nursing* 1993;(Oct):44.

Dennerstein AO, Franz CP. *New perspectives in the management of female sexual dysfunction.* Third Annual Female Sexual Function Forum. U.S. National Health and Social Life Survey. Boston, October 26–29, 2000.

Freeman MG. Introduction to the sexual history. In: Walker HK, Hall WD, Hurst JW, eds. *Clinical methods,* 2nd ed. Boston: Butterworth, 1980.

Good RS, Capone MA. Emotional considerations in the care of the gynecologic cancer patient. In: Youngs D, Ehrhardt A, eds. *Psychosomatic obstetrics and gynecology.* New York: Appleton-Century-Crofts, 1980:117.

Gould D. Hidden problems after a hysterectomy. *Nurs Times* 1986;(June 4):93.

Gross J. Our bodies, but my hysterectomy. *The New York Times,* June 1994.

Hammond C. Confronting aging and disease: the role of HRT. *http://www.medscape.com/Medscape/WomensHealth/TreatmentUpdate/1999/tu01/public/toc-tu01.html* (Hammond C, Love S. *Controversies in hormone replacement therapy.* ACOG 46th Annual Clinical Meeting, 4th Scientific Session. New Orleans, May 9–13, 1998.)

Health services research on hysterectomy and alternatives. Fact sheet. AHCPR Publication No. 97-R021. Rockville, MD: Agency for Health Care Policy and Research. *http://ahrq.gov/research/hysterec.htm*

Hufnagel V. *No more hysterectomies. http://s.topchoice.com/intercon/bookorder.html*

Incontinence and prolapse. *Treatment options for patients with vaginal vault prolapse.* Women's Surgery Group. *womenssurgerygroup.com/*

Kaplan HI, Sadock BJ. *Comprehensive textbook of psychiatry,* 5th ed. Baltimore: Williams & Wilkins, 1989:1563.

Kilpatrick DG, Edmunds CN, Seymour AK. *Rape in America: a report to the nation.* 1992.

Kritz-Silverstein D, Wingard DL, et al. Hysterectomy, oophorectomy, and depression in older women. *J Wom Health* 1994;3(4):255–263.

Lalinec-Michaud M, Engelsmann F. Depression and hysterectomy: a prospective study. *Psychosomatics* 1984;25:550.

Lamont JA, DePetrillo AD, Sargeant EJ. Psychosexual rehabilitative and exenterative surgery. *Gynecol Oncol* 1978:6:236.

Lepine LA, Hillis SD, Marchbanks PA, et al. Hysterectomy Surveillance—United States, 1980–1993. *MMWR CDC Surveillance Summaries* 1997;46:1–15.

Love S, Lindsey K, Williams M. *Dr. Susan Love's breast book.* Reading, MA: Addison Wesley Longman, 1990.

Love S, Lindsey K. *Dr. Susan Love's hormone book.* New York: Random House, 1997.

Mamelok AE. Psychiatry and other specialties. In: Kaplan HI, Sadock BJ, eds. *Comprehensive textbook of psychiatry,* 5th ed. Baltimore: Williams & Wilkins, 1989.

Maslow A. A theory of human motivation. *Psychol Rev* 1984;50:370–396.

Massler DJ, Devansan MM. Sexual consequences of gynecologic operations. In: Comfort A, ed. *Sexual consequences of disability.* Philadelphia: George F. Stickley, 1978.

Moth I, Andreasson B, Jensen SB, et al. Sexual function and somatopsychic reactions after vulvectomy. *Dan Med Bull* 1983;30(2):27.

Mull DJ. Cross-cultural communication in the physician's office. *West J Med* 1993;159:609.

Nolen-Hoeksema, Larson J, Grayson C. Explaining the gender differences in depressive symptoms. *J Personality Soc Psychol* 1999;77(5):1061–1072.

Novack DH, Plumer R, Smith RL, et al. Changes in physician's attitude toward telling the cancer patient. *JAMA* 1979;241:897–900.

Paul CP. Cited in *OBGYN.net*. Special Pelvic Pain Symposium Report, Denver, CO. April 3–4, 1998.

Peters AAW, Trimbos-Kemper GCM, Admiraal C, et al. A randomized clinical trial on the benefit of adhesiolysis in patients with intraperitoneal adhesions and chronic pelvic pain. *Br J Obstet Gynaecol* 1992;99:59–62.

Plourde Elizabeth L. *The ultimate rape: what every woman should know about hysterectomies and ovarian removal.* Irvine, CA: New Voice, 1998.

Ratliff CR, Gershenson DM, et al. Sexual adjustment of patients undergoing *Gracilis myocutaneous* flap vaginal reconstruction in conjunction with pelvic exenteration. *Cancer* 1996;78(10):2229–2235.

Roeske NCA. Hysterectomy and other gynecologic surgeries: a psychological view. In: Notman MT, Nadelson CC, eds. *The woman patient: medical and psychological interfaces.* New York: Plenum, 1978.

Roovers JPWR, van der Vaart CH, et al. Correspondence re: urinary incontinence after hysterectomy. *Lancet* 2000;356:9246–2012.

Schain WS. Sexual functioning, self-esteem and cancer care. In: Vaeth JM, Blomberg RC, Adler L, eds. *Body image, self-esteem, and sexuality in cancer patients.* New York: Karger, 1980.

Sherwin BB. Estrogen and cognitive functioning in women. *Proc Soc Exp Biol Med* 1998;217:17–22.

Shountz T, Kasselman JP, et al. MHC genotype controls the capacity of ligand density to switch T Helper(Th)-1d/Th-2 priming in vivo. *J Immunol* 1996;157(9):3893–3901.

Shute Nancy. Menopause is no disease. Interview 3/24/97 with Susan Love. *U.S. News & World Report.* *http://www.usnews.com*

Smart surgical probe licensed to fight breast cancer. NASA Ames Research Center, Moffett Field, CA: Computational Sciences Division. Press release, December 22, 2000.

Snyder H, Sickmund M. *Juvenile offenders and victims: 1999 national report.* Washington, DC: Office of Juvenile Justice and Delinquency Prevention, *http://www.buildingblocks foryouth.org/justiceforsome/conclusion.html*

Stress incontinence. *http://health.yahoo.com/health/dc/000891/0.html*

Tanskanen A, et al. Cholesterol, depression and suicide. Br J Psychiatry 2000; 176: 398–399.

Tjaden P, Thoennes N. Tull report of the prevalence, incidence, and consequences of violence against women: findings from the National Violence Against Women survey. Washington, DC: US Department of Justice, Office of Justice Programs, National Institute of Justice, 2000.

Ufema J. Helping loved ones say goodbye. *Nursing* 1991;(Oct):42.

Wagner JR, Russo P. Urologic complications of major pelvic surgery. *Surg Oncol* 2000;18:216–228.

Wagner JR, Russo P. Urologic complications of major pelvic surgery. *Semin Surg Oncol* 2000:18:216–228.

Warga Claire. *Menopause and the mind: the complete guide to coping with memory loss, foggy thinking, verbal confusion, and other cognitive effects of perimenopause and menopause.* New York: Simon & Schuster, 1999.

Webb C, Wilson-Barnett J. Hysterectomy: a study in coping with recovery. *J Adv Nurs* 1983;8:311.

Women's Surgery Group. *Research notes about state-of-the-art gynecologic practices: adhesions notes. http://www.womens surgerygroup.com*

Youngs DD, Ehrhardt AA, Wise TN. Psychological sequelae of elective gynecologic surgery. In: *Psychosomatic obstetrics and gynecology.* New York: Appleton-Century-Crofts, 1980:255.

Te Linde's Operative Gynecology, ninth edition, edited by John A. Rock and Howard W. Jones, III. Lippincott Williams & Wilkins, Philadelphia, © 2003.

CHAPTER
4

▼

Professional Liability and Risk Management for the Gynecologic Surgeon

CHARLES J. WARD

As we enter the new millennium the gynecologic surgeon, both in the United States and Europe, continues to be faced with increasing pressures from the threat of malpractice litigation. This chapter outlines practical steps that should reduce the exposure to malpractice claims. It also discusses the litigation process and its emotional impact on the physician. This chapter is neither to be considered a substitute for legal counsel nor a source of legal advice. A bibliography is furnished for those who wish to explore this subject further.

The history of liability suits extends back to the 14th century. The first recorded malpractice suit in English law occurred in 1374. This case involved an action brought before the King's Bench against a surgeon, J. Mort. The plaintiff sustained an injury to the hand, and treatment of this injury left the hand maimed. The defendant surgeon was found not liable because of a legal technicality in the writ of complaint. But the rule was clearly laid down that if negligence were proven, the law would provide a remedy. The court further held that, "if the surgeon does well as he can and employs all his diligence to the cure, it is not right that he should be held culpable."

The civil liability of surgeons arises out of the rule laid down in 1534 by the English jurist, Sir Anthony Fitzherbert, which stated, "it is the duty of every artificer to exercise his art right and truly as he ought."

The first recorded malpractice suit in the United States occurred in Connecticut in 1794 and was also against a surgeon. In this case, *Cross v. Guthrey,* the patient's husband sued the surgeon, Dr. Guthrey, after the patient died from postoperative mastectomy complications. The suit alleged the doctor was guilty of negligence in operating on the plaintiff's wife

> . . . in the most unskillful, ignorant, and cruel manner, contrary to all the well-known rules and principles of practice in such cases, that the patient survived by but three hours, and that the defendant had wholly broken and violated his undertaking and promise to the plaintiff to perform said operation skillfully and with safety to his wife.

The jury found the surgeon liable and awarded damages of £40.

The 1970s and 1980s found the United States engulfed in a malpractice crisis. The 1990s have continued this trend, which had now spread to Europe. The millennium continues to bring additional pressures to bear on the gynecologic surgeon. These pressures arise from areas such as the transformation of the practice from a fee-for-service (FFS) reimbursement to various managed care programs, third-party payer interventions, declining incomes yet increasing overhead costs, longer work hours, and sizable malpractice premiums. Because the obstetrician/gynecologist performs six of the 10 most common surgical procedures, it is not surprising to find this specialty to be the most frequently sued. The 1999 survey of the American College of Obstetricians and Gynecologists membership found that 76.5% of all fellows have been sued at least one time. The obstetricians/gynecologists surveyed had an average of 2.53 claims filed against them during their career. Even resident physicians in training reported that 27.8% had at least one professional liability claim filed against them during their training. Gynecologic care involved 41.1% of all the claims filed. Of the gynecologic claims, patient injury accounted for the most frequent primary allegation and represented 25.8% of these claims. Failure to diagnose was the second most common allegation and accounted for 25.1% of gynecologic claims. Of these, failure to diagnose breast cancer amounted to 63.3%, failure to diagnose cervical cancer 18.1%, and failure to diagnose ovarian cancer accounted for 5.9% of the gynecologic claims. On average, 4.2 years elapsed from the onset of the claim to its closing. Fifty-four percent of all the claims were dropped or settled without any payment on behalf of the physician. Obstetricians/gynecologists won 65.5% of those claims that went to arbitration or a jury verdict.

Contrary to popular impressions that "bad doctors" are the cause of most malpractice actions, studies have shown that physicians who possessed higher qualifications, were board certified, and had more experience were more likely to be sued. This is in part because of the fact that such physicians manage higher-risk patients; therefore, they are more likely to encounter adverse outcomes that can be a source of litigation.

Medical malpractice occurs when the treatment rendered is constituted to be below the degree of care exercised by physicians generally under the same or similar set of circumstances. Today most communities are held to a national standard of care that is defined as a duty to exercise the degree of care and skill expected of a reasonably competent practitioner in the same specialty acting under similar circumstances. *Maloccurrence,* or a poor outcome, is not malpractice unless the outcome arises from a direct effect of a breach of the standard of care. Substandard care per se does not always imply malpractice. There must exist a *direct cause-and-effect relationship* between the breach of the standard of care and the outcome to constitute malpractice.

RISK MANAGEMENT

Risk management refers to those medical practices and procedures that are designed to reduce patient injury and improve clinical outcomes. Risk management is an approach to the practice of medicine that minimizes the risk of lawsuits by practicing in a manner that reduces the possibility of human error, increasing the likelihood of obtaining desired results and providing a medical record that clearly outlines the treatment rendered, which in turn makes such a record very defensible. Risk management, whether in an office or hospital setting, must be a team effort. Each member of the health care team must understand that his or her actions can lead to liability for the others. This means that each member of the health care team must not only understand his or her responsibilities and duties, but also be capable of carrying out those responsibilities and duties.

Many hospitals now employ risk managers. Among their duties is the investigation of incident reports and adverse outcomes. The risk manager should be able to establish appropriate targeted audits that help the institution identify its risks. With this knowledge, the staff and appropriate departments then can develop procedures and policies to correct the identified problems. Risk management should never be considered a punitive exercise, but rather an approach that will improve the quality of care rendered by all health care professionals.

Risk management cannot always prevent a lawsuit; however, frequently it can protect against a nonmeritorious claim or at least improve the outcome of a malpractice claim. Risk management also has been shown to decrease malpractice premiums in states where it was actively employed. The four cornerstones to solid risk management for the gynecologic surgeon are good surgical technique, appropriate knowledge of current developments and therapy, adequate documentation, and good patient communication. The former two are discussed throughout this book; the latter two are discussed in this chapter.

Documentation

Documentation, or its absence, is a major problem in malpractice claims. The finest care given under the best of circumstances, if not documented, may be difficult if not impossible to defend in a court of law. Documentation should be made contemporaneously so that significant facts or incidents are not forgotten. Records should contain adequate documentation to provide sufficient reasons why a procedure was indicated or undertaken. Typed reports are preferred to handwritten reports because they are more legible and open to less question of interpretation. Physician notes should be factual, complete, and relevant. They should neither embellish nor appear grandiose. Only appropriate and widely accepted abbreviations are to be used. It is prudent to document both important negative findings and positive findings, especially in complicated cases. In court, those findings, positive or negative, not documented are often presumed to never have been established. Detrimental statements about the patient should be avoided, but it is prudent to document inappropriate patient behavior. This includes noncompliant behavior, such as failure to get requested tests or follow given advice. Broken or missed appointments also should be recorded. Medical records, especially operative notes, should avoid the words *unin-*

tentionally, inadvertently, accidentally, unfortunately, and *unexplainable* because they imply negligent behavior. For example, in the case of ureteral injury, the surgeon can state that the ureter was cut, and the injury recognized and repaired. However, it is important to detail difficult dissections, the presence of extensive adhesions, or any event that makes a surgical case more difficult. It is always wise to outline a plan of therapy. The surgeon should be aware that *judgmental decisions* supported by either literature or common use, are defensible and are not malpractice, even if they result in a less than desirous outcome.

There is a proper way to correct a record. Draw a single line through the error, but never obliterate the error. Write the correction either in the margin or on a separate page. Then date and initial the correction. Never change a record after a suit has been filed, because such behavior can lead to loss of credibility and generally makes a case indefensible.

Office Setting

The office frequently can be the catalyst of a malpractice claim. It can begin with the telephone, which some consider to be the most dangerous of liability risks. Misunderstanding and miscommunication easily can occur over the telephone. Improper telephone etiquette may change a disgruntled patient into an angry one who contemplates the instigation of a malpractice claim. Make sure that messages that require a reply by the physician are delivered in a timely manner and that the advice given is documented. Telephone calls of an urgent or emergency nature not only should be responded to in a timely manner, but also documented in the office chart with the date, time of call, time of response, and advice given. Prescription refills as well as patient instructions given over the telephone should be contemporaneously entered in the chart. Only standard abbreviations should be used in the medical chart. A protocol should be established to make sure that after-hour phone calls, problems, advice rendered, and prescriptions are documented in the patient's record.

Employees of the surgeon's office should be encouraged to provide a warm, courteous, and caring environment for patients who, for the most part, will be under considerable stress as they anticipate surgery or encounter the postoperative limitations that the surgery places on them.

New patients should be told of office policies regarding type of examination, laboratory work, and expected charges. This may be accomplished through written material. Owing to the time constraints that are often placed on the physician by managed care plans, the initial intake information is often obtained by forms filled out by the patient or a member of the office staff. The information should include not only the patient's complaint and pertinent history, but also her past medical, surgical, social, and family history. Drug allergies, identified risk factors, and current medications should be noted. The physician should review this information with the patient to clarify any questionable areas and be sure that the information is adequate for the appropriate management of the patient. Because the gynecologist is now taking care of an aging population, it is extremely important that the gynecologist be aware of all medications the patient is taking. This knowledge can decrease the risk of drug interactions and adverse reactions as new medications are added to the patient's regimen. In this regard, it would be prudent for the physician to have the names of the patient's current practitioners, so that the gynecologist can consult with them as needed. It also is prudent for the gynecologist to have access to a pharmacist, who may be more qualified to check for drug interactions, so that he or she can discuss any questions in this area when new medications are prescribed.

Appointments should be scheduled so that long delays are avoided and overbooking should be discouraged. Remember that the patient's time is as valuable to her as yours is to you. Records should be kept of broken or missed appointments. This type of information is extremely helpful in establishing a noncompliant behavioral pattern. A protocol should be established for the follow-up on patients who fail to keep appointments.

The patient's confidentiality cannot only be broken by employee gossip, but also by inadequate soundproofing in examination and consultation rooms. A simple test can be conducted by the surgeon by going into an examination room during working hours to see if he or she can hear conversation by the staff in the halls or other areas of the office. If such a problem exists, the staff should be made aware of it. Some simple solutions, such as background music and keeping up-to-date reading materials in the examination room to absorb the attention of patients awaiting the physician, may help to alleviate this potential breech of the patient's confidentiality.

A protocol should be in place so that reports, such as laboratory and x-ray studies, are seen and initialed by the physician prior to filing. Patients should be encouraged to call for the results of their tests (especially mammograms, because such results can be lost in the mail); yet, the physician may be held responsible for such reports. The patient can be made aware of this responsibility through verbal reminders as well as written notices posted conspicuously in the office.

Because the failure to diagnosis breast cancer is a leading cause of malpractice claims, it is prudent for the gynecologist to have a clear and sound approach to any patient who presents with a breast mass or complaint. Chapter 40 outlines the risk factors, diagnosis, and treatment of breast diseases. From a risk management approach, documentation is critical. It is prudent that the patient's medical record document the date the patient first noticed the change, the symptoms noted and a detailed description of the physician's findings. Drawings of the mass showing the location and exact measurements of the change are most helpful. Recommended referrals, as well as follow-up and return visits should be recorded. A system of in-office chart follow-up for these high-risk patients is prudent. Reports of mammograms or other studies should exhibit evidence of review by the physician. If the patient fails to follow advice, the office records should note this along with all attempts to contact the patient.

Billing and financial records have no place in the medical records. They must be kept separate. A confidential area should be made available for the patient to discuss the fees, insurance matters, or the bill. It is strongly advisable that the physician should review every bill before it is turned over to a collection agency. The act of turning a bill over to a collection agency has been the start of many malpractice claims.

When records are requested, make sure to send only copies and only after the appropriate patient authorization has been obtained. Most states have laws that prohibit the transfer of records that deal with drug and alcohol abuse or mental illness without the express authorization of the patient. If the physician sends such information without proper authorization, a separate cause of action can be brought against the physician. Therefore, it is important to be aware of the individual state's laws. Always retain the original copy for as long as your state requires or the statute of limitation exists. Information of this nature usually can be obtained from the state medical board or medical society.

Hospital Setting

The hospital setting is the source of most events that lead to malpractice claims involving the surgeon. Patients entering the hospital are under considerable stress and may not comprehend the full scope of their therapy. Patients should be made aware that perfect outcomes cannot be guaranteed. They should be made to understand that the chance of an unfavorable outcome is not necessarily related to the quality of care but can occur virtually in any medical encounter. Results should never be guaranteed, especially when performing corrective surgery, such as procedures for the treatment of urinary incontinence.

The hospital chart is an important vehicle for communicating significant information needed by the entire health team. Because what is not written in a medical record may be legally presumed to not have occurred, it is critical that the chart is complete, thorough and that documentation be recorded contemporaneously. The chart should reflect the outline for the plan of management, both current and future, using only approved abbreviations. By clearly writing out the plan of management, especially in complicated cases, the entire health team is able to understand the approach to the treatment and respond in a positive and appropriate manner.

Daily progress notes are generally advisable; however, more frequent notes are appropriate in complicated cases. Progress notes should not only be dated, but also timed. The timing of notes can be most beneficial from a risk management point of view. When a change in the patient's condition develops and the surgeon is notified of the patient's status, the response time may be critical in establishing the standard of care. The surgeon should develop the habit of timing all notes so that the habit becomes well established. Thus, the surgeon is less likely to forget to time a note in a critical situation.

Consultation should be encouraged, especially in complicated cases. Most patients appreciate this concern and understand that it is impossible with today's rapidly expanding advances in technology for one physician to have complete and superior knowledge in all situations. When consultation is obtained, to avoid confusion and lack of direction in the patient's therapy, one physician should be appointed to coordinate therapies and supervise critical orders.

The surgeon should carefully review all nursing notes on a daily basis. When there is a discrepancy between the observations of the physician and the nurse, the differences should be discussed. Then both parties should write clarifying notes that reflect the discrepancy in observations and its resolution in an appropriate chronological order.

The physician should review all laboratory reports. It is prudent to write progress notes about any significant or abnormal findings in the intended plan of action so that the subsequent members of the health team can understand the therapy and react in a positive manner.

It is imperative that derogatory remarks not be made in a patient's record. Physicians should never criticize the care rendered by another physician in front of the patient, nurse, or in an area where others may hear the discussion. There are proper avenues to take if one is dealing with an incompetent physician. To avoid breaching patient's confidentiality, idle discussions with other health care providers on elevators, in halls, or in the operating theater are to be avoided.

Follow-up and discharge care should be explained thoroughly to the patient. In an outpatient surgical center, at the time of discharge, many patients may still be under the influence of anesthesia or drugs that cloud their memories. Therefore, it is prudent not only to give verbal but also written discharge instructions. These instructions should cover medication, activity, diet, wound care, and follow-up appointments. The dose of any medication as well as the duration of its use should be noted clearly. Abbreviations that may not be understood by the patient are to be avoided. The physician's answering service and emergency phone numbers should be provided. A copy of the discharge instructions should be given to the patient and one retained in the chart.

When a complication or less than desirous outcome occurs, the surgeon should promptly have a frank discussion concerning the matter with the patient and other significant family members. Spending the time and providing quality information in an honest and thorough manner is appreciated by the patient and the family and often diffuses a potential malpractice claim. Saying that you are sorry is not an admission of guilt. Most patients, when given a reasonable explanation of a less than desirable outcome, accept our human limitations, but disgruntled patients sue. It is important to convey the fact that medicine remains an art and is not an exact science.

Hospital rules and protocols are established to insure uniform quality of care. The physician or nurse's failure to comply with them subsequently can be interpreted as a violation of the standard of care. Therefore, it behooves all members of the health team to know and understand the appropriate rules and protocols. If the surgeon feels that he or she needs to alter a rule or protocol for a patient's benefit, he or she should document the reason contemporaneously in the hospital chart.

Surgeons must stay abreast of current technological advances; however, before using these advances, they must be adequately trained. A borderline skilled surgeon who is learning new procedures on private patients without the patient's knowledge or approval is not only risking a malpractice suit, but also may be accused of practicing under questionable ethical standards.

The resident or house officer adds another potential risk to malpractice exposure. All residents or house officers practice as trainees under the supervision of the training institution and the staff of the hospital. Those who supervise—be they attending, clinical faculty, or full-time faculty—are usually held accountable for residents' acts. Residents and house officers, however, also can be held accountable for their own actions. Thus, it is important for the surgeon in a supervisory role to not only review the chart, but also assess the patient. If the supervising physician disagrees with a resident's evaluation, a discrete discussion of the matter should be held with the resident. Then the surgeon and resident should document the appropriate findings and note the rationale behind his or her change in observations or therapy.

On initial contact with the patient, residents, or house officers should convey the fact that they are trainees or residents. The patient has the right to refuse treatment by a resident, but most accept the advantage of such supervised training. It is prudent to document the acceptance or refusal of medical care from the resident or house officer, especially in an institution that is not directly connected with a medical school. When the patient is admitted to hospital under the care of a resident, the resident should go over the reason for hospitalization. They should discuss the recommended therapy, appropriate alternatives, potential benefits, risks, and complications of the proposed therapy. The resident should only perform those procedures, without supervision, for which he or she has been fully trained. If a patient's condition requires more expertise than the resident possesses, the resident must inform the supervisory physician of the nature of the patient's condition and the need for procedures beyond the resident's expertise. If a complication arises, the resident in the presence of a nurse or other medical witness should take time to thoroughly and openly discuss the complication and its impact on the patient's subsequent treatment and hospital stay. This conversation should then be documented in the chart.

Managed Care and Socialized Medicine

Managed care was created in an effort to control the rapidly rising U.S. health care costs. The ideal goals of managed care were to reduce cost, improve clinical outcomes, and control the utilization of resources; however, these goals have not always been achieved. Managed care

has become the dominant form of health care delivery in the United States and has had a tremendous impact on physicians as various types of managed care programs have rapidly replaced FFS. Managed care continues to evolve in an effort to meet the demands of the health care industry. At present the major types of plans include: (a) health maintenance organization (HMO), which also includes independent practice associations (IPA); (b) preferred provider organizations (PPO); and (c) point-of-service (POS) plans.

HMO plans provide or arrange coverage of specific health-care services for a fixed prepaid fee. In-network providers required by the members then provide the service. In the IPA type HMO, the plan contracts with individual physicians who maintain their own independent practice, offices, medical records, and staff but see HMO members.

PPO plans contract with independent providers who provide services at a discounted rate. Members in this plan, generally use in-network providers, but are permitted to use out-of-network providers as long as the member is willing to pay a higher out-of-pocket fee.

POS plans generally offer the cost control of an HMO plan with the choice of the FFS plans. This is accomplished by allowing members in the plan to choose from an HMO, PPO, or indemnity plan at the time the service is rendered. At present, POS plans have become the fastest growing managed care type plan.

In any managed care plan, financial conflicts can give rise to risks and liabilities for the physician, not seen in an FFS form of medicine. Problems can potentially arise when a physician is paid through a *capitation* scheme, receives year-end bonuses or other monetary rewards for under utilization of services. In capitation, the physician receives a fixed dollar amount to cover the cost of health care services for enrolled members of the plan. This per capita rate is paid on a periodic basis whether the physician does or does not provide service to all members of the plan. This is intended to reduce overuse of services. Although this system of payment is a powerful incentive for the physician to manage patient care as efficiently as possible, conflicts can arise when services provided by the physician exceed the financial reimbursement from the plan. Such conflicts of interest can impair the physician's moral judgment, threaten the patient's health and well-being, and threaten the physician's professional credibility. The physician cannot jeopardize the patient's care because of financial constraint placed on him or her by the managed care plan. Physicians must make patient-care decisions based on what is best for the patient even if such decisions adversely impact on the physician's financial status. The physician must discuss the appropriate alternatives to treatment that are available, even if the plan does not cover the cost of the preferred method of treatment, drug, test, or device. In such cases, the physician must become the patient's advocate and provide the care required to meet the patient's needs, even if the physician is not compensated for the care rendered. Legal precedents have established that the physician should act as a patient advocate in disputes over the financial cost of appropriate treatment and should attempt to convince the managed care plan administrators that the care is not only warranted, but that the care is the most appropriate for the patient's condition. Failure to practice within the standard of care because of the financial constraints of a managed care plan is *never a defense* should a malpractice suit arise from such an incident.

Under managed care plans in the United States and socialized medical plans in Europe, certain fundamental ethical values have become endangered owing to the financial constraints placed on the access to certain treatments, tests, or drugs, and the limitation to the availability of these treatments in a timely manner. These include *fiduciary beneficence* (the physician's obligation to act for the benefit of the patient), patient *autonomy* (the patient's right to make informed judgments regarding her care), and *justice* (the right to an adequate level of health care that is both available and accessible to all individuals). The physician must remain a strong advocate for the patient. The physician must have input into the decision-making process to be sure that resources are allocated in a proper and just way so that cost containment and economic efficiency are morally legitimate goals that enhance rather than undermine the quality of health care. Physicians must continue to inform the patient of the best treatment options available, whether or not these options are covered by the managed care plan or socialized medicine. They must remain a strong advocate for their patient's rights and should refuse to participate in medical plans or schemes that have policies that are deemed unethical.

Communication

Good communication is a major key to preventing malpractice claims. It has often been stated that satisfied patients are less likely to sue, but disgruntled patients will sue. It has been shown that even physicians with borderline skills but excellent bedside manners are less likely to be sued than well-trained board-certified specialists who lack communication skills. Initial impressions usually are long lasting. Therefore, it is important on the first visit to convey the physician's philosophy and the nature of his or her practice. It is prudent to explain what the physician expects from the patient in this relationship because expectations and responsibilities exist for both the patient and physician. Patients are generally looking for a physician who is easy to talk to, will answer questions, be accessible, be fair, show respect, and provide good care for a reasonable cost. Inattention, indignation, and injury can be not only the cause for a suit, but in combination also dramatically increase the potential for a suit.

Surgeons should be aware that the majority of what a patient perceives is obtained through nonverbal communications. Patients generally retain only 30% of verbal communication. Body language, posture, and facial expressions all convey strong messages. For example, the surgeon who stands with his or her hand on the door and asks, Do you have any questions? sends a strong message that he or she really does not have the time to answer questions; that his or her time is more important than the concerns of the patient. Simple things such as sitting in a relaxed position when the physician discusses a patient's condition or treatment generally convey a feeling of caring and concern. If notes or prescriptions are written in the examination room, the surgeon should make every attempt to face the patient while performing this task. The surgeon's back does not convey a sense of caring or concern.

In the hospital, the physician has to write daily progress notes and orders. The patient's bedside is an excellent place to write them. The surgeon then can explain the orders and therapy as they are written. Patients who are medicated have a slower reaction time and tend to easily forget things that are important to them. The silence that may ensue as the surgeon writes a note or thinks about the management gives the patient time to recall those important questions. This type of interaction builds trust and gives the patient the feeling that she is actively participating in her care and therapy.

Surgeons often do not realize the significant degree of stress a patient undergoes while she lies on the operating table prior to being anesthetized. The simple act of holding the patient's hand at this time can not only have a calming effect, but also demonstrate the physician's concern and care for the patient's well-being. In the office, little things such as warming speculums on a heating pad in the examination table drawer, providing adequate areas to dress and undress, and having mirrors in the examination room all help to convey a sense of caring for the patient's needs.

Good communication encourages questions and involvement of family members, especially partners. Therefore, it is important that the physician (preferably) or a designated nurse or physician assistant take the necessary time to answer the patient's questions and address concerns in a setting where respect and confidentiality can be maintained easily. Beware of the patient with the "great expectation syndrome." Physicians have greatly oversold their abilities and have created false expectations that have led to unjustified expectations. If the surgeon feels that the patient expects more than he or she can reasonably provide, it is prudent to refer this patient to another physician.

When it becomes necessary to terminate the doctor–patient relationship, the surgeon must remember that this relationship is a contract, be it informal or implied, and certain steps are required to break the contract. The patient should be sent a letter by certified mail, return receipt requested. The letter should state a specific date for the termination to occur, usually 30 days from the date of mailing. The letter should contain a release for the patient's records. The patient should be instructed to sign and return the release prior to forwarding any of the patient's records. Always send a *copy of the records,* and never the original records, to the physician of her choice. The physician may include a list of other gynecologists in the patient's area or refer her to the local medical society for appropriate referral. These letters of termination need not go into great detail as to why the contract is being terminated. It is perfectly acceptable to say that, owing to a personality conflict, the surgeon does not feel that he or she can provide the quality of care the patient should receive. Thus, the physician is requesting that the patient seek care elsewhere. The physician is required to treat any emergency that might arise prior to the specified termination date.

Improper communication can result in physicians getting other physicians sued. Negative comments made about other physicians continue to be a major source of problems. As Pogo the cartoon character once stated, "I have met the enemy and he is us." Nonprofessional opinions written in the medical record can open the treating surgeon, hospital, or other health-care members to malpractice actions. Careless talk, second-guessing colleagues, and open debate, carried out in public areas, regarding the patient's treatment or status can all lead to unwarranted malpractice claims.

In situations involving multiple physicians, such as a group practice, communication between those physicians is extremely important. The medical records must be a complete and thorough source of this information. The records should reflect clear and factual accounts so that confusion does not arise regarding the patient's treatment or status. Lack of such communication can increase the risk of liability claims. In group practices, it is prudent to have set aside a specific time each day to discuss patients, especially those with complicated courses.

A physician should know his or her limitations and not let an inflated or unrealistic ego prevent appropriate consultations when the patient's condition may exceed his or her expertise. Continuous and appropriate communication with the consulting physicians ensures that the patient receives the highest quality of care, the goal all physicians strive to achieve.

INFORMED CONSENT

Informed consent is a legal doctrine that requires physicians to obtain consent for treatment, whether it is diagnostic or therapeutic, medical or surgical, invasive, or noninvasive. Without informed consent the physician can be held liable for violating the patient's rights regardless of whether the treatment was appropriate and rendered within the standard of care. Although failure to provide informed consent is seldom the primary charge in a malpractice claim, it has been found to be a secondary issue in almost one third of malpractice claims. Informed consent is an ongoing process that includes the exchange of information and the development of choices. Informed consent is a process of ongoing-shared information. It provides for the development of choices and requires active participation from both the patient and the physician. It involves respect for the patient's bodily integrity and right to self-determination; thus, it respects the patient's autonomy. Informed consent should never be confused with the mere signing of a consent sheet. Without informed consent, a physician may be held liable of violating the patient's rights even if

the treatment was appropriate and administered within the standards of care. Failure to obtain informed consent can result in the physician being accused of "battery" under common law.

Since the 1947 Nuremberg Code, valid consent has consistently been described as having four characteristics: voluntary, competent, informed, and understanding. The American College of Obstetricians and Gynecologists, in its statement of May 1992 on "Ethical Dimensions of Informed Consent" explores the concept of voluntary or free consent and understanding or comprehension.

The concept of freedom implies both an ability to choose as well as an ability to refuse treatment. Freedom also implies a lack of coercion, manipulation, or infringement on the patient's decision-making process. Recognition of different values, preferences, and alternatives is important in the process of free consent.

Courts have recognized and states have adopted three different degrees of disclosure in informed consent. The first, *the professional or reasonable physician standard,* was prevalent prior to the 1970s. This degree of disclosure was based on the type and amount of information that a reasonable physician would tell the patient about the risks and benefits of a particular treatment. This paternalistic approach began to give way in the 1970s to the second type of disclosure, *The materiality or reasonable patient viewpoint standard.* This gave patients more input into the decision-making process. Under this standard, the physician had to disclose what a "reasonable person" would want to know under similar circumstances concerning the risks and benefits of a particular treatment. This concept is based on the patient's need rather than the professional perception of what the patient should know.

The third, but not widely held, disclosure is the *subjective patient viewpoint.* Under this disclosure, physicians must disclose varying amounts of information based on the individual's personal needs and peculiar requirements. This form renders a standard extremely difficult for physicians to understand and apply.

The need for informed consent can be suspended in an emergency situation, but specific criteria must be met for a situation to be declared an emergency. The patient must be unconscious or incapacitated and suffering from a life-threatening or serious health-threatening condition requiring immediate medical treatment. It is important in these situations for the physician to document the following: a description of the patient's condition at the time of the emergency, the reason the emergency existed, and an explanation for the need for immediate attention.

Patients have the right to refuse treatment after receiving informed consent. Under these circumstances, for legal protection, the physician should document the reason the patient gave for refusal of the proposed treatment, the reason that the physician felt that the proposed treatment was indicated, and the possible jeopardy to the future health and well-being of the patient that might occur from the refusal of the treatment. It would be prudent to have the patient sign a statement acknowledging

INFORMED CONSENT AND REQUEST FOR SURGERY

I, _____, request Dr._____ _and
his/her associates / assistants to perform upon me (name of procedure):
_____

Diagnosis and Procedure: The following has been explained to me in general terms and I
understand that:

My condition has been diagnosed as: _____
The nature of the procedure is: _____
The purpose of this procedure is to: _____

General Risks of Surgery: As a result of the performance of this procedure there may be
general risks involved such as: INFECTION, ALLERGIC REACTION, DISFIGURING SCAR,
SEVERE LOSS OF BLOOD, LOSS OR FUNCTION OF ANY LIMB OR ORGAN,
PARALYSIS, PARAPLEGIA OR QUADRIPLEGIA, BRAIN DAMAGE, CARDIAC
ARREST, OR DEATH. In addition to these general risks, there may be other possible risks
involved in this procedure. These risks and/or complications may include but are not limited to
such complications as: _____

Likelihood of Success: The likelihood of success of the above procedure is: () Good () Fair
() Poor

Prognosis: If I choose not to have the above procedure, my prognosis (future medical condition)
is: _____

Alternative Forms of Treatment, such as: _____
have been explained to me and I have chosen this surgical procedure as my method of treatment.

I understand and accept that during the procedure unexpected or unforeseen circumstances may
make it necessary to do an extension of the original procedure or another procedure that is not
named above. I request Dr. _____ and his/her associates or
assistants of his/her choice to perform those procedures that they judge to be necessary.

BY SIGNING THIS FORM, I ACKNOWLEDGE THAT I HAVE READ OR HAD THIS
FORM READ AND EXPLAINED TO ME AND THAT I FULLY UNDERSTAND ITS
CONTENTS.

I HAVE BEEN GIVEN AMPLE OPPORTUNITY TO ASK QUESTIONS AND ANY
QUESTIONS I HAVE ASKED HAVE BEEN ANSWERED OR EXPLAINED IN A
SATISFACTORY MANNER.   ALL   BLANKS   OR   STATEMENTS   REQUIRING
COMPLETION WERE FILLED IN AND ALL STATEMENTS WITH WHICH I DISAGREE
WERE MARKED OUT BEFORE I SIGNED THIS FORM.

I accept that medicine is not an exact science and understand that no guarantees can be given as
to the results. Understanding these limitations, I request that Dr. _____
and his/her associates/assistants to proceed with surgery.

_____   _____
Witness   Person giving consent
                                   Relationship to patient if not the patient_____

                                   Patient unable to sign because of:
Date: _____

                                   _____

Additional materials used, if any, during the informed consent process for this procedure include:
_____
_____
_____

Date: _____ Witness: _____

FIGURE 4.1. Informed consent and request for surgery.

the refusal for treatment and listing the potential adverse consequences that might occur.

The office setting provides the best environment for providing informed consent for several reasons. In this setting, the time for adequate consideration and ade-quate discussion is provided. Family members who have a definite influence on the patient's decision can attend or be encouraged to attend. If the physician lacks the ability or time to provide the necessary adequate in-formed consent, the physician can delegate this responsibility to a nurse practitioner or physician assistant who has been previously trained to provide informed consent and is able to answer the patient's questions. Pamphlets, audiovisual, and even interactive visuals can greatly assist in this process. Because people rarely retain more than 30% of verbal communications, the average patient leaves the physician's office having forgotten or not understanding most of what was shown and explained. Thus, the more the patient receives in writing or by audiovisual instruction, the better is her understanding.

Once the process of informed consent is complete, the physician can document the record to reflect when it took place, what was disclosed, that the patient had time to ask questions and have her questions answered to her satisfaction, and that the patient then requested the proposed treatment. Well-informed patients are more likely to overlook less than desirable outcomes and accept that medicine is still an art and not an exact science. Less-well informed patients are more likely to have unrealistic expectations and sue when these expectations are not met. Therefore, the best protection to a malpractice claim may come from taking full advantage of the legal doctrine of informed consent.

The degree of disclosure in informed consent varies from state to state. Some states require elaborate consent, others much less. When a complication develops that was disclosed in the informed consent; however, there is no cause for legal action so long as the complication did not arise from a negligent act.

There is almost universal agreement that informed consent should encompass the following six areas:

1. Diagnosis
2. Nature and purpose of the procedure
3. Risks of the procedure
4. Likelihood of success
5. Reasonable alternatives
6. Prognosis if the treatment is refused

Figure 4.1 is a general surgical informed consent meeting these requirements. There are several points to note regarding this particular form. First, throughout the form, the words "I request" or "request for surgery" are included. These words are used to place greater emphasis on the patient's responsibility for her choice in selecting the proposed procedure. Next, a list of the "general risks of surgery" is provided. This list covers those risks that can arise from any surgical procedure as well as anesthesia. In describing the risks and complications of the procedures, the words "may include but are not limited to such complications as" have been added and are used to indicate that the physician did not attempt to list every potential complication but rather those that a reasonable patient would expect to know before making a decision. In the section on alternative forms of treatment, the words "such as" indicate that only those alternatives considered to be appropriate need to be listed. Finally, space is provided to list any additional materials that the patient was given or might have reviewed in making her decision. If a claim arises, the physician can then explain to a jury the situation surrounding the alleged act of negligence and use the same material in his

or her defense to show that a reasonable person was properly informed.

Figures 4.2 through 4.6 are informed consents covering the five most common gynecologic operative procedures. These forms describe each procedure in words that a patient can comprehend easily. A reading specialist has reviewed each of these forms, as well as the general surgery consent form described in the preceding. The language used has been placed at the level of an individual with a sixth-grade education, which is generally that used by daily newspapers. Each of these forms covers the risks and complications as well as alternatives that apply to the specific procedure along with the "general risks of surgery."

Figure 4.2, the informed consent and request for dilatation and curettage, cervical biopsy, and hysteroscopy, lists the most common complication seen, namely perforation of the uterus. It also notes that the procedure can have an adverse impact on subsequent pregnancies.

Figure 4.3, the informed consent and request for hysterectomy, covers complications seen, including injuries to the genitourinary tract, the most frequently seen complication. It also discusses the risk associated with blood transfusion.

Figure 4.4, the informed consent and request for sterilization, clearly states that the procedure is not designed to be reversible. Many patients have a sterilization procedure performed in their twenties and in this age of divorce and remarriage, later request that the sterilization be reversed. When the procedure cannot be reversed, patients may sue with a claim of "lost opportunities." This statement in the informed consent is designed to cover that particular area. Ectopic pregnancy, one of the known and accepted risks of any sterilization procedure, is clearly spelled out.

Figure 4.5, the informed consent and request for diagnostic and therapeutic laparoscopy, reviews the more commonly seen complications of injury to the gastrointestinal, or genitourinary tracts and vascular injury. The form also notes the risk of exploratory laparotomy. This provides an opportunity for the physician to discuss this potential extension of a laparoscopy procedure so that the physician is not hesitant to proceed with laparotomy when the findings require this procedure.

Figure 4.6, the informed consent for repair of relaxation of pelvic organs and/or the correction of urinary incontinence problems, notes that recurrence of urinary incontinence is a potential complication. This is designed so that false expectations from the surgical procedure are not created.

These procedure-specific informed consent forms are detailed but have been found to be accepted by patients. They also have made the defense of surgical complications much easier, especially when there is no negligence.

The legal requirements of informed consent vary from state to state and jurisdiction to jurisdiction. The surgeon should be aware of the degree of disclosure required as well as any specific laws on informed consent that exist in his or her state. County or state medical societies are usually able to assist in providing this necessary information. (text continues on p. 61)

INFORMED CONSENT
And
REQUEST FOR DILATION & CURETTAGE,
HYSTEROSCOPY, OR CERVICAL BIOPSY

I, _____ , request Dr._____ and his/her associates / assistants to perform upon me (Circle procedure to be performed):

1.   Dilation & Curettage--stretch open the canal of my uterus and scrape the lining of my uterus to obtain tissue for study.
2.   Hysteroscopy--look inside my uterus with a small telescope and possibly remove any abnormal tissue, such as fibroid tumors, polyps, or scar tissue.
3.   Cervical Biopsy--remove tissue from tip of my uterus for tissue study.

Diagnosis and Procedure: The following has been explained to me in general terms and I understand that:

My condition has been diagnosed as: _____
The nature of the procedure is: _____
The purpose of this procedure is to: _____

General Risks of Surgery: As a result of the performance of this procedure there may be general risks involved such as: INFECTION, ALLERGIC REACTION, DISFIGURING SCAR, SEVERE LOSS OF BLOOD, FUNCTION OF ANY LIMB OR ORGAN, PARALYSIS, PARAPLEGIA or QUADRIPLEGIA, BRAIN DAMAGE, CARDIAC ARREST, or DEATH. In addition to these general risks, there may be other possible risks involved in this procedure. These risks and/or complications may include but are not limited to such complications as:

1.   Perforation of my uterus (womb)--that is, one of the instruments might go through the wall of the uterus and make it necessary to do an immediate or future operation that could include the removal of my uterus and/or tubes and ovaries
2.   Biopsy of my cervix--which may make it difficult for me to get pregnant or carry a pregnancy to term (9 months)
3.   Injury to my cervix, uterus, tubes, and bowel--which could make necessary immediate and/or future surgical procedures

Likelihood of Success: The likelihood of success of the above procedure is: () Good () Fair () Poor

Prognosis: If I choose not to have the above procedure, my prognosis (future medical condition) is:

FIGURE 4.2.   Informed consent and request for dilation and curettage, hysteroscopy, or cervical biopsy.

Alternative Forms of Treatment such as:

1.   Office biopsy of the lining of my uterus (endometrial biopsy) or cervix (cervical biopsy)
2.   Hormone therapy
3.   Do-nothing and accept the consequences of my present condition

These alternative treatments have been explained to me, and I have elected this surgical procedure as my method of treatment.

I understand and accept that during the procedure unexpected or unforeseen circumstances may make it necessary to do an extension of the original procedure or another procedure that is not named above.   I request that Dr. _____ and associates or assistants of his/her choice to perform those procedures that they judge to be necessary.

BY SIGNING THIS FORM, I ACKNOWLEDGE THAT I HAVE READ OR HAD THIS FORM READ AND EXPLAINED TO ME AND THAT I FULLY UNDERSTAND ITS CONTENTS.

I HAVE BEEN GIVEN AMPLE OPPORTUNITY TO ASK QUESTIONS AND ANY QUESTIONS I HAVE ASKED HAVE BEEN ANSWERED OR EXPLAINED IN A SATISFACTORY MANNER.   ALL BLANKS OR STATEMENTS REQUIRING COMPLETION WERE FILLED IN AND ALL STATEMENTS WITH WHICH I DISAGREE WERE MARKED OUT BEFORE I SIGNED THIS FORM.

I accept that medicine is not an exact science and understand that no guarantees can be given as to the results. Understanding these limitations, I request that Dr. _____ and his/her associates/assistants to proceed with surgery.

_____   _____
Witness   Person giving consent
                                                                 Relationship to patient if not the patient_____

                                                                 Patient unable to sign because of:

Date: _____   _____

Additional materials used, if any, during the informed consent process for this procedure include:

_____
_____
_____

Date: _____ Witness: _____
_____

FIGURE 4.2. *Continued*

INFORMED CONSENT And REQUEST FOR HYSTERECTOMY

I, _____ , request Dr._____ __ and his/her associates / assistants to perform upon me: (Circle procedure of choice)

1.   Removal of uterus (womb)
2.   Possible removal of tubes and/or ovaries
3.   Possible removal of appendix

Diagnosis and Procedure: The following has been explained to me in general terms and I understand that:

My condition has been diagnosed as: _____
The nature of the procedure is: _____
The purpose of this procedure is to: _____

General Risks of Surgery: As a result of the performance of this procedure there may be general risks involved such as: INFECTION, ALLERGIC REACTION, DISFIGURING SCAR, SEVERE LOSS OF BLOOD, FUNCTION OF ANY LIMB OR ORGAN, PARALYSIS, PARAPLEGIA or QUADRIPLEGIA, BRAIN DAMAGE, CARDIAC ARREST, or DEATH. In addition to these general risks, there may be other possible risks involved in this procedure. These risks and/or complications may include but are not limited to such complications as:

1.   Injury to bowel, bladder, or ureter, which could result in a fistula formation, an opening between bowel, bladder, ureter, vagina and/or skin
2.   Need for a colostomy or a second operation to repair any of the above injuries
3.   Possible need for hormones
4.   Blood loss necessitating transfusion, which carries the risk of exposure to AIDS or the hepatitis virus
5.   Pelvic pain due to adhesions, scar tissue, or residual ovary

Likelihood of Success: The likelihood of success of the above procedure is: () Good, () Fair, () Poor

Prognosis: If I choose not to have the hysterectomy, my prognosis (future medical condition) is:

_____

Alternative Forms of Treatment such as:

1.   Do nothing and accept the consequences of my present condition
2.   Dilatation & Curettage procedure, laser treatment, or removal of fibroid tumors
3.   Hormone therapy

FIGURE 4.3. Informed consent and request for hysterectomy.

These alternative treatments have been explained to me, and I have elected this surgical procedure as my method of treatment.

I understand and accept that during the procedure unexpected or unforeseen circumstances may make it necessary to do an extension of the original procedure or another procedure that is not named above. I request that Dr. _____ and associates or assistants of his/her choice perform those procedures that they judge to be necessary.

BY SIGNING THIS FORM, I ACKNOWLEDGE THAT I HAVE READ OR HAD THIS FORM READ AND EXPLAINED TO ME AND THAT I FULLY UNDERSTAND ITS CONTENTS.

I HAVE BEEN GIVEN AMPLE OPPORTUNITY TO ASK QUESTIONS AND ANY QUESTIONS I HAVE ASKED HAVE BEEN ANSWERED OR EXPLAINED IN A SATISFACTORY MANNER.   ALL BLANKS OR STATEMENTS REQUIRING COMPLETION WERE FILLED IN AND ALL STATEMENTS WITH WHICH I DISAGREE WERE MARKED OUT BEFORE I SIGNED THIS FORM.

I accept that medicine is not an exact science and understand that no guarantees can be given as to the results. Understanding these limitations, I request that Dr. _____ and his/her associates/assistants to proceed with surgery.

_____   _____
Witness   Person giving consent

                                                             Relationship to patient if not the patient_____

                                                             Patient unable to sign because of:

Date: _____   _____

Additional materials used, if any, during the informed consent process for this procedure include:
_____
_____
_____

Date: _____ Witness: _____

FIGURE 4.3. *Continued*

INFORMED CONSENT And REQUEST FOR STERILIZATION

I, _____, request Dr._____
_____ and his/her associates/assistants to perform upon
me: (Circle procedure of choice)

    1.   Removal of a portion of the tubes through an incision in my lower abdomen
    2.   Laparoscopy ("band-aid" incision or incisions)
            a. Coagulation technique
                1. Bipolar   b. Bands
                2. Unipolar   c. Clips

Diagnosis and Procedure: The following has been explained to me in general terms and I understand that:
This procedure is **NOT** designed to be reversible, and that I am intentionally giving up my ability to become pregnant.
The nature of the procedure is: _____
The purpose of this procedure is to: _____

General Risks of Surgery: As a result of the performance of this procedure there may be general risks involved such as: INFECTION, ALLERGIC REACTION, DISFIGURING SCAR, SEVERE LOSS OF BLOOD, FUNCTION OF ANY LIMB OR ORGAN, PARALYSIS, PARAPLEGIA or QUADRIPLEGIA, BRAIN DAMAGE, CARDIAC ARREST, or DEATH. In addition to these general risks, there may be other possible risks involved in this procedure. These risks and/or complications may include but are not limited to such complications as:
1.   Failure to become sterile--that is, I could become pregnant either in my uterus (womb) or have an ectopic pregnancy (in my tube or other site)
2.   Injury to bowel, bladder, ureter or blood vessel by way of burn and/or perforation, fistula formation (which is an opening that develops between the bowel, bladder, ureter and the vagina and/or or skin), requiring a second operation to repair the fistula
3.   Major surgery--requiring colostomy or possible removal of uterus, tubes and/or ovaries
4.   Necessity for an exploratory laparotomy (opening the abdomen) to either complete the laparoscopy procedure or repair any injury
5.   Blood loss necessitating transfusion, which carries the risk of exposure to AIDS or the hepatitis virus

Likelihood of Success: The likelihood of success of the above procedure is: () Good () Fair () Poor
Prognosis: If I choose not to have the above procedure, my prognosis (future medical condition) is: _____

Alternative Forms of Treatment such as:
    1   Diaphragm _____

FIGURE 4.4. Informed consent and request for sterilization.

2   Birth control pills
3   Intrauterine devices (IUD)
4   Barrier methods (use of foams, condoms, etc.)
5   Rhythm method
6.   Abstinence
7.   Vasectomy (male sterilization)

These alternative treatments have been explained to me, and I have elected this surgical procedure as my method of treatment.

I understand and accept that during the procedure unexpected or unforeseen circumstances may make it necessary to do an extension of the original procedure or another procedure that is not named above. I request that Dr. _____ and associates or assistants of his/her choice perform those procedures that they judge to be necessary.

BY SIGNING THIS FORM, I ACKNOWLEDGE THAT I HAVE READ OR HAD THIS FORM READ AND EXPLAINED TO ME AND THAT I FULLY UNDERSTAND ITS CONTENTS.

I HAVE BEEN GIVEN AMPLE OPPORTUNITY TO ASK QUESTIONS AND ANY QUESTIONS I HAVE ASKED HAVE BEEN ANSWERED OR EXPLAINED IN A SATISFACTORY MANNER.   ALL BLANKS OR STATEMENTS REQUIRING COMPLETION WERE FILLED IN AND ALL STATEMENTS WITH WHICH I DISAGREE WERE MARKED OUT BEFORE I SIGNED THIS FORM.

I accept that medicine is not an exact science and understand that no guarantees can be given as to the results. Understanding these limitations, I request that Dr. _____ and his/her associates/assistants to proceed with surgery.

_____   _____
Witness   Person giving consent

                                         _____
                                         Relationship to patient if not the patient_____

                                         Patient unable to sign because of:

Date: _____

                                         _____

Additional materials used, if any, during the informed consent process for this procedure include:
_____
_____
_____

Date: _____ Witness: _____

FIGURE 4.4. *Continued*

INFORMED CONSENT And REQUEST FOR LAPAROSCOPY

I, _____ , request Dr._____

_____ and his/her associates/ assistants to perform upon me:

      Laparoscopy--which involves inserting a telescope-like instrument into my abdomen through one or more small ("band-aid") size incisions to diagnose and/or repair any problems

Diagnosis and Procedure: The following has been explained to me in general terms and I understand that:

My condition has been diagnosed as: _____

The nature of the procedure is: _____

The purpose of this procedure is to: _____

I understand that treatment may require the use of laser and/or electrocautery during the performance of this surgery.

General Risks of Surgery: As a result of the performance of this procedure there may be general risks involved such as: INFECTION, ALLERGIC REACTION, DISFIGURING SCAR, SEVERE LOSS OF BLOOD, FUNCTION OF ANY LIMB OR ORGAN, PARALYSIS, PARAPLEGIA or QUADRIPLEGIA, BRAIN DAMAGE, CARDIAC ARREST, or DEATH. In addition to these general risks, there may be other possible risks involved in this procedure. These risks and/or complications may include but are not limited to such complications as:

1.   Injury to blood vessels, bowel, bladder, ureter (tube that connects kidney to bladder) by way of puncture and/or burn
2.   Fistula formation, which is an opening between the bowel, bladder, or ureter and the vagina and/or skin, that requires a second operation to repair.
3.   Colostomy
4.   Embolism, which is the spreading of a gas or other fluid into other parts or organs of the body
5.   Hernia in the incision site
6.   Injury to the cervix, uterus, or tubes that might require additional surgery or might affect my ability to get pregnant or carry a pregnancy to full term (9 months)
7.   Necessity for an exploratory laparotomy, which is the making of a larger incision through which the necessary surgery can be performed
8.   Blood loss necessitating transfusion, which carries the risk of exposure to AIDS or the hepatitis virus

Likelihood of Success: The likelihood of success of the above procedure is: () Good () Fair () Poor

Prognosis: If I choose not to have the above procedure, my prognosis (future medical condition) is: _____

FIGURE 4.5. Informed consent and request for laparoscopy.

Alternative Forms of Treatment such as:
1. Do nothing and accept the consequences of my present condition
2. Performance of surgery through a larger incision in my abdomen
3. Drug therapy

These alternative treatments have been explained to me, and I have elected this surgical procedure as my method of treatment.

I understand and accept that during the procedure unexpected or unforeseen circumstances may make it necessary to do an extension of the original procedure or another procedure that is not named above. I request that Dr. _____ and associates or assistants of his/her choice to perform those procedures that they judge to be necessary.

BY SIGNING THIS FORM, I ACKNOWLEDGE THAT I HAVE READ OR HAD THIS FORM READ AND EXPLAINED TO ME AND THAT I FULLY UNDERSTAND ITS CONTENTS.

I HAVE BEEN GIVEN AMPLE OPPORTUNITY TO ASK QUESTIONS AND ANY QUESTIONS I HAVE ASKED HAVE BEEN ANSWERED OR EXPLAINED IN A SATISFACTORY MANNER.   ALL BLANKS OR STATEMENTS REQUIRING COMPLETION WERE FILLED IN AND ALL STATEMENTS WITH WHICH I DISAGREE WERE MARKED OUT BEFORE I SIGNED THIS FORM.

I accept that medicine is not an exact science and understand that no guarantees can be given as to the results. Understanding these limitations, I request that Dr. _____ and his/her associates/assistants to proceed with surgery.

Witness _____

Person giving consent _____

Relationship to patient if not the patient_____

Patient unable to sign because of:

Date: _____

_____

Additional materials used, if any, during the informed consent process for this procedure include:

_____

_____

_____

Date: _____   Witness: _____

FIGURE 4.5. *Continued*

INFORMED CONSENT
And
REQUEST FOR REPAIR OF RELAXATION OF PELVIC ORGANS
And/Or
CORRECTION OF URINARY INCONTINENCE

I, _____, request Dr._____
_____ and his/her associates/ assistants to perform upon
me: (Circle procedure to be performed)

      1.   Anterior and/or posterior repair, that is, "tack up" the bladder and/or rectum
      2.   Enterocele repair, a repair to a hernia at the top of the vagina
      3.   Surgical correction of urinary incontinence problem by the following procedure(s)
           _____

Diagnosis and Procedure: The following has been explained to me in general terms and I
understand that:
      My condition has been diagnosed as: _____

      The nature of the procedure is: _____

      The purpose of this procedure is to: _____

General Risks of Surgery: As a result of the performance of this procedure there may be
general risks involved such as: INFECTION, ALLERGIC REACTION, DISFIGURING SCAR,
SEVERE LOSS OF BLOOD, FUNCTION OF ANY LIMB OR ORGAN, PARALYSIS,
PARAPLEGIA or QUADRIPLEGIA, BRAIN DAMAGE, CARDIAC ARREST, or DEATH. In
addition to these general risks, there may be other possible risks involved in this procedure.
These risks and/or complications may include but are not limited to such complications as:

1.   Injury to bowel, bladder, ureter (the tube from the kidney to the bladder) and urethra
      (tube from bladder to outside of body)
2.   Fistula formation, an opening between the bowel, bladder, ureter and the vagina and/or
      skin, which would require a second operation to repair
3.   Colostomy
4.   Reoccurrence of my loss of control of urine
5.   No improvement in my control of urine
6.   Prolonged need of a catheter to drain my bladder
7.   Discomfort with intercourse

Likelihood of Success: The likelihood of success of the above procedure is: () Good () Fair
                           () Poor

FIGURE 4.6. Informed consent and request for repair of relaxation of pelvic organs and/or
correction of urinary incontinence.

Prognosis: If I choose not to have the above procedure, my prognosis (future medical condition) is: _____

Alternative Forms of Treatment such as:
a.   Exercise
b.   Use of artificial supports (pessary)
c.   Do nothing and accept my present condition and its potential risks

These alternative treatments have been explained to me, and I have elected this surgical procedure as my method of treatment.

I understand and accept that during the procedure unexpected or unforeseen circumstances may make it necessary to do an extension of the original procedure or another procedure that is not named above. I request that Dr. _____ and associates or assistants of his/her choice perform those procedures that they judge to be necessary.

BY SIGNING THIS FORM, I ACKNOWLEDGE THAT I HAVE READ OR HAD THIS FORM READ AND EXPLAINED TO ME AND THAT I FULLY UNDERSTAND ITS CONTENTS.

I HAVE BEEN GIVEN AMPLE OPPORTUNITY TO ASK QUESTIONS AND ANY QUESTIONS I HAVE ASKED HAVE BEEN ANSWERED OR EXPLAINED IN A SATISFACTORY MANNER.   ALL BLANKS OR STATEMENTS REQUIRING COMPLETION WERE FILLED IN AND ALL STATEMENTS WITH WHICH I DISAGREE WERE MARKED OUT BEFORE I SIGNED THIS FORM.

I accept that medicine is not an exact science and understand that no guarantees can be given as to the results. Understanding these limitations, I request that Dr. _____ and his/her associates/assistants to proceed with surgery.

_____   _____
Witness   Person giving consent

                                                       Relationship to patient if not the patient_____

                                                       Patient unable to sign because of:
Date: _____

                                                       _____

Additional materials used, if any, during the informed consent process for this procedure include:
_____
_____

Date: _____   Witness: _____

FIGURE 4.6. *Continued*

LITIGATION PROCESS

The Claim

Several occurrences can forewarn a physician that a legal action may be impending. These include a complication or poor outcome, a disgruntled patient or dissatisfied family member, a request for medical records, or direct contact by the plaintiff's attorney. Under no circumstances should the physician ever discuss a potential case with the plaintiff's attorney unless he or she has been so advised by their attorney or insurance carrier claim investigator. Some plaintiff attorneys have been known to

call a physician and ask for the physician's opinion about an alleged incident. The attorney may tape this conversation or later in a courtroom allege that on the date of such a contact the physician said something different from what the physician is now alleging occurred. This situation could possibly lead to the jury questioning a physician's credibility. Thus, it is best for the physician never to respond to a plaintiff's attorney except through his or her own defense team.

A lawsuit actually begins when a plaintiff's attorney files a formal Complaint or Declaration. This is a legal document that lists the allegations to support a claim of medical malpractice. Some states require that an affidavit from an expert witness supporting the contention of malpractice be filed with the Complaint or Declaration. Once the filing occurs, the court serves the defendant physician with a summons. The summons is attached to the complaint and may contain questions to be answered by the physician. Responses to the complaint must be filed within a specified period of time, usually within 20 to 30 days. The defendant physician must respond within that period of time or he or she can be found guilty by default. Thus, it is critical that the physician immediately contact his or her insurance carrier and/or attorney on receiving the summons. The physician should send the original summons by certified mail or hand deliver these documents to the insurance carrier. Keep a photocopy of the summons in a separate file. Most insurance carriers require that the physician notify them of any incidence that might result in a claim. Failure to do so could negate the physician's policy. It is prudent to know what the requirements of the insurance carrier are in this regard.

Once a suit has been filed, do not communicate with the patient, her family, or her attorney. When records are requested, be sure that a proper authorization from the patient has been received and then send a complete *copy* of the chart. Never change or alter a record once the suit has been filed, because there are many methods by which a plaintiff's attorney can prove that records have been tampered with or altered.

Prepare a thorough chronological account of all events surrounding the incident. Include any oral communications that the physician had with the patient or her family. Gather all records, radiographs, laboratory tests, and consultant's reports and maintain these documents along with the complaint in a *separate file*.

The physician's defense attorney will know all aspects of the law but may not be knowledgeable about the specific medical condition. Thus, it is imperative that the physician take an active role in educating the attorney in all medical aspects of the case, discussing not only the positive aspects of the therapy, but also any questionable areas. The defense attorney should thoroughly understand all medical aspects of the case and the physician's reasoning behind the particular treatment chosen. The physician should research literature for articles by authors who completely support the treatment rendered. The physician should help select expert witnesses who can support his or her views on the treatment that was rendered in the case.

During the discovery process, both parties submit questions called *interrogatories* that are to be answered under oath within a specific period of time. The defendant physician should help prepare answers to these interrogatories.

If a physician has only peripheral involvement in a case and receives a summons requesting records, it is prudent that he or she notify the insurance carrier as well as his or her attorney before any response is given. There are times when poorly worded answers result in the physician who has only a peripheral involvement being named in the actual suit. The physician should not take unnecessary chances, but rather exercise his or her legal right and have appropriate counsel before responding to any questions. The defendant physician should not discuss the suit with any other physicians unless so advised by his or her attorney or the insurance claims representative. Idle conversation in a surgical dressing room may be overheard by a physician who could become the plaintiff's expert. The only people with whom it is safe to discuss a case are the defense attorney and the insurance claims representative.

The Deposition

The deposition is a standard legal process that takes place as part of the discovery process. A deposition is taken under oath in front of a court reporter and is generally admissible during the trial phase of the lawsuit. The deposition is serious in that what a defendant physician states is cast in stone and if not properly articulated can end up as a millstone about the physician's neck. Thus, adequate preparation cannot be overemphasized. The physician should be familiar with all of the records—both office and hospital—including office and hospital protocols, rules, and regulations. The physician should insist on considerable preparation and education from the attorney about this important legal process before the deposition.

The deposition has many purposes, including to: (a) discover facts; (b) lock in testimony; (c) narrow and clarify issues; (d) discover additional witnesses; and (e) provide an opportunity for settlement if appropriate. The deposition is primarily taken so that each side can learn the opinions, theories, and strategies of the opposing experts and those involved in the case. The opposing attorneys can thus prepare their cases for trial with the knowledge gained.

The demeanor of the physician is important. He or she should be professional, honest, and confident. Boredom, frustration, and hostility should not be shown. Anger can disrupt a physician's ability to concentrate, and under those circumstances, the physician may divulge things that should not be discussed. The physician should neither attempt to teach nor lecture during a deposition, remembering that the plaintiff already has an expert who stated that the physician committed malpractice. Therefore, any attempt to educate the lawyer is a frivolous and potentially dangerous act. During the deposition phase, the defendant physician is not acting as his or her own expert and thus should confine answers to short factual statements with no elaboration unless requested by further questioning. Answers should be specific and simple. Do not bring into a deposition any personal notes or records that include the physician's predeposition preparation. Such records are discoverable by the plaintiff's attorney if they are in the room. However, the physician should have a complete set of records to refer to. *Never guess about an answer.* If the physician does not understand the question, then simply state, "I do not understand the question," or "I do not know," or "I cannot recall." Avoid complex questions. Make the attorney break the questions down into simple ones by stating, "I do not understand the question. Would you please rephrase it?" Avoid repetitive questions by noting, "I have already answered that." When a question is asked, listen attentively, think, and organize your thoughts before responding. Then respond slowly, clearly, and as concisely as possible.

Given a *hypothetical question*, the physician should be sure the facts are consistent with his or her case and reply only as it applies to the case. If the hypothetical situation is not applicable to the physician's case, the physician should qualify the response and so state that the given facts are not applicable to the case. Again, remember that you are defending yourself and not acting as your own expert witness.

If the defense attorney objects to a question or its phrasing, do not answer the question until instructed to do so by the defense attorney. The physician should listen carefully to the objection raised by the defense attorney so that he or she can appropriately word the response. The physician should know the various alternative methods of therapy that might have been employed. The physician should have reasons why he or she selected the chosen therapy and be prepared to explain them in the courtroom. The deposition, however, is not the time to divulge any literature research that took place.

Avoid the word *authoritative*. Legally, it implies that every single statement in a book or journal is absolute fact. Because medicine is an art rather than an exact science, experts may have different opinions on the same subject. The physician can admit that a book is scholarly or written by intelligent, respected people, but should never concede that every statement in the text is absolutely correct, which would make such a text authoritative by legal definition.

Do not engage in bantering or make comments that could be overheard by the plaintiff's attorney during a recess or off-the-record moment. If the plaintiff's attorney overhears things stated during the recess, he or she has the right to come back on record and bring up such topics.

Do not accept the plaintiff's attorney's statement regarding prior testimony as being factual unless you are sure that the statements accurately reflect the stated facts. If you are not sure, state, "I do not know," or "I do not have sufficient experience in that matter to be able to give an honest answer." When a deposition is over, the physician should politely excuse himself or herself, leave the room and wait for further instructions from the defense attorney. Prepare for a deposition as if it were a trial. Although the setting may be more casual and appear friendlier, your answers are given under oath and carry the same weight as if they were given before a jury in a courtroom.

After the deposition is completed, the physician is given an opportunity to read and correct his or her testimony. The physician has the right to correct the deposition, even change the meaning of an entire sentence, as long as this is accomplished during the specified time, usually 30 days. Because this is the only time the physician has the right to change his or her testimony, it is extremely important that the physician read and correct the deposition before it is used in legal proceedings.

The Trial

The trial is an adversarial experience during which allegations are made and facts are presented. In a courtroom, the plaintiff's attorney states his or her perception of the facts that are beneficial to the client. This perception may not always correlate with the defense's understanding of the facts. The jury, however, is instructed to judge a case by the facts, as they understand them and not by what an attorney alleges. Often sharp, even bitter controversy develops over the interpretation of significant facts. Legal maneuvering can distort or even suppress the presentation of some facts. This is an emotionally draining experience.

Preparation for the trial is critical and should cover even demeanor and dress. Dress should be plain, conservative, and neat. Flashy or casual clothes project the wrong image. The physician wants to present himself or herself to the jury as a kind, considerate, compassionate person who projects warmth and sincerity, as well as a voice of authority. The defendant physician should go to the court before the trial to become familiar with the surroundings. He or she may even want to sit in on a trial to get a feel for this new and foreign environment. The physician should discuss in great detail any questions that he or she has regarding the trial, its proceedings, or the defense. Listen to your attorney's advice! The more familiar a physician is with the court and its proceedings, the more confident and less frightened he or she will be as the trial proceeds.

There are several things a physician should do when called to the stand to testify. The physician should make and keep eye contact with the jury throughout the testimony. Physicians generally tend to focus their attention on the plaintiff's attorney as he or she asks questions; however, this is not helpful to the physician. Physicians are trained to read people's facial expressions. By maintaining eye contact with the jury, the physician can closely observe whether the jurors comprehend the testimony. If the physician feels that the jury does not understand an area of the testimony, he or she can elaborate further on a simpler level of explanation. Physicians must remember that the jury, not the plaintiff's attorney, reaches the verdict; therefore, it is critically important that the physician employ all of his or her talents to be sure that the jury understands the testimony. Be polite and humble. Important words in the courtroom are *Sir* and *Madam*. When a physician uses these words, they generate an air of humility that is pleasing to a jury. When a question is asked, be sure to take time to think before a response is given. Respond in nontechnical language that a 12-year-old child could understand. Listen carefully, and then speak clearly and audibly. Jurors like a physician who really tries to explain what he or she did step by step. Unlike during the deposition, in the courtroom the physician should be a teacher, using a blackboard or other audiovisual aids to explain complex issues. If the plaintiff's attorney tries to be overbearing and abrasive, react by being humble yet dignified. Repeat significant facts often so that the jury will remember them.

There are also several things a defendant physician *should not do* on the stand. Do not be arrogant, pompous, or overbearing. Never try to outsmart or manipulate the plaintiff's attorney; this is the way attorneys make their living. Never instigate a fight or argue with an attorney because it will cause you to lose dignity and respect in front of the jury. Never belittle the patient's injury or pain, but show compassion and understanding. Never guess at an answer. If you do not know, then state, "I do not know," or "I do not recall." The physician should not worry if he or she misspeaks. The defense attorney, with further appropriate questions, generally is able to correct the mistake. Never get angry or show anger because anger breaks your concentration and often leads you to say things that should not be said.

Answer the plaintiff's questions as simply and briefly as possible. Use a yes-or-no answer whenever possible. The defense attorney, on direct examination, can have the physician elaborate in detail those issues that are important to the defense. It is important that the physician stay in the courtroom during the entire trial. The physician can help the defense attorney during the cross-examination of expert witnesses and reveal where the experts are inconsistent with known and accepted facts. The physician's very presence and demeanor can greatly influence the jury's perception. This can play a major role in the final outcome.

The trial begins with opening statements. The plaintiff's attorney proceeds first because he or she has the burden to prove the existence of malpractice and causation of injury. Then the trial testimony phase begins. Again, the plaintiff's attorney begins with testimony and expert witnesses to try to establish that the defendant is negligent and the negligence caused the plaintiff's injury. During this initial presentation, the plaintiff's attorney has the right to (and frequently does) call the defendant physician to the stand. At this stage of the trial, the defendant's attorney cannot question or cross-examine the physician to clarify any response made by the physician, so it is extremely important that the physician take the time to understand the plaintiff's attorney's questions and then formulate and give a *complete response* so that the jury can understand the physician's position on the matter in question. Do not leave any questionable areas unexplained, because at this stage, the plaintiff's attorney is trying to establish points that are beneficial to their case. If the plaintiff's attorney asks a series of short questions that only require a yes-or-no answer and do not seem to give the physician time to explain his or her position completely, it is very important that the physician break such a sequence and take as much time as needed to clarify the answer. The physician can simply say to the plaintiff's attorney, "Sir or Madam, I did not finish my response to the last question."

During the testimony phase, the plaintiff's attorney usually employs one of four basic forms of attack on the defendant's reputation. The plaintiff may challenge the physician's competence; accuse the physician of being careless; allege that the physician is not compassionate but rather an indifferent, uncaring, wealthy person; and finally, attack the physician's credibility, especially if records were altered or if the physician contradicted testimony given under oath during the deposition. This is why it is so important for a physician to know exactly what he or she said in the deposition. The physician should outline the deposition, noting significant facts and any figures he or she might have used. Again, as in preparation for the deposition, the physician should have a thorough knowledge of the office and hospital records, including any rules, protocols, or policies that have any bearing on the case. Ignorance of any of these rules, protocols, policies, or records may provide all the evidence a plaintiff's attorney needs to raise a question of the physician's competence.

If at the end of the presentation, the plaintiff has not produced sufficient evidence to establish the cause-and-effect relationship, the defense may request and be granted a *directed verdict*, and the suit is over.

Next, through testimony, expert witnesses, and medical documents, the defense tries to prove that the allegation of negligence is false and that the injuries were not a direct result of the defendant's negligence. After the defense finishes its presentation, the plaintiff has the chance to rebut any new evidence brought out during this defense presentation.

Following this, each side presents closing arguments. During this phase each side summarizes the major facts supporting their position. The plaintiff's attorney begins with his or her initial closing arguments. After the defense gives its closing arguments, the plaintiff's attorney responds with their final closing arguments. In other words, the plaintiff's attorney has the last word before the jury. Once this is completed, the judge instructs the jurors on the applicable laws for the case. The jury is then given the case and retires to the jury room to begin deliberations. The formal decision or finding made by the jury or the judge is called the *verdict*.

Emotional Impact

The practice of medicine in general, and of obstetrics and gynecology in particular, is filled with daily stresses uncommon to other professions. Physicians must deal with pain and suffering, problem patients, intense interpersonal relationships, and often-unrealistic expectations. A relatively new, but unfortunately rather frequent, stress is the threat of malpractice litigation. The stress of a malpractice suit has been equated to the stress and emotional reaction one undergoes during the loss of a loved one. Unlike other professionals, a physician is unable to accept that a malpractice suit is part of the risk of doing business owing to the very nature of the doctor–patient relationship.

Part of the intense anger the physician experiences at the onset of a suit arises because of the shock that he or she experiences when a bond built on trust has been broken. The physician feels betrayed. The accusation of being incompetent or at least practicing one's job badly challenges the very core of one's professional integrity and stirs strong feelings of anger. This anger may be so intense that it spills out in all directions, frequently in an inappropriate manner that may strain many personal and professional relationships.

In a study of physicians who had been sued, conducted by psychiatrist Dr. Sarah Charles, 96% of physicians reported not only emotional reactions, but also physical problems related to the suit. Eight percent had the onset of physical ailments, of which one fourth were life-threatening, such as coronaries, strokes, ulcers, and hypertension. Forty percent showed symptoms suggestive of major depressive disorders. Commonly experienced reactions were anger, mood changes, depression, tension, frustration, insomnia, fatigue, and alcohol and drug abuse. Fifteen percent of physicians lost confidence in themselves. Nineteen percent lost confidence in certain clinical situations. Fear is another common emotion experienced by sued physicians. They fear the loss of their patient's respect and confidence. They fear the loss of their own self-confidence and, in this day of excess awards, they fear the loss of financial security. The physician's reputation, ego, and self-worth are challenged. Professional training demands that the physician hold his or her reactions in check. This training becomes counterproductive at the time of a malpractice suit.

The physician's marriage also is put under considerable stress. The spouse carries a great part of the emotional burden of litigation. There are many sleepless nights and interrupted plans as depositions and trials are scheduled, postponed, and rescheduled by a seemingly uncaring legal system. Mood changes and periods of irritability have to be handled by the spouse. These stressful situations can be the downfall of a weak or borderline marriage. Children are often disturbed by the knowledge that a parent is legally accused of malpractice. They may indeed feel that their parent has deceived or shamed them. Younger children especially may misunderstand the nature of the accusation and believe the allegation as fact, especially if broadcast on the radio, television, or in the newspaper. Physicians must take action to protect their mental health during this major period of stress, realizing that we live in a litigious environment and that the stress surrounding malpractice suits not only affects physicians, but also adversely impacts all professions and occupations. Physicians need to discuss their *feelings* with their spouse, loved ones, mentors, or counselor.

Physicians and their spouses should become active in support groups. These groups have received the support of the American College of Obstetricians and Gynecologists and American Academy of Pediatrics as outlined in their December 1998 issue, "Coping with Malpractice Litigations Stress." Such forums are not intended to provide psychiatric therapy, but rather are safe and informal groups where participants can share their common stresses and experiences in a sympathetic environment. The physician should not hesitate to seek counseling if the stress becomes so great that daily function becomes impaired.

An open discussion with your children that shares their feelings and concerns as well as yours, often relieves their anxiety. This type of communication often strengthens the family relationship and ultimately results in a positive effect from the terrifying ordeal of a malpractice suit.

BIBLIOGRAPHY

American College of Legal Medicine. *Legal medicine: legal dynamics of medical encounters.* St Louis: CV Mosby, 1988

American College of Obstetricians and Gynecologists. *Litigation assistant: a guide for the defendant physician,* 2nd ed. Washington, DC: American College of Obstetricians and Gynecologists, 1998.

American College of Obstetricians and Gynecologists, Department of Professional Liability. *Managed care liability. The assistant,* No. 1. Washington, DC: American College of Obstetricians and Gynecologists, 1997.

American College of Obstetricians and Gynecologists, Department of Professional Liability. *Informed consent. The assistant,* No. 4. Washington, DC: American College of Obstetricians and Gynecologists, 1998.

American College of Obstetricians and Gynecologists, Department of Professional Liability. *Informed consent forms. The assistant,* No. 5. Washington, DC: American College of Obstetricians and Gynecologists, 1998.

American College of Obstetricians and Gynecologists, Department of Professional Liability. *Record keeping. The assistant,* No. 6. Washington, DC: American College of Obstetricians and Gynecologists, 1998.

American College of Obstetricians and Gynecologists, Department of Professional Liability. *Risk management in the office setting. The assistant,* No. 9. Washington, DC: American College of Obstetricians and Gynecologists, 1999.

American College of Obstetricians and Gynecologists, Department of Professional Liability. *Risk Management in the hospital setting. The assistant,* No. 10. Washington, DC: American College of Obstetricians and Gynecologists, 1999.

American College of Obstetricians and Gynecologists. *Ethical dimensions of informed consent.* ACOG Committee Opinion 108. Washington, DC: American College of Obstetricians and Gynecologists, 1992.

American College of Obstetricians and Gynecologists. *Physicians Responsibility under managed care.* ACOG Committee Opinion 170. Washington, DC: American College of Obstetricians and Gynecologists, 1996.

American College of Obstetricians and Gynecologists. *Cost containment in medical care.* ACOG Committee Opinion 171. Washington, DC: American College of Obstetricians and Gynecologists, 1996.

American College of Obstetricians and Gynecologists. *Sterilization of women, including those with mental disabilities.* ACOG Committee Opinion 216. Washington, DC: American College of Obstetricians and Gynecologists 1999.

American College of Obstetricians and Gynecologists. *Coping with the stress of malpractice litigation.* ACOG Committee Opinion 236. Washington, DC: American College of Obstetricians and Gynecologists 2000.

American College of Obstetricians and Gynecologists. *Informed refusal.* American College of Obstetricians and Gynecologists Committee Opinion 237. Washington, DC: American College of Obstetricians and Gynecologists 2000.

American College of Obstetricians and Gynecologists. *Ethical decision-making in obstetrics and gynecology.* Technical Bulletin, No. 136, November 1989.

American College of Obstetricians and Gynecologists. *Stress in the practice of obstetrics and gynecology.* Technical Bulletin, No. 149, November 1990.

American College of Obstetricians and Gynecologists, Department of Professional Liability. *Coping with malpractice litigation stress.* Washington, DC: American College of Obstetricians and Gynecologists, 1998.

American College of Obstetricians and Gynecologists. *Professional liability and its effects: report of a 1999 survey of ACOG's membership.* Washington, DC: American College of Obstetricians and Gynecologists, 1999.

Beauchamp TL, Childress JA. *Principles of biomedical ethics,* 3rd ed. New York: Oxford University Press, 1989.

Belli MM Sr, Carlova J. *Belli for your malpractice defense.* Oradell, NJ: Medical Economics, 1986.

Burns CR. Malpractice suits in American medicine before the Civil War. *Bull Hist Med* 1969;43(1):42.

Charles SC. The physician and malpractice litigation. *J Med Pract Man* 1985;1(2):123.

Charles SC, Wilbert JR, Kennedy EC. Physician's self-reports of reactions to malpractice litigation. *Am J Psychiatry* 1984;141:4.

Charles SC. How to handle the stress of litigation. *Clin Plast Surg* 1999;26:69.

Chin S. Delay in gynecologic surgical treatment: a comparison of patients in managed care and fee-for-service plans. *Obstet Gynecol* 1999;93:922.

Crane M. Malpractice wars: our national survey confirms even the best doctors are targets. *Medical Economics, Obstet Gynecol* 1999;August 29.

Danner D. *Medical malpractice: a primer for physicians.* Rochester, NY: The Lawyers Co-operative Publishing Co, 1988.

Elkins TE, Brown D. Informed consent: commentary on the ACOG Ethics Committee statement. *Women's Health Issues* 1993;3(1):31.

Emanuel EJ, Goldman L. Protecting patient welfare in managed care: six safeguards. *J Health Politics, Policy Law* 1998;23(4):635.

Faden RR, Beauchamp TL. *A history and theory of informed consent.* New York: Oxford University Press, 1986.

Frisch PR, Charles SC, Gibbons RP, et al. Role of previous claims and specialty on the effectiveness of risk management education for office-based physicians. *West J Med* 1995;163:346.

Furrow BR, Greaney TL, Johnson SH, et al. *Health law cases, materials and problems.* St Paul: West Publishing Co, 1997.

Furrow BR, Greaney TL, Johnson SH, et al. *Health law,* 3rd ed. St Paul, MN: West Group, 2000.

Gunderson M. Eliminating conflicts of interest in managed care organizations through disclosure and consent. *J Law Med Ethics* 1997;25:192.

Kennedy I, Grubb A. *Medical law,* 3rd ed. London: Butterworth, 2000.

King JH. *The law of medical malpractice.* St Paul, MN: West Publishing Co, 1986.

Lavery JP. The physician's reaction to a malpractice suit. *Obstet Gynecol* 1988;71:138.

Martin CA, Wilson JF, Fiebelman ND, et al. Physicians' psychologic reactions to malpractice litigation. *South Med J* 1991;84:1300.

Nora PF, ed. *Professional liability risk management: a manual for surgeons.* Chicago: Professional Liability Committee, American College of Surgeons, 1991.

Powers MJ, Harris N. *Clinical negligence,* 3rd ed. London: Butterworth, 2000.

Ransom SB, ed. *Practical strategies in obstetrics and gynecology.* Philadelphia: WB Saunders, 2000.

Rozovsky FA. *Consent to treatment: a practical guide,* 2nd ed. Boston: Little, Brown, 1990.

Sandor AA. The history of professional liability suits in the United States. *JAMA* 1957;163:459.

Terry K. Managed care. *Obstet Gynecol* 2000;(May):17.

Walker LM. The income slide continues for ob-gyns. *Obstet Gynecol* 2000;(Oct):63.

Ward CJ. Analysis of 500 obstetric and gynecologic malpractice claims: causes and prevention. *Am J Obstet Gynecol* 1991;165:298.

PRINCIPLES OF ANATOMY AND PERIOPERATIVE CONSIDERATIONS

Te Linde's Operative Gynecology, ninth edition, edited by John A. Rock and Howard W. Jones, III. Lippincott Williams & Wilkins, Philadelphia, © 2003.

CHAPTER

5

▼

Surgical Anatomy of the Female Pelvis

JOHN O. L. DE LANCEY

VULVA AND ERECTILE STRUCTURES

The bony pelvic outlet is bordered by the ischiopubic rami anteriorly and the coccyx and sacrotuberous ligaments posteriorly. It can be divided into anterior and posterior triangles, which share a common base along a line between the ischial tuberosities. The tissues filling the anterior triangle have a layered structure similar to that of the abdominal wall (Table 5.1). There is a skin and adipose layer (vulva) overlying a fascial layer (perineal membrane) that lies superficial to a muscular layer (levator ani muscles).

Subcutaneous Tissues of the Vulva

The structures of the vulva lie on the pubic bones and extend caudally under its arch (Fig. 5.1). They consist of the mons, labia, clitoris, vestibule, and associated erectile structures and their muscles. The mons consists of hair-bearing skin over a cushion of adipose tissue that lies on the pubic bones. Extending posteriorly from the mons, the labia majora are composed of similar hair-bearing skin and adipose tissue, which contain the termination of the round ligaments of the uterus and the obliterated processus vaginalis (canal of Nuck). The round ligament can give rise to leiomyomas in this region, and the oblit-

erated processus vaginalis can be a dilated embryonic remnant in the adult.

The labia minora, vestibule, and glans clitoris can be seen between the two labia majora. The labia minora are hairless skin folds, each of which splits anteriorly to run over, and under, the glans of the clitoris. The more anterior folds unite to form the hood-shaped prepuce of the clitoris, whereas the posterior folds insert into the underside of the glans as the frenulum.

Unlike the skin of the labia majora, the cutaneous structures of the labia minora and vestibule do not lie on an adipose layer but on a connective-tissue stratum that is loosely organized and permits mobility of the skin during intercourse. This loose attachment of the skin to underlying tissues allows the skin to be easily dissected off the underlying fascia during skinning vulvectomy in the area of the labia minora and vestibule.

In the posterior lateral aspect of the vestibule, the duct of the major vestibular gland can be seen 3 to 4 mm outside the hymenal ring. The minor vestibular gland openings are found along a line extending anteriorly from this point, parallel to the hymenal ring and extending toward the urethral orifice. The urethra bulges slightly around the surrounding vestibular skin anterior to the vagina and posterior to the clitoris. Its orifice is flanked on either side by two small labia. Skene ducts open into the inner aspect of these labia and can be seen

---

TABLE 5.1.
Layers of the Anterior Triangle of the Perineum

Skin
Subcutaneous tissue
   Camper's fascia
   Colles fascia
Superficial space
   Clitoris and its crura
   Ischiocavernous muscle
   Vestibular bulb
   Bulbocavernous muscle
   Greater vestibular gland
   Superficial transverse perineal muscle
Deep space-perineal membrane
   Compressor urethrae
   Urethrovaginal sphincter

---

as small, punctate openings when the urethral labia are separated.

Within the skin of the vulva are specialized glands that can become enlarged and thereby require surgical removal. The holocrine sebaceous glands in the labia majora are associated with hair shafts, and in the labia minora they are freestanding. They lie close to the surface, which explains their easy recognition with minimal enlargement. In addition, lateral to the introitus and anus,

there are numerous apocrine sweat glands, along with the normal eccrine sweat glands. The former structures undergo change with the menstrual cycle, having increased secretory activity in the premenstrual period. They can become chronically infected, as in hidradenitis suppurativa, or neoplastically enlarged, as in hidradenomas, both of which may require surgical therapy. The eccrine sweat glands present in the vulvar skin rarely present abnormalities, but on occasion they can form palpable masses as syringomas.

The subcutaneous tissue of the labia majora is similar in composition to that of the abdominal wall. It consists of lobules of fat interlaced with connective tissue septa. Although there are no well-defined layers in the subcutaneous tissue, regional variations in the relative quantity of fat and fibrous tissue exist. The superficial region of this tissue, where fat predominates, has been called Camper's fascia, because it is on the abdomen. In this region there is a continuation of fat from the anterior abdominal wall, called the digital process of fat.

In the deeper layers of the vulva there is less fat, and the interlacing fibrous connective tissue septa are much more evident than those in Camper's fascia. This more fibrous layer is called Colles fascia and is similar to Scarpa's fascia on the abdomen. Its interlacing fibrous septa of the subcutaneous tissue attach laterally to the ischiopubic rami and fuse posteriorly with the posterior edge of the perineal membrane (i.e., urogenital diaphragm). Anteriorly, however, there is no con-

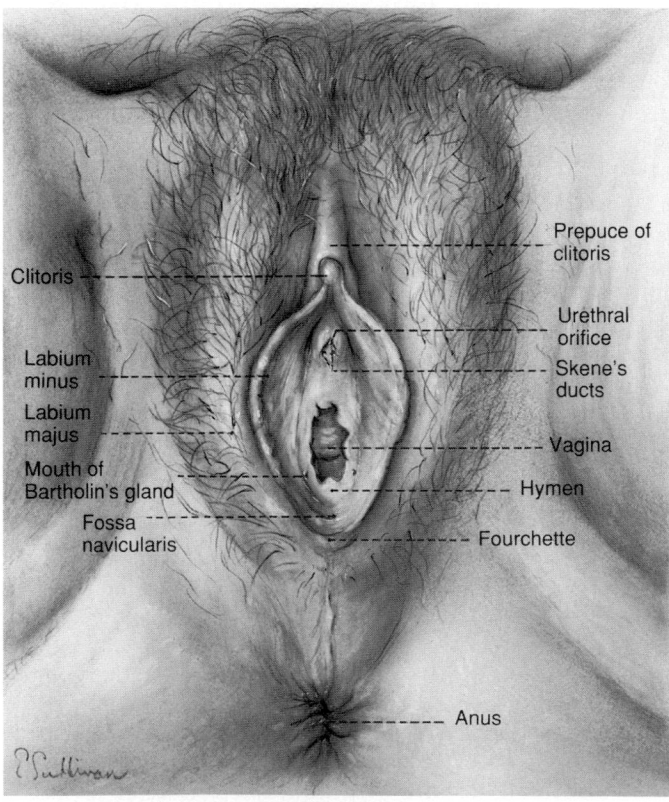

FIGURE 5.1. External genitalia.

nection to the pubic rami, and this permits communication between the area deep to this layer and the abdominal wall. These fibrous attachments to the ischiopubic rami and the posterior aspect of the perineal membrane limit the spread of hematomas or infection in this compartment posterolaterally but allow spread into the abdomen. This clinical observation has led to the consideration of Colles fascia as a separate entity from the superficial Camper fascia, which lacks these connections.

Superficial Compartment

The space between the subcutaneous tissues and perineal membrane, which contains the clitoris, crura, vestibular bulbs, and ischiocavernous and bulbocavernous muscles, is called the superficial compartment of the perineum (Fig. 5.2). The deep compartment is the region just above the perineal membrane; it is discussed later.

The erectile bodies and their associated muscles within the superficial compartment lie on the caudal surface of the perineal membrane. The clitoris is composed of a midline shaft (body) capped with the glans. This shaft lies on, and is suspended from, the pubic bones by a subcutaneous suspensory ligament. The paired crura of the clitoris bend downward from the shaft and are firmly attached to the pubic bones, continuing dorsally to lie on the inferior aspects of the pubic rami. The ischiocavernous muscles originate at the ischial tuberosities and the free surfaces of the crura, to insert on the upper crura and body of the clitoris. A few muscle fibers, called the superficial transverse perineal muscles, originate in common with the ischiocavernous muscle from the ischial tuberosity and lie medial to the perineal body.

The paired vestibular bulbs lie immediately under the vestibular skin and are composed of erectile tissue. They are covered by the bulbocavernous muscles, which originate in the perineal body and lie over their lateral surfaces. These muscles, along with the ischiocavernous muscles, insert into the body of the clitoris and act to pull it downward.

The Bartholin greater vestibular gland is found at the tail end of the bulb of the vestibule and is connected to the vestibular mucosa by a duct lined with squamous epithelium. The gland lies on the perineal membrane and beneath the bulbocavernous muscle. The intimate relation between the enormously vascular erectile tissue of the vestibular bulb and the Bartholin gland is responsible for the hemorrhage associated with removal of this latter structure.

The perineal membrane and perineal body are important to the support of the pelvic organs. They are discussed in the section on the pelvic floor.

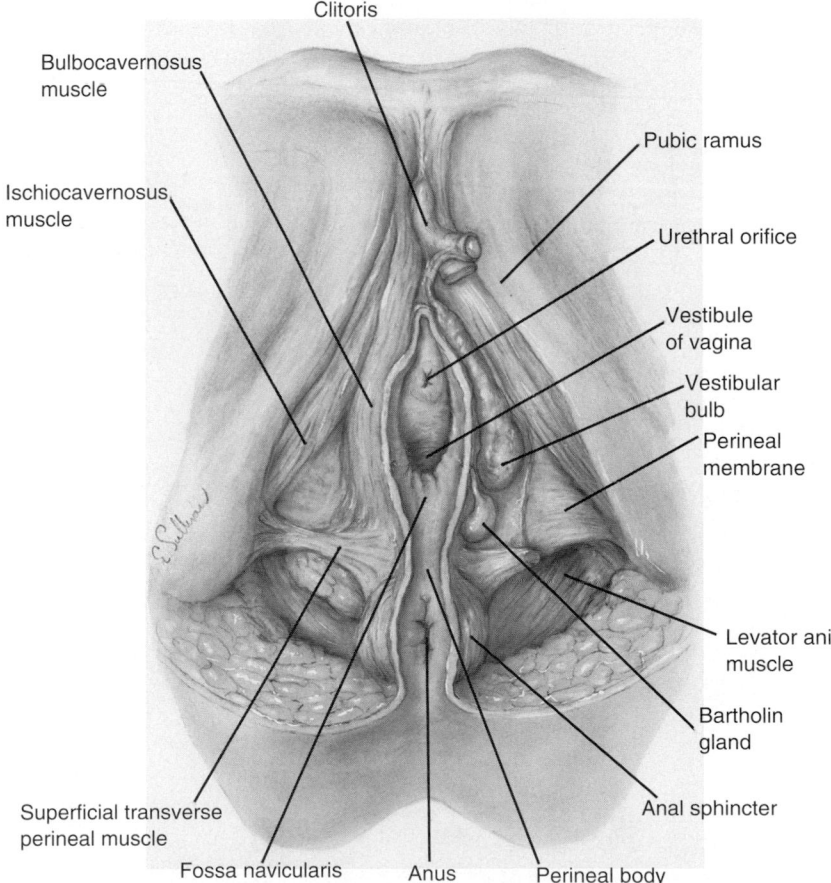

FIGURE 5.2. Superficial compartment and perineal membrane.

Clitoris
Bulbocavernosus muscle
Ischiocavernosus muscle
Pubic ramus
Urethral orifice
Vestibule of vagina
Vestibular bulb
Perineal membrane
Levator ani muscle
Bartholin gland
Anal sphincter
Superficial transverse perineal muscle
Fossa navicularis
Anus
Perineal body

Pudendal Nerve and Vessels

The pudendal nerve is the sensory and motor nerve of the perineum. Its course and distribution in the perineum parallel the pudendal artery and veins that connect with the internal iliac vessels (Fig. 5.3). The course and division of the nerve are described with the understanding that the vascular channels parallel them.

The pudendal nerve arises from the sacral plexus (52–54), and the vessels originate from the anterior division of the internal iliac artery. They leave the pelvis through the greater sciatic foramen by hooking around the ischial spine and sacrospinous ligament to enter the pudendal (Alcock) canal through the lesser sciatic foramen.

The nerve and vessels have three branches: the clitoral, perineal, and inferior hemorrhoidal. The clitoral branch lies on the perineal membrane along its path to supply the clitoris. The perineal branch (the largest of the three branches) enters the subcutaneous tissues of the vulva behind the perineal membrane. Here it supplies the bulbocavernous, ischiocavernous, and transverse perineal muscles. It also supplies the skin of the inner portions of the labia majora, labia minora, and vestibule. The inferior hemorrhoidal branch goes to the external anal sphincter and perianal skin.

Lymphatic Drainage

The pattern of the vulvar lymphatic vessels and drainage into the superficial inguinal group of lymph nodes has been established by both injection studies and clinical observation. It is important to the treatment of vulvar malignancies; an overview of this system is provided here. This area is described and illustrated in more detail in Chapter 33.

Tissues external to the hymenal ring are supplied by an anastomotic series of vessels in the superficial tissues that coalesce to a few trunks lateral to the clitoris and proceed laterally to the superficial inguinal nodes (Fig. 5.4). The vessels draining the labia majora also run in an anterior direction, lateral to those of the labia minora and vestibule. These lymphatic channels lie medial to the labiocrural fold, establishing it as the lateral border of surgical resection.

Injection studies of the urethral lymphatics have shown that lymphatic drainage of this region terminates in either the right or left inguinal nodes. The clitoris has been said to have some direct drainage to deep pelvic lymph nodes, bypassing the usual superficial nodes, but the clinical significance of this appears to be minimal.

The inguinal lymph nodes are divided into two groups—the superficial and the deep nodes. There are 12 to 20 superficial nodes, and they lie in a T-shaped distribution parallel to and 1 cm below the inguinal ligament, with the stem extending down along the saphenous vein. The nodes are often divided into four quadrants with the center of the division at the saphenous opening. The vulvar drainage goes primarily to the medial nodes of the upper quadrant. These nodes lie deep in the adipose layer of the subcutaneous tissues, in the membranous layer, just superficial to the fascia lata.

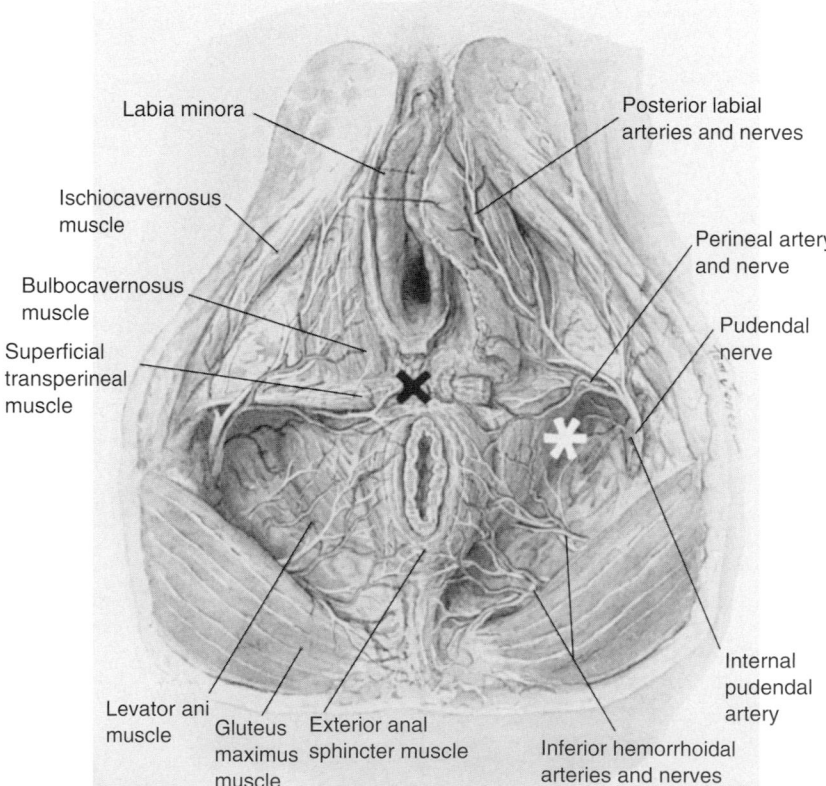

FIGURE 5.3. Pudendal nerve and vessels, with the position of the ischiorectal fossa *(asterisk)* and the perineal body *(cross)* indicated. (From: Anson BJ. *An atlas of human anatomy.* Philadelphia: WB Saunders, 1950, with permission.)

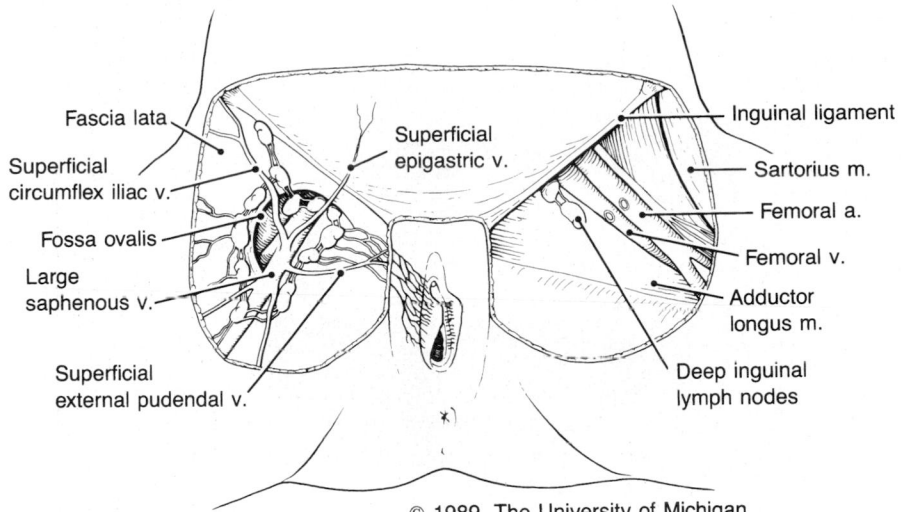

FIGURE 5.4. Lymphatic drainage of the vulva and femoral triangle. Superficial inguinal nodes are shown in the right thigh, and deep inguinal nodes are shown in the left thigh. Fascia lata has been removed on the left.

© 1989, The University of Michigan

The large saphenous vein joins the femoral vein through the saphenous opening. Within 2 cm of the inguinal ligament, several superficial blood vessels branch from the saphenous vein and femoral artery. They include the superficial epigastric vessels that supply the subcutaneous tissues of the lower abdomen; the superficial circumflex iliac vessels that course laterally to the region of the iliac crest; and the superficial external pudendal vessels that supply the mons, labia majora, and clitoral hood.

Lymphatics from the superficial nodes enter the fossa ovalis and drain into one to three deep inguinal nodes, which lie in the femoral canal of the femoral triangle. They pass through the fossa ovalis (saphenous opening) in the fascia lata that lies approximately 3 cm below the inguinal ligament, lateral to the pubic tubercle, along with the saphenous vein on its way to the femoral vein. The membranous layer of the subcutaneous tissues spans this opening as a trabeculate layer called a fascia cribrosa, pierced by lymphatics. The deep nodes are found under this fascia in the femoral triangle.

The femoral triangle is the subfascial space of the upper one third of the thigh. It is bounded by the inguinal ligament, sartorius muscle, and adductor longus muscle. Its floor is formed by the pectineal, adductor longus, and iliopsoas muscles. The femoral artery bisects it vertically between the anterosuperior iliac spine and pubic tubercle. The femoral vein lies medial to the artery; the femoral nerve is lateral to it.

As these vessels pass under the inguinal ligament, they carry with them an extension of the transversalis fascia, which is the extraperitoneal connective tissue deep to the rectus abdominis muscle called the femoral sheath. These sheaths extend about 2 to 3 cm below the inguinal ligament before fusing with the vascular adventitia. Besides the two parts of the femoral sheath that accompany these vessels, a third portion—the femoral canal—can be found in the space medial to the vein. The abdominal opening of this is the femoral ring. The femoral canal contains the deep inguinal lymph nodes. Lymph channels from these nodes pierce the membrane filling the femoral ring to communicate with the external iliac

nodes. Also within this region, the femoral vessels give rise to the deep external pudendal vessels. The external pudendal vessels run deep to the femoral vein over the pectineal muscle to pierce the fascia lata. Here they become subcutaneous and form anastomoses with branches of the internal pudendal vessels as well as the deep femoral and lateral circumflex femoral arteries.

THE PELVIC FLOOR

When humans assumed the upright posture, the opening in the bony pelvis came to lie at the bottom of the abdominopelvic cavity. This required the evolution of a supportive system to prevent the pelvic organs from being pushed downward through this opening. In the female, this system must withstand these downward forces but allow for the passage of the large and cranially dominant human fetus. The supportive system that has evolved to meet these needs consists of a fibromuscular floor that forms a shelf spanning the pelvic outlet and that contains a cleft for the birth canal and excretory drainage. A series of visceral ligaments and fasciae tethers the organs and maintains their position over the closed portions of the floor. The floor consists of the levator ani muscles and perineal membrane. The openings in these structures for parturition and elimination have required the development of ancillary fibrous elements that are concentrated over open areas in the muscular floor to support the viscera in these weak areas. This section discusses the structures of the pelvic floor; the fibrous supportive system is described in the section on the pelvic viscera and cleavage planes and fascia.

Perineal Membrane (Urogenital Diaphragm)

The perineal membrane forms the inferior portion of the anterior pelvic floor. It is a triangular sheet of dense, fibromuscular tissue that spans the anterior half of the pelvic outlet (see Fig. 5.2). It was previously called the

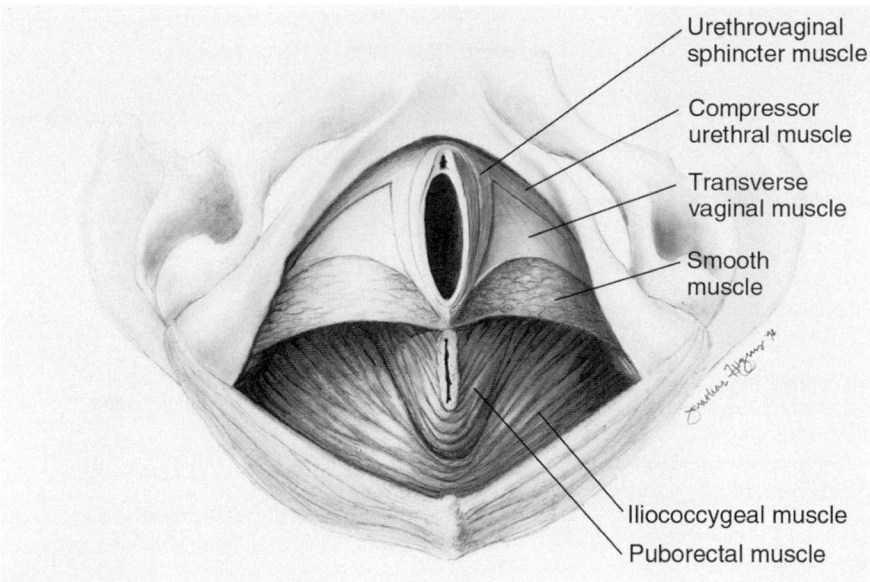

FIGURE 5.5. Structures visible after removal of the perineal membrane and superficial perineal muscles. (From: DeLancey, copyright 1995, with permission.)

urogenital diaphragm, and this change in name reflects the appreciation that it is not a two-layered structure with muscle in between, as was previously thought. It lies just caudal to the skeletal muscle of the striated urogenital sphincter (formerly the deep transverse perineal muscle). Because of the presence of the vagina, the perineal membrane cannot form a continuous sheet to close off the anterior pelvis in the female, as it does in the male. It does provide support for the posterior vaginal wall by attaching the perineal body and vagina and perineal body to the ischiopubic rami, thereby limiting their downward descent. This layer of the floor arises from the inner aspect of the inferior ischiopubic rami above the ischiocavernous muscles and the crura of the clitoris. The medial attachments of the perineal membrane are to the urethra, walls of the vagina, and perineal body.

Just cephalad to the perineal membrane lie two arch-shaped muscles that begin posteriorly to arch over the urethra (Fig. 5.5). These are the compressor urethrae and the urethrovaginal sphincter. They are a part of the striated urogenital sphincter muscle in the female and are continuous with the sphincter urethrae muscle. They act to compress the distal urethra. Posteriorly, intermingled within the membrane are skeletal muscle fibers of the transverse vaginal muscle and some smooth muscle fibers. The dorsal and deep nerve and vessels of the clitoris are also found within this membrane and are described later.

The primary function of the perineal membrane is related to its attachment to the vagina and perineal body. By attaching these structures to the bony pelvic outlet, the perineal membrane supports the pelvic floor against the effects of increases in intraabdominal pressure, and against the effects of gravity. The amount of downward descent that is permitted by this mechanism can be assessed by placing a finger in the rectum, hooking it forward, and pulling the perineal body downward. If the perineal membrane has been torn during parturition, then an abnormal amount of descent is detectable, and the pelvic floor sags and the introitus gapes.

Perineal Body

Within the area bounded by the lower vagina, perineal skin, and anus is a mass of connective tissue called the perineal body (see Fig. 5.3). The term *central tendon of the perineum* has also been applied to this structure and is descriptive, suggesting its role as a central point into which many muscles insert.

The perineal body is attached to the inferior pubic rami and ischial tuberosities through the perineal membrane and superficial transverse perineal muscles. Anterolaterally, it receives the insertion of the bulbocavernous muscles. On its lateral margins, the upper portions of the perineal body are connected with some fibers of the pelvic diaphragm. Posteriorly, the perineal body is indirectly attached to the coccyx by the external anal sphincter that is embedded in the perineal body, and it is attached at its other end to the coccyx. These connections anchor the perineal body and its surrounding structures to the bony pelvis and help to keep it in place.

Posterior Triangle: Ischiorectal Fossa

In the posterior triangle of the pelvis, the ischiorectal fossa lies between the pelvic walls and the levator ani muscles (see Fig. 5.3). It has an anterior recess that lies above the perineal membrane. It is bounded medially by the levator ani muscles and anterolaterally by the obturator internus muscle. The main portion of the fossa is lateral to the levator ani and external anal sphincter, and it has a posterior portion that extends above the gluteus maximus. Traversing this region is the pudendal neurovascular trunk.

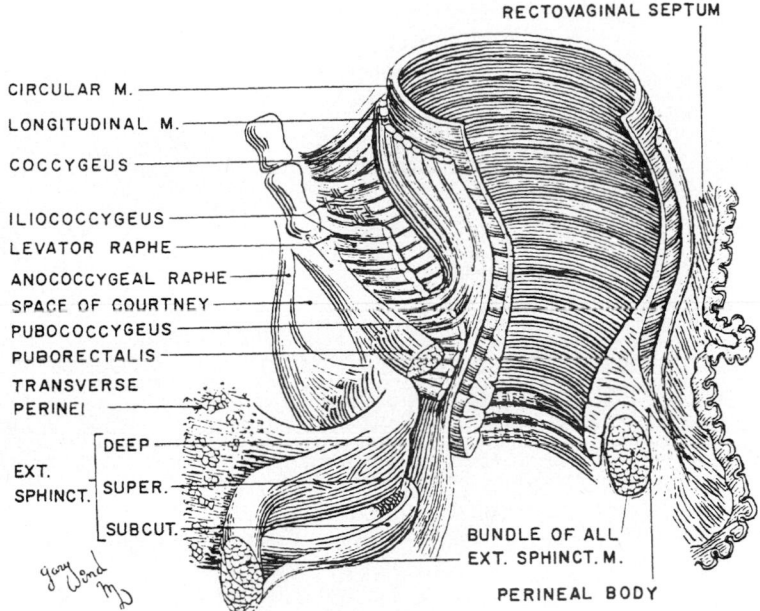

FIGURE 5.6. Semidiagrammatic dissection of the anorectal region in the female with the external sphincter cut in the anterior midsagittal plane and reflected posteriorly (mucosa removed). The origin of the anterior muscle-bundle is clarified and the remaining anterolateral portions of the external sphincters are interdigitated into the transverse perinei. (From: Oh C, Kark AE. Anatomy of the external anal sphincter. *Br J Surg* 1972;59:717–772, with permission.)

Anal Sphincters

The external sphincter lies in the posterior triangle of the perineum (see Fig. 5.6). It is a single mass of muscle, which has traditionally been divided into superficial and deep portions. The subcutaneous portion lies attached to the perianal skin and forms an encircling ring around the anal canal. It is responsible for the characteristic radially oriented folds in the perianal skin. The superficial part attaches to the coccyx posteriorly and sends a few fibers into the perineal body anteriorly and forms the bulk of the anal sphincter seen separated in third-degree midline obstetric tears. The fibers of the deep part generally encircle the rectum and blend indistinguishably with the puborectalis, which forms a loop under the dorsal surface of the anorectum and which is attached anteriorly to the pubic bone (see Fig. 5.6).

The internal anal sphincter is a thickening in the circular smooth muscle of the anal wall. It lies just inside the external anal sphincter and is separated from it by a visible intersphincteric groove. It extends downward inside the external anal sphincter to within a few millimeters of the external sphincter's caudal extent. The internal sphincter can be identified just beneath the anal submucosa in repair of a chronic fourth-degree laceration of the perineum as a rubber white layer that is often erroneously been referred to as fascia. The longitudinal smooth muscle layer of the bowel, along with some fibers of the levator ani, separates the external and internal sphincters as they descend in the intersphincteric groove.

Levator Ani and Pelvic Wall

Unfortunately, the extreme abdominal pressures generated during embalming greatly distort the levator ani muscles by forcing them downward. Most anatomy at-

lases therefore fail to give a true picture of the horizontal nature of this strong supportive shelf of muscle. Examination of the normal standing patient is the best way to appreciate the nature of this closure mechanism, because the lithotomy position causes some relaxation of the musculature. During routine pelvic examination of the nullipara, the effectiveness of this closure can be appreciated, because it is often difficult to insert a speculum if the muscles are contracted and not relaxed.

The opening between the bones and muscles of the pelvic wall is spanned by the muscles of the pelvic diaphragm: the pubococcygeal, iliococcygeal, puborectal, and coccygeal muscles (Fig. 5.7). The most medial of these muscles is the puborectal–pubococcygeal complex. The pubococcygeal portion of these muscles has an insertion into the anococcygeal raphe and the superior surface of the coccyx, whereas the puborectal portion represents those inferior fibers that pass behind and insert into the rectum. Both portions arise from the inner surface of the pubic bones and pass the urethra without attaching to it. Some fibers attach to the lateral vaginal wall and external anal sphincter and form a sling around the rectum before returning to a similar course on the other side. The pubococcygeal portion passes posteriorly from its origin ventral to the iliococcygeal muscle, where its fibers insert between the internal and external anal sphincter muscles in the intersphincteric groove, and form a sling behind the rectum. A few fibers also run on the cephalic surface of the iliococcygeal muscle to reach the inner surface of the sacrum and the coccyx.

The iliococcygeal muscle arises from a fibrous band overlying the obturator internus called the arcus tendineus levatoris ani. From these broad origins, the fibers of the iliococcygeal muscle pass behind the rectum and insert into the midline anococcygeal raphe and the coccyx. The coccygeal muscle arises from the ischial

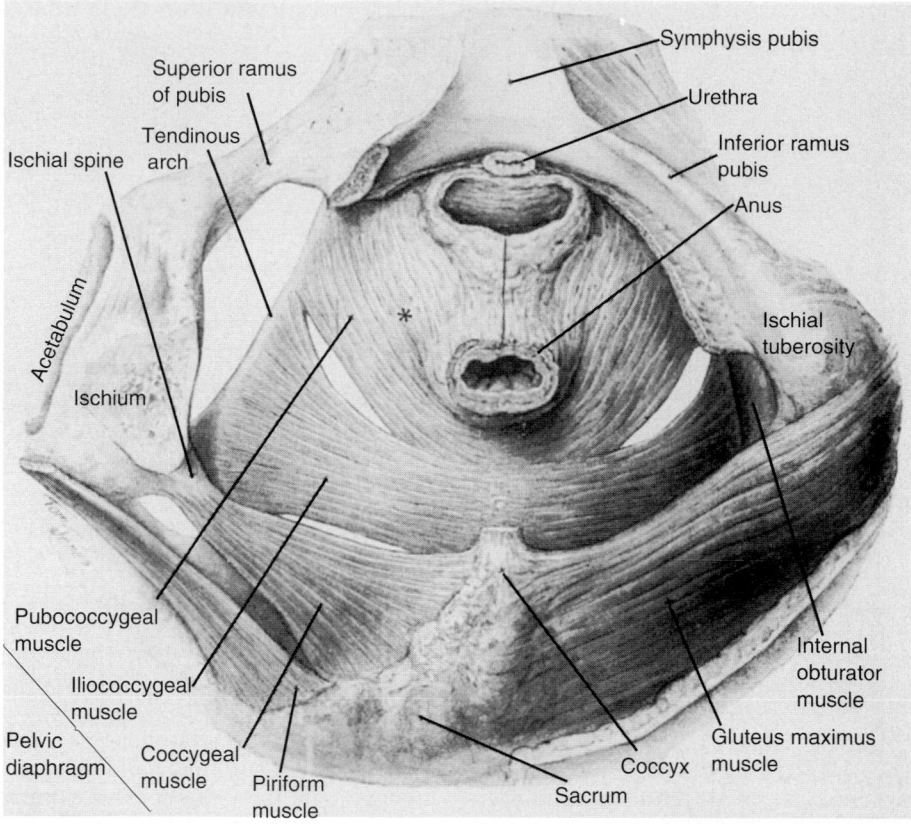

FIGURE 5.7. Anatomy of the pelvic floor. The asterisk indicates the puborectalis portion of the pubococcygeal muscle. (From: Anson BJ. *An atlas of human anatomy.* Philadelphia: WB Saunders, 1950, with permission.)

spine and sacrospinous ligament to insert into the borders of the coccyx and the lowest segment of the sacrum.

These muscles are covered on their superior and inferior surfaces by superior and inferior fasciae. When the levator ani muscles and their fasciae are considered together, they are called the pelvic diaphragm, not to be confused with the urogenital diaphragm (perineal membrane).

The muscle fibers of the pelvic diaphragm form a broad U-shaped layer of muscle with the open end of the U directed anteriorly. The open area within the U through which the urethra, vagina, and rectum pass, is called the urogenital hiatus. The normal tone of the muscles of the pelvic diaphragm keep the base of the U pressed against the backs of the pubic bones, keeping the vagina and rectum closed. The region of the levator ani between the anus and coccyx formed by the anococcygeal raphe (see previous discussion) is clinically called the levator plate. It forms a supportive shelf on which the rectum, upper vagina, and uterus can rest. The relatively horizontal position of this shelf is determined by the anterior traction on the fibrous levator plane by the pubococcygeal and puborectal muscles and is important to vaginal and uterine support.

The iliococcygeal and coccygeal muscles receive their innervation from an anterior branch of the ventral ramus of the third and fourth sacral nerves, whereas the medial portions of the puborectal and pubococcygeal muscles are probably supplied by the pudendal nerve.

THE PELVIC VISCERA

This section on the pelvic viscera discusses the structure of the individual pelvic organs and considers specific aspects of their interrelations (Fig. 5.8). Those aspects of blood supply, innervation, and lymphatic drainage that are idiosyncratic to the specific pelvic viscera are covered here. However, the section on the retroperitoneum, where the overall description of these systems is given, provides the general consideration of these latter three topics.

Genital Structures

Vagina

The vagina is a pliable hollow viscus whose shape is determined by the structures that surround it and by its attachments to the pelvic wall. These attachments are to the lateral margins of the vagina, so that its lumen is a transverse slit, with the anterior and posterior walls in contact with one another. The lower portion of the vagina is constricted as it passes through the urogenital hiatus in the levator ani. The upper part is much more

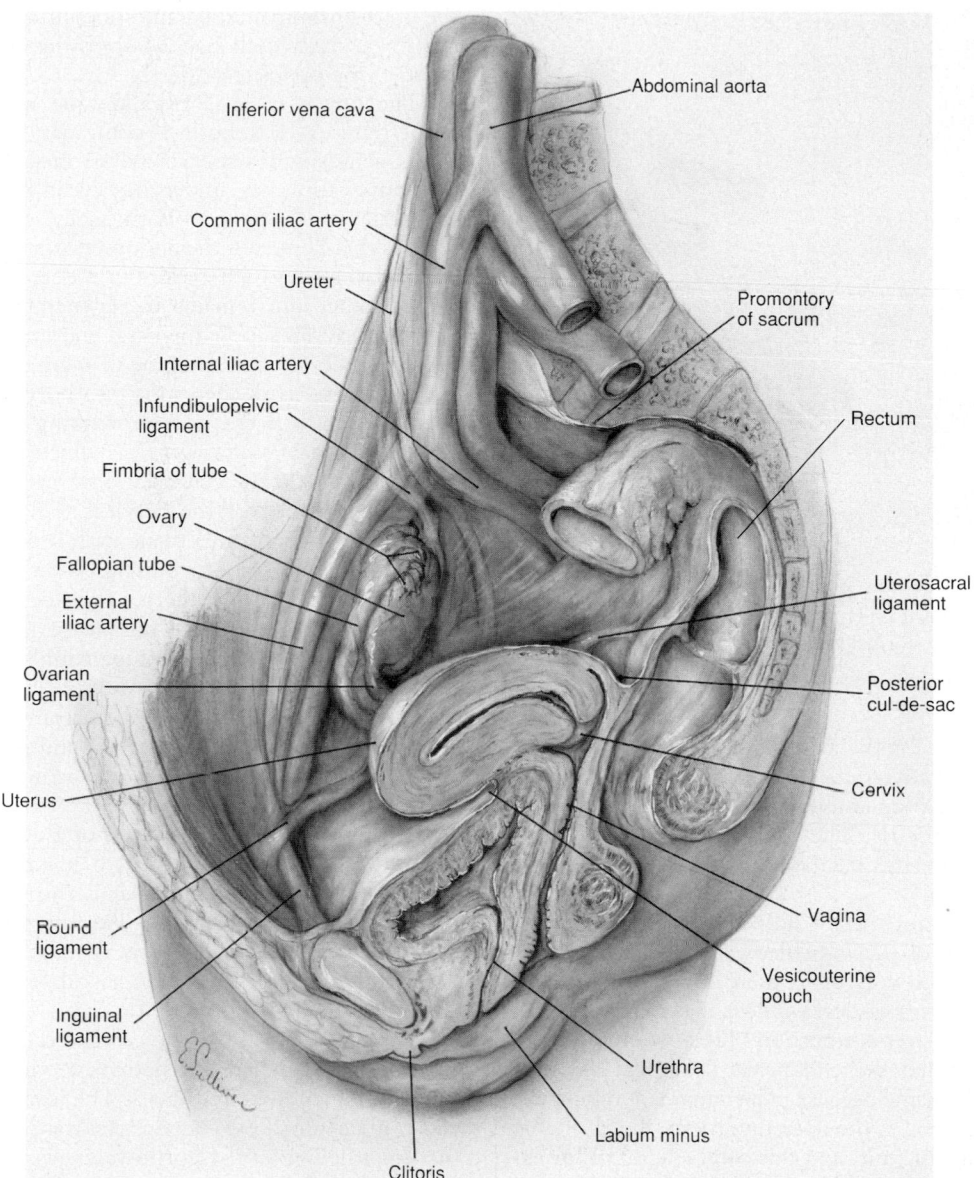

FIGURE 5.8. The pelvic viscera.

capacious. The vagina is bent at an angle of 120 degrees by the anterior traction of the levator ani muscles at the junction of the lower one third and upper two thirds of the vagina (Fig. 5.9). The cervix lies within the anterior vaginal wall, making it shorter than the posterior wall by about 3 cm. The former is about 7 to 9 cm in length, although there is great variability in this dimension.

When the lumen of the vagina is inspected through the introitus, many landmarks can be seen. The anterior and posterior walls have a midline ridge, called the anterior and posterior columns, respectively. These are caused by the impression of the urethra and bladder and the rectum on the vaginal lumen. The caudal portion of the anterior column is distinct and is called the urethral carina. The recesses in front of and behind the cervix are commonly called the anterior and posterior fornices of

the vagina, and the creases along the side of the vagina, where the anterior and posterior walls meet, are called the lateral vaginal sulci.

The vagina's relations to other parts of the body can be understood by dividing it into thirds. In the lower third, the vagina is fused anteriorly with the urethra, posteriorly with the perineal body, and laterally to each levator ani by the "fibers of Luschka." In the middle third are the vesical neck and trigone anteriorly, the rectum posteriorly, and the levators laterally. In the upper third, the anterior vagina is adjacent to the bladder and ureters (which allow these latter structures to be palpated on pelvic examination), posterior to the cul-de-sac, and lateral to the cardinal ligaments of the vagina.

The vaginal wall contains the same layers as all hollow viscera (i.e., mucosa, submucosa, muscularis, and ad-

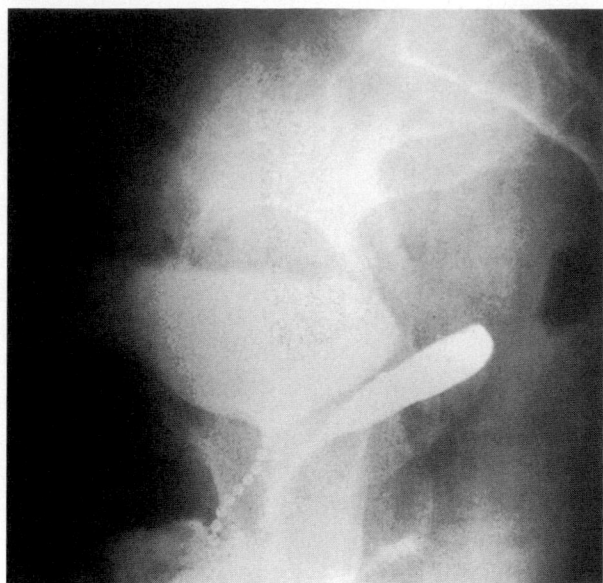

FIGURE 5.9. Bead chain cystourethrogram with barium in the vagina showing normal vaginal axis in a patient in the standing position.

ventitia). Except for the area covered by the cul-de-sac, it has no serosal covering. The mucosa is of the nonkeratinized stratified squamous type and lies on a dense, dermislike submucosa. The similarity of these layers to dermis and epidermis has resulted in their being called the "vaginal skin."

The vaginal muscularis is adherent to the submucosa, and the pattern of the muscularis is a bihelical arrangement. Outside the muscularis there is an adventitia that has varying degrees of development in different areas of the vagina. This layer is a portion of the connective tissue in the pelvis called the endopelvic fascia and has been given a separate name because of its unusual development. When it is dissected in the operating room, the muscularis is usually adherent to it, and this combination of specialized adventitia and muscularis is the surgeon's "fascia," which might better be called the fibromuscular layer of the vagina, as Nichols suggested in *Vaginal Surgery*.

Uterus

The uterus is a fibromuscular organ whose shape, weight, and dimensions vary considerably, depending on both estrogenic stimulation and previous parturition. It has two portions, an upper muscular corpus and a lower fibrous cervix. In a woman of reproductive age, the corpus is considerably larger than the cervix, but before menarche, and after the menopause, their sizes are similar. Within the corpus, there is a triangularly shaped endometrial cavity surrounded by a thick muscular wall. That portion of the corpus that extends above the top of the endometrial cavity (i.e., above the insertions of the fallopian tubes) is called the fundus.

The muscle fibers that make up most of the uterine corpus are not arranged in a simple layered manner, as is true in the gastrointestinal tract, but are arranged in a more complex pattern. This pattern reflects the origin of the uterus from paired paramesonephric primordia, with the fibers from each half crisscrossing diagonally with those of the opposite side.

The uterus is lined by a unique mucosa, the endometrium. It has both a columnar epithelium that forms glands and a specialized stroma. The superficial portion of this layer undergoes cyclic change with the menstrual cycle. Spasm of hormonally sensitive spiral arterioles that lie within the endometrium causes shedding of this layer after each cycle, but a deeper basal layer of the endometrium remains to regenerate a new lining. Separate arteries supply the basal endometrium, explaining its preservation at the time of menses.

The cervix is divided into two portions: the portio vaginalis, which is that part protruding into the vagina; and the portio supravaginalis, which lies above the vagina and below the corpus.

The substance of the cervical wall is made up of dense fibrous connective tissue with only a small (about 10%) amount of smooth muscle. What smooth muscle there is lies on the periphery of the cervix, connecting the myometrium with the muscle of the vaginal wall. This smooth muscle and accompanying fibrous tissue are easily dissected off the fibrous cervix and form the layer reflected during intrafascial hysterectomy. It is circularly arranged around the fibrous cervix and is the tissue into which the cardinal and uterosacral ligaments and pubocervical fascia insert.

The portio vaginalis is covered by nonkeratinizing squamous epithelium. Its canal is lined by a columnar mucus-secreting epithelium that is thrown into a series of V-shaped folds that appear like the leaves of a palm and are therefore called plicae palmatae. These form compound clefts in the endocervical canal, not tubular racemose glands, as formerly thought.

The upper border of the cervical canal is marked by the internal os, where the narrow cervical canal widens out into the endometrial cavity. The lower border of the canal, the external os, contains the transition from squamous epithelium of the portio vaginalis to the columnar epithelium of the endocervical canal. This occurs at a variable level relative to the os and changes with hormonal variations that occur during a woman's life. It is in this active area of cellular transition that the cervix is most susceptible to malignant transformation.

There is little adventitia in the uterus, with the peritoneal serosa being directly attached to most of the corpus. The anterior portion of the uterine cervix is covered by the bladder; therefore, it has no serosa. Similarly, as discussed in the following, the broad ligament envelops the lateral aspects of the cervix and corpus; therefore, it has no serosal covering there. The posterior cervix does have a serosal covering.

Adnexal Structures and Broad Ligament

The fallopian tubes are paired tubular structures 7 to 12 cm in length (Fig. 5.10). Each has four recognizable portions. At the uterus, the tube passes through the cornu as an interstitial portion. On emerging from the corpus, a narrow isthmic portion begins with a narrow lumen and thick muscular wall. Proceeding toward the

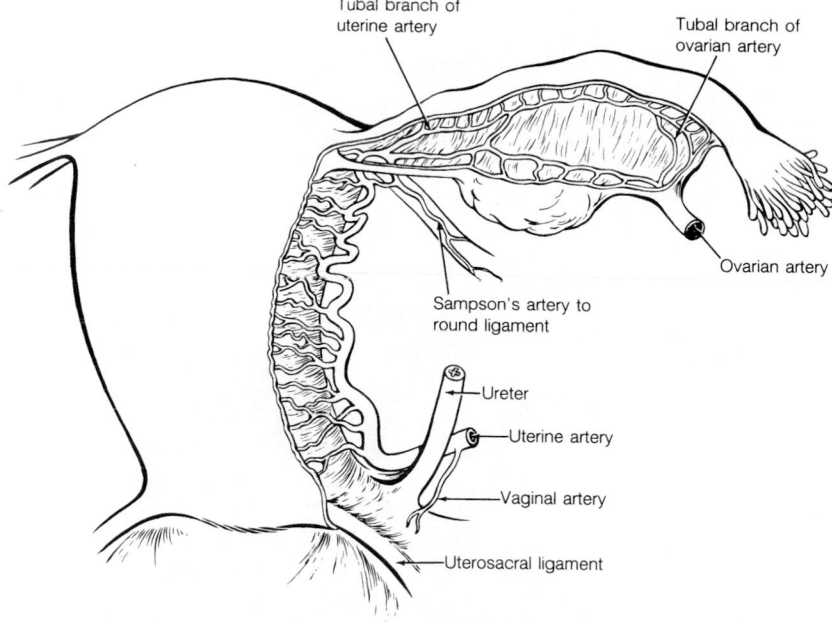

FIGURE 5.10. Uterine adnexa and collateral circulation of uterine and ovarian arteries. The uterine artery crosses over the ureter in the cardinal ligament and gives off cervical and vaginal branches before ascending adjacent to the wall of the uterus and anastomosing with the medial end of the ovarian artery. Note the small branch of the uterine or ovarian artery that nourishes the round ligament (Sampson artery).

abdominal end, next is the ampulla, which has an expanding lumen and more convoluted mucosa. The fimbriated end of the tube has many frondlike projections to provide a wide surface for ovum pickup. The distal end of the fallopian tube is attached to the ovary by the fimbria ovarica, which is a smooth muscle band responsible for bringing the fimbria and ovary close to one another at the time of ovulation. The outer layer of the tube's muscularis is composed of longitudinal fibers; the inner layer has a circular orientation.

The lateral pole of the ovary is attached to the pelvic wall by the infundibulopelvic ligament and the ovarian artery and vein contained therein. Medially, it is connected to the uterus through the uteroovarian ligament. During reproductive life, it measures about 2.5 to 5 cm long, 1.5 to 3 cm thick, and 0.7 to 1.5 cm wide, varying with its state of activity or suppression, as with oral contraceptive medications. Its surface is mostly free but has an attachment to the broad ligament through the mesovarium, as discussed in the following.

The ovary has a cuboidal to columnar covering and consists of a cortex and medulla. The medullary portion is primarily fibromuscular, with many blood vessels and much connective tissue. The cortex is composed of a more specialized stroma, punctuated with follicles, corpora lutea, and corpora albicantia.

The round ligaments are extensions of the uterine musculature and represent the homolog of the gubernaculum testis. They begin as broad bands that arise on each lateral aspect of the anterior corpus. They assume a more rounded shape before they enter the retroperitoneal tissue, where they pass lateral to the deep inferior epigastric vessels and enter each internal inguinal ring. After traversing the inguinal canal, they exit the external ring and enter the subcutaneous tissue of the labia majora. They have little to do with uterine support.

The ovaries and tubes constitute the uterine adnexa. They are covered by a specialized series of peritoneal folds called the broad ligament. During embryonic development, the paired müllerian ducts and ovaries arise from the lateral abdominopelvic walls. As they migrate toward the midline, a mesentery of peritoneum is pulled out from the pelvic wall from the cervix on up. This leaves the midline uterus connected on either side to the pelvic wall by a double layer of peritoneum.

Within the upper layers of these two folds, called the broad ligaments, lie the fallopian tubes, round ligaments, and ovaries (Fig. 5.11). The cardinal and uterosacral ligaments are at the lower margin of the broad ligament. These structures are visceral ligaments; therefore, they are composed of varying amounts of smooth muscle, vessels, connective tissue, and other structures. They are not the pure ligaments associated with joints in the skeleton.

The ovary, tube, and round ligament each have their own separate mesentery, called the mesovarium, mesosalpinx, and mesoteres, respectively. These are arranged in a constant pattern, with the round ligament placed ventrally, where it exits the pelvis through the inguinal ligament, and the ovary placed dorsally. The tube is in the middle and is the most cephalic of the three structures. At the lateral end of the fallopian tube and ovary, the broad ligament ends where the infundibulopelvic ligament blends with the pelvic wall. The cardinal ligaments lie at the base of the broad ligament and are described under the section on supportive tissues and cleavage planes.

Blood Supply and Lymphatics of the Genital Tract

The blood supply to the genital organs comes from the ovarian arteries and uterine and vaginal branches of the internal iliac arteries. A continuous arterial arcade con-

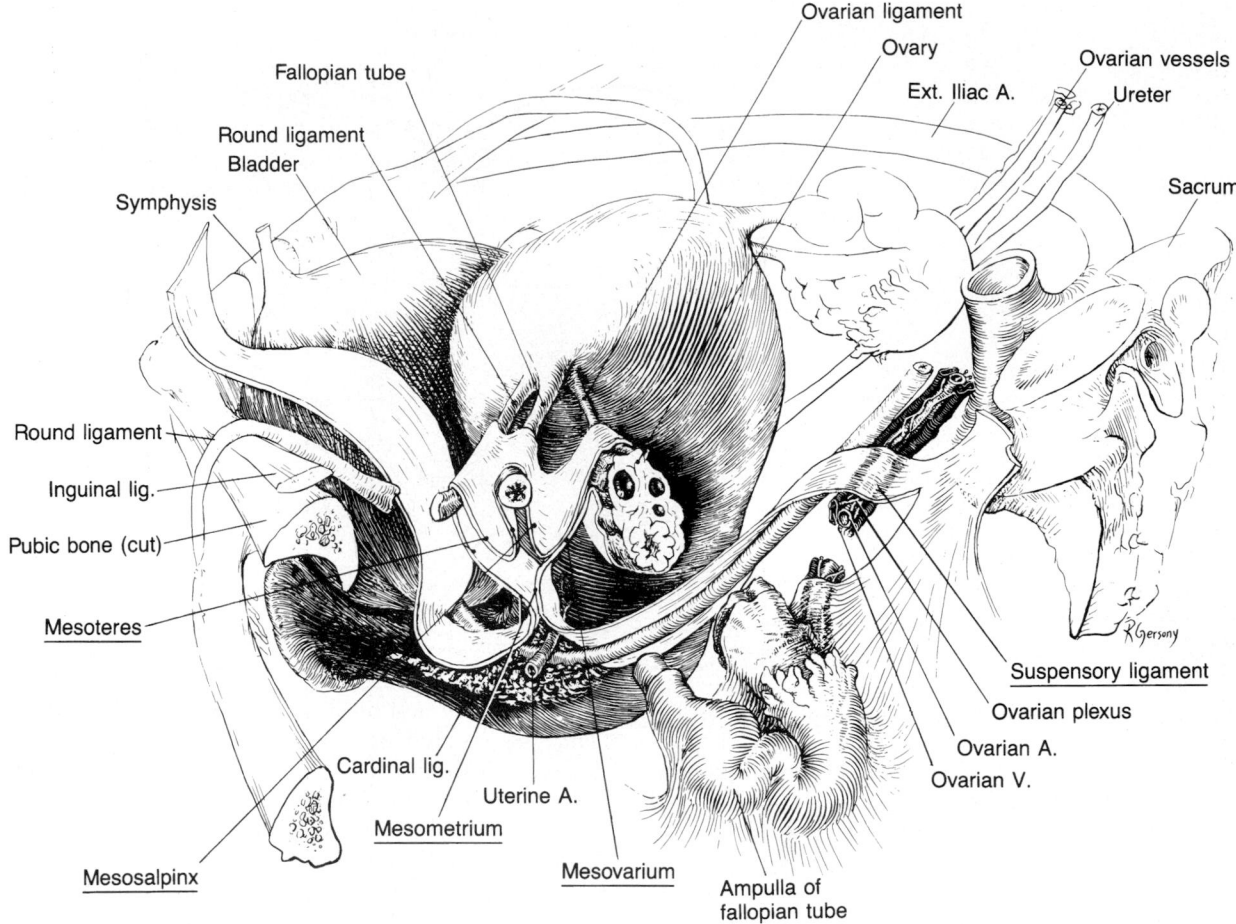

FIGURE 5.11. Composition of the broad ligament.

nects these vessels on the lateral border of the adnexa, uterus, and vagina (see Fig. 5.10).

The blood supply of the upper adnexal structures comes from the ovarian arteries that arise from the anterior surface of the aorta just below the level of the renal arteries. The accompanying plexus of veins drains into the vena cava on the right and the renal vein on the left. The arteries and veins follow a long, retroperitoneal course before reaching the cephalic end of the ovary. They pass along the mesenteric surface of the ovary to connect with the upper end of the marginal artery of the uterus. Because the ovarian artery runs along the hilum of the ovary, it not only supplies the gonad but also sends many small vessels through the mesosalpinx to supply the fallopian tube, including a prominent fimbrial branch at the lateral end of the tube.

The uterine artery originates from the internal iliac artery. It usually arises independently from this source but can have a common origin with either the internal pudendal or vaginal artery. It joins the uterus near the junction of the corpus and cervix, but this position varies considerably, both with the individual and the amount of upward or downward traction placed on the uterus. Ac-

companying each uterine artery are several large uterine veins that drain the corpus and cervix.

On arriving at the lateral border of the uterus (after passing over the ureter and giving off a small branch to this structure), the uterine artery flows into the side of the marginal artery that runs along the side of the uterus. Through this connection it sends blood both upward toward the corpus and downward to the cervix. Because the marginal artery continues along the lateral aspect of the cervix, it eventually crosses over the cervicovaginal junction and lies on the side of the vagina.

The vagina receives its blood supply from a downward extension of the uterine artery along the lateral sulci of the vagina and from a vaginal branch of the internal iliac artery. These form an anastomotic arcade along the lateral aspect of the vagina at the 3- and 9-o'clock positions. Branches from these vessels also merge along the anterior and posterior vaginal walls. The distal vagina also receives a supply from the pudendal vessels, and the posterior wall has a contribution from the middle and inferior hemorrhoidal vessels.

Lymphatic drainage of the upper two thirds of the vagina and uterus is primarily to the obturator and internal and external iliac nodes, and the distal-most vagina drains with the vulvar lymphatics to the inguinal nodes. In addition, some lymphatic channels from the uterine corpus extend along the round ligament to the superficial inguinal nodes, and some nodes extend posteriorly along the uterosacral ligaments to the lateral sacral nodes. These routes of drainage are discussed more fully in the discussion of the retroperitoneal space.

The lymphatic drainage of the ovary follows the ovarian vessels to the region of the lower abdominal aorta, where they drain into the lumbar chain of nodes (paraaortic nodes).

The uterus receives its nerve supply from the uterovaginal plexus (Frankenhäuser ganglion) that lies in the connective tissue of the cardinal ligament. Details of the organization of the pelvic innervation are contained in the section on retroperitoneal structures.

Lower Urinary Tract

Ureter

The ureter is a tubular viscus about 25 cm long, divided into abdominal and pelvic portions of equal length. Its small lumen is surrounded by an inner longitudinal and outer circular muscle layer. In the abdomen, it lies in the extraperitoneal connective tissue on the posterior abdominal wall, crossed anteriorly by the left and right colic vessels. Its course and blood supply are described in the section on the retroperitoneum.

Bladder

The bladder can be divided into two portions; the dome and base (Fig. 5.12). The musculature of the spherical bladder does not lie in simple layers, as do the muscular walls of tubular viscera such as the gut and ureter. It is best described as a meshwork of intertwining muscle

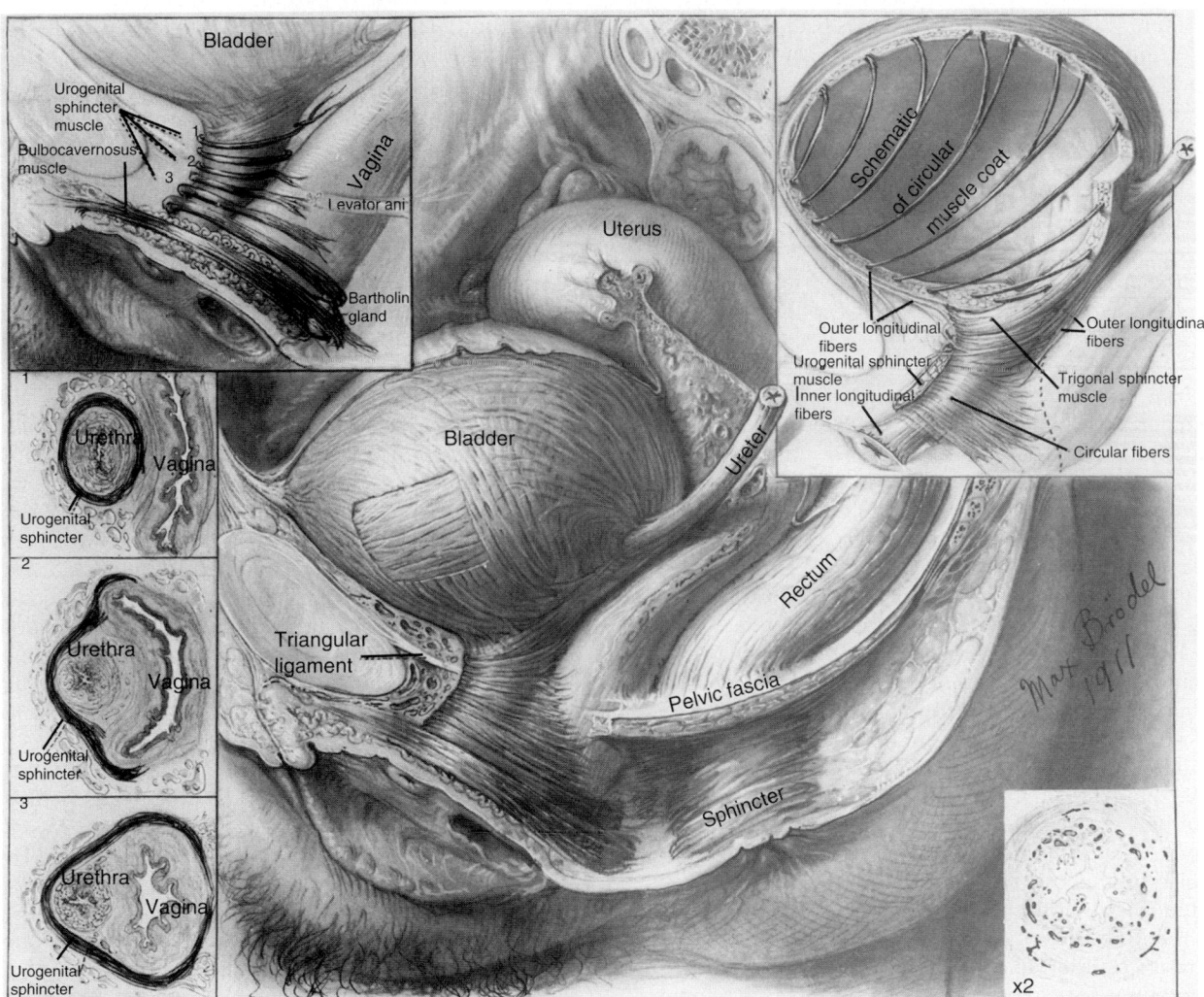

FIGURE 5.12. Lateral view of the pelvic organs showing the urethra and bladder. **Inset 3:** Two portions of the striated urogenital sphincter muscle, namely, the urethrovaginal sphincter and the urethral sphincter. The compressor urethra is not seen. (From: The Brödel Collection, Department of Art as Applied to Medicine, Johns Hopkins Medical Institution, Baltimore, MD, with permission.)

bundles. The musculature of the dome is relatively thin when the bladder is distended. The base of the bladder, which is thicker and varies less with distention of the dome, consists of the urinary trigone and a thickening of the detrusor, called the detrusor loop. This is a U-shaped band of musculature, open posteriorly, that forms the bladder base anterior to the intramural portion of the ureter. The trigone is made of smooth muscle that arises from the ureters that occupy two of its three corners. It continues as the muscle of the vesical neck and urethra. There it rests on the upper vagina. The shape of the bladder depends on its state of filling. When empty, it is a somewhat flattened disk, slightly concave upward. As it fills, the dome rises off the base, eventually assuming a more spherical shape.

The distinction between the base and dome has functional importance, because they have differing innervations. The bladder base has alpha-adrenergic receptors that contract when stimulated and thereby favor continence. The dome is responsive to beta or cholinergic stimulation, with contraction that causes bladder emptying.

Anteriorly, the bladder lies against the lower abdominal wall. It lies against the pubic bones laterally and inferiorly and abuts the obturator internus and levator ani. Posteriorly, it rests against the vagina and cervix. These relations are discussed further in consideration of the pelvic planes and spaces.

The blood supply of the bladder comes from the superior vesical artery, which comes off the obliterated umbilical artery and inferior vesical artery, which is either an independent branch of the internal pudendal artery or arises from the vaginal artery.

Urethra

The urethral lumen begins at the internal urinary meatus and has a series of regional differences in its structure. It passes through the bladder base in an intramural portion for a little less than a centimeter. This region of the bladder, where the urethral lumen traverses the bladder base, is called the vesical neck.

The urethra itself begins outside the bladder wall. In its distal two thirds it is fused with the vagina (see Fig. 5.12), with which it shares a common embryologic derivation. From the vesical neck to the perineal membrane, which starts at the junction of the middle and distal thirds of the bladder, the urethra has several layers. An outer, circularly oriented skeletal muscle layer (urogenital sphincter) mingles with some circularly oriented smooth muscle fibers. Inside this layer is a longitudinal layer of smooth muscle that surrounds a remarkably vascular submucosa and nonkeratinized squamous epithelium that responds to estrogenic stimulation.

Within the submucosa is a group of tubular glands that lie on the vaginal surface of the urethra. These paraurethral (or Skene's) glands empty into the lumen at several points on the dorsal surface of the urethra, but two prominent openings on the inner aspects of the external urethral orifice can be seen when the orifice is opened. Chronic infection of these glands can lead to urethral diverticula, and obstruction of their terminal duct can result in cyst formation. Their location on the

dorsal surface of the urethra reflects the distribution of the structures from which they arise.

At the level of the perineal membrane, the distal portion of the urogenital sphincter begins. Here the skeletal muscle of the urethra leaves the urethral wall to form the urethrovaginal sphincter (see Fig. 5.5) and compressor urethrae (formerly called the deep transverse perineal muscle). Distal to this portion, the urethral wall is fibrous and forms a nozzle for aiming the urinary stream. The mechanical support of the vesical neck and urethra, which are so important to urinary continence, is discussed in the section of this chapter devoted to the supportive tissues of the urogenital system.

The urethra receives its blood supply both from an inferior extension of the vesical vessels and from the pudendal vessels.

Sigmoid Colon and Rectum

The sigmoid colon begins its S-shaped curve at the pelvic brim. It has the characteristic structure of the colon, with three tenia coli lying over a circular smooth muscle layer. Unlike much of the colon, which is retroperitoneal, the sigmoid has a definite mesentery in its midportion. The length of the mesentery and the pattern of the sigmoid's curvature vary considerably. It receives its blood supply from the lowermost portion of the inferior mesenteric artery, the branches called the sigmoid arteries.

As it enters the pelvis, the colon straightens its course and becomes the rectum. This portion extends from the pelvic brim until it loses its final anterior peritoneal investment below the cul-de-sac. It has two bands of smooth muscle (anterior and posterior). Its lumen has three transverse rectal folds that contain the mucosa, submucosa, and circular layers of the bowel wall. The most prominent fold, the middle one, lies anteriorly on the right about 8 cm above the anus, and it must be negotiated during high rectal examination or sigmoidoscopy.

As the rectum passes posterior to the vagina, it expands into the rectal ampulla. This portion of the bowel begins under the cul-de-sac peritoneum and fills the posterior pelvis from the side. At the distal end of the rectum, the anorectal junction is bent at an angle of 90 degrees where it is pulled ventrally by the puborectalis fibers' attachment to the pubes and posteriorly by the external anal sphincter's dorsal attachment to the coccyx.

Below this level, the gut is called the anus. It has many distinguishing features. There is a thickening of the circular involuntary muscle called the internal sphincter. The canal has a series of anal valves to assist in closure, and at their lower border the mucosa of the colon gives way to a transitional layer of non–hair-bearing squamous epithelium before becoming the hair-bearing perineal skin.

The relations of the rectum and anus can be inferred from their course. They lie against the sacrum and levator plate posteriorly and against the vagina anteriorly. Inferiorly, each half of the levator ani abuts its lateral wall and sends fibers to mingle with the longitudinal involuntary fibers between the internal and external sphincters. Its distal terminus is surrounded by the external anal sphincter.

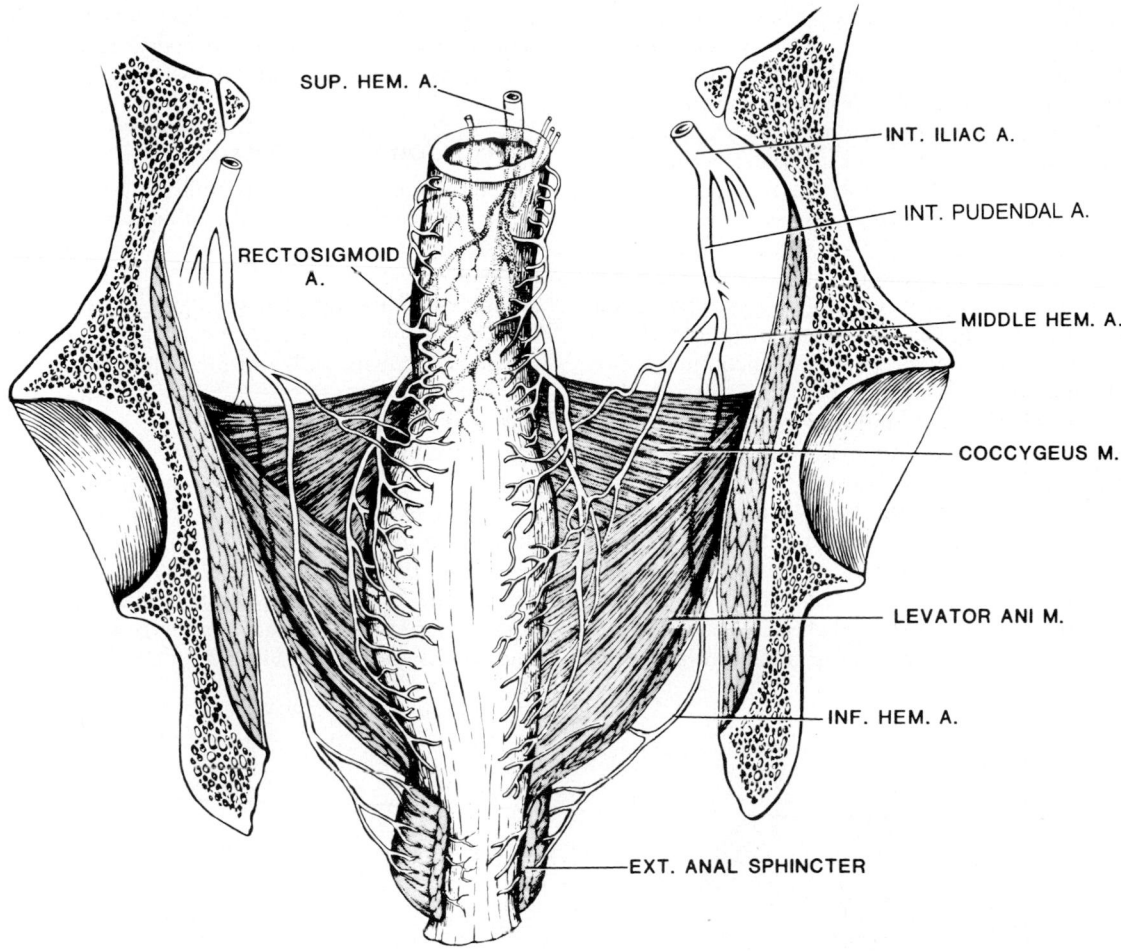

FIGURE 5.13. Rectosigmoid colon and anal canal, showing collateral arterial circulation from superior hemorrhoidal (inferior mesenteric), middle hemorrhoidal (hypogastric or internal iliac), and inferior hemorrhoidal (internal pudendal) arteries.

The anorectum receives its blood supply from a number of sources (Fig. 5.13). From above, the superior rectal (hemorrhoidal) branch of the inferior mesenteric artery lies within the layers of the sigmoid mesocolon. As it reaches the beginning of the rectum, it divides into two branches and ends in the wall of the gut. A direct branch from the internal iliac artery arises from the pelvic wall on either side and supplies the rectum and ampulla above the pelvic floor. The anus and external sphincter receive their blood supply from the inferior rectal (hemorrhoidal) branch of the internal pudendal artery, which reaches the terminus of the gastrointestinal tract through the ischiorectal fossa.

PELVIC CONNECTIVE TISSUE AND CLEAVAGE PLANES

The pelvic viscera are connected to the lateral pelvic wall by their adventitial layers and thickenings of the connective tissue that lie over the pelvic wall muscles (Fig. 5.14). These attachments, as well as the attachments of one organ to another, separate the different surgical

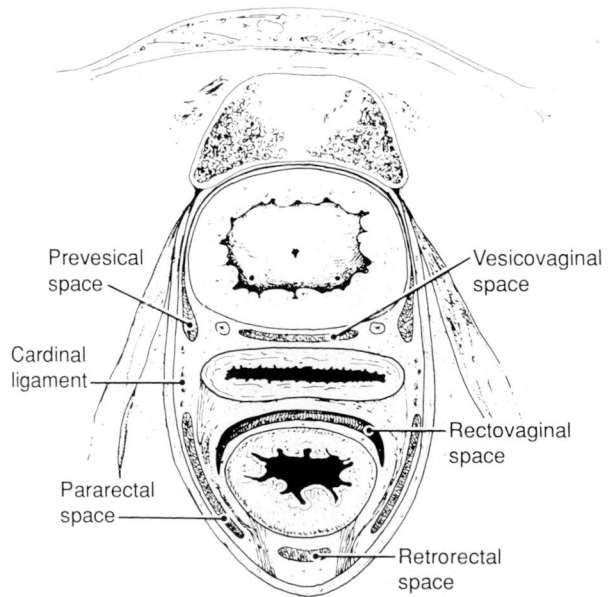

FIGURE 5-14. Cross section of the pelvis showing cleavage planes.

cleavage planes from one another. These condensations of the adventitial layers of the pelvic organs have assumed supportive roles, connecting the viscera to the pelvic walls, in addition to their role in transmitting the organs' neurovascular supply from the pelvic wall. They are somewhat like a mesentery that connects the bowel, for example, to the body wall. It has a supportive function as well as a role in carrying vessels and nerves to the organ. An understanding of their disposition is important to both vaginal and abdominal surgery.

The tissue that connects the organs to the pelvic wall has been given the special designation of endopelvic fascia. It is not a layer similar to the layer encountered during abdominal incisions (rectus abdominis "fascia"). It is composed of blood vessels and nerves, interspersed with a supportive meshwork of irregular connective tissue containing collagen and elastin. These structures connect the muscularis of the visceral organs to pelvic wall muscles. In some areas there is considerable smooth muscle within this tissue, as is true in the area of the uterosacral ligaments. Although surgical texts often speak of this fascia as a specific structure separate from the viscera, this is not strictly true. These layers can be separated from the vis-

cera, just as the superficial layers of the bowel wall can be artificially separated from the deeper layers, but they are not themselves separate structures.

Pelvic Connective Tissue

The term *ligament* is most familiar when it describes a dense connective tissue band that links two bones, but it also describes ridges in the peritoneum or thickenings of the endopelvic fascia. The ligaments of the genital tract are diverse. Although they share a common designation (i.e., ligament), they are composed of many types of tissue and have many different functions.

Uterine Ligaments

The broad ligaments are peritoneal folds that extend laterally from the uterus and cover the adnexal structures. They have no supportive function and were discussed in the section on the pelvic viscera.

Within the broad ligament, beginning just caudal to the uterine arteries, there is a thickening in the endopelvic fascia that attaches the cervix and upper vagina to the pelvic side walls (Fig. 5.15), consisting of the car-

A

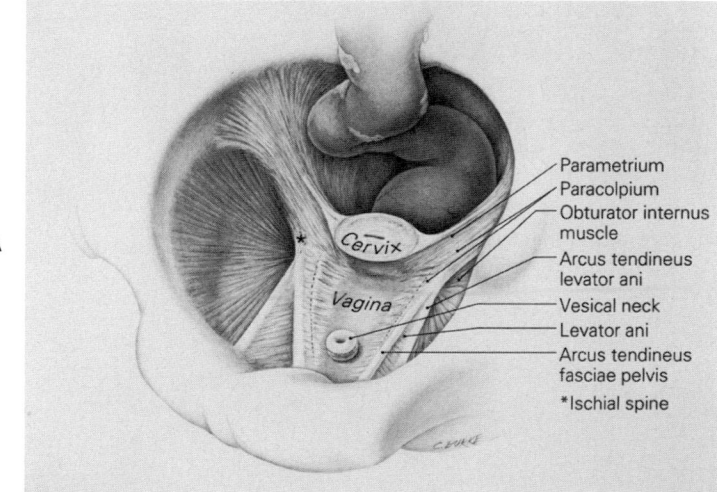

B

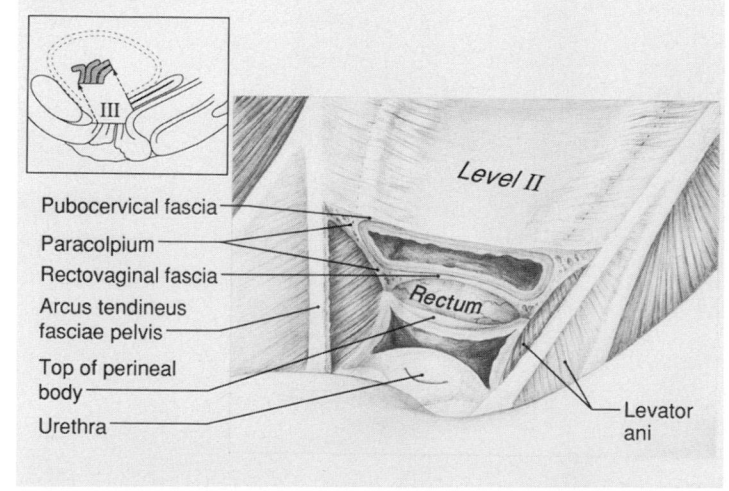

FIGURE 5.15. A: Suspensory ligaments of the female genital tract seen with the bladder removed. B: Close-up of the lower portion of the middle vagina (level II) shows how the lateral attachments of the vagina result in an anterior layer under the bladder (pubocervical fascia) and a posterior layer in front of the rectum (rectovaginal fascia). The cephalic surfaces of the transected distal urethra and vagina (level III) are shown. (From: DeLancey JOL. Anatomic aspects of vaginal eversion after hysterectomy. *Am J Obstet Gynecol* 1992;166:1717, with permission.)

dinal and uterosacral ligaments (parametrium). The term *uterosacral ligaments* refers to that portion of this tissue that forms the medial margin of the parametrium and that borders the cul-de-sac of Douglas. The term *cardinal ligament* is used to refer to that portion that attaches the lateral margins of the cervix and vagina to the pelvic walls. The cardinal and uterosacral ligaments, therefore, are simply two parts of a single body of suspensory tissue. The term *parametrium* refers to all of the tissue that attaches to the uterus (both cardinal and uterosacral ligaments), and the term *paracolpium* refers to the portion that attaches to the vagina (cardinal ligament of the vagina). The uterosacral ligament portion of the parametrium is composed predominantly of smooth muscle, the autonomic nerves of the pelvic organs, and some intermixed connective tissue and blood vessels, whereas the cardinal ligament portion consists primarily of perivascular connective tissue and the pelvic vessels. Although they are often described as extending laterally from the cervix to the pelvic wall, in the standing position they are almost vertical as one would expect for a suspensory tissue. Near the cervix, they are discrete, but they fan out in the retroperitoneal layer to have a broad, if somewhat ill-defined, area of attachment over the second, third, and fourth segments of the sacrum. These ligaments hold the cervix posteriorly in the pelvis over the levator plate of the pelvic diaphragm.

The cardinal ligaments lie at the lower edge of the broad ligaments, between their peritoneal leaves, beginning just caudal to the uterine arteries. They attach to the cervix below the isthmus and fan out to attach to the pelvic walls over the piriformis muscle in the area of the greater sciatic foramen. Although when placed under tension they feel like ligamentous bands, they are composed simply of perivascular connective tissue and nerves that surround the uterine artery and veins. Nevertheless,

these structures have considerable strength, and the lack of a separate "ligamentous band" in this area does not detract from their supportive role. They provide support not only to the cervix and uterus but also to the upper portion of the vagina (paracolpium) to keep these structures positioned posteriorly over the levator plate of the pelvic diaphragm and away from the urogenital hiatus.

Vaginal Fasciae and Attachments

The attachments of the vagina to the pelvic walls are important in maintaining the pelvic organs in their normal positions. Failure of these attachments, along with damage to the levator ani muscles, result in the clinical conditions of uterine prolapse, cystocele, rectocele, and enterocele.

The cervix and upper one third of the vagina are suspended within the pelvis by the downward extension of the cardinal ligaments (see Fig. 5.15). Anterior to the vagina in this area is the vesicovaginal space; posterior to it is the cul-de-sac and rectovaginal space. In its middle third, the vagina is attached laterally to the arcus tendineus fasciae pelvis. The arcus tendineus fasciae pelvis is a fibrous band that extends from its ventral attachment at the pubic bone to its dorsal attachment to the ischial spine. These lateral attachments suspend the anterior vaginal wall across the pelvis and prevent its downward descent with increases in abdominal pressure. The structural layer formed by the vaginal wall and its lateral attachments to the arcus tendineus is clinically referred to as the pubocervical fascia.

Support of the posterior vaginal wall prevents the rectum from bulging forward in the clinical condition known as rectocele. This support varies in different levels of the vagina. In the distal 2 or 3 cm of the posterior vaginal wall, attachments of the perineal body to the ischiopubic rami hold the perineal body in place and prevent protrusion of the distal rectum (Fig. 5.16). In the mid-

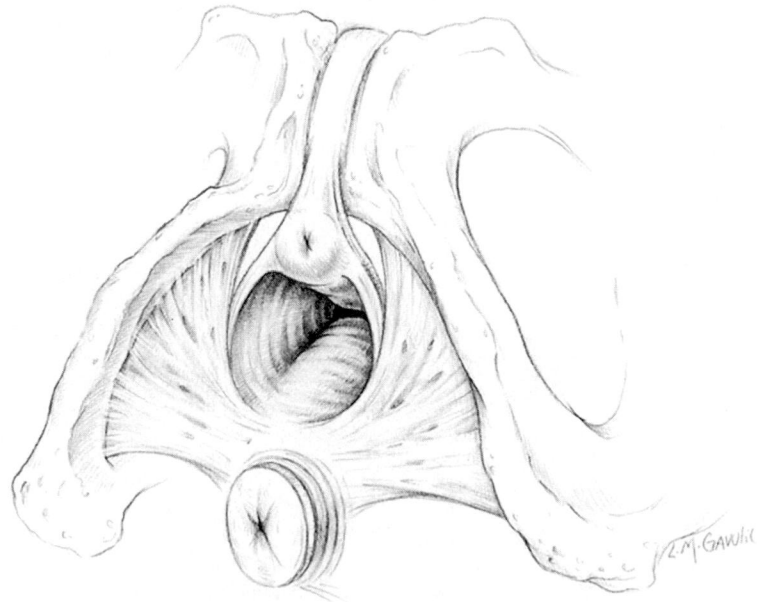

FIGURE 5.16. The peripheral attachments of the perineal membrane to the ischiopubic rami and direction of tension on fibers uniting through the perineal body. (From: DeLancey JOL. Structural anatomy of the posterior compartment as it relates to rectocele. *Am J Obstet Gynecol* 1999;180:815–823, with permission.)

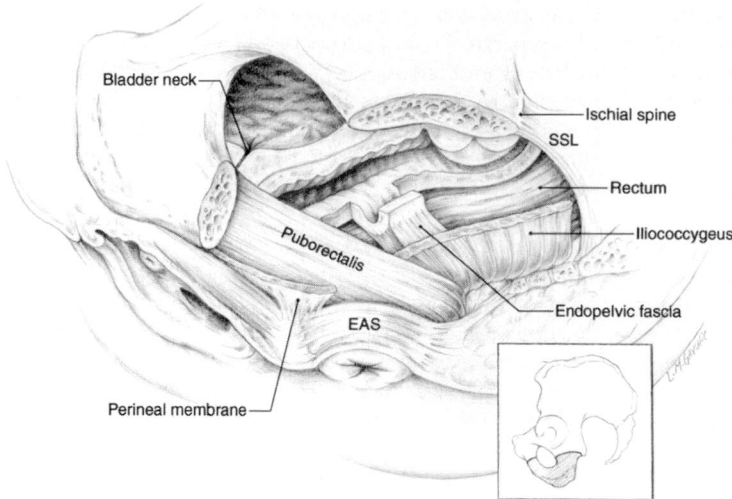

FIGURE 5.17. Lateral view of the pelvic organs after removal of the left ischial bone and ischial tuberosity. The bladder, vagina, and cervix have been cut in the sagittal plane to reveal their lumens. The rectum has been left intact. A strip of the posterior/lateral vaginal wall with its attached endopelvic fascia are shown indicating their position relative to the levator ani muscle and this fascia's course and attachment. The two portions of the levator ani muscle (puborectalis and iliococcygeus) are visible. The ischial spine and the intact sacrospinous ligament are above the level of the removed ischial tuberosity. The left half of the perineal membrane (urogenital diaphragm) is shown just caudal to the puborectalis portion of the levator ani muscle after its detachment from the inferior pubic ramus that has been removed. (From: DeLancey JOL. Structural anatomy of the posterior compartment as it relates to rectocele. *Am J Obstet Gynecol* 1999;180: 815–823, with permission.)

vagina above this, the vaginal is attached laterally to the fascia covering the inside of the levator ani muscles (Fig. 5.17). This connection prevents the middle of the posterior vaginal wall from moving forward and downward during increases in abdominal pressure. The combination of these attachments results in a structural layer that has been referred to by the term "fascia of Denonvilliers." Detailed histologic studies of this area, however, have failed to reveal a separate layer in the midline between the muscularis of the vagina and the rectovaginal space except in the distal vagina where the dense connective tissue of the perineal body separates these structures.

Urethral Supports
The support of the proximal urethra is important in the maintenance of urinary continence during times of increased abdominal pressure. The distal portion of the urethra is inseparable from the vagina, because of their common embryologic derivation. These tissues are fixed firmly in position by connections of the periurethral tissues and vagina to the pubic bones through the perineal membrane (Fig. 5.18). A hammocklike layer composed of the endopelvic fascia and anterior vaginal wall provides the support of the proximal urethra. This layer is stabilized by its lateral attachments both to the arcus tendineus fasciae pelvis and the medial margin of the levator ani muscles. The arcus tendineus fasciae pelvis is a fibrous band stretched from a ventral attachment at the lower portion of the pubic bones about 1 cm above the lower margin of the pubic bones and 1 cm from the midline to the ischial spine. The muscular attachment of the endopelvic fascia allows contraction and relaxation of the levator ani muscles to elevate the urethra and to let it descend.

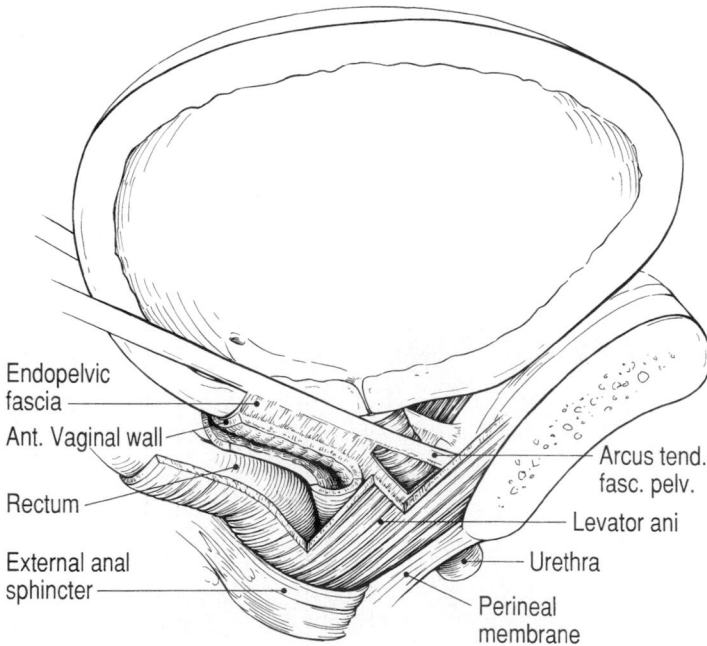

FIGURE 5.18. Lateral view of the urethral supportive mechanism transected just lateral to the midline. The lateral wall of the vagina and a portion of the endopelvic fascia have been removed so that one can see the deeper structures. (Redrawn from: DeLancey JOL. Structural support of the urethra as it relates to stress urinary incontinence: the hammock hypothesis. *Am J Obstet Gynecol* 1994;170:1713, with permission.)

During increases in abdominal pressure, the downward force caused by increased abdominal pressure on the ventral surface of the urethra compresses the urethra closed against the hammocklike supportive layer, thereby closing the urethral lumen against the increases in intravesical pressure. The stability of the fascial layer determines the effectiveness of this closure mechanism. If the layer is unyielding, it forms a firm backstop against which the urethra can be compressed closed; however, if it is unstable, the effectiveness of this closure is compromised. Therefore, the integrity of the attachment to the arcus tendineus and the levator ani is critical to the stress continence mechanism.

The muscular attachment is responsible for the voluntary control of vesical neck position visible during vaginal examination or fluoroscopy when the pelvic muscles are contracted and relaxed. Relaxation of these muscles with descent of the vesical neck is associated with the initiation of urination and contraction with arrest of the urinary stream. The limit of downward vesical neck motion is determined by the connective tissue elasticity in the attachments to the arcus tendineus fasciae pelvis.

Cul-de-sacs, Cleavage Planes, and Spaces

Each of the pelvic viscera can expand somewhat independently of its neighboring organs. The ability to do this comes from their relatively loose attachment to one another, which permits the bladder, for example, to expand without equally elongating the adjacent cervix. This allows the viscera to be easily separated from one another along these lines of cleavage. These surgical cleavage planes are called spaces, although they are not empty but rather are filled with fatty or areolar connective tissue. The pelvic spaces are separated from one another by the connections of the viscera to one another and to the pelvic walls.

Anterior and Posterior Cul-de-sacs

Properly termed the vesicouterine and rectouterine pouches, the anterior and posterior cul-de-sac separate the uterus from the bladder and rectum.

The anterior cul-de-sac is a recess between the dome of the bladder and the anterior surface of the uterus (Fig. 5.19). The peritoneum is loosely applied in the region of the anterior cul-de-sac unlike its dense attachment to the upper portions of the uterine corpus. This allows the bladder to expand without stretching its overlying peritoneum. This loose peritoneum forms the vesicouterine fold that can easily be lifted and incised to create a bladder flap during abdominal hysterectomy or Caesarean section. It is the point at which the vesico-cervical space is normally accessed during abdominal surgery.

The posterior cul-de-sac is bordered ventrally by the vagina anteriorly, the rectosigmoid posteriorly and the uterosacral ligaments laterally. Its peritoneum extends for approximately 4 cm along the posterior vaginal wall below the posterior vaginal fornix where the vaginal wall

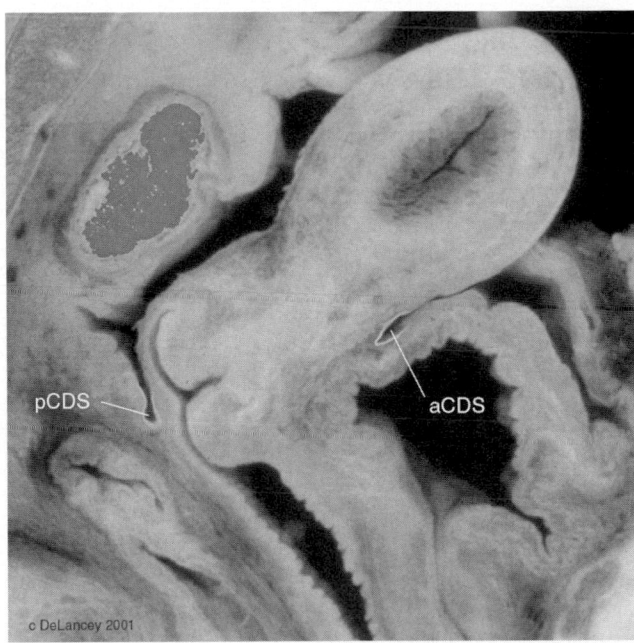

FIGURE 5.19. Sagittal section from a 28-year-old cadaver showing the anterior cul-de-sac (aCDS) and the posterior cul-de-sac (pCDS). Note how the posterior cul-de-sac peritoneum lies on the vaginal wall, whereas the anterior cul-de-sac lies several centimeters from the depth of the peritoneum in this area. (Peritoneum digitally enhanced in photograph to aid visibility.) (From: DeLancey, copyright 2001, with permission.)

attaches to the cervix. This allows direct entry into the peritoneum from the vagina when performing a vaginal hysterectomy, culdocentesis, or colpotomy. The anatomy here contrasts with the anterior cul-de-sac. Anteriorly, the peritoneum lies several centimeters above the vagina where posteriorly the peritoneum covers the vagina. Keeping this anatomic difference in mind facilitates entering both the anterior and the posterior cul-de-sacs during vaginal hysterectomy.

Prevesical Space

The prevesical space of Retzius (see Fig. 5.14) is separated from the undersurface of the rectus abdominis muscles by the transversalis fascia and can be entered by perforating this layer. Ventrolaterally, it is bounded by the bony pelvis and the muscles of the pelvic wall; cranially, it is bounded by the abdominal wall. The proximal urethra and bladder lie in a dorsal position. The dorsolateral limit to this space is the attachment of the bladder to the cardinal ligament and the attachment of the pubocervical fascia to the arcus tendineus fasciae pelvis. These separate this space from the vesico-vaginocervical space. This lateral attachment is to the arcus tendineus fasciae pelvis, which lies on the inner surface of the obturator internus and pubococcygeal and puborectal muscles.

Important structures lying within this space include the dorsal clitoral vessels under the symphysis at its lower border and the obturator nerve and vessels as they enter the obturator canal. A branch to the obturator canal often comes off the external iliac artery and lies on the pubic bone; therefore, dissection in this area should be performed with care (Fig. 5.20). Lateral to the bladder and vesical neck is a dense plexus of vessels that lie at the border of the lower urinary tract. They are deep to the pubovesical muscle, and although they bleed when sutures are placed here, this venous ooze usually stops when the sutures are tied. Also within this tissue, lateral to the bladder and urethra, lie the nerves of the lower urinary tract. The upper border of the pubic bones that form the anterior surface of this region has a ridgelike fold of periosteum called the iliopectineal line. This is sometimes used to anchor sutures during urethral suspension operations.

Vesicovaginal and Vesicocervical Space

The space between the lower urinary tract and the genital tract is separated into the vesicovaginal and vesicocervical spaces (see Fig. 5.14). The lower extent of the space is the junction of the proximal one third and distal two thirds of the urethra, where it fuses with the vagina, and it extends to lie under the peritoneum at the vesicocervical peritoneal reflection. It extends laterally to the pelvic side walls, separating the vesical and genital aspects of the cardinal ligaments

Rectovaginal Space

On the dorsal surface of the vagina lies the rectovaginal space (see Fig. 5.14). It begins at the apex of the perineal body, about 2 to 3 cm above the hymenal ring. It extends upward to the cul-de-sac and laterally around the sides of the rectum to the attachment of the rectovaginal septum to the parietal endopelvic fascia. It contains loose areolar tissue and is easily opened with finger dissection.

At the level of the cervix, some fibers of the cardinal-uterosacral ligament complex extend downward behind the vagina, connecting it to the lateral walls of the rectum and then to the sacrum. These are called the rectal pillars. They separate the midline rectovaginal space in this region from the lateral pararectal spaces. These pararectal spaces allow access to the sacrospinous ligaments (mentioned afterward). They also form the lateral boundaries of the retrorectal space between the rectum and sacrum.

Region of the Sacrospinous Ligament

The area around the sacrospinous ligament is another region that has become more important to the gynecologist operating for problems of vaginal support. The sacrospinous ligament lies on the dorsal aspect of the coccygeal muscle (see Fig. 5.20). The rectal pillar separates it from the rectovaginal space.

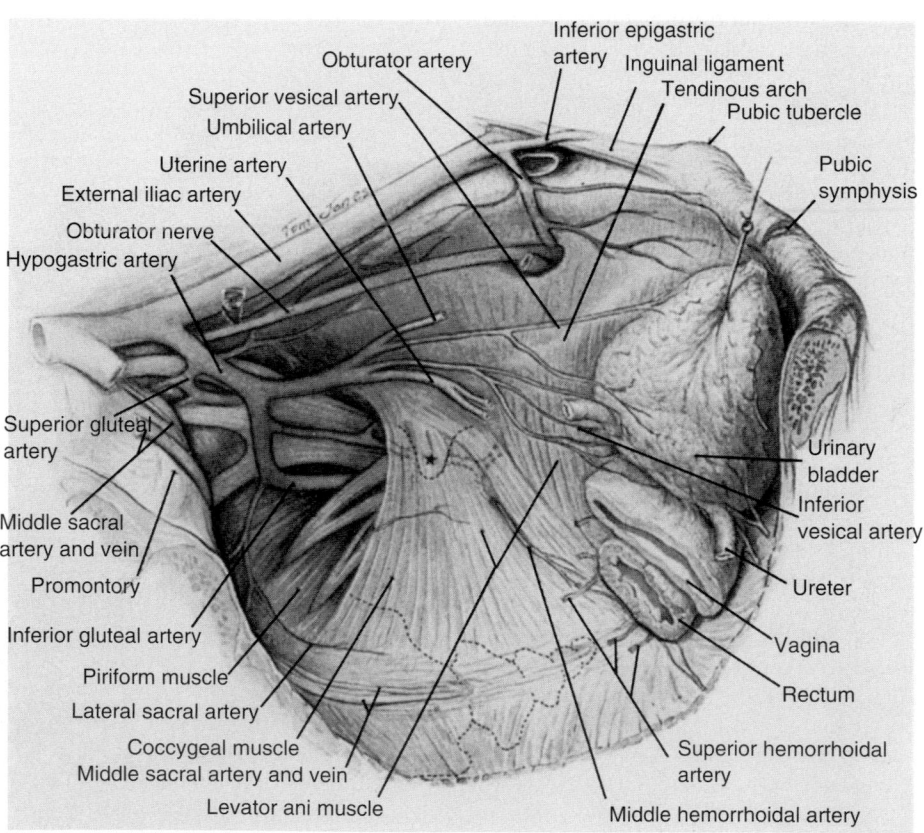

FIGURE 5.20. Structures of the pelvic wall. (From: Anson BJ. *An atlas of human anatomy.* Philadelphia: WB Saunders, 1950, with permission.)

As its name implies, the sacrospinous ligament courses from the lateral aspect of the sacrum to the ischial spine. In its medial portion it fuses with the sacrotuberous ligament and is a distinct structure only laterally. It can be reached from the rectovaginal space by perforation of the rectal pillar to enter the pararectal space or by dissection directly under the enterocele peritoneum. This area is covered in more detail in Chapter 35.

Many structures are near the sacrospinous ligament, and their location must be remembered during surgery in this region. The sacral plexus lies immediately next to the ligament on its cephalic border and comes to lie on its lateral surface as the nerve passes through the greater sciatic foramen. Just before its exit, the plexus gives off the pudendal nerve, which, with its accompanying vessels, passes lateral to the sacrospinous ligament at its attachment to the ischial spine. The nerve to the levator ani muscles lies on the inner surface of the coccygeal muscle in its midportion. In developing this space, the tissues that are reflected medially and cranially to gain access contain the pelvic venous plexus of the internal iliac vein, as well as the middle rectal vessels. If they are mobilized too vigorously, they can cause considerable hemorrhage.

RETROPERITONEAL SPACES AND LATERAL PELVIC WALL

The retroperitoneal space of the posterior abdomen, presacral space, and pelvic retroperitoneum contain the major neural, vascular, and lymphatic supply to the pelvic viscera. These areas are explored during operations to identify the ureter, interrupt the pelvic nerve supply, arrest serious pelvic hemorrhage, and remove potentially malignant lymph nodes. Because this area is free of the adhesions from serious pelvic infection or endometriosis, it can be used as a plane of dissection when the peritoneal cavity has become obliterated. The structures found in these spaces are discussed in a regional context, because that is the way they are usually approached in the operating room.

Retroperitoneal Structures of the Lower Abdomen

The aorta lies on the lumbar spine slightly to the left of the vena cava, which it overlies. The portion of this vessel below the renal vessels is encountered during retroperitoneal dissection to identify the paraaortic lymph nodes (Fig. 5.21). The renal blood vessels arise at the second lumbar vertebra. The ovarian vessels also arise from the anterior surface of the aorta in this region. In general, the branches of the vena cava follow those of the aorta, except for the vessels of the intestine, which flow into the portal vein, and the left ovarian vein, which empties into the renal vein on that side.

Below the level of the renal vessels and just below the third portion of the duodenum, the inferior mesenteric artery arises from the anterior aorta. It gives off ascending branches of the left colic artery and continues caudally to supply the sigmoid through the three or four sigmoid arteries that lie in the sigmoid mesentery. These vessels follow the bowel as it is pulled from side to side, so that their position can vary, depending on retraction.

Inferiorly, a continuation of the inferior mesenteric artery forms the superior rectal artery. This vessel crosses over the external iliac vessels to lie on the dorsum of the lower sigmoid. It supplies the rectum, as described in the section concerning that viscus.

The aorta and vena cava have segmental branches that arise at each lumbar level and are called the lumbar arteries and veins. They are situated somewhat posteriorly to the aorta and vena cava and are not visible from the front. When the vessels are mobilized, as is done in excising the lymphatic tissue in this area, they come into view.

At the level of the fourth lumbar vertebra (just below the umbilicus), the aorta bifurcates into the left and right common iliac arteries. After about 5 cm, the common iliac arteries (and the medially placed veins) give off the internal iliac vessels from their medial side and continue toward the inguinal ligament as the external iliac arteries. These internal iliac vessels lie within the pelvic retroperitoneal region and are discussed afterward.

The aorta and vena cava in this region are surrounded by lymph nodes on all sides. Surgeons usually refer to this lumbar chain of nodes as the paraaortic nodes, reflecting their position. They receive the drainage from the common iliac nodes and are the final drainage of the pelvic viscera. In addition, they collect the lymphatic drainage from the ovaries that follows the ovarian vessels and does not pass through the iliac nodes. The nodes of the lumbar chain extend from the right side of the vena cava to the left of the aorta and can be found both anterior and posterior to the vessels.

The ureters are attached loosely to the posterior abdominal wall in this region, and when the overlying colon is mobilized, they remain on the body wall. They are crossed anteriorly by the ovarian vessels, which contribute a branch to supply the ureter. Additional blood supply to the abdominal portion comes from the renal vessels at the kidney and the common iliac artery.

This region can be exposed either by a midline peritoneal incision to the left of the small bowel mesentery or, retroperitoneally, by reflection of the colon. During embryonic development, the colon and its mesentery fuse with the abdominal wall. A cleavage plane exists here that allows the colon and its vessels to be elevated to expose the structures of the posterior abdominal wall. Because the ureter and ovarian vessels originally arise in this area, they are not elevated with the colon.

Presacral Space

The presacral space begins below the bifurcation of the aorta and is bounded laterally by the internal iliac arteries (Figs. 5.22 and 5.23). Lying directly on the sacrum are the middle sacral artery and vein, which originate from the dorsal aspect of the aorta and vena cava (and

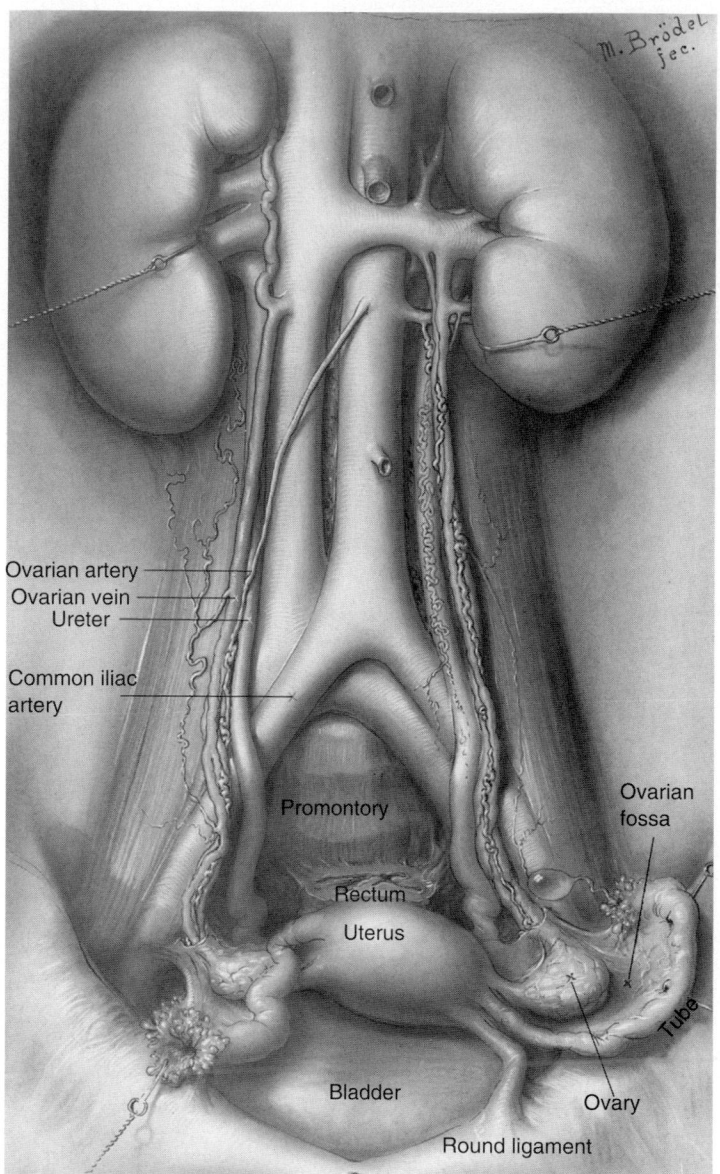

Ovarian artery
Ovarian vein
Ureter

Common iliac
artery

Promontory

Ovarian
fossa

Rectum

Uterus

Tube

Bladder

Ovary

Round ligament

FIGURE 5.21. Structures of the retroperitoneum. Note the anomalous origin of the left ovarian artery from the left renal artery rather than from the aorta. (From: The Brödel Collection, Department of Art as Applied to Medicine, Johns Hopkins Medical Institution, Baltimore, with permission.)

not from the point of bifurcation, as sometimes shown). Caudal and lateral to this are the lateral sacral vessels. The venous plexus of these vessels can be extensive, and bleeding from it can be considerable.

Within this area lies the most familiar part of the pelvic autonomic nervous system, the presacral nerve (superior hypogastric plexus). The autonomic nerves of the pelvic viscera can be divided into a sympathetic (thoracolumbar) and parasympathetic (craniosacral) system. The former is also called the adrenergic system, and the latter is called the cholinergic system, according to their neurotransmitters. Alpha-adrenergic stimulation causes increased urethral and vesical neck tone, and cholinergic stimulation increases contractility of the detrusor muscle. Similarly, adrenergic stimulation in the colon and rectum favors storage, and cholinergic stimulation favors evacuation. β-adrenergic agonists, which are used for tocoly-

sis, suggest that these influence contractility of the uterus. As is true in the male, damage to the autonomic nerves during pelvic lymphadenectomy can have a significant influence on orgasmic function in the female.

How these autonomic nerves reach the organs that they innervate has surgical importance. The terminology of this area is somewhat confusing, because many authors use idiosyncratic terms. However, the structure is simple: It consists of a single ganglionic midline plexus overlying the lower aorta (superior hypogastric plexus) that splits into two trunks without ganglia (hypogastric nerves), each of which connects with a plexus of nerves and ganglia lateral to the pelvic viscera (inferior hypogastric plexus).

The superior hypogastric plexus lies in the retroperitoneal connective tissue on the ventral surface of the lower aorta and receives input from the sympathetic chain ganglia through the thoracic and lumbar splanchnic

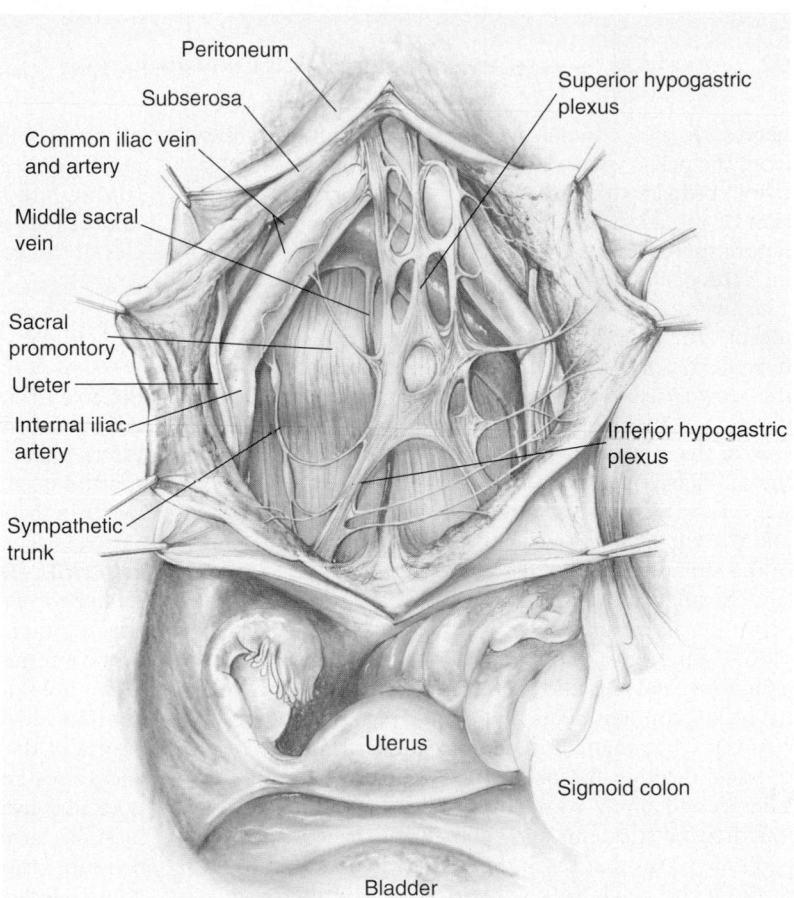

FIGURE 5.22. Presacral nerve plexus, showing passage of sympathetic trunk over bifurcation of aorta. Observe the division of the trunk into left and right presacral nerves. (Redrawn from: Curtis AH, Anson BJ, Ashley FL, et al. The anatomy of the pelvic autonomic nerves in relation to gynecology. *Surg Gynecol Obstet* 1942;75:743, with permission.)

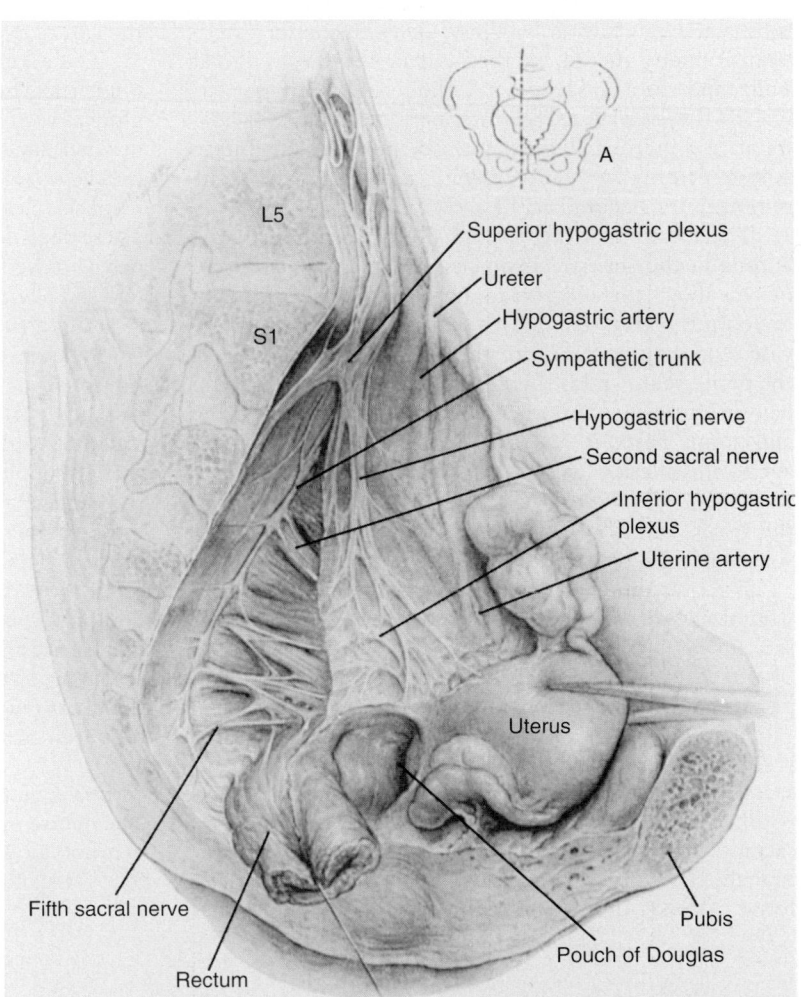

FIGURE 5.23. Nerves of the female pelvis. (From: Anson BJ. *An atlas of human anatomy.* Philadelphia: WB Saunders, 1950, with permission.)

nerves. It also contains important afferent pain fibers from the pelvic viscera, which makes its transection effective in primary dysmenorrhea. It passes over the bifurcation of the aorta and extends over the proximal sacrum before splitting into two hypogastric nerves that descend into the pelvis in the region of the internal iliac vessels. The hypogastric nerves end in the inferior hypogastric plexus. The hypogastric plexi are broad expansions of the hypogastric nerves. Their sympathetic fibers come from the downward extensions of the superior hypogastric plexus and pelvic splanchnic nerves from the continuation of the sympathetic chain into the pelvis. Parasympathetic fibers come from sacral segments 2 through 4 by way of the pelvic splanchnic nerves (nervi erigentes) to join these ganglia. They lie in the pelvic connective tissue of the lateral pelvic wall, lateral to the uterus and vagina.

The inferior hypogastric plexus (sometimes called the pelvic plexus) is divided into three portions: the vesical plexus anteriorly, uterovaginal plexus (Frankenhäuser ganglion), and the middle rectal plexus. The uterovaginal plexus contains fibers that derive from two sources. It receives sympathetic and sensory fibers from the tenth thoracic through the first lumbar spinal cord segments. The second input comes from the second, third, and fourth sacral segments and consists primarily of parasympathetic nerves that reach the inferior hypogastric plexus through the pelvic splanchnic nerves. The uterovaginal plexus lies on the dorsal (medial) surface of the uterine vessels, lateral to the sacrouterine ligaments' insertion into the uterus. It has continuations cranially along the uterus and caudally along the vagina. This latter extension contains the fibers that innervate the vestibular bulbs and clitoris. These nerves lie in the tissue just lateral to the area where the uterine artery, cardinal ligament, and uterosacral ligament pedicles are made during a hysterectomy for benign disease, and within the tissue removed during a radical hysterectomy.

The location of the sensory fibers from the uterine corpus in the superior hypogastric nerve (the presacral nerve) allows the surgeon to alleviate visceral pain from the corpus by transecting this structure. It does not provide sensory innervation to the adnexal structures or to the peritoneum and is therefore not useful for alleviating pain in those sites. Another important way in which the autonomic nervous system is involved is through damage to the inferior hypogastric plexus during radical hysterectomy. The extension of the surgical field lateral to the viscera interrupts the connection of the bladder and sometimes the rectum to their central attachments.

The ovary and uterine tube receive their neural supply from the plexus of nerves that accompany the ovarian vessels and that originate in the renal plexus. These fibers originate from the tenth thoracic segment, and the parasympathetic fibers come from extensions of the vagus.

As the lumbar and sacral nerves exit from the intervertebral and sacral foramina, they form the lumbar and sacral plexuses. The lumbar nerves and plexus lie deep within the psoas muscle on either side of the spine. The sacral plexus lies on the piriformis muscle, and its major branch, the sciatic nerve, leaves the pelvis through the lower part of the greater sciatic foramen. The sacral plexus supplies nerves to the muscles of the hip, pelvic diaphragm, and perineum, as well as to the lower leg (through the sciatic nerve). The femoral nerve from the lumbar plexus is primarily involved in supplying the muscles of the thigh.

Pelvic Retroperitoneal Space

Division of the internal and external iliac vessels occurs in the area of the sacroiliac joint. Just before passing under the inguinal ligament to become the femoral vessels, the external iliac vessels contribute the deep inferior epigastric and deep circumflex iliac arteries. There are no other major branches of the external iliac artery in this region.

Internal Iliac Vessels

Unlike the external iliac artery, which is constant and relatively simple in its morphology, the branching pattern of the internal iliac arteries and veins is extremely variable (Figs. 5.24 and 5.25). A description of a common variant is included here. The internal iliac artery supplies the viscera of the pelvis and many muscles of the pelvic wall and gluteal region. It usually divides into an anterior and posterior division about 3 to 4 cm after leaving the common iliac artery (Table 5.2). The vessels of the posterior division (the iliolumbar, lateral sacral, and superior gluteal) leave the internal iliac artery from its lateral surface to provide some of the blood supply to the pelvic wall and gluteal muscles. Trauma to these hidden vessels should be avoided during internal iliac artery ligation as the suture is passed around behind vessels.

The anterior division has both parietal and visceral branches. The obturator, internal pudendal, and inferior gluteal vessels primarily supply muscles, whereas the uterine, superior vesical, vaginal (inferior vesical), and middle rectal vessels supply the pelvic organs. The internal iliac veins begin lateral and posterior to the arteries. These veins form a large and complex plexus within the pelvis, rather than having single branches, as do the arteries. They tend to be deeper in this area than the arteries, and their pattern is highly variable.

Ligation of the internal iliac artery has proved helpful in the management of postpartum hemorrhage. Burchell's arteriographic studies showed that physiologically active anastomoses between the systemic and pelvic arterial supplies were immediately patent after ligation of the internal iliac artery (see Fig. 5.25). These anastomoses, shown in Table 5.2, connected the arteries of the internal iliac system with systemic blood vessels either directly from the aorta, as is true for the lumbar and middle sacral artery, or indirectly through the inferior mesenteric artery, as with the superior hemorrhoidal vessels. These *in vivo* pathways were quite different from the anastomoses that had previously been hypothesized on purely anatomic grounds.

Pelvic Ureter

The course of the ureter within the pelvis is important to gynecologic surgeons and is fully considered in Chapter 37. A few of the important anatomic landmarks are considered here (see Fig. 5.24). After passing over the bi-

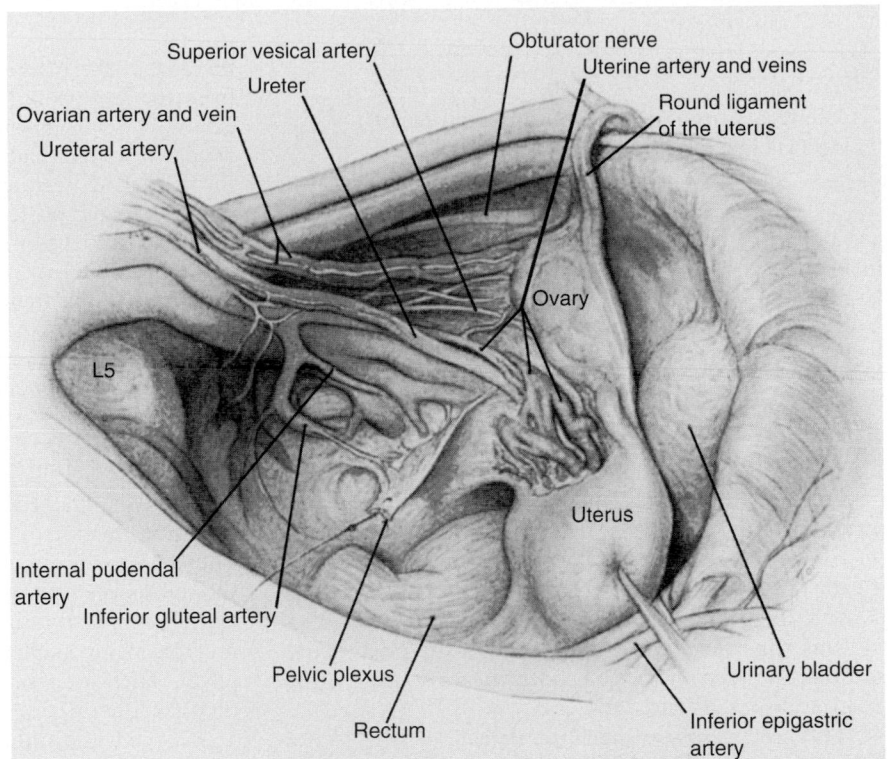

FIGURE 5.24. Arteries and veins of the pelvis. (From: Anson BJ. *An atlas of human anatomy.* Philadelphia: WB Saunders, 1950, with permission.)

Labels in figure 5.24:
Ovarian artery and vein
Ureteral artery
Superior vesical artery
Ureter
Obturator nerve
Uterine artery and veins
Round ligament of the uterus
Ovary
L5
Uterus
Internal pudendal artery
Inferior gluteal artery
Pelvic plexus
Rectum
Urinary bladder
Inferior epigastric artery

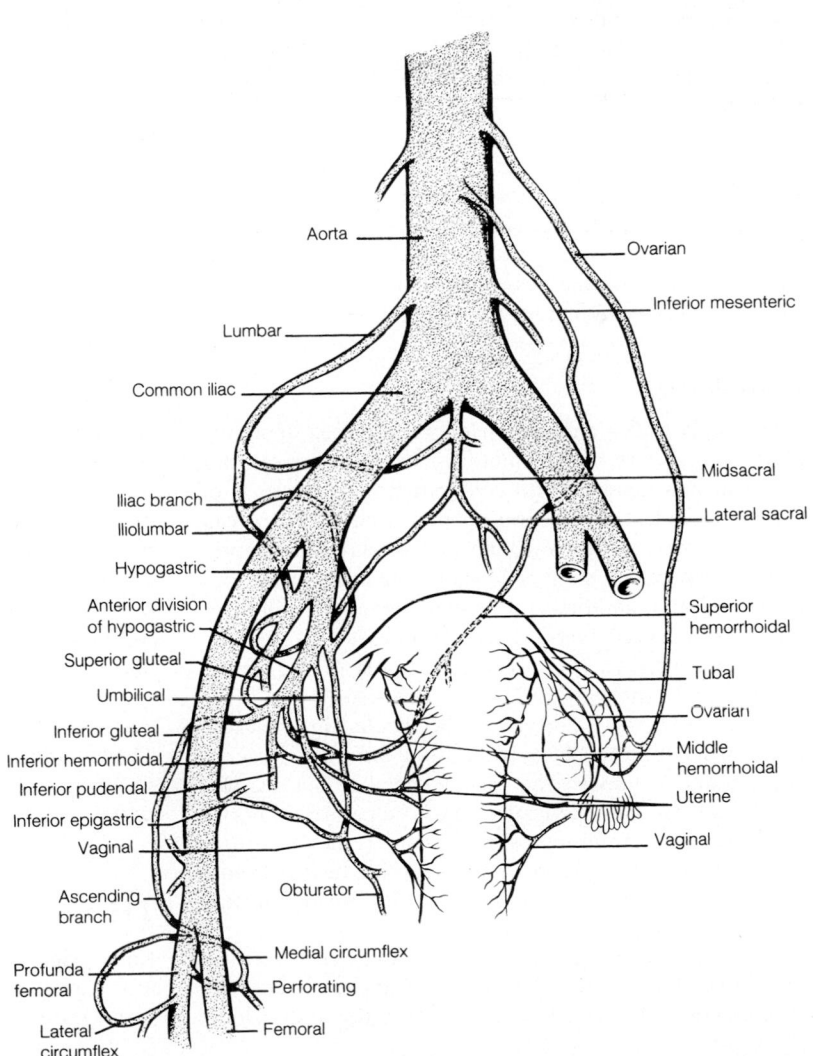

FIGURE 5.25. Collateral circulation of the pelvis.

Labels in figure 5.25:
Aorta
Ovarian
Inferior mesenteric
Lumbar
Common iliac
Midsacral
Lateral sacral
Iliac branch
Iliolumbar
Hypogastric
Anterior division of hypogastric
Superior gluteal
Umbilical
Inferior gluteal
Inferior hemorrhoidal
Inferior pudendal
Inferior epigastric
Vaginal
Ascending branch
Profunda femoral
Lateral circumflex
Medial circumflex
Perforating
Femoral
Obturator
Superior hemorrhoidal
Tubal
Ovarian
Middle hemorrhoidal
Uterine
Vaginal

TABLE 5.2.
Collateral Circulation After Internal Iliac Artery Ligation

Internal Iliac Systemic
Iliolumbar
Lateral sacral
Middle hemorrhoidal
Lumbar
Middle sacral
Superior hemorrhoidal

furcation of the internal and external iliac arteries, just medial to the ovarian vessels, the ureter descends within the pelvis. Here it lies in a special connective tissue sheath that is attached to the peritoneum of the lateral pelvic wall and medial leaf of the broad ligament. This explains why the ureter still adheres to the peritoneum and does not remain laterally with the vessels when the peritoneal space is entered.

The ureter crosses under the uterine artery ("water flows under the bridge") in its course through the cardinal ligament. There is a loose areolar plane around it to allow for its peristalsis here. At this point it lies along the anterolateral surface of the cervix, usually about 1 cm from it. From there it comes to lie on the anterior vaginal wall and then proceeds for a distance of about 1.5 cm through the wall of the bladder.

During its pelvic course, the ureter receives blood from the vessels that it passes, specifically the common iliac, internal iliac, uterine, and vesical arteries. Within the wall of the ureter, these vessels are connected to one another by a convoluted vessel that can be seen running longitudinally along its outer surface.

Lymphatics

The lymph nodes and lymphatic vessels that drain the pelvic viscera vary in their number and distribution, but they can be organized into coherent groups. Because of the extensive interconnection of the lymph nodes, spread of lymph flow, and thus malignancy, is somewhat unpredictable. Therefore, some important generalizations about the distribution and drainage of these tissues are still helpful. Distribution of the pelvic lymph nodes is discussed further in Chapter 46 on invasive carcinoma of the cervix. Figures 46.22 through 46.25 show this anatomy.

The nodes of the pelvis can be divided into the external iliac, internal iliac, common iliac, medial sacral, and pararectal nodes. The medial sacral nodes are few and follow the middle sacral artery. The pararectal nodes drain the part of the rectosigmoid above the peritoneal reflection that is supplied by the superior hemorrhoidal artery. The medial and pararectal nodes are seldom involved in gynecologic disease.

The internal and external iliac nodes lie next to their respective blood vessels, and both end in the common iliac chain of nodes, which then drain into the nodes along the aorta. The external iliac nodes receive the drainage from the leg through the inguinal nodes. Nodes in the external iliac group can be found lateral to the artery, between the artery and vein, and on the medial aspect of the vein. These groups are called the anterosuperior, intermediate, and posteromedial groups, respectively. They can be separated from the underlying muscular fascia and periosteum of the pelvic wall along with the vessels, thereby defining their lateral extent. Some nodes at the distal end of this chain lie in direct relation to the deep inferior epigastric vessels and are named according to these adjacent vessels. Similarly, nodes that lie at the point where the obturator nerve and vessels enter the obturator canal are called obturator nodes.

The internal iliac nodes drain the pelvic viscera and receive some drainage from the gluteal region along the posterior division of the internal iliac vessels as well. These nodes lie within the adipose tissue that is interspersed among the many branches of the vessels. The largest and most numerous nodes lie on the lateral pelvic wall, but many smaller nodes lie next to the viscera themselves. These nodes are named for the organ by which they are found (e.g., parauterine).

Not only is it difficult in the operating room to make some of the fine distinctions mentioned in this anatomic discussion, but also there is little clinical importance in doing so. Surgeons generally refer to those nodes that are adjacent to the external iliac artery as the external iliac group of nodes and to those next to the internal iliac artery as the internal iliac nodes. This leaves those nodes that lie between the external iliac vein and internal artery, which are called interiliac nodes.

The direction of lymph flow from the uterus tends to follow its attachments, draining along the cardinal, uterosacral, and even round ligaments. This latter connection can lead to metastasis from the uterus to the superficial inguinal nodes, whereas the former connections are to the internal iliac nodes, with free communication to the external iliac nodes and sometimes to the lateral sacral nodes. The anastomotic connection of the uterine and ovarian vessels makes lymphatic connections between these two drainage systems likely, and metastasis in this direction possible.

The vagina and lower urinary tract have a divided drainage. Superiorly (upper two thirds of the vagina and the bladder), drainage occurs along with the uterine lymphatics to the internal iliac nodes, whereas the lower one third of the vagina and distal urethra drain to the inguinal nodes. However, this demarcation is far from precise.

The common iliac nodes can be found from the medial to the lateral border of the vessels of the same name. They continue above the pelvic vessels and occur around the aorta and the vena cava. These nodes can lie anterior, lateral, or posterior to the vessels.

THE ABDOMINAL WALL

Knowledge of the layered structure of the abdominal wall allows the surgeon to enter the abdominal cavity with maximum efficiency and safety. A general summary

TABLE 5.3.
Table of Abdominal Wall Layers

Skin
Subcutaneous layer
   Camper's fascia
   Scarpa's fascia
Musculoaponeurotic layer
   Rectus sheath-formed by conjoined aponeuroses of the
     external oblique muscle
Internal oblique muscle: fused in lower abdomen
Transverse abdominal muscle
Transversalis fascia
Peritoneum

of these layers is provided in Table 5.3. The abdomen's superior border is the lower edge of the rib cage (ribs 7 through 12). Inferiorly, it ends at the iliac crests, inguinal ligaments, and pubic bones. It ends posterolaterally at the lumbar spine and its adjacent muscles.

Skin and Subcutaneous Tissue

The fibers in the dermal layer of the abdominal skin are oriented in a predominantly transverse direction following a gently curving concave upward line. This predominance of transversely oriented fibers results in more tension on the skin of a vertical incision and in a wider scar.

Between the skin and musculoaponeurotic layer of the abdominal wall lie the subcutaneous tissues. It is made of globules of fat held in place and supported by a series of branching fibrous septa. In the more superficial portion of the subcutaneous layer, called Camper's fascia, the fat predominates, and the fibrous tissue is less apparent. Closer to the rectus sheath, the fibrous tissue predominates relative to the fat in the region known as Scarpa's fascia. Camper's and Scarpa's fasciae are not discrete or well-defined layers but represent regions of the subcutaneum. Scarpa's fascia is best developed laterally and is not seen as a well-defined layer during vertical incisions.

Musculoaponeurotic Layer

Deep to the subcutaneous tissue is a layer of muscle and fibrous tissue that holds the abdominal viscera in place and controls movement of the lower torso (Figs. 5.26 and 5.27). Within this area are two groups of muscles: vertical muscles in the anterior abdominal wall and oblique flank muscles. The rectus abdominis muscle is found on either side of the midline, and the pyramidalis muscle is located just above the pubes. Lateral to these are the flank muscles: the external oblique, internal oblique, and transverse abdominal. The broad, sheet-like tendons of these muscles form aponeuroses that unite with their corresponding member of the other side, forming a dense white covering of the rectus abdominis muscle properly called the rectus sheath (rectus "fascia").

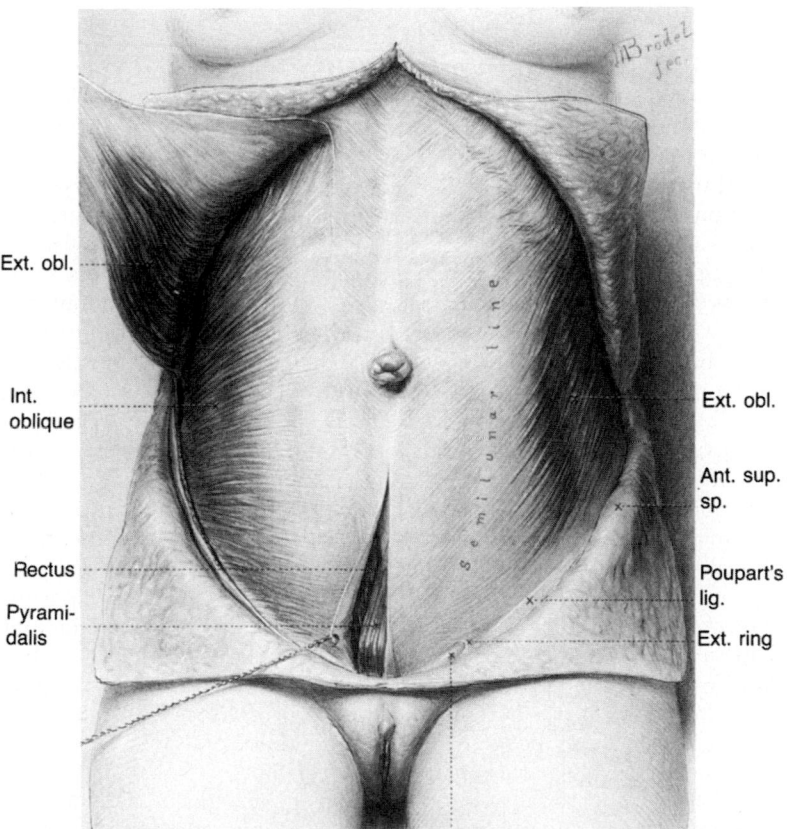

FIGURE 5.26. External oblique, internal oblique, and pyramidal muscles. (From: Kelly HA. *Gynecology.* New York: Appleton, 1928, with permission.)

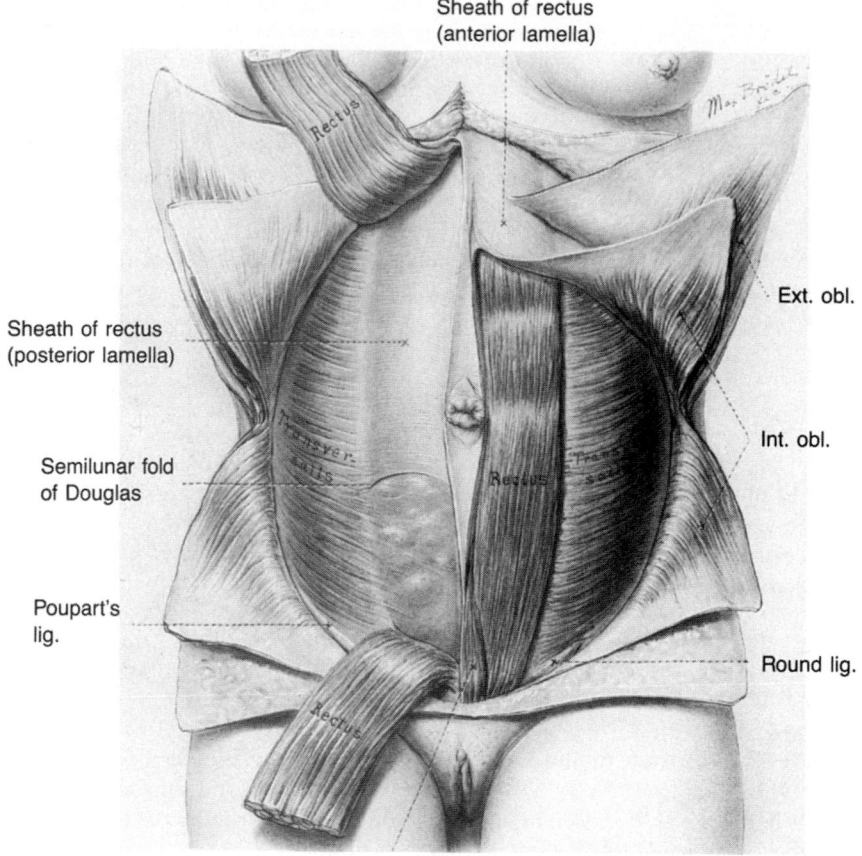

FIGURE 5.27. Transverse abdominal and rectoabdominal muscles. (From: Kelly HA. *Gynecology.* New York: Appleton, 1928, with permission.)

Rectus Abdominis and Pyramidal Muscles

Each paired rectus abdominis muscle originates from the sternum and cartilages of ribs 5 through 7 and inserts into the anterior surface of the pubic bone. Each muscle has three tendinous inscriptions. These are fibrous interruptions within the muscle that firmly attach it to the rectus abdominis sheath. In general, they are confined to the region above the umbilicus, but they can be found below it. When this happens, the rectus sheath is attached to the rectus muscle there, and these two structures become difficult to separate during a Pfannenstiel incision.

The pyramidal muscles arise from the pubic bones and insert into the linea alba in an area several centimeters above the symphysis. Their development varies considerably among individuals. Their strong attachment to the midline makes separation of their attachment here difficult by blunt dissection.

Flank Muscles

Lateral to the rectus abdominis muscles lie the broad, flat muscles of the flank. The aponeurotic insertions of these muscles join to form the conjoined tendon, or rectus sheath, which covers the rectus abdominis. Because of its importance, it is discussed separately subsequently.

The most superficial of these muscles is the external oblique. Its fibers run obliquely anteriorly and inferiorly from their origin on the lower eight ribs and iliac crest. Unlike the external oblique muscle's fibers, which run obliquely downward, the fibers of the internal oblique muscle fan out from their origin in the anterior two thirds of the iliac crest, the lateral part of the inguinal ligament, and the thoracolumbar fascia in the lower posterior flank. In most areas, they are perpendicular to the fibers of the external oblique muscle, but in the lower abdomen, their fibers arch somewhat more caudally and run in a direction similar to those of the external oblique muscle.

As the name transversus abdominis implies, the fibers of the deepest of the three layers have a primarily transverse orientation. They arise from the lower six costal cartilages, the thoracolumbar fascia, the anterior three fourths of the iliac crest, and the lateral inguinal ligament. The caudal portion of the transverse abdominal muscle is fused with the internal oblique muscle. This explains why, during transverse incisions of the lower abdomen, only two layers are discernible at the lateral portion of the incision.

Although the fibers of the flank muscles are not strictly parallel to one another, their primarily transverse orientation and the transverse pull of their attached muscular fibers place vertical suture lines in the rectus sheath under more tension than transverse ones. For this reason, vertical incisions are more prone to dehiscence.

Rectus Sheath (Conjoined Tendon)

The line of demarcation between the muscular and aponeurotic portions of the external oblique muscle in the lower abdomen occurs along a vertical line through the anterosuperior iliac spine (Fig. 5.28). The internal oblique and transverse abdominal muscles extend farther toward the midline, coming closest at their inferior margin, at the pubic tubercle. Because of this, fibers of the internal oblique muscle are found underneath the aponeurotic portion of the external oblique muscle during a transverse incision. In addition, it is between the internal oblique and transverse abdominal muscles that the nerves and blood vessels of the flank are found and their injury avoided.

In forming the rectus sheath, the conjoined aponeuroses of the flank are separable lateral to the rectus muscles but fuse near the midline. As they reach the midline, these layers lose their separate directions and fuse. Many specialized aspects of the rectus sheath are important to the surgeon. In its lower one fourth, the sheath lies entirely anterior to the rectus muscle. Above that point, it splits to lie both ventral and dorsal to it. The transition between these two arrangements occurs midway between the umbilicus and the pubes and is called the arcuate line. Cranial to this line, the midline ridge of the rectus sheath, the linea alba, unites these two layers. Sharp dissection is usually required to separate these layers during a Pfannenstiel incision. A vertical peritoneal incision cuts the posterior sheath.

The lateral border of the rectus muscle is marked by the semilunar line of the rectus sheath. Above the arcuate line, this is the level at which the anterior and posterior layers of the sheath split. Below it the transversalis fascia fuses with the sheath. The semilunar line is not always where the three layers of flank muscles join. During a transverse lower abdominal incision, the external and internal oblique aponeuroses are often separable near the midline.

The inguinal canal lies at the lower edge of the musculofascial layer of the abdominal wall. Through the inguinal canal, in the female, the round ligament extends to its termination in the labium majus. In addition, the ilioinguinal nerve and the genital branch of the genitofemoral nerve pass through the canal.

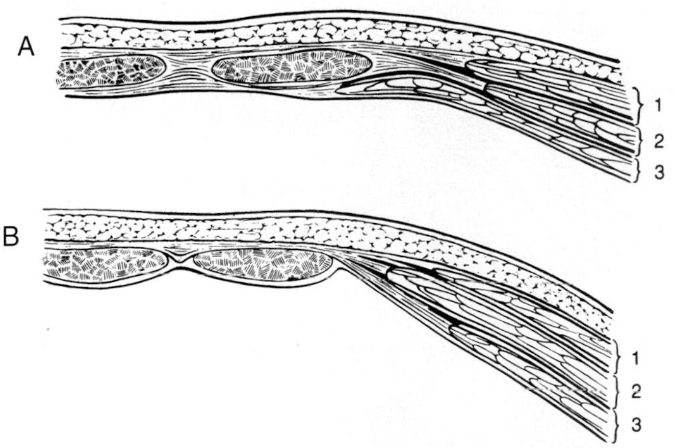

Transversalis Fascia, Peritoneum, and Bladder Reflection

Inside the muscular layers, and outside the peritoneum, lies the transversalis fascia, a layer of fibrous tissue that lines the abdominopelvic cavity. It is visible during abdominal incisions as the layer just underneath the rectus abdominis muscles suprapubically. It is separated from the peritoneum by a variable layer of adipose tissue. It is frequently incised or bluntly dissected off the bladder to take the tissues in this region "down by layers."

The peritoneum is a single layer of serosa. It is thrown into five vertical folds by underlying ligaments or vessels that converge toward the umbilicus. The single median umbilical fold is caused by the presence of the urachus (median umbilical ligament). Lateral to this are paired medial umbilical folds that are raised by the obliterated umbilical arteries that connected the internal iliac vessels to the umbilical cord in fetal life, and the corresponding lateral umbilical folds caused by the inferior epigastric arteries and veins.

The reflection of the bladder onto the abdominal wall is triangular in shape, with its apex blending into the medial umbilical ligament. Because the apex is highest in the midline, incision in the peritoneum lateral to the midline is less likely to result in bladder injury.

Neurovascular Supply of the Abdominal Wall

Vessels of the Abdominal Wall

Knowing the location and course of the abdominal wall blood vessels helps the surgeon anticipate their location during abdominal incisions and during the insertion of laparoscopic trocars (Fig. 5.29). The blood vessels that supply the abdominal wall can be separated into those that supply the skin and subcutaneous tissues and those that supply the musculofascial layer. Although there is only one set of epigastric vessels in the subcutaneous tissues (superficial epigastric), there are both superior and inferior epigastric vessels in the musculofascial layer, so care must be taken in using these terms to avoid confusion.

The superficial epigastric vessels run a diagonal course in the subcutaneum from the femoral vessels toward the umbilicus, beginning as a single artery that branches extensively as it nears the umbilicus. Its position can be anticipated midway between the skin and musculofascial layer, in a line between the palpable femoral pulse and the umbilicus. The external pudendal artery runs a diagonal course from the femoral artery medially to supply the region of the mons pubis. It has many midline branches, and bleeding in its territory of distribution is heavier than

FIGURE 5.28. Cross section of lower abdominal wall. **A:** The anterior fascial sheath of the rectus muscle from external oblique (1) and split aponeurosis of internal oblique (2) muscles. The posterior sheath is formed by aponeurosis of the transverse abdominal muscle (3) and split aponeurosis of the internal oblique muscle. **B:** Lower portion of the abdominal wall below arcuate line (linea semicircularis) with absence of a posterior fascial sheath of the rectus muscle and all of the fascial aponeuroses (1,2,3) forming the anterior rectus muscle sheath.

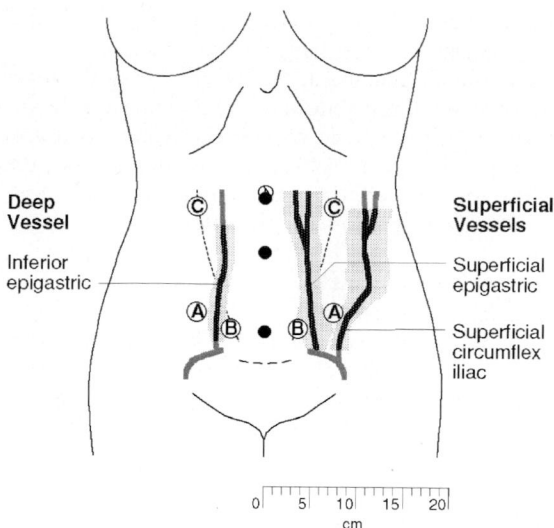

FIGURE 5.29. Normal variation in epigastric vessels. A, B, and C designate safe spots for laparoscopic trocar insertion. Dotted lines indicate lateral border of rectus muscle. (From: Hurd WW, Bude RO, DeLancey JOL, et al. The location of abdominal wall blood vessels in relationship to abdominal landmarks apparent at laparoscopy. *Am J Obstet Gynecol* 1994;171:642, with permission.)

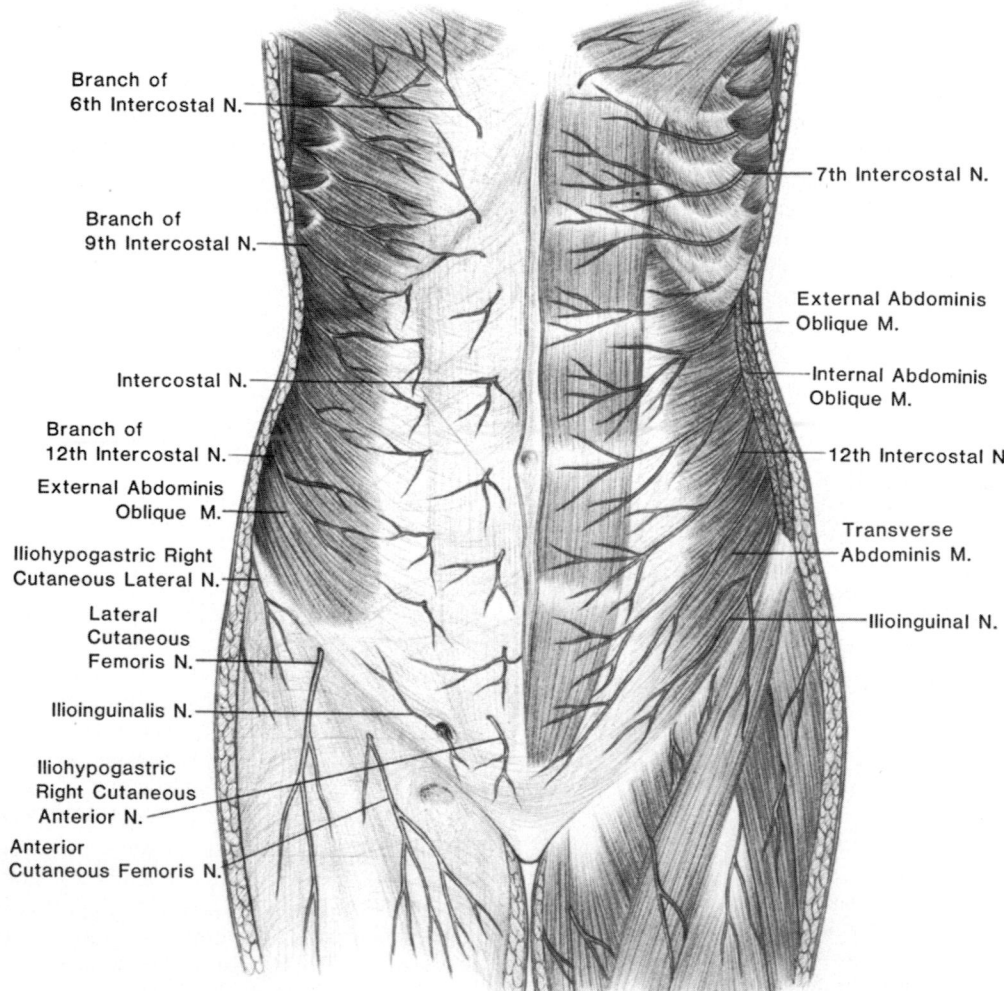

FIGURE 5.30. Nerve supply to the abdomen. **Right:** Deep innervation of T6BT12 to the transverse abdominal, internal oblique, and rectal muscles. **Left:** Superficial distribution, including cutaneous nerves, after penetration and innervation of the external oblique muscle and fascia. Innervation of the groin and thigh also is shown.

that from the abdominal subcutaneous tissues. The superficial circumflex iliac vessels proceed laterally from the femoral vessels toward the flank.

The blood supply to the lower abdominal wall's musculofascial layer parallels the subcutaneous vessels. The branches of the external iliac, the inferior epigastric, and the deep circumflex iliac arteries parallel their superficial counterparts (see Fig. 5.29). The circumflex iliac artery lies between the internal oblique and transverse abdominal muscle. The inferior epigastric artery and its two veins originate lateral to the rectus muscle. They run diagonally toward the umbilicus and intersect the muscle's lateral border midway between the pubis and umbilicus. Below the point at which the vessels pass under the rectus, they are found lateral to the muscle deep to the transversalis fascia. After crossing the lateral border of the muscle, they lie on the muscle's dorsal surface, between it and the posterior rectus sheath. As the vessels enter the rectus sheath, they branch extensively, so that

they no longer represent a single trunk. The angle between the vessel and the border of the rectus muscle forms the apex of the Hesselbach triangle (inguinal triangle), whose base is the inguinal ligament.

Lateral laparoscopic trocars are placed in a region of the lower abdomen where injury to the inferior epigastric and superficial epigastric vessels can occur easily. The inferior epigastric arteries and the superficial epigastric arteries run similar courses toward the umbilicus. Knowing the average location of these blood vessels helps in choosing insertion sites that will minimize their injury and the potential hemorrhage and hematomas that this injury can cause. Just above the pubic symphysis, the vessels lie approximately 5.5 cm from the midline, whereas at the level of the umbilicus, they are 4.5 cm from the midline (Fig. 5.30). Therefore, placement either lateral or medial to the line connecting these points minimizes potential vascular injury. In addition, the location of the inferior epigastric vessel can often be seen (Fig. 5.31) by

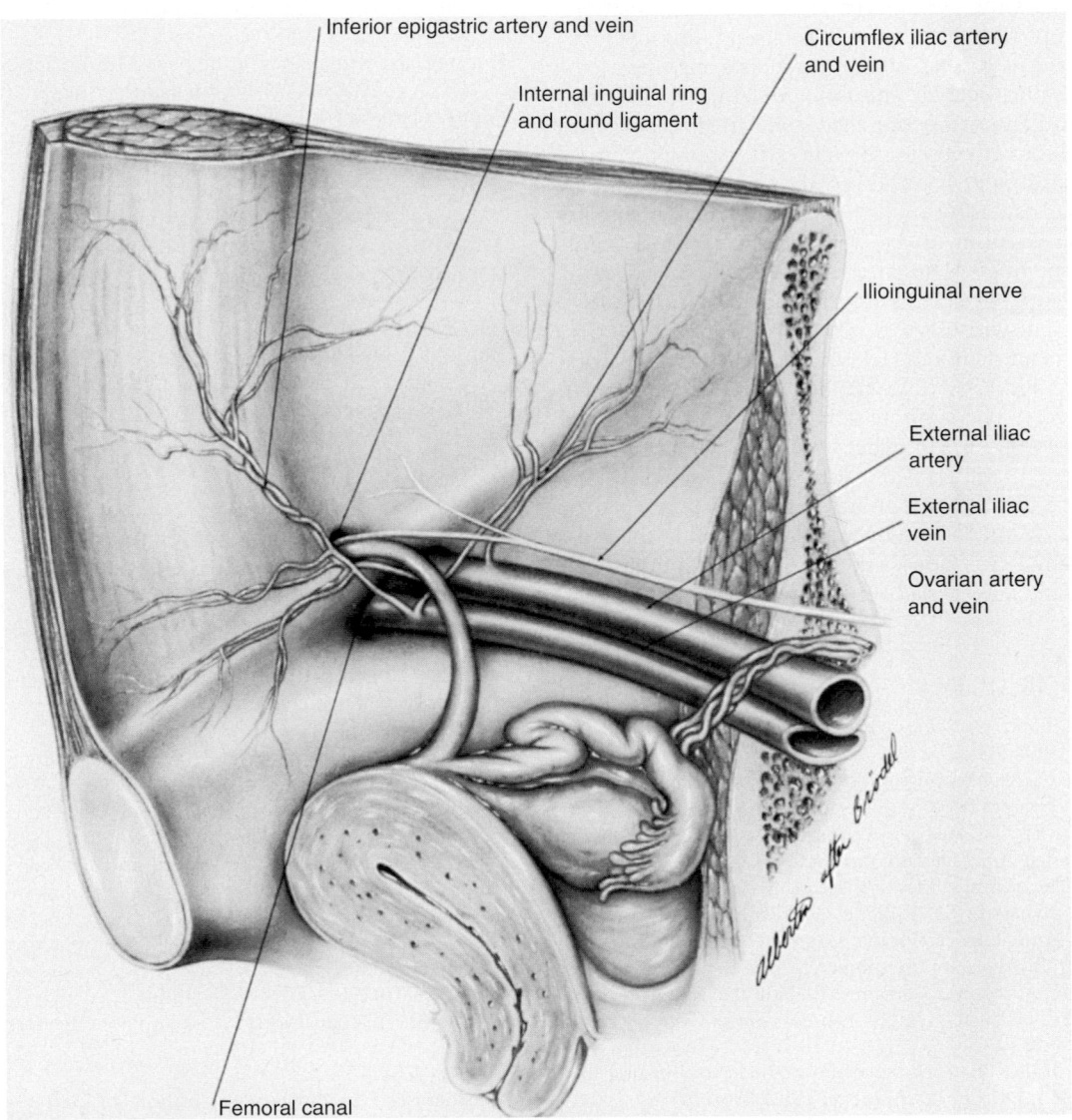

FIGURE 5.31. Sagittal view of female pelvis, showing inguinal and femoral anatomy.

following the round ligament to its point of entry into the inguinal ring, recognizing that the vessel lies just lateral to this point.

Nerves of the Abdominal Wall

The innervation of the abdominal wall (see Fig. 5.30) comes from the abdominal extension of intercostal nerves 7 through 11, subcostal nerves (T12), iliohypogastric nerves (T12 and L1), and ilioinguinal (L1) nerves. Dermatome T10 lies at the umbilicus.

After giving off a lateral cutaneous branch, each intercostal nerve pierces the lateral border of the rectus sheath. There it provides a lateral branch that ends in the rectus muscle. The anterior branch then passes through the muscle and perforates the rectus sheath to supply the subcutaneous tissues and skin as the anterior cutaneous branches. Incisions along the lateral border of the rectus lead to denervation of the muscle, which can render it atrophic and weaken the abdominal wall. Elevation of the rectus sheath off the muscle during the Pfannenstiel incision stretches the perforating nerve, which is sometimes ligated to provide hemostasis from the accompanying artery. This may leave an area of cutaneous anesthesia.

The iliohypogastric and ilioinguinal nerves pass medial to the anterosuperior iliac spine in the abdominal wall. The former supplies the skin of the suprapubic area. The latter supplies the lower abdominal wall, and by sending a branch through the inguinal canal, it supplies the upper portions of the labia majora and medial portions of the thigh. These nerves can be entrapped in the lateral closure of a transverse incision and may lead to chronic pain syndromes.

The genitofemoral (L1 and L2) and femorocutaneous (L2 and L3) nerves can be injured during gynecologic surgery. The genitofemoral nerve lies on the psoas muscle (see Fig. 5.31), where pressure from a retractor can damage it and lead to anesthesia in the medial thigh and lateral labia. The femoral cutaneous nerve can be compressed either by a retractor blade lateral to the psoas or by too much flexion of the hip in the lithotomy position, causing anesthesia over the anterior thigh.

BIBLIOGRAPHY

Anson BJ. *An atlas of human anatomy.* Philadelphia: WB Saunders, 1950:241.

Burchell RC. Arterial physiology of the human female pelvis. *Obstet Gynecol* 1968;31:855.

Campbell RM. The anatomy and histology of the sacrouterine ligaments. *Am J Obstet Gynecol* 1950;59:1.

Cox HT. The cleavage lines of the skin. *Br J Surg* 1941;29:234.

Curry SL, Wharton JT, Rutledge F. Positive lymph nodes in vulvar squamous carcinoma. *Gynecol Oncol* 1980;9:63.

Dalley AF. The riddle of the sphincters. *Am Surg* 1987;53:298.

Daseler EH, Anson BJ, Reimann AF. Radical excision of the inguinal and iliac lymph glands. *Surg Gynecol Obstet* 1948;87:679.

DeLancey JOL. Anatomic aspects of vaginal eversion after hysterectomy. *Am J Obstet Gynecol* 1992;166:1717.

DeLancey JOL. Correlative study of paraurethral anatomy. *Obstet Gynecol* 1986;68:91.

DeLancey JOL. Structural aspects of the extrinsic continence mechanism. *Obstet Gynecol* 1988;72:296.

DeLancey JOL. Structural support of the urethra as it relates to stress urinary incontinence: the hammock hypothesis. *Am J Obstet Gynecol* 1994;170:1713.

DeLancey JOL, Toglia MR, Perucchini D. Internal and external anal sphincter anatomy as it relates to midline obstetric lacerations. *Obstet Gynecol* 1997;90:924–927.

DeLancey JOL. Structural anatomy of the posterior compartment as it relates to rectocele. *Am J Obstet Gynecol* 1999;180:815–823.

Fernstrom I. Arteriography of the uterine artery. *Acta Radiologica Stockholm* 1955;122(Suppl):21.

Fluhmann CF, Dickmann Z. The basic pattern of the glandular structures of the cervix uteri. *Obstet Gynecol* 1958;11:543.

Forster DS. A note on Scarpa's fascia. *J Anat* 1937;72:130.

Funt MI, Thompson JD, Birch H. Normal vaginal axis. *South Med J* 1978;71:1534.

Goerttler K. Die architektur der muskelwand des menschlichen uterus und ihre funktionelle bedeutung. *Morph Jarb* 1930;65:45.

Goff BH. The surgical anatomy of cystocele and urethrocele with special reference to the pubocervical fascia. *Surg Gynecol Obstet* 1948;87:725.

Hudson CN. Lymphatics of the pelvis. In: Philipp EE, Barnes J, Newton M, eds. *Scientific foundations of obstetrics and gynecology,* 3rd ed. London: Heinemann, 1986:1.

Huffman J. Detailed anatomy of the paraurethral ducts in the adult human female. *Am J Obstet Gynecol* 1948;55:86.

Hughesdon PE. The fibromuscular structure of the cervix and its changes during pregnancy and labour. *J Obstet Gynaecol Br Commonw* 1952;59:763.

Huisman AB. Aspects on the anatomy of the female urethra with special relation to urinary continence. *Contrib Gynecol Obstet* 1983;10:1.

Hurd WW, Bude RO, DeLancey JOL, et al. The location of abdominal wall blood vessels in relationship to abdominal landmarks apparent at laparoscopy. *Am J Obstet Gynecol* 1994;171:642.

Hutch JA. *Anatomy and physiology of the bladder, trigone and urethra.* New York: Appleton-Century-Crofts, 1972.

Klink EW. Perineal nerve block: an anatomic and clinical study in the female. *Obstet Gynecol* 1953;1:137.

Krantz KE. The anatomy of the urethra and anterior vaginal wall. *Am J Obstet Gynecol* 1951;62:374.

Krantz KE. Innervation of the human uterus. *Ann NY Acad Sci* 1959;75:770.

Kuhn RJ, Hollyock VE. Observations on the anatomy of the rectovaginal pouch and septum. *Obstet Gynecol* 1982;59:445.

Lawson JON. Pelvic anatomy. I. Pelvic floor muscles. *Ann R Coll Surg Engl* 1974;54:244.

Lawson JON. Pelvic anatomy. II. Anal canal and associated sphincters. *Ann R Coll Surg Engl* 1974;54:288.

Milley PS, Nichols DH. The relationship between the pubourethral ligaments and the urogenital diaphragm in the human female. *Anat Rec* 1971;170:281.

Milloy FJ, Anson BJ, McAfee DK. The rectus abdominis muscle and the epigastric arteries. *Surg Gynecol Obstet* 1960;110:293.

Morley GW, DeLancey JOL. Sacrospinous ligament fixation for eversion of the vagina. *Am J Obstet Gynecol* 1988;158:872.

Muellner SR. Physiology of micturition. *J Urol* 1951;65:805.

Nesselrod JP. An anatomic restudy of the pelvic lymphatics. *Ann Surg* 1936;104:905.

Nichols DH. Sacrospinous fixation for massive eversion of the vagina. *Am J Obstet Gynecol* 1982;142:901.

Nichols DH, Milley PS, Randall CL. Significance of restoration of normal vaginal depth and axis. *Obstet Gynecol* 1970;36:251.

Nichols DH, Randall CL. *Vaginal surgery,* 3rd ed. Baltimore: Williams & Wilkins, 1989.

O'Connell HE, Hutson JM, Anderson CR, et al. Anatomical relationship between urethra and clitoris. *J Urol* 1998;159:1892–1897.

Oelrich TM. The striated urogenital sphincter muscle in the female. *Anat Rec* 1983;205:223.

Oh C, Kark AE. Anatomy of the external anal sphincter. *Br J Surg* 1972;59:717–723.

Oh C, Kark AE. Anatomy of the perineal body. *Dis Colon Rectum* 1973;16:444.

Parry-Jones E. Lymphatics of the vulva. *J Obstet Gynecol Br Emp* 1963;70:751.

Plentl AA, Friedman EA. *Lymphatic system of the female genitalia.* Philadelphia: WB Saunders, 1971.

Ramsey EM. Vascular anatomy. In: Wynn RM, ed. *Biology of the uterus.* New York: Plenum Press, 1977:60.

Range RL, Woodburne RT. The gross and microscopic anatomy of the transverse cervical ligaments. *Am J Obstet Gynecol* 1964;90:460.

Reiffenstuhl G. The clinical significance of the connective tissue planes and spaces. *Clin Obstet Gynecol* 1982;25:811.

Ricci JV, Lisa JR, Thom CH, et al. The relationship of the vagina to adjacent organs in reconstructive surgery. *Am J Surg* 1947;74:387.

Ricci JV, Thom CH. The myth of a surgically useful fascia in vaginal plastic reconstructions. *Q Rev Surg Obstet Gynecol* 1954;2:253.

Richardson AC, Edmonds PB, Williams NL. Treatment of stress urinary incontinence due to paravaginal fascial defect. *Obstet Gynecol* 1981;57:357.

Roberts WH, Habenicht J, Krishingner G. The pelvic and perineal fasciae and their neural and vascular relationships. *Anat Rec* 1964;149:707.

Roberts, WH, Harrison CW, Mitchell DA, et al. The levator ani muscle and the nerve supply of its puborectalis component. *Clin Anat* 1988;1:256–283.

Roberts WH, Krishinger GL. Comparative study of human internal iliac artery based on Adachi classification. *Anat Rec* 1967;158:191.

Sampson JA. Ureteral fistulae as sequelae of pelvic operations. *Surg Gynecol Obstet* 1909;8:479.

Sato K. A morphological analysis of the nerve supply of the sphincter ani externus, levator ani and coccygeus. *Acta Anat Nippon* 1980;44:187–223.

Schreiber H. Konstruktionsmorphologische Betrachtungen uber den Wandungsbau der menschlichen Vagina. *Arkiv fur Gynaekologie* 1942B43;174:222.

Skandalakis JE, Gray SW, Rowe JS. *Anatomical complications in general surgery.* New York: McGraw-Hill, 1983:297.

Stulz P, Pfeiffer KM. Peripheral nerve injuries resulting from common surgical procedures in the lower portion of the abdomen. *Arch Surg* 1982;117:324.

Tobin CE, Benjamin JA. Anatomic and clinical re-evaluation of Camper's, Scarpa's and Colles' fasciae. *Surg Gynecol Obstet* 1949;88:545.

Uhlenhuth E, Nolley GW. Vaginal fascia, a myth? *Obstet Gynecol* 1957;10:349.

Zacharin RF. The anatomic supports of the female urethra. *Obstet Gynecol* 1968;32:754.

Te Linde's Operative Gynecology, ninth edition, edited by John A. Rock and Howard W. Jones, III. Lippincott Williams & Wilkins, Philadelphia, © 2003.

CHAPTER

6

▼

Preoperative Care

SANFORD M. MARKHAM   JOHN A. ROCK

The preoperative care and management of women prior to gynecologic surgery has proven to be a critical factor in achieving anticipated and successful outcomes of both emergent and scheduled gynecologic surgical procedures. Although the importance of a thorough history and physical examination remain key elements in the preoperative evaluation of all gynecologic patients, the use of "routine" preoperative laboratory evaluation and imaging procedures have undergone considerable change since the last edition of this textbook. This is because of the impact of recent patient care outcome reviews that have focused on indicated preoperative testing compared to "routine" testing. Cost effectiveness and evidence-based medicine are terms that are now commonly used by both the medical professionals and by managed care organizations (MCOs) when ordering and approving preoperative laboratory assessment and imaging tests. This approach makes essential the understanding of what constitutes necessary and essential preoperative testing based on current evidence from both prospective and retrospective studies.

A thorough review of medical sources does not yet provide sufficient controlled trial data to make evidence-based decisions on most preoperative laboratory and imaging testing for gynecologic surgery. Sources such as the Cochrane Library do not currently contain controlled trial studies that relate to cost effectiveness of any gynecologic preoperative testing or procedures. However, significant other case series data do exist that support the need for minimal preoperative testing in the uncomplicated gynecologic patient as well as specific preoperative testing and imaging for the complicated case.

This chapter is designed to provide to gynecologic surgeons an in-depth understanding of the essential features of preoperative care from the preoperative examination in the office, or emergency room, to the time of surgery. Included are suggestions relating to appropriate preoperative testing and evaluation based on the experience of gynecologic surgeons and anesthesiologists. Also included are accumulated data that demonstrate the benefits of preoperative evaluation to patient care. Foremost, it is essential to keep in mind that each woman must be considered individually, based on her medical findings and needs, and that no suggestions can be completely adapted to all women preparing for gynecologic surgery.

IMPORTANCE OF PREOPERATIVE CARE

Successful surgical outcomes of operative gynecologic procedures occur as the result of several factors in addition to good surgical skills and techniques. These factors include:

1. An appropriate preoperative evaluation (the ability to accurately assess and diagnose gynecologic pathology, defects, and injury)

2. An appropriate patient selection (the ability to determine when surgical intervention is a necessary course of action)
3. An appropriate discussion with the patient regarding the benefits and risks of the surgery (the ability to communicate to the patient both short- and long-term complications in a manner that can be understood)
4. An ability to work with MCO organizations in terms of obtaining preoperative approval and complying with individual health care plan guidelines.

Once a gynecologic pathology or defect has been detected and surgical intervention is thought to be the appropriate course of action, surgical planning should be instituted. In nonemergent cases this planning should include a specific time for preoperative evaluation. The purpose of the preoperative evaluation is to accomplish the following tasks as described by Fischer: (a) decrease surgical morbidity; (b) minimize expensive delays and cancellations on the day of surgery; (c) evaluate and optimize patient health status; (d) facilitate the planning of anesthesia and perioperative care; (e) reduce patient anxiety through education; and (f) obtain informed consent. Although these objectives were presented in the context of accomplishing the tasks in a setting of a preoperative evaluation clinic, they are equally applicable to surgical planning in smaller communities where preoperative evaluation clinics are not yet available, provided that the major components of the operating team, specifically the gynecologist, anesthesiologist, and consultants are available.

The importance of effective preoperative evaluations should not be underestimated. Many studies have repeatedly shown that preoperative patient conditions are significant predictors of postoperative morbidity. It is essential that all women undergoing preoperative assessment have a complete history and thorough physical examination as a key element in their work-up. This examination is important to determine factors that could affect surgical outcome. Where medical status questions arise that can not be answered by the gynecologist, then laboratory testing and imaging procedures, as well as consultations, become important to promote optimal outcomes.

In the past, preoperative testing developed around the use of a history and physical examination. Batteries of "routine" individual and multiphasic laboratory tests and imaging procedures were used to detect subclinical or presymptomatic medical problems that might affect the outcomes of the surgical procedure. Additionally, it was felt that less than desirable outcomes of gynecologic surgical procedures could be minimized through the use of a wide battery of tests to prove or disprove normalcy prior to surgery. This reduction in less-than-desirable outcomes might also provide some legal protection.

Unfortunately, the use of multiple "routine" tests has resulted in considerable additional costs for surgery and has created a problem as to what should be done when preoperative test results are found to be unexpectedly abnormal. It has been reported that data from the last two decades indicate 60% to 70% of laboratory tests ordered preoperatively are not required based on a review of the history and/or physical examination. Other studies suggest that only 1% or less of routinely ordered preoperative tests revealed abnormalities that might have influenced perioperative management. Furthermore, between 30% and 60% of all unexpected abnormalities detected by preoperative laboratory tests were not actually noted or investigated before surgery. This fact alone suggests that not only does the ordering of multiple "routine" tests not provide legal protection but quite possibly it also sets up an opportunity for increased legal liability. Finally, the cost of accomplishing these unnecessary preoperative "routine" tests adds many millions of dollars to health-care costs each year without any proven benefit to patient care.

Using this information and applying it to the preoperative assessment of gynecologic surgery patients in the future, a preoperative evaluation should strive to answer the following three questions as outlined by Roizen.

1. Is the patient in optimal health?
2. Can, or should, the patient's physical or mental condition be improved before surgery?
3. Does the patient have health problems or use any medications that could unexpectedly influence perioperative events?

Therefore, all preoperative assessment and care should be directed toward answering these questions, using only those preoperative testing modalities that are expected to give information that leads to answers, as opposed to the random "routine" batteries of tests used in the past.

It is most important to dedicate a portion of the preoperative care time to a discussion with the patient of options for management of her gynecologic problem, including both short- and long-term potential complications. All patients must be given sufficient medical information to allow them to make an educated decision about whether to proceed with the planned surgery. Examples of gynecologic issues that require informed decisions include the recently reported significant increase in urinary incontinence following hysterectomy (60%), or the higher than previously reported failure rate of tubal sterilization (CREST [Collaborative Review of Sterilization] study: 10-year accumulative failure rate of 18.5 per 1,000), or the common recurrence of abnormal uterine bleeding leading to a subsequent hysterectomy in women with a history of abnormal uterine bleeding controlled by oral contraceptive pills who elect to undergo a tubal sterilization (relative risk 1.8). Not only is the discussion time useful in fostering a good physician–patient relationship, but it becomes extremely important if outcomes of surgery are less than expected, particularly if the discussion was documented in the patient's record.

HISTORY AND PHYSICAL EXAMINATION

History

Preoperative care of a patient always begins by carefully taking a complete history and doing a thorough preoperative examination. For the surgeon, the process of history and physical examination are fundamental to good surgical results. The physical and mental preparation of the patient are key to patient satisfaction after surgery. It is essential that the operating gynecologist personally take the history. This personal contact with the patient is of value to both the patient and surgeon. During this time the gynecologist can gain an individual perspective of not only the gynecologic problems but also the patient's general status. The patient can, in turn, ask direct questions relating to the surgical procedure as well as express her concerns. This interchange gives the surgeon a unique impression of the problem and allows the surgeon to better assess the pathology or defect that requires surgery. This places the gynecologist in a much better position to arrive at an accurate diagnosis, determine the essential preoperative testing that will be needed, and select the most appropriate surgery to manage the problem.

Good history taking and a thorough physical examination require time and patience, neither of which is easily available given the expanded demands of gynecologic practice. However, the reward for the gynecologist who takes the time to listen to the patient and accomplish a complete physical examination is the avoidance of unnecessary surgery. Unnecessary operations, particularly for patients already troubled by some difficult problem of life, may prove to be unsuccessful in relieving the patient's symptoms and also concentrate attention unnecessarily on the pelvic organs. If the condition is not urgent, do not make a firm decision regarding recommendation for major pelvic surgery on the first consultation.

Emergent and urgent conditions by necessity require a different approach of rapid assessment and action. In most gynecologic cases, however, the patient is counseled on the need for surgery only after all physical and psychological aspects of her case are thoroughly evaluated. The surgeon who does not ask questions and offer explanations, and who does not carefully consider choices, usually has less than desirable outcomes.

A patient's history should be concise, but accuracy should not be sacrificed for the sake of brevity. It has become a common practice to use a preprinted form when obtaining a history. Unfortunately, no medical form is applicable to every case. Maximum efficiency can be achieved by using a standard patient-completed history form (Fig. 6.1) along with a physician-completed history and physical examination form (Fig. 6.2). The physician can use the patient-completed form to efficiently assimilate the information and direct the history and physical examination process. The physician's history and physical examination form serve as a structured reminder of the essentials of the history-taking process as well as summarize the patient's medical history to facilitate the decision to accomplish surgery. This form additionally serves as a record for Current Procedural Terminology (CPT) coding documentation, as well as for later clinical research. Experience has shown that important omissions are much less frequent when information is compiled on a standard form. Care should be taken, however, to not allow such a form to restrict the accurate recording of the present illness. Forms always can be expanded to document an event in the patient's history that might have an important bearing on the present illness.

A few points should be stressed concerning proper gynecologic history taking. The menstrual history must be accurate and detailed. The clue to a correct diagnosis of the gynecologic condition for which surgery is being considered often appears in the pattern of menstrual irregularity, whether the menstrual disturbance results from an organic lesion or a dysfunctional cause. In fact, differentiation between dysfunctional and early organic disease is one of the most common and difficult clinical distinctions that must be made prior to surgery. Accurate dates of the last and previous menstrual periods are of major importance. When there is a discrepancy between menstrual dates and pelvic findings in a patient of reproductive age, pregnancy should be suspected and a pregnancy test accomplished. A discrepancy between menstrual dates and pelvic findings in a patient with suspected pregnancy requires quantitative human chorionic gonadotropin (hCG) testing to identify appropriate progression of the pregnancy along with a pelvic ultrasound when the pelvic examination and hCG test results are at odds.

Good gynecologic history taking can also provide valuable clues relating to findings in the physical examination. In a woman younger than 50 years of age with a history of maternal diethylstilbestrol (DES) exposure, attention should be paid to the potential presence of a variety of anatomical defects such as a "T-shaped" uterus, vaginal adenosis, or cervical defects ("cock's comb" cervix). A documented history of Type II herpes simplex viral infection of the lower genital tract has long-term implications for future recurrences and symptomatology. Of equal importance to postmenopausal women is obtaining an accurate date of the menopause. Some women are now cycling well into their fifties. Variations in vaginal bleeding in these patients may be of far different importance than vaginal bleeding in a woman 10 to 15 years postmenopausal.

The patient's reproductive history is also of great importance, particularly a history of previous pregnancies and complications of pregnancy such as dystocia, Cesarean section, postpartum infection, abortion, urinary tract infections, excessive infant size, vaginal lacerations, deep vein thrombophlebitis, and pulmonary embolization. A well-taken marital history may reveal dyspareunia and/or unsatisfactory sexual relations, which may explain some symptoms that resemble organic pelvic disease.

Because the symptoms of urinary tract disease so closely resemble those of reproductive tract disease, a complete urologic history is important along with laboratory investigation of the urinary tract before a final diagnosis is determined and a decision made regarding surgery. Too often the symptoms of urinary frequency, urgency, and dysuria are diagnosed as a mechanical support defect of the urinary bladder and treated by surgical repair with plication of the bladder neck, although the real problem of chronic urinary tract infection or neurogenic dysfunction of the bladder remains undiagnosed. Put in another way, a disorder of the lower uri-

B-1b DEPARTMENT OF OBSTETRICS AND GYNECOLOGY
Patient Self History

| DATE |
| HOSP. NO. |
| NAME |
| BIRTH DATE |
| ADDRESS |

● File most recent sheet of this number ON BOTTOM ●

IF NOT IMPRINTED, PLEASE PRINT DATE, HOSP. NO., NAME AND LOCATION

The University of Iowa Hospitals and Clinics requests this information for the purpose of providing patient care. Some questions may seem personal or appear to have no relationship to your care, but your responses are important. This information will help your health care providers to better understand how your health problems are affecting your daily life, and to find out how they can best help to improve your overall health. Your responses will be held in strict confidence. If you have questions or concerns about information on the form, please talk with your health care provider. If you choose not to respond to these items, patient care may be compromised/influenced.

GYNECOLOGIC/OBSTETRIC HISTORY

1. AGE _____
2. When was the first day of your last period? _____/_____/_____
3. Date of most recent pelvic exam? _____/_____/_____ normal / abnormal (please circle)
4. Date of most recent Pap smear? _____/_____/_____ normal / abnormal (please circle)
5. Date of most recent mammogram? _____/_____/_____ normal / abnormal (please circle)
6. ☐ No ☐ Yes   Have you ever been told you had an abnormal Pap smear? If *yes*, when? _____
        If treated, what kind of treatment was done? _____
7. How old were you when you first started your periods? _____
8. Usually, your periods come (came) every _____ days, and last(ed) _____ days.
9. Are/Were your periods usually: ☐ Regular   ☐ Light   ☐ Very painful
             ☐ Irregular   ☐ Moderate   ☐ A little painful
             ☐ Heavy   ☐ Painless
10. ☐ No ☐ Yes   Do you have bleeding between periods? (If *yes*, describe) _____
11. Describe any problems you are currently having (or had) with your periods. _____
12. ☐ No ☐ Yes   Do you need a birth control method today? (For gynecology appointment only)
    (If *no*, move on to question 14)
13. Which method do you want today? _____
14. List current/past birth control methods below:

Methods used	Year started	Year quit	Problems	Reason you stopped using this method

15. Total number of pregnancies _____ Number of living children _____ Age at first pregnancy _____

Year	Length of pregnancy	Losses	Delivery	Complications	
	D-Around due date P-Premature L-Late	A-Abortion M-Miscarriage S-Stillbirth E-Ectopic/(Tubal)	V-Vaginal CS-C-section	**Mother** DM-Diabetes BP-Blood Pressure BL-Bleeding S-Seizures	**Baby** J-Jaundice BD-Birth Defect MR-Mentally Retarded B-Breech
1.					
2.					
3.					
4.					
5.					
6.					
7.					
8.					

16. ☐ No ☐ Yes ☐ Undecided   Are you trying to become pregnant? (For gynecology appointment only)
17. ☐ No ☐ Yes ☐ Undecided   Is it possible you want to have children in the future? (For gynecology appointment only)
18. ☐ No ☐ Yes   Have you had any difficulty becoming pregnant?
         If *yes*, describe _____
19. ☐ No ☐ Yes   Are you currently breast feeding?

76339/4-97   **THE UNIVERSITY OF IOWA HOSPITALS AND CLINICS**

Side tab labels: B -1b | C LABORATORY | D X-RAY EXAM | E CONSULTATION | F SPEC. EXAM | G THERAPY | H PATHOLOGY | I DIAGNOSIS

FIGURE 6.1. Patient history (Hx) form. (From: University of Iowa Hospitals and Clinics, with permission.)

nary tract can produce symptoms suggestive of reproductive tract disease and vice versa. For this reason basic urologic training is advocated for every gynecologist. The gynecologist who is adept with a urologic workup, including cystoscopy and cystometrics, can evaluate a case better than one who must depend entirely on consultation and urology reports.

Symptomatology of gastrointestinal tract disease can also mimic disease of the reproductive tract. Thus, a proper gastrointestinal tract history along with labora-

tory investigation make a significant contribution toward arriving at a correct diagnosis and treatment plan prior to surgical intervention. Constipation, irritable bowel syndrome, colitis, Crohn's disease, and diverticulitis can cause abdominal and pelvic pain that is not dissimilar to the pain of endometriosis, pelvic adhesions, or ovarian neoplasms. Therefore, basic gastrointestinal training is also advocated for all gynecologists. The gynecologist experienced in accomplishing sigmoidoscopy is better prepared to assess gynecologic cases being con-

B-1b PATIENT SELF HISTORY P. 2   Pt. Name _____   Hosp. No. _____

20. Have you had any of the following? Please give approximate dates.

Dates	No	Yes		Dates	No	Yes	
_____	☐	☐	Vaginal infection	_____	☐	☐	Genital herpes
_____	☐	☐	Vaginal itching/dryness/discharge/odor	_____	☐	☐	Gonorrhea
_____	☐	☐	Unusual vaginal bleeding	_____	☐	☐	Chlamydia
_____	☐	☐	Pain/bleeding with intercourse	_____	☐	☐	Syphilis
_____	☐	☐	Hot flashes	_____	☐	☐	Genital warts
_____	☐	☐	Uterine fibroids	_____	☐	☐	HIV / AIDS
_____	☐	☐	Involuntary loss of urine		☐	☐	Group B Strep
_____	☐	☐	Bladder/kidney infection	_____	☐	☐	Partner with any of the above infections
_____	☐	☐	Pelvic inflammatory disease				

MEDICAL/SURGICAL HISTORY

21. Have you **ever had** or do you **currently have** any of the following?

No	Yes		No	Yes	
☐	☐	Diabetes	☐	☐	Blood transfusions (year _____)
☐	☐	High blood pressure	☐	☐	Blood diseases
☐	☐	Chest pain/heart attack	☐	☐	Sickle cell disease
☐	☐	Rheumatic fever	☐	☐	Trauma (such as fractures, concussion)
☐	☐	Heart murmur	☐	☐	Surgery(s) (If yes, what kind?)
☐	☐	Blood clots (in your lungs, brain or heart)			_____ date _____
☐	☐	Stroke			_____ date _____
☐	☐	Anemia	☐	☐	Hospitalization in the last 5 years?
☐	☐	Kidney/Bladder problems			For what reason: _____
☐	☐	Epilepsy/Convulsions			For what reason: _____
☐	☐	Hepatitis/Jaundice	☐	☐	Gall bladder problems
☐	☐	Liver problems	☐	☐	Stomach problems/vomiting
☐	☐	Varicose veins	☐	☐	Blood in stools
☐	☐	Thyroid problems	☐	☐	Constipation/Diarrhea
☐	☐	Tuberculosis	☐	☐	Cancer (If yes, what kind?)
☐	☐	Lived with someone who had Tuberculosis			_____ date _____
☐	☐	Asthma	☐	☐	Physical abuse
☐	☐	Depression	☐	☐	Alcohol dependency
☐	☐	Mental illness and/or suicide attempts	☐	☐	Drug dependency
☐	☐	Breast disease	☐	☐	Intravenous drug use
☐	☐	Migraine headaches	☐	☐	Sexual abuse
☐	☐	Frequent headaches			

IMMUNIZATION HISTORY

☐ No ☐ Yes ☐ Not sure   Have you had the Chicken Pox (Varicella-zoster)?
☐ No ☐ Yes ☐ Not sure   Are you immune to rubella (German measles)?
☐ No ☐ Yes ☐ Not sure   Have you had a hepatitis B vaccination? (3 shots)?
☐ No ☐ Yes ☐ Not sure   Have you had a tetanus shot in the last 10 years?
☐ No ☐ Yes ☐ Not sure   Have you had a recent skin test for TB?

FAMILY HISTORY

22. ☐ No ☐ Yes   Are you adopted?   *If yes, skip and go on to next section (General).*

23. Has anyone in your family had trouble with the following [include mother (M), father (F), brother (B), sister (S), grandfather (GF), grandmother (GM), aunt (A), uncle (U), son (SN), or daughter (D)]. (Place the appropriate initials in any categories that apply.)

No	Yes		Who	No	Yes		Who
☐	☐	Breast cancer	_____	☐	☐	Birth defects	_____
☐	☐	Female organ cancer	_____	☐	☐	Multiple gestation (twins, triplets)	_____
☐	☐	Other cancer	_____	☐	☐	Mother used DES (a medicine	
		If yes, what? _____				to prevent miscarriage)	_____
☐	☐	Diabetes	_____	☐	☐	Hereditary disease	_____
☐	☐	Stroke	_____			If yes, what? _____	
☐	☐	High blood pressure	_____			_____	
☐	☐	Heart attack	_____	☐	☐	Cystic Fibrosis	_____
☐	☐	High cholesterol	_____	☐	☐	Sickle cell disease	_____
☐	☐	Osteoporosis (bone thinning)	_____	☐	☐	Pre eclampsia (high blood pressure in pregnancy)	_____

FIGURE 6.1. *(Continued)*

sidered for surgery than the gynecologist who lacks such experience.

Because abnormal uterine bleeding can result from a variety of endocrine and metabolic disorders, a history of hypothyroidism, hyperprolactemia, insulin metabolism errors, as well as other endocrine and metabolic defects in the patient and in her family are of considerable importance in assessing and treating menorrhagia and metrorrhagia. A positive history followed by appropriate endocrine testing can give physicians significant insight into the etiology of the problem and allow them to institute proper management without always requiring surgery.

Finally, musculoskeletal and neurologic defects of the low back, pelvis, and hips can result in pain similar to that found in gynecologic pathology and disease. Therefore, an orthopedic and neurologic history is an important addition to a thorough gynecologic history.

B-1b DEPARTMENT OF OBSTETRICS AND GYNECOLOGY Patient Self History Page 3	DATE HOSP. NO. NAME BIRTH DATE ADDRESS
● File most recent sheet of this number ON BOTTOM ●	IF NOT IMPRINTED, PLEASE PRINT DATE, HOSP. NO., NAME AND LOCATION

CURRENT MEDICATION HISTORY

24. Please list medications used during the last three months on a routine basis

Name of Medication	Date started	Currently Taking Yes	No	Reason for Taking Medication

25. List any allergies to medications/Latex/Iodine _____

GENERAL HEALTH QUESTIONS

26. ☐ No ☐ Yes   Are you concerned about your eating habits?
27. ☐ No ☐ Yes   Are you concerned with your weight?
28. ☐ No ☐ Yes   Do you currently use WIC (Women's, Infant's and Children's Nutrition program)?
29. ☐ No ☐ Yes   Are you currently using vitamins (or prenatal vitamins)?
30. ☐ No ☐ Yes   Do you drink caffeine (like coffee, colas)?
                   If *yes*, how many cups per day? _____
31. ☐ No ☐ Yes   Do you exercise regularly?
32. ☐ No ☐ Yes   Have you been taught how to do self breast exam?
33. ☐ No ☐ Yes   Do you examine your breasts monthly?
34. ☐ No ☐ Yes   Have you had your cholsterol checked?
                   Year/Results _____
35. ☐ No ☐ Yes   Do you smoke cigarettes?
                   If *yes*, # _____ packs per day for _____ years.
36. ☐ No ☐ Yes   Do other people in your house smoke?
                   If *no*, are you an ex-smoker ☐ No ☐ Yes   Quit _____ years ago.
37. ☐ No ☐ Yes   Do you drink alcohol?
                   If yes, how many drinks, glasses of wine, or beers do you have in one week?
                   (Circle one)   1-2 drinks   3-6 drinks   7-25 drinks   over 25 drinks
38. If you had a baby before, how did you adjust emotionally after delivery of other children?
    ☐ No problem   ☐ Crying, Mood swings   ☐ Depressed   ☐ Never been pregnant
39. If pregnant, how has your mood been so far during pregnancy?
    ☐ No problem   ☐ Have felt depressed, sad, blue or anxious for more than two weeks at a time?
    ☐ Never been pregnant
40. How much help/support do you get from others in your house for day to day activities (for example, housework and childcare)?
    ☐ a lot of help   ☐ Some help   ☐ Little, if any

PLEASE CHECK ANY OF THE FOLLOWING TOPICS TO RECEIVE MORE INFORMATION:

☐ birth control methods   ☐ sexually transmitted disease   ☐ stopping smoking
☐ safer sex practices   ☐ getting pregnant and having   ☐ substance abuse
☐ depression   a healthy baby   ☐ menopause
☐ stress/anxiety reduction   ☐ sexual abuse, incest, or rape   ☐ sexual problems
☐ nutritional counseling   ☐ osteoporosis (bone thinning)   ☐ incontinence (loss of urine)
☐ weight control   ☐ cholsterol
☐ mammograms   ☐ other _____

Patient Signature _____   Date: _____

THE UNIVERSITY OF IOWA HOSPITALS AND CLINICS

(Right margin tabs: B -1b, C, LABORATORY, D, X-RAY EXAM, E, CONSULTATION, F, SPEC. EXAM, G, THERAPY, H, PATHOLOGY, I, DIAGNOSIS)

FIGURE 6.1. *(Continued)*

General Health Examination

Experience has shown that the gynecologist/obstetrician often is the only physician whom a patient consults, particularly if the symptoms of her problem seem to involve the reproductive tract. As such, preoperative care requires a complete physical examination and not just a focused examination on the lower abdomen and pelvis. This complete physical examination should include blood pressure assessment, weight and height measurement, temperature recording, thyroid and neck examination, auscultation of the heart and lungs, examination of the breasts, neurologic and orthopedic assessment, and examination of the abdomen and pelvis. During the physical examination particular attention should be given to evidence of abnormal sexual development; abnormal growth of hair on the face, chest, abdomen, extremities, back, and pubic regions; and to sexual ambiguity of the

B-1b PATIENT SELF HISTORY P. 4   **Pt. Name** _____   **Hosp. No.** _____

It is extremely important that we be able to contact you so that we may notify you of test results, return appointments, or schedule changes. So that we may efficiently do this and maintain confidentiality for you, please check the boxes below that apply to you.

_____ You may send letters to my home.

_____ You may phone me at home and leave messages. My phone number is _____

_____ You may phone me at home, but leave no messages.

_____ You may phone me at work and leave messages. My work phone number is _____

_____ You may phone me at work, but leave no messages.

_____ You may phone me at a number other than home or work. Phone number _____

May we leave messages at this number? _____

Whose number is this? _____

_____ An alternative address that would allow mail to get to me is _____

_____

The best time of day to phone me is _____

Other comments _____

_____

Patient Signature _____   Date _____

FIGURE 6.1. *(Continued)*

external and internal female genitalia. In addition, it is the responsibility of the gynecologist to carry out a critical evaluation of cardiac and pulmonary function prior to the accomplishment of any surgery. The need for additional medical and/or anesthesia consultation must be determined before surgical scheduling to complete the preoperative care assessment.

In any patient who presents with gynecologic disease and has symptoms remotely suggestive of urinary tract infection and/or disease, a meticulously collected, midstream clean-catch, or catheterized urine specimen should be examined and cultures obtained. Past data have suggested that complications of a single catheterization in terms of urinary tract infection or significant bacteriuria is minimal, whereas the complication of performing a gynecologic surgery in the presence of an undetected preexisting urinary tract infection offers a somewhat higher risk. Doing a transurethral catheterization in gynecologic patients with urinary tract symptoms is not considered to be a hazard to the normal bladder and can provide valuable information for the total assessment of gynecologic symptoms.

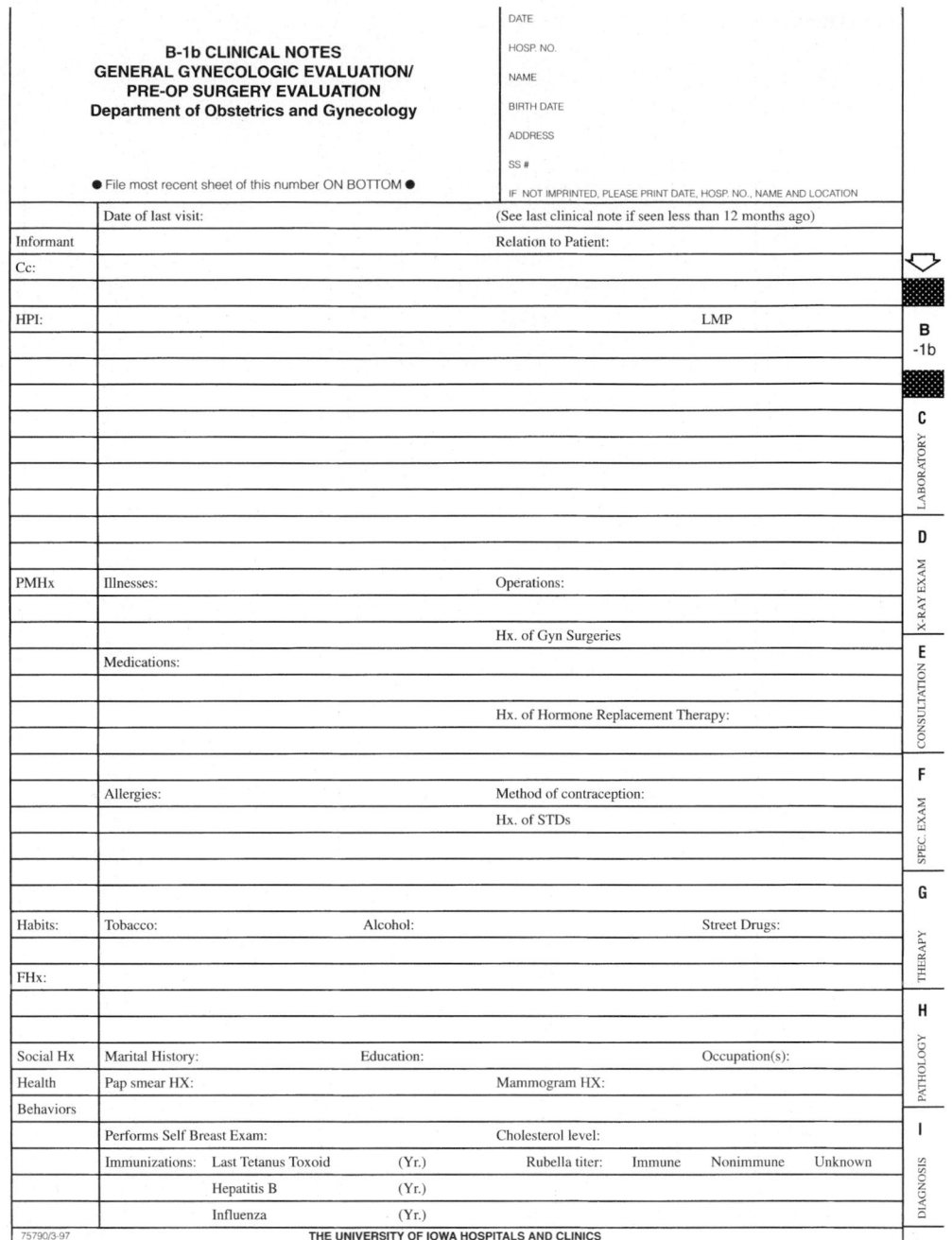

FIGURE 6.2. Physician's history (Hx) and physical examination (PE) form. (From: University of Iowa Hospitals and Clinics, with permission.)

Gynecologic Examination

The gynecologic examination includes a thorough inspection and palpation of the breasts, abdomen, pelvis, and rectum. Ample time should be dedicated to this portion of the preoperative evaluation because defects detected during this examination affects surgical planning. This examination should be completed by the gynecologist performing the surgery rather than by other physicians or staff. In some institutions a gynecologic team approach is used in the preoperative care process, and in such cases the operating gynecologist may not always be the preoperative evaluation gynecologist. In this situation the evaluating and the operating surgeon together must review the completed preoperative evaluation and plan, along with the patient's concerns and wishes. The operating surgeon must then make time before the surgery to meet the patient, review the plan of management with her, and respond to all of her questions.

Gynecology Evaluation (cont'd.)		Pt. Name	Hosp. #
DATE		CLINICAL NOTES	
ROS			
PE	Temp:	Pulse:	BP:
	HEENT		
	Neck		
	Lungs		
	Cardiac		
	Breasts		
	Abdomen		
	Extremities		
	Other		
	Pelvic - External Genitalia		
	Bartholin/Urethra/Skene		
	Vagina		
	Cervix		
	Uterus		
	Adnexa		
	Rectovaginal		
LABS			
	IMPRESSION:		
	PLAN:		
	Date:_____	Signature: _____ M.D.	
	Date:_____	Signature: _____ M.D.	

FIGURE 6.2. *(Continued)*

Breast Examination

The breasts are inspected for symmetry, size, condition of the nipples, the presence of gross lesions, and the presence of discharge. Normal breast tissue, which feels rather shotty to the fingertips, is often erroneously suspected to be tumorous by the patient and is sometimes even misjudged by the physician who is unfamiliar with the proper method of breast palpation. The breasts are examined in both the upright and supine positions for symmetry, contour, and a palpable mass. The supine shoulder of the breast being examined should be raised slightly to bring the lateral aspect of the breast tissue level with the remaining portion of the breast. The arm is then raised above the head to flatten the breast against the thoracic cage. This action permits easy examination of the full thickness of the breast tissue. Examination using the flat ventral surface of the fingers and palm almost always allows identification of an existent significant lesion. Any suspicious lesion is evaluated by mammography, ultrasonography, aspiration, and/or biopsy to confirm or discount the existence of a significant breast pathology. The nipples and adjacent areolar tissue are gently compressed to detect the presence of discharge or secretion (galactorrhea).

Cytologic examination of breast secretions has been reported in the past to be useful in the diagnosis of very early breast carcinoma before the clinical detection of a gross lesion. Current imaging techniques, along with fine needle biopsy offer diagnostic accuracy before abnormal breast secretion is usually experienced, however. Nonetheless, the observation of bilateral secretion showing only the presence of fat cells on an unstained microscopic examination is reassuring and can be accomplished in an office setting. Minimal galactorrhea is not uncommon, particularly in parous women and those in early pregnancy. Other causes of galactorrhea must be considered and include prolactin-secreting tumors of the pituitary, dopamine-agonist medications, birth control pills, and primary hypothyroidism. In these cases galactorrhea is usually found to be bilateral. Unilateral secretion should be evaluated by placing a drop of the secretion on a slide and sending the slide to cytology for examination and diagnosis. The importance of a thorough breast examination is not only to detect a previously undiagnosed breast pathology but also to detect other medical problems (galactorrhea) that could affect the outcome of a planned gynecologic surgery.

Abdominal Examination

Examination of the abdomen requires both visual inspection and palpation. Percussion and auscultation also may be useful. Bulging of the flanks suggests free abdominal fluid, but thin-walled ovarian cysts and irregularly shaped uterine leiomyomas can give a similar clinical picture. Although large ovarian cysts and leiomyomas most often cause protrusion of the anterior abdominal wall, there are a number of confusing exceptions. Palpation for a fluid wave through the lateral quadrants of the abdomen is useful. Percussion for areas of flatness or tympany and for shifting dullness can help determine whether distention is due to intraperitoneal fluid or to intestinal gas. Auscultation is especially useful to differentiate between a large tumor, a distended bowel, or an advanced pregnancy as the cause of abdominal enlargement. When physical findings are conflicting or inconclusive, imaging procedures such as abdominal-pelvic ultrasound or abdominal computed tomography scan or magnetic resonance imaging are quite helpful in completing the assessment of an abnormal abdominal examination.

Areas of tenderness and acute pain should be noted along with the consistency of the pain and whether the pain is experienced with palpation and/or rebound. Location may give some insight into the abdominal organ or tissues involved. Palpation tenderness is more commonly related to pathology of a specific organ, whereas rebound tenderness would suggest peritoneal involvement.

Pelvis and Rectum Examination

An accurate evaluation of the female reproductive tract is essential to establish the underlying cause of gynecologic symptoms. Although a detailed description of a pelvic examination is not provided in this chapter, it is important to stress a few of the steps necessary for proper evaluation of the female pelvis. Before an adequate pelvic examination can be performed, the bladder must be emptied by voiding. A clean-catch specimen is obtained for complete urinalysis and for culture and antibiotic sensitivity studies, if indicated. On the other hand, complaints of urinary incontinence requires examination with a full bladder in the lithotomy and in the erect positions to demonstrate stress incontinence of the urethral sphincter. Inspection of the vulva for gross lesions includes examination of the Bartholin and Skene glands for evidence of cyst formation and purulent exudate as sources of gynecologic infection. Particular attention is given to the mons pubis and labia majora and minora for subtle changes in skin pigmentation, for vesicle formation, and for small, raised lesions that may be evidence of viral or bacterial infection or of early neoplasia. The outlet is closely inspected for relaxation of the anterior and posterior vaginal walls and for uterine descensus. The vaginal mucosa is observed for any visible lesions, evidence of infection, and for estrogen effect. The patient is asked to bear down and cough without the use of a tenaculum to demonstrate the degree of relaxation of the anterior and posterior vaginal walls and the extent of uterine descensus. The urethra is compressed along its entire length to assess the possibility of a suburethral diverticulum, which often is manifested by a purulent discharge from the urethral meatus or a tender suburethral mass.

The cervix is evaluated for abnormal gross pathology, particularly ulceration, neoplastic growths, inflammation, and abnormal discharge. A Papanicolaou smear is obtained by a combined sampling of cells taken from the portio of the cervix by means of a flat stick, and from the endocervical canal by means of a small circular brush. This type of combined cytologic smear is extremely valuable in detecting cervical and endocervical lesions and is always a part of a complete gynecologic examination. Pelvic surgery always should be preceded by a recent cytologic study of the cervix. Patients with abnormal Papanicolaou smears showing repeated mild dysplasia or moderate to severe squamous cell dysplasia should be evaluated by colposcopy and suspicious lesions should be biopsied. Abnormal smears showing glandular cell dysplasia require both an endocervical and endometrial evaluation such as an endocervical curettage and endometrial biopsy before proceeding to pelvic surgery. A negative Papanicolaou smear does not, however, exclude the possibility of a cervical, endocervical, or endometrial neoplasm. False-negative cervical smears have been reported. Because 80% to 90% of all preclinical malignancies of the cervix demonstrate no significant gross lesion, it is impossible to be certain of the condition of the cervix without a Papanicolaou smear or a colposcopy and a colposcopically directed cervical biopsy if lesions are identified. The use of 3% acetic acid or Lugol's (strong iodine solution) staining of the cervix may be beneficial in identifying lesions for biopsy.

The uterus is examined bimanually by the abdominal-vaginal route for position, size, mobility, irregularity, and tenderness to motion. Both adnexal regions are evaluated vaginally and by rectovaginal examination. The rectal examination should never be omitted from the routine pelvic examination. Rectal examinations provide information that cannot be obtained through the vaginal examination alone. The rectal examination provides insight into the competence of the anal sphincter as well the presence of lesions of the anal canal and lower rectum. The rectal and vaginal examinations together are an effective method for detecting pelvic pathology and are especially useful for evaluating the broad and uterosacral ligaments, cul-de-sac of Douglas, uterus, and adnexa. The index finger is inserted into the vagina while the middle finger is inserted into the rectum to a higher level than is possible with the vaginal index finger (see Fig. 6.3). This method offers the most effective opportunity of evaluating the ovaries, posterior cul-de-sac, and posterior aspect of the broad ligament. When pelvic findings are doubtful or inconclusive, imaging techniques may be helpful in determining the preoperative diagnosis. When imaging techniques are inconclusive or unavailable, however, a more adequate examination may be performed under general anesthesia before a final decision for or against gynecologic surgery is made. Indeed, a complete pelvic examination always should precede any gynecologic surgery, whether it be major or minor. The pelvic organ findings of this examination should be described carefully in the operative note for future reference. Suspected pelvic pathology frequently can be ruled in or out after a thorough preoperative pelvic examination, and needless laparotomy or laparoscopy can be avoided. The most common area of clinical confusion occurs in determining the presence of an ovarian cyst, which can be confused with bowel, bladder, or uterine leiomyomas. If a normal ovary is palpated and a cyst not identified by imaging techniques such as pelvic ultrasound, an unnecessary operative procedure frequently can be spared.

LABORATORY ASSESSMENT

Prior to the era of evidence-based medicine most patients undergoing gynecologic surgery were assessed by a thorough history and physical examination followed by a battery of laboratory tests, the purpose of which was to detect a medical disease or defect that could adversely affect surgical outcome. These tests were accomplished on almost all patients, irrespective of age or concurrent medical or surgical pathologies, and might include: (a) blood count with hemoglobin and hematocrit; (b) urinalysis; (c) coagulation studies; (d) chemistry panel; (e) chest x-ray; and (f) electrocardiogram. This relatively universal use of "routine" preoperative testing has not proven to be beneficial in terms of good patient care and, additionally, it has added significantly to the cost of medical care. In one study an average of 72.5% of preoperative tests ordered by surgeons were considered unnecessary based on a review of the patient's history and physical examination. This same study suggested a medical care savings of between 4 and 10 billion dollars per year in the United States by eliminating these unnecessary tests with no adverse effect on outcome.

Over the last 10 years data has surfaced allowing gynecologists to better assess needed preoperative tests from those that in the past were labeled as "routine" tests. Because of information such as this and because of pressures from MCOs, the volume of preoperative testing has been reduced. With this reduction in the ordering of unnecessary tests, however, comes a reduction in the ordering of necessary tests. This finding emphasizes the need to accurately differentiate between indicated preoperative testing and the past practice of routine blanketed testing of gynecologic patients preparing for surgery. A large portion of the remainder of this chapter focuses on the best case series data to help guide the gynecologist when ordering appropriate preoperative tests

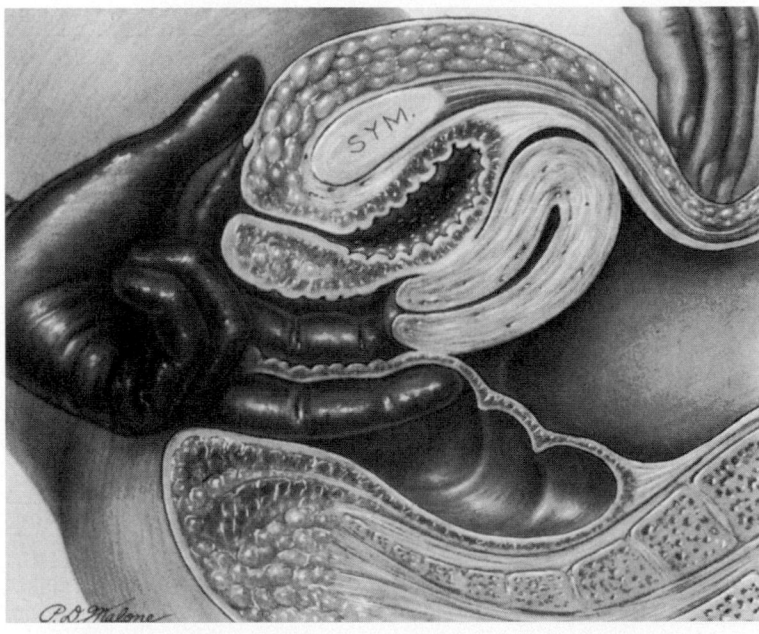

FIGURE 6.3. Rectovaginal-abdominal examination.

TABLE 6.1.

Classification of Physical Status, Established by the American Society of Anesthesiologists

Class	Description
P1	A normal healthy patient
P2	A patient with mild systemic disease
P3	A patient with severe systemic disease
P4	A patient with severe systemic disease that is a constant threat to life
P5	A moribund patient who is not expected to survive without the operation
P6	A declared brain-dead patient whose organs are being removed for donor purposes

From: *ASA Manual for Anesthesia Department Organization and Management, American Society of Anesthesiologists,* Park Ridge, Ill., 1995, with permission.

based on the individual patient's history and physical examination.

Key to the understanding of appropriate preoperative testing is an understanding of: (a) the risk category of the patient; and (b) the degree of complexity of the planned surgery. The risk category of any preoperative gynecology patient may be divided into one of six different classes as established by the American Society of Anesthesiologists (Table 6.1). The degree of complexity of the planned surgery may be divided into one of three separate types (Table 6.2). Therefore, preoperative testing should be planned around the assessed risk of the patient based on her age, history and physical examination, and the degree of complexity based on the invasiveness of the proposed surgery. Therefore, current data as well as experience suggest that, rather than a routine set of tests, all preoperative testing should be inextricably related to the type and complexity of the proposed gynecologic surgery and to the presence of the confounding medical or surgical condition.

Asymptomatic Patients

In an extensive review of currently available evidence on the value of routine preoperative testing in healthy or asymptomatic patients, Monro (1997) found that there were no controlled trials assessing the value of basic tests previously thought to be essential in presurgical evaluation and care. These tests included chest x-ray, electrocardiogram, blood counts and hemoglobin, coagulation studies, blood chemistries, and urinalysis. The authors further noted that all currently available evidence on preoperative testing of healthy or asymptomatic patients came only from case series studies. After reviewing all of the available case series data they concluded that the power of preoperative tests to predict adverse postoperative outcomes in asymptomatic patients is either weak or nonexistent.

Conclusions such as this have resulted in: (a) a marked reduction in the recommendation of routine testing; and (b) the suggestion that the amount of routine testing of preoperative healthy asymptomatic patients be related to the patient's age. Currently, in this category of patients, it has been recommended that a hemoglobin or hematocrit be accomplished on all patients over the age of 6 months; an electrocardiogram (ECG) on all patients over the age of 40; and a blood urea nitrogen (BUN) test and a glucose test on all patients over the age of 65. Additionally, a pregnancy test should be accomplished on all reproductive-age women who are at risk of early pregnancy (sexually active, no contraception, or questionably effective contraception) (Table 6.3).

TABLE 6.2.

Types of Surgical Procedures for Which Anesthesia May Be Administered

Type	General Definition	Special Examples
Type A	*Minimally invasive* procedures that have little potential to disrupt normal physiology and are associated with only rare periprocedural morbidity related to anesthesia. These procedures rarely require blood administration, invasive monitoring, and/or postoperative management in critical care setting.	Cataract extraction, diagnostic arthroscopy, postpartum tubal ligation
Type B	*Moderately invasive* procedures that have a modest or intermediate . potential to disrupt normal physiology. These procedures may require blood administration, invasive monitoring, or postoperative management in a critical care setting.	Carotid endarterectomy, transurethral resection of the prostate, and laparoscopic cholecystectomy
Type C	*Highly invasive* procedures that typically produce significant disruption of normal physiology. These procedures commonly require blood administration, or postoperative management in a critical care setting.	Total hip replacement, open aortic aneurysm, aortic valve replacement, and posterior fossa craniotomy for aneurysm

From: Roizen MF, Foss JF, Fischer SP. Preoperative evaluation. In: Miller RD, ed. *Anesthesia,* 5th ed. Philadelphia: Churchill Livingstone, 2000:843, with permission.

TABLE 6.3.
Recommended Preoperative Testing for
Healthy Asymptomatic Gynecologic Patients

Above Age 6 Months[a]	Above Age 40[a]	Above Age 65[a]
Hct or Hbg	Hct or Hbg	Hct or Hbg
	ECG	ECG
		BUN/glucose

All Women in Reproductive Age, Sexually Active, Questionable Contraception
Pregnancy test

[a] Recommendation of MF Roizen, Preoperative evaluation. In: Miller RD, ed. *Anesthesia*, 5th ed. Philadelphia: Churchill Livingstone, 2000:854, with permission.

Symptomatic Patients and Patients with Medical or Surgical Pathologies or Defects

Women considered for gynecologic surgery who are symptomatic and/or have other medical or surgical pathologies or defects must be considered in a different light from asymptomatic, healthy women during their preoperative evaluation and testing. Preoperative testing should be accomplished to determine the current status of medical or surgical pathologies and provide data on the potential effect that the compounding problem will have on the outcome of the proposed surgery. This would allow, if possible, for necessary medical correction or improvement of the problem prior to surgery in an attempt to minimize adverse outcomes of surgical intervention.

Despite the lack of an evidence-based, preoperative evaluation plan to guide preoperative testing, experience supports adopting a diagnosis-based preoperative testing protocol when planning any gynecologic surgery. A number of diagnosed-based or clinical condition-based protocols have been suggested. Because the diagnosed-based preoperative testing evaluation recommended by Fischer considers both clinical outcomes as well as cost-effectiveness, it is most appropriate in the preoperative evaluation of gynecologic patients who are other than healthy and asymptomatic (Table 6.4). This approach links necessary preoperative laboratory and imaging testing with concurrent medical disease, including cardiovascular, pulmonary, and endocrine pathologies, as well as with malignancies, and the use of many common drug therapies.

PREOPERATIVE EVALUATION: OVERVIEW

The outcome of pelvic surgery depends largely on four preoperative factors.

1. The skill and judgment of the gynecologic surgeon
2. The surgical correctability of the gynecologic abnormality or disease process
3. The severity, stability, and reversibility of concurrent medical/surgical pathologies
4. The availability of experienced support professionals for consultation as indicated, specifically from anesthesia, medicine, and surgery

Preoperative evaluation and care of the women undergoing gynecologic surgery must include not only a thorough physical assessment but also correction or stabilization of any concurrent medical or surgical pathologies that could adversely affect the surgical outcome. A skilled and appropriate gynecologic surgical procedure can have an undesirable outcome because of an unstable condition or incompletely prepared patient.

For this reason, when the preoperative history, physical examination, or laboratory testing reveals instability of the cardiovascular, pulmonary, renal, or hematologic systems, a consultation should be considered. The intent is to achieve maximal stabilization before surgery. If the patient can not be stabilized, then delaying or postponing the surgery must be considered based on the risk and benefit of the surgical procedure for the patient. A preoperative diminished cardiac, pulmonary or renal reserve, a blood coagulopathy, or dehydration and/or hypovolemia can play a critical role in the outcome of the surgery.

Particular attention must be given to the senior gynecologic patient. Not only does this group of women represent the fastest growing segment of gynecologic patients, but they also are more frequently prone to have other medical issues that can affect the outcome of gynecologic surgery. The US Department of Health and Human Services has recently noted that the US population over the age of 65 was growing faster than the population as a whole. They stated that currently 13 out of every 100 Americans are 65 years of age or older, and in 2030 this number will increase to 20 out of 100. They additionally noted that there were significantly more women than men in this older population, with women comprising 59% of the group aged 65 years and older and 71% of those aged 85 years and older. Considerable data as well as experience have shown that this group of senior gynecologic patients has significantly greater health care problems and therefore will require a greater effort in the preoperative evaluation in terms of laboratory evaluation and consultation.

With this increase in concurrent medical and surgical problems, and the resulting increase in operative risks of gynecologic surgery in the senior population, it is important to note that chronologic age, by itself, is not always an accurate indicator of organ function. Atheromatous changes of the cardiovascular system are uncommon in women until well past menopause. This biologic phenomenon is just one of the many factors that promote female (compared with male) longevity. The average female life expectancy in 1997 was just under 80 years. As a consequence of increased longevity, a high percentage of women are in the postmenopausal period of their life when gynecologic disease becomes more prevalent and surgery becomes more necessary. In spite

TABLE 6.4.
Diagnosed-based Preoperative Testing

Preoperative Diagnosis	ECG	CXR	Hct/Hb	CBC	Lytes	Renal	Glucose	Coag	LFTs	Rx Levels	Ca+
Cardiac disease											
MI history	X				±						
Stable angina	X				±						
CHF	X	±				±					
HTN	X	±			X[a]	X					
Chronic atrial fib	X									X[b]	
Periph vascular disease	X										
Valvular heart disease	X	±									
Pulmonary disease											
Emphysema	X	±								X[c]	
Asthma											
Chronic bronchitis	X	±		X							
Diabetes	X				±	X	X				
Hepatic disease											
Infectious hepatitis								X	X		
Alcohol/drug induced								X	X		
Tumor infiltration								X	X		
Renal disease			X		X	X					
Hematological disorders				X							
Coagulopathies				X				X			
CNS disorders											
Stroke	X			X	X		X			X	
Seizures	X			X	X		X			X	
Tumor	X			X							
Vascular/aneurysms	X		X								
Malignancy				X							
Hyperthyroidism	X		X		X						X
Hypothyroidism	X		X		X						
Cushing's syndrome				X	X		X				
Addison's disease				X	X		X				
Hyperparathyroidism	X		X		X						X
Hypoparathyroidism	X										X
Morbid obesity	X	±					X				
Malabsorption/poor nutrition	X			X	X	X	X	±			
Select drug therapies											
Digoxin (Digitalis)	X				±					X	
Anticoagulants			X					X			
Dilantin										X	
Phenobarbital										X	
Diuretics					X	X					
Steroids				X			X				
Chemotherapy				X							
Aspirin/NSAID											
Theophylline										X	

X = Obtained.

± = Consider.

[a] Patients on diuretics.

[b] Patients on digoxin.

[c] Patients on theophyilline.

From: Fischer SP. Cost-effective preoperative evaluation and testing. *Chest* 1999;115:98S, with permission.

of the increased concurrent medical and surgical problems and greater operative risks, excellent surgical skills, meticulous medical control of concurrent disease, and anesthesia carefully attuned to the physiologic requirements of the senior gynecologic patient have kept the risk of surgery at a level not much greater than that for the premenopausal patient.

Guidelines for the preoperative evaluation of the gynecologic patient may be divided into three separate areas.

1. Uncomplicated gynecologic pathology with an uncomplicated medical/surgical status
2. Complicated gynecologic pathology with uncomplicated medical/surgical status

3. Uncomplicated or complicated gynecologic pathology with a complicated medical/surgical status

The following preoperative evaluation recommendations are made based on the most current data from case series studies, evidence-based medical data, and consensus opinions of gynecologic preoperative care.

PREOPERATIVE EVALUATION, UNCOMPLICATED GYNECOLOGIC PATHOLOGY, UNCOMPLICATED MEDICAL/SURGICAL STATUS

A gynecologic patient who has an uncomplicated gynecologic pathology and no concurrent medical or surgical conditions that would affect surgical outcome should undergo the following preoperative evaluation.

1. Thorough history
2. Complete physical examination
3. Hematocrit or hemoglobin if over 6 months of age
4. Electrocardiogram if over 40 years of age
5. Blood urea nitrogen and glucose if over 65 years of age
6. Pregnancy test if in the reproductive age, sexually active and not on contraception or if using questionably effective contraception
7. Sexually transmitted diseases testing (chlamydia, gonococcus, syphilis, hepatitis, and human immunodeficiency virus [HIV]) with suspected or documented exposure
8. Blood type and screen if the potential exists for more than minimal surgical blood loss

PREOPERATIVE EVALUATION, COMPLICATED GYNECOLOGIC PATHOLOGY, UNCOMPLICATED MEDICAL/SURGICAL STATUS

A gynecologic patient who has a complicated gynecologic pathology and no concurrent medical or surgical conditions that would additionally affect surgical outcome should undergo the following preoperative evaluation (complicated gynecologic pathology includes past abdominal/pelvic surgery with evidence of or anticipation of pelvic adhesive disease, tumors, or cysts of a size making surgery more difficult or complicated; suspected or proven cancerous lesions; concurrent infection of the reproductive tract; active or chronic bleeding from the reproductive tract resulting in a demonstrated or highly probable hematologic instability).

1. Thorough history
2. Complete physical examination
3. Laboratory testing listed under uncomplicated gynecologic pathology
4. White blood cell (WBC) count with suspected or evidence of pelvic infection
5. Prothrombin time (PT) and partial thromboplastin time (PTT) with hemorrhage or anemia

6. Platelet count with hemorrhage or anemia or with a recent history of radiation or chemotherapy
7. Liver function tests and renal tests with any suspected hepatic or renal pathology
8. Type and cross match in an anticipated bloody surgery, otherwise only a type and screen
9. Anesthesia consultation

PREOPERATIVE EVALUATION, UNCOMPLICATED OR COMPLICATED GYNECOLOGIC PATHOLOGY, COMPLICATED MEDICAL/SURGICAL STATUS

A gynecologic patient who has either an uncomplicated or complicated gynecologic pathology and a concurrent medical or surgical problem offers the greatest risk for gynecologic surgery (concurrent medical or surgical problem includes cardiac, pulmonary, vascular, renal, intestinal, endocrine, neurologic, orthopedic pathologies as well as use of medications for these defects). These patients should undergo the following preoperative evaluation.

1. Thorough history
2. Complete physical examination
3. Laboratory testing listed under uncomplicated gynecologic pathology
4. Laboratory testing listed under complicated gynecologic pathology
5. WBC with suspected infection outside of the pelvis or with immunosuppressive therapy, anemias, white blood cell pathologies, steroid therapy, or collagen diseases
6. PT/PTT with any suspected or known coagulation defect, history of thrombosis or embolization, anticoagulation therapy, liver or intestinal disease
7. Platelet count with any suspected or known platelet pathology, leukemia, or splenic defect
8. Liver function tests, renal function tests, electrolytes, and/or blood sugars in women with renal, liver, or intestinal disease, on diuretics, with an unexplained fever, with endocrine disease, including diabetes, hypoglycemia, parathyroid disease, adrenal and pituitary disease, or with a recent history of radiation or chemotherapy
9. Electrocardiogram with suspected or known cardiac pathology
10. Anesthesia consultation
11. Medicine, cardiology, pulmonary medicine, endocrinology, urology, and surgery consultation as indicated

PREOPERATIVE MANAGEMENT AND PREPARATION

Preoperative care includes not only preoperative evaluation and laboratory testing, but also any medical or gynecologic management in the months preceding the surgical procedure to help achieve maximal physical status.

Achieving this goal is rewarded by a less complicated surgical procedure with better outcomes. Examples of this medical or gynecologic management includes a number of options. Ovarian suppression through the use of a gonadotropin-releasing hormone agonist in the 3 months before surgery has proven to be beneficial in hysteroscopic resection of uterine submucous leiomyomas larger than 2 cm in size and in myomectomies when the uterine volume is equivalent to or larger than a 12-week pregnant uterus size. A similar suppression is also useful in decreasing the thickness of the endometrial lining in an endometrial ablation, although an endometrial suction curettage can achieve a somewhat similar result. Perioperative antibiotic treatment of postmenopausal women undergoing reparative surgery for genital prolapse can be beneficial in reducing recurrent cystitis but has not been shown to significantly alter the outcome of surgery.

Use of preoperative vaginal estrogen cream starting 4 to 6 weeks before surgery may help in controlling uropathogens as well as thickening the vaginal mucosa, which results in an easier dissection of the vagina and in reducing postoperative morbidity. Routine preoperative endometrial sampling before hysterectomy has not been found to be cost effective unless there is suspicion of endometrial pathology such as manifested by abnormal perimenopausal or menopausal bleeding or the presence of abnormal glandular cells on Papanicolaou smear. In the latter case endocervical sampling additionally is necessary.

Another area of preoperative planning requiring an experienced decision by the gynecologist and possibly the anesthesiologist is the regulation of medications taken by the patient prior to surgery. When and how to modify insulin in diabetic women, surgery on women taking anticoagulants, and continuation or discontinuation of birth control pills are examples of issues that must be addressed in the preoperative period and conveyed to the patient in a manner that she understands. Because of the uniqueness of each patient it is not possible to provide a table of preoperative medication management that can be applied to every patient. However, some general suggestions serve as guidelines in the preoperative management of the more common concurrent diseases.

Preoperative insulin control in patients with diabetes is thought to be essential to achieve good surgical outcome. Older animal data has shown a relationship between hyperglycemia and wound healing with reduced tensile strength and wound failure. Experience has suggested a similar relationship in the gynecologic patient. It is therefore important to co-manage each diabetic woman undergoing gynecologic surgery with her primary care physician or internist to achieve this optimal control, and once achieved to continue the insulin regime right up to the time of surgery. Every attempt should be made to schedule the diabetic patient's surgery as a first morning case to minimize the time period between the patient's last oral intake and the onset of the surgical procedure. A protocol for patient preoperative management of insulin regulation may be found in Table

---

TABLE 6.5.
Recommendation for Preoperative Insulin Management
Classic "Nontight Control" Regimen of Roizen

1. Day before surgery: Patient should be given nothing by mouth after midnight; a 13-ounce glass of clear orange juice should be at the bedside or in the car for emergency use.
2. At 6 a.m. on the day of surgery, institute intravenous fluids using plastic cannulae and a solution containing 5% dextrose, infused at a rate of 125 mL/h/70 kg body weight.
3. After institution of intravenous infusion, give one-half the usual morning insulin dose (and usual type of insulin) subcutaneously.
4. Continue 5% dextrose solutions through operative period, giving at least 125 mL/h/70 kg body weight.
5. In recovery room, monitor blood glucose concentration and treat on a sliding scale.

Roizen MF. Anesthetic implications of concurrent diseases. In: Miller RD, ed. *Anesthesia*, 5th ed. Philadelphia: Churchill Livingstone, 2000:903, with permission.

6.5. Patients who are scheduled for gynecologic surgery who are on coumadin (warfarin), heparin or low-molecular-weight heparin (LMWH) represent another preoperative management issue. A number of options are available for converting the patient from warfarin to heparin. Experience has suggested that stopping the warfarin 4 to 5 days prior to the planned gynecologic surgery and at the same time converting to low dose heparin 5,000 U subcutaneously every 12 hours provides satisfactory anticoagulation protection. The low-dose heparin can be continued postoperatively until the patient is back on oral feeding, at which time the warfarin can be reinitiated. It is further suggested that these women use elastic stockings or intermittent pneumatic compression (IPC) at the beginning of the surgery and continue with this mechanical support through to the point of full postoperative ambulation.

Another preoperative medication issue involves the continuation or discontinuation of oral contraceptive pills prior to gynecologic surgery. Studies in the 1970s suggested a relationship between use of preoperative oral contraceptive pills and intraoperative or postoperative venous thrombosis. For this reason it has been the practice to discontinue oral contraceptive pills 2 to 4 weeks before surgery and convert to mechanical contraception. This practice, however, is unsupported by any current prospective controlled studies and places the patient at risk for unwanted pregnancy as well as menstrual irregularities. Therefore, routine discontinuation of oral contraception prior to gynecologic surgery is not recommended, but instead mechanical venous support such as elastic stockings or intermittent pneumatic compression be used at the time of surgery.

The immediate preoperative preparation of the patient includes the preoperative examination by the gynecologic surgeon and the anesthesia assessment in the anesthesia preoperative clinic or by an individual anesthesiologist. In most cases the assessment for anesthesia risks is accomplished before the day of surgery. If significant anesthesia risk is present, such as cardiovascular or pulmonary pathology, this allows time for relevant information to be obtained, additional testing accomplished, other consultation carried out, and treatment instituted in an attempt to have the patient in optimal condition on the day of surgery. In some cases involving low-risk ambulatory procedures, however, the anesthesia assessment is accomplished on the day of surgery. Experience suggests that an open dialog between the gynecologic surgeon and the anesthesiologist regarding the planned surgery is an essential element in achieving a successful outcome with the lowest patient risk.

Most gynecologic surgical patients are admitted on the day of surgery. Because of this, preoperative guidelines and instructions for patient activity and actions at home are important and need to be made clear to every patient. The goal is to have the patient rested and in the optimal physical condition with an empty stomach and reduced contents in the lower gastrointestinal tract at the time of surgery. There is no evidence to support the idea that marked reduction of activity on the day before surgery is beneficial; however, it would be reasonable to recommend planning activities so that the patient is not overstressed. Food intake on the day before surgery need not be restricted except for the evening meal before the morning of surgery, which should be light and easily digestible. An overloaded intestinal tract during surgery is particularly hazardous not only because it poses an anesthetic risk but also because it increases postoperative nausea and gas formation. The patient should be instructed to not eat or drink after midnight on the evening before surgery unless the surgery is scheduled for the late afternoon. Some exceptions to this rule might occur with the taking of indicated medications with water. Such an exception should be discussed between the gynecologist and the anesthesiologist in the preoperative evaluation sessions. Women who are scheduled for a late afternoon surgery may have a light breakfast of a liquid diet if taken no fewer than 6 hours preoperatively.

Women undergoing major abdominal surgery in which bowel entry or injury is anticipated (or is a high probability) should undergo a complete bowel prep. This bowel preparation should consist of the single use of a commercially available cleansing preparation such as GoLYTELY or NuLYTELY (Braintree Laboratories, Inc., Braintree, MA). In all other major abdominal cases the lower colon should be cleansed by a preoperative enema the evening before surgery. If the colon is not completely emptied, then a repeat enema may need to be given prior to performing the operation, allowing adequate time for evacuation. The patient needs to be given careful instructions for the use of enemas at home and the possible need for a repeat enema in the hospital prior to surgery. This issue is often overlooked in preoperative care and results in a more difficult surgical procedure because of space limitation and a less comfortable patient in the postoperative period. An adequate night's rest before surgery is also important for the patient. In some cases the use of a mild sedative is advisable.

Preoperative prophylactic broad-spectrum antibiotics or surgical antimicrobial prophylaxis has frequently been used in gynecologic surgery on the basis of the potential for vaginal flora contamination of the operative field and because of the close proximity of the rectum and intestinal tract. Data do not support the routine use of preoperative broad-spectrum antibiotics in uncomplicated, noninfected gynecologic surgery except in the case of vaginal hysterectomy or possibly abdominal hysterectomy. In these procedures the occurrence of postoperative cuff cellulitis and pelvic abscess has been significantly reduced with use of a preoperative antibiotic. First-, second-, or third-generation cephalosporins (e.g., cefazolin, cefotetan, or cefotaxime, 2 g i.m./i.v.) are effective as a prophylactic coverage, as are many of the semisynthetic penicillin family (e.g., ampicillin 1g i.m./i.v.) or the semisynthetic broad spectrum B-lactamase penicillin combinations (e.g., piperacillin tazobactam 3.75 g i.v. or ticarcillin clavulanate 3.1 g i.v.). When used, the prophylactic antibiotic should be given as a single dose approximately 1 to 2 hours prior to beginning surgery and may be repeated if the operation lasts longer than 3 hours or if there is significant blood loss (in excess of 1,500 mL). If the preoperative examination and testing identifies vaginal infections such as bacterial vaginosis, treatment prior to surgery with metronidazole intravaginal gel (0.75%) or clindamycin vaginal cream (2%) should be accomplished. In like manner, any sexually transmitted disease discovered during preoperative examination and testing should be fully treated prior to surgery.

Infections occurring after surgery in the female reproductive tract arise from the introduction of normal vaginal flora into the surgical field. Surgery on the reproductive tract accomplished through a bacteriologically contaminated field (e.g., the vagina), seeds bacteria into the pedicles and surgical margins of pelvic tissues and provides an excellent nidus for infection in devitalized tissue beds. Therefore, pelvic surgery provides an ideal condition for aerobic (principally polymicrobial rather than monomicrobial) infections. Tissue destruction and sutures lowers the tissue oxidation-reduction (redox) potential. Lower tissue oxygen levels enhance the growth of facultative anaerobes that normally inhabit the vagina. As tissue hypoxia progresses, primary anaerobic bacteria survive and proliferate. Therefore, the usual postoperative infection in the vaginal vault, although initially polymicrobial, usually can be prevented with the use of the preoperative prophylactic antibiotic when the vaginal apex has been opened during a vaginal or abdominal hysterectomy.

Although prophylactic antibiotics are effective in reducing the incidence of postoperative infectious morbidity, they should never be used as a substitute for the time-honored principles of adequate hemostasis and gentle handling of tissue. Despite Wangensteen's disparaging statement that, "antibiotics will turn a third-class surgeon into a second-class surgeon, but will never turn a second-class surgeon into a first-class surgeon," current data suggest that even in the hands of a highly skilled surgeon prophylactic preoperative antibiotics offer improved outcomes in gynecologic pelvic surgery such as vaginal and abdominal hysterectomy.

PREOPERATIVE PROCEDURES IN THE OPERATING SUITE

Just prior to surgery the patient is brought to the operating theater and transferred either directly to the operating table in the operating room or to an operating table in the anesthesia room adjoining the surgical suite. Preoperative preparation includes any trimming of pubic hair, preparation of abdominal and vaginal skin, and placement of a catheter, if indicated. Preoperative shaving of pubic and abdominal hair prior to gynecologic surgery is generally not recommended; in fact, preoperative shaving is associated with a significantly higher surgical site infection (SSI) rate, particularly if completed the night before the operation. These guidelines note studies showing SSI rates of 5.6% in patients who had hair removed by shaving compared to 0.6% in those who had no hair removed. Furthermore, shaving the night before surgery resulted in a significantly higher rate of SSI than shaving just before the operative procedure (7.1% versus 3.1%). Experience has shown that in some gynecologic procedures removal of pubic and abdominal hair is useful, and in these situations hair clipping is recommended immediately before the surgery.

After hair trimming and catheterization, the patient is usually sufficiently anesthetized for a careful bimanual pelvic examination, at which time the surgeon can obtain very valuable information not easily obtainable when the patient is awake. Detection of reduced mobility, identification of cysts or masses not previously known, and determination of the position of pelvic organs not appreciated in past examinations may persuade the gynecologist to alter the planned surgical approach or incision type. After the pelvic examination, the perineum and vagina are cleansed, followed by the abdominal preparation.

The pelvic cleansing should be accomplished before all pelvic or abdominal surgery. There is always the possibility that findings at the time of operation may make a total abdominal hysterectomy advisable, even when the preoperative plan did not include such an extensive procedure. It is extremely disconcerting to find that a total abdominal hysterectomy must be performed at the time of a laparotomy if the vagina is not properly prepared. For this reason it is strongly recommended that preoperative vaginal preparation be accomplished as a routine procedure. To clean the perineum and vagina, the vulva and perineum are first scrubbed by a nurse or surgical assistant with a sponge soaked in surgical soap or an iodophor (povidone-iodine) solution using a gloved hand. Prior to this preparation Kelly pads should be placed under the buttocks and low back to catch wash and preparation solutions, and the perineum and vulva

washed and wiped free of gross contamination (mucus, blood, bowel content). These pads should be removed prior to draping the patient to prevent contaminated fluids and concentrated iodine wash solutions from pooling and remaining under the buttocks during the operative procedure. After the perineal and vulvar preparation, the vagina is next scrubbed with a soapy sponge held in the gloved hand. After the vaginal scrub the nurse or operative assistant inserts his or her fingers in the vagina and spreads the fingers to enlarge the vaginal outlet. At the same time the perineum is depressed to allow the soapy water or povidone-iodine solution to run out of the vagina. This solution is then flushed away with sterile water poured into the vagina. After this the remaining cleanup is accomplished with a sterile sponge on a sponge forceps, which is used several times to clean the vagina with an appropriate antiseptic solution.

After the vaginal, vulvar, and perineal cleanup, the abdomen is prepared with a 5-minute scrub using a povidone-iodine or similar solution. Particular attention should be paid to cleansing the umbilicus with a Q-tip/cotton swab applicator. The surgically prepared area should extend superiorly from the inferior rib cage to the midthigh, inferiorly. The lateral margins of the skin preparation should extend to the anterior iliac crest and the anterior axillary line. The actual skin washing and preparation should be accomplished using concentric circles moving toward the periphery. To additionally protect the incision from contamination many surgeons use a clear plastic adhesive (3M Steri-Drape Ioban 2 or similar product) placed over the skin at the site of the incision.

The Hospital Infection Control Practices Advisory Committee of the Centers for Disease Control and Prevention has published *Guidelines for Prevention of Surgical Site Infection* (1999), which are important in gynecologic surgery and should be noted (Table 6.6).

UNIVERSAL PRECAUTIONS FOR THE PREVENTION OF SEROPOSITIVITY FOR ACQUIRED IMMUNODEFICIENCY SYNDROME

Because surgeons are at risk for acquiring seropositivity for the acquired immunodeficiency syndrome through contamination from body fluids and blood products, certain precautions should be taken at the time of surgery. In 1988, the Centers for Disease Control and Prevention published a document recommending that blood and other body fluid precautions be consistently used for all patients, regardless of their blood-borne infectious status. This extension of blood and other body fluid precautions to all patients is referred to as Universal Blood and Fluid Precautions, or simply Universal Precautions. Under universal precautions, blood and body fluids of all patients are considered potentially infectious for HIV, hepatitis B virus (HBV), and other blood-borne pathogens.

Universal precautions are intended to prevent parenteral, mucous membrane, and nonintact skin exposure

TABLE 6.6.
Recommendations for Preoperative Preparation of the Patient to Prevent Surgical Site Infections

1. Whenever possible, identify and treat all infections remote to the surgical site before elective operation and postpone elective operations on patients with remote site infections until the infection has resolved.
2. Do not remove hair preoperatively unless hair at or around the incision site will interfere with the operation.
3. If hair is removed, remove immediately before the operation, preferably with electric clippers.
4. Adequately control serum blood glucose levels in all diabetic patients and particularly avoid hyperglycemia perioperatively.
5. Encourage tobacco cessation. At a minimum, instruct patients to abstain for at least 30 days before elective operation from smoking cigarettes, cigars, pipes, or other form of tobacco consumption.
6. Do not withhold necessary blood products from surgical patients as a means to prevent surgical site infections.
7. Require patients to shower or bathe with an antiseptic agent on at least the night before the operative day.
8. Thoroughly wash and clean at and around the incision site to remove gross contamination before performing antiseptic skin preparation.
9. Use appropriate antiseptic agent for skin preparation.
10. Apply preoperative antiseptic skin preparation in concentric circles moving toward the periphery. The prepared area must be large enough to extend the incision or create new incisions or drain sites, if necessary.
11. Keep preoperative hospital stay as short as possible while allowing for adequate preoperative preparation of the patient.
12. No recommendation to taper or discontinue systemic steroid use (when medically permissible) before elective operation. (unresolved issue)
13. No recommendation to enhance nutritional support for surgical patients solely as a means to prevent surgical site infection. (unresolved issue)
14. No recommendation to preoperatively apply mupirocin to nares to prevent surgical site infection. (unresolved issue)
15. No recommendation to provide measures that enhance would space oxygenation to prevent surgical site infections. (unresolved issue)

Hospital Infection Control Practices Committee. Centers for Disease Control and Prevention (CDC). *Am J Infect Control* 1999;27:266–267, with permission.

of the surgeon to blood-borne pathogens. Immunization with HBV vaccine is also recommended as an important adjunct to the universal precautions for surgeons who are exposed to the risks. Protective barriers reduce the risk of exposure of the surgeon's skin or mucous membrane to potentially infectious materials. In the operating room, protective barriers include gowns, gloves, masks, and protective eyewear. Masks and protective eyewear or face shields reduce the incidence of contamination of mucous membranes of the mouth, nose, and eyes. Gloves reduce the incidence of contamination of the hands, but they cannot prevent penetrating injuries such as puncture by a needle or other sharp instrument. Special care must be taken to prevent any injury by needles, scalpels, or other sharp instruments or devices. Should a contamination occur in spite of these precautions, immediately and thoroughly wash the hands and other skin surfaces that have been contaminated and institute the medical institution's policy on rapid antigen testing to determine if the surgeon should consider prophylaxis for HIV.

SUMMARY

Gynecologic surgery encompasses a wide variety of surgical procedures from minimally invasive operations to radical and extensive dissections of pelvic pathology. No matter what the extent of the procedure all gynecologic surgery should be considered to have three separate parts: (a) the preoperative care and management phase; (b) the surgical procedure itself; and (c) postoperative care and the management phase. Each part is inextricably related to the others and each part is vital in the overall outcome of the gynecologic pathology being managed. Preoperative care and management sets the stage for a successful surgical procedure. Best outcomes are linked to a patient being in optimal physical and medical status prior to surgery. The preoperative process begins with an accurate diagnosis and an appropriate decision to operate. The preoperative evaluation of each gynecologic patient serves to identify other pathologies that could interfere with optimal surgical outcome and to implement corrections prior to surgery. As a result, both the gynecologic surgeon and the patient arrive in the operating room with little doubt as to the pathology, the overall medical status, and the plan for surgical correction.

BIBLIOGRAPHY

ACOG Educational Bulletin. *Antibiotics and gynecologic infections.* ACOG Educational Bulletin 1997;237.

Bonnar J. Can more be done in obstetric and gynecologic practice to reduce morbidity and mortality associated with venous thromboembolism? *Am J Obstet Gynecol* 1999;180:784–791.

Brown JS, Sawaya G, Thom DH, et al. Hysterectomy and urinary incontinence: a systematic review. *Lancet* 2000;356:535–539.

Centers for Disease Control. Universal precautions for prevention of transmission of human immunodeficiency virus, Hepatitis B virus, and other blood-borne pathogens in healthcare settings. *MMWR* 1988;37:377.

Centers for Disease Control and Prevention. Hospital Infection Control Practices Advisory Committee. Guidelines for prevention of surgical site infections, 1999. *Am J Infect Control* 1999;27:250–277.

Chen BH, Giudice LC. Dysfunctional uterine bleeding. *West J Med* 1998;169:280–284.

Eagle KA, Brundage BH, Chaitman BR, et al. Guidelines for perioperative cardiovascular evaluation for noncardiac surgery. Report of the American College of Cardiology/ American Heart Association Task Force on Practice Guidelines (Committee on Perioperative Cardiovascular Evaluation for Noncardiac Surgery). *JACC* 1996;27:910–948.

Fischer SP. Cost-effective preoperative evaluation and testing. *Chest* 1999;115:96S–100S.

Golub R, Cantu R, Sorrento JJ, et al. Efficacy of preadmission testing in ambulatory surgical patients. *Am J Surg* 1992;163:565–571.

Goodson WH, Hunt TK. Studies of wound healing in experimental diabetes mellitus. *J Surg Res* 1977;22:221–227.

Greene GR, Sartwell PE. Oral contraceptive use in patients with thromboembolism following surgery, trauma, or infection. *Am J Public Health* 1972;62:680–685.

Hammond CB. *Therapeutic options for menopausal health.* Monograph. Durham, NC: Duke University School of Medicine, 2000.

Hillis SD, Marchbanks PA, Ratliff Taylor S, et al. For the U.S. Collaborative Review of Sterilization Working Group. Tubal sterilization and long-term risk of hysterectomy: findings from the United States Collaborative Review of Sterilization. *Obstet Gynecol* 1997;89:609–614.

Kramarow E, Lentzner H, Rooks R, et al. *Health, United States, 1999, with health and aging chartbook.* Hyattsville, MD: National Center for Health Sciences, US Dept Health & Human Resources, 1999.

Kaplan EB, Sheiner LB, Boeckmann AJ, et al. The usefulness of preoperative laboratory screening. *JAMA* 1985;253:3576–3581.

Macario A, Roizen MF, Thisted RA, et al. Reassessment of preoperative laboratory testing has changed the test-ordering patterns of physicians. *Surg Gynecol Obstet* 1992;175:539–547.

Masukawa T, Levinson EF, Forst JK. The cytologic examination of breast secretions. *Acta Cytol* 1966;10:261–265.

Mittendorf R, Aronson MP, Berry RE, et al. Avoiding serious infections associated with abdominal hysterectomy: a meta-analysis of antibiotic prophylaxis. *Am J Obstet Gynecol* 1993;169:1661–1666.

Monro J, Booth A, Nicholl J. Routine preoperative testing: a systemic review of the evidence. *Health Tech Assess* 1997;1:1–63.

Narr BJ, Hansen TR, Warner MA. Preoperative laboratory screening in healthy Mayo patients: cost-effective elimination of tests and unchanged outcomes. *Mayo Clin Proc* 1991;66:155–159.

Ross AF, Tinker JH. Anesthesia risk. In: Miller RD, ed. *Anesthesia,* 3rd ed. New York: Churchill Livingstone, 1990:715–742.

Roizen MF. Anesthetic implications of concurrent diseases. In: Miller RD, ed. *Anesthesia,* 5th ed. Philadelphia: Churchill Livingstone, 2000:903–1015.

Roizen MF, Foss JF, Fischer SP. Preoperative evaluation. In: Miller RD, ed. *Anesthesia,* 5th ed. Philadelphia: Churchill Livingstone, 2000:824–883.

Roizen MF. More preoperative assessment by physicians and less by laboratory test (editorial comment). The value of routine preoperative medical testing before cataract surgery. *N Engl J Med* 2000;342:168–175.

Scher KS. Studies on the duration of antibiotic administration for surgical prophylaxis. *Am Surg* 1997;63:59–62.

Velanovich V. Preoperative laboratory screening based on age, gender, and concomitant medical diseases. *Surgery* 1994;115:56–61.

Vessey MD, Doll R, Fairbairn AS, et al. Postoperative thromboembolism and the use of oral contraceptives. *Br Med J* 1970;3:123–126.

Vogt AW, Henson LC. Unindicated preoperative testing: ASA physical status and financial implications. *J Clin Anesthesiol* 1997;9:437–441.

Westhoff C, Davis A. Tubal sterilization: focus on the U.S. experience. *Fertil Steril* 2000;73:913–922.

Te Linde's Operative Gynecology, ninth edition, edited by John A. Rock and Howard W. Jones, III. Lippincott Williams & Wilkins, Philadelphia: © 2003.

CHAPTER

7

Postanesthesia and Postoperative Care

IRA R. HOROWITZ   JACK B. BASIL

The most critical period of a patient's postoperative course occurs within the first 72 hours of surgery. Precise monitoring of the cardiovascular, renal, and respiratory systems provides the most valuable information about the patient's postoperative condition. Postoperative morbidity can be decreased with an appropriate preoperative evaluation of the surgical candidate. Emphasis should be placed on identifying those patients at risk for developing venous thrombosis and administering appropriate prophylaxis. Improved nutritional status in the preoperative and postoperative periods also has been shown to improve wound healing and decrease the postoperative recovery time.

VASCULAR COMPLICATIONS

Venous Thrombosis

About half a million hospitalizations are associated with deep venous thrombosis (DVT) or pulmonary embolism (PE). A fatal outcome occurs in about 50,000 of these patients. The incidence of venous thrombosis in the gynecology patient is 15%, with a range of 5% to 45%, depending on the procedure performed and associated risk factors. PE is responsible for 40% of the postoperative deaths in the gynecologic patient. The sudden occurrence of respiratory distress in a postoperative patient, followed by hypotension, chest pain, cardiac arrhythmias, and death, is a complication that converts a successful operative procedure into a postoperative mortality. In only 70% of patients who die of PE is it considered in the differential diagnosis. In recent years, diagnostic studies have provided more accurate information on the frequency of this vascular complication and have identified those patients with DVT who are at risk of shedding emboli. Preoperative and postoperative prophylaxis with heparin, dextran, antiembolic stockings, and intermittent pneumatic compression devices for moderate- and high-risk patients has reduced the incidence of pulmonary emboli. Clarke-Pearson and coworkers, using univariate and regression analysis, designed a prognostic model to evaluate the risks of postoperative DVT for an individual patient. The preoperative prognostic factors identified in a prospective study of 411 gynecology patients were type of surgery, age, leg edema, nonwhite patients, severity of venous varicosities, prior radiation therapy, and prior history of DVT.

Essentially all of the major factors contributing to postoperative venous thrombosis were described by Virchow more than 125 years ago. These factors include an increase in blood coagulability, venous stasis, and trauma to the vessel wall. Tissue injury activates blood coagulation by the extrinsic and intrinsic pathways (Fig. 7.1) by exposing the blood to increased levels of tissue

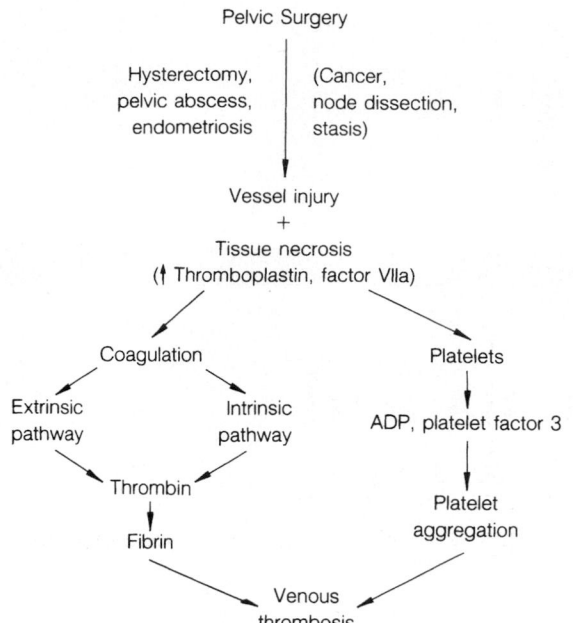

FIGURE 7.1. Formation of venous thrombus following various surgical procedures with the activation of clotting factors and aggregation of platelets.

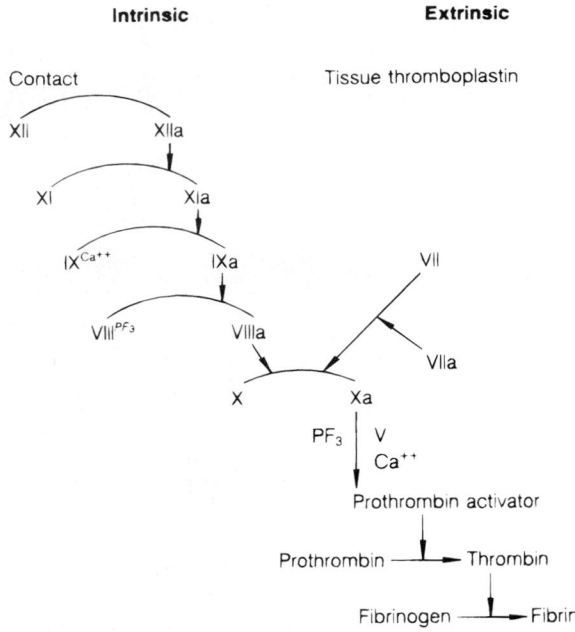

FIGURE 7.2. Schematic representation of the cascade clotting mechanism, illustrating the role of extrinsic and intrinsic factors. Increases in tissue thromboplastin-like substance and collagen-activated factor XII initiate the formation of fibrin through the extrinsic and intrinsic pathways, principally by the activation of factor X.

thromboplastin (extrinsic) or to subendothelial collagen in the vessel wall, which activates factor XII (intrinsic). Venous damage is particularly prevalent in patients undergoing radical surgery in which skeletonization of the pelvic vasculature is performed. When postoperative infection and pelvic cellulitis occur, there is an acceleration of the clotting mechanism caused by the release of tissue thromboplastin (extrinsic) and the activation of factor VII (intrinsic) by collagen. The activation of both extrinsic and intrinsic pathways results in the conversion of factor X to an active form that, in turn, interacts with factor V, calcium, and phospholipid from platelet factor III to convert prothrombin to thrombin (Fig. 7.2). Thrombin is the rate-regulating proteolytic enzyme that controls the conversion of fibrinogen to fibrin, the basic component of a venous thrombus. Other coagulation factors that are known to be increased after surgery are, principally, factors XI, IX, and VIII, which increase as a result of activation of the intrinsic pathway, and factor XII, which is activated by tissue collagen. There also is an increase in circulating platelets, platelet adhesiveness, and platelet aggregation within 72 to 96 hours of surgery. In addition, there is an increase in fibrinogen and in circulating fibrinolysin inhibitors. Normally, the fibrinolytic system, which is mostly plasmin formed from its inactive precursor, plasminogen, balances the clotting mechanism by digesting fibrin and fibrinogen and inactivating factors V and VIII. An acceleration of the clotting mechanism leads to a thrombus in either the venous or the arterial system. An excess of fibrinolytic activity causes failure of blood clotting and can produce serious hemorrhage. A proper balance of both is required for normal circulation.

Venous stasis is known to be the cornerstone of postoperative thrombus formation. Venous stasis in the lower extremities and pelvis results in platelet aggregation and the adhesion of platelets to the vein wall, with the release of a thromboplastin-like substance that forms a platelet-fibrin-red cell network with resultant thrombus formation. These physiologic changes in venous hemodynamics occur in the preoperative, operative, and postoperative periods. Many investigators have found it advisable to perform the preoperative studies on high-risk patients on an ambulatory basis or, if the patient has been hospitalized for a significant period of time, to discharge her home for several weeks to increase her physical activity before elective surgery. Doran and others have shown that venous return from the lower extremities is decreased to one half its normal rate during the operative procedure. The decrease results from the loss of muscle tone that is caused by muscle relaxation from anesthetic agents. ^{125}I-labeled fibrinogen scanning studies have demonstrated that venous clot is initiated during the operative procedure in 50% of the patients who develop thrombosis in the postoperative period. Blood flow from the lower extremity has been shown to undergo further reduction to about 75% of the normal drainage flow immediately after surgery. This reduced flow rate persists for 10 to 14 days because of the loss of pump action of the leg muscles. The major site of clot formation is in the soleal venous sinuses of the calf, a portion of the venous arcade that joins the posterior tibial and peroneal veins that drain the soleal muscle. Thrombi from these sinuses often occur behind the valves that are located at the point at which the sinuses drain into the collecting veins. Thrombi often form in these large sinuses or valve cusps in bedridden patients.

Another factor contributing to venous stasis is prolonged surgery with tight packing of the intestines in the upper abdomen and obstruction of the underlying vena cava. The type and length of operation are directly related to the incidence of postoperative venous thrombosis, as outlined in Table 7.1.

Diagnosis of Venous Thrombosis

The traditional clinical methods used to diagnose venous thrombosis of the lower extremity are of limited value. Such methods may be in error in 50% of the cases and provide both false-positive and false-negative information. This diagnostic problem results from the silent and insidious nature of the venous thrombus formation process, which takes place principally in the deep soleal veins in the lower extremity. Because the clinical diagnosis of this vascular complication is so inaccurate, more objective methods of diagnosis were required. In recent years, venography, ^{125}I-labeled fibrinogen scanning, Doppler ultrasound, and impedance plethysmography (IPG) have been used along with a variety of other imaging techniques. Venography is regarded as the most

definitive method for the diagnosis of venous thrombosis and has been used as the reference source against which other techniques are measured (Table 7.2).

Venography

The venogram has had the widest clinical use of all available techniques in the study of venous thrombosis, with the most extensive clinical correlation in the large veins of the lower extremities. Venography generally is reserved for cases in which there is clinical suspicion of venous thrombosis or a pulmonary embolus. Venography has limited usefulness as a screening procedure because it is an invasive technique.

[125]I-Labeled Fibrinogen Scanning

Recent studies have used scintillation counter scanning of the lower extremities following the administration of ^{125}I-labeled fibrinogen. The incorporation of iodinated fibrinogen into a developing thrombus was first tested by Hobbs and Davies in 1960. The large, collaborative English study by Kakkar and associates was one of the first to give clear evidence of the clinical accuracy of this technique in a collaborative, randomized study of more than 4,000 patients. This study demonstrated a 93% correlation of the fibrinogen scanning technique with venography in the identification of a developing venous thrombus in the lower extremity. Preoperative monitor-

TABLE 7.1.
Levels of Thromboembolism Risk in Surgical Patients Without Prophylaxis

Level of Risk Examples	Calf DVT, %	Proximal DVT, %	Clinical PE, %	Fatal PE, %	Successful Prevention Strategies

Low risk
  Minor surgery in patients <40 yr
    with no additional risk factors
	2	0.4	0.2	0.002	No specific measures
					Aggressive mobilization

Moderate risk
  Minor surgery in patients with
    additional risk factors; nonmajor
    surgery in patients aged 40–60 yr
    with no additional risk factors;
    major surgery in patients <40 yr
    with no additional risk factors
	10–20	2–4	1–2	0.1–0.4	LDUH q12h, LMWH, ES, or IPC

High risk
  Nonmajor surgery in patients
    >60 yr or with additional risk
    factors; major surgery in patients
    >40 yr or with additional risk
    factors
	20–40	4–8	2–4	0.4–1.0	LDUH q8h, LMWH, or IPC

Highest risk
  Major surgery in patients >40 yr
    plus prior VTE, cancer, or
    molecular hypercoagulable state;
    hip or knee arthroplasty, hip
    fracture surgery; major trauma;
    spinal cord injury
	40–80	10–20	4–10	0.2–5	LMWH, oral anticoagulants,
					IPC/ES + LDUH/LMWH, or
					ADH

Modified from Gallus et al. and International Consensus Statement.
Source: Geerts WH, Heit JA, Clagett GP, et al. Prevention of venous thromboembolism. [Sixth ACCP Consensus Conference on Antithrombotic Therapy] *Chest* 2001;119(Suppl 1):132S–175S.

TABLE 7.2.
Diagnosis of Deep Venous Thrombosis (DVT)

Method	Sensitivity and Specificity	Indication and Comments
Clinical history and physical examination		Classic symptoms often absent in proven DVT <60% with suggestive symptoms proven to have DVT Absence of symptoms does not exclude pulmonary embolism
D-dimer ELISA (plasma)	Sensitivity 97% Specificity: poor	Useful to exclude the diagnosis if D-dimer (ELISA) is <500 mug/mL Many conditions increase D-dimer levels (false-positive results)
B-mode compression ultrasonography ± Doppler	Symptomatic proximal DVT: Sensitivity 93%–97% Specificity 98% Asymptomatic DVT: Sensitivity 38%–59% Specificity: high	Noninvasive test First-line modality for confirming diagnosis in symptomatic patients Not useful for screening of asymptomatic patients Compression component best for thigh DVT
Impedance plethysmography	Symptomatic DVT: Sensitivity 90% Specificity 95% Asymptomatic DVT: Sensitivity 22% Specificity 98%	Noninvasive test Limited to *serial* examination in symptomatic patients with proximal DVT Insensitive to calf-vein thrombi and nonocclusive thrombi
MR venography	Proximal DVT: Sensitivity 100% Specificity 96% Calf-vein DVT: Sensitivity 87% Specificity 97%	Noninvasive but expensive Ability to screen for DVT in asymptomatic patients Can also image lungs for pulmonary embolism in same setting
Contrast-enhanced CT venography	Distal and proximal DVT: Sensitivity 100% Specificity 96%	Noninvasive test Superior to venography in evaluating the great vessels Expensive Less contrast than conventional venography Can image lungs for pulmonary embolism in same setting
Ascending contrast venography phlebography	Reference standard	Invasive test Reference standard but expensive Risk for contrast nephropathy and allergic reactions Risk for thrombogenicity (usually superficial veins) Negative test does not exclude pulmonary embolism Equivocal results in recurrent DVT

Source: De Wet CJ, Pearl RG. Venous thromboembolism: deep-vein thrombosis and pulmonary embolism. *Anesthesiol Clin North Am Clin* 1999;17(4):895–922.

ing is initiated 24 hours after the i.v. injection of 100 µCi of ^{125}I-labeled fibrinogen; subsequently, monitoring is performed in the immediate postoperative period and daily thereafter. An iodine preparation is administered to prevent ^{125}I uptake by the thyroid. Scintillation readings along the lower leg at 2-in. intervals that monitor the venous flow in the deep veins of the calf are compared with precordial readings, and a percentage of the heart count is plotted graphically for each leg. Venous thrombosis is suspected when the level of radioactivity at any point in the leg is 20% greater than either the reading taken 24 hours earlier at the same point or the reading taken at the same point in the other leg. A diagnosis of venous thrombosis can be made if the scan remains abnormal for more than 24 hours. However, the test has specific limitations. It is unreliable in the upper thigh because of the close proximity of the bladder, where the iodine is excreted in the urine, and because of the large veins and arteries in the pelvis, which increase the background noise. It is relatively insensitive in the diagnosis of established venous thrombosis, being positive in only 70% of the cases. Furthermore, as many as 72 hours may be required before enough iodinated fibrinogen is deposited in the formed thrombus to give a positive result. Therefore, its major use is in the prophylactic screening of high-risk patients to detect the earliest stage of deep venous thrombus formation.

Impedance Plethysmography

Impedance plethysmography is based on the measurement of electrical resistance in a specific area of the body, such as the lower extremities. When blood flow has been reduced by venous outflow obstruction, such as with venous thrombosis, there is a marked reduction in the electrical resistance over the involved vessel. IPG is most specific in venous occlusion in the larger veins of the thigh (i.e., the lower iliac, femoral, and popliteal), having an overall accuracy of 95% in comparison to venography. It is much less useful for the detection of small calf vein thrombi because of the caliber of the small soleus sinuses and the subtle changes in blood flow through these vessels. The ability of this technique to detect asymptomatic venous thrombi in the calf veins has been found to be less than 50% that of venography.

Huisman and colleagues evaluated 471 outpatients clinically suspected of having acute DVT. Four sequential impedance plethysmograms were obtained on days 1, 2, 5, and 10 of the study. Of the 137 patients with abnormal results, 117 (85%) had abnormal results on day 1, with the remaining 20 patients turning positive on subsequent days. When compared with venograms, serial IPG had a specificity of 92% and sensitivity of 100%. By performing serial studies, the authors were able to improve their ability to diagnose DVT. In a similar study involving 252 patients, Vaccaro and coworkers reported a sensitivity of 84.2% and a specificity of 78.2% when attempting to diagnose DVT with a single study.

Doppler Ultrasound

The use of Doppler ultrasound, a noninvasive technique, has become more prevalent during the past decade for the diagnosis of venous thrombosis. Its major physiologic use is the measurement of the velocity of blood flow in large vessels. With this technique, a reflected signal is converted to the audible range and directed through a loudspeaker. In the case of venous thrombosis, the absence of the signal signifies an obstructed vein. When used in the upper thigh, the technique is highly sensitive to venous thrombosis in the lower iliac, femoral, or popliteal vessels. However, sensitivity decreases rapidly in smaller vessels, particularly in the soleal sinuses of the calf, where the accuracy range, in most series, is less than 60%. The technique is of limited value as a routine screening test for high risk patients.

Real-Time Ultrasound

Real-time ultrasound diagnosis of DVT has recently been compared with venography. Aitken and Godden demonstrated a sensitivity of 94% and a specificity of 100% in evaluating a group of 46 patients with real-time ultrasound. In a similar study evaluating 121 patients, Appelman and colleagues found real-time ultrasound to have a sensitivity of 96% and a specificity of 97%. Hillner and coworkers suggested that real-time ultrasound and anticoagulation were an optimal cost-effective approach to diagnosing and treating patients with DVT.

Duplex Doppler Imaging

Real-time ultrasound and Doppler examination have been combined in a procedure known as duplex B-mode imaging or duplex Doppler imaging, which enables the radiologist to visualize the thrombus and measure blood flow through the vessels. Langsfeld and associates examined 431 patients and diagnosed thrombi in 86. They reported a sensitivity of 100% and observed two false positives, which resulted in a specificity of 78%. On further evaluation, they found that one of these patients, early in the protocol, had an incorrect reading of the duplex B-mode imaging; the second patient had a term pregnancy, and the observed decreased blood flow was a result of aortocaval compression from the pregnant uterus. An accurate study could have been obtained by positioning the patient on her side. Kristo and associates compared ipsilateral ultrasonic duplex imaging, contrast venography, and single bilateral IPG. The sensitivity and specificity were as follows: ultrasonography, 92% and 100%; venography, 100% and 75%; and IPG, 50% and 83%, respectively. Duplex B-mode imaging is a noninvasive procedure and has replaced venography as the gold standard for diagnosing DVT.

Light Reflection Rheography

Arora and colleagues evaluated 69 limbs in patients with gastrointestinal problems who were suspected of having DVT. All patients received a venogram and light reflection rheography (LRR). With this technique, infrared light is directed at the skin and backscattered rays are measured. This is used to estimate the volume of blood present. A venous emptying rate of 0.35 or less is considered positive for DVT. The sensitivity, specificity, positive predictive value, and negative predictive value for LRR are 96.4%, 82.9%, 79%, and 97.1%, respectively. LRR may prove to be a low-cost, highly sensitive tool for diagnosing DVT. Future studies are required to further evaluate this method.

Four hundred and one asymptomatic pregnant women in their second and third trimester were evaluated by Nolan and associates with LRR. All patients were asymptomatic for DVT. Twenty-five percent of scans were abnormal and 19% were inadequate. In light of these results, and because of the overall specificity of 45%, this test should not be used in the pregnant patient for diagnosing DVT.

Indium 111

Fibrinogen I 125 is of limited value in detecting thrombi in the proximal femoral vein and diagnosing pelvic thrombosis or pulmonary emboli. Clarke-Pearson and colleagues advocated using indium 111 (^{111}In) platelet imaging to diagnose DVT and pulmonary emboli. When compared with diagnostic tests such as pulmonary angiography, lung scans, venograms, and ^{125}I fibrinogen counting, ^{111}In platelet imaging was found to have a sensitivity of 100% and a specificity of 90%. In recent animal studies, Oster and coworkers suggested using [111]In- or iodine 123-radiolabeled monoclonal antiplatelet antibodies for thrombus identification with radioimmunoscintigraphy. Honkanen and associates evaluated 33 patients with signs and symptoms of DVT with venography and technetium-99m hexamethylpropyleneamineoxime (^{99m}Tc-HMPAO)–labeled autologous platelets. The sensitivity and specificity were 65% and 100%, respectively, in all patients, versus 83% and 100%, respectively, in patients not anticoagulated. Peters and colleagues used ^{111}In-radiolabeled monoclonal antibodies in platelets in six patients, three of whom had thrombus formation. Two patients were positive, and the third had a negative chronic radioimmunoscintigraphy. Radiolabeled monoclonal antibodies are easier to produce than ^{111}In-radiolabeled platelets and do not have the risk of hepatitis and human immunodeficiency virus transmission that donor ^{125}I fibrinogen and ^{111}In platelets have. Additional trials in humans are needed.

D-dimer

Studies by Wells and associates compared whole-blood D-dimer assay and IPG with contrast venography. A negative D-dimer and IPG have a negative predictive value of 97% and 99%, respectively, of proximal DVT. The combination of a positive IPG and D-dimer has a positive predictive value of 93% of any DVT and a positive predictive value of 90% of proximal DVT.

Dale and associates compared the NycoCard (Axis-Shield PoC, Oslo, Norway) D-dimer, latex, and D-dimer enzyme-linked immunosorbent assays with venography. The NycoCard had a sensitivity, negative predictive value, specificity, and positive predictive value of 100%, 100%, 40%, and 57%, respectively.

Magnetic Resonance Imaging

Magnetic resonance imaging (MRI) has been used to evaluate venous clot formation. Rapoport and colleagues demonstrated with *in vitro* studies that acute clot, when compared with stagnant blood, resulted in a marked reduction in relaxation time for both T1 and T2 measurements. The relaxation time was also reduced as the clot aged. Spritzer and associates prospectively evaluated 16 patients and 17 extremities to compare limited-flip-angle, gradient-refocused MRI with venography. By pulsing, flowing blood is excited while the adjacent tissue becomes saturated and therefore produces a signal of lower intensity. Stasis of blood flow would act in a manner similar to that in the adjacent tissues with decreased intensity. The authors were able to correctly locate the thrombus in 16 of 17 lower extremities. The 17th extremity was correctly diagnosed to have iliac and femoral vein clots; however, MRI also suggested the presence of calf and popliteal thrombi that were not confirmed on venography. Using the GRASS (gradient-recalled acquisition in a steady state)

images, Mintz and coworkers reported MRI diagnosis of puerperal ovarian vein thrombosis. MRI thrombus diagnosis is in its infancy. As our understanding of this technique increases and technology improves, MRI will prove to be a valuable noninvasive tool to diagnose thrombus formation. The advantage of MRI over computed tomography (CT) is that it does not require the use of i.v. contrast. Spritzer and associates (1995) diagnosed DVT in pregnant patients using MRI with a gradient-recalled echo technique. Several authors, including Evans and associates, found no statistical difference when diagnosing DVT with either contrast venography or MRI.

Risk Factors for Vascular Complications

Several factors have been observed that present a clinical profile of the patient who is prone to venous thrombosis and PE (Table 7.3). Among the many clinical factors that predispose to venous thrombosis in women, the following are the most prevalent: age greater than 40 years; obesity greater than 20% above ideal weight; prolonged surgery; and immobility in the preoperative, operative, and postoperative periods. Pelvic malignancy, previous thromboembolism, severe diabetes, heart failure, previous radiation therapy, and chronic pulmonary disease also increase the risk of vascular thrombi.

Age

In autopsy studies by Sevitt and Gallagher, the incidence of DVT was greatest in patients older than 60 years of age. Many additional studies have demonstrated a linear increase in fatal pulmonary emboli as patient age increases. The major correlation in such patients relates to degenerative changes in the vascular tree. The incidence of PE after major surgery increases sharply in women over 40 years of age.

Obesity

The risk of thromboembolism is decidedly increased in the obese patient. Breneman recognized obesity as one of the most significant factors in thromboembolic disease in the operative patient. His study of patients with thromboembolic disease demonstrated that they were 21.6% above their ideal weight. The major way that obesity influences thrombus formation is by venous stasis, which is aggravated by postoperative immobility.

Immobility

Prolonged inactivity in the preoperative patient causes an impairment in the venous circulation of the lower extremities. Preoperative immobilization, such as that required for prolonged diagnostic evaluation, produces a decrease in muscle tone of the lower extremity with diminished venous flow. These hemodynamic changes result in sludging of the platelets and red cells and set the stage for venous thrombosis during the operative period. Flane and associates and Kemble have clearly demonstrated this fact using ^{125}I-labeled fibrinogen scanning before and immediately after surgery. They observed that in 50% of patients who ultimately devel-

TABLE 7.3.
Profile of Patient at High Risk for Venous Thrombosis

Factor	Condition
Age	>40 Major surgery
Age	>60 Non-major surgery
Obesity	
Moderate	75–90 kg or >20% above ideal weight
Morbid	≥115 kg or >30% above ideal weight with reduced fibrinolysin and immobility
Immobility	
Preoperative	Prolonged hospitalization; venous stasis
Intraoperative	Prolonged operative time; loss of pump action of calf muscles; compression of vena cava
Postoperative	Prolonged bed confinement; venous stasis
Trauma	Damage of wall of pelvic veins
Radical pelvic surgery	
Malignancy	Release of tissue thromboplastin[a]
Activation of factor X; reduced fibrinolysin	
Radiation	Prior radiation therapy
Medical diseases	Diabetes mellitus
Cardiac disease; heart failure	
Severe varicose veins	
Previous venous thrombosis with or without embolization[a]	
Chronic pulmonary disease	
Molecular hypercoagulable state	

[a] Highest risk.

oped postoperative thrombosis, the onset of the clot formation was during the operative procedure. Similarly, the patient who has undergone prolonged anesthesia with generalized muscle relaxation has an increased incidence of venous stagnation of the lower extremities and a higher incidence of thromboembolism postoperatively. It is important to reemphasize the fact that the nidus for venous thrombosis is frequently initiated either before or, more commonly, during the operative procedure. Consequently, prophylactic treatment for the high-risk patient should be initiated before surgery and should be continued until the patient is fully ambulatory.

Postoperative immobilization provides an added physiologic insult to preexisting venous stasis. As many as 66% of patients who develop postoperative venous thrombosis have evidence of thrombosis within 48 hours of surgery, as detected by ^{125}I-labeled fibrinogen scanning. Such anatomic positions as sitting with the legs crossed, sitting with the legs dangling from the bed, and the exaggerated Fowler position produce impairment in venous return from the lower extremities. The high-risk patient (Table 7.3), in particular, should be ambulated vigorously. When confinement to bed is necessary, the legs and trunk should be elevated approximately 15 degrees above the horizontal. Sharnoff has demonstrated that immobilization in bed is perhaps more hazardous than the physiologic impact of advancing age.

Other Factors

Factors that lead to an increased risk of thrombosis and PE include varicose veins, previous thromboembolism, severe diabetes, cardiac failure, and chronic pulmonary disease. All of these produce impairment of circulation with resultant stasis and an increased frequency of venous thrombosis. Malignancy also is a recognized factor in venous thrombosis, although the exact mechanism is not fully understood. Many tumors undergoing tissue breakdown are known to elaborate a thromboplastin-like substance that may predispose to increased thrombosis. Hypercoagulable states, both congenital and acquired, increase the risk of thromboembolism in the gynecologic patient (Table 7.4).

It is evident that a clinical profile can be developed for the high-risk patient. The paradigmatic high-risk patient is a woman who is older than 40 years of age, is morbidly obese (greater than twice her ideal weight), is diabetic, has varicose veins or heart disease (or both), has been in the hospital for a prolonged period for medical evaluation or treatment, and has a malignant tumor. Regardless of the nature of the pelvic disease, the greater the number of risk factors, the longer the operation, and the more difficult the surgical procedure, the more frequent is the occurrence of venous thrombosis and pulmonary embolus. Patients who embody one or more of these surgical risks should have intensive monitoring and prophylactic treatment for venous thrombosis.

TABLE 7.4.
Risk of Thromboembolism

Deficiency/dysfunction
   Antithrombin
   Protein C
   Protein S
   Heparin cofactor II
Factor V Leiden
Prothrombin variant 20210A
Antiphospholipid antibodies
   Lupus anticoagulant
   Anticardiolipin
Hyperhonocystireria
Dysfibrinogenemia
Decreased levels of plasminogen
Decreased levels of plasminogen activators
Heparin-induced thrombocytopenia

Treatment of Venous Thrombosis

Prophylaxis

The most effective treatment of venous thrombosis is prevention. In view of the evidence that between 5% and 45% of patients undergoing major gynecologic surgery develop venous thrombosis of the lower extremity, a prophylactic method of preventing this complication should be considered before surgery. In about 20% of cases, venous thrombi in the calf veins extend to the popliteal or femoral vessels, and in an estimated 40% of these, the patient develops pulmonary emboli. These facts are sufficient to warrant the prophylactic treatment of the high-risk patient in an effort to avoid this life-threatening sequence of events (Table 7.5).

The Sixth ACCP (American College of Chest Physicians) Consensus Conference estimated the rate of pulmonary embolism (PE) in 7,000 gynecologic surgery patients enrolled in prospective studies. With the use of thromboprophylaxis, they observed a 75% reduction in fatal PE (Table 7.6).

LOW-DOSE HEPARIN

Many randomized prospective studies document the reduction of DVT from an incidence of 35% to 45% in untreated high-risk patients to about 7% in similar patients treated prophylactically with low-dose heparin. These studies were conducted during the past two decades and were verified by Kakkar and colleagues in a multicenter study of more than 4,000 surgical patients older than 40 years of age (Table 7.7). This study evaluated the effectiveness of low-dose heparin given prophylactically at doses of 5,000 United States Pharmacopeia units of calcium heparin, s.c., 2 hours before surgery and every 8 hours after for the subsequent 7 postoperative days. The study demonstrated the benefit of low-dose heparin in reducing the incidence of thrombi from 25% in the untreated control group to 8% in the low-dose heparin-treated control group. The most significant observation

from this study was that 16 patients in the control, untreated group and only two patients in the low-dose heparin-treated group died of acute massive PE, as revealed at autopsy. Of interest is the fact that there is no significant alteration of clotting time in the prophylactic use of low-dose heparin. As a consequence, there is no increase in operative or postoperative bleeding. This phenomenon is attributed to the mechanism of action of heparin, which binds to antithrombin III and exerts its major anticoagulant effect in combination with this naturally occurring inhibitor. Together they inhibit the activated coagulation factors XIIa, XIa, Xa, and thrombin. Low doses of heparin interfere with the early stages of coagulation before thrombin is formed, thereby preventing thrombus formation without significantly altering the clotting factors in the plasma. These results, as well as those from other studies recorded in Table 7.8, indicate that this method of prophylactic heparin therapy has been extremely successful in reducing venous thrombosis in surgical patients. Low-dose s.c. heparin, administered at a reduced dose of 5,000 units 2 hours preoperatively and every 12 hours postoperatively for 5 days, has proved efficacious in preventing thromboembolism. For the highest-risk patient, 5,000 units every 8 hours should be considered.

LOW-DOSE HEPARIN/DIHYDROERGOTAMINE

Nine years after Kakkar's landmark study, Sasahara and associates evaluated dihydroergotamine (DHE)-heparin prophylaxis in the prevention of DVT. Dihydroergotamine mesylate, 0.5 mg, exerts a selective constrictive effect on the veins and venules with a minimal effect on arteries and arterioles. By combining heparin with DHE, it is possible to alter the coagulability of blood with heparin and decrease venous stasis and accelerate peripheral venous return with DHE. The incidence of DVT was significantly decreased in patients treated with 5,000 units of DHE-heparin sodium every 12 hours until postoperative day 5 (Table 7.9). DHE is contraindicated in patients with severe vascular disease, severe hypertension, sepsis, or impaired liver or kidney function. The results of collaborative studies of prophylactic doses of DHE-heparin (5,000 units two times daily) are comparable to those of studies mentioned in this chapter in which doses of heparin (5,000 units three times daily) or intermittent pneumatic compression devices were used. These products are no longer available in the United States.

DEXTRAN 70/DEXTRAN 40

In 1972, Bonnar and Walsh suggested using dextran 70 to prevent thrombosis after pelvic surgery. Bernstein and associates decreased the incidence of leg vein thrombosis from 33% to 5% in patients undergoing radical hysterectomies who received dextran 70 prophylaxis. Dextran's mechanism in preventing thrombosis is through an effect on decreasing platelet function, coagulation factors V and VII, and fibrinolysis. To obtain adequate prophylaxis, dextran 70 is initiated during the operative procedure or immediately at its conclusion. Infusion of 1 L of dextran 70 over 6 to 8 hours should provide protection

TABLE 7.5.
Agents Used in Venous Thromboembolism

Agent	Mechanism of Action	Comments
Heparin	Combines with AT-III and neutralizes activated factors: IIa (thrombin activity) Xa (responsible for thrombin generation) XIIa, XIa, IXa	Prevention and treatment of venous thromboembolism Risk of heparin-induced thrombocytopenia Requires monitoring (aPTT) when used for treatment
LMWH Ardeparin Dalteparin Enoxaparin	Combines with AT-III and prevents thrombin generation through its anti-factor Xa effect	Prevention and treatment of venous thromboembolism Risk of heparin-induced thrombocytopenia No anti-IIa activity (if molecular weight <5.6 kDa) aPTT does not reflect anticoagulation state More predictable pharmacokinetic profile Renal failure and dehydration increase effective plasma concentration
Heparinoid Danaparoid	Same as LMWH High anti-Xa/IIa ratio	Prevention and treatment of venous thromboembolism Similar to LMWH but may be used for anticoagulation when heparin-induced thrombocytopenia is present
Direct thrombin inhibitors and hirudin	Directly inhibits thrombin activity	Prevention and treatment of venous thromboembolism May be used for heparin-induced thrombocytopenia
Plasminogen activators: Nonselective Streptokinase Urokinase	Activates plasminogen, which leads to the formation of plasmin, which dissolves fibrin clot (no effect on polymerized fibrin clot) Also degrades fibrinogen, which leads to fibrinogen degradation products and decreases in plasma fibrinogen	Treatment of life-threatening DVT or pulmonary embolism High risk of bleeding Many contraindications such as recent surgery or trauma
Thrombus-selective tissue plasminogen activator	Activates fibrin-bound plasminogen Degrades fibrinogen (to a lesser extent)	
Warfarin	Inhibits correct synthesis of vitamin K–dependent coagulation factors (II, VII, IX, X) These factors cannot bind calcium and therefore remain inactive Inhibits protein C (vitamin K–dependent)	Long-term treatment and prevention of venous thromboembolism Contraindicated in pregnancy (teratogenic) High risk of bleeding Requires anticoagulation monitoring Numerous drug interactions
Inferior vena caval filters	Trap larger emboli	Used as prevention of pulmonary embolism when anticoagulation fails or is contraindicated Used prior to pulmonary embolectomy or pulmonary endarterectomy
External pneumatic leg compression	Prevents venous stasis Stimulates fibrinolytic system	Used as prophylaxis for DVT Possibly contraindicated in peripheral arterial disease

Source: De Wet CJ, Pearl RG. Venous thromboembolism: deep-vein thrombosis and pulmonary embolism. *Anesthesiol Clin North Am* 1999,17(4):895–922.

TABLE 7.6.
Prevention of Deep Venous Thrombosis (DVT) After Gynecologic Surgery[a]

Regimen	No. of Trials	No. of Patients	Incidence of DVT, %	95% CI	Relative % Reduction
Untreated control subjects	12	945	16	14–19	—
Oral anticoagulants	5	183	13	8–18	22
IPC	3	253	9	6–13	44
LDUH	11	1,092	7	6–9	56
ES	1	104	0	0–3	"99"

[a] Pooled data from randomized trials that used routine FUT as the primary outcome.
Source: Geerts WH, Heit JA, Clagett GP, et al. Prevention of venous thromboembolism. [Sixth ACCP Consensus Conference on Antithrombotic Therapy] *Chest* 2001;119(1)Suppl:132S–175S.

TABLE 7.7.

Pulmonary Embolism and Deep Venous Thrombosis in Patients on Low-Dose Heparin and in Controls

	Low-Dose Heparin	Control
Number of patients	2,045	2,076
Number of deaths from all causes	80	100
Deaths caused by pulmonary embolism (verified at autopsy)	2	16
Deep venous thrombosis	8%	25%

Source: Kakkar W, Corrigan TP, Fossard DP. Prevention of postoperative pulmonary embolism by low dose heparin. *Lancet* 1975;2:45.

for 5 days. However, dextran 40 is cleared rapidly and should be administered at a continuous infusion rate of 20 mL/h. Alternatively, 500 mL of dextran 40 may be transfused over a period of 4 to 6 hours daily. Dextran 70 has been found to be as efficacious as low-dose heparin in preventing thromboembolism in patients undergoing major surgical procedures. Dextran was two to four times less efficacious than low-dose unfractionated heparin. This has resulted in the Sixth ACCP Consensus Conference not recommending dextran for prophylaxis in this population.

LOW-MOLECULAR-WEIGHT HEPARIN

The low-molecular-weight heparin (LMWH) fragment potentiates the inhibition of factor Xa and should have less of an effect than heparin in prolonging the partial thromboplastin time. Bergqvist and coworkers compared low-dose heparin, 5,000 units twice daily, with LMWH (kabi 2165), 5,000 units once daily, in a randomized, prospective, double-blind multicenter trial. Thrombus formation was observed in 4.3% of the patients receiving low-dose heparin and 6.4% receiving LMWH. Hemorrhagic complications were much more prevalent in the group treated with LMWH (11.6% versus 4.7% of those treated with heparin). These results were supported by a large multicenter study in France comparing subcutaneous (s.c.) heparin at a dose of 5,000 units three times daily with LMWH (enoxaparin) at doses of 20, 40, or 60 mg once daily. The authors did not find any of the preceding regimens to be significantly superior. Twenty milligrams per day of enoxaparin was found to be as safe and efficacious as 5,000 units of s.c. unfractionated heparin three times a day in preventing postoperative thrombus formation. Sasahara and colleagues evaluated LMWH and heparin sodium with the addition of DHE, 0.5 mg, to each. No significant difference was observed when comparing the ability of LMWH-DHE and heparin-DHE to prevent postoperative DVT. In addition, the hemorrhagic complications of LMWH-DHE every day and heparin-DHE twice a day were comparable. The authors believe that the once-daily regimen of LMWH-DHE gains greater patient and nursing staff acceptance and proves cost effective.

TABLE 7.8.

Results of Prophylactic Treatment of Venous Thrombosis After Gynecologic Surgery[a]

Investigators	Year	Type of Surgery	Number of Patients	Venous Thrombosis (%)					
				Control	Heparin	LMWH	Dextran	AC	Pneumatic Calf Compression
Bonnar et al.	1973	Simple hysterectomy	260	15.0	—	—	0.1	—	—
		Radical malignant	62	33.0	—	—	5.0	—	—
Ballard et al.	1973	Major gynecologic, age 40	110	29.0	3.6	—	—	—	—
McCarthy et al.	1974	Major gynecologic	130	—	10.9	—	16.2	—	—
Baertschi et al.	1975	Major gynecologic	458	—	2.3	—	—	4.7	—
Gjonnaess and Abildgaard	1976	Major gynecologic, age 50	95	8.0	2.0	—	—	—	—
Adolf et al.	1978	Major gynecologic	454	29.3	7.0	—	—	—	—
Taberner et al.	1978	Major gynecologic	146	23.0	6.0	—	—	6.0	—
Clarke-Pearson et al.	1983a	Gynecologic malignant	185	12.4	14.8	—	—	—	—
Clarke-Pearson et al.	1984	Gynecologic malignant	107	34.6	—	—	—	—	12.7
Borstad et al.	1992	Major gynecologic malignant	141	—	0.00	0.00[b]	—	—	—

[a] Detected by ^{125}I-labeled fibrinogen scan.

[b] One patient had pulmonary embolism 3 days after discontinuation of LMWH.

AC, anticoagulants; LMWH, low-molecular-weight heparin.

TABLE 7.9.
Thrombosis Prevention With Dihydroergotamine Mesylate Prophylaxis[a]

Treatment and Dose	Numbers of Patients Treated	Patients With DVT	Patients Without DVT	P Value[b]
DHE/heparin sodium, 5,000 IU	214	18 (8.4%)	196 (91.6%)	—
DHE/heparin sodium, 2,500 IU	226	32 (14.2%)	194 (85.8%)	.0396
Heparin sodium, 5,000 IU	222	32 (14.4%)	190 (85.6%)	.0341
DHE mesylate, 0.5 mg	110	18 (16.4%)	92 (83.6%)	.0263
Placebo	108	22 (20.4%)	86 (79.6%)	.0024

DHE, dihydroergotamine mesylate; DVT, deep venous thrombosis.

[a] All treatment modalities administered 2 hours before surgery and every 12 hours postoperatively for 5 days.

[b] P level compares with DHE–heparin sodium, 5,000 IU.

Source: Sasahara AA, DiSerio FJ, Singer JM, et al. Dihydroergotamine-heparin prophylaxis of postoperative deep vein thrombosis: a multicenter trial. *JAMA* 1984;251:2960.

Reiertsen and associates compared enoxaparin and dextran as DVT prophylaxis in gastrointestinal surgery. Enoxaparin was superior to dextran. In another study, Garcea and colleagues compared LMWH and calcium heparin. Although equally efficacious in prophylaxis, the latter group consumed more blood and blood products. Kaaja and coworkers found similar results when administering LMWH (enoxaparin, 20 mg) with and without DHE and unfractionated heparin. All three groups had a similar ability to provide prophylaxis. However, there was less bleeding in the LMWH regimens. The Sixth ACCP Consensus Conference on Antithrombotic Therapy did not identify trials using LMWH for gynecologic surgery that met their inclusion criteria. LMWH was felt to provide protection comparable to unfractionated heparin, although uncontrolled case studies were suggestive of protection. Maxwell and colleagues recently published a randomized study comparing pneumatic compression devices and low-molecular-weight heparin in the gynecologic oncology patient. Both were comparable in preventing DVT. LMWH did not appear to increase blood loss. The authors recommended either modality and do not require both for the prevention of DVT in the gynecologic oncology surgical patient.

Fricker and colleagues compared low-dose heparin, 5,000 units every 8 hours for 10 days, with LMWH (kabi 2165, Fragmin), 5,000 anti-Xa units every morning for 10 days. On postoperative day 0, the latter group received 2,500 anti-Xa units 2 hours before surgery and 12 hours after the initial injection. All patients in the study underwent primary or secondary surgery for an abdominal or pelvic carcinoma. Both regimens were equally effective in preventing DVT. Two patients in the heparin group had a PE, and two receiving LMWH had positive ^{125}I fibrinogen tests and negative phlebography. A second study compared kabi 2165 (Fragmin) and unfractionated heparin in 141 patients undergoing gynecologic surgery. Four of 70 patients receiving unfractionated heparin and six of 71 receiving LMWH had a gynecologic malignancy. Unfractionated heparin was administered in a 5,000-unit dose twice a day in this study.

No patients in the study developed DVT. One of the LMWH patients had a PE 3 days after prophylaxis was stopped.

COMPRESSION MODALITIES
Initial studies in 1944 by Stanton and colleagues used static compression to decrease venous stasis. By decreasing the luminal diameter, blood flow velocity was increased. Sigel and associates showed an increase in blood velocity of 20% (1973) using graduated elastic compression stockings versus an increase of 200% with intermittent sequential pneumatic compression. When comparing intermittent sequential pneumatic compression with uniform intermittent calf compression, Mittleman and coworkers found the former to be more effective in increasing blood flow in the thigh region. It is accepted that compression modalities decrease at least one component of Virchow's triad—stasis. Several investigators believe that compression modalities may have a marked effect on a second component in Virchow's triad—coagulability. Intermittent pneumatic compression (IPC) has been shown by several authors (Allenby and colleagues, Tarnay and associates, and Caprini and coworkers) to stimulate fibrinolysis. The role of IPC in increasing prostaglandin production has been suggested in two recent studies. Guyton and colleagues identified an increased production of 6-keto prostaglandin F1 in patients undergoing IPC when compared with controls. Frango and associates demonstrated in human endothelial cell cultures a 16-fold increase in prostacyclin production in cells under conditions of pulsatile shear stress versus a twofold increase with constant shear stress when compared with controls.

Graduated Compression Stockings. Initial studies evaluating antiembolic stockings were inconclusive and relied on several different methods to diagnose thrombosis (clinical DVT and PE versus ^{125}I fibrinogen uptake). In 1975, Sigel and colleagues designed a graduated compression thromboembolism-deterrent (TED) stocking with pressures of 18, 14, 8, 10, and 8 mm Hg from the ankle to the upper thigh. Scurr and associates evaluated the efficiency of TED hose in 75 patients older than 40 years of age undergoing major abdominal surgery with only one leg covered by the TED hose. During clinical evaluation of ^{125}I fibrinogen testing, 19 patients developed DVT in the control leg, and only 1 patient developed DVT in the stockinged leg. An additional 110 patients were evaluated by Inada and colleagues, with each patient wearing TED hose on one leg. DVT was found in 14.5% of the control legs and in 3.6% of the legs with stockings. Malignancy has been shown to predispose patients to the formation of DVT, secondary to stasis and plasminogen production by the tumor. Allan and coworkers demonstrated the efficacy of graduated compression stockings in preventing DVT formation in patients undergoing major abdominal surgery for benign and malignant diseases. In patients with benign disease, DVT was present in 24.5% of the control limbs and 6.1% of the stockinged limbs. In patients with malignancy, 27.9% of the control limbs and 11.5% of the stockinged limbs demonstrated the presence of DVT by ^{125}I fibrinogen testing. The Sixth ACCP Consensus Conference on Antithrombotic therapy suggested that graduated compression stockings with early ambulation would provide sufficient prophylaxis in the low-risk gynecologic operative candidate.

External Intermittent Pneumatic Compression. External compression of the lower extremities decreases stasis and improves fibrinolysis. Nicolaides and associates (1980) compared intermittent sequential pneumatic compression, nonsequential (one-chamber) pneumatic compression, and heparin in the prevention of postoperative DVT. Using pressures of 35, 30, and 20 mm Hg sequentially for 12 seconds at the ankle, calf, and thigh, Nicolaides and associates observed a 240% increase in the peak blood velocity. When using a single chamber inflated at 35 mm Hg for 12 seconds, the peak blood velocity increased 180%. Using the ^{125}I fibrinogen test, the authors demonstrated that the intermittent sequential pneumatic compression device was as effective as heparin, 5,000 units every 12 hours, in preventing DVT. The sequential device was also found to be more effective than the single chamber in preventing thrombosis of the lower extremities. In addition, intermittent sequential pneumatic compression increased the time interval for clot formation proximal to the calf when compared with heparin. In another study, Nicolaides and coworkers (1983) compared electrical calf stimulation, low-dose s.c. heparin, and intermittent sequential compression and the use of TED stockings in 150 patients older than 30 years of age undergoing major abdominal surgery. The incidence of ^{125}I fibrinogen-detected DVT was 18%, 9%, and 4%, respectively. In a prospective study, Clarke-Pearson and colleagues (1981) showed the efficacy of external pneumatic calf compression in preventing postoperative venous thromboembolism in patients undergoing surgery for a gynecologic malignancy. All 107 patients were prospectively screened for DVT with impedance plethysmography and ^{125}I fibrinogen testing. The control group did not receive thromboembolic prophylaxis, but nonsequential external

pneumatic pressure cuffs with pressures of 40 to 45 mm Hg every 12 seconds were placed on the lower extremities of the remaining patients. DVT or PE was present in 34.6% of the controls, compared with 12.7% of those who received external pneumatic calf compression devices intraoperatively and for 5 postoperative days ($p < .005$). The National Institutes of Health Consensus Development Conference on Prevention of Venous Thrombosis and Pulmonary Embolism recommended external pneumatic compression as a prophylactic measure in patients at moderate and high risk. Patients with a malignancy were believed to benefit from a combination of low-dose heparin and external pneumatic compression.

Thrombosis in Malignancies

Since its initial description in 1868, Trousseau's syndrome of migratory thrombotic disease in neoplasias has been described in conjunction with a multitude of primary tumors. The predominant histology is an adenocarcinoma. In a comprehensive review of the literature in 1977, Sach and colleagues at the Johns Hopkins Hospital identified 123 patients with Trousseau's syndrome. The patients presented with thrombus formation in several locations: venous, arterial, and cardiac. Nusbacher, in a series of 68 patients presenting with carcinoma, noted that 75% initially presented with migratory thrombophlebitis before the diagnosis of neoplasia, and 50% had a PE. In 128 patients who had PE documented by angiography, Gore and associates showed an increased incidence in the diagnosis of malignancies after a PE. The increased hypercoagulable state of a malignancy predisposes the patient to embolic processes, including PE.

Treatment of patients with Trousseau's syndrome consists of identification of the malignancy and appropriate treatment. Anticoagulation with i.v. heparin followed by oral coumadin (warfarin) compounds is required to decrease the thrombosis and the consumption of platelets and clotting factors. Several patients have been found to be resistant to coumadin and require daily maintenance with heparin. Sach and colleagues noted that all patients not responding to heparin were not sensitive to coumadin compounds. However, most who were resistant to coumadin responded to heparin. Proponents of coumadin therapy suggest that coumadin is a small nonpolar molecule that can diffuse out of the vascular space and act directly at the tumor site or intravascularly as an anticoagulant. Heparin is a large, charged compound unable to diffuse out of the vascular compartment and as such may not have a direct effect on the third-spaced tumor cells that produce a procoagulant. Heparin should be used as first-line therapy in patients with migratory thrombophlebitis. When the patient is fully anticoagulated, attempts should be made to administer an oral agent such as coumadin. Patients resistant to coumadin should be treated with s.c. or i.v. heparin on an outpatient basis.

After identification of a primary malignancy, patients with Trousseau's syndrome are treated by decreasing fibrin degradation, decreasing platelet consumption, and decreasing clot migration and embolization. Physical examination findings consistent with thrombophlebitis, arterial emboli, and bleeding may herald the presence of a malignancy. In addition to managing coagulopathy, identifying its etiology should include evaluating for a malignancy. As mentioned, an embolus is frequently the result of the hypercoagulable state of a malignancy that may be present. Hematologic changes, including increased fibrinopeptide A, increased fibrin split products, increased turnover rate of fibrinogen, prolonged prothrombin time, and microangiopathic hemolytic anemia, often present as a result of intravascular coagulation and fibrinolysis in patients with neoplasias.

Trousseau's syndrome in patients with gynecologic malignancies has not been addressed extensively in the gynecologic literature. Intravascular coagulation, fibrinolysis, and migratory thrombosis in the form of venous and arterial emboli as well as pulmonary embolism continue to present the gynecologist with a clinical dilemma.

Anticoagulant Therapy

There is general agreement that DVT should be treated initially with i.v. heparin, using 5,000 to 10,000 IU as an i.v. bolus. This produces therapeutic levels for anticoagulation in most patients. Because the major effect of an i.v. bolus of heparin will be cleared from the plasma within 4 hours, maintenance doses of heparin should be given either by intermittent i.v. injections at intervals of 4 to 6 hours or, preferably, by continuous i.v. infusion at a rate of 1,000 to 1,200 international units (IU) per hour. We prefer to use a constant-infusion i.v. pump that is reliable in delivering small continuous doses of heparin, because when heparin is administered by intermittent i.v. bolus, 15% to 25% of patients receive either an inadequate or excessive dose. A weight-based nomogram partial thromboplastin time (PTT) has been found to achieve therapeutic anticoagulation faster than dosing. Continuous heparinization by the i.v. route prevents the rise and fall of the heparin level and avoids recurrent thrombosis during the period of inadequate anticoagulation and potential bleeding complications when heparin levels are increased. The level of anticoagulation should be carefully monitored 30 min before each scheduled intermittent bolus. In patients receiving continuous i.v. infusion, the level of anticoagulation may be assessed at any time. An anticoagulation level equivalent to a Lee-White clotting time that is two to three times the control level is considered adequate. Alternatively, an activated PTT of 1.5 to 2 times the control level indicates adequate anticoagulation. The monitoring method should be in accordance with the local preference of the clinical laboratory being used. Once optimal levels are established, clotting studies can be done at 24-hour intervals to determine proper maintenance doses of heparin. The duration of i.v. treatment is difficult to specify, but treatment should be continued for at least 5 to 7 days, until there has been resolution of the thrombus in the leg veins or until thrombi have become firmly organized and attached to the vessel wall. If clinical signs of improvement are not clearly demonstrated, more than 7 days of treatment may be required. The symptomatic patient with acute thrombophlebitis also should be maintained at bed rest until the symptoms of pain and fever have subsided. The patient's leg should be maintained in an elevated position until the edema has completely subsided, at which time progressive ambulation is permitted. It is our policy to restrict ambulation until the leg edema has subsided. Oral anticoagulation is initiated after 5 to 7 days of heparin therapy. The combination of oral coumadin and tapered doses of heparin is used for about 48 to 72 hours, after which coumadin therapy is continued alone. Proper coumadin therapy is aimed at maintaining a prothrombin time approximately 2.5 times the normal control. Coumadin therapy is usually continued for 4 to 6 weeks.

The rationale for the treatment of asymptomatic DVT of the lower extremity has been questioned by many surgeons. In brief, some simply ignore this subclinical diagnosis and consider this vascular phenomenon to be an innocuous sequela of pelvic surgery. However, if patients with established venous thrombosis are not treated, the risk of serious morbidity or, possibly, mortality must be considered. The major risk is extension of the venous thrombus into the popliteal and proximal veins of the thigh, which reportedly occurs in about 20% of cases. A Doppler scan, plethysmogram, or venogram is required to identify a proximal thrombosis. It is estimated that 40% of these patients, or 8% of the group with thrombosis of the calf veins, will have pulmonary emboli and, more important, recurrent embolization. On the conservative side, one might question the advisability of treating the 80% of patients who do not have proximal migration of the venous clot into the thigh to protect the 20% who do. If the 8% risk of pulmonary embolization is not sufficient reason for treatment, one should consider that once extension of the thrombosis into the proximal vessels has occurred, nearly two thirds of the patients have residual disease in the venous system of the leg, with loss of valve function and impairment of venous return. This complication often leads to the postphlebitic syndrome of chronic pain and lymphedema of the lower extremity. Because of these unhappy consequences, the prudent surgeon should consider the brief treatment of documented DVT to be a relatively cost-effective method of managing this vascular complication of pelvic surgery.

Acute iliofemoral thrombosis is one of the most serious and hazardous complications of venous thrombosis of the lower extremity. An estimated 40% of patients with this condition develop pulmonary emboli. This condition is difficult to misdiagnose because in the acute stage, commonly called phlegmasia cerulea dolens, the leg becomes exquisitely tender, edematous, and cyanotic. During the acute stage there may be high morbidity from gangrene as well as high mortality from PE. This condition also results in a high incidence of chronic postphlebitic venous obstruction with chronic pain and peripheral edema. Effective therapy requires immediate anticoagulation as outlined. If complete occlusion occurs, then surgical treatment is usually required. Unless the clot is removed from the iliofemoral vessels, propagation into the vena cava and PE may occur in as many as 50% of cases, according to Mavor.

Venography is useful in confirming the diagnosis of iliofemoral thrombosis and is essential in evaluating the extent of involvement of the contiguous deep veins. When a pulmonary embolus has occurred, venography also is helpful in determining the presence of nonocclusive contralateral thrombosis in the opposite leg, which may be the site of origin of the embolus.

Most cases of iliofemoral thrombosis are insidious in origin and can be treated medically with heparin therapy if diagnosed early, thereby avoiding complete vascular occlusion leading to massive swelling of the leg with pooling of blood, which may produce hypovolemia. Although the risk of mobilization of an embolus is always present, when gangrene has set in it is urgent that immediate thrombectomy be performed, with clearance of the iliofemoral segments. With the use of i.v. heparin therapy and early thrombectomy, the incidence of pulmonary emboli has been extremely low. In these acutely ill patients, i.v. heparin must be maintained continuously until there is complete resolution of the leg edema, inflammation, and pain in the calf and thigh. Only then can the patient be ambulated and the process of oral anticoagulation be initiated. These patients require not only early and aggressive management, both medical and surgical, but continuation of the anticoagulation therapy for 6 to 9 months for complete vascular canalization and prevention of recurrent thrombosis.

PULMONARY COMPLICATIONS

Hypoventilation

Hypoventilation is one of the most common and dangerous complications in the immediate postoperative period, even in patients with normal lungs. To assess ventilation, the expired gas can be collected, and the volume expired per minute (minute volume, V_E) can be determined. However, a portion of this gas ventilates non–gas-exchanging areas of the lung, namely, conducting airways, referred to as dead space. This ventilation is wasted, because it does not participate in gas exchange. The normal dead space volume is about equal in pulmonary milliliters to the person's ideal weight in pounds (i.e., a 150-lb woman has a dead space volume of 150 mL). To calculate the effective or alveolar ventilation, the dead space must be subtracted from the tidal volume and the difference multiplied by the respiratory rate. Gross errors in the estimation of ventilation can be made if only V_E is considered. If tidal volume decreases from 500 to 250 mL but respiratory rate doubles from 14 to 28 respirations per minute, minute volume remains at 7.0 L. However, assuming a dead space of 150 mL, the alveolar ventilation under these conditions decreases from 4.9 to 2.8 L, resulting in a significant alteration in blood gases. This type of respiratory pattern is common in the patient with abdominal surgery, who tends to decrease tidal volume to

avoid pain. Hypoventilation is defined as a level of alveolar ventilation that is insufficient to prevent accumulation of carbon dioxide. The causes include depression of central respiratory control from obesity, neuromuscular disease, pain, restrictive dressings, immobility, hypomobility, and increased carbon dioxide production. Patients with obstructive and restrictive respiratory impairment are much more likely to develop hypoventilation during this critical early postoperative period.

Inadequate ventilation may not be clinically obvious unless an estimate of alveolar ventilation is made. Ultimately, arterial blood gas studies are the most accurate measure of alveolar ventilation. Table 7.10 shows the effect of decreasing alveolar ventilation on the arterial blood gases. From these data, it can be seen that although the arterial carbon dioxide tension ($PaCO_2$) rises almost linearly as alveolar ventilation decreases, changes in oxygenation (arterial oxygen saturation, SaO_2) are modest until respiratory acidosis is severe. Thus, the best indicator of adequate ventilation is the $PaCO_2$. A normal arterial oxygen tension (PaO_2) in the presence of a severe respiratory acidosis (elevated $PaCO_2$) would implicate the administration of oxygen as a causative factor in the hypoventilation.

Acute Ventilatory Failure

The treatment of acute ventilatory failure manifested by hypoventilation and a $PaCO_2$ greater than 50 mm Hg is mechanical ventilatory support until the causative factors can be alleviated. This may require several hours to several days. It is important, therefore, to leave the endotracheal tube in place after surgery until adequate spontaneous ventilation and arterial blood gas levels have been demonstrated. The adequacy of respiratory mechanics can be determined by measuring tidal volume and inspiratory effort. The tidal volume should exceed 10 mL/kg, and inspiratory pressure should be greater than -20 cmH$_2$O. The tidal volume alone is not a reliable indicator of respiratory adequacy in a patient with abnormal lungs because of changes in physiologic dead space. Under these circumstances, $PaCO_2$ is used as a guide, because an elevated or rising $PaCO_2$ is the best clinical indicator of inadequate alveolar ventilation and progressive respira-

TABLE 7.10.
Effect of Decreasing Alveolar Ventilation on Arterial Blood Gases

Alveolar Ventilation (L/min)	Arterial Blood Gases			
	PaO_2 (mm Hg)	SaO_2 (%)	$PaCO_2$ (mm Hg)	pH
5.0	100	96	40	7.40
4.0	82	94	50	7.32
3.0	68	87	75	7.20
2.0	30	40	105	7.05

tory acidosis. Weaning is accomplished either by taking the patient off the ventilator with supplemental oxygen and periodic monitoring of arterial blood gas levels or by intermittent mandatory ventilation (IMV). The latter technique allows the gradual reduction of ventilator support with the advantage of providing a known minimum minute ventilation and the security of the monitoring systems of the ventilator. The addition of pressure support (PS) ventilation to IMV or PS alone reduces the work of breathing and can facilitate the weaning process. These methods are particularly helpful in patients who have poor ventilatory reserve or who have been intubated for prolonged periods. After extubation, treatment can be continued with supplemental oxygen and intermittent positive pressure breathing (IPPB) until the patient's respiratory status is stabilized.

Acute Respiratory Distress Syndrome

Ashbaugh and colleagues were the first to describe acute respiratory distress syndrome (ARDS). Since that report in 1967, our understanding of the pathophysiology and treatment of ARDS has progressed considerably. The patients included in that first report had dyspnea, refractory hypoxemia, decreased lung compliance, and diffuse alveolar infiltrates. These authors also noted that a variety of causes could result in the clinical presentation of ARDS.

The American-European Consensus Conference Committee on ARDS was formed to address the overall lack of uniformity in the definition of ARDS and bring about international coordination in the study of ARDS and its treatments. This committee defined ARDS as a syndrome of inflammation and increased permeability through a process of nonhydrostatic pulmonary edema and hypoxemia associated with a variety of etiologies. They suggested the term acute lung injury (ALI) be used to describe the continuum of pathologic responses to parenchymal lung injury. ARDS is differentiated from the less severe ALI by the degree of disturbance in oxygenation level. These definitions are shown in Table 7.11. These definitions allow scientists and clinicians to discuss acute ventilatory failure in a more consistent manner.

ARDS has a reported annual incidence of about 150,000 cases in the United States. ARDS carries an extremely high morbidity rate. The mortality rate from ARDS has declined over the last two decades, but still remains relatively high, between 40% and 68%, despite extensive study with many therapeutic modalities. A multitude of factors have been implicated in the development of ARDS. These are shown in Table 7.12 and can be divided into direct and indirect causes.

Clinically, there are four stages patients experience with ARDS. The first phase is that of acute lung injury; the only manifestation may be a respiratory alkalosis. Patients then enter a latent phase lasting up to 48 hours, characterized by rales on physical examination and patchy infiltrates on chest radiograph. The next stage is acute respiratory failure with tachypnea, dyspnea, hypoxemia refractory to oxygen, and decreases in lung compliance. During this third stage chest radiograph commonly shows diffuse patchy infiltrates and air bronchograms. The last clinical stage is intrapulmonary shunting that leads to worsening hypoxemia despite conventional oxygen therapy. Severe physiologic derangements may occur, including simultaneous respiratory and metabolic acidosis.

On the cellular level changes that occur are quite complex and cause diffuse alveolar injury. Initially, the permeability of both the pulmonary endothelium and epithelium is increased causing a leakage of protein-rich fluid into the alveoli and interstitium. There is an increase in surface tension and an influx of neutrophils and monocytes as well as a release of numerous inflammatory mediators and complement activation. Fibrin and plasma proteins accumulate to form hyaline membranes. A fibroproliferative phase ensues over several days with continued infiltration of inflammatory cells. Fibrosis and scarring are the end results.

The cornerstone of therapy for ARDS is mechanical ventilatory support with low tidal volumes and high levels of positive end-expiratory pressure (PEEP). This lung-protective ventilation strategy limits peak airway pressures, and has been shown to decrease mortality and increase the number of days without ventilator use. A recently published study revealed a significant decrease in mortality (31% versus 40%), when ventilation with low tidal volumes was compared to traditional tidal volumes

TABLE 7.11.
Definitions of Acute Lung Injury (ALI) and Acute Respiratory Distress Syndrome (ARDS)[a]

ALI	200 mm Hg < PaO_2/FiO_2 ≤ 300 mm Hg
ARDS	PaO_2/FiO_2 ≤ 200 mm Hg

PaO_2/FiO_2 is the ratio of the partial pressure of oxygen to the inspired oxygen concentration.
[a] These terms were defined by the American-European Consensus Committee on ARDS.

TABLE 7.12.
Risk Factors for the Development of Acute Respiratory Distress Syndrome

Direct Causes	Indirect Causes
Pneumonia	Shock
Aspiration	Sepsis or Infection
Toxic inhalation	Trauma or burns
Pulmonary contusion	Drug overdose
Coagulation	Disseminated intravascular Pancreatitis
	Amniotic fluid or fat embolism
	Eclampsia

in treatment of patients with ALI and ARDS. Changing the body position of the patient from supine to lateral decubitus or prone has been studied in the treatment of ARDS. Results are extremely variable and the proning maneuver itself may introduce technical difficulties; therefore, this treatment modality has not gained widespread acceptance. Inverse ratio ventilation (usual ratio of inspiratory time to expiratory time is reversed) to improve ventilation has shown no survival advantage in treating patients with ARDS. General summary guidelines for mechanical ventilatory support for patients with ARDS includes use of PEEP with low tidal volumes (6 to 8 mL/kg) to keep plateau pressure <32 cmH$_2$O.

The use of antiinflammatory agents such as corticosteroids has been studied in patients with ARDS. Current data do not support their regular use in the treatment of ARDS. Future investigation with corticosteroids in patients with ARDS, especially those with persistent or late ARDS, is ongoing. Nitrous oxide has been shown to improve oxygenation in ARDS patients by reversing pulmonary vasoconstriction, but its use has revealed no survival benefit. Additional areas of study in the treatment of ARDS include partial liquid ventilation using perfluorocarbons, exogenous surfactant, and various combinations of the described modalities.

The prognosis of ARDS has improved with an increasing understanding of the mechanisms of ARDS, early recognition, and aggressive intervention. The long-term outlook is variable, but most patients who survive are left with surprisingly few pulmonary sequelae.

Atelectasis

The majority of patients who receive general anesthesia experience some degree of postoperative pulmonary dysfunction. Atelectasis, which is the collapse of the peripheral airways in the lung, is caused by hypoventilation. Additionally, obstruction of the bronchioles causing distal gas absorption can contribute to atelectasis. The functional residual capacity (FRC), which can be decreased up to 2 weeks after general anesthesia, is a major component of small airway patency.

The clinical manifestations of atelectasis are common in the first several days after surgery. These manifestations include decreased breath sounds (especially in the lung bases), rales, cyanosis, hypoxia, and tachycardia. Fever is one of the most common signs attributed to atelectasis. The question of whether atelectasis causes fever is controversial one. Traditionally fever, defined as a temperature of $>38°C$, in the immediate postoperative period without any obvious source of infection has been attributed to atelectasis. This common textbook axiom has little scientific support in human and animal studies. Engoren even reported data revealing a lack of association between atelectasis and postoperative fever. Nonetheless, this is a controversial issue; the routine postoperative care of patients often includes steps to prevent and treat atelectasis.

Prophylaxis against atelectasis should begin preoperatively with patient education. This includes instruction in the use of incentive spirometry and deep breathing and coughing exercises. Postoperatively the patient should be encouraged to use incentive spirometry and early and frequent ambulation. Frequent change in patient positioning along with deep breathing and coughing exercises may minimize atelectasis postoperatively. Adequate pain control should not be overlooked. Poor pain control may lead to a decrease in respiratory effort from the patient. Other measures, such as mucolytic agents and bronchodilators, have been used to treat postoperative atelectasis. As atelectasis becomes more widespread, positive pressure ventilation and hyperinflation may be necessary to reverse this process. For extensive atelectasis, bronchoscopy to remove mucus plugs may be necessary.

Pneumonia

Postoperative pneumonia has become less common with the introduction of early ambulation and intensive respiratory therapy in the immediate postoperative period. Because pneumonia is frequently associated with atelectasis and hypoventilation, prevention or prompt reversal of these conditions is the best prophylactic measure. Animal studies have shown that even with instillation of infected material directly into the lower respiratory tract, pneumonia could not result without such additional factors as atelectasis and hypoventilation. A decrease in the activity of cilia caused by drugs or altered humidity may interfere significantly with bacterial clearing. This is particularly true in patients with obstructive lung disease. In patients with an endotracheal tube in place, the normal protective mechanisms of the upper respiratory system are abolished. Infection is much more likely to develop in this group and is directly related to the duration of intubation. Gram-negative organisms, usually *Proteus* or *Pseudomonas,* are most often encountered under these circumstances. Deep tracheal secretions should be aspirated into a sterile sputum trap for culture and antibiotic susceptibility studies. Pathogenic organisms are invariably isolated, but it must be emphasized that a positive sputum culture cannot be equated with pulmonary infection requiring antibiotic therapy. Patients at risk for developing postoperative pneumonia are patients with an American Society of Anesthesia status of 3 or greater, a history of smoking, a preoperative hospital stay of 2 days or more, surgery lasting 3 hours or longer, or a surgical site in the upper abdomen or thorax. Treatment must be based on such additional criteria as fever, persistence of purulent sputum, leukocytosis, positive blood culture, and physical and roentgenographic signs of pneumonia. Prophylactic antibiotic therapy rarely has a place in the treatment of patients on assisted ventilation except in emergency situations, such as acute aspiration or fulminating infection, in which the Gram-stained sputum smear should be used as a guide for initial therapy. Meticulous aseptic technique must be used in suctioning to prevent the introduction of infection. Adequate humidification is essential to facilitate the removal of secretions.

CARE OF THE URINARY BLADDER

The most common postoperative problem in the female bladder is atony caused by overdistention and the reluctance of the patient to initiate the voluntary phase of voiding. After abdominal surgery, the patient is often unwilling to contract the abdominal muscles to produce sufficient intraabdominal pressure against the dome of the bladder to initiate the voiding reflex. After anterior colporrhaphy, spasm, edema, and tenderness of the pubococcygeal muscles may obstruct the process of voiding. The operative trauma from plication of the pubovesicocervical fascia causes edema of the urethral wall and submucosa, especially at the urethrovesical junction, thus contributing to the urinary obstruction.

For spontaneous voiding to occur, the parasympathetic function of the bladder detrusor must be coordinated with the voluntary motor function of the abdominal wall and the levator muscles. In the past, it was customary to insert an indwelling urethral catheter for 5 or more days after vaginal plastic surgery. Although this technique is still used in many clinics, a suprapubic catheter has proved to be very effective in urinary drainage. The suprapubic technique was developed and introduced to the gynecologic literature in 1964. When inserted at the time of surgery, the suprapubic Silastic tube eliminates the necessity for repeated bladder catheterization until spontaneous voiding occurs. Although used preferentially after anterior vaginal colporrhaphy, suprapubic bladder catheterization also is useful when the need for prolonged bladder drainage is anticipated, such as after radical Wertheim hysterectomy. A suprapubic catheter also can be inserted when a Marshall-Marchetti-Krantz urethral suspension is performed.

The procedure for suprapubic bladder drainage is performed either before or after the operative procedure. Catheter placement consists of insertion of a 12F Silastic (silicone) catheter into the bladder through a needle trocar (Fig. 7.3). A 12F pigtail (Bonnano) Teflon catheter and other modifications also have been used by many surgeons. The bladder is filled with 300 mL of sterile water, and the needle trocar is inserted through the surgically cleaned anterior abdominal wall about 2 cm above the symphysis pubis. When the stylet is removed from the trocar, clear fluid should pass from the bladder under pressure. About 10 cm of the suprapubic catheter is threaded through the trocar, after which the trocar is removed by sliding it over the indwelling tube. The opposite end of the Silastic catheter is connected to a sterile 1-L drainage bottle or to a sterile closed drainage urinometer bag. The tubing should be filled with fluid at all times and should be anchored to the skin with silicone paste or sutured to the skin to avoid accidental removal. A two-way stopcock is inserted between the catheter and drainage tubing for easy opening and closing of the system. The system is not irrigated unless there is plugging of the bladder catheter and failure of drainage.

Alternatively, at the Emory University Hospital, a Foley catheter is placed through the abdominal wall. Af-

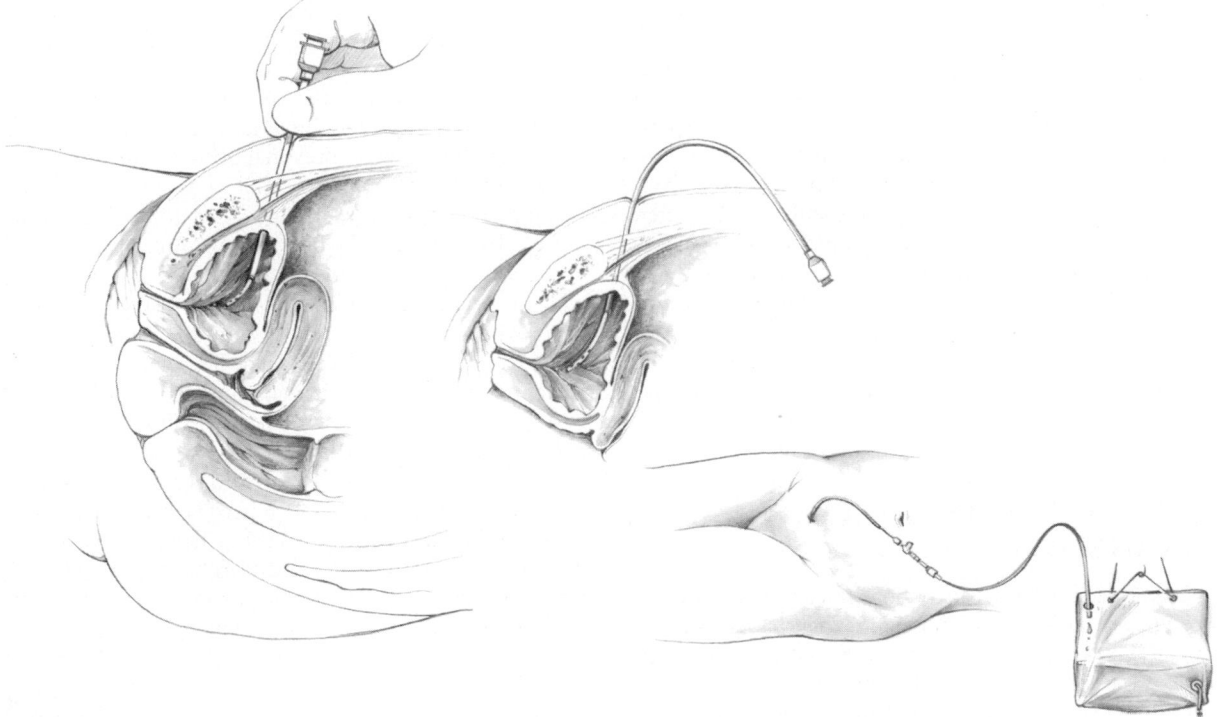

FIGURE 7.3. Method of inserting a suprapubic tube into the bladder through a needle, with resultant drainage into a bottle. Suprapubic catheterization avoids the trauma to the urethra caused by repeated catheterization of an indwelling catheter.

ter placing a Kelly clamp through the urethra and elevating the dome of the bladder, an incision is made in the abdominal wall superior to the Kelly clamp. A 14F Foley catheter is then pulled into the bladder and connected to gravity drainage. If a suprapubic urethropexy is performed, a 2- to 3-cm opening is made in the dome of the bladder and the bladder is inspected to ensure that no sutures penetrated the mucosa. The Foley catheter is placed in the bladder and sutured in place with a no. 2.0 absorbable pursestring suture. Using the preceding techniques for insertion of a suprapubic Foley catheter, we have decreased the frequency of catheter obstruction.

At the Emory University Hospital, suprapubic catheters are often used after vaginal reconstruction for ambiguous genitalia and suprapubic urethropexies. Transurethral Foley catheters, however, have replaced suprapubic catheters in most patients undergoing abdominal or vaginal hysterectomy and anterior colporrhaphy with Kelly urethral plication. Seven to 10 days postoperatively, the catheters are removed and postvoid residuals are evaluated. Patients with more than 100 mL of residual urine after spontaneous voiding require an extended period of transurethral catheterization, suprapubic catheterization, or intermittent self-catheterization. The gynecologic oncologists at our institution advocate the use of transurethral Foley catheters in patients undergoing radical hysterectomy. The catheter is routinely removed 14 to 21 days postoperatively, and residuals are evaluated as mentioned. Alternatively, we discharge the patient on postoperative day 4 or 5 with self-catheterization. The patient discontinues intermittent self-catheterization when postvoid residuals are less than 100 mL.

We believe, as do other authors, that prophylactic antibiotics given during the use of an indwelling bladder catheter are ineffective in preventing urinary tract infection. Although urinary tract symptoms may be delayed with the use of prophylactic antibiotics, it is our experience that the incidence of infection is unchanged and that a subsequent urinary tract infection may result from resistant organisms that are more difficult to treat later. Therefore, we prefer to treat only patients who have significant bacteriuria and pyuria, which includes about 10% to 15% of the patients with suprapubic drainage. This incidence of bladder infection is a significant improvement from the common rate of 70% to 90% (Kass and Sossen) when a urethral catheter is retained for more than 72 hours.

GASTROINTESTINAL TRACT MANAGEMENT

Dysfunction of the gastrointestinal tract remains a challenge in postoperative management. Each patient should be treated as an individual and not placed on a standard protocol for advancing diets. Patients who have had uncomplicated surgery may be given clear liquids on the first postoperative day if bowel sounds are present, if abdominal examination reveals no distention, and if the patient is no longer nauseated from her anesthesia. After fla-

tus is passed, the diet should be accelerated as tolerated to a regular diet. Seriously ill or malnourished patients or patients requiring extensive bowel surgery benefit from preoperative and postoperative parenteral nutrition.

Patients requiring extensive bowel manipulation, dissection, and excision undoubtedly experience a delay in the return of bowel function and require the placement of a nasogastric tube at the time of surgery. Nasogastric tubes may have a single or double lumen. Single-lumen tubes such as Levin-type tubes or Cantor tubes are connected to a source of low intermittent suction. Although either tube is acceptable in a patient with a small bowel obstruction, some surgeons prefer the long Cantor tube, which passes through the small intestines with the assistance of a mercury-filled balloon attached to its distal port. Double-lumen tubes, such as the Salem sump, have a second lumen that functions as a pressure valve. This tube can be connected to a source of low constant suction or high intermittent suction. If the second port is occluded, it should be managed as a single-lumen tube. It is imperative that all gastric contents be replaced equally with normal saline or half normal saline containing 20 to 40 mEq KCl/L. Patients on nasogastric suction also should have an electrolyte panel obtained daily to ensure adequate replacement.

It is important to differentiate between postoperative ileus and postoperative obstruction (Table 7.13) if proper therapy is to be initiated promptly with beneficial results. The distinction may be difficult. This is because partial bowel obstruction is often accompanied by a secondary ileus as part of the clinical picture. Only by close clinical monitoring of the bowel sounds, serial abdominal radiographic studies, and frequent white blood cell counts can one clearly separate these two postoperative complications. Adynamic ileus is the more common clinical entity, a fact that may mislead the surgeon into a false sense of security unless he or she remains acutely aware of the distinguishing features of intestinal obstruction. Serial monitoring of the white blood cell count and differential count is an important method for differentiating between bowel obstruction and paralytic ileus. A key feature of advancing bowel obstruction is necrosis of the bowel wall, which causes progressive leukocytosis, along with distention and peritonitis. The most common gynecologic disease process associated with both ileus and intestinal obstruction is severe pelvic inflammatory disease (PID). Notoriously, acute exacerbation of PID or rupture of a pelvic abscess is associated with prolonged ileus. Occasionally, fibrous adhesions form and secondary bowel obstruction occurs. Postoperative pelvic peritonitis from any cause, including cellulitis resulting from hematoma formation and secondary infection of the vaginal cuff, is often associated with ileus, whereas intestinal obstruction only rarely results from such a complication.

In contrast to pelvic surgery for benign disease, any cancer surgery, including pelvic exenteration for cervical carcinoma, can be complicated either by postoperative adynamic ileus or intestinal obstruction. When radical surgery is preceded by preoperative irradiation, the small bowel often is compromised by a protracted ileus.

TABLE 7.13.
Differential Diagnosis Between Postoperative Ileus and Postoperative Obstruction

Clinical Feature	Postoperative Ileus	Postoperative Obstruction
Abdominal pain	Discomfort from distention but not cramping pains	Cramping progressively severe
Relation to previous surgery	Usually within 48–72 h of surgery	Usually delayed, may be 5–7 d for remote onset
Nausea and vomiting	Present	Present
Distention	Present	Present
Bowel sounds	Absent or hypoactive	Borborygmi with peristaltic rushes and high-pitched tinkles
Fever	Only if related to associated peritonitis	Rarely present unless bowel becomes gangrenous
Abdominal radiographs	Distended loops of small and large bowels; gas usually present in colon	Single or multiple loops of distended bowel (usually small bowel) with air–fluid levels
Treatment	Conservative with nasogastric suction, enemas, cholinergic stimulation	Conservative management with nasogastric decompression Surgical exploration

TOTAL PARENTERAL NUTRITION

Nutritional support has proved efficacious in patients undergoing major surgery and in patients with impaired bowel function, inadequate oral intake, or cancer. A few patients require total parenteral nutrition (TPN) for prolonged periods secondary to their inability to obtain adequate calories orally. Parenteral nutrition may be administered through a peripheral or central access, depending on the patient's initial nutritional status and the time required on TPN.

Hospitalized patients may require TPN for disease processes such as gastrointestinal tract obstruction, prolonged ileus, short-bowel syndrome, radiation enteritis, intraabdominal abscess, pancreatitis, regional enteritis, and enterocutaneous fistula. A patient with any condition that prevents oral intake of adequate amounts of food for more than 7 to 10 days probably requires central parenteral nutrition. Because it is much easier to maintain an adequate nutritional state than to improve a poor one, the decision to use TPN should not be delayed.

Peripheral alimentation is used in patients who are not in a catabolic state and require nutritional support for less than 7 days. Peripheral total hyperalimentation solution (THAS) typically has an osmolality of 800 versus 1,850 mOsm for standard THAS and 2,050 mOsm for concentrated THAS (Table 7.14). Alternatively, central THAS is used in patients requiring prolonged nutritional support for more than 1 week or for the promotion of anabolism.

Total parenteral nutrition is not without complications. Many of these pertain to the need for central venous access. Catheter tip infection is one of the more frequently encountered problems. Meticulous aseptic technique when placing the central venous catheter and adherence to aseptic technique when using the catheter minimizes the risk of infection. Antibiotic-coated central venous catheters have been around for more than a decade, and are coming more into favor as compelling data surface suggesting decreased infection rates with their use. At The Emory University Hospital central venous catheters coated with chlorhexidine and silver sulfasalazine are being utilized. Other potential problems with central venous catheters include catheter or air embolism and pneumothorax or hemothorax. TPN itself can cause fluid overload, electrolyte abnormalities, or metabolic disturbances. The appropriate monitoring of these parameters is discussed later in this chapter.

Starvation and Stress

The starvation seen in severely ill, hospitalized patients is different from simple starvation in the way it affects the metabolic benefits of infused nutrients. Most patients can tolerate a weight loss of 5% to 10%. But a 40% loss of body weight is uniformly fatal. In addition to the fat supplies and skeletal muscle, vital body proteins are depleted, affecting the liver, spleen, and pancreas.

Even though a human weighing 70 kg stores about 100,000 kcal as fat for energy, the enzymes required to convert fat to glucose are not intrinsic; consequently, the body must make glucose from protein. This protein degradation is then used for gluconeogenesis to form glucose, which serves as a principal energy source in several vital organs, including the central nervous system (CNS), and in red and white blood cells.

An adaptive process to conserve vital body proteins must take over. After 3 weeks of starvation, nitrogen output in the urine will fall to 3 g/d from the normal level of 10 to 15 g/d, indicating a lesser rate of protein breakdown and conservation of body cell mass. Physical activity decreases, and the basal metabolic rate falls by about 12% to 20%.

The body's adaptation to starvation involves many parts of the metabolic process. The CNS converts to us-

TABLE 7.14.
Parenteral Nutrition Formulas[a]

Formula	Unit Volume (mL)	Amino Acids (g)	Nitrogen (g)	Dextrose (g)	Total kcal	Sodium (mEq)	Potassium (mEq)	Magnesium (mEq)	Calcium (mEq)	Phosphate[b] (mM)	Chloride (mEq)	Acetate (mEq)	mOsm	Calories (%)	Calories to Nitrogen
Standard THAS	1,000	41 (4.25%)	6.5	250 (25%)	1,020	30	20	5	5	5	30	67	1,850	16.7	157:1
Concentrated THAS	1,000	58 (6%)	9.2	280 (28%)	1,190	6	—	—	—	6	—	53	2,050	20	130:1
Hi-Pro THAS	1,000	72 (7.5%)	11.5	175 (17.5%)	885	7.5	—	—	—	7.5	2	67	1,700	32.6	77:1
Hi-Cal THAS	1,000	41 (4.25%)	6.5	350 (35%)	1,360	5	—	—	—	5	—	37	2,200	12.5	209:1
Peripheral THAS[c]	1,000	29 (3%)	4.6	70 (7%)	360	35	24.5	5	4	3.5	40	44	800	33	78:1
Low-nitrogen THAS	1,000	29 (3%)	4.6	50 (5%)	290	3	—	—	—	3	—	27	600	40.6	63:1
Fat emulsion 10%	500	—	—	—	550	—	—	—	—	7.5	—	—	280	—	—
Fat emulsion 20%	500	—	—	—	1,000	—	—	—	—	7.5	—	—	330	—	—

THAS, total hyperalimentation solution.
[a] Formulas used at the Johns Hopkins Hospital.
[b] 1 mM phosphate = 2 mEq phosphate.
[c] Peripheral parenteral nutrition is always coinfused with 1,000 mL 10% fat emulsion.

ing ketones and ketoacid substrates for energy, which allows the breakdown rate of protein to drop by about 70%. Another adaptive process decreases the use of glucose by muscle tissue; when insulin levels fall, muscle uses an energy substrate of fatty acids and, therefore, less glucose. Later in the starvation process, the elevated levels of ketoacids and ketones directly depress gluconeogenesis further.

Most of the endocrine systems are involved in the response to starvation. The insulin level falls rapidly, but levels of glucagon, growth hormone, and catecholamines increase, generating more glucose from protein substrate, which depletes the body cell mass rapidly. Later in the starvation process, glucagon returns to normal, growth hormone levels remain elevated, catecholamines decrease, and gluconeogenesis is slowed.

The kinds of changes that allow for conservation of body cell mass during simple starvation do not operate after injury, trauma, or infection. Afferent information, such as pain and other nerve responses to injury, along with hypovolemia and hypotension, is integrated in the CNS and hypothalamus, causing efferent responses that adjust the body to the stress condition. Levels of catecholamines and glucocorticoids become elevated, accentuating gluconeogenesis and preventing decreases in basal metabolic rates. Antidiuretic hormone levels are increased and the rennin-angiotensin system is activated. These processes allow fluid retention, which prevents early detection of the degree of weight loss.

During stress, urinary nitrogen levels may increase to 20 g or more in 24 hours, corresponding to a loss of 600 g of hydrated body protein. Body weight decreases because proteins, carbohydrates, and fats are all being degraded for energy, but the adaptive responses seen in simple starvation do not operate in the different hormonal milieu created by the stress condition.

Provision of nutrients can offset some of this nitrogen loss and even produce positive nitrogen balance. During starvation, the provision of 150 g of glucose (the amount in 3 L of 5% dextrose i.v. solution) reduces nitrogen loss even further than the maximum physiologic adaptive mechanisms, because glucose prevents much of the obligatory gluconeogenesis, creating a protein-sparing effect. As Moore explained in his concise review, if high levels of glucose are supplied (up to 750 g/d), protein sparing can be optimized and nitrogen output decreased to 1.8 g/m²/d.

During periods of injury and stress, patients must receive energy intake at least equal to energy expenditure, and to attain positive nitrogen balance, they must receive amino acid nitrogen in excess of urinary losses. Although fat alone cannot provide this energy intake, a combination of glucose and fat is effective.

Initiating Total Parenteral Nutrition

Safe venous access is required for initiating TPN. A reliable i.v. catheter should be placed into a large central vein with the catheter tip located so that blood flow dilutes the highly concentrated nutritional fluids. The insertion site also should allow easy fixation of the catheter at the entrance site, minimum catheter movement during body movements, and easy dressing changes. A subclavian vein approach satisfies the requirements for safe catheter placement, but neither internal jugular vein nor antecubital fossa placement is optimal. The internal jugular vein should be used only if the subclavian approach has failed. Movement of the head and neck results in an increased incidence of occluding venous access when the internal jugular vein has been cannulated.

Anatomy of Infraclavicular Subclavian Vein

In 1952, Aubaniac, a French physician, was among the first to advocate use of the subclavian vein for i.v. infusions. JN Wilson and colleagues cannulated the superior vena cava through a percutaneous puncture of the subclavian vein. They reported a high percentage of successful cannulations and a low incidence of complications.

As Figure 7.4 shows, the subclavian vein is located within the costoclavicular-scalene triangle, which is bounded anteriorly by the medial end of the clavicle, posteriorly by the upper surface of the first rib, and laterally by the anterior scalene muscle. The anterior scalene muscle separates the subclavian vein from the subclavian artery, which lies beneath and along the lateral aspect of the muscle. The subclavian vein is covered by 5 cm of the clavicle medially and joins the internal jugular vein near the medial border of the anterior scalene muscle to form the innominate vein. The innominate vein descends behind the sternum and joins with the opposite innominate vein to form the superior vena cava. The subclavian vein, which is about 3 or 4 cm long, continues as the axillary vein below the clavicle, en route to the axilla. Several other significant structures occupy this region. The phrenic nerve courses across the anterior surface of the anterior scalene muscle near its attachment to the first rib and courses medially to lie posterior to the subclavian vein. It can be injured if the posterior wall of the vessel is penetrated. The internal thoracic nerve and apical pleura are in contact with the posterior surface of the subclavian vein at its junction with the internal jugular vein. The roots of the brachial plexus formed by the fifth, sixth, seventh, and eighth cervical and first thoracic nerves lie lateral to the anterior scalene muscle on the lateral side of the subclavian artery. If a cannulating needle is directed too far laterally, the brachial nerve plexus could be injured or the subclavian artery could be punctured. The thoracic duct on the left side and the lymphatic duct on the right cross the anterior scalene muscle on either side of the thorax to enter the superior aspect of each subclavian vein near its junction with the internal jugular vein. These lymphatic vessels are rarely encroached on during subclavian catheterization.

Subclavian Catheter Placement

As illustrated in Figure 7.5A, the subclavian catheter is inserted with the patient in the supine position, with the foot of the bed elevated 6 to 12 inches to increase the pressure in the subclavian vein and produce venous distention. After meticulous aseptic preparation of the skin with povidone-

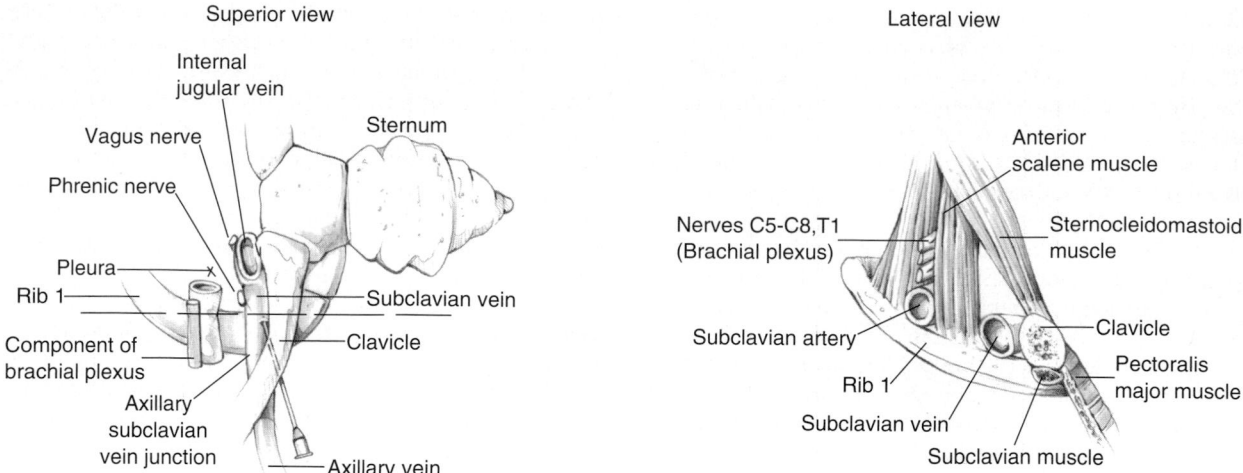

FIGURE 7.4. Anatomic relations of the subclavian vein. The broken line represents the location of the transverse section for lateral view. (Adapted from: Moosman DA. The anatomy of infraclavicular subclavian vein catheterization and its complications. *Surg Gynecol Obstet* 1973;136:71, with permission.)

iodine (Betadine), the skin and s.c. tissues are infiltrated with a 1% solution of lidocaine (xylocaine) if the patient is awake. The point of needle insertion is about 1 cm below the junction of the inner and middle third of the clavicle. Most central venous catheter units include an external in-

troducer catheter (Teflon) and an internal (silicone) infusion catheter. The outer, Teflon sheath accommodates a no. 12 needle, which fits snugly into and protrudes beyond the end of the Teflon catheter. The needle and sheath are introduced into the skin with the shaft of the needle held

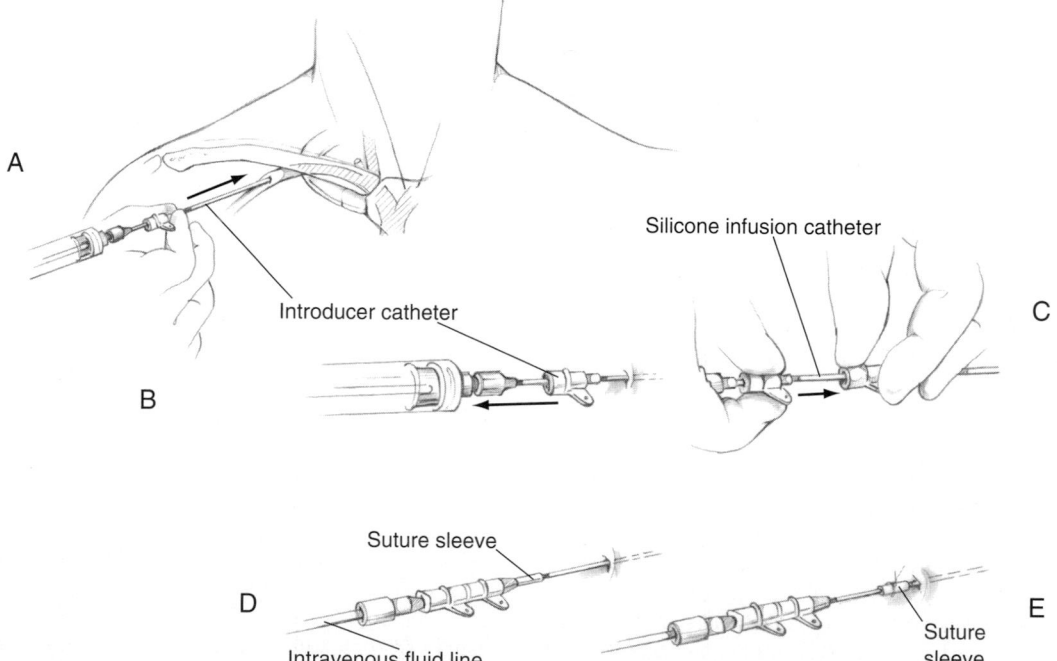

FIGURE 7.5. Insertion of subclavian catheter for monitoring central venous pressure. **A:** After locally anesthetizing the puncture site, the needle with overlying introducer catheter is directed medially between the first rib and the clavicle at the junction of the middle and inner third of the clavicle. The needle is held parallel to the anterior chest wall and advanced along the undersurface of the clavicle. Entry into the vein is evident with aspiration of blood in the attached syringe. **B:** The needle and syringe are removed from the Teflon sheath, and a finger is held over the end of the open catheter to prevent entry of air. **C:** The silicone infusion catheter is inserted through introducer catheter until the two connectors meet and lock firmly. **D:** The i.v. fluid line is connected to the silicone infusion catheter. **E:** The suture sleeve is advanced to the skin surface, where the catheter is sutured firmly to the skin.

almost parallel with the anterior chest wall (see Fig. 7.5A). The needle is directed medially and advanced along the undersurface of the clavicle. It is not necessary to scrape the posterior surface of the clavicle to ensure that the pleura is protected from puncture. By applying suction constantly, the needle passes beneath the skin and immediately aspirates dark red blood, which confirms entry into the vein. If the vein is not entered, the needle is withdrawn and readvanced in a similar manner but in a slightly more cranial or caudal direction. As soon as a free flow of blood is obtained, the introduced Teflon sheath is advanced far enough to be certain that it is securely placed within the vein. The sheath is held in place by the connector, the finger is placed over the end of the needle to prevent air embolism, and the internal needle is replaced (see Fig. 7.5B) by the silicone infusion catheter that accompanies the central venous pressure kit (see Fig. 7.5C). A thin wire stylet inside the infusion catheter allows the catheter to be advanced easily; occasionally, the stylet must be withdrawn slightly to advance the catheter as far as possible into the innominate vein and superior vena cava. The silicone infusion catheter is advanced until the attached connector can be securely wedged into the connector of the Teflon sheath (see Fig. 7.5C). After the infusion catheter is connected to an i.v. fluid line, the Teflon sheath is carefully withdrawn from the vein, remaining partially in the s.c. tissue while leaving an ample length of the infusion catheter in the vena cava (see Fig. 7.5D). A suture sleeve on the introducer sheath is slid down to the puncture site and sutured to the skin (see Fig. 7.5E). The tip of the catheter is preferably positioned in the superior vena cava and should not be advanced into the right atrium or ventricle, where it could cause accidental trauma to the heart wall or cardiac arrhythmias. To ensure its continued sterility and proper function, the subclavian vein catheter should not be used to replace fluids or withdraw blood for laboratory studies, if it is at all possible to avoid these uses. A central venous line for hyperalimentation is an exception to this rule. The dressing should be changed daily and the catheterization site cleaned with povidone-iodine or a similar antimicrobial solution.

Patient Evaluation

A complete medical history and physical examination must be obtained before parenteral nutrition is initiated. Particular attention should be paid to identifying patients with cardiovascular or renal disease, hyperlipidemia, diabetes, and thyroid disease. THAS modification can include decreasing or eliminating fat emulsion in patients with severe cardiovascular disease or hyperlipidemia, administering low-nitrogen THAS to patients with renal failure (see Table 7.14), and increasing the insulin dosage in patients with diabetes mellitus.

The patient's degree of malnutrition should be assessed by taking measurements of several physical indicators, such as actual body weight (ABW) and ideal body weight (IBW), usual body weight (UBW; preillness), creatinine to height index, triceps skin fold thickness (TSFT), and arm circumference (AC). At Emory University Hospital, the arm muscle circumference (AMC) is calculated and used as an index of nutritional status.

$$AMC = AC - (TSFT \times 3.14)$$

Fat stores are reflected in the triceps skin fold measurement, whereas somatic proteins are evaluated by measuring muscle mass such as the AMC. The Frisancho standards (1984) are used to interpret body weight (kg), triceps (mm), and bone-free arm muscle area (cm²). Patients found to be in the fifth to tenth percentiles are severely malnourished and require an anabolic environment. Weight loss is considered significant when the $(UBW - ABW)/UBW \times 100$ is >10%. Weight loss during starvation occurs at a rate of 0.4 kg/d. Survival also is compromised when the ABW falls below the 70th percentile of the IBW. In addition to the preceding physical measurements, a thorough evaluation of chemical indicators is required (Table 7.15) before initiating TPN. Extensive monitoring is required while the patient is receiving TPN (Table 7.16).

The physical and chemical measurements of malnutrition are subject to many influences during illness and should be treated as confounding variables. For example, albumin values less than 3.2 g/dL are frequently used to indicate malnutrition. Starker and colleagues observed that in hospitalized patients, albumin and body weight measurements in conjunction provided better indica-

---

TABLE 7.15.
Pretreatment Screening

Laboratory Evaluation

Complete blood count with differential
Prothrombin time/partial thromboplastin time
Electrolytic panel
Chemistry panel
Albumin
Transferrin
Total lymphocyte count
Triglycerides
Magnesium
Phosphorus
Copper
Zinc
Selenium

TABLE 7.16.
Treatment Monitoring

Test	Frequency
Electrolyte panel	Twice weekly
Chemistry panel	Weekly
Magnesium	Weekly
Transferrin	Weekly
Triglycerides	Monthly, or as needed
Zinc	Monthly, or as needed
Copper	Monthly, or as needed
Selenium	Monthly, or as needed

TABLE 7.17.
Trace Minerals

Minerals and Levels	Deficiency		Toxicity	
	Symptoms	*Etiology*	*Symptoms*	*Etiology*
Zinc, 55–150 mg/dL	Diarrhea, mental depression, alopecia, night blindness, dermatosis, impaired taste, hypogonadism, impaired wound healing	Gastrointestinal (failure of ingestion, absorption, retention) Large wounds Protein-energy malnutrition Cancer	Vomiting Diarrhea Neurologic damage ("zinc shakes")	Increased ingestion from galvanized containers Metal fume fever
Selenium, 90–150 µg/dL (synergism with vitamin E)	Myositis with muscle weakness Cardiomyopathy with arrhythmias and congestive heart failure	Unsupplemented TPN	Liver cirrhosis Alopecia Pathologic loss of nails Dermatitis	Increased ingestion (rare)
Chromium, 50–200 µg/d	Neuropathy Encephalopathy New insulin–dependent diabetes mellitus	Unsupplemented TPN Increased renal loss secondary to injury Gastrointestinal losses	Respiratory Lung cancer	Workers manufacturing products containing hexavalent chromium
Phosphorus, 3.0–4.5 mg/dL	Nausea, vomiting, anorexia, dysarthria, paresthesia, hemolytic anemia, peripheral neuropathy, respiratory depression, congestive heart failure, renal glycosuria	Gastrointestinal (failure of ingestion, absorption, retention) Cellular anabolism Respiratory or metabolic alkalosis Al(OH)$_3$ antacids Alcoholism	Neurotoxicity secondary to compensatory hypocalcemia	Renal failure Hypoparathyroidism
Magnesium, 136–145 mEq/L	Nausea, vomiting, muscle weakness, lethargy, tetany, muscle tremor, personality changes	Gastrointestinal (failure of ingestion, absorption, retention) Cellular catabolism, acidosis, K$^+$ depletion Glomerular dysfunction	Hyporeflexia, lethargy, respiratory depression, cardiac arrest	Magnesium supplementation in patients with renal compromise
Copper, 70–155 µg/dL	Hypochromic anemia not responsive to iron, neutropenia	THAS without copper or high amino acids Gastrointestinal (failure of ingestion, absorption, retention) Pregnancy, lactation (increased requirements) Renal losses	Jaundice—hepatic necrosis Intravascular hemolysis Gastric hemorrhage Tremors, choreoathetoid movements, dementia, rigidity, dysarthria	Iatrogenic Wilson's disease Absorption of copper nitrate salves in burn patients

THAS, total hyperalimentation solution; TPN, total parenteral nutrition.

tions of sodium balance and extracellular fluid volume. In addition, albumin serum levels are required for maintenance of the intravascular colloid oncotic pressure and as a carrier protein.

The half-life of albumin is 20 days and thus reflects a depletion of visceral proteins of at least 3 weeks' duration. Transferrin, with a half-life of 8 to 9 days, provides the clinician with a measurement of recent protein status changes. Because transferrin is required to bind Fe^{2+}, its level is affected by intravascular iron status and can increase during pregnancy, in patients with hepatitis, and in patients receiving estrogen supplementation. Serum protein content can be reduced in protein-losing enteropathy, nephropathy, chronic infections, uremia, and during catabolism. Transferrin reflects recent losses and therefore remains a better indicator of protein status and change than albumin. Total lymphocyte counts of less than 1,500 μL are indicative of an immunocompromised patient. Immunologic skin testing for recall antigens and total lymphocyte counts have been correlated with both nutritional status and morbidity and mortality. Its usefulness in the assessment of nutritional status is limited to confounding variables such as cancer, side effects of cancer treatment protocols, stress of trauma or surgery, and infection. Phosphorus and the trace elements are thoroughly evaluated before initiating TPN and during TPN because they are often depleted with many disease states and are required when alimenting (Tables 7.7 through 7.17).

Nutritional Requirements

Total parenteral nutrition consists of six components: carbohydrates, fat, protein, electrolytes, vitamins, and trace elements. The Harris-Benedict basal energy expenditure (BEE) accounts for two thirds of the total daily energy requirements, with the remaining one third obtained from protein. Daily requirements for protein are between 1.5 and 2.5 g/kg per day. Patients receiving TPN who are severely malnourished and stressed require larger amounts of protein daily.

The BEE is calculated as follows.

$$cal/d = 655.0955 + 9.5634 \, (wt) \\ + 1.8496 \, (ht) - 4.6756 \, (A)$$

where wt = weight (in kg), ht = height (in cm), and A = age (in years)

Once the patient has reached the estimated daily calorie goal, a 24-hour nitrogen balance study is performed by obtaining a 24-hour urine collection and an AM electrolyte panel. If a large quantity of fluid from the nasogastric tube, ileostomy, fistula, or wound is present, this also should be collected and sent for nitrogen measurements.

$$N_2 \, (g) \, balance = N_2 \, (g) \, in - N_2 \, (g) \, out$$

Adding 4 to the N_2 out value accounts for nitrogenous losses in the stool and skin. This does not include an estimate of the losses from the gastrointestinal tract and wound, as previously described.

$$N_2 \, (g) \, balance = N_2 \, (g) \, in \times [N_2 \, (g) \, out + 4] \\ N_2 \, (g) \, out = urine \, volume \, (mL) \\ \times \, urine \, urea \, N_2 \, (mg/dL) \\ N_2 \, (g) \, in = amino \, acids \, per \, day/6.24 \\ 6.24 = g \, protein/g \, nitrogen$$

Patients with normal renal and liver function are started on standard THAS (see Table 7.14). Each liter provides a total of 1,020 kcal, including 41 g of amino acids and 250 g of dextrose. The osmolality of this solution is 1,850 mOsm, which therefore necessitates a central venous access. The calories-to-nitrogen ratio of this solution is 157:1 and is optimal in nonstressed patients.

The addition of lipids also is effective in promoting a positive nitrogen balance. The total daily sodium concentration should be equivalent to that of normal saline (150 mEq/L). This can be altered to accommodate patients who require sodium restriction or loading. Table 7.18 outlines the recommendation for daily electrolyte requirements. It should be noted that acetate serves as a precursor to bicarbonate, because the latter is not compatible in the THAS solution. Multivitamins are added daily to 1 L of THAS, whereas trace elements are divided equally in the volume to be infused during a 24-hour period. The recommended daily allowances for both fat and water soluble vitamins are outlined in Table 7.19.

Blood glucose levels in patients receiving TPN should be between 100 and 200 mg/dL. A minimum of 10 IU should be added to each liter when required. This permits about 50% to adhere to the plastic tubing. This can be supplemented with s.c. doses of regular insulin to obtain the desired blood glucose level. About one half to two thirds of the previous day's requirements are added in divided doses to the THAS solutions.

Intravenous lipids provide a nonprotein source of energy and serve as a source of essential fatty acids. Ten percent fat emulsions (550 kcal/500 mL) and 20% fat emulsions (1,000 kcal/500 mL) are commercially available. In patients receiving standard THAS, 500 mL of 10% fat emulsion are infused twice weekly at a rate of 42 mL/h. However, when fat emulsion is used with peripheral THAS, the patient requires 2 L of peripheral THAS and 1 L of 10% fat emulsion daily. Twenty percent fat emulsions also can be used for calories in patients with glucose intolerance or patients who require a decreased protein-calorie percentage.

Patients deficient in fatty acids present with dermatitis, hemolytic anemia, thrombocytopenia, elevated liver enzymes, and poor wound healing.

To improve glucose tolerance, the first liter should be started at a rate of 42 mL/h. On the second day, the solution can be increased to 84 mL/h, and on day 3 it can be increased to 124 mL/h. If the patient is unable to tolerate this schedule, increments can be decreased to 21 mL/h each day. Treatment monitoring is outlined in Table 7.16. Total nitrogen balance should be recalcu-

TABLE 7.18.
Daily Electrolyte Requirements for Parenteral Nutrition

Electrolyte	Dosage (mEq/d)
Sodium	60–150
Potassium	60–240
Phosphate	30–45
Calcium	10–15
Magnesium	8–26
Acetate	80–120
Chloride	60–150

TABLE 7.19.
Recommended Dietary Allowances[a]

Age (Years) or Condition	Weight[b] (kg)	Weight[b] (lb)	Height[b] (cm)	Height[b] (in)	Protein g	Vitamin A >mg RE[c]	Vitamin D IU[d]	Vitamin E IU[e]	Vitamin K >mg	Ascorbic Acid (C) mg
Females 11–14	46	101	157	62	46	800	400	12	45	50
15–18	55	120	163	64	44	800	400	12	55	60
19–24	58	128	164	65	46	800	400	12	60	60
25–50	63	138	163	64	50	800	200	12	65	60
51+	65	143	160	63	50	800	200	12	65	60

[a] The allowances, expressed as average daily intakes over time, are intended to provide for individual variations among most normal persons as they live in the United States under usual environmental stresses. Diets should be based on a variety of common foods in order to provide other nutrients for which human requirements have been less well defined.

[b] Weights and heights of Reference Adults are actual medians for the US population of the designated age, as reported by NHANES II. The median weights and heights of those under 19 years of age were taken from Hamill PV et al. *Am J Clin Nutr* 1979;32:607–629. The use of these figures does not imply that the height-to-weight ratios are ideal.

[c] Retinol equivalents. 1 retinol equivalent = 1 mg retinol or 6 mg β-carotene.

[d] As cholecalciferol. 10 mg cholecalciferol = 400 IU of vitamin D.

[e] α-Tocopherol equivalents. 1 mg d-α-tocopherol = α-TE = 1.49 IU.

Source: National Academy of Sciences. *Recommended Dietary Allowances*, 10th ed. Washington, DC. National Academy Press, 1989.

lated if there is a marked change in the patient's condition or in the parenteral nutrition administered.

Recent data in the surgical literature suggest that supplementing TPN with glutamine dipeptides improves nitrogen balance, preserves intestinal permeability and absorption, and improves recovery of lymphocytes. These authors also demonstrated a shorter hospital stay in postoperative patients receiving glutamine dipeptide-enriched TPN compared to controls receiving TPN alone.

Cardiac and Respiratory Insufficiency

Patients with congestive heart failure require decreased sodium and decreased total fluid volume. The best solution can be prepared from the most concentrated solutions of glucose, amino acid, and fat available. Fluid-restricted solutions also may be beneficial for patients with respiratory failure, who should receive less total glucose in favor of more fat because the respiratory quotient (CO_2/O_2) of glucose (1.00) is greater than that of fat (0.70) and because excess glucose will increase the load of CO_2 the lungs must excrete. Excessive total caloric intake resulting in fat synthesis from glucose substrate may severely compromise respiratory function because large amounts of CO_2 are released (respiratory quotient 8.0).

Discontinuing Total Parenteral Nutrition

Before discontinuing TPN, the patient should tolerate an enteral diet that provides adequate calories. It is permissible to aliment patients with an enteral diet before decreasing the THAS solution. An abrupt discontinuation of central parenteral nutrition results in rebound hypoglycemia. Our recommendation is to decrease the

THAS stepwise to 42 mL/h before discontinuation. Some institutions recommend that the patient receive 10% dextrose for an additional 12 hours once central parenteral nutrition has been discontinued.

The Team Approach to Total Parenteral Nutrition

Total parenteral nutrition can now be safely administered to patients in many hospitals because of the existence of a team of physicians, nurses, and health care professionals. Although the composition and exact function of the team members vary between hospitals, most teams consist of a physician, nurse, pharmacist, and nutritionist. The role of the team varies in each institution from consultation to complete management of the patient's nutritional needs. The team approach by either method is highly beneficial because it provides a high concentration of personnel with knowledge, expertise, and interdisciplinary communication at the patient's bedside. Team members can provide continuing education on nutrition therapy, can continuously audit and collect quality control data, and can investigate ways to improve the safety and efficacy of TPN as a treatment modality. Most teams operate with a standardized protocol that covers patient assessment, catheter insertion techniques, solutions used, and monitoring functions performed.

ENTERAL NUTRITION

Enteral nutrition is preferable to TPN. The old adage "if the gut works, use it," applies for several reasons. Ease of administration, economic considerations, and decreased

Water-Soluble Vitamins						Minerals						
Thiamine (B$_1$) mg	Ribo-flavin (B$_2$) mg	Niacin (B$_3$) mg	Pyrido-xine (B$_6$) mg	Folate >mg	Cyano-cobalamin (B$_{12}$) >mg	Calcium mg	Phos-phorus mg	Magne-sium mg	Iron mg	Zinc mg	Iodine >mg	Sele-nium >mg
1.1	1.3	15	1.4	150	2	1,200	1,200	280	15	12	150	45
1.1	1.3	15	1.5	180	2	1,200	1,200	300	15	12	150	50
1.1	1.3	15	1.6	180	2	1,200	1,200	280	15	12	150	55
1.1	1.3	15	1.6	180	2	800	800	280	15	12	150	55
1	1.2	13	1.6	180	2	800	800	280	10	12	150	55

number of complications are all advantages of enteral feeding over parenteral nutrition. Several studies have shown TPN and enteral nutrition equally efficacious in achieving nitrogen balance. Patients with good bowel function should receive enteral feedings. Relative contraindications to enteral feeding include gastrointestinal bleeding, diarrhea, and intestinal obstruction. Small-bore nasal feeding tubes are placed in the stomach, duodenum, or jejunum. An abdominal radiograph should be obtained to confirm placement. Failure to obtain appropriate studies may result in tube placement in the trachea. Alternatively, a gastrostomy or jejunostomy tube could be placed for long-term enteral nutrition (Table 7.20). Several products are commercially available (Table 7.21). Enteral tube feedings are routinely administered by pump, with either bolus feeds to the stomach or continuous feeds to the small bowel and should be administered by pump at 25 to 30 mL/h with gastric residuals evaluated every 4 hours. Table 7.22 shows the essential and nonessential amino acids.

ROUTINE ORDERS

When the patient has fully recovered from the anesthetic and is ready for return to the nursing floor and routine postoperative care, we have found the basic postoperative orders shown in Figure 7.6 to be useful. They are only a general outline. This list should be expanded to include the special needs of each postoperative patient.

It is imperative that each patient be evaluated before being transferred from the recovery room. If the patient is not ready for transfer, additional efforts are made to stabilize the patient or transfer her to an intensive care bed. On transferring, the frequency of physicians' rounds should be based on the severity of the patient's condition. All patients should be evaluated on the evening of surgery and appropriate documentation made in the chart. A thorough evaluation of the vital signs, catheter drainage (nasogastric, peritoneal, and Foley), and pulmonary status is required, and abdominal examination is performed. Each physician has a desired proto-

TABLE 7.20.
Protocol for Enteral Tube Feeding

Nasogastric route: Use small-bore, flexible tube (8F preferred); obtain radiograph after placement to confirm position.

Elevate head of bed at least 30 degrees.

Use feeding pump for continuous feeding.

Begin with full-strength formula at 25–30 mL/h and, if tolerated, increase by 25–30 mL/h at 12-h intervals until desired total volume is reached.[a]

Check gastric residuals every 4 h; if greater than 100 mL, hold feeding and repeat at hourly intervals until residuals are less than 100 mL before resuming feeding.

Irrigate with 30–50 mL of water after each residual check or after any medications are given. (If patient requires additional free water, use greater volumes of water for irrigation.)

If patient experiences diarrhea or intestinal cramping, slow rate of feeding or decrease concentration of formula.

[a] When using hypertonic formulas or feeding into the jejunum with a naso-jejunal or jejunostomy tube, diluting the formula to one-half or three-quarter strength may improve tolerance initially. The concentration then can be increased after the desired volume is reached.

TABLE 7.21.
Emory University Hospital Enteral Nutrition Guidelines

	Product							
	Osmolite HN	Ultracal[a]	Perative	Respalor[a]	Two-Cal HN	Reabilin HN	Peptamen	AlitraQ[a]
Tube feedings								
Calories (per mL)	1.06	1.06	1.3	1.52	2.0	1.33	1.0	1.0
Protein (g/L)	44	44	67	76	84	58	40	53
Fat (g/L)	36	45	37	71	91	52	39	16
CHO (g/L)	141	123	177	148	217	158	127	165
Osmolality	300	310	385	580	690	490	270	575
Sodium, mEq (mg/L)	40 (930)	40 (930)	45 (1,040)	55 (1,270)	57 (1,310)	43 (1,000)	22 (500)	43 (1,000)
Potassium, mEq (mg/L)	40 (1,570)	41 (1,610)	44 (1,730)	38 (1,480)	63 (2,456)	43 (1,661)	32 (1,252)	31 (1,200)
Indications	Standard tube feeding, intact gastrointestinal	Fiber containing	Stress or wound	Fluid restriction, high protein	Fluid restriction	Trauma or gastrointestinal dysfunction	Gastrointestinal disorders	IBD/Crohn's disease
Price ratio (per 1,000 kcal)[b]	1	1.2	3	1.4	0.6	10.9	10.0	9.2

	Ensure	Sustacal	Gluceana	Ensure Plus	Nepro[a]	Suplena	Nutrihep[a]	Vital HN[a]
Oral supplements and disease-specific formulas								
Calories (per mL)	1.06	1.01	1.0	1.5	2.0	2.0	1.5	1.0
Protein (g/L)	37	61	42	55	70	30	40	42
Fat (g/L)	37	23	56	53	96	96	21	11
CHO (g/L)	145	139	94	200	215	255	290	185
Osmolality	470	650	375	690	635	600	690	500
Sodium, mEq (mg/L)	37 (846)	40 (930)	40 (930)	46 (1,050)	36 (829)	34 (783)	14 (320)	25 (566)
Potassium, mEq (mg/L)	40 (1,564)	54 (2,100)	40 (1,560)	50 (1,940)	27 (1,057)	29 (1,116)	34 (1,320)	36 (1,400)
Indications	Meal supplement	Supplement, high protein	Diabetic	High kcal needs	Dialysis	Predialysis	Liver failure	IBD/Crohn's disease
Price ratio (per 1,000 kcal)[b]	0.9	0.9	2.9	0.7	3.1	2.2	14.3	5.5

IBD, inflammatory bowel disease.

[a] Orally or by tube.

[b] Price ratio refers to relative cost of formulas, with the house formula (Osmolite HN) cost defined as 1, for the purpose of facilitating cost-effective formula selections.

Source: Emory University Hospital Food and Nutrition Services Enteral Formulary, 1995–1996.

TABLE 7.22.
Amino Acids

Essential
  Arginine
  Histidine
  Isoleucine
  Leucine
  Lysine
  Methionine
  Phenylalanine
  Threonine
  Tryptophan
  Valine
Nonessential
  Alanine
  Asparaginine
  Aspartic acid
  Cysteine
  Glutamic acid
  Glutamine
  Glycine
  Proline
  Serine
  Tyrosine

col for postoperative management. The routine orders outlined in this chapter provide the clinician with a framework to design patient care plans that address the individual patient's requirements. Laboratory and radiographic evaluation of the postoperative patient also is tailored to the individual patient. Unfortunately, many physicians are predominantly concerned with quantitative test values. However, it is just as important to develop a close rapport with the patient, the patient's family, and the nursing staff. Only through good communication can the gynecologic surgeon deliver optimum medical care.

ESTROGEN REPLACEMENT THERAPY

During the past decade, few subjects in medicine have engendered greater controversy than the use of estrogen by postmenopausal women. In the postoperative patient who has undergone bilateral oophorectomy at the time of pelvic surgery, important metabolic changes occur as a result of estrogen deficiency. The most significant effects include vasomotor symptoms, genitourinary atrophy, osteoporosis, cardiovascular disease, and cognitive

---

BASIC POSTOPERATIVE ORDERS

Patient's Name: _____.

1. Admit to Unit #____
2. Diagnosis:
3. Allergies:
4. Condition:
5a. Vital signs:
   ____ q 15 minutes until stable
   ____ q 2 hours for 24 hours
   ____ q 8 hours, if stable
5b. Notify House Officer (H.O.) if
   BP < 90/60, > 160/100
   Pulse <60, >120
   Temp >38.0°C
6. Activity:
   ____ Bed rest
   ____ Ambulate
   ____ Other (specify)
7. Diet:
   ____ NPO
   ____ Other (specify)
8. Intravenous fluids:
9. Incentive inspirometer q 2 hours while awake
10. Encourage deep breathing
11. Drains:

Type	Location	Drainage
____ Nasogastric	____ Stomach	____ Low/intermittent suction
____ Peritoneal	____ Pelvis	____ Bulb suction
____ Foley catheter	____ Bladder	____ Gravity

12a. Fluid intake and output chart.
12b. Notify H.O. if urine output <30 cc/h.
13. Pain medication: Specify
   (a) route of administration
   (b) dosage
14. Antiemetic medication: Specify
   (a) route of administration
   (b) dosage
15. Antibiotics
16. Venous thrombosis prophylaxis
17. Other medications
18. Catheterize q 6 hours, or sooner, if bladder is full and patient unable to void.

FIGURE 7.6. Sample of basic postoperative orders.

disturbances. In counseling the patient about the advisability or the necessity of oophorectomy and surgical castration at the time of surgery, it is important that the surgeon take the time to explain all the benefits and risks of postoophorectomy estrogen replacement.

In most cases, the uterus is removed with any gynecologic disease that requires bilateral oophorectomy. This prophylactic oophorectomy is reasonable if the patient is approaching menopause, because ovarian cancer is the major cause of death from gynecologic malignancy, and its cure rate has remained unchanged for the past three decades. These facts have encouraged many gynecologists to remove the ovaries at the time of hysterectomy in patients who are 45 years of age or older and approaching menopause. The ease of oral estrogen replacement has made this surgical approach quite acceptable.

Estrogen preparations may be administered in a variety of ways including orally, vaginally, and transdermally. The equivalent and usual doses for daily replacement are listed in Table 7.23. All of these estrogen preparations have demonstrated effectiveness for alleviating most menopausal symptoms. Conjugated equine estrogen at a dose of 0.625 mg/d for 25 days each month is one of the more common agents used. The prophylactic use of estrogen must be decided on an individual basis. Each patient must be counseled regarding the risk:benefit ratio and informed consent should be obtained and documented in the patient record. There are a select group of patients in which estrogen replacement has been considered contraindicated. Those patients with a history of thromboembolic disease or significant liver function impairment should avoid estrogen use. Endometrial cancers have long been considered a contraindication to estrogen use, presumably because these neoplasms are considered estrogen-dependent. However, three different studies involving early-stage endometrial cancer patients who received postoperative estrogen replacement therapy revealed no increased incidence of recurrent disease or decrease in overall survival when compared to controls.

One of the most important sequelae of castration or of natural menopause is bone demineralization or osteoporosis. With the sudden decrease in plasma estrogen af-

ter oophorectomy, there is bone reabsorption without change in the chemical composition of the bone. This reabsorption involves the entire skeleton, although the soft cancellous bone undergoes the demineralization process before the hard cortical bone. For this reason, the earliest effects of advancing osteoporosis are seen in spontaneous fracture of the distal radius, the weight-bearing vertebral bodies, and the neck of the femur.

In 1979, more than 125,000 women in the United States suffered a fracture of the proximal femur, and 12% died as a direct result. Of white women older than 60 years of age, 25% have radiographic or clinical evidence of vertebral crush injuries. Although bone loss is a normal aging process for both men and women, the most significant physiologic event associated with skeletal fractures in women is the loss of ovarian function, whether owing to oophorectomy or spontaneous menopause. Although there are apparently no estrogen receptors in bone, estrogen plays an important role in calcium metabolism. Osteoporosis is perhaps the most significant abnormality resulting from estrogen deficiency and is a major cause of morbidity and mortality.

Several theories have been proposed to explain the mechanism of action of estrogen in retarding bone reabsorption. Estrogen is known to suppress the action of parathyroid hormone at the osteoclastic cellular level and thereby suppress the effect of parahormone on bone reabsorption. A diminished plasma level of estrogen results in an increased sensitivity in these cells to parathyroid hormone stimulation, which in turn results in an acceleration of bone reabsorption. As a result of the estrogen deficiency, bone demineralization causes an increase in serum calcium. This, in turn, suppresses parathyroid hormone secretion. Consequently, the beneficial effect of parathyroid hormone on renal tubular reabsorption of calcium and the formation of the active, dihydroxy form of vitamin D is diminished. The low level of 1,25-dihydroxyvitamin D results in an increased renal excretion of calcium and a diminished calcium absorption from the gastrointestinal tract. If low-dose estrogen is provided on a continued basis, the action of the parathyroid hormone on bone reabsorption is decreased. This, in turn, lowers the serum calcium level. The lowered serum calcium level enhances parathyroid hormone release, which has a positive effect on calcium metabolism by increasing renal tubular reabsorption of calcium. Calcium absorption from the gastrointestinal tract also is increased because activated vitamin D levels are higher.

Although the foregoing may be a plausible explanation of the role of estrogen in bone reabsorption, the exact mechanism is by no means fully understood. Many investigators believe that estrogen does not affect osteoclast activity directly, because estrogen receptors have not been shown to be present in bone. There is some evidence that the effect of estrogen on bone metabolism is mediated by its control of calcitonin secretion. Calcitonin, a peptide hormone synthesized by the C cells of the thyroid gland, is decreased in the postmenopausal patient; calcitonin is known to reduce both the number of osteoclasts and their physiologic activity. The admin-

TABLE 7.23.
Daily Dosing Equivalents of Estrogen Replacement Therapy

Estrogen Type	Daily Dose
Conjugated equine estrogen	0.625 mg
Ethinyl estradiol	5.0 μg
Micronized estradiol	1.0 mg
Transdermal estradiol	50 μg
Mestranol	30 μg

mg, milligram; μg, microgram.

istration of estrogen not only prevents bone loss but also raises the plasma level of calcitonin to premenopausal levels. Therefore, another possible explanation of the pathogenesis of postmenopausal osteoporosis is the accelerated decline in calcitonin secretion that is associated with loss of ovarian function.

Photon absorptiometry studies have made it eminently clear that premature castration and the cessation of ovarian function at menopause are both associated with a dramatic and continued decline in bone density. Lindsay and colleagues (1978) showed that when oophorectomized perimenopausal patients were treated with estrogen for periods of up to 8 years, significant bone loss did not occur. When estrogen was withdrawn, bone mineral content fell at a normal postmenopausal rate, demonstrating the long-term prevention of bone loss by estrogen. This group also demonstrated a significant reduction in height loss among postoophorectomized women who were treated prophylactically with small doses of mestranol (mean dosage was 20 µg/d). It seems evident, therefore, that bone demineralization can be delayed with estrogen replacement therapy. Although no therapy now available can restore bone mass in a patient with osteoporosis, women who have premature ovarian failure or bilateral oophorectomy before 50 years of age would benefit if treated prophylactically with estrogen. At particular risk of osteoporosis are slender white or Asian women who smoke, have early menopause, have a low calcium intake, drink alcohol excessively, and are physically inactive. Kriska and associates identified an association between historical physical activity and bone density.

Patients receiving sequential or continuous therapy with estrogen and progesterone have demonstrated decreased vertebral bone loss. Savvas and colleagues used estradiol, 50 mg, and testosterone, 100 mg, in s.c. implants and were better able to prevent osteoporosis in these patients than in patients receiving sequential estrogen and progesterone therapy. Calcitonin and fluoride also have been shown to be efficacious in decreasing bone loss. Pak and associates demonstrated an increase in mineralized bone, an increase in vertebral bone mass, and a reduced frequency of vertebral fractures when using intermittent sodium fluoride treatment without 1,25-dihydroxyvitamin D_3. Future estrogen supplementation protocols to decrease osteoporosis may include agents such as calcitonin and fluoride.

The remaining major physiologic changes associated with loss of estrogen, namely, vasomotor symptoms and genitourinary atrophy, may or may not be clinically symptomatic. Although a hot flush appears to occur in synchrony with a pulsatile surge of luteinizing hormone, the change in hormone level is not the major causative factor. The major defect is in the heat regulatory mechanism in the intact hypothalamus. It has been postulated that gonadotropin-releasing hormone and the heat regulatory center are affected concomitantly by adrenergic stimulation. This stimulation produces a secondary autonomic response that causes a hot flush. Although the precise stimulatory mechanism is as yet incompletely ex-

plained, estrogen replacement has a dampening effect on both the pulsatile gonadotropin release mechanism and the thermogenic center. The treatment for vasomotor symptoms and genitourinary atrophy, however, may be given on a very temporary basis until the patient has adjusted to the change in circulating estrogen level. Genitourinary symptoms are less common and have a delayed onset. A troublesome clinical problem of estrogen deprivation is the urethral syndrome. This is a recurrent sterile urethritis that causes dysuria, nocturia, and urinary frequency and urgency. The syndrome is usually well controlled with estrogen replacement therapy, with the most immediate response being produced by local vaginal estrogen.

The atrophic changes of the vagina are late sequelae of the diminished plasma estrogen level and do not occur for many months or years after removal of the ovaries. Such changes as vaginal dryness, dyspareunia, irritation, and, occasionally, postcoital bleeding are associated with atrophy of the vaginal epithelium. Use of estrogen helps maintain the tissue integrity of the vaginal epithelium and may have a profound effect on improving these symptoms. Although vasomotor and genitourinary symptoms are troublesome, they produce no serious long-term health hazards to the patient.

Postmenopausal women receiving estrogen supplements have a marked reduction in cardiovascular disease and mortality. Estrogen supplementation has been shown to exert this protective effect through a variety of mechanisms. These include increasing serum levels of high-density lipoproteins (HDL), decreasing serum levels of low-density lipoproteins (LDL), decreasing fibrinogen levels, direct arterial vasodilation, and increased perfusion, and by way of its intrinsic antioxidant properties.

Some studies have suggested that norethindrone, megestrol acetate, medroxyprogesterone acetate, and levonorgestrel decrease HDL levels. Wren and Garrett demonstrated that low-dose levonorgestrel (30 mg) and low-dose estrogen therapy in postmenopausal women do not affect HDL levels. Additional studies by Ravnikar and colleagues evaluating medroxyprogesterone acetate sequentially administered with estrogen did not show a decrease in HDL serum levels. The Postmenopausal Estrogen/Progestin Intervention (PEPI) trial demonstrated a favorable affect on cardiovascular risk factors in women taking both estrogen and progestins. This multicenter controlled trial included 875 women over a 3-year period and randomized them to one of the following five groups: placebo, estrogen alone, sequential estrogen and micronized progesterone days 1 to 12, sequential estrogen and medroxyprogesterone days 1 to 12, or continuous combined estrogen and medroxyprogesterone daily. All patients receiving estrogen alone or estrogen plus a progestin were noted to have an increase in HDL and a decrease in LDL when compared to the placebo group. This favorable effect on the serum lipoprotein profile was greatest in the estrogen only and estrogen plus micronized progesterone groups, but was also demonstrated to a lesser degree in the estrogen plus medroxyprogesterone group. Other prospective studies are in progress, but it appears that postmenopausal estrogen and progesterone supplementation diminishes the risk of cardiovascular disease and death and also prevents bone demineralization with resultant osteoporosis.

Alzheimer's disease or senile-associated dementia has become an increasingly recognized problem in society today. Improved memory and cognitive function have been demonstrated in patients taking estrogen. As this topic is more extensively studied, this may become an important benefit to consider in postoophorectomy patients.

Finally, another potential benefit of estrogen replacement therapy is a reduction in the risk of colon cancer. Nanda and coworkers, in a metaanalysis of 42 studies, reported a 33% reduction in the risk of colon cancer in current and recent users of hormone replacement therapy. The authors found no association between hormone replacement therapy and rectal cancer.

The Women's Health Initiative (WHI) has discontinued the conjugated equine estrogen (CEE) 0.625 mg/day plus medroxyprogesterone acetate (MPA) 2.5 mg/day vs placebo arm. The study enrolled 16,608 women between the ages of 50 and 79 years. Each participant was randomized to the CEE/MPA or placebo arm. After an average 5.2 years of observation, the Data and Safety Monitoring Board halted participation in this arm of the WHI Study. Patients receiving CEE/MPA had a significantly increased risk of developing: breast cancer (26%), stroke (41%), coronary artery disease (29%), and thromboembolic events (110%). Advantages to patients in the ECC/MPA arm include a decrease in hip fractures (34%) and colon cancer (37%) when compared with placebo.

ACKNOWLEDGMENT

Sections of this chapter were written by Doctors Richard Mattingly, Edward J. Quebbeman, and Donald P. Schlueter, as in previous editions of this text.

BIBLIOGRAPHY

Adam S, Williams V, Vesse MP. Cardiovascular disease and hormone replacement treatment: a pilot case-control study. *Br Med J* 1981;282:1277.

Adami HO. Long-term consequences of estrogen and estrogen-progestin replacement. *Cancer Causes Control* 1992;3:1:83.

Adar R, Papa MZ, Amsterdam E, et al. Antithrombosis routines and hemorrhagic complications: a seven year survey comparing vascular and general surgical operations. *J Cardiovasc Surg (Torino)* 1985;26:275.

Adolf J, Buttermann G, Weidenbach A, et al. Optimization of postoperative prophylaxis of thrombosis in gynecology. *Geburtshilfe Frauenheilkd* 1978;38:98.

Aitken AGF, Godden OJ. Real-time ultrasound diagnosis of deep vein thrombosis: a comparison with venography. *Clin Radiol* 1987;38:309.

Allan A, Williams JT, Bolton JP, et al. The use of graduated compression stockings in the prevention of postoperative deep vein thrombosis. *Br J Surg* 1983;70:172.

Allenby F, Pflugg JJ, Boardman L, et al. Effects of external pneumatic intermittent compression on fibrinolysis in man. *Lancet* 1973;2:1412.

Almond DJ, Guillou PJ, McMahon MJ. Effect of i.v. fat emulsion on natural killer cellular function and antibody-dependent cell cytotoxicity. *Hum Nutr Clin Nutr* 1985; 39:227.

Aloia JF, Vaswani A, Yeh JK, et al. Calcitrol in the treatment of postmenopausal osteoporosis. *Am J Med* 1988;84:401.

AMA Department of Foods and Nutrition. Guidelines for essential trace element preparation for parenteral use. *JAMA* 1979;241:2051.

Anderson S. Thermography and plethysmography in the diagnosis of deep venous thrombosis: a comparison with phlebography. *Acta Med Scand* 1986;219:359.

Angus RM, Eisman JA. Osteoporosis: the role of calcium intake and supplementation. *Med J Aust* 1988;148:63.

Apelgren KN. Triple lumen catheters: technological advance or setback? *Am Surg* 1987;53:113.

Appelman PT, DeJong TE, Lampmann LE. Deep venous thrombosis of the leg: US findings. *Radiology* 1987;163: 743.

Aronen HJ, Pamilo M, Suoranta HT, et al. Sonography in differential diagnosis of deep venous thrombosis of the leg. *Acta Radiol* 1987;28:457.

Arora S, Lam DJ, Kennedy C, et al. Light reflection rheography: a simple noninvasive screening test for deep vein thrombosis. *J Vasc Surg* 1993;18:767.

Ashbaugh DG, Bigelow DB, Petty TL, et al. Acute respiratory distress in adults. *Lancet* 1967;2:319.

Askanazi J, Carpentier YA, Elwyn DH, et al. Influence of total parenteral nutrition on fuel utilization in injury and sepsis. *Ann Surg* 1980;191:40.

Askanazi J, Elwyn DH, Silverberg PA, et al. Respiratory distress secondary to a high carbohydrate load. *Surgery* 1980; 87:596.

Athanasoulis CA. Therapeutic applications of angiography: part 1. *N Engl J Med* 1980;302:1117.

Aubaniac R. L'injection intraveineuse sousclaviculaire: advantages et technique. *Presse Med* 1952;60:1456.

Ausman RK, Quebbeman EJ, Altmann CL. Liver malfunction associated with parenteral nutrition. In: Johnston IDA, ed. *Advances in clinical nutrition.* Boston: MTP Press, 1983.

Baertschi U, Schaer A, Bader P, et al. A comparison of low dose heparin and oral anticoagulants in the prevention of thrombophlebitis following gynaecological operations. *Geburtshilfe Frauenheilkd* 1975;35:754.

Bain C, Willett W, Hennekens CH, et al. Use of postmenopausal hormones and risk of myocardial infarction. *Circulation* 1981;64:42.

Baker JP, Detsky AS, Wesson DE, et al. Nutritional assessment: a comparison of clinical judgment and objective measurements. *N Engl J Med* 1982;306:969.

Baker WH, Mahler DK, Foldes MS, et al. Pneumatic compression devices for prophylaxis of deep venous thrombosis (DVT). *Am Surg* 1986;52:371.

Baker WL. Hypophosphatemia. *Am J Nurs* 1985;85:998.

Ballard RM, Bradley-Watson PJ, Johnstone FD, et al. Low doses of subcutaneous heparin in the prevention of deep vein thrombosis after gynaecological surgery. *J Obstet Gynaecol Br Commonw* 1973;80:469.

Baran GW, Frisch KM. Duplex Doppler evaluation of puerperal ovarian vein thrombosis. *Am J Radiol* 1987;149:321.

Barbul A, Fishel RS, Shimazu S, et al. Intravenous hyperalimentation with high arginine levels improves wound healing and immune function. *J Surg Res* 1985;38:328.

Bates GW. On the nature of hot flash. *Clin Obstet Gynecol* 1981;24:231.

Becker DM. Venous thromboembolism: epidemiology, diagnosis, prevention. *J Gen Intern Med* 1986;1:402.

Bell WK, Starksen NF, Tong S, et al. Trousseau's syndrome: devastating coagulopathy in the absence of heparin. *Am J Med* 1985;79:423.

Bellantani MF, Blackman MR. Osteoporosis: diagnostic screening and its place in current care (clinical conference). *Geriatrics* 1988;43:63.

Bergqvist D. Dextran in the prophylaxis of deep-vein thrombosis. (Letter) *JAMA* 1987;258:324.

Bergqvist D, Burmark US, Frisell J, et al. Low molecular weight heparin once daily compared with conventional low-dose heparin twice daily: a prospective double-blind multicentre trial on prevention of postoperative thrombosis. *Br J Surg* 1986;73:204.

Bernard GR, Artigas A, Brigham KL, et al. Report of the American-European Consensus conference on acute respiratory distress syndrome: definitions, mechanisms, relevant outcomes, and clinical trial coordination. Consensus Committee. *J Crit Care* 1994;9:72.

Bernstein K, Ulmsten U, Astedt B, et al. Incidence of thrombosis after gynecologic surgery evaluated by an improved ^{125}I-fibrinogen uptake test. *Angiology* 1980;3:606.

Bistrian BR, Blackburn GL, Hallowell E, et al. Protein status of general surgical patients. *JAMA* 1974;230:858.

Bjorson HS, Colle R, Bower RH, et al. Association between microorganism growth at the catheter site and colonization of the catheter in patients receiving total parenteral nutrition. *Surgery* 1982;92:20.

Black P MCL, Crowell RM, Abbott WM. External pneumatic calf compression reduces deep venous thrombosis in patients with ruptured intracranial aneurysms. *Neurosurgery* 1986;18:25.

Blackburn GL, Bistrian BR, Maini BS, et al. Nutritional and metabolic assessment of the hospitalized patient. *J Parenter Enteral Nutr* 1977;1:11.

Blackburn GL, Etter G, Mackenzie T. Criteria for choosing amino acid therapy in acute renal failure. *Am J Clin Nutr* 1978;31:1841.

Body JJ, Borkowski A. Nutrition and quality of life in cancer patients. *Eur J Cancer Clin Oncol* 1987;23:127.

Bonnar J. Venous thromboembolism and gynecologic surgery. *Clin Obstet Gynecol* 1985;28:432.

Bonnar J, Walsh J. Prevention of thrombosis after pelvic surgery by British Dextran 70. *Lancet* 1972;1:614.

Bonnar J, Walsh J, Haddon M, et al. Coagulation system changes induced by pelvic surgery and the effect of dextran 70. *Bibl Anat* 1973;12:351.

Borstad E, Urdal K, Handeland G, et al. Comparison of low molecular weight heparin vs. unfractionated heparin in gynecological surgery: II. reduced dose of low molecular weight heparin. *Acta Obstet Gynecol Scand* 1992;71:471.

Bower RH, Talamini MA, Sax HC, et al. Postoperative enteral versus parenteral nutrition: a randomized controlled trial. *Arch Surg* 1986;121:1040.

Breneman JC. Postoperative thromboembolic disease: computer analysis leading to statistical prediction. *JAMA* 1965;193:576.

Brenner DA. Total parenteral nutrition at home. *Outpatient Ther Med* 1987;2:1.

Brismar B, Hardstedt C, Jacobson S. Diagnosis of thrombosis by catheter phlebography after prolonged central venous catheterization. *Ann Surg* 1981;194:779.

Brown CE, Battocletti JH, Sprinivasan R, et al. In vivo 31P nuclear magnetic resonance spectroscopy of bone mineral for evaluation of osteoporosis. *Clin Chem* 1988;34:1431.

Brown JG, Ward PE, Wilkinson AJ, et al. Impedance plethysmography: a screening procedure to detect deep-vein thrombosis. *J Bone Joint Surg Br* 1987;69:264.

Brown R, Bancewicz J, Hamid J, et al. Delayed hypersensitivity skin testing does not influence the management of surgical patients. *Ann Surg* 1982;196:672.

Brun-Buisson C, Brochard L. Corticosteroid therapy in acute respiratory distress syndrome: Better late than never? *JAMA* 1998;280.182.

Burch JC, Byrd BF, Vaughn WK. The effects of long-term estrogen on hysterectomized women. *Am J Obstet Gynecol* 1974;118:778.

Bush TL, Barrett Connor E, Cowan DK, et al. Cardiovascular mortality and noncontraceptive use of estrogen in women: results from Lipid Research Clinics Program Follow-up Study. *Circulation* 1987;75:1102.

Buzby GP, Mullen JL, Mathews DC, et al. Prognostic nutritional index in gastrointestinal surgery. *Am J Surg* 1980;139:160.

Calle EE, Miracle-McMahill HL, Thun MJ, et al. Estrogen replacement therapy and risk of fatal colon cancer in a prospective cohort of postmenopausal women. *J Natl Cancer Inst* 1995;87:517.

Caprini JA, Chuckler JL, Zuckerman L, et al. Thrombosis prophylaxis using external compression. *Surg Gynecol Obstet* 1983;156:599.

Carpenter JP, Holand GA, Baum RA, et al. Magnetic resonance venography for the detection of deep venous thrombosis: comparison with contrast venography and duplex Doppler ultrasonography. *J Vasc Surg* 1993;18:734.

Carpentier YA. Indications for nutritional support. *Gut* 1986;27:14.

Cauley JA, La Porte RE, Sandler RB, et al. The relationship of physical activity to high density lipoprotein cholesterol in postmenopausal women. *J Chronic Dis* 1986;39:687.

Celli BR, Rodriguez KS, Snider GL. A controlled trial of intermittent positive pressure breathing, incentive spirometry, and deep breathing exercises in preventing pulmonary complications after abdominal surgery. *Am Rev Respir Dis* 1984;130:12.

Chapman JA, DiSaia P, Osann K, et al. Estrogen replacement in surgical stage I and II endometrial cancer survivors. *Am J Obstet Gynecol* 1996;175:1195.

Chory ET, Mullen JL. Nutritional support of the cancer patient: delivery systems and formulations. *Surg Clin North Am* 1986;66:1105.

Chow R, Harrison JE, Notarius C. Effect of two randomised exercise programmes on bone mass of healthy postmenopausal women. *Br Med J* 1987;295:6611.

Clarke-Pearson DL, Coleman RE, Siegel R, et al. Indium 111 platelet imaging for the detection of deep venous thrombosis and pulmonary embolism in patients without symptoms after surgery. *Surgery* 1985;98:98.

Clarke-Pearson DL, Coleman RE, Synan IS, et al. Venous thromboembolism prophylaxis in gynecologic oncology: a prospective controlled trial of low-dose heparin. *Am J Obstet Gynecol* 1983a;145:606.

Clarke-Pearson DL, Creasman WT. Diagnosis of deep venous thrombosis in ob-gyn by impedance phlebography. *Obstet Gynecol* 1981;58:52.

Clarke-Pearson DL, DeLong ER, Synan IS, et al. Complications of low-dose heparin prophylaxis in gynecologic oncology surgery. *Obstet Gynecol* 1984;64:689.

Clarke-Pearson DL, DeLong ER, Synan IS, et al. Variables associated with postoperative deep venous thrombosis: a prospective study of 411 gynecology patients and creation of a prognostic model. *Obstet Gynecol* 1987;69:146.

Clarke-Pearson DL, Jelovsek FR, Creasman WT. Thromboembolism complicating surgery for cervical and uterine malignancy: incidence, risk factors, and prophylaxis. *Obstet Gynecol* 1983b;61:87.

Clayton JK, Anderson JA, McNicol GP. Effect of cigarette smoking on subsequent postoperative thromboembolic disease in gynecological patients. *Br Med J* 1978;2:402.

Clinical Nutrition Cases. Is chromium essential for humans? *Nutr Rev* 1988;46:17.

Cogo A, Lensing AW, Well P, et al. Noninvasive objective tests for the diagnosis of clinically suspected deep vein thrombosis. *Haemostasis* 1995;25:27.

Colditz GA, Taden RL, Oster G. Rates of venous thrombosis after general surgery: combined results of randomised clinical trials. *Lancet* 1986;2:143

Colditz GA, Willett WC, Stampfer MJ, et al. Menopause and the risk of coronary heart disease in women. *N Engl J Med* 1987;316:1105.

Collaborative Group on Hormonal Factors in Breast Cancer. Breast Cancer and hormone replacement therapy: collaborative reanalysis of data from 51 epidemiological studies of 52,705 women with breast cancer and 108,411 women without breast cancer. *Lancet* 1997;350:1047–1059.

Colley R, Wilson J, Kapusta E, et al. Fever and catheter-related sepsis in total parenteral nutrition. *J Parenter Enteral Nutr* 1979;3:32.

Collins CG. Suppurative pelvic thrombophlebitis. *Am J Obstet Gynecol* 1970;108:681.

Comerota AJ, Katz M, Grossi RJ, et al. The comparative value of noninvasive testing for diagnosis and surveillance of deep vein thrombosis. *J Vasc Surg* 1988;7:40.

Common HH, Seaman AJ, Rosch J, et al. Deep vein thrombosis treated with streptokinase or heparin: follow-up of a randomized study. *Angiology* 1976;27:645.

Cooper HA, Bowie EJW, Owen CA. Evaluation of patients with increased fibrinolytic split products (FSP) in their serum. *Mayo Clin Proc* 1974;49:654.

Cranley JJ, Canos AJ, Sull WJ. The diagnosis of deep vein thrombosis. *Arch Surg* 1976;111:34.

Creasman WT, Henderson D, Hinshaw W, et al. Estrogen replacement therapy in the patient treated for endometrial cancer. *Obstet Gynecol* 1986;67:326.

Czer LSC, Appel P, Shoemaker WC. Pathogenesis of respiratory failure (ARDS) after hemorrhage and trauma: II. cardiorespiratory patterns after development of ARDS. *Crit Care Med* 1980;8:513.

Dale S, Gogstad GO, Brosstad F, et al. Comparison of three D-dimer assays for the diagnosis of DVT: ELISA, latex and an immunofiltration assay (NycoCard D-dimer). *Thromb Haemost* 1994;7:270.

Dalen N, Lamke B, Wallgren A. Bone-mineral losses in oophorectomized women. *J Bone Joint Surg* 1974;56:1235.

D'Alonzo WA, Alavi A. Detection of deep venous thrombosis by indium-111 leukocyte scintigraphy. *J Nucl Med* 1986;27:631.

Dalsky GP, Stocke KS, Ehsani AA, et al. Weight-bearing exercise training and lumbar bone mineral content in postmenopausal women. *Ann Intern Med* 1988;108:824.

Dark DS, Pingleton SK, Kerby GR. Hypercapnia during weaning: a complication of nutritional support. *Chest* 1985;88:141.

Davis RB, Theologides A, Kennedy BJ. Comparative studies of blood coagulation and platelet aggregation in patients with cancer and nonmalignant diseases. *Ann Intern Med* 1969;71:69.

De Boer K, Buller HR, Tencate JW, et al. Deep vein thrombosis in obstetrics patients: diagnosis and risk factors. *Thromb Haemost* 1992;67:4.

Delafosse B, Bouffard Y, Viale JP, et al. Respiratory changes induced by parenteral nutrition in postoperative patients undergoing inspiratory pressure support ventilation. *Anesthesiology* 1987;66:393.

Dempsy DT, Mullen JL, Buzby GP. The link between nutritional status and clinical outcome: can nutritional intervention modify it? *Am J Clin Nutr* 1988;47:352.

Devor M, Barrett-Connor E, Renvall M, et al. Estrogen replacement therapy and the risk of venous thrombosis. *Am J Med* 1992;92:275.

Dihydroergotamine-heparin to prevent postoperative deep vein thrombosis. *Med Lett Drugs Ther* 1985;27:45.

Dillon JD, Schaffner W, Van Way CW, et al. Septicemia and total parenteral nutrition: distinguishing catheter-related from other septic episodes. *JAMA* 1973;223:1341.

Dinsmore RE, Wedeen V, Rosen B, et al. Phase-offset technique to distinguish slow blood flow and thrombus on MR images. *AJR* 1987;148:634.

DiSerio FJ, Sasahara AA, Singer JM, et al. United States trial of dihydroergotamine and heparin prophylaxis of deep vein thrombosis. *Am J Surg* 1985;150:25.

Djokovic JL, Headley-Whyte J. Prediction of outcome of surgery and anesthesia in patients over 80. *JAMA* 1979;242:2301.

Doran FSA. Prevention of deep vein thrombosis. *Br J Hosp Med* 1971;6:773.

Dripps R, Deming M. Postoperative atelectasis and pneumonia: diagnosis, etiology, and management based on 1240 cases of upper abdominal surgery. *Ann Surg* 1946;24:94.

Duxbury B, Duxbury BM. Therapeutic quality control leading to further clinical assessment of oral anticoagulation. *Acta Haematol* 1986;76:65.

Elwyn DH. Nutritional requirements of adult surgical patients. *Crit Care Med* 1980;8:9.

Endl VJ, Auinger W. Early detection of postoperative deep-vein thrombosis in gynaecological patients by the ^{125}I-fibrinogen test. *Wien Klin Wochenschr* 1977;89:304.

Engoren M. Lack of association between atelectasis and fever. *Chest* 1995;107:81.

Evans AJ, Sostman HD, Knelson MH, et al. Detection of deep venous thrombosis: prospective comparison of MR imaging with contrast venography. *AJR* 1993;161:131.

Everett HS, Ridley JH. *Female urology.* New York: Harper-Horber, 1968.

Felmlee JP, Ehman RL. Spatial presaturation: A method for suppressing flow artifacts and improving depiction of vascular anatomy in MR imaging. *Radiology* 1987;164:559.

Fischer JE. *Surgical nutrition.* Boston: Little, Brown, 1983.

Flane C, Kakkar VW, Clarke MB. The detection of venous thrombosis of the legs using ^{125}I-labeled fibrinogen. *Br J Surg* 1958;55:742.

Fletcher JP, Little JM. A comparison of parenteral nutrition and early postoperative enteral feeding on the nitrogen balance after major surgery. *Surgery* 1986;100:21.

Francis DMA, Shenton BK. Fat emulsion adversely affects lymphocyte reactivity. *Aust NZ J Surg* 1987;57:323.

Francis RM, Peacock M. Local action of oral 1,25-dihydroxycholecalciferol on calcium absorption in osteoporosis. *Am J Clin Nutr* 1987;46:315.

Frango JA, Eskin SG, McIntire LV. Flow effects on prostacyclin production by cultured human endothelial cells. *Science* 1985;227:1477.

Fricker JP, Vergnes Y, Schach R, et al. Low dose heparin versus low molecular weight heparin (kabi 2165, Fragmin) in the prophylaxis of thromboembolic complications of abdominal oncological surgery. *Eur J Clin Invest* 1988;18:561.

Frisancho AR. New standards of weight and body composition by frame size and height for assessment of nutritional status. *Am J Clin Nutr* 1984;40:808.

Frisancho AR. Nutrition anthropometry. *J Am Diet Assoc* 1988;88:553.

Furman RH. Coronary heart disease and the menopause. In: Ryan KJ, Gibson DC, eds. *Menopause and aging.* DHEW Publication No. (NIH) 1971;73:319.

Gallagher JC, Nordin BEC. Estrogens and calcium metabolism. In: Curry AS, ed. *Biochemistry of women.* Cleveland: CRC Press, 1974.

Gallagher JC, Nordin BEC. Estrogens and calcium metabolism. In: van Keep PA, Lauritzen C, eds. *Frontiers of hormone research, vol 2: ageing and estrogens.* Basel: S Karger, 1973.

Garcea D, Martuzzi F, Santelmo N, et al. Post-surgical deep vein thrombosis: prevention, evaluation of the risk/benefit ratio of fractionated and unfractionated heparin. *Curr Med Res Opin* 1992;12:572.

Garibaldi RA, Britt MR, Coleman MI, et al. Risk factors for postoperative pneumonia. *Am J Med* 1981;70:677.

Gazzaniga AB, Day AT, Sankary H. The efficacy of a 20 per cent fat emulsion as a peripherally administered substrate. *Surg Obstet Gynecol* 1985;160:387.

Gebara OC, Mittleman MA, Sutherland P, et al. Association between increased estrogen status and increased fibrinolytic potential in the Framingham Offspring Study. *Circulation* 1995;91:83.

Geerts WH, Heit JA, Clagett G, et al. Prevention of venous thromboembolism (Sixth ACCP Consensus Conference on Antithrombotic Therapy). *Chest* 2001;119(1 Suppl): 132S–175S.

Genton E. Pulmonary embolism and infarction. In: Chung ED, ed. *Cardiac emergency care.* Philadelphia: Lea & Febiger, 1979.

Genton E, Turpie AGG. Venous thromboembolism associated with gynecologic surgery. *Clin Obstet Gynecol* 1980; 23:209.

Gever LN. Embolex: to prevent a double postop danger. *Nursing* 1986;16:73.

Gjonnaess H, Abildgaard U. Bleeding in gynecological surgery: influence of low dose heparin. *Int J Gynaecol Obstet* 1976;14:9.

Goldberg RJ, Seneff M, Gore JM, et al. Occult malignant neoplasm in patients with deep venous thrombosis. *Arch Intern Med* 1987;147:215.

Goodnight SH Jr. Bleeding and intravascular clotting in malignancy: a review. *Ann NY Acad Sci* 1974;230:271.

Gordon GS. Postmenopausal osteoporosis: cause, prevention and treatment. *Clin Obstet Gynecol* 1977;4:169.

Gordon SG, Franks JJ, Lewis B. Cancer procoagulant A: a factor X activating procoagulant from malignant tissue. *Thromb Res* 1975;6:127.

Gordon T, Kannel WB, Hjortland MC, et al. Menopause and coronary heart disease: The Framingham Study. *Ann Intern Med* 1978;89:157.

Gore JM, Appelbaum JS, Greene HL, et al. Occult cancer in patients with acute pulmonary embolism. *Ann Intern Med* 1982;96:556.

Gray LA, Christopherson WM, Hoover RN. Estrogens and endometrial carcinoma. *Obstet Gynecol* 1977;49:385.

Griffin MR, Stanson AW, Brown ML, et al. Deep venous thrombosis and pulmonary embolism: risk of subsequent malignant neoplasms. *Arch Intern Med* 1987;147: 1907.

Grubner UF, Saldeen T, Brokopt T, et al. Incidences of fatal post-operative pulmonary embolism after prophylaxis with dextran 70 and low dose heparin: an international multicenter study. *Br Med J* 1980;280:69.

Guyton DP, Khayat A, Schreiber H. Pneumatic compression stockings and prostaglandin synthesis: a pathway to fibrinolysis? *Crit Care Med* 1985;13:266.

Guyton DP, Khayat A, Schreiber H, et al. Endogenous plasminogen activator and venous flow: therapeutic implications. *Crit Care Med* 1987;15:122.

Hammond CB, Jelovsek FR, Lee KL, et al. Effects of long-term estrogen replacement therapy: I. metabolic effects. *Am J Obstet Gynecol* 1979;133:525.

Hammond CB, Ory SJ. Endocrine problems in the menopause. *Clin Obstet Gynecol* 1982;25:19.

Hands LJ, Royle GT, Kettlewell MGW. Vitamin K requirements in patients receiving total parenteral nutrition. *Br J Surg* 1985;72:665.

Hart DM, Farish E, Fletcher DC, et al. Ten years' postmenopausal hormone replacement therapy: effect on lipoproteins. *Maturitas* 1984;5:271.

Hauser CJ, Shoemaker WC, Turpin I, et al. Oxygen transport responses to colloids and crystalloids in critically ill surgical patients. *Surg Gynecol Obstet* 1980;150:881.

Haydock DA, Hill GL. Improved wound healing response in surgical patients receiving i.v. nutrition. *Br J Surg* 1987;74:320.

Heijboer H, Ginsberg JS, Buller HR, et al. The use of the D-dimer test in combination with non-invasive testing versus serial non-invasive testing alone for the diagnosis of deep vein thrombosis. *Thromb Haemost* 1992;67:510.

Heird WC, Grundy SM, Hubbard VS. Structured lipids and their use in clinical nutrition. *Am J Clin Nutr* 1986; 43:320.

Helgason S. Estrogen replacement therapy after the menopause. *Acta Obstet Gynecol Scand Suppl* 1982;107:1.

Hilgard P. Experimental vitamin K deficiency and spontaneous metastases. *Br J Cancer* 1975;35:391.

Hillner BE, Philbrick JT, Becer DM. Optimal management of suspected lower-extremity deep vein thrombosis: an evaluation with cost assessment of 24 management strategies. *Arch Intern Med* 1992;152:165.

Hirsh J, Deykin D, Poller L. "Therapeutic range" for oral anticoagulant therapy. *Chest* 1986;89:11S.

Hirsh J, Genton E, Hull R. *Venous thromboembolism.* New York: Grune & Stratton, 1981.

Hirsh J, Hull RD, Raskob GE. Clinical features and diagnosis of venous thrombosis. *J Am Coll Cardiol* 1986;2:4B.

Hirvonen E, Malkonen M, Manninen V. Effects of different progestogens on lipoproteins during postmenopausal therapy. *N Engl J Med* 1981;304:560.

Hoak JC, Connor WE, Warner ED. The antithrombotic effects of sodium heparin and sodium warfarin. *Arch Intern Med* 1966;117:25.

Hobbs JT, Davies JW. Detection of venous thrombosis with ^{131}I-labeled fibrinogen in the rabbit. *Lancet* 1960;2: 134.

Hodgkinson CP, Hodari AA. Trocar suprapubic cystostomy for postoperative bladder drainage in the female. *Am J Obstet Gynecol* 1966;96:773.

Honkanen T, Jauhola S, Karppinen K, et al. Venous thrombosis: a controlled study on the performance of scintigraphy with 99mTc-HMPAO-labelled platelets versus venography. *Nucl Med Commun* 1992;13:88.

Hoover JC, Ryan JP, Anderson EJ, et al. Nutritional benefits of immediate postoperative jejunal feeding of an elemental diet. *Am J Surg* 1980;139:153.

Hoshal VL. Total intravenous nutrition with peripherally inserted silicone elastomer central venous catheters. *Arch Surg* 1975;110:644.

Huisman MV, Buller HR, Ten Cate JW, et al. Serial impedance plethysmography for suspected deep venous thrombosis in outpatients. The Amsterdam General Practitioner Study. *N Engl J Med* 1986;314:823.

Hull RD, Raskob GE, Hirsh J. Prophylaxis of venous thromboembolism: an overview. *Chest* 1986;89:3745.

Inada K, Koike S, Shirai N, et al. Effects of intermittent pneumatic leg compression for prevention of postoperative deep venous thrombosis with special reference to fibrinolytic activity. *Am J Surg* 1988;155:602.

Ireton-Jones CS, Turner WW Jr. The use of respiratory quotient to determine the efficacy of nutrition support regimens. *J Am Diet Assoc* 1987;87:180.

Irving M. ABC of nutrition. *Br Med J* 1985;291:1403.

Iverson L, Ecker R, Fox H, et al. A comparative study of IPPB, the incentive spirometer and blow bottles: the prevention of atelectasis following cardiac surgery. *Ann Thorac Surg* 1978;25:197.

Jacobs EJ, White E, Weiss NS. Exogenous hormones, reproductive history, and colon cancer. *Cancer Causes Control* 1994;5:359.

Jeffcoate TNA, Tindall VR. Venous thrombosis and embolism in obstetrics and gynecology. *Aust NZ J Obstet Gynaecol* 1965;5:119.

Joist JH, Sherman LA, eds. *Venous and arterial thrombosis: pathogenesis, diagnosis, prevention and therapy.* New York: Grune & Stratton, 1979.

Joseph RR, Day HJ, Sherwin RM, et al. Microangiopathic haemolytic anaemia associated with consumption coagulopathy in a patient with disseminated carcinoma. *Scand J Haematol* 1967;4:271.

Judd HL, Cleary RE, Creasman WT, et al. Estrogen replacement therapy. *Obstet Gynecol* 1981;58:267.

Kaaja R, Lehtouirta P, Venesmaa P, et al. Comparison of enoxaparin, a low-molecular-weight heparin, and unfractionated heparin, with or without dihydroergotamine in abdominal hysterectomy. *Eur J Obstet Gynecol Reprod Biol* 1992;47:141.

Kadakia SC, Sullivan HO, Starnes E. Percutaneous endoscopic gastrostomy or jejunostomy and the incidence of aspiration in 79 patients. *Am J Surg* 1992;164:114.

Kakkar W, Corrigan TP, Fossard DP. Prevention of postoperative pulmonary embolism by low dose heparin. *Lancet* 1975;2:45.

Kaminski MV. Enteral hyperalimentation. *Surg Gynecol Obstet* 1976;32:1112.

Kass EH, Sossen HS. Prevention of infection of urinary tract in presence of indwelling catheters. *JAMA* 1959;169:1181.

Kemble JVH. Incidence of deep vein thrombosis. *Br J Hosp Med* 1971;6:721.

King CR, Daly JW. The prevention of postoperative pulmonary emboli with low-molecular-weight dextran. *Am J Obstet Gynecol* 1975;123:46.

Kiriloff LH, Owens GR, Rogers RM, et al. Does chest physical therapy work? *Chest* 1985;88:436.

Kline A, Hughes LE, Campbell H, et al. Dextran 70 in prophylaxis of thromboembolic disease after surgery: a clinically oriented randomized double-blind trial. *Br Med J* 1975;2:109.

Knight LC, Maurer AH, Ammar IA, et al. Evaluation of indium-111 labeled anti-fibrin antibody for imaging vascular thrombi. *J Nucl Med* 1988;29:494.

Kotz KL, Geelhoed GW. Lethal thromboembolism and its prevention in pelvic surgery: a review. *Gynecol Oncol* 1981;12:271.

Kriska AM, Sandler RB, Cauley JA, et al. The assessment of historical physical activity and its relation to adult bone parameters. *Am J Epidemiol* 1988;12:1053.

Kristo DA, Perry ME, Kollef MH. Comparison of venography, duplex imaging and bilateral impedance plethysmography for diagnosis of lower extremity deep vein thrombosis. *South Med J* 1994;87:55.

Langsfeld M, Hershey FB, Thorpe L, et al. Duplex B-mode imaging for the diagnosis of deep venous thrombosis. *Arch Surg* 1987;122:587.

Leiter LA, Marliss EB. Survival during fasting may depend on fat as well as protein stores. *JAMA* 1982;248:2306.

Lieberman JS, Borrero J, Urdaneta E, et al. Thrombophlebitis and cancer. *JAMA* 1961;177:542.

Lindhagen A, Bergqvist A, Bergqvist D, et al. Late venous function in the leg after deep venous thrombosis occurring in relation to pregnancy. *Br J Obstet Gynaecol* 1986;93:348.

Lindquist O. Relationship between menstrual status and development of osteoporosis. *Acta Obstet Gynecol Scand Suppl* 1982;110:22.

Lindsay R. Prevention of osteoporosis. *Clin Orthop* 1987; 222:44.

Lindsay R, Aitken JM, Anderson JB, et al. Long-term prevention of postmenopausal osteoporosis by oestrogen. *Lancet* 1976;1:1038.

Lindsay R, Hart DM, Forrest C, et al. Prevention of spinal osteoporosis in oophorectomised women. *Lancet* 1980; 2:1151.

Lindsay R, Hart DM, MacLean A, et al. Bone response to termination of estrogen treatment. *Lancet* 1978;1:1325.

Longerbeam JK, Vannix R, Wagner W, et al. Central venous pressure monitoring. *Am J Surg* 1965;110:220.

Lueg MC. Postmenopausal osteoporosis: treatment with low-dose sodium fluoride and estrogen. *South Med J* 1988;81:597.

MacIntyre I, Stevenson JC, Whitehead MI, et al. Calcitonin for prevention of postmenopausal bone loss. *Lancet* 1988;1:900.

Maki DG, Weise CE, Sarafin HW. A semiquantitative culture method for identifying intravenous-catheter-related infection. *N Engl J Med* 1977;296:1305.

Malluche HH, Faugere MC, Friedler RM, et al. 1,25-dihydroxy vitamin D_3 corrects bone loss but suppresses bone remodeling in ovariohysterectomized beagle dogs. *Endocrinology* 1988;125:1998.

Mamelle N, Meunier PJ, Dusan R, et al. Risk benefit ratio of sodium fluoride treatment in primary vertebral osteoporosis. *Lancet* 1988;2:361.

Mammer EF, ed. Venous thromboembolism. *Semin Thromb Hemost* 1976;2:4.

Marini JJ, Pierson DJ, Hudson LD. Acute lobar atelectasis: a prospective comparison of fiberoptic bronchoscopy and respiratory therapy. *Am Rev Respir Dis* 1979;119:971.

Markwardt F. Pharmacological approaches to thrombin regulation. *Ann NY Acad Sci* 1986;485:204.

Marshall DH, Horsman A, Nordin BEC. The prevention and management of post-menopausal osteoporosis. *Acta Obstet Gynecol Scand Suppl* 1977;65:49.

Mattingly RF, Moore DE, Clark DO. Bacteriologic study of suprapubic bladder drainage. *Am J Obstet Gynecol* 1972;114:732.

Mavor GE. Surgery of deep vein thrombosis. *Br J Hosp Med* 1971;6:755.

Maxwell GL, Synan I, Dodge R, et al. Pneumatic compression versus low molecular weight heparin in gynecologic oncology surgery: a randomized trial. *Obstet Gynecol* 2001; 98:989.

McCarthy TG, McQueen J, Johnstone FD, et al. A comparison of low dose subcutaneous heparin and intravenous dextran 70 in the prophylaxis of deep venous thrombosis after gynaecological surgery. *J Obstet Gynaecol Br Commonw* 1974;81:486.

McDevitt E. Thromboembolic complications following gynecologic operations: role of prophylactic anticoagulant therapy. In: Sherry S, Brinkhous KM, Genton E, et al, eds. *Thrombosis.* Washington, DC: National Academy of Sciences, 1969.

McGee CD, Ostro MJ, Kurran R, et al. Vitamin E and selenium status of patients receiving short-term total parenteral nutrition. *Am J Clin Nutr* 1985;42:432.

Meema HE, Bunker ML, Meema S. Loss of compact bone due to menopause. *Obstet Gynecol* 1965;26:333.

Mikkola T, Turunen P, Avela K, et al. 17 β-estradiol stimulates prostacyclin, but not endothelin-1, production in human vascular endothelial cells. *J Clin Endocrinol Metab* 1995;80:1832.

Miller SP, Sanchez-Avalos J, Stefanski T, et al. Coagulation disorders in cancer: I. clinical and laboratory studies. *Cancer* 1967;20:1452.

Mintz UC, Le DW, Axel A, et al. Puerperal ovarian vein thrombosis: MR diagnosis. *Am J Radiol* 1987;149:1273.

Mirtallo JM, Schneider PT, Mauko K, et al. A comparison of essential and general amino acid infusions in the nutritional support of patients with compromised renal function. *J Parenter Enteral Nutr* 1982;6:109.

Mittleman JS, Edwards WS, McDonald JB. Effectiveness of leg compression in preventing venous stasis. *Am J Surg* 1982;144:611.

Mobin-Uddin K, Callard GM, Bolooki H, et al. Transcaval interruption with umbrella filter. *N Engl J Med* 1972;286:55.

Mohr DN, Ryu JH, Litin SC, et al. Recent advances in the management of venous thromboembolism. *Mayo Clin Proc* 1988;63:281.

Moore FD. Energy and the maintenance of the body cell mass. *J Parenter Enteral Nutr* 1980;4:228.

Moosman DA. The anatomy of infraclavicular subclavian vein catheterization and its complications. *Surg Gynecol Obstet* 1973;136:71.

Morlion BJ, Stehle P, Wachtler P, et al. Total parenteral nutrition with glutamine dipeptide after major abdominal surgery: a randomized, double-blind, controlled study. *Ann Surg* 1998;227:302.

Moser KM, LeMoine JR. Is embolic risk conditioned by location of deep venous thrombosis? *Ann Intern Med* 1981;94:439.

Mullin TJ, Kirkpatrick JR. The effect of nutritional support on immune competency in patients suffering from trauma, sepsis, and malignant disease. *Surgery* 1981;90:610.

Munk-Jensen N, Pors Nielsen S, Obel EB, et al. Reversal of postmenopausal vertebral bone loss by oestrogen and progesterone: a double-blind placebo controlled study. *Br Med J* 1988;296:1150.

Nanda K, Bastian LA, Hasselblad V, et al. Hormone replacement therapy and the risk of colorectal cancer: a meta-analysis. *Obstet Gynecol* 1999;93:880.

Need AG, Horowitz M, Morris HA, et al. Effects of nandrolone therapy on forearm bone mineral content in osteoporosis. *Clin Orthop* 1987;225:273.

Nicolaides AN, Fernandes IF, Pollock AV. Intermittent sequential compression of the legs in the prevention of venous stasis and postoperative deep venous thrombosis. *Surgery* 1980;87:69.

Nicolaides AN, Miles C, Hoare M, et al. Intermittent sequential pneumatic compression of the legs and thromboembolism-deterrent stockings in the prevention of postoperative deep venous thrombosis. *Surgery* 1983;94:21.

Nolan TE, Banias BB, Devoe LD, et al. Antepartum assessment of the maternal peripheral venous system with light reflection rheology. *J Reprod Med* 1992;37:251.

Nordenstrom J, Carpentier YA, Askanazi J, et al. Metabolic utilization of intravenous fat emulsion during total parenteral nutrition. *Ann Surg* 1982;196:221.

Notelovitz M, Johnston M, Smith S, et al. Metabolic and hormonal effects of 25-mg and 50-mg 17 beta-estradiol implants in surgically menopausal women. *Obstet Gynecol* 1987;70:749.

Nusbacher J. Migratory venous thrombosis and cancer. *NY State J Med* 1964;64:2166.

O'Donohue WJ. National survey of the usage of lung expansion modalities for the prevention and treatment of postoperative atelectasis following abdominal and thoracic surgery. *Chest* 1985;87:76.

O'Keefe SJD, Bean E, Symmonds K, et al. Clinical evaluation of a '3-in-1' intravenous nutrient solution. *S Afr Med J* 1985;68:82.

Olson DL, Krubsack AJ, Stewart ET. Percutaneous enteral alimentation: gastrostomy versus gastrojejunostomy. *Radiology* 1993;187:105.

Oster G, Tuden RL, Colditz GA. Prevention of venous thromboembolism after general surgery: cost effectiveness analysis of alternative approaches to prophylaxis. *Am J Med* 1987;82:889.

Oster MW. Thrombophlebitis and cancer: a review. *Angiology* 1976;27:557.

Oster ZH, Srivastava SC, Som P, et al. Thrombus radioimmunoscintigraphy: an approach using monoclonal antiplatelet antibody. *Proc Natl Acad Sci USA* 1985;82:3465.

Ottosson UB, Johansson BJ, von Schoultz B. Subfractions of high-density lipoprotein cholesterol during estrogen replacement therapy: a comparison between progestogens and natural progesterone. *Am J Obstet Gynecol* 1985; 151:746.

Pacifici R, McMurty C, Vered I, et al. Coherence therapy does not prevent axial bone loss in osteoporotic women: a preliminary comparative study. *J Clin Endocrinol Metab* 1988;66:747.

Padberg FT, Ruggiero J, Blackburn GL, et al. Central venous catheterization for parenteral nutrition. *Ann Surg* 1981;193.264.

Pak CYC, Sakhaee K, Zerwekh JE, et al. Safe and effective treatment of osteoporosis with intermittent slow release sodium fluoride augmentation of vertebral bone mass and inhibition of fractures. *J Clin Endocrinol Metab* 1989;68:150.

Pangrazzi J, Abbadini M, Zametta M, et al. Antithrombotic and bleeding effects of a low molecular weight heparin fraction. *Biol Pharmacol* 1985;34:3305.

Peters AM, Lavender JP, Needham SG, et al. Imaging thrombus with radiolabelled monoclonal antibody to platelets. *Br Med J* 1986;293:1525.

Peterson CE, Kwaan HC. Current concepts of warfarin therapy. *Arch Intern Med* 1986;146:581.

Petitti DB, Wingard J, Pellegrin F, et al. Risk of vascular disease in women: smoking, oral contraceptives, non contraceptive estrogens, and other factors. *JAMA* 1979;242:1150.

Petty TL, Fowler AA. Another look at ARDS. *Chest* 1982;82:98.

Peuscher FW, Cleton FJ, Armstrong L, et al. Significance of plasma fibrinopeptide A (FPA) in patients with malignancy. *J Lab Clin Med* 1980;96:5.

Poller L, McKernan A, Thomson JM, et al. Fixed minidose warfarin: a new approach to prophylaxis against venous thrombosis after major surgery. *Br Med J* 1987;295:1309.

Polley KJ, Nordin BE, Baghurst PA, et al. Effect of calcium supplementation on forearm bone mineral content in post-menopausal women: a prospective sequential controlled trial. *J Nutr* 1987;117:1929.

Poulose KP, Kapcar AJ, Reba RC. False positive ^{125}I fibrinogen test. *Angiology* 1976;27:258.

Prevention of venous thrombosis and pulmonary embolism. N.I.H. consensus development conference on prevention of venous thrombosis and pulmonary embolism. *JAMA* 1986;256:744.

Proudfit CM. Estrogens and menopause. *JAMA* 1976;236:939.

Quebbeman EJ. Estimating energy requirements in patients receiving parenteral nutrition. *Arch Surg* 1982;117:1281.

Quebbeman EJ. A re-evaluation of energy expenditure during parenteral nutrition. *Ann Surg* 1982;195:282.

Quick AJ. Modern concepts of venous thrombosis. *Practitioner* 1951;166:213.

Quigley MM, Hammon CB. Estrogen replacement therapy: help or hazard? *N Engl J Med* 1979;301:646.

Ramchandani P, Soulen RL, Fedullo LM, et al. Deep vein thrombosis: significant limitation of noninvasive tests. *Radiology* 1985;156:47.

Rapoport S, Sostman HD, Pope C, et al. Venous clots: evaluation with MR imaging. *Radiology* 1987;162:527.

Ravnikar V, Murin V, Nutkik J, et al. *Blood lipid levels in postmenopausal women on hormone replacement therapy.* 35th Annual Meeting, Society of Gynecologic Investigation, 1988 (Abstract no. 422).

Rayburn W, Wolk R, Mercer N, et al. Parenteral nutrition in obstetrics and gynecology. *Obstet Gynecol* 1986;41:200.

Reginster JY, Denis D, Albert A, et al. 1-year controlled randomised trial of prevention of early postmenopausal bone loss by intranasal calcitonin. *Lancet* 1987;2:1481.

Reiertsen O, Larsen S, Storkson R, et al. Safety of enoxaparin and dextran-70 in the prevention of venous thromboembolism in digestive surgery: a play-the-winner-designed study. *Scand J Gastroenterol* 1993;28:1015.

Reilly JJ, Gerhardt AL. Modern surgical nutrition. *Curr Probl Surg* 1985;22:1.

Rickles FR, Edwards RL. Activation of blood coagulation in cancer: Trousseau's syndrome revisited. *Blood* 1983;62:14.

Rickles FR, Edwards RL, Barb C, et al. Abnormalities of blood coagulation in patients with cancer: fibrinopeptide A generation and tumor growth. *Cancer* 1983;51:301.

Riis BJ, Christiansen C. Measurement of spinal or peripheral bone mass to estimate early postmenopausal bone loss? *Am J Med* 1988;84:646.

Rinaldo JE, Rogers RM. Adult respiratory distress syndrome. *N Engl J Med* 1982;306:900.

Rivlin RS. Osteoporosis: nutrition. *Public Health Rep* 1987;Jul–Aug(Suppl):131.

Rose D, Yarborough MF, Canizaro PC, et al. One hundred and fourteen fistulas of the gastrointestinal tract treated with total parenteral nutrition. *Surg Gynecol Obstet* 1986; 163:345.

Rosenow EC. 3rd venous and pulmonary thromboembolism, an algorithmic approach to diagnosis and management. *Mayo Clin Proc* 1995;70:45.

Rosner NH, Doris PE. Diagnosis of femoropopliteal venous thrombosis: comparison of duplex sonography and plethysmography. *AJR* 1988;150:623.

Ross RK, Paganini-Hill A, Mack TM, et al. Menopausal oestrogen therapy and protection from death from ischaemic heart disease. *Lancet* 1981;1:858.

Rudman D, Williams PJ. Nutrient deficiencies during total parenteral nutrition. *Nutr Rev* 1985;43:1.

Ryan DA. Hazard associated with the use of a common pathway for infusion and vascular monitoring. *Anaesthesia* 1985;40:1134.

Sach GH, Levin J, Bell WR. Trousseau's syndrome and other manifestations of chronic disseminated coagulopathy in patients with neoplasms: clinical pathophysiologic and therapeutic features. *Medicine* 1977;S6:1.

Salvian AJ, Baker JD. Effects of intermittent pneumatic calf compression in normal and postphlebitic legs. *J Cardiovasc Surg (Torino)* 1988;29:37.

Samama M, Bernard P, Bonnardot JP, et al. Low molecular weight heparin compared with unfractionated heparin in prevention of postoperative thrombosis. *Br J Surg* 1988;75:128.

Sanders RA, Sheldon GF. Septic complications of total parenteral nutrition: a five year experience. *Am J Surg* 1976;132:214.

Sandler DA, Martin JF. Liquid crystal thermography as a screening test for deep-vein thrombosis. *Lancet* 1985;1:665.

Sandstedt S, Lennmarken C, Symreng T, et al. The effect of preoperative total parenteral nutrition on energy-rich phosphates, electrolytes and free amino acids in skeletal muscle of malnourished patients with gastric carcinoma. *Br J Surg* 1985;72:920.

Sasahara AA, DiSerio FJ, et al. Dihydroergotamine-heparin prophylaxis of postoperative deep vein thrombosis: a multicenter trial. *JAMA* 1984;251:2960.

Sasahara AA, Koppenhagen K, Haring R, et al. Low molecular weight heparin plus dihydroergotamine for prophylaxis of postoperative deep vein thrombosis. *Br J Surg* 1986;73:697.

Savvas M, Studd JW, Fogelman I, et al. Skeletal effects of oral oestrogen compared with subcutaneous oestrogen and testosterone in postmenopausal women. *Br Med J* 1988;297:331.

Schiff MJ, Feinberg AW, Naidich JB. Noninvasive venous examinations as a screening test for pulmonary embolism. *Arch Intern Med* 1987;147:505.

Schlueter DP. High-risk gynecology: pulmonary risks. *Clin Obstet Gynecol* 1973;16:91.

Scurr JH, Ibrahim SZ, Faber RG, et al. The efficacy of graduated compression stockings in the prevention of deep vein thrombosis. *Br J Surg* 1977;64:371.

Seem E, Stranden E, Stiris MG. Computed tomography in deep venous thrombosis with limb oedema. *Acta Radiol Diag* 1985;26:727.

Seiden AM, Pensak ML. Postoperative deep venous thrombosis and pulmonary embolism: diagnosis, management and prevention. *Am J Otol* 1986;7:377.

Semmens IP, Wagner G. Effects of estrogen therapy on vaginal physiology during menopause. *Obstet Gynecol* 1985;66:15.

Sevitt S, Gallagher NG. Venous thrombosis and pulmonary embolism: a clinical pathological study in injured and burned patients. *Br J Surg* 1961;48:475.

Sharnoff JG. Results in prophylaxis of postoperative thromboembolism. *Surg Gynecol Obstet* 1966;123:303.

Shils ME, Young VR, eds. *Modern nutrition in health and disease,* 7th ed. Philadelphia: Lea & Febiger, 1988.

Shoemaker WC, Appel P, Czer LSC, et al. Pathogenesis of respiratory failure (ARDS) after hemorrhage and trauma: I. cardiorespiratory patterns preceding the development of ARDS. *Crit Care Med* 1980;8:504.

Sibbald WJ, Anderson RR, Reid B, et al. Alveolo-capillary permeability in human septic ARDS: effect of high dose corticosteroid. *Ther Chest* 1981;79:133.

Sigel B, Edelstein AL, Felix WR, et al. Compression of deep venous system of the lower leg during inactive recumbency. *Arch Surg* 1973;106:38.

Sigel B, Edelstein AL, Savitch L, et al. Type of compression for reducing venous stasis: a study of lower extremities during inactive recumbency. *Arch Surg* 1975;110:171.

Sitges-Serra A, Puig P, Jaurrieta E, et al. Catheter sepsis due to *Staphylococcus epidermidis* during parenteral nutrition. *Surg Gynecol Obstet* 1980;151:481.

Smith DC, Prentice R, Thompson DJ, et al. Association of exogenous estrogen and endometrial carcinoma. *N Engl J Med* 1975;293:1164.

Sobel S. Osteoporosis: regulatory view. *Public Health Rep* 1987;Jul–Aug(Suppl):136.

Soong BCF, Miller SP. Coagulation disorders in cancer: III. fibrinolysis and inhibitors. *Cancer* 1970;25:867.

Speroff L, Glass RH, Kase NG. *Clinical gynecologic endocrinology and infertility,* 4th ed. Baltimore: Williams & Wilkins, 1989.

Spritzer CE, Eans AC, Kay HH. Magnetic resonance imaging of deep venous thrombosis in pregnant women with lower extremity edema. *Obstet Gynecol* 1995;88:603.

Spritzer CE, Sussman SK, Blinder RA, et al. Deep venous thrombosis evaluation with limited-flip-angle, gradient-refocused MR imaging: preliminary experience. *Radiology* 1988;166:371.

Sproul EE. Carcinoma and venous thrombosis: the frequency of association of carcinoma in the body or tail of the pancreas with multiple venous thrombosis. *Am J Cancer* 1938;34:566.

Stamp TC, Jenkins MV, Loveridge N, et al. Fluoride therapy in osteoporosis: acute effects on parathyroid and mineral homeostasis. *Clin Sci* 1988;75:143.

Stampfer MJ, Colditz GA. Estrogen replacement therapy and coronary heart disease: a quantitative assessment of the epidemiologic evidence. *Prev Med* 1991;20:47.

Stampfer MJ, Willett WC, Colditz GA, et al. A prospective study of postmenopausal estrogen therapy and coronary heart disease. *N Engl J Med* 1985;313:1044.

Stanton JR, Freis ED, Wilkins RW. Acceleration of linear flow in deep veins with local compression. *J Clin Invest* 1944;28:553.

Starker PM, Gump FE, Askanazi J, et al. Serum albumin levels as an index of nutritional support. *Surgery* 1982;91:194.

Starker PM, LaSala PA, Askanazi J, et al. The influence of preoperative total parenteral nutrition on morbidity and mortality. *Surg Gynecol Obstet* 1986;162:569.

Stevenson JC, Whitehead MI, Padwick M, et al. Dietary intake of calcium and postmenopausal bone loss. *Br Med J* 1988;297:15.

Stewart RD, Sanislow CA. Silastic intravenous catheter. *N Engl J Med* 1961;265:1283.

Stiller KR, Munday RM. Chest physiotherapy for the surgical patient. *Br J Surg* 1992;79:745.

Stock MC, Downs JB, Gauer PK, et al. Prevention of postoperative pulmonary complications with CPAP, incentive spirometry and conservative therapy. *Chest* 1985;87:151.

Sturdee DW, Wilson KA, Pipili E, et al. Physiological aspects of menopausal hot flush. *Br Med J* 1978;2:79.

Sue-Ling HM, Johnston D, McMahon MJ, et al. Pre-operative identification of patients at high risk of deep venous thrombosis after elective major abdominal surgery. *Lancet* 1986;1:1173.

Sugimura K, Yamasaki K, Kitagaki H, et al. Bone marrow diseases of the spine: differentiation with T1 and T2 relaxation times in MR imaging. *Radiology* 1987;165:541.

Summaria L, Caprini JA, McMillan R, et al. Relationship between postsurgical fibrinolytic parameters and deep vein thrombosis in surgical patients treated with compression devices. *Am Surg* 1988;54:156.

Sun NCJ, Bowie EJW, Kazmier FJ, et al. Blood coagulation studies in patients with cancer. *Mayo Clin Proc* 1974;49:636.

Sun NCJ, McAfee WM, Hum GJ, et al. Hemostatic abnormalities in malignancy: a prospective study of one hundred eight patients. *Am Soc Clin Pathol* 1979;71:10.

Sy WM, Seo IS. Radionuclide venography: imaging monitor in deep vein thrombosis of the pelvis and lower extremities. *Br J Radiol* 1986;59:325.

Szklo M, Tonascia J, Gordis L, et al. Estrogen use and myocardial infarction risk: a case-control study. *Prev Med* 1984;13:510.

Taberner DA, Poller L, Burslem RW, et al. Oral anticoagulants controlled by the British. Comparative thromboplastin versus low-dose heparin in prophylaxis of deep vein thrombosis. *Br Med J* 1978;1:272.

Tang M, Subbiah R. Estrogens protect against hydrogen peroxide and arachidonic acid induced DNA damage. *Biochim Biophys Acta* 1996;1299:155.

Tarnay TJ, Rohr PR, Davidson AG, et al. Pneumatic calf compression, fibrinolysis and the prevention of deep venous thrombosis. *Surgery* 1980;88:489.

Taussig FJ. Bladder function after confinement and after gynecological operations. *Trans Am Gynecol Soc* 1915;40:351.

Tenghorn L, Palmblad S, Wojciechowski J, et al. D-dimer and thrombin/antithrombin III complex: diagnostic tools to deep venous thrombosis? *Haemostasis* 1994;24:344.

The Acute Respiratory Distress Syndrome Network. Ventilation with lower tidal volumes as compared with traditional tidal volumes for acute lung injury and the acute respiratory distress syndrome. *N Engl J Med* 2000;342: 1301.

Thomas D, ed. Thrombosis. *Br Med Bull* 1978;2:34.

Thommi G. Nasal CPAP in treatment of persistent atelectasis. *Chest* 1991;99:1551.

Tice DA. Low dosage of heparin. *Surg Gynecol Obstet* 1976;143:970.

Torosian MH, Daly JM. Nutritional support in the cancer-bearing host: effects on host and tumor. *Cancer* 1986;58(Suppl 8):1915.

Tracey KJ, Legaspi A, Albert JD, et al. Protein and substrate metabolism during starvation and parenteral refeeding. *Clin Sci* 1988;74:123.

Trousseau A. *Phlegmasia alba dolens: clinique medicale de l'Hotel Dieu de Paris,* vol 3. London: New Sydenham Society, 1868:695.

Turner GM, Cole SE, Brooks JH. The efficacy of graduated compression stockings in the deep vein thrombosis after major gynaecological surgery. *Br J Obstet Gynaecol* 1984;91:588.

Turpie AGG, Hirsh J, Jay RM, et al. Double-blind randomised trial of Org 10172 low-molecular weight heparinoid in prevention of deep-vein thrombosis in thrombotic stroke. *Lancet* 1987;1:8523.

Twombly GH. Hemorrhage in gynecologic surgery. *Clin Obstet Gynecol* 1973;16:135.

Underwood SR, Firmin DN, Klipstein RH, et al. Magnetic resonance velocity mapping: clinical application of a new technique. *Br Heart J* 1987;57:404.

Utian WH. *Menopause in modern perspective.* New York: Appleton-Century-Crofts, 1980.

Vaccaro P, Van Aman M, Miller S, et al. Shortcomings of physical examination and impedance plethysmography in the diagnosis of lower extremity deep venous thrombosis. *Angiology* 1987;38:232.

Valerio D, Hussey JK, Smith FW. Central vein thrombosis associated with i.v. feeding: a prospective study. *J Parenter Enteral Nutr* 1981;5:240.

Van den Brande PM. The efficacy of dextran 40 in preventing early postoperative thrombosis following difficult lower extremity bypass. *J Vasc Surg* 1985;2:643.

Van Ooijen B. Subcutaneous heparin and postoperative wound hematomas: a prospective, double-blind, randomized study. *Arch Surg* 1986;121:937.

Vernet O, Christin L, Schutz Y, et al. Enteral versus parenteral nutrition: comparison of energy metabolism in lean and moderately obese women. *Am J Clin Nutr* 1986;43:194.

Vinton NE, Laidlaw SA, Ament ME, et al. Taurine concentrations in plasma and blood cells of patients undergoing long-term parenteral nutrition. *Am J Clin Nutr* 1986; 44:398.

Virchow R. *Handbuch der speciellen Pathologie and Therapie,* vol II. Erlangen and Stuttgart: F Enke, 1854.

Von Schulthess GK, Augustiny N. Calculation of T2 values versus phase imaging in the distinction between flow and thrombus in MR imaging. *Radiology* 1987;164:549.

Wakefield TW, Greenfield LJ. Diagnostic approaches and surgical treatment of deep venous thrombosis and pulmonary embolism. *Hematol Oncol Clin North Am* 1993;7:1251.

Walsh JJ, Bonnar J, Wright FW. A study of pulmonary embolism and deep leg vein thrombosis after major gynaecological surgery using labelled fibrinogen-phlebography and lung scanning. *J Obstet Gynaecol Br Commonw* 1974;81: 311.

Wardlaw G. The effects of diet and life-style on bone mass in women. *J Am Diet Assoc* 1988;88:17.

Weinstein MC. Estrogen use in post-menopausal women: costs, risks, and benefits. *N Engl J Med* 1980;303:308.

Weiss NS, Szekely DR, Austin DF. Increasing incidence of endometrial cancer in the United States. *N Engl J Med* 1976;294:1259.

Welch GW, McKeel DW, Silverstein P, et al. The role of the catheter composition in the development of thrombophlebitis. *Surg Gynecol Obstet* 1974;138:421.

Wells PS, Byill-Edwards P, Stevens P, et al. A novel and rapid whole-blood assay for D-dimer in patients with clinically suspected deep vein thrombosis. *Circulation* 1995; 91:2184.

Wheeler HB, Anderson FA Jr. Diagnostic methods for deep vein thrombosis. *Haemostasis* 1995;25:6.

Willatts SM. Nutrition. *Br J Anaesthesiol* 1986;58:201.

Williams TJ, Julian CG. Tidal drainage in the postoperative bladder. *Am J Obstet Gynecol* 1962;83:1313.

Wilson JE. Diagnostic methods for deep venous thrombosis. (editorial) *Arch Intern Med* 1980;140:893.

Wilson JN, Grow JB, Demony CV, et al. Central venous pressure in optimal blood volume maintenance. *Arch Surg* 1962;85:563.

Wilson PWF, Garrison RJ, Castelli WP. Postmenopausal estrogen use, cigarette smoking, and cardiovascular morbidity in women over 50: the Framingham Study. *N Engl J Med* 1985;313:1038.

Wren B, Garrett D. The effect of low-dose piperazine oestrogen sulphate and low-dose levonorgestrel on blood lipid levels in postmenopausal women. *Maturitas* 1985;7: 141.

Writing Group for the Women's Health Initiative. Risks and benefits of estrogen plus progestin in healthy postmenopausal women: principal results from the Women's Health Initiative randomized controlled trial. *JAMA* 2002;288:321–333.

Wu JJ, MacFall JR, Sostman HD, et al. Clot-blood contrast in fast gradient-echo magnetic resonance imaging. *Invest Radiol* 1993;28:586.

Yoda Y, Abe T. Fibrinopeptide A (FPA) level and fibrinogen kinetics in patients with malignant disease. *Thromb Haemost* 1981;46:706.

Young GP, Thomas RJS, Bourne DWF, et al. Parenteral nutrition. *Med J Aust* 1985;143:597.

Zacharski LR, Rickles FR, Henderson WG, et al. Platelets and malignancy: rationale and experimental design for the VA cooperative study of RA-233 in the treatment of cancer. *Am J Clin Oncol* 1982;5:593.

Ziel HK, Finkle WD. Increased risk of endometrial carcinoma among users of conjugated estrogens. *N Engl J Med* 1975;293:1167.

Te Linde's Operative Gynecology, ninth edition, edited by John A. Rock and Howard W. Jones, III. Lippincott Williams & Wilkins, Philadelphia: © 2003.

CHAPTER

8

▼

Water, Electrolyte, and Acid–Base Metabolism

JACK B. BASIL   CYRIL O. SPANN, JR.

Proper management of fluids and electrolytes in the gynecologic surgical patient is of extreme importance. Gynecological surgical patients can differ in age, baseline nutritional status, and in the complexity of medical problems that they possess. The stresses of surgery and the bodies' complex responses to that stress need to be understood to best care for these patients. The tendency to standardize postoperative care for all patients should be avoided.

The human body is about 60% water by weight (Table 8.1). An exchange of approximately 2 liters of fluid per day exists normally. This is a balance between an intake of 1,500 mL orally and 500 mL from foodstuffs, and an output of between 750 and 1,500 mL of urine, 500 mL in insensible losses, and 300 mL in stool. Thus, total body water, body weight, osmolality, and oncotic pressure, are critical concepts if one is to understand water metabolism. Comprehension of renal physiology, electrolytes, and acid–base metabolism is also important. This chapter discusses these concepts in detail.

RENAL PHYSIOLOGY

Blood enters the glomerulus by way of afferent arterioles. The filtration process begins with the filtrate passing into Bowman's space. Filtration depends on hydro-static pressure, which forces the filtrate out of the capillary, and oncotic pressure, which holds the filtrate in. The oncotic pressure in the glomerulus usually is negligible, resulting in net flow into Bowman's space. The filtrate then passes into the proximal tubule, where an isoosmotic solution of sodium bicarbonate, glucose, water, and amino acids is absorbed. The filtrate (urine) en-

TABLE 8.1.
Body Water Compartments in Health

Parameter	Total Body Water	Intra-cellular Water	Extra-cellular Water[a]
Total body water (%)	100	67	33
Body weight (%)	60	40	20
Actual volume in a 60-kg person (L)	36	24	12
Osmolality (mOsm/kg of water)	290	290	290

[a]The intravascular water space is about one-fourth of the extracellular water space. The intravascular volume is substantially larger than the intravascular water space because of the additional space occupied by blood cell and plasma proteins. The intravascular volume (blood volume) is about 7% of body weight or slightly more than 4 L in a 60-kg person.

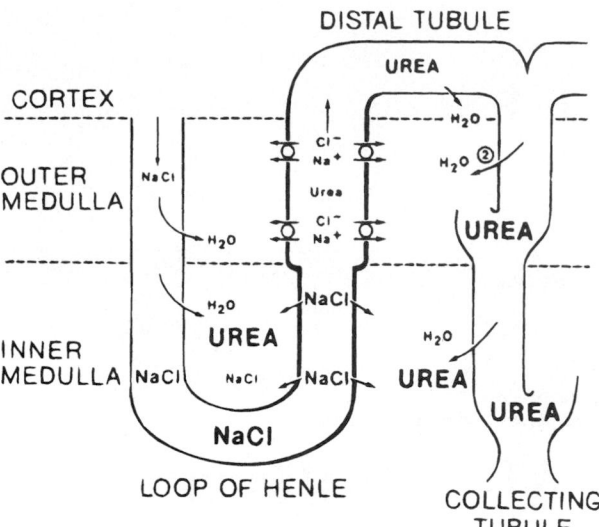

FIGURE 8.1. Passive model of the concentrating mechanism in the inner medulla. Arrows indicate movements of water (H_2O), sodium chloride (NaCl), and urea between the tubule and the interstitium. In the vasa recta, there is perfect exchange between the two limbs. (From: Jamison RL, Buerkert J. The urinary concentrating mechanism. *N Engl J Med* 1976;295: 1059, with permission.)

ters the descending portion of the loop of Henle, where it becomes hyperosmotic secondary to absorption of water into the interstitium. As urine flows up the ascending limb, sodium and chloride are absorbed, making the urine more dilute. Urine then enters the distal convoluted tubule, where active absorption of sodium occurs with exchange of potassium. Under the control of antidiuretic hormone (ADH), water is absorbed from the urine (in the collecting tubule and duct) into the interstitium, causing concentration of urine. Hydrogen ions secreted from tubular cells into the lumens of the tubules help maintain pH balance. Carbonic anhydrase in the renal tubular cells causes the transformation of water and carbon dioxide to bicarbonate and free hydrogen ion (Fig. 8.1). In acidotic states, bicarbonate is reabsorbed into the bloodstream and hydrogen ions are excreted into the tubular lumen. In alkalotic states, the opposite occurs.

OSMOTIC FORCES (OSMOLALITY AND OSMOTIC PRESSURE)

If a solute is added to pure water, then the presence of the second molecular species interferes with the normal activity of water molecules. As a result, water diffuses more slowly through the solution, and the solution has a higher boiling point and lower freezing point. These effects of solute on the colligative properties of water are related principally to the number of molecules present per unit volume rather than to the specific kind of molecule or the total weight of solute present. The determination of osmolality is a measure of the number of

molecules in the solution that is effective in reducing the concentration and, therefore, the chemical properties of water. The slower rate of diffusion of water caused by the solute accounts for the fact that water diffuses from zones of low osmolality (high water concentration) to zones of high osmolality (low water concentration). The hydrostatic pressure that must be applied to the zone of high osmolality to oppose exactly osmotic pressure is equal to the osmotic pressure between the zones of high and low osmolality. The effect of solute concentration on the freezing point vapor pressure of water is the basis for the clinical measurement of osmolality in body fluids.

The osmolality of normal extracellular fluid (ECF) is determined almost entirely by sodium and its accompanying anions. Under certain conditions, other substances (e.g., glucose, mannitol, alcohol, urea) can accumulate and contribute highly to plasma osmolality. Increased blood levels of glucose can artificially lower the serum concentration of serum sodium and thus serum osmolality. Serum sodium is lowered by 1.6 mEq/L for every increase in serum glucose of 100 mg/dL. The contribution of each of these solutes to plasma osmolality can be directly determined in the clinical laboratory by measuring freezing point depression or by calculation. Calculation of plasma osmolality (P_{osm}) from the known concentration of solutes is as follows:

$$P_{osm} = 2 \times [Na]\ mEq/L + glucose\ mmol/L$$
$$+\ urea\ mmol/L$$
$$+\ osmolar\ concentration\ of\ other\ solutes$$

For normal plasma,

$$P_{osm} = 2 \times 140\ mEq/L$$
$$+ \frac{(900\ mg\ glucose/L)}{(180\ mg\ glucose/mOsm)}$$
$$+ \frac{(140\ mg\ urea\ nitrogen/L)}{(28\ mg\ urea\ nitrogen/mOsm)}$$
$$+\ other\ solutes\ (negligible\ in\ normal\ plasma)$$
$$=\ 290\ mOsm/L$$

Most laboratories use different units, and the formula can be shortened to:

$$P_{osm} = 2 \times Na^+\ (mEq/L)$$
$$+ \frac{glucose\ (mg/dL)}{18} + \frac{BUN\ (mg/dL)}{2.8} = mOsm/L$$

The osmolalities of intracellular fluid (ICF) and ECF are equal because cell walls (except for the collecting duct of the kidney) are always freely permeable to water. Potassium is the major intracellular cation and is found in concentrations of about 150 mEq/L of cell water. Thus, potassium and its accompanying anions—principally phosphate and protein—account for almost all of the osmolality of ICF. In health, Na^+ is excluded from cells and K^+ is maintained in cells in most cases because of the cellular Na^+-K^+ pump.

ONCOTIC FORCES (ONCOTIC PRESSURE AND COLLOID OSMOTIC PRESSURE)

Just as crystalloids in solution, such as Na^+, Cl^-, and urea, reduce the concentration of water, so do colloids, such as albumin and globulins. In biologic solutions, however, the contribution of proteins in lowering the effective concentration of water is far less than that of crystalloids, because there are far fewer protein molecules than crystalloid molecules. One gram of albumin (molecular weight [MW] 68,000) theoretically yields 0.015 mOsm ([1,000 mg/68,000 mg mmol/L] $\times$ 1 mOsm mmol/L), whereas 1 g of sodium chloride theoretically yields 34.3 mOsm ([1,000 mg/58.5 mg mmol/L] $\times$ 2 mOsm mmol/L). Thus, gram for gram, sodium chloride is theoretically 2,300 times more effective in increasing the osmolality of a solution than albumin. The oncotic pressure of solutions is expressed in millimeters of mercury (mm Hg) for the same reason that osmotic forces are expressed in units of hydrostatic pressure.

Although oncotic forces are small in relation to osmotic forces, they are important in biologic systems because plasma proteins are selectively retained in the intravascular space. Thus, the effective concentration of water and electrolytes is selectively reduced in the intravascular space compared with the interstitial space. All other things being equal, this results in diffusion of water and electrolytes from the interstitial to the intravascular space. At the capillary level, however, where these oncotic forces are at work, the capillary blood hydrostatic pressure opposes an inward diffusion of water and electrolytes. At the arterial end of the capillary, the effect of capillary blood hydrostatic pressure ($\sim$35 mm Hg) pushing fluid outward is greater than the effect of capillary blood oncotic pressure (equivalent to 25 mm Hg) causing outward diffusion of fluid. Therefore, net outward movement of water and electrolytes occurs. At the venous end of the capillary the capillary blood oncotic pressure (equivalent to $\sim$25 mm Hg) exceeds capillary blood hydrostatic pressure (now $\sim$15 mm Hg); therefore, net inward movement of water and electrolytes occurs. In health, the rate of fluid outflow from the arterial end of the capillary equals the rate of uptake at the venous end of the capillary.

REGULATION OF WATER AND ELECTROLYTE DISTRIBUTION BETWEEN INTRACELLULAR AND EXTRACELLULAR COMPARTMENTS

Osmotic forces regulate the distribution of water between ECF and ICF. Under all steady-state conditions, ECF osmolality equals ICF osmolality. The implications of these principles when water or solute is added to body fluids are discussed in the following sections.

Effect of Addition of Water on Extracellular and Intracellular Fluid Volume and Osmolality

The ingestion of water or the intravenous (i.v.) infusion of water, as 5% solution of dextrose in water (D_5W), results in expansion of all body fluid compartments. Because the osmolality of all body compartments is the same, the water is distributed in the body water compartments in proportion to their size. For example, 1,000 mL of D_5W is infused into a normal 60-kg person with a plasma osmolality of 290 mOsm/L and a serum sodium level of 140 mEq/L. Assuming that no excretion of water occurs, the change in volume of the body water compartments (see Table 8.1) when complete mixing has occurred is as follows. The ICF is increased by about 666 mL, and the ECF is increased by about 333 mL. The intravascular water, which is 25% of the ECF, is increased by only about 83 mL. Plasma osmolality decreases by about 2%. This is sufficient to completely suppress ADH release and cause a maximum water diuresis in a normal person.

Effect of Addition of Solute on Extracellular and Intracellular Fluid Volume and Osmolality

If solutes that penetrate cells slowly (e.g., glucose) are ingested, infused, or actively excluded from cells (e.g., Na^+), water is obligated to remain with these solutes in the ECF so that conditions of osmotic equilibrium between ICF and ECF are met. If these solutes are given in isotonic solutions (i.e., if the osmolality of the solution equals that of body fluids), conditions of osmotic equilibrium are met without shifts of water between ICF and ECF. Thus, the ECF is selectively expanded. On the other hand, if these solutes are ingested without water or given as hypertonic solutions, ECF osmolality rises as these solutes move into the ECF, and water diffuses from ICF to ECF until osmolality in the two compartments is equal. Thus, the ECF expands as the ICF contracts.

Although certain other solutes, such as urea and ethyl alcohol, increase plasma osmolality, they do not affect the steady-state distribution of water between ECF and ICF because these solutes readily penetrate cells and rapidly distribute throughout the body water space. Nevertheless, in non–steady states, such as rapid removal of urea by hemodialysis, transient redistribution of water between ECF and ICF does occur. Such shifts of fluid in brain tissue can lead to significant changes in brain function.

Regulation of Water and Electrolyte Distribution Between the Intravascular and Interstitial Compartments

As discussed, the regulation of fluid and electrolyte transfer at the capillary level is determined by the balance among oncotic forces, hydrostatic forces, and capillary permeability to plasma proteins. These forces can be perturbed in the following ways.

Decrease in plasma albumin
↓
Decrease in plasma oncotic pressure
↓
Capillary outflux exceeds influx
↓
Intravascular volume decreases, interstitial volume increases
↓
Renal sodium and water retention develops
↓
Edema develops when a large interstitial fluid volume is needed to raise interstitial pressure enough to prevent the excessive capillary outflux caused by hypoalbuminemia

FIGURE 8.2. Sequence of events leading to edema formation in hypoalbuminemia.

Hypoalbuminemia results in a fall in plasma oncotic pressure, a rise in the effective concentration of water and electrolytes into the intravascular space, and, all other things being equal, net movement of water and electrolytes into the interstitial space. As a consequence, intravascular volume (IVV) decreases, and the kidney responds by retaining sodium and water in an attempt to restore IVV to normal. If the hypoalbuminemia is sufficiently pronounced (<2.5 g/dL) and the expected renal retention of sodium and water occurs, edema develops before a new equilibrium between outflux and influx of fluid at the capillary level is achieved.

The sequence of events that leads to edema formation is depicted in Figure 8.2. The stimulus to renal sodium and water retention in hypoalbuminemia is a decrease in IVV. In many hypoalbuminemic patients, the retention of sodium and water does not completely restore IVV to normal. In fact, in some patients with marked hypoalbuminemia, massive edema (expansion of the interstitial volume) may be present, yet the IVV may be dangerously low, even to the point of shock.

Marked edema also can develop in the presence of extensive lymphatic obstruction, distal to a venous obstruction, or because of ischemic injury. In these situations, the edema seldom accumulates at such a rate that a serious decrease in IVV becomes clinically evident. Once the edema in such patients is established, the IVV and the renal, endocrine, and hemodynamic factors regulating the IVV usually return to normal. Thus, if diuretic therapy is used to reduce the lymphedema, it can do so, but IVV is decreased below normal, possibly adversely affecting hemodynamics.

REGULATION OF WATER AND SODIUM EXCHANGES WITH THE EXTERNAL ENVIRONMENT

The following discussion focuses on the normal response of the kidney to perturbations of sodium or water balance because an examination of the state of renal sodium and water excretion often is key to the understanding of the pathogenesis of a disorder of fluid and electrolyte balance and usually provides the basis for planning appropriate fluid and electrolyte therapy.

Water Balance

Water balance equals water intake minus water output. Sometimes it is assumed that the measurement of fluid intake and output, as it is performed clinically, is a measure of water balance. The difficulty in assessing the state of water balance based on the measurement of intake and output is indicated in Table 8.2, which lists all the sources of intake and output of water from the body. It is evident from this table that only a few of the important components of water balance are included in the measurement of intake and output. For this reason, some serious disturbances of water balance may not be reflected in the intake and output record. Fortunately, the accurate measurement of water balance does not require that special techniques be used to measure the various sources of intake and output of water from the body. Instead, in most clinical situations, changes in water balance can be assessed simply by following changes in body weight. In the management of a compromised postoperative patient, it is imperative to follow daily weights.

In most clinical situations, changes in water balance occur secondarily to changes in sodium balance. For example, in the pathogenesis of fluid retention in congestive heart failure, the primary event is positive sodium balance because of a decreased renal capacity to excrete sodium. The ingested water is retained as a secondary event to maintain plasma osmolality at some level set by the thirst mechanism. If sodium had not been retained, water would not have been retained. For this reason, the key to preventing fluid retention in such patients is the regulation of sodium intake and output, not water intake.

Less commonly, a change in water balance is the primary event, and changes in sodium balance are secondary to the change in water balance. To recognize such situations, it is necessary to understand the normal renal response to primary changes in water balance. Because the capacity of the kidneys to concentrate and dilute the urine is commonly evaluated by measurement of the specific gravity of urine, it is first necessary to consider the relation between urine osmolality (U_{osm}) and specific gravity.

$$\text{specific gravity} = W_s/WH_2O$$

where: WH_2O = weight of an equal volume of water; and W_s = weight of the solution.

On the average, in normal urine, a linear relation exists between urine osmolality and specific gravity, as shown in Figure 8.3. This relation is disturbed when molecules that have molecular weights much higher than the predominant normal urinary solutes are excreted in large amounts. Thus, in the presence of large numbers of molecules with high molecular weight, specific gravity is no longer a reliable index of osmolality. The normal,

TABLE 8.2.
Components of Water Balance[a]

Sources	Measured Clinically	Comments
Water intake		
Oral intake of liquids, intravenous fluids	Yes	
Water in solid food	Rarely	Water content of solid food in diet of normal adult averages 800–1,000 mL/d
Metabolic water	No	The average adult forms about 200–300 mL of water daily by oxidation of carbohydrate and fat to water and CO_2
Water absorbed by way of respiratory tract during use of gases hydrated by ultrasonic nebulizer	No	Up to 350 mL of water can be absorbed daily at respiratory volumes of 10 L/min
Water output		
Sensible losses		
Urine	Yes	Output variable in health, depends on water intake. Usual range is 600–2,500 mL/d. With renal insufficiency and loss of renal concentrating capacity, urine flow rate depends principally on rate of solute excretion.
Sweat	No	In hot environments, several liters of water can be lost daily.
Stool	Rarely	A normally formed stool contains 80–100 mL of water. Diarrheal stools are principally water: diarrheal losses can be quantitated by collecting and weighing the feces.
Other sensible losses		
Gastric drainage, transudation from skin, etc.	Variable	
Insensible losses		
Evaporation from skin	No	Normally 450 mL is lost daily. In an average-sized adult with fever, losses increase about 10% per degree Fahrenheit.
Evaporation from lung surfaces	No	Normally 450 mL is lost daily. Losses increase by 50% with doubling of ventilatory rate.

[a] Water balance = water intake − water output.

predominant urinary solutes are sodium, potassium, chloride ions, and urea, which have molecular weights of 23, 39, 35, and 60, respectively. The commonly encountered urinary solutes that cause large increases in specific gravity but small increases in urine osmolality are glucose (MW 180), mannitol (MW 181), dextran (MW 20,000 to 40,000), iodine-containing radiographic contrast (MW 600 to 800), and protein (but only with heavy proteinuria). If these substances are absent, urine specific gravity can be relied on to reflect urine osmolality. If these substances are present, urine osmolality must be measured directly to determine the true extent to which the kidneys have concentrated or diluted the urine.

Normal Renal Response to Water Deprivation

The permeability of the collecting duct to water is markedly increased when ADH is released. Thus, as the tubular fluid enters the collecting duct, water diffuses

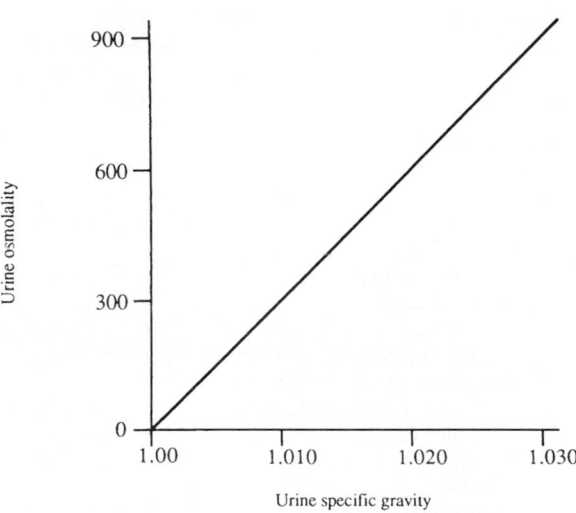

FIGURE 8.3. Approximate relation between specific gravity and osmolality in normal urine.

from the collecting duct into the hypertonic medullary interstitium, resulting in a marked reduction in urine volume and a marked increase in urine osmolality. In health, the osmolality of the medullary interstitium is 900 to 1,200 mOsm/L. Thus, in states of maximum water conservation, the urine osmolality approaches 900 to 1,200 mOsm/L. In such circumstances, urine flow rates approximate 0.5% or less of the normal glomerular filtration rate (GFR), resulting in urine flow rates of about 20 mL/h, or 500 mL/d, when kidneys function normally. Elderly people are unable to concentrate their urine, with maximum osmolalities among the aged often below 800 mOsm/L.

Normal Response to Water Loading

The administration of water or hypotonic solutions results in a reduction in the osmolality of body fluids. A 2% reduction in plasma osmolality (e.g., plasma osmolality from 290 to 284 mOsm/L, serum sodium from 140 to 137 mEq/L) is sufficient to completely suppress ADH secretion. In an average, healthy adult, the ingestion of 1 L of water is more than enough to elicit such a response and to cause the formation of a maximally dilute urine. When ADH secretion is inhibited and renal function is normal, urine specific gravity usually is less than 1.005, urine osmolality is less than 100 mOsm/kg, and urine flow rates approach 15% to 20% of the GFR (i.e., 10 to 15 mL/min, 600 to 900 mL/h). Elderly patients also cannot dilute their urine as well as young persons, with the minimum osmolality being 200 mOsm/L or slightly higher.

Sodium Balance

Sodium balance equals sodium intake minus sodium output. The components of sodium balance are shown in Table 8.3. From this table, it is evident that the kidneys play the central role in the regulation of sodium balance by adjusting sodium excretion to match sodium intake. Unless there are abnormal losses of sodium through the skin or gut, sodium balance can be assessed simply by determining dietary sodium intake and by measuring the urinary excretion of sodium. These measurements usually are not necessary because if the patient has free access to water and an intact thirst mechanism, water is ingested and retained in proportion to the level of sodium retention. Thus, changes in sodium balance are reflected by changes in body weight. Occasionally the measurement of urine sodium excretion is useful. For example, when body weight and serum sodium concentration are stable and there are no abnormal extrarenal sodium losses, the measurement of the 24-hour urinary excretion of sodium accurately reflects sodium intake.

Normal Renal Response to Sodium Restriction and Sodium Loading

When sodium intake is abruptly reduced from a normal level (e.g., 170 mEq/24 h) to a very low level (e.g., 10 mEq/24 h), it takes 3 or 4 days until maximal renal sodium conservation occurs. During this period of adjustment, renal sodium output exceeds intake, and water is lost with sodium in isosmotic proportion from the ECF. One to two liters of ECF usually is lost in the

TABLE 8.3.
Components of Sodium Balance[a]

Sources	Comments
Sodium intake	
Dietary	Normal adults intake of salt is about 10 g NaCl daily ($\sim$170 mEq Na$^+$ and Cl$^-$ or 4 g Na$^+$). Restricted dietary salt intake usually is 2 g sodium (87 mEq NaCl) daily
Parenteral	1,000 mL normal saline (0.9% saline) = 9 g NaCl = 155 mEq Na$^+$ + 155 mEq Cl$^-$
Sodium output	
Urine	Variable. In health, reflects intake, since virtually all ingested NaCl is excreted in urine
Skin	Neglible except with sweating. Sweat contains 50–60 mEq Na$^+$/L and several liters of sweat may be lost each day in hot environments.
Gastrointestinal secretion	
Normally formed stool	Na$^+$ $\sim$1 mEq/24 h
Diarrheal stool	
Secretory (infectious)	Na$^+$ $\sim$130 mEq/L
Fermentative (malabsorption)	Na$^+$ $\sim$50 mEq/L
Vomitus or gastric aspirate	
Normally acid gastric juice	Na$^+$ $\sim$40 mEq/L
Achlorhydria	Na$^+$ $\sim$130 mEq/L
All other secretions (bile, pancreatic juice, small bowel secretions)	Na$^+$ $\sim$130 mEq/L

[a]Sodium balance = sodium intake − sodium output.

change from a normal to a very low sodium intake. Thus, normal people come into balance on a low sodium intake, but the ECF volume then may be regulated at a suboptimal level. This is potentially dangerous because the patient may be vulnerable to the potential hypotensive effects of anesthesia or additional volume losses that can occur during surgery.

The normal renal response to salt loading is analogous to that of salt restriction, in that it takes several days for the renal excretion of sodium to increase in response to the higher level of sodium intake. Thus, when balance is finally achieved, ECF volume is being regulated at an expanded level, which can be undesirable. For example, a patient with underlying heart disease who achieves sodium balance on a high intake of sodium chloride is more vulnerable to the development of congestive heart failure if additional fluids are administered.

CLINICAL ASSESSMENT OF DISORDERS OF WATER AND ELECTROLYTE METABOLISM

Disorders of ECF electrolyte composition may be detected by measurement of the serum electrolyte concentrations. Identification of the process (or processes) behind the disturbance of electrolyte composition and the planning of subsequent therapy are critically dependent on the clinician's ability to accurately assess whether the disturbance in ECF electrolyte composition is associated with volume expansion, volume contraction, or a normal volume.

In the evaluation of a patient's ECF volume status, it must be kept clearly in mind that the critical volume is that portion of the IVV that is effective in determining the filling pressure of the ventricles and, hence, the cardiac output. Hereafter, this theoretic volume is referred to as the *effective IVV*.

In light of this definition, the most effective IVV is that which maintains an optimal cardiac output and thus maximizes tissue perfusion. Although the actual IVV and the effective IVV are the same in many clinical situations and can be expected to change in direct proportion, in a number of important clinical states, the actual IVV is different from the effective IVV. For example, in acute metabolic acidosis, increased venoconstriction can develop, resulting in an abnormal increase in central venous pressure (CVP) and cardiac output. Under this circumstance, the actual IVV could be less than normal, whereas the effective IVV is greater than normal. That is, because of the increase in venous tone, an IVV that is lower than normal can maintain a normal effective IVV.

Acute changes in venous tone induced by drugs (e.g., morphine, furosemide, norepinephrine), changes in acid–base status, and the presence of bacterial endotoxin also can disrupt the normal relation between the actual IVV and the effective IVV.

The most reliable clinical means for assessing the status of the effective IVV is the pulmonary capillary wedge pressure. This measurement is an estimate of the pulmonary capillary pressure, which is a measure of the filling pressure of the left ventricle. Factors that increase pulmonary capillary wedge pressure tend to increase cardiac output by increasing capillary outflux. When effective IVV is considered within these constraints, it becomes clear that under virtually any physiologic or pathophysiologic circumstance, an optimal effective IVV is one that results in a pulmonary capillary wedge pressure that is high enough to promote optimal cardiac output but low enough to prevent pulmonary edema.

Fortunately, in most clinical situations, it is not necessary to resort to measuring pulmonary wedge pressure to assess whether a disturbance of ECF composition is associated with an effective IVV that is abnormally high, abnormally low, or normal. Instead, an accurate assessment of the effective IVV usually can be made by a careful clinical assessment using the criteria listed in Table 8.4. This table lists the bedside and laboratory means to assess volume status according to whether the findings are consistent with an effective IVV that is less than normal or an effective IVV that is nearly normal or expanded.

Also shown in Table 8.4 are the conditions under which the given means for evaluating the IVV must be qualified (i.e., the conditions that may render the meaning of the finding indeterminate with respect to the evaluation of IVV). For example, the relation between an increase in weight and a change in IVV is rendered indeterminate if, at the same time, the patient has developed a third space, as in bowel obstruction. In this instance, the entire weight gain could be caused by the accumulation of fluid outside the IVV. Thus, the finding of weight gain in this setting cannot be used as evidence of an increase in effective IVV.

We suggest that the evaluation of effective IVV, using the criteria in Table 8.4, be approached in the following manner. First, whenever a finding can be significantly qualified, it should not be used in arriving at a final decision. Second, as many independent means as practical should be used to assess the effective IVV to minimize the effect of possible error on the final decision. The greater the number of independent, unqualified findings that agree in favor of a given clinical decision, the more likely it is that the decision is correct. If such a systematic approach to clinical decision making is used, it should be possible to arrive at an accurate evaluation of volume status in most circumstances.

DATABASE FOR ASSESSMENT OF EFFECTIVE INTRAVASCULAR VOLUME

Body Weight

All patients should be weighed on admission to the hospital and then periodically during their hospital stay. In patients undergoing surgery, or in whom problems in fluid and electrolyte balance are anticipated, weight must be measured daily.

TABLE 8.4.
Assessment of Effective Intravascular Volume (IVV)

Suggestive Evidence	Qualifying Conditions[a]
Significantly decreased effective IVV	
History of fluid and electrolyte deprivation or loss (e.g., vomiting, diarrhea)	Difficulty in establishing by history whether the magnitude of loss or deprivation is sufficient to result in negative balance of water and electrolytes
Decrease in body weight below normal not explained by inadequate caloric intake	None
Blood pressure less than usual for patient with orthostatic hypotension	1. Patient receiving methyldopa (Aldomet), prazosin (Minipress), minoxidil (Loniten), or other drugs that interfere with vascular α-receptors 2. Autonomic insufficiency as in diabetics, quadriplegics, and after prolonged bed rest
Elevated serum creatinine associated with concentrated urine ($U_{osm}/P_{osm} > 1.5$), and Na^+ conservation: ($U_{Na} < 20$ mEq/L) or $\%E/F_{Na} < 1\%$	Decreased renal perfusion owing to: (a) severe hepatic failure (hepatorenal syndrome); (b) severe cardiac failure. Acute, high-grade urinary tract obstruction (see text)
Low central venous pressure or pulmonary capillary wedge pressure	See text
Decreased tissue turgor	See text
Hematocrit above normal	Presence of conditions that may cause erthrocytosis
Nearly normal or expanded effective IVV (i.e., absence of significant intravascular volume depletion)	
Hypertension with patient in sitting or standing position and no orthostatic fall in blood pressure	None
Presence of cardiac failure: Left ventricular failure: audible third heart sound or pulmonary edema	Patients with markedly reduced cardiac output and very large left ventricles may have decreased effective IVV despite an audible third heart sound
Right ventricular failure: peripheral edema with increased venous pressure (neck vein distention, increased intravenous pressure)	Right ventricular failure but normal left ventricular function (see text)
Increase in weight above normal not explained by increased caloric intake	1. Significant hypoalbuminemia 2. Development of third spaces (e.g., ascites, bowel obstruction)
Increased central venous pressure	See text
Increased pulmonary capillary wedge pressure	See text
Edema, ascites, or pleural effusion	See text
Hematocrit less than normal	Presence of conditions that can cause loss, destruction, or decreased production of red blood cells

$\%E/F_{Na}$, percentage of excretion of filtered sodium (see text).

[a] Qualifying conditions are circumstances that can render the meaning of the finding indeterminate with respect to the evaluation of the effective IVV.

Alterations in body weight are the result of changes in body water content plus solid tissue content (fat, protein, bone). Gains or losses of solid tissue are almost always related to changes in caloric intake and seldom exceed 0.25 kg/24 h. For example, a patient who takes no calories for 24 hours is forced to consume her endogenous stores of fat and protein to meet the energy requirements for continued life. The complete oxidation of fat yields 9 cal/g, and protein yields 4 cal/g. It can be readily calculated that the complete oxidation of 0.25 kg of solid tissue (in starvation, a mixture of about 87% fat, 13% protein) yields enough calories to meet basal daily energy needs. Thus changes in weight exceeding 0.25 kg/24 h are almost always attributable to changes in water balance. Although the relation between body weight and effective IVV can be variable, usually the relation between changes in body weight and IVV can be correctly assessed by the application of the two guidelines. The first is that a decrease in body weight below normal (for the patient), and not explained on the basis of inadequate caloric intake, can be assumed to be accompanied by a decrease in IVV. The second is that an increase in body weight above normal not explained by increased nutrition can be assumed to be accompanied by an increase in IVV except when the weight gain develops in association with the following conditions.

- Significant hypoalbuminemia: serum albumin less than 2.5 g dL
- Venous obstruction or congestion

- Development of third spaces (e.g., obstructed or ischemic bowel)

Under these three general conditions, an increase in body weight may not reflect an increase in the effective IVV.

Renal Function

Creatinine, a byproduct of muscle energy metabolism, is produced at a constant rate that is related to muscle mass. Normal men produce 20 to 25 mg/kg (ideal body weight)/24 h, and women produce 15 to 20 mg/kg (ideal body weight)/24 h. Nearly all of the creatinine produced is excreted by glomerular filtration. Therefore, changes in the concentration of serum creatinine reflect changes in the GFR, and the clearance of creatinine (C_{cr}) is an index of the GFR.

$$C_{cr} = U_{cr}V/S_{cr} \sim GFR$$

where: S_{cr} = serum creatinine; U_{cr} = urinary creatinine concentration; V = urine volume per unit time.

Thus, by rearranging this equation:

$$S_{cr} \sim U_{cr}V/GFR$$

Normally, as muscle mass (which is proportional to $U_{cr}V$) increases, the GFR increases proportionately less. Therefore, on the average, children have lower serum creatinine values than do adults, and large adults have higher serum creatinine levels than do small adults. Because of these considerations, a single range of serum creatinine values cannot be applied to everyone. The suggested normal ranges of serum creatinine for adults, according to ideal body weight, are shown in Table 8.5. Creatinine clearance for men can be estimated, using the formula derived by Cockcroft and Gault, from the patient's age, body weight, and serum creatinine level as follows.

$$C_{cr} \text{ in mL/min} = \frac{[(140 - \text{age}) \times \text{weight in kg}]}{[72 \times S_{cr} \text{ in mg/dL}]}$$

This result multiplied by 0.85 provides a better estimate for women because of their relatively smaller muscle mass. Azotemia is arbitrarily defined here as a serum creatinine level greater than the upper limit of normal for body size, as shown in Table 8.5. The blood urea nitrogen level is influenced by dietary protein intake, tissue metabolism, and urine flow rate, in addition to GFR, and should not be relied on to assess changes in GFR.

The following guidelines are suggested for the evaluation of the IVV in light of the state of renal function. The azotemia can be assumed to result from decreased renal perfusion if the serum creatinine level is elevated, the urine is concentrated (U_{osm}:P_{osm} ratio greater than 1.5; specific gravity higher than 1.015), and renal sodium conservation is present (U_{Na} level less than 20 mEq/L) on a random and untimed urine sample. The

TABLE 8.5.
Normal Relation Between Body Size and Serum Creatinine Level

Ideal Body Weight	Expected Range of Serum Creatinine Level[a] (mg/dL)
<55 kg (120 lb)	0.6–1.0
55–80 kg (120–175 lb)	0.8–1.2
>80 kg (175 lb)	1.0–1.4

[a]Autoanalyzer picric acid method.

fractional excretion of sodium is based on serum and random urine concentrations of sodium and creatinine. If below 1%, azotemia can be attributed to decreased IVV, unless the patient has severe liver or cardiac disease.

$$\%E/F_{Na} = \text{percentage of fractional excretion}$$
$$\text{of filtered sodium}$$
$$(\text{excreted Na}^+) \times 100/(\text{filtered Na}^+)$$
$$\frac{(U_{Na} \times S_{cr} \times 100)}{(S_{Na} \times U_{cr})}$$

where: S_{cr} = serum creatinine concentration in mg/dL; S_{Na} = serum Na^+ concentration in mEq/L; U_{cr} = urine creatinine concentration in mg/dL; and U_{Na} = urinary Na^+ concentration in mEq/L.

If severe cardiac failure and severe liver failure (hepatorenal syndrome) can be excluded, the decreased renal perfusion can be assumed to be caused by a decreased effective IVV.

Edema, Ascites, and Pleural Effusion

Effective IVV is increased when edema, pleural effusion, or ascites occurs in the setting of congestive heart failure (CHF). Increased effective IVV cannot be assumed in the presence of edema, ascites, or pleural effusion if there is significant hypoalbuminemia or venous obstruction, or if the accumulation of fluid is in a relatively small area of capillary injury (e.g., pleural effusion caused by pulmonary infarction).

Tissue Turgor

Tissue turgor is a function of the elasticity of the solid components of tissue and the degree of distention of the tissues by interstitial fluid. If tissue is depleted of interstitial fluid, it becomes less elastic (i.e., it less readily returns to its original shape after being deformed). Skin turgor is best assessed on the forehead and anterior chest. In patients less than 50 years of age, the turgor of the dorsum of the hand also can be used. In older patients, the elasticity of the solid components of tissue is decreased, and the turgor of the skin becomes unreliable in interpreting changes in interstitial volume.

Central Venous Pressure

The measurement of CVP is a relatively simple but useful means for monitoring cardiac function and cardiovascular status. For the valid measurement of CVP, the catheter must be placed in the large intrathoracic veins near the right atrium (as assessed by chest radiograph) and the catheter must be patent (as assessed by the cyclic variation of CVP with ventilatory movements: decreased CVP during inspiration, increased CVP during expiration).

In normal adults, CVP is about 5 to 12 cm H_2O. CVPs below 3 cm H_2O are commonly seen in children and young adults who have no evidence of a decreased effective IVV. In older adults and elderly persons, CVP of less than 3 cm H_2O can be assumed to reflect a significant decrease in effective IVV.

CVP is an index of the filling pressure of the right atrium, which, in turn, is an index of the filling pressure of the right ventricle. In uncomplicated circumstances, expansion of the IVV results in increased CVP, whereas contraction of the IVV results in decreased CVP. CVP cannot be used to assess the adequacy of left ventricular function in patients in whom left ventricular function may be impaired relative to right ventricular function. CVP also is unreliable when lung disease is present, because it is commonly falsely elevated. In such patients, left ventricular function can be monitored by observing for signs and symptoms of left ventricular failure (dyspnea, development of an audible third heart sound, or pulmonary edema), or by direct measurement of pulmonary capillary wedge pressure. Under normal circumstances, the pulmonary capillary wedge pressure is about equal to the CVP plus 6 mm Hg.

Pulmonary Capillary Wedge Pressure

Technical refinements of the Swan-Ganz catheter make it possible to measure pulmonary artery systolic and diastolic pressure, CVP, pulmonary wedge pressure, and cardiac output using the thermodilution technique with the same catheter. This permits a definitive assessment of the volume status of the patient, because it can be determined whether the cardiac output is appropriate for a given pulmonary wedge pressure. Specific guidelines for the interpretation of the relation between pulmonary wedge pressure and cardiac output are discussed in the following sections.

Patients with Normal Volume Status

Pulmonary wedge pressure can be expected to be between 8 and 12 mm Hg in a patient with a normal cardiopulmonary system and a normal effective IVV. Cardiac output is normal. Pulmonary wedge pressure can be less than 8 mm Hg without indicating volume contraction; in this circumstance, the cardiac output is normal despite the unusually low pulmonary wedge pressure.

Patients Who Are Volume Contracted

Patients who have a normal cardiopulmonary system but who are significantly volume depleted usually have a pulmonary wedge pressure below 8 mm Hg and their cardiac output is less than normal. In patients with chronic pulmonary hypertension (e.g., those with chronic left ventricular failure), a higher than normal pulmonary wedge pressure is needed to drive a satisfactory cardiac output. Thus, in such patients, pulmonary wedge pressure can be above the normal range but be inappropriately low for the patient. This situation can be identified by showing that: (a) cardiac output is less than normal, despite the elevated pulmonary wedge pressure; (b) volume infusion causes an increase in cardiac output toward a more favorable range; and (c) despite further increase in pulmonary wedge pressure with volume expansion, pulmonary function does not deteriorate. (PaO_2 does not decrease, $PaCO_2$ does not increase, and pulmonary compliance does not worsen.)

Patients Who Are Volume Expanded

In patients with a normal cardiopulmonary system, pulmonary wedge pressure usually is above 18 mm Hg when volume expansion is substantial. Cardiac output is above normal. If cardiac function is impaired, cardiac output will be inappropriately low for the level of pulmonary wedge pressure.

When a given pulmonary wedge pressure is being interpreted, the serum albumin level also should be taken into consideration, because this opposes the effect of capillary hydrostatic pressure to cause migration of fluid from the capillary lumen to the interstitial space. Thus, at any given elevated pulmonary wedge pressure, pulmonary edema develops more rapidly in a patient who is hypoalbuminemic than in one who has a normal serum albumin concentration. In some patients, it is not possible to obtain a reliable pulmonary wedge pressure. In most of these patients, the pulmonary artery diastolic pressure is a good estimate of the pulmonary wedge pressure. If pulmonary hypertension is present, then pulmonary vascular resistance is increased; thus, pulmonary artery diastolic pressure may not be a good index of the pulmonary wedge pressure. In such patients, it is important to be able to obtain a wedge pressure. Finally, in patients who are being ventilated with high levels of positive end-expiratory pressure, pulmonary wedge pressure may become an unreliable index of left atrial filling pressure because the high intrapulmonary pressures may cause obstruction of the catheter orifice. Patients must be briefly taken off the ventilator for accurate measurements. Other circumstances in which pulmonary artery wedge pressure measurements may be inaccurate include the presence of mitral stenosis or pulmonary venous obstruction.

Blood Pressure

The following guidelines are suggested for the evaluation of the effective IVV from measurement of blood pressure.

1. A nearly normal or expanded effective IVV can be assumed in patients with hypertension that is demonstrated in the sitting or standing position.
2. Effective IVV may be decreased in patients who previously were hypertensive but who have become normotensive.

3. Effective IVV may be decreased in patients who develop orthostatic hypotension (a drop in systolic pressure greater than 10 mm Hg in changing from the supine to the sitting or standing position).

Orthostatic hypotension also can be present, in the absence of volume contraction, as a result of prolonged bed rest, during the use of such antihypertensive agents as methyldopa (Aldomet) or of vasodilators (Prazosin, Minoxidil). If the pulse rate does not rise as blood pressure falls when a patient stands, autonomic neuropathy should be considered as a cause of postural hypotension.

Systemic Vascular Resistance

Other measurements of hemodynamic importance derived from Swan-Ganz readings include calculations of resistance across the pulmonary and systemic vascular beds. The calculations are as follows:

$$PVR = \frac{P_{\overline{PA}} \ P_{\overline{PAW}} \times 80}{\dot{Q}T}$$

$$SVR = \frac{PSA - PRA \times 80}{\dot{Q}T}$$

where: $P_{\overline{PA}}$ = mean right atrial pressure; $P_{\overline{PAW}}$ = mean pulmonary artery wedge pressure; PVR = pulmonary vascular resistance; P_{SA} = mean systolic arterial pressure; $\dot{Q}T$ = cardiac output in liters per minute; and SVR = systemic vascular resistance.

Normal values are 50 to 150 dyne-s/cm for pulmonary vascular resistance and 800 to 1,200 dyne-s/cm for systemic vascular resistance. Pulmonary vascular resistance is elevated in hypovolemic shock, cardiogenic shock, pulmonary embolism, or airway obstruction; it is diminished in septic shock. Systemic vascular resistance is elevated in hypovolemic shock, cardiogenic shock, pulmonary embolism, and sometimes in right ventricular infarct and cardiac tamponade; it is decreased in end-stage liver disease and septic shock.

CLINICAL ASSESSMENT OF DISORDERS OF EXTRACELLULAR FLUID COMPOSITION

Hyponatremia

The schema for the evaluation of a hyponatremic patient depends on the assessment of volume status. That is, it must first be determined whether the patient's hyponatremia is associated with an effective IVV that is decreased, normal, or increased. Once this is decided on the basis of the assessment of IVV, a further separation, based only on the state of renal sodium and water excretion, is made. Each of the final categories contains relatively few diagnostic possibilities, and the presence or absence of each of these conditions in a given patient usually can be readily determined. The scheme for the evaluation of a hypernatremic patient is analogous, except that it depends on the assessment of the state of renal water excretion.

Clinical Assessment

In the discussion that follows, only patients with true hyponatremia are considered (i.e., hyponatremia in which serum osmolality is decreased in proportion to the reduction in serum sodium concentration, after appropriate correction for any elevation in the plasma urea nitrogen). By making this distinction, hyponatremia caused by accumulation of ECF solutes such as glucose or mannitol can be excluded. In this type of hyponatremia, the decreased concentration of ECF sodium is the result of the shift of water from cells to the ECF in response to the osmotic gradient caused by the accumulation of the solute. As a consequence, the hyponatremia is associated with an increased plasma osmolality. These patients also can be readily identified either by the presence of hyperglycemia sufficient to explain the decrease in serum sodium concentration or by a history of administration of large amounts of mannitol (>100 g in adults) usually in the presence of a decreased capacity to excrete mannitol (decreased GFR).

Also to be excluded are patients with spurious hyponatremia that results from the abnormal accumulation of plasma lipids or proteins. In such circumstances, the concentration of sodium in plasma water is normal; however, the concentration of sodium expressed per liter of whole plasma is reduced because an abnormally large volume of whole plasma is occupied by the lipids or proteins, which do not contain plasma water and electrolytes. Thus, when aliquots of hyperlipemic or hyperproteinemic plasma are analyzed, a lower amount of sodium is determined to be present in a given volume of whole plasma. Plasma osmolality, however, is normal because lipids and proteins do not contribute importantly to plasma osmolality (see section on osmotic forces). Patients with spurious hyponatremia can be readily identified by the presence of markedly elevated total serum protein levels (e.g., multiple myeloma) or grossly lipemic serum. The distinction can be readily made if lipemic serum is subjected to centrifugation and the lipoprotein layer is removed before evaluation, if flame photometry is being used for measurement of serum Na^+. Spurious hyponatremia is no longer a consideration in most laboratories, because serum Na^+ concentration is determined by ion-specific electrodes and increased levels are not affected by lipemic serum. Symptoms of hyponatremia include increased tendon reflexes, lethargy, mental confusion, and muscle twitching, which are followed by convulsions, coma, and possibly death if levels fall beneath 115 mEq/L.

Hyponatremia and Volume Depletion Associated with Renal Sodium Wasting

The normal renal response to volume depletion and hyponatremia is the virtual elimination of sodium from the urine (Fig. 8.4; see section on Sodium Balance). Thus, the presence of an excessive amount of urinary sodium under these conditions indicates that renal sodium loss is

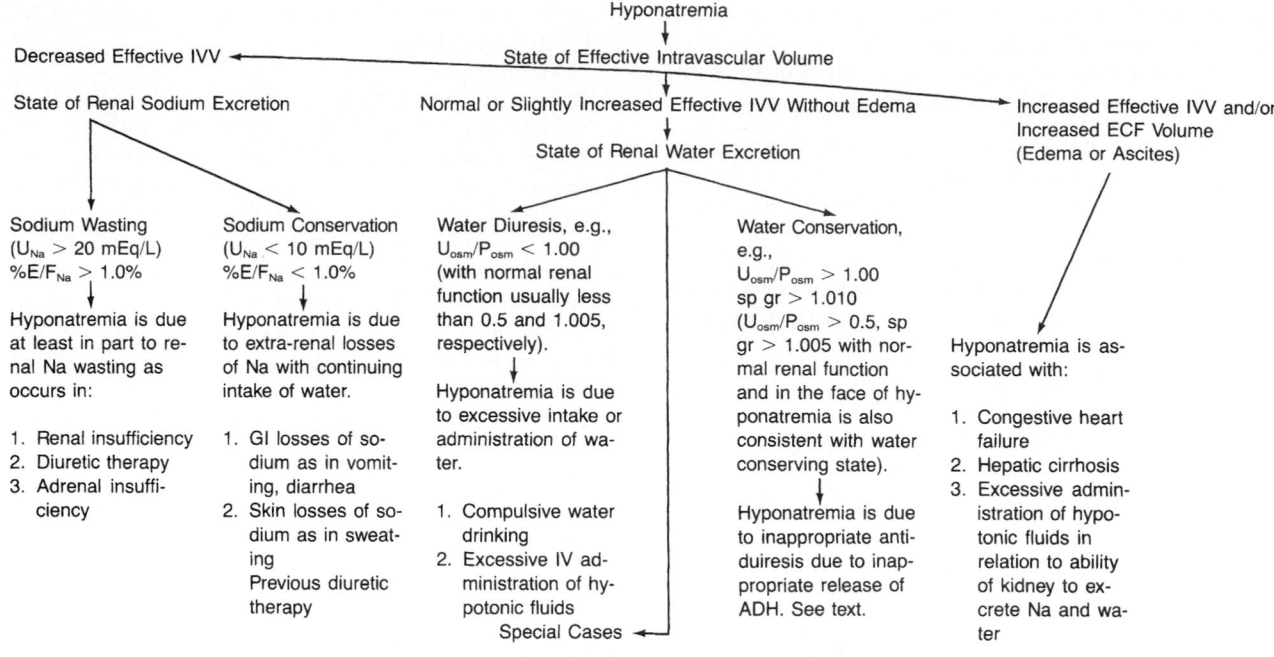

FIGURE 8.4. Approach to the assessment of a hyponatremic patient. This approach considers only patients with true hyponatremia (i.e., in nonazotemic patients, serum osmolality is reduced in proportion to the decrease in serum sodium). Thus, patients are excluded who have lowered concentrations of serum sodium because of hyperlipidemia, hyperproteinemia, or the abnormal accumulations of solutes in the extracellular fluid, such as glucose or mannitol. ADH, antidiuretic hormone; $\%E/F_{Na}$, fractional excretion of sodium; GI, gastrointestinal; IVV, intravascular volume.

the cause or a major contributing factor to the state of sodium depletion. A spot urine sodium concentration greater than 40 mEq/L, a $\%E/F_{Na}$ over 1%, or a urinary sodium excretion rate greater than intake indicates such renal sodium wasting. The conditions discussed in the following sections are associated with hyponatremia, IVV depletion, and renal sodium wasting.

CHRONIC RENAL DISEASE. All types of renal disease can be associated with renal salt wasting. In adults with such a disorder, the serum creatinine level is virtually always above 2 mg and usually much higher before a significant salt leak develops. These azotemic patients usually require 85 to 170 mEq of sodium daily (5 to 10 g of sodium chloride) to maintain salt balance at a normal effective IVV. Thus, if sodium intake is decreased in azotemic patients by anorexia or vomiting, or if additional sodium losses occur (e.g., diarrhea or diuretic therapy), the inability of the diseased kidneys to conserve sodium and water normally may rapidly lead to the development of significant sodium and water deficits. Water intake usually continues; therefore, sodium balance is

more adversely affected than water balance. As a consequence, the patient becomes volume contracted with hyponatremia. With the onset of congestive heart failure or the nephrotic syndrome, the salt leak of chronic renal failure usually disappears, and salt intake must be restricted.

DIURETIC THERAPY. The diuretics include thiazide agents or loop diuretics such as furosemide, bumetanide, and ethacrynic acid. Diuretics induce a renal salt-wasting state, and if the urinary output of sodium exceeds intake, sodium depletion ensues. Rarely, diuretics cause hyponatremia without evidence of volume depletion if severe potassium depletion has resulted from their use (see Fig. 8.4).

ADRENAL INSUFFICIENCY (ADDISON'S DISEASE). Destruction of the adrenal gland or sudden withdrawal of chronic, daily glucocorticoid therapy results in inadequate adrenal function. The lack of mineralocorticoid causes wasting of renal salt but retention of renal potassium, and leads to sodium depletion. The lack of glucocorticoid results in a decreased capacity to excrete a water load and leads to hyponatremia but not to volume depletion or hyperkalemia.

Hyponatremia and Volume Depletion Associated with Renal Sodium Conservation

A spot urine sodium concentration of less than 20 mEq/L or a %E/F_{Na} below 1% in a hyponatremic, volume-contracted patient is evidence of normal renal sodium conservation and indicates that the cause of the sodium depletion is nonrenal in origin or that it occurred during previous diuretic therapy. The fact that the serum sodium concentration is lower than normal indicates that water balance is less negative than sodium balance. The conditions discussed in the following sections can result in volume depletion and hyponatremia as a result of extrarenal losses of sodium.

GASTROINTESTINAL LOSSES. If losses of fluid from the upper gastrointestinal tract (e.g., vomiting, gastric aspiration) cause the hyponatremia, and if the gastric juice is normally acid, metabolic alkalosis is present. If diarrheal losses cause the hyponatremia, metabolic acidosis may be present. In patients with gastric achlorhydria, upper gastrointestinal losses also can lead to metabolic acidosis.

LOSSES OF SODIUM FROM THE SKIN. Sweat contains about 50 mEq/L of sodium and is a hypotonic fluid. If sweat losses are not replaced, then hypernatremia can develop. In most situations, the water losses from the skin are replaced more adequately than the sodium losses. Thus, most patients with significant sodium losses due to sweating become hyponatremic. Skin losses of fluid and electrolytes also can occur after burns or other skin injuries. These are isotonic losses of sodium and lead to hyponatremia if the water losses are more adequately replaced than the sodium losses.

LOSSES OF SODIUM FROM PRIOR DIURETIC THERAPY. The natriuretic action of most diuretics lasts less than 24 hours. Hyponatremia is made worse if water intake is excessive.

Hyponatremia and Normal Volume Status Associated with Water Diuresis

In a patient with normal renal function who has become hyponatremic as a result of the administration or ingestion of excessive amounts of water, intravascular and ECF volume are normal to slightly expanded, and high rates of urine flow in association with maximally, or nearly maximally, dilute urine can be expected (see section on water balance). In a patient with preexisting renal functional impairment, water loading also increases urine flow rate and dilution of the urine; however, maximally dilute urine cannot be formed. Hyponatremia secondary to water loading may occur in compulsive water drinkers, who usually are severely neurotic or psychotic, or after excessive i.v. administration of hypotonic fluids. Many of these patients also have high levels of ADH for various reasons (e.g., drugs, psychosis). Without this elevation of ADH, presuming normal renal function, con-

sumption of 20 L of water a day would be necessary for development of frank hyponatremia.

Hyponatremia and Normal to Slightly Elevated Volume Status Associated with Water Conservation

As discussed, it is appropriate to observe a brisk water diuresis in a patient with normal renal function who is hyponatremic and has evidence of normal or slightly elevated IVV without edema. When high flow rates of hypotonic urine are not observed, the patient is exhibiting an inappropriate antidiuresis. This may result from the inappropriate release of ADH, although other mechanisms also can be involved (e.g., decreased renal blood flow, certain drugs). Another characteristic of such patients is that administered sodium is promptly excreted in the urine, perhaps because of the effect of atrial natriuretic factors. On the other hand, when sodium intake is curtailed, renal sodium conservation is observed. These patients also exhibit normal adrenal and renal function, and are not edematous. The syndrome of inappropriate antidiuresis has been associated with various clinical states, including malignant tumors (e.g., in the lung or pancreas), central nervous system (CNS) disorders (e.g., head trauma, meningitis), infections (e.g., tuberculosis, bacterial pneumonias), the postoperative state, hypopituitarism, and myxedema, as well as with many drugs (Table 8.6). Infusion of oxytocin to induce uterine contraction also can cause hyponatremia because of the antidiuretic effects of oxytocin.

Within the category of hyponatremia associated with normal IVV are three special categories. The feature that sets these apart is that patients may exhibit evidence of water conservation when water is withdrawn or an appropriate or nearly appropriate water diuresis when water is administered. That is, it appears that osmoregulation has been reset to "defend" a lowered plasma osmolality. The first special category includes patients who have an unusual response to diuretic therapy, characterized by hyponatremia, severe potassium depletion,

TABLE 8.6.
Antidiuretic Drugs

Sulfonylureas (chlorpropamide, tolbutamide)
Cytotoxic agents (vincristine, cyclophosphamide)
Nicotine
Morphine
Barbiturates
Carbamazepine
Psychotropics (tricyclics)
Clofibrate
Isoproterenol
Nonsteroidals
Salicylates
Acetaminophen
Vasopressin
Oxytocin

and metabolic alkalosis. Despite the hyponatremia and normal IVV, exchangeable sodium is nearly normal, suggesting intracellular movement of sodium. Potassium replacement must be accomplished before specific treatment of hyponatremia. The second category involves patients with an unusual manifestation of a chronic illness, such as pulmonary tuberculosis, that resets the osmostat. The third category includes patients with sodium depletion resulting from any cause in whom the decrease in effective IVV is minimized by excessive water intake and retention. This effect of excessive water intake can occur in any of the causes of sodium depletion.

Hyponatremia Associated with Increased Effective Intravascular Volume or Increased Extracellular Fluid Volume (Edema or Ascites)

CONGESTIVE HEART FAILURE. When hyponatremia develops spontaneously in the course of chronic congestive heart failure (i.e., is not the result of excessive water administration or diuretic therapy), it usually is indicative of severe cardiac insufficiency and has a poor prognosis. The cause of the hyponatremia in such patients has been ascribed to a decreased capacity to increase renal free water clearance perhaps because of: (a) increased fractional reabsorption of glomerular filtrate proximal to the renal diluting sites of the distal nephron; and (b) an elevated ADH level.

CIRRHOSIS OF THE LIVER. Patients with cirrhosis and ascites have a decreased capacity to excrete a water load, possibly because of the same mechanisms at work in patients with congestive heart failure.

EXCESSIVE ADMINISTRATION OF HYPOTONIC FLUIDS. This usually is an iatrogenic situation and must be especially guarded against in postoperative patients whose ADH levels are elevated because of stress, pain, hypovolemia, or drugs, as well as in elderly patients who are unable to maximally dilute their urine.

Hypernatremia

All patients with hypernatremia are volume contracted except those in whom the disorder develops as a result of excessive administration of hypertonic saline or sodium bicarbonate and the rare patients with essential hypernatremia (Fig. 8.5). The following discussion considers only the first group of patients; the latter section on treatment discusses all forms of hypernatremia. Patients with hypernatremia usually have CNS deficits, and they may also have confusion and neuroseizures. Autopsy findings often reveal hemorrhages or thromboses of brain tissue.

Hypernatremia Associated with Formation of Concentrated Urine

The normal renal response to decreased intake of water or increased extrarenal losses of water is the formation of maximally concentrated urine (see section on water balance). In most clinical situations in which hypernatremia is the result of water depletion, the expected renal response is a $U_{osm}:P_{osm}$ ratio greater than 1.5 and a specific gravity above 1.015. Thus, the finding of hypernatremia with evidence of renal conservation of water indicates that the hypernatremia is caused by excessive nonrenal losses of water or solute diuresis.

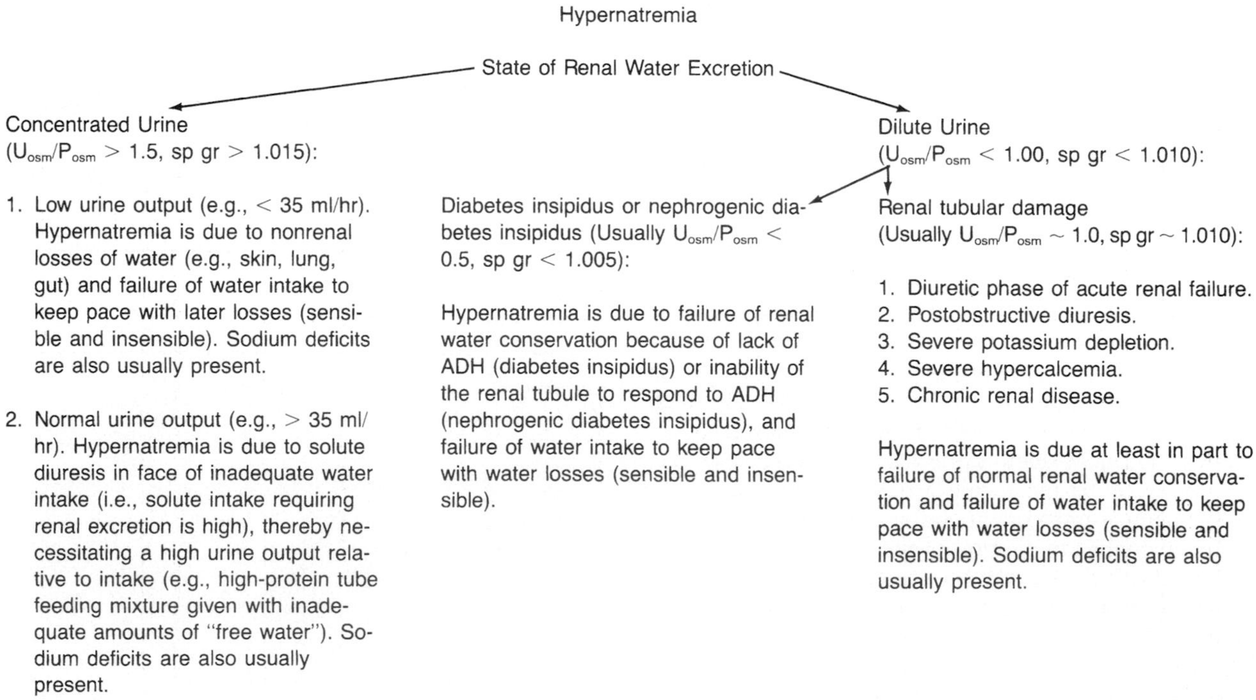

Hypernatremia

State of Renal Water Excretion

Concentrated Urine
($U_{osm}/P_{osm} > 1.5$, sp gr > 1.015):

1. Low urine output (e.g., < 35 ml/hr). Hypernatremia is due to nonrenal losses of water (e.g., skin, lung, gut) and failure of water intake to keep pace with later losses (sensible and insensible). Sodium deficits are also usually present.

2. Normal urine output (e.g., > 35 ml/hr). Hypernatremia is due to solute diuresis in face of inadequate water intake (i.e., solute intake requiring renal excretion is high), thereby necessitating a high urine output relative to intake (e.g., high-protein tube feeding mixture given with inadequate amounts of "free water"). Sodium deficits are also usually present.

Diabetes insipidus or nephrogenic diabetes insipidus (Usually $U_{osm}/P_{osm} < 0.5$, sp gr < 1.005):

Hypernatremia is due to failure of renal water conservation because of lack of ADH (diabetes insipidus) or inability of the renal tubule to respond to ADH (nephrogenic diabetes insipidus), and failure of water intake to keep pace with water losses (sensible and insensible).

Dilute Urine
($U_{osm}/P_{osm} < 1.00$, sp gr < 1.010):

Renal tubular damage
(Usually $U_{osm}/P_{osm} \sim 1.0$, sp gr ~ 1.010):

1. Diuretic phase of acute renal failure.
2. Postobstructive diuresis.
3. Severe potassium depletion.
4. Severe hypercalcemia.
5. Chronic renal disease.

Hypernatremia is due at least in part to failure of normal renal water conservation and failure of water intake to keep pace with water losses (sensible and insensible). Sodium deficits are also usually present.

FIGURE 8.5. Approach to the assessment of a hypernatremic patient. This approach does not consider patients with hypernatremia secondary to excessive administration of hypertonic saline.

EXCESSIVE NONRENAL WATER LOSS. Hypernatremia typically develops in patients with accelerated rates of nonrenal water loss owing to a hot environment, fever, or hyperventilation and in whom water losses are not replaced because the patient cannot perceive or communicate thirst. Despite the hypernatremia, sodium deficits usually are present because initially, as water deficits develop, renal sodium excretion increases to maintain normal plasma osmolality and serum sodium concentration. When more than about 15% of ECF volume is lost, renal conservation of sodium occurs; if the water losses continue, hypernatremia develops. The presence of volume deficits is indicated by the signs of IVV depletion, as previously described. Urine flow rate usually is less than 35 mL/h.

SOLUTE DIURESIS. The amount of water that must accompany the excretion of a given amount of solute in the urine is determined by the osmolality of the renal medullary interstitial fluid (with which the collecting duct fluid must equilibrate) and the plasma level of ADH activity (which determines the permeability of the collecting duct to water and, therefore, the rate at which water moves from the collecting duct to medullary interstitial fluid to achieve osmotic equilibrium). Hypernatremia results if water intake does not keep pace with renal water losses, because although renal sodium excretion also is increased in solute diuresis, renal sodium reabsorption is affected proportionally less than water reabsorption. Large amounts of mannitol infused intravenously or high-protein mixtures fed by nasogastric tube (each gram of protein yields 8 mOsm as urea, phosphate, and potassium) can cause a solute diuresis sufficient to cause hypernatremia if water intake is inadequate. In solute diuresis, urine volume usually is greater than 35 mL/h.

Hypernatremia Associated with Formation of Dilute Urine

The finding of hypernatremia in combination with isotonic or hypotonic urine indicates that, at least in part, the hypernatremia results from failure of normal renal conservation of water. Failure to concentrate the urine under these conditions may result from the lack of ADH (hypothalamic–pituitary diabetes insipidus) or impaired renal tubular function that interferes with the development of a hypertonic medullary interstitium (renal tubular damage).

Central diabetes insipidus or nephrogenic diabetes insipidus should be suspected immediately in a patient with hypernatremia when the urine is very dilute (a $U_{osm}:P_{osm}$ ratio less than 0.5, or specific gravity <1.005).

In patients with renal tubular damage, the ability to concentrate and dilute the urine is decreased. As a result, under all conditions, the urine is isotonic or nearly isotonic with plasma. Hypernatremia can supervene when water losses exceed sodium losses and water intake does not keep pace with water losses. Despite the hypernatremia, significant sodium deficits usually are present because renal sodium wasting also usually is a feature of

these disorders. The following sections are examples of clinical situations in which renal tubular damage can be associated with hypernatremia.

DIURETIC PHASE OF ACUTE RENAL FAILURE. Occasionally, in a patient recovering from acute renal injury, tubular function is more severely affected than glomerular function. Thus, an inordinately large fraction of the glomerular filtrate escapes reabsorption, resulting in high urine flow rates. The period of inappropriate diuresis can persist for a few days to several weeks.

POSTOBSTRUCTIVE DIURESIS. The sudden release of chronic urinary tract obstruction often is followed by several days or weeks in which urine flow rates are abnormally high. Short-lived nephrogenic diabetes insipidus develops in some patients.

MANAGEMENT OF WATER AND ELECTROLYTE BALANCE

Water requirements should be carefully monitored, especially in hospitalized patients. Patients with known fluid deficits or excesses should be approached as demonstrated in Tables 8.7 and 8.8. Maintenance requirements can be calculated from two simple formulas.

The first is the 4-2-1 rule (Table 8.9). A more simplified method of calculation using this formula in adults would be to administer 60 mL/h of fluid for the first 20 kg of body weight. Subtract 20 from the patient's weight (in kg) and add this difference to calculate the hourly rate. For example, a patient who weighs 65 kg has a maintenance requirement of 105 mL/h.

The second method is to calculate the body surface area and multiply by 1,000. A patient with a body surface area of 1.5 m^2 would require 1,500 mL of fluid daily.

Intraoperative Fluid Administration

The guidelines for fluid replacement during the perioperative period are dictated by (maintenance) basal requirements, deficits, intraoperative losses, and third-space losses. The basal requirement has been discussed. Deficits include actions of general or spinal anesthesia on effective blood volume, intestinal losses (bowel obstruction or diarrhea), perspiration, and blood loss. In some cases, a CVP or Swan-Ganz catheter may be needed to assess IVV.

Intraoperative losses of fluid occur through several routes. Evaporation from peritoneal surfaces occurs, but quantifying it is difficult. The most obvious source of fluid loss, blood loss, is first assessed by looking into the suction canister. Fluid from irrigation should be subtracted. A soaked lap pad contains about 50 mL of blood, and a 4 × 4 pad contains about 5 mL. These are crude approximations. For instance, a moistened lap pad absorbs less than a dry one. Most researchers recommend a replacement rate of three to one for blood

TABLE 8.7.
General Guidelines for Planning Fluid and Electrolyte Therapy in Complicated Cases

Volume-Contracted Patients (from Water and Electrolyte Loss)

Deficit Replacement

Moderate volume contraction (e.g., decreased effective IVV causing azotemia but not hypotension). Plan to replace deficits in about 24 h (e.g., 0.9% saline at 200–250 mL/h). If patient is hypernatremic, 0.9% and 0.45% saline can be alternated.

Severe volume contraction (e.g., decreased effective IVV causing hypotension). Give 0.9% saline as rapidly as practicable until the hypotension is corrected.

Estimate maintenance needs and add this amount to the fluids used to correct the preexisting water and electrolyte deficits.

For patients with normal renal function and no abnormal losses:

Maintenance	*Equivalent Intravenous Fluid Orders*
Water: 2,500–3,000 mL/24 h	Alternate:
Sodium: 150 mEq/24 h	5% dextrose in 0.45% saline with
Potassium: 40 mEq/24 h	5% dextrose in 0.25% saline
	Each day add:
	Multivitamins to first liter
	Potassium chloride 20 mEq to first and second liters
	Infuse at 100–125 mL/h

Nutrition (Short Term)

At least 400 carbohydrate calories/24 h

For patients with acute renal failure with no urine output and no abnormal losses:

Maintenance	*Equivalent Intravenous Fluid Orders*
Water: 600 mL/24 h	600 mL 20% glucose in water and multivitamins per 24 h
Sodium: 0	
Potassium: 0	

Nutrition (Long Term)

At least 400 carbohydrate calories/24 h

See Table 8.8. if patients have abnormal losses of water and electrolytes.

Monitor patient frequently:

Weigh daily.

Measure serum creatinine and electrolyte levels daily or more frequently if necessary.

Measure CVP or pulmonary wedge pressure in complicated cases. If patient has normal cardiopulmonary function, CVP is sufficient. If cardiac disease or pulmonary hypertension is suspected, pulmonary wedge pressure measurement is preferred.

Evaluate water and electrolyte needs daily or more frequently in patients with high rates of abnormal losses.

Volume-Expanded Patients (Increased Effective IVV)

Correct volume excess:

Mild (e.g., simple edema): Decrease NaCl intake.

Moderate (e.g., mild pulmonary vascular congestion): Induce diuresis with diuretic and allow the sodium and water losses to go unreplaced.

Severe volume excess (e.g., severe pulmonary edema): Steps 1 and 2 and phlebotomy or ultrafiltration (if the patient is anemic) and/or digitalis, vasodilators, if heart disease is present.

Estimate ongoing losses (as above) and begin replacing when volume excesses have been corrected.

Monitor patient frequently.

CVP, central venous pressure; IVV, intravascular volume.

loss using crystalloid suspension and one to one using colloid suspension. While anesthetized, patients experience third-space loss. This phenomenon is the movement of isotonic fluid from the intravascular space to the interstitial space. A replacement of 2 to 4 mL/kg/h is usually adequate to accommodate third-space losses. Actual total intraoperative losses may be difficult or impossible to monitor during long and difficult surgical procedures. Monitoring of vital signs and urine output (optimal, 0.5 mL/kg/h) is extremely important. Sometimes invasive monitoring can be used to guide the clinician.

Crystalloid solutions contain only sugars and electrolytes (Table 8.10). Lactated Ringer solution is usually used because its composition more closely resembles the extracellular component than does normal saline. Generally, solutions that contain less sodium than lactated Ringer solution does should not be used in the perioperative setting. Although D_5W solutions have an osmolality greater than 250, they are unsuitable as routine perioperative replacement because the sugar is metabolized. Normal saline is another popular crystalloid solution. It is preferred over lactated Ringer solutions in the perioperative period when the patient is hypona-

TABLE 8.8.
Major Sources, Loss Rates, and Replacement Fluids in Abnormal Water and Electrolyte Loss

Sources	Rate of Loss	Replacement Fluid
Fever	Insensible water losses (normally 450 mL/24 h from skin and 450 mL/24 h from lung) increase by about 10% per degree Fahrenheit or 20% per degree Celsius for each degree of temperature above normal.	Replace with 5% dextrose in water
Hyperventilation	Doubling alveolar ventilation (i.e., 50% reduction in $PaCO_2$)increases insensible water losses from lung by 50%. Thus, the increase in alveolar ventilation required to reduce $PaCO_2$ from 40 to 20 mm Hg increases insensible loss from lungfrom 450 to 675 mL/24 h.	Replace with 5% dextrose in water
Gastric fluid	Rates of loss from nasogastric suction usually are 1–2 L/24 hbut can be much greater. Normal composition of gastric juice is about H^+ 100 mEq/L; sodium 40 mEq/L; potassium10 mEq/L; and chloride 150 mEq/L.	Replace with 0.45 normal saline and potassium chloride (usually 20–40 mEq/L) as needed[a]
Diarrheal fluid	Losses can vary from trivial to several liters daily. In adults, diarrheal fluid usually resembles extracellular fluid except that the bicarbonate concentration is higher (about 30–50 mEq/L) and chloride concentration is lower (about 80 mEq/L). Potassium concentration is variable (10–40 mEq/L)	Replace with 0.45 normal saline and 50 mEq of sodium bicarbonate/L and potassium chloride (usually 20 mEq/L), as needed[a]
Urine in acute renal failure	Because of tubular injury, urine sodium concentration usually is between 40 and 80 mEq/L and is largely independent of urine flow rate.	Replace with 0.45 normal saline and potassium chloride, as needed[a]

[a]The rate of potassium replacement usually is determined by the serum potassium concentration rather than the rates of potassium loss. For example, even though a patient in acute renal failure may be losing 30 mEq/24 h potassium in the urine, it may not be necessary to replace this amount, since potassium may be entering the extracellular fluid at an even faster rate because of catabolism of cellular proteins. On the other hand, the potassium losses in gastric fluid may amount to only 10 to 20 mEq/24 h, yet far greater amounts of potassium may have to be administered to maintain a normal serum potassium level, since gastric aspiration may lead to metabolic alkalosis, causing renal potassium wasting and extensive diffusion of potassium into intracellular fluid.

tremic or if brain injury is present. Hypertonic saline is rarely used in the perioperative setting. Because water tends to follow sodium, its theoretic advantage is that water is drawn into the intravascular space from the interstitial space; hence, smaller volumes of hypertonic solution than isotonic solution are needed to provide the same intravascular expansion. Crystalloid solutions are preferentially used over colloid solutions for perioperative fluid replacement.

Colloid solutions include albumin, hetastarch, and dextran. Blood is also a colloid but is discussed in another chapter. Colloids are used primarily when patients have a low colloid oncotic pressure or when large amounts of crystalloids have been infused. For example, if a patient has suffered a significant protein loss from ascites secondary to pelvic malignancy, colloids should be used early in the fluid replacement process. If a patient's blood pressure becomes difficult to maintain after infusion of sufficient crystalloid, colloids should be used.

Albumin, hetastarch, and dextran are three commonly used colloid solutions. Albumin is the most popular of the colloid solutions. It is a blood product but has the advantage of complete absence of infectious agents. In addition, it is treated with heat, eliminating the possibility of transmission of hepatitis or human immunodeficiency virus (HIV). It comes in 5% and 25% concentrations. Hetastarch consists of large polymer molecules and comes in a solution of saline. It is synthetic; therefore, its use does not affect the blood supply. There is no risk for viral transmission. Hetastarch is metabolized by the kidney and so must be used judiciously in those who have renal disease. Other disadvantages include potential volume overload, dilution hypoproteinemia, and decreased coagulation. The half-life of hetastarch can be as long as 13 days. Dextran is similar to hetastarch in mode of action. Additional problems with this substance are interference with cross-matching and histamine release. Dextran and hetastarch should be carefully monitored. Usually no

TABLE 8.9.
Maintenance Requirements by 4-2-1 Rule[a]

Body Weight Category	Fluid Rate (mL/kg)	Weight Category (kg)	Fluid (mL/h)
0–10	4	10	40
11–20	2	10	20
21 +	1	40	40

[a]Patient weighs 60 kg. Fluid requirement would be 100 mL/h.

TABLE 8.10.
Composition of Parenteral Fluids[a]

Solutions	Cations				Anions		
	Na	K	Ca	Mg	Cl	HCO₃	Osmolality (mOsm)
Extracellular fluid	142	4	5	3	103	27	280–310
Lactated Ringer solution	130	4	3	—	109	28[b]	273
0.9% sodium chloride	154	—	—	—	154	—	308
D₅ 45% sodium chloride	77	—	—	—	77	—	407
D₅W	—	—	—	—	—	—	253
3% sodium chloride	513	—	—	—	513	—	1,026

[a]Electrolyte count in mEq/L.
[b]Present in solution as lactate that is converted to bicarbonate.

more than 1,500 mL of hetastarch or 1,000 mL of dextran should be infused during a 24-hour period.

In summary, crystalloids should be used primarily for perioperative volume replacement. Colloid solutions should be used under the following conditions.

1. Large amounts of crystalloid are needed to maintain normal hemodynamics.
2. Assessment of circulatory status is difficult.
3. The patient has an elevated pulmonary capillary wedge pressure.
4. The colloid pressure is below 12.

Colloid oncotic pressure may be difficult to ascertain in a routine clinical setting; therefore, total protein or albumin levels can be used to give a rough approximation of colloid pressure. If blood loss is over 25% of total blood volume (in an otherwise healthy patient), transfusion of red cells must be considered. Hemoglobin concentrations can help. If the patient is elderly or suffers from lung, heart, or renal disease, then the transfusion trigger point is higher.

Experience has shown that hemoglobin levels between 7 and 8 are generally well tolerated in healthy adults. Primate experiments have demonstrated adequate perfusion of tissues with hemoglobin levels of 5 as long as the blood pressure, urine output, and pulse are satisfactory.

Correction of Volume Deficits

Estimating the Magnitude of Sodium or Water Deficits

If the patient has been weighed daily, the magnitude of the water deficit owing to external losses of water can be estimated from the decrease in body weight. The coexisting sodium deficits can be estimated by examining the weight deficits in light of the serum sodium concentration. For example, if the patient has acutely lost 3 kg and the serum sodium concentration is within 10% either way of normal serum sodium concentration (i.e., 126 to 154 mEq/L), little error is incurred by assuming that the patient has lost 3 L of ECF (i.e., isotonic saline); therefore, replacement therapy should be about 3 L of 0.9% saline (155 mEq/L). Using an equivalent amount

of lactated Ringer solution offers no advantage, because the kidneys adjust electrolyte excretion to make up for small differences between the composition of the ECF and the isotonic saline.

In patients in whom sodium and water deficits cannot be documented by changes in body weight, or in whom the losses are from the IVV into internal third spaces, approximate but useful guidelines are available to estimate the magnitude of the IVV deficit. These guidelines are as follows.

1. A loss equivalent to 15% of ECF volume (about 2 to 3 L in the average adult) results in a decrease in tissue turgor, but blood pressure and renal function, as judged by serum creatinine level, usually are normal.
2. Losses of sodium and water in excess of 15% of ECF volume usually are accompanied by decreased tissue turgor, orthostatic or frank hypotension, and significant elevation of serum creatinine level.

Correction Rates and Criteria for Assessment

Sodium and water losses great enough to result in hypotension represent a medical emergency, and rapid i.v. administration of isotonic saline is indicated until the hypotension is reversed. Thereafter, the rate of i.v. therapy is guided by the adequacy of the IVV as assessed by other criteria, particularly the measurement of blood pressure and pulse in the supine and sitting positions, urine flow rate, and CVP or pulmonary wedge pressure. In patients with less severe degrees of volume depletion, salt and water deficits often can be corrected by increasing oral intake. Salt can be added to food (the salt packets commonly present on hospital trays provide slightly more than 1 g of sodium chloride), or plain sodium chloride tablets can be given, with unrestricted water allowance, letting the patient's thirst mechanism dictate water intake. As a guide to the amount of sodium chloride that should be added to the diet to restore the deficits, 1 L of ECF contains 140 mEq of sodium, or about 9 g of sodium chloride. The adequacy of replacement therapy can be assessed over the ensuing days by measurement of change in body weight and blood pressure and by the decrease in serum creatinine level.

Correction of Volume Excess

Expansion of effective IVV sufficient to precipitate pulmonary edema is a medical emergency and requires the usual treatment of pulmonary edema, including placement of the patient in the sitting position or elevation of the head of the bed and administration of oxygen, vasodilators—such as nitrates, hydralazine, or angiotensin-converting enzyme inhibitors (e.g., captopril, enalapril, lisinopril)—digitalis, and loop diuretics, as needed. If the pulmonary edema does not improve, then phlebotomy may be required to relieve the vascular congestion. If the volume excess is less severe (e.g., simple edema), the problem usually can be controlled by decreasing salt intake, adding a diuretic drug, or both. The effectiveness of treatment can be guided by the decrease in body weight and periodic measurement of serum electrolyte and creatinine levels.

Correction of Hyponatremia

The approach to the correction of hyponatremia depends on: (a) whether the patient has significant CNS symptoms as a result of the hyponatremia (coma or seizures); and (b) the cause of the hyponatremia. If the patient has coma or seizures as a result of hyponatremia, the serum sodium level is commonly below 125 mEq/L and the reduction usually has occurred rapidly, over a few hours to days. In these situations, regardless of the cause of the hyponatremia, the serum sodium level should be rapidly raised toward normal by the i.v. administration of 3% saline. The serum sodium level should be raised to 125 mEq/L at a rate of 1 to 2 mEq/h. The rate of replacement can be slowed once the serum sodium level reaches 125 mEq/L, because neurologic symptoms are rare above this concentration. Rapid elevation of the serum sodium concentration to normal or hypernatremic levels must be avoided, because it may cause central pontine myelinolysis. The correction using 3% saline (513 mEq/L) can be calculated as follows:

volume TBW = 0.6 H total body weight in kg
volume TBW × (desired [Na⁺] − actual [Na⁺])
= total Na⁺ (mEq)

where: [Na⁺] is expressed in mEq/L; and TBW = total body water.

The total amount of sodium required can then be replaced at a rate of 2 mEq/h using hypertonic saline. For example, if a 71-kg woman with neurologic symptoms has a serum sodium level of 113 mEq/L, correction to a serum sodium level of 125 mEq/L can be achieved as follows.

volume TBW = 0.6 × 71 = 42.6
42.6 × (125 − 113) = 511 mEq Na⁺

Therefore, this patient requires 1 L of 3% saline to raise her serum sodium level by 12 mEq. The liter of hypertonic saline is administered over 6 to 12 hours. Serum electrolyte levels should be checked every few hours and

rates of replacement readjusted as necessary. The infusion of hypertonic saline results in diffusion of water from ICF to ECF until isosmotic conditions are restored. This results in reduction of cell volume and an increase of ICF osmolality toward normal as well as in an expansion of ECF volume. The expansion of the ECF by the hypertonic saline may precipitate or worsen congestive heart failure. Therefore, patients who receive hypertonic saline should be carefully observed for signs of pulmonary edema and, if such signs are present, vigorously treated with a loop diuretic.

Hyponatremia Associated with Volume Depletion

The administration of isotonic saline in amounts sufficient to replace existing sodium deficits usually results in complete correction of the hyponatremia, as discussed, in connection with the treatment of volume depletion, because restoration of effective IVV toward normal allows a water diuresis. If specific disease states, such as adrenal insufficiency or diarrhea, are associated with the development of the hyponatremia and volume depletion, these also require treatment.

Hyponatremia Associated with Normal Intravascular Volume

If the hyponatremia is associated with excessive intake of water, restricting water intake to normal corrects the problem. If the hyponatremia is owing to an inappropriate antidiuresis, water intake must be restricted below normal—for example, to about 800 mL of measured liquid intake daily in an average-sized adult (see Table 8.2). This usually results in negative water balance, a fall in body weight, and a rise in serum sodium concentration toward normal. Excess total body water can be calculated as follows.

actual TBW = 0.6 × total body weight in kg
$\frac{\text{actual serum } [Na^+]}{\text{desired serum } [Na^+]}$ × actual TBW
= desired TBW
actual TBW − desired TBW = excess TBW in L
where: [Na⁺] is expressed in mEq/L.

If a specific cause for the inappropriate antidiuresis can be identified, it should be eliminated (see Table 8.6).

Hyponatremia Associated with Expanded Intravascular Volume and Extracellular Fluid

The spontaneous development of hyponatremia in the course of severe congestive heart or liver failure is an ominous sign. The hyponatremia usually does not cause any clinical symptoms, and although it can be successfully treated by water restriction, clinical improvement usually does not follow. Furthermore, during such treatment, patients complain bitterly of thirst. Thus, water restriction sufficient to raise the serum sodium concentration to normal is not indicated. Water intake should be restricted, however, to prevent the serum sodium concentration from decreasing to less than 120 mEq/L in an effort to prevent possible CNS symptoms of hyponatremia.

Correction of Hypernatremia

Hypernatremia Secondary to Water Depletion

The amount of water needed to correct the serum sodium concentration toward normal is given in the following equation.

$$actual\ TBW = 0.6 \times total\ body\ weight\ in\ kg$$

$$\frac{actual\ serum\ [Na^+]}{desired\ serum\ [Na^+]} \times actual\ TBW$$

$$= desired\ TBW$$

$$desired\ TB - actual\ TBW$$

$$= water\ necessary\ to\ lower\ serum\ [Na^+]$$

where: $[Na^+]$ is expressed in mEq/L.

The rate of correction usually is 1 to 2 mEq/h. This deficit usually would be corrected with administration of hypotonic fluid over 24 to 48 hours along with the water and electrolytes needed to maintain day-to-day water and electrolyte balance. The underlying cause of the hypernatremia also must be corrected if possible.

Hypernatremia Secondary to Excessive Administration of Hypertonic Saline

In the rare instance of hypernatremia secondary to excessive administration of hypertonic saline, which occurs when intraamniotic infusion of hypertonic saline is used to induce abortion, hypernatremia is owing solely to positive sodium chloride balance. Therefore, treatment involves simply inducing a state of negative sodium chloride balance while maintaining a slightly positive water balance. If the hypernatremia is associated with impairment of CNS function (Na^+ usually exceeds 160 mEq/L), 2 to 3 L of 5% solution of glucose in water should rapidly be given i.v., along with sufficient furosemide to induce a urine flow rate of about 10 to 20 mL/min. About 100 mg of i.v. furosemide is an appropriate initial dose. This results in the excretion of urine containing about 140 mEq/L of sodium and chloride and 10 mEq/L of potassium. If, at the same time, only the water and potassium are replaced (e.g., replacement of each 1,000 mL of urine with 1,000 mL of 5% solution of glucose in water plus 10 to 20 mEq of potassium chloride, given i.v.), the patient is selectively depleted of sodium chloride, and plasma electrolytes can be restored to normal within several hours. During this period of correction, serum and urine electrolyte levels must be monitored frequently to assess the adequacy of i.v. replacement therapy, particularly the rate of potassium administration.

POTASSIUM METABOLISM

Disorders of potassium metabolism frequently coexist with disorders of sodium and water balance. For example, sodium and potassium losses often accompany gastrointestinal losses of water and electrolytes. The recognition and management of potassium depletion under these circumstances were discussed earlier in connection with the management of disorders of sodium and water balance. Even small movements of potassium into and out of cells can cause significant changes in the serum potassium since over 90% of potassium resides intracellularly. It also is important to recognize disorders in which disturbances of potassium balance are the primary abnormality or the major feature of the electrolyte disturbances.

Hyperkalemia

Hyperkalemia is defined as a serum potassium level greater than 5 mEq/L. Serum potassium levels between 5 and 6 mEq/L usually cause little or no functional abnormality, but such levels indicate that an abnormality of potassium regulation is present. This sign should be heeded and its cause investigated, because further small elevations in serum potassium concentration can seriously impair cardiac and skeletal muscle function. At a serum potassium level of 6 or 7 mEq/L, the electrocardiogram (ECG) begins to show tall, peaked T waves and skeletal muscle weakness may be present. At a serum potassium level greater than 7 mEq/L, severe ECG abnormalities may be present, including complete suppression of atrial activity and an idioventricular rhythm that can then lead to ventricular tachycardia and fibrillation. Profound skeletal muscle weakness leading to respiratory arrest also may develop. If serious hyperkalemia is suspected, an ECG should be obtained immediately along with a blood specimen for potassium measurement. The ECG findings establish whether life-threatening hyperkalemia is present. Table 8.11 lists the principal clinical conditions associated with hyperkalemia.

Pseudohyperkalemia can result from hemolysis of red blood cells as a result of the mechanical trauma of venipuncture. Such pseudohyperkalemia should be readily recognized, because both potassium and hemoglobin are released by the damaged cells. If the serum potassium level has been significantly raised by *in vitro* hemolysis, the serum is visibly pink because of the presence of free hemoglobin. Patients with extraordinarily high white blood cell counts or platelet counts also can exhibit pseudohyperkalemia as the result of excessive traumatic *in vitro* lysis of these cells. Pseudohyperkalemia can be avoided by drawing venous blood samples under low pressure into a heparinized syringe.

Management

LIFE-THREATENING HYPERKALEMIA. ECG shows sine waves or loss of atrial activity and a broad QRS complex. Serum potassium level usually is higher than 7 mEq/L.

1. Infuse 10 mL of 10% calcium gluconate intravenously over a few minutes with ECG monitoring to observe for reversal of ECG changes toward normal. The same infusion of 10 mL of 10% calcium gluconate can be repeated once. Calcium ion directly antagonizes the effects of potassium on myocardial metabolism. The onset of action is a few minutes. If the patient is tak-

TABLE 8.11.
Causes of Hyperkalemia

Cause	Effect
Excessive intake of potassium Transfusion of blood stored for prolonged periods	Shortened life span of stored RBCs after transfusion leads to excessive release of RBC potassium to ECF. Plasma potassium of stored blood also is increased (30 mEq/L) after 14 days of storage.
Excessive oral or intravenous intake of potassium	Acute ingestion of 500 mEq potassium chloride can cause fatal hyperkalemia with normal renal function. If renal function is impaired, even normal potassium intake can cause severe hyperkalemia.

Excessive release of intracellular stores of potassium
    Chemotherapy of malignancies
    Catabolism of hematomas
    Rhabdomyolysis
    Succinylcholine action on muscle
    Sepsis with excessive catabolism of muscle protein
    Acute digitalis poisoning
    Familial hyperkalemic periodic paralysis
    Intravenous hypertonic glucose or mannitol
    Intravenous arginine
    Metabolic acidosis
	The potential for any of these conditions to cause serious hyperkalemia is greatly increased when they coexist with impaired renal function.
	
	H^+ displaces K^+ from intracellular sites, causing increased diffusion of K^+ into ECF.

Impaired renal capacity to excrete potassium Grossly reduced glomerular filtration rate	Almost all of filtered potassium is reabsorbed. Excreted potassium represents almost exclusively potassium secreted by the tubules. Nevertheless, grossly reduced glomerular filtration rate is associated with grossly reduced tubular function and hence the tendency to hyperkalemia.
Impaired tubular function Hyperkalemic renal tubular acidosis	Some patients with normal or mildly reduced glomerular filtration rate can have substantial impairment of potassium secretion (e.g., lupus patients with interstitial nephritis, mild obstructive uropathy)

Decreased aldosterone secretion
    Addison's disease
    Primary hypoaldosteronism
    Hyporeninemic hypoaldosteronism
	Alosterone is necessary for normal potassium and H^+ secretion and normal Na^+ absorption in the distal renal tubule.
	
	Common in patients with diabetes mellitus or obstructive uropathy.

Drugs that suppress angiotension formation
    β-blocking agents (e.g., propranolol)
    Prostaglandin synthetase inhibitors (e.g., indomethacin, ibuprofen)
    Angiotensin-converting enzyme inhibitors (e.g., captopril, enalapril, lisinopril)
	Angiotensin II causes aldosterone secretion; β-blockers and nonsteroidal antiinflammatory drugs directly suppress angiotensin formation by suppressing renin production. Captopril prevents angiotensin II formation by blocking conversion of angiotensin I.

Drugs that interfere with renal potassium secretion	Spironolactone competitively inhibits the action of aldosterone. Triamterene and amiloride block potassium secretion even in the absence of aldosterone.
Ureteral implantation into jejunal loop	Increased reabsorption of potassium from jejunum causes predisposition to hyperkalemia.

ECF, extracellular fluid; RBCs, red blood cells.

ing digitalis, consider not giving the calcium and proceed on to the next step.

2. Infuse 50 g of glucose, 10 units of regular insulin, and 50 mEq of sodium bicarbonate. The onset of action is about 15 minutes. Additionally, an i.v. infusion of glucose, insulin, and sodium bicarbonate (e.g., 500 mL of 10% dextrose in water plus 15 units of regular insulin plus 50 mEq of sodium bicarbonate) may be started. Infuse over several hours. This maneuver causes potassium to move intracellularly. The amount of glucose infused must be altered or omitted in hyperglycemic diabetic patients.

3. Nebulized albuterol at a dose of 10 to 20 mg is recommended. The peak action is approximately 90 minutes.
4. As soon as practical, give sodium polystyrene sulfonate (Kayexalate) by mouth, nasogastric tube, or retention enema (e.g., 20 to 50 g of Kayexalate every 2 to 4 hours). An equal number of grams of sorbitol should be given if the Kayexalate is administered into the upper gastrointestinal tract. Sorbitol, a sugar that is poorly absorbed from the intestine, causes an osmotic diarrhea and prevents concretions of Kayexalate from forming within the gut. Kayexalate is an ion-exchange resin that removes potassium by binding potassium and releasing sodium into body fluids.
5. Hemodialysis may be required in patients in whom these measures fail.

MODERATE HYPERKALEMIA. ECG shows only peaked T waves; serum potassium level usually is below 7 mEq/L.

1. Reduce potassium intake (normal potassium intake is 60 to 100 mEq/24 h). Reducing dietary potassium to 50 to 60 mEq/24 h usually is sufficient to correct mild hyperkalemia.
2. Kayexalate may be needed periodically to control the serum potassium level.
3. Correct metabolic acidosis if present.
4. Stop administration of medications that can contribute to hyperkalemia, such as angiotensin-converting enzyme inhibitors, nonsteroidal antiinflammatory drugs, and potassium-sparing diuretics.

Hypokalemia

Hypokalemia is defined as a serum potassium level below 3.5 mEq/L (Table 8.12). Significant symptoms usually do not result from hypokalemia unless the serum potassium level is less than 3 mEq/L. An important exception is in patients who are receiving digitalis preparations. In such patients, hypokalemia, or even low-normal serum potassium levels, can increase myocardial irritability and lead to serious arrhythmias. In addition to increasing myocardial irritability, hypokalemia can cause profound muscle weakness and ileus. Chronic severe hypokalemia also can cause metabolic alkalosis and decreased capacity to concentrate the urine. The ECG in hypokalemia often shows U waves, although this finding is not diagnostic of hypokalemia.

Management

MILD ASYMPTOMATIC HYPOKALEMIA. This usually can be corrected simply by eliminating the cause of the potassium wasting or by increasing potassium intake. If the hypokalemia is caused by diuretic therapy, potassium depletion usually can be avoided by administering spironolactone or triamterene. Potassium supplementation also can be used, but if the patient is on a low sodium chloride intake, the potassium supplement must be given as potassium chloride. The use of other, more palatable potassium salts (e.g., gluconate, citrate, acetate) and all forms of potassium in food is much less effective in correcting hypokalemia, and this treatment is used primarily in patients on a normal sodium chloride intake.

SEVERE OR SYMPTOMATIC HYPOKALEMIA. This usually requires i.v. administration of potassium chloride. In general, the use of i.v. solutions that contain more than 40 mEq/L of potassium should be avoided, because infusing high concentrations of potassium can cause hyperkalemia or cardiac disturbance. In correcting even severe potassium deficits, it is seldom necessary to infuse more than 120 to 160 mEq/24 h of potassium chloride. When higher rates are used, frequent monitoring of the patient's ECG and serum potassium level is essential. Intravenous replacement of potassium should never run at a rate of greater than 10 mEq/h. The oral route of potassium replacement should be used whenever possible.

Calcium

Approximately 99% of body calcium is contained in bone. Up to 40% of the extracellular calcium that circulates in the bloodstream is bound to plasma proteins. However, the unbound or ionized form of calcium is the form that exerts physiologic activity. Total calcium is a measure of both the bound and unbound or ionized form. Serum albumin levels affect the total serum calcium, as albumin is the plasma protein to which the majority of calcium is bound.

corrected calcium in mg/dL =
measured calcium + [(4 − albumin in g/dL) × 0.8]

Ionized or unbound calcium can be measured if specifically requested. Its concentration is affected by the serum pH. With alkalosis when the pH is increased, a decrease in ionized calcium results from the increased protein binding of calcium. Conversely, with acidosis a decrease in protein binding causes an increase in ionized calcium.

The homeostasis of calcium is quite complex and calcium serves many important functions. Calcium plays a role in regulation of muscle contraction and nerve conduction. Additionally, it functions in the coagulation cascade. The majority of calcium is stored in bone; however, calcium is under the control of several other organ systems including the integument, endocrine, and renal. Parathyroid hormone (PTH) appears to be the major hormone effecting calcium homeostasis. Vitamin D must be present, however, for it to exert its maximal effect. PTH causes the following.

- Mobilization of calcium and phosphorus from bone
- Increased renal tubular reabsorption of calcium
- Increased intestinal absorption of calcium
- Decreased renal tubular reabsorption of phosphorus

Hypocalcemia

Clinical manifestations of hypocalcemia (defined as a calcium level below 8 to 8.5 mg/dL) are characterized by neuromuscular irritability. Symptoms can include numb-

TABLE 8.12.
Causes of Hypokalemia

Cause	Comments on Pathogenesis
Decreased potassium intake	With 0 mEq potassium intake, stool potassium is about 10 mEq/2 h, urinary potassium is <30 mEq/24 h or is <20 mEq/L
Excessive renal losses of potassium	Urinary potassium usually greater than 30 mEq/24 h or 20 mEq/L.
Diuretic therapy	All diuretics except for spironolactone, triameterene, and amiloride cause renal potassium wasting. *Mechanism:* Diuretics cause increased sodium delivery to distal tubular sites where sodium is reabsorbed in exchange for potassium or hydrogen ion.
Diuretic phase of acute tubular necrosis and other causes of osmotic diuresis	*Mechanism:* Same as above
Metabolic alkalosis	*Mechanism:* Renal tubular cell potassium concentration increased resulting in enhanced potassium secretion.
Gentamicin or amphotericin B nephrotoxicity	Renal tubular damage presumably causes increased back flux of potassium into renal tubules in the case of amphotericin.
Increased renal mineralicorticoid effects Mineralocorticoid therapy (DOCA, 9 α-fluodrocortisone) Primary aldosteronism Secondary aldosteronism (e.g., cirrhosis of the liver, renal artery stenosis, malignant hypertension) Cushing's syndrome Excessive licorice or chewing tobacco (glycyrrhizic acid) Bartter's syndrome	Increased activity of distal tubular site, which reabsorbs sodium in exchange for potassium or H$^+$
Renal tubular acidosis	*Mechanism:* Distal: Possibly increased renal potassium secretion in exchange for sodium at the distal tubular site because of decreased availability of H$^+$ for secretion Proximal: Increased bicarbonate excretion leads to increased renal potassium excretion.
Excessive gastrointestinal losses of potassium Vomiting, gastric drainage, diarrhea, laxative abuse	Renal potassium excretion also increased in the case of vomiting or gastric drainage.
Villous adenoma of rectum	Loss of potassium-rich mucus per rectum.
Shift of potassium from the extracellular to the intracellular fluid	
Correction of metabolic acidosis	H$^+$ leaves cells, K$^+$ enters cells during correction of metabolic acidosis.
Correction of hyperglycemia	K$^+$ enters cells with glucose to provide cation to balance anion that forms during metabolism of glucose.
Hypokalemic periodic paralysis	Unexplained familial disorder.
Miscellaneous Ureterosigmoidostomy	Colonic secretion of HCO$_3^-$ and K$^+$ with absorption of Na$^+$ and Cl$^-$ results in hypokalemic metabolic acidosis.

ness, muscle cramping, paresthesias, Chvostek's (twitching of facial muscles) and Trousseau's (carpal spasm) signs, tetany, and seizures. Patients can also experience psychosis and memory loss. On physical examination patients may have hyperactive deep tendon reflexes. ECG findings of hypocalcemia include a prolonged QT interval, which can lead to heart block or ventricular fibrillation. Causes of hypocalcemia are shown in Table 8.13.

Treatment of hypocalcemia should be directed at its underlying cause. A low total calcium level with a normal ionized calcium level signifies a low level of plasma pro-

TABLE 8.13.
Causes of Hypocalcemia

Deficiency or absence of parathyroid hormone
Vitamin D deficiency—decreased intestinal absorption
Septic shock—suppression of parathyroid hormone products
Renal failure—decreased 1:25 dihydroxycholecalcifral
Hypomagnesemia—decreased parathyroid hormone release and decreased organ response to calcium
Hyperphosphatemia

teins. These patients usually are asymptomatic and calcium replacement in this setting usually is not necessary.

For patients with acute symptomatic hypocalcemia, calcium gluconate or chloride should be given intravenously. These may cause a local cellulitis or tissue necrosis if infiltration occurs. If infiltration occurs, especially with the chloride solution in emergent situations, 10 mL of 10% calcium gluconate can be administered intravenously over 15 minutes. In addition, 10 to 20 mL of calcium gluconate can be placed in 1 L of D_5W and administered over 24 hours. If the serum albumin level is below 2 mg/dL, then it may be prudent to replace albumin, especially if the urine output is low. Because albumin is heat treated, there is no risk of hepatitis or HIV exposure. In cases of symptomatic hypocalcemia magnesium levels must be checked and corrected if necessary. In those patients with metabolic acidosis and hypocalcemia, the hypocalcemia should be treated initially followed by the correction of the acidosis.

Long-term treatment of hypocalcemia involves adequate nutritional supplementation of calcium, vitamin D, or both. If the serum phosphorus level is high, hypoparathyroid disease must be suspected and the patient treated accordingly. If the serum phosphorus is normal or low, then primary bone disease (hungry bone) must be considered. It is imperative that magnesium levels be checked because replenishment of calcium cannot be accomplished in a patient who is hypomagnesemic.

Hypercalcemia

The clinical manifestations of hypercalcemia usually are seen when the total serum calcium is greater than 12 mg/dL. Common presenting symptoms include weakness, fatigue, nausea, vomiting, constipation, polyuria, polydipsia, lethargy, and confusion. Psychiatric disturbances and coma can be seen in severe cases of hypercalcemia. ECG changes include prolongation of PR and QRS intervals with a shortening of the QT interval. Complete heart block and cardiac arrest can occur in profound hypercalcemia. Additional laboratory abnormalities can include elevations in serum amylase and creatinine levels. The phosphorus level is critical in establishing the cause of hypercalcemia. A phosphorus level below 3.5 mg/dL suggests hyperparathyroidism, whereas an elevated phosphorus level suggests an underlying malignancy.

Hypercalcemia, unlike many other electrolyte disturbances, is rarely iatrogenically induced. There are several causes of hypercalcemia. The majority of hospitalized patients with hypercalcemia have an underlying malignancy, whereas the most common etiology of hypercalcemia in the ambulatory setting is hyperparathyroidism. Additional causes of hypercalcemia include thiazide diuretics, lithium, vitamin D intoxication, hyperthyroidism, and sarcoidosis. In the setting of gynecology, hypercalcemia is most often seen with malignancy. In patients with cancer, hypercalcemia results from increased bone resorption and decreased renal excretion. Metastasis to the bony skeleton causes an increase in osteoclastic activity that increases bone resorption. Some gynecologic tumors, however, may cause hypercalcemia by production of a substance similar to PTH, causing bone resorption without evidence of bony metastasis.

Volume expansion is crucial in the treatment of acute hypercalcemia. Replacement with normal saline solution decreases calcium reabsorption in the proximal renal tubule, thus improving renal function. Initial i.v. fluid therapy should be aggressive with rates of 250 to 500 mL/h, as most patients are volume contracted. Addition of loop diuretics such as furosemide may aid in increasing urinary calcium excretion, but caution must be used because these drugs may result in volume contraction and hypokalemia. After initial volume is restored, 3 to 6 L/d of normal saline solution should be given. Close monitoring of daily patient weights, intake and output, and frequent monitoring of serum electrolytes is necessary in patients with hypercalcemia.

Bisphosphates are commonly used for the treatment of hypercalcemia. This class of drugs inhibits osteoclast precursors and induces osteoclast cytotoxicity, thereby decreasing serum calcium levels. Etidronate disodium (Didronel) is given at a dose of 7.5 mg/kg i.v. over 2 hours daily for 3 to 7 days. Alternatively, pamidronate (Aredia) is given as a single dose of 60 to 90 mg i.v. over 4 to 24 hours. Peak onset of action with these medications is usually seen in 48 to 96 hours and may last 2 to 3 weeks. The single dose of 90 mg i.v. of pamidronate is recommended for severe cases of hypercalcemia because of its effectiveness. The bisphosphonates may be repeated if hypercalcemia recurs. Pamidronate can cause a low-grade temperature elevation and etidronate should not be given to patients with a serum creatinine level of greater than 2.5 mg/dL because it may cause an elevation in serum creatinine.

Calcitonin increases renal excretion of calcium and inhibits osteoclastic activity. In patients with hypercalcemia, calcitonin can be given at a dose of 4 to 8 IU/kg i.m. or s.c. every 6 to 12 hours. Commercial calcitonin preparations are generally from salmon. It has a rapid onset of action and serum calcium levels may decrease within several hours. Its effect usually subsides after several days, but may be potentiated by concomitant glucocorticoid administration. Calcitonin has minimal side effects. Tachyphylaxis is seen with calcitonin limiting its repeated usage, causing it to be less consistently effective compared to other available hypercalcemic treatments.

Glucocorticoids decrease the intestinal absorption of calcium, promote urinary excretion of calcium, and may lower calcium levels by a direct cytolytic effect on some tumor cells. Lowering of serum calcium levels with glucocorticoids may take 5 to 10 days. Dosages may vary from 20 to 100 mg of oral prednisone or its i.v. equivalent per day. Side effects limit the long-term use of glucocorticoids for hypercalcemia.

Another potent inhibitor of bone resorption is gallium nitrate. Its onset of action is usually seen in 1 to 2 days with a peak at 5 to 10 days after administration. Gallium nitrate is administered in a dose of 100 to 200 mg/kg per day for 5 days in a continuous drip. It is important to maintain a saline diuresis of at least 2 L/d during this therapy. Side effects are relatively uncommon, but renal toxicity may be seen. Gallium nitrate in early studies was significantly more effective than calcitonin with or without the addition of corticosteroids. Its obvious disadvantage over the biphosphates is that it requires continuous i.v. infusion over 4 or 5 days.

Oral and i.v. phosphorus has been used successfully to treat hypercalcemia. It has fallen out of favor, however, because it causes decreased excretion of calcium from the kidneys. Intravenous phosphorus can also lead to soft-tissue deposition of calcium compounds and renal failure. It was used in patients with serum phosphorus levels less than 3 mg/dL and normal renal function. For patients with extremely high calcium levels and severe symptoms (e.g., coma, arrhythmia), renal dialysis may be necessary for rapid correction of hypercalcemia.

Plicamycin (Mithramycin) is an antibiotic that blocks bone resorption, thus lowering serum calcium. The recommended dose of plicamycin in the treatment of hypercalcemia is 25 μg/kg i.v. over 4 to 6 hours and may be repeated every 24 to 48 hours. Its onset of action is relatively quick and peak action is usually noted in 2 to 3 days. Side effects can be severe and include nausea, vomiting, bleeding, thrombocytopenia, renal failure, and hepatotoxicity. These side effects are more common with repeated doses of plicamycin. Because of these side effects, plicamycin usually is reserved for hypercalcemia of malignancy or hypercalcemia refractory to other therapies.

Magnesium

Magnesium has several functions in the human body. Its primary role is in neuromuscular function, but it also serves as an enzyme cofactor in protein and carbohydrate metabolism. The majority (60%) of magnesium in the body is contained within the bone. Most of the remainder is found intracellularly, with only about 1% found in the extracellular fluid. Normal serum magnesium levels are between 1.2 and 2.2 mEq/L. Magnesium metabolism depends on potassium and calcium levels. The kidney serves as the organ primarily responsible for magnesium homeostasis. Magnesium is filtered at the glomerulus and reabsorbed in the ascending loop of Henle and to a lesser degree in the proximal and distal tubules.

Hypomagnesemia

Hypomagnesemia is more common than hypermagnesemia. Hypomagnesemia results from decreased gastrointestinal absorption with conditions such as chronic diarrhea, malabsorption syndromes, and nasogastric suction. Increased renal and gastrointestinal losses from osmotic diuresis, hypercalcemia, and medications such as cisplatin, diuretics, and aminoglycosides also can cause hypomagnesemia. Hypomagnesemia can result from decreased intake in malnutrition. For example, 10% to 15% of hospitalized patients and over half of patients in intensive care units exhibit low magnesium levels. Lastly, patients with heavy alcohol use may have hypomagnesemia.

Symptoms and signs of hypomagnesemia are usually nonspecific but may be manifested by neuromuscular excitability. Hypomagnesemia is often seen in combination with hypokalemia, hypocalcemia, and metabolic alkalosis. Neurologic abnormalities include weakness, dizziness, lethargy, confusion, tremors, fasciculations, and seizures. Typical ECG findings are prolonged PR and QT intervals; however, atrial and ventricular arrhythmias can result.

The treatment of hypomagnesemia involves the replacement of magnesium. Mild or chronic cases may be treated with oral magnesium supplements. Oral repletion is also preferred in asymptomatic patients. This is accomplished by giving 240 mg of elemental magnesium one to four times a day. Diarrhea is the most common side effect. For severe or acute cases, i.v. magnesium is indicated. Obstetricians and gynecologists are familiar with the 4-g magnesium load mixed with 50 mL of D_5W to infuse over 30 minutes. Deep tendon reflexes should be evaluated frequently because hyperreflexia suggests hypermagnesemia. Long-term oral therapy can be provided with magnesium oxide, 300 mg/d. Patients should receive proper nutritional counseling and be warned to avoid alcohol. Any underlying medical disorder that may contribute to magnesium losses should be treated. Hydration status should be evaluated because overhydration can lead to mild forms of hypomagnesemia. Gastrointestinal tract losses and alcohol consumption also should be addressed in the evaluation of this disease process.

Hypermagnesemia

Hypermagnesemia is rare and usually iatrogenic. Causes of hypermagnesemia include therapy with magnesium-containing antacids or laxatives or secondary to administration of parenteral hyperalimentation. Often hypermagnesemia is seen in patients with some degree of renal insufficiency. Lastly, it can be seen in preeclamptic or preterm labor patients treated with i.v. magnesium.

Mild to moderate hypermagnesemia usually is asymptomatic, but patients with severe cases may present with several symptoms. Clinical manifestations are normally seen if magnesium levels are greater than 4 mEq/L. Signs and symptoms include nausea, vomiting, weakness, lethargy, and somnolence. A prolonged PR interval, widening of the QRS complex, and increased T-wave amplitude can be seen with levels greater than 5 mEq/L. Areflexia occurs at levels above 6 to 7 mEq/L. Respiratory arrest, bradycardia, and hypotension can be seen when levels are over 10 to 11 mEq/L. Finally, cardiac arrest can occur when serum magnesium is above 14 mEq/L.

Discontinuation of magnesium intake is the primary therapy for symptomatic hypermagnesemia. Patients with severe cases should be given 10% calcium gluconate, 10 to 20 mL i.v. over 10 minutes. The calcium therapy antagonizes the effects of magnesium and is cardioprotective. Supportive therapy and mechanical ventilation may be necessary in those with respiratory failure. Hemodialysis may be required in patients with hypermagnesemia and renal insufficiency.

Phosphorus

As with magnesium, the majority of phosphorus is contained with the bony skeleton and the intracellular space, and only 1% is found in the extracellular fluid. As a result, serum phosphate levels may not accurately reflect total body phosphate stores. A normal range for serum phosphorus is 3.0 to 4.5 mg/dL. Phosphorus serves as an important energy source by means of high-energy phosphates. It is a key component to protein and lipid structure, and is a vital component for carbohydrate metabolism.

Hypophosphatemia

Causes of hypophosphatemia defined as a serum phosphate below 2.5 mg/dL include a redistribution of phosphate into the cells, a decrease in intestinal absorption, or an increase in renal excretion. Several causes of hypophosphatemia are listed in Table 8.14. Most patients with mild hypophosphatemia are asymptomatic. Moderate to severe hypophosphatemia causes neuromuscular abnormalities including weakness, rhabdomyolysis, paresthesias, confusion, seizures, and coma. Erythrocyte, leukocyte, and platelet dysfunction also can be seen because of a depletion of cellular ATP and 2,3-diphosphoglycerate.

Most patients with serum phosphate levels between 1.0 and 2.5 mg/dL usually are asymptomatic. Treatment is aimed at the correcting the underlying cause. In cases of chronic hypophosphatemia oral repletion can be instituted at a dose of 500 to 1,000 mg of elemental phosphorus two to three times per day and the most common side effect is diarrhea. This can be given in the form of sodium/potassium phosphate tablets called Neutra-Phos or Neutra-Phos K (each contains 250 mg of elemental phosphorus). Parenteral administration of phosphorus is indicated when serum phosphorus levels are below 1.0 mg/dL. Infusion at a dose of 2.5 to 5 mg elemental phosphorus/kg given every 6 hours is recommended. When the serum levels are greater than 1.5 to 2 mg/dL, patients may be switched to oral supplements. Care must be taken to avoid hyperphosphatemia. Also, concomitant calcium supplementation often is needed to prevent hypocalcemia. Serum magnesium, calcium, and potassium levels should be monitored closely.

Hyperphosphatemia

Hyperphosphatemia is relatively rare and is seen with either an increased endogenous or exogenous phosphorus load or with a decrease in renal clearance of phosphorus. Renal failure is the most common cause of hyperphosphatemia. Elevated phosphorus levels also may be seen secondary to rhabdomyolysis, tumor lysis syndrome, hypoparathyroidism, and respiratory or metabolic acidosis. Clinical manifestations include numbness, tingling, muscle cramps, paresthesias, and tetany and are caused by hypocalcemia. Hyperphosphatemia causes hypocalcemia by decreasing calcium absorption from the gastrointestinal tract.

Addressing the underlying cause is the cornerstone of management for hyperphosphatemia. In acute cases saline diuresis can be used in patients with normal renal function. Additionally, administration of glucose and insulin causes a shift in phosphorus from extracellular fluid to the intracellular space. Dialysis may be required if renal failure is present. Oral phosphate binders such as calcium carbonate can be used in patients with chronic hyperphosphatemia.

DISORDERS OF ACID–BASE METABOLISM

The pH of normal human ECF ranges from 7.35 to 7.45. For normal bodily functions to be maintained, the pH must remain in this range. Humans have buffer systems to absorb excess acids or alkali in the face of an abnormal pH. The lungs correct for acid–base disorders in an acute setting until the kidneys can compensate. In acidotic states, patients hyperventilate to drive down the CO_2 levels in the blood; in alkalotic states, patients hypoventilate. The kidneys gradually increase compensation by retaining or regenerating bicarbonate and hydrogen ions. The bicarbonate system is the most important of the human buffer systems and is described by the Henderson-Hasselbach equation.

$$pH = \frac{6.1 + \log (HCO_3^-)}{(@[Pa_{CO_2}])}$$

where: $6.1 = pK$; $@ = 0.03$ mmol/L/mm Hg at 38°C (solubility coefficient).

Table 8.15 shows the directional changes in acid–base parameters for the primary acid–base disorders. If the kidney detects a respiratory acidotic state, CO_2 and H_2O in renal tubule cells are converted by carbonic anhydrase to carbonic acid (H_2CO_3). This

---

TABLE 8.14.
Causes of Moderate to Severe Hypophosphatemia (<1.5 mg/dL)

Respiratory alkalosis
Malabsorption
Vitamin D deficiency
Hyperalimentation
Treatment of diabetic ketoacidosis
Hyperparathyroidism
Excessive alcohol use

TABLE 8.15.
Primary Disorders of Acid–Base Regulation

Acid–Base Disturbance	Primary (Initiating) Event	Secondary (Compensatory) Event	Resultant Change in Blood H^+ and pH
Metabolic acidosis	↓ HCO_3^-	↓ Pco_2^-	H^+ ↑, pH ↓
Metabolic alkalosis	↑ HCO_3^-	↑ Pco_2 (Minimal and only with severe increase in HCO_3^-)	H^+ ↓, pH ↑
Respiratory acidosis			
Acute (24 h)	↑ $Paco_2$	Negligible ↑ HCO_3^-	H^+ ↑, pH ↓
Chronic (3–7 days or longer)	↑ $Paco_2$	Important ↑ HCO_3^-	
Respiratory alkalosis	↓ $Paco_2$	↓ HCO_3^-	H^+ ↓, pH ↑

dissociates into HCO_3^-, which is secreted back into ECF, and H+, which is exchanged for sodium from the renal tubule. This in effect causes excretion of the hydrogen ion into the urine, where it is buffered with ammonium and phosphate ions or acted on by carbonic anhydrase (in the tubule) to ultimately form CO_2 and H_2O. The CO_2 is absorbed back into the cell, where more bicarbonate can be generated to buffer ECF acidosis. If a patient has a respiratory alkalosis, available levels of CO_2 are low, causing a decrease in hydrogen excretion. Figure 8.6 shows the expected range of arterial pH, $Paco_2$, and bicarbonate concentrations for primary acid–base disturbances. Figure 8.7 shows a simplified means of determining the acid–base status of patient given pH and $Paco_2$. A line is drawn between the pH and $Paco_2$ lines and extended to the

line marked "fixed acids." If the patient has a pH of 7.1 and a $Paco_2$ of 70, she has a respiratory acidosis, because the line drawn falls within the normal range of fixed acids. If, however, she has a pH of 7.0 and a $Paco_2$ of 38, she would have a pure metabolic acidosis with no compensation. A pH of 7.5 with a $Paco_2$ of 27 characterizes a patient with respiratory alkalosis with metabolic compensation.

Primary Acid–Base Disorders

Metabolic Acidosis

Metabolic acidosis begins as a reduction in plasma HCO_3 and a rise in H+. In response to these changes, alveolar ventilation is increased, resulting in a decrease in $Paco_2$ and restoration of H+ toward normal (see Fig.

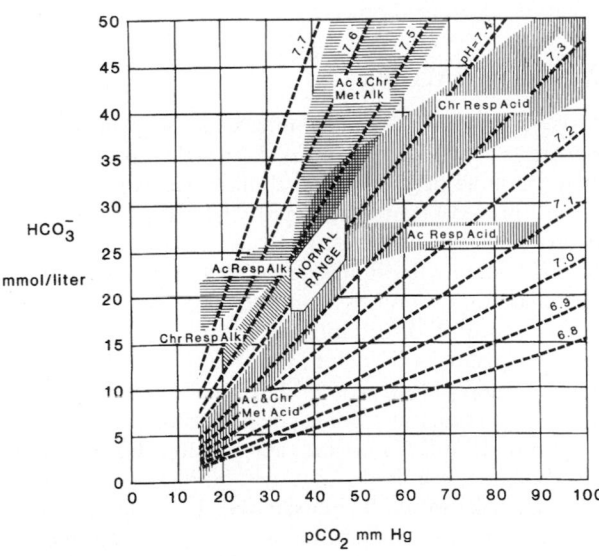

FIGURE 8.6. Range of arterial blood pH, Pco_2, and bicarbonate concentrations in the primary acid–base disturbances. The width of the bands indicates the 95% confidence limits of the range of variable. (From: Arbus GS. *Can Med Assoc J* 1973;109:291, redrawn and expanded to include chronic respiratory alkalosis, with permission.)

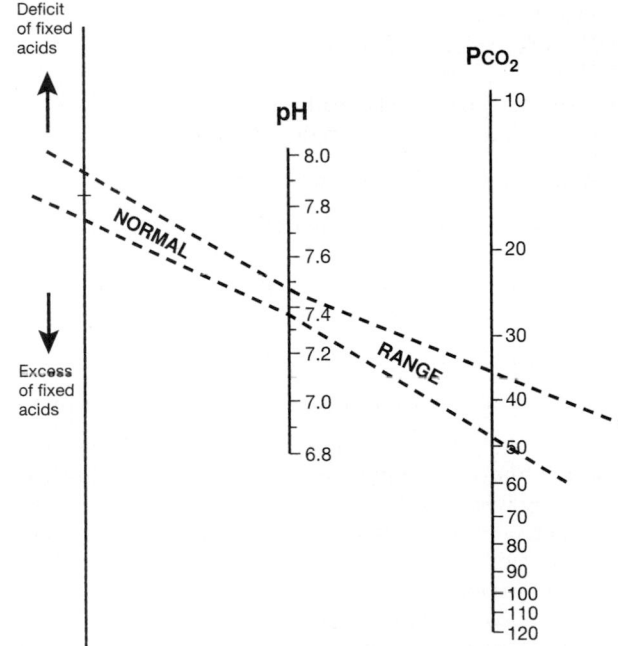

FIGURE 8.7. Normogram for acid–base disturbance.

8.6 for appropriate decrease in $PaCO_2$ for given HCO_3^- reduction in metabolic acidosis). The decrease in plasma HCO_3^- can result from the following:

- Excessive rate of production of nonvolatile acids requiring buffering by HCO_3^- (e.g., diabetic ketoacidosis, lactic acidosis, methanol ingestion)
- Normal rate of production of nonvolatile acids but a decreased ability of the kidney to regenerate the HCO_3^- consumed in the buffering reaction (e.g., chronic azotemic renal disease, distal renal tubular acidosis)
- Excessive losses of HCO_3^- (e.g., gastrointestinal losses from diarrhea, renal losses in proximal renal tubular acidosis)

CAUSES

Increase in Unmeasured Anions (Anion Gap Acidosis)

Mechanism: Increased nonvolatile acid production

- Diabetic ketoacidosis
- Alcoholic ketoacidosis
- Lactic acidosis
- Salicylate poisoning
- Ethylene glycol poisoning
- Paraldehyde poisoning
- Methanol poisoning

Mechanism: No increase in nonvolatile acid production

- Renal failure

No Increase in Unmeasured Anions (Non–Anion Gap Acidosis or Hyperchloremic Metabolic Acidosis)

Mechanism: Excessive HCO_3^- loss

- Diarrhea
- Drainage of pancreatic juice
- Ureterosigmoidostomy
- Proximal renal tubular acidosis
- Carbonic anhydrase inhibiting diuretics

Mechanism: Excessive HCl production

- Ammonium chloride, arginine HCl, or lysine HCl administration
- Intravenous hyperalimentation solution containing cationic amino acids

Mechanism: Decreased renal HCO_3^- production

- Distal renal tubular acidosis (classic and hyperkalemic)

Although classification based on rates of acid production and excretion is useful for teaching acid–base pathophysiology, it is not satisfactory as a diagnostic approach to a patient with metabolic acidosis because there are no readily available means to measure acid production or excretion. Instead, the diagnostic approach should be to determine whether the decrease in plasma HCO_3^- is associated with a normal or an increased concentration of unmeasured anion in the plasma, which is calculated as follows:

$$\text{unmeasured anion} = Na^+ \text{ in mEq/L} - (Cl^- + HCO_3^- \text{ in mEq/L})$$

Normal unmeasured anion concentration is 8 to 12 mEq/L. In health, the unmeasured anions are mostly protein anions along with small quantities of sulfate, phosphate, and organic acids. In metabolic acidosis associated with increased unmeasured anions, the increase in unmeasured anions can result from accumulation of sulfate and phosphate (as in renal failure) or nonvolatile organic acids (e.g., ketoacids, as in diabetic ketoacidosis).

In patients with metabolic acidosis, increased unmeasured anions, and increased acid production, the fall in serum bicarbonate level is a result of the rise in unmeasured anions. For example, in lactic acidosis, each lactic acid anion produced reacts with body buffers as follows:

$$H \text{ lactate} + NaHCO_3 \rightarrow Na \text{ lactate} + H_2CO_3$$
$$\downarrow$$
$$H_2O + CO_2$$

Thus, the rise in blood lactate level is accompanied by a fall in blood bicarbonate level.

In metabolic acidosis with increased unmeasured anion level and no increase in acid production (renal failure), the fall in bicarbonate level is caused by inadequate renal acid excretion (renal bicarbonate production). The rise in unmeasured anion level in renal failure is mostly the result of retention of sulfate and phosphate anions caused by the reduced renal capacity to excrete these ions by glomerular filtration.

MANAGEMENT

Moderate degrees of metabolic acidosis (plasma bicarbonate level >15 to 18 mEq/L) usually are well tolerated for short periods. If metabolic acidosis is acute and severe (plasma bicarbonate level <10 mEq/L), dyspnea, depressed cardiac function, and obtundation can result. In such a setting, it often is necessary to infuse sodium bicarbonate intravenously to correct the acidosis. The effective space of distribution of bicarbonate is approximately equal to body water (about 50% of body weight). Thus, for a 60-kg woman with severe metabolic acidosis in whom an acute increase in the plasma bicarbonate level from 6 to 10 mEq is desired, about 120 mEq of sodium bicarbonate is required (4 mEq/L H 30 L = 120 mEq). This normally would be infused over 1 to 2 hours. Bicarbonate could then be given at a slower rate until the acidosis was corrected. In general, the serum bicarbonate concentration should not be acutely raised to levels greater than 15 to 18 mEq/L. Too-rapid correction requires infusion of large amounts of sodium bicarbonate, which can cause overexpansion of the ECF and congestive heart failure. Finally, rapidly restoring the plasma bicarbonate level to normal may produce alkalosis because of persistence of a low $Paco_2$. That is, if plasma bicarbonate is rapidly restored to normal or above in the treatment of metabolic acidosis, alveolar ventilation frequently persists at elevated levels for an additional 24 to 48 hours. Thus, the low Pco_2 with normal plasma bicarbonate level can result in severe alkalosis, which, in turn, can cause cardiac arrhythmias, tetany, and seizures.

Metabolic Alkalosis
CAUSES

Mechanism: Chloride depletion and possibly ECF volume depletion (responds to sodium chloride and potassium chloride repletion)

- Vomiting
- Gastric drainage
- Certain diuretics
- Abrupt relief of hypercapnia
- Congenital chloride diarrhea
- Cystic fibrosis

Mechanism: Mineralocorticoid excess (responds to removal of mineralocorticoid or mineralocorticoid inhibition)

- Hyperaldosteronism
- Bartter's syndrome
- Cushing's syndrome
- Licorice ingestion

Mechanism: Increased renal acid excretion (responds to removal of offending mechanism)

- Milk-alkali syndrome
- Hypercalcemia

Mechanism: Massive alkali administration

- Massive blood or plasma transfusions
- Massive $NaHCO_3$ ingestion

Volume contraction with chloride depletion causes a metabolic alkalosis because of the active reabsorption of sodium and chloride. These electrolytes are exchanged for hydrogen and thus can presumably lead to alkalosis. Diuretics cause a metabolic alkalosis by inducing a sodium chloride excretion without bicarbonate, excretion of potassium, and secondary aldosteronism. The urine is usually more alkaline but may be paradoxically acidic secondary to potassium depletion. Persistent vomiting or gastric suctioning without replenishment leads to metabolic alkalosis.

Figure 8.8 depicts the normal handling of HCl and $NaHCO_3$ produced by the gastric mucosa. The initial reactants ($NaCl + H_2CO_3$, step 1) are the same as the final products ($NaCl + H_2CO_3$, step 4). Thus, gastric acid secretion normally has no net effect on acid–base regulation. If the gastric HCl is lost from the body and is not replaced, metabolic alkalosis will ensue (Fig. 8.9).

Step 1 HCl is formed and enters gastric fluid
Step 2 $NaHCO_3$ is formed and enters body fluids
Step 3 HCl moves to duodenum and reacts with $NaHCO_3$ (from bile or pancreatic fluid)
Step 4 NaCl and H_2CO_3 are formed

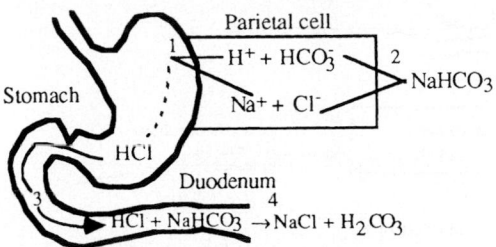

Summation: No net effect on acid–base balance since:
One H^+ and one HCO_3^- are formed in Steps 1 and 2.
One H^+ and one HCO_3^- are destroyed in Step 4.

FIGURE 8.8. Normal disposal of hydrochloric acid and sodium bicarbonate formed by gastric mucosa.

Severe potassium depletion alone also can cause metabolic alkalosis. Although the mechanism is not clearly established, severe potassium depletion appears to cause intracellular acidosis, which, at the renal tubular cell level, results in increased renal acid excretion (renal bicarbonate production) and an increased renal threshold for bicarbonate, so that the high filtered loads of bicarbonate can be retained by the kidney.

MANAGEMENT

Metabolic alkalosis can have serious consequences, such as tetany, major motor seizures, production of hypokalemia and cardiac arrhythmias (particularly in patients receiving digitalis), suppression of alveolar ventilation, and decrease in cerebral blood flow. Furthermore, the presence of metabolic alkalosis often is a sign that the patient is significantly volume contracted. For these reasons, it is important to treat metabolic alkalosis and its underlying causes. Effective treatment consists of replacing sodium, potassium, and chloride deficits as they occur, as discussed. Rarely, it is necessary to treat metabolic alkalosis with i.v. infusion of hydrochloric acid, ammonium chloride, arginine hydrochloride, or a carbonic anhydrase inhibitor (acetazolamide). This form of treatment is necessary in patients who cannot undergo the sodium bicarbonate diuresis necessary to correct the metabolic alkalosis. This inability usually is the result of severely impaired renal or cardiac function.

Respiratory Acidosis

Respiratory acidosis results from decreased alveolar ventilation, which causes decreased CO_2 excretion by the lungs and an increase in blood $Paco_2$. With acute rises in $Paco_2$, H+ rises linearly with increasing $Paco_2$ because there is little change in plasma HCO_3^- concentration. After 24 hours of hypercapnia, however, there is a significant increase in renal acid excretion (bicarbonate pro-

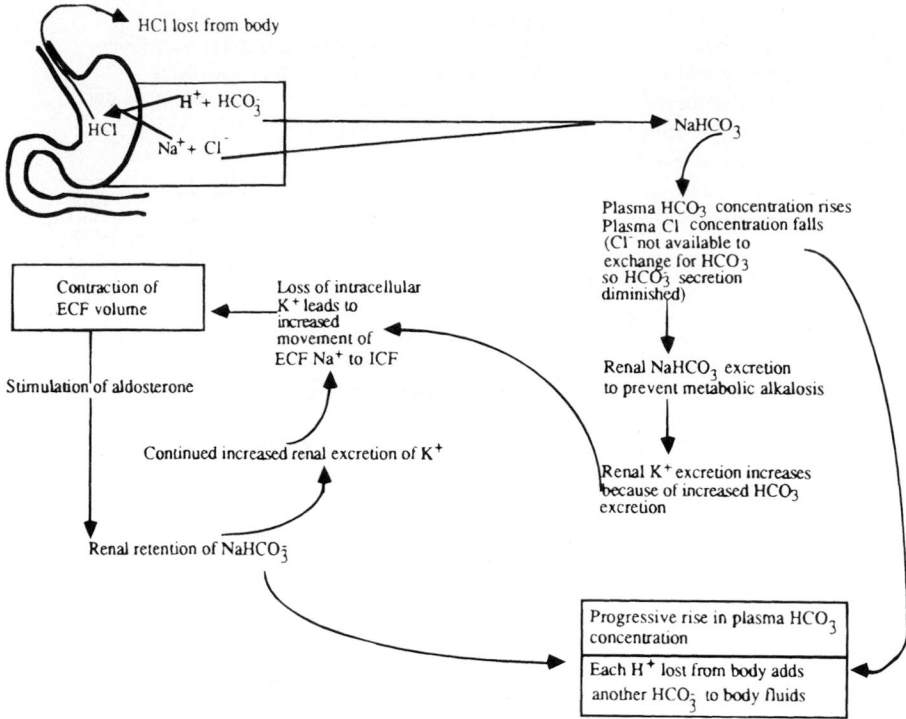

FIGURE 8.9. Pathogenesis of metabolic alkalosis from loss of gastric hydrochloric acid.

duction), which results in a rise in plasma HCO_3^- concentration and a fall in plasma $H+$. These plasma concentrations usually reach a steady state by 3 to 7 days. (See Figure 8.6 for HCO_3^- elevations appropriate for acute and chronic $Paco_2$ elevations.)

CAUSES

Mechanism: Any condition that decreases alveolar ventilation

- "Bellows" failure (e.g., respiratory muscle paralysis, fractured ribs)
- Obstructive pulmonary disease (e.g., asthma, pulmonary emphysema, foreign body in the trachea)
- Decrease in respiratory center drive (e.g., sedative drugs, oxygen therapy in chronic hypercapnia, pickwickian syndrome)

MANAGEMENT

The only way to manage respiratory acidosis is to increase alveolar ventilation (by endotracheal intubation, mechanical ventilation, or bronchodilation). Within minutes, severe respiratory acidosis can be reversed with adequate ventilation. In patients with chronic respiratory acidosis, severe posthypercapnic alkalosis develops if the $Paco_2$ is rapidly restored to normal and the patient is unable to initiate and sustain a bicarbonate diuresis. This inability usually results from sodium chloride or potassium chloride deficits. If sodium chloride or potassium chloride is provided to correct volume contraction and intracellular potassium deficits, a bicarbonate diuresis ensues and correction of metabolic alkalosis is achieved.

Respiratory Alkalosis

Respiratory alkalosis results from an increase in alveolar ventilation. This causes an increase in CO_2 excretion along with a fall in blood $Paco_2$. Concomitantly, plasma HCO_3^- is reduced primarily as a result of the action of intracellular buffers (see Fig. 8.6 for HCO_3^- concentrations appropriate for acute $Paco_2$ reductions). Symptoms of respiratory alkalosis include anxiety, paresthesia, and syncope. Blood calcium levels should be monitored because patients with respiratory alkalosis are subject to tetany from hypocalcemia.

CAUSES

Mechanism: Any condition that increases alveolar ventilation

- Hyperventilation syndrome—a manifestation of an anxiety reaction
- Hepatic failure
- Fever
- Aspirin intoxication
- CNS disorders (e.g., tumors, cerebrovascular accident, infection, trauma)
- Early sepsis
- Hypoxemia (heart failure, pulmonary emboli, restrictive lung disease, altitude, severe anemia)
- Iatrogenic causes (excessive ventilator therapy)

MANAGEMENT

The symptoms of acute respiratory alkalosis (e.g., paresthesia, light-headedness, tetany) can be rapidly controlled by raising $Paco_2$ to normal (e.g., by rebreathing into a paper bag). If the patient is being supported on a ventilator, the dead space can be increased or tidal volume and respiratory rate can be decreased while oxygenation is maintained. Definite treatment consists of removing the cause of hyperventilation. Respiratory alkalosis also can cause tetany and seizures and predispose to cardiac arrhythmias (by causing an intracellular shift of potassium), particularly in patients receiving digitalis. If the patient is septic, aggressive measures should be taken to alleviate this. She should be treated with appropriate antibiotics and adequate volume replacement. Surgery may be necessary if the patient has an abscess.

ACKNOWLEDGMENT

This chapter is based on material from: Water, Electrolyte, and Acid-Base Metabolism by Claire M. Fritsche, Lee A. Hebert, and Jacob LeMann, Jr, which appeared in the seventh edition of Te Linde's Operative Gynecology.

BIBLIOGRAPHY

Agus, Z. Hypomagnesemia. *J Am Soc Nephrol* 1999;10(7): 1616–1622.

Altura BT, Brust M, Bloom S, et al. Magnesium dietary intake modulates blood lipid levels and atherogenesis. *Proc Natl Acad Sci USA* 1990;87:1840.

American Diabetes Association. Magnesium supplementation in the treatment of diabetes. *Diabetes Care* 1992;14:1065.

Aono T, Kurachi K, Miyata M, et al. Influence of surgical stress under general anesthesia on serum gonadotropin levels. *J Clin Endocrinol Metab* 1976;42:144.

Arbus GS. An in vivo acid–base nomogram for clinical use. *Can Med Assoc J* 1973:109:291.

Arieff AI. Hyponatremia, convulsions, respiratory arrest, and permanent brain damage after elective surgery in healthy women. *N Engl J Med* 1986;314:1529.

Arieff AI, deFronzo RA. *Fluid, electrolyte and acid–base disorders.* New York: Churchill Livingstone, 1985.

Ayus JC, Krothapalli RK, Arieff AI. Treatment of symptomatic hyponatremia and its relation to brain damage: a prospective study. *N Engl J Med* 1987;317:1190.

Beutler B, Cerami A. Cachectin and tumor necrosis factor as two sides of the same biological coin. *Nature* 1986;320: 584.

Bilezikian JP. Management of acute hypercalcemia. *N Engl J Med* 1992;326:1196.

Breen, P. Arterial blood gas and pH analysis: clinical approach and interpretation. *Anesthesiol Clin North Am* 2001;19(4): 885–906.

Brown JM, Grosso MA, et al. Cytokines, sepsis and the surgeon. *Surg Gynecol Obstet* 1989;169:568.

Claes Y, Van Hemelrijck J, Van Gerven M, et al. Influence of hydroxyethyl starch on coagulation in patients during the perioperative period. *Anesthesiol Analg* 1992;75:24.

Claybaugh JR, Share L. Vasopressin, renin, and cardiovascular responses to continuous slow hemorrhage. *Am J Physiol* 1973;224:519.

Cockcroft DW, Gault MH. Prediction of creatinine clearance from serum creatinine. *Nephron* 1976;16:31.

Cohen JJ, Kassirer JP. *Acid base.* Boston: Little, Brown, 1982.

Dacey, M. Endocrine and metabolic dysfunction syndromes in the critically ill. Hypomagnesemic disorders. *Crit Care Clin* 2001;17(1):155–173.

Epstein FH. Signs and symptoms of electrolyte disorders. In: Maxwell MH, Kleeman CR, eds. *Clinical disorders of fluid and electrolyte metabolism.* New York: McGraw-Hill, 1980.

Fisken RA, Heath DA, Somers S, et al. Hypercalcemia in hospital patients: clinical and diagnostic aspects. *Lancet* 1981;1:202.

Fuss M, Cogan E, Gillet C, et al. Magnesium administration reverses the hypocalcaemia secondary to hypomagnesemia despite low circulating levels of 25-hydroxyvitamin D and 1,25-dihydroxyvitamin D. *Endocrinology* 1985;22:807.

Golzarian J, Scott WH. Hypermagnesemia induced paralytic ileus. *Dig Dis Sci* 1994;39:1138.

Harrington JL. Metabolic alkalosis. *Kidney Int* 1984;26:88.

Heinsimer JA, Lefkowitz RJ. Adrenergic receptors: biochemistry, regulation, molecular mechanisms and clinical indications. *J Lab Clin Med* 1982;100:641.

Kapoor M, Chan G. Fluid and electrolyte abnormalities. *Crit Care Clin* 2001;17(3):503–529.

Kendler KS, Weitzman RE, Fisher DA. The effect of pain on plasma arginine vasopressin concentrations in man. *Clin Endocrinol* 1978;8:89.

Klahr S. *The kidney and body fluids in health and disease.* New York: Plenum, 1984.

Klee GG, Kao PC, Heath H III. Hypercalcemia. *Endocrinol Metab Clin North Am* 1988;573:600.

Knochel JP. Neuromuscular manifestation of electrolyte disorder. *Am J Med* 1982;72:521.

Lennon EJ, Lemann J Jr. Fluid and electrolyte balance. In: Te Linde RW, Mattingly RF, eds. *Operative gynecology,* 6th ed. Philadelphia: JB Lippincott, 1985.

Leone BJ, Spahn DR. Anemia, hemodilution, and oxygen delivery. *Anesthesiol Analg* 1992;75:651.

Levi M, et al. Disorders of phosphate and magnesium metabolism. In: Coe FC, Favus, MJ, eds. *Disorders of bone and mineral metabolism.* New York: Raven, 1992:587.

Martinez F, Lash R. Intensive care unit complications: endocrinologic and metabolic complications in the intensive care unit. *Clin Chest Med* 1999;20(2):401–422.

Matthay MA. Invasive hemodynamic monitoring in critically ill patients. *Clin Chest Med* 1983;4:233.

Maxwell MH, Kleeman CR, Narins RG. *Clinical disorders of fluid and electrolyte metabolism,* 4th ed. New York: McGraw-Hill, 1987.

Narins RG. Therapy of hyponatremia: does haste make waste? *N Engl J Med* 1986;314:1573.

Narins RG, Emmett M. Simple and mixed acid–base disorders: a practical approach. *Medicine* 1980;59:161.

Ponce SP, Jennings AE, Madias NE, et al. Drug-induced hyperkalemia. *Medicine* 1985;64:357.

Riggs, JE. Neurologic manifestations of electrolyte disturbances. *Neurol Clin* 2002;20(1):227–239.

Roacha E, Silva M, Velasco IT, et al. Hypertonic saline resuscitation: saturated salt-dextran solutions are equally effective, but induce hemolysis in dogs. *Crit Care Med* 1990;18:203.

Robertson G, Aycinesa P, Zerbe R. Neurogenic disorders of osmoregulation. *Am J Med* 1986;2:339.

Schrier RW, ed. *Renal and electrolyte disorders,* 2nd ed. Boston: Little, Brown, 1980.

Schrier RW. Pathogenesis of sodium and water retention in high-output and low-output cardiac failure, nephrotic syndrome, cirrhosis and pregnancy. *N Engl J Med* 1988;319: 1065.

Skillman JJ, Lauler DP, et al. Hemorrhage in normal man: effect of renin, cortisol, aldosterone, and urine composition. *Ann Surg* 1967;166:865.

Slotman GJ, Burchard KW, et al. Thromboxane and prostacyclin in clinical acute respiratory failure. *J Eur Res* 1985;39:1.

Spiegel A. The parathyroid glands: hypercalcemia and hypocalcemia. In: Goldman L, ed. *Cecil textbook of medicine,* 21st ed. Philadelphia: WB Saunders 2000:1399–1406.

Steiner RW. Interpreting the fractional excretion of sodium. *Am J Med* 1984;77:699

Waters J, Miller L. Cause of metabolic acidosis in prolonged surgery. *Crit Care Med* 1999;27(10):2142–2146.

Williams SE. Hydrogen ion infusion for treating severe metabolic alkalosis. *BMJ* 1976;2:1189.

Ziegler, R. Hypercalcemic crisis. *J Am Soc Nephrol* 2001; 12(17 Suppl):S3–S9.

Te Linde's Operative Gynecology, ninth edition, edited by John A. Rock and Howard W. Jones, III. Lippincott Williams & Wilkins, Philadelphia: © 2003.

CHAPTER
9

Postoperative Infections: Prevention and Management

W. DAVID HAGER

Infection complicating surgical procedures has been the consternation of gynecologists since the first operations were performed. Even when medical and surgical care are beyond reproach, infectious morbidity can complicate the postoperative course. Unfortunately, using antibiotics prophylactically at the time of surgery does not eliminate this risk of infection.

It is imperative that the gynecologic surgeon understand basic infectious disease concepts to treat infected patients appropriately. Diagnosis and treatment are not guess work but depend on understanding basic principles.

An understanding of bacteria that are a part of the normal vaginal flora enables the gynecologist to recognize the pathogenic bacteria that contribute to postoperative infection. Certain risk factors play a role in increasing postoperative infection rates. A knowledge of these factors can enable the surgeon to take action to alter those risks. There are various types of postoperative infection, each with its own unique time of onset and usual bacterial etiology. Knowledge about likely causes of a disorder can facilitate decision making when an antibiotic is empirically selected to treat the patient.

Appropriate patient evaluation, including proper culturing techniques, is critical to this diagnostic process. Steps to prevent infection must become routine with every surgeon on every case. These steps are necessary not only for the operator, but also for all personnel participating in the surgical and medical treatment of the patient. These steps are described later in this chapter.

DEFINITIONS

In the evaluation of patients who have an elevated temperature in the postoperative period, it is important to recognize that all febrile morbidity is not infectious morbidity. Treating a fever without a definite cause of infection may do more harm than good.

Several different definitions of febrile morbidity have been used, and this may create confusion for the surgeon. The most frequent definition is a temperature of 38°C (100.4°F) or greater recorded on two occasions, at least 6 hours apart, more than 24 hours after the surgical procedure. This excludes a fever during the first 24 hours. Operative site infections during this time are unusual unless there is preexisting infection at the operative site or gross contamination of the site. Some investigators have used a definition of a single temperature elevation of 39°C (101°F) or greater recorded on any occasion in the postoperative period as indicative of febrile morbidity. We prefer the former definition.

Regardless of the choice of definition of febrile morbidity, it is important to treat infection and not fever. Fever may trigger sensitivity to the possibility of infection, but a positive culture or the presence of definite clinical criteria should be present before a diagnosis is made and treatment initiated.

INCIDENCE

In evaluating the incidence of postoperative infection in published studies, it is important to consider whether infectious morbidity or febrile morbidity was used to define infection, what the socioeconomic status of the population studied was, whether antibiotic prophylaxis was used, and whether there were other confounding variables that might have influenced infection rates (e.g., multiple surgical procedures, experience of the surgeon, or site of the study).

Prospective studies report the incidence of acute pelvic infection after abdominal hysterectomy to be 3.9% to 50%. The range for infection after vaginal hysterectomy is 1.7% to 64%. The incidence of septic pelvic thrombophlebitis (SPT) after gynecologic procedures is 0.1% to 0.5%.

VAGINAL FLORA

The most frequent source of bacteria that cause postoperative pelvic infection among women is the vagina. The vagina is colonized by large numbers of a variety of bacteria that normally exist in a symbiotic relationship. Several factors influence the vaginal flora, including age, sexual activity, stage of the menstrual cycle, use of antibiotic or immunosuppressive agents, and any invasive procedure.

Mean bacterial counts in vaginal secretions are 10^8 to 10^9 bacteria/mL, with three to six different species present. The most frequent aerobic bacteria are *Lactobacilli* sp, *Gardnerella vaginalis*, *Staphylococcus epidermidis*, *Corynebacterium* sp, *Enterococcus faecalis* species of *Streptococcus*, and *Enterobacteriaceae*. Anaerobes outnumber aerobes and include *Peptostreptococcus* sp, *Peptococcus* sp, *Prevotella biviua*, *Prevotella disiens*, and members of the *Bacteroides fragilis* group (Table 9.1). These same bacteria are frequently isolated from sites of pelvic infection among women who have undergone gynecologic surgery. This indicates, as Schottmueller proposed at the turn of the century, that pelvic infections are principally a result of endogenous sources of bacteria. The concepts of antibiotic prophylaxis and antiseptic douching before surgery or preoperative placement of antiseptic gel are related to reducing these large numbers of bacteria. Although investigators have found that colonization rates change in relation to the stage of the menstrual cycle, no data have supported the concept that timing of gynecologic surgery in relation to menses alters infection rates.

Surgery itself alters the numbers and types of bacteria in the vagina and cervix. After vaginal and abdominal hysterectomy, the number of lactobacilli decreases, and the number of facultative Gram-negative rods, *B fragilis* group species, and enterococci increases. Preoperative

TABLE 9.1.
Bacteria Composing Normal Vaginal Flora

AEROBES	ANAEROBES
Staphylococcus aureus	*Peptostreptococcus* sp
Staphylococcus epidermidis	*Peptococcus* sp
Group B streptococcus	*Bacteroides* sp
Streptococcus sp	*Fusobacterium* sp
Enterococcus faecalis	*Prevotella bivia*
Lactobacilli	*Prevotella disiens*
Corynebacterium sp	*Bacteroides fragilis* group
Escherichia coli	
Klebsiella sp	
Gardnerella vaginalis	

hospitalization before surgery on a gynecologic ward also alters the vaginal flora in a direction toward more virulent organisms.

RISK FACTORS FOR INFECTION

Several factors may increase the infectious morbidity of postoperative patients (Table 9.2). Of all the factors mentioned, the most basic appears to be immunocompromise. Anything that plays a role in altering the host's own defense mechanisms can result in a greater chance of infectious morbidity.

Some risk factors can be controlled by the surgeon, whereas others cannot be influenced by the surgeon or operative team and must be dealt with as they occur. Lower socioeconomic status is a risk factor for infection in gynecologic surgery. Although the focus is on economic condition, the greatest effect may be a result of inadequate nutrition and poor hygiene. Obesity is a risk factor for gynecologic infection, probably reflecting poor hygiene, altered nutrition, risk of diabetes, and prolonged operative time. These result in altered wound healing and greater possibilities for infection.

When a hysterectomy is performed through an infected operative site, there is an increased risk of postoperative infection. Likewise, contamination of the operative field by break in sterile technique or injury to the bowel promotes infection. Young age has been considered a risk factor for posthysterectomy infection, although the exact reason is unclear. This increased risk in younger patients may result from the presence of more virulent bacteria in the vagina or vascularity and difficulty in obtaining adequate hemostasis. Other factors are not as clear-cut and may result from interacting effects. For example, duration of surgery is considered to be a risk for infection in most studies, but this actually may reflect experience of the operating surgeon, complexity of the case, or a greater chance of inadequate hemostasis. Lack of adequate hemostasis increases the risk of undrained collections of blood and creates an ideal culture medium for contaminating bacteria. Low hemoglobin and hematocrit levels, preoperatively or postoperatively, have been

TABLE 9.2.
Risk Factors for Postoperative Infection

Altered immunocompetence
Premenopausal age
Obesity
Radical surgery
Bacterial vaginosis
Prolonged preoperative hospitalization
Excessive intraoperative blood loss
Operative inexperience
Lower socioeconomic status
Prolonged operative time
Poor nutrition
Excessive devitalized tissue
Diabetes mellitus
Failure to use prophylactic antibiotics
Surgery in an infected operative site

TABLE 9.3.
Pathogens Responsible for Infections After Gynecologic Surgery

AEROBIC GRAM-POSITIVE COCCI	ANAEROBES
Staphylococcus aureus	*Peptostreptococcus* sp
Staphylococcus epidermidis	*Peptococcus* sp
Streptococcus viridans group	*Prevotella bivia*
Group B streptococci	*Prevotella disiens*
Streptococcus faecalis	*Bacteroides melaninogenicus*
	Bacteroides capillosus
AEROBIC GRAM-NEGATIVE BACILLI	*Bacteroides fragilis* group
	B fragilis
Escherichia coli	*B ovatus*
Proteus mirabilis	*B thetaiotaomicron*
Klebsiella sp	*B distasonis*
Gardnerella vaginalis	*B vulgatus*
	Clostridium perfringens
	Fusobacterium sp

mentioned as factors in increased rates of postoperative infection, especially of abdominal incisions. No data, however, have indicated that raising the volume of red blood cells decreases the rate of infection. Leaving an excessive amount of devitalized tissue (e.g., large, ligated pedicles) can predispose to a greater risk of infection. Pedicles should be trim and dry, dead space should be closed, and hemostasis obtained.

Failure to use antibiotic prophylaxis in situations in which they have been shown to be beneficial may be a risk for pelvic infection. Prophylactic antibiotics should be used according to the accepted protocol for that procedure. The use of a vaginal cuff drain has been shown to have a significant beneficial effect on decreasing morbidity but has fallen out of favor because of the simplicity and effectiveness of antibiotic prophylaxis.

Bacterial vaginosis, characterized by increased vaginal concentrations of certain anaerobic and facultative bacteria, has been shown to increase the relative risk of postoperative infection in gynecologic procedures. The presence of increased concentrations of pathogenic bacteria adjacent to the site of incision in the vagina allows for ascending spread of these organisms in a susceptible host. Although treatment of bacterial vaginosis in pregnant women decreases their risk of preterm delivery and preterm, premature rupture of membranes, no studies have shown a decreased rate of postoperative infection in women treated before gynecologic surgery.

ETIOLOGY

All women have bacteria colonizing the vagina in greater or lesser numbers. Women without symptoms have a mean of 4.2 species present. It is these same bacteria normally existing in a symbiotic relationship that ultimately can invade tissue altered by surgery, leading to clinical infection. The virulence of the bacteria and the volume inoculated are countered by the host's immune defense mechanisms and may be aided by prophylactic antibiotics to combat the occurrence of infection.

The bacteria listed in Table 9.3, which are responsible for postoperative infection after gynecologic surgery, are the same organisms that can be recovered from vaginal cultures of women before hysterectomy, according to Hemsell. The volume of bacteria present and their proximity to the operative site promote a polymicrobial infection in women who experience posthysterectomy infectious morbidity. Aerobic bacteria may initiate the infectious process; as tissue is devitalized and the oxidation reduction potential is altered, anaerobes proliferate and add to the tissue damage. Large, necrotic tissue pedicles and undrained collections of blood are ideal sites for infection to occur. Once the infection has begun, the body's host immune defense mechanisms initiate an inflammatory response and attempt to wall off and localize the infection. Infected hematomas and abscesses can result.

CATEGORIES OF INFECTION

Not all women who have temperature elevation after gynecologic surgery are infected, and not all of those who are infected have the same clinical syndrome. It is important to categorize the infectious process because treatment can vary accordingly.

Cuff Cellulitis

Cuff cellulitis is an infection of the surgical margin in the upper vagina where the uterus was removed. Symptoms and signs of infection usually begin late in the hospital course or even after discharge from the hospital. These patients' immediate postoperative course may have been completely benign. There is always an element of induration, erythema, and edema in the vaginal cuff immediately after hysterectomy. If the patient becomes infected, she will often have initial complaints of lower abdominal pain, pelvic pain, back pain, fever, and abnormal vaginal discharge. Examination may reveal persistent hyperemia, induration, and tenderness of the vaginal cuff and possibly purulent discharge along with fever. The parametrial and adnexal areas are nontender. The white blood cell count usually is mildly to moderately elevated.

Gram-positive aerobes, facultative Gram-negative aerobes, and anaerobes can all contribute to the cause of cuff cellulitis. Single- or multiple-agent broad-spectrum coverage is effective in treating this infection, although single agents usually are preferred.

Infected Vaginal Cuff Hematoma or Cuff Abscess

Hysterectomy can result in small amounts of oozing from vascular pedicles or along the vaginal cuff. This bleeding may result in a walled-off collection of blood called a hematoma. If this localized mass above the vaginal cuff becomes infected, an abscess results. Bacteria, especially anaerobes, flourish in this environment.

Women with a vaginal cuff abscess present with fever early in the postoperative period. Other symptoms include chills, pelvic pain, and rectal pressure. Clinical findings include temperature elevation; lower abdominal and vaginal cuff tenderness; the presence of a tender, fluctuant mass near the cuff; and, occasionally, purulent drainage from the cuff. The pain and tenderness is often more predominant on one side.

An infected cuff hematoma actually can present later in the postoperative course than an abscess and usually is associated with a drop in the hemoglobin and hematocrit levels. The hematoma may not be readily palpable but can be delineated on pelvic ultrasound or computed tomographic (CT) scan.

Postoperative Ovarian Abscess

The patient who develops fever and abdominal and pelvic pain late in the postoperative hospital course or after hospital discharge may have a pelvic abscess, probably of ovarian origin. If there is a sudden increase in abdominal or pelvic pain, a rupture may have occurred. A ruptured abscess should be managed as a surgical emergency with a laparotomy and excision or drainage of the infected mass. The inciting site for an ovarian abscess is a place of recent follicle expulsion or a site of surgical trauma to an ovary in a premenopausal woman. Ovaries should not be aspirated or probed at the time of hysterectomy for fear that bacteria from the vagina may penetrate the ovary and initiate infection. Once again, anaerobes are the predominant bacteria in an ovarian abscess.

If an ovarian abscess is suspected, then a CT scan should be ordered. The CT scan not only identifies the size and location of the abscess but also allows for visualization and evaluation of the ureters, bladder, and colon. A pelvic ultrasound also may be useful to localize the abscess. Many abscesses respond to broad-spectrum antibiotic therapy; but if a tender, fluctuant mass persists, drainage is necessary. A radiologic interventionist may be able to accomplish percutaneous drainage with a needle or catheter using CT or ultrasound guidance, or colpotomy drainage may be possible. For colpotomy drainage to be accomplished safely, the abscess must be fluctuant, fixed in the cul-de-sac, and dissecting the upper third of the rectovaginal septum. With either approach, a closed-suction drain should be placed to ensure complete and continued evacuation during the next 2 to 3 days.

Septic Pelvic Thrombophlebitis

Septic pelvic thrombophlebitis complicates gynecologic surgery in 0.1% to 0.5% of procedures. It is a diagnosis of exclusion, made when a postoperative patient with febrile morbidity does not respond to appropriate parenteral antibiotic therapy in the absence of an undrained abscess or infected hematoma. The development of SPT is enhanced by venous stasis (e.g., obesity, diabetes), vascular injury, or bacterial contamination of pelvic vessels.

Two forms of SPT have been described. The *classic form* is seen in association with abdominal surgery. This form occurs 2 to 4 days after surgery and is characterized by fever, tachycardia, gastrointestinal distress, unilateral abdominal pain, and, in 50% to 67% of cases, a palpable abdominal cord resulting from acute thrombus formation. The *enigmatic form* complicates vaginal delivery or pelvic surgery and is characterized by spiking temperatures despite clinical improvement on antibiotics; tachycardia during the temperature spikes; and small, diffusely scattered thrombi in small pelvic vessels. Pelvic findings are minimal in both forms.

The diagnosis often may be confirmed by CT scan or magnetic resonance imaging.

The mainstay of treatment for SPT is anticoagulation with heparin for 7 to 10 days. Some experts recommend changing antibiotics or extending coverage before heparin is considered. All patients should be treated with antibiotics effective against heparinase-producing *Bacteroides* sp. Long-term anticoagulation is not required unless septic pulmonary emboli have occurred. Lysis of fever may occur 24 to 48 hours after starting heparin, yet other cases may require much longer for complete resolution. Treatment should be continued until the patient is afebrile for 48 hours and clinically well.

Osteomyelitis Pubis

Osteomyelitis pubis rarely complicates gynecologic procedures adjacent to the symphysis pubis, such as retropubic urethral suspension, radical vulvectomy, or pelvic exenteration. Direct or contiguous seeding of the periosteum from pelvic bacteria results in a delayed-onset infection 6 to 8 weeks after the original procedure. Patients complain of pain and tenderness along the symphysis pubis, especially with ambulation. Low-grade fever, an elevated erythrocyte sedimentation rate, and a moderate leukocytosis have been reported as well as positive cultures from blood or the bone itself. Aggressive antibiotic therapy covering *Staphylococcus aureus* and facultative Gram-negative bacilli is essential for adequate recovery. If the response is not adequate, surgical debridement of the pubis is necessary.

Wound Infection

Surgical wound infection is possible with any transabdominal gynecologic procedure, but especially with those that are contaminated. Extensive study of the epidemiology of wound infections resulted in a classification of operative wounds in relation to contamination and increasing risk of infection (Table 9.4). Because the vagina is entered during hysterectomy, even an uninfected hysterectomy is classified as a clean-contaminated operation.

The rates of wound infection according to case classification of the operative wound are summarized in Table 9.5. Culver and colleagues, using the National Nosocomial Infections Surveillance System, reported the percentage of operations in the United States by wound class and the surgical wound infection rate per 100 operations to be 2.1% for clean, 3.3% for clean-contaminated, 6.4% for contaminated, and 7.1% for dirty or infected cases. The more contaminated the operative site, the greater is the risk of wound infection. Fortunately, despite polymicrobial contamination by bacteria from the vagina when it is entered at the time of hysterectomy, prophylactic antibiotics, adequate host resistance, and good surgical technique result in most patients avoiding wound infection.

The Centers for Disease Control and Prevention (CDC) definitions of surgical wound infection were modified by Horan et al. This system divides infections into two major categories: (1) an organ/space surgical site infection (SSI), and (2) superficial and deep incision infection. A SSI is any anatomy that is opened or manipulated during a surgical procedure other than the incision itself. This would include most of the infections that develop after hysterectomy. It must develop within 30 days of the procedure and be accompanied by one of the following: diagnosis by a surgeon or attending physician; an abscess or other evidence of infection identified during re-operation or by radiologic or histopathologic examination; aseptically obtained organ/space fluid or tissue, the culture of which resulted in bacterial isolates; or purulent drainage from a drain placed through a stab wound into the organ/space.

Wound Cellulitis

Abdominal wound infections are categorized by their location and severity. The least severe are localized to the skin and adipose tissue above the fascia. Wound cellulitis is characterized by erythema, warmth, and swelling as well as tenderness. If there is no purulent drainage, antibiotic therapy alone with a cephalosporin or augmented penicillin often is effective. *Staphylococcus aureus,* coagulase-negative *Staphylococci,* and *Streptococci* cause most of these infections.

TABLE 9.4.
Classification of Operative Wounds in Relation to Contamination and Increasing Risk of Infection

CLEAN

Elective, primarily closed and undrained
Nontraumatic, uninfected
No inflammation encountered
No break in aseptic technique
Respiratory, alimentary, genitourinary tracts not entered

CLEAN-CONTAMINATED

Alimentary, respiratory, or genitourinary tract entered under controlled conditions and without unusual contamination
Appendectomy
Vagina entered
Genitourinary tract entered in absence of culture-positive urine
Minor break in technique
Mechanical drainage

CONTAMINATED

Open, fresh traumatic wounds
Gross spillage from gastrointestinal tract
Entrance of genitourinary tract in presence of infected urine
Major break in technique
Incisions in which acute nonpurulent inflammation is present

DIRTY OR INFECTED

Traumatic wound with retained devitalized tissue, foreign bodies, fecal contamination, or delayed treatment, or wounds from a dirty source
Perforated viscus encountered
Acute bacterial inflammation with pus encountered during operation

Source: Altemeier WA, Burke JF, Pruitt BA, et al. *Manual on control of infection in surgical patients,* 2nd ed. Philadelphia: JB Lippincott, 1984:28, with permission.

Wound Seroma

A collection of serous fluid beneath the skin surface is a seroma. A small amount of serous drainage may be managed with limited opening of the incision, drainage, and cleansing.

Deep Wound Infection

When purulent drainage is noted, the wound should be opened widely to allow drainage and removal of necrotic tissue. The incision should be probed gently to evaluate fascial integrity. If the fascia is intact, healing is hastened by mechanical debridement followed by loose, wet to dry packing with gauze moistened with saline; dilute hydrogen peroxide (1:1 mixture with saline) or Dakin's solution, 0.5%. Povidone-iodine is to be discouraged because it does not promote the development of granulation tissue. An antibiotic effective against anaerobes must be used.

Evisceration of bowel may occur if the infection involves the fascia. This is a surgical emergency requiring

TABLE 9.5.
Surgical Wound Infection Rates in 84,691 Operations by Traditional Wound Classification Score

Wound Class	Operations (%)	Surgical Wound Infection Rate (per 100 Operations)
Clean	58	2.1
Clean-contaminated	36	3.3
Contaminated	4	6.4
Dirty or infected	2	7.1

Source: Culver DH, Horan TC, Gaynes RP. Surgical wound infection rates by wound class, operative procedure and patient risk index. *Am J Med* 1991;91:152S, with permission.

identification of the defect, freshening of the fascial edges, placement of intraabdominal and subcutaneous closed suction drains, and reinforced closure of the fascia. Some surgeons would leave the skin open for delayed closure, others would close it primarily.

Necrotizing Fascitis

This severe complication results from synergistic bacterial infection of the fascia, subcutaneous tissue, and skin. It is seen more frequently in diabetic and immunocompromised patients. Patients present with severe pain in the area of involvement; clinical signs of sepsis; and a viscous, cloudy, malodorous drainage. The wound edges may be purple or even necrotic. If gangrene occurs in the area of fascitis, bullae of the skin and crepitus in the subcutaneous tissue may be seen. Treatment includes antibiotics effective against streptococci and anaerobes plus prompt and extensive resection of the tissue involved.

Urinary Tract Infection

Infection of the lower urinary tract is a frequent complication of gynecologic surgery. The patient can have low-grade fever, dysuria, frequency, and urgency, but in many situations has no symptoms. The criterion for defining a urinary tract infection (UTI) is more than 100,000 colonies/mL of a single pathogen. Appropriate insertion and management of indwelling catheters are important in preventing UTI. Catheters should be removed as soon as possible after surgery, and when bladder suspension procedures are done, self-catheterization should be taught. Treatment of a documented UTI should be with an appropriate oral or parenteral antibiotic. The quinolone antibiotics offer the broadest spectrum of coverage for urinary pathogens.

Bacteremia

Infection of the bloodstream can complicate any pelvic infection, but is seen more frequently in association with abscesses, peritonitis, and SPT. Antibiotics effective against the isolated organism should be used. Treatment beyond 5 to 7 days usually is not necessary to eradicate the offending pathogen.

Drug Fever

This diagnosis should be considered when appropriate parenteral antibiotics have been used, there are no localizing signs of infection and no undrained collection of fluid. Fevers are usually steady and not spiking in character. Most patients exhibit an eosinophilia. The antibiotic(s) should be discontinued.

EVALUATION OF THE PATIENT WITH SUSPECTED INFECTION

Fever is the most common sign of postoperative infection, but it is important to remember that fever is not always, or indeed not usually, caused by infection in the postoperative patient (Table 9.6). In a large study of 537 women who underwent major gynecologic surgery, Fanning et al. found that 39% developed postoperative fever, but only 17 patients (8%) actually had a documented infection. Other signs and symptoms of postoperative infection can include erythema, induration, and/or tenderness around the incision, drain, or intravenous infusion site, leg pain, tenderness or swelling, costovertebral angle (CVA) tenderness, cough, or dysuria. When any of these or other signs or symptoms alerts the surgeon to the possibility of a postoperative infection, an appropriate workup is indicated. A diagnosis of infection

TABLE 9.6.
Fever Evaluation in Gynecologic Patients

HISTORY

Time of onset
Surgical procedure
Risk factors
Antibiotic prophylaxis
Symptoms
Ancillary illnesses

PHYSICAL EXAMINATION

Upper respiratory
Lower respiratory
Gastrointestinal
Urinary tract
Wound
Pelvis

LABORATORY

Complete blood cell count with differential
Catheterized urinalysis
Chemistry panel
Cultures
    Urine
    Blood
    Surgical site

should be made or at least a high probability of infection should be present before antibiotics are started. The practice of treating a postoperative fever with broad spectrum antibiotics before a workup has been done or a diagnosis of infection made is to be condemned.

History

Careful history taking often can be the source of helpful clues to the cause of postoperative infection. The time of onset of the complicating infection is important. Ledger emphasized that the interval between surgery and the onset of fever is helpful in determining the cause of infection. For example, Garibaldi and colleagues suggested that most cases of early postoperative fever are not infectious in origin. Possible noninfectious causes include pulmonary atelectasis, hypersensitivity reactions to antibiotics or anesthetics, pyrogenic reactions to tissue trauma, or hematoma formation. Infectious causes of early postoperative fever include aspiration pneumonia, group A α-hemolytic streptococcal wound infection, or surgery in a previously infected site (e.g., pelvic inflammatory disease or recent D&C or cone biopsy). Other important aspects of history include the surgical procedures performed (e.g., abdominal versus vaginal approach, whether ovaries were invaded), risk factors encountered (pelvic abscess, bowel injury), use of antibiotic prophylaxis, symptoms, and whether the patient had any ancillary illnesses (smoking history, history of cardiac valvular disease, immunosuppression).

Physical Examination

Gynecologic surgeons tend to focus on the pelvis as the source of all postoperative infections. Instead, a comprehensive evaluation of the entire patient should be carried out. The upper respiratory tract should be examined to rule out otitis, pharyngitis, and bronchitis and the lower respiratory tract to rule out pneumonia. The gastrointestinal tract should be checked to evaluate bowel function, distention, and tenderness. Breast examination is usually only important in postpartum patients. The urinary tract should be evaluated, and the possibility of pyelonephritis must be considered. Intravenous needles, especially central lines or other indwelling foreign bodies, should be carefully inspected and palpated for evidence of infection. The surgical wound must be examined carefully, and if the site of infection has not been identified or symptoms suggest a pelvic infection, a pelvic examination should be carried out. The pelvic examination should evaluate the vaginal cuff for discharge, erythema, and induration. Palpation for tenderness and for masses should be done and cultures obtained if pus is identified.

Laboratory and Imaging Evaluation

In recent years, it has become clear that a routine postoperative "fever workup" including a variety of studies such as a complete blood count, urine analysis, chest x-ray, and multiple cultures is largely unrewarding in identifying the site of postoperative infections. A careful history and physical examination are the best guides to which laboratory tests, if any, are indicated. In a retrospective review of 257 patients who underwent major gynecologic surgery, Lyon et al. found that a urine culture was positive in only 9% of the patients who were cultured and less than 2% of all febrile patients. Fewer chest x-rays were ordered, and they were almost always negative with only 1.5% of all febrile patients having a significant finding. Similar results were described by Fanning who also noted that none of the 77 blood cultures in their series of 211 febrile postoperative patients was positive.

In a follow-up study, Schwandt, Andrews, and Fanning outlined a protocol for evaluating postoperative gynecological patients as follows: (a) record temperatures every 4 hours; (b) for temperatures greater than 38°C (100.4°F), evaluate the patient by history and physical examination; (c) when no significant signs or symptoms are identified, order no tests, and observe the patient. Antibiotics are not started at this point. A total of 105 consecutive postoperative patients were evaluated with this protocol. Twenty-eight patients (27%) had a fever of 38.5°C or higher on two occasions greater than 4 hours apart, excluding the night of surgery. Of these patients, only five had laboratory tests; five urine cultures, one chest x-ray, and two blood cultures. There were four documented urinary tract infections in the five urine cultures and one of those patients also had pneumonia with a positive chest x-ray. Neither of the blood cultures was positive. In addition, two women were diagnosed and successfully treated with oral antibiotics for urinary tract infections following discharge. The authors felt that this protocol of selectively ordering lab tests to evaluate a postoperative fever did not compromise patient care and saved considerable resources. Similar findings also have been reported in a retrospective review by McNally et al.

Although current practice discourages the use of "routine" testing to evaluate a postoperative fever, the clinician must be sensitive to special circumstances, unusual signs or symptoms, or persistent fever or other warning signs. Special circumstances could include a patient who was at high risk for infection because of immunosuppression, gross bacterial contamination at surgery, infection already present prior to surgery, or patient in such a frail or unstable condition that any postoperative infection could be fatal. Unusual signs or symptoms, which include evidence of necrotizing fasciitis or gasforming organisms and, most common of all, persistence of fever or other signs or symptoms of infection, definitely warrant a more exhaustive evaluation and, in most cases, prompt, aggressive therapy.

A complete blood count with differential usually is indicated, and electrolytes, renal function tests, and liver-associated tests may be useful if sepsis is anticipated, prior damage to these organs exists, and/or antibiotics excreted or metabolized by these organs may be used. Acute pancreatitis can be ruled out by a normal serum acid phophatase.

Blood cultures are rarely indicated; but in patients with high fever, those with persistent fever despite antibiotics, or the immunocompromised patient they may be useful. This is particularly true when patients have indwelling central lines for longer than a few days, especially if these lines have been used for several functions (blood transfusions, antibiotics, electrolytes, etc.), and/or the patient had bacteremia that could seed the tip of the line. In these cases, at least one culture should be taken through the central line catheter. Other cultures of pus from an abdominal incision, the vaginal cuff, or a drainage tube occasionally may be helpful in a patient who is not responding to antibiotics or in whom an unusual infection (actinomyces) is suspected. A sputum gram stain and culture is rarely useful but should be considered in a symptomatic, immunosuppressed patient who could have tuberculosis, coccidioidomycosis, or some other atypical pneumonia.

A number of different imaging techniques may be useful in special circumstances. A CT scan of the abdomen should identify an abscess. In many cases, CT-guided percutaneous catheter drainage in combination with intravenous antibiotics is the treatment of choice. Renal function always should be satisfactory before administering intravenous contrast for a CT or intravenous pyelogram. Ultrasound can be used to scan the abdominal incision for an abscess or hematoma. Ultrasound of the heart can diagnose valvular vegetations associated with bacterial endocarditis. It also is useful for evaluation of the leg vein for venous thrombosis. Pelvic or abdominal vein thrombosis can be diagnosed easily in most cases using CT scanning. Radioactive-tagged white blood cell scans can be useful for localizing occult infections, but these have largely been replaced by CT scans.

TREATMENT

The following factors must be considered when making antibiotic choices for the treatment of postoperative infections.

1. Pelvic infections are polymicrobial in etiology.
2. The most frequent causative organisms are aerobic, Gram-positive cocci (*streptococci, S. epidermidis, S. aureus*), facultative Gram-negative rods (*Escherichia coli, Klebsiella* sp, *Enterobacter* sp), anaerobic cocci (Peptostreptococci), and anaerobic rods (*Prevotella* sp, *Bacteroides* sp, *B. fragilis*).
3. Enterococci may occasionally cause sepsis or be a sole isolate but usually accompany other bacteria and are not principal pathogens.
4. The choice of an antibiotic is made empirically before culture results are available.
5. The timing of onset of the infection may be an indicator of pathogen group.
6. Resistance to frequently used antibiotics is developing.
7. Single agents may be as effective as multiple agents in treating postoperative infections.

The polymicrobial nature of postoperative pelvic infections results in about 20% aerobic, Gram-positive cocci, 20% Gram-negative rods, and 60% anaerobes. Infections that occur in the first 24 hours after surgery usually are caused by Gram-positive cocci or occasionally by facultative, Gram-negative rods. Infections that occur after the first 48 hours are more frequently anaerobic. The effect of timing should be considered in making the initial choice of an antibiotic because an extended-spectrum penicillin or cephalosporin may be the best choice in early-onset infections (Table 9.7).

The gold standard for treating gynecologic postoperative infections has been gentamicin, 2 mg/kg loading dose, followed by 1.5 mg/kg maintenance dose for patients with normal renal function, plus clindamycin, 900 mg administered parenterally every 8 hours. Unfortunately, increasing resistance among anaerobic rods to clindamycin is altering the effectiveness of this regimen. The fear of nephrotoxicity or ototoxicity when gentamicin is used for short treatment courses in young, healthy women has not been borne out. Aminoglycoside serum levels may be obtained if the treatment is expected to last more than 72 hours. The addition of ampicillin to the previous combination extends the spectrum of coverage to include enterococci.

To overcome the resistance of anaerobes to clindamycin, metronidazole may be used in combination with an aminoglycoside, ampicillin, or both. The dose of metronidazole is 500 mg every 6 hours. The oral absorption of this antibiotic is such that blood levels are equivalent to parenteral administration. Metronidazole is only effective against anaerobes and has minimal to no aerobic spectrum.

Investigators have studied various extended-spectrum penicillins and cephalosporins as single agents for the treatment of mild to moderately severe postoperative pelvic infections. These newer agents have an extended spectrum of *in vitro* antibacterial activity and β-lactamase stability. Single agents—such as cefoxitin, cefotetan, cefuroxime, ampicillin/sulbactam, ticarcillin/clavulanic acid, and piperacillin—avoid the problems of admixture with multiple agents and the potential for aminoglycoside toxicity. In our experience, persistence of infections despite these single agents usually is caused by anaerobic infection.

If an abscess is present and medical management is used to attempt to eradicate it or allow for stabilization before drainage is undertaken, imipenem-cilastatin, a carbapenem, is an excellent choice in a dose of 500 mg given i.v. every 6 hours. Metronidazole is a good option when anaerobes are suspected. If the patient has evidence of clinical improvement and decrease in size of the abscess, antibiotics should be continued; if there is no improvement by 48 to 72 hours, surgical drainage is indicated.

Parenteral antibiotics should be continued until the patient is afebrile and clinically well for 24 to 48 hours. At that point, antibiotics may be discontinued and the patient discharged. Several studies show no benefit to the continuation of oral antibiotics after successful parenteral therapy, or observing the patient for an additional 24 hours in the hospital.

If there is not a good response to appropriate antibiotic therapy within 72 hours, the patient should be completely

TABLE 9.7.
Treatment Choices for Gynecologic Infection

Postoperative Infection	Recommended Regimen	Failures	Penicillin Allergy
Mild to moderate	Extended-spectrum penicillin or cephalosporin (e.g., Piperacillin, 4.0 g/6 h; ampicillin/sulbactam, 3.0 g/6 h; ticarcillin/clavulanic acid, 3.1 g/4–6 h; ceftriaxone, 2.0 g followed by 1.0 g/24 h; cefoxitin, 2.0 g/6 h; cefotetan 2.0 g/12 h; cefotaxine, 1.0 g/8 h [i.v. doses]).	Clindamycin/gentamicin or metronidazole/gentamicin	Clindamycin/gentamicin
Severe	Clindamycin/gentamicin or metronidazole/gentamicin (e.g., Clindamycin, 900 mg/8 h or metronidazole, 500 mg/6 h plus gentamicin, 2.0 mg/kg followed by 1.5 mg/kg/8 h or a single daily dose of 5.0 mg/kg [Ampicillin, penicillin, or vancomycin may be added to cover enterococci.]).	Add ampicillin to clindamycin/ gentamicin; imipenem	Clindamycin/gentamicin
Pelvic abscess	Meropenem 500 mg-lg/IVq8h; clindamycin/gentamicin; metronidazole/gentamicin	Evaluate need for surgical drainage	NA
Septic pelvic thrombophlebitis	Meropenem 500 mg-lg/IVq8h; or metronidazole plus heparin		NA

NA, not applicable.

re-evaluated. After another review of the history and physical examination, imaging studies should be considered. Perhaps a chest x-ray may indicate new consolidation or an abdominal and pelvic CT scan may identify a collection or abscess or even septic thrombophlebitis. If a fever persists, antibiotics may be discontinued, and the patient recultured before new antibiotics are started if fever persists.

PREVENTION OF INFECTION

In this modern era of antibiotics, we have become somewhat lax in our efforts to prevent infection because we assume that if infection occurs, we can easily and effectively treat it. This ignores the potential for morbidity in the patient and the tremendous economic burden imposed by postoperative infections. In a 5-year study of wound infections after abdominal hysterectomy, Kandula and Wenzel found that women with infections were hospitalized an average of 3.55 days longer, resulting in a significant financial impact. It is important to implement specific strategies aimed at preventing postoperative infection and to use these with every patient. In doing so, a significant number of infections can be prevented. Identifying risk factors is important preoperatively. Major risks are: obesity, bacterial vaginosis, radical surgery, and excessive blood loss (>1,000 cc).

Some guidelines apply to all situations, and some are specific to certain types of infection. Careful hand washing, avoiding contact with septic patients before proceeding to the operating room, avoiding consecutive contact with two or more infected patients without vigorous hand washing, and minimizing the operating room exposure for infected personnel are a few of the seemingly obvious precautions that frequently are violated.

The skin is colonized with bacteria, some of which are transient and reside on the integument for only a short time and some of which are resident and are present continuously. One can effectively remove the transient microflora with routine hand washing with soap. The resident organisms require antimicrobial products for their inhibition of growth or elimination. It is not just the surgeon but also nursing personnel who can be the vectors of bacteria. Hand washing thus becomes the most important means of preventing the spread of infection (Table 9.8).

Prevention of Postoperative Pneumonia

All patients who undergo general endotracheal anesthesia are at risk for retention of pulmonary secretions, alveolar collapse, and in turn, atelectasis and possibly pneumonia. Atelectasis is frequently a cause of immediate postoperative fever. To help prevent this complication, all patients undergoing surgery, and especially those with chronic obstructive airway disease, should be encouraged to discontinue or decrease smoking and have any upper respiratory infections treated prior to operation. Postoperatively,

TABLE 9.8.
Recommendations for Hand Washing

In the absence of a true emergency, personnel should always wash their hands:

- before performing invasive procedures
- before taking care of particularly susceptible patients, such as patients who are severely immunocompromised and newborns
- before and after touching wounds, whether surgical, traumatic, or associated with an invasive device
- after situations during which microbial contamination of hands is likely to occur, particularly those involving contact with mucous membranes, blood, body fluids, secretions, or excretions
- after touching inanimate sources that are likely to be contaminated with virulent or epidemiologically important microorganisms
- after taking care of an infected patient or one who is likely to be colonized with microorganisms of special clinical or epidemiologic significance, such as multiple-drug resistant bacteria
- between contact with different patients in high-risk units

Most routine, brief patient care activities involving direct patient contact, other than those described, do not require hand washing.

Most routine hospital activities involving indirect patient contact do not require hand washing.

Source: Garner JS, Favero MS. Guideline for hand washing and hospital environmental control, 1985. In: *Guidelines for the prevention and control of nosocomial infections.* Washington, DC: US Department of Health and Human Services, PB82-9234401, 1985:7, with permission.

coughing, deep breathing, and devices to encourage alveolar expansions should be used. Adequate analgesia to control pain that interferes with respiratory effort should be administered. Early ambulation should be encouraged.

Prevention of Urinary Tract Infection

UTIs can complicate gynecologic surgery because of the proximity of the urethra to the operative site in the vagina. This effect is augmented by the placement of an indwelling urinary catheter. To limit UTIs, appropriate placement and management of catheters is essential. Personnel should be instructed in the proper sterile placement of catheters, maintained as a closed drainage system without traction on the device. Catheters should be placed only when necessary and should be removed as soon as feasible. Routine culture of terminal urine specimens when catheters are removed has not proved cost effective in our institution.

Prevention of Operative Site and Wound Infections

Other Considerations

Over the last decade or more, multiple studies have demonstrated that antibiotic prophylaxis significantly reduces infectious morbidity following both vaginal and abdominal hysterectomy. These results do not mean that the important surgical principles that have been shown to reduce morbidity can be ignored, but the use of prophylactic antibiotics in many gynecologic surgical procedures has reduced the incidence of postoperative surgical site infections from 30% to 50% to about 15% in most series.

Theory of Antibiotic Prophylaxis

At the time of hysterectomy, vaginal or cervical bacteria are inoculated into the surgical site, and it is hypothesized that antibiotics in these tissues at this time augment host defense mechanisms to reduce the incidence of clinical infections. In order for antibiotic prophylaxis to work effectively, several important criteria must be fulfilled. First, the operative procedure must have a significant risk of bacterial contamination and, in the absence of prophylactic antibiotics, an appreciable incidence of operative site infection. Hysterectomy or other gynecologic procedures involving the cervix, vagina, or vulva all qualify for the criterion. Second, the prophylactic antibiotic administered should be effective against expected pathogens and have a low rate of side effects. Although many antibiotic regimens have proven effective in prospective, randomized trials for gynecologic surgery, the cephalosporins have emerged as the generally recommended antibiotic because of their effectiveness, low incidence of side effects, and low cost. Finally, for effective antibiotic prophylaxis, the tissue levels of the chosen antibiotic need to be optimal at the time bacterial contamination of the surgical site occurs. This means that the antibiotic needs to be administered shortly before the start of surgery, usually at the time the patient is brought into the operating room and anesthesia is induced.

Choice of Antibiotics for Prophylaxis

As noted, the antibiotic selected for a given procedure should be effective, have few side effects, be administered in a way that results in a minimal risk of antibiotic-resistant infections, and be inexpensive. In a metaanalysis of 25 prospective, randomized trials of prophylactic antibiotics for abdominal hysterectomy, Mittendorf et al. reported a reduction of serious postoperative infections from 21.1% to 9.0%. The most commonly used antibiotic for hysterectomy is cefazolin, because it meets the preceding criteria and has a relatively long half-life of 1.8 hours. Recommended prophylactic antibiotic regimens for various gynecologic procedures are listed in Table 9.9.

Cephalosporins should not be given to patients with a history of penicillin allergy. The quinolones such as ciprofloxacin are a good alternative; metronidazole and clindamycin have been particularly effective when anaerobic contamination is anticipated in penicillin-sensitive patients.

In women with damaged or artificial heart valves or others at increased risk for bacterial endocarditis, combination antibiotics such as ampicillin (2 g) and gentamicin (1.5 mg/m^2) are recommended. If the patient is allergic to penicillin, vancomycin (1 g over 1 to 2 hours) is substituted for ampicillin. Unlike prophylactic antibiotics given for operative site infections where only a single

TABLE 9.9.
Antimicrobial Prophylactic Regimens by Procedure

Procedure	Antibiotic	Dose
Vaginal/abdominal	Cefazolin	1 or 2 single dose i.v.
Hysterectomy[a]	Cefoxitin	2 g single dose i.v.
	Cefotetan	1 or 2 single dose i.v.
	Metronidazole	500 mg single dose i.v.
Laparoscopy	None	
Laparotomy	None	—
Hysteroscopy	None	—
Hysterosalpingogram	Doxycycline[b]	100 mg twice daily/5 d orally
IUD insertion	None	—
Endometrial biopsy	None	—
Induced abortion/D&C	Doxycycline	100 mg orally 1 h before procedure and 200 mg orally after the procedure
	Metronizadole	500 mg twice daily orally for 5 d
Urodynamics	None	—

D&C, dilation and curettage; IV, intravenously; IUD, intrauterine device.

[a] A convenient time to administer antibiotic prophylaxis is just before induction of anesthesia.

[b] If hysterosalpingogram demonstrated dilated tubes. No prophylaxis indicated for a normal study.

Source: ACOG Practice Bulletin 2001;23:269, with permission.

dose is administered, it is recommended that a second dose be given 6 hours later.

Adverse Reactions

Although reactions to cephalosporins occur from 1% to 10%, severe side effects such as anaphylaxis have been reported in only about 0.02% of patients. The majority of reactions are skin rashes and urticaria, which usually are resolved by the time the patient has recovered from anesthesia postoperatively. Diarrhea secondary to pseudomembranous colitis associated with β-lactam antibiotics has been reported in up to 15% of patients, but it is probably not so common in women receiving only a single prophylactic dose. Although the induction of bacterial resistance to commonly used antibiotics has been a theoretical concern, this has not been a clinical problem when prophylactic antibiotic use is limited to a single dose of common cephalosporins. More potent "big gun" antibiotics should be reserved for specific indications and not used in a prophylactic setting to avoid induction of resistant organisms.

Surveillance for nosocomial infections must be carried out by the hospital infection control program so that surgeons are aware of their individual rates of postoperative infection. Several studies have shown that surgeon-specific wound infection rates can be reduced effectively by such reporting mechanisms.

The classic work of Cruse and Foord helped to delineate specific factors that influence wound infection rates. Others have added to this work so that preoperative and intraoperative management routines can be recommended even though they have not all been confirmed in controlled trials. Preoperative hospitalization should be limited as much as possible. Same-day admission is not just cost effective for third-party payers, it makes good sense from an infection control perspective. Hair removal should be avoided unless there is an abundance of hair at the operative site. Using a depilatory or clipping the hair is suggested if removal is necessary. Patients should be discouraged from shaving themselves at home before admission.

Because bowel entry is a major cause of contamination and subsequent wound or surgical site infection, having the bowel prepared whenever possible bowel involvement is suspected is beneficial. The Condon bowel prep includes adequate use of a cathartic plus oral neomycin and erythromycin in three doses the day before surgery. The use of a povidone-iodine douche or insertion of gel has been recommended for the night before admission or the day of surgery. Although this practice has been recommended for many years, and povidone-iodine solution and gel have been demonstrated to decrease vaginal bacterial counts to undetectable levels 10 minutes after application, the bacterial flora gradually return to approximately one half pretreatment levels in 2 hours. The benefit of vaginal cleansing with an antiinfective agent the night before, or even immediately prior to surgery, has not been evaluated in a prospective, randomized trial.

Bacterial vaginosis has been found to be a risk factor for postoperative infection when present before surgery in women undergoing hysterectomy. In a prospective study of 175 women who underwent major gynecologic surgery, Lin et al. found a 36% incidence of postoperative febrile morbidity in patients who had bacterial vaginosis preoperatively and only a 20% incidence of fever among the women who had a lactobacillus-predominant vaginal flora ($p = 0.045$). Although some data support the benefit of treating pregnant women with bacterial vaginosis to decrease the rates of preterm labor, premature rupture of the membranes, and intraamniotic infection, no data have shown a beneficial effect of preoperative treatment of hysterectomy patients. In light of the obstetric data, some gynecologists recommend screening hysterectomy patients preoperatively and treating those who are infected with metronidazole because anaerobes play such a significant role in postoperative gynecologic infections.

All gynecologists should employ careful hand-washing techniques preoperatively and when seeing patients. Appropriate gowns and eye coverings should be worn. Wearing double gloves is an effective way to decrease the chances of percutaneous injury. Careful surgical technique is essential to minimize postoperative infections. Adequate hemostasis should be obtained whenever possible. The amount of dead space should be limited. Large areas of necrotic tissue should be excised, and vascular pedicles should be short. Closing the subcutaneous space has no benefit, and using suture there can increase the rate of superficial wound infection. If the case is dirty, consideration should be given to delayed wound closure. If drains are used, they should be closed-suction drains, not gravity drains. Draining the subcutaneous space often is helpful in large patients to eliminate serous and bloody fluid.

UNIVERSAL PRECAUTIONS

The epidemics of acquired immunodeficiency syndrome and hepatitis B viral infection have brought to light the risks of lethal infection of the surgeon or other members of the operative team by blood or tissue fluids in association with surgery. Believing that all at-risk situations can be identified by history, physical examination, or laboratory data is naive and dangerous. To overcome this prevalent thought, universal blood and body fluid precautions were developed. This concept treats all patients' blood and certain other body fluids capable of transmitting blood-borne pathogens as potentially infectious. Universal precautions include the following requirements: (a) the use of gloves when touching blood and body fluids, mucous membranes, or broken skin, or when handling items or surfaces soiled with blood or body fluids; (b) the use of masks and eye protection during procedures that can generate splashing or droplets in the air; (c) the use of a gown or plastic apron if splashing of blood is anticipated; (d) careful hand washing if hands are contaminated with blood or body fluids; (e) extraordinary care in handling needles or other sharp objects, and proper disposal of sharp objects in puncture-resistant containers; (f) the availability of emergency resuscitation devices to minimize the need for emergency mouth-to-mouth resuscitation; and (f) the exclusion from patient care of personnel with exudative lesions or weeping dermatitis until these conditions are resolved.

Assuming that every patient is potentially infected, using specific protocols for the safe use of invasive procedures, and taking steps to avoid any and all risk-taking behavior by medical personnel can help to prevent nosocomial infections.

Multiple studies have shown that double gloving significantly reduces the risk of blood contamination to the surgeon and other members of the operative team. In a large study from Finland, Laine and Aarnio reported a 7.4% glove perforation rate for single gloves in 1,020 surgeon uses. When double gloves were used, the inner glove was perforated in only 0.52% of 1,148 uses. Overall, someone in the surgical team had a glove perforation during 18.9% of the operative procedures, and the literature quotes rates of up to 61% in orthopedics and trauma surgery. The most common site of perforation is the index finger of the left hand of the surgeon; but all members of the team are at risk, and gloves can be torn in clamps or retractors as well as punctured by needle stick injuries. Manufacturing defects in the gloves themselves are uncommon, but do occur and may go unnoticed until blood is seen on the finger or hand. Although double gloving does reduce dexterity and tactile sensation, it also reduces the potential for blood contamination almost tenfold. It is a good general practice and always should be used in high-risk situations.

BIBLIOGRAPHY

ACOG Practice Bulletin. *Antibiotic prophylaxis for gynecologic procedures.* 2001;23:269.

Brough SJ, Hunt TM, Barrie WW. Surgical glove perforations. *Br J Surg* 1988;75:317.

Brown CEL, Lowe TW, Cunningham FG, et al. Puerperal pelvic thrombophlebitis: impact on diagnosis and treatment using x-ray computed tomography and magnetic resonance imaging. *Obstet Gynecol* 1986;68:789.

Centers for Disease Control and Prevention. The 1997 USPHS/IDSA guidelines for the prevention of opportunistic infections in persons infected with human immunodeficiency virus. *MMWR* 1997;46(RR-12):1.

Centers for Disease Control and Prevention. Public Health Service guidelines for the management of health-care worker exposures to HIV and recommendations for postexposure prophylaxis. *MMWR* 1998;47(RR-7):1–33.

Classen DC, Evan RS, Pestotnik SL, et al. The timing of prophylactic administration of antibiotics and the risk of surgical-wound infection. *N Engl J Med* 1992;326:281.

Condon RE, Schulte WJ, Malongoni MA, et al. Effectiveness of a surgical wound surveillance program. *Arch Surg* 1983;118:303.

Cruse PJE, Foord R. The epidemiology of wound infection: a 10 year prospective study of 62,939 wounds. *Surg Clin North Am* 1980;60:27.

Cuchural GJ, Tally FP, Jacobus NV, et al. Susceptibility of the *Bacteroides fragilis* group in the United States: analysis by site of isolation. *Antimicrob Agents Chemother* 1988;32:717.

Culver DH, Horan TC, Gaynes RF. Surgical wound infection rates by wound class: operative procedure and patient risk index. *Am J Med* 1991;91:152S.

Dellinger EP, Gross PA, Barrett TL, et al. Quality standard for antimicrobial prophylaxis in surgical procedures. Infectious Disease Society of America [review]. *Clin Infect Dis* 1994;18:422.

Dinsmoor MJ. Imipenem-Cilastatin. *Obstet Gynecol Clin North Am* 1992;19:475.

Donowitz GR, Mandell GL. Beta lactam antibiotics. *N Engl J Med* 1988;318:490.

Duff P. Prophylactic antibiotics for hysterectomy. In: Mead PB, Hager WD, Faro S, eds. *Protocols for infectious diseases in obstetrics and gynecology,* 2nd ed. Malden, MA: Blackwell Scientific, 2000;476.

Duff P. The aminoglycosides. *Obstet Gynecol Clin North Am* 1992;19:511.

Evaldson GR, Frederici H, Jullig C, et al. Hospital-associated infections in obstetrics and gynecology, effects of surveillance. *Acta Obstet Gynecol Scand* 1992;71:54.

Fanning J, Neuhoff RA, Brewer JE, et al. Frequency and yield of postoperative fever evaluation. *Infect Dis Obstet Gynecol* 1998;6:252.

Gallup DC, Gallup DG, Nolan TE, et al. Use of a subcutaneous closed drainage system and antibiotics in obese gynecologic patients. *Am J Obstet Gynecol* 1996;175:358.

Garibaldi RA, Brodines, Mutsumiya S, et al. Evidence for the noninfectious etiology of early postoperative fever. *Infect Control* 1985;6:273.

Garner JS, Favero MS. Guideline for hand washing and hospital environmental control, 1985. *Guidelines for the prevention and control of nosocomial infections.* Washington, DC: US Department of Health and Human Services, 1985:7.

Grossman JH, Adams RL. Vaginal flora in women undergoing hysterectomy with antibiotic prophylaxis. *Obstet Gynecol* 1979;53:23.

Hager WD, Pascuzzi M, Vernon M. Efficacy of oral antibiotics following parenteral antibiotics for serious infections in obstetrics and gynecology. *Obstet Gynecol* 1989;73:326.

Hager WD, Rapp RP. Metronidazole. *Obstet Gynecol Clin North Am* 1992;19:475.

Haley RW, Culver DH, White JW, et al. The efficiency of infection surveillance and control programs in preventing nosocomial infections in U.S. hospitals. *Am J Epidemiol* 1985;121:182.

Harris WJ. Early complications of abdominal and vaginal hysterectomy. *Obstet Gynecol Surv* 1995;50:795.

Hemsell DL. Gynecologic postoperative infections in obstetric and gynecologic infectious disease. In: Pastorek JG, ed. *Obstetric and gynecologic infectious disease.* New York: Raven Press, 1994.

Hemsell DL, Bowden RE, Hemsell PG, et al. Single-dose cephalosporin for prevention of major pelvic infection after vaginal hysterectomy: cefazolin vs. cefoxitin vs. cefotaxime. *Am J Obstet Gynecol* 1987;156:1201.

Hemsell DL, Johnson ER, Bowden RE, et al. Ceftriaxone and cefazolin prophylaxis for hysterectomy. *Surg Gynecol Obstet* 1985;161:197.

Hemsell DL, Johnson ER, Heard MC, et al. Single-dose piperacillin vs. triple-dose cefoxitin prophylaxis at vaginal and abdominal hysterectomy. *South Med J* 1984;82:438.

Hemsell DL, Nobles B, Heard MC. Recognition and treatment of posthysterectomy pelvic infections. *Infect Surg* 1988;7:47.

Hill GB. Techniques for isolating pelvic bacterial pathogens. In: Mead P, Hager WD, Faro S, eds. *Protocols for infectious diseases in obstetrics and gynecology,* 2nd ed. Malden, MA: Blackwell Scientific, 2000;454.

Hoyme UB, Tamimi HK, Eschenbach DA, et al. Osteomyelitis pubis after radical gynecologic operations. *Obstet Gynecol* 1984;63:475.

Jenson SL, Kristensen B, Fabrin K. Double gloving as self protection in abdominal surgery. *Eur J Surg* 1997;163:163.

John JF. What price success? The continuing saga of the toxic therapeutic ratio in the use of aminoglycoside antibiotics. *J Infect Dis* 1988;158:1.

Kamat AA, Brancazio L, Gibson M. Wound infection in gynecologic surgery. *Infect Dis Obstet Gynecol* 2000;8:230.

Kandula PV, Wenzel RP. Postoperative wound infection after total abdominal hysterectomy: a controlled study of the increased duration of hospital stay and trends in postoperative wound infection. *Am J Infect Control* 1993;21:201.

Korn AP, Gullon K, Hessol N, et al. Does vaginal cuff closure decrease the infectious morbidity associated with abdominal hysterectomy? *J Am Coll Surg* 1997;185:404.

Laine T, Aarnio P. How often does glove perforation occur in surgery? Comparison between single gloves and a double-gloving system. *Am J Surg* 2001;181:564.

Lars P, Naver S, Gottrup F. Incidence of glove perforations in gastrointestinal surgery and the protective effect of double gloves: a prospective, randomised, controlled study. *Eur J Surg* 2000;166:293.

Leaper D, Ayliffe GA, Gilchrist B. Postoperative wound infection. *J Wound Care* 1996;5:330.

Ledger WJ. Infections following gynecologic operations. In: Faro S, ed. *Diagnosis and management of female pelvic infections in primary care medicine.* Baltimore: Williams & Wilkins, 1985.

Lin L, Song J, Kimber N, et al. The role of bacterial vaginosis in infection after major gynecologic surgery. *Infect Dis Obstet Gynecol* 1999;7:169.

Lyon DS, Jones JL, Sanchez A. Postoperative febrile morbidity in the benign gynecologic patient. *J Reprod Med* 2000;45:305.

Mage G, Masson FN, Canis M. Laparoscopic hysterectomy. *Curr Opin Obstet Gynecol* 1995;7:283.

McNally CG, Krivak TC, Alagoz T. Conservative management of isolated post hysterectomy fever. *J Reprod Med* 2000;45:572.

Mead PB, Hager WD, Faro S. *Protocols for infectious diseases in obstetrics and gynecology,* 2nd ed. Malden, MA: Blackwell Scientific, 2000.

Monif GR, Thompson JL, Stephens HD, et al. Quantitative and qualitative effects of povidone-iodine liquid and gel on the aerobic and anaerobic flora of the female genital tract. *Am J Obstet Gynecol* 1980;137:432.

Pastorek JG II. *Obstetric and gynecologic infectious disease.* New York: Raven Press, 1994.

Persson E, Bergstrom M, Larsson PG, et al. Infections after hysterectomy. A prospective, nation-wide Swedish study. *Acta Obstet Gynecol Scand* 1996;75:757.

Peters WA. Bartholinitis after vulvovaginal surgery. *Am J Obstet Gynecol* 1998;178:1143.

Sawyer RG, Pruett TL. Wound infections. *Surg Clin North Am* 1994;74:519.

Schwandt A, Andrews SJ, Fanning J. Prospective analysis of a fever evaluation algorithm after major gynecologic surgery. *Am J Obstet Gynecol* 2001;184:1066.

Shapiro M, Munoz A, Tager IB, et al. Risk factors for infection at the operative site after abdominal or vaginal hysterectomy. *NEJM* 1982;307:1661.

Soper DE. Bacterial vaginosis and postoperative infections. *Am J Obstet Gynecol* 1993;169:467.

Thomason JL, Gelbart SM, Scaylione NJ. Bacteria vaginosis: current review with indications for asymptomatic therapy. *Am J Obstet Gynecol* 1991;165:1210.

Weinstein L. Infection prevention in the gynecologic or obstetric patient. In: Sciarra JJ, ed. *Gynecology and obstetrics,* vol 1. Hagerstown, MD: Harper & Row, 1990.

Te Linde's Operative Gynecology, ninth edition, edited by John A. Rock and Howard W. Jones, III. Lippincott Williams & Wilkins, Philadelphia: © 2003.

CHAPTER

10

▼

Shock in the Gynecologic Patient

HARRIET O. SMITH   AUDREY A. ROMERO

Shock states are among the most formidable conditions that the gynecologist is likely to encounter. The morbidity and economic impact of shock—its primary treatment, multiorgan failure syndrome, the management of one of its worst sequelae, in addition to providing care for long-term disabilities that may result from partial or total loss of organ function—are enormous. In the United States annually, septic shock alone affects 100,000 to 300,000 patients at a cost of 5 to 10 billion dollars per year. Despite aggressive therapy and significant expenditure, 40% to 60% of those affected do not survive. In the field of obstetrics, two of the three most common causes of maternal mortality continue to be complications from hemorrhage and sepsis. An understanding of the pathogenesis, clinical signs and symptoms, and management of shock is paramount. In many instances prompt recognition of the early manifestations of shock followed by aggressive treatment significantly reduces the likelihood of morbidity and mortality.

Although shock can be defined as a metabolic defect, shock is best defined in practical terms as an acute clinical syndrome characterized by hypoperfusion and severe dysfunction of organs vital for survival. These manifestations result from an acute, generalized disturbance in the normal cardiovascular circulation. Cardiac output and circulatory blood volume may be compromised by direct myocardial injury or hypovolemia. Clinical manifestations include mean arterial hypotension and circulatory collapse. Severe hypovolemia can occur as a direct result of uncontrolled hemorrhage, or may result from the pathological redistribution of circulating volume as in septic shock.

CLASSIFICATION AND ETIOPATHOGENESIS

Based on the underlying cause, shock can be divided into four main categories (Table 10.1).

1. *Hypovolemic shock,* in which there is an inadequate circulating blood volume resulting from hemorrhage or acute volume depletion
2. *Distributive shock,* in which total body water is normal or slightly decreased, but is "pooled" into the interstitial fluid compartment, resulting in intravascular volume depletion
3. *Cardiogenic shock,* in which there is intrinsic pump failure
4. *Extracardiac obstructive shock,* in which the heart is intrinsically normal and total blood volume is adequate, but mechanical factors interfere with pump performance

TABLE 10.1.
Classification of Shock States

Classification	Conditions Encountered in Gynecology and Obstetrics
Hypovolemic	
Hemorrhagic	Obstetric hemorrhage, ectopic pregnancy, acute operative blood loss, retroperitoneal bleeding, trauma
Nonhemorrhagic	Vomiting, diarrhea, acute drainage of ascites, renal losses (diuretics, postobstructive diuresis, acute tubular necrosis), peritonitis
Distributive	Sepsis, anaphylaxis, preeclampsia, advanced ovarian cancer with ascites and/or pleural effusions, intestinal obstruction, adrenal insufficiency, cerebral or spinal cord injuries, toxic/pharmacologic (vasodilators, benzodiazepines), endocrinologic
Cardiogenic	Myocardial infarction, myocarditis, pharmacologic/toxic depression (anthracycline, beta-blockers, calcium channel blockers), cardiomyopathies, mechanical valve failure, arrhythmias
Extracardiac obstructive	Massive pulmonary embolism, cardiac tamponade, constrictive pericarditis, coarctation of the aorta, severe pulmonary hypertension, mediastinal tumors, tension pneumothorax, positive-pressure ventilation
Mixed	Sepsis, neurogenic shock, anaphylaxis, toxin poisoning, drug overdose, amniotic fluid embolism

Often, shock is the result of more than one of these circulatory disturbances, and the apparent cause of persistent cardiovascular dysfunction can change with time and intervening therapy. For example, septic shock generally is considered the result of tissue hypoperfusion caused by inadequate circulatory volume. However, endotoxins and mediators released from injured cells have direct myocardial depressant effects as well, and in this regard, are similar to cardiogenic shock from intrinsic cardiac disease.

Cardiogenic shock is characterized by a low systolic blood pressure (<80 mm Hg) associated with a severely reduced cardiac index (usually <1.8 L/min/m²) and a high left ventricular filling pressure (usually >18 mm Hg). Pulmonary edema may be present or absent. Extracardiac obstructive shock is characterized by the inability of the ventricle to fill during diastole. Consequently, stroke volume and cardiac output are severely reduced. In the gynecologic patient, massive pulmonary embolus is the most common example. Because the most common types of shock encountered in obstetrics and gynecology are hypovolemic (usually, resulting from hemorrhagic) and septic, this chapter focuses on the recognition and management of these forms of shock.

Regardless of the precipitating event, hypotension results from an inadequate circulatory volume caused by cardiac insufficiency, loss of sympathetic tone, inadequate plasma volume, or a combination of these factors (Fig. 10.1). Prolonged hypotension and organ hypoperfusion results in cellular injury that, if left unchecked, ultimately leads to organ system failure or cardiovascular collapse and death.

Hypovolemic Shock

Hemorrhagic shock often is subdivided into four classes, based on presenting signs and symptoms (Table 10.2). This classification schema is useful for estimating initial crystalloid or blood requirements and in understanding the pathophysiologic mechanisms responsible for the changes in clinical presentation associated with progressively greater increments of blood loss. Caution should be exercised, however, in basing clinical decisions solely on the initial estimate of intravascular volume. The clinical manifestations of hemorrhagic shock can vary greatly, depending on the rate and the total volume of blood loss. When the rate of loss has been gradual (as might be found with an unruptured ectopic pregnancy or a retroperitoneal bleed), plasma refill and other compensatory mechanisms can ensure an adequate circulating plasma volume despite substantial blood losses. In such cases, the resuscitative requirements can be severely underestimated. Thus, once initial fluid resuscitation is begun, close observation and frequent reassessment are required, because these patients remain at risk for circulatory collapse.

With losses of less than 15% of total volume (class I), there are no measurable changes in blood pressure, resting pulse, or respiratory rate. Transcapillary refill and other compensatory mechanisms usually restore plasma volume within 24 hours. With class II hypovolemia, or up to 1,500 mL blood loss, the most consistent clinical finding is tachycardia. The increase in heart rate is often associated with a narrowed pulse pressure (the difference between systolic and diastolic pressures). However, the resting blood pressure is generally preserved by compensatory mechanisms, including the renin-angiotensin system and the hypothalamic-hypophyseal-adrenal system. The juxtaglomerular cells release renin into plasma in response to a decrease in wall tension or sodium, or sympathetic activation. Renin converts angiotensinogen into angiotensin I, an inactive polypeptide, which is metabolized in the liver to angiotensin II, a potent vasoconstrictor that stimulates aldosterone secretion from the renal cortex. Aldosterone, along with the pituitary release of antidiuretic hormone, promotes sodium and water re-

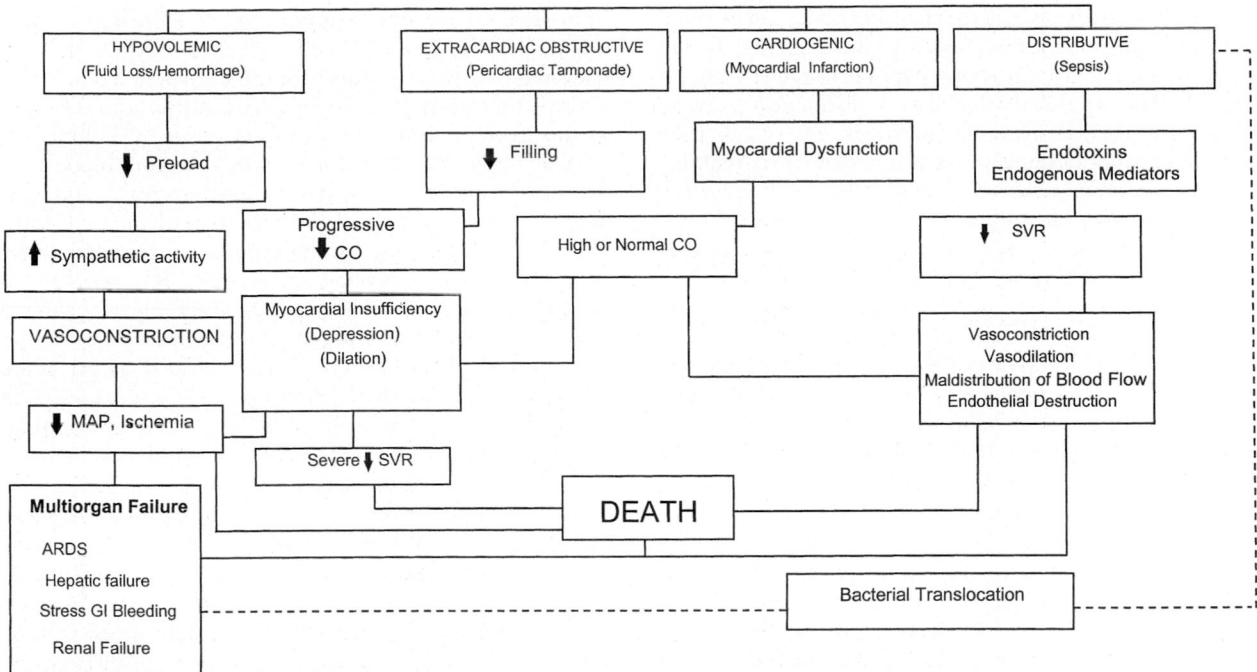

FIGURE 10.1. Pathogenesis of human shock. ARDS, adult respiratory distress syndrome; CO, cardiac output; GI, gastrointestinal; MAP, mean arterial pressure; SVR, systemic vascular resistance. (From: Hollenberg SM, Parrillo JE. Shock. In: Fauci AS, Martin JP, et al, eds. *Harrison's principles of internal medicine,* vol 1. New York: McGraw-Hill, 1997:217, with permission.)

tention. These mechanisms increase venous return and consequently, stroke volume, cardiac output, and blood pressure. Thus, oliguria is a common manifestation of hypovolemic shock. In response to hypovolemia, norepinephrine and epinephrine are locally and systemically released. Catecholamine-mediated effects are inotropic and chronotropic, resulting in increased cardiac output. Venoconstriction enhances venous return, which also increases stroke volume and cardiac output. In response to the catecholamine mediated increase in peripheral vascular resistance, the diastolic blood pressure is increased, which leads to a narrowed pulse pressure. Typically, the

TABLE 10.2.
Classification of Hypovolemic Shock[a]

	Class I	Class II	Class III	Class IV
Blood loss (mL)	up to 750	750–1,500	1,500–2,000	over 2,000
Blood volume (%)	up to 15	15–30	30–40	over 40
Heart rate (beats/minute)[b]	less than 100	over 100	over 120	over 140
Blood pressure[b]	Normal or increased	Normal (+ tilt)	Decreased (mean arterial pressure <60 mm Hg)	Decreased
Pulse pressure	Normal	Decreased	Decreased	Decreased
Capillary refill	Normal	May be delayed	Usually delayed	Always delayed
Respirations	Normal	Mildly increased	Moderate to marked tachypnea	Marked tachypnea; respiratory collapse
Urinary output (mL/h)	over 30	20–30	5–15	Essentially anuric
Mental status	Normal or anxious	Anxious	Confused	Lethargic, obtunded

[a] In a 70-kg, nonpregnant adult.

[b] Measure heart rate and blood pressure in standing, sitting, and recumbent positions with 5 min between measurements to permit equilibration. Orthostatic change (+ tilt) is a postural increase in pulse of 10 to 15 beats/min, or a drop in systolic blood pressure of at least 10 mm Hg.

Source: From *Advanced trauma life support® student manual,* American College of Surgeons, Chicago: 1997, second impression 1999:98, with permission.

resting blood pressure is normal; however, when blood pressure and pulse are recorded in the standing, sitting, or reclining position, postural hypotension is usually observed. This is the major clinical distinction between class I and class II hypovolemic shock. As long as these compensatory mechanisms remain intact, shock is almost always eventually reversible; hence, the frequently used descriptive term early shock.

Although patients with losses of 20% to 30% of their blood volume ultimately may require red blood cell replacement, crystalloid usually is adequate for immediate resuscitation. Crystalloid replacement is guided by the 3:1 rule: 300 mL crystalloid per 100 mL blood (plasma volume) lost. In normal adults, approximately two thirds of the total body water is intracellular, and the remaining one third in the extracellular fluid compartment is disproportionately distributed between the interstitial and intravascular compartments in a 3:1 ratio. Colloid oncotic pressure, the effective osmotic pressure between the intravascular and interstitial compartments, is dependent on transcapillary hydrostatic and oncotic pressures, and the relative permeability of capillary membranes that divide these spaces. Because of these forces, within 24 hours of intravenous (i.v.) crystalloid administration, approximately two thirds disperses into the interstitial compartments.

Although the principal determinant of oxygen delivery is hemoglobin, tissue oxygenation remains adequate despite major reductions in hemoglobin (<7 g/dL) as long as intravascular volume is adequate and cardiac output appropriately increases. However, with acute blood loss equivalent to 30% to 40% of the plasma volume (class III hypovolemic shock), the physiologic compensatory mechanisms previously described begin to fail. Patients almost always present with classic signs of insufficient perfusion, including marked tachycardia, tachypnea, severely diminished urinary output, and cold, clammy skin. Importantly, in uncomplicated shock, 1,500 to 2,000 mL is the smallest amount of blood loss that is consistently associated with a drop in the systolic blood pressure. Arterial hypotension and a fall in cardiac output diminish oxygen delivery to peripheral tissues. This is shown by the following formula:

$$\text{Oxygen delivery} = \text{cardiac output} \times \text{arterial oxygen content} ([O_2]a)$$

Oxygen consumption, the actual use of oxygen by the tissues, is defined by this formula:

$$\text{Oxygen consumption} = \text{cardiac output} \times ([O_2]a - [O_2]v)$$

where: $[O_2]v$ is the oxygen content in venous blood.

Tissues that can maintain their oxygen consumption accomplish this by increasing their *oxygen extraction,* the ratio of oxygen consumption to oxygen delivery. This results in an increase in the arterial and venous oxygen difference and a reduction in the mixed venous oxygen tension. Eventually, under conditions of increased oxygen demand (stress, sepsis) or insufficient oxygen delivery (severely reduced cardiac output, hypovolemia, profound anemia), these compensatory mechanisms fail, and tissue hypoxia and lactic acidosis ensue. Cerebral and cardiac functions are maintained by diverting blood flow from the skin, muscles, gastrointestinal tract, and kidneys. Complicated shock associated with loss of compensatory physiologic mechanisms is often called *intermediate shock.* In this phase, reversibility is dependent on prompt crystalloid and blood product replacement to avoid irreversible ischemia of vital organs.

Class IV hypovolemic shock, defined as an acute blood loss of more than 2,000 mL, or more than 40% of the circulating volume, is immediately life threatening. Survival depends on rapid transfusion of blood and crystalloid and immediate surgical intervention before cardiac and cerebral circulation fail, resulting in ischemia in these organs. When vital organs fail, total cardiovascular collapse, coma, and eventually, death or multiorgan failure is likely. The transition between the intermediate stage of shock and irreversible shock (late shock or cold shock) is dependent on the duration and severity of the hypovolemia; however, once cellular injury has occurred within the brain and cardiac muscle, shock is almost always irreversible and fatal.

Septic Shock

Sepsis represents a continuum from the preshock phase or early hyperdynamic phase to the late shock phase. The *early hyperdynamic phase* is characterized by a normal or slight decrease in blood pressure and tachycardia. The slight decrease in systemic vascular resistance (SVR) is offset by a marked increase in cardiac output. In contrast, the classic features of *late shock* include a low SVR and cardiac output, hypoperfusion, and lactic acidosis. When sepsis is recognized and treated in its early stages, survival and morbidity are significantly improved. A variety of terms lacking consistent definitions have appeared in the literature to describe early shock, including sepsis or septic syndrome, host septic response, and septicemia. In 1992, the American College of Chest Physicians/ Society of Critical Care Medicine Consensus Conference developed a set of clinical definitions to define the subsets of serious clinical infections (Table 10.3), and in this statement recommended that other arbitrary terminology no longer be used. The changes in terminology were made in an attempt to enhance the likelihood of detection of early infection, to standardize research protocols, and to facilitate reporting outcomes associated with new and investigational therapies. *Sepsis,* so defined, is a systemic response to infection manifested by two or more of the following: fever or hypothermia, tachycardia, tachypnea, and an elevated or severely depressed white blood cell count. *Septic shock* is defined as sepsis with hypotension that persists despite adequate fluid resuscitation, leading to derangements in cellular and organ system function. When the signs and symptoms of the early

TABLE 10.3.
Clinical Definitions of Infection Syndromes

Infection	Microbial phenomenon characterized by an inflammatory response to the presence of microorganisms or the invasion of normally sterile host tissue by those organisms
Bacteremia	Presence of viable bacteria in the blood
Systemic inflammatory response syndrome	Systemic inflammatory response to a variety of clinical insults. The response is manifested by two or more of the following conditions: temperature >38°C or <36°C; heart rate >90 beats/min; respiratory rate >20 breaths/min or a $PaCO_2$ <32 mm Hg; or WBC >12,000/μL, <4,000/μL, or >10% immature (band) forms.
Sepsis	The systemic response to infection. This response is manifested by two or more of the following conditions as a result of infection: temperature >38°C or <36°C; heart rate >90 beats/min; respiratory rate >20 breaths/min or $PaCO_2$ <32 torr (<4.3 kPa); WBC >12,000 μL or less than <4,000 μL, or more than >10% immature (band) forms
Severe sepsis[a]	Sepsis associated with organ dysfunction, hypoperfusion, or hypotension. Hypoperfusion and perfusion anomalies may include but are not limited to lactic acidosis, oliguria, or an acute alteration in mental status
Septic shock	Sepsis with hypotension despite adequate fluid resuscitation, along with the presence of perfusion abnormalities that can include, but are not limited to, lactic acidosis, oliguria, or an acute alteration in mental status *Patients who are on inotropic or vasopressor agents may not be hypotensive at the time that perfusion abnormalities are measured.*
Hypotension	A systolic blood pressure of <90 mm Hg or a reduction of >40 mm Hg from baseline, in the absence of other causes of hypotension
Multiple organ dysfunction syndrome	Presence of altered organ function in an acutely ill patient such that homeostasis cannot be maintained without intervention

bpm, beats per minute; WBC, white blood cell count.
[a] Sepsis with organ system dysfunction.
Source: American College of Chest Physicians/Society of Critical Care Medicine Consensus Conference. Definitions for sepsis and organ failure and guidelines for the use of innovative therapies in sepsis. *Crit Care Med* 1992;20:866, with permission.

hyperdynamic phase of shock are present but no site of infection can be found, the process is termed the *systemic inflammatory response syndrome.*

The incidence of sepsis, the precursor to septic shock and multiorgan failure, has continued to increase over the past several decades. It affects an estimated 300,000 to 400,000 hospitalized patients per year. In most institutions, Gram-negative organisms continue to account for over half of all episodes of bacteremia; the most commonly isolated microbes include *Escherichia coli, Klebsiella pneumoniae, Pseudomonas aeruginosa,* and *Enterobacter aerogenes.* Less frequent isolates include *Acinetobacter, Proteus, Serratia, Aeromonas, Xanthomonas, Citrobacter, Achromobacter, Salmonella,* and *Shigella* spp. The incidence of hospital-acquired bacteremia has increased coincident with the rise in predisposing risk factors. These include advanced age, underlying systemic disease (diabetes mellitus, cirrhosis, malignancy, lymphoproliferative disorders), use of indwelling catheters and other mechanical devices, burns, prolonged or indiscriminate use of broad-spectrum antibiotics, aggressive cytotoxic chemotherapy, and use of corticosteroids or other immunosuppressive agents. Nosocomial colonization of the oropharyngeal and digestive system of mechanically ventilated patients approaches 70% to 90% and is complicated by infection in over 60% of colonized patients.

Gram-negative microbes are by far the greatest offending organisms in obstetrics and gynecology, accounting for 75% to 80% of all septic episodes. Of these, *Escherichia coli* is responsible for approximately 50% of all cases; *Klebsiella, Serratia,* or *Enterobacter* spp. are identified in approximately 30% of patients. Gram-positive organisms (*Staphylococcus* and *Streptococcus* spp.) and obligate anaerobic infections (*Bacteroides fragilis, Peptostreptococcus, Clostridium perfringens, Clostridium sordellii,* and *Fusobacterium* spp.), respectively, account for 15% to 20% and less than 5% of the remaining cases.

The Gram-negative bacterial cell wall consists of an inner and outer cell membrane, the latter of which contains lipopolysaccharide (LPS), or bacterial endotoxin. LPS consists of three principal regions: the O antigen, the R core antigen, and lipid A. The lipid A region is responsible for most, if not all, of the toxicity of the compound. The lipid A portion of the LPS molecule mediates the binding of CD14 receptor (and perhaps other receptors) with lipopolysaccharide-binding protein (LBP). This coupling enables LPS to bind to mammalian cells. Depending on the involved cell type (monocyte, macrophage, leukocyte, endothelial cell), LPS-LBP-CD14 receptor binding induces the release of a variety of mediators. These include cytokines (tumor necrosis factor-α [TNF-α], interleukin-1 [IL-1], interleukin-6, interleukin-8, interferon-λ, prostaglandins, prostacyclins, thromboxane A_2, leukotrienes, other leukocyte granules that contain cytotoxic enzymes (cathepsin, elastase), complement protein fragments (especially C3a, C5a), platelet activating factor (PAF), and catecholamines. Other less-well characterized factors also may be responsible for the development of the charac-

teristic cellular and organ system derangements. Although the mechanisms are less well understood, it appears that the peptidoglycan and lipoteichoic acids of Gram-positive bacteria, certain polysaccharides, extracellular enzymes, and toxins are able to induce intracellular responses similar to those of LPS (Fig. 10.2). The in-

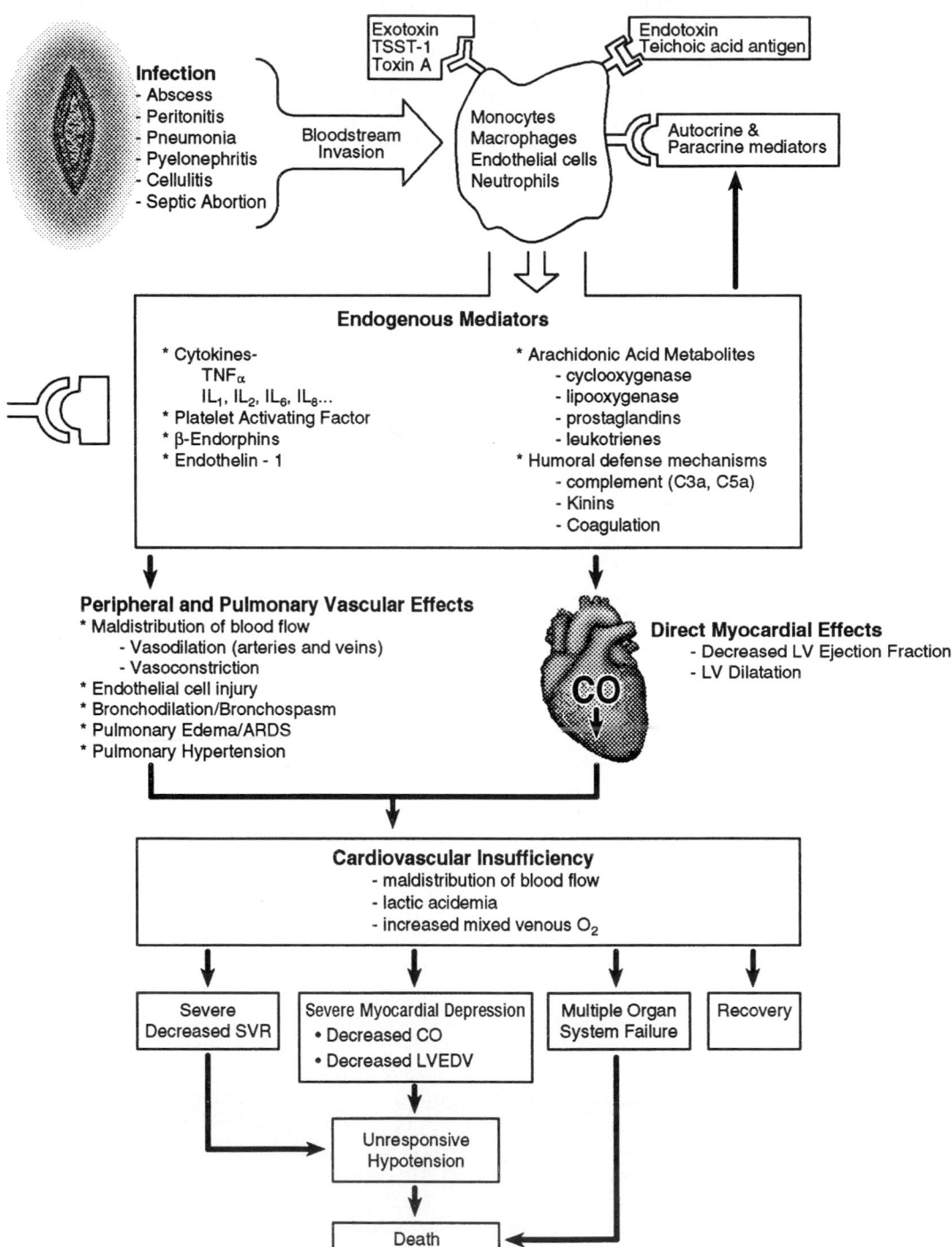

FIGURE 10.2. Pathogenesis of human septic shock. (Adapted from Parillo JE. Pathogenetic mechanisms of septic shock. *N Engl J Med* 1993;328:1471; and Cunnion RE, Parillo JE. Myocardial dysfunction in sepsis: recent insights. *Chest* 1989;95:941, with permission.)

flammatory cytokines interact by way of endocrine, paracrine, and autocrine mechanisms to stimulate leukocytes and vascular endothelial cells to release other cytokines, express cell-surface adhesion molecules, and increase production of arachidonic metabolites. Biologically, their effects appear to be synergistic. Available research suggests that TNF-α, in particular, plays an early, critical role in cellular activation and the propagation of the inflammatory response. Serum levels of TNF-α are elevated in severe sepsis, myocardial infarction, acute respiratory distress syndrome (ARDS), and multiorgan failure, and high levels correlate with increased mortality rates. In contrast, IL-1 levels are only slightly increased in humans with severe sepsis. Serum levels of IL-1 do not appear to correlate with severity or clinical outcome. In women with pelvic inflammatory disease interleukin-6 (IL-6) levels in cervical secretions were found to be significantly elevated compared with controls (median 317 versus 111 pg/dL, $p = 0.003$). Moreover, endometrial tissue IL-6 levels also were higher, suggesting that IL-6 eventually may be used as a clinical adjunct to pelvic inflammatory disease.

Hemostatic defects are common in sepsis and result from vascular endothelial cell injury thought to be caused by endotoxins and phospholipid-derived mediators. The net coagulation defects in sepsis are predominantly procoagulant and override the anticoagulant effects that concomitantly occur. Prostaglandin E_2 and prostacyclin are potent vasodilators, whereas thromboxane A_2 is a potent vasoconstrictor that, together with PAF, promotes platelet aggregation. Blood coagulation results from activation of the intrinsic (factor XII, prekallikrein, high-molecular-weight kininogen), extrinsic (factor VII), and common pathways, culminating in the generation of thrombin. Thrombosis is enhanced by impairment of antithrombin III and tissue plasminogen activator, as well as by plasminogen activator inhibitor-1, released by stimulated monocytes. Neutrophils, attracted by the injured vascular epithelium, release prostacyclins that inhibit thrombin formation, and elastases, free oxygen radicals, proteases, and leukotrienes that are responsible for fibrinolysis. Microcirculation is further impaired by the resulting microthrombi and the cytotoxic effects of cytokines released by inflammatory cells attracted to the damaged endothelium. This effect has been proposed as a possible mechanism for persistent organ system dysfunction. Thrombocytopenia is common. Although fulminant disseminated intravascular coagulation eventually can develop, the coagulation profile usually is consistent with compensated intravascular coagulation with fibrinolysis. That is, fibrinogen levels are normal or slightly decreased, prothrombin time and partial thromboplastin time are within the normal range, and the D-dimer assay is only weakly positive.

In addition to a severe systemic vascular response, patients with sepsis and septic shock also develop severe derangements in cardiac function. Although these effects have been attributed to global myocardial ischemia, recent studies support the hypothesis that myocardial depression occurs in response to circulating myocardial depressant substances, such as a soluble compound released by the pancreas and TNF-α. Initially, patients may present with a normal or slightly reduced cardiac output. This is caused by hypovolemia from arterial and venous dilatation and interstitial pooling. With adequate fluid resuscitation, the hemodynamic presentation is one with a marked increase in cardiac output (>11 L/min), a low SVR, and a severely reduced ventricular ejection fraction. In surviving patients, there is a compensatory increase in the left ventricular end-diastolic volume (LVEDV) secondary to ventricular dilatation. The initial cardiac effects of septic shock include decreased contractility, along with compensatory ventricular dilatation. Because stroke volume is maintained and tachycardia is pronounced, cardiac output is almost always dramatically increased. In this setting, cardiac output is a poor measure of myocardial performance. In the recovery phase, the SVR returns to normal over 24 hours or so, and the cardiac index drops to near normal levels. In studies that compared patients who died to survivors, little or no initial reduction in stroke volume or increase in LVEDV was found, suggesting that compensatory ventricular dilatation is absent in these patients. Consequently, there is no compensatory increase in stroke volume and cardiac output, which are essential to maintain arterial pressure and systemic vascular resistance. Depending on the severity of hypoperfusion and organ system reserve, cardiocirculatory collapse and death or multiorgan failure may ensue (see Fig. 10.2).

A major feature of the systemic inflammatory response, regardless of whether the initial insult is infection, pump failure, or hypovolemia, is the rapid loss of lean body mass associated with net nitrogen losses (20 to 30 g/d). The primary sites of total protein catabolism are the skeletal muscle, connective tissue, and gut mucosa. Hepatic uptake of amino acids is increased, with a concomitant increase in the synthesis of acute-phase proteins. Energy expenditure is often 1.5 to 2 times the basal rate, and is increased in proportion to the degree of injury by a process known as aerobic glycolysis. The net result is a significant increase in the production and release of lactate and pyruvate from muscles, wounds, and monocytes. Hepatic gluconeogenesis is increased, as well as glycogenolysis. As hypoperfusion worsens, lactic acid is generated by hypoxic tissue, resulting in metabolic acidosis. Initially, a blood gas analysis usually demonstrates a respiratory alkalosis; typically, a metabolic acidosis of multifactorial origin eventually develops. The decreases in bicarbonate are often in excess of the measured increase in lactic acid. Hyperglycemia can occur, especially in diabetics; however, impaired gluconeogenesis and excessive insulin release can lead to profound hypoglycemia. Lipolysis and ketogenesis are increased, and long-chain fatty acid deficiency develops in the absence of nutritional support.

In patients who develop irreversible organ failure, the systemic inflammatory response is maintained long after the initial injury and response have abated. Although the mechanisms for this process are poorly understood, undetected microcirculatory dysfunction may be a critical factor. More likely, at some critical point, the perpetuation of cellular and organ system hypermetabolism becomes independent of host regulatory mechanisms.

At the cellular level, differences in ionic composition between the cellular and extracellular compartment are normally maintained by semipermeable membranes, energy-dependent cell transport mechanisms, transmembrane differences in electrical potential, particle charge, and oncotic pressure. With the development of metabolic acidosis, coupled with a decreased production of intracellular cyclic adenosine triphosphate (the energy substrate for cell transport), the normal ionic composition within cells that is critical for mitochondrial function can no longer be maintained. There is an influx of sodium and water and an efflux of potassium, resulting in gradual hemoconcentration and hyponatremia. Although irreversible cellular injury and, ultimately, cell death can result from organ system dysfunction caused by these metabolic derangements, cell death, per se, is not an obligate precursor to organ system failure or demise.

CLINICAL FINDINGS AND THEIR PHYSIOLOGIC BASIS

The clinical presentation of shock varies considerably, depending on the severity of the perfusion defect, underlying etiology, and degree of preexisting organ dysfunction. Clinical signs and symptoms and systemic manifestations frequently are subdivided into early, usually reversible manifestations (Table 10.4) and late findings (Table 10.5). In early stages, the clinical findings of hypovolemic and septic shock are quite different, consistent with the differences in pathophysiology. However, in late or irreversible shock, as multiple organ systems become involved, the clinical features and systemic findings are essentially the same, in keeping with a final common pathway for organ system failure or patient demise, regardless of the precipitating insult.

When the cause of shock is reversible, early recognition and prompt therapy usually result in rapid and complete recovery. However, when there is a delay in diag-

TABLE 10.4.
Presenting Features of Shock: Early Signs and Symptoms

Organ System	Hypovolemic (Hemorrhagic) Shock		Septic Shock	
	Symptom or Sign	Cause	Symptom or Sign	Cause
Central nervous	Mental status changes[a]	Decreased cerebral perfusion	Subtle mental changes, septic encephalopathy	Decreased cerebral perfusion
				Cytokine-induced endothelial cell damage results in a leaky blood–brain barrier
Circulatory				Subtle mental changes, septic encephalopathy
Heart	Tachycardia, rapid thready pulse	Adrenergic stimulation increases contractility, increasing cardiac output and SVR. Cardiac output decreases with depressed contractility, decreased SVR	Tachycardia; bounding pulse	Myocardial ischemia, depressed cardiac function, cardiac output may be increased or decreased[a]; decreased SVR
Systemic	Normotensive or hypotensive,[a] decreased JVD;[a] narrow pulse pressure	Decreased SVR and venous return secondary to volume loss. Sympathetic stimulation increases vascular tone.	Normotensive or slightly hypotensive; widened pulse pressure	SVR decreased from reduced circulatory volume from extravascular pooling
Renal	Oliguria[a]	Decreased perfusion from decreased circulating volume	Oliguria	Afferent arteriolar vasoconstriction
Respiratory	Normal or tachypneic[a]	Sympathetic stimulation, acidosis	Tachypnea	Pulmonary edema, acidosis, muscle fatigue
Skin	Cold, clammy	Vasoconstriction, sympathetic stimulation	Warm	Increased cardiac output, peripheral vasodilation, febrile response
Other			Fever or hypothermia	Infection, endotoxins, cytokines

JVD, jugular neck vein distention; SVR, systemic vascular resistance.
[a]Variable in severity, depending on the rate and volume of loss.

TABLE 10.5.
Presenting Features of Shock: Late Signs and Symptoms

Organ System	Symptom or Sign[a]	Cause
Hypovolemic Shock or Septic Shock		
Central nervous	Disorientation, obtundation	Hypoxia, worsening cerebral edema
Circulatory		
Heart	Cardiac dysfunction, tachycardia, and other arrhythmias	Irreversible ischemia, decreased cardiac index, decreased ejection fraction
Systemic	Jugular neck vein distention may be increased or decreased; normotension or progressive hypotension	Right heart failure, extravascular pooling
Renal	Oliguria progressing to anuria	Acute renal failure
Respiratory	Tachypnea	Adult respiratory distress syndrome
Skin	Cold, clammy	Vasoconstriction, sympathetic stimulation
Other	Lactic acidosis	Anaerobic metabolism, hepatic dysfunction; endothelial cell injury, platelet deposition, vascular thrombosis; hepatic dysfunction
	Coagulopathy, thrombocytopenia, depressed platelet function	

[a] Variable in severity, depending on the rate and volume of loss.

nosis, or insufficient respiratory or cardiovascular support, shock can become irreversible, resulting in permanent organ dysfunction or death. As shock becomes irreversible, the patient may rapidly deteriorate and die, or, more commonly, may enter a chronic condition of continued malfunction of one or more organ systems, despite adequate volume restoration, the absence of persistent infection, and other identifiable insults (see Fig. 10.1). This condition has been termed *multiorgan failure syndrome.* Multiorgan failure, depending on the number of organ systems involved, carries a mortality of 30% to 100% and is the most common cause of death from shock. In addition to continued central nervous system, cardiac, and renal dysfunction, organ system failure in its classic presentation extends first to the lung (24 to 72 hours after the original injury), then the liver (5 to 7 days). Later, the gastrointestinal tract (10 to 15 days) is affected, and eventually the syndrome culminates with the development of renal failure (11 to 17 days). However, many variations in clinical presentation are seen. For example, patients can develop acute tubular necrosis without other organ system dysfunction.

Brain

Because the brain is able to compensate for moderate changes in perfusion pressure, unless the mean arterial pressure (MAP) falls below 60 to 70 mm Hg, cerebral perfusion usually remains intact. Symptoms range from subtle changes in mental acuity (class I and II hypovolemic shock; see Table 10.2) to confusion, lethargy, obtundation, and coma. Mental status changes depend on the severity and duration of hypovolemia.

Heart

Progressive cardiac dysfunction aggravates other systemic manifestations. Likewise, the rapid restoration of heart function frequently interrupts the progressive deterioration often associated with irreversible shock. Therefore, in shock states, preservation of cardiac function is critical. Mild to moderate losses in blood volume (up to 1,500 mL) result in a temporary decrease in cardiac output and SVR. Venoconstriction increases venous return, enhancing stroke volume and cardiac output. As shock worsens, cardiac output decreases and severe vasoconstriction develops, leading to hypotension and organ hypoperfusion. Coronary artery perfusion is reduced, leading to myocardial ischemia, dysrhythmias, and further evidence of cardiac dysfunction. With progressive heart failure, the left ventricular end-diastolic pressure rises, which may result in impairment of gas exchange, tissue hypoxia, and pulmonary edema. The most common clinical presentation of cardiac involvement is tachycardia. This may be associated with a wide pulse pressure and bounding pulses, as with the acute hyperdynamic phase of septic shock (systemic inflammatory response syndrome, warm shock, or early shock). Weak, thready pulses typically accompany severe hemorrhagic shock and advanced septic shock (cold shock or late shock). Signs and symptoms of coronary artery hypoperfusion include chest pain and dyspnea; clinical findings can include jugular neck vein distention, pulmonary rales and crackles, a new S3 or S4 gallop, and a mitral regurgitation murmur that signifies papillary muscle injury. ECG changes may be consistent with myocardial ischemia.

Kidney

The kidney, like the heart and brain, also has autoregulatory mechanisms (by way of the renin-angiotensin-aldosterone system) that compensate for mild to moderate hypovolemia. Oliguria is the most sensitive and reliable endpoint in assessing the magnitude of volume loss in a patient with normal renal function. The decrease in urinary output can be minimal or absolute, depending on the initiating insult, the rate of volume loss, and the severity of volume depletion. Early, reversible injury is termed oliguric prerenal azotemia. This phase is characterized by a urine-plasma creatinine ratio greater than 40, a urine sodium excretion of less than 20 mEq/L every 24 hours, a fractional excretion of sodium of less than 1%, and a high urine osmolality (>500 mOsm). Prolonged hypoperfusion can result in renal damage and, consequently, acute renal failure. Oliguric acute renal failure is characterized by a urine-plasma creatinine ratio of less than 20, an elevated urinary sodium (>40 mEq/L every 24 hours), a fractional excretion of sodium of more than 1%, and a decrease in the ability to concentrate urine. In this phase, urine osmolality is generally less than 350 mOsm.

In contrast to early hypovolemic shock, in the acute phase of septic shock the renovascular response is one of marked oliguria in association with reduced renal blood flow. Renal failure develops despite relative conservation of the mean arterial pressure and an intravascular volume that is normal or slightly reduced. Although the exact mechanisms leading to renal failure are not fully understood, potent vasoconstrictors, including endothelin, thromboxane A_2, and leukotriene D_4, may be responsible. In response to endotoxin-induced endothelial cell swelling, the peptide endothelin-1 is released from the endothelial cells lining the afferent arterioles. Severe vasospasm results, that subsequently reduces the glomerular filtration rate and the fractional excretion of sodium. Polymorphonuclear leukocytes attracted by endotoxin and endothelin-1 accumulate within the renovascular network, releasing cytokines and generating oxygen free radicals that injure the endothelial cell lining. In response to endothelin and leukotrienes, mesangial cells contract, resulting in interstitial edema and reduced glomerular capillary ultrafiltration. Damaged endothelial cells release another major vasoconstrictor, thromboxane A_2, by way of the cyclooxygenase pathway. Thromboxane A_2, a potent platelet activator, promotes platelet aggregation, resulting in renovascular thrombosis. The receptor for thromboxane A_2, or a closely related receptor, induces production of another major vasoconstrictor, a prostaglandin F_2 compound, 8-epi-prostaglandin $F_2\alpha$. This compound is formed by the oxidation of arachidonic acid by oxygen free radicals. Together, these vasoconstrictors selectively act on the renovascular system, progressively reducing renal blood flow. Depending on the severity of the perfusion defect and the redistribution of blood flow, the resulting perfusion defect can be partial or total, and tubular or cortical necrosis, or both, can result.

Skin and Mucous Membranes

When the skin is poorly perfused, its temperature falls and its color changes, so that it is cold to the touch and pale, dusky, or mottled in appearance. When hypoxemia is pronounced, the skin may become frankly cyanotic. Sympathetic stimulation results in increased sweat gland secretion; consequently, the skin may be moist, cold, or clammy. With mild hypovolemia, capillary refill, which is clinically assessed by compressing and then releasing pressure on the fingernail beds, remains normal. However, with losses of 30% or more of the circulating volume, patients nearly always demonstrate a positive capillary refill test (>2 sec). The lips and oral cavity may appear dry or chapped. The conscious patient usually experiences intense thirst.

Lung

The pulmonary vasculature is particularly susceptible to injury resulting from all forms of shock. Clinical manifestations include dyspnea, progressive hypoxemia, diffuse bilateral pulmonary infiltrates, and reduced compliance. This condition is referred to as ARDS. The combination of ARDS and Gram-negative sepsis is particularly ominous, with mortality rates of 80% to 90%. ARDS results from increased pulmonary capillary permeability and the accumulation of extravascular lung water. Inflammatory cells spill into the interstitium and alveoli, destroying the delicate type I alveolar cells. This is followed by proliferation of type II pneumocytes, thickening of the alveolar-capillary membranes, and subsequent fibrosis. Clinically, ARDS is characterized by intrapulmonary shunting, widening of the alveolar-arterial oxygen gradient, reduced pulmonary compliance, and functional residual capacity. Radiographic findings are consistent with pulmonary edema, despite a normal or low pulmonary capillary wedge pressure (PCWP). Arterial PaO_2 remains low (<65 mm Hg) even with supplemental oxygen, and assisted mechanical ventilation often is required.

Liver

Liver dysfunction is characterized by elevated bilirubin levels, rarely exceeding 10 mg/dL, approximately 80% of which is conjugated. Hyperbilirubinemia results from the breakdown of red blood cells and from hepatocellular dysfunction. Although alkaline phosphatase often is one to three times normal, more dramatic elevations are sometimes seen, especially in the elderly. Patients with hepatic failure secondary to sepsis continue to demonstrate progressively worsening abnormalities in glucose, fat, and amino acid metabolism. The amino acid profile is typically one of decreased branched chain and increased aromatic amino acids. The mechanism for these liver derangements remains uncertain. Liver biopsies in patients with certain forms of pneumonia (e.g., *Streptococcus pneumoniae*) have demonstrated hepatocellular injury with focal necrosis. In patients with other types of bacterial infection, liver biopsies that demonstrate extrahepatic cholestasis and Kupffer cell hyperplasia, but no evidence of hepatocyte necrosis, are more likely. It is well known that splanchnic ischemia can cause hepatocellular injury. In patients with shock, it has been postulated that bacteria and endotoxins released from the gastrointestinal tract and cleared by Kupffer cells within the liver may be responsible for the hepatic derangements associated with liver failure. Endotoxin stimulates the release of cytokines and other mediators from Kupffer cells that, in turn, act on hepatocytes in a paracrine fashion to modulate the synthesis of acute-phase proteins, as well as the changes in glucose and lipid metabolism. Regardless of the underlying mechanisms, in shock, metabolic processes are activated that, if left unchecked, result in hepatocellular injury.

Gastrointestinal Tract

Gastrointestinal failure presents as gastrointestinal stress bleeding, which is characterized clinically by "coffee-ground" staining of gastric aspirates, or frank, bright red bleeding. In addition to blood loss, the resulting mucosal injury increases the likelihood of translocation of bacteria to the blood and liver. In patients with other forms of shock, bacterial translocation, the movement of viable organisms from the gut lumen across intact epithelium into the mesenteric lymph nodes, liver, spleen, lungs, or blood has been postulated as a potential source of bacteria and sepsis. Normally, the gastrointestinal mucosa serves as an important mechanical barrier to systemic contamination by intraluminal microbes. Also, the normal gut flora consists predominantly of anacrobic bacteria that displace more pathogenic organisms such as *E. coli* and *Candida albicans* away from the gastrointestinal mucosa. This important host defense mechanism is termed *colonization resistance*. The source of Gram-negative bacteremia after trauma and hypovolemic shock is thought to be from mucosal endothelial cell injury or from bacterial translocation. The microvascular circulation of the mesenteric villi appears to be highly susceptible to mesenteric ischemia, which leads to further endothelial cell injury. As with the kidney and lung, inflammatory cells are attracted to the site of endothelial cell injury. Cytokines and oxygen free radicals are released that promote additional injury, that may result in mucosal ulceration or bleeding, or both.

MANAGEMENT OF SHOCK

Reversibility is dependent on severity, the underlying cause, the duration of cardiovascular collapse, and the presence of preexisting organ dysfunction. Survival and reduced morbidity are frequently dependent on the ability of the treating physician to respond quickly and logically. All immediate resuscitative efforts should be directed at maximizing oxygen delivery at the cellular level. Cellular oxygen content is dependent on the arterial oxygenation, circulatory volume, and hematocrit.

For the gynecologist who infrequently encounters a moribund, unstable patient in shock, it may be useful to remember to restore *ORDER*. The mnemonic, *ORDER*, outlined in Table 10.6, provides the appropriate sequence of resuscitative priorities. After immediate resuscitative measures are initiated, it is highly recommended that continued management of all but the least complicated cases be carried out in a modern critical care unit. A team approach with the benefit of staff trained in intensive care medicine can greatly improve the likelihood of survival as well as significantly reduce morbidity. General guidelines for managing shock are provided in Table 10.7.

Oxygenate

For patients with minimal or no respiratory distress, oxygen delivery at 1 to 6 L/min by nasal cannula may be sufficient. When respiratory distress is evident, oxygen delivery by face mask at the recommended flow rate (8 to 10 L/min) will increase the inspired oxygen concentrations to 80% to 100% with an oxygen reservoir compared to 40% to 60%, without a reservoir. For patients who are disoriented or obtunded, tiring, or unable to maintain sufficient arterial oxygenation ($PaO_2 < 60$ mm Hg), the airway must be protected. Immediate endotracheal intubation with positive pressure ventilation should be instituted. Oxygenation in patients with increased compliance and high intrapulmonary shunt fractions

---

TABLE 10.6.

Resuscitative Priorities in the Management of Overt Shock: Restore ORDER

O: *Oxygenate:* Assure adequate airway, tidal volume, 6 to 8 L/min of oxygen by closed mask, nasal catheter, or endotracheal tube

R: *Restore circulatory volume:* One or more intravenous lines, assess volume loss and replace with crystalloid; administer whole blood or packed red blood cells; with severe hemorrhage or disseminated intravascular coagulation replace clotting factors as indicated; sterile packing until hemodynamic stability is restored; central venous monitoring; obtain cultures if indicated with intravenous access

D: *Drug therapy:* Pharmacologic support of blood pressure, antibiotics, miscellaneous agents for specified conditions

E: *Evaluate response to therapy:* Identify etiology of shock; volume replacement based on right heart catheterization or central venous monitoring; reevaluate hemoglobin, coagulation profiles, serum chemistries (potassium, phospate, acid–base, PaO_2, creatinine); modify treatment plan/pharmacologic therapy; obtain culture results; radiographic studies—abdominal films, chest x-ray, CT—scan, ventilation—perfusion scan, as indicated by suspected underlying condition

R: *Remedy the underlying cause:* Surgical control of bleeding using selective interventional embolization or surgery; antibiotic therapy based on culture results

Source: Cavanagh D, Marsden DE. Hemorrhagic shock in the gynecologic patient. *Clin Obstet Gynecol* 1985;28:383, with permission.

TABLE 10.7.
General Guidelines for Managing Shock

Cardiovascular/hemodynamic	
Blood pressure	Maintain systolic blood pressure at least 90 mm Hg; mean arterial pressure at least 60 mm Hg
Pulmonary capillary wedge pressure	14–18 mm Hg
Central venous pressure	12–15 cm H_2O
Oxygen delivery	Maintain hemoglobin >8 g/dL; 10 g/dL in patients with cardiac compromise
Oxygen saturation	Arterial oxyhemoglobin saturation least 92% (pulse oximetry saturation does not reflect arterial PaO_2 with significant hypotension or compromised peripheral perfusion)
Cardiac index	>4.0 L/min/m² (septic shock)
	>2.2 L/min/m² (other shock states)
Pulmonary	Normalize alveolar-arterial gradient ($P\dot{a}O_2$ >30 mm Hg or $S\dot{a}O_2$ >55%)
Blood gases	Maintain:
	PaO_2 80–100 mm Hg
	$PaCO_2$ 30–35 mm Hg
	pH >7.35[a]
Renal	Maintain urine output of 20–30 mL/h (0.5 mL/kg/h); normalize blood urea nitrogen, creatinine
Hepatic	Bilirubin <3 mg/dL
Mental status	Restore/maintain orientation
Coagulation studies	Normalize
Serum lactate level	Should be 2.2 mMol/L; suspect tissue hypoperfusion when elevated

[a] Mild acidosis is preferable to alkalosis to maximize oxygen dissociation at the cellular level.
Source: Jimenez EJ. Shock. In: Civetta JM, Taylor RW, Kirby RR, eds. *Critical care*, 3rd ed., Philadelphia: Lippincott-Raven Publishers, 1997:89; and Hollenberg SM, Parrillo JE. Shock. In: Fauci AS, Martin JP, Braunwald E, Kasper DL, Isselbacher KJ, Hauser SL, Wilson JD, Longo DL, et al, eds. *Harrison's principles of internal medicine*, vol 1, New York: McGraw-Hill, 1997:220, with permission.

(e.g., ARDS, pulmonary edema) can be improved by the addition of positive end-expiratory pressure (PEEP) at physiologic or low levels (5 to 15 cm H_2O). Because high levels of PEEP can reduce venous return and consequently, reduce cardiac output, patients needing higher levels may benefit from invasive hemodynamic monitoring to determine the "best" PEEP to optimize oxygen delivery.

Restore Circulating Volume

Initial fluid therapy should consist of a 1- to 2-L fluid challenge with an isotonic electrolyte solution, preferably Ringer's lactate. Normal or half normal saline solution can also be infused; however, prolonged use of these infusions increases the risk of hyperchloremic acidosis, especially in a patient with impaired renal function. Because severe hypernatremia increases the risk of brain dehydration or death, hypertonic saline is not recommended except under special circumstances, and is not part of the initial management. Albumin and other colloidal solutions (high- or low-molecular-weight dextran, polyethyl starches) have been advocated to restore and maintain circulation, under the premise that these agents are more likely to remain in the intravascular compartment. In trauma and perioperative patients, hypoalbuminemia of some degree is almost universal, and results from crystalloid administration, increases in capillary permeability, and sequestration of albumin in the interstitial compartment. Hyperoncotic albumin has been used in edematous patients based on rationale that edema fluid may be "pulled" into the intracellular compartment and excreted. This practice is not supported by scientific data, and may actually be harmful. Colloids can eventually "leak" across damaged pulmonary capillary epithelium, promoting the development of pulmonary edema. Two recent metaanalyses of albumin administration versus crystalloid infusion found a 4% to 6% increase in the risk for death in those patients who received albumin. The choice of fluid replacement also has considerable cost implications, since colloid is considerably more expensive than crystalloid administration.

In most cases, hemorrhagic shock should be managed initially by inserting one or two large-bore (14- or 16-gauge) angiocatheters for volume replacement. Central venous catheterization is not recommended for most patients. Central venous access will not improve the rate of fluid administration and carries the risk of pneumothorax and other potentially life-threatening complications. Central circulation also can be improved by elevating the feet or by placing the patient in the Trendelenburg position. Blood can be drawn for initial laboratory assessment at the time that i.v. access is obtained and should include a complete blood count with differential and platelets, electrolytes, blood urea nitrogen (BUN), creatinine, calcium, magnesium, glucose, phosphate, and, where indicated, serum human chorionic gonadotropin-β, liver function studies, clotting profiles, serum lactate, and blood cultures.

In patients with distributive shock, or shock following ischemic injury from severe or prolonged hypovolemia, damage to the capillary endothelium results in increased capillary permeability and greater losses into the interstitium. Disproportionately larger volumes of fluid are required to restore circulatory volume than is immediately apparent by clinical estimation of the plasma volume. For example, 6 to 7 L of fluid may be required for what appears to be 1 to 1.5 L of plasma volume depletion. Most of these patients have some degree of cardiac dysfunction and are at high risk for lung injury from injudicious volume expansion. Because central venous pressure and PCWP are often discordant, right heart catheterization has been advocated after immediate fluid resuscitation. Additional volume replacement or pressure support may then be based on determinations of the pulmonary artery mean and occlusive pressures, cardiac output, cardiac index, and SVR. Mixed venous oxygen content also can be obtained, so that oxygen delivery at the cellular level may be estimated. For patients with pulmonary injury, shunt fractions and alveolar-arterial oxygen differences can be calculated, and may be used to guide adjustment in ventilatory support or the need for red blood cell transfusion. Connors and colleagues, in a prospective study of 52 critically ill patients with multiorgan system disease, found that clinical estimates of volume status were frequently not reflective of right heart catheterization findings. In this series, after right heart catheterization, major changes in therapy (altering the rate of fluid administration, or starting or stopping a pressor agent, or both) were necessary in 48.4% of patients.

Many cardiologists and critical care physicians believe that therapy guided by pulmonary artery catheterization leads to improved patient outcomes. However, the "routine" use of Swan-Ganz catheters in patients with sepsis is controversial. One or more randomized controlled clinical trials could clarify this issue; however, attempts at randomized controlled trials have failed, because physicians, convinced that the procedure is or is not beneficial, have refused to allow randomization of their patients. In the absence of controlled trials, observational studies, where placement of right heart catheters is at the discretion of the physician, are being used in an attempt to clarify the risk:benefit ratio. An obvious limitation of observational studies is that more critically ill patients are more likely to undergo right heart catheterization, and in turn, are more likely to die. This treatment selection bias has been termed "confounding by indication." In one observational study of 5,735 critically ill patients in five teaching hospitals, pulmonary artery catheterization was found to be associated with increased mortality and cost, with no proven benefit. The Pulmonary Artery Catheter (PAC) Consensus Conference: Consensus Statement concluded that evidence is insufficient to support the routine use of pulmonary artery catheterization in septic patients (Table 10.8). For patients with myocardial infarction complicated by cardiogenic shock and

right ventricular infarction, it was the consensus of the committee that right heart catheterization improves outcome. In patients with respiratory failure (i.e., adult respiratory syndrome versus pulmonary edema), determinations of pulmonary artery mean and occlusive pressures, cardiac output, cardiac index, and systemic vascular resistance may be useful to determine the underlying cause and to guide fluid therapy. Even in this clinical situation, it is inconclusive that pulmonary artery catheters improve survival.

Specific blood component therapy has virtually replaced whole blood transfusion as the standard of care. Packed red blood cells (PRBC) have a volume of 200 to 250 mL and a hematocrit of 70%, and, combined with normal saline, are the component of choice for hemorrhagic shock. Loss of approximately 20% of blood volume is equivalent to a 1,500-mL blood loss, and in a previously healthy 70-kg individual is not associated with a significant reduction in oxygen-carrying capacity or ventricular filling pressures when adequate crystalloid resuscitation is given. Because the oxygen-carrying capacity is met in most healthy patients with a hemoglobin of 7 g/dL, empiric transfusion for moderate anemia (hemoglobins of 8 to 10 mg/dL) is no longer recommended. It should be noted, however, that because most of the oxygen transported in the blood is by hemoglobin, correction of anemia is an important component in optimizing oxygen delivery at the cellular level (see Table 10.7).

In general, these recommendations regarding red blood cell transfusion have been derived from the management of trauma victims that were in normal health prior to an acute event. In critically ill patients and those with significant underlying cardiac disease, red cell transfusions have been used liberally to maintain hemoglobin levels between 10 and 12 g/dL, in order to reduce the potential adverse effects of oxygen debt. The importance of weighing the benefits of red blood cell transfusion against potential adverse effects, has received considerable attention in the recent literature. Known risks include hepatitis C (one in 30,000 to 250,000), human immunodeficiency virus (one in 200,000 to 2,000,000), human T-cell lymphotrophic virus (one in 250,000 to 2,000,0000), bacterial contamination (one in 500,000) acute hemolytic reactions (one in 250,000 to 1,000,000), delayed hemolytic reactions (one in 1,000) and transfusion-related lung injury (one in 5,000). Allogenic blood transfusion also increases the risks of immunosuppression, presumably secondary to exposure and sensitization of leukocytes. This has been associated with increased risks for postoperative infection, and in some series, increased risks for cancer recurrence. Despite these risks, the benefit of leukocyte reduction of cellular blood components is unproved, and this practice is unlikely to be adopted without proven benefit because the cost of universal leukodepletion is in excess of $500,000,000. In a multicenter, randomized controlled clinical trial of critically ill patients, there were no differences in mortality rates when hemoglobin levels were maintained between 7 and 9 mg/dL, compared with

TABLE 10.8.
Pulmonary Artery Catheter (PAC) Consensus Conference: Consensus Statement

Indications	Evidence[a]	Recommendations
MI and progressive hypotension or cardiogenic shock	Level IV or V	Based on expert opinion, management by guided by PAC is indicated, but no conclusive proof; prospective trials needed
Mechanical complications of acute MI	Level IV or V	Based on expert opinion, management by guided by PAC indicated, but no conclusive proof; prospective trials recommended
Refractory CHF	Level III	Benefit uncertain, may be indicated, studies needed to determine if outcome improved
Pulmonary hypertension	Levels IV or V	Benefits uncertain, may be indicated, studies needed to determine if outcomes are improved
Shock or hemodynamic instability	Levels IV or V	Benefits uncertain; may be useful in patients unresponsive to fluid resuscitation and vasopressors; clinical trials needed to determine if outcomes are improved over less invasive monitoring
Cardiac surgery	Level II	No benefit in low-risk patients; uncertain in high-risk patients; may be important in patients with left ventricular dysfunction
Peripheral vascular surgery	Level III	Perioperative complications are reduced, but effect on mortality uncertain
Perioperative care of geriatric patients	Level IV or V	Routine perioperative use not indicated
Preeclampsia	Level IV or V	Routine use not supported; may be beneficial in patients with oligouria unresponsive to fluid administration, pulmonary edema, or resistant hypertension
Sepsis or septic shock	Level III	No improvement in an observational study of patients with septic shock; benefits uncertain; may be useful in the absence of a response to initial aggressive fluid resuscitation and low-dose inotropic/vasoconstrictors
Augmentation of systemic oxygen delivery to supranormal levels	Level I	Not recommended
Respiratory failure	Level IV or V	May alter treatment and correct misdiagnosis. Patients with acute lung injury and acute respiratory distress syndrome who are hypotensive may benefit; clinical trials with carefully defined groups needed
Critically ill infants and children	Level IV or V	Beneficial in children with pulmonary hypertension, refractory shock, severe respiratory failure, multiple organ dysfunction. Relatively few pediatric patients require PACs.
Accuracy of measurements (venous oximetry, ejection fractions, cardiac output)	Level III	"Specialized" catheters accurately measure these parameters; comparisons of "standard" versus "specialized" catheters in specific clinical settings are needed
Reduction of complications	Level IV or V	PAC is a monitoring device, not a therapeutic modality, and should be placed only when used to guide therapy. Training, credentialing, and continuing quality improvement issues should be intensified.

[a] Levels of evidence: *Level I:* Large randomized trials with clear-cut results. *Level II:* Small randomized trials with uncertain results. *Level III:* Nonrandomized, contemporaneous controls. *Level IV:* Nonrandomized, historical controls and expert opinion. *Level V:* Case series, uncontrolled studies, and expert opinions. CHF, congestive heart failure; MI, myocardial infarction.

scheduled transfusions to maintain levels between 10 and 12 mg/dL. Significantly, among younger (<55 years) and less acutely ill patients, mortality rates were appreciably lower among those who were not transfused. Using lower hemoglobin values of 7 to 9 mg/dL as the threshold, the number of packed red cell transfusions and exposure to blood products was reduced by 54% and 33%, respectively.

Alternatives to PRBC transfusion are increasing in popularity and acceptance. Preoperative autologous donation, the practice of donating blood prior to surgery, accounted for one of every 12 units donated in the United States in 1992. Unfortunately, the practice of au-

tologous donation is inherently wasteful. Up to half of the blood donated for this purpose in the United States is ultimately discarded, because use of surplus autologous donations in other patients is not recommended. The risk of virus transmission, which spawned the wide acceptance of this practice, has dramatically declined in recent years, and autologous blood donation actually may be harmful to patients. Acute normovolemic hemodilution entails the removal of whole blood from a patient immediately before surgery, and volume is restored with crystalloid or colloid. After major bleeding is controlled, the blood is reinfused. Advantages are a reduction in the red-cell volume lost; the units procured require no testing and the possibility of an ABO-incompatible blood transfusion is theoretically eliminated because the blood never leaves the operating room. Acute normovolemic hemodilution also is less expensive. Cell-saving devices allow intraoperative recovery of red cells; survival of the red cells that are recovered appears to be similar to that of transfused allogeneic red cells. Relative contraindications include infection, malignancy, and contaminants (amniotic fluid/gastrointestinal contents/ascites/pus) within the operative field.

Epoetin alfa (Procrit; Ortho Biotech Inc., Raritan, NJ) is currently approved in the United States for the treatment of anemia in patients with nonmyeloid malignancies who receive concomitant chemotherapy. In patients with cancer who received chemotherapy independent of tumor response, epoetin alfa, 10,000 U given three times weekly (and increased to 20,000 U three times weekly, depending on hemoglobin response at 4 weeks) resulted in an improvement in patient-reported functional capacity and quality of life. Epoetin alpha is a valuable adjunct to transfusion in patients adverse to transfusion, or with underlying conditions that are associated with reduced erythropoiesis. This form of therapy should not be initiated unless iron intake is tolerated. Finally, red-cell substitutes that approximate the oxygen-carrying and oxygen-delivery capacity of red cells are in various stages of clinical development, and may become life-saving alternatives in military and trauma settings or for patients who refuse other transfusion options.

When blood loss exceeds 25% of the blood volume, whole blood or, in the presence of bleeding consistent with coagulopathy, packed red blood cells and fresh frozen plasma (FFP) in a 4:1 ratio is usually preferred. Whenever possible, the underlying coagulopathy should be determined, and platelets and FFP should be judiciously given based on clotting profiles/platelet counts. Cryoprecipitate is concentrated fresh frozen plasma in a small volume of 10 to 15 mL (one bag per 5 kg in a 70-kg individual). Because cryoprecipitate consists of pooled factor components from multiple donors, risk of infection is significantly increased. Therefore, cryoprecipitate should be reserved for deficiencies in factor VIII, von Willebrand factor, fibrinogen factor XIII, and /or fibronectin. When disseminated intravascular coagulation is suspected based on massive transfusion and the persistence of significant oozing or bleeding, FFP instead of cryoprecipitate is the component of choice. To avoid the risks of hemolysis, agglutination, and clotting, all blood products should be administered through filtered lines with normal saline without electrolyte or drug additives. To prevent hypothermia, warming of blood products is indicated when the volume infused exceeds 50 mg/kg per hour.

When transfusion is massive (10 U PRBC/24 h), platelets in addition to packed cell transfusion becomes critical, to replace platelets dilutionally depleted. One unit of platelet concentrate increases the count by 5,000 to 10,000/µL. Although not absolute, another indication for platelet transfusion is a preoperative or intraoperative platelet count of 50,000/µL or less. FFP is indi-

cated for patients with disseminated intravascular coagulation, severe liver disease, or massive transfusion, and for specific clotting disturbances when the factor concentrate is not available. However, FFP is not indicated for volume expansion or nutritional support, and should not be given empirically with PRBC transfusions.

Drug Therapy

Pharmacologic Support of Blood Pressure

Inotropic agents and vasopressors recommended in the management of hypotensive shock are outlined in Table 10.9. Except for the newer agents (inamrinone, milrinone acetate), all of these sympathomimetic agents have both inotropic and vasoconstrictive effects. Because of their cardiotropic effects, dopamine hydrochloride and dobutamine hydrochloride are the preferred agents in the initial treatment of shock. Epinephrine and norepinephrine, which are potent vasoconstrictors, usually are reserved for refractory hypotension. It is important to bear in mind that these vasoactive drugs are not indicated until adequate volume replacement has been given, and are seldom of benefit in the management of hemorrhagic shock. Use of vasopressors in the face of inadequate volume resuscitation can worsen preexisting ischemia, increasing cellular and organ system injury. However, the judicious use of sympathomimetic agents after adequate fluid repletion may be useful to correct inadequate cardiac function and persistent hypoperfusion after sufficient hydration.

Because they reduce myocardial oxygen requirements and improve myocardial performance, vasodilators (nitroglycerin, nitroprusside) are generally preferred in the management of patients with cardiogenic shock who have mean arterial pressures over 70 mm Hg. In these patients, myocardial oxygen requirements may be reduced and myocardial performance improved. Vasodilators are not indicated in the setting of hypovolemic and septic shock associated with low arterial pressures secondary to peripheral vasodilatation. Under these circumstances, vasodilators serve to further reduce venous return, and may intensify hypotension and further reduce coronary artery perfusion.

Dopamine is the preferred catecholaminergic agent in the management of the hypotensive patient whose MAP is less than 60 mm Hg. Dopamine stimulates dopaminergic, α-adrenergic, and β-adrenergic receptors in a dose-dependent fashion. At low doses (1 to 3 µg/kg per minute), dopamine stimulates cerebral, renal, and mesenteric dopaminergic receptors, resulting in vasodilatation and an increase in urinary output. At these doses, heart rate and blood pressure are usually not affected. At moderate doses (2 to 10 µg/kg per minute), both α-adrenergic and β-adrenergic receptors are stimulated, but the $\beta1$-adrenergic effects predominate. The $\beta1$-adrenergic cardiac effects are inotropic, increasing myocardial contractility, sinoatrial rate, and impulse conduction, thereby increasing cardiac output. Myocardial oxygen consumption is also increased, with no compensatory increase in coronary artery blood flow. In a patient

TABLE 10.9.
Pharmacologic Support of the Cardiovascular System

Agent	Usual Dose Range	Adrenergic Effects			Peripheral Vascular Effects	Clinical Setting
		α	β	Dopamine		
INOTROPHIC AGENTS						
Dopamine	1–2 μ/kg/min	+	+	+++	Vasodilation (+)	Oligouria, hypotension
	2–10 μ/kg/min	++	++	+++	Vasoconstriction (++)	Hypotension, bradycardia
	10–30 μ/kg/min	++	++	+++	Vasoconstriction (+++)	Hypotension, bradycardia
Dolbutamine	2.5–15 μg/kg/min (usual); 2–30 μg/kg/min	+	+++	0	Vasodilation (++)	Cardiogenic shock; cardiac pulmonary edema with marginal blood pressure
Isoproterenol	1–10 μg/min	0	+++	0	Vasodilation (++++)	Refractory bradycardia, refractory torsade de pointes
VASOPRESSORS						
Phenylephrine		+++	0	0	Vasoconstriction (+++)	Distributive shock, when no cardiac effect desired
Levarterenol (norepinephrine)	2–20 μg/min (usual); 0.5–89 μg/min	+++	++	0	Vasoconstriction (++++)	Initial emergency treatment of hypotension of any cause
Epinephrine	0.5–1 mg (1:10,0000)	+	++	0	Vasoconstriction (++++)	Cardiac arrest
	1–200 μg/min	++	+++		Vasodilation (+++)	Severe hypotension and bradycardia
	0.3–0.5 mg s.c. (1:1,000)					Anaphylaxis
Inamrinone (formerly, amrinone)	Load: 0.75 mg/kg IV bolus, then 5–10 μg/kg/min (up to 40 μg/kg/min)	0 0	0	Direct myocardial effect, at least in part secondary to inhibition of cardiac cyclic AMP	Vasodilation (++)	Congestive heart failure, cardiogenic shock, usually used combined with dolbutamine
Milrinone lactate	Load 50 μg/kg over 3 min; then 0.375–0.75 μg/kg/min	0 0	0	Direct myocardial effect, at least in part secondary to inhibition of cardiac cyclic AMP	Vasodilation (++)	Congestive heart failure, cardiogenic shock, usually used combined with dolbutamine
Metaraminol bitartrate	Load: 0.5–5 mg, then 15–100 mg infusion	+++	+	0	Vasoconstriction (++++)	Reversal of hypotension from spinal anesthesia; adjunctive treatment for hypotension from hemorrhage, drug reactions, and brain trauma or tumor

with myocardial ischemia, these effects further compromise cardiac function. At higher rates of infusion, there is some stimulation of the α-adrenergic receptors, resulting in vasoconstriction and a rise in blood pressure. At doses above 20 μg/kg per minute, the α-adrenergic effects predominate, resulting in renal, mesenteric, and peripheral arterial vasoconstriction. Dopamine has little β2-adrenergic activity, that is, systemic vasodilator effects.

Dobutamine, a direct-acting inotropic agent with both β1-adrenergic and β2-adrenergic effects, is the pharmacologic treatment of choice in patients with cardiogenic shock. The systemic vasodilatory effects from stimulation of the β2-adrenergic receptors effectively reduce afterload, and thus pulmonary congestion, without increasing oxygen consumption or causing clinically significant tachycardia. Tachycardia is a frequent, undesired side effect of dopamine in this clinical setting. Because cardiogenic shock, and often septic shock as well, are associated with myocardial depression, an elevated left ventricular end-diastolic volume, and an abnormally high pulmonary artery catheter wedge pressure, dobutamine may be preferred or needed in addition to dopamine. Used together at moderate doses, dopamine and dobutamine can maintain arterial pressure with less of an increase in pulmonary artery occlusive pressure and pulmonary congestion than when dopamine alone is used.

Inamrinone, formerly known as amrinone, is a phosphodiesterase inhibitor with positive inotropic and vasodilator activity. The mechanism of action is different from other inotropic agents. Its effects are not blocked by use of α-, β-, cholinergic, or ganglionic blocking agents. In part, inamrinone acts by inhibiting myocardial cyclic adenosine monophosphate phosphodiesterase (AMP) activity, thereby increasing cardiac cyclic AMP levels. Inamrinone has been demonstrated to improve lung compliance in mechanically ventilated patients with severe cardiogenic pulmonary edema, and is currently recommended in the setting of severe acute congestive heart failure with a systolic blood pressure greater than 100 mm Hg. In the treatment of acute refractory congestive heart failure and cardiogenic shock, the pharmacologic effects of inamrinone and milrinone are synergistic with dobutamine, and these agents often are used together.

Isoproterenol is a synthetic sympathomimetic amine with nearly pure β-adrenergic effects. Although its potent inotropic and chronotropic properties increase cardiac output despite a reduction in mean arterial pressure from peripheral vasodilatation, isoproterenol significantly increases tachycardia and oxygen consumption and can induce or exacerbate myocardial ischemia. For this reason, isoproterenol is seldom used to treat shock. The vasopressors (phenylephrine, norepinephrine, and epinephrine) are used for refractory shock. Although epinephrine and norepinephrine have both β- and α-adrenergic effects, they differ in that epinephrine has more potent α-adrenergic activity. These potent agents increase blood pressure predominantly by increasing systemic and peripheral vascular resistance. They must be used with great caution in patients with shock because they may induce or exacerbate myocardial ischemia. In addition to peripheral vasoconstriction, epinephrine and norepinephrine increase coronary artery vasoconstriction; myocardial ischemia and infarction has been reported in the presence of increasing oxygen consumption and tachycardia that is induced or aggravated by the use these agents.

Antibiotic Therapy

When shock is thought to be a result of sepsis, or infection may be a contributing factor, antibiotic therapy should be initiated immediately, as soon as samples of blood and other suspected sites of infections have been obtained for culture. The agents selected should be based on the likely pathogens at the probable site of infection, recent antibiotic use, and the patterns of antimicrobial resistance within the hospital or community (Table 10.10). Empiric broad-spectrum antibiotic therapy should be used and should cover both Gram-positive and -negative organisms. Anaerobic coverage is also indicated when a pelvic source is suspected (tuboovarian abscess or septic abortion). Agents should be given at maximum doses, with dose modification for impaired renal function. Acceptable regimens include an extended-spectrum penicillin (azlocillin, mezlocillin, piperacillin) or third-generation cephalosporin (cefotaxime, ceftazidime) combined with an aminoglycoside. Klastersky and colleagues found that extended-spectrum penicillins combined with aminoglycoside therapy were more effective than cephalosporin-aminoglycoside combinations for Gram-negative sepsis; thus, in the absence of a penicillin allergy, broad-spectrum β-lactam antibiotic–β-lactamase inhibitor combinations such as ticarcillin-clavulanate may be preferable. If *Pseudomonas aeruginosa* is the suspected organism, then coverage must include two agents: an aminoglycoside with either an appropriate third-generation cephalosporin (ceftazidime) or a β-lactam antibiotic β-lactamase inhibitor combination, to prevent the rapid development of resistance. Anaerobic coverage may consist of clindamycin or metronidazole (Flagyl), although dose modifications are required for hepatic failure. Because of the emergence of clindamycin-resistant B fragilis, β-lactam antibiotic–β-lactamase inhibitor combinations and metronidazole are better agents for the empiric treatment of *B. fragilis;* clindamycin can be substituted after drug sensitivity is verified. The only available coverage for methicillin-resistant *Staphylococcus aureus* is vancomycin, which requires dose adjustments in patients with renal compromise. When the suspected source of infection is a peripheral or central venous access site, vancomycin should be added to cover for *Staphylococcus* spp., pending culture results.

Empiric broad-spectrum antibiotic therapy should be replaced with specific therapy as soon as possible because of the significant adverse effects. These include disruption of the normal gut mucosal barrier that, as previously described, increases the risk for opportunistic infections, including yeast sepsis *(C. albicans)*, enterococcus infection, and pseudomembranous enterocolitis. *Clostridium difficile*-induced colitis (CDIC) is a gastrointestinal disorder that results from colonization by and overgrowth of *C. difficile,* a Gram-positive, spore-forming anaerobic bacillus. Exposure to oral antibiotic therapy is the most common predisposing factor; an association with clindamycin use is well established, but anyone colonized with *C. difficile* who receives antibiotic therapy is at risk. Associated medical comorbidities include advanced age and diabetes, recent bowel preparation, admission to an intensive care unit, and chemotherapy. The spore form of *C. difficile* is extremely hearty, resistant to disinfectants routinely used in institutional settings. Hospital spread can be reduced by isolation precautions, use of

TABLE 10.10.
Empiric Antibiotic Selection

	Suspected Source of Sepsis				
	Lung	Abdomen	Skin/Soft Tissue	Urinary Tract	Central Nervous
Major community-acquired pathogens	*Streptococcus pneumoniae*[a] *Hemophilus influenzae* *Legionella* sp *Chlamydia pneumoniae* *Pneumocystis carinii*	*Escherichia coli* *Bacteriodes fragilis*	Group A streptococcus *Staphylococcus aureus* *Clostridium* sp Polymicrobial enteric Gram-negative rods *Pseudomonas aeruginosa* anaerobes staphylococci	*Escherichia coli* *Klebsiella* sp *Enterobacter* sp *Proteus* sp	*Streptococcus pneumoniae*[a] *Niesseria meningiditis* *Listeria monocytogenes* *Escherichia coli* *Haemophilus influenzae*
Empiric antibiotic therapy	Macrolide and third-generation cephalosporin or levofloxacin	Imipenem-cilastatin; pipercillin–tazobactam ± aminoglycoside	Vancomycin ± imipenem-cilastatin; pipercillin-tazobactam	Ciprofloxacin ± aminoglycoside	Vancomycin + third-generation cephalo-sporin; meropenem
Major nosocomial pathogens	Aerobic Gram-negative bacilli	Aerobic Gram-negative rods anaerobes *Candida* sp	*Staphylococcus aureus* aerobic Gram-negative rods	Aerobic Gram-negative rods enterococci	*Pseudomonas aeruginosa* *Escherichia coli* *Klebsiella* sp staphylococci species
Empiric antibiotic therapy	Cefipime; imipenem-cilastinin plus aminoglycoside	Imipenem-cilastatin ± amphotericin B	Vancomycin + cefipime	Vancomycin + cefipime	Cefipime or menopenem + vancomycin

[a] Empiric antibiotic selection for invasive pneumococcal disease should be based on known antibiotic susceptibility patterns in the community. High-level penicillin resistance among pneumococcal isolates is increasing, as has resistance to third-generation cephalosporins and quinolones.

Empiric antibiotic selection for hospital-acquired sepsis should be based on antibiotic resistance patterns for bacteria from each specific institution or intensive care unit. Antibiotic regimen may be modified 48 to 72 hours later, based on culture and antibiotic susceptibility.

Source: Simon D, Trenholme G. Antibiotic selection for patients with septic shock. *Crit Care Clin* 2000;16:217, with permission.

disposable gloves, attention to hand washing after contact with an infected patient, and environmental decontamination. *C. difficile* infection usually presents with mild to moderate diarrhea, sometimes associated with lower abdominal cramping; systemic symptoms usually are absent. Severe colitis without pseudomembrane formation is associated with profuse, debilitating diarrhea, abdominal pain, and distention. Systemic manifestations include fever, nausea, anorexia, malaise, and dehydration. Serum leukocytosis and fecal leukocytes are commonly found. Pseudomembranous colitis is characterized by more severe diarrhea, abdominal pain, and systemic symptoms; proctosigmoidoscopy reveals characteristic adherent yellow plaques. When colitis is life threatening, patients appear acutely ill, with abdominal tenderness and distention, fever, tachycardia, and hypotension or shock. Abdominal tenderness and distention may signify colonic perforation and peritonitis, and abdominal films may demonstrate dilated colon, paralytic ileus, or free air in association with perforation. The development of a paralytic ileus and colonic dilatation can result in a paradoxic decrease in diarrhea. The laboratory diagnosis is made by cytotoxin assay and stool culture.

Antibiotic therapy should be discontinued when *C. difficile* infection is suspected. Antidiarrheals, which decrease gastrointestinal peristalsis and increase the duration of toxin exposure, should be avoided. Oral metronidazole is the drug of choice; oral vancomycin is reserved for patients who cannot tolerate or do not respond to metronidazole. Metronidazole, but not vancomycin can be used i.v. in patients who cannot tolerate oral intake. Patients with systemic manifestations require aggressive replacement of fluid and electrolytes, and may require surgical intervention. If antibiotics must be continued, agents less likely to disrupt the normal colonic microflora, such as aminoglycosides, aztreonam, and fluoroquinolones, which have little or no activity against obligate anaerobes, are preferable.

Necrotizing fasciitis is a rare, potentially fatal infection of the subcutaneous tissue associated with progressive destruction and necrosis of fascia and fat. Culture results can differentiate between two distinct types: type 1, caused by mixed anaerobes and facultative bacteria (Enterobacteriaceae and non–group A streptococci); type 2, associated with group A streptococcus alone or in association with *Staphylococcus* spp. Risk factors include diabetes mellitus, peripheral vascular disease, i.v. drug use, obesity, underlying malignancy, malnutrition, renal failure, and trauma. The portal of entry usually is an open wound. Diabetes mellitus may predispose to necrotizing fasciitis of the vulva, which can begin as a simple abscess, and rapidly track along fascial planes to the inner thighs, mons pubis, and lower abdominal wall. Cutaneous manifestations of streptococcal necrotizing fasciitis include diffuse swelling of the affected area followed by the appearance of bullae filled with clear fluid, which rapidly take on a purplish or violaceous color. Without intervention, the lesions evolve into frank cutaneous gangrene, sometimes with myonecrosis. Systemic symptoms ensue as the inflammatory process advances along fascial planes, including shock, multiorgan failure, and coagulopathy It may be difficult to distinguish between cellulitis, which is amenable to antibiotic therapy; and surgical wound infections and necrotizing fasciitis, which require immediate surgical debridement in addition to antimicrobial therapy. The wound should undergo extensive debridement until viable, bleeding margins are obtained; repeat debridement often is necessary. Initial antibiotic therapy is empiric, and should consist of a combination of a β-lactam plus a β-lactamase inhibitor, plus clindamycin. Specific therapy directed at the offending organisms should be given, once identified by Gram stain or culture.

Other Therapy

The risks of stress-related ulceration of the gastric mucosa can be significantly reduced by the use of oral antacids, i.v. H_2-blocking agents, or oral sucralfate. A recently described predisposing risk factor for Gram-negative pneumonia and sepsis is a reduction in gastric acidity from the routine use of antacids or H_2-blockers, such as cimetidine and ranitidine, to prevent stress-induced bleeding. Driks and associates, in a prospective randomized trial, found that the use of sucralfate, which provides equivalent prophylaxis against stress bleeding without reducing gastric acid levels, was associated with approximately half of the rate of pneumonia found with H_2-blockers or antacid use. Evidence that sucralfate is preferable to antacids or H_2-blockers is far from conclusive. Nevertheless, one of these agents should be used to protect the gastrointestinal tract from stress ulceration. Kerver and colleagues (1988) demonstrated that antibiotic prophylaxis with oral tobramycin, amphotericin B, and polymyxin E in critically ill patients requiring ventilatory support significantly reduced the incidence of nosocomial infection rates and their associated mortality. Prophylactic use of nystatin "swish and swallow" with 5 to 10 mL of nystatin (100,000 U/mL) has been found to reduce the incidence of systemic candidiasis as well as local wound infections. Hypothermic patients should be treated with warming therapy by elevating the room temperature, using radiant heat, or using convective warming therapy. In three large prospective trials, steroid use was not associated with an improvement in the overall survival. For patients with severe, late septic shock, steroid use should be limited to select patients with specific indications, such as adrenal insufficiency.

Oral, enteric, or parenteral nutritional support should be based on laboratory assessment of preexisting nutritional status (albumin, transferrin, thyroxine-binding prealbumin, somatomedin-C). The usual rule of thumb is to provide between 25 and 35 nonprotein kcal/kg per day fairly equally distributed between fat and carbohydrate. Optimal assessment of caloric requirements in the patient with shock requiring mechanical ventilation is especially important. Although underfeeding can compromise pulmonary status, increased CO_2 production from excessive carbohydrate loads can exacerbate hypercapnia and complicate weaning efforts. Intralipid therapy should be used judiciously in neutropenic and immunosuppressed patients because of its depressive effects on mononuclear and polymorphonuclear monocytes. The goal of amino acid therapy is to reduce catabolic expenditure; usually, 1 to 1.5 g/kg is sufficient. Electrolytes, BUN, creatinine, glucose, liver function studies, calcium, magnesium, and phosphate levels should be monitored as frequently as clinically indicated to adjust carbohydrate, lipid, or protein loads and to correct specific electrolyte deficits. Trace elements (zinc, copper, chromium, and manganese) should be provided. Enteric nutrition is preferable to parenteral nutrition when the gastrointestinal tract is intact, in order to preserve the gut mucosal barrier. Recent reports suggest that outcomes can be improved by providing oral glutamine to patients with systemic inflammatory response syndrome. Glutamine is a nonessential amino acid that is unstable in aqueous solutions and cannot be provided by standard total parenteral nutrition solutions.

Investigational Agents

Several studies have looked at the clinical use of antibodies that would effectively neutralize bacterial endotoxin and mitigate its effects. Polyclonal antiserum directed against a mutant strain (J-5) of *E. coli* was the first of these agents subjected to clinical trial. In 1982, Ziegler and colleagues found that, in subgroups of patients with Gram-negative bacteremia with or without shock, immunization was associated with a significant reduction in mortality. In a subsequent study, Klastersky and associates found that J-5 antiserum was able to reduce not only mortality from septic shock but also the risk of developing septic shock. However, immunization provided protection only for patients with Gram-negative bacteremia or septic shock associated with Gram-negative septicemia and did not benefit patients with sepsis or shock from other causes. J-5 antiserum did not become available for clinical use because it is difficult to manufacture; also, it carries the risk of blood-borne infections because pooled donor serum is required.

The use of monoclonal antibodies also has been investigated. The first of these, IgG antibody purified from pooled plasma obtained from volunteers immunized with *E. coli*, did not demonstrate a significant difference in survival in patients with profound septic shock in clinical trials. Two additional monoclonal antibodies to endotoxin subsequently were developed with more optimistic results. One of these, E5, an IgM antibody with reactivity to lipid A, was developed from murine splenocytes immunized with J-5 mutant *E. coli* cells. A second, HA-1A, a human monoclonal IgM antibody that binds to the lipid A domain of endotoxin, also was developed from J-5 mutant cells. Both of these monoclonal antibodies were able to improve survival and mitigate organ system dysfunction in patients with Gram-negative sepsis. However, no protection was afforded to patients with nonbacteremic Gram-negative infections or other causes of sepsis. To significantly alter the outcome of septic shock in most patients, it appears that monoclonal antiendotoxin therapy will need to be combined with other approaches.

Other agents that have been investigated for the treatment of shock are cytokine antagonists, including antibodies to TNF-α, and a recombinant form of IL-1 receptor antagonist, a naturally occurring protein that binds to IL-1 receptors. Receptor antagonists offer special promise in that their use can be extended to patients with acute inflammatory response syndrome in the absence of an identifiable infectious etiology. Intravenous infusions of TNF-α in humans and animals produce many of the physiologic abnormalities associated with sepsis. These symptoms include fever, tachycardia, myalgias, leukocytosis, tachypnea, diarrhea, and somnolence. In animal models, high doses of TNF-α result in shock, coagulopathy, severe myocardial dysfunction, and death. Monoclonal antibodies to TNF-α, when given promptly after TNF-α infusion, can reduce the systemic response and prevent death in these animals. In a pilot clinical trial, Vincent and colleagues found that anti-TNF antibody improved left ventricular function in 10 patients with septic shock; however, only three of the 10 patients survived. The poor outcome was attributed to the fact that TNF-α is an early mediator of the sepsis response. To prevent an adverse outcome, anti-TNF antibody must be given early in the course of the disease. Unfortunately, trials using cytokine antagonists, including PAF- and TNF-receptor antagonists in the treatment of shock, have demonstrated little benefit.

Critically ill patients with acute renal failure are preferably treated with continuous renal replacement therapies such as hemofiltration or hemoultrafiltration. These systems are unique in that they can be used in patients with hemodynamic instability. The use of high permeability membranes in these systems allows the removal of measurable quantities of cytokines, although plasma levels do not seem to be affected by this process. At least theoretically, highly permeable membranes may have a limited capacity to remove molecules involved in the pathogenesis of sepsis. Continuous plasma filtration absorption (CPFA) is a modality of blood purification in which plasma is separated from whole blood and circulated in a sorbent cartridge. Its rationale is an attempt to remove molecules that are not removed by hemofiltration or other hemodialysis techniques. In an initial trial, CFPA was associated with increased systemic vascular resistances and significant reductions in the use of vasopressors. This suggests that CPFA may prove superior to conventional hemofiltration in patients with acute renal failure.

Evaluate Response to Therapy

Once oxygenation and restoration of the intravascular volume have been completed, it is important to reassess the patient's response to therapy (Table 10.11). Thorough investigation to determine the underlying cause should be performed so that definitive therapy may be implemented. In managing the patient with septic shock, right heart catheterization with hemodynamic monitor-

TABLE 10.11.
Evaluation of Response to Initial Attempts at Fluid Resuscitation[a]

	Rapid Response	Transient Response	No Response
Vital signs	Return to normal	Transient improvement; recurrence of decreased blood pressure or increased heart rate	Persistent tachycardia, hypotension, altered mental status
Estimated blood loss (%)	Minimal (10–20)	Moderate and ongoing (20–40)	Severe (>40)
Need for more crystalloid	Low	High	High
Blood preparation	Low	Moderate to high	Immediate
Need for operative intervention	Possibly	Likely	Very likely

[a]2,000 mL Ringer's lactate solution in adults, 20 mg/kg in children.
Source: Advanced trauma life support® student manual. American College of Surgeons, Chicago: 1997, second impression 1999:98, with permission.

ing may be considered, if not previously initiated (Table 10.8), especially in those patients who have not responded to resuscitative efforts, or who have evidence of pulmonary edema, myocardial infarction, or congestive heart failure. Arterial blood gases should be obtained to affirm adequate ventilation. Electrolyte, coagulation, and complete blood count results should be available now, and deficits may be corrected based on specific laboratory findings. In the face of specific organ system dysfunction (e.g., renal or hepatic failure), doses of antibiotics, vasopressors, and fluid support should be adjusted. Gastrointestinal losses should be replaced based on the electrolyte and acid–base composition of the site of loss.

Hyponatremia usually results from excessive crystalloid replacement, although renal losses can be increased secondary to a high protein intake, hyperglycemia, diuretic therapy, or acute failure. Although symptoms can include coma or seizures, hyponatremia generally is asymptomatic unless severe (serum sodium <125 mEq/dL), or corrective measures are excessive. The management of mild, asymptomatic hyponatremia associated with an expanded intravascular volume is fluid restriction. Severe hyponatremia should be corrected by raising the serum sodium level to 125 mEq/L at a rate of 1 to 2 mEq/hour. Hypernatremia usually is secondary to insufficient volume replacement and is corrected with the administration of an isotonic crystalloid solution such as half normal saline.

Hypokalemia usually occurs secondary to diuretic use, other medications (digitalis, beta-antagonists, aminoglycosides, some penicillins), and gastrointestinal losses. Severe hypokalemia (serum potassium <3.0 mEq/L), and in high-risk patients, even moderately reduced values can result in cardiac arrhythmias, cardiac arrest, muscular paralysis, and respiratory failure. Intravenous replacement may be safely accomplished with a 20 to 40 mEq of potassium/L of isotonic solution. When more rapid replacement is warranted, the rate may be increased to 10 mEq/h. In the intensive care setting, severe, life-threatening hypokalemia may be treated by giving i.v. KCl at a rate of 20 mEq/h, in as little as 25 to 50 mL of compatible solution.

Hyperkalemia can develop secondary to renal failure, excessive potassium administration, tissue destruction, and acidosis, which shifts intracellular potassium into the extracellular fluid compartment. Treatment can be directed toward shifting potassium into the intracellular compartment by infusing insulin with glucose (10 U regular insulin after one ampule of 50% glucose), or insulin with sodium bicarbonate or albuterol. For life-threatening hyperkalemia (serum potassium >7 mEq/L), calcium gluconate, 10 mL of 10% solution, can be given i.v. over 2 to 5 minutes, followed by a second dose, if needed. Finally, calcium exchange resins such as sodium polystyrene sulfonate (15 to 30 g in 50 to 100 mL of 20% sorbitol) bind potassium in exchange for sodium within the gastrointestinal tract and are commonly used in patients with chronic renal failure. When rapid correction of hyperkalemia is needed, these agents may not be appropriate. In enema form, calcium exchange resins have been associated with intestinal necrosis, and should be used with caution in patients with diverticular or other colorectal disease.

Metabolic acidosis usually is satisfactorily corrected with appropriate ventilatory, electrolyte, and crystalloid administration. The routine use of bicarbonate is not recommended for mild to moderate metabolic acidosis (pH 7.25 to 7.34). Bicarbonate use may shift the oxygen-hemoglobin dissociation curve and reduce oxygen delivery at the cellular level. Furthermore, excessive alkalinization can induce tetanus, seizures, cardiac arrhythmias, and increased lactate production. When acidosis is severe (pH < 7.2), i.v. bicarbonate is given by slow infusion (1 to 3 ampules of 7.5% $NaHCO_3$ [44.6 mEq/ampule] in 500 to 1,000 mL D_5W), with the dose based on calculation of the total deficit. Approximately one half of the deficit can be replaced in 3 to 4 hours. No further replacement is necessary once the pH is 7.2 or greater. Serum potassium and calcium levels should be monitored concomitantly, because these shift into the intracellular space as the acidosis is corrected, resulting in hypokalemia or hypocalcemia.

Remedy the Underlying Cause

Although some causes of bleeding, such as a retroperitoneal hematoma developing after hysterectomy, can resolve without surgical intervention, all patients with continued intraabdominal bleeding, and bleeding that is associated with persistent hemodynamic instability in spite of volume and blood product replacement require immediate surgical intervention. Vaginal or other lacerations, if present, should be repaired. Septic abortion requires prompt evacuation of the uterine contents immediately after adequate serum and tissue levels of broad-spectrum antibiotics are reached. Nonhemorrhagic causes of hypovolemic shock should be identified, and specific therapy should be directed at the underlying cause.

SUMMARY

The management of patients with systemic inflammatory response syndrome and shock states remains one of the most formidable challenges facing the practicing gynecologist. However, a satisfactory outcome is achievable in most cases with early recognition, prompt intervention, and continued aggressive surveillance. Thus, caring for the patient in shock, although challenging, may well be rewarding.

BIBLIOGRAPHY

Advanced trauma life support student manual. American College of Surgeons, Chicago: 1997, 2nd impression. 1999:89.

Allon M, Copkney C. Albuterol and insulin for treatment of hyperkalemia in hemodialysis patients. *Kidney Int* 1990; 38:869.

American College of Chest Physicians/Society of Critical Care Medicine Consensus Conference. Definitions for sepsis and organ failure and guidelines for the use of innovative therapies in sepsis. *Crit Care Med* 1992;20:864.

Astiz ME, Rackow EC, Weil MH. Pathophysiology and treatment of circulatory shock. *Crit Care Clin* 1993;9:299.

Badr KF. Sepsis-associated renal vasoconstriction: potential targets for future therapy. *Am J Kidney Dis* 1992;20:207.

Baumgartner J-D, Glauser MP, McCutchan JA, et al. Prevention of gram-negative shock and death in surgical patients by antibody to endotoxin core glycolipid. *Lancet* 1985;2:59.

Beutler B, Cerami A. Cachectin: more than a tumor necrosis factor. *N Engl J Med* 1987;316:379.

Billiar TR, Curran RD. Kupffer cell and hepatocyte interactions: a brief overview. *J Parenter Enteral Nutr* 1990;14:175S.

Bisno AL, Stevens DL. Streptococcal infections of skin and soft tissues. *N Engl J Med* 1996;334:245.

Blood component therapy. ACOG technical bulletin no. 199. Washington, DC: The American College of Obstetricians and Gynecologists, 1995.

Bone RC. A critical evaluation of new agents for the treatment of sepsis. (review) *JAMA* 1991;266:1686.

Bone RC, Fisher CJ Jr, Clemmer TP, et al. A controlled clinical trial of high-dose methylprednisolone in the treatment of severe sepsis and septic shock. *N Engl J Med* 1987;317:653.

Burke DJ, Alverdy JC, Aoys E, et al. Glutamine-supplemented total parenteral nutrition improves gut immune function. *Arch Surg* 1989;124:1396.

Carrico CJ, Meakins JL, Marshall JC, et al. Multiple-organ-failure syndrome. *Arch Surg* 1986;121:196.

Cavanagh D, Marsden DE. Hemorrhagic shock in the gynecologic patient. *Clin Obtstet Gynecol* 1985:28:383.

Cerra FB. Hypermetabolism, organ failure syndrome: a metabolic response to injury. *Crit Care Clin* 1989;5:289.

Cerra FB. Hypermetabolism, organ failure, and metabolic support. (clinical review) *Surgery* 1987;101:1.

Cerra FB, Siegel JH, Border JR, et al. The hepatic failure of sepsis: cellular versus substrate. *Surgery* 1979;86:409.

Chapnik EK, Abter EI. Necrotizing soft-tissue infections. *Infect Dis Clin North Am* 1996;10:835.

Cipolle MD, Pasquale MD, Cerra FB. Secondary organ dysfunction. *Crit Care Clin* 1993;9:261.

Clark SL, Horenstein JM, Phelan JP, et al. Experience with the pulmonary artery catheter in obstetrics and gynecology. *Am J Obstet Gynecol* 1985;152:374.

Connors Jr AF, McCaffree DR, Gray BA. Evaluation of right-heart catheterization in the critically ill patient without acute myocardial infarction. *N Engl J Med* 1983;308:263.

Connors Jr AF, Speroff T, Dawson NV, et al. The effectiveness of right heart catheterization in the initial care of critically ill patients. *JAMA* 1996;276:889.

Cochrane injuries group albumin reviewers. Human albumin administration in critically ill patients: systemic review of randomised controlled trials. *BMJ* 1988;317:235.

Cruse PJE, Foord R. A five-year prospective study of 23,649 surgical wounds *Arch Surg* 1973;107:206.

Cruse PJE, Foord R. The epidemiology of wound infection: a 10-year prospective study of 62,939 wounds. *Surg Clin North Am* 1980;60:27.

Cummins RO, ed. *Textbook of advanced cardiac life support.* Libertyville, IL: American Heart Association, 1994.

Cunnion RE, Parillo JE. Chest editorials: myocardial dysfunction in sepsis: recent insights. *Chest* 1989;95:941.

Dalen JE, Bone RC. Is it time to pull the pulmonary artery catheter? *JAMA* 1996;276:916.

Damas P, Reuter A, Gysen P, et al. Tumor necrosis factor and interleukin-1 serum levels during severe sepsis in humans. *Crit Care Med* 1989;17:975.

Danzl DF, Pozos RS. Current concepts: accidental hypothermia. *N Engl J Med* 1994;331:1756.

Deitch EA. The role of intestinal barrier failure and bacterial translocation in the development of systemic infection and multiple organ failure. *Arch Surg* 1990;125:403.

Deitch EA, Bridges W, Ma L, et al. Hemorrhagic shock-induced bacterial translocation: the role of neutrophils and hydroxyl radicals. *J Trauma* 1990;30:942.

Demetri GD, Kris M, Wade, et al. Quality-of-life benefit in chemotherapy patients treated with epoetin alfa is independent of disease response or tumor type: results from a prospective community oncology study. *J Clin Oncol* 1998;16:3412.

Desai MH, Rutan RL, Heggers JP, et al. Candida infection with and without nystatin prophylaxis: an 11-year experience with patients with burn injury. *Arch Surg* 1992;127:159.

Dixon AC, Parillo JE. Managing the cardiovascular effects of sepsis and septic shock. *J Crit Illness* 1991;6:1197.

Driks MR, Craven DE, Celli BR, et al. Nosocomial pneumonia in intubated patients given sucralfate as compared with antacids or histamine type 2 blockers. *N Engl J Med* 1987;317:1376.

Duchateau J. Complement activation in patients at risk of developing the adult respiratory distress syndrome. *Am Rev Respir Dis* 1984;130:1058.

Dunn DL. Gram-negative bacterial sepsis and sepsis syndrome. *Surg Clin North Am* 1994;74:621.

Fink MP. Why the GI tract is pivotal in trauma, sepsis, and MOF. *J Crit Illness* 1991;6:253.

Fisher CJ Jr, Dhainaut J-F A, Opal SM, et al. Recombinant human interleukin 1 receptor antagonist in the treatment of patients with sepsis syndrome: results from a randomized, double-blind, placebo-controlled trial. *JAMA* 1994;271:1836.

Fry DE. Postoperative pneumonia in the intensive care unit. *Surg Gynecol Obstet* 1993;177S:41.

Gallup DG, Nolan TE. Review: the gynecologist and multiorgan failure syndrome. *Gynecol Oncol* 1993;48:293.

Gerding DN, Johnson S, Peterson LR, et al. Clostridium difficile-associated diarrhea and colitis. (Shea position paper) *Infect Control Hosp Epidemiol* 1995;16:459.

Giroir BP. Mediators of septic shock: new approaches for interrupting the endogenous inflammatory cascade. *Crit Care Med* 1993;21:780.

Goldie AS, Fearon KCH, Ross JA, et al. Natural cytokine antagonists and endogenous antiendotoxin core antibodies in sepsis syndrome. *JAMA* 1995;274:172.

Goodnough LT, Brecher ME, Kanter MH, et al. Transfusion medicine: blood transfusion. (review articles) *N Engl J Med* 1999;340:438.

Grant JP, ed. *Handbook of total parenteral nutrition,* 2nd ed. Philadelphia: WB Saunders, 1992.

Greenman RL, Schein RMH, Martin MA, et al. A controlled clinical trial of E5 murine monoclonal IgM antibody to endotoxin in the treatment of Gram-negative sepsis. *JAMA* 1991;266:1097.

Hankins GDV. Acute pulmonary injury and respiratory failure during pregnancy. In: Clark S, Phelan J, eds. *Critical care obstetrics.* Oradell, NJ: Medical Economics, 1987:290.

Harris RL, Musher DM, Bloom K, et al. Manifestations of sepsis. *Arch Intern Med* 1987;147:1895.

Hayashi RH. Hemorrhagic shock in obstetrics. *Clin Perinatol* 1986;13:755.

Hebert PC, Wells G, Morris A, et al. A multicenter, randomized, controlled clinical trial of transfusion requirements in critical care. *N Engl J Med* 1999;340:409.

Henrich WL. Southwestern internal medicine conference: the endothelium, a key regulator of vascular tone. *Am J Med Sci* 1991;302:319.

Hinshaw L, Peduzzi P, Young E, et al. Effect of high-dose glucocorticoid therapy on mortality in patients with clinical signs of systemic sepsis. *N Engl J Med* 1987;317:659.

Hollenberg SM, Parrillo JE. Shock. In: Fauci AS, Martin JP, Braunwald E, et al, eds. *Harrison's principles of internal medicine,* vol 1. New York: McGraw-Hill, 1997:214.

Holman JM Jr. The role of fibronectin in severe surgical sepsis. *Infect Surg* 1988;7:135.

Houtchens BA, Westenskow DR. Oxygen consumption in septic shock: collective review. *Circ Shock* 1984;13:361.

Jimenez EJ. Shock. In: Civetta JM, Taylor RW, Kirby RR, eds. *Critical care,* 3rd ed. Philadelphia: Lippincott-Raven, 1997:359.

Kaminski MV Jr, Blumeyer TJ. Metabolic and nutritional support of the intensive care patient: ascending the learning curve. *Crit Care Clin* 1993;9:363.

Kaufman BS, Rackow EC, Falk JL. The relationship between oxygen delivery and consumption during fluid resuscitation of hypovolemic and septic shock. *Chest* 1984;85:336.

Kelly CP, Pothoulakis C, LaMont JT. *Clostridium difficile* colitis. *N Engl J Med* 1994;330:257.

Kemper M, Weissman C, Hyman AI. Caloric requirements and supply in critically ill surgical patients. *Crit Care Med* 1992;20:344.

Kerver AJH, Rommes JH, Mevissen-Verhage EAE, et al. Colonization and infection in surgical intensive care patients: a prospective study. *Int Care Med* 1987;13:347.

Kerver AJH, Rommes JH, Mevissen-Verhage EAE, et al. Prevention of colonization and infection in critically ill patients: a prospective randomized study. *Crit Care Med* 1988;16:1087.

Klastersky J, Glauser MP, Schimpff C, et al. Prospective randomized comparison of three antibiotic regimens for empirical therapy of suspected bacteremic infection in febrile granulocytopenic patients. *Antimicrob Agents Chemother* 1986;29:263.

Leor J, Goldbourt U, Reicher-Reiss H, et al. Cardiogenic shock complicating acute myocardial infarction in patients without heart failure on admission: incidence, risk factors, and outcome. *Am J Med* 1993;94:265.

Lillemoe KD, Romolo JL, Hamilton SR, et al. Intestinal necrosis due to sodium polystyrene (Kayexalate) in sorbitol enemas: clinical and experimental support for the hypothesis. *Surgery* 1987;101:267.

Lowe TW. Hypovolemia due to hemorrhage. *Clin Obstet Gynecol* 1990;33:454.

Martin MA, Silverman HJ. Gram-negative sepsis and the adult respiratory distress syndrome. (review article) *Clin Infect Dis* 1992;14:1213.

Miller SB. Renal diseases. In: Woodley M, Whelan A, eds. *Manual of medical therapeutics.* Boston: Little, Brown, 1992:216.

Moore FA, Moore EE, Jones TN, et al. TEN versus TPN following major abdominal trauma: reduced septic morbidity. *J Trauma* 1989;29.916.

Munford RS. Sepsis and septic shock. In: Isselbacher KJ, Braunwald E, Wilson JD, eds. *Harrison's principles of internal medicine.* New York: McGraw-Hill, 1994: 511.

Natanson C, Fink MP, Ballantyne HK, et al. Gram-negative bacteremia produces both severe systolic and diastolic cardiac dysfunction in a canine model that simulates human septic shock. *J Clin Invest* 1986;78:259.

Nathan L, Peters MT, Ahmed AM, et al. The return of life-threatening puerperal sepsis caused by group A streptococci. *Am J Obstet Gynecol* 1993;169:571.

National Institutes of Health consensus conference. Fresh-frozen plasma: indications and risks. *JAMA* 1985;253: 551.

Ognibene FP, Parker MM, Natanson C, et al. Depressed left ventricular performance: response to volume infusion in patients with sepsis and septic shock. *Chest* 1988;93: 903.

O'Shea MH. Fluid and electrolyte management. In: Woodley M, Whelan A, eds. *Manual of medical therapeutics.* Boston: Little, Brown, 1989:42.

Parker MM, Parillo JE. Septic shock: hemodynamics and pathogenesis. *JAMA* 1983;250:3324.

Parillo JE. Pathogenetic mechanisms of septic shock. *N Engl J Med* 1993;328:1471.

Parillo JE, Burch C, Shelhamer JH, et al. A circulating myocardial depressant substance in humans with septic shock. *J Clin Invest* 1985;76:1539.

Parillo JE, Parker MM, Natanson C, et al. NIH conference. Septic shock in humans: advances in the understanding of pathogenesis, cardiovascular dysfunction, and therapy. *Ann Intern Med* 1990;113:227.

Pulmonary artery catheter consensus conference: consensus statement. *Crit Care Med* 1997;25:910.

Pine RW, Wertz MJ, Lennard ES, et al. Determinants of organ malfunction or death in patients with intra-abdominal sepsis. *Arch Surg* 1983;118:242.

Prentice CRM. Acquired coagulation disorders. *Clin Haematol* 1985;14:413.

Priest BF, Brinson DN, Schroeder DA. Treatment of experimental Gram-negative bacterial sepsis with murine monoclonal antibodies directed against lipopolysaccharide. *Surgery* 1989;106:147.

Rackow EC, Astiz ME. Pathophysiology and treatment of septic shock. *JAMA* 1991;266:548.

Rao PS, Cavanagh D. Endotoxic shock in the primate: some effects of dopamine administration. *Am J Obstet Gynecol* 1982;144:61.

Reed RL II. Antibiotic choices in surgical intensive care unit patients. *Surg Clin North Am* 1991;71:765.

Richter HE, Holley RL, Andrews WW, et al. The association of interleukin 6 with clinical and laboratory parameters of acute pelvic inflammatory disease. *Am J Obstet Gynecol* 1999;181:940.

Ronco C, Brendolan A, Dan M, et al. Adsorption in sepsis. *Kidney Int* 2000;58:148S.

Roumen RM, Hendriks T, Wevers RA. Intestinal permeability after severe trauma and hemorrhagic shock is increased without relation to septic complications. *Arch Surg* 1993;128:453.

Ruokonen E, Takala J, Kari A, et al. Regional blood flow and oxygen transport in septic shock. *Crit Care Med* 1993;21:1926.

Rush BF Jr, Sori AJ, Murphy TF, et al. Endotoxemia and bacteremia during hemorrhagic shock. The link between trauma and sepsis? *Ann Surg* 1988;207: 549.

Schlichtig R, Ayres SM. Nutritional assessment of the critically ill. In: *Nutritional support of the critically ill.* Chicago: Year Book Medical Publishers, 1988:75.

Septic shock. *ACOG technical bulletin no. 204.* Washington, DC: The American College of Obstetricians and Gynecologists, 1995.

Shires GT, Canizaro PC. Fluid and electrolyte management of the surgical patient. In: Sebastian DC Jr. *Textbook of surgery,* 14th ed. Philadelphia: WB Saunders, 1991:57.

Shoemaker WC, Appel PL, Kram HB. Hemodynamic and oxygen transport effects of dobutamine in critically ill general surgical patients. *Crit Care Med* 1986;14:1032.

Shoemaker WC, Appel PL, Kram HB, et al. Comparison of hemodynamic and oxygen transport effects of dopamine and dobutamine in critically ill surgical patients. *Chest* 1989;96:120.

Simon D, Trenholme G. Antiobiotic selection for patients with septic shock. *Crit Care Clin* 2000; 16:215.

Snyder HS. Lack of a tachycardiac response to hypotension with ruptured ectopic pregnancy. *Am J Emerg Med* 1990;8:23.

Sori AJ, Rush BF Jr, Lysz TW, et al. The gut as source of sepsis after hemorrhagic shock. *Am J Surg* 1988;155:187.

Sprung CL, Caralis PV, Marcial EH, et al. The effects of high-dose corticosteroids in patients with septic shock. A prospective, controlled study. *N Engl J Med* 1984;311:1137.

Sprung CL, Peduzzi PN, Shatney CH, et al. Impact of encephalopathy on mortality in the sepsis syndrome. *Crit Care Med* 1990;18:801.

Suffredini AF, Harpel PC, Parillo JE. Promotion and subsequent inhibition of plasminogen activation after administration of intravenous endotoxin to normal subjects. *N Engl J Med* 1989;320:1165.

Taylor RW, Norwood SH. The adult respiratory distress syndrome. In: Civetta JM, Taylor RW, Kirby RR, eds. *Critical care.* Philadelphia: JB Lippincott, 1988:1057.

Tracey KJ, Cerami A. Tumor necrosis factor: an updated review of its biology. *Crit Care Med* 1993;21:S415.

Vincent J-L, Bakker J, Marecaux G, et al. Administration of anti-TNF antibody improves left ventricular function in septic shock patients: results of a pilot study. *Chest* 1992;101:810.

Wenzel RP. Anti-endotoxin monoclonal antibodies: a second look. (editorial) *N Engl J Med* 1992;326:1151.

Wiernik KA, Jarstrand C, Julander I. The effect of intralipid on mononuclear and polymorphonuclear phagocytes. *Am J Clin Nutr* 1983;37:256.

Wilmore DW, Smith RJ, O'Dwyer ST, et al. The gut: a central organ after surgical stress. (clinical review) *Surgery* 1988;104:917.

Young MJ, Woolliscroft JO, Billi JE. Steroids and septic shock. *Infect Surg* 1987;7:173.

Zaloga GP, Prielipp RC, Butterworth JF, et al. Pharmacologic cardiovascular support. *Crit Care Clin* 1993; 9:335.

Ziegler EJ, Fisher CJ Jr, Sprung CL, et al. Treatment of Gram-negative bacteremia and septic shock with HA-1A human monoclonal antibody against endotoxin: a randomized, double-blind, placebo-controlled trial. *N Engl J Med* 1991;324:429.

Ziegler EJ, McCutchan JA, Fierer J, et al. Treatment of Gram-negative bacteremia and shock with human antiserum to a mutant *Escherichia coli. N Engl J Med* 1982;307:1225.

Te Linde's Operative Gynecology, ninth edition, edited by John A. Rock and Howard W. Jones, III. Lippincott Williams & Wilkins, Philadelphia: © 2003.

CHAPTER

11

Wound Healing, Suture Material, and Surgical Instrumentation

GARY H. LIPSCOMB   FRANK W. LING

WOUND HEALING

Ideally, organic tissue lost by destruction or injury would be replaced with tissue identical in form and function. This process is known as regeneration. Although tissue regeneration does occur in lower animals (e.g., salamanders), humans have lost this ability for the most part. With the exception of the epidermis of the skin, mucosa of the intestinal tract, and liver, damaged human tissue heals by the laying down of collagen, a repair process better know as scarring. This process is responsible for emergently sealing the wound and ultimately providing long-term structural support for the injured organ, but is unable to reproduce other functions of the replaced tissue. As a result, the healing process also leads to disease if an organ becomes unable to function properly owing to extensive replacement of functioning tissue by nonfunctioning scar. Heart failure following a massive myocardial infarction is an example. In other cases, the healing process itself directly produces disease (e.g., postoperative adhesion formation following surgical procedures or tubal occlusion after pelvic inflammatory disease).

Physiology of Wound Healing

The healing of a wound involves several distinct biological processes: (a) inflammation; (b) epithelialization; (c) fibroplasia; (d) wound contraction; and (e) scar maturation. Although considered distinct, these processes do not occur in a strict sequence, but often occur simultaneously with each other. These repair mechanisms are also nonspecific. They are activated whether a wound is made with a surgical scalpel and sutured closed, or is a traumatic wound that is allowed to heal without surgical closure. However, the nature of the wound influences the degree to which each individual process is involved, and this in turn can affect the ultimate success of the repair.

Inflammation

The inflammatory phase of healing is the initial response to any injury involving more than an epithelial surface. This phase can be divided into two separate but simultaneously occurring responses: a vascular and a cellular response. Both are initiated by amines, most notably histamine as well as the kinins and proteolytic enzymes released by the injured tissue. Immediately after injury, a transient vasoconstriction of the local vasculature lasts for 5 to 10 minutes. Vasoconstriction is followed by vasodilatation and an increase in vascular permeability. Edema caused by the escape of plasma through altered vessel walls becomes clinically apparent at this point.

The cellular response is characterized by the migration of leukocytes into the injured area. Although the agents responsible for this active migration of leukocytes remain unclear, chemotactic factors are thought to play a major role. Initially, the polymorphonuclear leukocytes and monocytes in the wound are present in the same concentration as in the systemic circulation. As a result, polymorphonuclear leukocytes predominate for the first 3 days. Because polymorphonuclear leukocytes are relatively short-lived compared with monocytes, the latter stages of the inflammatory phase are characterized by a predominance of monocytes that transform into macrophages. These leukocytes actively phagocytize bacteria, foreign proteins, and necrotic debris. As polymorphonuclear leukocytes die, their intracellular enzymes and debris are released into the wound and become part of the wound exudate. These released enzymes also facilitate the breakdown of material not phagocytized by the leukocytes. This accumulated exudate or pus develops even in the absence of bacteria. Even when this exudate is sterile, the presence of proteolytic enzymes, including collagenase, can interfere with epithelialization and fibroplasia, and thus, interfere with continued wound healing. Poor wound healing, however, is more common in wounds contaminated with bacteria and foreign material. In these cases the inflammatory response may persist for long periods of time.

Epithelialization

By virtue of their exposed location, the epithelial surfaces of the gastrointestinal, urogenital, and respiratory tract as well as the skin itself are continually subjected to the physical and chemical trauma associated with the activities of daily living. As a result, these surfaces are constantly replacing damaged or destroyed cells through a process known as epithelialization. Epithelialization occurs by migration and subsequent maturation of immature epithelial cells from the deeper basal layers of surrounding areas. If the cellular damage is confined entirely to the epithelium, the healing response is merely an exaggerated form of the basic normal replacement process.

If an injury involves the supporting connective tissue beneath the epithelium, however, the other components of the healing processes, in addition to epithelialization, become involved. If the injury severs blood vessels, the vessels retract and the process of hemostasis is initiated. If bleeding is not too severe, a blood clot soon forms. This clot subsequently contracts, dehydrates, and becomes a scab. Within 12 hours, basal cells from the surrounding epithelial surfaces begin migrating onto the injured surface. Epithelial cells move beneath the scab, detaching it from the wound and sealing the surface. In incised and sutured wounds, epithelialization generally produces a watertight seal within 24 hours of injury. This new layer of epithelial cells is initially thin and poorly attached to the underlying surface, rendering it susceptible to injury from even minor trauma. Final epithelial healing is accomplished by differentiation and maturation of the migrated cells and by scar formation through fibroplasia.

Fibroplasia

The process by which wounds regain strength is termed fibroplasia. Fibroplasia results in the production of the collagen necessary to form a fibrous scar, and ultimately determines the final strength of the healed wound. This process begins with the differentiation of mesenchymal cells into fibroblasts. Fibroblasts then migrate into the wound, apparently along fibrin strands produced during clot formation. Once at the injury site, fibroblasts proliferate and manufacture the glycoproteins and mucopolysaccharides that make up the ground substance of connective tissue. Ground substance is an amorphous matrix that is believed to induce aggregation of collagen subunits and influences the final orientation of the fibers.

Once the ground substance is produced, fibroblasts begin to synthesize the basic building block of collagen-tropocollagen. Tropocollagen is a stiff elongated macromolecule of three helically intertwined chains of amino acids consisting of two identical $\alpha 1$ chains and one $\alpha 2$ chain. Within the ground substance and at the proper pH, osmolality, and temperature, tropocollagen molecules polymerize into collagen fibrils by forming covalent bonds with their neighbor. These fibrils bond with other fibrils to form collagen bundles. It is not until 4 to 5 days after injury that the wound produces enough collagen to result in a measurable increase in wound tensile strength. Prior to this time, the wound is held together only by fibrous adhesion. This time frame between wounding and an increase in tensile strength originally was referred to by Howes and Harvey as the "lag period" of wound healing.

Wound Contraction

The manner in which tissue heals is dependent on whether tissue integrity is simply interrupted (as in a surgical incision), or if tissue is removed (as in an avulsion injury). In both types of injury, tissue seals itself, begins to reepithelialize and synthesize collagen for structural support. However, when large amounts of tissue are missing, the edges of the wound must be brought closer together so that the previously noted tissue responses can repair the defect. This process is known as contraction. Contraction of wound margins begins about 5 days after injury, and corresponds with the fibroplasia phase of healing. Because this process can be inhibited by cytochrome poisons, such as potassium cyanide and by smooth muscle relaxants, older theories attributing wound contraction to passive collagen changes have been discarded. Instead, wound contraction appears to be an active process produced by contractile proteins within the fibroblasts. If the area is too large for contraction to bring the edges together, the wound remains covered with granulation tissue or if small enough, it is covered with epithelium only. Epithelialization of such a wound prevents weeping, but without the normal underlying supporting stroma, remains too fragile to provide lasting protection. Pathologic progression of skin contraction ultimately may result in restriction of joint or limb mobility. This deformity is termed contracture and should not be confused with contraction.

Scar Maturation

The bulky scar formed during the fibroplasia phase consists of randomly oriented soluble collagen fibers. This scar has little tensile strength. During scar maturation, the disordered fibers are replaced with fibers arranged in a more orderly fashion producing a denser and stronger scar. Collagen fibers also continue to form covalent bonds within fibrils as well as between adjacent fibrils and fibers, resulting in a continued increase in wound tensile strength over time. This maturation process may continue for years.

During scar maturation and remolding, the breakdown of old disordered collagen slightly exceeds production of new organized collagen fibers. The resulting new scar is softer and less bulky than the original scar but also is stronger because of its more organized and extensively cross-linked nature. However, if collagen production exceeds breakdown, then a keloid or hypertrophied scar results.

Surgical Wound Healing

Depending on the manner of wound closure, three types of surgical wound healing are recognized: primary, secondary, and third intention. Figure 11.1 illustrates these types of wound healing.

Primary Intention

Healing occurs by primary intention if the wound layers are reapproximated following injury. This apposition of tissue layers allows healing to occur in a minimum of time, with no separation of wound edges and with minimum scar formation. This is the desired mode of healing for surgical incisions.

Secondary Intention

It has been known for centuries that a wound has a higher resistance to infection when left open rather than closed. This was demonstrated experimentally in dogs by Bilroth, who applied dressings soaked in liquid feces and pus to wounds. Wounds left open remained healthy in appearance, whereas those that were subsequently closed became infected. As a result, contaminated or infected surgical wounds often are left unapproximated and allowed to close spontaneously. This type of wound healing is referred to as healing by secondary intention. This healing process obviously is more complicated and prolonged than that of primary intention. The wound eventually heals by a combination of contraction and the formation of granulation tissue with the wound gradually filling in from the raw surfaces. This type of healing is slow, and frequently characterized by formation of excessive scar tissue. Granulation tissue from the healing wound also may protrude above the wound margin during this process. This can prevent final epithelialization of the surface and require further treatment for complete healing.

Third Intention

Wound healing by third intention, also known as delayed primary closure, refers to the technique of wound closure after a period of delay. This method often is used after postoperative wound breakdown, or as an alternative to healing by secondary intention of wounds that should not be closed primarily, such as grossly contaminated or infected wounds. The timing of closure is important. Af-

Primary Intention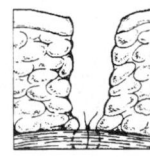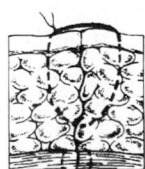

Secondary Intention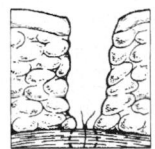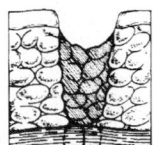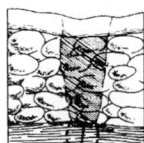

Third Intention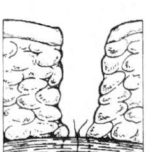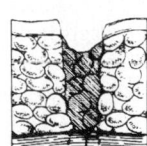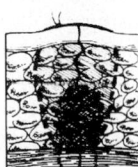

FIGURE 11.1. Types of wound healing.

ter delays of 7 to 8 days, the wound edges become increasingly difficult to approximate because of the increasing collagen content. Edlich and colleagues have suggested that closure on or after the fourth day appears to be ideal. This concept also is supported by Lowery and Curtis, who showed that wounds closed after a delay of between 3 and 6 days have the lowest infection rates. Furthermore, studies by Fogdestam revealed that wounds closed during this time frame also have greater wound strength at 20 days than wounds closed primarily.

Methods of Wound Closure

Wound dehiscence with evisceration is a serious complication of abdominal surgery. This complication is associated with prolonged morbidity and high mortality. Published mortality figures range from 18% to 35%, with a mean of 20%. Wound dehiscence occurs in 0.5% to 5% of all abdominal surgeries, but is less frequent (0.1% to 0.7%) with gynecologic abdominal procedures. Potential reasons for the decreased rate of dehiscence associated with gynecologic surgery include the use of transverse incisions, healthier patients, lower infection rates, and a lower rate of bowel enterotomies.

Traditionally, gynecologic surgeons have been taught that vertical incisions are associated with a greater likelihood of dehiscence than transverse incisions. Critical review of the earlier data supporting this conclusion reveals that significant confounding variables often were ignored. In general, vertical incisions often were performed emergently on sicker patients or those who had other risk factors for dehiscence, such as cancer. Transverse incisions typically were performed on relatively healthy patients undergoing elective surgery. At least two randomized studies by Greenwall and colleagues and Stone and associates have shown no difference in hernia formation or dehiscence between vertical and transverse incisions.

Proper suture selection is critical in preventing wound dehiscence. The wound may break down if the suture has too little initial tensile strength or if the suture is absorbed too quickly before the wound regains enough strength to resist normal stress. The suture also is only as strong as the knots placed in it. If the knot is tied using an improper technique or too few knots are placed, the knot can slip and the suture line fail. The issues involved with proper suture selection and knot security are discussed in detail later in this chapter. Proper surgical technique is one of the most critical factors in preventing wound dehiscence. Several studies have indicated that the most common cause of wound dehiscence is intact sutures pulling through fascia. Animal studies have confirmed that incisions closed with wide loose fascial bites have greater tensile strength than those closed using smaller fascial bites. Sanders and DiClementi also have shown that tightly tied fascial sutures result in fascial necrosis beneath the sutures. Thus, the old adage that one should "approximate and not strangulate fascia" is well taken.

Although the use of loose, wide fascial bites appears to reduce the likelihood of suture pull through, the optimum distance sutures should be placed from the fascial edge is unknown. However, data obtained by Campbell and colleagues can provide some guidelines. When the pullout force and pullout energy of sutures placed in cadaver fascia were plotted against bite size, bites of 0.9 cm yielded the maximum pullout force, but maximum pullout energy was obtained with bite sizes of 1.2 to 1.5 cm. Unfortunately, it is unknown whether pullout energy or pullout force is more clinically relevant.

Tera and Aberg, working with human cadavers, has shown that the strength of a sutured midline incision is approximately doubled if sutures are placed lateral enough to include the edge of rectus muscle. Normally a bite of approximately 1.5 to 2.0 cm is required to include rectus muscle in a midline closure. From these studies, it appears that fascia sutures should be placed at least 1.0 cm from the fascia edge, and that bites of 1.5 cm or larger are probably preferable.

The use of large tissue bites may be responsible, in part, for the success of mass closure techniques, such as retention sutures, or the Smead-Jones closure, in which wide sutures are passed through fascia, muscle, and peritoneum. The Smead-Jones mass closure consists of a combination "far" mass closure bite at least 2.5 cm from the fascial edge on each side of the incision with a second "near" bite through the fascial edge. This far-far/near-near technique is considered the gold standard for vertical closure because it has been shown consistently to be more secure than simple layered closure.

Unfortunately, the Smead-Jones technique is time consuming and requires a large number of sutures. One solution to this problem has been the use of a continuous running mass closure. In gynecologic surgery, abdominal incisions traditionally have been closed in layers with interrupted sutures. The belief that interrupted sutures provide greater wound security than a continuous suture is not well documented, and there are several well performed studies using both general surgery and gynecologic oncology patient populations showing continuous closure to be comparable to Smead-Jones closure provided that adequate tissue bites are taken. A recent metaanalysis of available randomized trials suggest that a continuous technique also is associated with decrease in subsequent ventral hernia formation. The continuous technique is not only the most rapid of all the mass closure methods, it also is more rapid than traditional interrupted layer techniques. One theoretical advantage of a continuous suture line is that any stress on the incision is distributed along the entire suture line and not confined to one loop of suture, thereby potentially decreasing the likelihood of suture pullout.

Mass closure techniques classically have used a nonabsorbable permanent suture. The use of nonabsorbable sutures occasionally produces painful palpable knots, or results in the formation of suture sinuses. The development of slowly absorbed synthetic sutures has allowed the use of these sutures for running continuous closures, thus avoiding the potential complications of nonabsorbable sutures. Several studies are now available showing excellent results using a continuous absorbable suture line for fascial closure even in high-risk patients. Although the use of continuous polyglycolic acid and polyglactin 910 sutures to close vertical midline incisions has been discouraged by some surgeons, others have obtained good results in patients at low risk for dehiscence. Since these initial studies, other synthetic absorbable sutures (polydioxanone and polyglyconate) that retain their tensile strength much longer than polyglycolic acid and polyglactin 910 have become available. Because of this delayed loss of tension strength compared to other absorbable suture material, polydioxanone and polyglyconate sutures are especially well suited for continuous fascial closure and should be considered the absorbable sutures of choice for mass closure of patients at high risk for dehiscence.

The manner in which the incision is made also may influence the dehiscence rate. Although no good data are available, it has been suggested that the shearing produced when scissors are used to incise the fascia results in increased fascia necrosis and an increased breakdown rate when compared to incisions produced by a scalpel. Likewise, the use of electrosurgery to incise the fascia has been implicated by some data to result in an increase in the dehiscence rate. These factors are magnified if the fascia then is closed improperly. Because such fascia necrosis generally occurs only at the cut edge of the fascia, the use of generous fascia bites during fascial closure probably is more important in preventing fascial dehiscence than the manner of opening the fascia.

SUTURE MATERIAL

It is unknown when humankind first learned to use strings or animal sinews to ligate bleeding vessels or approximate tissue. Any material used for this purpose is commonly referred to as suture, whereas the act of reapproximating tissue with suture is known as suturing. The first recorded use of suture and suturing dates to the 16th century B.C. in the Edwin Smith papyrus, the oldest record of a surgical procedure. Over the centuries, many different materials have been used as sutures. These materials include metals (gold, silver, and tantalum wire), plant material (linen and cotton), and animal products (horsehair, tendons, intestinal tissue, and silk). The United States Pharmacopeia (USP) is the official compendium that defines the various classes of suture as well as sets standards for dimensions and minimum tensile strength for each class of suture marketed in the United States. Most sutures today significantly exceed the minimum tensile strength required by the USP (Table 11.1).

Sutures are divided into size categories based on diameter as defined by the USP. Sutures progressively larger than 0 are numbered in increasing numerical order; that is, 1, 2, etc. Sizes progressively smaller than 0

TABLE 11.1.
US Pharmacopeia–Required Knot-Pull Tensile Strength (lb)

| Size | Absorbable Sutures | | Nonabsorbable Sutures | | |
	Natural	Synthetic	Class I	Class II	Class III
4-0	1.7	2.4	1.3	1.0	1.8
3-0	2.7	3.9	2.1	1 5	3.0
2-0	4.4	6.2	3.2	2.3	4.0
1-0	6.1	8.8	4.8	3.2	7.5
1	8.4	11.6	6.0	4.0	10.5

are indicated by an increasing number of zeros; that is, 0, 00, 000. The smaller the suture, the more zeros. For simplicity, the smaller numbers often are written numerically as 1-0, 2-0, etc., where the first numeral refers to the number of zeros.

The USP characterizes suture based on their rate of absorption by bodily tissues. Sutures initially are classed as either absorbable or nonabsorbable. Absorbable sutures lose the majority of their tensile strength before 60 days when implanted in body tissues. Absorbable sutures are further subdivided by the USP into natural and synthetic sutures. Figure 11.2 illustrates the percentages of tensile strength remaining for common absorbable sutures at various postoperative time intervals.

Nonabsorbable sutures are defined as sutures that maintain the majority of their tensile strength for more than 60 days in body tissue. These sutures are further subdivided by the USP into three classes: class I is composed of silk or synthetic fibers; class II is composed of cotton or linen fibers or coated natural or synthetic fibers with the coating forming a casting of significant thickness but not contributing appreciably to strength (these coatings typically are added to improve handling characteristics or resist degradation); and class III sutures are composed of monofilament or multifilament metal wire.

Natural Absorbable Sutures

Plain and Chromic Catgut
One of the oldest suture materials is plain catgut. Catgut consists of highly purified strands of collagen obtained from the submucosa of animals. Despite its name, catgut normally is obtained from sheep intestines. The name is believed to have originated from the Arabic term "kitgut," which referred to the strings of a musical instrument known as a kit. Kitgut was made from sheep intestines and probably served as a readily available source of suture material. Over the years the term has evolved into catgut.

Because plain catgut is a foreign protein, it elicits a marked inflammatory response in tissue. It is rapidly degraded by proteolytic enzymes released by white blood cells. This suture loses over 70% of its tensile strength in

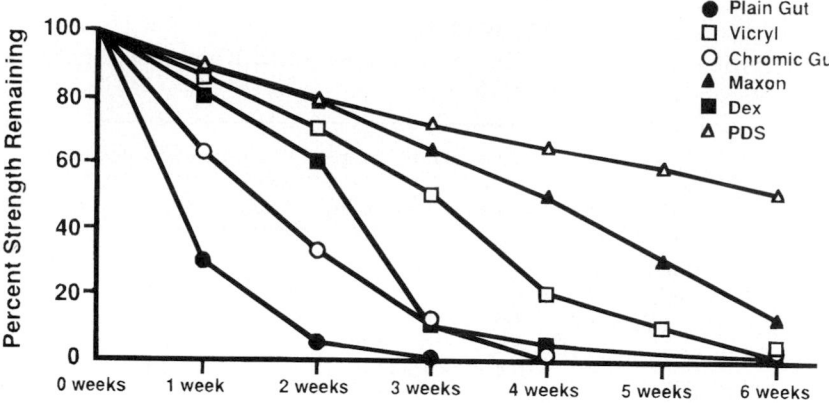

FIGURE 11.2. Percentage of *in vivo* tensile strength of absorbable sutures remaining at various postoperative times.

7 days and is totally digested by 70 days. Plain gut is used in tissue where strength is needed for very short periods of time. It is ideal for Pomeroy tubal ligations because it dissolves rapidly, and thus allows the severed ends to fall apart. Less rapidly absorbed sutures, particularly permanent suture, are associated with higher failure rates, probably because of fistula formation.

Chromic gut is treated with chromic acid salts that bind to the antigen sites in the collagen. The resulting suture elicits less inflammatory response and subsequently is more resistant to degradation. Chromic catgut maintains more than half of its tensile strength at 7 to 10 days, with some measurable strength up to day 21. It is suitable for tissue where long-term strength is not needed. Examples of such tissue include serosal, visceral, and vaginal tissues. This suture should not be used in skin because the inflammatory response can cause scarring, and the suture often serves as a nidus for infection. Because natural absorbable sutures are degraded by the proteolytic enzymes released by inflammatory cells, these sutures lose strength more rapidly in infected tissue.

Synthetic Absorbable Sutures

Polyglycolic Acid and Polyglactin 910

During the 1970s, two synthetic absorbable sutures (polyglycolic acid and polyglactin 910) became available in the United States. These sutures were designed to be stronger, longer-lasting, and less reactive than catgut. Both sutures are composed of braided filaments of a synthetic polymer. Polyglycolic acid (Dexon: Sherwood/Davis & Geck, St. Louis, MO) is a copolymer of glycolic acid, whereas polyglactin 910 (Vicryl: Ethicon, Somerville, NJ) is a copolymer of lactic and glycolic acid. The two sutures have very similar biologic properties. Breakdown is by hydrolysis rather than digestion by proteolytic enzymes. The result is minimal inflammatory reaction and a constant absorption rate. There essentially is no loss in tensile strength in the first 7 to 10 days after implantation. Approximately 50% to 60% of tensile strength remains after 14 days, 20% to 30% after 21 days, and almost no tensile strength at 28 days. The initial tensile strength of both these sutures is significantly greater than catgut suture of equal size. In fact, the tensile

strength of the synthetic absorbable sutures is almost equal to the tensile strength of a catgut suture one size larger.

One disadvantage of the synthetic absorbable sutures is that they do not handle as well as catgut suture. To counter this difficulty, manufacturers have attempted to enhance the handling qualities of their products by offering versions with various surface coatings or variations with finer and more tightly woven filaments. Although these refinements improve handling characteristics, they increase the tendency of knots to slip. As a result, additional throws may be needed when using these versions of polyglycolic acid or polyglactin 910.

These sutures can be used in most situations that chromic catgut would be used and have replaced catgut almost entirely for many surgeons. Because they retain tensile strength longer than natural absorbable sutures, they are acceptable for fascial closure in patients at low risk for fascial dehiscence.

Polyglyconate and Polydioxanone

Sutures of polyglycolic acid and polyglactin are by necessity composed of braided filaments because the inherent rigidity of the polymers produces a monofilament suture too stiff for general surgical use. A newer class of polymers allow the production of pliable monofilament sutures. This type of suture is represented by polyglyconate (Maxon) and polydioxanone (PDS). Although subtle differences exist between the two sutures, they are similar enough to consider them together when discussing the biologic properties of this suture class.

The initial tensile strength of these monofilament sutures is comparable to that of the multifilament absorbable sutures. However, this class of suture undergoes absorption at a much slower rate than other absorbable sutures. As a result, tensile strength is maintained for a longer period of time. More than 90% of initial tensile strength is maintained by the end of the first postoperative week, 80% at 2 weeks, 50% at 4 weeks, and 25% at 6 weeks. As with the other synthetic sutures, inflammatory response is minimal. An additional advantage is that these monofilament sutures lack interstices that could serve as a nidus for bacterial infection. As a result, chronic inflammation is rarely seen with this class of monofilament sutures. In comparison, infected absorbable braided sutures have been shown experimentally by Buckall to contain bacteria even after 70 days of implantation.

Because of their delayed absorption profile, both polyglyconate and polydioxanone are excellent choices for fascial closure. Because these sutures are composed of only one fiber, care must be taken to insure that the strand is not inadvertently damaged by instruments, needles, or other sharp-edged material. Such damage may not be easily recognized in the operating room but can seriously weaken a monofilament suture and may result in suture line disruption postoperatively. This precaution is even more critical when a continuous suture line is used.

Poliglecaprone 25 and Polyglactin 910 (Rapide)

With recent advances in polymer chemistry, it is now possible to manufacture the synthetic equivalent of surgical gut. First introduced in 1993, poliglecaprone 25 (Monocryl) has the absorption similar to chromic catgut. Unlike natural collagens, poliglecaprone 25 produces highly uniform and predictable absorption patterns. Like the other synthetic sutures, poliglecaprone 25 is absorbed by hydrolysis and thus does not induce the inflammatory response of catgut. This monofilament suture retains approximately 50% to 60% of its original tensile strength at 7 days postoperatively, 20% to 30% at 14 days, and by 21 days has lost essentially all tensile strength. This particular suture has the advantages of chromic catgut suture, but without many of the disadvantages (i.e., intense inflammatory response and somewhat unpredictable absorption rate). Although it is similar to chromic catgut in tensile strength and actually maintains its tensile strength longer than chromic catgut, it is not recommended by the manufacturer for use for fascial closure or in any tissue where approximation under stress is required.

Polyglactin 910 Rapide (Vicryl Rapide) is identical in chemical structure to polyglactin 910 but is of lower molecular weight. The result is a braided suture with performance characteristics similar to plain catgut. Absorption is rapid with 70% of tensile strength lost in the first 7 days. After 10 to 14 days, essentially no strength remains. It is intended for use in the superficial soft tissue where only short-term support is needed. It can be used for skin closure because of its rapid absorption and minimal inflammatory response. The sutures typically begin to fall off at 7 to 10 days. Because sutures remaining in skin longer than 7 days may cause scarring, any suture remaining at this time can be wiped off with sterile gauze or, if necessary, cut. In Europe, this suture also is promoted for episiotomy closure. Although this suture does not meet USP strength requirements for synthetic absorbable sutures, its tensile strength exceeds the tensile strength specifications for similar size natural collagen suture.

Nonabsorbable Sutures

By definition, nonabsorbable sutures are suitably resistant to the action of living mammalian tissue. These sutures, however, are not completely resistant to absorp-

tion. Over time, these sutures also lose tensile strength and in the case of natural fiber sutures eventually are completely absorbed or digested. Despite beliefs to the contrary, the initial tensile strength of many nonabsorbable sutures is less than comparable size absorbable suture (see Table 11.1). Nonabsorbable sutures, however, have the advantage of maintaining tensile strength for long periods of time. Disadvantages of nonabsorbable sutures include the potential suture-related pain, palpable sutures, and occasionally the formation of suture sinuses.

Natural Nonabsorbable Sutures

Modern nonabsorbable natural fiber sutures are composed of either surgical silk or cotton. Silk suture is one of the best handling sutures. The handling and knot tying characteristics of silk suture remains the standard against which other sutures are judged. This suture has little "memory;" that is, it does not tend to return to its original form after being bent or twisted. As a result, it handles well, ties easily, and possesses excellent knot security. Silk suture loses over half of its tensile strength after 1 year of implantation and frequently cannot be found after 2 years. In this respect, it can be viewed as a delayed absorbable suture. Because silk is a foreign animal protein, it initiates the greatest inflammatory response of the nonabsorbable sutures. The multifilament nature and the capillary action of this suture, makes it unsuitable in contaminated tissue or in tissues where the potential for infection is high.

Cotton is the other natural nonabsorbable natural suture material still available today. It is rarely used in modern surgical practice. Cotton is the weakest of the nonabsorbable sutures. Cotton loses 50% of its original tensile strength within 6 months of implantation, but still has 30% to 40% remaining at the end of 2 years. Unlike silk, which loses tensile strength when exposed to moisture, wet cotton is 10% stronger than dry cotton. Because wet cotton also is easier to handle, it is commonly moistened prior to use.

Synthetic Nonabsorbable Sutures

A wide variety of nonabsorbable synthetic sutures exist. Nylon is a synthetic polyamide polymer derived from coal, air, and water. It is available both as a braided polyfilament suture (Neurolon, Surgelon) and as a monofilament suture (Dermalon, Ethilon). Monofilament nylon has slightly greater tensile strength than braided nylon, but braided nylon handles better and has better knot security than the monofilament nylon suture. Monofilament nylon suture incites less inflammatory reaction and is less prone to infection than the braided nylon sutures. However, because nylon is relatively inert, all types of nylon suture produce minimal tissue reaction. Nylon undergoes slow hydrolysis in tissue over extended periods of time. It loses approximately 15% to 20% of tensile strength each year.

Polyester sutures are produced only in braided forms. Most differences in the properties of these sutures are determined by whether they are coated, and by the type of coating. The uncoated forms (Mersilene, Dacron) generally offer the best knot security. As with synthetic absorbable suture, coatings can improve the handling characteristics of the polyester sutures. Knot security of coated polyester sutures is generally poorer than that of uncoated sutures. Coatings currently used include polytetrafluoroethylene, also known as Teflon (Polydek, Ethiflex, and Tevdek) polybutilate (Ethibond), and silicone (Ti-Cron).

Polypropylene (Prolene, Surgilon) is a monofilament suture composed of a linear hydrocarbon polymer. It has the least tissue reactivity of all nonabsorbable sutures. Although polypropylene has a high memory it also exhibits a small degree of plasticity. If it is tied carefully and the knots set firmly, a flattening occurs where the strands cross. This flattening helps lock the knot, and thus provides somewhat greater knot security than is possible with many other monofilament nonabsorbable sutures. As with the absorbable monofilament sutures, the same precautions to prevent damage to the suture must be observed with the monofilament nonabsorbable sutures.

Metal Sutures

Although silver wire was used by Sims for closure of vesico-vaginal fistulas, metal sutures are rarely used in gynecologic surgery today. Historically, metal sutures have been used in infected sites or for repair of wound dehiscence and evisceration. Stainless steel once was used routinely by the military for closure of battle wounds of the abdomen. Metal sutures have the highest tensile strength of all suture material. They are also particularly nonreactive. Metal sutures, however, are difficult to handle, require the use of special instruments, and tend to puncture gloves and tissue. With the availability of other nonabsorbable suture materials that also offer high tensile strength and low reactivity but are easier to handle, little reason exists to use these sutures in gynecologic surgery today.

Choice of Suture for Fascial Closure

Tensile strength is critical, although many factors are important in choosing a suture for fascial closure. As noted, the most common cause of dehiscence is sutures pulling through fascia. Because a fascial closure can only be as strong as the weakest component, suture for fascial closure should maintain a tensile strength greater than that of the fascia through the critical healing period. Because the incidence of wound infection is related to the amount of suture material placed in the wound, it would also seem reasonable to use the smallest suture able to provide this necessary tensile strength.

All sutures marketed in the United States must meet minimum tensile strength requirements as defined by the USP. The tensile strength measurement required by USP is knot-pull tensile strength. In measuring knot-pull tensile strength, the suture is tied around a plastic tube using a flat surgeon's knot with one end held in place and the opposite end attached to a tensilometer. Although these data are easily obtained from the various suture

manufacturers and are frequently used in suture advertisements, knot-pull tensile strength is not particularly applicable to actual surgical situations. A more useful measurement of strength is obtained using the knotted loop model as suggested by Herman. In this model, a loop is formed by tying a suture around a glass rod using sufficient square knots to prevent slippage. The rod is removed and the loop placed over two right angle rods gripped in the jaws of a tensilometer. The jaws are then separated at a constant rate until breakage occurs. This model stresses the material and the knot more comparably to actual *in vivo* situations and also allows estimation of knot security. Assuming no slippage at the knot, tensile strength calculated using the knotted loop model is approximately twice the knot-pull tensile strength.

The force required to pull a loop of suture through intact fascia (pull-out force) is frequently cited as 8.3 lbs. This figure is derived from work on the fascia of dogs by Howes and Harvey in 1929 and does not necessarily apply to humans. Fortunately, several studies are now available that have measured the strength of human fascia (Campbell, Tera, Boerema). Two of these studies by Campbell and colleagues and Tera and Alberg were performed using human cadavers. The third study by Boerema measured the pull-out force of fascia at the time of surgery on living patients. All three produced data that indicated the pull-out force for human fascia was approximately 15.2 to 24.2 lbs.

Fascial incisions regain their strength slowly, achieving approximately 10%, 25%, 30%, and 40% of original strength by postoperative week one, two, three, and four, respectively (Fig. 11.3). The point at which fascia has regained enough strength to resist the stress of daily activities is unknown. Some estimation of this time frame can be obtained from available data on fascial dehiscence. The majority of fascial dehiscence occurs between 2 and 12 days postoperatively with a mean occurring around day 7 to 8. Dehiscence rarely occurs after postoperative day 12 but has been reported up to day 18. This would suggest that in most patients, fascia has regained enough strength by 2 weeks after surgery to resist reasonable stresses, but that in a limited number of patients, fascia may not regain sufficient strength to prevent dehiscence until 3 weeks postoperatively.

Using the fascia pull-out data, tensile strength as measured by the knotted loop model following various lengths of implantation in animals and dehiscence data, the appropriate size absorbable suture for fascial closure can now be estimated. As can be seen by Figure 11.4, both 1 and 0 polydioxanone and polyglyconate retain tensile strength greater than the fascial pull-out force for 4 to 6 weeks, but polyglycolic acid sutures of the same size maintain adequate tensile strength only for 7 to 14 days. Based on this model, a 1 or 0 polydioxanone or polyglyconate suture appears to be the most appropriate absorbable suture for fascial closure. Unfortunately, although these types of data are theoretically appealing, there are little clinical data to support these conclusions. It must be realized that in most healthy patients, fascial dehiscence does not occur, even when rapidly absorbed

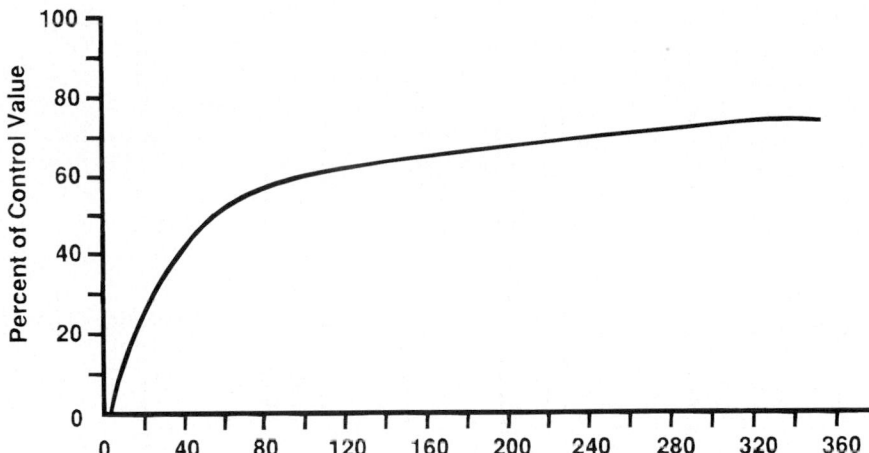

FIGURE 11.3. Fascial tensile strength after surgery. (Adapted from Howes EL, Sooy JW, Harvey SC. The healing of wounds as determined by their tensile strength. *JAMA* 1929;92:42.)

sutures are used. Prior to the development of the synthetic absorbable sutures, 1 and 0 chromic catgut sutures were frequently used for fascial closure. In fact, based on a survey of Ob/Gyn residency programs, chromic catgut still was being used for fascial closure in 16.1% of vertical fascial incisions and 23.4% of transverse fascial incisions as of 1979. Although fascial dehiscence in healthy patients remained uncommon after fascial closure with chromic catgut, dehiscence rates of up to 11% were reported for other patient populations. Likewise, polyglycolic acid and polyglactin 910 sutures have been used for fascial closure with good success, even in patients at risk for dehiscence.

Surgical Needles

Needles are necessary to carry suture material through tissue. The specific needle required for a procedure is determined by the tissue type, its location and accessibility, as well as the surgeon's personal preference. All surgical needles have three basic components: the eye, the body, and the point.

The eye of the needle is the point of attachment for suture. Eyes may be classed as closed, French, or swaged. Closed eyes are similar to those on household sewing needles, whereas French eye needles have a slit with ridges inside the slit to catch and hold the suture. Swaged or eyeless needles have the suture mechanically attached to the end of the needle to form a continuous unit. Eyed needles have several disadvantages over swaged needles, including difficulties with threading and the need to pull a double loop of suture through the tissue. Swaged needles are available with either the suture permanently attached or attached in such a manner that it can be removed from the needle by a slight straight tug on the suture. These controlled-release needles, also known as "pop-off" needles increase the speed at which interrupted sutures can be placed.

The shape of the body or shaft of a needle determines how easily the needle performs in different appli-

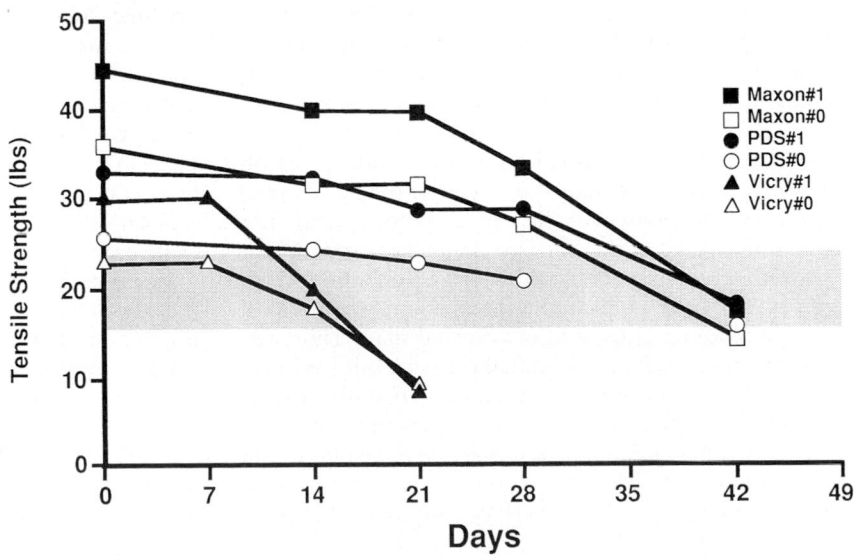

FIGURE 11.4. The tensile strength of various implanted suture materials over time and the point at which tensile strength is less than fascial pull-out strength (14.5 to 24.2 lb).

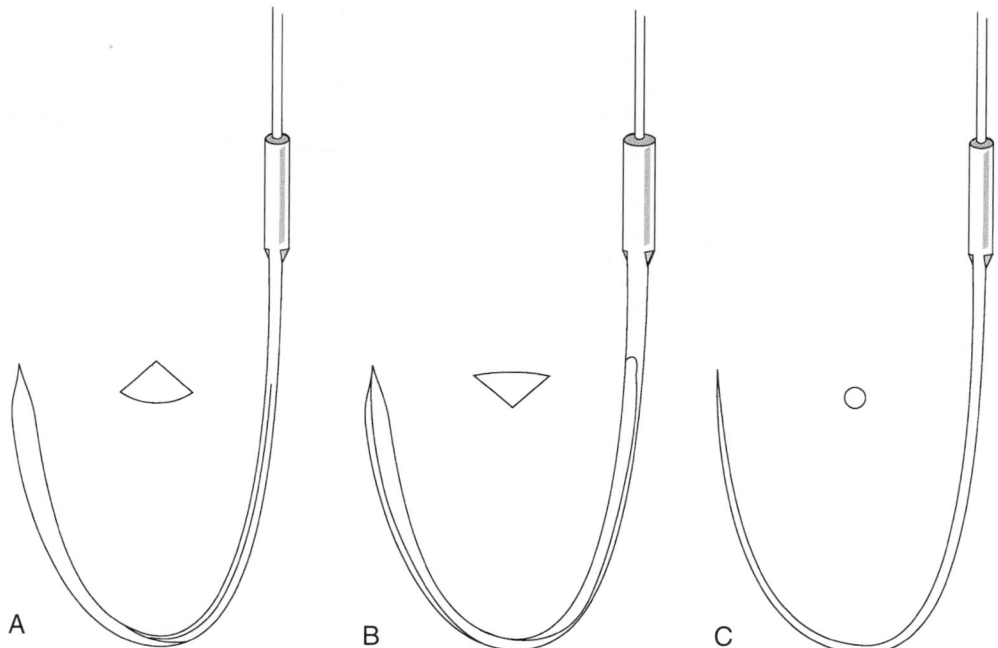

FIGURE 11.5. Common points and body shapes for curved needles.

cations (Fig. 11.5). The longitudinal shape of the body may be straight, half-curved, curved, or compound. Straight needles are used commonly when tissue is easily accessible. This type of needle is rarely used by gynecologists except for skin closure. Half-curved, or ski, needles may be used to close skin, but have primarily been used in gynecology to facilitate laparoscopic suturing. Curved needles require less space for maneuvering than other needles; thus, are ideally suited for most surgical procedures. Curved needles are commonly named based on the percentage of a circle they complete; that is, a 1/2 circle needle is one half of a full circle. Curved needles are available in various curvatures with the 3/8 circle the most commonly used. The less of an arc the needle completed, the more shallow a bite the needle takes. For example a 5/8 needle is useful in deep wounds where deep, narrow bite is required. Compound curve needles were originally developed for anterior segment ophthalmic surgery and are not used in gynecologic surgery.

The point of the needle begins at the widest part of the needle body and extends to the extreme tip. The two types of needle points are the cutting point and the tapered point (Fig. 11.5). Tapered points are used in easily penetrated tissue such as bowel or peritoneum. A variation of the taper point is the blunt point, which has a rounded blunt tip at the end of a tapered shaft. This needle tip was designed for use in friable tissue, but has been advocated by some surgeons for use with other tissues because of its reduced likelihood to penetrate the surgeon's gloves or skin. Cutting needles are used in tough tissue such as skin. The most common cutting needle is the reverse cutting needle. Its sharp edge is on the out-

side of the outer curvature of the needle. Conventional cutting points have the sharp edge on the inside of the curvature. Variations of the cutting point include spatula and lancet points and are used for specialized applications such as ophthalmology.

Needle Holders

Straight needles can be held and pushed through tissue with the fingers. Straight needles can be used only to sew in a straight line, and only then when the tissue is easily accessible. When straight needles are used, sewing is done in a direction away from the operator.

In the depths of a wound, curved needles are needed. A needle holder is required when curved needles are used. All needle holders have a broad head with a variety of surfaces to prevent the needle from slipping or rotating. Needle holders may be large and heavy, or small and delicate, depending on the size needle to be used. Many needle holders have ring finger grips and locking mechanisms. Two common types of basic needle holders used in gynecology are Wagensteen (straight) or Heaney (angled) (Fig. 11.6). Curved needle holders are especially useful in vaginal surgery where the angled head allows easier needle placement. The needle is loaded so that the angled tip is pointed toward the needle eye and not the tip. Sewing, using needle drivers, is performed toward the operator.

Surgical Knots

The surgical knot has been described as the weakest link in any knotted suture, regardless of the knot configura-

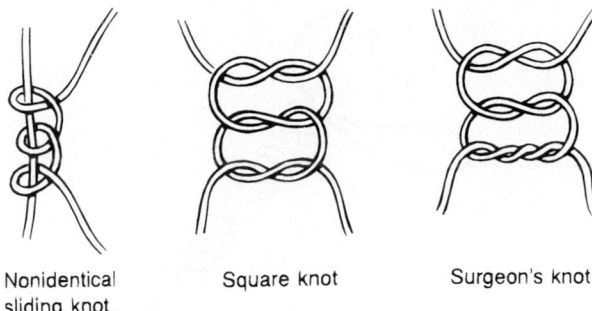

Nonidentical   Square knot   Surgeon's knot
sliding knot

FIGURE 11.7. Flat and sliding knots.

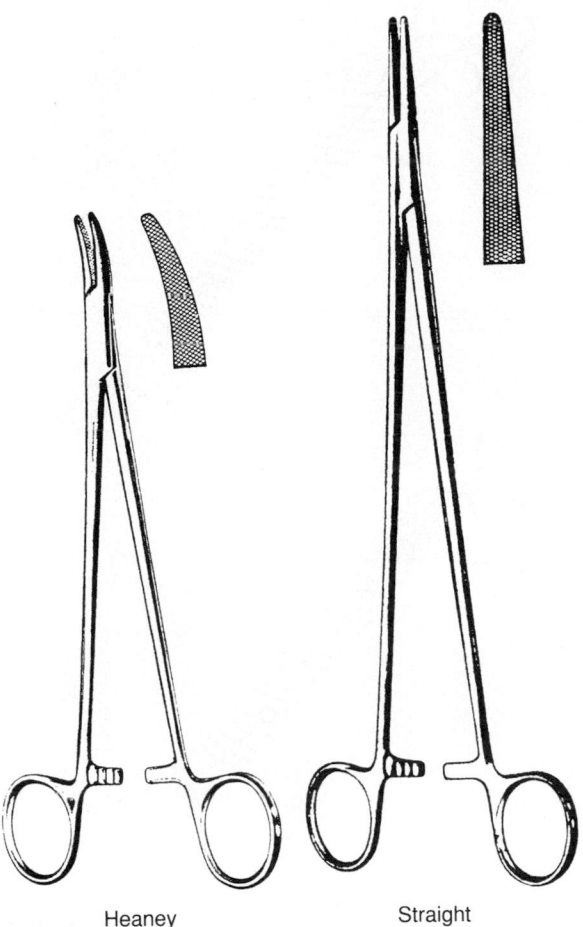

Heaney   Straight

FIGURE 11.6. Needle holders. (Courtesy of Zinnati Surgical Instruments, Inc., Chatsworth, CA)

tion and the type of suture used. If tied improperly, a surgical knot will fail before the tensile strength of the suture is reached. Even when performed perfectly, the mere placement of a knot in suture reduces its overall tensile strength by 30% to 35%. Therefore, some knowledge of surgical knots is imperative for all surgeons.

All surgical knots can be divided into two basic groups: flat knots (square, surgeon's, and granny) and sliding knots (identical and nonidentical) (Fig. 11.7). Flat knots are formed with half hitches tied with equal tension on the ends of the suture. Surgeon's knots are formed by adding an additional loop to the first throw of the half hitch. Sliding knots are two half hitches either nonidentical (square knot) or identical (granny knot), tied with greater tension on one segment than the other.

The term sliding knot suggests the tendency of the knot to slip compared to the flat, but this is not completely true. Simple sliding knots of two or three throws do slip often and should not be used as surgical knots. Brouwers has shown, however, that flat knots with only two throws also tend to slip rather than break.

The flat square knot is the most secure of all the surgical knots and theoretically the most desirable knot for tying suture. However, in a study by Trimbos, sliding knots are used more commonly by gynecologists than are square knots. It has been shown also that many surgeons actually tie sliding knots despite being convinced they tie flat knots. Sliding knots frequently are used in actual surgical practice for two reasons. The crossing of the surgeon's hands needed to tie square knots unavoidably releases tension on the knot, and this can lead to knot slippage. The tying of deep ligatures is most easily performed by keeping constant tension on one suture. Thus, sliding knots may be preferable to square knots in certain situations. Whichever knot is used, the operator should be aware of the knot being used and the number of throws needed to obtain maximum knot-capacity.

The number of throws required for knot security is frequently debated. Too few throws and the knot is weaker than the suture, additional throws above that needed to equal the sutures tensile strength adds unneeded suture to the wound and may increase the infection rate. When flat square knots are used, Brown has shown that maximum knot-holding capacity was achieved with four throws in all noncoated suture tested. In fact, three throws were sufficient to achieve maximum knot-holding capacity except for sutures composed of nylon (both monofilament and braided). The addition of coating to improve handling characteristics also decreases knot security. In a 1983 study, Rodeheaver and colleagues showed that coated suture required two additional flat throws to equal the maximum knot-holding capacity of uncoated suture. In a similar study by Van Rijssel and colleagues the knot-holding capacity of a sliding knot with one extra throw equaled that of square knots in smaller gauge (3-0) suture. In larger sutures (0), square knots remained stronger than sliding knots with an extra throw, but sliding knots with more than five throws were not tested. From these studies, it appears that a surgical knot of four to six throws is adequate for most sutures. The exact number of throws required, of course, depends on the type of suture and whether a flat or sliding knot is formed.

It is common practice for some surgeons to leave suture tails long to prevent knot disruption should the knot slip. As might be expected, the usefulness of this practice is dependent on the type of suture involved. It has been shown that any knot slippage in nylon, poly-

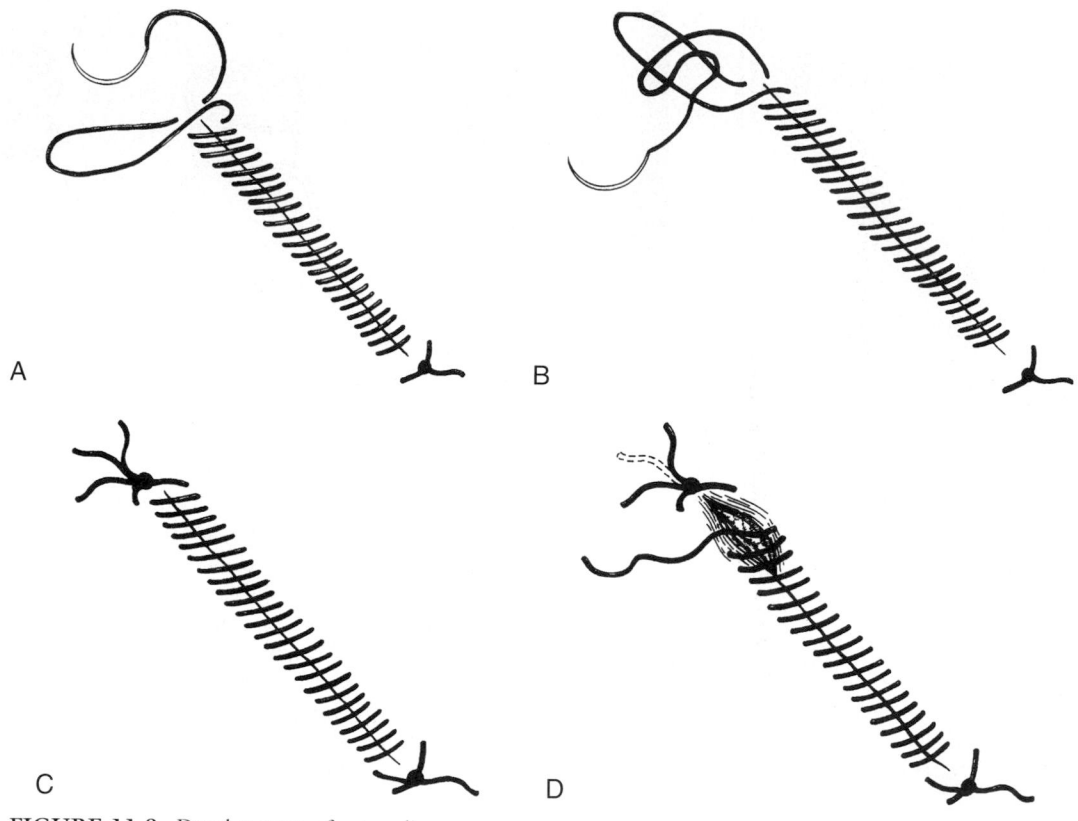

FIGURE 11.8. Development of suture line.

dioxanone, and polypropylene sutures results in total knot disruption. In other sutures (polyglyconate and polyglactin) initial knot slippage is followed by knot recomposition. The reconstituted knot remains intact until greater force is applied. A long suture tail is only helpful in preventing knot disruption in this latter class of suture.

Knot security is of utmost importance when using a continuous suture line. It is common practice for many surgeons to form the terminal knot in a continuous suture line by tying the ending single strand to the last loop of suture. This "loop-to-strand" knot is a potentially weak configuration. Unless multiple square knots are used, the single strand may slip from the knot when placed under tension. As a result, the entire suture line disrupts. At reoperation, the strand may appear broken but, in fact, one of the three terminal knot ends has slipped through what appears to be an intact knot (Fig. 11.8). A safer method for tying continuous suture is to run two sutures to the midpoint of the incision and tie the two single strands to each other, thus avoiding the "loop-to-strand" knot.

SURGICAL INSTRUMENTATION

A multitude of surgical instruments are designed to perform one unique function or slightly improve on the performance of another instrument. This section is not intended to be a comprehensive list of all instruments available, but to review the basic surgical instrumentation needed for most common gynecologic procedures.

Scalpel

The scalpel is the first instrument used in most surgeries and remains the best instrument for dividing tissue with minimal trauma to surrounding tissue. Scalpel blades come in various sizes and shapes to allow performance of different tasks (Fig. 11.9). The basic scalpel blade has a straight ribbed back and an oval cutting surface. This basic blade is commonly available in sizes 10, 15, 20, and 22. The 10 scalpel blade is the most versatile and the most commonly used size. The smaller blades are use for fine dissection and when precise turns are required in making the incision; that is, plastic surgery, although the larger blades are used to rapidly perform an incision. Blades such as the 11 and 12 are designed for specific purposes. The 11 blade is bayonet-shaped and use to perform stab incisions for drains and in draining abscesses. The 12 blade is hook-shaped and originally used for myringotomies. It is infrequently used by gynecologists.

Scissors

The scissors are the second most commonly used instrument to divide tissue. In addition to cutting, scissors also can be used for blunt dissection by opening the scissors

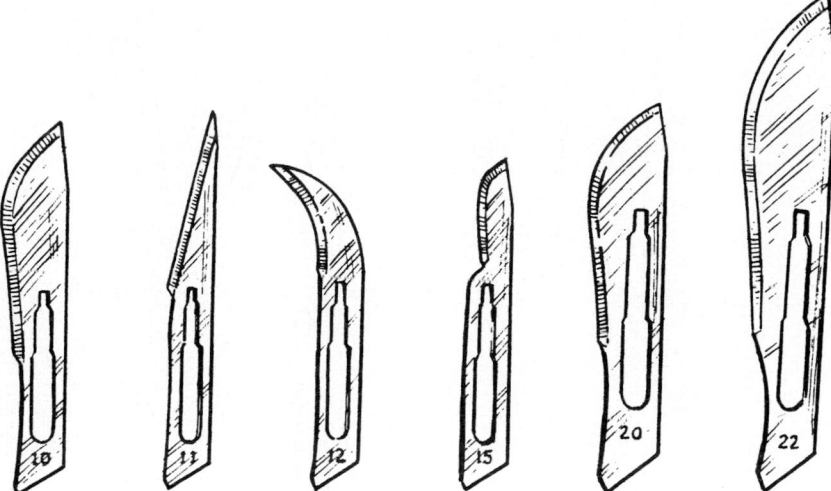

FIGURE 11.9. Surgical scalpel blades.

after the tips have been inserted into a tissue plane. The basic scissors designs used in gynecology surgery are the Mayo, Metzenbaum, and Iris scissors. All come in both straight and curved versions (Fig. 11.10). Curved scissors allow horizontal cutting deep in a wound and thus improve visibility. Curved scissors also are used to cut tissue in a smooth curve, such as for incising the vaginal cuff in an abdominal hysterectomy.

Mayo scissors are used when dividing tough tissue, such as the rectus fascia, parametrial tissue, or vaginal cuff. Metzenbaum scissors are more delicate than the heavier Mayo scissors and are used for cutting thinner tissue, such as peritoneum and adhesions. Metzenbaum scissors are frequently use for retroperitoneal dissection or for developing tissue planes in adhered or distorted tissue.

Iris scissors are small scissors used for delicate dissection. Originally designed for ophthalmic surgery, they are used in gynecology for precise vulvar and vaginal surgery, such as fistula repair or colporrhaphy.

Suture scissors are used only to cut suture and never tissue. Suture scissors are general-purpose scissors with blunt ends to avoid the possibility that the tips will injure structures distal to the suture.

Tissue Forceps

Tissue or thumb forceps consist of two strips of metal joined at one end (Fig. 11.11). The opposable ends of the forceps are used to grasp and hold tissue during dissection, suturing, or cutting. These ends are of varying

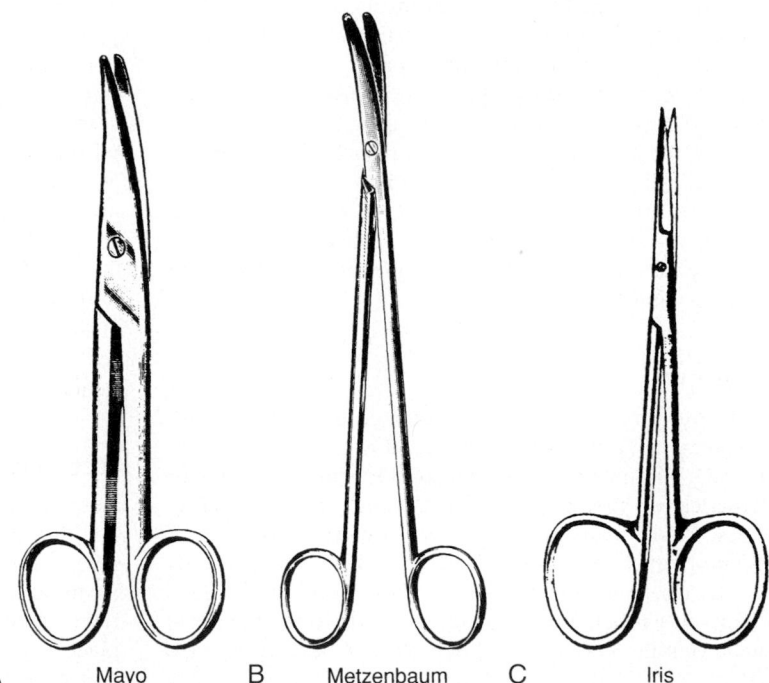

FIGURE 11.10. Surgical scissors. (Courtesy of Zinnati Surgical Instruments, Inc., Chatsworth, CA)

A   Mayo   B   Metzenbaum   C   Iris

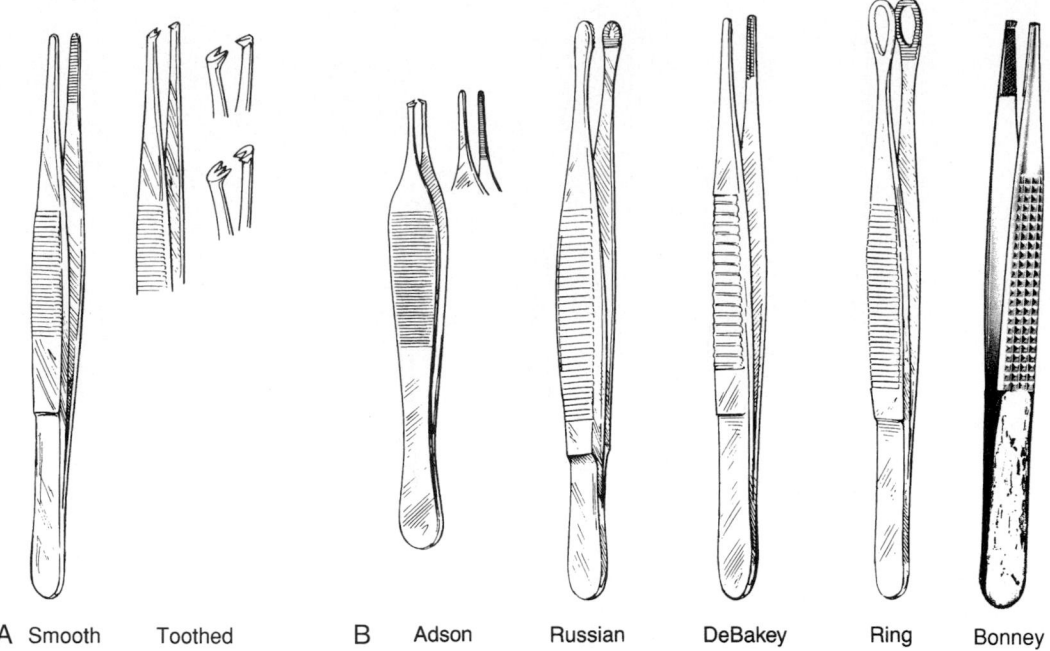

| A | Smooth | Toothed | B | Adson | Russian | DeBakey | Ring | Bonney |

FIGURE 11.11. Tissue (thumb) forceps. (Courtesy of Zinnati Surgical Instruments, Inc., Chatsworth, CA)

shapes and configuration, depending on the purpose for which the forceps are intended. The most common alteration to the ends is the addition of teeth. Smooth forceps without teeth are used when handling friable or delicate tissue. DeBakey forceps have long fine smooth tips that provide precise control of small or delicate tissue deep in the wound. They are commonly used in vascular surgery or retroperitoneal node dissection. Toothed forceps bite into tissue providing a firm grip with minimal pressure. The teeth can vary from one to many and be fine or large. Adson forceps are equipped with fine teeth and are commonly used to approximate skin for staple or suture placement. Ring-tipped and Russian forceps increase the grasping force without using teeth by increasing the surface area of the grasping tips. These forceps are used when a secure hold is needed on structures that would be traumatized by toothed forceps. Bonney tissue forceps are heavy-toothed forceps with serrations along the shaft for maximum gripping power. They are used when sewing fascia.

Clamps

Grasping forceps, commonly referred to as clamps, are designed to grasp and apply traction to tissues (Fig. 11.12). All have finger rings and a locking mechanism. Babcock clamps have no teeth and are atraumatic. These clamps can grasp and hold delicate tissues such as fallopian tube or bowel without causing damage. Allis clamps have serrated edges with short teeth. This clamp has much more grasping power than the Babcock clamp. Kocher/Oschner clamps have transverse

ridges along the shaft and interlocking teeth at the tip. Because of their design, tissue within the clamp is unlikely to slip. These clamps are frequently used to grasp heavy tissue such as fascia, and occasionally as hysterectomy clamps. Ring forceps can be used like ring-tipped tissue forceps, but more commonly are used to hold folded sponges. In this fashion, they can be used to retract tissue, sponge fluid or blood, or apply solutions to the skin in preparation for surgery. Renal stone forceps were designed to remove stones from the renal pelvis but are commonly used by the gynecologic surgeon to explore the uterine cavity for polyps or retained tissue. When used in this capacity, they are inserted, opened, rotated 180 degrees, closed, and withdrawn.

Heaney, Heaney-Ballentine, and Masterson clamps are the commonly used clamps for clamping the parametrial and paracervical tissue during hysterectomy (Fig. 11.13). Hysterectomy clamps are heavy crushing clamps with ridged shafts. The classic clamps (Heaney, Heaney-Ballentine) also have toothed tips. The more recent Masterson clamp lacks a toothed tip and was designed to generate the least amount of crushing force.

Retractors

Retractors are used to hold tissue out of the operative field to improve exposure during surgical procedures (Fig. 11.14). Retractors are either held by an assistant (manual retractors) or use counter-pressure from other tissue (self-retaining retractors) to hold themselves in place.

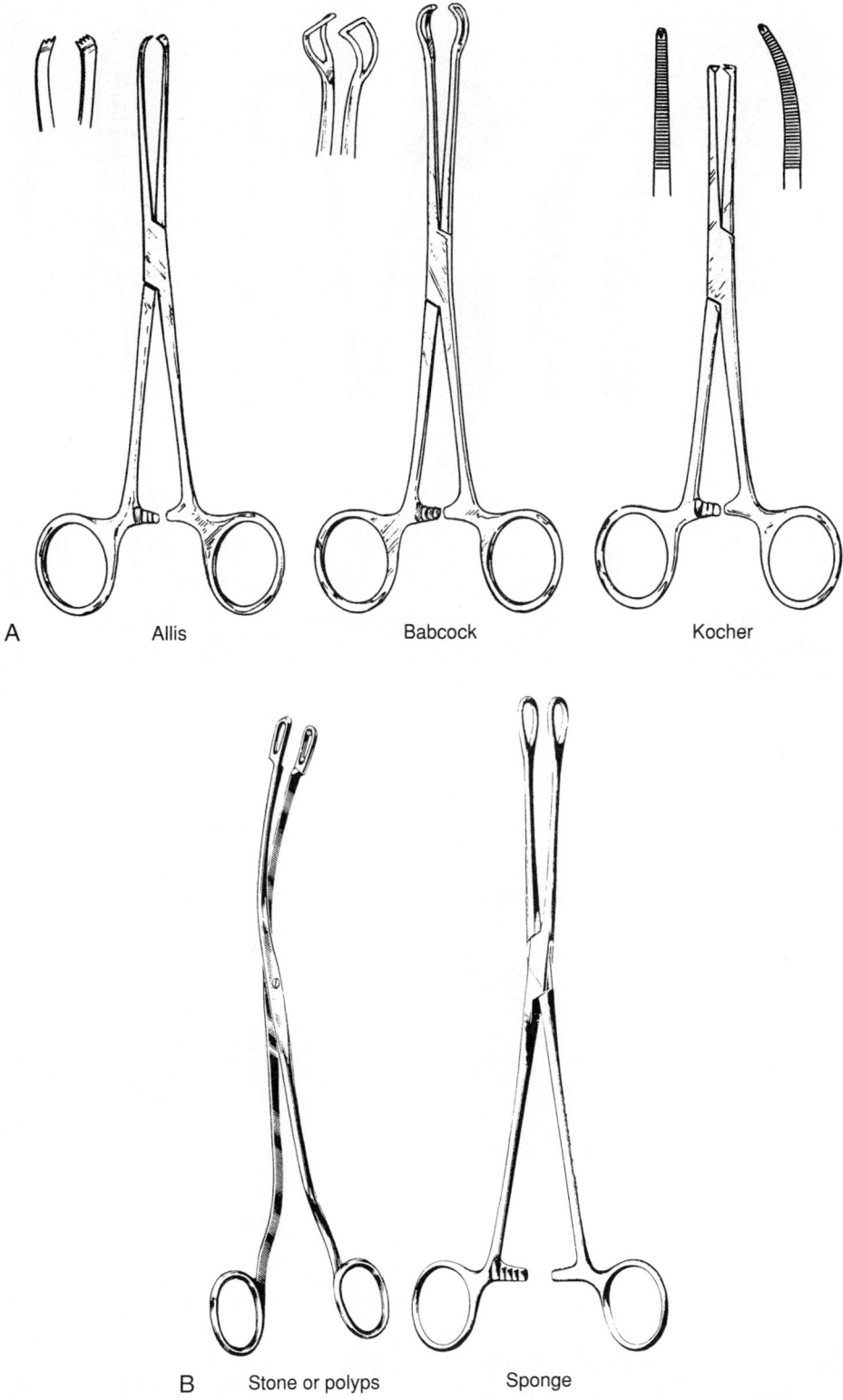

FIGURE 11.12. Tissue clamps. (Courtesy of Zinnati Surgical Instruments, Inc., Chatsworth, CA)

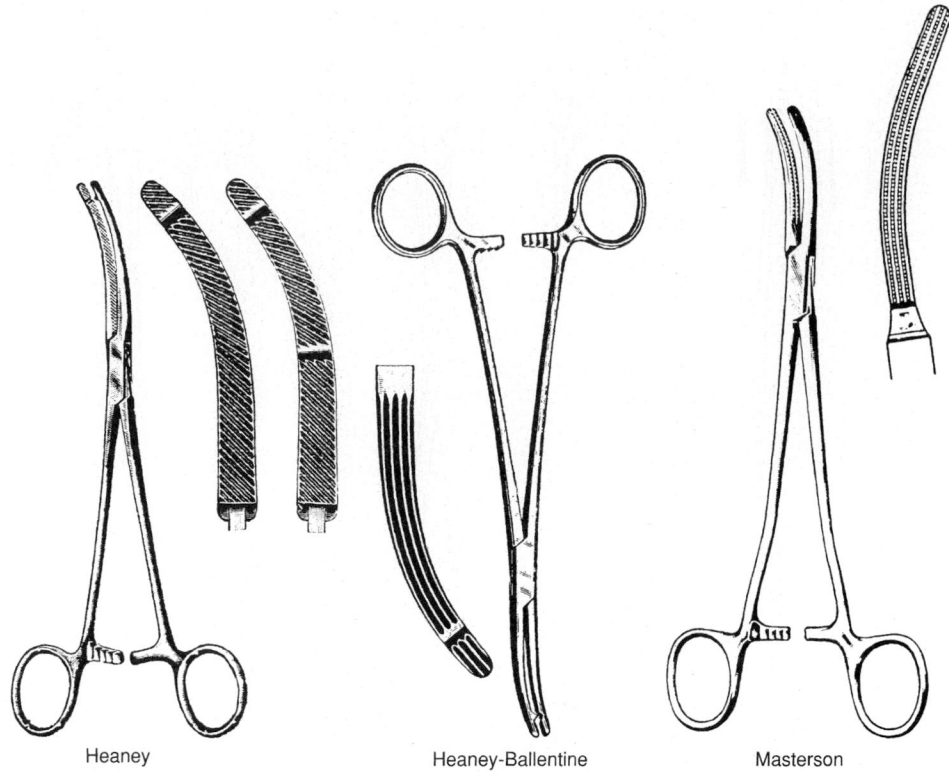

Heaney   Heaney-Ballentine   Masterson

FIGURE 11.13. Hysterectomy clamps. (Courtesy of Zinnati Surgical Instruments, Inc., Chatsworth, CA)

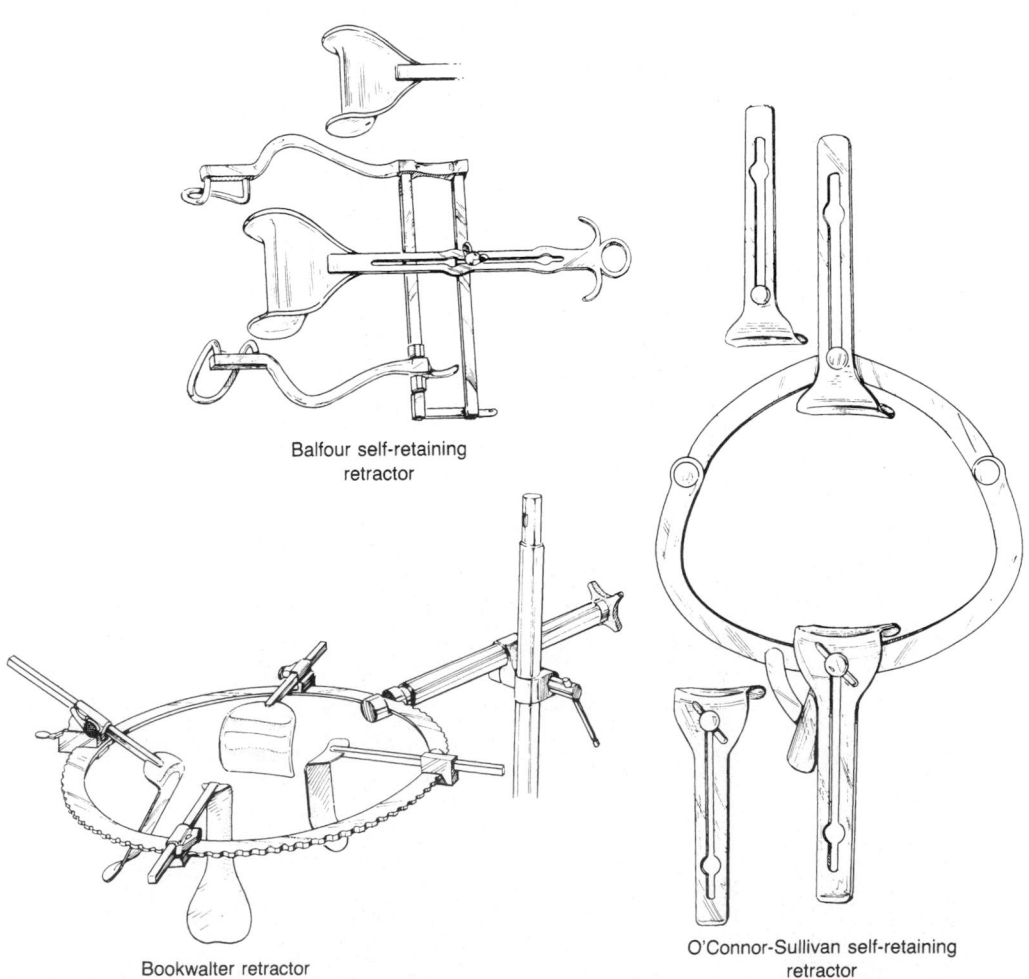

Balfour self-retaining
retractor

Bookwalter retractor

O'Connor-Sullivan self-retaining
retractor

FIGURE 11.14. Retractors. (Courtesy of Zinnati Surgical Instruments, Inc., Chatsworth, CA)

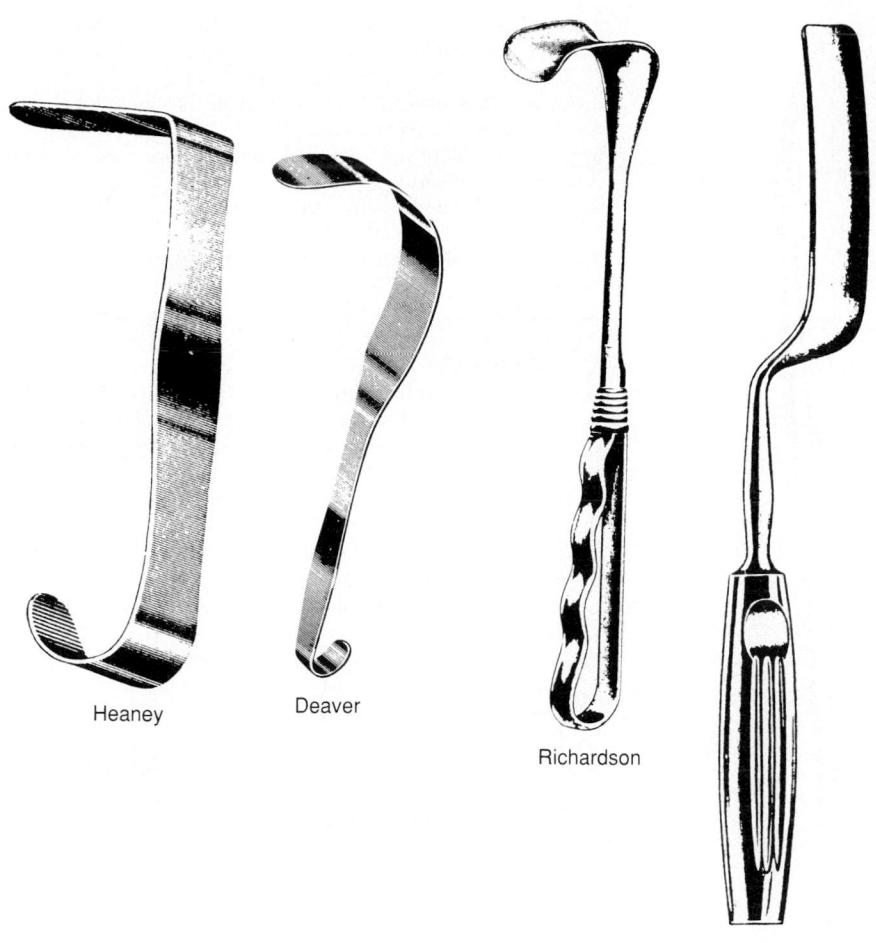

Heaney   Deaver

Richardson

Breisky

FIGURE 11.15. Manual retractors. (Courtesy of Zinnati Surgical Instruments, Inc., Chatsworth, CA)

Self-retaining retractors frequently are used to hold the sides of the incision apart during gynecologic surgery. Gynecologists seem to favor the O'Conner-O'Sullivan retractor when performing pelvic surgery. General surgeons, on the other hand, prefer the Balfour retractor. The O'Conner-O'Sullivan is a circular retractor with four blades, two permanently attached lateral retractors to retract the sidewalls, and a removable upper and lower blade to retract the bowel and bladder, respectively. This retractor is available with large or small lateral blades, whereas the removable blades come in several sizes. The Balfour retractor also has two lateral blades but only one additional retractor blade. This blade normally is employed as an upper blade with a manual retractor used for bladder retraction if needed. However, if the bowel is carefully packed away with laparotomy packs, the third blade can be used as a bladder retractor. All blades of the Balfour retractor are removable and available in different sizes.

The Bookwalter retractor is the most versatile of retractors, providing excellent exposure to the operative field. It consists of a circular metal ring to which a wide variety of retractors can be attached at any point. Its best use is during radical pelvic surgery or when operating on massively obese patients. In extremely obese patients, it may necessary to attach the Bookwalter retractor to the operating table.

Manual retractors allow maximum flexibility in providing exposure (Fig. 11.15). They can be used alone or as a supplement to self-retaining retractors. Common manual retractors include the Heaney, Deaver, and Richardson retractors. Specialized retractors include the Briesky-Navratil (used during sacrospinous vault suspension), Army-Navy, and Parker retractors (used for skin and subcutaneous tissue).

Dilators

Dilators are metal or plastic cylinders used to dilate the cervical os to sufficient size to admit other surgical instruments (Fig. 11.16). Dilators may have tapered (Hank and Pratt) or rounded tips (Hegar). Dilators with tapered tips require less force to perform dilatation than dilators with rounded tips. The sizes are measured either by diameter or by circumference. The unit of measurement for diameter is millimeters, whereas the unit of measurement for circumference is in French calibration. The relationship of the two measurements can be calculated by the formula for the circumference of a circle where the diameter times pi (3.14) equals the circumfer-

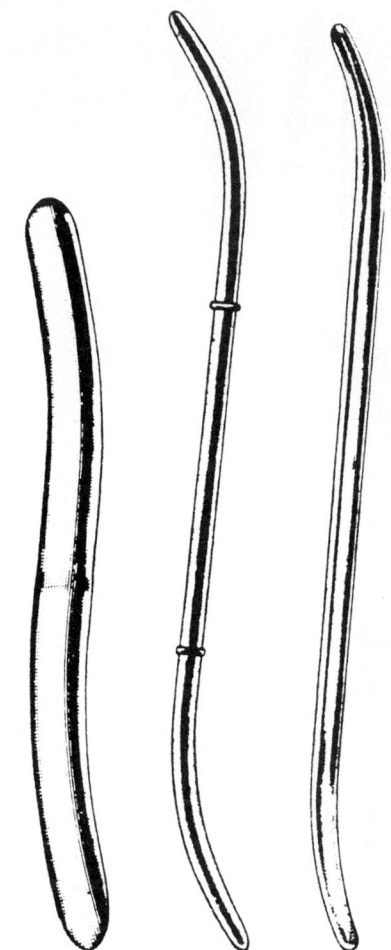

FIGURE 11.16. Common cervical dilators. (Courtesy of Zinnati Surgical Instruments, Inc., Chatsworth, CA)

ence. For comparison purposes, approximately 3 French equals 1 mm of diameter.

CONCLUSION

This chapter has attempted to present an introduction to the mechanisms of wound healing, wound closure, suture material, and instrumentation. It is hoped that this chapter will be a useful resource not only for those embarking on a surgical career but also for experienced surgeons as well.

BIBLIOGRAPHY

Alexander HC, Prudden JF. The causes of abdominal wound disruption. *Surg Gynecol Obstet* 1966;124:1223–1229.

Archie JP, Feltman RW. Primary abdominal wound closure with permanent, continuous running monofilament sutures. *Surg Gynecol Obstet* 1981;153:721.

Bilroth T. Beobachtungs-studien über wundfieber und accidentelle wundkrankheiten. *Achr Klin Chir* 1866;6:443–444.

Boerema I. Cause and repair of large incisional hernias. *Surgery* 1971;69:111–116.

Bourne RB, Bitar H, Andreae PR, et al. In-vitro comparison of four absorbable sutures: Vicryl, Dexon Plus, Maxon and PDS. *Can J Surg* 1988;31:43–45.

Brouwers JE, Oosting H, Haas D, et al. Dynamic loading of surgical knots. *Surg Gynecol Obstet* 1991;173:443–448.

Brown RP. Knotting material and suture. *Br J Surg* 1992;79:399–400.

Bryant WM. Wound healing. In: Bekiesz, ed. Ciba clinical symposia. *Ciba-Geigy* 1977;29:2–36.

Buckall TE. Abdominal wound closure: choice of suture. *J R Soc Med* 1981;74:580–585.

Campbell JA, Temple WJ, Frank CR, et al. A biomechanical study of suture pullout in linea alba. *Surgery* 1989;106:888–892.

Corman ML, Veidenheimer MC, Coller JA. Controlled clinical trial of three suture materials for abdominal wall closure after bowel operations. *Am J Surg* 1981;141:510–513.

Douglas DM. The healing of aponeurotic incisions. *Br J Surg* 1952;40:79–84.

Edlich RF, Rogers W, Kasper G, et al. Studies on the management of the contaminated wound. I. Optimal time for closure of contaminated open wounds. *Am J Surg* 1969;117:323–329.

Ethicon. *Wound closure manual.* Somerville, NJ: Ethicon Inc, 1985.

Ethicon. *Wound closure manual.* Somerville, NJ: Ethicon Inc, 1994.

Fagniez PL, Hay JM, Lacaine F, et al. Abdominal midline incision closure. *Arch Surg* 1985;120:1351–1353.

Fogdestam I. A biomechanical study of healing rat skin incisions after delayed primary closure. *Surg Obstet Gynecol* 1981;153:191–199.

Gallup DG, Talledo EO, King LA. Primary mass closure of midline incisions with a continuous running monofilament suture in gynecologic patients. *Obstet Gynecol* 1989;73:675–676.

Greenburg AG, Salk RS, Peskin GW. Wound dehiscence: pathology and prevention. *Arch Surg* 1979;114:143–146.

Greenall MJ, Evans , Pollack AV, et al. Midline or transverse laparotomy? A random controlled clinical trial. *Br J Surg* 1980;67:180.

Hartko WJ, Ghanekar G, Kemmann E. Suture materials currently used in obstetric-gynecologic surgery in the United States: a questionnaire survey. *Obstet Gynecol* 1982;59:241–246.

Herman JB. Tensile strength and knot security of surgical suture materials. *Am Surg* 1971;37:209–217.

Higgns GA, Antkowiak JG, Esterkyn SH. A clinical and laboratory study of abdominal wound closure and dehiscence. *Arch Surg* 1969;98:421–427.

Hodgson NC, Malthaner RA, Ostbye T. The search for an ideal method of abdominal fascial closure: a metaanalysis. *Ann Surg* 2000;231:436–442.

Hoffman MS, Villa A, Roberts WS, et al. Mass closure of the abdominal wound with delayed absorbable suture in surgery for gynecologic cancer. *J Reprod Med* 1991;36:356–358.

Howes EL, Harvey SC. The strength of the healing wound in relation to the holding strength of the chromic catgut suture. *NEJM* 1929;200:1285–1291.

Hunter J. *Treatise on blood, inflammation and gunshot wounds.* London: Nichol, 1794:216–220.

Katz AR, Mukherjee DB, Kagnanov AL, et al. A new synthetic monofilament absorbable suture made from polytrimethylene carbonate. *Surg Gynecol Obstet* 1983;161:213–222.

Kim YB, DuBeshter, Nilaoff JM. Continuous single-layer closure of midline abdominal incisions in high-risk gynecologic patients. *J Gynecol Surg* 1992;8:15–19.

Knight JP, Fewldman RW. Primary abdominal wound closure with permanent, continuous running monofilament sutures. *Arch Surg* 1983;118:1305.

Lichtenstein IL, Herzoikoff S, Shore JM, et al. The dynamics of wound healing. *Surg Gynecol Obstet* 1970;130:685–690.

Lowery KF, Curtis GM. Delayed suture in the management of wounds: analysis of 721 traumatic wounds illustrating the influence of time interval in wound repair. *Am J Surg* 1950;80:280–287.

Orr JW, Orr P, Barrett JM, et al. Continuous or interrupted fascial closure: a prospective evaluation of No. 1 Maxon in 402 gynecologic procedures. *Am J Obstet Gynecol* 1990; 163:1485–1489.

Paterson-Brown S, Dudley HAF. Knotting in continuous mass closure of the abdomen. *Br J Surg* 1986;73;679–680.

Peacock EE. Wound healing. In: Schwartz SI, Shircs GT, Spenser FC, et al, eds. *Principles of Surgery,* 3rd ed. New York: McGraw-Hill, 303–324.

Ray JA, Doddi N, Regula D, et al. Polydioxanone (PDS), a novel monofilament synthetic absorbable suture. *Surg Gynecol Obstet* 1981;151:497–507.

Reul GJ. The role of sutures in the complications in vascular surgery and their relationship to pseudoaneurysm formation. In: Bernham VM, Town JB, eds. *Complications in vascular surgery.* New York: Grune & Stratton, 1981: 615–637.

Rodeheaver GT, Tacker JG, Edlich RF, Mechanical performance of polyglycolic acid and polyglactin-910 synthetic absorbable suture. *Surg Gynecol Obstet* 1981;153:835–841.

Rodeheaver GT, Tacker JG, Edlich RF, et al. Knotting and handling characteristics of coated synthetic sutures. *J Surg Res* 1983;35:525–530.

Sanders RJ, DiClementi D, Ireland K. Principles of abdominal wound closure: I. Animal studies. *Arch Surg* 1977;112: 1184–1187.

Sanders RJ, DiClementi D. Principles of abdominal wound closure: II. Prevention of dehiscence. *Arch Surg* 1977; 112:1188–1191.

Sanz LE. Wound management: technique and suture material. In: Sanz LE, ed. *Gynecologic surgery.* Oradell, NJ: Medical Economics, 1988:21–38.

Sanz LE, Patterson JA, Kamath R, et al. Comparison of Maxon suture with Vicryl, chromic catgut, and PDS sutures in fascial closure in rats. *Obstet Gynecol* 1988;71:418–422.

Sanz LE. Sutures: a primer on structure and function. *Contemp Obstet Gynecol* 1990;33:99–106.

Sloop RD. Running synthetic absorbable suture in abdominal closure. *Am J Surg* 1981;141:572–573.

Stone HH, Hoefling SJ, Strom PR, et al. Abdominal incisions: transverse vs vertical placement and continuous vs interrupted closure. *South Med J* 1983;76:1106–1112.

Stone IK, Fraunhofer, Masterson BJ. The biomechanical effects of tight suture closure upon fascia. *Surg Obstet Gynecol* 1986;163:448–452.

Tera H, Aberg C. Tissue strength of structures involved in musculo-aponeurotic layer sutures in laparotomy incisions. *Acta Chir Scand* 1976;142:349–355.

Trimbos JB. Security of various knots commonly used in surgical practice. *Obstet Gynecol* 1984;64:274–280.

Trimbos JB, Van Rijssel EJC, Klopper PJ. Performance of sliding knots in monofilament and multifilament suture material. *Obstet Gynecol* 1986;68:425–430.

The United States Pharmacopeia, 23th rev. Taunton, MA: Rand McNally, 1994.

Van Rijssel EJC, Trimbos JB, Booster MH. mechanical performance of square knots and sliding knots in surgery: a comparative study. *Am J Obstet Gynecol* 1990;162:93–97.

Wasiljew BK, Winchester DP. Experience with continuous absorbable suture in the closure of abdominal incisions. *Surg Obstet Gynecol* 1982;154:375–380.

Wilhelm DL. Inflammation and healing. In: Anderson WA, Kisssane JM, eds. *Pathology,* 7th ed. St Louis: CV Mosby, 25–87.

PRINCIPLES OF GYNECOLOGIC SURGICAL TECHNIQUES

Te Linde's Operative Gynecology, ninth edition, edited by John A. Rock and Howard W. Jones, III. Lippincott Williams & Wilkins, Philadelphia © 2003.

CHAPTER

12

▼

Incisions for Gynecologic Surgery

JAMES J. BURKE II   DONALD G. GALLUP

One of the lasting marks of any abdominal surgery, and most noticeable to the patient, is the scar made by the incision. In selecting an incision, the gynecologist must take into consideration the underlying pathology prompting the surgery, the suspicion of malignancy, the absence or presence of upper abdominal disease, and the underlying comorbid state of the patient. Although there are many types of incisions for gynecological surgery, selection of any incision must be highly individualized. However, selection of an incision *should not* be dictated by patient choice to preserve cosmesis if it may compromise the surgical approach. Conversely, unduly large or poorly positioned incisions may increase the likelihood of infection, herniation, or dehiscence, as well as unsightly cosmesis. During the surgical consenting process, the patient should be counseled on the location of the incision, the rationale for the particular incision, and any possible complication that may arise from the planned incision. In gynecologic oncology patients, the need for urinary diversion, colostomy, or an extraperitoneal approach to node-bearing areas will dictate the type of incision to be made. This chapter presents the classic incisions used by gynecologists to perform most gynecologic surgery. In addition, incisions used for gynecologic oncology will be shown. Finally, discussion and management of common complications associated with abdominal incisions will be presented.

ANATOMY OF THE ANTERIOR ABDOMINAL WALL

To avoid injury to vessels and nerves and to close any incision with minimal chance of dehiscence, abdominal wall anatomy should be thoroughly understood. The abdominal wall protects the visceral organs and vasculature within the abdominal cavity. Cephalad, the anterior abdominal wall extends to the costal margins and the xiphoid process. The costal cartilages of the seventh, eighth, ninth, and tenth ribs form a portion of the cephalad boundary. Lateral boundaries include the iliac crests, and inferiorly, the abdominal wall is delineated by the inguinal ligaments, the pubic crests, and the superior border of the symphysis pubis. The principal anatomic structures of the abdominal wall include the overlying skin, subcutaneous tissue, muscles, fascia, and the nerves and vascular supply to these structures. Many factors—such as age, muscle mass and tone, obesity, intraabdominal pathology, previous pregnancies, and posture—can result in variation in the contour of the abdominal wall. These variations in contour affect abdominal wall topography and may present problems in the correct choice and placement of incisions.

Skin and Lymphatics

The skin contains small vessels, lymphatics, and nerves. A minimal loss of skin sensation can result from any ab-

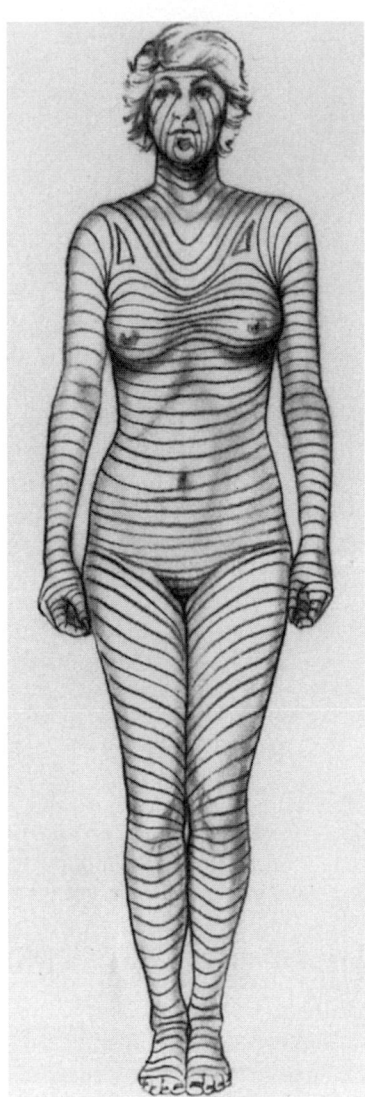

FIGURE 12.1. Langer lines run horizontally across the lower abdomen. A transverse incision cuts parallel to the Langer lines and usually heals with a fine scar.

dominal incision. Numbness below a transverse incision frequently occurs. As stated in the discussion on nerve supply, laterally extended transverse abdominal incisions can result in numbness of the skin on the anterior thigh.

The lymphatic drainage of the upper abdominal wall passes directly to the axillary lymph nodes. The lymphatic drainage of the lower abdomen passes to the inguinal nodes and then to the iliac chain. Some lymphatics around the umbilicus drain toward the liver through the falciform ligament. When an incision is placed transversely in the lower abdomen, lymphatic drainage of the abdominal wall above the incision site is interrupted. Some tissue swelling may develop temporarily until collateral lymphatic drainage can be established. Patients should be counseled about this possible swelling before undergoing surgery.

In 1861, Langer, working with cadavers, described cleavage lines of the skin that pull the skin edges apart when cut across. These have become known as *Langer lines* (Fig. 12.1). These lines usually run horizontally across the abdomen. A vertical incision in the skin of the abdomen cuts perpendicular to Langer lines, whereas a horizontal incision cuts parallel to them. Thus, transverse incisions heal with a relatively fine scar, and vertical incisions can heal with a broad scar, particularly in the lower abdomen.

Muscles and Fascia

The abdominal muscles assist in respiration, defecation, urination, coughing, and childbirth by increasing intraabdominal pressure. They work synergistically with the muscles of the back to flex, extend, and rotate the trunk and pelvis. There are two groups of muscles that form the musculature of the anterior abdominal wall. The *flat muscles* include the external oblique, the internal oblique, and the transversalis. Their fibers basically run diagonally or transversely. The second group, composed of the rectus muscles and the paired pyramidalis muscles, have fibers that run vertically (Fig. 12.2). The recti, with their thin investing fascia, are muscles of locomotion and posture. The paired pyramidalis muscles arise from the crest of the pubic symphysis and insert into the lower linea alba. Preservation of the pyramidalis muscles is not essential when making incisions. The integrity of the anterior abdominal wall is not really associated with this second group of muscles.

A cross section of the lower abdominal wall shows that the fascia of the abdominal muscles envelop the anterior and posterior surfaces of the rectus muscles and anchor the external oblique, internal oblique, and transversalis muscles to the vertical (rectus) muscles (Fig. 12.3). There is excellent fascial support anteriorly and posteriorly to the rectus muscles above the arcuate (semicircular) line. In this location, the fascial aponeurosis of the external oblique and the split fascial aponeurosis of the internal oblique fuse together anterior to the rectus muscle and insert in the midline (linea alba). Above the arcuate line, the posterior lamella of the internal oblique aponeurosis fuses with the aponeurosis of the transversalis muscle, passes posterior to the rectus muscle, and inserts in the midline. The lower half of the lower abdominal wall is weakened below the arcuate line, at a level about horizontal to the anterior superior iliac spine, where the posterior division of the rectus sheath disappears. In this location, the divided lamella of the internal oblique muscle combines and passes anterior to the rectus muscle. From this lower portion of the lower abdominal wall to the pubic rami, only the attenuated transversalis fascia and the peritoneum lie adjacent to the posterior surface of the muscle. It is in this weakened section of the lower abdomen that most incisional hernias occur after pelvic surgery through lower midline incisions. In the lower abdomen, the force required to approximate edges of a vertical incision is 30 times greater than the force required to approximate edges of a transverse incision.

The external oblique muscle and its aponeurosis form the most anterior layer of the flat muscles. The ex-

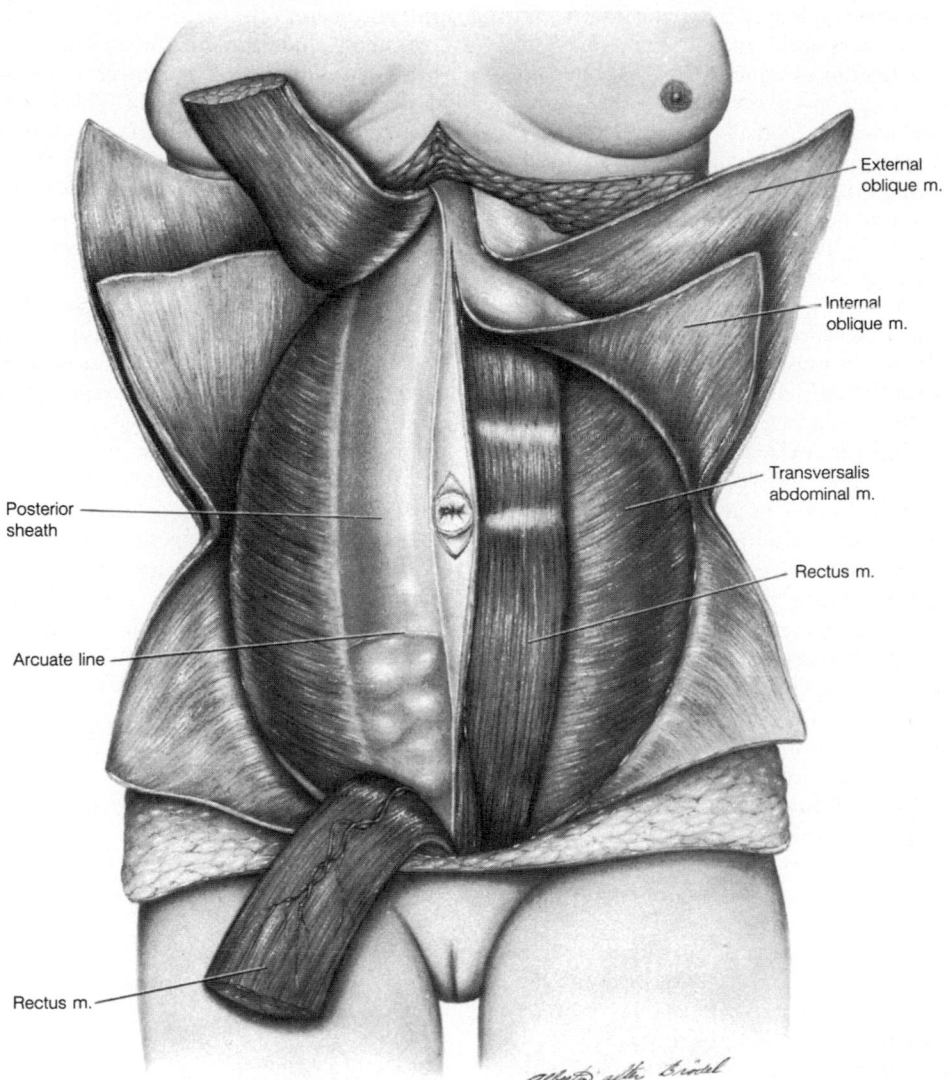

External
oblique m.

Internal
oblique m.

Transversalis
abdominal m.

Rectus m.

Posterior
sheath

Arcuate line

Rectus m.

FIGURE 12.2. Musculature of the abdominal wall **(left),** showing reflection of external and internal oblique muscles along with anterior division of rectus sheath, which exposes the transversalis and rectus muscles. Tendinous inscriptions in rectus sheath are visible above the umbilicus. The rectus muscle has been reflected **(right)** to demonstrate the posterior rectus sheath and the abrupt cessation of the posterior lamella of the internal oblique at the linea semicircularis (*arcuate line*). Below the *arcuate line,* the intestines are separated from the abdominal wall by the peritoneum and the attenuated fascia of the transversalis muscle.

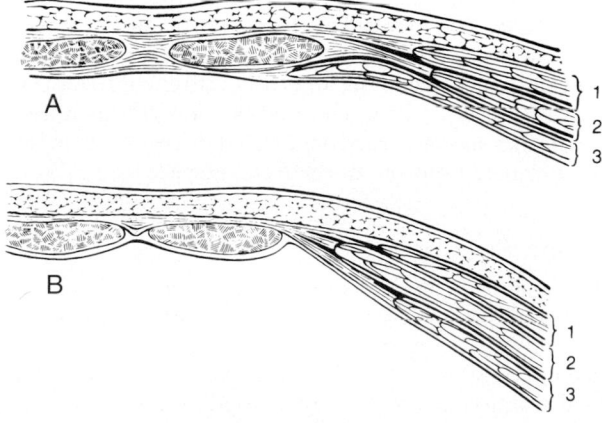

A

B

FIGURE 12.3. Cross section of lower abdominal wall. **A:** The anterior fascial sheath of the rectus muscle from external oblique muscle (*1*) and split aponeurosis of internal oblique muscle (*2*). The posterior sheath is formed by aponeurosis of transversalis muscle (*3*) and split aponeurosis of internal oblique muscle. **B:** Lower portion of abdominal wall below arcuate line (linea semicircularis) with absence of a posterior fascial sheath of the rectus muscle and all of the facial aponeuroses (*1–3*) forming the anterior rectus sheath.

ternal oblique muscle originates from the lower eight ribs. Superiorly, the fibers of this muscle run transversely; inferiorly, they assume an oblique downward course. A portion of the muscle gives rise to a broad fibrous aponeurosis, which courses medially, anterior to the rectus muscle. The next posterior fanlike muscle is the internal oblique, which originates primarily from the iliac crest, the thoracolumbar fascia, and the inguinal ligament. The mid-portion of the muscle runs an upward oblique course and gives rise to the aponeurosis of the internal oblique. As noted, at the lateral border of the rectus musculature, the aponeurosis splits and forms a sheath around the rectus muscle, rejoining medial to the rectus to help form the linea alba. The third flat muscle, the transverse abdominis, arises from the lower six costal cartilages, thoracolumbar fascia, and internal lip of the iliac crest. It has a truly transverse course. Above the midway point between the umbilicus and pubis, the aponeurosis of this muscle passes behind the rectus muscle and contributes to the posterior rectus sheath. Below this point, the aponeurosis passes anterior to the rectus muscle, contributing to the anterior rectus sheath. Medial to the rectus muscle, the fascia of all three flat muscles insert to form the linea alba.

The major functions of the flat muscles are to assist with respirations and to assist in increasing intraabdominal pressure. Each time these muscles contract, they pull at the linea alba. Because the linea alba represents the insertion of six major abdominal muscles (three on each side), cutting it, as with lower midline incisions, actually interrupts the major portion of the insertion of these six muscles. Thus, contractions of these muscles in the postoperative period can result in considerable tension on a suture line in the linea alba and can cause considerable discomfort.

The rectus abdominis muscle arises from the pubic crest. It courses superiorly and inserts into the xiphoid process with the upper attachments being three times as broad as its pubic insertion. It has three or four fibrous insertions. One is at the level of the umbilicus; two are usually halfway between the umbilicus and the insertions, superiorly and inferiorly. Of note, the fibrous insertions are tightly adherent to the anterior rectus sheath. These limit the retraction of the muscle when it is cut. Thus, when performing a transverse-muscle cutting incision, it is not necessary to reapproximate the rectus muscle. The pyramidalis, a triangular muscle, usually lies anterior to the rectus and arises from the anterior portion of the symphysis, inserting into the inferior portion of the linea alba. The mid-portion of this muscle usually has an avascular raphe, which can easily be incised for adequate exposure of the Retzius space.

Blood Supply

The abundant blood supply to the anterior abdominal wall comes from several sources. The main arterial supply consists of the superior epigastric, musculophrenic, deep circumflex iliac, and inferior epigastric vessels. The medial abdominal wall receives blood from the epigastric arteries, whereas the lateral wall is supplied by the musculophrenic and deep circumflex iliac arteries. The lateral wall is also supplied by the lower intercostal and lumbar arteries (T-8 to T-12 and L-1). This freely anastomosing vascular system provides one continuous arterial and venous channel on both sides of the anterior abdominal wall, extending from the subclavian artery and vein cephalad to the external iliac vessels caudad (Fig. 12.4). Because of the rich anastomosis, vascular deficiency is usually not a complication of abdominal wall surgery. The linea alba is relatively bloodless. The limited vascular supply in this area of fascial fusion can impair wound healing when lower midline incisions are used. Thus, a secure closure is mandatory to avoid incisional hernias or eviscerations.

Conversely, the epigastric vessels are subject to injury, particularly when a muscle-splitting incision is used. Also, the deep circumflex or musculophrenic vessels can be injured when an extraperitoneal approach is chosen.

The superior epigastric artery is a continuation of the internal thoracic (mammary) artery. It enters the sheath of the rectus from behind the seventh costal cartilage and descends posterior to the rectus. It has multiple branches in the substance of the rectus muscle and anas-

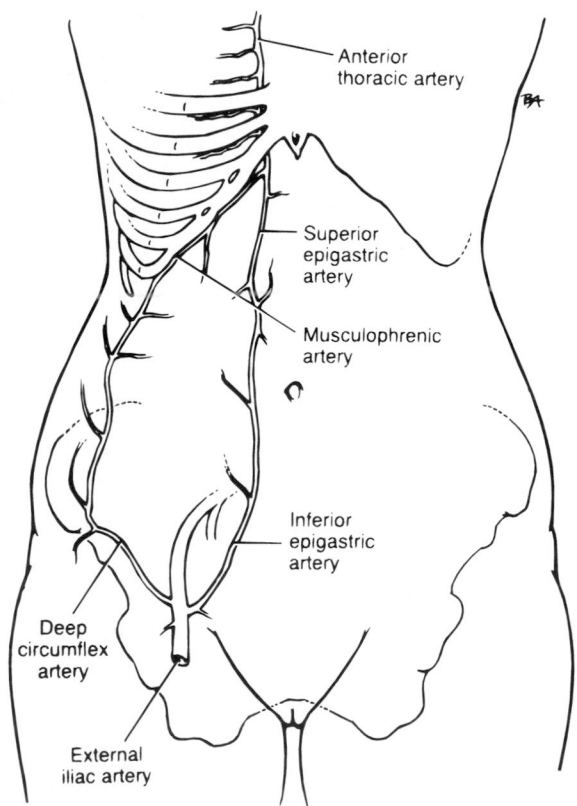

FIGURE 12.4. The major arterial blood supply of the anterior abdominal wall consists of four major vessels. Two lateral and two medial contribute to the rich anastomosis. (From Gallup DG. Opening and closing the abdomen and wound healing. In: Gershenson D, Curry S, DeCherney A, eds. *Operative gynecology.* Philadelphia: WB Saunders, 1993:127, with permission.)

tomosis to the inferior epigastric artery. In the upper abdomen, cephalad to the umbilicus, the main branch of the artery tends to lie posterior to the *mid-portion* of the rectus muscle (Fig. 12.5). The inferior epigastric artery arises from the external iliac artery near the mid-inguinal point. It continues in a cephalad course along the posterior *lateral* portion of the rectus muscle and has an anastomosis with the superior epigastric arteries. The lower a transverse incision is made, the more lateral the inferior epigastric arteries are encountered. Bleeding from branches of the inferior epigastric vessels beneath the rectus muscle can dissect cephalad or caudad along the entire length of the posterior sheath. Below the arcuate line, bleeding can dissect laterally and inferiorly along the retroperitoneal planes and spaces, resulting in extensive

hematomas of the abdominal wall and pelvis. Such bleeding can produce confusing acute abdominal signs in the postoperative patient, and large quantities of blood may be lost in these loose tissues and spaces.

The musculophrenic artery, arising from the internal thoracic, courses along the costal margin behind the cartilages. It has an anastomosis with the deep circumflex artery, which originates from the external iliac at about the same level as the inferior epigastric artery. The deep circumflex courses behind the inguinal ligament and along the iliac crest, eventually piercing the transversus muscle and digitating between that muscle and the internal oblique. Before its anastomosis with the musculophrenic, it can be relatively large. Care must be taken when these muscles are incised laterally.

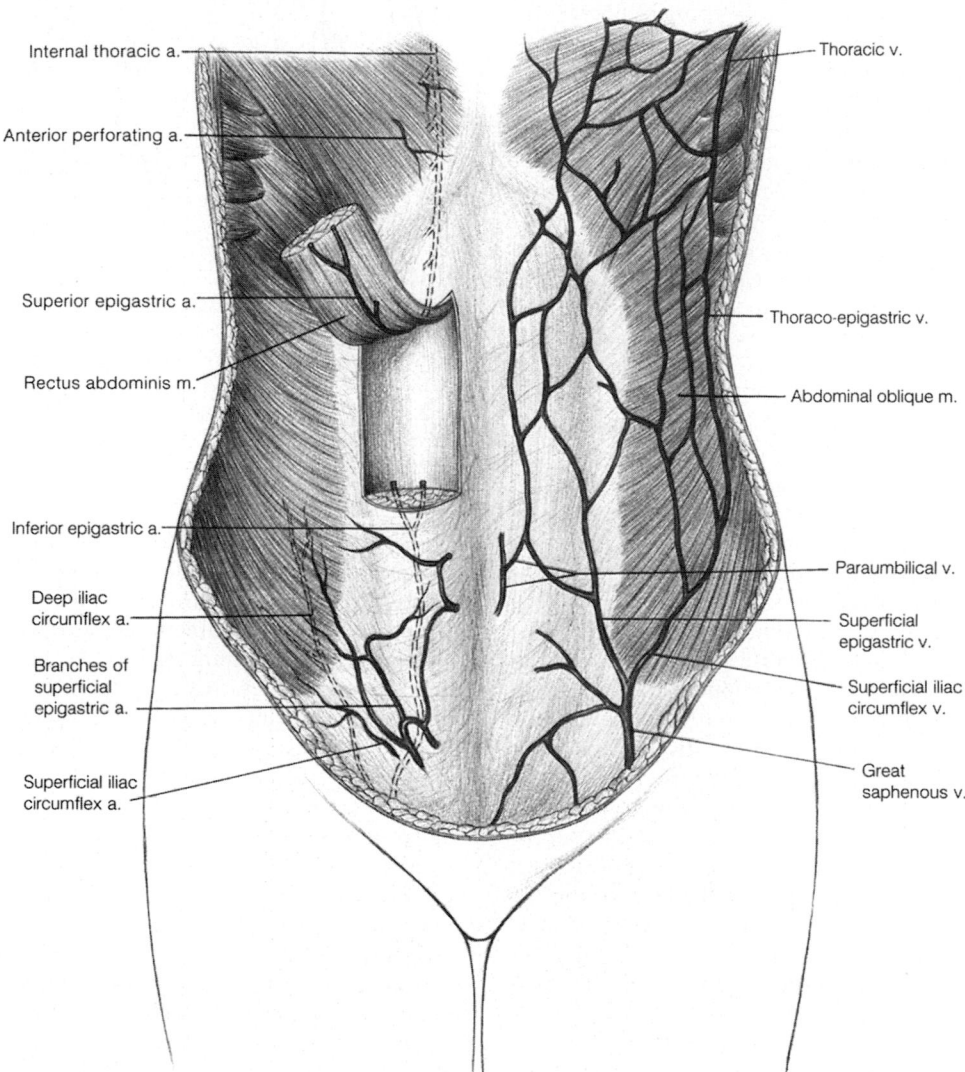

FIGURE 12.5. Arterial and venous circulation of abdominal wall. The superior and inferior epigastric arteries provide a rich arcade for the rectus muscles, arising superiorly from the internal thoracic artery and inferiorly from the external iliac artery. The venous system has a similar origin, with the exception that the superficial inferior epigastric vein communicates with the saphenous vein of the leg.

The venous drainage of the abdominal wall accompanies the arteries. The veins of the abdominal wall may be dilated in patients with obstruction of blood flow through the liver and porta hepatis.

Innervation

The nerve supply to the anterior abdominal wall is easily damaged by some incisions. The anterior abdominal wall is supplied by the thoracoabdominal nerves, the iliohypogastric nerves, and the ilioinguinal nerves. The thoracoabdominal nerves, which are the seventh to eleventh intercostal nerves, leave the intercostal spaces and travel caudad and anterior between the transversus and internal oblique. They supply these muscles and the external oblique. They enter the sheath of the rectus, and their branches supply the rectus and the overlying skin. Most of the nerves are supplied by several trunks. Any one nerve in the anterior abdominal wall contains fibers from the last two to three intercostal nerves. When an incision is made lateral to the midline, a transverse type is least likely to cause injury to nerves. In the upper abdomen, an obliquely caudad and laterally directed incision is least likely to cause significant nerve injury. In the lower part of the abdomen, an obliquely directed cephalad and laterally directed incision is relatively nerve sparing.

A vertical incision that passes lateral to the rectus muscle or through the muscle itself can denervate medially lying tissue. Depending on the length of the incision, atony or atrophy of the muscle can occur. A midline incision in the linea alba or a transverse incision (even through the rectus muscle), however, does not interfere with motor innervation of the abdominal musculature.

A minimal loss of skin sensation can result from abdominal incisions and is unavoidable in most cases. The iliohypogastric and ilioinguinal nerves are sensory in function (Fig. 12.6). Injury to the former, when wide transverse incisions are used, can result in sensation changes in the skin over the mons, whereas injury to the latter can result in sensation changes to the labia majora. A widely placed transverse incision can result in numbness of the skin over the upper anterior thigh. Both nerves are chiefly derived from the first lumbar nerve root. Although they lie for a distance between the internal oblique and the transversus, they do not enter the rectus sheath. They do not supply the external oblique or the rectus muscle. Both nerves supply the lower fibers of the internal oblique and transversus. If damage occurs to these nerves at the level of the anterosuperior iliac spine, these muscle fibers are denervated. A weakening of the normal canal-controlling mechanism can occur, predisposing the patient to an inguinal hernia.

PHYSIOLOGY OF WOUND HEALING

Wound complications are a psychological and economic problem for the patient and include infections, dehiscence, and evisceration, as well as late-occurring prob-

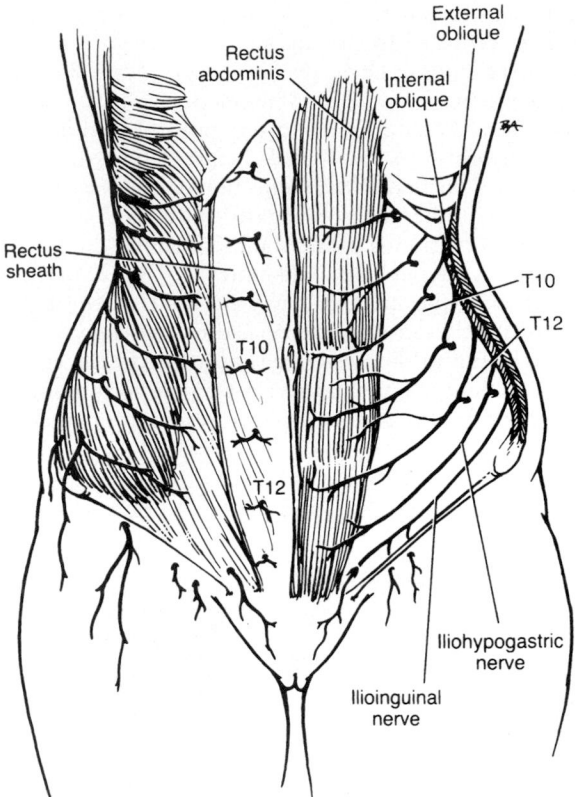

FIGURE 12.6. Major innervation of the anterior abdominal wall. The iliohypogastric nerves and ilioinguinal nerves supply the sensory innervation of the lower abdominal wall. (From Gallup DG. Opening and closing the abdomen and wound healing. In: Gershenson D, Curry S, DeCherney A, eds. *Operative gynecology.* Philadelphia: WB Saunders, 1993:127, with permission.)

lems such as incisional hernias and wound sinus formation. Factors negatively affecting proper wound healing include diabetes, malnutrition, prior irradiation or chemotherapy, older patient age, alcoholism, preoperative shaving the evening before the operation, longer duration of preoperative hospitalization, longer duration of the operation, use of Penrose-type drains brought out through the incision, ascites, malignancy, immunosuppression (including long-term corticosteroid therapy), and obesity. In addition, factors affecting wound disruption that usually occur in the absence of infection include choice of suture material, closure technique, occurrence of excessive coughing caused by pulmonary disease, retching and vomiting, and intestinal obstruction.

The four phases of wound healing are inflammation, migration, proliferation, and maturation. Breaks in the normal cycle of wound healing can occur anywhere, depending on preexisting conditions. Increases in fibroblasts during the proliferation phase, which occurs from day 5 through day 20, provide most of the strength to the wound. By day 21, most wounds have regained almost 30% of their original tensile strength. Any wound contamination or the presence of foreign bodies can cause chronic inflammation, wound sinuses, delayed in-

TABLE 12.1.
Wound Classification

Class	Category	Definition	Wound Infection Rate (%)
I	Clean	Wounds are made under ideal operating room conditions. The procedures are usually elective, and no entry is made into the oropharyngeal cavity or lumen of the respiratory, alimentary, or genitourinary tract. Inflammation is not encountered, and no break in technique occurs. The wounds are always primarily closed and seldom drained. Almost 75% of all operations are included in this group.	<5
II	Clean-contaminated	Wounds occur from entry into the oropharyngeal cavity, respiratory, alimentary, or genitourinary tract without significant spillage. Clean wounds are included in this category when there is a minor break in surgical technique. These procedures include about 16% of all operations.	2–10
III	Contaminated	This category includes open, fresh, and traumatic wounds; operations with a major break in sterile technique; and incisions encountering acute, nonpurulent inflammation, such as in cholecystitis or cystitis.	15–20
IV	Dirty	Old (>4 h) traumatic wounds, perforated viscera, or operations involving clinically evident infections are included in this category. Wounds containing foreign bodies or devitalized tissue are also considered dirty.	>30

cisional hernias, or the early postoperative problems of infection and dehiscence.

The risks of wound infections are directly related to the classification of wounds (Table 12.1). Obviously, few surgeons would primarily close a dirty wound. Many of the abdominal procedures performed by gynecologists include a hysterectomy. Whenever the vagina is entered, the procedure is then classified as a clean-contaminated procedure with attendant risk.

SUTURES

Suture choice is basically a surgeon's prerogative, but the characteristics of suture material intended for fascial closure should be well known to the surgeon. Additionally, suture choice should be based on the patient's condition, the type of incision, and the strength and reaction of the suture (Table 12.2). In general, the ideal suture material should have the following characteristics: knot security,

TABLE 12.2.
Commonly Used Sutures for General Closure

Suture Type	Tissue Reaction	Relative Strength	Knot Security
Absorbable			
Monofilament			
Plain gut	4	1	2
Chronic gut	3	2	3
Polydioxanone (PDS)	1	4	2
Polyglyconate (Maxon)	1	3	2
Polyglecaperone 25 (Monocryl)	1	2	2
Vicryl Rapide	2	2	2
Braided			
Polyglycolic acid (Dexon, Dexon 2)	2	3	2
Polyglactin 910 (Vicryl)	2	3	2
Poly (L-actide/glycolide) (Panacryl)	2	3	3
Nonabsorbable			
Monofilament			
Polypropylene monofilament (Surgilene, Novofil, Prolene)	1	4	1
Stainless-steel wire (Flexon)	1	4	4
Nylon (Dermalon, Ethilon, Surgilon)	1	3	2
Braided			
Natural (silk, cotton)	4	2	3
(Dacron, Mersilene, Ti-Cron, Ethibond, Tevdeck)	2	3	3

Scale on 1, least; 4, most.

inertness, adequate tensile strength, flexibility, ease in handling, smooth passage through tissue, nonallergenicity, resistance to infection, and absorbability at a predictable rate. Neither plain catgut nor chromic catgut maintains tensile strength during the critical time of wound healing. They should not be used for fascial closure of the abdominal wall, irrespective of the type of incision used. Estimation of tensile strength of chromic suture after 14 days is 34%, whereas plain gut has none.

In general, sutures are classified as nonabsorbable if they maintain tensile strength for more than 60 days. In the permanent suture group, monofilament sutures yield less inflammation than that of polyfilament sutures. Wire has been the traditional suture used by surgeons for decades in high-risk patients, particularly when infection was an associated operative finding. However, wire is difficult to tie and breaks easily if bent sharply. If placed too closely to the incisional edges, it may cut through tissues. In some patients, wire can cause a prickling sensation. Also, wire ends may penetrate the surgeon's gloves, exposing the surgeon to body fluid–borne pathogens. Furthermore, in animal models, both monofilament nylon and monofilament polypropylene sutures have elicited less infection in contaminated tissue and may be more durable than wire. Both cotton and silk are highly tissue-reactive sutures. Although silk and cotton are considered nonabsorbable sutures, silk loses all of its tensile strength after 1 year, and cotton loses half of its tensile strength after 1 year. If a permanent suture is chosen for closure, one of the monofilament polypropylene sutures or monofilament nylon should be used.

During the past two decades, synthetic absorbable sutures have been added to the surgeon's armamentarium. Polyglycolic acid and polyglactin have been extensively studied. They maintain an estimated 55% of their original tensile strength at 14 days, but lose all their tensile strength by 30 days. A newer polyglycolic acid suture, Dexon 2, appears to have better knot security. Many surgeons use one of these for various types of transverse incision closures. In 1984, Fagniez and colleagues reported few cases of fascial dehiscence in a large series of patients who had midline incisions closed with polyglycolic acid sutures.

Polyglyconate (Maxon) and polydioxanone (PDS) represent a new class of monofilament absorbable sutures, sometimes referred to as a "delayed-absorbable" suture. In animal studies, both of these sutures were observed to have a much less inflammatory response than that of polyglactin sutures. In addition, these investigators estimated that Maxon and PDS retain about 90% of their tensile strength by postoperative day 14 and retain 50% by postoperative day 30. In one study of degradation patterns of Maxon and PDS in rabbit fascia, PDS was noted to be superior. Rodeheaver and associates found no significant difference in knot-breaking strength in these two sutures, but Maxon appeared to have less stiffness in handling. Another study in rabbits also revealed the tensile strength superiority of Maxon and PDS compared with polyglycolic acid and polyglactin. In this study, Maxon was thought to have the best knot se-

curity. These investigators also observed that the most consistent knot security was achieved when six square knots were used. Alternatively, two surgeon's knots and two square knots can be used. Our clinical impression is that there is little difference in suture handling and knot security when Maxon and PDS II are compared. When wound healing is anticipated to take longer than 2 weeks, particularly for fascial closure of midline incisions, one of these two delayed-absorbable sutures should be highly considered. In addition, usage of one of these sutures should be considered in the presence of infection or contamination.

Finally, knot security will depend on suture size and the tissue needing approximation. Although sliding knots can be safely used for pelvic viscera, sutures used to close abdominal wall fascia should be tied with square knots. Van Rissel and colleagues observed poor knot performance when a surgeon's knot plus a square knot was made with monofilament sutures. We have not noticed this problem with knots tied similarly.

DRAINS

Sometimes, drainage of the abdominal cavity is appropriate after an operation for a tuboovarian abscess or some other type of pelvic infection. In addition, intraperitoneal drainage may be helpful for oozing peritoneal surfaces after complicated hysterectomies or other pelvic surgery. Although used in the past for prevention of lymphoceles or ureteral fistulae, retroperitoneal drains are not routinely used after radical pelvic surgery.

The use of prophylactic drains in the subcutaneous space or "wet" subfascial space remains controversial. Some investigators suggest that the lowest clean-wound infection rate is found in patients who have no drains. However, most surgeons use some type of closed drainage system when an unavoidable large potential space remains, for example, in dissection of a large incisional hernia or when mesh or a fascial or myocutaneous graft is used. Drainage may also be necessary to prevent subsequent hematoma formation when persisting defects in blood coagulation result in persistent "oozing." As discussed later, two published series on pelvic-abdominal surgery in obese patients indicate an advantage with the use of subcutaneous drains. On the other hand, Scott and coworkers operated on 56 patients whose panniculi measured 6 to 11 cm in thickness. They used systemic and oral antibiotics, transverse incisions, copious lavage, and tape to close the skin. No drains were used, and only one patient had a wound infection. Few randomized prospective studies with significant numbers of patients exist. In some series, only patients at high risk for wound infection were drained subcutaneously or subfascially, which clearly results in noncomparable groups for evaluation. Farnell and associates, in a prospective study, analyzed 3,282 incisions of the wound varieties listed in Table 12.1. When patients with clean-contaminated or contaminated wounds received subcutaneous closed-drainage systems, alone or with antibiotics or saline irrigation, no significant advantage was noted compared with primary closure without drainage. However, a trend favoring subcutaneous drainage and antibiotic irrigation was seen in patients with contaminated wounds.

Although the adage "the solution to pollution is dilution" is used quite often during wound irrigation, irrigation with bactericidal agents may be detrimental. In one study, irrigating solutions *in vitro* and in laboratory animals—such as 1% povidone-iodine, 0.25% acetic acid, or 0.5% sodium hypochlorite—were shown to have cytotoxic effects when applied to human fibroblasts. In the same study, hydrogen peroxide did not retard wound healing but had minimal bactericidal potency.

Drains can be classified into two basic categories: passive and active. The former function primarily by overflow, sometimes being assisted by gravity. The latter are connected to some type of suction device. The use of passive drains in wounds may be one reason that wound drainage has been associated with increased infection rates. The two types of passive drains used—whether Penrose or cigarette (a Penrose drain with gauze placed inside it to enhance capillary activity), if used at all—should never be brought out through the incision because of the risk of wound infection or seroma formation. We prefer a closed drainage system such as a Jackson-Pratt or a Blake. Both have small reservoir systems (100 mL) that are relatively easy for paramedical personnel to manage on the ward. In our experience, the Blake drain, with its longitudinal ridges, offers less chance of obstruction from small tissue fragments or clots than does the Jackson-Pratt drain. However, no large prospective trials comparing these systems are available.

In patients who undergo a clean-contaminated procedure without prophylactic antibiotics, closed-suction drainage of the wound may be beneficial. When antibiotics are used, prophylactic drainage may not be advantageous. To avoid clot formation and subsequent obstruction, the drain is placed on suction early, usually while completing closure of the incision. In addition, the nursing staff should be instructed to "strip" the drain catheter each shift while the drain is in place. Drains in the subfascial or subcutaneous space should be removed, not advanced, when the drainage is less than 50 mL per 24 hours, usually by postoperative day 2 or 3.

PREVENTION OF WOUND COMPLICATIONS

Wound infection, dehiscence, and evisceration usually occur early in the postoperative period, whereas suture sinuses and incisional hernias are late manifestations of impaired primary wound healing. Management of these problems is discussed later in this chapter.

The usual rate of significant wound infections is 5% or less for all abdominal operations and is related to many factors, including surgeon experience, the population operated on, the procedure performed, and the comorbid condition of the patient. Large series, such as those by Cruse and Foord, have added to current knowledge about wound infections and their causes. Preoperative showering with hexachlorophene lowered the infection rate in clean wounds (1.3%) compared with the rate with no showering (2.3%). In addition to others, Cruse and Foord also observed that clip preparation of abdominal and/or pubic hair versus shave preparation the evening before surgery resulted in fewer wound infections. Truthfully, the only reason to remove hair is to prevent interference with wound approximation in some incisions. Other methods of hair removal, including the use of depilatories, have been advocated by some surgeons, but they are relatively expensive. In the series reported by Seropian and Reynolds, the wound infection rates for depilatory preparations versus no hair removal were equal (0.6%). We prefer to use an electric razor, clipping the hair, in the operating room, when it is necessary to remove pubic hair.

Skin preparations and draping do not need to be complex. In one study of 2,253 consecutive general surgical procedures, the use of disposable gown and drape systems, rather than reusable cotton material, reduced postoperative infection incidence from 6.4% to 2.3%. Plastic adhesive drapes have been shown to be disadvantageous in preventing wound infections, and may actually increase infection rates if the adhesive loosens and the drape detaches from the skin. As shown in earlier studies, operative procedures that exceeded 90 minutes had much higher infection rates than did shorter-length procedures. This study from Duke University also revealed a relatively higher wound infection rate in women older than 60 years of age compared with men.

Newer antiseptic scrub techniques have been developed, including povidone-iodine (Betadine), 4% chlorhexidine gluconate (Hibiclens), and 3% hexachlorophene (pHisoHex). Of the three, Hibiclens produced the best immediate and persistent reduction in normal hand flora. A 3-minute skin preparation is adequate. Furthermore, the time-honored 10-minute scrub of the surgeon's hands is unnecessary. Galle and coworkers observed no difference in infection rates between a 5-minute versus a 10-minute scrub time. A lesser time obviously decreases total operative time and water usage.

Incisions of the skin or fascia should not be made with cautery. In one study, Kenady found the wound infection rate doubled when a Bovie device was used compared with a knife. Discarding the skin knife has not been shown to reduce wound infection rates, but instead leaves an extra "sharp" on the operative field that may injure the health care team. In a randomized prospective study, the rate of postoperative wound infections was not significantly different after the use of one or two scalpels for the incision (Hasselgren et al. 1984). The same scalpel can be safely used for superficial and deep incisions. The incision should be made in a bold strike to minimize dead space. In general, subcutaneous sutures should be avoided because the subcutaneous tissue does not provide support. In some patients, a fine (4-0) running polyglycolic acid suture in the subcutaneous layer may diminish tension from the approximated skin edges.

Chromic catgut should never be used to close the fascia and should not be used in subcutaneous closure. In general, delayed closure should be used for contaminated or dirty wounds. Alternatively, intermittent staples can be placed in the skin with intervening saline moistened "wicks" into the subcutaneous spaces. When a bacteria-containing organ is opened (the unprepped bowel or abscessed gynecological organs) and delayed closure is not used, copious saline irrigation of all layers for closure should be instituted. In addition, a monofilament delayed or nonabsorbable suture should be used in the closure. Systemic antibiotics can help control wound infections when pelvic infection is encountered. To be of benefit, they should be administered at least 30 minutes before the skin incision and readministered if the operation is prolonged. Currently, first-generation and second-generation cephalosporins are the most popular antibiotics used in the prophylactic setting.

ABDOMINAL INCISIONS

In general, abdominal incisions used for most gynecologic procedures can be divided into transverse or vertical incisions. For extraperitoneal incisions and access to organs not associated with the female genital tract, modifications of oblique incisions are sometimes used. Because of the ease and rapid entry, the abdomen was originally routinely opened by a longitudinal incision in the linea alba. One of the first successful abdominal operations was performed by McDowell in 1809. In the early days of abdominal surgery, transverse incisions were generally avoided because they were more time-consuming. Also, an unfounded fear was that transection of the rectus muscle would leave a defect because of retraction of the muscle. As previously stated in the section on anatomy, the adherence of the recti to the anterior rectus fascia by several transverse inscriptions prevents retraction. In the late 1800s and early 1900s, several transverse incisions were developed, such as the Küstner, Pfannenstiel, Maylard, and Cherney incisions. Most of the transverse incisions used for pelvic surgery are identified by the name of the surgeon who first described them, whereas the few vertical abdominal incisions have no such eponyms.

Transverse Incisions

Transverse incisions for pelvic surgery are attractive because they produce the best cosmetic results. Additionally, low transverse incisions are as much as 30 times stronger than midline incisions, are less painful, and result in less interference with postoperative respirations. Wound dehiscence is allegedly more common with vertical incisions. The older literature suggests that wound evisceration was three to five times more common and hernia occurrence was two to three times more common when vertical incisions were used compared with transverse incisions. Many earlier studies reported an increased incidence of eviscerations with midline incisions that could be associated with inappropriate closures. More recent studies, however, have shown no difference in the risk of wound dehiscence or even a slight advantage for midline incisions. A large study, completed at Hutzel Hospital in Detroit by Hendrix et al. found that there was no difference in fascial dehiscence between transverse (Pfannenstiel) and vertical incisions.

Transverse incisions have certain associated disadvantages. They are relatively more time-consuming and relatively more hemorrhagic. Occasionally, nerves are divided, and division of multiple layers of fascia and muscle can result in formation of potential spaces with subsequent hematoma formation. Ability to explore the upper-abdominal cavity adequately is compromised with most low transverse incisions.

Pfannenstiel Incision

Most surgeons would agree that the Pfannenstiel incision provides the best wound security of all gynecologic incisions. The cosmetic results are excellent, but exposure is limited. Thus, it should not be used for patients with known gynecologic malignancies. It should not be used when pelvic exposure is needed in operating on patients with nonmalignant conditions, such as severe endometriosis or large leiomyomas with distortion of the lower uterine segment, or when reoperating on a patient for hemorrhage.

The original, true Pfannenstiel incision is described as a transverse incision that is slightly curved (concavity upward) and may be made at any level suitable to the surgeon (Fig. 12.7A). It is usually 10 to 15 cm long and extends through the skin and subcutaneous fat to the level of the rectus fascia. The rectus fascia is incised transversely on either side of the linea alba, which is cut separately, joining the two lateral incisions but leaving the rectus fascia intact across the midline (Fig. 12.7B). The rectus sheath is separated from the underlying muscle by inserting the fingers on either side of the cut edge of the sheath and pulling the fascia in opposite directions, with one hand toward the head and the other hand toward the feet. This maneuver frees the fascia from the anterior surface of the rectus muscle as far as desired between the symphysis and the umbilicus (Fig. 12.7C). The rectus muscles are then separated in the midline, and the peritoneum is opened vertically (Fig. 12.7D). This procedure avoids the necessity of dissecting the subcutaneous fat away from the anterior rectus fascia, as is done in the Küstner incision. It separates the perforating nerves and small blood vessels that enter the fascia from the underlying muscles and nourish the fascia, although possibly weakening the incision.

If the Pfannenstiel incision is extended laterally beyond the edge of the rectus muscles and into the substance of the external and internal oblique muscles, injury to the iliohypogastric or ilioinguinal nerves can occur, with resulting neuroma formation. In addition, closure of this extended fascial incision can entrap these nerves in either the closing suture or surrounding scar tissue. To avoid these nerve injuries in laterally extended incisions, including a Cherney or Maylard incision, the

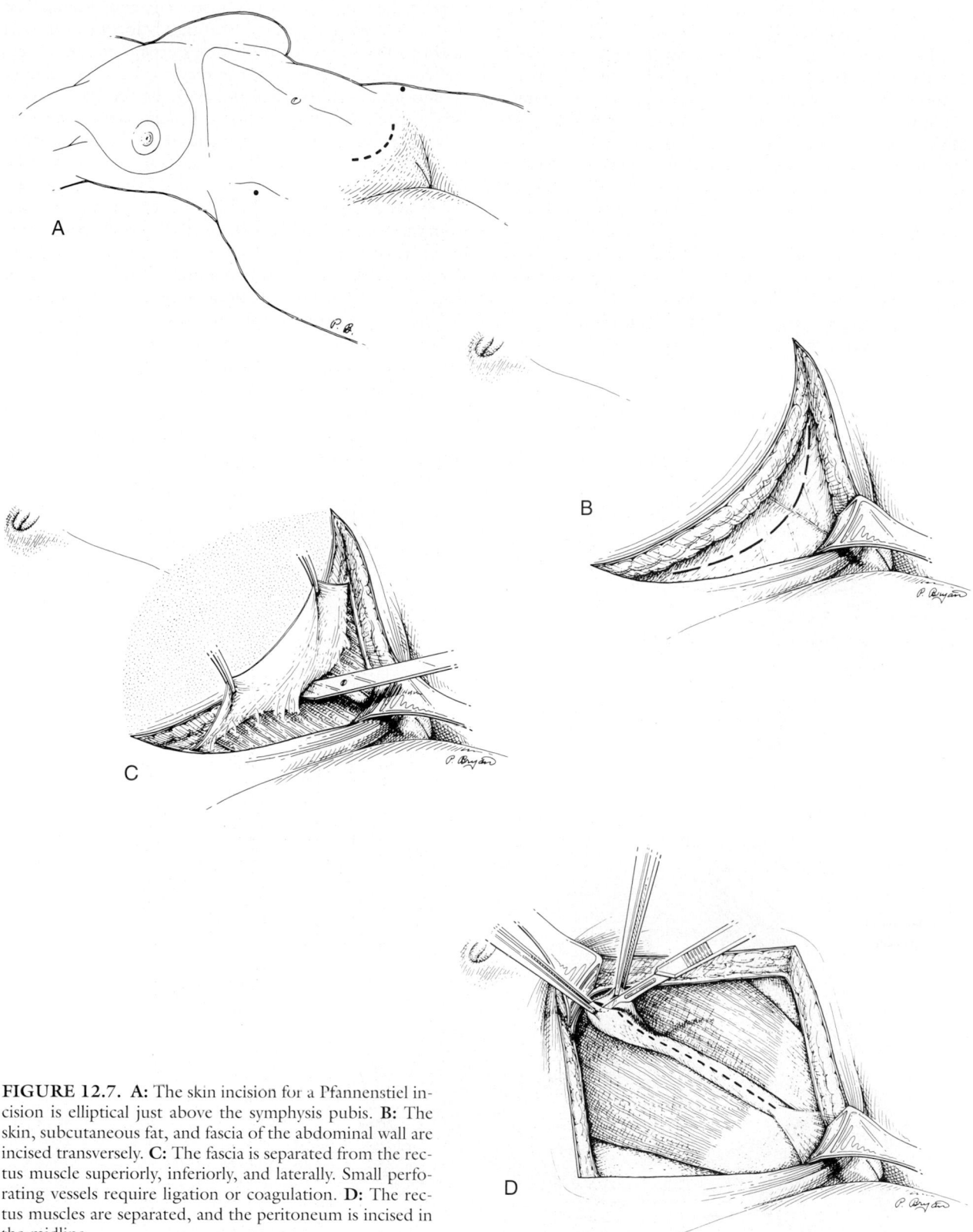

FIGURE 12.7. A: The skin incision for a Pfannenstiel incision is elliptical just above the symphysis pubis. **B:** The skin, subcutaneous fat, and fascia of the abdominal wall are incised transversely. **C:** The fascia is separated from the rectus muscle superiorly, inferiorly, and laterally. Small perforating vessels require ligation or coagulation. **D:** The rectus muscles are separated, and the peritoneum is incised in the midline.

lateral extensions should have sutures placed only in the external oblique fascia.

The incision may be wet and require subfascial drainage. The fascia can be closed with a running technique in patients with clean wounds or clean-contaminated wounds. Polyglycolic acid, polyglactin 910, or one of the delayed-absorbable sutures can be used. In assessing the use of running versus interrupted polyglycolic acid sutures in midline incisions, Fagniez and colleagues observed no difference in fascial dehiscence in a randomized prospective trial of 3,135 patients.

Subcutaneous sutures are usually unnecessary (unless they are being used as tension releasing sutures for the skin closure), and the skin is closed with a subcuticular suture (preferably monofilament), reinforced surgical tape (e.g. Steri-Strips), skin glue, or staples.

Küstner Incision

Some surgeons advocate a Küstner incision, incorrectly referred to as a modified Pfannenstiel incision. The slightly curved transverse skin incision begins below the level of the anterior superior iliac spine and extends just below the pubic hairline, through subcutaneous fat, down to the aponeurosis of the external oblique muscle and the anterior sheath of the recti in the same manner as all other transverse incisions (Fig. 12.8A). The superficial branches of the inferior epigastric artery and vein may be encountered in the subcutaneous fat at the lateral margin of the incision. When encountered, they can be ligated or sealed with Bovie cautery. The fascia is cleaned superiorly and inferiorly until a sufficient area is exposed from the region of the umbilicus to the symphysis to permit an adequate vertical incision in the linea alba. Excessive separation of the fat from the fascia in the lateral margins of the incision is unnecessary and can provide sites for small postoperative hematomas. Separation of the rectus muscles and entrance into the peritoneum are performed in the same manner in the ordinary midline incision (Fig. 12.8B). Because of the importance of obtaining adequate hemostasis in the subcutaneous fat of the skin flaps, this incision is definitely more time-consuming than the low midline incision or the Pfan-

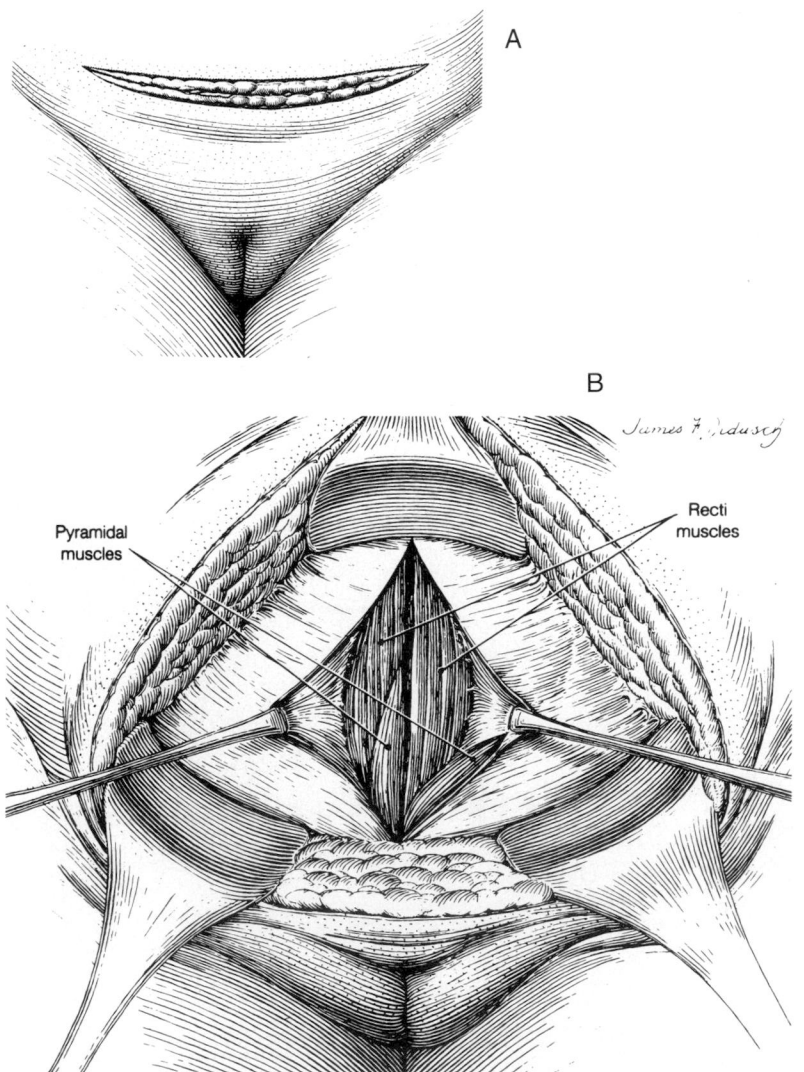

A

B

Pyramidal muscles

Recti muscles

FIGURE 12.8. Küstner incision. **A:** Skin incision just below hairline. **B:** Midline incision through fascia, exposing rectus and pyramidalis muscles. The rectus muscles are retracted laterally, and the peritoneum is incised in the midline.

Symphysis

Space of Retzius

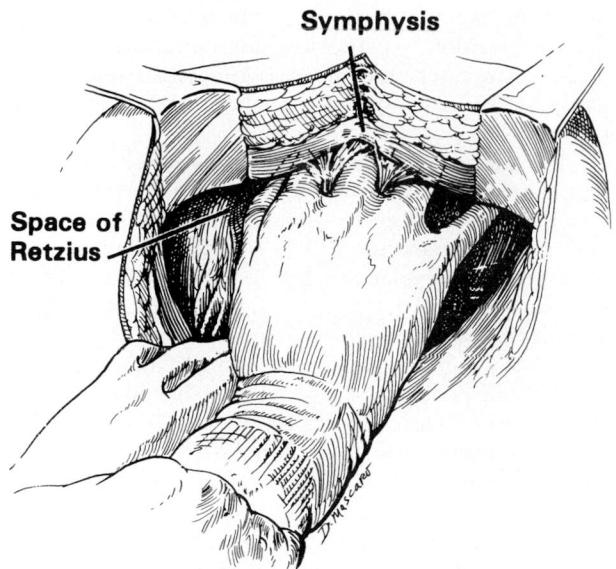

FIGURE 12.9. Developing the space of Retzius. The weight of the hand of the operator easily separates the bladder from the overlying symphysis in the relatively bloodless midline. (From Gallup DG. Opening and closing the abdomen. In: Phelan JP, Clark SL, eds. *Cesarean delivery*. New York: Chapman & Hall, 1988:449, with permission.)

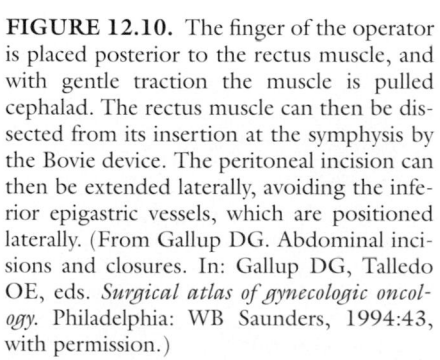

nenstiel incision. It offers little or no advantage, and its extensibility is severely limited. If this incision is used, strong consideration of subcutaneous, closed-suction drainage should be given.

Cherney Incision

The Cherney differs from the muscle-dividing Maylard incision by the location of transection of the recti. In both incisions, the skin and fascia are divided transversely

as with a Pfannenstiel, but Cherney advocated freeing the rectus muscles at their tendinous insertion into the symphysis pubis. The recti are then retracted cephalad to improve exposure. The transverse Cherney incision is about 25% longer than a midline incision, from the umbilicus to the symphysis.

The Cherney incision provides excellent access to the space of Retzius for urinary incontinence procedures. It provides excellent exposure of the pelvic side wall when needed, that is, in patients who require hypogastric artery ligation. Occasionally, the surgeon who uses a Pfannenstiel incision finds the incision inadequate for exposure for hemostasis or not large enough to expose areas of associated abnormal conditions. Under these circumstances, the safe approach is not to transect the rectus muscles halfway but to perform a Cherney incision. Partial incision of the rectus muscle can lead to injury to the inferior epigastric vessels. Also, if conversion to a Maylard is attempted after a previous Pfannenstiel, the anterior rectus sheath will have already been widely separated from the rectus muscles. The ends of the muscle are likely to retract and will not reunite when the edges of the aponeuroses are later reapproximated. In this situation, it may be necessary to reapproximate the rectus muscle ends with horizontal mattress sutures.

Even if the peritoneum is opened, the space of Retzius can be bluntly dissected (Fig. 12.9). The inferior epigastric vessels, which course more laterally in the caudad portion of the abdominal wall, are identified. The pyramidal muscles are sharply dissected. The fibrous tendinous rectus muscles are then dissected sharply from their insertion into the symphysis pubis (Fig. 12.10). Bleeding is negligible in this area, and the inferior epigastric vessels do not need to be ligated. The peritoneal incision can be extended laterally about 2 cm cephalad to the bladder while the vessels are visualized.

Deep inferior epigastric vessels

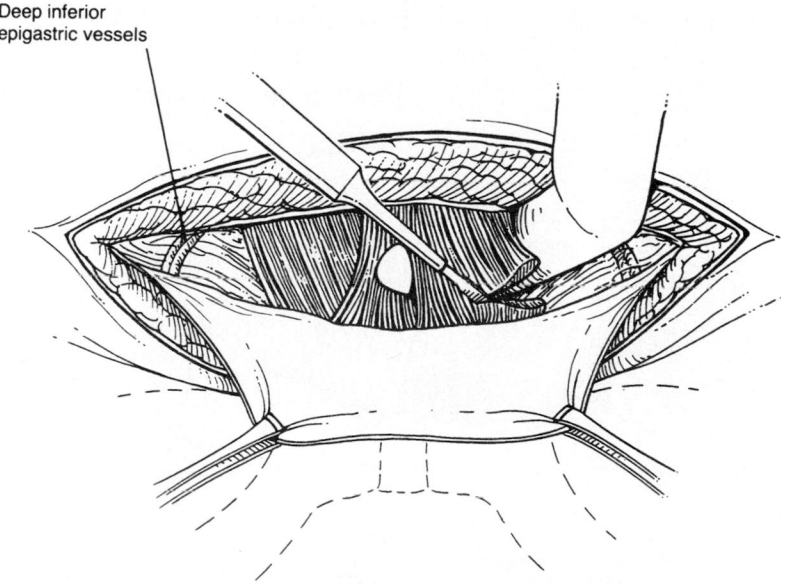

FIGURE 12.10. The finger of the operator is placed posterior to the rectus muscle, and with gentle traction the muscle is pulled cephalad. The rectus muscle can then be dissected from its insertion at the symphysis by the Bovie device. The peritoneal incision can then be extended laterally, avoiding the inferior epigastric vessels, which are positioned laterally. (From Gallup DG. Abdominal incisions and closures. In: Gallup DG, Talledo OE, eds. *Surgical atlas of gynecologic oncology*. Philadelphia: WB Saunders, 1994:43, with permission.)

As stated earlier, transverse incisions, particularly the Cherney and the later-described Maylard, can result in nerve injury. The femoral nerve is particularly at risk when a self-retaining retractor with deep lateral blades is used in these widely extended incisions. If a self-retaining retractor is used with either of these incisions, the lateral blades should be only deep enough to fit under the edges of the incision. They should not rest on the psoas muscle.

In closing a Cherney incision, we prefer to close the peritoneum separately with a running polyglycolic acid suture. Drainage of the subfascial space may be necessary. The ends of the rectus tendons are united to the inferior portion of the lower flap of the rectus sheath with five or six interrupted delayed-absorbable or permanent sutures, in horizontal mattress configuration (Fig. 12.11). To avoid osteomyelitis, the rectus muscles should not be sutured to the periosteum of the symphysis pubis. Fascial closure is then accomplished with a running continuous suture of delayed-absorbable suture, as in the Pfannenstiel. Although the lines of tension favor transverse incisions as opposed to vertical incisions, running sutures should be placed at least 1.5 cm from the fascial edge and 1.5 cm from one another. The remainder of the closure is similar to the Pfannenstiel closure, depending on the surgeon's preference.

Maylard Incision

The Maylard incision is a true transverse muscle-cutting incision in which all layers of the lower abdominal wall are incised transversely. This incision was originally described by Ernest Maylard in 1907. The incision provides excellent pelvic exposure and is used by many surgeons for radical pelvic surgery, including radical hysterectomy with pelvic lymph node dissection and pelvic exenteration. Although we prefer midline incisions for patients with suspicious adnexal masses, young patients with adnexal masses that are questionable for malignancy by radiographic and serological studies may be candidates for this cosmetic incision. Patients must be informed that if malignancy is found, the transverse incision will take the form of a "hockey stick" (i.e., a J-shaped incision; see Incisions for Extraperitoneal Approaches), or a separate upper-abdominal incision will be used to evaluate the upper-abdominal cavity and retroperitoneal paraaortic nodes.

The Maylard-Bardenheuer incision has been modified in several aspects since its original description. Before the skin incision is made, a series of three to four perpendicular markings with a sterile marking pen are made across the planned line of the incision. These markings help in later approximation of the skin edges. The transverse skin incision is made about 3 to 8 cm above the symphysis, depending on the indications for surgery and patient age and weight. The skin incision should never be made in a deep skin crease or beneath a large panniculus. The fascia is incised transversely, and the aponeurosis is *not* detached from the underlying muscle.

After a transverse fascial incision, lateral to the borders of the rectus muscles, the inferior epigastric vessels, lying on the posterior lateral border of each muscle, are identified. (Some surgeons suggest preservation of these vessels even when the rectus muscles are transected.) The vessels are teased away from their attachments by using a gentle finger dissection. The vessels are ligated *before* incising the rectus muscles, to avoid tearing of the vessels, vessel retraction, and hematoma formation (Fig. 12.12). The fingers of the surgeon tease the overlying rectus muscle from the peritoneum, and the muscles are sectioned between the fingers by using a Bovie cautery.

For better approximation of the muscles during closure, we prefer to suture the underlying muscle to the overlying fascia before entering the peritoneum. A 2-0 delayed-absorbable "U" suture is used, and the knots are placed anterior to the fascia. The peritoneum is incised transversely.

Closure of the fascia is similar to the running technique for other transverse incisions. The muscles do not need to be reapproximated with individual sutures (exception noted above), although some surgeons prefer to close the parietal peritoneum with a running polyglycolic

Deep Epigastric Vessels

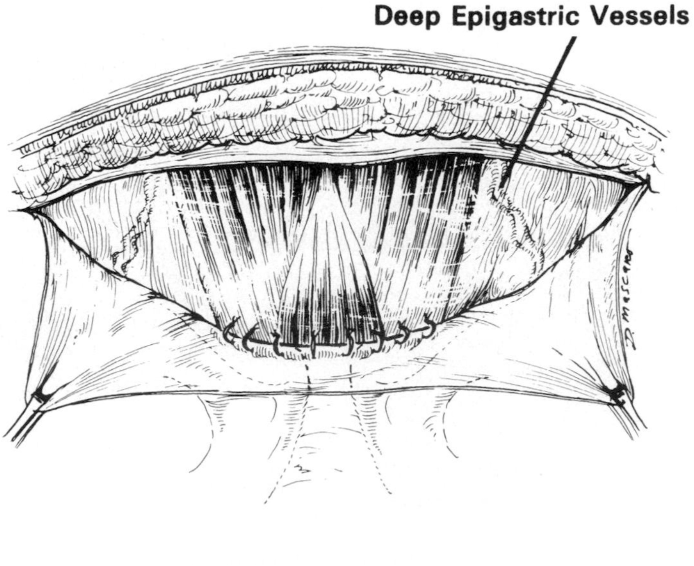

FIGURE 12.11. Reuniting of the rectus tendons to the inferior portion of the lower flaps. The deep inferior epigastric vessels are positioned laterally in the caudad portion of the abdomen. (From Gallup DG. Opening and closing the abdomen. In: Phelan JP, Clark SL, eds. *Cesarean delivery.* New York: Chapman & Hall, 1988:449, with permission.)

Deep Epigastric Vessels

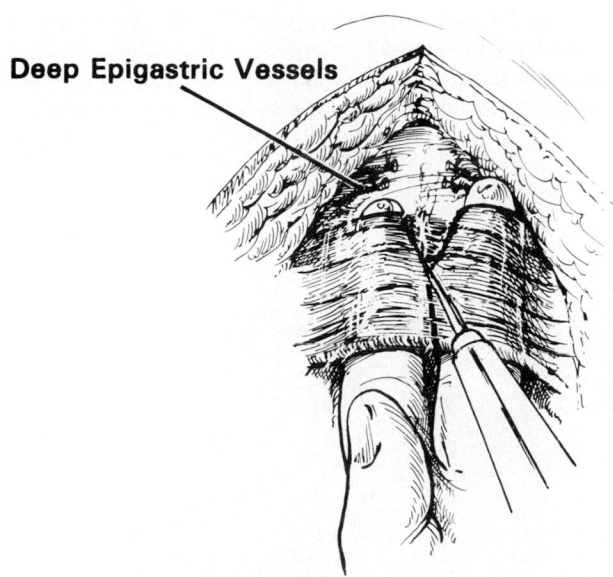

FIGURE 12.12. Maylard incision. The rectus muscles are incised with a knife or a Bovie device. The hand of the surgeon is withdrawn as the muscle is cut. The inferior epigastric vessels were previously isolated, sectioned, and ligated. (From Gallup DG. Opening and closing the abdomen. In: Phelan JP, Clark SL, eds. *Cesarean delivery.* New York: Chapman & Hall, 1988:449, with permission.)

suture. A subfascial drain is indicated if hemostasis is not absolute (Fig. 12.13).

Caution should be exercised in using the Maylard incision in patients with impaired circulation to the leg secondary to obstruction of the common iliac arteries or terminal aorta. In this situation, blood flow from the inferior epigastric artery may provide the only additional collateral circulation to the lower extremity. Ligation of this artery could result in lower-extremity ischemia and a real vascular surgical emergency. In the gynecologic patient with clinical evidence of impaired circulation in the lower extremity, a midline incision should be used.

Vertical Incisions

Generally, vertical incisions afford excellent exposure. They can be easily extended and provide rapid entry to the abdominal cavity. Whether midline or paramedian, the resulting scar may be wide. Thus, they are not cosmetic incisions and leave the skin portion of the incision for the patient to see.

Midline (Median) Incision

As stated in the section on anatomy, the midline incision is the least hemorrhagic incision, as well as the incision that affords rapid entry into the abdominal/pelvic cavity. Exposure is excellent, and minimal nerve damage occurs. However, dehiscence and hernias are said to be more common, particularly in the area inferior to the arcuate line. Abdominal wound disruption is one of the most serious postoperative problems associated with gynecologic surgery. The "burst abdomen," or evisceration, seen more frequently in general surgery patients, occurs with a frequency of 0.3% to 0.7% in gynecologic patients and is associated with a mortality of 10% to 35%. The type of incision is only one factor associated with evisceration, and wound infection is present in over half the cases. Use of chromic catgut for fascial closure is associated with a higher incidence of dehiscence compared with that for any other class of suture. Mechanical factors—such as wound hematomas, paroxysmal coughing associated with chronic lung disease, and gastrointestinal problems (retching, vomiting, ileus)—can lead to evisceration. Newer closure techniques have been shown to have lower wound infection, dehiscence, and hernia rates and are discussed later in the chapter.

The midline incision is the most easily mastered gynecologic incision because the fascial area is relatively bloodless and the rectus muscles are usually separated in parous women. If the patient has a prior midline incision, the surgeon should incise the peritoneum more cephalad to the earlier incision in order to avoid injury to possibly adherent bowel. In patients undergoing radical pelvic surgery or surgery for deep-seated, adherent pelvic masses, we prefer

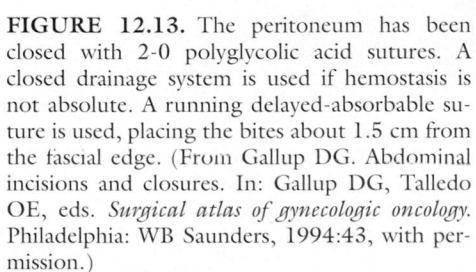

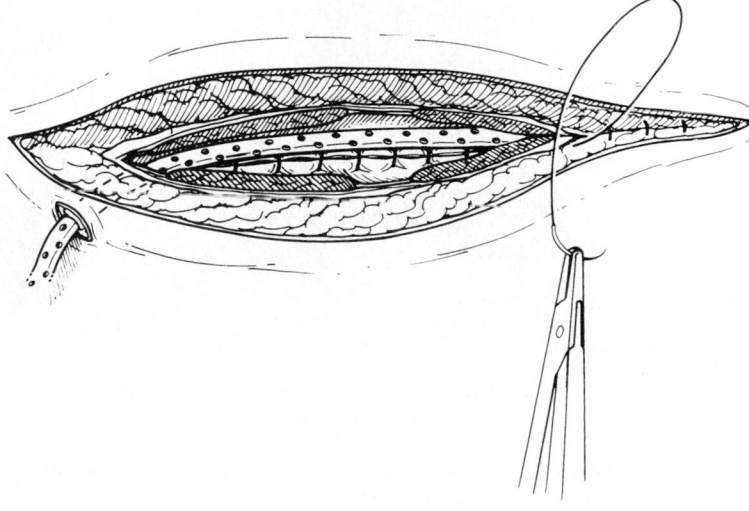

FIGURE 12.13. The peritoneum has been closed with 2-0 polyglycolic acid sutures. A closed drainage system is used if hemostasis is not absolute. A running delayed-absorbable suture is used, placing the bites about 1.5 cm from the fascial edge. (From Gallup DG. Abdominal incisions and closures. In: Gallup DG, Talledo OE, eds. *Surgical atlas of gynecologic oncology.* Philadelphia: WB Saunders, 1994:43, with permission.)

to develop the space of Retzius to allow extension of the incision between the pyramidal muscles, providing better exposure in the deep pelvis. In nulliparous women, the midline separation between the rectus muscles may not be obvious. In such cases, the pyramidalis muscles are useful landmarks in directing the surgeon to the midline. Because this incision can easily be extended, the midline incision is the most versatile of all incisions used by gynecologists.

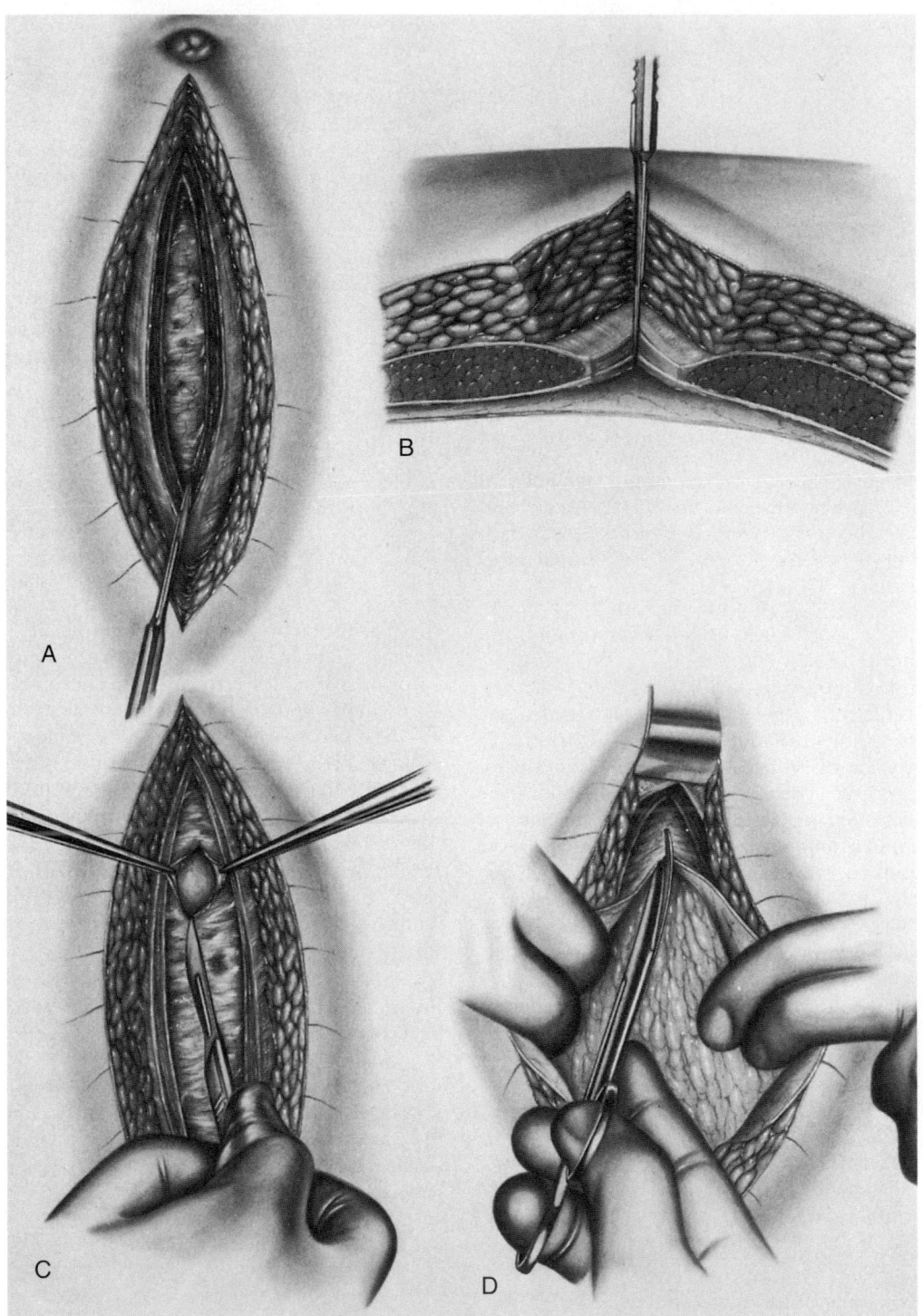

FIGURE 12.14. A: Cutting of linea alba in low midline incision with scalpel. **B:** Cross section of abdominal wall showing skin, subcutaneous fat, anterior and posterior rectus sheaths, and underlying peritoneum. **C:** Opening of peritoneum with knife, and demonstration of small bowel protruding into peritoneal opening. **D:** Enlargement of peritoneal opening to the region of the umbilicus with Mayo scissors.

Hemostasis from incision of more anterior layers should always be complete before the peritoneum is entered (usually done with the scalpel) (Fig. 12.14). Once the abdomen is explored (in a repetitive systematic fashion), the bowel must be carefully packed out of the pelvis. Seldom are more than two or three moist laparotomy packs needed to accomplish exposure of the pelvis. If more packs are required or there is a struggle to pack the upper abdominal contents cephalad, anesthesia may be inadequate. The more packs used, the more likely the small-bowel terminal nerve endings will be damaged, resulting in postoperative adynamic ileus. Use of more modern table-fixed retractors, such as the Bookwalter retractors, not only improves exposure in vertical and transverse incisions but also limits the use of excessive packs.

Paramedian Incision

Paramedian incisions have been advocated over midline incisions because of alleged greater strength. In a prospective study, Guillou and coworkers found no significant difference in respiratory complications, wound infection, and dehiscence when comparing midline, medial paramedian, and lateral paramedian incisions. None of the patients with lateral paramedian incisions developed an incisional hernia. The incidence of hernia in midline and medial paramedian incisions was the same. In a randomized prospective study, however, Cox and colleagues found 22 incisional hernias in patients with midline incisions, compared with two hernias in the patients who had paramedian incisions. Like the midline or median incision, the paramedian incision has excellent extensibility and exposure, particularly on the side of the pelvis where the incision is made. For example, a left paramedian incision can be useful when operating for disease that involves the sigmoid colon and/or the left pelvic sidewall.

Although advantageous in some situations, paramedian incisions have many potential problems, including increased infection rates, increased intraoperative bleeding, increased operating time, and the possibility of nerve damage with resultant atrophy to the rectus muscle. Long paramedian incisions can increase pain with respiration during the immediate postoperative period. If a paramedian incision is placed parallel to a previous midline incision, or vice versa, the blood supply between the two incisions can be inadequate, resulting in tissue slough, delayed healing, and/or incisional herniae formation.

Closure of Vertical Incisions

Although closure of transverse incisions (discussed previously) raises little controversy because of the inherent relative strength of the incision, the closure of vertical incisions is controversial. Three general comments about closure can be made:

1. Paramedian incisions, because of their location, may require layered closure. However, we tend to use a mass running closure with a looped delayed-absorbable suture. No data exist to guide closure technique in these incisions.
2. With the advent of modern suture materials and knowledge about suturing techniques, retention sutures are almost never needed, except in some cases of evisceration.
3. With midline incisions, rectus muscles should not be sutured together unless there is sufficient diastasis to cause symptoms.

In closing midline incisions, some surgeons prefer a layered closure (Fig. 12.15). However, two metaanalyses (Weiland et al. and Hodgson et al.) have shown that mass closures are superior to layered closures with respect to postoperative incisional herniae, wound dehiscence, suture sinuses, infection, and wound pain. If a layered closure is used, sutures should always be loosely tied because the major cause of wound evisceration is too many sutures placed too closely together, placed too close to the fascial edge, and tied too tightly (remember, "approximate; not strangulate"). Often, at reoperation for evisceration, the sutures and knots are intact, but the

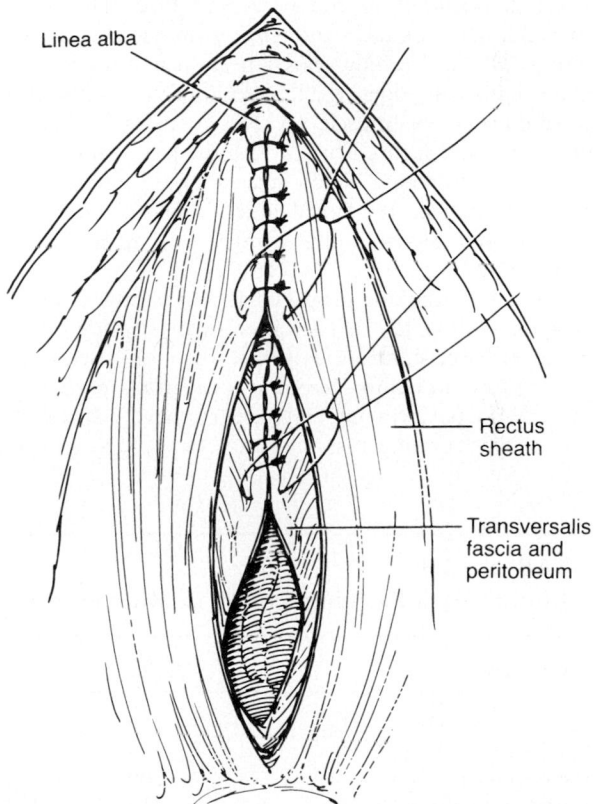

FIGURE 12.15. Layered closure of a midline incision. The peritoneum can be closed with a continuous 2-0 absorbable suture. The posterior and anterior fasciae can be closed with interrupted No. 0 delayed-absorbable suture. Figure-of-eight sutures also work for fascial closure. (From Gallup DG. Opening and closing the abdomen and wound healing. In: Gershenson D, Curry S, DeCherney A, eds. *Operative gynecology.* Philadelphia: WB Saunders, 1993:127, with permission.)

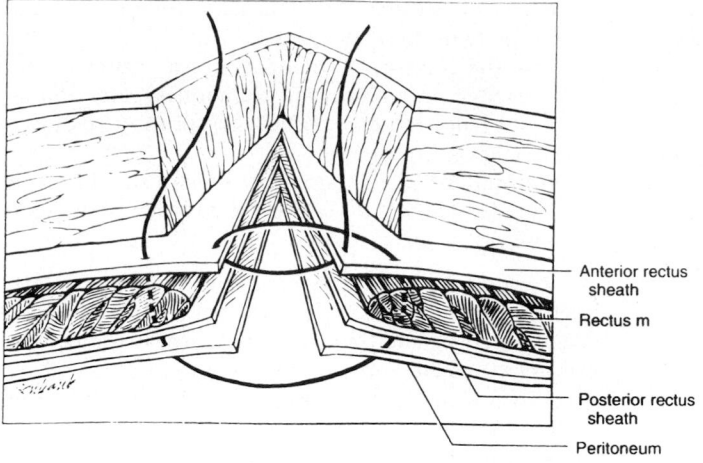

Anterior rectus sheath

Rectus m

Posterior rectus sheath

Peritoneum

FIGURE 12.16. Smead-Jones layered closure. This is a far–far, near–near suturing technique, with the anterior fascia being included in the near–near bite. A No. 1 nylon or No. 1 polypropylene suture (or some other delayed-absorbable suture) is used, with the key to the success of this closure being widely spaced far–far bites. (at least 1.5 to 2 cm from the fascial edges). This closure technique may be performed in an interrupted fashion or as running suture. (From Morrow CP, Curtin JP. Incisions and wound healing. In: *Gynecologic cancer surgery.* Churchill Livingstone, 1996:152, with permission.)

suture has simply torn through the fascia. To avoid wound disruptions in high-risk patients, several investigators have advocated a Smead-Jones closure technique (Fig. 12.16). This is a far–far, near–near mass closure technique. The first (far–far) bite includes both the fascia and peritoneum on each side, and only the anterior fascia is included in the near–near bite. The widely spaced initial pass takes the tension off the healing incision, and the carefully placed near–near bites approximate the fascial edges to allow good healing without intervening fat or muscle. A No. 1 nylon or No. 1 polypropylene suture is used, with the key to the success of this closure being widely spaced far–far bites (at least 1.5 to 2 cm from the fascial edges). The main disadvantage to the Smead-Jones closure is that it is time-consuming.

In 1976, Jenkins proposed that bursting of an abdominal wound can be prevented by using wide bites of nonabsorbable continuous suture through fascia, muscle, and peritoneum. Some investigators, particularly those who perform general surgery, have advocated a single-layer running mass-closure technique as an expedient, yet safe, technique for closing the abdomen. A study performed by Gallup and colleagues reported the use of this technique in high-risk patients in 1989, demonstrating no fascial dehiscence in 210 patients. However, one patient in their series later developed an incisional hernia.

Several studies using running mass closure of the abdomen have been published and are listed in Table 12.3. These studies show a fascial dehiscence rate of 0.4% with this closure technique. The patient with the fascial dehiscence reported by Sutton and Morgan eviscerated after the closure suture was transected by a Kevorkian curette during wound debridement. In a randomized prospective study, Stone and colleagues found no difference in dehiscence rates between interrupted and mass closures.

Gallup and colleagues closed the midline incisions in their study with a continuous No. 2 polypropylene suture, placing the bites 1.5 to 2 cm from the fascial edge and including all anterior abdominal wall layers (the peritoneum, if easily located, the fascial layers, and the intervening muscle) (Fig. 12.17). One suture should be

TABLE 12.3.
Closure With Running Sutures in Midline Incisions

Investigators	Patients	Material	Patients With Fascial Dehiscence
Archie and Feldman 1981	120	MFPP (No. 1)	1
Murray and Blaisdell 1978	255	PGA (No. 1)	1
Shepherd et al. 1983	200	MFPP (No. 2)	0
Knight and Griffen 1983	419	MFPP (No. 1)	4
Gallup et al. 1989	210	MFPP (No. 2)	0
Montz et al. 1991[a]	231	MFPG (0)	0
Sutton and Morgan 1992[b]	154	MFPB (0)	1
TOTALS	1589		(0.4%)

MFPP, monofilament polypropylene; PGA, polyglycolic acid; MFPG, monofilament polyglyconate; MFPB, monofilament polybuster.

[a]Looped suture with running Smead-Jones technique.

[b]Looped suture.

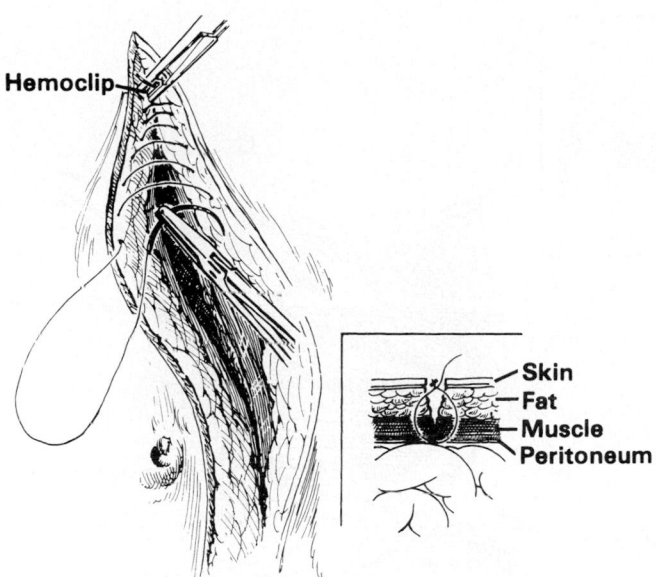

Skin
Fat
Muscle
Peritoneum

FIGURE 12.17. Closure of a midline incision using a No. 2 polypropylene, running mass closure. The anterior fascia, muscle, posterior fascia, and peritoneum are included in the bites **(inset),** which are taken 1.5 to 2 cm from the fascial edge and about 1 cm apart. With permanent polypropylene suture, a hemoclip can be used on the short end to avoid suture unraveling. (From Gallup DG. Opening and closing the abdomen. In: Phelan JP, Clark SL, eds. *Cesarean delivery.* New York: Chapman & Hall, 1988:449, with permission.)

started from each end of the incision, tying the ends in the middle and securing the suture with three square knots (six throws). In the original series, a small hemoclip was placed above each knot to prevent unraveling. Several caveats must be kept in mind with this closure technique: (a) a double-strand suture should never be tied to a single strand, and (b) the sutures should not be pulled too tightly, as this distributes tension unequally over the incision and negates the major advantage of this closure. Not all investigators include the peritoneum in the closure, but they still report excellent results. As shown by Ellis and Heddle in 1977, closure of the peritoneum as a separate layer appears to play no significant role in wound healing when midline incisions are used.

One problem with the use of large-bore, permanent suture for mass closure is occasional, late-occurring wound sinus formation. However, with the development of monofilament (delayed) absorbable sutures (Maxon and PDS), the risk of wound sinus formation is significantly reduced. Again, Gallup and colleagues changed their running closure technique, to avoid this problem of sinus formation, by using No. 1 Maxon suture. This suture was selected because of its relatively easier handling and knot security. The closure technique (running mass closure) was similar to the closure with polypropylene suture; however, seven throws were used for each knot and each knot was buried. Most of the 285 patients with midline incisions closed with the No. 1 Maxon were at high risk for wound disruption. Of

these, seven developed superficial wound infections, one developed a ventral hernia, and one had an evisceration on postoperative day 4. At reexploration of this last patient, the central knot of the intact suture had untied, and later questioning of the surgeons revealed that only four throws had been used per knot. Montz and colleagues also reported no eviscerations or hernias in their series. Most of the recent running mass closure articles, however, have no long-term follow-up to assess later hernia formation.

Oblique Incisions

Oblique incisions can be used for a transperitoneal or an extraperitoneal approach.

Gridiron (Muscle-Splitting) Incision of McBurney

The McBurney incision is an excellent choice for an uncomplicated appendectomy and can be used for the extraperitoneal drainage of an abscess from pelvic inflammatory disease. In pelvic inflammatory disease, when drainage becomes necessary for an indolent broad ligament abscess that does not respond to antibiotics and does not point into the cul-de-sac for drainage, drainage through a gridiron incision is most effective. The incision is constructed as for an appendectomy, except that it is made a little lower, and the peritoneal cavity is not entered. Similarly, if drainage of the pelvis is required during a pelvic laparotomy, the drain should not exit through the midline incision, but rather through a small gridiron (stab-wound) incision in the lower abdomen. In treating a large tuboovarian abscess that extends out of the pelvis and does not respond to antibiotic therapy, extraperitoneal drainage through a McBurney incision is also possible by approaching the abscess laterally. This permits entrance into the site of infection without soiling the peritoneal cavity.

The gridiron incision is made obliquely downward and inward over the McBurney point (Fig. 12.18A). The location can be varied when the incision is performed for appendectomy during pregnancy or when it is used for abscess drainage, as mentioned above. The incision in the skin can be made at a lower level to preserve the cosmetic appearance of the abdominal wall. The incision is carried through the skin and subcutaneous fat to the external oblique muscle. The fibers of the muscle are separated in the direction in which they run (Fig. 12.18B). The internal oblique and the transverse abdominis are separated in the line of their fibers (Fig. 12.18C). At this point, the internal oblique and the transversus abdominis course in the same direction and are closely fused. Retractors are avoided, if possible. Instead, the peritoneum should be gently reflected away from the abdominal wall inferiorly and the abscess entered beneath the round ligament for extraperitoneal drainage. Thickened indurated tissue may make this step difficult. If the parietal peritoneum is adherent to the peritoneal surface of the abscess, drainage still may be possible without transversing free space in the peritoneal cavity. The surgeon should

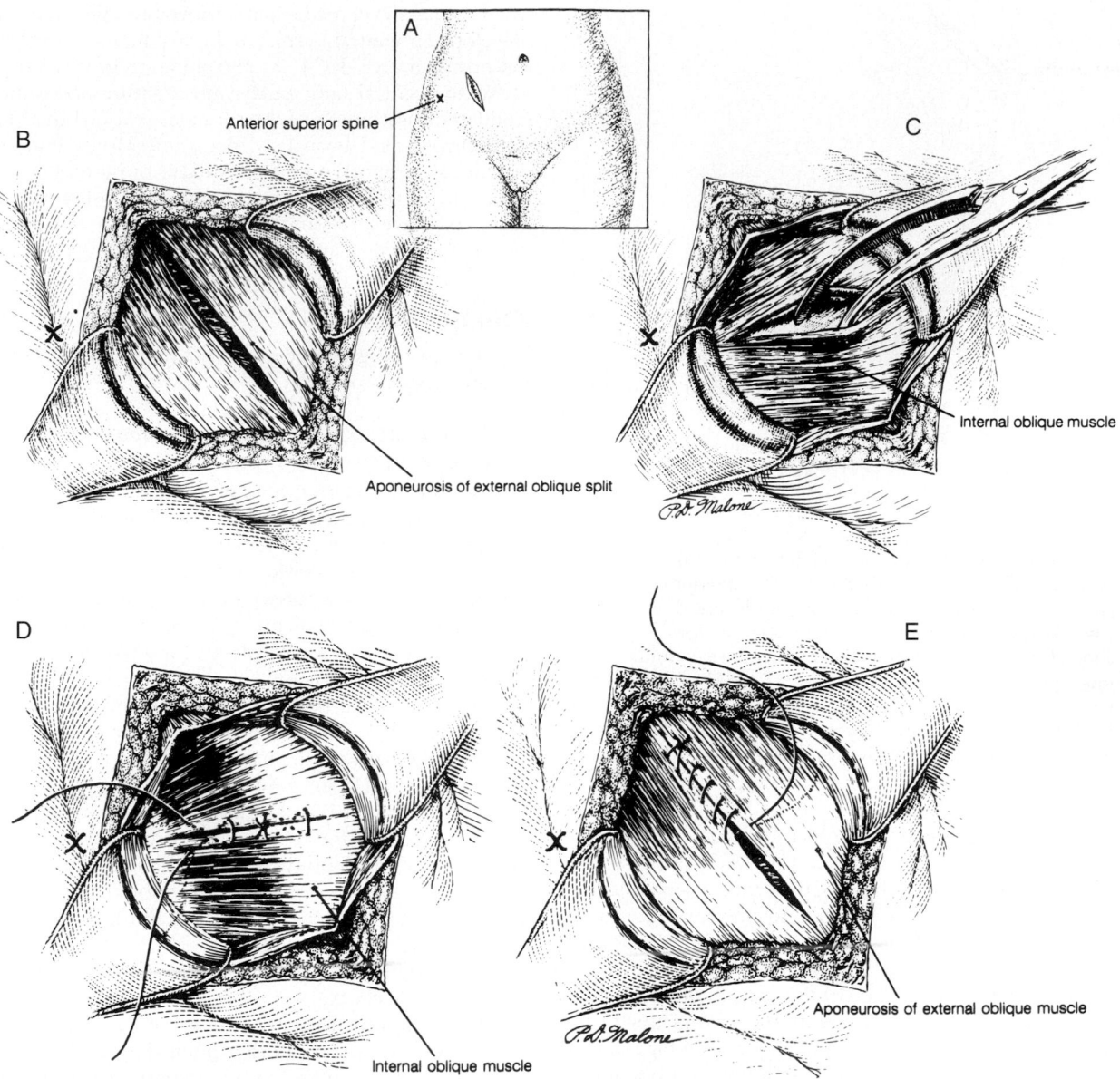

FIGURE 12.18. Gridiron incision. **A:** Position of incision. **B:** Fibers of external oblique have been split. **C:** Internal oblique muscle being split with a Kelly clamp. **D:** In closing, internal oblique fibers are approximated with figure-of-eight No. 0 delayed-absorbable sutures. **E:** Aponeurosis of external oblique is closed with continuous or interrupted No. 0 delayed-absorbable sutures.

avoid contaminating the peritoneal cavity with pus, if possible.

The gridiron incision can be used in the left lower quadrant to drain an abscess on the left side of the pelvis as well as to perform sigmoid colostomy. Closure is depicted in Fig. 12.18D,E and is best made with a delayed-absorbable suture.

Rockey-Davis Incision

An alternative to the McBurney incision is the Rockey-Davis (or Elliot) incision. It is a transverse incision placed at the junction of the middle and lower thirds of a line extending from the anterosuperior iliac spine to the um-

bilicus. Medially, the incision extends to the border of the rectus muscle. The aponeurosis of the external oblique muscle is split in the line of its fibers. The internal oblique and transversus muscle fibers can be separated by blunt finger dissection. The peritoneum is incised transversely. This incision has provided satisfactory exposure to pathology in either lower-abdominal quadrant. A similar incision made lower on the abdomen preserves the cosmetic appearance of the abdominal wall.

Incisions for Obese Patients

Obesity, especially when the condition is morbid (>130% of ideal body weight or body mass index of greater than 30 kg/m²), presents problems with incision placement and closure. Obesity is a recognized high-risk factor for wound infections and complications. Pitkin observed a 4% wound complication rate in nonobese women undergoing abdominal hysterectomy compared with a 29% rate in obese patients. Krebs and Helmkamp reported a wound infection rate of 24% in massively obese patients when a periumbilical transverse incision was used. Because muscle cutting may be needed for this transverse incision, entry time can be lengthy and the resulting incision relatively bloody. If any transverse incision is chosen for obese patients, it should be far removed from the anaerobic moist environment of the subpannicular fold.

In 1977, Morrow and colleagues suggested modifications of preoperative care, intraoperative techniques, and postoperative care in obese gynecologic patients and observed only a 13% wound infection rate. Gallup and colleagues subsequently modified Morrow's techniques. They operated on a group of 97 mostly high-risk obese patients and then compared them with obese patients not operated on by the modified protocol. The wound infection rate in obese patients not operated on by protocol was 42% compared with a 3% rate in protocol-operated obese patients.

Gallup's original protocol, which we still use for obese patients on our service, has only been modified by fascial closure techniques. All patients have careful cleansing of the umbilicus and undergo preoperative showering. Minidose subcutaneous heparin, 5,000 to 8,000 U, is administered 2 hours before surgery and every 12 hours after surgery, continuing until the patient is fully ambulatory. In addition, sequential compression devices (SCDs) are used in these high risk patients. Prophylactic antibiotics are routinely given, and clip preparation of abdominal hair (rather than shaving) is used. The midline incision is made by first retracting the pan-

niculus caudad, below the inferior margins of the symphysis, to avoid an incision in the anaerobic subpannicular fold (Fig. 12.19). The skin incision is a periumbilical incision because it is usually extended around the umbilicus. The fascial incision is always extended to the symphysis.

Once the uterus and other organs are removed, the pelvic peritoneum is not reapproximated. However, the vaginal cuff is closed. Fascia may be closed with a Smead-Jones or running mass closure (our preference). Subcutaneous sutures are not used, but a Jackson-Pratt or Blake drain is placed anterior to the fascia, after irrigating the tissues with normal saline. This drain is removed in 72 hours, or when the output is less than 50 mL per 24 hours. The skin is closed with staples, which are left in place for 2 weeks. Although controversial, a nasogastric tube may be inserted during surgery and left in place for 24 hours to avoid abdominal distention. Gallup's relatively low wound infection rate in obese patients supports this type of operative management.

Panniculectomy and Abdominoplasty

An alternate surgical approach in the massively obese patient is to remove the large panniculus *before* the intended pelvic surgery. As observed by Kelly in 1910, wound complications can be avoided and cosmesis can be achieved by this procedure. Exposure to the pelvic organs is certainly improved. In 1978, Pratt and Irons reported on 126 panniculectomies, and 85 of these were performed to facilitate exposure to the surgical field. The average hospital stay was only 14 days, but 34.5% of the patients had some degree of morbidity. In the series by Voss and colleagues, five of 76 (6.6%) patients undergoing panniculectomy and hysterectomy developed pulmonary embolism. In another series, investigators encountered excessive blood loss and acknowledged the need for transfusion in combined surgery. More recently,

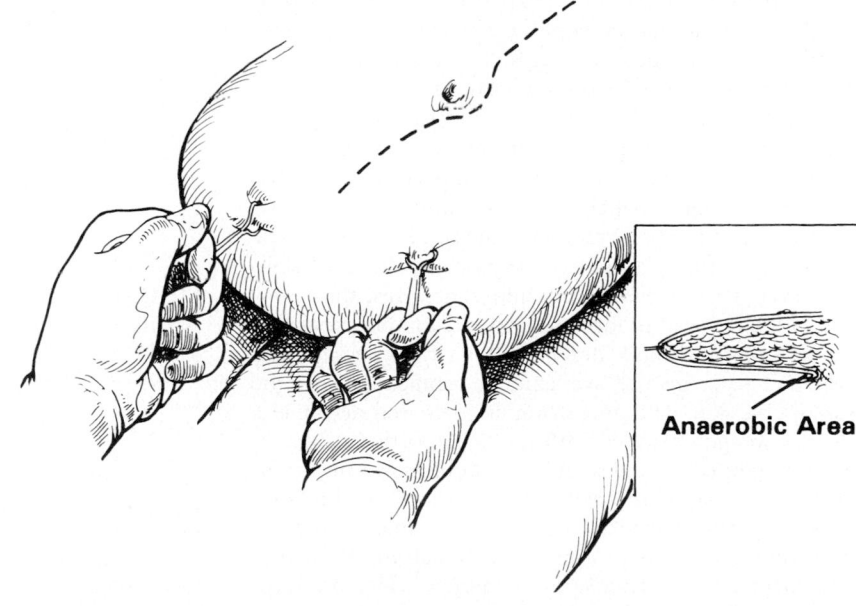

FIGURE 12.19. Midline incision in an obese patient. The panniculus is retracted inferiorly and the incision avoids the moist anaerobic environment *(inset)* beneath the subpannicular fold. (From Gallup DG. Opening and closing the abdomen. In: Phelan JP, Clark SL, eds. *Cesarean delivery.* New York: Chapman & Hall, 1988:449, with permission.)

Anaerobic Area

several series have noted the relative safety of combining abdominoplasty with other surgical procedures. Hopkins and colleagues performed a retrospective review of patients who underwent panniculectomy at the time of gynecological surgery. They identified 78 patients (average weight, 278 lb) on whom the procedure was performed. Their infection rate was a laudable 2.6%, with an equally impressive average blood loss of 71 mL. Four of the patients had minimal incisional separations.

As more sophisticated monitoring, better antibiotics, better suture material and techniques, and a safer blood supply have become more available, selective use of combined gynecologic procedures and plastic surgical removal of the panniculus is increasing. In a study of patients who had a mean weight of 261 lb, Morrow et al. found no operative mortality and a mean hospital stay of 8.2 days. Only 11% of the patients required transfusion. The investigators in this series emphasized that the panniculectomy should be performed initially to improve exposure.

Although removal of a large panniculus results in better exposure, patient selection for this potentially morbid procedure should be carefully considered. Also, the patient must be counseled and must be strongly motivated to lose weight and change her nutritional habits. If the patient is not committed to these life-style changes, it seems impractical to perform an extensive abdominoplastic procedure and incur the associated morbidity. If the surgical procedure is not urgent, an alternative would be to defer the procedure until the patient has achieved 40% to 50% of the planned weight loss.

Patients who have large diastasis recti in association with the panniculus are also candidates for this procedure, at which time plication of the rectus fascia should be performed, either directly or using a "vest-over-pants" layered technique. In many instances, the rectus abdominoplasty is as much a cosmetic and therapeutic benefit to the patient as is the panniculectomy. When both anatomic conditions coexist, the panniculectomy alone does not give a satisfactory surgical result.

Of the various operative techniques available for panniculectomy and abdominoplasty, the elliptical transverse incision, originally described by Kelly, has proved to be the procedure of choice. Two modifications of the transverse panniculectomy can be useful. The most common procedure includes an elliptical "watermelon" incision (Fig. 12.20A), extending from the lateral aspect of the lumbar regions to about 3 to 4 cm above the umbilicus. If the patient requests the preservation of the umbilicus, it can be excised and transplanted to the upper pedicle of skin. However, as shown by Cosin and colleagues, this transplantation can lead to increased wound complications. Inferiorly, the transverse incision follows the concave skinfold that separates the overhanging panniculus from the suprapubic skin. The underlying fat is excised deeply in a slightly wedged manner, with the deep portion of the fat extending outward and slightly beyond the skin margin to avoid ischemia of the skin edge. Meticulous attention must be given to absolute hemostasis (a time-consuming procedure) to avoid postoperative hematoma formation and infection. The *excessive* use of cautery, which produces

a favorable environment for bacterial growth in devitalized tissue, should be avoided. The lateral angles of the incision may require separate "V" incisions to avoid the unsightly folds of redundant fat (Fig. 12.20B). When these V-shaped wedges are closed, the angle of the incision is converted into a Y-shaped configuration, which eliminates the excessive skin in the lateral aspects of the abdominal wall. After the removal of the large panniculus, the abdomen can be opened either transversely or vertically. A vertical incision has been advocated to improve exposure. If an abdominoplasty is required to approximate widely separated rectus muscles, a midline incision is necessary. In this way, a tight closure of the rectus fascia or a vest-over-pants repair, as shown in Fig. 12.20D,E, gives additional

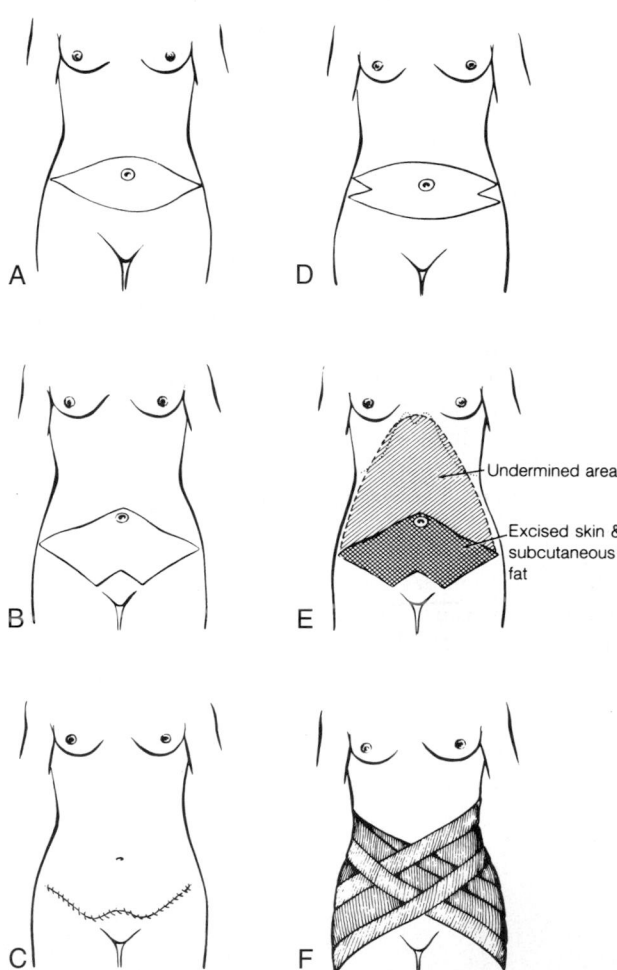

FIGURE 12.20. Panniculectomy incisions. **A:** Elliptical transverse incision extending from region of iliac crest passes above and below umbilicus. **B:** V-shaped incision in lateral angles eliminates folds of skin in abdominal wall. **C:** W-shaped incision over the mons pubis extends along the inguinal ligament to the iliac crest. **D:** The upper incision passes above the umbilicus. Wide mobilization of the upper skin flap is carried to the sternum and rib margins. **E:** After removal of panniculus and skin, the upper skin flap is sutured without tension to the lower skin margin. **F:** A firm elastic dressing is criss-crossed over the abdominal wall for abdominal support and prevention of seroma formation.

strength to the abdominal wall. If the rectus fascia is of poor quality and does not provide adequate support to the abdominal wall, a mesh graft can be inserted at the completion of the procedure, either anterior or posterior to the rectus muscle (discussed below). If the fascia of the rectus sheath can be plicated in the midline, wide plication and anchoring of the medial margins of the rectus muscle can be used to close the diastasis, resulting in a firm abdominal wall.

A second type of transverse panniculectomy is a "W" technique, initially described by Regnault in 1975 and shown in Fig. 12.20C. The incision is outlined before the operative procedure in the form of a "W" over the symphysis pubis, inside the hairline. The incision is started in the center of the mons pubis and extended laterally and downward on each side to the inguinal fold near the external inguinal ring. The line then follows above the inguinal ligament in the panniculus skin crease to the region of the iliac crest on each side of the pelvis. The upper margin of the incision is drawn above the umbilicus to the upper margin of the redundant fat. If the umbilicus is to be relocated, the new umbilical site is drawn in the upper skin flap before the incision is made and the umbilicus is transposed to the upper skin flap after the incision is closed.

In closing the W-shaped incision of Regnault after the abdominal or pelvic operation is completed, the upper flap of the abdominal skin is mobilized superficial to the fascia as far as necessary to the region of the xiphoid process and to the inferior margin of the costochondral junctions of the rib cage (Fig. 12.20D). A thin layer of fat is left attached to the fascia to facilitate the postoperative absorption of serous fluid. As shown in Fig. 12.20E, the upper skin flap is sutured to the W-shaped pubic skin margins, using interrupted sutures of 2-0 delayed-absorbable suture for the subcutaneous fat. Multiple fine sutures are used to anchor the skin flap to the fascia to prevent seroma formation and loculation. Closed-suction drainage is always used beneath the upper skin flap and left in place until the drainage is less than 50 mL per day. If the upper skin flap cannot reach the pubic skin without excessive tension, the patient is placed in a slightly jackknife position on the operating table by having the upper portion of the table elevated and the legs maintained in a straight horizontal position. When the skin margins have been approximated over the pubis and along the inguinal ligament, additional V-shaped incisions can be taken from the lateral angles of the incision when redundant skin is present.

The skin is closed with staples or 3-0 polypropylene interrupted sutures, which are left in place for at least 2 weeks. Rather than being removed all at once, alternate staples can be removed over a period of several days and replaced with adhesive reinforced surgical tape (e.g., Steri-Strips). A firm elastic-based tape dressing (e.g., Elastoplast) tape dressing is applied under tension over the abdominal wall in a criss-cross manner, beginning at the rib cage and extending to the thighs (Fig. 12.20F). This abdominal support relieves tension on the suture line and also prevents seroma and hematoma formation

beneath the skin flaps. Another technique is to use an abdominal binder (or multiple binders, placed end to end) to support the anterior abdominal wall and prevent seroma and hematoma formation.

INCISIONS FOR EXTRAPERITONEAL APPROACHES

Although controversial as a routine surgical procedure, the value of a staging laparotomy to assess paraaortic lymph nodes in patients with advanced stage (IIB to IV) cervical cancer has been studied extensively over the past two decades. As the stage of disease increases, the incidence of positive paraaortic nodes is progressively higher and has prompted organizations such as the Gynecologic Oncology Group to require paraaortic node sampling before placing patients with advanced cervical cancer on some phase III studies. Serious bowel complications have been observed in cervical cancer patients who have had operative evaluation through a transperitoneal approach followed by radiotherapy. When extraperitoneal approaches to evaluate paraaortic lymph nodes are compared with transperitoneal approaches before radiation therapy, more serious, later-occurring small bowel problems are associated with the latter approach (Wharton et al. 1977). To avoid these complications, an extraperitoneal approach has been advocated by means of bilateral superior groin incisions, a unilateral J-shaped incision, or an upper-abdominal incision.

We use the J-shaped incision or the "sunrise" incision for staging. If bulky pelvic nodes are evident or paraaortic nodes contain metastases, these can be removed without entering the peritoneum and may improve patient response to therapy (Downey et al. 1989). Irradiation with concurrent chemotherapy can then be safely used, starting almost immediately.

J-Shaped Incision

A modification of the extraperitoneal inguinal incision (a modified Gibson incision) was described in the gynecologic literature by Berman and colleagues in 1977. These investigators prefer to make the skin incision on the left, because the left paraaortic lymphatic channels are lateral and posterior to the aorta. They believe that it is technically more feasible to dissect the precaval nodes from a left-sided incision if a single incision is to be used for extraperitoneal paraaortic node sampling. We prefer to make the incision on the right, as discussed later.

Access is gained by a vertical incision, starting just cephalad to the umbilicus and 3 cm medial to the right iliac crest. Caudad to the crest, the incision is carried medially, about 3 cm cephalad and parallel to the inguinal ligament (Fig. 12.21). The fascial layers are incised separately (Fig. 12.22). Exposure of the extraperitoneal space is achieved by rolling the peritoneum medially and cephalad (Fig. 12.23). The round ligament and inferior epigastric vessels can be ligated and transected to improve exposure. The paraaortic area is exposed by blunt dissection, and

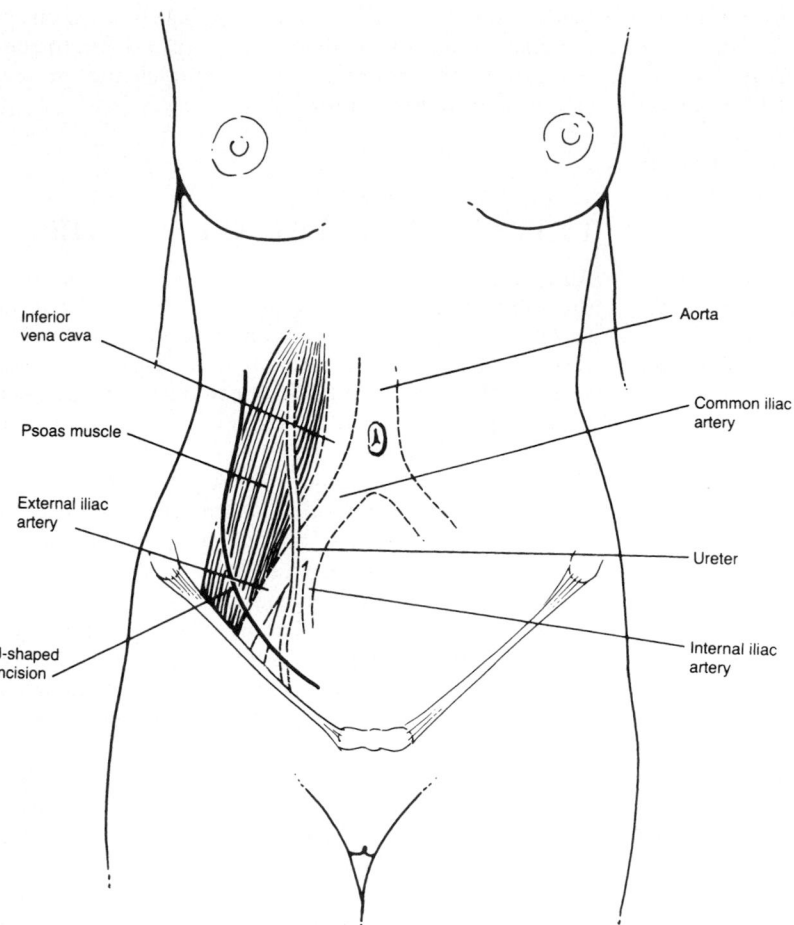

FIGURE 12.21. J-shaped incision on the right is shown in relation to deeper structures, the ureter, iliac vessels, and great vessels. It is initiated about 3 cm cephalad to the umbilicus and is carried inferiorly parallel to the round ligament. (From Gallup DG. Abdominal incisions and closures. In: Gallup DG, Talledo OE, eds. *Surgical atlas of gynecologic oncology.* Philadelphia: WB Saunders, 1994:43, with permission.)

node sampling is performed by removing the precaval fat pad over the vena cava. With a Deaver retractor on the medial and cephalad portion of the incision, paraaortic nodes can be sampled to the level of the inferior mesenteric artery, directly anterior and lateral to the aorta.

In the left-sided approach, left paraaortic node dissection is more easily accomplished. Berman and colleagues described lifting the peritoneum from the underlying vena cava to resect the precaval fat pad. They cautioned that gentle traction must be used when dissecting the precaval nodes to avoid injury to the inferior mesenteric vessels and also suggested that the table should be tilted toward the patient's right to facilitate dissection.

The inferior vena cava lies relatively posterior to the aorta, and we have experienced technical difficulties in removing precaval nodes through a left-sided approach. In a later updated report from the same institution, Ballon and associates observed that two of 95 patients had avulsion of the inferior mesenteric artery (repaired without sequelae). In addition to the relative difficulty in sampling right-sided nodes, the lower portion of a J-shaped incision lies in future radiation fields in some patients.

Sunrise Incision

Because there is a delay in initiation of irradiation by some radiation oncologists when a midline incision is used for staging, Gallup and colleagues have subsequently used a supraumbilical incision to remove paraaortic nodes extraperitoneally. In this small reported series, the mean number of paraaortic nodes removed was 12.2, and the mean operating time was 111 minutes. All but two of 20 patients underwent external-beam irradiation within 2 weeks of the operative procedure (Fig. 12.24).

The sunrise skin incision is initiated in a transverse manner about 4 to 6 cm cephalad to the umbilicus (Fig. 12.25). It is carried laterally in a downward fashion to the level of the iliac crests. Preoperatively, the site of the supraumbilical incision can be estimated and varied by placing a radioopaque object at the level of the umbilicus during intravenous contrast computed tomography (CT) to estimate the level of the bifurcation of the aorta. In thin patients, a unilateral incision, usually performed on the right side, can be used, and adequate exposure to both sides of the aorta can be obtained. In the event of bulky disease in the lower common iliac or pelvic nodes, the incision can be extended in a caudad fashion to remove these nodes. The advantage of pelvic node debulking in cervical cancer patients, who were later irradiated, has been reported by Downey and associates.

Once the skin and subcutaneous tissue are incised, the fascia is also incised transversely. After the rectus muscles are dissected free from their attachments to the anterior fascia, they are transected with a Bovie device. In relatively

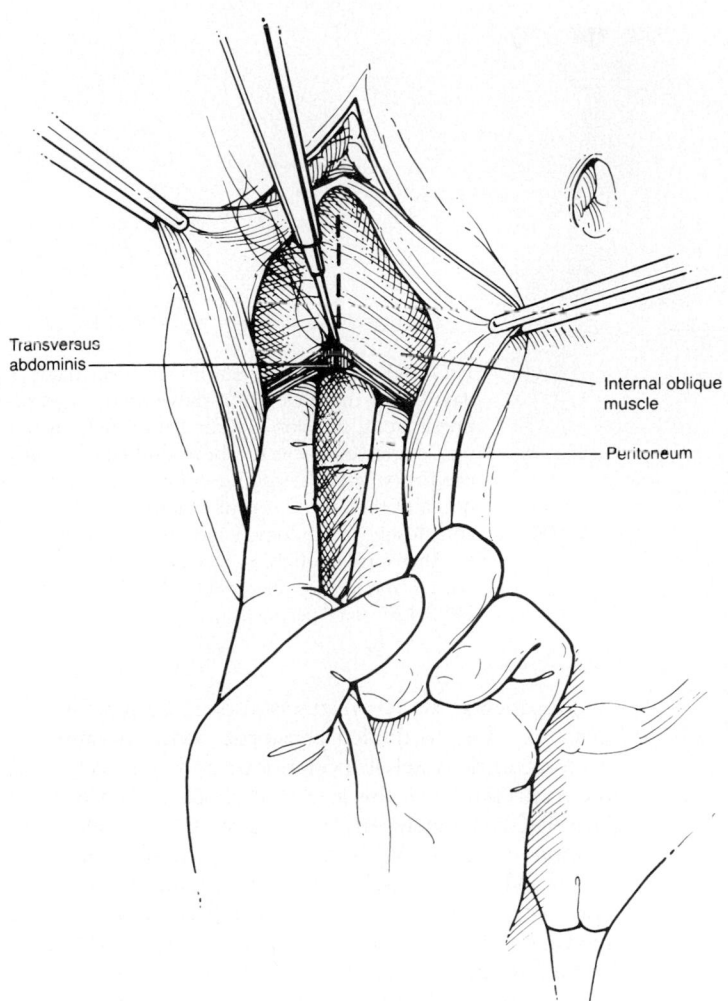

Transversus abdominis

Internal oblique muscle

Peritoneum

FIGURE 12.22. The previously incised external oblique fascia is shown retracted with small clamps. The internal oblique muscle and transversus abdominis are then sectioned. The fingers of the operator push the peritoneum medial and posterior while these two muscles are sharply incised. The Bovie device is used to transect these muscles, with the fingers of the operator protecting the underlying peritoneum. (From Gallup DG. Abdominal incisions and closures. In: Gallup DG, Talledo OE, eds. *Surgical atlas of gynecologic oncology.* Philadelphia: WB Saunders, 1994:43, with permission.)

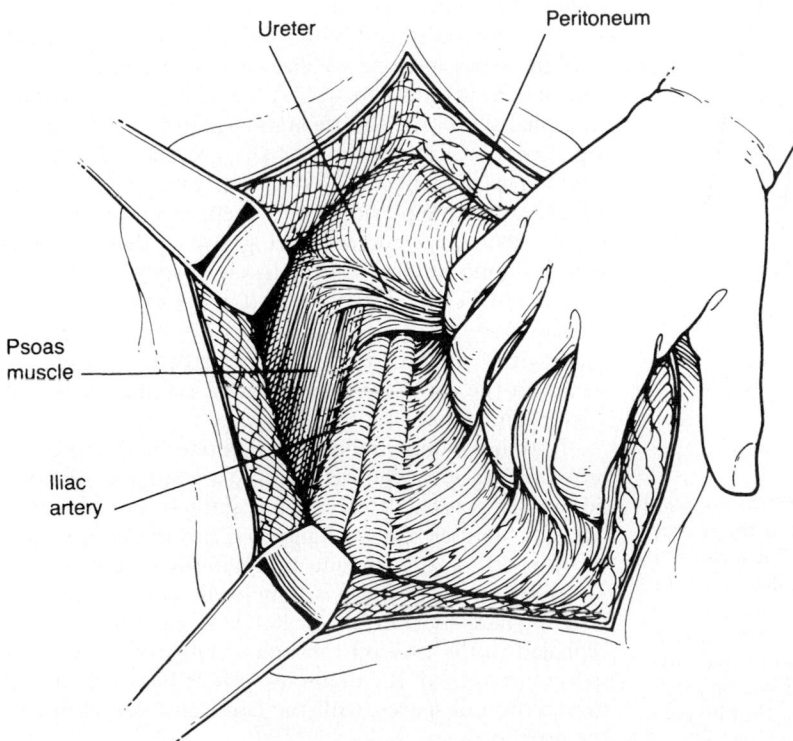

Ureter

Peritoneum

Psoas muscle

Iliac artery

FIGURE 12.23. With the round ligament sectioned, the peritoneum is bluntly dissected by the hand of the operator. The psoas muscle is palpated, as is the external iliac artery lying medial to the psoas. The peritoneum is gently swept from lateral and caudad to medial and cephalad. This maneuver easily exposes the psoas muscle and the pelvic vessels. The ureter remains on the medial left of the retracted peritoneum. (From Gallup DG. Abdominal incisions and closures. In: Gallup DG, Talledo OE, eds. *Surgical atlas of gynecologic oncology.* Philadelphia: WB Saunders, 1994:43, with permission.)

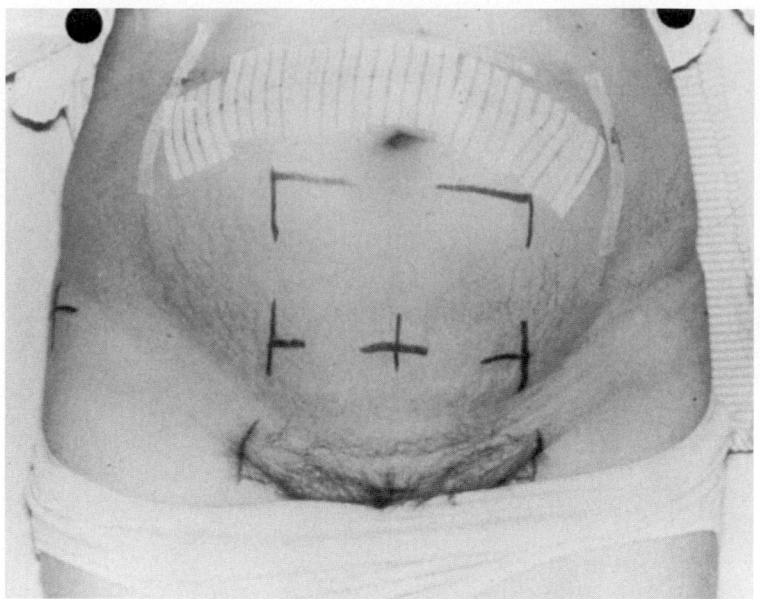

FIGURE 12.24. The sunrise incision made 3 days before this illustration shows Steri-Strips approximating the skin. The radiation field in this postoperative patient has been outlined for early irradiation after a staging procedure for carcinoma of the cervix. (From Gallup DG. Opening and closing the abdomen and wound healing. In: Gershenson D, Curry S, DeCherney A, eds. *Operative gynecology.* Philadelphia: WB Saunders, 1993:127, with permission.)

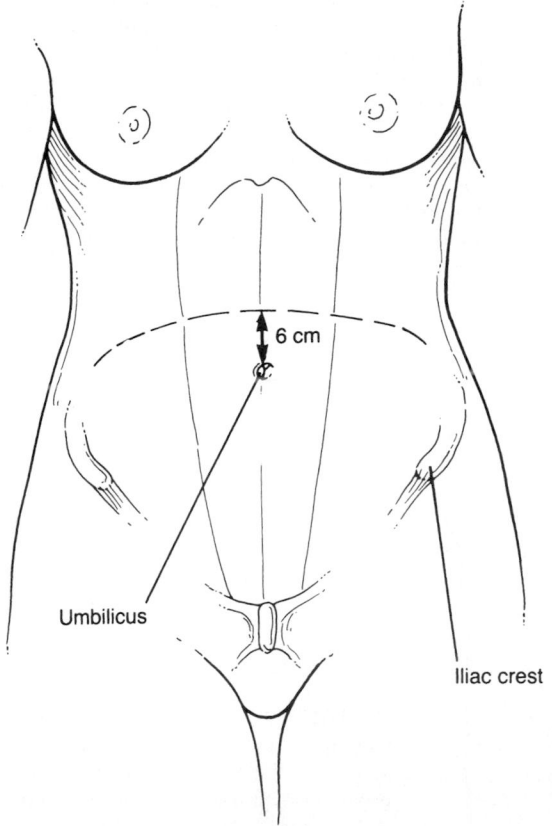

FIGURE 12.25. For an extraperitoneal approach to paraaortic nodes, we prefer to use the sunrise incision. In the center, this incision is about 6 cm above the umbilicus. The incision is carried laterally and downward to the level of the iliac crests. In the event of palpable bulky disease in the lower common iliac or pelvic nodes, the incision can be extended caudad to remove the nodes. (From Gallup DG. Abdominal incisions and closures. In: Gallup DG, Talledo OE, eds. *Surgical atlas of gynecologic oncology.* Philadelphia: WB Saunders, 1994:43, with permission.)

obese patients, the left rectus is also transected for adequate exposure to the left paraaortic nodes. Because the deep epigastric vessels lie posterior to, and in the center of, the rectus muscle at this level, the vessels do not need to be isolated separately. Any bleeding can be controlled with ligation or cautery. With the rectus transected, the transversus abdominis muscle is located on the right and is incised with scissors or cautery. The peritoneum is retracted medially and cephalad by the hand of the surgeon. The incision into the transversus is extended more inferiorly and laterally to complete the transection of this muscle without entering the peritoneum. The fingers of the surgeon stretch the wound to ensure adequate exposure.

The surgeon's hand is inserted deep into the incision until the psoas and external iliac vessels are palpated. The peritoneum is bluntly dissected from caudad and lateral to cephalad and medial, separating it from the underlying common iliac vessels until the great vessels are exposed. This maneuver is similar to that illustrated in Fig. 12.23, except the peritoneum is swept more cephalad. If the peritoneum is entered during any of these maneuvers, it should be closed immediately. A self-retaining retractor can be inserted to retract the right ureter and ovarian vessels to avoid injury. The precaval nodes, located within the fat pad over the vena cava, are then resected in the usual manner by using vascular clips and scissors and a "clip-cut" technique.

In thin patients, the paraaortic nodes lateral and anterior to the aorta can be removed through a right abdominal approach. If exposure is limited, however, the left rectus muscle can be transected and the peritoneum mobilized from the left side as previously described.

When node dissection is completed, a closed drainage system (Jackson-Pratt or Blake) may be brought out cephalad to the incision through a stab wound. If both spaces are opened, the drains are placed bilaterally in the extraperitoneal spaces, with the fascia and skin closed in the usual manner.

DELAYED PRIMARY CLOSURE AND SECONDARY CLOSURE

The value of delayed primary wound closure in managing possible contaminated wounds has been recognized by military surgeons for many years. In 1968, Grosfeld and Solit reported that patients with perforating appendicitis had a reduction in wound infection rates from 34.1% to 2.3% when delayed closure was used. Similarly, in a high-risk group of patients—which included patients with obesity, cancer, possible contamination from above-and-below procedures, infection, and bowel content contamination—Brown and colleagues found a marked reduction in wound infection rates when delayed primary closure was used compared with immediate closure in matched patients. The infection rate for the former group was 2.1%; for the latter, 23.3%. Possible candidates for such a closure include patients with suppurative appendicitis, ruptured tuboovarian abscess, extensive bowel injury in the unprepared bowel, or diverticulitis with contamination. Delayed closure can also be of value in select patients who have groin incisions associated with radical vulvectomy procedures.

After closure of the fascia, the wound is irrigated with copious amounts of saline. Some investigators prefer to then spray the wound with a combined broad-spectrum antibiotic spray. Vertical interrupted mattress sutures of No. 3 nylon or No. 3 monofilament polypropylene are placed 2 to 3 cm apart. They are loosely tied over dilute povidone-iodine dressing gauze. The wound dressing sponges are changed two to three times a day with a wet-to-dry technique, using sterile saline. Some surgeons use bridges, consisting of rolled gauze on the lateral borders of the incision, to support these sutures. In 4 to 5 days, depending on the appearance of granulation tissue in the subcutaneous tissues, the previously placed sutures are tied to approximate the skin edges. Tincture of benzoin is placed at the lateral edges of the closed incision, and Steri-Strips are used to approximate uneven skin edges.

Alternatively, the skin edges of the incision can be closed with widely spaced staples, "wicking" the intervening spaces with saline soaked gauze (e.g., Nu-gauze or Kerlex strips). Once adequate granulation tissue is present, the skin edges can be reapproximated with nonabsorbable monofilament sutures and local lidocaine at the patient's bedside before discharge from the hospital.

Superficial separation of layers anterior to the fascia is usually associated with wound infections or hematomas. Many centers suggest opening the wound, usually the entire length; obtaining appropriate cultures for antibiotic choice; and allowing healing by second intention. Although most cleansing in a second-intention scenario is accomplished by home health care personnel, patients are inconvenienced by this method. A trend in many centers and practices has been to perform delayed closure after a period of 2 to 5 days. In 1988, in a prospective randomized study, Hermann and associates found that secondary closure, performed 2 days after wound drainage had ceased, resulted in a significant reduction in healing time when compared with healing by second intention.

In a larger series of patients on an obstetrics and gynecology service, Walters and colleagues found a similar advantage in delayed closure of wounds. In 35 patients who underwent reclosure, 85.7% had their wounds successfully closed. Patients in this study had abdominal incisions that had been opened owing to infection, hematoma, or seroma. The fascia was intact in all patients, and all patients had wound debridement and cleansing for a minimum period of 4 days. All patients in this series had reclosure performed in the operating room and received three doses of cefazolin. The closure was done by an en bloc technique, using No. 2 monofilament nylon sutures. In a series from the University of Mississippi (Dodson et al.), patients with extrafascial wound dehiscence were randomized to en bloc closure with No. 1 polypropylene versus a superficial closure through the skin using No. 2 polypropylene vertical mattress sutures. There was no statistical difference in the number of days needed to complete wound healing. However, the en bloc group required longer time for closure, and these patients experienced more pain. Of note, none of these patients received prophylactic antibiotics, and all wounds were reclosed under local anesthesia in the patient care area 2 to 6 days after reopening the wound.

Our technique for reclosing wounds is similar to that reported by Dodson and associates. After reopening the wound in patients with extrafascial dehiscence, the subcutaneous tissues are debrided daily, and wet-to-dry dressings using sterile saline are placed in the wound two to three times daily. Antibiotics are generally not used unless the patient has a concomitant infection (e.g., cellulitis or cuff infection). The wound is closed when a healing bed of granulation tissue without exudate or necrotic debris is present. Many wounds require sharp debridement, but most can still be closed within 5 days of reopening.

Wounds are closed in the treatment room on the ward or in the office with local 1% lidocaine anesthesia after premedication with 50 mg of intramuscular meperidine hydrochloride or similar narcotic. The skin is then prepped with a povidone-iodine solution, and the sutures are placed 1 cm from the skin edges and 2 cm apart. The suture of choice is a No. 0 polypropylene suture or a similar permanent or delayed absorbable suture. We leave the sutures in for 2 weeks.

COMPLETE WOUND DEHISCENCE AND EVISCERATION

Technically, wound dehiscence means separation of all layers of the abdominal incision, but wound dehiscence has been subdivided based on the layers of tissue that have separated. Incomplete or partial dehiscence (superficial dehiscence) means separation of the skin and all tissue layers posterior to the skin, sometimes including the fascia. However, if the disruption includes the peritoneum, the disruption is called a complete dehiscence. Should the intestine protrude through the wound, the term *evisceration* (also a *burst abdomen*) is used. The frequency of fascial dehiscence range between 0.3% and 3% of all cases of pelvic surgery.

Evisceration is one of the most feared and dangerous postoperative complications. The mortality rate associated with evisceration has been to be reported as high as 35%, and is usually associated with other complications, such as sepsis. However, Helmkamp's 10-year study noted a mortality rate of only 2.9% in 70 cases, which may reflect improved supportive care available for these patients in recent years. Evisceration is less likely to occur in gynecology patients than in general surgery patients.

Older studies reported that the type and location of the incision and the type of suture used were major causative factors in evisceration. However, many of the predisposing factors for complete wound disruption or evisceration are metabolic and include malnutrition, poorly controlled diabetes, corticosteroid use, and older age. Mechanical factors associated with dehiscence and evisceration include obesity, intraabdominal distention (including rapid postoperative reaccumulation of ascites), infection, retching, and coughing. In addition, any process that can impair wound healing, such as radiotherapy or chemotherapy, can contribute to an increased risk for wound disruption. As noted, complete wound dehiscence and evisceration are usually problems associated with tissue failure and not suture failure. Rollins and associates noted that about half of their patients with serious wound complications had prior abdominal or pelvic surgery. In the series reported by Jurkiewicz and Morales, 88% of eviscerated wounds had tearing of suture through the fascia, with knots and suture intact. Thus, large loose sutures with secure knots are always preferable to tight strangulating sutures that cause ischemia of the incision margin.

Eviscerations usually occur from day 5 to 14 after operation, with a mean of about 8 days. One of the early signs of complete dehiscence and impending evisceration is the seepage of serosanguineous pink discharge from an apparently intact wound. It can be present for several days before evisceration occurs. Although occult hematomas are usually the cause of such discharge, these wounds need to be examined carefully by probing with a cotton-tipped swab to assess the integrity of the fascial closure. Frequently, the patient is conscious of something giving way, "tearing" or "popping" immediately before the burst abdomen becomes clinically apparent.

With few exceptions, complete dehiscence or eviscerations should be closed as soon as they are recognized. In case of evisceration, when a delay of several hours is anticipated because of a recent meal, the bowel can be replaced by using sterile gloves, gently packing it in place with lap pads soaked in povidone-iodine, and securing it with an abdominal binder. Broad-spectrum antibiotics should be initiated, and baseline blood counts and serum electrolyte studies should be obtained.

Closing an evisceration should be performed in the operating room (never on the floor) and always under general anesthesia so that the extent of the dehiscence may be determined. Necrotic tissue, clots, and suture material should be removed, and aerobic and anaerobic cultures should be obtained. The bowel and omentum should be inspected and thoroughly cleansed with several liters of warm normal saline. If the fascial margins can be located and are not ragged, a Smead-Jones closure (Fig. 12.16) with large-bore polypropylene or nylon can be used. The subcutaneous tissue and skin are packed open for later delayed closure.

If the wound edges are ragged or the patient's condition is poor, a through-and-through retention suture of No. 2 nylon or polypropylene is used. The sutures are placed at least 2.5 to 3 cm from the skin edges and are passed through all layers. To allow for edema, they are placed 2 cm apart (Fig. 12.26). To prevent inclusion of the underlying intestine in a suture, all sutures are held up before the first one is tied. Skin edges unopposed between the through-and-through sutures can be approximated with interrupted 3-0 polypropylene. The through-and-through sutures should be left in place for 3 weeks. A nasogastric tube should be used in the immediate postoperative period to avoid abdominal distention, and broad-spectrum antibiotics should be continued and modified according to culture results.

INCISIONAL HERNIA

Incomplete healing of an operative wound will result in an incisional hernia. In this situation, the peritoneum remains intact, and the fascial margins and adjacent muscles separate, leaving a defect beneath the subcutaneous tissue, into which the bowel may herniate.

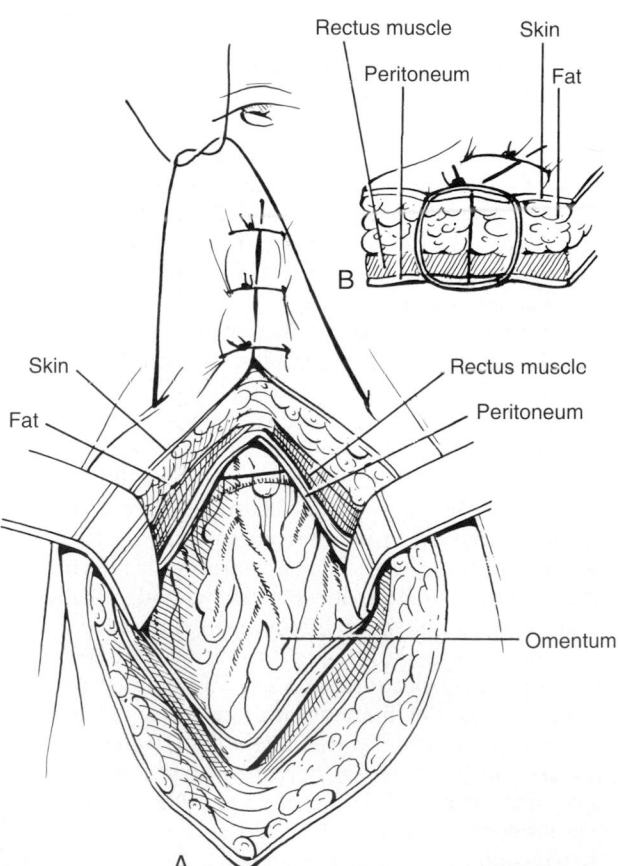

FIGURE 12.26. A: Secondary closure of an evisceration with through-and-through silver wire and preferably No. 2 polypropylene sutures. **B:** All layers are incorporated.

Causes of herniation are similar to those of evisceration; however, the skin, subcutaneous tissue, and peritoneum remain intact. Most cases of ventral hernia follow an incisional infection, weakening the supporting tissues. Increased intraabdominal pressure from coughing and vomiting, along with necrosis of the fascial margins, permits the sutures to pull through the edge of the fascia. These changes result in separation of the wound edges and failure of fibroblastic bridging of the fascia. This complication occurs more frequently in lower-abdominal incisions because of the anatomic deficit of the posterior fascial sheath beneath the rectus in the area inferior to the semicircular line. Ventral hernias occur after low midline incisions in about 0.5% to 1% of all gynecologic operations, with the incidence rising to about 10% after a wound infection. Similarly, reclosure after dehiscence increases the chance of hernia formation to about 25%.

Although the initial fascial defect may be small, the size of the resultant hernia can assume varying proportions and involve the entire length of the lower-abdominal wall. The size of the hernia depends on the mobility of the bowel and omentum and the final aperture size in the ventral defect. A large amount of small bowel and omentum can escape from a small fascial defect into an easily expandable subcutaneous space. The smaller the fascial defect through which small bowel has herniated, the greater is the frequency of incarceration, obstruction, and infarction.

Patients with ventral hernias often complain of lower-abdominal discomfort, and with large ventral hernias, the abdominal wall is distended to varying degrees (Fig. 12.27). Patients with large hernias may note bowel peristalsis beneath the skin, and report that the bulge becomes smaller when they are in a recumbent position. The hernia is more noticeable during coughing and straining and can increase in size over time, because of enlargement of the hernial ring or incorporation of additional segments of bowel into the hernial sac. Rarely, a ventral hernia produces acute symptoms of visceral torsion, incarceration, and infarction. Repair of the hernia is preferably done on an elective basis.

Surgical Management of Small Hernias

The principles of ventral hernia repair include (a) dissection of the hernia sac from the subcutaneous fat, rectus fascia, and peritoneal margin; (b) excision of the redundant hernia (peritoneal) sac; and (c) closure of the abdominal wound, using a layer-for-layer closure, an overlap repair of the rectus fascia, or the placement of a synthetic mesh prosthesis, such as polypropylene (Prolene) or Gore-Tex.

The low midline incisional scar is excised, and the underlying subcutaneous fat is mobilized free from the adjacent hernia sac. Sharp dissection is used to separate the skin and underlying fat widely from the margins of the hernia sac (Fig. 12.28A). The surgeon should defer opening the sac until the boundaries of the hernia have been delineated and dissected, because this aids in identifying the various tissue planes. To identify the margins of the fascial ring, it is advisable to open the sac and separate any underlying bowel from the peritoneal surface of the sac

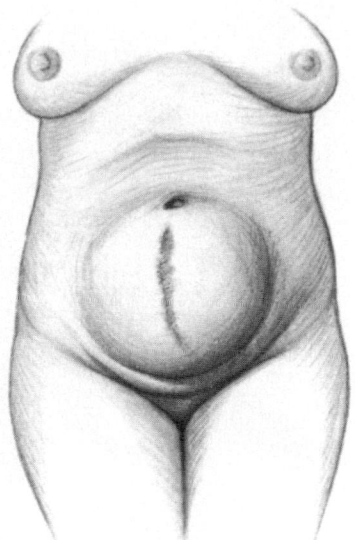

FIGURE 12.27. A ventral hernia in a low midline incision.

(Fig. 12.28B). Loops of small bowel and adherent omentum frequently obscure the true identity of the sac, and many pockets of the peritoneal lining are formed by fibrous bands that anchor the bowel to the peritoneum. After releasing the omentum and bowel, with particular attention given to hemostasis, it is important to determine whether the hernia defect can be adequately closed with the adjacent fascia before excising the line of the sac. If adequate fascial tissue remains after the dissection, either a layer-for-layer or an overlap fascial closure should be done. If inadequate fascia is available to close, the defect must be bridged with Prolene or Gore-Tex mesh. However, most incisional hernias can be closed without the use of a mesh support. When there has been failure of an initial hernia repair, when the hernia defect is so large that the edges cannot be adequately approximated, or when the tissues of the abdominal wall are attenuated, the use of synthetic mesh is strongly advised.

The layer-for-layer closure is accomplished after closure of the peritoneum as the initial layer. The fascial margins of the anterior rectus sheath are then sutured with nonabsorbable No. 0 (polypropylene or nylon) suture (Fig. 12.28C). Interrupted far–near, near–far pulley sutures (modified Smead-Jones) that include the inner margin of the abdominal musculature are placed to avoid subsequent pull-through of the suture from the edge of the incision. These sutures serve as internal stay sutures and increase the tensile strength of the wound while healing takes place.

When there is adequate fascial margin of good strength, a vest-over-pants closure gives extra support to the defect and produces a double-layer closure of the fascia (Fig. 12.28D). The surgeon should separate the peritoneum and posterior rectus sheath from the hernia margins to permit an overlap of the anterior fascia. The peritoneum is closed separately with a continuous suture of No. 2-0 delayed-absorbable suture of polyglactin material. The anterior rectus sheath of the hernia margins is separated widely on each side of the wound. Horizontal mattress sutures of a permanent suture (such as polypropylene)

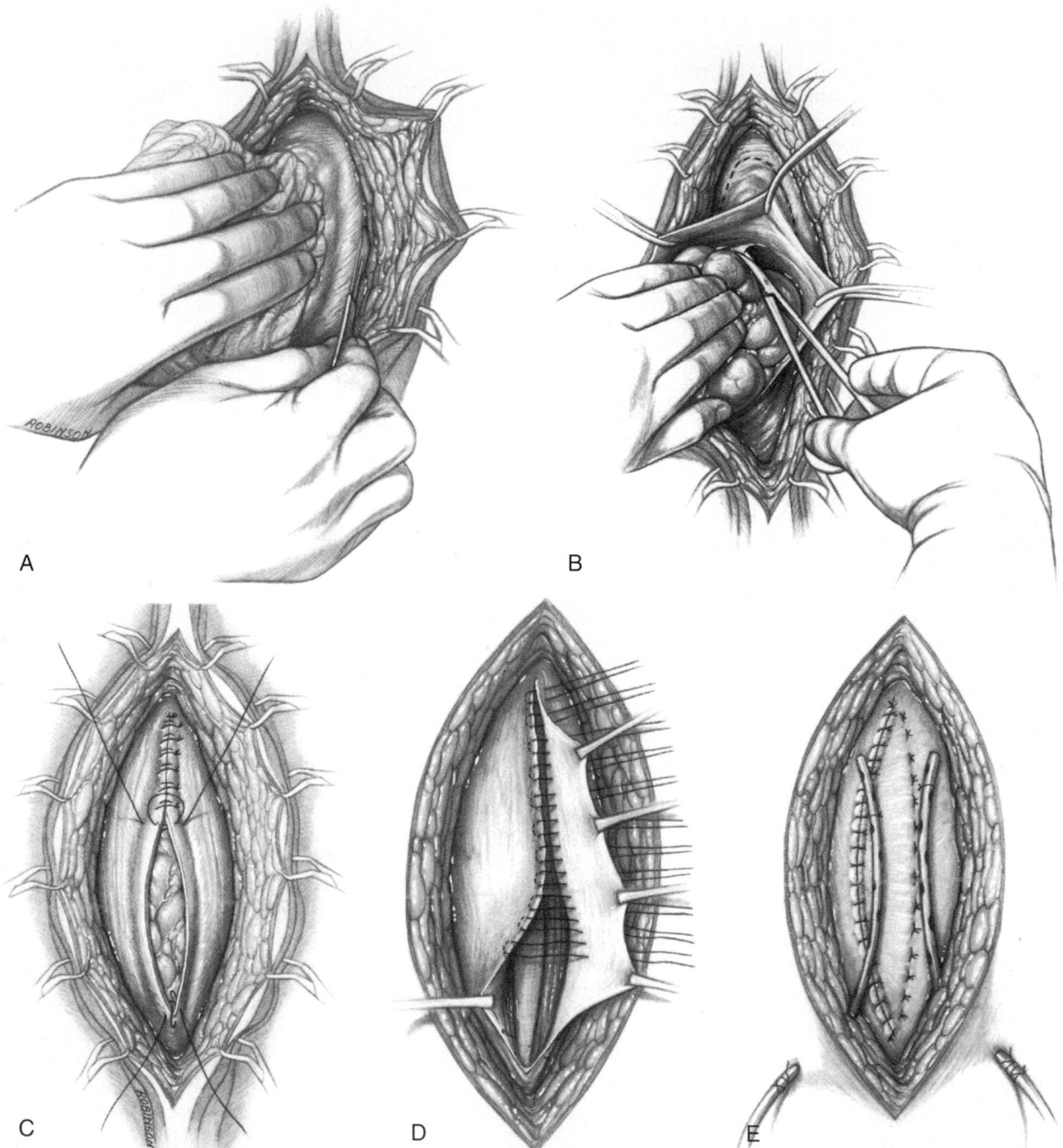

FIGURE 12.28. Repair of ventral hernia. **A:** Wide dissection of subcutaneous fat from the lateral boundaries of the hernia. **B:** The hernial sac is opened, and adherent bowel and omentum are released from the peritoneal surface. The superior margin of the fascial defect is indicated by a *dashed line*. **C:** Layer-for-layer closure of midline ventral hernia. Redundant hernial sac has been excised, and the fascial margins are sutured by far–near, near–far technique. A crown stitch at the lower pole anchors the apex of the defect to the lateral fascial margins. When possible, the peritoneum is closed as a separate layer. **D:** The vest-over-pants technique of midline hernia repair. The peritoneum is separated from hernia and closed. The anterior rectus fascia is dissected widely, and horizontal mattress sutures are placed distant from fascial edge and passed through the opposite fascial margin. When the sutures are tied, the fascial margins are drawn firmly beneath the opposite layer, producing a double fascial layer closure of hernia. **E:** Completion of a vest-over-pants closure of midline ventral hernia, showing suture of the free margin of the fascial flap to the underlying fascial surface. Perforated plastic closed-suction drainage tubes are sutured to the fascia to permit adequate drainage.

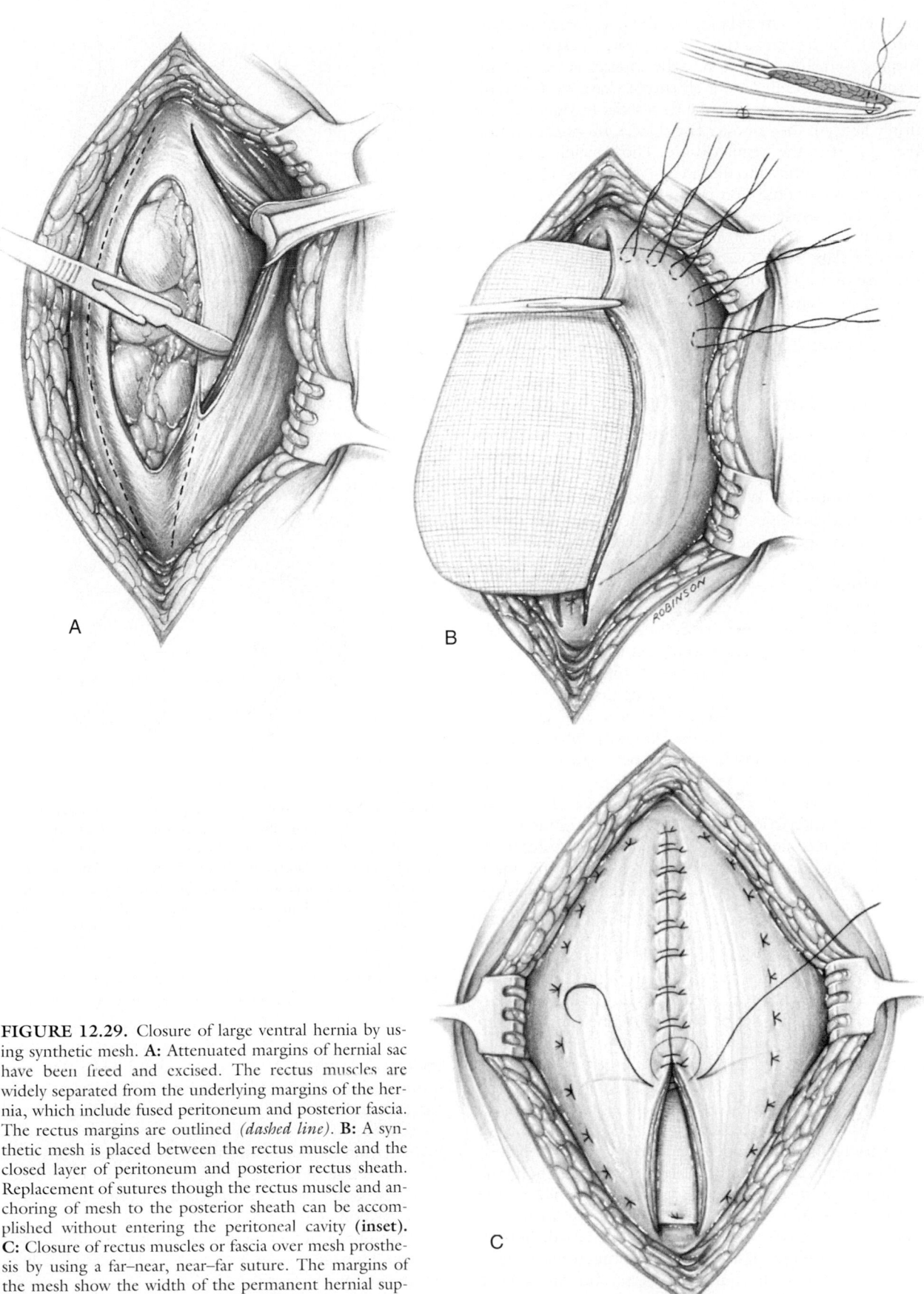

FIGURE 12.29. Closure of large ventral hernia by using synthetic mesh. **A:** Attenuated margins of hernial sac have been freed and excised. The rectus muscles are widely separated from the underlying margins of the hernia, which include fused peritoneum and posterior fascia. The rectus margins are outlined *(dashed line)*. **B:** A synthetic mesh is placed between the rectus muscle and the closed layer of peritoneum and posterior rectus sheath. Replacement of sutures though the rectus muscle and anchoring of mesh to the posterior sheath can be accomplished without entering the peritoneal cavity **(inset).** **C:** Closure of rectus muscles or fascia over mesh prosthesis by using a far–near, near–far suture. The margins of the mesh show the width of the permanent hernial support.

are placed 3 to 4 cm distant from the fascial edge and pass through the free margin of the opposite fascia before returning to the distal portion of the anterior fascia. The sutures are held untied until all sutures have been placed. When the sutures are tied, the free fascial margin is drawn firmly beneath the opposite fascial layer, producing a double support to the hernia closure. The remaining free fascial margin is sutured to the fascial surface (Fig. 12.28E) to complete the double-layer closure.

When closure of the fascial margins is complete, Jackson-Pratt or Blake drains can be inserted beneath the skin flaps for subsequent drainage (Fig. 12.28E). Penrose drains do not provide a satisfactory method for wound drainage and should not be used. The drains should exit through a separate stab incision in the skin several centimeters away from the primary incision.

Surgical Management of Large Hernias

In repairing a ventral hernia with a large fascial defect and poor abdominal tissue, it may be necessary to reinforce the hernia defect with a polypropylene prosthetic mesh or Gore-Tex. When using mesh, it is important to dissect the hernia sac as previously described and to define the layers of the abdominal wall carefully (Fig. 12.29A). Because of the placement of a foreign body in the abdominal incision, meticulous hemostasis and aseptic technique are essential. The implanted mesh must completely bridge the entire defect, with adequate margins for suturing to the adjacent rectus muscles.

After the hernia sac is removed and the margins of the fascial defect are freed, the rectus muscle is released from the underlying posterior fascial sheath and peritoneum (Fig. 12.29A). The fascia and peritoneum beneath the rectus muscle should be dissected widely around the margins of the defect to permit closure of the peritoneum without tension. A large piece of mesh or Gore-Tex is then inserted between the rectus muscle and the closed peritoneum (Fig. 12.29B). Lateral sutures are placed to anchor the mesh to the fascia so that the mesh does not buckle when the overlying rectus muscles are approximated in the midline. Nonabsorbable No. 0 polypropylene or nylon sutures are used to anchor the mesh to the rectus abdominis muscle. Closure of the rectus fascia over the mesh is then attempted, using the far–near, near–far closure technique (Fig. 12.29C).

If the rectus muscles or fascia cannot be approximated in the midline without undue tension, several other approaches may be used to repair these large herniae. These surgical techniques use a series of relaxing incisions in the anterior abdominal wall fascia to allow the surgeon to reapproximate the fascial edges over the defect. Again, when using these techniques, careful attention to hemostasis is paramount. In the fascial partition method, the subcutaneous tissue is widely dissected, anterior to the rectus fascia and lateral to the rectus musculature. Parasagittal incisions (Fig. 12.30A) are then made in both the external oblique fascia (several centimeters lateral to the rectus musculature) and transverse abdominis fascia (just lateral to the rectus musculature—care must be taken not to injure the inferior epigastric vasculature in this re-

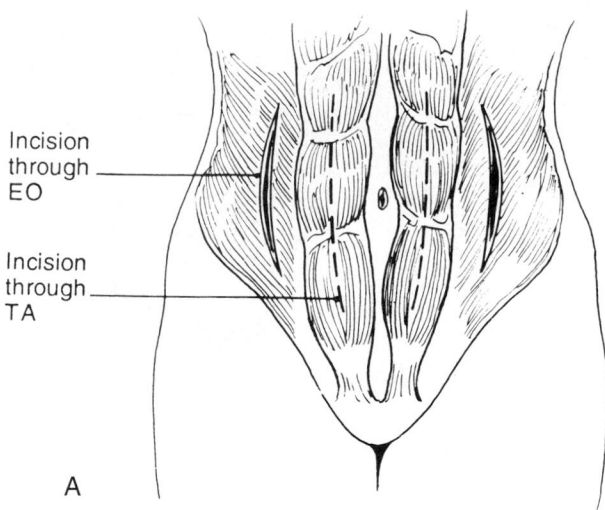

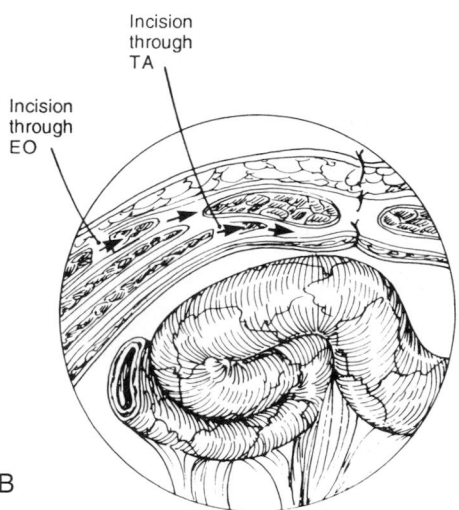

FIGURE 12.30. In the fascial partition method, relaxing incisions are made that allow wide mobilization of the fascia. **A:** Parasagittal relaxing incisions are placed through the external oblique (EO), lateral to the rectus muscles. The *dotted line* denotes similarly placed incisions in the transverse abdominis (TA) muscles. **B:** This cross-sectional view demonstrates location of the incisions with a closure of either an interrupted or Smead-Jones type.

gion) to mobilize tissue lateral to the fascial defect. The fascia may then be closed with either running mass closure or interrupted Smead-Jones sutures (Fig. 12.30B).

The sliding myofascial flap uses relaxing incisions in the external oblique fascia only (Fig. 12.31A). These relaxing incisions are made lateral to the rectus musculature, from the level of the lowest rib to the inguinal ligament. Further dissection laterally is completed with a combination of blunt and sharp dissection and carried as far as possible (Fig. 12.31B). Once adequately mobilized, the peritoneum and fascia are closed in a Smead-Jones fashion (Fig. 12.31C).

Should the subcutaneous tissues be "wet," a closed-suction drainage system may be placed longitudinally on either side of the fascial incision, and the subcutaneous fat and skin closed separately. Suction is applied to the drainage tubes to give negative pressure beneath the skin

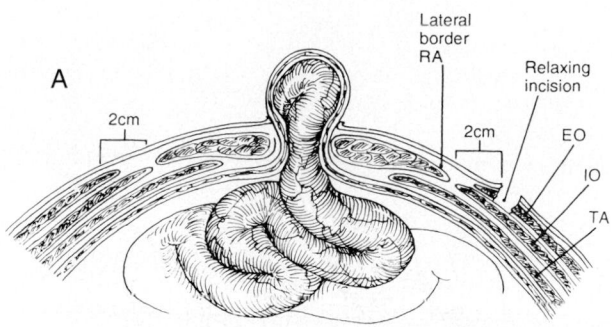

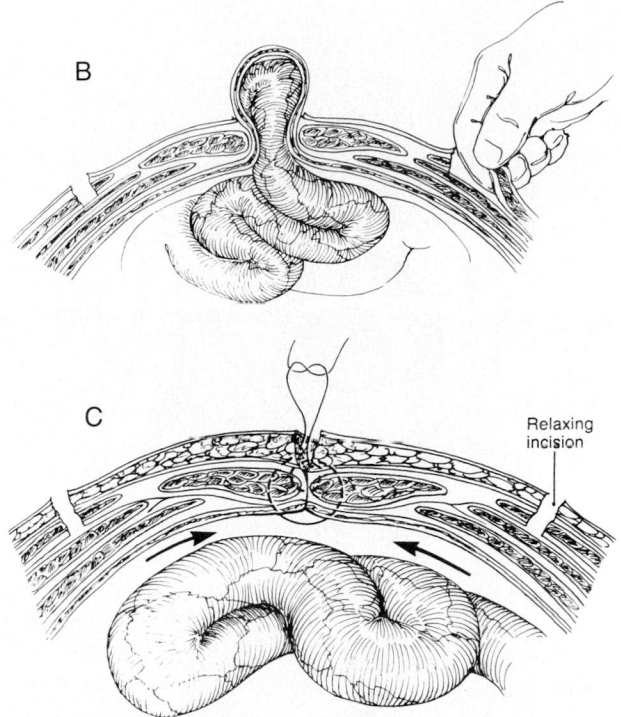

FIGURE 12.31. The sliding myofascial flap. **A:** Initially, the subcutaneous tissues must be sharply and widely dissected from the underlying fascia. A vertical relaxing incision is made in the external oblique (EO) only. This incision is made from the level of the lowest ribs to just cephalad to the inguinal ligament. The internal oblique (IO) and the transverse abdominis (TA) are not incised. **B:** A combination of blunt and sharp dissection is used to separate the EO from the IO as far laterally as possible. **C:** A cross-sectional view of the closure of the anterior abdominal wall, after performing the sliding myofascial flap. The closure shown is a Smead-Jones type, although an interrupted mass closure may be used.

and prevent elevation of the skin flaps by serum or blood. The drains may be removed by day 5 but must be left in place until there has been complete cessation of incisional drainage.

Postoperatively, the patient is ambulated on the day after surgery, without prolonged bed rest. The abdominal incision should be protected from excessive strain (e.g., coughing) by use of an elastic abdominal binder. If the bowel becomes distended, the use of nasogastric tube decompression should be considered. Prophylactic antibiotics are used perioperatively to prevent secondary infection in the operative site and are particularly useful in patients in whom mesh has been used for closure of a large hernia defect.

PERINEOTOMY INCISIONS

Adequate exposure is just as important with vaginal surgery as it is with abdominal surgery. When exposure is not adequate with abdominal operations, the incision is extended, or some other measure is used to improve exposure. Certain measures also can improve exposure with vaginal operations. A tight vaginal introitus may restrict exposure of the upper vagina, but can be enlarged at the beginning of the operation by making a midline or mediolateral episiotomy incision. A mediolateral incision can be made on one or both sides of the vaginal introitus. If a midline episiotomy is made and closed transversely, the vaginal introitus can be made larger than before, if that is deemed advisable. These incisions can be closed with 2-0 or 3-0 delayed-absorbable suture.

Sometimes, the entire vagina is small in caliber because of virginity or nulliparity, atrophic shrunken vaginal mucosa, previous colporrhaphy, or previous irradiation or disease. The vaginal vault may be fixed in a relatively high position, with relatively little descensus. Because adequate exposure through the vagina may be impossible, some operations may require an abdominal approach. On the other hand, required exposure may be obtained by making a Schuchardt incision. The entire vagina can be enlarged with this incision, achieving remarkable improvement in exposure of the upper vagina. Therefore, a patient whose problem might otherwise have necessitated an abdominal approach can have the advantage of a perfectly satisfactory vaginal operation if a Schuchardt incision is made.

According to Speert (1958), Langenbeck made a deep relaxing incision into the perineal body in attempting vaginal hysterectomy for uterine cancer in 1828. Similar incisions were used by Olshausen in 1881 and Duhrssen in 1891. Karl Schuchardt described his incision in 1893:

to make more accessible from below a uterus whose mobility is limited. . . . With the patient in the lithotomy position and her buttocks elevated, a large, essentially sagittal incision is made, somewhat convex externally, beginning between the middle and posterior third of the labium majus, . . . extending posterior toward the sacrum, and stopping two fingerbreaths [sic] from the anus. The wound is deepened only in the fatty tissue of the ischiorectal fossa, leaving the funnel of the levator ani muscle, the rectum behind it, and the sacral ligaments intact. Internally, the sidewall of the vagina is opened into the ischiorectal fossa and the vagina divided in its lateral aspect by a long incision extending up to the cervix. There thus results a surprisingly free view of all the structures under consideration.

The incision is ordinarily made on the patient's left side by a right-handed operator (Fig. 12.32). A left-handed operator may find it technically easier to make the incision on the patient's right side. Bilateral incisions have

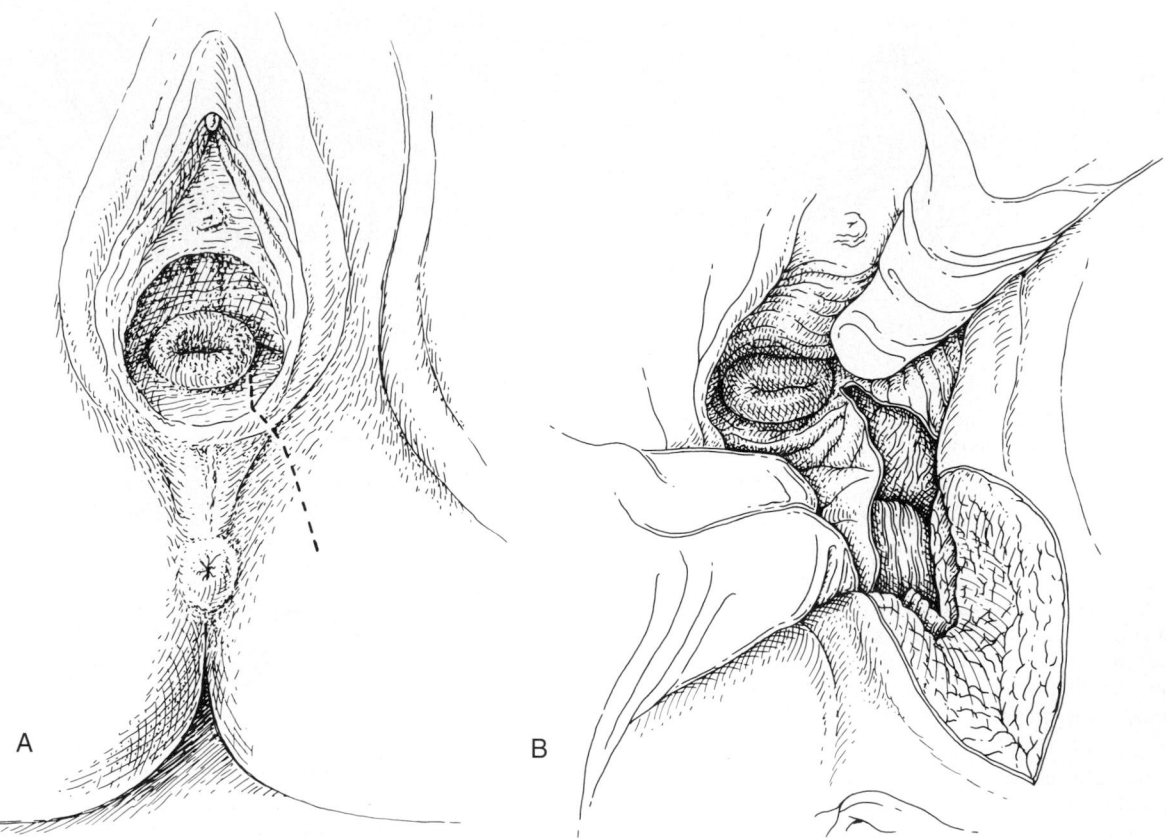

FIGURE 12.32. A: The Schuchardt incision begins at the 4-o'clock position in the vaginal introitus and extends into the buttock and up the posterolateral wall of the vagina to the cervix. **B:** The ischiorectal fossa fat is exposed. The puborectalis muscle is divided. The left paravesical and pararectal spaces can be exposed through the incision.

been advocated in extreme cases. The side on which the incision is made may be dictated by the location of the pathology to be removed. Injection of the tissues to be incised with sterile saline solution can be helpful, especially beneath the vaginal mucosa in the line of the incision. The assistant pulls upward to the left with the index finger placed as deep as possible in the vagina just to the left of the urethra. The operator makes countertraction by placing two fingers in the vagina and pulling downward to the right. This pull and counter-pull in opposite directions stretches the left vaginal wall. The incision is made with the electrosurgical unit beginning at the 4-o'clock position at the introitus and extending downward in the skin of the buttock to the level of the anus. The incision is then carried upward through the vaginal mucosa into the upper third of the vagina. As the incision is deepened, the fingers of the operator's left hand are used to displace the rectum medially to protect it from injury. The ischiorectal fossa fat is visible below the puborectalis muscle which is incised with the electrosurgical knife (Fig. 12.32). If necessary, the left paravesical space can be developed. For the best possible exposure, the apex of the vaginal incision should intersect any incision made around the cervix, achieving hemostasis by coagulation or ligation.

At the end of the operation, the Schuchardt incision is closed with 2-0 and 3-0 delayed-absorbable sutures, attempting to reapproximate the puborectalis muscle

edges and to obliterate the dead space in the ischiorectal fossa. Drainage of these incisions is usually not necessary.

The Schuchardt incision most often is used for extensive vaginal hysterectomy for early invasive cervical cancer. We also have used it when performing extensive dissections to remove endometriosis in the vaginal vault, to gain better exposure for difficult vaginal hysterectomy or vesicovaginal fistula repair, to repair injuries to the lower ureter, to remove organized hematomas just above the puborectalis muscle, to drain lymphocysts vaginally, or to remove benign cystic teratomas in the lower presacral area behind the rectum. It can convert a technically difficult, complicated, and dangerous vaginal operation into one that is simple, easy, and safe. It is difficult to understand why perineotomy incisions are so quickly performed for obstetric operations and so reluctantly for gynecologic operations.

BIBLIOGRAPHY

Alexander HC, Prudden JF. The causes of abdominal wound disruption. *Surg Gynecol Obstet* 1966;122:1223.

Alexander JW, Aerni S, Plettner JP. Development of a safe and effective one-minute preoperative skin preparation. *Arch Surg* 1985;120:1367.

Archie JP, Feldman RW. Primary wound closure with permanent continuous running monofilament sutures. *Surg Gynecol Obstet* 1981;153:721.

Averette HE, Dudan RC, Ford JH. Exploratory celiotomy for surgical staging of cervical cancer. *Am J Obstet Gynecol* 1972;133:1090.

Ballon SL, Berman ML, Lagasse LD, et al. Survival after extraperitoneal pelvic and paraaortic lymphadenectomy and radiation therapy in cervical carcinoma. *Obstet Gynecol* 1981;57:90.

Balthazar ER, Colt JD, Nicols RL. Preoperative hair removal: a random prospective study of shaving versus clipping. *South Med J* 1982;75:799.

Berman ML, Lagasse LD, Watring WG, et al. The operative evaluation of patients with cervical carcinoma by an extraperitoneal approach. *Obstet Gynecol* 1977;50:658.

Bourne RB, Bitar H, Andrese PR, et al. *In-vivo* comparison of four absorbable sutures: Vicryl, Dexon Plus, Maxon and PDS. *Can J Surg* 1988;31:43.

Brown SE, Allen HH, Robins RN. The use of delayed primary wound closure in preventing wound infections. *Am J Obstet Gynecol* 1977;127:213.

Cherney LS. A modified transverse incision for low abdominal operations. *Surg Gynecol Obstet* 1941;72:92.

Cosin JA, Powell JL, Donovan JT, et al. The safety and efficacy of extensive abdominal panniculectomy at the time of pelvic surgery. *Gynecol Oncol* 1994;55:36.

Cox PJ, Ausobsky JR, Ellis H, et al. Towards no incisional hernias: lateral paramedian versus midline incisions. *J R Soc Med* 1986;79:711.

Cruse PJE. Infection surveillance: identifying the problem and the high-risk patient. *South Med J* 1977;70[Suppl 1]:40.

Cruse PJE, Foord R. A five year prospective study of 23,649 surgical wounds. *Arch Surg* 1973;107:206.

Cruse PJE, Foord R. The epidemiology of wound infection: a 10-year prospective study of 62,939 wounds. *Surg Clin North Am* 1980;60:27.

Daversa B, Landers D. Physiologic advantages of the transverse incision in gynecology. *Obstet Gynecol* 1961;17:305.

Dineen P. A critical study of 100 conservative wound infections. *Surg Gynecol Obstet* 1961;113:91.

Dodson MK, Magann EF, Sullivan DL, et al. Extrafascial wound dehiscence: deep en bloc closure versus superficial skin closure. *Obstet Gynecol* 1994;83:142.

Dougherty SH, Simmons RL. The biology of surgical drains. *Curr Probl Surg* 1992;9:648.

Downey GO, Potish RA, Adcock LL, et al. Pre-treatment surgical staging in cervical carcinoma: therapeutic efficacy of pelvic lymph node dissection. *Am J Obstet Gynecol* 1989;160:1055.

Edlich RF, Panek RH, Rodeheaver GT, et al. Physical and chemical configuration of suture in the development of surgical infection. *Ann Surg* 1973;177:679.

Ellis H, Heddle R. Does the peritoneum need to be closed at laparotomy? *Br J Surg* 1977;64:733.

Fagniez P, Hay JM, Lacaine F, et al. Abdominal midline incisions closure: a randomized prospective trial of 3,135 patients, comparing continuous vs. interrupted polyglycolic acid sutures. *Arch Surg* 1984;120:1351.

Farnell MB, Worthington-Self S, Mucha P Jr, et al. Closure of abdominal incisions with subcutaneous catheters. *Arch Surg* 1986;126:641.

Fletcher HS, Joseph WL. Bleeding into the rectus abdominis muscle. *Int Surg* 1973;58:97.

Galle PC, Homesley HD, Rhyne AL. Reassessment of the surgical scrub. *Surg Gynecol Obstet* 1978;147:214.

Gallup DG. Modification of celiotomy techniques to decrease morbidity in obese gynecologic patients. *Am J Obstet Gynecol* 1984;150:171.

Gallup DG. Extraperitoneal and transperitoneal approaches for removal of retroperitoneal pelvic and paraaortic lymph nodes. In: Thompson JP, Rock JA, eds. *Te Linde's operative gynecology updates*, eighth edition. Philadelphia: JB Lippincott Co, 1993:1.

Gallup DG, Jordan GH, Talledo OE. Extraperitoneal lymph node dissections with use of a midline incision in patients with female genital cancer. *Am J Obstet Gynecol* 1986;155:559.

Gallup DG, Talledo OE, King LA. Primary mass closure of midline incisions with a continuous running monofilament suture in gynecologic patients. *Obstet Gynecol* 1989;73:67.

Gallup DG, Nolan TE, Smith RP. Primary mass closure of midline incisions with a continuous polyglyconate monofilament absorbable suture. *Obstet Gynecol* 1990;76:872.

Gallup DG, King LA, Messing MJ, et al. Paraaortic lymph node sampling by means of an extraperitoneal approach with a supraumbilical transverse "sunrise" incision. *Am J Obstet Gynecol* 1993;169:307.

Greenburg G, Salk RP, Peskin GW. Wound dehiscence: pathophysiology and prevention. *Arch Surg* 1979;114:143.

Grosfeld JL, Solit RW. Prevention of wound infection in perforated appendicitis: experience with delayed primary wound closure. *Ann Surg* 1968;168:891.

Guillou PJ, Hall TJ, Donaldson DR, et al. Vertical abdominal incisions: a choice? *Br J Surg* 1980;67:359.

Hamilton HW, Hamilton KR, Lone FJ. Preoperative hair removal. *Can J Surg* 1977;20:269.

Hasselgren AO, Harbery E, Malmer H, et al. One instead of two knifes for surgical incision. *Arch Surg* 1984;118:917.

Helmkamp BF. Abdominal wound dehiscence. *Am J Obstet Gynecol* 1977;128:803.

Helmkamp BF, Krebs HB, Amstey MS. Correct use of surgical drains. *Contemp OB/GYN* 1984;23:123.

Hendrix SL, Schimp V, Martin J, et al. The legendary superior strength of Pfannenstiel incision: a myth? *Am J Obstet Gynecol* 2000;182:1446.

Hermann GG, Bagi P, Christofferson I. Early secondary suture versus healing by second intention of incisional abscesses. *Surg Gynecol Obstet* 1988;167:16.

Higson RH, Kettlewell MGW. Parietal wound drainage in abdominal surgery. *Br J Surg* 1978;65:326.

Hodgson NC, Malthaner RA, Ostbye T. The search for an ideal method of abdominal fascial closure: a meta-analysis. *Ann Surg* 2000; 231:3: 436.

Hopkins MP, Shriner AM, Parker MG, et al. Panniculectomy at the time of gynecologic surgery in morbidly obese patients. *Am J Obstet Gynecol* 2000; 182: 1502.

Jenkins TPN. The burst abdominal wound: a mechanical approach. *Br J Surg* 1976;63:873.

Jurkiewicz MJ, Morales L. Wound healing, operative incisions, and skin grafts. In: Hardy JD, ed. *Hardy's textbook of surgery*. Philadelphia: JB Lippincott Co, 1983:108.

Küstner O. Der suprasymphysare kreuzschnitt, eine methode der coeliotomie bei wenig umfanglichen affektioen der weiblichen beckenorgane. *Monatsschr Geburtsh Gynakol* 1896;4:197.

Keill RH, Keitzer WF, Henzel J, et al. Abdominal wound dehiscence. *Arch Surg* 1973;106:573.

Kelly HA. Excision of the fat of the abdominal wall: lipectomy. *Surg Gynecol Obstet* 1910;10:229.

Kenady DE. Management of abdominal wounds. *Surg Clin North Am* 1984;64:803.

Knight CD, Griffen FD. Abdominal wound closure with a continuous monofilament polypropylene suture. *Arch Surg* 1983;118:1305.

Krebs HB, Helmkamp F. Transverse periumbilical incision in the massively obese patient. *Obstet Gynecol* 1984;63:241.

Krupski WC, Sumchai A, Effeney DJ, et al. The importance of abdominal wall collateral blood vessels. *Arch Surg* 1984;119:854.

Langer K. Cleavage of the cutis (the anatomy and physiology of the skin): presented at the Meeting of the Royal Academy of Sciences, April 25, 1861. *Clin Orthop* 1973;91:3.

Lineweaver W, Howard R, Soucy D, et al. Topical antimicrobial toxicity. *Arch Surg* 1985;120:1985.

Macht SC, Krizek TJ. Sutures and suturing: current concepts. *J Oral Surg* 1978;36:240.

Maylard AE. Direction of abdominal incision. *Br Med J* 1907;2:895.

McBurney C. The incision made in the abdominal wall in cases of appendicitis, with a description of a new method of operating. *Ann Surg* 1894;20:38.

McDowell E. Three cases of extirpation of diseased ovaria: 1817 *Am J Obstet Gynecol* 1995;172:1632.

McMinn RMH, Hutchings RJ, Logan BM. *Color atlas of applied anatomy.* Chicago: Mosby–Year Book, 1984:110.

Mead PB. Managing infected abdominal wounds. *Contemp OB/GYN* 1979;14:69.

Mendenez MA. The contaminated wound. In: O'Leary JP, Waltering EA, eds. *Techniques for surgeons.* New York: John Wiley and Sons, 1985:36.

Metz SA, Chegini N, Masterson BJ. *In vivo* tissue reactivity and degradation of suture materials: a comparison of Maxon and PDS. *J Gynecol Surg* 1989;5:37.

Montz FJ, Creasman WT, Eddy G, et al. Running mass closure of abdominal wounds using an absorbable looped suture. *J Gynecol Surg* 1991;7:107.

Morris DM. Preoperative management of patients with evisceration. *Dis Colon Rectum* 1982;25:249.

Morrow CP, Hernandez WL, Townsend DE, et al. Pelvic celiotomy in the obese patient. *Am J Obstet Gynecol* 1977;127:335.

Moss JP. Historical and current perspective on surgical drainage. *Surg Gynecol Obstet* 1981;152:517.

Mowat J, Bonnar J. Abdominal wound dehiscence after cesarean section. *Br Med J* 1971;2:256.

Moylan JA, Kennedy B. The importance of gown and drape barriers in the prevention of wound infection. *Surg Gynecol Obstet* 1980;151:465.

Murray DH, Blaisdell FW. Use of synthetic absorbable sutures for abdominal and chest wound closures. *Arch Surg* 1978;113:477.

Nelson JH, Boyce J, Macasaet M, et al. Incidence, significance, and follow-up of para-aortic lymph node metastases in late invasive carcinoma of the cervix. *Am J Obstet Gynecol* 1977;128:336.

Olson M, O'Connor MO, Schwartz ML. A 5-year prospective study of 20,193 wounds at Minneapolis VA Medical Center. *Ann Surg* 1984;199:253.

Parsons L, Ulfelder H. *Atlas of pelvic surgery,* second ed. Philadelphia: WB Saunders, 1968:156.

Peterson AF, Rosenberg A, Alatary SO. Comparative evaluation of surgical scrub preparation. *Surg Gynecol Obstet* 1978;146:63.

Pfannenstiel JH. Uber die vortheile des suprasymphysaren fascienguerschnitt fur die gynaekologischen koeliotomien. *Samml Klin Vortr Gynaekol (Leipzig) Nr 268,* 1900;97:1735.

Pitkin RM. Abdominal hysterectomy in obese women. *Surg Gynecol Obstet* 1976;142:532.

Postlethwait RW. Long-term comparative study of nonabsorbable sutures. *Ann Surg* 1970;171:892.

Pratt JH. Wound healing: evisceration. *Clin Obstet Gynecol* 1973;16:126.

Pratt JH, Irons B. Panniculectomy and abdominoplasty. *Am J Obstet Gynecol* 1978;132:165.

Rees VL, Coller FA. Anatomic and clinical study of the transverse abdominal incision. *Arch Surg* 1943;47:136.

Regnault P. Abdominoplasty by the W technique. *Plast Reconstr Surg* 1975;55:265.

Richards PC, Balch CM, Aldrete JS. Abdominal wound closure. *Ann Surg* 1983;197:238.

Rodeheaver GT, Powell TA, Thacker JG, et al. Mechanical performance of monofilament synthetic absorbable sutures. *Am J Surg* 1987;154:544.

Rollins RA, Corcoran JJ, Gibbs CE. Treatment of gynecologic wound complications. *Obstet Gynecol* 1966;28:268.

Sanz LE, Smith S. Mechanism of wound healing, suture material, and wound closure. In: Buchsbaum HJ, Walton LA, eds. *Strategies in gynecologic surgery.* New York: Springer-Verlag, 1986:53.

Sanz LE, Patterson JA, Kamath R, et al. Comparison of Maxon suture with Vicryl, chromic catgut, and PDS sutures in fascial closure in rats. *Obstet Gynecol* 1988;71:918.

Savage RC. Abdominoplasty combined with other surgical procedures. *Plast Reconstr Surg* 1982;70:437.

Schuchardt K. Eine neue Methode der Gebarmutterexstirpation. *Sentralbl Chir* 1893;20:1121.

Scott HW, Law HD, Sandstead HH, et al. Jejunoileal shunt in surgical treatment of morbid obesity. *Ann Surg* 1970;171:770.

Seropian R, Reynolds BM. Wound infections after preoperative depilatory versus razor preparation. *Am J Surg* 1971;121:251.

Shepherd JH, Cavanagh D, Riggs D, et al. Abdominal wound closure using a nonabsorbable single-layer technique. *Obstet Gynecol* 1983;61:248.

Shull BL, Verheyden CN. Combined plastic and gynecologic procedures. *Ann Plast Surg* 1988;20:252.

Speert H. *Obstetric and gynecologic milestones.* New York: Macmillan, 1958:630.

Stone HH, Hester TR. Topical antibiotic and delayed primary closure in the management of contaminated surgical incisions. *J Surg Res* 1972;12:70.

Stone HH, Holfling SJ, Strom PR, et al. Abdominal incisions, transverse vs. vertical placement and continuous vs. interrupted closure. *South Med J* 1983;76:1106.

Sutton G, Morgan S. Abdominal wound closure using a running, looped monofilament polybuster suture: comparison to Smead-Jones closure in historical controls. *Obstet Gynecol* 1992;80:650.

Thompson JB, Maclean KF, Collier FA. Role of the transverse abdominal incision and early ambulation in the reduction of postoperative complications. *Arch Surg* 1949;59:1267.

Thorek P. *Anatomy in surgery,* third ed. New York: Springer-Verlag, 1985:368.

Tollefson DG, Russell KP. The transverse incision in pelvic surgery. *Am J Obstet Gynecol* 1954;68:410.

van Rissel EJC, Trimbos BJ, Booster MH. Mechanical performance of square knots and sliding knots in surgery: a comparative study. *Am J Obstet Gynecol* 1990;162:93.

Voss SC, Sharp HC, Scott JP. Abdominoplasty combined with gynecologic surgical procedures. *Obstet Gynecol* 1986;67:181.

Wallace D, Hernandez W, Schlaerth JB, et al. Prevention of abdominal wound disruption utilizing the Smead-Jones closure technique. *Obstet Gynecol* 1980;56:226.

Walters MD, Dombroski RA, Davidson SA, et al. Reclosure of disrupted abdominal incisions. *Obstet Gynecol* 1990;76:597.

Weiland DE, Bay RC, Del Sordi S. Choosing the best abdominal closure by meta-analysis. *Am J Surg* 1998; 176:6: 666-70.

Weiser EB, Bundy B, Hoskins WJ, et al. Extraperitoneal versus transperitoneal selective paraaortic lymphadenectomy in the pre-treatment surgical staging of advanced cervical carcinoma: a Gynecologic Oncology Group study. *Obstet Gynecol* 1989;33:283.

Wharton JT, Jones HW, Day TG, et al. Preirradiation celiotomy for invasive carcinoma of the cervix. *Obstet Gynecol* 1977;49:333.

Te Linde's Operative Gynecology, ninth edition, edited by John A. Rock and Howard W. Jones, III. Lippincott Williams & Wilkins, Philadelphia © 2003.

CHAPTER

13

▼

Principles of Electrosurgery as Applied to Gynecology

RICHARD SODERSTROM

Usually, little attention is paid to the applied principles of electrophysics when surgeons receive their formal training. Most training programs consider electrosurgery a skill acquired by the student through hands-on exposure, and the average professor's knowledge in electrophysics is awarded through a "grandfather" process of credentials. As a result, many myths about the risks of electrosurgery have been perpetuated during the past decades. Modern electrical generators are finely tuned instruments that offer many versatile variables for the contemporary surgeon to harness, allowing the surgeon to deliver energy to tissue in either a discrete or broad manner to obtain a desired effect and outcome.

HISTORY OF ELECTROSURGERY

Dating back to antiquity, applying heat to wounds has been a part of the medical armamentarium. Neolithic skulls unearthed in France revealed evidence of thermal cauterization. Hippocrates used heat to destroy growths and to treat phthisis and epilepsy; his aphorism that fire succeeds when other methods fail influenced medicine and surgery for centuries. Albucasis in 980 BC described using a hot iron to stem bleeding; this approach is true cautery.

Electrosurgery is frequently erroneously referred to as electrocautery. Because the physical mechanisms and, consequently, the possible physiologic effects and potential hazards of the two methods are different, it is important to keep these two techniques separated by precise terminology. *Surgical diathermy,* a term more commonly used in Europe than in the United States, means "through heating," which is not a feature of monopolar electrosurgery but may be applicable to bipolar surgical techniques.

Most historians credit Arsenne d'Arsonval, in 1893, as the first to use high-frequency currents for medical therapy. In 1907, Riviere described "white coagulation" at low voltages without a spark. In 1925, Ward showed that a continuous sine wave from a vacuum-tube oscillator was most effective for cutting and that a damped sinusoidal waveform from a spark-gap oscillator produced more effective coagulation. Harvey Cushing, a neurosurgeon, and William T. Bovie, a physicist, were the most effective promoters of electrosurgery, using it with success during brain surgery to control hemorrhage. Cushing and Bovie published their results in 1928, describing the three distinct effects of electrosurgery: desiccation, cutting, and coagulation. Since then, manufacturers of electrosurgical units have provided medicine with an array of electrosurgical generators, each improving, with time, in output characteristics and safety features.

In the early 1970s, electrosurgery was the main energy source used in laparoscopy, and it was used with great success, although most procedures performed were sterilizations and lysis of simple adhesions. Reports of bowel injuries presumed to be secondary to "sparking" of monopolar energy prompted several investigators to develop bipolar instruments, as they claimed these tools would reduce the bowel injuries caused by the monopolar technique. By 1980, bipolar electrosurgery had caught the fancy of most endoscopic surgeons. At the same time, laser instruments designed for endoscopic procedures became available, and laser endoscopic postgraduate courses became commonplace, leaving electrosurgery as a back-up method. During the past two decades, the same surgical injuries formerly attributed to monopolar energy have persisted, and no study has demonstrated a reduction in laparoscopic injuries, especially bowel injuries, by the change to bipolar or laser technology.

Near the end of the 1980s, general surgeons recognized the advantages of intraabdominal endoscopic surgery, especially for laparoscopic cholecystectomy, but they quickly became frustrated by several limitations of contemporary lasers and returned to electrosurgical generators for more versatility and power. The manufacturers responded quickly with solid-state generators designed specifically for endoscopic use. Each energy source capable of destroying tissue can, in specific circumstances, lead to a surgical complication that may be unique to that energy source. But a watt is a watt, and when the output of energy of any source is matched for power density, power output in wattage, and the same amount of time (joules), the same tissue injury occurs. Although many hazards attendant to an energy source such as electrosurgery can be reduced and managed, not all can be eliminated. Surgeons are expected to be familiar with their surgical tools and appreciate the variables inherent in this technology.

BASIC ELECTRICAL DEFINITIONS

Electrons are particles of energy that, when pushed (or passed) through human tissue, create heat and sometimes destruction. *Voltage* is the pressure force required to push electrons. The standard unit of measure of this electrical pressure is 1 V. Thus, in drawing the analogy of electricity to water, an electron is to a molecule of water what voltage is to water pressure.

Whereas volume of water may be measured in cubic centimeters, the volume of electrons is measured in *coulombs*. If we push a volume of water through a conduit at a given pressure during a specific period, we create *current*. In electricity, current (measured in *amperes*, or coulombs per second) means the passage of a given quantity of electrons through a conductor during a given period of time. With either water or electricity, as resistance increases, the flow of current decreases (given constant pressure or voltage). The difficulty of pushing the electrons through tissue or other material can be defined as *resistance* and is measured in *ohms* (Ω).

Electrical power (*watts*) is the energy produced. The electrical power may be defined as pressure times current, volts times current, or volts times electron flow per second. The total energy consumed during a period of time is measured in *joules* (Table 13.1). For a complete list of terms used in electrosurgery, see the Glossary at the end of this chapter.

FUNDAMENTALS OF ELECTROSURGERY

Electrocautery is a term frequently used improperly when physicians actually mean electrosurgery. *Electrocautery* involves use of a direct electrical current to heat up a metal conductor with a high impedance to flow so that the metal becomes physically hot. Tissue is then cauterized by touching the hot metal object to tissue. In contemporary surgery, few instruments employ the principles of electrocautery. *Electrosurgery* involves manipulating electrons through living tissue by using an alternating current with enough current concentration (current density) to create heat within a tissue cell to destroy tissue. *Electrogenerators* or *electrosurgical units* are machines that produce an alternating current of electricity at a frequency that does not stimulate muscle activity (500,000 to 3 million cycles per second). Whereas direct current flows in one direction only, alternating current flows to and fro, first increasing to a maximum in one direction and then increasing to a maximum in the other direction. This *sinusoidal waveform* can be interrupted or varied, thus creating different surgical effects.

TABLE 13.1.
Electrophysics Definitions Equated to a Hydraulic Analogue

Electrical Concept	Electrical Unit	Equation	Hydraulic Analogue
Energy	Joule	—	Energy
Charge	Coulomb	$(6.3 \times 1,018$ electrons)	Volume (mass)
Power	Watt	Joules/second	Power
Voltage	Volt	Joules/coulomb	Pressure difference
Current	Ampere	Coulombs/second	Flow
Impedance	Ohm	Volts/ampere	Resistance

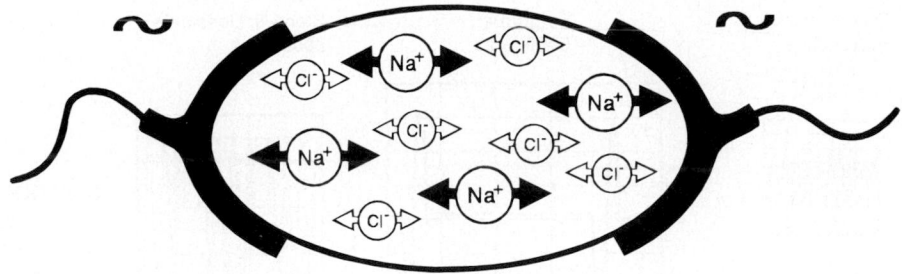

FIGURE 13.1. The sine wave of negative or positive polarity of an alternating current creates intracellular heat as it passes through each cell.

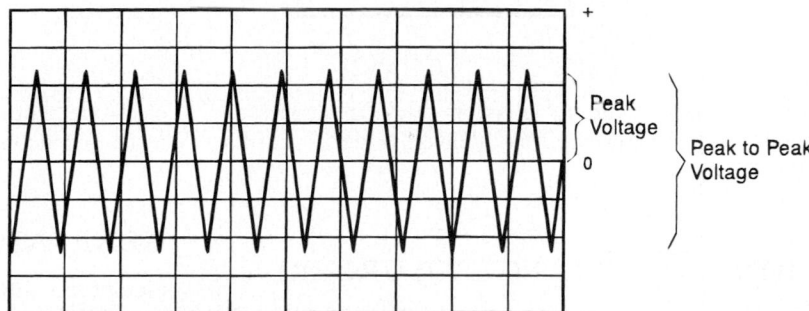

FIGURE 13.2. An undamped (or *CUT*) waveform is a continuous delivery of energy.

The waveform of alternating current has a negative and a positive excursion, or peak. As it passes through each cell, the electrolytic polarity is agitated, creating cellular heat (Fig. 13.1). The measurement from zero polarity to positive or negative polarity is called the *peak voltage* of the waveform (the relation is the same for peak current). The measurement from plus peak to negative peak, which is twice peak voltage, is called *peak-to-peak voltage*. A pure cutting/desiccation (CUT) waveform is a simple sinusoidal, undamped, or nonmodulated waveform and is generally produced by continuous energy (Fig. 13.2). An output waveform that is interrupted or varied (modulated or damped) is called a coagulating (COAG) waveform (Fig 13.3).

When there is a continuous flow or waveform, the peak voltage need not be as high as with the COAG waveform to create the same wattage. However, when a coagulation effect must be enhanced, the damped wave-

form is preferable and is created by pushing bursts of electrons through the tissue. The cooling effect of the off time between bursts allows for the coagulation effect. For an instant, with the damped waveform, a higher voltage than that with an undamped waveform is present within the electrical circuit. Most generators provide a blended current, which does not result from combined CUT and COAG waveforms, as is commonly thought. Instead, the blended waveform interrupts the current at variable intervals, delivering variable degrees of coagulating and cutting properties (Fig. 13.4). The degree to which the blended mode cuts or coagulates depends on the relative time interval that the current flow is on or

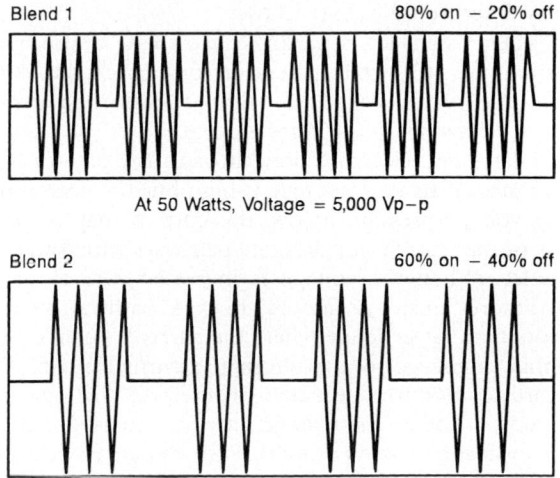

FIGURE 13.4. *BLEND* settings can vary as to the percentage of time the generator delivers the energy.

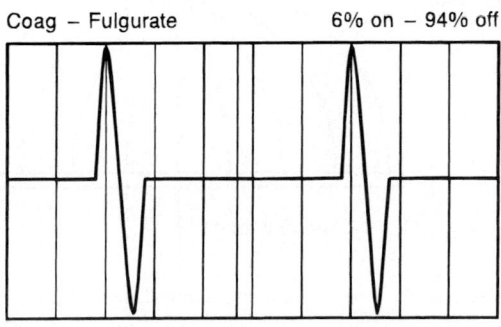

FIGURE 13.3. The damped or interrupted waveform (or *COAG*) delivers energy less than 10% of the time.

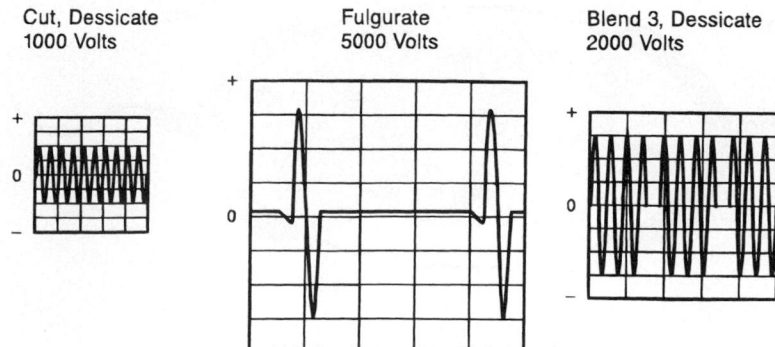

Cut, Dessicate
1000 Volts

Fulgurate
5000 Volts

Blend 3, Dessicate
2000 Volts

FIGURE 13.5. A pure cutting/desiccation (CUT), interrupted electrical current (COAG), and BLEND set at 50 W. As the generator is switched from one waveform to another, the voltage must change to match the designated power output. The voltage increases from CUT to BLEND to COAG.

off. Thus, one of the tissue effects of electrosurgery depends on the various modes of delivering electric current (Fig. 13.5).

MONOPOLAR ELECTROSURGERY

As electrons, pushed with a given voltage, are concentrated in one specific location, heat within the tissue increases rapidly. This concentration phenomenon is defined as *current density*. The diathermy generator, an example of equipment that uses this principle, is familiar to most physicians. Electrons are passed through the body by applying two large metal conductors or plates on opposite sides of the body part to be heated. The electrons are pushed through the plate called the *active electrode*. Electrons are received on the other plate, the *return (neutral) electrode* or ground plate, after they leave the body. Once the electrons enter the body (conductor), they are dispersed through the tissue toward the pathway of least resistance to the return electrode. Because current is dispersed over the entire surface area of both plates (low current density), the heat generated is of low intensity. If either plate is markedly reduced in size, however, current density (and thus heat) is increased accordingly (Fig. 13.6).

Thus, a small active electrode can create a burn (high current density) where the electrons enter the body. Also, the electrons that leave the body through a small return electrode can produce a burn.

Like water, electrons flow through the path of least resistance. If tissue resistance is high but the corresponding voltage pressure is low, the current may cease to flow or may search out alternate pathways with lower resistance. When the voltage is increased, the electrons have more "push" to find an alternate pathway, such as through a vital structure where the current is condensed, or they might seek out an alternate return electrode, like a cardiac monitor electrode. Therefore, the operator should use the lowest voltage necessary to accomplish a given job and should ensure that the dispersive electrode is in good contact with the patient and is broad enough to reduce current density far below the level of tissue destruction. Isolated ground circuitry systems or return-

electrode sentinel systems are preferable when an ineffective or incomplete return path is present.

GENERATORS

Significant differences exist among electrogenerators available for electrosurgical use. In general, generators that are set by a number dial are calibrated to peak voltage output rather than to power output, as is found in generators that have a digital liquid-crystal display window showing the output in watts. To determine the wattage output with the dial-a-number generators, the operator must refer to an output graph found in the manufacturer's manual; some generators have these output curves imprinted on the top of the generator box (Fig. 13.7). The power output set by the company is the power available at the start of the electrosurgical process,

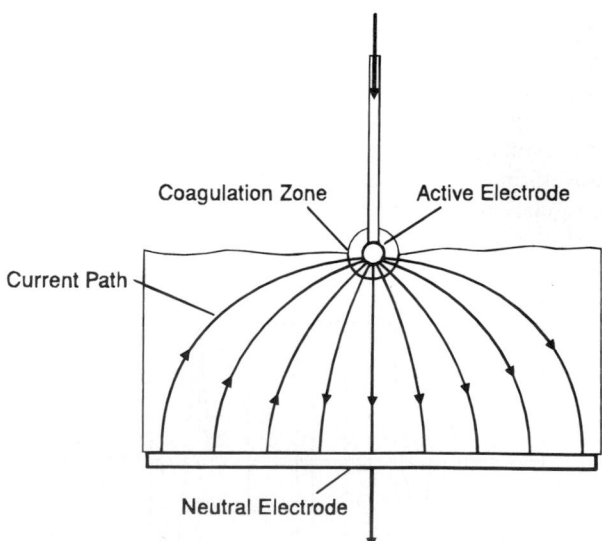

Coagulation Zone   Active Electrode

Current Path

Neutral Electrode

FIGURE 13.6. Distribution of current flow in the tissue during monopolar HF surgical technique. When one electrode pole is reduced in size, the tissue in contact with the smaller electrode is heated rapidly because of a high current (power) density.

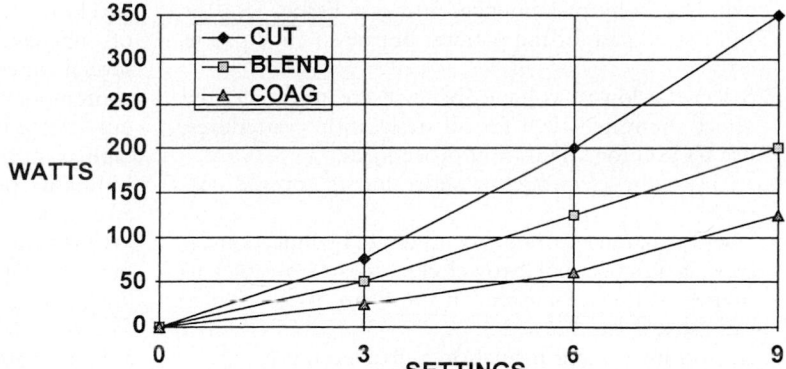

FIGURE 13.7. The characteristics of the monopolar power output curves in a generator with dial settings to a maximum of 350 W against a 500-Ω load. The power in each waveform chosen is different for the same setting.

but this power falls off as tissue impedance increases during the heating of cellular fluids. The output measurements of each generator are calibrated against a fixed resistance. For unipolar use, most generators are calibrated against a 500-Ω load; for bipolar use, the load is usually set at 100 Ω (Fig. 13.8). Each generator has its own power output characteristics; the proper settings can be found with attention to the manual and with experience.

For general surgical use, most generators can produce a maximum of 8,000 V in the COAG mode. An 8,000-V pressure can push electrons 3 mm through room air under certain atmospheric conditions, which means that arcing to distant tissue is improbable; most of the time, these generators are used in the 1,000- to 3,000-V range. The waveform frequency is set above 350,000 cycles per second to prevent muscle stimulation. At frequencies below 100,000 cycles per second, muscle contraction can occur, which is known as the *faradic effect* and is undesirable. The higher the radiowave frequency of a generator, the more leakage of current occurs that can enhance a capacitance effect, especially worrisome in certain endoscopic procedures.

Most contemporary generators offer an *isolated ground circuitry* system to reduce the risk of monopolar energy seeking an alternative pathway to ground; older-model generators are known as *ground-referenced generators*. With an isolated or "floating" ground system, the electricity delivered to the patient and returned to the

generator is created by an induction of current in transformers that are insulated or isolated from the frame of the generator. When a break in the circuit occurs, the electrons do not seek ground, and thus, no current flows. This also reduces the risk of an aberrant burn to the surgeon, *unless* the surgeon is leaning against the patient, thus becoming part of the isolated circuit.

Return-electrode safety systems use disposable return electrodes (called *ground pads*), which are usually two conductive pads placed side by side. Built-in monitors, through low-impedance feedback to the generators, measure pad-to-skin contact stability and power-density contact by measuring the balance of contact between the two pads. If there is an imbalance or poor contact to the patient, an alarm sounds and the generator does not function. The return electrode should be orientated so that each pad is at equal distance from the operating site and in close proximity.

The basic principles of safety during electrosurgery include the following:

1. Avoid arcing electrosurgical energy to a hemostat: Always touch the hemostat first, then initiate the energy. Place electrode pencils in their safety holster when not in use.
2. Use a monitored return-electrode system (frequently referred to as a REM system). Place return electrodes close to the operative site on a clean, dry, shaved area,

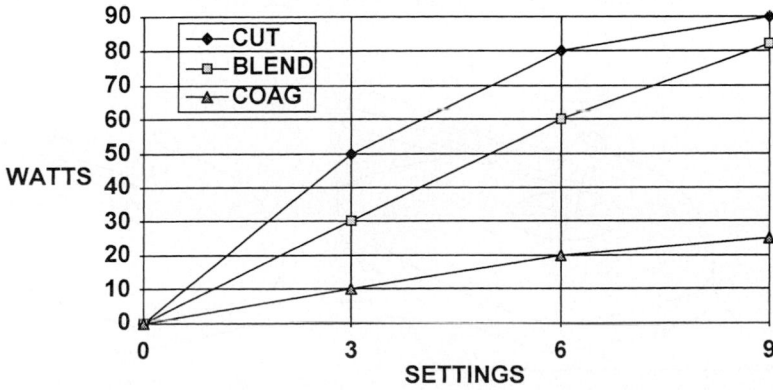

FIGURE 13.8. The characteristics of bipolar power output curves in a generator with dial settings to a maximum of 100 W against a 100-Ω load. Note that the power in each waveform chosen is different for the same setting.

avoiding bony prominences and scar tissue. Use the right-sized pad for the patient, but never cut a pad to size.

3. Select the lowest voltage that will create the desired effect. Activate CUT for all desiccation procedures; use COAG for fulguration procedures.

4. Activate the electrode in short bursts (over 3 seconds).

5. Use the manufacturer's recommended connection cables. Never use metal towel clips to attach cables to drapes, as leakage current in the form of capacitance can cause a skin burn.

6. Inspect instrument insulation before each use.

7. If the patient has a pacemaker, get advice from the pacemaker representative before using unipolar energy. Consider using bipolar methods.

8. If the usual power settings are inadequate, do not increase the power until the circuit is checked, especially the return electrode.

BIPOLAR ELECTROSURGERY

As mentioned earlier, in unipolar or monopolar electrosurgery, a ground plate or return electrode carries the flowing electrons back to the generator after the electrons have passed through the patient. The electrons that spread out after leaving a high density of energy at the point of tissue contact, by the active or efferent electrode, are dispersed over the broad surface of the return electrode, which lowers the power (current) density too low to cause significant tissue heating.

The bipolar system incorporates an active (efferent) electrode and a return (afferent) electrode into a two-poled instrument, such as forceps or scissors. This eliminates the need for a ground plate, allowing the instrument to produce a high power density at each pole of the forceps (Fig. 13.9). This permits a discrete amount of desiccation that is confined primarily to the shape and size of the forceps in contact with the tissue, and eliminates the chance of stray or alternate pathways for current flow that can occur with monopolar activation if the ground plate is improperly applied or if there is a break in the return lead.

Although these advantages over monopolar electrosurgery seem obvious, several restrictions unique to bipolar electrosurgery need to be appreciated. First, the load of impedance used to calibrate power output is usually several times lower than that with monopolar modes in contemporary generators. In a generator that has an output-selection knob measuring volts rather than watts, the bipolar output of energy is many watts less than the same setting in the monopolar side of the generator. In generators that read power output in watts, the impedance load is three to five times less than the load used to calibrate monopolar output, so the tissue effect may be much less than the same output reading for monopolar. Therefore, in most situations, bipolar applications are limited to a discrete area held between the forceps or scissor poles, with a restricted power output but with high power density. For sterilization and other laparoscopic procedures, the manufacturer's advice should be followed because each instrument can differ in design and ability to desiccate completely. With bipolar electrosurgery, only a CUT or continuous waveform should be used. As we learn more about how to apply bipolar energy, new instruments will be developed that will broaden its applications.

BIOLOGIC BEHAVIOR OF ELECTROSURGERY

Electrosurgery may be used to cut (*vaporize*) and to coagulate deeply (*desiccate*) or superficially (*fulgurate*). These frequently misused terms stand for specific functions of electrosurgery that should be familiar to the surgeon. As mentioned earlier, at the end of an electrode, the performance depends on the shape and size of the electrode, the frequency and wave modulation, the peak voltage, and the current coupled against output impedance. The tissue may be cut in a smooth deliberate fashion without arcing, or it can be burned and charred. This great variation of tissue effects is frequently ignored or misunderstood, which is why, in the past, some surgeons claimed that the laser provided better control of energy and promoted better wound healing.

Electrocoagulation may be performed in many different forms, from slow delicate contact coagulation (*desiccation*) to the charring effects of the spray coagulation mode (*fulguration*), at times leading to carbonization. The temperature differences can vary from 45°C to more than 500°C.

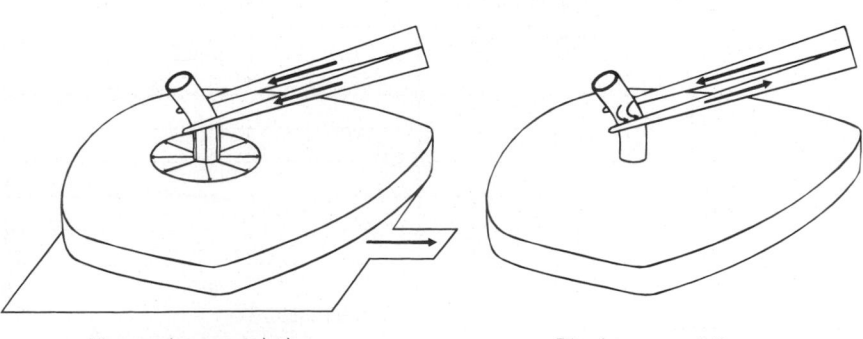

Monopolar coagulation   Bipolar coagulation

FIGURE 13.9. Bipolar instruments eliminate the need for a large return electrode (ground plate) and confine the energy delivered to the tissue between the two poles of the instrument.

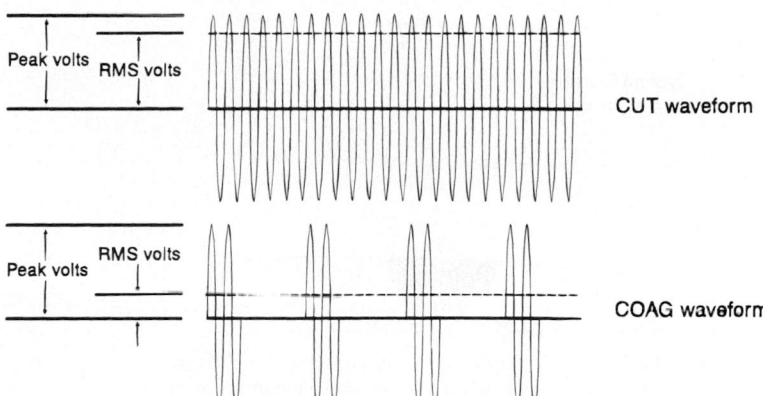

FIGURE 13.10. When the voltage is the same between pure cutting/desiccation (CUT) and interrupted electrical current (COAG), the amount of power delivered in COAG is only one third that of CUT. RMS, root mean square.

The essential characteristic of CUT waveforms is that they are continuous sine waves. That is, if the voltage output of the generator is plotted over time, a pure CUT waveform is a continuous sine wave alternating from positive to negative at the operating frequency of the generator, 500 to 3,000 kHz. The COAG waveform consists of short bursts of radio-frequency sine waves. With the sine wave frequency of 500 kHz, the COAG bursts occur 31,250 times per second. The important feature of the COAG waveform is the pause between each burst. Suppose that a COAG waveform had the same peak voltage as the CUT waveform, the average power delivered (heat per second) would be less because the COAG is turned off most of the time (Fig. 13.10). Then suppose that the COAG waveform had the same average voltage (root-mean-square voltage) as the CUT waveform and thus could deliver the same heat per second. Because the COAG is turned off most of the time, it can only produce the same root-mean-square voltage as the CUT by having large peak voltages and currents during the periods when the generator is on (Fig. 13.11).

A high-voltage COAG waveform can spark to tissue without significant cutting effect because the heat is more widely dispersed by the long sparks and because the heating effect is intermittent. The temperature of the water in the cells does not get high enough to flash into steam. In this way, the cells are dehydrated slowly but are not torn apart to form an incision. Because the high peak voltage is a quality of the COAG waveform, it can drive

a current through high resistances. In this way, it is possible to fulgurate long after the water is driven out of the tissue and to actually char it to carbon.

Coagulation is a general term that includes both desiccation and fulguration. Fulguration can be contrasted with desiccation in several ways. First, sparking to tissue with fulguration *always* produces necrosis anywhere sparks land. This is not surprising because each cycle of voltage produces a new spark, and each spark has an extremely high current density. In desiccation, the current is no more concentrated than the area of contact between the electrode and the tissue (Fig. 13.12). As a result, desiccation may or may not produce necrosis, depending on the current density. For an equal level of current flow, fulguration is always more efficient at producing surface necrosis; however, the depth of tissue injury is superficial compared with that of contact desiccation. With fulguration, the sparks jump from one spot to another in a random fashion, and the energy is "sprayed" rather than concentrated (Fig. 13.13).

In general, fulguration requires only one fifth the average current flow of desiccation. For example, if a ball electrode is pressed against moist tissue, the electrode begins in the desiccation mode, regardless of the waveform (Fig. 13.12). The initial tissue resistance is low, and the resulting current is high, typically 0.5 to 0.8 A (root mean square). As the tissue dries out, its resistance rises until the electrical contact is broken. Because moist tissue is no longer touching the electrode, sparks jump to the nearest areas of moist tissue in the fulguration mode,

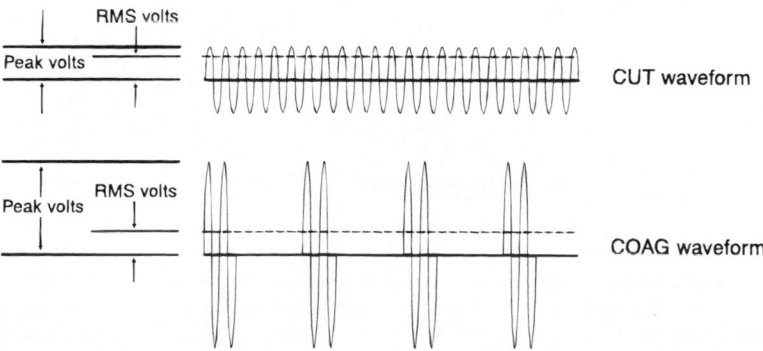

FIGURE 13.11. When the power settings are equal between pure cutting/desiccation (CUT) and interrupted electrical current (COAG), the peak voltage of COAG is about three times higher than that of CUT.

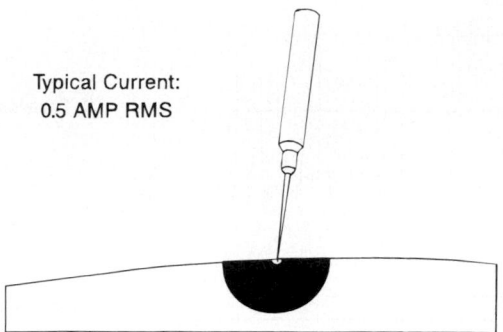

Typical Current:
0.5 AMP RMS

FIGURE 13.12. Desiccation occurs by touching the tissue before keying the generator, which creates deep penetration of heat and minimal charring of the surface tissue.

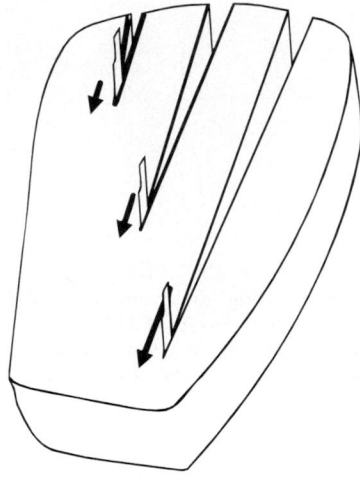

FIGURE 13.14. The tissue effect (influence on the degree of coagulation) of increasing the speed of passage of a cutting electrode of the same size and at the same depth of cut.

as long as the voltage is high enough to make a spark. Eventually, the resistance of desiccated tissue stops the flow of electrons, limiting the depth of coagulation.

Electrosurgical electrodes can be sculpted to perform certain tasks. A microneedle, a knife, a wire loop, or even a scissors can be shaped and sized to a specific duty. When the waveform variables are added, cutters can be made to coagulate, and coagulators can be made to cut. The faster an electrode passes over or through tissue, the less is the coagulation effect, leading to more cutting. If the power setting and the electrode size remain constant, more desiccation of the adjacent tissue occurs the slower the electrode is passed through the tissue (Fig. 13.14). The more broad the electrode is, the less cutting and more coagulation effect there are (Fig. 13.15). If the electrode is touched to the tissue before keying the generator, desiccation occurs, but with more lateral charring in the COAG mode than in the CUT mode. There is a point at which the desiccation effect is limited in depth by the impedance to flow at a fixed power setting. Interwoven into these acts are the output intensity and output impedance characteristics of the different electrosurgical generators. If a constant voltage can be maintained at a given power setting, which is variable as tissue re-

sistance changes, lateral thermal damage is controlled, giving the surgeon a predetermined surgical effect. Using a constant voltage controls the depth of coagulation independent of the cutting rate.

INCISIONS

High electrical current that is delivered with a fine electrode yields a high power density, which generates intense intracellular heat, causing the intracellular water to boil and thereby vaporizing the cell. The vaporization of the cell dissipates heat, a cooling effect that prevents thermal damage to adjacent tissue. This cooling effect, however, allows for little heat transfer to deeper tissue, resulting in minimal or no coagulation effects when electrosurgery is used at the pure cutting mode. To further enhance the vaporizing effects of the cutting waveform, the electrode should be activated just before touching the tissue (Fig. 13.16). The low-voltage sparks, by their high power density, produce a plume of steam and car-

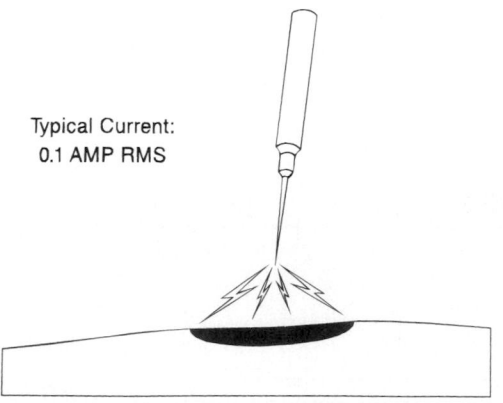

Typical Current:
0.1 AMP RMS

FIGURE 13.13. Fulguration sprays spark to the surface of tissue, causing a rapid surface char with minimal heating of the deeper layers.

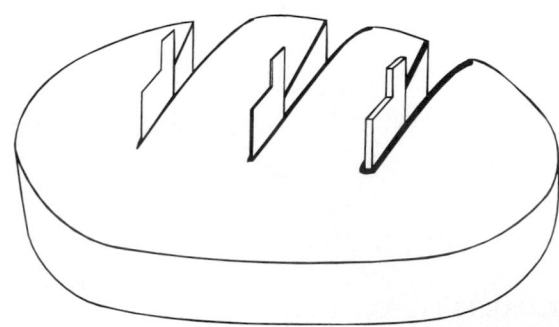

FIGURE 13.15. The tissue effect (influence on the degree of coagulation) of increasing the size of a cutting electrode if the speed and depth of cut are constant.

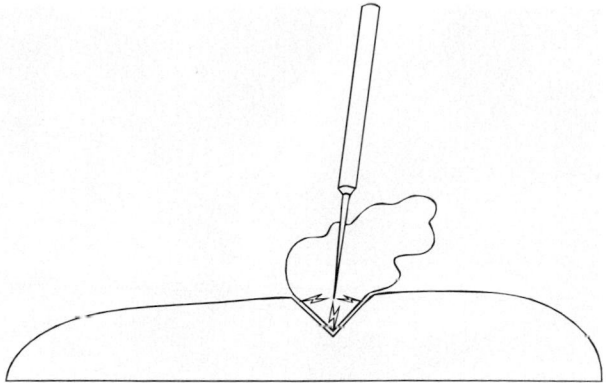

FIGURE 13.16. Electrosurgical cutting. Because of the continuous flow of low-voltage energy in the pure cutting/desiccation (CUT) mode, the high-power density of each spark vaporizes the cells into steam. The cutting effect is enhanced by allowing a needle or blade electrode to glide along the layer of steam, letting the sparks do the cutting.

bon particles between the electrode and the impacted tissue through which the current is rapidly conducted. This highly focused electrical energy yields the maximum power density, resulting in the most efficient cutting effects and the least thermal damage. Therefore, to incise tissue, cutting current should be used with a small or thin electrode that is activated just before making contact with the target tissue. The electrode "glides" on a layer of steam as the sparks do the cutting.

Because speed of passage and electrode size and shape determine the heat effect on tissue to be incised, the amount of desired thermal effect decides what electrode to use and how fast the incision should be made. In addition, the chosen waveform can play a role. To compound the decision, the natural resistance of the tissue to be incised should be considered.

In cutting, the voltage must exceed about 200 peak V. Although most choose a scalpel to incise the skin, a knife or needle electrode can mimic the incision if the surgeon applies the principle of speed of passage and waveform. With either electrode, the speed of passage is coupled with a CUT waveform. Because a needle electrode has the highest power density, if the speed of passage is swift and the waveform is set at pure CUT, no visible desiccation of tissue occurs, but like a knife, the skin bleeds without coagulation effect. A slow deliberate sweep of the electrode causes some desiccation effect, and the skin may blister and heal poorly. For that reason, only the experienced electrosurgeon should cut the skin with electrodes.

In fat, which has a high impedance, a blade electrode, passing a COAG waveform (high fulguration) into the tissue, cuts because of its edge density. The small bleeders, however, are fulgurated quickly. When larger vessels are exposed, such as the superficial epigastric vessels, the blade can be rotated 90 degrees to desiccate the vessel with its broad surface before it is severed. Thus, mixing the electrode size and shape with the chosen waveform can produce a variety of results.

DESICCATION TECHNIQUE

The most common desiccation maneuver used in surgery is the coaptation of blood vessels. Coaptive coagulation involves clamping a bleeding vessel with a conductive clamp and applying a cutting or desiccating current to coagulate and promote a collagen weld of the vessel. To prevent unnecessary overdesiccation of surrounding tissue, the low-voltage, undamped waveform (CUT/desiccation) should be used. It is important that the generator not be activated until the electrode is in contact with tissue. With monopolar energy, deep desiccation of the tissue in the grasp of the instrument, such as a hemostat, is uniform throughout the thickness of the tissue; with bipolar energy, the output characteristics are such that the surface is heated first, leaving the center of the tissue mass to be heated last. For this reason, most newer models of bipolar generators have a current flow meter (ammeter) to ensure that desiccation is complete, and most are preset in the CUT mode. If the tissue is too thick, the bipolar current may cease to flow before deep desiccation is complete; thus, if the tissue coagulated is cut, it may bleed briskly.

CUT techniques can be used to amputate large tissue pedicles with either monopolar or bipolar modes if the amount of energy is enough. The monopolar snare-electrode, common to intracolonic surgery, can be used to amputate an ovarian pedicle with ease and with minimal lateral spread if the power setting is kept low. In addition, time must be allowed to first desiccate the tissue to be cut. Then, by increasing the pressure to tighten the snare, the cutting effect of the waveform and the wire loop transect the tissue with ease. The coagulation waveform should not be used because, as previously mentioned, the voltage is increased threefold and the generator runs at less than 10% efficiency.

OPEN CIRCUITRY

If the surgeon keys the generator when an electrode is not in touch with tissue, open circuitry occurs. Because the electrons cannot move to ground, there is a pressure buildup of voltage. A water analogy would be holding a finger over the end of a garden hose with the faucet valve open. When the finger is released from the end of the hose, for a moment the water pressure buildup projects the water well beyond the point of projection when the current flows continuously under steady pressure.

In general, open circuitry should not be used except to initiate a fulguration of tissue or to start an incision. A common accident that occurs during routine surgery is when the surgeon keys the generator before touching a hemostat for coaptation of a blood vessel. Because of the high voltage created by open circuitry, especially in the COAG mode, the voltage drives the energy through the surgical glove of the person holding the hemostat. Before this was understood, the glove was usually blamed as being defective.

FULGURATION TECHNIQUES

The fulguration or COAG waveform is frequently used at the wrong time and for the wrong reasons. The generator manufacturers introduced terms that in the beginning seemed to simplify the waveform choices available to surgeons. For the most part, however, the assigned labels COAG and CUT have confused the surgeon about the science of their purposes. If the surgeon grasps tissue with a grasping electrode, either waveform begins to desiccate tissue. If, however, the tissue shrinks away from the electrode contact point, sparking (fulguration) occurs, creating surface char that acts as an insulator against deeper desiccation.

If an electrode is held off the surface of the tissue and the generator is activated, sparking to tissue occurs, sending each spark in a random fashion to char the surface only because the char acts as an insulator. Surface charring is desirable to stop surface oozing, such as liver bleeding of a venous nature. Because blood is saline-rich, a bloody field is hard to coagulate. Irrigating with a non-electrolyte solution or removing the blood from the bleeders by using suction improves the task. For arterial vessels larger than 1 to 2 mm, fulguration is usually not effective, and desiccation, staples, or ligatures are required.

Because the tissue effect of fulguration is owing to the high power density of each spark, the effect of a single spark is probably the same, independent of voltage (at least within the voltage range of current generators). Thus, during fulguration techniques, the higher output settings can be used with more efficiency, reducing the chance of touching the electrode to the tissue, which might cause an undesirable desiccation effect. It is this feature of fulguration that encouraged the development of the argon beam coagulator.

ARGON BEAM COAGULATOR

The argon beam coagulator is a monopolar electrode device that is housed inside a cannula through which argon gas is dispelled at 12 L per minute for open laparotomy and 4 L per minute for laparoscopy (Fig. 13.17). The ionization properties of argon gas flowing over the electrode enhance the distance the spark can travel to complete the circuit to the tissue surface. Because the electrons prefer to stay in the stream of argon gas rather than pass through room air or carbon dioxide (CO_2), each having a higher resistance to electron flow, the collimation of the sparks leaves a more uniform surface coagulation effect. These properties create a bright bluish hue to the sparks, which makes them easy to see and aim at the bleeding surface. The gas, expelled under pressure, blows the pooled blood away from the surface bleeders, making coagulation more discrete and efficient. Flooding the field with glycine while fulgurating the tissue adds another dimension to efficient surface coagulation (see below). To create the planned fulguration effect, the wand must move like a paint brush to prevent deep tissue damage.

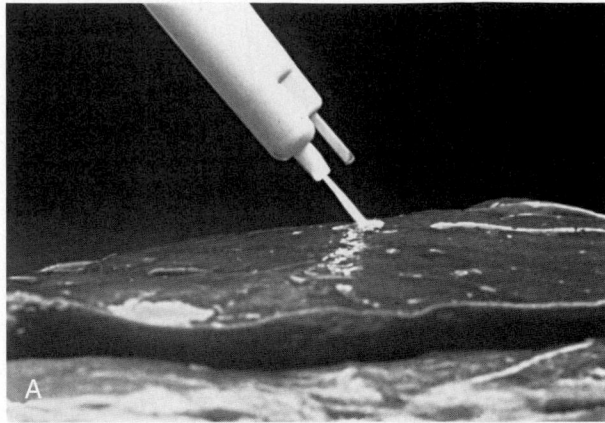
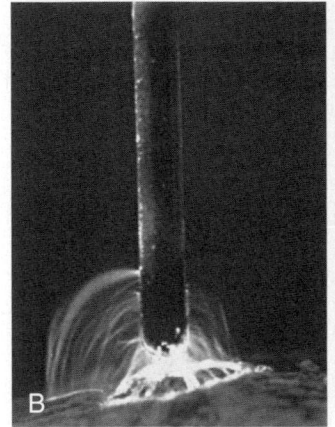
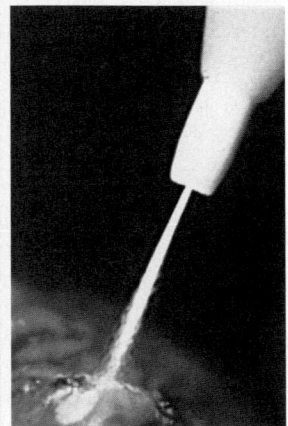

FIGURE 13.17. The argon beam coagulator enhances the electrosurgical technique of fulguration by injecting argon gas over a monopolar electrode inside of a narrow cannula. The ionization characteristics of the gas lengthen the distance a spark can be maintained. Because electrons choose to flow the path of least resistance, they stay collimated in the flow of gas, so the enhanced flow of sparks can be directed with efficiency. The ionized gas has its own unique blue hue that makes the sparks easily visible for accurate fulguration. **A:** The argon beam coagulator at work. **B:** Sparking effect of standard electrode (L) compared with argon beam coagulator (R). (From Valleylab, Inc., Boulder, CO, with permission) (See color figure 16.17.)

ELECTROSURGERY DURING PREGNANCY

No data indicate that using electrosurgical techniques in a pregnant patient has any untoward effect on the fetus at any stage of development. Owing to the dispersion effect, the fetus, bathed in electrolyte-rich amniotic fluid, is protected from any concentration of electrical current. Just as the radiowave frequency of all generators is above the faradic effect (the level that stimulates muscle contraction) for adult electrosurgery, the same is true for the fetus.

During a Caesarean section, the only concern is the accidental touching of an activated electrode to the fetus, which causes tissue heating. This does not mean that the usual technique of making an incision in the uterus would preclude using an electrosurgical incision, but rather that a "backstop" under the incision line, between the amniotic membrane and the muscle wall, should be in place. Although using a nonconductive material, such as a plastic suction tip, may seem wise, a metal ribbon retractor also can be used because it has a large surface area. Caution should be exercised when using the gloved finger of the surgeon as a backstop because if open circuitry is used, the voltage may create a hole in the glove.

VULVECTOMY

For a skinning vulvectomy, a blade electrode works well, but the pace of dissection should be deliberate and at an even speed, or deep desiccation can occur. The blade may be used to push the fat away from the skin, much like a snowplow. When doing a full-thickness vulvectomy, turn up the fulgurating waveform (COAG) and use a thick needle electrode to cut and fulgurate at the same time. At times, a bipolar thumb forceps can be used by an assistant to desiccate and seal individual bleeders while the surgeon uses the monopolar side of the generator for the incision.

NONELECTROLYTIC IRRIGATION FLUIDS

As with operative hysteroscopy and cystoscopy, nonelectrolytic fluids, such as glycine (a nonelectrolytic solution with pH 6.1, similar to lactated Ringer solution) and sorbital (pH 5.2) can be used during other surgical procedures to allow electrical energy to desiccate or fulgurate tissue. Blood does not mix well with these fluids, leaving a stream of blood easily seen in the nonelectrolytic fluid. Electricity seeks out the electrolytic-rich blood, and its ability to coagulate is enhanced because the energy is not dispersed, as it would be in an irrigation fluid, such as lactated Ringer solution. This is particularly helpful during microsurgical procedures and in attempts at surface fulguration of broad oozing surfaces.

To use the fluid properly as an irrigation media, the fluid does not have to be delivered under great pressure, as with some laparoscopic irrigation systems. A slow low-pressure flooding of the field helps in identifying the individual bleeders for pinpoint coagulation and fulguration. The flooding has a cooling effect on all fluids, so the power setting may need to be increased about 20% more than that needed for dry-surface coagulation. Within the fluid, as hydrogen gas is released from the vaporized cell, the surgeon's field of view can be impaired because of bubble formation. To prevent intravascular water excess, residual nonelectrolytic fluids should be removed from body cavities.

APPLIED PHYSICS IN LAPAROSCOPY

Because the tissue effect of electrophysics depends on the size and shape of each electrode, the chosen waveform, and the power output, the challenge facing the laparoscopist is to properly match and mix the electrodes and generators. For instance, because of the difference in the power density of the forceps as they grasp the tissue, a 5-mm grasping forceps desiccates tissue much slower than does a 3-mm forceps of similar design. A knife electrode can be used to incise tissue, yet when coagulation is needed, the surgeon can place the flat side of the electrode on the tissue and, with a CUT waveform, desiccate the tissue. Regardless of the waveform, a ball-shaped electrode desiccates when pressed against tissue, but if the surgeon holds the ball electrode away from an oozing surface and delivers a high-voltage coagulation waveform, the bleeding area can be fulgurated without deep tissue penetration.

As one electrode is changed to another, the surgeon should adjust the generator output to match the task at hand. This is especially important when needle electrodes are used after a more blunt electrode. If not, the tissue touched by the high current density of the needle electrode can be severely damaged, and passive heat transfer can destroy the needle electrode.

When bipolar instruments are used, if a coagulation waveform is used, a sticking phenomenon is common; in general, an undamped waveform should be used with bipolar instruments. When performing tubal sterilization with bipolar forceps, if the coagulation or damped waveform for bipolar sterilization is being used, the center of the tube may not be destroyed because the surface of the tube is charred too quickly, rapidly increasing tissue impedance. The same problem can happen when blood vessels surrounded by fat (e.g., mesenteric vessels) are coagulated with a bipolar instrument delivering a damped waveform; if the desiccated vessel is cut, it may bleed briskly. When using an undamped waveform, an in-line ammeter is a valuable accessory to ensure that all of the tissue between the forceps has been coagulated before the tissue is transected.

As with laser surgery during operative laparoscopy, smoke accumulation can occur if fulguration techniques are used; for the most part, desiccation techniques create steam. Smoke can be reduced or eliminated by irrigating the field to be coagulated with glycine rather than with saline or lactated Ringer solution because the energy can be applied while irrigating. If the surgeon floods the field as electrical energy is being delivered, the energy is not dissipated within the solution, as it is with electrolyte-rich fluids; in a liquid media, smoke does not develop. Several accessory instruments have been designed to allow the simultaneous delivery of glycine and electricity through an irrigation/aspiration cannula, which contains an insulated internal electrode that can protrude beyond the tip of the cannula. At the end of the procedure, any intraabdominal glycine is aspirated.

Glycine has another characteristic that is helpful. As the surgeon flushes the bleeding area, the individual bleeder streams through the irrigating solution, giving the appearance of red "snakes." The port of bleeding can be seen with ease and quickly fulgurated by using the snake of blood as a conductor. Unlike with hysteroscopy or cystoscopy, these nonelectrolytic solutions are not delivered at a pressure high enough to cause an intravascular infusion that could lead to a water intoxication syndrome.

In the early 1980s, it was thought that the occasional bowel perforation after a laparoscopy was the result of sparking or arcing to the bowel when electrodes were used. Because the physics of fulguration do not allow an arc to be maintained in one spot, it is now understood that at the worst, only a surface charring of the bowel could occur. To burn a hole in the bowel, the electrode must touch the bowel during the delivery of electroenergy and remain in contact with the bowel wall long enough to coagulate deep into the bowel wall. For this reason, it is best to disconnect electrodes from the generator when they are not needed for the delivery of electroenergy. To prevent accidentally touching the bowel with an active electrode, the surgeon should withdraw the laparoscope from the operating field before keying the generator, to create a wide panoramic view.

CAPACITANCE IN MONOPOLAR ELECTROSURGERY

Capacitance is a physical property of monopolar energy whereby two conductors in close proximity, each insulated from one another, can induce an electrical current from one to the other (Fig. 13.18). The amount of this induced transfer of energy is influenced by the length of the conductors (the longer the distance, the more effect), the distance between the conductors (the shorter the distance, the more the effect), the character of the waveform (a damped, or COAG, waveform increases the effect), and the frequency of the waveform (the higher the frequency of the generator, the more the capacitance effect). The operating laparoscope becomes a capacitor when monopolar energy with a high-voltage damped current is transmitted through a long insulated electrode, especially if the electrogenerator emits high-frequency radiowave cycles. Because the operating channel is eccentrically located in the shell of the laparoscope, thus in close proximity, the induced current in the shell can be 50% to 80% of that current flowing through the active electrode into the laparoscope shell (Fig. 13.19).

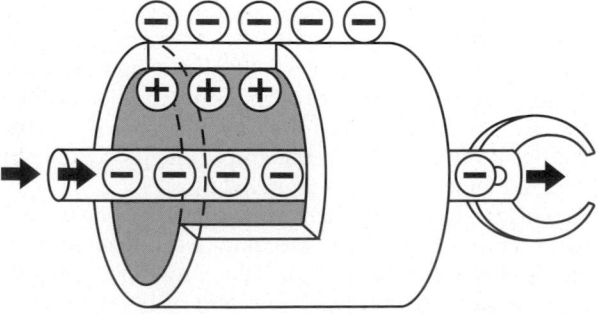

FIGURE 13.18. Capacitance is the induction of electrical current between two conductors separated by insulation; one conductor carries the active current and induces, by high-frequency radiowaves, a separate current in the nearby conductor.

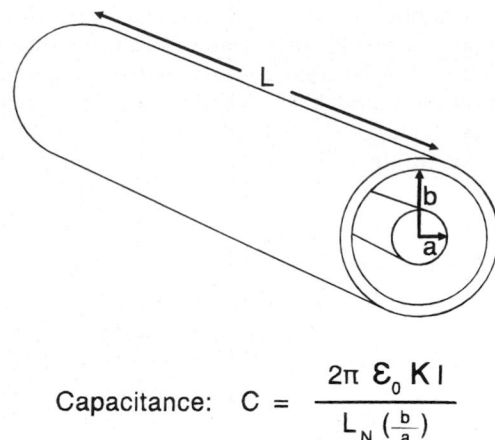

$$\text{Capacitance:} \quad C = \frac{2\pi\, \varepsilon_0\, K\, l}{L_N\left(\frac{b}{a}\right)}$$

FIGURE 13.19. Part of the formula that increases the capacitance effect in endoscopic surgery is the length (L) of the capacitor plus the diameter of the electrode (**a**), divided by the distance of separation or insulation (**b**).

If a metal trocar sleeve is used to transport the operating laparoscope into the abdomen, the induced current is quickly transferred through the metal sleeve, through the patient, to the return electrode. Because the current (power) density is broad (low) where the trocar sheath contacts the abdominal wall, no harmful heat occurs. If the trocar sheath is nonconductive (e.g., fiberglass) or radiolucent, or if a plastic securing collar is used (with either a metal or nonconductive trocar sleeve), the laparoscope cannot deliver the induced energy to ground. In this scenario, if a vital structure, such as bowel, touches the laparoscope (especially a small portion of its surface) while energy is being activated, the energy induced into the laparoscope can burn the organ; this may occur outside of the view of the laparoscopist. This same problem can occur when a secondary trocar sleeve is made of metal and uses a plastic securing collar (*hybrid laparoscopic trocar sleeve*), if that sleeve is used to transport a monopolar electrode. In this situation, the metal trocar sleeve becomes an active electrode by the capacitance effect. The best way to reduce this risk is to use all-metal trocar sleeves and metal securing collars; the next best way is to use all-plastic sleeves and collars. *Never mix plastic with metal.*

Unintended electrical injuries also can result from *direct coupling* or insulation failure. Direct coupling occurs when the active electrode touches other metal instruments within the abdomen, transferring the energy to the second instrument, which can injure tissue with which it comes in contact. For example, the active electrode touches the laparoscope, which then touches and burns bowel or other organs. The only way to avoid injuries from direct coupling is never to activate the electrode until the operative field is in full panoramic view.

Electroscope, Inc. (Boulder, CO) has the Electroshield, a device that eliminates the risk of capacitance regardless of the type of trocar sleeve used (Fig. 13.20). The device is a cannula that shrouds the electrode shaft and shunts all capacitance-coupled current directly to the

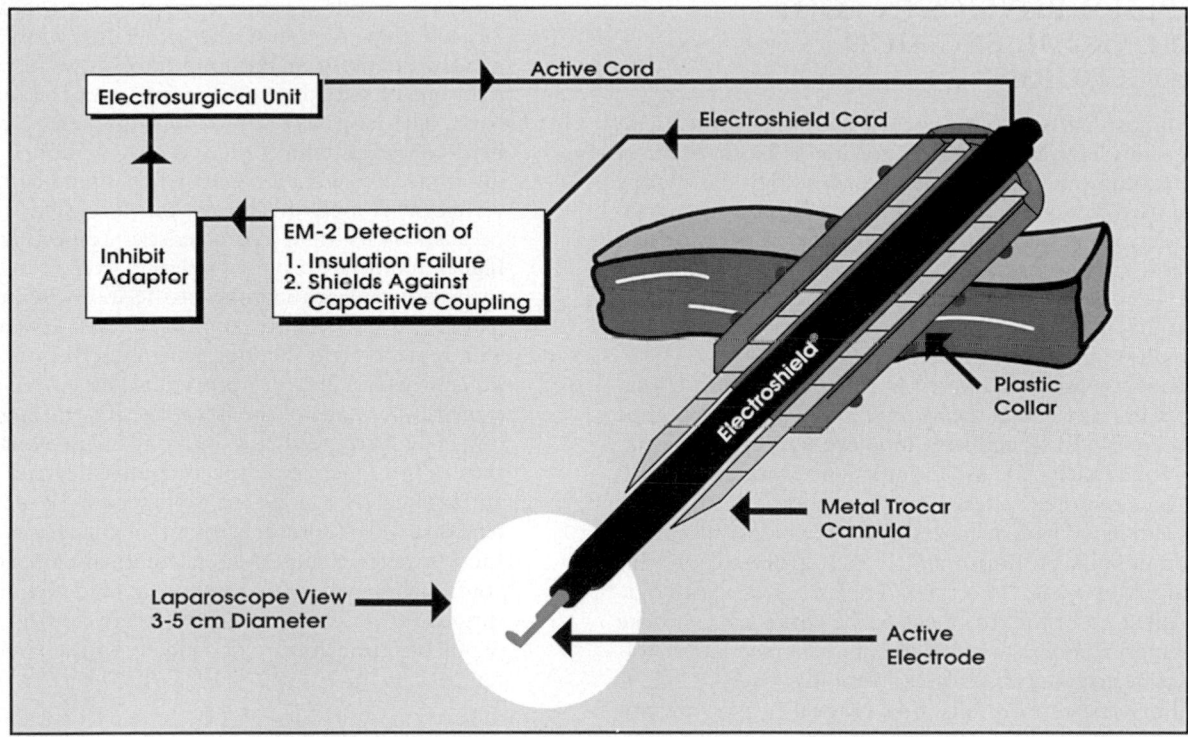

FIGURE 13.20. The Electroshield device eliminates the threat of an inadvertent capacitance injury during laparoscopy by returning the capacitance-induced current back to the generator. If an insulation breakdown occurs, it alerts the surgeon.

return plate of the generator, thereby avoiding transmission to biologic tissue. In addition, if there is a break in the insulation of the active electrode, which could promote direct coupling of the primary current to other metal instruments or adjacent tissue, this device alerts the surgeon with an audible alarm. Insulation failures occur when the insulation shield of the electrode is compromised from high voltage, abuse, poor handling, or mechanical accidents. The defect in the insulation, often too small to be recognized, can divert the full current from the generator to unintended tissue proximal to the end of the electrode. Sometimes, the defect is on the part of the electrode that is within the trocar sleeve.

ELECTROPHYSICS APPLIED TO OPERATIVE HYPEROSCOPY

With endometrial ablation, the resectoscope cutting loop and a roller electrode or coagulating loop are used. Some surgeons shave the endometrial lining with the cutting loop electrode; others desiccate the endometrial lining with the roller ball or bar. A few surgeons shave first and then "paint" the shaved myometrium with the roller electrode or coagulation loop. Unfortunately, studies on the tissue effects of different techniques, electrodes, and waveforms are few in number. Even the pressure applied to the endometrial surface changes the current (power) density; the more the pressure, the broader is the contact surface of the electrode, creating a de-

creased current density. Because the speed of passage of the electrode unique to each surgeon is another variable, only the outcome statistics can be evaluated with any reasonable scrutiny. Some surgeons use a coagulation-only waveform at a low wattage of 30 W; others report success with a pure cutting waveform at 100 W.

Our preference is to shave the endometrium first. We use a pure undamped waveform and drag the wire loop in a slow deliberate motion to a depth of 4 mm through the tissue, so there is some coagulation effect in addition to the cutting. By using the cutting waveform, bubble formation on the anterior surface of the endometrial cavity is less than that in the coagulation mode. We do not shave the lateral sulcus of the cavity near the uterine vessels.

During the painting phase, we continue to use an undamped waveform with a light contact of the coagulation loop electrode set at 100 W. Unlike the roller electrode, which can trap dead tissue in its axle and increase the impedance of electron flow, the coagulation loop electrode avoids that impedance. By not rolling, the surface of the electrode in contact with tissue stays clean, much like an eraser cleans itself. If the roller electrode is a bar or barrel, we either slow up the rolling motion or increase the power output, because the electrode current density is lower. At the end of the ablation procedure, we switch to a coagulation waveform at 75 W. With the increased peak voltage of this waveform, skipped areas are sought out by the electrons under higher pressure, ensuring complete surface coagulation.

APPLIED PHYSICS IN LOOP ELECTRODE EXCISION PROCEDURES

For almost half a century, circular and other shaped wire electrodes have been available for use as biopsy tools in dermatology and gynecology. In gynecology, these loops were used for cervical and hot-cone biopsies. After such biopsies, anecdotal case histories of severe scarring led gynecologists to choose nonelectrical methods of cervical biopsy by the 1950s. Although the rate was not established, infertility after hot-cone cervical biopsy occurred because of cervical stenosis.

Today, a renewed interest in electrosurgical wire loop biopsy has surfaced in the form of loop electrode excision procedure (LEEP) and large loop excision of transformation zone (LLETZ). As an outpatient procedure, LEEP or LLETZ surgery offers a one-time approach to a pesky problem plus an adequate and complete biopsy specimen. Made popular by British and French gynecologists, this excisional approach to cervical dysplasia gives a histologic confirmation of the treatment of the entire lesion, unlike the random approach of colposcopic-directed biopsy followed by cryosurgery or laser ablation.

The long-term results after cervical healing are not available. No publication has evaluated different electrode loops matched with different electrogenerators, exploring their thermal effects on the tissue left behind the remaining viable cervix. Performing LEEP procedures is a complete exercise in the applied principles of electrosurgery. The following features of LEEP procedures should be appreciated:

Electrode size: The thinner the wire is, the higher the power density, giving a better cutting effect. Electrode wires thicker than 0.20 mm in diameter can cause deep coagulation, up to a 10-mm depth, depending on speed of excision and waveform.

Waveform: There is an increasing depth of coagulation as the waveform is blended from a pure undamped waveform to a 50:50 ratio of undamped-to-damped waveform.

Power density: In addition to the diameter or gauge of the wire used, the size and depth of the biopsy must be considered. As the electrode loop sinks deeper into the cervical tissue, the power density, as measured by the length and total surface area of wire loop penetrating the cervical tissue, decreases rapidly, losing the cutting effect created by a high power density. To compensate for this change, the operator must increase the power output from the generator during the incision process *or* increase the speed of the electrode incision process. If the power output is adequate (usually at 60 W) but the loop is passed through the tissue at a slow pace, deep coagulation of the cervix may occur. When possible, it is preferable to use a generator with a low-output impedance because this keeps the energy fluctuations created by different tissue densities to a minimum.

Speed of incision: It is easier to increase the speed of incision than to adjust the generator with one hand while pressing the loop into, through, and then out of the area to be excised with the other hand. The loop wire should be rigid; a loop that bends or flexes reduces the speed of incision, leading to deep coagulation even when a pure cutting waveform is used. It appears that tungsten wire, because of its rigid characteristics (especially at higher temperatures), is preferred over stainless-steel wire, unless the yoke of the loop electrode handle can be shaped so that the stainless-steel wire remains rigid. Several generators that are especially helpful in LEEP procedures have been designed. They control the flow of energy through a low-impedance feedback by controlling voltage; the effect is much like a speed-control device in an automobile. If a constant voltage can be maintained at a given power setting that changes as tissue resistance changes, lateral thermal damage is controlled, giving the surgeon a predetermined surgical effect. Using constant voltage controls the depth of coagulation independent of the cutting rate.

Because the vaginal fluids are rich in electrolytes, the vagina and cervix should be rinsed with a nonelectrolytic fluid before biopsy; the acetic acid solution used during colposcopy is adequate. The generator should be keyed or activated *before* the electrode touches the tissue, and the energy should be delivered in a continuous mode until the biopsy is complete. If the operator turns the energy off during the excisional biopsy, deep coagulation will occur when the generator is restarted.

Care should be taken to not touch the metal speculum with the active electrode. Because the surface area of the metal speculum (in contact with the patient) is large, the current density is too low to cause a burn, but the effective frequency of the radiowave delivered through the speculum is altered to a much lower frequency, which may stimulate involuntary muscle contractions of the patient. This is not painful, but it is startling and disconcerting to both patient and operator. The use of an insulated metal speculum is preferable.

It is better to cut and excise with minimal coagulation during the biopsy process and then use fulguration, not desiccation, to control spot bleeding. Use a large ball electrode held close to, yet off of, the bleeding site, and switch to a damped (coagulation) waveform with high-voltage output. If the operative field is obscured with electrolyte-rich blood, reduce the amount of blood with suction during the fulguration process. As an alternative, slow irrigation with a nonelectrolytic solution (e.g., sterile or distilled water) also allows effective spot fulguration with the ball electrode.

Again, with LEEP or LLETZ procedures, it is best to choose a rigid loop electrode with a steady pace of transfer through the tissue to be excised. Choose an undamped waveform with minimal, if any, damped characteristics. A pure undamped waveform delivered through an electrode, transecting tissue at a slower rate, creates some coagulation effect. The latter is preferable to a partially damped waveform passed through a loop electrode that may "stall" because of inadequate power as it tries to pass through the cervical tissue.

NEW ELECTRODE DEVICES

Bipolar Vessel Sealing

Using a feedback technology called Instant Response, the type of tissue held in a bipolar forceps is diagnosed, and the appropriate amount of energy is delivered to effectively seal arterial blood vessels up to 7 mm in size (Fig. 13.21). The forceps are available in a 7-inch pean-style clamp, a 9-inch Heaney-style clamp, and a 5-mm laparoscopic Maryland-style grasper. The vessel to be sealed is grasped in the jaws of the instrument, and a calibrated force is applied to the tissue. Early experience in abdominal and vaginal hysterectomy shows promise once the learning curve has settled.

Bipolar Endometrial Ablation

The NovaSure Global Endometrial Ablation System consists of a single-use, three-dimensional bipolar device and radio-frequency generator that enables a controlled endometrial ablation in an average of 90 seconds without the need of a hysteroscope or hysteroscopic skills (Fig. 13.22). The device is inserted transcervically into the uterine cavity; the sheath is retracted by deploying a fan-shaped bipolar electrode that conforms to the uterine cavity. Unlike the balloon concept of other devices designed for endometrial ablation, vacuum is used to ensure good electrode tissue contact. This also allows removal of blood, endometrial debris, and steam, eliminating any uncontrollable steam ablation effect. A form of "pretreatment" of the endometrium is not necessary.

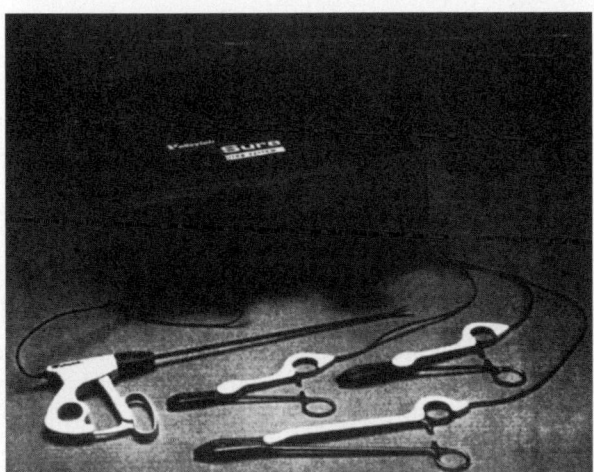

FIGURE 13.21. The LigaSure Vessel Sealing System with an assortment of bipolar forceps that can seal arterial blood vessels up to 7 mm in diameter.

The electrode consists of a conformable bipolar metallized porous fabric, mounted on an expandable frame. An integral component of the handheld endometrial device is an intrauterine measuring device to evaluate uterine cavity width. Once the length is evaluated by sounding, the values are keyed into the generator, which automatically calculates the needed output power to ensure a confluent lesion within the uterine cavity.

A perforation detection system is an integral part of the NovaSure System. Delivered at a slow flow rate and pressure, CO_2 pressure is monitored within the uterine cavity, with the generator sensing a maintained pressure over a known period of time. Once the proper pressure is maintained, confirming good uterine wall integrity, the generator proceeds with the ablation in an automatic or semiautomatic mode.

Using a constant power output generator, the maximum power delivered is 180 W. The depth of ablation is controlled by monitoring tissue impedance during the procedure. A shorter center-to-center distance between electrodes provides a shallower depth of desiccation at the cornual area and lower uterine segment, and a deeper ablation in the uterine mid-body. Once the tissue impedance reaches 50 Ω, or after 2 minutes, the NovaSure Global Endometrial Ablation System terminates the process.

Preliminary results in Europe and North America suggest that the NovaSure Global Endometrial Ablation System can be an effective method of endometrial ablation. At present, a Food and Drug Administration–approved multicenter randomized clinical trial is underway.

COMPLICATIONS DURING ELECTROSURGERY

The most common complication during electrosurgery is return-electrode burns owing to improper application of the electrode. Because these total two thirds of such electrosurgical accidents, each manufacturer provides specific recommendations for skin preparation and site application. Alternate site burns, such as to cardiac leads, usually result from improper grounding, use of too much power, and high-voltage application.

Intraoperative complications during laparotomy are rare. Following the principles of electrosurgery should prevent such occurrences.

With laparoscopy, claims of sparking to adjacent organs causing burns or perforation can be refuted if one understands the principle of fulguration. Because human tissue cannot maintain an arc as metal can, the tissue effect is one of surface charring without the consequences of deep penetration. An exception is the use of the argon beam coagulator, which if held in one spot can cause deeper penetration than that of the random scatter of high-voltage fulguration. Although capacitance, described above, can lead to a serious injury when unipolar energy is used, the variables that must be present are such that the incidence is uncommon. Although unipolar energy can be used safely, the surgeon must have a

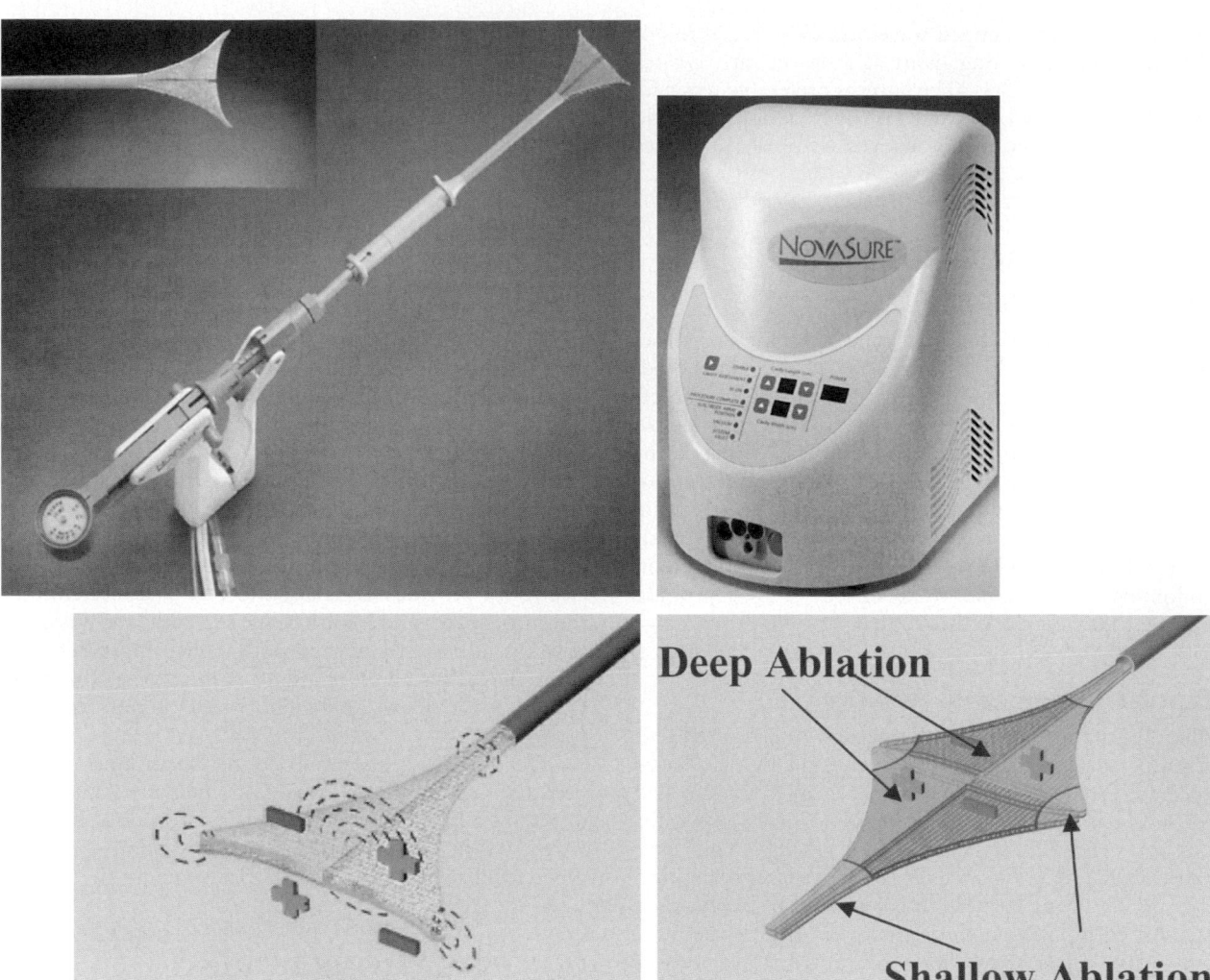

FIGURE 13.22. The NovaSure Global Endometrial Ablation System is a bipolar device for endometrial ablation using a metallized mesh electrode, vacuum for firm tissue contact, and a controlled generator designed to create a shallower depth of desiccation at the cornual area and lower uterine segment, with a deeper ablation in the uterine mid-body.

thorough grasp of electrosurgical principles. Bipolar energy, with its reduced power output, can give a false sense of security. If one studies the energy physics of each tool, the adage "a watt is a watt is a watt" rings true.

With operative hysteroscopy, uterine perforation with the active electrode is the most common complication. Using proper technique, never activating the electrode in a forward motion, can reduce this to only a few cases. Understanding the tissue effect of different shaped electrodes, coupled with the principle of using the lowest power necessary to perform the task, reduces such risks.

SUMMARY

Electrosurgery provides the surgeon with a wide range of options: type of current, power level, unipolar or bipolar systems, and electrodes of various shapes and sizes. With the proper equipment and a basic understanding of the electrosurgical principles, the reproductive surgeon can use electrosurgery in many useful ways. Faulty or improper equipment or a lack of understanding by the surgeon can result in poor surgical outcome and unnecessary complications. Just as physicians are expected to understand and prescribe drugs in a precise and logical manner, so should they have a working knowledge of the energy sources they choose to use in surgery.

GLOSSARY

Active electrode monitoring Technique of placing a sleeve around the electrode to detect stray energy and to carry the induced energy to ground. Stray energy generally occurs from breaks in insulation or capacitive coupling.

Ammeter Device that measures the amount of current flowing through a conductor at a specific moment.

Ampere Quantity of electrons that move through a conductor over time (coulombs per second).

Bipolar Type of electrode or electrical delivery system in which the active and passive electrodes are of similar sizes and, thus, similar current densities. The bipolar generators are usually calibrated against a 100-Ω load of resistance.

BLEND Term used when the electrical current is interrupted between 20% and 50% of the time.

Capacitance or **Capacitive coupling** Ability of two conductors to transmit or receive electrical flow while separated by an insulator; one conductor carries the active current and induces a separate current in the nearby conductor. In general, it occurs in monopolar circuits consisting of two metal plates or tubes separated by air or another insulator. It does not occur during bipolar electrosurgery.

COAG Term used to describe an interrupted electrical current. In some generators, the period of interruption of current flow can be adjusted from 10% to 50%. At the same power settings, the voltage of the waveform is always higher than it is with CUT waveforms.

Coulomb Measure of a quantity of electrons.

Current (power) density Surface area of an electrode in contact with tissue during electrical flow. The smaller the spot of contact, the greater is the heat effect for the same amount of time, increasing by the square root of the area of contact.

Current rate (amperes) Flow rate of a quantity (coulombs) of electrons.

CUT Term used when referring to a continuous or undamped electrical current. At the same power settings, the voltage of the waveform is always lower than it is with COAG waveforms or BLEND.

Desiccation Act of coagulating tissue *after* making contact with an active electrode. Either CUT or COAG waveforms may be used, but CUT waveform is preferable. Intracellular temperature stays below 100°C, which leads to cell shrinkage and dehydration.

Direct coupling Occurs when two conductive materials in the same circuit touch during electrical activation or are close enough that arcing can occur. A break in the insulation of an electrode that allows sparking to tissue is an example of direct coupling.

Edge density Affinity of electrons to concentrate at the edges of flat or irregularly shaped electrodes as they exit the electrode. This feature enhances the cutting ability of blade-shaped electrodes.

Electricity Movement of electrons between two oppositely charged poles, positive and negative.

Electrocautery Transfer of energy by heat, such as a hot wire. Electrons do not move into the affected tissue; only heat is transferred.

Electrosurgery Transfer of energy from an electrosurgical generator to tissue by means of energy packets (electrons).

Energy (joules) Quantity of work produced over time. Energy (joules) equals work (watts) multiplied by time (seconds).

Faradic effect Electrical stimulation of muscle responding to a frequency of electrical current that is less than 100,000 cycles per second.

Fulguration Intentional application of sparks to tissue surface to coagulate surface bleeding. The COAG waveform is preferable.

Heat (thermal energy) Produced as electrons move from the low resistance of an electrosurgical probe to the high resistance of tissue. This energy may boil (vaporize) or denature (coagulate) tissue, depending on the extent and rapidity with which heat is generated.

Hybrid laparoscopic trocar sleeve Conductive trocar sleeve used in laparoscopy that is covered by an outer nonconductive locking sleeve.

Impedance (ohms) Resistance to flow of electrons through a conductor. Although resistance refers to direct current through a uniform wire, such as copper, it is generally substituted for impedance. Impedance is correctly applied with changes in voltage (alternating or fluctuating), frequency (modulating or demodulating), or tissue type (lipid membranes, soft tissue, fibrous tissue, fat, muscle, bone, or artificial appliances). It can measure the combination of tissue resistance and capacitance. Impedance in human tissue is generally 100 to 1,000 Ω; in the fallopian tube, it is 400 to 500 Ω.

Isolation ground circuitry Safety feature that uses transformers not in contact with the parent generator so that the induced electrical flow "floats" its own separate circuit. If a break in the floating circuit occurs, all energy within that circuit stops and does not seek ground.

Kilohertz (kHz) Measure representing 1,000 cycles of radiowaves per second.

Monopolar Type of electrode or electrical system in which the active electrode is small (high current density) and the passive electrode is large (low current density). Most monopolar generators are calibrated against a 500-Ω load of resistance.

Open circuit State in which a generator is activated before the active electrode touches tissue. This promotes higher voltage, especially in the COAG mode, than activating the generator after touching the tissue. Open circuitry is used to start fulguration.

Patient return electrode (grounding pad) Large pad (low current density) placed on the patient to complete an electrosurgical pathway.

Return-electrode monitoring Dual-padded patient return-electrode system designed to monitor irregular separation of the ground pad.

Sparking (arcing, fulguration) Result of electrical flow through gas (air, argon).

Vaporizing Raising the cellular temperature rapidly above 100°C, which causes cell rupture, releasing steam.

Voltage (volts) Force (pressure) driving current.

Watts (work) Amount of work produced by electron flow (current). Work (watts) equals force (volts) multiplied by current rate (amperes).

Waveform Oscillation characteristic of an alternating electrical current from positive to negative.

Waveform frequency Number of oscillations of an alternating electrical current, usually between 350,000 and 4 million cycles per second in electrosurgery.

BIBLIOGRAPHY

Luciano AA, Whitman GF, Maier DB, et al. A comparison of thermal injury, healing patterns and postoperative adhesion formation following CO_2 laser and electromicrosurgery. *Fertil Steril* 1987;48:1025.

Luciano AA, Frishman GN, Kratka SA, et al. A comparative analysis of adhesion reduction, tissue effects, and incising characteristics of electrosurgery, CO_2 laser, and Nd-Yag laser at operative laparoscopy. *J Laparoendosc Surg* 1992;2:305.

Odell RC. Biophysics of electrical energy. In: Soderstrom RM, ed. *Operative laparoscopy: the master's techniques.* New York: Raven Press, 1993:35.

Pearce JA. *Electrosurgery.* London: Chapman & Hall, 1986.

Reich H, Vancaillie TG, Soderstrom RM. Electrical techniques. In: Martin DC, ed. *Manual of endoscopy.* Baltimore: Port City Press, 1990:105.

Voyles CR, Tucker RD. Education and engineering solutions for potential problems with monopolar electrosurgery at laparoscopy. *Am J Surg* 1992;164:57.

Te Linde's Operative Gynecology, ninth edition, edited by John A. Rock and Howard W. Jones, III. Lippincott Williams & Wilkins, Philadelphia © 2003.

CHAPTER
14

▼

Ultrasonic Surgery

MARK D. ADELSON

The technique of ultrasonic surgery for anatomic dissection and excision is not new. In recent years, sufficient experience has been reported documenting improved efficacy in performing surgical procedures by using ultrasonic energy. The effect of ultrasound on tissue is still being studied. This knowledge will help us avoid adverse effects by providing a model to predict tissue trauma.

The ability to preserve cell architecture is an important attribute of a surgical technique. Histopathologic interpretation of surgical specimens is often the foundation for clinical decision making. At times, this knowledge is required before surgical therapy; at other times, a histopathologic diagnosis is needed to guide or fine-tune surgical therapy intraoperatively. After surgery, the pathologic interpretation of specimens is used to validate therapeutic decisions and to plan future or adjunct therapy.

Blood loss has been reduced by 70% because the Cavitron ultrasonic surgical aspirator (often referred to as the CUSA) can coagulate vessels as large as 1 mm and can skeletonize larger vessels for control by other means. Tactile sensation is preserved, because the handpiece tip touches the tissue, unlike cautery techniques and carbon dioxide (CO_2) laser. Tissue does not stick to the instrument, as it does with cryosurgery and electrocautery. Visual control is maintained because the instrument continuously irrigates and aspirates, removing tissue debris. In addition, smoke is not produced and therefore does not obscure the field as it may when electrocautery and laser are used. Also, the depth of injury is significantly shallower compared with that of the argon beam coagulator (25 μ compared with 1,000 to 3,000 μ, respectively). This increases the margin of safety, reducing the potential for delayed tissue necrosis. Finally, unlike other techniques, the action of the CUSA is selective. Tissue with a high water content (i.e., tumor) is preferentially removed, and tissue with a high collagen and elastin content (i.e., serosa, vasculature, muscle) is preferentially spared.

In this chapter, the effects on tissue structure and function produced by ultrasonic surgical devices will be reviewed. The two dominant devices include the CUSA and the harmonic scalpel (often referred to as the ultrasonic dissector, the ultrasonic knife, or the ultrasonic scalpel). Discussion of surgical technique, indications, and results will follow. The final result will be an appreciation and understanding of the impact of ultrasonic surgery on treatment outcome.

BASIC SCIENCE
Mechanics of Ultrasound

The CUSA, a surgical device, should not be confused with diagnostic ultrasound. The ultrasonic irradiation produced by the CUSA differs in several ways from the irradiation patients are exposed to during a diagnostic ultrasound exam. The maximum power output of the original CUSA was 100 W, and the working tip of the instrument was 2 mm in diameter. This produced an energy output that was many orders of magnitude greater than that produced during a clinical ultrasound exam (25×10^5 mW/cm² versus less than 10 mW/cm², respectively). The frequency of the original CUSA was much lower, at 23 kHz (or 0.023 MHz), than the 3 MHz used for a diagnostic exam. The distance between the irradiation source and the tissue was much shorter (i.e., the source contacts the tissue) during CUSA use than for diagnostic ultrasound, so that more energy was delivered to a smaller volume of tissue. Another difference was that the duration of irradiation to a localized tissue region could be much greater during surgical CUSA use. All of these differences provided more opportunities to exceed the *in vitro* threshold for cavitation (3 W/cm²), resulting in tissue damage necessary for therapeutic effect.

Mechanism of Action

The *in vivo* mechanism of action on cells produced by this ultrasonic frequency continues to be studied. Ultrasonic irradiation has been shown to affect tissue by three mechanisms *in vitro*: viscous stress, heating, and cavitation. Viscous stress, or acoustic microstreaming, is a phenomenon of small-scale fluid motion. It occurs primarily in liquid or "soft-solid" media (i.e., in substances with a high water content, such as cellular cytoplasm found in living systems). It is thought to occur primarily at tissue interfaces between media of different viscosity, and results from the vibration of gas bodies or bubbles (micrometer size), giving rise to liquid or particle movement (so-called radiation pressure or torque). This results in a circulatory flow. This phenomenon occurs at lower irradiation intensities than does the more violent cavitation. It has been described in fruit fly larvae, in plant tissues, and in fish. If a critical shear stress is exceeded, cell-membrane breakage and hemolysis can occur.

Thermal effects occur when the ultrasound wave is propagated through tissue by a transfer of energy from the beam to the tissue (absorption) to overcome internal frictional forces. This energy is degraded into heat. The higher the frequency of the irradiation, the more rapidly the molecules must move. The greater the energy expended in overcoming friction, the greater the attenuation of beam energy. This results in poorer penetration of the beam into the tissues, and greater heat production. The temperature produced in the tissue is modified by tissue heat conduction and perfusion. More rigid tissues and those with a higher collagen content (i.e., more viscous tissues) absorb more of the ultrasonic energy, resulting in a greater heating effect. Absorption in bone, for instance, is 10 times that in soft tissue, which is 10 times that in bodily fluids. In addition, bone causes greater attenuation of the beam. Because the absorption coefficient is higher, the half-value layer (the distance the beam travels when one half of its energy is absorbed) is shorter, and the concentration of beam energy results in greater heat production. An additional mechanism of heat production, unique to bone, is the occurrence of mode conversion to rapid shear-wave absorption. In bone, both longitudinal (molecules vibrate parallel to the direction of propagation) and transverse (vibration perpendicular to the direction of propagation) waves occur. In contrast, only longitudinal waves occur in other tissues. One last source of heat production is that produced within the transducer or surgical tip, which is in contact with the tissue, from contact friction.

Acoustic cavitation requires the presence of microscopic gaseous bubbles in the tissue. This was first demonstrated *in vitro* by Hill in 1969 and in the guinea pig leg model *in vivo* by Ter Haar in 1982. These bubbles may be preexisting or may develop from preexisting nuclei by rectified diffusion. When exposed to low-frequency sound, bubble oscillation gives rise to fluid motion and highly localized shear stress in the fluid near the bubbles. When driven at resonance, the bubbles may intercept, reradiate, and absorb much more acoustic power than that which passes through their geometric cross section. This is termed stable cavitation. It occurs at moderate sound levels, and the bubbles pulsate over an indefinite period of time.

Bubbles can also undergo violent expansion and collapse, resulting in inertial (collapse) cavitation (formerly known as transient cavitation). This occurs only at relatively high ultrasound levels. As the trough, or rarefaction, of the ultrasonic wave traverses the tissue, the local tissue pressure decreases below that of the vapor pressure of the liquid in that tissue, allowing conversion of the liquid to gas. When the local pressure rises, as the peak or condensation of the sound wave traverses, the gas in the bubble once again becomes liquid and the cavity collapses. This transient collapse results in micropockets (a cubic millimeter or less) of high-temperature (many thousands of degrees centigrade) high-pressure (many thousands of atmospheres) cells, causing release of toxic products and disruption of the cell. Even though the temperature of the bubble region is so high, the bubble is so small that the heat dissipates quickly, and the temperature of the larger fluid or tissue area does not change. Suslick estimated that the heating and cooling rates during cavitation are more than a billion degrees centigrade per second. The intense heat generated decomposes water (H_2O) into the extremely reactive hydrogen atoms (H^+) and hydroxyl radicals (OH^-). During the quick cooling phase, hydrogen atoms and hydroxyl radicals recombine to form hydrogen peroxide (H_2O_2) and molecular hydrogen (H^2). As a result, organic compounds are highly degraded, and inorganic compounds can be oxidized or reduced. Changes to cell organelles and DNA can occur. Theoretic calculations predict that the pressure can reach 5,175 millibar (75,000 psi), and the temperature can reach 7,200°C (13,000°F). With isolated pulses of ultrasound, the probability of cavitation increases with the pulse length and decreases as the frequency increases to greater than 2 MHz (i.e., the frequency range used for diagnostic ultrasound). Millions of cavitation events can occur each second. Harmful cavitation-mediated effects have not been clinically noted with diagnostic ultrasound; yet, they are thought to represent the dominant mechanism of tissue destruction by the ultrasonic surgical aspirator and dissector.

Verdaasdonk studied CUSA-induced cavitation *in vitro* by using high-speed imaging techniques. A stroboscopic flashlight was used to emit a 1-microsecond pulse at 50 Hz for illumination of the tip, while recording the images in real-time video. In addition, Schlieren's techniques were applied to capture the cavitational phenomenon and to verify the presence of shockwaves. This was accomplished by subtracting the background light from an image, leaving light that interacted with the ultrasound probe. Using light flashes of 10-nanosecond duration at 5 kHz, generated by a copper vapor laser, density waves traveling through the medium at sonic speeds were "frozen" into an image. A transparent hydrated polyacrylamide gel was used to simulate soft biologic tissues. The start of the duty cycle for ultrasonic action on tissue was the hollow handpiece tip moving forward. On CUSA tip retraction (at up to 20 m per second), a cylindrical cavity was left behind as the water does not immediately follow the ultrasonic motion of the titanium tip. Next, the cavity fell apart into smaller, collapsing cavitational bubbles, because the water filled the "vacuum" left behind by the tip. When the tip slowed down toward its starting position, the smaller cavitation bubbles detached from the tip and imploded rapidly. The momentum of the water mass focused at the center of the collapsing bubble was associated with such extreme forces that within each individual bubble crater, a shock wave expanded at supersonic speed through the water. The centers of collapse occurred 100 to 200 μm in front of the rim of the tip. The selective tissue action of the CUSA may be explained, in part, by more elastic tissue (relatively resistant to CUSA action), only partially following the "low"-speed segment of the expansion and implosion, and deforming without breaking but remaining intact. Hard tissue does not deform but might be fragmented by the jet streams formed by the momentum of the accelerated fluid at the surface of the tissue.

In Vitro Cellular Damage

Because of concern about the impact of high-frequency ultrasound irradiation produced by the vibrating tip on the cellular integrity of remaining tissue, we initiated a prospective study. We tested (a) whether the ultrasound produced at the CUSA tip caused alterations in cell structure or cell physiology in adjacent areas, and (b) the suitability of tumor specimens aspirated through the CUSA handpiece into the specimen trap for clinical and research use, including the establishment of cell cultures. The structural integrity of CUSA tissue fragments also was demonstrated by evaluating sections prepared with hematoxylin and eosin staining for pathologic diagnosis by light microscopy. All CUSA specimens contained easily recognizable tissue fragments, in addition to cell debris and necrotic tumor. Histologic sections prepared from CUSA-trap tissue fragments were almost identical to those from the specimens dissected by sharp knife. Some mechanical distortion was present in a portion of the CUSA specimens, but this was not significant.

Flow cytometric DNA analysis confirmed that both surgical methods produced matched specimens, and that the CUSA material still contained the normal complement of genetic material. The index correlation between pairs was excellent. Assessment of initial tumor-cell viability (trypan blue exclusion staining) and of viability in short-term tissue culture verified intact synthetic and metabolic apparatus, without demonstrable damage from CUSA irradiation.

A major concern regarding use of this surgical instrument in anatomic areas supporting reproduction is the residual effect of ultrasonic irradiation on tissues remaining *in situ*. Tissue left *in situ* (i.e., adjacent to that removed) is exposed to even less irradiation than is the aspirated tissue, and if any injury occurs, it should be of a lower magnitude. This is consistent with our observation that tissue healing occurred without obvious scar formation when the CUSA was used for tumor reduction from intestines and serosal surfaces.

In Vivo Cellular Damage

The minimal impact on neighboring tissue has also been demonstrated *in vivo*, both histologically and functionally. Minimal residual tissue injury has also been demonstrated in studies of wound healing. Rader and colleagues (1992) compared the CUSA with the CO_2 laser by using a porcine skin model, which histologically resembles human skin. Tissue damage and wound repair were assessed histologically. The laser-ablated site immediately showed destruction of the epidermis, dermal collagen, and appendages. Adnexal and vascular damage did not extend beyond the zone of detectable collagen damage at the mid-dermis. The CUSA-aspirated specimen revealed that the epidermis was removed with destruction of dermal collagen and damage to appendages. In some cases, tissue destruction extended through the dermis into the subcutaneous tissue (full thickness). The depth of tissue injury with the CUSA was not different from the depth of injury with the laser. The lateral injury of the CUSA site was significantly less than the injury from the laser. Epidermal regeneration had begun by 48 hours in both the CUSA and the laser groups. All specimens were reepithelialized by 3 weeks. The peak inflammation, depth of collagen denaturation, and reepithelialization at 28 days were similar in both groups. No clinical difference in healing was noted.

Using a porcine model, Hambley and colleagues compared wound healing of skin incisions caused by a conventional scalpel, electrosurgery, a CO_2 laser, and an ultrasonically vibrating knife (10-W power; Energy and Mineral Research Company, Exton, PA). The ultrasonic knife incisions caused less tissue damage and resulted in more rapid healing than did either electrosurgery or the CO_2 laser. Scalpel incisions had the least tissue injury and fastest healing. The discrepancy between this study and that of Rader and associates can be explained in part by different instrumentation, wounding, and assessment intervals.

Albright and Sclabassi found that using the CUSA and monitoring evoked potentials when resecting central nervous system (CNS) tumors in children resulted in more complete tumor removal with less risk of permanent neurologic deficit. The CUSA dissection temporarily diminished the evoked potentials in some cases, although these recovered within 15 minutes. No neurologic deficit has been attributable clinically to CUSA use in the human CNS. Perhaps the limited exposure time and low power used clinically contribute to the lack of injury.

CLINICAL EFFECT

Instrumentation

The initial prototype of the CUSA was first introduced into clinical use as the Cavitron dental scaler (1949), which was used to remove plaque and tarter from teeth. The Phacoemulsifier was introduced in 1967 by Kelman for fragmentation and removal of cataracts. The more powerful version (CUSA NS-100) was introduced in 1976 for use in neurosurgery. About 30% more power was obtained from the model 200 Macro-Dissector (ValleyLab, Inc., Boulder, CO), which was introduced in 1986. The third generation system, the CUSA Excel, was introduced December 1998.

CUSA functions are controlled at the console. Aspiration, irrigation, and amplitude (power) to the handpiece can be adjusted incrementally from one-tenth to full power. A foot-pedal control contains the on-off pedal for vibrating the handpiece, in addition to a pedal for the fast flush mode. When the power to the handpiece is interrupted, suction is automatically stopped, and the hollow tip is backflushed to prevent suction injury to tissue and to dislodge any attached tissue (Fig. 14.1). In addition, the handpiece can be fitted with the

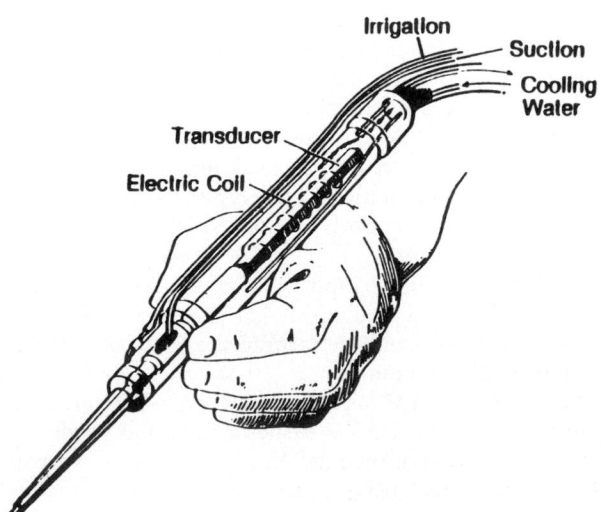

FIGURE 14.1. Diagram of the Cavitron ultrasonic surgical aspirator handpiece. (From Courtesy of ValleyLab, Inc, Boulder, CO, with permission.)

Cavitron electrosurgical module (CEM) hand-switching nose cone. This provides fingertip control of conventional electrosurgical cutting and coagulation, delivered through the titanium tip. The ValleyLab CUSA System 200 provides improvement in power output, electrosurgical capability, and the cavipulse mode. Cavipulse increases the safety of use in delicate tissue by intermittently interrupting the ultrasonic output, reducing the rapidity and degree of tissue damage. The cavipulse mode eliminates the need to reduce power settings. The cavipulse mode is replaced by the tissue select mode in the CUSA Excel.

An alternative to the magnetostrictive transducer for this conversion is the piezoelectric crystal, used by Sharplan Lasers, Inc. (Allendale, NJ), in the Ultra ultrasonic aspirator and in the Selector Integra ultrasonic surgical aspirator (Integra NeuroSciences, Plainsboro, NJ). The piezoelectric crystal, naturally occurring as quartz, is now a synthetic ceramic crystal (i.e., barium titanate and lead zirconate titanate). The crystal is housed in the hollow titanium horn, converting the high voltage to motion of the tip at a 300μ amplitude. Less heat is generated by this method, so a lighter handpiece and power cord are needed for air cooling only. This is contrasted with the CUSA, which must be cooled with water. In addition to a standard preset mode, the Ultra ultrasonic aspirator has a linear mode that gives the surgeon control over the rate of tissue fragmentation, which is varied by the pressure applied to the foot switch. The handpiece vibrates at 23 kHz.

The UltraCision harmonic scalpel (Ethicon Endo-Surgery, Cincinnati, OH) is a variation of the ultrasonic surgical aspiration device (Fig. 14.2). It uses piezoelectric technology. It consists of a knife blade that vibrates at 55.5 kHz, with a linear motion of 50 to 100 μ, depending on the type of blade and power level. In addition to the sharp hook, other tip options include a dissecting hook, a ball coagulator, and a coagulating spatula. Most recently, the laparosonic coagulating shears (LCS), a scissor-like device, has been introduced. These fit the laparosonic handpiece for laparoscopic surgery. Although little heat is produced and the bladelike configuration may provide better cutting action, the instrument functions like the ultrasonic aspirator (without aspiration) and provides a greater degree of hemostasis than the steel scalpel. Vessels up to 5 mm experimentally, and up to 3 mm clinically, may be sealed coaptively by denatured protein coagulum. The zone of thermal injury, charring, and desiccation has been shown to be less than that with other powered techniques. Vessels less than 0.5 mm can be coagulated and transected simultaneously with the hook blade (Fig. 14.3). Larger vessels must be coapted first with a blunt side of the blade, coagulated, and then transected.

The ultrasonic energy is propagated only in the direction in which the force of the blade or ball is applied. Hambley and associates studied wound healing after use of an ultrasonic scalpel in the porcine skin model, and Tulandi and coworkers studied adhesion formation in the rat uterine horn model. The lateral zone of coagula-

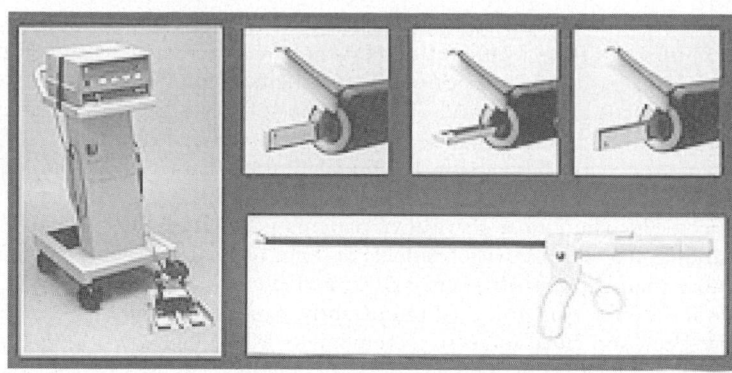

FIGURE 14.2. **Top left:** UltraCision console and foot pedal. **Right:** The laparosonic coagulating shears (LCS) attachment **(bottom)** and three positions of the tip of the LCS **(top).** The rounded, flat (maximal coagulation), or sharp titanium blade edge (maximal cutting) (pictured **left** to **right**) are rotated to oppose the passive (not ultrasonically activated) tissue pad at the top of the scissor-like tip. (From Ethicon Endo-Surgery, Inc, Cincinnati, OH, with permission.)

tion measured was 0 to 1,000 μ. No lateral tissue damage occurred when dissecting in a tissue plane. The mechanism of cutting is mechanical (e.g., the moderately sharp blade vibrating at 55.5 kHz) and cavitational. The mechanical action facilitates incision of high-protein density and collagen-rich tissue such as muscle, peritoneum, and fibrous connective tissues. Tissue planes are opened by the selective cavitational effect that disrupts low-density tissue such as fat and parenchyma.

The LCS was developed to cut and coagulate unsupported vessels more easily. This device consists of a stationary ultrasonically activated blade and a side-clamping tissue pad (Fig. 14.2). Cutting speed and coagulation are inversely related and are controllable by the surgeon. Power, blade sharpness, tissue tension, and grip force and pressure are varied. The LCS has five power levels. At the highest level, blade excursion (100 μ) and cutting are maximized, and coagulation decreases. Reducing tissue tension and grip force and pressure improves coagulation. In the experimental animal model, tissue injury and adhesion formation were greater and the rate of healing was slower with the ultrasonic dissector compared with the steel scalpel.

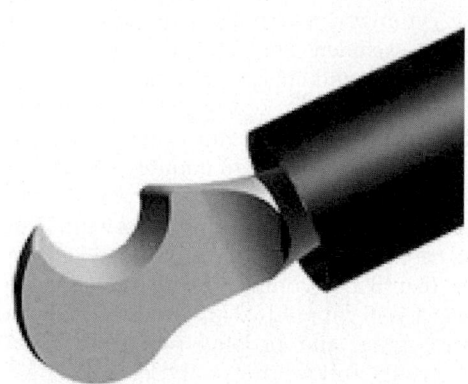

FIGURE 14.3. The dissecting hook blade attachment for the UltraCision. The sharp concave inner radius **(top)** is angled for cutting. The flat convex outer radius **(bottom)** is dull and used for dissection when more coagulation is required. The flat blade surface (widest side) is used for dissection and maximal coagulation. (From Ethicon Endo-Surgery, Inc, Cincinnati, OH, with permission.)

Schemmel et al. compared the degree of tissue injury and adhesion formation caused by the ultrasonic scalpel, the CO_2 laser, electrosurgery, and the sharp steel knife. Ovarian wedge resection and removal of the distal uterine horn were performed in New Zealand white rabbits. The depth and degree of coagulation necrosis was similar for the power techniques. Adhesion formation was the same for all techniques. In a letter to the editor, Miller and Amaral stated that the instrument was effective for myomectomy, showing a decreased incidence of adhesions and improved outcome in terms of fertility.

An instrument similar to the harmonic scalpel is the SonoSurg (Olympus Optical, Tokyo, Japan). The reusable SonoSurg scissors vibrate at 23.5 kHz, with an amplitude of 200 μ.

CYTOREDUCATION

Ovarian Cancer

In women with ovarian cancer, several studies have shown that survival benefits depend on the degrees of cytoreduction that can be achieved at the initial operation. Surgical cytoreduction is the removal of as much grossly visible disease as is possible. There are many theoretical benefits to tumor cytoreduction. The Goldie-Coldman hypothesis describes tumor burden in relation to tumor kinetics, genetics, and treatment response. The larger the tumor burden, the larger the cell population within the resting phase, or G_0, which is resistant to injury by chemotherapy and radiotherapy. In addition, a larger bulk of tumor has a larger number of genetically different clones, which increases the chance of having *de novo* resistance to chemotherapy. Cytoreduction removes the large tumors with hypoxic, poorly vascularized areas, which are relatively resistant to radiotherapy and into which chemotherapy agents may not diffuse. Also, because each treatment of chemotherapy destroys a constant fraction of the cell population, starting with a smaller population should increase the likelihood of killing all the cells. Fewer courses of therapy may then be required.

Clinical evidence of the benefit of surgical cytoreduction stems from retrospective and uncontrolled prospective studies. In 1983, Young and colleagues reported patients with residuals of 3 cm or less and residuals of more than 3 cm and demonstrated a differential complete pathologic response rate to chemotherapy of 69% versus 11%, respectively. The median survival of patients with a residual disease diameter of 2 cm or less, compared with those with a residual disease diameter greater than 2 cm, is 36 months versus 11 months, respectively. The 2-year survival of patients with stage III (abdominal) disease with residuals of 2 cm or less versus more than 2 cm is 40% versus 20%, and the 5-year survival is 20% versus 0%. Most importantly, patient survival has been shown to increase incrementally as the diameter of maximal residual disease decreases below 2 cm, approaching zero residuum. Hacker and associates demonstrated a median survival of 40 months for a disease residuum less than 5 mm, compared with 18 months for a residuum of 5 to 15 mm and 6 months for a residuum greater than 15 mm. In addition, the success of techniques such as intraperitoneal therapy and whole-abdomen radiotherapy depends on a tumor residuum less than 6 mm.

A more urgent reason to perform cytoreduction is palliation of symptoms. Removal of large masses distending the abdomen or compressing the periosteum or retroperitoneal nerves will afford rapid relief of pain. Removal of tumor compressing or encasing the bowel will improve the patient's ability to eat. Bulk removal of tumor will decrease the production of ascites, which in most cases will not return to presurgical volumes. This will afford relief from abdominal distention, gastroesophageal reflux, and early satiety and will permit more normal bowel peristalsis. After vigorous cytoreduction and removal of ascites, lower-extremity edema may improve, perhaps from reduction of intraperitoneal pressure on veins and lymphatics. Standard cytoreduction techniques, as reported from referral centers by physicians with specialized training and expertise (e.g., gynecologic oncologists), result in cytoreduction below 2 cm in 55% of patients (range, 23% to 87%). These techniques are reviewed in Chapter 48.

In 1993, Eisenkop and colleagues evaluated the importance of eliminating small-volume residual disease in patients with untreated stage IIIC ovarian cancer by using a variety of cytoreductive techniques, including the CUSA. This was not a study of the contribution of the CUSA per se. Villena-Heinsen and associates reported using the ultrasonic aspirator for secondary tumor reduction in two patients with ovarian cancer that was recurrent after aggressive surgery and chemotherapy. In 1992, Rose reported a retrospective series of 22 patients undergoing primary cytoreduction and three patients undergoing secondary cytoreduction with the CUSA. Pretreatment tumor dimensions were not given, and residual disease of the CUSA patients was not stated. The rate of optimal cytoreduction in a larger group of 45 patients, including these patients, was 86%; 48% of patients had a residuum of less than 0.5 cm. Five of 22 (23%) CUSA patients and eight of 23 (35%) non-CUSA patients required bowel resection, and two patients required bladder resection. The high rate of visceral resec-

tion (33% of patients) brings into question whether the investigators took full advantage of the capabilities of the CUSA.

Donovan and associates reported a retrospective series of 19 patients in whom the CUSA was used for cytoreduction. This study evaluated the development of coagulopathy in CUSA-treated patients, so few surgical details were provided. Five of 19 CUSA patients developed coagulopathy, compared with none of the 14 non-CUSA patients ($p < 0.04$). The duration of use of the CUSA correlated with the risk of coagulopathy ($p < 0.001$), although the relation between the CUSA time and the total operative time was not stated. All patients with coagulopathy had grade III tumors. Thus, coagulopathy may have been triggered by a paraneoplastic syndrome. Extent and volume of disease were not evaluated by Donovan et al., but increasing disease volume is known to be associated with increasing grade. In the correlation between CUSA time and coagulopathy, this time may simply be a dependent variable, the significant (independent) variable being extent of disease. In addition, the presence or absence of ascites was not noted; ascites is associated with coagulopathy. Patients with coagulopathy had greater blood loss and fluid replacement volumes, either of which could have resulted in coagulopathy, instead of being a consequence of coagulopathy. Although this retrospective analysis is severely compromised by small numbers and a lack of data and control, some laboratory evidence does support the hypothesis of increased coagulopathy risk. Ultrasonic irradiation can produce fibrinolysis and clot dissolution, as well as cavitation-mediated hemolysis *in vitro*.

van Dam et al. reported a randomized prospective trial of CUSA debulking. Forty patients with stage IIc to IV ovarian cancer were randomized to "ultraradical cytoreduction" by using CUSA (group 1) or standard techniques (group 2). The two groups were comparable with regard to patient age, tumor stage, histology, and grade and percentage of primary and interval debulking. Patients with liver or distant metastases (except positive pleural cytology), and those requiring emergency surgery were excluded. Standard procedures were used for organ removal, and an attempt at optimal cytoreduction by standard techniques was applied to both groups. The CUSA was then used in group 1 only, for a mean time of 22 minutes (range, 12 to 53 minutes). Ninety percent of patients in the CUSA group had cytoreduction to less than 1 cm maximal residual compared with 75% in group 2. No patient in the CUSA group had residual disease greater than 5 cm (compared with 10% in group 2) and 10% had 1 to 5 cm residual (15% in group 2). Blood loss, operative time, and hospital stay were lower in the CUSA group. Intraoperative and postoperative complications occurred half as often in the CUSA group (12% versus 23%, $p < 0.05$, respectively). Overall survival was better for optimal versus suboptimal cytoreduction, but not with respect to CUSA versus non-CUSA groups. Treatment cost per patient was lower in the CUSA group. Parenchymatous organ and bowel resection were performed in 30% of each group. Because of the small number of patients involved, the differences in optimal/suboptimal cytoreduction rates were not statistically significant.

Technique

The CUSA has been used in women with ovarian cancer for aggressive cytoreduction, short of visceral resection, at our institution since 1986. The goal of cytoreduction is to remove as much disease as is feasible so that no residual disease larger than 5 mm remains. Tumor that can be eliminated manually by blunt dissection, such as disease involving the peritoneum or surrounding the ovaries, is removed. When tumor masses include the small or large intestine, which often occurs by extension of the ovarian tumor within the pelvis, an intratumoral plane is developed to avoid injury to the bowel and to facilitate removal of the bulk of tumor, leaving reduction of the disease adherent to the bowel for the end of the case. Sharp and cautery dissection are used to remove nonvital structures such as the ovaries, tubes, and uterus; greater and lesser omentum; and accessible peritoneal masses, excluding the diaphragm. Retroperitoneal disease, such as disease beneath the pericolic gutters and in the nodal spaces, is removed by use of standard techniques wherever the risk to vital structures is not prohibitive, such as in the high periaortic nodes. Resection of the bladder, ureters, small or large intestine, diaphragm musculature, and spleen is avoided if possible. Hepatic resection is not performed by standard means.

After the surgical staging and standard cytoreduction are completed, the CUSA is used. The straight CUSA handpiece is used in all cases. The power is set at 10 for most applications, delivering the full 100 W of power output. In high-risk areas, such as over blood vessels and around the spleen, the power setting is reduced to three. The irrigation is adjusted to deliver sufficient saline to keep the field clean but to avoid producing visible spray from the tip. The settings range from 7 to 15 mL per minute, averaging 10 mL per minute. The aspiration is set high enough to keep the field clean by aspirating debris, but not so high as to lacerate tissue to be spared, such as mesenteric blood vessels or bowel wall. The aspiration is usually set at 10 in Hg (range, 5 to 17). A plastic Yankauer's tip attached to wall suction is needed on occasion.

The Cavitron generally is applied with a gentle stroking motion, in a plane parallel to the tissue surface along its long axis, such as along bowel serosa, vessels, or peritoneum. Depth of penetration is controlled both visually and tactilely. Occasionally, a plunging motion in and out of the tissue plane is used when the volume of tissue to be removed is large. Because very fibrotic tissue is relatively resistant to cavitation injury, it can be removed most successfully with a plunging motion in a plane parallel to and along the surface of the tissue to be preserved, coagulating this fibrotic tumor with the ball-tip cautery or argon beam coagulator before removing it with the Cavitron facilitates Cavitron removal. This maneuver is especially useful on the diaphragm and for ex-cising large masses from flat surfaces, rather than using the more tedious piecemeal aspiration of the entire mass. Hemostasis is obtained with standard techniques after vessels are skeletonized with the Cavitron.

When nodes are grossly uninvolved by malignancy, and minimal fatty and areolar tissue surrounds them, either blunt or CUSA dissection can be used. Nodes that are adherent to the vessels, grossly positive, or surrounded by an abundance of fat are removed safely and more easily with CUSA dissection. Cytoreduction is crucial to improve treatment response and survival for patients with adenocarcinoma of the ovary. We have used CUSA to improve cytoreduction in 58 patients; of whom 46 had adenocarcinoma of the ovary, two had mesenchymal sarcoma of the ovary, one had a germ-cell tumor of the ovary, two had adenocarcinoma of the fallopian tube, four had papillary peritoneal serous tumor, and one each had peritoneal mesothelioma, appendiceal carcinoma, and breast carcinoma. All patients presented with bulky disease greater than 15 mm in diameter. After the use of standard cytoreduction techniques (blunt and sharp dissection and coagulation), 53 patients still had suboptimal disease. After use of the CUSA, only four patients had suboptimal residual disease, whereas 53 patients had a disease residuum less than 6 mm in diameter.

Small Intestine

The CUSA was used to reduce the volume of small intestine metastases in 37 patients. To shorten the length of the procedure, the CUSA was used at full power in most cases. When working around high-risk areas, such as mesenteric vessels, the power was reduced to one third. A dragging technique, moving the handpiece tip in a plane parallel to the surface of the bowel or mesenteric serosa or vasculature, provides the greatest security against injury. Longitudinal and circular muscle layers can be seen as tumor is removed, if tumor invasion of the bowel wall has occurred. Defects left in the serosal or outer muscular layer were generally not repaired if the intestinal wall remained pink and viable. Deeper defects (including those down to or through the mucosa) that were caused by removal of tumor penetrating these structures were repaired with interrupted polyglycolic acid sutures. Hemostasis was obtained with cautery coagulation.

Thirty-four patients had epithelial carcinoma of the ovary, and one each had tubal adenocarcinoma, papillary peritoneal tumor, and mesothelioma. Thirty-one patients had stage IIIC disease; six patients, stage IV disease. Initially, 18 patients had small bowel disease (of any single nodule) greater than 15 mm in diameter, and 10 had disease 6 to 15 mm in diameter. After cytoreduction with use of standard means, 18 patients had disease greater than 15 mm in diameter, and nine patients had disease 6 to 15 mm in greatest diameter. After use of the CUSA, 13 patients had no gross residual disease, and 24 patients had disease 1 to 5 mm in diameter. The CUSA is invaluable for obtaining minimal residual disease of small bowel metastases while avoiding intestinal resection.

Diaphragm

The CUSA was used to reduce the volume of the diaphragmatic metastases in 33 patients. A midline incision was extended to the xiphoid process, if needed, for exposure of the diaphragm. Further access to the diaphragm was obtained by mobilizing the liver dorsally and by resecting the falciform, triangular, and coronary ligaments as needed. Standard techniques were used first, including manual blunt removal of the tumor and sharp knife and cautery excision.

The CUSA was used at full power. A dragging technique, moving the handpiece tip in a plane parallel to the surface of the diaphragm, provides the greatest security against full-thickness injury to the diaphragm. Muscle fiber bundles can be seen as tumor is removed. Very fibrotic tumors, and tumors invading the muscle that are subperitoneal, must be approached with a thrusting motion, moving the handpiece in a plane perpendicular to the surface of the diaphragm. In some cases, the peritoneum and fibrous tissue can be opened sharply or with the use of cautery to gain access to the tumor. Hemostasis in these patients was obtained with cautery coagulation.

Thirty patients had epithelial carcinoma of the ovary, and one each had tubal adenocarcinoma, papillary peritoneal tumor, and mesothelioma. Twenty-seven patients had stage IIIC disease, and six had stage IV disease. Initially, 13 patients had diaphragmatic disease (of any single nodule) greater than 15 mm in diameter, and two had disease 6 to 15 mm in diameter. After cytoreduction with standard means, 11 patients still had disease greater than 15 mm in diameter and two patients had disease 6 to 15 mm in greatest diameter. After use of the Cavitron, one patient had no gross diaphragmatic residual disease, and 30 patients had disease 1 to 5 mm in diameter. No complication resulted from cytoreduction of diaphragm disease with use of the Cavitron. The CUSA is invaluable for obtaining minimal residual disease of diaphragmatic metastases.

Spleen

The CUSA also has been used to reduce the volume of splenic metastases in seven patients. Our results confirm those of a smaller series reported by Patsner and Rose. Standard techniques were used first and included manual blunt removal of the tumor and sharp knife and cautery excision.

The CUSA was used at one-third power to reduce the chance of injury to the numerous hilar splenic vessels and the splenic capsule. A dragging technique, moving the handpiece tip in a plane parallel to these vessels and to the splenic capsule, provided the greatest security against laceration. Tumor invading the spleen beyond the capsule was debulked, leaving a thin shell of tumor to avoid bleeding from the splenic pulp. Very fibrotic tumors must be approached with a thrusting motion, moving the handpiece with short strokes in a plane perpendicular to the surface of the tissue. Cautery may be used as an adjunct to CUSA cytoreduction when the cancer is very fibrotic. Bleeding from minor abrasion or laceration of the splenic capsule was controlled by application of topical hemostatic agents and pressure. Injury to small splenic vessels was controlled with Ligaclips.

Six patients had epithelial carcinoma of the ovary, and one had peritoneal mesothelioma. All patients had stage IIIC disease. Initially, six patients had disease (of any single nodule) greater than 15 mm in diameter, and one had disease 6 to 15 mm in diameter. To avoid resection of the spleen, cytoreduction could not be performed by standard means. After use of the CUSA, three patients had no gross residual disease, and four patients had disease 1 to 5 mm in diameter. No complication resulted from cytoreduction of splenic disease with the CUSA, and splenectomy was not performed in any case. The CUSA is invaluable for obtaining minimal residual disease of splenic metastases without performing splenectomy.

Liver Resection

Hodgson (1979) developed the technique for liver resection in dogs and described it first in 1979. Schroder and coworkers compared the suction knife, CUSA, and Nd:YAG laser in liver resection in pigs and revealed a similar outcome for all three techniques. Tranberg and associates demonstrated the superiority of CUSA versus blunt dissection or Nd:YAG laser in liver resections in dogs. Putnam published the CUSA surgical technique for humans in 1983. In 1984, Hodgson described removal of a large cavernous hemangioma of the liver with use of the CUSA in a 52-year-old patient. Ottow and colleagues compared four different transection techniques in pigs: ultrasonic dissection, suction dissection, electrocautery, and sharp dissection. Ultrasonic dissection was the only technique that had lowered blood loss (because medium-size and large-size vessels were dissected free and ligated before transection) and a hemostatic effect on small vessels. The histology was preserved without necrosis and with a smooth resection line. Savvina and associates demonstrated improved hemostasis, the ability to preserve normal structures, and rapid wound healing by using an ultrasonic aspirator for liver resection in dogs.

Debulking of liver metastases from ovarian cancer is made possible by use of the CUSA. The malignancy can be removed from within the parenchymal liver bed, leaving a rim of fibrosis, with very little blood loss. Abundant literature documentation supports decreased morbidity and mortality when the CUSA is used to perform liver resection for a variety of benign and malignant conditions. Farid and O'Connell demonstrated a 71% decrease in blood loss, a 50% decrease in operative time, and a 50% decrease in hospital stay when the CUSA and the liver clamp were added to their routine. Segawa and coworkers reported on a series of 143 patients and cited a reduction in morbidity and mortality with use of the CUSA and the microwave tissue coagulator. Fasulo and colleagues reported a decrease in blood loss and morbidity and mortality, compared with conventional techniques, when using the CUSA for 34 liver resections. Andrus and Kaminski reported a favorable outcome in 13 patients undergoing segmental hepatic resection with the CUSA. Giordano and associates demonstrated improvements in technique and outcome with the addition of the CUSA and the argon laser. Storck and colleagues compared 14 major liver resections with a conventional technique to 14 resections with the CUSA; they demonstrated reduced blood loss, shorter duration of operation, lower morbidity and mortality, and shorter intensive care unit and hospital stays in the CUSA group. Snajdauf and coworkers demonstrated reduced mortality and improved survival when the CUSA and Nd:YAG laser were used for liver resection in children.

The harmonic scalpel was compared with the CUSA in a small study of hepatectomy for carcinoma by Ouchi et al. Reduced blood loss and shortening of the operative time was noted with the harmonic scalpel. The harmonic scalpel was used with less blood loss, safer isolation of bile ducts, and more anatomic dissection in 24 patients by Vyhnanek et al. Thirty-six resections were reported by Aliev et al. A new modification of hepatic portoenterostomy (Kasai operation) using the CUSA for biliary atresia was reported by Hashimoto et al.

Nerve-Sparing Radical Hysterectomy

Radical hysterectomy is the primary treatment for early (stage IB) invasive cancer of the cervix. In 1991, Yabuki and colleagues published an improved understanding of the anatomy of the cardinal ligament (Figs. 14.4 and 14.5). They demonstrated the feasibility of division of the cardinal ligament into the ventral pars vasculosa (containing the vascular and lymphatic drainage to the cervix) and the dorsal pars nervosa (containing the vascular supply and drainage for the rectum and the pelvic splanchnic nerves to the bladder and rectum). This ventral resection now provides another solution to the bladder (and rectal) denervation that occurs with a traditional Meigs' radical hysterectomy. Yabuki and associates compared 21 patients treated with anatomic dissection by using the CUSA with removal of the pars vasculosa to 20 patients treated with the standard Meigs' approach. They noted a reduction in blood loss and a shorter operating time in the ultrasonic aspirator group, and equivalent survival. Bladder function was not evaluated. Possover et al. performed this nerve-sparing dissection during 38 laparoscopic-assisted radical hysterectomies. Compared with 28 patients who had a standard type III laparoscopic-assisted dissection ("non–nerve sparing"), the nerve-sparing group had a significantly shorter time to return of bladder function (11 versus 21 days, respectively; $p = 0.0007$).

Although they did not use this same technique, Villena-Heinsen and coworkers reported a case of dissection and mobilization of the ureter with the ultrasonic

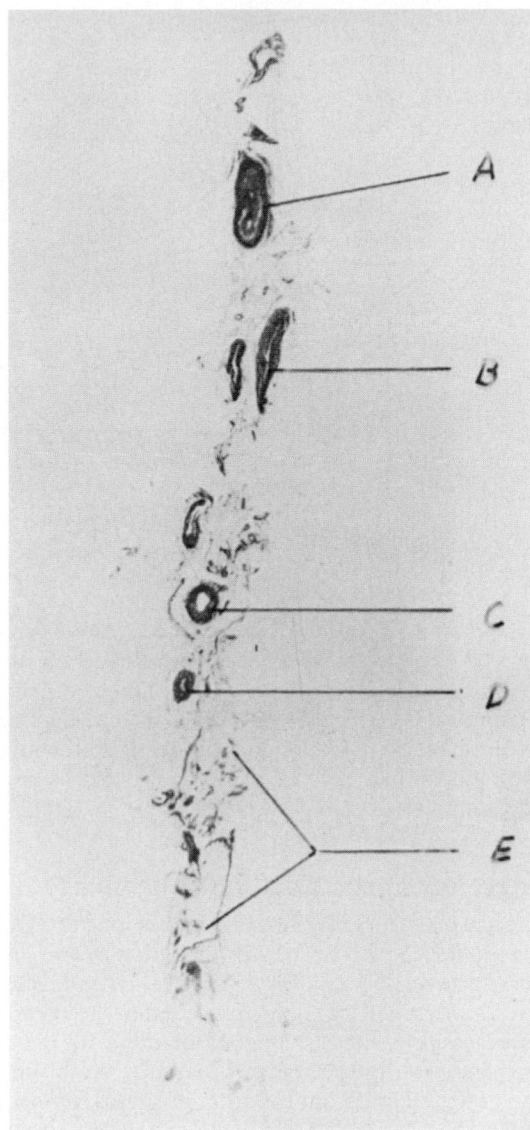

FIGURE 14.4. Histologic cross section of a resected cardinal ligament showing the uterine artery (**A**), deep uterine vein (**B**), middle rectal artery (**C**), middle rectal vein (**D**), and pelvic splanchnic nerves (**E**). Elastica van Gieson stain, H1. (From Yabuki Y. Dissection of the cardinal ligament in radical hysterectomy for cervical cancer with emphasis on the lateral ligament. *Am J Obstet Gynecol* 1991;164:7, with permission.)

aspirator during radical hysterectomy for a stage IIB cancer of the cervix. Shiina and colleagues evaluated vesicourethral function after radical hysterectomy in 13 patients in whom the CUSA was used and in 15 patients in whom it was not used. No mention was made of the surgical technique used or the role the CUSA played. They reported no difference in bladder function between the two groups. Szantho and colleagues reported good results using the CUSA during radical hysterectomy to remove parametria infiltrated with cancer; unfortunately, few details were given. Szantho reported 86 patients with cervical cancer treated with radical hysterectomy by using the CUSA. Niwa evaluated postoperative vesi-

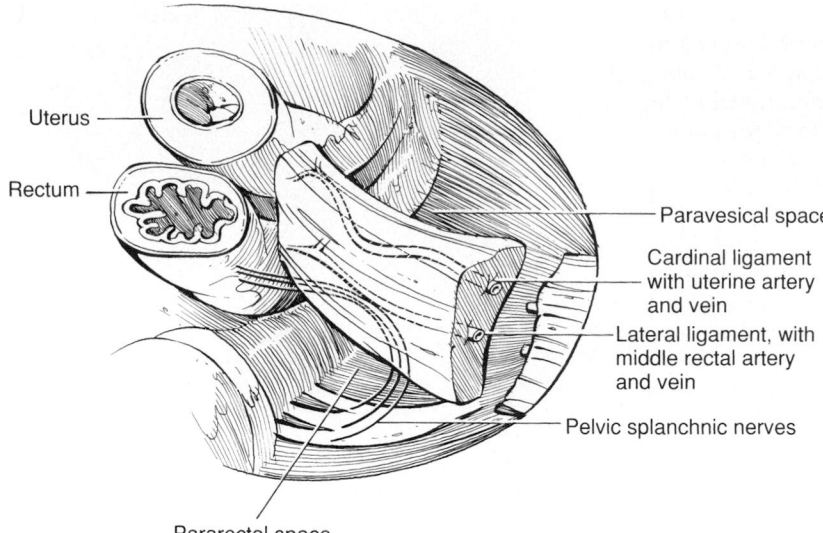

Uterus

Rectum

Paravesical space

Cardinal ligament with uterine artery and vein

Lateral ligament, with middle rectal artery and vein

Pelvic splanchnic nerves

Pararectal space

FIGURE 14.5. Diagram of the cardinal ligament and pelvic anatomy. (Redrawn from Yabuki Y. Dissection of the cardinal ligament in radical hysterectomy for cervical cancer with emphasis on the lateral ligament. *Am J Obstet Gynecol* 1991;164: 7, with permission.)

courethral function after CUSA-assisted radical hysterectomy in 275 patients. They found that the percentage of patients complaining of dysuria, the number of patients with abnormally large residual urine, and the number of days until recovery of bladder function was better in these patients than in those with surgery that used standard techniques.

Dissection of the Cardinal Ligament

The technique for ultrasonic aspiration of the cardinal ligament for the nerve-sparing operation begins in accordance with the standard radical hysterectomy technique as described in Chapter 46. After the pararectal and paravesical spaces are opened bluntly with finger or sharp dissection in the standard manner, the bladder is taken down sharply from the anterior uterus, cervix, and vagina. The uterosacral ligaments are skeletonized, repeatedly clipped (large clips), and transected. The uterine artery is identified, skeletonized, doubly clipped (medium-size clips) at its hypogastric origin, and transected. The ureter is bluntly and sharply dissected out of the tunnel in the cardinal ligament.

The ultrasonic aspirator is set at full power and applied in a gentle stroking motion parallel to the cardinal ligament. Dissection continues from the uterus, cervix, and vaginal wall to the pelvic wall, with removal of connective and areolar tissue and small vessels. The deep uterine vein, which can be identified at the level of the ischial spine, is removed. The dorsal limit of the dissection is the middle hemorrhoidal artery, which courses from the common trunk of the inferior gluteal and internal pudendal arteries of the posterior division of the hypogastric artery to the rectum. At the completion of resection, all vascular and lymphatic tissue draining the cervix is removed. One or two nodes are consistently identified at the termination of the cardinal ligament at the pelvic wall. These are sent for histologic analysis and are believed to be the sentinel nodes of the cardinal ligament, which are

positioned last in the chain just before the lymphatics enter the pelvic wall system. The blood supply to the rectum, and the pelvic splanchnic nerve supply to the rectum and the bladder, located in the dorsal portion of the cardinal ligament, are largely left uninjured (Fig. 14.6). The radical hysterectomy is completed in standard fashion without use of the ultrasonic aspirator.

Patients operated on by using the ultrasonic applicator had a shorter operative time, less estimated blood loss, and fewer transfusions compared with levels for patients whose surgery was performed with the standard Meigs' technique. Postoperatively, the median time to recovery of gastrointestinal function and the number of postoperative days until discharge was less in women in whom the CUSA was used. Voiding function and residual urine volume also were better in the group of patients treated with the nerve-sparing technique.

Retroperitoneal Lymphadenectomy

For lymphadenectomy, the Cavitron is used in a gentle stroking motion in a direction parallel to the vessels. Movement in a piston motion perpendicular to the vessels should be avoided, because vessel injury (especially venous) may occur. Generally, full power is used, but reduced power (decreased up to two thirds) should be considered for small vessels and when working over veins, especially the inferior vena cava. Control of small vessels and lymphatics, after ultrasonic skeletonization, is obtained with the use of cautery or medium clips. The dissection is often assisted by retracting pelvic vessels with a vein retractor, and by distracting the nodal specimen by holding it with a right-angled camp (Fig. 14.7). Great care should be taken when dissecting over the right common iliac vein and the vena cava. Small perforating veins often course at right angles from these vessels into the underside of the nodal pad. Avulsion can occur, resulting in laceration of the vessel and profuse bleeding.

FIGURE 14.6. Completion of resection of the ventral part of the right cardinal ligament. The uterine artery has been transected, and two medium clips can be seen on the stump of the uterine artery, next to the origin of the superior vesical artery coursing to the upper left. The inferior vesical artery runs to the left at the edge of the narrow Deaver retractor. The middle rectal artery can be seen medially, with its origin just under and cephalad to the uterine artery. In the curved tonsil clamp is the sentinel node, which has just been removed from the lateral extent of the cardinal ligament at the right pelvic wall, lateral and deep to the hypogastric vessels. The bifurcation of the right common iliac artery into the external and internal iliac arteries can be seen between the fourth and fifth fingers.

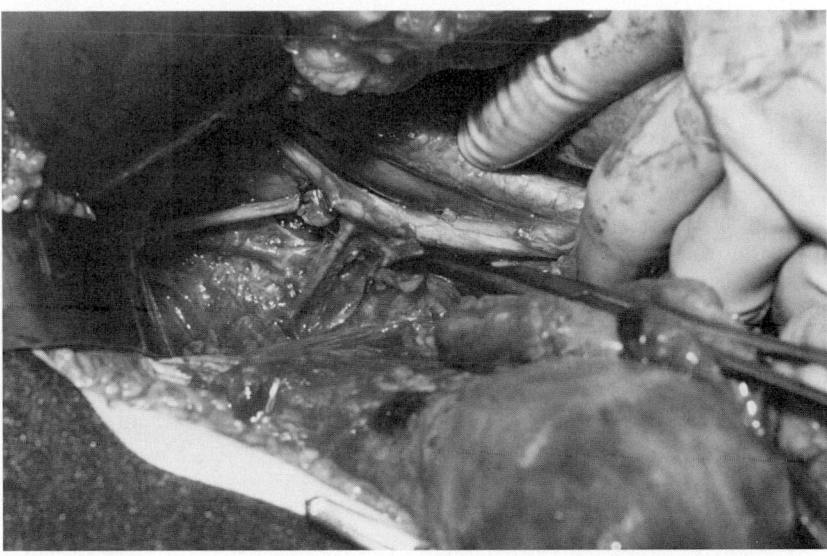

VULVAR CANCER

Intraepithelial Neoplasia

In 1991, Rader and colleagues evaluated the CUSA as a cytoreductive modality to treat vulvar intraepithelial neoplasia (VIN). Ultrasonic removal of the epithelium of the vulvar lesions was performed in 18 patients with condyloma, and in nine patients with VIN, under general anesthesia. Repeated passes over the tissue were required to obtain a depth of removal of 2 to 2.5 mm. Recurrent or persistent disease was diagnosed in 22% of patients, although the true persistence-recurrence rate may have been higher because colposcopy was not used for follow-up. The histology of the tissue removed was adequate in most cases, and all patients had a good cosmetic result.

Complete preoperative assessment by colposcopy and adequate biopsy is essential when this technique is used because the shallow and fragmented nature of the CUSA-obtained biopsy specimens may render them insufficient to diagnose invasive malignancy. Obtaining an adequate depth of tissue removal is also important. We demonstrated that a depth of destruction of up to 2.5 mm was required when using the laser to encompass 95% of appendageal disease from vulvar intraepithelial neoplasia. Laser vaporization of condyloma and VIN is precise and highly effective, and any new technique should be compared with this in a randomized prospective fashion.

Radical Vulvectomy and Inguinal Lymphadenectomy

We have found no advantage to using the CUSA for vulvar dissection compared with knife or electrosurgical resection. However, Patsner reported CUSA resection of massive recurrent vulvar cancer to facilitate surgical removal and rotational flap repair. We debulked

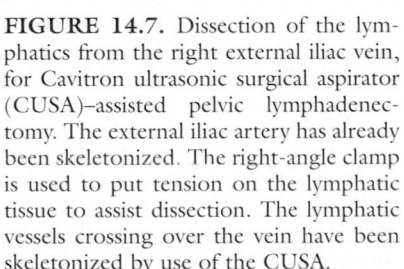

FIGURE 14.7. Dissection of the lymphatics from the right external iliac vein, for Cavitron ultrasonic surgical aspirator (CUSA)–assisted pelvic lymphadenectomy. The external iliac artery has already been skeletonized. The right-angle clamp is used to put tension on the lymphatic tissue to assist dissection. The lymphatic vessels crossing over the vein have been skeletonized by use of the CUSA.

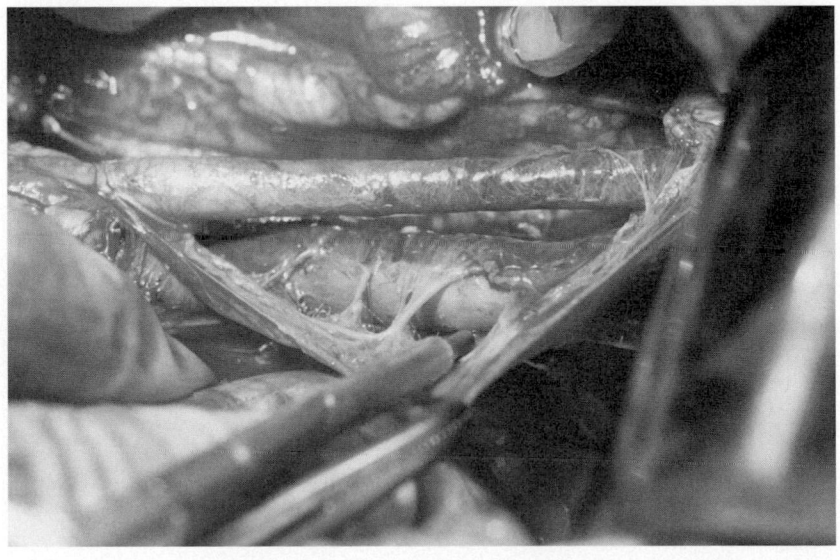

malignant/necrotic vulvar tissue in two patients. The first had recurrent vulvar cancer after prior surgery involving the anus. The CUSA was used to aspirate/dissect all gross disease, including disease involving the anus. The rectal sphincter was preserved by using this technique. Interstitial template radiation was then used. The second patient had been treated by primary surgery for vulvar cancer. A secondary excision was followed by radiation for recurrent disease. The CUSA was used to debride necrotic tissue that persisted despite conservative treatment. The perirectal tissues were also involved. The rectal wall and sphincter were skeletonized and preserved. The histology of multiple biopsies and the CUSA-aspirated fluid fragments were benign. The wound was left to heal by granulation.

Inguinal Lymphadenectomy

We have found the ultrasonic aspirator useful in performing inguinal lymphadenectomy. The technique has been shown to result in less thermal and mechanical tissue damage than that of standard lymphadenectomy. It has also been shown to permit precise tissue dissection and sparing of vessels.

The operation begins with an 8-cm inguinal skin incision made along Langer lines or within 1 cm of the inguinal crease. The scalpel is used to incise the skin and Scarpa fascia. The CUSA is used to dissect nodal tissue from surrounding structures. The CUSA power is set from 70% to 100%. An attempt is made to spare all superficial vessels (e.g., external pudendal, superficial epigastric, superficial circumflex iliac) and the saphenous vein. Fat surrounding the nodes is removed by the CUSA, resulting in dissection and skeletonization of the nodes. Afferent and efferent lymphatic vessels are skeletonized with the CUSA. They are controlled with unipolar coagulation or small or medium titanium clips. Clamping and tying of pedicles is not performed (Fig. 14.8).

OBSTETRICS

Lopoo et al. reported two cases of umbilical cord transection for selective termination of a monochorionic twin. This was performed under ultrasonic guidance via one trocar by using the harmonic scalpel.

ULTRASONIC DEBRIDEMENT

Debridement of necrotic, fibrinoid, and infected tissue is often difficult because of the bleeding that results and the delicate nature of the inflamed or infected underlying tissue. Successful use of an ultrasonic device for debridement is predicted by analyzing the histologic effect and susceptibility to enzymatic digestion. We have successfully debrided extensive fibrinoid exudate from pelvic visceral serosa and peritoneum in patients with pelvic inflammatory disease. This technique permits complete removal of the infected devitalized tissue without injury to underlying viable tissue. Ultrasonic aspiration of purulent soft-tissue cavities in children, suppurative wounds in diabetic patients, and trophic ulcers of the lower extremities has been reported. More rapid healing was noted with this technique than with conventional methods.

LAPAROSCOPIC APPLICATIONS

Grochmal and associates reported several gynecologic laparoscopic uses. They performed pelvic adhesiolysis in six cases and presacral neurectomy in 11 cases, taking advantage of the dissection capabilities of ultrasonic aspiration. In 17 of 21 cases of laparoscopic hysterectomy, they were able to identify and dissect the uterine artery, and in seven of these, they dissected the ureter to the psoas muscle. In 15 cases of endometriosis, the instrument was helpful in extracting small superficial peritoneal and uterosacral implants less than 5 mm in diameter. They

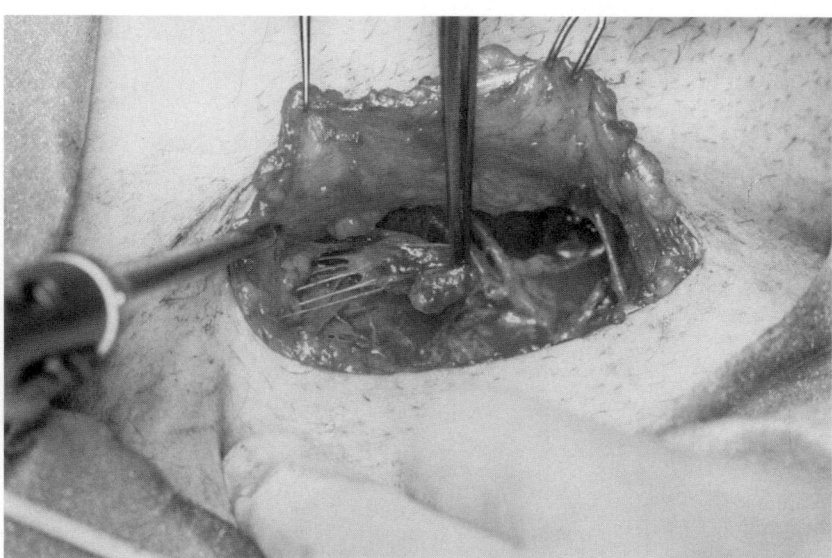

FIGURE 14.8. Superficial left inguinal lymphadenectomy performed with the Cavitron ultrasonic surgical aspirator. A bundle of dissected nodes is grasped by the forceps, still attached by the skeletonized lymphatic vessels. Preserved superficial epigastric vessels (crossing under the forceps) and superficial circumflex artery (at right edge of incision) can be seen. The superficial pudendal artery is not yet dissected.

encountered difficulty with lesions larger than 5 mm and with those that were flat and plaquelike. Vasquez reported successful ablation of endometriosis in 15 patients by using the CUSA. Robbins reported on 14 patients who had excision of endometriosis by using the harmonic scalpel. Stefanidis reported 30 cases of laparoscopic tubal sterilization with the harmonic scalpel without complication. The average operative time was 7 minutes. Four cases of laparoscopic excision of interstitial pregnancy by using the harmonic scalpel were reported by Dalkalitsis et al. Laparoscopic myomectomy using the harmonic scalpel was reported in 25 consecutive cases by Stringer, who noted improved hemostasis and less tissue sticking to the instrument compared with electrosurgical methods. Laparoscopic Burch procedure for stress urinary incontinence using the harmonic scalpel for dissection of the space of Retzius was performed in 50 patients. This resulted in a bloodless dissection.

Laparoscopic-assisted vaginal and total laparoscopic hysterectomy with the harmonic scalpel have been reported in 10 papers, comprising more than 80 patients. Laparoscopic supracervical hysterectomy with the harmonic scalpel has been reported in two papers describing 19 cases. Richards compared laparoscopic supracervical hysterectomy with the harmonic scalpel and Endostapler. He found that both instruments resulted in similar outcomes, but the harmonic scalpel resulted in less patient cost. Holub et al. reported a randomized study of laparoscopic hysterectomy with the harmonic scalpel (36 patients) and electrosurgery. They found no significant differences in intraoperative and postoperative variables. Electrosurgery was superior to the harmonic scalpel in cases of larger fibroids and in cost effectiveness. The advantages of the ultrasonic technique included better visualization and less charring and plume. Minami et al. reported the first two cases of laparoscopic hysterectomy/oophorectomy with the harmonic scalpel for pyometra in dogs.

DISADVANTAGES

The disadvantages of the CUSA for cytoreduction are few. The technique can be tedious because of the small diameter of the handpiece tip. Even though the length of time the CUSA must be used is short, operator fatigue is often high at the end of an aggressive cytoreduction surgery, when the CUSA would be used to complete the cytoreduction. The same is true for the harmonic scalpel technique, which is generally slower than other standard techniques.

An additional concern is that cells contained within the Cavitron specimen that is aspirated into the suction trap are viable, as demonstrated by Thompson and associates for ovarian cancer cells, by Oosterhuis and colleagues for Lewis lung carcinoma grown in mice, and by Oakes and coworkers for medulloblastoma. It is likely, then, that cells in the spray thrown off by the tip also contain viable cells. This spray can often be seen grossly. Nahhas demonstrated cytologically intact ovarian cancer

cells within this spray. In contrast, Nduka et al. assessed the viability of colon cancer cells grown in mice, generated by an ultrasonically activated scalpel and by electrosurgery. They demonstrated no viable cells from the plume of either device, by using either trypan blue staining or *in vitro* culture. Ott et al. also confirmed the presence of blood and tissue particles of respirable size in the plume of the harmonic scalpel.

The potential of hepatitis transmission has been reported. Matsumata and associates demonstrated hepatitis B surface antigen in the aspirated irrigating solution of seven of eight patients with hepatocellular carcinoma, at almost the same level as that in the patients' serum, when the CUSA was used for liver surgery. Higashi and colleagues demonstrated hepatitis C virus RNA in the irrigating solution aspirated by an ultrasonic dissector that was used in liver surgery in 12 seropositive patients. The potential risk to operating personnel might be reduced by the appropriate use of protective eyewear or a face shield attached to the surgical mask. Use of an efficient smoke/plume evacuator should be considered. Of even greater concern to the operator is the potential for infective human immunodeficiency virus (HIV) or human papillomavirus DNA that could be carried in the spray.

CONCLUSION

The addition of ultrasonic tissue aspiration, dissection, and excision enriches our armamentarium of standard surgical techniques. The patient benefits from lowered morbidity and mortality. In some cases, lowered blood loss may be the tangible benefit, or there may be a reduction in injury of normal tissue. Subjective and objective improvements in recovery often occur. Survival owing to improved response to adjunctive treatment may be attained.

The surgeon must be well versed in whichever technique might prove most beneficial to the patient in any given situation. At times, a marriage of techniques, such as sharp and blunt resection augmented with CUSA dissection and argon beam coagulation, may be most beneficial. It has been said that a miracle is simply an occurrence that we do not completely understand and is not completely studied. Only with an open and questioning mind can we find new treatments or adapt treatments used in other specialties to improve the outcome of gynecologic care.

BIBLIOGRAPHY

Adelson MD. The pelvic mass and ovarian cancer. Surgical techniques for the treatment of gynecologic malignancy. *Clin Pract Gynecol* 1991;3:105.

Adelson MD. Ultrasonic surgical aspirator in the treatment of vulvar disease. *Obstet Gynecol* 1991;78:477.

Adelson MD. Avoidance of splenectomy by cytoreduction of splenic metastases using the Cavitron ultrasonic surgical aspirator. *J Reprod Med* 1992;37:917.

Adelson MD. The Cavitron ultrasonic surgical aspirator in gynecologic oncology: ovarian cancer. In: Gershenson DM, ed. *Advances in gynecologic oncology*. Philadelphia: WB Saunders, 1992:84.

Adelson MD. Future directions in the surgical management of ovarian carcinoma. In: Rubin SC, Sutton GP, eds. *Ovarian cancer.* New York: McGraw-Hill, 1993:465.

Adelson MD. The role of laparoscopy in the gynecologic oncology patient. In: Rock JA, Faro S, Gant NF, et al., eds. *Advances in obstetrics and gynecology,* Vol. 1. Chicago: Mosby–Year Book, 1994:283.

Adelson MD. Cytoreduction of intraperitoneal malignancy using the Cavitron ultrasonic surgical aspirator: I. Technique and efficacy. 2000 (in preparation).

Adelson MD. Nerve-sparing radical hysterectomy using the ultrasonic aspirator. 2000 (in preparation).

Adelson MD. Cytoreduction of diaphragmatic metastases using the Cavitron Ultrasonic Surgical Aspirator. *Gynecol Oncol* 1991;41:220–222.

Adelson MD. Cytoreduction of small intestine metastases using the Cavitron Ultrasonic Surgical Aspirator. *J Gynecol Surg* 1995;11:197–200.

Adelson MD. The ultrasonic aspiration technique for inguinal lymphadenectomy. 2000 (in preparation).

Adelson MD, Baggish MS, Seifer DB, et al. Cytoreduction of ovarian cancer with the Cavitron ultrasonic surgical aspirator. *Obstet Gynecol* 1988;72:140.

Adelson MD, Jozefczyk MA. Cytoreduction of peritoneal mesothelioma using the Cavitron Ultrasonic Surgical Aspirator. *J Gynecol Surg* 1992;8:95–101.

Adelson MD, Jozefczyk MA, Reece, MT. Pathologic interpretation of the ultrasonic specimen. In: Rader JS, ed. *Ultrasonic surgical techniques for the pelvic surgeon.* New York: Springer-Verlag, 1995.

Adelson MD, Mazur MT. Cytoreduction of urethral carcinoma using the ultrasonic surgical aspirator. *J Gynecol Surg* 1992;8:37–41.

Adelson MD, Thompson MA. Cytoreduction of intraperitoneal malignancy using the Cavitron ultrasonic surgical aspirator: II. Operative morbidity, mortality and survival. 2000 (in preparation).

Albright AL, Sclabassi RJ. Use of the Cavitron ultrasonic surgical aspirator and evoked potentials for the treatment of thalamic and brain stem tumors in children. *Neurosurgery* 1985;17:564.

Aliev MA, Sultanaliev TA, Seisembaev MA, et al. Optimization of diagnosis and methods of liver resection in alveolar echinococcosis. *Khirurgiia (Mosk)* 1999;5:11.

Amaral JF. The experimental development of an ultrasonically activated scalpel for laparoscopic use. *Surg Laparosc Endosc* 1994;4:92.

Andrus CH, Kaminski DL. Segmental hepatic resection utilizing the ultrasonic dissector. *Arch Surg* 1986;121:515.

Barrett SB, ter Haar GR, Ziskin MC, et al. Current status of research on biophysical effects of ultrasound. *Ultrasound Med Biol* 1994;20:205.

Bond LJ, Cimino WW. Physics of ultrasonic surgical tissue fragmentation. *Ultrasonics* 1996;34:579.

Carstensen EL. Acoustic cavitation and the safety of diagnostic ultrasound. *Ultrasound Med Biol* 1987;13:597

Crum LA, Roy RA, Dinno MA, et al. Acoustic cavitation produced by microsecond pulses of ultrasound: a discussion of some selected results. *J Acoust Soc Am* 1992;91:1113.

Dalkalitsis N, Stefanidis K, Paschopoulos M, et al. Laparoscopic treatment of interstitial pregnancy using the harmonic scalpel. *Clin Exp Obstet Gynecol* 1998;25:49.

Deppe G, Malviya VK, Malone JM. Use of Cavitron ultrasonic surgical aspirator (CUSA) for palliative resection of recurrent gynecologic malignancies involving the vagina. *Eur J Gynaecol Oncol* 1989;10:1.

Deppe G, Malviya VK, Malone JM, et al. Debulking of pelvic and para-aortic lymph node metastases in ovarian cancer with the Cavitron ultrasonic surgical aspirator. *Obstet Gynecol* 1990;76:1140.

Donovan JT, Veronikis DK, Powell JL, et al. Cytoreductive surgery for ovarian cancer with the Cavitron ultrasonic surgical aspirator and the development of disseminated intravascular coagulation. *Obstet Gynecol* 1994;83:1011.

Eisenkop SM, Nalick RH, Wang H, et al. Peritoneal implant elimination during cytoreductive surgery for ovarian cancer: impact on survival. *Gynecol Oncol* 1993;51:224.

Farid H, O'Connell T. Hepatic resections: changing mortality and morbidity. *Am Surg* 1994;60:748.

Fasulo F, Giori A, Fissi S, et al. Cavitron ultrasonic surgical aspirator (CUSA) in liver resection. *Int Surg* 1992;77:64.

Giordano G, Margari A, Scattarella M, et al. Aspetti tecnici nella chirurgia resettiva epatica: contributo d'esperienza. *Giornale di Chirurgia* 1994;15:284.

Grochmal SA, Weekes A, Garratt D, et al. Applications of the laparoscopic ultrasonic aspirator for advanced gynecologic operative endoscopic procedures. *J Am Assoc Gynecol Laparosc* 1993;1:43.

Hacker NF, Berek JS, Lagasse LD, et al. Primary cytoreductive surgery for epithelial ovarian cancer. *Obstet Gynecol* 1983;61:413.

Hambley R, Hebda PA, Abell E, et al. Wound healing of skin incisions produced by ultrasonically vibrating knife, scalpel, electrosurgery, and carbon dioxide laser. *J Dermatol Surg Oncol* 1988;14:1213.

Hashimoto T, Otobe Y, Shimizu Y, et al. A modification of hepatic portoenterostomy (Kasai operation) for biliary atresia. *J Am Coll Surg* 1997;185:548.

Higashi H, Matsumata T, Hayashi J, et al. Detection of hepatitis C virus RNA in the ultrasonic dissector irrigating solution used in liver surgery. *Br J Surg* 1994;81:1346.

Hill CR. Ultrasonic exposure thresholds for changes in cells and tissues. *J Acoust Soc Am* 1972;52:667.

Hodgson WJB. The technique of ultrasonic dissection in cavernous hemangiomas of the liver. *Surg Rounds* 1984b;7:30.

Hodgson WJB, Aufses A. Surgical ultrasonic dissection of the liver. *Surg Rounds* 1979;2:68.

Holub Z, Voracek J, Jun L, et al. Laparoscopic hysterectomy: randomized study of harmonic scalpel and electrosurgery. *J Gynecol Surg* 2000;16:33.

Hurst BS, Thompson LK, Awoniyi CA, et al. Application of the Cavitron ultrasonic surgical aspirator (CUSA) for gynecological laparoscopic surgery using the rabbit as an animal model. *Fertil Steril* 1992;58:444.

Kauko M. New techniques using the ultrasonic scalpel in laparosonic hysterectomy. *Curr Opin Obstet Gynecol* 1998;10:303.

Konno R, Akahira J, Igarashi T, et al. Conization of the cervix using the harmonic scalpel. *Tohuku J Exp Med* 1999;189:171.

Lejbkowicz F, Salzberg S. Distinct sensitivity of normal and malignant cells to ultrasound *in vitro. Environ Health Perspect* 1997;105:1575.

Lopoo JB, Paek BW, Maichin GA, et al. Cord ultrasonic transection procedure for selective termination of a monochorionic twin. *Fetal Diagn Ther* 2000;15:177.

Matsumata T, Kanematsu T, Okadome K, et al. Possible transmission of serum hepatitis in liver surgery. *Surgery* 1991;109:284

McCarus SD. Physiologic mechanism of the ultrasonically activated scalpel. *J Am Assoc Gynecol Laparosc* 1996;3:601.

Minami S, Okamoto Y, Eguchi H, et al. Successful laparoscopy assisted ovariohysterectomy in two dogs with pyometra. *J Vet Med Sci* 1997;59:845

Miller CE, Amaral JF. Harmonic scalpel: pros and cons? *Fertil Steril* 1994;62:1094.

Nahhas WA. Case report: a potential hazard of the use of the surgical ultrasonic aspirator in tumor reductive surgery. *Gynecol Oncol* 1991;40:81.

Nduka CC, Poland N, Kennedy M, et al. Does the ultrasonically activated scalpel release viable airborne cancer cells? *Surg Endosc* 1998;12:1031.

Niwa K, Imai A, Hashimoto M, et al. Postoperative vesicourethral function after ultrasonic surgical aspirator-assisted surgery of gynecologic malignancies. *Eur J Obstet Gynecol Reprod Biol* 2000;89:169.

Oakes WJ, Friedman HS, Bigner SH, et al. Successful laboratory growth and analysis of CUSA-obtained medulloblastoma samples. *J Neurosurg* 1990;72:821.

Oosterhuis JW, Lung PFL, Verschueren RCJ, et al. Viability of tumor cells in the irrigation fluid of the Cavitron ultrasonic surgical aspirator (CUSA) after tumor fragmentation. *Cancer* 1985;56:368.

Ott DE, Moss E, Martinez K. Aerosol exposure from an ultrasonically activated (harmonic) device. *J Am Assoc Gynecol Laparosc* 1998;5:29.

Ottow RT, Barbieri SA, Sugarbaker PH, et al. Liver transection: a controlled study of four different techniques in pigs. *Surgery* 1985;97:596.

Ouchi K, Mikuni J, Sugawara T, et al. Hepatectomy using an ultrasonically activated scalpel for hepatocellular carcinoma. *Dig Surg* 2000 17:138.

Patsner B. CUSA resection of massive recurrent vulvar carcinoma. *Eur J Gynaecol Oncol* 1998;19:19.

Patsner B, Rose PG. CUSA splenorrhaphy for ovarian cytoreductive surgery. *Gynecol Oncol* 1991;41:28.

Piver M, Lele S, Marchetti D, et al. The impact of aggressive debulking surgery and cisplatin-based chemotherapy on progression-free survival in stage III and IV ovarian carcinoma. *J Clin Oncol* 1988;6:983.

Possover M, Stober S, Plaul K, et al. Identification and preservation of the motoric innervation of the bladder in radical hysterectomy type III. *Gynecol Oncol* 2000;79:154.

Putnam CW. Techniques of ultrasonic dissection in resection of the liver. *Surg Gynecol Obstet* 1983;157:474.

Rader JS, Leake JF, Dillon MB, et al. Ultrasonic surgical aspiration in the treatment of vulvar disease. *Obstet Gynecol* 1991;77:573.

Rader JS, Rest MS, Farmer ER, et al. A comparison of wound healing after epithelial resection by ultrasonic surgical aspiration and ablation by the carbon dioxide laser. *Gynecol Oncol* 1992;46:351.

Richards SR, Simpkins S. Laparoscopic supracervical hysterectomy versus laparoscopic-assisted vaginal hysterectomy. *J Am Assn Gynecol Laparosc* 1995;2:431.

Richards SR, Simpkins S. Comparison of the harmonic scissors and endostapler in laparoscopic supracervical hysterectomy. *J Am Assn Gynecol Laparosc* 1995;3:87.

Robbins ML. Excision of endometriosis with laparosonic coagulating shears. *J Am Assoc Gynecol Laparosc* 1999;6:199.

Robinson JB, Sun CC, Bodurka-Bevers D, et al. Cavitational ultrasonic surgical aspiration for the treatment of vaginal intraepithelial neoplasia. *Gynecol Oncol* 2000;78:235.

Rose PG. The cavitational ultrasonic surgical aspirator for cytoreduction in advanced ovarian cancer. *Am J Obstet Gynecol* 1992;166:843.

Rose PG, Piver MS. Primary resection of vaginal metastases with the Cavitron ultrasonic surgical aspirator in stage III endometrial carcinoma. *Gynecol Oncol* 1990;39:264.

Savvina TV, Vishnevskii VA, Ikramov RZ, et al. Dinamika morfologicheskikh izmenenii pecheni pri ee rezektsiiakh s po-moshch'iu otechestvennogo ul'trazvukovogo khirurgicheskogo aspiratora. *Biull Eksp Biol Med* 1991;111:311.

Schemmel M, Haefner HK, Selvaggi SM, et al. Comparison of the ultrasonic scalpel to CO2 laser and electrosurgery in terms of tissue injury and adhesion formation in a rabbit model. *Fertil Steril* 1997;67:382.

Schroder T, Hasselgren PO, Brackett K, et al. Techniques of liver resection: comparison of suction knife, ultrasonic dissector, and contact neodymium-YAG laser. *Arch Surg* 1987;122:1166.

Schwartz RO. Total laparoscopic total hysterectomy with the harmonic scalpel. *J Gynecol Surg* 1994;10:33.

Segawa T, Tsuchiya R, Furui J, et al. Operative results in 143 patients with hepatocellular carcinoma. *World J Surg* 1993;17:663.

Shiina H, Ehara S, Ishibe T. Vesicourethral function after surgery for uterine cancer: predictive value of postoperative maximum urethral closure pressure on residual urine. *Urol Int* 1993;51:125.

Shiozawa H, Miki M, Tochimoto M. Newly developed ultrasonic aspirator and its application for endoscopic surgery. *J Endourol* 1994;8:285.

Silverman JF, Douglas Jones F, Unverferth M, et al. Cytopathology of neoplasms obtained by the Cavitron ultrasonic surgical aspirator. *Acta Cytol* 1989;33:576.

Snajdauf J, Zeman L, Horn M, et al. Chirurgicka taktika v lecbe neuroblastomu retroperitonea. *Rozhl Chir* 1994;73:31.

Stanojevic D, Scepanovic R, Perunovic R, et al. An ultrasonic scalpel for laparoscopic gynecologic surgery. *Srp Arh Celok Lek* 1998;126:214.

Stefanidis K, Paschopoulos M, Dalkalitsis N, et al. Laparoscopic sterilization with the Harmonic scalpel. *J Gynecol Surg* 1999;15:41.

Storck BH, Rutgers EJ, Gortzak E, et al. The impact of the CUSA ultrasonic dissection device on major liver resections. *Neth J Surg* 1991;43:99.

Stringer NH. Laparoscopic myomectomy with the harmonic scalpel: a review of 25 cases. *J Gynecol Surg* 1994;10:241.

Suslick KS. The chemical effects of ultrasound. *Sci Am* 1989;260:80.

Szantho A, Konrad S, Hidvegi J, et al. The use of CUSA (Cavitron ultrasonic surgery aspirator) in the surgery of gynecologic malignancies. *Magy Onkol* 1993b;37:37.

Ter Haar G, Daniels S, Eastaugh KC, et al. Ultrasonically induced cavitation in vivo. *Br J Cancer* 1982;45:151.

Thompson MA, Adelson MD, Jozefczyk MA, et al. Structural and functional integrity of ovarian tumor tissue obtained by ultrasonic aspiration. *Cancer* 1991;67:1326.

Tranberg KG, Rigotti P, Brackett KA, et al. Liver resection: a comparison using the Nd-YAG laser, an ultrasonic surgical aspirator, or blunt dissection. *Am J Surg* 1986;151:368.

Tulandi T, Chan KL, Arseneau J. Histopathological and adhesion formation after incision using ultrasonic vibrating scalpel and regular scalpel in the rat. *Fertil Steril* 1994;61:548.

van Dam PA, Coppens M, van Oosterom AT, et al. Is there an increased risk for tumor dissemination using ultrasonic surgical aspiration in patients with vulvar carcinoma? *Eur J Obstet Gynecol Reprod Biol* 1994;55:145.

van Dam PA, Tjalma W, Weyler J, et al. Ultraradical debulking of epithelial ovarian cancer with the ultrasonic surgical aspirator: a prospective randomized trial. *Am J Obstet Gynecol* 1996;174:943.

Vanderburgh E, Nahhas WA. Case report: debridement of vaginal radiation ulcers using the surgical ultrasonic aspirator. *Gynecol Oncol* 1990;39:103.

Vasquez JM, Eisenberg E, Osteen KG, et al. Laparoscopic ablation of endometriosis using the cavitational ultrasonic surgical aspirator. *J Am Assoc Gynecol Laparosc* 1993;1:36.

Verdaasdonk R, Balgobind D, van Swol C, et al. The mechanism of action of the ultrasonic tissue resectors disclosed using high-speed and thermal imaging techniques. *SPIE* 1999;3594:221.

Villena-Heinsen C, Alloussi S, Schmidt W. Bisherige erfahrungen mit dem ultraschalldissektor in der gynakologischen onkologie. *Geburtshilfe Frauenheilkd* 1992;52:360.

Vyhnanek F, Fanta J, Denemark L, et al. Liver resection using the harmonic scalpel. *Rozhl Chir* 2000;79:241.

Winter ML, Mendelsohn SA. Total laparoscopic hysterectomy using the harmonic scalpel. *JSLS* 1999;3:185.

Wu AY, Sherman ME, Rosenshein NB, et al. Pathologic evaluation of gynecologic specimens obtained with the Cavitron ultrasonic surgical aspirator (CUSA). *Gynecol Oncol* 1992;44:28.

Yabuki Y, Asamoto A, Hoshiba T, et al. Dissection of the cardinal ligament in radical hysterectomy for cervical cancer with emphasis on the lateral ligament. *Am J Obstet Gynecol* 1991;164:7.

Young RC, Decker DG, Wharton JT, et al. Staging laparotomy in early ovarian cancer. *JAMA* 1983;250:3072.

Te Linde's Operative Gynecology, ninth edition, edited by John A. Rock and Howard W. Jones, III. Lippincott Williams & Wilkins, Philadelphia © 2003.

CHAPTER
15

▼

Application of Laser in Gynecology
JAMES H. DORSEY

HISTORY OF THE LASTER

The term laser is an acronym for *l*ight *a*mplification by *s*timulated *e*mission of *r*adiation. In 1917, Albert Einstein predicted and described the process of stimulated emission of radiation, but it was not until 1953 that Charles Townes and coworkers produced a device called a maser, which amplified microwaves by stimulated emission of radiation. In 1958, Schawlow and Townes published a hypothesis that described the laser in general terms. In 1960, Maiman constructed the first working laser, which consisted of a ruby crystal that was stimulated to emit laser energy by pumping with light from a xenon flash lamp. The carbon dioxide (CO_2) laser was developed by Patel in 1964; this laser was used for the first time in experimental surgery in 1965. In 1973, the laser was first used in gynecology by Kaplan and colleagues, who reported CO_2 laser vaporization of infected cervical tissue.

Over the past 25 years, there have been numerous reports concerning laser usage in many different medical and surgical specialties. In gynecology, lower reproductive tract surgery and endoscopic surgery have provided enormous opportunity for laser energy to be used for surgical tasks and to achieve desired goals quickly and safely and in the most conservative manner possible.

LASER PHYSICS
Stimulated Emission

Laser light is most often described in terms of its wave characteristics or wavelength. Wavelength is the distance between two successive crests or troughs, and wavelength determines the color of the light. Wavelengths are usually measured in microns or nanometers. One micron (μm) equals $1/1,000$ mm, and 1 nanometer (nm) equals $1/1,000,000$ mm. Electromagnetic waves are often referred to as light, although visible light occupies only a small portion of the electromagnetic spectrum. CO_2 laser energy in the far infrared portion of the spectrum, although invisible to the eye, may therefore be correctly thought of as light energy (Table 15.1).

An atom is composed of a positively charged nucleus surrounded by electrons that orbit this nucleus. Each electron orbit can be described in terms of energy levels.

TABLE 15.1.
Laser Colors and Wavelengths

Name	Color	Wavelength (nm)
Excimers	Ultraviolet	200–400
Argon	Blue-green	488 nm/515
KTP 532	Green	532
Krypton	Green-yellow	532 nm/568
Dye laser	Yellow-green-red	577 nm/630
Helium neon	Red	632
Gold vapor	Red	630
Krypton	Red	647
Ruby	Deep red	694
Nd:YAG	Infrared	1,064 nm/1,318
CO_2	Infrared	10,600

As orbital distance from the nucleus increases, energy level increases. As described by the laws of quantum mechanics, when an electron moves from a higher-energy orbit to a lower-energy orbit, the atom loses a specific amount of energy in the form of a photon, which also has a specific wavelength.

Lasers contain what is referred to as an active lasing medium, a collection of atoms or molecules that are housed in an optically resonant cavity. This cavity, often cylindrical, is designed so that light of a specific wavelength will resonate between the closed ends of the cavity, much as sound will resonate in a properly constructed chamber. The active medium is stimulated, or "pumped," by an external energy source such as electricity or light, which stimulates the active lasing medium to higher energy levels. As decay back to resting energy levels occurs, photons of energy are released into the optical cavity. Electrons that are still in excited higher orbital energy levels can also be stimulated by bombardment with these newly released photons so that they undergo identical decay and emit an identical photon. This is called stimulated emission, because one photon has stimulated the production of another photon. The optical cavity of the laser tube is closed at each end by a mirror. One of these mirrors is totally reflective, but the other is semitransparent. Although photon direction in the tube is random, a certain number of photons will be emitted in the axis of the optical cavity, and the others are focused by the mirrors so that most are resonating or bouncing back and forth along the axis of the cavity. Some of these photons emerge through the semitransparent mirror and are emitted from the laser as the monochromatic parallel coherent laser beam. Coherent means that the waves are all in phase or perfectly aligned. The laser thus creates a light that travels in a tight beam over long distances.

Laser power is measured in terms of watts, and laser energy is expressed in terms of joules. One joule equals 1 W of power applied for 1 second. Lasers are named for the active medium contained in their optical cavities. Many different lasers have been constructed for diverse uses. In gynecologic surgery, the CO_2 and YAG lasers are the most commonly used, with the argon and KTP lasers following as distant seconds. Despite many efforts, fiber-

optic delivery systems have never been satisfactorily adapted to CO_2 laser energy. However, the three other lasers produce wavelengths that are conducted along quartz fibers. The use of the fiber is of great advantage in endoscopic surgery because it can be passed down the channel of an operative telescope, suction irrigator probe, or other hollow instrument.

Power Density and Transverse Electromagnetic Mode

When laser energy passes from the laser, the photons are coherent and parallel and theoretically could travel in space in this form to infinity. All this changes when laser light is focused through a lens or directed into a quartz fiber. CO_2 laser energy is usually focused by a lens to a relatively small spot, the focal point of that lens. Focal spot size varies directly with the focal length of the lens. In surgical usage, however, additional lenses or mechanical devices allow the surgeon to change the spot-size diameter with ease. For any given power setting of the CO_2 laser, the concentration or density of the power is greater as the spot size becomes smaller, and conversely, as the spot size (tissue impact area) is enlarged, the power density decreases. Power density is expressed as watts per square centimeter. Because the calculation of power density is relatively complicated, most surgeons prefer to note the power setting on the laser and the effective spot size used for surgery. Obviously the biologic effect and type of surgical injury are varied by changing spot size.

Although the photons of laser light are parallel, laser energy is not completely uniform throughout the cross-sectional diameter of the beam (Fig. 15.1). The term transverse electromagnetic mode (TEM) refers to the energy distribution of the cross-sectional diameter. For example, in most CO_2 surgical lasers, the energy distribution is greatest at the center of the beam and decreases toward the periphery. If one graphs the energy distribution of the cross-sectional beam diameter of the CO_2 laser, the resultant curve is bell-shaped. This gaussian distribution does not hold true in fiber-optic lasers, YAG, KTP, and argon in which energy distribution tends to be more uniform. However, when energy from these lasers enters a quartz fiber, conduction alters parallelism and

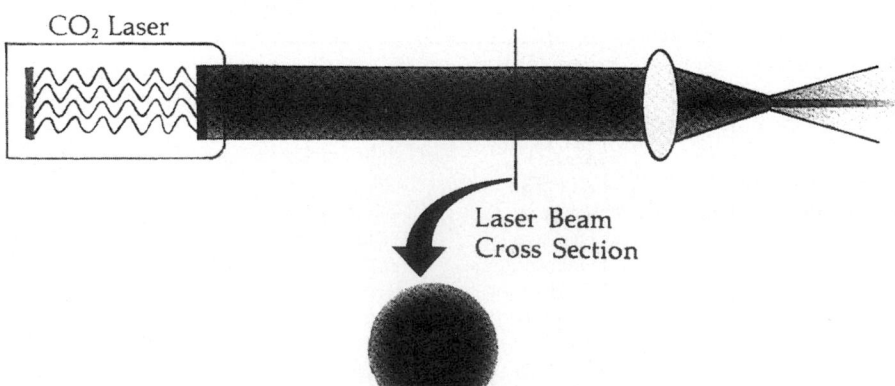

CO_2 Laser

Laser Beam
Cross Section

FIGURE 15.1. Transverse electromagnetic mode. Laser energy distribution is not uniform throughout the cross section of the beam. Energy concentration is highest at the beam center and decreases toward the periphery.

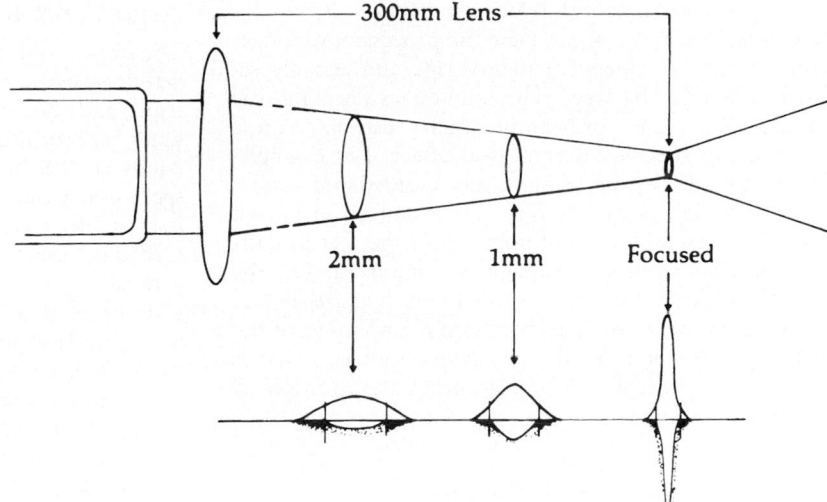

FIGURE 15.2. Beam profile variations. For any given power setting, beam profile (the shape of the gaussian curve) can be altered by changing spot size diameter. The small spot size results in a steep curve, which is used for cutting. Larger spot sizes produce flatter curves suitable for vaporization. Tissue damage and crater shape mirror the energy distribution.

beam divergence of approximately 15 degrees occurs at the fiber tip. Thus, laser energy emerging from a fiber-optic conductor is not coherent, and the greatest concentration of this energy exists at the fiber–air or tissue interface where the spot size is smallest, that is, the same diameter as the conductor.

LASER TISSUE INTERACTION

The primary tissue effects of the surgical lasers used in gynecology are produced by laser heat energy. The water content of soft tissue is about 80% by volume, and if latent heat or vaporization of water is delivered by the beam, the tissue crater shape reflects the intensity profile of the incident energy (Fig. 15.2). In the case of the CO_2 laser, because of the gaussian distribution of energy in the beam, some of the tissue at the periphery of the lesion that does not receive enough energy to become vaporized will still be damaged by heat. When tissue tem-

perature is elevated to about 57°C, irreversible damage occurs and the cell dies. Thus, between 57° and 100°C, there will be tissue death without vaporization. Additional tissue damage also results from lateral conduction of heat away from the laser impact site. The amount of damage caused by heat conduction is directly proportional to the amount of time spent in lasing. Therefore, there are three zones of laser tissue damage that can be defined: the area vaporized, the area of tissue death that results from heating tissue short of vaporization, and the area of tissue damage caused by conduction of heat away from the lased site (Fig. 15.3).

CO_2 Laser Effects on Tissue

CO_2 laser energy is almost completely absorbed by a very thin layer of water. Because of the high water content of our cells, deep penetration of this laser energy into tissue is minimal as long as intracellular and extracellular water remains to be vaporized. Tissue can therefore be de-

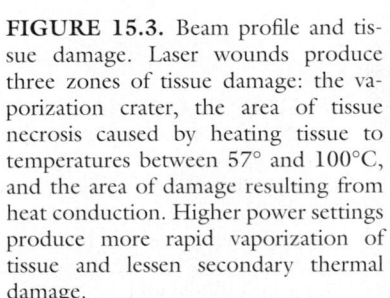

FIGURE 15.3. Beam profile and tissue damage. Laser wounds produce three zones of tissue damage: the vaporization crater, the area of tissue necrosis caused by heating tissue to temperatures between 57° and 100°C, and the area of damage resulting from heat conduction. Higher power settings produce more rapid vaporization of tissue and lessen secondary thermal damage.

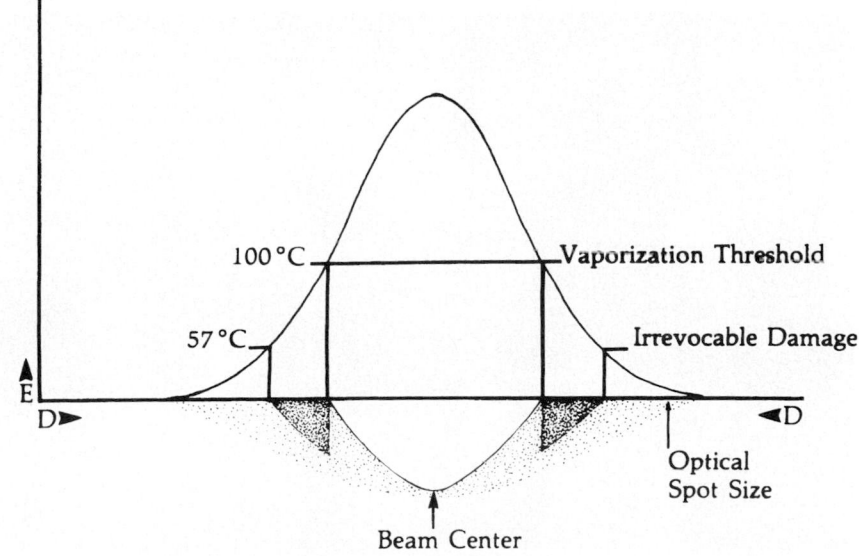

stroyed very accurately in relatively small or shallow increments. The surgeon can view the process of vaporization through an operative microscope and actually remove cells layer by layer. This minimizes deeper tissue damage. Knowledge of beam geometry also plays a role in achieving specific laser surgical effect. For example, the sharply focused beam has a very narrow spot diameter with a high power density and produces an impact crater that resembles a drill hole. This is perfect for cutting, and lateral tissue damage is minimized. On the other hand, enlarging the spot diameter by partially defocusing the beam reduces the central amplitude of the gaussian curve and results in a larger spot size that is more easily controlled when accurate vaporization of larger target areas is desired.

YAG Laser Effects on Tissue

YAG laser energy, because it is poorly absorbed by water, is able to penetrate human tissue to depths of 4 mm or more. Additionally there is scatter in the tissues, and damage is much greater than that with CO_2 laser. Therefore YAG is not a good laser for vaporization procedures. This laser energy serves better as a coagulator of tissue than as a vaporizer and is often deliberately used to cause deeper destruction, as in endometrial ablation.

The tissue penetration and the effect of YAG laser energy can be altered by applying artificial sapphire tips to the end of the fiber-optic cable. The sapphire is heated by laser energy, and depending on the configuration of the sapphire tip, a fine incision or a broad area of coagulation may be produced. Most of the YAG energy is absorbed by the sapphire, and little actual laser light is delivered to the tissue. Thus, tissue damage is greatly reduced, except where the sapphire actually touches the target. Development of the various sapphire tips has greatly increased the precision with which this laser can be used. The YAG laser can now be used very safely and effectively in laparoscopic surgery (Fig. 15.4).

Argon and KTP Tissue Effects

The argon and the KTP laser both produce energy at wavelengths that are close on the electromagnetic spectrum, and their effects on tissue are very similar. The argon laser produces a blue-green light that has two distinct bands at 488 nm and 515 nm on the electromagnetic spectrum. Colored lasers traverse water very well. This laser is also a photocoagulator because its energy is absorbed preferentially by its opposite color, red or black. In general, argon is located somewhere between CO_2 and YAG in its ability to produce vaporization and coagulation. The laser will vaporize tissue, but not as rapidly as the CO_2 laser. Coagulation extends deeper into tissues than with CO_2 because of the penetrability of its beam.

The KTP/532 laser derives its name from the potassium (K), titanyl (T), and phosphate (P) crystal that is used to double the frequency and halve the wavelength ($\frac{1}{2} \times 1,064$ nm $= 532$ nm) of the YAG laser. The 532-nm wavelength is emerald green, and its tissue effects are very similar to those produced by the argon laser. The KTP/532 can be used to vaporize or to coagulate, and energy emerging from the end of the fiber can be used to cut tissue. Because of its penetration, its tissue effects often extend 1 to 2 mm into the irradiated target. In general, although these fiber-optic lasers have been used by some surgeons on the lower reproductive tract, their greatest application has been in endoscopic surgery, because the delivery systems for their energy can be passed down the operative channel of an endoscope.

LASER ENERGY DELIVERY SYSTEMS AND BEAM MANIPULATION

The CO_2 laser beam is delivered through a tubular arm, and the direction of the beam is changed by mirrors. CO_2 laser energy has not been effectively transmitted by

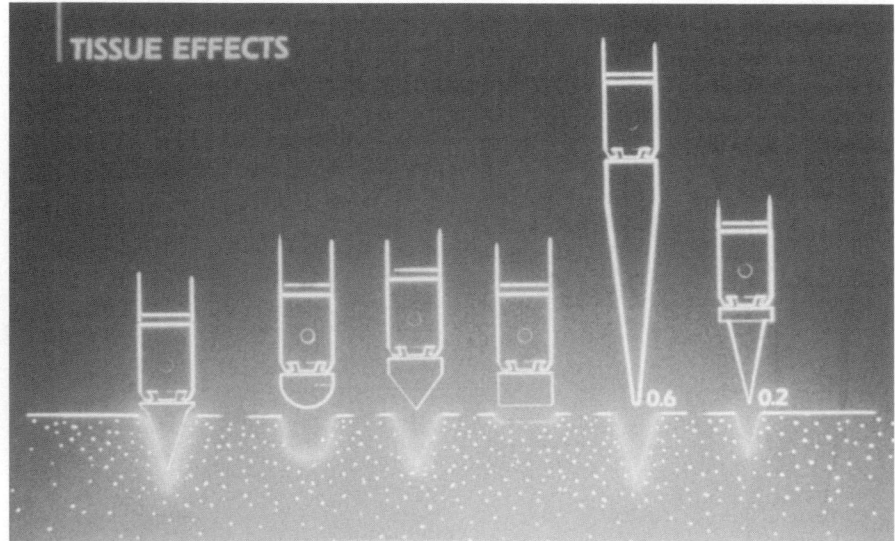

TISSUE EFFECTS

FIGURE 15.4. Sapphire tips for the Nd:YAG laser. Sapphire tips alter the energy egress from the YAG quartz fiber. Here, tissue effects are shown to vary with changes in sapphire design. Sharp tips make good scalpels; rounded tips are used for vaporization.

a fiber-optic system, and in most surgical procedures, the beam is propagated through air to the target site. The coherent beam is focused (or made to converge) by lenses mounted on several different useful devices, which are mentioned below.

Micromanipulator: A joystick is used to move a mirror that is located past the focusing lens, and the beam is thus directed to the target. Micromanipulators are mounted on colposcopes or operative microscopes and provide a highly accurate method of directing the beam.

Laser handpiece: The focusing lens is actually located in the handpiece. The handpiece houses a lens with a short focal length, which is thus capable of producing the smallest focal spot sizes. This makes the handpiece ideal for fine incisions.

CO_2 laser operative laparoscope and laser laparoscopic probes: The longer focal length lenses required in laparoscopic delivery systems make small spot sizes a bit more difficult to achieve. Incisions that are smallest in width (i.e., the finest incision) are, of course, made by the focused beam.

Defocusing the beam is achieved by moving the lens farther away from the target tissue. This results in either a broader incision or a larger spot size with which to vaporize.

Micromanipulators can be fitted with focusing lenses that are very similar to the zoom lens of a camera, so the spot can be varied in size without changing the optical focus for the surgeon.

Fiber-optic lasers are much easier to use in endoscopes and handpieces because beam delivery is through fibers 100 to 600 μm in diameter. The beam diverges from the cable at about 15 degrees, so power density is greatest just off the tip of the fiber, and the beam can be defocused by moving the tip of the fiber further away from the target tissue.

LOWER REPRODUCTIVE TRACT LASER SURGERY

Most lower reproductive tract laser surgery has been directed at the treatment of intraepithelial neoplasia and human papilloma virus (HPV) infection. Because certain HPV types are more likely to produce significant dysplastic changes, some laser surgeons have treated even subclinical evidence of HPV infection with laser. It is now apparent that although the laser provides a highly effective and accurate method of treating intraepithelial neoplasia and condylomas, the laser does not eradicate the virus from all of the infected areas of the lower reproductive tract. It follows that cytologic evidence of HPV infection without pathologic proof of dysplasia or clinical manifestation of the disease does not serve as an indication for laser surgery.

Laser Selection and Advantages

Colposcopy provides the most accurate means of visually identifying the lesions of intraepithelial neoplasia and HPV. Laser surgery for this spectrum of disease has most often been performed with a CO_2 laser coupled to a micromanipulator that is mounted on a colposcope. The colposcope then becomes an operative microscope, and the CO_2 laser beam, which can be directed by the micromanipulator with unparalleled precision, can be used to produce a wide variety of tissue effects, from fine deep incisions to broad shallow vaporization.

It is this microsurgical approach to the lower reproductive tract and the great versatility of the CO_2 laser that have made this laser so effective in dealing with intraepithelial neoplasia.

Cervical intraepithelial neoplasia (CIN) has been treated successfully by both *in situ* destruction and excisional biopsy. In either case, the transformation zone (TZ) must be included in the ablation. In 1968, Palucek and Townsend reported a series in which cryosurgery was used to destroy dysplasia and the TZ. Many subsequent studies have shown excellent results with cryotherapy for the treatment of smaller CIN lesions.

From the beginning, however, the use of destructive procedures that did not produce a pathologic specimen evoked strong criticism by colposcopists, who feared that lack of a complete pathologic examination of the target tissue would result in a missed diagnosis of true invasion. In the late 1960s, Cartier in Paris developed a cutting loop electrode with a wire diameter of 200 μm that, when properly used, produced only a very small amount of thermal damage in the excised specimen. These loops were very similar to the loop electrodes used today for electrosurgical coagulation.

Both cryotherapy and loop electrode excision have had adequate time to prove that they are excellent methods for treating some cases of CIN. We have continued to use CO_2 lasers to accurately tailor excisional and vaporization operations to fit the individual geometric requirements of each case. We have also combined these two procedures, electrosurgical excisional conization with the loop electrode or laser excision conization with the finely focused laser beam followed by vaporization with expanded laser spot size, for the large or multifocal lesions of the lower reproductive tract. These combination procedures have yielded excellent results and have proved to be particularly effective in avoiding excessive deep tissue loss.

Laser Surgery of the Cervix

Although CIN has been described as a noninvasive surface phenomenon, it is well known that the process involves the endocervical crypts. The work of Te Linde, Danforth, Flumen, Burghardt, and others pointed out that the endocervical crypts were involved in CIN, but it was Anderson and Hartley in 1980 who really emphasized the therapeutic implications; namely, adequate depth of destruction or excision is required to achieve satisfactory results. Anderson and Hartley measured the depth of crypt involvement and found that 99% of CIN extends no further than 4 mm from the surface into the cervical crypt. A logical assumption can then made. If an area of intraepithelial neoplasia on the cervix was either excised or vaporized to a depth greater than 4 mm, virtually all of the neoplastic process would be irradiated. This concept of depth of crypt involvement is extremely important to the surgeon, for it dictates a measurable depth of destruction to be achieved by vaporization of the TZ if a surgical specimen is not to be removed by conization.

There are several constant findings that explain the diagnostic accuracy of colposcopically directed biopsies.

1. Atypical epithelial changes almost always start in the TZ.
2. Intraepithelial neoplasia is almost always found in contact with the original squamous epithelium of the cervix.
3. The neoplastic process does not arise in isolated foci of metaplasia found elsewhere in the TZ or in the endocervical canal.
4. Multifocal CIN or skip lesions (lesions not in contact with the main focus of CIN) are very rare.

It follows that if the lesion of intraepithelial neoplasia is visualized in its entirety (i.e., if the borders of the lesion are clearly seen on the cervix, and the lesion does not extend up into the canal), then it can be biopsied and correctly diagnosed as intraepithelial neoplasia. This assumption provides the justification for all nonexcisional ablative procedures used to destroy cervical intraepithelial disease.

The reserve cells and columnar cells of the TZ constitute the cell population at risk for the development of atypical squamous metaplasia and CIN. In the early days of laser surgery, we attempted to destroy only the visible lesion and not the entire TZ. Unfortunately, this practice has been associated with a high rate of persistence or recurrence of the CIN. Therefore, it is necessary to destroy the entire TZ, including the visible lesion to a measured depth of 5 mm, if satisfactory results are to be anticipated.

Cervical conization is defined as an operation that removes a volume of tissue from the central longitudinal axis of the cervix. This includes the external os and a certain length of endocervical canal. The actual shape of the volume of tissue removed should be determined by the distribution of the lesion and not by some preconceived geometric design. Conization, then, is a generic term and does not necessarily imply that a perfect cone-shaped defect has been produced in the cervix. Cones can certainly be asymmetric and can be short, long, thin, cylindrical, or any other shape that accomplishes the intended goal of complete removal of the lesion and the tissue at risk. A number of different techniques have been used to perform conization operations. In laser surgery, the instrument can be used as a scalpel to excise. The end results for both excisional laser conization and laser vaporization for CIN are essentially the same. There is a central defect in the longitudinal axis of the cervix surrounding the cervical canal that has been created by the laser, and the cervical stroma has been coagulated for hemostasis by laser heat energy. The term vaporization conization is therefore often used to describe the laser vaporization procedure performed on the cervix for the treatment of CIN.

CIN that involves the endocervical canal (which means it cannot be entirely visualized) or a neoplastic lesion that cannot be properly diagnosed for some reason must not be treated by a destructive, nonexcisional ablative procedure. Although the visible lesion may be intraepithelial, the nonvisualized lesion in the canal may be invasive. The requirements for vaporization conization are listed in Table 15.2.

Vaporization Conization

Vaporization conization can be performed in the office, the clinic, or the operating room. We have used the CO_2 laser coupled to the colposcope by micromanipulator for most cervical conizations. This method continues to produce the most satisfactory results. General anesthesia is usually not required for cervical vaporization, particularly if the patient has been carefully reassured about the laser surgery and the nature of her disease. Preoperative medication may include antiprostaglandins; this sometimes reduces the cramping that accompanies the laser ablation. Local anesthesia may be directly injected into the cervix. We use a 10-mL syringe and inject 1% lidocaine into the cervix in 1-mL aliquots around the circumference and into the stroma. Patients who request general anesthesia are treated on an outpatient basis.

The patient is placed in the dorsal lithotomy position, and a bivalve speculum is inserted into the vagina. No drapes are used, and no prep is necessary. The cervix is cleaned with a 4% acetic acid solution, and the lesion is again identified. The margin is outlined by a series of dots by using short bursts of laser energy (Fig. 15.5A). The entire TZ is included in the area to be vaporized, and a margin of at least 2 mm is allowed peripheral to the lesion.

The dots are then connected so that the cone is completely outlined (Fig. 15.5B). A spot size of about 2 mm is appropriate for this vaporization operation. We prefer a power setting of about 25 W. The laser surgeon, however, should select a power setting that is comfortable to use. Very high power settings require that the surgery be performed very quickly, whereas lower power settings mean greater ease of vaporization and very accurate ob-

---

TABLE 15.2.
Vaporization Conization Requirements

The lesion must be completely visualized.
The transformation zone must be completely seen.
There must be no doubt as to the intraepithelial nature of the disease.
Adenocarcinoma of the endocervical canal must be ruled out.

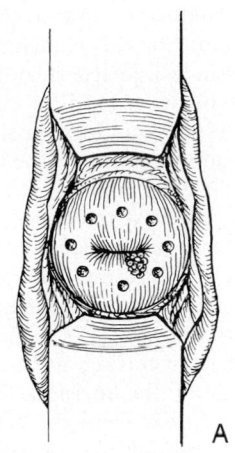 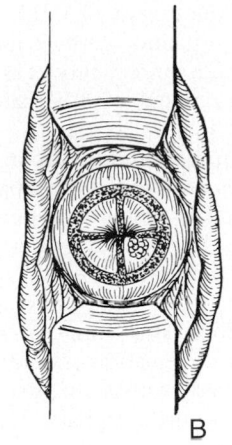 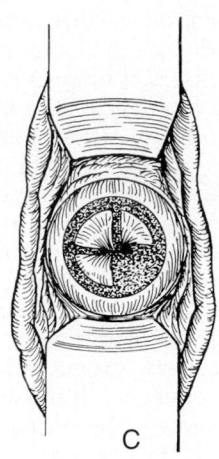

FIGURE 15.5. Cervical vaporization for cervical intraepithelial neoplasia. The cervix is reexamined with the colposcope and the margin of the vaporization conization is outlined by a series of dots (**A**), the dots are connected and the cervix is divided into four quadrants (**B**), and the tissue is vaporized quadrant by quadrant to a depth of 7 mm (**C**).

servation of the depth of the defect. The defect is carried to 7 mm, and the surgeon should make an attempt to measure the depth accurately. Often, the cervix and the area of the external os are not flush, and an accurate measurement of depth of vaporization may be difficult. For this reason, it seems more accurate to divide the cervix into four quadrants and then destroy the tissue quadrant by quadrant (Fig. 15.5C). In this way, part of the normal cervical anatomy is preserved throughout the operation, and even though the topography of the cervix

may change, the exact depth of destruction can always be measured for each quadrant. When all four quadrants have been vaporized to 7 mm, we then vaporize an additional 2 to 3 mm up into the endocervical canal. This technique has been used to avoid prolapse of the endocervical canal, which is often seen when the vaporization defect is totally cylindrical with a very flat base (Fig. 15.6). It is desirable to place the new squamocolumnar junction just inside the external os so that the metaplastic epithelium is not constantly bathed in the same vagi-

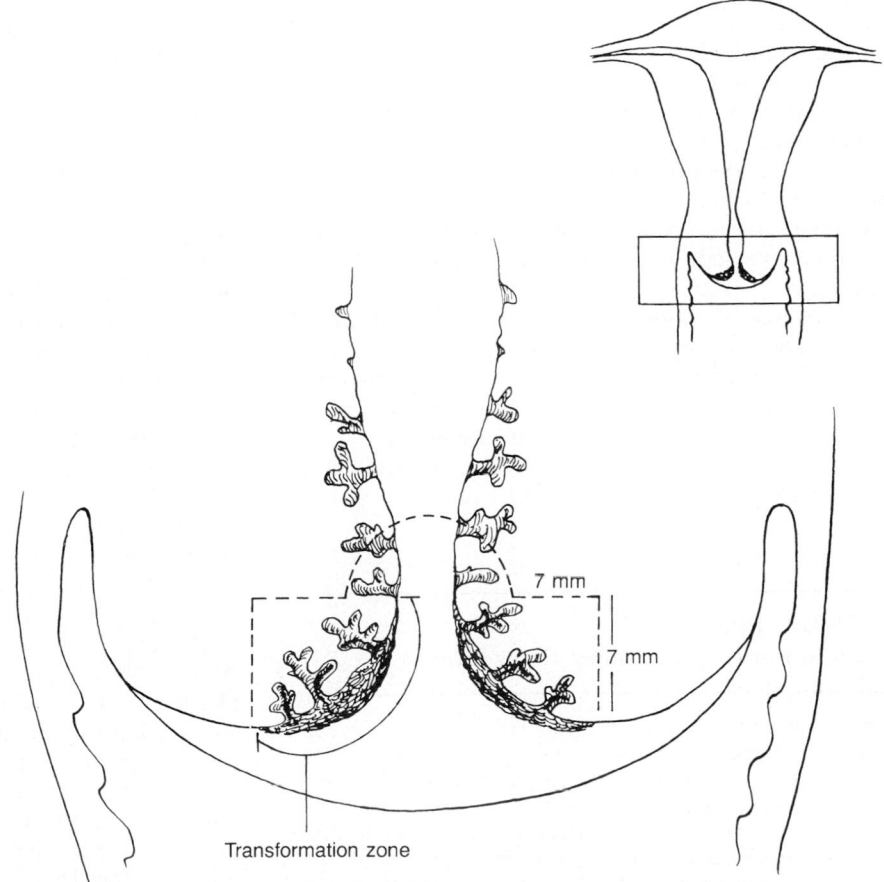

FIGURE 15.6. Cervical vaporization defect. After the cervix has been vaporized to the appropriate depth, an additional 3 mm of endocervical canal is vaporized to avoid endocervical prolapse and to ensure that the new squamocolumnar junction is just inside of the external os.

7 mm

7 mm

Transformation zone

nal milieu that initiated the development of CIN. Although the location of the new squamocolumnar junction is at times unpredictable, laser surgery produces an end result that is much more predictable than that of other methods of destruction.

Bleeding is not usually encountered during vaporization procedures. If bleeding does occur, a cotton-tipped applicator is used to tamponade the vessel. The power density is lowered by defocusing the beam or by slightly reducing the power, and the bleeding point is coagulated by using a rapid circular motion to surround the vessel. If bleeding is more active or if there is a pumper in the cervical stroma, other forms of coagulation should be considered. If bleeding is particularly worrisome, a small figure-of-eight stitch with a fine suture material will ensure hemostasis.

Excisional Conization of the Cervix

The goals of excisional conization are to produce a conization biopsy specimen that is adequate for pathologic examination and, if possible, to excise all disease. The indications for laser excisional conization are the same as those for cold-knife conization and are listed in Table 15.3.

The average excisional conization penetrates cervical stroma more deeply than does vaporization conization, and the patient may experience more discomfort and more bleeding with this procedure. Although excisional conization may often be satisfactorily performed with local anesthesia, we do not hesitate to perform this procedure on an outpatient basis under general anesthesia. Before starting an excisional conization, the surgeon must decide on the size and shape of the cone. These are tailored to fit the patient and the lesion. Some surgeons who are adept at endoscopy believe that the lesion in the canal can be evaluated by contact hysteroscopy. In any case, the endocervical canal should be sounded. Severe dysplasia with obvious worrisome canal involvement will require a larger and deeper cone specimen.

A weighted posterior retractor is placed in the vagina, and the anterior lip of the cervix is grasped with a single-toothed tenaculum. The cervix is painted with 4% acetic acid, and the patient is recolposcoped. The visible borders of the lesion are again carefully noted, and the external cervical margin of the cone is outlined. In the excisional procedures, high power and small spot size

are used for cutting so that the hemostatic effect is minimized. For this reason, a dilute solution of 1.5% vasopressin is injected through a 25-gauge needle at 1-mL increments around the cervix. With the CO_2 laser set for 25 to 50 W and a spot size of 0.5 to 1 mm, the incision is made straight into the cervical stroma and deepened to 3 to 4 mm. Superpulse for the CO_2 laser can also be effectively used to reduce lateral thermal damage. Smoke evacuation is performed by an assistant who holds a suction wand close to the target zone. The stromal edge of the incision is grasped with a single-toothed forceps or a laser conization hook. Gentle traction is applied to facilitate laser cutting and to allow the surgeon to view the depth of the incision. The cone specimen is actually peeled away from the cervical stroma as the laser beam slices through the tissue and works toward the canal. After removal of the cone specimen, the spot size is enlarged to 2 mm, and the stroma is coagulated superficially to prevent delayed hemorrhage.

Laser Combination Conization Procedures

The greatest benefits of CO_2 laser surgery are appreciated when vaporization procedures and excisional conization are performed together for the diagnosis and treatment of certain cases of CIN. Large areas of intraepithelial neoplasia and multifocal lesions that involve much of the cervix (including the endocervical canal) and then extend into the vagina or even involve the vulva are best treated by combination laser procedures. The endocervical lesion must be removed by laser excisional conization, but the peripheral portions of the lesion that were previously biopsied and proved benign may be vaporized. Thus, the indications for both excisional and vaporization conization have been met, and a conservative procedure has been performed. Baggish and Dorsey have shown that the volume of tissue removed by a combination of vaporization and excision is far less than that removed by excision alone. Combination procedures are the most conservative procedures possible because the operation is microsurgical and tailored to destroy the smallest amount of tissue. Of course, the pathologist must be aware that the peripheral margin of the excisional cone may be positive for intraepithelial disease and that the remaining margins of the excisional operative procedure have been vaporized.

Postoperative Instructions

Patients undergoing cervical vaporization or excisional procedures usually require very little postoperative care. We instruct our patients to avoid coitus for at least 4 weeks and to report any unusual fever or bleeding. About 15% of these patients will have some vaginal bleeding. The amount is significant, however, in only about 2% of the patients. The patient is requested to inform her physician if the bleeding becomes heavier than that associated with a normal menstrual period. She is allowed to return to work within 48 hours. The very definite advantages associated with laser conization are listed in Table 15.4.

TABLE 15.3.
Indications for Excisional Conization

The lesion disappears into the canal.
The entire transformation zone cannot be visualized.
Abnormal cytologic smear in the absence of positive colposcopic findings cannot be explained.
The endocervical curettage is indicative of disease in the canal.
Invasive cancer has not been ruled out by biopsy.

TABLE 15.4.
Advantages of Laser Conization

There is less bleeding than with a scalpel.

There is less tissue damage than with the electric cautery.

The procedure has advantages over cryosurgery in that it can be done with much more precision, and the results are better for lesions of all sizes.

Morbidity is low.

All types and extents of intraepithelial neoplasia can be treated.

The most conservative procedures can be performed by using combinations of vaporization and excision.

Results of Laser Surgery of the Cervix

In the early days of laser surgery, before 1982, a number of authors reported disappointing results with laser surgery for intraepithelial neoplasia. As techniques of laser surgery became better defined and understood, the results have improved. Baggish and Dorsey reported a series of over 4,000 cases of CIN treated by laser with an overall success rate between 96% and 97%. In those patients monitored by colposcopy, cytology, and biopsy for 1 year or more, vaporization procedures and excisional conization procedures seem to produce about the same cure rate. In addition, cure rates do not vary when degree of CIN is taken into consideration. Other authors, such as Burke and colleagues, Reid (1987), and Wright, report success rates between 95% and 98%.

Cure is a somewhat difficult term to define. Most laser surgeons have used colposcopy and cytology to evaluate the cervix at the end of 1 year. If no intraepithelial neoplasia can be demonstrated, cure is presumed. On the other hand, it has become very obvious in our own large series that although intraepithelial neoplasia may not be present, evidence of HPV has certainly not disappeared from the lower reproductive tract as a result of the lasing. Therefore, the number of patients who will once again develop intraepithelial neoplasia from viral persistence or repeat exposure remains to be determined. It appears that placing the TZ higher in the endocervical canal reduces the incidence of CIN recurrence.

Laser Surgery of the Vulva

Unlike the cervix, the vulva is often the site of multifocal disease. There is no doubt that the concepts of accurate identification of disease and proper depth of destruction must also be applied to the therapy of VIN. Vulvar laser surgery should be done with the aid of the colposcope, and we usually prefer to use the micromanipulator. It is also imperative that the surgeon performing laser surgery on the vulva or the vagina have a working knowledge of vulvovaginal histology and of the variations in thickness of normal and abnormal neoplastic vulvovaginal epithelium.

Vulvar skin is composed of two layers, epidermis and dermis (Fig. 15.7). The margin between epidermis and dermis is an irregular one because of the rete ridges. Be-tween the rete ridges are projections of dermis known as dermal papillae. The dermis can be divided into two layers, the superficial papillary layer and the deeper reticular layer. There are also skin appendages, such as pilosebaceous follicles, eccrine sweat glands, and apocrine glands, which project deep into the dermis. VIN, as well as HPV, may involve skin appendages and epidermis. Although the thickness of the epidermis may be a fraction of a millimeter, the dermis may measure 7 to 8 mm in thickness, and skin appendages may penetrate the full thickness. It is the goal of the laser surgeon to remove the involved epidermis and a portion of the skin appendage that may also be involved in the disease process.

When the epidermis is removed by the plastic surgeon's knife in obtaining a split thickness graft or when the epidermis is removed by the laser surgeon during a vaporization procedure for intraepithelial neoplasia, the donor site or the vaporization site heals without replacement by a skin graft because the remaining skin appendages located in the dermis have not been completely destroyed. Each skin appendage serves as a source of squamous epithelium, so that when reepithelialization takes place, the process proceeds from the skin appendages. On the other hand, if the entire thickness of the dermis is taken and the skin appendages are completely destroyed, the operative site must be grafted or closed. It is important for the surgeon to review vulvar biopsies in order to judge the extent, if any, of disease into the skin appendages.

Unlike cervical vaporization, the depth of vaporization on the vulva cannot be measured. The expert laser microsurgeon is able to recognize the depth of ablation and can remove epidermis so accurately that the papillary dermis is not entirely destroyed. The papillary dermis can be identified at colposcopic magnifications. Reid has suggested that four surgical planes can be recognized. The first surgical plane represents the epidermis down to the basement membrane. The second surgical plane is described as extending into the papillary layer of the dermis so that the laser surgeon removes both the epidermis and the papillary dermis. The third surgical plane reaches well into the reticular dermis and uncovers the coarse collagen bundles that can be seen through the colposcope as grayish white fibers. The fourth surgical plane involves complete removal of the skin right down to the underlying subdermal fat. If this level is reached, healing must take place from the periphery, or a graft must be supplied.

Condylomata Acuminata

The papilloma virus involves the epidermis and may also involve the superficial portions of skin appendages. One of the common mistakes of the novice surgeon is to go too deeply into the dermis in an attempt to destroy condylomas. Although only the warty lesion itself plus the surrounding epidermal margin need to be destroyed, a power density that is sufficient to accomplish this maneuver without creating excessive carbonization at the impact site must be used. Power densities below 600 W/cm^2 cause excessive carbonization, and irradiance of

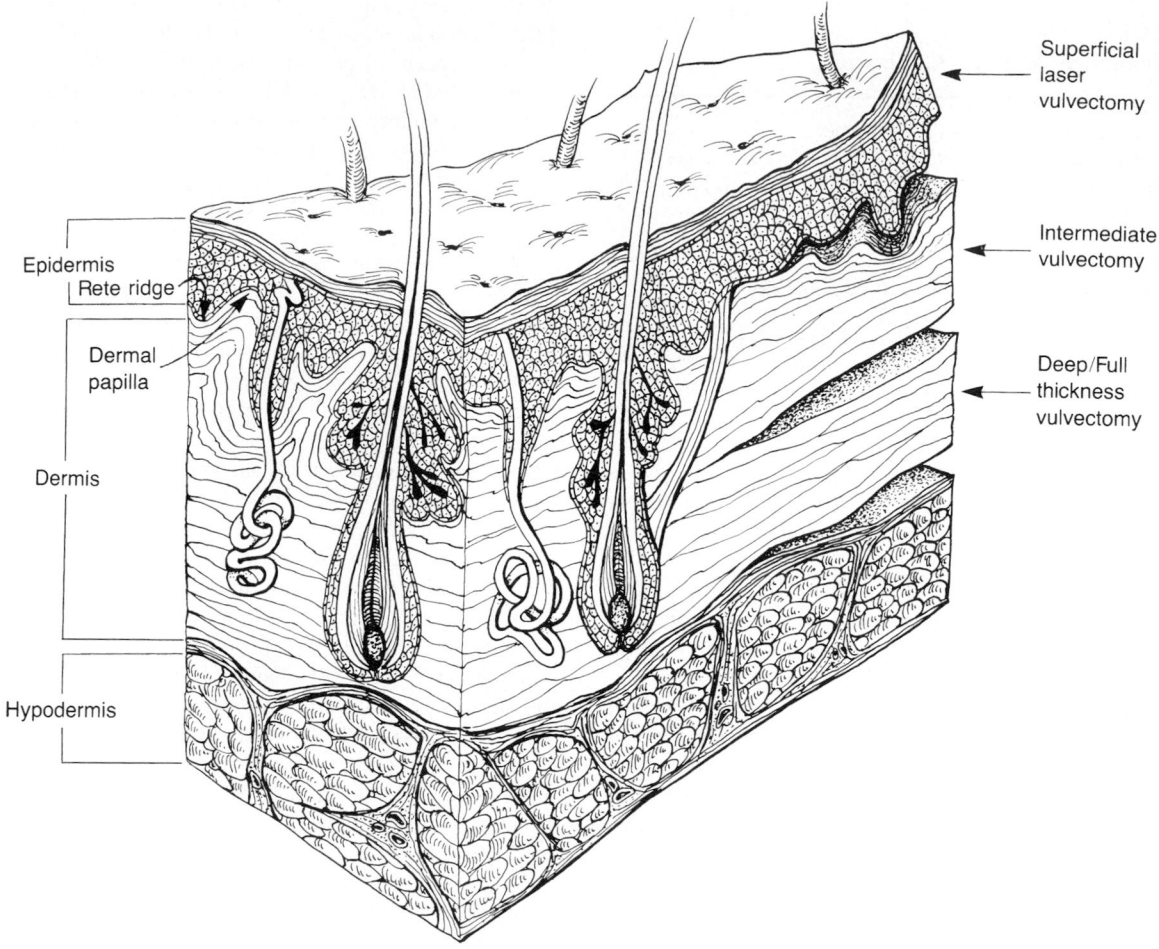

FIGURE 15.7. Vulvar skin. Vulvar skin is composed of epidermis and dermis plus the skin appendages. Complete removal of the epidermis and partial removal of the dermis still results in reepithelialization of the wound because of squamous recolonization from the skin appendages.

the carbonized surface of the vulva will raise laser-impact-site temperatures to more than 600°C. The power densities that we like to use are between 600 and 1,500 W/cm², and a 2- to 3-mm focal spot size with a power setting of 15 to 30 W will accomplish this. Each condyloma should be identified and the laser beam directed to the center of this target. Laser heat energy collapses the tissues inwardly as vaporization occurs. The surrounding skin is then again very rapidly brushed with the beam. The char and debris are wiped away, and the proper surgical level is colposcopically identified. Vaporization is taken to the papillary dermis (second surgical plane). Cold saline is used to cool the vulvar skin, because cooling helps reduce the heat diffusion and, therefore, the resultant tissue injury lateral to the laser impact site.

Vulvar Intraepithelial Neoplasia

It is impossible to colposcopically differentiate between some forms of HPV lesions that occur on the vulva and significant vulvar intraepithelial neoplasia. Therefore, it is extremely important to obtain a biopsy specimen of the vulva in as many areas as necessary to correctly identify the pathology before laser surgery. Local or general anes-

thesia may be used for vulvar laser surgery. In the case of multiple lesions or very large areas of involvement, general anesthesia is more practical. Despite extensive vulvar laser surgery, patients usually are allowed to return home on the day of the operation.

The vulva is recolposcoped, and 4% acetic acid is applied to demonstrate areas and borders of neoplastic or viral involvement. The larger areas are outlined in the manner described for CIN. If a lesion is very large, it may be divided into smaller areas for lasing, because this provides a more accurate approach. As soon as the laser beam is passed over the surface of the tissue, all landmarks disappear. Proper identification and marking of the limits of the disease by the laser is a highly necessary step in treatment. Again, a spot size of 2 to 3 mm and a power setting of 15 to 50 W may be used, depending on the surgeon's skill in manipulating the beam and spot size. Although destruction must be carried to the third surgical plane (i.e., the reticular dermis), the first step in vulvar laser surgery always involves identifying the papillary dermis. When the tiny micropapules of this layer are seen, the laser surgeon again ablates through this most superficial dermis, wiping away char and identifying the underlying reticular dermis. Often intermittent pulses of laser energy can improve surgical control of the laser beam. Instead of reducing the power of the beam, it is possible to use the mechanical timer on the laser console to reduce exposure by delivering one-tenth-second to one-twentieth-second bursts of laser energy. This technique allows the surgeon time to react to the microsurgical review of the tissue and more easily control the rate of energy delivery, thus too deep penetration, char, and residual thermal damage are also reduced to a minimum.

Postoperative Care

If the lasing has been extensive, a Foley catheter may be required to avoid the immediate discomfort caused by urinary salts on the denuded vulvar surface. Catheters can be placed either through the urethra or suprapubically. Suprapubic drainage avoids the deposit of urinary salts on the wound, reducing pain and possible infection.

Customarily, an antibacterial cream or ointment, such as sulfadine cream or bacitracin ointment, is applied to the laser wound to protect the raw surface from agglutination and to help prevent superficial infection. The patient must be given instructions to keep the vulvar folds separated, and the application of this medication helps in this respect. An ice pack is placed on the vulva when the patient leaves the operating room. Sitz baths begin the first day after laser surgery and are continued three times a day until the patient is no longer uncomfortable and the vulvar area is well on the way to reepithelialization. The patient should be seen in a week to ensure there is no agglutination of vulvar folds. Because it is possible for new lesions to appear during the healing period, weekly colposcopic inspection helps identify this problem immediately so that adjunctive therapy may begin.

Results of Vulvar Laser Surgery

In general, the results of laser surgery on the vulva have been quite satisfactory, and it appears that there are some definite advantages to using the CO_2 laser for this disease as opposed to using conventional skinning vulvectomy. These again include accurate ablation of relatively large areas and a more controlled depth of removal because of colposcopically identifiable tissue planes. Rapid healing usually occurs because of relatively little residual thermal damage. In our own series of over 100 patients with intraepithelial neoplasia, 1-year cure rates have been over 90%. Other lower reproductive tract laser surgeons report similar figures. One of the greatest benefits of vulvar laser surgery is that normal vulvar anatomy, particularly the labia minora and clitoris, is maintained. This may not be possible when skinning vulvectomy is performed.

Laser Surgery of the Vagina

Vaginal intraepithelial neoplasia (VAIN) and associated HPV infections are among the most difficult lower reproductive tract intraepithelial neoplasias to treat for a number of reasons:

1. The vagina has a large surface area, which is difficult to screen colposcopically.

2. There are many rugae and folds in the vagina.
3. The angle of the vaginal axis makes it difficult to treat by perpendicular beam impact.
4. The vaginal fornices are difficult to stabilize because they are quite distensible and the cervix may hide portions of the fornix.
5. The colposcopic appearance of VAIN varies greatly and often goes unrecognized even by the expert colposcopist.

On colposcopy, VAIN does not demonstrate mosaic patterns except in areas of adenosis. Often one does see coarse punctation, but the lesion may vary in color from a pale grayish white to the intense whiteness produced by hyperkeratosis. Most often the lesions are multifocal and the borders are usually distinct, although the lesions may be somewhat serpiginous.

The laser microsurgeon must be particularly aggressive in obtaining adequate biopsy specimens for VAIN. If the patient has had a hysterectomy, the lateral fornix may contain a dimple that must be everted for adequate visualization and biopsy. Often, a laser hook or skin hook can be used to evert this area and stabilize the tissue so that appropriate biopsy can be obtained. Once again, it must be emphasized that the surgeon should be absolutely sure of the noninvasive nature of the disease before vaporization is performed.

Technique for Vaporization of VAIN

The squamous epithelium of the mucous membrane of the vagina rests on a basement membrane. Below this is the lamina propria of the vagina, and this layer corresponds to the dermis of the vulvar skin. Below the lamina propria is a layer of muscle, loose connective tissue, and fat. When the vaginal epithelium is destroyed, there must be visual identification of the underlying lamina propria because, as in the case of the vulva, it is impossible to accurately measure the depth of destruction in this very irregular area. Because the vaginal squamous epithelium is only a fraction of a millimeter thick and there are no skin appendages in the vagina, ablation is a very superficial operation.

Lasing the vagina is painful for most patients, and although occasional small lesions in the vaginal vault can be vaporized without anesthesia, the chances of producing pain with vaginal laser surgery are very high. The manipulation of the speculum can also be very painful to the patient. In an effort to manipulate the target into a position that is perpendicular to the laser beam, the surgeon often cocks the speculum to one side and shoots through the open sides. The vaginal rugae must also be ironed out to ensure even laser energy application. All of this is most uncomfortable. For this reason, most of our patients with VAIN have undergone general anesthesia on an outpatient basis.

The micromanipulator is preferred because it eliminates bulky and unnecessary instrumentation from the vagina. We prefer to use a spot size of 2 mm and power settings of 15 to 30 W. Large areas are subdivided so that more accurate ablation can be performed. The laser beam is rapidly passed over the area, and the epidermis is lifted away from the underlying lamina propria. A wet sponge or cotton swab is used to wipe away char and coagulated epithelium. Often the surgeon will find that the tops of rugae have been removed, but the troughs or valleys in between still contain viable dysplastic epithelium. With proper use of the speculum and other instruments, this problem is easily overcome. Adequate margins of 5 mm or more are always planned.

Postoperative Care for Vaginal Laser Surgery

Much of the discomfort encountered in postoperative vaginal laser surgery stems from laser wounds in the vaginal introitus. Because VAIN and VIN are so often multifocal diseases, many of these patients will have had extensive laser surgery of the entire lower reproductive tract. In addition to sitz baths and protective vulvar creams, we also use daily vaginal applications of either estrogen or sulfa cream or of some other bacteriostatic preparation. The patient should also be examined on a weekly basis to make sure that vaginal coaptation is not occurring. Vaginal healing usually takes place from the periphery of the wound because of the lack of skin appendages in vaginal mucosa. If the laser surgeon has been thorough and the denuded area is large, healing is often delayed and granulation tissue may result. This granulation tissue may be removed and the wound then treated with a silver nitrate stick.

Results of Laser Vaporization of VAIN

Over 80 patients have been treated in our clinic with CO_2 laser for VAIN. Although Townsend and colleagues have reported very satisfactory cure rates in the laser therapy of this disease, our recurrence rates for multifocal HPV-associated VAIN are about 30% within the first year. On the other hand, unicentric VAIN has a better than 90% chance of cure with one laser surgery. As in vulvar cases, if both patient and physician are willing to retreat and use some adjunctive therapeutic measures, the 1-year cure rates are about 90%.

Indications for Laser Surgery and HPV Infection

Although 1-year cure rates produced by laser surgery for lower reproductive tract intraepithelial neoplasia have been very satisfactory, particularly in cervical cases, the persistence or recurrence of wart virus lesions has been discouraging to patients and physicians alike. Our inability to cure HPV manifestations has led many laser surgeons to question the indications for laser surgery for this disease. Most agree that intraepithelial neoplasia should be treated; however, disagreement concerning the advisability or necessity of therapy for minor HPV infection prevails. For example, patients who have evidence of HPV infection found on a cytologic smear or who have a whitish change in the vaginal introitus after application of acetic acid are dubious candidates for laser surgery. Because recurrence or persistence of subclinical HPV is so common, a more logical approach is to monitor these patients carefully but not subject them to surgery unless significant change occurs.

Adjunctive Therapy in Laser Surgery

Because of the disappointing recurrence rates of clinically evident wart virus infection, other methods of treating the disease are often combined with laser surgery. We often use local applications of trichloroacetic acid (TCA) and 5-fluorouracil (5-FU). Trichloroacetic acid is a caustic agent that precipitates the proteins in the epithelium at the site of application. Our patients are colposcoped on a weekly basis during the healing period, and obvious persistent or recurrent lesions are carefully touched with 90% TCA. The application is limited to a very small area and often needs to be repeated on a weekly basis until success is achieved. If the patient complains of burning, sodium bicarbonate on a cotton swab is applied to the area. This immediately neutralizes the acid.

5-FU has been used by dermatologists to treat superficially invasive neoplasms since the early 1960s. As reported by Krebs, topical 5-FU is available in a 5% cream in a hydrophilic base (Efudex creams). After vulvovaginal laser surgery in patients with extensive disease, the 5-FU cream is applied to the vulva and vagina with a vaginal applicator once a week for 10 weeks. Most patients are able to tolerate this treatment. Some patients will tolerate an application twice a week. This type of aggressive adjunctive therapy seems to eliminate clinical disease in a high percentage of patients. The use of 5-FU in women of reproductive age is of some concern because of possible teratogenic effects. It is therefore necessary to warn the patient and have her sign an informed consent form, acknowledging the possible untoward effects of this therapy.

Interferon alfa has also been used as adjuvant therapy to laser cytoreductive surgery in the attack on refractive condylomas. Interferons are immunostimulatory proteins that possess antiviral and antiproliferative properties. These substances have been used by direct intralesional injections, as well as systemically. Unfortunately, intralesional injection is tedious, and the number of condylomas able to be injected during one treatment is rather limited. Systemic injection carries with it significant toxicity. Thus far, interferon alfa therapy remains costly and of marginal benefit.

Anal Intraepithelial Neoplasia

Because of the high frequency of multifocal disease, colposcopic examination is not complete without inspection of the perianal tissue and the anal canal. The same techniques that were described earlier are used for the diagnosis and treatment of intraepithelial neoplasia and HPV in this region. A pediatric speculum can be used to inspect the anal canal. The surgeon should be careful to avoid lasing into hemorrhoids, but if bleeding does occur it is usually easily controlled by laser or by a stitch. A theoretic hazard of laser surgery in this region is the ignition or possible explosion of methane gas from the bowel. We often insert a wet gauze sponge in the rectum to keep stool out of the field. This also guards against methane gas explosion. In more than 4,000 cases treated in our clinic, we have never experienced this complication.

Lower Reproductive Tract Laser Surgery With Fiber-Optic Lasers

Although fiber-optic lasers have less bulky delivery systems than those of CO_2 lasers, they have not gained universal acceptance in the treatment of lower reproductive tract intraepithelial neoplasia for several reasons:

1. Wavelengths of the fiber-optic lasers available for clinical use (argon, KTP/532, YAG) penetrate tissue more deeply than does the wavelength of the CO_2 laser, thus producing more thermal damage and subsequent delayed healing.
2. Vaporization of tissue does occur but, in general, it is slower, less accurate, and more difficult than with the CO_2 laser because of the deeper penetration of the beam and the coagulation of underlying tissue.
3. The beam diverges at the quartz/air interface so that power density is greatest just at the end of the fiber. Incision of tough connective tissue, such as the cervix, is therefore best done in the contact mode. This means that, unlike the CO_2 laser mounted in the colposcope, the field is cluttered by a handpiece and other instruments that must be introduced into the operative field.

After thoroughly testing both the KTP/532 and the YAG laser on the lower reproductive tract in a variety of clinical situations, we concluded that the advantages of the fiber-optic delivery systems were far outweighed by the disadvantages for lower reproductive tract surgery.

Some surgeons, particularly urologists, continue to coagulate large condylomas with YAG laser energy and then wait for the necrotic debris to slough. This result does not seem to be as satisfactory as the results seen with CO_2 vaporization because of the obvious delay in attaining the end result and because of the deeper tissue damage caused by raw YAG laser energy.

INTRAABDOMINAL LASER SURGERY

Intraabdominal laser surgery in gynecology has been performed both at laparotomy with the abdomen open and at laparoscopy by passing laser energy down an operative laparoscope or through a laparoscopic laser handpiece.

In open abdominal surgery, the CO_2 laser can be coupled to the micromanipulator, which is mounted on an operative microscope. Just as in lower reproductive tract laser surgery, this instrument is able to vary the focal spot size of the beam and to direct the energy to target tissue with great accuracy. Alternatively, any laser, CO_2 or fiber-optic, can be used with a handpiece in conjunction with either the microscope or surgical loops. Al-

though this approach seems logical and promising, no convincing data have yet been presented that show a definite benefit or superiority of open abdominal laser surgery over the usual conventional surgical techniques.

On the other hand, laser laparoscopy has provided an extremely versatile and safe alternative to the use of laparoscopic unipolar electrical instruments. Numerous reports by gynecologic laparoscopists attest to the efficacy of laser in both reproductive and reconstructive surgery. Laparoscopy continues to offer the most challenging and accepted use of laser in the abdominal cavity.

In our clinic, open abdominal laser surgery is now a relatively rare event. This is the result of two factors: Most intraabdominal laser operations are now performed laparoscopically, and we are not convinced that laser has any benefit over electrosurgery for open abdominal surgery.

Open Abdominal Laser Surgery

Most laser laparotomies reported in the literature have been performed by surgeons using the CO_2 laser. Safety, small residual thermal damage, and great variability of focal spot size contribute to the appeal of this instrument.

In the abdominal cavity, laser surgery and conventional techniques go together. The laser surgeon uses the same microsurgical instrumentation as in conventional microsurgery but has added some special instruments for use with the laser. Although the laser has been used for many types of intraabdominal procedures, it seems most useful for adhesiolysis, particularly the filmy types of adhesions that often obstruct the adnexa; ablation of endometriosis; and certain types of tubal reconstructive procedures such as neosalpingostomy.

General Principles of Intraabdominal Laser Surgery

Paper drapes should not be used by the laser surgeon as they could burst into flames by a misdirected laser beam. The newer disposable laparotomy drapes are flame resistant, although the drape may literally melt with resulting burn. Protective wet cotton packs are always used for the wound edges, bowel, and other exposed organs. Laser energy may be reflected from polished instruments, so all delicate surfaces should be protected.

The proper power density must be selected for each laser procedure. In general, power densities used in intraabdominal laser surgery are relatively low, varying between 5 and 30 W. Superpulse is often used for cutting to further limit lateral thermal damage, but the use of continuous-wave gated pulses also may give greater control for the laser surgeon when either vaporizing or cutting.

Because laser energy continues to travel and damage tissue once it cuts through the target, the surgeon must often select an appropriate backstop. Various microsurgical dissecting rods are available to use as both dissecting tools and laser backstops. In general, glass, Pyrex, and quartz rods should be avoided because they shatter under the intense heat of the laser. The surgeon must always keep the temperature of the dissecting rod at appropriate levels by constant irrigation and cleansing of char. Titanium or very smooth blackened rods serve as excellent backstop dissectors.

Although the laser is superb for coagulating tiny bleeders, vessels larger than 0.5 mm in diameter may be difficult to coagulate with the CO_2 laser. If it is not immediately apparent that the laser is achieving hemostasis without significant damage to tissue, conventional methods of hemostasis should be used. The surgeon should not hesitate to use a bipolar electrode or precise atraumatic microsurgical suturing to minimize tissue damage. Char must always be cleared or washed away from lased tissue. Not only are carbon particles incorporated into the peritoneal scar, but scorched tissue impedes healing and decreases the surgeon's ability to visually recognize tissue planes. Wet cotton-tipped applicators help in the gentle removal of char and often serve as excellent backstops.

The laser mirror is also an instrument that may allow the surgeon to operate in inaccessible areas. For example, an ovary that is adherent to the lateral pelvic wall may often be freed by visualizing the adherent surface in the mirror and then directing the laser beam from the mirror to the adhesion. The best mirrors have polished-gold reflecting surfaces. Dental mirrors cannot be used because of the possibility of shatter. Mirrors tend to be clouded very rapidly by laser smoke and other debris, so constant polishing and wiping of this instrument are required.

Removal of the laser plume is extremely important because the smoke is unpleasant to breathe and may carry some health hazards.

CO_2 Laser Adhesiolysis

Adhesiolysis with the laser has been performed mainly by reproductive surgeons to enhance fertility. There are few studies that compare the results of laser adhesiolysis to those of conventional surgical methods. Unfortunately, very few surgeons actually use a system of grading adhesions; therefore, it is difficult to accumulate statistically meaningful numbers of equivalent patients in study subsets. Differences in surgeons' techniques and abilities also make comparisons less meaningful.

A number of techniques are useful in laser adhesiolysis. The operation varies with the type of adhesion. In general, three maneuvers are used:

1. Laser incision of thick adhesions is performed with use of a small spot size and high power density. Dense adhesive bands are usually cut with spot sizes of 0.2 mm to 1 mm, and power settings are in the range of 20 to 30 W.
2. Filmy adhesions are vaporized and divided with much lower power density. The defocused beam is often used, and when the appropriate backstop is applied, the adhesion can literally be made to disappear without damage to underlying structures.
3. Thick adhesions between delicate structures such as tube and ovary may be lased with intermediate power

density and spot size. A good assistant who is knowledgeable in the use of the dissecting rods and backstops can present the adhesions to the surgeon, and with gentle traction applied, the adhesion can be vaporized with minimal or no residual tissue damage.

Laser Laparotomy for Endometriosis

Small endometrial implants can be effectively vaporized by CO_2 laser energy. However, to excise larger implants and ovarian endometriomas, the surgeon needs a precise knowledge of excisional depth. Incomplete vaporization often results in persistence of disease. Excision offers a more complete and accurate method of removal. Endometrial ovarian cysts resected with a CO_2 laser may require suturing, and raw surfaces of the peritoneum and other structures should be closed by conventional microsurgical technique when possible. The results of laser surgery for patients with endometriosis seem comparable to the results produced by other careful operative procedures using conventional techniques. Pregnancy rates and recurrence rates are essentially the same; however, many laser surgeons feel that laser surgery speeds the operative procedure.

Laser Surgery of the Tube

The adaptation of microsurgical principles to tubal surgery has greatly improved the outcome of fertility enhancement procedures. Undoubtedly, laser vaporization and excision have added some new dimensions to the practice of microsurgery. As with conventional microsurgery, three types of laser tubal microsurgical procedures are usually described, depending on the anatomic region of the tube involved. These are terminal tuboplasty, tubotubal anastomosis, and tubouterine anastomosis.

Terminal salpingostomy is often suitable for laser surgery. The success of this procedure is related to the amount of terminal tube that has to be removed to cause satisfactory neostomy. The best result depends on identifying the original site of the tubal ostium, opening this area with the focused laser beam, and freeing what is left of the fimbria. The tube is gently distended by intrauterine injection of dilute indigo-carmine solution so that use of a backstop is not necessary. As laser incision of this area proceeds, the lumen is immediately identified as the dye appears. Three or four radial incisions may be made in the closed tube so that satisfactory eversion of mucosa results. The defocused laser beam may also be applied to the tubal serosa, which contracts, thereby producing mucosal eversion. This technique was first described by Bruhat and is often referred to as Bruhat's procedure. This operation may also be accomplished at laparoscopy by using exactly the same technique. If the surgeon prefers a contact laser such as the YAG with a sapphire tip, the side of the sapphire is applied to the serosa of the tube and the handpiece is gently rolled. In either case, it is heat and the resultant contraction of desiccated tissue that cause the eversion of the fimbria. We have found that it is sometimes necessary to use no. 9-0 nylon sutures to effect a permanent eversion of the fimbria or ampullary mucosa.

Although tubotubal anastomosis and tubouterine anastomosis have been successfully accomplished with laser in the open abdomen, we believe that less tissue damage occurs with the knife, scissors, or even the microelectrode. For this reason, laser has not recently been used in our operating rooms for these procedures.

The results of CO_2 laser surgery are often compared with the results of tubomicrosurgery with microelectrodes. Bellina (1983) reported excellent results with the CO_2 laser that are certainly comparable to those achieved by conventional microsurgical methods. He also believes that operative time has been reduced by using the CO_2 laser. On the other hand, it certainly appears that expert microsurgeons who champion a particular method have developed a tremendous confidence with their favorite tool. Superiority of one modality over the other remains to be established. It appears that microsurgical technique and a competent surgeon, plus extent of the disease, are the most important factors in tubal reconstructive surgery.

Laser Myomectomy

Both the CO_2 laser and fiber-optic lasers have been used for myomectomy, as a substitute for electrocautery. The superficial vessels on the leiomyoma can be coagulated by the defocused beam. Whether one uses the CO_2 laser or the KTP, argon, or YAG laser scalpel, hemostasis may be enhanced by the use of laser energy to perform the dissection. Again, there is no benefit to laser over electrosurgery for open myomectomy.

Summary

The use of the laser in open abdominal surgery, when used by experienced laser microsurgeons, certainly produced results equivalent to those of other conventional approaches, but convincing data on laser benefits are still lacking. Perhaps one of the best reasons for gaining expertise with open abdominal laser surgery is that it schools the laser surgeon for the much more demanding task of advanced laparoscopic laser surgery.

GYNECOLOGIC LASER LAPAROSCOPY

In the United States, operative laparoscopy really began in the late 1960s when unipolar electrical instruments were used with the laparoscope to effect tubal sterilization. During the 1970s, Semm described the techniques of laparoscopic vessel ligation and tissue suturing, and in 1978 Bruhat used the CO_2 laser with an operative laparoscope to treat ectopic pregnancy. The ability to cut and vaporize tissue, and to control bleeding as well, provided gynecologic surgeons with the tools necessary to effect complicated surgical procedures with laparoscopic

instrumentation. Because the laser alone is not adequate to ensure the hemostasis so often needed for major laparoscopic surgery, the conventional methods for achieving hemostasis, including suturing and ligation of vascular pedicles, and electrical coagulation must also be mastered by the laser laparoscopist (Table 15.5). The laser is a surgical tool that assists the informed and skilled operator to safely perform a given task. It is by no means a complete system of laparoscopy and must be viewed only as an instrument that forms a part of our laparoscopic armamentarium.

Advantages of Laser Laparoscopy

In operative laparoscopy, the energy source with which the laser is most commonly compared, and for which it most often substitutes, is electricity. Electricity delivered through an insulated instrument that has been passed down the operative channel of a telescope or through a trocar sheath is an efficient and inexpensive coagulator, as well as an excellent cutting tool. Unfortunately, because of the different manner in which electrical energy is delivered into the abdominal cavity (i.e., through long insulated instruments passing through trocar sheaths), the use of electricity in laparoscopy is not as safe as when the abdomen is open. This problem is compounded by the fact that the laparoscopic surgeon seldom views more than about 15% to 20% of the operative field while performing a surgical task. The dangers of electrical bowel injury were first appreciated by laparoscopists whose patients sustained bowel injuries while undergoing tubal sterilization procedures in the early days of laparoscopic surgery. There are several important electrical phenomena that any surgeon using electricity must thoroughly understand. It is these characteristics of radiofrequency electrical currents that may make electricity difficult to control in laparoscopic surgery.

1. Electricity follows the path of least resistance, and that pathway may not be immediately apparent to the operator.
2. Breaks in the insulation surrounding the conductor in a laparoscopic instrument may allow electricity to directly flow into an area not under observation by the laparoscopist. Disruption of insulation may also pro-

---

TABLE 15.5.
Methods for Achieving Laparoscopic Hemostasis

Unipolar electrocoagulation
Bipolar electrocoagulation
Laser coagulation
Extracorporeal ligatures
Extracorporeal sutures
Intracorporeal sutures
Endocoagulation (Semm)
Hemoclip

duce direct coupling of the current to another laparoscopic instrument, such as a trocar sheath. A metallic trocar sheath may then become an electrode in contact with intraabdominal organs.

3. Capacitive coupling may occur even though insulation is completely intact when current flows through one insulated conductor that has been passed through another conductor. An example of capacitive coupling is appreciated when a well-insulated needle electrode is passed down the channel of an operative microscope, and up to 80% of the current is found to be induced in the barrel of the telescope. The laparoscopist cannot see the telescopic trocar sheath or the barrel of the scope that may be transmitting electrical energy.

4. Even bipolar coagulation may be dangerous if the operator is not aware that although the current is flowing through the tissue between the jaws of the bipolar forceps, significant heat is being produced and significant lateral tissue damage may occur by thermal spread.

Laser energy may provide a safer type of surgery for the laparoscopist. With the laser, there is no path of least resistance, direct and capacitive coupling does not occur, and, depending on the wavelength of the laser used, lateral thermal damage is usually minimal and can be accurately predicted by a surgeon who understands the characteristics of the wavelength.

In our operating room, laser is commonly used as the primary energy for incision and vaporization during laparoscopic surgery. It is particularly useful to use laser energy with the operative laparoscope for several reasons:

1. The operative laparoscope provides a straight-on shot at a pelvic target, which is not possible when a laser handpiece is passed into the pelvis from a secondary lateral port.

2. The operative scope provides another port of entry for laser energy. If only a diagnostic telescope is used, an additional trocar over and above the ones inserted for laparoscopic instrumentation must be used.

3. The operative scope may also provide an additional channel for the longer bipolar forceps.

We believe that bipolar forceps are the safest of the electrical instruments available to the laparoscopist because capacitive coupling does not occur with this instrument, and the electrical current flows between the two jaws of the forceps. When used with laser to achieve hemostasis, it became an indispensable instrument for the laser surgeon. Again, the operator must always be aware of the possibility of spreading lateral thermal damage and must be sure of the anatomic structures such as the ureter that may lie adjacent to the point of application.

CO_2 Laser Laparoscopy

The CO_2 laser can be connected to an operative laparoscope or to laparoscopic handpieces through a laser coupler that transmits the beam through a focusing lens and then down a special channel in the instrument. Laser couplers may be direct or may require adjustment of the beam by means of a joystick that is then fixed in position once the beam has been aligned with the operative channel. Usually there are interchangeable lenses that provide focal lengths commensurate with the length of the laparoscope or the handpiece. Focal spot sizes produced by these systems are usually a bit less than a millimeter in diameter. The CO_2 laser is an excellent laser for laparoscopic usage because it cuts quickly, produces very little thermal damage, and can be used for vaporization, coagulation, or excision. It is very safe in the hands of a knowledgeable surgeon because of its almost complete absorption in a thin layer of water. On the other hand, there are some definite disadvantages to CO_2 laser laparoscopy. These are listed in Table 15.6.

The mirrors in the CO_2 laser arm must be very carefully aligned or the arm will lack rotational stability (i.e., when the arm is rotated, the aiming beam and the CO_2 beam will become misaligned). The resultant reflection of the beam within the arm itself produces distortion of the CO_2 laser and distortion of the helium-neon aiming beam so that the latter is often difficult to see, particularly in a brightly lit peritoneal cavity. In general, the more the laser is moved from room to room and used by many different surgeons, the more difficult it becomes to keep the arm adjusted. Because of these difficulties, efforts to develop a fiber that will carry CO_2 laser energy have continued.

KTP/532 and Argon Laser Laparoscopy

The fiber-optic lasers have some great advantages over CO_2 lasers because the laser energy passes down a quartz fiber, and endoscopic delivery is greatly simplified (Table 15.7). The deeper penetration of these wavelengths, however, must always be kept in mind.

TABLE 15.6.
CO_2 Laser Laparoscopy Disadvantages

Poor hemostatis
Cumbersome equipment
Difficult to align beam
Often difficult to identify helium-neon beam
Too much laser plume produced

TABLE 15.7.
Advantages of Fiberoptic Laser Surgery

Equipment less cumbersome
Contact modes of cutting, vaporizing, coagulating
Very accurate targeting
Less plume
Better hemostasis
Smaller channel needed for fibers

The blue or green aiming beams of these lasers are more easily seen against the reddish background of the abdominal organs than is the helium–neon beam. The quartz laser fibers will pass through an 18-gauge or smaller needle, so handpieces designed for suction and irrigation also may have a central channel that accommodates the fiber. This enables the surgeon to use suction, irrigation, and laser energy through one handpiece, and these handpieces fit easily through a 5-mm trocar sheath. The disadvantages of fiber-optic lasers are that they do not cut quite as well as CO_2 lasers and are less safe because of their penetration of both tissue and water.

YAG Laser Laparoscopy

YAG laser energy was first used through the laparoscope in 1982. Most laser surgeons have considered the delivery of YAG energy by bare fiber too dangerous for use in the abdominal cavity because YAG energy penetrates up to 4 mm into tissue. However, by attaching an artificial sapphire tip to the end of the quartz fiber, the egress of laser energy from the fiber is blocked, and most of the energy is absorbed by the sapphire tip. Thus, YAG energy heats the tip, and cutting, coagulation, and vaporization are accomplished by the heated sapphire. Because the sapphire tip may become too hot, it is continuously cooled by the flow of CO_2 delivered through a hollow plastic tubing that holds the fiber. A number of different sapphire tips are available and can be selected, depending on their intended use (Fig. 15.8). Little laser energy is passed into the tissue, and the hot sapphire accomplishes the job at hand. The YAG laser is the device most often used in our operating rooms for laparoscopy. It provides contact cutting with the target tissue that is similar to, but safer than, that of a monopolar electrode. It is important to note that the clad fiber with its CO_2 delivery

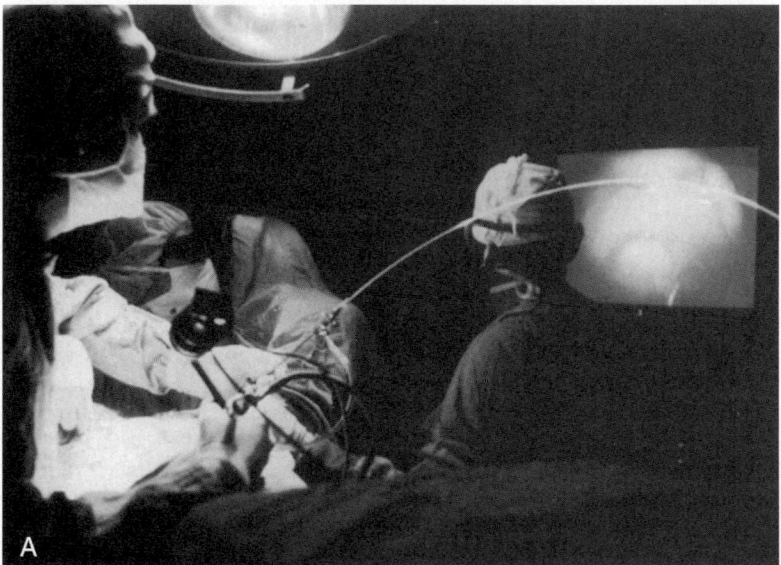

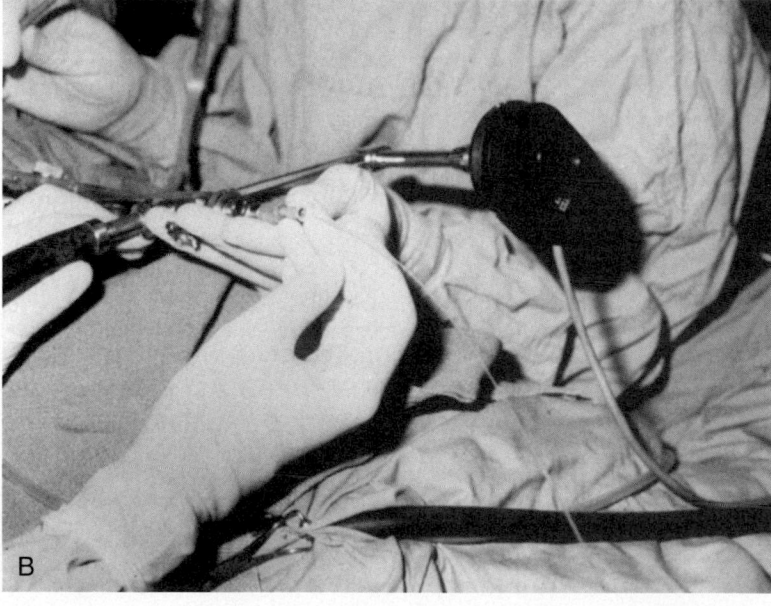

FIGURE 15.8. Fiber-optic laser laparoscopy. Some of the advantages of fiber-optic lasers are the ease with which the fiber is used in either the operative laparoscope or through a suction irrigation handpiece (**A**) and the uncluttered area surrounding the operative site (**B**). Here a quartz fiber of a KTP laser is passed into the laparoscope, which is equipped with an optical filter. The video camera will be attached over this filter.

system is never used in hysteroscopy because of the probability of gas embolization.

Techniques of Operative Laparoscopy

Irrespective of the type of laser used, the surgeon will need to remove laser plume effectively. Often clotted blood may occlude the suction cannula so that a superior suction-irrigation device with adequate trumpet valves that do not constantly obstruct is needed. The new rapid-fill automatic insufflators are highly desirable because they can be set to maintain a constant intraabdominal pressure and will deliver a flow of CO_2 of up to 6 L per minute and will simultaneously record intraabdominal pressure. A high-intensity light source is also of great importance. A high-quality video camera is attached to the laparoscope, and all operative endoscopy in our clinic is performed while the surgeon views the video monitor. The advantages of video usage are that the entire operating room becomes a team. The assistant is always aware of the progress of the operation, and the surgeon is able to stand erect while inspecting all parts of the abdominal cavity.

The patient is placed in a modified lithotomy position so that the thigh is almost level with the patient's abdomen. This enables the surgeon to direct the laparoscope cephalad. This maneuver may be important not only for exploration but also for operating at the pelvic brim. If the hip is flexed and the thighs are elevated, the scope and perhaps the accessory instrumentation cannot be manipulated freely because they will be in contact with the patient's thighs. After preparation and draping, an intrauterine manipulating device is placed into the uterus for two purposes: to elevate or maneuver the uterus during surgery without having to use intraabdominal instruments for this task, and to perform chromopertubation when necessary.

Most of our advanced operative laparoscopic procedures require three incisions. The laparoscope is inserted through a transverse incision in the umbilicus, and two other incisions are made in the lower abdomen on either side of the midline. The anterior abdominal wall is viewed from the inside, and the inferior epigastric vessels are identified so that they are not damaged by the secondary trocar insertions. We insert a 22-gauge spinal needle through the anterior abdominal wall at the intended site of trocar insertion, and we note its position in relation to the inferior epigastric vessels and the iliac vessels. This helps us ensure that the trocar will miss these vessels, and it also indicates the angle of approach that the instruments will take to the target. Needless to say, the entrance of secondary trocars into the abdominal cavity is carefully watched through the laparoscope.

Trocar diameters are selected depending on the intended use. If stapling devices are to be used, a 11.5-mm trocar will be inserted in both lower quadrants. Laparoscopic needle holders and curved needles are able to be passed without difficulty through these sleeves.

In our operating rooms, more than 2,000 operative laparoscopies are performed each year. Since the last edition of this text, the number of procedures and their complexity have increased. Table 15.8 lists the more common procedures that have been aided by the use of laser.

Fulguration or Excision of Endometriosis

Smaller implants of mild-to-moderate endometriosis can be effectively vaporized, coagulated, or excised with either the CO_2 or the fiber-optic laser. Even small endometrial implants are surrounded by subclinical endometriosis, so a margin of vaporization or coagulation is planned around the endometrial implant. Implants that are located over the ureter may be vaporized safely by a variety of methods. The ureter is always identified by the laparoscopic surgeon. Often, in cases of severe endometriosis, preoperative cystoscopy is performed and ureteral catheters placed. It is usually easier to visualize the ureter at the bifurcation of the common iliac artery as it passes into the pelvis. The ureter is then traced down to the cardinal ligament, where it is more difficult to identify. Often the ureter can be moved beneath the peritoneum by manipulating the ureteral catheter so that its position is more easily seen. Injection of the irrigating fluid retroperitoneally into the broad ligament or the lateral pelvic side wall will provide a watery backstop that helps with dissection and also increases safety, particularly if CO_2 energy is used. This is not protective for fiber-optic laser energy; however, hydrodissection does often separate the ureter from the implant so that excision with scissors or a sapphire tip is safely expedited.

The laser surgeon rapidly develops the ability to excise peritoneum. This is a technique that may be used for the removal of endometriomas. The peritoneum is perforated by laser energy, and the opening is enlarged with the suction irrigator. Dissection can be performed bluntly by the instrument or with the aid of the irrigating fluid. Forceps are used to elevate the peritoneum, and the laser is used to complete the excision. The small

---

TABLE 15.8.
Laser Laparoscopy Procedures

Procedure	Percentage
Fulguration or excision of endometriosis	68
Lysis of adhesions	62
Ovarian cystectomy	31
Division of uterosacral ligaments	30
Presacral neurectomy	10
Salpingo-oophorectomy and variations	22
Removal of ectopic pregnancy	10
Myomectomy	4
Neosalpingostomy	4
Laparoscopically assisted vaginal hysterectomy	18
Retropubic urethropexy	10
Sacral colpopexy	3

blood vessels usually encountered in this type of dissection are effectively sealed by laser. Results of reported early series of endometriosis treated laparoscopically have been compiled by Martin and Diamond. These compare favorably to results produced by conventional surgery at laparotomy (Table 15.9). More recent reports by Sutton and associates of controlled, randomized trials of CO_2 laser laparoscopy for the treatment of endometriosis and pelvic pain have continued to emphasize favorable outcomes.

Ovarian Cystectomy

Resection of an ovarian cyst at laparoscopy is a controversial subject. Many surgeons believe that spillage of a stage I malignant neoplasm or an epithelial tumor of borderline malignancy may result in spread of the disease. Unfortunately, most ovarian malignancies are not discovered when they are at an early stage. Because most young women who have cystic adnexal masses will not have ovarian malignancies, it seems desirable to make an attempt at diagnosis and extirpation by the laparoscopic approach. To minimize mistakes, the cystic mass should always be evaluated by noninvasive means, such as sonography or magnetic resonance imaging. Tumor markers are also obtained, and finally, a laparoscopic diagnosis is attempted.

Ovarian endometriomas should be excised rather than vaporized. We have experienced a high incidence of recurrence when endometriomas larger than 2 cm have been opened and vaporized rather than excised. Then, too, the universal rule of laser surgery applies to the laparoscopic surgeon, as well as to the lower reproductive tract surgeon. Vaporization should never be performed in the absence of a pathologic diagnosis. Therefore, we prefer to evacuate the ovarian endometrioma and remove it by stripping the cystic capsule away from the ovarian stroma. Two forceps are placed through the two lower abdominal 5-mm trocar sheaths, and while one forceps holds the ovarian cortex, the other gently strips away the cyst wall. After the cyst has been removed, the ovarian stroma is coagulated. Hemostasis is usually achieved very easily in this fashion. We try to avoid suturing the ovary because suture material often produces adhesions. If hemostasis is not obtained with the laser, then the endocoagulator or bipolar electrode may be used.

Other ovarian cysts that appear to be benign may be handled in a similar fashion. After percutaneous tap of

---

TABLE 15.9.
CO_2 Laser Laparoscopy for Endometriosis

Investigator	Patients Number	Patients Pregnant	Minimal or Mild Number	Minimal or Mild Pregnant	Moderate Number	Moderate Pregnant	Severe or Extensive Number	Severe or Extensive Pregnant
ENDOMETRIOSIS IN ALL PATIENTS								
Kelly and Roberts, 1983	10	6 (60%)	3	3 (100%)	7	3 (43%)	0	0 (0%)
Feste, 1983	140	82 (59%)	106	62 (58%)	31	18 (58%)	3	2 (67%)
Daniell, 1985	48	26 (54%)	24	16 (67%)	15	7 (47%)	9	3 (33%)
Martin and Diamond, 1986	115	54 (47%)	56	23 (41%)	45	22 (49%)	14	9 (64%)
Davis, 1986	64	37 (58%)	31	20 (65%)	26	15 (58%)	7	2 (29%)
Nezhat, 1986	102	65 (64%)	24	18 (75%)	51	32 (63%)	27	15 (56%)
Adamson, 1986	156	86 (55%)	133	77 (58%)	20	7 (33%)	3	0 (0%)
Bowman, 1986	35	18 (51%)	19	12 (63%)	13	4 (31%)	3	2 (67%)
Donnez, 1987	70	40 (57%)	42	26 (62%)	21	11 (52%)	7	3 (43%)
Paulsen, 1987	431	225 (52%)	257	144 (56%)	174	81 (47%)	0	0 (0%)
Gast, 1988	122	57 (47%)	105	49 (47%)	17	8 (47%)	0	0 (0%)
Nezhat, 1989	243	168 (69%)	39	28 (72%)	86	60 (70%)	118	80 (68%)
TOTALS	1,536	864 (56%)	839	478 (57%)	506	268 (53%)	191	116 (61%)
ENDOMETRIOSIS AS AN ISOLATED FACTOR								
Feste, 1985	60	42 (70%)	44	3 (70%)	14	10 (71%)	2	1 (50%)
Martin, 1985	34	23 (67%)	13	9 (69%)	11	6 (55%)	10	8 (80%)
Nezhat, 1986	102	65 (64%)	24	18 (75%)	51	32 (63%)	27	15 (56%)
Adamson, 1986	60	39 (65%)	47	31 (66%)	11	7 (61%)	2	0 (0%)
Paulsen, 1987	228	169 (74%)	140	109 (78%)	88	60 (68%)	0	0 (0%)
Gast, 1988	27	7 (26%)		NA		NA	0	0 (0%)
Nezhat, 1989	243	168 (69%)	39	28 (72%)	86	60 (70%)	118	80 (68%)
TOTALS	754	513 (68%)	307	226 (74%)	261	175 (67%)	159	104 (65%)

NA, not available.

(Adapted from: Martin DC, Diamond MP. Operative laparoscopy: comparison of lasers with other techniques. *Curr Probl Obstet Gynecol Fertil* 1986;9:564.)

the cysts with a 22-gauge needle, the fluid is sent for cytology. A small incision can be made in the cyst wall with the laser, and a 5- or 3-mm scope can actually be placed into the cyst cavity and the wall of the cyst inspected. If papillary projections are seen, the surgeon has the choice of immediately proceeding to laparotomy or removing the ovary laparoscopically by endoloop ligation of the adnexal blood supply. Expert aspiration of the cyst with a 22-gauge needle seldom results in significant leakage, and lavage of the pelvic cavity with copious quantities of lactated Ringer solution further reduces the chance of spread of disease. Bruhat reports use of a protocol similar to ours and, in more than 600 ovarian cystectomies, has encountered only three low-malignant-potential tumors. None of these have spread. We have now performed hundreds carefully selected cystectomies in our clinic and have not encountered a problem with spread of a malignancy.

Lysis of Adhesions

Adhesions between omentum and anterior abdominal wall are usually handled very rapidly and efficiently by laser energy. One of the great benefits of using laser energy through the operative scope is that most omental adhesions to the anterior abdominal wall may be separated with laser and scope alone without insertion of other trocars (Fig. 15.9). Often we have cleaned off all adhesions that lie directly under intended sites of secondary trocar incision with this single puncture method. We also often use the Hasson's open technique when inserting the umbilical trocar in cases that may involve significant adhesions. Blood vessels that are seen in the adhesions can often be coagulated slowly with the laser beam or sapphire tip before cutting.

Bowel adhesions prove a more difficult problem. If a backstop can be manipulated between loops of bowel, or if the loop of bowel can be held gently apart so the laser energy is directly applied to the adhesion without fear of bowel damage, then laser adhesiolysis is feasible. On the other hand, sharp and blunt dissection with laparoscopic

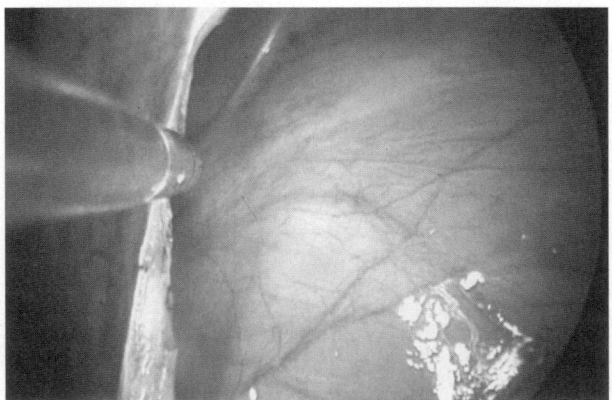

FIGURE 15.9. Laser through the operative scope often provides an excellent tool for cutting adhesions that may interfere with the insertion of secondary trocars. See color version of figure.

forceps, scissors, or microscissors is often a safer procedure. When thick bands of adhesions are attacked with any of the lasers, the power should be turned up. The laser surgeon rapidly becomes accustomed to the effects of various power settings on a chosen laser. It is particularly helpful if the laparoscopic surgeon is familiar with open laser laparotomy techniques.

One of the rare complications of laser surgery has been bowel perforation. In general, the small bowel should not be subjected to the laser beam. The wall of this organ is too thin, and delayed postoperative perforation may occur. The large bowel is much thicker, and the expert laser surgeon comes to appreciate how much laser dissection is possible on areas such as the rectosigmoid.

Uterosacral Ligament Division

Very little has been written about uterosacral ligament division for the treatment of pelvic pain. Pain stimuli originating from the cervix are usually registered through the sacral sympathetic chain and conducted through the uterosacral ligaments to the sacral sympathetic plexus by way of nerve roots S-2, S-3, and S-4. Feste has reported relief of dysmenorrhea in more than 70% of the women who underwent CO_2 laser division of the uterosacral ligaments and who were monitored for over a year. Lichten in 1987, in a well-controlled series, reported a success rate of more than 80% in patients followed for more than a year. In our series of 60 patients undergoing uterosacral ligament division for either primary dysmenorrhea or dysmenorrhea associated with endometriosis, 70% of the women monitored over the course of the year claimed complete or significant pain relief.

The uterosacral ligament can sometimes be confused with the ureter, so the latter structure must always be positively identified. We identify the ureter at the bifurcation of the common iliac artery and trace it into the pelvis to a point at which it disappears in the cardinal ligament. At the same time that the uterosacral ligament is identified, the division is planned close to its insertion into the uterus. Uterosacral ligaments vary tremendously in size and structure. The division should begin at the posterior uterine wall, and a section of about 1 cm of uterosacral ligament should be removed in its entire thickness. Just lateral to the uterosacral ligament lies a branch of the uterine artery as well as the ureter, so one should make an attempt to stay medial. Power settings of 20 W may be used on the CO_2 laser, and on fiber-optic lasers, 10 to 15 W will suffice.

Presacral Neurectomy

Presacral neurectomy has been performed laparoscopically in our operating rooms since 1993. The approach to the presacral space demands greater care because the superior border of the space is formed by the bifurcation of the aorta, and the lateral borders are represented by the iliac vessels and the ureters. The bowel must be moved away from the peritoneum over the promontory

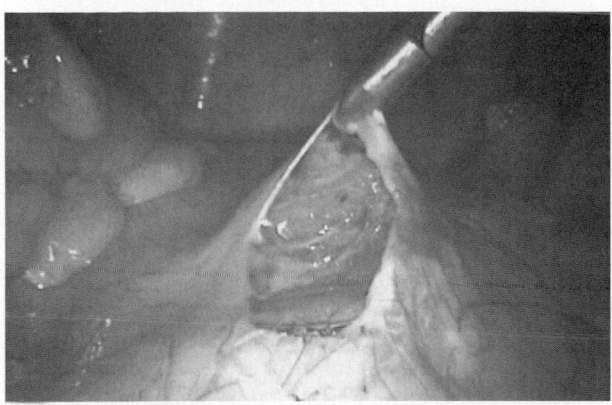

FIGURE 15.10. Presacral neurectomy. The peritoneum has been incised vertically. The tissue over the sacral promontory is seen. To either side, irrigating fluid can be seen beneath the peritoneum. See color version of figure.

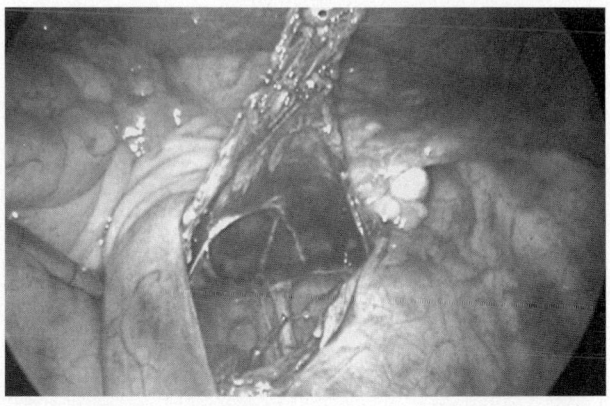

FIGURE 15.12. Most of the neural trunk is now mobilized and will be excised with the laser. Ureter and great vessels have been carefully identified. See color version of figure.

of the sacrum. This is often aided by placing the patient in a relatively steep Trendelenburg position and tilting the table to the left. The peritoneum is carefully palpated and then lifted over the sacral promontory, and a small incision is made (Fig. 15.10). Hydrodissection gently lifts the peritoneum from the underlying tissue, and a vertical incision is carefully made with laser energy through the operative scope. The nerve branches are then dissected as described elsewhere in this text (Fig. 15.11). Laser is used to sever the nerve trunks, and clips, ligatures, or bipolar current is used to obtain hemostasis (Fig. 15.12). Our results with this procedure have been exactly the same as when the operation is performed through the open abdomen.

Terminal Salpingostomy

Laser laparoscopy for terminal salpingostomy is performed in a fashion very similar to that already described for laser laparotomy. We use a CO_2 laser with a very small spot size or a YAG laser with a sapphire tip. Linear inci-

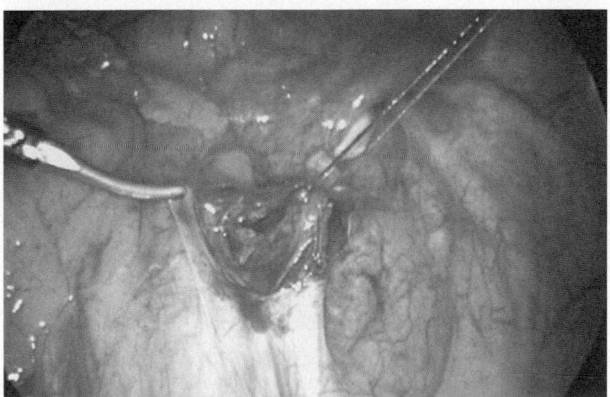

FIGURE 15.11. Nerve bundles and connective tissue are elevated as the periosteum is cleaned of the overlying tissue. A suture ligature serves as traction. See color version of figure.

sions are made as described after the tube has been filled with a dilute solution of indigo-carmine dye, which is injected through an intrauterine cannula. The ampulla is distended by the solution, and the scar marking the previous ampullary opening is identified. Linear incisions are then used to open the tube. The CO_2 laser is used at 20 to 40 W, whereas the YAG setting is 15 to 15 W. The tubes can be held gently with atraumatic forceps while the laser beam is applied through either the operative scope or one of the secondary puncture sites. In 1988, Fayez and colleagues reported a postoperative patency rate of 31% in 19 patients monitored over 1 year by hysterosalpingography. Two of the 19 patients conceived; both of these were ectopic gestations. Daniell and Herbert (1984) reported that better results were obtained with the CO_2 and KTP lasers. Tubal patency at 6 weeks in 140 patients treated by either CO_2 or KTP laser was 83%; the overall intrauterine pregnancy rate was 28%, the tubal pregnancy rate was 13%, and the abortion rate was 12%.

Myomectomy

The indications for a laparoscopic myomectomy are the same as the indications for myomectomy in general. Significant size, rapid growth, selected cases of infertility or pressure symptoms, and heavy bleeding have all been acceptable indications for surgical intervention. Pedunculated leiomyomas can often be easily removed at laser laparoscopy, but intramural myomas that are deeply imbedded in the myometrium may pose a real challenge.

Laparoscopic myomectomy is a controversial procedure because of the need to perform careful uterine reconstruction if the patient desires future childbearing. This operation should not be attempted by any laparoscopist who is not familiar with advanced suturing techniques or able to close the myometrium in layers.

Our technique uses percutaneous injection of a dilute solution of vasopressin to the base of the leiomyoma and the surrounding myometrium. Three lower abdominal accessory punctures are used. The myometrium over the leiomyoma is incised with the laser. Two lateral forceps are used to grasp the myometrium, and this is gently stripped away from the underlying myoma much in the way that an orange is peeled. The laser is used to coagulate vessels on the surface of the leiomyoma and, as the base is approached, to coagulate and cut vessels in that area. If excessive bleeding is encountered, laser coagulation is attempted, but if this fails, bipolar coagulation or endoscopic suturing will usually control the bleeding. Additional methods of controlling hemorrhage include the placement of rubber tourniquets around the lower uterine segment so that the uterine arteries are temporarily occluded. Constant traction can be placed on the leiomyoma as it is being removed through the third 5-mm accessory incision, which is usually located near the midline. A small myoma corkscrew instrument can be used through this trocar to stabilize and exert the necessary traction.

We have removed intramural leiomyomas 6 to 8 cm in size by using these techniques. The surgery must be carefully performed, and hemostasis must be complete at the end of the procedure. The possibility of excessive blood loss during this operation is always present, and both patient and surgeon must be prepared for immediate laparotomy.

The specimen can be removed through a colpotomy incision by morcellation and a large trocar (Fig. 15.13).

Tubal Pregnancy

Laparoscopic laser surgery for tubal pregnancy was reported by Bruhat in 1978. Ampullary ectopic pregnancies are usually intramural rather than intraluminal, and this is the perfect setting for a laser incision. Once again, a dilute solution of vasopressin can be delivered percutaneously to the tube, and the laser is used for the linear salpingostomy. Hemostasis is achieved by any of the lasers; however, bipolar coagulation may be necessary for very active bleeding. Usually the pregnancy is extruded from the tube as the incision is made. Gentle traction

with an atraumatic forceps may help. It is not necessary or desirable to curette the tube in an effort to remove the contents. It is always necessary to monitor any conservatively treated tubal pregnancy with postoperative human chorionic gonadotropin titers to rule out persistent trophoblastic disease.

Partial salpingectomy is sometimes necessary. This may be particularly true for isthmic tubal pregnancies. Pregnancies in this region of the tube are usually intraluminal, and although they are not encountered as frequently as are ampullary pregnancies, segmental rupture may occur earlier, and recanalization of the tube is infrequent. For this reason, excision of the segment may be desirable. This can be performed by coagulation on either side of the ectopic pregnancy and then excision with laser or laparoscopic scissors. Bipolar coagulation may be necessary because of the bleeding despite the use of vasopressin.

Salpingectomy is used when the tube is destroyed or when future pregnancy is not desired.

Salpingo-oophorectomy and Laparoscopically Assisted Hysterectomy

These procedures are now well known to most laparoscopic surgeons, and we have found the laser to be of assistance in their performance. These operations involve securing large vascular pedicles. Laser energy, usually delivered through the operative laparoscope, has been used mainly for:

- Dividing large pedicles that have either been coagulated with bipolar forceps or suture ligated.
- Accomplishing division of adhesions, ablating endometrial implants, and performing other tasks related to removal of the specimen.
- Dividing the peritoneum over the bladder, mobilizing the bladder off of the cervix (Fig. 15.14), finding uterosacral ligaments, and entering the vagina from

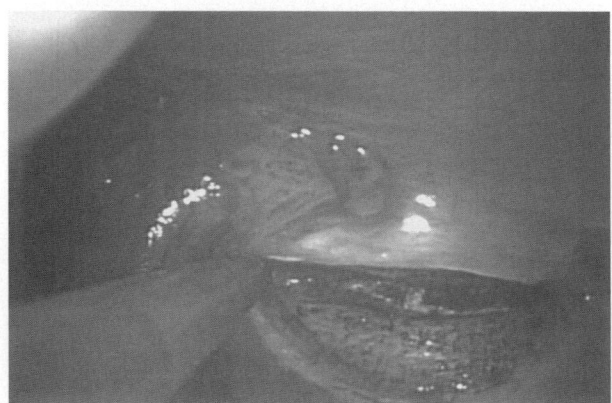

FIGURE 15.13. The laser through the operative scope is used to open the cul-de-sac over a wet sponge that has been inserted into the vagina. Care is taken to stay between the uterosacral ligaments. See color version of figure.

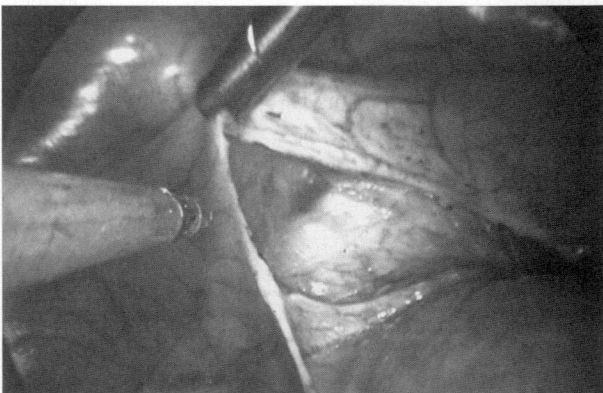

FIGURE 15.14. Bladder peritoneum is incised using the YAG sapphire tip during laparoscopically assisted hysterectomy. The uterus is visible in the lower right corner of the figure. Note the absence of bleeding. Lateral uterine attachments down to the uterine vessels have been taken with the EndoGIA (Autosuture, Norwalk, CT). See color version of figure.

above all of these specifically in laparoscopically assisted hysterectomy.

Again, laser through the operative laparoscope allows for rapid and safe performance of these steps without the need for constantly introducing or removing instruments through the trocar sleeves.

Laparoscopic Procedures for Pelvic Support Defects

One of the newest and most challenging areas now being explored by the laparoscopic surgeon involves operations for the correction of pelvic support defects and genuine stress incontinence. During the past 5 years, we have performed a relatively large number of intraabdominal repairs such as retropubic urethropexy (Burch's procedure), Moschcowitz culdoplasty, and sacral colpopexy with laparoscopic instrumentation and laser.

These operations usually involve a combined vaginal and laparoscopic approach, and laser energy has been used through the laparoscope for dissection of spaces suprapubically (Fig. 15.15) and in the presacral area, as well as for myriad other required maneuvers. Again, the ability to safely divide and coagulate without the need for constant introduction and removal of laparoscopic instrumentation speeds these often long and tedious operations.

HYSTEROSCOPIC LASER SURGERY

Fiber-optic lasers have been used successfully through the hysteroscope. Hysteroscopic laser surgery includes YAG endometrial ablation, metroplastic procedures such as division of uterine septa and destruction of synechiae, and other miscellaneous procedures such as laser excision

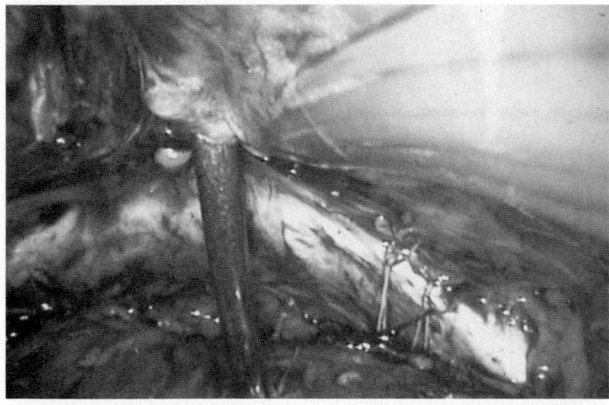

FIGURE 15.15. Final laparoscopic view of a retropubic urethropexy is shown. A CO_2 laser beam directed through the operative laparoscope was used to dissect the space. Two permanent sutures on each side have been taken through the Cooper ligament, the full thickness of the pubovesical fascia, and the vaginal mucosa at the appropriate level near the vesicle neck. A suprapubic catheter is placed under laparoscopic direction. See color version of figure.

of submucous leiomyomas. Again, laser competes with electrosurgery as an energy source to use in the endometrial cavity. Over the past 5 years, we have increasingly turned to electrosurgery to perform operations such as endometrial ablation and resection of submucous myomas. The continuous-flow resectoscope with either the rollerball or the loop electrode is almost always faster and easier than is the fiber-optic laser. Division of intrauterine septa continues to be a relatively easy procedure for either electrosurgery or the laser.

On the other hand, there are still some enthusiastic users of laser for endometrial ablation. Garry and associates have reported a modern series of more than 600 endometrial ablations accomplished without complications and with an overall success rate of more than 80%.

YAG Endometrial Ablation

YAG laser endometrial ablation was reported by Goldrath and coworkers in 1981. Because of its ability to penetrate tissue, the YAG represents an ideal laser for this purpose. Myometrium is normally about 2 to 3 cm in thickness except at the cornu, where it may be significantly less. Endometrial thickness can usually be measured in terms of a few millimeters. Because YAG laser energy delivered by the unclad laser fiber penetrates about 4 mm, the YAG can be used to effectively coagulate the endometrium and the inner layers of the myometrium. The risk of damage to tissues outside the myometrium is minimal.

All patients who are candidates for endometrial ablation must have prior recent microscopic examination of the endometrium to rule out malignancy or premalignant lesions. Adenomatous hyperplasia should not be ablated with the YAG. Patients are usually given 2 months of either danazol or leuprolide to suppress the endometrium. At the time of laser surgery, the cervix is dilated so that the distending medium, saline, is able to flow out of the cervix past the hysteroscope. Note that one of the advantages of hysteroscopic laser surgery is that the saline distending medium avoids some of the dangers associated with nonionic solutions used in electrosurgery. This rapid flow of saline in and out of the uterine cavity makes visualization very easy, even in the presence of active bleeding. The endometrium is ablated by use of the touch technique; that is, the endometrium is actually in contact with the fiber. Fifty watts of power are used, and an effort is made to destroy all endometrium. The ablation is performed with a system of wavy strokes that completely cover the endometrial cavity. The destruction is taken to just past the level of the internal os.

In more than 100 YAG endometrial ablations that have been performed in our clinic, satisfactory results have been achieved in about 70%. Of the 30% of patients in the unsatisfactory result group, most had a decrease in menstrual flow but were unhappy because they wished for a complete cessation of uterine bleeding. These results are comparable to the many electrosurgical ablations done in our clinic.

Laser Metroplasty

Any of the fiber-optic lasers can be used for removal of uterine septa and synechiae. Although KTP/532 and argon do not penetrate the endometrium and myometrium far enough for satisfactory ablation, contact cutting with these fibers produces good results. The YAG unclad fiber can also be used. It should be emphasized that when septa are divided, concomitant laparoscopy should be performed to ensure that perforation does not occur.

Pedunculated myomas may be removed by laser division of the pedicle. Deeper submucous myomas are more easily handled by resectoscopic surgery.

LASER SAFETY

Many volumes have been written about the safe use of surgical lasers. The hazards of laser usage can be divided into two categories, those common to lasers in general and those associated with the specific wavelength and power output of the laser. The most common cause of injury with lasers is careless or uninformed use by surgeons or operating room personnel. Education is the most important step in the avoidance of laser injury. All lasers produce heat and are therefore capable of producing fire. Flammable liquids, paper drapes, and other flammable material may be ignited. Because electricity is used to produce laser energy in many surgical lasers, electrical hazards from the high voltages generated in the instruments are always possible.

There has been concern about viral DNA sequences identified in laser smoke. The possibility of transmission of HPV or human immunodeficiency virus by way of laser plume continues to be investigated. Although several studies show the harmful effects of laser smoke on lung tissue, actual infection by transmitted viral particles has certainly not been conclusively proven. Careful evacuation and filtration of laser smoke should reduce this health hazard. It has been conclusively shown that the effectiveness of smoke evacuation is inversely proportional to the distance of the suction device from the target tissue. An effort should be made to collect smoke no farther than 2 cm from the target site. It is particularly important to remove smoke from the closed abdominal cavity during laparoscopic surgery not only to allow the surgeon to see clearly but also to remove noxious products of combustion such as carbon monoxide and char.

Various types of thermal injury result from specific wavelengths. CO_2 laser energy can produce eye injury by damaging the cornea. Protective glasses, colposcopes, and the operative lenses of laparoscopes shield the laser surgeon's eyes from CO_2 laser injury. The fiber-optic lasers that penetrate water and clear glass also penetrate the eye, however, so retinal damage may occur when eye protection is not used. Each of these lasers is absorbed by a specific color. Therefore, in each case, special glasses or filters are used to protect the eye. Endoscopic surgery with fiber-optic lasers usually involves the use of an optical filter coupled to the eyepiece of the telescope. This filter is activated when the surgeon steps on the laser foot switch.

SUMMARY

It has now been more than 25 years since the lasers were first used in gynecologic surgery, and many applications of laser have been recognized and better defined. The laser is another excellent tool that has been added to our armamentarium. However, it is not a magic wand that can be used to accomplish all surgical tasks. Laser energy is often used to best advantage when applied in conjunction with other conventional techniques or energy sources. A good example of this beneficial combination is afforded by the skilled laparoscopist who achieves an economy of time and motion when cutting and vaporizing with laser, coagulating larger bleeders with bipolar forceps, and suturing and ligating with endoscopic graspers.

In the literature concerning laser surgery, there are numerous references on how to establish a laser program for hospitals and outpatient facilities. Although it is certainly mandatory to develop and enforce safety rules, credentialing guidelines, and service records for lasers, all of these tasks can very logically be incorporated into a much larger approach to modern endoscopic surgery. Laser surgery involves the use of various types of scopes, cameras, video equipment, suction irrigation devices, smoke evacuators, and other sophisticated instrumentation. In addition to a physician director and a laser safety officer, in our clinic, a team of nurses and technicians are assigned the tasks of maintaining and setting up all audio visual equipment, as well as the lasers and other specialized instrumentation used endoscopically. This dedicated team approach often makes the difference between success and frustration in the operating room. Obviously, in a large clinic, it would be difficult and impractical for all operating room personnel to be trained in these special duties. The number of team members will vary with the characteristics of the facility. However, at least one team member is always on call at night so that all emergencies requiring endoscopy have the necessary equipment available and a skilled technician in attendance.

For many procedures, the long-term results of the specific benefits of endoscopic laser surgery—indeed for many advanced operative laparoscopic techniques—such as the repair of fascial support defects and the extensive pelvic dissections of the gynecologic oncologist, remain to be documented by carefully designed randomized clinical trials. The concept of replacing many open abdominal operations with advanced laparoscopic procedures is appealing, because the advantages of reduced

---

TABLE 15.10.
Criteria for the Evaluation of New Surgical Procedures

Obvious advantages
Comparable or improved results
Low risk, great benefit
Technically mastered by most surgeons

(Modified from: Rock JA, Katayama KP, Martin EJ, et al. Pregnancy outcome following uterotubal implantation: a comparison of the reamer and sharp wedge excision techniques. *Fertil Steril* 1979;31:634.)

operative time, recovery time, cost, and magnitude of surgery seem obvious. Before enthusiasm leads to the replacement of tried and proven operations; however, certain criteria should be applied to make a more valid judgment (Table 15.10). One of the most compelling questions involves the need for subsequent surgery after the advanced laparoscopic procedure. Only time will establish the ultimate position of this type of surgery.

BIBLIOGRAPHY

Adamson GD, Lu J, Subak LL. Laparoscopic CO_2 laser vaporization of endometriosis compared with traditional treatments. *Fertil Steril* 1988;50:704.

American College of Obstetricians and Gynecologists Committee. *Committee on Gynecological Practice Report on Carbon Dioxide Laser.* Washington, DC: April 1994.

Anderson MC, Hartley RB. Cervical crypt involvement by cervical intraepithelial neoplasia. *Obstet Gynecol* 1980;55:546.

Apfelberg DB, Mittleman H, Chadi B. Carcinogenic potential of *in vitro* carbon dioxide laser exposure of fibroblast. *Obstet Gynecol* 1989;61:493.

Baggish MS. Management of cervical intraepithelial neoplasia by carbon dioxide laser. *Obstet Gynecol* 1982;60:479.

Baggish MS. Treating viral venereal infection with CO_2 laser. *J Reprod Med* 1982;27:737.

Baggish MS. Status of the carbon dioxide laser for infertility surgery. *Fertil Steril* 1983;40:442.

Baggish MS, Baltoyannis P. Carbon dioxide laser treatment of cervical stenosis. *Fertil Steril* 1987;48:24.

Baggish MS, Chong AP. Carbon dioxide laser microsurgery of the uterine tube. *Obstet Gynecol* 1981;58:111.

Baggish MS, Chong AP. Intraabdominal surgery with the CO_2 laser. *J Reprod Med* 1983;28:269.

Baggish MS, Dorsey JH. CO_2 laser for the treatment of vulvar carcinoma in situ. *Obstet Gynecol* 1981;57:371.

Baggish MS, Dorsey JH. The laser combination cone. *Am J Obstet Gynecol* 1985;151:23.

Baggish MS, Sze E, Badawy S, et al. Carbon dioxide laser laparoscopy by means of a 3.0 mm diameter rigid waveguide. *Fertil Steril* 1988;50:419.

Bellina JH. Microsurgery of the fallopian tube with the carbon dioxide laser: analysis of 230 cases with a two-year follow-up. *Lasers Surg Med* 1983;3:555.

Bellina JH, Hemmings R, Voros JI, et al. Carbon dioxide laser and electrosurgical wound study with an animal model: a comparison of tissue damage and healing patterns in peritoneal tissue. *Am J Obstet Gynecol* 1984;158:327.

Bellina JH, Voros JI, Fick AC, et al. Surgical management of endometriosis with the carbon dioxide laser. *Microsurgery* 1984;5:197.

Bruhat MA, Mage G. Use of CO_2 laser in salpingotomy. In: Kaplan I, ed. *Laser surgery III.* Jerusalem: Jerusalem Academic Press, 1979:271.

Burke L, Covell L, Antonioli D. Laser therapy of cervical intraepithelial neoplasia: factors determining success rate. *Lasers Med Surg* 1980;1:113.

Buttram VC Jr. Evolution of the revised American Fertility Society classification of endometriosis. *Fertil Steril* 1985;43:347.

Byrne MA, Taylor-Robinson D, Wickenden C, et al. Prevalence of human papillomavirus types in the cervices of women before and after laser ablation. *Br J Obstet Gynaecol* 1988;95:201.

Choe JK, Dawood MY, Andrews AH. Conventional versus laser reanastomosis of rabbit ligated uterine horns. *Obstet Gynecol* 1983;61:689.

Chong AP. Infertility amenable to laser surgery. *Basic Adv Laser Surg Gynecol* 1985;279:296.

Chong AP, Baggish MS. The use of carbon dioxide laser in tubal surgery. *Int J Fertil* 1983;28:24.

Daniell JF, Brown DH. Carbon dioxide laser laparoscopy: initial experience in experimental animals and humans. *Obstet Gynecol* 1982;59:761.

Daniell JF, Herbert CM. Laparoscopic salpingostomy utilizing the CO_2 laser. *Fertil Steril* 1984;41:558.

Daniell JF, Kurtz B, Gurley L. Laser laparoscopic management of large endometriomas. *Fertil Steril* 1991;55.

Daniell JF, Pittaway DE. Use of the CO_2 laser in laparoscopic surgery: initial experience with the second puncture technique. *Infertility* 1982;5:15.

Davis GD, Brooks RA. Excision of pelvic endometriosis with the carbon dioxide laser laparoscope. *Obstet Gynecol* 1988;72:816.

David SS. Microsurgical management of distal tube disease. In: Reyniak JV, Lauersen NH, eds. *Principles of microsurgical techniques in infertility.* New York: Plenum, 1982:161.

Department of Health, Education and Welfare/Food and Drug Administration Report on Laser Products. Federal Register 40(148): part II, July 1975.

Diamond E. Microsurgical reconstruction of the uterine tube in sterilized patients. *Fertil Steril* 1977;28:1203.

Diamond NP, Daniell JF, Martin DC, et al. Tubal patency in pelvic adhesions at early second look laparoscopy following intraabdominal use of the carbon dioxide laser: initial report of the Intraabdominal Laser Study Group. *Fertil Steril* 1984;42:717.

Dlugi AM, Saleh WA, Jacobsen G. KTP/532 laser laparoscopy in the treatment of endometriosis-associated infertility. *Fertil Steril* 1992;57.

Dorsey JH. Recurrent cervical intraepithelial neoplasia (CIN) and the endocervical button. *Colpos Gynecol Laser Surg* 1984;1:221.

Dorsey JH. The evolution of operative colposcopy. *Colpos Gynecol Laser Surg* 1986;2:65.

Dorsey JH. Marsupialization techniques with the CO_2 laser: methods and case reports. *Colpos Gynecol Laser Surg* 1986;2:113.

Dorsey JH. Endometrial ablation. *Obstet Gynecol Clin North Am* 1991;15:637.

Dorsey JH. Indications and general techniques for lasers in advanced operative laparoscopy. *Obstet Gynecol Clin North Am* 1991;15:555.

Dorsey JH. The role of lasers in advanced operative laparoscopy. *Obstet Gynecol Clin North Am* 1991;15:545.

Dorsey JH, Baggish MS. Initiating a CO_2 laser program. *Basic Adv Laser Surg Gynecol* 1985;373:381.

Dorsey JH, Baggish MS. Vaginal intraepithelial neoplasia, II: indications and technique for total vaginectomy with split thickness graft replacement. *Colpos Gynecol Laser Surg* 1984;1:149.

Dorsey JH, Cundiff G. Laparoscopic procedures for incontinence and prolapse. *Curr Opin Obstet Gynecol* 1992;166:1062.

Dorsey JH, Sharp HT. *Laparoscopic surgery and ovarian disorders: diagnosis and management of ovarian disorders.* New York: Igaku-Shoin, 1995:350.

Dorsey JH, Sharp HT, Chovan J, et al. Laparoscopic knot strength: a comparison with conventional knots. *Obstet Gynecol* 1995;86:536.

Doughtery TJ, Kaufman JE, Goldfarb A, et al. Photoradiation therapy for the treatment of malignant tumors. *Cancer Res* 1978;38:2628.

Fayez JA, Collazo LM, Vernon C. Comparison of different modalities of treatment for minimal and mild endometriosis. *Am J Obstet Gynecol* 1988;159:927.

Feste JR. Laser laparoscopy: a new modality. *Fertil Steril* 1984;41:74S.

Fuller TA, Nadkarni VJ, et al. Carbon dioxide laser fiber optics. *Bio-Laser News* 1985;4:1.

Garry R, Shelley-Jones D, Mooney P, et al. Six hundred endometrial laser ablations. *Obstet Gynecol* 1995;85:24.

Giles JA, Gafar A. The treatment of CIN: do we need lasers? *Br J Obstet Gynaecol* 1991;98:3.

Goldrath M, Fuller T, Segal S. Laser photovaporization of endometrium for the treatment of menorrhagia. *Am J Obstet Gynecol* 1981;140:14.

Gomel V. Causes of failure of reconstructive infertility microsurgery. *J Reprod Med* 1980;24:239.

Gordon HK, Duncan ID. Effective destruction of cervical intraepithelial neoplasia (CIN) 3 at 100°C using the Semm cold coagulator: 14 years' experience. *Br J Obstet Gynaecol* 1991;98:14.

Gordts S, Boeckx W, Brosens I. Microsurgery of endometriosis in infertile patients. *Fertil Steril* 1984;42:520.

Grosspietzsch R. Microtubular reanastomosis in animal model and very early human results. In: *Gynecological laser surgery*. New York: Plenum, 1981.

Grosspietzsch R, et al. Experiments on operative treatment of tubal sterility by CO_2 laser technique. *Proceedings of the Third International Congress on Laser Surgery* Tel-Aviv, 1979:256.

Gurgan T, Urman B, Aksu T, et al. Laparoscopic CO_2 laser uterine nerve ablation for treatment of drug-resistant primary dysmenorrhea. *Fertil Steril* 1992; 58.

Hagen B, Skjeldestad FE. The outcome of pregnancy after CO_2 laser conization of the cervix. *Br J Obstet Gynaecol* 1993;100:717.

Helkjaer PE, Eriksen PS, Thomsen CF, et al. Outpatient CO_2 laser excisional conization for cervical intraepithelial neoplasia under local anesthesia. *Acta Obstet Gynecol Scand* 1993;72:302.

Hoffman MS, Pinelli DM, Finan M, et al. Laser vaporization for vulvar intraepithelial neoplasia III. *J Reprod Med* 1992;37.

Hulka JF, Omran K, Bergen GS. Classification of adnexal adhesions: a proposal and evaluation of its prognostic value. *Fertil Steril* 1978;30:661.

Jordan JA. Laser treatment of cervical intraepithelial neoplasia. *Obstet Gynecol* 1979;34:831.

Kaplan I, Goldman J, Ger R. The treatment of erosions of the uterine cervix by means of the CO_2 laser. *Obstet Gynecol* 1973;41:795.

Kelly RW. Laser surgery for adhesions. *Basic Adv Laser Surg Gynecol* 1985;323:329.

Kelly RW, Diamond MP. Intra-abdominal use of the carbon dioxide laser for microsurgery. *Obstet Gynecol Clin North Am* 1991;15:537.

Kelly RW, Roberts DK. Experience with the carbon dioxide laser in gynecologic microsurgery. *Am J Obstet Gynecol* 1983;146:586.

Keye WR Jr, Hansen LW, Astin M, et al. Argon laser therapy of endometriosis: a review of 92 consecutive patients. *Fertil Steril* 1987;47:208.

Klink F, Grosspietzsch F, Klitzing LV, et al. Animal *in vivo* studies and *in vitro* experiments with human tubes for end-to-end anastomotic operation by a CO_2 laser technique. *Fertil Steril* 1978;30:100.

Krebs HB. The use of topical 5-fluorouracil in the treatment of genital condylomas. *Obstet Gynecol Clin North Am* 1987;559.

Larsson G, Alm P, Grundsell H. Laser conization versus cold knife conization. *Surg Gynecol Obstet* 1982;154:59.

Lomano JM. Photocoagulation of early pelvic endometriosis with the Nd:YAG laser through the laparoscope. *J Reprod Med* 1985;30:2.

Lomano JM. Ablation of the endometrium with the Nd:YAG laser: a multi-center study. *Colpos Gynecol Laser Surg* 1986;4:203.

Lopes A, Morgan P, Murdoch J, et al. The case for conservative management of "incomplete excision" of CIN after laser conization. *Obstet Gynecol* 1993;49:247.

MacLean AB, Murray EL, Sharp F, et al. Residual cervical intraepithelial neoplasia after laser ablation. *Lasers Surg Med* 1987;7:278.

Mage G, Canis M, Pouly JL, et al. CO_2 laser laparoscopy: a ten-year experience. *Eur J Obstet Gynecol Reprod Biol* 1988;28:120.

Mage G, Chany Y, Bruhat MA. Intraabdominal conservative surgical treatment for endometriosis by CO_2 laser. *Contrib Gynecol Obstet* 1987;16:297.

Mage G, Pouly JL, Bruhat MA. Laser microsurgery of the oviducts. *Basic Adv Laser Surg Gynecol* 1985;299:321.

Maiman TH. Stimulated optical radiation in the ruby. *Nature* 1960;157:493.

Martin DC. Laparoscopic and vaginal colpotomy for the excision of infiltrating cul-de-sac endometriosis. *J Reprod Med* 1988;33:806.

Martin DC. Laser techniques for pelvic adhesions. *Basic Adv Laser Surg Gynecol* 1985;331:340.

Martin DC, Diamond MP. Operative laparoscopy: comparison of lasers with other techniques. *Curr Probl Obstet Gynecol Fertil* 1986;9:564.

Murdoch JB, Morgan PR, Lopes A, et al. Histological incomplete excision of CIN after large loop excision of the transformation zone (LLETZ) merits careful follow up, not retreatment. *Br J Obstet Gynaecol* 1992;99: 990.

Mylotte MJ, Allen JM, Jordan JA. Regeneration of cervical epithelium following laser destruction of intraepithelial neoplasia. *Obstet Gynecol Surg* 859.

Nezhat C, Crowgey SR, Garrison CP. Surgical treatment of endometriosis via laser laparoscopy and videolaparoscopy. *Contrib Gynecol Obstet* 1987;16:303.

Nezhat C, Winer WK, Nezhat F, et al. Smoke from laser surgery: is there a health hazard? *Lasers Surg Med* 1987;7: 376.

Ott DE, Carboxyhemoglobinemia due to peritoneal smoke absorption from laser tissue combustion at laparoscopy. *J Clin Laser Med Surg* 1998; 16:309.

Patel CKN. High-power carbon dioxide lasers. *Sci Am* 1968;219:23.

Pegues RF, Dorsey JH. Gynecologic laparoscopy. *Complications Laparosc Surg* 1995;12:313.

Pittaway DE, Maxson WS, Daniell JF. A comparison of the CO_2 laser and electrocautery on postoperative intraperitoneal adhesion formation in rabbits. *Fertil Steril* 1983;40:366.

Polanyi TG, Bredemeir HC, Davis TW. A CO_2 laser for surgical research. *Med Biol Eng* 1970;8:541.

Reid R. Physical and surgical principles governing expertise with the carbon dioxide laser. *Obstet Gynecol Clin North Am* 1987;14:513.

Reid R. Laser surgery of the vulva. *Obstet Gynecol Clin North Am* 1991;15:491.

Rettenmaier MA, Berman ML, DiSaia PJ, et al. Photoradiation therapy of gynecologic malignancies. *Gynecol Oncol* 1984;17:206.

Rock JA, Katayama KP, Martin EJ, et al. Pregnancy outcome following uterotubal implantation: a comparison of the reamer and sharp wedge excision techniques. *Fertil Steril* 1979;31:634.

Schawlow AL. Advances in optical masers. *Sci Am* 1963;209:36.

Schawlow AL, Townes CH. Infrared and optical masers. *Physiol Rev* 1958;112:1940.

Semm K. Tissue punches and loop ligation: new aids for surgical-therapeutic pelviscopy. *Endoscopy* 1978;10:119.

Semm K. New methods of pelviscopy for myometry, ovariectomy, tubectomy, and adnectomy. *Endoscopy* 1979;2:85.

Sesti F, DeSantis L, Farne C, et al. Efficacy of CO_2 laser surgery in treating squamous intraepithelial lesions. *J Reprod Med* 1994;39:441.

Spitzer M, Krumholz BA. Photodynamic therapy in gynecology. *Obstet Gynecol Clin North Am* 1991;15:649.

Surrey MW, Hill DL. Treatment of endometriosis by carbon dioxide laser during gamete intrafallopian transfer. *J Am Coll Surg* 1994;179:440.

Sutton CJG, Ewen SP, Whitelaw N, et al. Prospective, randomized, double-blind, controlled trial of laser laparoscopy in the treatment of pelvic pain associated with minimal, mild, and moderate endometriosis. *Fertil Steril* 1994;62:699.

Sutton CJG, Pooley AS, Ewen SP, et al. Follow-up report on a randomized controlled trial of laser laparoscopy in the treatment of pelvic pain associated with minimal to moderate endometriosis. *Fertil Steril* 1997;68:1070.

Tadir Y, Kaplan I, Zuckerman Z, et al. New instrumentation and technique for laparoscopic carbon dioxide laser operations: a preliminary report. *Obstet Gynecol* 1984;63:582.

Townsend DE, Smith LH, Kinney WK. Condylomata acuminata: roles of different techniques of laser vaporization. *J Reprod Med* 1993;38:362.

Trofatter KF Jr. Interferon. *Obstet Gynecol Clin North Am* 1987:569.

Turner RJ, Cohen RA, Voet RL, et al. Analysis of tissue margins of cone biopsy specimens obtained with "cold," CO_2 and Nd:YAG lasers and a radio frequency surgical unit. *J Reprod Med* 1992;37:607.

Ueki M, Kitsuki K, Miksaki O, et al. Clinical evaluation of contact Nd:YAG laser conization for cervical intraepithelial neoplasia of the uterus. *Acta Obstet Gynecol Scand* 1992;71:465.

Vergote IG, Makar AP, Kjorstad KE. Laser excision of the transformation zone as treatment of cervical intraepithelial neoplasia with satisfactory colposcopy. *Obstet Gynecol* 1992;44:235.

Woodruff JD, Paurstein CJ. *The fallopian tube,* first ed. Baltimore: Williams & Wilkins, 1969:336.

Wright VC. Laser vaporization of the cervix for the management of cervical intraepithelial neoplasia. *Basic Adv Laser Surg Gynecol* 1985;207:215.

Te Linde's Operative Gynecology, ninth edition, edited by John A. Rock and Howard W. Jones, III. Lippincott Williams & Wilkins, Philadelphia © 2003.

CHAPTER

16

Diagnostic and Operative Laparoscopy

ANNE BRAWNER NAMNOUM   ANA ALVAREZ MURPHY

Laparoscopy has had a remarkable impact on the field of gynecology over a short period of time. The use of the laparoscope to make safe and accurate diagnoses in a variety of settings has been well recognized for years. The acceptance of the laparoscope as an operative tool, other than for sterilization, has lagged significantly. Only since the 1980s have the potential applications of operative laparoscopy been recognized. Advances in technology, instrumentation, and surgical skills have led to the successful laparoscopic treatment of various gynecologic conditions.

HISTORY

Endoscopy evolved rapidly in various medical fields. The first description of endoscopy is attributed to Phillip Bozzini, who in 1805 attempted to observe the interior of the urethra with a simple tube and candlelight. Hysteroscopy was the first gynecologic endoscopic procedure to be attempted. In 1869, Pantaleoni of Ireland used a cystoscope to identify polyps in a patient complaining of irregular vaginal bleeding. It was not until 1910 that Jacobaeus of Sweden introduced a Nitze cystoscope into the peritoneal cavity and coined the term laparoscopy. Kalk of Germany was principally responsible for developing laparoscopy into an effective diagnostic

and surgical procedure in the early 1930s. It enjoyed a modest success in Europe. In the United States, Ruddock introduced a biopsy forceps with diathermy coagulation and reported on 500 cases with a mortality rate of 0.2%. In 1937, Hope emphasized the utility of laparoscopy in the differential diagnosis of ectopic pregnancy, and Anderson suggested tubal sterilization by diathermy coagulation during peritoneoscopy. Despite these reports in the late 1930s, laparoscopy did not gain much acceptance in the United States.

In 1947, Raoul Palmer of France published his first 250 cases in which he used the lithotomy Trendelenburg position and created a gaseous distention; he also described using a uterine cannula to elevate the uterus. Introduction of the "cold light" concept by Fourestier, Gladu, and Valmiere and the use of fiberoptics by Kampany and Hopkins were undisputed breakthroughs for endoscopy. Before development of the cold-light system in 1952, the source of light consisted of a lamp introduced into the cavity. This improvement allowed the light source to remain entirely outside the body, which removed the dangers of accidents owing to electrical faults and heat, and permitted intense light to be concentrated so that photographs and cinematographic films could be taken.

In Europe, the broad acceptance of laparoscopy in the late 1950s was owing to the efforts and writings of

Palmer in France, Frangenheim in Germany, and Albano and Cittadini in Italy. In 1967, Steptoe, of England, published the first English-language monograph, and Cohen published the first North American text in 1968.

The recognition that laparoscopy could be a safe, simple, and effective means of sterilization revived American interest in laparoscopy. In 1962, Palmer published his initial experience with destruction of the isthmic and proximal ampulla of the fallopian tube with unipolar electrosurgery. The search for safe and effective methods of sterilization led to bipolar electrosurgery, thermocoagulation, and the use of rings and clips. Semm of Germany reported the performance of salpingectomy, myomectomy, oophorectomy, ovarian cystectomy, and salpingostomy through the laparoscope in 1974. In 1977, Gomel reported sharp dissection and neosalpingostomy in nine patients, eight with previous tuboplasties. Four of these patients subsequently achieved intrauterine pregnancies. Multiple reports followed that attested to the successful use of laparoscopy for operative and diagnostic purposes.

In the 1980s, many simultaneous developments led to the further expansion of operative laparoscopy. Laparoscopy for oocyte retrieval allowed many reproductive endocrinologists to become comfortable with the operative procedures. As vaginal ultrasound replaced laparoscopy for this indication, other new indications were emerging. Procedures involving resection of severe endometriosis requiring side-wall and posterior cul-de-sac dissections were performed. Various laparoscopic approaches to hysterectomy were also developed. The availability of new instruments and improvements on old instruments made many of these expanding indications for laparoscopic surgery possible. Additionally, technologic advancements such as fiberoptic light sources and chip cameras became available. Miniaturization led to the adoption of the television for monitoring the operation and for recording. Because laparoscopic techniques offer shorter hospitalization, less postoperative pain and morbidity, and shorter recuperation time than does laparotomy, operative laparoscopy has gained widespread acceptance.

INDICATIONS FOR LAPAROSCOPY

Diagnostic Laparoscopy

Diagnostic laparoscopy is an important tool in the evaluation of the patient presenting with acute or chronic pelvic pain. Ectopic pregnancy, pelvic inflammatory disease, endometriosis, adnexal torsion, and other intrapelvic pathology can be diagnosed in a timely manner with use of the laparoscope. A significant reduction in complications owing to delay in diagnosis is an apparent benefit. Laparoscopy also permits evaluation of tubal and peritoneal factors in the infertile patient. A thorough evaluation of the severity of pelvic adhesions or the extent of endometriosis allows selection of the appropriate treatment. In some instances, anomalies of the müllerian or wolffian ducts may require visualization to further elucidate the anatomy.

Operative Laparoscopy

In addition to providing diagnostic accuracy, the laparoscope may be used to safely perform many surgical procedures. The indications for these procedures are the same as if the procedures were to be performed through a laparotomy incision. Laparoscopy may have a more limited place in the primary diagnosis and treatment of patients with gynecologic malignancies, but radical hysterectomies, pelvic and paraaortic lymphadenectomies, and other oncologic procedures are being performed laparoscopically.

CONTRAINDICATIONS TO LAPAROSCOPY

Contraindications to diagnostic and operative laparoscopy generally relate to the laparoscopic approach to the procedure. Contraindications to laparoscopy include bowel obstruction, ileus, peritonitis, intraperitoneal hemorrhage, diaphragmatic hernia, and severe cardiorespiratory disease. The first three contraindications are due to the unacceptably high risk of bowel perforation in patients with distended bowel. Although diffuse peritonitis may be considered a contraindication, the laparoscope is useful to diagnose pelvic inflammatory disease and tuboovarian abscesses. In addition, patients with an ectopic pregnancy may have signs of peritonitis although they are cardiovascularly stable, and these patients are candidates for laparoscopy. Patients with diaphragmatic hernias and severe cardiorespiratory disease may experience acute exacerbation of symptoms induced by the pneumoperitoneum raising the diaphragm, the Trendelenburg position, and the decrease in venous return from gaseous compression of the large vessels. Similarly, unstable patients with brisk intraperitoneal bleeding may have further exacerbation of their already compromised cardiorespiratory status induced by the procedure. The speed with which bleeding can be controlled is also predicated on the experience of the laparoscopist.

Other, more relative contraindications include extremes of body weight, inflammatory bowel disease, the presence of a large abdominal mass, and advanced intrauterine pregnancy. Massive obesity is a contraindication because it may be difficult to insert the instruments into the peritoneal cavity, and it is difficult to manipulate instruments through second puncture sites. Obese patients may also have cardiorespiratory compromise owing to the pneumoperitoneum and Trendelenburg position. Small thin patients require a modification in technique to ensure safety. The Veress needle and trocar should be inserted almost parallel to the abdominal wall because the distance between the anterior abdominal wall and the abdominal aorta is often quite small in these patients. Adhesive bowel disease and fistula formation increase the risk of bowel perforation in patients with Crohn's disease or ulcerative colitis. A large intraabdominal mass and advanced pregnancy may make visualization impossible and increase the risk of puncturing the mass or gravid uterus.

Previous abdominal surgery should not be considered a contraindication to operative laparoscopy. Patients with previous bowel surgery or those known to have severe adhesions should be evaluated on an individual basis. With use of the direct trocar technique, several studies have found no increase in the rate of complications or bowel perforations in patients with previous surgery. Laparoscopy should not be performed if appropriate instrumentation is not available, particularly instruments necessary for obtaining hemostasis. Lack of availability of general anesthesia and insufficient experience of the surgeon should deter physicians from performing operative laparoscopy without adequate supervision.

EQUIPMENT FOR LAPAROSCOPY

Laparoscopes

Diagnostic laparoscopes are available with different angles of view, either straightforward (0-degree deflection) or fore-oblique. The selection is the surgeon's choice, but the straightforward view requires less adjustment and is used more often. Diagnostic and operative laparoscopes also come in a variety of sizes, ranging from 4 to 12 mm. The smaller laparoscope is satisfactory for diagnostic purposes and may be useful in patients at higher risk of trocar injuries because less force is required to penetrate the abdomen. Operating laparoscopes are of greater caliber than are diagnostic ones because the operating channel through which the instruments must pass varies in diameter from 3 to 8 mm (Fig. 16.1). In addition, the laparoscope has a magnification system. The degree of magnification varies with the distance of the laparoscope from the object (Table 16.1), a concept that the surgeon must consider when estimating size through the laparoscope.

Most laparoscopists do not use an operating laparoscope but prefer instead to insert the ancillary instruments through separate incision sites. They claim improved depth perception and a wider field of vision. Proponents of the operating laparoscope, however, believe that the advantages gained from the additional angle of operation outweigh these disadvantages. The operating laparoscope is most often used with ancillary puncture sites as well.

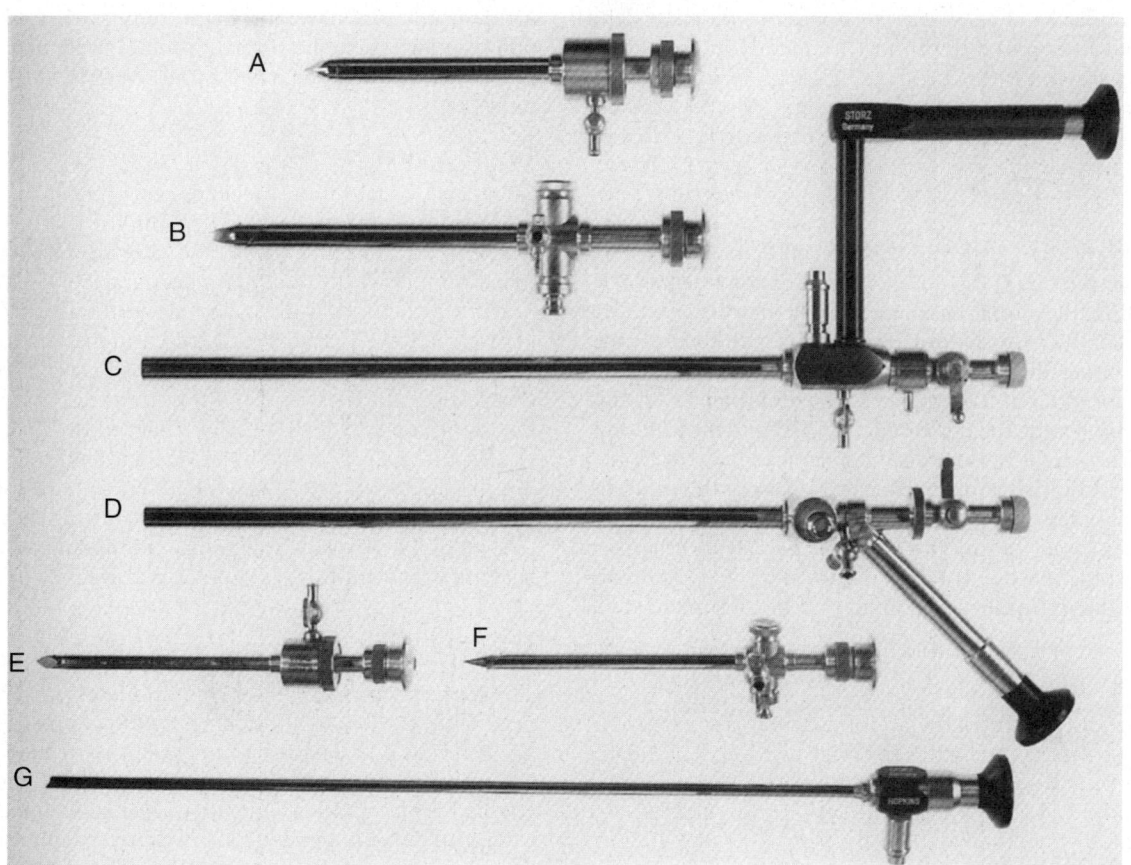

FIGURE 16.1. Laparoscopes and trocars: trocar sleeve with flapper valve (**A, E**), trocar sleeve with trumpet valve (**B, F**), Jacobs-Palmer operating laparoscope (**C**), 45-degree-angle operating laparoscope (**D**), and straightforward diagnostic laparoscope (**G**). (Instruments made by Karl Storz Co, Endoscopy-America, Culver City, CA.)

TABLE 16.1.

Differences in Magnification in Relation to the Distance of the Laparoscope from the Object[a]

Working Distance (mm)	Magnification		
	Wolf[a]	Olympus[a]	Storz[a]
3		8.2	10
5		5.7	6
10	3.19	3.2	3
15		2.2	2
20	1.71	1.7	1.5
30		1.2	1
50	0.73	0.7	0.6

[a] Studies were performed with a 10-mm operating laparascope with a 3-mm channel.

(Personal communication from Richard Wolf Medical Instruments Vernon Hills, IL, Olympus New Hyde Park, NY, and Karl Storz, Endoscopy-America Culver City, CA)

Microlaparoscopy

Refinements in fiberoptic technology have led to the production of "microlaparoscopes" as small as 1.8 mm, which have been used in the office setting with the patient under local anesthesia or conscious sedation. This procedure has been used most frequently in the evaluation of patients with chronic pelvic pain or infertility. As technology progresses and pressures for cost containment continue, these instruments may continue to gain wider use.

Pneumoperitoneal Needle

Carbon dioxide (CO_2) passes through the pneumoperitoneal needle after it has pierced the abdominal wall. The most common needle for insufflation is the Veress needle. This needle has a spring that allows retraction of the blunt inner point as it traverses the abdominal wall, and the blunt point springs out to protect the intraabdominal structures when the needle encounters the decreased pressure of the abdominal cavity. Disposable and reusable Veress needles are available. A Tuohy needle, which is used for epidural anesthesia, may also be used for insufflation but is rarely used today. Some surgeons prefer direct trocar insertion and do not insufflate at all.

Trocars

The trocar punctures the abdominal wall after appropriate insufflation and carries the sleeve with it. The laparoscope is then inserted through the sleeve after the trocar is removed. The two basic models are the flapper valve and the trumpet valve. The flapper valve model allows the laparoscope and other instruments to be inserted or withdrawn without loss of gas. The more traditional instrument is the trumpet valve model. The trocar tip may be pyramidal or cone-shaped, but it is important that the

trocar be sharp. The increased force necessary to insert a dull trocar is more likely to cause damage. Disposable trocars have the advantage of always being sharp but are more expensive. A spring mechanism similar to that of the Veress needle is present on most disposable safety-shield trocars, which may provide an added measure of safety. The "direct view" optical trocars are also available and allow visualization of tissue as the trocar passes through the anterior abdominal wall. Trocars may be anchored into the incision with screw-type sheaths, or some disposable trocars have an inflatable balloons at the internal end of the trocar to anchor the trocar in place.

Gas Insufflator

A gas insufflator is used to produce a controlled pneumoperitoneum. For safety, a series of gauges monitor pressure and flow. Laparoscopic surgery is possible only if adequate pneumoperitoneum with CO_2 can be maintained, despite multiple instrument changes. Operative procedures require multiple puncture sites, which may become sources of gas leaks. Irrigation with subsequent aspiration can also contribute to gas loss. It is therefore imperative that a high-flow insufflator be available for operative procedures. To maintain the high flow necessary for laparoscopic surgery, a high-flow setting must be used that will produce up to 10 to 20 L per minute. Most insufflators have automatic sensors that will shut off gas flow when the intraabdominal pressure reaches 15 to 20 mm Hg, which will avoid overinflation.

Light Sources

Adequate visualization depends on the quality and power of the light delivered. High-intensity light sources use xenon or mercury halide, and provide excellent illumination for visualization and photography. Most of the heat from the light is dissipated along the length of the light cable, but there may still be enough heat to cause thermal injury or ignite paper drapes if precautions are not taken. The beam of light is transmitted through fiberoptic cables, which must be intact to obtain optimal visualization. Broken fibers can be identified by examining the lighted end for dark spots. These dark spots indicate broken cables that are not transmitting light. Liquid light cables provide superior illumination and do not have this problem but are more expensive.

Cameras

The camera consists of two components, the camera head with its cable and the camera control unit. The image is received through the camera lens (attached to the laparoscope), converted by the high-resolution charged-coupled device (CCD) chips to an electronic image, and transmitted to the camera control unit through the camera cables. The image is then sent to the monitor, where it is converted from an electronic image back into an optical image. The newer cameras have multiple small, lightweight CCD chips. A high-resolution color monitor is necessary to permit adequate operation from the screen. Improvements in camera and monitor allow proper assistance and the ability to perform the most exacting microsurgical procedures.

ANCILLARY INSTRUMENTS

Multiple ancillary instruments produced for use through a second puncture site or through the operating channel of the laparoscope provide great versatility in operative procedures. Broad categories of instruments are considered here.

Probes

The simplest and most commonly used instrument is the blunt probe. It is essential for visualization of structures that require manipulation, such as the ovaries. It is often used to stabilize structures atraumatically. Other instruments such as closed biopsy forceps or grasping forceps are often used as blunt probes, but they should truly be blunt to reduce the possibility of trauma. Probes that are marked in centimeters are useful because the magnification of the laparoscopic lens can make estimation of size difficult.

Forceps

The ability to stabilize a structure atraumatically is the key to many procedures. A range of forceps of different sizes and designs is essential in an operative laparoscopy set (Fig. 16.2). Atraumatic grasping tongs and forceps are used most often. Small grasping forceps can be used to delicately hold the fallopian tube as the tongs gently separate fimbriae or dilate the distal fallopian tube at fimbrioplasty. Traditional grasping forceps with springs are generally too traumatic for use on the fallopian tube, but they can be used safely on the uteroovarian ligament to stabilize the ovary. Right-angle graspers or more delicate graspers that resemble hemostats can be used to control bleeding, allowing more precise coagulation or suturing. Ridged instruments with and without teeth can be used to provide traction for dissection of tissue or adhesions and are less traumatic than claw forceps. Tissues that are to be removed, such as myomas or adnexa, can also be grasped with large claw forceps or toothed forceps. The hinged jaws of these forceps are particularly effective in stabilizing tissue during use of the morcellator or during morcellation with scissors.

Punch-biopsy forceps are constructed with a single sharp tooth on one or both jaws that helps keep tissues from slipping. The edges of these forceps should be kept sharp, so that tissue is cut, and not avulsed, during

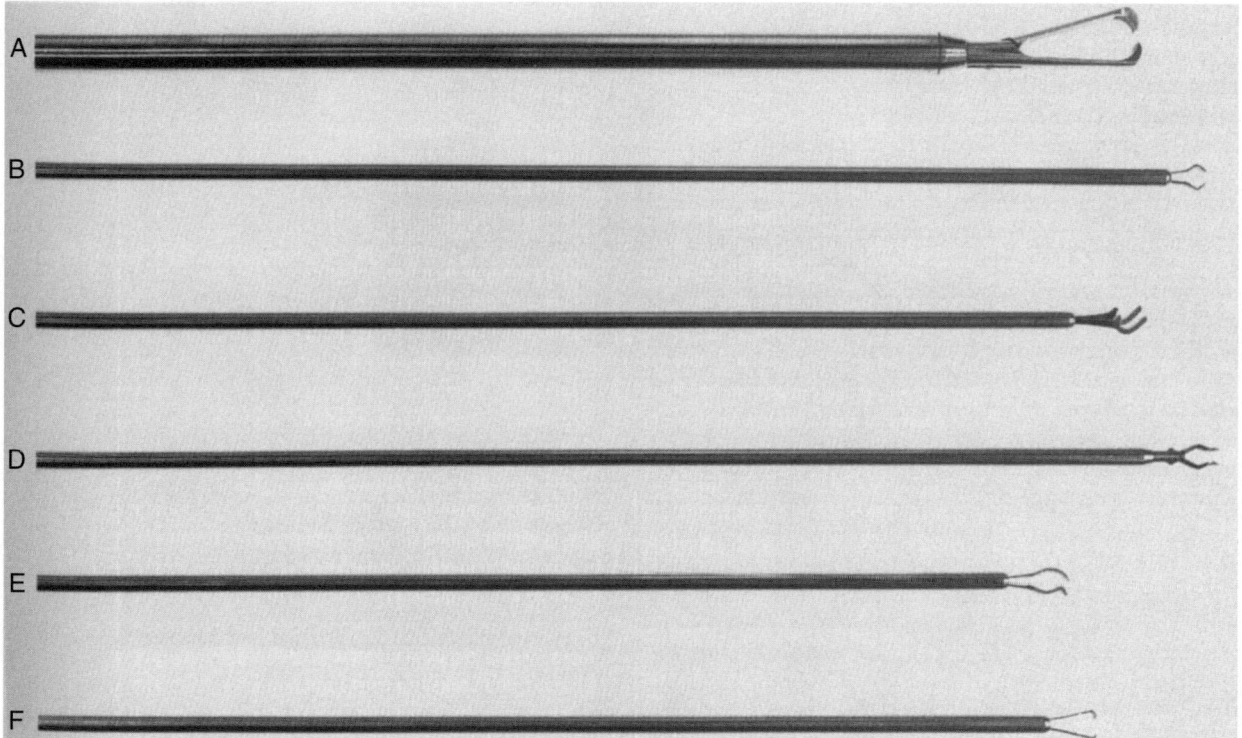

FIGURE 16.2. Traumatic and atraumatic grasping forceps: traumatic claw forceps **(A),** atraumatic grasping forceps for fixation of tissue **(B),** atraumatic grasping forceps **(C),** atraumatic grasping forceps or tongs **(D),** atraumatic grasping forceps for fallopian tube **(E),** and traumatic forceps to hold sponges **(F).** (Instruments made by Karl Storz Co, Endoscopy-America, Culver City, CA.)

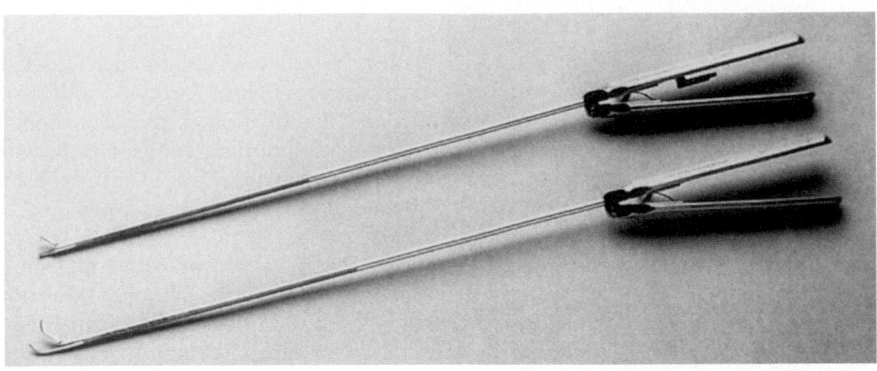

FIGURE 16.3. Straight and curved needle holders. (Instruments made by Karl Storz Co, Culver City, CA.)

biopsy. Hemostasis should be obtained after the tissue has been removed from the jaws so that histologic detail is not lost as a result of electrosurgical damage. The drill forceps are capable of obtaining a large cylindrical core of material from the ovary. An incisional biopsy with scissors or knife is often more precise and easier to perform.

Various needle holders are available, both straight and curved (Fig. 16.3). Some have a spring that facilitates the laparoscopic use of a curved needle.

Scissors and Scalpels

Scissors are commonly used and come in many designs, including toothed, serrated, micro, and hooked (Fig. 16.4). It is essential that they be kept sharp. Scissors that avulse, rather than cut, can be damaging. Hook scissors can be used for large tissue dissection or to cut tissue after loop ligation. These should be used cautiously because the tips may overlap even when closed and may cause inadvertent damage. Microscissors are quite delicate and are the most practical tool for fine dissection. Serrated scissors tend to "chew" through tissues because they are difficult to sharpen; therefore, they are used less often. They can be used to cut suture.

Scalpels of different sizes and shapes are available for use through the operating channel of the laparoscope or through an ancillary port. Unipolar electrosurgical units can be attached to scissors and to laparoscopy scalpels. This combines cutting with coagulation and is useful for both adhesiolysis and linear salpingostomy.

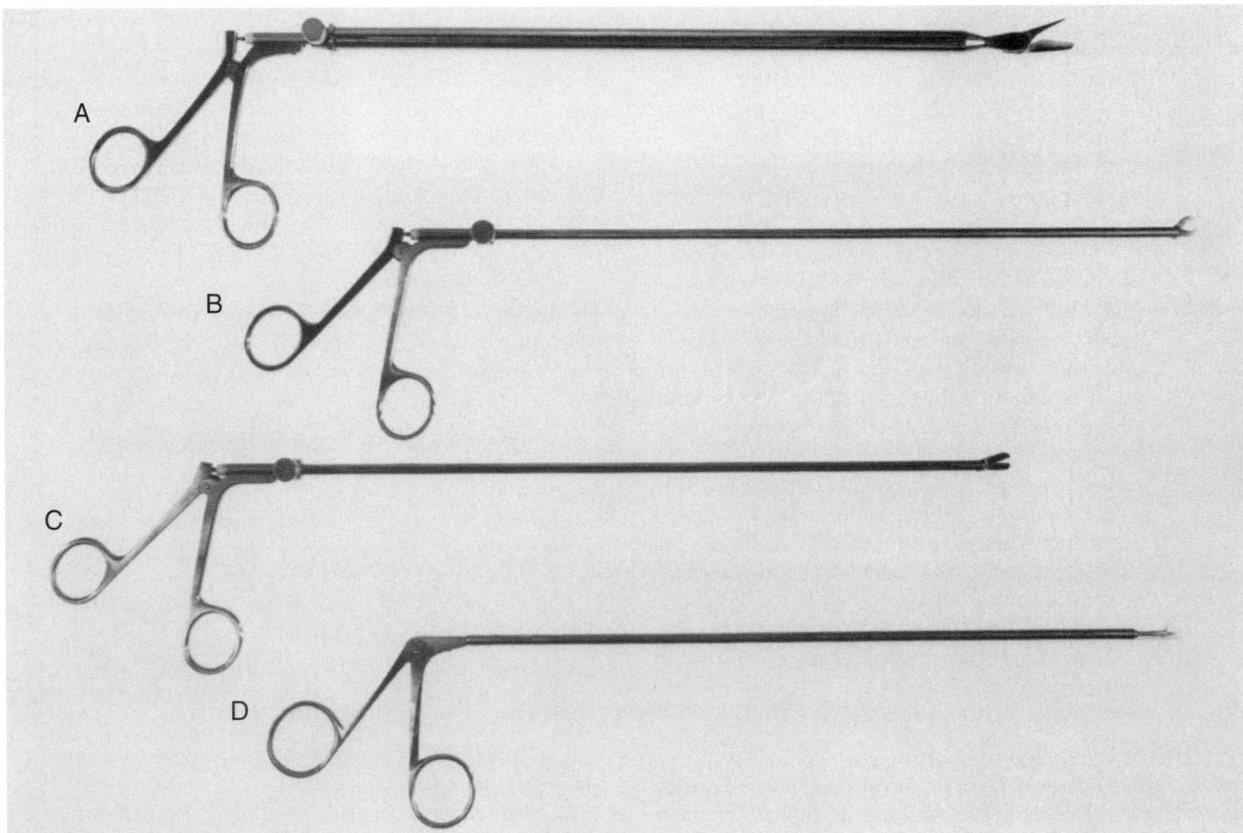

FIGURE 16.4. Scissors: large (A), hook (B), serrated (C), and micro (D). (Instruments made by Karl Storz Co, Culver City, CA.)

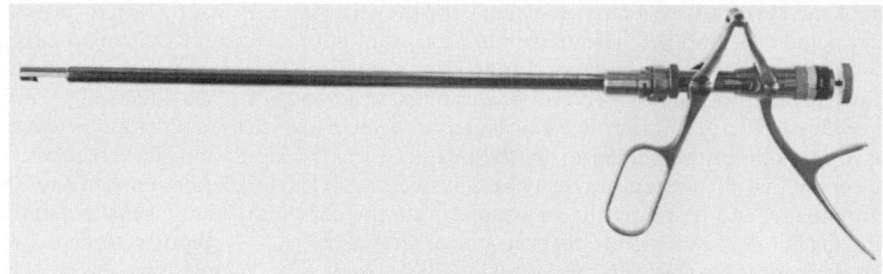

FIGURE 16.5. Morcellator. (Instrument made by Wisap, Tomball, TX.)

The ultrasonically vibrating scalpel is a cutting and coagulating tool that uses high-frequency vibrations as its energy source. It can be used in place of scissors, the laser, or the electrosurgical scalpel to incise tissue.

Aspirators and Irrigators

Endoscopic aspiration of simple-appearing ovarian cysts, cul-de-sac fluid for bacteriologic and cytologic examination, and intraabdominal blood can be effected by way of endoscopic blunt and needle-tipped aspirators. Aspiration can be regulated mechanically by suction devices or manually with a large syringe. The ability to quickly evacuate a hemoperitoneum is essential. Automatic irrigation/aspiration units are available commercially and are an essential part of operative laparoscopy procedures.

Morcellators

Morcellation is commonly performed during myomectomy and is occasionally necessary with oophorectomy, salpingectomy, or removal of gestational tissue after conservative endoscopic surgery for ectopic pregnancy. Pieces of tissue too large to be removed intact from the pelvis can be cut into smaller pieces and removed through the laparoscopic sleeve. Alternatively, morcellation can be performed with a tissue punch device containing an automatic storage sheath that is capable of collecting numerous tissue specimens (Fig. 16.5). This procedure can be time-consuming and exhausting. The sheath may need to be emptied several times. Electromechanical morcellators have been developed that may make morcellation of tissue faster and more efficient, but these require large trocars.

HEMOSTATIC INSTRUMENTS

The ability to achieve hemostasis is integral to any endoscopic procedure. The method selected usually depends on instrument availability, type of proposed surgical procedure, and physician preference. Physician preference usually is related to the degree of familiarity the surgeon has with a particular method.

Electrosurgical Units

Most good modern electrosurgical units are much safer than the early generators, which were "spark gap" units. These modern generators are low-voltage, high-frequency, solid-state units with insulated circuitry. Unipolar and bipolar modes may be used. In a unipolar system, the current passes from the generator through the instrument to a ground plate and then back to the generator. The ground plate must be covered with a conductive jelly to obtain appropriate contact with the patient. Most units will stop automatically and emit a warning sound if the sensor part of the plate recognizes any change in the resistance of the tissue.

Current is provided in two modes: coagulating and cutting. Cutting and coagulating current can be used in "pure" form (Fig. 16.6). Cutting current provides a constant high-energy waveform. The coagulating waveform creates an initial high-voltage peak that quickly dissipates and results in desiccation of the outer layer of the tissue and increased tissue resistance. A "blend" current consists of coagulating current combined with cutting current usually dispensed through the cut mode. The inten-

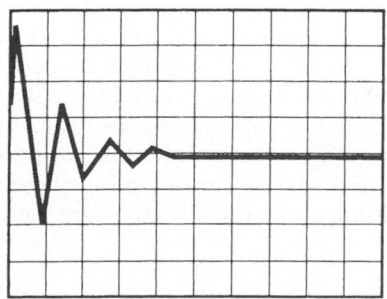

Coagulating Wave Form

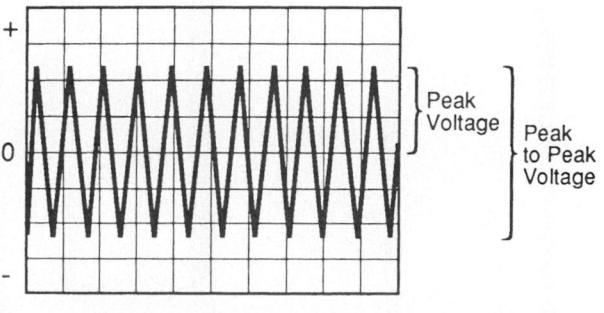

Cutting Wave Form

FIGURE 16.6. Coagulating and cutting waveforms.

sity of the current is regulated separately for the cutting and coagulating modes. The maximum and minimum power output may vary with each unit. The numerical setting needed to achieve a certain power output can be determined by a graph that is often taped or welded to the top or side of the generator by the manufacturer. It is essential that the current intensity be adjusted properly before usage, and that only the surgeon activate the current. Proper usage demands that the tip of the instrument be kept in view of the surgeon while the current is activated. The surgeon must also be aware of the lateral spread of current, which may result in tissue necrosis at a distant site. Tissue damage can be seen as far as 2 to 3 cm away from an area of unipolar coagulation.

Many different terms are used to describe the action of electrosurgical instruments. Fulguration refers to heating the target tissue without actually contacting it. This is beneficial for superficial hemostasis with minimal tissue penetration. Coagulation leaves the tissue blanched. The tissue is heated to the extent that the protein loses its innate configuration and becomes solid. Desiccation of tissue occurs when the liquid component of the tissue is evaporated and the tissue becomes dry.

Many instruments can be combined with unipolar current, most commonly scissors, point coagulators, and scalpels (Fig. 16.7A–C). A combination point coagulator and irrigation instrument permits irrigation of a specific site to facilitate localization and coagulation of a bleeding point.

The bipolar system uses the two insulated jaws of the instrument to carry the current to and from the generator. The tissue between the jaws completes the circuit, and the tissue is heated (coagulated) by passage of the current. Bipolar forceps use high-frequency, low-voltage "cutting" current to coagulate vessels and other tissue. The power density achieved is lower with coagulating current than with cutting current because the coagulation current desiccates the surface of the tissue, increasing tissue impedance. Therefore, cutting current should be used to achieve full coagulation of the fallopian tube during tubal sterilization, because the coagulating mode is insufficient to drive the electrons through the already coagulated muscularis into the endosalpinx. Tubal destruction can be achieved with the bipolar system set at the cutting mode (25 W). Peripheral damage with bipolar coagulation is less extensive than with unipolar coagulation. Nevertheless, there can be about 1 to 2 cm of coagulation damage around the point coagulated, particularly if too much tissue is grasped at one time.

Bipolar forceps are available as paddlelike instruments that were developed for sterilization (Fig. 16.7D,E). Their use has been generalized, and they are now widely used to achieve hemostasis during operative laparoscopic procedures. Microbipolar forceps can be used for more precise coagulation. Bipolar forceps coagulate and desiccate but do not achieve the power density needed to vaporize or cut tissue. (Further discussion of electrosurgical techniques can be found in Chapter 13.)

Thermocoagulation

For decades, high-frequency coagulation was the only means of achieving hemostasis during endoscopic procedures. Because of the well-documented accidents that occurred during the use of high-frequency current, a safer method that does not use electrical current to heat the tissue was sought. This system coagulates tissue by increasing the temperature through heat convection. Electricity is used to heat the metal inside the instrument that delivers the heat. At no time does electricity come into contact with the target tissue. Consequently, thermocoagulation can be applied with good results to wet tissue. Hemostasis is achieved by heating the tissue to 100° to 120°C. As the temperature in the tissue rises slowly, the color changes to white.

Laser

The laser is a device that produces and amplifies light, creating intense coherent electromagnetic energy. The energy can be brought to the target site by reflection off of mirrors. A lens in this path can focus the spot size and

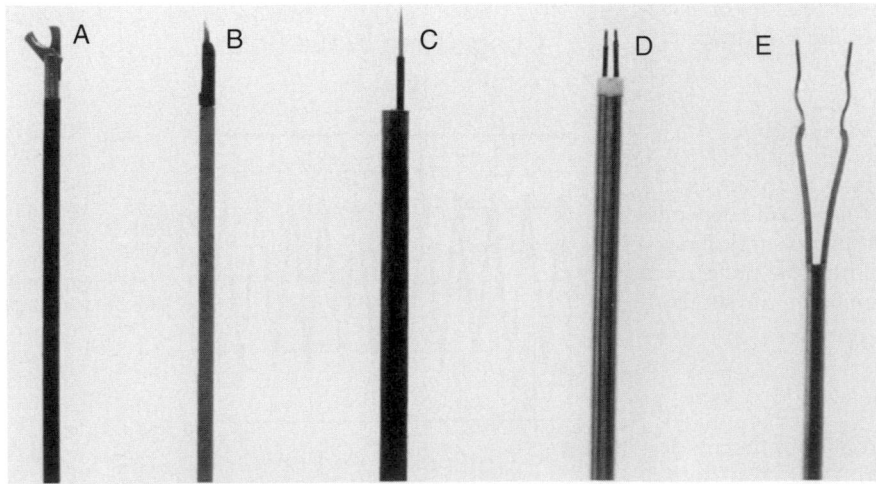

FIGURE 16.7. Laparoscopic hemostatic instruments. **A:** Scissors with monopolar coagulation attachment. **B:** Scalpel with monopolar cautery attachment. **C:** Microtip monopolar cautery. **D:** Microtip bipolar forceps. **E:** Bipolar paddle forceps or Kleppinger forceps. (**A, B:** Instruments made by Richard Wolf Medical Instruments, Vernon Hills, IL; **C–E:** Instruments made by Karl Storz Co, Culver City, CA.) (From: Rock JA, Murphy AA, Jones HW, eds. *Female reproductive surgery.* Baltimore: Williams & Wilkins, 1992:53, with permission.)

increase the power density. The beam from a fiber, however, is divergent and thus more powerful at the tip of the fiber. In general, the major types of lasers used in surgery are the CO_2, argon, 532-nm potassium-titanyl-phosphate (KTP/532), and neodymium:yttrium-aluminum-garnet (Nd:YAG) lasers. Power density is the most important single factor in the effective operation of any laser. The power density determines the ability of the laser to vaporize, excise, and coagulate various tissues. Power density is expressed in watts per centimeter squared. The surface area of the spot size and power (watts) determine the power density. The ability of the target tissue to absorb the beam determines the area of destruction. The biologic effects depend on power density, not power in watts as read from a power meter. The optimum power density for laser ablation or vaporization is the highest value that can be safely controlled by the surgeon. This restricts the damage to healthy tissue in the vicinity of the impact by limiting the time of exposure of the beam. The pulse or superpulse mode of the CO_2 laser is an attempt to increase power density without decreasing control, and to thereby decrease thermal spread and damage.

The CO_2 laser is the laser most commonly combined with laparoscopy. Special modification of the operating channel allows the focusing lens and gas to flow through the same channel. The laser can also be carried by an ancillary port. The need to evacuate the plume is a drawback, and a pneumoperitoneum may be difficult to maintain. The CO_2 laser is highly absorbed by nonreflective solids and liquids, especially water. The laser energy is absorbed at a depth of 100 mm from the surface, with no significant scatter from the target point. Fine focusing (high power density) results in cutting, whereas a defocused beam (low power density) has coagulating properties. The CO_2 has the ability to seal off blood flow in vessels up to 0.5 to 2.0 mm in diameter. Bipolar coagulation should be readily available in the event that larger vessels are encountered.

The CO_2 laser is used primarily to vaporize tissue. The argon, KTP/532, and Nd:YAG lasers have greater coagulative effects. They are of greater use in cutting through vascular tissue, such as myomas. The efficacy of these lasers as cutting instruments can be increased by using fibers or sapphire tips that convert the properties of the laser beam to characteristics similar to those of the CO_2 laser. The depth of penetration of the argon and KTP/532 lasers is 0.4 to 0.8 mm, much deeper than that of the CO_2 laser. The depth of the Nd:YAG laser is 0.6 to 4.2 mm. The argon laser beam is preferentially absorbed by reddish pigment, so its widest use has been for the treatment of endometriosis. Because of its depth of penetration, the Nd:YAG laser is used for endometrial ablation, although it has also been used in the treatment of endometriosis. The KTP/532 laser has uses similar to those of the CO_2 laser. (An in-depth discussion of the laser can be found in Chapter 15.)

Suture

Suturing has added a new dimension to operative laparoscopy. Although suturing is often unnecessary, certain procedures are facilitated by its use. Several new instruments have been created to make intracorporeal suturing and knot tying technically simpler. The loop ligature is a modification of a tonsillectomy or rectal polyp snare and is now available in several suture types (Fig. 16.8). The loop can be placed around a structure and tightened, thereby ligating the tissue and blood vessels. The slip-knot of the loop is introduced, along with its applicator sleeve, through a 5-mm trocar. Forceps are used to position the slipknot until the suture can be tightened. In procedures such as oophorectomy, salpingectomy, and salpingo-oophorectomy, three sutures are typically placed. Simple bleeding sites usually need only one suture ligature.

Any type of suture material or needle can be used laparoscopically. Straight needles are introduced more easily through a trocar sleeve, but curved needles make suture placement simpler. The suture and needle are introduced into the peritoneal cavity through a trapless trocar or introducer cannula. The needle is placed through the tissue as desired with a 3- or 5-mm needle holder, and the suture is drawn through the tissue. If an extracorporeal knot is to be used, the suture is brought back out of the peritoneal cavity so that both ends of the suture extend from the trocar or cannula. A single-throw knot (half hitch) can be tied, and a metal knot pusher can

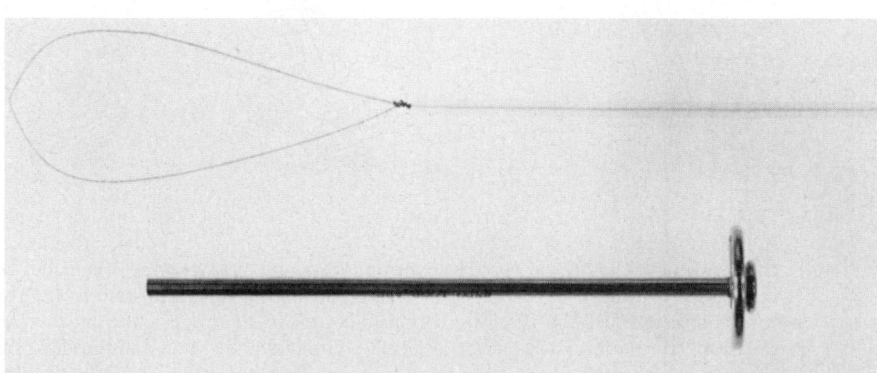

FIGURE   16.8. Introducer   and endoloop   ligature.   (Instrument made by Ethicon, Somerville, NJ.)

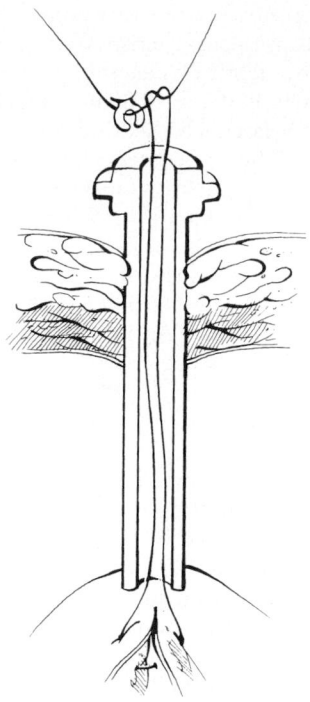

FIGURE 16.9. Extracorporeal knot tying with the Clarke knot pusher. (Modified from: Hulka JF, Reich H. *Textbook of laparoscopy,* second edition. Philadelphia: WB Saunders, 1994:202, with permission.)

be applied to push the knot through the trocar or cannula (Fig. 16.9). The knot pusher thus acts as an extension of the surgeon's fingers to tighten the knot in the desired location. The knot pusher is then removed, and two additional half hitches are placed and tightened. Alternatively, a slipknot can be tied extracorporeally and tightened (Fig. 16.10).

Intracorporeal knot tying can be used to ligate blood vessels, reconstruct organs, or perform any suturing that might be required. The suture and needle are introduced as above, the desired stitch is taken, and the suture is drawn through the tissue until the tail is 3 to 4 cm long. The grasper and the needle holder are used to make an instrument tie, with two loops (a surgeon's knot) placed for the initial throw (Fig. 16.11). Two additional knots are thrown and tightened, and the suture is cut. The needle is carefully removed through the trocar, or it can be "parked" in the anterior abdominal wall or another safe area if additional sutures are required. Other suturing devices have been developed that simplify endoscopic suturing.

Clips and Staples

Hemostatic clips can be used for large vessels after the vessel has been skeletonized, as an alternative to bipolar coagulation. Automatic clip applicators can be introduced through a large trocar sleeve.

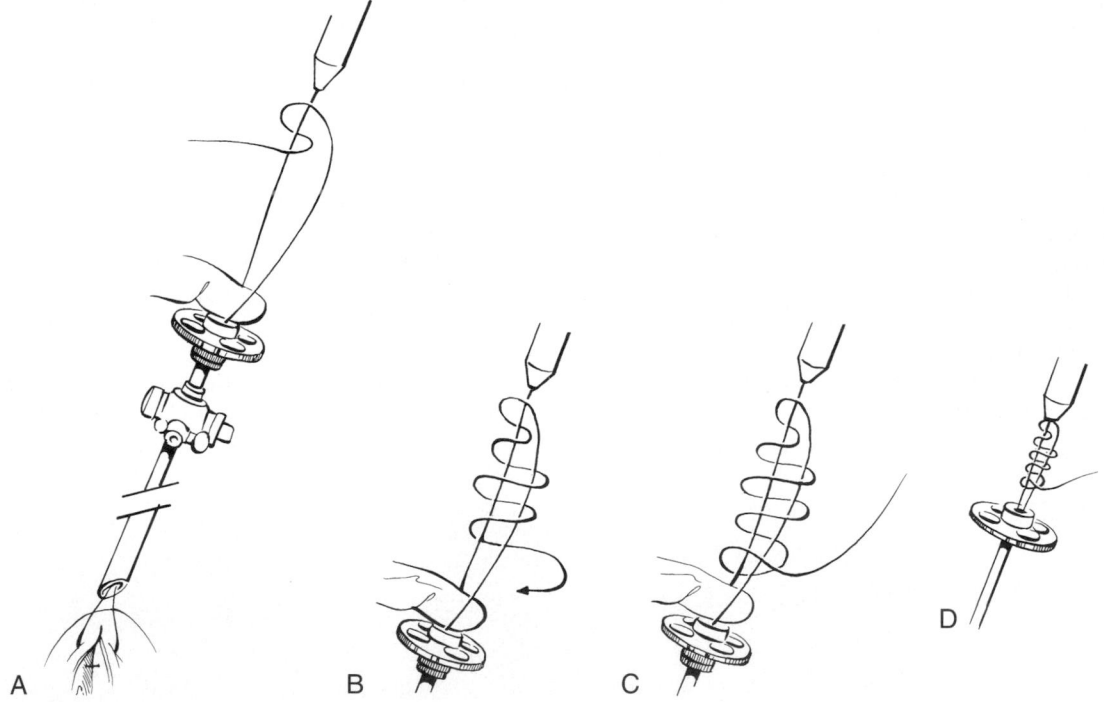

A   B   C   D

FIGURE 16.10. Extracorporeal knot tying with Endoknot (Ethicon, Somerville, NJ). **A:** With both suture ends outside the body, the suture is cut below the needle, and a finger is placed over the introducer channel to prevent loss of peritoneum. A single throw is made. **B:** With the free end of the suture, three revolutions are made around both suture strands. **C:** The tail of the suture is inserted through the lowest loop (adjacent to the finger covering the channel). **D:** The tail is pulled to tighten the knot, the suture is cut above the knot, and the slipknot is pushed with the applicator to the desired position. (Modified from: Murphy AA. Operative laparoscopy. *Fertil Steril* 1987;47:1, with permission.)

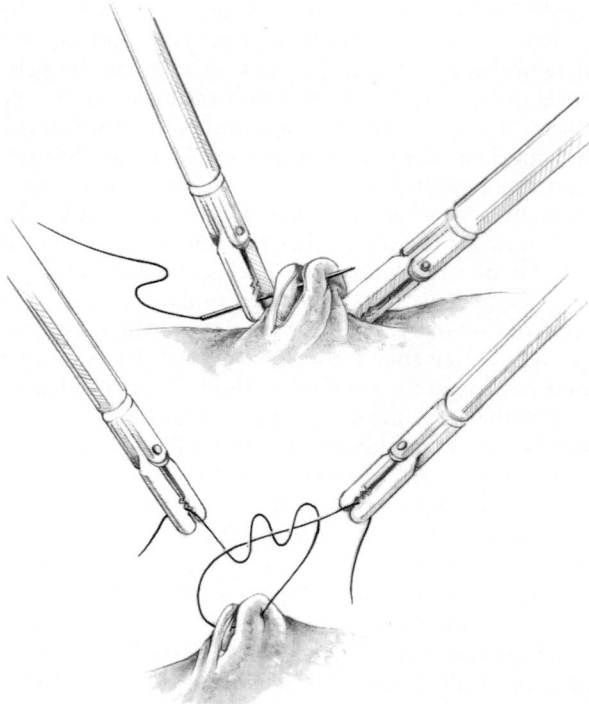

FIGURE 16.11. Intracorporeal knot tying. **A:** The needle is passed through the tissue. **B:** A surgeon's knot is made with the instruments and pulled tight.

Multiple-staple applicators that apply several rows of staples and divide the tissue between the staples (similar to those used for open gastrointestinal anastomoses) have been developed for laparoscopic use. These can be used for division of the infundibulopelvic ligament or other pedicles. These place several rows of clips on either side of the area to be divided. When fired, the instrument automatically staples and incises. These staplers can be wide, and care must be taken to avoid damage to adjoining structures such as the ureter during laparoscopic hysterectomy. Laparoscopic staplers are also available for bowel anastomoses.

Chemical Substances

A dilute solution of vasopressin can be used with caution before a myomectomy or linear salpingostomy for an ectopic pregnancy. Care should be taken to avoid intravascular injection or excessive use of the vasopressin, as is the case in open procedures. Substances used for hemostasis in open cases, such as Surgicel or Avitene, can be applied laparoscopically to achieve hemostasis in areas such as a myoma bed after myomectomy.

TECHNIQUES OF LAPAROSCOPY

Before beginning any operative procedure, a careful preoperative evaluation is essential. Indications for the procedure and its appropriateness must be reviewed. Contraindications to endoscopic surgery must be ruled out.

Informed consent should be obtained in such a manner that the patient understands the nature of the procedure, the risks, the complications, and the alternatives, if any. It is important that the patient understand what circumstances would lead to a laparotomy.

Although sterilization and microlaparoscopy procedures can be performed under local anesthesia, it is generally preferable that general anesthesia with good muscle relaxation be used for traditional diagnostic and operative procedures. These cases require meticulous inspection of the peritoneal cavity, and complex operative cases may take several hours to perform. General anesthesia offers greater comfort to both the patient and surgeon and increases safety. Patients should be intubated and should receive assisted ventilation. The Trendelenburg position and pneumoperitoneum increase the risk of hypercarbia.

Operating Room Equipment

The operating room table should be electric for rapid reversals of angles for irrigation and aspiration. The table should also be capable of achieving the steep Trendelenburg position, preferably up to 30 degrees. The arm on the surgeon's side, and preferably both arms, should be tucked and well cushioned to allow the surgeon and assistant greater freedom of movement for manipulation of instruments. If both arms are tucked, shoulder braces may become necessary to keep the patient from slipping. These must be placed carefully over the acromioclavicular joint to prevent brachial plexus damage.

Stirrups that support the foot and knee while the patient is in the lithotomy position are necessary for laparoscopic procedures. Allen stirrups (Allen Medical Systems, Inc., Mayfield, OH) or other similar stirrups support the heel and therefore should cause no pressure points. The thigh should be at the abdominal level or only slightly elevated, thus facilitating manipulation of instruments in the lower quadrants. Handles near the foot allow easy adjustments to the patient's position during surgery. This facilitates laparoscopic surgery and procedures that require a combined laparoscopic and vaginal approach.

Most pelvic surgeons prefer to have the video monitor at the foot of the table, which affords the surgeon and the assistant an equally good view. More importantly, it also eliminates the hand–eye coordination problem that results from having the monitor placed across the table or at the head (for an assistant who is standing between the patient's legs). The video monitor and video-cassette recorder are placed in a cart, which also has the insufflator and light source. Permanent mounting in a movable holder overhead saves the equipment from considerable wear and tear, but this cannot be achieved unless endoscopy has a dedicated room. The electrosurgical unit and the suction irrigator can come from behind the surgeon or assistant. The laser is usually placed above the operative field and cephalad. The many demands for space lead to a variety of practical spatial arrangements that take into consideration the space in the room and the surgeon's needs and desires.

Positioning of the Patient

Positioning the patient appropriately can save time as it can facilitate the operation. As noted previously, on the surgeon's side, the patient's arm should always be placed by his or her side rather than on an extended arm support. This results in greater freedom of movement for the surgeon. The lithotomy position greatly facilitates manipulation of the uterine cannula and also provides access to the vagina. The patient's buttocks should slightly protrude from the table, further facilitating uterine manipulation. A pelvic examination to assess uterine size, position, and mobility is performed before insertion of the uterine cannula. Pelvic anomalies are noted, and changes in insufflation technique can be made if needed. Although manual manipulation can be used in rare cases, uterine manipulators are mandatory, especially for long operative cases. Manipulators can be placed in the rectum and vagina to help identify structures in the posterior cul-de-sac.

Pneumoperitoneum

Insufflation and trocar insertion should be performed only after it is ensured that the patient's stomach and bladder are empty. A nasogastric tube can be passed to assess whether the stomach may have become distended with gas during intubation. It is common practice to ensure an empty bladder by asking the patient to void before induction of anesthesia. If any doubt exists, it is safer to catheterize the patient. An indwelling Foley catheter is usually inserted at the beginning of all operative cases and removed immediately after surgery.

Pneumoperitoneum allows visualization of abdominal and pelvic structures. CO_2 is generally used because it is rapidly absorbed by blood and is therefore less likely to lead to embolism than is nitrous oxide. Pneumoperitoneum is usually achieved by insertion of the Veress or Tuohy needle in an incision in or at the inferior rim of the umbilicus. The lower abdominal wall is grasped and elevated as the needle is aimed toward the hollow of the sacrum (Fig. 16.12). In obese patients, a more vertical angle of the needle may be necessary to reach the peritoneal cavity. The correct insertion of the Veress needle is a critical step in avoiding major complications. Patients with previous surgical scars, a mass, or organ enlargement may require selection of an alternate site, depending on the area at risk. Alternate sites of entry include the lower-quadrant puncture sites and above the umbilicus in the midline. Patients who have undergone multiple surgeries, patients who are known to have extensive adhesive disease of the pelvis, or patients in whom insufflation is not attainable in the conventional spaces may be good candidates for entrance in the left upper-quadrant beneath the costal margin (ninth intercostal space) at the edge of the lateral rectus or anterior axillary line.

Intraperitoneal pressures should not exceed 10 mm Hg on entry. Appropriate positioning of the needle can be verified by placing a drop of saline on the opening of the needle and observing its disappearance when the abdominal wall is lifted. Proper placement can also be confirmed with the syringe test. About 2 to 3 mL of saline is injected through the needle and aspirated. If the needle is correctly placed, the saline cannot be retrieved; only gas bubbles will be seen as the plunger is elevated. If fluid returns, the surgeon may conclude that the saline is contained in bowel, bladder, or preperitoneal space. Loss of liver dullness after passage of 1 L of CO_2 into the abdominal cavity is also reassuring. Patients can vary widely in their pressure and volume requirement. A small thin patient with strong abdominal muscles will require less volume (about 1 to 2 L) than will an obese parous patient with lax abdominal muscles (3 to 6 L). Intraabdominal pressure should never exceed 20 to 25 mm Hg because these higher pressures may interfere with diaphragmatic excursion or with central venous return owing to compression of the vena cava. Operative laparoscopy requires delivery systems capable of high rates of insufflation to compensate for leaks during instrument changes and suction evacuation of smoke.

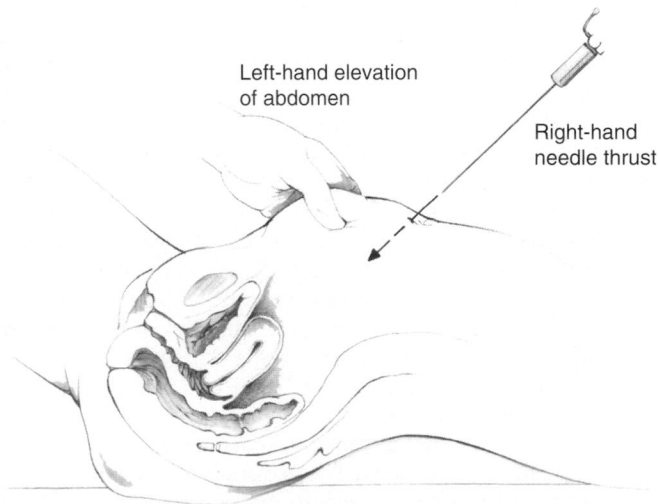

Left-hand elevation of abdomen

Right-hand needle thrust

FIGURE 16.12. Insertion of the Veress needle.

Insertion of the Primary Trocar

When adequate insufflation has been achieved, the Veress needle is removed, and the trocar is inserted. The skin of the lower abdomen is elevated while a sharp trocar is inserted through the umbilical incision, aimed toward the hollow of the sacrum or the uterus. When the trocar is felt to pass through the fascia and peritoneum, the sleeve of the trocar is advanced several centimeters before the trocar is removed. Correct placement of the trocar is confirmed by the escape of gas when the trocar is removed from the sleeve. The laparoscope is then inserted, and correct intraperitoneal placement is confirmed.

Open Laparoscopy

The technique of open laparoscopy was developed by Hasson in 1971 to decrease the risk of complications associated with the "blind" insertion of the Veress needle and trocars. A small incision is made at the umbilicus, and Allis clamps are used to expose the fascia. The fascia is incised, and a 1-cm incision is made in the peritoneum. The special cannula is inserted in the incision and is sutured to the peritoneum and fascia. The obturator is withdrawn, and CO_2 is attached to the cannula to establish pneumoperitoneum. The laparoscope is then inserted.

Ancillary Trocar Placement

An ancillary puncture site is usually necessary to perform a thorough examination of the pelvis. Multiple ancillary puncture sites are necessary for extensive laparoscopic procedures. Proper placement of the second, third, and even fourth puncture sites is necessary to manipulate, cut, and suture tissue. Generally, the surgeon needs one to two sites for stabilization and another site for manipulations. The ancillary trocars are placed slightly superior and lateral to the operative site for optimal visibility and maneuverability. These recommendations are, of course, generalizations, and the surgeon's approach should be tailored to the individual patient. Careful assessment of the operative site and the appropriate placement of ancillary puncture sites are critical to safe laparoscopic surgery.

After ensuring that the bladder is empty, the site of secondary puncture should be indented with the finger, and its placement should be checked to ensure that it provides the access required and avoids trauma to the abdominal structures. The surgeon should try to directly visualize the inferior epigastric vessels through the laparoscope and confirm that the puncture site avoids these vessels. Significant blood loss may occur if these vessels are damaged, and transillumination often does not demonstrate their position. The abdominal course of these vessels usually begins lateral to the insertion of the round ligament, running parallel and lateral to the umbilical ligaments. The exact entry point can be established by pressing down on the abdominal wall with a finger while watching through the laparoscope. Direct visualization will also help avoid injury to the bladder, bowel, side-wall vessels, and other pelvic organs.

Diagnostic Examination of the Pelvis

After insertion of the laparoscope, the surgeon should carefully examine the abdomen to ensure that inadvertent damage was not caused by the Veress needle or trocar. A systematic inspection of the upper and lower abdomen should also be performed. The patient can then be placed in the Trendelenburg position to facilitate visualization of the pelvis. A panoramic inspection gives a general impression of the state of the pelvis. The laparoscope is then advanced and a systematic careful assessment is performed. The uterus is lowered, and the anterior uterus and the uterovesical reflection are examined. Endometriotic implants can be missed if the uterus is not lowered and these areas are not examined. The uterus is raised, and the posterior surface examined. The right adnexa is then thoroughly viewed. The medial and lateral surfaces of the ovary are seen. With use of the ancillary probe or graspers, the ovary can be raised to examine the lateral surface. If the procedure is not performed in the early or mid follicular phase, a preovulatory follicle or corpus luteum may be encountered. Ovarian manipulation should be carefully performed to prevent damage to these fragile vascular structures. If the ovary is adherent, gentle pressure from the blunt probe may free the ovary from its attachment. The ovary and pelvic side wall should be carefully examined for the presence of endometriosis. The fallopian tube is then carefully inspected. The proximal portion is examined for nodules, which may be indicative of salpingitis isthmica nodosa. The tube is viewed in its entirety for the presence of endometriosis or adhesions. The fimbriae are carefully manipulated and assessed to rule out prefimbrial phimosis or fine fimbrial adhesions that may impede ovum pickup. The other adnexa is then similarly assessed. The posterior cul-de-sac and uterosacral ligaments are carefully examined. Endometriosis can be present and may be associated with distortion of the anatomy. If fluid in the posterior cul-de-sac obscures the view, the fluid should be aspirated through the operative site on the laparoscope or the ancillary puncture site. If active infection is suspected, the fluid may be sent for culture.

Chromopertubation may be performed by injecting leukomethylene blue or indigo carmine into the uterine cavity through the uterine cannula. It is essential that a watertight seal be achieved with the uterine cannula. Passage of dye can be observed from the fimbriated end. Lack of tubal filling may be owing to obstruction, spasm, or leakage from the cervix.

Assistance

The assistant is an integral part of the operating team. The surgeon may have both hands occupied with ancillary instruments, and it is critical that instruments be held steadily. With a video camera, an experienced assistant can actively assist the operator.

Assisting an experienced laparoscopic surgeon and operating under direct supervision is the best way to achieve competence in laparoscopic techniques. Laparoscopic surgery should not be attempted by surgeons who have not mastered diagnostic laparoscopy and received further training and experience.

OPERATIVE LAPAROSCOPIC PROCEDURES

Laparoscopic Lysis of Adhesions

Pelvic adhesions can be associated with infertility and chronic pelvic pain. Laparoscopy can be used to diagnose and treat pelvic adhesive disease in many cases. The results of these procedures are comparable with the results obtained at laparotomy. Good results depend on the use of microsurgical technique. This approach uses the philosophy of gentle technique with small instruments and delicate tissue handling. Precise hemostasis should be obtained with minimum coagulation. Magnification is provided by the laparoscope.

Both laparoscopic surgery and laparotomy microsurgery can be time-consuming and technically difficult. These procedures are best performed by expert laparoscopists and microsurgeons. Despite lengthy laparoscopic procedures (2 to 4 hours), most patients are discharged on the day of surgery, have minimal complications, and return to full activity within about 1 week of surgery.

Blunt Dissection

Blunt dissection is the most rudimentary form of adhesiolysis. Traction placed on an adhesion during stabilization of the involved structures can cause separation. This technique may be used for avascular adhesions and filmy adhesions. Virtually any laparoscopic instrument can be used: the suction-irrigator, a blunt probe, forceps, or a closed pair of scissors. If bleeding is encountered, this method should be abandoned, and electrosurgery or a laser should be used. In most cases, sharp dissection is preferable.

Sharp Dissection

Sharp dissection is the preferred method of adhesiolysis and is useful for thin avascular adhesions and thicker bands. The adhesion should be placed on tension, and all aspects of the adhesion should be inspected to ensure that no vital structures are involved. With the adhesion on stretch, scissors can be used to lyse the band. The tips of the scissors should be turned to give the best view of the tissue being incised. If the adhesion bleeds after it is cut, bipolar forceps may be used to achieve hemostasis.

Aquadissection

The suction-irrigator has many functions in laparoscopy. It can be used for blunt dissection, for irrigation, and for suctioning clot, debris, and smoke. The hydraulic pressure delivered can be used to create tissue planes. The multidirectional force of the fluid can create a cleavage plane by way of the path of least resistance, which should be between the two adherent structures. Tissue damage may occur owing to high pressures; thus, aquadissection should be used cautiously.

Electrodissection

Unipolar and bipolar electrosurgery are used in laparoscopy for coagulation and dissection. Vascular adhesions can be desiccated before being divided with scissors. With use of a fine unipolar needle, adhesions can be lysed, but the unpredictable nature of current arcing makes unipolar coagulation unwise around the bowel and ureter. Cold scissor dissection is preferable in these areas, if possible.

Laser Dissection

The small spot size of a laser makes it a useful tool in laparoscopy. The beam can be positioned with precision. With use of a probe, forceps, or the suction irrigator, the adhesion can be placed on tension, and the laser can be used to cut and coagulate in one step. The laser can be introduced through the operating channel of the scope or through an ancillary site.

Salpingo-ovariolysis

Adhesions involving the fallopian tube and ovary should be incised at both ends and removed from the peritoneal cavity. Adhesiolysis is best achieved by placing the adhesion on tension by manipulating the uterus or using a probe or forceps through an ancillary site. Microscissors, a knife, or the laser can be introduced through the operating channel or an ancillary port. Once the adhesion is lysed on one side, it can be grasped and rolled on the forceps to provide traction.

Pelvic adhesions vary from thin and avascular to thick, multilayered, and vascular. Multilayered adhesions should be divided one layer at a time to prevent trauma to underlying structures. It is imperative that the surgeon identify pelvic organs such as the bowel and ureter before embarking on extensive resection. Vascular adhesions can be spot-coagulated before sharp excision. It is important to consider the surrounding area of tissue damage associated with the various modalities of hemostasis and to use minimum coagulation. A dilute solution of vasopressin can be instrumental in obtaining spot hemostasis.

Fimbrioplasty and Salpingostomy

Proximal obstruction of the fallopian tube is usually approached hysteroscopically or radiographically with selective catheterization. If this is unsuccessful, *in vitro* fertilization is the preferred mode of therapy, but resection and tubal anastomosis is an alternative.

Phimotic or clubbed fimbriae can be released through the laparoscope. The distal portion of the tube must first be freed of adhesions. The tube is distended by chromopertubation to identify the lumen, and the fallopian tube is stabilized with atraumatic forceps. Occasionally, the anterior cul-de-sac and uterus can be used to provide a platform for dissection. If the fimbriae are agglutinated, forceps or tongs in the closed position may be introduced into the tubal ostium and then gently withdrawn. This can be repeated several times in different directions. Gentleness is necessary to avoid excessive trauma and bleeding. Intrafimbrial adhesions should be carefully lysed.

If a neosalpingostomy is to be performed, the end of the tube must first be freed of adhesions. After the tube is distended by chromopertubation, the area of the dimple is incised sharply with scissors, electrosurgery, or the laser (high power density). Relaxing incisions in areas of scar are then made, as is commonly performed at laparotomy (Fig. 16.13). This may be all that is necessary to expose the fimbriated end. Eversion can be accomplished by grasping the luminal surface gently and using another forceps to evert the edges. Sutures of No. 4-0 polydioxanone or Vicryl can be placed with the use of intraabdominal or extracorporeal knot-tying techniques (Fig. 16.14). The CO_2 laser technique consists of applying a defocused beam of low power density to the serosal surface. The beam is moved continuously over the serosal area to limit damage to the tube. Absorption of water causes contraction of the serosal surface and a "flowering" effect, which exposes more mucosal area.

Reports of pregnancy rates after laparoscopic neosalpingostomy in the literature range from 0% to

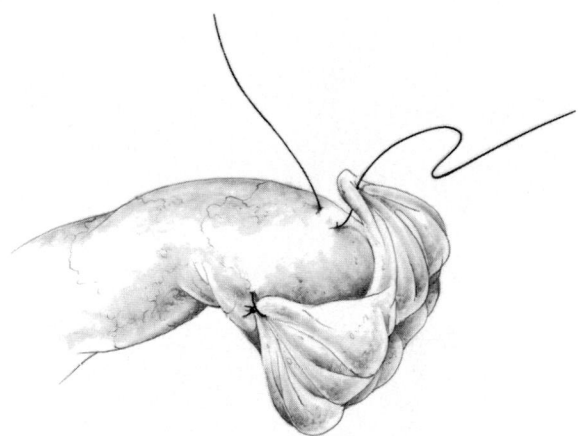

FIGURE 16.14. Eversion of the fimbria with fine sutures.

44%, with ectopic pregnancy rates of 0% to 14%. As with neosalpingostomy at laparotomy, the preexisting condition of the fallopian tube(s) is the most important prognostic factor. Patients with mild-to-moderate tubal disease have significantly higher intrauterine pregnancy rates than do those with severe disease. There are no randomized controlled studies comparing pregnancy rates after laparoscopic neosalpingostomy with pregnancy rates after microsurgery by way of laparotomy, but results from nonrandomized series appear comparable.

Pelvic Side-Wall Dissection

It is often necessary to locate and trace the course of the ureters and iliac vessels in gynecologic surgery. Dissection of the pelvic side wall is performed to confirm the location of normal anatomic structures and avoid their injury, or to remove endometriosis or adhesions that involve the peritoneum overlying the pelvic side wall.

The peritoneum overlying the pelvic side wall is grasped and carefully opened with scissors or laser (Fig. 16.15). If the anatomy is distorted by endometriosis or adhesions, the dissection should begin at the pelvic brim or in a region not affected by endometriosis or adhesions. Aquadissection can be used to elevate the peritoneum from the underlying structures and to aid in dissection. The ureter is identified, and its course is traced deep into the pelvis, where it crosses under the uterine artery.

When the course of the ureter has been confirmed, adhesions to the pelvic side wall from the ovaries, rectosigmoid, or small intestine can be carefully lysed with scissors or a CO_2 laser. Hemostasis is achieved with bipolar coagulation as necessary.

Salpingectomy

Salpingectomy is the treatment of choice for an ectopic pregnancy when preservation of fertility is not an issue, or when the fallopian tube has been markedly damaged by rupture or adhesive disease. Salpingectomy may also

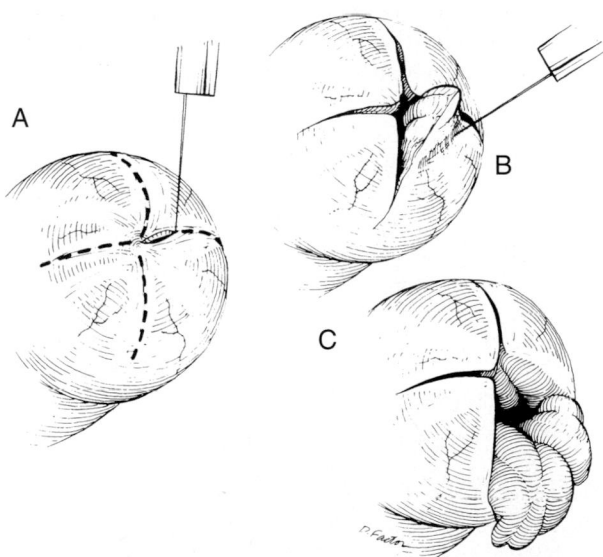

FIGURE 16.13. Neosalpingostomy with use of the CO_2 laser. **A:** The initial incision is made in the area of the dimple. The relaxing incisions are made along the areas of scar. This may be all that is necessary to expose the fimbriae. **B:** A defocused beam of low power density may be "swept" along the serosal surface to effect eversion. **C:** The fimbriae are everted all the way around as the serosa contracts. (From: Roseff SJ, Murphy AA. Helpful techniques in laser laparoscopy. *Contemp Obstet Gynecol* 1988;32:164, with permission.)

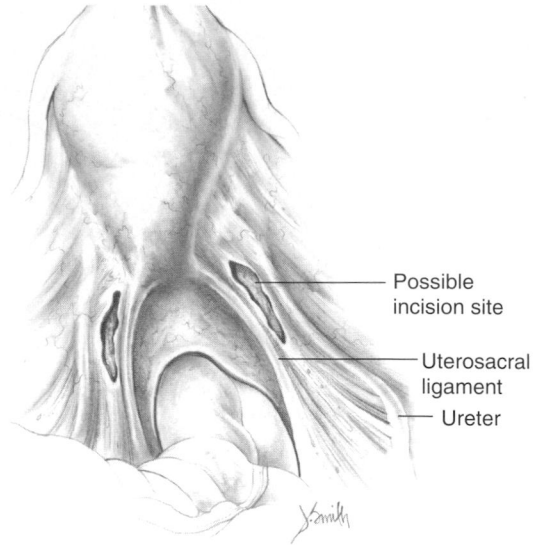

FIGURE 16.15. Pelvic side-wall dissection. The peritoneum has been incised so that the retroperitoneal structures can be visualized.

be indicated for chronic pelvic pain in the presence of a large hydrosalpinx. Many procedures for salpingectomy through the laparoscope have been described. A salpingectomy can be performed by successive electrosurgical coagulation of the mesosalpinx and subsequent cutting with scissors or a knife. Coagulation and cutting can begin at the proximal or fimbriated end of the fallopian tube (Fig. 16.16). Unipolar coagulation combined with scissors allows minimal instrument changes, but care must be taken to avoid excessive coagulation near the ovary and its vasculature. Coagulation and cutting must

be as close to the fallopian tube as possible to avoid damage to the ovary and its blood supply.

A loop ligature can also be used to perform the salpingectomy. Two or three loops are placed around the fallopian tube and tightened; the tube is then transected distal to the loops. The mesosalpinx may need to be dissected partially to allow placement of the loops on the isthmic portion of the tube. An automated stapling device can also be used after the tube has been mobilized. The resected fallopian tube is removed from the abdomen through one of the trocars, or as discussed in the section on tissue removal.

Partial Salpingectomy

The conservative procedure of choice for some proximal isthmic and interstitial pregnancies is a partial salpingectomy. It can also be performed for a ruptured ectopic pregnancy, depending on the extent of tubal damage. A failed salpingostomy procedure can be converted to a partial salpingectomy.

Segmental resection may be accomplished with electrosurgery, thermocoagulation, laser, or loop. Thorough coagulation of the tube proximal and distal to the ectopic pregnancy is achieved. The tube is incised in the area of coagulation. The tubal segment containing the ectopic pregnancy is grasped with forceps and elevated. A series of burns and cuts are placed progressively along the mesosalpinx, beneath the tubal segment being excised (Fig. 16.17). The mesosalpinx is inspected carefully, and any bleeding points are coagulated.

A variation of the technique for Pomeroy tubal sterilization can be performed with the loop ligature. The loop is placed around the ectopic gestation. Then the intervening tube containing the ectopic pregnancy is resected.

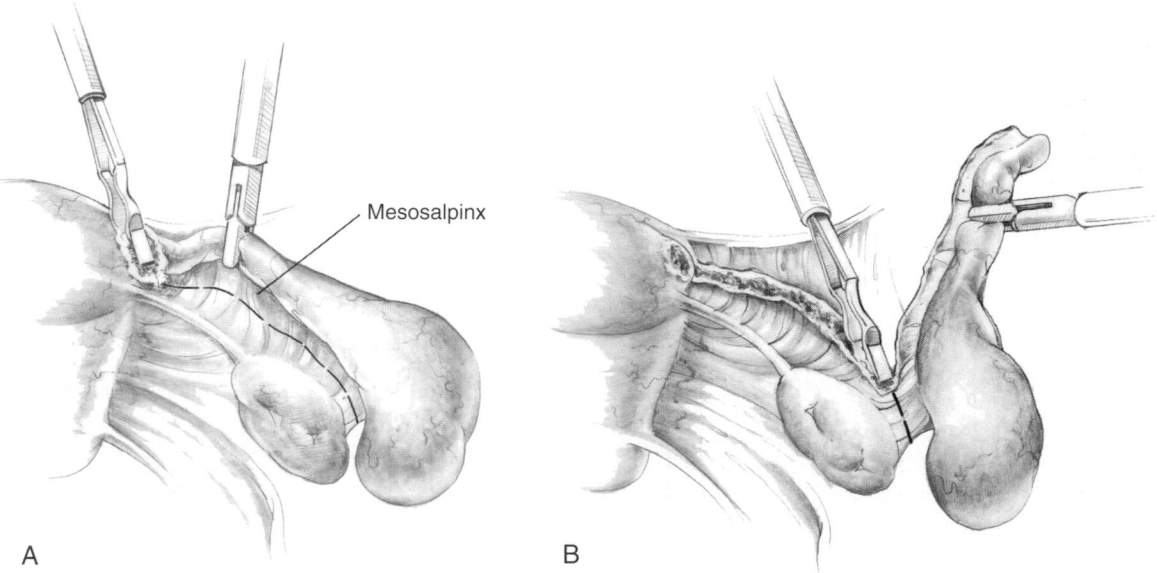

A

B

FIGURE 16.16. Salpingectomy with use of bipolar electrocoagulation. **A:** Coagulation of the proximal fallopian tube with bipolar forceps. **B:** Bipolar coagulation of the mesosalpinx is followed by excision of the fallopian tube with scissors or laser.

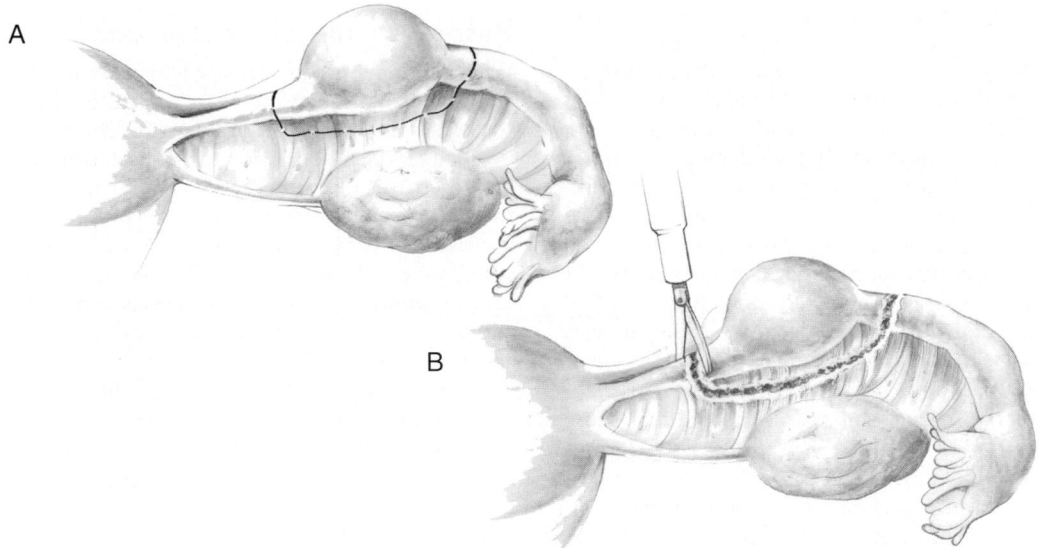

FIGURE 16.17. Partial salpingectomy with use of bipolar electrocoagulation. **A:** The fallopian tube proximal and distal to the ectopic gestation, and the underlying mesosalpinx are coagulated with bipolar forceps. **B:** The tube and mesosalpinx are cut in the coagulated areas, and the segment of fallopian tube is removed.

Linear Salpingostomy

Unruptured ampullary and selected isthmic ectopic pregnancies can be treated with linear salpingostomy. An incision is made along the antimesenteric border of the ectopic pregnancy at the point of maximal bulging. This can be accomplished with unipolar needlepoint coagulation, laser, scissors, or a knife (Fig. 16.18). Before incision with the scissors, the area can be coagulated. To decrease blood loss, the mesosalpinx below the ectopic pregnancy can be infiltrated with a dilute solution of vasopressin. Alternatively, if a vessel can be seen supplying the area of the fallopian tube containing the ectopic pregnancy, bipolar coagulation can be used selectively to decrease blood loss.

Atraumatic forceps are used to hold the edges of the salpingostomy incision. The conceptual debris is removed with an aspirator or forceps. The bed is observed closely for bleeding and to ensure that no trophoblastic tissue remains. The salpingostomy incision is usually not closed. Fistula formation at the operative site is a possible complication but does not appear to be common. If the defect is large or if marked eversion of mucosa occurs, then a suture can be used to approximate the tubal edges. The suture is tied with instruments inside the peritoneal cavity or is tied outside the cavity with use of a slipknot as previously described. The trophoblastic tissue can usually be removed through one of the puncture sites. (See Chapter 22 for a further discussion of ectopic pregnancy.)

Resection and Ablation of Endometriosis

Small superficial implants of endometriosis can be electrosurgically coagulated (unipolar or bipolar), thermocoagulated, or vaporized. When using bipolar electro-

surgery, the operator can grasp the lesion before coagulation or can apply open blades to the surface area to be coagulated. Because the CO_2 laser is accurate in depth of penetration and because it creates small lateral spread, it permits safe vaporization. Small implants are ablated. The argon laser, with its selective absorption by hemo-

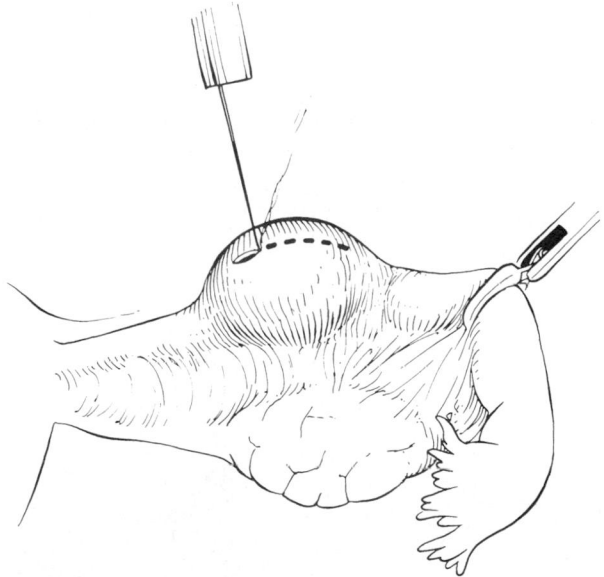

FIGURE 16.18. Linear salpingostomy with use of the CO_2 laser. An incision on the antimesenteric border over the ectopic gestation is made. The contents are removed. Hemostasis is obtained, and the tube is usually left to heal by second intention. (From: Roseff SJ, Murphy AA. Helpful techniques in laser laparoscopy. *Contemp Obstet Gynecol* 1988;32:159, with permission.)

globin-pigmented lesions, has also been used. Flexible-fiber lasers such as the KTP/532 are easier to master.

Laser or scissors can be used to excise the lesions, especially if histologic confirmation of endometriosis is desired. An incision is made in a nearby normal area of peritoneum. The peritoneum is pulled medially, and a blunt probe is used to separate the lesion from the underlying loose connective tissue. This technique is particularly helpful in vascular areas because sharp dissection with scissors or laser may inadvertently divide vessels. For deeper lesions, excision can be taken down to the level of healthy tissue, but this usually requires excision with laser or scissors and electrosurgical energy. This technique is useful for lesions suspected of being deeply penetrating. Fulguration and vaporization techniques cause tissue distortion, which can be confusing. Deep lesions may be incompletely destroyed, especially with the bipolar technique. Carbon can be easily confused with endometriosis at second-look laparoscopy; thus, excision may be helpful in deciding whether there is recurrence. Use of high–power density superpulse may decrease carbonization by facilitating vaporization and decreasing lateral spread. Carbon should be removed as much as possible with lavage or by the use of a pusher sponge.

When endometriosis involves the peritoneum overlying the bladder or ureter, a laparoscopic technique similar to that for laparotomy is used. An incision is made in uninvolved peritoneum away from the ureter. The peritoneum is pulled toward the midline, and the ureter is bluntly dissected from the peritoneum. It should be pushed away easily with a blunt probe. Difficulty with this procedure may indicate that the ureter is infiltrated with endometriosis, and the laparoscopic procedure should be abandoned. Alternatively, saline can be injected below the peritoneum to achieve separation of tissues and facilitate dissection. Electrosurgery, laser, or thermocoagulation should be used very cautiously on or near the ureter. Direct injury to the ureter or injury owing to spread of current or heat may result.

Posterior Cul-de-Sac Dissection

When endometriosis or pelvic adhesions partially or completely obliterate the posterior cul-de-sac and are associated with pelvic pain or infertility, a surgical approach is usually indicated. Cul-de-sac obliteration secondary to endometriosis often involves deep fibrotic endometriosis that may involve the rectum, rectovaginal septum, or uterosacral ligaments. Dissection of the posterior cul-de-sac may be necessary and can be performed laparoscopically by skilled laparoscopic surgeons. The goal is to lyse adhesions, excise large or deep endometriotic lesions, and resect or vaporize small superficial lesions.

Before surgery, the patient should undergo a thorough bowel preparation. A uterine manipulator is used to antevert the uterus, and a rectal probe is placed in the rectum to delineate and retract the rectum posteriorly. A sponge stick placed in the vagina can further help delineate rectum from vagina (Fig. 16.19). The anterior rectum is carefully dissected from the posterior aspect of the uterus or vagina with scissors or the CO_2 laser. Aquadissection may also be helpful. Dissection should continue until the loose areolar tissue of the rectovaginal space is reached. If a ureter is near the site of dissection, the position of the ureter should be confirmed before any dissection is performed. The fibrotic endometriosis can then be excised from the posterior vagina or uterosacral ligaments. If the endometriosis extends through to the vaginal mucosa, this is excised and the posterior vagina is closed vaginally or laparoscopically. Palpation of the endometriotic nodule before and after removal is helpful to ensure complete excision.

If the endometriotic lesion involves the lower rectal muscularis, the nodule can be excised with the help of the surgeon's or assistant's finger in the rectum. Defects in the rectal muscularis are repaired with the suturing techniques described earlier. Potential complications of this procedure include rectal injury or perforation, ureteral injury, and recurrent pain or symptoms.

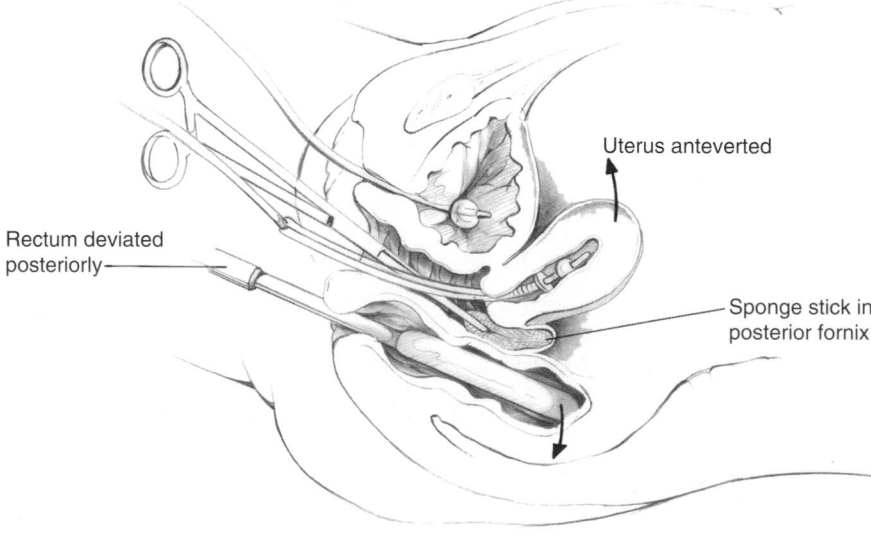

Uterus anteverted

Rectum deviated
posteriorly—

Sponge stick in
posterior fornix

FIGURE 16.19. Dissection of the posterior cul-de-sac. Instruments in the uterus, posterior fornix of the vagina, and rectum help define the anatomy.

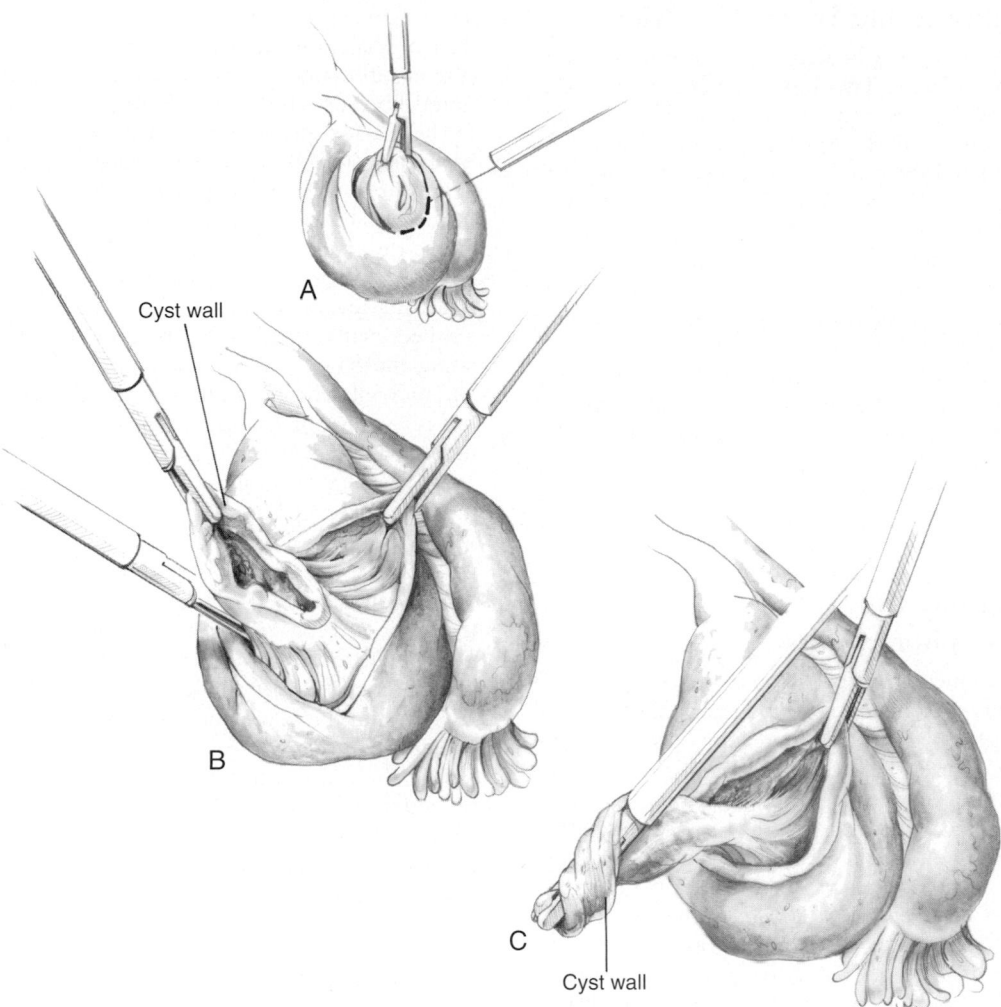

Cyst wall

A

B

C

Cyst wall

FIGURE 16.20. Ovarian cystectomy. **A:** The cyst has been drained, the cyst wall is grasped, and a plane is developed between the cyst wall and normal ovarian tissue. **B:** The cyst wall is further dissected with blunt and sharp dissection. **C:** The cyst wall is twisted to assist in dissection.

Ovarian Cystectomy

Surface endometriomas smaller than 1 cm can be "decapitated" at the ovarian endometrioma junction, and the base can be coagulated or vaporized. The cyst wall is often difficult to resect in these cases. The resulting defect is not closed. Endometriomas that are 3 to 5 cm in size are resected in a manner similar to that used at laparotomy. Endometriomas larger than 5 cm can be difficult to handle at laparoscopy, although resection can be accomplished.

The cyst is drained and lavaged. The ovarian endometrioma is opened on its axis in the most dependent portion. The lining is inspected, and a relaxing incision is made. The plane of the pseudocapsule is identified. Atraumatic grasping forceps are used to hold the ovary and provide countertraction. The cyst wall lining is grasped, and dissection is performed with laser, scissors, or blunt probe (Fig. 16.20). Incompletely resected areas can be further coagulated or vaporized. Extreme care

must be taken when working near the hilar vessels. An alternative method involves coagulation or vaporization of the lining rather than resection, but resection is preferable. Simple drainage of endometriomas should be avoided because the recurrence rate is very high.

A persistent simple cyst that is shown on sonography to have no external excrescences or adhesions can be aspirated. The cyst is opened, and the wall is closely inspected. If the cyst wall is not suspicious, then cystectomy is performed in the same manner as that described for endometrioma. Alternatively, if the cyst wall is suspicious, multiple biopsy specimens of the wall can be obtained and sent for frozen section. Ovarian cysts with features suspicious for malignancy are not good candidates for laparoscopic cystectomy (see Chapter 26). Solid tumors or tumors with a solid component can be carefully evaluated through the laparoscope, and the procedure can be converted to a laparotomy when appropriate. Solid/cystic tumors that are thought to be benign cystic teratomas are commonly treated laparoscopically.

Ovarian Biopsy and Wedge Resection

Biopsy of the ovary may be necessary to confirm or identify suspicious lesions. Two instruments are available: a punch biopsy forceps and drill forceps. These instruments are described in the Ancillary Instruments section. Wedgelike resections can be performed with use of a knife or scissors. Coagulation can be obtained subsequently with electrocoagulation or thermocoagulation.

Therapeutic multiple biopsies, wedge resection, or ovarian "drilling" with electrocoagulation or laser has been recommended for patients with polycystic ovarian disease that is resistant to standard ovulation-induction regimens (see Chapter 26). Therapeutic multiple biopsies consist of puncturing and coagulating all visible follicles on the cortex. Success in restoring ovulation has been reported in 45% to 92% of patients after ovarian "drilling," but periovarian adhesions may occur, and long-term effects await further study.

Oophorectomy and Salpingo-oophorectomy

Several techniques for laparoscopic oophorectomy or salpingo-oophorectomy have been described. One procedure involves the placement of three loop ligatures around the ovary or adnexa. Before placement of the loops, the structures must be free of adhesions. Incisions in the mesosalpinx are sometimes necessary to facilitate placement. The ovary or adnexa is cut distal to the three loops. Small bleeding points can be coagulated on the stump, but care must be taken not to coagulate the suture.

Alternatively, the peritoneum is opened, and the ureter is identified (Fig. 16.21A,B). Lactated Ringer solution or saline can be injected into the retroperitoneal space to help push the ureter away from the site of coagulation and increase the margin of safety. The uteroovarian ligament is coagulated with bipolar coagulation and transected, and the infundibulopelvic ligament is then coagulated with bipolar forceps and transected. Pedicles are examined for hemostasis, and the ovary is then removed from the abdominal cavity by one of the described methods of tissue removal. If the fallopian tube is to be removed with the ovary, the proximal fallopian tube and uteroovarian ligament are coagulated before transection (Fig. 16.21C–E). After coagulation and transection of the infundibulopelvic ligament, the mesosalpinx is coagulated and cut in the same manner that is used for salpingectomy. Laparoscopic stapling devices can also be used on the pedicles, but care must be taken to avoid injury to the ureter. Adnexal tissue is removed from the pelvis by any of the methods described below.

Myomectomy

Some women with symptomatic leiomyomata may prefer myomectomy to hysterectomy because they want to preserve fertility or retain the uterus. In properly selected cases, laparoscopic myomectomy may be feasible. Patients should understand that a myomectomy can be more difficult and time-consuming than a hysterectomy, and myomectomy can be associated with greater blood loss, postoperative adhesions, and a risk of uterine rupture in subsequent pregnancies. Patients with large intramural fibroids who desire pregnancy in the future may be better served by a myomectomy through a laparotomy incision, because the uterine defect is more difficult to repair laparoscopically. Gonadotropin-releasing hormone (GnRH) analogs are commonly used to decrease the size and vascularity of fibroids preoperatively. In cases that are suited to a laparoscopic approach, the following techniques can be used.

Pedunculated myomas are easily resected by coagulating the base. The myoma is transected from its base and morcellated or cut if necessary (Fig. 16.22). The defect is usually not sutured. For an intramural fibroid, the incision is made with scissors, laser, or the knife electrode. A dilute solution of vasopressin can be injected into the myometrium with use of a long spinal needle. When the characteristic whorled white appearance of the myoma is seen, the edges of the incision are held open with atraumatic graspers, and the myoma is grasped with traumatic forceps or a corkscrew for good traction (Fig. 16.23). Dissection of the myoma from the myometrium is performed bluntly and sharply as needed. If the CO_2 laser is used, bipolar electrocoagulation should be available to obtain hemostasis when large vessels are encountered. The defect can be closed with the previously described suturing technique and usually requires several layers. Submucosal myomas should be approached through the hysteroscope rather than through the laparoscope. Patients with large myomas are not good candidates for the laparoscopic approach when visualization is obscured because of the size or location of the myomas. Adhesion formation after laparoscopic myomectomy has not been adequately studied. Intrauterine pregnancy rates after laparoscopic myomectomy appear to be comparable to those after laparotomy.

An alternative that is less technically difficult and less time-consuming is the laparoscopically assisted myomectomy. The myomas are removed laparoscopically as noted above, and the uterine defect is sutured through a minilaparotomy incision. The benefit is the ability to perform a multiplayer closure with less coagulation, which would presumably decrease the risk of uterine rupture. This technique may be useful for patients with multiple myomas and/or deep intramural myomas that require a multiplayer closure.

Alternatives to myomectomy include laparoscopic myolysis and cryomyolysis. GnRH analogs are used before therapy and may be continued after surgery. Generally this therapy maintains or slightly reduces the size of myomas to post-GnRH analog size. A nonsurgical alternative for the treatment of symptomatic uterine fibroids, uterine artery embolization, is currently under study and shows some promise in selected cases.

Other Laparoscopic Procedures

Laparoscopy-assisted vaginal hysterectomy, laparoscopic appendectomy, and other laparoscopic procedures are discussed in the appropriate chapters.

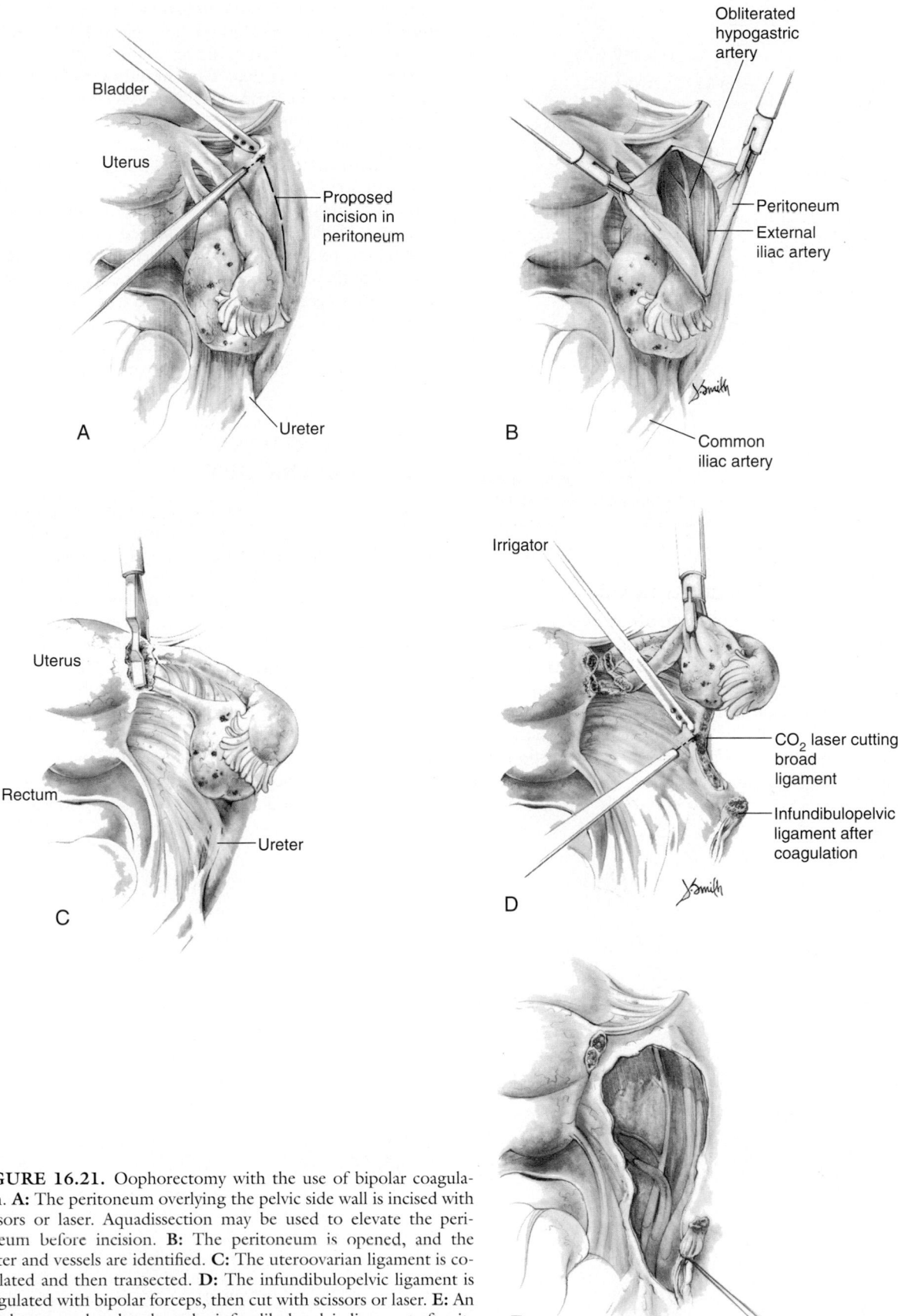

FIGURE 16.21. Oophorectomy with the use of bipolar coagulation. **A:** The peritoneum overlying the pelvic side wall is incised with scissors or laser. Aquadissection may be used to elevate the peritoneum before incision. **B:** The peritoneum is opened, and the ureter and vessels are identified. **C:** The uteroovarian ligament is coagulated and then transected. **D:** The infundibulopelvic ligament is coagulated with bipolar forceps, then cut with scissors or laser. **E:** An endoloop may be placed on the infundibulopelvic ligament after its transection for an added measure of hemostasis.

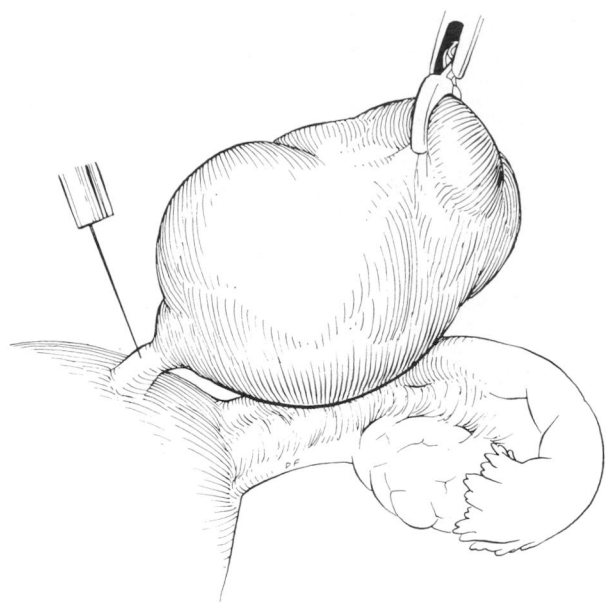

FIGURE 16.22. Excision of pedunculated myoma. The base is thoroughly coagulated and cut. (From: Roseff SJ, Murphy AA. Helpful techniques in laser laparoscopy. *Contemp Obstet Gynecol* 1988;32:168, with permission.)

Techniques for Tissue Removal

As an increasing number of expirative surgeries are being performed laparoscopically, it has become necessary to remove large volumes of tissue. Morcellators can be used as described earlier. Specimens can also be removed by way of a small suprapubic incision (or enlargement of the suprapubic ancillary trocar incision) or a colpotomy incision. If a colpotomy is to be performed, a wet sponge is placed in the posterior vagina just behind the cervix while the uterus is anteverted. When it is certain that the

rectum is posterior to the incision site, laser or electro-surgery is used to make a transverse incision in the posterior cul-de-sac over the sponge. This technique is often more hemostatic than is the traditional colpotomy incision through the vagina. This should be the last step of the procedure because the pneumoperitoneum will be more difficult to maintain, and laparoscopic visualization may be more difficult thereafter.

Impermeable sacs can be introduced abdominally or through a colpotomy incision for the removal of tissue. The sacs are of differing sizes to accommodate varied amounts of tissue. Some are attached to an expandable metal ring to simplify the placement of tissue into the sac. Once the tissue is placed inside the sac, a drawstring closes the sac and the sac is removed from the peritoneal cavity. If the tissue is too large to be pulled through the port, the trocar can be removed and the sac brought through the skin incision or colpotomy incision.

COMPLICATIONS OF LAPAROSCOPY

Complications occur with laparoscopic procedures as with all surgical procedures. Surgical experience and meticulous adherence to proper technique are essential to prevent complications. Nevertheless, some complications, such as those associated with blind insertion of the trocar, may be unavoidable. A laparoscopic surgeon should be aware of the potential complications and know how to manage them.

Pneumoperitoneum

Extraperitoneal insufflation occurs when the Veress needle fails to enter the peritoneal cavity. When the incorrect placement is recognized, CO_2 should be allowed to es-

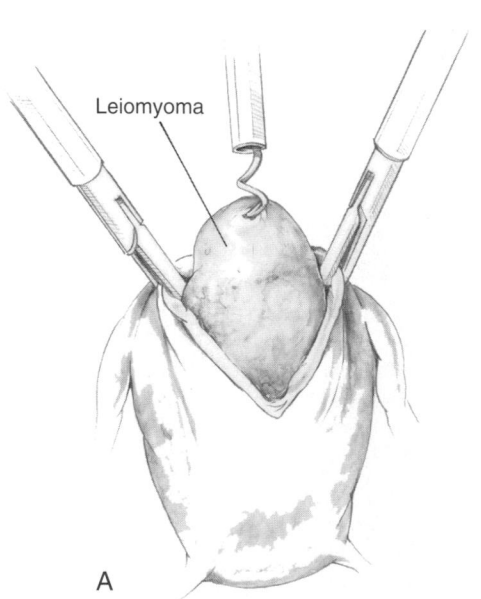

Leiomyoma

A

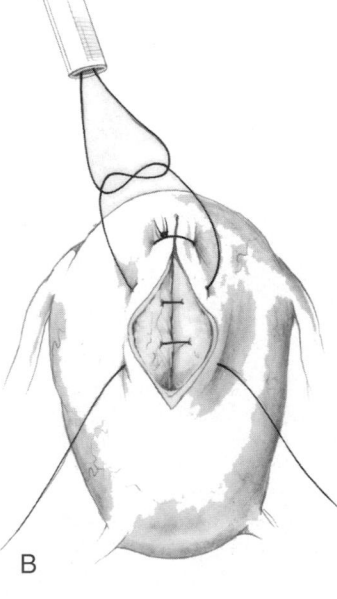

B

FIGURE 16.23. Myomectomy. A: The leiomyoma is grasped with forceps or a corkscrew and is dissected from the myometrium with careful blunt and sharp dissection. B: The defect, if large, is closed with sutures in two layers.

cape and the needle reinserted. The emphysema will resolve spontaneously. If the preperitoneal insufflation extends to the mediastinum, mediastinal emphysema can be seen. Mediastinal emphysema is usually recognized by the anesthetist, who will have difficulty ventilating the patient. As much gas as possible should be allowed to escape, and the patient carefully monitored. Severe cases may require assisted ventilation. Pneumothorax is a rare complication and occurs with inadvertent insufflation of the pleural cavity when an upper abdominal site is chosen for insufflation. Emphysema of the omentum is usually a self limited problem but may make visualization of the abdominopelvic structures more difficult. Rarely, a penetrating injury to blood vessels is not recognized at the time of insufflation and may lead to gas embolism and death. The anesthesiologist may recognize the classic "mill-wheel" murmur that can be heard over the precordium. If a gas embolism is suspected, the patient should be hyperventilated with 100% oxygen and given cardiovascular support. A central venous catheter can be placed in the right atrium or the superior vena cava in an attempt to aspirate the CO_2 gas.

Vessel Injury

The Veress needle or trocar may traumatize omental or mesenteric blood vessels or any of the major abdominal or pelvic arteries or veins. Thin or small patients are at particular risk. Elevating the anterior abdominal wall and directing the needle or trocar toward the pelvic area may avoid most of these serious complications. Injury to small vessels, such as omental vessels, may require coagulation. Major vessel injury usually requires immediate laparotomy, transfusion, and vascular repair. Injury to mesenteric vessels may also lead to compromise of a segment of bowel and bowel resection. Rarely, injury to retroperitoneal vessels may not be diagnosed intraoperatively. Elevated abdominal pressures created by pneumoperitoneum can tamponade vessels. Once the pneumoperitoneum is released, these vessels may bleed and cause hypovolemic shock.

Both pairs of epigastric vessels can be injured during placement of accessory trocars. The superficial epigastric vessels can usually be identified by transillumination and avoided. The inferior epigastric vessels are deeper, making transillumination difficult. Direct laparoscopic visualization of the inferior epigastric vessels and insertion of trocars lateral to the edge of the rectus muscle (6 to 7 cm lateral to the midline) will decrease the risk of vessel laceration. Bleeding from superficial vessels can often be controlled by pressure. The trocar sleeve may tamponade bleeding if left in place during the case. Turning the sleeve occasionally helps compress a bleeding vessel. If the trocar sleeve does not completely stop the bleeding, an additional port can be placed, and instruments can be used to achieve hemostasis intracorporeally. The bipolar forceps can be used to coagulate the vessel cephalad and caudad to the sleeve. Alternatively, sutures can be placed through the anterior abdominal wall. A straight needle or a curved urologic needle can facilitate the passage of sutures through the anterior abdominal wall. Another approach is to wedge an inflated Foley catheter balloon into the puncture site. The Foley can be taped or clamped to the skin to secure its position. If a hematoma forms, the hematoma should be evacuated, the incision explored, and the vessel identified and ligated.

Laceration of the fallopian tube, mesosalpinx, or infundibulopelvic ligament may occur during dissection or as a result of efforts to stabilize the structure. Medium-vessel injury is best controlled with bipolar electrocoagulation. Minimal damage is caused if the vessel walls are grasped before coagulation. Irrigation may be necessary to pinpoint the source. Alternatively, a suture or loop ligature can be placed. The CO_2 laser is not an effective coagulator for vessels that are larger than 2 mm. Laparotomy should be required only if the techniques mentioned earlier are not successful in achieving hemostasis or if a large-vessel injury has occurred.

Bowel Injury

Gastric injury is uncommon, but the risk is increased by gastric distention after intubation. If the intubation is difficult, it may be wise to have a nasogastric tube placed to decompress the stomach before placement of the Veress needle. Some prefer to have a nasogastric tube placed routinely. If gastric juice is obtained after placement of the Veress needle or if gastric perforation by the Veress needle is suspected, the stomach should be decompressed, the Veress needle removed and replaced, and the site of gastric perforation assessed laparoscopically. If the site is hemostatic, injuries less than 5 mm will usually heal spontaneously. Larger lacerations will require closure.

Injury to the intestines can occur during insertion of the Veress needle or trocars, or at the time of operative laparoscopic procedures. Injuries are more common in patients who have had previous abdominal surgery or pelvic adhesive disease. Perforation of the bowel with the Veress needle often goes undiagnosed because the area of perforation usually seals off spontaneously. The "syringe test" usually permits early recognition of stomach or bowel penetration, but the test is not infallible. If penetration is suspected, the needle is withdrawn and insufflation is attempted at another site. Once the laparoscope is inserted, the site of penetration is carefully examined. Most needle injuries do not require laparotomy but should be closely monitored. A hemostatic injury to the bowel serosa does not need to be repaired. Trocar insertion more often results in injury that must be surgically corrected. If the laparoscope enters the lumen, it should be left in place to limit peritoneal soiling and facilitate identification of the injured site. In some cases, small perforations of the bowel can be repaired laparoscopically with interrupted sutures tied intracorporeally or externally. Large bowel injuries may be repaired laparoscopically if the patient has undergone a bowel preparation or if there is minimal fecal spill. If the surgeon is not experienced in laparoscopic suture technique or if the injury is extensive, a laparotomy should be performed. A colostomy is sometimes necessary, depending on the site and nature of the injury.

Extensive bowel dissection may lead to postoperative ileus, which resolves in a few days. Symptoms include nausea, vomiting, and abdominal distention. Patients who have undergone extensive lysis of bowel adhesions may be admitted for observation of possible ileus or unsuspected bowel injury.

Thermal injury can be caused by direct contact of electrical, thermal, or laser energy with an organ or tissue. Some accidents occur because the field of vision is incomplete, and bowel may come in contact with a charged or heated instrument without the surgeon's knowledge. With electrical injury, the full extent of damage may not become obvious immediately, and patients may be asymptomatic for up to 3 days. Abdominal pain and signs of peritonitis in a patient who has recently undergone operative laparoscopy should raise the question of a thermal bowel injury. Significant thermal bowel injury should be treated with wide resection and reanastomosis.

Laser-induced injury to organs can result from accidental activation of the laser while it is aimed at the wrong target, penetration past the actual target, and striking targets close to the true target. Exposure to carbon plume should be avoided because it is an irritant, and it has been shown to be mutagenic in *Salmonella*.

Bladder Injury

The bladder can be injured as the trocar is inserted. This is more common in patients who have had previous pelvic surgery. All patients should have their bladder drained after anesthesia is induced. If the procedure is expected to take longer than 30 minutes, a catheter should be inserted for continuous bladder drainage. The size of the bladder injury will dictate treatment. Veress needle perforations can be managed expectantly. Lacerations smaller than 5 mm may heal spontaneously if the bladder is drained continuously for 4 to 5 days postoperatively. Larger injuries require suturing. This can be attempted laparoscopically by surgeons who are experienced at laparoscopic suturing techniques.

Ureteral Injury

The ureter is injured less frequently than is the bladder. It is particularly susceptible to injury when adhesions or endometriosis involves the pelvic side wall. Ureteral stents can sometimes be helpful in locating the ureters if the anatomy is severely distorted. If a ureteral injury is suspected, indigo carmine solution can be injected intravenously; cystoscopic examination will reveal dye from the ureteral orifices in about 5 minutes. If ureteral injury is suspected postoperatively, an intravenous pyelogram should be obtained. The location of the injury will determine the type of reparative procedure needed.

Trocar Hernias

Although rare, bowel can herniate through laparoscopic incisions and become incarcerated. The Z-track method can lessen the risk of herniation. Trocars larger than 7 mm create an increased risk, and the use of these larger ports often mandates closure of the fascia with sutures. Bowel can also be trapped in the incisions at the time of trocar removal secondary to increased abdominal pressure. Consequently, accessory sleeves should be removed under direct visualization. These should be covered, and the CO_2 gas should be expelled through the umbilical port. The laparoscope should then be reinserted, and the sleeve and laparoscope should be removed as a single unit under direct visualization.

Incidence of Complications

The most recent published survey of the American Association of Gynecologic Laparoscopists reported on more than 80,000 laparoscopic procedures performed in 1993; 49,697 of these were operative laparoscopy cases. Table 16.2 presents the complications reported. The rate of bowel and urinary tract injuries appears to have increased substantially since 1991. This may be associated with the increased performance of laparoscopically assisted vaginal hysterectomies and other complex operative procedures. Another study in 1999 of all hospitals performing operative gynecologic laparoscopy in Finland showed a total complication rate of 4.0 per 1,000 procedures, 0.6 per 1,000 in diagnostic procedures, 0.5 per 1,000 in sterilization procedures, and 12.6 per 1,000 in operative laparoscopies. Intestinal injuries were reported in 0.7 per 1,000, incisional hernias in 0.3 per 1,000, urinary tract injuries in 2.5 per 1,000, major vascular injuries in 0.1 per 1,000, and other injuries in 0.5 per 1,000 gynecologic laparoscopies. Seventy-five percent of the major complications in operative laparoscopies occurred during laparoscopic hysterectomies, with a 1% incidence of ureteral injuries with laparoscopic hysterectomies.

TABLE 16.2.
Complications Associated With Laparoscopy

Complication	1993 Rate/1,000[a]	1991 Rate/1,000
Hospitalization >24 h	36.7	30.3
Hospital readmission	3.2	4.2
Unintended laparotomy	8.5	8.9
Hemorrhage	7.9	6.8
Transfusion for hemorrhage	3.2	2.7
Bowel or urinary tract injury	5.5	2.8
Nerve injury	0.3	0.5
Death	0.0	0.018

[a] The 1991 survey did not include diagnostic laparoscopies and laparoscopic sterilizations as did the 1993 survey; thus, the 1993 rate may be underestimated.

(Modified from Levy BS, Hulka JF, Peterson HB, et al. Operative laparoscopy: American Association of Gynecologic Laparoscopists, 1993 membership survey. JAAGL: Journal of the American Association of Gynecologic Laparoscopists 1994;1:301)

TRAINING IN LAPAROSCOPY

There is no formal certification required to perform laparoscopic procedures. Residency training has evolved to incorporate more laparoscopic training in its curriculum, but many surgeons currently performing laparoscopic surgery were not trained in these approaches during their residencies. Before attempting the advanced techniques described in this chapter, a thorough knowledge of the pelvic anatomy and a well-developed appreciation for three-dimensional spatial relationships are necessary. Short courses in laparoscopic techniques should be followed by ongoing clinical association with surgeons who are experienced in these techniques.

CONCLUSION

The evolving role of laparoscopy in the field of operative gynecology has had a dramatic effect on clinical practice. The advantages of a laparoscopic procedure include a shorter hospital stay and decreased recovery time. The benefits of laparoscopic procedures appear to be at least equivalent to those of laparotomy in many cases, but well-controlled studies are lacking. There is general agreement that operative laparoscopy is an important technique in the armamentarium of the gynecologic or reproductive surgeon.

BIBLIOGRAPHY

Bahig CS. Electrosurgical burn injuries and their prevention. *JAMA* 1968;204:1025.

Beretta P, Franchi M, Ghezzi F, et al. Randomized clinical trial of two laparoscopic treatments of endometriomas: cystectomy versus drainage and coagulation. *Fertil Steril* 1998;70:1176.

Borten M. *Laparoscopic complications: prevention and management.* Toronto: BC Decker, 1986.

Bruhat MA, Goldchmit R. Minilaparoscopy in gynecology. *Eur J Obstet Gynecol Reprod Biol* 1998;76:207.

Bruhat MA, Manhes H, Mage G, et al. Treatment of ectopic pregnancy by means of laparoscopy. *Fertil Steril* 1980;33:411.

Daniell JF, Herbert CM. Laparoscopic salpingostomy utilizing the CO_2 laser. *Fertil Steril* 1984;41:558.

Daniell JF, Miller W. Polycystic ovaries treated by laparoscopic laser vaporization. *Fertil Steril* 1989;51:232.

DeCherney AH, Boyers SP. Isthmic ectopic pregnancy: segmental resection as the treatment of choice. *Fertil Steril* 1985;44:307.

DeCherney AH, Kase N. The conservative management of unruptured ectopic pregnancy. *Obstet Gynecol* 1979;54:451.

Dubuisson JB, Aubriot FX. Laparoscopic salpingectomy for tubal pregnancy. *Fertil Steril* 1987;47:225.

Dubuisson JB, Fauconnier A, Chapron C, et al. Reproductive outcome after myomectomy in infertile women. *J Reprod Med* 2000;45:23.

Dubuisson JB, Fauconnier A, Deffarges JV, et al. Pregnancy outcome and deliveries following laparoscopic myomectomies. *Human Reprod* 2000;15:869.

Esposito JM. The laparoscopist and electro-surgery. *Am J Obstet Gynecol* 1976;126:633.

Fauconnier A, Dubuisson JB, Ancel PY, et al. Prognostic factors of reproductive outcome after myomectomy in infertile women. *Human Reprod* 2000;15:1751.

Fayez JA. An assessment of the role of operative laparoscopy in tuboplasty. *Fertil Steril* 1983;39:476.

Feste JR. Laser laparoscopy: a new modality. *J Reprod Med* 1985;30:413

Gant NF. Infertility and endometriosis: comparison of pregnancy outcomes with laparotomy versus laparoscopic techniques. *Am J Obstet Gynecol* 1992;166:1072.

George SM Jr, Fabian TC, Voeller GR, et al. Primary repair of colon wounds: a prospective trial in nonselected patients. *Ann Surg* 1989;209:728.

Gomel V. Laparoscopic tubal surgery in infertility. *Obstet Gynecol* 1975;46:47.

Gomel V, Taylor PJ, Yuzpe AA, et al. Indications, contraindications, complications. In: Gomel V, Taylor PJ, Yuzpe AA, et al., eds. *Laparoscopy and hysteroscopy in gynecologic practice.* Chicago: Mosby–Year Book, 1986:56.

Grimes DA. Frontiers of operative laparoscopy: a review and critique of the evidence. *Am J Obstet Gynecol* 1992;166:1062.

Harkki SP, Sjoberg J, Kurki T. Major complications of laparoscopy: a follow-up Finnish study. *Obstet Gynecol* 1999;94:94.

Harris WJ. Uterine dehiscence following laparoscopic myomectomy. *Obstet Gynecol* 1992;80:545.

Hasson HM, Rotman C, Rana N, et al. Laparoscopic myomectomy. *Obstet Gynecol* 1992;80:884.

Hulka JF, Reich H. *Textbook of laparoscopy,* second edition. Philadelphia: WB Saunders, 1994.

Hurst BS, Stackhouse DJ, Matthews ML, et al. Uterine artery embolization for symptomatic uterine myomas. *Fertil Steril* 2000;74:855.

Johns DA, Hardie RP. Management of unruptured ectopic pregnancy with laparoscopic carbon dioxide laser. *Fertil Steril* 1986;46:703.

Jones HW Jr, Rock JA. *Reparative and constructive surgery of the female generative tract.* Baltimore: Williams & Wilkins, 1983.

Lauritsen JG, Pagel JD, Vangsted P, et al. Results of repeated tuboplasties. *Fertil Steril* 1982;37:68.

Levine RL. Economic impact of pelviscopic surgery. *J Reprod Med* 1985;30:655.

Levy BS, Hulka JF, Peterson HB, et al. Operative laparoscopy: American Association of Gynecologic Laparoscopists, 1993 membership survey. *J Am Assoc Gynecol Laparosc* 1994;1:301.

Martin DC. CO_2 laser laparoscopy for endometriosis associated with infertility. *J Reprod Med* 1986;31:121.

Martin DC, Diamond MP. Operative laparoscopy: comparison of lasers with other techniques. *Curr Probl Obstet Gynecol Fertil* 1986;9:564.

McLaughlin DS. Metroplasty and myomectomy with CO_2 laser for the preservation of normal tissue and minimizing blood loss. *J Reprod Med* 1985;30:1.

Mettler L, Giesel H, Semm K. Treatment of female infertility due to tubal obstruction by operative laparoscopy. *Fertil Steril* 1979;32:384.

Mirhashemi R, Harlow BL, Ginsburg ES, et al. Predicting risk of complications with gynecologic laparoscopic surgery. *Obstet Gynecol* 1998;92:327.

Murphy AA. Operative laparoscopy. *Fertil Steril* 1987;47:6.

Nezhat C, Nezhat FR. Safe laser endoscopic excision or vaporization of peritoneal endometriosis. *Fertil Steril* 1989;52:149.

Nezhat CR, Nezhat FR, Luciano AA, et al. *Operative gyneco-logic laparoscopy: principles and practice.* New York: McGraw-Hill, 1995.

Olive DL, Martin DC. Treatment of endometriosis-associated infertility with CO_2 laser laparoscopy: the use of one- and two-parameter exponential models. *Fertil Steril* 1987;48:18.

Palter SF. Microlaparoscopy under local anesthesia and conscious pain mapping for the diagnosis and management of pelvic pain. *Curr Opin Obstet Gynecol* 1999;11:387.

Palmer R. Sterilisation per-coelioscopique (avec film). *Presse Med* 1962;70:1106.

Portuondo JA, Melchor JC, Neyro JL, et al. Periovarian adhesions following ovarian wedge resection or laparoscopic biopsy. *Endoscopy* 1984;16:143.

Pouly JL, Manhes H, Mage G, et al. Conservative laparoscopic treatment of 321 ectopic pregnancies. *Fertil Steril* 1986;46:1093.

Pring DW. Inferior epigastric haemorrhage, an avoidable complication of laparoscopic clip sterilization. *Br J Obstet Gynaecol* 1983;90:480.

Reich H, McGlynn F. Laparoscopic oophorectomy and salpingo-oophorectomy in the treatment of benign tubo-ovarian disease. *J Reprod Med* 1986;31:609.

Reich H, McGlynn F. Treatment of ovarian endometriomas using laparoscopic surgical techniques. *J Reprod Med* 1986;31:577.

Schwartz RO, Martin JB. Laparoscopic salpingectomy for ectopic pregnancy. *South Med J* 1985;78:1341.

See WA, Cooper CS, Fisher RJ. Predictors of laparoscopic complications after formal training in laparoscopic surgery. *JAMA* 1993;270:2689.

Semm K. New methods of pelviscopy for myomectomy, ovariectomy, tubectomy and adnectomy. *Endoscopy* 1979;2:85.

Semm K, Mettler L. Technical progress in pelvic surgery via operative laparoscopy. *Am J Obstet Gynecol* 1980;138:121.

Shapiro HI, Adler DH. Excision of an ectopic pregnancy through the laparoscope. *Am J Obstet Gynecol* 1973;117:290.

Smith S. Minimizing, recognizing, and managing laparoscopic complications. In: Azziz R, Murphy AAM. *Practical manual of operative laparoscopy and hysteroscopy,* second edition. New York: Springer-Verlag New York, 1997:248.

Soderstrom RM. Unusual uses of laparoscopy. *J Reprod Med* 1975;15:77.

Stangel JJ, Gomel V. Techniques in conservative surgery for tubal gestation. *Clin Obstet Gynecol* 1980;23:1221.

Steptoe PC. *Laparoscopy in gynecology.* Edinburgh, Scotland: E & S Livingstone, 1967.

Sulewski JM, Curcio FD, Bronitsh TC, et al. The treatment of endometriosis at laparoscopy for infertility. *Am J Obstet Gynecol* 1980;138:128.

Tarasconi JC. Endoscopic salpingectomy. *J Reprod Med* 1981;26:541.

Taylor RC, Berkowitz J, McComb PF. Role of laparoscopic salpingostomy in the treatment of hydrosalpinx. *Fertil Steril* 2001;75:594.

Yuzpe AA, Gomel V, Taylor PJ, et al. Instruments for laparoscopy and hysteroscopy. In: Gomel V, Taylor PJ, Yuzpe AA, et al., eds. *Laparoscopy and hysteroscopy in gynecologic practice.* Chicago: Mosby–Year Book, 1986:7.

Zullo F, Pellicano M De Stefano R, et al. A prospective randomized study to evaluate leuprolide acetate treatment before laparoscopic myomectomy: efficacy and ultrasonographic predictors. *Am J Obstet Gynecol* 1998;178:108.

CHAPTER

17

▼

Operative Hysteroscopy

MICHAEL S. BAGGISH

Hysteroscopy has become a standard part of the gynecologic surgeon's armamentarium and is now routinely taught as part of residency training curriculums and postgraduate seminars. As gynecologists have grown better acquainted with the benefits and techniques of operative hysteroscopy, and as hysteroscopy increasingly has become the method of choice for treatment of intrauterine pathology, the number of complications has also risen. Most of these complications are caused by operator error and inexperience.

Hysteroscopic procedures were first described by Pantaleoni in 1869, but the technique did not excite substantial interest within the specialty until the late 1970s. There has been concern that hysteroscopy performed as a routine office procedure to diagnose the causes of abnormal uterine bleeding might spread undiagnosed endometrial carcinoma transtubally. The most vocal opponents of hysteroscopy continue to perform blind dilatation and curettage (D&C) rather than hysteroscopy to diagnose, among other things, endometrial carcinoma. However, Roberts et al. documented the presence of malignant cells in inferior vena cava blood immediately after vigorous curettage of the endometrium, and the disparaging rhetoric against hysteroscopy seems to have little basis in fact. Indeed, during the mid-1980s, hysteroscopy replaced blind D&C as the standard procedure for precise diagnosis of intrauterine pathology.

The advantages of hysteroscopy as an accurate diagnostic technique are that it not only allows direct visual observation and accurate localization of pathology but also provides a means to sample the site most likely to yield positive results. During the 1980s and 1990s, gynecology has shifted heavily toward endoscopy as a specialty.

The philosophy of least-invasive surgery is driven by the positive outcomes of shortened hospital stays and diminished recovery times and by good performance in a competitive free-market environment. Operative hysteroscopy has, in many instances, superseded even laparoscopy in meeting these strategic criteria. Hysteroscopy generally is a low-risk technique that uses the endocervical canal, the natural passageway of the body, to gain entry into the intrauterine environment. Refinements of optical and fiberoptic light instrumentation and of operative accessories allow high-resolution and excellent visual documentation by hysteroscopy, and tremendous advances still are being made. Nonhysteroscopic techniques to treat intrauterine septa and adhesions are obsolete. Ablation or resection of the endometrium is considered an acceptable alternative to hysterectomy for the management of abnormal uterine bleeding. Submucous myomata no longer require hysterectomy because they can be satisfactorily managed conservatively by operative hysteroscopy. Cornual and interstitial tubal obstruction also are now managed hysteroscopically. Office-based, low-skill techniques for rapidly managing abnormal uterine bleeding by means of thermal catheters are now a reality. Hysteroscopy in the 21st century has finally found its proper niche, and every gynecologist is required to learn the skills of hysteroscopy, just as every urologist must be an accomplished cystoscopist.

INSTRUMENTATION

Telescopes

The 4-mm telescope (lens) gives the sharpest, clearest image and the smallest outside diameter. The most desirable optics provide a large field that subtends an angle of about 105 degrees. Contemporary 3-mm-diameter telescopes coupled to endoscopic video systems with zoom lenses are highly satisfactory for office hysteroscopy and for operative hysteroscopy. Telescopes are usually available with a 0-degree straight-on or a 30-degree fore-oblique view (Fig. 17.1A). The major advantage of the 0-degree lens is that it allows the operator to see the operative devices as a relatively distant panorama, whereas this view is lost when the 30-degree lens is used. The telescope has three parts: the eyepiece,

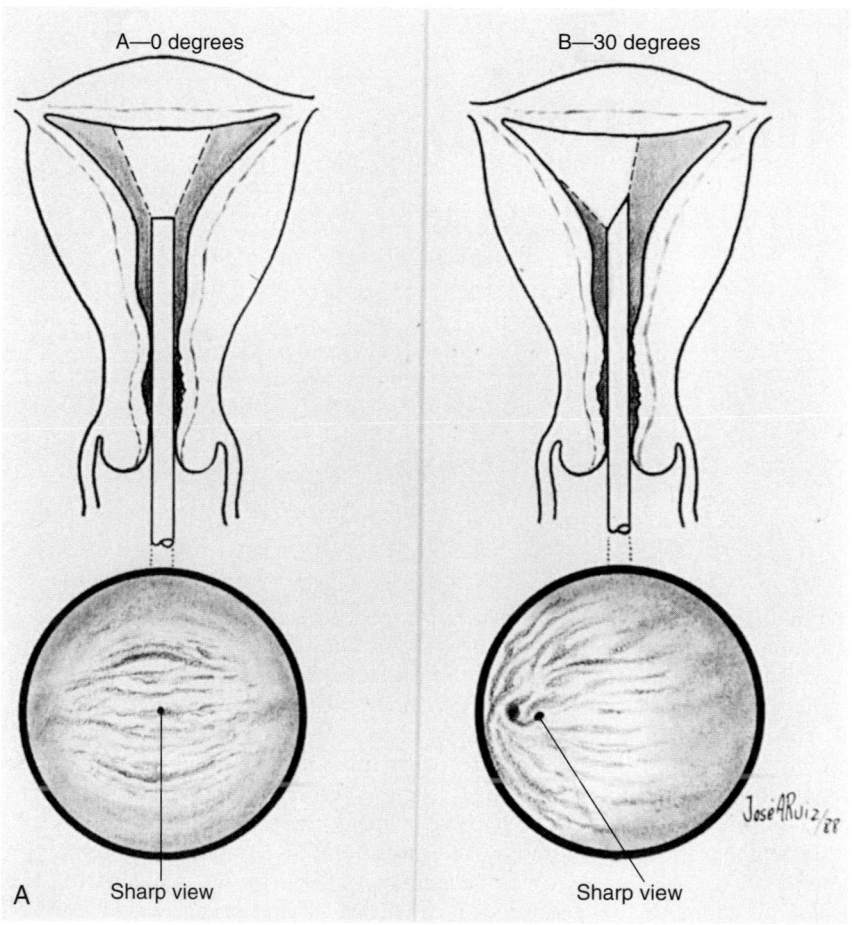

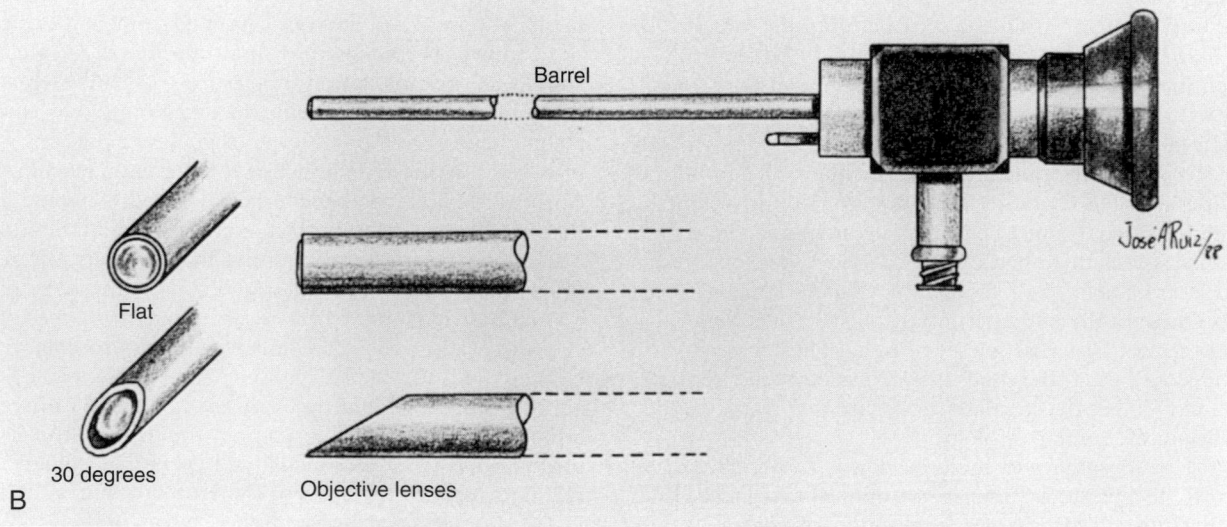

FIGURE 17.1. A: Telescopes are available with either straight-on (0 degrees) or fore-oblique (30 degrees) viewing objective lenses. B: A telescope can be conveniently subdivided into three parts: eyepiece, barrel, and objective lens. (From Baggish MS, Barbot J, Valle RF. *Diagnostic and operative hysteroscopy.* Chicago: Mosby–Year Book, 1989, with permission.)

the barrel, and the objective lens (Fig. 17.1B). Surrounding the optics are numerous small-diameter incoherent fiberoptic bundles that provide intense cold illumination to the operative field. Although a few manufacturers provide focusing telescopes that permit contact hysteroscopy, the standard telescope has fixed optics. The contact hysteroscope is a highly specialized device used largely in research settings. Although magnifying hysteroscopes reached a peak of popularity in the 1980s, their full practical value has never been realized.

Light Generators

The quality and power of light delivered to the telescope depend on the wattage and characteristics of the remote light generator and the type and structural integrity of the connecting fiberoptic light cable. Three general types of light generators are available: tungsten, metal halide, and xenon. The simplest and cheapest generator is the tungsten generator, which produces an orange-yellow light; the xenon white light is a powerful generator that provides the best shower for video imaging (Fig. 17.2). The xenon light generator is well worth the additional cost because of its superior color and intensity.

Fiberoptic light cables must be intact to convey the optimal light from the generator to the telescope. Broken fibers can be easily identified by viewing the stretched-out cable against a dark background and looking for light emitting through the sides of the cable. The liquid cable conducts light effectively and, when combined with a xenon generator, provides superior light.

Diagnostic and Operative Sheaths

A diagnostic sheath is required to deliver the distending medium into the uterine cavity. The telescope fits into the sheath and is secured by means of a watertight seal that locks into place. The sheath is 4 to 5 mm in diameter, depending on the outer diameter of the telescope, with a 1-mm clearance between the inner wall and the telescope, through which either carbon dioxide or liquid distending medium is transmitted. Medium instillation into the sheath is controlled by means of an external stopcock. Even the 5-mm instrument allows easy access through the narrow endocervical canal past the point of maximal constriction (i.e., the internal os). Therefore, diagnostic hysteroscopy can be performed without cervical canal dilatation. If the hysteroscope is inserted into the canal under direct vision (as it should be), and if the axes of the cervical and uterine canals are carefully followed until the corpus is reached, there should be no risk of perforation. Imprecise or loose coupling between the telescope and sheath will result in leakage of the medium at that interface.

Operative sheaths have a larger diameter than do diagnostic sheaths (Fig. 17.3). They range in size from 7 to 10 mm and average 8 mm in diameter. The operative sheath allows space for instillation of the medium, for the 3- to 4-mm telescope, and for the insertion of operating devices. The operating channel is sealed with a rubber nipple or gasket to prevent leakage of the distending medium. The standard operating sheath consists of a single common cavity shared by the medium, telescope, and operating tools. The major disadvantages of this type of sheath are that the uterine cavity cannot be flushed with the distending medium, and the operative tools cannot be accurately placed and manipulated within the cavity (Fig. 17.4A). Hysteroscopes with isolated channels overcome the problems inherent to the common cavity sheath (Fig. 17.4B). The dual operating channels permit flushing of the cavity and precise placement of operating accessories. The most recently introduced isolated-channel sheath consists of a double-flushing sheath (Fig. 17.4C) that permits media instillation by way of the innersheath and media return by way of the perforated outersheath. The constant flow of medium in and out of the cavity creates a very clear operative field. The single isolated operating channel has a diameter sufficiently large (3 mm) to permit an entirely new generation of larger, sturdier op-

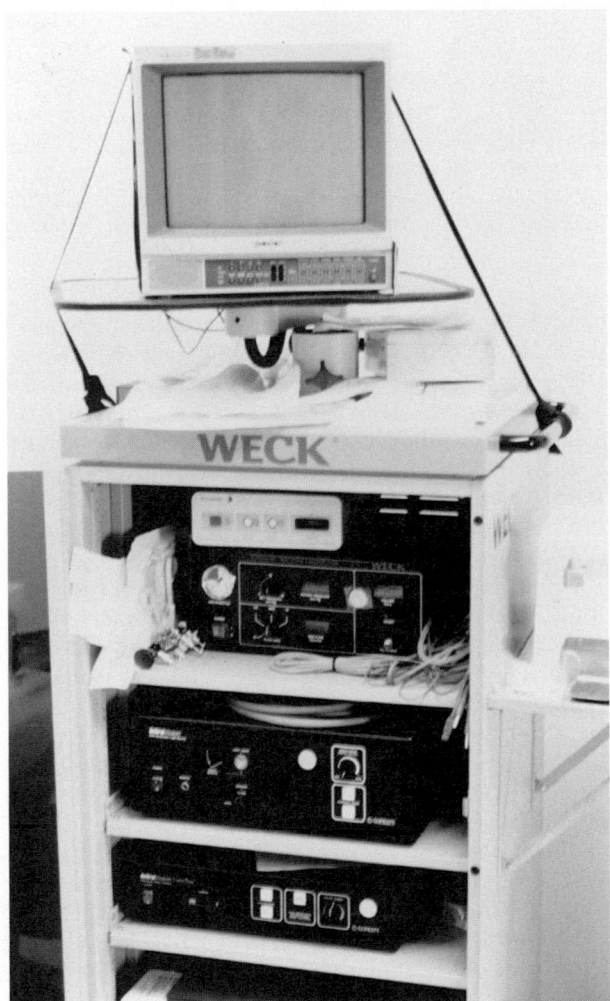

FIGURE 17.2. This surgical cart is adaptable for either the office or the operating room. It contains a television monitor, a light source, a recording unit, a television control unit, and an electrosurgery generator. The light is a xenon source, which provides clear white light.

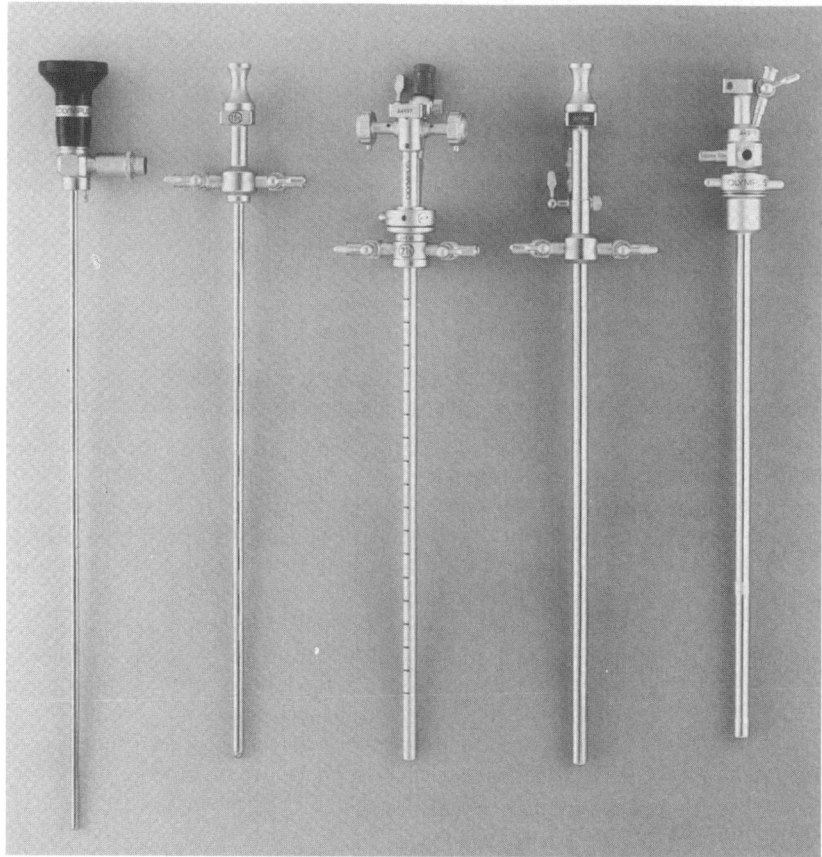

FIGURE 17.3. Instrumentation for hysteroscopic procedures. From **left:** a 4-mm telescope, a 5-mm diagnostic sheath, an operating sheath with a deflecting bridge, and a standard single-channel operating sheath (shown in two views).

erating tools to be used (Fig. 17.4D). The new sheath combines the advantages of the resectoscope with the facility of the operating hysteroscope.

The resectoscope is a specialized electrosurgical (monopolar) endoscope that consists of an innersheath and outersheath (Fig. 17.5A). The outersheath is for medium return as described above. The innersheath has a common channel for the telescope, medium, and electrode. The double-armed monopolar electrode is fitted to a trigger device that pushes the electrode out beyond the sheath and then pulls it back within the sheath. The operating tools consist of three basic electrodes: a ball, barrel, and cutting loop (Fig. 17.5B). Most resectoscopes are equipped with a 30-degree telescope. The lens is angled toward the electrode to permit a clear view of the near operative field. Clarity is lost when the electrode is fully extended outward. The classic operating sheaths measure at least more than 8 mm in diameter, and dilatation is usually required for insertion. A new smaller diameter resectoscope uses a 3-mm telescope and a 7.5-8 mm sheath.

ACCESSORY INSTRUMENTS

During the 1990s, many new accessory devices appeared on the market. The standard accessories are the 7F (2.3 mm) alligator grasping forceps, biopsy forceps, and scissors. The small size of these fragile semirigid instru-

ments is a disadvantage, and excessive torque at the junction of the shaft and handle frequently leads to breakage. Development of the large isolated-channel sheath has made the use of totally flexible 3-mm operating instruments feasible. The scissors and graspers are substantially heavier and almost indestructible (Fig. 17.6).

A variety of monopolar and bipolar electrodes are also now available for operative hysteroscopy. Monopolar balls, needles, shaving loops (3 mm), and ridged (vaporizing) loops can be inserted through the large operating channel (Fig. 17.7). Bipolar needles for myolysis, as well as bipolar ball electrodes, have been manufactured (Fig. 17.7C), together with bipolar scissors and cutting needles.

The hysteroscopic sheath has an advantage over the resectoscopic sheath, allowing insertion of an aspirating cannula (2.3 or 3 mm), which permits the operator to selectively clear the field of bubbles and debris that cannot be removed by way of the return second sheath (Fig. 17.8). Nevertheless, the resectoscope is generally easier to use for the average gynecologist.

An intriguing new bipolar system marketed under the trade name of Versapoint (Gynecare, Ethicon, Somerville, New Jersey) permits cutting and ablation via operative hysteroscopes or via a dedicated bipolar resectoscope. The mechanism for the bipolar current flow through the electrode is illustrated in Fig. 17.9. The electrodes measure 5F diameter (i.e. <2 mm) and therefore can be accommodated by standard and isolated hysteroscopic channels.

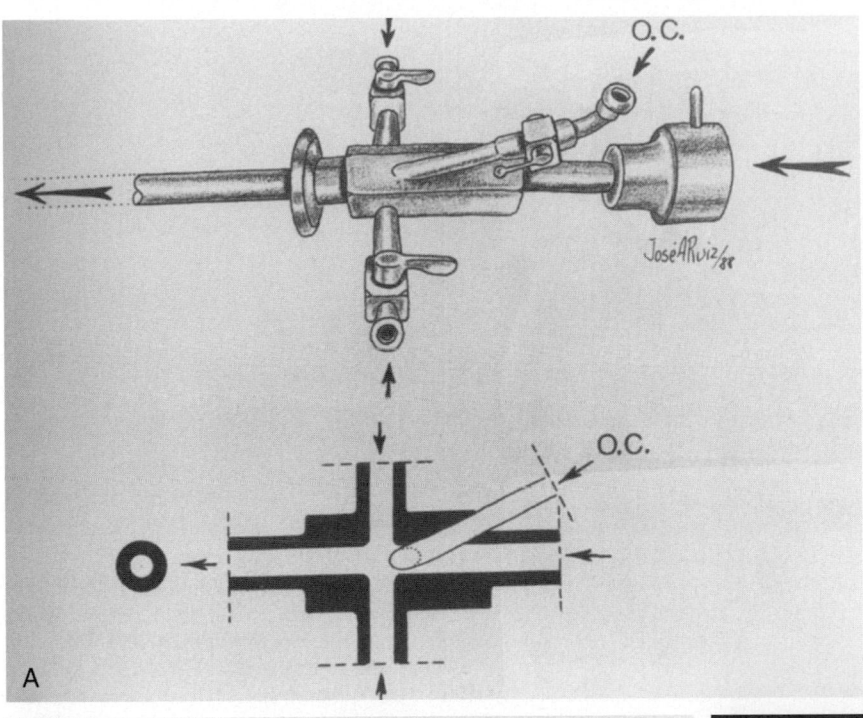

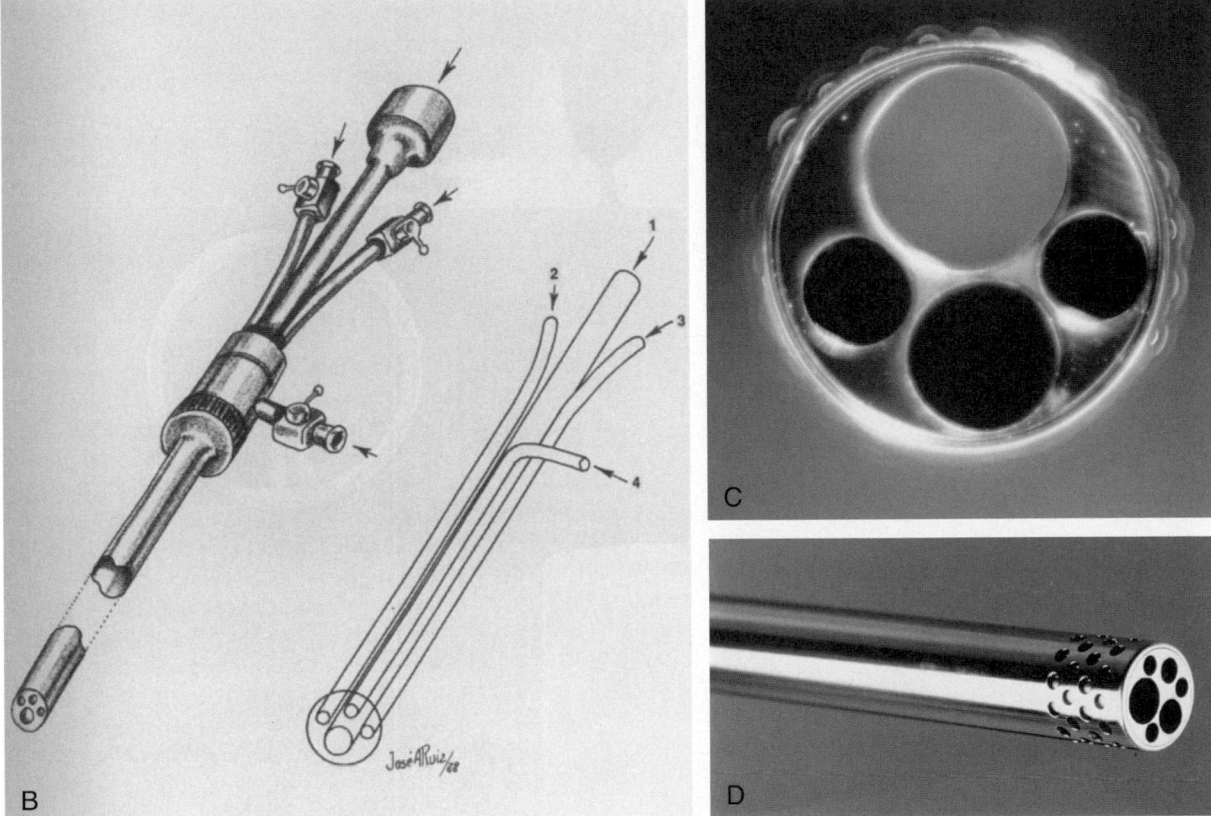

FIGURE 17.4. A: A single-channel operating sheath consists of a single cavity that the telescope, distending medium, and operating instruments share. O.C., operating channel. **B:** A dual-channel operating sheath is constructed with isolated channels for *(1)* a telescope, *(2* and *3)* two operating devices, and *(4)* distending medium. **C:** The terminal portion of the second-generation isolated-channel hysteroscope shows the channel for the 4-mm optic **(top)** and a 3-mm operating channel for a variety of large accessory instruments **(bottom).** The two channels at either side are the fluid intake channels. **D:** The double-sheath mechanism of the isolated-channel hysteroscope. The perforations in the outersheath are for fluid return. The uterus is continuously flushed. (A and B: From Baggish MS, Barbot J, Valle RF. *Diagnostic and operative hysteroscopy.* Chicago: Mosby–Year Book, 1989, with permission; C and D: From Bryan Corporation, Woburn, MA, with permission.)

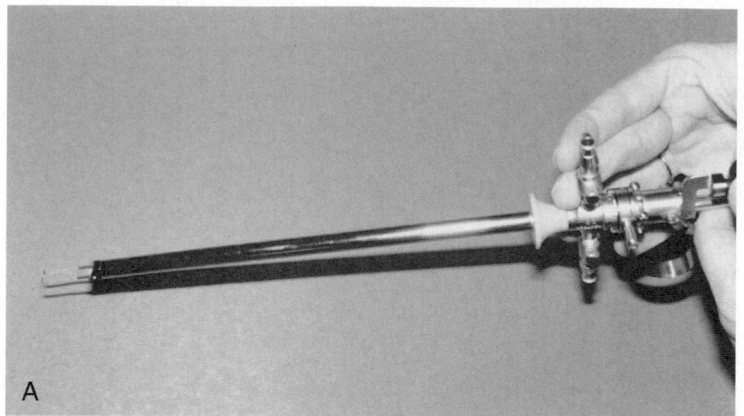

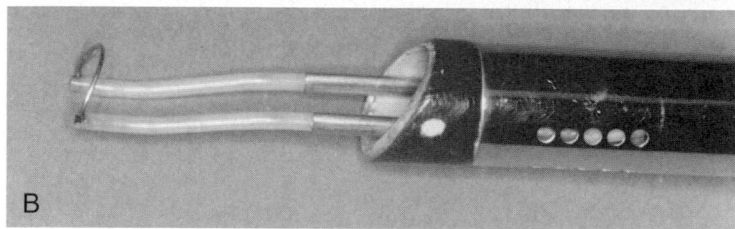

FIGURE 17.5. A: A panoramic view of a resectoscope. This consists of an innersheath for fluid entry and an outersheath for fluid return. **B:** This photo details the monopolar electrode of the resectoscope. The resecting loop electrode is shown. In other cases, a ball or barrel electrode may be used.

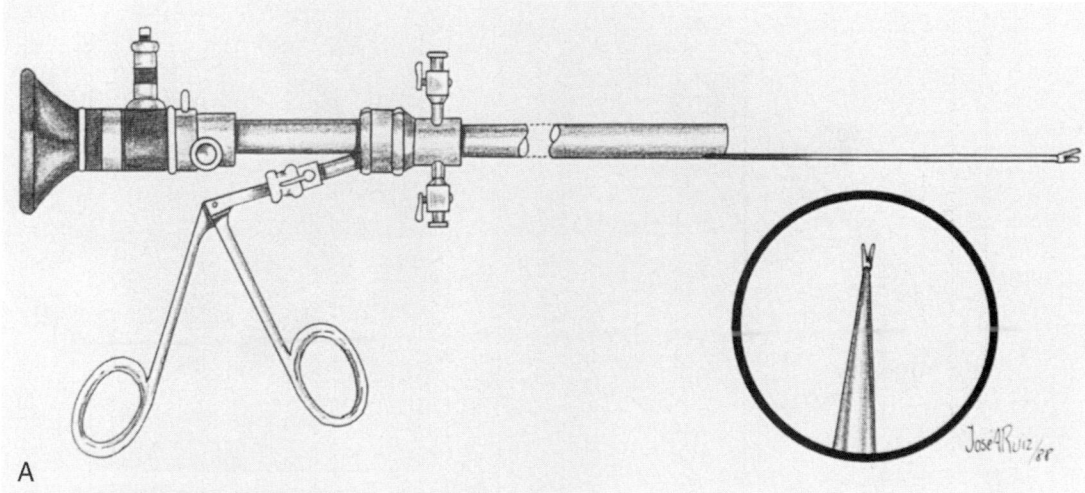

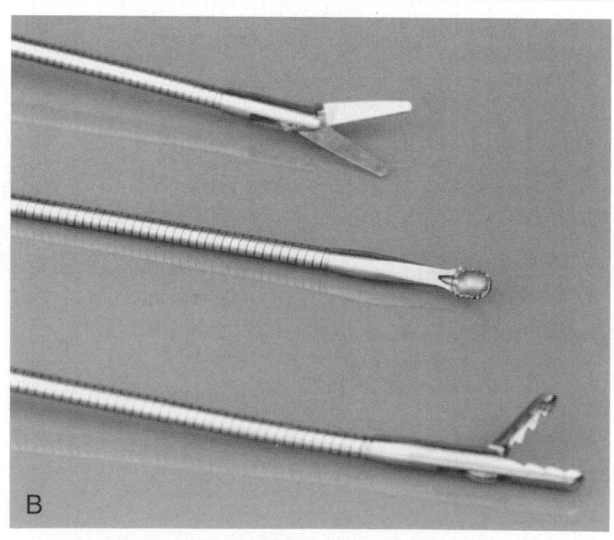

FIGURE 17.6. A: A flexible or semirigid operating instrument can be delivered to the operative site by way of the operating channel. **Inset** is hysteroscopic view of device. (From Baggish MS, Barbot J, Valle RF. *Diagnostic and operative hysteroscopy.* Chicago: Mosby–Year Book, 1989, with permission.) **B:** A variety of flexible 3-mm accessory instruments is shown: large dual-action scissors **(top),** curette to allow sampling under direct vision **(middle),** and alligator forceps **(bot-**

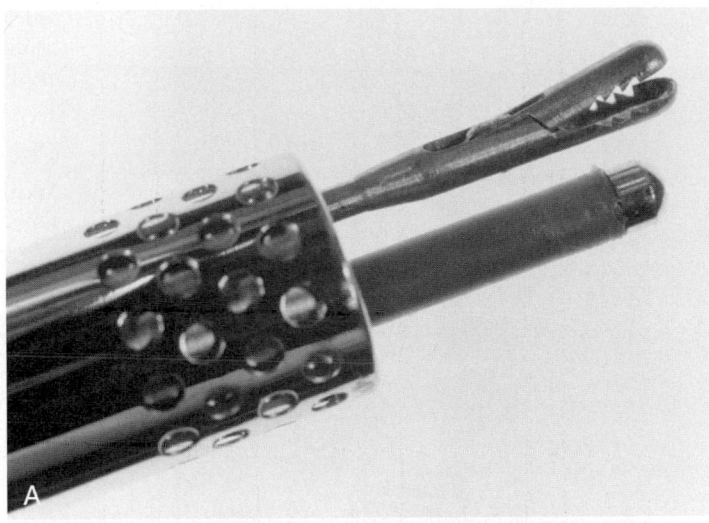

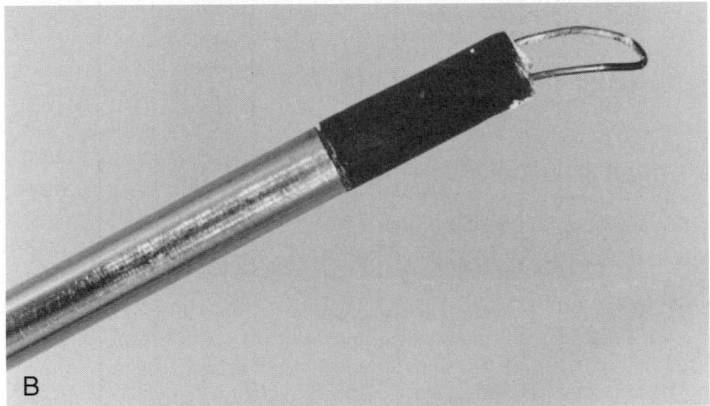

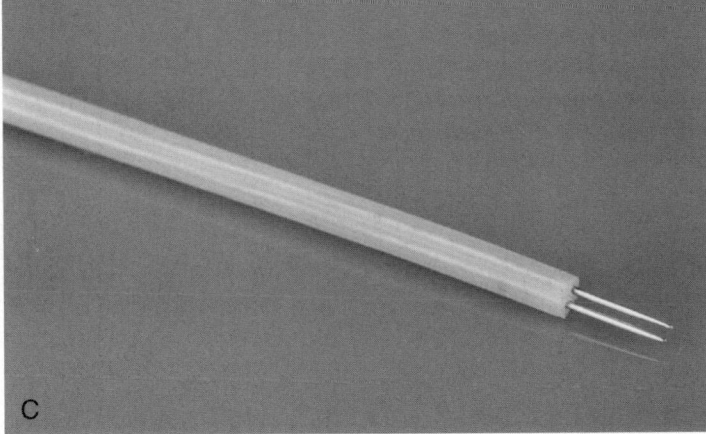

FIGURE 17.7. A: An isolated-channel flushing hysteroscope. In one channel is a 3-mm ball electrode, and in the other channel is an alligator grasping forceps. B: A 3-mm resecting loop that can be inserted through the large channel of the isolated-channel hysteroscope. C: A 3-mm bipolar needle that can be inserted into submucous myomas for myolysis. (From Unimed, Largo, FL, with permission.)

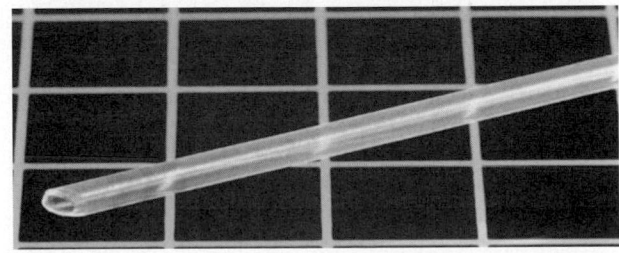

FIGURE 17.8. A 9F aspirating cannula (Cook OB/GYN). The cannula can be inserted through the large 3-mm channel of the operating hysteroscope for aspiration of either debris or fluid, or for endometrial sampling.

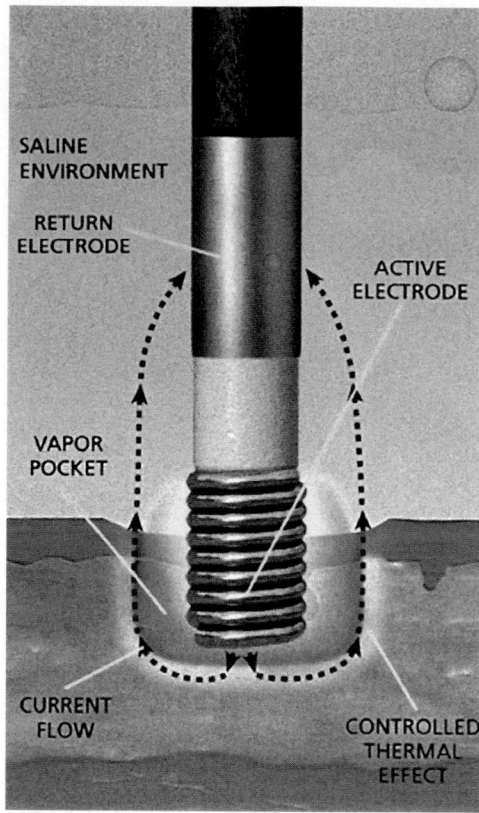

FIGURE 17.9. The mechanism of action for the Versapoint bipolar electrode is illustrated. The coiled bottom portion is the active electrode, and the upper (separately illustrated) metal portion serves as the return electrode. The saline medium facilitates the conduction of current between the two poles. See color version of figure.

The biggest advantage of this bipolar technology is the same that exists for the Nd-YAG laser; that is, saline may be used as the distending medium for the operative hysteroscopy. This obviates the risk of hyponatremia (see sections on media and complications).

The Contact Hysteroscope

Among all modern hysteroscopes, only the contact hysteroscope (Fig. 17.10A) does not require a sheath or a distending medium. This is a unique instrument that is available just for diagnostic purposes, as described by Baggish and Dorsey and by Barbot and associates. The contact hysteroscope traps and transmits ambient light directed onto a special light-trapping mechanism. Because actual contact is made with the mucosa, and the cavity of the endocervix and endometrium is viewed in its natural collapsed state, bleeding will not interfere with vision when this instrument is used. Unique procedures such as embryoscopy are ideally performed with the contact hysteroscope (Fig. 17.10B).

The view obtained with the contact hysteroscope lies between panoramic vision and microscopy. Diagnosis is based on color, architectural pattern, contour, and touch. Compared with other hysteroscopic techniques, contact hysteroscopy is the easiest to perform but the most difficult to interpret.

The Microhysteroscope

Another specialized endoscope is the microhysteroscope. This instrument converts a panoramic hysteroscope into a high-powered microscope by switching the lens to 150×. Light contact is made with the mucous membrane in a fashion analogous to that of the oil-immersion lens of a microscope. A type of *in vivo* cytology can then be performed, as described in two reports by Hamou. The exact application of this instrument and the technique of microcolpohysteroscopy have eluded American endoscopists to date, and the instrument has been relegated to a position of historical interest.

The Flexible Hysteroscope

A 4.8-mm-diameter soft and rigid fiberoptic hysteroscope designed by Fujinon consists of three sections: a soft flexible front section, a rigid rotating middle section, and a semirigid rear section. In 1990, Lin and colleagues reported their experiences with this instrument in 153 procedures, including transcervical tubocornual recanalization, chorionic villus sampling, and retrieval of lost intrauterine devices (IUDs). The flexible hysteroscope has a particular advantage in its ease of aligning the catheter for tubal canalization.

DISTENDING MEDIA

Under normal circumstances, the uterine cavity is a potential space, and the anterior and posterior walls are in close if not actual opposition. To achieve a panoramic view within the uterus, the walls must be forcibly separated. The thick muscle of the uterine wall requires a minimum pressure of 40 mm Hg to distend the cavity sufficiently to see with a hysteroscope. The endometrium is so richly endowed with blood vessels that touching it with the sheath of the hysteroscope invariably produces bleeding. However, the walls of the uterus usually are held more widely apart during operative hysteroscopy. Although a variety of distending media can be used to attain this desired degree of distention, it usually requires pressures approximating 70 mm Hg, which at the same time propel the medium through the oviducts into the peritoneal cavity. Overdilatation of the cervix with a loosely applied hysteroscopic sheath permits leakage of medium, suboptimal pressure, and poor expansion of the uterine cavity. Additionally, the lower pressure produced by the leakage allows blood to flow through damaged subendometrial vessels. In contrast, a tight application of the sheath maintains the medium within the cavity, keeps intrauterine pressure above mean arterial pressure, and maintains a clear operative field. Media may be conveniently divided into gaseous or liquid. The latter may be

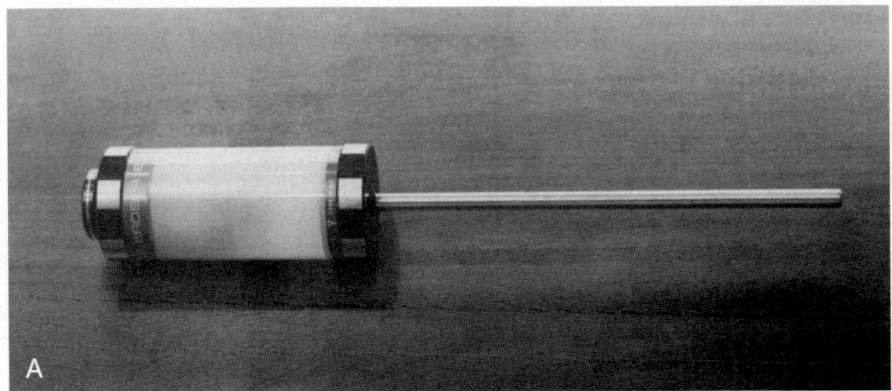

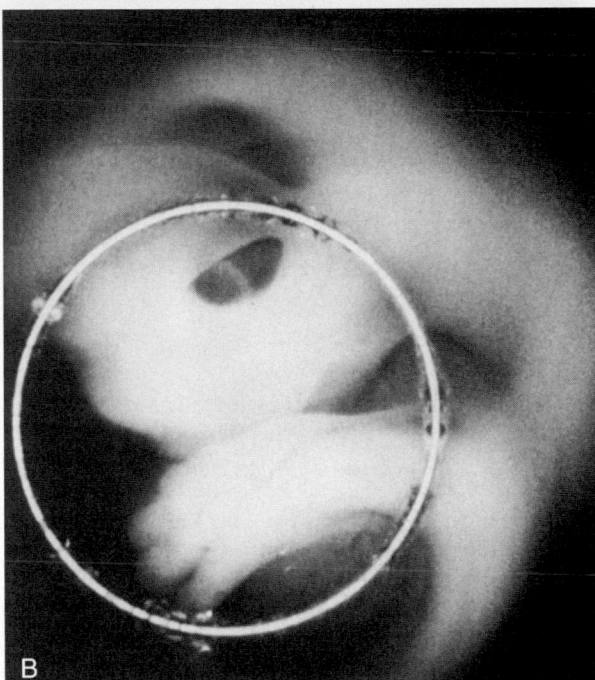

FIGURE 17.10. **A:** The contact hysteroscope is a specialized instrument used for diagnosis only. The cylindrical white chamber traps and transmits ambient light. **B:** A 6-week living embryo viewed by contact hysteroscope. The diameter of the focus circle is 6 mm.

further subdivided into high-viscosity and low-viscosity fluids.

GASEOUS MEDIA

Carbon Dioxide

Carbon dioxide (CO_2) is a colorless gas that is highly soluble when mixed with blood. It can be used to safely distend the uterus when instilled with a proper insufflation apparatus, as described by Lindemann. This distention medium is ideal for office hysteroscopy. The hysteroscopic insufflator delivers CO_2 into the uterus at a flow rate measured in cubic centimeters per minute, in contrast to the laparoscopic insufflator, in which CO_2 flows in at the rate of liters per minute. The laparoscopic insufflator is both unsuitable and unsafe for hysteroscopic insufflation. The rate of flow of CO_2 into the uterus should never exceed 100 mL per minute, and pressure should be adjusted below 150 mm Hg

(Fig. 17.11). Before CO_2 is infused, the hysteroscopic tubing and the hysteroscope must be purged of air. Additionally, the Trendelenburg position should be avoided.

When CO_2 flow is excessive, bubbles appear and obscure the field. Bleeding and CO_2 gas are incompatible; the gas and blood mix, producing an obscuring bubbling foam. CO_2 tends to flatten the endometrium, and this artifact can obscure pathology. When CO_2 is improperly instilled, emboli form and can produce severe derangements in cardiovascular physiology.

The best feature in favor of CO_2 is its neatness. It does not foul instruments, it does not mess up the office or operating room, and it allows entry evaluation of the endocervical canal. CO_2 is therefore an excellent diagnostic medium, perhaps the best according to Siegler and Kemmann. However, the liquid media are superior in most aspects for operative hysteroscopy. CO_2 cannot be used to flush the cavity of debris, and if the pressure drops sufficiently to allow the walls of the uterus to

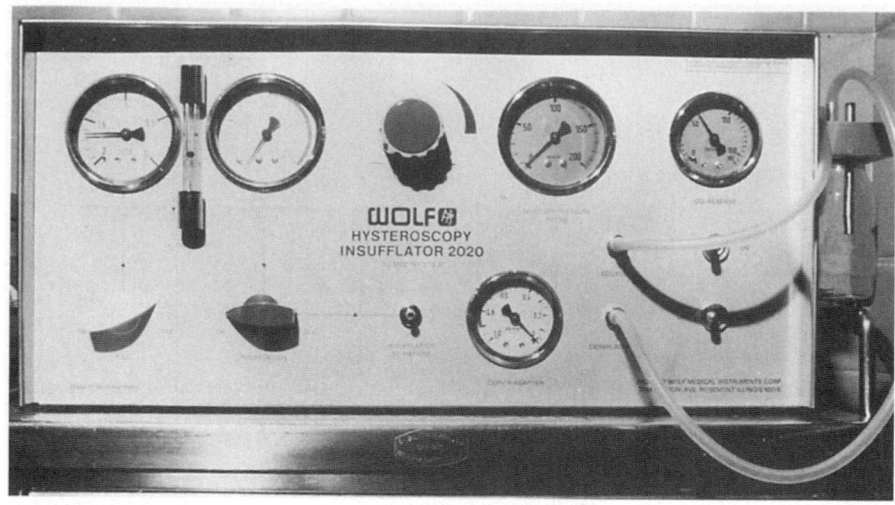

FIGURE 17.11. CO_2 must be infused by a special insufflator that measures flow rate (not to exceed 100 mL per minute) and uterine pressure (not to exceed 150 mm Hg).

coapt, bleeding will ensue, making this medium less than advantageous.

LIQUID MEDIA

High Viscosity

Hyskon (32% dextran 70 in dextrose) is a colorless, viscid solution that is an excellent medium for both diagnostic and operative hysteroscopy. Baggish and colleagues (1992) published data on blood levels of Hyskon attained during a variety of operative procedures. Hyskon blood levels were not directly correlated with either the volume of instilled medium or the operative time. The blood levels did correlate with the degree of uterine damage created. The mean intrauterine pressure measured during Hyskon infusion was 76 mm Hg. Ruiz and Neuwirth monitored Hyskon reactions in nearly 2,000 hysteroscopies and reported a rate of pulmonary edema of 0.11% and anaphylactoid reaction of 0.05%. Although no significant correlation between volume and reaction was demonstrated, the investigators cautioned that when more than 500 mL of Hyskon were instilled, the incidence of pulmonary edema increased to 1.4%. They recommended that 500 mL represent the upper limits for Hyskon infused during a single case. Hyskon is a safe medium and has properties that other media do not share. A major advantage of Hyskon is its immiscibility with blood, which permits excellent visualization, even during active bleeding, and permits the surgeon to pinpoint the site of bleeding.

Because Hyskon is so viscid, it is difficult to instill during diagnostic hysteroscopy when the 5-mm sheath with the 1-mm clearance between the lens and sheath is used. Up to 650 mm Hg pressure may be required to push it through the sheath–lens interface. With the addition of a simple hand pump (Cook OB/GYN, Spencer, Indiana), a 60-mL syringe of Hyskon is easy to instill and is ideal for diagnostic office hysteroscopy (Fig. 17.12A). Most diagnostic hysteroscopies can be satisfac-

torily completed with less than 100 mL of Hyskon, whereas most operative procedures usually require 200 to 500 mL of Hyskon (Fig. 17.12B). Interestingly, Hyskon interaction with heat induced by Nd:YAG laser at about the 100°C level appears to complement the thermal action of the laser.

A disadvantage of Hyskon is that dried residue tends to harden and clog hysteroscopic sheath channels. This clogging is easily prevented by immediately flushing the scope and sheath with hot water after completion of the surgery.

As we have mentioned, two types of Hyskon reactions have been reported. The rare idiosyncratic anaphylactoid reaction should be managed like any acute allergic reaction. The second reaction is caused by excessive vascular uptake of dextran, which allows a more general manifestation of its physiologic actions, including fibrinoplastic action, stearic exclusion, alteration of platelet adhesiveness, and interference with von Willebrand's factor (factor VIIIR). The end result is a bleeding diathesis. The osmotic activity of dextran is such that for each gram of Hyskon instilled into the vascular space, 20 mL of interstitial water will be pulled into the circulation; 100 mL of Hyskon will expand the plasma volume by 640 mL. As the volume of intravascular Hyskon increases, a critical level is reached and pulmonary edema occurs. Finally, dextran 70 (Hyskon) is a mixture of macromolecules ranging from 25 to 125 kd. Although the lower-weight molecules are rapidly excreted, the larger molecules can interfere with glomerular filtration and will remain in the bloodstream for 4 to 6 weeks, as detailed in the report by Mishler. Seven case reports of Hyskon-related pulmonary edema were published between 1985 and 1990. The pathogenesis of the Hyskon reaction has been incorrectly described as an example of noncardiogenic pulmonary edema, and this incorrect description has unfortunately been propagated from report to report. No evidence whatsoever supports this hypothesis. The Hyskon-induced pulmonary edema reaction is fully understood, and its actions are cardiogenic, as de-

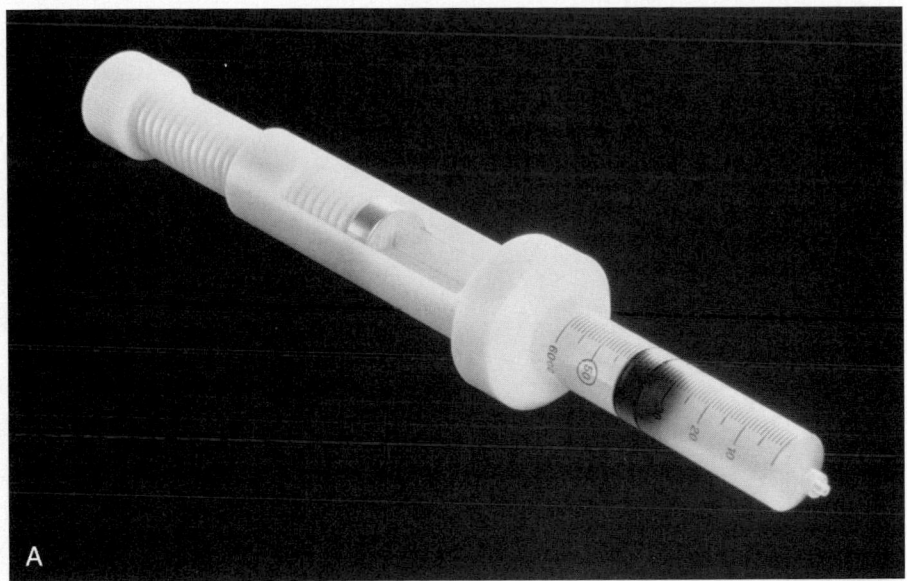

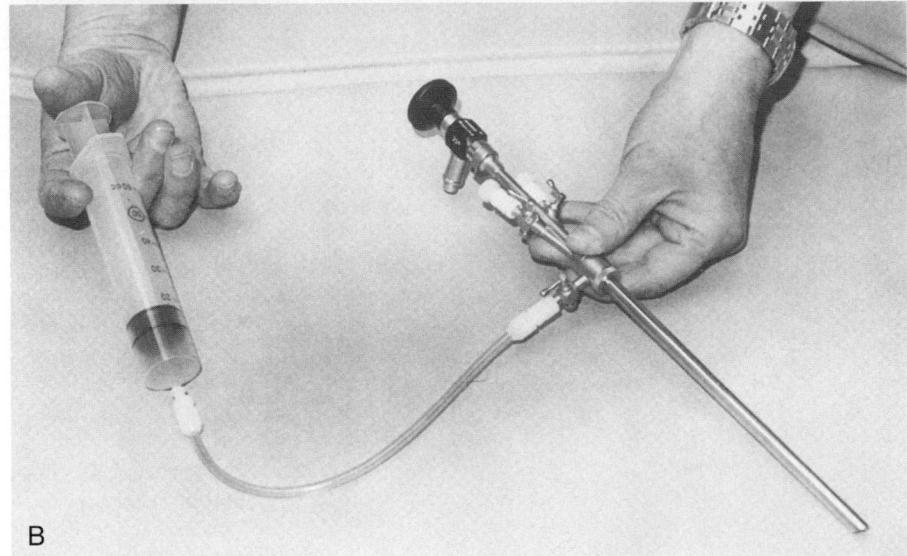

FIGURE 17.12. A: A simple Hyskon Pump (Cook OB/GYN). This syringe driver allows Hyskon to be administered through even a diagnostic sheath with ease. **B:** Hyskon is delivered directly by syringe through an operating sheath. The connecting tube allows easy instillation of the viscid medium.

scribed earlier. Hyskon can be used universally with electrosurgical devices, lasers, and conventional equipment.

Low Viscosity

Low-viscosity distention media may be delivered by hanging the usual 2- to 3-L bag or bottle of fluid 6 to 8 feet above the operating table, permitting the fluid to infuse by gravity feed. A newer technology for instilling low-viscosity fluid is by rotary pump. The newest pumps weigh the fluid in real time and give the surgeon a constant read out of flow rate and total volume of fluid infused.

Normal Saline

Normal (physiologic) saline (0.9% sodium chloride) is perhaps the safest of the hysteroscopic media. The worst results of excessive vascular absorption are fluid overload and pulmonary edema, which are managed by diuresis

and support. The medium is readily available in a 3-L sterile bag that can be mounted on an intravenous pole or given via an infusion pump (Fig. 17.13). Garry and colleagues (1992) reported excellent safety results and precise maintenance of uterine pressure by using a hysteromat pump, which was combined with one of the operating channels of the dual-channel operating sheath to provide an outflow tract and thus a constant flow rate through the uterine cavity.

Unfortunately, because saline is an efficient conductor of electrons, it does not permit a current density that is high enough for tissue action. Saline is therefore not suitable for monopolar electrosurgery, although it is effective when the Nd:YAG laser, the KTP/532 laser, bipolar electrodes, and mechanical devices such as scissors are the hysteroscopic accessories of choice.

In contrast with the Hyskon medium, saline leaks easily out of the uterus. Constant infusion and high flow

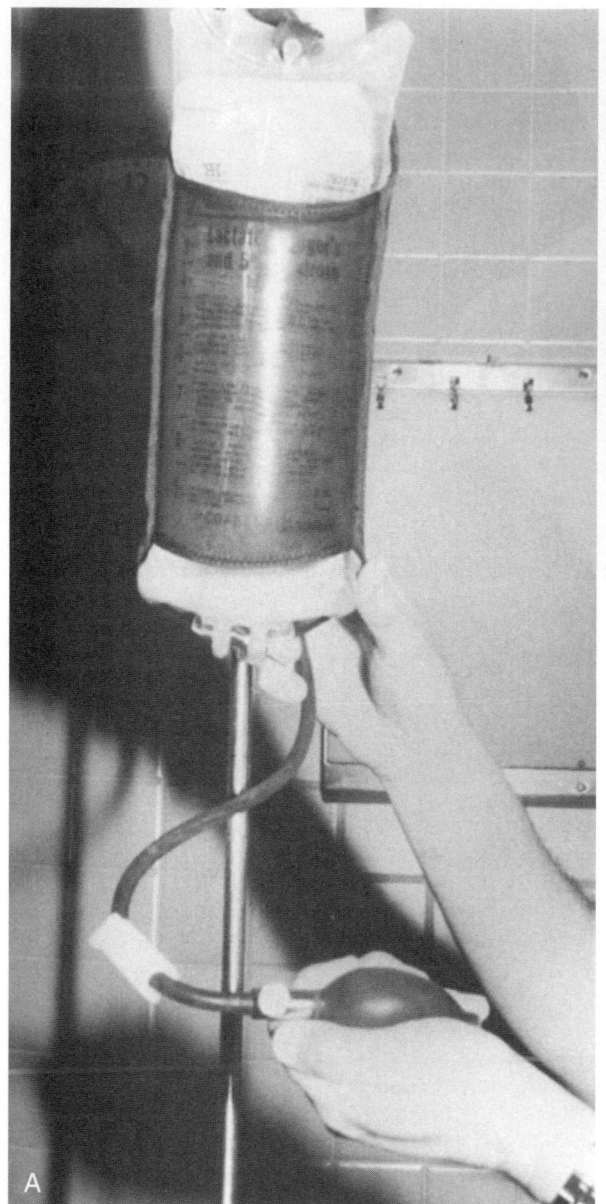

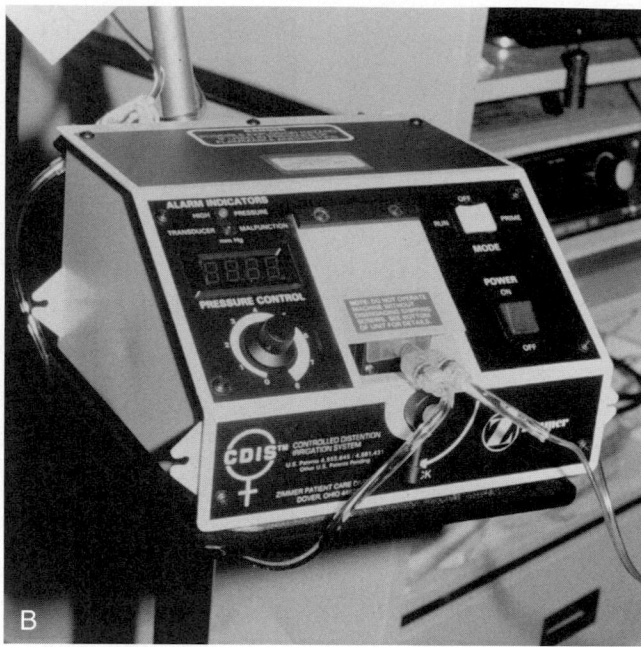

FIGURE 17.13. A: Saline, mannitol, glycine, or lactated Ringer solution is enclosed with a pressure cuff and delivered to the medium (intake) port of the hysteroscopic sheath by intravenous tubing. **B:** Shown is a pump to maintain a constant intrauterine pressure of nonviscid medium. This pump is a roller type and presents no risk to the patient, unlike pumps that are driven by gas.

rates are required to maintain distention. This medium also mixes easily with blood, which further necessitates constant flow of the medium through the operative field for flushing. The large volumes of fluid required make this medium less than ideal for office use.

The best drape for the operating room is the urologic type with a plastic reservoir pocket into which the outflow fluid can be collected and quantified to determine the fluid deficit (i.e., the difference between instilled fluid and returned fluid). The surgeon should be given a running account by a nurse or surgical assistant of the volume of fluid instilled (i.e., liters of fluid hung on the intravenous pole minus volume of return fluid). Whenever any significant fluid deficit is calculated, the procedure should be discontinued and scheduled for completion at a later date. For purposes of this chapter, a

significant overload of isotonic sodium chloride could be quantitated at 1.5 to 2.0 L

1.5% Glycine and 3.% Sorbitol

Glycine (1.5%) and sorbitol (3%) solutions were first used in urologic surgery, principally for male patients. They were adopted later by gynecologists for use with monopolar electrosurgical devices (e.g., the resectoscope). Both glycine and sorbitol are used for hysteroscopic distention, but both have several disadvantages inherent to their composition. Clearly, better and safer alternatives exist for uterine distention. Both solutions are hypo-osmolar (sorbitol, 178 mOsmol/L; glycine, 200 mOsmol/L). When delivered by a high-pressure infusion pump, glycine has been reported to cause disturbances in oxygenation and coagulation. However, the

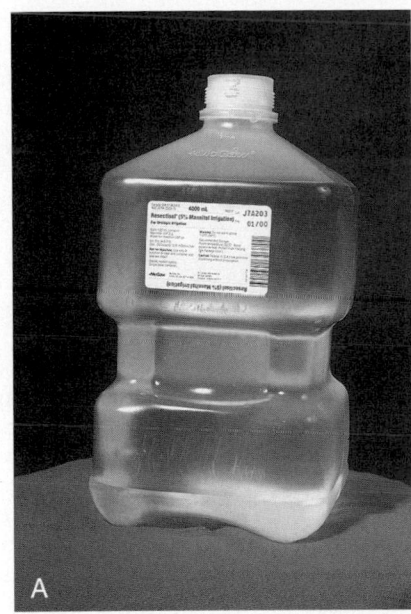

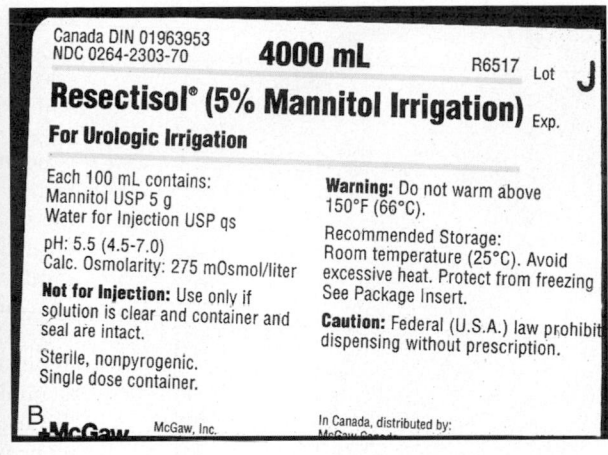

Canada DIN 01963953
NDC 0264-2303-70   **4000 mL**   R6517 Lot J

Resectisol® (5% Mannitol Irrigation) Exp.
For Urologic Irrigation

Each 100 mL contains:
Mannitol USP 5 g
Water for Injection USP qs

pH: 5.5 (4.5-7.0)
Calc. Osmolarity: 275 mOsmol/liter

Not for Injection: Use only if
solution is clear and container and
seal are intact.

Sterile, nonpyrogenic.
Single dose container.

Warning: Do not warm above
150°F (66°C).

Recommended Storage:
Room temperature (25°C). Avoid
excessive heat. Protect from freezing
See Package Insert.

Caution: Federal (U.S.A.) law prohibit
dispensing without prescription.

B McGaw   McGaw, Inc.

In Canada, distributed by:
McGaw Canada

FIGURE 20-14. A: A 4-L bottle of sterile 5% mannitol solution for infusion into the uterus. **B:** Magnified view of the label detailing the content of the solution. Note the osmolarity is 275 mOsmol/L.

principal hazard of these media relates to their vascular absorption and the creation of an acute hyponatremic state. A fluid deficit equal to or greater than 500 mL should alert the surgeon to a likelihood of hyponatremia and hypoosmolality. Two reports have presented data concerning significant complications secondary to hyponatremia. In one series of four women, two died (50% mortality); in the other, one of four women died (25% mortality). Absorption of hypo-osmolar solutions produces a gradient between the circulating blood and the brain cells. The brain cells respond by pumping cation out to diminish the positive infusion of water into the brain. Unfortunately, the cation pumping mechanism of the brain is deficient in women, secondary probably to the actions of progesterone, and women are at significantly greater risk for the development of life-threatening cerebral edema when a hypo-osmolar state exists. When sorbitol or glycine are used as uterine distension media, we refer the reader to the papers of Arieff and Ayus and of Baggish for a detailed discussion of the treatment of acute severe hyponatremia.

Minimally, preoperative, intraoperative, and 4-hour postoperative serum sodium determinations should be requested on a stat basis. A fact that all hysteroscopists should bear in mind is the consistent overfilling of the medium bags by the manufacturer. Typically, the bags have 150 mL more fluid than indicated.

5% Mannitol and 2.2% Glycine

Mannitol (5%) and glycine (2.2%) are safer than the former two solutions because they may be used with electrosurgical devices and are approximately isoosmolar. Mannitol has an osmolality of 285 mOsmol and is an osmotic diuretic (Fig. 17.14A,B). Its optical characteristics are equivalent to glycine and sorbitol; however, it is an infinitely safer medium. In a study of 181 hysteroscopic examinations using isotonic 2.2% glycine, although there

was a mean decrease in sodium of 9 mmol/L in patients absorbing 1,000 mL, the serum osmolality remained normal with no significant adverse sequelae.

Regardless of the medium used, the exact volume of fluid infused (taking into account the overfilling) must be accurately measured and recorded. In a similar fashion, the operating room nurse must empty collection canisters to accurately measure the medium return volume; less compulsion about these measurements is unacceptable. Finally, the type and volume of intravenous fluids infused by the anesthesiologist must be factored into the intake portion of the equation. Typically, anesthesiologists infuse lactated Ringer's solution, which is hyponatremic.

DIAGNOSTIC HYSTEROSCOPY TECHNIQUES

Diagnostic hysteroscopy can be performed in an office setting under local anesthesia. Injection of lidocaine 1%, 10 to 15 mL, directly into the cervix produces excellent anesthesia for this easy operation, and discomfort for the patient can be diminished by ibuprofen (Motrin), 600 to 800 mg, administered 30 minutes before the procedure. Patients who require cardiac prophylaxis (e.g., for prolapsed mitral valve) should be covered by appropriate antibiotics. Patients should be given suitable information for informed consent.

Accurate knowledge of the position of the uterus is critical to facilitate the examination. The best view of the uterus is obtained during the proliferative phase of the menstrual cycle. The patient is placed in the dorsal lithotomy position. The perineum and vagina are gently swabbed with povidone-iodine or another suitable antiseptic solution. A Sims retractor is placed in the posterior vagina and retracted downward. The edge of the cervix

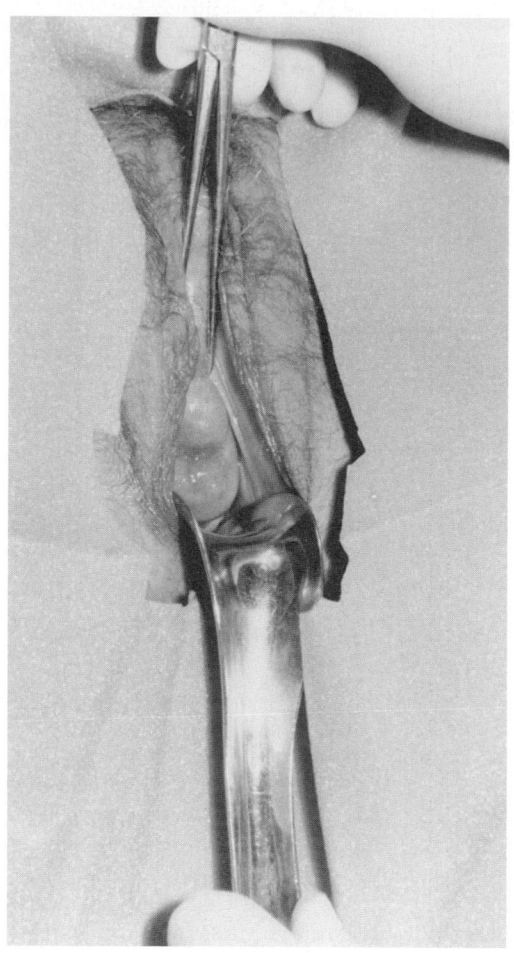

FIGURE 17.15. The Sims retractor is most convenient for retraction of the posterior vaginal wall. This brings the edge of the cervix into view, and it can be easily grasped with the single-toothed tenaculum. This provides an excellent view for office and operative hysteroscopy.

comes into view and is grasped with a single-toothed tenaculum (Fig. 17.15). A suitable telescope is selected and checked by the operator for clarity of the eyepiece and objective lens. If necessary, the lens is cleansed with a soft saline-soaked or water-soaked sponge. The light generator is switched on, and the fiberoptic cable is attached to the telescope. The telescope is inserted into the diagnostic sheath, and the selected medium is flushed through the sheath to expel any air within the sheath (Fig. 17.16). At Good Samaritan Hospital in Cincinnati, 60 mL of Hyskon, delivered by a Cook OB/GYN handheld pump, is routinely used for office hysteroscopy. Typically, one full syringe of this medium is ample for completion of a diagnostic examination of the uterus. The flow of Hyskon starts as the hysteroscope is engaged into the external os of the cervix.

If CO_2 is the selected medium, the flow rate is adjusted to deliver 30 mL per minute. The hysteroscope is engaged into the external cervical os. As the endoscope is advanced, the gas separates the walls of the endocervix to allow an excellent view of the endocervical folds and crypts. The internal os is seen above as the endoscope is manipulated along the axis of the canal and through the os under direct vision. Flow is adjusted to a rate of 60 mL per minute when the isthmus is entered (Fig. 17.17).

Routine dilatation of the cervix should be avoided, because even careful and gentle insertion of cervical dilators will traumatize the endocervix and endometrium. Typically, the endocervical canal shows longitudinal folds, papillae, and clefts. The vascular pattern of the normal endocervix reveals branching treelike vessels. These are especially well observed with a focusing hysteroscope. The internal os appears as a narrow constriction at the top of the endocervical canal. The isthmus is a cylindrical extension above the os. The corpus is a capacious cavity above the isthmus. The central point of müllerian duct fusion is seen projecting down from the

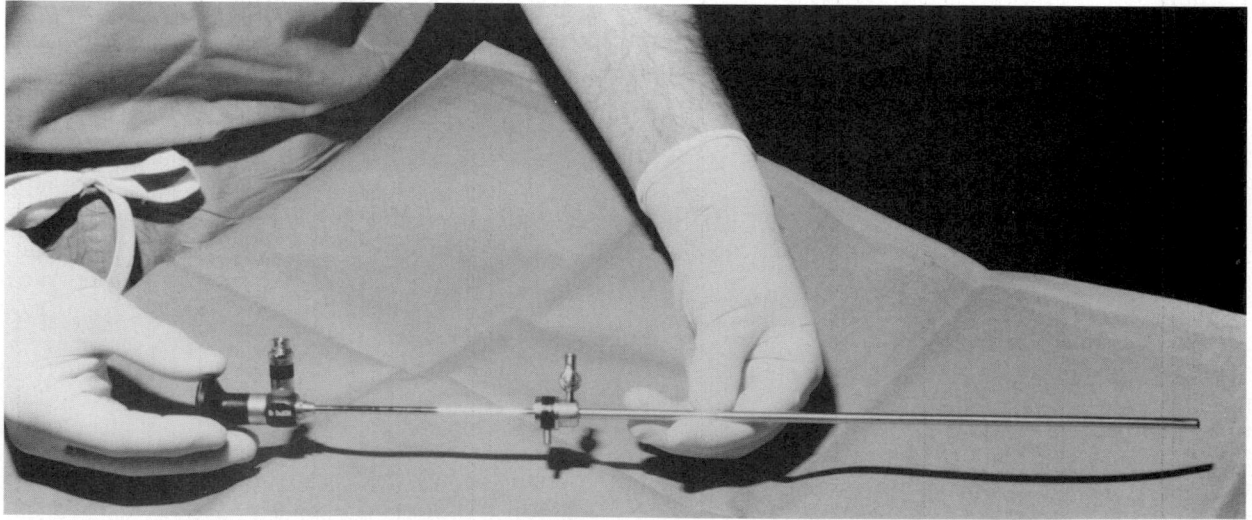

FIGURE 17.16. The telescope is engaged in the 5-mm diagnostic sheath. This is the ideal hysteroscopic setup for office and other diagnostic hysteroscopy procedures.

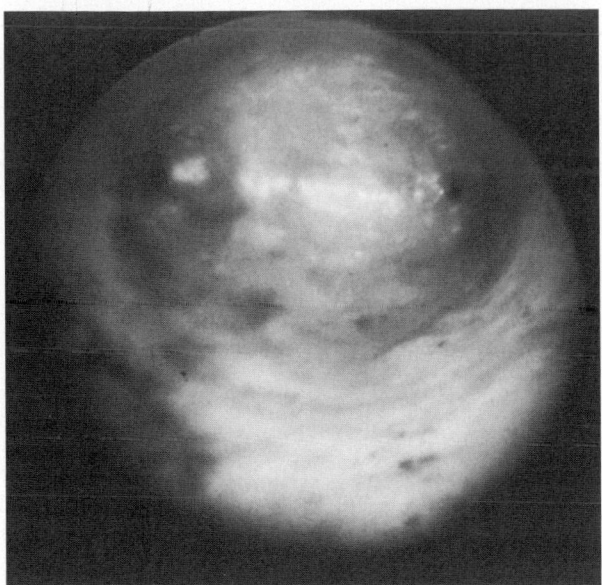

FIGURE 17.17. CO_2 hysteroscopy details the capacious corpus above the narrow isthmus. The tubal ostia are seen at the right and left extremes in the fundus.

fundus. The cornua occupy either side of this fused area. The tubal ostia are visible at the upper extremities of the fundal cornua and show great variation in their appearance and angle of entry into the uterine cavity. The uterine mucosa (endometrium) is smooth and pink-white in color during the proliferative phase. The gland openings appear as white-ringed elevations surrounded by netlike vessels. During the secretory phase of the cycle, the endometrium is lush and velvety; it protrudes into the cavity irregularly and can be easily mistaken for small polyps. The hue of secretory endometrium is magenta. The interior of the cavity, particularly when liquid media are used, first appears cloudy with fine debris floating in the medium.

When CO_2 is the distending medium, the endometrium is artificially flattened. Although the cornua are easily recognized, the tubal ostia may not be seen during the latter phase of the menstrual cycle. The

thickness of the endometrium can be easily appreciated by placing pressure on the telescope and pushing on the posterior wall of the uterus. This maneuver creates a groove in the endometrium.

OPERATIVE HYSTEROSCOPY TECHNIQUES

The telescope is inserted into the operative or resectoscope sheath. If the operative sheath is used, a proper nipple is selected and attached to the opening of the operating channel (Fig. 17.18). The sheath is flushed with the distending medium, and a light cable is attached. Careful dilatation with Pratt dilators should be performed until the operative sheath negotiates a tight passage through the cervix. With the medium flowing, the hysteroscope can be inserted into the uterine cavity under direct vision or coupled to the television camera. The uterine cavity is scanned, and the operator mentally notes landmarks (e.g., the tubal ostia, depth of the cornua, the location and attachments of the lesion, the proximity of the internal cervical os). The flow of debris with the liquid medium will also help the operator locate the tubal ostia. If there is difficulty viewing the cavity clearly, the hysteroscope has probably been inserted too deeply, and the telescope has come in contact with the uterine wall. When the view is blocked, the most prudent first maneuver is to pull the instrument back into the medium flowing into the uterus.

After a clear view is obtained, the operating instrument is inserted into the cavity and advanced to make contact with the endometrium for relative calibration and spatial orientation within the cavity. The knowledgeable and skilled endoscopist at this point inserts an aspirating cannula to further clear the cavity of debris. The cavity can also be further distended with a constant flow sheath by closing off the return-valve stopcock. The valve is then opened, and the cavity is flushed clear. No operative procedure can be performed unless an absolutely unobstructed view is obtained.

In certain cases, it is advantageous to perform a simultaneous laparoscopy to permit an assistant to view the serosal surface of the uterus to provide some addi-

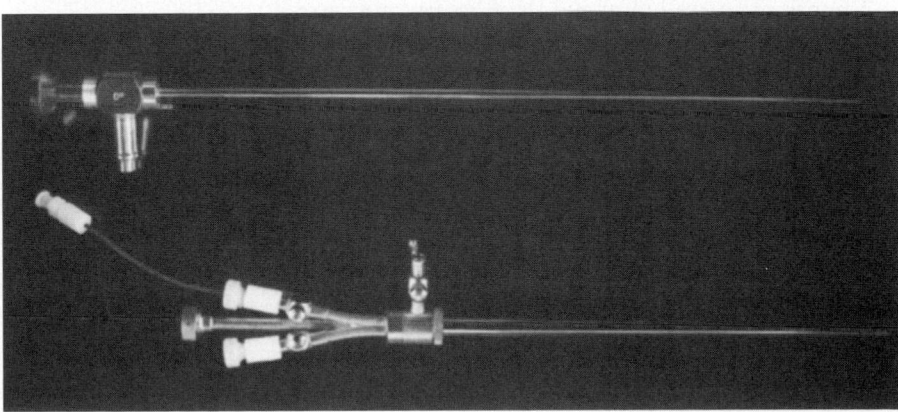

FIGURE 17.18. Two Luerlock leaf valves are screwed into position (**bottom**) before operative hysteroscopy is performed.

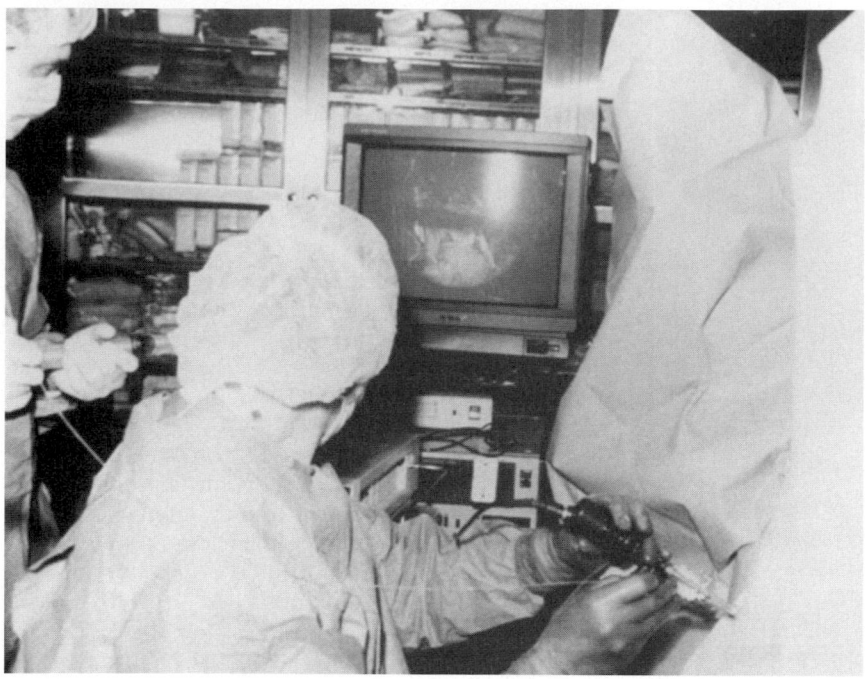

FIGURE 17.19. Contemporary operative hysteroscopy is performed with a microchip video camera attached to the eyepiece of the telescope. The operator and assistants view the field by way of a high-resolution video monitor.

tional insurance against inadvertent perforation. Laparoscopy is recommended during the cutting of septa, during lysis of uterine adhesions, and during excisions for large submucous myomata.

Most experienced hysteroscopic surgeons use the endoscopic microchip camera coupled directly to the telescope. Performance of hysteroscopic surgery by video monitoring has the following advantages (Fig. 17.19):

1. Some camera lenses permit sufficient magnification of the operative field for the image to fill the entire video monitor screen.
2. The video camera eliminates one source of operator fatigue by allowing the endoscopist to sit upright rather than hunched over.
3. An image projected clearly on the video screen helps residents, nurses, and students maintain interest throughout the procedure; enables them to learn more about the technique; and allows them to render better assistance than is possible with conventional procedures.
4. The risk of an eye injury and the need for protective eyewear are obviated.

Endoscopic video camera lenses range in focal length from 25 to 38 mm. A 28- to 30-mm lens provides satisfactory magnification. The operator should first view the cavity by direct vision and should then attach the camera to the eyepiece of the lens. The view with the coupled camera provides magnification comparable to that obtained during microsurgery. If a video recorder is available, a permanent record of the procedure can be captured on tape. A xenon light generator provides the best illumination for video techniques, although less-expensive light sources may be satisfactory when coupled to newer cameras, which are highly light sensitive.

LASERS AND ELECTROSURGICAL DEVICES

The Nd:YAG laser, which works by thermal energy, is the preferred laser for hysteroscopic surgery. Electrosurgical devices exert their tissue actions in a similar fashion: Light energy from lasers is transformed to thermal energy by electron flow (Fig. 17.20A). Lasers and electrosurgical devices both produce coagulation at 60° to 70°C and vaporization at 100°C (Table 17.1), and both require sufficient power density to exert the desired action. Similar tissue actions can be produced by raising the power density or by keeping the power constant and increasing the tissue exposure time. A 1-mm laser fiber delivering 30 W of power to tissue will create a power density of 3,000 W/cm². A 3-mm ball electrode will need to generate 300 W of power to create a similar power density (Fig. 17.20B).

The Nd:YAG laser beam can be transmitted equally well with any distending medium, whereas monopolar electrosurgical devices operate most effectively in an electrolyte-free medium.

Uterine perforation by either a laser fiber or an electrode is much more serious than perforation by scissors or another mechanical device, because the thermal energy can inflict great damage to surrounding structures (e.g., bowel or bladder). The injury may not attain its maximum damage until 2 or 3 days after surgery. Therefore, either laparoscopy or laparotomy is indicated in such cases to determine the extent of injury.

The surgeon must be familiar with the physics governing the actions of lasers or electrosurgical tools and with the tissue actions exerted by these energized devices. A knowledgeable surgeon would not use a ball device to cut or a loop electrode to coagulate tissue. Proper

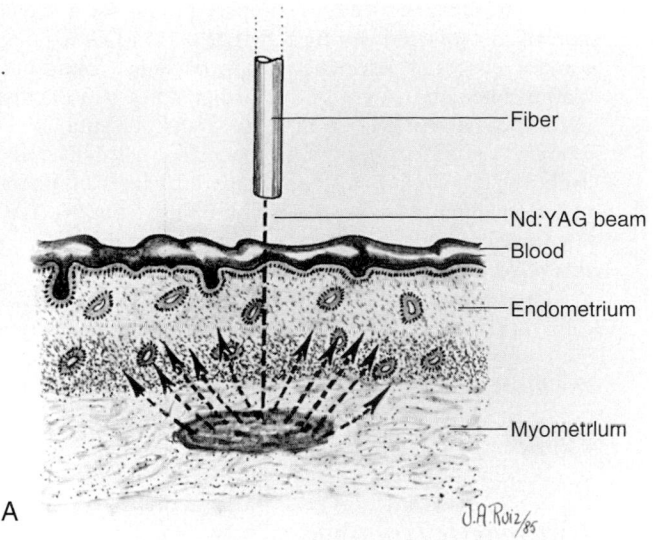

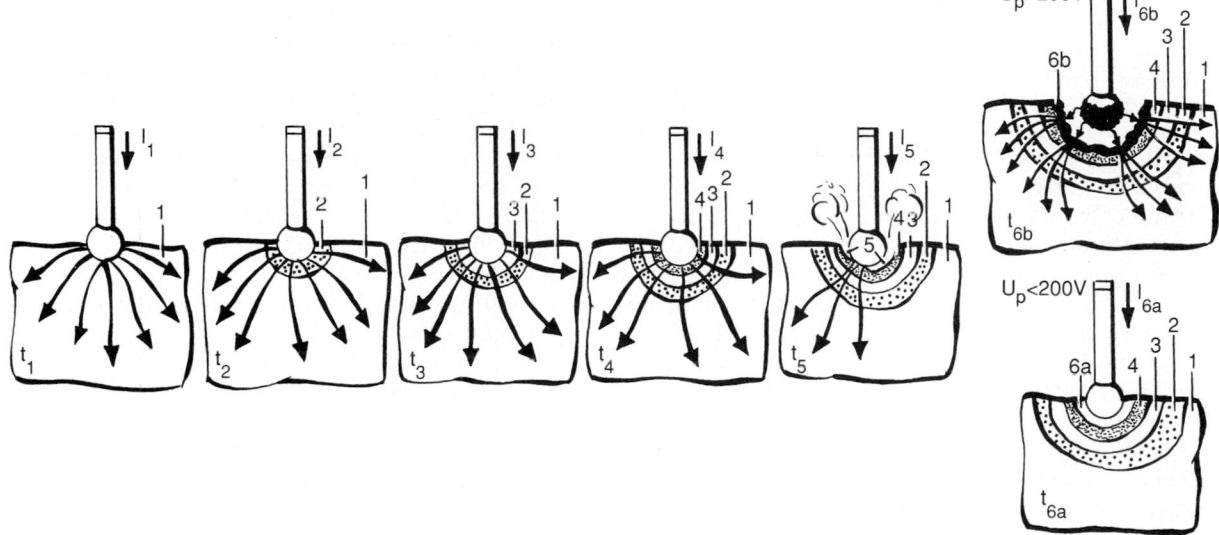

FIGURE 17.20. A: This schematic drawing illustrates the front scatter of the Nd:YAG laser. The initial lesion occurs a few millimeters below the surface of the endometrium. Backscatter then lifts the surface of the endometrium off as the tissue is ablated. **B:** Electrosurgery coagulation of the endometrium with a ball electrode. As the time increases, the temperatures in the vicinity of the electrode are raised to 100°C or vaporization temperature. A vapor barrier is formed, and current ceases to flow unless high voltage penetrates the insulating barrier. (From ERBE, Tubingen, Germany, with permission.)

selection of wattage depends on disease pathology and location. High power applied for a long period of time is risky, is inappropriate, and will inevitably lead to unwanted tissue injury.

Regardless of whether a laser, resectoscope, or handheld electrode is used, depth of tissue action is extremely important; transmural injury is possible at high-power densities or with prolonged exposure. One must keep in mind that the thickness of the distended uterine wall (0.5 to 1 cm) is considerably less than that of the nondistended uterine wall (1.5 to 2 cm) (Fig. 17.21 A,B).

THE PROCEDURES OF HYSTEROSCOPIC SURGERY

Septate Uterus

Modern hysteroscopy has rendered the correction of septate uterus relatively simple and straightforward by the transcervical route, as documented by DeCherney and associates (1986) and by March and Israel (1987). Uterine septa are a treatable factor contributing to pregnancy wastage, usually secondary to premature labor and late

TABLE 17.1.
Gross Effects of Thermal Injury as Caused by Both Laser and Electrosurgery Apparatus

Approximate Degree of Heat	Thermal Damage Caused
<40°C	No significant cell damage.
>40°C	Reversible cell damage, depending on the duration of exposure.*
>49°C	Irreversible cell damage (denaturation).*
>70°C	Coagulation (Latin: coagulatio = clotting). Collagens are converted to glucose.
>100°C	Phase transition from liquid to vapor of the intracellular and extracellular water. Tissue rapidly dries out (dessication) (Latin: ex sico = dehydration). Glucose has an adhesive effect after dehydration.
>200°C	Carbonization (Latin: carbo = coal). Medical pathologic burns of the 4th degree.

*According to Bender and Schramm, 1968.

second trimester abortion. The diagnosis of a uterine septum is usually made at hysterosalpingography or during a diagnostic hysteroscopy. Unfortunately, neither of the studies mentioned above differentiates between septate and bicornuate uteri. A diagnostic laparoscopy is most helpful for an accurate differential diagnosis. A laparoscopic view of a septate uterus will reveal a wide but otherwise normal fundus, whereas the bicornuate uterus typically appears heart-shaped. A bicornuate uterus should be treated by the Jones or Strassman procedure. A septate uterus should be treated hysteroscopically. The standard technique, reported by March et al. (1978), is to cut the septum with scissors under direct hysteroscopic view.

Cararach and colleagues compared hysteroscopic incision of septate uteri during a 5-year period (81 women) using a scissors or resectoscope approach and found only marginal benefit in favor of the former. Choe and Baggish used the Nd:YAG laser fiber to transect septa in 14 women. Of 13 patients who conceived, 10 delivered a liveborn, term infant (87%), compared with a preoperative term pregnancy rate of 11%. Clearly, the Nd:YAG laser, resectoscope, and needle electrode are more appropriate for the broad and usually vascular septum.

Uterine rupture during pregnancy and more specifically in labor has been reported after hysteroscopic metroplasty with and without uterine perforation. It would be prudent to inform the patient who will undergo metroplasty of the subsequent risk so that she is knowledgeable and can inform her obstetrician should she become pregnant.

Hysteroscopic Technique

The uterine septum is viewed from the level of the internal cervical os. The endoscope is moved into each chamber of the divided uterine cavity, and the locations of the tubal ostia are marked. The hysteroscope is again withdrawn to a level just above the internal os. The appropriate operating instrument is inserted through the sheath, and the septum is cut from below and upward, as described by March (Fig. 17.22). As the fundus is approached, the operator depends on a signal from the assistant to indicate when the quality of the hysteroscope light demonstrates transmission through the intact uterine wall. A dialog between the hysteroscopist and laparoscopist prevents perforation. A new technique permits the operator to scan the uterus ultrasonographically to determine whether the myometrium has been entered and to monitor the amount of space existing between the operating device and the serosal surface of the uterus. It is unnecessary to excise the septum completely. Transection eliminates the septum and unites the uterus

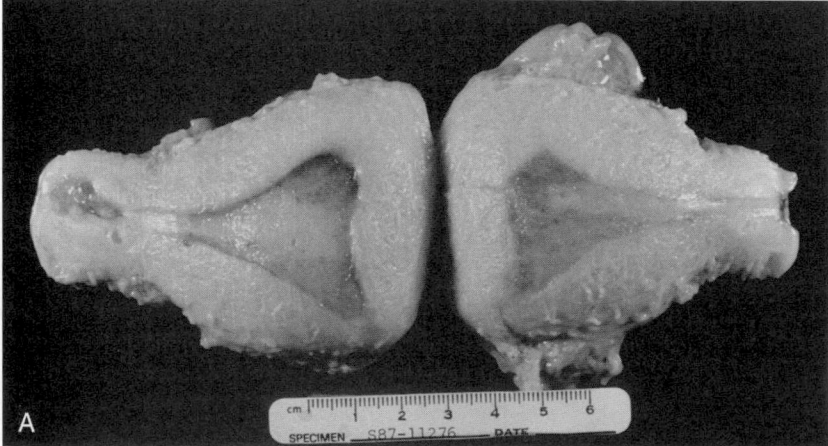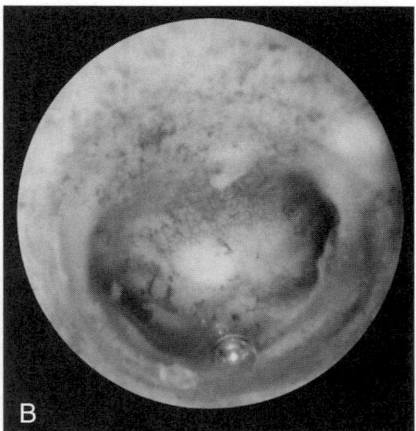

FIGURE 17.21. A: A uterus that is removed at hysterectomy shows the thick walls of the myometrium. These walls average about 1.5 cm in thickness, with the exception of the cornu, where the myometrium is thinner. **B:** The uterus is distended with the liquid medium. The walls of the uterus are now much thinner, averaging 0.5 to 1 cm in thickness.

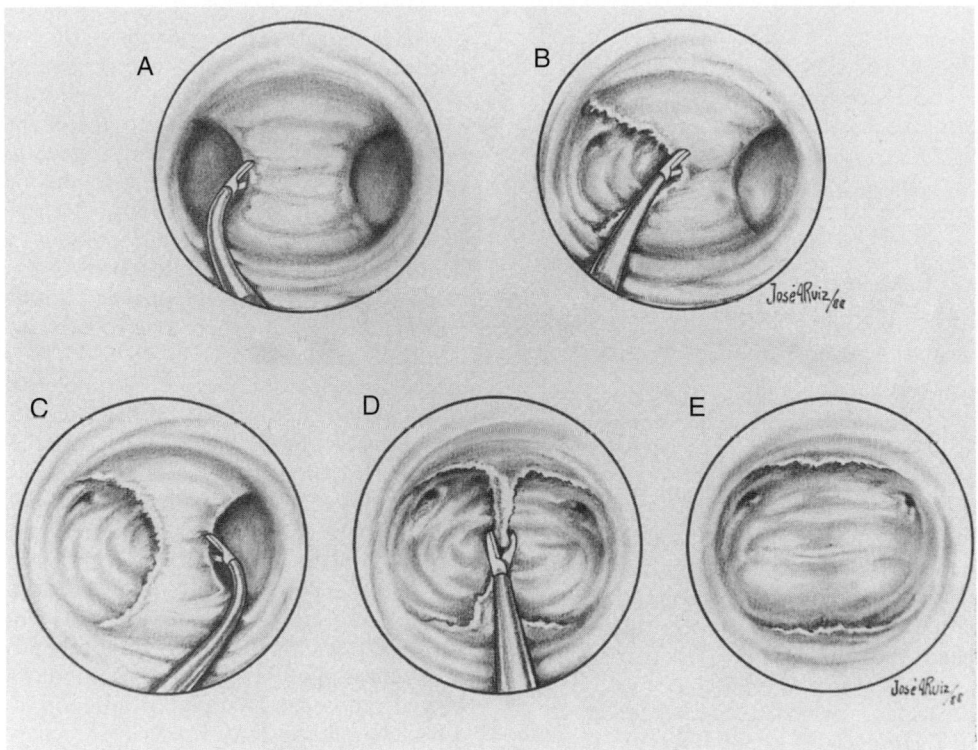

FIGURE 17.22. During this technique for a hysteroscopic section of a uterine septum, the operator cuts the septum from below and moves upward **(A–D)** until a single cavity is seen **(E).** (From Baggish MS, Barbot J, Valle RF. *Diagnostic and operative hysteroscopy.* Chicago: Mosby–Year Book, 1989, with permission.)

into a single cavity. We take the opportunity here to stress an important technical point. The surgeon should be aware of the common tendency of the cutting instrument to drift posteriorly and should clip the septum squarely in the middle. When the drift goes unnoticed, the operating instrument invariably cuts into the myometrium and causes pulsatile bleeding. Similarly, correcting the septum too perfectly at the level of the fundus results in deep penetration into the myometrium and subsequent hemorrhage (Fig. 17.23). If a multichannel hysteroscope is used, a 3-mm ball electrode can be used to coagulate the bleeding vessel. The double-needle bipolar electrode is a safe alternative method for electrocoagulation.

If bleeding does ensue, a Foley catheter with a 10-mL balloon is inserted into the endometrial cavity at the terminus of the operation and inflated to 5 to 6 mL. The pressure exerted by the bag on the uterine walls is sufficient to control the bleeding promptly. The bag is deflated 6 to 12 hours postoperatively and is removed if no further bleeding ensues. Overinflation of a catheter bag can lead to uterine rupture; therefore, one should add increments of water, 1 to 2 mL at a time, to the catheter bag until bleeding ceases. Patients are usually advised to take 2.5 mg of estrogen daily by mouth for 30 days after surgery. Antibiotics are not routinely administered.

Uterine Synechiae

Adhesions form between the anterior and posterior walls of the uterus as a result of trauma or infection in a milieu of estrogen deprivation. Classically, this problem follows an abortion or postpartum hemorrhage for which a vigorous curettage was performed to control the bleeding, as reported by March and associates. Friedler and associates report the incidence of adhesions after one abortion to be 16.3%. This figure rises to 32% after three or more abortions. The severity of adhesions also typically rises as the number of abortions increases. Microscopic sections obtained from the curettage invariably reveal fragments of myometrium interspersed with inflamed decidua and glands. Historically, the patient does not resume menstruation; however, a minority of patients continues to menstruate normally. Because the patient is subsequently infertile or amenorrheic, a hysterogram is performed. The radiograph reveals filling defects that vary from minimal to severe (i.e., virtually obliterating the endometrial cavity). Past treatment of uterine synechiae consisted of blind curettage; the results were predictably poor. With the advent of operative panoramic hysteroscopy, treatment has progressed to identification of adhesions and sharp incision of the adhesions with scissors.

Adhesiolysis surgery is probably the most difficult of the hysteroscopic operations. Because numerous

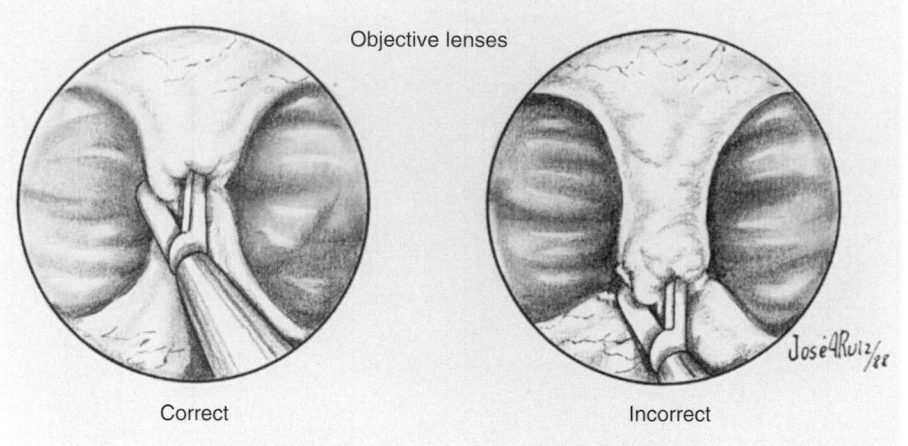

Objective lenses

Correct   Incorrect

FIGURE 17.23. The scissors or laser fiber should be maintained in the center of the septum to avoid bleeding. (From Baggish MS, Barbot J, Valle RF. *Diagnostic and operative hysteroscopy.* Chicago: Mosby–Year Book, 1989, with permission.)

vascular channels are opened up, the risk of intravascular absorption of the medium is high. Rock et al. report a technique of laparoscopically injecting the uterus with leukomethylene blue dye to help identify the junction at which the anterior and posterior walls are adhered.

Hysteroscopic Technique

A thorough diagnostic hysteroscopy is performed to assess the degree of adhesion formation and deformity of the cavity. Small openings in the curtain of adhesions in which there are flow patterns of tiny blood fragments and tissue debris are helpful and should be sought out, as are any normal anatomic landmarks. Photographs, videotapes, and detailed drawings are helpful reminders in planning the strategy for cutting these adhesions.

Simultaneous laparoscopy is a prudent measure to prevent perforation of the uterus. Flexible or semirigid scissors and the Nd:YAG laser are the operating instruments of choice, although some operators use the monopolar needle electrode at 40 to 50 W of cutting power, blend 1 or 2. The laser is initially set to deliver 30 to 50 W of power. The medium is instilled into the cavity by way of an operating sheath. Continuous maintenance of distention is one key to success. Filmy and central adhesions should be cut first, always following the fluid flow. Marginal and dense adhesions should be tackled last, always cutting from below and moving upward. A second key to success is to maintain the hysteroscope in midchannel relative to the uterine walls. The cavity can usually be restored to reasonably normal architecture. Bleeding is not uncommon during this operation, particularly when cutting marginal adhesions, because the border between adhesion and myometrium is blurred. Hyskon provides an advantage here.

The patient should be placed on conjugated estrogens, 2.5 mg daily, during postoperative recovery. Placement of an IUD within the cavity to keep the walls from adhering is clearly not based on scientific fact but has been used for so many years that it is a standard postoperative procedure.

Cannulation of the Fallopian Tube

Novy et al. described a technique for passing a special catheter into the tubal ostium and through the obstructed interstitial portion of the tube. This procedure was successful in 92% of cases. Dumesic and Dhillon reported a tubal cannulation procedure in which they used a flexible guiding insert to facilitate passage of the cornual cannulation catheter. These techniques are useful for treating interstitial obstruction secondary to cellular debris and tubal spasm. The obvious advantage of this cannulation technique is its usefulness in treating cases that might otherwise require tubocornual anastomosis. Pregnancy rates range from 25% to 54% in 6 months.

Hysteroscopic Technique

A 5.5F Teflon cannula with a metal obturator (Cook OB/GYN) is introduced through the operating channel of the hysteroscopic sheath. The obturator is removed. A 3F catheter with a guide cannula wire is introduced into the 5.5F cannula by way of a Y-adapter on the end of the cannula, engaged into the tubal ostium, and gently advanced into the tube. When the cornual portion of the tube is negotiated or when resistance is encountered, the guide wire is withdrawn and leukomethylene blue or indigo carmine dye is injected through the 3F catheter. Simultaneous laparoscopy allows one to see the dye exit the fimbriated end of the tube and to confirm patency. Alternatively, one can place a radiologic plate beneath the patient and inject radiopaque dye.

Uterine Polyps

Functional and nonfunctional polyps produce intermenstrual bleeding, as reported by Barbot. Functional polyps tend to be smaller than nonfunctional polyps. If a hysterogram is performed, then a focal filling defect will be seen. Diagnosis is directly and readily made by hysteroscopy. Polyps protrude into the endometrial cavity. A functioning polyp has a lining identical to the surrounding endometrium. A nonfunctioning polyp presents as a white protuberance covered with branching surface vessels; thick-walled vessels are usually seen within the depths of the polyp. Polyps are relatively easy to diagnose and to treat.

Hysteroscopic Technique

A multichannel operating hysteroscope is inserted into the uterine cavity, and a retractable electric snare loop is inserted through the 3-mm channel of the operating sheath. The polyp is encircled by the loop such that the loop encompasses the polyp base as it is tightened. The polyp is cut off at the base with 30 to 40 W of power for cutting current. The snare is then removed, and an alligator jaw forceps is inserted. The polyp is grabbed by the forceps. The hysteroscope is withdrawn, removing with it the freed polyp, which is sent to the pathology lab for histologic evaluation. The site of removal is inspected again, and the procedure is terminated. If any bleeding is observed, a 3-mm ball electrode is applied to the site for coagulation (40 to 50 W).

Myomata Uteri

Submucous myomas characteristically appear as white spherical masses covered with a network of fragile thin-walled vessels when viewed by hysteroscopy. Myomas typically are sessile or pedunculated. A hysterogram shows a filling defect that is not dissimilar to that produced by a polyp. Unfortunately, blind D&C is a grossly inaccurate method of diagnosing this disorder. Although subserous and intramural myomas rarely produce alarming symptoms, even when they attain relatively large size, smaller lesions in the submucous location invariably cause considerable bleeding. Additionally, submucous myomas are commonly associated with chronic endometritis, which interferes with implantation of the fertilized ovum and becomes a factor contributing to subfertility.

In the past, a diagnosis of submucous myoma was usually followed by a recommendation for hysterectomy. Today, hysteroscopic surgery offers a therapeutic alternative to that radical approach. Various regimens of drug therapy (e.g., danazol [Danocrine] and gonadotropin-releasing hormone analogs such as leuprolide acetate [Lupron] or goserelin acetate [Zoladex]) have been recommended as supplementary preoperative medical therapy. The general plan is to treat symptomatic patients for 2 to 3 months preoperatively in order to reduce the size and vascularity of the lesion during surgery. All patients should be given detailed information concerning the need for typing and holding blood and the possibility of hysterectomy if intractable bleeding occurs.

Valle (1990) reported data on 59 cases of abnormal bleeding, dysmenorrhea, and infertility that were diagnosed as submucous myomas. Hysteroscopy eliminated or markedly decreased bleeding in 52 of these cases. Baggish and Sze treated 71 patients with symptomatic myomas and four patients with incidental submucous myomas. The treatment methods used with the multichannel hysteroscope were Nd:YAG laser ($n = 41$), monopolar loop ($n = 6$), monopolar needle ($n = 6$),

bipolar needles ($n = 10$), and electrosurgery or scissors and laser ($n = 12$). As with Valle's series, results were excellent; 65 of 75 (87%) returned to normal menses postoperatively. Barbot and Parent (*personal communication,* 1994) performed resectoscopic myomectomies in 825 women, of whom 83% were relieved of abnormal bleeding and suffered no recurrence.

Hysteroscopic Technique

Several variations of hysteroscopic procedures are now available to manage submucous myomas. Current resectoscopic techniques differ little from those described by Neuwirth (1978) and by DeCherney and Polan (1983). However, the resectoscopic instrumentation has vastly improved compared with those earlier instruments. Self-flushing sheaths, straight and offset cutting loops, and diminished-diameter, low-profile scopes are among these recent improvements. In addition, electrosurgical generators have been modernized and are safer devices than instruments from 1970s and 1980s (Fig. 17.24A,B). Under video control, the resectoscopic technique consists of progressive shaving of the myoma and harvesting the pieces of tissue for subsequent histologic evaluation. For fundal myomas, the straight electrode is the most ef-

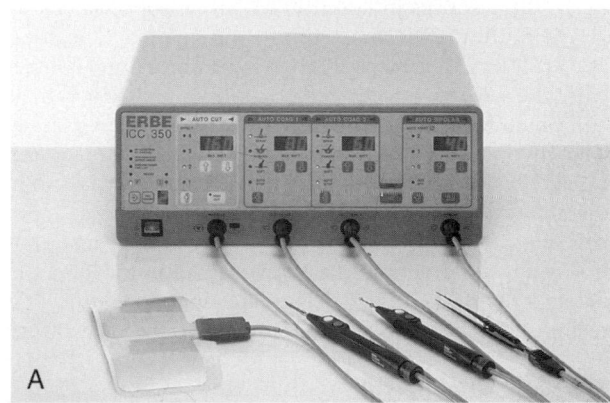

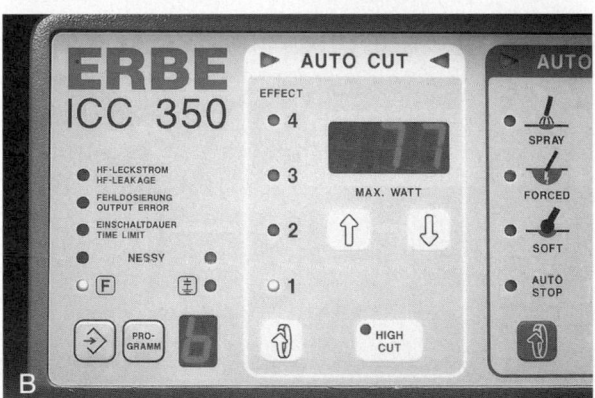

FIGURE 17.24. A: A modern, state-of-the-art, computerized, constant-voltage electrosurgical generator. This apparatus is divided into cut, coagulation, monopolar, and bipolar functions. It incorporates numerous and sophisticated safety features. **B:** Close-up of the electrosurgical generator panel. The high cut feature is for bipolar cutting (vaporization).

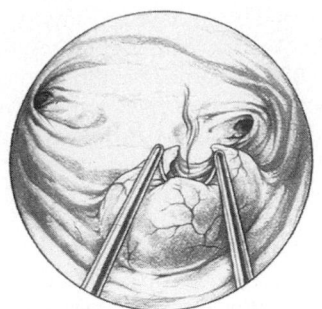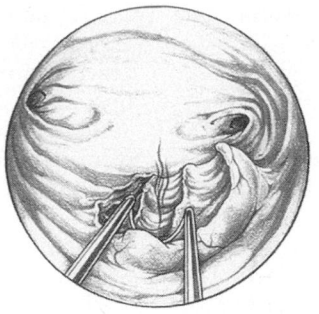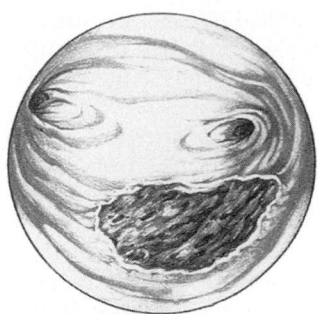

FIGURE 17.25. The shaving technique for the elimination of a submucous myoma is shown using an angulated loop electrode via the resectoscope. (From Baggish MS, Barbot J, Valle RF. *Diagnostic and operative hysteroscopy,* second edition. St. Louis: Mosby–Year Book, 1999, with permission.)

fective device, whereas the angulated electrode is preferred for lesions located on the anterior or posterior walls (Fig. 17.25A–C). (The electrode should be activated only while returning toward the hysteroscope, never while advancing outward away from the lens.)

The four Nd:YAG laser techniques described by Baggish and associates (1999) use power levels of 30 to 60 W. The first uses a hysteroscopic needle inserted through the operating channel, through which about 5 to 10 mL of 1:100 vasopressin solution (1 mL vasopressin in 99 mL sterile water) is injected into the myoma. The conical, sculpted, 1-mm laser fiber is brought into contact with the myoma to cut across its base. Scissors can be combined with the laser to free the myoma from its base. The myoma is extracted intact by way of the cervical canal. This technique is useful for myomas up to 3 cm in diameter. The second Nd:YAG technique uses a 1-mm ball of sculpted fiber that is drawn over the myoma multiple times for ablation of the myoma until it is level and flat in relation to the surrounding endometrium. This technique is used for 1- to 2-cm myomas. The third

technique is similar to that used with the resectoscope. Layer upon layer of the myoma is sliced off until the base is reached. The fourth technique is used for a large (2- to 5-cm) lesion. The laser is used to devascularize the myoma by making multiple punctures into its substance. The large myoma can then be quartered with the laser and extracted piece by piece (Fig. 17.26A–C).

Other electrosurgical techniques are now performed with the large isolated-channel, flushing hysteroscope. The 3-mm needle, shaving loop, and bipolar electrodes may be used to perform all of the optional operations described above for the resectoscope and laser. The fine-needle electrode can be substituted for the laser fiber to excise pedunculated or section sessile myomas. The 3-mm retractable cutting loop can perform shaving procedures in a fashion similar to that of the resectoscope loop. The bipolar needles can be plunged many times into the substance of a submucous myoma of any size to coagulate the interior of the myoma (myolysis).

If postoperative bleeding occurs, a 10-mL Foley balloon is placed in the cavity and blown up to 5 mL for 6

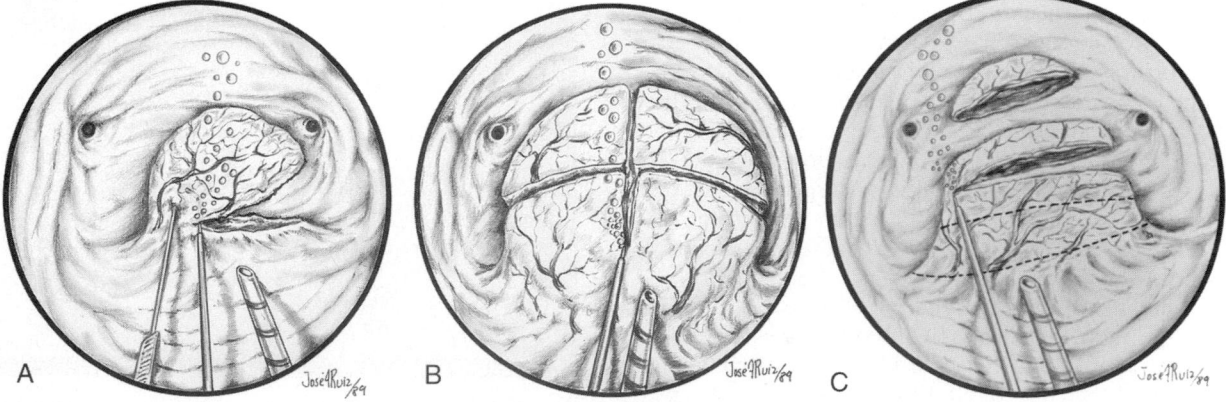

FIGURE 17.26. A: Several Nd:YAG laser techniques are for the treatment of submucous myoma. Here the laser fiber cuts the small sessile myoma across its base. **B:** A large myoma is quartered by the laser fiber and then extracted in pieces. **C:** Layered cleaving of the myoma can be accomplished with a resectoscope or a laser. (From Baggish MS, Barbot J, Valle RF. *Diagnostic and operative hysteroscopy,* second edition. St. Louis: Mosby–Year Book, 1999, with permission.)

to 12 hours. If the cavity is large, a 30-mL balloon inflated with 10 to 15 mL of water can be used. We prefer to do a simultaneous laparoscopy when large myomas (2 to 5 cm) are resected and extracted. Regardless of myoma size, a simultaneous laparoscopy should be performed whenever concern for perforation exists. The central fundal myoma is associated with the greatest risk of uterine perforation.

Reports caution that uterine rupture can occur during pregnancy after hysteroscopic myomectomy. This is particularly the case when the operator attempts to resect the intramural portion of the submucous myoma.

Endometrial Ablation

More than 600,000 hysterectomies are performed annually in the United States, although the advent and growth of integrated health care will target this largely elective operation for reduction because of its substantial cost. The numbers will be further reduced because 40% of hysterectomies are unnecessary and 20% show no pathology; hence, cheaper alternatives are continuously sought. According to a recent study of hysterectomy by the New York State Department of Health, 30,065 hysterectomies were performed in that state during 1986, 10% of which were performed for the principal diagnosis of disorders of menstruation. Endometrial ablation or resection is the hysteroscopic alternative to hysterectomy as treatment for abnormal uterine bleeding. Two earlier reports by Droegemueller et al. describe blind procedures such as cryocoagulation that were used in an attempt to control dysfunctional uterine bleeding by creating physical destruction of the endometrium without sacrificing the uterus. Unfortunately, either the techniques themselves were associated with significant side effects or the endometrium promptly regenerated.

Since the first practical method of hysteroscopic ablation was described in 1981, several thousand procedures have been performed by a variety of techniques, including the Nd:YAG laser, the resectoscopic roller ball or loop, and, most recently, the long hysteroscopic ball electrodes. Garry and associates (1995) reported 600 endometrial laser ablations performed on 524 women. No major operative morbidity was reported. The success rate (mean age, 43 years) was 83.4%. Baggish and Sze have performed 568 ablations; 401 of these were performed with the Nd:YAG laser, 167 by electrosurgery. Excellent results were obtained in 89% of the women treated, and amenorrhea was achieved in 58%. Again, no major operative complications were observed. Magos and coworkers reported 250 cases of endometrial resection with a 92% improvement in abnormal bleeding. However, data obtained from the Royal College of Obstetricians and Gynaecologist's Mistletoe (Minimally Invasive Surgical Technique Laser, Endothermal or Endoresection) Study in 1997 revealed a 6.4% rate of significant complications associated with endometrial resection alone and a rate of rate of 11.4/1,000 for emergency hysterectomy. This compares to complication rates of 2.7% and 2.1% for laser and rollerball, respectively. The latter two techniques had emergency hysterectomy rates of 1.3/1,000 (i.e., 11 times less than endometrial resection).

Two large controlled, randomized studies compared hysterectomy with hysteroscopic ablation-resection. Dwyer et al. prospectively compared 100 cases of endometrial resection and 100 cases of abdominal hysterectomy for menorrhagia. Postoperative morbidity, length of hospital stay, and time to return to work, normal daily activities, and sexual intercourse were significantly lower for the endometrial resection group. Dysmenorrheic premenstrual symptoms were significantly higher in the endometrial resection group. Pinion et al. randomized 204 patients to abdominal or vaginal hysterectomy ($n = 99$), endometrial laser ablation ($n = 53$), or endometrial resection ($n = 52$). Women treated by ablation or resection had less morbidity and a shorter recovery time. After 12 months, 89% of the hysterectomy group and 78% of the hysteroscopy group were very satisfied with the effect of surgery; 95% in the first group and 90% in the second reported acceptable improvement in symptoms. Equal numbers in each group stated that they would recommend the same operation to others. Several published reports confirm the cost effectiveness and efficacy of endometrial ablation for the control of abnormal uterine bleeding compared with hysterectomy.

Hysteroscopic Technique

All patients who might be candidates for endometrial ablation should be managed first by hormonal treatment in an attempt to control the abnormal uterine bleeding. If this strategy fails, and if the woman does not desire to bear children, then she is a candidate for endometrial ablation. A preoperative diagnostic hysteroscopy, endometrial sampling, or both should be performed to exclude endometrial carcinoma or atypical hyperplasia, and all pertinent hematologic studies and consultations should be performed. All patients are pretreated to atrophy the endometrium. The drugs available to accomplish this effect include Danocrine, Lupron, Zoladex, Megace, and Depo-Provera. It is our experience that the best endometrial suppression is seen after 6 weeks of drug therapy.

A simultaneous laparoscopy is not performed during endometrial ablation unless a perforation or other transmural injury is suspected. Depending on the technique selected, either 5% mannitol or 0.9% saline is used as the distending medium. The operating hysteroscope or resectoscope is inserted into the uterine cavity. With the hysteroscope, a 9F aspirating cannula (Cook OB/GYN) is inserted, and blood and debris are evacuated until the cavity is clear. We prefer to treat the fundus by dragging the laser fiber or the ball electrode from side to side (cornu to cornu) (Fig. 17.27). The anterior and lateral walls are ablated next, before the posterior wall. Ablation should not be extended below the internal os into the cervix. Power settings for the electrosurgical generator range from 50 to 150 W, depending on the size of the ball, barrel, or loop electrode (Figs. 17.28 and 17.29). Laser power is set at 40 to 60 W. The goal of the abla-

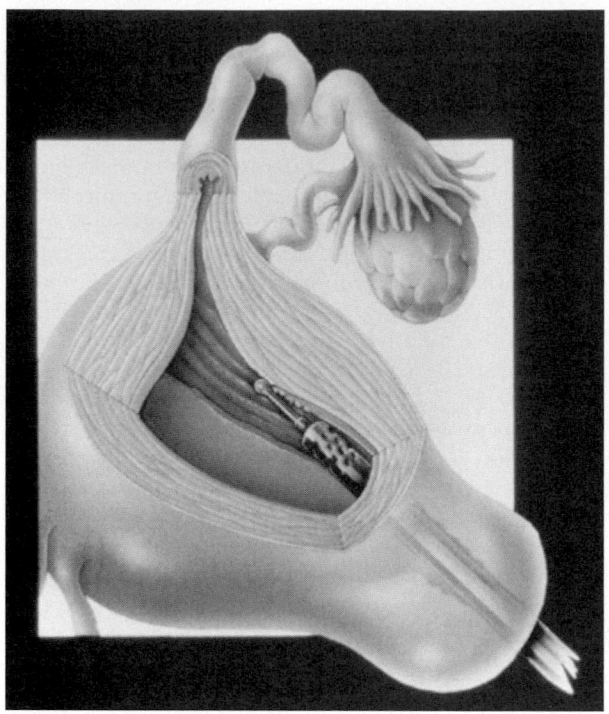

FIGURE 17.27. Endometrial ablation can be performed by use of a ball electrode in direct contact with the endometrium. The energized ball is pulled down to create a 1- to 2-mm furrow of endometrium. The conduction injury can extend down another 1 to 2 mm.

tion operation is to destroy the visible endometrium, including the cornual endometrium, to a depth of 1 to 2 mm. The conduction heat will actually spread deeper, usually to 3 to 5 mm, depending on how long the device remained on the tissue. This penetration translates into extensive superficial myometrial destruction and coagu-

lation of the radial branches of the uterine artery (Fig. 17.30). When the endometrium sloughs, regeneration is prevented because basal and spiral arterioles do not survive the 100°C heat exposure. Over a period of 6 to 8 weeks, the uterine walls scar and shrink. Subsequent sampling or hysteroscopy is possible after endometrial ablation. The mean duration of the operation is about 30 minutes. Patients usually are sent home on the day of surgery. The operation is usually completed with little or no blood loss (Fig. 17.31).

Nonhysteroscopic Minimally Invasive Techniques for Endometrial Ablation

Although these new techniques are not hysteroscopic in the strictest sense, they are nonetheless closely related and should be included in this chapter.

This basis for these methods encompass the following logic:

1. Removal of the skill factor as a variable for endometrial ablation.
2. Elimination of requirement for a distending medium.
3. Reduction in the time required to perform the operation.
4. Equivalency of efficacy compared with hysteroscopic ablation.
5. Performance in an office setting.

The first practical technique described by Phipps et al. (1990) used a microwave technique of heating the endometrium by a probe inserted into the uterine cavity, exposing the endometrium to temperatures of 60° to 65°C for 15 minutes. Thijssen reported a large multicenter study using the technique. The report described a number of serious complications, including fistula formation and third-degree burn injuries. Several techniques using balloons containing hot water, balloons covered with

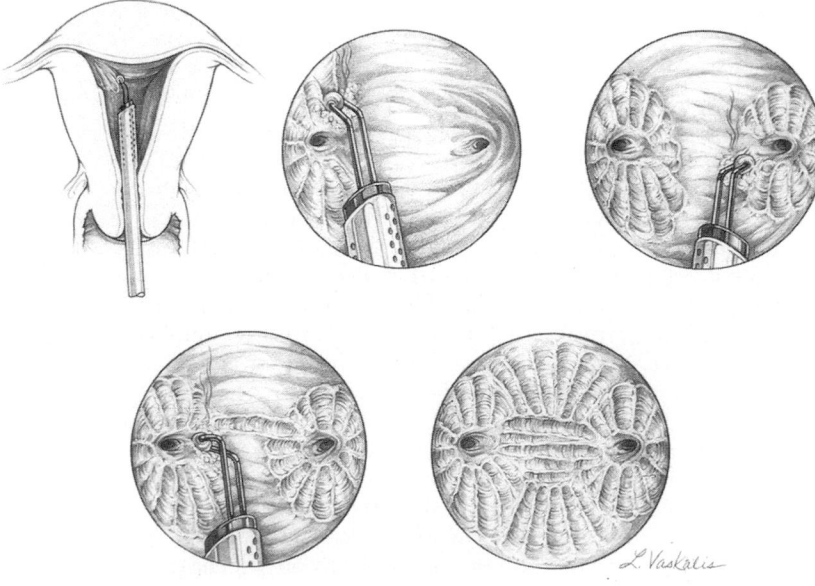

FIGURE 17.28. The resectoscope with ball electrode attached is inserted into the uterine cavity. Initially, the cornu and fundus are carefully ablated taking care to keep dwell time low in order to reduce the risk of deep heat-conduction injury. Next, the anterior wall is ablated, followed by the posterior wall. (From Baggish MS, Barbot J, Valle RF. *Diagnostic and operative hysteroscopy*, second edition. St. Louis: Mosby–Year Book, 1999, with permission.)

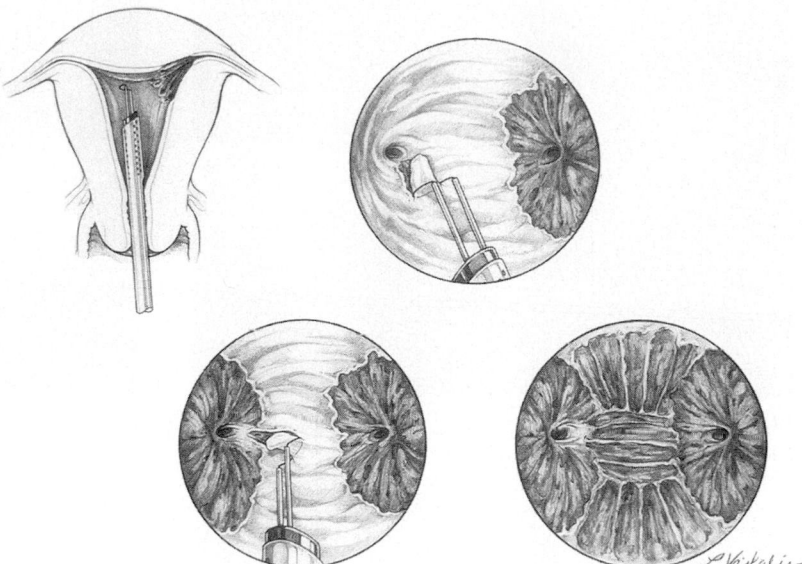

FIGURE 17.29. Endometrial resection is performed in a manner similar to ablation; however, instead of a ball electrode, a cutting loop is substituted. This is clearly a riskier procedure compared with ablation by either laser or ball electrode, particularly relative to deep myometrial resection and the accompanying risks of hemorrhage and/or perforation. (From Baggish MS, Barbot J, Valle RF. *Diagnostic and operative hysteroscopy*, second edition. St. Louis: Mosby–Year Book, 1999, with permission.)

monopolar electrodes, computerized continuously circulating *in situ* hot saline, and cryosurgical and photochemical techniques have been reported (Figs. 17.32–17.34). The only device which has been practically used in the current marketplace has been the Thermachoice balloon technique (Ethicon Endo-Surgery, Cincinnati, Ohio) which was developed by Neuwirth. A cannula fitted with a terminal balloon is placed in the uterine cavity (Fig. 17.35). Sterile water distends the balloon and is heated *in situ* to 80° to 90°C. Thermistors mounted on the balloon give a continuous readout of temperature within the uterine cavity (Fig. 17.36). NaDH diaphorase staining showed destruction to a depth of 3.3 to 5 mm. The published data show efficacy to be lower than that for hysteroscopic ablation, and cost to be no less than that for hysteroscopic ablation. The dream of an office-based procedure has not yet been realized.

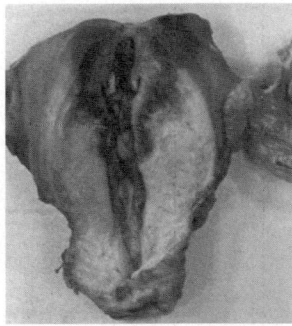

FIGURE 17.30. The uterus was removed 5 days after a Nd:YAG laser ablation. Note the extensive laser injury involving about half the thickness of the myometrium. Laser penetration depends not only on power but also on the length of time the laser beam remains in contact with the tissue.

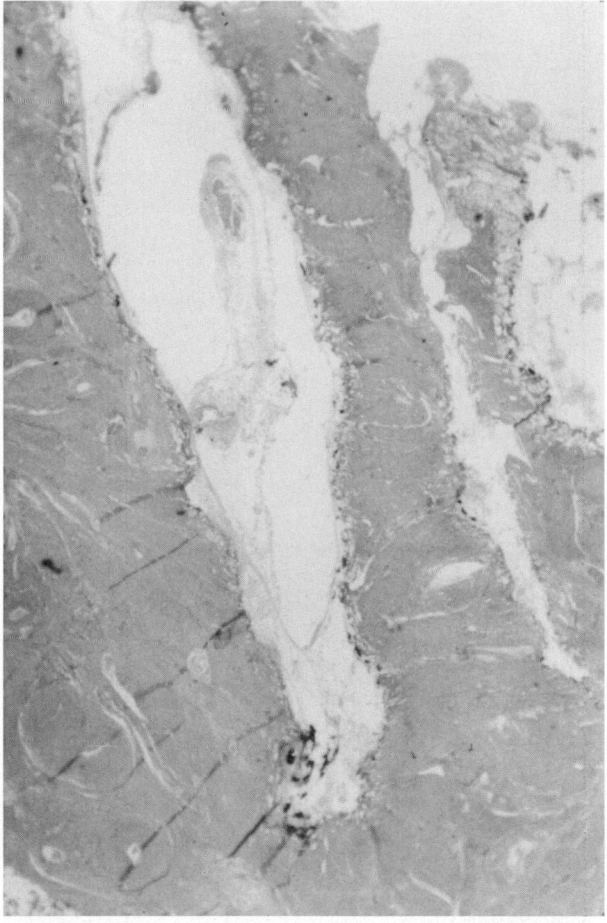

FIGURE 17.31. Photomicrograph of a section of endometrium that was ablated by a Nd:YAG laser. The troughs represent places in which the laser fiber has cut into the tissue. The tissue between the troughs, as well as at the lower extremity, is necrotic.

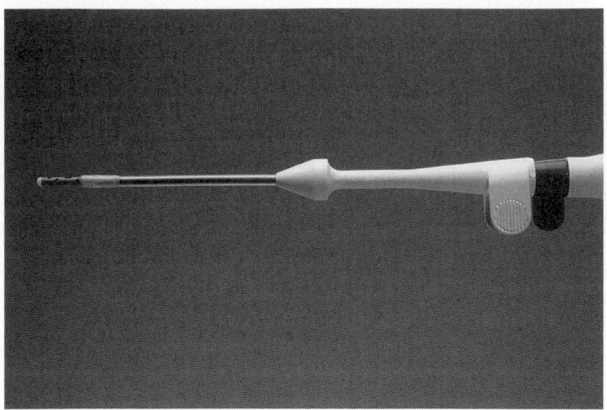

FIGURE 17.32. Innerdyne (Tyco) "Enable" cannula. The terminal mushroom fitting and the acorn seal the cervix and isolate the corpal cavity from the cervical canal. The apparatus contains an *in situ* heater and thermistors.

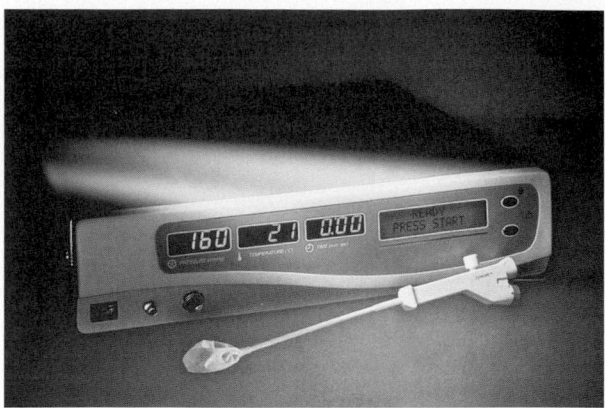

FIGURE 17.35. The Gynecare balloon cannula and control equipment. The cannula is inserted into the uterus. The balloon is inflated with water, which in turn is heated to 80° to 90°C.

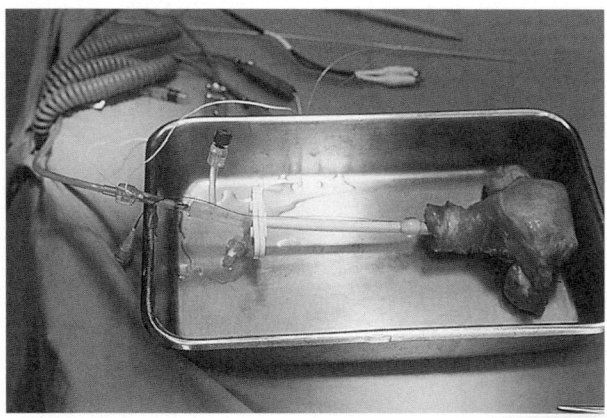

FIGURE 17.33. The "Enable" computerized continuously circulating hot saline cannula is engaged into a uterus and will ablate the endometrium at 80° to 90°C for 15 minutes.

Miscellaneous Procedures

IUD Removal

Although the number of IUD insertions has diminished over recent years, the gynecologist is occasionally called on to search for and remove a device with an indicator string that is not seen in the cervix. In such circumstances, the operating hysteroscope is a vital tool with which to locate the device and remove it under direct vision, according to Valle et al. The hysteroscope is inserted, and the device is viewed. If a string is seen, an alligator-jaw forceps is inserted, and the string is grasped. The hysteroscope is withdrawn, pulling the device through the uterine cavity and the cervix to the exterior. If the IUD is embedded, then a rigid grasping forceps is required. The IUD is located, and the large jaws of the rigid instrument grab the extruded portion of the IUD itself. Strong pressure is exerted on the jaws as the sheath of the hysteroscope is slowly withdrawn from the uterus, into the cervix, and out of the vagina.

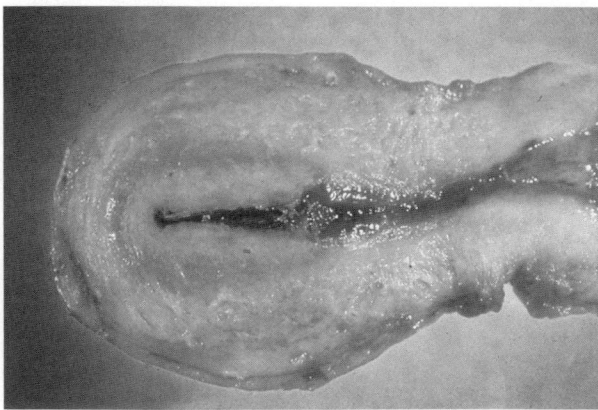

FIGURE 17.34. Hemiresection of a uterus removed at hysterectomy after "Enable" 15-minute ablation. Notice the brown, "cooked" appearance of the endometrium. See color version of figure.

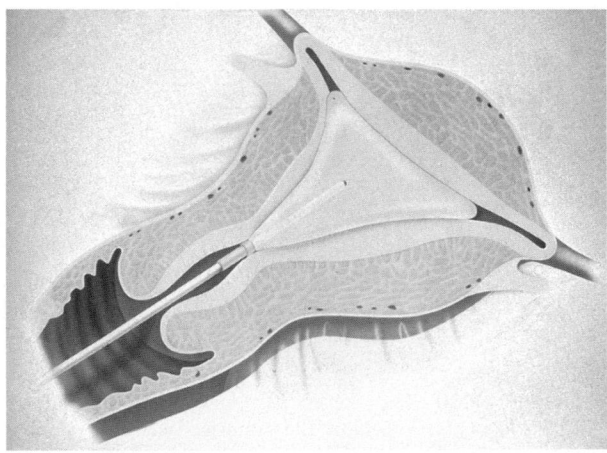

FIGURE 17.36. Schematic view of the inflated Gynecare hot-water balloon. See color version of figure.

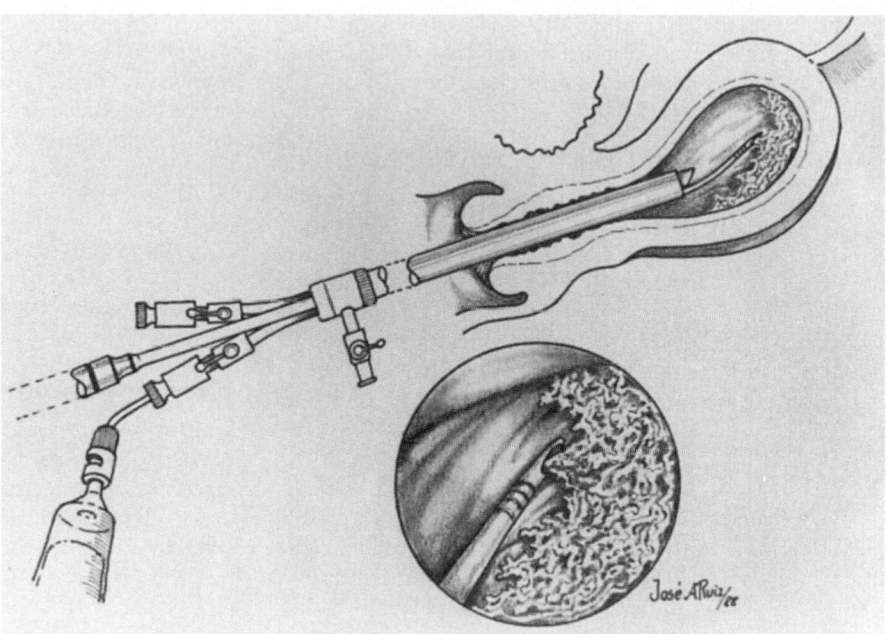

FIGURE 17.37. Direct sampling of an intrauterine lesion can be accomplished with a plastic cannula attached to a 30-mL syringe.

Biopsy of Intrauterine Lesions

When a tumor is suspected, the operative hysteroscope is inserted into the cavity, a 9F biopsy forceps is directed to the tumor site, and multiple biopsy specimens are obtained in a fashion analogous to that used with colposcopic biopsies. A 9F plastic cannula is inserted by way of the operating channel, and strong suction is applied to the mouth of the cannula by means of a 30-mL syringe (Fig. 17.37). The cannula is removed, and the contents are flushed out with saline into a bottle of fixative. Similarly, a 9F curette can be inserted under direct vision. Alternatively, a diagnostic hysteroscope can be inserted into the uterus. The site of pathology is noted. The endoscope is withdrawn, a Novak curette is inserted into the cavity, and biopsy specimens are taken at the previously located site. Finally, the hysteroscope is pulled back to the level of the internal cervical os, a small Novak curette is inserted alongside the hysteroscope, and a directed biopsy specimen is obtained.

Hemangiomas and Arteriovenous Malformations

Hemangiomas and arteriovenous malformations can be diagnosed by their characteristic hysteroscopic appearance and by a history of massive unresponsive bleeding. Historically, women with these conditions are young and of low parity. Hysteroscopic examination shows the subsurface of the endometrium to be covered with irregular bluish purple vessels that form an abnormal tangle of distended channels that differ markedly from the normal fine-capillary net pattern. The abnormal channels are not unlike the vessels that cover the surface of submucous myomas. The Nd:YAG fiber is inserted through the operating channel, and the fiber is held several millimeters above the vascular abnormality at a

power up to 50 to 60 W. The laser is discharged without touching the vessels or the surface of the endometrium. The laser energy causes the vessels to collapse and coagulate and the surface to blanch white. The endometrium neighboring the abnormality is also treated and coagulated. The fiber is then withdrawn, the field is aspirated clear, and the hysteroscope is withdrawn. Similar treatment is repeated two or three times at 1-month intervals or until all evidence of the abnormality is obliterated.

Complications

Unfortunately, accurate data concerning complications are hard to obtain, although one simple fact is clear: As greater numbers of gynecologists have begun to perform operative hysteroscopy, the rate of complications has increased. Voluntary surveys are worthless. Only state-mandated reports, such as those that are required for laparoscopic cholecystectomy in New York, have rendered any useful information. The exception to this is an excellent report by Smith et al., which details complications encountered by 42 gynecologists performing 257 endoscopic procedures (operative laparoscopy and hysteroscopy) in 218 patients (mean, 5.4 cases per surgeon) over a period of 15 months at the Swedish Hospital Medical Center in Seattle. Of 43 endometrial ablations, perforation was observed in three, fluid imbalance in two, and technical failure to complete in two. Myomectomy was performed in 30 and ablation plus myomectomy in 13. Perforation occurred in two, fluid imbalance in four, and fistula, sepsis, or both in three. Lysis of septa or synechiae was performed in 14 women, with perforation or hemorrhage in six patients. The overall complication rate ranged from 12% to 43%.

Similarly, the MISTLETOE data cited in the Endometrial Ablation section are useful accurate data relative to endometrial ablation/resection complications.

Intraoperative and Postoperative Bleeding

The most common complications inherent to hysteroscopic surgical procedures are intraoperative and postoperative bleeding. Generally speaking, intraoperative bleeding can be managed by aspirating the blood and by increasing the pressure of the distending medium so that it exceeds arterial pressure and compresses the walls of the uterus sufficiently to stop bleeding. Then the bleeding vessel can be coagulated with a 3-mm ball electrode with the use of forced coagulation at 30 to 40 W of power or by multiple jabs with bipolar needles at 20 to 30 W of power with the generator set for automatic bipolar. If the counterpressure of the medium is relaxed (at the termination of the procedure) and bleeding continues, then control is best obtained by inserting an intrauterine balloon initially inflated to 2 to 5 mL. If this pressure does not promptly stop the bleeding, then a larger balloon can be distended to 10 mL until the bleeding has stopped. More distention may be required for larger uteri. Care must be taken because overinflation of an intrauterine balloon can itself rupture the uterus. The balloon remains in place for 6 to 8 hours, is partially deflated for 6 hours, and, finally, is totally deflated before removal. When the bleeding is pulsatile, the source is arterial rather then venous. If this type of bleeding is not immediately controlled by balloon compression, then

hysterectomy will usually be required. Delayed postoperative bleeding is most commonly associated with endometrial slough (after ablation), chronic endometritis, or spontaneous extrusion and expulsion of the intramyometrial portion of a previously resected submucous myoma (Figs. 17.38 and 17.39). Bleeding-clotting studies should be obtained in cases of late postoperative bleeding, particularly if these studies were not performed preoperatively in women with a diagnosis of abnormal uterine bleeding (preoperative endometrial ablation or myomectomy).

Uterine Perforation

Uterine perforation can occur during any operative hysteroscopy procedure but is most common during septum resection, myomectomy operations, and adhesion takedown. The best insurance against this complication is simultaneous laparoscopy. Among novice operators, perforation can occur even during insertion of the hysteroscope. With appropriate care, this sort of perforation should not happen, because the cervix and internal os should be negotiated under direct vision, and the cavity should likewise be entered under direct vision. Examination under anesthesia is also simple and lets the operator know the direction of the uterine axis.

As we noted above, the most dangerous perforations are those associated with lasers and electrosurgical devices. The risk of this type of injury can be reduced by not activating the energy device during a thrusting or forward movement. The foot pedal is activated only dur-

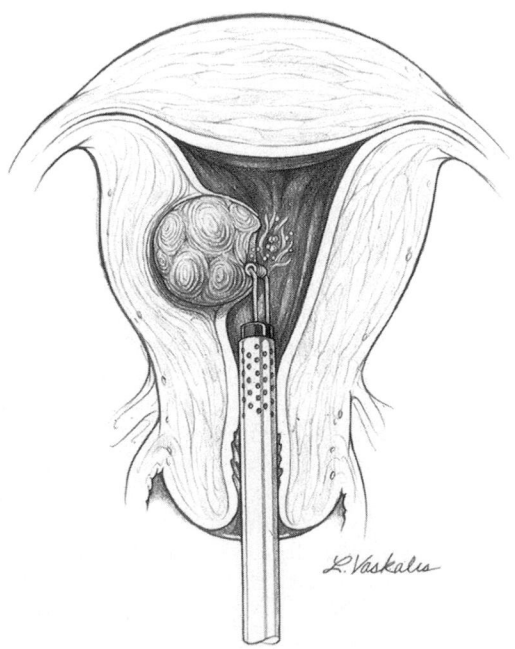

FIGURE 17.38. A new method for ablating a myoma via a ridged electrode or vaportrode, which develops very high power densities. (From Baggish MS, Barbot J, Valle RF. *Diagnostic and operative hysteroscopy,* second edition. St. Louis: Mosby–Year Book, 1999, with permission.)

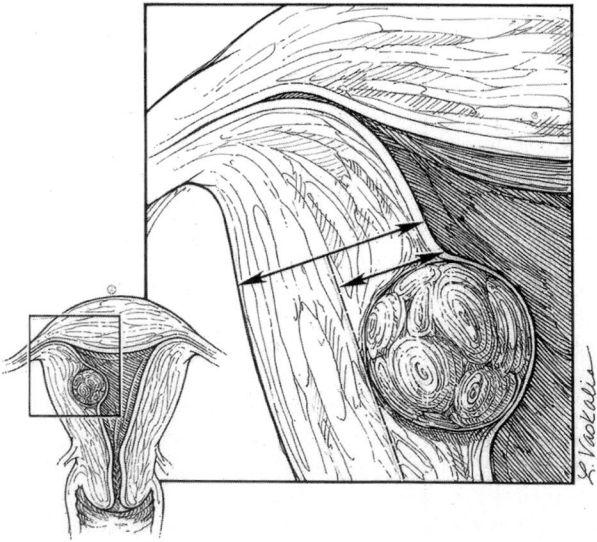

FIGURE 17.39. The part of the myoma protruding into the uterine cavity (submucous portion) is destroyed by either resection or vaporization. That portion remaining within the myometrium may be sufficiently devascularized so as to subsequently extrude itself into the cavity and be expelled via the cervix. (From Baggish MS, Barbot J, Valle RF. *Diagnostic and operative hysteroscopy,* second edition. St. Louis: Mosby–Year Book, 1999, with permission.)

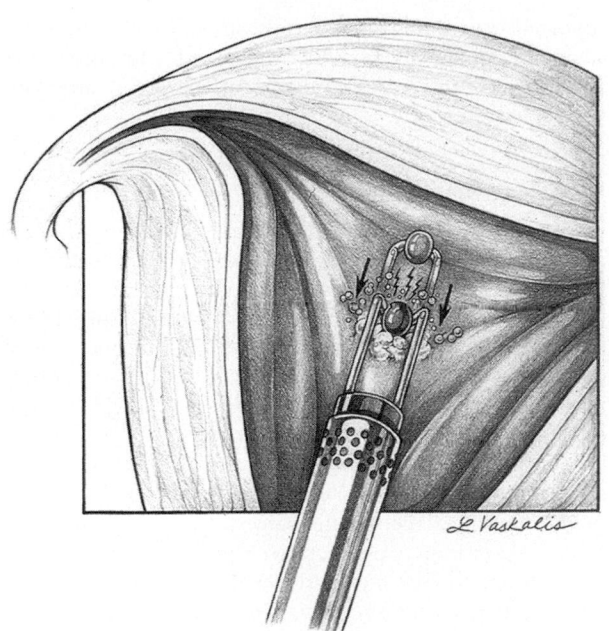

FIGURE 17.40. The operator should never apply power to an energy device while advancing the electrode. The power can safely be applied as the electrode returns toward the sheath. (From Baggish MS, Barbot J, Valle RF. *Diagnostic and operative hysteroscopy,* second edition. St. Louis: Mosby–Year Book, 1999, with permission.)

ing the return phase of the laser fiber or electrosurgical electrode. If a perforation does happen with an energy device, then laparotomy is required to ensure that no injury has been inflicted on the intestine, bladder, or ureter (Fig. 17.40).

A risk of perforation is associated with septum transection in its final phase at the level of the uterine fundus because the operator may have some difficulty determining where the septum ends and the myometrium begins. This risk is constant regardless of the cutting instrument used. The operator rapidly becomes aware that uterine perforation has occurred because distention becomes difficult to maintain and the flow of the distending medium exits at the perforation site. An alert assistant viewing by laparoscope should warn the hysteroscopist of impending perforation the moment any increasing intensity of light transmission through the thinning uterine wall is observed. If perforation is unnoticed and if simultaneous laparoscopy is not performed, a serious complication is even possible with a nonenergy instrument, but this is far less common than those occurring with lasers or electrodes. Nevertheless, if a perforation is suspected, the patient should be carefully observed in the hospital. Injuries to the iliac vessels can occur as the result of uterine perforation. An unexplained falling blood pressure, together with medium leakage, should alert the surgeon to this possibility. Perforation of the uterus during hysteroscopy can place a woman at an increased risk for uterine rupture during a future pregnancy (Fig. 17.41).

Poor Visibility in the Operative Field

Inability to see the operative field is a common problem. The usual cause of this problem is deep insertion of the hysteroscope so that the telescope lies directly in contact with the endometrium. The surgeon will see nothing but a red blur. The natural tendency is to push the hysteroscope deeper in. This strategic mistake invariably leads to perforation. Another cause of visibility problems is blood within the uterine cavity secondary to dilatation. The fastest way to deal with a bloody cavity is rapid flushing with the hysteroscopic medium combined with aspiration using a cannula placed into the cavity via the operating channel.

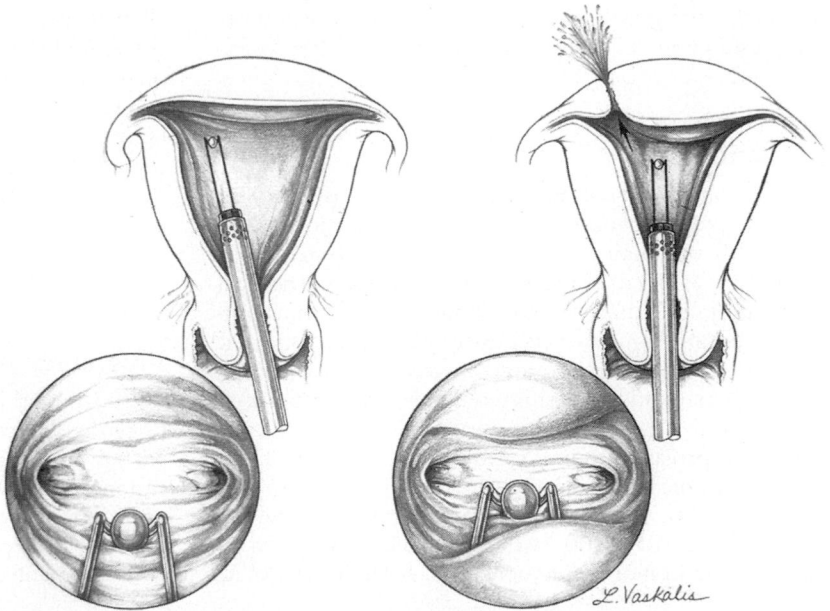

FIGURE 17.41. Perforation should be immediately suspected when the endometrial cavity depressurizes and collapses around the hysteroscope, creating a compromised view of the cavity.

Overdilatation of the cervix is an equally common mistake that results in excessive leakage of distending medium and an inability to maintain distention, with the resultant inability to perform the operative hysteroscopy. Blood and debris can cloud the field to such a degree that accurate operative endoscopy is impossible. Overdilatation is a less common occurrence when Hyskon is selected as the distending medium. If the operator cannot clearly see the field, it is better to discontinue the procedure than to press on and risk a catastrophic error. It is easy to become disoriented in the uterine cavity if normal anatomic landmarks cannot be recognized.

Gas Embolus

CO_2 embolism may occur during diagnostic or operative hysteroscopy. This will happen if an inappropriate method (e.g., laparoscopic insufflator) is used to infuse CO_2 into the uterus. However, this complication may also occur when a proper CO_2 hysteroscopic insufflator is used. The diagnosis is made by the presence of a cogwheel murmur accompanied by a rapid fall in expired CO_2.

Brundin and Thomasson observed 70 women during CO_2 hysteroscopy and reported the presence of the mill (cog)-wheel murmur in seven (10%). When the hysteroscopy was stopped, the murmur disappeared. Corson et al. infused CO_2 gas directly into the circulation of ewes. At 90 cc per minute, the P_{CO_2} dropped; however, at lower flow rates only transient drops in P_{CO_2} were observed. The investigators concluded that CO_2 clearance is very efficient owing to its high solubility in blood.

Air embolism is exceedingly dangerous and has been reported to occur during hysteroscopy. Corson et al. and Perry and Baughman have reported this type of complication. These investigators recommended avoiding the Trendelenburg position, purging air from all tubing and sheaths, and careful dilatating to avoid opening venous channels. Baggish and Daniell reported air embolism that resulted in death secondary to the use of gas-cooled coaxial Nd:YAG laser fibers.

Infection

The endometrium seems to be peculiarly resistant to infection, and infection is an unlikely complication associated with or coming after hysteroscopy. Hysteroscopy should be avoided in the presence of gross cervical infection, uterine infection, or salpingitis. Infection is otherwise uncommon after even extensive intrauterine surgery (e.g., adhesiolysis or myomectomy). Prophylactic antibiotics should be administered only when indications such as a history of rheumatic carditis, congenital heart defect, or prolapsed mitral valve exist, or in cases of suspected chronic endometritis (submucous myoma or embedded IUD). Baggish et al. (1999) observed only 13 infections out of 5,000 cases that could be casually related to the hysteroscopic operation. Salat-Baroux et al. reported seven mild infections out of 4,000 hysteroscopic examinations. On the other hand, McCausland et al. reported three cases of tuboovarian abscess after operative hysteroscopy.

Operator Technique

The most serious complications happen because of operator error. Most often, these are the result of inexperience and are avoidable. Difficult cases beyond the capabilities of the primary care gynecologist should be referred to an expert hysteroscopist. Skill in one area of endoscopy (e.g., operative laparoscopy) does not confer similar expertise in operative hysteroscopy. Indeed, the opposite may be more true.

During the postoperative period, operative complications should be the initial exclusion diagnosis for any patient who is not recovering according to the usual pattern. Worsening postoperative pain, fever, nausea, distention, and free intraperitoneal air are the signals of bowel injury. Diminished urinary output, fever, and distention suggest bladder or ureteral trauma. Falling blood pressure and rapid thready pulse, with or without distention, should raise concerns of a vascular problem and third-space hemorrhage.

Most negligence cases adjudicated in favor of the plaintiff have involved delayed initiation of appropriate treatment for an operative complication. Cases involving injury recognized at the time of surgery and correctly managed in a timely fashion do not usually become medicolegal problems.

Cancer After Ablation

Valle and Baggish reported on eight patients who had an endometrial ablation and who were found to have carcinoma of the endometrium between 5 months and 5 years (one patient diagnosed at endometrial resection) later. The authors identified risk factors for carcinoma in all patients, including obesity, hypertension, and diabetes. Additionally, five out of eight showed hyperplasia on preoperative biopsy. The investigators considered that women with abnormal uterine bleeding who fall into the high-risk category might be better served by hysterectomy rather than by endometrial ablation.

The risk of leiomyosarcoma is less than 1%. Nevertheless, any myoma or part of a myoma that is excised should be sent to the pathology laboratory for evaluation. This, of course, includes resectoscopic fragments.

Pregnancy After Hysteroscopic Ablation

Fortunately, this is not a common complication after hysteroscopic endometrial ablation. Rogerson et al. reported on four cases of pregnancy after ablation of the endometrium, with pregnancy loss of 75%. Two of the cases were associated with adherent placentas, including the one viable pregnancy that ended in the delivery of a preterm infant.

BIBLIOGRAPHY

A randomized trial of endometrial ablation versus hysterectomy for the treatment of dysfunctional uterine bleeding: outcome at four years. Aberdeen Endometrial Ablation Trials Group. *Br J Obstet Gynaecol* 1999;106:360.

Arieff AI, Ayus C. Endometrial ablation complicated by fatal hyponatremic encephalopathy. *JAMA* 1993;270: 1230.

Baggish MS. Contact hysteroscopy: a new technique to explore the uterine cavity. *Obstet Gynecol* 1979;54:350.

Baggish MS. Hysteroscopic media: a two-edged sword. *J Gynecol Surg* 1992;8:197.

Baggish MS. A new laser hysteroscope for Nd-YAG endometrial ablation. *Lasers Surg Med* 1988;8:248.

Baggish MS, Baltoyannis P. New techniques for laser ablation of the endometrium in high risk patients. *Am J Obstet Gynecol* 1988;159:287.

Baggish MS, Barbot J, Valle RF. *Diagnostic and operative hysteroscopy: a text and atlas.* Chicago: Mosby–Year Book, 1989.

Baggish MS, Brill AI, Rosensweig B, et al. Fatal acute glycine and sorbitol toxicity during operative hysteroscopy. *J Gynecol Surg* 1993;9:137.

Baggish MS, Davauluri CH, Rodriguez F, et al. Vascular uptake of Hyskon (dextran 70) during operative and diagnostic hysteroscopy. *J Gynecol Surg* 1992;8:211.

Baggish MS, Dorsey JH. Contact hysteroscopic evaluation of the endocervix as an adjunct to colposcopy. *Obstet Gynecol* 1982;60:107.

Baggish MS, Paraiso MF, Breznock EM, et al. A computer controlled, continuously circulating, hot irrigating system for endometrial ablation. *Am J Obstet Gynecol* 1995;173:1842.

Baggish MS, Ringgenberg E, Sze EHM. Adenocarcinoma of the corpus uteri following endometrial ablation. *J Gynecol Surg* 1995;11:91.

Baggish MS, Sze EHM. Experience with 568 endometrial ablation procedures. *Am J Obstet Gynecol* 1996;174:908.

Baggish MS, Sze EHM, Morgan G. Hysteroscopic treatment of symptomatic submucous myomata uteri with the Nd-YAG laser. *J Gynecol Surg* 1989;5:127.

Barbot J. Hysteroscopy for abnormal bleeding in diagnostic and operative hysteroscopy. In: Baggish MS, Barbot J, Valle RF, eds. *Diagnostic and operative hysteroscopy: a text and atlas.* Chicago: Mosby–Year Book, 1989:147.

Barbot J, Parent B, Doeler B. Hysteroscopie de contact et cancer de pendometre. *Acta Endosc* 1978;8:17.

Barbot J, Parent B, Dubuisson JB. Contact hysteroscopy: another method of endoscopic examination of the uterine cavity. *Am J Obstet Gynecol* 1980;136:721.

Brink DM, DeJong P, Fawcus S, et al. Carbon dioxide embolism following diagnostic hysteroscopy. *Brit J Obstet Gynaecol* 1994;101:717.

Brundin J, Thomasson K. Cardiac gas embolism during carbon dioxide hysteroscopy: risk and management. *Eur J Obstet Gynecol Reprod Biol* 1989;33:241.

Burnet JE. Hysteroscopy-controlled curettage for endometrial polyps. *Obstet Gynecol* 1964;24:621.

Bustos-Lopez H, Baggish MS, Valle RF, et al. Assessment of the safety of intrauterine instillation of heated saline for endometrial ablation. *Fertil Steril* 1998;65:155.

Cameron IM, Mollison J, Pinion SB, et al. A cost comparison of hysterectomy and hysteroscopic surgery for the treatment of menorrhagia. *Eur J Obstet Gynecol Reprod Biol* 1996;70:87.

Cararach M, Penella J, Ubeda A, et al. Hysteroscopic incision of the septate uterus: scissors versus resectoscope. *Hum Reprod* 1994;9:87.

Choe JK, Baggish MS. Hysteroscopic treatment of septate uterus with neodymium YAG laser. *Fertil Steril* 1992;57:81.

Corson SL, Brooks PG, Soderstrom RM. Gynecologic endoscopic gas embolism. *Fertil Steril* 1996;65:529.

Corson SL, Hoffman JJ, Jackowski J, et al. Cardiopulmonary effects of direct venous CO_2 insufflation in ewes. *J Reprod Med* 1988;33:440.

Creinin M, Chen M. Uterine defect in a twin pregnancy with a history of hysteroscopic fundal perforation. *Obstet Gynecol* 1992;79:879.

DeCherney AH, Cholst I, Naftolin F. The management of intractable uterine bleeding utilizing the cystoscopic resectoscope. In: Siegler AM, Lindemann HJ, eds. *Hysteroscopy: principles and practice.* Philadelphia: JB Lippincott Co, 1984:140.

DeCherney AH, Polan ML. Hysteroscopic management of intrauterine lesions and intractable uterine bleeding. *Obstet Gynecol* 1983;61:392.

DeCherney AH, Russell JB, Graebe RA, et al. Resectoscopic management of mullerian fusion defects. *Fertil Steril* 1986;45:726.

Droegemueller W, Greet BE, David JR, et al. Cryocoagulation of the endometrium at the uterine cornua. *Am J Obstet Gynecol* 1978;131:1.

Droegemueller W, Greet BE, Makowski E. Cryosurgery in patients with dysfunctional uterine bleeding. *Obstet Gynecol* 1971;38:256.

Dumesic DA, Dhillon SS. A new approach to hysteroscopic cannulation of the fallopian tube. *J Gynecol Surg* 1991;7:7.

Dwyer N, Hutton J, Stirkat GM. Randomized controlled trial comparing endometrial resection with abdominal hysterectomy for surgical treatment of menorrhagia. *Br J Obstet Gynecol* 1993;100:237.

Edstrom K, Fernstrom I. The diagnostic possibilities of a modified hysteroscopic technique. *Acta Obstet Gynecol Scand* 1970;49:327.

Fisher JC. Principles of safety in laser surgery and therapy. In: Baggish MS, ed. *Basic and advanced laser surgery in gynecology.* Norwalk, CT: Appleton-Century-Crofts, 1985: 85.

Friedler S, Margalioth EJ, Kafka I, et al. Incidence of post-abortion intrauterine adhesions evaluated by hysteroscopy: a prospective study. *Hum Reprod* 1993;8:442.

Gabriele A, Zanetta G, Pasta F, et al. Uterine rupture after hysteroscopic metroplasty and labor induction. *J Reprod Med* 1999;44:642.

Garry R, Hasham F, Kokri MS, et al. The effect of pressure on fluid absorption during endometrial ablation. *J Gynecol Surg* 1992;8:1.

Garry R, Shelley-Jones D, Mooney P, et al. Six hundred endometrial laser ablations. *Obstet Gynecol* 1995;85:24.

Goldenberg M, Zolti M, Seidman DS, et al. Transient blood oxygen desaturation, hypercapnia and coagulopathy after operative hysteroscopy with glycine used as the distending medium. *Am J Obstet Gynecol* 1994;170:25.

Goldrath MH. Vaginal removal of the pedunculated submucous myoma: the use of laminaria. *Obstet Gynecol* 1987;70:670.

Goldrath MH, Fuller T, Segal S. Laser photovaporization of endometrium for the treatment of menorrhagia. *Am J Obstet Gynecol* 1981;140:14.

Gonzales R, Brensilver JM, Rovinsky JJ. Post hysteroscopic hyponatremia. *Am J Kidney* Dis 1994;23:735.

Halvorson LM, Aserkoff RD, Oskowitz SP. Spontaneous uterine rupture after hysteroscopic metroplasty with uterine perforation. *J Reprod Med* 1993;38:236-8.

Hamou JE. Hysteroscopic et microhysteroscopic avec un instrument nouveau: le microhysteroscope. *Endosc Gynecol* 1980;2:131.

Hamou JE. Microhysteroscopy: a new procedure and its original application in gynecology. *J Reprod Med* 1981;26:375.

Harris WJ. Uterine dehiscence following laparoscopic myomectomy. *Obstet Gynecol* 1992;80:545.

Hidlebaugh DA, Orr RK. Long-term economic evaluation of resectoscopic endometrial ablation versus hysterectomy for the treatment of menorrhagia. *J Am Assoc Gynecol Laparosc* 1998;5:351-6.

Howe RS. Third trimester uterine rupture following hysteroscopic uterine perforation. *Obstet Gynecol* 1993;81:827.

Jones HW, Seegar-Jones G. Double uterus as an etiological factor in repeated abortion: indications for surgical repair. *Am J Obstet Gynecol* 1953;65:325.

Kivnick S, Kanter MH. Bowel injury from rollerball ablation of the endometrium. *Obstet Gynecol* 1992;79:833.

Lin BL, Iwata Y, Liu KH, et al. Clinical applications of a new Fujinon operating fiberoptic hysteroscope. *J Gynecol Surg* 1990;6:81.

Lin JC, Chen YO, Lin BL, et al. Outcome of removal of intrauterine devices with flexible hysteroscopy in early pregnancy. *J Gynecol Surg* 1993;9:195.

Lindemann HJ. The use of CO_2 in the uterine cavity for hysteroscopy. *Int J Fertil* 1972;17:221.

Lindemann HJ, Mohr J. CO_2 hysteroscopy, diagnosis, and treatment. *Am J Obstet Gynecol* 1976;124:129.

Lobaugh ML, Bammel BM, Duke D, et al. Uterine rupture during pregnancy in a patient with a history of hysteroscopic metroplasty. *Obstet Gynecol*, 1994;83:838.

Lomano JM. Photocoagulation of the endometrium with the Nd-YAG laser for the treatment of menorrhagia: a report of 10 cases. *J Reprod Med* 1986;31:26.

Magos AL, Baumann R, Lockwood GM, et al. Experience with the first 250 endometrial resections for menorrhagia. *Lancet* 1991;337:1074.

March CM. Hysteroscopy for infertility in diagnostic and operative hysteroscopy. In: Baggish MS, Barbot J, Valle RF, eds. *Diagnostic and operative hysteroscopy: a text and atlas.* Chicago: Mosby–Year Book, 1989:136.

March CM, Israel R. Gestational outcome following hysteroscopic lysis of adhesions. *Fertil Steril* 1981;36:455.

March CM, Israel R. Hysteroscopic management of recurrent abortion caused by septate uterus. *Am J Obstet Gynecol* 1987;156:834.

March CM, Israel R, March AD. Hysteroscopic management of intrauterine adhesions. *Am J Obstet Gynecol* 1978;130:65.

McCausland VM, Fields GA, McCausland AM, et al. Tuboovarian abscess after operative hysteroscopy. *J Reprod Med* 1993;38:198.

Mishler JM. Synthetic plasma volume expanders: their pharmacology, safety, and clinical efficacy. *Clin Haematol* 1984;13:75.

Neuwirth RS: Endometrial ablation using a thermal balloon system. *Contemp Obstet Gynecol* 1995;40:35.

Neuwirth RS. Hysteroscopic management of symptomatic submucous fibroids. *Obstet Gynecol* 1983;62:509.

Neuwirth RS. Hysteroscopic resection of submucous leiomyoma. *Contemp Obstet Gynecol* 1985;25:103.

Neuwirth RS. A new technique for and additional experience with hysteroscopic resection of submucous fibroids. *Am J Obstet Gynecol* 1978;131:91.

Neuwirth RS, Amin HK. Excision of submucous fibroids with hysteroscopic control. *Am J Obstet Gynecol* 1976;126:95.

Neuwirth RS, Duran AA, Singer A, et al. The endometrial ablater: a new instrument. *Obstet Gynecol* 1994;83:792.

Novy MJ, Thurmond AS, Patton P, et al. Diagnosis of cornual obstruction by transcervical fallopian tube cannulation. *Fertil Steril* 1988;50:434.

Overton C, Hargreaves J, Maresh M. A national survey of complications of endometrial destruction for menstrual disorders: the Mistletoe study. *Brit J Obstet Gynaecol* 1997;104:1351.

Pantaleoni D. On endoscopic examination of the cavity of the womb. *Med Press Circ* 1869;8:26.

Perry CP, Daniell JF, Gimpelson RJ. Bowel injury from Nd-YAG endometrial ablation. *J Gynecol Surg* 1990;6:199.

Perry PM, Baughman VL. A complication of hysteroscopy: air embolism. *Anes* 1990;73:546.

Phipps JH, Lewis BV, Roberts T, et al. Treatment of functional menorrhagia with radio-frequency endometrial ablation. *Lancet* 1990;335:374.

Pinion SB, Parkin DE, Abramoukh DR, et al. Randomized trial of hysterectomy, endometrial laser ablation, and transcervical endometrial resection for dysfunctional uterine bleeding. *BMJ* 1994;309:979.

Porto R, Gaujoux J. Une nouvelle methode d'hysteroscopic instrumentation et technique. *J Gynecol Obstet Biol Reprod (Paris)* 1972;7:691.

Propst AM, Liberman RF, Harlow BL, et al. Complications of hysteroscopic surgery: predicting patients at risk. *Obstet Gynecol* 2000;96:517.

Quinones RG. Hysteroscopy with a new fluid technique. In: Siegler AM, Lindemann HJ, eds. *Hysteroscopy: principles and practice.* Philadelphia: JB Lippincott Co, 1984:41.

Reed TP, Erb RA. Hysteroscopic tubal occlusion with silicone rubber. *Obstet Gynecol* 1983;61:388.

Roberts S, Long L, Jonasson O. The isolation of cancer cells from the bloodstream during uterine curettage. *Surg Gynecol Obstet* 1960;111:3.

Rock JA, Singh M, Murphy A. A modification of technique for hysteroscopic lysis of severe uterine adhesions. *J Obstet Gynecol* 1993;9:191.

Rogerson L, Gannon MJ, Donovan PJ. Outcome of pregnancy following endometrial ablation. *J Gynecol Surg* 1997;13:155-160.

Romer T. Benefit of GnRH analogue pre-treatment for hysteroscopic surgery in patients with bleeding disorders. *Gynecol Obstet Invest* 1998;45[Suppl 1]:12.

Ruiz JM, Neuwirth RS. The incidence of complications associated with the use of Hyskon during hysteroscopy: experience in 1793 consecutive patients. *J Gynecol Surg* 1992;8:219.

Salat-Baroux J, Hamou JE, Maillard G, et al. Complications from micro-hysteroscopy. In: Siegler A, Lindemann H, eds. *Hysteroscopy.* Philadelphia: JB Lippincott Co, 1984.

Schmitz MJ, Nahhas WA. Hysteroscopy may transport malignant cells into the peritoneal cavity: case report. *Eur J Gynaecol Oncol* 1994;15:121.

Siegler AM, Kemmann EK. Hysteroscopic removal of occult intrauterine contraceptive device. *Obstet Gynecol* 1975;46:604.

Siegler AM, Kemmann EK. Hysteroscopy: a review. *Obstet Gynecol Surv* 1975;30:567.

Singer A, Almanza R, Gutierrez A, et al. Preliminary clinical experience with a thermal balloon endometrial ablation method to treat menorrhagia. *Obstet Gynecol* 1994;83:732.

Smith DC, Donohue LR, Waszak SJ. A hospital review of advanced gynecologic endoscopic procedures. *Am J Obstet Gynecol* 1994;170:1635.

Strassman EO. Plastic unification of double uterus. *Am J Obstet Gynecol* 1952;64:25.

Sullivan B, Kenney P, Seibel M. Hysteroscopic resection of fibroid with thermal injury to sigmoid. *Obstet Gynecol* 1992;80:546.

Tapper AM, Heinonen PK. Experience with isotonic 2.2% glycine as distension medium for hysteroscopic endomyometrial resection. *Gynecol Obstet Invest* 1999;47:263.

Thijssen RFA. Radio-frequency induced endometrial ablation: an update. *Br J Obstet Gynaecol* 1997;104:608.

Valle RF. Hysteroscopic evaluation of patients with abnormal uterine bleeding. *Surg Gynecol Obstet* 1981;153.521.

Valle RF. Hysteroscopic removal of submucous leiomyomas. *J Gynecol Surg* 1990;6:89.

Valle RF. Hysteroscopy for gynecologic diagnosis. *Clin Obstet Gynecol* 1983;26:253.

Valle RF, Baggish MS. Endometrial carcinoma after endometrial ablation: high-risk factors predicting its occurrence. *Am J Obstet Gynecol* 1998;179:569-72.

Valle RF, Sciarra JJ, Freeman DW. Hysteroscopic removal of intrauterine devices with missing filaments. *Obstet Gynecol* 1977;49:55.

Valle RF, Sciarra U. Hysteroscopy: a useful diagnostic adjunct in gynecology. *Am J Obstet Gynecol* 1975;122:230.

Vilos GA. Intrauterine surgery using a new coaxial bipolar electrode in normal saline solution (Versapoint): a pilot study. *Fertil Steril* 1999;4:740.

Vilos GA, Vilos EC, Pendley E. Endometrial ablation with a thermal balloon for the treatment of menorrhagia. *J Am Assoc Gynecol Laparosc* 1996;3:383.

Yaron Y, Shenhav M, Jaffa AJ, et al. Uterine rupture at 33 weeks' gestation subsequent to hysteroscopic uterine perforation. *Am J Obstet Gynecol* 1994;170:786.

Te Linde's Operative Gynecology, ninth edition, edited by John A. Rock and Howard W. Jones, III. Lippincott Williams & Wilkins, Philadelphia © 2003.

CHAPTER
18

▼

Control of Pelvic Hemorrhage

HOWARD W. JONES, III WILLIAM A. ROCK, JR.

The successful performance of any surgical procedure involves control of pain, control of bleeding, and control of infection. The subject of this chapter is control of bleeding. Recognition and correction of an abnormal hemostatic mechanism, and the prevention and control of bleeding are fundamental to the success of any operation. Preoperative, intraoperative, and postoperative hemorrhage are potential complications in every patient undergoing gynecologic surgery. Preoperative hemorrhage is encountered in a variety of circumstances, such as in patients with intraperitoneal bleeding from a ruptured tubal pregnancy or in patients taking heparin who have a massive intraperitoneal hemorrhage with ovulation. Intraoperative and postoperative hemorrhage can result from vascular injury and failure to control bleeding during surgery, and postoperative bleeding is often a carryover from bleeding, owing to reflex vasoconstriction or hypotension, that was not apparent when the abdomen was closed. In all settings (preoperative, intraoperative, and postoperative), the bleeding can be caused or aggravated by a systemic bleeding diathesis that may or may not be related to the patient's other reason for hemorrhage.

Many benign gynecologic conditions are associated with an increase in menstrual blood loss (menorrhagia), an increase in the duration of menstrual flow (metrorrhagia), an increase in the frequency of menstrual periods (polymenorrhea), or combinations of all three. Repeated small menstrual hemorrhages, such as those that occur with menorrhagia, will reduce the iron stores in the body over time. The daily dietary intake of iron usually is sufficient to replace the iron lost with normal menstruation, but it is inadequate to replace the increased loss of iron associated with heavy menstruation. In gynecologic patients with a history of heavy or prolonged menstrual blood loss, it is a good idea to check the hematocrit or hemoglobin before setting a date for elective surgery. Preoperative iron supplementation is indicated in these women because a good hemoglobin level and adequate iron stores are the first step in managing perioperative hemorrhage. Transfusion before elective gynecologic surgery is rarely if ever indicated in women with chronic blood loss anemia. Menstrual blood loss may be controlled with hormonal therapy while surgery is delayed and iron supplementation given to enable the patient to replete her own hemoglobin stores.

The preoperative use of epoetin alfa (recombinate erythropoietin) for correction of preoperative anemia has been used successfully in orthopedics. Its application in gynecologic surgery remains unclear. It is probably most applicable in gynecologic patients with chronic renal failure, nonmyeloid (hematopoietic) leukemia, or human immunodeficiency virus (HIV). Occasionally, other forms of anemia will be encountered that require a more extensive evaluation and treatment before elective surgery. On the other hand, some women who present with acute blood loss from a ruptured ectopic pregnancy or malignancy may require urgent transfusion even as preparations are being made for surgical intervention.

413

FUNDAMENTAL CONCEPTS OF NORMAL COAGULATION

Every surgeon should understand at least the basic mechanisms of normal hemostasis that can be relied on when surgical injury to tissue is inflicted. Bleeding during gynecologic surgery usually results from cutting or lacerating small or large vessels, but occasionally it may result from or be complicated by some preexisting or intraoperative defect in the clotting mechanism. The surgeon should be able to recognize when normal hemostasis is interdicted, so that available remedies to protect against or remedy excessive bleeding can be found. Hemostasis is a complex, intricate, integrated, complementary, and countervailing system that maintains a delicate balance between normal coagulation and hypocoagulation or hypercoagulation. Unusual clinical situations can arise that require hematologic consultation for resolution. A specialist in coagulation disorders can provide invaluable assistance in the diagnosis and treatment of many rare disorders of coagulation.

The following is a discussion of the principles and concepts of normal hemostasis, abnormal hemostasis (congenital and acquired), and management techniques.

Effective hemostasis is the result of all aspects of the coagulation system functioning together to stop bleeding. Coagulation is the working interrelation of five aspects of a complex biochemical and vascular system that causes the formation and dissolution of the fibrin platelet plug. These five components are (a) vasculature; (b) platelets; (c) plasma clotting proteins; (d) fibrinolysis and clot inhibition; and (e) the hypercoagulable response. How these five components interrelate in the normal setting must be understood before one can appreciate how the five relate to bleeding or abnormal clotting in disease states.

Vasculature

The vasculature presents an endothelial-lined flexible conduit through which red cells, white cells, platelets, and all of the plasma proteins flow. At the interface between the flowing blood and vessel wall are several inhibitory biochemical systems that prevent the generation of the platelet–thrombin clot. The antiplatelet substance prostacyclin, produced in the vessel wall, inhibits platelet adhesion to the vessel wall. The surface antithrombin III–heparan sulfate complex inhibits deposition of thrombin and fibrin.

A tear in the vessel wall removes the endothelial cell layer, exposing the basement membrane, smooth muscle, collagen, and supporting adventitia. These substances are biochemical activators of platelets and have their own thromboplastic activity, which initiates fibrin generation and deposition. Therefore, the disruption in the vessel wall removes the protective covering of the endothelial cells, exposing platelet clumping and clot-initiating substances that produce a platelet–fibrin mass that will plug the tear in the vessel wall. A disease or medication that interferes with or intensifies this process can cause bleeding or inappropriate clotting. The vessel wall is diagrammed in Fig. 18.1.

Congenital diseases associated with inadequate connective tissue and vascular dysfunction associated with bleeding are rare. The more frequently seen conditions are hereditary hemorrhagic telangiectasia, Ehlers-Danlos' syndrome, and Marfan's syndrome, which are characterized by defects in the quality of collagen. Defective collagen is responsible for poor clot formation and platelet activation at the injured site. No disease is known to be associated with excessive inappropriate clotting related to the vasculature as a structure. The congenital diseases closest to that definition are a predisposition to atherosclerosis owing to abnormalities in lipid metabolism, such as hypercholesterolemia, homocystinemia, and diabetes mellitus.

Acquired diseases of the vessel associated with bleeding include deficiencies in vitamin C, Cushing's syndrome, acute and chronic inflammatory diseases such as infectious vasculitis and immune vasculitis, pyrogenic purpura, embolic purpura, and anaphylactoid reactions from drugs. Myeloproliferative disorders, such as multiple myeloma and Waldenström's macroglobulinemia, produce abnormal proteins that interfere with vascular function and therefore permit bleeding.

Routine laboratory assessment of vascular function is extremely primitive. The capillary fragility test, the only routinely available test used to assess vascular function, has limited value. It is sensitive to only the severest vascular structure abnormalities. More in-depth studies include vascular biopsies and skin window testing procedures, which are research procedures. There are no routinely available methods for assessing increased vascular activity in the area of inappropriate clotting.

Platelet Function

Platelets are disk-shaped fragments of the large multinucleated megakaryocytes released from the bone marrow on a daily basis (normal count is $150 \times 10^3/\mu L$ to $400 \times 10^3/\mu L$) (Fig. 18.2). Their life span is 8 to 10 days.

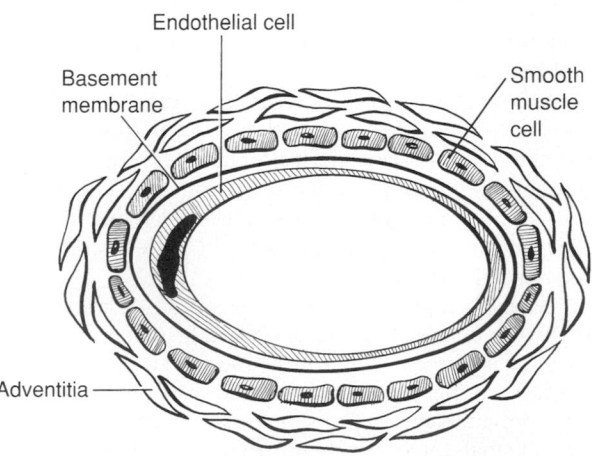

FIGURE 18.1. Vessel cross section.

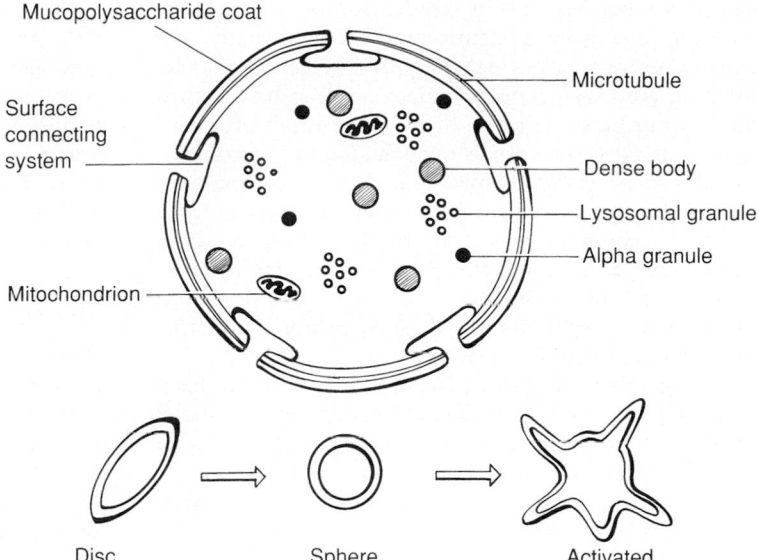

FIGURE 18.2. Platelet cross section.

These microscopic fragments have a well-defined substructure that can be directly correlated with platelet function.

The surface activation of the receptor sites on the platelet causes it to change first to a sphere and finally to a spider-like structure, with pseudopods in all directions. This release reaction is the summation of biochemical and structural changes in the platelet, which are characterized as follows. The surface receptor sets up a biochemical chain reaction, resulting in the generation of thromboxane A_2. This causes contraction of the protein thrombosthenin, which causes the ejection of the platelet contents. Of great importance are the dense granules with nonmetabolic adenosine diphosphate (ADP). ADP is a potent platelet-aggregating agent that, in a domino-like sequence, stimulates more platelets, generating a large platelet plug.

The congenital diseases associated with poor platelet function are divided into four types of dysfunction: (a) adhesion to collagen, (b) adhesion to subendothelium, (c) release reaction defects, and (d) ADP aggrega-

tion defects. With the exception of von Willebrand's disease, a defect in the adhesion to subendothelium, all the congenital defects are rare and not essential to this discussion. von Willebrand's disease (Table 18.1) is a classically autosomal, dominantly inherited disorder resulting from absence, decreased production, or abnormal function of a large multimeric protein synthesized by megakaryocytes and vascular endothelium. This protein is responsible for the proper binding of platelets to the collagen surface exposed in vascular trauma. Its absence results in the failure of platelets to bind normally to disruptions in the vasculature, preventing formation of the platelet plug necessary for normal hemostasis. The condition remains undetected in most patients until some form of vascular trauma occurs or surgery is performed. In addition, such patients are particularly sensitive to aspirin or other antiplatelet medications, and bleed excessively in surgery while taking this kind of medication. von Willebrand's disease is the most common congenital platelet disorder and is the disease most likely to go undetected until surgery. This disorder is particularly

TABLE 18.1.
More Commonly Seen Rare Congenital Clotting Disorders

Name	Incidence (per million)	Treatment
Factor VIII (classic hemophilia A, sex-linked)	60–80	FVIII concentrate
Factor IX (classic hemophilia B, sex-linked)	15–20	FIX concentrate
von Willebrand's disease (dominant; autosomal)	5–10	Cryoprecipitate (DDAVP), factor VIII concentrate with von Willebrand factor

DDAVP, Deamino-D-arginine vasopressin.

The remainder of the known congenital clotting factors are very rare and occur with such low frequency that their discussion, diagnosis, and management can be found elsewhere. (See Harker LA, *Hemostasis manual,* second edition, Philadelphia: FA Davis, 1974; Corriveau DM, Fritsma GA, *Hemostasis and thrombosis,* Philadelphia: JB Lippincott Co, 1988; Triplett DA, ed. *Laboratory evaluation of coagulation.* Chicago: ASCP Press, 1982.)

dangerous because, in its milder forms, a history of bleeding in surgery is negative and the preoperative co-agulation screen is normal. Acquired defects in platelet function are much more common and can be classified into two groups: (a) those that are the result or conse-quence of a disease, such as renal failure, myeloprolifera-tive disorders (polycythemia vera, chronic myelogenous leukemia), and increased fibrin split products in con-sumptive coagulopathies; and (b) those that are iatro-genic, such as defects caused by medications (aspirin, nonsteroidal antiinflammatory drugs, antibiotics, anti-histamines, tricyclic antidepressants, dextran) and car-diopulmonary bypass surgery.

Congenitally increased platelet function has not been described. Acquired disorders associated with increased platelet function, however, are common. The stress of routine surgery or trauma (fractured hip, femur, or pelvis) can create a hypercoagulable state with thrombo-cytosis and increased platelet activity.

The laboratory assessment of platelet function has been expanded from the research laboratory and is more readily available to the surgeon. The routine analysis of platelet function should begin with a platelet count and PFA-100. In special cases, platelet adhesion and platelet aggregation are useful in identifying the inadequate or overstimulated platelet. In addition, biochemical mark-ers for increased platelet use or turnover can be demon-strated with platelet factor IV and β-thromboglobulin assays. Recent studies by Gewirtz et al. confirm previous studies that the bleeding time is not a good prediction of surgical bleeding.

Plasma-Clotting Proteins

Plasma-clotting proteins are a group of serine proteases and cofactors that interact in a synergistic system to gen-erate fibrin. The activation of the clotting system can be initiated in two ways: either by contact activation with factor XII or through thromboplastin activation of factor VII. The clotting cascade is diagrammed in Fig. 18.3. As we will see later in the discussion of fibrinolysis and an-tithrombin systems, anticoagulation forces are initiated at the inception of clotting. The tear in the vessel wall, described earlier, begins the orderly activation of the

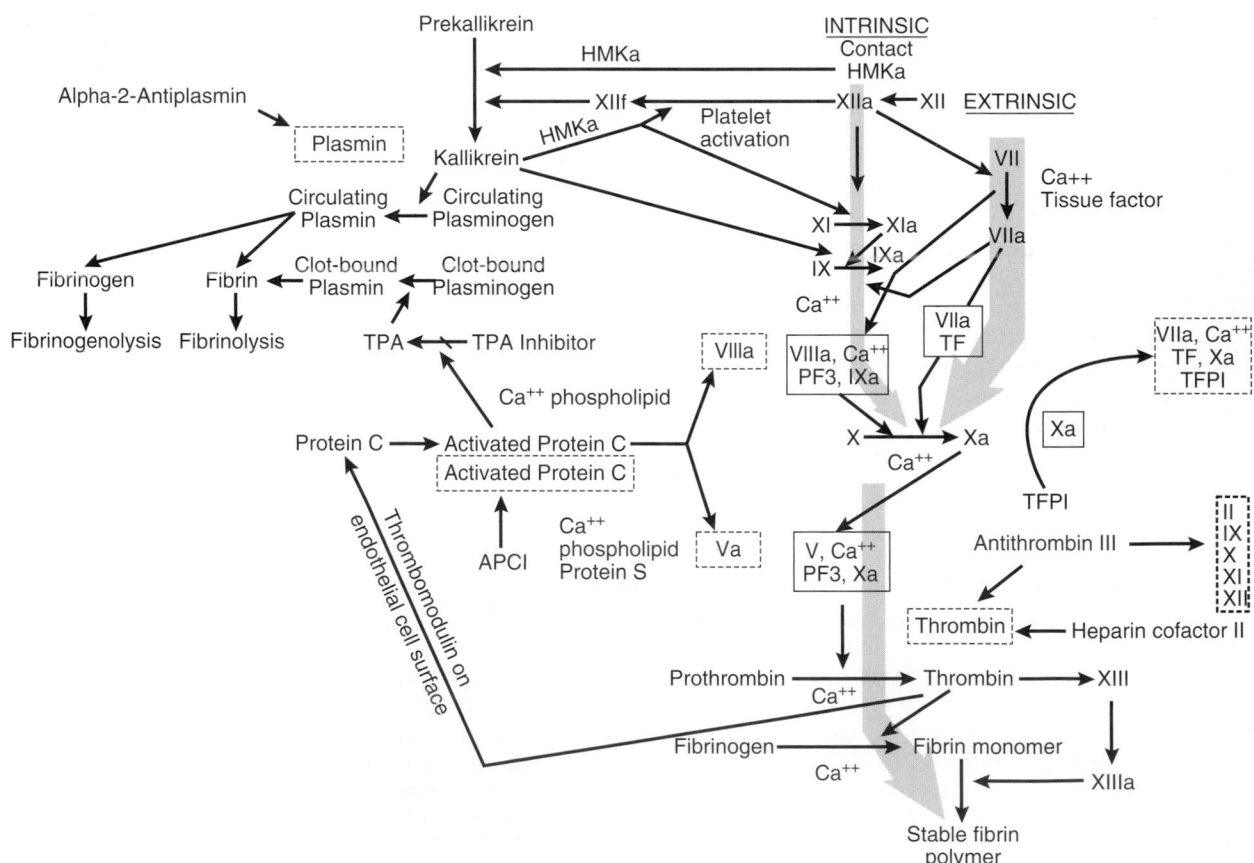

FIGURE 18.3. Coagulation system. Dashed boxes indicate destruction of factors. HMKa, high-molecular-weight kininogen; PF3, platelet factor 3; TPA, tissue plasminogen activator; TFPI, tissue factor pathway inhibitor.

plasma-clotting system. The fibrin contribution to the platelet—fibrin plug is initiated with the activation of factor XII by collagen and of factor VII by tissue juice (thromboplastin). Any congenital or acquired disorder of the clotting factors can lead to inadequate or no generation of fibrin. Each clotting factor has a different role and significance in the overall generation of fibrin. This also is true with abnormal increases in some clotting factors that are associated with inappropriate clotting.

The congenital-factor deficiencies associated with bleeding are either relatively common or rare. The relatively common group includes hemophilia A (factor VIII deficiency) and hemophilia B (factor IX deficiency). Both are seen in the male and rarely in the female disorders with sex-linked inheritance patterns. The rare group includes all the remaining factors that have an autosomal recessive inheritance pattern or a dominant pattern with variable penetrance.

The acquired factor deficiencies are common. Multiple deficiency is usually owing to iatrogenic vitamin K deficiency with loss of factors II, VII, IX, and X. This deficiency often is the result of multiple-antibiotic therapy, which kills the vitamin K–producing bacterial flora in the intestine, and the nothing-by-mouth status of many critically ill patients, which results in the loss of food sources of vitamin K. Other common acquired multifactor deficiencies are seen in acute and chronic liver disease, as in viral hepatitis and alcoholic cirrhosis; consumptive coagulopathies, as in sepsis and placenta abruptio; washout coagulopathies, as in multiple-transfusion patients after severe blood loss (such as from ruptured abdominal aneurysms); and major trauma, as from automobile accidents or gunshot wounds.

The laboratory assessment of the plasma clotting factors has traditionally begun with the prothrombin time (PT; factors V, VII, and X, prothrombin, and fibrinogen) and the activated partial thromboplastin time (APTT; factors VIII, IX, XI, and XII). Specific factor assays also can identify the exact deficiencies. One must remember that a factor deficiency as low as 30% can generate a normal PT and APTT. This relation is important in investigating minimal prolongations of the PT or APTT that appear insignificant but could be hiding a moderately severe deficiency. The tissue factor pathway inhibitor modulates activated factors X and VIII but is not apparently significant in disease.

The sensitivity of the PT and APTT reagents is essential to the appreciation of the proper use of these tests as preoperative screening tests, or in monitoring warfarin and heparin anticoagulant therapy. Recent publications from Europe and the United States stress the importance of and need for a standardized prothrombin reagent system in the United States. The lack of sensitivity of the rabbit brain thromboplastin used in the United States has led to the over-coumarinization of some patients. The original value of 2.0 to 2.5 times the control was based on the more-sensitive human thromboplastin. Current recommendations have lower ratios (Table 18.2). These ratios are applicable only in stable, coumarinized patients. Studies of different APTT

TABLE 18.2.
Therapeutic Ranges for the International Normalized Ratios

Condition	Therapeutic Ranges
Prophylaxis for venous thromboembolism in high-risk surgery and in hip surgery	2.0–3.0
Treatment of venous thrombosis and pulmonary embolism	2.0–3.0
Prevention of systemic embolism	
Tissue heart valves	
Acute myocardial infarction	
Valvular heart disease	
Atrial fibrillation	
Bileaflet mechanical value in aortic position	
Treatment for mechanical prosthetic heart valves (high risk)	2.5–3.5
Prevention of recurrent systemic embolism	
Prevention of recurrent myocardial infarction	

From: Hirsh J, Dalen JE, Anderson DR, et al. Oral anticoagulants: mechanism of action, clinical effectiveness, and optimal therapeutic range. *Chest* 2002;119:8S.

reagents have revealed a similar variability of sensitivity to heparin.

Fibrinolysis

The activation of the fibrinolytic system begins with the activation of the plasma substrate plasminogen. This substrate is converted by naturally occurring activators such as urokinase, kallikrein, and clot-activated proteases to the active enzyme plasmin. Plasmin is the active enzyme that, if free or clot-bound, lyses fibrin clots and destroys fibrinogen. This enzyme is modulated by α_2-antiplasmin and antitrypsin, which destroy the active enzyme plasmin.

This enzymatic conversion of fibrinolysis normally is initiated by clot formation or by a direct activator such as urokinase or tissue plasminogen activator (tPA). tPA released from the endothelium activates tissue plasminogen and is neutralized by PAI-1 inhibitor. Sometimes direct activation is seen in liver disease and during extracorporeal bypass. This activation also can be secondary to disease, as in a consumptive coagulopathy, such as bacterial sepsis, or a large abdominal aneurysm.

Hypercoagulable State

With physiologic stress, such as emotional stress and surgical stress, there is a response of fright or flight. This response to stress is evident in the coagulation system. The plasma-clotting proteins, such as fibrinogen and factor VIII, increase, and the platelet count and stickiness can increase as well. This normal response is important in ensuring hemostasis at the time of increased need. When this process is exaggerated, uncontrolled, or unmodulated, inappropriate clotting can occur, which produces venous and arterial clots and all their sequelae. In gynecologic surgery, the normal physical hypercoagulable state, as well as the inappropriate state, must be understood to appreciate the diagnosis, intervention, and management of postoperative vascular occlusive complications. Virchow, in 1845, was the first to conceptualize the triad of blood flow, vessel wall, and content of blood itself as a basis for inappropriate clotting. An understanding of the relation of the three parts is essential to explain what has occurred in the problem patient.

CONGENITAL CAUSES OF INAPPROPRIATE CLOTTING

The congenital etiology of inappropriate arterial and venous clotting has long been ill defined. Only recently has it been more completely elucidated (Tables 18.3 and 18.4). Procoagulants, when increased on a congenital basis, have been associated with a propensity to generate clots. These procoagulants include fibrinogen and factor VIII; however, they are not present frequently enough to warrant testing every suspect case. Naturally occurring

---

TABLE 18.3.
Risk Factors for Arterial Thrombosis

INHERITED

Elevated cholesterol, triglycerides, lipoprotein (a), decreased high-density lipoprotein
Diabetes
FVII polymorphism
Hyperhomocysteinemia
Methylenetetrahydrofolate reductase mutation C677T
PLA_2 glycoprotein IIb/IIIa
Gender, male > female

ACQUIRED

Antiphospholipid antibodies
Lupus anticoagulant
Hypertension
Diet with increased fat
Infection: chlamydia, cytomegalovirus
Heparin-induced thrombocytopenia
Social class, body mass index

MIXED HEREDITARY/ACQUIRED

Factor VIII
Fibrinogen
FVII
Homocysteine
C-reactive protein
Von Willebrand factor

From: Triplett DA. Thrombophilia: laboratory evaluation. *ASCC Clinical Laboratory News* 2002;28:12.

TABLE 18.4.
Risk Factors for Venous Thrombosis

INHERITED

Common
Factor V Leiden (R506Q)
Factor II Mutation (G21201A)
Factor VIII
Rare
Antithrombin III deficiency
Protein C deficiency
Protein S deficiency
PAI-1 polymorphism
Dysfibrinogenemia
Factor XII deficiency
Prekalikrein (Fletcher factor) deficiency
Plasminogen deficiency
Tissue plasminogen activator deficiency

ACQUIRED

Surgery and trauma
Prolonged immobilization
Older age
Cancer
Myeloproliferative disorders
Previous venous thrombosis
Pregnancy/puerperium
Contraceptives/hormone replacement
APC resistance not due to FV Leiden
Antiphospholipid antibodies
Mild-to-moderate hyperhomocysteinemia
Obesity

From: Seligsohn U, Lubetsky A. Genetic susceptibility to venous thrombosis. *N Engl J Med* 2001;344:1222.

---

inhibitors of clotting are defined as those factors that actively destroy clotting factors or substrates as they are formed. The more common of these rare deficiencies are antithrombin III, protein C, protein S, factor V Leiden (R506Q), factor II mutation (G21201A), and methylenetetrahydrofolate reductase mutation (C677T).

IMPAIRED FIBRINOLYSIS

A congenital decrease in the plasma substrate plasminogen results in inadequate fibrinolysis of thrombi. This deficiency can be qualitative and quantitative, with similar effects.

A congenital decrease in tPA that normally is released from the vascular endothelium is associated with impaired fibrinolysis. An abnormal increase in plasminogen activator inhibitor also will reduce the level of tPA, resulting in inappropriate clotting.

The decrease or absence of Fletcher factor (prekallikrein) and factor XII also can result in impaired fibrinolysis because of a decrease in activation of circulating plasminogen at the time of clot activation.

ACQUIRED CAUSES OF INAPPROPRIATE CLOTTING

The number of acquired causes of inappropriate clotting is much greater than the number of congenital causes and is expanding every day because the same chemistry found in the congenital mechanism can be identified as a deficiency in an ongoing disease process.

Factor VIII has been shown to determine the rate of thrombin production and is a cause of thrombogenesis and coronary artery disease. Increases in dietary fat also increase factor VIII:C levels, resulting in an increased aggregability of platelets, which causes platelet thrombi to increase. Also noteworthy is the fact that smoking as a cause of coronary artery disease may be mediated through a rise in fibrinogen.

Natural physiologic states also can increase the levels of plasma-clotting factors. Instead of a single factor being the cause of inappropriate clotting, in these cases, it is likely that the complementary activity of all factors working synergistically produces inappropriate clotting. In pregnancy, factor VIIIc and fibrinogen are increased. A common reaction to trauma such as a leg fracture or surgery is an increase in factor VIIIc and fibrinogen levels and in the platelet count.

Disease states associated with inappropriate clotting include both acute and chronic forms. The acute forms are seen in diseases such as thrombotic thrombocytopenic purpura (owing to the acquired or congenitally absent von Willebrand factor cleaving protease) and nephrotic syndrome, with loss of antithrombin III in the urine along with other plasma proteins. The chronic forms are seen in diseases such as diabetes mellitus (endothelial hyperplasia of smaller arterioles, reduced prostaglandin I_2 production, and hypersensitivity of platelets), heavy cigarette smoking, and diets high in fat and cholesterol. Neoplastic diseases such as carcinoma of the lung, colon, and prostate are associated with severe thromboembolic complications. Myeloproliferative diseases, including polycythemia vera, chronic myelogenous leukemia, and essential thrombocythemia, are associated with inappropriate clotting. The lupuslike inhibitor and the anticardiolipin antibodies seen in lupus patients and in patients with infectious diseases and other autoimmune diseases are associated with inappropriate clotting and spontaneous abortions.

Iatrogenic causes of inappropriate clotting are common findings in the hospital setting and generate great concern. Such causes include the postsurgical state, medication, vascular prosthetic devices, and immobilization for any reason.

As a physiologic acute-phase response to surgical stress, an exaggerated outpouring of clotting factors and platelets in combination with a decrease in physiologic inhibitors can result in clot formation. This often occurs in deep leg veins, particularly in association with venous stasis.

Prosthetic devices such as grafts, shunts, and artificial heart valves can provide a clottable surface that will form a nidus for initial thrombosis quickly followed by further clot formation, resulting in obstruction or embolization.

The vascular component of acquired thrombotic disease has only recently been described in detail. It appears that decreased blood flow through a vein can decrease the contact between thrombin and thrombomodulin, diminishing the contact with protein C and predisposing the vein to thrombosis. However, the arterial side with high blood flow rates has a rich capillary bed with greater contact with protein C, lysing clots more efficiently. Local thrombus formation can be generated by direct mechanical disruption of the vascular endothelium, traumatic damage to the vessel wall, infectious or chemical damage to the vessel wall, and vasculitis.

PREOPERATIVE COAGULATION SCREENING

For the preoperative evaluation, gynecologic patients must of necessity be divided into two categories: those having routine or elective surgery and those having emergency surgery.

Elective Surgery

The elective gynecologic surgical patient must be evaluated in two ways: general medical history and specific nature of the surgery. The medical history taken at bedside, with review of the medical chart when available, is an excellent place to begin. Table 18.5 highlights the most important positive and negative findings to be identified.

Preoperative coagulation screening is of limited value without complete knowledge of the patient's past and current history. It does not replace a good history and physical examination. One should not expect this screening to reveal the estimated blood loss in a routine surgical procedure. It is essential, however, for resolving and eliminating risk factors that can affect postoperative bleeding (Tables 18.6 and 18.7).

Risk factors such as unknown history, or known history in an emergency surgical procedure; positive personal or family history of bleeding or bleeding with or without surgery; and known history of taking medications that can affect coagulation, such as antiplatelet

---

TABLE 18.5.
Pertinent Medical History to Screen for Coagulation Problems

History of spontaneous bruising or bleeding
History of unusual bruising or excessive bleeding after surgery
Family history of bruising or bleeding after surgery
Medication associated with bruising or bleeding
Current medication within past week
Previous coagulation testing
Current coagulation testing

TABLE 18.6.
Tests to Indicate Coagulation Status

Test	Reference Range*	Level of Alarm	Significance
Hematocrit (%)	37–47	25	Tissue anoxia
White cell count (μL)	4×10^3—12×10^3	3×10^3–25×10^3	Susceptibility to infection, leukemia
Platelet count (μL)	140×10^3–400×10^3	100×10^3–700×10^3	Bleeding, myeloproliferative disorder
Fibrinogen (mg/dL)	150–400	100	Bleeding, liver disease, intravascular consumption
Prothrombin time (s)	10–13	14	Bleeding factor deficiency
Activated partial thromboplastin time (s)	28–38	40	Bleeding factor deficiency, inhibitor
Clot retraction	Complete clot in 60 min: retraction complete in 120 min	No clot / Clot lysis	Low platelets or fibrinogen / Fibrinolysis
PFA-100	Collagen–epinephrine	Prolonged closure time	Screen for medication effect Bleeding (will not predict surgical bleeding)

*Reference ranges may vary in each laboratory, reflecting method, instrumentation, and reagents.

medication, acquired vitamin K deficiency (nothing-by-mouth status with long use of antibiotics), and fibrinolytic therapy (decreased fibrinogen), are assessed by preoperative screening.

Preoperative coagulation screen is not usually indicated unless the medical history and physical examination reveal suspicious or explained findings that suggest a risk of surgical bleeding. Items such as a history of unexplained surgical bleeding, family history of bleeding, bleeding after medication, or evidence of bruising or bleeding on examination to mention only a few.

The decision to transfuse blood and blood components must be made with all the current knowledge of the patient's status. The surgeon must actively seek the patient's past history, hematology and coagulation test results, and chemistry results as appropriate (Fig. 18.4). The surgeon must be aware of the patient's hematologic and coagulation status throughout the case. Then, and only then, does the proper selection of blood components solve problems. The surgeon's surgical dictation

and progress notes also should reflect the observations, test results, and course of action taken.

The risk of bloodborne infections and adverse reactions is always present, but the documented need for blood as a life-saving substance will validate the decision. When blood is transfused when indicated but is not justified in writing, this life-saving substance becomes a liability to all who use it. The routine preoperative orders for blood require knowledge of the specific needs of the patient and the surgeon's usual transfusion requirements for a specific surgical procedure. For the routine gynecologic procedure, such as simple hysterectomy in an otherwise healthy woman, a type and antibody screen are appropriate. With the type and antibody screen, the patient's blood is screened for unexpected antibodies. No specific blood units are set aside, but blood is available from the general inventory in an emergency. If an unexpected antibody is identified, the blood bank should notify the ordering physician and set aside 2 U of antigen-negative crossmatched compatible blood for use in an emergency situation.

In an emergency, the blood bank can release blood immediately (with a type and match to follow) with a 99.99% safety factor when the previous screen for unexpected antibodies was negative. Additionally, when the surgeon can wait 10 to 15 minutes, an immediate spin crossmatch can be performed to further verify ABO compatibility between donor and recipient. The value of the type and antibody screen is in monetary savings for the patient, and there is no undue or unnecessary risk to the patient.

In more complex procedures, such as pelvic exenteration for cancer, where there usually is significant blood loss, a type and crossmatch for the average number of units used is appropriate. With extremely difficult procedures or other complicating diseases, additional blood, fresh-frozen plasma, and platelets may be required during the procedure and should be requested preoperatively.

TABLE 18.7.
Coagulation Profiles

Brief Coagulation Profile	Complete Coagulation Profile
CBC (includes WBC differential)	CBC (includes WBC differential)
Platelet count	Platelet count
Prothrombin time	Prothrombin time
Partial activated thromboplastin time	Partial activated thromboplastin time
	Fibrinogen
	Bleeding time

CBC, complete blood count; WBC, white blood cell.

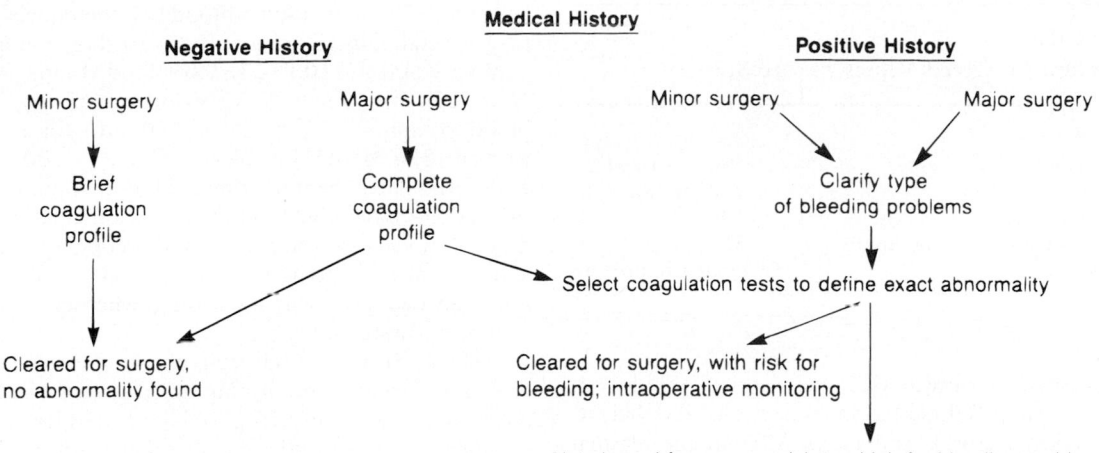

FIGURE 18.4. Evaluation of candidate for elective surgery.

Ideal or time-proven guidelines are difficult to establish for every operative case. Each surgical experience will benefit the surgeon, and over time he or she will establish usual transfusion requirements for both type and antibody screen, as well as type and crossmatch. The hospital quality assurance program, in planning with the transfusion service or blood bank and transfusion committee, should establish guidelines to assist the surgeon in identifying the usual blood transfusion needs. The use of either *Guidelines for Transfusion Therapy* (Boral) or *Maximal Surgical Blood Order Schedule* (Judd) is helpful in developing hospital guidelines.

Emergency Surgery

As the emergency procedure is begun, decisions regarding blood replacement must be made. A direct approach to blood replacement therapy and the complications of such therapy depends on a clear understanding of the following concepts.

1. As bank blood replacement with just packed red cells corrects the blood loss problem, it may create an acquired bleeding disorder. Thrombocytopenic hemophilia. Platelets and fresh-frozen plasma may be indicated.
2. The patient's bleeding potential is dynamic and will change rapidly and frequently with the loss of blood and replacement therapy.
3. Direct monitoring before, during, and after surgery offers the best chance to diagnose and manage the bleeding. Direct monitoring also allows formulation of plans and adjustment of the replacement therapy program.

COMPONENT THERAPY FOR REPLACEMENT BEFORE SURGERY

With surgery planned, the preoperative data can be evaluated. Assuming the patient does not have hemophilia, von Willebrand's disease, severe liver disease, or liver failure, a prolonged PT and APTT may suggest a less common acquired or congenital bleeding disorder. (The blood sample must be properly drawn and mixed well and must not be taken from an A-line containing heparin or from an infusion site.) Assistance from a clinical pathologist or hematologist should be requested if an intrinsic bleeding disorder is suspected.

von Willebrand's disease is the most common hereditary bleeding disorder transmitted predominately as an autosomal dominant defect. Effecting men and women equally, this disease often undiagnosed at the time of surgery can be a cause of increased morbidity and mortality. von Willebrand's disease presents commonly with a history of mucosal bleeding, such as epistaxis, or with a history of easy bruising or menorrhagia. A familial history of this kind of bleeding in many female members of a family is also a clue to the possible presence of von Willebrand's disease. This missing von Willebrand factor is manufactured in the vessel endothelial cell Weibel-Palade bodies and megakaryocytes. This factor has a major role in hemostasis, including (a) binding platelets to subendothelial collagen, and (b) joining with and stabilizing circulating factor VIII. Without von Willebrand factor, platelets adhere poorly to damaged endothelium, and clotting factor VIII can be significantly reduced.

Treatment will evolve around the type, severity of the disease, and the nature of the surgical procedure. The more common type I and some of the rarer variants can be managed with DDAVP (deamino-D-arginine vasopressin; a vasopressor analog) that increases the release of the stores of von Willebrand factor in epithelial Weible-Palade bodies. This is contraindicated in most cases of type IIB. Cryoprecipitate and the manufactured Humate P (fractionated FVIII) are sources of von Willebrand factor that are infused before, during, and after a surgical procedure. The amount and frequency of replacement will depend on the type of surgery, blood loss, and risk of bleeding in a critical tissue or structure. Diagnosis and management of this disorder is often complex and difficult. Consultation with a clinical pathologists or hematologist should be considered.

If the patient is bleeding before surgery, packed red blood cells should be given. If bleeding is severe, fresh-

TABLE 18.8.
Minimum Preferred Values Before Surgery

Hematocrit	>25%
Platelet count	>150 × 10³/μL
Fibrinogen	>150 mg/dL
Prothrombin time	<13 s
Activated partial thromboplastin time	<39 s
Clot reaction	Clot at 1 h, no lysis

frozen plasma, cryoprecipitate, or platelets should be given as indicated. Whole blood (8 days old) is deficient in coagulation factor V and factor VIII in the plasma portion, as well as in platelets. Although the levels of these factors can produce normal PT and APTT readings, they are insufficient for a patient undergoing surgery and blood loss. (Mild hemophilia also can produce a normal APTT reading.) When packed red blood cells and fresh-frozen plasma are not available, whole blood can be used, although it may create a greater coagulation deficit when given in large amounts, making intraoperative monitoring even more critical. The goals of emergency preoperative screening are as follows:

- To determine whether a coagulation defect exists before surgery is begun and possibly to identify the cause
- To establish a baseline for assessing the changes owing to massive blood replacement and the success of specific component therapy
- To establish immediate component therapy needs

The minimum preferred values to be achieved before surgery are listed in Table 18.8.

Packed red cells are given as needed, and 2 U of fresh-frozen plasma may be given with every 6 to 8 U of packed red blood cells to begin normalizing the PT and APTT. Platelet transfusions should not be given routinely until a deficiency is documented during surgery and the surgical procedure is nearly completed. The fibrinogen level should not be corrected until the intraoperative monitoring results are seen. The transfusion of fresh-frozen plasma may correct the fibrinogen deficiency. Poor clot retraction may be owing to deficient platelets and fibrinogen, and the presence of clot lysis suggests intravascular coagulation. Cryoprecipitate is suggested for rapid correction of a fibrinogen deficiency. Additional investigative procedures (with specialty input) are suggested for further evaluating and managing complex cases.

COMPONENT THERAPY FOR REPLACEMENT DURING SURGERY

According to Schifman and Steinbronn, when intraoperative blood loss exceeds 15% of the patient's estimated blood volume, the surgeon should consider red blood cell transfusion to replace the acute blood loss. As a general rule, 15% of an adult's blood volume equals the patient's weight (in kilograms) times 10. For example, for a 50-kg woman (110 lb), 15% of blood volume = 50 × 10 = 500 mL; for a 75-kg woman (165 lb), 15% of blood volume = 75 × 10 = 750 mL; for a 100-kg woman (220 lb), 15% of blood volume = 100 × 10 = 1000 mL. The patient's estimated blood volume, the estimated intraoperative blood loss, the anticipation of additional blood loss, the presence of preoperative anemia, and the risk of hypoxic complications must all be taken into consideration when deciding whether or not to transfuse (Table 18.9).

When massive blood replacement therapy is under way, intraoperative monitoring of coagulation at 2-hour intervals, or after every 10 U of blood transfused, usually is sufficient. One should remember that a patient bleeding during a surgical procedure has a higher demand for clotting factors and platelets than does a patient at bed rest. In many oncology cases in which the patient is undergoing chemotherapy, a platelet count of 50 × 10³/μL is adequate; in a surgical case in which the patient is bleeding, a 50 × 10³/μL platelet count is not adequate to achieve a good platelet plug. The use of blood and blood components in the management of massive bleeding due to a major vessel rupture has the following objectives:

1. To maintain sufficient blood volume and circulating red cells to sustain life
2. To replace blood sufficiently to achieve adequate coagulation and hemostasis, assuming there was extensive loss of plasma-clotting factors and platelets
3. To avoid falling so far behind in replacement that management involves not only bleeding from a vascular tear but also bleeding at the microvascular level because of insufficient clotting factors and platelets

Each of these objectives requires repeated assessment of the patient throughout the surgical procedure. Care-

TABLE 18.9.
Evaluation of Intraoperative Bleeding

KNOWN MEDICAL HISTORY

Positive
  Manage according to preoperative plan
Negative
  Intraoperative coagulation profile: assess amount of blood loss, transfuse up to 6 U packed red blood cells. After sixth unit, repeat coagulation profile and prepare to transfuse components.
  Determine whether cause of bleeding is surgical or nonsurgical.

UNKNOWN MEDICAL HISTORY

Attempt to acquire history.
Intraoperative coagulation profile: assess amount of blood loss, transfuse up to 6 u packed red blood cells. After sixth unit, repeat coagulation screen and prepare to transfuse components.

ful monitoring by established routine policies often is the best way to handle a crisis situation created by massive bleeding.

Formulas for blood transfusion that are applied ritualistically without the benefit of laboratory data may resolve the need to treat but do not answer the needs of the patient. The formulas described below are designed to initiate the marshaling of blood bank resources. They do not replace the thoughtful analysis of laboratory data coupled with the selection of a specific blood component to correct a specific deficit. The following guidelines are recommended for component therapy in clinical situations requiring massive blood replacement to maintain normal hemostasis.

For every 6 to 8 U of packed red blood cells, 2 U (500 mL) of fresh-frozen plasma should be given. The size and age of the patient affect blood replacement. If the patient's blood volume can accommodate an additional 500 mL of fresh-frozen plasma, this amount should be transfused and the PT and APTT monitored.

Platelets should be given when the platelet count falls below $100 \times 10^3/\mu L$ in massive hemorrhage. (Measurement error of a platelet count can be high as $\pm 20 \times 10^3/\mu L$ in a bleeding patient.) When a long surgical procedure is anticipated, or when more than 6 U of blood are given, 6 U of platelets in a volume of 300 mL should be given toward the end of the surgical procedure or when surgical hemostasis is achieved. This amount should be administered once to provide a maximum bolus effect. Because platelets are often difficult to obtain, their use should be reserved until near the end of the procedure. Otherwise, they may be lost and therefore unavailable when needed because of continued blood loss and replacement during extensive surgical repair. Pooling and transporting the platelets can take up to an hour, so the blood bank should be given sufficient notice to have them available in surgery when needed. In assessing the patient's coagulation status, it should be remembered that clotting factors are constantly changing. Six units of platelets will achieve maximum bolus effect in an average patient (3 U in a child or small adult) and will also enable evaluation of platelet use. A platelet count of 40×10^3 to $60 \times 10^3/\mu L$ should be expected in a 70-kg person after transfusion of 6 U of platelets. Monitoring the platelet count after transfusion and for the next several hours will reveal the success of replacement, consumption, and life of the platelets.

When the PT and APTT are prolonged (more than 14 seconds and 40 seconds, respectively) after replacement therapy, intrinsic disease must be considered initially, if only to be ruled out later. A borderline hemophiliac or patient with liver disease may manifest excessive bleeding after stress, trauma, or blood replacement because of the increased coagulation needs. A mild hemophilia or liver disease is rare as an unknown, but it is possible. Therefore, administration of fresh-frozen plasma in these 2-U (500 mL) doses should begin to correct the deficiencies caused by massive red blood cell replacement. If oozing continues despite the rapid transfusion of 6 U of fresh-frozen plasma, a clotting problem or other ongoing bleeding disorder should be suspected and additional support sought.

When the fibrinogen level falls below 100 mg/dL, transfusion of 20 U of cryoprecipitate will provide about 150 mg/dL fibrinogen in a 70-kg person. A low fibrinogen level is rare because fibrinogen is stable and present in fresh-frozen plasma. Liver disease or intravascular consumption must be suspected if the fibrinogen level is initially less than 100 mg/dL and remains low throughout surgery and recovery. The 20 U of cryoprecipitate will achieve therapeutic levels quickly and permit monitoring over several hours.

The goals of intraoperative monitoring are as follows:

- To assess changes in the coagulation mechanism resulting from blood loss and replacement therapy
- To identify the coagulation components affected and determine the correct components to initiate therapy
- To determine the success of replacement component therapy in an extensive operative procedure
- To enable selection of components to achieve the following values: PT less than 14 seconds, APTT less than 40 seconds, fibrinogen more than 100 mg/dL, and platelets more than $80 \times 10^3/\mu L$. If surgical hemostasis appears to have been achieved from a technical viewpoint and bleeding is present but mild, one can "wait to see" for 2 hours. If bleeding is profuse and worsening, 2 to 4 U of fresh-frozen plasma and a 10-U dose of platelets are given, and then packed red cells are given as needed. The patient is monitored when the transfusion is completed. Laboratory monitoring is repeated after 1 to 2 hours, whether the patient is bleeding or not, to determine the success of replacement.

COMPONENT THERAPY FOR POSTOPERATIVE REPLACEMENT

The presurgical and intrasurgical alarm levels for hematocrit, platelet count, PT, APTT, fibrinogen, and clot retraction also apply postoperatively, and a comparison of these values provides an accurate assessment of the bleeding patient. Significant clinical bleeding with good postoperative coagulation values suggests surgical bleeding. When laboratory values are abnormal, however, further surgery can be delayed until an attempt at aggressive specific component therapy is made. We have found that when abnormal coagulation studies exist, the following causes predominate, in order of frequency (most frequent first):

1. Low platelet count owing to transfusion of only packed red cells or fresh-frozen plasma.
2. Prolonged PT and APTT owing to replacement with packed red cells without fresh-frozen plasma. In administering aggressive replacement therapy, it should be remembered that some patients have a meager blood volume. Careful monitoring of venous and arterial pressure, as well as cardiac output, should be

considered in blood component therapy. Often a slower rate of administration can achieve hemostasis without cardiovascular overload. In rare cases, phlebotomy may be required to create needed space for transfusion. If nearly normal coagulation values are achieved but bleeding continues, surgical causes for bleeding should be considered.

3. Low fibrinogen level owing to dilution with plasma expanders, or concurrent development of a disseminated intravascular coagulation.

The goals of postoperative monitoring are as follows:

- To determine whether a coagulopathy was created by blood replacement, and to determine current status.
- To determine the success of specific component therapy and identify the need for additional components.
- To enable the surgeon to distinguish surgical from nonsurgical bleeding.

The routine use of postoperative monitoring, whether the patient is bleeding or not, will achieve these goals. As the surgeon reviews the results of each case, he or she will develop a valuable assessment of the patient's usual postoperative coagulation states. With this knowledge, the unexpected is recognized and resolved in a more timely manner.

RISKS OF BLOOD TRANSFUSION

Transfusions of whole blood were given sporadically before 1900, usually to treat specific diseases rather than to replace lost blood volume. Indeed, heavy bleeding was thought to be beneficial and therapeutic for many diseases. Even as late as World War I, the importance of blood loss and replacement was not recognized, because shock was thought to be owing to toxins released from traumatized tissue. It was the work of Cannon and Bayliss in 1919 and of Blalock in 1930 that proved that the important factors in shock were the loss of circulating blood volume and the decreased return of venous blood to the right heart.

Landsteiner discovered the four major blood groups in 1900. Banking and storage of donated blood became possible with refrigeration and the addition of sugar and later sodium citrate as an anticoagulant. In World War II, a remarkable program was organized to collect and store large quantities of type O (so-called universal donor) blood for shipment to U.S. military hospitals throughout the world. Many lives were saved by the use of this banked blood to treat the shock associated with battle casualties. This experience firmly established the need for blood banks and the importance of blood transfusions in combatting hypovolemic shock from hemorrhage before, during, and after surgery.

To be safe, homologous blood must be collected from carefully selected volunteer donors and properly matched to the potential recipient. Although many lives have been saved by properly administered transfusions, gynecologic surgeons must be aware of the potential hazards of perioperative transfusions. The risks of red blood cell transfusion were recently reviewed by a National Institutes of Health and Food and Drug Administration Consensus Development Conference on Perioperative Red Cell Transfusion and published in 1988. The following excerpt is taken directly from their report.

In deciding whether to use red blood cell transfusion in the perioperative period, the need for possibly improved oxygenation must be weighed against the risks of adverse consequences, both short-term and long-term. The disadvantages are of two general types: transmission of infection and adverse effects attributable to immune mechanisms.

Any infectious agent that is present in the blood of a donor at the time of donation is potentially transmissible to a susceptible recipient. The consequence may be seen as clinical morbidity and mortality after an incubation period characteristic of the agent or recognized only by serological or other types of laboratory testing. If the agent produces chronic infection, clinical mortality may not be seen until years after the transfusion (Table 18.10).

In modern blood banking practice, bacterial contamination of red blood cell units is rare. For practical pur-

TABLE 18.10.
Blood Transfusion Risks

Disease or Situation	Risk
Viral infection	
HIV	1:1.9 million
HTLV	1:250,000–1:2.0 million
Hepatitis B	1:180,000
Hepatitis C	1:1.6 million
Bacterial contamination	
Platelet packs (stored at room temperature)	1:12,000
Packed or whole red blood cells	1:5 million
Fatal red-cell hemolytic reaction	1:250,000–1:1.1 million
Delayed red-cell hemolytic reaction	1:1,000–1:1,500
TRALI	1:5,000
Febrile red-cell nonhemolytic reaction	1:100
Allergic (urticarial reaction)	1:100
Anaphylactic reaction	1:150,000

HIV, human immunodeficiency virus; HTLV, human t-cell lymphotropoic virus; TRALI, transfusion-related acute lung injury.
From: Zoon KC, Ten years after: what has been achieved by Consent Decrees: The FDA View. *Fifth Annual FDA and the Changing Paradigm for Blood Regulation,* January 16–18, 2002, New Orleans, Louisiana; Schreiber GB, Busch MP, Kleinman SH, et al. The risk of transfusion-transmitted viral infections: the retrovirus epidemiology donor study. *N Engl J Med* 1996;334:1685; Dziecxkowski JS, Anderson KC, Transfusion biology and therapy. In, *Harrison's principles of internal medicine,* fourteenth edition. Fauci AS, Martin JB, Braunwald E, et al., eds. New York: McGraw-Hill, 1998:718; Goodnough LT, Breacher ME, Kanter MH, et al. Transfusion medicine: first of two parts—blood transfusion. *N Engl J Med* 1999;340;438.

poses, the transmissible agents of greatest concern are viruses.

Cytomegalovirus infection occurs with moderate frequency among those recipients without prior infection. Most of these infections are asymptomatic, except among immunocompromised people. The use of the newer leukocyte reduction filters (less than 5×10^6) is under extensive clinical study and application as an alternative to cytomegalovirus negative blood.

Human T-cell lymphotropic viruses occur with low but not negligible frequency among donor populations in the United States. It is not known whether transfusion-transmitted infection with these viruses among adults results in T-cell leukemia/lymphoma and/or neurological disease several to many years later.

On rare occasions, other microbial agents—including paroviruses, malaria, *Toxoplasma*, Epstein-Barr virus, and *Babesia*—cause infection and disease.

It is known for the human hepatitis viruses that the incidence of infection in recipients increases with the number of donor exposures. This relationship is probably true for other transfusion-transmitted infections. If homologous transfusion is to be used, therefore, the number of units administered should be kept to a minimum.

HIV about which there is the greatest public concern, presently poses only a remote hazard because of donor selection and laboratory screening procedures. The consequences of HIV infection are rarely seen until 2 or many more years have elapsed, but ultimately morbidity and mortality are extremely high.

Immunologic consequences also complicate homologous red blood cell transfusion. Hemolytic and nonhemolytic reactions are largely caused by alloimmunization to red blood cell and leukocyte antigens. Compatibility testing virtually has eliminated immediate hemolytic transfusion reactions; when they occur, they are largely owing to human error. Nonhemolytic febrile reactions occur in 1% to 2% of recipients owing to sensitization to leukocyte antigens. This may be reduced by the use of leukocyte reduction filters (less than 5×10^6).

Although blood transfusions are and will remain an essential component of perioperative gynecologic care, an awareness of their associated risks is important in every patient before electing their use. There is every reason to carefully consider the risk:benefit ratio of giving "just one bottle of blood." Indeed, it is the rare clinical situation in which this action can be justified.

The growing public concern about transfusion-associated infections should make gynecologic surgeons aware of the importance of being selective in their use of transfusion therapy. The public has been greatly sensitized by the transfusion-associated transfer of acquired immunodeficiency syndrome (AIDS). The most common transfusion-related viral infection, however, is non-A, non-B hepatitis, which accounts for 90% to 95% of cases of previous transfusion-acquired hepatitis and possibly as many as 3,000 deaths per year in the United States. Ultimately, on further testing, many of these cases will be found to have hepatitis C. When mortality or significant morbidity occurs with blood transfusion, the gy-

necologic surgeon must be able to show that the transfusion was indicated.

There are alternatives to blood and blood component transfusion that may be considered in critically ill patients such as those with sepsis and deseminated intravascular coagulation. The drug activated protein C, drotrecogin alfa (Xigris), is recombinant human activated protein C (drotrecogin alfa, activated). It is used in replacement therapy in sepsis and holds a great promise in the management and survival in sepsis. By replacing this essential naturally occurring anticoagulant, there is reversal of the bleeding and thrombosis seen with sepsis. Its specific application in septic gynecological surgical patients has not been reported in any large study.

Recombinant activated FVII (NovoSeven) has been clinically demonstrated to successfully manage patients with FVIII and FIX inhibitors. It has also been used in management of bleeding in cardiovascular surgery, liver failure and coumadin overdose, and disseminated intravascular coagulation. It has significantly reduced the use of blood components in these disorders, and although expensive, it has the potential to greatly improve the outcomes with these disorders.

By reducing the need for blood and blood components with the use of activated protein C, drotrecogin alfa, and recombinant activated FVII, you can reduce the infectious disease exposure of blood, as well as the generation of allogenic antibodies. Not only may there be improved survival, but also there should be a substantial reduction of blood and blood components used in the treatment of similar complications in gynecological surgery.

According to Friedman et al., in every age range the mean hematocrit of men is higher than that of women. Women adapt to this relative state of anemia physiologically by a variety of mechanisms. Their red blood cells have a greater capacity than those of men to release oxygen. The erythrocyte oxygen dissociation curve of women is right-shifted when compared with that of men. Levels of 2,3,-diphosphoglycerate, adenosine triphosphate (ATP), and glucose-6-phosphate are higher in the red blood cells of women than in those of men. Because of these physiologic adaptations, Friedman et al. suggest that a lower hematocrit support level to govern the blood transfusion of female surgical patients be considered.

There are a variety of methods to support circulating volume, but there is no available material to support oxygen transport. Future research may be successful in developing modified hemoglobin solutions and perfluorochemical emulsions for oxygen transport, but there currently is no substitute for red blood cells for this purpose.

In a comprehensive discussion of perioperative interventions to decrease transfusion of allogeneic blood products, Ereth et al. suggest that an increased awareness of transfusion-related morbidity from allogeneic blood products has resulted in increased development and application of alternatives to allogeneic transfusion. As an indication of what can be accomplished, a program instituted by the Transfusion Committee of the Methodist

Hospital of Indianapolis modified transfusion practice in the hospital by establishing new transfusion guidelines based on national standards rather than on local practices and by implementing educational and monitoring systems. As reported by Rosen et al., over a 3-year period, the total decrease in donor exposures for patients was 42,072. Overall savings amounted to $1,627,348. This program was able to effect substantial cost and patient risk reductions, even though hospital services involving blood transfusion increased. A comprehensive update entitled "Transfusion Medicine in Obstetrics and Gynecology" was published recently by Santoso et al.

AUTOLOGOUS BLOOD TRANSFUSION

Blood collected from a patient for retransfusion at a later time into the same patient is called autologous blood. Autologous blood transfusions have been endorsed by the Council on Scientific Affairs of the American Medical Association and by the Committee on Hospital Transfusion Practice of the American Association of Blood Banks. If established guidelines are followed, autologous blood is the safest type of blood for transfusion. It does not eliminate all risks associated with red blood cell transfusion, because there is still the possibility of a hemolytic reaction caused by the rare clerical error or bacterial contamination. It does eliminate the risk of alloimmunization and the risk of transferring such infections as hepatitis, malaria, cytomegalovirus, and AIDS. In patients with rare blood types who have antibodies to common blood antigens, it may be the only blood available for transfusion. Autologous blood transfusion is acceptable to most Jehovah's Witnesses who have a religious objection to transfusion with homologous blood or blood products. The use of autologous blood decreases the need for banked blood, which may then be reserved for other purposes. Given the improved safety of allogeneic transfusions today, the increased protection afforded by donating autologous blood is limited and may not justify the increased cost. This choice may be presented to the patient who has concerns about blood transfusion.

Intraoperative Autologous Transfusion

The frequency of autologous transfusion has increased appreciably in the past decade, especially for cardiovascular operations. Keeling et al. reported on the use of the Haemonetics Cell Saver for autologous intraoperative transfusion in 725 consecutive general hospital patients. Seventy-five percent were cardiovascular patients, but a variety of other patients, including gynecology–obstetric patients, were represented.

A general subject review of intraoperative autologous transfusion was published by Popovsky et al. in 1985. These investigators stated that although the technology of the earlier experiences was comparatively crude and associated with technical problems and complications, better methods have been developed in recent years to eliminate problems in the operation and maintenance of the machinery and to make intraoperative autologous transfusion safe. Our experience in gynecologic surgery reported by Shapiro and Toledo, although limited at this point to a series of 25 myomectomy operations, has demonstrated to our satisfaction that intraoperative autologous transfusion is convenient to use and does not in any way interfere with the performance of the procedure.

The Haemonetics Cell Saver operates by retrieving blood from the operative site by suctioning it into a double-lumen catheter, in which it is immediately anticoagulated with heparin. It is then collected in a cardiotomy reservoir, where a filter removes gross debris. The blood is then pumped to a spinning centrifuge bowl, where the red blood cells are separated, washed with normal saline solution, and then concentrated to a hematocrit of about 50%. The supernatant waste that is subsequently collected contains saline, anticoagulant, activated coagulation factors, platelets, leukocytes, free hemoglobin, and other small debris. The washed packed red blood cells are pumped into a reinfusion bag. The blood is then directly transfused to the patient through a filter. The reagents and the collecting system are sterile and disposable. The entire process takes 8 to 10 minutes to process about 250 mL of packed cells. The machine is maintained and operated by a trained technician.

At least until additional data are available to the contrary, intraoperative autologous transfusion is contraindicated in patients with malignant disease and in patients with bacterial contamination of blood in the operative field. Although the addition of antibiotic agents to the cell-washing system can reduce or eliminate contaminating bacteria, some bacteria with the potential of causing systemic infection if retransfused may remain. There is a theoretical concern that malignant cells contained in retransfused blood may be responsible for generalized seeding of the malignant process. Although there are no data to support or deny this position—for medicolegal reasons at least—intraoperative autologous transfusion should be considered contraindicated in a patient with cancer unless the need is desperate. It is difficult to distinguish the hematologic changes induced by intraoperative autologous transfusion from the changes induced by hemorrhage and massive transfusion with homologous blood. Guidelines for the use of component therapy are the same for both groups.

Merrill et al. reported the use of intraoperative autotransfusion in 38 patients with ruptured ectopic pregnancy. Transfusion-related morbidity occurred in six patients; two patients developed clinical coagulopathy, two patients developed pulmonary edema, and two patients developed minor transfusion reactions from concomitantly used bank blood. The total amount of retransfused blood was 49,475 mL, or 59% of the total amount of blood administered. This saved about 90 U of banked blood.

It must be remembered that both autologous (intraoperative) and homologous blood are essentially packed red blood cells. One risk with autologous blood transfusions is forgetting that only the patient's packed cells are transfused. The patient still will need fresh-frozen plasma and platelets when massive transfusion of autologous blood is used.

Predeposit Autologous Blood Transfusion

With increasing frequency, gynecologic patients scheduled for elective surgery are asking to predeposit their own blood in the blood bank just in case a blood transfusion is needed. Experience has shown that such autologous blood can be collected and stored as whole blood, red blood cells, plasma, or platelets for retransfusion into the same patient during surgery if needed or at some other time. Donation can be scheduled at weekly intervals up to 3 days before surgery. Oral iron therapy is administered, and the hematocrit and hemoglobin levels must not be low. The American Association of Blood Banks' standards for elective preoperative autologous blood donation include the following guidelines:

- A hemoglobin of no less than 11 g/dL or a packed cell volume of no less than 34%.
- Phlebotomy no more frequently than every 3 days and not within 72 hours of surgery.

If a patient's condition is stable enough to allow elective surgery, then preoperative donation for autologous transfusion is not contraindicated. Mann et al. studied the safety of autologous blood donation before elective surgery for a variety of potentially high-risk patients. Of 300 patients in the study, 46 were at least 70 years old. Four percent of patients experienced a minor reaction to blood donation. This method of providing autologous blood should have applicability in gynecologic surgery. Experience suggests that it should be encouraged when practical.

The number of centers providing autologous blood transfusion programs will probably continue to increase as a result of AIDS and public knowledge of the possibility of spread of this disease by homologous blood transfusion, even though rare. Programs encouraging selected patients to donate their own blood before surgery are becoming increasingly popular, despite the numerous logistical problems that must be solved. Only 2% of the blood collected in the United States is for predeposit autologous transfusion.

Much of gynecologic surgery is elective, and many patients are comparatively healthy. Elective gynecologic surgery often is scheduled 3 to 4 weeks in the future. During this time, many patients can have blood predeposited for use during operation. Axelrod and associates suggest that 2 U of predeposited blood is sufficient for patients scheduled for hysterectomy. Only 10% to 20% of patients undergoing elective hysterectomy require blood transfusion, depending on the skill of the operator and the extent and nature of the gynecologic pathology.

Goodnough et al. have found that the administration of recombinant human erythropoietin increases the amount of autologous blood that can be collected before surgery. The volume of red cells donated by patients treated with erythropoietin during the study was 41% greater than that donated by patients given placebo.

BASIC SURGICAL PRINCIPLES TO AVOID EXCESSIVE BLEEDING IN PELVIC SURGERY

Bleeding caused by coagulation disorders is at the microvascular level. All the blood components used in replacement therapy cannot plug up holes in larger arteries and veins. Techniques of avoiding or controlling bleeding from pelvic vessels are most essential in efforts to reduce the risk of pelvic hemorrhage.

The following discussion will be of little importance to the seasoned pelvic surgeon, but it may be helpful to those who are learning the basic techniques of gynecologic surgery. Assuming that the patient has been properly evaluated and prepared for surgery, the judgment and skill of the surgeon will determine, to a great extent, the amount of blood that will be lost during the operation. A good medical history and physical examination are still good screening tools to assess the patient's risk for bleeding. Regardless of the thoroughness of the preoperative evaluation, visual inspection of the first and any subsequent incision alerts the surgeon to the possibility of excessive bleeding. There should be no hesitation to seek specialty support if clinically indicated.

Among the many contributions to surgery made by William S. Halsted, first chief of surgery at Johns Hopkins Hospital, was a surgical technique that emphasized meticulousness in dissection, gentleness in the handling of tissues, accuracy in hemostasis, precision in wound approximation, and absolute asepsis. This meticulous technique has become widely known in the United States as the Halstedian technique. It promotes good tissue healing by reducing tissue damage and wound infection. The accuracy of dissection, hemostasis, and tissue approximation is emphasized rather than speed, but wasting time with unnecessary hesitation, indefiniteness, and indecision can increase blood loss and infection. The experienced surgeon will be able to finish procedures in a deliberate, purposeful, timely, and precise manner. The speed with which the dissection is performed should be varied from one phase of the operation to the other, but the operation should progress in an orderly manner. For example, the incision can be fashioned with some haste, but dissection around deep pelvic veins must be performed with great caution to avoid injury and bleeding.

Although shorter operative procedures are generally associated with less blood loss and lower rates of infection, the pace of the procedure should be governed by the difficulty of the surgery and the skill and experience of the surgeon. Too much haste will sooner or later result in excessive blood loss or injury to adjacent organs or structures, which will ultimately prolong the operation. It is impossible to place too much emphasis on the need for optimum exposure to limit blood loss. During vaginal operations, a contracted pelvic outlet will limit exposure for vaginal hysterectomy. A leiomyomatous uterus may require morcellation to allow sufficient exposure for safe vaginal removal. A Schuchardt incision may be required to improve exposure during vaginal operations (see Fig. 12.32). If exposure is inadequate, bleeding from vessels in the upper broad ligament may not be controllable from below, and an abdominal incision may be necessary to achieve final hemostasis from above. During abdominal operations, the exposure achieved will depend on the choice of incision, the method of retracting, the placement and intensity of the lights, and the presence of willing and skilled assistants. Suction should be available to keep the field as free of blood as possible and is preferred over sponges for two reasons. First, sponges can cause damage to delicate serosal surfaces. Second, a determination of the amount of blood lost can be more accurate if the largest percentage has actually been suctioned into a calibrated bottle and measured. One can then add to this exact amount an estimate of the amount of blood lost on the drapes, sponges, and lap packs. The record of the amount of blood lost should be as accurate as possible and can be of great value in making correct decisions subsequently about the patient's care, especially regarding the need for blood replacement in case there is a suspicion of hypovolemia.

For pelvic laparotomy, the patient usually is placed in a modest Trendelenburg position. In this position, the packs required to keep the intestines displaced in the upper abdomen tend to stay in place better, thereby enhancing exposure. An anesthetic or muscle relaxant is needed to keep the patient from pushing her bowels into the operative field, especially when the dissection is tedious, and good exposure is mandatory for safe performance of the operation. If a hypotensive anesthetic technique is used, the amount of blood lost will be decreased. The effect of the hypotensive anesthesia on the reduction of blood loss will be enhanced if the operative field is elevated above the level of the heart, as in the Trendelenburg position. Hypotensive anesthesia, although useful in extensive operations, usually is not needed for routine major gynecologic surgery and should never be used as a substitute for hemostasis.

It usually is possible, and always desirable, to keep the number of clamps in the operative field to an absolute minimum. If the field is cluttered with clamps, the operators cannot see as well to operate. The length of the instruments must vary, depending on the thickness of the abdominal wall, the depth of the pelvis, and other variables. Pedicle clamps, tissue forceps, dissecting scissors, needle holders, and all other instruments must be longer for operations on obese patients and for extensive operations in a deep pelvis. The handles of the instruments must come all the way out and above the level of the incision so as not to interfere with the operator's view of the pelvis. There is an unfortunate tendency for gynecologic surgeons to use instruments that are too short. The operator must stand high enough to see down into the pelvis. The patient's abdominal wall should be at about the level of the operator's umbilicus, not too high or too low.

Cushing, a neurosurgeon, introduced the hemostatic silver metal clip in 1908 to occlude cranial vessels inaccessible to ligation. More recently, clips have been made of stainless steel, tantalum, and the new synthetic absorbable nonopaque polydioxanone polymer. The latter has the advantage of not causing the streaked artifact of metal clips when subsequent computed tomography (CT) of the pelvis is performed. Clips cause little tissue reaction, usually are easily and rapidly applied, and provide secure control of bleeding vessels in relatively inaccessible places in the pelvis where ligation would be more difficult. A small vessel can be quickly occluded with a clip even before the vessel is cut, thus keeping the field dry and the tissues to be dissected free of blood staining. Clips are especially useful in retroperitoneal dissections. They are available in several sizes. Disposable applicators loaded with multiple clips are available, obviating the need for reloading and facilitating rapid use. If appropriately used, clips can reduce blood loss, facilitate dissection, and reduce operating time.

Working with Bovie, Cushing also pioneered the use of electrocautery for surgical hemostasis. Modern electrosurgical units are radiofrequency generators that supply 500,000 to 2 million Hz of alternating current to the tip of the electrode. The amount of current is preselected by the surgeon. It rapidly dissipates throughout the body and returns to the unit through the ground plate, which provides a large surface area of contact over a heavy muscle mass, usually the anterior surface of the thigh. Failure to properly secure the ground plate can cause burns at the grounding pad or other sites, as the current is inefficiently grounded resulting in thermal effects.

The surgeon can use the electrocautery for dissection of tissues by setting it on the "cutting" current and for hemostasis by setting it on the "coagulation" current. The needle-point electrode can be used for precise monopolar cautery of small vessels. The tissue surrounding the site of monopolar cautery, however, is damaged to a greater extent than necessary. If the vessel is grasped with a fine-pointed clamp or forceps, hemostasis is achieved by a low-current bipolar cautery and excess tissue necrosis is avoided, because the current will pass between the two points of the forceps or clamp grasping the vessel. This method of hemostasis is quick and convenient. Used properly, it can cause less tissue necrosis than that of ligatures. Experience in its use will result in maximum efficiency with minimum tissue damage, and a shorter operating time. The principles of electrosurgical technique are discussed fully in Chapter 13.

With a thorough knowledge of pelvic anatomy, the surgeon, during dissection, should emphasize the development of pelvic planes and spaces. This will avoid unnecessary bleeding and allow more accurate placement of clamps on vessels. Certain parts of the dissection can be delayed until later, especially if they are not needed now and blood loss is likely to be increased. For example, when abdominal hysterectomy is performed, dissection of the bladder away from the cervix and vagina may be associated with blood loss and should not be performed at the beginning of the operation. Exposure of the anterior lower uterine segment and cervix is not required until the uterine vessels and broad ligament need to be clamped. This is, therefore, the time to "take the bladder down."

Even simple maneuvers can reduce blood loss. When a cervical conization is performed, the cervical stroma should be injected with a vasoconstrictive agent such as dilute epinephrine, pitressin, or plain sterile saline solution. If a quantity sufficient to actually distend and blanch the cervix is used, an internal tourniquet is created, constricting and compressing small vessels and reducing the amount of blood loss. The posterior cervical incision should be made first. If the anterior incision is made first and bleeding is profuse, it will be difficult to see the posterior cervical lip and to make an accurate incision, which may further increase blood loss. When vaginal hysterectomy is performed, dilute epinephrine or saline can be injected beneath the vaginal mucosa to decrease persistent mucosal bleeding and to help identify the correct plane for dissection. A needle-point attachment to the electrosurgical unit can be used to make the incision and to precisely coagulate any small bleeding vessels as they are encountered. When the incision in the posterior vagina is finished, the same technique can be used to incise the anterior vaginal mucosa behind the anterior cervical lip. The same technique will reduce the amount of blood lost in anterior colporrhaphy. This operation is a good example of a procedure in which the amount of blood lost will depend, to a large extent, on the time required to complete the procedure, because bleeding from paravesical veins cannot always be controlled with sutures or coagulation. In this situation, the surgeon is encouraged to finish the operation quickly and to control the continued venous oozing with a pack placed tightly in the vagina against the anterior wall. The pack should be removed in 24 hours.

In the early days of abdominal pelvic surgery, in the 19th century, postoperative hemorrhage was common because an effective technique of hemostasis was not known. The usual method of performing abdominal hysterectomy involved use of a ligature en masse around the lower uterus. This mass ligature saved time and was used to occlude both uterine and ovarian vessels simultaneously. The uterine corpus with adnexa attached was simply amputated above the ligature. The stump thus formed was such a large mass of tissue that it could not be safely returned to the peritoneal cavity because of the danger of intraperitoneal bleeding. Therefore, sometimes the stump was fixed extraperitoneally in the incision, so that it was available for hemostatic clamping if the need arose. It was not until 1889 that Stimson published a technique for secure individual ligation of the uterine and ovarian vessels that was responsible for significantly reducing the incidence of postoperative hemorrhage. Kelly published a similar technique with illustrations in 1891.

In abdominal operations today, all major vascular pedicles should be individually ligated twice. Delayed-absorbable sutures should be used and the knots firmly tied. Catgut suture knots tend to swell and come apart

in tissue fluid. If vessels can be skeletonized (as with uterine vessels), ligation will be more secure. A vascular pedicle where the tip of the clamp is free, such as the infundibulopelvic ligament, should always be ligated first with a free tie to occlude the vessels. Hemostasis is then secured with a transfixion suture ligature placed between the previous free tie and the clamp. This technique avoids hematoma formation and the rare occurrence of a traumatic arteriovenous fistula. If a suture ligature is to be held long for traction or later identification, there is a danger that it will become loosened or be pulled off, with a resulting hematoma or bleeding. Sutures used to ligate vessels should be cut and never held for traction for that reason. During vaginal hysterectomy, the upper broad ligament containing the uteroovarian ligament and the fallopian tube should be doubly clamped. The lateral-most clamp is replaced by a free tie completely around the pedicle. Tied tightly, this ligature compresses the vessels in the pedicle so that the most medial clamp (the one closest to the uterus) can then be replaced with a suture ligature placed through the pedicle, passed around the tip of the clamp both ways and tied tightly around the pedicle. This is one vascular ligature that can be held long for identification and traction with minimal risk of bleeding.

"The finer the suture, the finer the surgeon" is an aphorism that is associated with meticulous surgical technique. The aphorism is good advice, up to a point. The newer delayed-absorbable sutures are strong, and smaller-gauge sutures are strong enough to ligate vessels. However, it is dangerous to use suture that is too small to maintain its tensile strength long enough to ensure permanent hemostasis, and newer absorbable sutures cause relatively little tissue reaction. Fine needle with small sutures are useful for controlling venous or arterial bleeding, but larger suture with bigger bites are less likely to pull through infected or malignant tissue. Proper suture selection for the specific technique and patient is an important part of obtaining the best result from any given surgical procedure.

The use of microfibrillar collagen for the local control of diffuse venous oozing that is usually associated with malignancy or infection has been used with some success. This bovine collagen material can be applied directly and compressed against an area of a small bleeding vessel. It acts as a fibrin nidus to accelerate thrombus formation on the surface of the vessel. It will only control bleeding from a small arteriole or venule. Caution must be exercised in the use of this material because it can produce secondary fibrosis in the pelvis and even a persistent palpable mass. There have been reports of retroperitoneal fibrosis and ureteral obstruction secondary to the use of this material. These sequelae have cautioned the pelvic surgeon against applying this agent near the ureter. When it is used in other sites, we have found fewer adverse reactions. If a localized hemostatic agent is considered necessary, the use of Gelfoam or topical thrombin may prove more efficacious with less fibrosis. More important, the surgeon should not rely on any agent for control of a significant amount of arterial or venous bleeding. Instead, every effort should be made to identify the bleeding vessel and to occlude it with either a hemoclip or a ligature.

In one case of severe bleeding from deep pelvic veins, we were successful in finally controlling the bleeding with multiple layers (sandwiches) of Gelfoam and Avitene cut to appropriate size from sheets and stacked one on top of the other. If coagulation factors have been depleted because of multiple transfusions, the Gelfoam can be soaked in thrombin. When the material is applied, the field should be as dry as possible. Constant pressure can be applied by placing sutures that can be tied on top of the sandwiches.

Malviya and Deppe have reported the successful use of fibrin glue, a biodegradable tissue adhesive and sealant and topical hemostatic agent, to control life-threatening hemorrhage in one obstetric and two gynecologic patients. The fibrin glue is prepared from equal amounts of cryoprecipitate (highly concentrated human fibrinogen) and bovine thrombin. It imitates the last stages of physiologic coagulation at the local site. Equal volumes are drawn into separate syringes and applied directly to the bleeding site in a field as dry as possible. A firm rubbery clot is formed in 2 minutes. This technique has been used successfully in microvascular, cardiovascular, and thoracic surgical procedures and has recently been effective in controlling hemorrhage in liver transplantation. It should be helpful in extensive pelvic dissections for gynecologic cancer, especially to control low-pressure pelvic vein bleeding that is not controllable by other standard measures.

Gynecologic surgeons usually do not have the luxury of using tourniquets to control bleeding. There are, however, two special procedures in which tourniquets have been used to advantage. These are myomectomy and uterine unification operations. The tourniquet is fashioned in the manner used by vascular, thoracic, and trauma surgeons to occlude major vessels. A medium-sized soft plastic tube or rubber drain is used and threaded through a 4-in length of a 22F or 24F soft red rubber catheter. A tourniquet loop can be placed around the uterine isthmus through a small hole made in the broad ligament just lateral to the uterine vessels. Loops also can be placed around both infundibulopelvic ligaments through the same hole in the broad ligament. When these are snugged down tightly and held with a Kelly clamp, the entire circulation to the uterus can be occluded. The sterile Doptone can be used to ensure that arterial pulsations have disappeared completely. This technique can reduce blood loss to a minimum in these two procedures, especially when hypotensive anesthesia is used. Similarly, vessel loops can be used when repairing defects in the walls of large pelvic vessels.

Unnecessary bleeding in the area of dissection stains tissues, obscures visibility, restricts technical freedom, and gradually adds up to a significant amount of blood loss that may require replacement. Reducing the circulation to the operative field by deliberate induction of hypotension is a safe and effective anesthetic technique in properly selected patients. Hypotensive anesthesia is not recommended for most routine gynecologic surgery. The technique requires planning and cooperation between the surgeon and the anesthesiologist. A reduction in arteriolar resistance will lower blood pressure and reduce, to a certain degree, bleeding in the operative field. The main mechanism for control of operative field bleeding with hypotensive anesthesia is the reduction of venous tone, which reduces ventricular filling and cardiac output, the major determinants of blood pressure. The desired reduction in venous tone is achieved by one or more of the following anesthetic techniques: ganglionic blockade; spinal or epidural anesthesia; specific venodilating agents, such as sodium nitroprusside or glyceryl trinitrate; and some anesthetic agents. Induced hypotension is more effective if the operative field is raised above the level of the heart to encourage local venous emptying by gravity. For this purpose, a modest Trendelenburg position should be used.

Deliberate hypotension is now an established practice, although some anesthesiologists are more enthusiastic about its use than others, and they must be trained in the technique to use it safely. It has been most effective in operations on the head, face, neck, and upper thorax. Our experience with its use in extensive pelvic dissections for malignant disease has been uniformly favorable. The blood loss in radical hysterectomy can be reduced by 50% or more, and the need for blood replacement can be reduced by a corresponding amount. In a report by Powell et al., a deliberate hypotensive technique using nitroglycerin and general anesthesia decreased the blood loss in extensive hysterectomy and pelvic lymphadenectomy by 70% when compared with a control group. The percentage of patients requiring blood transfusion was reduced from 81% to 11.5%. Also, according to Yamasaki et al., the simultaneous use of autotransfusion and autologous blood transfusion was effective in reducing the need for homologous blood transfusion. There is no doubt that deliberate hypotension is a valuable technique, but it cannot be a substitute for careful surgical hemostasis. "Reactionary hemorrhage," bleeding that occurs after the blood pressure returns to normal, will present problems unless hemostasis is meticulous.

Whenever an extensive pelvic dissection is anticipated, preparations should be made in advance in case pelvic hemorrhage is suddenly encountered. Adequate quantities of blood should be available to replace lost volume. More blood should be requested in advance of its need. A responsible member of the operating team or anesthesia team should be asked to monitor blood loss, blood replacement, and urine output. In the excitement of the moment, it is possible to lose count of the number of units of whole blood, blood components, crystalloids, and other fluids that have been given, and how much blood has been lost. A dependable route for administering blood must be maintained. Without it, blood replacement is not possible. All other physiologic functions (e.g., blood pressure, pulse, central venous pressure, blood gases, hematocrit values) should be carefully monitored. If massive hemorrhage occurs, or even if a possibility of its occurrence exists, a Swan-Ganz catheter should be placed for better control of volume replacement. For extreme cases in which no other vessels are available intraoperatively, transfusions can be given under pressure directly into the common iliac artery or aorta.

INTRAOPERATIVE MEASURES TO CONTROL PELVIC HEMORRHAGE

Despite adequate technical skills and careful dissection, serious hemorrhage can suddenly complicate almost any operative procedure. These occasions call for a maximum use of a surgeon's knowledge, technical ability, and leadership to produce a happy outcome. The first task is to control the hemorrhage. A finger should immediately be placed on the bleeding point for prompt, atraumatic control with pressure. When the blood has been suctioned out and the fingertip exposed, it may be gently rolled off the bleeding point while a fine tipped clamp of adequate length is poised to clamp the bleeding vessel and suction is ready to provide exposure. In most instances, this will adequately control the hemorrhage, although it is often necessary to place another clamp, clip or suture adjacent to the first clamp in order to control the other side of the lacerated vessel or other nearby bleeders. It is most important to avoid placing too many clamps in the area because this will obscure the bleeding site and cause additional trauma to the vessels. Multiple sutures and/or clips may also cause more bleeding and can injure adjacent structures such as the ureter, bladder, pelvic vessels, and nerves. Cautery should not be used to attempt to control significant bleeding. It will only cause increased bleeding and more tissue injury.

If an immediate attempt to control the hemorrhage by simple means is unsuccessful, the bleeding should be controlled again with pressure, either with a fingertip, a sponge forceps, or occasionally by packing. The surgeon should step back, take a deep breath, and carefully consider the situation. The anesthesiologist should be made aware of the situation and consulted about the patient's stability, blood loss up to this point, availability of blood for transfusion, intravenous lines, and so forth. The anesthesiologist will play an important role in fluid and blood replacement, monitoring coagulation factors and ensuring perfusion of vital organs. Therefore, it is important that he or she be fully aware of the situation and an active participant in such decisions as how long to safely continue surgery. The anticipated difficulty in controlling the hemorrhage must be honestly evaluated, and the patient's overall condition and the planned operative procedures should be considered and discussed with the surgical team. If additional suction or instruments are needed, they should be requested. If additional or more experienced assistants or additional scrub and/or circulating nurses are needed, they should be requested. Would it be helpful to have your partner, a gynecologic oncologist, a urologist, a general surgeon, or a vascular surgeon scrub in? They are probably not immediately available, so it is important to request their help sooner rather than later.

If the patient is stable and any necessary equipment such as a second suction, deeper retractors, or hemoclips have been readied, it is reasonable to reconsider the anatomy, obtain good exposure, and have another try at controlling the bleeding. If you are lucky, the 10 minutes or so that the hemorrhage has been controlled by pressure will result in a substantial reduction in the bleeding. Perhaps the vessel or bleeding site can be more clearly seen and controlled with a clamp and a few small sutures or a clip or two. Arterial bleeding in the pelvis usually is easily controlled. The vessels have thick walls and are not easily torn further. Blood spurting from the vessel leads to its easy identification. If the artery can be clamped, it usually can be ligated, a clip can be applied, or both. If an artery has mostly retracted from view with only one small edge still visible, that edge may be grasped with a clamp and gently twisted, thus decreasing the amount of bleeding sufficiently to allow clipping or ligation. Venous hemorrhage in the pelvis may be a much more difficult problem. Such bleeding can vary in magnitude from a trivial ooze to life-threatening hemorrhage. Pelvic veins can be fragile, tortuous, hidden from view, and distended. Blood returning through the lacerated vein can come from multiple deeper sources that are unavailable for ligation. Placing clamps and sutures blindly is dangerous and can even make the problem worse. Electrocoagulation of a laceration in a large vein should not be attempted because it will inevitably result in a larger hole that will be even more difficult to secure. Sometimes the best procedure is to hold a finger against the bleeding site for a minimum of 7 minutes, after which the bleeding may stop or be easily controlled in other ways. Digital pressure to control venous bleeding takes advantage of the fact that the pressure in pelvic veins is very low. The initial use of digital pressure also is less likely to cause further tearing and trauma to the vein. Sometimes additional careful dissection in the area is required to free the vessel above and below, to allow more precise ligation or clipping. A long, finely pointed instrument is used to clamp the vessel, and clips are placed on each side. If the vessel can be sufficiently liberated, another instrument is gently slipped beneath the first one so that its point is free. Then a fine ligature is placed around the clamp. If necessary, clips can also be placed on each side of the tie.

If the bleeding has still not been controlled at this point or if bleeding cannot be controlled by pressure on the bleeding site, consultation should be requested to get additional help or expertise. By this time, the surgeon may feel frustrated, and it is important to maintain control of the operation and the surgical team. Blood and clotting factors should be replaced as discussed earlier in this chapter, the patient kept warm, and the whole situation reevaluated with input from all members of the team. The surgeon must maintain a positive outlook and exert good judgment and leadership. Good leadership involves using the skills and ideas of each member of the surgical team. Good judgment involves knowing which ideas to use, when to use them, and when to ask for help.

SPECIAL SITUATIONS AND TECHNIQUES

Pararectal Space

When dissecting in the pelvis, one should avoid making a deep hole with a bottom that cannot be exposed, in case a deep vein might be lacerated. For example, development of the pararectal space must be done carefully because of the danger of injuring deep veins. The space is developed between the ureter and the hypogastric artery. The dissection is directed posteriorly at first but soon changes to a more caudal direction. Failure to make this directional change results in laceration and bleeding from veins in the bottom of the space. If development of the pararectal space is difficult, it should not be forced.

Aortic Area

The removal of lymph nodes around the aorta and vena cava can result in serious hemorrhage from either vessel if not done carefully and with adequate exposure. An incision that provides sufficient exposure for a routine pelvic operation is not ordinarily sufficient for dissection around the aorta and vena cava unless it can be extended. A laceration in the aorta must be repaired. The aorta cannot be ligated without serious consequences. Although the vena cava usually can be ligated without serious problems, a laceration in the vena cava should be repaired by placing a finger over it and gaining the necessary exposure by retraction and suctioning. Continuous no. 5-0 Prolene suture is used to close the laceration from side to side as the finger is slowly withdrawn. The same technique can be used to repair lacerations in other large veins, such as the common and external iliac veins. These two veins usually can be ligated with no untoward results, but we prefer to repair the laceration if possible, and it usually is possible. Lacerations of the common and external iliac arteries must always be repaired. These vessels cannot be ligated without serious consequences. If the laceration is not repairable, the artery must be replaced.

Iliac Vessels

One of the most dangerous places in the pelvis to dissect is in the region of the bifurcation of the common iliac artery and vein. This is the "axilla" of the pelvis, where many lymph nodes that drain the cervix are found. The hypogastric vein and its branches are at risk of injury when dissecting between the distal common iliac artery and the psoas muscle and deeper in the area of lumbosacral nerve trunks. When the surgeon pulls on surrounding areolar tissue, a relatively loose and thin-walled vein may inadvertently be pulled into the scissor dissection. The vein wall may not be distinct, especially when the tissue is blood-stained. One is wise to proceed cautiously. Furious hemorrhage threatening exsanguination can result from laceration of either the external iliac vein or the hypogastric vein where they join together, or from laceration of their major branches in the area. On the medial side of these veins, the lateral sacral veins disappear into the sacral foramina. Fatal hemorrhage can result from laceration of these vessels. They cannot be clamped and ligated. They cannot be clipped. They are kept open by their attachment to the walls of the foramina. Extreme measures usually are needed to control the bleeding. One can try to pack the foramen with bone wax, but this usually is not successful. Alternatively, multiple layers (sandwiches) of absorbable gelatin sponge (Gelfoam) and microfibrillar collagen (Avitene) can be tightly sewn over the foramen. This area deserves its reputation as the "corona mortis" of the pelvis.

Numerous variations in the branches of the hypogastric artery and vein are encountered in dissecting the obturator fossa, especially in the floor of the fossa. The "web" of paracervical tissue separating the paravesical and pararectal spaces contains branches of the hypogastric artery and vein. These vessels must be carefully ligated with clips or sutures during a radical hysterectomy. The dissection can be carried to the depths of the paravesical space and pararectal space by carefully ligating or clipping each vessel encountered. The obturator artery and vein are usually found just below the obturator nerve. In a radical hysterectomy or even a pelvic exenteration, these vessels are usually not disturbed. If injured, they may be ligated or clipped. If these vessels are allowed to retract through the obturator foramen into the upper thigh without being ligated, bleeding into the thigh may be a significant problem.

In the presacral region, bleeding usually can be avoided by choosing a plane of dissection that is superficial to the anterior sacral artery and vein. The retrorectal space is easily entered and developed inferiorly to the tip and lateral margins of the sacrum without appreciable bleeding, provided the dissection is carefully made with the hand and in the correct plane superficial to the presacral fascia and the vessels that overlie the periosteum of the sacrum. Timmons et al. and Khan and Fang have recommended using metal thumbtacks to control presacral hemorrhage when the usual methods fail. Sterilized metal thumbtacks are placed directly over the bleeding point in the presacral fascia and pushed all the way into the sacrum with the thumb. An intercommunicating network of presacral veins is protected by a covering layer of presacral fascia. Bleeding from the veins can be aggravated by clips, ligatures, or cautery. Packs, hemostatic agents, and thumbtacks are more effective in controlling the bleeding in this area.

Laparoscopic Vascular Injury

In a prospective series of 1,033 patients who underwent gynecologic laparoscopy, the most frequent complication (48%) was vascular injury. Many of these injuries occurred during blind insertion of the laparoscopic trocar. Although the majority of these injuries are minor hematomas in the abdominal wall or mesentery, major injury to the vena cave, aorta, and pelvic vessels have been reported including several fatalities. Although experienced laparoscopic surgeons may be able to manage bleeding from the ovarian vessels or more minor vascular injuries via laparoscopy, major injuries require immediate exploratory laparotomy with appropriate vascular repair techniques and consultation as necessary. As noted earlier, immediate pressure on the aorta, vena cava, or iliac vessels will usually control bleeding and provide time for the patient to be stabilized. These major vessels should not be ligated but repaired or, if necessary, replaced by a graft.

In rare cases, standard techniques of pressure, clipping, ligation, or application of hemostatic agents is unsuccessful for controlling bleeding. Several techniques may be considered in these cases. Trauma surgeons will occasionally pack persistent venous bleeding and close the abdomen when the procedure has been prolonged and/or the patient is unstable. The patient is then operated on again in 24 to 48 hours when coagulation factors and blood volume have been normalized and everyone is refreshed. In some cases, the packing can be brought out through a large, hollow, soft rubber drain placed in a separate incisions in the abdominal walls. The packing can then be removed through the drain in 48 hours under a light general anesthesia without opening the abdomen. If bleeding persists, it can sometimes be controlled by vascular embolization by the interventional radiologist.

POSTOPERATIVE BLEEDING

With normal hemostasis and proper surgical technique, postoperative hemorrhage is a rare occurrence. Every patient, however, should be carefully monitored postoperatively for signs of occult bleeding. The intensity and duration of the monitoring will depend on the type of surgery and the medical condition of the patient. In addition to measuring the vital signs such as pulse, blood pressure, and urine output, the abdominal incision and/or the perineum should be inspected for bleeding. Any sign of restlessness in the patient may be an indication of blood loss. A hematocrit can be checked if there is a suspicion of postoperative bleeding or anemia. Because the risk of postoperative hemorrhage is so low, many experts do not recommend routinely checking the hematocrit or hemoglobin postoperatively; but a hematocrit 8 to 12 hours postop may be helpful for radical surgery, patients with intraoperative hemorrhage, or patients who were not "dusty dry" when the abdomen was closed.

Occult intraperitoneal bleeding is one of the most serious postoperative complications after abdominal or vaginal surgery. It usually does not become evident suddenly in the recovery room. The vital signs in the recovery room may remain stable. Indeed, the vital signs may be stable for 12 to 18 hours after the operation is completed, and then suddenly severe hypotension, tachycardia, tachypnea, restlessness, and abdominal distention lead to a diagnosis of intraperitoneal hemorrhage that has actually been developing slowly since surgery. In most cases, a small vessel has been slowly bleeding since surgery; only after a significant blood loss has occurred, do changes in the vital signs or symptoms of abdominal distention alert the clinician to a problem.

The diagnosis of intraperitoneal bleeding in the postoperative patient can be difficult. Peritoneal signs are subtle and can be masked by incisional pain and analgesic medications. Unfortunately, the initial examination of the abdomen may be quite benign. The peritoneal cavity has an enormous capacity for occult blood loss without appreciable abdominal distention. As much as 3,000 mL of blood (about 65% of the total blood volume of a 70-kg person) can be hidden in the peritoneal cavity, with only a 1-cm increase in the radius of the abdomen. Occult intraperitoneal hemorrhage is even more serious when one considers that the postoperative patient may not have had replacement of all the blood that was lost at the initial operation and may already be hypovolemic when she reaches the recovery room. Although peritoneal lavage can be performed with a blunt Tuohy needle placed through the abdominal wall in a lower abdominal quadrant of a distended abdomen in the recovery room or on the ward, abdominal ultrasound is a rapid, noninvasive, readily available method of confirming the diagnosis of intraperitoneal bleeding.

Sometimes it is difficult for the surgeon who performed the original operation to convince himself or herself that bleeding is persistent and intervention is urgently needed. Sometimes a consult with a colleague will be helpful. There may be a temptation to blame the coagulation system and look for some defect in clotting factors. A routine coagulation profile, ordered at the first suspicion, or even simple observation of clot formation in a tube of blood at the bedside will eliminate this possibility. However, the experienced surgeon knows that the most common reason for intraperitoneal blood and postoperative shock is loss of surgical hemostasis—a vessel has become disligated. The question now becomes should the patient be immediately operated on again to identify and control the bleeding vessels or taken to the radiology suite in an attempt to control the bleeding by intraarterial embolization. Both techniques are highly effective, and we have generally used the stability of the patient as a guide. For instance, if the patient is unstable with a rapid pulse, falling blood pressure, and/or low urine output, or if the interval since surgery is short, suggesting fairly rapid hemorrhage, we would prefer to quickly return to the operating room where we have a team of anesthesiologists and often other personnel to monitor the patient, assist with blood replacement, and treat hemorrhagic shock. On the other hand, if the patient is stable and bleeding does not appear too brisk based on time from surgery and the volume of blood in the abdomen or retroperitoneal space by ultrasound estimate, then it is reasonable to try to identify the bleeding vessel and embolize the arterial supply by transcatheter interventional radiological techniques.

Whichever plan is selected, one or more large bore intravenous lines should be started, and fluid replacement should begin with packed red blood cells ordered and started as indicated and available. A Foley catheter should be inserted and urine output monitored. Broad-spectrum antibiotics should be started. If the patient is not in the recovery room, she should be transferred there or to a monitored bed with easy access to the operating room. Preop labs should be obtained, and the operating room and anesthesia service should be notified, as well as the interventional radiology team if appropriate.

Arterial Embolization

In 1969, Nusbaum et al. described this method to control bleeding from esophageal varices by selectively cannulating the superior mesenteric artery and infusing small doses of vasopressin into terminal vessels. The subsequent use of particulate matter to achieve hemostasis within bleeding viscera developed rapidly. Its use in the control of pelvic and postoperative bleeding was popularized by Anthanasoulis and associates. It has been used effectively to treat patients with severe bleeding after hysterectomy (Sproule et al.; Teichmann et al.) and patients with a variety of other gynecologic problems, including gestational trophoblastic disease (Pearl and Braga), uterine arteriovenous malformation, vulvar hemangioma, and ovarian vein syndrome (Abbas et al.). It has been used by Simon et al. to control bleeding from cervical pregnancy and by Martin et al. to control bleeding from abdominal pregnancy. Its use in the management of bleeding in patients with recurrent and advanced gynecologic cancer is well documented by Harima et al., Pisco et al., Anthanasoulis and coworkers, and many others. It was formerly used as the initial procedure in patients who were bleeding and were poor surgical risks for additional major surgery while in the hypotensive state. In particular, patients with cardiopulmonary compromise or debilitating disease and elderly patients can develop more serious complications if another surgical procedure is undertaken when they are in a precarious hemodynamic state. Experience has shown that selective pelvic artery embolization is a comparatively simple and safe procedure. Dramatic results can be seen. Clinical success rates of more than 90% are routinely reported when embolization is used for postsurgical and posttraumatic hemorrhage. Therefore, embolization rather than surgery ligation is appropriately selected as the primary procedure to control bleeding in patients who are stable or who cannot tolerate another operation.

After embolization, patients usually have no complications or evidence of the effects of local ischemia. Those who have not had a hysterectomy will resume normal menstruation. Some patients will exhibit evidence of a mild postembolization syndrome, including discomfort, fever, leukocytosis resulting from vascular thrombosis, and tissue necrosis. A few isolated cases of more serious problems have been reported, including bladder necrosis, vesicovaginal fistula, neuropathies, and renal toxicity from the contrast medium. The overall complication rate should be less than 10%.

The method of intravascular embolization is quite simple, although it requires the expertise of a skilled interventional radiologist. Percutaneous catheterization of the femoral artery under local anesthesia provides direct

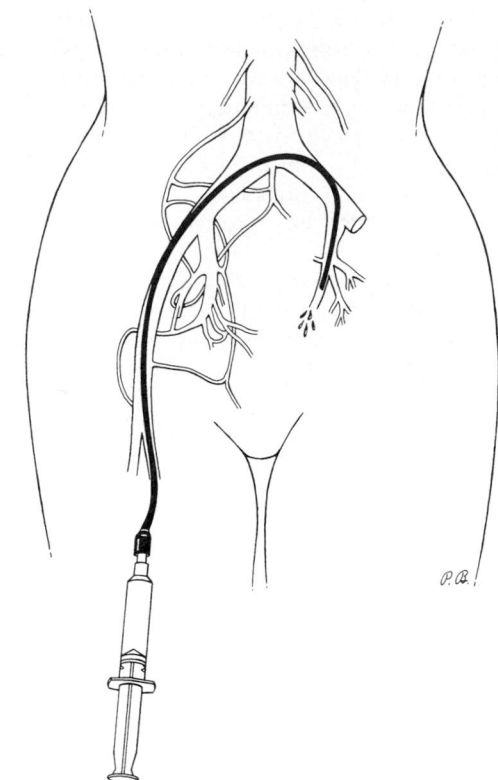

FIGURE 18.5. The femoral artery can be catheterized under local anesthesia to provide access to the hypogastric artery and its branches.

access in a retrograde manner to the hypogastric artery (Fig. 18.5). The brachial artery can also be used for access to the vascular system. If prior hypogastric artery ligation has obstructed this pathway, arteriography of the pelvic vasculature through one of the collateral arteries usually localizes the specific bleeding vessel or vessels, although with greater difficulty. The site of bleeding can be accurately identified with angiography and fluoroscopy if the rate of bleeding is 2 to 3 mL per minute or more at the bleeding site. The hypogastric artery or the specific collateral vessel is cannulated for injection (Fig. 18.6). If the bleeding vessel is a vein, venous access for embolization can be obtained through the femoral vein or antecubital vein.

A variety of materials can be used for embolization, including small pieces of Gelfoam, metal coils, autologous clot, subcutaneous tissue, small Silastic spheres, and other hemostatic materials. Gelfoam is one of the most practical and easily injected materials. It is sterile, is nonantigenic, remains in the vessel for 20 to 50 days, and forms a fibrin mesh framework on which blood clots can develop. Its immediate effect is to obstruct the distal artery or arteriole and reduce pulse pressure in the bleeding vessel, thereby permitting clot formation and cessation of bleeding. Material is injected under angiographic observation. When it becomes evident by repeat angiography that the bleeding vessel has been occluded, the catheter is removed and the patient is carefully monitored for evidence of further bleeding.

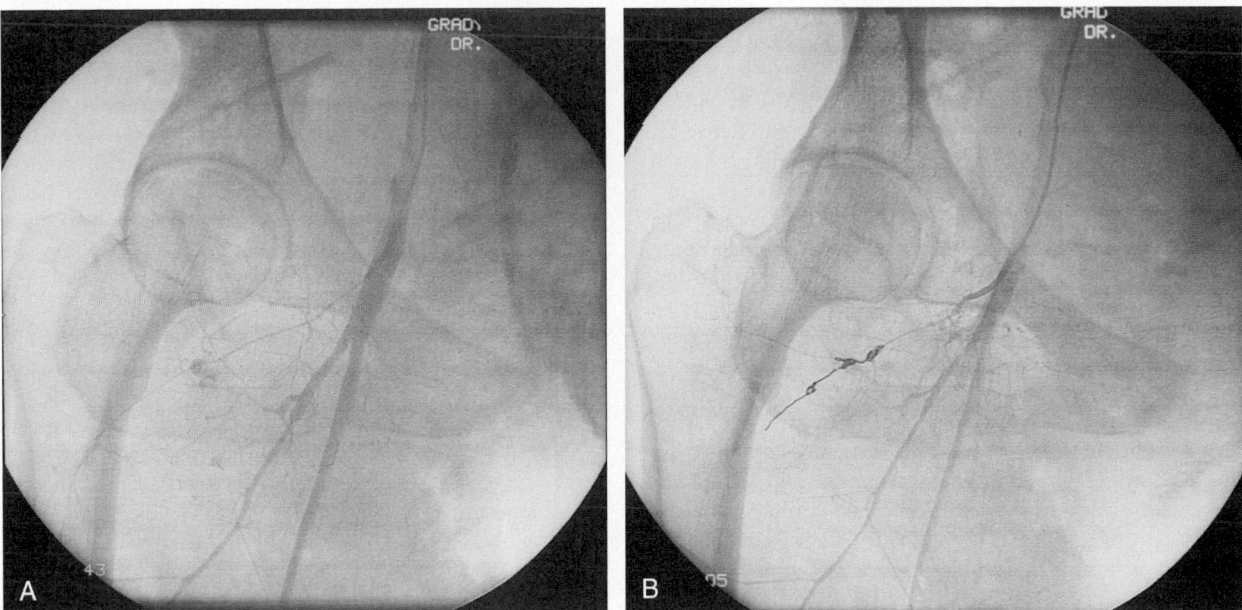

FIGURE 18.6. A: Pelvic angiography demonstrates bleeding from the obturator artery. **B:** Embolization of the artery stops the bleeding.

Selective angiographic arterial embolization has been used to control hemorrhage after abdominal and vaginal hysterectomy and other gynecologic operations, hemorrhage from cervical cancer and gestational trophoblastic disease, postpartum hemorrhage, hemorrhage from abdominal pregnancy, and retroperitoneal hemorrhage. In 1989, O'Hanlan et al. reported the results of embolotherapy in six patients whose postoperative hemorrhage was associated with pelvic surgery. The arterial embolization achieved hemostasis in three patients. The remaining three patients required reoperation for final hemostasis. The investigators point out that in each of the cases that required reoperation, the information obtained by arteriography directed the surgeon immediately and precisely to the site of bleeding, thus expeditiously facilitating the control of bleeding. Posttreatment fever with positive blood cultures in two patients suggested the advisability of prophylactic antibiotics.

Life-threatening pelvic hemorrhage from multiple sites and uncontrollable by standard means can be promptly controlled by direct intraoperative embolization of the hypogastric artery on one side, or on both sides if the bleeding is bilateral, as reported by Saueracker et al. (Fig. 18.7).

Reoperation

If reoperation is selected, the patient should be as stable as possible, with blood running or at least available in the room. Two suctions should be ready and an adequate staff and assistants involved. If the patient has previously had an abdominal operation, the incision should be reopened. A preoperative ultrasound should have identified the bleeding as intraperitoneal or retroperitoneal. The previous procedure should be mentally reviewed to

identify any possible ligatures that were tentative or any troublesome bleeding sites that may have continued to bleed. When the abdomen is opened, the clots should be evacuated and a search instituted for the bleeding sites, starting with the most likely locations. Care should be taken when removing clots from the pelvic area.

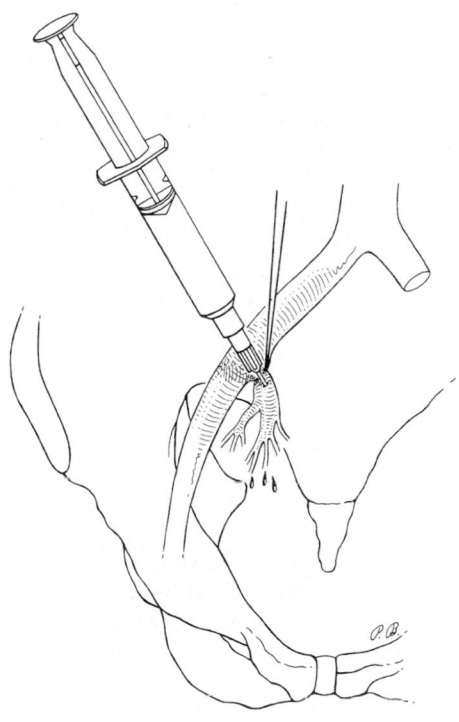

FIGURE 18.7. After the hypogastric artery is ligated, embolization of distal bleeding vessels can be accomplished by direct intraarterial injection below the site of ligation.

Bleeding sites should be carefully ligated, sutured, or clipped. It is not unusual to reopen the abdomen and find no active bleeding sites. This is somewhat disconcerting because of the concern that the problem will repeat itself after the abdomen is again closed. Every attempt should be made to get the pelvis and abdomen completely dry before closing.

During reoperation, patients are at increased risk of ureteral injury. In addition to exercising care in clamping and ligating blood-stained tissue with distorted anatomy, it may be wise to prove ureteral integrity at the end of the operation. This can be done by injecting 5 mL of indigo carmine dye intravenously and observing efflux of dye from each ureteral orifice through the cystoscope or by opening the bladder dome (see Chapter 38). After reoperation, such patients are at increased risk of developing postoperative complications, such as pulmonary atelectasis, abdominal distention from ileus, postoperative infection, incisional complications, and coagulation disorders from multiple transfusions. The anticipation of these complications allows the adoption of measures to prevent or manage them correctly should they occur.

Postoperative hemorrhage from the vaginal vault usually comes from the vaginal artery in the lateral vaginal fornix, or from one of its branches. Most often, the lateral vaginal angle, including the vaginal artery, is not properly secured or becomes disligated. To prevent such bleeding, the lateral vaginal angle stitch should be anchored in tissue lateral to the angle so that the angle cannot slip out. This stitch should not be held for traction because it can become loose. Excessive vaginal bleeding may be noted in the recovery room or after the patient has returned to her room. Every attempt should be made to establish an objective measurement of the amount of blood lost, and to follow vital signs and changes in hematocrit values. One must realize that the vagina is a distensible organ. If a clot occludes the vaginal introitus, a large amount of blood—sometimes several hundred milliliters—can distend the vagina behind it and not be evident on a perineal pad. When significant vaginal bleeding is present, the patient should be returned to the operating room. Sometimes adequate examination can be performed with analgesia alone, but anesthesia should be used if necessary. The vaginal apex should be inspected. If the bleeding point can be seen, it should be clamped and ligated from below. Figure-of-eight no. 0 or 00 delayed-absorbable transfixion sutures should be placed to include the vaginal mucosa and underlying paravaginal tissue. Care must be taken to avoid the inadvertent placement of a suture into the musculature of the bladder wall, the ureter, or the underlying rectum. If bleeding is not controlled by this technique, it is unwise to continue to add suture on suture in a frantic effort to control the vaginal bleeding. In such cases, it is probable that the bleeding vessels have retracted well above the vaginal apex and cannot be reached by this approach.

If surgical hemostasis cannot be achieved transvaginally, laparotomy may be necessary. A vaginal pack will not control significant bleeding from the vaginal vault that has already required a return to the operating room, although a temporary pack may be used while the patient is prepared for laparotomy. In some patients, the hemorrhage will be delayed until 10 to 14 days after surgery, when the sutures lose their tensile strength. Posthysterectomy disruption of the vaginal vault with hemorrhage also can result from coitus, as reported by Hacker et al. Their two cases occurred 2 and 8 weeks after total abdominal hysterectomy. In one case, the blood loss was 2,500 mL, and ligation of the hypogastric, ovarian, and uterine vessels was required to control the hemorrhage.

Bleeding from anterior and posterior colporrhaphy usually is from veins that have not been secured. A fairly tight vaginal pack effectively compresses these vessels and controls the bleeding. It seldom is necessary to reexplore an anterior or posterior colporrhaphy to locate and ligate a specific bleeding vessel. The patient will feel an uncomfortable sensation of urgency of urination that will be relieved when the pack is removed in 24 to 48 hours.

A postoperative pelvic hematoma can cause serious morbidity, especially if it is large and becomes infected. Hematomas can develop above the vaginal vault, along the pelvic side wall, in the paravesical space, in the abdominal wall, and in the ischiorectal fossa and vulva. A hematoma in the ischiorectal fossa and on the vulva may be obvious on examination when the patient complains of discomfort in the area. If it is below the puborectalis muscle attachment to the vagina, it will not dissect into the pelvis above but will be limited to the perineum and buttocks. A pelvic hematoma may be recognized in a patient whose postoperative discomfort and anemia exceed what is normally expected, whose temperature is progressively increasing, and whose postoperative abdominal distention is slow to resolve. If a patient is on anticoagulant therapy, even simple coughing can spontaneously cause a tremendous postoperative pelvic hematoma. Abdominal and pelvic examinations reveal a mass. A definitive diagnosis can be made by ultrasound or CT scan which is helpful in delineating its exact size and location. An extended, morbid, and complicated postoperative course may be alleviated if the hematoma can be drained. Sometimes simple drainage through the vaginal vault can be accomplished by probing with a uterine dressing forceps. A small Penrose drain can be inserted through the drainage tract and left in place for a day or so. If drainage cannot be achieved in this simple way, drainage with guidance of CT or through an abdominal incision may be necessary. In our experience, if the hematoma can be drained, the patient's recovery will be expedited. But in some cases, drainage is difficult or contraindicated and infection is not a serious problem, so it may be preferable to allow the hematoma to gradually resolve over a few months. Unfortunately, sometimes a hematoma will not resolve completely, and residual fibrosis will persist and continue to cause pain. We have removed large pieces of an organizing hematoma as late as 1 year after operation. For these reasons, we prefer to drain pelvic hematomas initially whenever possible.

There are a few other special circumstances. Hemorrhage after uterine curettage is extremely rare, even with perforation of the uterus. The perforation is usually caused by the uterine sound and occurs through the corpus. The curettage should be stopped and the patient's vital signs checked for several hours. If she is not already in the hospital, she can be admitted for overnight observation. It is extremely unlikely that any problem will develop, and hospital admission as a precautionary measure may be unnecessary. However, if the perforation was caused by a wide, blunt instrument, such as a curet or a suction device; if the patient is pregnant; or if fatty tissue appears in the curettage specimen, the patient must be hospitalized and closely observed for intraperitoneal bleeding. Ultrasound, CT scan, or laparoscopy also may be performed in high-risk cases to assess the damage and determine if a hematoma or active bleeding is present. A misdirected cervical dilator can lacerate the uterine artery and vein, with subsequent intraperitoneal bleeding or broad ligament hematoma formation. In such cases, laparotomy is required to control the bleeding and evacuate the hematoma. A hysterectomy may or may not be necessary, depending on the damage to the uterus.

Hemorrhage from cervical conization can occur in the first 24 hours or 7 to 14 days later, when cervical sutures lose their tensile strength. If the patient is bleeding heavily at any time after conization, the cervix should be inspected. Measures to control the bleeding include resuturing, cautery, and Monsel's solution. If bleeding is not profuse, Monsel's solution, Gelfoam, and/or a small pack can be tried. In taking the conization specimen, one must be certain that the apex of the cone intersects the endocervical canal. If the cervical incision is misdirected to one side or the other, the uterine vessels are in danger of laceration. Serious hemorrhage or broad ligament hematoma will result. To prevent this problem, the cervix should first be sounded to ascertain the direction of the endocervical canal and the incision planned accordingly.

Hypogastric Artery Ligation

One of the methods of controlling severe pelvic hemorrhage is ligation of both hypogastric arteries. In 1893 at the Johns Hopkins Hospital, Howard Kelly performed bilateral hypogastric artery ligation to control hemorrhage during hysterectomy for uterine cancer. Hypogastric artery ligation was later introduced by Mengert and colleagues and was then extensively investigated by Burchell. Burchell demonstrated that the pulse pressure in the artery just distal to the point of ligation was decreased significantly (77%) on the same side. If both hypogastric arteries are ligated, the pulse pressure is decreased 85%. This reduction in pulse pressure presumably allows blood clots to form at the site of bleeding from damaged vessels. Blood flow in vessels distal to the point of ligation is decreased by only 48%.

Because of the major collateral circulation with the aorta and femoral artery—including the lumbar, iliolumbar, middle sacral, lateral sacral, superior and middle hemorrhoidal, and gluteal arteries—it is important to ligate the anterior division of the hypogastric artery dis-

tal to the posterior parietal branch, as demonstrated in Fig. 18.8. When the hypogastric artery is ligated *proximal* to the posterior division, flow can still occur distal to the point of ligation by reversed flow through the iliolumbar and lateral sacral collateral arteries. When the hypogastric artery is ligated *distal* to the posterior division, flow can still occur distal to the point of ligation, but only by reversed flow in middle hemorrhoidal arteries, and flow in the iliolumbar and lateral sacral arteries above the point of ligation will continue to be normal.

In ligating the hypogastric artery, the peritoneum is opened on the lateral side of the common iliac artery near its bifurcation, with the ureter left attached to the medial peritoneal reflection to avoid disturbing its blood supply. The posterior branch of the hypogastric artery must be clearly identified before double ligation of the anterior division is performed. The artery is dissected and carefully mobilized free from the underlying hypogastric vein. Nonabsorbable suture is passed around the artery with an Adson or right-angle clamp and tied. A second free-tie suture is placed distal to the initial ligature to avoid recanalization. Transfixion or division of the vessel is not essential or desirable in this procedure. The major advantages of ligating the anterior division of the hypogastric artery are isolation of the collateral arterial circulation from the pelvis and reduced pulse pressure in the bleeding artery, as demonstrated by Burchell. This reduction in pulse pressure permits thrombosis of the bleeding vessel to occur. When possible, we believe that the arterial branch closest to the bleeding point should be ligated. Because the uterine artery is the first visceral branch of the hypogastric artery, it may be feasible to identify this artery and ligate it separately, if this vessel is the origin of the pelvic bleeding. This may be a somewhat more difficult procedure than ligating the en-

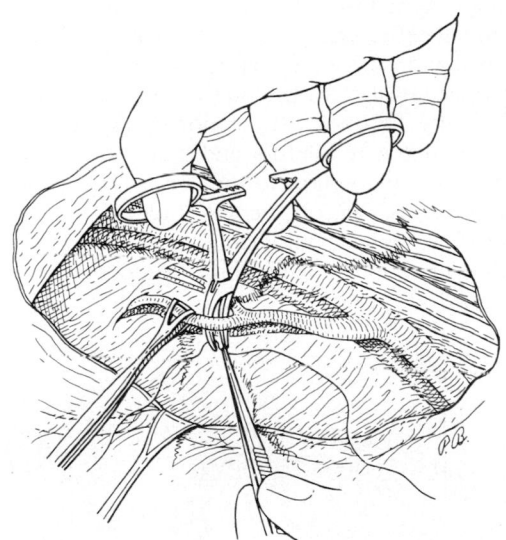

FIGURE 18.8. Ligation of right hypogastric artery, showing peritoneal reflection with attached ureter from bifurcation of iliac artery, and ligature placed around anterior division of hypogastric artery.

tire anterior division of the hypogastric artery and should not be attempted in the face of massive pelvic bleeding, distorted pelvic anatomy, or shock.

When massive bleeding is present but the uterus has not been removed (as may occur in certain obstetric operations), it is important to separately identify and ligate each ovarian artery after each hypogastric artery has been ligated because of the important collateral communication of the aorta with the ovarian and uterine arteries. This procedure is easily accomplished by extending the lateral peritoneal incision above the pelvic brim and the bifurcation of the common iliac artery, being careful to remain lateral to the ureter and to avoid traumatizing the ovarian vessels. If there is difficulty in distinguishing the artery from the ovarian vein, ligation of both the ovarian artery and vein within the infundibulopelvic ligament is acceptable. Even though ligating both the arterial and venous circulation to the ovary leads to a high incidence of postoperative cystic enlargement of the ovary, this complication is preferable to the risk of recurrent pelvic bleeding when the ovarian arteries are not ligated. Each ovarian artery should be dissected free from its retroperitoneal position at or above the pelvic brim and free-tied. Only one ligature is necessary for each. The artery should not be cut. This avoids the need for multiple ligatures and the risk of retraction and retroperitoneal bleeding of the vessel. A single hemoclip also can be placed on each ovarian artery as a quicker and easier method of occlusion. Care must be taken to avoid injury to the ovarian vein when the artery is being freed for ligation. If injury occurs, control of bleeding may be troublesome. The left ovarian vein can be particularly troublesome; if it retracts beneath the peritoneum, its drainage into the left renal vein makes it difficult to trace. The ureter runs medially, and it should be carefully identified to prevent injury or ligation.

As an alternative to ligating the ovarian artery in the infundibulopelvic ligament, Cruikshank and Stoelk have described a technique of ligating this artery at the point of its anastomosis with the uterine artery in the medial mesosalpinx. This point of ligation allows maintenance of the blood flow to the tube and ovary but occludes the ovarian artery blood flow to the uterus (Fig. 18.9).

In cases of life-threatening uterine hemorrhage, Fehrman prefers bilateral ligation of the uterine arteries as primary treatment. When this method was used in 66 patients with post-Caesarean delivery hemorrhage, emergency hysterectomy to achieve final hemostasis was necessary in six patients. If bilateral uterine ligation is not effective in controlling the uterine bleeding, Fehrman recommends supplementary ligation of the round ligaments and the ovarian ligaments at their junction with the uterine corpus. He also believes that bilateral uterine artery ligation is a more effective treatment for life-threatening uterine hemorrhage than is bilateral hypogastric artery ligation.

The vaginal artery can originate as a separate branch from the hypogastric artery. Uncontrollable bleeding from the vagina may not be stopped by hysterectomy or by ligation of the uterine arteries. Hypogastric artery ligation is required.

Amazingly, there are many reports of full-term deliveries after bilateral hypogastric artery ligation with and without bilateral ovarian artery ligation. This is ample testimony to the abundant collateral blood supply to the uterus that can develop over time. According to Burchell, the blood flow to the pelvis is reduced by as much as 50%, and yet there remains an adequate reserve to nourish a term pregnancy. Ischemic necrosis of pelvic tissues does not occur unless additional collateral pathways are destroyed.

The collateral circulation of the female pelvis is extensive and provides a variety of intercommunicating sources of arterial blood from various sites along the arterial tree. These collateral vessels anastomose with the hypogastric artery and the blood supply to the uterus through a number of circuitous arterial pathways in the pelvis. During a difficult hysterectomy, the collateral circulation can create problems in achieving adequate hemostasis. Therefore, it is important to have a clear understanding of the various extrapelvic arteries that communicate with the pelvic circulation.

The collateral circulation of the pelvis can be divided into three main arterial groups: (a) those vessels that communicate with branches from the aorta, (b) those that communicate with branches from the external iliac artery, and (c) those that communicate with branches from the femoral artery (Fig. 18.10).

Hypogastric artery ligation is a more conservative surgical procedure than is hysterectomy in patients with a variety of pelvic hemorrhage problems. There is less morbidity, and reproductive function can be preserved in some patients. However, it must be pointed out that bi-

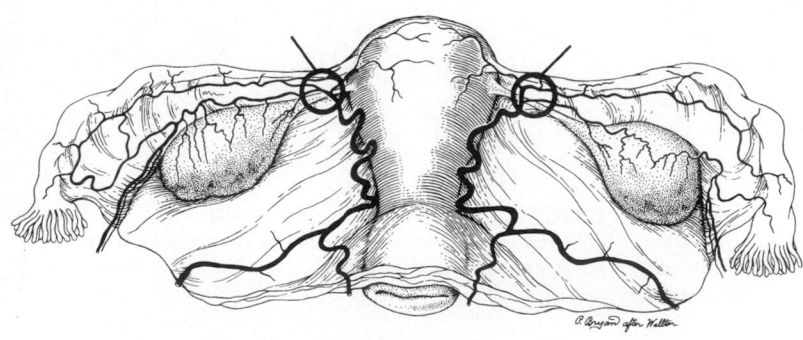

FIGURE 18.9. In addition to ligation of the anterior division of the hypogastric artery, the blood flow to the uterus through the ovarian artery can be ligated in the medial mesosalpinx without interfering with the blood flow to the tube and ovary.

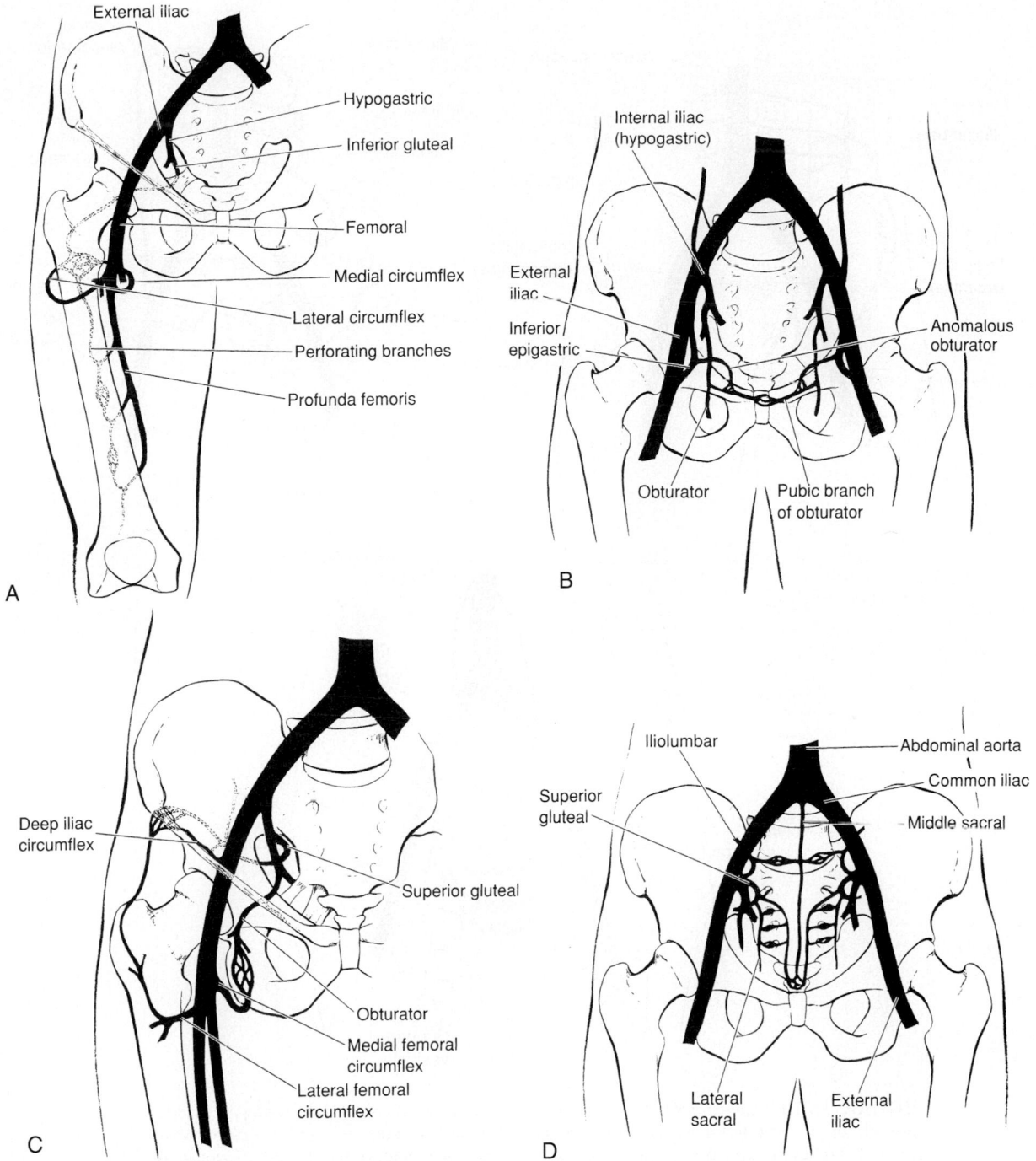

FIGURE 18.10. A: Anastomoses of deep medial and lateral femoral circumflex arteries around hip joint to posterior division (inferior gluteal) of hypogastric artery. **B:** Anastomosis of external iliac and hypogastric arteries through obturator originating anomalously from inferior epigastric artery. **C:** Collateral arterial circulation between external iliac and hypogastric arteries through anastomoses with iliolumbar and superior gluteal arteries. Note anastomoses from medial and lateral femoral circumflex vessels with obturator and superior gluteal branches of hypogastric artery. **D:** Anastomosis of middle sacral artery from aorta with hypogastric branches, including lateral sacral and iliolumbar arteries.

lateral hypogastric artery ligation is not uniformly successful in controlling bleeding. Clark et al. found that hypogastric artery ligation was successful in only eight of 19 patients with obstetric hemorrhage. Bleeding continued in the remaining 11 patients and hysterectomy was required. Evans and McShane performed hypogastric artery ligation in 18 patients and had a failure rate of 57%. Fahmy reported a similar experience. Some improvements in the technique mentioned above may improve the success rate. However, one major disadvantage

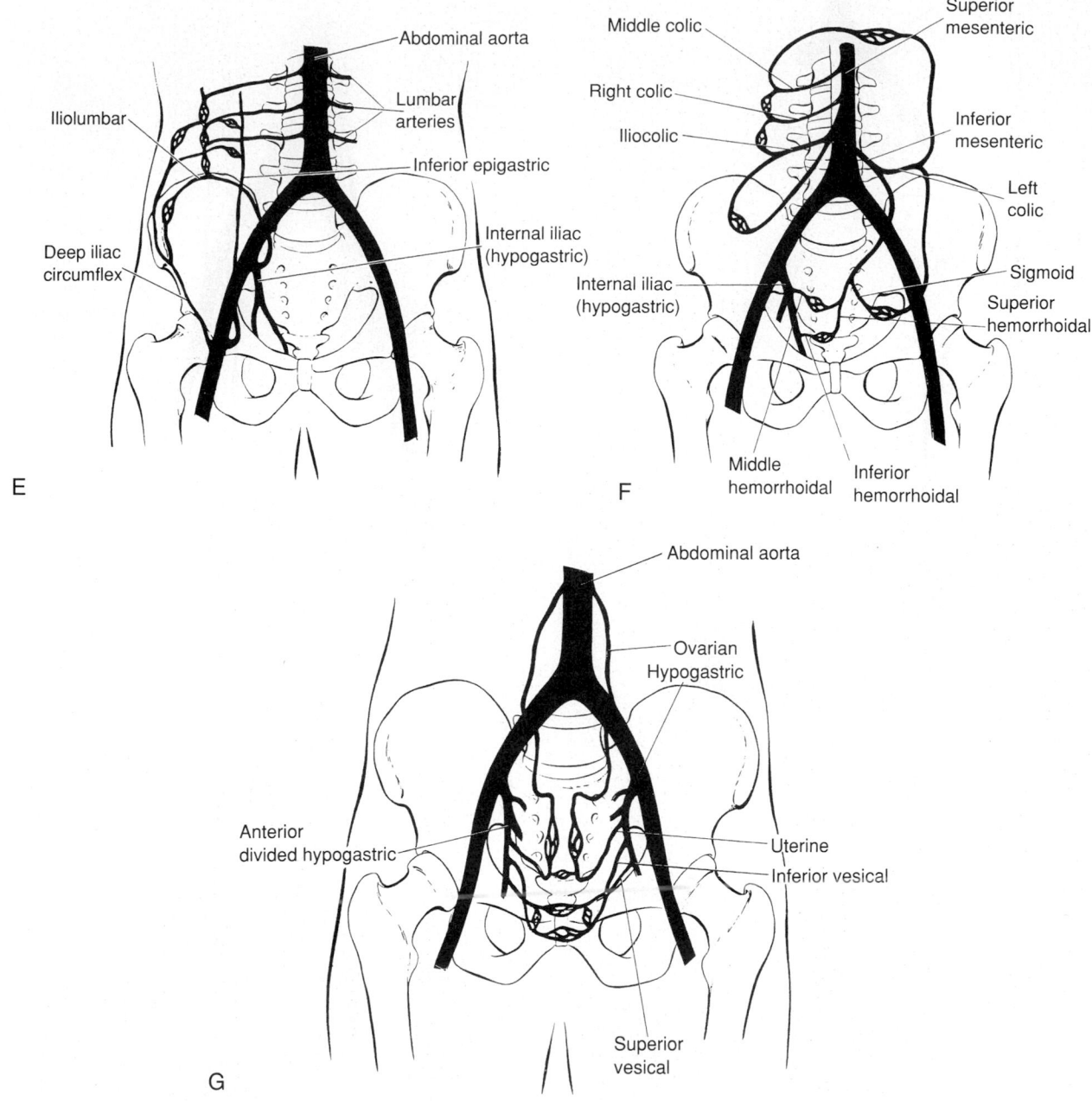

FIGURE 18.10 *(Continued).* **E:** Collateral circulation of aorta and hypogastric arteries through lumbar and iliolumbar anastomoses. **F:** Collateral circulation of inferior mesenteric artery to branches of hypogastric artery, from superior hemorrhoidal to middle and inferior hemorrhoidal arteries. **G:** Arterial arcade and anastomosis between ovarian and uterine arteries.

should be mentioned. If a bilateral hypogastric artery ligation is performed, selective arterial catheterization and embolization of peripheral bleeding arterial branches in the pelvis are made much more difficult and perhaps even impossible. Before deciding to ligate the hypogastric arteries, the gynecologic surgeon would be well advised to consult with a vascular radiologist familiar with the technique of embolization before deciding which technique to use.

UNUSUAL METHODS OF CONTROLLING PELVIC HEMORRHAGE

Antishock Trousers

The principle of external counterpressure was originally described by Crile in 1903. He used an inflatable rubber suit to counter the postural hypotension that developed in patients who were operated on in the semirecumbent or sitting position. It was subsequently used in the Korean War to transport casualties from the battlefield to the hospital. According to Gardner and Storer, its usefulness in patients with intraabdominal bleeding was discovered serendipitously.

External counterpressure by means of an inflatable garment wrapped around the legs and abdomen (sometimes called the MAST suit or G suit, or pneumatic antishock garment) has been used for the temporary control of acute, profuse intraabdominal hemorrhage while the patient is being prepared for surgery. In some cases, the bleeding can be controlled and surgery can be avoided. This technique has been used in more than 175 cases of surgically uncontrollable hemorrhage, as reported in the literature, and in all cases, it resulted in temporary or complete control of the hemorrhage.

The suit is made of polyvinyl, wraps around the patient, and secures with loop-and-hook fasteners. It contains an abdominal pneumatic bladder that extends from the xiphoid to the pubis, and it has two separate leg bladders. It is inflated to a pressure of 25 to 40 mm Hg (some clinics have used pressures of 100 mm Hg or higher). There are definite disadvantages and dangers in the use of an inflatable garment for external counterpressure. Absolute contraindications to the use of the garment include pulmonary edema, known rupture of the diaphragm, and left ventricular dysfunction. Abdom-

inal examination is not possible unless the garment is removed. Likewise, pelvic examination is impossible. If pressures are not carefully monitored, circulation to the lower extremities can be impaired sufficiently to cause progressive muscle necrosis, crush syndrome, and death. It is rarely used today.

Logothetopulos Pack

Some surgeons have found the Logothetopulos pack, or umbrella pack, to be of assistance in compressing the retracted, bleeding vessels in the pelvis. This technique involves the formation of a large pack of loose gauze within an outstretched, opened piece of gauze or plastic sheet. This can be used in an umbrella manner within the pelvic cavity by tying the four corners of the opened gauze together, creating a ball or bag, and placing traction on the free end of the pack when it is pulled through the vaginal vault. This approach attempts to compress the bleeding vessels against the pelvic floor by the downward traction and pressure exerted with the pack. It can be used after pelvic exenteration or abdominal–perineal resection for compression of bleeding vessels that cannot be controlled by other means. The pack can be left in place with perineal traction for 24 to 48 hours until the bleeding has ceased. It is removed vaginally by first withdrawing the internal gauze and then the outside bag (Fig. 18.11).

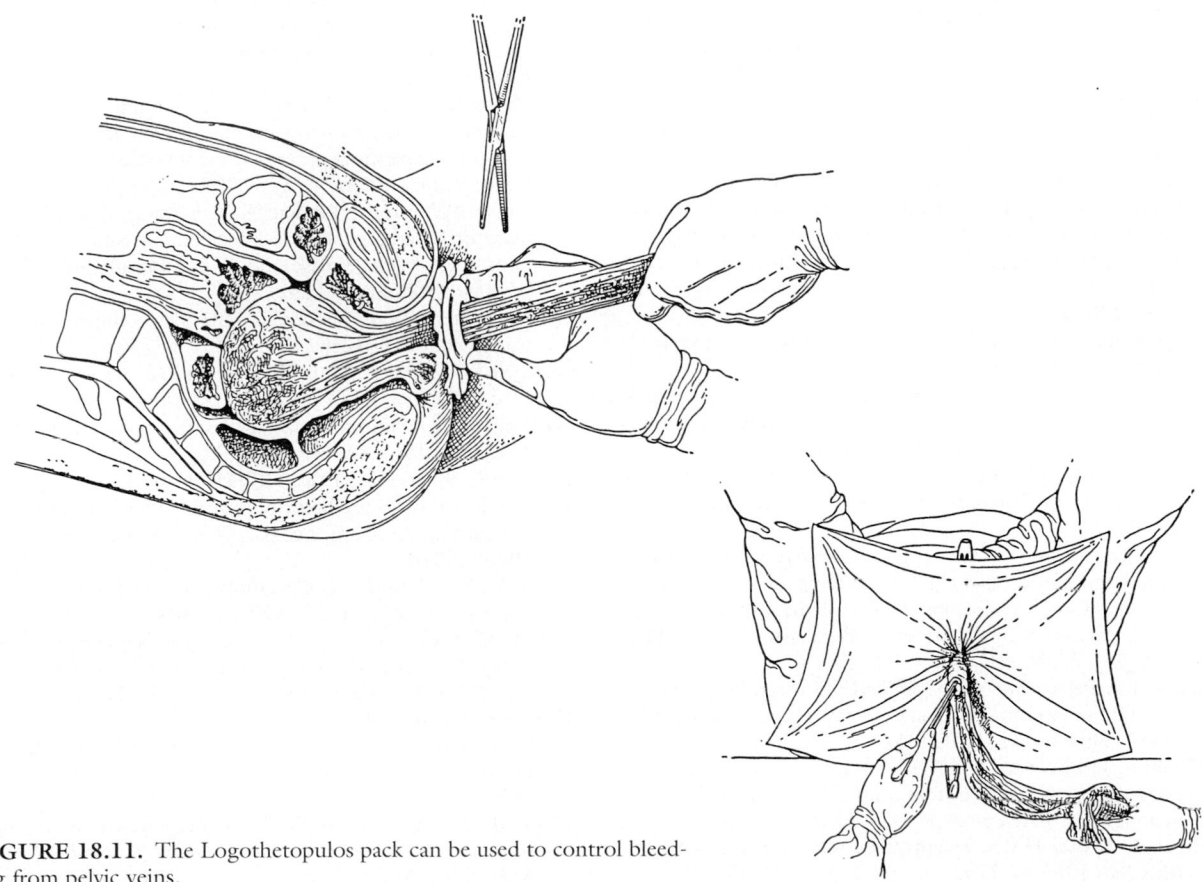

FIGURE 18.11. The Logothetopulos pack can be used to control bleeding from pelvic veins.

Aortic Compressor

An instrument such as the one described by Conn et al. to temporarily compress and stop circulation through the aorta to the pelvis may be useful in special cases to control pelvic hemorrhage. It is used by vascular surgeons in operations for aortic aneurysms and by trauma surgeons to control traumatic hemorrhage from the aorta or large pelvic vessels. When massive arterial bleeding in the pelvis is difficult to control, temporarily occluding the aorta by compressing it against the lumbar vertebrae may be helpful. It is less effective in hemorrhage from pelvic veins. Because the vena cava also is compressed, pelvic veins can temporarily become distended. The aortic compressor may be helpful when excessive blood loss from extensive myomectomy is anticipated, especially if a tourniquet cannot be fitted around the lower uterus. It is also useful in removing large pelvic tumors with blood supply that is difficult to isolate or control. It is a temporary expedient to control an urgent problem. The operator can simply compress the aorta with his or her hand until the aortic compressor arrives.

When the aorta is occluded for more than a few minutes, clots may form in vessels at distal sites. This can be avoided by injecting heparin distal to the point of occlusion and by releasing the compressor periodically to allow the blood to flow.

BIBLIOGRAPHY

Abbas FM, Currie JL, Mitchell S, et al. Selective vascular embolization in benign gynecologic conditions. *J Reprod Med* 1994;39:492.

Al-Mondhiry H. Disseminated intravascular coagulation: experience in a major cancer center. *Thrombos Diathes Haemorrh* 1975;34:181.

Alvarez M, Lockwood CJ, Ghidini A, et al. Prophylactic and emergent arterial catheterization for selective embolization in obstetric hemorrhage. *Am J Perinatol* 1992;9:441.

Amrein PC, Ellman L, Harris WH. Aspirin-induced prolongation of bleeding time and perioperative blood loss. *JAMA* 1981;245:1825.

Anthanasoulis CA. Therapeutic applications of angiography. *N Engl J Med* 1980;302:1117.

Anthanasoulis CA, Waltman AC, Barnes AB, et al. Angiographic control of pelvic bleeding from treated carcinoma of the cervix. *Gynecol Oncol* 1976;4:144.

Anthanasoulis CA, Waltman AC, Ring EJ, et al. Angiographic management of postoperative bleeding. *Radiology* 1974; 113:37.

Ashley FL, Anson BJ. The hypogastric artery in American whites and Negroes. *Am J Phys Anthropol* 1941;28:381.

Autologous blood transfusions: report of the Council on Scientific Affairs of the American Medical Association. *JAMA* 1986;256:2378.

Axelrod FB, Pepkowitz SH, Goldfinger D. Establishment of a schedule of optimal preoperative collection of autologous blood. *Transfusion* 1989;29:677.

Behnam K, Jarmolowski CR. Vesicovaginal fistula following hypogastric embolization for control of intractable pelvic hemorrhage. *J Reprod Med* 1982;27:304.

Bennet B, Towler HMA. Haemostatic response to trauma. *Br Med Bull* 1985;67:274.

Benson RE, Isbister JP. Massive blood transfusion. *Anaesth Intensive Care* 1980;8:152.

Bergqvist D, Bergqvist A. Vascular injuries during gynecologic surgery. *Acta Obstet Gynecol Scand* 1987;66:19.

Beris P, Miescher PA. Hematological complications of antiinfectious agents. *Semin Hematol* 1988;25:123.

Bernard GR, Vincent JL, Laterre PF, et al. Efficacy and safety of recombinant human activated protein C for severe sepsis. *N Engl J Med* 2001;344:699-709.

Bertina RM, Koeleman BPC, Koster T, et al. Mutation in blood coagulation factor V associated with resistance to activated protein C. *Nature* 1994;369:64.

Bickell WH, Pepe PE, Wyatt CH, et al. Effect of antishock trousers on the trauma score: a prospective analysis in the urban setting. *Ann Emerg Med* 1985;14:218.

Bickell WH, Wall MJ, Pepe PE, et al. Immediate versus delayed fluid resuscitation for hypotensive patients with penetrating torso injuries. *N Engl J Med* 1994;331:1105.

Boral LI, Dannemiller FJ, Stanford W, et al. A guideline for anticipated blood usage during elective surgical procedures. *Am J Clin Pathol* 1979;71:680.

Boral LI, Henry JB. The type and screen: a safe alternative and supplement in selected surgical procedures. *Transfusion* 1977;17:163.

Bowie EJ, Owen CA. Hemostatic failure in clinical medicine. *Semin Hematol* 1977;14:341.

Bowie EJW, Owen CA. The significance of abnormal preoperative hemostatic tests. In: Spaet TH, ed. *Progress in hemostasis and thrombosis*, vol. 5. New York: Grune & Stratton, 1980:170.

Braf ZF, Knootz WWJ. Gangrene of bladder: a complication of hypogastric artery embolization. *Urology* 1979;9:670.

Breen JL, Gregori CA, Kindzierski JA. Hemorrhage in gynecologic surgery. In: Schaefer G, Graber EA, eds. *Complications in obstetric and gynecologic surgery*. New York: Harper & Row, 1980.

Brinkhous K, Smith H, Warner E, et al. Inhibition of blood clotting: an unidentified substance which acts in conjunction with heparin to prevent the conversion of prothrombin to thrombin. *Am J Physiol* 1939;125:683.

Brockman AW, van der Linden IK, Velt Kamp JJ, et al. Prevalence of isolated protein C deficiency in patients with venous thrombotic disease and in the population. *Thromb Haemost* 1983;50:350(abst).

Buonassisi V. Sulfated mucopolysaccharide synthesis and secretion in endothelial cell cultures. *Exp Cell Res* 1973;76:363.

Burchell RC. Physiology of the internal iliac artery ligation. *J Obstet Gynaecol Br Commonw* 1968;75:642.

Burchell RC. The umbrella pack to control pelvic hemorrhage. *Conn Med* 1968;32:734.

Burns ER, Billet HH, Frater RWM, et al. The preoperative bleeding time as predictor of postoperative hemorrhage after cardiopulmonary bypass. *J Thorac Cardiovasc Surg* 1986;92:310.

Cass RM, Blumberg N. Single-unit blood transfusion: doubtful dogma defeated. *JAMA* 1987;257:628.

Chung AF, Menon J, Dillon TF. Acute postoperative retroperitoneal fibrosis and ureteral obstruction secondary to the use of Avitene. *Am J Obstet Gynecol* 1978;132:908.

Ciavarella S, Reed RL, Counts RB, et al. Clotting factor levels and the risk of diffuse microvascular bleeding in the massively transfused patient. *Br J Haematol* 1987;67:365.

Clark SL, Phelan JP, Yeh SY, et al. Hypogastric artery ligation for obstetric hemorrhage. *Obstet Gynecol* 1985;66:353.

Collection, transport, and preparation of blood specimens for coagulation testing and performance of coagulation assays. Wayne, PA: National Committee for Clinical Laboratory Standards; 1991; H21-A.

Collins JA, Murawski K, Shafer AW. Massive transfusion in surgery and trauma. *Prog Clin Biol Res* 1982;108:1.

Comp P, Nixon R, Esmon C. A functional assay for protein C, and antithrombotic protein, using a thrombomodulin complex. *Blood* 1984;63:15.

Conard J, Brosstad F, LieLarson M, et al. Molar antithrombin III concentration in normal human plasma. *Haemostasis* 1983;13:363.

Conn J Jr, Trippel OH, Bergan JJ. A new atraumatic aortic occluder. *Surgery* 1968;64:1158.

Consensus Conference. Fresh frozen plasma indications and risks. *JAMA* 1985;253:551.

Consensus Conference. Perioperative red blood cell transfusion. *JAMA* 1988;260:2700.

Consensus Conference. Platelet transfusion therapy. *JAMA* 1987;257:1777.

Corriveau DM, Fritsma GA. *Hemostasis and thrombosis: in the clinical laboratory.* Philadelphia: JB Lippincott Co, 1988.

Cowley RA, Trump BF, eds. *Pathophysiology of shock, anoxia, and ischemia.* Baltimore: Williams & Wilkins, 1982.

Crile GW. *Blood pressure in clinical surgery: an experimental and clinical research.* Philadelphia: JB Lippincott Co, 1903:288.

Crisp WE. One pint of blood. *Obstet Gynecol* 1956;7:216.

Cruikshank SH, Stoelk EM. Surgical control of pelvic hemorrhage: bilateral hypogastric artery ligation and method of ovarian artery ligation. *South Med J* 1985;78:539.

Cushing H. The control of bleeding in operations for brain tumors: with description of silver "clips" for occlusion of vessels inaccessible to the ligature. *Ann Surg* 1911;54:1.

Dahlback B, Carlsson M, Svensson PH. Familial thrombophilia due to a previously unrecognized mechanism characterized by poor anticoagulant response to activated protein C: prediction of a cofactor to activated protein C. *Proc Natl Acad Sci USA* 1993;90:1004.

Dahlback B, Hildebrand B. Inherited resistance to activated protein C is corrected by anticoagulant cofactor activity found to be property of factor V. *Proc Natl Acad Sci USA* 1994;91:1396.

Dehaeck CMC. Transcatheter embolization of pelvic vessels to stop intractable hemorrhage. *Gynecol Oncol* 1986;24:9.

DiScipio R, Hermodson M, Yates S, et al. A comparison of human prothrombin, factor IX (Christmas factor), factor X (Stuart factor), and protein S. *Biochemistry* 1977;16:698.

Dodd RY. The risk of transfusion transmitted infections. *N Engl J Med* 1992;327:419.

Dubay ML, Holshausen CA, Burchell RC. Internal iliac artery ligation for postpartum hemorrhage: recanalization of vessels. *Am J Obstet Gynecol* 1980;136:689.

Edmunds LH, Addonizio VP. Massive transfusion. In: Colman RW, Hirsh J, Marder VJ, et al, eds. *Hemostasis and thrombosis: basic principles and clinical practice,* second edition. Philadelphia: JB Lippincott Co, 1987:913.

Egeberg O. Inherited antithrombin III deficiency causing thrombophilia. *Thrombos Diathes Haemorrh* 1965;13:513.

Ereth MH, Oliver WC, Santrach PJ. Perioperative interventions to decrease transfusion of allogenic blood products. *Mayo Clin Proc* 1994;69:575.

Esmon CT, Owen W. Identification of an endothelial cell cofactor for thrombosis catalyzed activation of protein C. *Proc Natl Acad Sci USA* 1981;78:2249.

Esmon NL, Owen W, Esmon C. Isolation of a membrane bound cofactor for thrombin catalyzed activation of protein C. *J Biol Chem* 1982;257:859.

Etchason J, Petz L, Keeler E, et al. The cost effectiveness of pre-operative autologous blood donations. *N Engl J Med* 1995;332:719.

Evans S, McShane P. The efficacy of internal iliac artery ligation in obstetric hemorrhage. *Surg Gynecol Obstet* 1985;160:250.

Fahmy K. Internal iliac artery ligation and its efficacy in controlling pelvic hemorrhage. *Int Surg* 1969;51:244.

Fehrman II. Surgical management of life threatening obstetric and gynecologic hemorrhage. *Acta Obstet Gynecol Scand* 1988;67:125.

Ferraris VA, Swanson E. Aspirin usage and perioperative blood loss in patients undergoing unexpected operations. *Surg Gynecol Obstet* 1983;156:439.

Friedman BA, Oberman HA, Chadwick AR, et al. The maximum surgical blood order schedule and surgical blood use in the United States. *Transfusion* 1976;16:380.

Gardner WJ, Storer J. The use of the G-suit in control of intra-abdominal bleeding. *Surg Gynecol Obstet* 1966;123:792.

Gewirtz AS, Miller ML, Keys TF. The clinical usefulness of the preoperative bleeding time. *Arch Pathol Lab Med* 1996;120:353.

Gilbert WM, Moore TR, Resnik R, et al. Angiographic embolization in the management of hemorrhagic complications of pregnancy. *Am J Obstet Gynecol* 1992;166:493.

Given FT, Gates HS, Morgan BE. Pregnancy following bilateral ligation of the internal iliac (hypogastric) arteries. *Am J Obstet Gynecol* 1964;89:1078.

Godbout B, Burchard KW, Slotman GJ, et al. Crush syndrome with death following pneumatic antishock garment application. *J Trauma* 1984;24:1052.

Goldfinger D. Safety of autologous blood donation prior to elective surgery for a variety of potentially "high-risk" patients. *Transfusion* 1983;23:229.

Goodnough LT, Rudnick S, Price TH, et al. Increased preoperative collection of autologous blood with recombinant human erythropoietin therapy. *N Engl J Med* 1989;321:1163.

Greenwood LH, Glickman MG, Schwartz PE, et al. Obstetric and non-malignant gynecologic bleeding: treatment with angiographic embolization. *Radiology* 1987;164:155.

Grindon AJ, Tomasulo PA, Bergin JJ, et al. The hospital transfusion committee: guidelines for improving practice. *JAMA* 1985;253:540.

Hacker NF, Charles EH, Savage EW. Postcoital posthysterectomy vaginal vault disruption with haemorrhagic shock. *Aust NZ J Obstet Gynaecol* 1980;20:182.

Halal F, Quenneville G, Laurin S, et al. Clinical and genetic aspects of antithrombin III deficiency. *Am J Med Genet* 1983;14:737.

Hall M III, Marshall JR. The gravity suit: a major advance in management of gynecologic blood loss. *Gynecol Obstet* 1979;53:247.

Hare WSC, Holland CJ. Paresis following internal iliac artery embolization. *Radiology* 1983;147:47.

Harima Y, Shiraishi T, Harima K, et al. Transcatheter arterial embolization therapy in cases of recurrent and advanced gynecologic cancer. *Cancer* 1989;63:2077.

Harker LA. *Hemostasis manual,* second edition. Philadelphia: FA Davis Co, 1974.

Hillyer CD, Emmens RK, Zago-Novaretti M, et al. Methods for the reduction of transfusion-transmitted cytomegalovirus infection: filtration versus the use of seronegative donor units. *Transfusion* 1994;34:929.

Hirsh J, Dalen JE, Deykin D, et al. Oral anticoagulants: mechanism of action, clinical effectiveness, and optimal therapeutic range. *Chest* 1992;102[Suppl]:3125.

Hirsh J, Deykin D, Poller L. "Therapeutic range" for oral anticoagulant therapy. *Chest* 1986;89[Suppl]:11.

Hirsh J, Levine M. Review article: confusion over the therapeutic range for monitoring oral anticoagulant therapy in North America. *Thromb Haemost* 1988;59:129.

Hirsh J, Poller L, Deykin D, et al. Optimal therapeutic range for oral anticoagulants. *Chest* 1989;95:55.

Iberti TJ. Thrombocytopenia following peritonitis in surgical patients. *Ann Surg* 1986;204:341.

Jespersen J, Munkvad, Gram J. Induction of coagulant activity and increase of t-PA and PAI-1 in plasma after thrombolysis in patients with myocardial infarction. *Fibrinolysis* 1990;4[Suppl 3]:95(abst).

Johnson H, Knee-Ioli S, Butler TA, et al. Are routine preoperative laboratory screening tests necessary to evaluate ambulatory surgical patients? *Surgery* 1988;104:639.

Judd WB. Pretransfusion testing in clinical laboratory medicine. In: McClatchey KD, ed. *Clinical laboratory medicine.* Baltimore: Williams & Wilkins, 1994:1733.

Kanji S, Devlin J, Piekos K, et al. Recombinant human activated protein C, drotrecogin alfa (activated): a novel therapy for severe sepsis. *Pharmacotherapy* 2001;21:1389.

Kaplan EB, Sheiner LB, Boeckmann AJ, et al. The usefulness of preoperative laboratory screening. *JAMA* 1985;253:3576.

Keeling MM, Gray LA Jr, Brink MA, et al. Intraoperative autotransfusion: experience in 725 consecutive cases. *Ann Surg* 1983;197:536.

Kelly HA. Ligature of the trunks of the uterine and ovarian arteries as a means of checking hemorrhage from the uterus and broad ligaments in abdominal operations. *Johns Hopkins Hosp Rep* 1891;2:220.

Kelly HA. Ligation of both internal iliac arteries for hemorrhage in hysterectomy for carcinoma uteri. *Bull Johns Hopkins Hosp* 1894;5:53.

Kelton, JG, Moore JC, Warkentin TE, Hayward CPM, Isolation and characterization of cysteine protinase in thrombotic thrombocytopenic purpura. *Br J Haematol* 1996;93:421.

Khan FA, Fang DT, Nivatvongs S. Management of presacral bleeding during rectal resection. *Surg Gynecol Obstet* 1987;165:275.

Kisiel W, Canfield W, Ericsson L, et al. Anticoagulant properties of bovine plasma protein C following activation by thrombin. *Biochemistry* 1977;16:5824.

Kitchens CS. Concept of hypercoagulability: a review of its development, clinical application, and recent progress. *Semin Thromb Hemost* 1985;11:293.

Kivikoski AI, Martin C, Weyman P. Angiographic arterial embolization to control hemorrhage in abdominal pregnancy: a case report. *Obstet Gynecol* 1988;71:456.

Krieger JN, Hilgartner MW, Redo SF. Surgery in patients with congenital disorders of blood coagulation. *Ann Surg* 1977;185:290.

Lee VS, Tarassenko L, Bellhouse BJ. Platelet transfusion therapy: platelet concentrate preparation and storage. *J Lab Clin Med* 1988;111:371.

Leonard F, Lecuru F, Rizk E, et al. Perioperative morbidity of gynecological laparoscopy: a retrospective monocenter observational study. *Acta Obstet Gynecol Scand* 2000; 79:129.

Leparc CF, Schmidt PJ. Autologous transfusion: a community blood bank experience. *South Med J* 1987;80:320.

Levy GG, Nichols WC, Lian EC, et al. Mutations in a number of the ADAMTS gene family cause thrombotic thrombocytopenic purpura. *Nature* 2001:413:488.

Loeliger EA, Poller L, Samama M, et al. Questions and answers on prothrombin time standardization in oral anticoagulant control. *Thromb Haemost* 1985;54:515.

Loffer FD, Pent D. Indications, contraindications and complications of laparoscopy: a review. *Obstet Gynecol* 1975;30:407.

Logothetopulos K. Eine absolut sichere Blutstillungsmethode bei vaginalen Und. *Zentralbl Gynakol* 1926;50:3202.

Malar RA, Kleiss AJ, Griffin JH. An alternative extrinsic pathway of human blood coagulation. *Blood* 1982;60:1352.

Malar R, Kleiss A, Griffin J. Human protein C: inactivation by factor V and VIII in plasma by the activated molecule. *Ann NY Acad Sci* 1981;370:303.

Malviya VK, Deppe G. Control of intraoperative hemorrhage in gynecology with the use of fibrin glue. *Obstet Gynecol* 1989;73:284.

Mann M, Sacks HJ, Goldfinger D. Safety of autologous blood donation prior to elective surgery for a variety of potentially "high-risk" patients. *Transfusion* 1983;23:229.

Mannucci PM. Desmopressin (DDAVP) in the treatment of bleeding disorders: the first 20 years. *Blood* 1997;90:2515.

Mannucci PM, Tenconi PM, Gastaman G, et al. Comparison of four virus-inactivated plasma concentrates for treatment of severe von Willebrand disease; a cross-over randomized trial. *Blood* 1992;79:3130.

Mannucci PM, Tripodi A. Laboratory screening of inherited thrombotic syndromes. *Thromb Haemost* 1987;57:247.

Martin JN, Ridgway LE III, Connors JJ, et al. Angiographic arterial embolization and computed tomography–directed drainage for the management of hemorrhage and infection with abdominal pregnancy. *Obstet Gynecol* 1990;76:941.

Meade TW. The epidemiology of hemostatic and other variables in coronary artery disease. In: Verstraete M, Vermylen J, et al, eds. *Thrombosis and hemostasis 1987: International Society on Thrombosis and Haemostasis.* Belgium: Leuven University Press, 1987:37.

Mengert WF, Burchell RC, Blumstein RW, et al. Pregnancy after bilateral ligation of the internal iliac and ovarian arteries. *Obstet Gynecol* 1969;34:664.

Merrill BS, Mitts DL, Rogers W, et al. Autotransfusion: intraoperative use in ruptured ectopic pregnancy. *J Reprod Med* 1980;24:14.

Miletich J, Sherman L, Broze G. Absence of thrombosis in subjects with heterozygous protein C deficiency. *N Engl J Med* 1987;317:991.

Miller N, Hultin MB, Gounder M, et al. Hereditary antithrombin III deficiency: case report and review of recent therapeutic advances. *Am J Hematol* 1986;21:215.

Mintz PD, Henry JB, Boral LI. The type and antibody screen: symposium on blood banking and hemotherapy. *Clin Lab Med* 1982;2:169.

Mitty HA, Sterling KM, Alavarez M, et al. Obstetric hemorrhage: prophylactic and emergency arterial catheterization and embolotherapy. *Radiology* 1993;188:183.

Morgan CH, Penner JA. Bleeding complications during surgery: part I. Defects of primary hemostasis and congenital coagulation. *Lab Med* 1986;17:207.

Morgan CH, Penner JA. Bleeding complications during surgery: part II. Acquired hemorrhagic disorders. *Lab Med* 1986;17:262.

Moscardo F, Perez F, de la Rubia J, et al, Successful treatment of severe intra-abdominal bleeding associated with disseminated intravascular coagulation using recombinant activated FVII. *Br J Haematol* 2001;114:174.

Myrhe BA, Bove JR, Schmidt PJ. Wrong blood: a needless cause of surgical deaths. *Anesth Analg* 1981;609:777.

Nagy I, Losonczy H. Three types of hereditary antithrombin III deficiency. *Thromb Haemost* 1979;42:187.

National Institutes of Health and Federal Drug Administration Consensus Conference on perioperative red blood cell transfusion. *JAMA* 1988;260:2700.

Nordestgaard AG, Bodily KC, Osborne RW, et al. Major vascular injury during laparoscopic procedures. *Am J Surg* 1995;169:543.

Nusbaum M, Baum S, Balkemore WS. Clinical experience with the diagnosis and management of gastrointestinal hemorrhage by selective mesenteric catheterization. *Ann Surg* 1969;170:506.

O'Hanlan KA, Trambert J, Rodriguez-Rodriguez L, et al. Arterial embolization in the management of abdominal and retroperitoneal hemorrhage. *Gynecol Oncol* 1989;34:131.

Oliver JA Jr, Lance JS. Selective embolization to control massive hemorrhage following pelvic surgery. *Am J Obstet Gynecol* 1979;135:431.

Pais SO, Glickman M, Schwartz P, et al. Embolization of pelvic arteries for control of postpartum hemorrhage. *Obstet Gynecol* 1980;55:754.

Pearl ML, Braga CA. Percutaneous transcatheter embolization for control of life-threatening pelvic hemorrhage from gestational trophoblastic disease. *Obstet Gynecol* 1992;80:571.

Pearse CS, Magrina JF, Finley BE. Use of the MAST suit in obstetrics and gynecology. *Obstet Gynecol Surg* 1984;39:416.

Pelligra R, Sandberg EC. Control of intractable abdominal bleeding by external counterpressure. *JAMA* 1979; 241:708.

Peterson HB, Greenspan JR, Ory HW. Death following puncture of the aorta during laparoscopic sterilization. *Obstet Gynecol* 1982;59:133.

Pineo GF, Regoeczi E, Hatton MW, et al. The activation of coagulation by extracts of mucus: a possible pathway of intravascular coagulation accompanying adenocarcinomas. *J Lab Clin Med* 1973;82:255.

Pisco JM, Martins JM, Correia MG. Internal iliac artery: embolization to control hemorrhage from pelvic neoplasms. *Radiology* 1989;172:337.

Poller L, Hirsh J. Special report: a simple system for the derivation of international normalized ratios for the reporting of prothrombin time results with North American thromboplastin reagents. *Am J Clin Pathol* 1989;92: 124.

Poller L, McKernan A, Thomson JM. Fixed minidose warfarin: a new approach to prophylaxis against venous thrombosis after major surgery. *Br Med J* 1987;295:1309.

Poon MC, Use of recombinate FVIIa in hereditary bleeding disorders. *Curr Opin Hematol* 2001;8:312.

Popovsky MA, Devine PA, Taswell HF. Intraoperative autologous transfusion. *Mayo Clin Proc* 1985;60:125.

Powell JL, Mogelnicki SR, Franklin EW III, et al. A deliberate hypotensive technique for decreasing blood loss during radical hysterectomy and pelvic lymphadenectomy. *Am J Obstet Gynecol* 1983;147:196.

Rabkin B, Rabkin MS. Individual and institutional liability for transfusion-acquired diseases. *JAMA* 1986;256:2242.

Rao LM, Rapaport SI. Factor VIIa catalyzed activation of factor X independent of tissue factor: its possible significance for control of hemophilic bleeding by infused factor VIIa. *Blood* 1990;75:1069.

Rao LM, Rapaport SI. Studies of a mechanism inhibiting the initiation of the extrinsic pathway of coagulation. *Blood* 1987;69:645.

Rapaport SI. Preoperative hemostatic evaluation: which tests, if any? *Blood* 1983;61:229.

Reich NE, Hoffman CG, de Wolfe VG, et al. Recurrent thrombophlebitis and pulmonary emboli in congenital factor 5 deficiency. *Chest* 1976;69:113.

Reich WJ, Nechtow MJ. The iliac arteries: a gross anatomical study based on dissection of seventy-five fresh cadavers: Clinical and surgical correlation. *J Int Coll Surg* 1964;41:53.

Reich WJ, Nechtow MJ. Ligation of the internal iliac (hypogastric) arteries: a life-saving procedure for uncontrollable gynecologic and obstetric hemorrhage. *J Int Coll Surg* 1961;36:157.

Rickles FR, Edwards R. Activation of blood coagulation in cancer: Trousseau's syndrome revisited. *Blood* 1983;62:14.

Rock WA Jr, Meeks GR, Managing anemia and blood loss in elective gynecologic surgery patients, *J Reprod Med* 2001;46:507.

Rodgers CRP, cd. A critical reappraisal of the bleeding time. *Semin Thromb Hemost* 1990;16:1.

Rodgers GM, Shuman MA. Congenital thrombotic disorders. *Am J Hematol* 1986;21:419.

Rohrer MJ, Michelotti MC, Nahrwold DL. A prospective evaluation of the efficacy of preoperative coagulation testing. *Ann Surg* 1988;208:554.

Root HD, Hauser CW, McKinley Cr, et al. Diagnostic peritoneal lavage. *Surgery* 1965;57:633.

Rosen NR, Bates LH, Herod G. Transfusion therapy: improved patient care and resource utilization. *Transfusion* 1993;33: 341.

Rosenthal DM, Harkins JL, Garzo G, et al. Management of postoperative vaginal hemorrhage. *Obstet Gynecol* 1983;61:425.

Salzman EW. Hemostatic problems in surgical patients. In: Colman RW, Hirsh J, Marder VJ, et al., eds. *Hemostasis and thrombosis: basic principles and clinical practice,* second edition. Philadelphia: JB Lippincott Co, 1987:920.

Santoso JT, Lin DW, Miller DS. Transfusion medicine in obstetrics and gynecology. *Obstet Gynecol Surg* 1995;50:470.

Sas G, Peto I, Banhegyi D, et al. Heterogeneity of the "classical" antithrombin III deficiency. *Thromb Haemost* 1980;43:133.

Saueracker AJ, McCroskey BL, Moore EE, et al. Intraoperative hypogastric artery embolization for life threatening pelvic hemorrhage: a preliminary report. *J Trauma* 1987;27: 1127.

Schafer M, Lauper M, Krahenbuhl L. Trocar and Veress needle injuries during laparoscopy. *Surg Endosc* 2000: 15:275.

Schifman RB, Steinbronn KK. Estimating intraoperative blood loss: when to transfuse autologous units. *JAMA* 1988;260:704.

Seegers W, Marciniak E. Inhibition of autoprothrombin C activity in plasma. *Nature* 1962;193:1188.

Seyer AE, Seaber AV, Dombrose FA. Coagulation changes in elective surgery and trauma. *Ann Surg* 1981;193:210.

Shapiro S, Toledo AA. *Evaluation of patients undergoing myomectomy operations utilizing the Haemonetics Cell Saver.* Resident Research Day, Emory University School of Medicine, Department of Gynecology and Obstetrics, 1988.

Shinagawa S. Extraperitoneal ligation of the internal iliac arteries as a life and uterus saving procedure for uncontrollable postpartum hemorrhage. *Am J Obstet Gynecol* 1964;88: 130.

Shinagawa S, Nomura Y, Kudoh S. Full-term deliveries after ligation of bilateral internal iliac arteries and infundibulopelvic ligaments. *Acta Obstet Gynecol Scand* 1981;60:439.

Sieber PR. Bladder necrosis secondary to pelvic artery embolization: case report and literature review. *J Urol* 1994;151:422.

Siegal T, Seligsohn U, Aghai E, et al. Clinical and laboratory aspects of disseminated intravascular coagulation (DIC): a study of 118 cases. *Thromb Haemost* 1978;39:122.

Siegel P, Mengert WF. Internal iliac artery ligation in obstetrics and gynecology. *JAMA* 1961;178:1059.

Simon PH, Conner C, Delcour C, et al. Selective uterine artery embolization in the treatment of cervical pregnancy: two case reports. *Eur J Obstet Gynecol Reprod Biol* 1991;40:159.

Slate WG. Internal iliac ligation. *Am J Obstet Gynecol* 1966;95:326.

Smith DC, Wyatt JF. Embolization of the hypogastric arteries in the control of massive vaginal hemorrhage. *Obstet Gynecol* 1977;49:317.

Sproule MW, Bendomir AM, Grant KA, et al. Embolisation of massive bleeding following hysterectomy, despite internal iliac artery ligation. *Br J Obstet Gynaecol* 1994;101:908.

Stead NW, Bauer KA, Kinny TR, et al. Venous thrombosis in a family with defective release of vascular plasminogen activator, and elevated FVIII/von Willebrand factor. *Am J Med* 1983;74:33.

Stenflow J. A new vitamin K–dependent protein: purification from bovine plasma, and preliminary characterization. *J Biol Chem* 1976;251:355.

Stimson LA. On some modifications in the technique of abdominal surgery, limiting the use of the ligature en masse. *Trans Am Surg Assoc* 1889;7:65.

Stirling Y, Woolf WRS, North MJ, et al. Haemostasis in normal pregnancy. *Thromb Haemost* 1984;51:176.

Svensson PJ, Dahlback B. Resistance to activated protein C as a basis for venous thrombosis. *N Engl J Med* 1994;330:517.

Tawes RL Jr, Scribner RG, Duval TB, et al. The cell-saver and autologous transfusion: an under-utilized resource in vascular surgery. *Am J Surg* 1986;152:105.

Teichmann AT, Korber HJ, Schuster R, et al. Embolization therapy in patients with severe arterial bleeding after hysterectomy. *Int J Gynecol Obstet* 1989;28:289.

Thaler E, Lechner K. Antithrombin III deficiency and thromboembolism. *Clin Haematol* 1981;10:369.

Thompson JD. Anemia due to gynecologic disease: its correction by the use of iron orally. *South Med J* 1957;50:679.

Timmons MC, Kohler MF, Addison WA. Thumbtack use for control of presacral bleeding, with description of an instrument for thumbtack application. *Obstet Gynecol* 1991;78:313.

Toy PTCY, Strauss RG, Stehling LC, et al. Predeposited autologous blood for elective surgery: a national multicenter study. *N Engl J Med* 1987;316:517.

Triplett DA, ed. *Laboratory evaluation of coagulation.* Chicago: ASCP Press, 1982.

Triplett DA, Brandt JT. Lupus anticoagulants: misnomer, paradox, riddle, epiphenomenon. *Hematol Pathol* 1988;2:121.

Twombley GH. Hemorrhage in gynecologic surgery. *Clin Obstet Gynecol* 1973;16:135.

Walker F. The regulation of activated protein C by a new protein: a possible function for bovine protein S. *J Biol Chem* 1980;255:5521.

Walker F. Regulation of activated protein C by protein S: the role of protein C in factor Va inactivation. *J Biol Chem* 1981;256:1128.

Werner EJ, Broxson EH, Tucker EL, et al. Prevalence of von Willebrand disease in children: a multiethnic study. *J Pediatr* 1993; 1123: 893-898.

Winman B. Altered fibrinolysis as a risk factor in cardiovascular disease. *Fibrinolysis* 1990;4[Suppl 3]:111(abst).

Yamasaki M, Sawada M, Urabe T, et al. The simultaneous use of autologous blood transfusion and hypotensive anesthesia to the radical hysterectomy for uterine carcinomas. *Asia Oceania J Obstet Gynaecol* 1989;15:317.

Yamashita Y, Harada M, Yamamoto H, et al. Transcatheter arterial embolization of obstetric and gynaecological bleeding: efficacy and clinical outcome. *Br J Radiol* 1994;67:530.

Yates AJ. Intra-arterial balloon tamponade. *Surgery* 1969;66:634.

Zimmerman L, Veith L. *Great ideas in the history of surgery.* Baltimore: Williams & Wilkins, 1961:130.

SURGERY FOR FERTILITY AND BENIGN GYNECOLOGIC CONDITIONS

Te Linde's Operative Gynecology, ninth edition, edited by John A. Rock and Howard W. Jones, III. Lippincott Williams & Wilkins, Philadelphia © 2003.

CHAPTER

19

▼

Evolving Aspects of Reparative Surgery

HOWARD W. JONES, JR.

By the 1970s, it had been established that the application of then-standard operative techniques by open laparotomy had a certain usefulness in treating infertility caused by obstructed fallopian tubes, congenital anomalies of the müllerian ducts, endometriosis, polycystic disease of the ovaries, pelvic adhesive disease, and other conditions. Microsurgical technology with a compound microscope or surgical loupes was developed during the 1970s and widely practiced in the early 1980s and through the 1990s. Assisted reproduction technologies (ARTs), that is, *in vitro* fertilization (IVF) and its associated techniques, began to play a role in the early 1980s and heavily influenced reparative surgery in the late 1980s. Also in the 1980s, surgical manipulation through the laparoscope became popular as an approach to pelvic diseases and as a substitute for open operation. Grafted onto this in the late 1980s was the use of laser technology, particularly through the laparoscope and, to a lesser extent, by an open operation, as an approach to conditions in the pelvis amenable to surgery. This chapter attempts not only to evaluate the medical benefits of competing therapies for the solution of impairments to reproduction but also to point out the change in surgical approaches to standard surgical procedures caused by the availability of IVF. In the real world for practical reasons, it is sometimes necessary to choose a therapy that is less than best to solve the problem. Among such prac-

tical reasons are specified insurance coverage, provider capability and bias, and patient choice.

In this discussion, these practical reasons are minimized, and the emphasis is on what seems to be the best for the patient.

IN VITRO FERTILIZATION AND ALLIED TECHNOLOGIES

To accomplish the purpose of this chapter and this volume, it is not necessary to dwell on the minute details of the technology of IVF or the now-obsolescent allied procedures of gamete intrafallopian transfer, zygote intrafallopian transfer, or other procedures. Rather, it is more useful to emphasize those factors that allow estimations of the probabilities of a pregnancy and term delivery by IVF for a particular patient. Only in this way can a judgment be made whether the best interests of the patient can be served by a surgical procedure or by some form of ART.

Procedures

Essentially all programs of ART imply ovarian stimulation with the aim of harvesting multiple eggs because increasing pregnancy rates are directly related to the transfer of increasing numbers of fertilized eggs up to a point. Using British data, Templeton and Morris found that there was no increase in pregnancy rates with the transfer of more than two eggs, but Shieve et al., using American data, found no increase after the transfer of three eggs. However, as the number of transferred eggs increases, so does the multiple-pregnancy rate. To prevent high-order multiple births, many programs limit the number of transferred preembryos. Many sovereign nations limit by law the number of eggs that may be transferred. Other nations, including the United States, have no laws but operate under guidelines. In the United States under guidelines issued by the American Society for Reproductive Medicine, the number to transfer varies from two to five eggs, depending on age and other factors.

The transfer of concepti allowed to proceed in culture to a blastocyst seems to offer improvement of the implantation rate so that an excellent pregnancy rate can be achieved with the use of two, or even one, blastocyst, thus eliminating the possibility of triplets except for the rare spontaneous splitting of a blastocyst after transfer. Gardner et al. have championed this approach.

Ovarian stimulation usually is accomplished by the use of clomiphene citrate, human menopausal gonadotropins in a 1:1 mixture of follicle-stimulating hormone (FSH) and luteinizing hormone (LH) or by FSH alone. Biosynthetic gonadotropins are in common use and will in time probably replace the material derived from menopausal urine. There has been increasing concomitant use of either a gonadotropin-releasing hormone agonist (GnRHa) or an antagonist (GnRHantag). The GnRHa and GnRHantag improve the control of ovarian stimulation by suppressing pituitary gonadotropin output, although GnRHa causes an initial flare. These GnRHa products have a slightly different effect. GnRHa allows for improved synchrony of nuclear oocyte maturation while blocking any premature and, therefore, detrimental LH surge. GnRHantag does not seem to affect maturation synchrony but does block the LH surge. Overall, one or two fewer oocytes seem to be harvested after the antagonists.

The patient's response to stimulation is monitored by serum estradiol (E_2) values and ultrasound examination with a vaginal transducer. After suitable follicular growth and proper elevation of the serum E_2, final maturation of the oocytes can be induced by administration of biosynthetic LH or exogenous human chorionic gonadotropin as a surrogate for the LH surge, which is suppressed by the agonists or antagonists and exogenous gonadotropins. Mature oocytes are collected about 34 to 36 hours after LH or human chorionic gonadotropin administration.

All programs now use ultrasound-directed transvaginal needle aspiration of the follicles as the method of oocyte collection.

Oocytes in meiosis II can be inseminated as soon as convenient after harvest. Oocytes in meiosis I or prophase need to be allowed to mature to meiosis II before insemination (Fig. 19.1). Centrifugation and a "swim-up" technique are used to prepare the sperm if the semen examination is normal. The insemination cul-

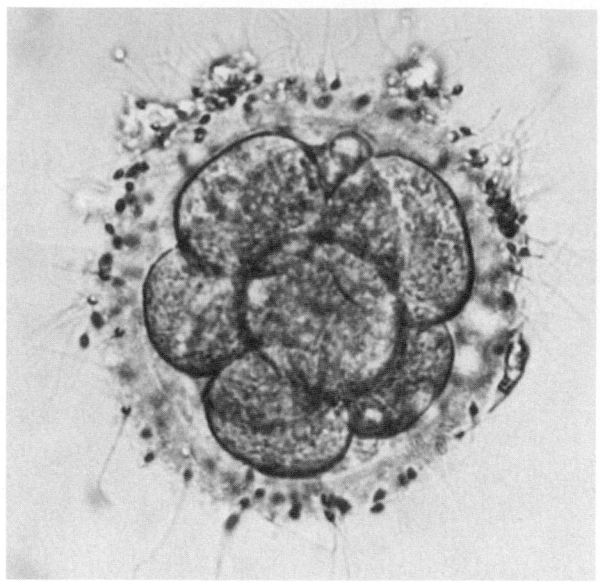

FIGURE 19.1. An eight-cell preembryo just before transfer. Note the large number of sperm adherent to the outer surface of the zona pellucida.

ture medium is supplemented with protein support, such as fetal cord serum, or other protein. With a normal semen examination, 50,000 motile sperm per milliliter of culture medium is adequate, but with compromised sperm examination, a larger number of sperm is helpful. Transfer by the transcervical route occurs 48 to 72 hours after insemination, when the preembryos are in the four-cell to eight-cell stage. A preembryo that has developed to eight cells by 48 hours seems to have an enhanced chance to result in a pregnancy. Blastocyst transfer is usually done on day 5 after aspiration.

PROGNOSTIC FACTORS FOR PREGNANCY

The Male

For both surgery and ART, an adequate semen specimen is essential. It is no longer appropriate to eliminate from the evaluation of surgical results those patients with a complicating "male factor." Such patients can and should be identified preoperatively, and appropriate alternate therapy should be used. If treatment of the male is unsuccessful—as it usually is—IVF is helpful in patients with oligospermia, provided that the total motile sperm population in the original ejaculate is not less than 1.5 million. With an extremely low count, pregnancy should be attempted by injection of sperm into the oocyte by intracytoplasmic sperm injection (ICSI) because such techniques have become highly successful.

Age

A number of investigators have observed that the IVF pregnancy rates decrease and abortion rates increase in patients older than 40 years of age. This is probably true of surgical results as well, although reported surgical results are seldom stratified by age.

Patient Response

It was observed early in the IVF experience that patients responded differently to the same gonadotropin stimulation. This led to the classification of patients as low, intermediate, or high responders. Further study revealed that standardized basal FSH values correlate well with response—the higher the basal FSH value, the lower the response. With the use of agonists or antagonists, larger numbers of better synchronized oocytes are harvested in the intermediate-responder and high-responder groups. This has led to substantially enhanced pregnancy and take-home baby rates in these groups. Proper stimulation in the low-responder group remains a problem.

Pregnancy Rates

There is no overall IVF pregnancy rate against which surgical results can be compared. If the male is compromised to the point at which pregnancy is unlikely to occur if all else is normal, IVF (including ICSI) should be recommended, regardless of the surgical problem. The importance of an expert andrologic evaluation of the male partner before undertaking therapy of any kind cannot be overemphasized. Among husbands with normal sperm, however, there are categories of patients with well-determined prognostic characteristics that enable the observer to estimate with considerable accuracy the expectancy of pregnancy in a good IVF program. This anticipated take-home baby rate varies from about 11% in patients older than 40 years of age to more than 60% per cycle and higher among intermediate and high responders who use cryopreservation. Pregnancy rates are also enhanced by selection of the best oocytes and pre-embryos for transfer. Those not selected are sometimes discarded or cryopreserved. It is against this individualized prognosis that the choice of surgery or ART must be made.

THE OPERATION OF SALPINGECTOMY

For many years, it was taught and practiced that salpingectomy, as for ectopic pregnancy or pyosalpinx, was performed by excising a generous portion of the intramural part of the tube and closing the myometrium with interrupted stitches. The purpose of this technique was to prevent a postoperative interstitial abscess when operating for a pyosalpinx or to prevent a postoperative interstitial pregnancy. Both of these are well-recognized conditions in the older literature. With the widespread use of perioperative antibiotics, postoperative interstitial abscesses have disappeared, and interstitial pregnancies are so rare that a reevaluation of interstitial excision was the subject of a review. The difficulty is that after deep

cornual resection, there is a measurable incidence of uterine rupture at that point, with a subsequent intrauterine pregnancy. This problem can be aggravated by the widespread use of ART when intrauterine pregnancies occur after bilateral salpingectomy. Therefore, the technique of salpingectomy probably should be modified for whatever indication, and for the reasons mentioned earlier, if salpingectomy is performed, a traditional cornual resection is not appropriate. A superficial resection at the uterine attachment, removing none of the myometrium, is all that is required, with closure of the peritoneal defect by two or three interrupted stitches of fine caliber.

SURGERY FOR INFLAMMATORY TUBAL OBSTRUCTION

End Results

Because the evaluation of end results from tubal surgery is subject to many variables, it is exceedingly difficult to be confident that any end result is a consequence of the procedures being tested. There are at least four major concerns: diagnosis, clinical material, operative technique, and presentation of end results.

Diagnosis

How is the diagnosis of tubal obstruction made? Neither hysterosalpingogram nor laparoscopy with hydrotubation is free from technical problems or misinterpretations. As a general rule, one should be hesitant to offer or perform an operative procedure based on a single diagnostic technique at a single examination. This caution about diagnostic dependability applies particularly to obstruction at the proximal end of the tube, especially when the tube appears otherwise normal at laparoscopic examination. A false-positive outcome can result from thickened endometrium in the premenstrual period, technical details with the apparatus, transient debris in the uterus or isthmic portions of the tube, or other conditions, which can be different at a second examination, with completely different findings.

Clinical Material

It is difficult to be confident in a test and control series that the clinical material is similar. In 1988, the then American Fertility Society suggested a classification, but it seems to have had only limited appreciation in subsequent publications. Pelvic disease is so variable in its manifestations that no two cases are exactly alike. Furthermore, certain populations are more prone to reinfection, which influences end results.

Operative Technique

Many times, an operative technique is the variable being tested in one of the two arms of a study population. It is not unusual, however, for the procedure itself to evolve during the course of a test, so that the results often do not express the technique. In this connection, ancillary matters often creep in, such as a change in the prophylactic antibiotics or change in size of the suture material, any of which can influence the end results.

Presentation of End Results

Of all the variables, the method of the presentation of end results is the most troublesome. It can be stated without question that the only meaningful methods for the evaluation of end results are by a cumulative pregnancy rate per month of year of exposure (a modified life-table analysis) or the calculation of a fecundity rate (i.e., pregnancy per menstrual cycle of exposure). Despite this, even contemporary clinical trials often present results as a percentage of patients who are pregnant after a follow-up of some arbitrary minimum interval, usually 1 year. This has only limited value. The bibliography at the end of this chapter gives preference to those articles in which the end results are presented in a meaningful manner. It is not always possible to do this, simply because the data are not available.

Operations for Inflammatory Obstruction at Specific Areas

Cornual Obstruction

As mentioned earlier, diagnosis of cornual obstruction is tricky, and a single hysterogram or a single laparoscopic examination with apparent cornual obstruction is not reliable. When cornual obstruction is identified, if the distal tube appears normal by laparoscopy and operative relief is considered, the diagnosis is almost always salpingitis isthmica nodosa. Because of poor results, the time has passed when surgical relief for a tube with both distal and cornual obstructions should be undertaken. Results from ART are far superior to results obtained by surgery when the obstruction is at more than one site in the fallopian tube. An understanding of the causes of cornual obstruction can be obtained by a review of the histopathologic findings after excision of the obstruction. Several of these studies have found either no demonstrable lesion obstructing the lumen, or endosalpingosis or a related condition. The cases with no demonstrable obstruction or other pathologic lesion attest to the fickleness of the diagnostic accuracy of cornual obstruction.

For many years, the reamer technique, with excision of the obstructed part of the proximal portion of the tube, was performed. The results from this type of macrosurgery were reasonably acceptable, even by contemporary standards, with a cumulative pregnancy rate of about 40% after 4 years and an even higher rate if the isthmic portion of the tube was sacrificed and the ampullary portion of the tube was introduced through the reamer defect. Despite these good results, uterine rupture after tubal reimplantation was a troubling complication. For this reason, this procedure must be considered of historical interest only. An alternate surgical technique wherein tubocornual anastomosis is performed avoids the complication of uterine rupture. One of the preoperative variables in this condition is the question of visualization of the intramural tube by hysterosalpingography before surgery. In an informative study, Donnez and Casanas-Roux pointed out that the best results could be obtained if the intramural portion was visualized before surgery. Unfortunately, these results are not presented by life-table analysis, but the gross pregnancy rate was 44%. The practical point is that Donnez and Casanas-Roux advocated a surgical attempt even if the intramural portion could not be visualized preoperatively, pointing out that most often after amputation of the tube, patency in the intramural portion proved to be satisfactory despite preoperative information to the contrary.

Transuterine catheterization of the tube has been advocated as a method of overcoming proximal tubal obstruction. Despite its use for several years, the method remains controversial. A study of the histopathologic material from cornual obstruction would lead to the suspicion that transuterine tubal catheterization would be likely to succeed when there was no intrinsic pathologic lesion. It would be difficult to imagine that permanent relief of obstruction owing to endosalpingosis or infection could be overcome by catheterization even if it were accompanied by dilation. Honare et al. report good results. All of these techniques must be evaluated against the prospects of pregnancy by IVF.

Midtubal Obstruction

Midtubal obstruction of an inflammatory nature is often owing to unusual etiological agents, for example, tuberculosis. Urman et al. have reported on 16 women with this condition. Operation was possible in eight (50%), with three term deliveries.

From a practical and overall view, ART is most likely to give the best result in this condition.

Distal Tubal Obstruction

Distal tubal obstruction represents the major portion of tubal obstructive disease. There are various alternate applicable techniques: macrosurgery, microsurgery, laparoscopic surgery with or without laser, and ART. Data are simply not available to show a clear superiority of any one method of surgical treatment, but certain general facts have emerged.

MACROSURGERY. Macrosurgery necessarily forms the base against which subsequent techniques must be compared. A number of series of salpingostomy using macrosurgical techniques have resulted in similar pregnancy rates of about 30% after 4 to 5 years.

MICROSURGERY. Microsurgical techniques have likewise resulted in pregnancy rates of about 30%. Tulandi and Vilos showed that with open microsurgery, carbon dioxide (CO_2) laser salpingostomy results in essentially the same pregnancy rate as microdiathermy. Other groups have shown the same results.

OPERATIVE LAPAROSCOPY. There are few references to good studies for terminal salpingostomy using operative laparoscopic techniques. There are some reports in non–peer-review journals; the results indicate that the expectancy of pregnancy is not too different from that reported using macrosurgical and microsurgical techniques. Dlugi et al. in a good study (1994) reported a 9% cure rate with unilateral neosalpingostomy and a 34.2% rate with bilateral salpingostomy. Prapas et al. reported results with laparoscopy that were as good as with laparotomy in a small series. With open surgical procedures, however, there is little case selection, whereas laparoscopic operative techniques are selectively applied. It follows that laparoscopic operative procedures are being performed in the most favorable cases, and the results must be viewed with this in mind.

PREGNANCY OUTCOME IN RELATION TO EXTENT OF DISEASE. A number of studies of open operative techniques have related the pregnancy rates to the extent of tubal disease. They are in agreement, although it is difficult to compare one study with another because of varying techniques in classifying the extent of disease. In a study of 87 cases, Rock et al. found a pregnancy rate of 87% in patients with mild disease, 30% in those with moderate disease, and only 5% in those with severe disease. About half of the patients (45) had mild or moderate disease. Mage et al. showed essentially the same results. Although these investigators divided the grades of disease into four categories, 55% of cases (42 of 76) were in the lesser grades, with a pregnancy rate of 43% (18 of 42), whereas in the more severe categories, only two of 34 patients became pregnant.

SOCIOLOGICAL INDICATIONS FOR THERAPY. In this era of managed care and third-party payers, the physician is often forced to select a treatment that is not in the best interest of the patient. This usually revolves around the approach of payment for a surgical procedure, whereas the more efficacious IVF is disallowed. When relative costs have been carefully examined, it turns out that costs for IVF are comparable or less than for surgery. For example, Lilford and Watson studied the problem in Great Britain and concluded that "insurers should make IVF more widely available. They should purchase this service rather than tubal microsurgery for most patients with tubal blockage."

Haan and van Steen studied the problem in the Netherlands and concluded that "IVF and tubal surgery can be regarded as equivalent alternatives for couples with tubal pathology with regard to medical and economical aspects of treatment."

Studies of cost comparisons in the United States for obstructive tubal disease have not been published, but some studies have compared the purely medical outcomes of the two methods. IVF fares well in such comparative studies, which generally include all cases of tubal blockage. It should be possible by proper selection to tailor treatment to provide the best for each patient.

RECOMMENDATIONS IN REGARD TO DISTAL SALPINGOTOMY. Evidence fails to indicate any superiority of any one surgical technique on an end-result basis. Laparoscopic approaches can have some advantage in length

of hospital stay, hospital costs, quick return to work, and so on. It cannot be concluded that laparoscopic salpingostomy offers the patient the best possible chance to get pregnant. This, after all, should be the main goal of reparative surgery of the tubes. The data indicate that success, as measured by pregnancy outcome from operative treatment of tubal disease, is related more to extent of disease than to operative technique. Furthermore, in severe tubal disease, surgical treatment yields results that are inferior to those obtainable by IVF. For these reasons, it is not difficult to recommend that, in distal tubal obstruction, considerable care be exercised in the selection of patients for operative treatment. Patients with severe tubal disease should be offered IVF as primary therapy. This recommendation applies to more than half of all patients with distal obstruction.

Fimbrioplasty and Salpingolysis
By definition, the tubes in this group of patients are open when examined by hysterosalpingography or by hydrotubation at laparoscopy. There are pelvic adhesions of various degrees, however, and many times there is phimosis impeding the free motion of the fimbria. Thus, these conditions are considered together because one seldom occurs without at least some degree of the other. In these patients, there is a choice between open operation, laparoscopic surgery with or without the laser, and ART.

It is not easy to determine past and current experience by a review of the literature. In the older literature, with open operative procedure in which results are not expressed by life-table analysis, a postsalpingolysis pregnancy rate of 50% to 60% or somewhat higher was common. Lavy et al. found that in five series using macrosurgery, reporting a total of 465 patients, there was a pregnancy rate of 42%. When microsurgery was used among 271 patients, there were 142 pregnancies, or 52%. With laparoscopic techniques in about 100 patients, the pregnancy rate was 61%. There were no statistically significant differences among any of these series.

With results in the 50% to 60% range, an operative procedure with one of the techniques discussed earlier would be a reasonable choice in this particular situation, provided the patient was young. For patients in their mid-30s or older, IVF is the first choice.

Reiterative Surgery for Tubal Disease
Second operations in patients who have failed to conceive after a primary tuboplasty have yielded poor results. For this reason, with few exceptions, failed tuboplasty is a strong indication for the use of ART.

REANASTOMOSIS AFTER SURGICAL INTERRUPTION

Of all the therapeutic options available for various types of tubal disease, open surgical reanastomosis after surgical tubal interruption is perhaps the least controversial. It is the shining example of the best there is of microsurgical technique. Tubal anastomosis is not a single operative procedure. The technique used depends on the type of anastomosis required, for example, isthmic–isthmic, ampullary–isthmic, or ampullary–ampullary.

Isthmic–Isthmic Anastomosis

The isthmic–isthmic anastomosis is one of the most satisfactory of the tubal procedures. With this situation, there is no tubal or muscular disparity, and the operative procedure seldom takes more than 30 or 40 minutes for each tube. After excision of the stump of the tubes and identification of the adequacy of the two lumina, the mesosalpinx can be brought together with a few interrupted stitches of 8-0. The tubal ends can be approximated by three or four muscle-to-muscle stitches, with care being taken not to enter the lumen of the tube because this can result in an undesirable endosalpingian reaction with postoperative obstruction. After approximation of the muscularis, the serosa can be brought together with three or four interrupted fine stitches. The operative procedure can be performed either with or without a stent introduced through the lumen of the tube. Most surgeons prefer to remove the stent at the end of the procedure, but for a number of years, we have left a coiled stent within the endometrial lumen, removing it a few weeks after the primary operation.

Isthmic–Ampullary Anastomosis

Isthmic–ampullary anastomosis requires the approximation of lumina with different diameters. There are various techniques to accomplish this. One commonly used method is to open the isthmic end longitudinally for a short distance, thus artificially increasing the lumen of the proximal stump. With this technique, it usually is necessary for the suture to penetrate the lumen of the distal stump because of the thickness of the muscularis at this point. Despite this theoretical disadvantage, this technique has given excellent results. Although the sudden change in luminal size would appear to predispose to ectopic pregnancy, this concern is not borne out in fact.

Ampullary–Ampullary Anastomosis

As mentioned earlier, it is undesirable to enter the tubal lumen with the fine suture. The muscularis in the ampullary portion of the tube often is so thin that a good bit of tearing occurs unless the endosalpinx or serosa is involved in the suture. Because results are satisfactory, one should not hesitate to do this in indicated situations. Indeed, through-and-through sutures in the ampullary portion of the tube often are required because of the delicacy of the tissues. In this technique, a minimum bite should be taken on both sides of the anastomosis to prevent a diaphragm-like effect at the site. Seven or eight interrupted stitches are required around the circumference of the lumen for a satisfactory anastomosis. The results of this surgery are reasonably good, but the number of cases in which this is required is small because this is an undesirable place to interrupt the tube. Thus, the procedure most often is used after the occasional interruption by an operator or under special circumstances.

Use of the Microscope

Microsurgical techniques involve more than the use of magnification; they involve meticulous handling of tissue, use of special light instruments, and use of fine suture 8-0 and smaller. In a randomized trial of end results comparing a compound microscope with an optic visor and loupe, no difference in success rates could be shown in terms of subsequent pregnancies. In this connection, it is of interest that in an early series using fine suture material, a high pregnancy rate was obtained without the use of either loupe or microscope.

Contraindications to Tubal Reanastomosis

Tubal reanastomosis after surgical interruption is an extremely satisfactory operation. With the availability of ART; however, there are certain situations in which it should not be recommended. The principal situation has to do with the residual length of the ampullary portion of the tube. A number of studies have indicated that if the residual ampulla is less than 4 cm, the expectancy of pregnancy is greatly diminished. The conclusion is obvious: Unless one can have at least 4 cm of ampulla after anastomosis, the patient should seek to solve her problem with IVF.

Some evidence suggests that reanastomosis after interruption for more than 5 years has a decreased chance of success. Personal experience casts doubt on this conclusion. Thus, prolonged surgical interruptions may not be an absolute contraindication to surgical reanastomosis, provided there is adequate tubal length and provided the patient is less than 35 years of age. The younger the patient, the better.

Some evidence also suggests that the technique by which the tube is interrupted is reflected in ultimate pregnancy rates. Thus, interruption by cautery carries an ultimate pregnancy rate inferior to that of interruption by clips or bands. Although these data state the facts, interruption by cautery can result in a shortened ampullary length on reanastomosis, and the inferior results may be related to the length of the residual tube rather than to the technique of interruption. Nevertheless, if interruption has been by cautery, special attention needs to be paid to the residual length of the tube. If one has doubts in surveying the patient before recommending a technique for overcoming the tubal obstruction, IVF may represent a more reliable alternative to surgical reanastomosis.

Techniques have been advocated for tubal reanastomosis by laparoscopic means. The few scattered data available from such procedures present results comparable to those for open operation. However, the reports are few, and it is easy to argue that only successes are reported. Except in expert and experienced hands, such efforts cannot be considered in the best interests of the patient.

OVARIAN PLACEMENT AT PELVIC LAPAROTOMY

Operations because of pain caused by extensive pelvic disease often involve not only the release of pelvic adhesions but also removal of one or both fallopian tubes. At the end of the operative procedure, the surgeon has certain options in the placement of the ovary. Clearly, if both tubes have been removed or if one is removed and the other is nonfunctional, ART offers the patient an opportunity to achieve her family goals. In the interval when laparoscopic egg harvest was routinely being performed, there were persuasive reasons to locate the remaining ovary as high in the pelvis as possible. In fact, a location in the region of the cornua of the uterus was far better than having the ovary in its normal position against the lateral pelvic wall.

The widespread use of transvaginal ultrasonic-guided oocyte retrieval makes the high placement of the ovary a disadvantage. It is much better to locate the ovary low in the pelvis, in the cul-de-sac region, attached with one or two sutures to the posterior surface of the uterus in the neighborhood of the uterosacral ligaments, so that it is immediately adjacent to the cul-de-sac for oocyte retrieval (Fig. 19.2).

TREATMENT OF ENDOMETRIOSIS

The optimum treatment for endometriosis is still uncertain. It has been difficult to show that treatment of stage I and II (American Fertility Society classification) endometriosis is beneficial. Sometimes, it has been concluded from such data that minimal endometriosis is not associated with infertility. An alternate and more likely conclusion is that the treatment of minimal endometriosis is not efficacious. This conclusion is supported by the fact that patients with mild endometriosis, treated or untreated, have a low fecundity level, which is probably explained on the basis of the endometriosis.

For more advanced disease, treatment apparently needs to be modulated according to whether there are endometriomas; it usually is agreed that endometriomas larger than 1 or 2 cm are not favorably influenced by standard hormonal treatment for endometriosis. Therefore, with ovarian involvement, some type of surgical approach is useful. This has traditionally been by open operation, but in more recent years, operative laparoscopy has been considered an alternative.

Nevertheless, surgical therapy or medical treatment is not always successful. In that circumstance, ART, especially IVF, offers the possibility of therapy. An additional point is that although fertility lessens with patient age, particularly past 35 years of age, the expectancy of pregnancy with IVF does not diminish much until 40 years of age. In view of the delay that is necessarily involved in the medical management of endometriosis and, to a lesser extent, in the surgical management, consideration needs to be given to the use of ART as the primary method of therapy in patients older than 35 years of age.

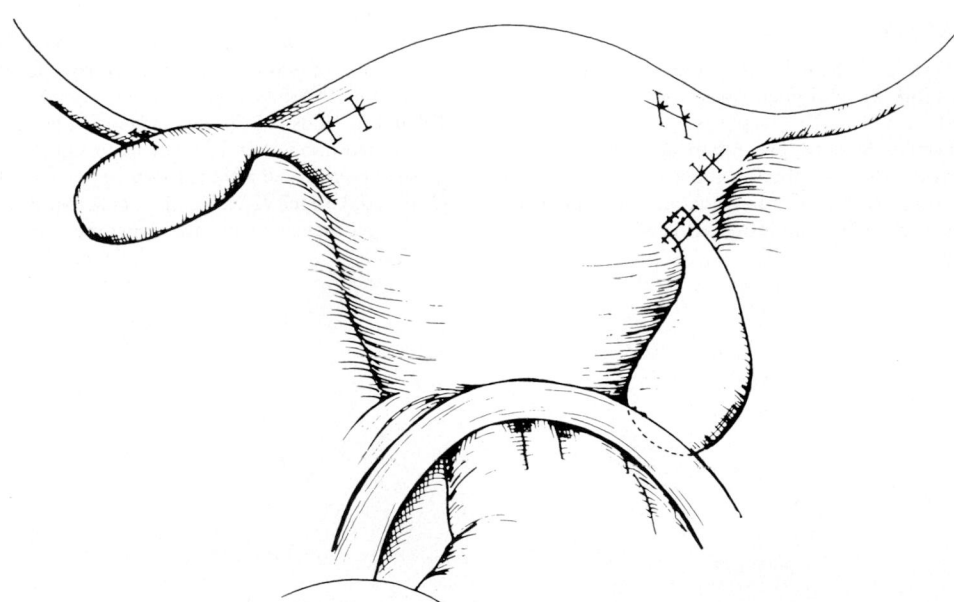

FIGURE 19.2. Pelvis after a bilateral salpingectomy. **Left:** The uteroovarian ligament is undisturbed, but the ovary is suspended to the round ligament to provide maximum access for laparoscopic approach. With anticipated transvaginal ultrasound-guided oocyte aspiration, this is no longer a desirable operative procedure. **Right:** The uteroovarian ligament has been divided and the ovary placed low in the pelvis for easy access from the vagina. It is not always necessary to sever the uteroovarian ligament.

CHANGING INDICATIONS FOR HYSTERECTOMY

For many years, it was considered good practice to perform a prophylactic hysterectomy when removing both fallopian tubes or when it otherwise appeared that future reproduction was impossible. The reason for this was to prevent the subsequent development of uterine cancer. The use of IVF has shown that fallopian tubes are not required for normal intrauterine pregnancies. Therefore, in deciding whether a hysterectomy should be performed prophylactically in association with operations for benign pelvic disease, the future reproductive potential of the patient and her partner must be considered. In our litigious society, malpractice suits have been brought against surgeons who have performed a hysterectomy under these circumstances, wherein the plaintiff has taken the position that the surgeon should have realized that IVF would have made it possible for her to achieve a pregnancy. This thought can be extended, even to patients in whom oophorectomy or removal of streak ovaries is necessary, for whatever reason. With donor eggs and exogenous hormonal stimulation, reproduction is possible if the uterus is in place. Therefore, hysterectomy must be carefully evaluated before surgery in all patients, and a clear understanding should be reached about whether the uterus will be retained. These considerations should be clearly set forth in the operative permit, so that there is little opportunity for misunderstanding after the operative procedure.

BIBLIOGRAPHY

The American Fertility Society. Revised American fertility society classification of endometriosis: 1985. *Fertil Steril* 1985;43:351.

The American Fertility Society. The American Fertility Society classifications of adnexal adhesions, distal tubal occlusion, tubal occlusion secondary to tubal ligation, tubal pregnancies, müllerian anomalies and intrauterine adhesions. *Fertil Steril* 1988;6:944.

American Society for Reproductive Medicine. *Guidelines on number of embryos transferred. A Practice Committee Report.* Birmingham, AL: November 1999.

Dlugi AM, Reddy S, Saleh W, et al. Pregnancy rates after operative endoscopic treatment of total (neosalpingostomy) or near total (salpingostomy) distal tubal occlusion. *Fertil Steril* 1994;62:913.

Donnez J, Casanas-Roux F. Prognostic factors in fimbrial microsurgery. *Fertil Steril* 1986;46:200.

Gardner DK, Lane M, Schoolcraft WB. Culture and transfer of viable blastocysts: a feasible proposition for human IVF. *Hum Reprod* 2000;15:9.

Haan G, van Steen R. Costs in relation to effects of in-vitro fertilization. *Hum Reprod* 1992;7:982.

Honore GM, Holden AEC, Schenken RS. Pathophysiology and management of proximal tubal blockage. *Fertil Steril* 1999;71:785.

Jones HW Jr, Rock JA. On the reanastomosis of the fallopian tubes after surgical sterilization. *Fertil Steril* 1978;29:702.

Lavy G, Diamond MP, DeCherney AH. Ectopic pregnancy: its relationship to tubal reconstructive surgery. *Fertil Steril* 1987;47:543.

Lilford RJ, Watson AJ. Has in-vitro fertilization made salpingostomy obsolete? *Br J Obstet Gynaecol* 1990;97:557.

Mage G, Pouly JL, Coulet de Joliniere Jr., et al. Preoperative classification to predict intrauterine and ectopic pregnancy rates after distal tubal microsurgery. *Fertil Steril* 1986;46:807.

Prapas Y, Prapas N, Papanicolaou A, et al. Laparoscopic tubal surgery: a retrospective comparative study of open microsurgery versus laparoscopic surgery. *Acta Eur Fertil* 1995;26:81.

Rock JA, Katayama KP, Martin EJ, et al. Factors influencing the success of salpingostomy techniques for distal fimbrial obstruction. *Obstet Gynecol* 1978;52:591.

Schieve LA, Peterson HB, Meikle SF et al. Live-birth rates and multiple-birth risk using *in vitro* fertilization. *JAMA* 1999;282:1832.

Templeton , Morris JK. Reducing the risk of multiple births by transfer of two embryos after *in vitro* fertilization. *N Engl J Med* 1998;339:573.

Tulandi T, Vilos GA. A comparison between laser surgery and electrosurgery for bilateral hydrosalpinx: a 2-year follow-up. *Fertil Steril* 1985;44:846.

Urman B, Gomel V, McComb P, et al. Midtubal occlusion: etiology, management, and outcome. *Fertil Steril* 1992;57:747.

Te Linde's Operative Gynecology, ninth edition, edited by John A. Rock and Howard W. Jones, III. Lippincott Williams & Wilkins, Philadelphia, © 2003.

CHAPTER
20

Normal and Abnormal Uterine Bleeding

WILLIAM J. BUTLER

Reproductive capability in a young woman begins at the point of menarche, which is the beginning of cyclic uterine bleeding in the anatomically and physiologically normal female. Menarche marks the beginning of an important stage in a young woman's physical reproductive maturation and development. Even before the onset of this entirely natural but potentially disturbing function, a young woman's early psychological reactions to menstruation, and probably also her lifelong view, can be influenced by the accuracy of her information and the degree of empathy with which this knowledge has been conveyed to her.

Many women, perhaps appropriately, conclude that any departure from their personal menstrual experience is abnormal, and they will seek treatment for these departures. Conversely, some women accept or perhaps ignore even significant variations in their menstrual function, sometimes to the extent that serious health impairment occurs (e.g., severe iron-deficiency anemia).

Clinical experience has led to empiric definitions of variations in menstrual pattern that constitute abnormal or dysfunctional uterine bleeding (DUB). Various terms are in general use to facilitate description and record-keeping regarding patterns of uterine bleeding. We define here some of the terms used in this discussion.

Polymenorrhea—a menstrual cycle interval of less than 21 days

Amenorrhea—the absence of menstrual bleeding for more than 6 months

Dysmenorrhea—painful menstruation

Interval bleeding—bleeding between menstrual cycles

Oligomenorrhea—a menstrual cycle interval of more than 37 days

Metrorrhagia—a period of menstrual bleeding longer than 7 days, or interval bleeding

Menorrhagia—excessive menstrual bleeding

Postmenopausal bleeding—uterine bleeding occurring more than 12 months after the last menstrual period of a menopausal woman

Break-through bleeding—intermenstrual bleeding that is the result of exogenous hormones

Current medical therapies are quite effective in the management of most of the disturbances of menstrual function that occur in the absence of infection, gestation, or uterine tumor. The success of these therapies depends on a complete understanding of normal menstrual physiology and of the effects of the various agents available for treatment. New surgical diagnostic and therapeutic technologies are becoming available to aid in the management of patients who fail to respond to conventional endocrine manipulation by medical therapies.

NORMAL MENSTRUAL PHYSIOLOGY

Menstruation is the physiologic shedding of the endometrium associated with uterine bleeding that occurs at monthly intervals from menarche to menopause. In the years between these two physiologic landmarks, menstruation will occur 400 to 500 times in the average female. According to the classical theory of the physiology of menstruation, it is the superficial functional layer of the endometrium that is shed during menstruation, and regeneration proceeds from the remaining intact basalis. This process of monthly shedding and regeneration can occur as often as it does without producing permanent tissue damage possibly because most of the functional endometrium is conserved during menses and because the metamorphosis from proliferative to secretory endometria is controlled not only by processes of cell desquamation and reproliferation but also by dynamic and interactive processes of the endocrinologic and reproductive systems involving many organs. Any interruption of these normal but quite complex cyclic processes can lead to irregularities in endometrial breakdown and to DUB.

ENDOCRINOLOGY

The endometrium is an endocrine organ that responds to circulating blood levels of estrogen and progesterone. These two steroids alone are sufficient to induce growth and maturation of an endometrium that can support blastocyst implantation, as has been demonstrated by their sequential administration to patients with ovarian failure to prepare for the transfer of donated embryos. Estradiol (E_2) production by the developing follicle stimulates metabolic activity in the endometrium. E_2 has multiple effects that are mediated through binding to estrogen receptors. There are two estrogen receptors, alpha and beta. The estrogen receptors are members of a hormone receptor family that includes not only the other steroid receptors but also receptors for vitamin D and thyroid hormone. All receptors in this family have three domains. The regulatory domain at the amino acid terminal binds regulatory protein factors. The hormone-binding domain on the carboxy terminal, with its contiguous hinge region, undergoes conformational changes when a steroid hormone binds to it, allowing DNA binding. The DNA-binding domain binds to the hormone-responsive elements in the target gene. The conformation of the DNA-binding domain consists of the highly conserved zinc finger structures that interact with complementary patterns in the DNA.

Steroid hormones have relatively low molecular weights and are rapidly transported into cells by passive diffusion. Binding of a steroid hormone to the intranuclear receptors transforms and activates the hormone receptor complex to allow DNA binding to specific hormone response elements and initiates subsequent transcription. Both estrogen and progesterone receptors bind to their response elements as dimers. After gene activation, the hormone receptor complex undergoes processing with dissociation and loss of activity.

Transcription of target genes with mRNA synthesis leads to translation with synthesis of proteins on ribosomes in the cytoplasm. The biologic effects of E_2 are mediated through this protein synthesis.

Estrogen and Progesterone Receptor Induction

One important function of estrogen is the induction of synthesis of its own and other steroid hormone receptors, called replenishment. Estrogen receptors reach a maximum concentration in the middle-to-late proliferative phase of the menstrual cycle. Progesterone receptors are also induced, and their concentration peaks in the late proliferative phase. Progesterone then blocks the estrogen replenishment mechanism, possibly by accelerating receptor turnover and inhibiting E_2-induced gene transcription. Enough progesterone receptors persist throughout the luteal phase, however, to maintain endometrial responsiveness and induction of deciduation.

Estrogen and Progesterone Target Genes

Target genes of the E_2 receptor complex code for the synthesis of numerous proteins, including structural proteins, enzymes, and growth factors. The relative roles played by the alpha and beta estrogen receptors in the endometrium have yet to be completely elucidated. The net effect of estrogenic stimulation is to induce DNA synthesis and mitotic activity with proliferation of the endometrial glands and stroma. The results are cessation of menstrual flow and an increase in the thickness of the endometrium.

Progesterone also has multiple biologic effects mediated through its receptors. It actively inhibits synthesis of both its own receptors and estrogen receptors, although sufficient progesterone receptors remain throughout the luteal phase of the cycle to mediate maturation and secretory differentiation of the endometrium. The net effect is to antagonize estrogenic metabolic activity with suppression of DNA synthesis in endometrial cells, which results in dynamic inhibition of cell mitosis. Progesterone is also responsible for the active induction of synthesis of various cytoplasmic enzymes, the secretion of proteins such as prolactin-dependent and progesterone-dependent endometrial peptide from decidualized stromal cells, and the stabilization of lysosomes, all of which may play an important role in the onset of menstruation.

Histology and Physiology

The postmenstrual endometrium that remains after collapse and partial shedding during menstruation consists of a thin but stable layer of basalis cells and the dense irregular remnants of the stromal cell–derived stratum spongiosum. The glands are narrow and lined by low cuboidal epithelial cells with few mitoses. The glandular stromal cells are small and spindly with little cytoplasm or mitotic activity. Protein synthesis and secretory activity are minimal. It is on this substrate of basal and stromal cells that estrogen induces a proliferative response.

Early Proliferative Phase

Mitotic activity results in growth and pseudostratification of the glandular epithelial cells. With development and elongation of the glands, the epithelial cells assume a more columnar shape, with secretory granules in the cytoplasm, and glycogen begins to collect in the basal vacuoles. Arteriolar vessels grow up into the endometrium as part of the general proliferative response. The stromal cells also proliferate and expand from a dense compact state to an expanded matrix by transient edema. The combined effects of proliferation and expansion cause the endometrium to grow in this phase to a thickness of 3 to 5 mm.

The increased mitotic activity that results in proliferation is mediated by way of estrogen induction of various peptide growth factors. Epidermal growth factor and insulin-like growth factor I (IGF-I) are two potent mitogens with synthesis that is stimulated by estrogen in endometrial epithelial and stromal cells. Endothelin-1 is a vasoactive peptide with mitogenic activity; its synthesis is induced by both estrogen and growth factors, and its metabolism is enhanced by progesterone. Endothelin-1 may play a role in proliferation and in menstruation. The various peptides that are secreted from stromal and epithelial cells to form the extracellular matrix of the endometrium can be either induced or suppressed by both estrogen and progesterone. Fibronectin, for example, is suppressed by progesterone, whereas several integrin subtypes are stimulated by progesterone. These peptides may have a functional role in proliferation, differentiation, and embryo implantation.

Angiogenesis allows both repair of the endometrium after menstruation and supports cellular proliferation for regrowth during the follicular phase. It is supported and promoted by multiple growth factors. An important role is played by vascular endothelial growth factor (VEGF). VEGF mRNA expression is induced by E_2 and increases from the early proliferative phase through the secretory phase (Torry and Torry). VEGF is produced by the glandular epithelial cells, although some stromal expression is evident in the secretory phase. The increased expression throughout the cycle supports a possible role of VEGF in expansion and coiling of the spiral arterials. Changes in VEGF expression have been detected in women with abnormal uterine bleeding, supporting a possible role in the pathogenesis of menorrhagia (Kooy et al.).

E_2 induces several enzymes (alkaline phosphatase, 5α-reductase, and possibly phospholipase A_2). Phospholipase A_2, which releases arachidonic acid from phospholipid esters, controls the rate-limiting step in prostaglandin synthesis. E_2 also stimulates cyclooxygenase synthesis of prostaglandin $F_{2\alpha}$ ($PGF_{2\alpha}$) and prostaglandin E_2 (PGE_2), both of which have a role in menstrual function. $PGF_{2\alpha}$ has vasoconstrictive and muscle contraction effects. PGE_2 is generally a vasodilator but can also cause contractions in uterine smooth muscle. Alterations in the relative levels of $PGF_{2\alpha}$ and PGE_2 are known to change menstrual bleeding patterns.

Late Proliferative Phase

Ovulation with corpus luteum formation and significant progesterone secretion leads to secretory transformation in the late proliferative-phase endometrium. Progesterone inhibits both estrogen and progesterone receptor synthesis and inhibits DNA synthesis and mitosis. This inhibition process is accompanied by the development of RNA-filled channels between the nucleoli and nuclear membranes that are responsible for the progesterone-induced active synthesis of cytoplasmic enzymes during the secretory phase of the cycle.

The Secretory Phase

The cytoplasmic enzymes 17β- and 20α-hydroxysteroid dehydrogenase (HSD) are induced by progesterone and modulate steroid activity. The enzyme 17β-HSD catalyzes the conversion of E_2 to the relatively weaker estrogen estrone, which, when sulfated by estrogen sulfotransferase, can no longer bind to estrogen receptors. The enzyme 20α-HSD alters progesterone receptor binding and activity. Cytoplasmic lytic enzymes such as acid phosphatase are also induced by progesterone but are kept inactive within Golgi-derived lysosomes, the membranes of which are stabilized by progesterone. Insulin-like growth factor II (IGF-II) is synthesized locally by middle-to-late secretory-phase endometrium and appears to be involved in the differentiation response of the endometrium to progesterone. Insulin-like growth factor binding protein I also appears at this time and is regulated by the insulin-like growth factors and by relaxin. Other autocrine or paracrine agents secreted locally by decidual cells are relaxin, progesterone-dependent endometrial peptide, and prolactin.

Progesterone has also been shown to induce the activity of metalloendopeptidase, which degrades the endothelin-1 peptide. Withdrawal of progesterone can lead to increased endothelin-1 activity with vasospasm and initiation of menstrual bleeding. Several investigators have described increased levels of protease inhibitors such as α_1-antitrypsin and antithrombin III in secretory-phase uterine fluid, which may also be involved in the mechanism of menstrual bleeding.

The Luteal Phase

Morphologically, secretory transformation of the endometrium results in coiling of the spiral arterioles and endometrial glands. The endometrium reaches its maximum thickness of 5 to 6 mm and maintains this thickness throughout the luteal phase. The subnuclear intracytoplasmic glycogen vacuoles in the basal glandular cells transpose to the apex and are expelled into the glandular lumen. The stromal cells subsequently flatten into a low cuboidal form. Stromal cell differentiation from reticular spindle-shaped cells into plump predecidual cells and phagocytic granulated cells defines two layers in the functional endometrium known as the superficial compactum and the deeper spongiosum. The spongiosum has a loose edematous matrix that is the consequence of increased capillary permeability, mediated possibly by prostaglandins. The predecidual, late secretory-phase stromal cells produce several metabolically active substances, as previously described, and are infiltrated by migratory leukocytes. The release of lysosomal enzymes from endometrial cells and possibly also from leukocytes may be involved in the initiation of menstruation.

Menstruation

Menstruation is controlled by many complex, interrelated, and incompletely understood factors. Normal menstruation results from progesterone withdrawal from the estrogen-primed endometrium. Changes that occur in the endometrium during menstruation were described by Markee by observation of endometrial tissue transplanted to the anterior chamber of the eyes of Rhesus monkeys. Markee described cyclic changes in endometrial vascularity and the development of coiled vessels supplying the superficial two thirds of the endometrium. The estrogen-primed endometrium of the follicular phase is compact, with relatively underdeveloped vasculature. Progesterone converts this endometrium into a thick, edematous, secretory lining that is glycogen-enriched and prepares the metabolically active stroma and glands with an increased vasculature to receive and nourish a fertilized ovum.

If implantation does not occur, estrogen and progesterone levels fall, prostaglandin synthesis occurs, and lysosomal membranes rupture, causing constriction of the spiral arterioles, ischemic necrosis, and sloughing of the endometrium superficial to the basalis layer. This process begins in the premenstrual phase of the cycle with cessation of synthesis and inspissation of ground substance and supporting tissues by lytic enzymes released from lysosomes, which causes loss of fluids and compression of the endometrium, tonic contractions of spiral arterioles with reduction of blood flow to the tissues, loss of stromal edema, and kinking of the coiled spiral arterioles caused by the reduction in endometrial thickness.

A generalized state of ischemia develops in the superficial layers of endometrium, and bleeding into the stroma begins. Acid phosphatase and prostaglandin substances released from autolyzed cells, together with increased endothelin-1 activity, cause more intense vasoconstriction of spiral arterioles, and devitalized tissues finally slough as small hemorrhages in the stroma coalesce. According to Beller, coagulation factors are decreased in normal menstrual discharge. Fibrinogen is absent, plasminogen is converted to plasmin by released peptidases, and the amount of plasmin inhibitor is decreased. Menstrual blood generally does not clot, but it can form red blood cell aggregates with mucoid substances, mucoproteins, and glycogen as it collects in the vagina. These red cell aggregates may appear to be blood clots, but they contain no fibrin. In the presence of very heavy flow, however, clotting can occur.

According to classical theory, during menstruation the superficial compacta and the intermediate stratum spongiosum layers of the endometrium are shed, leaving only the basalis layer intact. New endometrium is regenerated from the basalis. Regeneration of new capillaries from the basalis has been observed by Markee, and restoration of the endometrial circulation has been correlated with the cessation of menstrual bleeding. Blood loss from the process of normal menstruation is limited by recovery of tone in the myometrium and endometrial vasculature, cessation of cellular autolysis, eventual clotting over the endometrial surface, and eventual active regeneration of glands, stroma, and vessels in the basalis layer in response to rising estrogen levels in the new cycle. The retained basalis endometrium is protected from destruction by lysosomal enzymes by a mucinous carbohydrate coat that covers the free surfaces of endometrial cells. This mechanism for retention of some endometrium during menstruation may explain the lack of permanent damage during the years of menstruation.

Endometrial regression during menstruation is described by classical theory as the result of four processes: autophagia, heterophagia, extrusion of secretory products, and elimination of fluids with some, but not complete, shedding of tissue. Autophagia and heterophagia are the kindred processes of intracellular lytic digestion of debris in vacuoles and of extracellular lytic digestion of debris taken up by phagosomes. Both processes eliminate damaged tissue to allow regeneration of normal endometrial cells. With fluid loss and secretion, the functionalis (the remaining functional basalis) regresses to a resting state, ready to regenerate in the next cycle. These two processes can only partially explain the observation that initial endometrial regeneration occurs in the absence of estrogen. This initial lack of estrogen dependence can also be secondary to the lesser proliferative response required after regression, compared with complete endometrial shedding. Much work remains to be done to define the complex processes involved in menstruation.

ABNORMALITIES OF THE MENSTRUAL CYCLE

Given the complexities and varieties of possible alterations of the systems that control menstruation, it is not surprising that abnormal uterine bleeding should occur even in the absence of obvious disease. Prolonged estrogen stimulation can result in endometrium that outgrows its blood supply and has asynchronous development of endometrial glands, stroma, and blood vessels. Any failure of progesterone production can also profoundly affect endometrial glands, stroma, and blood vessels. Abnormal synthesis of acid mucopolysaccharides can result in the release of excessive amounts of hydrolytic enzymes into the stroma. Lysosome release from endometrial glands, influenced by plasma progesterone levels, can affect menstrual flow. The endometrium and myometrium of patients with menorrhagia produce altered types of prostaglandins. Smith and associates have shown that the amount of menstrual flow is influenced by a change in the endometrial conversion of prostaglandin endoperoxide from PGF_2 to PGE_2, and that women with menorrhagia synthesize mainly the vasodilator PGE_2 in the endometrium.

Menstruation has three clinical characteristics: the menstrual interval or cycle length, the duration of flow, and the amount of flow. The mean cycle length is 28 to 29 days, although a menstrual interval of 21 to 37 days can be considered normal. A menstrual interval shorter than 21 days is defined as polymenorrhea. A menstrual interval longer than 37 days is defined as oligomenorrhea. Amenorrhea is the absence of menses for 6 months or longer. The menstrual interval can vary from month to month by several days. Regularity of the menstrual cycle is more important than exact approximation to the 28-day mean menstrual interval. Variation in the length of the menstrual interval in regular ovulatory cycles usually occurs in the preovulatory (proliferative) phase of the cycle and is more frequent among postmenarchal teenagers and in women approaching menopause.

A duration of flow of 7 days or less is considered normal. A patient bleeding beyond 7 days enters the intermenstrual phase of the cycle, which is defined as metrorrhagia. Regardless of the length of the menstrual flow, 70% of the blood loss usually occurs by the second day and 90% by the third day. A total blood loss of 20 to 80 mL, representing 10 to 35 mg iron, is considered to be within normal limits.

The mean menstrual blood loss for a normal period is about 40 mL. Signs of iron deficiency are present in a significant proportion of women who lose more than 60 mL of blood with each menstrual flow, however. Hallberg and associates found that iron deficiency is common among women who lose more than 80 mL of menstrual blood. Unfortunately, objective measurement of menstrual blood loss is rarely accomplished for women complaining of heavy menstruation or for women with unexplained iron-deficiency anemia. A patient's self-described history of normal or heavy menstrual blood loss is not an accurate indicator of the amount of flow. It is also difficult to accurately estimate the amount of blood loss by counting the number of days of menstrual flow or the number of pads and tampons used, as emphasized by Grimes.

Iron-deficiency anemia is a late manifestation of excessive menstruation. Serum iron (ferritin) levels are more sensitive than hematocrit and hemoglobin levels for detection of iron depletion before anemia develops, as shown by Guillebaud et al. We believe that development and routine use of a convenient, standardized, objective method for measuring menstrual blood loss would significantly improve the clinical practice of gynecology. One fifth of women have a problem with excessive menstrual blood loss sometime during their reproductive years. The method of Hallberg and Nilsson for quantification of iron and blood loss is based on the simultaneous use of tampons and pads for the collection of menstrual blood. Menstrual blood is extracted with 5% sodium hydroxide, which converts hemoglobin to alkaline hematin. The concentration is then determined spectrophotometrically. The method is simple and gives accurate results but is not widely used.

DYSFUNCTIONAL UTERINE BLEEDING

DUB is a symptom complex that includes any condition of abnormal uterine bleeding in the absence of pregnancy, neoplasm, infection, or other intrauterine lesion. Such bleeding is most often the result of endocrinologic dysfunction that inhibits normal ovulation.

Chronic Anovulation and DUB

The state of chronic anovulation is the result of unopposed estrogen stimulation of the endometrium with consequent irregular breakdown and bleeding. Chronic anovulation syndrome is a "wastebasket" diagnosis for multiple endocrine etiologies. Hyperthyroidism and hypothyroidism, hyperprolactinemia, hormone-producing ovarian tumors, and Cushing's disease are all endocrine syndromes that can induce anovulation, but the primary etiology of DUB is chronic anovulation syndrome, often commonly described as the polycystic ovary or Stein-Leventhal's syndrome. Any imbalance in hypothalamic pulsatile release of gonadotropin-releasing hormone (GnRH), in pituitary synthesis or release of follicle-stimulating hormone (FSH) or luteinizing hormone (LH), or in ovarian follicular production of E_2, androgens, or progesterone can upset the delicate balances that induce cyclic ovulation and normal menstrual function. Exogenous androgen production in the adrenal glands and estrone production in adipose tissue produce identical clinical pictures.

Abnormal bleeding associated with ovulatory cycles thus requires careful differential diagnosis. Patients at the extremes of reproductive function, both perimenarchal and perimenopausal, require evaluations modified to recognize their unique clinical situations. A clear understanding of the diverse etiologies of DUB will lead to easier and more practical diagnostic schemes and more effective therapeutic interventions.

Abnormal Ovulation and DUB

Although the most frequent cause of DUB is anovulation, histologic studies consistently show that 15% to 20% of DUB patients have secretory endometrium, indicative of at least intermittent, if not regular, ovulation. The differential diagnosis of abnormal bleeding with ovulation differs from that of anovulation. Ovulatory patients with abnormal bleeding are more likely to have an underlying organic pathology and are not, therefore, true DUB patients by strict definition.

Aksel and Jones studied endometria of patients with dysfunctional bleeding and found hyperplasia in 63% of cases; secretory endometrium was observed in 17%, and nonsecretory endometrium of the interval, postmenstrual, or atrophic type made up the remaining 20%. Thus, at least 17% of patients in this series had normal cyclic hormonal function and ovulation before the endometrium was examined, and it is possible that many patients with the postmenstrual type of endometria would have shown secretory changes if curettage had been performed somewhat later. In addition to histologic confirmation of ovulation by the presence of secretory endometrium, ovulation can be documented by basal body temperature charting, urinary LH surge detection, or prospective hormonal evaluation. In some cases, the prospective hormonal studies using daily serum estrogen and progesterone levels are more accurate for defining ovulatory status than are the historically accepted studies of endome-trial histology, which can be misleading because of previous hormonal therapy. A serum progesterone concentration exceeding 3 ng/mL in the luteal phase of the cycle indicates ovulation.

Diagnostic Imaging Techniques

Diagnostic vaginal ultrasound can be particularly useful in cases of ovulatory abnormal uterine bleeding. A non-randomized study of 45 otherwise unselected patients with abnormal uterine bleeding demonstrated anatomic pathology in 31% by vaginal ultrasound, compared with 9% by clinical examination. Pathologic findings included leiomyoma uteri, polyps, and abnormal endometrial architecture. If these data are confirmed by later studies, the implication is that true DUB in ovulatory patients may be even more rare than the currently accepted figure of 15% to 20%. Endovaginal ultrasound is also of particular value in cases of perimenopausal and postmenopausal abnormal bleeding, which will be discussed later (Fig. 20.1).

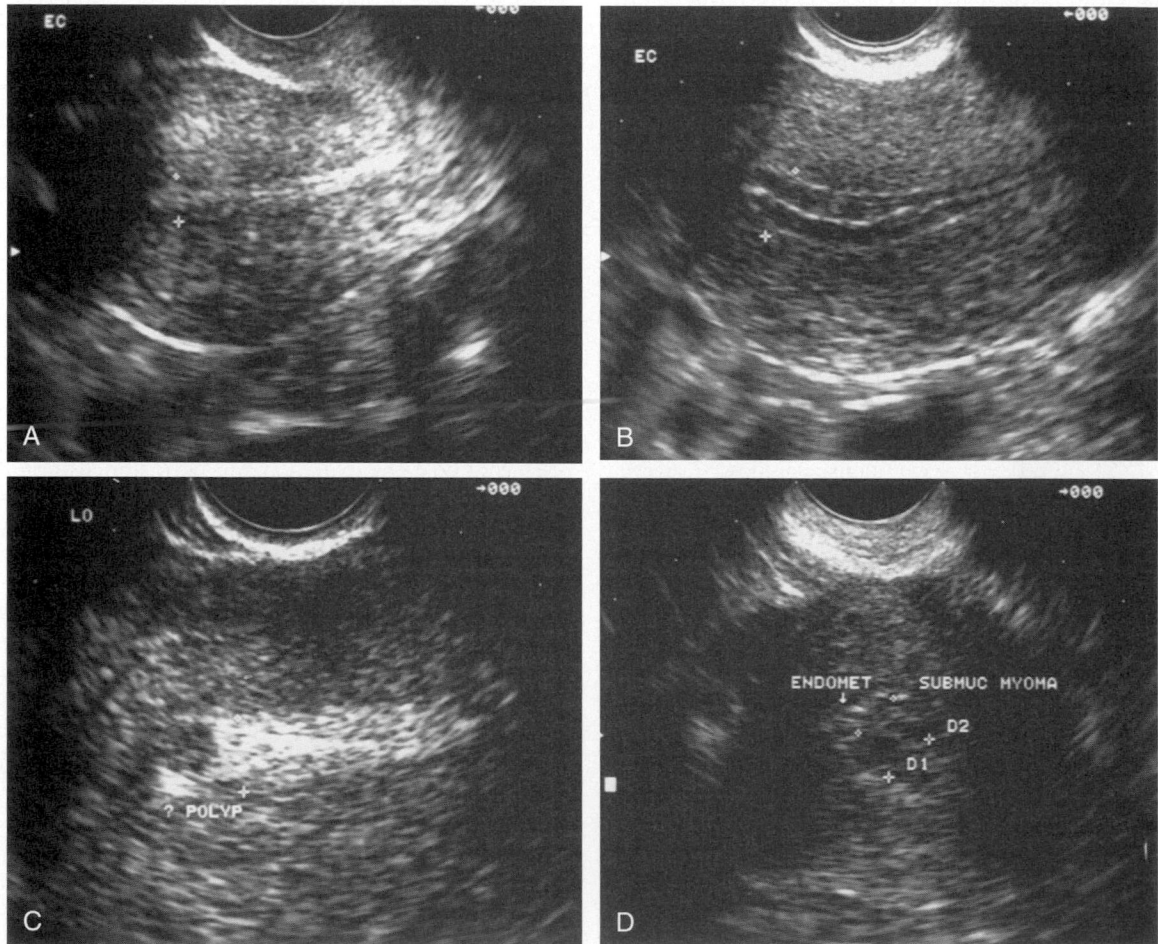

FIGURE 20.1. A: Single-line endometrium consistent with postmenstruation, early proliferation, and postmenopause. **B:** Three-line endometrium from estrogen stimulation, late follicular phase. **C:** Endometrial polyp in hyperechoic thickened endometrium consistent with luteal phase or hyperplasia–neoplasia. **D:** Submucous myoma with distortion of endometrial cavity marked by single-line endometrium.

Saline infusion sonography (SIS) is a technique to improve visualization of the endometrial cavity during transvaginal ultrasonography. The technique involves a pelvic examination with placement of an open-sided bivalve speculum. The cervix is prepared with antiseptic solution, and a small catheter is inserted through the cervical os for instillation of sterile saline. A number of catheters are available both with and without small balloons, which are useful in the case of a parous cervix. The speculum is then removed, and the endometrial cavity is distended with sterile saline during transvaginal ultrasonography. Dueholm et al. compared the accuracy of saline infusion sonography with transvaginal sonography, hysteroscopy, and magnetic resonance imaging (MRI). In 108 patients with abnormal uterine bleeding, pain, endometriosis, or myomas, SIS had an overall sensitivity comparable to the gold standard of hysteroscopy and better than either MRI or transvaginal sonography. MRI had the highest sensitivity for submucous myomas, but a relatively low sensitivity for other intrauterine pathology such as polyps. As SIS is a less invasive procedure than a surgical technique such as hysteroscopy and is much less expensive than MRI, it should be the procedure of choice for imaging of the endometrial cavity in patients with abnormal uterine bleeding.

Proper evaluation of abnormal bleeding in the ovulatory patient demands assessment for other less common causes of bleeding. According to Claessens and Cowell, bleeding dyscrasias are particularly common in perimenarchal patients, up to 19% of whom have a primary coagulation disorder such as idiopathic thrombocytopenic purpura or von Willebrand's disease. Hemorrhagic diatheses can occur with leukemia, with chemotherapy treatment, or as secondary to oral anticoagulant therapy or ingestion of foods or drugs that inhibit platelet aggregation. Infection has been shown to cause abnormal uterine bleeding. *Mobiluncus* species identified in cases of abnormal bleeding respond to oral metronidazole therapy. *Chlamydia* has been implicated in abnormal bleeding, particularly with concurrent use of oral contraceptives. Menorrhagia has been described as an early symptom in patients with subclinical hypothyroidism before diagnosis of overt disease. Thyroid replacement in a normal physiologic dosage will resolve the abnormal bleeding.

Arteriovenous malformation is a very rare cause of ovulatory bleeding. In a report by Fleming et al., only two cases were diagnosed before definitive surgery; the diagnosis was by pelvic angiography.

The reported association between tubal ligation and new onset of abnormal uterine bleeding should also be noted. Although numerous anecdotal reports exist, no underlying pathologic changes in anatomy or hormone production have ever been documented. Long-term follow-up studies do not confirm an increased incidence of abnormal bleeding in these patients but do implicate biased patient perception. Patients who discontinue oral contraceptive use after tubal ligation have heavier and more painful bleeding, whereas patients who have intrauterine devices removed after sterilization have improved menstrual symptomatology.

DUB Pathophysiology

As stated earlier, the most common etiology for DUB is estrogen withdrawal or estrogen break-through bleeding in an anovulatory patient. In the absence of progesterone exposure to cause inhibition of DNA synthesis and mitosis, the estrogenic proliferative response causes stromal cell growth to exceed the structural integrity of its stromal matrix, and the endometrium breaks down with irregular bleeding. Unopposed estrogen results in vascular endometrial tissue with relatively scant stroma, giving glands a back-to-back appearance. The endometrium is fragile and undergoes repetitive spontaneous breakdown. In the absence of normal control mechanisms to limit menstrual blood loss, bleeding can be prolonged and excessive.

Other contributing factors are the lack of coordinated vasoconstriction and the release of lytic enzymes, which occurs in a normal progesterone-stimulated endometrium. The absence of progesterone stimulation of metalloendopeptidase increases endothelin-1 activity, which contributes to vasospasm. Lysosomal enzymes inappropriately released in the absence of progesterone stabilization of the lysosomal membrane further contribute to structural breakdown.

Hemostasis in a bleeding endometrium depends both on coagulation, with thrombus formation forming plugs in superficial blood vessels, and on vasoconstriction of spiral arterioles; generalized endometrial collapse with compression of bleeding vessels can also contribute. The lack of coordinated vasoconstriction and the irregular structural collapse lead to irregular and often heavy bleeding. The amount of bleeding correlates directly with the level of estrogen stimulation. The chronic high estrogen milieus seen in cases of obesity and chronic anovulation, and in perimenarchal and perimenopausal patients, cause the greatest amount of DUB blood loss.

Unopposed estrogen stimulation can, over time, induce a hyperplastic response in the proliferating endometrium (Fig. 20.2A). Such hyperplasia can eventually develop the cytologic changes associated with neoplasia: atypical adenomatous hyperplasia or even low-grade adenocarcinoma. Such cellular transformation takes time, as much as 10 to 20 years; a young patient with DUB has a low risk of hyperplasia or neoplasia and generally does not require endometrial sampling. The perimenopausal patient has a substantially higher risk, however, and sampling is mandated.

Making the Differential Diagnosis

DUB occurs most frequently at the extremes of menstrual life, but it can develop at any intervening time. The characteristics of DUB are variable, from infrequent heavy flow (oligomenorrhea) to almost continuous spotting or bleeding. The age of onset and duration of irregularity can provide important clues to etiology. Anovulation is common in the perimenarchal girl. More than 50% of cycles are anovulatory in the first 2 years after menarche. Complications of pregnancy are also common in this age group and must be ruled out before initiation of treatment for

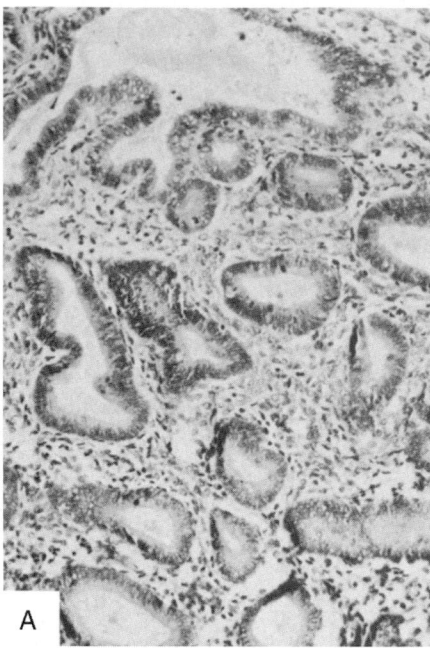 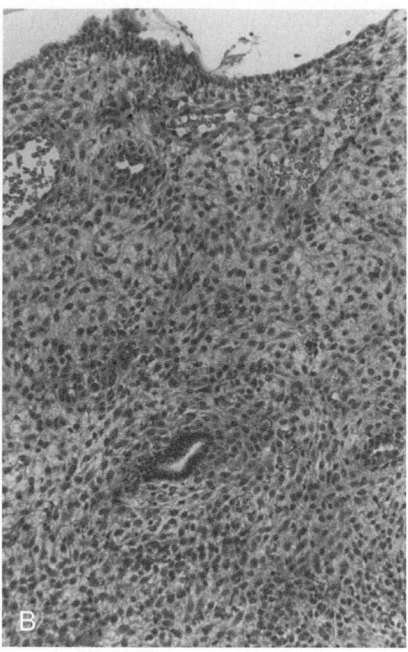

FIGURE 20.2. A: Endometrial hyperplasia before treatment showing hyperplastic cellular changes of glands. **B:** Hyperplastic endometrium after continuous progestin treatment.

DUB. New sensitive radioimmunoassays for the beta subunit of human chorionic gonadotropin are accurate for evaluating the possibility of pregnancy without invasive tissue sampling. Although relatively rare, endocrinologically active ovarian neoplasms do occur and should be particularly excluded in prepubertal vaginal bleeding. Other causes of irregular bleeding in the adolescent include genital trauma and coagulopathies such as idiopathic thrombocytopenic purpura and von Willebrand's disease. As previously mentioned, the Claessens and Cowell review of children's hospital admissions for menorrhagia reports an overall 19% incidence of primary coagulation disorders and a 50% incidence in patients presenting at the time of menarche. Although newer studies have demonstrated a lower risk of 5%, coagulopathies are still considered a significant cause of DUB in adolescents (Falcone et al.). The most common diagnosis is idiopathic thrombocytopenic purpura, but platelet disorders such as von Willebrand's and Glanzmann's diseases, thalassemia, and leukemia are also found.

The adult patient with DUB can have either an acute or a chronic history of menstrual irregularity. Onset at menarche and persistence into adulthood is a classic history for chronic anovulation syndrome, but nonclassical adrenal hyperplasia must be differentiated when there is coexistent androgen excess. The differential diagnosis can be made by obtaining a baseline 17α-hydroxyprogesterone level. A level less than 200 ng/dL rules out partial adrenal 21-hydroxylase enzyme deficiency. An elevated baseline 17α-hydroxyprogesterone requires a cosyntropin stimulation test to confirm the nonclassical adrenal hyperplasia diagnosis. A more acute history requires a differential diagnosis of other endocrinologic causes of anovulation, for example, thyroid and prolactin disorders, complications of pregnancy, neoplastic processes such as fibroids or hormone-producing ovarian tumors, in-

trauterine lesions such as polyps and synechiae, and coagulopathies. Adult patients with menorrhagia are at higher risk than previously thought to have a bleeding diathesis. Dilley et al. identified coagulopathies in 10.7% of 121 patients in a case control study. The majority of cases were von Willebrand's disease. Women over the age of 30 years with a history consistent with chronic anovulation should undergo endometrial sampling because of their greater risk of hyperplasia and neoplasia. Perimenopausal women with DUB have an even higher risk of hyperplasia and neoplasia and should always undergo extensive endometrial sampling, in most cases by dilatation and curettage (D&C).

Several years before menopause, menstrual cycles usually shorten secondary to a decreased proliferative phase, with resultant moderate elevation of FSH and subsequent frequent anovulatory cycles. This unopposed estrogen environment is conducive to the development of both DUB and hyperplasia. Appropriate evaluation of the perimenopausal and postmenopausal patient will be thoroughly discussed later in this chapter.

A diagnosis of DUB is often a diagnosis of exclusion. Problems of pregnancy such as incomplete or missed abortion, subinvolution of the placental site, placental polyp, trophoblastic disease, and extrauterine pregnancy must be ruled out. All gynecologic malignancies can cause abnormal bleeding. Common epithelial tumors of the ovary can produce estrogen and cause uterine bleeding. Submucous leiomyomata and endometrial polyps can be present in older women but are not a problem in the differential diagnosis of adolescents. Excessive anovulatory bleeding is common with polycystic ovarian disease, with functional cysts of the ovary, and perhaps in some cases of luteal phase deficiency.

The patient workup for abnormal uterine bleeding should include a complete history and physical examination. Pelvic examination may disclose an adnexal mass, evidence of genital trauma or laceration, or a fibroid uterus. Laboratory studies should include thyroid function tests and the evaluation of levels of human chorionic gonadotropin, FSH, LH, prolactin, and serum androgens if indicated. A significant increase in dehydroepiandrosterone sulfate indicates a need to screen for nonclassical adrenal hyperplasia. A serum progesterone level measurement is useful for assessment of ovulatory status. A complete blood count with platelet and coagulation studies is appropriate, and a bleeding time may be indicated to assess platelet function. As mentioned earlier, endovaginal ultrasound and SIS are valuable adjuncts to pelvic examination. They are particularly informative for assessment of intrauterine or extrauterine pregnancies and pelvic masses detected on examination. Occasionally, they may also reveal anatomic pathology not detected by other means (Fig. 20.1). Invasive tissue-sampling procedures include endometrial sampling and D&C. A D&C is preferable in the perimenopausal or postmenopausal patient and may also be indicated when there is clinical suspicion of an abnormal pregnancy. A D&C is relatively contraindicated in the adolescent. Hysterosalpingography and hysteroscopy also have potential benefit and will be reviewed later in this chapter.

Treatment of DUB

Because most patients with DUB have an underlying etiology of chronic anovulation with unopposed estrogen stimulation of the endometrium, medical treatment with progestational compounds is the mainstay of therapy. Precise amounts can differ depending on the patient's age, but adequate progestin stimulation will decrease DNA synthesis and cell proliferation, deplete estrogen receptors, and increase the conversion of E_2 to the less potent estrone sulfate. These effects will induce maturation of the endometrium, healing of superficial breaks, enhancement of the stromal matrix with increased structural stability, and cessation of bleeding. Withdrawal of the progestin after adequate exposure results in orderly and uniform shedding of the endometrium with a finite self-limited bleed. The progestin dosage and duration of therapy must induce a complete secretory transformation; otherwise, complete inhibition of all estrogenic effects will fail and islands of proliferative endometrium will remain.

Whitehead has shown that postmenopausal estrogen replacement mimics the unopposed estrogen environment of chronic anovulation, and that 4% of patients develop endometrial hyperplasia with only 7 days of progestin exposure, 2% with 10 days of exposure, and 0% with 12 days of exposure. He recommends 12 days of progestin every month to counteract the estrogen proliferative effects. Medroxyprogesterone acetate, 10 mg, or norethindrone acetate, 5 mg per day, may be prescribed. After initial control of the dysfunctional bleeding, the 12-day course can be repeated at monthly intervals to prevent the development of hyperplasia. It is convenient to start each new course on the first day of each month. A

regular withdrawal can be expected to start either during the last 2 days of progestin or within several days of the last dose. Failure to withdraw could signify pregnancy, development of a hypoestrogenic state, or, rarely, induction of ovulation by progestin stimulation of the estrogen-primed patient. In such a case of endogenous progesterone production, the menses can be delayed 2 weeks. A word of caution: This regimen is not contraceptive.

An alternative method for delivery of a progestin to control dysfunctional bleeding and menorrhagia is local administration with a progestin-impregnated intrauterine device (IUD). Irvine et al. performed a randomized trial of 44 women with menorrhagia, comparing a levonorgestrel IUD with cyclic progestin therapy. The mean menstrual blood loss was reduced by 90% in the IUD group, with 76% patient satisfaction with the treatment compared with only 22% satisfaction with cyclic progestin therapy. In another study, Istre and Trolle compared the levonorgestrel IUD with endometrial resection and demonstrated a lower treatment success for the IUD (67% versus 90%) and an increased incidence of side effects, with six of 30 patients discontinuing treatment because of irregular bleeding, pain, and acne. Although further studies are needed, the progestin IUD may be an effective therapy in carefully selected patients.

Chronic unopposed estrogen can produce a very lush endometrium that can bleed heavily during progestin withdrawal. Speroff recommends treatment using combination oral contraceptives in a step-down regimen. Two to four pills are given daily, one every 6 to 12 hours, for 5 to 7 days for acute control of bleeding. This will usually control acute bleeding within 24 to 48 hours, allowing time to complete the diagnostic evaluation. Withdrawal of medication will result in a heavy bleed. On the fifth day of this bleed, a low-dose cyclic oral contraceptive is started and repeated for three cycles to allow orderly regression of the excessive proliferative endometrium. Alternatively, the dosage of combination pills can be tapered (four times a day, then three times a day, then two times a day) over 3 to 6 days and then continued at one pill every day. Combination oral contraceptives induce atrophy of the endometrium because the chronic estrogen–progestin exposure suppresses pituitary gonadotropins and inhibits endogenous steroidogenesis. They are useful for long-term management of DUB in patients without contraindications and have the added benefit of pregnancy prevention. Particularly in perimenarchal patients, heavy prolonged bleeding can denude the basal endometrium and make it unresponsive to progestins. Curettage for control of hemorrhage is contraindicated because of a high risk of development of intrauterine synechiae (Asherman's syndrome) if the basalis is curetted. High-dose intravenous estrogen (conjugated estrogens 25 mg every 4 hours until bleeding abates) will give acute control by proliferative repair of the endometrium and by direct effects on coagulation, including increased fibrinogen and platelet aggregation. A progestin alone or oral conjugated estrogens in combination with a progestin can then be used to induce orderly withdrawal bleeding.

Hysteroscopy of patients who fail to respond to hormonal therapy may reveal previously missed pathology such as a submucous myoma or polyp. These diagnoses are particularly common in patients with ovulatory dysfunctional bleeding. If a diagnostic curettage has not been previously performed, one can be performed in conjunction with the hysteroscopy, both for diagnosis and for temporary therapy. If atypical hyperplasia has been identified and preservation of fertility is desired, more aggressive progestin therapy is recommended. Medroxyprogesterone acetate, 30 mg, or megestrol, 20 to 40 mg, daily for 3 months should be monitored by repeat endometrial sampling to assess the efficiency of the medical treatment (Fig. 20.2B). If atypical hyperplasia persists, very high-dose progestin protocols can be tried, but hysterectomy must be considered.

Menorrhagia can be reduced when prostaglandin E_2 and prostacyclin synthesis are decreased by nonsteroidal antiinflammatory medications. These drugs inhibit the cyclooxygenase enzyme necessary for endometrial production of prostaglandin under estrogen stimulation and thus alter the relative production of the proaggregation vasoconstrictor thromboxane A_2 and the antiaggregation vasodilator prostacyclin. Pathology studies have confirmed that this improves both platelet aggregation and vasoconstriction. Fraser et al. (1981) demonstrated these compounds to be most effective when given in therapeutic dosages for 7 to 10 days before the expected onset of the next menstrual period in ovulatory DUB patients, but they are commonly started with the onset of menses and continued throughout the bleeding episode with good success.

For coagulation disorders, 1-desamino-8-D-arginine vasopressin (also known as desmopressin, or simply DDAVP) increases coagulation factor VIII with a therapeutic effect lasting about 6 hours. It is best administered intravenously, 0.3 μg/kg in 50 mL saline over 15 to 30 minutes, but can be used intranasally. Antifibrinolytic agents such as ε-aminocaproic acid and tranexamic acid can decrease blood loss up to 50%, but their significant central nervous system and gastrointestinal side effects and the risk of intracranial arterial thrombosis limit their applicability. Ergot derivatives are ineffective for treatment of menorrhagia. Local delivery of progestational agents by way of an intrauterine device has been demonstrated by Milsom et al. to be extremely effective, with more than a 90% reduction in bleeding in some patients. This has the potential to provide long-term therapy for patients with chronic bleeding unresponsive to other therapies.

Long-acting derivatives of GnRH agonists downregulate pituitary synthesis of FSH and LH and induce "medical castration." Withdrawal of endogenous steroid stimulation will result in endometrial atrophy. Various delivery options are available, including intranasal delivery, daily subcutaneous delivery, monthly intramuscular depot, and subcutaneously implanted pellet analog. GnRH agonists are not effective in acute control of abnormal bleeding. At least 2 to 4 weeks are required for adequate suppression of gonadotropin production and inhibition of steroidogenesis. Long-term therapy can effectively control blood loss with chronic DUB secondary to chronic systemic illness, thrombocytopenia, or other coagulopathies. Because of the profoundly hypoestrogenic state induced by these drugs, there is accelerated bone resorption and the risk of development of significant osteoporosis. Therefore, long-term therapy requires "add-back" treatment with an estrogen-progestin combination to prevent bone loss. GnRH agonists can also be used as adjuncts for endometrial preparation before endometrial ablation.

Ablation or destruction of the endometrium has been advocated for treatment of chronic abnormal bleeding unresponsive to medical management in the presence of a normal endometrial cavity and the absence of submucous leiomyomata, endometrial hyperplasia, or neoplasia. Although there has been significant disagreement regarding the appropriate indications for this procedure, it has been widely applied with varying success. The original methods included use of hysteroscopy with the Nd:YAG laser, electrosurgical rollerball cauterization, or endomyometrial resection using a loop electrode. These hysteroscopic surgical techniques require special training. More recently, new techniques have been described to ablate the endometrial cavity without the requirement for hysteroscopy. These include thermal balloon ablation, direct instillation of heated saline, cryoablation with a cryoprobe, microwave endometrial ablation, and use of radio frequency electromagnetic energy (Corson et al.; O'Connor and Magos; Rutherford et al.; Sharp et al.; Singer et al.; Weisberg et al.). Success rates reported with the various techniques have ranged from 60% to 95% of patients achieving either hypomenorrhea or amenorrhea. Pretreatment with danazol, GnRH analogs, or suction curettage to thin the endometrium appears to improve long-term success rates (Brooks; Donnez et al.). Seeras and Gilliland reported resumption of menstruation in 44% of women after ablation if they had not received preoperative endometrial suppression.

A number of comparison studies have looked at success rates of the various techniques in order to determine relative efficacy, complication rates, and relative cost. Meyer et al. compared rollerball ablation with thermal balloon ablation in a prospective, randomized trial. A greater percentage of women in the roller ball group (27.2%) were amenorrheic at their 12-month follow-up than were women in the uterine balloon group (15.2%). The rates of hypomenorrhea plus amenorrhea were not significantly different (balloon, 80.2%; roller ball, 84.3%). Overall patient satisfaction was equivalent. The complication rate was 3.2% in the hysteroscopic rollerball group with no significant intraoperative complications in the thermal balloon group. Endomyometrial resection has been reported to have higher amenorrhea rates compared with rates for other techniques (Kooy et al.). Vercellini et al. compared myometrial resection with endometrial ablation using a vaporizing electrode similar to a roller ball. Amenorrhea rates were 48% for the endomyometrial resection group and 36% for the ablation group, although overall patient satisfaction rates were equivalent. Difficulty of surgery and mean fluid deficit were both described as greater in the resection group. Comparison of endometrial ablation with laser versus endomyometrial resection showed equivalent amenorrhea rates of approximately 45%, with overall patient satisfaction rates of 90%. (Battacharya et al.) There are no comparative data available for the newer techniques, but preliminary results are comparable.

Operative hysteroscopic techniques require specialized training, and complications, although relatively infrequent, can be significant. A multihospital survey in The Netherlands reported an overall complication rate for hysteroscopy of 0.28%. (Jansen et al.) Diagnostic hysteroscopy had a significantly lower complication rate than that of operative hysteroscopy (0.13% versus 0.95%). The most frequent surgical complication was uterine perforation (0.76%). Reported complication rates for hysteroscopic ablation procedures are significantly higher. O'Connor et al. followed 525 women for up to 5 years after endometrial resection. They reported a 6% incidence of intraoperative complications and a 3% incidence of postoperative complications. They also reported a 15% complication rate in patients who required a repeat ablative procedure. The "Mistletoe" survey from the Royal College of Obstetricians and Gynaecologists recorded endomyometrial resection complication rates of 7.2% but only 4% for roller ball and laser ablations. (Overton et al.) A prospective trial of thermal balloon versus rollerball ablation reported intraoperative complications in 3.2% of the rollerball patients but no significant intraoperative complications in the thermal balloon patients. (Meyer et al.) Reported complications include uterine perforation with hemorrhage, laser or electrosurgical damage to the bowel, excessive absorption of distending medium with fluid overload, hyponatremia and pulmonary edema, and persistence of bleeding requiring repeat ablation or hysterectomy. The reported complication rates do compare favorably with reported morbidity rates for women undergoing hysterectomy, which range from 7% to 15%. (Summitt et al.)

Another concern has been possible obliteration of warning signs heralding the development of endometrial carcinoma, with subsequent delay in diagnosis. Endometrial ablation procedures usually result in a narrowed tubular uterine cavity without the obliteration seen in Asherman's syndrome, but are rarely expected to result in total ablation of all endometrial tissue. Several cases of postablation endometrial carcinoma have now been reported. (Brooks-Carter et al.; Copperman et al.) The cost of endometrial ablation does compare favorably with that of hysterectomy, with hysterectomy reported as 58% more expensive when all costs, including lost work time, are considered (Vilos et al.).

D&C is both diagnostic and therapeutic. Removal of the structurally fragile bleeding endometrium allows restoration of normal hemostatic events, with regeneration of the integrity of the endometrium and restoration of the normal proliferative response. If the patient fails to respond to medical therapy, repeated curettage, or even

endometrial ablation, then more definitive therapy such as hysterectomy should be considered, taking into account the age of the patient and her desire for future childbearing. It has been estimated that 2 million women in the United States are seen annually with complaints of excessive uterine bleeding, and about 150,000 undergo hysterectomy, which accounts for 20% to 30% of all hysterectomies performed.

In general, the ovulatory type of bleeding has the poorest response to replacement hormonal therapy and the highest incidence of recurrence. Although a hysterectomy can be considered an admission of therapeutic defeat, it is frequently an expeditious method of resolving this refractory and recurrent type of DUB. When bleeding persists after repeated curettage and cyclic hormonal therapy, hysterectomy may be required. If other conditions are present that should be corrected surgically, such as a relaxed vaginal outlet, rectocele, cystocele, or uterine descensus, we recommend vaginal hysterectomy with support of the vaginal vault and repair of the vaginal wall relaxation. When hysterectomy is indicated in premenopausal women younger than 50 years of age, normal ovarian tissue is conserved. In a patient younger than 30 years of age, radical surgical treatment should be strongly avoided; one can almost always control uterine bleeding by repeated curettage or by increasing amounts of cyclic hormone therapy. Today, the availability and use of estrogen and progesterone have changed the need for hysterectomy to treat DUB. Hysterectomy is not indicated in young women but may be indicated in older women when hormonal therapy and repeated curettage have failed.

Blood transfusions are seldom required when DUB is associated with anemia, but they may be given if the anemia is so severe that symptoms are present. Oral iron therapy should be started at the first sign of heavy menstruation to prevent depletion of iron stores, and it should be given for 3 to 6 months after normal hemoglobin and hematocrit levels have been restored in patients with iron-deficiency anemia.

PERIMENOPAUSAL AND POSTMENOPAUSAL BLEEDING

When uterine bleeding occurs more than 12 months after the last regular menstrual period, it is defined as postmenopausal bleeding. For a period varying from months to years before menopause, the individual patient may experience irregular patterns of bleeding. Often the first sign is a shortening of the menstrual interval secondary to premature elevation in FSH, followed by intermittent periods of amenorrhea alternating with heavy bleeding consistent with oligo-ovulation or anovulation. With this clinical picture, special consideration must be given to ruling out a neoplastic process as the source of the bleeding. The first diagnostic consideration is to ensure that the bleeding originates from the uterus. In elderly women especially, bleeding from the urethra or rectum may be reported as vaginal bleeding. Vaginal or cervical

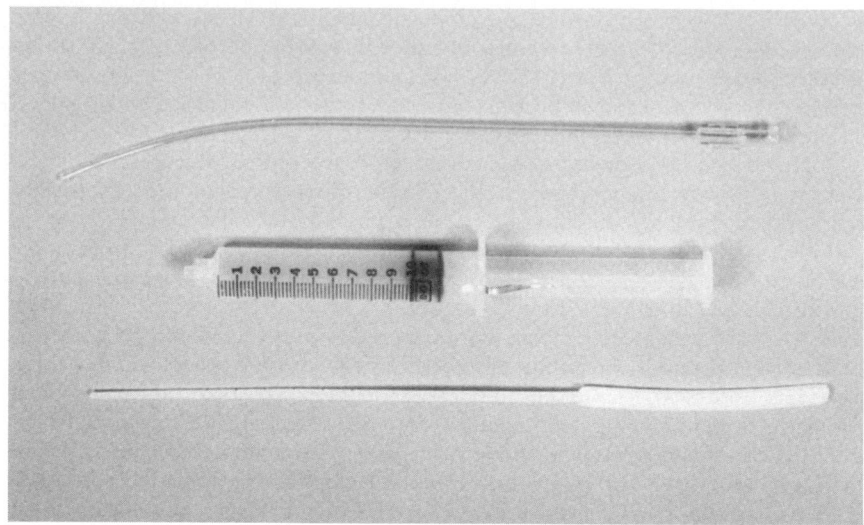

FIGURE 20.3. An endometrial suction sampling (UTER CYTE) instrument with syringe vacuum.

lesions causing the bleeding should be diagnosed readily with careful inspection or biopsy. Cancers of the vagina or cervix or cervical polyps can also be readily diagnosed and appropriate treatment rendered.

When the source of the bleeding is determined to be the uterine cavity, sampling of the endometrium for pathology examination is usually considered to be mandatory. Although D&C continues to be a commonly performed procedure for both its diagnostic and therapeutic benefits, office endometrial biopsy can often expedite appropriate evaluation and therapy. Many instruments have been devised for the sampling of endometrial tissue and evaluation of the endometrial cavity. The standard instrument used for many years has been the Novak curet. Although this curet was initially devised to obtain a sample of the endometrium by suction and aspiration, it is most commonly used as a miniature curet that contains a serrated edge surrounding its biopsy aperture. The curet is about 5 mm in diameter and can usually be passed without dilatation through a small cervical canal, even in nulliparous women. Occasionally, the postmenopausal cervical canal is stenotic and difficult to penetrate. Because of the discomfort associated with passage of the Novak curet, newer Silastic curets have been developed. These have a smaller diameter (3 mm), are flexible, and are often better tolerated by patients. They can be difficult to pass through a truly stenotic cervix be-

cause of their pliability. Often there is an accompanying syringe that attaches and develops effective vacuum pressure to improve the size of the sample obtained (Fig. 20.3). A four-quadrant endometrial biopsy with passes along the anterior and posterior and both lateral walls of the endometrial cavity is recommended for diagnosis of abnormal bleeding. Another potentially useful device not requiring a syringe to develop negative pressure is a disposable plastic tube with a 3.1 mm outer diameter, an aspiration port, and solid plastic obturator at its tip. The obturator fits so closely that its slow withdrawal from the uterine cavity causes sufficient suction to obtain an adequate endometrial specimen (Fig. 20.4). Because of the small aperture of this device and its almost total reliance on suction to obtain a specimen, the architecture of the obtained biopsy may be somewhat distorted.

Vacuum suction curettage has gained some popularity as an office procedure for endometrial sampling that does not require general anesthesia. A small metal or plastic cannula, with an outside diameter of 3 mm, that has a slightly curved tip and an opening on the concave surface for easier insertion through a small endocervical canal is connected to a plastic tubal chamber containing a cylindrical plastic filter. At the opposite end of the chamber, a plastic spout is connected to a negative pressure source. The apparatus is prepackaged in a sterile disposable container, and the vacuum source can be ei-

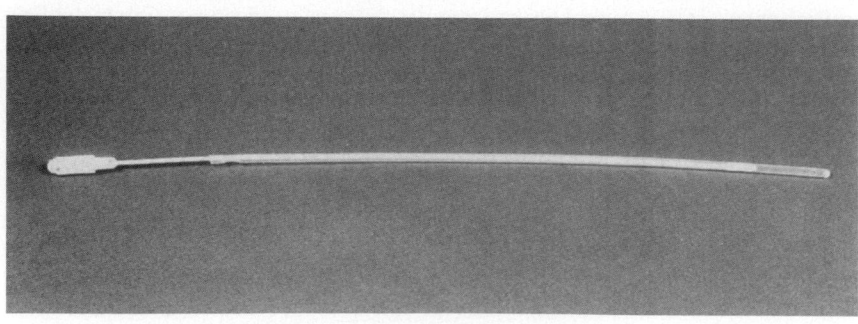

FIGURE 20.4. A useful suction endometrial sampling Pipelle instrument, with 3.1 mm in outside diameter, and no pump or syringe required.

ther a commercial pump or a faucet in which about 60 mL of negative water pressure is developed for proper suction through the curet. Several improvements have been made in the technology. Aspirators today have the convenience of being completely prepared and disposable, but they have the disadvantage of high cost, which must be borne by the patient. Several studies have compared the results of suction curettage with those of regular curettage under anesthesia in the same patient. Cohen et al. studied 98 patients; in 93, they found identical histologic patterns with both methods. In five patients, there was no correlation between the results of the two techniques, and none of these had cancer. At the Medical University of South Carolina, Lutz et al. found suction curettage to be 98% accurate in evaluating high-risk women with abnormal bleeding for endometrial malignant disease.

These new tools require little or no cervical dilatation and permit almost painless endometrial sampling. A quick-acting, nonsteroidal antiinflammatory drug (e.g., 550 mg naproxen sodium) administered 15 to 30 minutes before curetting provides satisfactory analgesia for most patients. If dilatation of the cervix is required, paracervical block anesthesia can be initiated by injecting 4 to 5 mL of 1% lidocaine at the 3-o'clock and 9-o'clock positions in the paracervical tissues, exercising care to avoid intravascular injection.

The principal value of an endometrial biopsy is that a formal D&C under anesthesia has been avoided if the removed tissue contains adenocarcinoma. If the cause of postmenopausal bleeding is not identified in a screening endometrial biopsy, however, then a standard curettage is obligatory. In office biopsies of the endometria of more than 20,000 patients of all ages, Hofmeister detected 273 cases of endometrial carcinoma, 32 of which (14.28%) were totally asymptomatic. The endometrial carcinoma detection rate was 1.76% of the total group of 23,202 patients. Hofmeister's routine office endometrial biopsies using a modification of the Novak and Randall curet provide one of the largest clinical experiences of this instrument to date. Unfortunately, only patients who had continued uterine bleeding or who demonstrated an atypical pattern in the office biopsy were subjected to a complete curettage. Therefore, the true-negative and false-negative rate for the Novak type of curet in the detection of endometrial cancer has not been determined accurately. In other studies, summarized by Cohen et al., the accuracy of detection of endometrial cancer by endometrial curettage varied from 76% to 92%. However, a thorough endometrial curettage under anesthesia is also not infallible in the detection of endometrial cancer.

Vaginal ultrasound has been investigated as a screening tool in patients with postmenopausal bleeding. The average thickness of the postmenopausal endometrial stripe has been reported as 2.3 ± 1.8 mm, with a range of 0 to 10 mm, in a series of 300 asymptomatic women. Twenty-two had endometrial stripes of 5 mm or larger, and all had benign pathology. In a series of 51 cases of postmenopausal bleeding, Nasri et al. reported that if the

endometrial thickness was less than 5 mm, the pathology would show either inactive or no endometrial tissue. Karlsson et al. reported on 1168 women with postmenopausal bleeding. Patients with an endometrial echo of less than 4 mm had a sensitivity of 96% and a specificity of 68% for detecting endometrial pathology. If a 5-mm cutoff was used, two endometrial carcinomas would have been missed. In another study by Gull et al., 198 women screened for postmenopausal bleeding had an endometrial thickness of 5 mm or greater. Endometrial sampling diagnosed 36 primary endometrial cancers, one metastatic breast cancer, and three cases of atypical endometrial hyperplasia. Of 163 women with an endometrial stripe of 4 mm or less, only one was found to have endometrial cancer. Other series have shown that an endometrial thickness of greater than 8 mm is an indication for endometrial sampling, regardless of whether or not there is a complaint of bleeding. This will detect most, if not all, endometrial cancers. Although the exact indications for patient screening and parameters for follow-up need to be more precisely defined, vaginal ultrasound appears to have promise as a noninvasive method for evaluating the postmenopausal patient.

Office hysteroscopy using new smaller-diameter flexible or rigid hysteroscopes is growing in popularity because it enables selective biopsy of the areas of visualized endometrium that appear most likely to contain a neoplastic process. A blind endometrial biopsy that reveals benign endometrial histology does not absolutely preclude the presence of a malignant process elsewhere within the endometrium. A neoplastic transformation in the endometrium is often a focal abnormality. Another major advantage of hysteroscopy is the diagnosis of endometrial polyps, submucous myomas, or other sources of bleeding that may not always be identified by endometrial biopsy or conventional curettage. In a series of 110 cases of postmenopausal bleeding, the causes of 95 were identified as endometrial polyps or submucous myomas. Only two cases of early adenocarcinoma were identified. Operative hysteroscopy, endometrial ablation, or both successfully controlled bleeding in most cases of benign disease. In cases of postmenopausal uterine bleeding, the recommended diagnostic procedures may or may not produce a tissue sample of endometrium. It is not uncommon to obtain no tissue from patients with marked hypertension or from patients undergoing chronic anticoagulant therapy. This lack of tissue is also consistent with bleeding from an atrophic endometrium, which is a benign condition. When endometrium is present, a wide range of histology can be observed. Occasionally, simple proliferative endometrium is found. The endometrium can exhibit simple hyperplasia, more marked adenomatous hyperplasia, or hyperplasia with atypical cells, resulting in a diagnosis of atypical endometrial hyperplasia. Later in the menopausal years, it is not uncommon for the endometrium to have the characteristics of cystic hyperplasia, often referred to in the older literature as "Swiss cheese hyperplasia."

Hormone-induced postmenopausal uterine bleeding can be the result of endogenous or exogenous hormonal effects. The proliferation of endometrium in a patient who is not receiving exogenous hormonal therapy is generally attributed to endogenous production of estrone. Estrone is the peripheral conversion product of the weak androgenic precursor androstenedione (85% from adrenal, 15% from ovary), and its synthesis occurs primarily in adipose tissue. In the absence of exogenous hormonal therapy, one must also exclude the possibility of an estrogen-producing ovarian tumor (granulosis cell tumor).

Management of perimenopausal bleeding in the absence of significant hyperplasia or neoplasia is essentially the same as for DUB in a younger patient. One recently accepted method that in the past was proscribed is the use of low-dose oral contraceptives. The Food and Drug Administration has approved them for patients older than 40 years of age in the absence of specific contraindications, such as hypertension, hyperlipidemia, and smoking. They provide excellent cycle control with a monthly withdrawal bleed and suppression of the endometrium. Oral contraceptives can be continued until an FSH level greater than 40 IU/L during the week of placebo pills confirms ovarian failure. Standard postmenopausal hormone replacement can then be used. A sequential program of 12 days of progestin, 5 to 10 mg medroxyprogesterone acetate, or 5 mg norethindrone acetate on a monthly basis is an alternative and is continued until failure of withdrawal bleeding occurs, indicating the need for estrogen replacement. Because recent studies indicate that perimenopausal patients are relatively hypoestrogenic and can be at risk for accelerated bone loss before the actual onset of menopause, some clinicians recommend concurrent estrogen replacement even in the perimenopausal patient.

Endometrial hyperplasia requires a more aggressive progestational regimen. Atypical adenomatous endometrial hyperplasia is considered by most to be the equivalent of an intraepithelial malignancy, and hysterectomy is often advised. Management of several types of endometrial hyperplasia other than atypical adenomatous hyperplasia can generally be accomplished by monthly administration of a progestin such as medroxyprogesterone acetate, 10 mg per day for 12 days, or norethindrone acetate, 5 mg per day for 12 days. Another endometrial biopsy should be obtained within 3 to 6 months to assess for resolution of the hyperplasia. A more aggressive hormonal regimen uses continuous high-dose progestin for 3 to 6 months (i.e., megestrol, 20 to 160 mg per day).

Any of the regimens currently in use for postmenopausal hormonal replacement therapy can cause uterine bleeding. Unopposed estrogen is no longer recommended for postmenopausal hormone replacement in the case of an intact uterus because hyperplasia develops in 18% to 32% of cases and because unopposed estrogen has an up to seven-fold increased risk of endometrial carcinoma. Cyclic estrogen-progestin regimens significantly decrease this risk to less than 1% with 12 days of progestin. There are numerous dosage regimens for the use of conjugated estrogens, 0.625 to 1.25 mg; micronized E_2, 1 to 2 mg; esterified estrogens, 0.625 to 1.25 mg; and E_2 patches. Although estrogen replacement therapy performs well if used for only 21 to 25 days of the month, there is no clinical reason for its discontinuance, and recent recommendations are to continue it throughout the entire cycle. The progestin regimens are those that have already been outlined. The bleeding that accompanies these commonly used continuous-estrogen and cyclic-progestin regimens should occur predictably, at the conclusion of the progestin phase of the cyclic administration. Most investigators of the subject now agree that the predictable and appropriately timed withdrawal bleeding that occurs with these regimens does not require sampling for endometrial histology. Continuous daily regimens of estrogen and low-dose progestin replacement therapy (i.e., conjugated estrogen, 0.625 mg, and medroxyprogesterone acetate, 2.5 mg) are commonly accompanied by irregular bleeding patterns for at least 4 to 8 months after initiation of the regimen. They are used with the anticipation that over months of use, the proportion of women becoming completely amenorrheic will increase, and for most women, the long-term benefits with these regimens will outweigh those of the conventional cyclic regimen, in which most women bleed regularly at the conclusion of the progestin phase of the cycle for at least 6 to 24 months. As a general rule, just as intermenstrual bleeding during the regular menstruating years dictates investigation and management, so do patterns of postmenopausal bleeding not following an anticipated schedule require investigation and management.

The most important point about the significance of postmenopausal bleeding is its frequent association with gynecologic malignancy, particularly endometrial carcinoma. Although the incidence of malignancy to explain postmenopausal bleeding has decreased in recent decades, diagnostic efforts must carefully consider and rule out possible malignancy by use of appropriate diagnostic procedures, especially careful pelvic examination and uterine curettage. An endometrial biopsy is helpful for the diagnosis of suspected endometrial carcinoma only if the biopsy is positive. The definitive method for obtaining adequate histology for diagnosis is D&C.

DILATATION OF THE CERVIX

Recamier invented the curet in 1943. Since then, dilatation of the cervix with curettage of the endometrial cavity has become the second most frequently performed gynecologic procedure in the United States. Curettage is used to diagnose uterine malignancy, to complete an incomplete or missed abortion, to evaluate the causes of infertility, to relieve dysmenorrhea, and to control DUB. Improved medical therapies for DUB and dysmenorrhea have made dilatation of the cervix and curettage of the uterus less necessary for these two problems, especially in young women.

Dilatation of the cervix is performed as a preliminary step to curettage of the uterine cavity. As a therapeutic measure, it is used for acquired or congenital cervical stenosis, for dysmenorrhea, for introduction of intracervical and intrauterine radium or cesium, occasionally for insertion of an intrauterine contraceptive device, or for allowing drainage of the uterine cavity in the presence of pyometra, as well as a part of other operations on the cervix.

Most indications for cervical dilatation are obvious. In connection with primary dysmenorrhea, however, there is room for controversy. It is a recognized fact that many cases of primary dysmenorrhea are not cured by cervical dilatation. Because of frequent failures, some gynecologists have almost abandoned it as a therapeutic technique. We do not subscribe totally to this pessimistic point of view. Unfortunately, in most instances, it is impossible to detect those cases of dysmenorrhea that will be relieved by cervical dilatation. Often the operation must be performed as a therapeutic test, but it is fortunately such a minor procedure that its performance is justified on that basis. In nulliparous women in whom pain is greatest just before or during the early part of the menstrual flow, there is a possibility of relief from the pain by cervical dilatation. The result is unpredictable, however, and we advise permitting the patient to decide whether menstrual pain is sufficiently severe to justify an operation that is of limited or possibly no benefit.

Ibuprofen, naproxen sodium, and mefenamic acid have proved to be so effective in the management of dysmenorrhea that a thorough trial of these agents is indicated. It is now evident that endometriosis can occur much earlier than was once believed; dysmenorrhea unrelieved by these nonsteroidal antiinflammatory drugs or oral contraceptives should be considered an indication for laparoscopy.

Postmenopausal Cervical Stenosis

In cases of postmenopausal cervical stenosis, pyometra may be discovered by uterus sounding. The pus should be cultured for anaerobic and aerobic organisms, and the cervix should be dilated. A short, soft, rubber or plastic tube can be sutured in place to keep the cervical canal open while the uterine cavity is draining. Although antibiotics may not be strictly necessary in all cases, fever and pelvic pain and tenderness herald the onset of spreading pelvic infection.

Curetting a pyometra can produce parametritis or wider pelvic cellulitis. Because the risk of perforation, with the potential for development of serious peritonitis is increased during curettage, it should be delayed until adequate drainage has occurred (3 to 10 days, depending on the magnitude of the pyometra), and antibiotic therapy should be used. Curettage is mandatory to exclude the endocervical or endometrial malignancies frequently associated with pyometra.

Technique of Cervical Dilatation

The patient is placed on the table in the lithotomy position. A careful pelvic examination locates the position of the uterine corpus, and the vagina and the perineum are

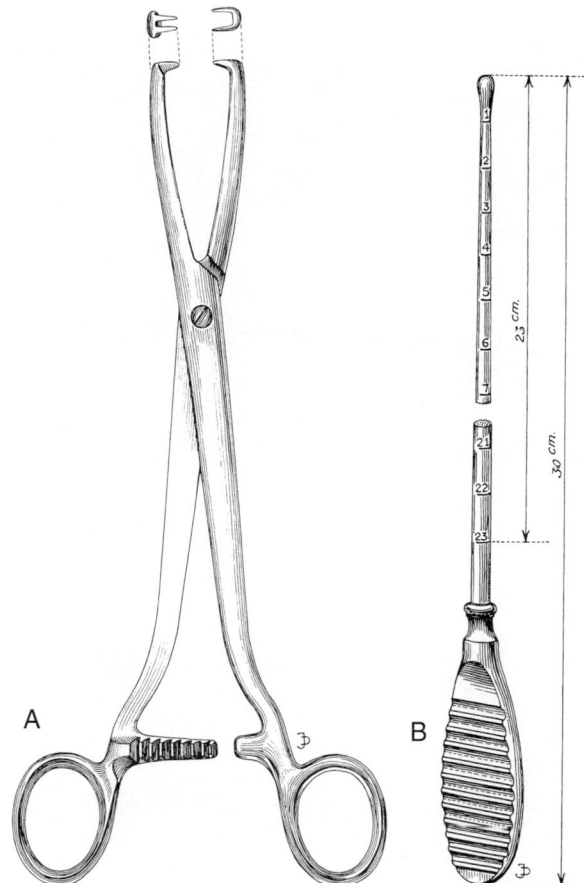

FIGURE 20.5. A: Straight Jacobs clamp, used for pulling down cervix when performing curettage. **B:** Uterine sound.

cleaned with the usual vaginal preparation of povidone-iodine (Betadine). The cervix is grasped with a four-pronged tenaculum (Fig. 20.5A) and gently drawn toward the vaginal outlet. We favor the straight Jacobs clamp, especially when difficult dilatation is either anticipated or encountered. It is much less likely to cause cervical laceration than is the single-tooth tenaculum. A sound (see Fig. 20.5B) is passed carefully through the cervical canal into the uterine cavity to avoid creating a false passage. Resistance is greatest at the internal cervical os. Occasionally, a fine silver probe is needed for finding the proper passage if the canal is stenotic. Passing the uterine sound provides confirmatory information about the position of the uterus, the length of the uterine cavity, and the angulation between the cervical canal and the uterine cavity. The degree of stenosis of the cervical canal can be detected in this manner. Sounding the uterus is contraindicated in the presence of a pregnancy because of the increased risk of perforating the soft myometrium.

The cervical canal is dilated with a small Hegar dilator (Fig. 20.6). The uterine wall can be perforated by improper passage of the dilator; the cause usually is lack of knowledge or disregard of the position of the uterus. When acute anteflexion is present, the dilator can perforate posteriorly (Fig. 20.7). When retrodisplacement

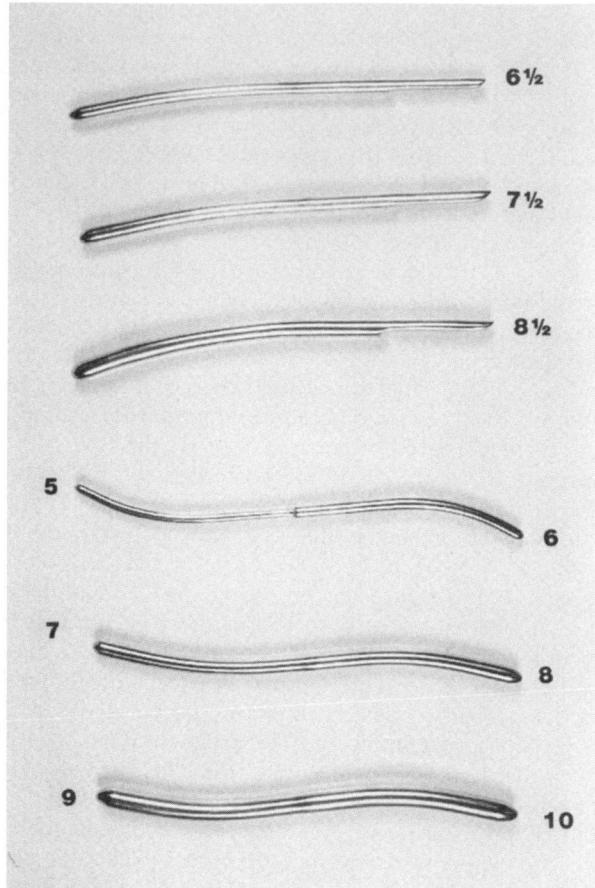

FIGURE 20.6. Graduated Hegar dilators and "half-size" Hegar dilators.

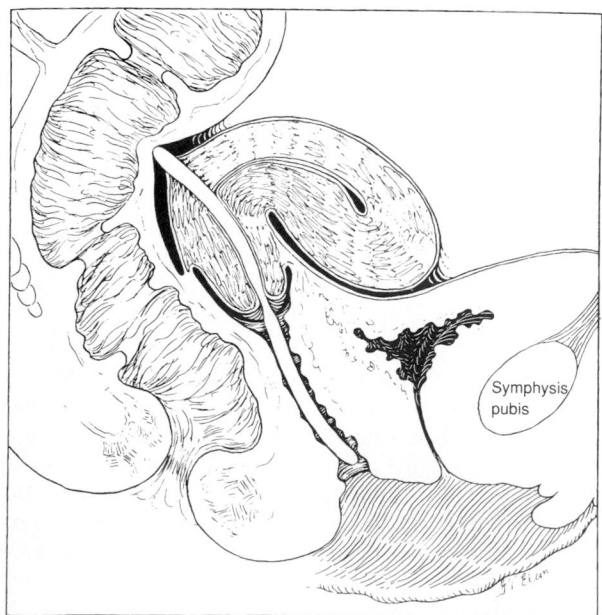

FIGURE 20.7. Perforation of the acutely anteflexed uterus. The uterus was thought to be in retroposition, and the Hegar dilator was erroneously directed posteriorly.

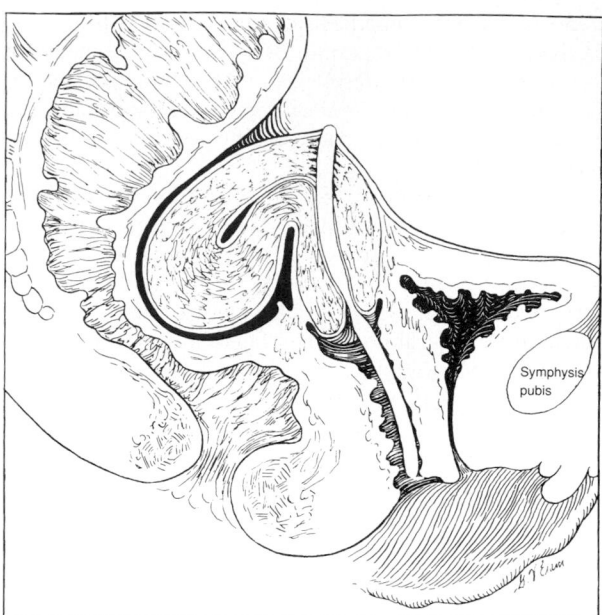

FIGURE 20.8. Perforation of the retroflexed uterus. The uterus was thought to be in anteposition, and the Hegar dilator was erroneously directed anteriorly.

exists, the perforation usually occurs anteriorly (Fig. 20.8). These two complications can be avoided by sounding the uterine cavity before dilating the cervix and by following the direction of the endocervical canal and uterine cavity indicated by the sound. The dilator rarely perforates the fundus except when there is an atrophic postmenopausal uterus or when an invasive tumor or pregnancy has softened the uterine wall. After either the 3- or 4-mm Hegar dilator is passed, successively larger ones are used. For ordinary curettage, dilatation to 8 or 9 mm suffices. When the dilatation is for dysmenorrhea, we prefer to carry the dilatation up to 10 mm. Be aware of concerns that excessive dilatation can be associated with an incompetent cervix in a subsequent pregnancy. If cervical dilatation is difficult, half-size Hegar dilators with incremental diameters of 0.5 mm are useful (Fig. 20.6).

The Hank-Bradley dilator has the shape and contour of the Hegar dilator but has a more tapered shank (Fig. 20.9), with the advantage of a hollow center, which prevents any piston effect that might force air into the uterine cavity during progressive dilatation of the cervix. The positive pressure created within the uterine cavity by passing a Hegar dilator can cause blood, endometrium, fragments of neoplastic tissue, or infected material to be forced into the fallopian tubes or peritoneal cavity. Beyth et al. have demonstrated that significant numbers of patients have endometrial tissue in their peritoneal fluid after curettage, and there is a possibility of reflux of endometrial carcinoma cells into the peritoneal cavity with forceful dilatation of a postmenopausal cervix harboring endometrial carcinoma. In the small postmenopausal uterus, however, it is quite easy for the tip of the Hank-Bradley dilator to perforate the uterine fundus when one

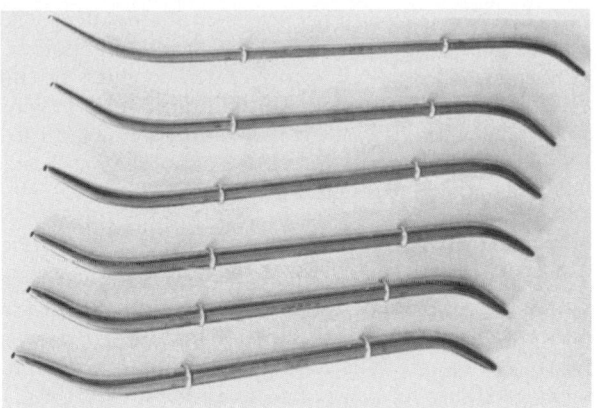

FIGURE 20.9. Hank-Bradley dilators in graduated sizes. Note central canal that extends through length of dilator.

is attempting to achieve the maximum dilating effect from the widest portion of the instrument.

The Hank-Bradley dilator is used more commonly during curettage for an incomplete abortion because it permits the release of blood through the dilator while the cervix is being dilated. When dilatation is for removal of placental tissue, dilatation up to no. 19 or 20 Hank-Bradley (the equivalent of a 9- or 10-mm Hegar dilator) is often necessary to permit the introduction of a large blunt curet and placental forceps. The cervix is most resistant to dilatation at about 8 mm. Cervical injury is a potential problem when the cervix is forcefully dilated to a larger diameter. The cervical tenaculum can lacerate the cervix, or the internal cervical os can be damaged. Tapered Pratt dilators require less force than blunt Hegar dilators.

The incidence of cervical incompetence can be related to the degree of cervical dilatation. Insertion of *laminaria* into the cervical canal several hours before cervical dilatation can make the procedure less difficult and traumatic, as suggested by Manabe and Manabe.

CURETTAGE OF THE UTERUS
Indications and Contraindications

It is important that D&C be performed for the proper indications, be performed correctly to obtain the most useful information, and be performed safely. A curettage performed properly and with aseptic technique involves little risk, but if precautions are disregarded, complications and even death can result.

The chief purpose of curettage of the uterus is the removal of endometrial or endocervical tissue for histologic study of cases of abnormal uterine bleeding. Although classical curettage of the uterus continues to be a useful procedure, new practices and instrumentation permit the procurement of endometrium as a screening diagnostic test under many circumstances. Appropriate use of such procedures can reduce significantly the need for operating room curettage. Careful pelvic examina-

tion under relaxation anesthesia has been an important adjunctive diagnostic aid to conventional D&C, but the precision and availability of ultrasound and other imaging techniques have brought them to the forefront of importance in diagnosis.

Outpatient Curettage

Over the years, there have been efforts to lower the cost of D&C by making it an outpatient procedure. In 1957, Vermeeren et al. presented a series of 10,000 minor gynecologic operations performed on an outpatient basis on the gynecology service at the Johns Hopkins Hospital. The results were more than satisfactory. These women were usually operated on under general anesthesia and were discharged after recovery from anesthesia. D&C was the operation most frequently performed. The success and safety of such a program depend, of course, on the careful selection of patients and the willingness of the practitioner to admit a patient for observation should complications occur. Today, D&C is often performed satisfactorily on an outpatient basis or in an ambulatory surgery center. Reports by Sandmire and Austin and by Martin and Rust are among many that record favorable experiences with this procedure.

As mentioned earlier, endometrial sampling today is often performed by biopsy, suction, or D&C as an office procedure. Although these relatively easy outpatient techniques for evaluating endometrium histology can often provide a correct diagnosis, they do not fulfill the requirement of a thorough curettage for absolute determination of the etiology of uterine bleeding. One can have total confidence in the biopsy or office curettage findings only if they show frank adenocarcinoma. If the histology of the office procedures is negative, one cannot rule out this serious condition. Even in the most experienced hands, endometrial carcinoma can be quite elusive. A further note of caution is that none of the office endometrial sampling methods can ensure the removal of an endometrial polyp. Therefore, endometrial carcinoma in a polyp could be missed, as could a polyp that is a source of benign bleeding. Office sampling techniques are used only as screening procedures; if the results are negative, a more thorough D&C under anesthesia is indicated. Office hysteroscopy can sometimes be an alternative to D&C to identify missed pathologies, such as a polyp or a submucous myoma, or to allow directed biopsy of a suspicious endometrium.

Indications for obtaining endometrial histology by one or more of the aforementioned methods include the following:

- Abnormal bleeding at any premenopausal age, especially when not corrected promptly by medical management, in women older than 35 years of age, or if a submucous myoma is suspected (include hysteroscopy or hysterosalpingography).
- Postmenopausal bleeding of any amount, regardless of a finding of atrophic vaginitis, polyp, or urethral caruncle.

- Prehysterectomy in the postmenopausal woman to exclude endocervical or endometrial carcinoma.
- Postmenopausal vaginal surgery without hysterectomy.

When office procedures fail to establish the diagnosis, it is preferable to use a general anesthetic during D&C. The procedure is more comfortable for the patient and easier to perform with the patient fully relaxed, and most patients will opt for a general anesthetic for this procedure. A D&C under general anesthesia also provides an ideal opportunity for thorough examination of the pelvic organs. Before the examination, the bladder should be empty and an enema should have been given and expelled. The pelvic examination should be performed after the anterior abdominal wall is relaxed from the anesthesia and before the patient is draped. Occasionally, new and important pelvic findings will be discovered. In a study of 2,666 women requiring curettage, McElin et al. found unanticipated adnexal masses in 30 women during pelvic examination under anesthesia before D&C. Twenty-eight masses were benign, and two were malignant. When women who are serious medical risks require curettage for postmenopausal bleeding, the operation is performed without anesthetic other than hypodermic or intravenous administration of a sedative combined with paracervical nerve block.

A single curettage will not remove all of the surface endometrium completely from the uterine cavity. Repeated studies have demonstrated the inability of a thorough curettage to remove more than 50% to 60% of the endometrium when the procedure has been performed by experienced gynecologists immediately before a planned hysterectomy. Stock and Kanbour, from McGee Hospital in Pittsburgh, observed that in 60% of hysterectomy specimens studied, less than 50% of the endometrial surface had been removed by a prehysterectomy curettage. They also found 26 cases of endometrial carcinoma that had been classified as clinically normal-appearing tissue on prehysterectomy curettage; six of these carcinomas were reported as benign on frozen section. These facts and other similar experiences indicate that it is difficult to be certain of the histology of the endometrium by gross examination of the curetting. If the symptoms warrant a curettage, then the endometrium deserves a full histologic diagnosis.

Curettage is also performed for bleeding from a cervical stump and is frequently performed as part of a cervical conization to rule out extension of cervical carcinoma into the endometrium. Helmkamp et al. found no evidence of endometrial abnormality in any of 114 curettage specimens removed at the time of 114 cervical conizations. These investigators recommend that curettage at the time of cervical conization should not be performed routinely but should be performed selectively in postmenopausal and perimenopausal patients when the cytology smear shows abnormal glandular cells or when an intrauterine abnormality is suspected.

The chief contraindication to curettage is infection. Acute endometritis and salpingitis are conditions under which curettage should be avoided. If curettage is necessary for removal of infected placental tissue, it should be preceded by a period of parenteral antibiotic therapy adequate to achieve therapeutic tissue levels of antibiotics. Endometritis associated with retained products of conception will remain unresolved until the infected necrotic material is cast off spontaneously or until it is removed by the curet. Curettage is also contraindicated when pyometra is present.

Technique of Curettage of the Uterus

I am increasingly using the abortion suction apparatus to perform diagnostic and therapeutic endometrial evacuations. The connecting tubing is flushed with normal saline to ensure recovery of all tissue fragments. Overall, the use of suction should cause less trauma to the uterine wall and provide a more complete sample of the endometrium. The perineum need not be shaved before uterine curettage, but an enema given before surgery should be expelled before the patient comes to the operating room so that hard stool in the rectum and sigmoid will not interfere with the accuracy of the pelvic examination under anesthesia. After the patient is anesthetized and placed in the lithotomy position, the bladder is emptied with a catheter. The pelvic organs are examined thoroughly before the patient is prepped and draped. The procedure includes a bimanual rectovaginal–abdominal examination. The examination under anesthesia is one of the most informative features of this operation because it can provide anatomic details of the reproductive tract that are unrecognizable without anesthesia. The vagina and perineum are cleaned with the usual technique.

Fractional curettage is an attempt to remove tissue samples from the endocervical canal apart from tissue removed from the endometrial cavity. The cervical canal should be curetted before dilatation of the cervical canal and curettage of the endometrial cavity. The special shape of the small Gusberg curet makes it particularly useful for curetting the endocervix. Differential curettage of the endocervix, separate from the endometrium, is important for diagnosis of endometrial carcinoma that may have extended to the endocervix. All cases of perimenopausal bleeding should be fractionally curetted; this procedure is too often neglected. If the endocervical curettage is not performed, a second fractional curettage is required to determine the anatomic boundaries of endometrial carcinoma. The value of fractional curettage has been questioned, but Chen and Lee and others have emphasized the importance of cervical stromal invasion, rather than the finding of tumor tissue, as the crucial criterion in endocervical curetting affecting staging and prognosis.

The uterine cavity is then sounded to determine its size and to confirm the position determined from examination under anesthesia. The cervical canal is dilated with the Hegar or Hank-Bradley dilator. A dilatation to 8 or 9 mm by a Hegar dilator is sufficient for the usual diagnostic curettage. A gauze is placed in the posterior vaginal fornix along the posterior retractor so that the blood and the endometrium removed from the uterus can fall on it (Fig. 20.10). Before the curettage is per-

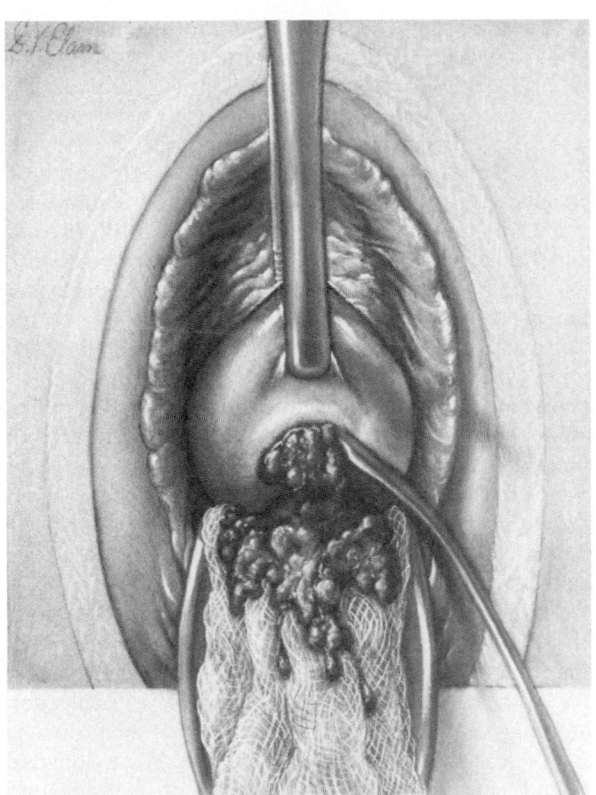

FIGURE 20.10. Method of collecting curettings and blood on gauze.

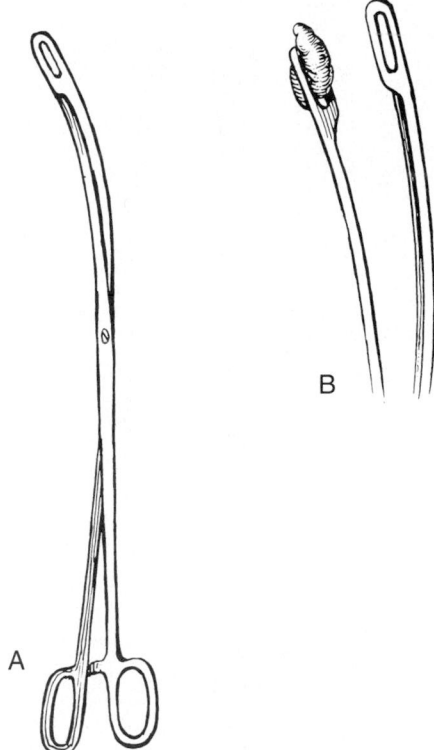

FIGURE 20.11. A: Ureteral stone forceps, an excellent instrument for removing endometrial polyps. **B:** A polyp, grasped in forceps, that was missed at curettage.

formed, the uterine cavity is explored for endometrial polyps by use of a narrow stone forceps (Fig. 20.11). This forceps can be opened and closed as the tip of the forceps is moved systematically across the dome of the uterus and the anterior and posterior walls. An endometrial polyp can be easily missed with an ordinary curet, and unnecessary hysterectomies have been performed because of supposed persistent or recurrent dysfunctional bleeding after a curettage (Fig. 20.12). If polyp forceps are routinely used, such operations can be avoided. It is easier to identify and remove an endometrial polyp if the uterine cavity is explored with the stone forceps before the uterus is curetted. In a 28-month period during which forceps were used routinely at the Johns Hopkins Hospital, Josey found that endometrial polyp was diagnosed 130 times. In 83 of these cases, the polyp was removed by forceps. Although the sessile form of a submucous myoma is diagnosed easily by noting an irregularity of the uterine wall with the curet, the pedunculated variety, like the endometrial polyp, can escape detection because of its narrow stalk. Often, such a leiomyoma can be grasped with the polyp forceps. A uterine septum can also be detected with the forceps.

A small-sized or medium-sized, malleable, bluntly serrated curet (Fig. 20.13) is then introduced into the uterus, and the entire uterine cavity is systematically curetted. The anterior, lateral, and posterior walls are scraped gently but firmly, and finally, the top of the cavity is scraped with a side-to-side movement (Fig. 20.14). The handle of the curet should never be held against the

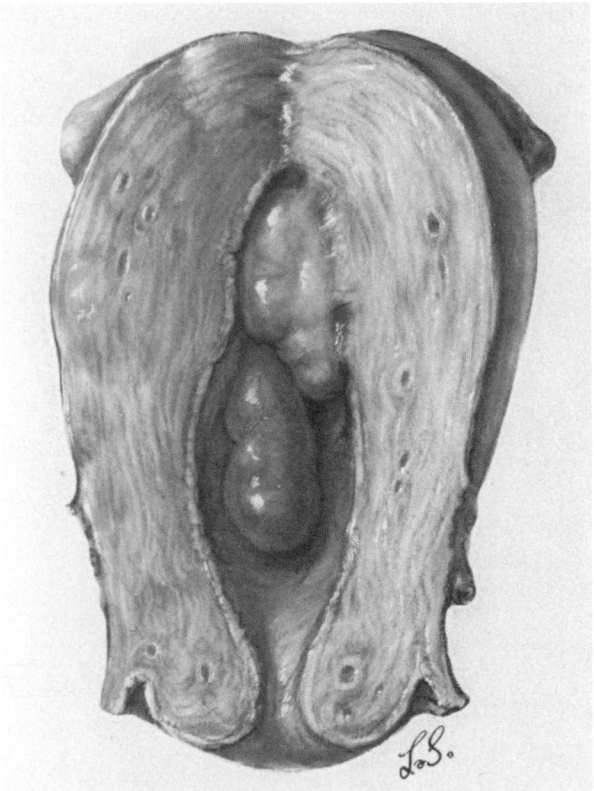

FIGURE 20.12. Opened uterus, showing two separate endometrial polyps.

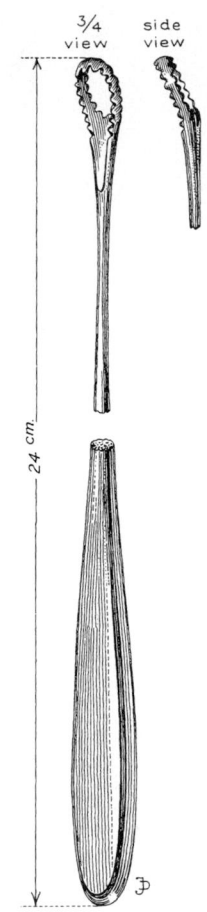

FIGURE 20.13. Small serrated curet for routine curettage.

its curvature can be changed to conform to the contour of the uterine cavity. A uterine "cry," vibrations felt in the hand holding the curet, is often used as a sign that adequate tissue has been removed.

The unclotted blood is absorbed quickly by the gauze sponge, leaving the relatively clean endometrium to be placed in a prepared container with appropriate fixative. Again, the curettings should never be mashed or scraped but should be picked carefully from the sponge with a smooth-tip forceps and placed immediately in the fixative. The curettings should be examined carefully at this time for fatty tissue or other unusual tissue. Fragments of hyperplastic endometrium sometimes appear tan or yellow.

When curettage is performed as a curative measure for removal of placental tissue, a large, blunt, smooth curet is used to lessen the possibilities of perforation and endometrial sclerosis. The larger and softer the uterus, the larger the curet should be and the more care one should exercise to avoid these complications. When large masses of placental tissue are present, ovum forceps are most useful when used in conjunction with the curet. High vacuum suction is now used almost routinely for placental tissue removal.

Routine blind biopsy of the cervix is usually unrewarding if a negative cytologic smear has been obtained and there is no suspicious cervical lesion. We no longer do a blind biopsy of the cervix at the time of curettage unless an abnormal lesion is present. If a patient's recent cytologic results are normal and she has a profuse, recurrent, mucous discharge associated with cervicitis and nabothian cysts, cervical cauterization or laser vaporization can be done at the time of curettage, but biopsy confirmation to exclude occult malignancy should be obtained.

Complications of Cervical Dilatation and Uterine Curettage

If the position and the consistency of the uterus are carefully observed on bimanual examination under

palm of the hand. Instead, it should be held gently as one would hold a pencil. The instrument is held loosely as it is inserted for the full distance. Pressure is then exerted against the uterine wall as the curet is drawn in an outward direction. Because the instrument is malleable,

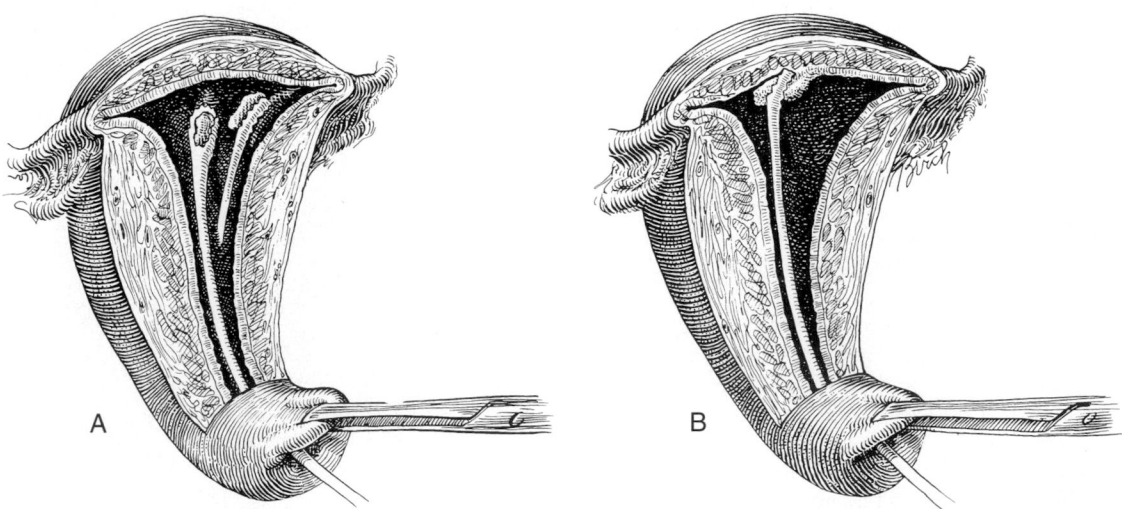

FIGURE 20.14. Method of curetting the uterine cavity systematically. **A:** The anterior, posterior, and lateral walls of the cavity are curetted systematically. **B:** The top of the cavity is then curetted thoroughly.

anesthesia before curettage is begun, perforation will rarely occur. When the position of the uterus is not known to the operator, perforation occurs with remarkable ease. Special care should be exercised with a uterus that is acutely anteflexed or retroflexed. With cervical stenosis, pregnancy, or intrauterine malignancy, perforation is more likely. The postmenopausal atrophic uterus can be perforated with only slight force applied to the uterine sound or the curet. Perforation is discovered when the sound or the curet fails to encounter resistance where it normally should, as judged by the palpated size of the uterus.

Perforation by the uterine sound or cervical dilator causes less damage than perforation by the sharp curet or suction cannula. Sharp curettage for legally induced abortion has a major complication rate that is two to three times higher than that for suction curettage, according to Grimes and Cates. The two principal dangers of uterine perforation are bleeding and trauma to the abdominal viscera. Lateral perforation through the uterine vessels is especially dangerous from the standpoint of intraperitoneal hemorrhage and broad ligament hematoma formation. Damage can occur to the bowel, omentum, mesentery, ureter, and fallopian tube. Perforation of the anterior or posterior wall of the uterus by a small curet in performing a diagnostic curettage is usually not a serious accident. However, it is usually necessary to discontinue curettage. One must watch carefully for signs of hemorrhage or infection. If signs of hemorrhage develop, the abdomen should be opened and the uterine wound sutured. If signs of infection occur, broadspectrum antibiotics should be given. If a pelvic abscess develops, the abscess should be drained if possible. Serious hemorrhage or infection occurs only rarely. When serious damage from perforation is suspected, laparoscopy can be performed to assess the extent of the damage and the needed repair. According to MacKenzie and Bibby, complications occurred in 1.7% of cases of D&C. McElin et al. reported that 0.5% of cases had postoperative febrile morbidity after D&C. Uterine perforation occurred in 0.63% of cases.

One should be absolutely certain that the endometrial cavity has been entered when D&C is performed for postmenopausal bleeding. A relatively stenotic internal cervical os and a fear of uterine perforation can prevent entry into the uterine cavity above the internal cervical os, resulting in failure to curet the uterine cavity and consequent failure to diagnose the cause of the bleeding.

Perforation of a pregnant uterus is a more serious complication than is perforation of the nonpregnant uterus. First, there is the requirement that all remaining pregnancy tissue be completely removed to prevent sepsis. To accomplish this blindly when there is a defect in the uterine wall is unsafe. Second, the pregnant uterus is a much more vascular organ than is the nonpregnant uterus, and intraperitoneal bleeding can be profuse without significant external bleeding. Third, it often is difficult to be certain when the perforation occurred. If a high-vacuum suction vacuret has passed through the myometrium and the vacuum has been activated, major bowel injury can be present. These con-

siderations have led to the following protocol for D&C of the pregnant uterus:

1. Never activate the vacuum suction if there is any question about the safe location of the vacuret within the uterine cavity.
2. Laparoscope any pregnant uterus that is possibly perforated. With the laparoscope in place, a second operator can evacuate remaining placental tissue while the laparoscopist monitors safety. Many perforations in which no other visceral damage has occurred are fundal. If laparoscopic observation confirms that bleeding is minimal, the perforation can be managed conservatively with antibiotics and serial hematocrit determination for 24 to 48 hours. If there is no evidence of continued bleeding or developing infection, the patient can be discharged.
3. During laparoscopy, if there is any evidence of intestinal injury or any suspicion of such injury, or if bleeding is significant, then laparotomy is mandatory. Unfortunately, bowel injury by high-vacuum suction may require bowel resection and anastomosis.

Fig. 20.15 shows a uterus removed immediately after a perforation because of intraperitoneal bleeding. Word analyzed 70 accidental uterine perforations. Among these, an unplanned hysterectomy was performed on seven unprepared patients. In none of these cases did the intraperitoneal findings indicate the need for hysterectomy. In fact, hysterectomy compounded the surgical error. Fifty-five patients were treated conservatively, and only one developed a complication, in the form of a pelvic abscess that was drained by colpotomy. Forty-one of the 70 perforations occurred in postmenopausal women.

When a large, boggy, postabortion or puerperal uterus is perforated by a large curet or placental forceps in removing placental tissue, there is more danger of hemorrhage, infection, or injury to bowel. The treatment protocols and the procedures for these serious complications are discussed elsewhere in this textbook.

Asherman's syndrome is a pathologic condition of intrauterine adhesions that can cause secondary amenorrhea, other menstrual irregularities, infertility, or recurrent abortion. Numerous investigators have shown a strong association between puerperal D&C and the formation of synechiae that can partially or completely obliterate the endometrial cavity. No incidence figures are available because no prospective studies have been performed, but factors other than pregnancy that increase the risk of endometrial sclerosis after D&C are infection, scant endometrium that exposes the basalis to trauma, and a hypoestrogenic state. Rarely, significant synechiae are seen in the absence of an antecedent curettage. Cases have been reported after severe endometritis, tuberculosis, myomectomy, and Caesarean section. Diagnosis is made by clinical history, hysterosalpingography, or hysteroscopy. Therapy requires lysis of adhesions by repeat curettage or, preferably, by hysteroscopic scissors or KTP laser.

Patency of the uterine cavity is maintained with an intrauterine device or balloon catheter, and endometrial

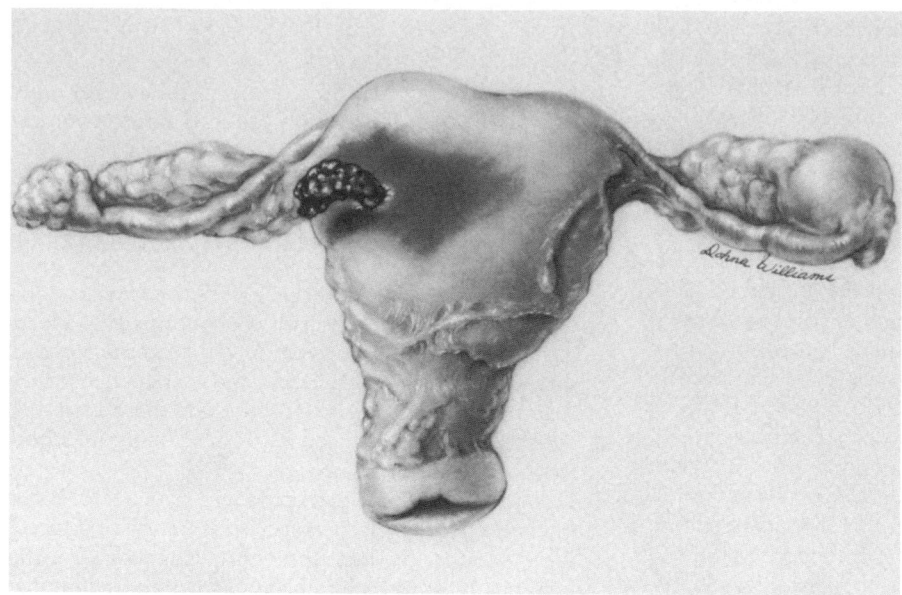

FIGURE 20.15. Result of uterine perforation. Specimen removed directly after perforation.

regeneration is stimulated by oral estrogen therapy. The prognosis with significant adhesions is poor. Only 40% of patients will become pregnant, and about half of these will undergo spontaneous abortion or premature delivery. Consideration should be given to the risks of adhesion formation before the curettage of a pregnant or infected uterus, and possibly a less vigorous scraping should be performed in an attempt to minimize endometrial trauma.

BIBLIOGRAPHY

Aksel S, Jones GS. Etiology and treatment of dysfunctional uterine bleeding. *Obstet Gynecol* 1974;44:1.

Anderson ABM, Haynes PJ, Guillebaud J, et al. Reduction of menstrual blood loss by prostaglandin synthesis inhibition. *Lancet* 1976;1:774.

Andolf E, Dahlander K, Aspenberg P. Ultrasonic thickness of the endometrium correlated to body weight in asymptomatic postmenopausal women. *Obstet Gynecol* 1993;82:936.

Asherman J. Amenorrhea traumatica (atretica). *J Obstet Gynecol Br Emp* 1948;55:23.

Atwood JT, Toth TL, Schiff I. Abnormal uterine bleeding in the perimenopause. *Int J Fertil* 1993;38:261.

Azziz R, Zacur HA. 21-Hydroxylase deficiency in female hyperandrogenemia. *J Clin Endocrinol Metab* 1989;69:577.

Barnett JM. Suction curettage on unanesthetized outpatients. *Obstet Gynecol* 1973;42:672.

Battacharya S, Cameron IM, Parkin DE, et al. A pragmatic randomized comparison of transcervical resection of the endometrium with endometrial laser ablation for the treatment of menorrhagia. *Br J Obstet Gynaecol* 1999;106:360.

Bayer SR, DeCherney AH. Clinical manifestations and treatment of dysfunctional uterine bleeding. *JAMA* 1993;269:1823.

Beller FK. Observations on the clotting of menstrual blood and clot formation. *Am J Obstet Gynecol* 1971;3:535.

Beyth Y, Yaffe H, Levii I, et al. Retrograde seeding of endometrium: a sequela of tubal flushing. *Fertil Steril* 1975;26:1094.

Brooks PG. Complications of operative hysteroscopy: how safe is it? *Clin Obstet Gynecol* 1993;35:256.

Brooks PG. Hysteroscopic surgery using the resectoscope: myomas, ablation, septae and synechiae: does pre-operative medication help? *Clin Obstet Gynecol* 1993;35:249.

Brooks PG, Serden SP. Endometrial ablation in women with abnormal uterine bleeding aged fifty and over. *J Reprod Med* 1992;37:682.

Brooks-Carter GN, Killackey MA, Neuwirth RS. Adenocarcinoma of the endometrium after endometrial ablation. *Obstet Gynecol* 2000;96:836.

Cameron IT, Haining R, Lumsden M-A, et al. The effects of mefenamic acid and norethisterone on measured menstrual blood loss. *Obstet Gynecol* 1990;76:85.

Chen SS, Lee L. Reappraisal of endocervical curettage in predicting cervical involvement by endometrial carcinoma. *Obstet Gynecol* 1986;31:50.

Chiazze L Jr, Brayer FT, Macisco JJ Jr, et al. The length and variability of the human menstrual cycle. *JAMA* 1968;203:377.

Claessens EA, Cowell CA. Acute adolescent menorrhagia. *Am J Obstet Gynecol* 1981;139:227.

Cohen CJ, Gusberg SB, Koffier D. Histologic screening for endometrial cancer. *Gynecol Oncol* 1974;2:279.

Copperman AB, DeCherney AH, Olive DL. A case of endometrial cancer following endometrial ablation for dysfunctional uterine bleeding. *Obstet Gynecol* 1993;82:640.

Corson SL, Brill AI, Brooks PG, et al. Interim results of the American VESTA trial of endometrial ablation. *J Am Assoc Gynecol Laparosc* 1999;6:45.

Coulam CB, Annegers JF, Kranz JS. Chronic anovulation syndrome and associated neoplasia. *Obstet Gynecol* 1983;61:403.

Crosignani PG, Vercellini P, Mosconi P, Oldani S, et al. Levonorgestrel-releasing intrauterine device versus hysteroscopic endometrial resection in the treatment of dysfunctional uterine bleeding. *Obstet Gynecol* 1997;90:257-63.

Davies AJ, Anderson ABM, Turnbull AC. Reduction by naproxen of excessive menstrual bleeding in women using intrauterine devices. *Obstet Gynecol* 1981;57:74.

Denis R Jr, Barnett JM, Forbes SE. Diagnostic suction curettage. *Obstet Gynecol* 1973;42:301.

DeVore G, Owens O, Case NL. Use of intravenous Premarin in the treatment of dysfunctional uterine bleeding: a double-blind randomized control study. *Obstet Gynecol* 1982;59:285.

Dickson RB, Johnson MD, el-Ashry D, et al. Breast cancer: influence of endocrine hormones, growth factors and genetic alterations. *Adv Exp Med Biol* 1993;330:119.

Dickson RB, Lippman ME. Estrogenic regulation of growth and polypeptide growth factor secretion in human breast carcinoma. *Endocr Rev* 1987;8:39.

Dilley A, Drews C Miller C, et al. Von Willebrand disease and other inherited bleeding disorders in women with diagnosed menorrhagia. *Obstet Gynecol* 2001;97:630.

Dodson MG. Use of transvaginal ultrasound in diagnosing the etiology of menometrorrhagia. *J Reprod Med* 1994;39:362.

Donnez J, Vilos G, Gannon MJ, et al. Goserelin acetate (Zoladex) plus endometrial ablation for dysfunctional uterine bleeding: a large randomized double-blind study. *Fertil Steril* 1997;68:29.

Dueholm M, Lundorf E, Hansen ES, et al. Evaluation of the uterine cavity with magnetic resonance imaging, transvaginal sonography, hysterosonographic examination, and diagnostic hysteroscopy. *Fertil Steril* 2001;76:350.

Economos K, MacDonald PC, Casey ML. Endothelin-1 gene expression and protein biosynthesis in human endometrium: potential modulator of endometrial blood flow. *J Clin Endocrinol Metab* 1992;74:14.

Evans RM. The steroid and thyroid hormone receptor family. *Science* 1988;240:889.

Falcone T, Desjardins C, Bourgue J, et al. Dysfunctional uterine bleeding in adolescents. *J Reprod Med* 1994;39:761.

Fleming H, Oster AG, Pickel H, et al. Arteriovenous malformations of the uterus. *Obstet Gynecol* 1989;73:209.

Fraser IS, Baird DT. Blood production and ovarian secretion rates of estradiol-17, 3 and estrone in women and dysfunctional uterine bleeding. *J Clin Endocrinol Metab* 1974;38:727.

Fraser IS, Michie EA, Wide L, et al. Pituitary gonadotropins and ovarian function in adolescent dysfunctional uterine bleeding. *J Clin Endocrinol Metab* 1973;37:407.

Fraser IS, Pearse C, Shearman RP, et al. Efficacy of mefenamic acid in patients with a complaint of menorrhagia. *Obstet Gynecol* 1981;58:543.

Friedman AJ, Juneau-Norcross M, Rein MS. Adverse effects of leuprolide acetate depot treatment. *Fertil Steril* 1993;59:448.

Fritsch N. Ein Fall von volligen Schwund der gebarmutter Hohle nach Auskratzung. *Zentralbl Gumsrl* 1894;18:1337.

Garry R, Shelly-Jones D, Mooney P, et al. Six hundred endometrial ablations. *Obstet Gynecol* 1995;85:24.

Gregg RII. The praxiology of the office dilatation and curettage. *Am J Obstet Gynecol* 1981;140:179.

Grimes D. Estimating vaginal blood loss. *J Reprod Med* 1979;22:190.

Grimes D, Cates W Jr. Complications from legally-induced abortion: a review. *Obstet Gynecol Surv* 1979;34:177.

Guidice LC, Dsupin BA, Jin IH, et al. Differential expression of messenger ribonucleic acids encoding insulin-like growth factors and their receptors in human uterine endometrium and decidua. *J Clin Endocrinol Metab* 1993;76:1115.

Guillebaud J, Barnett MD, Gordon YB. Plasma ferritin levels as an index of iron deficiency in women using intrauterine devices. *Br J Obstet Gynaecol* 1979;86:51.

Gull B, Carlsson SA, Karlsson B, et al. Transvaginal ultrasonography of the endometrium in women with postmenopausal bleeding: Is it always necessary to perform an endometrial biopsy? *Am J Obstet Gynecol* 2000;182:509.

Hallberg L, Hogdahl A, Nilsson L, et al. Menstrual blood and iron deficiency. *Acta Med Scand* 1966;180:639.

Hallberg L, Nilsson L. Constancy of individual menstrual blood loss. *Acta Obstet Gynecol Scand* 1964;43:352.

Hallberg L, Nilsson L. Determination of menstrual blood loss. *Scand J Clin Lab Invest* 1964;16:244.

Handwerger S, Richards RG, Markoff E. The physiology of decidual prolactin and other decidual protein hormones. *Trends Endocrinol Metab* 1992;3:91.

Haynes PJ, Hodgson H, Anderson ABM, et al. Measurement of menstrual blood loss in patients complaining of menorrhagia. *Br J Obstet Gynaecol* 1997;84:763.

Healy DL, Hogden GD. The endocrinology of human endometrium. *Obstet Gynecol Surv* 1983;38:509.

Helmkamp BF, Denslow BL, Boufiglio TA, et al. Cervical conization: when is dilatation and curettage indicated? *Am J Obstet Gynecol* 1983;146:893.

Hofmeister FJ. Endometrial biopsy: another look. *Am J Obstet Gynecol* 1974;118:773.

Hofmeister FJ. Endometrial curettage. In: Symmonds CM, Zuspan FT, eds. *Clinical and diagnostic procedures in obstetrics and gynecology.* New York: Marcel Dekker, 1984.

Hunt JS, Chen H-L, Hu X-L, et al. Tumor necrosis factor-α messenger ribonucleic acid and protein in human endometrium. *Biol Reprod* 1992;47:141.

Istre O, Trolle B. Treatment of menorrhagia with the levonorgestrel intrauterine system versus endometrial resection. *Fertil Steril* 2001; 76:304.

Jansen FW, Vredevoogd CB, Van Ulzen K, et al. Complications of hysteroscopy: a prospective multicenter study. *Obstet Gynecol* 2000;96:266.

Jensen JA, Jensen JG. Abragio mucosae uteri e aspiratione. *Ugeskr Laeger* 1968;130:2121.

Jensen JG. Vacuum curettage. Outpatient curettage without anesthesia: a report of 350 cases. *Dan Med Bull* 1970;17:199.

Josey WE. Routine intrauterine forceps exploration at curettage. *Obstet Gynecol* 1958;11:108.

Joshi SG. Progestin-regulated proteins of the human endometrium. *Semin Reprod Endocrinol* 1983;1:221.

Karlsson B, Granberg S, Wikland M, et al. Transvaginal ultrasonography of the endometrium in women with postmenopausal bleeding: a Nordic multicenter study. *Am J Obstet Gynecol* 1995;172:1488.

Kelly HA. Curettage without anesthesia on the office table. *Am J Obstet Gynecol* 1925;9:78.

King RJB. Structure and function of steroid receptors. *J Endocrinol* 1987;114:341.

Klein SM, Garcia CR. Asherman's syndrome: a critique and current review. *Fertil Steril* 1973;24:722.

Kooy J, Taylor NH, Healy DL, Rogers PA. Endothelial cell proliferation in the endometrium of women with menorrhagia and in women following endometrial ablation. *Hum Reprod* 1996;11:1067.

Krettek JE, Arkin SI, Chaisilwattana P, et al. *Chlamydia trachomatis* in patients who used oral contraceptives and had intermenstrual spotting. *Obstet Gynecol* 1993;81:728.

Kubrinsky NL, Tulloch H. Treatment of refractory thrombocytopenic bleeding with desamino-8-D-arginine vasopressin (desmopressin). *J Pediatr* 1988;112:993.

Larsson PG, Bergman BB. Is there a causal connection between motile curved rods, *Mobiluncus* species and bleeding complications? *Am J Obstet Gynecol* 1986;154:107.

Laufer MR, Mitchell SR. Treatment of abnormal uterine bleeding with gonadotropin-releasing hormone analogues. *Clin Obstet Gynecol* 1993;36:668.

Leather A, Studd J, Watson N, et al. The prevention of bone loss in young women treated with GnRH analogues with "add-back" estrogen therapy. *Obstet Gynecol* 1993;81:104.

Lessey BA, Castelbaum AJ, Sawin SW, et al. Further characterization of endometrial integrins during the menstrual cycle and in pregnancy. *Fertil Steril* 1994;62:497.

Lessey BA, Damjanovich L, Cautifaris C, et al. Integrin adhesion molecules in the human endometrium: correlation with normal and abnormal menstrual cycle. *J Clin Invest* 1992;90:188.

Lomano JM. Photocoagulation of the endometrium with the Nd:YAG laser for the treatment of menorrhagia: a report of 10 cases. *J Reprod Med* 1986;31:149.

Lutz MH, Underwood PB Jr, Kreutner A, et al. Vacuum aspiration: an efficient outpatient screening technique for endometrial disease. *South Med J* 1977;70:393.

MacKenzie IZ, Bibby JG. Critical assessment of dilatation and curettage in 1,029 women. *Lancet* 1978;2:566.

Manabe Y, Manabe A. Nelaton catheter for gradual and safe cervical dilatation: an ideal substitute for laminaria. *Am J Obstet Gynecol* 1981;140:465.

March CM. Hysteroscopy. *J Reprod Med* 1992;37:293.

Markee JE. Menstruation in intraocular endometrial transplants in the rhesus monkey. *Contr Embryol Carneg Justn* 1940;28:219.

Martin PL, Rust JA. Surgical gynecology for the ambulatory patient. *Clin Obstet Gynecol* 1974;17:205.

McElin TW, Burd CC, Reeves BD, et al. Diagnostic dilatation and curettage. *Obstet Gynecol* 1969;33:807.

Mengert WF, Slate WG. Diagnostic dilatation and curettage as an outpatient procedure. *Am J Obstet Gynecol* 1960;79:727.

Meyer WR, Walsh BW, Grainger DA, et al. Thermal balloon and roller ball ablation to treat menorrhagia: a multicenter comparison. *Obstet Gynecol* 1998;92:98-103.

Milsom I, Andersson K, Andersch B, et al. A comparison of flurbiprofen, tranexamic acid and a levonorgestrel-releasing intrauterine contraceptive device in the treatment of idiopathic menorrhagia. *Am J Obstet Gynecol* 1991;164:879.

Mishell DR Jr, Connel E, Haney A, et al. Oral contraception for women in their 40s. *J Reprod Med* 1990;35:447.

Mularoni A, Mahfoudi A, Beck L, et al. Progesterone control of fibronectin secretion in guinea pig endometrium. *Endocrinology* 1992;131:2127.

Narula RK. Endometrial histopathology in dysfunctional uterine bleeding. *J Obstet Gynecol India* 1967;17:614.

Nasri MN, Shepherd JH, Setchell ME, et al. The role of vaginal scan in measurement of endometrial thickness in postmenopausal women. *Br J Obstet Gynaecol* 1991;98:470.

Nilsson L, Rybo G. Treatment of menorrhagia. *Am J Obstet Gynecol* 1971;110:713.

Novak E. Relation of hyperplasia of endometrium to so-called functional uterine hemorrhage. *JAMA* 1920;75:292.

Novak E. A suction curette apparatus and endometrial biopsy. *JAMA* 1935;104:1497.

O'Connor H, Magos A. Endometrial resection for the treatment of menorrhagia. *N Engl J Med* 1996;335:151.

Osmers R. Transvaginal sonography in endometrial cancer. *Ultrasound Obstet Gynecol* 1991;2:2.

Overton C, Hargreaves J, Maresh M. A national survey of the complications of endometrial destruction for menstrual disorders: the "the Mistletoe" study. *Br J Obstet Gynaecol* 1997;102:1351.

Pacheco JC, Kempers RD. Etiology of postmenopausal bleeding. *Obstet Gynecol* 1968;32:40.

Reyniak JV. Dysfunctional uterine bleeding. *J Reprod Med* 1976;17:293.

Rodgers WH, Osteen KG, Matrisian LM, et al. Expression and localization of matrilysin, a matrix metalloproteinase, in human endometrium during the reproductive cycle. *Am J Obstet Gynecol* 1993;168:253.

Rubin MC, Davidson AR, Philliber SG, et al. Long-term effect of tubal sterilization on menstrual indices and pelvic pain. *Obstet Gynecol* 1993;82:118.

Rutherford TJ, Zreik TG, Troiano RN, et al. Endometrial cryo ablation, a minimally invasive procedure for abnormal uterine bleeding. *J Am Assoc Gynecol Laparosc* 1998;5:23.

Sandmire HF, Austin SD. Curettage as an office procedure. *Am J Obstet Gynecol* 1974;119:82.

Seeras RC, Gilliland GB. Resumption of menstruation after amenorrhea in women treated by endometrial ablation and myometrial resection. *J Am Assoc Gynecol Laparosc* 1997;4:305.

Sharp NC, Cronin N, Feldberg I, et al. Microwaves for menorrhagia: a new fast technique for endometrial ablation. *Lancet* 1995;346:1003.

Singer A, Almanza R, Rutierrez A, et al. Preliminary clinical experience with a thermal balloon ablation method to treat menorrhagia. *Obstet Gynecol* 1994;83:732.

Smith SK, Abel MH, Kelly RW, et al. Prostaglandin synthesis in the endometrium of women with ovular dysfunctional uterine bleeding. *Br J Obstet Gynaecol* 1981;88:434.

Smith SK, Abel MH, Kelly RW, et al. A role for prostacyclin (PGI_2) in excessive menstrual bleeding. *Lancet* 1981;1:522.

Southam AI, Richard RM. The prognosis for adolescents with menstrual abnormalities. *Am J Obstet Gynecol* 1966;94:637.

Speroff L, Glass RH, Kase NG. Dysfunctional uterine bleeding. In: *Clinical gynecologic endocrinology and infertility,* sixth edition. Baltimore: Lippincott Williams & Wilkins, 1999:575-593.

Stock RJ, Kanbour A. Pre-hysterectomy curettage: an evaluation. *Obstet Gynecol* 1975;45:537.

Summitt RJ Jr, Stovall TG, Steege JF, Lipscomb GH. A multicenter randomized comparison of laparoscopically assisted vaginal hysterectomy and abdominal hysterectomy candidates. *Obstet Gynecol* 1998;92:321.

Swartz DP, Jones GES. Progesterone in anovulatory uterine bleeding: clinical observations. *Fertil Steril* 1957;8:103.

Taylor PJ, Graham G. Is diagnostic curettage harmful in women with unexplained infertility? *Br J Obstet Gynaecol* 1982;89:296.

Teare AJ, Rippey JJ. Dilatation and curettage. *S Afr Med J* 1979;55:535.

Torry DS, Torry RJ. Angiogenesis and the expression of vascular endothelial growth factor in endometrium and placenta. *Am J Reprod Immunol* 1997;37:21-9.

Townsend DE, Fields G, McCausland A, et al. Diagnostic and operative hysteroscopy in the management of persistent postmenopausal bleeding. *Obstet Gynecol* 1993;82:419.

Tseng L, Gusberg SB, Gurpide E. Estradiol receptor and 17β-dehydrogenase in normal and abnormal human endometrium. *Ann NY Acad Sci* 1977;286:190.

VanEijkeren MA, Christiaens GC, Geuze JH, et al. Effects of mefenamic acid on menstrual hemostasis in essential menorrhagia. *Am J Obstet Gynecol* 1992;166:1419.

VanEijkeren MA, Christiaens GC, Haspels AA, et al. Measured menstrual blood loss in women with a bleeding disorder or using oral anticoagulant therapy. *Am J Obstet Gynecol* 1990;162:1261.

VanEijkeren MA, Christiaens GC, Sixma JJ, et al. Menorrhagia: a review. *Obstet Gynecol Surv* 1989;4:421.

Vercellini P, Oldani S, Yaylayan L, et al. Randomized comparision of vaporizing electrode and cutting loop for endometrial ablation. *Obstet Gynecol* 1999;94:521.

Vermeeren J, Chamberlain RR, Te Linde RW. Ten thousand minor gynecologic operations on an outpatient basis. *Obstet Gynecol* 1957;9:139.

Vilos GA, Pispidkis JT, Botz CK. Economic evaluation of hysteroscopic endometrial ablation versus vaginal hysterectomy for menorrhagia. *Obstet Gynecol* 1996;88: 241.

Weisberg M, Goldrath MH, Berman J, et al. Hysteroscopic endometrial ablation using free heated saline for the treatment of menorrhagia. *J Am Assoc Gynecol Laparosc* 200;7:311.

Whitehead MI, Frazier D. The effects of estrogens and progestogens on the endometrium. *Obstet Gynecol Clin North Am* 1987;14:299.

Whitehead MI, King RJ, McQueen J, et al. Endometrial histology and biochemistry in climacteric women during estrogen and estrogen/progestogen therapy. *J R Soc Med* 1979;72:322.

Wilansky DL, Greisman B. Early hypothyroidism in patients with menorrhagia. *Am J Obstet Gynecol* 1989;160:673.

Wilborn WH, Flowers CE Jr. Cellular mechanisms for endometrial conservation during menstrual bleeding. *Semin Reprod Endocrinol* 1984;2:307.

Word B. Current concepts of uterine curettage. *Postgrad Med* 1960;28:450.

Word B, Gravlee LC, Wideman GL. The fallacy of simple uterine curettage. *Obstet Gynecol* 1958;12:642.

Te Linde's Operative Gynecology, ninth edition, edited by John A. Rock and Howard W. Jones, III. Lippincott Williams & Wilkins, Philadelphia © 2003.

CHAPTER
21

▼

Management of Abortion

DAVID A. GRIMES

The management of abortion remains a principal focus of gynecology. On a national scale, the scope of the challenge posed by spontaneous and induced abortion is broad. Several million spontaneous abortions occur annually, and more than 1 million induced abortions are performed each year in the United States. Induced abortion is one of the most frequently performed operations in gynecology, and one of the most thoroughly studied. This chapter summarizes the medical and surgical management of abortion. It reviews the incidence, risk factors, and treatment of spontaneous, illegal, and legal abortion.

Two important advances in abortion practice have occurred since publication of the eighth edition of this text. First, in 2000, mifepristone received approval by the Food and Drug Administration (FDA) for use as an early abortifacient in combination with misoprostol. Second, growing use of misoprostol for cervical preparation has made suction curettage easier for the patient and physician. Readers should keep in mind that medical abortion technology is rapidly evolving, and new protocols may supplant those described here.

SPONTANEOUS ABORTION

Incidence

The true incidence of spontaneous abortion is uncertain because of the difficulty in recognizing early conceptions and losses. An estimated 78% of conceptions fail to result in a live birth. When Edmonds et al. monitored urine β-human chorionic gonadotropin (β-hCG) in a cohort of volunteers attempting to conceive, 62% of conceptuses died before 12 weeks' gestation. Most (92%) of these losses occurred before the woman was aware of the pregnancy. Others have confirmed the high rate of loss of unsuspected pregnancies; two thirds occurred before clinical detection. These estimates did not include the unknown, but presumably sizable, proportion of fertilized ova lost before implantation.

Most studies of spontaneous abortion have addressed only pregnancies recognized by the woman. Overall, reported spontaneous abortion rates are about 15% to 17%. These data support the clinical maxim that about one in six women who recognize they are pregnant experience a spontaneous abortion. From a biological perspective, early pregnancy loss is the most common outcome in human reproduction.

Risk Factors

Spontaneous abortion has several important risk factors. The risk increases with advancing maternal age, particularly for women older than 35 years. Likewise, the risk increases with advancing paternal age. Race also plays a role. At each stage of pregnancy, women of minority races in the United States have higher rates of spontaneous abortion than do white women. The racial discrepancy in rates is greatest at 12 to 19 weeks' gestation.

Independent of the effect of age, the risk of spontaneous abortion increases with increasing gravidity. In addition, a history of one or more spontaneous abortions increases the risk of recurrence. This effect is seen at all gestational ages. The risk of spontaneous abortion increased linearly with increasing numbers of prior spontaneous abortions in one recent study. On the other hand, the length of the interval between pregnancies appears to have little impact.

Both gestational age and the aging of sperm and egg appear to influence the likelihood of spontaneous abortion. The probability of spontaneous abortion is inversely related to gestational age. Rates are presumably high in the first weeks of pregnancy, although they are not well quantified. Assuming a total fetal loss of 22%, one study estimated gestational age-specific rates of spontaneous abortion to be 8% at 4 to 7 weeks' gestation, 8% at 8 to 11 weeks, 5% at 12 to 19 weeks, and 2% at 20 or more weeks. Although spontaneous abortion occurs predominantly in the first 12 weeks of pregnancy, with the mean being 9 weeks, some losses do occur later in pregnancy. Conceptions that do not occur near the shift in basal body temperature may be more likely to fail than those that occur near the shift.

Smoking also appears to increase the risk of spontaneous abortion. In one study, the risk doubled; in other studies, the increase in risk was slight. Because smoking is not teratogenic, its effect on spontaneous abortion rates may be through abortion of normal conceptuses.

Fever in early pregnancy can lead to spontaneous abortion. In one study, rates of spontaneous abortion of euploid conceptuses increased two-fold to three-fold if fever had preceded the abortion. External stress also may increase the likelihood of such abortions. Heavy occupational lifting and effort may increase rates of spontaneous abortion. Infection with *Chlamydia trachomatis,* mycoplasmas, or other organisms does not appear to influence spontaneous abortion.

The season of the year does not influence spontaneous abortion rates. The number of spontaneous abortions, however, fluctuates significantly. The incidence of spontaneous abortion peaks in the spring and again in the late fall; this pattern reflects the marked seasonal variation in numbers of conceptions. The proportion of conceptions that end in spontaneous abortion, however, varies little from month to month.

Role

Spontaneous abortion serves primarily as a quality-control mechanism. Human reproduction tolerates a broad diversity of conceptions; more exacting criteria, however, determine survival to viability.

An extensive literature supports this teleologic role for spontaneous abortion as a screening device for abnormal pregnancies. The frequency of chromosomal abnormalities in aborted conceptuses is high, ranging from 30% to 61%. In decreasing order of frequency, the most common abnormalities are trisomy, sex chromosome monosomy, and triploidy. The earlier the gestational age at abortion, the higher is the frequency of chromosomal anomaly. Almost all anomalies, including some that would not appear to handicap survival (such as cleft lip), increase the likelihood of spontaneous abortion.

Multiple gestations, common in other species, are atypical in humans and appear to carry high risk of fetal death. For example, loss of one twin without apparent adverse effect on its partner is well documented. Most fetuses with abnormalities are identified and rejected by the body (high sensitivity). The incidence of chromosomal or other abnormalities in fetuses that survive this selection process is low.

Prevention

Although an abnormal karyotype is the most important risk factor for spontaneous abortion, others probably have a role. These include endocrine defects, environmental toxins, and immunologic factors. In addition, several surgically correctable conditions can influence spontaneous abortion. Uterine synechiae (intrauterine adhesions) are associated with spontaneous abortion. When synechiae occur in this clinical setting, lysis of adhesions by hysteroscopy may be advisable.

Abnormalities of müllerian fusion also can influence spontaneous abortion. Although no effect occurs in the first trimester, the incidence of abortion after 13 weeks' gestation may be 20% to 25%. Septate and bicornuate uteri appear to have more adverse effects than do uterus bicornis bicollis. Women with müllerian anomalies who experience spontaneous abortions at 13 weeks' gestation or later may be candidates for reconstructive operations, described elsewhere in this text.

Leiomyomas, a common condition, may cause spontaneous abortion. The evidence supporting this association, however, is scanty. Submucous leiomyomas may have more effect than intramural or subserosal tumors. Women with leiomyomas who experience abortions at 13 weeks' gestation or later may be candidates for myomectomy. Myomectomy, if performed only because of infertility, may help little; the effect of myomectomy on spontaneous abortion rates is unknown.

How to reduce the risk of spontaneous abortion is largely unknown. Indeed, one small cohort study of women with a history of three or more consecutive spontaneous abortions in early pregnancy found no treatment to be as effective as conventional treatments in achieving subsequent live births.

Management
Threatened Abortion

The traditional approach to threatened abortion, characterized by uterine bleeding without cervical dilation or expulsion of tissue, has been watchful waiting. The likelihood of spontaneous abortion under these circumstances appears to be about 50%. Reliably predicting fetal outcomes in such situations may spare couples substantial anguish.

Fetal well-being early in pregnancy often involves monitoring β-hCG. In addition, ultrasonography is useful for prognosis. To be clinically useful in predicting spontaneous abortion, a sonogram must have high sensitivity and predictive value of an abnormal pregnancy. Specificity and predictive value of a normal scan are of little consequence. If ultrasonography incorrectly identifies a woman as destined to have a spontaneous abortion, curettage performed on the basis of this error would abort a viable pregnancy. On the other hand, if ultrasonography incorrectly predicts a normal outcome, no intervention ensues from the diagnostic error.

Two sonographic criteria have high specificity: a gestation sac at least 25 mm mean diameter without an embryo, and distorted sac shape. On the other hand, the sensitivity of these criteria appears low. Repeating the ultrasonography examination improves the diagnostic accuracy of this procedure. Fetal heart motion is more accurate in predicting spontaneous abortion than are morphologic criteria. Several reports concur that once fetal cardiac activity is documented by ultrasonography in the first 12 weeks of pregnancy, the likelihood of spontaneous abortion is low, about 2%.

Increasing use of vaginal ultrasound has improved diagnostic validity, especially at early gestational ages. When an embryo is visible, management is straightforward. Regrettably, most abnormal pregnancies stop developing before an embryo is visible by sonography. If an embryo has a crown–rump length of more than 5 mm on vaginal sonography (or more than 10 mm on transabdominal sonography) but no heart activity, the pregnancy is not viable. Given the lack of medical need for intervention in early pregnancy failure, physicians should not act on a single abnormal clinical finding, such as a falling β-hCG level or failure to observe fetal cardiac activity.

Medical or Surgical Intervention

For women with inevitable abortion (characterized by progressive cervical dilation without expulsion of products of conception) and for those with threatened abortion in whom the pregnancy has been judged nonviable, several options are available. Patient preferences should generally determine the management. One option is to await spontaneous expulsion of the pregnancy. A randomized, controlled trial by Nielson and Hahlin compared expectant versus surgical management of spontaneous abortion. Most women randomized to expectant management (79%) had completed abortions within 3 days; other outcomes were similar, except for more infections in the group having curettage. Another option is to expedite the expulsion by giving oral or vaginal misoprostol. A randomized controlled trial by Chung et al. found that this medical management was safer than surgical evacuation, although half of those receiving misoprostol subsequently required suction curettage. However, many women faced with the disappointing diagnosis of a failed pregnancy prefer prompt surgical evacuation. Unless concurrent problems such as uterine infection or anemia exist, evacuation of the uterus can be handled like an elective abortion (described later). In summary, no evidence supports the necessity or advantage of routine suction curettage for spontaneous abortion.

However, if suction curettage is elected, then two other decisions must be made: where the curettage is to occur and by what technique. The choice between outpatient curettage in the physician's office or curettage in an emergency room may depend on the time of day and available equipment. For uncomplicated cases, curettage in an operating room adds to the costs, inconvenience, and emotional burden yet offers no medical benefits over outpatient curettage. The choice of evacuation technique depends on the state of the cervix, gestational age, and availability of equipment. Suction curettage is both faster and safer than sharp curettage; sharp curettage for spontaneous abortion is suboptimal management. A flexible Karman cannula with syringe as a source of suction is portable, inexpensive, and convenient for outpatient use.

Distinguishing between incomplete and complete abortion is frequently difficult. The woman's description of tissue may not be helpful, and not all women are aware that they should save expelled tissue for the physician's inspection. Likewise, dilation of the cervix, size of the uterus, and presence or absence of bleeding may not indicate whether the abortion is complete or incomplete. Ultrasonography, however, may provide information about the completeness of abortion.

Spontaneous abortion is a potentially sensitizing event for Rh-negative women at risk. Rates of use of Rh immunoglobulin (RhIG) after spontaneous abortion are significantly lower than after induced abortion. RhIG candidates at 12 weeks' gestation or earlier should receive a 50-μg dose; later abortions mandate a 300-μg dose. A Cochrane systematic review found the evidence insufficient to evaluate the potential benefit of prophylactic antibiotics after spontaneous abortion.

The profound grief that frequently accompanies spontaneous abortion often receives insufficient attention. Women and, to a lesser extent, men experience the usual stages of grief. Guilt may be the most difficult stage to resolve without help, and counseling plays an important role.

Complications

Attentive gynecologic care has reduced the risk of complications. Nevertheless, women continue to die from spontaneous abortions. The Centers for Disease Control and Prevention identified 62 maternal deaths from spontaneous abortion in the United States between 1981 and 1991. This represented a case-fatality rate of 0.7 deaths per 100,000 spontaneous abortions. Infection, hemorrhage, and embolism were the leading causes of death. The mortality risk increased with gestational age; women who were older and of minority races also were at increased risk of death.

FETAL DEATH

Definitions

Physicians categorize fetal death by gestational age and length of retention of the dead fetus. Death before the twentieth week of gestation is *spontaneous abortion;*

thereafter, *antepartum fetal death*. If the dead fetus remains in the uterus for 8 or more weeks (or a prolonged period), then the term becomes *missed abortion*. However, many misuse this term to refer to any failed pregnancy that is not promptly expelled.

The proliferation of terms related to fetal death is both unnecessary and confusing. For example, *fetal death in utero* is a tautology because the uterus is the only site where a fetus could die. These diagnostic categories all should be viewed as variations of a single obstetric entity: a *nonviable* or *failed pregnancy*.

Incidence

Fetal death is uncommon after the first trimester. The incidence of fetal death is about 10 per 1,000 live births, and about nine per 1,000 live births require hospitalization.

Management

Data on the natural history of fetal death are scarce. The uterus ejects most dead fetuses within 3 weeks of death. The gestational age, however, influences the probability of expulsion within a given interval: the more remote from term, the longer is the time required.

After confirmation of fetal death, the next—and perhaps most important—step is to counsel the parents (Fig. 21.1). Helping the couple to grieve appropriately can minimize psychological sequelae from this often devastating loss. After these two initial steps, subsequent clinical management is largely discretionary. The risk of coagulation defects within 5 weeks is minimal, as is the risk of infection, provided the membranes are intact. The emotional burden of carrying a dead fetus, however, often for weeks, can compound the misery experienced by the parents. Thus, although either watchful waiting or uterine evacuation are appropriate, most women seem to opt for intervention. Because there is no compelling medical indication for one course over the other, the woman should choose after counseling about the alternatives.

Before uterine evacuation, the physician should confirm that the woman's coagulation system is intact. Two approaches to evacuation exist: surgery or labor induction. The choice between surgery and labor induction should reflect the skill and experience of the physician, the size of the fetus and uterus, the availability of equipment and drugs, and the preference of the woman. Before dilation and evacuation (D&E), accurate determination of fetal size by ultrasonography is helpful.

Suction curettage is a safe and easy way to evacuate early pregnancies. If the pregnancy is more advanced and if the physician chooses not to perform a D&E procedure, then labor induction can be accomplished in several ways. These include use of misoprostol, vaginal prostaglandin E_2 suppositories, high-dose oxytocin, or intrauterine balloon catheters. Misoprostol and oxytocin are less noxious and less expensive than are prostaglandin suppositories. However, data are inadequate to establish the preferable means of medical management.

Intraamniotic hypertonic abortifacients are inappropriate in this setting of fetal death. For example, instillation of hypertonic saline may be hazardous because of rapid uptake into the woman's circulation owing to altered membrane permeability.

A suction or sharp curet check of the uterine cavity to confirm complete evacuation may be advisable after any of these evacuation techniques, although evidence is limited. As with all pregnancy terminations, physicians must identify all RhIG candidates and give them an appropriate dose of RhIG.

Complications

Fetal death carries risks of both morbidity and mortality for the woman. The risks of coagulation disorders and infection have received the most attention, yet recent data on their incidence are lacking. The risk of maternal death associated with fetal death is small, although no recent data are available. In the 1970s, the maternal case-fatality rate was estimated to be 4.5 deaths per 100,000 fetal deaths.

The risk of maternal death from fetal death increases with maternal age. The risk for women age 35 years and older was 3.6 times that for women age 15 to 24 years. The most frequent causes of maternal death from fetal death were uterine perforation and coagulopathy.

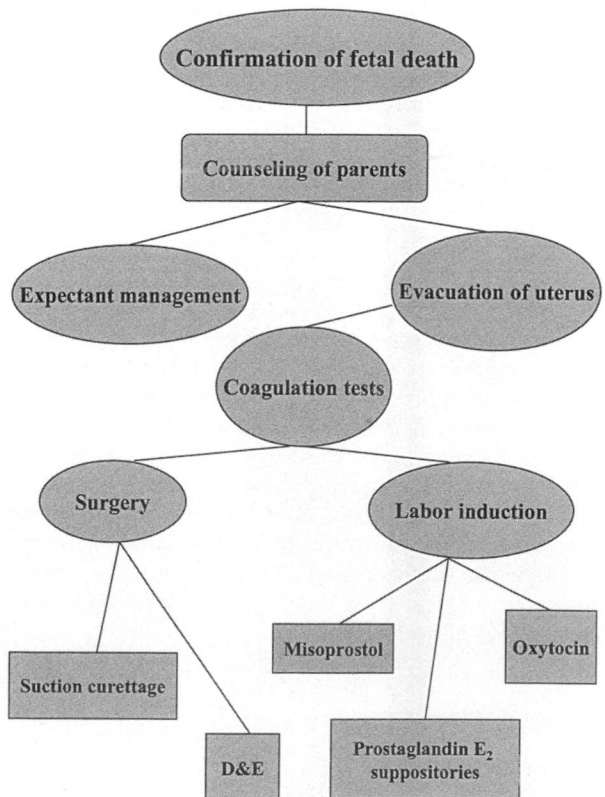

FIGURE 21.1. Algorithm for managing fetal death.

CERVICAL INCOMPETENCE

Incidence

Cervical incompetence is a nebulous and objectionable term used to explain spontaneous abortions thought to be owing to cervical factors. The term itself is derogatory: Women who receive this diagnosis may feel that they are unfit or incompetent as mothers and as women. Hence, we should purge the term from obstetric terminology. *Premature cervical dilation without labor* is both more descriptive and less pejorative to women.

Equally unfortunate is the disagreement about the case definition and diagnostic criteria. Many reported cases of premature cervical dilation without labor are inconsistent with the classic picture: repetitive, acute, painless abortion in midpregnancy without associated bleeding or uterine contractions. Some physicians base their diagnoses on asymptomatic cervical dilation observed in midpregnancy, whereas others rely on tests of unknown validity performed on nonpregnant women. These include passage of an 8-mm Hegar dilator, traction on an intrauterine Foley catheter, or hysterography. Some have used ultrasonography to diagnose premature cervical dilation without labor. This technique appears to have poor validity.

Moreover, the correlation between anatomic measurements and function of the cervix in pregnancy is unknown, and no valid diagnostic test of cervical incompetence exists. The history of unexplained spontaneous abortion in midpregnancy may be the most useful diagnostic criterion, yet its sensitivity and specificity remain unknown. This diagnostic imprecision appears in reported incidence rates. Rates range from 0.05 to one per 100 pregnancies. Differences in diagnosis, rather than differences in women, probably account for most of this variation.

Risk Factors

The cause of premature cervical dilation without labor is unknown but may be multifactorial. Early theories about this problem focused on cervical trauma, such as conization, laceration, or excessive mechanical dilation. Data are lacking, however, to confirm or refute these hypothetical risk factors. The occurrence of this condition in primigravidas suggests alternative causes. These may include associated uterine anomalies, prenatal exposure to diethylstilbestrol, or abnormal histology of the cervix. In addition, premature cervical dilation without labor may be inheritable.

Premature cervical dilation without labor may reflect asynchrony between the uterine corpus and cervix. In normal pregnancy and delivery, biochemical and biophysical changes in the cervix in late pregnancy allow cervical dilation and effacement to occur synchronously with labor contractions. At one extreme of asynchrony, the corpus contracts, yet cervical dilation and effacement do not occur; this may account for cervicovaginal fistulae during instillation abortions with older abortifacients, such as intraamniotic prostaglandin $F_{2\alpha}$ ($PGF_{2\alpha}$). At the other extreme, progressive dilation and effacement occur prematurely and without perceptible contractions. The underlying pathophysiology for many cases may be biochemical; that tying a noose around the cervix is the best available treatment suggests how limited is our understanding of the problem.

Management

Three serious problems in published studies prohibit conclusions about the treatment of choice. First, without a precise and reproducible definition of premature cervical dilation without labor, comparison of success rates in published reports is impossible.

Second, some of the benefit attributed to cerclage operations may not be owing to the operation itself but rather to a phenomenon termed *regression to the mean*. A variable (e.g., pregnancy outcome) that is extreme or unusual when first measured (e.g., fetal expulsion at 20 weeks' gestation) tends to be nearer the mean of the population distribution at a subsequent observation (e.g., another pregnancy). Although methods exist for estimating the effect of this phenomenon in studies without comparison groups, only one study of cerclage has even considered this problem.

Third, new operations frequently are adopted into clinical practice without appropriate evidence of their efficacy. In the largest randomized controlled trial, performed in the United Kingdom, the policy of early cerclage had an important benefit for one in 25 women treated. On the other hand, this policy was associated with increased medical intervention and a doubling in the incidence of postpartum fever. Overall, the trial suggested that early cervical cerclage is appropriate for women at high risk, such as those with three prior pregnancy losses.

A variety of approaches have been used to treat premature cervical dilation without labor. Among the more innocuous, bed rest has been suggested as primary therapy, as well as adjunctive therapy after cerclage. This may be a reasonable approach in terms of hydraulics, although data concerning efficacy are lacking, as is true for most obstetrical uses of bed rest.

A Smith-Hodge pessary can displace the cervix in a posterior direction. Although this approach has received little attention in the United States, it has the appeal of exerting a mechanical effect without requiring an operation.

Surgery is the principal form of therapy for premature cervical dilation without labor in the United States. Two strategies have been used: primary repair of an anatomic defect and reinforcement of the cervix with a circumferential suture. The repair approach, the Lash procedure, is appropriate only for nonpregnant women who have a demonstrable anatomic defect of the cervix. Moreover, the suggestion of diminished fertility after this operation is worrisome. Hence, the Lash procedure is rarely used.

Several types of cerclage procedures are used; the McDonald and Shirodkar are the most common. Contraindications to cerclage include rupture of membranes, uterine bleeding, uterine contractions, chorioamnionitis, cervical dilation of more than 4 cm, polyhydramnios, or known fetal anomaly.

The McDonald procedure places a reinforcing purse-string suture around the proximal cervix. Unlike the Shirodkar procedure, however, the McDonald suture is not buried entirely (Fig. 21.2). Instead, several deep penetrations into the cervical stroma are made with a nonabsorbable suture, such as Mersilene. The advantages of this approach compared with the Shirodkar procedure are simplicity, ease of removal, and usefulness when the cervix is effaced or when fetal membranes are bulging. A notable disadvantage is the vaginal discharge associated with the exposed suture material. Because the McDonald and Shirodkar procedures have been reported to have similar efficacy, the simplicity and versatility of the McDonald operation make it preferable for most patients in need of cerclage.

The Shirodkar operation places a reinforcing band around the cervix beneath the mucosa at the level of the internal os (Figs. 21.3 and 21.4). Spinal or epidural anesthesia is recommended; the Trendelenburg position and adequate retraction facilitate placement of the suture. The original operation used aneurysm needles to place a band of fascia lata around the cervix; then the knot was tied anteriorly. In recent years, many physicians have used a wide (e.g., 5-mm) Mersilene band swaged onto large atraumatic needles, with the knot tied posteriorly to avoid erosion into the bladder. The cervical canal

should remain open 3 to 5 mm. After the band is tied, the band and knot can be secured with several interrupted sutures of silk or other permanent material; the incisions in the mucosa are then closed with absorbable suture, thus burying the band.

Opinions are divided as to whether the cerclage procedure is best performed during or between pregnancies. Most studies suggest that the timing of cerclage during pregnancy influences outcome. Cerclage at about 14 weeks' gestation appears preferable. If substantial dilation or bulging of fetal membranes has occurred, then the likelihood of a successful cerclage is lessened. An attempt can be made, however, to replace the protruding forewaters by means of a sterile Foley catheter. Thereafter, the suture is placed and tied down, and the Foley balloon is deflated and withdrawn.

Postoperative care after cerclage for pregnant women has not been uniform. Although most investigators advise bed rest for several days, and some advocate prophylactic antibiotics, tocolytic drugs, or progesterone, the usefulness of these measures has not been established. The cerclage suture can be removed at 38 weeks' gestation or when fetal pulmonary maturity has been confirmed; it should be removed immediately if membranes rupture or labor starts. Although some physicians leave a well-placed Shirodkar suture in place and deliver infants by Caesarean, evidence supporting this course of action is limited.

Intraabdominal cerclage may be appropriate in rare instances. Indications include traumatic cervical lacera-

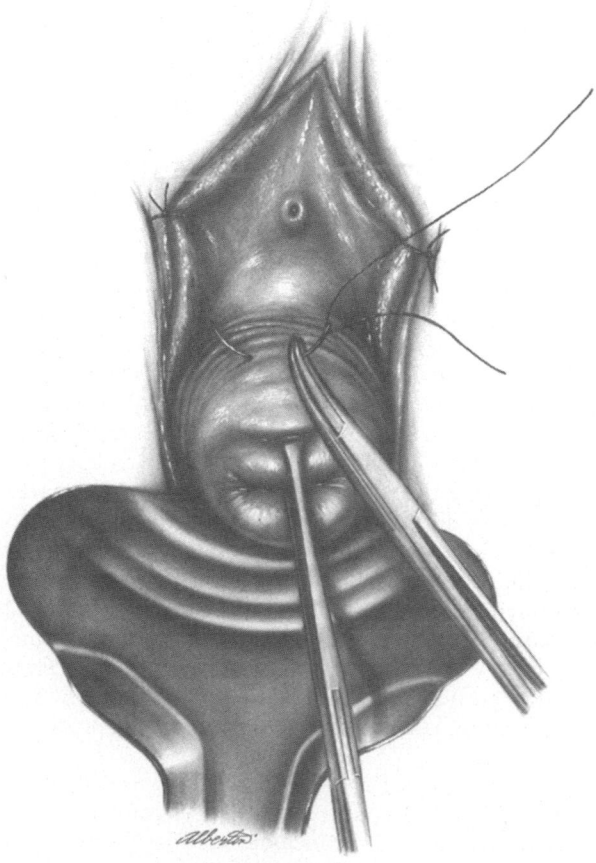

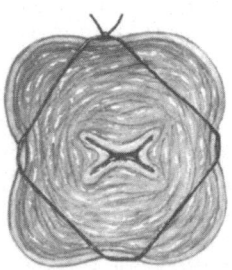

FIGURE 21.2. McDonald cerclage operation. **A:** Four bites taken at the junction of vaginal mucosa and cervix. **B:** A cross section of the cervix with the cerclage in place.

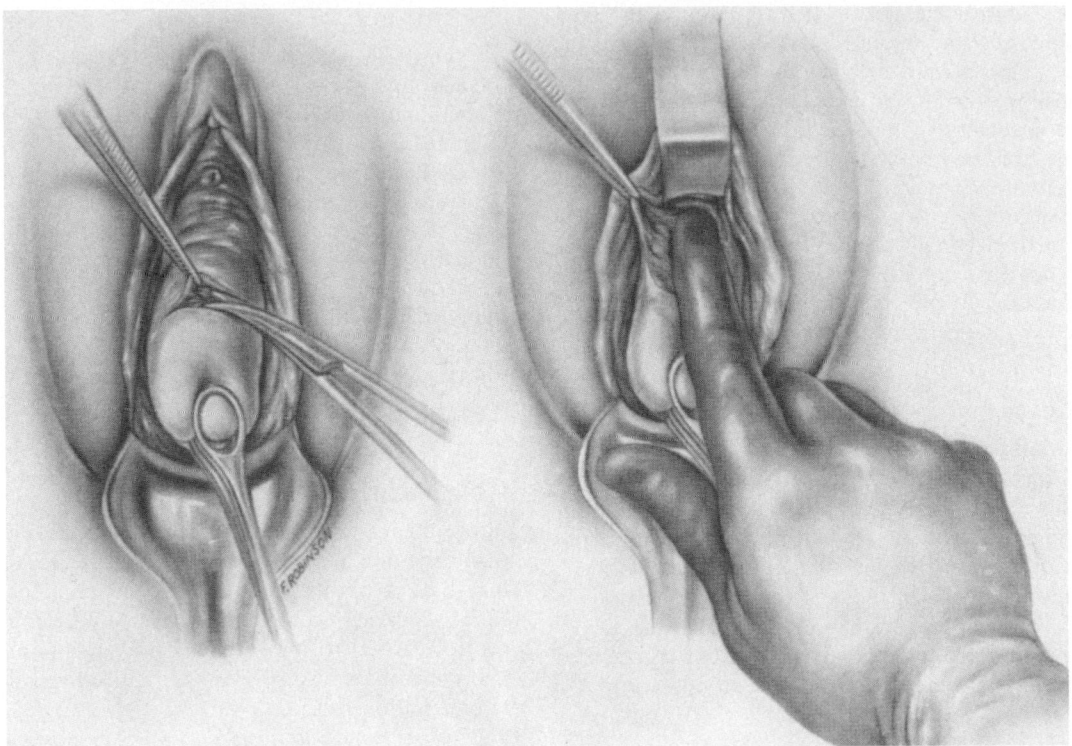

FIGURE 21.3. Shirodkar cerclage operation. **Left:** A transverse incision through the anterior vaginal mucosa at its junction with the cervix. **Right:** The surgeon pushes the bladder cephalad to enable high placement of the suture.

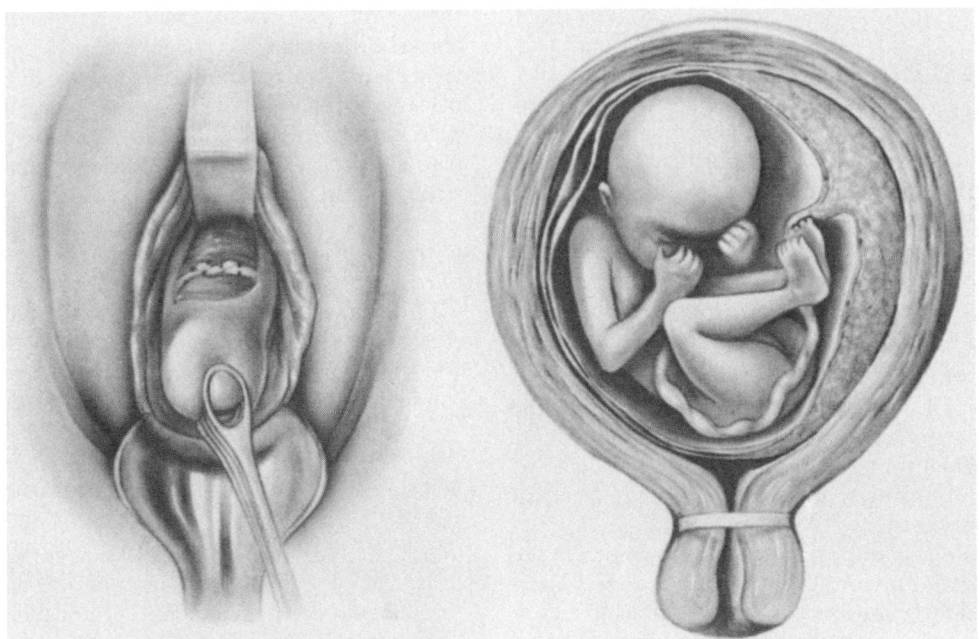

FIGURE 21.4. Shirodkar cerclage operation. **Left:** The encircling suture leaves the cervix with an opening of 3 to 5 mm. The surgeon anchors the suture anteriorly with fine silk. **Right:** Cross section with suture in place.

tion, congenital shortening of the cervix, previous failed vaginal cerclage, and advanced cervical effacement. This procedure places a band around the cervix at the level of the internal os in an avascular space between the branches of the uterine artery. Compared with the vaginal cerclage operations, this procedure has several important disadvantages: two abdominal operations are needed (one to place the suture, one for Caesarean delivery), the surgery is performed in a highly vascular area adjacent to the ureters, and the complication rate is higher than with vaginal cerclage. Hence, this approach should be used only when vaginal cerclage has failed or is not feasible.

Complications

Complications of cerclage range from annoying to fatal. A partial inventory of reported complications includes hemorrhage; rupture of membranes; infection, including chorioamnionitis, abscess, and death; cervical dystocia; uterine rupture; vesicovaginal fistula; and fetal death. Although the incidence of most of these complications is unknown, one report documented rates of chorioamnionitis ranging from 15 to 39 per 100 patients, depending on gestational age at the time of operation.

ILLEGAL ABORTION
Incidence

Despite the availability of legal abortions, small numbers of illegal procedures continue to occur. Estimates of the incidence of illegal abortion in the United States before 1970 ranged from 200,000 to 1.2 million per year; estimates for the late 1970s ranged from 5,000 to 23,000 per year. More recent estimates are not available. However, illegal abortions occur in large numbers in developing countries, where, according to World Health Organization estimates, 50,000 to 100,000 women die of illegal abortion complications each year.

Risk Factors

Lack of access to safe, legal abortion is the most important risk factor in the world today. After liberalization of restrictive abortion laws in the United States, septic abortion wards in municipal hospitals emptied, then closed. The reverse phenomenon was seen in Romania when the government restricted access to abortion and contraception: the maternal mortality ratio rose to the highest in Europe, as women resorted to unsafe abortions again. When the Romanian dictator Ceaucescu was deposed and abortion access again provided, maternal mortality plummeted.

Little is known about characteristics of women in the United States who obtain illegal abortions. Some inferences can be drawn, however, from the characteristics of 17 women who died from illegal abortion in the United States from 1975 to 1979. These women were older, of higher parity, and more likely to be black or Hispanic than were women who died from legal abortion during these years. Slightly more than half lived in the South.

Techniques

Although a wide variety of illegal abortion methods are used around the world, two methods dominate in the United States: oral abortifacients and intrauterine instrumentation. The most frequently used method in New York City in the 1960s was orally administered substances, including turpentine, laundry bleach, and large doses of quinine. The misconception that quinine is a safe and effective oral abortifacient persists. Intrauterine techniques were less common; these ranged from intrauterine injection of soap or phenol disinfectants to insertion of foreign objects. As reported by the women surveyed, intrauterine techniques successfully aborted pregnancy much more often than did oral substances.

Complications

Although intrauterine techniques have greater efficacy than early oral abortifacients, the intrauterine techniques may have a higher risk of complications. In countries such as Brazil, recent black-market availability of misoprostol has led to important improvements in abortion safety, because misoprostol has reduced reliance on instrumentation of the cervix.

Transcervical administration of toxic substances carries a high risk of serious complications. Other important variables influencing the likelihood of morbidity include the skill of the provider, gestational age, and availability of gynecologic care. The most frequently reported complication of illegal abortion is retained products of conception, although the incidence of such complications is unknown.

The number of illegal abortion deaths in the United States declined dramatically during the 1970s. During the 1975 to 1979 interval, women in both extremes of the reproductive age span had higher death rates from illegal abortion than did other women. The racial discrepancy in death rate is more striking: the mortality rate for black and Hispanic women is more than 10 times greater than for white women.

As with morbidity, the likelihood of mortality is strongly related to the abortion technique. Of the 17 illegal abortion deaths from 1975 to 1979, only one followed ingestion of an abortifacient (pennyroyal oil). The other deaths were related to intrauterine techniques, ranging from injection of cleaning solutions to insertion of foreign bodies (e.g., catheters, cotton swabs, thermometers, and coat hangers). Sepsis (10 cases) and air embolism (three cases) accounted for most of these deaths.

Management of Septic Abortion

Most women with septic abortion respond rapidly to uterine evacuation plus broad-spectrum antibiotics. Before beginning treatment, intrauterine and blood cultures should be obtained. An upright radiograph of the abdomen may identify a residual foreign body, gas bubbles in the uterus, or free air under the diaphragm; these findings change management.

Antibiotic administration should begin in the emergency department. Coverage should include Gram-positive, Gram-negative, and anaerobic bacteria. If the woman's condition is stable, then she can go directly from the emergency department to the operating room. Peak serum levels of antibiotics will be present within an hour of their administration. Further delay of uterine evacuation is unwarranted and can compromise recovery. Prompt elimination of the necrotic infected tissue is critical. Tissue obtained during curettage should quickly go for microbiologic cultures. The yield of organisms, especially anaerobes, is often higher from a tissue specimen than from a swab inserted into the uterus.

Subsequent management is governed by the response of the woman and by microbiologic findings. All women with septic abortions should be closely observed after surgery, with special attention to vital signs and urine output, to detect incipient shock. Prompt aggressive therapy is essential if septic shock develops. Administration of glucocorticoids is not helpful in this setting.

Postabortal sepsis from *Clostridium perfringens* has become rare. When this infection occurs, however, it can be catastrophic. In the absence of hemolysis, *C. perfringens* bacteremia can be managed by curettage and antibiotics. In the presence of hemolysis, hysterectomy and more aggressive medical therapy are indicated.

LEGAL ABORTION

Incidence

Legal abortion is one of the most frequently performed operations in the United States. In 1997, 1.2 million induced abortions were reported to the Centers for Disease Control and Prevention. The national abortion ratio was 306 abortions per 1,000 live births in that year. The abortion rate was 20 abortions per 1,000 women age 15 to 44 years. Stated alternatively, about one in four recognized pregnancies ends in induced abortion, and each year, 2% of all women of reproductive age in the United States have an abortion. The numbers of induced abortions performed in the United States declined steadily from 1990 to 1997, the most recent year for which data are available.

Demographic Characteristics

Women who have induced abortions in the United States tend to be young, white, single, and of low parity. Most (55%) abortions took place at 8 weeks' gestation or earlier; 88% occurred at 12 weeks' gestation or earlier. Nearly all abortions (99%) involved curettage, although FDA approval of mifepristone for medical abortion will likely change this pattern.

Techniques

All methods of abortion fall into two broad categories: surgical and medical. Surgical evacuation includes suction curettage (vacuum aspiration), sharp curettage, D&E (defined as transcervical evacuation at 13 menstrual weeks' gestation or later), hysterotomy, and hysterectomy. Medical abortifacients in the United States include uterotonic drugs, such as prostaglandins and oxytocin; the antiprogestin mifepristone; and intrauterine instillation of hypertonic agents, such as saline or urea. In addition, several adjuncts, such as cervical preparation with misoprostol or osmotic dilators, have an important role in abortion practice. This section reviews the principal methods of abortion in use; comprehensive descriptions of these techniques have been published recently in a comprehensive text by Paul et al.

Surgical Evacuation

Suction curettage is the most important and frequently used method of abortion in the United States. The preoperative evaluation should include counseling, informed consent, a brief history, and a limited physical examination. The history taking should focus on only relevant data, such as gynecologic problems (e.g., leiomyomas) or medical problems (e.g., cardiac valvular disease, asthma, or drug sensitivities) that might influence the conduct of the operation. Physical examination should include the heart, lungs, abdomen, and pelvis. Although ultrasonography is not warranted on a routine basis, it is useful if the size, shape, or position of the uterus are unclear.

Few laboratory tests are necessary. Determination of the hematocrit (or hemoglobin) and Rh type are appropriate. Many physicians perform a urine pregnancy test on all patients requesting abortion. Screening for chlamydial infection or gonorrhea should not be routine, but should be targeted.

Menstrual Regulation

Menstrual regulation, menstrual extraction, and *minisuction* are euphemisms for early suction curettage. This technique uses a flexible plastic cannula 4 to 6 mm in diameter, with a self-locking syringe as a source of suction (Fig. 21.5). The upper gestational age limit for this procedure ranges from 42 to 50 days from last menstrual period. Extensive literature has documented the simplicity and safety of the technique.

Menstrual regulation differs from traditional suction curettage in several ways. First, anesthesia may not be necessary, although analgesia can ease the cramping that occurs toward the end of the evacuation. Second, dilation is often unnecessary for menstrual regulation. If a given cannula does not slide into the uterus, the physician can use smaller flexible cannulas in the set as dilators. After insertion of the appropriate cannula, the physician attaches the syringe and releases the pinch valve to begin the suctioning. Blood and tissue flow into the syringe. Alternatively, some physicians connect the cannula to the syringe before insertion. The abortion involves rotary and in-and-out cannula movement until the gritty feel of the endometrium occurs. Bubbles appear in the syringe. The physician should not remove the cannula from the uterus while a vacuum exists in the syringe, because the endocervical canal should not be aspirated; likewise, the physician must never advance the plunger of the syringe while the cannula is connected and is within the uterus. Air embolism can result. The syringe and cannula are disposable, although some physi-

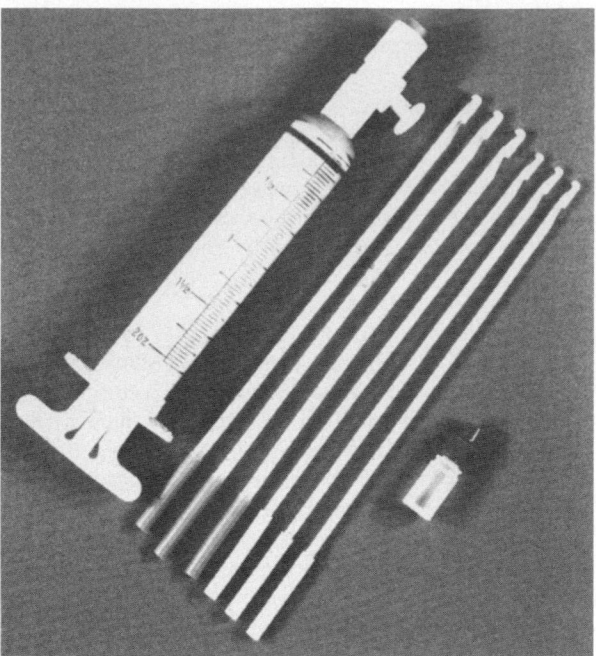

FIGURE 21.5. Karman cannulas, self-locking syringe with pinch valve, and bottle of silicone lubricant. (From: IPAS, Chapel Hill, NC, with permission.)

cians clean and disinfect the syringe and use it multiple times.

Some physicians have begun to offer suction curettage with a 7-mm rigid cannula at less than 6 weeks' gestation. In addition to routine tissue inspection, the protocol used by Edwards and Carson uses vaginal ultrasonography before and immediately after the aspiration. While early clinical experience has been encouraging, further formal study of this approach is needed.

Suction Curettage

Suction curettage involves dilation of the cervix followed by vacuum aspiration at 12 weeks' gestation or earlier. Sharp curettage, which is slower and less safe, is analogous to diagnostic dilation and curettage. Sharp curettage is obsolete as an abortion method.

Preparing the patient for surgery is simple. Some physicians ask the woman to avoid oral intake on the day of surgery, while others allow light meals before local anesthesia. The patient should bring someone with her to the facility to take her home. She should empty her bladder before being placed in the dorsal lithotomy position; catheterization is unnecessary. Most physicians wash the vagina with a povidone-iodine or chlorhexidine solution, although the benefit of this practice is uncertain. Likewise, routine sterile precautions (e.g., drapes, caps, masks, and gowns) are unnecessary. The physician should use a "no-touch" technique: He or she wears sterile gloves and does not touch those portions of the sterile instruments inserted into the uterus. Either local or general anesthesia is appropriate; use of local anesthesia predominates in the United States. Although local

anesthesia does not completely relieve discomfort, it is less expensive and safer than general anesthesia.

To perform a paracervical block safely, the physician should use the smallest volume of the lowest concentration of local anesthetic. Local anesthetics vary in their toxicity; for example, chloroprocaine is substantially less toxic than lidocaine, although lidocaine is less expensive. With lidocaine, a 0.5% concentration is safer than a 1% solution and is equally effective. The total dose of lidocaine should not exceed 2 mg/lb (lean weight) or 300 mg, whichever is less. Alternatively, use of local anesthesia with vasoconstrictor (e.g., epinephrine 1:200,000) slows systemic absorption of anesthetic and allows a larger total dose, although many women find the epinephrine unpleasant. Some physicians buffer the lidocaine solution with sodium bicarbonate to make it less irritating.

The site of injection of paracervical anesthesia appears to matter little; injection at almost any site next to the cervix results in excellent anesthesia. Common regimens include infiltration of the cervix at the 12-o'clock position (for application of the tenaculum), then injection at four sites (at the 3-, 5-, 7-, and 9-o'clock positions) or two sites (at the 3- and 9-o'clock positions) at the junction of cervix and vagina. Submucosal injection precludes inadvertent intravascular injection.

The physician can minimize the pain of inserting the needle by placing the tip of a 21-gauge spinal needle against the mucosa and having the woman cough, while the needle is held still. The Valsalva maneuver "pops" the vaginal epithelium over the needle point, frequently without any sensation of pain. This technique seems to work better at the 3- and 9-o'clock positions than at the 5- and 7-o'clock positions. Slow injection is less painful than rapid injection.

Suction curettage requires few instruments. Most physicians prefer to use a bivalve speculum. A speculum with standard-length blades, however, prevents the cervix from being drawn toward the introitus during the procedure and makes the operation more difficult. The commercially available Moore modification of the Graves speculum, which has 1-inch shorter blades of standard width, is excellent. Some physicians prefer an atraumatic tenaculum. Alternatively, having an extra single-toothed tenaculum can sometimes be helpful. If difficulty during dilation occurs, then the physician can place the second tenaculum on the posterior cervix to stabilize it. Sounding the uterus provides no important information for routine abortions and may perforate the uterus. For this reason, many experienced physicians have abandoned its use for abortion.

If the direction of the cervical canal is in question, then the physician can gently probe with a small dilator. Pratt dilators are preferable to Hegar dilators for abortion because they require less force to dilate the cervix. A useful modification of the Pratt dilators is the Denniston dilator; this is similar to the Pratt dilator but is plastic. Hence, it is light, slightly flexible, and inexpensive, yet it is capable of being autoclaved. Other instruments required for suction curettage include the vacuum machine, hose, swivel handle, and a cannula. Some physicians use a sharp curette to check for completeness at the end of the operation, although use of small (e.g., 8-mm-diameter) Karman-type double-port cannulas provides the same gritty sensation as a metal curette.

Traction on the cervix is important during suction curettage; it both stabilizes the uterus and straightens the angle between cervix and corpus, which should reduce the risk of perforation. The tenaculum should have a firm purchase on the cervix. High vertical placement at the 12-o'clock position, with one tooth in the canal and one on the anterior cervix, almost eliminates the risk of the tenaculum tearing through during dilation. In contrast, a superficial horizontal application of the tenaculum is more likely to allow the tenaculum to pull off. If the uterus is retroverted, some physicians prefer to place the tenaculum on the cervix at the 6-o'clock position (Fig. 21.6). If the puncture site on the cervix bleeds after tenaculum removal, direct pressure for a brief time stops the bleeding. Application of silver nitrate or Monsel's solution should not be done.

Gentleness is the key to safe cervical dilation. Dilation should allow insertion and rotation of the desired cannula. Pratt dilators are measured in French units, or mm of circumference. Hence, to determine the diameter, the physician needs to divide by π, or approximately three. For example, to insert an 8-mm cannula, dilation to 25F allows free rotation. The physician should hold the dilator between the thumb and index finger to limit the force applied. In addition, the other fingers can remain extended to prevent plunging forward in case of sudden loss of resistance. Dilation need not start with the smallest dilator on the set; starting with a larger size (e.g., 15F instead of 13F) may reduce the risk of perforating the uterus or creating a false channel.

If more than two fingers of force is necessary during dilation, the physician should stop and reassess the situation, rather than risk injuring the cervix. One option is to use a smaller cannula than originally planned. Alternatively, the physician can pack the cervix with one or more osmotic dilators, interrupt the procedure, then complete the operation several hours later, by which time adequate dilation will have been achieved. Another treatment option is to administer oral or vaginal misoprostol and complete the procedure in several hours. Performance of the procedure in two stages is far preferable to forceful dilation.

Osmotic dilators help to prepare the cervix for curettage abortions (Fig. 21.7). Laminaria are hygroscopic sticks of seaweed that dilate the cervix over several hours. The mode of action is not well understood, but the principal mechanism appears to be desiccation of the cervix. This drying can alter the ratio of collagen to ground substance, thus changing collagen cross-linkages. Alternatively, laminaria can alter the elaboration, release, or degradation of uterine prostaglandins. Laminaria cause the cervix to dilate the areas not in physical contact with the laminaria; whatever the mechanism, it is more complex than mere passive stretching, as used to be thought.

One synthetic osmotic dilator is currently marketed in the United States. Lamicel is a cylinder of polyvinyl alcohol sponge impregnated with magnesium sulfate. It works within several hours and has the advantage of uniform size (either 5 or 3 mm diameter), assured sterility, and easy insertion and removal. Unlike laminaria, the Lamicel device does not assume a rigid hourglass shape that hinders removal.

Osmotic dilators are convenient in an outpatient setting. Placement of laminaria or Lamicel for 3 to 4 hours

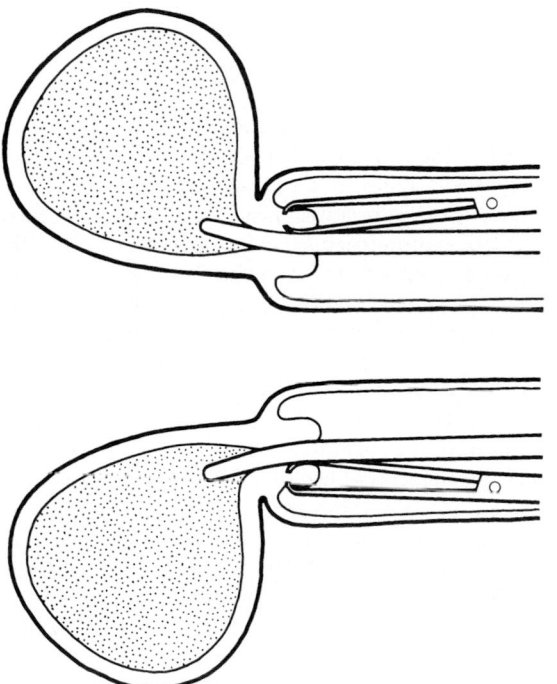

FIGURE 21.6. Traction on cervix during dilation. **(Top)** Tenaculum placed vertically on the anterior lip. **(Bottom)** Tenaculum placed vertically on the posterior lip for a retroverted uterus. Note posterior direction of dilator.

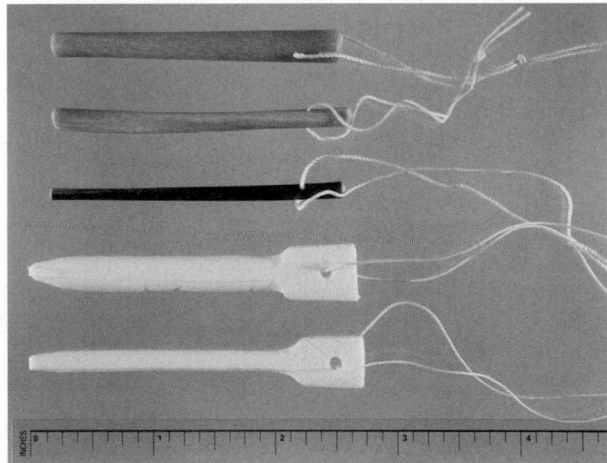

FIGURE 21.7. Osmotic dilators. **Top:** Laminaria of various sizes. **Bottom:** Lamicel in 5- and 3-mm sizes.

before abortion frequently dilates the cervix sufficiently for abortion. Compared with use of metal dilators, use of laminaria dramatically reduces the risk of cervical injury requiring suturing and of uterine perforation compared with use of metal dilators. This protection against trauma can be especially important for young teenagers with immature cervices who are at increased risk for cervical injury. Disadvantages include the cost, inconvenience, and occasional cramping involved.

Preoperative preparation of the cervix with misoprostol can facilitate abortion. Misoprostol, a prostaglandin E derivative, is safe, inexpensive, stable at room temperature, and effective in improving the Bishop score of the cervix. The drug can be given either orally or vaginally. In general, misoprostol is more effective and better tolerated when given by the vaginal route; this probably relates to different pharmacokinetics when absorbed through the vagina versus through the gut, as shown by Zieman et al. On the other hand, women often prefer oral to vaginal administration. When placed in the vagina by the physician at the end of the pelvic examination, most patients find this acceptable. A randomized controlled trial by Singh et al. suggests that misoprostol 400 μg per vagina 3 to 4 hours before the operation may be the optimal dose. Afterwards, the cervix is often dilated sufficiently to operate without further dilation. Disadvantages of cervical preparation with misoprostol include the delay required, spotting and cramping, and occasional abortion in the waiting room.

After adequate dilation, the physician inserts the cannula. In general, the diameter of the cannula in millimeters should be about one less than the weeks of gestation from last menses. For example, an 8-mm cannula is adequate for evacuating a pregnancy of 9 weeks' gestation. Skilled physicians often prefer to use even smaller cannulas than this guideline suggests; the physician must weigh the advantage of needing less dilation against the potential disadvantages of longer operating time and an increased risk of incomplete abortion.

The most frequently used cannulas in the United States are clear plastic, with a slight angulation (Fig. 21.8). The physician should insert the cannula into the lower uterine segment. The physician then turns on the suction machine and aspirates the uterus with the can-

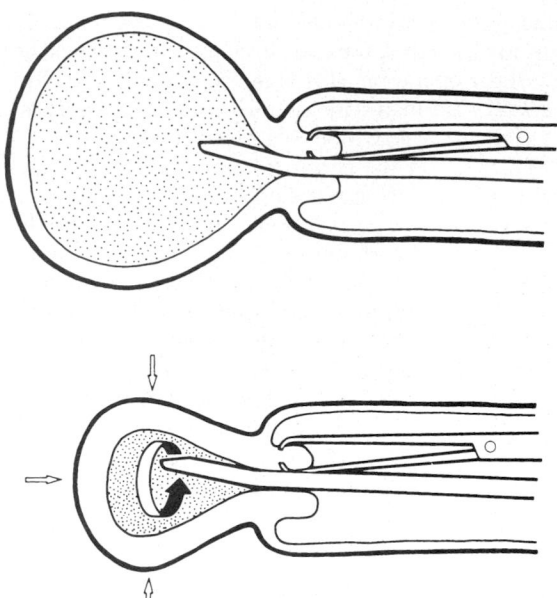

FIGURE 21.9. Uterine aspiration. **(Top)** Cannula inserted just beyond internal os. **(Bottom)** Aspiration with rotating motion.

nula (Fig. 21.9). When bubbles appear in the cannula and the interior of the cavity feels empty, some physicians use a sharp curette to confirm the completeness of evacuation. The flexible plastic cannula in Fig. 21.8 suctions opposite sides of the cavity simultaneously and provides a distinct gritty sensation when the evacuation is complete. While no contemporary studies have compared rigid versus flexible cannulas, the flexible cannulas may be more efficient and seem to provide better tactile sensation.

The operation is not finished until the physician or another trained observer has examined the aspirated tissue. This is to confirm the presence of fetal tissue, which usually excludes the possibility of an ectopic pregnancy. Since 1972, more than 20 women in the United States have died from ectopic pregnancies undetected at the time of attempted suction curettage. This tissue inspection will not detect the rare twin ectopic pregnancy, commonly (and incorrectly) termed "heterotopic."

Pregnancies of 9 weeks' gestation and later will have recognizable fetal parts; earlier pregnancies may not. Identification of chorionic villi and membranes in these earlier pregnancies is essential. The physician rinses the aspirated tissue in a fine-mesh kitchen strainer under tap water to remove blood and clots. A glass baking dish or a plastic basin is useful for examining the tissue suspended in water. For early pregnancies, white vinegar (instead of water) may facilitate the recognition of villi. Back lighting from a horizontal x-ray viewing box is especially useful (Fig. 21.10). Villi appear soft, fluffy, and feathery, with discernible finger-like projections; in contrast, decidua appears coarse and shaggy (Fig. 21.11). Amnion and chorion are filmy and transparent; decidua is translucent. With early pregnancies, a magnifying

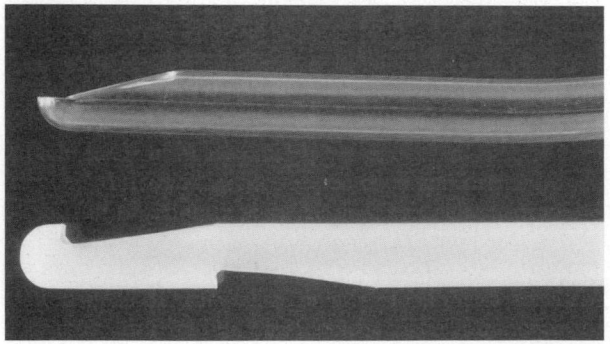

FIGURE 21.8. Distal ends of rigid curved 8-mm cannula and flexible 8-mm cannula with twin whistle-tip ports.

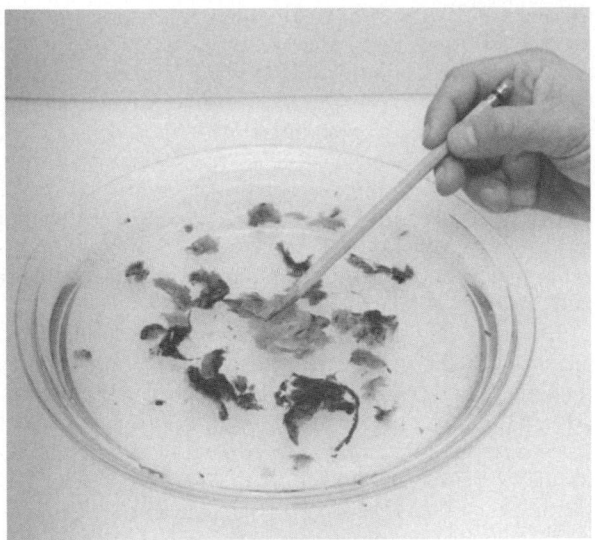

FIGURE 21.10. Examination of aspirated tissue over x-ray viewing box for back lighting.

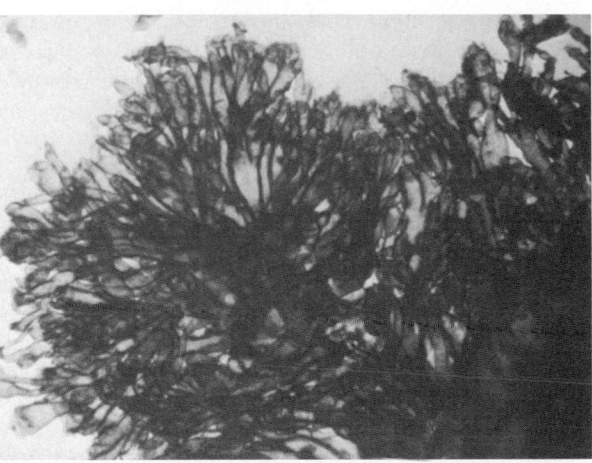

FIGURE 21.12. Wet-mount microscopic appearance of placental villi. (From: Munsick RA. Clinical test for placenta in 300 consecutive menstrual aspirations. *Obstet Gynecol* 1982;60:738, with permission.)

glass, dissecting microscope, colposcope, or standard microscope ($\times 100$) can help identify villi (Fig. 21.12).

When the physician cannot confirm fetal tissue, he or she should reevaluate the patient, with special attention to the adnexa. Repeat aspiration is often appropriate. A sensitive urine pregnancy test or a quantitative β-hCG can be helpful. Ultrasound can sometimes identify a gestational sac. Failure to identify villi in the presence of a positive pregnancy test suggests several possibilities: recent spontaneous abortion, failed attempted abortion, perforation with aspiration outside the uterus, or ectopic pregnancy. The physician must carefully evaluate these possibilities.

Women with uterine anomalies, such as a bicornuate uterus, have a high risk of failed attempted abortion. One useful approach is to perform the aspiration under ultrasound guidance. If the physician can insert a bent

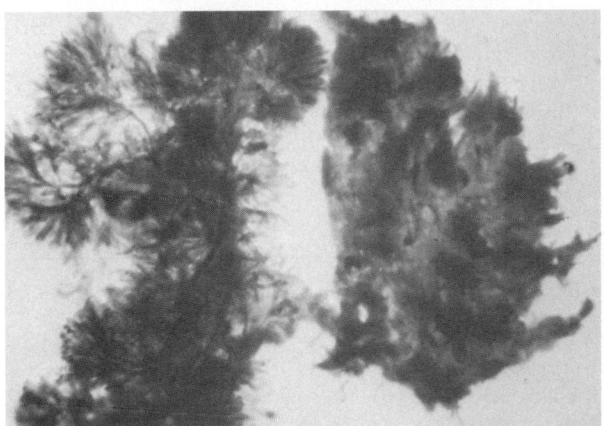

FIGURE 21.11. Left: Typical fluffy villi of placenta. **Right:** Shaggy decidua. (From: Munsick RA. Clinical test for placenta in 300 consecutive menstrual aspirations. *Obstet Gynecol* 1982;60:738, with permission.)

sound into the cavity with the pregnancy, he or she can then place the bent sound inside a flexible 8-mm plastic cannula as a stent or guide. With ultrasound guidance, the physician then inserts the cannula into the cavity and removes the sound, connects the cannula adapter, and then aspirates the cavity. Another alternative is to use medical abortion. Rarely, hysterotomy may be needed if curettage and medical abortion fail in the setting of müllerian anomalies.

Use of Oxytocic Agents

The usefulness of administering oxytocic agents during suction curettage is unclear, although administering oxytocin or ergot derivatives reduces blood loss from suction curettage performed under general anesthesia. Although statistically significant, the reduction in blood loss is clinically unimportant. Because blood loss is less with local anesthesia, oxytocic agents probably are not necessary. Although physicians commonly give ergot derivatives by mouth for several days after suction curettage, evidence of the benefit of this practice is lacking, and the drugs cause painful uterine cramping in some women.

Prophylactic Antibiotics

Induced abortion patients should receive prophylactic antibiotics. A metaanalysis of the randomized, controlled trials on this topic by Sawaya et al. showed benefit for women deemed low- and high-risk for infection.

Administration of drugs such as doxycycline to anxious, fasting pregnant women before surgery can cause nausea and vomiting. Hence, the most practical approach may be to begin a short-course antibiotic with food promptly after the abortion. The choice of antibiotic and duration of therapy is unclear. However, if one administers antibiotics for more than 24 hours, prophylaxis ends and presumptive treatment of *C. trachomatis* begins. In high-risk populations, presumptive treatment of all patients for chlamydia may be a reasonable course of action.

Medical Abortion in Early Pregnancy

The marketing of the antiprogestin mifepristone has opened a new chapter in abortion practice. The regimen recommended by the distributor and approved by the FDA (for use up to 49 days' gestation) calls for a single oral dose of mifepristone 600 mg, followed in 48 hours by misoprostol 400 μg orally. Success rates with this regimen range from 92% to 97%.

However, several randomized, controlled trials have shown that a single oral dose of mifepristone 200 mg is as effective as 600 mg (and considerably less expensive); this is owing to the nonlinear pharmacokinetics of the drug. Increasing doses in this range do not translate into increasing blood levels or efficacy. Moreover, Schaff and others have challenged the practice of delaying the misoprostol administration. In a randomized, controlled trial in pregnancies up to 56 days' gestation, they found similar, high success rates (96% to 98%) with misoprostol 800 μg taken vaginally at home 1, 2, or 3 days after having received mifepristone 200 mg by mouth.

The National Abortion Federation protocols note that mifepristone 200 mg is equivalent to 600 mg when combined with misoprostol 400 μg orally in pregnancies up to 49 days. Regimens using misoprostol 800 μg vaginally have fewer gastrointestinal side effects and a higher proportion of abortion within 4 hours of misoprostol administration than do regimens using misoprostol 400 μg orally. When mifepristone 200 mg is followed in 48 hours by misoprostol 800 μg vaginally, complete abortion rates >95% can be achieved through 63 days' gestation. Self administration of vaginal misoprostol is both safe and highly acceptable to U.S. women. The initial follow-up evaluation after medical abortion can occur sooner than 2 weeks if ultrasonography or serial β-hCG levels are used.

Compared with suction curettage, medical abortion is technically simpler and logistically more complex. Follow-up is important to ensure that the abortion has been successful. Women need to be evaluated about 2 weeks later to confirm by ultrasonography or serum β-hCG that the pregnancy has ended.

Medical abortion is safe, effective, and well-tolerated. With current regimens, cramping and bleeding are common, but infection and bleeding heavy enough to require transfusion are rare. In the few percent of women who fail to abort or who have incomplete abortions, completion of the process with a hand-held syringe and cannula (Fig. 21.5) works well. No additional dilation is usually required with this regimen.

Before the marketing of mifepristone in the United States, physicians relied on other medical abortifacient regimens. One regimen includes a single intramuscular injection of methotrexate, 50 mg/m² body surface area,

followed 3 days later by vaginal administration of misoprostol, 800 μg. In a randomized, controlled trial, this regimen proved superior to the same dose of misoprostol given alone. The efficacy of the combined regimen was 90%. At 49 days' gestation or less, methotrexate and misoprostol can achieve success rates similar to those with mifepristone and misoprostol, but the process is slower with methotrexate. From 20% to 30% of women require 1 to 5 weeks to complete the abortion. On the other hand, methotrexate is much less expensive than is mifepristone.

Another alternative is use of misoprostol alone. Varying success rates have been reported with different doses, frequency, and routes of administration. The success rates with misoprostol alone appear lower than with when misoprostol is used as an adjunct with mifepristone or methotrexate. In addition, the potential benefit of wetting the tablets before placing them in the vagina remains unclear. Protocols that have achieved a high success rates with misoprostol alone have had high rates of side effects as well, including nausea, vomiting, and diarrhea.

Medical approaches may be especially useful for challenging abortions. These include patients with müllerian anomalies, large cervical leiomyomas, prior failed attempted abortion, or obesity (e.g., 150 kg and more). Should the medical regimen not effect abortion, surgical completion is made substantially easier by this preparation of the cervix.

Dilation and Evacuation

Dilation and evacuation is the generic term for curettage abortions at 13 weeks' gestation or later. During the 1970s, D&E emerged as the most frequently used method for second-trimester abortions. The proportion of abortions performed by curettage techniques is inversely related to gestational age (Table 21.1): even at

TABLE 21.1.

Percentages of Reported Legal Abortions at 13 Menstrual Weeks' Gestation and Greater, by Method and Gestational Age, Selected States, United States, 1997

	Weeks of Gestation		
Type of Procedure	13–15	16–20	>21
Curettage (D&E)	98.6	93.7	85.0
Intrauterine saline instillation	0.0	0.3	0.7
Intrauterine prostaglandin instillation	0.2	2.9	2.9
Medical (nonsurgical)	0.2	0.6	0.9
Other	1.0	2.5	10.5
TOTAL	100.0	100.0	100.0

From Koonin LM, Strauss LT, Chrisman CE, et al. Abortion surveillance: United States, 1997. In: *CDC surveillance summaries*, December 8, 2000. MMWR 2000;49 (no. SS-11):1, with permission.

gestations greater than 20 weeks, D&E remains the dominant method of abortion in the United States.

Based on data from the 1970s, D&E is clearly safer than alternative methods through 16 weeks' gestation. At later gestational ages, the distinction blurs between D&E and labor induction methods in terms of morbidity and mortality. Hence, the choice of abortion method at this later stage usually hinges on nonmedical considerations: cost, convenience, comfort, and compassion. Errors in estimating gestational age, especially underestimation, can have serious consequences during a D&E procedure. Hence, confirmation of gestational age by ultrasonography is important before D&E.

D&E differs from suction curettage in two principal ways: D&E requires wider cervical dilation, and physicians need forceps to evacuate more advanced pregnancies. To achieve adequate dilation, many physicians insert osmotic dilators several hours to several days before D&E (Fig 21.13). For example, five laminaria placed overnight result in 1.5- to 2-cm dilation with minimal or no discomfort for most women. Use of a single Lamicel for about 4 hours produces as much dilation as do several laminaria at 14 to 16 weeks' gestation.

Patients must understand that once osmotic dilators have been inserted, the abortion needs completion. Rarely, a patient changes her mind about abortion after placement of an osmotic dilator. Although some women have continued their pregnancies uneventfully after removal of the devices, others have developed severe chorioamnionitis and aborted.

Dilating the cervix to a large diameter over several minutes can damage the cervix. Indeed, the first large study of this question revealed a higher incidence of low-birthweight infants in subsequent desired pregnancies. Hence, in the absence of evidence to the contrary, D&E procedures beyond about 14 weeks' gestation should use osmotic dilators.

In the 13- to 16-week interval, vacuum alone is adequate; thereafter, forceps extraction predominates. Although some physicians have advocated administering feticidal agents such as digoxin or potassium chloride under ultrasound guidance, a randomized, controlled trial by Jackson et al. found no benefit of this intrusive practice. A cannula 14 mm in diameter can evacuate pregnancies through about 16 menstrual weeks' gestation. For later pregnancies, the cannula primarily drains amniotic fluid at the beginning of the evacuation and draws tissue into the lower uterus for forceps extraction. Specially designed forceps for D&E are far superior to standard sponge forceps. As with suction curettage, extraction should occur from the lower uterus to minimize the risks of perforation. Some physicians use a flexible 8-mm cannula to confirm complete evacuation.

The physician must confirm completion by identifying all major fetal parts (extremities, spine, and calvarium). The calvarium is the component most frequently missed during the initial evacuation. Gentle exploration of the fundal and cornual areas with a large curette or forceps usually enables location and removal of the calvarium. Intraoperative ultrasonography can be helpful. If ultrasonography is not available, the physician may be able to remove the speculum and insert one digit into the uterine cavity to locate the missing part.

If the abortion cannot be completed with ease, the physician should interrupt the procedure. A safe and simple remedy is to discontinue the operation and administer intravenous oxytocin to the woman for 2 to 3 hours in the recovery room. After the patient returns to the operating room, the physician usually finds the retained tissue at the internal os, from which it can be removed in a few seconds. No D&E abortion needs to finish in a single session; time often helps. Once membranes rupture, the uterus contracts to expel its contents.

In D&E abortions, unlike medical abortion, the skill of the physician is critical. D&E abortion is an eclectic area of gynecology. Physicians should not dabble in these activities. This is not to say that D&E is too difficult for most physicians to learn. On the contrary, residents can quickly learn to do D&E procedures skillfully. For example, in a number of institutions, residents learn to perform D&E abortions with local anesthesia and ultrasound guidance up to 22 weeks' gestation. A before–after study from San Francisco General Hospital found use of ultrasound guidance for residents learning D&E was associated with a dramatic lowering of the perforation rate and a reduction in operating time.

Facility with suction curettage is a prerequisite to learning to perform D&E abortions. The physician should study operative technique. He or she should then observe and assist skilled physicians and then perform D&E procedures only under direct supervision. The gestational age range can advance as skill grows. In summary, D&E is not a trivial undertaking. However, like vaginal hysterectomy, it can be learned.

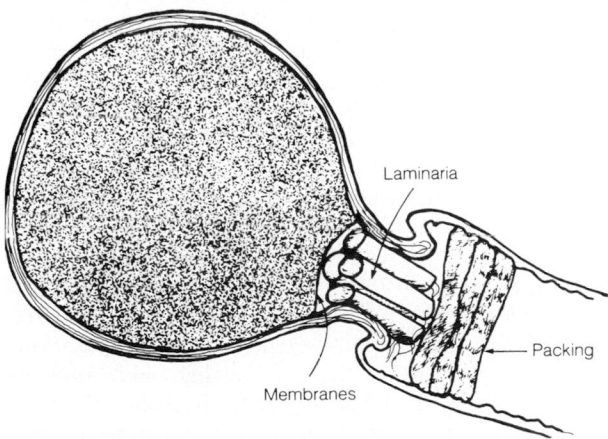

FIGURE 21.13. Laminaria in place after overnight preparation of the cervix. (From: Grimes DA, Hulka JF. Midtrimester dilatation and evacuation abortion. *South Med J* 1980;73:448, with permission.)

Labor Induction

Although D&E has supplanted many labor-induction abortions, the need for such abortions continues, particularly at later gestational ages. In contrast to D&E, the proportion of abortions performed by labor induction increases with gestational age (Table 21.1).

Abortifacients include two broad groups: hypertonic solutions (e.g., saline or urea) and uterotonic agents (e.g., oxytocin or misoprostol). The mechanism of action of hypertonic solutions is unclear, but these agents usually result in fetal death from osmotic insult; labor then usually ensues. Uterotonics act directly on the myometrium to stimulate contractions. Common doses of hypertonic solutions include 200 mL of 20% saline or 80 g of urea. Prostaglandins available in the United States include misoprostol, prostaglandin E_2 (PGE_2) vaginal suppositories, and 15-methyl $PGF_{2\alpha}$ for intramuscular injection.

Instillation of the abortifacient requires amniocentesis. Some physicians prefer a "blind" insertion in the midline, several centimeters inferior to the level of the fundus. Others mark on the woman's abdomen the location of a pocket of amniotic fluid identified at ultrasonography. Still others use real-time ultrasonography during the needle insertion.

Preparation for the amniocentesis is similar to that for diagnostic amniocentesis. The bladder should be empty. Aseptic technique should apply. The physician infiltrates the full thickness of the abdominal wall with several milliliters of local anesthetic. After needle insertion, a free flow of clear amniotic fluid should occur. Nitrazine paper or urine dipsticks for protein can differentiate amniotic fluid from urine if necessary. Blood-tinged fluid that clears does not present a problem; grossly bloody fluid that does not clear is a contraindication to injection of hypertonic solutions. If the uterus is small, lifting the uterus anteriorly with two fingers in the vagina can facilitate amniocentesis.

Draining amniotic fluid is unnecessary before the injection of abortifacient: withdrawing fluid does not shorten the induction-to-abortion time. On the other hand, withdrawing several hundred milliliters of fluid (and the corresponding decrease in the size of the uterus) may displace the needle tip. Hence, remove only enough fluid to confirm free flow.

Gravity-drip infusions should administer hypertonic solutions. If the physician loses correct needle placement during the injection, the flow stops. On the other hand, with syringe injection, the physician can inject hypertonic solutions into the myometrium in this situation.

Careful observation of the patient is necessary during instillation. The patient should not receive a sedative or narcotic. She should be alert and watchful for any symptom (e.g., burning abdominal pain, severe thirst, headache, or nausea) that might indicate faulty administration or rapid systemic uptake of the abortifacient. Any such symptom dictates immediate cessation of the infusion and close observation of the patient. If the symptom persists, the instillation should stop, and the physician should choose an alternative method or agent for the abortion.

Administration of prostaglandins has the advantage of simplicity. Amniocentesis is unnecessary, and inadvertent intravascular administration of hypertonic solutions cannot occur. Disadvantages of prostaglandins alone for

abortion include a high frequency of nausea, vomiting, and diarrhea. Routine prophylactic use of antiemetics and antidiarrheal drugs can reduce but not eliminate these noxious side effects. Fever occurs in about one-third to one-half of patients given prostaglandin E_2. Another serious drawback of prostaglandins alone for abortion is that these drugs are not inherently feticidal.

Vaginal PGE_2 suppositories appear to be more effective, but more noxious than intramuscular 15-methyl $PGF_{2\alpha}$. With the 20-mg vaginal suppositories given every 3 hours, the mean abortion time is about 13 hours, and 90% of abortions occur within 24 hours. With intramuscular 15-methyl $PGF_{2\alpha}$, mean abortion times are longer, and about 80% of abortions occur within 24 hours. Hypertonic solutions are useful in combination with uterotonic agents such as vaginal or parenteral prostaglandins.

The discovery of the uterotonic effects of misoprostol led to trials of this drug for midtrimester abortion. Regimens with vaginal administration of misoprostol ranging from 100 to 200 µg vaginally every 12 hours have achieved success rates of about 90% within 48 hours. A randomized, controlled trial found the efficacy of 200 µg every 12 hours to be comparable to that achieved with vaginal PGE_2 20 mg suppositories given every 3 hours. On the other hand, the misoprostol regimen was much less expensive and less noxious. Another trial found that 15-methyl $PGF_{2\alpha}$ 2.5 mg injected in the amniotic fluid resulted in a higher success rate at 24 hours than did misoprostol 200 µg administered vaginally twice, 12 hours apart. However, misoprostol use does not require amniocentesis.

Interest in high-dose oxytocin infusion for abortion has renewed. Small comparative studies have suggested that this method may be a safe alternative to vaginal PGE_2 suppositories given every 4 hours. The frequency of fever, vomiting, and diarrhea was significantly lower with oxytocin. One regimen includes oxytocin, 50 U in 500 mL of dextrose and normal saline administered intravenously over 3 hours; maintenance fluid (dextrose in normal saline) then follows for 1 hour. In stepwise fashion, the concentration of oxytocin increases by 50 U every 4 hours to a maximum of 300 U/500 mL. The investigators administered oxytocin in isotonic fluid and interrupted the oxytocin infusion every 4 hours for diuresis. With prolonged high-dose oxytocin infusion in hypotonic solutions, water intoxication and death can result.

Much of the morbidity (and mortality) associated with labor-induction abortion is preventable. Women in labor with abortions need the same meticulous, attentive obstetric care as do women in labor with childbirth. Induction-to-abortion times of 13 to 24 hours appear to have the lowest complication rates; thus, abortion within this interval should be the goal. Serious complications increase significantly with increasing induction-to-abortion times. If labor is ineffective, the physician should stimulate labor. If the membranes rupture, then labor must conclude within a reasonable period. Similarly, active management of a retained placenta after abortion prevents morbidity. A passive approach to desultory labor in the presence of ruptured membranes exposes the woman to unnecessary risk of complications.

Ancillary Measures

Several adjuncts can expedite instillation abortions. Administering intravenous oxytocin shortens induction-to-abortion times with saline instillation. Similarly, prostaglandins can augment labor; these agents are the pharmacologic treatments of choice for slow or failed instillation abortions.

Direct cervical dilation is also useful. Osmotic dilators shorten induction-to-abortion times and protect against cervicovaginal fistulae, although this protection is not absolute. Sequential packing of dilators can be useful if uterotonic agents do not achieve adequate dilation. Alternatively, if progress stalls, a metreurynter can accomplish abortion. The physician inserts a sterile Foley catheter with a 30- to 75-mL balloon into the uterus, inflates the balloon with a sterile solution (not air), and ties the catheter to 0.5-kg orthopedic traction at the foot of the bed. A liter bag of intravenous fluids hung over the foot of the bed and tied to the catheter by a string also suffices. This method has the disadvantage of placing a foreign body in the uterus.

In many cases, the preferred means of concluding a slow induction abortion is D&E. Twenty-four hours is a reasonable limit for labor-induction abortions. Frequently, the cervix is open several centimeters, and D&E proceeds quickly.

Hysterotomy and Hysterectomy

Neither hysterotomy nor hysterectomy should be a primary method of abortion. The morbidity, mortality, expense, and pain associated with these operations are greater than with alternative methods. Hysterotomy for abortion is an archaic operation that should be used only when usual surgical and medical approaches fail. Fig. 21.14 depicts a hysterotomy to evacuate a 14-week preg-

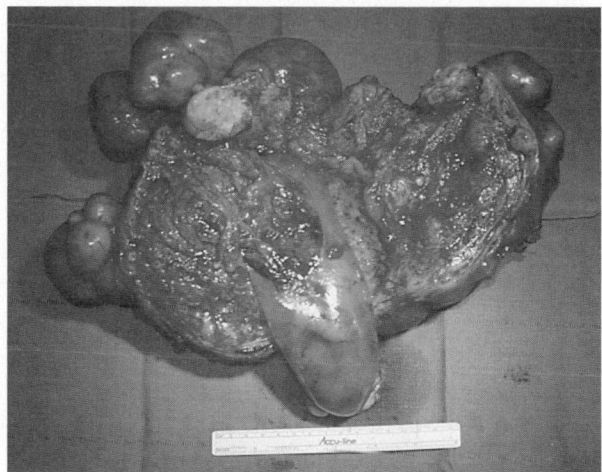

FIGURE 21.15. Total abdominal hysterectomy for abortion at 15 weeks' gestation in a patient with multiple symptomatic leiomyomas with resultant anemia. Gestational sac and fetus visible *in situ*. **Bottom:** 15-cm ruler.

nancy in the left horn of a bicornuate uterus; both labor induction and attempts to enter to pregnant horn through the cervix with ultrasonography and laparoscopy guidance had failed in this primigravida. Hysterectomy is appropriate in rare cases in which preexisting pathology, such as large leiomyomas (Fig. 21.15) or carcinoma *in situ* of the cervix, justify hysterectomy.

Complications

Morbidity

Legal abortion in the United States is safe. Fewer than one woman in 100 develops a serious complication, and fewer than one in 100,000 dies as a result of the operation.

Gestational age is one of two important determinants of the likelihood of morbidity. In Table 21.2, which lists

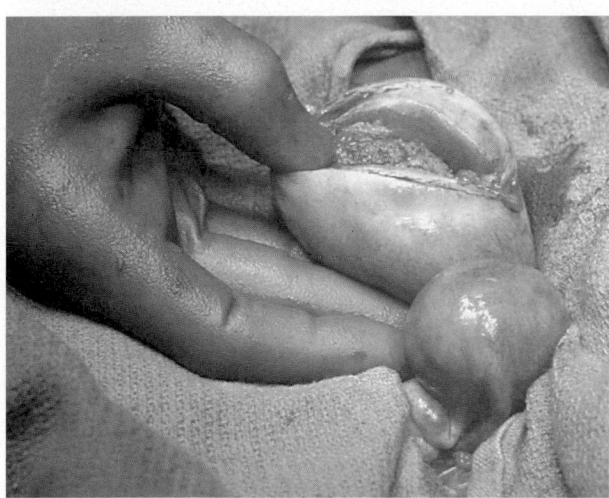

FIGURE 21.14. Hysterotomy incision in left uterine cavity, 14 weeks' gestation, after failed labor-induction abortion and failed attempted dilation and evacuation. Patient had a single cervix and two cavities. Non-pregnant cavity seen at right.

TABLE 21.2.

Serious Complication Rates for Legal Abortions by Gestational Age: United States, 1975–1978*

Gestational Age (wk)	Rate†
≤6	0.4
7–8	0.2
9–10	0.1
11–12	0.3
13–14	0.6
15–16	1.3
17–20	1.9

* For women with follow-up and without concurrent sterilization or preexisting conditions. Serious complications include temperature of 38°C or higher for 3 days or more, hemorrhage requiring blood transfusion, and any complication requiring unintended surgery (excluding curettage).

† Per 100 abortions.

serious complication rates for abortion by gestational age, the term *serious complication rates* refers to the percentage of women who had fever of 38°C or higher for 3 or more days, hemorrhage requiring transfusion, or unintended surgery. These data, derived from a 1970s multicenter study including 84,000 abortions, relate to those women without concurrent sterilization or preexisting medical conditions and for whom follow-up information was available. Abortions performed at the 7 to 10 weeks' gestation interval had the lowest incidence of serious complications. Thereafter, complications increased progressively with advancing gestational age. The finding that serious complications are more frequent at or before 6 weeks' gestation than at later gestational ages is consistent with two previous large studies in the United States.

The method of abortion is the second principal determinant of the likelihood of complications. Table 21.3, derived from the same study as Table 21.2, demonstrates that suction curettage is the safest available abortion method. The risk of serious complications with D&E at 13 weeks' gestation or later is higher than that with suction curettage and lower than that with labor-induction abortion.

Abortion complications have three temporal categories: immediate, delayed, and late complications. Immediate complications are those that develop during or within 3 hours of the operation. Delayed complications occur more than 3 hours and up to 28 days after the procedure. Late complications develop thereafter.

Immediate Complications

HEMORRHAGE. Reported rates of hemorrhage vary widely, reflecting both diverse definitions (100 to 1000 mL blood loss) and imprecision in estimating volumes of blood loss. Rates of hemorrhage range from 0.05 to 4.9 per 100 abortions in large case-series reports. The best index of clinically important hemorrhage is probably the rate of blood transfusion. The rate of transfusion associated with suction curettage in a large multicenter study was 0.06 per 100 abortions. For abortions performed

later in pregnancy, investigators have reported rates of 0.26 for D&E, 0.32 for urea-prostaglandin, and 1.72 for saline.

Vasopressin administered with paracervical anesthesia decreases blood loss with D&E abortion after 14 weeks' gestation. As little as 4 U (0.2 mL) mixed in with the anesthetic lowers the blood loss significantly; overall, vasopressin lowers four-fold the risk of a hemorrhage of 500 mL or more.

When hemorrhage occurs after suction curettage, administration of uterotonic agents and manual compression usually resolve the problem. In addition to oxytocic agents, the physician can inject vasopressin in the paracervical tissue to slow bleeding. Should bleeding persist, assessment of the endometrial cavity by hysteroscopy and internal compression of the cavity by a large Foley catheter balloon or a vasopressin-soaked pack can be helpful.

With the increasing cohort of women who have had Caesarean deliveries, the risk of encountering placenta accreta during abortion is increasing as well. In a series of more than 16,000 D&E abortions, the incidence of placenta accreta leading to hysterectomy was four per 10,000 cases.

CERVICAL INJURY. Cervical injury encompasses a broad spectrum of trauma. The most common type is a superficial laceration caused by the tenaculum tearing off during dilation. At the other extreme are the cervicovaginal fistula and the longitudinal laceration ascending to the level of the uterine vessels. Rates of cervical injury range from 0.01 to 1.6 per 100 suction curettage abortions. In older studies, the incidence of cervical injury requiring sutures was about one per 100 suction curettage abortions.

Several risk factors for cervical injury during suction curettage have emerged. Among factors within the control of the physician, use of laminaria and performance of the abortion by an attending physician (rather than a resident) lower the risk significantly, whereas use of general anesthesia raises the risk significantly. Among factors beyond the control of the physician, a history of a prior abortion lowers the risk, and age of 17 years or under increases the risk. Use of laminaria and performance of the abortion under local anesthesia by an attending physician together yield a 27-fold protective effect. Cervical preparation with misoprostol may confer similar benefits as laminaria, although more extensive experience will be needed to confirm this.

ACUTE HEMATOMETRA. Also termed the *postabortal syndrome* or the *redo syndrome*, acute hematometra is an important complication of suction curettage; its cause is unknown. The incidence of this syndrome ranges from 0.1 to one per 100 suction curettage abortions, according to the available literature.

Women with this condition develop severe cramping, usually within 2 hours of the abortion. Vaginal bleeding is less than expected. The woman may be weak and sweaty, and her uterus is large and markedly tender. Treatment consists of prompt repeat curettage, usually

---

TABLE 21.3.
Serious Complication Rates for Legal Abortions by Method: United States, 1975–1978*

Method	Rate†
Suction curettage	0.2
Dilation and evacuation	0.7
Saline instillation	2.1
Prostaglandin instillation	2.5
Urea—prostaglandin instillation	1.3

* For women with follow-up and without concurrent sterilization or preexisting conditions. Serious complications include temperature of 38°C or higher for 3 days or more, hemorrhage requiring blood transfusion, and any complication requiring unintended surgery (excluding curettage).

† Per 100 abortions.

without anesthesia or dilation. Evacuation of both liquid and clotted blood leads to rapid resolution of the symptoms. The physician can aspirate the blood with a suction cannula, a Karman cannula and syringe, or even a catheter attached to wall suction. Administration of an oxytocic after the repeat evacuation is standard. Whether routine prophylactic use of an oxytocic would reduce the incidence of acute hematometra is unknown.

ANESTHESIA COMPLICATIONS. Pain experienced during abortion relates not only to the choice of anesthesia but also to the characteristics of the patient. Young women (age, 13 to 17 years) and those with depression before the abortion report more pain than do other women.

Local anesthesia is safer than general anesthesia for both first- and second-trimester abortions. In an Italian study, use of general anesthesia had a relative risk for all complications combined of 1.8 (95% confidence interval, 1.4 to 2.5). The largest effect occurred with hemorrhage. Similarly, use of general anesthesia for D&E abortion in the United States increases the risk of serious complications. Overall, the attributable risk related to general anesthesia is low, and many women are willing to assume incremental risks in order to have no discomfort during the operation.

PERFORATION. Perforation is a potentially serious, but infrequent complication of abortion. According to most reports, the incidence of perforation is about 0.2 per 100 suction curettage abortions.

Several risk factors for perforation exist. Performance of a curettage abortion by a resident rather than by an attending physician increases the risk more than five-fold; on the other hand, cervical dilation by laminaria decreases the risk about five-fold. The risk of perforation increases significantly with advancing gestational age. Multiparous women have three times the risk of nulliparous women.

The two principal dangers of perforation are hemorrhage and damage to the abdominal contents. Lateral perforations in the cervico–isthmic region are particularly hazardous because of the proximity of the uterine vessels. Perforations of the fundus are more likely to be innocuous. Indeed, most perforations are not suspected or detected. In a series of patients undergoing combined abortion and sterilization by laparoscopy, the investigators found a six-fold higher rate of uterine perforation than they had suspected clinically (20 versus three per 1,000 abortions).

Not all perforations require treatment. Many suspected or documented perforations require only observation. Perforation with a dilator or sound is unlikely to damage abdominal contents. On the other hand, a suction cannula or forceps in the abdominal cavity can be devastating.

If the physician suspects a perforation, the procedure should stop immediately. If unmanageable hemorrhage, expanding hematoma, or injury to abdominal contents occurs, prompt laparotomy is necessary. Laparoscopy can be useful in documenting perforation and assessing dam-

age; if necessary, the physician can complete the abortion under laparoscopic visualization. Any woman with severe pain within hours after the abortion should be evaluated for possible perforation with bowel injury.

Delayed Complications

RETAINED TISSUE. Although retained tissue after abortion can pass without incident, retained tissue can lead to hemorrhage, infection, or both. This complication occurs infrequently, however. Its incidence after suction curettage abortion is less than one per 100 abortions.

This complication usually manifests itself within several days of the abortion. Cramping and bleeding can be accompanied by fever. When women develop pain, bleeding, and low-grade fever after abortion, retained tissue may be present. Prompt outpatient suction curettage usually resolves the symptoms, but close follow-up is advisable.

INFECTION. Postabortal infection can result from retained tissue. The likelihood of febrile morbidity after abortion depends on the method used. The incidence of fever of 38°C or higher for one or more days is usually less than one per 100 abortions by suction curettage. Corresponding figures for D&E are 1.5 per 100 abortions; for urea-prostaglandin, 6.3; and for hypertonic saline, 5.0. The organisms responsible for postabortal infection are similar to those responsible for other gynecologic infections.

A number of risk factors for infection exist. Women are at increased risk if they have untreated endocervical gonorrhea or chlamydial infection. Late abortions also increase the risk. Likewise, use of labor-induction abortion instead of D&E and use of local rather than general anesthesia for suction curettage increase the risk. Administration of broad-spectrum antibiotics and, if needed, uterine curettage are the cornerstones of therapy.

Late Complications

RH SENSITIZATION. Legal abortion is a potentially important cause of Rh sensitization for women at risk. The likelihood of sensitization increases with advancing gestational age (and, hence, larger volumes of fetal erythrocytes). One study has quantified the risk of Rh sensitization from first-trimester suction curettage without RhIG prophylaxis. A total of 3.1% of secundigravidas whose first pregnancy terminated by suction curettage without RhIG prophylaxis had antibodies in their second pregnancy. Subtracting 0.5% (the percentage of women estimated to have become sensitized primarily during the second pregnancy), the investigators estimated the risk of sensitization from suction curettage to be 2.6%. Thus, on a nationwide basis, the clinical impact of failure to administer RhIG to candidates after abortion may be substantial. Candidates should receive 50 µg of RhIG after abortions performed at 12 weeks' gestation or earlier or 300 µg after abortions performed later in pregnancy.

ADVERSE PREGNANCY OUTCOMES. Investigators have linked induced abortion with a broad array of adverse reproductive outcomes, ranging from infertility to ectopic pregnancy. Most published reports, however, suffer from serious methodologic shortcomings that limit their usefulness. To examine the potential association between first-trimester induced abortion and subsequent reproductive performance, epidemiologists have performed an exhaustive review and analysis of the world literature. This includes more than 150 epidemiologic studies published in 11 languages.

The findings of this analysis are largely reassuring. No increase in the risk of secondary infertility and ectopic pregnancy appears, even in studies with substantial power to detect differences in rates. Midtrimester spontaneous abortion is no more common among women who have had one previous abortion than among women pregnant for the first time. Similarly, the risk of premature delivery does not increase for women having undergone induced abortion.

On the other hand, low birthweight is more frequent in first births after abortion by sharp curettage performed under general anesthesia compared with first-pregnancy births. This does not occur after other methods of abortion, such as suction curettage. The questions of the effect of repeat induced abortion and second-trimester abortion remain unresolved, but repeat sharp curettage may carry increased risks. First-born infants of women who had one induced abortion have risks of morbidity and mortality similar to those of other first-born children.

Additional studies have corroborated the absence of adverse effects of induced abortion on subsequent reproduction. Outcomes studied included infertility, ectopic pregnancy, spontaneous abortion, and adverse obstetric outcomes. One unresolved issue is placenta previa. Sophisticated studies have found either no or a marginally significant increase in the risk (relative risk, 1.3; 95% confidence interval, 1.0 to 1.6), which was comparable to that with spontaneous abortion.

Induced abortion does not threaten a woman's emotional health. In contrast, the dominant emotional reaction to induced abortion is a sense of relief. In several studies, abortion appeared to improve the emotional well-being of women by resolving an intense personal crisis. Specifically, claims of a *postabortion trauma syndrome* lack scientific merit.

The putative association between induced abortion and breast cancer remains controversial. Although a number of case-control studies have found an association, this appears because of recall bias among controls. Women who are well (controls) are less likely to report prior induced abortions than are women with breast cancer (cases). This type of information bias has been documented in studies from Sweden. Two large cohort studies, which are less likely to be biased than are case-control studies, have shown either no effect or a protective effect of induced abortion on later breast cancer. No firm evidence links abortion to other cancers.

Mortality

Since 1972, when the Centers for Disease Control and Prevention first began nationwide surveillance of abortion deaths, the safety of abortion has improved dramatically. As shown in Figure 21.16, the case-fatality rate fell

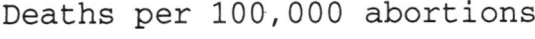

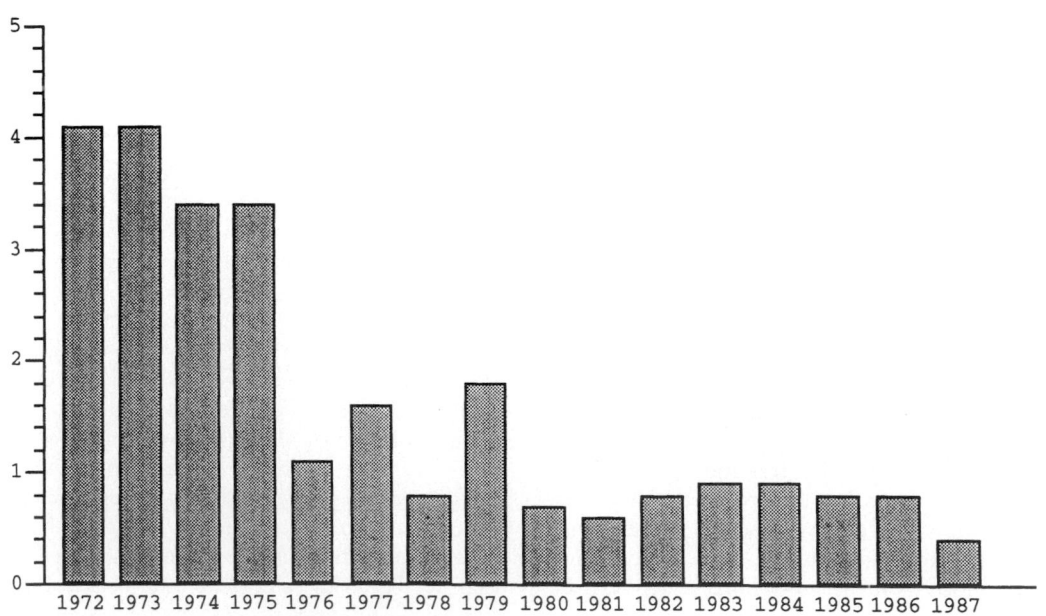

FIGURE 21.16. Case-fatality rates from legal abortion by year, United States, 1972 to 1987. (From: Lawson HW, Frye A, Atrash HK, et al. Abortion mortality, United States, 1972 through 1987. *Am J Obstet Gynecol* 1994;171:1365, with permission.)

from 4.1 deaths per 100,000 abortions in 1972 to 0.4 in 1987.

The causes of death from legal abortion have changed as well. From 1972 to 1977, infection and hemorrhage were the leading causes of death. Thereafter, complications of anesthesia (usually general anesthesia) became more important, emerging in 1983 as the leading cause of death from abortion. Most of these deaths were owing to hypoventilation or loss of airway resulting in hypoxia. The message from these deaths is clear: people administering general anesthesia for abortion must be skilled in airway management and observant for signs of hypoxia.

The risk of death from legal abortion increases with gestational age: the earlier the abortion, the safer the abortion. As shown in Table 21.4, which includes deaths from 1972 to 1987, the death-to-case rate for abortions at 8 weeks' gestation or earlier was 0.4 per 100,000 abortions. The risk was nearly eight times higher in the 13- to 15-week interval. For abortions at 21 weeks and later, the risk of death was more than 30 times that for abortions at 8 weeks' gestation or earlier.

Curettage abortion (which includes suction curettage and D&E) is the safest method overall (Table 21.4). The risk of death for curettage abortions was 0.5 per 100,000 abortions, whereas that for D&E was nearly

TABLE 21.4.
Legal Abortion Case-Fatality Rates and Relative Risks by Selected Categories: United States, 1972–1987

Risk Category	Rate*	Relative Risk and 95% Confidence Interval
AGE GROUP (Y)		
≤19	1.0	Referent
20–24	1.3	1.3 (0.9–1.8)
25–29	1.2	1.2 (0.8–1.8)
30–34	1.6	1.5 (1.0–2.4)
35–39	2.5	2.3 (1.4–3.8)
≥40	3.1	3.0 (1.5 6.0)
RACE		
White	0.9	Referent
Black and other	2.3	2.4 (1.9–3.2)
PARITY†		
0	0.9	Referent
1	1.1	1.3 (0.9–1.9)
2	1.1	1.3 (0.8–1.9)
≥3	2.5	2.8 (2.0–4.0)
GESTATIONAL AGE (WK)‡		
≤8	0.4	Referent
9–10	0.8	2.1 (1.3–3.3)
11–12	1.4	3.7 (2.3–5.8)
13–15	2.9	7.7 (5.0–11.7)
16–20	9.3	24.5 (18.6–32.3)
≥20	12.0	31.5 (22.2–44.5)
PROCEDURE§		
Curettage	0.5	Referent
Dilation and evacuation	3.7	6.8 (4.9–9.5)
Labor induction	7.1	13.0 (9.7–17.5)
Hysterotomy or hysterectomy	51.6	95.0 (69.6–129.5)
Other	1.9	3.6 (1.5–8.3)

* Number of legal abortion deaths per 100,000 abortions.

† Denominators for calculating rates by parity use previous live-birth data from abortion surveillance. Deaths with unknown parity are excluded.

‡ Deaths with unknown gestational age are excluded.

§ Figures for 1972 and 1973 are excluded because data necessary to calculate rates by procedure were not collected. Deaths with unknown procedure are excluded.

(Lawson HW, Frye A, Atrash HK, et al. Abortion mortality, United States, 1972 through 1987. *Am J Obstet Gynecol* 1994;171:1365)

TABLE 21.5.
Case-Fatality Rates* for Dilation and Evacuation and Labor Induction at 13 Weeks' Gestation or Later, by Method and Gestational Age: United States, 1972–1987

Method	Gestational Age (wk)			
	13–15	16–20	≥21	All
Dilation and evacuation	2.0	6.5	11.9	3.7
Labor induction	3.8	7.9	10.3	7.1

* Per 100,000 abortions.

(Lawson HW, Frye A, Atrash HK, et al. Abortion mortality, United States, 1972 through 1987. *Am J Obstet Gynecol* 1994;171:1365)

seven times higher. Labor-induction abortions had a rate 13 times higher than that of curettage. Hysterotomy and hysterectomy had a rate 95 times higher, although this rate reflects only 10 deaths. Women of minority race, those of advanced maternal age, and multiparas also had higher risks of death from abortion. At 13 to 15 weeks' gestation, D&E carries about half the risk of death as does labor induction (Table 21.5). At later gestational ages, the risks of death associated with both methods are similar. Because of the large number of D&E abortions performed at 13 to 15 weeks' gestation, the overall safety of D&E at 13 weeks' gestation or later is superior to that of labor induction.

CONCLUSION

Abortion is the most frequent outcome of human conception; thus, management of abortion and its complications is an important responsibility for physicians. Chromosomal anomalies are the single most important cause of spontaneous abortion. For women with threatened abortion, use of ultrasonography and β-hCG monitoring can help predict the outcome of the pregnancy. Evacuation of the uterus in cases of fetal death is primarily for psychological rather than medical indications; either curettage or labor induction may be appropriate. Premature cervical dilation without labor is a poorly understood cause of spontaneous abortion. There is no uniform case definition and no valid diagnostic test. Randomized clinical trials reveal modest benefit of cervical cerclage on obstetric outcomes.

Small numbers of illegal abortions continue to occur in the United States. Legally induced abortion, however, is one of the most frequently performed—and one of the safest—operations in contemporary practice. Fewer than one per 100 of those having an abortion suffer a major complication, and fewer than one per 100,000 die from causes associated with the procedure. The marketing of mifepristone in the United States for early abortion has broadened the options available to women, and use of misoprostol for cervical preparation before curettage represent important advances in gynecology.

BIBLIOGRAPHY

Adler NE, David HP, Major BN, et al. Psychological responses after abortion. *Science* 1990;248:41.

Atrash HK, MacKay HT, Hogue CJR. Ectopic pregnancy concurrent with induced abortion: incidence and mortality. *Am J Obstet Gynecol* 1990;162:726.

Blanchard K, Winikoff B, Ellertson C. Misoprostol used alone for the termination of early pregnancy. Review of the evidence. *Contraception* 1999;59:209.

Borgiba AF, Rodis JF, Hanlon W, et al. Second-trimester abortion by intramuscular 15-methyl-prostaglandin F₂ or intravaginal prostaglandin E₂ suppositories: a randomized trial. *Obstet Gynecol* 1995;85:697.

Bugalho A, Bique C, Almeida L, et al. Pregnancy interruption by vaginal misoprostol. *Gynecol Obstet Invest* 1993;36:226.

Chung TK, Lee DT, Cheung LP, et al. Spontaneous abortion: a randomized, controlled trial comparing surgical evacuation with conservative management using misoprostol. *Fertil Steril* 1999;71:1054.

Creinin MD, Vittinghoff E. Methotrexate and misoprostol vs. misoprostol alone for early abortion: a randomized controlled trial. *JAMA* 1994;272:1190.

Edmonds DK, Lindsay KS, Miller JF, et al. Early embryonic mortality in women. *Fertil Steril* 1982;38:447.

Edwards J, Carson SA. New technologies permit safe abortion at less than six weeks' gestation and provide timely detection of ectopic gestation. *Am J Obstet Gynecol* 1997;176:1101.

El-Refaey H, Rajasekar D, Abdalla M, et al. Induction of abortion with mifepristone (RU-486) and oral or vaginal misoprostol. *N Engl J Med* 1995;332:983.

Jackson RA, Teplin VL, Drey EA, et al. Digoxin to facilitate late second-trimester abortion: a randomized, masked, placebo-controlled trial. *Obstet Gynecol* 2001;97:471.

Jain JK, Mishell DR Jr. A comparison of intravaginal misoprostol with prostaglandin E₂ for termination of second-trimester pregnancy. *N Engl J Med* 1994;331:290.

Koonin LM, Strauss LT, Chrisman CE, et al. Abortion surveillance: United States, 1997. In: *CDC Surveillance Summaries*, December 8, 2000. MMWR 2000;49 (no. SS-11):1.

Lawson HW, Frye A, Atrash HK, et al. Abortion mortality, United States, 1972 through 1987. *Am J Obstet Gynecol* 1994;171:1365.

Levi CS, Lyons EA, Zheng XH, et al. Endovaginal US: demonstration of cardiac activity in embryos of less than 5.0 mm in crown-rump length. *Radiology* 1990;176:71.

MRC/RCOG Working Party on Cervical Cerclage. Final report of the Medical Research Council/Royal College of Obstetricians and Gynaecologists Multicentre Randomized Trial of Cervical Cerclage. *Br J Obstet Gynaecol* 1993;100:516.

National Abortion Federation. *Early medical abortion with mifepristone or methotrexate: overview and protocol recommendations.* Washington, D.C.: National Abortion Federation, 2001.

Neilson S, Hahlin M. Expectant management of first-trimester spontaneous abortion. *Lancet* 1995;345:84.

Newhall EP, Winikoff B. Abortion with mifepristone and misoprostol: regimens, efficacy, acceptability and future directions. *Am J Obstet Gynecol* 2000;183:S44.

Osborn JF, Arisi E, Spinelli A, et al. General anaesthesia, a risk factor for complication following induced abortion? *Eur J Epidemiol* 1990;6:416.

Owen J, Hauth JC, Winkler CL, et al. Midtrimester pregnancy termination: a randomized trial of prostaglandin E₂ versus concentrated oxytocin. *Am J Obstet Gynecol* 1992;167:1112.

Paul M, Lichtenberg ES, Borgatta L, et al. *A physician's guide to medical and surgical abortion.* New York: Churchill Livingstone, 1999.

Peyron R, Aubeny E, Targosz V, et al. Early termination of pregnancy with mifepristone (RU-486) and the orally active prostaglandin misoprostol. *N Engl J Med* 1993;328: 1509.

Rashbaum WK, Gates EJ, Jones J, et al. Placenta accreta encountered during dilation and evacuation in the second trimester. *Obstet Gynecol* 1995;85:701.

Remennick LI. Induced abortion as cancer risk factor: a review of epidemiological evidence. *J Epidemiol Commun Health* 1990;44:259.

Saraiya M, Green CA, Berg CJ, et al. Spontaneous abortion–related deaths among women in the United States: 1981–1991. *Obstet Gynecol* 1999;94:172.

Sawaya GF, Grady D, Kerlikowske K, et al. Antibiotics at the time of induced abortion: the case for universal prophylaxis based on a meta-analysis. *Obstet Gynecol* 1996;87: 884.

Schaff EA, Fielding SL, Westhoff C, et al. Vaginal misoprostol administered 1, 2, or 3 days after mifepristone for early medical abortion: A randomized trial. *JAMA* 2000;284: 1948.

Schaff EA, Wortman M, Eisinger SH, et al. Methotrexate and misoprostol when surgical abortion fails. *Obstet Gynecol* 1996;87:450.

Singh K, Fong YF, Prasad RN, et al. Randomized trial to determine optimal dose of vaginal misoprostol for preabortion cervical priming. *Obstet Gynecol* 1998;92:795.

Stephenson P, Wagner M, Badea M, et al. The public health consequences of restricted induced abortion: lessons from Romania. *Am J Public Health* 1992;82:1328.

Stotland NL. The myth of the abortion trauma syndrome. *JAMA* 1992;268:2078.

Taylor VM, Kramer MD, Vaughan TL, et al. Placenta previa in relation to induced and spontaneous abortion: a population-based study. *Obstet Gynecol* 1993;82:88.

Townsend DE, Barbis SD, Mathews RD. Vasopressin and operative hysteroscopy in the management of delayed postabortion and postpartum bleeding. *Am J Obstet Gynecol* 1991;165:616.

Ulmann A, Silvestre L, Chemama L, et al. Medical termination of early pregnancy with mifepristone (RU-486) followed by a prostaglandin analogue: study in 16,369 women. *Acta Obstet Gynecol Scand* 1992;71:278.

Winkler CL, Gray SE, Hauth JC, et al. Mid-second-trimester labor induction: concentrated oxytocin compared with prostaglandin E_2 vaginal suppositories. *Obstet Gynecol* 1991;77:297.

World Health Organization. *Medical methods for termination of pregnancy.* WHO technical report series 871. Geneva: World Health Organization, 1997.

Yapar EG, Senoz S, Urkutur M, et al. Second trimester pregnancy termination including fetal death: comparison of five different methods. *Eur J Obstet Gynecol Reprod Biol* 1996;69:97.

Zieman M, Fong SK, Benowitz NL, et al. Absorption kinetics of misoprostol with oral or vaginal administration. *Obstet Gynecol* 1997;90:88.

Te Linde's Operative Gynecology, ninth edition, edited by John A. Rock and Howard W. Jones, III. Lippincott Williams & Wilkins, Philadelphia © 2003.

CHAPTER

22

Ectopic Pregnancy

MARK A. DAMARIO   JOHN A. ROCK

Ectopic pregnancy was first recognized in 1693 by Busiere, when he was examining the body of a prisoner executed in Paris. Gifford of England made a more complete report in 1731 that described the condition of a fertilized ovum implanted outside the uterine cavity. Ectopic pregnancy has since become recognized as one of the more serious complications of pregnancy. One of the leading causes of maternal morbidity and mortality in the United States, it still accounted for 9% of all maternal deaths from 1990 to 1992, according to the Centers for Disease Control. Even despite significant advances in diagnosis and treatment, ectopic pregnancy remains the leading cause of maternal death in the first trimester.

Today, early diagnosis of ectopic pregnancy is possible with highly sensitive and rapid β-human chorionic gonadotropin (β-hCG) assays and the aid of advanced vaginal ultrasonographic equipment. The benefit of early diagnosis is that expectant medical therapy or conservative surgery becomes possible. Conservative management in the case of a small ectopic pregnancy that is present without rupture is usually successful when preservation of the oviduct to maintain or enhance fertility is important. Physicians should maintain a high index of suspicion for ectopic pregnancy and should be cognizant of the importance of early diagnosis and early intervention. This chapter summarizes the contemporary methods for diagnosis and treatment of ectopic pregnancy.

EPIDEMIOLOGY OF ECTOPIC PREGNANCY

Although the total number of pregnancies has declined over the past three decades, the rate of ectopic pregnancy has continued to increase in most western nations. In the United States, the incidence of ectopic pregnancy has increased from 4.5 per 1,000 pregnancies in 1970 to 19.7 per 1,000 pregnancies in 1992. In Norway, an increase from 12.5 to 18.0 per 1,000 pregnancies was reported from 1976 to 1993. One contributing factor for the rising ratio of extrauterine to intrauterine pregnancies is felt to be the rising incidence of sexually transmitted diseases as well as the efficacy of modern antibiotic treatments for pelvic inflammatory disease (PID). A second factor may be the increased ability to detect the disease. Although the risk of death from ectopic pregnancy continues to decline among all races and ages in the United States, women of black and other minority races remain at significantly increased risk of death from ectopic pregnancy compared with white women. Although the overall incidence of ectopic pregnancy in the United States during 1970 to 1989 increased approximately five-fold, the risk of death from ectopic pregnancy declined by 90%. This decline in mortality from ectopic pregnancies may be related both to the increased awareness of the condition as well as improved diagnostic and therapeutic methods.

PATHOLOGY

A tubal gestation traditionally has been defined as one that implants and grows within the tubal lumen. Budowick and associates have suggested that tubal implantation actually occurs in the lumen but is soon followed by penetration into the lamina propria and muscularis to become extraluminal. Pauerstein, Hodgson and Kramen demonstrated that trophoblastic infiltration can be predominantly intraluminal or predominantly extraluminal, or, occasionally, mixed. It is impossible to ascertain in the operating room the predominant pattern of growth of a given tubal pregnancy. In any event, fimbrial expression usually is an unacceptable method for removal of ectopic pregnancy. Not only is the method traumatic, but it frequently does not remove all of the trophoblastic tissue. The resultant persistent ectopic pregnancy may therefore require additional therapy.

ETIOLOGY OF ECTOPIC PREGNANCY

Tubal Damage Secondary to Inflammation

Both the increased incidence of sexually transmitted disease resulting in salpingitis and the efficacy of antibiotic therapy in preventing total tubal occlusion after an episode of salpingitis are related to the increasing incidence of ectopic pregnancy. Levin and associates have demonstrated that the risk of ectopic pregnancy is increased in women with a primary history of PID. Westrom compared women with PID confirmed by laparoscopy with healthy women, matched by age and parity, and found a six-fold greater incidence of ectopic pregnancy in women with PID, an alarming rate of 1 ectopic pregnancy out of every 24 gestations. Similar statistics have been reported by other authors. Many of the patients in these studies had received antibiotic treatment for salpingitis.

Before antibiotics became available for the treatment of PID, salpingitis was usually so acute that the inflamed tube became totally occluded, and permanent sterility was the result. Women who attempted to conceive after a pelvic infection were successful less than 40% of the time. Today, the rate of pregnancy exceeds 60% for patients adequately treated with antibiotics. After initial appropriate treatment of an infection with antibiotics, agglutination of the cilia can still occur and synechial bands can form within the tubal lumen to cause partial tubal obstruction. Westrom has demonstrated by laparoscopy that bilateral tubal occlusion occurs in approximately 12.8% of patients after treatment for the first tubal infection, in 35% after two infections, and in 75% after three or more infections. In addition, Westrom found that approximately 4% of all pregnancies subsequent to salpingitis were ectopic.

Fallopian tubes containing a gestation are frequently normal on macroscopic visualization and gross histologic examination. Vasquez, Winston and Brosens using scanning electron microscopy and light microscopy studies of tubal biopsies from five groups of women, discovered marked differences in their ciliated surfaces. The proportion of ciliated cells was significantly lower in biopsy specimens taken from 25 women with tubal pregnancies as compared to biopsy specimens from seven women with intrauterine pregnancies at the same stage of gestation. Marked deciliation was likewise seen in eight women who had undergone biopsies during tubal reconstructive surgery. In another study, Gerard and colleagues found that seven of ten fallopian tube samples from patients with ectopic pregnancy were PCR-positive for *C. trachomatis* DNA. Therefore, the increased occurrence of sexually transmitted diseases contributing to subclinical tubal epithelial damage may be an important contributor to ectopic pregnancy. Comprehensive programs to prevent sexually transmitted diseases undertaken in Sweden and Wisconsin have been found to not only decrease the incidence of *C. trachomatis* infections and other sexually transmitted diseases but also the rate of ectopic pregnancies.

Contraceptive Devices

The use of IUDs has been associated with an increased incidence of ectopic pregnancy. In a summary of published reports on ectopic pregnancy, Tatum and Schmidt observed that 4% of the pregnancies that occurred with an IUD in place were ectopic. In a recent meta-analysis, Mol and associates reported a range of odds ratios from 4.2 to 45.0 from heterogenous studies of IUD use and ectopic pregnancy. Subtle tubal epithelial damage or actual PID episodes are likely responsible for the observed association between IUDs and ectopic pregnancy.

Oral Contraceptives

The overall risk of an ectopic pregnancy is lowered in women using oral contraceptives. When oral contraceptives fail, however, the risk of an ectopic pregnancy is slightly increased. This increase is presumed secondary to the inhibitory progestin effect on tubal motility. This hypothesis is supported by several studies implicating progestin-only oral contraceptives in the etiology of ectopic pregnancies.

Prior Tubal Surgery

An operative procedure on the oviduct, whether a sterilization procedure or tubal reconstructive surgery, can cause an ectopic pregnancy. The incidence of ectopic pregnancies occurring after neosalpingostomy for distal tubal obstruction ranges from 2% to 18% (Table 22.1). The rate of ectopic pregnancy after a microsurgical reversal of a sterilization procedure is only about 4%, presumably because the tubes have not been damaged by prior infection.

The United States Collaborative Review of Sterilization Working Group followed a total of 10,685 women undergoing tubal sterilization in a multicenter, prospec-

TABLE 22.1.
Summary: Ectopic Pregnancy After Tubal Surgery

Procedure	Technique	Total Pregnancy (%)	Pregnancy Range (%)	Ectopic (%)	Ectopic Range (%)
Salpingoscopy	Macrosurgery	42	35–65	3.4	1–20
	Microsurgery	52	31–69	1.8	0–16
Fimbrioplasty	Macrosurgery	42	36–50	14	10–18
	Microsurgery	59	26–68	6	4–11
Neosalpingostomy	Macrosurgery	27	20–38	4.2	2–10
	Microsurgery	26	17–44	7.7	0–18
Tubal anastomosis	Macrosurgery	44	25–83	9.2	0–15
	Microsurgery	62	35–78	2.3	1–6.2
Removal of ectopic pregnancy	Salpingectomy	42	38–49	12	8–17
	Salpingostomy	57	39–73	11	0–20

(Lavy G, Diamond MP, DeCherney AH. Ectopic pregnancy: relationship to tubal reconstructive surgery. *Fertil Steril* 1987;47:543–556.)

tive cohort study. The overall cumulative probability of pregnancy in the study cohort 10 years after sterilization was 18.5 per 1000 procedures (failure rate of 1.85%). The 10-year cumulative probability of ectopic pregnancy for all methods of tubal sterilization was 7.3 per 1000 procedures. From these data, one can therefore estimate that in the setting of a positive pregnancy following tubal sterilization, there is an approximately 40% risk that the pregnancy will be ectopic. The type of sterilization procedure and age of the patient at the time of sterilization appear to be relevant factors. Women sterilized by bipolar tubal coagulation before the age of 30 years had a probability of ectopic pregnancy that was 27 times as high as that of women of similar age who underwent postpartum partial salpingectomy (31.9 versus 1.2 ectopic pregnancies per 1000 procedures). In addition, ectopic pregnancy was often seen many years after the sterilization procedure. The annual rates of ectopic pregnancy in the fourth through tenth years after sterilization were no lower than that seen in the first three years.

The pathophysiology of ectopic pregnancy after elective tubal sterilization is not clear. It is possible that a tuboperitoneal fistula in a previously coagulated segment of fallopian tube may allow spermatozoa to escape and reach the oocyte. Such fistulas have been demonstrated radiographically by Shah and colleagues in 11% of 150 women after laparoscopic electrocoagulation. Improper surgical technique (such as incomplete coagulation or misplacement of a mechanical device) may also influence the sterilization failure rate and incidence of ectopic pregnancy, although their likelihood is presumably low.

Assisted Reproductive Technologies

Ectopic pregnancies are known to occur with increased frequency after in vitro fertilization (IVF) and related techniques. The Society for Assisted Reproductive Technology (SART) reported that 2.1% of pregnancies established after IVF in the United States during 1997 were ectopic. Several theories have been proposed regarding the occurrence of ectopic implantation after transcervical intrauterine embryo transfer. Potential factors include the possibility of direct injection of embryos into the fallopian tube, uterine contractions provoked by the transfer catheter that propel the embryos retrograde, position or depth of the transfer catheter in the uterine cavity, and the volume of transfer medium. Verhulst and colleagues reported that tubal damage was a major risk factor. These researchers found that the ectopic pregnancy rate after IVF was significantly greater in patients with tubal disease (3.65% of pregnancies) than in those without tubal disease (1.19% of pregnancies). Strandell, Thorburn and Hamberger found that a history of a previous ectopic pregnancy and a history of a previous myomectomy also appear to be risk factors for ectopic pregnancies following IVF.

Tummon and coworkers reported a 2% risk of heterotopic pregnancy in women undergoing IVF who had distorted tubal anatomy. This is about 100 to 200 times the reported incidence of combined intrauterine and extrauterine pregnancies occurring spontaneously. These authors also found that the risk of heterotopic pregnancy appeared to increase proportionately with the number of embryos transferred.

Developmental Anomalies

Intramural polyps and tubal diverticula can block or alter tubal transport of fertilized ova. Congenital absence of segments of the fallopian tube with peritoneal fistulas can also predispose to tubal pregnancy. Women exposed to diethylstilbestrol (DES) in utero are at higher risk of ectopic pregnancy. These women may have absent or minimal fimbriae and fallopian tubes that are shorter and thinner than normal.

Other Causal Factors

Several studies have demonstrated that cigarette smoking seems to be an independent, dose-related risk factor for

---

TABLE 22.2.
Risk Factors for Ectopic Pregnancy

Chronic pelvic inflammatory disease
Prior tubal surgery
Surgical sterilization
Use of an intrauterine device
Previous ectopic pregnancy
DES exposure
Progestin-only contraceptives
Assisted reproductive technologies
Infertility
Developmental tubal anomalies
Multiple sexual partners
Early age at first intercourse
Cigarette smoking
Vaginal douching

---

ectopic pregnancy. Other lifestyle factors such as multiple sexual partners and early age at first intercourse are associated with an increased risk. Vaginal douching has also been associated with a slightly increased risk of ectopic pregnancy, probably by increasing the overall risk of pelvic infections and resultant tubal damage. A summary of risk factors related to ectopic pregnancy is summarized in Table 22.2.

SITES OF ECTOPIC PREGNANCY

About 95% of extrauterine implantations occur in the oviduct. About 55% of these tubal implantations occur in the ampulla, the most common site: implantation in the isthmic portion accounts for 20% to 25%, implantation in the infundibulum and fimbria account for 17%, and implantation in the interstitial segment (cornua) accounts for 2% to 4%. Ectopic implantations occur less often in the ovary, the cervix, and the peritoneal cavity (Fig. 22.1).

Walters, Eddy, and Pauerstein reported that 16% of tubal pregnancies result from a contralateral ovulation. Transmigration of the ovum in the peritoneal cavity can occur because the oviducts and ovaries may be situated close together in the cul-de-sac. Alternatively, this phenomenon could also result from transmigration of the embryo through the endometrial cavity into the opposite oviduct.

EFFECTS OF ECTOPIC PREGNANCY ON FUTURE REPRODUCTION

Tubal pregnancy is associated with a poor prognosis for subsequent reproduction. In most cases, an extrauterine pregnancy represents an impairment of the fertilized ovum's ability to migrate through the deep rugae of the oviduct as a result of altered tubal function. The morphologic abnormality is usually bilateral, irreversible and can produce repeated ectopic pregnancies or permanent sterility. In a 1975 study, Shoen and Nowak concluded that about 70% of patients who have an ectopic first pregnancy are unable to produce a living child. As many as 30% of the patients who have an ectopic first pregnancy will have a repeat ectopic pregnancy, which compares with the total repeat ectopic rate of 10% to 15% for the overall population of reproductive-age women. More than half of the subsequent extrauterine pregnancies will occur within a 2-year period, and 80% will occur within 4 years of the initial ectopic pregnancy. In reviewing the experience of the Kaiser Foundation hospitals, Hallatt reported a 9.2% overall incidence of repeat ectopic pregnancies among 1330 women who had extrauterine pregnancies. The potential reproductive capacity for a patient who has had an ectopic pregnancy therefore depends on her reproductive history. If an ectopic pregnancy was the result of her first reproductive effort, then the prognosis for future pregnancies is much worse than if the complication occurred after one or more successful pregnancies.

Mueller and associates have estimated that 92% of infertility in women who have had a tubal pregnancy results from tubal damage due to the tubal pregnancy itself or other factors that had predisposed to its occurrence. A history of infertility itself is a risk factor for ectopic pregnancy. A two-fold increase in the risk of tubal pregnancy exists among infertile women with no evident abnormality during infertility evaluation.

TUBAL ECTOPIC PREGNANCY

The morbidity and mortality associated with extrauterine pregnancy are directly related to the length of time required for diagnosis. In a Centers for Disease Control survey, two thirds of all patients who were later proven to have an ectopic pregnancy were previously seen by a physician, and either the diagnosis was deferred or the condition was incorrectly assessed. The mortality rate from an ectopic pregnancy is higher in rural areas, where patients are less likely to receive early medical care.

For a successful outcome, an ectopic pregnancy must be diagnosed early. In some clinics where the condition is treated frequently, more than 50% of cases are diag-

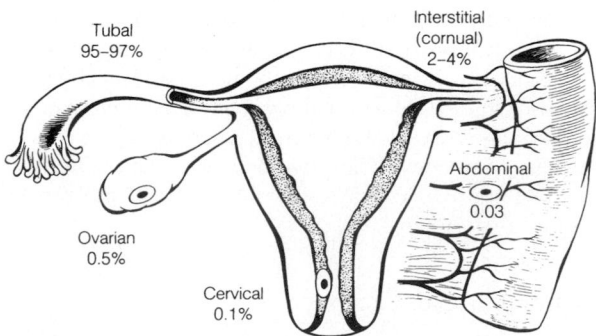

FIGURE 22.1. Sites and incidence of ectopic pregnancy.

nosed and treated before tubal rupture occurs. In some cases, however, the symptoms that bring a patient to seek medical care are caused by an already leaking or ruptured ectopic pregnancy. As many as 15% of all tubal pregnancies rupture before the first missed menstrual period, particularly if a patient's usual menstrual pattern is very irregular.

Diagnostic accuracy is often improved in repeat ectopic pregnancies. The vast majority of patients with repeat ectopic pregnancies will be diagnosed and treated before tubal rupture. A difference with a repeat ectopic pregnancy is that the patient herself often raises the question of an extrauterine pregnancy. Being suspicious, the patient may seek medical care earlier and provides a more specific medical history than does a patient experiencing her first ectopic pregnancy. The result is often an earlier diagnosis and an improved chance for a successful outcome.

Some form of vaginal bleeding occurs around the expected time of menses in more than 50% of women with an ectopic pregnancy, so that many patients and their physicians are unaware that a pregnancy has occurred. The vaginal bleeding may be followed by a period of amenorrhea. Clinical symptoms of an ectopic pregnancy usually appear 6 to 10 weeks after the last normal menstrual period.

DIAGNOSIS

Classic Symptoms: Pain, Bleeding, and Adnexal Mass

The classic presentation of pain and uterine bleeding with the finding of an adnexal mass has been the clinical hallmark of an extrauterine pregnancy, but even classic presentations can be misleading. Schwartz and DiPietro observed that of the patients who presented with the classic signs and symptoms, only 14% had an ectopic pregnancy. The severity of the symptoms and signs depends on the stage of the condition, but in the early stages of an ectopic gestation, symptoms are less predictive than in the more advanced stages of the disease. A discrete, unilateral mass separate from the adjacent ovary has been detected in less than one third of all proven ectopic pregnancies. Locating a mass depends on many factors, including the diagnostic skill of the examiner, the degree of pelvic peritonitis present, the presence or absence of tubal rupture, and the degree of stoicism and cooperation of the patient. Even when all factors are optimal, an adnexal mass can be felt in only half of the cases.

Diagnostic Studies

Three major advances have made early diagnosis of extrauterine pregnancy possible: (1) the development of highly sensitive and rapid β-hCG assays; (2) the ability to use ultrasound to evaluate the uterus and the adnexa (vaginal sonography further increases the accuracy of diagnosis); and (3) the application of laparoscopy as a di-

agnostic tool. Culdocentesis or suction curettage, or both, can be useful under certain circumstances (e.g., to help establish the presence of a hemoperitoneum or a nonviable intrauterine pregnancy, respectively). Other newer diagnostic methods, such as serum progesterone assays or color Doppler flow analyses, can also provide useful information.

β-hCG Assays

The principal endocrine marker of pregnancy is human chorionic gonadotropin (hCG), which is synthesized by the trophoblast. Human chorionic gonadotropin is a glycoprotein consisting of two subunits: α and β. The α subunit has significant homology with other glycoprotein hormones, such as follicle-stimulating hormone, luteinizing hormone and thyroid-stimulating hormone. The β-subunit, on the other hand, is specific to hCG, and antibodies against the β-subunit form the basis for current radioimmunoassay and monoclonal antibody laboratory assays. A radioimmunoassay for β-hCG can detect levels of hCG as low as 5 to 10 IU/L of serum with less than a 0.5% incidence of false-negative results. β-hCG can be detected in maternal serum as early as 7 to 8 days after ovulation, or approximately the day after blastocyst implantation. One-step qualitative urinary pregnancy tests, which positively identify a threshold level of hCG of 20 to 50 IU/L, have also become available and have been successfully used in an emergency department setting as the initial step in triaging women of reproductive age who present with abdominal pain or abnormal vaginal bleeding.

The quantification of serum β-hCG levels is useful in determining the viability of pregnancy. To optimally use β-hCG data in treating a patient with a problematic pregnancy, one should first have a thorough understanding of the particular assay used. The World Health Organization has established reference standards for β-hCG assays. The Third International Standard (Third IS) is the most commonly used reference standard used by the available commercial kits of today. This standard is roughly equivalent to the First International Reference Preparation (First IRP), but is quite a bit different from the Second International Standard (Second IS). The Second IS contains about 20% intact hCG and was initially developed for use in hCG bioassays. One international unit of β-hCG based on the First IRP is equal to approximately 0.58 IU of β-hCG using the Second IS. Fortunately, the Second IS has been exhausted and is no longer used but can still be found in some studies and publications. The First IRP and Third IS are highly purified preparations that were developed to overcome the deficiencies seen in the use of a heterogeneous standard.

Serum hCG concentrations increase in an exponential fashion in early pregnancy. During the period of gestation in which the hCG concentration is less than 10,000 IU/L (First IRP), or about 25 to 30 days postovulation, the time required for doubling of hCG levels remains constant, with a mean of 1.9 days. Kadar, Caldwell and Romero reported that 87% of women with ectopic pregnancies and 15% of women with normal intrauterine pregnancies could expect to have hCG doubling times of more than 2.7 days when the hCG concentration measured less than 6000 IU/L. The lower limits of the increase in serum hCG for viable intrauterine pregnancies have also been established in the authors' laboratory by use of the First IRP. Serum quantitative β-hCG levels appear to increase between 30% and 50% (mean, 39.1%) for an interval of 24 hours in a normal intrauterine pregnancy. A more meaningful interval determination is at 48 hours with a minimum 66% (range, 65% to 100%) increase over preceding hCG values expected. Interval β-hCG determinations interpreted within the context of several values can therefore be of prognostic significance in the differentiation between normal intrauterine versus extrauterine pregnancies. A normal rise in hCG production, however, does not always differentiate an ectopic from a viable intrauterine pregnancy. Shepherd and associates reported that, in their experience, a normal rise in hCG production did not reliably differentiate an ectopic from a viable intrauterine pregnancy in the symptomatic patient. Early ectopic pregnancies can initially secrete appropriate amounts of hCG because of a well-vascularized placental bed.

Serum Progesterone Assay

Serum progesterone levels reflect the production of progesterone by the corpus luteum in early pregnancy. During the first 8 to 10 weeks of gestation, serum progesterone concentrations change little; as pregnancy fails, the levels decrease. Matthews, Coulson and Weld reported progesterone levels in 29 patients with ectopic pregnancy using a direct radioimmunoassay that offers results within 4 hours. Patients with normal intrauterine pregnancies had serum progesterone levels greater than 20 ng/mL, and all patients with ectopic pregnancies had progesterone levels less than 15 ng/mL. Yeko and associates proposed that all ectopic pregnancies could be potentially diagnosed at the first emergency visit with a single serum progesterone determination using a discriminatory value of 15 ng/mL. Other authors, however, have demonstrated some overlap in the serum progesterone concentrations in ectopic and normal intrauterine pregnancies. One large study by Gelder, Boots, and Younger reported that 98% of patients with a normal intrauterine pregnancy had progesterone levels greater than 10 ng/mL, and that 98% of patients with ectopic pregnancies not associated with ovulation induction had progesterone levels less than 20 ng/mL. Unfortunately, 31% of viable intrauterine pregnancies, 23% of abnormal intrauterine pregnancies, and 51% of ectopic pregnancies in this series had progesterone levels that fell between 10 and 20 ng/mL, which greatly limited the clinical usefulness of the test. Hahlin, Sjoblom and Lindblom reported that a serum progesterone value of less than 9.4 ng/mL combined with an abnormal hCG increase had a positive predictive value of 1.0 for pathologic pregnancy. In 1992, Stovall and colleagues reported that in a group of more than 1,000 first-trimester pregnant patients, the lowest serum proges-

terone level associated with a viable pregnancy was 5.1 ng/mL. Therefore, these investigators established the lower cutoff limit of serum progesterone levels of 5 ng/mL; patients below this threshold had a nonviable pregnancy with 100% certainty and therefore underwent curettage. Patients with serum progesterone levels greater than 25 ng/mL had a 97% likelihood of having a viable intrauterine pregnancy in this study.

Transvaginal Ultrasonography

Pelvic ultrasound has revolutionized the diagnostic process of ectopic pregnancy. Transvaginal ultrasonography, in particular, may identify masses in the adnexa as small as 10 mm in diameter and can provide more detail about the character of the mass than clinical exam (Fig. 22.2). At the same time, transvaginal ultrasonography can evaluate the contents of the endometrial cavity and can document the presence of a viable intrauterine pregnancy with great accuracy. In addition, transvaginal ultrasonography allows for the simultaneous assessment for the presence of free peritoneal fluid.

Transvaginal ultrasonography is usually considered superior to transabdominal ultrasonography in the diagnosis of ectopic pregnancy. Although the latter provides a broader perspective of the abdominal cavity and pelvis, transvaginal ultrasonography generally provides better resolution of the internal female genitalia. A 5-MHz transvaginal transducer allows for a deeper penetration of the pelvis than transducers of higher frequency, whereas a 7.5 MHz transvaginal transducer provides for better near-resolution at the cost of shallower penetration. On rare occasions, an ectopic pregnancy may be located beyond the reach of the transvaginal transducer's scanning field. On these particular occasions, incorporation of transabdominal ultrasonography may be an important adjunctive step.

Jain, Hamper and Sanders compared endovaginal and transabdominal ultrasound results in 90 patients

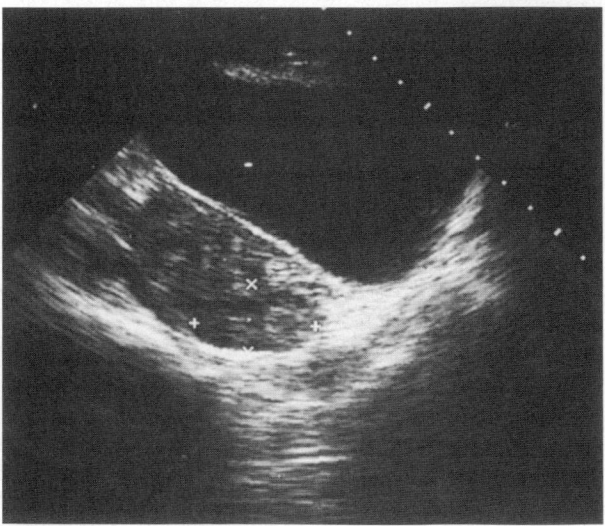

FIGURE 22.2. Tubal ectopic pregnancy documented by endovaginal sonography.

with a positive serum pregnancy test (Table 22.3). The specific diagnosis of ectopic pregnancy was impossible utilizing only transabdominal ultrasound before 7 gestational weeks. Normal intrauterine pregnancies could be detected earlier with endovaginal ultrasound because the yolk sac, fetal pole, and fetal heart motion could be seen sooner. Fetal heart motion was detected as early as 34 days after the last menstrual period in patients with identifiable fetal poles at the time the crown to rump length was 0.3 cm.

Although diagnosis by transvaginal ultrasound can be quite useful, it may at times be confusing. One problem is that a "pseudo" gestational sac due to a decidual cast can be mistaken for an amniotic sac. A useful differentiating feature is the "double-line" image, caused by the faint hypoechoic decidual lining of the uterus and the hyperechogenic rim of the trophoblast surrounding the gestational sac. The "double-line" image can be seen as early as 5 weeks after the last menstrual period. Even in the presence of the "double-line" image, however, it is important to further follow the course of pregnancy and subsequently confirm a viable intrauterine pregnancy with the ascertainment of ultrasonographically-imaged intrauterine cardiac motion.

Although not always seen, Frates and Laing reported that the presence of a non-cystic extraovarian adnexal mass, extrauterine cardiac motion, or a "tubal ring" by transvaginal ultrasonography is highly specific for ectopic pregnancy (98.9%), with a high positive predictive value

TABLE 22.3.
Pregnancy Earliest Seen with Ultrasonography

Early Intrauterine Pregnancy	Endovaginal	Transabdominal
GESTATIONAL SAC SEEN		
Gestational sac size	0.5 cm	0.5 cm
Gestational sac age	4.3 wk	4.3 wk
DOUBLE DECIDUAL OUTLINE		
Gestational sac size	0.6–0.7 cm	1.0 cm
Gestational sac age	4.4 wk	5.0 wk
YOLK SAC SEEN		
Gestational sac size	0.7 cm	1.0 cm
Gestational sac age	4.6 wk (34 d)	5.0 wk (35 d)
FETAL POLE SEEN		
Gestational sac size	0.7 cm	1.7 cm
Gestational sac age	4.6 wk	6.0 wk
FETAL HEART MOTION SEEN		
Crown-rump length	0.3 cm	0.6 cm
Gestational sac age	4.6 wk (34 d)	6.5 wk (47 d)

(Jain K, Hamper VM, Sanders RC. Comparison of transvaginal and transabdominal sonography in the detection of early pregnancy and its complications. *Am J Radiol* 1988;151:1139–1143.)

(96.3%). These authors described that the direct imaging of the ectopic pregnancy utilizing any of these differentiating features is possible in 84% of cases.

Many authors have reported on correlations between threshold levels of hCG above which an intrauterine gestational sac is expected by ultrasonography in a normal pregnancy (discriminatory zone). Early on, Kadar, DeVore and Romero described a threshold level of hCG above which an intrauterine gestational sac was expected by abdominal sonography in a normal pregnancy (discriminatory zone). This threshold hCG level was initially characterized as a titer of 6500 IU/L or higher using the First IRP. Presently, transvaginal ultrasonography reliably detects intrauterine gestations as early as 1 week after missed menses (β-hCG $\geq$ 1500 IU/L ; 5-6 weeks gestation). Barnhart and associates reported that with a β-hCG concentration of 1500 IU/L or higher, an empty uterus on transvaginal ultrasonography indentified an ectopic pregnancy with 100% accuracy. Even using a discriminatory serum β-hCG concentration of 1000 IU/L, Cacciatore, Stenman and Ylostalo indentified an intrauterine gestation in all intrauterine pregnancies and in none of the ectopic pregnancies. Furthermore, these investigators reported that the detection of an adnexal mass in combination with an empty uterus had a sensitivity of 97%, specificity of 99%, positive predictive value of 98% and negative predictive value of 98% provided serum β-hCG concentrations exceeded 1000 IU/L. The coupling of hCG titers with transvaginal ultrasonographic findings has therefore greatly facilitated the early diagnosis of ectopic gestation. It must be stressed, however, that considering the variations in β-hCG assays, ultrasound equipment and sonographer experience, each institution must determine their own discriminatory thresholds for the sonographic detection of an intrauterine pregnancy.

The advent of color-flow Doppler technology may even further improve the accuracy of noninvasive diagnostic methods. Kurjak, Zalud and Schulman reported that ectopic pregnancies are characterized by the identification of peritrophoblastic flow associated with an adnexal mass by color Doppler techniques. Kirchler and coworkers showed that color Doppler qualitative blood flow analyses of the tubal arteries can help localize the side of a tubal ectopic pregnancy. These investigators reported a between-side difference in tubal blood flow of 20% to 45%, with increased blood flow seen on the side of the ectopic pregnancy. Emerson and colleagues demonstrated that color flow Doppler capability can help differentiate between viable intrauterine pregnancy, completed abortion, incomplete abortion, and ectopic pregnancy by analyzing uterine color Doppler appearance, intrauterine venous flow, the presence or absence of intrauterine peritrophoblastic flow, corpus luteal flow, and the presence or absence of peritrophoblastic flow in the adnexa. Pellerito and associates reported that color flow imaging increased the sensitivity of detecting an ectopic pregnancy. Of 65 patients with surgically confirmed ectopic pregnancies, 36 (sensitivity, 54%) cases were detected by endovaginal sonography alone, whereas 62 (sensitivity, 95%) cases were detected by a combination of endovaginal sonography and color flow imaging.

Dilation and Curettage

At one time, the histologic changes in the endometrium that accompany an ectopic gestation were routinely confirmed by dilatation and curettage (D&C). Today, more accurate diagnostic methods, such as the radioimmunoassay for β-hCG, transvaginal ultrasonography and laparoscopy exist. In this setting, a D&C may therefore not always be necessary. If, however, the plateau level of β-hCG is low, a D&C can be helpful to establish the presence of degenerating villi, and if a patient is bleeding excessively, a D&C may also be required. In either case, assessment of the removed material and findings of decidua without chorionic villi suggests the diagnosis of ectopic pregnancy. Such findings do not provide absolute proof, however, because they also occur with spontaneous abortion.

A frozen section may be obtained immediately after curettage, providing an opportunity to confirm the diagnosis within minutes while the patient is still in the operating room under anesthesia. If no chorionic villi is present, further assessment and treatment by laparoscopy may be undertaken. In a recent report of 87 consecutive frozen section samples taken from uterine curettings, Spandorfer and colleagues found that 93.1% of these specimens were identified correctly after further analyses of the tissue by permanent section.

The atypical epithelial changes of the gestational endometrium in a case of tubal pregnancy were first described by Polak and Wolfe in 1924 and were further expanded upon by Arias-Stella in 1954 (Fig. 22.3). These comprise a highly controversial set of histologic criteria which depends for its accuracy on the precise definition of the particular cell type involved in the morphologic change, together with ill-defined physiologic events that reportedly produce the changes. Arias-Stella and others were convinced that these histologic changes are a progressive phenomenon resulting from the exaggerated proliferative and secretory endometrial responses to the elevated hormonal levels of pregnancy. Fienberg and Lloyd disagreed, maintaining that these endometrial changes are regressive, involutional and are the result of declining hormonal levels. Whichever hypothesis is ultimately proven, similar endometrial changes may be seen with a normal pregnancy, spontaneous abortion or ectopic pregnancy. Histologic endometrial criteria, therefore, seems to have limited value in the specific diagnosis of extrauterine pregnancies.

Culdocentesis

Culdocentesis is a diagnostic tool for identifying the presence of intraperitoneal bleeding. This simple procedure of inserting an 18-gauge spinal needle attached to a 50 mL aspirating syringe into the cul-de-sac between the uterosacral ligaments (Fig. 22.4) provides immediate clinical information when unclotted blood is aspirated from the cul-de-sac. The procedure cannot be used for a definitive diagnosis, of course, because a tubal pregnancy may not have ruptured or leaked into the peritoneal cavity. In addition, a culdocentesis does not provide information concerning whether the blood is from an ectopic pregnancy or from some other cause of intraabdominal

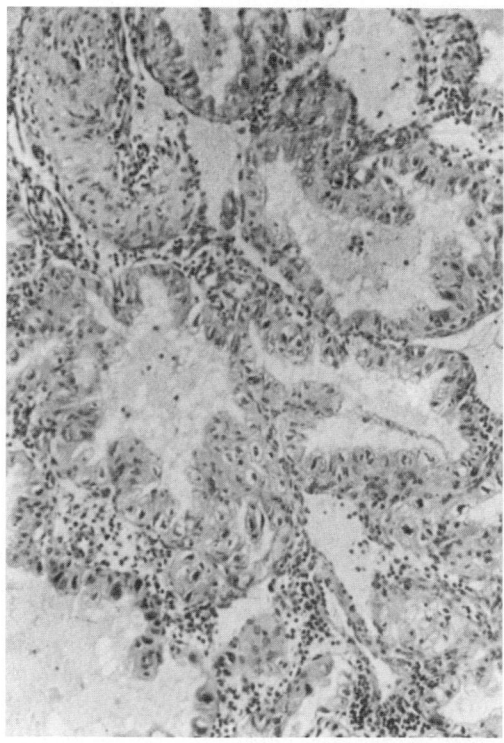

FIGURE 22.3. Arias-Stella reaction in endometrial cells associated with ectopic pregnancy, showing nuclear enlargement, irregularity, and hyperchromasia with cytoplasmic vacuolation.

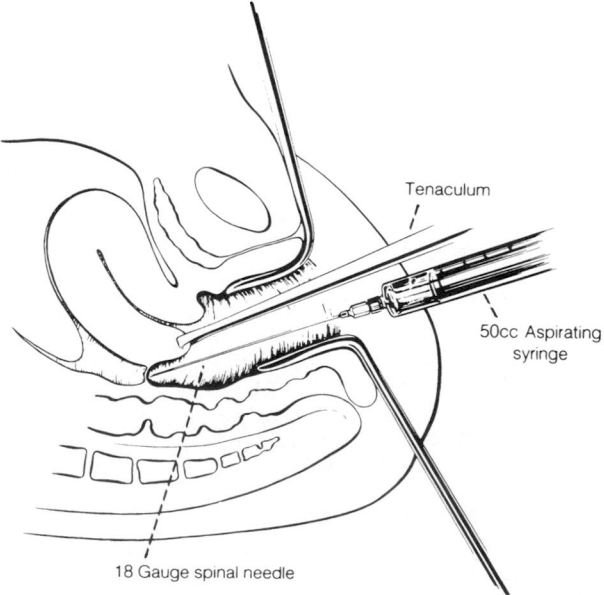

Tenaculum

50cc Aspirating syringe

18 Gauge spinal needle

FIGURE 22.4. Culdocentesis. An 18-gauge spinal needle is inserted through the posterior fornix and enters the cul-de-sac between the uterosacral ligaments.

bleeding. The rupture of a corpus luteal hemorrhaghic cyst, for instance, may cause a similar bleeding pattern.

The availability of sensitive transvaginal ultrasonographic technology presently limits the specific usefulness of the culdocentesis procedure. Free intraperitoneal blood has a characteristic ultrasonographic appearance and can be seen in nearly all cases in which a significant intraperitoneal hemorrhage has occurred. In the absence of the immediate availability of transvaginal ultrasonography or in an emergency setting, however, culdocentesis can still be of significant value.

Laparoscopy

Laparoscopy remains the "gold standard" in the detection of ectopic pregnancy, although non-invasive diagnostic methods continue to improve. In addition to permitting the diagnosis of an ectopic pregnancy, it enables surgical treatment. Laparoscopy also provides an opportunity to visualize the entire pelvis and other peritoneal organs. In particular, the condition of the unaffected fallopian tube can be assessed, as well as the presence of pelvic adhesions and endometriosis. This information may be particularly valuable for those patients interested in future fertility. The disadvantage of laparoscopy is that it is an invasive procedure which carries some risk of complications. Utilizing standard methods, it requires general anesthesia and an operating room setting, thereby contributing to increased medical costs. Recent investigators, however, have been exploring the potential of "microlaparoscopy," in which improved optics and smaller diameter laparoscopes and trocars allow for a definitive diagnosis and possible treatment in the non-operating room setting. Several authors have reported the encouraging use of "microlaparoscopy" in the office setting, utilizing primarily local rather than general anesthesia. The specific utility of "microlaparoscopy", however, for the primary evaluation and treatment of ectopic pregnancy remains to be established.

Laparoscopy may be useful when an ectopic pregnancy is suspected but no signs of an ultrasonographically visualized extrauterine gestational sac is evident. This includes situations in which there is an inability to visualize an intrauterine gestational sac and serial β-hCG determinations are rising inappropriately. This also includes situations in which a D & C fails to indentify products of conception. One must be careful, however, in settings in which the β-hCG determinations are very low or the gestational age is limited. In these settings, the ectopically implanted gestational mass may be so small that it is not able be seen at laparoscopy. The clinician and patient might therefore be falsely reassured by negative laparoscopic findings. All patients without a definitive diagnosis established at laparoscopy should be followed closely.

Other Potential Diagnostic Aids

Gleicher, Parilli and Pratt described the use of hysterosalpingography and selective salpingography in differentiating early (biochemical) intrauterine from failing intratubal gestations. A characteristic tubal opacification pattern was seen in the cases of early tubal pregnancy. Confino and coworkers reported that selective salpingography was useful in diagnosing early tubal pregnancies in some patients with equivocal clinical, laboratory, and sonographic findings. In addition, these investigators injected a single dose of methotrexate through the selective salpingography catheter after cannulation of the tubal ostia and identification of a characteristic ampullary radiolucency in seven patients. Each had subsequent complete resolution of the pregnancy without complication. Risquez and colleagues reported the successful visualization of two ectopic pregnancies by transcervical tubal cannulation and falloposcopy. The falloposcope is a microendoscopic instrument 0.5 mm in external diameter that is introduced by a 1 mm coaxial catheter. Although limited by the presence of blood in the tubal lumen, direct visualization of the ectopic pregnancies was accomplished in both cases and confirmed by concurrent laparoscopy. Other investigative teams have explored the potential of other imaging methods, such as magnetic resonance imaging (MRI), in the diagnostic work-up for ectopic pregnancy. MRI might be useful if the sonographic image is inconclusive, although it is likely to be rarely needed, particularly if laparoscopy is generally considered in uncertain cases.

Summary of Diagnostic Methods for Detecting Tubal Ectopic Pregnancy

When a patient is seen with a clinical history suggestive of ectopic pregnancy, a careful examination is performed (Fig. 22.5). Quantitative serum β-hCG and rapid serum progesterone levels (if available) are obtained. If the β-hCG titre is positive, a transvaginal ultrasound is performed. If an intrauterine sac is visualized with fetal heart activity, then the diagnosis of intrauterine pregnancy is established. If, however, there are no intrauterine sacs or there is a questionable intrauterine sac without fetal heart activity, then the asymptomatic patient may be expectantly treated awaiting further testing. If the serum progesterone level is, with certainty, below the threshold level for viability, then a uterine curettage can be performed. The subsequent failure to find chorionic villi on curettage is very suggestive, but not diagnostic, of an ectopic pregnancy. If the serum progesterone level is more than 25 ng/mL in the absence of ovulation induction, then there is a strong likelihood that a viable pregnancy is present. If the quantitative serum β-hCG level is above the discriminatory zone for a particular institution and no intrauterine gestational sacs are apparent using transvaginal ultrasonography, then an ectopic pregnancy is likely. The level of hCG at which a intrauterine gestational sac should be visible varies, however, depending on the β-hCG assay and the method of pelvic ultrasonography. Most contemporary investigators report that with transvaginal ultrasonography, an intrauterine gestational sac should be identified at a β-hCG level of 1500 IU/L (Third IS) with high sensitivity and specificity.

Commonly, results from initial testing are equivocal. The ectopic pregnancy can produce a low level of

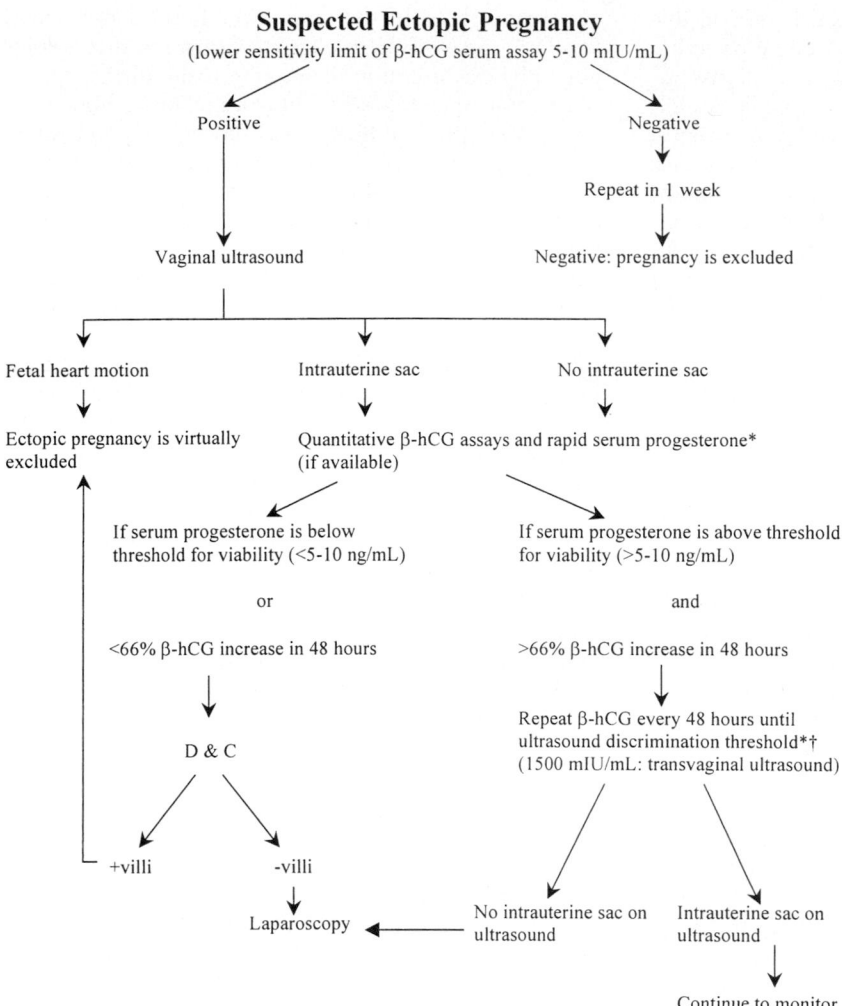

Suspected Ectopic Pregnancy
(lower sensitivity limit of β-hCG serum assay 5-10 mIU/mL)

Positive

Negative

Repeat in 1 week

Vaginal ultrasound

Negative: pregnancy is excluded

Fetal heart motion

Intrauterine sac

No intrauterine sac

Ectopic pregnancy is virtually excluded

Quantitative β-hCG assays and rapid serum progesterone*
(if available)

If serum progesterone is below threshold for viability (<5-10 ng/mL)

If serum progesterone is above threshold for viability (>5-10 ng/mL)

or

and

<66% β-hCG increase in 48 hours

>66% β-hCG increase in 48 hours

D & C

Repeat β-hCG every 48 hours until ultrasound discrimination threshold*†
(1500 mIU/mL: transvaginal ultrasound)

+villi

-villi

Laparoscopy

No intrauterine sac on ultrasound

Intrauterine sac on ultrasound

Continue to monitor

FIGURE 22.5. Evaluation of the stable patient with suspected ectopic pregnancy. Hormonal parameters can vary depending on the assay technique and reference standard used. The discriminatory threshold for sonographic detection of an intrauterine gestational sac must be established by each institution.

β-hCG from the aborting or degenerating trophoblast. The differential diagnosis should include spontaneous abortion or blighted ovum. When the diagnosis is uncertain and the patient is in an unstable condition or significant intraperitoneal fluid is seen, then evaluation should proceed immediately by laparoscopy and, if necessary, by laparotomy. If the patient is in stable condition, tests for serial β-hCG levels should be taken at 48-hour intervals and the assays should be correlated with the patient's previous values. If the hCG level increases more than 66% within a 48-hour period, then the patient probably has a normal intrauterine pregnancy, and nonsurgical care is indicated. If the increase in the serial hCG level is less than 66% of the original value, then an ectopic pregnancy should be suspected. Ultrasound can often then corroborate the diagnosis, with the demonstration of a gestational sac in the adnexa or fluid in the cul-de-sac.

Initially, a normal increase in the β-hCG level may be observed. Over time, however, the level may slowly fall, never reaching the discriminatory zone. If a possible in-

trauterine pregnancy is thought to be nonviable, then a D&C can be performed. If there is any question of viability, however, laparoscopy is preferred to rule out ectopic pregnancy first. Once fetal heart motion is observed within the uterine cavity, the possibility of a tubal ectopic pregnancy is virtually excluded. Certain patients should continue to be observed closely, however, particularly after a superovulation regimen, which is associated with an increased risk of a simultaneous intrauterine and ectopic pregnancy. Nevertheless, the overall risk of the two existing simultaneously even after a superovulation regimen is quite small.

The use of vaginal ultrasonography with improved resolution and the addition of color Doppler flow analysis will invariably further define a lower discriminatory zone in the future. Both modalities appear to complement each other in attaining improved sensitivity and specificity in the diagnosis of ectopic pregnancy. Other investigative diagnostic techniques, such as selective salpingography and falloposcopy, should be considered strictly experimental.

TREATMENT FOR ECTOPIC PREGNANCY

Expectant Therapy

Prior to the advent of effective therapy for ectopic pregnancy, it was noted that the condition was not uniformly fatal and that some patients had spontaneous resolution of the ectopic gestation, either through spontaneous regression or tubal abortion. The natural history of ectopic pregnancy therefore suggests that a number of tubal pregnancies can resolve without treatment. In 1988, Fernandez and associates observed a spontaneous resolution of ectopic pregnancy in 64% of carefully selected patients. The mean time for resolution was 20 ± 13 days. Spontaneous resolution occurred more frequently when the initial hCG concentration was less than 1000 IU/L. The authors observed that a β-hCG threshold of 1000 mIU/mL and a hemoperitoneum of less than 50 mL with a hematosalpinx of less than 2 cm appeared to be most compatible with successful expectant management.

Subsequent larger studies have demonstrated similar results with expectant therapy. Korhonen, Stenman and Ylostalo have published the largest series to date. Criteria for patient selection included decreasing β-hCG levels, an absent intrauterine pregnancy by transvaginal ultrasonography, and an adnexal mass of less than 4 cm without an embryonic heartbeat. Seventy-seven (65%) of 118 patients had spontaneous resolution of the ectopic pregnancy. The remaining patients had laparoscopy for either increasing abdominal pain, increasing cul-de-sac fluid volume or plateauing or increasing β-hCG levels. One patient required a salpingectomy for a ruptured ectopic pregnancy. Similar to other reports, these authors also noted an increased expectant management success rate with lower initial β-hCG concentrations.

Medical Treatment

Systemic Medical Therapy

Methotrexate (MTX) is a folic acid antagonist that can be administered to eradicate trophoblastic tissue in an ectopic pregnancy. MTX is the chemotherapeutic agent of choice in the treatment of gestational trophoblastic disease. Long-term follow-up of women who have taken MTX for gestational trophoblastic disease has failed to demonstrate an increase in congenital malformations, spontaneous abortions, or second tumors after chemotherapy.

Tanaka and colleagues reported the first use of systemic MTX for an ectopic pregnancy in 1982. This group successfully treated an interstitial pregnancy with a course of systemic MTX. Shortly thereafter, Farabow and coworkers described the use of systemic MTX in the treatment of a cervical pregnancy. Ory and associates reported the use of high-dose, short-course MTX therapy (plus citrovorum factor) to resolve small unruptured ectopic pregnancies without the need for conservative surgery. Six patients with ampullary pregnancies were treated, and resolution of the ectopic pregnancy was achieved in five patients. Surgical intervention was required in the sixth patient. Two of the five patients who experienced resolution, however, had protracted courses and required blood transfusions. Sauer and associates also reported the use of systemic MTX and citrovorum factor (CF) in 21 patients with ectopic pregnancy. Inclusion criteria included β-hCG levels that were reaching a plateau or slightly rising, laparoscopic confirmation of the ectopic pregnancy, and a tubal diameter of less than 3 cm with the tubal serosa intact and no evidence of bleeding. Treatment consisted of 1.0 mg/kg MTX administered intramuscularly on postoperative days 1, 3, 5, and 7, along with 0.1 mg/kg CF administered intramuscularly on postoperative days 2, 4, 6, and 8. Twenty of 21 pregnancies resolved without the need for laparotomy. Two patients required blood transfusions, including one patient who required laparotomy and salpingectomy for a hemoperitoneum. In both of these cases, fetal heart activity in the adnexa was identified initially on ultrasound examination. This led the authors to suggest that MTX+CF can be safely used in selected cases of unruptured ectopic pregnancies that have not formed fetal elements that can be visualized by ultrasound.

In 1991, Stovall and colleagues reviewed the results of several series of tubal ectopic pregnancies treated with MTX + CF. Of 100 cases, 50 were diagnosed by laparoscopy, and 50 were diagnosed by a nonlaparoscopic algorithm. Complete resolution was achieved in 96 patients over a range of 14 to 92 days. In four patients, laparotomy was necessary because of tubal rupture; in one case, rupture occurred as late as 23 days after MTX administration. In five patients, cardiac activity was observed on ultrasound, and treatment was successful in four of them. Three patients experienced minor side effects. In 49 of 58 (84%) women who underwent subsequent hysterosalpingograms, tubal patency was demonstrated on the ipsilateral side. Of 56 patients desiring to conceive, 37 subsequently became pregnant; 33 of these were intrauterine pregnancies and 4 were repeat ectopic pregnancies.

Stovall and Ling later studied the efficacy and safety of a simplified regimen of single-dose systemic methotrexate. All patients were diagnosed with a nonlaparoscopic algorithm by the use of serial hCG titers, serum progesterone, transvaginal ultrasonography, and curettage. Patients were treated with a single dose of 50 mg/m² MTX intramuscularly if they were hemodynamically stable and the unruptured ectopic pregnancy did not exceed 3.5 cm in diameter. In the initial report, one hundred twenty patients were treated, including 14 (11.7%) with visualized cardiac activity. One hundred thirteen (94.2%) patients had compete resolution with treatment, with a mean time to resolution of 35.5 days. Four (3.3%) of the successfully treated patients required a second course of MTX on day 7. Seven (5.8%) patients required surgical management of the ectopic pregnancy, including two of the patients with cardiac activity. No major chemotherapy-related side effects were seen. Posttreatment hysterosalpingograms demonstrated tubal patency on the ipsilateral side in 51 of 62 (82.3%) patients. Of those attempting pregnancy, 79.6% subsequently became pregnant; 87.2% of these were intrauterine and 12.8% were ectopic.

Lipscomb and colleagues further reported on the expanded Memphis cohort of patients treated with "single-dose" methotrexate. They utilized similar inclusion criteria, with the exception of further allowing pregnancies up to 4.0 cm in diameter provided that ectopic cardiac activity was not present. In this series, 287 of 315 (90.1%) patients were successfully treated with methotrexate. Forty-four patients with positive ectopic cardiac activity were treated with an 87.5% success rate. Of note, however, is that approximately 20% of these patients required more than one cycle of treatment. The authors' protocol reported that following the methotrexate dosing on day 1, serum chorionic gonadotropin was measured on days 1, 4 and 7. In many patients, they noted that β-hCG levels frequently continued to rise until day 4. If the chorionic gonadotropin levels then declined less than 15% between days 4 and 7, the MTX protocol was repeated. If the levels declined 15 percent or more between days 4 and 7, serum β-hCG was measured weekly until the level was less than 15 IU/L. If the chorionic gonadotropin level declined less than 15% during any subsequent week of follow-up, the MTX protocol was also then repeated. Other potentially difficult issues with "single-dose" methotrexate therapy include the management of "resolution pain" (which may occur in 20% of patients) and the prolonged time to resolution sometimes seen.

A further review of the variables related to the success of single-dose methotrexate in the treatment of singleton ectopic pregnancy has been compiled. In this review, logistic regression analysis demonstrated that the serum chorionic gonadotropin level before treatment was the only factor that contributed significantly to the failure rate (Table 22.4). Interestingly, the size and volume of the mass, the volume of hematoma, and the presence or absence of free peritoneal blood in the pelvis were not associated with a significant risk of treatment failure.

Methotrexate has also been used to treat persistent ectopic pregnancy after conservative surgery. In these patients, persistent ectopic pregnancy results from proliferation of residual trophoblastic tissue remaining after a conservative surgical procedure. The trophoblast can be located within the muscular layer of the oviduct or between the muscularis and the serosa such that at the time of salpingotomy, only the portion of the trophoblast within the tubal lumen is removed. In those patients with persistent ectopic pregnancy described in the literature, the majority have been managed by a second operation and salpingectomy. Some patients, however, have been treated with either expectant management or methotrexate. Hoppe, Bekkar and Nager have reported the largest methotrexate experience to date for persistent ectopic pregnancy. These authors noted successful treatment in all 19 patients treated following linear salpingotomy. All patients should therefore have a follow-up β-hCG titer 1 to 2 weeks after conservative surgery. If the titer is elevated, then serial β-hCG titers are indicated. If the titer then continues to fall, the patient can be treated expectantly. If the β-hCG level remains the same or increases, however, consideration should be given to a single dose of MTX or perhaps further surgery to remove the remaining portion of the ectopic pregnancy.

Systemic MTX is an alternative that can be used for the treatment of patients with small unruptured ectopic pregnancies or patients with persistant ectopic pregnancies following conservative surgery. Safeguards are necessary to enhance the success and minimize the toxicity of therapy. Patients should be carefully monitored with hematologic indices and liver chemistries. A history of active hepatic, renal, or peptic ulcer disease, elevated baseline liver enzyme concentrations, and thrombocytopenia or neutropenia are contraindications to therapy. Patients should avoid exposure to the sun, because photosensitivity can be a complication. Patients should refrain from sexual intercourse during therapy. Patients should also avoid folate-containing vitamins. Appropriate candidates for systemic medical therapy should also be willing to accept a small risk of tubal rupture and participate in closely monitored follow-up.

Medical Therapy By Local Injection

In 1987, Feichtinger and Kemeter reported the direct injection of MTX under transvaginal ultrasound guidance into an ectopic gestational sac. They instilled 10 mg of MTX and observed resolution of the pregnancy within 2 weeks. Other investigators, including Kojima and colleagues, have reported the successful application of local MTX administered by direct injection at the time of laparoscopy. In 1993, Fernandez and colleagues reported a large series of patients who underwent intratubal MTX at a dose of 1 mg/kg under transvaginal sonographic control. Eighty-three of 100 patients were successfully cured; however, 28 of the 83 successfully cured patients required additional MTX, which was subsequently given intramuscularly.

TABLE 22.4.

Success Rates of Methotrexate Treatment With Ectopic Pregnancies as a Function of Their Initial Serum Chorionic Gonadotropin Concentrations

Serum Chorionic Gonadotropin Concentration (IU/L)	Success Rate (95% confidence interval)
<1000	98 (96–100)
1000–1999	93 (85–100)
2000–4999	92 (86–97)
5000–9999	87 (79–98)
10,000–14,999	82 (65–98)
≥15,000	68 (49–88)

(Modified from Lipscomb GH, McCord ML, Stovall TG, et al. Predictors of success of methotrexate treatment in women with tubal ectopic pregnancies. *N Engl J Med* 1999;341:1974–1978.)

Direct injection of MTX has theoretic advantages over systemic treatment. The concentration of MTX at the site of implantation is many times higher after local injection than after systemic administration. With less systemic distribution of the drug, a smaller therapeutic dose might be necessary and toxicity would be less. Schiff and associates, however, evaluated the pharmacokinetics of MTX after local tubal injection and found that the peak serum level of MTX after local injection was not significantly lower than that of patients who were treated systemically with a similar dose of the drug. In addition, the success rates in practice appear to be unacceptably low. A review by Carson and Buster revealed that only 83% of the direct tubal injection procedures reported were successful.

Several trials have been conducted evaluating other intratubal agents administered for the treatment of ectopic pregnancy. Studies utilizing prostaglandins (prostaglandin $F_{2\alpha}$, 15-methyl-prostaglandin $F_{2\alpha}$) were discouraging due to poor efficacy and serious adverse effects, including cardiac arrhythmia, malignant hypertension, and gastrointestinal symptoms. Other investigators have studied the use of hyperosmolar glucose, a less toxic agent, injected locally into the gestational sac of the ectopic gestation by either laparoscopy or transvaginal ultrasound-guided needle puncture. Lang and colleagues reported a 92% success rate utilizing hyperosmolar glucose by laparoscopic puncture. Gjelland and associates reported successful treatment in 32 (82%) of 39 patients utilizing local hyperosmolar glucose administered by transvaginal ultrasound guidance.

They noted an inverse relationship between initial serum hCG concentrations and successful outcomes. Further larger trials are needed, however, to determine the precise clinical role, if any, of local injection therapies for ectopic pregnancy.

Surgical Treatment

Conservative Surgical Treatment

Conservative management of an unruptured ectopic pregnancy usually consists of one of two possible procedures: linear salpingotomy or segmental resection. A conservative surgical approach is possible when the diagnosis of ectopic pregnancy is made sufficiently early so that rupture of the oviduct has not yet occurred.

LINEAR SALPINGOTOMY. In women who wish to preserve their fertility, conservative surgery by linear salpingotomy is considered the gold standard for the management of a distal tubal pregnancy. Recent studies have reported that the uninvolved tube may be abnormal, either grossly or subclinically, in at least 50% of cases of ectopic pregnancy. Although there have been no randomized studies comparing the fertility outcome after conservative and radical surgery for ectopic pregnancy, most of the available information suggests that the subsequent intrauterine pregnancy rate is higher after conservative surgery (linear salpingotomy).

In 1898, Kelly was among the first to advocate conservative surgery for tubal gestation. He recommended

drainage of the pregnancy per vaginam, particularly for chronic hemorrhage and formation of a pelvic hematoma. More than half a century elapsed before Stromme reported the first successful use of salpingotomy to treat a patient with tubal pregnancy. In 1973, Stromme reported his surgical experience with 36 cases of unruptured tubal pregnancy, 21 of which were treated by conservative salpingotomy. Five were performed when there was only one tube remaining. Only one term pregnancy ensued from the five single-tube procedures, but Stromme's work led to the development of more effective conservative surgical procedures. Stromme reported a rate of 13.5% repeat ectopic pregnancies, which was no higher than the repeat ectopic rate at the time for more radical procedures.

Since the time of Stromme's report, physicians have achieved good success with conservative linear salpingotomy. According to the review by Yao and Tulandi, of the 1,514 patients attempting to conceive following linear salpingotomy, 61.2% had a subsequent intrauterine pregnancy, whereas 15.5% had an ectopic recurrence. On the other hand, only 38.1% of the 3584 patients attempting to conceive following salpingectomy had a subsequent intrauterine pregnancy, although the ectopic recurrence risk was likewise lower (9.8%). In 1993, Silva and colleagues reported a prospective cohort study in which the intrauterine pregnancy rates were 60.0% and 53.8%, and recurrent ectopic rates were 18.3% and 7.7%, in the conservative and radical surgery groups, respectively. Many of the available reports on linear salpingotomy unfortunately do not describe the condition of the uninvolved oviduct. Langer and associates (1982) did include a description of the uninvolved oviduct in their report of 30 patients undergoing salpingotomy. Of the patients in whom the contralateral tube was normal, 80% subsequently had normal pregnancies. When the contralateral tube was damaged or contained peritubal adhesions, only 11 (55%) patients later achieved a viable pregnancy.

Among recent reports of salpingotomy performed on a single remaining oviduct, an intrauterine pregnancy rate of about 50% has been achieved by several investigators, although the results are quite variable and some reports have only a limited number of patients treated. The repeat ectopic pregnancy rate in the single-tube salpingotomy patients appears to be about 20%, a slightly higher rate than that in series of patients with both oviducts.

In general, conservative salpingotomy is the preferred treatment for patients who desire further pregnancies. For results to be optimal, the oviduct should be unruptured and without serosal invasion, and the patient in a surgically stable condition.

TRANSABDOMINAL CONSERVATIVE PROCEDURE. The procedure for linear salpingotomy starts by exposing, elevating, and stabilizing the tube. A linear incision is then made over the distended segment of the tube (Figs. 22.6 and 22.7). The incision is extended through the antimesenteric wall until entry is made into the lumen of

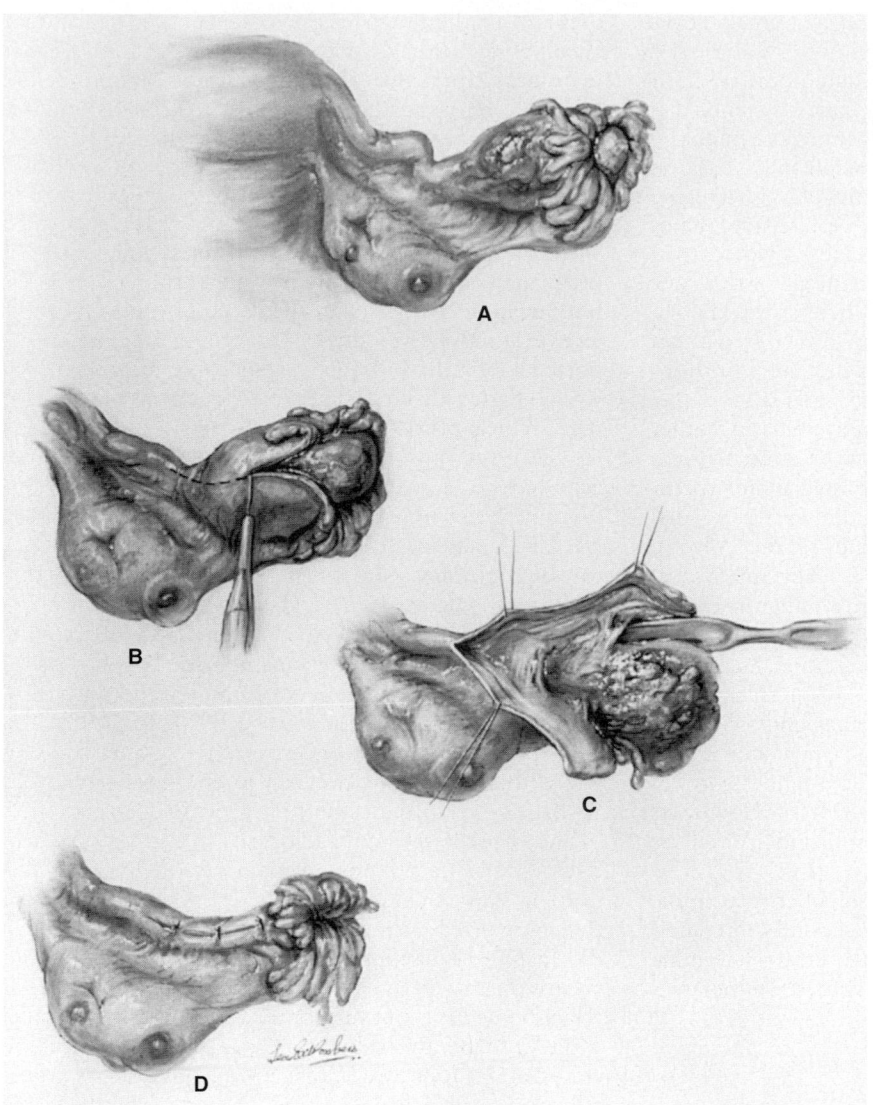

FIGURE 22.6. Removal of ectopic pregnancy of the distal ampulla. **A:** Distal ampulla involved with ectopic pregnancy. **B:** Initial incision on the antimesenteric border. **C:** The gestational contents are carefully removed by use of blunt dissection. **D:** Tubal serosa and muscularis are closed as a single layer with 5-0 nonreactive suture material.

the distended oviduct. When gentle pressure is exerted from the opposite side of the tube, the products of gestation are gently expressed from the lumen. Because a certain amount of separation of the trophoblast has usually occurred, the conceptus generally can be easily removed from the lumen. Gentle traction by suction or by forceps teeth can be used if necessary, but care should be taken to avoid trauma to the mucosa. Any remaining fragments of the anchoring trophoblast should be removed by profuse irrigation of the lumen with warm Ringer's lactate solution to prevent further damage to the mucosa.

Care must be taken to provide complete hemostasis in the tubal mucosa; failure to do so results in troublesome postoperative bleeding, which can lead to the formation of intraluminal adhesions. The small tubal vessels are easily identified while the tube is being irrigated, and loupe magnifying glasses can be used if necessary for better resolution. An operating microscope is usually not needed. Bleeding points can be easily identified with 2 to 4 × magnification.

The mucosal margins are then closed with interrupted sutures, taking care that only the serosa and muscularis are approximated and that there is no undue tension. Care should be taken also to ensure that no suture material is retained on the mucosal surface, because even a small amount can produce a secondary inflammatory reaction with subsequent adhesion formation.

LAPAROSCOPIC CONSERVATIVE PROCEDURE. Currently, most ectopic pregnancies may potentially be treated by laparoscopic surgery. In fact, most studies have suggested that laparoscopic surgery is superior to laparotomy in hemodynamically stable patients. Advantages of laparoscopy include lower cost, shorter hospital stay, less surgical blood loss, less analgesia requirement and a shorter post-operative convalescence. Not all patients, however, may be suitable for laparoscopic treatment. These include patients with an unstable hemodynamic status, those with severe pelvic adhesions as well as those with a specific contraindication to laparoscopy.

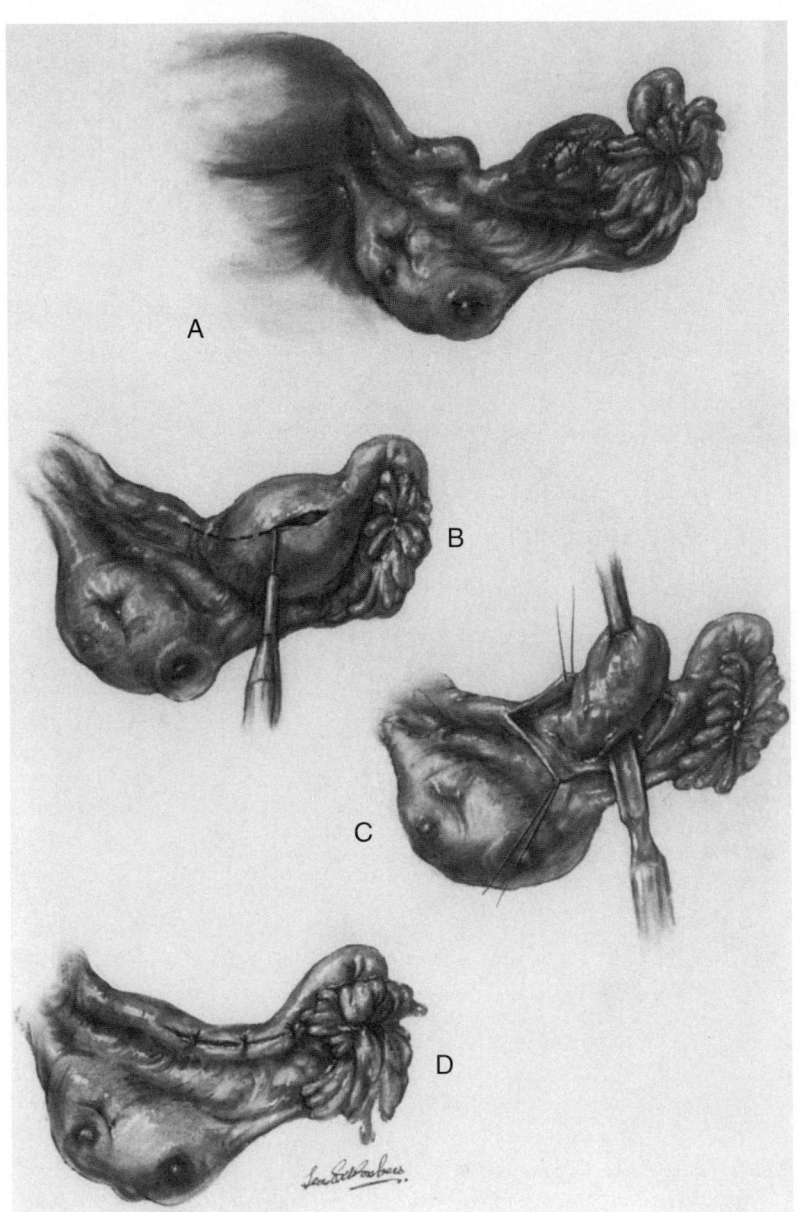

FIGURE 22.7. Removal of a midampullary ectopic pregnancy. **A:** Midampullary ectopic pregnancy. **B:** Antimesenteric incision with fine microdiathermy needle. **C:** The pregnancy is carefully removed by grasping the tissue and lifting while bluntly teasing the trophoblastic tissue away from the endosalpinx. **D:** The serosa and muscularis are closed with interrupted 5-0 nonreactive suture material.

The presence of a hemoperitoneum should not preclude laparoscopic treatment. Utilizing a large-bore suction irrigator, the blood can be evacuated, and the pelvic organs irrigated with a crystalloid solution. Once the ectopic has been documented, two auxiliary puncture sites are made suprapubically to allow manipulation of the fallopian tube (Fig. 22.8). Using a 22-gauge injection needle inserted either directly through the abdominal wall or through a 5-mm portal, a dilute solution of vasopressin (prepared by mixing 20 U of vasopressin with 100 ml of physiologic saline) is injected into the tubal wall at the area of maximal bulge. This step is crucial and allows for minimal bleeding and the precise removal of the ectopic pregnancy without damaging the surrounding mucosa. Either laser, unipolar needle electrocautery, or scissors can than be used to make the salpingotomy

incision. It is important to make the incision along the antimesenteric wall of the tube in the area of maximal distension and large enough to allow for complete extrusion of the products of conception without difficulty. It is also important to keep the fallopian tube taut. If the products of conception do not spontaneously extrude following completion of the incision, either hydrodissection or gentle tubal compression with a blunt probe or suction irrigator will usually work. The tissue is then placed in an endoscopic bag and removed from the abdominal cavity. Special care is taken to remove all of the placental tissue as it is known that persistent peritoneal implants of trophoblastic tissue following laparoscopic salpingotomy may occur. After the tissue is removed, the tube is irrigated carefully and checked for hemostasis. The tube is then either left to heal by secondary inten-

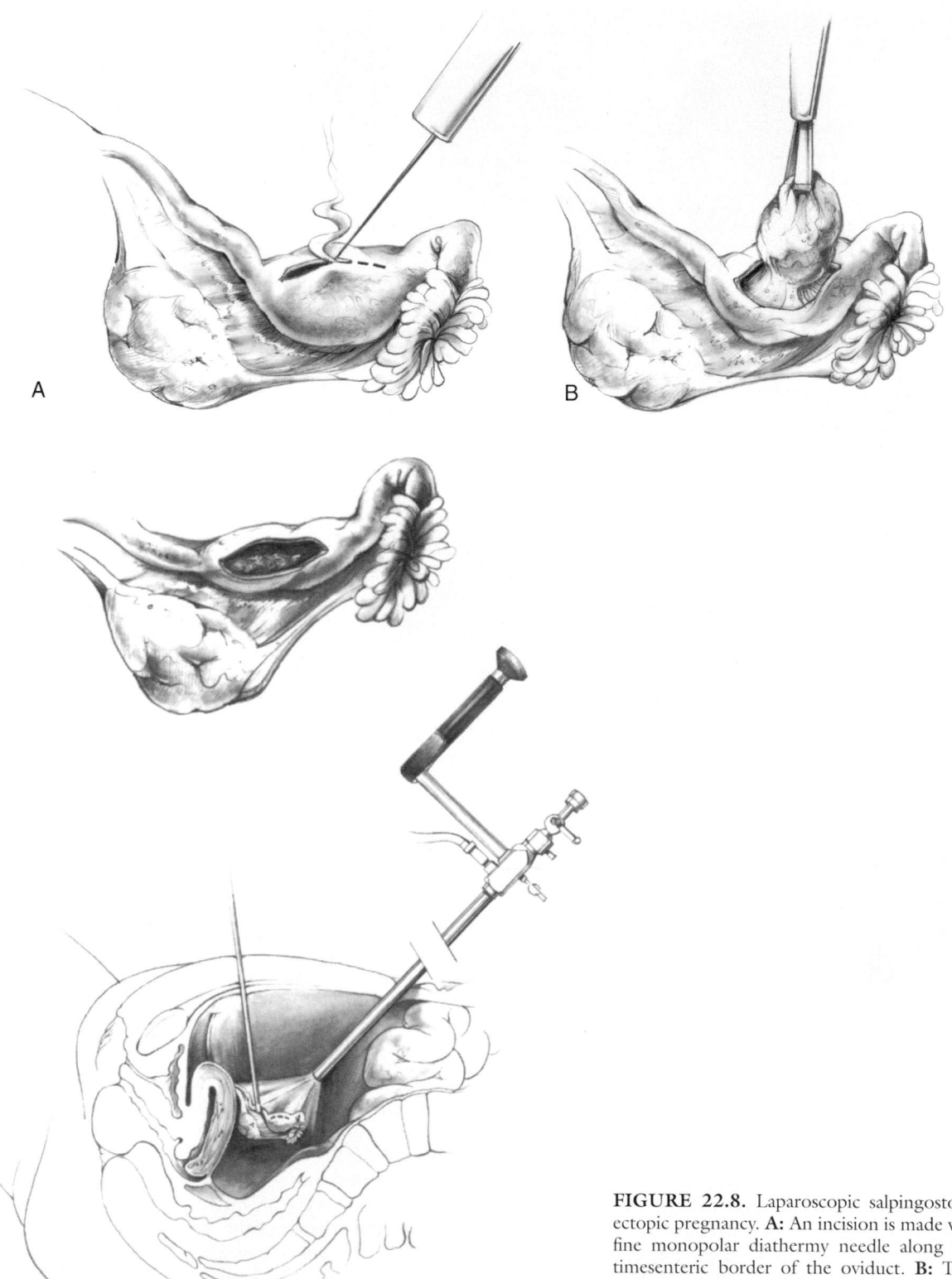

FIGURE 22.8. Laparoscopic salpingostomy for ectopic pregnancy. **A:** An incision is made with the fine monopolar diathermy needle along the antimesenteric border of the oviduct. **B:** The trophoblastic mass is removed with forceps. **C:** The lumen is allowed to heal by secondary intention.

tion or sutured, with secondary intention being appropriate for most cases.

The results of salpingotomy are very similar, whether performed by either laparotomy or laparoscopy. Yao and Tulandi reported that among the 811 patients attempting to conceive after the laparotomy approach, the intrauterine pregnancy rate was 61.4% and the recurrent ectopic pregnancy rate was 15.4%, Similarly, of the 703 patients attempting to conceive following laparoscopy, 61.0% had an intrauterine pregnancy and 15.5% had a repeat ectopic.

PERSISTENT TUBAL ECTOPIC GESTATION. Persistent trophoblastic tissue can remain after linear salpingotomy. Although there can be an initial decrease in the β-hCG level after surgery, the level can then slowly rise, ultimately resulting in symptoms. For this reason, it is recommended to obtain weekly β-hCG measurements after linear salpingotomy. Yao and Tulandi reported that persistent ectopic pregnancy was encountered in 8.3% of patients treated by laparoscopic salpingotomy and in 3.9% of patients treated by a similar procedure at laparotomy. The incidence of persistent ectopic pregnancy following laparoscopy, however, was quite variable, ranging from 3.5% to 20.0%. Pouly and colleagues achieved a relatively low 3.5% incidence of recurrent ectopic pregnancy in the largest series of patients treated to date by laparoscopic salpingotomy. Indeed, in many current practices, the incidence of persistent ectopic pregnancy appears to be low. There is a tendency for persistent trophoblastic tissue to be found in the proximal portion of the tube; therefore, special attention to this area is important. The use of hydrodissection to flush out the gestational products rather than removal of trophoblastic tissue piecemeal with forceps is recommended. One must, however, never assume that the chance for persistent trophoblast is entirely mitigated by the characteristics and ease of the procedure.

Risk factors for persistent ectopic pregnancy include small ectopic pregnancies (< 2 cm diameter), early therapy (< 42 days from last menstrual period) and high concentrations of β-hCG (< 3,000 IU/L by the third IRP) preoperatively. In high-risk cases, a single dose of methotrexate (1 mg/kg) can be administered postoperatively for prophylaxis. Gracyzykowski and Mishell demonstrated that the rate of persistent ectopic pregnancy was reduced to a rate of 1.9% utilizing methotrexate prophylaxis in comparison to a rate of 14.5% amongst controls. Spandorfer and associates suggested that the postoperative day 1 serum β-hCG concentration can be used as a predictor of persistent ectopic pregnancy. They reported that a day 1 serum β-hCG decrease of < 50% from preoperative levels may be predictive of persistent ectopic pregnancy. If day 1 serum β-hCG concentrations decreased ≥ 50% of the preoperative value, there was a greater than 85% probability that a persistent ectopic pregnancy would not occur.

Options for treatment of persistent ectopic pregnancy include re-operation and medical therapy. The choice of treatment can also include expectant therapy if the patient is asymptomatic and β-hCG levels are not rapidly increasing. Methotrexate appears to be particularly effective in the setting of persistent ectopic pregnancy following linear salpingotomy. In the largest series reported to date, all 19 patients with persistent ectopic pregnancies were successfully treated with a single intramuscular dose of systemic methotrexate (50 mg/m^2).

The patient's reproductive prognosis does not appear to be particularly lessened following a persistent ectopic pregnancy. In a review of 50 cases, Seifer and colleagues reported that after 36 months of follow-up, there were 19 (59%) intrauterine pregnancies and no recurrent ectopic pregnancies in 32 such women attempting to conceive.

Due to the chance for persistent ectopic pregnancies to present relatively late following initial appropriate decreases in β-hCG concentrations, it is recommended to obtain weekly β-hCG measurements until they return to the normal range.

SEGMENTAL RESECTION. The optimal surgical approach to the isthmic ectopic pregnancy remains controversial. Three conservative operations have been described: segmental resection of the involved portion of oviduct with primary microsurgical anastomosis, segmental resection with reanastomosis at a later operation, and linear salpingotomy. In Sweden, Swolin initially advocated for segmental resection in 1967. Subsequently, other surgeons, including Stangel and Gomel as well as DeCherney and Boyers have found segmental resection to be preferable to salpingotomy in most cases of isthmic pregnancy. In the isthmus, the tubal lumen is narrower and the muscularis is thicker than in the ampulla. Thus, the isthmus is more predisposed to severe post-operative damage and the rate of proximal tubal obstruction seems to be higher following linear salpingotomy.

With segmental resection and end-to-end reanastomosis, the implantation site is removed so that it cannot be involved in a subsequent tubal pregnancy. A more normal architecture for the oviduct is consequently achieved. The anatomic restoration is a time-consuming process requiring special expertise and extensive microsurgical experience; *it should not be undertaken by an inexperienced surgeon*. The success of future pregnancies depends on the skill and precision of technique used in the procedure, and, once begun, the only alternative is total salpingectomy.

Segmental resection is best performed with loupe magnification or the operating microscope; the required microsurgical techniques are identical to those discussed elsewhere in this text. Care must be taken to avoid trauma to the very vascular oviduct; only patients with minimal bleeding should be considered for the operation. The adjacent mesosalpinx must be incised and removed with care to avoid the formation of a hematoma in the broad ligament (Fig. 22.9). The seromuscular sutures are placed with use of magnification and no. 6-0 or 7-0 delayed-absorbable material, and the serosa is secondarily supported by additional interrupted sutures. Patency of the oviduct is tested by insufflation of the uterine cavity with indigo carmine dye.

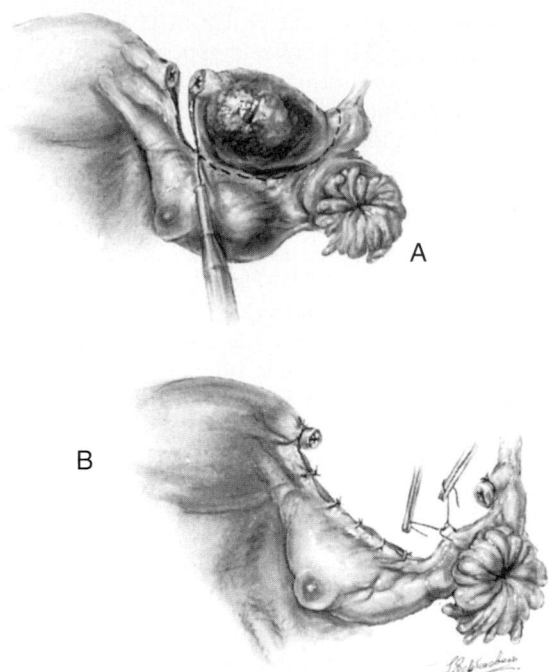

FIGURE 22.9. Segmental resection of midtubal ectopic pregnancy. **A:** A needle cautery is useful to resect the pregnancy. **B:** Care should be taken to approximate the mesosalpinx. Reanastomosis can be performed either immediately or in 3 to 5 months.

Radical Surgical Treatment

Total salpingectomy is required when a tubal pregnancy has ruptured and a substantial hemoperitoneum has occurred. In these cases, the intraabdominal hemorrhage must be quickly controlled and a conservative operation should not be attempted. Extensive hemoperitoneum places a patient in serious jeopardy of cardiopulmonary crises.

A salpingectomy may also be indicated for other reasons. These include a recurrent ectopic pregnancy in the same fallopian tube, an ectopic pregnancy in a severely damaged tube and an ectopic pregnancy in a women who has completed her family.

Some earlier reports advocated for the combined use of a prophylactic oophorectomy with salpingectomy. Theoretically, removal of the ipsilateral ovary would cause the other ovary to ovulate more frequently, perhaps favoring future pregnancy. In reality, the benefits of removal of the contralateral ovary are outweighed by the consideration that any future procedure would then mean castration. The high success rate of IVF is a further incentive to maintain functioning of both ovaries.

As stated earlier, most patients with an ectopic pregnancy currently are candidates for laparoscopic surgery. Radical surgical procedures, such as salpingectomy, are also easily adapted to laparoscopic surgery. Of course, certain patients remain non-candidates for laparoscopic surgery, including those with unstable hemodynamic status or severe pelvic adhesions. The latter patients are still best treated by laparotomy.

At laparotomy, total salpingectomy with partial cornual resection has been criticized for providing a residual sinus tract that allows development of a subsequent interstitial pregnancy. This problem may not lie in the procedure per se, but rather the surgeon's performance of the procedure. Complete peritonealization of the cornual incision and advancement of the round and broad ligaments over the uterine cornua (the modified Coffey technique of uterine suspension) should provide complete protection from recurrent interstitial pregnancy (Fig. 22.10). A too vigorous resection of the uterine cornua can also cause problems. A residual myometrial defect can cause uterine rupture, interstitial recanalization, or placental encroachment during a subsequent intrauterine pregnancy and should be avoided by making certain that the interstitial resection includes less than one third the thickness of the cornual portion of the myometrium.

Dubuisson, Aubriot, and Cardone reported the first large series of patients treated by total salpingectomy at laparoscopy for ampullary ectopic pregnancies. They utilized a three-puncture laparoscopic technique. They thermocoagulated the tubal isthmus, mesosalpinx, and tubal-ovarian ligament, followed by excision with hook scissors. The tube was subsequently removed with polyp forceps through one of the suprapubic punctures. They reported no immediate complications in 98 patients successfully treated at laparoscopy, although one patient experienced a post-operative deep venous thrombosis. Two patients initially intended for laparoscopy, however, required laparotomy either due to severe pelvic adhesions or significant intraperitoneal blood. In a later report, Dubuisson and associates advised opening the tube first in order to aspirate the trophoblast in cases in which the tube is large, in order to more easily remove the tissue through a 12 mm trocar.

TECHNIQUE OF SALPINGECTOMY AT LAPAROTOMY. A suprapubic Pfannenstiel or low midline vertical abdominal incision is used, and the distended tube is elevated. The mesosalpinx is clamped with a succession of Kelly clamps as close to the tube as possible (see Fig. 22.10A). The tube is then excised by cutting a small myometrial wedge at the uterine cornu (see Fig. 22.10B). Care should be taken to avoid a deep incision into the myometrium. A figure-of-eight mattress suture of no. 0 delayed-absorbable material is used to close the myometrium at the site of the wedge resection. The mesosalpinx is closed with interrupted ligatures of no. 2-0 delayed-absorbable suture. Complete hemostasis is essential to avoid a hematoma of the broad ligament.

The fundus is held forward and the round and broad ligaments are sutured over the uterine cornu (see Fig. 22.10C). This procedure, the modified Coffey suspension, accomplishes complete peritonealization. Mattress sutures anchor the broad ligament to the uterus. The no. 0 delayed-absorbable suture first penetrates the broad ligament from its anterior surface, just below the round ligament, at a distance of 2 to 3 cm from the cornu. The next "bite" is taken into the fundus of the uterus, a little posterior and superior to the uterine incision. The suture

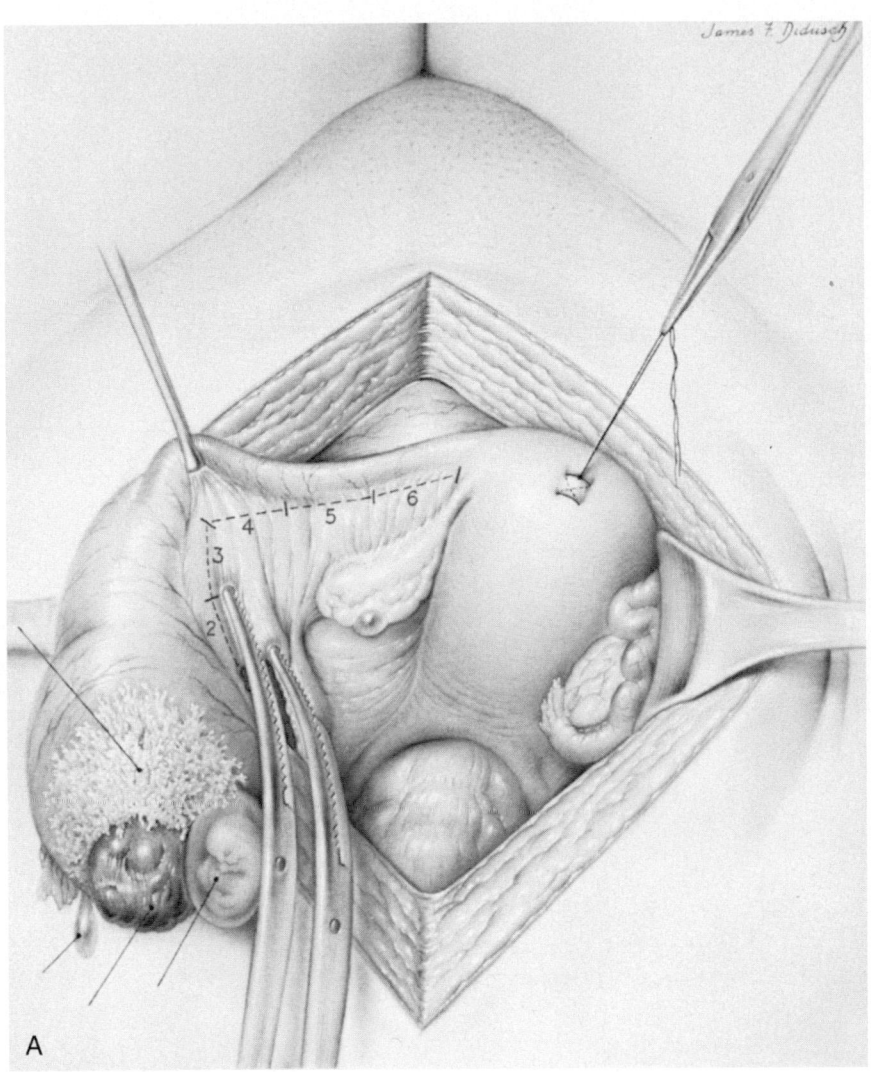

FIGURE 22.10. Salpingectomy for tubal pregnancy. **A:** The tube has been delivered, and the mesosalpinx is being clamped and cut with a succession of Kelly clamps.   *Continued*

is then placed through the posterior aspect of the broad ligament, about 1 cm lateral to the previous suture. When this suture is tied, the cornual incision and the mesosalpinx are covered with mesothelium (see Fig. 22.10D). If there is excessive tension on this suture, or if peritonealization is incomplete, then supporting sutures can be placed in the myometrium and the round ligament to ensure that the peritonealization suture will remain in place.

TECHNIQUE OF SALPINGECTOMY AT LAPAROSCOPY. Several methods have been successfully utilized for laparoscopic salpingectomy, including endoscopic stapling devices, endocoagulation, bipolar cautery, as well as pre-tied endoscopic ligatures. Following placement of laparoscopic trocar ports (usually three-puncture technique), irrigation of the pelvis, and the evacuation of all blood clots, the involved tube is then grasped with a toothed grasper. One method then includes cauterizing the tubal-ovarian ligament first with bipolar forceps followed by transection with scissors (Fig. 22.11). The mesosalpinx is similarly cauterized and transected, taking care to stay as close as possible to the fallopian tube. The

proximal tubal isthmus is then cauterized and transected. Care should be taken such that excess cauterization of the uterine cornua does not occur, due to concerns about the potential of interstitial sinus tracts or diminished myometrial integrity. The specimen is then placed in an endoscopic specimen retrieval bag and removed through a 12-mm port. Alternatively, the tube can be excised distal to two no. 0 chromic catgut endo-loop ligatures secured proximal to the ectopic implantation site, although this technique works optimally if the entire mesosalpinx is transected such that the endo-loop ligatures can be placed precisely at the tubal insertion at the cornua. Consideration may also be given to covering the proximal tubal pedicle with an absorbable adhesion prevention barrier.

Comparisons of Surgical and Medical Therapy

Several studies have compared conservative laparoscopic treatment with systemic methotrexate in the management of ectopic pregnancy. Saraj and associates reported a randomized trial comparing single-dose intramuscular

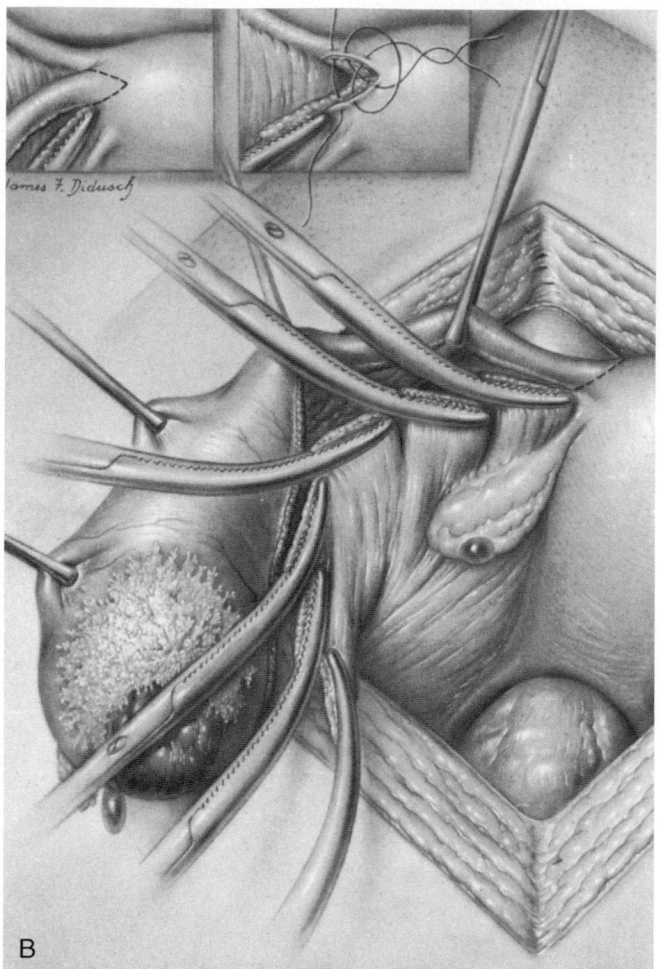

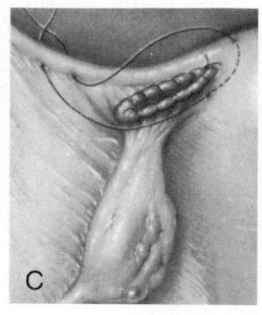

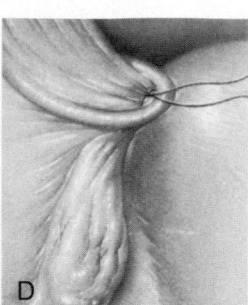

FIGURE 22.10, *Continued.* **B:** The mesosalpinx has been completely clamped and cut. The dashed line indicates the line of excision of the tube at the cornu. Inset shows the superficial wedge resection of the interstitial tube and the suture of the cornu. **C:** The method of placing mattress suture for peritonealization is shown with anchoring of the medial portion of the broad ligament to the uterus, a little posterior and superior to the uterine incision. **D:** Peritonealization is completed by tying mattress sutures, which brings the broad and the round ligaments over the uterine cornu.

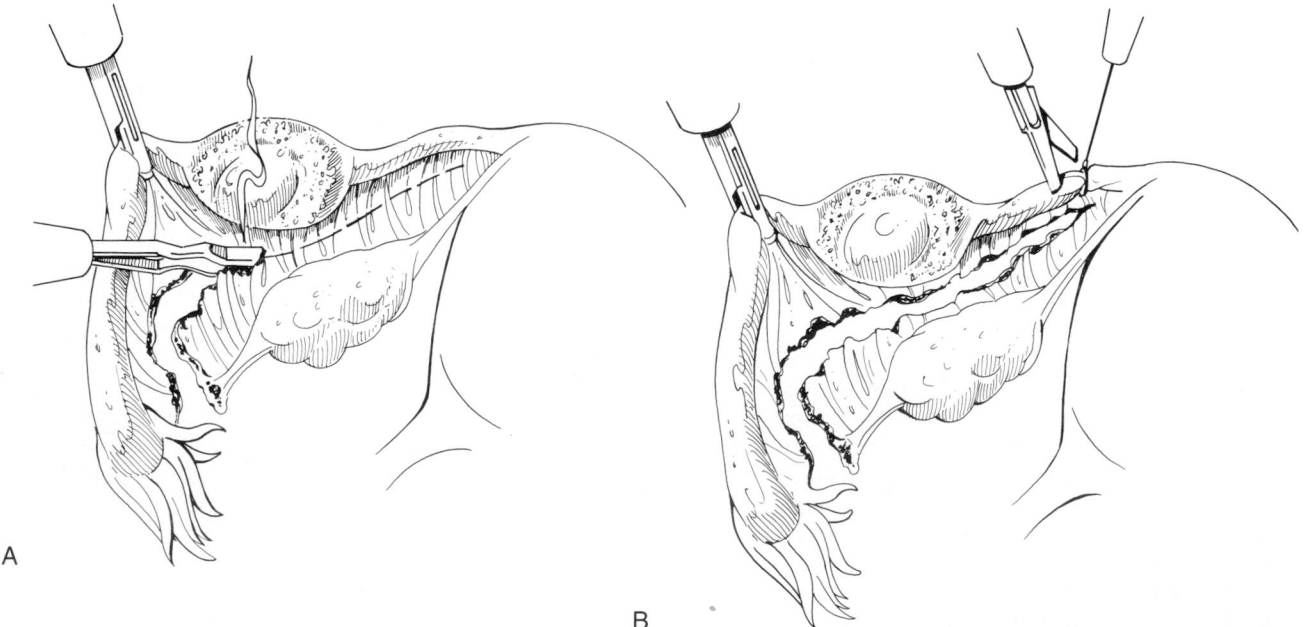

FIGURE 22.11. Techniques of laparoscopic salpingectomy utilizing bipolar cautery and excision.

methotrexate (1 mg/kg) with laparoscopic salpingotomy. They reported similar immediate treatment success rates: 94.7% for methotrexate and 91.4% for laparoscopic salpingotomy. Additional methotrexate injections were required in 15.8% of women who were randomized to the single-dose methotrexate group. Initial serum hCG titres were higher for the patients who required additional methotrexate doses than for those who required only one dose. The mean times for serum progesterone and hCG concentrations to decrease to less than 1.5 ng/mL and 15 IU/L, respectively, were significantly less for laparoscopic salpingotomy. Fernandez and colleagues also reported a randomized trial of conservative laparoscopic treatment and methotrexate administration (by either transvaginal or intramuscular injection) and found similar immediate treatment success. Additional studies have also suggested that despite the increased number of post-treatment visits that are necessary, methotrexate therapy results in appreciable costs-savings in comparison to laparoscopic treatment.

Hemodynamically stable patients who meet strict criteria, without excessively large or advanced ectopic pregnancies, may therefore be offered either medical or conservative surgical therapy. The immediate clinical and long-term outcomes in these selected patients appear to be similar.

INTERSTITIAL PREGNANCY

Interstitial (cornual) pregnancy is a rare condition that accounts for no more than 2% to 4% of all tubal pregnancies. The condition occurs once for every 2500 to 5000 live births. An interstitial pregnancy should be differentiated from an angular pregnancy. The latter entity was first described by Kelly in 1898. It occurs when an embryo implants in the lateral angle of the uterine cavity medial to the internal ostium of the fallopian tube. The clinical course of an angular pregnancy varies, although in many instances leads to asymmetric and symptomatic enlargement of the uterus.

The gestational sac is better protected in the interstitial than in other portions of the tube; thus, symptoms manifest later and pregnancies are often more advanced before they present. After 2 to 3 months of amenorrhea, vaginal spotting commonly begins. The developing chorionic villi may eventually erode into the blood vessels of the uterine cornu, causing a severe hemorrhage. Because the pregnancy occurs at the most richly vascularized area of the female pelvis, the junction of the uterine and ovarian vessels, rupture usually causes profound and sudden shock.

Before 1893, the only available reports on interstitial pregnancies were from autopsies. Since then, numerous cases have been reported. Most of the same risk factors for interstitial pregnancy are similar to those for ectopic pregnancy in general, including pelvic inflammatory disease, previous pelvic surgery and the use of ART. Ipsilateral salpingectomy may be a unique risk factor for interstitial pregnancy, occurring in approximately 25% of their patients. Earlier diagnosis and more experience in treating this disorder have reduced the present maternal mortality rate to approximately 2% to 2.5% of all interstitial pregnancies.

The diagnosis of interstitial pregnancy is made by critical evaluation of all the criteria used for other types of tubal pregnancy. Symptoms are acute abdominal pain, intraperitoneal bleeding, a low hematocrit, and a positive serum or urine pregnancy test. Diagnostic tests include the sensitive β-hCG radioimmunoassay, culdocentesis, and ultrasonography.

Asymmetry of the uterus, often indicative of an interstitial pregnancy, can be misinterpreted as a pregnancy in a bicornuate uterus or a myoma in a pregnant uterus instead of an interstitial pregnancy. Knowledge of the previous shape of the uterus can help to confirm or exclude the existence of a bicornuate or myomatous uterus. A firm protrusion on the uterus suggests a myoma; a soft, tender asymmetric enlargement suggests an interstitial pregnancy.

Timor-Trisch and colleagues established transvaginal ultrasonic criteria for interstitial pregnancy. These criteria include: a) an empty uterine cavity, b) a chorionic sac seen separately and < 1 cm from the most lateral edge of the uterine cavity, and c) a thick myometrial layer surrounding the chorionic sac. All of these parameters were relatively specific (88% to 93%), but lacked high sensitivity (only about 40%) for the diagnosis of interstitial pregnancy. Other investigators have described an "interstitial line sign." This sign refers to the visualization of an echogenic line extending from the endometrial cavity into the cornual region and abutting the interstitial mass or gestational sac. Ackerman and associates reported that the "interstitial line sign" was 80% sensitive and 98% specific for the diagnosis of interstitial pregnancy.

Often the difference between an interstitial pregnancy and an angular pregnancy is subtle. In addition, it may be easy to confuse an angular pregnancy with a pregnancy in a septated or bicornuate uterus. Because ultrasound cannot always confirm the position of the pregnancy, laparoscopy may be required to confirm the diagnosis. In cases of massive intraabdominal bleeding, an immediate laparotomy should be performed.

Treatment for Interstitial Pregnancy

The choice of treatment for an interstitial (cornual) pregnancy depends on the extent of trauma that has occurred in the uterine wall and on the interest of the patient in preserving her childbearing function. Systemic methotrexate has been used in a limited number of patients with unruptured interstitial pregnancies. Tanaka and coworkers reported the first successful treatment of an interstitial pregnancy with systemic methotrexate. Since this report, according to Lau and Tulandi, there have been 40 additional published cases of interstitial pregnancies treated with the use of systemic or local methotrexate, or a combination of both. An overall success rate of 83% was reported.

If an interstitial pregnancy is observed when it is still small, it might be excised utilizing conservative laparoscopic techniques. In their review, Lau and Tulandi noted 22 successful cases of laparoscopic treatment of interstitial pregnancy. Techniques utilized varied from cornuostomy with careful extraction of the products of conception to a more formal cornual resection. In only one case was bleeding severe enough to require a transfusion. Hemostatic methods have include ligation of the ascending branches of the uterine vessels, intracorporeal and extracorporeal suturing as well as the endo GIA stapler. Although the immediate efficacy of laparoscopic conservative procedures for interstitial pregnancy is high, the risk of uterine rupture in a subsequent pregnancy is unknown. Uterine rupture can occur at the site of a previous interstitial pregnancy. Patients treated by conservative laparoscopic techniques should therefore be carefully counseled about this risk. The risk of uterine rupture also emphasizes the importance of proper suturing of the uterine cornu during conservative surgical treatment of an interstitial pregnancy.

For many surgeons, cornual resection and repair of the defect by laparotomy remains the standard conservative surgical procedure for interstitial pregnancy. Provided that uterine rupture has not occurred, this is technically feasible in most cases. Unfortunately, in many cases in which uterine rupture has occurred or a very large interstitial pregnancy is present, a hysterectomy may be required. Hysterectomy remains the treatment of choice for pregnancies advanced to such a stage that repair of the cornu would be technically difficult and medically hazardous.

Excision of Interstitial Pregnancy by Cornual Resection and Salpingectomy

Whenever possible, the ovary should be saved. A cornual resection and salpingectomy is performed by first ligating the ascending uterine vessels where they approach the cornu (Figure 22.12). Each is ligated separately with a figure-of-eight suture. One may also consider the use of a dilute solution of vasopressin (prepared with mixing 20 U of vasopressin with 30 ml of physiologic saline) injected in the intended myometrial incisional line in order to further optimize intraoperative hemostasis. The interstitial pregnancy is excised in a V-shaped manner, and the myometrium is approximated with a figure-of-eight closure using no. 0 delayed-absorbable suture (see Fig. 22.12B). The remainder of the fallopian tube is excised. If it becomes necessary, the round ligament can be cut and resutured to the cornu and the uterine serosa by use of interrupted sutures (see Fig. 22.12C). The round and broad ligaments are brought over the incision with mattress sutures (once again, the modified Coffey suspension) (see Fig. 22.12D), and additional interrupted sutures of no. 2-0 or no. 3-0 delayed-absorbable material can be used to secure the serosa of the round ligament to the serosa of the uterus to maintain the operative site in a permanent retroperitoneal position.

OVARIAN ECTOPIC PREGNANCY

Because IUDs protect the endometrium and, to a lesser extent, the proximal oviducts from implantation, it was expected when IUDs were introduced that future reports of extrauterine pregnancies might show an in-

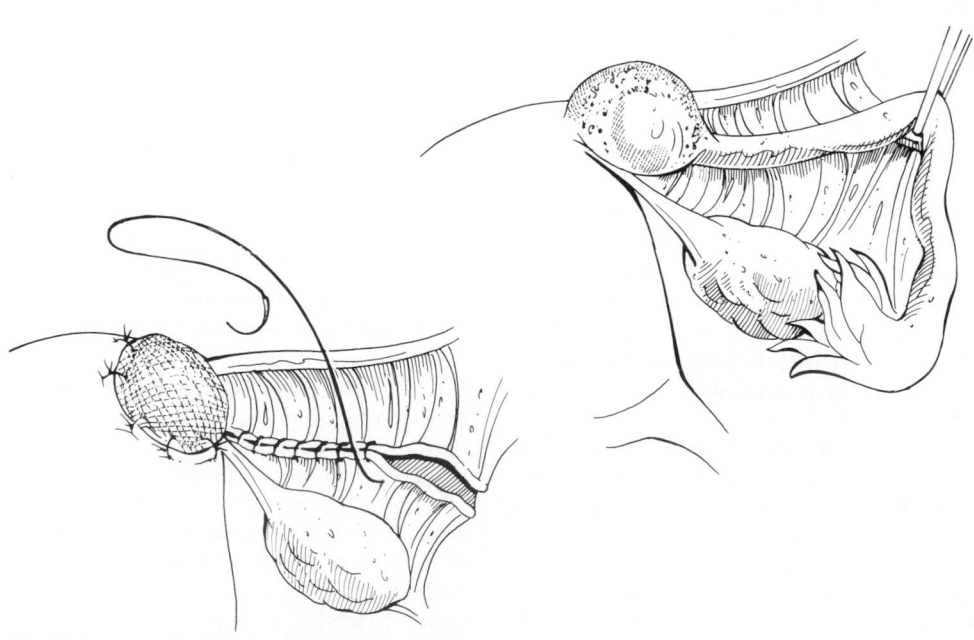

FIGURE 22.12. Technique of corneal resection and salpingectomy.

creased rate of ovarian involvement. Data from the Co-operative Statistical Program of the Population Council show that 1 of every 9 ectopic pregnancies among IUD users is an ovarian pregnancy. Of total pregnancies among IUD users, 4.3% are extrauterine.

There are several reviews in the English literature on the subject of primary ovarian pregnancy. Boronow and associates summarized 62 cases in a review of the literature between 1950 and 1963. Campbell and associates brought the list up to date through 1973 with 91 cases, including 3 new cases of their own. Pratt-Thomas, White, and Messer reported an additional 10 new cases in 1974. Grimes, Nosal, and Gallagher summarized the major reviews through 1980 and added 18 previously unreported cases of primary ovarian pregnancy from the records of six hospitals. Their combined data from this review, the hospital cases, and four other recent reports totaled 34 cases of primary ovarian pregnancy among 236,983 deliveries, a rate of 1 ovarian pregnancy in 7,000 deliveries.

In an intrafollicular ovarian pregnancy, the second stage of meiosis, ovum capacitation, and fertilization each occur within the follicle. Only 15% of cases of ovarian pregnancy are intrafollicular in origin. In an intrafollicular pregnancy, a well-preserved corpus luteum can be identified in the wall of the gestational sac. Four other criteria presented by Spiegelberg for identifying an intrafollicular pregnancy are that the tube, including the fimbria ovarica, is intact and is clearly separate from the ovary, that the gestational sac definitely occupies the normal position of the ovary, that the sac is connected to the uterus by the uteroovarian ligament, and that ovarian tissue is unquestionably demonstrated in the wall of the sac.

Diagnosis of Ovarian Pregnancy

Early diagnosis of an ovarian pregnancy, of all the diagnoses relating to extrauterine gestations, is perhaps the most difficult. As stated previously, the classic symptoms of a tubal gestation are abdominal pain, amenorrhea, and bleeding; however, chronic pelvic pain alone, a symptom not always easily related to its cause, is the most frequent clinical manifestation of an ovarian gestation. Although an adnexal mass is palpable in as many as 60% of ovarian pregnancies, the mass is frequently confused with a leaking corpus luteum hematoma.

All of the test criteria used for diagnosing a tubal pregnancy are helpful in diagnosing a primary ovarian pregnancy. In particular, the highly sensitive β-hCG radioimmunoassay is effective for identifying the presence of low hCG levels. The test can confirm the presence of a gestational process, but knowing the β-hCG level does not help to precisely locate the gestation. Incomplete spontaneous abortion with a leaking corpus luteum hematoma, one of the most common complications of pregnancy, mimics an ovarian pregnancy. In such cases, a D&C will often show the remnants of trophoblastic villi responsible for the low levels of β-hCG.

A tubal pregnancy can easily be ruled out with laparoscopy, but an ovarian pregnancy is sometimes difficult to differentiate from a leaking corpus luteum hematoma by gross appearance. Ultrasonography can be helpful, but only in advanced ovarian pregnancy will the ultrasound image show a discrete gestational sac, therefore confirming the clinical suspicion of an ovarian pregnancy.

Critical evaluation of all of the diagnostic studies, particularly the sensitive β-hCG radioimmunoassay and vaginal ultrasonography, is necessary in making the diagnosis. When the β-hCG is positive, ultrasonography shows no intrauterine gestational sac and free blood exists in the peritoneal cavity, a laparoscopy should be performed to confirm or refute a diagnosis of suspected ovarian pregnancy.

Treatment for Ovarian Pregnancy

Raziel and Golan as well as Chelmow, Gates and Penzias reported cases in which an intact ovarian pregnancy was diagnosed by laparoscopy and systemic methotrexate treatment was successful. In many cases, an ovarian pregnancy is diagnosed after a significant hemoperitoneum has occurred and medical therapy is contraindicated. An ovarian pregnancy is easily confused with a leaking corpus luteum hematoma. For this reason, a safe approach is to proceed with localized surgical resection of the bleeding mass with conservation of the ovary, if possible. Unless the diagnosis is made late, the ovary can usually be preserved. In 1997, Seinera and colleagues reported successful laparoscopic treatment of ovarian pregnancy in eight patients over a 12 year time span. Einenkel and associates even reported the successful conservative resection of an ovarian pregnancy in a patient with ovarian hyperstimulation. The concomitant increased ovarian size, fragility and vascularity presented an additional surgical challenge for these authors, although the use of intra-operative ultrasound greatly facilitated the precise localization of the ectopic pregnancy within the ovary.

Only rarely is the hemorrhage so profuse that oophorectomy is required to control bleeding. Even if the last trophoblastic villus cannot be removed in the ovarian resection, the ovary should be preserved. Any remaining trophoblastic tissue will usually degenerate rapidly or respond to postoperative methotrexate therapy and therefore produce no long-standing clinical problem.

ABDOMINAL ECTOPIC PREGNANCY

An abdominal pregnancy is perhaps both the rarest and the most serious type of extrauterine gestation. Reports of the frequency of abdominal pregnancy vary, ranging from 1 in 3371 deliveries to greater than 1 in 10,200 deliveries. Stafford and Ragan reported an incidence of 1 abdominal pregnancy in 7269 deliveries, a figure that is representative of the reports in the literature.

Abdominal pregnancies are classified as primary or secondary. Most are secondary, the result of early tubal abortion or rupture with secondary implantation of the pregnancy into the peritoneal cavity. To be considered a primary abdominal pregnancy, the pregnancy must meet the three criteria defined by Studdiford in 1942:

1. Both tubes and ovaries must be in normal condition with no evidence of recent or remote injury.
2. No evidence of uteroperitoneal fistula should be found.
3. The pregnancy must be related exclusively to the peritoneal surface and be early enough to eliminate the possibility that it is a secondary implantation following a primary implantation in the tube.

Secondary abdominal pregnancy occurs when a tubal gestation attaches itself to other viscera as the enlarging placenta spreads through the wall of the tube or is aborted through the fimbriated end. The placenta probably retains some tubal attachment, which supplies blood for the gestation to continue developing in the new peritoneal site. Rare types of secondary abdominal pregnancies have occurred after spontaneous separation of an old cesarean section scar, after uterine perforation during a therapeutic or elective abortion, and after subtotal or total hysterectomy.

Diagnosis of Abdominal Pregnancy

Early diagnosis of an abdominal pregnancy is difficult but critical, because a catastrophic hemorrhage can result from separation of the placenta. A history of recurrent abdominal discomfort, fetal movement beneath the abdominal wall, and the presence of fetal movements high in the upper abdomen should alert the clinician to the possibility of an abdominal implantation. Other clinical clues include cessation of fetal movement, vomiting late in pregnancy, fetal malposition, a closed and uneffaced cervix or the failure of oxytocin to stimulate the gestational mass.

Confirmation of the diagnosis requires demonstration of the fetus outside the uterine cavity. In their review of 199 cases, Costa and colleagues reported that only in 68 cases (40.2%) was a mass adjacent to or distinct from the uterus found. The radiologic finding of fetal small parts in the lateral position overlying the maternal spine was first noted by Weinberg and Sherwin in 1956; this finding is a fairly reliable sign of an abdominal pregnancy. A radiologic examination of the abdomen, including anterior, posterior, and lateral views, is also helpful in defining malposition of the fetus, which is most often discovered to be in the transverse position. Ultrasound, however, is the most effective method for diagnosing an abdominal pregnancy. Ultrasound can usually identify an abdominal gestation as separate from the nonpregnant uterus. Ultrasonography can be expected to enhance diagnostic accuracy in more than two thirds of cases. In those cases in which ultrasonography is equivocal, MRI may be useful.

The maternal mortality risk from abdominal pregnancy in the United States is 7.7 times greater than the maternal mortality risk from tubal ectopic pregnancy and 90 times greater than that with intrauterine pregnancy.

Reported maternal mortality rates in the literature have varied in the past from 4% to 29%. Maternal morbidity can also be substantial, with high incidences of pelvic abscess, peritonitis, and sepsis caused by retained placental remnants. Rare instances of massive rectal bleeding or rectal passage of fetal bones secondary to the formation of celointestinal fistulae have also been reported. Fetal mortality is notoriously high, ranging from 75% to 95% of all cases.

Management of Advanced Abdominal Pregnancy

Recent techniques of fetal monitoring served as diagnostic adjuncts to the management of the abdominal pregnancy. Fetal assessment, including repeated sonography to measure biparietal diameter, non-stress testing, monitoring of fetal movements, and biophysical profiles, can provide clinical evidence of fetal maturity and fetal welfare. Despite the use of these diagnostic tools, fetal death occurred in all of the 15 cases of abdominal pregnancy reported by Martin and associates. Clark and Jones reported a fetal salvage rate of only 11.4% in a study of 35 advanced abdominal pregnancies.

One of the major factors in fetal survival is the condition of the fetal membranes. If the membranes rupture, the fetus usually dies from respiratory distress in the peritoneal cavity within a short time of the rupture. When the volume of amniotic fluid is significantly decreased or absent, the incidence of fetal malformations increases significantly, pressure deformities occur and pulmonary hypoplasia precludes the possibility of delivering a viable fetus. In situations where the pregnancy is advanced and there is sufficient volume of amniotic fluid, there exists a reasonable possibility of a good fetal outcome. In rare instances, there may be justification for postponed surgery to allow for further fetal maturity and a better perinatal prognosis.

Preoperative preparation of a patient with an advanced abdominal pregnancy should include an adequate supply of compatible blood and blood products and appropriate intravenous infusion lines that can deliver large amounts of fluid quickly. The use of a cell-saver or MAST (Military Antishock Trouser) Suit has been reported in management of patients experiencing massive hemorrhage and shock. A surgical team should be standing by that is capable of handling the possible bowel, vascular or genitourinary complications that may arise.

Following incision into the amniotic sac and delivery of the fetus, the management of the placenta still remains a controversial issue. Most clinicians believe the best treatment is to clamp the cord, to leave the placenta in situ, and to close the abdomen, but to allow retroperitoneal drainage if possible. The placenta can be removed after complete cessation of function is demonstrated by quantitative hCG titers. The placenta should be removed during laparotomy only if it is accessible and if its removal can be accomplished without excessive blood loss. When all functioning stops, the circulation has undergone fibrosis. In case of doubt, the placenta should be left in place. Thompson has reported leaving the placenta in the peritoneal cavity for a period of 13 years without physical harm to the patient. Methotrexate has been used occasionally to hasten trophoblastic degeneration, but leads to the accelerated accumulation of necrotic placental tissue which may become infected. For this reason, it is currently felt best not to administer methotrexate in this clinical setting.

CERVICAL ECTOPIC PREGNANCY

The cervix is a rare but hazardous site for placental implantation because the trophoblast can penetrate through the cervical wall and into the uterine blood supply. Cervical gestations have, until recently, received little attention in the literature, but increased awareness of the condition has resulted in a number of recent reports. The following three criteria for the diagnosis of cervical pregnancy were established by Rubin in 1911:

1. Cervical glands must be opposite the placental attachment.
2. Placental attachment to the cervix must be situated below the entrance of the uterine vessels or below the peritoneal reflection of the anterior and posterior surfaces of the uterus.
3. Fetal elements must be absent from the corpus uteri.

Because strict anatomical and histological criteria necessitate a hysterectomy for a complete study of the entire uterus, Paalman and McElin proposed five more clinically practical criteria for the diagnosis of this condition:

1. Uterine bleeding without cramping pain following a period of amenorrhea
2. A soft, enlarged cervix equal to or larger than the fundus (the "hourglass" uterus)
3. Products of conception entirely confined within and firmly attached to the endocervix
4. A closed internal cervical os
5. A partially opened external os

The incidence of this rare entity varies. The Mayo Clinic reported 1 in 16,000 pregnancies. The highest incidence, 1 in 1000 pregnancies, was reported from Japan. The high incidence of elective abortion in Japan is probably a factor in the higher rates. Dilatation and curettage (D & C) seems to be a predisposing factor for cervical pregnancy. Shinagawa and Nagayama noted that in 18 of 19 cases of cervical pregnancy there was a history of legal abortion. In the review by Ushakov and associates, 68.6% of patients with a cervical pregnancy had a previous uterine curettage. It has also suggested that a previous cesarean section may play a role in the etiology of cervical pregnancy.

Cervical gestation is frequently confused with a neoplastic process because of the marked vascularity and friable appearance of the cervix. Profuse bleeding can occur if the placenta is mistaken for a tumor and a biopsy is taken. A cervical gestation also can be mistaken for a spontaneous abortion in which the products of conception were retained within the cervical canal (Fig. 22.13).

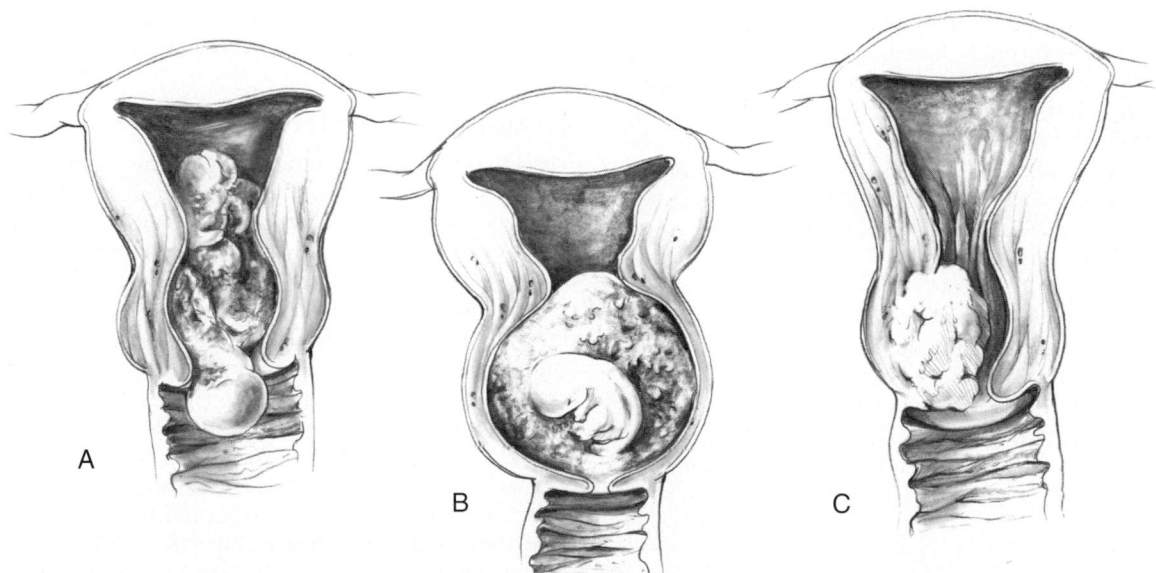

FIGURE 22.13. Differential diagnosis of cervical pregnancy. **A:** In the cervical phase of uterine abortion, the placenta is mainly within the expanded cervix, and the external and internal ora are dilated. **B:** In a cervical abortion (abortion into the cervix) due to stenosis of the external os, spontaneous rupture of the cervical wall can cause severe hemorrhage. **C:** Ragged, friable cervix seen in cervical pregnancy mimics carcinoma of the cervix. (Redrawn from Rothe DJ, Birnbaum SJ. Cervical pregnancy: diagnosis and management. *Obstet Gynecol* 1973;42:675–680.)

Treatment for Cervical Pregnancy

The treatment for a cervical pregnancy is surgical, and the condition often requires an abdominal hysterectomy. In selected patients, conservative evacuation of an early cervical pregnancy may be accomplished by skillful D&C, although the procedure has the potential to be complicated by profuse hemorrhage. Further preoperative preparations directed to reduce the vascularity of the uterine cervix, such as transvaginal ligation of cervical branches of the uterine arteries, a Shirodkar type cerclage, angiographic uterine artery embolization, or intracervical vasopressin injection, may reduce operative morbidity. In a review by Ushakov and colleagues, of the 16 cases in which one of these methods was employed, 15 had minimal (50-200 ml) blood loss, one patient had a hemorrhage of 1200 ml requiring transfusion and no patient required laparotomy or hysterectomy. Among 41 cases in which D & C was performed without cervical preparation, minimal bleeding occurred in just 5 cases (12.2%), massive bleeding (1200–5000mL) occurred in 70.7% and hysterectomy was performed in seven cases (17.1%). Laparotomy with bilateral internal iliac artery ligation or bilateral uterine artery ligation was also required in an additional five (12.2%) of these patients. In order to control postevacuation bleeding, several authors, including Kuppuswami and colleagues as well as Werber, Prasadarao and Harris have described the successful use of a Foley catheter balloon to tamponade the cervical implantation site in patients who continued to have blood loss after cervical pregnancy evacuation. A 26-French Foley catheter with a 30-ml balloon is preferably used and left inflated for 0.5 to 6 days, as clinically indicated.

Medical therapy can also be considered for the primary treatment of cervical pregnancy or as an adjunct to surgical therapy through decreased vascularization of the mass. Kung and Chang reviewed the use of methotrexate (MTX) administration for cervical ectopic pregnancy from 1983 to 1997. Among 35 cases of viable cervical ectopic pregnancies < 12 weeks gestation, 63% of patients received either systemic MTX alone or a combination of systemic MTX with a local (intra-amniotic or intracervical) injection of either MTX or potassium chloride. Among the 23 cases of nonviable cervical pregnancy < 12 weeks gestation, 96% of women required systemic MTX alone. The ultimate success rate of uterine preservation was similar (94% for the viable pregnancy group; 91% for the non-viable pregnancy group), although the patients in the viable pregnancy group required a significantly higher number of concomitant additional surgical procedures (43% versus 13%).

HETEROTOPIC PREGNANCY

Heterotopic pregnancy (coexistence of intra- and extrauterine pregnancies) is rare. The incidence has been estimated to be about 1 in 30,000 spontaneous pregnancies. With the use of assisted reproductive technologies, the incidence is higher, as high as 0.75-1.5% of pregnancies.

Although the precise cause of a combined pregnancy is frequently obscured, most of the factors are the same as those associated with ectopic pregnancy. The use of ovulation-inducing agents has greatly increased the incidence of multiple gestations and heterotopic pregnancies. Berger and Taymore reported an incidence of combined pregnancy in as many as 1 in 100 stimulated patients. The most common predisposing anatomic finding associated with heterotopic pregnancies is pre-existing tubal disease.

Abdominal pain, an adnexal mass, peritoneal irritation, and an enlarged uterus together constitute the major clinical features associated with a heterotopic pregnancy. Additional diagnostic findings include the presence of two corpora lutea found at the time of laparotomy or laparoscopy, hemoperitoneum, acute abdominal pain after the termination of an intrauterine pregnancy, and the persistence of an enlarged uterus with amenorrhea after excision of an ectopic pregnancy.

As opposed to solely extrauterine pregnancies, which are presently diagnosed and treated electively at an early preclinical stage, heterotopic pregnancies are still mostly diagnosed after clinical signs develop. In their review, Rojansky and Schenker report that nearly half of the cases present with rupture, hemorrhage and emergency intervention. This is due to the fact that serial β-hCG determinations and transvaginal ultrasonography are often not helpful in establishing an early diagnosis of heterotopic pregnancy.

The majority of heterotopic pregnancies consist of a single tubal gestation combined with an intrauterine pregnancy. Rarer varieties include combined cervical-intrauterine, ovarian-intrauterine, abdominal-intrauterine and interstitial-intrauterine pregnancies.

Treatment for Heterotopic Pregnancy

Laparoscopy has been employed with reasonable success for the treatment of combined tubal and intrauterine pregnancies. Louis-Sylvestre and associates reported treating thirteen patients laparoscopically, ten by salpingectomy and three by salpingostomy. Subsequently, 60% of the patients with a viable intrauterine pregnancy at the time or surgery had a favorable outcome. On the other hand, in cases in which hemodynamic instability or an interstitial-intrauterine pregnancy is present, a laparotomy is indicated. Expectant management does not seem to have a role in the care of a patient with a heterotopic pregnancy. This is due to the fact that the specific course of the extrauterine component can not be monitored by serial β-hCG determinations. Likewise, either local or systemic methotrexate therapy would be contraindicated in the presence of a viable intrauterine gestation. The use of a local injection of potassium chloride into the extrauterine gestational sac, however, has been used successfully in a few cases. There are very rare cases in which extrauterine abdominal pregnancies progress simultaneously with intrauterine pregnancies to viability. In their review of the world's literature, Reece and associates found only 13 cases in which both pregnancies reached term and both infants were delivered and survived the neonatal period. In the absence of such rare circumstances, the outcome for the intrauterine pregnancy is optimized by immediate therapy of the extrauterine pregnancy.

RH IMMUNOGLOBULIN USE AFTER ECTOPIC PREGNANCY

Grimes has reported that Rh-negative mothers were recognized and administered Rh immunoglobulin in only 23% of cases. Fetomaternal hemorrhage associated with ectopic pregnancy can sensitize Rh-negative women at risk. A dose of 50 μg Rh immunoglobulin is usually sufficient to prevent Rh sensitization.

BIBLIOGRAPHY

Ackerman TE, Levi CS, Dashefsky SM, et al. Interstitial line: sonographic finding in interstitial (cornual) ectopic pregnancy. *Radiology* 1993;189:83–87.

Ankum WM, Mol BWJ, Van der Veen R, et al. Risk factors for ectopic pregnancy: A meta-analysis. *Fertil Steril* 1996;65:1093–1099.

Arias-Stella J. Atypical endometrial changes associated with the presence of chorionic tissue. *Arch Pathol* 1954;58: 112–128.

Atrash HK, Friede A, Hogue CJ. Ectopic pregnancy mortality in the United States: 1970–1983. *Obstet Gynecol* 1987;70: 817–822.

Atrash HK, Friede A, Hogue CJR. Abdominal pregnancy in the United States: frequency and maternal mortality. *Obstet Gynecol* 1987;69:333–337.

Auslender R, Arodi J, Pascal B, et al. Interstitial pregnancy: Early diagnosis by ultrasonography. *Am J Obstet Gynecol* 1983;146:717–718.

Barnhart K, Mennuti M, Benjamin J, et al. Prompt diagnosis of ectopic pregnancy in an emergency department setting. *Obstet Gynecol* 1994;84:1010–1015.

Berger MJ, Taymor ML. Simultaneous intrauterine and tubal pregnancies following ovulation induction. *Am J Obstet Gynecol* 1972;113:812–813.

Boronow RC, McElin TW, West RH, et al. Ovarian pregnancy: a report of 4 cases and a 13-year survey of the English literature. *Am J Obstet Gynecol* 1965;91:1095–1106.

Budowick M, Johnson TRB Jr, Genadry R, et al. The histopathology of the developing tubal ectopic pregnancy. *Fertil Steril* 1980;34:169–171.

Cacciatore B, Stenman U, Ylostalo P. Diagnosis of ectopic pregnancy by vaginal ultrasonography in combination with a discriminatory serum hCG level of 1000 IU/L (IRP). *Br J Obstet Gynecol* 1990;97:904–908.

Campbell JS, Hacquebard S, Mitton DM, et al. Acute hemoperitoneum, IUD, and occult ovarian pregnancy. *Obstet Gynecol* 1974;43:438–442.

Carson SA, Buster JE. Ectopic pregnancy. *N Engl J Med* 1993;329:1174–1181.

Chelmow D, Gates E, Penzias AS. Laparoscopic diagnosis and methotrexate treatment of an ovarian pregnancy: a case report. *Fertil Steril* 1994;62:879–881.

Clark JF, Jones SA. Advanced ectopic pregnancy. *J Reprod Med* 1975;14:30–33.

Confino E, Binor Z, Molo MW, et al. Selective salpingography for the diagnosis and treatment of early tubal pregnancy. *Fertil Steril* 1994;62:286–288.

Costa SD, Presley J, Bastert G. Advanced abdominal pregnancy. *Obstet Gynecol Surv* 1991;46:515–525.

De Voe RW, Pratt JH. Simultaneous intrauterine and extrauterine pregnancy. *Am J Obstet Gynecol* 1948;56: 1119–1123.

DeCherney AH, Boyers SP. Isthmic ectopic pregnancy: segmental resection as treatment of choice. *Fertil Steril* 1985;44:307–312.

Dor J, Seidman DS, Levran D, et al. The incidence of combined intrauterine and extrauterine pregnancy after in vitro fertilization and embryo transfer. *Fertil Steril* 1991;55: 833–834.

Dubuisson JB, Aubriot FX, Cardone V. Laparoscopic salpingectomy for tubal pregnancy. *Fertil Steril* 1987;47: 225–228.

Dubuisson JB, Morice P, Chapron C, et al. Salpingectomy: the laparoscopic surgical choice for ectopic pregnancy. *Hum Reprod* 1996;11:1199–1203.

Ectopic pregnancy-United States, 1990–1992, *JAMA* 1995; 273:533.

Egger M, Low N, Smith GD, et al. Screening for chlamydia infections and the risk of ectopic pregnancy in a county in Sweden: ecological analysis. *BMJ* 1998;316:1776–1780.

Einenkel J, Baier D, Horn LC, et al. Laparoscopic therapy of an intact primary ovarian pregnancy with ovarian hyperstimulation syndrome: case report. *Hum Reprod* 2000;15: 2037–2040.

Emerson DS, Cartier MS, Altieri LA, et al. Diagnostic efficacy of endovaginal color Doppler flow imaging in an ectopic pregnancy screening program. *Radiology* 1992;183:413–420.

Faber BM, Coddington CC. Microlaparoscopy: a comparative study of diagnostic accuracy. *Fertil Steril* 1997;67:952–954.

Farabow W, Fulton J, Fletcher V, et al. Cervical pregnancy treated with methotrexate. *N C Med J* 1983;44:91–93.

Feichtinger W, Kemeter P. Conservative treatment of ectopic pregnancy by transvaginal aspiration under sonographic control and methotrexate injection. *Lancet* 1987;1: 381–382.

Fernandez H, Benifla J-L, Lelaidier C, et al. Methotrexate treatment of ectopic pregnancy: 100 cases treated by primary transvaginal injection under sonographic control. *Fertil Steril* 1993;59:773–777.

Fernandez H, Capella S, Vincent AY, et al. Randomized trial of conservative laparoscopic treatment and methotrexate administration in ectopic pregnancy and subsequent fertility. *Hum Reprod* 1998;13:3239–3243.

Fernandez H, Rainhorn JD, Papiernik E, et al. Spontaneous resolution of ectopic pregnancy. *Obstet Gynecol* 1988;71: 171–174.

Fienberg R, Lloyd HE. The Arias-Stella reaction in early normal pregnancy: an involutional phenomenon. The ovary-placenta changeover as a possible cause. *Hum Pathol* 1974;5:183–190.

Frates MC, Laing FC. Sonographic evaluation of ectopic pregnancy: an update. *AJR* 1995;165:251–259.

Gelder MS, Boots LR, Younger JB. Use of a single random serum progesterone value as a diagnostic aid for ectopic pregnancy. *Fertil Steril* 1991;55:497–500.

Gerard HC, Branigan PJ, Balsara GR, et al. Viability of Chlamydia trachomatis in fallopian tubes of patients with ectopic pregnancy. *Fertil Steril* 1998;70:945–948.

Giuliani A, Panzitt T, Schoell W, et al. Severe bleeding from peritoneal implants of trophoblastic tissue after laparoscopic salpingostomy for ectopic pregnancy. *Fertil Steril* 1998;70:369–370.

Gjelland K, Hordnes K, Tjugum J, et al. Treatment of ectopic pregnancy by local injection of hyperosmolar glucose: A randomized trial comparing administration guided by transvaginal ultrasound or laparoscopy. *Acta Obstet Gynecol Scand* 1995;74:629–634.

Gleicher N, Parrilli M, Pratt DE. Hysterosalpingography and selective salpingography in the differential diagnosis of chemical intrauterine versus tubal pregnancy. *Fertil Steril* 1992;57:553–558.

Goldner TE, Lawson HW, Xia Z, et al. Surveillance for ectopic pregnancy-United States, 1970–1989. *MMWR CDC Surveill Summ* 1993;42:73–85.

Graczykowski JW, Mishell DR. Methotrexate prophylaxis for persistent ectopic pregnancy after conservative treatment by salpingostomy. *Obstet Gynecol* 1997;89:118–122.

Grimes DA, Geary FH Jr., Hatcher RA. Rh immunoglobulin utilization after ectopic pregnancy. *Am J Obstet Gynecol* 1981;140:246–249.

Grimes DA. The morbidity and mortality of pregnancy: Still risky business. *Am J Obstet Gynecol* 1995;170:1489–1494.

Grimes HG, Nosal RA, Gallagher JC. Ovarian pregnancy: a series of 34 cases. *Obstet Gynecol* 1983;61:174–180.

Hahlin M, Sjoblom P, Lindblom B. Combined use of progesterone and human chorionic gonadotropin determinations for differential diagnosis of very early pregnancy. *Fertil Steril* 1991;55:492–496.

Hallatt JG. Tubal conservation in ectopic pregnancy: a study of 200 cases. *Am J Obstet Gynecol* 1986;54:1216–1221.

Hillis SD, Nakashima A, Amsterdam L, et al. The impact of a comprehensive chlamydia prevention program in Wisconsin. *Fam Plann Perspect* 1995;27:108–111.

Hoppe DE, Bekkar BE, Nager CW. Single-dose systemic methotrexate for the treatment of persistent ectopic pregnancy after conservative surgery. *Obstet Gynecol* 1994;83:51–54.

Jain K, Hamper VM, Sanders RC. Comparison of transvaginal sonography in the detection of early pregnancy and its complications. *Am J Radiol* 1988;151:1139–1143.

Jauchler GW, Baker RL. Cervical pregnancy: Review of the literature and a case report. *Obstet Gynecol* 1970;35:870–874.

Kadar N, Caldwell BV, Romero R. A method of screening for ectopic pregnancy and its indications. *Obstet Gynecol* 1981;58:162–166.

Kadar N, DeVore G, Romero R. Discriminatory hCG zone: its use in the sonographic evaluation for ectopic pregnancy. *Obstet Gynecol* 1981;58:156–161.

Kataoka ML, Togashi K, Kobayashi H, et al. Evaluation of ectopic pregnancy by magnetic resonance imaging. *Hum Reprod* 1999;14:2644–2650.

Kelly H. *Operative gynecology*, vol 2. New York, Appleton, 1898:453.

Kirchler HC, Seebacher S, Alge AA, et al. Early diagnosis of tubal pregnancy: changes in tubal blood flow evaluated by endovaginal color Doppler sonography. *Obstet Gynecol* 1993;82:561–565.

Kojima E, Abe Y, Morita M, et al. The treatment of unruptured tubal pregnancy with intratubal methotrexate injection under laparoscopic control. *Obstet Gynecol* 1990;75:723–725.

Korhonen J, Stenman UH, Ylostalo P. Serum human chorionic gonadotropin dynamics during spontaneous resolution of ectopic pregnancy. *Fertil Steril* 1994;61:632–636.

Kung F-T, Chang S-Y. Efficacy of methotrexate treatment in viable and nonviable cervical pregnancies. *Am J Obstet Gynecol* 1999;181:1438–1444.

Kuppuswami N, Vindekilde J, Sethi CM, et al. Diagnosis and treatment of cervical pregnancy. *Obstet Gynecol* 1983;61:651–653.

Kurjak A, Zalud I, Schulman H. Ectopic pregnancy: transvaginal color Doppler of trophoblastic flow in questionable adnexa. *J Ultrasound Med* 1991;10:685–689.

Lang PF, Tamussino K, Honigi W, et al. Treatment of unruptured tubal pregnancy by laparoscopic instillation of hyperosmolar glucose solution. *Am J Obstet Gynecol* 1992;166:1378–1381.

Langer R, Bukovsky I, Herman A, et al. Conservative surgery for tubal pregnancy. *Fertil Steril* 1982;38:427–430.

Lau S, Tulandi T. Conservative medical and surgical management of interstitial ectopic pregnancy. *Fertil Steril* 1999;72:207–215.

Lavy G, Diamond MP, DeCherney AH. Ectopic pregnancy: relationship to tubal reconstructive surgery. *Fertil Steril* 1987;47:543–556.

Lecuru F, Robin F, Chasset S, et al. Direct cost of single dose methotrexate for unruptured ectopic pregnancy. Prospective comparison with laparoscopy. *Eur J Obstet Gynecol Reprod Biol* 2000;88:1–6.

Levin AA, Schoenbaum SC, Stubblefield PG, et al. Ectopic pregnancy and prior induced abortion. *Am J Public Health* 1982;72:253–256.

Lipscomb GH, Bran D, McCord ML, et al. Analysis of three hundred fifteen ectopic pregnancies treated with single-dose methotrexate. *Am J Obstet Gynecol* 1998;178:1354–1358.

Lipscomb GH, McCord ML, Stovall TG, et al. Predictors of success of methotrexate treatment in women with tubal ectopic pregnancies. *N Engl J Med* 1999;341:1974–1978.

Louis-Sylvestre C, Morice P, Chapron C, et al. The role of laparoscopy in the diagnosis and management of heterotopic pregnancies. *Hum Reprod* 1997;12:1100–1102.

Marcus SF, Macnamee M, Brinsden P. Heterotopic pregnancies after in-vitro fertilization and embryo transfer. *Hum Reprod* 1995;10:1232–1236.

Martin JN Jr, Sessums JK, Martin RW, et al. Abdominal pregnancy: current concepts of management. *Obstet Gynecol* 1988;71:549–557.

Matthews CP, Coulson PB, Weld RA. Serum progesterone levels as an aid in the diagnosis of ectopic pregnancy. *Obstet Gynecol* 1986;68:390–394.

Mol BMJ, Ankum WM, Bossuyt PMMM, et al. Contraception and the risk of ectopic pregnancy: A meta-analysis. *Contraception* 1995;52:337–341.

Morlock RJ, Lafata JE, Eisenstein D. Cost-effectiveness of single-dose methotrexate compared with laparoscopic treatment of ectopic pregnancy. *Obstet Gynecol* 2000;95:407–412.

Mueller BA, Daling JR, Weiss NS, et al. Tubal pregnancy and the risks of subsequent infertility. *Obstet Gynecol* 1987;69:722–726.

Ory SJ, Villanueva AL, Sand PK, et al. Conservative treatment of ectopic pregnancy with methotrexate. *Am J Obstet Gynecol* 1986;154:1299–1306.

Paalman R, McElin T. Cervical pregnancy. *Am J Obstet Gynecol* 1959;77:1261–1270.

Pauerstein CJ, Hodgson BJ, Kramen MA. The anatomy and physiology of the oviduct. *Obstet Gynecol Annu* 1974;3:137–201.

Pellerito JS, Taylor KJW, Quedens-Case C, et al. Ectopic pregnancy: evaluation with endovaginal color flow imaging. *Radiology* 1992;183:407–411.

Peterson HB, Xia Z, Hughes JM, et al. The risk of ectopic pregnancy after tubal sterilization. *N Engl J Med* 1997;336:762–767.

Peterson HB, Xia Z, Hughes JM, et al. The risk of pregnancy after tubal sterilization: findings from the U.S. Collaborative Review of Sterilization. *Am J Obstet Gynecol* 1996;174:1161–1170.

Polak JO, Wolfe SA. A further study of the origin of uterine bleeding in tubal pregnancy. *Am J Obstet Gynecol* 1924;8:730–738.

Pouly JL, Mahnes H, Mage G, et al. Conservative laparoscopic treatment of 321 ectopic pregnancies. *Fertil Steril* 1986;46:1093–1097.

Pratt-Thomas HR, White L, Messer HH. Primary ovarian pregnancy: presentation of ten cases including one full-term pregnancy. *South Med J* 1974;67:920–925.

Raziel A, Golan A. Primary ovarian pregnancy successfully treated with methotrexate [letter; comment]. *Am J Obstet Gynecol* 1993;169:1362–1363.

Reece EA, Petrie RH, Sirmans MF, et al. Combined intrauterine and extrauterine gestations: a review. *Am J Obstet Gynecol* 1983;146:323–330.

Risquez F, Pennehoaut G, McCorvey, et al. Diagnostic and operative microlaparoscopy: a preliminary multicentre report. *Hum Reprod* 1997;12:1645–1648.

Risquez F, Pennehouat G, Foulot H, et al. Transcervical tubal cannulation and falloposcopy for the management of tubal pregnancy. *Fertil Steril* 1992;7:274–275.

Rojansky N, Schenker JG. Heterotopic pregnancy and assisted reproduction. An update. *J Assist Reprod Genet* 1996;13:594–601.

Rothe DJ, Birnbaum SJ. Cervical pregnancy: diagnosis and management. *Obstet Gynecol* 1973;42:675–680.

Rubin IC. Cervical pregnancy. *Surg Gynecol Obstet* 1911;13:625–633.

Sandberg EC, Pelligra R. The medical antigravity suit for management of surgically uncontrollable bleeding associated with abdominal pregnancy. *Am J Obstet Gynecol* 1983;146:519–525.

Saraiya M, Berg CJ, Kendrick JS, et al. Cigarette smoking as a risk factor for ectopic pregnancy. *Am J Obstet Gynecol* 1998;178:493–498.

Saraj AJ, Wilcox JG, Najmabadi S, et al. Resolution of hormonal markers of ectopic gestation: a randomized trial comparing single-dose intramuscular methotrexate with salpingostomy. *Obstet Gynecol* 1998;92:989–994.

Sauer MV, Gorrill MJ, Rodi LA, et al. Nonsurgical management of unruptured ectopic pregnancy: an extended clinical trial. *Fertil Steril* 1987;48:752–755.

Schiff E, Shalev E, Bostan M, et al. Pharmacokinetics of methotrexate after local tubal injection for conservative treatment of ectopic pregnancy. *Fertil Steril* 1992;57:688–690.

Schwartz RO, DiPietro DL. Beta-hCG as a diagnostic aid for suspected ectopic pregnancy. *Obstet Gynecol* 1980;56:197–203.

Seifer DB, Silva PD, Grainger DA, et al. Reproductive potential after treatment for persistent ectopic pregnancy. *Fertil Steril* 1994;62:194–196.

Seinera P, DiGregorio A, Arisio R, Decko A, Crana F. Ovarian pregnancy and operative laparoscopy: report of eight cases. *Hum Reprod* 1997;12:608–610.

Shah A, Courey NG, Cunanan RG. Pregnancy following laparoscopic tubal electrocoagulation and excision. *Am J Obstet Gynecol* 1977;129:459–460.

Shepherd RW, Patton PE, Novy MJ, et al. Serial beta-hCG measurements in the early detection of ectopic pregnancy. *Obstet Gynecol* 1990;75:417–420.

Shinagawa S, Nagayama M. Cervical pregnancy as a possible sequela of induced abortion. Report of 19 cases. *Am J Obstet Gynecol* 1969;105:282–284.

Shoen JA, Nowak RJ. Repeat ectopic pregnancy: a 16-year clinical survey. *Obstet Gynecol* 1975;45:542–546.

Silva PD, Schaper AM, Rooney B. Reproductive outcome after 143 laparoscopic procedures for ectopic pregnancy. *Obstet Gynecol* 1993;81:710–715.

Smith M, Vessey MP, Bounds W, et al. Progestogen-only oral contraception and ectopic gestation. *Br Med J* 1974;4:104–105.

Society for Assisted Reproductive Technology and American Society for Reproductive Medicine. Assisted reproductive technology in the United States: 1997 results generated from the American Society for Reproductive Medicine/Society for Assisted Reproductive Technology Registry. *Fertil Steril* 2000;74:641–653.

Spandorfer SD, Menzin A, Barnhart KT, et al. Efficacy of frozen section evaluation of uterine curettings in the diagnosis of ectopic pregnancy. *Am J Obstet Gynecol* 1996;175:603–605.

Spandorfer SD, Sawin SW, Benjamin I, et al. Postoperative day 1 serum human chorionic gonadotropin level as a predictor of persistent ectopic pregnancy after conservative surgical management. *Fertil Steril* 1997;68:430–434.

Spiegelberg O. Zur Casuistik den Ovarial-Schwangerschaft. *Arch Gynaek* 1878;13:73.

Stafford JC, Ragan WD. Abdominal pregnancy: review of current management. *Obstet Gynecol* 1977;50:548–552.

Stangel JJ, Gomel V. Techniques in conservative surgery for tubal gestation. *Clin Obstet Gynecol* 1980;23:1221–1228.

Storeide O, Veholmen M, Eide M, et al. The incidence of ectopic pregnancy in Hordaland county, Norway 1976–1993. *Acta Obstet Gynecol Scand* 1997;76:345–349.

Stovall TG, Ling FW, Carson SA, et al. Serum progesterone and uterine curettage in differential diagnosis of ectopic pregnancy. *Fertil Steril* 1992;57:456–457.

Stovall TG, Ling FW, Gray LA, et al. Methotrexate treatment of unruptured ectopic pregnancy: a report of 100 cases. *Obstet Gynecol* 1991;77:749–753.

Stovall TG, Ling FW. Single-dose methotrexate: an expanded clinical trial. *Am J Obstet Gynecol* 1993;168:1759–1762.

Strandell A, Thorburn J, Hamberger L. Risk factors for ectopic pregnancy in assisted reproduction. *Fertil Steril* 1999;71:282–286.

Stromme WB. Conservative surgery for ectopic pregnancy: a twenty-year review. *Obstet Gynecol* 1973;41:215–223.

Stromme WB. Salpingotomy for tubal pregnancy: report of a successful case. *Obstet Gynecol* 1953;1:472–475.

Studdiford WE. Primary peritoneal pregnancy. *Am J Obstet Gynecol* 1942;44:487–491.

Swolin K, Fall M. Ectopic pregnancy;recurrence, postoperative fertility and aspects of treatment based on 182 patients. *Acta Eur Fertil* 1972;3:147–157.

Tanaka T, Hayashi J, Kutsuzawa T, et al. Treatment of interstitial ectopic pregnancy with methotrexate: report of a successful case. *Fertil Steril* 1982;37:851–852.

Tatum HJ, Schmidt FH. Contraceptive and sterilization practices and extrauterine pregnancy: a realistic perspective. *Fertil Steril* 1977;28:407–421.

Thompson LR. Abdominal pregnancy at term with later removal of placenta. *Am J Surg* 1966;111:272–273.

Timor-Tritsch IE, Monteagudo A, Matera C, et al. Sonographic evolution of cornual pregnancies treated without surgery. *Obstet Gynecol* 1992;79:1044–1049.

Tummon IS, Whitmore NA, Daniel SAJ, et al. Transferring more embryos increases risk of heterotopic pregnancy. *Fertil Steril* 1994;61:1065–1067.

Ushakov FB, Elchalal U, Aceman PJ, et al. Cervical pregnancy: past and future. *Obstet Gynecol Surv* 1996;52:45–59.

Vasquez G, Winston RML, Brosens IA. Tubal mucosa and ectopic pregnancy. *Br J Obstet Gynaecol* 1983;90:468–474.

Verhulst G, Camus M, Bollen N, et al. Analysis of the risk factors with regard to the occurrence of ectopic pregnancy after medically assisted procreation. *Hum Reprod* 1993;8:1284–1287.

Walters MD, Eddy C, Pauerstein CJ. The contralateral corpus luteum and tubal pregnancy. *Obstet Gynecol* 1987;70:823–826.

Weinberg A, Sherwin AS. A new sign in roentgen diagnosis of advanced ectopic pregnancy. *Obstet Gynecol* 1956;7:99–101.

Weissman A, Fishman A. Uterine rupture following conservative surgery for interstitial pregnancy. *Eur J Obstet Gynecol Reprod Biol* 1992;44:237–239.

Werber J, Prasadarao PR, Harris VJ. Cervical pregnancy diagnosed by ultrasound. *Radiology* 1983;149:279–280.

Westrom L. Effect of acute pelvic inflammatory disease on fertility. *Am J Obstet Gynecol* 1975;121:707–713.

WHO Task Force. A multinational case-control study of ectopic pregnancy. *Clin Reprod Fertil* 1985;3:131–143.

Yao M, Tulandi T. Current status of surgical and nonsurgical management of ectopic pregnancy. *Fertil Steril* 1997;67:421–433.

Yeko TR, Gorrill MJ, Hughes LH et al. Timely diagnosis of early ectopic pregnancy using a single blood progesterone measurement. *Fertil Steril* 1987;48:1048–1050.

Te Linde's Operative Gynecology, ninth edition, edited by John A. Rock and Howard W. Jones, III. Lippincott Williams & Wilkins, Philadelphia: © 2003.

CHAPTER
23

▼

Tubal Sterilization

HERBERT B. PETERSON   AMY E. POLLACK

JEFFREY S. WARSHAW

In proposing the concept of tubal sterilization in 1842, James Blundell suggested the following:

> . . . the operator . . . ought to remove a portion, say one line, of the Fallopian tube, right and left, so as to intercept its caliber—the larger blood vessels being avoided. Mere divisions of the tube might be sufficient to produce sterility, but the further removal of a portion of the tube appears to be surer practice. I recommend this precaution, therefore, as an improvement of the operation.

Samuel Smith Lungren of Toledo, OH, is credited with having performed the first tubal sterilization in 1880, after having performed a Caesarean section for a woman whose previous child was also born by Caesarean section because of a contracted pelvis. During the second Caesarean section, Lungren intended to remove the woman's ovaries to prevent future pregnancy, but instead decided that ". . . the risk would be lessened and the same result would be accomplished by tying both Fallopian tubes with strong silk sutures about one inch from the uterus." At the time of Lungren's successful tubal sterilization, laparotomy was a life-threatening procedure; thus, the performance of tubal sterilization at the time of Caesarean section to prevent future pregnancy was potentially lifesaving. In 1919, Madlener reported on 85 tubal sterilizations performed at the time of lapa-

rotomy for other reasons, including Caesarean section; three of the 85 women died postoperatively from infection. Because of the extreme risks, performing a laparotomy for the sole purpose of tubal sterilization remained an unpopular idea until the mid-20th century. Indeed, when three deaths occurred from 1936 to 1950 among 1,022 women who had postpartum Pomeroy sterilization, the investigators concluded that the risk for sterilization was comparable to that for multiparity and that "sterilization because of great multiparity alone cannot be justified on medical grounds" (Prystowsky and Eastman).

In addition to concerns about safety, the early history of tubal sterilization included debate about the appropriateness of tubal sterilization for fertility control. At the twenty-first Annual Meeting of the American Gynecological Society in 1886, participants debated a woman's right to undergo surgical sterilization. During this debate, Edward P. Davis said, "I hold it [sterilization] to be the right of a woman who is in a condition to which natural delivery is impossible . . . ." H.J. Garrigues objected by saying,

> We must leave that to Nature or to God. . . . I do not think that the woman has a right of that kind. . . . The mere fact that she does not want to have more children should not decide the question. (Speert)

The availability and acceptability of tubal sterilization as a method of fertility control remained limited until the mid-20th century, and, accordingly, tubal sterilization remained uncommon in the United States and around the world until the 1960s. In the 1970s, the worldwide popularity of tubal sterilization increased dramatically. Between 1970 and 1980, the estimated number of tubal sterilizations increased markedly in Europe, China, India, other parts of Asia, and Latin America. In the United States, the number of tubal sterilizations increased nearly fourfold—from about 200,000 in 1970 to about 700,000 in 1977. Among the factors affecting this increase were the availability and acceptability of two new surgical approaches—minilaparotomy and laparoscopy. In contrast to laparotomy for sterilization, these approaches were safer, allowed for surgery without hospitalization, reduced recovery time, and gave a better cosmetic result. Minilaparotomy has been used in many developing countries, and laparoscopy has been used in many developed countries, as well as in the United States.

Minilaparotomy for interval sterilization (i.e., sterilization at a time unrelated to pregnancy) requires a 2.5- to 3.0-cm suprapubic incision. The technique was first described by Uchida and colleagues in Japan in 1961. It was used in the early 1970s in Thailand by Vitoon and associates and then rapidly gained acceptance worldwide. Laparoscopy for tubal sterilization was first proposed by Anderson (1937) and later described by Power and Barnes (1941). The use of laparoscopy in Europe was encouraged by the work of Palmer (France), Steptoe (Britain), and Frangenheim (Germany), and use of the technique rapidly gained popularity in the 1970s, particularly in Europe and the United States.

In the United States, the increased use of tubal sterilization in the 1970s occurred concurrently with the widespread availability and acceptability of laparoscopy. In 1970, less than 1% of sterilizations were performed with a laparoscope, but by 1975, more than one third of the 550,000 women who had tubal sterilization had the procedure performed laparoscopically. This transition was associated with a marked reduction in length of hospital stay for tubal sterilization—from 6.5 nights in 1970 to 4 nights in the years 1975 to 1978. By 1987, one third of tubal sterilizations in the United States required no overnight hospital stay, and 79% of these were performed by way of laparoscopy.

Sterilization is now the method of family planning most commonly used in the world. In 1990, about 191 million married women of reproductive age used sterilization (of themselves or their spouses) for contraception; 169 million of these women were in developing countries, and 22 million were in developed countries. The corresponding percentage of married women of reproductive age who used sterilization was 22% in developing countries and 11% in developed countries; these women represented 44% and 18% of all contraceptive users in developing and developed countries, respectively.

Thus, the developing world accounts for most of the use of sterilization. Nearly half of all users are in China, and more than one fourth are in India. Vasectomy accounts for only a small percentage of sterilization procedures in developing countries except for China, India, and South Korea. In nearly all countries, the prevalence of tubal sterilization exceeds that of vasectomy. Worldwide, the ratio of female to male sterilization is 3 to 1.

In the United States, more than 1 million sterilizations are performed each year. In 1987, about 640,000 tubal sterilizations were performed. Most (66%) were inpatient procedures, and most of these (90%) were performed by laparotomy. Of the outpatient procedures (34%), 79% were performed by laparoscopy. The percent distribution of sterilizations by timing with respect to pregnancy interval (concurrent with Caesarean section or occurring postpartum or postabortion) is not available from national data, but most inpatient laparotomy sterilizations were presumably associated with pregnancy or delivery.

In the United States, sterilization has also become the most commonly used method of contraception among married couples. The proportion of couples who used sterilization for contraception more than doubled from 1973 (16%) to 1995 (39%). Most of this increase was in female sterilization—from 9% in 1973 to 28% in 1995; the increase in male sterilization was from 8% in 1973 to 11% in 1995. Among U.S. women using contraception in 1995, 17% 25 to 29 years old, 29% 30 to 34 years old, and 41% 35 to 44 years old had undergone tubal sterilization.

TIMING OF STERILIZATION

Tubal sterilization can be performed at the time of Caesarean section, shortly after delivery or induced abortion, or at a time unrelated to pregnancy. About one half of tubal sterilizations in the United States are performed at a time unrelated to pregnancy. The timing of tubal sterilization can influence the choice of anesthetic, surgical approach, and method of tubal occlusion. For example, most sterilizations performed concurrently with Caesarean section require no separate anesthesia and involve partial salpingectomy as the method of tubal occlusion. Most tubal sterilizations performed after vaginal delivery are done by minilaparotomy with subumbilical incisions and partial salpingectomy. Tubal sterilization not associated with birth usually is performed by laparoscopy (with use of coagulation, silicone rubber band application, or spring clip application) or minilaparotomy (with use of partial salpingectomy).

PREOPERATIVE EVALUATION

The candidate for sterilization should be extensively counseled. The intended permanence of the procedure, alternatives to sterilization, and risks of surgery should be discussed. For couples desiring sterilization, no such discussion is complete without consideration of vasectomy as an alternative. Women also should be made aware that sterilization failure can occur and that the relative likelihood of ectopic pregnancy is increased when sterilization failure does occur.

The work-up of women who are to undergo tubal sterilization includes a history and physical examination and a laboratory evaluation, as indicated. Consideration should be given to whether the woman might be pregnant at the time of sterilization, and pregnancy testing should be ordered as necessary.

A careful gynecologic history and examination also are necessary before sterilization. Women with gynecologic disease or complaints may require additional diagnostic or therapeutic measures. Some ultimately may be better served by other surgical procedures, either instead of or in addition to sterilization. For example, some women with enlarged and symptomatic uterine leiomyomata and women with symptomatic pelvic relaxation may benefit more from hysterectomy than from tubal sterilization. Others, such as women with abnormal cervical cytology, need careful evaluation before a decision can be made about preventing or treating invasive cervical cancer.

ANESTHESIA

Complications of general anesthesia are the leading cause of death attributed to sterilization in the United States. The risks inherent in general anesthesia are exacerbated by its use postpartum and during laparoscopy. The special requirements of general anesthesia for laparoscopy have been well described.

Except for the use of conduction anesthesia postpartum, general anesthesia is the technique most often used for female sterilization in the United States. A 1988 survey of members of the American Association of Gynecologic Laparoscopists revealed that the number of providers of tubal sterilization who used local anesthesia for laparoscopic sterilization had increased from 4% (in the 1982 survey) to 8%. Worldwide, more than 75% of tubal sterilization procedures are performed under local anesthesia. A discussion of the technology and regimen for administering general or conduction anesthesia is beyond the scope of this chapter. Instead, we focus on local anesthesia because of its increasing use in outpatient settings for many types of surgery.

Sterilization by laparoscopy or minilaparotomy can be performed safely under local anesthesia. The patient avoids the risks associated with general anesthesia, spends less time sedated or anesthetized, and has a more rapid recovery. Nausea and vomiting are less likely to occur, and the patient is awake to report symptoms that can indicate the occurrence of a complication. Television technology has made it possible for the patient to observe the procedure if she desires. Furthermore, the overall expense often is reduced compared with procedures done under general anesthesia.

In the United States, the overall morbidity rate for female sterilization is so low that it is difficult to obtain a sample large enough to demonstrate a comparative

safety advantage for local versus general anesthesia. One U.S. study randomly assigned 100 women to either local or general anesthesia for laparoscopic sterilization. Serious or life-threatening events did not occur in either group. However, women who had general anesthesia were more likely to have intraoperative hypotension, hypertension, or tachycardia, which suggests that these women were hemodynamically less stable and may have been at increased risk for cardiovascular complications. In another study, 125 women were randomly allocated to the use of local or general anesthesia for laparoscopic sterilization. Women who had general anesthesia were more likely to develop hypotension; hypertension was more common in the local anesthesia group. No women in either group had tachycardia.

Operating under local anesthesia incurs several possible disadvantages. The patient's anxiety may be increased; therefore, the surgeon must use a decisive and gentle surgical technique while talking with the patient. The patient may feel discomfort; thus, the physician must have a thorough understanding of the use of sedative and analgesic drugs. Although obesity can complicate the use of local anesthesia, several studies indicate that local anesthesia can be used successfully for obese women. Women with a history of multiple abdominal or pelvic surgical procedures or peritonitis may need additional anesthesia if the procedure is difficult or prolonged. Additional anesthesia also may be required during minilaparotomy if the abdominal incision needs to be extended. One U.S.-based, retrospective study reviewed 2,827 outpatient laparoscopic sterilizations performed under local anesthesia and mild sedation from 1980 to 1988. The mean operating time was 10.0 ($\pm$5.1) minutes, and the mean anesthesia time was 23.3 ($\pm$6.9) minutes. The hospital cost to the patient was reduced 65% to 85%. Another U.S. study reported on 358 minilaparotomies for interval sterilization performed under local anesthesia. The average operating time was 21 minutes, and no complications were reported. In both series, the local anesthetic was 0.5% bupivacaine hydrochloride used alone or in combination with lidocaine. In one series, midazolam hydrochloride and fentanyl citrate were used for mild intravenous sedation; in the other series, meperidine hydrochloride and diazepam were used.

For local infiltration and paracervical block, agents of intermediate intrinsic potency (defined as the minimum concentration required to produce a block within 5 to 10 minutes), such as lidocaine or mepivacaine, have been found suitable. Both are amides with good stability and low toxicity. Onset of analgesic effects is rapid, even when a low concentration of medication is used, and the duration of the effect is sufficient for the procedure but not prolonged (about 1.5 hours when the medication is given in plain solution). Bupivacaine, a more potent and a longer-acting amide, is frequently used in the United States. However, the short duration of action provided by lidocaine or mepivacaine is preferred by some because it allows for awareness of any abnormal degree of persistent pain and early diagnosis of complications, such as hematoma formation.

SURGICAL APPROACH

Minilaparotomy

The minilaparotomy approach to tubal occlusion can be used in the interval or postpartum period. Although interval sterilization by minilaparotomy is the sterilization procedure most frequently performed in many countries, it is not a common procedure in the United States. Minilaparotomy in the United States often is used preferentially among women considered to be at increased risk for laparoscopy.

Interval minilaparotomy is performed with use of a 2- to 3-cm midline vertical or transverse suprapubic incision. In patients with an enlarged uterus resulting from uterine leiomyomata or other benign conditions, the minilaparotomy incision should be made at the level of the uterine fundus to ensure access to the fallopian tubes. A uterine manipulator is placed through the cervix just before surgery and is used to bring the uterus toward the incision. Placement of a paracervical block before insertion of the uterine manipulator reduces discomfort for patients having surgery under local anesthesia. The abdomen is then entered with the approach that is used for laparotomy; small hand-held retractors and the Trendelenburg position are used to enhance exposure. Once the uterus is identified, a tubal hook or a finger is placed posteriorly at the top of the fundus and moved along the uterus. The fallopian tube is identified first by the fimbriated end, and then the midportion of the fallopian tube is grasped with a small Babcock clamp and elevated through the abdominal incision. Tubal occlusion most often is performed by use of the modified Pomeroy or Parkland technique. However, clips or rings can be applied through the minilaparotomy incision with modified instruments originally developed for use through the operating laparoscope.

Postpartum minilaparotomy is performed in a manner similar to that of interval minilaparotomy. It is ideally performed before the onset of postpartum uterine involution while the uterine fundus is high in the abdomen (within 48 hours of delivery). A 2- to 3-cm subumbilical vertical or semicircular incision is made in the midline where the abdominal wall is thin. Because of the proximity of the enlarged uterus to the incision, access to the fallopian tubes is easier than it is with an interval approach. A uterine manipulator is unnecessary when minilaparotomy is performed in the postpartum period.

Laparoscopy

> The magic is in the magician, not in the wand. . . .
> Entering the abdomen is the most dangerous part of
> the laparoscopic procedure. (Hulka and Reich)

The laparoscopic instrumentation, including laparoscope, light cables and light source, insufflator and tubing, and video camera and television, if used, should be set up and tested for proper functioning before any incisions are made. If a Veress needle is to be used, it is good practice to attach it to the insufflation tubing and test that gas flows freely through it. High line pressures (3 mm Hg or higher) during low-flow insufflation (1 L/min) through a Veress needle that has yet to be inserted into the abdominal cavity suggest that the needle has some occlusion. Checking for occlusion before inserting the needle can avoid the multiple attempts at needle placement that might occur in the belief that incorrect placement, rather than needle occlusion, is the cause of resistance to flow. It is convenient, while waiting for surgery, to have the end of the laparoscope bathing in warm sterile fluid to prevent it from fogging when it is inserted into the abdominal cavity.

A no. 11 scalpel blade is used to make a single vertical incision in the lower rim of the umbilicus. This must be done carefully because the aorta can lie just a few centimeters beneath the abdominal wall, particularly in a thin patient. The abdominal wall is lifted away from the aorta by pinching the skin beneath the umbilicus between thumb and index finger. The umbilicus is elevated with one hand while the surgeon's other hand makes the controlled incision.

The Veress needle is disconnected from the insufflation tubing before insertion. The stopcock on the needle then is placed in the open position, and the spring action of the needle is tested for smooth operation. Elevating the abdominal wall and using the Veress needle with the stopcock open allows air to rush into the previously gas-free abdominal cavity when the end of the needle penetrates the peritoneal layer. The in-rushing air, if heard, is one of the first indicators that successful abdominal entry has occurred. Outflow of blood likewise can serve as an immediate indicator of vessel injury. Allowing air to rush in also can cause the bowel to fall away from the abdominal wall.

The terminal aorta is palpated, even in a moderately obese patient, through the abdominal wall in the midline, just above or at the umbilicus. The pulsations of the aorta are lost in the midline just beneath the umbilicus, corresponding to the sacral hollow. The aorta bifurcates at the level of L4, which corresponds to the summits of the iliac crests. This is a more reliable landmark for bifurcation of the aorta than the umbilicus. The Veress needle is placed through the umbilical incision and is directed at an angle toward the sacral hollow or uterine fundus (to avoid the aorta) and in the midline (to avoid the iliac vessels). Elevating the abdominal wall during this placement increases the distance between the Veress needle and major vessels. While placing the Veress needle, the surgeon should hold the needle like a dart, being careful not to impede the action of the spring mechanism. Resistance at the tip of the needle causes the blunt cannula inside the needle to be pushed back, and the spring mechanism at the hub of the needle extends. When resistance at the tip of the advancing needle is lost, as occurs with successful penetration of the peritoneal cavity, the blunt cannula inside the needle advances back out to the tip, and the spring mechanism at the hub of the needle snaps back in. Observing the spring mechanism for this snap can serve as a sign to test for successful placement. Often there are two snaps—the first when the fascia is penetrated and the second with peritoneal penetration. Continuing to advance the needle tip much beyond the point of penetration of the parietal peritoneum risks placing the needle tip between loops of bowel or under the omental apron, both of which can cause resistance to flow and can result in reinsertion of the needle. Continued advancement of the Veress needle also risks vascular injury. The needle tip should not be moved laterally once the tip is inserted in the abdomen; any simple vascular puncture could be transformed into a major laceration if the needle tip is moved from side to side. Once abdominal penetration is made with the Veress needle, the needle should be stabilized carefully until the safety checks have been completed. The needle should not be moved, and a laparotomy should be performed immediately if major vascular injury is suspected.

The distance between skin and fascia can increase with increasing patient obesity. A given angle of entry of the Veress needle that successfully penetrates the peritoneal cavity in a thin patient might fall far short of the peritoneum in an obese patient. To bring the peritoneal cavity within the physical length of the Veress needle, it is often necessary to pursue entry with a trajectory closer to the vertical. However, this also directs the Veress needle toward the aorta and therefore should be attempted only by experienced surgeons, and with extreme care. Alternatively, open laparoscopy can be performed.

Several safety checks for correct intraabdominal placement can be performed while the Veress needle is held steady. The instillation of 5 to 10 mL of sterile saline through the needle, followed immediately by aspiration, can be helpful. The fluid should meet little resistance, and, more important, scant fluid should return on reaspiration. Reaspiration of fluid suggests that the needle tip is in a small enclosed space that does not allow immediate dispersion of the instilled fluid. Reaspiration of feculent fluid or bloody fluid suggests bowel or vascular penetration, respectively. Simple penetration of the bowel with a Veress needle does not mandate immediate exploratory laparotomy. Depending on the setting and the skill level of the surgeon, reinsertion of the needle or open laparoscopy, followed by laparoscopic visualization of the intestine, can be pursued.

A second safety check consists of attaching a filled 10-mL syringe to the hub of the Veress needle and then removing the plunger. Elevation of the abdominal wall at this point should cause an increased negative intraperitoneal pressure, which allows the fluid in the syringe to drain passively into the abdominal cavity through an open stopcock. Alternatively, a drop of saline can be placed on the hub of the Veress needle, and, with the stopcock open, elevation of the abdominal wall should result in the drop flowing downward freely.

Once these safety checks are performed, insufflation is begun at 1 L/min or less. Initial insufflation pressures often are 5 mm Hg or less in thin patients and, even with correct needle placement, can be 10 mm Hg or more in obese patients. An intraabdominal pressure greater than 15 mm Hg during insufflation generally is avoided to prevent respiratory compromise and decreased venous return secondary to vena caval compression. Abdominal distention increases the distance between the abdominal wall and major pelvic vessels, and this increases the safety buffer when the trocar is inserted. However, the abdomen should not be so distended that it is difficult to elevate it for trocar insertion.

During insufflation, a shift from dullness to tympany with percussion over the liver is indicative of pneumoperitoneum formation. It also is prudent for the surgeon to pay attention to the ECG rhythm during insufflation, because the sudden appearance of premature ventricular contractions can be an indicator of intravascular insufflation. Sudden vascular collapse during insufflation can be caused by a gas embolism in the right side of the heart. Rapidly turning the patient onto her left side and advancing a Swan-Ganz catheter into the right heart for aspiration can be life-saving.

Once insufflation is complete, the Veress needle is removed, and the umbilical incision is widened to accommodate the trocar and sleeve. An incision that is too large can result in leakage of gas around the sleeve. An incision that is too small can restrict access. The trocar should be checked before insertion to ensure that it is sharp; a dull trocar potentially is dangerous because it requires increased force for abdominal entry.

The trocar is grasped as shown in Fig. 23.1. The middle finger serves as a stopper, preventing the forward momentum following fascial puncture from carrying the

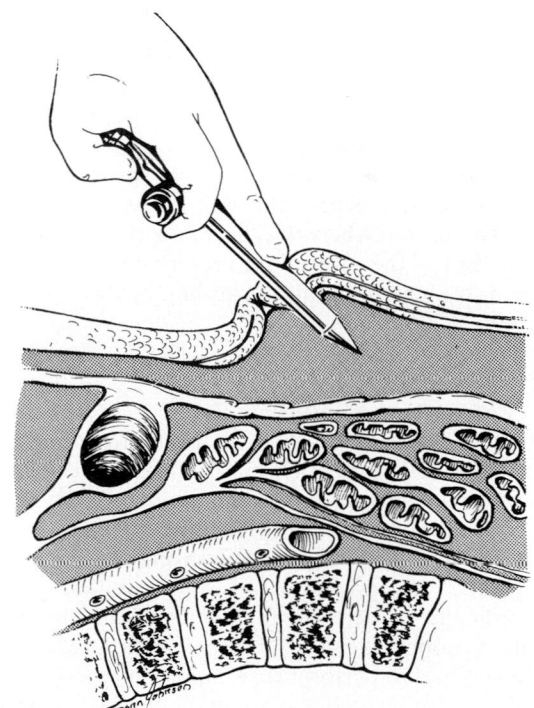

FIGURE 23.1. Trocar entry. When inserting the trocar through the abdominal wall, the trocar is "palmed" in the surgeon's dominant hand, with the extended middle finger serving as a stopper to deep abdominal penetration. If the surgeon's hand is too small to accomplish this, open laparoscopy should be considered.

trocar deep into the pelvis. The precautions for insertion of the Veress needle pertain even more to insertion of the trocar; the abdominal wall is elevated and the trocar is directed toward the hollow of the sacrum or the uterine fundus, and a midline trajectory is followed.

Open laparoscopy is performed without previous creation of a pneumoperitoneum. A transverse fold of skin beneath the umbilicus is elevated with two Allis clamps about 4 cm apart. The skinfold is then incised transversely about 1.5 cm with use of a scalpel, and the incision is carried down to the fascia. The skin is released and the fascia is grasped and elevated with the two Allis clamps. The fascia is then incised in the midline, and the opening is stretched with a hemostat. Next, the peritoneum is identified, elevated, and incised. Each angle of the fascial incision is sutured with a no. 0 absorbable stitch but not tied. The Hasson blunt cannula and sleeve are then placed through the opening of the peritoneum. The blunt cannula then is removed and the abdomen is insufflated through the port found on the sleeve.

METHOD OF TUBAL OCCLUSION

All tubal sterilization methods rely on correct identification of the fallopian tube for success. With any of the methods, the tube should be followed out to its fimbriated end to confirm that the correct structure has been identified.

Theoretically, the risk of tuboperitoneal fistula formation can be reduced by preserving a proximal tubal segment 1 to 2 cm in length. It is possible that the proximal tubal stump serves as a distensible reservoir for the small amount of uterine fluid that is normally forced through the interstitial portion of the tube by uterine contractions. The capacitance of the proximal stump might serve to dissipate the fluid pressure emanating from the uterus. Otherwise, this direct fluid pressure on the cut end of the tube might prevent complete closure of the tubal lumen during the healing process.

Irving Procedure

In 1924, and later, in 1950, Irving reported on his method of achieving tubal sterilization. He attempted to reduce the risk of tuboperitoneal fistulae by extensively dissecting the ligated ends of the tubes and burying the proximal tubal segment. Although the extra dissection in this technique likely enhances effectiveness, it also carries the potential for greater blood loss as well as increases the difficulty of performing the technique through a minilaparotomy incision. The procedure also takes slightly longer to perform than simpler methods.

The Irving technique is accomplished by first using a hemostat or scissors to create a window in the mesosalpinx just beneath the tube, about 4 cm from the uterotubal junction (Fig. 23.2A). Then the tube is twice ligated (no. 1 chromic) and divided between the ties at this location. The free ends of the proximal stump ligature are held long. A 1-cm incision is made in the serosa

of the posterior uterine wall near the uterotubal junction. A hemostat, or similar pointed instrument, is then used to bluntly deepen the incision, creating a pocket in the uterine musculature about 1 to 2 cm deep (Fig. 23.2B). The two free ends of the proximal stump ligature, previously held long, are then individually threaded onto a curved needle and brought deep into the myometrial tunnel and out through the uterine serosa (Fig. 23.2C). Traction on the sutures then draw the ligated proximal stump deep into the myometrial tunnel, and tying the free sutures fix the tube in this buried location (Fig. 23.2D). Often this can be accomplished without incising the mesosalpinx, but if extra mobilization of the proximal stump is needed, or if the proximal stump mesosalpinx appears in danger of being torn when traction is applied, then the mesosalpinx under the proximal tubal segment can be incised partly back toward the uterus. The serosal opening of the myometrial tunnel is then plicated closed around the tube with use of a fine absorbable suture, but great care should be exercised to avoid compromising the tube as it enters the tunnel. Strangulation or damage to the tube with this stitch could cause necrosis and fistula formation in the extramyometrial portion of the proximal tube. No treatment of the distal tubal stump is necessary, but some surgeons choose to bury that segment in the mesosalpinx.

Modified Pomeroy Procedure

Bishop and Nelms, colleagues of Pomeroy, reported on the Pomeroy technique for tubal occlusion in 1930. They were careful to point out the importance of using absorbable suture as opposed to permanent suture.

In this method, the tube is grasped in its midportion, usually with a small atraumatic clamp such as the Babcock, and a loop of tube is elevated (Fig. 23.3A). The base of the loop is ligated with no. 1 plain catgut, and the sutures are held long. A 1- to 2-cm portion of tube in the ligated loop is transected and removed with scissors (Fig. 23.3B). Bishop and Nelms, in the original report on this method, pointed out that ligation was performed with a double strand of absorbable chromic catgut suture to allow the cut tubal ends to quickly separate after surgery. It was their belief that this would allow the ends to naturally fibrose and peritonealize without fistulization or communication. This also is the rationale for the common modification of the Pomeroy technique, in which the original chromic suture is replaced by plain catgut because of the more rapid degradation of the latter. Surgeons have a tendency to strenuously tighten the catgut ligature around the tube (as though the tighter the ligature, the better the occlusion), but this appears to go against the very principles of the procedure. This tightening can result in greater strangulation and necrosis of the adjoining tubal segments, potentially increasing the risk of fistula formation and failure. Taking time to identify the muscular tube, which is often seen pouting from each of the severed limbs of the ligated tube, is a good habit to develop, as is checking the tubal stumps for hemostasis. Resection of

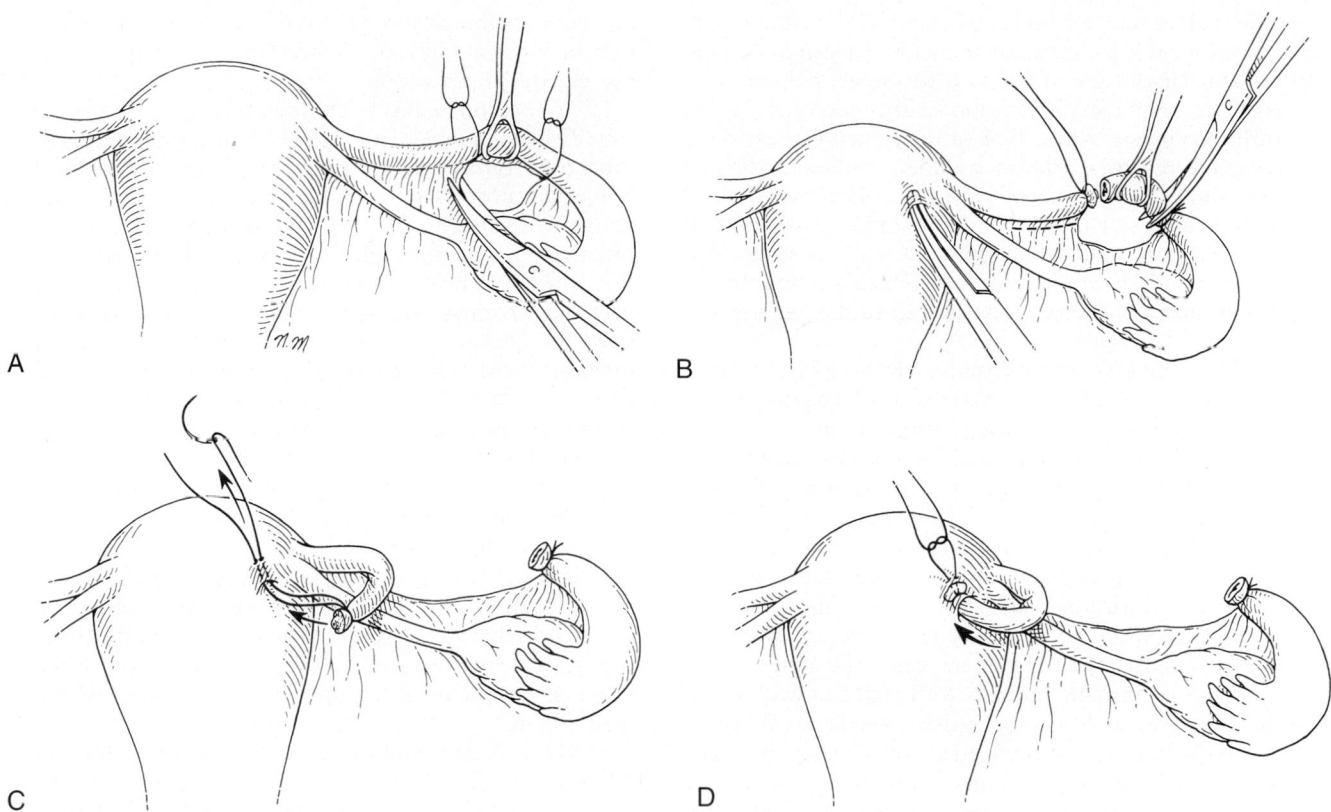

A

B

C

D

FIGURE 23.2. Irving method. **A:** A fenestration is made beneath the tube about 4 cm from the uterotubal junction using scissors or a hemostat. **B:** The tube is then twice ligated and a portion resected. A deep pocket is created in the myometrium on the posterior uterus. The dashed line shows the line of incision if added mobilization of the proximal tube is necessary to bury the end of the tube in the myometrium. **C:** The tagged ends of the tube are sutured deep into the myometrial tunnel and out through the uterine serosa. **D:** Tying these sutures secures the cut end of the proximal tube deep in the myometrial pocket.

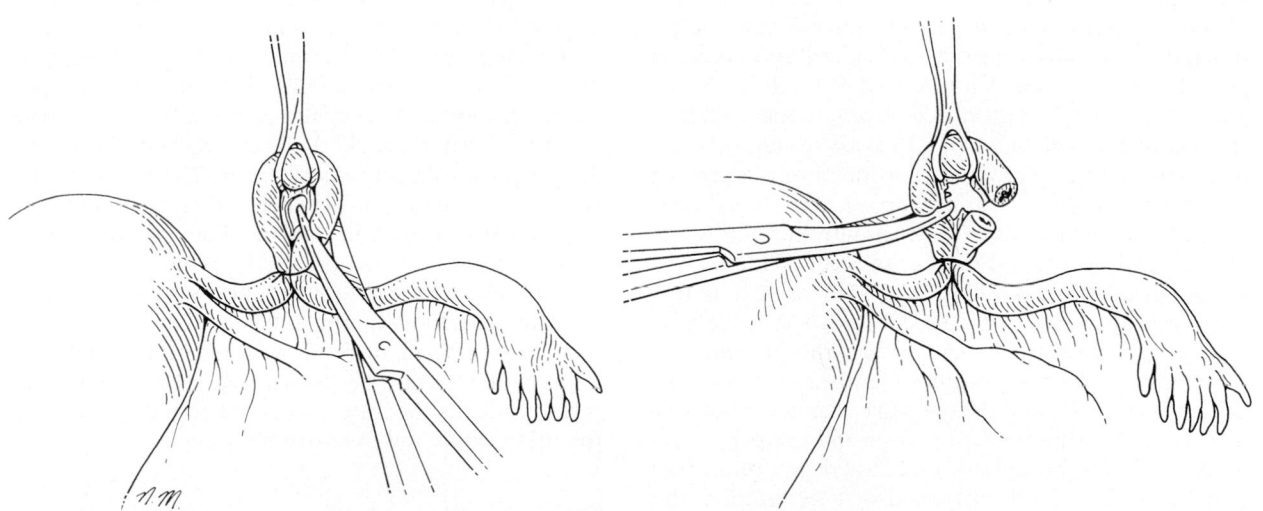

FIGURE 23.3. Pomeroy method. **A:** A loop of the isthmic portion of the tube is elevated and ligated at its base with one or two ties of no. 1 plain catgut suture. If performed through a minilaparotomy incision, these ties should be held long to prevent premature retraction of the tubal stumps into the abdomen when the loop of tube is transected. **B:** A fenestration is bluntly created through the mesentery within the tubal loop, and each limb of the tube on either side of this fenestration is individually cut. The cut ends of the tube are inspected for hemostasis and allowed to retract into the abdomen.

a limited amount of tube, restricted to the isthmic section, is ideal if future anastomosis is requested. Making the knuckle of tube in the loop too small, however, can result in only a shave excision of the side of the tube, with incomplete transection of the lumen. To avoid incomplete resection, the mesosalpinx within the ligated loop should be perforated with scissors before the tubal limb on each side of this window is individually cut. It is important not to cut the loop so close to the suture that only short distal segments of tube remain beyond the tie. These short limbs can easily slip out of the ligature and cause delayed bleeding.

The Pomeroy method minimizes bleeding by compressing and sealing the vascular mesosalpinx before tubal transection. It is not unusual when performing tubal sterilization at the time of Caesarean section to find the mesosalpinx greatly engorged with distended veins. Elevation of the uterus often facilitates tubal occlusion by allowing the vessels to drain and decompress. It is important when replacing the uterus into the peritoneal cavity to lead with one adnexa at a time while protecting the tubal ligation site on that side. Otherwise, when the uterus is replaced, a tight fit can cause the adnexa to be squeezed against the incision with resultant avulsion of the ligature and postoperative bleeding. When a Pomeroy ligation is performed through a minilaparotomy incision, the ligation sutures are held while the tube is cut. This prevents retraction of the cut tubal stumps into the peritoneal cavity before they can be adequately examined and before hemostasis can be ensured. After examination is complete, the sutures are cut and the tubal stumps are allowed to retract into the abdomen.

It is also possible to perform a modified Pomeroy tubal ligation as a laparoscopic interval procedure. In this technique, a laparoscope with an operating channel is placed through the umbilical port, and a 5-mm midline suprapubic cannula is introduced under direct vision. A plain gut Roeder loop is introduced through the 5-mm port. A grasper is introduced through the operative channel of the laparoscope and passed through the suture loop, and the appropriate portion of tube is grasped and elevated while the suture loop is passed over the tissue and tightened. Scissors are then introduced through the operative scope, and the suture is cut. With use of a grasper through the 5-mm port, the loop is held on tension while the scissors are used through the operative channel to transect the tube. When the procedure is complete and the tubal segment has been resected, the grasper is used through the operative channel to hold the specimen while the operative scope and grasper are removed together through the umbilical sleeve. In contrast to most other methods of laparoscopic sterilization, this technique has the advantage of producing a surgical specimen for evaluation.

Uchida Method

Originally reported on in 1961, and reported on in revised form in 1975, the Uchida method, like the Irving procedure before it, recognized the role of fistula formation in tubal sterilization failures and included steps to prevent this complication.

This method begins by having the surgeon grasp the tube in its midportion, about 6 to 7 cm from the uterotubal junction. A 1:1,000 epinephrine in saline solution is injected subserosally, creating a bleb over the tube that is then incised (Fig. 23.4A). The muscular tube, which often can be seen springing up through the serosal incision, then is divided between two hemostats. The serosa over the proximal tubal segment is dissected bluntly toward the uterus, exposing about 5 cm of the proximal tubal segment (Fig. 23.4B). The tube then is ligated with no. 0 chromic suture near the uterotubal junction, and this 5-cm segment of exposed tube is resected. The shortened proximal stump is allowed to retract into the mesosalpinx (Fig. 23.4C). The serosa around the opening in the mesosalpinx is sutured in a pursestring fashion with a fine absorbable stitch. Simultaneous ligation of the distal tube and gathering of the mesosalpinx around the distal stump are accomplished when the pursestring suture is tied (Fig. 23.4D). This step also fixes the distal stump in a position open to the peritoneal cavity while burying the proximal stump within the leaves of the mesosalpinx.

Uchida added fimbriectomy to the procedure in 1975 to enhance effectiveness. Some surgeons omit this step, and in addition excise only 1 to 2 cm of tube (rather than the recommended 5 cm) to permit future tubal anastomosis.

Parkland Method

In this method, made popular during the 1960s at Parkland Memorial Hospital, the tube is grasped in its midportion with a Babcock clamp, and a hemostat or scissors are used to create a window in an avascular area of the mesosalpinx just beneath the tube (Fig. 23.5A). The window is stretched to about 2.5 cm in length by opening the hemostat. Two ligatures of no. 0 chromic material are passed through the window, and the tube is ligated proximally and distally (Fig. 23.5B). The intervening segment of tube between the ties then is resected (Fig. 23.5C). In contrast to the Pomeroy method, in which the resected portions of the tubes are ligated together and later separate when the suture weakens, immediate separation of the tubal ends is accomplished with the Parkland method. Care should be taken to avoid undue traction on the ligatures while resecting the tubal segments, because this could result in tearing of the mesosalpinx and excessive bleeding.

Unipolar Coagulation

Unipolar coagulation was the first method of laparoscopic tubal occlusion to achieve widespread use. However, reports of electrical complications, particularly thermal bowel injury, resulted in a significant decline in this method's popularity as soon as alternative methods of laparoscopic tubal occlusion became available in the

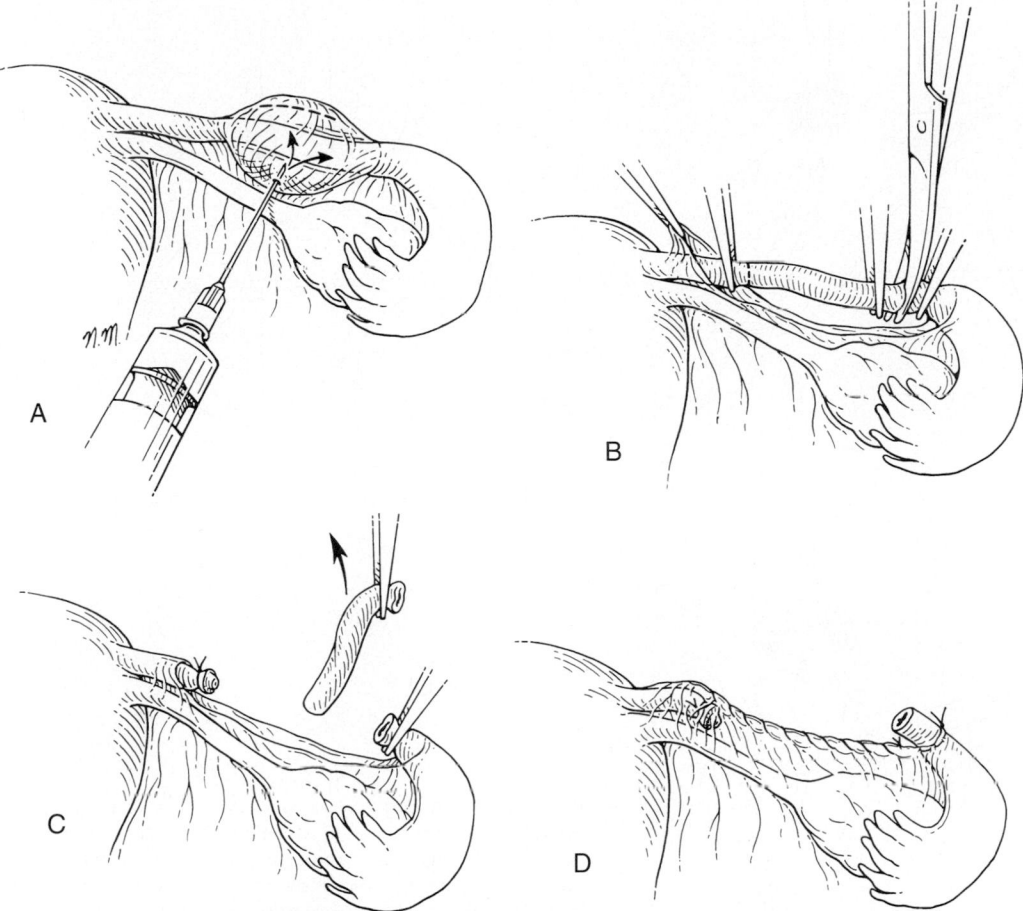

FIGURE 23.4. Uchida method. **A:** Injection of vasoconstricting solution beneath the serosa of the tube about 6 cm from the uterotubal junction. The serosa is then incised *(dashed line)*. **B:** The antimesenteric edge of the mesosalpinx is pulled back toward the uterus, exposing about 5 cm of the tube. **C:** The tube is ligated proximally and cut, and the tied stump is allowed to retract into the mesosalpinx. The hemostat on the distal stump remains attached to facilitate exteriorization of this portion of the tube. **D:** The mesosalpinx is closed. A pursestring stitch of the mesosalpinx around the exteriorized tubal stump secures it in a position open to the abdomen, whereas the ligated proximal stump is buried within the mesosalpinx. Once the pursestring suture is tied, the hemostat can be removed.

mid-1970s. In unipolar coagulation, a specially designed insulated grasping forceps is introduced through the operating channel of the laparoscope or independently through a 5-mm second puncture port. As a safety precaution, attachment of the electric cable to the grasping forceps should be delayed until the surgeon is ready to coagulate the fallopian tube.

With unipolar coagulation, as much as 3 to 5 cm of tube can be destroyed with a single burn, with occult damage occurring beyond the visual zone of desiccation. For this reason, the isthmic–ampullary portion of the tube should be carefully identified and grasped about 5 cm from the uterus to preserve some length of proximal tube. The jaws of the grasping forceps should completely encircle the fallopian tube and include a portion of the mesosalpinx as well. The tube should be elevated away from adjacent structures, such as bowel and blad-

der, before current is applied for about 5 seconds. If a second burn is required, it should be applied to the proximal rather than the distal portion of the tube. The current should be turned off before the tube is released and the grasping forceps are retracted into the laparoscope. Both jaws of the grasping forceps serve as active electrodes and will burn any structure they touch while current is applied.

The thermal injuries to abdominal viscera that are seen with unipolar coagulation are, in some cases, likely attributable to the phenomenon of capacitive coupling. The current flowing down the unipolar probe creates an electromagnetic field that can transfer an electric charge to any conductor surrounding the probe. The greater the voltage being used with the probe, the greater this capacitive effect. In the case of laparoscopic unipolar coagulation for sterilization, the conductor surrounding

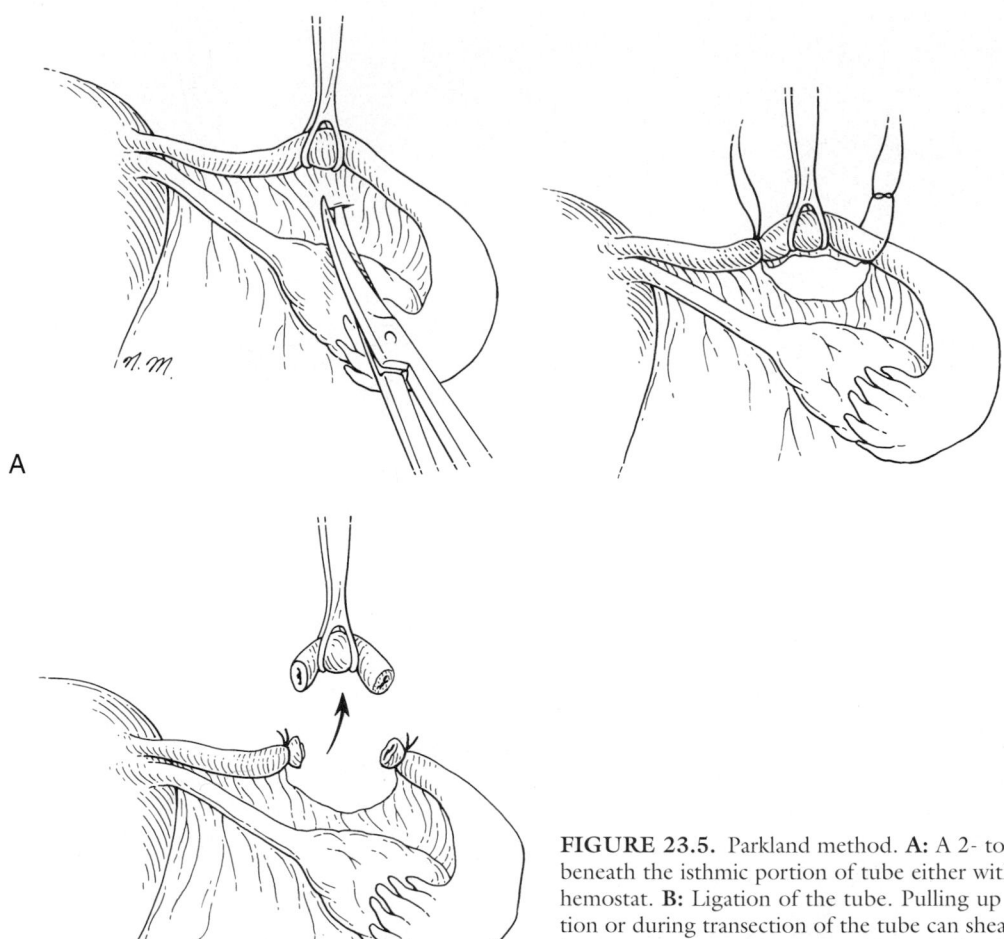

FIGURE 23.5. Parkland method. **A:** A 2- to 3-cm fenestration is made beneath the isthmic portion of tube either with scissors or bluntly with a hemostat. **B:** Ligation of the tube. Pulling up on the suture during ligation or during transection of the tube can shear the tube off the underlying mesentery, resulting in troublesome bleeding. **C:** Portion of tube removed.

the insulated unipolar probe is the operative laparoscope itself. As long as the operative laparoscope is safely grounded (usually by contact with a metal trocar sleeve that, in turn, is in contact with the abdominal wall over a large surface area), then the capacitive charge on the laparoscope can be harmlessly dissipated. If, however, the laparoscope is prevented from safely grounding into the abdominal wall by a nonconducting trocar sleeve, or by a nonconducting barrier around the trocar sleeve (e.g., a plastic collar with threads), then the capacitive charge that builds up on the scope discharges when and wherever any portion of that instrument touches the patient's tissues. Depending on the surface area of contact, the discharging current from the scope into the patient's tissues has either a high current density (small contact surface) or a low current density (large contact surface), resulting in either a large thermal effect or a minimal thermal effect, respectively. In the case of contact with bowel, this thermal effect easily can result in delayed necrosis and peritonitis. If the unipolar probe is brought into the abdomen by way of a second puncture trocar sheath, then it is the sheath itself that is capacitively charged (if it is made of a conducting material). If the charge on the conducting trocar sleeve is prevented from grounding through the abdominal wall (as could occur if

a plastic collar with threads is being used around the trocar sleeve), then any bowel or other grounded tissue touching the trocar sleeve again has capacitive current flowing into it.

If thermal injury to the intestine is noticed during the laparoscopic procedure, then it is important to recognize that the injury can extend well beyond the visibly damaged area. Small burns of the bowel serosa may not require repair, but hospitalization for 5 to 7 days is recommended so the patient can be observed for delayed peritonitis. A laparotomy is required if peritonitis occurs. A large area of superficial thermal bowel injury, or one that is thought to extend beyond the serosa, requires resection of that portion of intestine with a 5-cm margin on either side of the lesion. Oversewing the damaged area can result in stitches being placed in bowel that appears healthy visually but in reality is destined to necrose from occult thermal or electrical injury.

Further potential for thermal injury with the use of unipolar coagulation is related to the ground plate. With unipolar coagulating systems, the patient's body is used as an essential element of the electrical circuit. Current flows into the patient in a high density (and over a small surface area) at the interface between the unipolar instrument and the patient's tissues and exits the body in a low density (and over a large surface area) at the interface between the patient's body and the ground plate (return electrode). If the ground plate is only partly attached to the patient, then this exiting current might achieve sufficient power density to result in thermal damage at the point of contact. Some electrosurgical generators have built-in circuitry that disables the unit if there is incomplete contact with the ground plate.

Bipolar Coagulation

The use of bipolar coagulation for tubal sterilization was reported by Rioux and Cloutier in 1974. With bipolar coagulation, current flows from one jaw of the grasper to the other, requiring only the intervening tissue of the patient within the jaws of the instrument to complete the circuit. This eliminates the need for a distant ground plate. Compared with unipolar coagulation, which uses the patient's body to complete the circuit, bipolar coagulation applies current in a more discrete manner (a 1.5- to 3-cm zone of thermal injury) and with an increased element of safety. Capacitive coupling does not occur with bipolar forceps because the field effects from the equal but opposite currents that flow in both directions along the shaft of the instrument cancel out one another.

Once the fallopian tube is carefully identified, it is grasped in the distal isthmic section with the bipolar forceps in such a way that the tube is completely encircled, including a portion of the mesosalpinx (Fig. 23.6). The tube then is elevated away from any adjacent structures and current is applied. Two additional contiguous areas similarly are coagulated to ensure at least a 3-cm area of desiccation. As with unipolar coagulation, an effort should be made to leave the proximal 2 cm of tube undisturbed to reduce the risk of tuboperitoneal fistula formation.

The visual end points of tubal blanching and swelling noted with bipolar coagulation cannot be used to ensure destruction of the endosalpinx. Desiccation of the outer one third of the fallopian tube can occur without desiccation of the inner one third. The use of an optical flow meter has been recommended to evaluate cessation of

current flow through the tube as an end point. Presumably, when complete desiccation occurs, there will be no further electrolytes in solution to carry current through the dehydrated tissue. Soderstrom and coworkers have demonstrated that complete desiccation of the fallopian tube with bipolar systems is more likely when a cutting waveform, as opposed to a coagulation or blended waveform, is used and when the power output is at least 25 W against a 100-Ω load.

Silicone Rubber Bands

High complication rates with the use of unipolar coagulation led to the pursuit of safer, nonthermal methods that could be applied laparoscopically. The first of these methods to gain popularity was the silicone rubber band, developed by Yoon and coworkers in the early 1970s.

The band is introduced with a specially designed endoscopic applicator that can be delivered either through the operating channel of a laparoscope or a separate second puncture port. The band is first stretched over the distal end of the applicator barrel (immediately before use to avoid extended deformation of the band). A transcervical uterine manipulator can be used to help achieve proper exposure. After the device is introduced into the abdominal cavity, grasping tongs are extended from within the applicator barrel. One of the tongs is used to gently hook and elevate the isthmic portion of the tube about 3 cm from the uterus. The tongs then are retracted into the applicator, which closes both arms of the tongs around the grasped tube while pulling the loop of tube up into the barrel (Fig. 23.7). The surgeon must take care in ensuring that the tube is completely encircled by the tongs as they are retracted into the applicator. Failure to do this can result

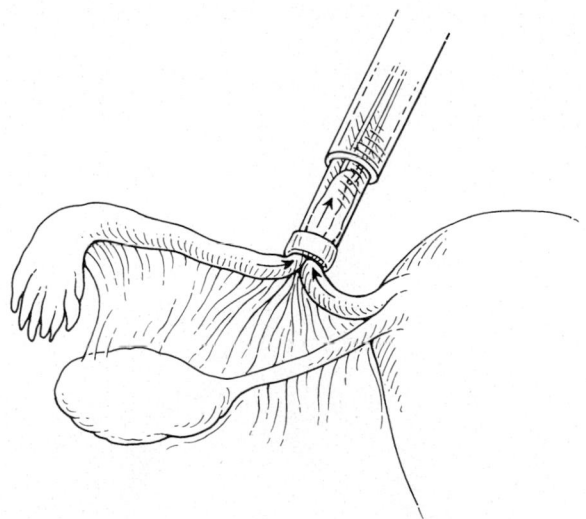

FIGURE 23.7. Silicone band method. The isthmic portion of the tube is retracted into the applicator barrel using grasping tongs, which should completely surround the tube. The applicator barrel is advanced toward the tube during this retraction process to avoid excessive traction on the tube and its mesentery.

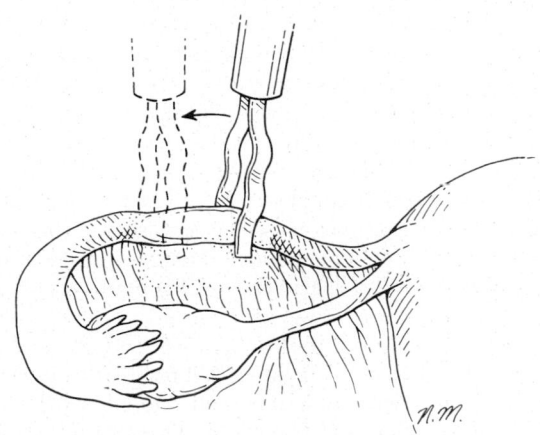

FIGURE 23.6. Bipolar method. A 3-cm minimum zone of isthmic tube is desiccated with bipolar forceps. The paddles of the forceps extend across the tube onto the mesosalpinx.

in a band that is only tangentially applied to the tube (failing to occlude its lumen), or applied only to the mesosalpinx.

It is important to avoid excessive traction on the tube during retraction of the tongs. The surgeon should slowly advance the entire applicator toward the tube while gradually retracting the tongs and tube up into the applicator. Failure to do this can result in mesosalpingeal hemorrhage and tubal laceration. Once the loop is fully retracted into the device, the band is slid off the applicator barrel and onto the base of the loop.

About 1.5 to 2 cm of tube is contained in the constricted loop. After devascularization, this portion of tube becomes anoxic and resorbs over time. Eventually, the band no longer encircles any tube, and later it is often found in the mesosalpinx. Apart from the 2-cm loop of encircled tube, very little destruction is caused by the band, and 2 mm lateral to the area of constriction of the tube is relatively undisturbed.

It is difficult to apply a band to edematous or thickened fallopian tubes successfully. Tubal adhesions can reduce the mobility of the tube and preclude pulling an adequate loop of tube into the applicator. Additional rings can be applied to the cut edges if transection of the mesosalpinx or tube with accompanying hemorrhage occurs. Bipolar or unipolar coagulation can be used if this is unsuccessful.

Spring Clip

The use of a spring clip for tubal sterilization was reported by Hulka and colleagues in 1973. The introducer for the clip can be delivered into the abdomen through the operative channel of the laparoscope or a second puncture cannula (Fig. 23.8). Because the clip must be applied exactly perpendicular to the long axis of the fallopian tube, it is helpful at times to use the two-puncture method—placing the tube on stretch by use of a trans-

cervical uterine manipulator and a grasping forceps inserted through the operating channel of the laparoscope, and introducing the applicator through the second puncture port.

The clip is held in a cradle by the applicator and can be closed and opened on the tube multiple times until an acceptable application is achieved. At this point, further pressure on the thumb device of the applicator drives the spring mechanism over the jaws of the clip, locking it closed. If improper application is determined at this point, the clip cannot be removed, and another clip has to be placed. To be effective, the clip must be applied to the isthmic portion of the tube, about 2 cm from the uterus and exactly at right angles to the long axis of the tube. It must be applied fully advanced over the tube, with the hinge of the clip pressing against the tube and with the tips of the jaws of the clip extending beyond the tube onto the mesosalpinx, creating a characteristic fold in the mesosalpinx when the clip is closed. The tube is not elevated when applying the clip, in contrast to the techniques used in coagulation and band application.

The clip, like the silicone rubber band, is most likely to be successful when applied to a normal tube. Tubal distortion, thickening, and adhesions make correct application difficult and often impossible.

A considerable advantage to the clip method of sterilization is that only 3 mm of tube is compressed by the clip, and minimal collateral damage occurs in the adjacent tissue. As a result, anastomosis procedures after clip sterilization often are highly successful.

Filshie Clip

The Filshie clip was first introduced in Europe in 1975 and the hinged Mark VI model was approved for use in the United States by the Food and Drug Administration in 1996. The device has titanium jaws lined with silicone rubber and is used with specially designed applicators that are available in both single- and double-puncture versions for use with laparoscopy or minilaparotomy. The Filshie clip has a hinge on one end and a small curve on the other and is designed to be placed on the isthmic portion of the fallopian tube approximately 1 to 2 cm from the cornua (Fig. 23.9).

To be effective, the jaws of this clip, as with the spring clip, must include the entire circumference of the tube. Only one properly applied clip needs to be applied to each fallopian tube. Once the tube is occluded, both the tube and the silicone rubber lining of the clip are compressed. Over time, about 3 to 5 mm of the compressed tissue undergoes avascular necrosis and the compressed silicone rubber expands. Eventually, plical attenuation and fibrosis of the adjacent tubal segments occurs and the clips are peritonealized.

The clip is placed into the applicator and the applicator and clip then are introduced through the cannula with the jaws of the clip in a partially closed position, so that the instrument with the clip in place can be used to manipulate the fallopian tube into proper position. The clip may close prematurely if too much pressure is placed

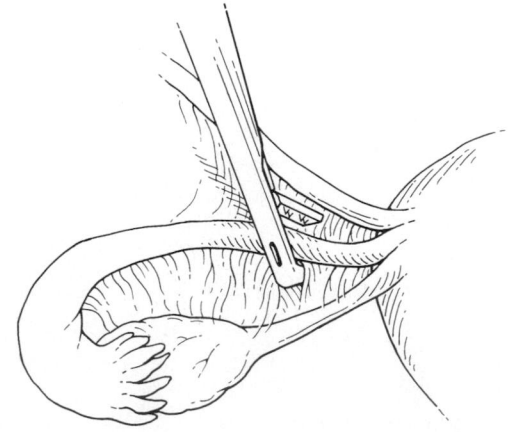

FIGURE 23.8. Spring clip method. The clip is applied to the midisthmus (about 2 cm from the cornua) at a 90-degree angle to the long axis of the tube. The hinge of the clip should be pressed against the tube, and the tips of the clip should extend onto the mesosalpinx.

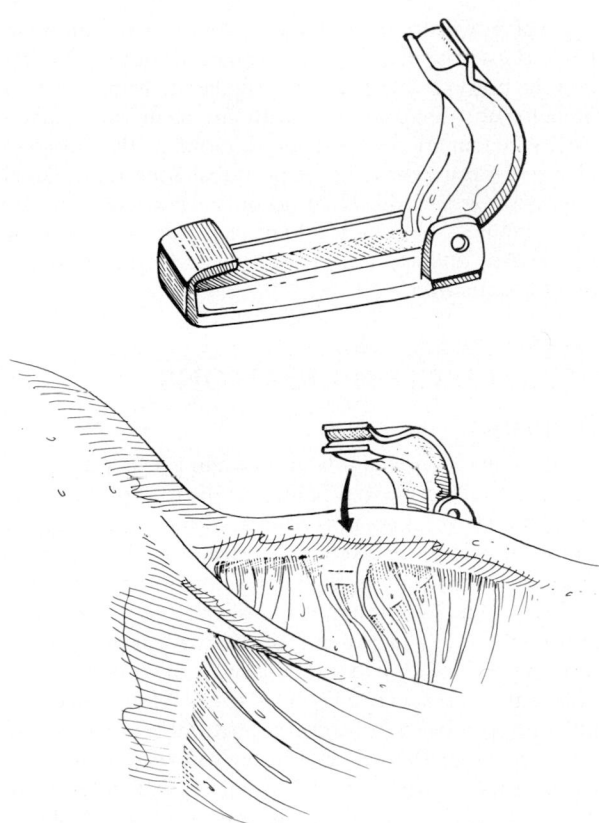

FIGURE 23-9. Filshie clip method. The clip is applied to the mid isthmus (about 1 to 2 cm from the cornua) with the lower jaw of the clip being visible in the mesosalpinx to assure that the entire circumference of the tube is included.

on the handle of the applicator. The lower jaw of the clip, with its small curve at the tip, should be seen through the mesosalpinx to assure that the clip includes the entire circumference of the isthmic portion of the tube before the clip is applied. Because of the clip's hinge, and the silicone lining of the jaws, the tubes can be manipulated and released several times for better positioning of the clip. Gentle pressure is placed on the applicator handle once desired placement is obtained, which causes the upper jaw of the clip to flatten and lock under the curved tip of the lower jaw. The clip should be closed slowly to avoid transection of the fallopian tube, which is more likely with edematous tubes. A clip can be placed on each transected end if transection occurs. Many surgeons recommend the use of a double-puncture technique to assure proper placement.

IMMEDIATE COMPLICATIONS

Mortality

In an international study of 41,834 sterilizations performed from 1971 to 1979 in 28 countries, the estimated case-fatality rate was 13.4 per 100,000 interval tubal sterilization procedures, 53.3 per 100,000 postabortion sterilization procedures, and 43.4 per 100,000 sterilizations after vaginal delivery. At least some of the differences in case-fatality rates between interval tubal sterilization and sterilization associated with pregnancy were likely attributable to complications of pregnancy termination or delivery rather than tubal sterilization per se.

The potential health impact of tubal sterilization in countries that have a high rate of maternal mortality can be assessed by analyzing sterilization-attributable deaths in Bangladesh. In the first of two epidemiologic investigations, 28 deaths were attributed to tubal sterilization in two geographic areas; the case-fatality rate was 19 deaths per 100,000 tubal sterilizations. In the second investigation, 19 deaths were identified nationwide, for a case-fatality rate of 12.4 deaths per 100,000 procedures. Anesthesia overdosage, tetanus, and hemorrhage were the leading causes of death in both investigations. On the basis of an estimated maternal mortality rate of 570 per 100,000 live births, more than 1,000 maternal deaths for each 100,000 tubal sterilizations performed would have been averted during the reproductive years of the cohort.

In the United States, deaths attributable to tubal sterilization are rare. Based on an assessment of tubal sterilizations performed in U.S. hospitals in 1979 and 1980, the estimated case-fatality rate for tubal sterilization is one to two per 100,000 procedures. Complications of general anesthesia are the leading cause of sterilization-attributable death. In a survey of deaths attributable to tubal sterilization in the United States from 1977 to 1981, 29 deaths were identified: 11 followed complications of general anesthesia, seven were caused by sepsis, four were caused by hemorrhage, three were caused by myocardial infarction, and four were related to other causes.

At least some of these deaths are preventable. Safer use of general anesthesia or use of local anesthesia, particularly for interval laparoscopic and minilaparotomy procedures, should reduce the risk of death from anesthesia. Of the seven identified deaths caused by sepsis from 1977 to 1981, three were associated with the use of unipolar electrocoagulation. Safer use of unipolar coagulation or alternative methods of tubal occlusion reduces the risk of thermal bowel injury. Three of the four deaths attributable to hemorrhage occurred after major vessel laceration during abdominal entry for laparoscopy. Safer insertion of the Veress needle and trocar, or use of alternative techniques, such as open laparoscopy or minilaparotomy, should reduce the risk of such laceration.

Morbidity

Morbidity attributable to tubal sterilization is uncommon but not rare. The risks for and types of morbidity vary somewhat by surgical approach and method of tubal occlusion. Direct comparisons of minilaparotomy and laparoscopy for tubal sterilization are limited, but studies suggest several differences. In a nonrandomized study in 23 countries, 7,053 women who had silicone rubber band application by way of laparoscopy were compared with 3,033 women who had silicone rubber band application by minilaparotomy and 5,081 women who had modified Pomeroy ligation by minilaparotomy. The surgical complication rates were 2.04%, 1.45%, and 0.79% for the three groups, respectively. In a smaller but randomized study in eight centers, 791 women who had modified Pomeroy occlusion by minilaparotomy were compared with 819 women who had occlusion from electrocoagulation (technique not specified) by way of laparoscopy. Major complications occurred in 1.5% of the women in the minilaparotomy group and 0.9% of the women in the laparoscopy group. Minor complications, which are more common, occurred in 11.6% of women in the former group and 6.0% in the latter group.

In a U.S. multicenter, collaborative study, major complications were more common among women who had minilaparotomy (3.5%) than among those who had interval laparoscopic sterilization (1.6%). However, women in the study were not randomly assigned to groups, and the sterilization procedures were performed in institutions where most interval tubal sterilizations were done by way of laparoscopy. Thus, minilaparotomy sterilizations may have been performed selectively for women at increased risk for complications.

Although the overall complication rates are similar for minilaparotomy and laparoscopy, the types of complications appear to vary. Complications of minilaparotomy usually are not serious and typically include minor wound infection, longer operating time, slightly longer postoperative convalescence, and greater postoperative pain. Laparoscopic complications are more likely to include rare but life-threatening hemorrhage and viscus perforations during abdominal entry, and thermal bowel injury during electrocoagulation. A study of 100,000 laparoscopies in France suggests that major vessel laceration occurs in three of 10,000 procedures. In a study conducted in the United Kingdom, major vessel laceration occurred in nine of 10,000 laparoscopies.

Some of the most serious complications of both interval minilaparotomy and laparoscopy occur during abdominal entry. Bladder laceration during suprapubic minilaparotomy can occur, but usually it is recognized during surgery and is repaired easily. Major vessel and bowel laceration during needle or trocar insertion for laparoscopy are more difficult to recognize or repair, and delayed treatment of these injuries can be fatal. Meticulousness is required to reduce the risks of abdominal entry. Comparative studies of open versus conventional laparoscopy are limited and have insufficient power to assess the risk of life-threatening complications, but use of open laparoscopy should markedly reduce the risk of major vessel laceration and should reduce, to a lesser extent, the risk of bowel laceration. The use of open laparoscopy can be particularly advantageous for women known or strongly suspected to have multiple abdominal or pelvic adhesions. However, even open laparoscopy can result in bowel injury if the bowel is adherent to the anterior abdominal wall.

The method of tubal occlusion chosen influences the risk for and type of complications during laparoscopy.

Thermal bowel injury is more common with unipolar than bipolar coagulation, but it can occur during the latter if the bowel is grasped and coagulated. Transection of the fallopian tube can occur with any technique, particularly when an attempt is made to mobilize the fallopian tube in the presence of thick peritubal adhesions. Tubal transection is most likely to occur when silicone rubber bands are used, but any resultant bleeding usually can be managed by the application of a second ring or by the use of coagulation.

DELAYED COMPLICATIONS

Pregnancy

Tubal sterilization is highly effective in preventing pregnancy. A frequently cited failure rate is four pregnancies per 1,000 sterilization procedures. However, a range of failure rates is more likely to portray the risk of pregnancy after sterilization. The determinants of that range are likely to include the method of tubal occlusion, surgical technique, and the age of the woman at sterilization. In the U.S. Collaborative Review of Sterilization, a multicenter, prospective, cohort study, 10,685 women undergoing tubal sterilization in medical centers in nine U.S. cities from 1978 to 1987 were followed for up to 8 to 14 years. A total of 143 sterilization failures were identified with the 10-year cumulative probability of failure ranging from 7.5 per 1,000 procedures (for unipolar coagulating procedures and postpartum partial salpingectomy procedures) to 36.5 per 1,000 (for spring clip application procedures). The failure rates for most methods of tubal occlusion were higher for women aged 18 to 27 years at sterilization (as high as 54.3 and 52.1 per 1,000 bipolar coagulation and spring clip applications, respectively) than for women aged 34 to 44 years at sterilization (as low as 1.8 and 3.8 per 1,000 unipolar coagulation and postpartum partial salpingectomy procedures, respectively).

This large U.S. multicenter study, along with two smaller studies in Thailand and Belgium have dispelled the widely held belief that nearly all pregnancies after sterilization occur in the first year or two after the procedure. In the Thai study, 418 women were followed for 6 to 10 years after sterilization, and only one of four pregnancies identified occurred within 2 years of the procedure. In the Belgian study, of 17 pregnancies after 1,437 sterilizations by bipolar coagulation, none occurred within 12 months of electrocoagulation, and eight occurred more than 24 months after the procedure. In the U.S. study, the 10-year cumulative probability of pregnancy after bipolar coagulation (24.8 per 1,000 procedures) was about 10 times the probability (2.3 per 1,000) at one year. Further, pregnancies occurred in the tenth year after all four methods of laparoscopic sterilization studied (bipolar and unipolar coagulation, silicone rubber band application, and spring clip application).

The fact that the risk of pregnancy after sterilization only can be determined after long-term follow-up creates a dilemma in interpreting published failure rates. For example, the failure rates in the U.S. Collaborative Review of Sterilization for six methods of tubal occlusion were based on procedures performed in the late 1970s and 1980s when laparoscopic sterilization was fairly new. Whether failure rates for procedures performed in the past reflect the risk for current procedures is unclear. In an analysis of bipolar coagulation procedures in the U.S. Collaborative Review of Sterilization, the 5-year cumulative probability of pregnancy for women sterilized in 1978 to 1982 (19.5 per 1,000 procedures) was significantly greater than that for women sterilized in 1985 to 1987 (6.3 per 1,000 procedures). Further, most of the procedures evaluated in that study were performed in teaching institutions; it is unclear whether procedures performed in teaching institutions can be generalized outside such settings.

Luteal phase pregnancy, or pregnancy diagnosed after sterilization but conceived prior to sterilization, is estimated to occur in two to three per 1,000 sterilization procedures. The most effective strategy for reducing the risk for luteal phase pregnancy is to time the sterilization procedure to occur during the follicular phase of the menstrual cycle. Reliance on dilatation and curettage at the time of sterilization is substantially less effective. The likelihood of luteal phase pregnancy occurring also depends on the method of contraception used before tubal sterilization. Women who use steroid hormonal contraceptives or intrauterine devices are at substantially lower risk for luteal phase pregnancy than are women who use barrier methods or no method of contraception. Testing for pregnancy by using an enzyme-linked immunosorbent assay pregnancy test on the day of sterilization also reduces the risk for luteal phase pregnancy.

The likelihood of ectopic pregnancy occurring is increased when pregnancy occurs after sterilization. In the U.S. Collaborative Review of Sterilization, the highest proportion of ectopic pregnancies among all pregnancies after sterilization was among women who underwent bipolar coagulation (65%), followed by interval partial salpingectomy (43%), silicone rubber band application (29%), postpartum partial salpingectomy (20%), unipolar coagulation (17%), and spring clip application (15%). The proportion of pregnancies that were ectopic increased over time; for all methods combined, the proportion of ectopic pregnancies was three times greater in the fourth through tenth years after sterilization (61%) than in the first 3 years (20%). The pregnancies that occurred in the tenth year after unipolar and bipolar coagulation, silicone rubber band application, and spring clip application were all ectopic. All but one (an ovarian pregnancy after bipolar coagulation) of the 47 ectopic pregnancies identified in the study were tubal pregnancies. The index of suspicion for ectopic pregnancy should be high when pregnancy is suspected after tubal sterilization. Pregnancy should be confirmed by use of a highly sensitive pregnancy test as soon as feasible.

A woman's individual risk for ectopic pregnancy can be considered in both absolute and relative terms. Her absolute risk is determined by the likelihood that the sterilization procedure can fail to prevent pregnancy and the likelihood that a resulting pregnancy will be ectopic. This risk is also relative to the risk for ectopic pregnancy that a woman had before tubal sterilization. Depending on the method of contraception used before sterilization, some women may be at greater risk for ectopic pregnancy after tubal sterilization. In a report from a case-control study in Seattle, both postpartum sterilization and interval sterilization were associated with a lower risk of ectopic pregnancy than was use of no contraception. However, women who had interval tubal sterilization had a higher risk of ectopic pregnancy than did women who were using oral contraceptives or barrier methods of contraception. In contrast, the risk for ectopic pregnancy was similar between women who had postpartum tubal sterilization and those who used oral contraceptives or barrier contraception.

Careful attention to surgical technique is required to maximize sterilization effectiveness. To reduce the risk of pregnancy after bipolar coagulation, Soderstrom and colleagues identified determinants of complete electrocoagulation. In the U.S. Collaborative Review of Sterilization, women undergoing bipolar coagulation later in the study who had three or more sites of coagulation had a 5-year cumulative probability of failure of 3.2 per 1,000 procedures. This is similar to the 5-year probability for unipolar coagulation (2.3 per 1,000) and substantially lower than that for women undergoing bipolar coagulation with fewer than three sites of coagulation (12.9 per 1,000). Stovall and coworkers reported on the use of silicone rubber bands and spring clips in a residency training program; all of 20 sterilization failures were associated with improper application of the occlusive device on gross and microscopic evaluation after subsequent bilateral salpingectomy. In the U.S. Collaborative Review of Sterilization, the risks of pregnancy were significantly increased among women who had a silicone rubber band applied solely to the distal one-third of at least one fallopian tube and among women who had a spring clip applied to a site other than the proximal one-third of at least one tube.

The likelihood of sterilization failure depends not only on the sterilization technique but also on patient and physician factors. For example, proper application of silicone rubber bands and spring clips generally is difficult in the presence of thickened tubes or dense pelvic adhesions; under such circumstances, alternative techniques usually are preferred. As noted, failure rates generally are higher for women sterilized at younger ages, not only because they are more fecund at the time of sterilization than older women, but also because they have a longer period after sterilization during which it would be feasible for pregnancy to occur. The latter consideration, which is an issue because it is now clear that pregnancy can occur for many years after sterilization, also applies to any temporary method of contraception that a woman chooses to use. For example, based on data from the U.S. Collaborative Review of Sterilization, a woman sterilized at 28 to 33 years old has a 10-year chance of pregnancy of less than 1% to about 3%, depending on the method of tubal occlusion. The comparable risk for 10 years of use of the Copper T 380 intrauterine device is about 2%, but the typical failure rate for oral contraceptive use is about 6% to 8% in just the first 12 months of use.

Menstrual Changes

After nearly a half century of debate, questions regarding the existence of a posttubal ligation syndrome of menstrual abnormalities appear to be largely resolved. Questions arose initially when Willliams and colleagues reported in 1951 that sterilized women had a higher than expected occurrence of menorrhagia and metrorrhagia. Studies in the 1970s appeared to support the existence of a poststerilization syndrome, but most of those studies had major methodologic shortcomings, including failure to account for factors other than sterilization per se that might have influenced poststerilization menstrual changes. One such factor was the use of oral contraceptives; in the United States, as many as 30% of women may use oral contraceptives immediately before tubal sterilization and many of these women have menstrual changes after sterilization attributable solely to cessation of oral contraceptive use. Although one well-controlled study (Shain et al., 1989) in the 1980s identified poststerilization menstrual changes, nearly all other studies reported in the 1980s that controlled for factors such as cessation of oral contraceptive use found little or no evidence of a poststerilization syndrome at 1 to 2 years after sterilization.

Until the 1990s, questions remained about whether menstrual changes attributable to sterilization may occur several years after the procedure. Two U.S. multicenter, prospective, cohort studies argue strongly against such an occurrence. In the first, reported in 1993, 500 women were evaluated at 6 to 10 months and 3 to 4.5 years after sterilization. When women who were taking oral contraceptives were excluded, no significant differences in seven menstrual parameters were found between sterilized women and two groups of nonsterilized women.

In the second, reported in 2000, 9,514 sterilized women enrolled in the U.S. Collaborative Review of Sterilization were compared with 573 women whose husbands underwent vasectomy. All women were asked the same questions about six menstrual parameters before tubal sterilization or the husband's vasectomy and again at annual follow-up interviews for up to 5 years. The sterilized women were no more likely than the nonsterilized women to report changes in intermenstrual bleeding or cycle length. The sterilized women were more likely than the nonsterilized women to have decreases in the number of days of bleeding and the amount of bleeding and menstrual pain; they were also more likely to have cycle irregularity. When the risk of menstrual abnormalities was evaluated by method of tubal occlusion, there were no significant differences between the women sterilized by any of six methods and the women whose husbands underwent vasectomy

in amount or duration of menstrual bleeding, intermenstrual bleeding or menstrual pain. Women undergoing three methods of sterilization (silicone rubber band application, interval partial salpingectomy, and thermocoagulation) were more likely than nonsterilized women to have an increase in cycle irregularity, whereas women undergoing two other methods (unipolar and bipolar coagulation) were more likely to have decreases in cycle irregularity. This latter observation suggests strongly that the differences between sterilized and nonsterilized women in the likelihood of cycle irregularity and other menstrual features were attributable to chance or unmeasured differences between the study groups. Finally, sterilized women were compared with nonsterilized women for risk of a syndrome consisting of either persistent increases or decreases in amount of bleeding, days of bleeding, or intermenstrual bleeding; no significant differences were identified.

Although sterilization procedures have been hypothesized to adversely affect ovarian function, laboratory studies have identified no consistent abnormalities that reflect ovarian dysfunction. Further, the biological plausibility of such an occurrence is uncertain. The tubal branch of the uterine artery, which often is occluded during sterilization, connects with the ovarian branch of the uterine artery; thus, interrupting the tubal branch could affect the blood supply to the ovary. However, blood also is supplied to the ovary by the ovarian artery, which branches directly off the aorta and is remote from the site of tubal occlusion. The possibility has been raised that tubal occlusion could damage the ovary by acutely increasing pressure in the uteroovarian arterial loop. However, as noted, neither laboratory nor epidemiologic studies find changes consistent with acute injury to the ovary and there is now strong evidence against the occurrence of sterilization-attributable menstrual abnormalities within 5 years of the procedure.

Some women who have no menstrual abnormalities before sterilization have them later, and for other women, menstrual abnormalities before sterilization resolve. To consider the former group as having a syndrome is inappropriate unless the latter group is considered to have an opposing syndrome. Although menstrual abnormalities are common among sterilized women, they also are common among nonsterilized women of similar ages. The balance of the evidence to date suggests strongly that sterilized women are no more likely than comparable nonsterilized women to have menstrual abnormalities.

Hysterectomy

Tubal sterilization and hysterectomy are common procedures in the United States, and any relation between the two has important consequences. Tubal sterilization could increase the risk for hysterectomy by increasing either the reality or the perception that a poststerilization syndrome occurs. As noted, the evidence against such a syndrome is now strong; thus, it should not be an indication for hysterectomy. Alternatively, the fact that a woman has had tubal sterilization could affect decision making about further surgery. At least three studies suggest that this effect can occur. Cohen studied 4,374 women 25 to 44 years old who had tubal sterilization in 1974 while enrolled in a universal health insurance plan in Canada. Women 25 to 29 years old at the time of sterilization were 1.6 times more likely than nonsterilized women to have a hysterectomy at a later time. However, women 30 years or older at the time of sterilization were no more likely than nonsterilized women to have a hysterectomy subsequently. Goldhaber and colleagues, who studied 39,502 women sterilized from 1971 to 1984, found that women sterilized at 20 to 24 years old were 2.4 times more likely than nonsterilized women to have a hysterectomy subsequently. For other sterilized women, the risk for hysterectomy steadily decreased with increasing age; women sterilized at 40 to 49 years old had no increased risk. Stergachis and associates studied 7,414 women sterilized from 1968 to 1983 and found that women sterilized at 20 to 29 years old were 3.4 times more likely than nonsterilized women to subsequently have a hysterectomy. Women sterilized at 30 years old or older had no increased risk for hysterectomy.

The fact that the increased risk for hysterectomy was concentrated among women sterilized at a young age in the noted studies suggests that any increased risk for hysterectomy after tubal sterilization is not biologic in etiology but attributable to other factors, such as removal of fertility preservation as a factor in decision making. In the U.S. Collaborative Review of Sterilization, women sterilized at 34 years old and younger were four to five times more likely to undergo hysterectomy than women the same age whose husbands underwent vasectomy. However, women sterilized at 35 years old and older were also four to five times more likely to undergo hysterectomy than women whose husbands underwent vasectomy, suggesting that fertility preservation does not explain all differences in decision-making between sterilized and nonsterilized women.

In the U.S. Collaborative Review of Sterilization, the cumulative probability of undergoing hysterectomy within 14 years after sterilization was 17%. Although women with gynecologic disorders at the time of sterilization were at greater risk of hysterectomy, most women who reported gynecologic disorders at sterilization did not undergo hysterectomy within the follow-up period. For example, women who reported having endometriosis at sterilization were 2.5 times more likely to undergo hysterectomy than women without endometriosis; the probability of women reporting endometriosis undergoing hysterectomy within 14 years was 35%, versus 15% for women without endometriosis. Similarly, women who reported having uterine leiomyomata at sterilization were 2.7 times more likely to undergo hysterectomy than women without leiomyomata; the 14-year cumulative probability of hysterectomy among women reporting leiomyomata was 27% versus 14% for women without leiomyomata.

Regret

The decision to undergo sterilization is serious to both men and women because the intent is to permanently terminate fertility. Although new and refined microsurgical methods of reversal are available, these methods require special skill, the procedures are complicated and lengthy, the costs are high, and none of the methods guarantees success.

Findings from studies of poststerilization regret provide useful information for presterilization counseling. Sterilization regret is a complex condition that is often causally linked to unpredictable life events. The risk factors for regret described here should not be used as reasons for restricting access to sterilization. Instead, they should be used to identify persons who may need extensive counseling. Presterilization counseling has been shown to correlate with poststerilization satisfaction.

Poststerilization regret can arise from several factors, including preexisting patient characteristics, subsequent changes in the patient's social situations or attitudes, and dissatisfaction resulting from adverse side effects caused or perceived to be caused by the procedure. Estimates of the prevalence of sterilization regret vary widely by measure of indication of regret and geographic region. During the last two decades, U.S.-based studies have reported rates of poststerilization regret ranging from 0.9% to 26.0%. The wide range reflects, in part, differences in study design and questions asked of respondents. In general, the likelihood of a woman expressing regret after sterilization appears to increase over time. In the U.S. Collaborative Review of Sterilization, the cumulative probability of regret increased from 4% at 3 years after sterilization to 8% at 7 years and 13% at 14 years.

In the 1982 National Survey of Family Growth, about 10% of women who had been sterilized reported that they would have the sterilization reversed if it were safe to do so. In the U.S. Collaborative Review of Sterilization, 14% of sterilized women reported that they had sought information about tubal reanastomosis at least once within 14 years of sterilization; only 1% actually obtained a reversal.

At least five studies have identified young age at sterilization as the strongest predictor of later regret of sterilization. In the U.S. Collaborative Review of Sterilization, young age at sterilization also was a strong predictor of regret, regardless of parity or marital status. After adjusting for other risk factors, women 30 years of age or younger at sterilization were about twice as likely as older women to express regret within 14 years of sterilization. Similarly, the cumulative probability of expressing regret within 14 years was 20% for women 30 years old or younger versus 6% for women over 30 years old at sterilization. Likewise, the 14-year cumulative probability of requesting information about reversal was 40% among women sterilized at 18 to 24 years old and, after adjustment for other risk factors, women 18 to 24 years old were almost four times as likely as women 30 years old or older to request information about reversal. Although low parity has been identified as a risk factor for regret in some studies, it was not an independent risk factor in other studies after control for factors such as young age at the time of sterilization.

Timing of the procedure in relation to pregnancy has been reported as a risk factor for regret. Several studies found that women who had tubal sterilization concurrent with Caesarean section, or following vaginal delivery or abortion were more likely to regret sterilization, but studies have been inconsistent in this regard. In the U.S. Collaborative Review of Sterilization, the 14-year cumulative probability of regret was nearly identical for women whose sterilizations were concurrent with Caesarean section (16%), after vaginal delivery (18%), and within 1 year of pregnancy (18%).The probability of regret decreased with time since the birth of the youngest child; women with 8 or more years since the birth of the youngest child had a probability of only 5%, a rate similar to that for women with no previous births (6%).

In summary, indicators of regret can vary significantly by cultural and individual circumstances. Most studies have found that age younger than 30 years is an independent risk factor for regret. The presterilization counseling for women in this age group should place special emphasis on the risk for regret. Other risk factors, such as time in relation to an obstetric event, ambivalence, or unstable life circumstances, should be assessed with each patient on an individual basis.

Cancer

One large study found no effect of tubal sterilization on breast cancer risk. Several studies identified a reduced risk of ovarian cancer after tubal sterilization. Hankinson and colleagues reported on the first large prospective cohort study of this relation; the risk of ovarian cancer for women who had tubal sterilization was one third that of nonsterilized women. In a pooled analysis of case-control studies, Whittemore and coworkers found a reduced risk of ovarian cancer after tubal sterilization.

Whether the observed reduction in risk is a real protective effect or is attributable to some other factor remains unclear. However, there is reason for optimism that tubal sterilization may provide an important noncontraceptive health benefit.

VASECTOMY AS A SURGICAL ALTERNATIVE

Some couples who have chosen surgical sterilization for permanent contraception have difficulty in deciding whether vasectomy or tubal sterilization is most appropriate. Although numerous individual- or couple-related concerns can influence the decision, many couples include considerations about safety and effectiveness in their decision making. To assist such couples, we provide a brief overview of the health effects of vasectomy.

In regard to immediate surgical complications, vasectomy is a remarkably safe procedure. Serious morbidity and death are extremely rare. Fairly minor complications, such as scrotal swelling, ecchymosis, and pain, occur in up to 50% of men who have a vasectomy, but these symptoms usually resolve spontaneously within 1 to 2 weeks. Vasectomy generally has been performed through two incisions in the scrotum, one overlying each vas. Hematoma formation occurs in about 2% of such procedures; infections occur in less than 2%. In 1985, a new vasectomy technique was introduced, referred to as no-scalpel vasectomy. It reduced the already-low rate of minor complications. In most reports, pregnancy rates after vasectomy are less than 1%. Unlike tubal sterilization, vasectomy is not immediately effective. Three months or 20 ejaculations are required to flush the vasa of viable sperm. This should be confirmed by a postvasectomy semen analysis.

In 1978, questions about the long-term health effects of vasectomy were raised when an increased risk for atherosclerosis was found among monkeys that had had a vasectomy. At least nine subsequent epidemiologic studies in men found no such increased risk, and later findings in monkeys did not support an increased risk. Thus, vasectomy does not affect the risk for subsequent cardiovascular disease.

More recently, questions have been raised about the risk of prostate cancer after vasectomy. A 1998 meta-analysis of 14 observational studies concluded that the evidence for an association between vasectomy and prostate cancer was of low quality because of biases that overestimate the effect of vasectomy, and that the association is likely not a causal one. The results of studies of the relationship between vasectomy and prostate cancer are inconsistent, the observed associations in most positive studies are weak, and the biological arguments for a harmful effect of vasectomy on prostate cancer risk are no more plausible than those for a beneficial effect. Pending further studies, a scientific panel convened by the National Institutes of Health concluded that

> Because the results of research to date on vasectomy and prostate cancer are inconsistent, and the associations that have been found are weak, there is insufficient basis for recommending a change in clinical and public health practice at this time.

BIBLIOGRAPHY

Allyn DP, Leton DA, Westcott NA, et al. Presterilization counseling and women's regret about having been sterilized. *J Reprod Med* 1986;31:1027.

Anderson ET. Peritoneoscopy. *Am J Surg* 1937;35:36.

Bernal-Delgado E, Latour-Perez J, Pradas-Arnal F, et al. The association between vasectomy and prostate cancer: a systematic review of the literature. *Fertil Steril* 1998;70:191.

Bhiwandiwala PP, Mumford SD, Feldblum PJ. A comparison of different laparoscopic sterilization occlusion techniques in 24,439 procedures. *Am J Obstet Gynecol* 1982;144:319.

Bhiwandiwala PP, Mumford SD, Kennedy KI. Comparison of the safety of open and conventional laparoscopic sterilization. *Obstet Gynecol* 1985;66:391.

Bishop E, Nelms WF. A simple method of tubal sterilization. *NY State J Med* 1930;30:214.

Bordahl PE, Raeder JC, Nordentoft J, et al. Laparoscopic sterilization under local or general anesthesia? A randomized study. *Obstet Gynecol* 1993;81:137.

Boring CC, Rochat RW, Becerra J. Sterilization regret among Puerto Rican women. *Fertil Steril* 1988;49:973.

Chamberlain G, Brown JC, eds. *Gynaecological laparoscopy: the report of the confidential inquiry into gynaecological laparoscopy.* London: The Royal College of Obstetricians and Gynaecologists, 1978.

Cheng MCE, Cheong J, Ratnam SS, et al. Psychosocial sequelae of abortion and sterilization: a controlled study of 200 women randomly allocated to either a concurrent or interval abortion and sterilization. *Asia Oceania J Obstet Gynaecol* 1986;12:193.

Chi I-C, Feldblum PJ. Luteal phase pregnancies in female sterilization patients. *Contraception* 1981;23:579.

Cohen MM. Long-term risk of hysterectomy after tubal sterilization. *Am J Epidemiol* 1987;125:410.

DeStefano F, Greenspan JR, Ory HW, et al. Demographic trends in tubal sterilization: United States, 1970–1978. *Am J Public Health* 1982;72:480.

DeStefano F, Perlman JA, Peterson HB, et al. Long-term risks of menstrual disturbances after tubal sterilization. *Am J Obstet Gynecol* 1985;152:835.

Dueholm S, Zingenburg HJ, Sandgren G. Late sequelae after laparoscopic sterilization in the pregnant and nonpregnant woman. *Acta Obstet Gynecol Scand* 1987;66:227.

Emens JM, Olive JE. Timing of female sterilization. *BMJ* 1978;2:1126.

Escobedo LG, Peterson HB, Grubb GS, et al. Case-fatality rates for tubal sterilization in U.S. hospitals, 1979 to 1980. *Am J Obstet Gynecol* 1989;160:147.

Filshie GM, Casey D, Pogmore JR, et al. The titanium/silicone rubber clip for female sterilization. *Br J Obstet Gynaecol* 1981:88:655.

Fishburne JI. Anesthesia for laparoscopy: considerations, complications, and techniques. *J Reprod Med* 1978;21:37.

Gentile GP, Kaufman SC, Helbig DW. Is there any evidence for a post-tubal sterilization syndrome? *Fertil Steril* 1998;69:179.

Goldhaber MK, Armstrong MA, Golditch IM, et al. Long-term risk of hysterectomy among 80,007 sterilized and comparison women at Kaiser Permanente, 1971–1987. *Am J Epidemiol* 1993;138:508.

Grimes DA. Primary prevention of ovarian cancer. *JAMA* 1993;270:2855.

Grimes DA, Peterson HB, Rosenberg MJ, et al. Sterilization-attributable deaths in Bangladesh. *Int J Gynaecol Obstet* 1982;20:149.

Grimes DA, Satterthwaite AP, Rochat RW, et al. Deaths from contraceptive sterilization in Bangladesh: rates, causes, and prevention. *Obstet Gynecol* 1982;60:635.

Grubb GS, Peterson HB. Luteal phase pregnancy and tubal sterilization. *Obstet Gynecol* 1985;66:784.

Handa VL, Berlin M, Washington AE. A comparison of local and general anesthesia for laparoscopic tubal sterilization. *J Women's Health* 1994;3:135.

Hankinson SE, Hunter DJ, Colditz GA, et al. Tubal ligation, hysterectomy, and risk of ovarian cancer: a prospective study. *JAMA* 1993;270:2813.

Healy B. From the National Institutes of Health: does vasectomy cause prostate cancer? *JAMA* 1993;269:2620.

Henshaw SK, Singh S. Sterilization regret among U.S. couples. *Fam Plann Perspect* 1986;18:238.

Hillis SD, Marchbanks PA, Tylor LR, et al. Tubal sterilization and the long-term risk of hysterectomy: findings from the United States Collaborative Review of Sterilization. *Obstet Gynecol* 1997;89:609.

Hillis SD, Marchbanks PA, Tylor LR, et al. Higher hysterectomy risk for sterilized than nonsterilized women: findings from the U.S. Collaborative Review of Sterilization. *Obstet Gynecol* 1998;91:241.

Hillis SD, Marchbanks PA, Tylor LR, et al. Poststerilization regret: findings from the United States Collaborative Review of Sterilization. *Obstet Gynecol* 1999;93:889.

Holt VL, Chu J, Daling JR, et al. Tubal sterilization and subsequent ectopic pregnancy: a case-control study. *JAMA* 1991;226:242.

Hulka JF, Fishburne JI, Mercer JP, et al. Laparoscopic sterilization with a spring clip: a report of the first fifty cases. *Am J Obstet Gynecol* 1973;116:715.

Hulka JF, Peterson HB, Phillips JM. American Association of Gynecologic Laparoscopists' 1988 membership survey on laparoscopic sterilization. *J Reprod Med* 1990;35:584.

Hulka JF, Reich H. *Textbook of laparoscopy,* 2nd ed. Philadelphia: WB Saunders, 1994:85.

Irving FC. Tubal sterilization. *Am J Obstet Gynecol* 1950;60:1101.

Irwin KL, Lee NC, Peterson HB, et al. Hysterectomy, tubal sterilization and the risk of breast cancer. *Am J Epidemiol* 1988;127:1192.

Jamieson DJ, Hillis SD, Duerr A, et al. Complications of interval laparoscopic sterilization: Findings from the United States Collaborative Review of Sterilization. *Obstet Gynecol* 2000;96:997–1002.

Kjer JJ, Knudsen LB. Ectopic pregnancy subsequent to laparoscopic sterilization. *Am J Obstet Gynecol* 1989;160:1202.

Koetsawang S, Gates DS, Suwanichati S, et al. Long-term follow-up of laparoscopic sterilizations by electrocoagulation, the Hulka clip, and the tubal ring. *Contraception* 1990;41:9.

Layde PM, Peterson HB, Dicker RC, et al. Risk factors for complications of interval tubal sterilization by laparotomy. *Obstet Gynecol* 1983;62:180.

Leader A, Galan N, George R, et al. A comparison of definable traits in women requesting reversal of sterilization and women satisfied with sterilization. *Am J Obstet Gynecol* 1983;145:198.

Levinson CJ, Daily HJ, Skinner SJ. Pathologic changes in the fallopian tube after Silastic ring occlusion. In: Phillips JM, ed. *Endoscopy in gynecology.* Downey, CA: American Association of Gynecologic Laparoscopists, 1978:180.

Lichter ED, Laff SP, Friedman EA. Value of routine dilation and curettage at the time of interval sterilization. *Obstet Gynecol* 1986;67:763.

Lipscomb GH, Spellman JR, Ling FW. The effect of same-day pregnancy testing on the incidence of luteal phase pregnancy. *Obstet Gynecol* 1993;82:411.

Liskin L, Pile JM, Quillin WF. Vasectomy—safe and simple. *Pop Rep D* 1983;4:D61.

Liskin L, Rinehart W. Minilaparotomy and laparoscopy: safe, effective, and widely used. *Pop Rep C* 1985;9:c-127.

Madlener M. Über sterilisierende operationen an den tuben. *Zentralbl Gynakol* 1919;20:380.

Makar AP, Vanderheyden JS, Schatteman EA, et al. Female sterilization failure after bipolar electrocoagulation: a six-year retrospective study. *Eur J Obstet Gynecol Reprod Biol* 1990;37:237.

Marcil-Gratton N. Sterilization regret among women in metropolitan Montreal. *Fam Plann Perspect* 1988;20:222.

Marquette CM, Koonin LM, Antarsh L, et al. Vasectomy in the United States 1991. *Am J Public Health* 1995;85:644.

Mintz M. Risks and prophylaxis in laparoscopy: a survey of 100,000 cases. *J Reprod Med* 1977;18:269.

Mumford SD, Bhiwandiwala PP, Chi I-C. Laparoscopic and minilaparotomy female sterilisation compared in 15,167 cases. *Lancet* 1980;2:1066.

Nirapathpongporn A, Huber DH, Krieger JN. No-scalpel vasectomy at the King's birthday vasectomy festival. *Lancet* 1990;335:894.

Nisanian A. Outpatient minilaparotomy sterilization with local anesthesia. *J Reprod Med* 1990;35:380.

Penfield AJ. The Filshie clip for female sterilization: a review of world experience. *Am J Obstet Gynecol* 2000;182:485.

Peterson HB, DeStefano F, Rubin GL, et al. Deaths attributable to tubal sterilization in the United States, 1977 to 1981. *Am J Obstet Gynecol* 1983;146:131.

Peterson HB, Greenspan JR, DeStefano F, et al. The impact of laparoscopy on tubal sterilization in United States hospitals, 1970 and 1975 to 1978. *Am J Obstet Gynecol* 1981;140:811.

Peterson HB, Huber DH, Belker AM. Vasectomy: an appraisal for the obstetrician-gynecologist. *Obstet Gynecol* 1990;76: 568.

Peterson HB, Hulka JF, Spielman FJ, et al. Local versus general anesthesia for laparoscopic sterilization: a randomized study. *Obstet Gynecol* 1987;70:903.

Peterson HB, Xia Z, Hughes JM, et al. The risk of pregnancy after tubal sterilization: Findings from the U.S. Collaborative Review of Sterilization. *Am J Obstet Gynecol* 1996;174:1161.

Peterson HB, Xia Z, Hughes JM, et al. The risk of ectopic pregnancy after tubal sterilization. *N Engl J Med* 1997;336:762.

Peterson HB, Xia Z, Wilcox LS, et al. Pregnancy after sterilization with bipolar electrocoagulation. *Obstet Gynecol* 1999;94:163

Peterson HB, Xia Z, Wilcox LS, et al. Pregnancy after tubal sterilization with silicone rubber band and spring clip application. *Obstet Gynecol* 2001;97:205–210.

Peterson HB, Jeng G, Folger SG, et al. The risk of menstrual abnormalities after tubal sterilization. *N Engl J Med* 2000;343:1681.

Peterson HB. Howards SS. Vasectomy and prostate cancer: the evidence to date. *Fertil Steril* 1998;70:201.

Piccinino LJ, Mosher WD. Trends in contraceptive use in the United States: 1982–1995. *Fam Plann Perspect* 1998;30:4.

Pitaktepsombati P, Janowitz B. Sterilization acceptance and regret in Thailand. *Contraception* 1991;44:623.

Poindexter AN, Abdul-Malak M, Fast J. Laparoscopic tubal sterilization under local anesthesia. *Obstet Gynecol* 1990;75:5.

Power FH, Barnes AC. Sterilization by means of peritoneoscopic tubal fulguration. *Am J Obstet Gynecol* 1941;41: 1038.

Prystowsky H, Eastman NJ. Puerperal tubal sterilization: report of 1,830 cases. *JAMA* 1955;158:463.

Rennie AL, Richard JA, Milne MK, et al. Post-partum sterilisation—an anaesthetic hazard? *Anaesthesia* 1979;34:267.

Rioux JE, Cloutier D. A new bipolar instrument for tubal sterilization. *Am J Obstet Gynecol* 1974;119:737.

Rochat RW, Bhiwandiwala PP, Feldblum PJ, et al. Mortality associated with sterilization: preliminary results of an international collaborative observational study. *Int J Gynaecol Obstet* 1986;24:275.

Ross JA, Frankenberg E. Sterilization. In: Ross JA, Frankenberg E, eds. *Findings from two decades of family planning research.* New York: Population Council, 1993:57.

Rulin MC, Davidson AR, Philliber SG, et al. Long-term effect of tubal sterilization on menstrual indices and pelvic pain. *Obstet Gynecol* 1993;82:118.

Rulin MC, Turner JH, Dunworth R, et al. Post-tubal sterilization syndrome—a misnomer. *Am J Obstet Gynecol* 1985;151:13.

Schmidt JE, Hillis SD, Marchbanks PA, et al. Requesting information about and obtaining reversal after tubal sterilization: findings from the U.S. Collaborative Review of Sterilization. *Fertil Steril* 2000;74:892.

Schwartz D, Wingo PA, Antarsh L, et al. Female sterilizations in the United States, 1987. *Fam Plann Perspect* 1989;21:209.

Shain RN, Miller WB, Holden AEC. Married women's dissatisfaction with tubal sterilization and vasectomy at first-year follow-up: effects of perceived spousal dominance. *Fertil Steril* 1986;45:808.

Shain RN, Miller WB, Mitchell GW, et al. Menstrual pattern change one year after sterilization: results of a controlled, prospective study. *Fertil Steril* 1989;52:192.

Shy KK, Stergachis A, Grothaus LG, et al. Tubal sterilization and risk of subsequent hospital admission for menstrual disorders. *Am J Obstet Gynecol* 1992;166:1698.

Siegler AM, Grunebaum A. A short history of tubal sterilization. In: Phillips JM, ed. *Endoscopic female sterilization: a comparison of methods.* Downey, CA: American Association of Gynecologic Laparoscopists, 1983:3.

Soderstrom R. Electrical safety in laparoscopy. In: Phillips JM, ed. *Endoscopy in gynecology.* Downey, CA: American Association of Gynecologic Laparoscopists, 1978:306.

Soderstrom RM, Levy BS, Engel T. Reducing bipolar sterilization failures. *Obstet Gynecol* 1989;74:60.

Speert H. *Obstetrics and gynecology in America: a history.* Chicago: The American College of Obstetricians and Gynecologists, 1980:68.

Stergachis A, Shy KK, Grothaus LC, et al. Tubal sterilization and the long-term risk of hysterectomy. *JAMA* 1990;264: 2893.

Stovall TG, Ling FW, O'Kelley KR, et al. Gross and histologic examination of tubal ligation failures in a residency training program. *Obstet Gynecol* 1990;76:461.

Trussell J, Hatcher RA, Cates W, et al. A guide to interpreting contraceptive efficacy studies. *Obstet Gynecol* 1990;76:558.

Trussell J, Kost K. Contraceptive failure in the United States: a critical review of the literature. *Stud Fam Plann* 1987;18: 237.

Uchida H. Uchida tubal sterilization. *Am J Obstet Gynecol* 1975;121:153.

Whittemore AS, Harris R, Itnyre J, et al. Characteristics relating to ovarian cancer risk: collaborative analysis of 12 U.S. case-control studies. II. Invasive epithelial ovarian cancers in white women. *Am J Epidemiol* 1992;136:1184.

Williams EL, Jones HE, Merrill RE. The subsequent course of patients sterilized by tubal ligation: a consideration of hysterectomy for sterilization. *Am J Obstet Gynecol* 1951;61: 423.

World Health Organization Task Force on Female Sterilization, Special Programme of Research, Development and Research Training in Human Reproduction. Minilaparotomy or laparoscopy for sterilization: a multicenter, multinational, randomized study. *Am J Obstet Gynecol* 1982;143:645.

Wortman J. Female sterilization by minilaparotomy. *Pop Rep C* 1974;5:c-53.

Wortman J, Piotrow P. Laparoscopic sterilization—a new technique. *Pop Rep C* 1973;1:c-1.

Yoon IB, Wheeless CR, King TM. A preliminary report on a new laparoscopic sterilization approach: the silicone rubber band technique. *Am J Obstet Gynecol* 1974;120:132.

Te Linde's Operative Gynecology, ninth edition, edited by John A. Rock and Howard W. Jones, III. Lippincott Williams & Wilkins, Philadelphia © 2003.

CHAPTER

24

▼

Reconstructive Tubal Surgery

VICTOR GOMEL

The physiologic functions of the human oviduct include proovarian sperm transport to the site of fertilization, ovum pickup and prouterine transport of the ovum, ampullary retention of the ovum (approximately 72 hours), provision of a suitable environment for fertilization to occur and for the zygote to survive, and eventually transport of the zygote from the ampulla to the uterine cavity. Alterations in any of these functions (caused by either damage to the ciliated epithelium or tubal distortion or occlusion) can result in tubal implantation (owing to the lack of transport of the zygote to the uterus) or infertility (owing to the prevention of sperm meeting the oocyte).

TUBAL FACTOR INFERTILITY

Much of the increase in the incidence of both infertility and tubal pregnancy in the past three decades has been the result of tubal damage after sexually transmitted pelvic infections. The most commonly isolated organisms are *Chlamydia trachomatis* (identified most often), *Neisseria gonorrhoeae*, and *Mycoplasma hominis*. These organisms appear to account for most primary invasions; however in 15% to 60% of cases of acute pelvic inflammatory disease (PID), aerobic or anaerobic bacteria, or both can also be identified. The clinical picture can vary from an almost asymptomatic condition to a life-threatening event. Patients with a more severe clinical appearance often have both aerobic and anaerobic infection.

The classic clinical picture of PID, which includes pain, fever, and lower genital tract infection, occurs in less than 50% of affected patients. I have reported (1983a) that more than half of the patients who were investigated for infertility and were found to have a hydrosalpinx gave no previous history of acute PID. This observation has since been confirmed.

It has been estimated that acute PID occurs at a rate of 10 cases per 1,000 women per year in the age group 15 to 39 years, and at a rate of 20 cases per 1,000 women in the age group 15 to 24 years. A single episode of PID will leave a residue of tubal damage sufficient to cause infertility in nearly 20% of affected women.

Reconstructive tubal surgery, by open access, was at one time the only treatment option for infertile women with damaged fallopian tubes. This is no longer the case. Improvement in the outcomes, simplification of the techniques, and much wider availability of *in vitro fertilization* (IVF) and assisted reproduction technologies (ART) provide such couples with a realistic therapeutic alternative. In addition, tubal cannulation has been shown to have a role in women with apparent cornual occlusion. Furthermore, it has been demonstrated that many tubal reconstructive procedures can be performed by laparoscopic access. Thorough investigation of both the male and female partners will aid in the selection of the most appropriate treatment option.

Investigation

The investigation of the infertile couple should be concluded rapidly, accurately, and inexpensively, with as little invasion as possible. In addition, the emotional needs of the couple must be recognized and addressed. This chapter will discuss only investigations specific to tubal and peritoneal factors of infertility.

Tubal Insufflation

Tubal insufflation is a tubal patency test that is now rarely performed. The test was first described by Rubin in 1920, and although there have been modifications of the original technique; the test rightfully bears his name, Rubin's test. The procedure uses an endocervical cannula connected, by rubber tubing, to a mercury manometer and a source of carbon dioxide (CO_2). The rate of gas flow through the system is gradually increased to about 30 to 60 mL per minute. The cervix can be submerged in sterile water in the upper vagina to detect any leakage of the gas from the cervical canal. Tubal patency can be determined by one or more of the following: a written record of the rise and rapid fall of the gas pressure, auscultation of the lower abdomen for the gas passing through the tubes into the peritoneal cavity, or direct visualization of the pressure changes on a mercury manometer. Although normal fallopian tubes demonstrate patency by the rapid escape of gas at pressures below 100 mm Hg, the test is still considered in the normal range if patency is demonstrated below 180 mm Hg. A negative Rubin's test cannot be interpreted as conclusive for tubal obstruction. A study by Sweeney and Gepfert documented this fact by reporting an ultimate pregnancy rate of 50% in patients whose tubal insufflation test had recorded pressures greater than 180 mm Hg. The use of a smooth-muscle relaxant, such as inhaled amyl nitrate, or a mild sedative, such as Valium, 10 mg, before any tubal function test may be helpful in decreasing tubal spasm.

As with hysterosalpingography (HSG), which is discussed next, Rubin's test should be performed before ovulation, about the tenth day of the cycle.

Hysterosalpingography

HSG is a contrast study of the uterine cavity and fallopian tubes. It is a simple, inexpensive, safe, and rapid diagnostic procedure that, when performed properly, provides valuable information about the uterine cavity and tubal architecture.

Contraindications to HSG are possible pregnancy, uterine bleeding, lower genital tract infection, PID, and allergy to the contrast material. In women with a history of recurrent PID, or with any suggestion of a recent exacerbation, there is a significant risk of reactivation of quiescent PID. This occurs in about 3% of such patients. To combat this risk, some centers prophylactically administer antibiotics. During the preliminary history and physical examination, the physician must search for possible contraindications, and lower genital tract infection must be ruled out.

TECHNIQUE. HSG must be timed to occur between the complete cessation of menstruation and ovulation. This will avoid the risk of disturbing a luteal phase pregnancy. Such timing also avoids radiation exposure to the oocyte that will resume meiosis after the luteinizing hormone surge. Administration of one of the prostaglandin synthesize inhibitors before the procedure reduces the patient's discomfort and diminishes errors associated with hysterosalpingography. The latter is especially applicable to errors regarding cornual occlusion. This has been clearly demonstrated in a study by Lang and Dunaway.

There is continuing debate on the selection of oil-soluble versus water-soluble contrast medium. The patient better tolerates the water-soluble medium. In addition, this type of medium coats the surfaces without sticking to them and produces sharp and finely shaded images and greater visual detail of the lesions. These characteristics enable better assessment of the intraluminal architecture (Fig. 24.1). The contrast material is eliminated within 30 minutes.

After the patient has emptied her bladder, she is placed on the radiographic table. A bivalve speculum is inserted into the vagina, and the cervix and upper vagina are washed with an antiseptic solution. The appropriate cannula, which is filled with contrast material and emptied of any air, is attached to the cervix in such a way as to ensure a tight seal. The speculum is removed before the injection of contrast material. Removal of the speculum is important (especially if the metal variety is used), not only to decrease the patient's discomfort but also to avoid obscuring the cervical canal and vaginal fornices.

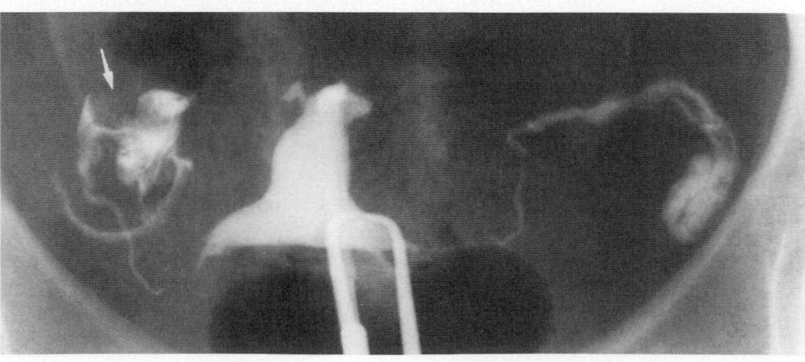

FIGURE 24.1. Hysterosalpingogram. Early film demonstrates a normal uterus and a left hydrosalpinx. On the **right** there is an ampullary defect (*arrow*) at the site of a previous tubal pregnancy, which was treated with parenteral methotrexate administration.

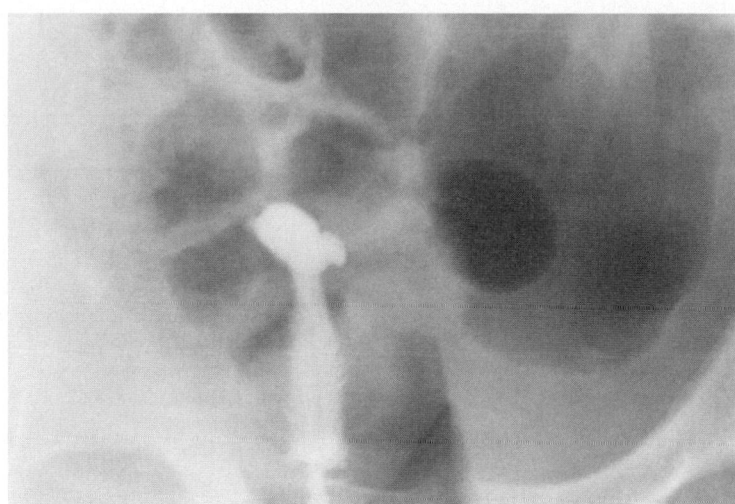

FIGURE 24.2. Hysterosalpingogram in a patient with Asherman's syndrome. Contrast material outlines the cervical canal and a part of the lower uterine cavity, the remainder of which is obliterated by synechiae. (From: Gomel V, Taylor PJ. *Diagnostic and operative gynecologic laparoscopy.* St Louis: Mosby, 1995, with permission.)

HSG must be performed under fluoroscopic control with use of an image intensifier. With the syringe attached to the cannula, the contrast material is injected very slowly to avoid discomfort, contraction of the uterus, spasm of the uterotubal junction, and obscuring lesions with a large quantity of contrast material. Films are taken to record salient features as they appear on the monitor. An average of three to five films are taken. Preliminary films are of limited value; they can be used to identify misplaced intrauterine contraceptive devices or areas of pelvic calcification. Such information can also be gained by examining the first film.

As the contrast material is injected slowly and intermittently, the endocervical canal, isthmus, and uterine cavity are visualized. To straighten the uterus, firm traction is maintained on the cervix. A film is taken at this point. It is essential to obtain films early during the procedure to record any intrauterine lesions and details of the intratubal architecture. Such details are obscured by larger amounts of contrast material in the uterus, tubes, and peritoneal cavity. Another film is taken when the contrast material starts to escape into the peritoneal cavity (Fig. 24.1). Injection of medium is continued slowly until tubal patency is unquestionably established. Manipulation of the uterus with the cannula may be necessary to display specific tubal segments. A film is obtained when abnormal findings are encountered. In certain cases, a true lateral film may provide useful information. When taking this exposure, the traction on the cervix is temporarily released to obtain information regarding the position of the uterus, the location of intrauterine lesions, and the course and configuration of the tubes.

The last phase of the procedure includes a delayed fluoroscopic examination and a film taken 10 to 20 minutes (when water-soluble contrast material is used) after removal of the cannula. This examination and film may yield information about the external contour of the internal genitalia, the shape of the ovarian fossa, and the presence of periadnexal adhesions.

With adherence to proper technique, complications are rare. Major complications include PID, uterine perforation, bleeding from the tenaculum site, and intolerance to iodine, especially if intravasation of contrast occurs.

HSG provides valuable information about the uterus and oviducts. Abnormal uterine findings include fusion anomalies, T-shaped uterus, submucous fibroids and endometrial polyps, intrauterine synechiae (Fig. 24.2), and other less commonly identified lesions, such as adenomyosis. Tubal abnormalities that can be observed are listed in Table 24.1 (Figs. 24.3 through 24.6).

It must be noted that HSG has limitations: (a) it often does not indicate the exact nature of intrauterine lesions, (b) it is associated with false-positive results with regard to cornual occlusion, and (c) it has a low positive predictive value in the diagnosis of periadnexal adhesions and endometriosis. For these reasons, laparoscopy and, when necessary, hysteroscopy are undertaken to elucidate the diagnosis. Indeed, HSG and laparoscopy are complementary, and not competitive, procedures in the investigation of infertility associated with tubal and peritoneal factors.

In many instances, HSG demonstrates the presence of severe tubal damage, or conditions deemed inoperable. Severe intratubal adhesions and distal tubal occlusion in association with cornual lesions, such as salpingitis isthmica nodosa, are examples of contraindications of reconstructive surgery. In such instances, the couple may be advised of the significance of the findings, and IVF may be recommended as primary treatment, without recourse to laparoscopy.

Selective Salpingography and Tubal Cannulation

Selective salpingography is the injection of contrast medium directly into the uterine tubal ostium with the use of a special radiopaque cannula inserted through the cervix. The increased pressure generated by the direct injection helps to overcome obstructions associated with mucus plugs or minor synechiae.

TABLE 24.1.
Abnormalities of the Oviduct

Abnormality	Signs	Comments
TUBOCORNUAL REGION		
Failure of contrast to enter tube	Simple obstruction	May be owing to tubal spasm; may be unilateral or bilateral
Salpingitis isthmica nodosa (SIN)	Appears as a simple obstruction or as spicules of contrast radiating from tubal lumen	May be unilateral or bilateral
Endometriosis	Similar to SIN, usually with more-pronounced punctate pattern	May be unilateral or bilateral
Polyps	Small globular or elongated vacuoles surrounded by contrast medium	
ISTHMUS		
Occlusion	Contrast outlines portion of the isthmic segment	Most commonly owing to prior surgical sterilization or tubal pregnancy; less commonly to SIN; and uncommonly to tuberculosis and endometriosis
AMPULLA		
Intraluminal adhesions	Patchy filling defects	Caused by endosalpingeal infection
Tubal pregnancy	Obstruction, stenosis, round defect, occasionally calcification	
INFUNDIBULUM		
Hydrosalpinx	Obstruction usually bilateral	Most common type of occlusion
Phimosis of distal tubal ostium	Intraluminal retention of contrast medium and slow intraperitoneal spill from stenosed tube	Both conditions are usually sequelae of pelvic inflammatory disease
INTRAPERITONEAL SPREAD		
Adhesions	Localized pooling and loculation of contrast medium around distal end of oviducts	

(Modified from: Gomel V, Taylor PJ. *Diagnostic and operative gynecologic laparoscopy.* St Louis: Mosby, 1995:105.)

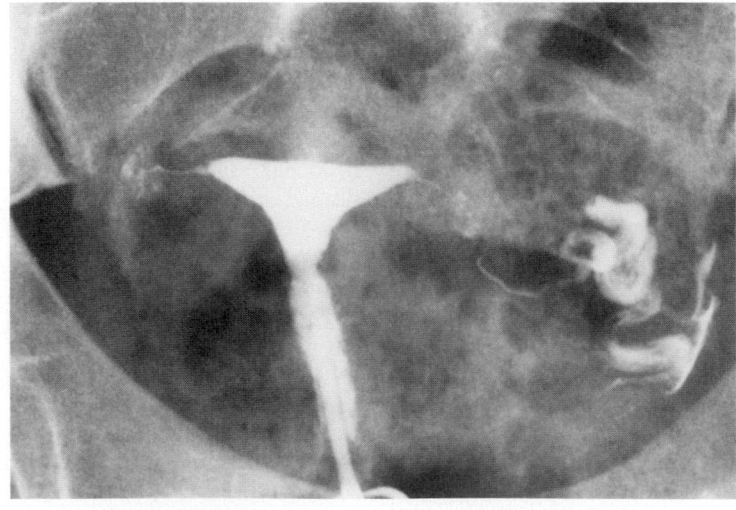

FIGURE 24.3. Hysterosalpingogram showing bilateral proximal isthmic lesions typical of salpingitis isthmica nodosa. The right tube is occluded, whereas the left is still patent. (From: Gomel V, Taylor PJ. *Diagnostic and operative gynecologic laparoscopy.* St Louis: Mosby, 1995, with permission.)

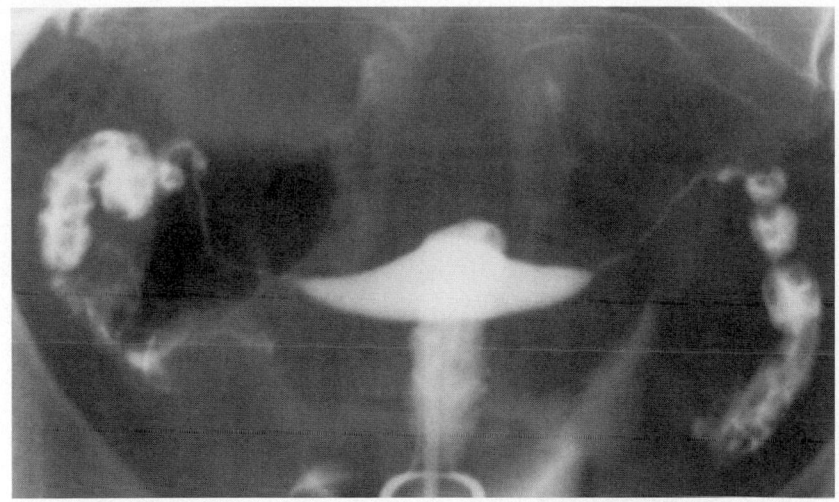

FIGURE 24.4. Hysterosalpingogram. Both tubes exhibit extensive intratubal adhesions. (From: Gomel V, Taylor PJ. *Diagnostic and operative gynecologic laparoscopy.* St Louis: Mosby, 1995, with permission.)

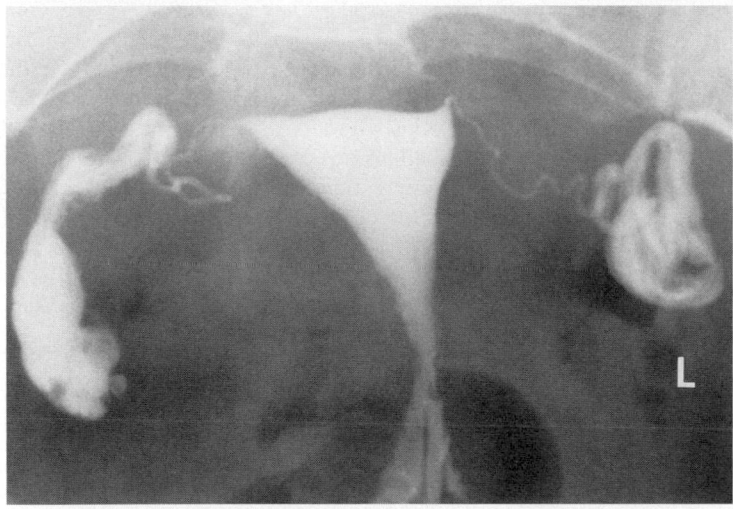

FIGURE 24.5. Hysterosalpingogram showing bilateral hydrosalpinx. The longitudinal epithelial folds are preserved in the left tube. (From: Gomel V, Taylor PJ. *Diagnostic and operative gynecologic laparoscopy.* St Louis: Mosby, 1995, with permission.)

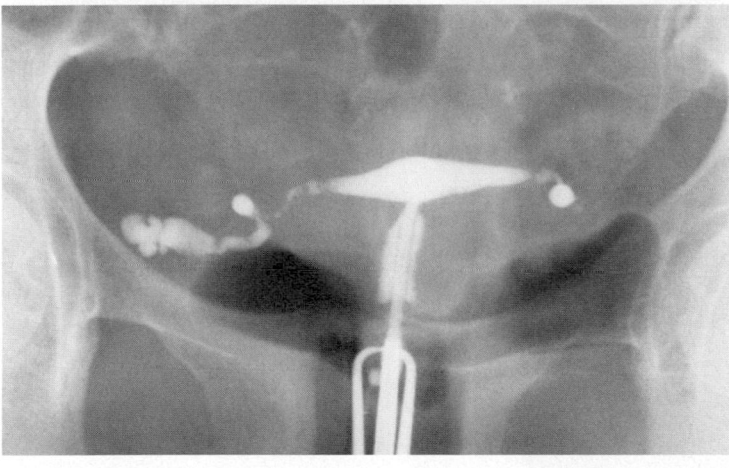

FIGURE 24.6. Hysterosalpingogram. The tubes exhibit findings typical of a prior tuberculous salpingitis. (From: Gomel V, Taylor PJ. *Diagnostic and operative gynecologic laparoscopy.* St Louis: Mosby, 1995, with permission.)

Cannulation of the tube requires the use of a special flexible guide wire and narrow-gauge cannula. This cannulation system is introduced through the larger cannula, which is used for selective salpingography.

If HSG demonstrates a cornual or proximal tubal obstruction (Fig. 24.7), selective salpingography with or without tubal cannulation (Fig. 24.8) should be the next step; this is ideally performed in the same setting. These techniques are useful in differentiating true from false cornual occlusion. The benefits of this approach have been shown for apparent cornual spasm, obstructions caused by amorphous material (tubal plugs), and tubal

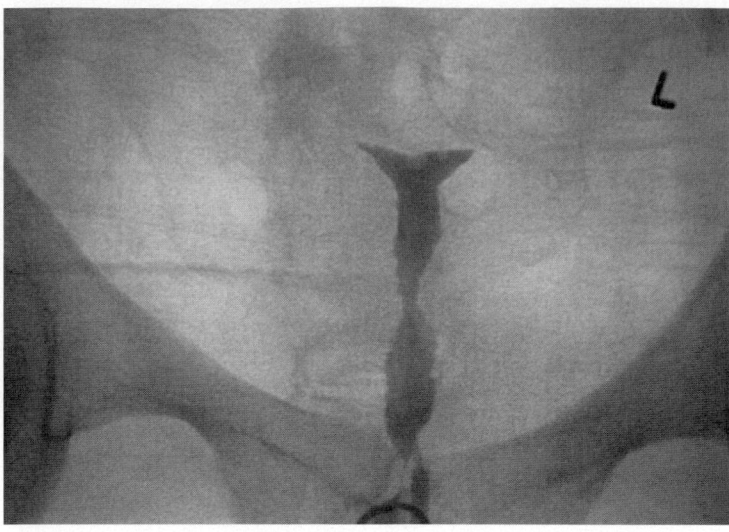

FIGURE 24.7. Hysterosalpingogram showing bilateral cornual occlusion. (From: Gomel V, Taylor PJ. *Diagnostic and operative gynecologic laparoscopy.* St Louis: Mosby, 1995, with permission.)

synechiae. It is doubtful that these techniques have a real therapeutic effect on occlusions owing to obliterative fibrosis, chronic follicular salpingitis, salpingitis isthmica nodosa, or endometriosis.

Salpingoscopy

Salpingoscopy is the endoscopic examination of the ampullary portion of the tubal lumen. This can be accomplished with a rigid or flexible hysteroscope during either laparoscopy or laparotomy. If the distal tube is totally occluded (hydrosalpinx), it is necessary to make a small opening at the fimbriated end to permit the introduction of the scope. The tubal lumen is visualized while distended with physiologic solution injected through the outer sheath of the rigid hysteroscope or the channel of the flexible hysteroscope. The distal end of the tube must be appropriately manipulated to bring it into the axis of the scope. Salpingostomy permits direct assessment of the tubal epithelium. The findings have been classified into five grades. Grade 1 refers to normal mucosal architecture. Grade 2 refers to tubes that demonstrate variable degrees of flattening of both major and minor mucosal folds, which are largely preserved. Grade 3 refers to tubes that demonstrate focal adhesions between mucosal folds. Grade 4 refers to tubes with extensive intraluminal adhesions or disseminated flattened epithelial areas. Grade 5 refers to tubes that are rigid and hollow with a complete loss of epithelial folds. Salpingoscopy appears to have a good prognostic predictive value, as demonstrated by Henry-Suchet et al., Brosens and Puttemans, Bowman and Cooke, and Marana et al.

Falloposcopy

Falloposcopy is a transvaginal microendoscopic technique aimed at exploring the entire length of the tube, especially the intramural and isthmic segments. A linear eversion catheter system has been used to perform falloposcopy without the need for preliminary hysteroscopy and anesthesia. The patient requires premedication to decrease the discomfort associated with the procedure.

The system includes a linear eversion catheter with an outer plastic polymer body 2.8 mm in diameter and a sliding stainless steel inner body 0.8 mm in diameter, containing a 0.48-mm fiberoptic endoscope. The tip of

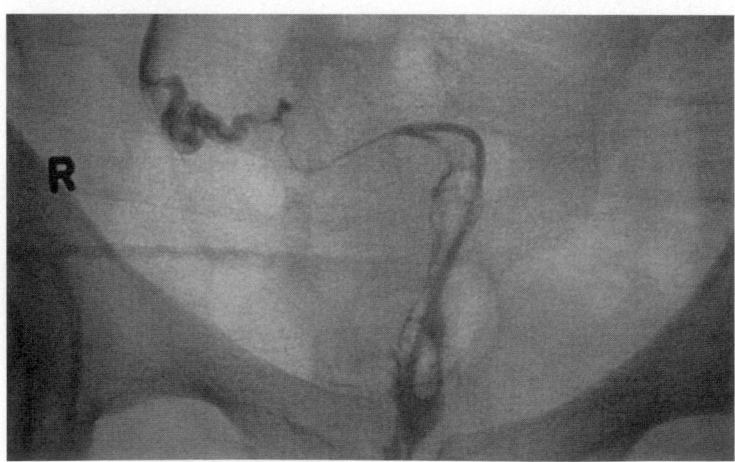

FIGURE 24.8. Tubal cannulation (same patient as in Fig. 24.7). The occlusion has been relieved, and the tube has opacified. (From: Gomel V, Taylor PJ. *Diagnostic and operative gynecologic laparoscopy.* St Louis: Mosby, 1995, with permission.)

the outer catheter is angulated so it can be directed toward the uterotubal junction. Once the tubal ostium is identified, the tip of the catheter is held against the ostium. The pressure within the eversion catheter is increased, and the membrane of the eversion catheter is introduced into the fallopian tube for a short distance. The endoscope is pushed down the lumen to the tip of the introduced catheter. The image obtained is displayed on a high-resolution color monitor. The eversion catheter and the endoscope it houses are advanced in the described manner, slowly and gradually, with the endoscope always maintained within the inverting membrane to prevent the tip of the endoscope from piercing the tubal wall.

Falloposcopy may be used as a means of tubal catheterization and has the added benefit of permitting assessment of the lumen of the tube, especially its intramural and isthmic segments. In 1992, Kerin proposed a classification based on a scoring system that takes into account the degree of tubal patency, tubal dilatation, epithelial and vascular changes, intratubal adhesions, and other abnormal findings.

This technique, which requires expensive disposable equipment, did not gain clinical acceptance. Technical improvements, amelioration of the image quality, and parallel reduction in cost may trigger reassessment of the cost effectiveness of this procedure in the future.

Tests Designed to Assess Tubal Function

Salpingography, salpingoscopy, and falloposcopy are designed to assess tubal morphology.

Procedures designed to assess function are being developed. Early attempts at using radioactive microspheres, as oocyte surrogates, to evaluate egg transport did not appear to be clinically valuable. Uher et al. have introduced biodegradable microspheres into the pouch of Douglas by either cul-de-sac puncture or laparoscopy. These microspheres, which were recognizable by fluorescence, were collected in a cervical cup 24 hours later. Microspheres were present in the cup in 66% of 69 patients with unexplained infertility and in 100% of 20 patients with male factor infertility.

RADIONUCLIDE HSG. Radionuclide HSG is a scintigraphic procedure designed to evaluate the spontaneous proovarian transport of microspheres in the genital tract. A solution containing ^{99m}Tc-labeled albumin microspheres is squirted toward the external cervical os of the cervix and upper vagina. The subsequent transport of the microspheres through the cervix, uterus, and tubes is monitored by a gamma camera equipped with a pinhole collimator. The proovarian transport of microspheres depends on both the anatomic patency and the functional integrity of the uterus and oviducts. This test is designed to assess primarily the sperm transport function of the uterus and tubes. This technique is still experimental.

Laparoscopy

Laparoscopy permits direct visualization of the peritoneal cavity, pelvis, and internal reproductive organs. It can also test tubal patency with the use of concomitant chromopertubation. Laparoscopy is an invasive procedure that usually requires a general anesthetic. It is the most accurate way to identify periadnexal adhesive disease and endometriosis.

There are those who argue in favor of an immediate laparoscopy bypassing HSG. An analysis of 18 published series demonstrates good congruence between laparoscopic and HSG findings. These collected data indicate that the sensitivity and specificity of HSG are around 76% and 83%, respectively. These studies represent a selected population of patients in whom the prevalence of tubal occlusion was 38%. This prevalence figure falls to 10% in studies of large numbers of unselected patients, which reflects more accurately the general population. If the sensitivity and specificity figures reported above are applied to a hypothetical group of patients with a 10% rate of tubal occlusion, 3% of those with a normal HSG will have an abnormal laparoscopy. Thus, the laparoscopy will be normal in about 97% of patients. These data support delaying endoscopy for 4 to 6 months in those with an apparently normal HSG, except in women of older reproductive age.

Based on the preceding information, a well-performed HSG should be the preliminary investigation for tubal factor infertility. This approach permits the identification of (a) uterine anomalies and lesions, (b) cornual occlusion or lesions even in the presence of cornual patency, (c) distal tubal occlusion, and (d) assessment of intratubal architecture. This information is of paramount importance to the surgeon at the time of laparoscopy, especially if the condition is amenable to laparoscopic surgery, which should be performed during at the same time.

LAPAROSCOPIC SURVEY. A thorough laparoscopic survey will identify any adhesions, along with their extent and nature; reveal the presence of endometriosis, its extent, and other abdominal and pelvic lesions; and permit assessment of the uterus, ovaries, and tubes. The information yielded by the prior HSG and this survey enables the surgeon to undertake reconstructive laparoscopic surgery and to recommend surgery by open access or the use of assisted reproductive technologies. These will be discussed later (see Selection of Treatment).

A bimanual pelvic examination is performed on the anesthetized patient. The cervix is then exposed, and a uterine cannula is attached to the cervix. In addition to permitting intraoperative chromopertubation, the cannula enables manipulation of the uterus and enhances laparoscopic visualization.

Once the laparoscope is inserted, the entire peritoneal cavity is inspected. Inspection commences in the upper abdomen and includes the liver and the under surface of the diaphragm, which are inspected in a clockwise fashion. Particular attention is then focused on the lower abdomen and pelvis. To improve access to the pelvis, the patient is placed in the Trendelenburg position. The bowel is displaced upward, initially by manipulating the uterus and thereafter by using the probe inserted through a second puncture, usually placed suprapubically in the midline, or in one of the lower quadrants.

A general panoramic inspection of the pelvis is performed with the laparoscope at some distance from the pelvic organs. This permits a general impression to be formed. Subsequently, a systematic survey is performed. The laparoscope is advanced; appropriate manipulation of the uterus, with the cervical cannula, and of the suprapubic probe enhances visibility of specific organs. The uterus is assessed, along with its anterior surface, the vesicouterine pouch, and the dome of the bladder. The uterus is then moved into anteversion. The fundus and the posterior surface of the uterus, the uterosacral ligaments, and the pouch of Douglas are thoroughly inspected. If fluid is present in the pouch, its nature is noted. It will be necessary to aspirate the fluid to inspect the underlying peritoneal surfaces. To aspirate the fluid, the probe is replaced by a suction cannula, which can also be used as a manipulating probe. The aspirated fluid can be sent for microbiologic or biochemical studies as deemed necessary. The cul-de-sac and the lateral peritoneal surfaces are inspected for any scarring or evidence of endometriosis.

The extent and type of pelvic and periadnexal adhesions are noted (Fig. 24.9). Each tube and ovary and the respective pelvic side walls are thoroughly scrutinized. Once the anterior surface of the ovary is inspected, the ovary is elevated and flipped upward with the probe, exposing its posterior surface, the fossa ovarica, and the pelvic side wall down to the level of the uterosacral ligament, which are assessed. The tube is inspected from the proximal to the distal end. Attention is paid to any evidence of fusiform swelling at the uterotubal junction (which is usually caused by salpingitis isthmica nodosa or endometriosis) and the presence of fimbrial phimosis or frank distal tubal occlusion (hydrosalpinx) (Fig. 24.10). The ovarian fimbrial relation is assessed, and the fimbriae are viewed *en face*. Once the other adnexa are similarly assessed, chromopertubation is performed by injection of dilute indigo carmine or methylene blue solution through the uterine cannula. The passage of the dye solution is followed through the tube, and the nature of the spill is examined by viewing the fimbriae to determine the presence of prefimbrial phimosis or fine fimbrial adhesions that may impede ovum pickup.

Abdominal, pelvic, and periadnexal adhesions may impede laparoscopic access to the pelvis and the adnexa, in which case preliminary adhesiolysis may be necessary.

SELECTION OF TREATMENT

Two treatment options for achieving pregnancy are available to the infertile woman with damaged fallopian tubes: reconstructive surgery and IVF. Surgery and IVF must not be regarded as competitive treatments but rather as complementary treatments necessary to achieve the desired goal. The choice of treatment is ideally dependent on various considerations, both technical and nontechnical.

Technical Considerations

In vitro fertilization is the only treatment option for women with inoperable fallopian tubes and tubal disease coincident with another important fertility factor, such as male factor infertility. Reconstructive tubal surgery should be the first treatment option in patients likely to benefit from this approach. IVF may be attempted if reconstructive tubal surgery proves unsuccessful.

The provision of accurate information regarding both IVF and tubal surgery is essential in the decision-making process of the couple. The couple must be given the live birth rate per cycle of IVF, the cumulative birth rate after multiple cycles of treatment, and the potential complication rates including multiple pregnancy, abortion, and ectopic pregnancy. In addition, the effect of frozen embryo replacement on the cumulative pregnancy rate must be considered in the analysis. Similar information must also be provided regarding reconstructive tubal surgery. It is imperative that such figures reflect the experience of the center in

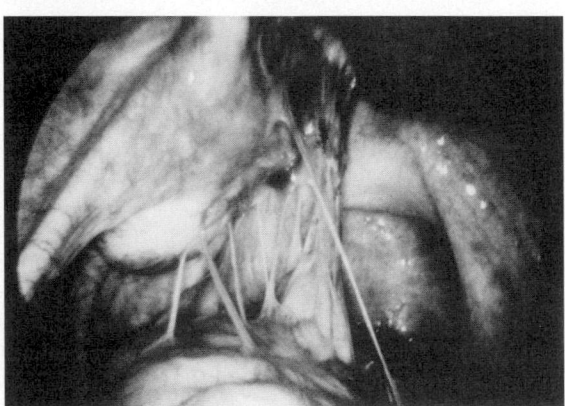

FIGURE 24.9. Laparoscopy. Periadnexal adhesions cover and fix the distal half of the fallopian tube. See color version of figure.

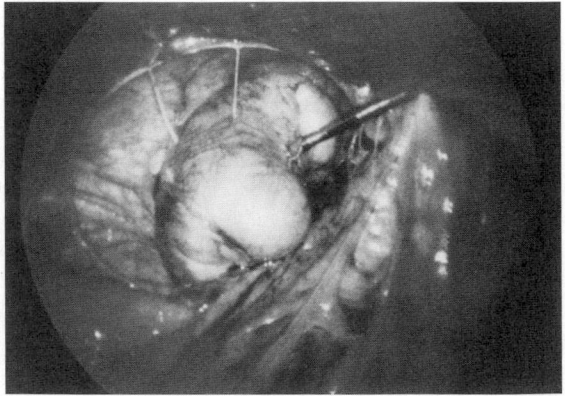

FIGURE 24.10. Laparoscopy. Thin-walled dilated hydrosalpinx with extensive pelvic and periadnexal adhesions. See color version of figure.

which treatment will be performed, and not those reported in international journals. However, in this chapter, by necessity, figures derived from the world literature will be used.

In Vitro *Fertilization and Embryo Transfer*

Data collected retrospectively for ART treatments during the whole year of 1997, from 335 programs in the United States provided the following outcome data, which was tabulated by the Society for Assisted Reproductive Technology (SART). There were 33,032 cycles of standard IVF initiated, 21.7% of which were canceled. Of the 25,878 cycles that had oocyte retrieval, 24,027 (92.8%) resulted in embryo transfer. These yielded 7,353 deliveries, representing delivery per retrieval and delivery per initiated cycle rates of 28.4% and 22.3%, respectively. It is interesting to note that for the year of 1993, the rate of delivery per initiated cycle was 16%, as was indicated in the last edition of this book.

Intracytoplasmic sperm injection (ICSI) represents a very important progress in ART, especially in the treatment of male infertility. There were 18,312 IVF plus ICSI cycles reported for the year 1997; 18,292 of these had oocyte retrieval, 17,243 (94.3%) of which had embryo transfers. There were 4,949 deliveries, which represents delivery per retrieval and delivery per initiated cycle rates of 27.1% and 27.0%, respectively. In both groups, the rate of pregnancy loss was 18.2% of clinical pregnancies; the rate of ectopic pregnancy was 2.1% of clinical pregnancies.

The outcome of IVF, both for standard and associated with ICSI, is adversely affected by the age of the female partner. In standard IVF, with couples who had no associated male factor infertility, the delivery per oocyte retrieval rates based on the age of the female partner were as follows; 34 years or less, 33.9%; 35 to 37 years, 29.4%; 38 to 40 years, 21.2%; and 41 years or more, 9.4%. The delivery per oocyte retrieval rates for IVF plus ICSI, in couples that had male factor infertility were approximately the same for each group, demonstrating a similar decline with increasing age. These rates were 33.8%, 30.7%, 20.0%, and 10.2%, respectively.

If the pregnancy rate were to remain relatively constant in successive cycles, on the basis of a delivery per initiated cycle rate of 23%, a cumulative delivery rate of 54.0% would be expected after three cycles of treatment. However, recent data have shown a steady decline in the success rate with consecutive failed IVF attempts. This decline appears to affect women of advanced reproductive age and those with polycystic ovarian disease.

Success with transfer of cryopreserved embryos has improved significantly. During 1997, there were 10,181 thaw cycles, resulting in 9,165 transfer procedures. These yielded 1,719 deliveries, for a delivery rate of 16.9% per thaw and 18.8% per transfer procedure. Replacement of frozen embryos improves the overall success rate of a stimulation cycle. However, the overall net effect remains limited because not all of the cycles provide spare embryos, and not all of the frozen embryos withstand the thawing process.

IVF and embryo transfer is not risk free, especially in stimulated cycles. Although uncommon, ovarian hyperstimulation, bleeding, and infection can occur. Pregnancies resulting from IVF have an abortion rate of about 20%. The overall tubal pregnancy rate is 2.1% of clinical pregnancies. A study from our center demonstrated a tubal pregnancy rate of only 2.6% (of clinical pregnancies) among IVF patients without tubal factor infertility. However, this rate was 12% in patients with prior tubal disease (these are the patients who must choose between IVF and tubal surgery). ART procedures, including transfer of cryopreserved embryos, are associated with a significant increase in the rate of multiple pregnancy. The SART report for 1997 indicated that of the resulting deliveries, only 62.0% were singleton; 31.7% were twins, 5.8% were triplets, and 0.5% were of higher order than triplets. The Caesarean section rate is over 35%, and about one fourth of the births are premature. It is significant that more than 10% of monofetal births are preterm. This rate is significantly greater among twins, triplets, and higher multiple births. The perinatal mortality rate is high (about 30 per 1,000). This rate is also increased among singletons (about 19 per 1,000).

Reconstructive Surgery

The overall risks of reconstructive tubal surgery are small and include the recognized complications of anesthesia and surgery. Surgery, if successful, offers multiple cycles in which to achieve conception and the opportunity to have more than one pregnancy. The abortion rate subsequent to reconstructive tubal surgery is not increased over that of the normal population. The live birth and ectopic pregnancy rates depend on the specific nature of the tubal disease and the extent of tubal damage.

After thorough investigation of the couple, a decision must be made regarding whether or not to proceed with reconstructive surgery. The preceding arguments and results yielded by IVF must be taken into consideration in this decision-making process. In addition, the results achieved by the center in which the patient will be treated must be considered. The results are dependent on the proper selection of patients and the technical expertise of the team and the surgeon.

Nontechnical Considerations

The nontechnical considerations include age, cost, and the wishes of the couple. Female fecundity is adversely affected by age. Fecundity begins to decline at about 31 years of age. This trend has been observed both in "normal" couples and in those with unexplained infertility. This decline becomes more evident after 37 years of age.

In women of advanced reproductive age, the marked decline of fecundity rate per cycle of IVF must be weighed against the fact that reconstructive surgery offers multiple cycles during which conception can occur. Therefore, although the younger woman may consider surgery first and IVF thereafter (if this becomes necessary), those between 37 and 40 years of age may be advised to consider IVF first.

Health insurance coverage and the cost of the procedure, depending on the jurisdiction, and the resources of the couple play important roles in the decision-making process. Another, often underestimated, potential factor is the economic impact of a multiple pregnancy, which occurs much more frequently with IVF.

The perceptions and wishes of the couple regarding treatment options depend on many influences, including their own values and ethical views. There may be disagreement between partners. The physician should provide detailed information for the couple as clearly and accurately as possible and should abstain from interfering with their decision making except to clarify misunderstandings and misinterpretations. The physician must advise against active treatment when the prognosis is poor because treatment with essentially no chance of success cannot be justified.

Selection

Periadnexal adhesive disease may be the only apparent lesion or may be present in addition to tubal occlusion. The tubes may be occluded at their outer end or proximally as the end result of disease processes, or the tubes may have been interrupted by a previous sterilization.

If *periadnexal adhesive disease* is the sole lesion, *laparoscopic salpingo-ovariolysis,* performed preferably at the time of the initial diagnostic laparoscopy, is the approach of choice. For patients who have undergone this procedure, the reported intrauterine pregnancy rates range from 51% to 62%, and the ectopic pregnancy rates range from 5% to 8%.

Agglutination of the fimbriae *(fimbrial phimosis)* necessitates a *fimbrioplasty,* which can also be performed laparoscopically. This condition often coexists with periadnexal adhesions, which are dealt with first. The reported intrauterine pregnancy rates after laparoscopic *fimbrioplasty* range from 40% to 48%, and the ectopic pregnancy rates range from 5% to 6%.

Distal tubal occlusion *(hydrosalpinx)* can be treated surgically. In major published series, the live birth rates after microsurgical *salpingostomy* range from 20% to 37%, and ectopic pregnancy rates range from 5% to 18%. The improved results achieved with the use of microsurgical techniques are much less impressive with salpingostomy than with other tubal procedures. Furthermore, salpingostomy, performed by laparoscopic access, yields almost similar results to those achieved by open access.

The factors that affect the outcome of salpingostomy include distal ampullary diameter, tubal wall thickness, nature of the tubal endothelium, extent of adhesions, and type of adhesions. These prognostic factors have been quantified in a numerical scoring system (approved by the American Fertility Society in 1988). In cases deemed favorable (mild), the reported live birth rates after microsurgical salpingostomy range from 40% to 60%. This rate drops to less than 20% in cases considered unfavorable (severe). In such cases, IVF may be the initial treatment of choice. If surgery is the initial treatment of choice, the decision of whether to proceed with an immediate laparoscopic salpingostomy or undertake reconstructive microsurgery must depend on local experience and success rates with both approaches.

In cases of *proximal tubal occlusion, selective salpingography* or transcervical fallopian tube *cannulation* may be useful in elucidating false-positive results obtained by HSG and in overcoming obstruction associated with a mucus plug or synechiae. True pathologic tubal occlusion resulting from salpingitis isthmica nodosa, endometriosis, or extensive postinflammatory fibrosis may be treated by *microsurgical tubocornual anastomosis.* The reported live birth rates after such procedures range from 33% to 56%, and ectopic pregnancy rates range from 5% to 7%.

Tubotubal anastomosis by laparoscopic access to reconstruct a previous tubal sterilization or a prior segmental excision for tubal pregnancy, is being performed in several centers. Whereas some investigators obtain satisfactory outcomes with this approach, others report significantly inferior results in comparison to open access. As is the case with other microsurgical reconstructive tubal procedures, tubotubal anastomosis is now performed through a *minilaparotomy incision* and on a daycare or short (24 hours or less) hospital stay basis.

Microsurgery is ideal for tubotubal anastomosis for reversal of sterilization and produces excellent results that are principally dependent on the length and status of the reconstructed tube. Live birth rates of 60% to 80% can be achieved, provided that the reconstructed tube is longer than 4 cm and the ampullary portion is more than 2 cm. The tubal pregnancy rates are usually low. Microsurgical reconstruction offers the opportunity to conceive more than once. This and the impressive results favor the choice of this approach over IVF.

Surgical correction of a Kroener's sterilization *(fimbriectomy)* is possible, but the outcome depends on the remaining ampullary length. Live birth rates of about 30% have been reported when more than 50% of the ampulla has been preserved. Tubal length, in such cases, can be determined by HSG, and in the absence of sufficient ampullary length, IVF should be recommended as the initial treatment. Fortunately, this type of sterilization is now rarely performed.

The choice of the primary treatment and any subsequent treatment depends on a careful consideration of both nontechnical and technical factors. These must be individualized for each patient. Information about success and complication rates of the available treatment options must accurately reflect local experience. Active involvement of the couple in the decision-making process is more likely to result in resolution of the conflict of infertility if treatment proves unsuccessful.

MICROSURGERY

Microsurgery has been defined as "surgery under magnification." In fact, magnification is only a single facet of microsurgery, which embraces a broad concept of tissue care designed to minimize tissue damage.

The basic principles of microsurgery include the following:

- Using a technique designed to minimize tissue injury. In addition to delicate handling of tissues and judicious use of electrical or laser energy, frequent intraoperative irrigation with heparinized lactated Ringer solution is performed to keep serosal surfaces moistened and prevent desiccation.
- Preventing foreign body contamination of the peritoneal cavity.
- Obtaining meticulous pinpoint hemostasis while minimizing adjacent tissue damage.
- Identifying proper cleavage planes.
- Completely excising abnormal tissues.
- Precisely aligning and approximating tissue planes.
- Using magnification, which permits prompt identification of abnormal morphologic changes, recognition and avoidance of surgical injury, and application of the preceding principles with the use of fine microsurgical instruments and suture materials.
- Performing a thorough pelvic lavage at the close of the procedure, to remove from the peritoneal cavity any blood clots, foreign body, or debris that may be present.

Thus, microsurgery is a surgical attitude as much as a technique.

In the late 1960s, Swolin used magnification together with electrosurgery for the reconstruction of distal tubal occlusion. In addition, he strived to reduce peritoneal trauma and kept the operative site wet by frequent irrigation. Magnification, the use of an operating microscope, and microsurgical techniques were subsequently expanded (largely in Vancouver) and used in the correction of pathologic cornual and midtubal occlusions and in reversal of sterilization. Microsurgery, in fact, finds its ultimate application in tubal anastomosis. The use of magnification, microsurgical instruments, and sutures enables the recognition of subtle abnormalities (even in the presence of tubal patency), the excision of abnormal tissues, and the correct alignment of the tubal segments and precise apposition of each layer. Indeed, the application of microsurgery has significantly improved the outcome of such procedures. However, in the treatment of distal tubal occlusion, any improvement attributable to the use of microsurgical techniques has been modest, despite the reduction in postoperative adhesions and improved tubal patency rates.

The introduction of microsurgery into gynecology has yielded benefits much greater than simple improvement in the outcome of certain fertility operations. It created a great awareness of the effects of peritoneal trauma and the resulting postoperative adhesions. It also promoted the use of conservative approaches that are now considered standard care for women undergoing surgical treatment for benign gynecologic disease. These are additional and important reasons to continue to teach reconstructive infertility surgery.

Thus, microsurgery is a surgical philosophy, a delicate surgical approach designed to minimize peritoneal trauma and tissue disruption and to prevent postoperative adhesions while increasing the accuracy of the procedure and improving the outcome.

Microsurgical techniques are equally applicable to both laparotomy and laparoscopic access. We demonstrated the applicability of microsurgical techniques by laparoscopy for adhesiolysis, salpingo-ovariolysis, fimbrioplasty, and salpingostomy as early as the mid-1970s. Microsurgical techniques must be used in all reproductive operations, irrespective of the mode of access. This is especially important today because most such procedures are performed by laparoscopy and minilaparotomy.

The laparoscope provides a degree of magnification. It is also possible to bring the distal end of the laparoscope close to the area of interest and achieve excellent visibility and illumination. There are microsurgical advantages inherent to laparoscopic access. Operating within a closed peritoneal cavity eliminates the need to use packs and prevents the introduction of foreign materials such as lint and talcum powder. The pressure effect of the pneumoperitoneum diminishes venous oozing and permits spontaneous coagulation of minor vessels. It is possible to perform intraoperative irrigation to expose any bleeding vessels and keep tissues moistened. Fine electrodes can also be used to achieve precise electrosurgical hemostasis. Like microsurgery, laparoscopic procedures are performed with few instruments. The instrument manufacturers have at last recognized the need for proper microsurgical instruments for laparoscopy; they are now readily available. We must stress, however, that the large volume of insufflation necessary in operative laparoscopy causes desiccation of the mesothelial cells that line the peritoneum. This phenomenon, which may enhance formation of postoperative adhesions, can be largely prevented by the use of warmed humidified gas, which can be accomplished with the introduction a special apparatus into the CO_2 line. There is also evidence that CO_2 pneumoperitoneum alters the protective mechanisms of cells against free radicals. This increases with the duration of the pneumoperitoneum, insufflation pressure, and flow rate. This deleterious effect may be partly overcome by frequent irrigation with lactated Ringer solution. Experimental data in animals suggest that the addition of a small percentage of oxygen to the pneumoperitoneum reduces these local effects, as well as the systemic effects of carbonemia and acidosis.

Major Equipment and Surgical Instruments

The major equipment includes an electrosurgical generator suitable for both general and microsurgical work and, depending on the access mode used, either an operating microscope or appropriate laparoscopic equipment.

Most of the good modern electrosurgical generators can be used for both general and microsurgical work. Such generators are now standard equipment in most operating rooms.

When access to the pelvis is achieved by laparotomy or minilaparotomy, magnification is obtained by the use of an operating microscope or loops. Loops provide low levels of fixed magnification. It is difficult to work with loops that provide magnification greater than 4×. They are suitable for use only in simple short procedures and are quite helpful when used to divide adhesions or excise endometriotic lesions located deep in the pelvis.

Magnification is best obtained with an operating microscope that provides magnification ranges from 2× to 40×; coaxial illumination of a constant visual field enables precise focusing and change of the level of magnification. In gynecologic microsurgery, an objective lens with a focal distance of 250 to 300 mm allows for a suitable working distance under the lens. The microscope can be mounted on the floor or ceiling. Focusing, varying the level of magnification, and other functions of the microscope can be manual or motorized. The latter version is preferable because changes can be readily accomplished through controls on a foot pedal while the surgeon's hands remain in the operative field. Most modern operating microscopes are equipped with beam splitters, which permit the fitting of two pairs of binoculars so that both the surgeon and the assistant can simultaneously view the operative field. A miniature television camera can also be fitted to the same beam splitter, which enables the operating room personnel to follow the surgery on the monitor and allows video recordings of the procedure to be made.

When laparoscopic access is used, a good laparoscope equipped with a high-resolution mini TV camera and monitor is required. The laparoscope does not offer the stereoscopic vision and the excellent depth of field that the operating microscope provides. Nonetheless, first generations of three-dimensional laparoscopic equipment and magnification devices have been produced. Progress is under way.

Good microsurgical instruments are now available from many manufacturers. Their shape is obviously different for open and laparoscopic procedures. However, their functions are similar. The basic microsurgical instruments are few and include plain and toothed platform microforceps, microscissors, microneedle holder, and straight scissors and/or a microblade to transect the tube (Fig. 24.11). The forceps have rounded tips with a shaft designed so that they, like the scissors and needle holder, have good ergonomics and can be used comfortably. Teflon-coated probes with variable rounded tips are used for retraction.

Electromicrosurgery requires the use of a true insulated microelectrode of 100 or 150 microns in diameter with a free pointed conical tip. The microelectrode is connected to the handle of the electrosurgical unit with an adaptor. A rocker switch mounted on the handle allows delivery of current in cutting, coagulating, or blend modes. Irrigation can be performed with an appropriate laparoscopic irrigator. For open procedures, a device with a fingertip control (Gomel irrigator, Fig. 24.12) is commercially available and enables accurate irrigation.

Immediate Preoperative Preparation

Before the induction of anesthesia, the surgeon must ensure that all necessary equipment and instruments are present and in working order. After the induction of anesthesia, the patient's bladder is catheterized with a Foley catheter, which is connected to continuous drainage. If intraoperative chromopertubation is required, either a pediatric Foley catheter or an appropriate uterine cannula is introduced through the cervix and fixed in place. The catheter or cannula is connected either directly or by means of an extension tube to a syringe filled with dilute dye solution.

When open surgical access is used, anteversion and elevation of the uterus can be achieved either by selecting a suitable uterine cannula or by packing the vagina. With the latter option, a pediatric Foley catheter should first be placed in the uterine cavity, if intraoperative chromopertubation is desired.

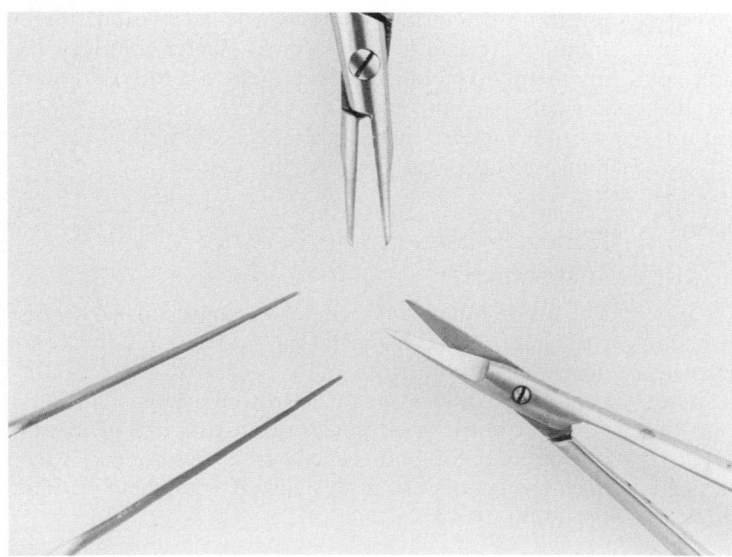

FIGURE 24.11. The working tips of the principal microsurgical instruments: plain forceps, scissors, and needle holder.

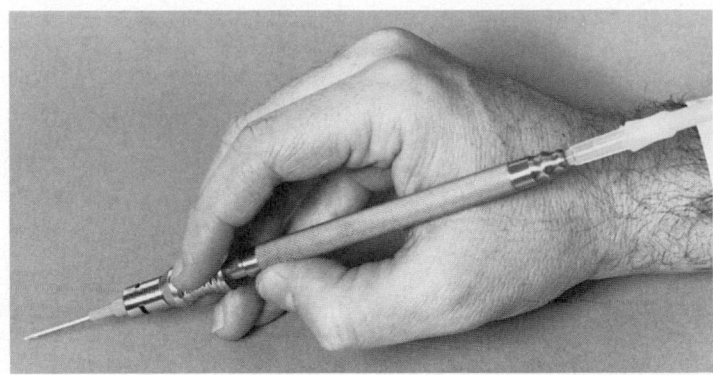

FIGURE 24.12. The Gomel microsurgical irrigator. An intravenous cannula has been attached to the tip of the irrigator. Fingertip control of the sliding valve permits one to initiate or stop irrigation.

Surgical Access

As indicated earlier in the text, many reconstructive tubal operations can be performed by laparotomy, minilaparotomy, or laparoscopic access. The selection of the specific access route depends on the nature of the lesion, the type of procedure required, and the skill of the surgeon. The aim is to select the access route that will yield the best outcome for the patient.

Many reconstructive operations, especially those for distal tubal disease, can be efficiently performed by laparoscopic access. Because of the advantages inherent in undertaking such a procedure at the time of the initial diagnostic laparoscopy, it is preferable that a surgeon trained in this type of surgery perform the laparoscopy.

Access by Laparoscopy

Once a proper pneumoperitoneum is obtained, the principal trocar and cannula are inserted (usually intraumbilically), the trocar is removed, and the laparoscope is introduced through the cannula. The details of performing a laparoscopy will not be described in this chapter. A thorough laparoscopic survey is performed as described earlier in this text, and the nature and extent of the tubal and pelvic lesions is assessed. The information yielded by the prior HSG, complemented by the laparoscopic findings and the status of the other fertility parameters, permits the surgeon to select the therapeutic approach that is best for the patient.

The laparoscopic survey requires the establishment of a secondary portal for the introduction of a probe or other appropriate instrument. This ancillary portal is placed suprapubically in the midline or in one of the lower abdominal quadrants. The undertaking of reconstructive surgery will necessitate the establishment of additional portals of entry. These are placed, depending on the clinical findings and the procedure to be performed, at sites that permit easy access to the operative field.

Abdominal Incision Minilaparotomy

In reconstructive tubal surgery, a transverse suprapubic incision is the type used most often. Since 1985, we have used a small, minilaparotomy, suprapubic transverse or vertical (if a midline or paramedian scar is present) incision to gain access to the pelvis. The length of this minilaparotomy incision is usually 5 to 6 cm. The prior pelvic findings and especially the depth of the patient's subcutaneous adipose layer determine the length of the incision. The site of the proposed incision is infiltrated with a long-acting anesthetic agent such as 0.25% bupivacaine (Marcaine) solution. A transverse suprapubic incision is made and extended down to the fascia. The subcutaneous fat is dissected over the fascia, in the midline upward and downward. The fascia is then incised vertically in the midline. The recti muscles are separated in the midline, and the peritoneum is incised vertically, with the incision curbed laterally at the lower end to avoid the bladder. The subcutaneous tissues are reinfiltrated with the same solution before closure of the skin incision. Thereafter, a bilateral inguinal nerve block is established. The small size of the incision; the lack of bowel manipulation, along with gentle handling of tissues during the procedure; and the use of local anesthesia reduce postoperative discomfort and analgesia requirements. This approach permits prompt mobilization of the patient and discharge from the hospital or surgicenter within 4–24 hours. These patients return to normal activity almost as rapidly as those who have had their procedures performed laparoscopically.

It is essential that the surgical personnel thoroughly wash their gloves after they have been put on and again before making the peritoneal incision. Once the peritoneal cavity is entered, a wound protector is introduced through the incision, and a small Dennis-Brown retractor is applied. Pads soaked in heparinized (5000 U/L) lactated Ringer solution can be introduced into the pouch of Douglas to further elevate the uterus and isolate the bowel already displaced by a mild (10- to 15-degree) Trendelenburg tilt.

A new disposable device, *Protractor*, combines the functions of wound protector and retractor, providing circumferential retraction with maximal exposure for the incision size. This device is easy to use and enhances access through minilaparotomy.

Once the surgical site is well exposed, the operating microscope is positioned. Although the operating microscope can be draped, we have not found this to be necessary, particularly if foot pedals control the microscope. Intraoperative irrigation is performed with heparinized lactated Ringer solution in an intravenous bag that is elevated and connected with intravenous tubing to a Gomel microsurgical irrigator (Fig. 24.12). This enables periodic irrigation of the exposed peritoneal surfaces and ovaries to prevent desiccation and to visualize individual bleeders.

Pelvic Lavage

At the close of a reconstructive procedure, irrespective of the type and the mode of access, the operative site is inspected to ensure that complete hemostasis has been achieved. Any bleeding vessels are electrodesiccated. A thorough pelvic lavage is then performed with the irrigation solution until the fluid remains clear. Pelvic lavage serves to remove from the peritoneal cavity any blood clots or other debris that may be present.

When laparoscopic access is used for the procedure, underwater examination of the operative site may be performed. When the irrigation fluid remains clear, the pneumoperitoneum pressure is reduced, and the region is inspected with the distal end of the laparoscope under the surface of the fluid. This permits prompt recognition of any small bleeding vessels, which can be desiccated with use of a microelectrode or microbipolar forceps.

Once the irrigation fluid is completely suctioned out of the pelvis, some investigators leave varying amounts of physiologic solution in the peritoneal cavity to reduce postoperative adhesions. We continue to use 200 to 300 mL of lactated Ringer solution containing 500 mg of hydrocortisone succinate. Hyskon, which was in vogue for many years, is no longer used. There are promising new products, that are easy to apply by both open and laparoscopic access, such as Intergel (Gynecare) and Spraygel (Confluent Surgical) that are undergoing clinical trials. The topic of ancillary measures for adhesion prevention is outside the purview of this chapter and will not be discussed further.

SURGICAL TECHNIQUE

In this chapter, the following procedures will be discussed: salpingo-ovariolysis, fimbrioplasty, salpingostomy, tubotubal anastomosis to repair midtubal disease or to reverse a prior sterilization, tubocornual anastomosis to treat proximal tubal disease, and other procedures performed rarely in unusual circumstances.

The techniques used in these procedures are essentially the same irrespective of the access route.

Whereas procedures for distal tubal disease are very amenable to laparoscopic access, anastomotic procedures are technically more difficult to accomplish by this route. Isthmic–isthmic and isthmic–ampullary anastomosis (usually used for sterilization reversal) have been performed with varying degrees of accuracy through laparoscopic access, but accomplishing other types of anastomoses (especially tubocornual) through this mode of access is much more difficult.

When I use microsurgical procedures, my aim has always been to keep the techniques as simple as possible in order that the results will be reproducible not only by surgical virtuosi but also by all physicians who practice in this field.

Our more recent technical modifications, including access through minilaparotomy incision and the use of a Protractor, were the result of the same thought process. Although we remain enthusiastic proponents of laparoscopic access, we do not let this enthusiasm blind us to the possibility that some procedures may still be performed better by improvements in traditional methods.

Salpingo-ovariolysis

Pelvic and periadnexal adhesions usually are the sequelae of PID. These adhesions may be broad or shallow; they are usually not too vascular and extend from one structure to another. In so doing, they tend to leave a space or potential space between the involved structures, an aspect that facilitates adhesiolysis (Fig. 24.13). Dense cohesive adhesions often result from prior surgery. In this case, adjacent structures are intimately conglutinated. The adherent area is devoid of the superficial mesothelial layer of peritoneum. In other words, the underlying stromal layers of the two structures coalesce. The lysis of such an adhesive process is technically difficult and is associated with a very high percentage of recurrence.

Periadnexal adhesions usually coexist with other types of tubal disease. Thus, salpingo-ovariolysis is often an integral part of other reconstructive procedures. However, periadnexal adhesive disease may be the sole apparent lesion, in which case, infertility depends on the severity and nature of these adhesions. Even in the presence of a patent tube, extensive adhesions may encapsulate the tube (especially the fimbriated end, the ovary, or both) and prevent ovum pickup (Fig. 24.9). By fixing the fimbriated end of the patent tube away from the ovary, adhesions could possibly distort the spatial relation and, hence, the functional relation that exists between these two organs. For example, the fimbriated end

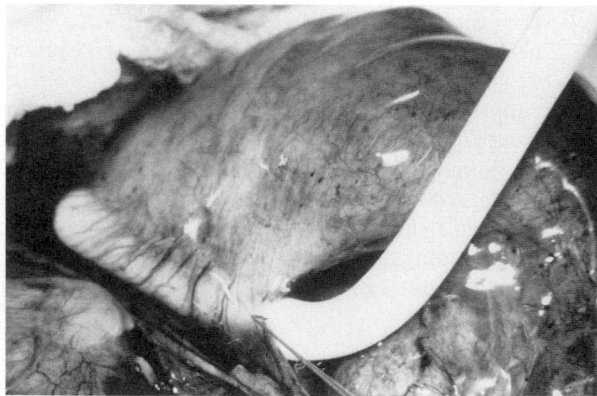

FIGURE 24.13. Salpingolysis. The space between the two involved structures facilitates division. See color version of figure.

of a patent tube may be adherent to the anterior abdominal wall or the uterine fundus, whereas the ovary is fixed in the pouch of Douglas. Periovarian adhesions may also affect follicular development, as has been demonstrated in both animal and human studies. Human studies were usually performed on patients undergoing IVF treatment.

When salpingo-ovariolysis is performed with an open abdomen (laparotomy or minilaparotomy), adhesiolysis is usually commenced by defining the distal margins of the adhesions. The division of adhesions at their distal attachment frees the adnexa, making it possible to elevate and bring them closer to the abdominal wall. This move facilitates the remainder of the procedure. Elevation of the adnexa is achieved by the use of inert pads soaked in the irrigation fluid. Adhesiolysis is then completed by systematically excising the adhesions from the tubal serosa or ovarian surface (Fig. 24.14). With laparoscopic access, it is usually preferable to reverse this order and commence the adhesiolysis in the adnexa.

Adhesions are put on tension with a toothed forceps, and the site of incision is exposed. Division is effected electrosurgically or with appropriate microsurgical scissors. It is imperative to divide adhesions one layer at a time, slightly lateral to their attachments to the organ in order to avoid damaging the adjacent peritoneum. Adhesions are often composed of two layers, even though they may initially appear as a single layer. They tend to attach to an organ at two different levels. It is essential to enter between the two layers first, which permits exposure of the demarcation line between the adhesion and the mesothelium of the adjacent structure. Each layer of adhesion is then put on a stretch with toothed forceps, the demarcation line is identified, and the adhesion is transected. With open access, placement of a Teflon rod under the incision line enhances exposure. Damage to the peritoneum or ovarian surface is avoided by keeping the transection line 1 mm away from these surfaces. Prominent vessels along the transection line are individually electrodesiccated.

When a microelectrode is used for this purpose, the electrosurgical unit is put on the blend setting, which on cut mode combines coagulating current with cutting current to provide concurrent hemostasis during the division of adhesions. Pure coagulating current (COAG mode) may be used to obtain hemostasis of individual bleeders, which are exposed under a jet of irrigation fluid. With open access, an elongating adaptor may be attached to the handle of the electrosurgical unit to facilitate adhesiolysis in the deeper parts of the pelvis.

All of the broad adhesions are excised and removed from the pelvis (Fig. 24.14). Shallow adhesions are simply divided. In this case, a small opening is made on the adhesion, through which a fine instrument or Teflon rod is introduced. This permits separation of the adjacent structures and better visualization of the adhesion, which is incised without damaging these structures. The procedure is completed with a thorough pelvic lavage with the irrigation solution mentioned earlier.

The technical principles are identical when laparoscopic access is used for the procedure. In this case, however, because there is no need to lift the adnexa close to the abdominal wall, the salpingo-ovariolysis is commenced with the tube and ovary. Once again, the performance of effective and safe salpingo-ovariolysis requires clear identification of each adhesive layer, which is grasped and retracted, permitting clear identification of the attachments to the organ of interest. The adhesions are incised parallel to the organ of interest and about 1 mm away to prevent damaging its mesothelial envelope (Figs. 24.15 and 24.16). Division is accomplished electrosurgically with a microelectrode, or mechanically with the use of proper scissors. We use scissors for laparoscopic salpingo-ovariolysis and electrodesiccation to secure obvious vessels or bleeders encountered along the incision line. As described earlier, shallow adhesions are simply divided, whereas broad adhesions are excised (by dissecting them free at all points of attachment) and removed through one of the ancillary portals (Fig. 24.16).

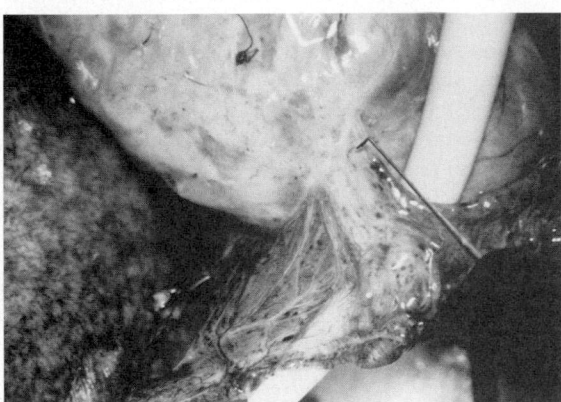

FIGURE 24.14. Ovariolysis. Broad adhesions that had already been divided at their distal margins are being excised from the ovary. See color version of figure.

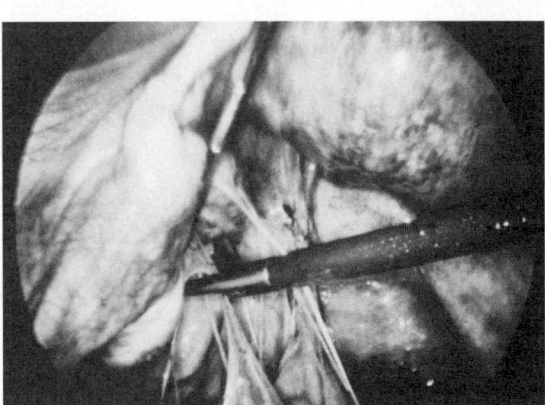

FIGURE 24.15. Salpingo-ovariolysis by laparoscopic access (same patient as in Figure 24.9). Division of adhesions parallel to the tube. See color version of figure.

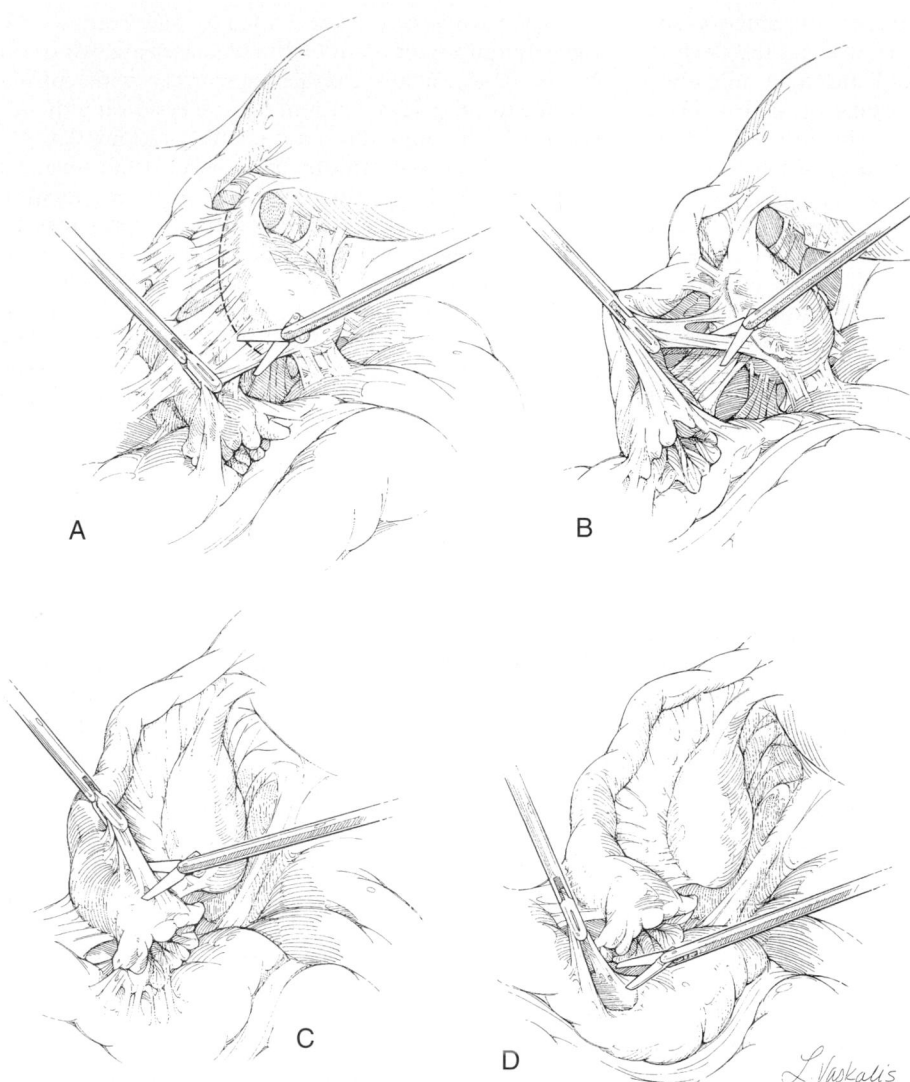

FIGURE 24.16. Salpingo-ovariolysis. **A:** Division of adhesions commences in a well-exposed area. **B:** Adhesions are stretched and are divided one layer at a time parallel to the organ of interest. **C:** Broad adhesions are freed at all points and removed from the peritoneal cavity. **D:** Salpingo-ovariolysis being completed. (From: Gomel V, Taylor PJ. *Diagnostic and operative gynecologic laparoscopy.* St Louis: Mosby, 1995:171, with permission.)

Cohesive adhesions require identification of the dissection plane. This is achieved by making a small incision and developing a tissue plane either by spreading the jaws of the scissors, by blunt dissection, or by hydrodissection (injecting irrigation solution into the site under pressure). It is important to abstain from using thermal energy in such cases because of the inherent danger.

It should not be necessary to do a laparotomy solely for the purpose of salpingo-ovariolysis. Our primary approach in such cases has been to perform the procedure by way of laparoscopy, usually at the time of the diagnostic survey.

Results of Salpingo-ovariolysis

The reported intrauterine pregnancy rates resulting from microsurgical salpingo-ovariolysis range from 41% to 57%. The rates for live births are 37% to 57%, and the rates for ectopic pregnancies are 5% to 8% of operated patients. In one of these studies, 33 of 63 (52.4%) patients who underwent microsurgical salpingo-ovariolysis achieved intrauterine pregnancies, and there were three (4.8%) ectopic pregnancies at 2-year follow-up. These 63 patients had been randomized to two cutting modalities: electrosurgery ($n = 33$) and CO_2 laser ($n = 30$). The results were identical in both subgroups. Indeed, there has been no demonstrable improvement in the outcome of such procedures with the use of lasers, in both clinical and experimental studies.

The preexisting tubal patency and the uncontrolled nature of the salpingo-ovariolysis series reported in the literature may cast doubt on the value of this procedure. The Canadian Infertility Evaluation Study Group addressed this issue by studying treatment-dependent and treatment-independent pregnancies in patients with periadnexal disease whose fallopian tubes were not completely occluded. This was a multicenter, controlled, randomized study. The cumulative pregnancy rates were 59% among 69 patients in the group who underwent microsurgical salpingo-ovariolysis and only 16% among the 78 control patients who were not treated. This study confirms that pregnancies may occur in a small proportion of women with periadnexal adhesions and patent tubes and proves the therapeutic value of salpingo-ovariolysis in such cases.

In the early stages of development of operative laparoscopy, we demonstrated that laparoscopic salpingo-ovariolysis yields results similar to those obtained by microsurgery. We also stressed the importance of adhering to microsurgical principles in the performance of such procedures by laparoscopic access. We reported later a series of 92 patients who underwent salpingo-ovariolysis by laparoscopy. The duration of involuntary infertility was longer than 20 months for all patients. Periadnexal adhesions were severe in 79 patients and moderate in 13. Moreover, the series included only those patients in whom ovum pickup by the tube on the side with lesser disease was deemed impossible or greatly hampered. At the time of the survey, the patients had been monitored postoperatively for a period of 9 months or longer. Of the 92 patients, 57 (62%) achieved at least one intrauterine pregnancy, 54 (59%) had one or more live births, and five (5.4%) had ectopic pregnancies. Ten of the patients who did not get pregnant had a second-look laparoscopy that demonstrated no significant residual adhesive process.

Similar results were corroborated by other centers in Europe and North America. This demonstrates that the results of laparoscopic salpingo-ovariolysis, as expected, depend on the severity of the adhesions. The reported intrauterine pregnancy rates after laparoscopic salpingo-ovariolysis range from 51% to 62%, and ectopic pregnancy rates range from 5% to 8% of operated cases. Although no prospective, randomized trials exist, these results appear similar to those yielded by laparotomy.

Fimbrioplasty

Fimbrioplasty is the reconstruction of the fimbriae or infundibulum in a tube that exhibits fimbrial agglutination or prefimbrial phimosis, and results in partial distal occlusion. Often, the tube and ovary are involved in adhesions, in which case, salpingo-ovariolysis must precede the fimbrioplasty. The technique of fimbrioplasty, which will be described further, is the same irrespective of the access route used. Our approach is invariably by laparoscopic access.

Fimbrial phimosis results from the agglutination of the fimbriae. A small opening is usually present at the distal end of the tube unless this opening is covered by fibrous tissue. The latter usually becomes evident when the tube is distended by transcervical chromopertubation. When the opening is covered by fibrous tissue, this tissue must be incised or excised to gain access to the fimbriae. Agglutination of the fimbriae can be corrected simply by introducing a fine forceps (mosquito forceps by way of laparotomy or a 2-mm grasping or alligator forceps by way of laparoscopy) with jaws closed through the phimotic fimbrial opening. The jaws of the forceps are opened within the tubal lumen, and the forceps are gently withdrawn with the jaws open. Deagglutination is achieved by repeating this movement a few times, varying the direction in which the jaws of the forceps are opened (Fig. 24.17). When sufficient gentleness is used during this manipulation, bleeding is usually negligible.

When the stenosis is located at the level of the true abdominal tubal ostium, which is located at the apex of the infundibulum, the fimbriae may have a normal appearance. However, when chromopertubation is performed, the ampullary portion of the tube distends before any exit

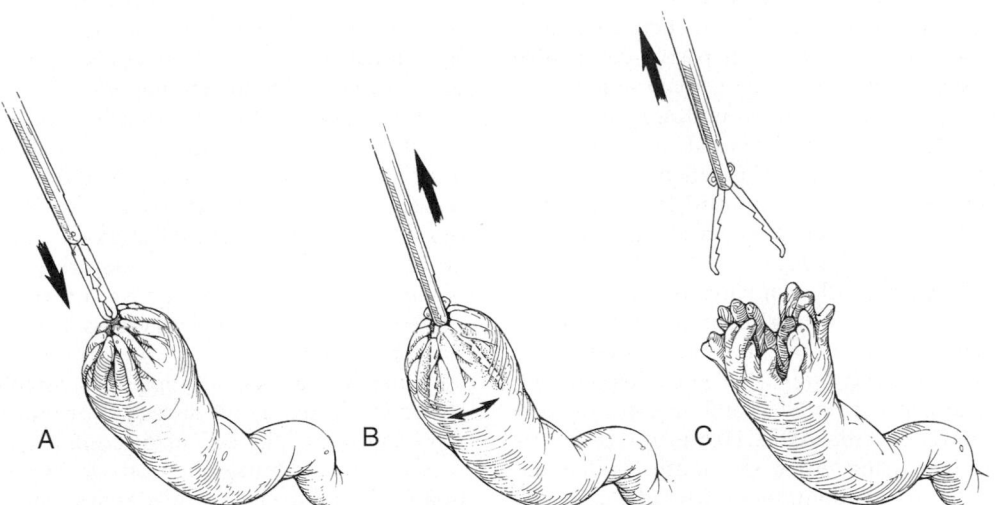

FIGURE 24.17. Fimbrioplasty: to free agglutinated fimbriae. **A:** The 3-mm alligator-jawed forceps is introduced through the stenosed opening. **B:** The jaws of the forceps are opened within the tube. **C:** The forceps is gently withdrawn while the jaws are kept open. (From: Gomel V, Taylor PJ. *Diagnostic and operative gynecologic laparoscopy.* St Louis: Mosby, 1995:173, with permission.)

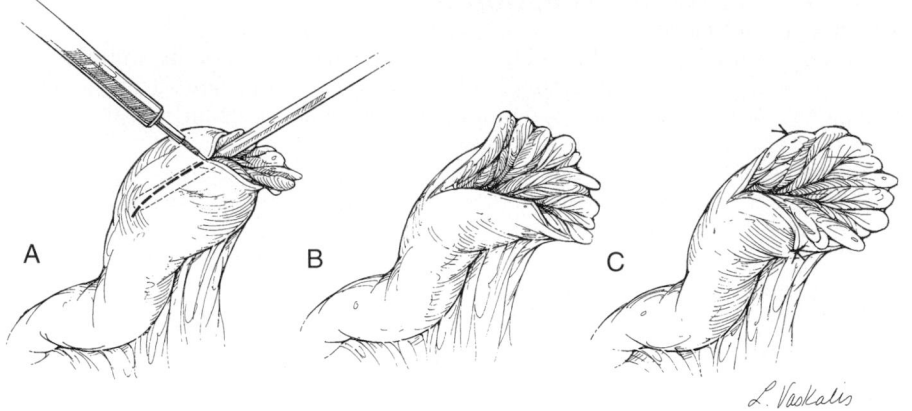

FIGURE 24.18. Fimbrioplasty: correction of prefimbrial phimosis. **A and B:** An incision is placed at the antimesosalpingeal border of the tube. **C:** Completed procedure with flaps everted. (From: Gomel V, Taylor PJ. *Diagnostic and operative gynecologic laparoscopy.* St Louis: Mosby, 1995: 173, with permission.)

of dye solution. In this instance, it is necessary to place an incision on the antimesosalpingeal border of the tube, which commences at the infundibulum and continues past the stenotic area into the distal ampulla. The tube is stabilized by introducing a thin Teflon probe, through the stenotic opening, into the distal ampulla, and the incision is made electrosurgically by using a microelectrode. This is the approach we generally use. Alternatively, the area can be injected with 1 mL of dilute vasopressin solution (1 IU in 10 mL of normal saline), and the incision made mechanically with microsurgical scissors. Bleeders are desiccated electrosurgically. The edges of the two flaps thus created are folded back either by securing them to the adjacent ampullary serosa with no. 7-0 or 8-0 polyglactin 910 (Vicryl) sutures or by electrosurgery (or a defocused CO_2 laser beam), which desiccates the serosal aspect of the flaps, causing them to fold backward (Fig. 24.18).

Results of Fimbrioplasty

Very few investigators have classified fimbrioplasty as an independent procedure. Most include such patients in their salpingostomy series. French and Belgian centers include fimbrioplasty (correction of partial distal tubal occlusion) as stage 1 in their salpingostomy series.

Patton et al., in a series of microsurgical fimbrioplasty procedures in 40 patients, reported total intrauterine and ectopic pregnancy rates of 63% (25 patients) and 5% (2 patients), respectively, after 24 months' follow-up. The outcome of the intrauterine pregnancies and the live birth rates were not provided.

In 1983, I reported 40 such patients, all treated by laparoscopic access. Live births occurred in 19 (48%), and two patients (5%) had tubal gestations. Mettler and associates reported a crude pregnancy rate of 31% among 51 women. The anatomic location and outcome of these pregnancies were not recorded. Dubuisson et al. reported 31 such patients. After 18 months' follow-up, eight patients (25.8%) had intrauterine pregnancies, and four (12.9%) had ectopic pregnancies. Donnez and colleagues, in a series of 100 patients, reported a total pregnancy rate of 61%. The location and outcome of these pregnancies were not provided. Canis et al. included 32 such patients with their salpingostomy patients; 16

(50%) of these achieved intrauterine pregnancies, but the outcome was not reported. Surprisingly, there were no tubal pregnancies.

There are no randomized trials for fimbrioplasty that compare the two access routes; however, the results appear similar in both groups.

Salpingostomy (Salpingoneostomy)

Salpingostomy, or salpingoneostomy, is the creation of a new stoma in a tube with a completely occluded distal end (hydrosalpinx). Salpingostomy can be terminal, ampullary, or isthmic, depending on the anatomic location at which the new stoma is fashioned. Isthmic and ampullary salpingostomy are of historic interest, except for the reversal of prior fimbriectomy (Kroener's sterilization), in which ampullary salpingostomy may have a place. We did demonstrate that success with ampullary salpingostomy in such cases is dependent on ampullary length, and suggested that reconstructive surgery should only be undertaken when more than one half of the ampulla is present. This recommendation is corroborated by a recent study, by Tourgeman et al., reporting on 41 women who had fimbriectomy reversal.

Distal tubal occlusion is usually associated with varying degrees of pelvic and periadnexal adhesions that must first be lysed. Thereafter, the distal end of the tube is examined to ensure that it is not adherent to the ovary or other structures. If the distal tube is adherent, it must be dissected free until the tuboovarian ligament is exposed (Fig. 24.19). Only by freeing the tube can the surgeon ensure that the neostomy is being performed at the appropriate site.

Once the salpingo-ovariolysis is completed and the tube is totally freed, it is distended by transcervical chromopertubation. The occluded terminal end of the tube is examined under magnification, which permits recognition of the relatively avascular zones that radiate from a central punctum. The tube is entered at this central point with use of the microelectrode or microsurgical scissors, and the incision is extended toward the ovary over an avascular line (Fig. 24.20). This incision fashions a new fimbria ovarica that maintains the tuboovarian relation.

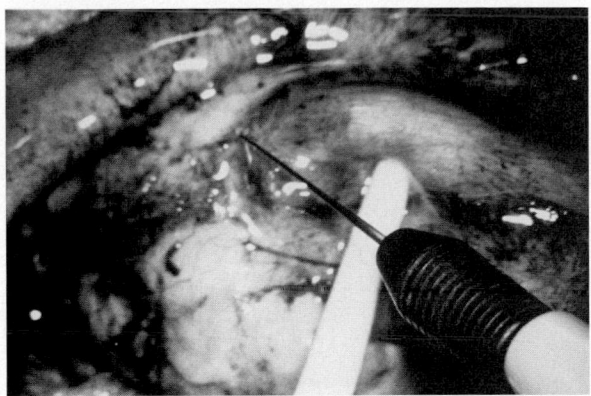

FIGURE 24.19. Dissection of the distal hydrosalpinx from the anterior surface of the ovary to which it is intimately adherent. See color version of figure.

At this point in the procedure, it becomes possible to view the tube from within when placing additional incisions along its circumference to complete the creation of a new stoma. These additional incisions are made between endothelial folds, over avascular areas. In so doing, one avoids cutting through vascular mucosal folds, which will be shaped as fimbriae, and bleeding is mini-

mized as a result. Any bleeding points that occur are exposed under a jet of irrigation fluid and desiccated individually with a microelectrode or microbipolar forceps. Once a satisfactory stoma is achieved, the flaps created in the process are everted either by securing them without tension to the ampullary seromuscularis with interrupted no. 8-0 Vicryl sutures (Fig. 24.20) or by desiccating their serosal surface, which causes them to fold backward. Desiccation is achieved either electrosurgically with a ball-shaped electrode and a low power density, or with CO_2 laser using a defocused beam. The procedure is concluded with a thorough pelvic lavage, as described earlier in this chapter.

If during the initial diagnostic laparoscopy, the surgeon decides to perform the salpingostomy by open access and if the adnexa are found to be fixed by periadnexal adhesions, these adhesions can be lysed laparoscopically at their distal margins, thus mobilizing the adnexa. Such an undertaking permits the subsequent salpingostomy to be readily performed through a mini-laparotomy incision.

Results of Salpingostomy

In the major published series, the live birth rate after microsurgical salpingostomy ranges from 20% to 37%, and

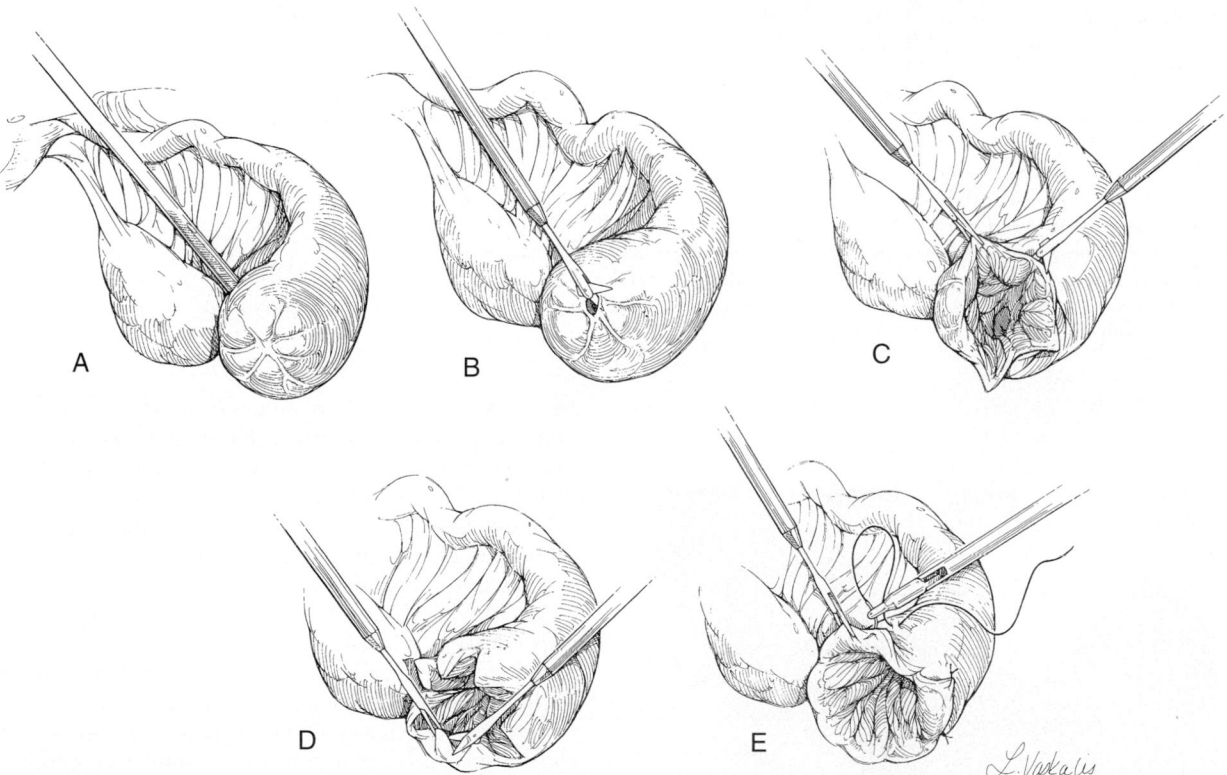

FIGURE 24.20. Salpingostomy. **A:** The occluded distal end of the tube usually has a centrally placed avascular area, from which avascular scarred lines extend in a cartwheel manner. **B:** The first incision is made along an avascular line toward the ovary. **C:** Avascular lines are incised by viewing from within the tube along the circumference of the initial opening. **D:** Cutting along the avascular lines is continued until a satisfactory stoma is fashioned. **E:** The flaps can be everted by placing two or three no. 6-0 absorbable synthetic sutures. (From: Gomel V, Taylor PJ. *Diagnostic and operative gynecologic laparoscopy.* St Louis: Mosby, 1995:174, with permission.)

TABLE 24.2.
Results of Microsurgical Salpingostomy

Investigators	Year	Patients	Intrauterine Pregnancies	Live Births	Ectopic Pregnancies
ACCESS BY LAPAROTOMY					
Swolin[a]	1975	33	9	8 (24.2%)	6
Gomel[b]	1978b	41	12	11 (26.8%)	5
Gomel[b]	1980b	72	22	21 (29.2%)	7
Larsson[c]	1982	54	21	17 (31.5%)	0
Verhoeven et al.[d]	1983	143	34	28 (19.6%)	3
Tulandi and Vilos[e]	1985	67	15	NS	3
Boer-Meisel et al.	1986	108	31	24 (22.2%)	19
Donnez and Casanas-Roux	1986a	83	26	NS	6
Kosasa and Hale	1988	93	37	34 (36.6%)	13
Schlaff et al.	1990	82	14	NS	6
Winston and Margara	1991	323	106	74 (22.9%)	32
ACCESS BY MINILAPAROTOMY					
Gomel	1990	90	27	23 (25.6%)	8
ACCESS BY LAPAROSCOPY					
Gomel	1977b	9	4	4	
Daniell and Herbert[g]	1984	22	4	3 (13.6%)	1
Dubuisson et al.	1990	34	10	NS	1
Canis et al.	1991	55	13	NS	6
McComb and Paleologou	1991	22	5	5 (22.7%)	1
Dubuisson et al.	1994	90	29	26 (29.9%)	4
Oh	1996	82	29	NS	8
Millingos et al.	2000	61	14	NS	2
Taylor et al.	2001	139	44	25 (18%)	23

NS, not stated.

[a] Follow-up period more than 8 years.

[b] Follow-up period more than 1 year.

[c] Follow-up period more than 4 years.

[d] Twenty-three of these were iterative procedures; only three of these patients (13%) had live births.

[e] Thirty-seven of these procedures were performed with the carbon dioxide laser.

[f] Eight of the nine patients had prior salpingostomy by conventional techniques that resulted in reocclusion.

[g] Performed with the carbon dioxide laser.

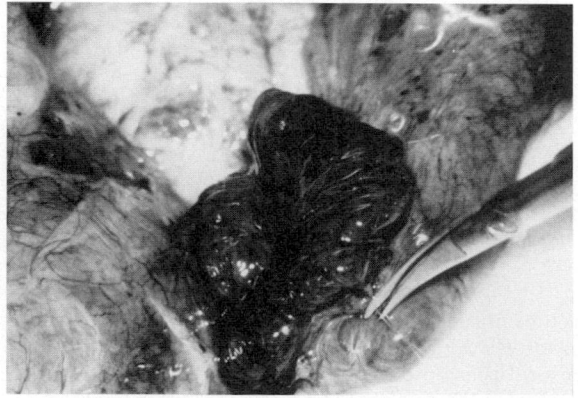

FIGURE 24.21. Microsurgical salpingostomy by open access. The tube is minimally dilated and has a well-preserved epithelium. See color version of figure.

the ectopic pregnancy rate ranges from 5% to 18% (Table 24.2). The factors that affect the outcome of salpingostomy were reviewed earlier in this chapter. Work performed in the past 30 years has made it evident that the major determinants of the outcome of salpingostomy are the degree of preexisting tubal damage and the extent and nature of periadnexal adhesions (Figs. 24.21 and 24.22). As stated earlier in this chapter, the reported live birth rate after microsurgical salpingostomy in favorable cases (mild) ranges from 40% to 60%. This rate drops to less than 20% in unfavorable (severe damage) cases.

I reported a series of 90 patients who underwent microsurgical salpingostomy with a minilaparotomy incision. Nineteen (21.1%) were lost to follow-up and were considered failures. Twenty-seven (30%) patients achieved one or more intrauterine pregnancies, and eight (8.9%) had tubal pregnancies. Ectopic gestations occurred in two additional patients who also had intrauterine pregnancies. Twenty-three (25.6%) women were successful in having one or more live births. These 90

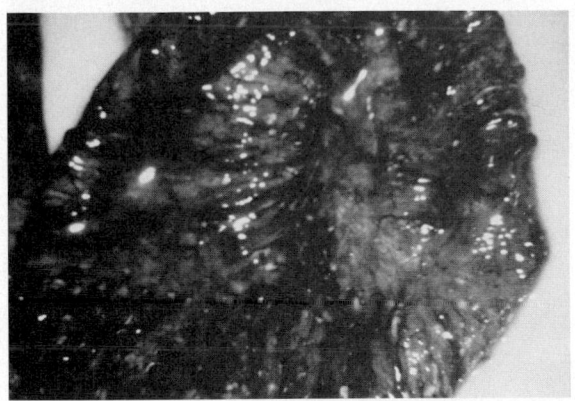

FIGURE 24.22. Microsurgical salpingostomy by open access. The tube is markedly dilated and exhibits a flat epithelium with poorly preserved folds. See color version of figure.

patients were assessed with the classification approved by the American Fertility Society. On the basis of this classification, 73 patients had extensive (severe) damage, and 17 had limited (mild) damage. In the group of 73 patients, 15 (20.5%) had one or more intrauterine pregnancies, and 13 (17.8%) had one or more live births. In the "mild" group of 17 patients, 12 (70.6%) had one or more intrauterine pregnancies, and 10 (58.8%) had one or more live births ($p < 0.05$) (Table 24.2). These observations emphasize the importance of a thorough preoperative investigation and proper patient selection.

On the surface, the results yielded by laparoscopic salpingostomy appear to be somewhat inferior to those obtained by open access. However, laparoscopic salpingostomy offers distinct advantages: It can be performed during the initial diagnostic laparoscopy, avoiding a second intervention and result in cost savings.

During the past decade, there have been many more reports about the deleterious effect of hydrosalpinx on the outcome of IVF treatment, than reports on surgical reconstruction of the condition. This deleterious effect is more evident when hydrosalpinges are large enough to be visible at sonography. In such cases, salpingectomy, before IVF, clearly improves the outcome of this treatment. The detrimental effect on IVF is thought to be a "wash-out effect" owing to the passage of the collected tubal fluid to the uterine cavity at the time when embryos are transferred. Indeed, the timing of embryo transfer to the uterus corresponds to the phase in the menstrual cycle when the tube assumes a prouterine transport. The assumption that the deleterious effect of large hydrosalpinges may be owing to a wash-out of the transferred embryos is supported by a study of Van Voorhis et al. They compared women with hydrosalpinges ($n = 34$) with women who had tubal disease but no hydrosalpinges ($n = 124$), undergoing IVF treatment. Women with hydrosalpinges were found to have a reduced clinical pregnancy rate (18% versus 37%, $p = 0.053$), a reduced ongoing pregnancy rate (15% versus 34%, $p = 0.051$), and reduced implantation rate (7% versus 18%, $p = 0.003$) after IVF procedures. Among

women who had hydrosalpinges, 16 had their hydrosalpinges aspirated at the time of oocyte retrieval, and 18 did not. Aspiration of hydrosalpinges was associated with a higher clinical pregnancy rate (31% versus 5%, $p = 0.07$), a higher ongoing pregnancy rate (31% versus 0%, $p = 0.015$), and a higher implantation rate (14 versus 1%, $p = 0.015$).

In cases with hydrosalpinges visible at sonography, salpingostomy may provide the same beneficial outcome with IVF, while offering the couple the potential of spontaneous pregnancy. This work remains to be done.

Tubotubal Anastomosis

The term tubotubal anastomosis refers to an anastomosis performed anywhere along the tube either to treat occlusions resulting from disease processes or to reverse a prior sterilization. The procedure used to repair proximal or cornual tubal disease is usually referred to as tubocornual anastomosis and will be discussed separately.

Microsurgery finds its ultimate application in tubotubal anastomosis. The precision afforded by this technique allows total excision of occluded or diseased portions, proper alignment, and excellent apposition of each layer of the proximal and distal tubal segments.

Tubotubal anastomosis is performed either to reverse a previous tubal sterilization or to reconstruct the tube after removal of lesions that are often occlusive and affect the tube at sites other than the fimbriated end. Depending on the tubal segments that are approximated, tubotubal anastomosis can be intramural–isthmic, intramural–ampullary, isthmic–isthmic, isthmic–ampullary, or ampullary–infundibular. This section first describes the fundamentals of tubotubal anastomosis and then the technical variations necessary to deal with each specific type of anastomosis.

Basic Principles of Tubotubal Anastomosis

When periadnexal adhesions are present, salpingo-ovariolysis is first completed. When access is achieved through laparotomy or minilaparotomy, the side to be worked on is elevated with the use of pads soaked in irrigation solution. The contralateral adnexa is left in its natural position to prevent desiccation. When access occurs by way of laparoscopy, the mesosalpinx under the site of anastomosis may be injected with 1 to 2 mL of dilute vasopressin solution to reduce oozing and facilitate hemostasis.

The principles of tubotubal anastomosis are the same, irrespective of the mode of access used. The proximal tubal segment is distended by transcervical chromopertubation. This helps identification of the site of occlusion. The tube is transected, with appropriate scissors, adjacent to the site of occlusion or, in the case of a previous tubal sterilization, near the occluded end. The occluded end or occluded segment of the tube is grasped with a strong-toothed forceps to expose the site and facilitate the transection (Fig. 24.23A), which is effected with straight scissors or a sharp microblade. It is essential to halt the incision at the mesosalpinx, in the immediate periphery of the tubal muscularis, to avoid damaging the

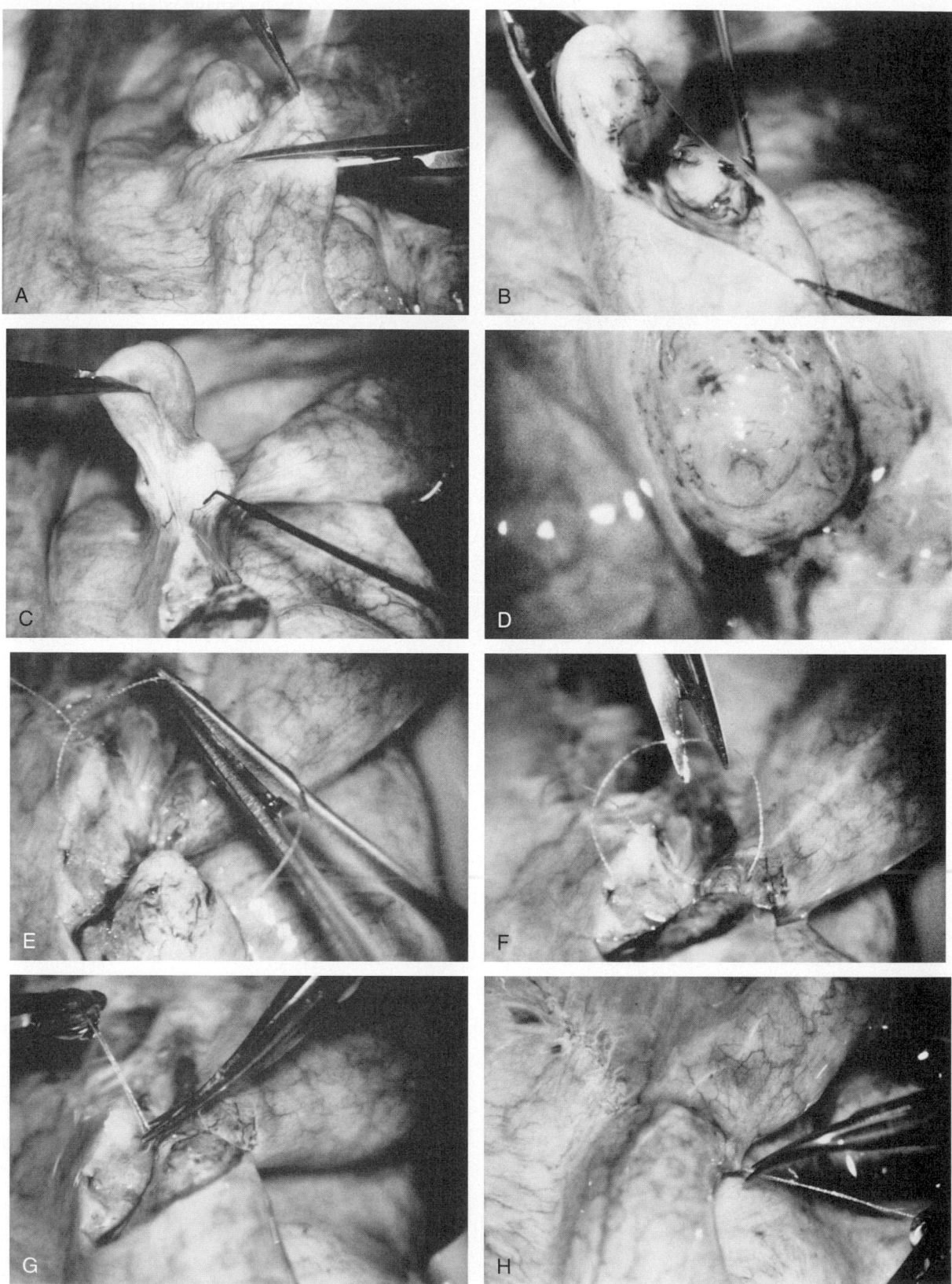

FIGURE 24.23. Microsurgical tubotubal anastomosis for reversal of Falope-ring sterilization.
A: The occluded end of the isthmus is grasped, and the tube is transected with scissors. **B:** Dye
solution escapes from the lumen. **C:** The occluded tubal segment is excised from the mesosalpinx
electrosurgically by use of a microelectrode. **D:** The cut surface of the patent tube is assessed under high magnification. **E:** Once the 6-o'clock suture is tied, subsequent sutures can be placed
with use of a single strand of suture as a continuous series of loops. **F:** Each suture is tied individually after the division of the loop between successive sutures. **G:** The apposition of the inner
musculoepithelial layer is complete. **H:** The anastomosis is completed with approximation of the
serosa. See color version of figure.

adjacent vascular arcade. Dye solution can now escape from the transected tubal lumen (Fig. 24.23B).

The occluded tubal segment is excised from the mesosalpinx electrosurgically or with scissors, the line of incision kept close to the tube to avoid damaging the vessels mentioned earlier (Fig. 24.23C). The cut surface is examined under high magnification to ensure that the tube is normal. Healthy tube is devoid of scarring and exhibits normal muscular and vascular architecture together with intact mucosal folds (Fig. 24.23D). Hemostasis is obtained by precise electrodesiccation of the more significant bleeders, which are located between the serosa and muscularis. Each is exposed by irrigation and desiccated with an insulated microelectrode. If open access is used, gentle compression of the tube between thumb and forefinger facilitates this process. Desiccation of minor bleeders is unnecessary because they stop spontaneously. Desiccation of the tubal epithelium must be avoided to prevent damaging it and adversely affecting future tubal function. Major tubal vessels (such as those composing the vascular arcade) may be divided inadvertently or by necessity. These can be electrodesiccated with monopolar or bipolar current. Overzealous electrodesiccation must be avoided to prevent devitalizing the anastomosis site.

When there is no significant luminal disparity between the two segments, the distal portion is prepared in a similar manner. Before transection, the distal segment is distended by descending hydropertubation, which consists of injecting a few milliliters of irrigation fluid or dilute dye solution through the fimbriated end to identify the distal limit of the occluded portion or, in the case of a prior sterilization, to identify the extremity of the stump. The tubal segments are approximated in two layers. The first of these joins the epithelium and muscu-laris, and the second joins the serosa. We generally use no. 8-0 Vicryl sutures swaged on a 130-micron-shaft, 4- or 5-mm-long, taper-cut needle for tubal anastomosis. The first suture of the inner musculoepithelial layer is always placed at the mesosalpingeal border (6-o'clock position) to ensure proper alignment of the two segments of tube. All of the sutures are placed in a way that positions the knots peripherally.

In exceptional circumstances when the distance between the two segments is great, the mesosalpinx adjacent to the cut ends of the two tubal segments can be approximated first, using a single interrupted no. 7-0 or 8-0 suture. This step brings the tubal segments into close proximity; thus, it facilitates placement of the sutures of the inner layer and reduces the tension that would have existed when tying these sutures.

Once the 6-o'clock suture is tied, the placement of three or more additional sutures (depending on the type of anastomosis) is required to appose the inner layer. These additional sutures can be placed by using a single strand of suture as a continuous series of loops, including the muscularis and the epithelium of the two segments (Figs. 24.23E and 24.24). The sutures are tied individually, after the division of the loop between each successive suture (Fig. 24.23F). This approach facilitates and speeds up suture placement. We advise against the use of a splint in the lumen of the tube because this does not facilitate the procedure and may traumatize the endothelium. Instead, if necessary, the cut surface may be stained with methylene blue or indigo carmine solution to accentuate the visibility of the individual layers.

After approximation of the inner layer, chromopertubation should demonstrate tubal patency and a watertight anastomotic site (Fig. 24.23G). The serosa is joined either with interrupted sutures or with two con-

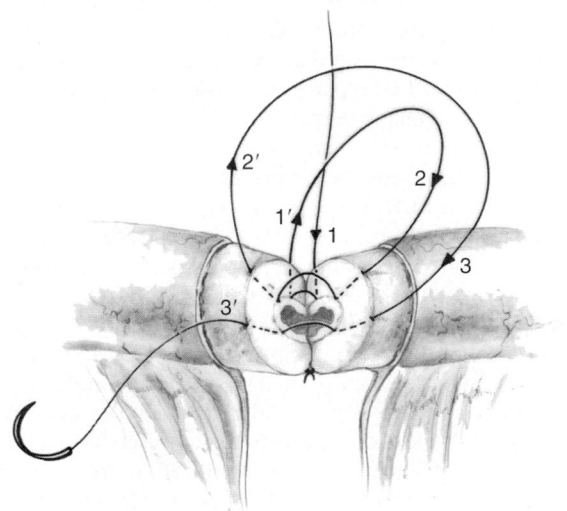
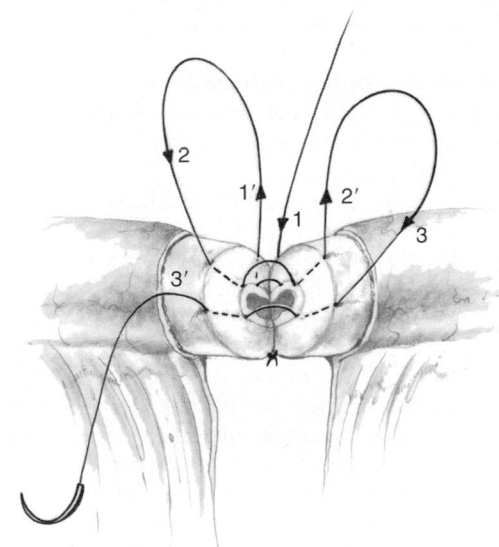

FIGURE 24.24. Microsurgical tubotubal anastomosis. Placement of sutures using a single strand of suture as a continuous series of loops.

tinuous sutures, one that runs anteriorly and the other posteriorly, starting at the antimesosalpingeal border (12-o'clock). Finally, the defect in the mesosalpinx is repaired (Fig. 24.23H).

Tubotubal Anastomosis to Repair Midtubal Disease

The most common reason to perform a tubotubal anastomosis is reversal of sterilization. Midtubal occlusions resulting from disease processes are rare. Such lesions usually affect the intramural or proximal isthmic segments and require a tubocornual type anastomosis.

The causes of midtubal occlusion include endometriosis and tubal pregnancy, usually undiagnosed or treated by observation. A tubal pregnancy treated medically with methotrexate administration or surgically by linear salpingotomy may result in tubal occlusion at the gestational site. Treatment of tubal pregnancy by segmental excision will leave the tube in two segments, as with tubal sterilization. Rare causes of occlusion include congenital absence of a midtubal segment and tuberculosis. In the later instance, reconstruction is contraindicated.

In an intact tube, the site of occlusion may be apparent on inspection; palpation of the tube may identify an indurated segment that is the likely site of occlusion. As mentioned earlier, transcervical chromopertubation distends the proximal segment up to the site of occlusion and helps the surgeon define its proximal limit. The tube is transected either immediately proximal to the occluded segment or in the occluded zone itself. Successive transection of the tube at 1- to 2-mm intervals helps identify the normal segments proximal and distal to the occlusion site.

Irrespective of the type of anastomosis, the basic steps of the procedure are the same. The luminal diameter of the tube is not uniform and is significantly greater in the ampullary segment. The technical variations required largely depend on the disparity of the luminal calibers of the two segments to be joined.

Intramural–Isthmic Anastomosis

Anastomosis between the intramural and isthmic segments is the type of anastomosis most often required to treat cornual disease.

In most cases of reversal of sterilization, a short segment of isthmus is usually present. This short segment is frequently adherent to the side of the uterus as a result of retraction of the adjacent mesosalpinx, thus giving the appearance of total absence of the proximal tube. The presence of a portion of isthmus would have been evident from HSG. Transcervical chromopertubation distends this small segment of isthmus, facilitating identification of its distal margin and its dissection from the uterus. The dissection must be effected carefully to avoid damaging the tube itself and the vessels supplying it. The conservation and appropriate preparation of this segment, even when very small, convert the anastomosis to an isthmic–isthmic type and facilitates the procedure.

In the absence of any isthmus (as may be the case subsequent to either a tubal sterilization or excision of an isthmic pregnancy), maintenance of uterine distention by chromopertubation will indicate the site where the intramural segment should be sought, between the uterine insertion points of the round and ovarian ligaments. Excision of the serosa and underlying scar tissue over the distended area may permit the dye solution to stream out of the intramural segment. In some instances, it is also necessary to dissect the muscularis of this segment from the surrounding uterine muscle for 1 or 2 mm with microscissors or a microelectrode. After this, the tube is transected with microscissors. This process may have to be repeated until the patent tube is reached, at which point dye solution should stream out of the lumen (see Fig. 24.30).

Because of extensive vascularity, dissection in the cornua usually causes significant oozing that hinders visibility. When more than superficial dissection of this region is anticipated, initial infiltration with dilute vasopressin solution (1 U of vasopressin in 10 mL of normal saline) significantly decreases capillary oozing and facilitates the procedure. With use of a 30-gauge needle on a 3-mL syringe, the cornual region of the uterus is injected with 2 mL of this solution in a circular fashion under the serosa 1 cm medial to the uterotubal junction. The resulting vasoconstriction is recognized by serosal blanching.

In this type of anastomosis, there is no significant luminal disparity between the two segments of tube. Hence, the isthmus is simply transected near the occluded end and prepared, as described earlier. A two-layer anastomosis is then performed. Once the inner layer has been joined, the serosa and superficial muscle of the cornual region are approximated to the serosa of the isthmus. The defect under the tube is repaired by suturing the mesosalpinx to the serosa of the lateral edge of the uterus.

Intramural–Ampullary Anastomosis

The salient feature of intramural–ampullary anastomosis is the considerable luminal disparity that exists between the intramural and ampullary segments. The key technical issue lies in the preparation of the occluded proximal end of the ampulla, where an opening into the ampullary lumen, which is not much larger than that of the intramural segment, must be fashioned.

The intramural segment is first prepared as described under intramural–isthmic anastomosis. To identify the occluded end of the ampulla, which may be buried between the leaves of the mesosalpinx, the tube is distended with a few milliliters of dye or irrigation solution introduced through the fimbriated end. Alternatively, a malleable blunt probe can be introduced through the infundibulum and gently threaded toward the occluded end. With the use of microscissors, the serosa over the tip of the ampullary stump is incised in a circular manner. The serosa and any scar tissue under it are then excised to expose the muscularis of the occluded end. The center point of the exposed muscularis is grasped with toothed microforceps, and a small incision is made into the ampullary lumen with the microscissors. This opening is enlarged, to correspond in size to the lumen of the

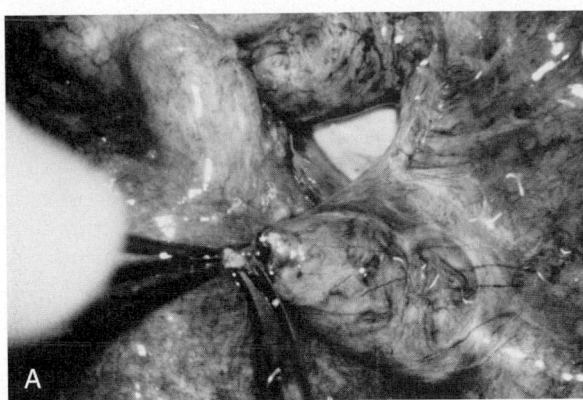 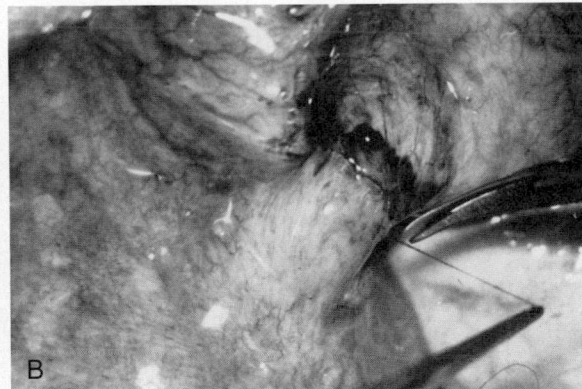

FIGURE 24.25. Microsurgical isthmic–ampullary anastomosis. **A:** Preparation of the ampullary segment. **B:** Approximation of serosa. (See Color Fig. 24.25.)

proximal tubal segment, by excising a tiny circular portion of muscularis and epithelium (Figs. 24.25A and 24.26). The resulting opening is slightly larger than the intramural lumen, but because of the absence of significant disparity, anastomosis of the two segments can be performed as described for isthmic–isthmic anastomosis.

Isthmic–Isthmic Anastomosis

Isthmic isthmic anastomosis is the simplest type of anastomosis to perform. The lumina are comparable in size. The technique is the same as that described earlier under the basic principles of tubotubal anastomosis.

Isthmic–Ampullary Anastomosis

The salient feature of this type of anastomosis is also the considerable luminal disparity that usually exists between the lumina of the isthmic and ampullary segments. The isthmic stump is prepared as described under the basic principles of tubotubal anastomosis. In most instances, the occluded end of the ampullary stump will be free, enabling a lumen of appropriate diameter (comparable in size to that of the isthmic segment) to be fashioned, as

described under intramural–ampullary anastomosis (Fig. 24.25A and 24.26). A two-layer anastomosis is then performed as described under the basic principles of tubotubal anastomosis (Fig. 24.25B). Although the muscularis of the ampulla is considerably thinner than that of the isthmus, this poses no problem in approximating the epithelium and muscularis of the two segments.

Occasionally, circumstances will not permit the use of the technique described earlier in the preparation of the occluded ampullary end. The ampullary stump may be occluded by a permanent suture or clip, and removal of this suture or clip may lead to the creation of an opening that is much larger than the isthmic lumen and through which lush epithelial folds will prolapse. The proximal end of the ampullary segment may have a fistulous opening that is similarly large.

If the opening into the ampullary lumen is made significantly larger than that of the isthmic segment (either inadvertently or by necessity), it will be necessary to either enlarge the isthmic lumen or narrow the ampullary lumen. To enlarge the lumen of the isthmic segment, a 2- to 3-mm slit is made with scissors at its antimesosal-

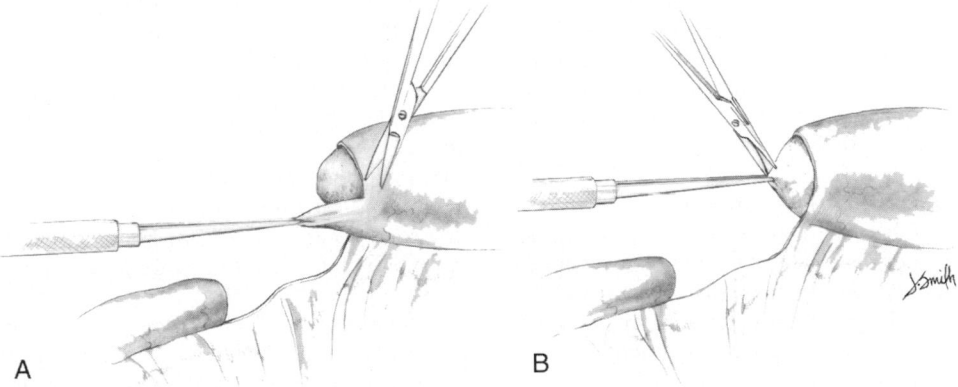

FIGURE 24.26. Preparation of the ampulla in intramural–ampullary or isthmic–ampullary anastomosis. **A:** The serosa over the tip of the ampullary stump is incised in a circular manner and excised. **B:** The center point of the exposed muscularis is grasped and a small opening is made into the lumen.

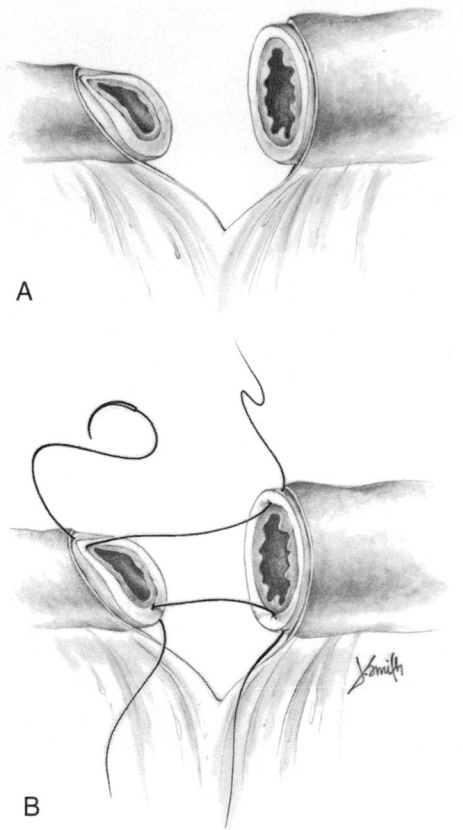

FIGURE 24.27. Isthmic–ampullary anastomosis in the presence of significant luminal disparity. **A:** Enlargement of the isthmic lumen. **B:** Placement of the 12-o'clock suture.

pingeal border. Partial excision of the corners thus created results in an enlarged oval opening (Fig. 24.27A). To approximate the inner musculoepithelial layer, the 6-o'clock suture is placed first and tied. Five additional sutures are usually required, and these are placed as described earlier. The 12-o'clock suture must incorporate the muscularis and epithelium of the ampulla and the same tissues at the apex of the isthmic slit (Fig. 24.27B). Approximation of the serosa and closure of the defect in the mesosalpinx complete the anastomosis. An alternative approach is to reduce the size of the large ampullary opening. This is achieved by plicating the muscular layer surrounding the opening with interrupted sutures, after which the prolapsing epithelium is invaginated.

Ampullary–Ampullary Anastomosis

The proximal ampullary segment is transected near the occluded end, which is then excised from the mesosalpinx as previously described. An opening that corresponds in size to the lumen of the proximal segment is made in the occluded end of the distal ampullary segment, as described under isthmic–ampullary anastomosis.

In this type of anastomosis, the major difficulty to be overcome is the propensity of the ampullary epithelium to prolapse through the lumen. Although investigators such as Winston have advocated excision of these epithelial fronds, we advise against this approach because there

could potentially be subsequent intratubal adhesion formation at this site. The epithelial fronds can be replaced with pressure from the irrigating solution or with the tip of the plain microforceps while the successive sutures of the inner layer are tied. One must be careful not to include these epithelial fronds within a suture or knot or between the segments that are being approximated. Because of the larger circumference of the ampulla, approximation of the two ampullary segments will require a greater number of interrupted sutures than in an isthmic–isthmic anastomosis.

Ampullary–Infundibular Anastomosis

An ampullary–infundibular anastomosis may be necessary when a distal ampullary portion of tube has been ablated or excised either during a prior sterilization or during removal of a tubal gestation, leaving distally the infundibular segment only. The occluded ampulla is prepared as described previously. To make anastomosis of the two segments possible, it is necessary to fashion an opening in the infundibular portion. To do so, a Teflon probe with a conical tip is introduced into the infundibulum from the fimbriated end, and a circular opening is fashioned with microscissors, from the medial side, corresponding in size to the lumen of the ampullary segment. A two-layer anastomosis is then performed.

Results of Tubotubal Anastomosis for Reversal of Sterilization

The major published series report live birth rates between 40% and 80% after microsurgical tubotubal anastomosis for reversal of sterilization (Table 24.3). The ectopic gestation rates are usually low but range from under 2% to 12.5%.

The factors that affect the outcome of such procedures are multiple and include the following: the type of prior sterilization, the site of anastomosis, and the length of the reconstructed tube or tubes, which are interrelated factors; the presence of single versus double reconstructed oviducts; the status of the tubes (presence or absence of disease); the extent and nature of adhesions and the presence of other pelvic disease; the age of the patient and the time interval between the sterilization and the tubal reconstruction, which may be interrelated factors; the status of other fertility parameters, especially that of the male partner; and, last but not least, the surgical technique used. Therefore, the outcome depends on the degree of rigor in selection criteria and the quality of the surgical technique. This is also corroborated by recent reports on sterilization reversal, which include two large series from Korea (Table 24.3).

The first report on laparoscopic tubotubal anastomosis was a case report; instead of microsurgical suturing for the apposition of the tubal segments, they used a biologic glue over a stent. Pregnancy outcome was not reported. Early reports on tubotubal anastomosis were on small series, performed with simplified techniques, and although most of the cases were simpler forms of sterilization reversal, the results were relatively poor.

TABLE 24.3.
Results of Microsurgical Tubotubal Anastomosis for Reversal of Sterilization

Investigators	Year	Patients	Intrauterine Pregnancies	Live Births	Ectopic Pregnancies
ACCESS BY LAPAROTOMY					
Gomel	1974	14	8	NS	1
Gomel	1980c	118	76	NS	1
Winston	1980	105	63	NS	3
Gomel[a]	1983b	118	96	93 (78.8%)	2
DeCherney et al.[b]	1983	124	84	72 (58.1%)	8
Schlosser et al.	1983	119	NS	44 (37%)	11
Silber and Cohen[c]	1984	48	33	31 (64.6%)	2
Henderson	1984	95	61	51 (53.7%)	5
Paterson	1985	147	93	87 (59.2%)	5
Spivak et al.[d]	1986	83	48	39 (47%)	6
Boeckx et al.	1986	63	44	NS	3
Rock et al.	1987	80	58	49 (61.3%)	10
Xue and Fa[e]	1989	117	98	95 (81.2%)	2
Putman et al.	1990	86	64	55 (64%)	
teVelde et al.	1990	215	156	137 (63.7%)	8
Kim JD et al.[f]	1997	387	329	295 (76.2%)[f]	6
Kim SH et al.[g]	1997	1118	505	366 (32.7%)[g]	42
Cha et al.	2001	44	31	NS	1
ACCESS BY LAPAROSCOPY					
Dubuisson et al.[h]	1998	32	17	13 (40.6%)	NS
Bisonette et al.[h]	1999	102	64	49 (50.5%)[i]	5
Yoon et al.[j]	1999	202	154	98 (48.5%)[k]	5
Mettler et al.[b,l]	2001	28	15	15 (53.6%)	2
Cha et al.[j,m]	2001	37	28	NS	1

NS, not stated.

[a] Resurvey of 1980 series; follow-up period more than 18 months.

[b] Follow-up period more than 18 months.

[c] Follow-up period more than 4 years.

[d] Follow-up period more than 1 year.

[e] Follow-up period more than 3.5 years.

[f] Follow-up period more than 2 years. There were eight ongoing pregnancies, in addition to the live births.

[g] Follow-up period more than 5 years. There were 31 ongoing pregnancies, in addition to the live births.

[h] Tubal anastomosis performed with "single-suture" technique.

[i] Tubal anastomosis performed by using two-layer microsurgical technique.

[k] There were 31 ongoing pregnancies, in addition to the live births.

[l] A screening laparoscopy was performed, and only those having a distal tubal segment of 4 cm and a proximal segment of 3 cm were included.

[m] Comparative study with 44 cases performed with open access.

Most surgeons, who attempted tubotubal anastomosis by laparoscopic access, using the microsurgical technique described earlier, found that operating times are prolonged. Many attempted to simplify the technique, by using glue as described above or using only two sutures for the apposition of the prepared tubal segments, as first reported by Dubuisson and Swolin. In this technique, the first suture (4/0 Vicryl) approximates the mesosalpinx immediately beneath the two segments of tube, and the second (6/0 Vicryl) the tube at 12-o'clock position. The second suture incorporates the serosa and muscularis of the two segments of tube. There are several recent reports in the literature on this technique. There are also publications reporting on the laparoscopic use of a truly microsurgical, two layer anastomosis technique. One of these is a large series by Yoon et al., from Korea, which includes 202 cases. Fifteen of these were lost to follow-up, and one had no partner. The remaining 186 were monitored for a minimum of 12 months. One hundred fifty-four achieved intrauterine pregnancies, a rate of 77% if we consider, as most series do, the 15 cases lost to follow-up as failures. Ninety-eight were delivered of healthy infants, 25 pregnancies ended in abortion, and 31 patients had ongoing pregnancies at the time of the survey. There were five cases of ectopic pregnancy. These results are not dissimilar to those achieved by open access, which supports the premise that what is important is the technique used and not the mode of access. Cha et al., also from Korea, further support this assumption in a recent study. In this study, they compare the fertility outcome in

81 women who had microsurgical reversal of sterilization, 37 by laparoscopic and 44 by open access. The outcomes, intrauterine and tubal pregnancy rates, were similar in both groups (Table 24.3).

Tubocornual Anastomosis for Proximal Tubal Disease

Various disease processes can affect the proximal tube and occlude the region of the uterotubal junction. On the basis of histologic studies on resected tubal segments, these occlusive lesions in order of frequency are as follows: obliterative fibrosis, chronic inflammation, salpingitis

isthmica nodosa, intratubal endometriosis, and, rarely, ectopic gestation and tuberculosis. All of the published series report a varying but usually low percentage of cases with no demonstrable lesions. This may be related to tubal spasm (at the time of HSG or laparoscopy) or to the presence of tubal plugs or synechiae. Such conditions, as opposed to occlusive disease, are amenable to treatment with selective salpingography or tubal cannulation, which were discussed earlier in this chapter.

The management strategy in proximal tubal occlusion must take into account other variables, including the condition of the distal tube, the extent and nature of pelvic adhesions, the presence of associated pelvic dis-

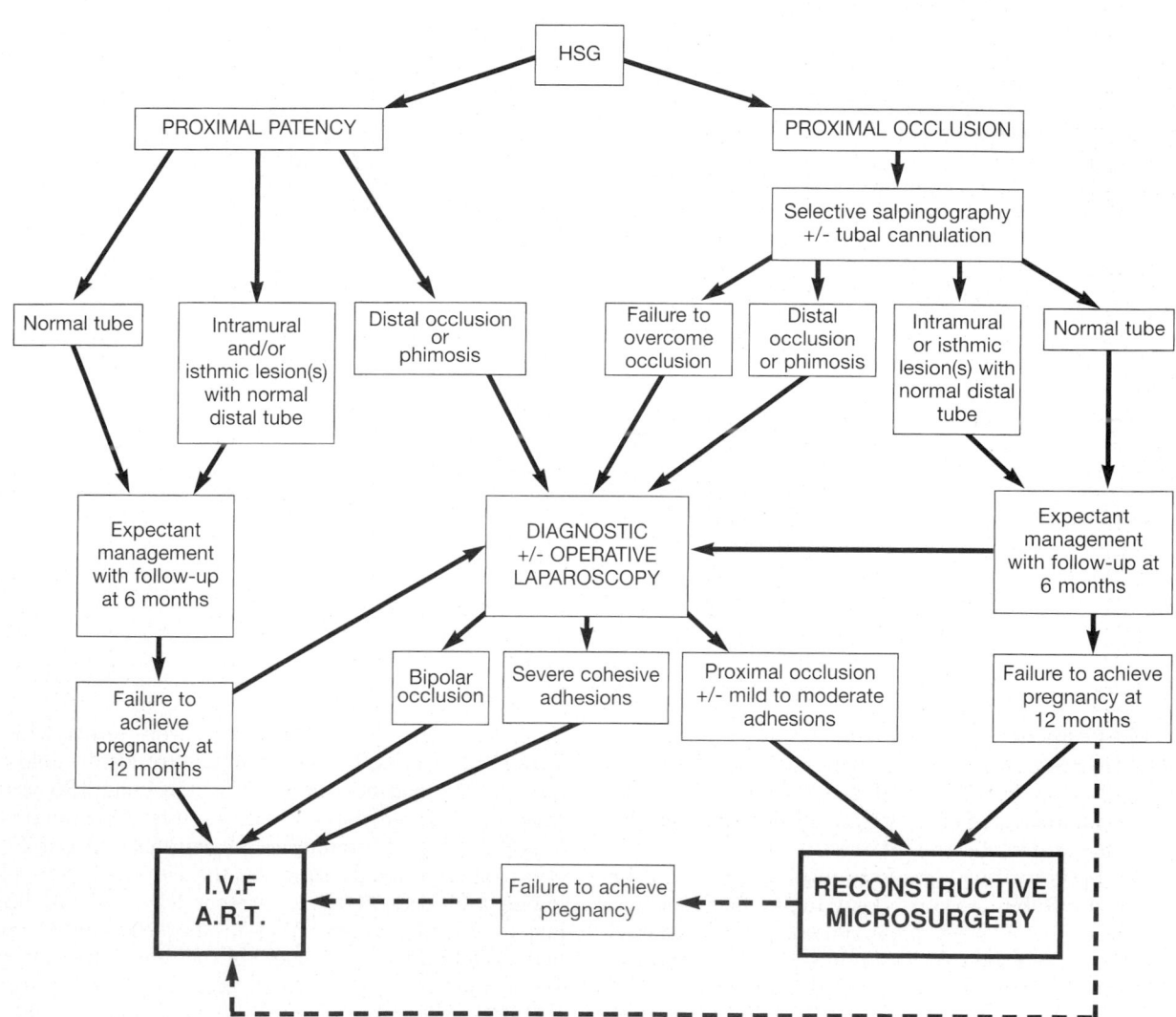

FIGURE 24.28. Management of proximal tubal occlusion. HSG, hysterosalpingogram; IVF, *in vitro* fertilization; ART, artificial reproductive technology. (Modified from: Gomel V, Dubuisson JB. *References en Gynecologie et Obstetrique*. September 1995:251, with permission.)

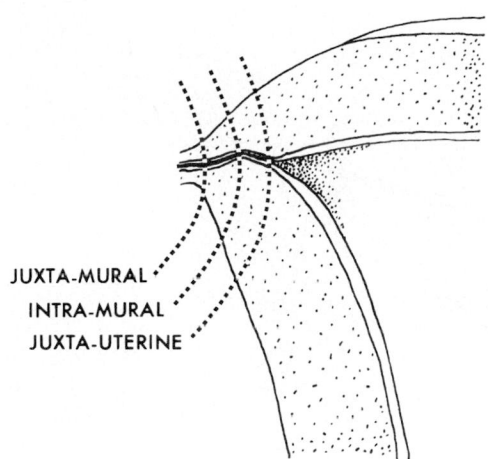

FIGURE 24.29. Types of tubocornual anastomosis.

ease, and the status of other fertility parameters, especially male factor infertility. This strategy must also respect the following principles: simplicity, reproducibility, and cost-effectiveness.

The selection of treatment must be individualized according to the investigative findings, the wishes of the couple, the expertise of the surgeon, and the results achieved by the center in which the couple will be managed. Fig. 24.28 diagrammatically summarizes the management of proximal tubal occlusion.

The traditional surgical treatment of occlusive proximal tubal disease was uterotubal implantation. The application of microsurgery has made it possible to perform an anastomosis instead, after removal of the affected tubal segment.

Central to this approach is the complete excision of the affected portion of tube, whether it is intramural or isthmic. In cases of pathologic occlusion, a portion of healthy intramural tube is usually spared, permitting the conservation of sometimes all but more often a part of this segment. In other instances, the whole intramural segment is involved in the disease process and must be excised. In such cases, microsurgery permits an anastomosis to be performed between the uterine tubal ostium and the healthy portion of isthmus. Depending on the extent of intramural tube that is excised and thus the site at which the anastomosis is performed, tubocornual anastomosis may be juxtamural, intramural, or juxtauterine (Fig. 24.29).

The cornual region of the uterus is infiltrated with dilute vasopressin solution. This is done by injecting 2 mL of this solution, in a circular fashion, under the serosa 1 cm medial to the uterotubal junction with use of a 30-gauge needle on a 3-mL syringe. Vasoconstriction is recognized by serosal blanching. The tube is then incised at the uterotubal junction, with care taken not to divide the arteriovenous arcade at its mesosalpingeal margin (Fig. 24.30). After transection of the tube, patency of the intramural segment is assessed by transcervical chromopertubation, and the normalcy of the cut surface is evaluated under high magnification.

If the intramural tube is found to be occluded or abnormal at this site, its musculature is dissected further from the surrounding uterine muscle, 1 to 2 mm at a time, toward the uterine cavity (Fig. 24.30A). The small portion of tube thus dissected is transected, and the cut surface is reassessed. If the intramural tube is still occluded or abnormal, the same procedure is repeated until normal patent tube is reached. Dye solution will spurt from the open lumen. It is essential that dissection of the intramural tube from the surrounding uterine muscle be effected at the level of the immediate periphery of the tubal muscularis (Fig. 24.30B). The preoperative HSG usually provides information about the length of the normal intramural segment and the extent of excision required. Transection of successive portions of the intramural tube can be achieved with either curved microscissors or especially designed cornual blade (Gomel cornual blade, Spingler-Tritt, Jestetten, Germany). By limiting the excised tissue to the intramural tube, there is little risk of creating a large defect at the cornu.

After the preparation of the cornual end, the occluded or abnormal isthmic segment is prepared by making serial cuts 1 to 2 mm apart, beginning at the initial transection site at the uterotubal junction and continuing until normal patent tube is identified (Fig. 24.30C,D). Patency of the distal segment is confirmed by descending hydropertubation, with injection of a few milliliters of dye or irrigation solution through the fimbriated end. Hemostasis of the cut end of the normal distal tube is obtained by precise electrocoagulation of bleeders located between the muscularis and serosa. The intervening abnormal tubal segments are excised from the mesosalpinx electrosurgically, avoiding the vascular arcade beneath the tube.

The intramural and isthmic segments are approximated in two layers as follows. The initial suture of the first layer, which incorporates the muscularis and epithelium of the two segments, is placed at the 6-o'clock position (Fig. 24.30E). If the anastomosis is superficial (juxtamural type), the suture is tied.

With anastomoses located deep in the cornua, as in intramural or juxtauterine types, the 6-o'clock suture is held with a clip until the remaining sutures have been placed, because tying this initial suture would make placement of the subsequent sutures difficult if not impossible. In such cases, the subsequent sutures are placed with use of a continuous strand of suture, as described earlier (Fig. 24.30). This approach facilitates suture placement and prevents the individual sutures from becoming tangled. Three additional sutures, placed at cardinal points, are usually sufficient to join the inner layer. If the cornual crater is deep and the placement of sutures is difficult, this task can be facilitated by making a coronal incision on the uterus, above the cornual crater. The edges of this incision must be approximated at the end of the procedure.

If the distance between the two segments of tube is significant or if there is undue tension, it is necessary to hold the distal tubal segment close to the intramural segment while tying the sutures. Alternatively, a single

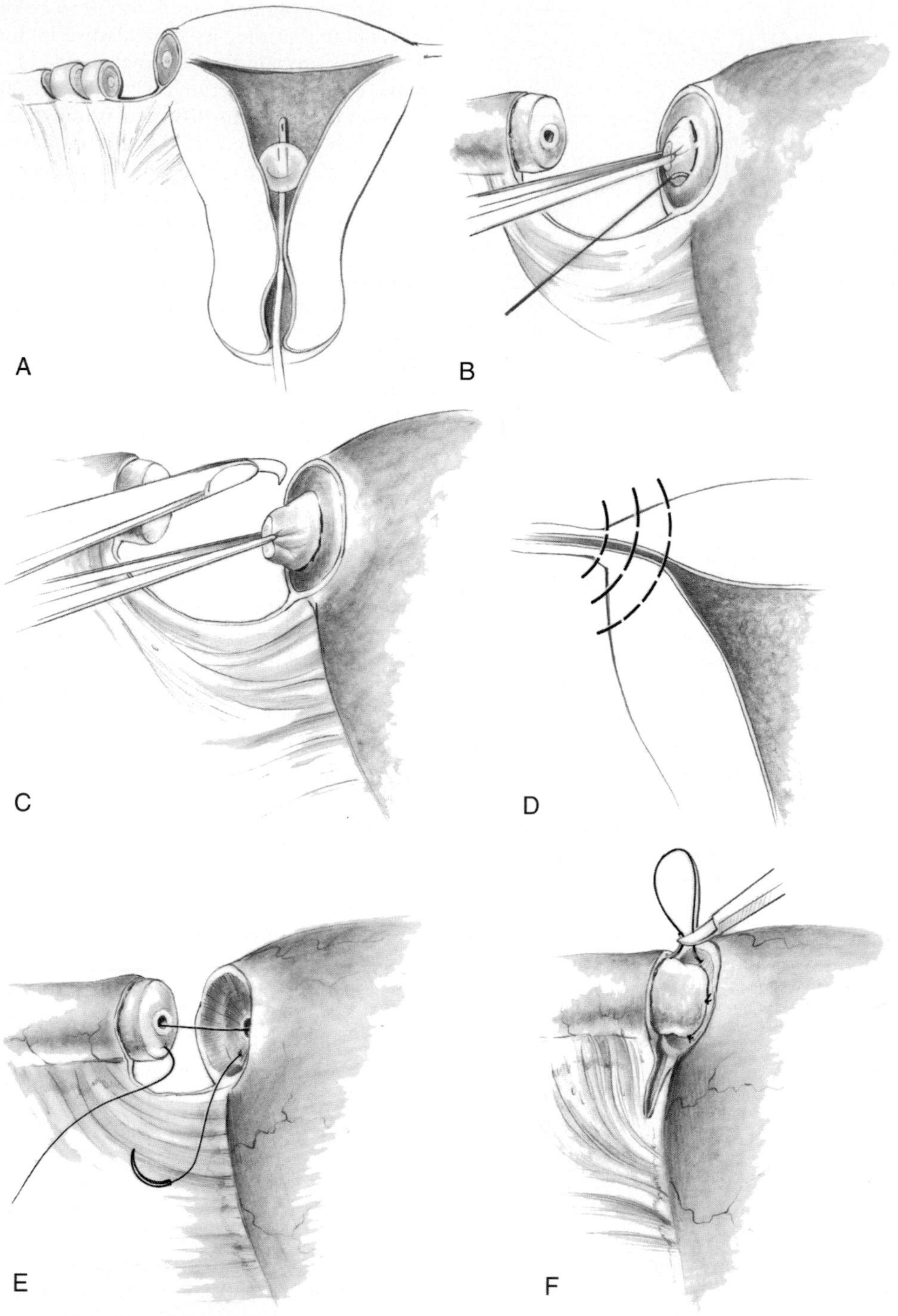

A

B

C

D

E

F

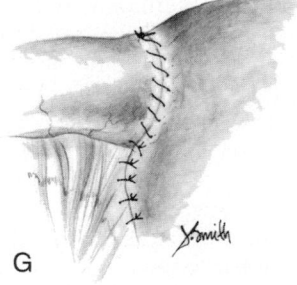
G

FIGURE 24.30. Microsurgical tubocornual anastomosis for proximal tubal disease. **A:** The tube is transected at the uterotubal function (UTF). Commencing at the UTF, serial cuts are made on the isthmus until patent and normal tube is identified. **B:** The intramural tube is dissected electrosurgically, by using a microelectrode, from the surrounding uterine muscle, 1 to 2 mm at a time, and (**C** and **D**) transected until patent and normal tube is reached. **E:** The first anastomotic suture of the inner musculoepithelial layer is placed at the 6-o'clock position. **F:** After the opposition of the inner layer, the seromuscularis of the uterus is joined to the serosa of the tube. **G:** The mesosalpinx is joined to the lateral aspect of the uterus.

no. 7-0 Vicryl suture is passed through the mesosalpinx below the cut end of the distal segment of tube and then through the border of the uterus immediately beneath the cornual crater. The suture is tied to bring the two segments into close proximity. The 6-o'clock suture is tied first. Then the loop between each succeeding suture is divided and tied in turn. After approximation of the first layer, the seromuscularis of the uterus is joined to the serosa of the tube with no. 8-0 sutures. The defect under the tube is closed by approximating the mesosalpinx to the lateral edge of the uterus (see Fig. 24.30F,G).

Compared with tubouterine implantation, microsurgical tubocornual anastomosis offers several advantages: It largely maintains the integrity of the uterine cornua; preserves a longer tube; obviates the need for a Caesarean section, except for obstetric reasons; and yields better results.

Results of Tubocornual Anastomosis

Microsurgical tubocornual anastomosis for the treatment of occlusive cornual disease yields fairly good results in centers experienced with this procedure. The published series report live birth rates between 33% and 56% and ectopic pregnancy rates between 5% and 7% (Table 24.4). This table makes it clearly evident that there has been a paucity of reports regarding this procedure for more than a decade.

Rare Procedures and Technically Difficult Cases

Rare circumstances may be encountered that are amenable to microsurgical correction. Some of these circumstances are discussed in this section.

The technical difficulty of a procedure must be differentiated from the prognosis that the procedure offers. Furthermore, difficulty is a relative term because what is commonplace work for some may be difficult or even impossible to achieve for others. From the patient's standpoint, what is important is the prognosis, the yield associated with the surgical procedure. Furthermore, the prognosis is not necessarily inversely proportional to the difficulty of the procedure. For example, microsurgical tubocornual anastomosis to treat occlusive cornual lesions is one of the technically more difficult reconstructive tubal operations. However, centers experienced in this procedure achieve excellent results. An even more technically difficult operation is tuboovarian transposition.

Tuboovarian Transposition

In the case of a unicornuate uterus without an ipsilateral tube and ovary, the contralateral tube and ovary, if present, may be transposed while preserving their vascular pedicle. We performed such a procedure in a woman with a single left unicornuate uterus whose ipsilateral tube and ovary were removed subsequent to a left tubal pregnancy. On the right side, placed high on the pelvic sidewall, were an ovary and a short oviduct, composed of infundibulum and ampulla (Fig. 24.31A).

The uterus was mobilized centrally as follows. The left round ligament was divided near its inguinal insertion and dissected from the broad ligament with its vascular supply intact (Fig. 24.31A). The divided end of the round ligament was then affixed to the right inguinal region (Fig. 24.31B). Microsurgical transposition of the right ovary and tube with preservation of their vascular supply permitted anastomosis between the left intramural and right ampullary tubal segments (Fig. 24.31C). The ovary was mobilized further to achieve the proper spatial relation with the fimbrial extremity of the tube (Fig. 24.31D). In the third postoperative cycle, the patient was successful in achieving an intrauterine pregnancy, which resulted in a normal live birth. She has since had two more children. Since the publication of this report in May 1985, there have been at least five case reports of successful transposition of the fallopian tube without the ovary. These reports clearly illustrate the potential of surgery, even though technically difficult, in restoring fertility in the face of unusual pelvic anatomy.

Correction of Bipolar Tubal Disease

The results associated with surgical correction of bipolar (both proximal and distal) tubal occlusion are dismal. A

TABLE 24.4.
Results of Microsurgical Tubocornual Anastomosis for Occlusive Proximal Tubal Disease

Investigators	Year	Patients	Intrauterine Pregnancies	Live Births	Ectopic Pregnancies
Gomel	1977c	13	NS	7 (53.8%)	1
Gomel	1980b	38	21	20 (52.6%)	2
Winston	1980	49	NS	16 (32.7%)	2
McComb	1986	26	15	14 (53.8%)	2
Donnez and Casanas-Roux	1986	82	NS	36 (43.9%)	6
Gillett and Herbison	1989	32	19	18 (56.3%)	2
Tomazevic et al.*	1996	59	NS	27 (45.8%)	NS

* Of the 32 operated patients who did not deliver within 2 years after surgery, 21 were treated with 66 cycles of *in vitro* fertilization; resulting in live births for 12.

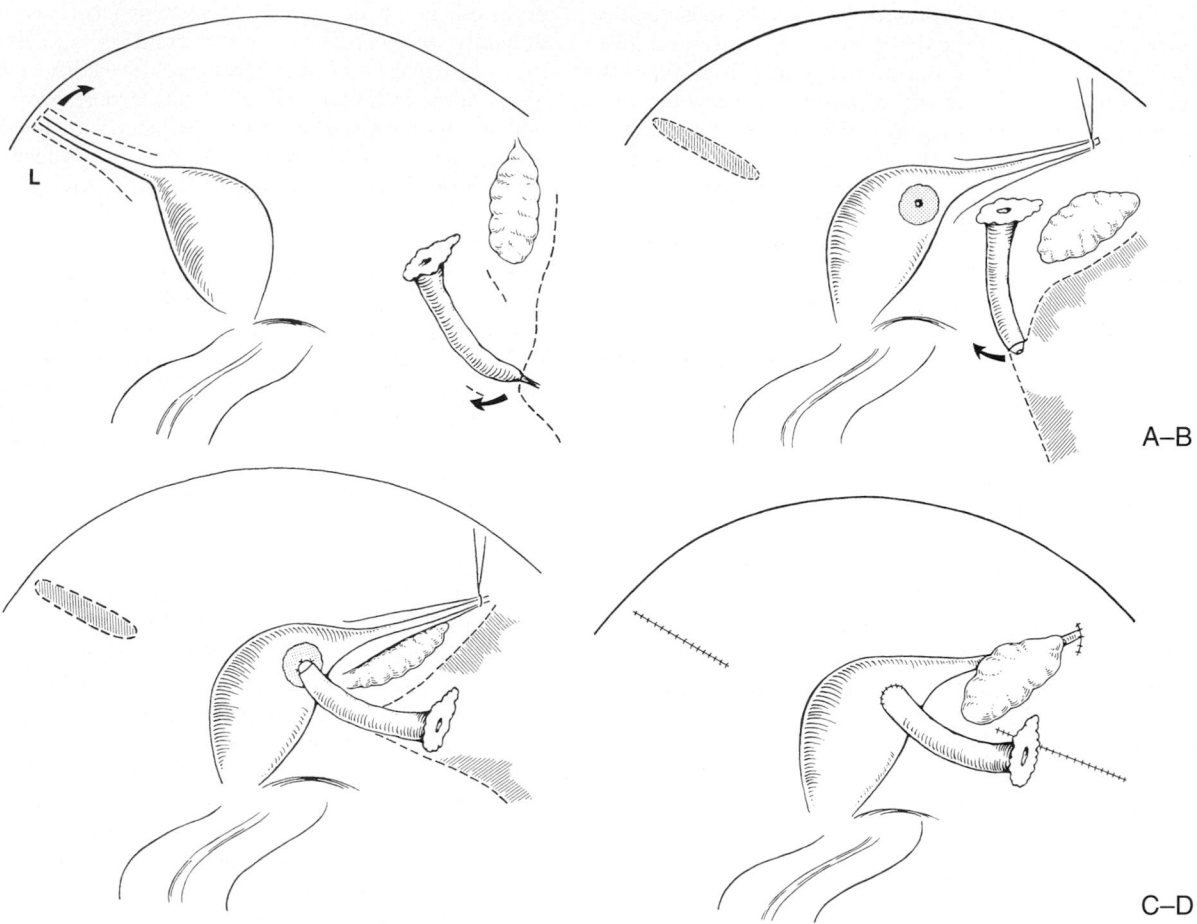

A–B

C–D

FIGURE 24.31. Microsurgical tuboovarian transposition. (From: Gomel V, McComb P. Microsurgical transposition of the human fallopian tube and ovary with subsequent pregnancy. *Fertil Steril* 1985;43:804, with permission.)

report from the Mayo Clinic included 31 such patients: bipolar tubal occlusion of both tubes ($n = 13$), or their only remaining tube ($n = 5$); bilateral distal and unilateral proximal occlusion ($n = 7$); and bilateral proximal and unilateral distal occlusion ($n = 6$). Despite a mean follow-up period of more than 3 years, pregnancies occurred in only three patients. Furthermore, two of these were ectopic, and one was a spontaneous abortion.

Anastomosis of Contralateral Tubal Segments

A patient may have a healthy proximal segment of tube on one side, whereas on the opposite side, an ampullary–infundibular segment exists. In such a circumstance, microsurgical reconstruction of one functional tube can be achieved by anastomosis of the contralateral tubal segments behind the uterus, maintaining the physiologic relation between the infundibulum and ovary. In the presence of both ovaries, the uteroovarian ligaments are first approximated with interrupted, nonabsorbable no. 4-0 or 5-0 nylon sutures. This brings the ovaries together and helps reduce tension in achieving the subsequent tubal anastomosis (Fig. 24.32). Successful delivery after such a procedure has been reported.

Approximation of the Fimbriated End of the Oviduct to the Contralateral Ovary

When a single ovary exists on the side opposite the patient's only tube, simple approximation of the fimbriated extremity of the tube to the ovary may be possible. The ovary is mobilized, and the mesovarium is fixed to the posterior surface of the uterus with nonabsorbable sutures. The contralateral oviduct is mobilized, and its mesosalpinx is sutured to the posterior aspect of the uterus. The nonabsorbable sutures are placed on the mesosalpinx about 1 cm from the tube. This will effectively place the infundibulum in close proximity to the ovary. Alternatively, the ovary can be transposed to the contralateral side with its vascular pedicle kept intact.

Iterative Reconstructive Surgery

Except in rare circumstances, there are no data to support the undertaking of an iterative surgical procedure when a prior reconstructive operation has failed.

Rare exceptions include cases of tubotubal anastomosis that failed for purely technical reasons, in which sufficient lengths of healthy tube is available for recon-

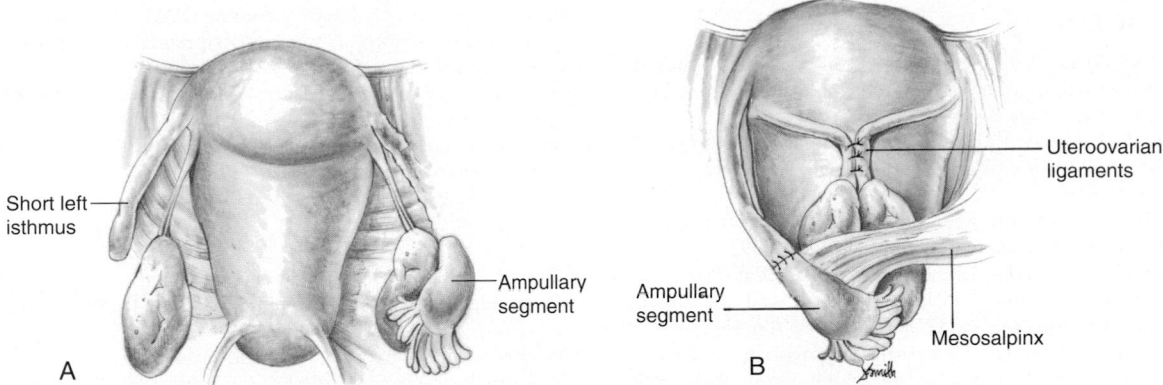

FIGURE 24.32. Microsurgical anastomosis of contralateral tubal segments. **A:** Isthmic segment of tube on left and ampullary–infundibular segment on right. **B:** The uteroovarian ligaments are approximated with nonabsorbable sutures behind the uterus; the left isthmic segment of tube is anastomosed to the right ampullary–infundibular segment.

struction. In such instances, an iterative microsurgical anastomosis may be undertaken if tubal cannulation fails to restore patency.

Tubal cannulation, performed at the time of the postoperative control HSG that demonstrates an obstruction at the anastomosis site, may prove beneficial in a small percentage of cases by breaking down synechiae or dislodging debris that may be present at this site.

Iterative surgery yields a modest success rate if the initial procedure was performed with the use of conventional techniques. However, the success rate of iterative procedures is disappointing when they are undertaken after a failed microsurgical intervention.

Most of the available data on iterative surgery concern salpingostomy. Of the 119 such cases reported in the literature, 18 (15.1%) achieved live births, six had spontaneous abortions, and seven (5.9%) had ectopic gestations. All of these 119 patients had their first procedure performed by conventional techniques and their second intervention performed by microsurgery.

My first report on laparoscopic salpingostomy included, except for one case, iterative procedures on patients who had previously undergone surgery with conventional techniques. This fact may explain the satisfactory rate of success that was obtained.

The conception rate after iterative microsurgical fertility-promoting procedures is significantly lower than that obtained with primary microsurgical interventions. Thie et al. reported a conception rate of 51% after various primary microsurgical procedures in 161 patients. This rate was only 18% at 3 years' follow-up in a similar group of 21 patients who had microsurgery after a failed primary operation performed by conventional techniques.

The preceding data strongly suggest that iterative surgery may be indicated in selected, rare instances and that most of these patients may be better served with IVF.

Observations on Current Practice

The enormous progress in IVF and ART, in the past 15 years, has been accompanied with the industrialization of this technology and its services, all over the world. In parallel fashion, there has been a significant decline in the practice and teaching of reconstructive surgery. There is a paucity of publications on this subject. IVF is offered now, as primary treatment option, in most cases of tubal factor infertility. These changes have occurred despite the greater acceptance of laparoscopic access to perform many of the reconstructive tubal operations and the use of minilaparotomy incision for more complex anastomotic procedures, which represent a major progress in gynecologic surgery. These changes have occurred despite the satisfactory results yielded by reconstructive surgery in appropriately selected cases, and despite the fact that surgery offers the couple the opportunity to attempt a pregnancy over a long period of time and to conceive more than once.

The evidence suggests that surgery should retain its place in the treatment of tubal infertility. Preservation of the place of surgery will require a concerted effort on the part of the teaching institutions. Surgery and ART are complementary approaches that can be used singly or in combination to improve the outlook of couples suffering from tubal infertility. In the preface of my book *Microsurgery in Female Infertility*, published in early 1983, I wrote

This manuscript has been completed during a time of rapid change and expansion with the understanding that it represents not an end point but merely an accounting at a given point in time. Further developments are also occurring in the area of IVF and embryo transfer (IVF & ET), which will undoubtedly produce improved results. Nonetheless, I do not consider the techniques of microsurgery on the one hand and IVF & ET on the other as competitive; on the contrary, I see them as complementary, enabling us to achieve a greater success rate among those patients presenting with complex fertility problems.

This statement is still valid today.

BIBLIOGRAPHY

Alper MM, Garner PR, Spence JEH, et al. Pregnancy rates after hysterosalpingography with oil- and water-soluble contrast media. *Obstet Gynecol* 1986;68:6.

Bisonette F, Lapensee L, Bouzayen R. Outpatient laparoscopic tubal anastomosis and subsequent fertility. *Fertil Steril* 1999;72:549.

Boeckx W, Gordts S, Buysse K, et al. Reversibility after female sterilization. *Br J Obstet Gynaecol* 1986;93:839.

Boer-Meisel ME, teVelde ER, Habbema JDF, et al. Predicting the pregnancy outcome in patients treated for hydrosalpinx: a prospective study. *Fertil Steril* 1986;45:23.

Bowman MC, Cooke ID. Comparison of fallopian tube intraluminal pathology as assessed by salpingoscopy with pelvic adhesions. *Fertil Steril* 1994;61:464.

Brosens IA, Puttemans PJ. Double-optic laparoscopy. Salpingoscopy, ovarian cystoscopy and endo-ovarian surgery with the argon laser. *Baillieres Clin Obstet Gyanecol* 1989;3:595.

Bruhat MA, Mage G, Manhes H, et al. Laparoscopy procedures to promote fertility ovariolysis and salpingolysis: results of 93 selected cases. *Acta Eur Fertil* 1983;14:113.

Brundin A, Dahlborn M, Ahlberg-Ahre E, et al. Radionuclide hysterosalpingography for measurement of human oviduct function. *Int J Gynecol Obstet* 1989;28:53.

Canis M, Mage G, Pouly JL, et al. Laparoscopic distal tuboplasty: report of 87 cases and a 4-year experience. *Fertil Steril* 1991;56:616.

Caspi E, Halperin V, Bukovsky I. The importance of periadnexal adhesions in tubal reconstructive surgery for infertility. *Fertil Steril* 1979;31:296.

Cha SH, Lee MH, Kim JH et al. Fertility outcome after tubal anastomosis by laparoscopy and laparotomy. *J Am Assoc Gynecol Laparoscp* 2001;8:348.

Cohen J. The efficiency and efficacy of IVF and GIFT. *Hum Reprod* 1991;6:613.

Collins JA, Rowe TC. Age of the female partner is a prognostic factor in prolonged unexplained infertility: a multicenter study. *Fertil Steril* 1989;52:15.

Dan U, Oelsner G, Gruberg L, et al. Cerebral embolization and coma after hysterosalpingography with oil-soluble contrast medium. *Fertil Steril* 1990;53:939.

Daniell JF, Herbert CM. Laparoscopic salpingostomy using the CO_2 laser. *Fertil Steril* 1984;41:558.

DeCherney AH, Mezer HC, Naftolin F. Analysis of failure of microsurgical anastomosis after mid-segment, non-coagulation tubal ligation. *Fertil Steril* 1983;39:618.

Dicker D, Ashkenazi J, Feldberg D, et al. Severe abdominal complications after transvaginal ultrasonographically guided retrieval of oocytes for *in vitro* fertilization and embryo transfer. *Fertil Steril* 1993;59:1313.

Donnez J, Casanas-Roux F. Prognostic factors of fimbrial microsurgery. *Fertil Steril* 1986a;46:200.

Donnez J, Casanas-Roux F. Prognostic factors influencing the pregnancy rate after microsurgical cornual anastomosis. *Fertil Steril* 1986;46:1089.

Donnez J, Nisolle M, Casanas-Roux F. CO_2 laser laparoscopy in infertile women with adnexal adhesions and women with tubal occlusion. *J Gynecol Surg* 1989;5:47.

Dubuisson JB, Bouquet de Joliniere J, Aubriot FX, et al. Terminal tuboplasties by laparoscopy: 65 consecutive cases. *Fertil Steril* 1990;54:401.

Dubuisson JB, Chapron C, Morice P, et al. Laparoscopic salpingostomy: fertility results according to the tubal mucosal appearance. *Hum Reprod* 1994;9:334.

Dubuisson JB, Chapron C. Single suture laparoscopic tubal reanastomosis. *Curr Opin Obstet Gynecol* 1998;10:307

Erenus M, Zouves C, Rajamahendran DVM, et al. The effect of embryo quality on subsequent pregnancy rates after *in vitro* fertilization. *Fertil Steril* 1991;56:707.

Fayez JA. An assessment of the role of operative laparoscopy in tuboplasty. *Fertil Steril* 1983;39:476.

Filmar S, Gomel V, McComb P. The effectiveness of CO_2 laser and electromicrosurgery in adhesiolysis: a comparative study. *Fertil Steril* 1986;45:407.

FIVNAT 1989 et bilan general 1986–1989. *Contracept Fertil Sex* 1990;18:588.

Gillett WR, Herbison GP. Tubocornal anastomosis: surgical considerations and coexistent infertility factors in determining the prognosis. *Fertil Steril* 1989;51:241.

Glazener CMA, Loveden LM, Richardson SJ, et al. Tubocornual polyps: their relevance in subfertility. *Hum Reprod* 1987;2:59.

Gomel V. Laparoscopic tubal surgery in infertility. *Obstet Gynecol* 1975;46:47.

Gomel V. Reconstructive surgery of the oviduct. *J Reprod Med* 1977;18:181.

Gomel V. Salpingostomy by laparoscopy. *J Reprod Med* 1977b;18:265.

Gomel V. Tubal anastomosis by microsurgery. *Fertil Steril* 1977c;28:59.

Gomel V. Profile of women requesting reversal of sterilization. *Fertil Steril* 1978;30:39.

Gomel V. Salpingostomy by microsurgery. *Fertil Steril* 1978b;29:380.

Gomel V. Causes of failure of reconstructive infertility microsurgery. *Clin Obstet Gynecol* 1980b;23:1269.

Gomel V. Clinical results of infertility microsurgery. In: Crosignani PG, Rubin BL, eds. *Microsurgery in female infertility*. London: Academic Press, 1980b:77.

Gomel V. Microsurgical reversal of sterilization: a reappraisal. *Fertil Steril* 1980c;33:587.

Gomel V. *Microsurgery in female infertility*. Boston: Little, Brown, 1983b.

Gomel V. An odyssey through the oviduct. *Fertil Steril* 1983a;39:144.

Gomel V. Salpingo-ovariolysis by laparoscopy in infertility. *Fertil Steril* 1983c;34:607.

Gomel V. Distal tubal occlusion. *Fertil Steril* 1988;49:946.

Gomel V. Operative laparoscopy: time for acceptance. *Fertil Steril* 1989;52:1.

Gomel V. From microsurgery to laparoscopic surgery: a progress. *Fertil Steril* 1995;63:464.

Gomel V, Erenus M. *The American Fertility Society, 46th Annual Meeting. Program Supplement* 1990:P-097, S-106(abst).

Gomel V, Filmar S. Arrested tubal pregnancy. *Fertil Steril* 1987;48:1043.

Gomel V, McComb P. Microsurgical transposition of the human fallopian tube and ovary with subsequent intrauterine pregnancy. *Fertil Steril* 1985;43:804.

Gomel V, McComb P. Unexpected pregnancies in women afflicted by occlusive tubal disease. *Fertil Steril* 1981;36:529.

Gomel V, Rowe TC. Microsurgical tubal reconstruction and reversal of sterilization. In: Wallach EE, Zacur HA, eds. *Reproductive medicine and surgery*. St Louis: Mosby, 1995:1074.

Gomel V, Swolin K. Salpingostomy: microsurgical technique and results. *Clin Obstet Gynecol* 1980;23:1243.

Gomel V, Taylor PJ. *In vitro* fertilization versus reconstructive tubal surgery. *J Assist Reprod Genet* 1992;9:306.

Gomel V, Taylor PJ. Reconstructive tubal surgery in the female. In: Insler V, Lunenfeld B, eds. *Infertility, male and female*. Edinburgh: Churchill Livingstone, 1993:481.

Gomel V, Taylor PJ. *Diagnostic and operative gynecologic laparoscopy.* St Louis: Mosby, 1995.

Gordts S, Boeckx W, Vasquez G, et al. Microsurgical resection of intramural tubal polyps. *Fertil Steril* 1983;40:258.

Gurgan T, Urman B, Yarali H, et al. Salpingoscopic findings in women with occlusive and nonocclusive salpingitis isthmica nodosa. *Fertil Steril* 1994;61:461.

Henderson SR. The reversibility of female sterilization with the use of microsurgery: a report on 102 patients with more than one year of follow-up. *Am J Obstet Gynecol* 1984;149:57.

Henry-Suchet J, Loffredo V, Tesquier L, Pez JP. Endoscopy of the tube (= tuboscopy): its prognostic value for tuboplasties. *Acta Eur Fertil* 1985;16:139.

Hulka JF. Adnexal adhesions: a prognostic staging and classification system based on a five-year survey of fertility surgery results at Chapel Hill, North Carolina. *Am J Obstet Gynecol* 1982;144:141.

Hull MGR, Glazener CMA, Kelly NJ, et al. Population study of causes, treatment, and outcome of infertility. *Br Med J* 1985;291:1693.

Jones HW Jr, Rock JA. On the reanastomosis of fallopian tubes after surgical sterilization. *Fertil Steril* 1978;29:702.

Kerin JF. Nonhysteroscopic falloposcopy: a proposed method for visual guidance and verification of tubal cannula placement for endotuboplasty, gamete and embryo transfer procedures. *Fertil Steril* 1992;57:1133.

Kerin JF, Williams DB, San Roman GA, et al. Falloposcopic classification and treatment of fallopian tube lumen disease. *Fertil Steril* 1992;57:731.

Kim JD, Kim KS, Doo JK, et al. A report on 387 cases of microsurgical tubal reversals. *Fertil Steril* 1997;68:875.

Kim SH, Shin CJ, Kim JG, et al. Microsurgical reversal of tubal sterilization: a report on 1118 cases. *Fertil Steril* 1997;68:865

Kosasa TS, Hale RW. Treatment of hydrosalpinx using a single incision eversion procedure. *Int J Fertil* 1988;33:319.

Lang EK, Dunaway HH. Recanalization of obstructed fallopian tube by selective salpingography and transvaginal bougie dilatation: outcome and cost analysis. *Fertil Steril* 1996;66:210.

Larsson B. Late results of salpingostomy combined with salpingolysis and ovariolysis by electromicrosurgery in 54 women. *Fertil Steril* 1982;37:156.

Lauritsen JG, Pagel JD, Vangsted P, et al. Results of repeated tuboplasties. *Fertil Steril* 1982;37:68.

Letterie GS, Luetkehans T. Reproductive outcome after fallopian tube canalization and microsurgery for bipolar tubal occlusion. *J Gynecol Surg* 1992;8:11.

Luber K, Beeson CC, Kennedy JF, et al. Results of microsurgical treatment of tubal infertility and early second-look laparoscopy in the post-pelvic inflammatory disease patient: implications for *in vitro* fertilization. *Am J Obstet Gynecol* 1986;154:1264.

Madlenat P, DeBrux J, Palmer R. L'etiologie des obstructions tubaires proximales et son róle dans le prognostic des implantations. *Gynecologie* 1977;28:47.

Mahadevan MM, Wiseman D, Leader A, et al. The effects of ovarian adhesive disease upon follicular development in cycles of controlled stimulation for *in vitro* fertilization. *Fertil Steril* 1985;44:489.

Marana R, Muscatello P, Muzii L, et al. Perlaparoscopic salpingoscopy in the evaluation of the tubal factor in infertile women. *Int J Fertil* 1990;35:211.

McComb P. Microsurgical tubocornual anastomosis for occlusive cornual disease: reproducible results without the need for tubouterine implantation. *Fertil Steril* 1986;46:571.

McComb P, Gomel V. Cornual occlusion and its microsurgical reconstruction. *Clin Obstet Gynecol* 1980;23:1229.

McComb PF, Lee NH, Stephenson MD. Reproductive outcome after microsurgery for proximal and distal occlusions in the same fallopian tube. *Fertil Steril* 1991;56:134.

McComb P, Paleologou A. The intussusception salpingostomy technique for the therapy of distal oviductal occlusion at laparoscopy. *Obstet Gynecol* 1991;78:443.

Medical Research International, Society for Assisted Reproductive Technology, The American Fertility Society. *In vitro* fertilization-embryo transfer (IVF-ET) in the United States: 1989 results from the IVF-ET Registry. *Fertil Steril* 1991;55:14.

Mettler L, Giesel H, Semm K. Treatment of female infertility due to tubal obstruction by operative laparoscopy. *Fertil Steril* 1979;32:384

Mettler L, Ibrahim M, Lehmann-Willenbrock E, et al. Pelviscopic reversal of tubal sterilization with the one- to two-stitch technique. *J Am Assoc Gynecol Laparosc* 2001;8:353.

Millingos SD, Kallipolitis GK, Loutradis DC, et al. Laparoscopic treatment of hydrosalpinx: factors affecting pregnancy rate. *J Am Assoc Gynecol Laparosc* 2000;7:355.

Molloy D, Martin M, Speirs A, et al. Performance of patients with a "frozen pelvis" in an *in vitro* fertilization program. *Fertil Steril* 1987;47:450.

Munro MG, Gomel V. Fertility-promoting laparoscopically-directed procedures. *Reprod Med Rev* 1994;3:29.

Musset R. *An atlas of hysterosalpingography.* Quebec: Les Presses de l'Universite Laval, 1979.

Navot D, Bergh PA, Williams MA, et al. Poor oocyte quality rather than implantation failure as a cause of age-related decline in female fertility. *Lancet* 1991;337:1375.

Novy MJ, Thurmond AS, Patton P, et al. Diagnosis of cornual obstruction by transcervical fallopian tube cannulation. *Fertil Steril* 1988;50:434.

Oh ST. Tubal patency and conception rates with three methods of laparoscopic terminal salpingostomy. *J Am Assoc Gynecol Laparosc* 1996;3:519.

Pabuccu R, Ulgenalp I, Baser I, et al. Microsurgical transposition of the human fallopian tube. *Gynecol Obstet Invest* 1991;31:51.

Patton PE, Williams TJ, Coulam CB. Results of microsurgical reconstruction in patients with combined proximal and distal tubal occlusion: double obstruction. *Fertil Steril* 1987;48:670.

Pauerstein CJ, Turner T, Eddy CA. A technique for evaluating functional patency of the oviduct. *Fertil Steril* 1977;28:777.

Putman JM, Holden AEC, Olive DL. Pregnancy rates following tubal anastomosis: Pomeroy partial salpingectomy versus electrocautery. *J Gynecol Surg* 1990;6:173.

Reich H, McGlynn F, Parents C, et al. Laparoscopic tubal anastomosis. *J Am Assoc Gynecol Laparosc* 1993;1:16.

Rock JA, Guzick DS, Katz E, et al. Tubal anastomosis: pregnancy success following the reversal of Falope ring or monopolar cautery sterilization. *Fertil Steril* 1987;48:13.

Rock JA, Katayama KP, Martin EJ, et al. Factors influencing the success of salpingostomy techniques for distal fimbrial obstruction. *Obstet Gynecol* 1978;52:591.

Rowe TC, Gomel V, McComb P. Investigations of tuboperitoneal causes of female infertility. In: Insler V, Lunenfeld B, eds. *Infertility, male and female.* Edinburgh: Churchill Livingstone, 1993:253.

Rubin IC. Non-operative determination of patency of fallopian tubes in sterility: intrauterine inflation with oxygen and production of a subphrenic pneumoperitoneum. *JAMA* 1920;74:1017.

Rubin IC. Roentgendiagnostik der uterus tumorens mit hilfe von intrauterine collargol injectionen vorlaeufige mitteilung. *Zentralbl Gynakol* 1914;38:658.

Rubin IC. Therapeutic aspects of uterotubal insufflation in sterility. *Am J Obstet Gynecol* 1945;50:621.

Rufat P, Olivennes F, deMouzon J, et al. Task force report on the outcome of pregnancies and children conceived by *in vitro* fertilization (France: 1987 to 1989). *Fertil Steril* 1994;61:324.

Schlaff WD, Hassiakos DK, Damewood MD, et al. Neosalpingostomy and distal tubal obstruction: prognostic factors and impact of surgical technique. *Fertil Steril* 1990;54:984.

Schlösser HW, Frantzen C, Mansour N, et al. Sterilisation Refertilisierung. Erfahrungen und Ergebnisse bei 119 microchirurgisch refertilisierten Frauen. *Geburtshilfe Frauenheilkd* 1983;43:213.

Sedbon E, Bouquet de la Joliniere J, Boudouris O, et al. Tubal desterilization through exclusive laparoscopy. *Hum Reprod* 1989;4:158.

Silber SJ, Cohen R. Microsurgical reversal of tubal sterilization: factors affecting pregnancy rate, with long-term follow-up. *Obstet Gynecol* 1984;64:679.

Singhal V, Li TC, Cooke ID. An analysis of factors influencing the outcome of 232 consecutive tubal microsurgery cases. *Br J Obstet Gynaecol* 1991;98:628.

Society for Assisted Reproductive Technology, American Society for Reproductive Medicine. Assisted reproductive technology in the United States and Canada: 1992 results generated from the American Fertility Society/Society for Assisted Reproductive Technology Registry. *Fertil Steril* 1994;62:1121.

Society for Assisted Reproductive Technology, American Society for Reproductive Medicine. Assisted reproductive technology in the United States and Canada: 1993 results generated from the American Society for Reproductive Medicine/Society for Assisted Reproductive Technology Registry. *Fertil Steril* 1995;64:13.

Society for Assisted Reproductive Technology and American Society for Reproductive Medicine. Assisted reproductive technology in the United States: 1997 results generated from the American Society for Reproductive Medicine/Society for Assisted Reproductive Technology Registry. *Fertil Steril* 2000;74:641.

Spivak MM, Librach CL, Rosenthal DM. Microsurgical reversal of sterilization: a six-year study. *Am J Obstet Gynecol* 1986;154:355.

Strandell A, Lindhard A, Waldenstrom U, et al. Hydrosalpinx and IVF outcome: a prospective, randomized, multicentre trial in Scandinavia on salpingectomy before IVF. *Hum Reprod* 1999;14:2762.

Strandell A, Lindhard A, Waldenstrom U, et al. Hydrosalpinx and IVF outcome: cumulative results after salpingectomy in a randomized, controlled trial. *Hum Reprod* 2001;16:2403.

Strandell A, Waldenstrom U, Nilsson L, et al. Hydrosalpinx reduces *in-vitro* fertilization/embryo transfer pregnancy rates. *Hum Reprod* 1994;9:863.

Stumpf PG, March CM. Febrile morbidity following hysterosalpingography: identification of risk factors and recommendations for prophylaxis. *Fertil Steril* 1980;33:487.

Sweeney WJ III, Gepfert R. The fallopian tube. *Clin Obstet Gynecol* 1965; 8:32.

Swolin K. Electro microsurgery and salpingostomy: long-term results. *Am J Obstet Gynecol* 1975;121:418.

Swolin K. Fertiltatsoperationen: Teil I and II. *Acta Obstet Gynecol Scand* 1967;46:204.

Tan SL, Royston P, Campbell S, et al. Cumulative conception and live birth rates after *in-vitro* fertilization. *Lancet* 1992;339:1390.

Taylor PJ, Collins JA. *Unexplained infertility*. New York: Oxford Medical Publications, 1992.

Taylor RC, Berkowitz J, McComb PF. Role of laparoscopic salpingostomy in the treatment of hydrosalpinx. *Fertil Steril* 2001;75:594.

Templeton AA, Mortimer D. The development of a clinical test of sperm migration to the site of fertilization. *Fertil Steril* 1982;37:410.

teVelde ER, Boer ME, Looman CWN, et al. Factors influencing success or failure after reversal of sterilization: a multivariate approach. *Fertil Steril* 1990;54:270.

Thie JL, Williams TJ, Coulam CB. Repeat tuboplasty compared with primary microsurgery for postinflammatory tubal disease. *Fertil Steril* 1986;45:784.

Thurmond AS. Selective salpingography and fallopian tube recanalization. *AJR Am J Roentgenol* 1991;156:33.

Tomazevic T, Ribic-Pucelj M, Omahen A, et al. Microsurgery and *in-vitro* fertilization and embryo transfer for infertility resulting from pathological proximal tubal blockage. *Hum Reprod* 1996;11:2613.

Tourgeman DE, Bhaumik M, Cooke GC, et al. Pregnancy rates following fimbriectomy reversal via neosalpingostomy: a 10 years retrospective analysis. *Fertil Steril* 2001;76:1041.

Trimbos-Kemper TCM. Reversal of sterilization of women over 40 years of age: a multicenter survey in the Netherlands. *Fertil Steril* 1990;53:575.

Tulandi T. Salpingo-ovariolysis: a comparison between laser surgery and electrosurgery. *Fertil Steril* 1986;45:489.

Tulandi T, Collins JA, Burrows E, et al. Treatment-dependent and treatment-independent pregnancy among women with periadnexal adhesions. *Am J Obstet Gynecol* 1990;162:354.

Tulandi T, Vilos GA. A comparison between laser surgery and electrosurgery for bilateral hydrosalpinx: a two year followup. *Fertil Steril* 1985;44:846.

Tureck RW, Garcia C-R, Blasco L, et al. Perioperative complications arising after transvaginal oocyte retrieval. *Obstet Gynecol* 1993;81:590.

Uher J, Rypacek F, Presl J. Transport of novel ovum surrogates in the human fallopian tube: a clinical study. *Fertil Steril* 1990;54:278.

Urman B, Gomel V, McComb P, et al. Midtubal occlusion: etiology, management, and outcome. *Fertil Steril* 1992;59:747.

Urman B, Zouves C, Gomel V. Fertility outcome following tubal pregnancy. *Acta Eur Fertil* 1991;22:205.

van Noord-Zaadstra BM, Looman CWN, Alsbach H, et al. Delayed childbearing: effect of age on fecundity and outcome of pregnancy. *Br Med J* 1991;302:1361.

Van Voorhis BJ, Sparks AE, Syrop CH, et al. Ultrasound guided aspiration of hydrosalpinges is associated with improved pregnancy and implantation rates after *in-vitro* fertilization cycles. *Hum Reprod* 1998;13:736.

Verhoeven HC, Berry H, Frantzen C, et al. Surgical treatment for distal tubal occlusion: a review of 167 cases. *J Reprod Med* 1983;28:293.

Westrom L. Effect of acute pelvic inflammatory disease on fertility. *Am J Obstet Gynecol* 1975;121:707.

Westrom L. Incidence, prevalence and trends of pelvic inflammatory disease and its consequences in industrialized countries. *Am J Obstet Gynecol* 1980;138:880.

Winston RML. Reversal of sterilization. *Clin Obstet Gynecol* 1980;23:1261.

Winston RML, Margara RA. Microsurgical salpingostomy is not an obsolete procedure. *Br J Obstet Gynaecol* 1991;98:637.

Xue P, Fa Y-Y. Microsurgical reversal of female sterilization. *J Reprod Med* 1989;34:451.

Yoon TK, Sung HR, Kang HG, et al. Laparoscopic tubal anastomosis: fertility outcome in 202 cases. *Fertil Steril* 1999: 72:1121.

Zouves C, Erenus M, Gomel V. Tubal ectopic pregnancy after *in vitro* fertilization and embryo transfer: a role for proximal occlusion or salpingectomy after failed distal tubal surgery? *Fertil Steril* 1991;56:691.

Zouves C, Gomel V. Gamete intrafallopian transfer (GIFT): procedure-dependent and procedure-independent pregnancy. *Infertility* 1990;13:163.

Te Linde's Operative Gynecology, ninth edition, edited by John A. Rock and Howard W. Jones, III. Lippincott Williams & Wilkins, Philadelphia © 2003.

CHAPTER
25

Endometriosis

JOHN S. HESLA   JOHN A. ROCK

Endometriosis is a clinical and pathologic entity initially described by von Rokitansky in 1860 that is characterized by the presence of tissue resembling functioning endometrial glands and stroma outside the uterine cavity. These ectopic implants can be located throughout the pelvic cavity, including the ovaries, uterine ligaments, rectovaginal septum, parietal peritoneum, intestinal serosa, and appendix. Less common sites of involvement include the cervix, hernial sacs, the umbilicus, laparotomy and episiotomy scars, and the pleural and pericardial cavities (Fig. 25.1).

Although endometriosis has been extensively investigated over the past century, it remains an enigmatic disease process. There are scant data to support the many hormonal and surgical therapies that have been proposed. In addition, the often subtle and varied appearances of endometriosis can make recognition and surgical staging difficult, thereby casting doubt on the utility of the classification systems currently used. Nevertheless, the findings of well-designed clinical trials and recent studies that have elucidated the pathogenesis of endometriosis have enabled a more rational approach to the medical and surgical management of this disease.

PREVALENCE

Although the exact prevalence of endometriosis in the general female population of reproductive age is not precisely known, it is believed to lie within the range of 3% to 10%. Jeffcoate reported that endometriosis was found in 10% to 25% of women undergoing laparotomy by gynecologists in the United Kingdom and the United States. In women with dysmenorrhea, the incidence of endometriosis ranges from 40% to 60%. The disease is diagnosed in 20% to 40% of infertile women. The frequency of endometriosis in multiparous women undergoing laparoscopic sterilization has been reported to range from 6% to 43%. Verkauf prospectively identified endometriosis in 38.5% of infertile women and 5.2% of fertile women. Other studies have confirmed the odds that infertile women are seven to 10 times more likely to have endometriosis than their fertile counterparts. However, any postmenarchal female is at risk, because endometriotic implants have been identified in postmenopausal women, in women with primary amenorrhea secondary to müllerian anomalies, and in 69.6% of teenagers who underwent diagnostic laparoscopy for chronic pelvic pain. The possibility of a familial tendency to endometriosis has been reported by several investigators. No studies have confirmed a human lymphocyte antigen linkage for the disease; a polygenic, multifactorial mode of inheritance has been suggested. Simpson and colleagues reported a 6.9% occurrence rate in first-degree female relatives, which compared with 1% for the non–blood-related control group.

HISTOGENESIS

The mechanism by which endometriosis develops is unknown, although there has been much discussion as to

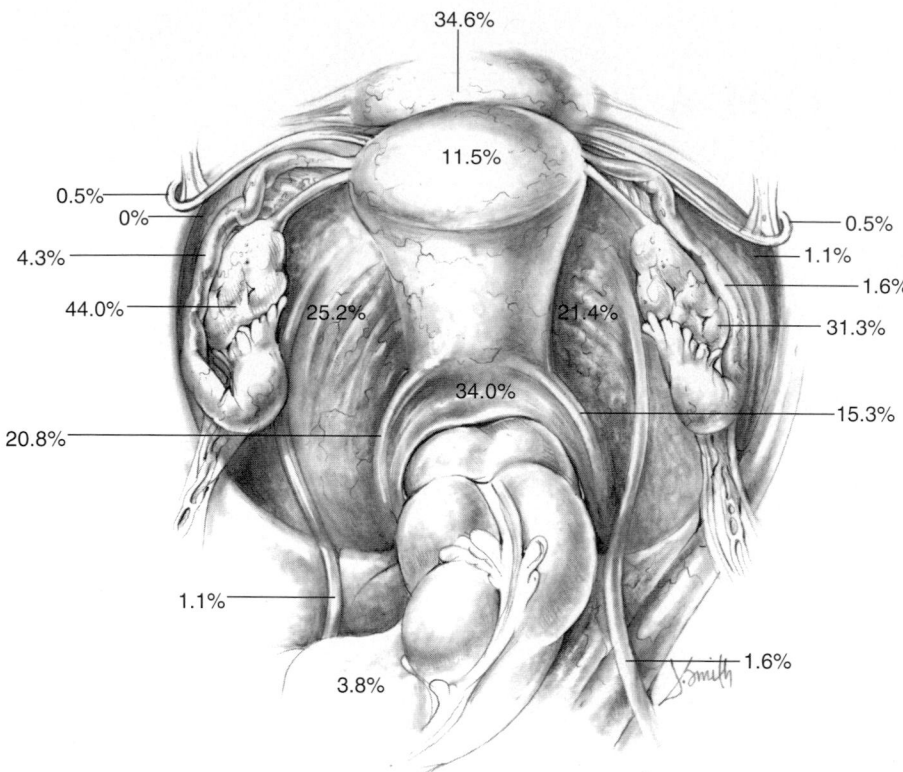

FIGURE 25.1. Anatomic locations of endometriosis implants in 182 consecutive infertility patients found to have endometriosis by laparoscopy. The rates shown indicate the percentage of all patients with implants in a given locale. (Redrawn from Jenkins S, Olive DL, Haney AF. Endometriosis: pathogenic implications of the anatomic distribution. *Obstet Gynecol* 1986;67:335)

its origin (Table 25.1). A complete understanding of the histogenesis of the aberrant endometrial cells has been compromised because of the variations of disease presentation. Four major theories have been proposed:

1. The reflux and direct implantation theory suggests that viable endometrial cells reflux through the fallopian tubes during menstruation and implant on surrounding pelvic structures.
2. The coelomic metaplasia theory suggests that the multipotential cells of the coelomic epithelium may be stimulated to transform into endometrium-like cells.
3. The vascular dissemination theory suggests that endometrial cells enter the uterine vasculature or lym-

phatic system at menstruation and are transported to distant sites.
4. The autoimmune disease theory suggests that endometriosis is a disorder of immune surveillance that allows ectopic endometrial implants to grow.

Reflux and Direct Implantation Theory

It was Sampson who postulated that endometriosis arose from retrograde flow of fragments of endometrial tissue through the oviducts and into the peritoneal cavity, and the evidence for the validity of this theory is conclusive. The anatomic distribution of endometriosis as noted at laparoscopy is consistent with a reflux pattern of development; the most common sites of disease in the infertile woman are the ovary and uterosacral ligament, followed by the posterior uterus, posterior cul-de-sac, and posterior broad ligament. Endometriosis developed in monkeys when the uterus was surgically inverted to cause menstruation to occur intraperitoneally. Exposure of abraded peritoneum to endometrial cells has resulted in the growth of endometriotic implants in rabbits and rats. In clinical studies performed at Grady Memorial Hospital in Atlanta, Ridley demonstrated that endometrium desquamated at the time of menstruation is viable tissue and capable of growth after implantation. Endometriosis has developed in laparotomy, episiotomy, and Caesarean section scars after surgical entrance into the endometrial cavity, and anomalies of the müllerian tract are associated with an increased occurrence of endometriosis. Epidemiologic data suggest that women

---

TABLE 25.1.
Theories for the Histogenesis of Endometriosis

Transtubal regurgitation or retrograde menstruation
Direct implantation of endometrial cells
Metaplasia of coelomic epithelium
Lymphatic dissemination
Hematogenous spread
Activation of embryonic cell rests
Activation of wolffian rests
Metaplasia of urothelium
Hereditary factor
Immunologic factor

who menstruate more frequently, more heavily, or for a longer duration have an increased likelihood of disease development. Endometriosis is a common finding in women with stenosis of the external cervical os.

Focal endometriosis has been identified in 16% to 63% of proximal tubal segments after cautery or Pomeroy tubal sterilization, perhaps as a consequence of recurrent bathing of the healing terminal area with menstrual products. Nevertheless, bloody peritoneal fluid has been observed in 90% of women with patent fallopian tubes undergoing laparoscopy during the perimenstrual time period, a figure much greater than the estimated 2% to 5% prevalence of symptomatic endometriosis in women of reproductive age. Additionally, peritoneal implants have been identified in women who had a prior tubal ligation procedure and were undergoing laparoscopy for the evaluation of pelvic pain. Hence, other factors evidently are present to promote the ectopic implantation.

Coelomic Metaplasia Theory

The germinal epithelia of the ovary, endometrium, and peritoneum all originate from the same totipotential coelomic epithelium. The metaplasia theory postulates that these totipotential cells are transformed by repeated exposure to hormonal or infectious stimuli. This may explain the development of endometriotic lesions in unusual locations and in the odd cases of male patients in whom endometriosis develops after prostatectomy, orchiectomy, or prolonged treatment with estrogen. Reports of endometriosis in women with primary amenorrhea and an absence of functioning uterine endometrium and of endometriosis identified in mature teratomas also lend support to the metaplasia theory. Metaplasia may account for the development of endometriomas from the invaginations of the mesothelial layer of the ovarian cortex.

Vascular Dissemination Theory

Endometrial cells can be transported to extrauterine sites by blood vessels or the lymphatic system, or by contamination of the pelvis or abdominal wall incision if the uterine cavity is surgically entered. Retroperitoneal endometriosis is hypothesized to arise from lymph vascular spread; 29% of patients with pelvic endometriosis documented on autopsy had pelvic lymph nodes that contained endometriosis. Theories of vascular dissemination help explain how endometriosis can develop in the lung or pericardium.

Autoimmune Disease

Alterations in cellular immunity can facilitate the successful implantation of translocated endometrial cells. Compared with control subjects, monkeys with spontaneous endometriosis had both a lowered cell-mediated response to autologous endometrial tissue, as determined by skin testing, and a decreased *in vitro* blastogenesis response. Similar studies performed in women demonstrated that lymphocytes obtained from control patients were significantly more efficient in cytolysis of isolated endometrial stromal cells than were lymphocytes obtained from patients with endometriosis. This decreased cytotoxic response to endometrial cells may be due to a defect in natural killer cell activity, such as a decreased lytic effect toward stroma that allows ectopic development of endometrial fragments. In addition, there may be an increased resistance of endometrium in women with endometriosis to natural killer cytotoxicity.

Promoting Factors

Clinical and laboratory studies support the concept that endometriosis is an estrogen-dependent condition. Estradiol concentrations greater than approximately 60 pg/mL have been identified as necessary for proliferation of endometriotic lesions. Nevertheless, estrogen and progesterone receptors are found in much lower concentrations in endometriotic tissue than in normal endometrium tissue; such endometriotic tissue also frequently fails to show cyclic variations of development in response to hormonal changes. In a mouse model of endometriosis, estrogen failed to stimulate *in vitro* cell proliferation of endometrial epithelial cells, although functional integrity of the estrogen receptor system was demonstrated by an increase in progesterone receptor synthesis. Early data from primate studies suggested that endometriosis required no steroidal supplementation to become initially established, but later studies demonstrated that chronic exposure to ovarian steroids is necessary for the survival of these experimentally induced endometrial plaques.

Growth factors can originate from the peritoneal environment to stimulate endometrial development. Platelet-derived growth factor, a macrophage secretory product, enhanced endometrial stromal cell proliferation in a dose-dependent manner. Similarly, macrophage-conditioned media promoted mouse endometrial stromal cell proliferation *in vitro*, and this activation was enhanced with the addition of estrogen. Increased concentrations of macrophage-derived growth factors, including vascular endothelial growth factor, have been identified in the peritoneal fluid of women with endometriosis.

Molecular alterations in steroidogenic enzyme function have been implicated in the pathogenesis of endometriosis. Endometrial tissue from patients with endometriosis expresses aromatase P-450, whereas endometrium from control women without identifiable endometriosis does not. The presence of aromatase within endometriosis results in higher local production of estrogen necessary to support the growth and metabolic activity of the lesion.

Hence, no single theory explains all cases of endometriosis, although the direct implantation mechanism seems the likely cause for most disease locations. Immunologic factors, inducing substances, or other mediators may explain the development of endometriosis in more distant sites.

NATURAL HISTORY

The natural history of endometriosis is not clearly understood. The disease appears to progress in most untreated patients, although spontaneous regression can occur in as many as 58% of milder cases. Surgical and medical therapies may prevent a temporal regression but may not effectively eliminate microscopic, retroperitoneal, and hormonally resistant disease. Dmowski and Cohen described persistent disease in 15% of patients treated with danazol, and Henzl and associates noted a progression of disease during the course of treatment in 4% to 8% of patients receiving danazol or an analog of gonadotropin-releasing hormone (GnRH). When conservative surgery was combined with danazol or GnRH agonist therapy, the overall recurrence rate at 36 months was between 13.5% and 33%.

The effect of pregnancy on the clinical course of endometriosis is uncertain. Although Sampson proposed that pregnancy induces involution of implants, other authors recently described a variable response of endometriosis to pregnancy. It is possible that endometriosis becomes temporarily suppressed during pregnancy. McArthur and Ulfelder analyzed the clinical effect of pregnancy on endometriosis in 24 patients. They found that the behavior of endometriosis during the gravid state was extremely variable and that the regression of disease appeared to be due to decreased tissue responsiveness to hormonal stimulation rather than to actual necrosis of the lesions. More patients in their series experienced disease persistence than permanent regression. Monkey studies have confirmed these findings; the response of endometrial implants to pregnancy varied from total regression to significant progression.

Approximately 2% to 4% of early postmenopausal women suffer from endometriosis. These cases are usually associated with exogenous intake of estrogens or tamoxifen. Nevertheless, there are reports of symptomatic endometriosis in women older than 60 years of age who have not received steroid replacement therapy. Such cases presumably are secondary to the responsiveness of the residual lesions to low levels of estrogens that arise from peripheral conversion of ovarian and adrenal androgens.

PATHOPHYSIOLOGY

Gross Appearance

Signs of endometriosis may be evident on physical examination. Endometriosis can form tender nodules on the uterosacral ligaments that are readily palpable on rectovaginal examination. It may infiltrate the rectovaginal septum and cause pain with defecation and, rarely, cyclic rectal bleeding. Lesions of endometriosis have been identified in the umbilicus, in the vulva, and in episiotomy scars. Complete ureteral obstruction has been reported. This can be temporarily reversed with the administration of danazol, GnRH agonists, and progestogens. Diaphragmatic involvement can lead to chronic, recurrent pneumothorax at the time of menstruation. Lesions have been identified in the upper and lower extremities, the pericardium, and the lung.

The gross appearance of endometriosis is extremely variable. On entering the abdomen, the surgeon may find a small, adherent mass in one or both sides of the pelvis, usually attached to the posterior cul-de-sac and posterior surface of the uterus. Frequently, release of these adhesions to mobilize the adnexa results in an egress of chocolate-colored or dark red fluid that is highly suggestive of endometriosis. Examination of the ovary may disclose a cyst that is rarely larger than 10 cm and has a dark, hemorrhagic lining. Endometriomas develop over a time span of a few months as a result of extensive intracystic hemorrhage. Reddish blue, fibrinlike areas that consist of small islands of endometriosis can be present on the ovarian surface. Peritoneal implants vary in appearance from black, puckered lesions, to red polypoid material, to clear vesicles. These implants can be located throughout the pelvic cavity. The fallopian tube is usually nonobstructed and free of gross disease, although peritubal adhesions can extend to adjacent structures, particularly in patients with extensive disease. Endometrial invasion of the rectal or sigmoidal wall can simulate malignancy or produce complete obstruction.

Microscopic Appearance

The essential diagnostic criterion is the presence of endometrial tissue, both stroma and glandular elements. This aberrant tissue resembles the uterine mucosa both histologically and physiologically. Secretory change and decidualization are seen in response to hormone influences in the luteal phase, and estrogen stimulates proliferation of the ectopic implants. Nevertheless, these functional changes are less uniform for implants than for the uterine mucosa.

The ultrastructural features of endometriosis are consistent with an incomplete response to the hormonal milieu; the tissue response to progesterone is dependent more on the extent of morphologic differentiation than on the degree of hormonal stimulation. Endometriotic implants contain lower concentrations of progesterone and estrogen receptors than does corresponding normal endometrium, so the histologic response to progesterone is less profound. Gould and colleagues reported that the nucleus of endometriotic stromal cells had a marked degree of estrogen binding throughout the menstrual cycle, whereas stromal binding sites in the uterine endometrium were present only during the proliferative phase and not the secretory phase of the cycle. The differing responses of the two tissue types to steroid hormones were reflected by the modulation of estrogen binding and changes in glandular histology. Estrogen receptors did not undergo downregulation during the luteal phase of the cycle in endometriotic foci, despite an increase in endogenous progesterone concentration. Alterations in the quantity, activation, or function of the progesterone receptor may be responsible for this lack of change in estradiol receptors, the abnormal response of the ectopic endometrium to progesterone, and the failure of hormonal therapy in some patients.

Because of the pressure of retained blood in the cyst cavities of endometriomas, a large concentration of endothelial leukocytes heavily laden with hemosiderin (pseudoxanthoma cells) may be found, and the glandular lining may be nearly absent and replaced by reactive connective tissue elements. Biopsy may fail to yield histologic proof of the endometrial glands and stroma in about one third of all cases of typical clinical endometriosis, even if many tissue sections are analyzed.

The "chocolate cyst" description of the ovary is used synonymously with endometrial cyst. Nevertheless, other types of ovarian cysts may have a similar fluid content, including the hemorrhagic follicle, corpus luteum, or cystadenoma. Pathologic confirmation of the diagnosis is always advised.

Approximately 0.7% to 1.0% of patients with endometriosis have lesions that undergo malignant transformation. Atypical glandular changes have been found in 3% to 6% of cases of ovarian endometriosis. Several histologic tumor types have been described (Table 25.2). Endometrioid adenocarcinomas account for 69% of reported lesions, with the ovary being the primary site in most cases. Rapidly enlarging endometriomas or those measuring greater than 10 cm should be sectioned carefully to search for malignant foci. Tumors arising in endometriosis are predominantly of low grade and confined to the site of origin. Progestogen therapy is recommended after surgical resection of these lesions.

Clinical Characteristics

The clinical features of endometriosis are varied, and the presentation depends on the site of growth and the severity of disease. The classic triad of dysmenorrhea, dyspareunia, and infertility has been described as characteristic of the disease (Table 25.3). Nevertheless, patients with extensive endometriosis may be clinically symptom-free, and women with only minimal involvement may manifest disabling pelvic pain. Dysmenorrhea is a common symptom that most likely is associated with endometriosis if it develops after age 20 years, is progressive, and is not well relieved by nonsteroidal antiinflammatory agents or oral contraceptives. Spasmodic pain beginning before the onset of menstrual bleeding is another common complaint of patients with endometriosis. When the rectovaginal septum or uterosacral region is involved, the pain is often referred to the rectum or lower sacral and coccygeal regions because of premenstrual and menstrual swelling of ectopic implants. Dyschezia and constipation may be present. Dyspareunia is common, especially in cases of uterosacral or vaginal infiltration, fixed retroversion of the uterus, or ovarian fixation by adhesions. Again, there is no absolute correlation between the amount of endometriosis and the extent of symptoms; minor disease involvement may result in severe pain, whereas massive areas of superficial endometriosis may cause no discomfort.

Other presenting complaints can include signs or symptoms of urinary tract involvement, such as hematuria or ureteral obstruction, unusual abdominal or adnexal masses, cyclic sciatica, catamenial pneumothorax or hemoptysis, and swollen and painful scars. Premenstrual

TABLE 25.2.
Histology of Tumors Arising in Endometriosis

Histology	Numbers[a]	Incidence (%)
Endometrioid carcinoma		
Adenocarcinoma	96	46.4
Adenoacanthoma	43	20.8
Adenosquamous carcinoma	4	1.9
Clear cell carcinoma	28	13.5
Sarcoma, including mixed mesodermal tumor	24	11.6
Serous cystadenocarcinoma	6	2.9
Squamous cell carcinoma	3	1.4
Mucinous cystadenocarcinoma	2	1.0
Mixed germ cell tumor and adenocarcinoma	1	0.5
TOTALS	207	100

[a] Two patients had two different histologic patterns.
From Heaps JM, Nieberg RK, Berek JS. Malignant neoplasms arising in endometriosis. *Obstet Gynecol* 1990;75:1023, with permission.

TABLE 25.3.
Symptoms Associated With Endometriosis

PELVIC
Dysmenorrhea
Dyspareunia
Chronic pelvic pain
Sciatica
Premenstrual spotting

GASTROINTESTINAL
Constipation
Diarrhea
Dyschezia
Tenesmus
Hematochezia

URINARY
Flank pain
Back pain
Abdominal pain
Urgency
Frequency
Hematuria

PULMONARY
Hemoptysis
Catamenial chest pain
Pneumothorax

spotting can occur for 3 to 7 days before the start of menses; this is a poorly recognized but relatively consistent sign of endometriosis. An endometrial cyst can leak, causing considerable pain, or it can rupture and produce a clinical picture much like that seen with a ruptured ectopic pregnancy or acute appendicitis. Nearly 10% of patients with endometriosis present with acute symptoms that may require exploration for diagnosis and treatment.

Twenty percent to 40% of women with endometriosis are infertile. When extensive pelvic scarring or large endometriomas are present in the patient with endometriosis, the associated infertility can be clearly attributed to anatomic distortion. However, the pathophysiology of infertility in patients with less advanced disease is more controversial.

Endometriotic implants within the fallopian tube or ovary can promote a local inflammatory response that has a direct, deleterious effect on tubal function (Table 25.4). Oocyte pickup by the fallopian tube can be prevented despite the normal process of oocyte maturation and ovulation. Chronic salpingitis was detected in 29 of 87 (33%) fallopian tubes of patients undergoing laparotomy for ovarian endometriosis; tubal obstruction was demonstrated in only one of these cases, although adhe-

sions were present in 24%. Endometriosis has been identified in the resected segments of fallopian tubes in women undergoing tubal-cornual anastomosis for proximal tubal obstruction when there was no evidence of implants elsewhere in the pelvis. Others have reported a correlation between tubal endometriosis and chronic salpingitis in similar cases, although data from Forrest and associates did not corroborate this relation.

Altered folliculogenesis or ovulation has been described in endometriotic patients. Doody and colleagues sonographically evaluated follicular development in 20 patients with mild endometriosis previously treated with diathermy or conservative surgery, in 46 patients who received clomiphene citrate, and in a control group of 20 fertile women. Linear regression analysis of increasing follicular diameter that demonstrated a lower rate of growth in all endometriotic patients gave them reason to speculate that an abnormal follicular growth rate and total growth period may disturb the normal synchronization of oocyte maturation, uterine receptivity, and ovulation. Tummon and co-workers reported that women with minimal endometriosis had more, yet smaller, follicles and lower preovulatory estradiol levels at the time of midcycle luteinizing hormone (LH) surge.

Luteinized unruptured follicle syndrome (LUF), a condition of normal ovulatory hormone secretion and luteinization of the follicle without the expected occurrence of ovulation, has been reported to be more common in patients with endometriosis. Donnez and Thomas were able to identify stigmata of ovulation in only 28% and 49% of patients with moderate and severe endometriosis, respectively, at the time of laparoscopy. These figures were significantly lower than the 91% and 85% stigma formation rates observed for the normal control and mild endometriosis groups, respectively. Schenken and associates also noted an increased rate of LUF and associated luteal phase deficiency in monkeys with surgically induced moderate to severe endometriosis. In another study, the incidence of LUF was significantly higher in patients with minimal or mild endometriosis (35%) compared with that in patients who did not have endometriosis (11%). An absence of sonographic evidence of midcycle follicular collapse in patients with mild endometriosis has ranged from 4% to 34% in the literature.

Luteal phase function has been evaluated by endometrial biopsy and peripheral progesterone concentrations. There is insufficient evidence to conclusively link endometriosis with a deficiency of corpus luteum activity, although some studies have suggested the existence of a shortened luteal phase and delayed increase in progesterone secretion after ovulation. Women with proven endometriosis demonstrated two distinct midcycle peaks of LH 2 to 3 days apart and delays in the maximum concentrations of urinary estriol-16-glucuronide and pregnanediol-3-glucuronide compared with those in control subjects, although no serum differences could be detected. Conversely, analyses of early follicular phase estradiol and progesterone concentrations in the peripheral and ovarian veins of patients with endometriosis

---

TABLE 25.4.
Possible Mechanisms by Which Endometriosis Causes Infertility

MECHANICAL INTERFERENCE

Pelvic adhesions
Chronic salpingitis
Altered tubal motility
Distortion of tuboovarian relations
Impaired oocyte pickup

ALTERATIONS IN PERITONEAL FLUID

Increased concentration of prostaglandins
Increased number of activated macrophages
Increased production of cytokines
Enhanced phagocytosis of sperm

ABNORMAL SYSTEMIC IMMUNE SYSTEM RESPONSE

Increased cell-mediated gamete injury
Increased prevalence of autoantibodies
Antiendometrial antibody production

HORMONAL OR OVULATORY DYSFUNCTION

Defective folliculogenesis
Luteinized unruptured follicle syndrome
Hyperprolactinemia
Luteal phase deficiency

FERTILIZATION OR IMPLANTATION FAILURE

EARLY SPONTANEOUS ABORTION

From Surrey ES, Halme J. Endometriosis as a cause of infertility. *Obstet Gynecol Clin North Am* 1989;16:79, with permission.

have suggested an increased frequency of inadequate luteolysis and prolongation of corpus luteum function into the subsequent menstrual cycle.

The effect of endometriosis on fertilization and preimplantation development is widely debated. Peritoneal fluid from patients with endometriosis had a deleterious effect on sperm-oocyte interaction in homologous mouse and hamster fertilization assays. *In vitro* studies involving human zona pellucida confirmed an adverse effect of peritoneal fluid on sperm binding in this patient population, although others reported that peritoneal fluid from women with low-stage endometriosis had no detrimental effect on sperm motility characteristics. Peritoneal fluid from women with moderate and severe endometriosis caused declines in sperm motility and velocity. Exposure of two-cell mouse embryos to the peritoneal fluid or serum of patients with endometriosis resulted in a decreased rate of cleavage and development to the blastocyst and hatching stages as compared with control, nonendometriotic specimens.

Integrins are ubiquitous cell adhesion molecules that undergo dynamic alterations during the normal menstrual cycle in the human endometrium. The $\alpha v\beta 3$ vitronectin receptor integrin is normally expressed in endometrium during the periimplantation period; such expression may be lost in women with mild endometriosis, which may result in decreased cycle fecundity due to defects in uterine receptivity.

A high frequency of abortions in infertile women with endometriosis has been reported, although the relation was questioned because of potential control group bias. Naples and co-workers found that patients with endometriosis who refused treatment had the same abortion rate before and after diagnosis (26% and 25.5%).

Mechanisms Influencing Symptoms

Because of the uncertain mechanisms causing infertility and pelvic pain in patients with minimal and mild endometriosis, many investigators have attempted to identify specific alterations in the peritoneal environment that would explain these symptoms. Significant increases or decreases in peritoneal fluid volume due to increased production by the ovaries, altered mesothelial permeability, or increases in the colloid osmotic pressure have been hypothesized to inhibit ovum capture by the fallopian tube or to adversely affect tubal transport. Koninckx and associates reported elevations in peritoneal fluid volume during cycle days 1 through 5 in patients with mild and moderate endometriosis. The quantity of fluid was comparable to that in control subjects during the remainder of the follicular phase. These authors described reduced volumes in the early luteal phase, which directly contrasts with findings reported by Oak and colleagues. Rock and associates evaluated patients during cycle days 8 through 12 and measured no difference in fluid volumes in patients with endometriosis compared with that in control subjects. Similar findings were noted by Rezai and associates. Hence, it appears unlikely that fluid volume alone plays a role in the establishment of infertility.

Peritoneal fluid from patients with minimal and mild endometriosis has been shown to increase macrophage proliferation *in vitro*. In addition, several studies have described increases in total macrophage number in the peritoneal fluid of patients with endometriosis. Hill and co-workers measured significant elevations in total leukocytes, macrophages, helper T cells, lymphocytes, and natural killer cells in women with stages I and II endometriosis. Activated macrophages can affect the reproductive process by altering sperm motility, fimbrial ovum capture, sperm-oocyte interaction, and early embryonic growth. Increased sperm phagocytosis by macrophages has been demonstrated by *in vivo* animal and *in vitro* human studies. Suginami and Yano have demonstrated the presence of an ovum capture inhibitor in peritoneal fluid from patients with endometriosis, which reduces fimbrial activity for ovum capture *in vitro*. This macromolecule may prevent contact between the fimbrial cells and cumulus oophorus.

Prostaglandins, interleukins, and other substances produced by macrophages may be harmful to reproduction. Fakih and colleagues demonstrated that interleukin-1 was present in the peritoneal fluid of almost all patients with endometriosis, but not in the fertile control group. Interleukins have been shown to adversely affect mouse embryo growth *in vitro*. In addition, interleukin-1 stimulated fibroblast proliferation, collagen deposition, and fibrinogen formation; hence, elevated concentrations of such lymphokines may account for the development of fibrosis and adhesions in advanced stages of endometriosis. Interleukin-6 secretion *in vitro* is upregulated in ectopic and eutopic endometrial stromal cells from women with endometriosis. Nevertheless, not all studies have confirmed the existence of a difference in interleukin activity between endometriosis patients and control groups. Decreased plasminogen activator activity in endometriotic implants may also be a cause for increased adhesion formation.

Chronic elevations in the level of peritoneal prostaglandins have been hypothesized to interfere with ovulation, to alter tubal mobility such that the embryo may arrive in the uterus at a suboptimal time for implantation, or to diminish corpus luteum function. Drake and associates measured the metabolites of prostacyclin and thromboxane A_2 in peritoneal fluid and noted a 10-fold increase in these levels in patients with endometriosis. Ylikorkla and colleagues confirmed these observations, although the increase in prostanoid metabolites in the patients with endometriosis was less than twice that of the controls. When cycle stage was experimentally controlled, Rock and co-workers, Rezai and associates, and others failed to demonstrate a significant change in prostaglandin levels in peritoneal fluid from patients with endometriosis as compared with control groups. In addition, prostaglandin concentrations did not vary between the follicular and luteal phase in either endometriosis patients or controls. Variations in collection of samples during the menstrual cycle, selection of control groups, and collection techniques have compromised the interpretation of data regarding the relative importance of prostanoid content in peritoneal fluid in the studies that have been published on this topic.

Alterations in the systemic immune response of endometriosis patients can influence fecundity. Cellular and humoral abnormalities have been reported in the peripheral blood and peritoneal fluid of women with endometriosis. Translocated endometrial cells may implant only in patients with an inherent defect in cell-mediated immunity. Functional changes in monocytes and macrophages, natural killer cells, cytotoxic T lymphocytes, and B cells suggest decreased surveillance, recognition, and destruction of misplaced endometrial cells and possible facilitation of their implantation. The endometrial proteins of menstrual fluid may be recognized as foreign by the host and trigger an autoimmune response. This host reaction can be variable, thus explaining why some women with a weak autoimmune response and varying extent of disease can conceive with no difficulty. Other investigators have confirmed a high prevalence of autoantibodies against endometrial and ovarian tissues in the sera and cervical and vaginal secretions of women with endometriosis.

In a study of 59 patients with endometriosis by Gleicher and associates, 29% had positive antinuclear antibody titers, 46% had positive lupus anticoagulant assays, and almost 50% demonstrated IgM and IgG antibodies, perhaps reflecting a polyclonal B-cell activation that is characteristic of autoimmune disease. Abnormal concentrations of IgG antiphospholipid and antihistone antibodies have been measured within the peritoneal cavity of endometriosis patients. Activated B cells may regulate this increased immunoglobulin production, because concentrations of T cells and B cells and the ratio of CD4 to CD8 lymphocytes were increased in the peritoneal fluid and peripheral blood of patients with endometriosis as compared with those in control subjects.

Matrix metalloproteinases play an important role in remodeling the extracellular matrix of many tissues. They appear to be involved in the marked cyclic changes of growth and tissue breakdown of the endometrium. Suppression of matrix metalloproteinase production by progesterone decreased ectopic implantation of endometrium in the nude mouse, implicating these proteinases in the pathogenesis of endometriosis.

Dioxin, a pollutant that is known to decrease cell-mediated cytotoxicity by reducing the number of helper T cells, has been suggested as a causative factor in the high incidence of endometriosis in Belgium and other developed countries. Women with endometriosis were reported to have increased concentrations of polychlorinated biphenyl compounds in their blood. Moreover, a dose-dependent relation existed between dioxin exposure and the subsequent development of and severity of endometriosis in the rhesus monkey after a latent period of more than 5 years.

Nevertheless, other studies have suggested that endometriosis may not promote immunologic alterations in the pelvis. In a retrospective analysis of the cell count and volume of peritoneal fluid in 135 infertile women with endometriosis, Haney and colleagues found a negative correlation between total cell numbers and extent of disease and no significant correlation between fluid volume and extent of disease. Similarly, in the rabbit model of endometriosis, there was no difference in peritoneal fluid volume, macrophage numbers, or macrophage activation in treated versus control animals.

Hence, the exact cause-and-effect relation between endometriosis and infertility in the absence of a distortion in pelvic anatomy remains unknown. In a recent study using an adhesion-free rabbit model of endometriosis, peritoneal implants did not adversely affect the number of corpora lutea, the oocyte recovery or fertilization rates, tubal transport, embryonic development and cleavage, or nidation index. Similarly, Mahmood and Templeton were unable to detect differences in hormonal patterns of the menstrual cycle, follicular growth, preovulatory peritoneal fluid volume and sex steroid concentration, rate of LUF, oocyte maturity, fertilization rate, or cleavage rate between patients with minimal and mild endometriosis and control women.

Little is known about the mechanisms by which endometriosis induces pain symptoms. Dyspareunia may be related to stimulation of pain fibers by stretching of scarred, inelastic tissue or by direct pressure on nodules of endometriosis embedded in fibrotic tissue. Endometriosis implants may secrete inflammatory substances such as prostaglandins, cytokines, and growth factors that initiate the sequence of events that results in the development of pain. Moreover, the extravasated debris and blood from endometriotic implants may stimulate an inflammatory reaction within the peritoneal cavity, with production of the aforementioned substances.

DIAGNOSIS

Symptoms

Dysmenorrhea, dyspareunia, and pelvic, back, and rectal pain, the more common symptoms of endometriosis, have been assumed to be caused by endometrial implants. However, the development of such symptoms is not diagnostic of the disease state. In one random survey of women in the general population, more than 60% reported dyspareunia at some point in their lives, and 33% had persistent discomfort. The prevalence of laparoscopically diagnosed endometriosis in patients with chronic pelvic pain has ranged from 4% to 52% in published series.

Some authorities have suggested that the symptoms may be dependent on the location of the implants, the presence of adhesions, distortion of ovarian anatomy by endometriosis, and involvement of other organs such as the ureter or rectum. However, Fedele and colleagues found no significant association between the American Fertility Society (AFS; now known as the American Society for Reproductive Medicine) classification of disease stage and the presence and severity of dysmenorrhea, pelvic pain, and dyspareunia in a prospective study of 160 women. The pain profiles of the patients with ovarian lesions were similar to those of the patients with peritoneal or ovarian and peritoneal disease. Conversely, in a later study by the same group, ovarian endometriomas were the only lesions significantly associated with severe dysmenorrhea and pelvic pain in infertile women. Koninckx and co-workers demonstrated that the presence of pelvic pain did not correlate with the total area of endometriosis, type of lesion, or volume of disease. The only significant discriminator proved to be the depth of infiltration; endometriotic lesions greater than 1 cm in depth were associated with severe discomfort (Fig. 25.2). This supports earlier data that strongly linked pain with deep infiltration of the fibromuscular tissue of the pelvis.

Pain symptoms generally correlate with fluctuations in steroid hormone concentrations. In response to cyclic stimulation by ovarian estradiol and progesterone, endometriotic lesions undergo epithelial and stromal proliferation, variable secretory changes, stromal pseudodecidual reaction, and periodic regression in a manner more disorganized than, yet similar to, that of normal endometrium. Surgical castration and ovarian suppressive therapy result in diminution of pain in most patients.

Physical Findings

Bimanual pelvic examination may reveal tender uterosacral ligaments, cul-de-sac nodularity, induration of the rectovaginal septum, fixed retroversion of the uterus, adnexal masses, and generalized or localized pelvic tenderness. The adherent tube and ovary may constitute a tender, irregular mass that is similar in characteristics to the mass palpated in cases of chronic salpingo-oophoritis. Uterosacral nodules occasionally reach 1 cm or more in size. Lesions implanted in the retrocervical area or rectovaginal wall are frequently more easily felt than seen and can be missed if the physical examination is omitted. A perceptible, painful swelling of the implant before and at menstruation remains a classic and reliable clinical sign of active rectovaginal or retrocervical endometriosis.

Cancer antigen-125 (CA-125), a high-molecular-weight glycoprotein expressed on the cell surface of some derivatives of embryonic coelomic epithelium, is often elevated toward the end of the luteal phase and during menstruation in patients with AFS stages II to IV endometriosis. Barbieri and colleagues reported that a value higher than 35 U/mL had a positive predictive value of 0.58 and a negative predictive value of 0.96 in establishing the presence of endometriosis. Many other conditions have been associated with an elevated CA-125 concentration, including acute pelvic inflammatory disease, adenomyosis, uterine leiomyoma, menstruation, pregnancy, epithelial ovarian cancer, pancreatitis, and chronic liver disease. Pittaway reported that 80% of women with pelvic pain and endometriosis had a CA-125 titer greater than 16 U/mL, whereas only 6% of patients with pelvic pain and without endometriosis had an increased serum concentration of this cell-surface antigen.

Increased concentrations of CA-125 and placental protein 14 (PP14) have been related specifically to the presence of endometriotic cysts and deep endometriosis.

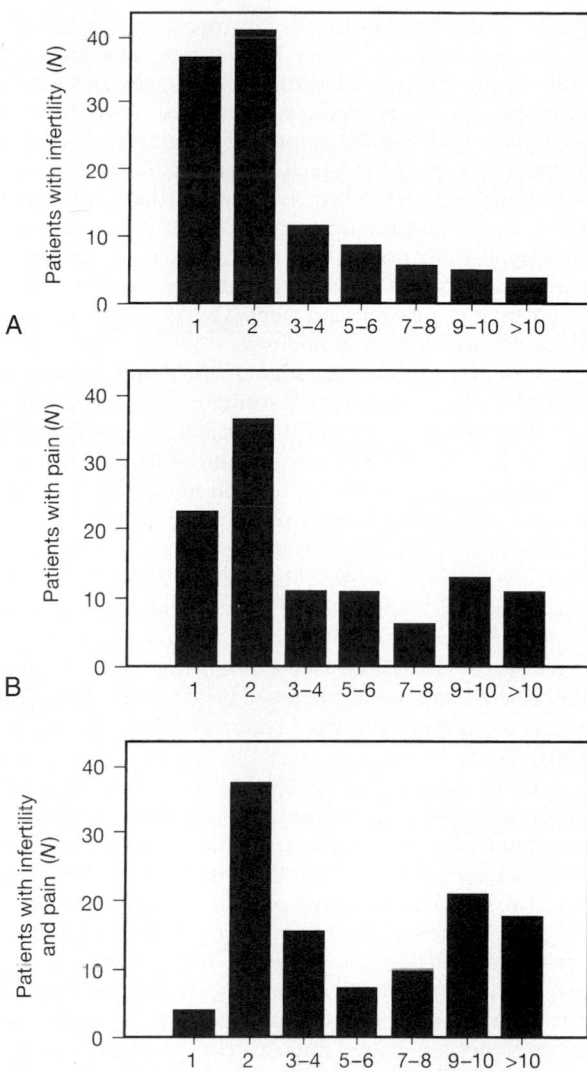

FIGURE 25.2. Frequency distributions of depth of infiltration of pelvic endometriosis in women with **(A)** infertility (N = 283), **(B)** pain (N = 119), or **(C)** infertility and pain (N = 48). (Redrawn from Koninckx PR, Mueleman C, Demeyere S, et al. Suggestive evidence that pelvic endometriosis is a progressive disease, whereas deeply infiltrating endometriosis is associated with pelvic pain. *Fertil Steril* 1991;55:759)

The results of most studies, however, suggest that CA-125 is not sufficiently sensitive to identify lesser stages of endometriosis and is therefore not reliable as a screening test. Doppler sonographic evaluation of resistance indices in the vessels of adnexal masses increases the sensitivity and negative predictive values of two-dimensional sonography and CA-125, but this yields many false-positive results because of the neovascularity of benign tumors.

The patient with unexplained lower abdominal pain or a presentation suggesting endometriosis requires laparoscopy for definitive diagnosis. Ultrasonography and other noninvasive procedures cannot provide the specific information needed to diagnose or classify the extent or severity of disease. For proper laparoscopic evaluation, a double puncture technique is essential. The ancillary probe or forceps placed through the lower abdominal sheath permits mobilization of the tubes and ovaries. A methodical, regimented approach should be used to thoroughly inspect the lateral side walls, all ovarian surfaces, both sides of the broad ligaments, the bladder and bowel serosa, and the inferior aspects of the cul-de-sac. Uterine manipulation with a cannula fixed to the cervix facilitates evaluation of the uterosacral ligaments and rectal serosa. Photography and videotape recording are useful for documentation of findings.

Awareness of the wide range of visual appearances of endometriosis is necessary for accurate diagnosis and appropriate surgical therapy of the disease. Although darkly pigmented lesions are readily recognizable and are considered a classic presentation of endometriosis, less discernible yet common forms of implants were described as early as the 1920s, when Sampson noted "red raspberries, purple raspberries, blueberries, blebs, and peritoneal pockets." The black or blue puckered "powderburn" implant is a late consequence of cyclic growth and regression of the lesion, to the point that bleeding and hemosiderin staining of the tissue have occurred. Biopsy of such areas reveals inactive endometrial glands and fibrous stroma.

Distinctive morphologic variations include vesicles, flat plaques, raised lesions, polypoid structures, areas of fibrosis and adhesion formation, and peritoneal defects (Table 25.5). Yellow, brown, blue, or black coloration is proportional to the amount of hemosiderin deposition. Red polypoid lesions share the closest histologic characteristics with native endometrium and are thought to have the greatest metabolic activity, as is suggested by their high concentrations of prostaglandin metabolites. Biopsy of nonpigmented implants (i.e., implants that are the same color as adjacent peritoneum) may reveal active endometriotic glands and stroma. White lesions are predominantly fibromuscular scarring with scattered glandular and stromal elements, and brown lesions are mainly hemosiderin deposits. Peritoneal defects and subovarian adhesions contain endometriosis in 40% to 70% of cases. Because other peritoneal lesions share morphologic features similar to those of endometriosis, the differential diagnosis is broad and includes old suture locations, epithelial malignancies, hemangioma, inflammatory reaction to infection or oil-based hysterosalpingogram dye, and carbon deposition from laser surgery. Rectovaginal endometriotic lesions consist of smooth muscle with active glandular epithelium and scanty stroma. They share similar characteristics to adenomyomas.

Small endometriotic lesions become more visible during the premenstrual and menstrual phases of the cycle, because during this time microfoci of peritoneal disease become congested with blood and debris. In addition, vascular dilatation, superficial hemorrhage, and ecchymosis formation cause accentuation of the more typical features of endometriosis. Performance of laparoscopy at a time when ovarian steroidogenesis is suppressed by medications such as danazol or GnRH analogs can lead to inaccuracies in the assessment of extent of disease.

Jansen and Russell reported the presence of nonpigmented lesions in 38% of their 202 patients with biopsy-proven endometriosis; 15% had only nonpigmented implants. Most areas of pigmented endometriosis are surrounded by nonpigmented endometriosis. These subtle lesions may represent the first stage of development of peritoneal disease. Recognition of nonpigmented endometriosis may be enhanced by "painting" the peritoneum with the patient's blood or by filling the pelvis with irrigation fluid and submerging the laparoscope to appreciate the three-dimensional configuration of clear lesions. Subtle lesions are likely to originate from microscopic glands; they appear and disappear like blebs on the peritoneal surface. With progressive fibrosis, these implants become the classic pigmented, scarred lesions, and finally, when fibrosis replaces the stroma, they appear as white, inactive disease.

The ability to detect subtle lesions of endometriosis increases with the experience of the surgeon and is reinforced by histologic confirmation. Although depth perception is impaired when the monocular lens of the laparoscope is used to view the pelvic cavity, the magnification ability of this lens when closely approximated to the peritoneum may allow identification of subtle surface irregularities present in occult disease. Magnification up to 10× power can be obtained with the laparoscope, depending on the working distance. Microscopic implants of endometriosis not visible even with 10× magnifica-

TABLE 25.5.
Histologic Confirmation of Lesions Categorized by Appearance

Investigators	Confirmation by Appearance (%)						
	Black	White	Red	Glandular	Subovarian Adhesions	Yellow-Brown Patches	Pockets
Jansen and Russell, 1986	—	81	81	67	50	47	47
Stripling et al, 1988	97	91	75	—	—	33	—
Martin et al, 1989	94	80	75	66	39	22	39

tion have been documented by scanning electron microscopy in peritoneal biopsies of patients with unexplained infertility who had no evidence of disease at the time of laparoscopy. Similarly, a scanning electron microscopic study of samples of supposedly normal tissue from endometriosis patients has documented the presence of endometriotic foci in 25% of cases. Lesions as small as 200 μm have been identified. Hence, surgical treatment of all visible disease is more accurately described as cytoreductive rather than ablative.

An ovarian endometrial cyst is usually formed by an inversion of the ovarian cortex. The frontal surface of the ovary in proximity to the hilus is the most common site for the invagination process to occur. Adhesions are common from the ovary to the fossa ovarica or to the posterior leaf of the parametrium. Recognition of deep ovarian endometriosis is necessary for correct surgical staging. Small endometriomas were diagnosed in 48% of infertile women with mildly enlarged ovaries (3.5 to 5 cm in diameter) when the ovaries were punctured with a 16-gauge needle. The ovarian surfaces were without gross disease in this series of patients. Preoperative sonographic evaluation is a useful screening test for the presence of small endometrial cysts; their identification may affect the disease categorization to which the patient is assigned. Sonographic patterns may indicate purely cystic features, cystic features with few septations or minimal debris, complex combinations of cystic and solid elements, and largely solid features. More recently, fat-saturated magnetic resonance imaging has been shown to be an acceptable tool for detecting endometriomas larger than 4 mm in diameter. Deep ovarian endometriosis is frequently associated with the presence of intestinal or more extensive pelvic disease.

Vercellini and colleagues studied the visual diagnostic parameters of ovarian endometriomas at laparotomy in 245 women with ovarian cysts. The gross characteristics that established the diagnosis included a size smaller than 12 cm in diameter; adhesions to the pelvic side wall, to the posterior broad ligament, or to both; the presence of powder-burn lesions; superficial endometriosis with adjacent puckering on the surface of the ovary; and tarry, thick, chocolate-colored fluid content. These criteria yielded a sensitivity of 97%, a specificity of 95%, and an accuracy of 96%.

An adnexal mass in a patient with known pelvic endometriosis cannot be assumed to be an endometrial cyst of the ovary. Ovarian malignancy must remain in the differential diagnosis; the size of the mass has been correlated with malignancy. In a study of 180 women, 1% of masses smaller than 5 cm, 11% of masses between 5 and 10 cm, and 72% of masses larger than 10 cm were malignant. In 1957, Thompson reported 20 cases of ovarian malignancy arising in ovarian endometriosis. Most of these malignant tumors were adenocarcinoma; one was a carcinosarcoma. Thompson also reported 17 cases of ovarian adenoacanthoma, 7 of which definitely arose from endometriosis.

The rules that apply to the management of all women in whom an adnexal mass develops also apply to patients with endometriosis with an adnexal mass. Among women of reproductive age, unilateral adnexal masses that are cystic and unilocular with regular borders on ultrasound examination are likely to be benign, whereas masses with solid areas, septa, papillations, or irregular borders have a greater likelihood of being malignant. Endometriomas vary in their appearance but usually have regular borders and slightly thickened and diffuse internal echoes unless fresh hemorrhage is present.

The depth of peritoneal infiltration by endometriosis cannot be evaluated by inspection alone. Deep endometriosis, which is almost exclusively localized to the posterior cul-de-sac and the uterosacral ligaments, is better detected by palpation and becomes even more apparent during excision. Deep endometriosis has been recognized to become smaller with increasing depth, although in some women the largest volume is hidden under an adhesion involving the bowel or is buried in the rectovaginal septum. Diagnosis is enhanced if clinical examinations are performed during menstruation in women with chronic pelvic pain, severe dysmenorrhea, or deep dyspareunia. In most cases, a nodule is more palpable at this time.

Koninckx and Martin have described three types of infiltrating endometriosis. Type I is characterized by a large pelvic area of typical or subtle lesions surrounded by white sclerotic tissue. During excision, deep disease becomes obvious and grows progressively smaller with deeper sectioning of tissue (like a cone). Type II is formed by retraction of the bowel and is recognized clinically as a small classic lesion associated with retraction. In some women, no implant is visible but induration is associated with the retraction. Excision usually reveals the presence of a nodule. Type III is nodular endometriosis of the rectovaginal septum. This category is clinically suspected at the time of rectovaginal examination when painful nodularities are noted. Occasionally, nodular endometriosis presents as small, typical lesions at laparoscopy or as dark blue cysts at the vaginal fornix during speculum examination. Type III disease is the most severe and often spreads laterally to involve the ureter.

CLASSIFICATIONS

Many endometriosis classification systems have been introduced to allow direct comparison of patient responses to medical and surgical treatments and to identify factors predictive of disease outcome. No system has yet been devised that is entirely satisfactory. The AFS organized a panel of experts in 1979 to develop a classification system that might serve as a basis for evaluating various therapies. By attempting to quantify the location and extent of endometriosis with a scalar rather than numeric terminology, the committee devised an innovative scheme based on the natural progression of the disease. Three anatomic areas—the peritoneum, ovary, and fallopian tube—were examined for the presence of endometriosis or adhesions, with allowances made for unilateral involvement. However, the system was not weighted for depth of infiltration of peritoneal implants. A point system instead assigned values to each area of disease involvement based on the presumption that implant area and adhesion characteristics were most often associated with disease prognosis. The stage of disease was determined by the cumulative score of the assigned points. This classification system was criticized for its arbitrary division of endometriosis into categories that did not necessarily reflect the true relative risk of disease sequelae, pain, and infertility.

The AFS classification was revised in 1985 to provide a more standard assessment of endometriosis for correlation of surgical treatment with distribution and severity of implants (Table 25.6). The point range of mild disease was expanded and greater weight was given to deep endometriosis, dense adhesions, and cul-de-sac obliteration by adhesive disease. Although the revised staging system appropriately acknowledges the importance of adhesive

disease and endometriomas, most women with extensive peritoneal disease in the absence of ovarian involvement, particularly deeply invasive implants, receive a very low score on laparoscopic inspection of the lesions.

This revised AFS classification has been widely used by investigators to categorize disease states. Nevertheless, direct comparison of treatment outcome is compromised by inconsistencies in the application of the staging criteria and by the great variations in medical and surgical therapeutic options being applied in the management of endometriosis. Evaluation of the extent of disease by laparoscopy may be limited by a lack of recognition of atypical implants, particularly if the patient is hypoestrogenic as a result of recent discontinuation of medical therapy for endometriosis. Furthermore, the divisions between stages of endometriosis remained arbitrary, the point score for ovarian involvement was weighted too heavily, and the classification scheme did not address disease involving the fallopian tubes, intestines, or urinary tract. Also, there were no parameters to indicate the present activity and state of evolution of the disease. Active endometrial tissue is usually found in the white lesions.

The Endometriosis Classification Subcommittee of the American Society for Reproductive Medicine released new recommendations in 1996 for the documentation of the extent and location of disease. One concern over the reproducibility of the scoring system was directed at the variability in assessing ovarian endometriosis and cul-de-sac obliteration. The subcommittee indicated that an endometriotic cyst should be confirmed by histology or by the presence of the following features: (1) cyst diameter less than 12 cm; (2) adhesion to pelvic side wall and/or broad ligament; (3) endometriosis on surface of ovary; (4) tarry, thick, chocolate-colored fluid content. Cul-de-sac obliteration should be considered partial if some normal peritoneum is visible below the uterosacral ligaments, but adhesions or endometriosis have obliterated part of the cul-de-sac. Complete obliteration exists when no peritoneum is visible below the uterosacral ligaments. Because information is accumulating to suggest that the morphologic appearance of the endometriotic implants may correlate with biologic activity and consequently fertility, the newly revised classification scheme requests the categorization of lesions as red, white, and black. The percentage of surface involvement of each implant type is to be documented.

The revised AFS (ASRM) classification system is oriented toward the infertile population. Muzii and colleagues, using a pain questionnaire administered to women before surgery, found a significant correlation between the severity of dysmenorrhea and total revised AFS score, partial score for deep disease, and partial score for adhesions. However, they found no correlation between the pain score for dysmenorrhea and the partial score for superficial disease, number of typical and atypical implants, or the total number of implants. Limited knowledge of the specific pathophysiologic alterations by which endometriosis can cause these symptoms has so far prevented any precise categorization of disease based on response to conventional therapies for these symptoms.

TABLE 25.6.
The American Fertility Society Revised Classification of Endometriosis[a]

Endometriosis	<1 cm	1–3 cm	>3 cm
Peritoneum			
Superficial	1	2	4
Deep	2	4	6
Ovary			
Right superficial	1	2	4
Right deep	4	16	20
Left superficial	1	2	4
Left deep	4	16	20

Posterior Cul-de-Sac Obliteration	Partial		Complete
	4		40

Adhesions	<1/3 Enclosure	1/3–2/3 Enclosure	>2/3 Enclosure
Ovary			
Right filmy	1	2	4
Right dense	4	8	16
Left filmy	1	2	4
Left dense	4	8	16
Tube			
Right filmy	1	2	4
Right dense	4[b]	8[b]	16
Left filmy	1	2	4
Left dense	4[b]	8[b]	16

[a] Determination of the stage or degree of endometrial involvement is based on a weighted point system. The following categories have been established: stage I (minimal disease) 1–5 points; stage II (mild disease) 6–15 points; stage III (moderate disease) 16–40 points; stage IV (severe disease) >40 points.

[b] If the fimbriated end of the fallopian tube is completely enclosed, change the point assignment to 16.

THERAPIES

Although women with endometriosis can present with a range of symptoms, therapy is usually initiated for the correction of pain, infertility, or a persistent pelvic mass. Pain and infertility can coexist in a patient; nevertheless, many women with endometriosis-associated infertility have relatively little or no discomfort. Treatment options vary depending on the clinical history and findings at the time of surgery.

Expectant Management

Treatment of mild and moderate endometriosis with hormonal preparations may not offer any advantage over expectant management in promoting conception. In studies by Seibel and colleagues, Hull and associates, and Telimaa, patients assigned to expectant management conceived earlier than the medically treated group, and the cumulative pregnancy rate was not higher for women receiving progestogens or danazol. This lack of enhancement of fecundity may be related to the lower number of estrogen, progesterone, and androgen receptors in endometriotic lesions as compared with normal endometrium. Nevertheless, patients with minimal or mild disease who have pelvic pain or dysmenorrhea do benefit from hormonal therapy.

The age of the patient and the duration of her infertility are important factors to consider in determining the appropriate therapy for the symptomatic individual. Laparoscopic laser ablation of milder stages of endometriosis appears to lessen the interval to conception, although the cumulative pregnancy rate may not be greater than that of women managed expectantly. Surgical therapy for more advanced disease results in a higher pregnancy rate than does expectant management or hormonal treatment, partly because of correction of mechanical factors that may be inhibiting ovulation or tubal function. There is no direct evidence to support the contention that surgical treatment of minimal or mild endometriosis in the asymptomatic patient will hinder future disease progression and sequelae. The potential benefits of cytoreductive therapy must be weighed against the risk of adhesion formation through surgical devitalization of peritoneal surfaces.

Medical Treatment

Mild pain symptoms associated with endometriosis may be effectively treated with nonsteroidal antiinflammatory agents and oral contraceptives. Additional endocrinologic therapies include progestogens, danazol, and GnRH agonists. These agents have similar degrees of efficacy in the relief of pain symptoms; side effects vary depending on their mechanism of action.

Progestogens

High-dose combination estrogen/progestogen regimens were introduced in the late 1950s for the symptomatic relief of moderate to severe pain associated with endometriosis. The rationale for this therapy was based on the observation that pregnancy provided subjective and objective improvement in many patients with extensive pelvic endometriosis. As is often seen in pregnancy, high doses of estrogens and progestogens are thought to transform endometrial tissue into decidua that ultimately undergoes necrosis and involution. Oral contraceptives with strongly progestational properties have been prescribed in the past. Typical regimens included an initial dose of 2 tablets daily; the dose was increased by 1 to 2 tablets at biweekly intervals until the patient was amenorrheic or was receiving the equivalent of 20 mg of norethynodrel. This dose was continued for 6 to 9 months. Although this combination therapy did relieve pelvic pain and dysmenorrhea in 50% to 80% of patients, significant side effects were encountered, including weight gain, mastalgia, nausea, headaches, and irregular bleeding. As a result, the discontinuation rate was high.

Because of these side effects and the potential risks of the high-dose administration of estrogen in some patients, progestogen-only regimens have gained favor over the continuous high-dose oral contraceptive schedule for creating a pseudopregnancy state. Progestogens inhibit the pituitary release of LH and thereby suppress ovarian steroidogenesis and promote secretory changes in the glandular epithelium and decidualization of the endometrial stroma. Progestogens oppose the growth-promoting effects of estrogens on the endometrial tissue by altering the clearance of the nuclear estrogen receptor and inducing 17β-hydroxysteroid dehydrogenase, which converts estradiol to the weaker estrone. Moreover, by eliminating cyclic bleeding and suppressing uterine contractility, progestogens prevent reflux menstruation, a potential stimulus for continued endometriosis development.

Luciano and colleagues administered medroxyprogesterone acetate, 50 mg daily for 4 months, to symptomatic women with moderate to severe endometriosis. Improvement of pain, pelvic nodularity, and tenderness on examination occurred in 80% of patients. Twenty percent of women experienced breakthrough bleeding, and an additional 10% reported persistent cyclic bleeding. Minor weight gain, edema, and increased irritability were other described side effects, which were generally well tolerated. A lower daily dose of 30 mg may provide equivalent relief of symptoms. Compared with the cost of danazol and GnRH agonists, which are the other commonly prescribed agents, the low cost of the medroxyprogesterone acetate is a notable advantage.

Parenteral depot medroxyprogesterone acetate has also been used to produce long periods of amenorrhea and elicit direct progestational changes of the endometrial tissue. A regimen of 150 mg intramuscularly every 3 months for 1 year has been used to manage endometriosis patients with moderate to severe pelvic pain. Twenty-nine of 40 subjects (72.5%) were satisfied with their pain relief after 1 year of therapy.

A similar response rate can be obtained with megestrol acetate. Doses of 40 mg per day for up to 24 months resulted in significant relief of dysmenorrhea, noncyclic pelvic pain, and dyspareunia in 86% of subjects.

The rate of recurrence of symptomatic endometriosis after progestogen therapy appears to be related to the length of follow-up. Riva and colleagues reported an 18% rate after an average of 11 months, whereas Moghissi and Boyce described a 42% recurrence rate during a 2-year interval after discontinuation of medication.

Relief of pelvic pain, particularly cramping associated with menstruation, can be achieved with cyclic administration of low-dose oral contraceptive pills. This line of therapy should be considered for the woman with mild symptoms who is not attempting to conceive. Low dose (20 to 35 µg ethinyl estradiol) combination oral contraceptives may be given daily for 6 to 9 months without break to relieve pain or more severe dysmenorrhea. The dose may be increased to 2 or more tablets per day for several days to alleviate episodes of breakthrough bleeding.

Danazol

Danazol is a synthetic (2,3-isoxazole) derivative of 17α-ethinyl testosterone that was introduced into clinical practice by Greenblatt and colleagues in 1971 after good performance in uncontrolled trials. The drug gained rapid acceptance because of its effectiveness in relieving pain associated with endometriosis and in enhancing fertility. All of the progestational and the weak androgenic effects of the drug result from retention of the methyl group in the 19 position of the steroid nucleus, whereas the oral activity of danazol is ascribed to the ethinyl group at position 17.

The pharmacologic action of danazol is complex. By directly inhibiting GnRH secretion, the midcycle LH surge is ablated, although basal gonadotropin concentrations are maintained. The drug interacts with endometrial androgen and progesterone receptors, suppresses the activity of multiple enzymes necessary for ovarian and adrenal steroidogenesis, and displaces androgens from sex hormone–binding globulin, thereby augmenting androgen action on endometrial receptors. The decline in sex hormone–binding globulin induced by danazol lowers estradiol binding, increases estradiol clearance, and promotes a decline in the circulating level of this hormone. Hence, the derivative has direct androgenic and antiprogestational action on endometrial implants and creates a hypoestrogenic, hypoprogestational environment antagonistic to endometriosis. Moreover, by producing amenorrhea, danazol prevents peritoneal seeding of refluxed endometrial tissue. In addition, danazol is capable of suppressing elevated autoantibodies in several autoimmune diseases and has been shown to decrease immunoglobulin and autoantibody levels in women with endometriosis. In contrast to GnRH agonists, danazol use maintains a normal estrogenic state and increases bone mineral density over baseline.

The adverse effects of danazol reflect its anabolic, androgenic, and antiestrogenic properties and may be dose-related (Fig. 25.3). Weight gain, muscle cramps, decreased breast size, and vasomotor symptoms are noted in 50% or more of patients maintained on doses of 400 to 800 mg per day. In Buttram's 1985 series, 41% of patients treated with the standard dose of 800 mg per day gained more than 10 pounds during the course of therapy. The threefold increase in free testosterone can cause acne, oily skin, and deepening of the voice in a small percentage of recipients. High-density lipoprotein (HDL) cholesterol declines by 50% or more in response to the altered steroid concentrations; an 80% decrease in the HDL_2 subfraction has been reported. Most series have described a concomitant increase in low-density lipoprotein (LDL) cholesterol; the alteration in the ratio of HDL to LDL cholesterol may be an unacceptable risk to some patients. Because danazol is metabolized by the liver, modest elevations in serum glutamic oxaloacetic transaminase and serum glutamate pyruvate transaminase may arise. Reported idiopathic drug reactions include gastrointestinal disturbances, weakness, dizziness, skin rashes, headaches, and muscle cramps. Bothersome side effects occur in as many as 85% of patients, and at least 10% of women receiving danazol discontinue pharmacologic treatment because the adverse effects are intolerable. Combining danazol therapy with aerobic exercise appears to reduce the incidence of many of these androgenic side effects. Preliminary data from trials using danazol rings suggest that this route of administration may result in symptomatic improvement of pain while avoiding the androgenic side effects noted with oral administration.

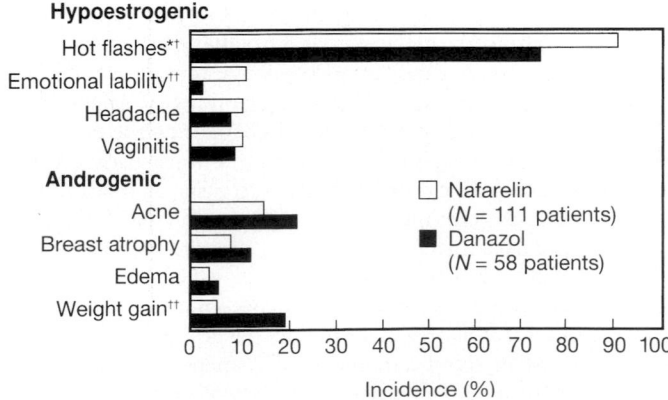

FIGURE 25.3. Summary of most frequent adverse effects associated with therapy in patients receiving danazol or nafarelin. *Women with hot flashes before treatment were excluded (one had danazol, five had nafarelin). + $p <$ .01 for between-treatment difference. ++ $p <$ .05 for between-treatment difference. (Redrawn from Burry KA. Nafarelin in the management of endometriosis: quality of life assessment. *Am J Obstet Gynecol* 1992;166:735)

Because of the potential androgenic action of this hormone on the developing fetus, the patient must not be pregnant when initiating therapy. Barrier contraception has been recommended for the entire course of treatment to eliminate the possibility of conception, although high doses of danazol usually cause anovulation.

The amenorrhea induced by danazol has been found to benefit patients with dysmenorrhea, dyspareunia, and cyclic pelvic pain associated with endometriosis. Young and Blackmore reviewed the effects of different dosages of danazol with respect to relief of symptoms in 452 patients. At a dose of 800 mg, 95% of patients noted relief of dysmenorrhea, and 89% reported relief of pelvic pain. At a dose of 400 mg, posttherapeutic relief was reduced by 10%. Moore and associates reported that pain associated with minimal and moderate pelvic endometriosis appeared to respond well to doses of danazol of 400 mg or less per day, whereas severe endometriosis was best treated with doses greater than 400 mg per day. A 6-year prospective study that evaluated the effectiveness of danazol at two doses (400 mg and 800 mg) in carefully classified patients concluded that there was no difference in side effects between the two doses and that gross resolutions of disease at second-look laparoscopy were similar. However, ovarian endometriosis greater than 1 cm did not respond as well to either dose of danazol as did peritoneal or ovarian disease less than 1 cm.

Recurrence of symptoms within 4 to 12 months of discontinuation of danazol therapy approaches 50% in most studies. Puleo and Hammond found that pain recurred in 38% of patients after a mean of 6.9 months; active disease was found within 1 year in 51% of women. Lower daily doses of medication or courses of treatment less than 4 months in duration may result in a shorter symptom-free interval.

Danazol has been extensively prescribed as therapy for endometriosis-associated infertility, although there are no well-controlled studies to support this indication. Pregnancy rates after the use of danazol as the sole therapy have ranged from 30.9% to 52.6% in mild endometriosis, 23.1% to 50% in moderate disease, and 0% to 100% in severe stages. Monthly fecundity rates range from 1.6% to 6.8%. The findings of many early studies have been questioned because of their lack of randomization, failure to include an expectant management control group, and failure to account for other infertility factors. Recent data concerning medical therapy of minimal, mild, and moderate stages of disease refute the notion that danazol may enhance conception. When all other infertility factors are excluded, the estimated monthly fecundity rate with expectant management of mild endometriosis is 8.7%. Furthermore, conception is delayed while the patient is receiving danazol.

Gonadotropin-Releasing Hormone Agonists

GnRH agonists are available for use in the treatment of estrogen-dependent diseases such as endometriosis. Some of the more frequently studied analogs include leuprolide, nafarelin, buserelin, and goserelin. Alteration of the amino acid at position 6 and ethylamide replacement of the C-terminal amino acid of the native decapeptide hormone results in a GnRH agonist with increased resistance to lysosomal degradation. Pituitary receptor binding is enhanced, resulting in a decline in the number of receptors available for further occupancy. Continued administration of the GnRH agonist leads to a desensitization of the pituitary gonadotrope receptor and a reversible downregulation of the pituitary-ovarian axis. Ovarian estrogen secretion may reach castrate levels.

The initial response to GnRH agonist administration is a markedly increased secretion of pituitary stores of follicle-stimulating hormone (FSH) and LH. If therapy is begun in the follicular phase of the menstrual cycle, the developing follicle may respond to the flare in circulating gonadotropin levels with a rapid increase in estradiol production. Estradiol levels may remain elevated for 3 weeks before declining. GnRH agonist administration in the luteal phase leads to a more rapid decline in estrogen secretion, although FSH and LH levels remain elevated for 1 and 4 weeks, respectively.

GnRH agonist treatment results in improvement or resolution of pain symptoms in all stages of disease. Lemay and colleagues reported resolution of pain in 70% and improvement in discomfort in 15% of 24 subjects after 2 to 4 months of treatment with the agonist buserelin. Dyspareunia improved in 9% and disappeared in 91% of patients studied. The depot formulation of leuprolide acetate has also been shown to significantly reduce dysmenorrhea, pelvic pain, and pelvic tenderness in patients with endometriosis.

Henzl and associates, in a double-blind, multicenter study, treated 213 patients with either danazol or nafarelin. After 6 months of treatment, more than 80% of patients in all groups experienced a significant reduction in visible implants. A 43% reduction in AFS score was noted for each treatment group; there was no difference in response among patients receiving the 0.4- and 0.8-mg daily dose of nafarelin. Most patients continued to demonstrate some visible implants at the time of follow-up laparoscopy, and, as with danazol, there was some diminution in size of endometriomas but no effect on preexisting adhesions.

The optimal interval of GnRH analog administration has been widely debated. Six months of medication has been traditionally prescribed, although a significant reduction in implant volume occurs as early as 2 weeks after initiation of treatment in the rat model. A maximal effect was measured after 4 weeks of therapy in this animal study, suggesting that short courses of drug may be as efficacious as 6 months of continuous therapy. The regrowth of lesions after estrogen therapy has been reported years after the menopause; hence, hypoestrogenism results in inactivation rather than resolution of the disease.

Response to therapy may be dependent on route of administration. Donnez and colleagues reported that buserelin administration by a long-acting subcutaneous implant led to a greater reduction in endometriosis score, mitotic index, and endometrial cyst diameter than when given in an intranasal form. This may have been due to a greater consistency in hormonal release by the injected preparation.

As occurs with danazol and progestogen regimens, symptoms recur at variable periods after discontinuation of GnRH analog therapy. Subjective return of pain occurred in 57% of patients within 6 months of discontinuing leuprolide, although 37% with moderate or severe pelvic pain at baseline were still improved at 1 year. Franssen and colleagues noted a lasting and significant amelioration of dysmenorrhea and dyspareunia 6 months after completion of treatment; however, scores for chronic pelvic pain had nearly reached their pretreatment level once this time had elapsed. Patients with a higher disease stage at the onset are more likely to experience recurrence and to experience it earlier than patients with minimal disease. One treatment option for such patients may be a second 3-month course of GnRH analog. Henzl reported a significant decrease in mean pain scores and essentially no change in compact bone density in most patients when nafarelin was readministered for 3 months after a treatment-free interval of 6 months or more.

The effect of GnRH analog on endometriosis-associated infertility is difficult to assess because of a lack of an expectant management control group in most clinical studies. The preliminary pregnancy rates, which range from 0% to 60%, are derived from trials that do categorize response based on stage of disease.

Most of the side effects associated with GnRH analog therapy are related to hypoestrogenism. Hot flashes are common and can lead to sleep disturbances and chronic fatigue in extreme cases (Fig. 25.3). Vaginal dryness, superficial dyspareunia, headaches, and depression have been reported. In general, these adverse effects are better tolerated than those experienced with danazol use. In addition, there are no undesirable changes in HDL, LDL, or total cholesterol throughout the prolonged period of hypoestrogenism induced by GnRH analog, unlike the changes accompanying danazol intake.

A decline in trabecular bone mineral content and an increase in urinary calcium excretion to menopausal levels occur during the course of GnRH analog therapy in about two thirds of patients. Quantitated computed tomographic studies consistently show significant loss of trabecular bone of the vertebrae and hip with GnRH analog exposure. Restoration of normal estrogen production after cessation of therapy appears to at least partially reverse these bone changes. In a study of the GnRH agonist goserelin, an 8.2% decline in density of the lumbar spine was measured after completion of 6 months of treatment; this improved to a mean loss of 5.4% at 6 months postcessation. Others found no significant change from baseline after a 6-month course of GnRH analog when bone density was assessed 6 months after treatment.

Concomitant administration of a progestogen during the course of GnRH analog therapy has been examined to ameliorate vasomotor symptoms and retard both urinary calcium excretion and radiologic evidence of loss of bone mineral density. Cedars and co-workers reported a diminution in the side effects mentioned earlier when medroxyprogesterone acetate was administered at a dose of 20 to 30 mg per day during the 6-month course of agonist therapy; however, laparoscopic evaluation after completion of therapy failed to reveal any improvement or suppression of active endometriosis with the combination regimen, and the regimen failed to significantly reduce symptoms of pelvic pain. Conversely, Makarainen and colleagues reported that medroxyprogesterone acetate, 100 mg per day, diminished hot flushes and the urinary excretion of calcium in women treated with goserelin acetate, 3.6 mg monthly, for 6 months. Second-look laparoscopy revealed equivalent diminution in extent of endometriosis when compared with the goserelin-progestin placebo group.

Norethindrone, a 19-nortestosterone progestin, has been shown to suppress both the painful symptoms of endometriosis and the extent of disease at laparoscopy when used in daily doses of 1.4 mg to 10 mg during GnRH agonist therapy. A recent randomized, double-blind study has demonstrated that GnRH agonist therapy may be safely and effectively extended for up to 1 year in the management of endometriosis-associated pelvic pain when prescribed in conjunction with low-dose sex steroid hormones. Hornstein et al. reported that norethindrone acetate, 5 mg, alone or in combination with conjugated equine estrogens, 0.625 mg daily, from the onset of depot leuprolide acetate therapy alleviated hypoestrogenic symptoms and preserved bone density while resulting in equivalent pain relief to that achieved by the placebo estrogen-progestin patient group.

The addition of calcium carbonate and alendronate or etidronate sodium, which are organic bisphosphonates, to the low-dose norethindrone acetate add-back therapy in patients with symptomatic endometriosis receiving prolonged GnRH agonist treatment may further minimize the adverse side effects of hypoestrogenism. Additional controlled studies will better establish the optimal medical management of this condition.

Conservative Surgery

Endoscopic assessment of the pelvis allows determination of the appropriate therapy for the patient with endometriosis. Surgery is indicated for correction of pain, infertility, or other symptoms in patients with extensive pelvic endometriosis, or when hormonal manipulation fails to adequately diminish pain symptoms in women with lesser stages of disease (Table 25.7). Surgery is successful in relieving pain in a very high percentage of cases and offers a better prognosis for pregnancy than does endocrine therapy in cases of advanced disease. The surgeon who has mastered the specialized techniques of operative laparoscopy can treat a wide range of pathologic findings at the time of diagnosis. Therapeutic planning depends on many factors, including the age of the patient, her desire for fertility or pain relief, the duration and intensity of her symptoms, the extent of disease, and previous treatments undertaken. Preoperative rectoscopy-

TABLE 25.7.
Treatment of Endometriosis

	Desires Childbearing		Childbearing Complete
Stage of Disease	Infertility	Pelvic Pain	Pelvic Pain
Stages I and II	1. Expectant Rx 2. Laparoscopic Rx 2. Medical Rx 3. CSEL ± PSN 3. IVF/ET	1. Laparoscopic Rx 2. Medical Rx 3. CSEL + PSN	1. Laparoscopic Rx 2. Medical Rx 3. TAH ± BSO 3. CSEL ± PSN
Stage III	1. Laparoscopic Rx 1. CSEL ± PSN 2. Medical Rx 3. IVF/ET	1. Laparoscopic Rx 2. CSEL ± PSN 3. Medical Rx	1. Laparoscopic Rx 2. Medical Rx 3. TAH ± BSO 3. CSEL + PSN

Stage IV	1. CSEL + perioperative
	    medical Rx
	2. CSEL alone
	3. Laparoscopic Rx +
	    postoperative medical RX
	4. IVF/ET
		1. CSEL + PSN + peripoerative
		    medical Rx
		2. Medical Rx
		3. Laparoscopic Rx + medical Rx
			1. TAH ± BSO
			1. CSEL + PSN + medical Rx
			1. Laparoscopic Rx + medical Rx

Modified from Wheeler JM. Macro- and microsurgical treatment of endometriosis. In: Thomas E, Rock JA, eds. *Modern approaches to endometriosis.* Boston: Kluwer Academic Publishers, 1991, with permission.

Rx, treatment; CSEL, conservative surgery for endometriosis at laparotomy; PSN, presacral neurectomy; TAH, total abdominal hysterectomy; BSO, bilateral salpingo-oophorectomy; IVF/ET, *in vitro* fertilization and embryo transfer; ±, adjunctive treatment option based on individual patient findings.

sigmoidoscopy and intravenous pyelography are recommended in patients with symptoms suggestive of deeply invasive endometriosis of the posterior cul-de-sac and rectovaginal septum.

The decision of whether to perform surgical resection of endometriosis through the laparoscope or open abdomen is not entirely dependent on the stage of disease encountered. Laparoscopy can be considered for all cases unless there is difficulty in establishing the appropriate tissue planes of dissection or unless improved access is necessary for atraumatic manipulation of the involved organs. Specific endoscopic procedures include ablation of endometriotic implants, adhesiolysis, ovarian cystectomy, oophorectomy, and salpingectomy. Although the results and complications are similar, the cost savings with respect to decreased hospital expenses and loss of work time favor laparoscopy over laparotomy when other factors regarding risks and outcome are equal. Laparoscopy provides superior visualization of the posterior cul-de-sac and allows a high degree of magnification of peritoneal surfaces, which aids in the identification of subtle disease.

Conservative resection of disease by laparotomy is most valuable in cases of extensive, dense pelvic adhesions or endometriomas greater than 5 cm in diameter. In addition, deep involvement of the rectovaginal septum with fibrotic extension into the perirectal fossa, invasion of the bowel muscularis, and endometriotic infiltration in the region of the uterine vessels and ureter are generally best approached through the open abdomen for all but advanced endoscopic surgeons. The objective of the laparotomy procedure is complete excision of all endometriosis and associated adhesive disease to restore normal functional anatomy of the reproductive tract. The usual surgical approach is through a transverse suprapubic incision. A Maylard incision provides adequate exposure for presacral neurectomy and reconstructive surgery of ovarian endometriomas of almost any size.

Principles of Microsurgery

Microsurgical technique, or the philosophy of gentle manipulation of tissue in an attempt to avoid trauma, is the major tenet of pelvic reconstruction. The inflammation, trauma, coagulation, and foreign materials associated with conventional macrosurgical technique lead to tissue ischemia and adhesion formation because of local failure of the intrinsic peritoneal fibrinolytic system. Adhesion formation can be reduced by the application of loupe magnification or use of the operating microscope, reconstruction with fine, nonreactive sutures, precise hemostasis, and continuous irrigation of tissues with warmed lactated Ringer solution, each liter of which is supplemented with 5,000 U of heparin. Nevertheless, there are no definitive data to suggest that use of the particularly costly, ancillary laser and the operating microscope has appreciably improved the reproductive prognosis in the surgical management of endometriosis through laparotomy.

Several basic techniques are available for the endoscopic ablation of endometriosis, including excision, coagulation, and vaporization. Coagulation can be achieved by monopolar or bipolar cautery, thermocoagulation, or, in some circumstances, laser, depending on the wavelength of energy applied. The extent of tissue penetration in electrocautery is related to the power and type of current, the duration of application, and the size of the electrode. Less tissue damage is achieved with bipolar than with monopolar cautery. The carbon dioxide (CO_2) laser is more precise than the fiber lasers, although CO_2 laser energy is strongly absorbed by water molecules and is rendered ineffective in the presence of blood. Meticulous technique that maintains serosal integrity may reduce the incidence of *de novo* adhesion formation.

Sites of Conservative Surgery
PERITONEUM
Small lesions of superficial peritoneal endometriosis less than 5 mm in diameter are easily treated with laser or bipolar coagulation while under a constant stream of irrigation. Deep lesions or more extensive peritoneal disease must be excised with a tissue margin of at least 2 to

4 mm, because, as noted previously, microscopic lesions are commonly present in tissue adjacent to visible implants (Fig. 25.4). Ablation of deep disease by monopolar microdiathermy or CO_2 laser vaporization rather than excision of the disease may result in inadequate resection and a greater amount of ischemic damage to the tissue, heightening the propensity toward adhesion formation. Immobilizing adhesions can be merely divided during the preparatory phase of the procedure; precise excision is more easily accomplished after the involved organs are freed. Before dissection of the pelvic side wall, the ureter must be identified and isolated; it frequently is displaced from its normal location by endometriotic adhesive disease. A Lucite, Teflon, or laparoscopic titanium probe can be used to isolate adhesions and protect adjacent structures during separation of the tissue planes. Suture placement can lead to foreign body reaction, tissue anoxia, and fibrosis and should therefore be avoided. Covering hemostatic, deperitonealized surfaces with an

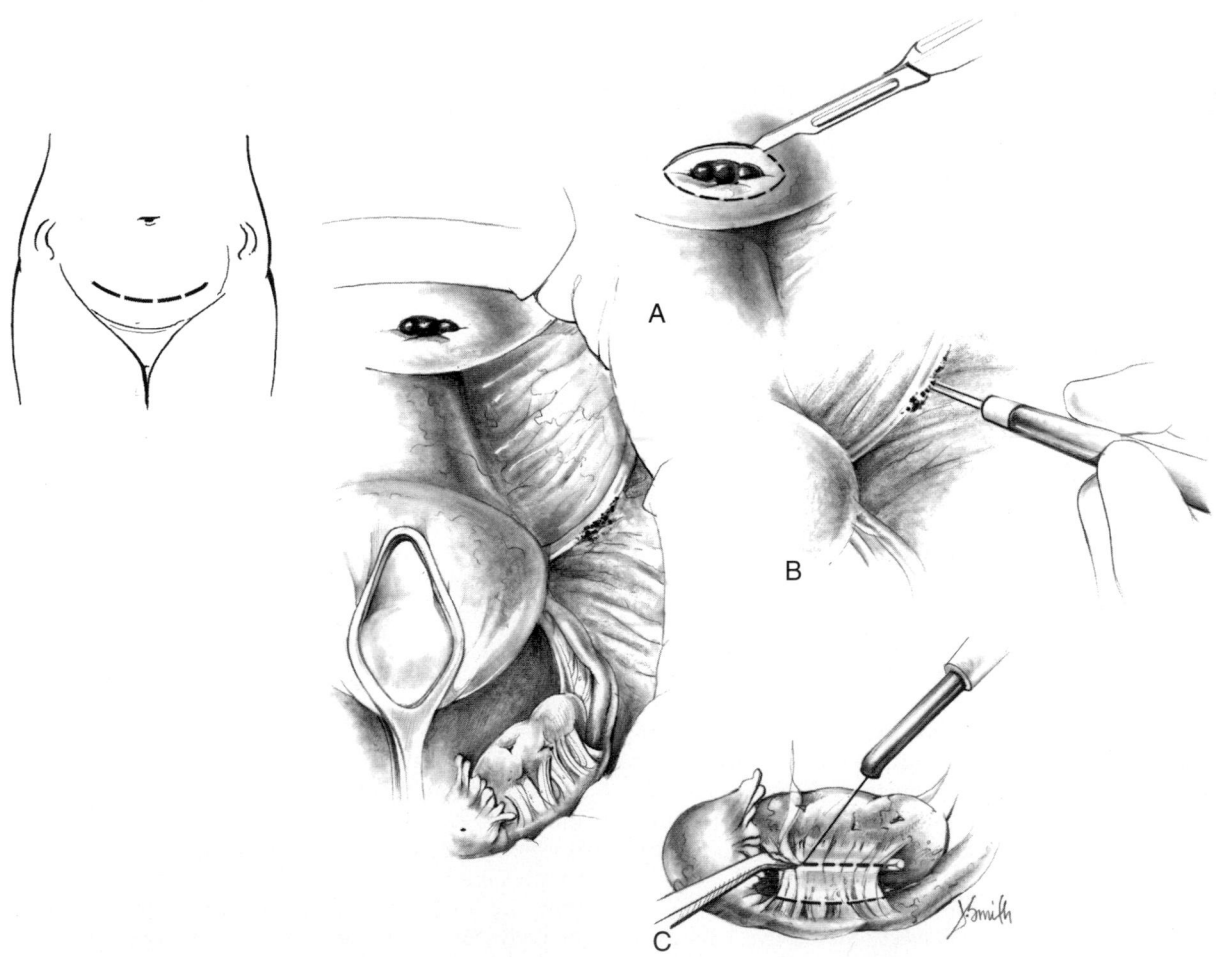

FIGURE 25.4. Excision or CO_2 laser vaporization of peritoneal implants. **A:** Superficial implants are vaporized by use of power densities between 1,000 and 3,000 W/cm^2, with a spot size of 0.8 to 1 mm, or they are cauterized with microbipolar forceps. More extensive peritoneal disease is excised. Very large defects can be closed with 5-0 or 6-0 polyglactin or polydioxanone sutures. Adhesion barriers can be placed. **B:** Endometriosis can be associated with extensive adnexal adhesions. **C:** Wide adhesion bands can be retracted with a glass rod and completely excised with a monopolar microelectrode.

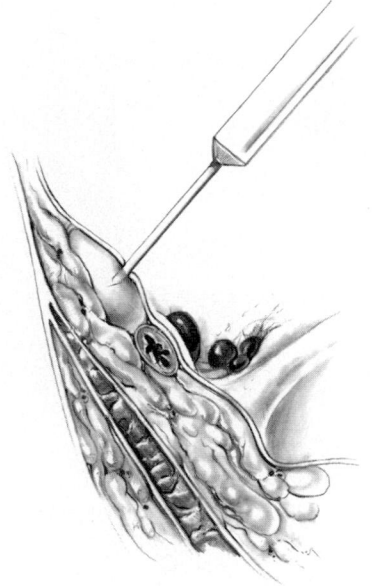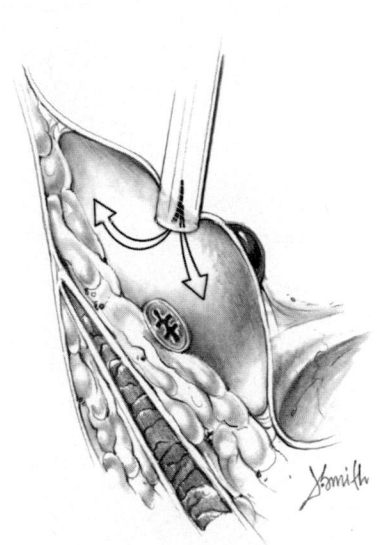

FIGURE 25.5. Hydrodissection.

absorbable, oxidized, regenerated cellulose barrier (Interceed) significantly reduces the incidence, extent, and severity of postsurgical pelvic adhesions, even in patients with severe endometriosis. Alternatively, application of the Gore-Tex surgical membrane has been shown to result in a statistical reduction in adhesion score; this barrier can be removed at the time of a second-look laparoscopic procedure if its presence would impair tuboovarian function.

Estimations of the depth of endometrial implants at the time of laparoscopic resection relate well with histologic measurements. Superficial implants can be destroyed by bipolar cauterization; however, 25% of patients have lesions greater than 5 mm in depth. Deep (greater than 5 mm) and very deep (greater than 10 mm) lesions represent an active form of the disease and occur almost exclusively in patients who complain of pain. The diagnosis of retroperitoneal endometriosis is suggested by preoperative digital rectovaginal palpation and laparoscopic blunt probe palpation. The depth of infiltration of deep lesions appears to correlate poorly with the visible surface area of involvement. The laparoscopic treatment of deep disease is often complicated by the proximity of implants to vital structures such as the ureter, bladder, and vessels. The superficial action of nonvaporizing modalities such as bipolar or thermal coagulation is not sufficient for deep disease.

Laparoscopic forceps are used to elevate and isolate the tissue to be excised. Instruments should be placed with care, because surgical manipulation of tissue that will not be resected may result in *de novo* adhesion formation. The diseased peritoneum may also be separated from underlying tissue by the technique of hydrodissection, which forcefully injects physiologic irrigant retroperitoneally through a small defect created in the peritoneum (Fig. 25.5). This retroperitoneal placement

of fluid acts to dissipate CO_2 laser energy and, in so doing, promotes safer dissection or vaporization of the peritoneal surface. Coagulation or vaporization of disease in the ovarian fossa or near the uterosacral ligament should be undertaken only after clear identification of the ureter. Uterine manipulation with a Valtchev retractor may be used while treating lesions of the posterior cul-de-sac.

Dissection of retroperitoneal disease can be facilitated by placing a bougie probe in the rectum and a sponge forceps in the vagina (Fig. 25.6). Traction in either direction opens the rectovaginal and perirectal spaces. Initial dissection of the anterior rectum provides a landmark of the retrovaginal space and permits posterior mobilization of the nodule. Subsequent lateral dissection is performed, followed by anterior dissection, which permits retrieval of the involved tissue.

It is difficult to evaluate the depth of tissue damage with electrocauterization; however, laser vaporization allows visualization of the three-dimensional boundaries of every lesion. The laser beam should be applied until the bubbling of retroperitoneal areolar tissue is noted. The zone of thermal necrosis is minimal with the CO_2 laser, particularly when applied in the superpulse mode. In the region of the ureter, urinary bladder, colon, or large blood vessels, a single or repeat pulse mode of 0.05 to 0.1 second allows a depth of penetration of 100 to 200 μm. Irrigation of the pelvis washes off debris and carbon deposition and better exposes the base of the site of laser impact. A 2- to 4-mm clear margin is desired around each lesion treated. Excision of the involved peritoneum is superior to vaporization of implants when the extent of tissue penetration cannot be recognized.

Resection of deep posterior cul-de-sac nodules requires great endoscopic expertise. A combined laparoscopic-vaginal approach may be necessary to effectively

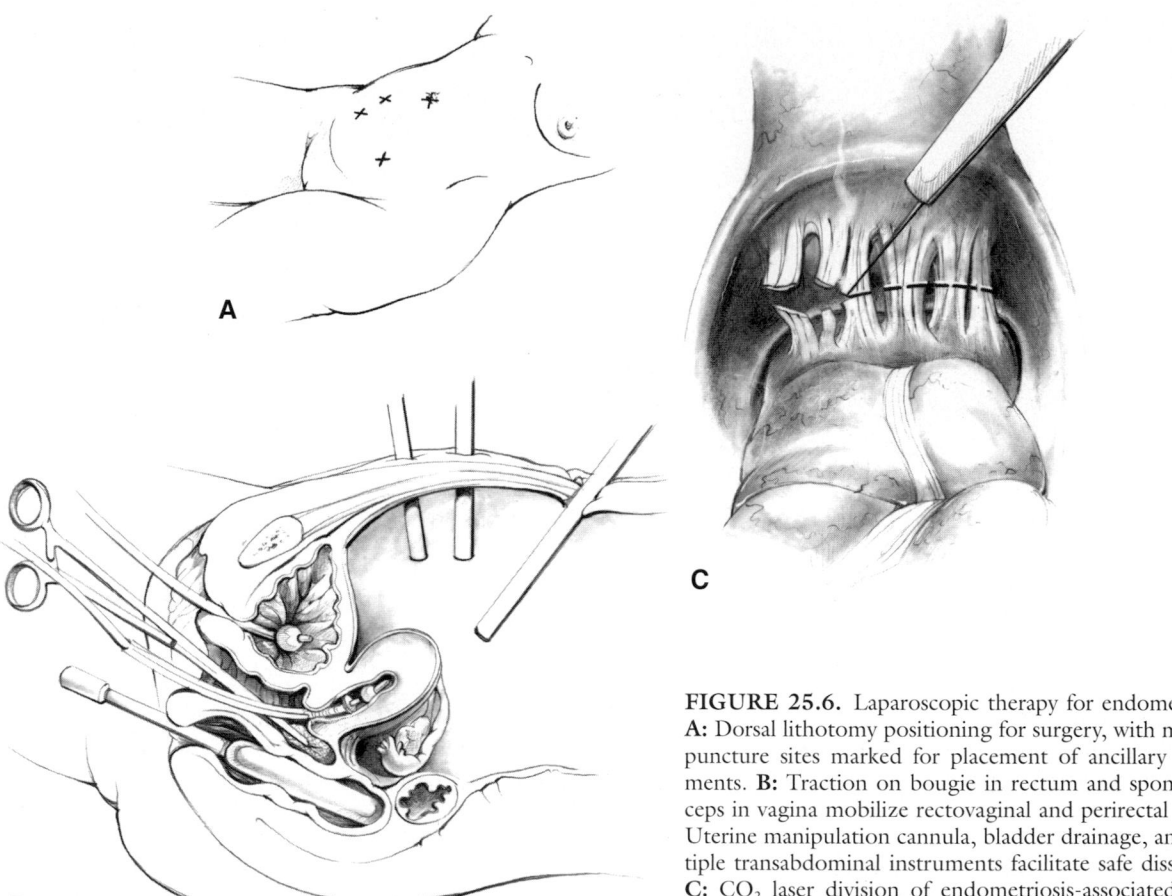

FIGURE 25.6. Laparoscopic therapy for endometriosis. **A:** Dorsal lithotomy positioning for surgery, with multiple puncture sites marked for placement of ancillary instruments. **B:** Traction on bougie in rectum and sponge forceps in vagina mobilize rectovaginal and perirectal spaces. Uterine manipulation cannula, bladder drainage, and multiple transabdominal instruments facilitate safe dissection. **C:** CO_2 laser division of endometriosis-associated adhesions extending from lower uterus to rectal serosa.

remove these implants (Fig. 25.7). It is often helpful to have an assistant place his or her fingers deep in the vaginal fornices or a bougie probe in the rectum to indicate the sites of the nodules to ensure their complete removal (Fig. 25.7). The direct palpation made possible through laparotomy may be required to recognize all indurated, deep lesions. A complete bowel preparation is mandatory in all cases of suspected deep endometriosis.

Defects in the peritoneal surface are frequently associated with endometriosis and are most commonly found in the posterior cul-de-sac region. These defects should be explored and ablated even if they appear grossly normal, because of the frequency of microscopic disease. Electrosurgery should be avoided when extensive dissection is performed because it may be associated with widespread thermal damage and difficulty in recognizing tissue planes. Superficial invasion of the muscularis of bowel or bladder can be treated with laser vaporization or endocoagulation because of the precision and lack of penetration of these energy sources. Anterior cul-de-sac treatment should be accompanied by continuous bladder drainage.

Tubal endometriosis may distort the normal anatomic relationship of the distal tube to the ovary and in severe cases may cause complete fimbrial obstruction. Short pulses of CO_2 laser may be used to vaporize lesions while

minimizing thermal damage. Endoscopic adhesiolysis of the distal tube may be accomplished with fine scissors or careful application of laser. Unipolar electrocautery should not be used on this tissue.

OVARY

Superficial endometriosis of the ovary usually presents as small, dark, punctate lesions immediately beneath the cortical surface. This disease can be readily treated with laser or bipolar forceps under constant irrigation. Occasionally, however, the small, visible lesion may be merely the tip of a large endometrial cyst. If there is any doubt, the implant should be excised and the ovary explored to determine the extent of disease. Care should be taken to minimize thermal injury to surrounding ovarian tissue. This is particularly important near the fimbria ovarica, because postoperative adhesion formation could compromise distal tubal function. Inability to elevate the ovary is usually a sign of adhesions and endometriotic implants of the inferolateral surface of the ovary and the peritoneum of the ovarian fossa.

Reconstruction by Laparotomy

Extensive ovarian endometriosis is often associated with periovarian and peritubal adhesions. These adhesions may become apparent while manipulating the ovary to visualize the lateral surface adjacent to the broad liga-

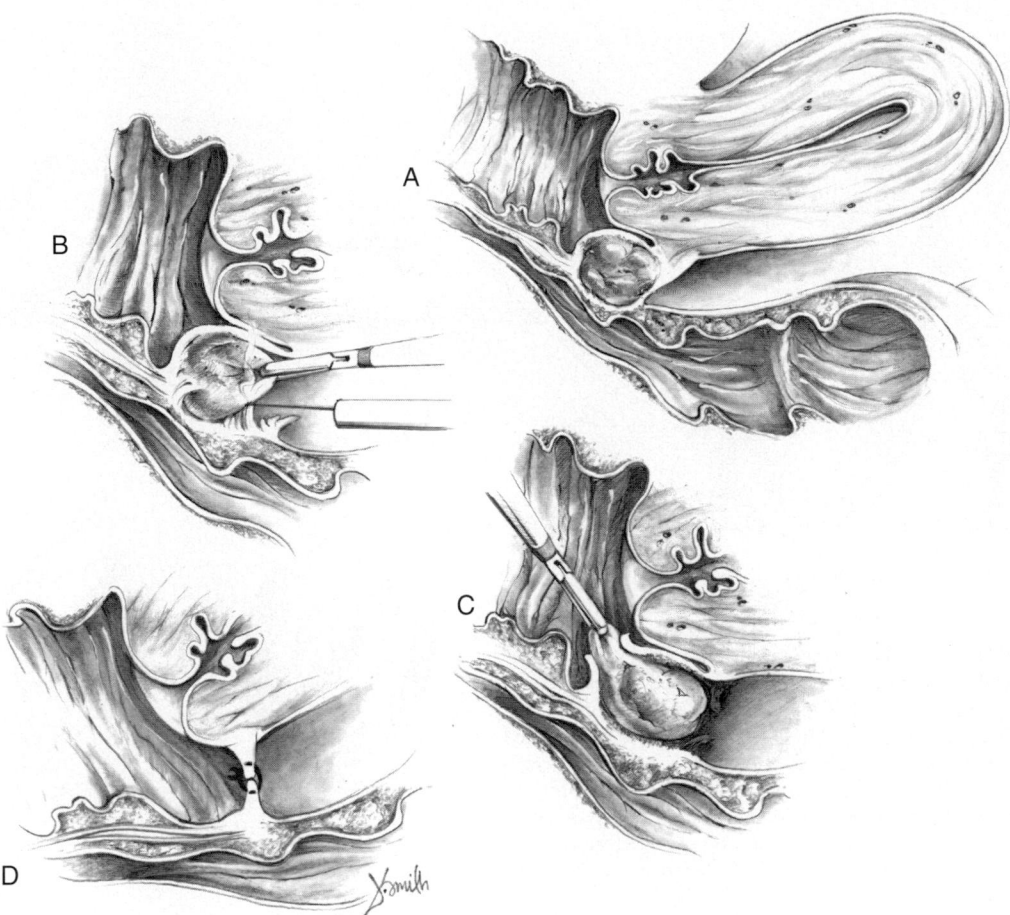

FIGURE 25.7. A: Deep laparoscopic dissection of the rectovaginal space, in combination with colpotomy, for the excision of a large endometriotic nodule of the rectovaginal septum. **B:** Initial laparoscopic dissection of nodule. **C:** Completion of dissection by way of colpotomy incision. **D:** Vaginal suture placement to reapproximate the rectovaginal septal defect.

ment. Filmy adhesions are elevated with delicate tissue forceps and can be resected with fine-needle cautery, a scalpel, or the laser. Care must be taken to maintain the integrity of the ovarian capsule. After the appropriate adhesiolysis is accomplished, the posterior cul-de-sac is packed with moist, lint-free packs, and a silicon surgical platform can be placed to stabilize the adnexa. The ovary should be carefully examined for extent of disease involvement before creation of the initial incision. Peritoneal spillage of the contents of the endometrioma can be avoided by placement of a lint-free pack around the platform.

The cortical incision should be made in a way that will preserve the normal anatomic relations of the ovary with the uteroovarian ligament and fimbria ovarica (Fig. 25.8). This is best accomplished by making a shallow longitudinal incision over the endometrioma with the monopolar microneedle, scalpel, or laser. The surgeon should attempt to remove the endometrioma in an intact state; however, if the cyst cavity is inadvertently entered, an elliptical incision around the site of rupture is useful for exposure. The intact endometrioma can be transfixed

with a traction suture of 2-0 nylon to facilitate creation of a cleavage plane between the cyst and normal ovarian tissue. Blunt, curved scissors or a flat probe or knife handle is used for dissection. Particular care must be taken when dissecting the hilar region to maintain hemostasis. An attempt should be made to preserve as much of the normal ovarian cortex as possible; pregnancies have been achieved with only a small fraction of remaining ovary.

The ovary is reconstructed by placing one or two pursestring sutures of 4-0 or 5-0 polyglactin, polyglycolic acid, or polydioxanone to eliminate the dead space and maximize hemostasis. This is followed by placement of a running subcortical 5-0 suture of the same delayed-absorbable material (Fig. 25.8). In some circumstances, less tissue distortion can be achieved by placing a deep layer of interrupted mattress sutures followed by additional layers of running sutures (Fig. 25.8). Suture on or extruding through the surface should be strictly avoided because of its adhesiogenic properties.

After the ovary has been carefully approximated, the posterior surfaces of the uterus and broad ligament are inspected for hemostasis wherever the ovary was previ-

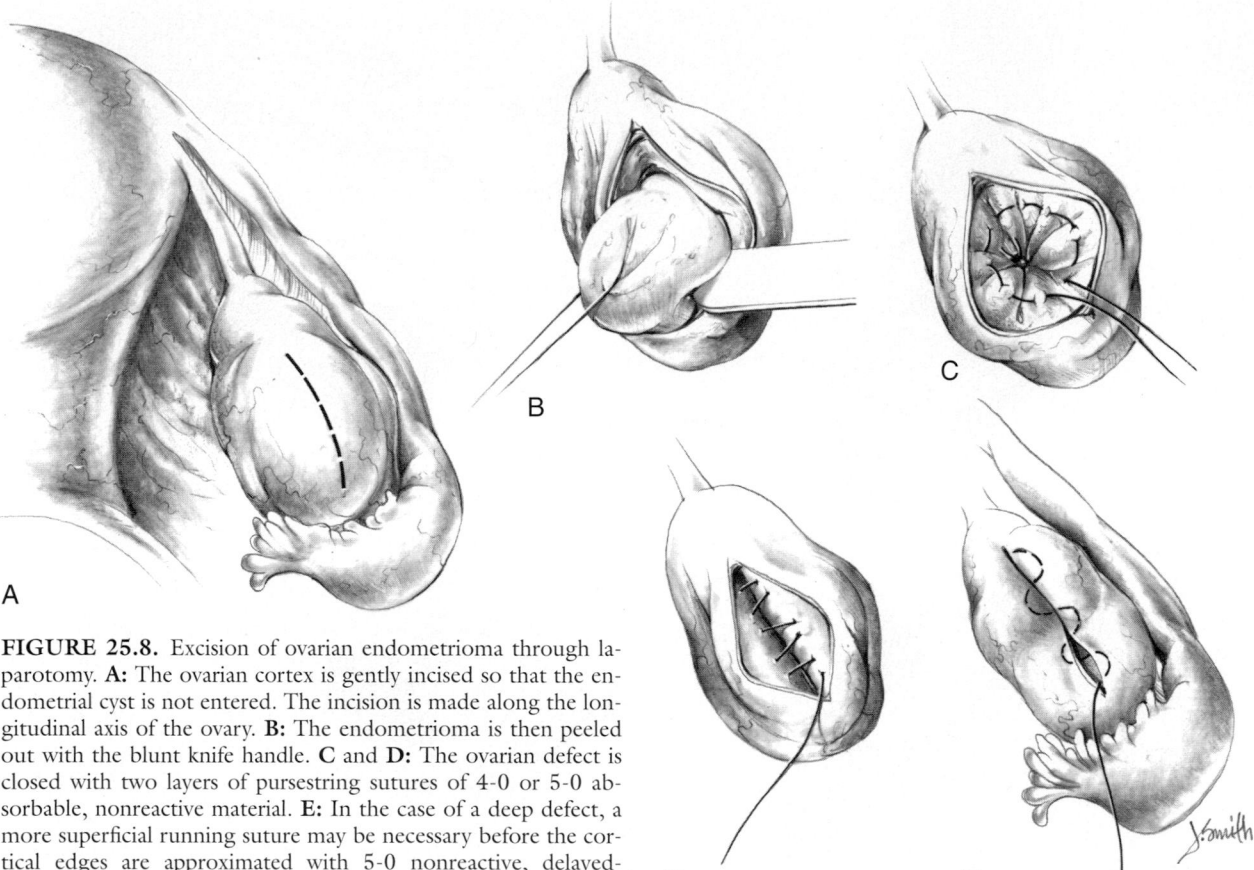

FIGURE 25.8. Excision of ovarian endometrioma through laparotomy. **A:** The ovarian cortex is gently incised so that the endometrial cyst is not entered. The incision is made along the longitudinal axis of the ovary. **B:** The endometrioma is then peeled out with the blunt knife handle. **C** and **D:** The ovarian defect is closed with two layers of pursestring sutures of 4-0 or 5-0 absorbable, nonreactive material. **E:** In the case of a deep defect, a more superficial running suture may be necessary before the cortical edges are approximated with 5-0 nonreactive, delayed-absorbable sutures.

ously adherent. Microbipolar cauterization may be necessary. Placement of an adhesion barrier is useful in separating raw peritoneal surfaces during the healing process.

Endoscopic Therapy of Ovarian Endometriosis

Surgical treatment of endometriosis less than 4 to 5 cm in diameter can be accomplished with relative ease; however, endoscopic resection of larger lesions may be compromised by the presence of dense, cohesive adhesions and by difficulties removing the entire cyst wall. The endometrioma can be excised in an intact or ruptured state during the laparoscopic procedure. In either case, the technique is initiated by longitudinally incising the cortex overlying the cyst after achieving full mobilization of the ovary by adhesiolysis. The incision is generally made along the inferior pole on the opposite side to the hilus in such a manner as to preserve the apposition of healthy ovarian tissue to the fimbria. The cyst contents are immediately drained with the suction cannula and the cavity is irrigated and inspected for papillary structures or other suspicious features. Very small endometriomas may be effectively treated by electrocoagulation of the mucosal lining. Because carbon dioxide laser is absorbed by fluid, complete ablation of the cyst wall with this energy source may be compromised in an environment rich in blood and hemosiderin. With larger endometriomas, the

normal ovarian cortex is stabilized with atraumatic forceps, and the cyst wall is grasped with biopsy forceps and stripped from the bed of normal ovarian tissue (Fig. 25.9). Hydrodissection may facilitate separation of the tissue planes. Remaining fragments of the cyst wall should be vaporized with laser or fulgurated by electrocautery. Hemostasis can be achieved with bipolar cautery.

An alternative technique involves sharp and blunt dissection to remove the cyst in an intact state. Hydrodissection is particularly useful with this approach. The cyst contents are carefully drained in a plastic laparoscopy pouch to facilitate clean removal from the peritoneal cavity.

The ovarian defect is usually left to heal spontaneously. Ischemia associated with suture placement can provoke adhesion formation after laparoscopic ovarian reconstruction. Low-power continuous carbon dioxide laser or bipolar coagulation can be applied to the inside wall of the redundant ovarian capsule to cause an inversion of the incised cortex. Most authors have reported excellent results with this no-suture technique. Rarely does the ovarian cortex need to be reapproximated with sutures. If fine, absorbable suture is used, the knot should be placed internally to minimize the possibility of it becoming a nidus for adhesion formation.

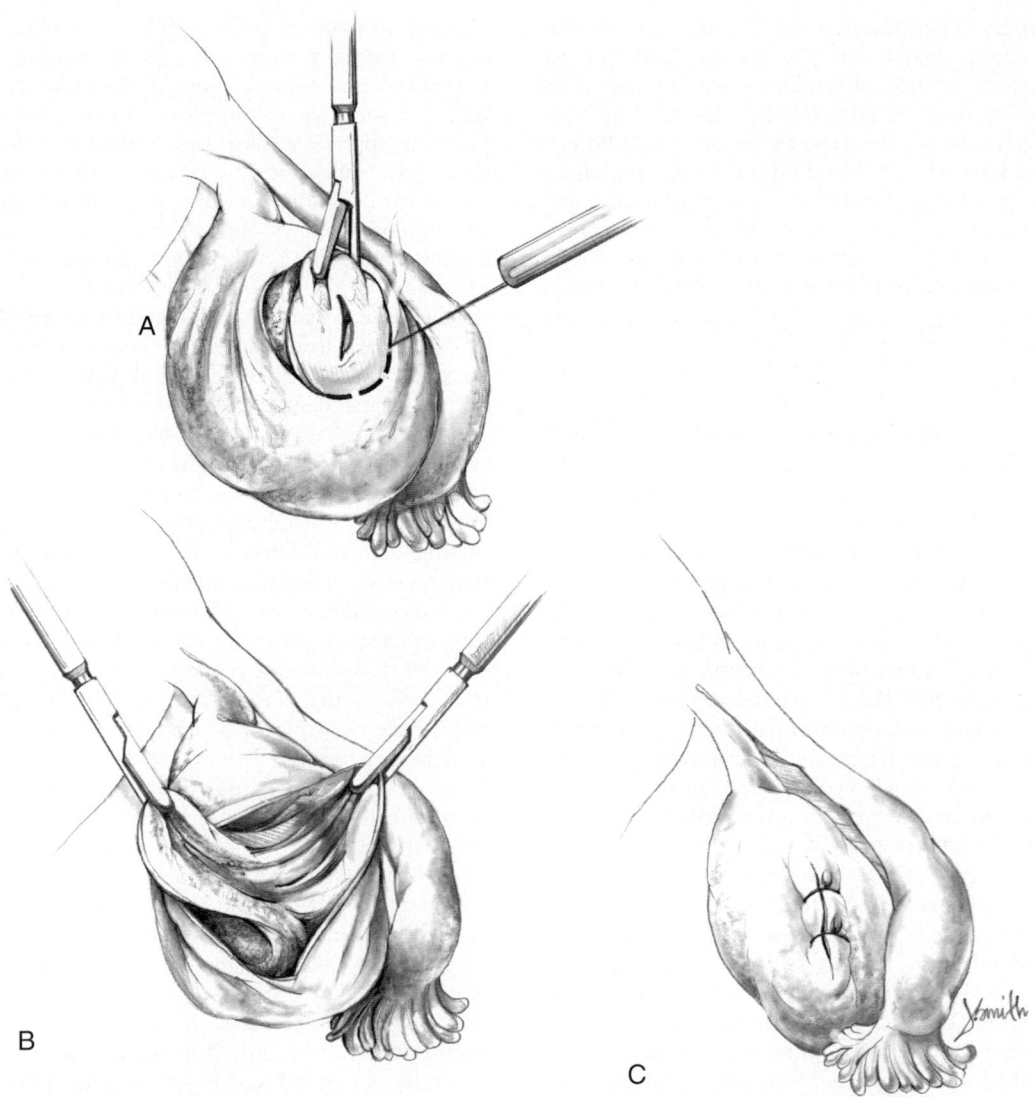

FIGURE 25.9. Laparoscopic ovarian cystectomy after fenestration of the cyst. **A:** The cut edges of the ovarian cortex and cyst wall are held and teased apart. **B:** The cyst wall can be stripped off by twisting it around the grasping forceps. Hydrodissection may be helpful. **C:** Large defects can be closed with laparoscopic suturing. Most incisions are left to heal by second intention.

Fayez and Vogel prospectively evaluated four laparoscopic methods for the treatment of endometriomas. Patients were treated postoperatively with danazol and underwent a second-look laparoscopy 8 weeks after their initial surgery. Complete excision with scissors successfully eliminated recurrence of the cysts, but adnexal adhesions had developed postoperatively in all cases. Mere incision and drainage of the cyst contents, followed by stripping or CO_2 laser vaporization of the lining, resulted in adhesion formation in only 25% to 37% of cases, but endometrioma cysts recurred in 21% to 22%. Other authors have used the KTP laser to photocoagulate or remove the cyst lining of large endometriomas and have reported a very low rate of recurrence at 6 months after the procedure.

In a prospective study by Beretta and colleagues, patients were randomly allocated at the time of laparoscopy to undergo either cystectomy or drainage of the endometrioma and bipolar coagulation of the inner lining. No preoperative or postoperative adjunctive medical therapies were administered. The excision technique resulted in a lower 24-month cumulative recurrence rate of dysmenorrhea, deep dyspareunia, and nonmenstrual pelvic pain. The median interval between the operation and the recurrence of moderate to severe pelvic pain was longer in the cystectomy group (19 months) versus the drainage and coagulation group (9.5 months). In addition, the 24-month cumulative pregnancy rate was statistically significantly higher in the former group than in the latter group (66.7% versus 23.5%, respectively).

If there is evidence of functional destruction of the ovary or if the patient has chronic, incapacitating pelvic pain secondary to ovarian endometriosis and has completed her family, appropriate therapy may consist of oophorectomy. The infundibulopelvic and uteroovarian ligaments can be ligated with Roeder loop suture, bipolar coagulation, or surgical staples before excision of the structure. The ovary is retrieved by morcellation or by posterior colpotomy. This type of surgery must be performed carefully when adnexal adhesions are present to avoid ovarian remnant syndrome. Screening sonography and sometimes CA-125 measurements are recommended before endoscopic therapy of larger endometriomas or adnexal masses in women older than 40 years to identify those with increased risk of a neoplastic process that should be treated by laparotomy.

INTESTINES

Intestinal involvement has been estimated to occur in 3% to 15% of women with endometriosis and in up to 50% of patients with severe disease. The most common areas of intestinal involvement are the rectum and rectosigmoid colon, followed by the sigmoid colon, cecum, terminal ileum, proximal colon, and appendix. The incidence of appendiceal endometriosis has been estimated at approximately 0.8% of all appendectomies; 3% to 5% of patients with endometriosis have appendiceal involvement. Symptoms that should arouse suspicion of colorectal involvement include constipation alternating with diarrhea, rectal pain, tenesmus, dyspareunia, and dysmenorrhea. Cyclic rectal bleeding is seen in as many as one third of females with rectosigmoid involvement, but the mucosa is rarely invaded. Small intestine disease accounts for up to 16% of gastrointestinal endometriosis and most often involves the terminal ileum. The most common symptom associated with disease in this location is midabdominal cramping pain. Ten percent of small bowel involvement presents with obstruction requiring surgery. The more common large bowel disease results in clinical obstruction in only 1% of cases.

The differential diagnosis of intestinal endometriosis includes primary carcinoma, metastatic carcinoma, diverticulitis, inflammatory bowel disease, irritable bowel syndrome, pelvic inflammatory disease, radiation colitis, and ischemic stricture. Endometrial adenocarcinomas have been reported in the colon and rectum but are exceedingly rare in comparison to the relatively large numbers of patients with colorectal endometriosis.

Preoperative or intraoperative rigid sigmoidoscopy may be helpful in ruling out primary colorectal malignancy. An intact mucosa effectively rules out primary colorectal malignancy. The greatest chance of diagnosing colorectal endometriosis occurs when the examination is performed at the time of menstruation. Although endometriosis rarely invades the intestinal mucosa, mucosal distortion is possible secondary to infiltration of the submucosa.

Pelvic and rectal pain are the major symptoms that lead to colorectal resection in patients with advanced endometriosis. Bowel resection should be undertaken in the symptomatic patient or when there is a suspicion of malignancy; however, the frequency of such indications is small. In a series authored by Prystowsky and colleagues of 1,573 consecutive patients with endometrio-

sis, only 11 women (0.7%) required bowel resection. Resection is usually undertaken for lesions producing partial obstruction because most of these lesions are fibrotic and unresponsive to hormonal manipulation. Recommended approaches for less extensive lesions include CO_2 laser vaporization of superficial serosal disease of the rectum or large intestine, excision without entering the mucosa, and oophorectomy or induction of hormonal menopause. Although oophorectomy can cause regression of the endometrial nodule, large implants of the bowel can scar and ultimately lead to obstruction. The use of electrocautery or fiber lasers should be avoided, because of their greater risk of causing transmural thermal damage.

A full mechanical and antibiotic bowel preparation is carried out preoperatively. In cases of large lesions that encroach on the mucosa, full-thickness excision of involved bowel can be undertaken either by disk excision of small, isolated lesions or by segmental resection for larger lesions. The anastomosis can be hand sewn with a continuous single layer of absorbable monofilament suture or created with surgical staples; however, patients with cul-de-sac disease must be in the lithotomy position to allow transanal placement of the stapler. These procedures have been performed by or with the assistance of general surgeons.

Appendectomy should be considered when there is physical evidence of peritonitis, when implants are large and active, when associated adhesive disease to adjacent bowel may result in partial or complete angulation and obstruction, or when the benign nature of the lesion is in doubt. Spontaneous perforation of the appendix due to endometriotic involvement is very rare. The technique of incidental endoscopic appendectomy is similar to that performed through laparotomy, although the stump need not be buried in the cecum. The tip of the appendix is grasped and elevated. The appendiceal vessels are bipolar cauterized or occluded with surgical clips near the base of the appendix before being excised. Two Endoloop ligatures are placed immediately next to each other at the base, and a third Endoloop is then secured approximately 5 mm distal to the first two. The appendix may then be transected between the second and third ligature and placed in a surgical pouch for safe retrieval from the abdominal cavity. Judicious application of bipolar cautery at the stump sterilizes the raw surface of the pedicle without causing damage to the adjacent cecum.

Coronado and colleagues reported a complete relief of pelvic symptoms in 49% and an improvement in 39% of patients who underwent full-thickness resection of the colon; 39% of patients in the series achieved a term pregnancy. In a later series by the same colorectal surgeons of 130 patients who underwent aggressive, conservative surgical management for advanced disease, the operative procedures performed included low anterior resection with anastomosis to the extraperitoneal rectum ($n = 109$), sigmoid resection ($n = 10$), disc excision of the rectum ($n = 7$), ileocecal resection ($n = 2$), and small bowel resection ($n = 2$). Twenty-four of 49 patients (49%) who attempted to conceive delivered a viable child.

The sequelae of intestinal endometriosis may not appear until the patient is postmenopausal. Although the endometriosis can become inactive, the resulting cicatrization can lead to a decrease in the bowel lumen and to symptoms of obstruction.

URINARY TRACT

Endometriosis involving the urinary tract is relatively rare. The spectrum of disease severity varies from incidental findings at laparoscopy, laparotomy, or cystoscopy to more significantly associated hematuria, flank pain, hypertension, and ureteral obstruction. Bladder and ureteral involvement represent 85% and 15% of cases, respectively. Cystoscopy and intravenous pyelography are helpful studies in documenting the extent of disease. Vesical endometriosis can be treated by hormonal suppressive therapy or partial cystectomy. These nodular lesions develop within the muscularis. Extrinsic ureteral compression by endometriosis presents four times more frequently than intrinsic involvement and is most likely to occur in the region of the ovarian fossa. Patients with paracervical and extensive uterosacral ligament disease are also at risk. The preferred treatment for ureteral obstruction is ureterolysis or resection of the involved segment followed by ureteroneocystostomy or ureteroureterostomy.

Involvement of peritoneum overlying the ureter is amenable to resection by laparotomy or laparoscopy. An incision is made in normal peritoneum adjacent to the involved area. The inferior margin of the incision is grasped and deviated medially, and the ureter is separated from the peritoneum bluntly or by hydrodissection. The peritoneal lesion can be excised or vaporized. Periureteral vessels must remain intact to prevent ischemia and resultant fistula formation. If the peritoneum is adhesed and the lesion cannot be dissected, the ureter is likely involved in the disease process. Ureteroneocystostomy should be considered.

INCISIONAL SCARS

Surgical scars are occasionally the sites of endometriotic implantation. Perineal, vaginal, and vulvar scars, particularly episiotomies, colporrhaphies, and Bartholin gland excisions, are likely areas for involvement by endometriosis. There is often a history of delayed wound healing of the incisional scar infiltrated with endometriosis. These implants typically appear as either deep-lying or subcutaneous nodules infiltrating the fascia and muscle. Bleeding into the tissues at the time of menstruation can cause cyclic local pain, tenderness, and discoloration; however, the nodule may lie too deep for detection of any color change through the skin. If the nodule is superficial, cyclic bleeding or ulceration may be apparent.

In most instances, incisional endometriomas have followed surgical procedures that violated the uterine cavity and allowed the endometrium to be transplanted. Wespi and Kletzhändler suggested that the frequency might approach 5% among patients having Caesarean section or hysterectomy. Metroplasty and myomectomy also increase the risk of incisional endometriosis. Indeed,

endometriosis has been reported along the needle tracts after amniocentesis or saline injection for abortion. Careful flushing and irrigation of the abdomen and of the incision during closure should minimize the chance of contamination when incision into the uterine cavity is required.

Episiotomy scars and cervical and vaginal lacerations also serve as implantation sites after delivery. The chance is significantly increased when postpartum curettage is performed. Paull and Tedeschi reported 15 instances in 2,208 deliveries when curettage was carried out, and no instances in 13,800 deliveries without curettage.

Management, usually best accomplished by local excision, is both diagnostic and curative. Various hormonal regimens may be appropriate if it is imperative to avoid surgery. However, malignancy can occur in each area of ectopic endometriosis, and histologic confirmation of the tentative diagnosis is recommended.

THORAX

Sixty-five cases of thoracic endometriosis were reported by Foster and associates in 1981. Pleural and lung parenchymal disease presented with different clinical findings. Ninety-three percent of women with pleural disease developed pain with right-sided pneumothorax or pleural effusion. Because numerous right diaphragmatic defects were noted in patients with pleural involvement, pleural implants are believed to be secondary to tubal regurgitation and transport of endometrial tissue through the diaphragmatic defects. Other symptoms may include upper quadrant abdominal pain or referred pain to the shoulder. Disease involving the lung parenchyma produced hemoptysis rather than the pleuritic symptoms. Previous pelvic surgery was more common among women who had parenchymal endometriosis; however, pelvic endometriosis was found more often in those with pleural disease.

Catamenial pneumothorax or hemoptysis should alert the physician to the possibility of thoracic endometriosis. The chest roentgenogram is usually of little value in diagnosing this disease; however, cytology, aspiration biopsy, and pleuroscopy may be useful. Massive effusion and bleeding can occur, but this presentation is more commonly associated with a malignancy. GnRH agonist or surgical treatment may be effective in the symptomatic patient. Surgical pleural abrasion may be superior to hormonal treatment in the long-term management of pneumothorax.

Adjunctive Procedures of Conservative Surgery
UTERINE SUSPENSION

Uterine suspension techniques have been devised to prevent adhesion formation at denuded peritoneal surfaces of the posterior cul-de-sac, uterine serosa, and broad ligament. Elevation of the adnexa can prevent adhesion reformation of the ovary or fallopian tube at a site where existing adhesions have been excised. This procedure may be particularly useful in the case of a posterior or retroflexed uterus. It is indicated in selected cases of dyspareunia after resection of posterior cul-de-sac en-

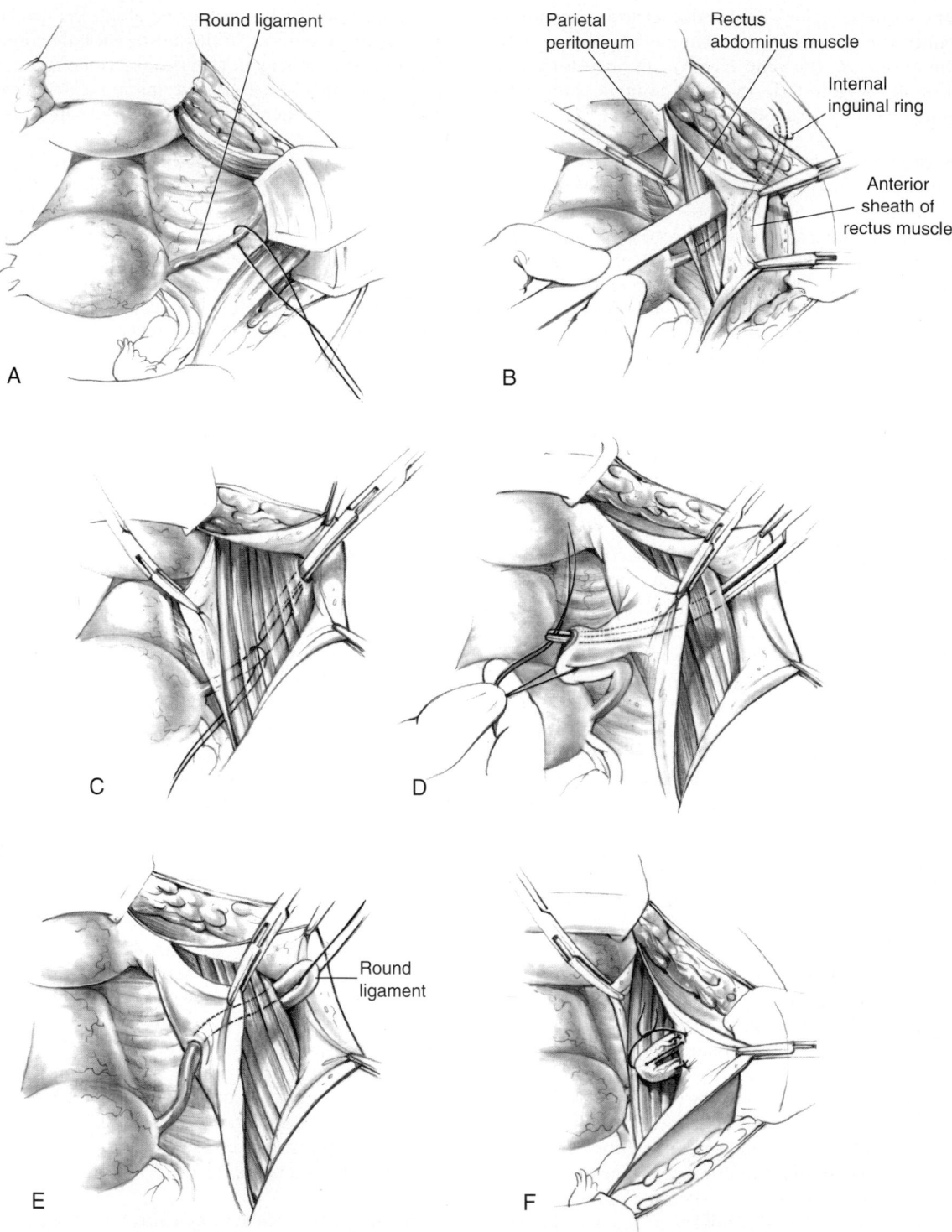

FIGURE 25.10. Modified Gilliam suspension. **A:** A chromic suture is placed around the round ligament about 3 to 4 cm from the uterine cornu. **B:** The rectus fascia is grasped with Kocher clamps and separated from the belly of the rectus muscle bluntly with the index finger or knife handle. **C:** The parietal peritoneum is grasped with Kelly forceps. A long Kelly forceps is introduced through the internal inguinal ring as it passes over the belly of the rectus. **D:** The Kelly clamp is brought through the internal inguinal ring and along the round ligament to a point adjacent to the chromic stay suture. A knife is used to open the peritoneum. The ends of the chromic suture are grasped by the Kelly clamp. **E:** As traction is applied to the suture, a knuckle of the round ligament passes through the internal ring. **F:** Three sutures of 2-0 delayed-absorbable or silk suture are placed, fixing the ligament to the rectus fascia in a manner that will not interrupt the blood supply.

dometriosis. There is no evidence to suggest that uterine suspension is detrimental to subsequent pregnancies, although it is of unproven efficacy in enhancing fertility. The modified Gilliam procedure offers certain advantages over other uterine suspensions because of its maintenance of normal anatomic relations. Shortening the round ligament through the internal inguinal ring eliminates the opening that is made lateral to the point of the ligament's attachment to the abdominal wall in the Olshausen suspension procedure.

When a modified Gilliam suspension is performed, the uterus is elevated and a 2-0 absorbable suture is placed around each round ligament about 3 to 4 cm from its insertion into the uterus (Fig. 25.10). The edge of the rectus fascia is grasped by a Kocher clamp at the level of the anterosuperior spine of the ileum. The adjacent peritoneal edge is grasped with a Kelly clamp. The rectus fascia is separated from the underlying musculature with blunt dissection. A long Kelly clamp is inserted between the fascia and muscle to the level of the inguinal ring, while displacing the peritoneum superiorly. This clamp is inserted through the ring and along the round ligament by gently opening and closing the instrument. The insertion is facilitated by placing traction on the suture to stabilize the round ligament. The peritoneum overlying the ligament is then incised at a point adjacent to the suture, and the suture is grasped by the Kelly clamp. By withdrawing the clamp, the round ligament is brought through the internal ring and outside of the peritoneal cavity; it can then be sutured to the rectus sheath with 2-0 interrupted delayed-absorbable sutures. These sutures must be placed through the round ligament without encircling the ligament and thus occluding its blood supply. This procedure is repeated on the opposite side.

At the end of the suspension, the surgeon's hands should be introduced into the abdomen to ascertain whether there is a loop of round ligament lateral to the point where the ligament has been withdrawn from the peritoneal cavity. If so, this should be corrected to prevent strangulation of the involved segment lying between the ligament and abdominal wall. In addition, the fallopian tube should be inspected to ensure that its course has not been disturbed. This can occur if the traction suture has been placed through a segment of round ligament too close to the uterus.

Laparoscopic suspension is possible after placement of a trocar and sheath approximately 5 cm lateral to the midline and 3 cm above the inguinal ligament. The anterior rectus fascia in this site is tagged with suture. The round ligament is grasped at the usual site with laparoscopic forceps to elevate the ligament to the tagged anterior fascia, where it is sutured in place with nonabsorbable suture. The desired positioning of the uterus is confirmed laparoscopically.

PRESACRAL NEURECTOMY

Presacral neurectomy, or division of the superior hypogastric plexus, is useful as an adjunctive procedure to eliminate the uterine component of dysmenorrhea that results from endometriosis. Sixty percent to 70% of patients with secondary dysmenorrhea experience complete relief of symptoms. There is no evidence that this procedure enhances fertility. A significantly greater relief of midline pelvic pain is achieved when endometriosis resection is combined with presacral neurectomy, compared with conservative resection alone. In a series by Tjaden and colleagues, all 17 patients undergoing presacral neurectomy noted a complete resolution of midline pelvic pain, and only two of these had a recurrence of pain within the 42-month follow-up period. Endometriosis rarely provokes exclusively midline pelvic pain, however, and lateralizing adnexal pain and deep dyspareunia are not affected by this procedure. Careful patient selection is necessary if the desired outcome is to be achieved.

The hypogastric plexus consists of fine strands of nerves embedded in a delicate areolar tissue. The plexus is formed as a continuation of the aortic and inferior mesenteric plexuses and passes over the bifurcation of the aorta. It then continues below the promontory of the sacrum before dividing into the right and left inferior hypogastric nerves. The presacral neurectomy procedure can be performed through a transverse Maylard incision or longitudinal incision that adequately exposes the region of the bifurcation of the aorta (Fig. 25.11). At the time of laparotomy, the descending colon is packed superiorly and to the left to expose the left margin of the hypogastric plexus. The posterior peritoneum overlying the sacrum is elevated and incised with the scalpel. The incision is extended caudally with scissors for about 5 cm to the third or fourth sacral vertebra, and cranially to just below the bifurcation of the aorta. The margin of the posterior peritoneum can be drawn upward and outward by a stay suture or an Allis clamp. A Kitner sponge is then used to dissect the areolar tissue and associated nerve fibers off the posterior aspect of the peritoneal flap. The right ureter is readily visible and can be retracted laterally, and the areolar tissue is dissected from it without disturbing its blood supply. The common iliac artery, which lies just below the ureter, is freed superiorly from the adjacent tissue. A right-angle clamp or probe can be introduced medially next to the promontory to elevate the sheath and allow blunt dissection underneath it. Care must be taken to avoid the middle sacral vessels that may be left intact on the surface of the promontory. Injury to the middle sacral vein can result in significant blood loss. Hemorrhage is controlled with cautery, suture ligation, hot packs, hypogastric vessel ligation, use of an absorbable gelatin sponge (Gelfoam) or microfibular collagen (Avitene), or packing with bone wax.

The areolar tissue is taken off the left flap of peritoneum until the superior hemorrhoidal vessels are exposed. These vessels should remain on the peritoneum but are bluntly freed from the overlying tissue. By elevating the sheath, several vessels that feed into the left common iliac vein can be identified. These branches are isolated, clamped, and tied as they are visualized. When the plexus has been isolated, a Babcock clamp can be used to elevate the sheath. Two 2-0 absorbable or silk

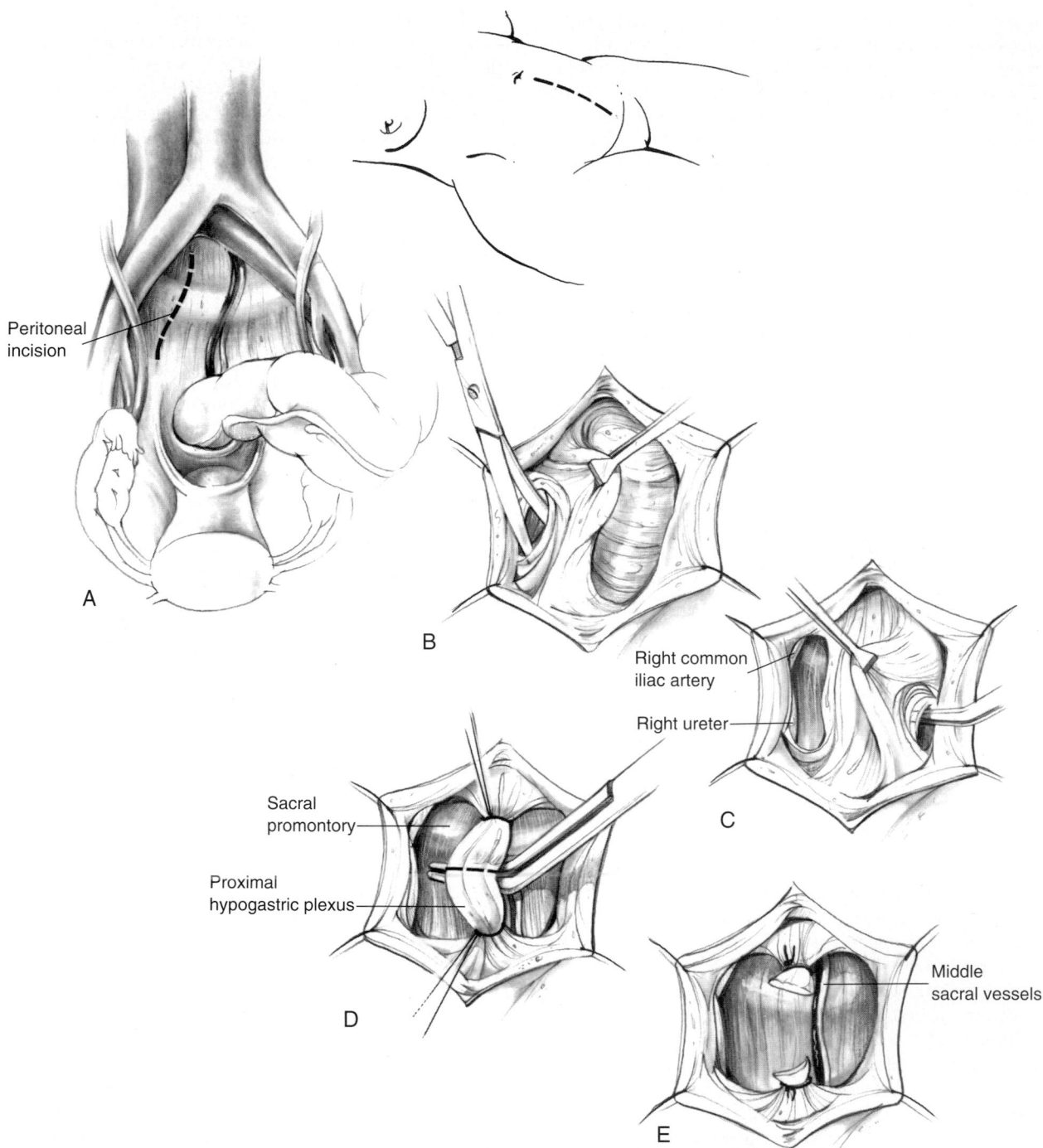

FIGURE 25.11. Presacral neurectomy. **A:** Location of incision in relation to anatomic landmarks. A Maylard incision can also be used in some cases. The descending colon is displaced superiorly and to the left for good exposure of the left margin of the hypogastric plexus. **B:** A Kitner sponge is used to dissect the areolar tissue medially and off the posterior aspect of the peritoneal flap. The right ureter can be identified easily. **C:** The areolar nerve-bearing tissue is dissected from the peritoneum on the left side, exposing the left internal iliac vessels and superior hemorrhoidal vessels. **D:** The plexus is isolated and elevated off the sacral promontory. A segment of plexus about 5 cm in length is isolated with 2-0 silk sutures. **E:** The plexus is excised. Note relation between pedicles of the nerve bundle and adjacent structures.

sutures are placed around the proximal and distal aspects of a 5-cm segment of the plexus and are loosely tied. The tonsil clamp is applied to each end of the nerve bundle. As the clamps are removed, the sutures are slipped down over the crushed areas and tied securely. The intervening portion of the plexus is then excised. The procedure is terminated by approximating the peritoneum with absorbable suture.

In less than 10% of cases, the pelvic mesocolon is inserted in front of the interiliac trigone and the nerve bundle cannot be reached by simple incision of the peritoneum. In these cases, the chief branches of the inferior mesenteric artery must be moved to the left to expose the triangular space between the two common iliac arteries. Unless there is adequate exposure and meticulous dissection, incomplete resection of the superior hypogastric plexus can occur, resulting in suboptimal denervation.

A laparoscopic approach to presacral neurectomy has been described, but its efficacy has yet to be conclusively established. This technique involves insertion of a 10-mm trocar sheath 3 cm above the symphysis pubis and placement of two accessory ports in each iliac fossa. Steep Trendelenburg position with a left lateral tilt is required to allow displacement of the intestines cephalad to expose the bifurcation of the aorta and sacral promontory. The parietal peritoneum overlying the sacral promontory is grasped and elevated to allow a transverse incision midway between the bifurcation of the aorta and the sacral promontory. The presacral nerve is isolated by developing the avascular space between the nerve and right internal iliac artery down to the periosteum. Segments of the superior hypogastric plexus are removed by sharp dissection after diathermy. The entire length of removed nerve plexus should not exceed 3 to 4 cm. Venous bleeding is controlled with bipolar cautery. Meticulous hemostasis must be ensured at the completion of the operation. This technique should only be performed by experienced laparoscopic surgeons because the vascular complications can be serious. In a review of 655 laparoscopic presacral neurectomy procedures, Chen and colleagues reported a 0.6% rate of major complications, including one case of injury of the right internal iliac artery and three cases of chylous ascites.

Polan and DeCherney reported that the combination of presacral neurectomy and conservative surgery in women with chronic pelvic pain, endometriosis, and pelvic inflammatory disease increased total postoperative pain relief from 26% to 75%, although only a small number of patients were included in this laparotomy series. In 1986, Lee and co-workers performed presacral neurectomy in 50 women with chronic pelvic pain. Dysmenorrhea resolved in 73% of the cases, dyspareunia lessened in 77%, and acyclic pain improved in 63%. The uterosacral ligaments were resected in half of the subjects in this study, but this did not seem to affect the overall rate of pain relief. In a randomized clinical trial of women with moderate to severe endometriosis and pelvic pain undergoing conservative surgical therapy, Candiani and colleagues reported a recurrence of midline menstrual pain in 23% of women who underwent presacral neurectomy versus a 42% recurrence in those who did not. This difference reached the limit of statistical significance ($p = .06$). In a recent uncontrolled laparoscopic study by Nezhat and associates of 100 women subjected to vaporization of endometriosis and presacral neurectomy, the symptoms of pelvic pain, dysmenorrhea, and dyspareunia were reduced by more than 50% in 74, 61, and 55 patients, respectively, over the 1-year follow-up period. The stage of endometriosis did not correlate with the degree of pain improvement achieved.

Two common side effects of the presacral neurectomy procedure have been observed. Constipation may require laxatives or stool softeners for a period of 3 to 4 months. The vaginal dryness that develops in as many as 10% to 15% of patients is transient and usually resolves within 6 months. Difficulty with micturition is an infrequent complication that rarely lasts for more than 1 or 2 months. A painless first stage of labor has been reported in women who have undergone presacral neurectomy.

UTERINE NERVE ABLATION

The technique of uterosacral neurectomy was initially described by Ruggi in 1899. Later popularized by Doyle, it has since been adapted for performance during laparoscopic procedures for the alleviation of dysmenorrhea. Sympathetic fibers T10 to L1 are contained within the inferior hypogastric plexus and course along the inferior vena cava and sacrum to enter the uterus through the nerves of the uterosacral ligaments and accompanying uterine arteries. The parasympathetic components of the paracervical nerves originate from S1 through S3 or S4, travel within the nervi erigentes, and emerge in the lateral pelvis to form the Frankenhäuser ganglia lateral to the cervix. Division of the uterosacral ligaments at a point approximately 1.5 cm distal to the cervix should interrupt many sensory nerve fibers of the cervix and uterine corpus.

In general, uterine nerve ablation by laser is preferable to electrocautery because it is less likely to cause undesirable thermal damage. The course of the ureters and adjacent vasculature should be noted before commencement of dissection. The uterosacral ligaments are exposed by manipulating the uterine cannula to anteflex the corpus and by applying pressure to the posterior cervix with an ancillary laparoscopic probe.

The initial incision is made on the medial aspect of the ligament at its junction with the uterus. A second incision is made just lateral to the uterosacral ligament and medial to the ureter. The ligament is then grasped with forceps and stretched toward the sidewall. The CO_2 laser is used to vaporize a 2- to 5-cm area of each ligament to a depth of approximately 1 cm. This division should be centered approximately 1.5 cm distal to the cervix. The posterior aspect of the cervix between the insertion of the uterosacral ligaments may be superficially vaporized to interrupt the sensory fibers crossing to the contralateral side. Because extension of the beam too far laterally or posteriorly from the ligament can result in considerable bleeding, the surgeon should have immediate access to bipolar cautery, endocoagulation, or hemostatic clips.

Fiber lasers such as the KTP/532 offer the advantages of increased hemostasis and lack of carbon plume, compared with the CO_2 instrument. If bipolar diathermy is used to fulgurate the uterosacral ligament, laparoscopic scissors are used to excise the segment of ligament in question.

Few published clinical trials exist that delineate the efficacy of the uterosacral neurectomy technique. Feste reported significant improvement in the symptoms of primary dysmenorrhea or dysmenorrhea associated with endometriosis in 71% of a series of 42 patients. In a similar series of 100 patients by Donnez, 50% experienced complete relief, 41% had mild to moderate relief, and 9% described no relief. Using the carbon dioxide laser, Davis observed a considerable improvement in dysmenorrhea in 135 of 146 women (92%) with endometriosis and an improvement in dyspareunia in 103 of 109 women (94%) with endometriosis who underwent uterine nerve ablation and vaporization of endometriosis. This therapeutic benefit did not seem to differ among revised AFS classification stages of endometriosis. Lichten and Bombard published a randomized, prospective, double-blind study of laparoscopic uterosacral nerve ablation for the treatment of severe or incapacitating dysmenorrhea unresponsive to oral contraceptives and nonsteroidal anti-inflammatory agents. None of the control patients noted improvement, whereas 9 of 11 in the treated group had almost complete relief at 3 months, and 5 of 11 described complete relief from dysmenorrhea 1 year after surgery. Patients with endometriosis were not included in this small series.

Uterine nerve ablation by laparotomy fell from favor before it was revived as an endoscopic technique. The potential neurologic, intestinal, orthopedic, and psychological components of pain should be considered before subjecting the patient to a procedure that, although now performed endoscopically, carries some surgical risk, and whose effectiveness has been questioned because of the small number of cases evaluated. Surgical resection of pelvic endometrial implants may be all that is necessary to alleviate discomfort in most endometriosis patients. Vercellini and colleagues could not demonstrate the efficacy of this laparoscopic technique. Complications associated with transection of the uterosacral ligaments include ureteral damage, bowel damage, and postoperative hemorrhage, which, if undetected, may result in death. Uterine prolapse has recently been described as a potential long-term side effect of the procedure.

Second-Look Laparoscopy

Second-look laparoscopy has been suggested as an appropriate procedure for additional lysis of pelvic adhesions in patients who have undergone a laparotomy or a laparoscopy for the resection of endometriosis. If scheduled 8 days to 6 weeks after the initial dissection, second-look laparoscopy allows separation of *de novo* adhesions that are still relatively filmy in consistency. In addition, laparoscopy after pelvic reconstructive surgery provides an opportunity to assess future prognosis for fertility.

Early second-look laparoscopy after endoscopic treatment of endometriomas has revealed a recurrence rate of endometriomas of 15% to 20%. Equally significant are the nearly 20% incidence of *de novo* adhesion formation and the 40% to 82% recurrence rate of dense adhesions. Second-look laparoscopy allows treatment of these findings; however, there is little direct evidence that this secondary surgical procedure will increase the cumulative pregnancy rate.

Surgical Outcomes

No classification schedule for endometriosis provides an accurate correlation between extent of disease and pregnancy rate. Nevertheless, point categorization through the revised AFS classification does provide a framework in which to report outcomes of therapy. The crude pregnancy rate after conservative surgery by laparotomy for mild endometriosis is 61%; this approximates the 58% rate derived from an accumulated series of patients with minimal and mild endometriosis treated by CO_2 laser laparoscopy (Table 25.8). The results of laparoscopic electrocoagulation of all stages of disease are presented in Table 25.9. Murphy and colleagues, using life-table analysis and the two-parameter exponential method, studied 72 patients with stage I or stage II endometriosis treated by laparoscopic electrocoagulation of endometrial implants. They reported a crude pregnancy rate of 74% for stage I and 57% for stage II during an average follow-up period of 7.9 months; however, the monthly fecundity rates were only 10.3% for stage I and 7.6% for stage II endometriosis.

A recent retrospective study by Tulandi and Al-Took that compared reproductive outcome after treatment of mild endometriosis with laparoscopic excision and electrocoagulation showed no significant difference between the two modalities. The total pregnancy rate was 53.5% in the excision group and 57.1% in the electrosurgery group. The mean interval between surgery and conception was 10.7 months in the electrosurgery group and 13.3 months in the excision group. Excision of tissue may result in more complete removal of infiltrating endometriosis, which should be of particular benefit to patients with deep nodules.

Expectant management of mild to moderate endometriosis after diagnosis by laparoscopy yields a crude pregnancy rate of about 50%, which has brought into question whether surgical therapy of lesser stages of disease enhances fertility. In a retrospective study comparing the efficacy of electrosurgical treatment of endometriosis with the efficacy of expectant management in minimal and mild endometriosis-associated infertility, Tulandi and Mouchawar reported that the cumulative probability of conception was significantly higher among patients treated surgically. In a more recent large prospective, multicenter, double-blind, controlled, randomized trial, resection or ablation of endometriosis during diagnostic laparoscopy resulted in a significantly higher fecundity rate after 36 weeks as compared with expectant management (Fig. 25.12). Electrosurgery or laser was used to treat implants and adhesions in this Canadian study by Marcoux and co-workers.

The performance of a laparotomy to excise minimal or mild stages of endometriosis is not warranted. In a

TABLE 25.8.
Pregnancy Rates After Laparoscopic CO_2 Laser Vaporization of Endometriosis[a]

Investigator	Number of Pregnancies/Number Treated (%)					Length of Follow-up (mo)
	Stage I	Stage II	Stage III	Stage IV	Combined	
Daniell and Brown	—	—	—	—	3/10 (30)	5
Daniell and Pittaway	—	—	—	—	3/15 (20)	6
Kelly and Roberts	3/3 (100)	3/7 (43)	—	—	6/10 (60)	6
Chong et al.	21/32 (66)[b]	—	—	—	21/32 (66)	12
Feste	24/47 (51)	4/6 (66)	2/5 (40)	—	30/58 (52)	12
Martin	7/27 (26)	3/9 (16)	1/4 (25)[c]	—	11/50 (22)	9
Martin	25/56 (45)[d]	22/45 (49)[d]	9/14 (64)[c]	—	56/115 (49)	12
Davis[e]	20/31 (65)	—	15/26 (58)	2/7 (29)	37/64 (58)	15
Olive and Martin[f]	23/59 (39)	22/48 (46)	10/20 (50)	—	55/127 (43)	—
Donnez[g]	26/42 (62)	11/21 (52)	3/7 (43)	—	40/70 (57)	18
Paulsen and Asmer[g]	109/140 (78)	60/88 (68)	—	—	169/228 (74)	8–32
Gast et al.[e]	36/70 (51)	12/33 (38)	9/19 (47)	—	50/122 (41)	10
Fayez et al.[e]	27/38 (71)	33/44 (75)	—	—	60/82 (73)	12
Nezhat et al.[g]	28/39 (72)	60/86 (70)	45/67 (67)	35/51 (69)	168/243 (69)	—
TOTALS	329/553 (59)	230/397 (58)	94/162 (58)	37/58 (64)	690/1,170 (59)	—

[a] The original American Fertility Society classification system is used unless noted.
[b] Postoperative danazol for 132 days.
[c] Postoperative danazol for 6 months.
[d] Three-month course of danazol 6 to 18 months postoperatively if not pregnant.
[e] Revised American Fertility Society classification system.
[f] Patients treated with either laser laparoscopy only or a combination of laser laparoscopy and preoperative or postoperative danazol.
[g] Patients with factors other than endometriosis excluded from study.
Cook AS, Rock JA. The role of laparoscopy in the treatment of endometriosis. *Fertil Steril* 1991;55:663, with permission.

comparison between laparotomy and laparoscopy for treatment of these categories of disease, life-table analysis showed similar pregnancy outcomes.

Operative treatment of more extensive disease does offer a greater likelihood of conception than does expectant management, in part because of correction of mechanical factors such as adhesions. The overall crude pregnancy rate reported by various studies of conservative laparotomy for endometriosis that stratified reproductive results by disease severity was 38%, with a monthly fecundity rate averaging 1.4% to 1.5% (Table 25.10). Laparoscopic treatment of severe endometriosis offers a mean crude pregnancy rate of 47.6%, although data from only a few series have been published (Table

TABLE 25.9.
Pregnancy Rates After Laparoscopic Electrocoagulation of Endometriosis

Investigator	Number of Pregnancies/Number Treated (%)					Length of Follow-up (mo)
	Minimal	Mild	Moderate	Severe	Combined	
Eward	4/7 (57)	10/18 (56)	—	—	14/25 (56)	13
Hasson	0/1 (0)	—	2/2 (100)	4/5 (80)	6/8 (75)	7
Sulewski et al.	—	20/42 (48)	20/58 (35)	—	40/100 (40)	37
Daniell and Pittaway	—	—	—	—	33/60 (55)	—
Reich and McGlynn	—	—	—	—	15/23 (65)	18
Seiler et al.	—	20/45 (44)	—	—	20/45 (44)	7
Nowroozi et al.	—	42/69 (61)	—	—	42/69 (61)	8
Murphy et al.	24/36 (67)	18/36 (50)	2/7 (29)	0/3 (0)	44/82 (54)	8
TOTALS	28/44 (64)	110/210 (52)	24/67 (36)	4/8 (50)	214/412 (52)	—

From Cook AS, Rock JA. The role of laparoscopy in the treatment of endometriosis. *Fertil Steril* 1991;55:663, with permission.

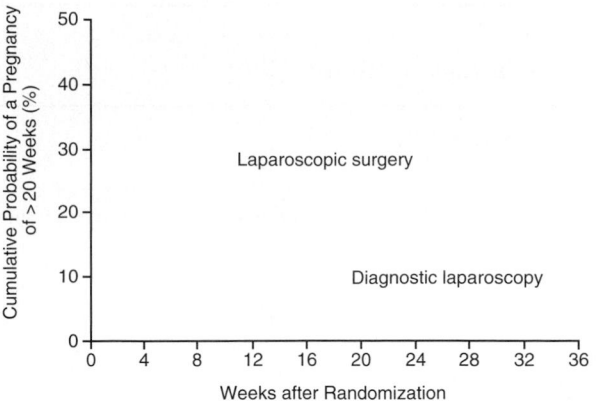

FIGURE 25.12. Cumulative probability of a pregnancy carried beyond 20 weeks in the 36 weeks after laparoscopy in women with endometriosis, according to study group. (Marcoux S, Maheux R, Béribé S. Laparoscopic surgery in infertile women with minimal or mild endometriosis. *N Engl J Med* 1997;337:217.)

25.8). Hence, expert laser laparoscopists have reported results that appear to be as good as those obtained through the open abdomen, although there are no substantive data for direct comparison of outcomes of the two surgical modalities, and the correct identification and classification of disease may vary between laparotomy and laparoscopy groups. The apparent equivalence of pregnancy rates for all stages of endometriosis after laparoscopic laser vaporization is noteworthy. Life-table analysis demonstrated that pregnancy is most likely to occur during the first 36 months after surgery. Furthermore, the duration of infertility and, perhaps, patient age may have a greater impact on cumulative pregnancy rates

than the actual stage (revised AFS stages I through IV) of the disease.

In a prospective, randomized double-blind, controlled trial of laser laparoscopy in the treatment of pelvic pain associated with minimal to moderate endometriosis, Sutton and associates found that 62.5% of the laser-treated women reported symptom improvement at 6 months, as compared with 22.6% of those treated expectantly. Treatment results were poorest for patients with stage I disease and best for those with stage III disease. Symptom relief continued at 1 year in 90% of those who initially responded. Deeply infiltrative endometriosis is frequently present in stage I disease, and an inadequate depth of incision may contribute to the lack of surgical response in this group.

Aggressive and complete excision of deep endometriosis is justified. Resection of deep endometriosis relieved dyspareunia in 40% and dysmenorrhea in 60% of cases. Nezhat and associates noted moderate to complete relief of pain in 162 of 175 women; however, some patients in this series had several surgical interventions. Preliminary analysis of the surgical results in 250 women in whom deep endometriosis had been excised with CO_2 laser showed a cure rate of pelvic pain in 70% and a recurrence rate of less than 5% over a 5-year follow-up period. Spontaneous pregnancy rates as high as 60% within 1 year of excision of deep endometriosis have been reported.

Rock and colleagues have shown that 13.5% of patients initially treated with conservative surgery required subsequent operative procedures. Wheeler and Malinak noted a cumulative recurrence rate at 3 and 5 years after conservative surgery of 13.5% and 40.3%, respectively. Neither the initial staging nor the ability to conceive after the initial surgery greatly affected the recurrence

TABLE 25.10.
Conservative Surgery by Laparotomy for Severe Endometriosis:
Effect on Conception According to the Literature

Investigators	Year	Procedures (N)	Pregnancies (N)	Incidence of Pregnancy (%)	Monthly Fecundity Rate
Acosta et al.	1973	39	13	33.3	—
Hammond et al.	1976	2	0	0.0	—
Sadigh et al.	1977	42	20	47.6	—
Garcia and David	1977	49	14	28.6	—
Schenken and Malinak	1978	21	6	28.6	—
Buttram	1979	68	32	47.1	—
Rock et al.	1981	81	39	48.1	0.015
Wheeler and Malinak	1981	119	36	30.3	—
Rantala et al.	1983	46	18	39.1	—
Chong and Baggish	1984	10	3	30.3	—
Gordts et al.	1984	57	20	35.1	—
Olive and Lee	1986	34	10	29.4	0.014
Candiani et al.	1986	8	3	37.5	0.012
Donnez et al.	1987	15	7	46.7	0.026
TOTALS		591	221	37.4	

From Candiani GB, Vercellini P, Fedele L, et al. Conservative surgical treatment for severe endometriosis in infertile women: are we making progress? *Obstet Gynecol Surv* 1991;46:490, with permission.

rates. In a study of patients who underwent laparoscopic cystectomy of ovarian endometriomas of greater than 3 cm in diameter, Busacca and colleagues reported a cumulative rate of ultrasonographic recurrence of 11.7% over 48 months. Laparoscopic excision of ovarian endometriomas by the stripping technique is associated with a lower reoperation rate than that of fenestration. Redwine reported a cumulative recurrence rate of 19% at 5 years after conservative laparoscopic excision of endometriosis by sharp dissection. A second cytoreductive procedure may benefit some infertile women who have undergone surgery in the past, if assisted reproductive technologies are not pursued. A cumulative pregnancy rate of 31% at 25 months was achieved after a second conservative laparotomy for recurrent endometriosis.

Combination Medical and Surgical Treatment

Preoperative and postoperative medical therapies have been proposed as treatment adjuncts to conservative resection of endometriosis to enhance fertility. Preoperative suppression of disease with hormonal agents may facilitate the surgical procedure by reducing tissue vascularity, and the greater ease in tissue dissection may decrease adhesion formation during the postoperative period. The preoperative hormonal agents also eliminate the corpus luteum that might otherwise be mistaken for an endometrioma. However, they may also reduce the size of endometriosis implants, making them less recognizable after short-term drug therapy. In a controlled clinical trial, a 3-month course of GnRH agonist treatment before laparoscopy for endometrioma excision failed to result in a reduction in operative time or recurrence rate of disease during a 1-year follow-up period.

Initiation of postoperative medical therapy may inhibit the activity of any residual disease, suppress ovulation, and decrease the possibility of adverse effects of peritoneal spillage of disease at the time of resection. Postoperative medical therapy has a serious drawback, however; the patient is unable to attempt conception for several months. Wheeler and Malinak demonstrated an improved pregnancy rate in patients with severe endometriosis treated with danazol in the immediate postlaparotomy period compared with patients treated with surgery alone. Nevertheless, in Buttram's 1985 series, the conception rate for severe disease treated by conservative surgery followed by a 6-month course of danazol was only 32% (7/22), compared with a 40% rate for surgery alone in the historical control group. Andrews and Larsen have noted that the best chance for postsurgical conception occurs during the first 6 months after conservative surgery by laparotomy. Thus, suppressing ovulation during that critical period may be counterproductive.

Preoperative danazol therapy has been shown to slightly improve fecundity rates when compared with rates achieved with surgery alone, although this result has been questioned because of the lack of treatment randomization. The addition of hormonal therapy has not been shown to be beneficial in less advanced stages of disease. Hence, the value of combination therapy in the treatment of endometriosis-associated infertility remains controversial. Because of the lack of substantive data to support its efficacy, a short postoperative course of danazol or GnRH analog of 3 months or less should be considered in infertile patients in cases of residual disease or peritoneal spillage of the contents of an endometrioma.

Contemporary management of women with endometriosis-associated pelvic pain involves both surgical and long-term medical therapy. When reductive laparoscopy is followed by a 6-month course of GnRH analog, there is a significant delay in the return of endometriosis symptoms requiring further treatment. In a randomized, prospective study, Hornstein and colleagues found that this interval was more than 24 months in those receiving nafarelin versus 11.7 months in the placebo group. Similarly, postoperative administration of low-dose, cyclic oral contraceptives for 6 months delayed the recurrence of pain symptoms and endometriomas at 12 months, but no significant differences were detected at 24 months or 36 months following laparoscopic excision. A shorter duration of hormonal therapy during the postoperative period may be inadequate in reducing recurrence risk. A 3-month course of nafarelin following surgical therapy of stage III and IV endometriosis was ineffective in reducing pain scores as compared with placebo.

Hysterectomy

The number and rate of hysterectomies performed for endometriosis increased steadily from the 1960s to the 1980s, more so than for other diagnoses. The reported rate for 1982 to 1984 was more than double the rate for 1965 to 1967, although the exact reasons for the increase remain uncertain. Endometriosis was the primary indication for 20% of white women and 9% of black women undergoing hysterectomy in the United States from 1988 to 1990. Because of concern over the risk of recurrence even after definitive surgical therapy, bilateral oophorectomy was performed at the time of hysterectomy in 52% of women 44 years of age or younger and in 81% of women 45 years of age or older.

Definitive surgery offers prompt, complete, and long-term relief of pain from endometriosis more often than do the various available medical regimens. Most hysterectomies are performed by the abdominal route; in selected cases, laparoscopy might reveal a free cul-de-sac or allow lysis of complicating adhesions, thus allowing safe vaginal hysterectomy. When the posterior cul-de-sac is obliterated and extensive fibrosis is present deep in the pelvis, subtotal hysterectomy may be indicated.

The recurrence of cyclic pain associated with endometriosis after hysterectomy with preservation of normal ovaries has been estimated at 3% to 7%. Nevertheless, in a study of 138 women who underwent hysterectomy with the diagnosis of endometriosis at the Johns Hopkins Hospital, ovarian conservation was associated with a 6.1 times greater risk of development of recurrent pain and an 8.1 times greater risk of reoperation as compared with oophorectomy at the time of hysterectomy. Laparoscopic resection of invasive peritoneal and intestinal disease that persists after castration may result in an improvement in pain symptoms. Hysterectomy does not improve symptoms in 25% of cases of chronic pelvic pain when the uterus is believed to be the source of the pain.

Minute, hormonally active ovarian fragments may be detected in women with symptomatic endometriosis, even after total abdominal hysterectomy and bilateral salpingo-oophorectomy. This ovarian remnant syndrome is the result of incomplete excision of cortical tissue at the time of extirpative surgery for endometriosis or pelvic inflammatory disease. Most ovarian remnants are retroperitoneal in location, and they are often densely adherent to pelvic side wall structures, including the ureter, hypogastric vessels, and bladder base. Complete surgical removal may be difficult.

Estrogen replacement therapy after total hysterectomy and bilateral oophorectomy is associated with less than a 10% rate of recurrence of endometriosis. A cause-and-effect relation between estrogen replacement and malignancy in endometriosis has not been established, suggesting that progestational agents need not be prescribed together with estrogens after hysterectomy for a diagnosis of endometriosis. However, it may be wise to administer both progestin and estrogen if the disease was incompletely resected or deeply invasive, contained atypical epithelial changes, or is recurrent. Women who begin estrogen replacement therapy immediately after total abdominal hysterectomy and bilateral salpingo-oophorectomy are at no greater risk of recurrent pain than those who delay estrogen therapy for more than 6 weeks postoperatively.

ENDOMETRIOSIS AND ASSISTED REPRODUCTIVE TECHNOLOGIES

If spontaneous conception is not achieved within 3 years of surgical resection of endometriosis or within 1 year of repair of tubal obstruction associated with endometriosis, the odds are poor that it ever will occur. Techniques in assisted reproduction have been widely used during the past decade for the management of endometriosis-associated infertility unresponsive to cytoreductive surgical or hormonal therapy. Endometriosis is the sole identifiable cause of infertility in 25% to 35% of women undergoing *in vitro* fertilization/embryo transfer (IVF/ET). The responses to gonadotropic stimulation, the numbers of preovulatory oocytes, the fertilization and cleavage rates, and the clinical pregnancy rates associated with endometriosis have been equivalent to rates associated with tubal disease and unexplained infertility. Loh and colleagues found that the ovarian follicular response to gonadotropins after laparoscopic cystectomy for endometriotic cyst was equivalent to that of normal ovaries. Moreover, the stage of disease does not appear to influence clinical outcome. However, one study has reported a significantly higher miscarriage rate with moderate or severe endometriosis; this is perhaps due to poor embryo quality or autoimmune phenomena.

The necessity of initial medical or surgical therapy before use of assisted reproductive technologies remains controversial. In a 1986 report by Wardle and co-workers, oocyte fertilization rates were markedly reduced in women with untreated endometriosis as compared with those with tubal infertility and endometriosis who were treated with danazol for 6 to 9 months before the IVF treatment cycle. Dicker and associates noted that 35 women with severe endometriosis who underwent 6 months of ovarian suppression with a GnRH analog had a higher clinical pregnancy rate per cycle and per transfer than did 32 women who received ovarian stimulation for IVF without prior GnRH treatment (per cycle, 25% versus 3.9%; per transfer, 33% versus 5.3%). Recent reports suggested that success with IVF was lower in women with endometriomas and that the spontaneous abortion rate may be higher. Hence, resolution or surgical therapy of the endometriomas before the IVF treatment cycle may enhance the ongoing pregnancy rate. Reports of infected endometriotic cysts secondary to oocyte aspiration for IVF also give support to surgical correction before commencing techniques of assisted reproduction.

Gamete intrafallopian transfer (GIFT) may overcome impairment of sperm transport to the fallopian tube, failed ovum capture, or abnormalities in the peritoneal environment associated with endometriosis, although the presence of any anatomic disorders of the fallopian tubes has negative prognostic significance for a successful outcome for this procedure. Hulme and colleagues performed GIFT on 46 infertile patients with minimal to moderately active endometriosis not previously treated by medical or surgical methods. The only prerequisite was patency of at least one fallopian tube. The pregnancy rate per GIFT cycle was 30.5% (18/59), which compared with a clinical pregnancy rate of 25.8% for all patients undergoing the procedure at their unit. One or more endometriomas were aspirated from the ovaries at the time of follicle aspiration in 11 patients; 4 of the 11 achieved live births with GIFT. Nevertheless, Guzick and associates, in a case-control study, found that pelvic endometriosis significantly impaired the efficacy of GIFT. Of 114 laparoscopic oocyte retrievals performed in the endometriosis group, there were 37 pregnancies (32.5%) and 25 deliveries (23.7%); of the 214 retrievals in the control group, there were 101 pregnancies (47.2%) and 76 deliveries (35.5%).

Controlled ovarian hyperstimulation (COH) with human menopausal gonadotropins or pure FSH together with intrauterine insemination (IUI) has been proposed as a method to increase cycle fecundity of patients with endometriosis, although few series have been published to date. By increasing the number of oocytes released at the time of ovulation and introducing a high concentration of spermatozoa into the female reproductive tract, the chance for conception is improved merely because of the larger number of gametes available for fertilization. In addition, subtle abnormalities of folliculogenesis, corpus luteum function, tubal motility, or sperm function may be corrected with this therapy. Cycle fecundity rates associated with COH/IUI therapy in patients with endometriosis-associated infertility have ranged from 9% to 13%, although these series did not include a nontreatment control group. One recent prospective randomized study found a higher pregnancy rate with COH/IUI following at least 6 weeks of GnRH agonist suppression in patients with advanced stages of endometriosis.

One report has suggested that controlled ovarian hyperstimulation does not enhance fecundity in women with minimal endometriosis undergoing timed IUI. In addition, Fedele and associates reported that superovulation with timed intercourse was not associated with a better cumulative pregnancy rate than expectant management in infertile women with endometriosis stages I and II, although the cycle fecundity rate was improved. However, a more recent randomized, controlled trial of controlled ovarian hyperstimulation (COH) and IUI for infertility associated with stage I and II endometriosis demonstrated a live birth rate of 11% in the treatment group and 2% in the control group. Hence, the clinical history must be carefully weighed when planning a sequence of therapy for the infertile patient with endometriosis.

ADENOMYOSIS

The disease called *adenomyosis* is defined as heterotopic endometrial glands and stroma located deep within the myometrium. Adenomyosis can be categorized as diffuse or local in its distribution. Diffuse adenomyosis can be relatively localized but is never encapsulated (Fig. 25.13). The uterus itself is usually mildly enlarged, rarely to more than twice-normal size, and is generally symmetric. Cut sections of the myometrium reveal a coarse trabecular pattern of interlacing musculature and fibrous tissue with small islands of endometrium that are often dark and hemorrhagic. Localized, encapsulated disease of the uterine wall is termed *adenomyoma*, to distinguish this manifestation of adenomyosis from the more usual diffuse pattern. An adenomyoma is always located mainly within the wall of the uterus but may project into the uterine cavity to become further known as a submucous adenomyoma. This encapsulated, submucous form of adenomyosis disease resembles the leiomyoma.

The most widely accepted theory of the origin of adenomyosis is that endometrial tissue within the myometrium is of müllerian origin. Its presence in this location is the result of a direct, downward extension of the endometrium of the uterine cavity. Serial sectioning of tissue has revealed a direct continuity between the basalis portion of the endometrium and the endometrial islands within the areas of adenomyosis. Endometrial extensions sometimes are present through the full thickness of the myometrium to the serosal surface of the uterus. Occasionally, only subserosal adenomyosis is seen. Subserosal adenomyosis is often associated with pelvic endometrio-

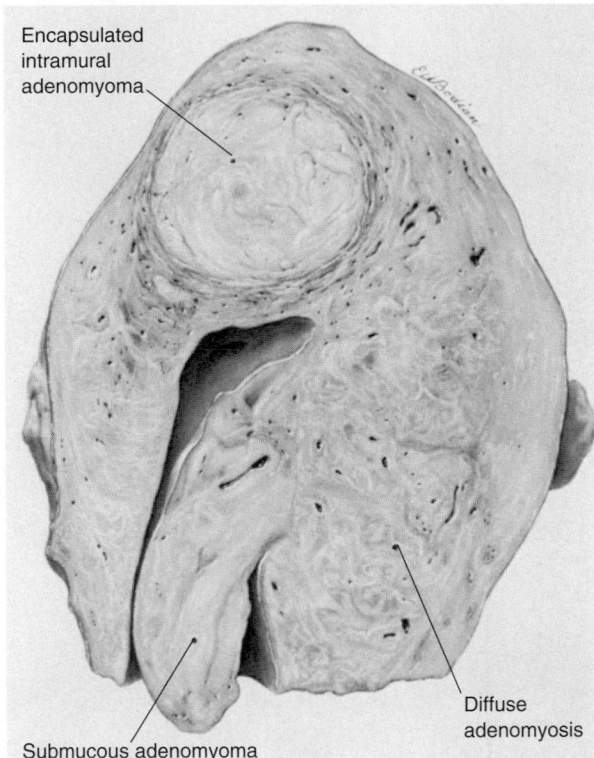

FIGURE 25.13. Uterus showing three types of adenomyomatous growth: encapsulated intramural adenomyoma, submucous adenomyoma, and diffuse adenomyosis of walls.

sis and may cause the lymphatic spread of endometrial fragments.

The intramural islands generally have the same histologic appearance as the basalis of the endometrium (Fig. 25.14) and often respond to estrogen stimulation by demonstrating a proliferative or, occasionally, cystic hyperplastic pattern. Cellular atypia is rare. The effect of progestational agents on the ectopic endometrium is less predictable. Secretory changes in the glands are uncommon except in pregnancy, when a decidual reaction of the stroma is anticipated. Unlike endometriosis, adenomyotic lesions are not characterized by a pronounced hemorrhagic tendency or inflammatory response. In the absence of hormonal stimulation, adenomyosis becomes atrophic. Adenocarcinomas involving adenomyosis are characterized by a history of prior exogenous estrogen use, by low histologic grades, and by an excellent prognosis. Adenomyosis can be definitively diagnosed only through histologic sections of myometrium. The reported incidence of the disease varies widely among institutions, from 8% to 62%, depending on the criteria used for diagnosis and on the thoroughness with which the excised uterine tissue is studied. By tradition, a histologic diagnosis is made when endometrial glands and stroma are found at least 1 low-power field beneath the endomyometrial junction (greater than 4 mm). A more rigid criterion suggested by Benson and Sneeden requires that ectopic endometrium extend into the myo-

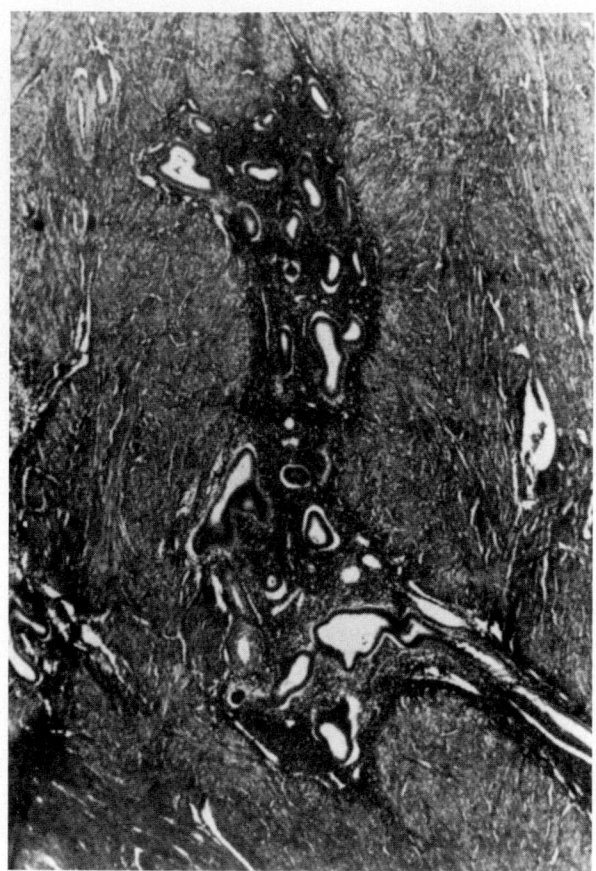

FIGURE 25.14. Area of adenomyosis. Compact stroma and proliferative, slightly hyperplastic glands surrounded by hypertrophied myometrium.

metrium at least 2 low-power fields (8 mm) from the basalis.

The incidence of adenomyosis peaks in the fifth decade. Infertility is not common, although most patients are multiparous. About 12% have coexisting external endometriosis. Adenomyosis is often discovered incidentally in patients undergoing surgery for uterine leiomyomas.

Symptoms

Adenomyosis is often an incidental pathologic finding and may be entirely asymptomatic. Dysmenorrhea is more likely to be reported when glandular invasion exceeds 80% or more of the myometrium. Pain can be severe, cramping, or knifelike. The pattern of dysmenorrhea is likely associated with bleeding episodes within the deep-lying islands of endometrium. Menorrhagia can be a consequence of the increased surface area of the enlarged uterine cavity. In addition, extensive involvement of the myometrium can interfere with the normal contractility of the uterine musculature and can lead to excessive bleeding. Nevertheless, data collected from 1,851 hysterectomies for the prospective, multicenter Collaborative Review of Sterilization study indicate that adeno-

myosis occurs as often in asymptomatic uteri removed for prolapse (19%) as in uteri removed for excessive bleeding (22%) or pain symptoms (15%).

Pelvic Findings

The uterus may be very firm to palpation and is usually enlarged to not more than twice its normal size. As it is classically described, the adenomyotic enlargement occurs in the anteroposterior dimension, a reflection of the more prominent involvement of the posterior uterine wall. In the more common diffuse type of adenomyosis, the uterus is a symmetrically enlarged, globular structure. Encapsulated adenomyomata may cause the uterus to be irregular or asymmetric, much as it is when leiomyomata are present. At times, particularly during menstruation, the enlarged uterus is tender on examination.

Diagnosis

Adenomyosis should always be suspected in a woman with dysmenorrhea and menorrhagia of increasing severity her fourth or fifth decade, particularly if the uterus is symmetrically enlarged, firm, and tender. An exact preoperative diagnosis is often difficult to establish because dysfunctional uterine bleeding and multiple small leiomyomas can present in a similar fashion. Gambone and colleagues reported that a presumptive diagnosis of adenomyosis was verified in only 38% of hysterectomy specimens. The diagnosis can be histologically established before hysterectomy only in the rare case in which excessive myometrium is removed during curettage or a polypoid submucous adenomyoma is excised. However, hysteroscopic myometrial biopsy of the posterior uterine wall with use of a 5-mm loop electrode has been shown to effectively establish the diagnosis in women with menorrhagia.

Hysterosalpingography of the adenomyomatous uterus with water-based media can occasionally demonstrate multiple spiculations or tuft defects leading from the uterine cavity to the myometrial wall; however, similar findings can occur in cases of vascular or lymphatic extravasation. Magnetic resonance imaging has proved to be highly accurate for distinguishing adenomyosis from leiomyomata; on T2-weighted images, adenomyosis appears as an ill-defined, relatively homogeneous, low-signal-intensity area embedded with sparse, high-intensity spots. The optimal junctional zone thickness value for establishing the diagnosis of adenomyosis is 12 mm or more. Recent studies have also suggested an important role for transvaginal ultrasound in distinguishing adenomyosis from leiomyomata. By using the diagnostic criterion of the presence of unencapsulated, heterogeneous, myometrial areas within round anechoic areas 1 to 3 mm in diameter, Fedele and colleagues noted a sensitivity of 80%, a specificity of 74%, a negative predictive value of 81%, and a positive predictive value of 73%. Nevertheless, when transvaginal sonography and magnetic resonance imaging have been prospectively compared, the latter has been significantly more accurate in correctly establishing the diagnosis.

Treatment

Hormone receptor studies have documented the presence of steroid receptors in adenomyotic foci. Estrogen receptors are more consistently present than are progesterone receptors, which are completely absent in 40% of cases evaluated. Progestins or cyclic estrogen-progestin combination preparations offer little aid in treatment, although one recent report indicated that adenomyosis-associated menorrhagia may be controlled with the insertion of a levonorgestrel-releasing intrauterine device. GnRH agonist therapy for 6 months resulted in the disappearance of pain symptoms and a decline in uterine volume in 65% of cases of biopsy-proven adenomyosis, but the dysmenorrhea and menorrhagia recurred at the end of treatment. Nevertheless, extended, intermittent use of these agonists can effectively relieve pain symptoms while having the significant advantage of preserving fertility between treatments.

Curettage does not aid in establishing the diagnosis of adenomyosis and is ineffective as treatment, although it may be required because of abnormal bleeding. The need for surgery, therefore, is based on continued menorrhagia and dysmenorrhea rather than on an estimation of uterine size or even the known presence of adenomyosis or leiomyomata. The definitive treatment for abnormal bleeding caused by adenomyosis is hysterectomy. The vaginal route is preferred if the size of the uterus is appropriate and no other pelvic abnormalities are present. Under certain circumstances, as with a younger patient who wishes to retain her reproductive capability, excision of an encapsulated adenomyoma should be considered instead of hysterectomy. Such situations arise infrequently because adenomyosis is generally diffuse and usually occurs in multiparous women who are no longer interested in childbearing. The precise efficacy of hysteroscopic endometrial resection, laparoscopic myometrial reduction, and myometrial excision as conservative surgical procedures for adenomyosis has yet to be proved. Endometrial ablation is ineffective as treatment for deep, subserosal adenomyosis. Hysterectomy should be considered when preoperative ultrasonography, magnetic resonance imaging, or myometrial biopsy demonstrates deep adenomyosis.

BIBLIOGRAPHY

Adamson DG, Subak LL, Pasta DJ, et al. Comparison of CO_2 laser laparoscopy with laparotomy for the treatment of endometriomata. *Fertil Steril* 1992;57:965.

Adamson GD, Hurd SJ, Pasta DJ, et al. Laparoscopic endometriosis treatment: Is it better? *Fertil Steril* 1993;59:35.

American Fertility Society. The classification of endometriosis. *Fertil Steril* 1979;32:633.

American Fertility Society. Revised American Fertility Society classification of endometriosis: 1985. *Fertil Steril* 1985;43:351.

American Society for Reproductive Medicine. Revised American Society for Reproductive Medicine classification of endometriosis: 1996. *Fertil Steril* 1997;67:817.

Andrews WE, Larsen GD. Endometriosis: treatment with hormonal pseudopregnancy and/or operation. *Am J Obstet Gynecol* 1974;118:643.

Ascher SM, Arnold LL, Patt RH, et al. Adenomyosis: prospective comparison of MR imaging and transvaginal sonography. *Radiology* 1994;190:803.

Awadalla SG, Friedman CI, Haq AU, et al. Local peritoneal factors: their role in infertility associated with endometriosis. *Am J Obstet Gynecol* 1987;157:1207.

Ayers JW, Birenbaum DL, Menon KM. Luteal phase dysfunction in endometriosis: elevated progesterone levels in peripheral and ovarian veins during the follicular phase. *Fertil Steril* 1987;47:925.

Badawy SZA, Cuenca V, Kaufman L, et al. The regulation of immunoglobulin production by B cells in patients with endometriosis. *Fertil Steril* 1989;51:770.

Bailey HR, Ott MT, Hartendorp P. Aggressive surgical management for advanced colorectal endometriosis. *Dis Colon Rectum* 1994;37:747.

Barbieri RL. Etiology and epidemiology of endometriosis. *Am J Obstet Gynecol* 1990;162:565.

Barbieri RL. Hormone treatment of endometriosis: the estrogen threshold hypothesis. *Am J Obstet Gynecol* 1992;166:740.

Barbieri RL. Stenosis of the external os: an association with endometriosis in women with chronic pelvic pain. *Fertil Steril* 1998;70:571.

Barbieri RL, Niloff JM, Bast RC Jr, et al. Elevated serum concentrations of CA-125 in patients with advanced endometriosis. *Fertil Steril* 1986;45:630.

Barbieri RL, Ryan KJ. Danazol: endocrine pharmacology and therapeutic applications. *Am J Obstet Gynecol* 1981;141:453.

Benson RC, Sneeden VD. Adenomyosis: a reappraisal of symptomatology. *Am J Obstet Gynecol* 1958;76:1044.

Beretta P, Franchi M, Ghezzi F, et al. Randomized clinical trial of two laparoscopic treatments of endometriomas: cystectomy versus drainage and coagulation. *Fertil Steril* 1998;70:1176.

Biberoglu KO, Behrman SJ. Dosage aspects of danazol therapy in endometriosis: short term and long term effectiveness. *Am J Obstet Gynecol* 1981;138:645.

Brosens IA, Koninckx PR, Corveleyn PA. A study of plasma progesterone, oestradiol-17β prolactin and LH levels and of the luteal phase appearance of the ovaries in patients with endometriosis and infertility. *Br J Obstet Gynaecol* 1978;85:246.

Brosens I, Vasquez G, Gordts S. Scanning electron microscopy study of the pelvic peritoneum in unexplained infertility and endometriosis. *Fertil Steril* 1984;41:215.

Brooks JJ, Wheeler JE. Malignancy arising in extragonadal endometriosis. *Cancer* 1977;40:3065.

Bruner KL, Mastrsian LM, Rodgers WH, et al. Suppression of matrix metalloproteinases inhibits establishment of ectopic lesions by human endometrium in nude mice. *J Clin Invest* 1997;99:2851

Busacca M, Marana R, Caruana P, et al. Recurrence of ovarian endometriomas after laparoscopic excision. *Am J Obstet Gynecol* 1999;180:519.

Buttram VC Jr, Reiter RC, Ward S. Treatment of endometriosis with danazol: report of a 6 year prospective study. *Fertil Steril* 1985;43:353.

Candiani GB, Fedele L, Vercellini P, et al. Presacral neurectomy for the treatment of pelvic pain associated with endometriosis: a controlled study. *Am J Obstet Gynecol* 1992;167:100.

Candiani GB, Fedele L, Vercellini P, et al. Repetitive conservative surgery for recurrence of endometriosis. *Obstet Gynecol* 1991;77:421.

Candiani GB, Vercellini P, Fedele L. Laparoscopic ovarian puncture for correct staging of endometriosis. *Fertil Steril* 1990;53:994.

Candiani GB, Vercellini P, Fedele L, et al. Conservative surgical treatment for severe endometriosis in infertile women: are we making progress? *Obstet Gynecol Surv* 1991; 48[Suppl 7]:490.

Candiani GB, Vercellini P, Fedele L, et al. Conservative surgical treatment of rectovaginal septum endometriosis. *J Gynecol Surg* 1992;8:177.

Canis M, Mage G, Wattiex A, et al. Second-look laparoscopy after laparoscopic cystectomy of large ovarian endometriomas. *Fertil Steril* 1992;58:617.

Carpenter SE, Markham SM, Rock JA. Exercise may reduce side effects of danazol. *Infertility* 1988;2:259.

Cedars MI, Lu JK, Meldrum DR, et al. Treatment of endometriosis with a long-acting gonadotropin releasing hormone agonist plus medroxyprogesterone acetate. *Obstet Gynecol* 1990;75:641.

Chaffkin LM, Nulsen JC, Luciano AA, et al. A comparative analysis of the cycle fecundity rates associated with combined human menopausal gonadotropin (hMG) and intrauterine insemination (IUI) versus either hMG or IUI alone. *Fertil Steril* 1991;55:252.

Cheesman KL, Ben-Nun I, Chatterton RT Jr, et al. Relationship of luteinizing hormone, pregnanediol-3-glucuronide and estriol-16-glucuronide in urine of infertile women with endometriosis. *Fertil Steril* 1982;38:542.

Cheesman KL, Cheesman SD, Chatterton RT, et al. Alterations in progesterone metabolism and luteal function in infertile women with endometriosis. *Fertil Steril* 1983;40:590.

Chen FP, Soong YK. The efficacy and complications of laparoscopic presacral neurectomy in pelvic pain. *Obstet Gynecol* 1997;90:974.

Chong AP, Luciano AA, O'Shaughnessy AM. Laser laparoscopy versus laparotomy in the treatment of infertility patients with severe endometriosis. *J Gynecol Surg* 1990;6: 179.

Coddington CC, Oehninger S, Cunningham DS, et al. Peritoneal fluid from patients with endometriosis decreases sperm binding to the zona pellucida in the hemizona assay: a preliminary report. *Fertil Steril* 1992; 57:783.

Confino E, Harlow L, Gleicher N. Peritoneal fluid and serum autoantibody levels in patients with endometriosis. *Fertil Steril* 1990;53:242.

Cornillie FJ, Oosterlynck D, Lauweryns JM, et al. Deeply infiltrating pelvic endometriosis: histology and clinical significance. *Fertil Steril* 1989;53:978.

Coronado C, Franklin RR, Lotze EC, et al. Surgical treatment of symptomatic colorectal endometriosis. *Fertil Steril* 1990;53:411.

Cullen TS. The distribution of adenomyomata containing uterine mucosa. *Arch Surg* 1919;80:130.

Czernobilsky B, Morris W. A histologic study of ovarian endometriosis with emphasis on hyperplastic and atypical changes. *Obstet Gynecol* 1979;53:318.

Czernobilsky B, Silverstein A. Salpingitis in ovarian endometriosis. *Fertil Steril* 1978;30:45.

Damewood MD, Hesla JS, Schlaff WD, et al. Effect of serum from patients with minimal to mild endometriosis on mouse embryo development *in vitro*. *Fertil Steril* 1990;54: 917.

Daniell JF. Fiberoptic laser laparoscopy. *Baillieres Clin Obstet Gynaecol* 1989;3:545.

Davis GD. Management of endometriosis and its associated adhesions with the CO_2 laser laparoscope. *Obstet Gynecol* 1986;68:422.

Davis GD, Brooks RA. Excision of pelvic endometriosis with the carbon dioxide laser laparoscope. *Obstet Gynecol* 1988; 72:816.

Dawood MY. Impact of medical treatment of endometriosis on bone mass. *Am J Obstet Gynecol* 1993;168:674.

Dawood MY, Kahn-Dawood FS, Wilson L Jr. Peritoneal fluid prostaglandins and prostanoids in women with endometriosis, chronic pelvic inflammatory disease, and pelvic pain. *Am J Obstet Gynecol* 1984;148:391.

DeLeon FD, Vijayakumar R, Brown M, et al. Peritoneal fluid volume, estrogen, progesterone, prostaglandin, and epidermal growth factor concentrations in patients with and without endometriosis. *Obstet Gynecol* 1986;68:189.

Dicker D, Feldberg D, Goldman JA, et al. The impact of long-term gonadotropin-releasing hormone analogue treatment on preclinical abortions in patients with severe endometriosis undergoing *in vitro* fertilization-embryo transfer. *Fertil Steril* 1992;57:597.

Dickey RP, Olar TT, Taylor SN, et al. Relationship of follicle number, serum estradiol, and other factors to birth rate and multiparity in human menopausal gonadotropin-induced intrauterine insemination cycles. *Fertil Steril* 1991;56:89.

diZerega G, Hodgen G. Endometriosis: role of ovarian steroids in initiation, maintenance, and suppression. *Fertil Steril* 1980;33:649.

Dlugi AM, Miller JD, Knittle J, et al. Lupron depot (leuprolide acetate for depot suspension) in the treatment of endometriosis: a randomized, placebo-controlled, double-blind study. *Fertil Steril* 1990;54:419.

Dmowski WP, Cohen MR. Treatment of endometriosis with an antigonadotropin, danazol. A laparoscopic and histologic evaluation. *Obstet Gynecol* 1975;46:147.

Dmowski WP, Radwanska E, Binor Z, et al. Mild endometriosis and ovulatory dysfunction: effect of danazol treatment on success of ovulation induction. *Fertil Steril* 1986;46: 784.

Dmowski WP, Steele RW, Baker GF. Deficient cellular immunity in endometriosis. *Am J Obstet Gynecol* 1981;141:377.

Döberl A, Berquist A, Jeppson S, et al. Regression of endometriosis following the shorter treatment with, or lower dose of, danazol. *Acta Obstet Gynecol Scand Suppl* 1984; 123:51.

Dodin S, Lemay A, Maheux R, et al. Bone mass in endometriosis patients treated with GnRH agonist implant or danazol. *Obstet Gynecol* 1991;77:410.

Dodson WC, Haney AF. Controlled ovarian hyperstimulation and intrauterine insemination for treatment of infertility. *Fertil Steril* 1991;55:457.

Donnez J, Nisolle M. Co_2 laser laparoscopic surgery: adhesiolysis, salpingostomy, laser uterine nerve ablation and tubal pregnancy. *Baillieres Clin Obstet Gynaecol* 1989;3:525.

Donnez J, Casanas-Roux F, Ferin J, et al. Tubal polyps, epithelial inclusions, and endometriosis after tubal sterilization. *Fertil Steril* 1984;41:56.

Donnez J, Nisolle-Pochet M, Clerckx-Braun F, et al. Administration of nasal buserelin as compared with subcutaneous buserelin implant for endometriosis. *Fertil Steril* 1989;52: 25.

Donnez J, Thomas K. Incidence of luteinized unruptured follicle syndrome in fertile women and in women with endometriosis. *Eur J Obstet Gynecol Reprod Biol* 1982;14:187.

Doody MC, Gibbons WE, Buttram VC Jr. Linear regression analysis of ultrasound follicular growth series: evidence for an abnormality of follicular growth in endometriosis patients. *Fertil Steril* 1988;49:47.

Doyle JB. Paracervical uterine denervation by transection of the cervical plexus for the relief of dysmenorrhea. *Am J Obstet Gynecol* 1955;70:11.

Drake TS, O'Brien WF, Ramwell PW, et al. Peritoneal fluid thromboxane B_2 6-keto-prostaglandin $F_{1\alpha}$ in endometriosis. *Am J Obstet Gynecol* 1981;140:401.

Dunselman GA, Dumoulin JC, Land JA, et al. Lack of effect of peritoneal endometriosis on fertility in the rabbit model. *Fertil Steril* 1991;56:340.

Evers JL. The second look laparoscopy for evaluation of the results of medical treatment of endometriosis should not be performed during ovarian suppression. *Fertil Steril* 1987; 47:502.

Fahaeus L, Larsson-Cohn U, Ljungberg S, et al. Profound alterations of the lipoprotein metabolism during danazol treatment in premenopausal women. *Fertil Steril* 1984;42: 52.

Fakih H, Baggett B, Holtz G, et al. Interleukin-1: a possible role in the infertility associated with endometriosis. *Fertil Steril* 1987;47:218.

Fakih HN, Tamura R, Kesselman A, et al. Endometriosis after tubal ligation. *J Reprod Med* 1985;30:939.

Fayez JA, Collazo LM. Comparison between laparotomy and operative laparoscopy in the treatment of moderate and severe endometriosis. *Int J Fertil* 1990;35:252.

Fayez JA, Vogel MF. Comparison of different treatment methods of endometriomas by laparoscopy. *Obstet Gynecol* 1991;78:660.

Fedele L, Bianchi S, Bocciolone L, et al. Pain symptoms associated with endometriosis. *Obstet Gynecol* 1992;79:767.

Fedele L, Bianchi S, Dorta M, et al. Transvaginal ultrasonography in the differential diagnosis of adenomyoma versus leiomyoma. *Am J Obstet Gynecol* 1992;167:603.

Fedele L, Bianchi S, Marchini M, et al. Superovulation with human menopausal gonadotropins in the treatment of infertility associated with minimal or mild endometriosis: a controlled randomized study. *Fertil Steril* 1992;58:28.

Fedele L, Parazzini F, Bianchi S, et al. Stage and localization of pelvic endometriosis and pain. *Fertil Steril* 1990;53:155.

Feste JR. Laser laparoscopy. A new modality. *J Reprod Med* 1985;30:413.

Forrest J, Buckley CH, Fox H. Pelvic endometriosis and tubal inflammatory disease. *Int J Gynecol Pathol* 1984;3:343.

Foster DC, Stern JL, Buscema J, et al. Pleural and parenchymal pulmonary endometriosis. *Obstet Gynecol* 1981;58: 552.

Franssen AM, Kaver FM, Chadha DR, et al. Endometriosis: treatment with gonadotropin-releasing hormone agonist buserelin. *Fertil Steril* 1989;51:401.

Gambone JC, Reiter RC, Lerich JB, et al. The impact of a quality assurance process in the frequency and confirmation rate of hysterectomy. *Am J Obstet Gynecol* 1990;163:545.

Gant NF. Infertility and endometriosis: comparison of pregnancy outcomes with laparotomy versus laparoscopic techniques. *Am J Obstet Gynecol* 1992;166:1072.

Gerhard I, Gunnebaum B. Grenzen der hormonsubstitution bei schadstoffbelastung und fertilitätsstörungen. *Zentralbl Gynakol* 1992;114, 593.

Glatt AE, Zinner SH, McCormack WM. The prevalence of dyspareunia. *Obstet Gynecol* 1990;75:433.

Gleicher N, El-Roeiy A, Confino E, et al. Is endometriosis an autoimmune disease? *Obstet Gynecol* 1987;70:115.

Gould SF, Shannon JM, Cunha GR. Nuclear estrogen binding sites in human endometriosis. *Fertil Steril* 1983;39:520.

Granberg S, Wikland M, Jansson I. Macroscopic characterization of ovarian tumors and the relation to the histologic diagnosis: criteria to be used for ultrasound evaluation. *Gynecol Oncol* 1989;35:139.

Greenblatt RB, Dmowski WP, Mahesh VB, et al. Clinical studies with an antigonadotropin danazol. *Fertil Steril* 1971;22:102.

Grow DR, Filer RB. Treatment of adenomyosis with long-term GnRH analogues: a case report. *Obstet Gynecol* 1991;78: 538.

Gruenwald P. Origin of endometriosis from the mesenchyme of the coelomic walls. *Am J Obstet Gynecol* 1942;44:470.

Guzick DS. Clinical epidemiology of endometriosis and infertility. *Obstet Gynecol Clin North Am* 1989;16:43.

Guzick DS, Yao YA, Berga SL, et al. Endometriosis impairs the efficacy of gamete intrafallopian transfer: results of a case-control study. *Fertil Steril* 1994;62:1186.

Habuchi T, Okagaki T, Miyakawa M. Endometriosis of bladder after menopause. *J Urol* 1991;145:361.

Halme J, Hammond MG, Hulka JK, et al. Retrograde menstruation in healthy women and in patients with endometriosis. *Obstet Gynecol* 1984;64:151.

Halme J, White C, Kauma S, et al. Peritoneal macrophages from patients with endometriosis release growth factor activity *in vitro. J Clin Endocrinol Metab* 1988;66:1044.

Haney AF, Jenkins S Weinberg JB. The stimulus responsible for the peritoneal fluid inflammation observed in infertile women with endometriosis. *Fertil Steril* 1991;56: 408.

Heaps JM, Nieberg RK, Berek JS. Malignant neoplasms arising in endometriosis. *Obstet Gynecol* 1990;75:1023.

Henzl MR. Gonadotropin-releasing hormone analogs: update on new findings. *Am J Obstet Gynecol* 1992;166:757.

Henzl MR, Corson SL, Moghissi K, et al. Administration of nasal nafarelin as compared with oral danazol for endometriosis. *N Engl J Med* 1988;318:485.

Hickman TN, Namnoum AB, Hinton EL, et al. Timing of estrogen replacement therapy following hysterectomy with oophorectomy for endometriosis. *Obstet Gynecol* 1998;91: 673.

Hill JA, Faris HM, Schiff I, et al. Characterization of leukocyte subpopulations in the peritoneal fluid of women with endometriosis. *Fertil Steril* 1988;50:216.

Hornstein MD, Hemmings R, Yuzpe AA, et al. Use of nafarelin versus placebo after reductive laparoscopic surgery for endometriosis. *Fertil Steril* 1997;68:860.

Hornstein MD, Surrey ES, Weisberg GW, et al. Leuprolide acetate depot and hormonal add-back in endometriosis: a 12-month study. *Obstet Gynecol* 1998;91:16.

Houston DE, Noller RL, Melton LJ III, et al. Incidence of pelvic endometriosis in Rochester, Minnesota 1970β1979. *Am J Epidemiol* 1987;125:959.

Hull ME, Moghissi KS, Magyar DF, et al. Comparison of different treatment modalities of endometriosis in infertile women. *Fertil Steril* 1987;47:40.

Hulme VA, van der Merwe JP, Kruger TF. Gamete intrafallopian transfer as treatment for infertility associated with endometriosis. *Fertil Steril* 1990;53:1095.

Ishimaru T, Masuzaki H. Peritoneal endometriosis: endometrial tissue implantation as its primary etiologic mechanism. *Am J Obstet Gynecol* 1991;165:210.

Jänne O, Kauppila A, Kukko E, et al. Estrogen and progestin receptors in endometriosis lesions: comparison with endometrial tissue. *Am J Obstet Gynecol* 1981;141:562.

Jansen RP, Russell P. Nonpigmented endometriosis: clinical, laparoscopic, and pathologic definition. *Am J Obstet Gynecol* 1986;155:1154.

Javert CT. Pathogenesis of endometriosis based on endometrial homeoplasia direct extension, exfoliation and implantation, lymphatic and hematogenous metastasis. *Cancer* 1949;2: 399.

Jeffcoate T. *Principles of gynecology.* London: Butterworth, 1975.

Jenkins S, Olive DL, Haney AF. Endometriosis: pathogenetic implications of the anatomic distribution. *Obstet Gynecol* 1986;67:335.

Johnson JV, Roxek MM, Moreno AC, et al. Surgically induced endometriosis does not alter peritoneal factors in the rabbit model. *Fertil Steril* 1991;56:343.

Killick S, Elstein M. Pharmacologic production of luteinized unruptured follicles by prostaglandin synthetase inhibitors. *Fertil Steril* 1987;47:773.

Kim CH, Cho YK, Mok JE. Simplified ultralong protocol of gonadotophin-releasing hormone agonist for ovulation induction with intrauterine insemination in patients with endometriosis. *Hum Reprod* 1996;11:398.

Koninckx PR, Braet P, Kennedy SH, et al. Dioxin pollution and endometriosis in Belgium. *Hum Reprod* 1994;9: 1001.

Koninckx P, Ide P, Vandenbroucke W, et al. New aspects of the pathophysiology of endometriosis and associated infertility. *J Reprod Med* 1980;24:257.

Koninckx PR, Martin DC. Deep endometriosis: a consequence of infiltration or retraction or possibly adenomyosis externa? *Fertil Steril* 1992;58:924.

Koninckx PR, Mueleman C, Demeyere S, et al. Suggestive evidence that pelvic endometriosis is a progressive disease, whereas deeply infiltrating endometriosis is associated with pelvic pain. *Fertil Steril* 1991;55:759.

Koninckx PR, Rittinen L, Seppälä M, et al. CA-125 and placental protein 14 concentrations in plasma and peritoneal fluid of women with deeply infiltrating pelvic endometriosis. *Fertil Steril* 1992;57:523.

Lamb K, Hoffman RG, Nichols TR. Family trait analysis: a case-control study of 43 women with endometriosis and their best friends. *Am J Obstet Gynecol* 1986;154:596.

Laufer MR. Identification of clear vesicular lesions of atypical endometriosis: a new technique. *Fertil Steril* 1997;68:739.

Laufer MR, Goitein L, Bush M, et al. Prevalence of endometriosis in adolescent girls with chronic pelvic pain not responding to conventional therapy. *J Pediatr Adolesc Gynecol* 1997;10:199.

Leach RE, Arneson BW, Ball GD, et al. Absence of antisperm antibodies and factors influencing sperm motility in the cul-del-sac fluid of women with endometriosis. *Fertil Steril* 1990;53:351.

Lee NC, Dicker RC, Rubin GL, et al. Confirmation of the preoperative diagnoses for hysterectomy. *Am J Obstet Gynecol* 1984;150:283.

Lee RB, Stone K, Magelssen D, et al. Presacral neurectomy for chronic pelvic pain. *Obstet Gynecol* 1986;69:517.

Lemay A, Maheux R, Faure N, et al. Reversible hypogonadism induced by a luteinizing hormone-releasing hormone (LH-RH) agonist (buserelin) as a new therapeutic approach for endometriosis. *Fertil Steril* 1984;41:863.

Lessey BA, Castelbaum AJ, Sawin SW, et al. Aberrant integrin expression in the endometrium of women with endometriosis. *J Clin Endocrinol Metab* 1994;79:643.

Lichten EM, Bombard J. Surgical treatment of primary dysmenorrhea with laparoscopic uterine nerve ablation. *J Reprod Med* 1987;32:37.

Loh FH, Tan AT, Kumar J, et al. Ovarian response after laparoscopic ovarian cystectomy for endometriotic cysts in 132 monitored cycles. *Fertil Steril* 1999;72:316.

Luciano AA, Hauser KS, Chapler FK, et al. Effects of danazol on plasma lipids and lipoprotein levels in healthy woman and in women with endometriosis. *Am J Obstet Gynecol* 1983;145:422.

Luciano AA, Turksoy RN, Carleo J. Evaluation of oral medroxyprogesterone acetate in the treatment of endometriosis. *Obstet Gynecol* 1988;72:323.

Mahmood TA, Arumugam K, Templeton AA. Oocyte and follicular fluid characteristics in women with mild endometriosis. *Br J Obstet Gynaecol* 1991;98:573.

Mahmood TA, Templeton A. Folliculogenesis and ovulation in infertile women with mild endometriosis. *Hum Reprod* 1991;6:225.

Mahmood TA, Templeton A. Pathophysiology of mild endometriosis: review of literature. *Hum Reprod* 1990;5:765.

Mahmood TA, Templeton A. Peritoneal fluid volume and sex steroids in the preovulatory period in mild endometriosis. *Br J Obstet Gynaecol* 1991;98:179.

Makarainen L, Ronnberg L, Kauppila A. Medroxyprogesterone acetate supplementation diminishes the hypoestrogenic side effects of gonadotropin-releasing hormone agonist without changing its efficacy in endometriosis. *Fertil Steril* 1996;65:29.

Marcoux S, Maheux, Bérubé S, et al. Laparoscopic surgery in infertile women with minimal or mild endometriosis. *N Engl J Med* 1997;337:217.

Marrs RP. The use of potassium-titanyl-phosphate laser for laparoscopic removal of ovarian endometriomas. *Am J Obstet Gynecol* 1991;164:1622.

Martin D. Laparoscopic treatment of ovarian endometriomas. *Clin Obstet Gynecol* 1991;34:452.

Martin DC, Hubert GD, Levy BS. Depth of infiltration of endometriosis. *J Gynecol Surg* 1989;5:55.

Martin DC, Hubert GD, Vander Zwaag R, et al. Laparoscopic appearances of peritoneal endometriosis. *Fertil Steril* 1989;51:63.

Max E, Sweeney WB, Bailey HR, et al. Results of 1,000 single-layer continuous polypropylene intestinal anastomoses. *Am J Surg* 1991;162:461.

McArthur JW, Ulfelder H. The effect of pregnancy upon endometriosis. *Obstet Gynecol* Surv 1965;20:709.

McCausland AM. Hysteroscopic myometrial biopsy: its use in diagnosing adenomyosis and its clinical application. *Am J Obstet Gynecol* 1992;166:1619.

Meldrum DR, Chang RJ, Lu J, et al. "Medical oophorectomy" using a long-acting GnRH agonist: a possible new approach to the treatment of endometriosis. *J Clin Endocrinol Metab* 1982;54:1081.

Metzger DA, Olive DL, Stohs GF, et al. Association of endometriosis and spontaneous abortion: effect of control group selection. *Fertil Steril* 1986;45:18.

Meyer R. über Stand der Frage der Adenomyositis und Adenomyome im Allgemeinen und ins Besondere über Adenomyositis seroepithelialis und Adenomyometritis sarcomatosa. *Zentralbl Gynakol* 1919;36:745.

Mio Y, Toda T, Harada T, et al. Pathophysiology of infertility associated with endometriosis: luteinized unruptured follicle in the early stages of endometriosis as a cause of unexplained infertility. *Am J Obstet Gynecol* 1992;167:251.

Mittal KR, Barwick KW. Endometrial adenocarcinoma involving adenomyosis without true myometrial invasion is characterized by frequent preceding estrogen therapy, low histologic grades, and excellent prognosis. *Gynecol Oncol* 1993;49:197.

Moen M, Bratlie A, Moen T. Distribution of HLA antigens among patients with endometriosis. *Acta Obstet Gynecol Scand Suppl* 1984;123:25.

Moghissi KS, Boyce CR. Management of endometriosis with oral medroxyprogesterone acetate. *Obstet Gynecol* 1976;47: 265.

Moore EE, Harger JH, Rock JA, et al. Management of pelvic endometriosis with low-dose danazol. *Fertil Steril* 1981; 36:15.

Moore JG, Binstock MA, Growdon WA. The clinical implications of retroperitoneal endometriosis. *Am J Obstet Gynecol* 1988;158:1291.

Moore JG, Hibbard LT, Growdon WA, et al. Urinary tract endometriosis: enigmas in diagnosis and management. *Am J Obstet Gynecol* 1979;134:162.

Morcos RN, Gibbons WE, Findlay WE. Effect of peritoneal fluid on *in vitro* cleavage of 2-cell mouse embryos: possible role in infertility associated with endometriosis. *Fertil Steril* 1985;44:678.

Murphy AA, Green WR, Bobbie D, et al. Unsuspected endometriosis documented by scanning electron microscopy in visually normal peritoneum. *Fertil Steril* 1986;46:522.

Murphy AA, Schlaff WD, Hassiakos D, et al. Laparoscopic cautery in the treatment of endometriosis-related infertility. *Fertil Steril* 1991;55:246.

Muscato JJ, Haney AF, Weinberg JB. Sperm phagocytosis by human peritoneal macrophages: a possible cause of infertility in endometriosis. *Am J Obstet Gynecol* 1982;144:503.

Muzii L, Marana R, Caruana P, et al. The impact of preoperative gonadotropin-releasing hormone agonist treatment on laparoscopic excision of ovarian endometriotic cysts. *Fertil Steril* 1996;65:1235.

Muzii L, Marana R, Pedulla S, et al. Correlation between endometriosis-associated dysmenorrhea and the presence of typical and atypical lesions. *Fertil Steril* 1997;68:19.

Muzii L, Marana R, Caruana P, et al. Postoperative administration of monophasic combined oral contraceptives after laparoscopic treatment of ovarian endometriomas: a prospective, randomized trial. *Am J Obstet Gynecol* 2000; 183;588.

Namnoum AB, Hickman TN, Goodman SB, et al. Incidence of symptom recurrence after hysterectomy for endometriosis. *Fertil Steril* 1995;64:898.

Naples JD, Batt RE, Sadigh A. Spontaneous abortion rate in patients with endometriosis. *Obstet Gynecol* 1981;57:509.

Nezhat C, Seidman DS, Nezhat F, et al. Laparoscopic surgical management of diaphragmatic endometriosis. *Fertil Steril* 1998;69:1048.

Nezhat CH, Seidman DS, Nezhat FR, et al. Long-term outcome of laparoscopic presacral neurectomy for the treatment of central pelvic pain attributed to endometriosis. *Obstet Gynecol* 1998;91:701.

Nezhat C, Nezhat F, Pennington E. Laparoscopic treatment of infiltrative rectosigmoid colon and rectovaginal septum endometriosis by the technique of video laparoscopy and the CO_2 laser. *Br J Obstet Gynaecol* 1992;99:664.

Nishida M. Relationship between the onset of dysmenorrhea and histologic findings in adenomyosis. *Am J Obstet Gynecol* 1991;165:229.

Noble AD, Letchworth AT. Medical treatment of endometriosis: a comparative trial. *Postgrad Med J* 1979;55:37.

Noble LS, Simpson ER, John A, et al. Aromatase expression in endometriosis. *J Clin Endocrinol Metab* 1996;81:174.

Oak MK, Chantler EN, Williams CA, et al. Sperm survival studies in peritoneal fluid from infertile women with endometriosis and unexplained infertility. *Clin Reprod Fertil* 1985;3:297.

Oehninger S, Acosta AA, Kreiner D, et al. *In vitro* fertilization and embryo transfer (IVF/ET): an established and successful therapy for endometriosis. *J Vitro Fert Embryo Transfer* 1988;5:249.

Ohtsuka N. Study on pathogenesis of adhesions in endometriosis. *Nippon Sanka Fujinka Gakkai Zasshi* 1980;32: 1758.

Olive DL, Haney AF. Endometriosis-associated infertility: a critical review of therapeutic approaches. *Obstet Gynecol Surv* 1986;41:1.

Olive DL, Henderson DY. Endometriosis and müllerian anomalies. *Obstet Gynecol* 1987;69:412.

Olive DL, Lee KL. Analysis of sequential treatment protocols for endometriosis-associated infertility. *Am J Obstet Gynecol* 1986;154:613.

Olive DL, Martin DC. Treatment of endometriosis-associated infertility with CO_2 laser laparoscopy: the use of one- and two-parameter exponential models. *Fertil Steril* 1987;48:18.

Olive DL, Montoya I, Riehl RM, et al. Macrophage-conditioned media enhance endometrial stromal cell proliferation *in vitro*. *Am J Obstet Gynecol* 1991;164:953.

Oosterlynck DJ, Cornillie FJ, Waer M, et al. Women with endometriosis show a defect in natural killer cell activity resulting in a decreased cytotoxicity to autologous endometrium. *Fertil Steril* 1991;56:45.

Parazzini F, Fedele L, Busacca M, et al. Postsurgical medical treatment of advanced endometriosis: results of a randomized clinical trial. *Am J Obstet Gynecol* 1994;171:1205.

Paull T, Tedeschi LG. Perineal endometriosis at the site of episiotomy scar. *Obstet Gynecol* 1972;40:28.

Pinkert T, Catlow C, Straus R. Endometriosis of the urinary bladder in a man with prostatic carcinoma. *Cancer* 1979;43:1562.

Pittaway DE. CA-125 in women with endometriosis. *Obstet Gynecol Clin North Am* 1989;16:237.

Pittaway DE, Daniell JF, Maxson WS. Ovarian surgery in an infertility patient as an indication for a short-interval second-look laparoscopy: a preliminary study. *Fertil Steril* 1985;44: 611.

Pittaway DE, Douglas JW. Serum CA-125 in women with endometriosis and chronic pelvic pain. *Fertil Steril* 1989;51: 68.

Pittaway DE, Vernon C, Fayez JA. Spontaneous abortions in women with endometriosis. *Fertil Steril* 1988;50:711.

Pokras R, Hufnagel VG. Hysterectomy in the United States, 1965–84. *Am J Public Health* 1988;78:852.

Polan ML, DeCherney A. Presacral neurectomy for pelvic pain in infertility. *Fertil Steril* 1980;34:557.

Prystowsky JB, Stryker SJ, Ujiki GT, et al. Gastrointestinal endometriosis. Incidence and indications for resection. *Arch Surg* 1988;123:855.

Puleo JG, Hammond CB. Conservative treatment of endometriosis externa: the effects of danazol therapy. *Fertil Steril* 1983;40:164.

Punnonen R, Soderstrom P, Alanen A. Isthmic tubal occlusion: etiology and histology. *Acta Eur Fertil* 1984;15:39.

Ranney B. Endometriosis IV: hereditary tendency. *Obstet Gynecol* 1971;37:734.

Rao B, Karim SM. *in vitro* effects of ICI 81008, a $PGF_{2\alpha}$ analogue on the human corpus luteum. *IRCS Med Sc Endocrinol Syst* 1985;3:339.

Redwine DB. Conservative laparoscopic excision of endometriosis by sharp dissection: life table analysis of reoperation and persistent or recurrent disease. *Fertil Steril* 1991;56:28.

Redwine DB. The distribution of endometriosis in the pelvis by age groups and fertility. *Fertil Steril* 1987;47:173.

Redwine DB. Endometriosis persisting after castration: clinical characteristics and results of surgical management. *Obstet Gynecol* 1994;83:405.

Redwine DB. Peritoneal blood painting: an aid in the diagnosis of endometriosis. *Am J Obstet Gynecol* 1989;161:865.

Redwine DB. Ovarian endometriosis: a marker for more extensive pelvic and intestinal disease. *Fertil Steril* 1999;72:310.

Rezai N, Ghodgaonkar RB, Zacur HA, et al. Cul-de-sac fluid in women with endometriosis: fluid volume, protein and prostanoid concentration during the periovulatory period—days 13 to 18. *Fertil Steril* 1987;48:29.

Ridley JH. The validity of Sampson's theory of endometriosis. *Am J Obstet Gynecol* 1961;82:777.

Rier SE, Martin DC, Bowman RE, et al. Endometriosis in rhesus monkeys (*Macaca mulatta*) following chronic exposure to 2,3,7,8-tetrachlorodibenzo-p-dioxin. *Fundam Appl Toxicol* 1993;21:433.

Riis BJ, Christiansen C, Johansen JS, et al. Is it possible to prevent bone loss in young women treated with luteinizing hormone-releasing hormone agonists? *J Clin Endocrinol Metab* 1990;70:920.

Riva HL, Kawasaki DM, Messinger AJ. Further experience with norethynodrel in treatment of endometriosis. *Obstet Gynecol* 1962;19:111.

Rivlin ME, Miller JD, Krueger RP, et al. Leuprolide acetate in the management of ureteral obstruction caused by endometriosis. *Obstet Gynecol* 1990;75:532.

Rock JA, Dubin NH, Ghodgaonkar RB, et al. Cul-de-sac fluid in women with endometriosis: fluid volume and prostanoid concentration during the proliferative phase of the cycle—days 8–12. *Fertil Steril* 1982;37:747.

Rock JA, Guzick DS, Jones HW Jr. The efficacy of accessory surgical intervention in conjunction with resection and fulguration of endometriosis. *Infertility* 1981;4:193.

Rock JA, Guzick DS, Sengos C, et al. Evaluation of pregnancy success with respect to extent of disease as categorized using contemporary classification systems. *Fertil Steril* 1981;35:131.

Rock JA, Parmley TH, King TM, et al. Endometriosis and the development of tuboperitoneal fistulas after tubal ligation. *Fertil Steril* 1981;35:16.

Ruggi G. Della sympatectamia al collo ed ale ad ome. *Policlinico* 1899;193.

Sakamoto A. Subserosal adenomyosis: a possible variant of pelvic endometriosis. *Am J Obstet Gynecol* 1991;165:198.

Saleh A, Tulandi T. Reoperation after laparoscopic treatment of ovarian endometriomas by excision and by fenestration. *Fertil Steril* 1999;72:322.

Sampson JA. Benign and malignant endometrial implants in peritoneal cavity, and their relation to certain ovarian tumors. *Surg Gynecol Obstet* 1924;38:287.

Sampson JA. Peritoneal endometriosis due to menstrual dissemination of endometrial tissue into the peritoneal cavity. *Am J Obstet Gynecol* 1925;14:422.

Schenken RS, Asch RH, Williams RF, et al. Etiology of infertility in monkeys with endometriosis: luteinized unruptured follicles, luteal phase defects, pelvic adhesions and spontaneous abortions. *Fertil Steril* 1984;41:122.

Schenken RS, Williams RF, Hodgen GD. Effect of pregnancy on surgically induced endometriosis in cynomolgus monkeys. *Am J Obstet Gynecol* 1987;157:1392.

Schlaff WD, Dugoff L, Damewood MD, et al. Megestrol acetate for treatment of endometriosis. *Obstet Gynecol* 1990;75:646.

Schmidt CL. Endometriosis: a reappraisal of pathogenesis and treatment. *Fertil Steril* 1985;44:157.

Schneider VL, Schneider A, Reed KL, et al. Comparison of Doppler with two-dimensional sonography and CA-125 for prediction of malignancy of pelvic masses. *Obstet Gynecol* 1993;81:983.

Schoysman R. Tubal microsurgery versus *in vitro* fertilization. *Acta Eur Fertil* 1984;15:5.

Schweppe KW, Wynn RM. Ultrastructural changes in endometriotic implants during the menstrual cycle. *Obstet Gynecol* 1981;58:465.

Schweppe KW, Wynn RM, Beller FK. Ultrastructural comparison of endometriotic implants and eutopic endometrium. *Am J Obstet Gynecol* 1984;148:1024.

Seibel MM, Berger MJ, Weinstein FG, et al. The effectiveness of danazol on subsequent fertility in minimal endometriosis. *Fertil Steril* 1982;38:534.

Sekiba K, Obstetrics and Gynecology Adhesion Prevention Committee. Use of Interceed (TC7) absorbable adhesion barrier to reduce postoperative adhesion reformation in infertility and endometriosis surgery. *Obstet Gynecol* 1992;79:518.

Serta RT, Rufo S, Seibel MM. Minimal endometriosis and intrauterine insemination: does controlled ovarian hyperstimulation improve pregnancy rates? *Obstet Gynecol* 1992;80:37.

Shook TE, Nyberg LM. Endometriosis of the urinary tract. *Urology* 1988;31:1.

Simpson JL, Elias S, Malinak LR, et al. Heritable aspects of endometriosis. I. Genetic studies. *Am J Obstet Gynecol* 1980;137:325.

Simpson JL, Malinak LR, Elias S, et al. HLA associations in endometriosis. *Am J Obstet Gynecol* 1984;148:395.

Spandorfer SD, Davis OK, Navarro J, et al. Endometrioma at the inception of an IVF-ET cycle: A negative predictor of outcome. *Am Soc Reprod Med* (abst P-216) Toronto, Canada, Sept 1999.

Steele RW, Dmowski WP, Marmer DJ. Immunologic aspects of human endometriosis. *Am J Reprod Immunol* 1984;6:33.

Stock RJ. Postsalpingectomy endometriosis: a reassessment. *Obstet Gynecol* 1982;60:560.

Stovall TG, Ling FW, Crawford DA. Hysterectomy for chronic pelvic pain of presumed uterine etiology. *Obstet Gynecol* 1990;75:676.

Strathy JH, Molgaard CA, Coulam CB, et al. Endometriosis and infertility: a laparoscopic study of endometriosis among fertile and infertile women. *Fertil Steril* 1982;38:667.

Stripling MC, Martin DC, Chatman DL, et al. Subtle appearance of pelvic endometriosis. *Fertil Steril* 1988;49:425.

Sueldo CE, Lambert H, Steinleitner A, et al. The effect of peritoneal fluid from patients with endometriosis on murine sperm–oocyte interaction. *Fertil Steril* 1987;48:697.

Suginami H, Yano K. An ovum capture inhibitor (OCI) in endometriosis peritoneal fluid: an OCI-related membrane responsible for fimbrial failure of ovum capture. *Fertil Steril* 1988;50:648.

Surgical Membrane Study Group. Prophylaxis of pelvic sidewall adhesions with Gore-Tex surgical membrane: a multicenter clinical investigation. *Fertil Steril* 1992;57:921.

Surrey ES, Gambone JC, Lu JK, et al. The effects of combining norethindrone with a gonadotropin-releasing hormone agonist in the treatment of symptomatic endometriosis. *Fertil Steril* 1990;53:620.

Surrey ES, Halme J. Effect of platelet-derived growth factor on endometrial stromal cell proliferation *in vitro*: a model for endometriosis? *Fertil Steril* 1991;56:672.

Surrey ES, Voigt B, Fournet N, et al. Prolonged gonadotropin-releasing hormone agonist treatment of symptomatic endometriosis: the role of cyclic sodium etidronate and low-dose norethindrone "add-back" therapy. *Fertil Steril* 1995;63:747.

Sutton CJ, Ewen SP, Whitelaw N, et al. Prospective, randomized, double-blind, controlled trial of laser laparoscopy in the treatment of pelvic pain associated with minimal, mild, and moderate endometriosis. *Fertil Steril* 1994;62:696.

Takahashi K, Okada S, Ozaki T, et al. Diagnosis of pelvic endometriosis by "fat-saturation" technique. *Fertil Steril* 1994;62:973.

Tamaya T, Motoyama T, Ohono Y, et al. Steroid receptor levels and histology of endometriosis and adenomyosis. *Fertil Steril* 1979;31:396.

Telimaa S. Danazol and medroxyprogesterone acetate inefficacious in the treatment of infertility in endometriosis. *Fertil Steril* 1988;50:872.

Te Linde RW, Scott RB. Experimental endometriosis. *Obstet Gynecol* 1978;130:569.

Thomas EJ, Lenton EA, Cooke ID. Follicle growth patterns and endocrinological abnormalities in infertile women with minor degrees of endometriosis. *Br J Obstet Gynaecol* 1986;93:852.

Thompson JD. Primary ovarian adenoacanthoma: its relationship to endometriosis. *Obstet Gynecol* 1957;9:403.

Tjaden B, Schlaff WD, Kimball A, et al. The efficacy of presacral neurectomy for the relief of midline dysmenorrhea. *Obstet Gynecol* 1990;76:89.

Togashi K, Ozasa H, Konishi I, et al. Enlarged uterus: differentiation between adenomyosis and leiomyoma with MR imaging. *Radiology* 1989;171:531.

Tseng JF, Ryan IP, Milam TD, et al. Interleukin-6 secretion *in vitro* is up-regulated in ectopic and eutopic endometrial stromal cells from women with endometriosis. *J Clin Endocrinol Metab* 1996;81:1118.

Tulandi T, Al-Took S. Reproductive outcome after treatment of mild endometriosis with laparoscopic excision and electrocoagulation. *Fertil Steril* 1998;69:229.

Tulandi T, Mouchawar M. Treatment-dependent and treatment-independent pregnancy in women with minimal and mild endometriosis. *Fertil Steril* 1991;56:790.

Tummon IS, Asher LJ, Martin JS, et al. Randomized controlled trial of superovulation and insemination for infertility associated with minimal or mild endometriosis. *Fertil Steril* 1997;68:8.

Tummon IS, Colwell KA, MacKinnoa CJ, et al. Abbreviated endometriosis-associated infertility correlates with *in vitro* fertilization success. *J Vitro Fert Embryo Transfer* 1991;8:149.

Tummon IS, Maclin VM, Radwanska E, et al. Occult ovulatory dysfunction in women with minimal endometriosis and unexplained infertility. *Fertil Steril* 1988;50:716.

Typhonas H, Luster MI, Schiffman G, et al. Effect of chronic exposure of PCB (Aroclor 1254) on specific and nonspecific immune parameters in the rhesus (*Macaca mulatta*) monkey. *Fundam Appl Toxicol* 1991;16:773.

Uchima FDA, Edery M, Iguchi T, et al. Growth of mouse endometrial luminal epithelial cells *in vitro*: functional integrity of the oestrogen receptor system and failure of oestrogen to induce proliferation. *J Endocrinol* 1991;128:115.

Uohara JK, Kovara TY. Endometriosis of the appendix: report of 12 cases and review of the literature. *Am J Obstet Gynecol* 1975;121:423.

Vaughan Williams CA, Oak MK, Elstein M. Cyclical gonadotrophin and progesterone secretion in women with minimal endometriosis. *Clin Reprod Fertil* 1986;4:259.

Vercellini P, Vendola N, Bocciolone L, et al. Reliability of visual diagnosis of ovarian endometriosis. *Fertil Steril* 1991;56:1198.

Vercellini P, Fedele L, Bianchi S, et al. Pelvic denervation for chronic pain associated with endometriosis: fact or fancy? *Am J Obstet Gynecol* 1991;165:745.

Vercellini P, De Giorgi O, Oldani S, et al. Depot medroxyprogesterone acetate versus an oral contraceptive combined with very-low-dose danazol for long-term treatment of pelvic pain associated with endometriosis. *Am J Obstet Gynecol* 1996;175:396.

Verkauf BS. The incidence, symptoms, and signs of endometriosis in fertile and infertile women. *J Fla Med Assoc* 1987;74:671.

Vernon MW, Beard JS, Graves K, et al. Classification of endometriotic implants by morphologic appearance and capacity to synthesize prostaglandin F. *Fertil Steril* 1986;46:801.

Vigano P, Vercellini P, Di Blasio AM, et al. Deficient antiendometrium lymphocyte–mediated cytotoxicity in patient with endometriosis. *Fertil Steril* 1991;56:894.

von Rokitansky C. Ueber Uterusdrusen-Neubildung im Uterus und Varialsarcomen. *Zkk Gesellsch d Aerzte zu Wien* 1860;37:577.

Wardle PG, Foster PA, Mitchell JD. Endometriosis and IVF: effect of prior therapy. *Lancet* 1986;1:256.

Wardle PG, Hull MG. Is endometriosis a disease? *Baillieres Clin Obstet Gynaecol* 1993;7:673.

Weed JC, Arquembourg PC. Endometriosis: can it produce an autoimmune response resulting in infertility? *Clin Obstet Gynecol* 1980;23:885.

Wentz AC. Premenstrual spotting: its association with endometriosis but not luteal phase inadequacy. *Fertil Steril* 1980;33:605.

Wespi HJ, Kletzhändler M. Uber Narbenendometriosen. *Mschr Geburtsh Gynakol* 1940;111:169.

Wheeler JM, Johnston BM, Malinak LR. The relationship of endometriosis to spontaneous abortion. *Fertil Steril* 1983;39:656.

Wheeler JM, Malinak LR. Postoperative danazol therapy in infertility patients with severe endometriosis. *Fertil Steril* 1981;36:460.

Wheeler JM, Malinak LR. Recurrent endometriosis: incidence, management, and prognosis. *Am J Obstet Gynecol* 1983;146:247.

Wilcox LS, Koonin LM, Pokras R, et al. Hysterectomy in the United States, 1988–1990. *Obstet Gynecol* 1994;83:549.

Wihemsson L, Lindblom B, Wiqvist N. The human uterotubal junction: contractile patterns of different smooth muscle layers and the influence of prostaglandin E_2, prostaglandin $F_{2\alpha}$ and prostaglandin I_2 *in vitro*. *Fertil Steril* 1979;32:303.

Wood C, Maher P, Hill D. Biopsy diagnosis and conservative surgical treatment of adenomyosis. *Aust NZ J Obstet Gynaecol* 1993;33:319.

Yaron Y, Peyser MR, Samuel D, et al. Infected endometriotic cysts secondary to oocyte aspiration for in-vitro fertilization. *Hum Reprod* 1994;9:1759.

Ylikorkla O, Koskimies A, Laathainen T, et al. Peritoneal fluid prostaglandins in endometriosis, tubal disorders, and unexplained infertility. *Obstet Gynecol* 1984;63:616.

Yanushpolsky EH, Best CL, Jackson KV, et al. Effects of endometriomas on oocyte quality, embryo quality, and pregnancy rates in *in vitro* fertilization cycles: a prospective, case-controlled study. *J Assist Reprod Genet* 1998;15:193.

Young MD, Blackmore WP. The use of danazol in the management of endometriosis. *J Int Med Res* 1977;5[Suppl 3]:86.

Zanagnolo VL, Beck R, Schlaff WD, et al. Time-related effects of gonadotropin-releasing hormone analog treatment in experimentally induced endometriosis in the rat. *Fertil Steril* 1991;55:411.

CHAPTER
26

▼

Surgery for Benign Disease of the Ovary

JOSEPH S. SANFILIPPO   JOHN A. ROCK

Significant progress has been made with regard to ovarian reconstruction for benign disease. It has been established that the ovaries and fallopian tubes are sensitive to ischemia from the trauma of surgery; secondary adhesions may develop, and the normal anatomic relationship between fallopian tubes, ovaries, and uterus may be altered. Knowledge regarding anatomy and embryology of the ovaries and other reproductive organs complemented by mastery of the principles and skills of microsurgery are the prerequisites for excellent results following ovarian reconstructive surgery. Embryology and anatomy are addressed in this chapter with emphasis on the importance of the anatomic relations of the ovary to other pelvic organs in the section on the evaluation and management of the adnexal mass. State of the art surgical procedures and techniques devised for the reconstruction of the ovary and for full restoration of normal pelvic anatomy are presented in the context of specific pathology or other abnormal conditions that require surgical intervention. This chapter also focuses on pediatric and adolescent surgical procedures that are performed when ovarian pathology is identified.

EMBRYOLOGY

Early in gestation, at about 4 to 5 weeks, two gonadal ridges arise in the developing embryo as thickening on the medial aspect of the coelomic cavity adjacent to the mesonephros. These gonadal outgrowths are composed of coelomic epithelium and underlying mesenchyme projecting into the future peritoneal cavity. The epithelial and mesenchymal cells of the gonadal primordia are of mesodermal origin (large, spherical ovoid germ cells that originate extragonadally in the wall of the yolk sac and migrate to the developing gonads). The gonads of the two sexes remain morphologically indistinguishable until the 6th week of gestation. The presumptive ovaries remain undifferentiated until the onset of meiosis at the end of the first trimester. The ovarian cortex is a single germinal epithelium. The tunica albuginea lies beneath the cortex and is composed of connective tissue. The stroma is made up of fibroblasts, smooth muscle, endothelium and interstitial cells, including undifferentiated theca cells and corpora albicans.

Sexual differentiation requires initiation by various genes along with a single gene determinant on the Y chromosome (TDF, testis-determining factor), which is necessary for testicular differentiation. In XX individuals (in the absence of a Y chromosome), the bipotential gonad develops into an ovary.

The mechanisms responsible for gonadal sex differentiation are largely unknown. Investigators have theorized the presence of a testicular determining factory (H-Y cell-surface antigen on the short arm of the Y chromosome) that is elaborated by a specific gene. Meiosis-inducing and preventing substances, both of which are produced by cells derived from mesonephric structures adjacent to the gonad, are the agents of regulation of ovarian and testicular germ cell differentiation. The balance between these two substances varies between the two sexes and at different stages of development. The meiosis-inducing substance predominates in the fetal ovary. Maternal ovarian hormone production is not required for differentiation of the germ cells or, apparently, for later development of the fetal reproductive tract. Various ultrastructural studies have shown no specific changes in fetal granulosa cells that can be definitely associated with steroid hormone secretion such as is identified in the fetal Leydig cells. Thecal cells play an essential role in steroid synthesis in the adult ovary, but they do not appear until later in gestation and even then retain a relatively undifferentiated appearance. Fetal pituitary gonadotropin production begins as early as 10 weeks' gestation and reaches peak levels at midgestation. Gonadotropins have a major influence on follicular development in the adult ovary, but evidence for a similar function in the fetus is lacking.

GENE EXPRESSION

Specific follicular cell receptors bind growth factors, which are locally synthesized with the ultimate effect of intracellular signaling and protein kinase activation. This activity affects transcription of targeted genes. Gene expression is involved in follicle development, ovulation, and corpus luteum and corpus albicans formation. Transcription factors include protooncogenes, C-myc, and CCAAT/enhancer binding protein.

FEMALE FETAL DEVELOPMENT

During the early prefollicular stage, the ovarian surface cortex is characterized by germ cells and granulosa cells organized in cords and sheets, but the cortex lacks specific conformation. The last distinctive change to occur in the fetal ovary is the onset of meiosis, at the 11th or 12th week of gestation. Meiosis is preceded by differentiation of primitive germ cells into actively dividing mitotic cells called *oogonia*. The mitotic divisions of the oogonia are associated with complete separation at telophase, leaving the daughter cells connected by intracellular bridges. After a series of mitotic divisions, there is progressive entry into meiosis by cell groups, beginning in the innermost cortex and gradually extending to the periphery. These cells passing through the various stages of the first meiotic prophase are then designated *oocytes*. By late gestation, all surviving oocytes have advanced to the diplotene stage. Further differentiation of the oocytes is arrested at this stage and does not resume until ovulation begins at menarche, about 12 years later.

Follicular formation begins at 18 to 20 weeks' gestation and continues throughout the remaining weeks of fetal development. All the surviving oocytes are surrounded by adjacent granulosa cells; oocyte and follicular growth are well established by the late fetal and early neonatal period. The constant degeneration and loss of oocytes before their incorporation into the follicles reduces their numbers to only 1 to 2 million (follicles) in the newborn ovary.

ANATOMY

The ovary is almond-shaped and is about half the size of a testis. The dimensions of the adult ovary vary from individual to individual but average 3 to 5 cm long, 2 to 3 cm wide, and 1 to 2 cm thick, with a weight of 3 to 8 g. The surface of the ovary is pinkish gray to white. The ovary normally is smooth in childhood, but its surface becomes pitted from follicular maturation and atresia, and the surface of the adult ovary can be markedly wrinkled.

The size, shape, and position of the ovary in the pelvis are somewhat variable, and both the consistency and the follicular changes taking place within the ovary vary with the stage of the menstrual cycle. The ovary typically is anchored to the side wall of the pelvis in the shallow peritoneal fossa of Waldeyer formed between the angle of proximity of the ovary to the ureter. This knowledge is important before dissecting the ovary off the pelvic side wall.

The ovary is connected to the uterus by the uteroovarian ligament, to the posterior aspect of the broad ligament by the mesovarium ligament, and to the lateral pelvic sidewall by the infundibulopelvic ligament (Fig. 26.1). The mesovarium ligament attaches to the mesentery of the ovary. The other two ligaments are attached at the hilum of the ovary.

The ovary, like the testis, migrates downward from high in the abdomen during embryonic life. The infundibulum of the fallopian tube extends onto the ovary and is attached to it at its most distal pole by a structure called the *fimbria ovarica*. The relation of the ovary to the fimbria ovarica and to the uteroovarian ligament is crucial, and they should be carefully maintained during ovarian reconstruction.

During embryogenesis, the ovary may assume an unusual appearance (i.e., it may be septate) or assume an unusual position (Fig. 26.2). An accessory ovary (Fig. 26.2A) contains ovarian tissue and usually is close to or is connected to a normally placed ovary. An accessory ovary also may be attached to the broad, uteroovarian or infundibulopelvic ligaments. Unlike the accessory ovary, a *supernumerary ovary* (Fig. 26.2B) must have an independent embryologic origin. It may develop from a primordium such as arrested migrating gonadocytes. A supernumerary ovary consists of typical ovarian tissue but has no direct or ligamentous connection with a normally placed ovary. A supernumerary ovary is thus a true third ovary that has independent function and is located at some distance from a normally placed ovary. Ovarian malposition (Fig. 26.2C) also may occur when the ovary fails to descend into the pelvis to assume its normal lo-

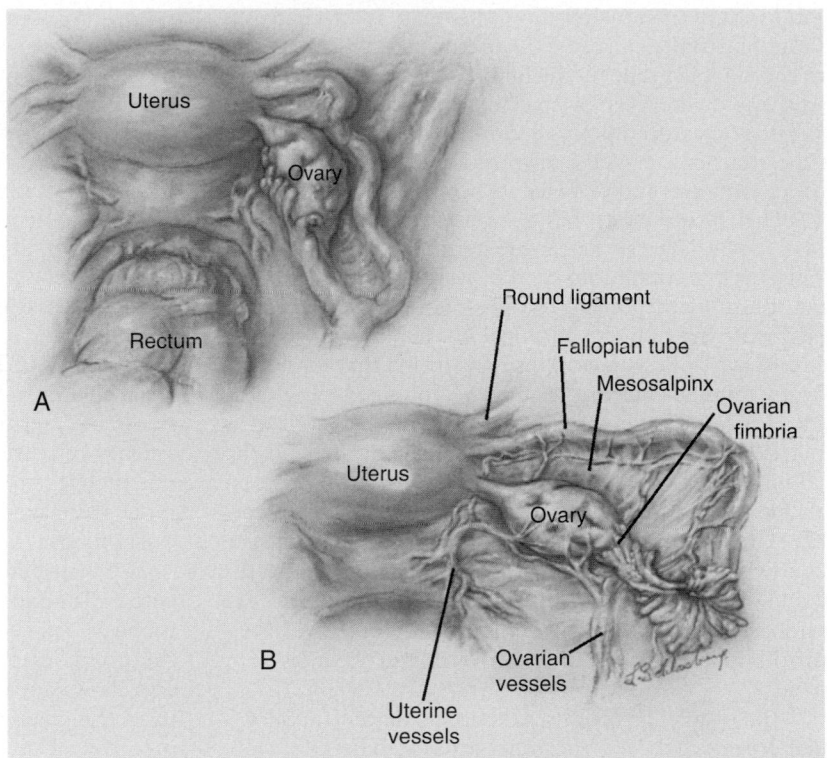

FIGURE 26.1. Normal anatomy of the ovary. **A:** Anatomic relations of the uterus, tube, and ovary. **B:** The infundibulum of the oviduct extends onto the ovary and is attached at its most distal pole (ovarian fimbria). The mesovarian is the mesentery of the ovary. Each ovary is attached at the hilum.

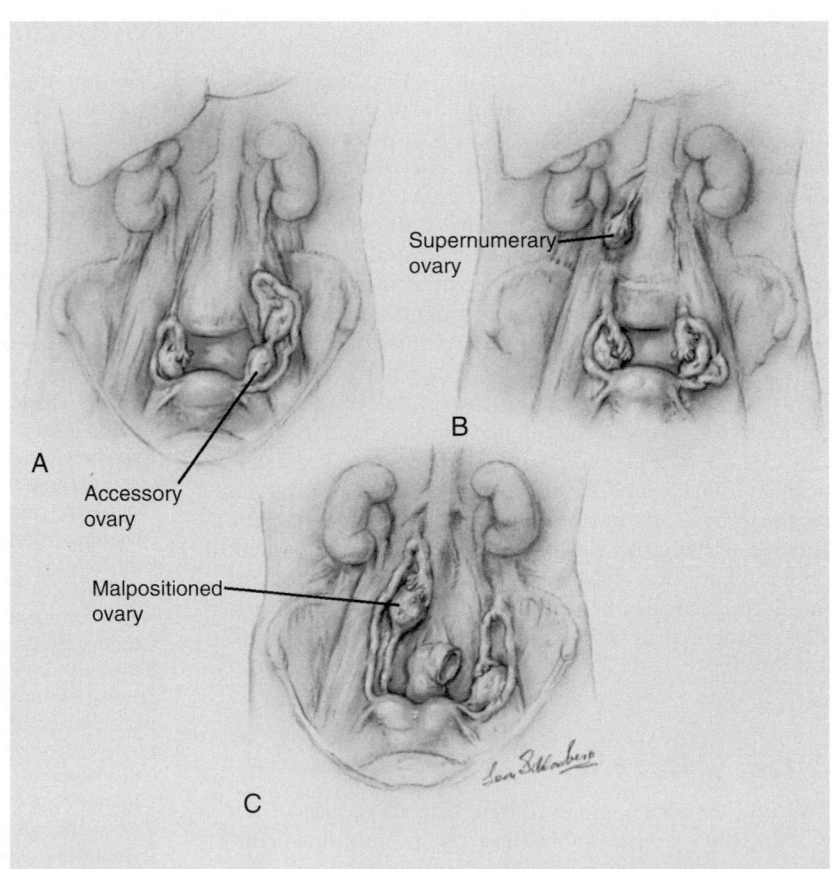

FIGURE 26.2. Ovarian anomalies. **A:** Accessory. **B:** Supernumerary. **C:** Malpositioned.

cation. In ovarian malposition, the ovary is attached as it should be to the uterus by the uteroovarian ligament and to the fallopian tube by the fimbria ovarica, but it may lie adjacent to the liver or spleen. The ovary is elongated and may measure up to 15 cm in length. The fallopian tube attaching to such a malpositioned ovary may be 20 to 26 cm long, almost twice its normal length.

The normal ovary has a surface covering composed of a single layer of flattened, germinal epithelial cells. This layer is contiguous at the ovarian hilum, with the peritoneal epithelium of the posterior leaf of the broad ligament. Beneath the germinal epithelium is a second, strong layer of condensed ovarian stroma that forms a fibrous capsule called the tunica albuginea. The area through which the vessels and nerves enter and exit is called the hilum of the ovary. Immediately around the hilum and extending into the substance of the ovary is an area known as the medulla, which is covered by the cortex. The medulla is composed of fibrous tissue unlike the condensed stroma of the ovarian cortex. The medulla contains no follicles; it has only blood vessels and the remnants of the tubular structure that would have developed into a testis (i.e., the rete ovarii) had the fetus been male.

The ovarian artery arises on each side of the abdominal aorta just below the renal arteries. The artery descends from the aorta and crosses the ureter obliquely to enter the infundibulopelvic ligament on its course to the ovary. When it reaches the broad ligament, the ovarian artery branches also to the fallopian tube and ovary before it finally anastomoses directly with the uterine artery to form a continuous arcade in the broad ligament. The ovarian veins are situated mainly in the mesosalpinx, where they give rise to the pampiniform plexus. At the outer end of the broad ligament, this plexus coalesces to form a single, large ovarian vein. The ovarian vein accompanies the ovarian artery to terminate in the inferior vena cava on the right and the renal vein on the left.

The lymphatic vessels of the ovary drain in three directions. The main group accompanies the ovarian vessels in the infundibulopelvic ligament and eventually reaches the periaortic nodes in the vicinity of the kidney. Other lymphatic channels communicate with channels of the opposite ovary by crossing the fundus of the uterus through the ovarian ligament. Some channels drain through the ovarian and round ligaments into the superficial inguinal lymph nodes in the groin. The ovary is supplied by both motor and sensory parasympathetic and sympathetic nerves, which accompany the ovarian vessels from the abdomen as they pass into the infundibulopelvic ligament to reach the hilum of the ovary. The segmented nerves supply the ovary from T-10 and T-11.

ADNEXAL MASS

The uterine adnexa (gynecologic origin) consist of the ovaries, the fallopian tubes, and the uterine ligaments. Although adnexal pathology often involves one of these structures, contiguous tissue of nongynecologic origin also may be involved. The bimanual examination is the most practical method of screening for an adnexal mass. When such a mass is found, its initial characteristics should be carefully described so that any subsequent change can be appreciated and the nature of the mass can be better ascertained. The description should include location, size (in centimeters), consistency, shape, mobility, tenderness, bilaterality, and associated findings (e.g., fever, ascites).

Adjunctive diagnostic techniques such as sonography, magnetic resonance imaging (MRI), and computed tomography (CT) may help delineate the nature of adnexal enlargement. Pelvic ultrasonography is an accurate means of determining the location, size, extent, and consistency of pelvic masses and is also useful for detecting obstructive uropathy, ascites, and metastasis. Other, more specialized diagnostic procedures also may be necessary for the evaluation of an adnexal mass (Table 26.1).

CT can detect and precisely measure pelvic masses with a diameter of 2 cm or more. It has been particularly useful in gynecologic oncology because it helps define the extent of paracervical and parametrial involvement and allows a reasonable determination of the resectability of malignant neoplasms. MRI has surpassed CT in the precision of measurement of adnexal masses. MRI also allows a clear definition of the relationship of adjacent organs.

OVARIOSCOPY

Evaluation and management has taken on a new parameter–ovarioscopy. This surgical technique provides endocystic visualization within the ovary. The surgeon can

---

TABLE 26.1.
Special Diagnostic Procedures for the Evaluation of an Adnexal Mass

---

Nonoperative Noninvasive
  Abdominal and pelvic radiography
  Barium enema
  Excretory urography
  Gastrointestinal series with small bowel follow-through
  Computed tomography scan
  Magnetic resonance imaging
  β-hCG
  CA-125
Nonoperative Invasive
  Culdocentesis
  Pelvic arteriography
Operative Noninvasive
  Abdominal and pelvic examination under anesthesia
Operative Invasive
  Culdoscopy
  Laparoscopy
  Exploratory posterior colpotomy
  Exploratory laparotomy

---

evaluate the cyst wall and any anatomic abnormality related to its blood supply. Ovarioscopy has proven to be one other means of further enhancing diagnostic acumen to distinguish benign from frankly malignant as well as borderline lesions. The procedure was performed in a series of 68 patients with unilateral or bilateral adnexal masses without clinical or sonographic evidence of suspected malignancy. Tumor markers [cancer antigen 125 (CA-125), carcinoembryonic antigen, and alpha fetoprotein] were obtained preoperatively. Intraoperative endocystic ovarioscopic evaluation and ovarioscopic-directed biopsy were performed before laparoscopy. In comparison with tumor markers and transvaginal ultrasonography, ovarioscopy proved to have the greatest specificity for detecting benign ovarian cysts. The positive predictive value of the technique was 50% in comparison to 5% for tumor markers and 6% for transvaginal ultrasound. Although the data are preliminary, ovarioscopy appears to be one possible additional step in distinguishing benign from malignant ovarian masses.

Although every adnexal mass requires individual evaluation and management, it is possible to make a number of useful general recommendations. Expectant management is justified only when an asymptomatic, physiologic cyst is suspected. Most cysts greater than 6 cm in diameter require a thorough evaluation. Imaging techniques are invaluable for characterizing the nature of the adnexal enlargement, but these procedures do not replace a careful medical history and thorough physical and pelvic examination.

In a study conducted by Timmerman and co-workers, assessment was made of the use of both ultrasound and circulating levels of CA-125 antigen. Multivariate logistic regression analysis algorithms were used to distinguish benign adnexal masses from a malignant process. Transvaginal ultrasonography with color Doppler imaging was recorded in the 191 patients evaluated, ages 18 to 93 years. Of interest, 26.7% of the cohort of patients studied had malignant tumors. The authors believed that regression analysis could be used to accurately discriminate malignant from benign adnexal masses preoperatively.

An intriguing aspect of ultrasound assessment is the prediction of malignancy in adnexal masses using an artificial neural network. Taylor and colleagues reported generating a neural network algorithm that enables computing of a probability of malignancy score for preoperative discrimination between malignant and benign adnexal masses. A retrospective analysis that included training in artificial neural network assessing transvaginal B-mode ultrasonography and color Doppler imaging was determined. The variables that were put into the artificial neural network included age, menopausal status, maximum diameter of the neoplasm, tumor volume, and papillary projections. The results identified four primary variables that were most effective in distinguishing benign versus malignant processes. These variables included age, time-average maximum velocity, papillary projection score, and maximum tumor diameter. The authors concluded that artificial neural networks are a useful clinical parameter to distinguish benign from malignant ovarian masses.

Surgery ultimately may be necessary to determine the nature of the adnexal mass. Laparoscopy may be useful to exclude benign ovarian or nonovarian neoplasms. Indications for visualization of an adnexal mass with laparoscopy or exploratory laparotomy include the following:

- Ovarian mass greater than 6 cm in diameter
- Adnexal mass greater than 10 cm in diameter
- Any mass first developing after menopause
- Failure to discover the nature of the mass (e.g., leiomyoma) with radiologic or sonographic imaging techniques

One of the major goals of the evaluation of the adnexal mass is to rule out malignancy. There is an age-dependent risk for a malignant adnexal mass. The incidence of malignant neoplasm increases significantly after age 50 years. Increased size of the adnexal mass is associated with an increased risk of malignancy.

Granberg and colleagues found that less than 1% of masses smaller than 5 cm were malignant, less than 11% of masses 5 to 10 cm were malignant, and 72% of masses larger than 10 cm were malignant. Sassone and associates, in an evaluation of women of all ages (mean age, 41 years) by transvaginal sonography, found that 3% of masses smaller than 5 cm and 7% of masses 5 to 10 cm were malignant; the incidence of malignancy for masses larger than 10 cm was 13%.

Endometriosis is a common cause of an adnexal mass. An endometrial cyst of the ovary may develop into an endometrioma. Leakage of blood from the cyst may cause peritoneal irritation, pelvic adhesions, and pelvic organ fixation.

Tuboovarian inflammatory complex usually is the result of incompletely treated or unresolved subacute, chronic pelvic inflammatory disease (PID) in the walled-off area surrounding the pelvic structure.

A hydrosalpinx may be unilateral or bilateral and is primarily a sequela of acute or chronic PID. A hydrosalpinx usually is asymptomatic; however, it may be associated with chronic pelvic pain, dyspareunia, and a sense of pelvic pressure.

Ectopic pregnancy may be the cause of a potentially serious, nonneoplastic, nonovarian mass. The physician should have a high index of suspicion in the case of any patient with irregular bleeding, pain, and an adnexal mass. More than 50% of women with tubal pregnancy have no palpable adnexal mass, and an adnexal mass is an unusual finding if the pregnancy is early.

Uterine leiomyomata cause nodularity and consequent irregular conformation of the uterus. The uterus may become enlarged and may present as an abdominal mass. The inability to distinguish a leiomyoma from an ovarian tumor on pelvic examination is an indication for further diagnostic evaluation.

Adnexal enlargement may be the result of carcinoma of the rectum, appendix, or bladder. Patients present with a variety of symptoms according to the organ involved. A complete and thorough evaluation is necessary to fully delineate the cause of a neoplasm. A barium enema before surgery for women older than 40 years of age with a left adnexal mass is recommended to address the possibility of cancer of the rectosigmoid.

An adnexal mass may be noted in cases of acute abdomen. The differential diagnosis should include adnexal torsion, ruptured hemorrhagic cyst, degenerating leiomyomata, ectopic pregnancy, unruptured tuboovarian abscess, acute appendicitis with or without abscess formation, and diverticular disease of the sigmoid colon. A careful history, pelvic examination, and appropriate imaging studies often allow a prompt diagnosis.

ADNEXAL MASS DURING PREGNANCY

The incidence of adnexal mass in pregnancy requiring surgical intervention has been reported to occur in 1 in 81 to 2,500 pregnancies. When an adnexal mass is noted incidentally on ultrasound during pregnancy, the majority of small, simple cysts do not pose a risk to the pregnancy. Furthermore, most large or sonographically complex masses spontaneously resolve as reported by Bernhard and colleagues. This study evaluated 18,391 ultrasound studies done in an obstetric population for which 432 women were identified with an adnexal mass. The rate of incident of adnexal masses was 2.3% in the pregnant population evaluated. In addition, the rate of torsion of the adnexal mass was 1% and the rate of malignancy was also reported as 1%.

Before operative intervention, a complete assessment of the fetus, including ultrasound to rule out a lethal anomaly and to document cardiac activity, is in order. The optimal time for elective surgery is during the second trimester. The patient should be informed of the increased risk of preterm labor and delivery. The patient should be placed in the left lateral tilt position to avoid inferior vena cava compression and associated uteroplacental insufficiency. Postoperatively, the fetus should be placed on continuous fetal heart rate monitoring.

The most effective approach in management of adnexal masses during pregnancy remains a point of controversy (i.e., laparoscopy versus laparotomy). In a series of 88 pregnant women who underwent 93 surgical procedures for suspected adnexal pathology, laparoscopy was performed during the first trimester in 39 patients. The remaining 54 patients underwent laparotomy, 25 during the first trimester and 29 during the second trimester. Neither intraoperative nor postoperative internal complications were reported in the series. Five of 39 women undergoing the first trimester surgery had a spontaneous abortion. During the first trimester, a Veress needle was used for insufflation and the procedure was in essence conducted in a manner virtually identical to that in the nonpregnant state (i.e., closed laparoscopy). It was concluded that laparoscopic gynecologic surgery is safe during pregnancy when conducted in the first trimester.

ULTRASOUND

Ultrasound is also useful in predicting malignancy (Table 26.2). Many authors have identified characteristic features of benign versus malignant neoplasms. Collated data from studies of ultrasound accuracy in the prediction of malignancy have an average positive predictive value of 74% and an average sensitivity of 88% (Table 26.3).

Weiner and co-workers have used transvaginal color flow imaging before exploratory surgery to study the impedance to blood flow in women with an adnexal mass. Intramural blood vessels consistently demonstrated low impedance to flow with a pulsatility index less than 1:16 in women with malignant tumors. The sensitivity and specificity of the preoperative pulsatility index in detecting malignant ovarian tumors were 94% and 97%, respectively. Kurjak and colleagues found that vessels with a low resistance index near the center of the mass or within papules or septa were highly correlated with malignancy. Therefore, transvaginal color flow imaging may be a useful clinical tool in the preoperative evaluation of ovarian masses.

Doppler resistance index has been used as a "vascular" scoring system. Color Doppler ultrasonography appears to be a reliable method in presurgically evaluating ovarian neoplasms.

Transvaginal color Doppler sonography has identified the following parameters as useful in determining malignant versus benign ovarian masses. The parameters include the number of vessels detected in each tumor, tumor vessel location (central versus peripheral), peak systolic velocity, lowest resistance index, mean resistance index, lower pulsatility index, and mean pulsatility index. Color Doppler signals were detected in 100% of malignant masses and 75% of benign masses, with the difference being statistically significant as reported by Alcazar and associates. Tumor vessel location appears to be cen-

---

TABLE 26.2.
Ultrasound Characteristics of the Ovary

Benign Pattern
   Simple cyst without internal echoes
   Simple cyst with scattered echoes
   Polycystic echoes
   Polycystic echoes with thick septum
   Sessile or polypoid smooth mural echoes
   Central dense round echoes
   Thin or thick multiple linear echoes
   Thin or thick multiple linear echoes with dense part
Malignant Pattern
   Cystic echoes with papillary or indented mural part
   Polycystic echoes with irregular thick septum and solid part
   Solid pattern (>50%) heterogeneous component with irregular cystic part
   Completely solid with homogeneous component
   Low impedance to flow (color Doppler)

TABLE 26.3.
Ultrasound Accuracy in Prediction of Malignancy

Author	Patients (*n*)	Malignancy Prevalence	Positive Predictive Value (%)	Negative Predictive Value (%)	Sensitivity	Specificity
Kobayashi et al. 1976	406	15	31	93	71	73
Meire et al. 1978	51	35	83	91	83	91
Pussell, 1980	25	48	83	91	83	84
Herrmann et al. 1987	241	21	75	95	82	93
Finkler et al. 1988	102	36	88	81	62	95
Benacerraf et al. 1990	100	30	72	91	80	87
Granberg et al. 1989	180	21.5	74	95	82	92
Sassone et al. 1991	143	10	87	100	100	83

tral in virtually all malignant masses. Overall the receiver operating characteristic curves generated can be used to predict malignant processes. The lowest resistance index was associated with the majority of malignant tumors.

Three-dimensional ultrasonographic technology has been used to evaluate adnexal masses. Images are dissected in XYZ planes and can be focused especially on areas suggestive of malignancy. Three-dimensional ultrasonography facilitates real-time analysis of acquired image data and allows reassessment of the findings at the time of the original ultrasound. Three-dimensional transvaginal ultrasonographic technology appears to enhance and facilitate morphologic assessment of benign as well as malignant ovarian masses.

TUMOR MARKERS

Tumor markers are substances that are identified in higher than normal amounts in blood, urine, or body tissues of patients with specific malignancies. The tumor marker is produced by the tumor per se or as a response to the presence of cancer. They are not unique to malignant processes and can be elevated with benign conditions. Tumor markers are not elevated in every patient with malignancy, especially in the early stages of the disease. Many (tumor markers) are not specific for a particular type of cancer; therefore, there are limitations to the use of tumor markers.

CA-125 is a tumor-associated antigen to an antibody expressed by about 80% of patients with epithelial ovarian cancer. It can be increased by nongynecologic malignancies with involvement of the pleura or peritoneum and by benign conditions that result in ascites. Because of the many medical diagnoses that give false-positive CA-125 results, CA-125 cannot be used for general population screening for ovarian cancer in either premenopausal or postmenopausal women. However, in menopausal women who present with a pelvic mass, CA-125 can help differentiate benign from malignant masses.

Because menopausal women have fewer gynecologic diseases that give false elevation of CA-125, the test is more sensitive and specific in this age group. Several authors have demonstrated that a panel of assays can improve both sensitivity and specificity in the detection of ovarian malignancies. For example, Soper and associates demonstrated 100% specificity and predictive value for CA-125 with TAG 72 or CA-15-3. Table 26.4 provides specific markers and their clinical application.

TABLE 26.4.
Tumor Markers-Adnexal Masses

Marker	Comments
CA-125	80% nonmucinous ovarian carcinomas have elevation of CA-125. Decreasing levels generally indicate response to therapy. Used to identify recurrences.
CEA	Primary use is to monitor recurrence of colon cancer. Oncofetal antigen-Ag complex glycoprotein, 20,000 d associated with plasma membrane of tumor cells. Increased with ovarian cancer and with melanoma, breast, pancreatic, stomach, cervical, bladder, kidney, thyroid, and liver cancer. Inflammatory bowel disease and smoking elevates CEA.
cMyc	Amplified in 30%–50% of ovarian tumors. The protein is simultaneously overexpressed.
CMycRA	Associated with aneuploidy in ovarian malignant cell progression.
BRCA-1	Associated with mutations of breast tumor related antigen. BRCA-1 tumor suppressor gene has been identified; 63% risk of developing ovarian cancer with positive BRCA-1 gene.

LAPAROSCOPIC MANAGEMENT OF AN OVARIAN MASS

The pelvic (adnexal) mass may be of gynecologic or nongynecologic origin (Table 26.5). Specific clinical findings are helpful to differentiate a malignant from a benign neoplasm (Table 26.6). It is important to establish whether the mass is of ovarian origin and to understand that a mass causing an ovary to enlarge to greater than 6 cm in diameter should be considered potentially malignant until proved otherwise. The most common ovarian mass is the physiologic ovarian cyst, which is caused by failure of a follicle to rupture or to regress. Physiologic ovarian cysts normally are less than 6 cm in diameter, smooth, mobile, and slightly tender to palpation. They usually contain straw-colored fluid and may be associated with menstrual irregularity. Physiologic ovarian cysts smaller than 6 cm usually regress by absorption of the fluid or spontaneous rupture. The premenopausal patient may be managed conservatively over two menstrual cycles. If regression fails to occur over two periods of observation or if enlargement is noted, reassessment is indicated.

Oral contraceptives have been suggested as an alternative treatment for functional cysts. The combination-type oral contraceptives send negative feedback to the pituitary gland to decrease gonadotropin stimulation of the ovary, which causes regression of the cyst. Steinkampf and colleagues noted that the rate of disappearance of functional ovarian cysts was not affected by estrogen-progestin treatment; nevertheless, a patient taking oral contraceptives with an adnexal mass should be thoroughly investigated.

Failure of the corpus luteum to regress (in the nonpregnant patient) may cause development of a corpus luteum cyst. The size of the corpus luteum cyst varies according to the amount of blood contained within the cyst. A large corpus luteum may rupture and cause intraperitoneal hemorrhage. Amenorrhea or irregular uterine bleeding may accompany the development of a corpus luteum cyst. A sensitive pregnancy test, ultrasonography, and laparoscopy can be used to differentiate an ectopic pregnancy from a persistent corpus luteum.

A theca-lutein cyst, which may be associated with gestational trophoblastic disease or pregnancy, is the result of luteinization of the ovary by human chorionic gonadotropin (hCG). Many of these cysts are bilateral and multicystic. A reduction in hCG levels usually leads to their spontaneous regression.

Polycystic ovarian disease is associated with bilaterally enlarged ovaries with a smooth surface. The ovaries contain multiple follicular cysts; many patients are obese and hirsute and have accompanying anovulation.

The clinical findings listed in Tables 26.3 through 26.6 are often helpful in differentiating a malignant from a benign neoplasm. All ovarian neoplasms larger than 6 cm in diameter *or with a solid* component should undergo investigation. The postmenopausal ovary is usually small and nonpalpable. Enlargement of the postmenopausal ovary requires immediate investigation. Symptoms of ovarian neoplasms usually depend on their size, rate of growth, and position in the pelvis or abdomen. Symptoms may include vague lower abdominal fullness or pressure discomfort. Larger masses rise out of the true pelvis and may cause abdominal enlargement with varicosities and edema of the lower extremities. Most ovarian neoplasms are asymptomatic until they enlarge or involve adjacent organs and structures.

Congenital anomalies of the müllerian system and vestigial remnants of the wolffian system are of gynecologic, if not strictly ovarian, origin. Müllerian anomalies

TABLE 26.6.
Clinical Findings Suggesting Benign or Malignant Adnexal Mass

Benign	Malignant
Unilateral	Bilateral
Cystic	Solid
Mobile	Fixed
Smooth	Irregular
No ascites	Ascites
Slow growth	Rapid growth
Young patient	Older patient

TABLE 26.5.
Classification of the Adnexal Mass

Gynecologic Origin	Nongynecologic Origin
Nonneoplastic	Nonneoplastic
Ovarian	Appendiceal abscess
Physiologic cysts	Diverticulosis
Follicular	Adhesions of bowel and
Corpus luteum	omentum
Theca-lutein cyst	Peritoneal cyst
Luteoma of pregnancy	Feces in rectosigmoid
Polycystic ovaries	Urine in bladder
Inflammatory cysts	Pelvic kidney
	Urachal cyst
Nonovarian	Anterior sacral meningocele
Ectopic Pregnancy	Neoplastic
Congenital anomalies	Carcinoma
Embryologic remnants	Sigmoid
Tubal	Cecum
Pyosalpinx	Appendix
Hydrosalpinx	Retroperitoneal neoplasm
Bladder	Presacral teratoma
Neoplastic	
Ovarian	
Nonovarian	
Leiomyomata	
Paraovarian cyst	
Endometrial carcinoma	
Tubal carcinoma	

Adapted from Hall DJ, Hurt WG. The adnexal mass. *J Fam Pract* 1982;14:135, with permission.

should be considered in the differential diagnosis of an adnexal mass. Uterine anomalies usually are associated with cyclic pain from development of hematometra, whereas an enlarged paraovarian cyst may be asymptomatic.

OVARIAN REMNANT SYNDROME

The ovarian remnant occurs in patients who have had previous oophorectomy with or without hysterectomy. The symptomatic patient may present with or without a palpable mass or with a palpable pelvic mass but no symptoms. Pathologic investigation confirms the presence of ovarian tissue when there should be none.

The ovarian remnant syndrome differs from the residual ovarian syndrome in that, with the latter, the ovary is purposely saved and a pathologic process subsequently develops in the ovary. The ovarian remnant syndrome follows oophorectomy.

Minke and associates demonstrated that devascularization of ovarian tissue can occur with reimplanting on intact or abraded peritoneal surfaces, where it may resume endocrine function. Thus, the authors suggest that great care should be exercised to remove all ovarian tissue, particularly when oophorectomy is performed through the laparoscope.

Ultrasonography remains a valuable tool in establishing the diagnosis of ovarian remnant syndrome. The use of both transabdominal sonography and transvaginal sonography with use of color Doppler identification of the mass acquire information with respect to both arterial and venous flow. This facilitates identification of ovarian tissue. With respect to diagnosis, use of gonadotropin-releasing hormone (GnRH) agonist stimulation test has specific utility. The patient often presents with chronic pelvic pain with or without a pelvic mass. Use of GnRH agonist stimulation test allows identification of the presence of functioning ovarian tissue in association with ovarian remnant syndrome. Associated chronic pelvic pain frequently responds to suppressive therapy. Initially, the gonadotropin flare results in increased production of estradiol and allows confirmation of the diagnosis. As treatment is continued, the GnRH agonist often proves efficacious in relief of pelvic pain.

Symmonds and Petit identified three major factors that may complicate the initial surgery and make it difficult or impossible for the surgeon to ascertain whether all ovarian tissue has been removed: increased pelvic vascularity, which renders hemostasis difficult; adhesions, which distort the anatomy and make dissection difficult; and neoplasms, which also distort the anatomy. The most common preexisting disease is endometriosis, followed in frequency by PID. Patients with ovarian remnant syndrome often present with both pelvic pain and a mass. The quality of the pain varies, often cyclically, and ranges from a sensation of pressure or dull aching to a severe stabbing pain.

The clinical diagnosis of ovarian remnant syndrome can be difficult. A finding of premenopausal levels of follicle-stimulating hormone (FSH) may facilitate the diagnosis. Sonography (especially vaginal) may be of some value, and a CT scan or MRI may be useful for defining the physical relation of the ovarian remnant to surrounding structures.

The treatment of choice is adequate excision of the ovarian remnant with removal of contiguous adherent tissue such as pelvic peritoneum, bowel serosa, the underlying involved ligament, and alveolar and vascular tissues (Fig. 26.3). Excision of ovarian tissue may require a retroperitoneal dissection to define the relation of the ureter to the bowel and ovary. Special care should be taken to carefully define all anatomic relations before extirpation of the remnant.

Laparoscopic excision of ovarian remnant ovaries is feasible. A laparoscopic retroperitoneal approach that allows dissection of the course of the ureters with coagulation and dissection of the infundibulopelvic ligament and the uterine vessels can be accomplished. Surgeons with appropriate laparoscopic skills can consider this surgical approach. There is potential for ureteral injury as well as cystotomy and bowel injury.

RESIDUAL OVARY

Based on the clinical circumstance, the gynecologic surgeon should consider the value of ovarian conservation at the time of hysterectomy for benign disease. Some authors have noted the incidence of malignant neoplasm in retained ovaries as a reason for prophylactic oophorectomy, and others have noted the presence of "residual ovary syndrome," characterized by either recurrent pelvic pain or a persistent pelvic mass (Fig. 26.4). However, Funt followed up 992 patients after conservation of one or both ovaries at the time of hysterectomy and reported that none developed ovarian malignancy and only 1.4% required subsequent surgical intervention for adnexal pathology. The benefits of preserved ovarian function thus appear to substantially outweigh the risk of subsequent ovarian pathology requiring further surgery. Before surgery, the gynecologic surgeon should discuss the various risks and benefits of castration and should encourage the patient to participate in any decision concerning the fate of her ovaries.

GnRH agonists have been used to assess response of residual ovaries with chronic pelvic pain followed by surgical intervention to remove the residual ovarian tissue. Resolution of pelvic pain in six treated patients occurred with the analog (GnRH agonist) and persisted with surgical extirpation of the ovarian tissue. Suppression of ovarian function by GnRH agonists allows differentiation of pelvic pain caused by residual ovary from other sources and thus should be a prerequisite to surgical intervention.

In a retrospective report of 20 years' experience with residual ovary syndrome in which 2,561 hysterectomies were performed, the incidence of residual ovary syndrome was 2.85%. Thus, 1 in 35 women who undergo hysterectomy become symptomatic, that is, they experi-

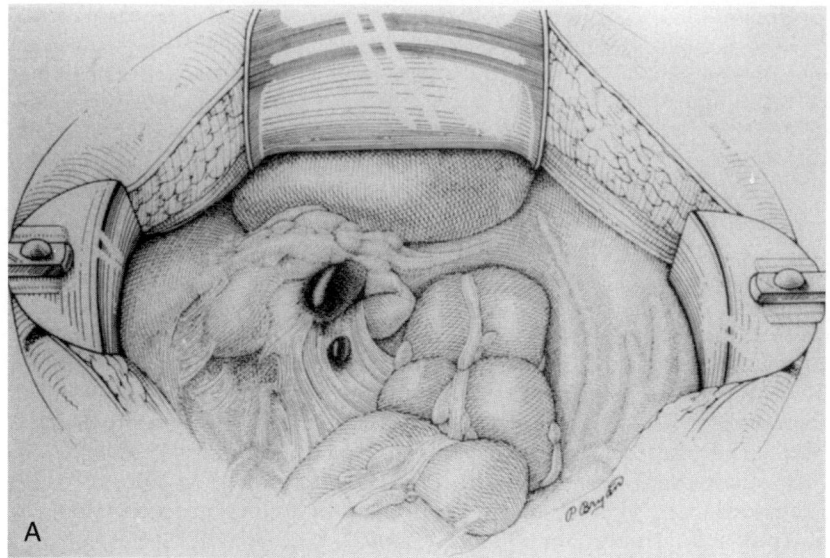

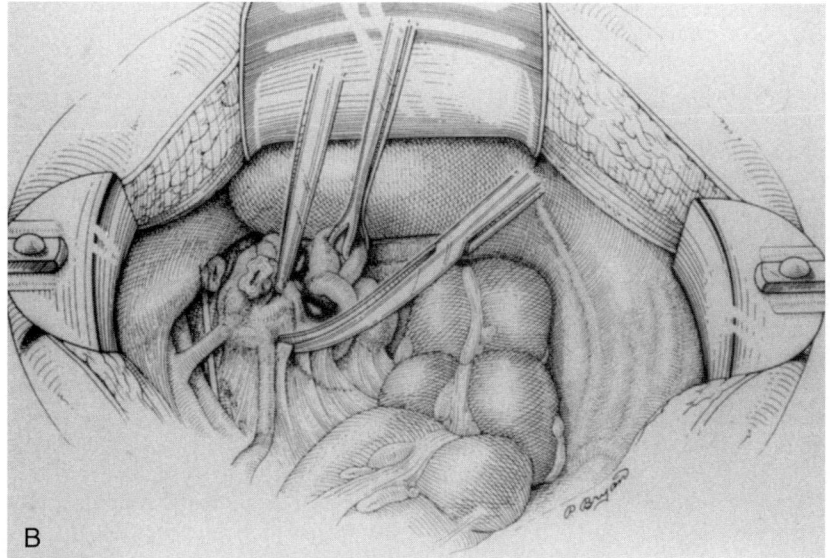

FIGURE 26.3. A: Not infrequently, the ovarian remnant may adhere to the bowel and the pelvic side wall peritoneum. **B:** The ureter must be visualized and its relation to the bowel and ovarian remnant established. This may require development of the pararectal and rectovaginal spaces.

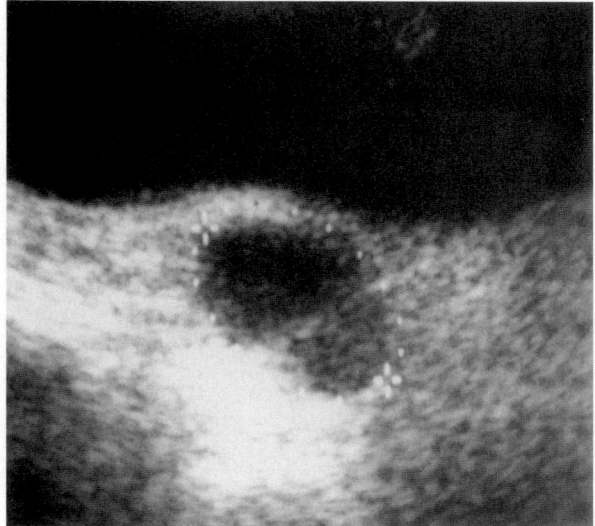

FIGURE 26.4. Abdominal sonogram showing a residual ovary with presumed follicular activity.

ence pelvic pain often with the presence of a benign cyst. Patients should be counseled preoperatively with respect to the potential for residual ovary syndrome when the initial surgical intervention is anticipated. In addition to chronic pelvic pain, a pelvic mass and dyspareunia include the "cluster of symptoms" that can occur in patients who have undergone previous hysterectomy.

ADNEXAL TORSION

Torsion of the adnexa is an infrequent cause of pain in the lower abdomen. However, torsion is a common gynecologic surgical emergency, with a prevalence of 2.7%. Treatment of adnexal torsion is considered an emergency because peritonitis and death can result. Any portion of the adnexa (tube or ovary) may undergo torsion. It may occur in neoplastic ovaries or as a consequence of hyperstimulation.

The clinical findings of torsion are usually nonspecific. For this reason, delays in diagnosis and surgical intervention may be substantial. The classic presentation is the acute onset of abdominal pain with clinical evidence of peritonitis and an adnexal mass. However, according to Bayer and Wiskind, the presenting findings in most patients are nonspecific and unimpressive. Torsion is more likely to occur during ovulation or as a premenstrual event associated with increased pelvic congestion; the authors found no correlation between the phase of the cycle and the onset of the symptoms.

Historically, the adnexa usually were removed because some authors suggested that untwisting the adnexa could increase the risk of thromboembolism and infection. There is growing evidence that unwinding the involved adnexa to observe for tissue reperfusion and viability is safe. Nevertheless, a significant delay in surgical intervention may result in irreversible necrosis requiring removal of the tube, ovary, or both.

The laparoscopic management of adnexal torsion has been increasing in efficacy. Mage and colleagues found that unwinding the adnexa was possible in most patients in their series and no further intervention was required. Likewise, Shalev and Peleg demonstrated that laparoscopic detorsion of the adnexa is safe and reliable as a primary treatment of this condition. Thus, the weight of evidence warrants conservation of the adnexa, if there is evidence of reperfusion and if significant delay has not resulted in irreversible tissue necrosis. In most instances, detorsion may be accomplished through the laparoscope.

SURGERY OF THE OVARIAN SURFACE

Surgery to remove adhesions or endometriosis from the ovarian surface is not unusual. *De novo* adhesions or adhesions between the medial surface of the ovary and the broad ligament may be filmy and vascular (Fig. 26.5A), and may be excised by fine electrocautery or vaporized with the use of a laser (Fig. 26.5B). More extensive adhesions that completely cover the ovarian surface may be thick and avascular (Fig. 26.5C and D). The plane of dissection between the broad ligament or pelvic side wall and the adherent ovarian surface must be developed with care so as not to remove or damage the peritoneum while excising the adhesion (Fig. 26.5D).

The removal of multiple, small adhesions distributed over the ovarian surface once coagulated can be gently

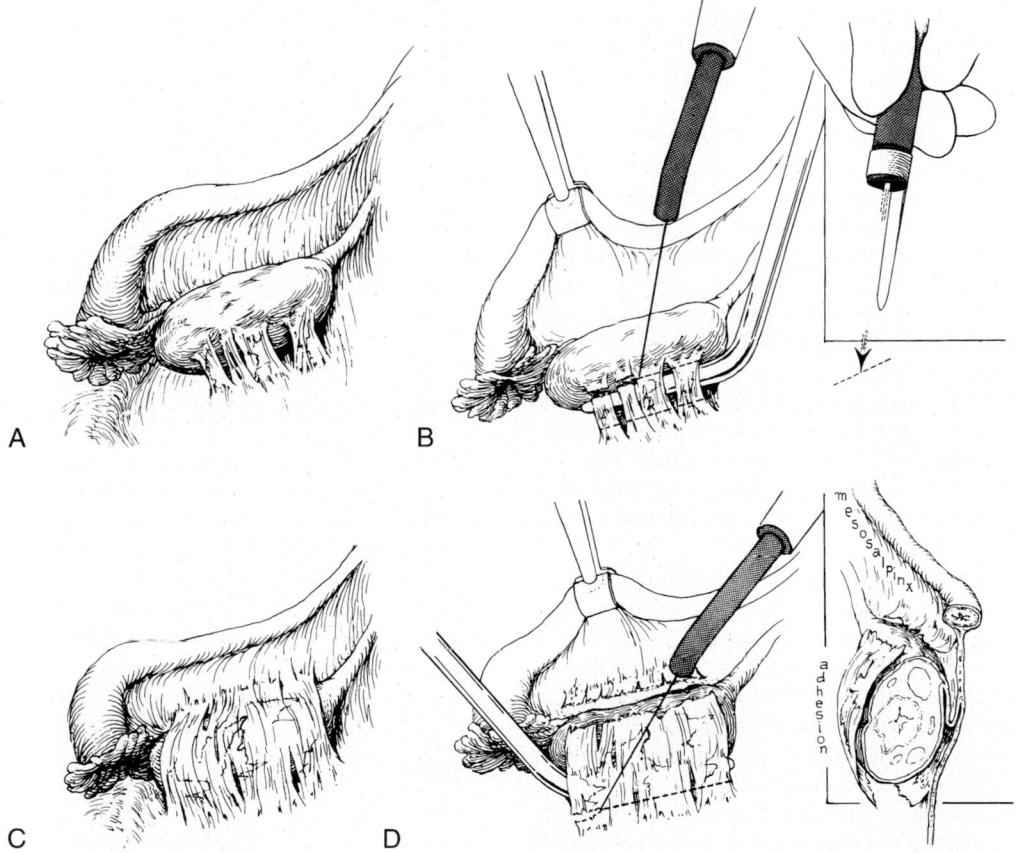

FIGURE 26.5. Ovarian adhesions. **A:** Filmy adhesions between the medial aspect of the ovary and the pelvic side wall. **B:** These may be removed with laser or fine electrocautery with use of a quartz or glass rod, respectively, as a backstop. **C:** The ovary may be enveloped by adhesions. **D:** Care should be taken to tent up the adhesions so that the peritoneum is not damaged or incised.

removed from the ovary without trauma to the ovarian cortex. Alternatively, such adhesions can be coagulated by monopolar cautery and then removed.

If the lateral aspect of the ovary is densely adherent to the broad ligament, it may be necessary to dissect the ovary free. Some cases require that a large area of the side wall or the broad ligament be denuded; reperitonealization can be accomplished with 7-0 fine, nonreactive suture material.

Small endometrial implants can be fulgurated or vaporized. The resulting small ovarian defect usually does not require closure. Care should be taken to ensure that the endometriosis is superficial and that the implant is not actually the tip of a large endometrioma within the substance of the ovary.

RECONSTRUCTION OF THE OVARY

Before ovarian reconstruction is begun, it is important that proper mobilization of the ovary be accomplished for reestablishment of normal anatomic relations. Once complete excision of the involved ovarian pathology has been accomplished, the main objectives of ovarian reconstruction are atraumatic closure of the stroma and cortex and prevention of adhesion formation. The principles for accomplishing this goal include gentle tissue handling, hemostasis, the use of fine (and ideally minimally reactive) suture material, and an effort to "bury knots" for the prevention of adhesions.

The restoration of normal-appearing anatomy is the most logical approach for creating maximal ovarian surface, which facilitates ovum pickup by the fallopian tube. Controversy continues as to whether it is more appropriate to completely excise or lyse paraovarian and peritubal adhesions.

The most important aspect of ovarian reconstruction is reapproximation of the cortex with the use of atraumatic techniques, including fine absorbable suture material. Large amounts of intraabdominal lavage should be used, ideally with a physiologic substance such as lactated Ringer's solution. Every effort should be made to remove all blood from the peritoneal cavity, preferably with the patient taken out of the Trendelenburg position.

The approach to resection of an ovarian cyst should be planned so as to minimize adhesion formation. The incidence of *de novo* adhesion formation appears to be decreased when the initial approach is through laparoscopy rather than laparotomy. The Operative Laparoscopy Study Group assessed the issue of frequency and severity of adhesion reformation and of *de novo* adhesions after operative laparoscopy. In a multicenter collaborative approach that included early second-look intervention, 68 patients underwent operative laparoscopic procedures, including adhesiolysis as well as ovarian cystectomy. The scoring of adhesions noted during the second-look laparoscopy occurred at nine sites (each ovary, each fallopian tube, omentum, cul-de-sac, pelvic side

wall, and large and small bowel). The study concluded that adhesion reformation is a frequent occurrence and that *de novo* adhesion formation occurred less frequently after initial operative laparoscopy.

A number of agents have been advocated for preventing adhesions, including oxidized regenerated cellulose [Interceed (TC7), Johnson & Johnson Medical, Arlington, TX], which is an absorbable barrier that promotes reepithelialization of the affected area. Pagidas and Tulandi compared Interceed with Ringer's lactate solution for adhesion prevention. Ringer's lactate solution was as effective as Interceed in decreasing adhesion formation. Haney and colleagues compared oxidized regenerated cellulose with expanded polytetrafluoroethylene (Gore-Tex surgical membrane). The results indicated that expanded polytetrafluoroethylene was associated with fewer postsurgical adhesions. Other agents include sodium hyaluronate carboxymethyl cellulose (Seprafilm).

Functional Ovarian Cysts

Physiologic cyst enlargement of the ovary may occur as a sequela of failure of either follicular rupture or corpus luteum regression. The latter is termed *Halban's syndrome*. The former has been associated with luteinized unruptured follicle syndrome in which "intraovarian ovulation" is thought to occur; this is a diagnosis usually established with ultrasound. In general, functional ovarian cysts regress spontaneously; however, they may persist and become symptomatic, reaching dimensions as large as 10 cm in diameter. The obvious and most feasible approach is observation, because most such cysts are self-limited. The cyst, however, may prove to be a source of continued pelvic pain or may adhere to the posterior broad ligament, producing persistent symptoms. The potential for adnexal torsion always exists with an ovarian cyst.

RESECTION OF BENIGN CYSTS

Surgical intervention often is initiated with a laparoscopic approach, which permits completion of fenestration of the nonneoplastic ovarian cyst. The cyst lining is stripped from the remaining "normal ovary," and ovarian reconstruction takes place. In several series of laparoscopic management of ovarian cysts, a simple follicular or luteal cyst was identified in most patients evaluated for pelvic pain. In a series by Kleppinger, 31 of 64 ovarian cysts were noted to fall into this category.

Surgical Techniques

Laparotomy

An elliptic incision is made through the thin ovarian cortex of a benign cyst (Fig. 26.6). The end of the knife handle is then inserted and a plane developed over the cyst wall. Alternatively, fine-needle electrocautery can be used to develop a plane, and microsurgical scissors can

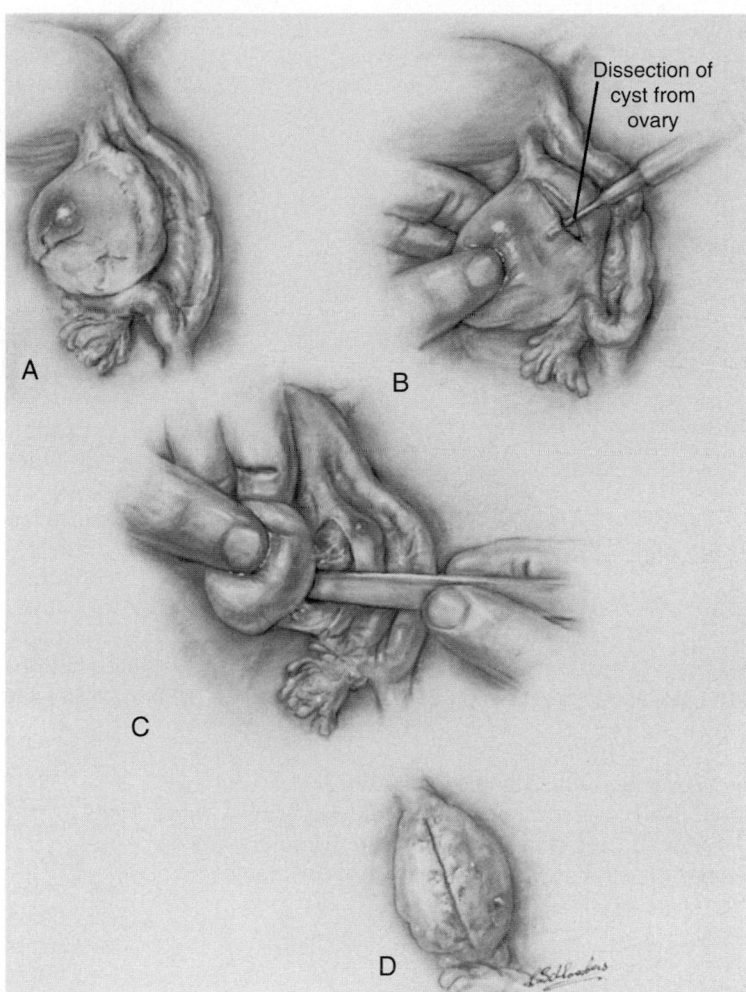

Dissection of cyst from ovary

A

B

C

D

FIGURE 26.6. Resection of benign cyst. **A:** Thin-walled ovarian cyst. **B:** An incision is made through the cortex. **C:** A plane is developed by the use of blunt dissection. The inner ovarian stroma may be approximated with a pursestring suture of 5-0 nonreactive material. **D:** The ovarian cortex is approximated with 7-0 nonreactive suture material.

be used to separate the cyst wall from the ovarian cortex. Low-power magnification (i.e., surgical loupes) often assists the surgeon in identifying the correct plane between the cyst wall and the ovarian parenchyma. After the cyst wall has been completely separated from its adherent attachments to the thin ovarian cortex, it can be shelled out without rupture. However, even with the gentlest technique, rupture can occur because of the friability of the cyst wall. Before the cyst is shelled out, it is important to pack the cul-de-sac with moist, lint-free pads so that, if rupture does occur, spillage does not contaminate the pelvic cavity. *After* the cyst has been removed, the dead space can be obliterated with a pursestring suture of 7-0 nonreactive material. Alternatively, 5-0 nonreactive vertical mattress sutures or figure-of-eight, or both, can be placed to approximate the lateral walls of the ovary. The ovarian surface is then neatly reapproximated with a subcortical running suture of 7-0 nonreactive material (Fig. 26.6D). If the cortex is quite friable, it may be necessary to place interrupted 7-0 sutures to achieve adequate approximation. Some authors advocate leaving the ovary open after cystectomy. To date, there have been no controlled trials evaluating postoperative adhesion for-

mation when the incised ovarian surface is or is not reapproximated.

In some instances, there is excessive redundant thin cortex, which may present a special problem in ovarian reconstruction. The amount of cortex removed depends on the position of the cyst as well as its overall size. Careful assessment of the ovary is necessary before the initial incision is made. The incision in the ovarian cortex should allow a symmetric reconstruction. The redundant cortex can be removed and the dead space obliterated with an internal closure, with care taken that suture material does not penetrate the ovarian cortex. This prevents ischemia and adhesion formation. The infolding technique recommended by Kistner and Patton may result in anatomic distortion and puckering of the ovarian cortex. The "baseball" closure allows careful approximation or cortical edges when redundancy is noted (Fig. 26.7).

Van der Watt reported concern over ovarian surgery. Of 36 young women operated on for an ovarian cyst, 45% were noted subsequently to be infertile. The author conveyed the importance of not interfering with functional cysts in "normal ovaries," because resulting adhe-

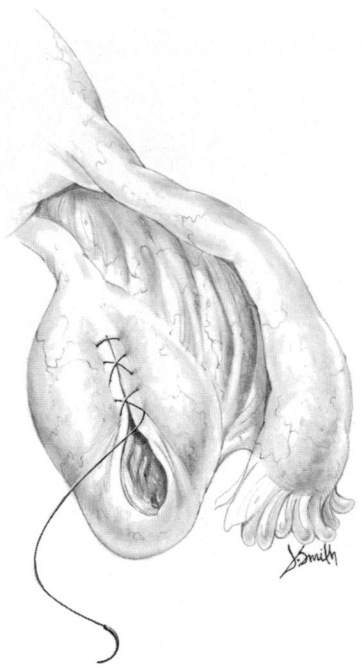

FIGURE 26.7. Closure of the ovary with a baseball stitch.

sion formation could compromise fertility. It was advocated that benign ovarian cysts should not be removed at the time of surgery for other indications unless they are sufficiently large to interfere with tubal function or cause discomfort to the patient.

Laparoscopy

Specific skill levels reflecting both the degree of operator expertise and appropriate instrumentation provide clinicians with four levels of training. Level I stands for equipment needs and potential surgical procedures for basic operative laparoscopy, including such entities as diagnostic laparoscopy, tubal sterilization, lysis of filmy adhesions, and biopsy. Level II reflects the clinician's ability to perform linear salpingostomy for ectopic pregnancy, salpingectomy, lysis of vascular adhesions, and elimination of endometriotic implants. Level III includes the ability to perform salpingo-oophorectomy, lysis of extensive adhesions (including bowel adhesions), ovarian cystectomy, appendectomy, myomectomy, laparoscopic-assisted hysterectomy, and neosalpingostomy, as well as the ability to treat tuboovarian abscess and uterine suspension. Level IV includes bowel resection, anastomosis, pelvic lymphadenectomy, presacral neurectomy, tubal reanastomosis, and excision of deep, infiltrating vaginal, paravaginal, and rectal endometriosis.

A number of principles should be followed as surgeons proceed with the correction of pelvic abnormalities that are amenable to a laparoscopic approach. The first is to restore normal anatomy. Once the ovary is stabilized, ideally with an atraumatic forceps, an appropriately planned ovarian incision can be made to correct the

pathology encountered. Every effort should be made not to spill the contents.

Large amounts of irrigation solution should be used. When necessary, hydrostatic pressure (aqua dissection) facilitates removal of the ovarian cyst lining from the cortex. In some instances, the cyst wall can be stripped (Fig. 26.8), electrocoagulated, or vaporized. The ovarian incision can then be either left open to heal by primary intention or reapproximated with sutures with either extracorporal or intracorporal suture-tying techniques. When this procedure is completed, the pelvis is irrigated with large amounts of irrigation solution (Ringer's lactate), and the patient is taken out of the Trendelenburg position to facilitate removal of any blood products that remain in the peritoneal cavity.

One alternative to suturing is to reapproximate incised segments of ovarian cortex with the use of bipolar coagulation to provide coaptation of the incised segment of the ovary. There is continued debate regarding the use of adhesion prevention materials.

A number of potential pitfalls continue to be of concern in the laparoscopic approach to ovarian lesions. These have been addressed by Seltzer and include the following:

- The potential for disruption of an ovarian malignancy
- Whether observation-recommended surgical intervention would be the most feasible alternative
- Potential for increased duration of the surgical procedure if done endoscopically
- Total cost
- Potential for incomplete resection of an ovarian lesion laparoscopically
- Education and credentialing of the gynecologic surgeon
- Overlooking the ultimate surgical goal

One can view laparoscopic approach to the adnexal mass based on age. Specifically, in the pediatric patient, problems such as torsion, hemorrhagic cysts, benign neoplasm (e.g., teratoma), as well as oophorectomy have been reportedly addressed via the laparoscope. One advantage over laparotomy is the ability to better visualize the entire lower abdomen and pelvis including the opposite ovary. In the adult, depending on the clinical circumstance, cyst aspiration, cystectomy, or oophorectomy can be accomplished laparoscopically.

Concern is expressed for an ovarian neoplasm subsequently noted to be malignant. In a countrywide survey in Austria, Wenzl and colleagues reported on 54,198 laparoscopies; 16,601 were performed for adnexal masses and 108 cases of ovarian tumors were subsequently found to be malignant. Of the 108 cases, 20 were managed laparoscopically, 22 by immediate laparotomy, and the rest by delayed laparotomy (3 to 1,415 days). The authors concluded that laparoscopic surgery with the finding of an ovarian malignancy is rare: 0.65% of all endoscopic surgical procedures. If a malignancy is identified, laparotomy is recommended for optimal staging and treatment.

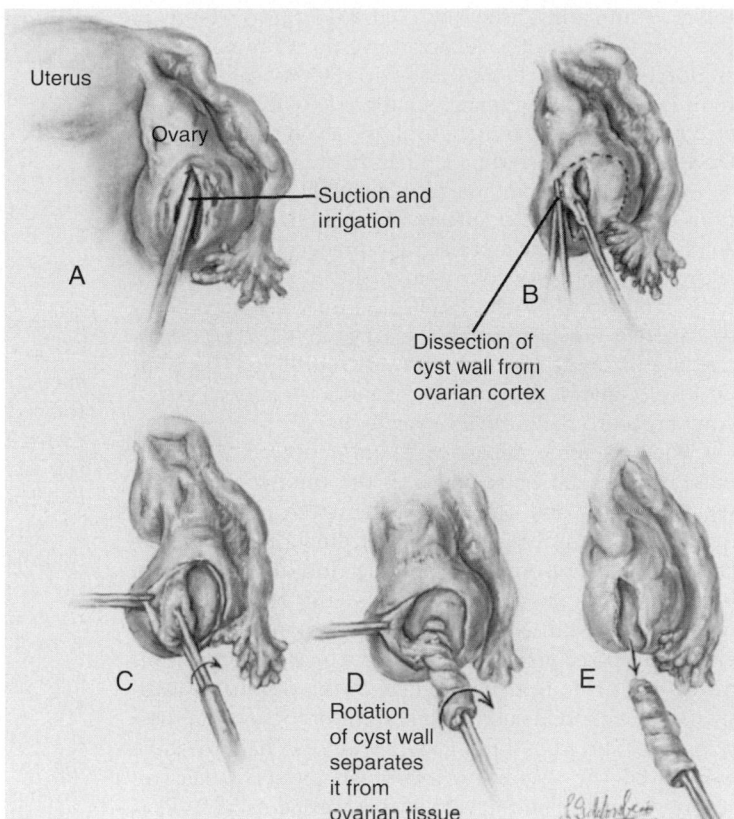

FIGURE 26.8. Removal of a small ovarian endometrial cyst through the laparoscope. **A:** After incision of the ovarian cortex, the contents of the endometrioma are removed with suction and irrigation. **B:** The plane between the ovary and the cyst wall is developed by using traction and twisting the forceps clockwise. **C:** The endometrial cyst wall is grasped with forceps. **D:** The cyst wall separates from the ovarian tissue by use of a twisting motion. The ovarian defect may be left open to heal by secondary intention or may be closed with vertical mattress sutures. **E:** The cyst wall is removed.

OVARIAN SURGERY FOR POLYCYSTIC OVARIAN DISEASE

Signs and symptoms of polycystic ovarian (PCO) syndrome begin at puberty. PCO is a sign, not a diagnosis. It is usually accompanied by a degree of hirsutism, infertility, and, in most cases, oligoovulation. The polycystic ovary may result from a virilizing ovarian or adrenal neoplasm or from congenital adrenal hyperplasia, or it may result from suboptimal hypothalamic-pituitary function at puberty. The exact mechanism for the development of ovulatory failure has been attributed to androgen overproduction and its effect on the hypothalamic-pituitary ovarian axis.

Stein and Leventhal, during the period 1902 to 1935, noted that a group of women had evidence for, what is currently called *polycystic ovaries*, at the time of laparotomy. Specifically, in 1935, Stein and Leventhal reported seven patients with the hallmarks of PCO.

The histologic findings in a polycystic ovary cover a broad spectrum, ranging from the typical Stein-Leventhal type of polycystic ovary with a large number of follicular cysts and few atretic cysts in which there is marked stromal hyperplasia and hyperthecosis, to a smaller ovary with a few follicular cysts and atretic follicles. The polycystic ovary may exhibit microscopic islands of luteinized thecal cells scattered in the stroma, but usually there is a thickened, fibrosed tunica with a large number of cystic follicles beneath this thickened capsule.

There are several hypotheses regarding the mechanism by which wedge resection of the polycystic ovary resolves ovulatory failure. The theory stating that the fibrous capsule acts as a mechanical barrier to the ovulatory follicle has been refuted. Evidence against this theory consists of the observation that if one ovary is removed, ovulation occurs from the other ovary. In addition, the use of clomiphene citrate results in ovulation through an intact capsule. Some have stated that neonatal androgens may cause an abnormal hypothalamic-pituitary axis, resulting in abnormal gonadal patterns. This theory is not widely accepted. Neonatal androgen treatment in rats is associated with masculinization of the hypothalamus and with ovulatory failure with polycystic ovaries.

The most popular theory explaining how wedge resection results in the resumption of ovulatory cycles notes that the removal of androgen-secreting stroma and theca reduces the amount of abnormal steroid production in the ovary. After wedge resection, there is usually a decrease in the mean level of 17α-hydroxyprogesterone, dehydroepiandrosterone, androstenedione, and testosterone, as well as a transitory decrease in estradiol. This reduction in the steroidogenesis of androgens, allowing normalization of the luteinizing hormone (LH):

follicle stimulating hormone (LH:FSH) ratio, results in the resumption of ovulatory cycles. Ovarian renin-angiotensin activity is enhanced with PCO. This system—renin-angiotensin—remains unaltered following ovarian electrocautery (i.e., ovarian drilling), even though serum levels of LH, testosterone, and androstenedione decline.

Sex hormone–binding globulin (SHBG) concentrations following electrocautery with PCO have been evaluated. Whereas there were significant decreases in serum androgens and gonadotropins, the concentration of SHBG increased in the serum. Gjonnaess has reported that there is no change with respect to dehydroepiandrosterone sulfate (DHEAS) with ovarian drilling. This is indicative of neural alteration in the pituitary-adrenal axis in comparison to the pituitary-ovarian axis.

There is some debate as to the amount of ovarian mass that should be removed at the time of wedge resection. Halbe and co-workers attempted to clarify this question by removing different amounts of ovarian cortex and medulla from a random selection of patients with polycystic ovarian disease. Thirty-eight of 62 patients were interested in conception. The 38 patients were divided into three groups, the first of which underwent removal of not more than one fifth of the original ovarian size. The second group had one third of the ovarian mass removed, and the third group had one half to three fourths of the original ovarian size reduced. The resumption of ovulatory cycles was recorded at 53%, 71%, and 91%, respectively. The authors concluded that the best ovulatory rate and the best pregnancy rate resulted after removal of at least half of the ovarian medulla.

Indications

The introduction of clomiphene citrate has changed the management of polycystic ovarian disease in patients who desire pregnancy. Johnson reported ovulation in 359 of 436 patients with Stein-Leventhal syndrome with the first course of therapy. An additional 58 patients ovulated after two or more cycles. The conception rate with clomiphene citrate (50% to 60%) is, however, less than 86% pregnancy rate reported by Stein and Leventhal for wedge resection. The incidence of post-clomiphene citrate birth defects (3.1%) is not increased over commonly quoted rates for populations at large.

Some patients may not want to accept the risks of multiple births or hyperstimulation with pure FSH or FSH and LH ovulation induction. The need for wedge resection of the polycystic ovary is much lower with the development of the newer reproductive technologies.

Antidiabetic agents have been advocated to reduce insulin resistance with PCO. Metformin has been shown to decrease insulin levels with resultant diminishing of circulating androgens. Hirsutism often improves. Metformin may enhance the efficacy of clomiphene and gonadotropin therapy with PCO. Metformin may also promote weight loss. Baseline and periodic liver function tests are recommended. Metformin is contraindicated with renal or hepatic disease. Patients have shown a response at dosages of 500 mg three times per day.

Surgical Technique of Laparoscopic Treatment of Polycystic Ovaries

The laparoscopic approach incorporates the use of monopolar cautery with a needlepoint applicator, laser, or bipolar cautery to drill holes several millimeters apart through the ovarian cortex (Fig. 26.9). Care should be exercised to avoid the hilum because bleeding could result if it is penetrated. It is important to achieve hemostasis over the drilled areas.

The ovarian drilling technique is performed with a 10-mm laparoscope coupled with a CO_2 laser. A 5-mm second puncture is placed suprapubically, through which suction irrigation or grasping of tissues can be performed. All visible subcapsular follicles are vaporized, and a 2- to 4-mm diameter crater is made randomly in the ovarian stroma. Hemostasis is accomplished with bipolar forceps.

Ovarian coagulation can be accomplished with unipolar punch biopsy forceps or a needle electrode. The power setting is 20 to 30 W in a cutting mode. The cortex is usually penetrated at 10 to 15 sites for a depth of 3 to 5 mm. Caution is exercised to minimize thermal damage. Smaller ovaries may require fewer cauterization sites.

There are no randomized controlled studies addressing the efficacy of the laparoscopic approach to ovarian drilling. Twenty-seven studies were evaluated by Donesky and Adashi and involved a total of 729 patients. The ovulation rate was 84.2% and the pregnancy rate was 55.7%. These authors emphasized that well-designed studies are needed in this area, which would encompass the PCO population proposed for laparoscopic drilling. This cohort of patients would require a well-documented clinical and biochemical finding of PCO, documented long-standing infertility (2 years or more), evidence for failure of clomiphene citrate, absence of correction of other infertility factors, randomization into a treatment group, and standardized documented follow-up, with particular attention to postovulatory patterns.

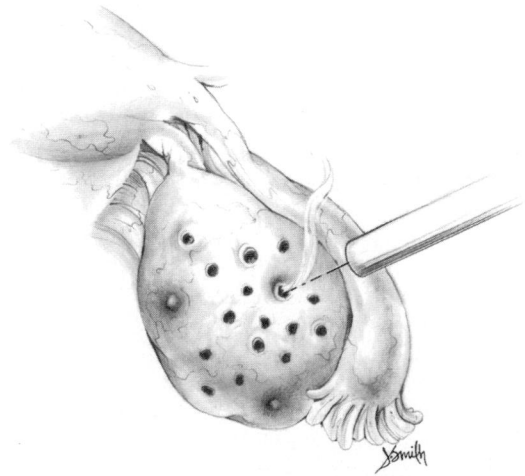

FIGURE 26.9. Laser drilling of ovary for surgical treatment of polycystic ovarian disease.

Complications

The major concern is that of adhesion formation after either wedge resection or laparoscopic drilling. Toaff and associates noted extensive peritubular and periovarian adhesions in a small series (seven) of patients who did not conceive after bilateral wedge resection. One other concern is that of bilateral ovarian atrophy, as a reflection of aggressive ovarian resection. This is a rare complication of the procedure. Thus, iatrogenic consequences of the surgical approaches must be discussed with the patient preoperatively. There is continued controversy as to whether a bilateral wedge resection approach results in suboptimal pregnancy rates because of postoperative adhesion formation. The principles of microsurgery must be reemphasized (e.g., gentle tissue handling, precise hemostasis, keeping tissues moist).

PARADOXICAL OOPHORECTOMY

Paradoxical oophorectomy is the removal of severely pathologic adnexa to improve fertility in patients with strictly unilateral tubal disease. Consideration of removal of the contralateral ovary when there is single tubal patency (i.e., paradoxical oophorectomy) has perhaps taken on a new perspective with the advent of assisted reproductive technology (ART). From a historical point of view, Jeffcoate advocated that a patient with one functional tube would benefit from paradoxical oophorectomy, thus ensuring that ovulation would occur repeatedly on the appropriate side. Scott and co-workers reported a series of 24 patients with unilateral tubal patency diagnosed by retrograde injection at laparotomy. Contralateral oophorectomy or salpingo-oophorectomy was performed on all patients, and 16 women subsequently had 21 pregnancies, for a pregnancy rate of 67%. The authors suggested that the frequency with which transperitoneal migration occurs may be a factor. Hallet noted that one in five tubal ectopic pregnancies has a corpus luteum. On the contralateral side, Jansen noted an intrauterine pregnancy rate of 18.7% ($n = 91$), contrasted with bilateral salpingostomy for hydrosalpinges in the presence of only one ovary wherein the pregnancy rate was 43.8% ($n = 16$). With unilateral salpingostomy or bilateral division of adhesions, pregnancy rates were comparable to those after bilateral salpingolysis. The mean surgery-pregnancy interval was longer after unilateral salpingostomy (104 weeks) than after bilateral salpingolysis (45 weeks). The author suggested that salpingo-oophorectomy may be preferable to salpingoncostomy for unilateral hydrosalpinx.

Perhaps the major concern is for the patient who presents with tubal ectopic gestation in which the opposite (i.e., normal-appearing) adnexa appears to be unaffected. The paradoxical salpingo-oophorectomy approach has been advocated with this circumstance by Scott and co-workers. It has been advocated to wait at least 2 years after diagnostic laparoscopy reveals extensive unilateral disease before proceeding with paradoxical oophorectomy.

Randomized, carefully controlled clinical trials are necessary to further evaluate the efficacy of paradoxical oophorectomy. The risks and benefits must be carefully considered both preoperatively and intraoperatively, especially if the patient is a candidate for ART. There is clear evidence that increased numbers of ova can be recovered when both ovaries are *in situ*. Increased pregnancy success after superovulation is a reflection of the number of ovaries (one versus two)—the total number of follicles available for stimulation.

Laparoscopic Oophorectomy

The general principles of laparoscopic oophorectomy include placing the patient in the Trendelenburg position, with appropriate planning of ports for the proposed procedure, and planning for removal of the affected adnexa. Pelvic washings and the use of frozen section may be germane to the task at hand. After restoration of normal anatomy and adhesiolysis as indicated, the adnexa are gently placed on stretch. They are approached from either the infundibulopelvic ligament or the insertion of the round ligament. Regardless of the approach chosen, identification of the ureter is mandatory. The infundibulopelvic ligament is identified, ligated with a loop ligature, or coagulated. Use of a suture ligament is an appropriate alternative to coagulation. The broad ligament is incised, beginning at the round ligament, and further dissection is performed with an irrigating dissecting probe into the retroperitoneal space. Every effort must be made to completely remove all ovarian tissue to prevent ovarian remnant syndrome.

Tissue Removal

Once the adnexa have been completely freed, if benign disease is extremely likely, desiccation of the tissue and thus segmental removal is appropriate. However, if there is concern for the pathology, use of either an endoscopic pouch or a culpotomy incision is appropriate. In this circumstance, every effort is made to remove the ovary intact. Careful inspection of the operative site and a check for any bleeding are recommended. In addition, the endpoint pressure of CO_2 insufflation should be reduced with suctioning of some of the CO_2 to check for any tamponade effect. As with all laparoscopic procedures, the patient should be monitored carefully after surgery for any signs of intraperitoneal bleeding.

OVARIAN TRANSPOSITION BEFORE RADIOTHERAPY

Lemevel and co-workers reported laparoscopic transposition in a patient being treated for Hodgkin's disease before receiving radiotherapy. The ovaries were laparoscopically suspended out of the field of radiation. Iatrogenic menopause did not occur in the four patients for which this was reported. Other authors have reported similar recommendations.

Fertility outcome following ovarian transposition and pelvic irradiation for pelvic cancer has been addressed in a total of 37 consecutive cases by Morice and colleagues. Patients were treated for clear cell adenocarcinoma of the vagina or cervix, ovarian dysgerminoma, and sarcoma. The pregnancy rate was 15% (4/27) in patients attempting pregnancy with clear cell adenocarcinoma of the vagina or cervix. In the dysgerminoma and sarcoma group, 80% pregnancy occurred (8/10). Thus, the prognosis for future fertility following ovarian transposition and irradiation should be considered for discussion in selected patients before radiotherapy.

LAPAROSCOPIC OVARIAN SURGERY IN THE PEDIATRIC OR ADOLESCENT PATIENT

A number of gynecologic problems from the neonatal period through adolescence can be addressed laparoscopically. Entities such as ovarian torsion, acute pelvic inflammatory disease (diagnosis and treatment complementing antimicrobial therapy), torsion, and benign neoplasms must be considered in this age group. In addition, gonadectomy for problems such as male pseudohermaphroditism is amenable to the laparoscopic approach.

Follicular cysts appear to be of particular concern in both the pediatric and adolescent patient because they present with abdominal pain. An abdominal or pelvic mass can be identified on physical examination. The clinician must always keep in mind the importance of appropriate preoperative assessment (with the use of ultrasound and other clinical parameters) in deciding which patients are candidates for operative intervention. Depending on the clinical circumstance, a conservative approach in this age group is advocated; appropriate concern must be given (especially in the pediatric patient) to the potential for malignancy with ovarian masses, particularly if a solid component is identified.

The literature attests to operative intervention of ovarian cysts that appear to be nonfunctional. One of these was reported in a 1.5-month-old infant in whom ultrasound showed evidence of an ovarian mass. At laparotomy, the mass proved to be consistent with right ovarian torsion and necrosis, and it required adnexectomy. In one other reported case, a follicular-appearing cyst seen on ultrasound was associated with rapidly progressive virilization and a markedly elevated plasma testosterone level (289 ng/dL); histologic evaluation identified a granulosa cell tumor with mild luteinization.

The feasibility of aspirating an ovarian cyst continues to be controversial. In two case reports, laparoscopic puncture and aspiration of a malignant ovarian cyst was performed. Preoperative ultrasound indicated that the involved adnexal mass had a benign nature. Cytologically negative fluid was obtained from the aspirate. Eight weeks after operation, extensive disseminated ovarian carcinoma was noted at laparotomy.

Endoscopic surgery continues to broaden its horizon with expansion into laparoscopic surgical care beginning with the neonate. The use of 2-mm laparoscopes with the addition of 2- to 3-mm instrumentation has facilitated the diagnostic and therapeutic aspects of laparoscopy in this age group. Miniaturized video camera systems are necessary when one uses the 2-mm laparoscope telescope. When a decision is made to proceed with laparoscopy in a neonate or infant, general endotracheal anesthesia is used. Ideally, prophylactic antibiotics are administered preoperatively. The stomach is emptied with a suction catheter when the patient is asleep, and the bladder is emptied by use of the Crede maneuver. The abdominal wall is thinner and more elastic in the child than in the adolescent or adult. One must take this into consideration when introducing instrumentation, because it may be easier to insufflate in the subcutaneous space of the child than in the subcutaneous space of an adult. A Veress needle can be used with insufflation of carbon dioxide at 0.5 L/min. In infants, the end point of peritoneal distending pressure should be set at 6 to 8 mm Hg; in the pediatric patient, 8 to 10 mm Hg; in the older child or adolescent, 10 to 12 mm Hg.

After surgery, the trocar sites can be sutured in children, whereas in neonates and infants the use of Steri-Strips (3M, St. Paul, MN) or other wound closure bandages is usually adequate for reapproximation of the incised skin edges. Waldschmidt and Schier reported a series of 136 laparoscopic surgical procedures in neonates and infants. The most frequent indications were lysis of adhesions, abdominal cysts and neoplasms, gonadectomy, appendectomy, and cholecystectomy. A 1,400-g preterm infant was the only one in the series who suffered a complication (hernia at the incision site). Thus, adnexal pathology in this age group appears to be amenable to a laparoscopic approach.

Procedures such as transposition of an ovary before radiotherapy, bilateral gonadal excision in a male pseudohermaphrodite (i.e., Y-bearing chromosomal analysis), adnexal torsion, suspected salpingitis, and endometriosis all have been identified in this age group. The authors concluded that because the morbidity is low and recovery is likely, the laparoscopic approach should be considered.

Although certain procedures in the child do not differ significantly from those in the adult, the early diagnosis of ovarian pathology (e.g., adnexal torsion) can result in a significant advantage in terms of managing the patient and preserving ovarian tissue.

BIBLIOGRAPHY

Aakvaag A, Gionnaess H. Hormonal response to electrocautery of the ovary in patients with polycystic ovarian disease. *Br J Obstet Gynaecol* 1985;92:1258.

Adashi EY, Rock JA, Guzick D, et al. Fertility following bilateral ovarian wedge resection: a critical analysis of 90 consecutive cases of the polycystic ovary syndrome. *Fertil Steril* 1981;35:320.

Adhesion Barrier Study Group. Interceed (TC-7). Prevention of post surgical adhesions by Interceed (TC-7). *Fertil Steril* 1989;51:933.

Alcazar J, Ruiz-Perez M, Errasti T. Transvaginal color-Doppler sonography in adnexal masses: which parameter performs best? *Ultrasound Obstet Gynecol* 1996;8:114–119.

Andolf E, Jorgensen C, Astedt B. Ultrasound examination for detection of ovarian carcinoma in risk groups. *Obstet Gynecol* 1990;75:106.

Anttila L, Tenttila T, Matinlauri I, et al. Serum total renin levels after ovarian electrocautery in women with polycystic ovary syndrome. *Gynecol Endocrinol* 1998,12.327–331.

Babaknia, A, Calfopoulos P, Jones HW Jr. The Stein-Leventhal syndrome and coincidental ovarian tumors. *Obstet Gynecol* 1976;47:223.

Bayer AI, Wiskind AK. Adnexal torsion: can the adnexa be saved? *Am J Obstet Gynecol* 1994;171:1506.

Benacerraf BR, Finkler NJ, Wojchiechowski C, et al Sonographic accuracy in the diagnosis of ovarian masses. *J Reprod Med* 1990;35:491.

Bernhard LM, Klebba PK, Gray DL, et al. Predictors of persistence of adnexal masses in pregnancy. *Obstet Gynecol* 1999;93:585–589.

Burns RK Jr. Hormones versus constitutional factors in the growth of embryonic sex primordia in the opossum. *Am J Anat* 1956;98:35.

Burns RK Jr. The origin and differentiation of the epithelium of the urogenital sinus in the opossum, with study of modifications induced by oestrogens. *Contrib Embryol* 1942;30:63.

Campo S, Gracia N, Carus A, et al. Effect of celioscopy ovarian resection in patients with polycystic ovaries. *Gynecol Obstet Invest* 1983;15:213.

Carey M, Slack M. GnRH analogue in assessing chronic pelvic pain in women with residual ovaries. *Br J Obstet Gynaecol* 1996;103 :150–153.

Caruso A, Caforio L, Testa A, et al. Transvaginal color Doppler ultrasonography in the presurgical characterization of adnexal masses. *Gynecol Oncol* 1996;63:184–189.

Casper RF, Greenblatt EM. Laparoscopic ovarian cautery for induction of ovulation in women with polycystic ovary disease. *Semin Reprod Endocrinol* 1990;8:209

Chan L, Lin W, Uerpairojkit B, et al. Evaluation of adnexal masses using three-dimensional ultrasonographic technology: preliminary report. *J Ultrasound Med* 1997;16:349–354.

Christ JE, Lotze EC. The residual ovary syndrome. *Obstet Gynecol* 1973;46:551.

Daniell JF, Miller W. Polycystic ovaries treated by laparoscopic laser vaporization. *Fertil Steril* 1989;51:232.

Darwish A, Amin A, El-Feky M. Ovarioscopy, a technique to determine the nature of cystic ovarian tumors. *J Am Assoc Gynecol Laparosc* 2000;7:539–546.

Davidoff AM, Hebra A, Kerr J, et al. Laparoscopic oophorectomy in children. *J Laparoendosc Surg* 1996;6[Suppl 1]:SIIS.

Dexel A, Efrat Z, Orvito R, et al. The residual ovary syndrome: a 20 year experience. *Eur J Obstet Gynecol Reprod Biol* 1996;68:159–64.

Diamond MP, Daniell JF, Feste J, et al. Adhesion reformation and de novo adhesion formation after reproductive pelvic surgery. *Fertil Steril* 1987;47:864.

Donesky BW, Adashi EY. Surgically induced ovulation in the polycystic ovary syndrome: wedge resection revisited in the age of laparoscopy. *Fertil Steril* 1995;63:439.

Einhorn N, Bast RC Jr, Knapp RC, et al. Preoperative evaluation of serum CA 125 levels in patients with primary epithelial ovarian carcinoma. *Obstet Gynecol* 1986;67:414.

Favez A, Jones HS. Assessment of the role of laparoscopic ovarian biopsy. *Obstet Gynecol* 1976;48:397.

Finkler NJ, Benacerraf B, Lavin PT, et al. Comparison of serum CA-125, clinical impression, and ultrasound in the postoperative evaluation of ovarian masses. *Obstet Gynecol* 1988;72:659.

Fleischer A, Tait D, Burnett L, Simpson J. Sonographic features of ovarian remnants. *J Ultrasound Med* 1998;17:551–555.

Ford CE. The cytogenetics of germ cells and testes in animals. In: *The human testis.* New York: Plenum Press, 1970.

Funt M. The residual adnexa: asset or liability? *Am J Obstet Gynecol* 1977;129:251.

Gillman J. The development of the gonads in man with a consideration of the role of fetal endocrine and the histogenesis of ovarian tumors. *Contrib Embryol* 1948;32:81.

Gjonnaess H. Polycystic ovarian syndrome treated by ovarian electrocautery through the laparoscope. *Fertil Steril* 1984;41:20.

Gjonnaess H. Late endocrine effects of electrocautery in women with polycystic ovary syndrome. *Fertil Steril* 1998;69:697–701.

Goldzieher JW. Polycystic ovarian disease. In: Lehrman SJ, Kistner RW, eds. *Progress in infertility.* Boston: Little, Brown, 1975:325.

Granberg S, Wickland M. A comparison between ultrasound and gynecologic examination for detection of enlarged ovaries in a group of women at risk for ovarian carcinoma. *J Ultrasound Med* 1988;7:59.

Granberg S, Wikland M. Jansson I. Macroscopic characterization of ovarian tumors and the relation to the histologic di agnosis: criteria to be used for ultrasound evaluation. *Gynecol Oncol* 1989;35:139.

Grogan RH. Reappraisal of the residual ovary. *Am J Obstet Gynecol* 1967;97:124.

Gurgan T, Yarali H, Urman B. Laparoscopic treatment of polycystic ovarian disease. *Hum Reprod* 1994;9:573.

Halbe HW, da Fonseca AM, Silva P deP, et al. Stein-Leventhal syndrome. *Am J Obstet Gynecol* 1972;114:280.

Hallet JC. Repeat ectopic pregnancy: a study of 123 consecutive cases. *Am J Obstet Gynecol* 1975;122:520.

Haney AF, Doty E. Murine peritoneal injury and de novo adhesion formation caused by oxidized-regenerated cellulose (Interceed [TC7] but not expanded to polytetrafluoroethylene (Gore-Tex surgical membrane). *Fertil Steril* 1992;57:202.

Haney AF, Hesla J, Hurst BS, et al. Expanded polytetrafluoroethylene (Gore-Tex surgical membrane) is superior to oxidized regenerated cellulose (Interceed TC7) in preventing adhesions. *Fertil Steril* 1995;63:1021.

Hasson HM. Laparoscopic management for ovarian cysts. *J Reprod Med* 1990;35:863.

Hasson HM. Ovarian surgery. In: Sanfilippo JS, Levine RL, eds. *Operative gynecologic endoscopy.* New York: Springer-Verlag, 1989:102.

Heinrich U. Eberlein-Gonska M, Benz G, et al. Late-onset 30-hydroxysteroid dehydrogenase deficiency with virilization induced by a large ovarian cyst. *Horm Res* 1993;40:227.

Heloury Y, Guiberteau V, Sagot P, et al. Laparoscopy in adnexal pathology in the child: a study of 28 cases. *Eur J Pediatr Surg* 1993;3:75.

Herrmann UJ Jr, Locher GW, Goldhirsch A. Sonographic patterns of ovarian tumors: prediction of malignancy. *Obstet Gynecol* 1987;69:777.

Hernandez E, Miyazawa K. The pelvic mass: patients' ages and pathologic findings. *J Reprod Med* 1988;33:361.

Hulka JF, Peterson HB, Phillips JM, et al. Operative hysteroscopy: American Association of Gynecologic Laparoscopists 1991 Membership Survey. *J Reprod Med* 1993; 38:572.

Jansen RP. Surgery pregnancy time intervals after salpingolysis, unilateral salpingostomy and bilateral salpingostomy. *Fertil Steril* 1980;34:222.

Jeffcoate TA. *Principles of gynecology*. London, Butterworths, 1975.

Johnson JE Jr. Outcome of pregnancies following clomiphene citrate therapy. In: *Proceedings of the Fifth World Congress on Fertility and Sterility*. Amsterdam: Excerpta Medica, 1967:101.

Kamprath S, Possover M, Schneider A. Description of a laparoscopic technique for treating patients with ovarian remnant syndrome. *Fertil Steril* 1997;68:663–667.

Killackey MA, Neuwirth RS. Evaluation and management of the pelvic mass: a review of 540 cases. *Obstet Gynecol* 1988;71 (Pt 1):319.

Kistner RW, Patton GW. Surgery of the ovary. In: *Atlas of infertility surgery*. Boston: Little, Brown, 1975;105:177.

Kleppinger RK. Ovarian cyst fenestration via laparoscopy. *J Reprod Med* 1978;21:16.

Kobal B, Omahen A, Fetih A, et al. Laparoscopic treatment of acute adnexitis; one step forward. *Acta Eur Fertil* 1990;21:225.

Kobayashi M. Use of diagnostic ultrasound in trophoblastic neoplasms and ovarian tumors. *Cancer* 1976;38:441.

Kojima E. Ovarian wedge resection with contract Nd:YAG laser irradiation used laparoscopically. *J Reprod Med* 1989;34:444.

Kurjak A, Predanic M, Kupesic-Urek S, et al. Transvaginal color and pulsed Doppler assessment of adnexal tumor vascularity. *Gynecol Oncol* 1993;50:3.

Larsen JF, Pedersen OD, Gregersen E. Ovarian cyst fenestration via the laparoscope. *Acta Obstet Gynecol Scand* 1986;65:539.

Laxman D, Burgman A, Sagi J, et al. The postmenopausal adnexal mass: correlation between ultrasonic and pathologic findings. *Obstet Gynecol* 1991;77:726.

Lemevel A, Bourdin S, Harousseau J, et al. Ovarian transposition by laparoscopy before radiotherapy in the treatment of Hodgkin's disease. *Cancer* 1998;83:1420.

Mage G, Canis M, Mandes H, et al. Laparoscopic management of adnexal torsion: a review of 35 cases. *J Reprod Med* 1989 Aug;34:520–4.

Maiman M, Seltzer V, Boyce J. Laparoscopic excision of ovarian neoplasms subsequently found to be malignant. *Obstet Gynecol* 1991;77:563.

McKay DG, Hertig AT, Adams EC, et al. Histochemical observations on germ cells of human embryos. *Anat Rec* 1953;117:201.

Malkasian G Jr, Knapp R, Lavin PT, et al. Preoperative evaluation of serum CA125 levels in premenopausal and postmenopausal patients with pelvic masses: discrimination of benign from malignant disease. *Am J Obstet Gynecol* 1988;159:341.

Mecke H, Hehmann-Willenbrock E, Ibrahim M, et al. Pelviscopic treatment of ovarian cysts in premenopausal women. *Gynecol Obstet Invest* 1992;34:36.

Meire HB, Farrant P, Guha T. Distinction of benign from malignant ovarian cysts by ultrasounds. *Br J Obstet Gynaecol* 1978:85:893.

Merritt DR. Torsion of the uterine adnexa: a review. *Adolesc Pediatr Gynecol* 1991;4:3.

Minke T., Depond W, Winkelmann T, et al. Ovarian remnant syndrome: study in laboratory rats. *Am J Obstet Gynecol* 1994:171:1440.

Morice P, Thiam-Ba R, Castaige D, et al. Fertility results after ovarian transposition for pelvic malignancies treated by external irradiation or brachy therapy. *Hum Reprod* 1998;13:660–663.

Nezhat F, Nezhat C, Welander C, et al. Four ovarian cancers diagnosed during laparoscopic management of 1011 women with adnexal masses. *Am J Obstet Gynecol* 1992;167:90.

Operative Laparoscopy Study Group. Postoperative adhesion development after operative laparoscopy: evaluation at early second-look procedures. *Fertil Steril* 1992;55:700.

Pagidas K, Tulandi T. Effects of Ringer's lactate, Interceed (TC7) and Gore-Tex surgical membrane on post-surgical adhesion formation. *Fertil Steril* 1992;57:199.

Parker W, Berek J. Management of selected cystic adnexal masses in postmenopausal women by operative laparoscopy: a pilot study. *Am J Obstet Gynecol* 1990;163:1574.

Pussell SJ, Cosgrove DO, Hinton J, et al. Carcinoma of the ovary-correlation of ultrasound with second look laparotomy. *Br J Obstet Gynaecol* 1980;87:11140.

Rane A, Ohiz Ray O. "Acute" residual ovary syndrome. *Aust N Z J Obstet Gynaecol* 1998:38:447–448.

Richards JS. Estradiol receptor content in rat granulosa cells during follicular development: modification by estradiol and sonadotropins. *Endocrinology* 1975;97:1176–11784.

Richards JS. Hormonal control of gene expression in the ovary. *Endocr Rev* 1994;15:725–751.

Sassone AM, Timor-Tritsch IE, Artner A, et al. Transvaginal sonographic characterization of ovarian disease: evaluation of a new scoring system to predict ovarian malignancy. *Obstet Gynecol* 1991;78:70.

Schwobel MG, Stauffer UG. Surgery of the female gonads. *Zeitschrift fur kinderchirurgie* 1988;43:289.

Scott JS, Lynch EM, Anderson JA. Surgical treatment of female infertility; value of paradoxical oophorectomy. *BMJ* 1976;1:631.

Scott RT, Beatse SN, Illions EH, et al. Use of the GnRH agonist stimulation test in the diagnosis of ovarian remnant syndrome. A report of three cases. *J Reprod Med* 1995;40:143–146.

Seltzer V. Laparoscopic surgery for ovarian lesions: potential pitfalls. *Clin Obstet Gynecol* 1993;36:402.

Seltzer V, Maiman M, Boyce J. Laparoscopic survey in the management of ovarian cysts. *Female Patient* 1992;17:19.

Shalev E, Mann S, Romano S, et al. Laparoscopic detorsion of adnexa in childhood: a case report. *J Pediatr Surg* 1991;26:1145.

Shalev E, Peleg D. Laparoscopic treatment of adnexal torsion. *Surg Obstet Gynecol* 1993;176:448.

Silva P, Ziff A. Polycystic ovary syndrome—an update. *Female Patient* 2000;25:33

Soper JT, Hunter VJ, Daly L, et al. Preoperative serum tumor-associated antigen levels in women with pelvic masses. *Obstet Gynecol* 1990;75:249.

Soriano D, Wefet Y, Seidman D, et al. Laparoscopy versus laparotomy in the management of adnexal masses during pregnancy. *Fertil Steril* 1999;71:955–960.

Stein I, Leventhal ML. Amenorrhea associated with bilateral polycystic ovaries. *Am J Obstet Gynecol* 1935;29:181–191.

Steinkampf MP, Hammond KR, Blackwell RE. Hormonal treatment of functional ovarian cysts: a randomized prospective study. *Fertil Steril* 1990;54:775.

Sumioki H, Utsunomyiya T, Matsuoka K, et al. The effect of laparoscopic multiple punch resection of the ovary on the hypothalamopituitary axis in polycystic ovary syndrome. *Fertil Steril* 1988;50:567.

Symmonds RE, Petit P. Ovarian remnant syndrome. *Obstet Gynecol* 1979;54:175.

Tawa K. Ovarian tumors in pregnancy. *Am J Obstet Gynecol* 1964;90:5111

Taylor A, Jurkovic D, Bourne T, et al. Sonographic prediction of malignancy in adnexal masses using an artificial neural network. *Br J Obstet Gynaecol* 1999;106:21–30.

Terz J, Barber H, Bronschwig A. Incidence of carcinoma in the retained ovary. *Am J Surg* 1967;113:511.

Timmerman D, Bourne T, Tailor A, et al. A comparison of methods for pre-operative discrimination between malignant and benign adnexal masses: the development of a new logistic regression model. *Am J Obstet Gynecol* 1999;181:57–65.

Toaff R, Toaff ME, Peyser MR. Infertility following wedge resection of the ovaries. *Am J Obstet Gynecol* 1976;124:92.

Trimbos JB, Hacer NF. Case against aspirating ovarian cysts. *Cancer* 1993;72:828.

Trimbos-Kemper TC, Trimbos JB, van Hall EV. Management of infertile patients with unilateral tubal pathology by paradoxical oophorectomy. *Fertil Steril* 1982;37:623.

Tulandi T, Al-Took S. Laparoscopic ovarian suspension before a radiation therapy. *Fertil Steril* 1998;70:381–383.

Turner CD, Asakawa H. Experimental reversal of germ cells in ovaries of fetal mice. *Science* 1964;143:1344.

Van der Watt J. The mutilated ovary syndrome. *S Afr Med J* 1970;44:687.

Waldschmidt J, Schier F. Laparoscopic surgery in neonates and infants. *Eur J Pediatr Surg* 1991;1:145.

Weiner Z, Thaler I, Beck D, et al. Differentiating malignant from benign ovarian tumors with transvaginal color flow imaging. *Obstet Gynecol* 1992;79:159.

Wenzl R, Lehner R, Husslein,P, et al. Laparoscopic surgery in cases of ovarian malignancy: an Austria-wide survey. *Gynecol Oncol* 1996;63:57

Westrom L. Incidence, prevalence and trends of acute pelvic inflammatory disease and its consequences in industrialized countries. *Am J Obstet* 1980;138:880.

Witschi E. Embryology of the ovary. In: *The ovary*. Baltimore: Williams & Wilkins, 1963:1.

Witschi E. Migration of the germ cells of human embryos from the yolk sac to the primitive gonadal folds. *Contrib Embryol* 1948;32:69.

Te Linde's Operative Gynecology, ninth edition, edited by John A. Rock and Howard W. Jones, III. Lippincott Williams & Wilkins, Philadelphia © 2003.

CHAPTER

27

▼

Persistent or Chronic Pelvic Pain

JOHN F. STEEGE

Chronic pelvic pain (CPP) is defined as pain present either intermittently or continuously for 6 months or more. Although much work remains to be done concerning the epidemiology of the disorder, preliminary surveys suggest that it may affect 5% to 15% of women at some time in their lives, predominantly during their reproductive years. The gynecologist confronts this problem on a regular basis. Many organic and functional disorders of the reproductive, gastrointestinal, urinary tract, and musculoskeletal systems may contribute nociceptive stimuli to the problem. In addition, by dysregulation of neurologic pathways, pain can become an illness in itself when it lasts longer than 4 to 6 months. This chapter reviews the common structural and functional components of CPP, describes the criteria for a chronic pain syndrome (CPS), and offer a theoretical model to explain the evolution of chronic pain over time.

DEFINITION

Many pain disorders are deemed "chronic" by virtue of their duration, that is, 6 months or longer. In practice, this usually connotes decreased function (perhaps even disability) as well as progressive behavioral and affective changes. Although this definition is useful as a benchmark, some victims of chronic pain may develop these characteristics sooner than 6 months into the problem, and others may endure severe pain for years while remaining surprisingly functional and well adjusted. As suggested later, it is therefore perhaps useful to employ additional behavioral and psychometric criteria to the chronologic definition of "chronic" in order to focus diagnostic and treatment efforts.

HISTORY

Over the past 50 years, the study of CPP has gone through significant changes in approach. Investigations undertaken before the development of laparoscopy focused on correlations between pelvic pain and psychologic distress. (These studies included an extensive literature dealing with the psychologic dimensions of dysmenorrhea, much of which has received less attention since the discovery of prostaglandins.) This approach was prompted by the fact that the two most common organic contributors to CPP—endometriosis and adhesions—can be difficult to diagnose by history and physical examination alone. In the absence of palpable pathology, the gynecologist of the 1950s and 1960s was understandably reluctant to subject a patient to laparotomy to investigate pain. During this era, the prevailing cartesian theory of pain perception suggested that pain should be somewhat proportional to the degree of tissue damage found. If the pathology was not big enough to palpate, it was seldom operated upon. Although this was sufficient to explain most acute pain, the cartesian model fails to explain the majority of chronic pain disorders, in gynecology as well as other areas of medicine. The gate control theory, promulgated by Melzack and Wall in 1965, allowed integration of physical and psychologic parameters, and explains how chronic pain can be quite different from acute pain. The model also suggests that information flows in two directions regarding pain: (1) nociceptive signals from peripheral tissue ascend through the spinal cord to higher centers, and (2) central centers can modulate, via descending signals altering spinal cord neurotransmitter and interneuron activity, the transmission of these nociceptive signals from the periphery. Deterioration of these regulatory processes were thought to potentially account for development of chronic pain states by allowing too many peripheral signals through the spinal cord "gates."

While these changes in pain theory were stimulating the field of pain research, gynecologists were busy developing laparoscopy. Previously cherished myths soon fell by the wayside, for example, endometriosis is seldom found in adolescents or African-Americans. With these observations came the hope that laparoscopic and medical treatment of this pathology would fix CPP. Reports of CPP from that era focused on "laparoscopy-negative" patients; indeed, some pelvic pain clinics required a negative laparoscopy as an entry criterion, implying that if some pathology were found, it must be a "real" cause for pain. Subsequent experience has shown that, even though treatment of laparoscopically diagnosed pathology is often helpful, the clinical reality is more complex:

1. In many instances, the organic pathology found at laparoscopy may be incidental, and not related to the pain.
2. In those with pathology that does contribute to nociception, the pain experienced by the patient may be the sum of this contribution plus signals from some or all of the disorders listed in Table 27.1.

Consider the research of the 1980s that documented a distressingly high prevalence of physical and sexual abuse. Epidemiologic surveys of community samples revealed that as many as 25% to 30% of adult women reported having experienced sexual abuse during childhood. Studies of women attending pelvic pain clinics, especially those based in psychiatric settings, showed that up to 60% of these women had been abused. These observations led to the speculation that the experience of abuse may make a person more vulnerable to the development of CPP or perhaps be a specific cause for pain. Currently, preliminary studies using positron-emission tomography and functional magnetic resonance imaging (MRI) methods suggest that the experience of abuse may indeed leave its neurophysiologic footprints: stressful stimuli produce different central response patterns in abused vs nonabused subjects. However, detection of abuse in a patient's history seems to prompt referral for tertiary care, whereas symptom levels in various pain dis-

TABLE 27.1.
Possible Causes of Pelvic Pain in Laparoscopy-Negative Patients

Gastrointestinal
  Constipation
  Irritable bowel syndrome
  Inflammatory bowel disease
  Diverticulitis
Urinary
  Urethral syndrome
  Interstitial cystitis
Musculoskeletal or Neurologic
  Pelvic floor tension myalgia
  Piriformis syndrome
  Nerve entrapment
  Ventral hernia
  Rectus tendon strain
  Myofascial pain
  Back or pelvic postural changes
Gynecologic
  Pelvic vascular congestion
  Cervical stenosis

From Steege JF, Stout AL, Somkuti SG. Chronic pelvic pain: toward an integrative model. *Obstet Gynecol Surv* 1993;48:95, with permission.

orders [e.g., irritable bowel syndrome (IBS)] are similar in referred and nonreferred patients. The presence of an abuse history means that the evaluating health professionals need to take this into account, but it does not necessarily imply that the abuse is causally involved in the development of the pain. The impact of a history of abuse on the outcome of treatment of organic pathology should be the subject of further research.

Finally, even the gate control theory is held to be inadequate to explain clinical manifestations of pain. The neuromatrix theory, described by Melzack, is an expansion that includes the notion of neuroplasticity, among other elements. The concept of neuroplasticity suggests that experience can change the neurophysiologic behavior of the central nervous system in a manner that influences the subsequent processing of nociceptive stimuli. It may explain the apparent development of pain responses to stimuli usually thought of as nonpainful (allodynia), as well as exaggerated responses to painful stimuli (hyperalgesia). Every practicing gynecologist has seen patients whose pain responses seem out of proportion to the pathology found. This may reflect the emotional meaning of the problem for the patient, as well as past or present emotional trauma, but it may also be the result of nociceptive mechanisms not yet understood (e.g., the mechanism of pain from endometriosis) or the result of sensitization of spinal cord interneurons that have become pain generators as a result of being on the receiving end of peripheral nociceptive stimuli for prolonged periods. The positive side of the neuroplasticity concept is that, perhaps, given enough time and the right treatment, even seemingly intractable chronic pain problems may ameliorate to the point of allowing substantially improved function.

This chapter reviews the various organic, psychologic, and physiologic factors that contribute to CPP, outlines methods of evaluation, gives suggestions for treatment, and finishes with a discussion of an integrated model of the development of CPP.

CONTRIBUTIONS OF TISSUE DAMAGE TO PAIN

Endometriosis

A recent review summarized laparoscopic findings from 2,615 patients in 15 studies (nine retrospective, six prospective). Endometriosis was found in 2% to 51% of patients, suggesting that referral biases lead to very skewed samples. Clearly, not every woman with pain has endometriosis, nor does every woman with endometriosis have pain, although women with the disease had pain more often than those without it. A number of previous studies of CPP either described only patients without organic laparoscopic findings or stratified patients according to the presence or absence of physical pathology. The description of atypical (nonpigmented) endometriosis by Jansen in 1986 calls these classifications into question. Laparoscopy studies published before that time reported that 11% of women with CPP had endometriosis, whereas three similarly conducted studies published since 1986 reported a 41% prevalence of endometriosis in women undergoing laparoscopy for CPP. The pre-1986 literature on pelvic pain must be reevaluated with this information in mind. Many studies may have included women with endometriosis in the anatomically normal group, thus generating erroneous conclusions about the entirely psychogenic nature of their pain.

The first symptom of significant endometriosis is often increased dysmenorrhea alone, but other pain often develops, and its duration and severity often progress as the disease advances, to the point that it can be present almost constantly. Again, the severity of the pain correlates poorly with the amount of diffuse peritoneal disease, but may vary more directly with deeply infiltrative cul-de-sac disease. Fear of worsened pain, impaired fertility, or recurrent disease after treatment can increase pain levels. Of the many women upon whom we have performed laparoscopy for recurrent pain following complete hysterectomy and adnexectomy for endometriosis, only a small minority (3% to 5%) proved to have recurrent disease. Most cases of postoperative pain have been attributable to a combination of postoperative adhesions, fear of recurrent disease, and functional problems such as levator spasm and IBS.

Hysterectomy and bilateral salpingo-oophorectomy relieve endometriosis-related pain in more than 90% of cases. When one or both ovaries are preserved, the recurrence rate is estimated to be 30% or higher, but this figure includes endometriosis of all stages. Some practitioners believe that if disease does not involve the ovaries, surgical excision of the disease, with ovarian conservation, results in an acceptable 5% to 10% recurrence rate over the subsequent 5 years. Further investigation of this unorthodox approach is warranted.

Pelvic Adhesions

In a review by Steege and colleagues, 6% to 55% of the 2,615 patients who underwent laparoscopy for pelvic pain had pelvic adhesions. As is the case for endometriosis, the site of adhesive disease correlated well with the site of pain, but the intensity of pain was unrelated to the extent of adhesions present. Nociceptive signals from the damaged tissue seem subject to modulation at the spinal cord level and interpretation in higher centers. Adhesions are most likely stable anatomically a few months after injury (e.g., surgery, infection), but the intensity of associated pain can progress. After about 6 months of pain experience, complex relationships among physical, emotional, and cognitive factors can exist that require comprehensive treatment.

Pelvic Support

Although problems with pelvic relaxation are common in women in their sixth or seventh decade of life, most patients at pain clinics are in their third or fourth decade. The implication is that cases of pain associated with pelvic support problems constitute the minority of pelvic pain problems.

Pelvic relaxation usually leads to complaints of heaviness, pressure, dropping sensations, or aching. In attempting to hold in prolapsing organs, the patient may be tensing the levator plate and contributing to tenderness during daily activities and intercourse. Fear of (or actual) loss of urinary control during coitus can add to the discomfort by impairing physiologic sexual response.

Excess mobility of the pelvic organs (universal joint or Allen-Masters syndrome) attributed to childbirth or other traumatic causes of ligament (especially broad ligament) tears in uterine supports has been implicated in CPP. Such highly subjective physical examination findings are difficult to document rigorously, and because surgery has been the traditional primary treatment, controlled studies of the association of pain with ligamentous tears have not been possible.

Uterine retroversion is another controversial potential etiology for CPP, particularly in the form of deep dyspareunia. Uncontrolled clinical series of uterine suspension procedures for pelvic pain suggest that the most frequent scenario involves a combination of uterine retroversion (most often innocent by itself) with new intrinsic uterine pathology (e.g., adenomyosis, myomas) or nearby cul-de-sac or adnexal pathology (e.g., endometriosis, adhesions, ovary prolapsed into the cul-de-sac). On occasion, these anatomic circumstances combined with a new partner of more generous penile dimensions produce new deep dyspareunia.

Pelvic Congestion

Overfilling (congestion) of the pelvic venous system has been implicated as a cause of dull chronic aching pain that usually is worse at the end of the day after prolonged standing, premenstrually, and after coitus not accompanied by orgasm. The pain is occasionally unilateral, is usually present in multiparous women, and is likely due to anatomic causes, at least in part. The high comorbidity with psychologic distress indicates that psychophysiologic factors may also contribute. Medroxyprogesterone can help (by eliminating the menstrual cycle), but the best long-term results have followed psychotherapy in conjunction with this medication. In any case, good radiologic studies in women who are awake during the procedure have documented increased pelvic venous diameter in those affected. Veins cannot be reliably evaluated during laparoscopy due to confounding effects of position, fluid load, etc.

Residual Ovary

When the uterus has been removed, with or without removal of one ovary, the remaining ovary or ovaries can become symptomatic in 1% to 4% of women. In many instances, benign functional ovarian cysts can form and can be transiently symptomatic. Pain from the ovary can be increased by confinement of the ovary within postoperative adhesions, rupture or leakage of a cyst prompting additional adhesion formation, or attachment of the ovary to the sigmoid colon or vaginal apex by postoperative adhesions. In the case of attachment to the vaginal apex, deep dyspareunia can result when the vaginal apex is struck. When this pain causes diminished sexual response, loss of the normal vaginal apex expansion and elongation that is part of sexual response can leave the ovary or ovaries closer to the introitus, thus aggravating the deep dyspareunia.

Ovarian Remnant

A more difficult situation can develop if a small fragment of ovarian tissue is left behind during attempted oophorectomy. In most instances, this happens when extensive pelvic adhesive disease or endometriosis made the dissection difficult. Within 1 to 3 years of the attempted oophorectomy, continued follicle-stimulating hormone (FSH) stimulation will result in growth of the ovarian fragment, often producing an intermittently symptomatic pelvic mass located along the course of the ovarian vascular supply. This problem is uncommon, but not rare, as implied by early case series. The prevalence of asymptomatic ovarian remnants is unknown. As in the case of the residual ovary, the remnant can produce dyspareunia if it is located close to the vaginal apex.

Musculoskeletal Problems

Musculoskeletal changes can become involved with CPP, either as the primary problem or as a secondary reaction to the pelvic pain. Dysmenorrhea can be referred to the midline of the low back, especially when the uterus is retroverted. Pain can also be referred to the midline of the low back in the presence of cul-de-sac endometriosis. An ovary fixed to the pelvic sidewall can refer pain to the ipsilateral low back.

The muscular problem that most often produces pelvic pain is pelvic floor tension myalgia. Intermittent or constant painful contraction of the levator plate can be

present as a primary psychophysiologic problem, but contraction is more often a reaction to some other source of pain. Even when the primary source of pain is successfully treated, the reactive muscle contraction can persist as a learned response, in much the same way that vaginal introital muscle spasm (vaginismus) can persist after transient but repeated painful vaginal events.

Lumbar musculature can become tender as a primary problem or in reaction to subtle changes in posture and motion. Trigger points can be present in the low back and gluteal areas, in the muscles best inspected by pelvic examination (e.g., levator plate, piriformis, obturator internus).

The piriformis muscle warrants additional mention because it is seldom appreciated as a possible source of pain. This muscle is an external rotator of the leg, and rotation against resistance can allow detection of tender spasm of the muscle during the pelvic examination. The sciatic nerve can traverse the belly of the piriformis as a normal anatomic variant, producing symptoms similar to sciatica when the muscle is in spasm.

Myofascial Pain

Focal lower quadrant abdominal wall pain can be produced by entrapment of the genitofemoral and ilioinguinal nerves, as described by Applegate. Such entrapment appears most often after Pfannenstiel abdominal incisions. Slocumb has advanced the theory that myofascial trigger points account for a large fraction of CPP. In my experience, abdominal wall components may be the primary cause for pain in some cases, but are more often a later reaction to the long duration of pain from some other source. Reiter and Gambone reported that 14% of 122 laparoscopy-negative women had myofascial pain probably related to a previous surgical incision.

Medical Comorbidity

The cause of chronic lower abdominal or pelvic pain often involves nongynecologic systems (Table 27.1). A careful history and close physical examination of gastrointestinal, urologic, musculoskeletal, and neurologic systems are needed to evaluate the contributions of nongynecologic systems to CPP. Most of the available literature examines these problems of other systems independently of each other and without reference to their relevance to CPP or to the overall prevalence of these disorders in CPP.

The gastrointestinal system is perhaps the most common nongynecologic source of pelvic pain. Constipation and IBS occur most frequently, although inflammatory bowel disease and diverticulitis can at times present with pain alone. Women with IBS may have increased relaxin levels (produced by a dysfunctional corpus luteum) as one of many possible contributing factors. Treatment with a gonadotropin-releasing hormone (GnRH) agonist may reduce symptoms of IBS.

Urologic problems, which are less easily confused with gynecologic disorders, are perhaps second in terms of prevalence. The urethral syndrome (frequency, urgency, and dysuria in the absence of bacteriuria), interstitial cystitis, and bladder spasms are all accompanied by significant anxiety and depression symptoms. The symptoms of these three disorders are very similar to those in a population of gynecologic CPP patients. A history (whether pain occurs during micturition, daily activities, or coitus) does not always reveal the involved system, but careful pelvic examination with stepwise gentle palpation of the urethra, bladder base, and bladder may help the physician identify from the patient's response the site of the pain she is experiencing.

Many patients do not experience the problems described here in pure form, but rather in varying degrees of intensity, with varying contributions to an individual's total discomfort. Close attention to such nuances of detail is warranted both in clinical management and in published reports.

PSYCHOLOGIC FACTORS

Personality

The links between chronic pain and individual psychology and personality style have been sought after and discussed in the psychiatric literature for many years. Some early reports implied that women who complained of CPP had a high prevalence of feminine identity problems related to conflicts about adult sexuality, psychiatric disturbance characterized by mixed character disorder with predominant schizoid features, high neuroticism, and unsatisfactory relationships. Although these initial studies were an important beginning, the high prevalence of psychopathology in some reported samples did not seem applicable to significant numbers of CPP patients seen in practice. The findings are difficult to interpret, partly because there is a lack of clarity concerning the operational definition of CPP that was used. Biases in patient selection and interviewer information, inadequate control groups, and the absence of diagnostic laparoscopy also contribute to the confusion. Despite these shortcomings, it seems apparent that disorders of personality, especially borderline personality, are overrepresented both in the general population of severe chronic pain patients and in the population of pelvic pain patients. In primary care, such patients usually are seen less often. In any case, a label of personality disorder should not be applied indiscriminately to every angry patient by her frustrated physician. People who have difficulties maintaining satisfactory relationships and function in life, even when these difficulties are caused in part by subsyndromal personality problems, can be more vulnerable to nociceptive signals from tissue damaged by endometriosis, infection, or surgery. Unmet dependency needs may lead them to seek external solutions such as medications and further surgery, rather than to rely on their own undeveloped coping skills.

Depression

Focusing specifically on a CPP sample that had been evaluated by diagnostic laparoscopy, Walker and associates found that women with CPP (with and without positive laparoscopic findings) met criteria for lifetime major depression, current major depression, lifetime substance abuse, adult sexual dysfunction, and somatization more often than did control subjects. Stout and Steege found that 59% of 294 women seeking evaluation at a pelvic pain clinic scored in the depressed range (greater than 16) on the Center for Epidemiologic Studies Depression Scale at the time of their initial visit. Slocumb and colleagues reported that patients with an abdominal pelvic pain syndrome scored higher as a group on scales of anxiety, depression, anger-hostility, and somatization on the Hopkins Symptom Checklist; however, 56% of the total sample scored within the normal range on all scales.

Because no study of CPP has assessed its association with depression over time, no statement can be made as to whether depressive symptoms are a predisposing factor leading to, or a reaction to, the pain condition. There seem to be two distinct groups of CPP patients: one in which pain and depression are common final presentations reached by a number of pathways and another in which depression develops in reaction to pain, as is the case with many other acute and chronic medical diseases.

History of Sexual Abuse

Women seeking treatment for CPP have a high prevalence of sexual trauma in their personal histories. In Reiter's study of 106 women with CPP, 48% had a history of major psychosexual trauma (molestation, incest, or rape), compared with 6.5% of 92 pain-free control subjects presenting for annual routine gynecologic examination ($p < .001$). The high prevalence of reports of psychosexual trauma elicited from pelvic pain patients supports the hypothesis that pelvic pain is specifically and psychodynamically related to sexual abuse. However, Rapkin did not find a higher prevalence of childhood or adult sexual abuse in a group of women with CPP compared with women with chronic pain in other locations, although women with CPP reported a higher incidence of childhood sexual abuse. These findings argue against a unique relation between sexual abuse and CPP and suggest that abusive experiences promote the chronicity of many different painful conditions. Morrison also reported an association between sexual abuse and a wide variety of pathologic conditions. Jamieson and Steege, in a survey of 581 women seen in primary care practices, found that 28% of women reported having been sexually abused as children, and 26% as adults. In this study, those abused only in childhood did not have an increased prevalence of CPP or other pain disorders, whereas those who had suffered abuse both as children and adults did.

When such a history is documented, the clinician and patient together must judge whether the feelings surrounding these events are intense enough to intrude upon the present. If so, psychotherapeutic help may be indicated. If not, although the memories may be painful, further emotional work on this area may not be beneficial. The treatment literature on the sequelae of abuse (and their treatment) is disappointing, especially when the abuse occurred in the distant past. In either case, it is difficult to judge whether these events are directly relevant to the present pain and hence demand attention, or whether they contribute to a psychologically vulnerable substrate acted upon by subsequent physical and emotional events. In these circumstances, it may be worthwhile to suggest further mental health evaluation as an exploratory measure, being careful not to imply that the patient is being referred because the physician is certain that the abuse is related to the development of the pain.

Sexual Dysfunction

In clinical practice, women presenting with CPP often report a high incidence of marital distress and sexual dysfunction, particularly dyspareunia. Stout and Steege found that 56% of 220 married women scored in the maritally distressed range (less than 100) on the Locke-Wallace Marital Adjustment Scale at the time of initial visit. A high level of marital distress has also been reported in other chronic pain patients and their spouses. Although some women report satisfactory sexual functioning before the onset of pain symptoms, others appear to have long-standing impairments in sexual response.

DIAGNOSTIC STRATEGIES

Recognizing a Chronic Pain Syndrome

Many women can experience pain for longer than 6 months without becoming debilitated; although their pain is chronic, such women are not described as having a CPS. The following are the common clinical hallmarks of true CPS:

1. Duration of 6 months or longer
2. Incomplete relief by most previous treatments
3. Significantly impaired physical function at home or at work
4. Signs of depression (sleep disturbance, weight loss, loss of appetite)
5. Pain out of proportion to pathology
6. Altered family roles

Of the signs of depression, sleep disturbance is usually the first to appear. Careful questioning is needed to distinguish awakening caused by pain from awakening that just happens. In the true vegetative sign, the person usually cannot get back to sleep even if pain is relieved (by medication or other means).

The alteration of family roles is perhaps the most important of those mentioned. This includes changed responsibilities for household, children, finances, and so forth. Initially intended as helpful, such changes may in the long run diminish the patient's self-esteem and progressively reduce her family's interactions with her to little more than checking on her pain. Over time, this covertly reinforces the complaint of pain and imparts to it unintended value as a major means of maintaining communication within the family.

Simultaneous Medical and Psychosocial Evaluation

When the aforementioned markers of CPS are present, one should surrender the need to immediately discover how much of the pain problem is physical and how much is psychologic. Rather than guess, it is useful to ask two separate questions: Is there physical disease that requires medical or surgical treatment? Is there emotional or psychological distress that requires treatment?

It is useful to directly state that the precise connection between these two cannot be measured; this can help diminish the patient's fear that she will be told "it's all in her head." The patient can then be more open to sharing her personal and emotional concerns. If this statement is made early in the evaluation, before all physical evaluations have been carried out, the patient is likely to be less defensive. At this stage, a mental health consultant has a better chance of developing rapport with the patient and will be a more helpful collaborator when needed.

History Taking

The site, duration, pattern during activities, relation to position changes, and association with bodily functions are all important elements of pain. For example, pain that is focal and positional is more often associated with adhesive disease; pain that is absent in the morning but worsens progressively during the day may be associated with pelvic congestion. The patterns of pain associated with endometriosis are discussed earlier.

The chronology of the pain is critical. As CPS develops, pain can be present over a progressively larger area despite stable organic pathology. Interpreting this as the breakdown or wearing out of physiologic systems that deal with pain signals has some biologic validity and may make sense to the patient.

From a cognitive perspective, it is invaluable to discern the patient's and her family's ideas about the causes of and future for her pain. Fears of cancer can be discovered even if this diagnosis was never even remotely considered by the clinician. Less dramatic, but equally powerful, attributions of cause can emerge, such as pelvic infection due to sexual acts remote in time, arguments with a spouse, divine retribution, and so forth.

Physical Examination

Guiding a patient through contraction-relaxation sequences of the abdominal, thigh, and vaginal introital muscles can reduce the discomfort of the examination and can indicate the patient's degree of control over muscle tension. Single-digit palpation of the levator plate and piriformis muscles can elicit tenderness compatible with the label of pelvic floor tension myalgia. This condition is often present as a sequel to some other pelvic pain, but it can become a problem in itself. Discomfort is usually felt as pelvic pressure and radiation pain to the sacrum, near the insertions of the levator plate muscles.

Adnexal thickening and mobility, pelvic relaxation, coccygeal tenderness, and foci of pain that reproduce dyspareunia should be noted. Gentle palpation with a cotton swab can detect areas of sensitivity compatible with vestibulitis in the introitus or trigger points higher in the vagina. On occasion, gentle fingertip palpation of the abdominal wall can detect such trigger points in the musculature.

Laboratory Tests

Imaging Studies

In the case of CPS, it has already been established that intensity of pain does not correlate well with extent of organic pathology. It follows that if the physical examination is relatively benign and is not severely limited by body habitus, extensive imaging usually adds little to the database needed before laparoscopy is performed. This is especially true in the case of organ-specific studies (intravenous pyelography, barium enema, colonoscopy) in the absence of symptoms or signs pointing to a specific organ system (e.g., blood in the stools). If the patient has had multiple previous surgeries, high-resolution studies such as MRI and computed tomography scans are often misleading because of postoperative artifact. "Cystic masses" seen on such studies often prove to be nothing more than pockets of adhesions or peritoneal inclusion cysts.

Blood Studies

Relatively few hematologic or chemical measures are of use in diagnosing CPP. An elevated leukocyte count and erythrocyte sedimentation rate may make the clinician suspect chronic pelvic inflammatory disease even when cervical cultures are negative for the most common sexually transmitted diseases. The cancer antigen-125 test is positive in advanced endometriosis but is not sufficiently sensitive to detect early stage disease or reliably monitor its response to treatment. If any remnant ovarian tissue is present, FSH and estradiol levels remain in premenopausal ranges in almost all instances. Replacement estrogen therapy should be withdrawn 3 weeks before these levels are measured.

Anesthetic Blocks

Injection of small volumes of a local anesthetic, 1 to 5 mL of 1% lidocaine or 0.5% bupivacaine, blocks pain from either an entrapped segmental nerve (e.g., ilioinguinal) or an abdominal wall trigger point. In the latter case, such blocks can be therapeutic as well as diagnostic. Many anesthesia pain clinics administer epidural or spinal anesthetics to distinguish pain arising from peripheral organs from pain that has become completely central in origin.

In some instances it is useful to attempt transvaginal blocks with the same local anesthetics. For example, the (posthysterectomy) vaginal apex may be focally intrinsically tender, suggesting a trigger point or other focal nerve root irritation. Again, local blocks can be therapeutic as well as diagnostic. A series of three or four blocks administered 1 to 2 weeks apart may give relief for months to years in some instances.

In most cases, a history and careful routine physical examination distinguishes central from lateral sources of pelvic pain. When this discrimination is difficult, it may be useful to administer a transvaginal uterosacral block (blocking most uterine innervation) and then repeat the pelvic examination. When this relieves the pain, the pain can be assumed to arise from the uterus, but if the pain is not relieved, one cannot distinguish a failed block from pain of nonuterine origin.

Psychologic Tests and Interviews

To distinguish physical from psychologic causes for pain, many studies of CPP have used traditional psychologic instruments that were developed to measure general psychopathology or personality factors. In some studies, more abnormalities are detected in women without physical pathology at laparoscopy. In other papers, women with organic disease who have had pain for a long time appear equally distressed in their questionnaire responses. These psychometric instruments generally have little face value for chronic pain patients, and their use often confirms the patient's fears that the health care provider thinks she is "crazy" or that the pain is "all in her head." Once again, the question of whether the emotional distress identified by these instruments is an antecedent to or a consequence of persistent pain remains unanswered. A more complete review of the psychometric instruments that have been used to study CPP is presented elsewhere.

Psychometric tests are most useful when they are interpreted by a psychologist who has interviewed the patient, and they serve best as a means to better understand the patient's strengths and weaknesses, rather than as a means to decide who needs surgery.

Laparoscopy

Great strides have been made in operative laparoscopy in the past 2 decades. New techniques and new terminology (e.g., pelviscopy) imply new "magic" to the physician and public alike. Laparoscopy should be liberally performed for diagnostic purposes, and ablation/excision of endometriosis and lysis of adhesions are no doubt useful procedures. However, the premature surgical procedure errs in the notion that pain is "hard-wired" to pelvic pathology. The available evidence clearly argues against this. When a CPS is clinically evident, results of laparoscopic treatment alone, despite comparable pathology, are much less impressive. For a patient with the clinical markers of CPS listed earlier, the complete workup as described should be performed before laparoscopy.

In some puzzling cases in recent years, we have performed laparoscopy under local anesthesia to "pain map" the pelvis. A 2-mm laparoscope and a small suprapubic probe are placed with the use of short-acting intravenous analgesia (remifentanyl), and local lidocaine 1%. Having been oriented to the procedure beforehand, as each organ is touched, she is asked (1) "Does this give you the pain you get?" and (2) "Please rate the pain." She responds with a number picked from a scale of 1 to 10, with 10 signifying the "worst pain you could imagine." This technique may make it possible to determine whether visualized pathology is causing nociceptive signals or to discriminate visceral from somatic pain.

It is possible in some cases to block the superior hypogastric plexus during pain mapping to better predict benefit from presacral neurectomy. In this approach, mapping is done before and after injecting 10 mL of 1% lidocaine just underneath the peritoneum over the sacrum, using a 7-inch, 22-gauge spinal needle.

MANAGEMENT

Physicians use specific treatments in chronic pain depending on the model of pain perception that they follow. The surgically oriented gynecologist often tacitly follows the cartesian model, attempting to eliminate organic tissue damage to diminish pain proportionately. The behaviorist, cognitive therapist, and insight-oriented psychotherapist use approaches consistent with each one's basic therapeutic orientation, whereas advocates of the gate control theory use medications and other treatments that make sense based on that theory. The following represents an eclectic treatment approach. The treatment literature is considerably more sparse than is the literature exploring the etiology of CPP.

General Principles

A complete evaluation of CPS often reveals a number of contributing factors, such as bladder irritability, irregular bowel function, poor posture, and emotional and relationship stresses, in addition to laparoscopically visualized pathology. Treating each component sequentially is common practice but often ends in frustration because each treatment addresses only a part of the problem. Simultaneous treatments often begin with disquieting multiple drug therapy but allow better relief. Close follow-up at regularly scheduled visits allows gradual tapering of medications over time. Planned visits also provide support and a coping mechanism for the patient. When the patient is essentially required to feel worse in order to be seen again, the pain may be tacitly reinforced.

Medication Use
Analgesics
Advocates of the operant conditioning model suggest that analgesics be taken continuously, in a non—pain-contingent fashion. This eliminates the need to demonstrate pain behaviors or voice pain complaints to justify the use of medication, thus eliminating the tendency of medication to act as a reinforcer of pain behaviors. This approach is benign enough when relatively nontoxic and nonaddicting medications such as acetaminophen are used, but it presents potential hazards when drugs such as the following are used: nonsteroidal antiinflammatory drugs (NSAIDs; gastric irritation, renal damage); aspirin or NSAIDs in combination with the milder narcotics, such as codeine, oxycodone, and pentazocine (constipation, sedation, habituation); and pure narcotics (addiction, diminished analgesic potency over time). When well tolerated, all three types of drugs can serve well in appropriate patients (without histories of substance abuse). Indeed, contrary to common perception, there is support for the notion that chronic low-dose opiate therapy may allow good return of function without adverse side effects in those who have failed intensive pain clinic treatments.

Antidepressants
This class of drugs, particularly the tricyclic antidepressants, can potentiate the effects of analgesics in CPS, even when given at doses less than those usually used in the treatment of depression. New agents such as fluoxetine (Prozac) show promise and have a low level of side effects. Few controlled trials of antidepressants have been carried out in CPP patients.

Anxiolytics
Anxiolytic drugs are certainly widely prescribed by gynecologists, although it is uncertain how often they are given for pain. In one study, alprazolam, a triazolobenzodiazepine with mixed anxiolytic and antidepressant effects, had a surprising degree of analgesic effect in moderate to high doses in patients with chronic pain of malignant origin and concomitant mood changes or anxiety. These patients were already receiving narcotics, which may suggest that alprazolam potentiates the analgesic effect of narcotics. Their role in conjunction with nonnarcotic analgesics is uncertain, and the addiction potential is obvious.

Other Medications
Nonanalgesic and nonpsychotropic drugs also have potential roles in the treatment of specific pelvic conditions. For example, medroxyprogesterone acetate treatment sufficient to suppress ovarian function may reduce the diameter of engorged pelvic veins and thus reduce the discomfort of pelvic congestion. However, the longest lasting relief was observed when psychotherapy was used as well.

The use of GnRH agonists has been recommended to distinguish gynecologic from nongynecologic sources of pain; however, these agents also relieve the symptoms of IBS, probably by reducing serum relaxin levels. When the differential diagnosis includes ovarian remnant syndrome, residual ovary syndrome, or any other disorder influenced by the menstrual cycle, the impact of GnRH agonists on pelvic pain must be interpreted with caution in anyone with symptoms at all compatible with bowel dysfunction. In addition, pain threshold has been shown to be lower premenstrually, even in asymptomatic women. The impact of the menstrual cycle itself in chronic pain patients has not been well explored, but it seems likely that it may impart some cyclicity even to conditions unrelated to the reproductive tract. Cyclicity of symptoms must therefore be interpreted with caution, and the obliteration of symptoms or of their cyclicity by pharmacologically obliterating the menstrual cycle does not demonstrate a gynecologic cause. To address the most common clinical circumstance: relieving pain with a GnRH agonist does not prove that the pain is due to endometriosis.

Surgery

Two basic surgical approaches have been used to treat CPP: removing pelvic organs and treating visible disease while leaving the pelvic organs in place. Only the former approach has been evaluated for efficacy to any degree.

In the United States, about 12% of hysterectomies are performed with pelvic pain as the primary indication. An additional 6.1% are performed for endometriosis or adenomyosis, and 5.1% are performed for pelvic inflammatory disease; no doubt many in these two categories also involve complaints of pain. In about one third of hysterectomies performed for pain, no pathology is found. Despite the frequency of pain as an indication for this procedure, data regarding efficacy are surprisingly sparse. One report notes relief in 78% of women after hysterectomy for pelvic pain of uterine etiology (women with adnexal or other pelvic disease were excluded). However, the presence or absence of uterine pathology (adenomyosis or leiomyomata) had no bearing on whether or not pain was relieved. It cannot be determined from the report (Table 27.1) whether failure to obtain relief was due to the presence of other pelvic conditions, postoperative adhesion formation, or psychologic reasons. Symptom substitution was not evaluated in the report. Relief of pain by removal of the normal uterus is even more puzzling; apparently this was not accounted for by concomitant procedures performed for deficient pelvic support. Some of these cases may have involved pelvic congestion or perhaps other mechanisms even less well understood. A 22% failure rate emphasizes the need for careful preoperative evaluation of all potentially contributing factors, both physical and emotional.

According to two recent reports, hysterectomy performed in primary care settings was very effective for the treatment of CPP. In a prospective observational study of private practices in Maine, Carlson and associates reported that at a 1-year follow-up, satisfaction with the outcome of surgical treatment was much higher than satisfaction with the outcome of medical therapy. However, about one third of women improved substantially on medical therapy, and perhaps women were more likely to undergo operation when organic pathology was demonstrable. In the Maryland Women's Health Study, 1,299 women were interviewed at length before hysterectomy for benign disease and at 3, 6, 12, and 24 months after surgery. In more than 90% of cases, the procedure was well tolerated and did not result in postoperative depression or a decline in sexual functioning. In the subset of women with pain as the primary indication for surgery, relief of pain occurred in more than 80%, indicating that the clinicians involved generally employed good judgment and technique. In general, women with preoperative depression or sexual dysfunction did not fare as well as their less symptomatic counterparts. Further analyses of these data are underway.

Adnexal and other intrapelvic diseases, usually endometriosis or adhesions due to either postoperative changes or chronic pelvic inflammatory disease, have been treated by both laparotomy and laparoscopy. Use of the CO_2 laser during laparotomy does not improve the results of standard infertility surgical techniques as evaluated by second-look laparoscopy and by pregnancy rate.

Laparoscopy is probably superior to laparotomy for treating adhesive disease. In the rabbit model, infliction of injuries with the laser by way of laparotomy resulted in adhesion formation, but no adhesions formed when identical damage was caused by laparoscopy. In the rabbit and the human, adhesiolysis is more effective with laparoscopy than with laparotomy. However, none of the large clinical trials of laparoscopic adhesiolysis evaluate the effects of the procedures on pain.

Although second-look verification of effective adhesiolysis is lacking, results of several studies on the treatment of pelvic adhesions for the relief of pain are encouraging. Even when treated by laparotomy, with the use of infertility techniques, 28 of 42 (65%) patients reported cure or improvement of pain. In a sample of mostly primary care patients, 84% of 65 patients had relief of pain after laser laparoscopic adhesiolysis with follow-up intervals of 1 to 5 years. In a sample of 42 patients with more severe adhesive disease, Daniell reported improvement in 67% at a 4-month follow-up. In Sutton's large series, 85% had pain relief at 1 year. Steege and Stout reported that 15 of 20 (75%) patients without a CPS who were undergoing laser laparoscopic adhesiolysis had good relief of pain at a follow-up 6 to 12 months after surgery. However, if a CPS was present, only 4 of 10 (40%) patients with equivalent adhesive disease obtained relief. The greater the emotional and behavioral disability, the greater the need for combined medical, surgical, and mental health management.

Several studies support an association between pelvic pain and endometriosis, although a strict quantitative relation is lacking. In terms of surgical treatment of pain from endometriosis, laser ablation results in relief of pain in about 60% of women at 1 year follow-up, compared with 96% treated by laparoscopic excision of the disease. A randomized trial comparing these two methods has not been done. The benefits of surgical excision may be prolonged by subsequent medical therapy; studies comparing the relative benefits of various medical therapies (continuous oral contraceptives, continuous progestins, GnRH agonist with/without add-back estrogens) following surgical treatment have not been performed. The more economical and less physiologically intrusive approach would seem to favor sex steroids over GnRH agonists.

Presacral neurectomy, as an adjunct to surgical excision of endometriosis, has been evaluated for its effect on pelvic pain. In a retrospective sample of 71 women undergoing conservative resection of endometriosis by way of laparotomy, 35 (50%) who also had presacral neurectomy enjoyed significantly greater improvement in both dysmenorrhea and dyspareunia, with 75% to 95% obtaining improvement. Two subsequent retrospective reports noted that similar percentages (about 75%) of women obtained pain relief after endometriosis surgery that included presacral neurectomy, compared with about 25% who obtained relief without neurectomy.

Two studies on the treatment of presacral neurectomy as adjunctive therapy along with conservative resection for stage III-IV endometriosis reached different conclusions about the additive value of presacral neurectomy. Tjaden and associates performed conservative resection by way of laparotomy and randomized eight women to receive or not receive presacral neurectomy. All the neurectomized women improved dramatically, whereas the others did not. The institutional review board mandated stopping the study because statistical significance had been reached. The authors then reported an open clinical series in which 15 of 17 women improved substantially after conservative resection with presacral neurectomy. Candiani and colleagues reached a different conclusion after randomizing 71 women to receive or not receive presacral neurectomy along with conservative resection of advanced endometriosis. They found that central dysmenorrhea improved slightly more in neurectomized women, but daily pain and dyspareunia were not improved by adding presacral neurectomy to the procedure. The literature is therefore inconclusive regarding the value of the neurectomy procedure.

Laparoscopic treatment of even severe endometriosis has a growing number of advocates. Again, the focus has been on fertility rates, but one prospective report notes prolonged pain relief in two thirds of patients. The ability to perform presacral neurectomy by way of laparoscopy should not provoke wide adoption of the procedure without careful consideration of these data.

An ovarian remnant should be removed if it is persistently symptomatic despite all reasonable attempts at medical suppression, and if menopause cannot be expected in the patient's near future. Whether performed by laparoscopy or laparotomy, the dissection should be detailed and should include all the peritoneum surrounding the mass. The ureter and pelvic side wall vessels should be exposed and carefully freed from the specimen. When a GnRH agonist has been used preoperatively for symptom control or to distinguish the relative contributions made by the remnant and other pelvic pathology, such as adhesions, the remnant tissue may become so small as to make it difficult to identify. Hence, if a palpable (or ultrasonically visible) mass disappears after GnRH agonist treatment, it may be wise to allow time for it to regrow before pursuing surgical excision. When the remnant is small, some surgeons have stimulated the remnant with clomiphene citrate to make it easier to find.

Finally, the peritoneal windows syndrome must be mentioned. Openings in the peritoneum covering the posterior broad ligament and the cul-de-sac of Douglas, or peritoneal "windows," have been noted since the 1950s and were associated with endometriosis by Chatman. Excision and closure of the windows have been anecdotally reported, but the value of these operations in treating pain associated with the disease remains to be demonstrated. It is this author's practice to excise the peritoneum involved with the window, but not to stitch the area closed. Microscopic endometriosis is found in the vast majority of cases.

Alternative Treatments

Biofeedback, transcutaneous electric nerve stimulation units, relaxation training, and individual and couples counseling all have their appropriate roles in individual cases, but none is so clearly applicable or effective that its automatic use is supported in cases of CPP. In keeping with the approach outlined in the earlier discussion of medications, problems requiring counseling should be addressed but should be treated as issues separate from the discussion of appropriate surgical approaches. Cause-and-effect relations are difficult to demonstrate even in retrospect when psychologic assistance works.

Management Overview

The most effective clinical approach requires simultaneous treatment of as many factors as possible: anatomic, musculoskeletal, functional bowel and bladder, psychologic, and so forth. Patient and physician must contract for the long term and work from a rehabilitation perspective, rather than hope that the latest single addition to the treatment will prove to be *the* answer. The physician, to prevent frustration and feelings of defeat, must often play the role of helping to manage and relieve the pain while helping to maximize function, even when pain persists. To the surgically trained gynecologist who prefers a clear-cut single answer to a clinical problem, this can be the most difficult part of dealing with the problem of CPP.

THE EVOLUTION OF A CHRONIC PAIN SYNDROME

As is apparent from this discussion, CPP is a heterogeneous problem, not a single diagnosis, and no single etiologic hypothesis is clearly supported. Most of the hypotheses reviewed here have some credible evidence supporting them; none have been sufficiently validated. Psychologic and neurologic mechanisms are proposed here to explain how the evolution of chronic pain may occur, regardless of the particular tissue damage or functional disorder that may first have provided nociceptive stimuli. We suggest the following elements (Fig. 27.1): biologic events sufficient to initiate nociception, alterations of lifestyles and relations over time, anxiety and af-

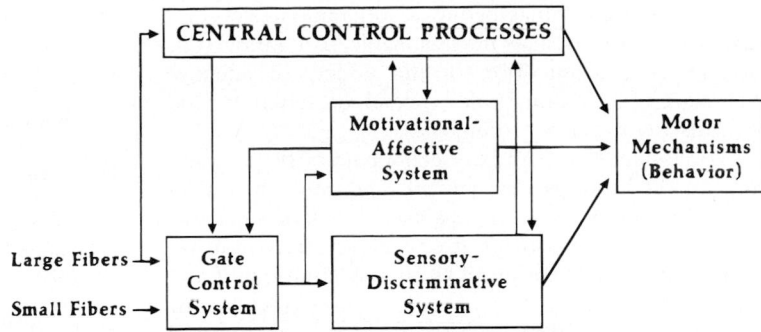

FIGURE 27.1. The gate control theory of pain perception.

fective disorders, and a circular interaction (vicious cycle) among these elements.

Biologic Events Sufficient to Initiate Nociception

Sexually transmitted diseases, endometriosis, recurrent bladder and vaginal infections, primary or secondary functional dyspareunia, alterations of bowel habit, pelvic congestion, and gynecologic or other abdominal surgeries (Table 27.1) may contribute individually or in combination.

Alteration of Lifestyle and Relations

Physical activities at home and recreational pursuits can suffer. Believing that rest usually helps in the treatment of most causes of acute pain, the patient may assume that the same applies to chronic pain and may thus restrict herself more than actual discomfort dictates. Family members start to regard the patient as sick and leave her out of many activities, thus reducing her roles within the family structure. With time, concern for and discussion of her pain can become the family's major pattern of communication with the pain victim. If sexual intimacy has been the major means of emotional sharing and smoothing over of differences and if this intimacy is reduced, then the altered pattern of interactions may take hold more quickly.

Anxiety and Affective Disorders

Depression can occur as a cumulative result of the disability suffered, or the pain can bring on an episode of depression in a patient already biologically vulnerable. The observation most relevant here is that pain patients with a family history of depression can derive the most benefit from tricyclic antidepressants.

The Vicious Cycle

Diminished activity, altered family roles and social supports, anxiety, and affective disturbances can influence nociception by a variety of central pathways, ultimately altering spinal cord "gating" of nociceptive signals. Cognitions about the pain can play an additional role.

Several important modifying influences can be present in addition to these major pathways (Fig. 27.2). Incest and other forms of sexual abuse have attracted the most attention as possible forerunners of CPP. However, CPP is clearly not a unique or specific sequel to sexual abuse, and a large proportion of CPP patients have not been abused in this manner. Victims of sexual abuse have many negative emotional sequelae; pain problems often occur after abuse, but they are not necessarily directly caused by the abuse.

Sexual abuse perpetrated by a family member is a clear indication of a psychologically detrimental environment of rearing that might have led to disturbances in character and personality development perhaps equal in importance to the terrible trauma of the abuse itself. Learning more about the factors that can mitigate the impact of sexual abuse in general will facilitate our understanding of the psychologic vulnerabilities that can make a particular person more susceptible to development of CPP or other chronic pain disorders.

A genetic predisposition to depression also allows the vicious cycle to become easily established and strengthened over time. Antidepressant medications play an important role in the overall therapeutic plan in such cases.

Several authors have suggested that the concept of perceived control best explains the development of affective changes accompanying chronic pain, regardless of the location of the pain. The individual who sees herself as having little control over the physical and emotional

Integrative Model for Chronic Pelvic Pain

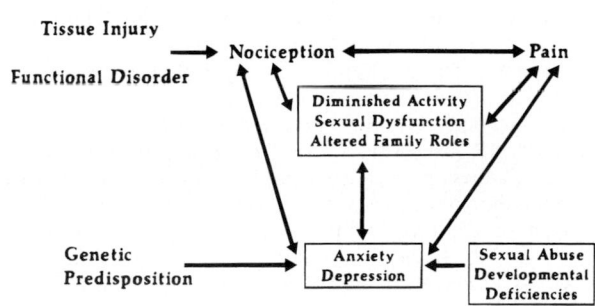

FIGURE 27.2. An integrative model for chronic pelvic pain, including elements of gate control theory, cognitive-behavioral theory, and the operant conditioning model.

events affecting her may be most vulnerable to development of a CPS. It may be reasonable to consider this variable as a culmination of the effects of affective change, activity, family roles, sexual dysfunction, and previous victimization experiences.

The longer that pain has been a part of the person's life, and the more psychologic vulnerabilities she carries forward to the present, the less likely it is that any treatment of the tissue damage itself will be effective in relieving pain and restoring physical and emotional function. However, as treatment studies show, the organic contribution to chronic pain can seldom be dismissed entirely. The more difficult task is the selection of an efficient and cost-effective combination of treatment approaches aimed at the most important factors acting in the present.

BIBLIOGRAPHY

Applegate WV. Abdominal cutaneous nerve entrapment syndrome. *Surgery* 1972;71:188.

Barbot J, Parent B, Dubuisson JB, et al. A clinical study of the CO_2 laser and electrosurgery for adhesiolysis in 172 cases followed by early second-look laparoscopy. *Fertil Steril* 1987;48:140.

Beard RW, Belsey EM, Lieberman BA, et al. Pelvic pain in women. *Am J Obstet Gynecol* 1977;128:566.

Beard RW, Highman JH, Pearce S, et al. Diagnosis of pelvic varicosities in women with chronic pelvic pain. *Lancet* 1984;2:946.

Candiani GB, Fedele L, Vercellini P, et al. Presacral neurectomy for the treatment of pelvic pain associated with endometriosis: a controlled study. *Am J Obstet Gynecol* 1992;167:100.

Carlson KJ, Miller BA, Fowler FJ. The Maine Women's Health Study: II. Outcomes of nonsurgical management of leiomyomas, abnormal bleeding, and chronic pelvic pain. *Obstet Gynecol* 1994;83:566.

Castelnuovo-Tedesco P, Krout BM. Psychosomatic aspects of chronic pelvic pain. *Int J Psychiatry Med* 1970;1:109.

Chan CLK, Wood C. Pelvic adhesiolysis: the assessment of symptom relief by 100 patients. *Aust NZ J Obstet Gynaecol* 1985;25:295.

Chatman DL, Zbella EA. Pelvic peritoneal defects and endometriosis: further observations. *Fertil Steril* 1986;46:711.

Crisson JE, Keefe FJ. The relationship of locus of control to pain coping strategies and psychological distress in chronic pain patients. *Pain* 1988;35:147.

Daniell JF. Laparoscopic enterolysis for chronic abdominal pain. *J Gynecol Surg* 1989;5:61.

Diamond MP, Daniell JF, Johns DA, et al. Postoperative adhesion development after operative laparoscopy: evaluation at early second-look procedures. *Fertil Steril* 1991;55:700.

Diamond MP, Daniell JF, Martin DC, et al. Tubal patency and pelvic adhesions at early second-look laparoscopy following intra-abdominal use of the carbon dioxide laser: initial report of the Intra-abdominal Laser Study Group. *Fertil Steril* 1984;42:717.

Dicker RC, Greenspan JR, Straus LT, et al. Complications of abdominal and vaginal hysterectomy among women of reproductive age in the United States: the collaborative review of sterilization. *Am J Obstet Gynecol* 1982;144:841.

Duncan CH, Taylor HC. A psychosomatic study of pelvic congestion. *Am J Obstet Gynecol* 1952;64:1.

Farquhar CM, Rogers V, Franks S, et al. A randomized controlled trial of medroxyprogesterone acetate and psychotherapy for the treatment of pelvic congestion. *Br J Obstet Gynaecol* 1989;96:1153.

Fedele L, Parazzini F, Bianchi S, et al. Stage and localization of pelvic endometriosis and pain. *Fertil Steril* 1990;53:155.

Fernandez F, Adams F, Holmes VF. Analgesic effect of alprazolam in patients with chronic, organic pain of malignant origin. *J Clin Psychopharmacol* 1987;7:167.

Fordyce WE. *Behavioral methods of control of chronic pain and illness.* St. Louis: CV Mosby, 1976.

Garcia C-R, David SS. Pelvic endometriosis: infertility and pelvic pain. *Am J Obstet Gynecol* 1977;129:740.

Gidro-Frank L, Gordon I, Taylor HC. Pelvic pain and female identity: a survey of emotional factors in 40 patients. *Am J Obstet Gynecol* 1960;79:1184.

Gross R, Doerr H, Caldirola D, et al. Borderline syndrome and incest in chronic pelvic pain patients. *Int J Psychiatry Med* 1980/81;10:79.

Haber J, Roos C. Effects of spouse abuse and/or sexual abuse in the development and maintenance of chronic pain in women. *Adv Pain Res Ther* 1985;9:889.

Hornstein MD, Hemmings R, Yuzpe AA, et al. Use of nafarelin versus placebo after reductive laparoscopic surgery for endometriosis. *Fertil Steril* 1997;68:860.

Howard FM, El-Minawi AM, Sanchez RA. Conscious pain mapping by laparoscopy in women with chronic pelvic pain. *Obstet Gynecol* 2000;96:934.

Jamieson DJ, Steege JF. The association of sexual abuse with pelvic pain complaints in a primary care population. *Am J Obstet Gynecol* 1997;177:1408–1412.

Jansen RPS, Russell P. Nonpigmented endometriosis: clinical, laparoscopic, and pathologic definition. *Am J Obstet Gynecol* 1986;155:1154.

Keye WR, Hansen LW, Astin M, et al. Argon laser therapy of endometriosis: a review of 92 consecutive patients. *Fertil Steril* 1987;47:208.

Kjerulff KH, Langenberg PW, Rhodes JC, et al. Effectiveness of hysterectomy. *Obstet Gynecol* 2000;95:319.

Kresch AJ, Seifer DB, Sachs LB, et al. Laparoscopy in 100 women with chronic pelvic pain. *Obstet Gynecol* 1984;64:672.

Lee RB, Stone K, Magelssen D, et al. Presacral neurectomy for chronic pelvic pain. *Obstet Gynecol* 1986;68:517.

Ling FW, for the Pelvic Pain Study Group. Randomized controlled trial of depot leuprolide in patients with chronic pelvic pain and clinically suspected endometriosis. *Obstet Gynecol* 1999;93:51.

Luciano AA, Maier DB, Koch EL, et al. A comparative study of postoperative adhesions following laser surgery by laparoscopy versus laparotomy in the rabbit model. *Obstet Gynecol* 1989;75:220.

Mathias JR, Clench MH, Roberts PH, et al. Serum relaxin levels detected in women with functional bowel disease and reduced by leuprolide acetate (LA) therapy. *Gastroenterology* 1993;104[Suppl 4]:A549.

Mattingly RF, Thompson JD. Leiomyomata uteri and abdominal hysterectomy for benign disease. In: *Te Linde's operative gynecology*, ed 6. Philadelphia: JB Lippincott, 1985:227.

Melzack R. From the gate to the neuromatrix. *Pain* 1999;82[Suppl 6]:121.

Melzack R. Neurophysiologic foundations of pain. In: Sternbach RA, ed. *The psychology of pain*. New York: Raven Press, 1986:1.

Melzack R, Wall PD. Pain mechanisms: a new theory. *Science* 1965;150:971.

Morrison J. Childhood sexual histories of women with somatization disorder. *Am J Psychiatry* 1989;146:239.

Nezhat CR, Nezhat FR, Metzger DA, et al. Adhesion reformation after reproductive surgery by videolaseroscopy. *Fertil Steril* 1990;53:1008.

Olive DL. Endometriosis. *N Engl J Med* 1993;328:1759.

O'Shaughnessy A, Check JH, Nowroozi K, et al. CA-125 levels measured in different phases of the menstrual cycle in screening for endometriosis. *Obstet Gynecol* 1993;81:99.

Portenoy RK, Foley KM. Chronic use of opioid analgesics in non-malignant pain: report of 38 cases. *Pain* 1986;25:171.

Rapkin AJ, Kames LD, Darke LL, et al. History of physical and sexual abuse in women with chronic pain. *Obstet Gynecol* 1990;76:92.

Raskin DE. Diagnosis in patients with chronic pelvic pain. *Am J Psychiatry* 1984;141:824(letter).

Redwine DB. Conservative laparoscopic excision of endometriosis by sharp dissection: life table analysis of reoperation and persistent or recurrent disease. *Fertil Steril* 1991;56:628.

Reiter RC. Occult somatic pathology in women with chronic pelvic pain. *Clin Obstet Gynecol* 1990;33:154.

Reiter RC, Gambone JC. Demographic and historic variables in women with idiopathic chronic pelvic pain. *Obstet Gynecol* 1990,75:428.

Rudy TE, Kerns RD, Turk DC. Chronic pain and depression: toward a cognitive-behavioral mediation model. *Pain* 1988;35:129.

Simons DG, Travell J. Myofascial trigger points: a possible explanation. *Pain* 1981;10:100.

Sinaki M, Merritt JL, Stillwell GK. Tension myalgia of the pelvic floor. *Mayo Clin Proc* 1977;52:717.

Slocumb J. Neurological factors in chronic pelvic pain: trigger points and the abdominal pelvic pain syndrome. *Am J Obstet Gynecol* 1984;149:536.

Slocumb JC, Kellner R, Rosenfeld RC, et al. Anxiety and depression in patients with the abdominal pelvic pain syndrome. *Gen Hosp Psychiatry* 1989;11:48.

Steege JF. Dyspareunia and vaginismus. *Clin Obstet Gynecol* 1984;27:750.

Steege JF. Ovarian remnant syndrome. *Obstet Gynecol* 1987;70:64.

Steege JF, Metzger DA, Levy BS. *Chronic pelvic pain: an integrated approach*. Philadelphia: WB Saunders, 1998.

Steege JF, Stout AL. Resolution of chronic pelvic pain following laparoscopic adhesiolysis. *Am J Obstet Gynecol* 1991;165:278.

Steege JF, Stout AL, Somkuti SG. Chronic pelvic pain: toward an integrative model. *Obstet Gynecol Surv* 1993;48:95.

Stout AL, Steege JF. Psychosocial and behavioral self-reports of chronic pelvic pain patients. Presented at the meeting of the American Society for Psychosomatic Obstetrics and Gynecology, Houston, TX, March 1991.

Stout AL, Steege JF, Dodson WC, et al. Relationship of laparoscopic findings to self-report of pelvic pain. *Am J Obstet Gynecol* 1991;164:73.

Stovall TG, Ling FW, Crawford DA. Hysterectomy for chronic pelvic pain of presumed uterine etiology. *Obstet Gynecol* 1990;75:676.

Summitt RL, Ling FW. Urethral syndrome presenting as chronic pelvic pain. *J Psychosom Obstet Gynaecol* 1991; 12(Suppl):77.

Sutton CJ, Ewen SP, Whitelaw N, et al. Prospective, randomized, double blind controlled trial of laser laparoscopy in the treatment of pelvic pain associated with minimal, mild, and moderate endometriosis. *Fertil Steril* 1994;62:696.

Sutton C, MacDonald R. Laser laparoscopic adhesiolysis. *J Gynecol Surg* 1990;6:155.

Sutton CJ, Pooley AS, Ewen SP, et al. Follow-up report on a randomized, controlled trial of laser laparoscopy in the treatment of pelvic pain associated with minimal to moderate endometriosis. *Fertil Steril* 1997;68:1070.

Tjaden B, Schlaff WD, Kimball A, et al: The efficacy of presacral neurectomy for the relief of midline dysmenorrhea. *Obstet Gynecol* 1990;76:89.

Tulandi T. Adhesion reformation after reproductive surgery with and without the carbon dioxide laser. *Fertil Steril* 1987;47:704.

Tulandi T. Salpingo-ovariolysis: a comparison between laser surgery and electrosurgery. *Fertil Steril* 1986;45:489.

Walker EW, Katon W, Harrop-Griffiths J, et al. Relationship of chronic pelvic pain to psychiatric diagnoses and childhood sexual abuse. *Am J Psychiatry* 1988;145:75.

Walters MD. Definitive surgery. In: Schenken RS, ed. *Endometriosis: contemporary concepts in clinical management*. Philadelphia: JB Lippincott, 1989:267.

Winkel CA, Bray M. Treatment of women with endometriosis using excision alone, ablation alone, or ablation in combination with leuprolide acetate. Proceedings of the 5th World Congress on Endometriosis, Yokohama, Japan, 1996:55.

Te Linde's Operative Gynecology, ninth edition, edited by John A. Rock and Howard W. Jones, III. Lippincott Williams & Wilkins, Philadelphia © 2003.

CHAPTER
28

▼

Pelvic Inflammatory Disease

MARK G. MARTENS

Pelvic inflammatory disease (PID) is one of the most serious infections facing women today. Untreated or unsuccessfully treated women may suffer life-threatening consequences, and even adequately treated women are at much higher risk for potentially serious sequelae. PID is a spectrum of diseases initially involving the cervix, uterus, and fallopian tubes. Acute PID, the acute clinical syndrome, is most often attributed to an ascending spread of microorganisms from the vagina and endocervix to the endometrium, fallopian tubes, and contiguous structures. The terms *acute PID* and *acute salpingitis* are often used interchangeably, but PID is not limited to tubal infection only. Recently, a more descriptive term to differentiate the severity and extent of various forms of PID was introduced by Hemsell and colleagues, termed *upper genital tract infection (UGTI)*. This is differentiated from *lower genital tract infection (LGTI)*, because response to treatment appears to be different in these two entities, which were previously grouped as inpatient or outpatient treatment regimens, sometimes at a conflict with diagnostic or severity of illness realities.

Sexually transmitted diseases (STDs) have been reported at epidemic proportions in the United States. Since the mid-1960s, the incidence of gonorrhea and chlamydia infections has been estimated at more than 2 million and 4 million cases, respectively, each year. For women, acute PID is the most common and important complication of STDs. Bell and Holmes estimated that 1 million women a year are treated for acute salpingitis in the United States. About 250,000 to 300,000 women are hospitalized each year with a diagnosis of salpingitis or PID. The disease generates nearly 2.5 million visits to physicians, and an estimated 150,000 surgical procedures are performed for complications every year. According to Westrom, the direct and indirect costs of PID and its sequelae totaled 4 billion dollars in the United States this past decade. In terms of overall incidence, acute PID occurs in about 1% to 2% of young, sexually active women each year. PID is the most common serious infection in women age 16 to 25 years, and the resultant morbidity exceeds that produced by all other infections combined for this age group.

ETIOLOGY

Although certain geographic areas with near epidemic rates of STDs have *Neisseria gonorrhoeae* as a common cause of PID, many cases of acute PID are the result of a polymicrobial infection caused by organisms ascending from the vagina and cervix to infect the mucosa of the endometrium and fallopian tube. About 85% of cases are naturally occurring infections in sexually active females of reproductive age. The remaining 15% of infections occur after procedures that break the cervical mucous barrier, such as placement of an intrauterine device (IUD), endometrial biopsy, or uterine curettage, which allow the vaginal flora to colonize the upper genital tract.

In the United States, nontuberculous acute PID was traditionally separated into gonococcal and nongonococcal disease, depending on the isolation of *N. gonorrhoeae* from the endocervix. A variety of organisms can be isolated from the endocervix, and it is difficult to determine which of these organisms are PID-related and which are normal cervicovaginal flora. Upper genital tract organisms are probably more indicative of the causative organisms but are difficult to obtain. Bacterial organisms cultured directly from tubal fluid commonly include *N. gonorrhoeae, Chlamydia trachomatis,* endogenous aerobic and anaerobic bacteria, and genital *Mycoplasma* species. Laparoscopic studies have demonstrated a correlation of no more than 50% between endocervical and tubal cultures, but the presence of *N. gonorrhoeae* is usually considered an important causative factor. However, endocervical gonorrhea does not necessarily indicate its sole pathogenic nature in all cases. Direct fallopian tube cultures have demonstrated that tubal infections are often polymicrobial. The type and number of species vary depending on the stage of the disease. Gonorrhea, for example, is often cultured from the cervix during the first 24 to 48 hours of the disease but is often absent later. Similarly, fewer organisms are cultured late in the disease, and anaerobic bacteria such as *Prevotella, Bacteroides, Peptococcus,* and *Peptostreptococcus* species tend to predominate. Whether these anaerobes play a causative role or increase in number and frequency as a result of the acute inflammatory response is uncertain. Sweet has summarized the literature by stating that in approximately one third of women with PID, *N. gonorrhoeae* is the only organism recovered by direct tubal or cul-de-sac culture. One third have a culture positive for *N. gonorrhoeae* plus a mixture of endogenous aerobic and anaerobic flora, and the remaining one third have only aerobic and anaerobic organisms. Chow and colleagues and Monif and colleagues have postulated that the gonococcus initiates acute PID and produces tissue damage. This damage changes the local environment, which in turn allows anaerobic and aerobic organisms from the vaginal and cervical flora to invade the upper genital tract. Eschenbach and Sweet have suggested that not all PID follows gonococcal infection, and that acute PID initially may also solely have a polymicrobial etiology.

According to Sweet and Gibbs, about 20% of all women with salpingitis have tubal cultures positive for *C. trachomatis. N. gonorrhoeae* and *C. trachomatis* are found in the same individual 25% to 40% of the time. Scandinavian studies by Eilard and co-workers have reported the recovery of *C. trachomatis* from the cervix in 22% to 47% of women with acute PID. *C. trachomatis* by itself produces a mild form of salpingitis with an insidious onset. In contrast to gonorrhea, *Chlamydia* can remain in the fallopian tubes for months or years after initial colonization of the upper genital tract. Svensson and colleagues found that women with *C. trachomatis* infection at laparoscopy had the most severe fallopian tube involvement, probably because of its clinically silent or minimally symptomatic nature, which results in difficult or delayed diagnosis and therefore delayed or absent treatment. The two major sequelae of acute PID are tubal infertility and ectopic pregnancy. These have been strongly associated with prior chlamydial infection as a consequence of intratubal and peritubal adhesions.

Although *C. trachomatis* is generally believed to be one of the most common causes of PID, along with *N. gonorrhoeae,* its etiologic role is very different. *N. gonorrhoeae* is a gram-negative diplococcus with rapid growth due to a growth cycle of about 20 to 40 minutes. This results in a great increase in the number of organisms once *N. gonorrhoeae* reaches an area such as the endometrium or fallopian tube, where growth is relatively unimpeded. This rapid increase in the number of gram-negative bacteria usually results in a rapid and intense inflammatory response by the woman's host defenses. The response to this rapid bacterial growth is proliferation and aggregation of white blood cells and their inflammatory products. Migration of this bacterial and leukocytic mixture through the fallopian tube to the ovary and peritoneal cavity, and back to the cervix and vagina, causes the symptoms that are pathognomonic of acute PID.

C. trachomatis, however, is a slow-growing intracellular organism. Its lack of mitochondria results in its obligatory intracellular existence and also causes its growth cycle to be extremely slow compared with *N. gonorrhoeae* and nonintracellular microorganisms. The growth cycle of *Chlamydia* is 48 to 72 hours; therefore, several weeks to months are required for the growth to reach numbers sufficient to cause acute symptoms, if at all. Its slow growth does not induce a rapid or violent inflammatory response. This explains the slow and insidious nature of the symptoms of acute *C. trachomatis* infections. However, because of its intracellular growth cycle, the release of the elementary bodies (its infectious vehicle) occurs by rupture of the cell that it has invaded. The repeated occurrence of elementary body infection of susceptible cells, and their subsequent destruction by rupture, is the major mechanism by which *C. trachomatis* causes disease in acute pelvic infections. Also, because of its slow growth and lack of acute inflammatory response and clinical symptoms, treatment is often delayed or not started at all, adding to the extended tissue destruction and PID sequelae.

The lack of acute symptoms does not lessen the importance of *Chlamydia* as a PID pathogen. Not only does the tissue destruction result in severe complications such as ectopic pregnancy and infertility, but also the tissue damage provides fertile ground for the growth of secondarily infecting aerobic and anaerobic bacteria. This necrotic tissue is an excellent growth medium, and the epithelial damage enhances the breakdown of the surface defense mechanisms. The importance of *Chlamydia* was documented during the 1980s when treatment of acute PID was initially believed to be successfully accomplished with regimens not active against *C. trachomatis.* However, although success was evident with short-term follow-up, long-term follow-up demonstrated that treatment of *C. trachomatis* was necessary.

PID regimens without *Chlamydia* coverage resulted in an increased incidence of long-term complications such as abscesses and chronic pelvic pain, with resultant increased surgical intervention. Therefore, modern treatment of PID includes *C. trachomatis* coverage, even though it may not be the cause of the acute symptoms.

Nongonococcal infections are believed to be the result of acute bacterial infections or possibly a preceding or previously treated *C. trachomatis* UGTI. This is confirmed by the high incidence of *Chlamydia* antibodies in patients with acute PID, ectopic pregnancy, and infertility.

In addition to *N. gonorrhoeae, Chlamydia,* and aerobic and anaerobic bacteria, other microorganisms have been implicated as etiologic agents in acute salpingitis. The genital tract mycoplasmas, *Mycoplasma hominis* and *Ureaplasma urealyticum,* have also been suggested as causal agents in acute salpingitis. However, their role remains controversial. Cervical cultures positive for both *M. hominis* and *U. urealyticum* have been recovered from women with PID. However, the rate of isolation is about 75%, which is not statistically different from that of women who are sexually active but without PID (baseline rate of about 50%), as found by Lemeke and Lsonka.

RISK FACTORS

Several factors that predispose to the development of acute PID have been identified. Risk factors are important considerations in both the clinical management and prevention of UGTIs. There is a strong correlation between exposure to STDs and PID. In the United States, recent studies have confirmed this association with the recovery of *N. gonorrhoeae* or *C. trachomatis* in about 50% of patients hospitalized with acute PID. Age at first intercourse, frequency of intercourse, number of sexual partners, and marital status are all associated with the frequency of exposure to STDs and thus are associated with PID. Women with multiple partners have an increased risk (four to six times normal) for development of acute salpingitis, compared with women who have monogamous sexual relations.

The incidence of acute PID decreases with advancing age. Adolescent females are at significant risk for development of acute salpingitis. Westrom reported that nearly 70% of females with PID were younger than 25 years of age, 33% experienced their first infection before the age of 19, and 75% were nulliparous. The risk for development of acute PID in a sexually active adolescent female patient was 1:8, whereas the risk was 1:80 for a sexually active woman 24 years of age or older. Several reasons have been suggested for this increased risk. The two microorganisms most commonly considered to be the inciting agents in cases of PID, *N. gonorrhoeae* and *C. trachomatis,* have a predilection for columnar epithelium. As suggested by Schaefer and by Sweet and colleagues, cervical columnar epithelium is exposed to a greater extent in younger individuals, and recedes into the cervical canal with increasing age.

Clinical and laboratory studies have documented that the use of contraceptives changes the relative risk for development of PID. Multiple case-controlled studies have shown an increased risk of acute PID in women who wear an IUD. It has been estimated that IUD users have a threefold to fivefold increased risk for development of acute PID. In a report by Tatum and colleagues of animal model investigations, it was suggested that multifilament strings may be a major contributing factor in the increased risk of PID. Barrier methods of contraception (condoms, diaphragms, and spermicidal preparations) are effective both as mechanical obstructive devices and as chemical barriers. A nearly 60% decrease in the risk of PID has been demonstrated among women using a barrier method of contraception. Nonoxynol 9, the material in spermicidal preparations, is both bactericidal and viricidal. Laboratory tests have demonstrated that nonoxynol 9 kills *N. gonorrhoeae,* genital *Mycoplasma* species, *Trichomonas vaginalis, Treponema pallidum,* herpes simplex virus, and human immunodeficiency virus (HIV), but has been removed from many vaginal products due to safety warnings.

Oral contraceptives have also been shown to reduce the risk of acute PID. The mechanism for such protection remains speculative. The thicker cervical mucus produced by the progestin component of oral contraceptives is believed to inhibit sperm and bacterial penetration into the upper genital tract. The decrease in duration of menstrual flow accompanying oral contraceptive use theoretically creates a shorter interval for bacterial colonization. Svensson and co-workers reported that, in addition to protecting against PID, the use of oral contraceptive pills was associated with a better prognosis for future fertility than was seen in women with acute PID using other contraceptive methods or no contraceptive methods.

Surgical procedures of the female genital tract also place the patient at risk for PID. About 15% of pelvic infections occur after procedures that break the cervical mucous barrier, allowing for colonization of the upper genital tract. Eschenbach and Holmes reported that these procedures include endometrial biopsy, curettage, IUD insertion, hysteroscopy, and hysterosalpingography. The incidence of UGTI associated with first-trimester abortions is about 1 in 200 cases. Recent practice has emphasized the use of prophylactic antibiotics in high-risk cases to attempt to decrease the incidence of iatrogenic acute PID. Acute salpingitis occurring in a woman with a previous tubal ligation was once believed to be rare. Phillips and D'Abling reported that acute PID developed in the proximal stump of previously ligated fallopian tubes in 1 of 450 women hospitalized for acute salpingitis. However, many cases may be undiagnosed because of the absence of peritoneal signs.

Previous acute PID is also a risk factor for future episodes of the disease. Another acute tubal infection develops in about 25% of women who have had acute PID. The exact mechanism for this increased susceptibility has not been determined, but it may be loss of the natural protective mechanisms of the fallopian tube against microorganisms. This increased risk may be related to the sexual habits of the woman involved, such as reinfection from an untreated male partner or genital tract damage from the initial infection. Eschenbach has documented that more than 80% of male contacts are not treated.

DIAGNOSIS

Acute PID presents with a broad spectrum of clinical symptoms. The differential diagnosis of acute PID includes acute appendicitis, endometriosis, torsion or rupture of an adnexal mass, ectopic pregnancy, and lower genital tract infection.

Common clinical manifestations include lower abdominal pain, cervical motion tenderness, and adnexal tenderness and may include fever, cervical discharge, and leukocytosis. Historically, the diagnosis of acute PID was not established unless the patient had the triad of lower abdominal and pelvic pain, fever, and leukocytosis. Jacobson and Westrom have shown that all three are present in only 15% to 30% of actual PID cases. In addition, about 50% of patients initially present with a normal temperature and white blood cell (WBC) count. Pain in the lower abdomen and pelvis is by far the most common symptom of acute PID. It occurs in more than 90% of patients at initial presentation. The pain is usually described as constant and dull and is accentuated by motion and sexual activity. Generally, the pain is of recent onset, usually less than 7 days. About 75% of patients with PID have an associated endocervical infection and coexistent purulent vaginal discharge. Nausea and vomiting are comparably late symptoms in the course of the disease. Abnormal vaginal bleeding, especially menorrhagia, or spotting, is noted in about 40% of patients. The Centers for Disease Control and Prevention (CDC) have established the criteria for making the diagnosis of salpingitis based on clinical grounds. The most recent update includes only selected tender signs as required for a diagnosis and eliminates leukocytosis and fever as essential criteria (Table 28.1).

Perihepatic inflammation and adhesions, more commonly known as the Fitz-Hugh-Curtis syndrome, develop in 1% to 10% of patients with acute PID. Signs and symptoms include right upper quadrant pain, pleuritic pain, and tenderness in the right upper quadrant when the liver is palpated. Usually the symptoms and signs of this syndrome are preceded by the clinical onset of acute PID. The condition is often mistakenly diagnosed as either acute cholecystitis or pneumonia. Fitz-Hugh-Curtis syndrome is believed to develop from vascular or transperitoneal dissemination of either *N. gonorrhoeae* or *C. trachomatis* to produce the perihepatic inflammation. Other organisms may be involved, but limited data exist on their causality.

Jacobson and Westrom attempted to correlate the clinical diagnosis of acute salpingitis with laparoscopic visualization. Of 814 women in whom laparoscopy was performed for presumed acute PID, 512 (65%) had visual evidence of salpingitis; 184 (23%) had normal visual findings; and 98 (12%) had other pelvic pathology. Because of the positive clinical findings, many of the patients with normal findings were suspected to have early

---

TABLE 28.1.
Criteria for the Diagnosis of Acute Salpingitis

Minimum Criteria
Empirical treatment of PID should be initiated in sexually active young women and others at risk for STDs if the following minimum criteria are present and no other cause for the illness can be identified:
    Uterine/adnexal tenderness or
    Cervical motion tenderness

More Elaborate Criteria
More elaborate diagnostic evaluation often is needed, because incorrect diagnosis and management might cause unnecessary morbidity. These additional criteria may be used to enhance the specificity of the minimum criteria. Additional criteria that support a diagnosis of PID include the following:

Routine Criteria for Diagnosing PID:
    Oral temperature >38.3°C (>101°F)
    Abnormal cervical or vaginal mucopurulent discharge
    Elevated erythrocyte sedimentation rate
    Elevated C-reactive protein
    Laboratory documentation of cervical infection with *Neisseria gonorrhoeae* or *Chlamydia trachomatis*
    Presence of WBCs on saline microscopy of vaginal secretions

Specific Criteria for Diagnosing PID:
    Histopathologic evidence of endometritis on endometrial biopsy
    Transvaginal sonography or MRI scan showing thickened fluid-filled tubes with or without free pelvic fluid or tuboovarian complex
    Laparoscopic abnormalities consistent with PID

MRI, magnetic resonance imaging; PID, pelvic inflammatory disease; STD, sexually transmitted disease.

PID with endometritis and endosalpingitis without visual evidence of tubal or pelvic damage. Thus, laparoscopy is limited as a method of diagnosing the early stages of PID, but it is important to rule out non-PID surgical emergencies such as appendicitis, and other entities requiring different treatment modalities, such as endometriosis.

Despite these shortcomings of early diagnosis, laparoscopic visualization of the pelvis is still the most accurate method of confirming the diagnosis of acute PID. However, it is logistically and economically impractical for all patients suspected of having acute PID to undergo diagnostic laparoscopy in the United States. Therefore, the diagnosis of most episodes of acute PID is often made on the basis of clinical history and physical examination. Although it is suggested that laparoscopy be offered to all patients with an uncertain diagnosis, it is strongly indicated for patients who are not responding to therapy, in an effort to confirm the diagnosis, obtain cultures from the cul-de-sac or fallopian tubes, and drain pus if necessary. In summary, laparoscopic studies have shown the following:

1. The clinical diagnosis of acute PID may be inaccurate.
2. Acute PID is sometimes found in patients undergoing laparoscopy for other causes of pelvic pain.

3. Laparoscopy is a relatively safe method for making the visual diagnosis of the latter stages of PID, and thus assessing future fertility prognosis and planning.
4. Laparoscopy is an excellent means of obtaining cultures directly from the tube.

The appearance of the pelvic organs can vary from erythematous, indurated, edematous oviducts, to pockets of purulent material, to a large pyosalpinx or tuboovarian abscess. However, although no disease may be evident in early stages, it is imperative to render treatment to all stages to avoid long-term sequelae.

Other less invasive methods of diagnosis have been suggested for verifying a clinical diagnosis of acute PID. Endometrial biopsy is one alternative to laparoscopy. Paavonen and associates reported a 90% correlation between histologic endometritis and laparoscopically confirmed salpingitis. However, results may be delayed up to 2 to 3 days, making its clinical applicability limited. Ultrasonography is of limited value for patients with mild or moderate pelvic PID. Thus, the routine use of sonography in patients with acute salpingitis does not appear to be indicated. Ultrasound is helpful in distinguishing an adnexal mass, especially in patients who demonstrate a lack of response to antimicrobial therapy in the initial 48 to 72 hours of therapy. Sonohysterography, an ultrasound examination using the instillation of saline to better define pelvic structures, is not indicated at this time for patients suspected of having PID, because no studies have been performed to demonstrate its safety in the event that pathogens are dispersed into the upper genital tract in the process of instilling the saline. Culdocentesis, with evidence of purulent peritoneal fluid, is helpful in the diagnosis of acute PID. With acute PID, the WBC count of peritoneal fluid is greater than 30,000 cells/mL, compared with a WBC count of 1,000 cells/mL in women without peritoneal inflammation. However, other infections, such as appendicitis and diverticulitis, among others, can also cause purulent pelvic fluid and a false diagnosis of PID.

Laboratory tests can be obtained, but their results lack sufficient sensitivity and specificity to make them an important factor in establishing the diagnosis. Leukocytosis is not a reliable indicator of acute PID, nor does it accurately correlate with the severity of tubal inflammation or need for hospitalization. Less than 50% of women with acute PID have a WBC count greater than 10,000 cells/mL. Similarly, the erythrocyte sedimentation rate (ESR), which for years was a laboratory test for women with acute PID, is nonspecific and is a crude indicator of severity of disease. The ESR is elevated higher than 15 mm/hr in about 75% of women with laparoscopically confirmed acute salpingitis. However, 53% of women with pelvic pain and normal-appearing pelvic organs have an elevated ESR. Plasma proteins, such as C-reactive protein and antichymotrypsin, have been studied to determine whether they help in the diagnosis of acute PID. They have been found to be more sensitive than the ESR. Other investigators have found that decreased or absent isoamylase in peritoneal fluid in cases of acute PID is the best nonculture laboratory test for the disease. The major disadvantages of this test are that it requires several hours to complete and that peritoneal fluid must be obtained.

Other evaluation has revealed various inflammatory cytokines to be associated with pelvic infections; however, these tests are not commercially available to a useful extent. Because most cases of UGTI are associated with, and preceded by, lower genital tract infection, examination of the endocervix for inflammation, Gram stain, and culture for both *N. gonorrhoeae* and *C. trachomatis* are all important for proper evaluation. A negative Gram-stained smear of the endocervix does not rule out upper tract infection. However, other studies have found that acute PID is rare without a concomitant increase in inflammatory cells in the vagina and the cervix.

SEQUELAE

Infertility

One fourth of all women who have had acute salpingitis experience one or more long-term sequelae. The most common is involuntary infertility, which occurs in about 20% of patients. PID ranks as one of the major causes of infertility. Before antibiotic therapy, 50% to 70% of women who had experienced UGTIs were sterile. The sequelae of infections vary from a patent oviduct, to peritubular and periovarian adhesions that may interfere with ovum pickup, to complete tubal obstruction. The infertility rate increases directly with the number of episodes of acute pelvic infection. Also, women with mild disease are seven times less likely to suffer tubal obstruction than women with severe PID.

Ectopic Pregnancy

The number of ectopic pregnancies has doubled over the past 10 years. This increased rate is directly proportional to the increase in cases of STD and acute PID. The chance of ectopic pregnancy is increased sixfold to 10-fold in patients with a previous episode of acute salpingitis. Pathologic studies estimate that at least 50% of ectopic pregnancies occur in fallopian tubes damaged by previous salpingitis. The mechanism for the increased rate is believed to be interference of ovum transport through the tube or entrapment of the ovum secondary to microscopic tubal damage.

Chronic Pelvic Pain

The chance that chronic pelvic pain will develop in a woman after acute salpingitis is four times that of control subjects without pelvic infection (20% versus 5%). Chronic pelvic pain can be caused by a hydrosalpinx. A hydrosalpinx is presumably the end-stage development of a pyosalpinx. The pain can also be related to adhesions surrounding the ovary. All patients with chronic pelvic pain believed to be caused by acute PID should undergo laparoscopy or laparotomy to establish the cause of the chronic pain and rule out other diseases such as endometriosis, which require different treatment.

A tuboovarian complex is a collection of pus within an anatomic space created by adherence to adjacent organs. The incidence of true adnexal abscess is about 10% in women with acute PID. Landers and Sweet noted a 20% rate of early treatment failure (after 48 to 72 hours) of antibiotic therapy as a result of persistent pain or enlargement of a tuboovarian abscess or complex. In addition, according to Landers and Sweet, 31% required an operation several weeks to months after their acute infections for persistent disease or pain.

MORTALITY

Before antibiotic therapy, the mortality rate associated with acute PID was 1%. Most of these deaths resulted from rupture of tuboovarian abscesses. Today, death associated with PID is rare, but the mortality rate can still be as high as 5% to 10% for ruptured tuboovarian abscesses, even with modern medical and operative therapy, mostly the result of subsequent development of adult respiratory distress syndrome (ARDS), a condition often associated with serious infection.

TREATMENT

The therapeutic goals in the management of acute PID include both elimination of the acute infection and symptoms and prevention of long-term sequelae such as infertility, ectopic pregnancy, chronic pelvic pain, and the residue of infection. Antibiotic treatment should be started as soon as cultures have been obtained and diagnosis is confirmed or strongly suspected. Treatment is based on the consensus that PID is polymicrobial in cause. Empirical antibiotic protocols should cover a wide range of bacteria, including *N. gonorrhoeae, C. trachomatis,* anaerobic rods and cocci, gram-negative aerobic rods, gram-positive aerobes, and *Mycoplasma* species. Despite general agreement that broad-spectrum therapy is appropriate, questions persist regarding optimal therapeutic regimens.

Controversy has arisen over the issue of outpatient treatment with oral antibiotics versus inpatient treatment with parenteral antibiotics. There are no data available to evaluate the efficacy of hospital versus ambulatory management of acute PID. In the United States, three of four women with acute pelvic infection are treated as outpatients for their disease. In Scandinavia, which has a different health care system, most women are treated as inpatients. In 2002, the CDC published recommended treatment guidelines for outpatient management of acute PID (Table 28.2). Some of the treatment regimens are based on the controversial premise that it may be adequate to cover just a few of the major etiologic agents (*N. gonorrhoeae* and *C. trachomatis*) involved in acute salpingitis. As a result, studies have documented a 10% to 20% treatment failure rate for women receiving oral an-

TABLE 28.2.
CDC-Recommended Treatment Regimens for Outpatient Therapy of Acute Pelvic Inflammatory Disease

Regimen A
Ofloxacin 400 mg orally twice a day or levofloxacin 500 mg orally once daily for 14 days, with or without metronidazole 500 mg orally twice a day for 14 days.

Oral ofloxacin has been investigated as a single agent in two well-designed clinical trials, and it is effective against both *Neisseria gonorrhoeae* and *Chlamdyia trachomatis.* Despite the results of these trials, ofloxacin's lack of anaerobic coverage is a concern; the addition of metronidazole provides this coverage.

Regimen B
Ceftriaxone 250 mg IM once, *or* cefoxitin 2 g IM plus probenecid 1 g orally in a single dose concurrently once, *or* other parenteral third-generation cephalosporin (e.g., ceftizoxime or cefotaxime), *plus* doxycycline 100 mg orally twice a day for 14 days with or without metronidazole 500 mg orally twice a day for 14 days.

The optimal choice of a cephalosporin for Regimen B is unclear; although cefoxitin has better anaerobic coverage, ceftriaxone has better coverage against *N. gonorrhoeae*. Clinical trials have demonstrated that a single dose of cefoxitin is effective in obtaining short-term clinical response in women who have pelvic inflammatory disease (PID); however, the theoretical limitations in its coverage of anaerobes may require the addition of metronidazole. The metronidazole also effectively treats BV, which also is frequently associated with BV. No data have been published regarding the use of oral cephalosporins for the treatment of PID.

Alternative Oral Regimens
Information regarding other outpatient regimens is limited, but one other regimen has undergone at least one clinical trial and has broad-spectrum coverage. Amoxicillin/clavulanic acid plus doxycycline was effective in obtaining short-term clinical response in a single clinical trial; however, gastrointestinal symptoms might limit the overall success of this regimen. Several recent investigations have evaluated the use of azithromycin in the treatment of upper reproductive tract infections; however, the data are insufficient to recommend this agent as a component of any of the treatment regimens for PID.

tibiotics as outpatients compared with a 5% to 10% failure rate for women receiving intravenous antibiotics as inpatients, where broader coverage is used. The inclusion of the quinolone arm, ofloxacin, and levofloxacin in the outpatient treatment regimen does permit broader coverage of pathogens, but this still may not be adequate for serious disease. It is important to reevaluate patients within 48 to 72 hours of initiating outpatient therapy to determine the response of the disease. If a poor response has been obtained, the patient should be hospitalized with parenteral antibiotics in the hope of preventing or limiting the sequelae of PID.

Ideally, every woman with acute PID should be hospitalized for the first few days for parenteral antibiotic treatment. Because this may not be practical because of limited economic or physical facility resources, the clinician who diagnoses acute salpingitis in the office or emergency department is faced with the question of which patient to hospitalize. Indications for the hospitalization of patients with acute salpingitis are also defined by the CDC in the 2002 guidelines (Table 28.3). However, it is suggested that all adolescents with salpingitis be hospitalized because of their high noncompliance rate and to optimize treatment to prevent damage to the reproductive tract, which could affect future fertility.

Another indication for hospitalization is the presence of an adnexal or pelvic abscess. Outpatient therapy may not provide antibiotic levels high enough to penetrate an abscess, and rupture of the abscess may have serious consequences. Women in whom the definitive diagnosis of acute PID is in question should also be hospitalized, and diagnostic measures should be instituted. As previously stated, at least 10% of all patients have other serious diagnoses, such as acute appendicitis, ectopic pregnancy, or adnexal torsion, and these should be ruled out. Patients with serious illness, patients with nausea and vomiting, patients who are unable to follow or tolerate outpatient therapy, and patients with a previously failed outpatient oral regimen also should be hospitalized and given parenteral antibiotics. The 2002 CDC guidelines for inpatient treatment of acute PID describe two regimens (Table 28.4). Regimen A is a combination of oral or parenteral doxycycline plus intravenous cefoxitin or cefotetan. Other third-generation cephalosporins can be substituted, such as ceftizoxime (Cefizox) or cefotaxime (Claforan). All of these agents are effective against penicillinase-producing *N. gonorrhoeae*, *Peptostreptococcus* and other anaerobic species and *Escherichia coli*, and other aerobic (facultative) species. Ceftriaxone is recommended by the CDC; however, its poor anaerobic activity and lack of trials do not make it an acceptable alternative for several investigators. Doxycycline can be given intravenously if the patient is unable to tolerate oral therapy, but it must be infused very slowly to prevent pain and sclerosis of the vein. Oral doxycycline has been demonstrated to be equally effective because of the slow

---

TABLE 28.3.
Criteria for Hospitalization of Patients With Acute Pelvic Inflammatory Disease

The following criteria for hospitalization are based on observational data and theoretical concerns:

- Surgical emergencies such as appendicitis cannot be excluded.
- The patient is pregnant.
- The patient does not respond clinically to oral antimicrobial therapy.
- The patient is unable to follow or tolerate an outpatient oral regimen.
- The patient has severe illness, nausea and vomiting, or high fever.
- The patient has a tuboovarian abscess

TABLE 28.4.
CDC-Recommended Treatment Regimens for Inpatient Therapy of Acute Pelvic Inflammatory Disease

Regimen A
Cefoxitin, 2 g intravenously every 6 hours
   or
Cefotetan, 2 g intravenously every 12 hours
   plus
Doxycycline, 100 mg intravenously or orally every 12 hours
Note: This regimen should be continued for at least 24 hours after the patient demonstrates substantial clinical improvement, after which doxycycline, 100 mg orally two times a day, should be continued for a total of 14 days. Doxycycline administered orally has bioavailability similar to that of the intravenous formulation and may be administered if normal gastrointestinal function is present. When tuboovarian abscess is present, many health care providers use clindamycin or metronidazole with doxycycline for continued therapy rather than doxycycline alone, because it provides more effective anaerobic coverage. Other cephalosporins (ceftizoxime, cefotaxime, and ceftriaxone) may be effective therapy for pelvic inflammatory disease (PID) as replacements for cefotetan or cefoxitin.

Regimen B
Clindamycin, 900 mg intravenously every 8 hours
   plus
Gentamicin, loading dose intravenously or intramuscularly (2 mg/kg of body weight), followed by a maintenance dose (1.5 mg/kg) every 8 hours (single daily dosing may be substituted)
Note: This regimen should be continued for at least 24 hours after the patient demonstrates substantial clinical improvement and then followed with doxycycline, 100 mg orally two times a day, or clindamycin, 450 mg orally four times a day, to complete a total of 14 days of therapy. When tuboovarian abscess is present, many health care providers use clindamycin for continued therapy rather than doxycycline because it provides more effective anaerobic coverage. Single daily dosing of gentamicin has not been evaluated for PID, but it has been efficacious in other analogous situations.

Alternative Parenteral Regimens
Limited data support the use of other parenteral regimens, but the following three regimens have been investigated in at least one clinical trial, and they have broad-spectrum coverage.
Ofloxacin 400 mg IV every 12 hours, or levofloxacin 500 mg IV once daily, with or without metronidazole 500 mg IV every 8 hours, *or*
Ampicillin/sulbactam 3 g IV every 6 hours, *plus* doxycycline 100 mg IV or orally every 12 hours
Ampicillin/sulbactam plus doxycycline has good coverage against *Chlamydia trachomatis, Neisseria gonorrhoeae,* and anaerobes, and appears to be effective for patients who have tuboovarian abscess. IV ofloxacin has been investigated as a single agent; however, because of concerns regarding the anaerobic coverage, metronidazole may be included.

---

growth cycle of *Chlamydia* and the requirement of prolonged treatment. A possible disadvantage of the cephalosporin-doxycycline combination is that these two antibiotics may be less than ideal for anaerobic infections or for a pelvic abscess. Regimen B is a combination of clindamycin and an aminoglycoside (gentamicin). This combination provides excellent activity against anaerobes, gram-negative aerobes, and gram-positive aerobes. Historically, it has been the preferred regimen for patients with an abscess, IUD-related infections, or pelvic infections after a diagnostic or operative procedure. However, there are few data to prove that it is significantly more effective than the cephalosporin regimens. A possible disadvantage of regimen B is that it may not provide optimal activity against *C. trachomatis* and *N. gonorrhoeae.* Clindamycin in high doses (900 mg in 8 hours) has good activity against *Chlamydia,* and *in vitro* studies by Martens and colleagues have demonstrated effectiveness against only 90% of *C. trachomatis* strains. Doxycycline is believed to be the most effective chlamydial agent, according to *in vitro* testing, and is often used for at least 7 days to complete treatment when the patient is switched from parenteral to post-hospitalization therapy. Also, the CDC recommendation of once daily dosing for gentamicin is not based on any data on PID patients, and should be used only if indicated for renal considerations.

Each regimen stresses two concepts: the polymicrobial etiology of acute pelvic infection and the necessity of protecting against *C. trachomatis* and *N. gonorrhoeae.* With both protocols, the CDC recommends a minimum of at least 24 hours of intravenous treatment after clinical improvement. Both protocols also require completion of a 14-day course of oral antibiotics (doxycycline or clindamycin) to eradicate slow-growing organisms such as *C. trachomatis.*

Alternative inpatient parenteral regimens are included in the 2002 CDC PID guidelines. While the CDC lists only the β-lactamase inhibitor combination ampicillin-sulbactam (Unasyn), piperacillin-tazobactam has been demonstrated by Hemsell, Sweet and colleagues, and others to have excellent *in vitro* and *in vivo* activity against PID and its pathogens (Table 28.4).

Management of acute PID should include treatment of the male partner and education for the prevention of reinfection, including the use of proper contraception. The importance of treating sexual partners cannot be overstressed. Eschenbach reported that 25% of gonococcal PID patients were readmitted to the hospital within 10 weeks of the initial treatment. A study of gonococcal PID noted that 13% of male partners screened were asymptomatic urethral carriers and that even higher rates for *C. trachomatis* were present. These partners should be treated with one of the regimens for uncomplicated gonorrhoeae and chlamydial infection (i.e., ceftriaxone, 125 mg intramuscularly, followed by oral doxycycline, 100 mg twice a day for 7 days, oral azithromycin in 1 g or ofloxacin 300 mg b.i.d. for 7 days orally). Women with acute PID often return to the same social situations they were in before treatment. Treating sexual partners and educating patients with regard to contraception would decrease the incidence of recurrent infections and hopefully affect the often poor prognosis for future fertility.

Following are the 2002 CDC guidelines for the management of male partners of women with PID.

MANAGEMENT OF SEX PARTNERS

Evaluation and treatment of sex partners of women from the previous 60 days who have PID is imperative because of the risk of reinfection and the likelihood of urethral gonococcal or chlamydial infection of the partner.

Sex partners should be treated empirically with regimens effective against both of these infections, regardless of the apparent etiology of PID or pathogens isolated from the infected woman.

Even in clinical settings in which only women are seen, special arrangements should be made to provide care for male sex partners of women with PID. When this is not feasible, health care providers should ensure that sex partners are appropriately referred for treatment.

HIV INFECTION

Treatment of HIV-infected patients diagnosed with PID has also been addressed by the CDC. Differences in the clinical manifestations of PID between HIV-infected women and uninfected women have not been described clearly. In recent studies, HIV-infected women with PID had similar symptoms to non–HIV-infected patients with PID, but they were more likely to have a tuboovarian abscess. HIV-infected women in whom PID develops should be managed aggressively but appear to respond equally well to antibiotic regimens. Hospitalization and inpatient therapy with one of the intravenous antimicrobial regimens is recommended by several experts, but is no longer considered mandatory by the CDC. Higher HPV infections and cytologic abnormalities were noted in HIV-positive PID patients and should be evaluated fully.

SURGICAL MANAGEMENT

Laparotomy should generally be reserved for patients with surgical emergencies such as ruptured abscesses or definitive treatment of failed medical management. Laparoscopy, however, is an underused but usually helpful procedure for diagnosis, prognosis, and possibly treatment of PID. Laparoscopic evaluation should be considered in all patients with a differential diagnosis of PID and without laparoscopic surgery contraindications. Laparoscopy is important not only to diagnose PID but also to rule out surgical emergencies, such as appendicitis and ruptured abscesses. It also prevents inappropriate management of patients with noninfectious problems, such as endometriosis. These patients need additional surgical and medical management, not antibiotic therapy. In addition, evaluation of the extent of the inflammatory process in confirmed PID is helpful in establishing a prognosis and further management plan, if initial treatment fails. Patients with evidence of current or previous abscesses have a higher failure rate with antibiotic therapy. Also, treatment of unilateral abscesses may necessitate surgical management to avoid the spread of the infection to the other, perhaps less damaged, tube and ovary.

Cultures obtained from the peritubal region or from the peritoneal cavity can also be helpful for identifying organisms resistant to initial management. This has become increasingly important in light of the increasing rate of clindamycin-resistant anaerobes and the elimination of metronidazole from the CDC-recommended inpatient guidelines in the 1980s. Laparoscopic management of PID that appears helpful includes copious drainage of the pelvis with normal saline or preferably Ringer's solution. Antibiotic inclusion in the lavage fluid has not been demonstrated to be helpful to date. Laparoscopic manipulation or drainage of documented pelvic abscesses has been attempted by several investigators.

Henry-Suchet and associates reported the successful use of laparoscopy to diagnose and drain tuboovarian abscesses in 50 women. Adhesions were lysed, and the abscesses were drained through the laparoscope. All patients received intravenous antibiotics. Forty-five of the 50 (90%) patients were cured. Reich and McGlynn had a similar experience in 25 women with pelvic abscesses treated laparoscopically. Four of seven women desiring pregnancy conceived, and two women had unplanned pregnancies. However, the diagnosis of abscesses is not uniform in these studies. Also, it is of concern that similar results will not necessarily be demonstrated in less experienced hands. Anatomically, drainage of abscesses within the pelvic cavity by laparoscope will not drain the entire abscess contents out of the pelvic cavity, and despite how extensive the lavage or laparoscopic removal is, pus and bacteria will be spilled and exposed to the pelvic cavity. This is contrary to the natural defense mechanism of the body of isolating and containing the inflammation-causing organisms within an abscess. Therefore, laparoscopic drainage of pelvic abscesses should be undertaken only by experienced laparoscopic surgeons, and with the patient's full understanding of all other options.

Laparotomy with extensive pelvic surgery was often recommended in the past, before the development of broad-spectrum antibiotics.

If a patient has been hospitalized on several occasions for acute exacerbation of PID with bilateral tuboovarian abscesses to the point where the future surgical risk increases significantly, definitive surgical intervention may be indicated. The operation should be done when the infection is quiescent, if possible. The surgery may still be difficult, but there will be fewer complications than when patients are operated on in the acute phase of the infection. The timing of the operative intervention is important. There should be complete absorption of the inflammatory exudate surrounding the focus of the infection, as seen radiologically. Bimanual pelvic examination should be possible without producing a marked or persistent febrile response. It has been suggested that definitive surgery be delayed for 2 to 3 months after the recent exacerbation for more complete resolution of the infection. Ideally, the patient should have a normal ESR, WBC count, and hematocrit, and relatively nontender pelvic organs, except with motion.

Kaplan and associates recommended more aggressive management in patients who exhibit either no clinical response or only partial response after 24 to 72 hours. Their approach included a total abdominal hysterectomy and bilateral salpingo-oophorectomy and was thought to reduce the protracted period of intensive medical therapy in a group of patients who would eventually require surgery. They noted that conservative management of their cases usually resulted in protracted periods of intensive care and repeated hospital admissions, and rarely in subsequent pregnancies. However, the early surgical intervention of Kaplan and colleagues was associated with six incidences of injury to the bowel and additional postoperative complications. Unfortunately, patients with acute pelvic abscess are frequently young, and future childbearing is often desired, even though it may be impossible for most patients. Conservation of ovarian function for these young women is an important benefit of medical management. Some differences in the percentage of patients responding to conservative management in different studies and different geographic locations might be explained by differences in the predominant microorganisms causing the infection at these locations and their sensitivity to the antibiotics used.

Older studies of the management of patients with pelvic abscess, which emphasized the early use of surgery, are no longer pertinent, because modern antibiotic drugs were not available then. Collins and Jansen in 1959 had an early failure rate of 10% for conservative medical therapy. However, 113 of their 174 patients required later surgery, which resulted in a late failure rate of 65%. Ginsburg and associates reviewed cases of 160 patients treated for tuboovarian abscess during the years 1969 to 1979. The early failure rate with broad-spectrum antibiotics was 31%, whereas the late failure rate was 21%. In an average follow-up period of 25.5 months, 48% did not require later surgery. Subsequent reports by Hager and by Landers and Sweet support conservative management.

When conservative management fails and a pelvic abscess is noted dissecting the rectovaginal septum, drainage by way of colpotomy may be possible.

POSTERIOR COLPOTOMY

In a classic article, Wharton described various techniques of vaginal drainage of pelvic abscess. Today, posterior colpotomy is done to evacuate pus and to establish drainage from a pelvic abscess that presents in the cul-de-sac.

There are three requirements for colpotomy drainage of a pelvic abscess.

1. The abscess must be midline or nearly so.
2. The abscess should be adherent to the cul-de-sac peritoneum and should dissect the rectovaginal septum to assure the surgeon that the drainage will be extraperitoneal and that pus will not be disseminated transperitoneally.
3. The abscess should be cystic or fluctuant to ensure adequate drainage.

Occasionally, a cul-de-sac abscess can be successfully drained without dissecting the septum. However, the serosal surface of the abscess should be adherent to the cul-de-sac peritoneum. Ultrasonography may be helpful in locating the pockets of pus.

After adequate anesthesia, the patient is placed in the lithotomy position. It is essential that a thorough examination of the pelvis be performed under anesthesia so that the operator knows the size and position of the mass that is to be drained.

After preparation and draping in the dorsal lithotomy position, the posterior lip of the cervix is grasped with a tenaculum and drawn down and forward. The vaginal mucosa of the posterior vaginal fornix is incised just below the reflection of the vaginal mucosa onto the cervix, and the transverse incision is widened with a pair of long scissors (Fig. 28.1A). The incision must be large enough

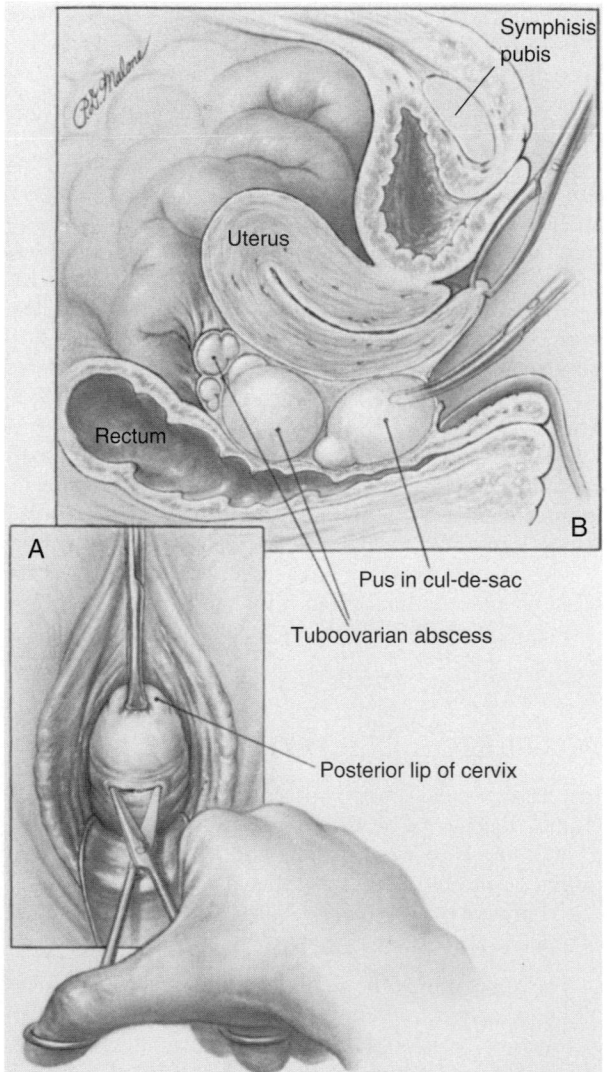

FIGURE 28.1. Posterior colpotomy. **A:** A transverse incision is made through the vaginal mucosa at the junction of the posterior vaginal fornix with the cervix. **B:** A Kelly clamp is thrust through the abscess wall.

to allow adequate exploration and drainage of the abscess cavity with the index finger. The cul-de-sac peritoneum and abscess wall are punctured with a long Kelly clamp (Fig. 28.1B). As the abscess wall is perforated, there is a definite sensation of puncturing a cystic cavity. If blood or pus is present, this is soon seen in the upper vagina. The jaws of the clamp are spread, and the flow of liquid from the cul-de-sac is increased. A sample of the purulent exudate is sent to the microbiology laboratory for appropriate culture and sensitivity. Collection of the specimen anaerobically with a capped syringe with rapid transport to the laboratory allows the more fastidious flora to be defined. A direct smear for Gram stain is also made from the pus and examined for predominating organisms.

There may be more than one compartment in an abscess cavity (Fig. 28.2). It is desirable to insert an index finger in the cavity and explore. Fibrous adhesions within the cavity can be gently broken. If another abscess wall is felt, it can often be cautiously and safely punctured under the guidance of a finger. Exploration and manipulation should be done carefully to avoid intraperitoneal rupture of the abscess or perforation of the bowel. To allow adequate drainage, the vaginal incision should be at least 2 cm wide. If pus has been obtained, one or two drains are inserted into the abscess cavity and anchored with fine absorbable suture to permit easy removal. Penrose or closed suction drainage systems can be used. These are left for several days or longer. Wharton has emphasized the importance of prolonged drainage. A suture or two may be required to control bleeding from the vaginal mucosa. However, if a mushroom (Malecot) catheter is used for drainage, it should be removed in 48 to 72 hours to prevent significant fibrosis that could hinder removal.

Patients in whom the abscess does not meet the criteria for colpotomy drainage often require laparotomy and direct drainage. Transabdominal or transvaginal drainage has been attempted to avoid the expense and complications of laparotomy and for patients in whom laparotomy is contraindicated.

Experience with percutaneous drainage of intraabdominal and pelvic abscesses under ultrasonographic or computed tomographic (CT) guidance has been reported by Olak and associates, and by others. Worthen and Gunning used percutaneous catheter drainage of 11 abscesses in nine patients and achieved a cure rate of 77%. Two patients required surgical intervention subsequently. In 19 patients, simple percutaneous aspiration of 23 abscesses was successful with a 94% cure rate. The attempt at aspiration failed in seven patients (Fig. 28.3). The Grady Memorial Hospital experience, as reported by Tyrrel and associates, is similar. CT-guided percutaneous drainage in eight patients with tuboovarian abscess resulted in recovery without surgery in seven. One patient had marked clinical improvement but still required a posterior colpotomy. No complications occurred. Loy and associates have reported that the simultaneous use of real-time pelvic ultrasonography can facilitate transvaginal drainage of a pelvic abscess. If pa-

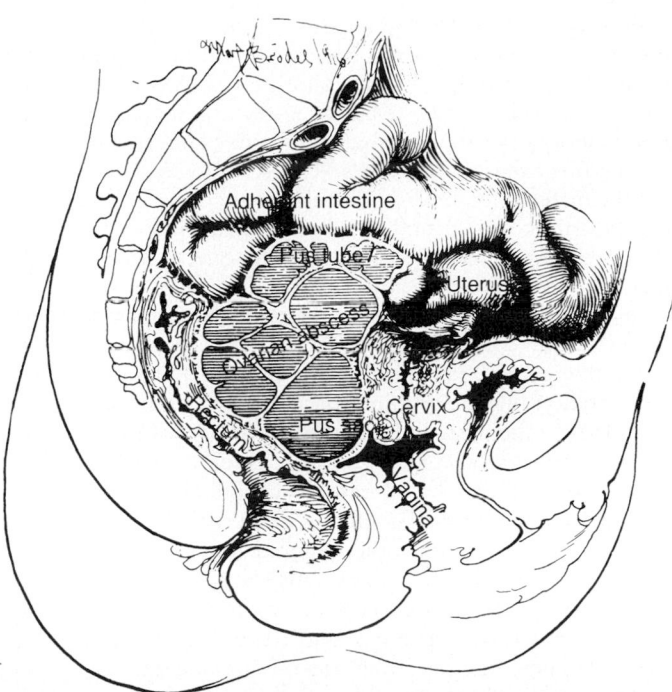

FIGURE 28.2. Pus may be contained within the tuboovarian abscess and within other pockets in the pelvic cavity.

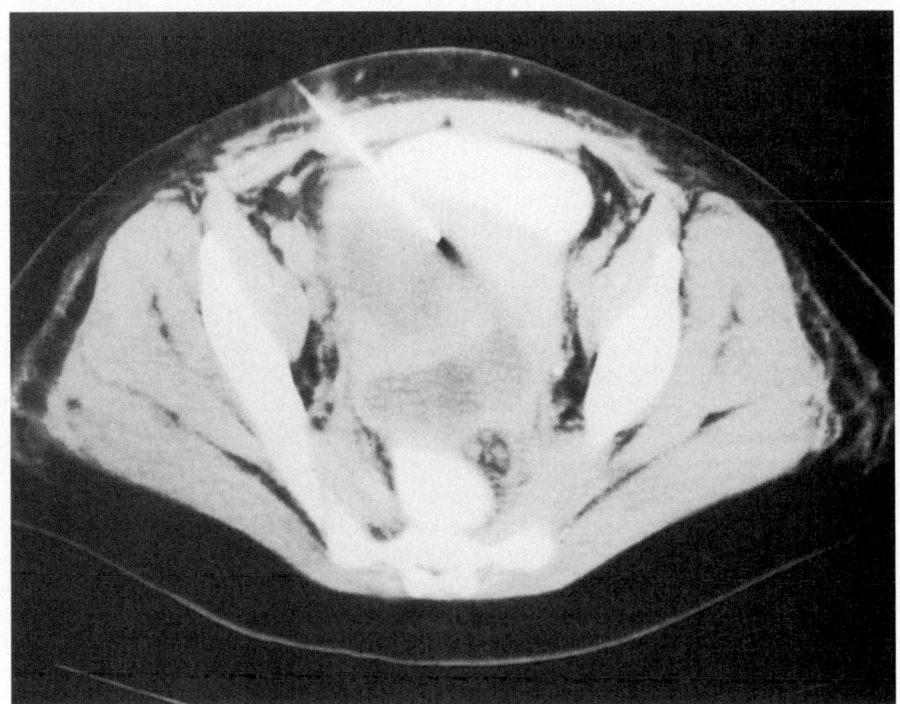

FIGURE 28.3. Transabdominal needle aspiration of a pelvic abscess under guidance of computed tomography. Drainage tube is also placed.

tients do not respond to intravenous antibiotics and percutaneous drainage or aspiration, surgical intervention is required.

The long-term effects of pus and organisms released into the pelvis from the puncture site are unknown. However, short-term success rates are good, and surgical drainage of acute abscess is a basic principle. Therefore, needle drainage can be considered with proper patient selection and appropriate informed consent, which includes other management options.

If exploratory laparotomy is necessary, the patient can be positioned in Allen universal stirrups. A lower abdominal transverse Maylard incision is ideal because it affords good exposure to the lateral adnexal pelvic organs and pelvic side walls. Pelvic adhesions should be released and the bowel should be packed off before the pelvic dissection commences. During the dissection, free pus is often spilled, and the upper abdomen should be isolated from this, if possible. When a ruptured abscess is encountered, the exudate is collected and sent immediately to the laboratory for anaerobic and aerobic cultures and antimicrobial sensitivity studies. The easiest way to obtain the material for anaerobic culture is simply to collect it in an airtight syringe and to submit a small piece of the abscess wall in an airtight container. The easiest place to begin the dissection is in the round ligament, which is the most consistently available and identifiable landmark. Following the round ligament medially always leads to the uterine corpus. Variations in the usual technique for the operation may be required because of extensive disease, dense adhesions, indurated and edematous tissue, and distorted anatomy. For example, it is sometimes convenient to perform the central dissection first (i.e., a subtotal hysterectomy). This allows more space and adequate exposure to perform the required adnexal surgery. Tuboovarian inflammatory masses may be found densely adherent in the cul-de-sac to the uterus, to the posterior surface of the broad ligament, and to the lateral pelvic side wall. There is risk of injury to the ureters, sigmoid, rectum, and small intestines. The method of dissection used depends on the nature of the adhesions. Soft, fresh adhesions can be broken gently and easily with finger dissection. Dense fibrotic adhesions must be carefully dissected and cut with scissors. The dissection can be especially difficult and risky if pelvic tissues are intensely indurated, as in ligneous pelvic cellulitis. If the infundibulopelvic ligament can be clamped, cut, and securely ligated, one can gain access to the lateral retroperitoneal space and identify the ureter. This facilitates a safe dissection of the abscess wall away from the ureter. In cases with extensive disease involving one or both adnexa, the use of preoperative ureteral catheterization may be helpful in identifying the location of the pelvic ureters. With tuboovarian abscess, the anatomic limits of the ovary may be difficult to define. If the ovary is to be removed, it should be removed completely to prevent subsequent development of ovarian remnant syndrome.

When both adnexa must be removed, a hysterectomy should usually be performed. In some cases, only a subtotal hysterectomy is feasible. The cervix can usually be excised after removal of the adnexa and the uterine corpus. The vaginal vault is left open for drainage. A Penrose drain can be inserted and then removed several days later. Suspension of the vaginal vault and reperitonization of the pelvis are accomplished in the usual manner, if possible. A routine closure of the abdominal incision is performed. Jackson-Pratt suction drains are often placed above the fascia and brought out through a separate incision.

Because the patient has been placed in the Allen universal stirrups for laparotomy, ureteral integrity can be confirmed as discussed elsewhere. Five milliliters of indigo carmine is given intravenously and a cystoscope is placed in the bladder. Blue dye can then be seen flowing from each ureteral orifice.

In the past, it was standard practice to do a bilateral salpingo-oophorectomy in almost all patients who had a laparotomy for acute pelvic abscess. This practice was based on the belief that the disease is almost always severe in both adnexa. Recent studies have suggested that as many as 25% to 50% of patients will have a relatively normal tube and ovary on one side. This may be especially true of patients whose infection is associated with IUD use. Golde and associates reported that 37 of 85 patients (44%) with tuboovarian abscesses confirmed at operation had unilateral abscesses; 20 were using an IUD. The studies of Landers and Sweet, Hager and Majmudar, and Ginsburg and co-workers also found a higher percentage of unilateral adnexal disease than was previously reported. In light of these findings, conservative adnexal surgery should be performed if possible. We have no hesitation in leaving a relatively normal tube and ovary at the time of hysterectomy with removal of the opposite adnexa for acute pelvic abscess. When the uterus is removed and the continuity between the conserved tube and the lower genital tract is interrupted, there is little risk of a new infection. If a strictly unilateral pelvic abscess is found at laparotomy, removal of the affected tube and ovary only, leaving in the uterus and the opposite adnexa, is acceptable in a patient who wishes to preserve fertility. However, *in vitro* fertilization techniques may be required to accomplish pregnancy. Such a patient does have a risk of recurrent tuboovarian abscess. It is especially important that her sexual partner be examined and receive treatment when indicated.

In recent years there have been advances in reproductive technology that allow infertile patients to conceive and carry pregnancies to term under the most extraordinary circumstances. It has been possible, for example, to accomplish a successful pregnancy in a woman who has a uterus but no ovaries by instillation of a donated fertilized ovum into a suitably prepared uterus. Such a sophisticated procedure is not available to a large number of patients. However, mostly for medicolegal reasons, the option of leaving in the uterus when lateral salpingo-oophorectomy is to be performed should be discussed with the patient, especially if she is young and nulliparous.

In summary, patients with an acute pelvic abscess should be hospitalized for treatment with parenteral broad-spectrum antibiotics. Surgery is indicated if the diagnosis is uncertain, if intraperitoneal rupture is diagnosed or suspected, or if the patient fails to respond to medical management.

RUPTURED PELVIC ABSCESS

A tuboovarian or pelvic abscess can rupture spontaneously into the rectum or sigmoid colon, into the bladder, or into the free peritoneal cavity. A pelvic abscess almost never ruptures spontaneously into the vagina unless the patient had a previous posterior colpotomy for drainage of an abscess. Under these circumstances, a recurrent pelvic abscess can dissect along the tract of the previous posterior colpotomy incision and drain spontaneously through the vagina.

Spontaneous drainage through the rectum or sigmoid colon usually occurs in a patient whose abscess is too high to drain with a posterior colpotomy. In other words, although the abscess is fluctuant and midline, it is not yet dissecting the rectovaginal septum. While waiting for the abscess to come down, a sudden unexpected improvement in the patient's condition is noted, and she will confirm that pus has begun to drain through the anus. Further improvement in her condition usually occurs. A posterior colpotomy is not needed and, indeed, is contraindicated because doing so could cause a rectovaginal fistula to form.

Spontaneous drainage through the bladder is rare. It occurs most commonly in elderly women with chronic abscesses developing from ruptured sigmoid diverticula. Only rarely does a chronic tuboovarian or pelvic abscess rupture and drain through the bladder, causing secondary infection of the bladder. When the abscess is removed with laparotomy, a defect in the bladder wall is noted. The indurated tissue around the defect should be removed and the defect closed with 3-0 delayed-absorbable suture in two layers. A Foley catheter can be left in place for 10 to 14 days while healing of the bladder wall takes place.

Of all the complications that can result from PID, intraabdominal rupture of a tuboovarian abscess is the most life-threatening. Mortality from this complication is due to septic shock and the complications of generalized peritonitis, and the mortality rate can approach up to 10% in patients with warm shock.

Abscesses can rupture spontaneously, after bimanual examination or accidental trauma. Bacteriologic study of the contents of the abscess has historically been unrewarding; a specific organism has been isolated in less than 50% of cases. The gonococcus is rarely identified in a pelvic abscess. Careful aerobic and anaerobic cultures often demonstrate the presence of a mixed infection that includes anaerobic organisms. McNamara and Mead reviewed the results of three separate studies that demonstrated 31 positive isolates of anaerobes in 30 patients with a pelvic abscess. Landers and Sweet have also confirmed similar findings in their series.

Diagnosis of Ruptured Tuboovarian Abscess

The major clinical symptom of ruptured tuboovarian abscess is acute, progressive pelvic pain that is usually so severe that the patient can accurately identify the time and place of its occurrence. In the series from the Johns Hopkins Hospital reported by Vermeeren and Te Linde, the average age of patients with a ruptured tuboovarian abscess was 33 years, which is at least 10 years older than the average age of patients with acute PID. About 2% of these patients are postmenopausal. To our knowledge, only two cases of ruptured tuboovarian abscess in a pregnant patient have been reported. Often, there is a history of recurrent attacks of PID, with a sudden increase in the severity and extent of abdominal pain during a recent exacerbation of infection. On examination, the patient appears seriously ill and dehydrated, with rapid, shallow respirations. The abdomen is distended and quiet, with diminished or absent bowel sounds. Signs of generalized peritonitis, direct and rebound tenderness, muscle rigidity, and shifting dullness may be noted. A pelvic mass is palpable in more than 50% of cases. Tachycardia is common. Shock can be present or can develop while the patient is under observation. It is due to accumulation of fluids in peripheral tissues and later failure of compensatory vasoconstrictor mechanisms. The patient's temperature is usually greater than 101°F, but it can also be normal and even subnormal late in the course. The leukocyte count is likely to be more than 15,000, but it also can be normal. Severe leukopenia is an ominous sign. A culdocentesis is a valuable diagnostic aid and was positive for purulent material in 70% of the cases in the Mickal and Sellmann series. An abdominal radiograph usually shows a paralytic ileus, sometimes evidence of free fluid in the peritoneal cavity, and atelectasis in the lung bases.

Treatment of Ruptured Tuboovarian Abscess

The longer the delay in the operative treatment of ruptured tuboovarian abscess, the greater the primary mortality rate. In the series by Vermeeren and Te Linde from the Johns Hopkins Hospital, death occurred less than 90 hours after the time of rupture in 88% of fatal cases, both operative and nonoperative.

As time passes after rupture of a tuboovarian abscess, septic peritonitis becomes more severe and generalized. The passage of time allows the development of septic shock from greater absorption of bacteria and bacterial endotoxins, and secretion of great quantities of fluid into the peritoneal cavity across inflamed peritoneal surfaces. Fluid shifts from the intravascular compartment to interstitial spaces as a result of the increased vascular permeability of the inflamed peritoneal membrane. This leads to hypovolemia, decreased cardiac output, decreased central venous pressure, hypotension, vasoconstriction, increased peripheral resistance, decreased tissue perfusion, metabolic acidosis, ARDS, decreased renal glomerular perfusion and filtration with decreased urine flow, severe hypoxemia, multiple organ system failure, and death. The prompt diagnosis and treatment of intraperitoneal rupture of a tuboovarian abscess is essential to minimize the risk of mortality of generalized peritonitis.

The treatment of patients with ruptured tuboovarian abscess can be divided into three phases: preoperative, operative, and postoperative.

Preoperative Phase

Operation should be undertaken after rapid but adequate preoperative preparation. The patient should be typed and crossmatched with 2 to 4 units of packed red blood cells. Monitoring of central venous pressure is essential for proper evaluation of the hemodynamics of this condition because many patients are dehydrated, in shock, and anemic. Swan-Ganz catheter placement may be preferable because it allows pulmonary capillary wedge pressure and pulmonary artery pressure determinations that are helpful in assessing the adequacy of fluid replacement and in detecting fluid overload. Variable amounts of fluid, sometimes tremendous amounts, are lost into the peritoneal cavity and intestinal tract because of peritonitis. Emergency blood chemistry determinations (e.g., serum electrolytes, creatinine, glucose, bilirubin, and alkaline phosphatase) are obtained, and intravenous fluids, preferably Ringer's lactate, are started immediately. Crystalloid solutions for fluid volume resuscitation are preferred for most patients with septic peritonitis. It may be advantageous to use partial colloid resuscitation in some patients with evidence of cardiopulmonary dysfunction because a smaller total volume is required. An excess of intravenous crystalloid solution may result in fluid overload.

Vigorous broad-spectrum intravenous antibiotic therapy should be instituted. An indwelling urethral catheter is used to monitor fluid intake with hourly urine output. Generally, it is advantageous to insert a Cantor or Miller-Abbott intestinal tube before operation to decompress the distended bowel. Combating shock is a primary concern throughout treatment. Clinical assessment of respiratory function should be made. A distended tender abdomen may cause rapid, shallow respirations and use of accessory muscles for ventilation. Arterial blood gases may indicate mild hypoxemia, in which case oxygen should be administered and ventilator support provided. Blood transfusion should be started before surgery. When the patient has been properly prepared, immediate surgery should be undertaken. The results of treatment are better if major metabolic and hemodynamic problems are corrected before operation, but one cannot waste time in treating a critically ill patient with septic peritonitis.

Operative Phase

The anesthetic of choice depends on the preference and experience of the anesthesiologist and the medical condition of the patient.

The operation should be performed as rapidly as possible. Because speed as well as access to the upper abdomen may be required, a lower midline incision should be used. It can be quickly extended above the umbilicus if necessary. The patient should not be put in the Trendelenburg position until the abdomen is packed off, and no more of a dependent position should be used than is needed to prevent further dissemination of pus into the upper abdomen. When the abdomen is opened, any odor that is present should be noted. An unpleasant putrid odor is indicative of infection with anaerobic organisms. Pus from the abdomen should be collected correctly for both aerobic and anaerobic culture and for Gram stain, and be promptly transported to the laboratory. Organisms grown should be tested for sensitivity to various antibiotics.

The operation of choice is removal of the free pus, together with the abscess, the uterus, the tubes, and usually the ovaries. Only occasionally is it possible to leave an ovary in a patient with a ruptured pelvic abscess. If rupture has occurred from a strictly unilateral tuboovarian abscess, with a relatively normal tube and ovary on the opposite side, a unilateral salpingo-oophorectomy can be performed, especially if the patient is young. However, the risk of a recurrent abscess in the opposite tube and ovary is high if the uterus is also left in place. When the uterus is removed along with the tuboovarian abscess, the risk of recurrent abscess in the opposite adnexa is reduced. When hysterectomy is performed, usually a total hysterectomy can be done. However, even in the best surgical hands, a subtotal hysterectomy is faster than a total one and is sometimes justified. It is probable that the mortality rate would be increased if total hysterectomies were always performed. Although we believe firmly in total hysterectomy, we do not believe in performing it when the danger of total hysterectomy exceeds the danger from a retained cervix. Except in the young patient, it is better to remove the corpus than to perform a unilateral adnexectomy alone. Furthermore, the opposite adnexa is significantly involved in most patients, and subsequent operation may be necessary if conservation of one side is practiced, as was required in 35% of Pedowitz and Bloomfield's cases. This is contrary to what has been described earlier in the surgical treatment of an unruptured abscess, because the risk of incomplete eradication of the immediate infection in an acutely ill patient with rupture, peritonitis, and possibly septic shock is much too risky; therefore, definitive surgical treatment is usually recommended in severely ill patients with ruptured abscess.

The technical performance of the procedure may be difficult, but is similar to that described earlier for laparotomy followed by failed colpotomy drainage or suspected rupture. Anatomy is distorted, dependable landmarks are obscured, and tissues are thick, edematous, friable, and inflamed. Loops of densely adherent intestine must be separated carefully to avoid injury. Injury to the serosa of distended bowel occurs commonly and sometimes requires repair. An entry into the lumen of the bowel must be recognized and repaired. The most dependable anatomic landmark is the round ligament. Followed medially, it always leads to the uterine corpus. Retroperitoneal planes of dissection can be used to advantage in identifying the ureters and removing inflammatory adnexal masses. Otherwise, it is likely that fragments of ovary will be left behind, which can subsequently cause signs and symptoms of the ovarian remnant syndrome. As much of the remaining abscess wall as possible should be removed without causing unnecessary additional bleeding. Pieces of the abscess wall can be left adherent to the pelvic side wall and culde-sac. Oozing of blood from all dissected tissue has been likened to "cinder bed bleeding" and is difficult to control.

In 1977, Rivlin and Hunt used conservative pelvic surgery combined with intraoperative and postoperative peritoneal lavage with antibiotics in 113 women with generalized peritonitis caused by a ruptured tuboovarian abscess. The uterus, ovaries, and tubes were retained whenever possible. Either one or both of the adnexa were retained in whole or in part, and hysterectomy was performed in only four cases. All loculations of pus were opened, and aggressive lavage of the peritoneal cavity with gentamicin was carried out for several days postoperatively. The mortality rate was 7.1%, and further surgery was required in only 17.5%.

Before the incision is closed, the abdominal cavity should be irrigated with copious quantities of sterile saline to remove remaining bacteria and debris. When generalized septic peritonitis is also present, large volumes of warm saline should also be used to irrigate the upper abdomen. There is always some fear of dissemination of the infection by copious irrigation. However, this disadvantage is far outweighed by the benefit of diluting and removing bacteria and necrotic debris. We do not add antiseptics or antibiotics to the irrigating solution. If hemostasis is poor or if considerable necrotic material is left behind, there may be some benefit from peritoneal drainage with closed suction catheters. Closed suction drains can be placed through a separate stab wound in the abdominal wall, through the cul-de-sac, or through the vaginal vault when a total hysterectomy has been done, but the drainage of free peritoneal exudate in the upper abdomen is of no therapeutic value.

The upper abdomen should be carefully explored for collections of pus in the subdiaphragmatic and subhepatic regions. If an upper abdominal abscess is found, it may be necessary to place a closed suction drain into the abscess cavity through the upper abdominal wall.

The abdominal incision is closed with a Smead-Jones technique or with a continuous suture taking large bites of tissue. A monofilament suture of polypropylene or nylon should be used. Retention sutures can be placed but are not usually necessary. The incision should be irrigated with warm saline. When there has been gross contamination of the incision, the subcutaneous fat and skin should be left open and packed lightly with gauze soaked in an antibiotic solution. The wound is repacked daily and inspected. In 4 to 5 days, if the tissues are healthy, the incision is closed secondarily with sutures. Alternatively, the edges can be drawn together with sterile adhesive strips.

Postoperative Phase

Postoperative care should consider shock, infection, ileus, and fluid imbalances. Complications of the late postoperative period include pelvic and abdominal abscesses, intestinal obstruction, intestinal fistulas, incisional breakdown with or without evisceration, pulmonary embolus, continued sepsis, and disseminated intravascular coagulation. Serious medical diseases such as uncontrolled diabetes or renal or pulmonary failure (ARDS) further complicate recovery from this potentially lethal disease.

Septic shock should be combated with blood (when indicated for a hemoglobin less than 7.0 g), Ringer's lactate, respiratory support, and, if necessary, vasoactive substances. Infection is controlled by the continued aggressive use of broad-spectrum intravenous antibiotics until the patient can take antibiotics orally. When the results of the antibiotic sensitivity studies on the operative specimen are available, a change to more effective agents should be considered, but only if the patient shows evidence of continued sepsis. Antibiotics should not necessarily be changed on the basis of sensitivity studies if the patient is improving clinically. Sometimes the patient's condition improves initially only to show signs of recurring intraabdominal infection the second week after operation. Under these circumstances, it is appropriate to change antibiotics. Antibiotics should be continued until the patient is afebrile with only a mild leukocytosis and is able to eat a regular diet. A long period of treatment with antibiotics may result in complications such as pseudomembranous enterocolitis.

The semi-Fowler position may help prevent subphrenic and subdiaphragmatic abscess formation. Patients with signs of continued intraabdominal sepsis should have CT scans to identify collections of pus. If found, CT-directed drainage may be possible.

Constant intestinal suction by means of a long intestinal tube is a very important feature of postoperative care. A dynamic ileus persists postoperatively for a variable period and is best treated with the long intestinal tube until there is evidence of peristalsis and the patient is passing flatus.

Close attention to fluid balance and blood chemistry determinations is mandatory. Frequently, patients with ruptured tuboovarian abscess have poor kidney function. The fluid output and serum creatinine should be followed closely.

The results of the preceding therapeutic measure have been gratifying. At Grady Memorial Hospital, the mortality rate for this formerly lethal disease is 3.5%.

PRIMARY OVARIAN ABSCESS

A primary ovarian abscess is an entity distinctly different from tuboovarian abscess. A tuboovarian abscess is one in which the abscess wall is composed of fallopian tube and ovarian parenchyma. A primary ovarian abscess, on the other hand, is one in which the infection occurs in the parenchyma of the ovary. Unlike tuboovarian abscess, it is an unusual condition. Interest in primary ovarian abscess was stimulated by the 1964 report of Willson and Black. According to a review by Wetchler and Dunn, 120 cases had been reported by 1985.

Although bacteria can gain access to the ovarian parenchyma by hematogenous or lymphatic spread, it is probable that most primary ovarian abscesses occur because bacteria present around the ovary gain access to the parenchyma through a break in the ovarian capsule. The capsule can be broken naturally by ovulation or it can be broken by a surgical procedure. Bacteria come from the fallopian tube, from the vagina during or after hysterectomy, from intrauterine infection associated with an IUD, or from appendicitis, diverticulitis, or any other condition that is associated with peritonitis. A primary ovarian abscess is usually unilateral. However, its occurrence simultaneously in both ovaries and during pregnancy seems to support the occasional hematogenous or lymphatic spread, or both. Primary ovarian abscess has been reported secondary to infections at distant sites (tonsillitis, typhoid, parotitis, and tuberculosis). A mixed flora of anaerobic and aerobic bacteria is usually present. *Actinomyces israelii* with sulfur granules has also been identified in a few cases.

Diagnosis of an unruptured primary ovarian abscess can be difficult because of the variable clinical presentation. Lower abdominal pain and fever are usually present. Lower abdominal and pelvic tenderness and an adnexal mass may be present, but the pelvic examination is sometimes not helpful. Although an event predisposing to primary ovarian abscess (e.g., surgery, IUD use, appendicitis, or systemic infection) may be uncovered in the history, the event is sometimes remote. Ultrasonography and CT can be helpful in identifying an abscess cavity. When the ovarian abscess ruptures, the clinical picture is much the same as in ruptured tuboovarian abscess, with abdominal distention, direct and rebound tenderness, ileus, and sometimes shock. The patient appears gravely ill, and the need for immediate surgery is usually obvious.

The management of patients with primary ovarian abscess is similar to the management of patients with acute tuboovarian abscess. If the abscess is not ruptured, medical management with antibiotics for both anaerobic and aerobic organisms plus supportive care is indicated. A failure to respond or deterioration in the patient's condition suggests alteration in antibiotic coverage or possible exploratory surgery, or both, to remove the abscess. Ruptured ovarian abscess requires immediate laparotomy after a brief but intense effort to stabilize the patient and start antibiotic therapy. At operation, only the affected ovary need be removed. The tubes and the uterus can be conserved. If both ovaries are involved, they should be removed. For a patient who is not interested in conception in the future, the uterus and both tubes can also be removed. If the patient is interested in pregnancy, the uterus and fallopian tubes can be left in place for possible implantation of a donated egg in the future.

SURGERY FOR CHRONIC PELVIC INFLAMMATORY DISEASE

Although the gonococcus may be responsible for initiating acute salpingitis, which is short-lived, the residual chronic salpingitis is usually due to secondary invaders, both aerobic and anaerobic, or perhaps to an initial infection with *C. trachomatis*. As a result of the initial infection or from subsequent secondary exacerbations, the fimbria can become occluded and the tubes bound to the ovaries with adhesions. In addition, the bowel can become adherent to the broad ligament and the adnexal structures, and the fascia and loose connective tissue of the broad ligament can be converted into an indurated, brawny structure typical of ligneous induration. This can extend to include tissues beneath the peritoneum on the lateral pelvic side wall, where ligneous pelvic cellulitis can cause ureteral obstruction. If the chronic infection persists, serious effusion from the inflammatory process within the endosalpinx produces a hydrosalpinx that can ignite periodically with secondary subacute pelvic infection or can progress to produce a pyosalpinx and tuboovarian abscess. If the subacute infection is left untreated or is treated inadequately, spontaneous intraabdominal rupture or leakage of an old tuboovarian abscess can occur. In a review of this subject, Heaton and Ledger identified this problem principally in premenopausal women, with only 1.7% of patients with a tuboovarian abscess being postmenopausal.

The signs and symptoms of chronic PID that most often require surgical treatment include severe, persistent, progressive pelvic pain, usually bilateral, although occasionally localized in one of the lower abdominal quadrants; repeated exacerbations of PID requiring multiple hospitalizations and recurrent medical treatment; progressive enlargement of a tuboovarian inflammatory mass, especially if it cannot be distinguished from a neoplastic tumor of the ovary; severe dyspareunia related to the chronic pelvic infection; and bilateral ureteral obstruction from ligneous cellulitis. It was formerly accepted that a history of previous colpotomy for drainage of a pelvic abscess was sufficient reason in itself to justify definitive abdominal surgery later for removal of the uterus and adnexa. We have seen several patients who have become pregnant after posterior colpotomy for drainage of a cul-de-sac abscess and who have remained relatively free of symptoms for long periods. Today, previous posterior colpotomy for pelvic abscess drainage is not a sufficient indication by itself for definitive abdominal surgery.

Selection of Operation

The final decision regarding the proper operation for the surgical management of chronic PID is usually made with the abdomen open. Consideration must be given not only to the pathologic lesions found at operation but also to the patient's age, parity, desire for children, previous history of pelvic disease, and other associated pelvic disease and symptoms. Because a knowledge of all these is essential to the best surgical judgment, the operator should be thoroughly familiar with the patient, her history, and her desires.

In the surgical management of chronic PID, the question of removal or retention of the ovary at the time of hysterectomy and salpingectomy has been left open to conjecture and individual surgical opinion in most instances. This question was the subject of a study by Weiner and Wallach of the ovarian histology in ovaries removed from patients with PID. In 40 consecutive women who underwent oophorectomy during surgical treatment of PID, nearly 50% of the removed ovaries were free of inflammatory disease and demonstrated normal follicular activity. The study concluded that ovarian histology was usually normal among patients who gave no history of dysfunctional uterine bleeding. Therefore, the menstrual history of such patients should be helpful in the decision regarding ovarian conservation or ablation. Kirtley and Benigno have reviewed our experience with ovarian conservation at the time of surgery for PID. In this series, 98 (82%) patients who required surgery had a total abdominal hysterectomy and bilateral salpingo-oophorectomy. In 22 patients (18%), either part or all of an ovary was retained. Of the 22 patients, 15 were available for follow-up hormonal assays. The mean follow-up time was 58 months. Cyclic ovarian function was confirmed in all but two patients. In the two patients with ovarian failure, other significant disease processes were also present. No patient suffered a complication as a result of adnexal conservation. We believe that normal ovarian tissue should be conserved at the time of definitive surgery for PID. A small hydrosalpinx on the same side as the normal ovary can also be left in place so that ovarian blood supply is not disturbed during an attempt to remove the tube.

The release of peritubal adhesions in mild chronic PID is indicated occasionally in women in whom future childbearing is desired, as long as the tubes can be shown to be patent, usually by transfundal chromotubation after the lower uterine isthmus is occluded by a Ziegler clamp. This type of procedure provides the most rewarding pregnancy rate of all types of tubal reconstructive surgery. More often, one tube is hopelessly closed and the opposite tube is patent after release of adhesions. In such a case, unilateral salpingectomy may be required if reconstructive surgery is not possible. Many other procedures are available in the treatment of this disease, including salpingo-oophorectomy with or without hysterectomy (Figs. 28.4 and 28.5).

In most instances of surgery for chronic PID, total abdominal hysterectomy and bilateral salpingo-oophorectomy are necessary to remove the primary tubal pathology because of inflammatory damage of both tubes and ovaries. Total abdominal hysterectomy and bilateral salpingo-oophorectomy (Fig. 28.6) have been performed for severe actinomycosis infection.

If the uterus is removed and an ovary is preserved, it may be preferable to leave the entire adnexa in place in the absence of active tubal infection rather than compromise the venous drainage or the arterial blood supply to the ovary, with subsequent cystic changes that may require an additional operative procedure later. Once the continuity of the tubal lumen from the uterine cavity is broken, the chronically inflamed tube does not usually produce subsequent symptoms, as shown by Falk in his series of cases with interstitial tubal resection. When it is considered advisable to remove both adnexa because of the extent of the tuboovarian disease, a total hysterectomy is also advisable unless the uterus is hopelessly encased in pelvic scar tissue and densely adherent to the pelvic viscera. Usually the uterus can be removed without difficulty, thus providing an easier opportunity to peritonize the operative site and avoid additional postoperative adhesions. However, there is a place for mature surgical judgment in this instance, and discretion dictates whether a subtotal hysterectomy rather than a total hysterectomy is surgically advisable.

In the optimum case, especially in a young woman who wishes to establish or maintain the possibility of future fertility, conservative surgery may be desirable, with the hope that pregnancy can be accomplished through *in vitro* fertilization techniques. In this situation, the uterus and one adnexa should be conserved, and the ovary should be positioned in the pelvis so an ovum can be harvested later through the laparoscope or through the vagina. As mentioned earlier, if the patient wishes, the uterus can be left in place even though both tubes and ovaries have been removed.

Salpingectomy for Chronic Salpingitis

At the time of surgery for the treatment of chronic PID, every effort should be made to retain uninvolved organs. Unilateral salpingectomy should be considered when the oviduct is hopelessly destroyed by the disease process and presents as a large hydrosalpinx.

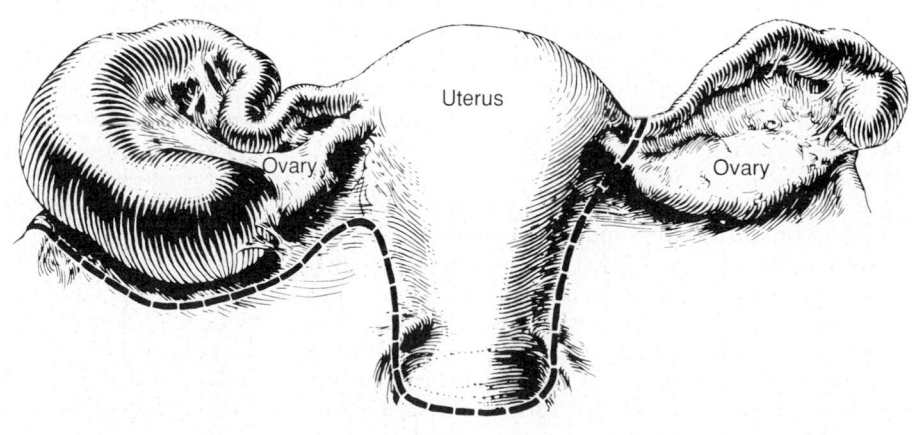

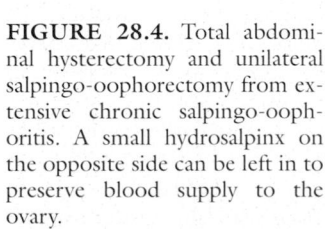

FIGURE 28.4. Total abdominal hysterectomy and unilateral salpingo-oophorectomy from extensive chronic salpingo-oophoritis. A small hydrosalpinx on the opposite side can be left in to preserve blood supply to the ovary.

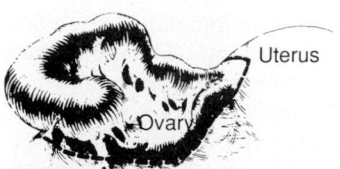

FIGURE 28.5. When significant chronic pelvic inflammatory disease involves only one adnexa and preservation of uterine function is indicated, a unilateral salpingo-oophorectomy can be performed.

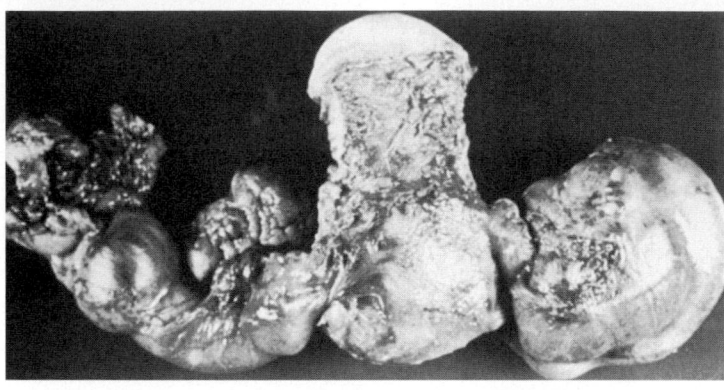

FIGURE 28.6. Total abdominal hysterectomy and bilateral salpingo-oophorectomy for severe pelvic actinomycosis.

The abdomen is entered through a transverse Maylard incision. The adhesions binding the tube are cut and the tube is freed. It is held by a Kelly clamp placed on the mesosalpinx just beneath the fimbriated end. The mesosalpinx is then clamped and cut, with a succession of small bites taken as close to the tube as possible (Fig. 28.7A).

Keeping the operative trauma as far as possible from the ovary that is to be retained lessens the danger of imperiling its blood supply. Experience has shown that the ovary whose tube has been removed is more apt to become cystic than the ovary whose tube has been left undisturbed. Therefore, it seems logical to interfere as little as possible with the blood supply of the ovary by hugging the tube closely when excising it.

The tube is excised at the uterine cornu in a wedge-shaped manner, as indicated in Figure 28.7B. A wide, figure-of-eight 2-0 delayed-absorbable suture is placed in the cornu before the wedge is excised and is tightened as the interstitial portion of the tube is removed. If there is palpable extension of the inflammation at the uterine cornu (so-called salpingitis isthmica nodosa), the wedge may be large.

The wound in the uterus is closed with one or more 2-0 delayed-absorbable figure-of-eight sutures (Fig. 28.7B). The vessels in the mesosalpinx are ligated with transfixion 3-0 delayed-absorbable sutures. The advantage of the transfixion suture is that it does not slip off the tissue when tied as the clamp is withdrawn (Fig. 28.7C).

A mattress suture of 3-0 delayed-absorbable material is used to bring the broad and round ligaments over the cornual wound (Fig. 28.7D). This suture passes just beneath the round ligament, so that the ligament is not strangulated when the suture is drawn tight. When this suture is tied, the cornual wound is covered with the broad ligament, and the uterus is suspended to some extent in a manner similar to that used in the Coffey sus-

pension. Usually, a second mattress or interrupted suture is necessary to cover the mesosalpinx completely, as shown in Figure 28.7E.

Salpingo-oophorectomy for Chronic Salpingitis

As in salpingectomy, the abdomen is entered through a transverse Maylard incision. The chronic tuboovarian inflammatory mass is first dissected free and the infundibulopelvic ligament is identified. It is doubly clamped with Ochsner clamps, and a third clamp is applied to control back-bleeding (Fig. 28.8A). The ureter must be identified before the infundibulopelvic ligament is clamped, cut, and ligated.

After the infundibulopelvic ligament is cut and ligated, the remainder of the broad ligament attachment of the tube and the ovary is clamped, cut, and ligated. The uterine end of the tube and the ovarian ligament are excised from the uterus in a wedge-shaped manner. The ascending uterine vessels are ligated just below the cornual wound, and the cornual incision is closed with a 2-0 delayed-absorbable figure-of-eight suture (Fig. 28.8B).

The infundibulopelvic ligament is doubly ligated with 2-0 delayed-absorbable sutures, and the vessels in the broad ligament are ligated with 3-0 delayed-absorbable sutures. The cornual wound is peritonized, and the uterus is suspended to some degree by bringing the round and the broad ligaments over the uterine cornu with a mattress suture of 2-0 delayed-absorbable material, as shown in Figure 28.8C. An attempt should be made to remove the tuboovarian inflammatory complex completely. If a fragment of ovary is left attached to the lateral pelvic peritoneum or the broad ligament, the ovarian remnant syndrome may develop later. To prevent this, a retroperitoneal approach may be required.

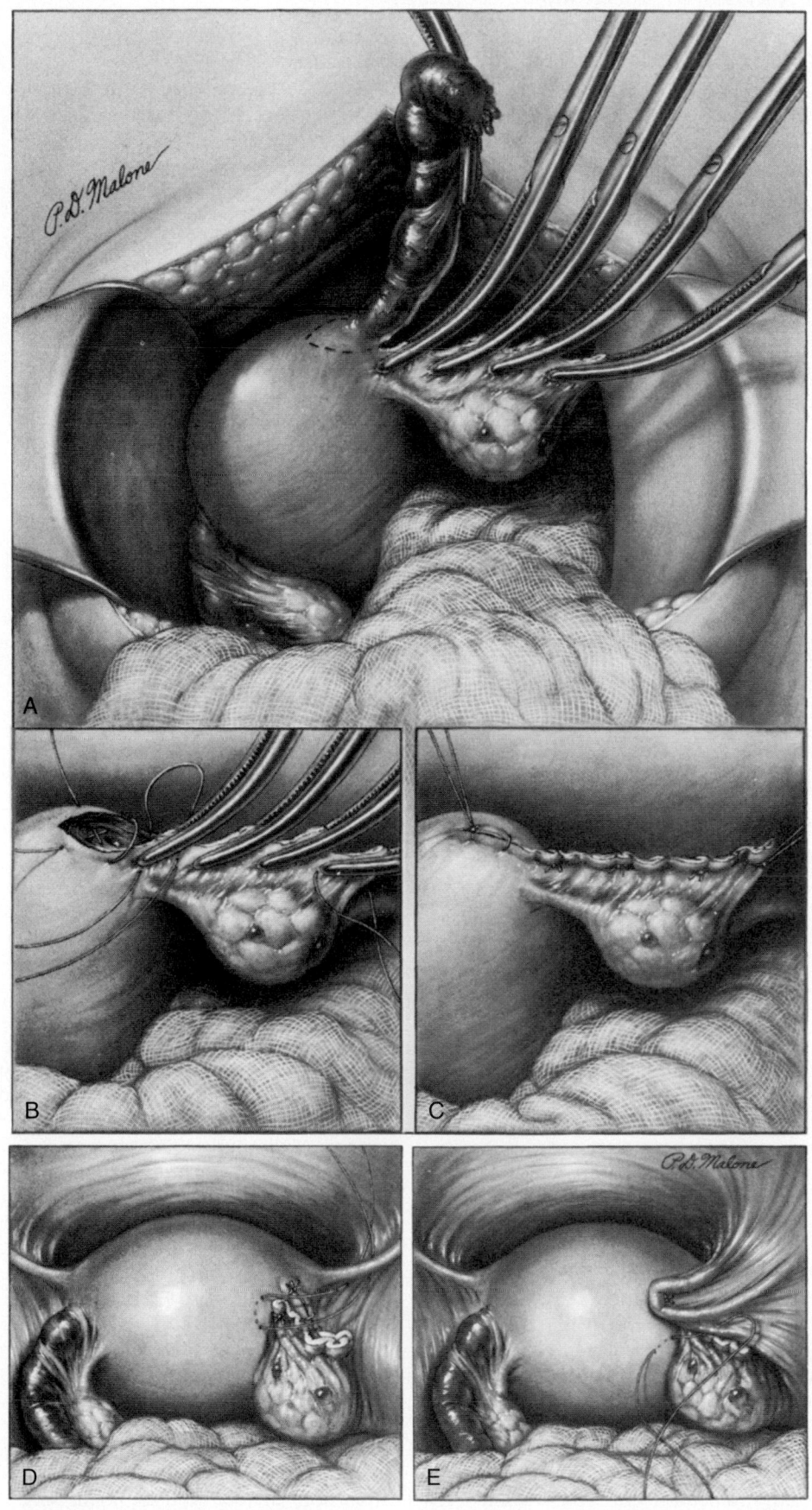

FIGURE 28.7. Salpingectomy. **A:** Mesosalpinx is clamped with multiple Kelly clamps and cut. Dotted lines indicate cornual excision, which is elective. **B:** Cornual wound is closed with 2-0 delayed-absorbable suture. **C:** Mesosalpinx vessels are transfixed. **D:** Mattress suture is placed to cover operative area. **E:** Round ligament and broad ligament cover operative area.

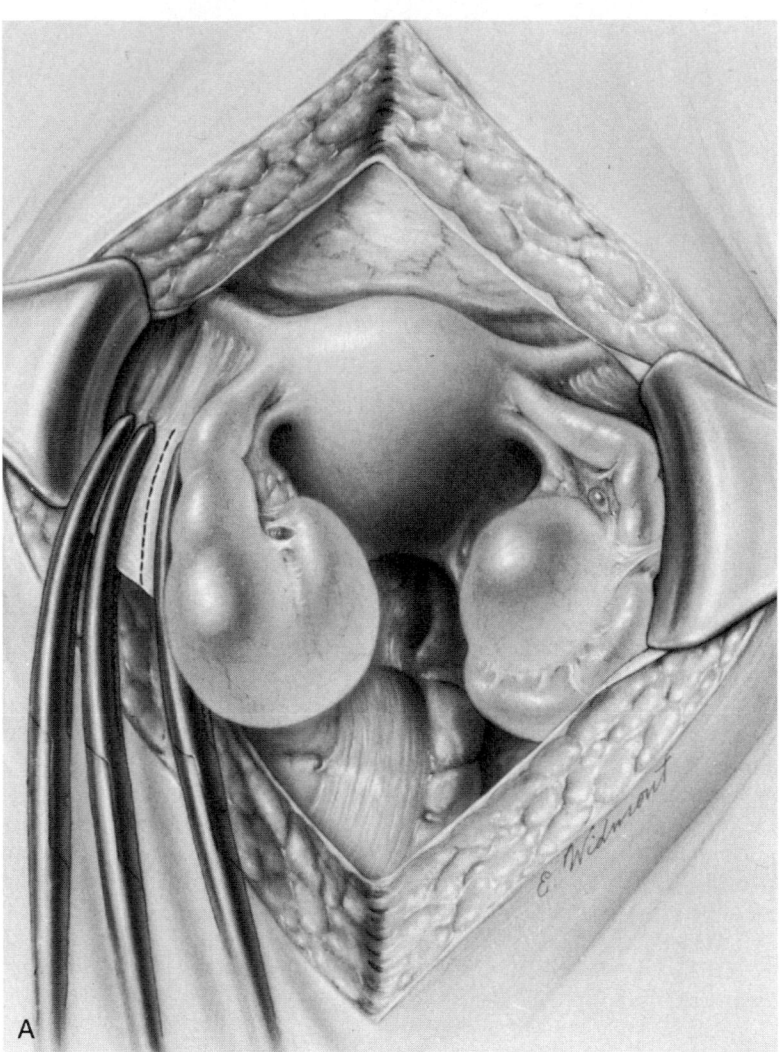

A

FIGURE 28.8. Salpingo-oophorectomy. **A:** The infundibulopelvic ligament is doubly clamped. Another clamp is placed to control back-bleeding. Dotted line indicates incision.

Identification of the Ureter

Identification of the course of the ureter in a pelvis in which the anatomy has become obliterated as a result of PID is one of the most important responsibilities of the gynecologist. In the surgical treatment of this disease, one may find a tuboovarian inflammatory mass that is located between the leaves of the broad ligament and extends to the lateral pelvic wall. It is not uncommon for the ligneous induration of the thickened parietal peritoneum to obscure completely the location and course of the pelvic ureter so that dissection of the diseased adnexa produces a surgical risk to the urinary tract, requiring great technical skill to avoid ureteral injury. Knowledge of the normal anatomic location of the pelvic ureters is essential so that these vital structures can be identified before an attempt is made to remove the adnexal masses. Division of the round ligament allows access to the lateral pelvic wall beneath the peritoneum. After the round ligament is divided, the peritoneum is incised inferiorly toward the internal cervical os and superiorly just lateral to the infundibulopelvic ligament. The peritoneum is easily reflected medially away from the pelvic side wall with finger dissection, and the ureter is identified. It remains attached to the peritoneum. If there is difficulty with this procedure, the ureter can usually be identified as it crosses over the common iliac artery just above its bifurcation, and it can be traced downward.

Such patients may have a preoperative ureteral catheterization when there is clinical evidence of large, adherent adnexal masses. However, if such an anatomic problem is encountered at the time of laparotomy, an incision can be made in the dome of the bladder that allows the passage of ureteral catheters. If the patient has been positioned in the Allen universal stirrups for operation, intraoperative cystoscopy with passage of ureteral stents is easily accomplished. At the end of the operation, 5 mL of indigo carmine is given intravenously. With a cystoscope in the bladder, the dye can be seen effusing from both ureteral orifices, confirming that the ureters have not been injured or compromised.

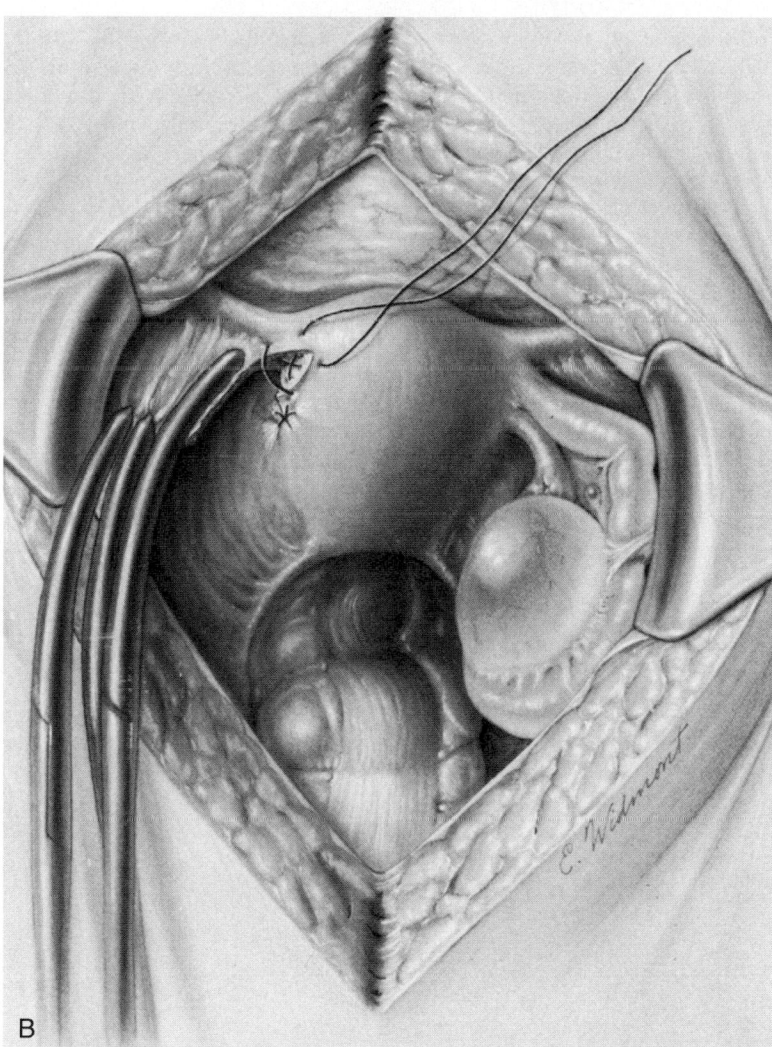

FIGURE 28.8. Salpingo-oophorectomy. **B:** A suture has been placed to ligate the ascending uterine vessels just below the cornual incision. The cornual incision is closed with a figure-of-eight suture of 2-0 delayed-absorbable material.

Drainage at Laparotomy for Pelvic Abscess

Views on drainage at laparotomy for PID have changed during the past several years. Whereas drainage was an everyday occurrence in gynecologic operating rooms in the 1950s, it is used only occasionally today. Several factors are responsible for this change. Operations for acute and subacute PID are avoided by aggressive medical management; hence, pus is encountered less frequently. Even when small pockets of pus are encountered, experience has shown that the pus can be suctioned away, the peritoneum irrigated thoroughly with saline, and the abdomen closed without drainage. Antibiotic therapy has also reduced drainage. The operator is justified in depending on postoperative antibiotics to combat the infection.

When an abscess is densely adherent to the bowel wall or the region of the ureter, thorough removal of all the abscess wall may result in bleeding and damage to a viscus. In such cases, small portions of the necrotic abscess wall can be left *in situ* and a closed suction drain placed against the area. The ideal exit for a drain is through the cul-de-sac, as shown in Figure 28.9. Sometimes the cul-de-sac is completely obliterated by adhesions between the anterior rectal wall and the cervix. In such instances, use of the posterior vaginal fornix for drainage may not be feasible. When drainage is indicated under such circumstances, it should be done through a small stab wound in whichever lower quadrant is most directly above the point to be drained (Fig. 28.10). We dislike drainage through the primary incision because of the danger of hernia formation and incisional infection. When the large bowel has been entered accidentally and a perfectly satisfactory closure has been effected, the abdomen is closed without drainage and the patient is placed on antibiotic therapy. If the condition of the large bowel wall is such that satisfactory closure cannot be done, temporary colostomy above the injury may be preferable to the risk of an abscess and an intestinal fistula.

When pus is spilled and gross contamination of the operative field is present, a closed suction drainage sys-

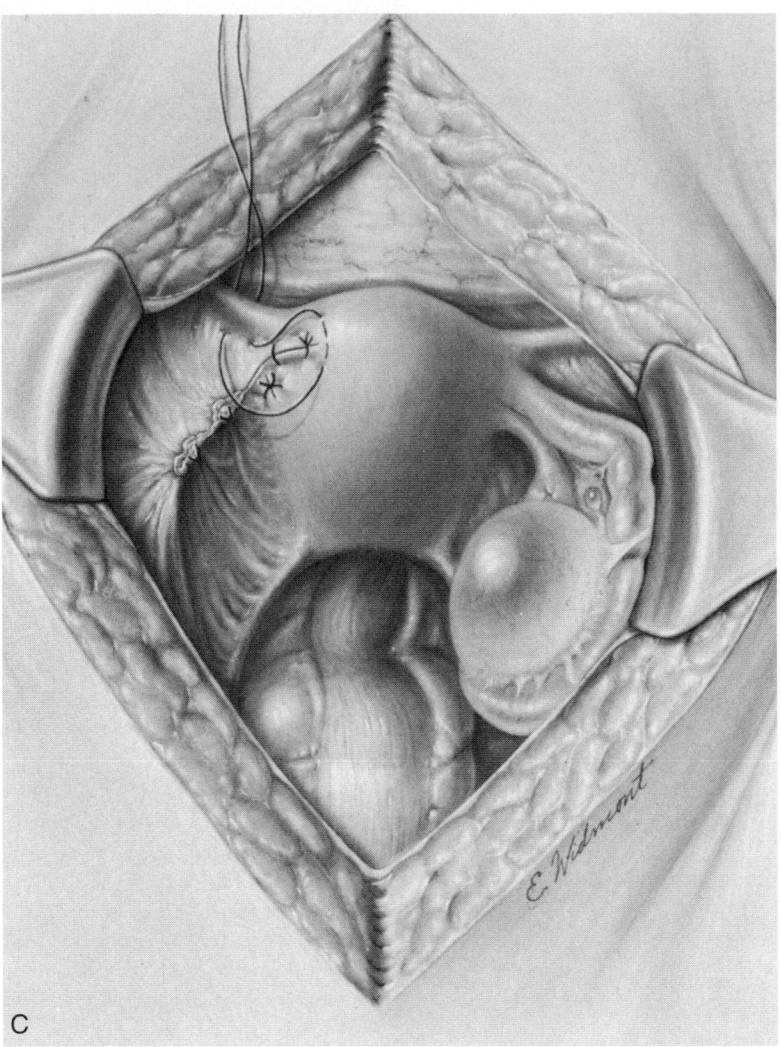

C

FIGURE 28.8. Salpingo-oophorectomy.
C: The infundibulopelvic ligament and the rest
of the broad ligament vessels have been ligated. The cornual wound is covered with the
round and the broad ligament using a mattress
suture of 2-0 delayed-absorbable material.

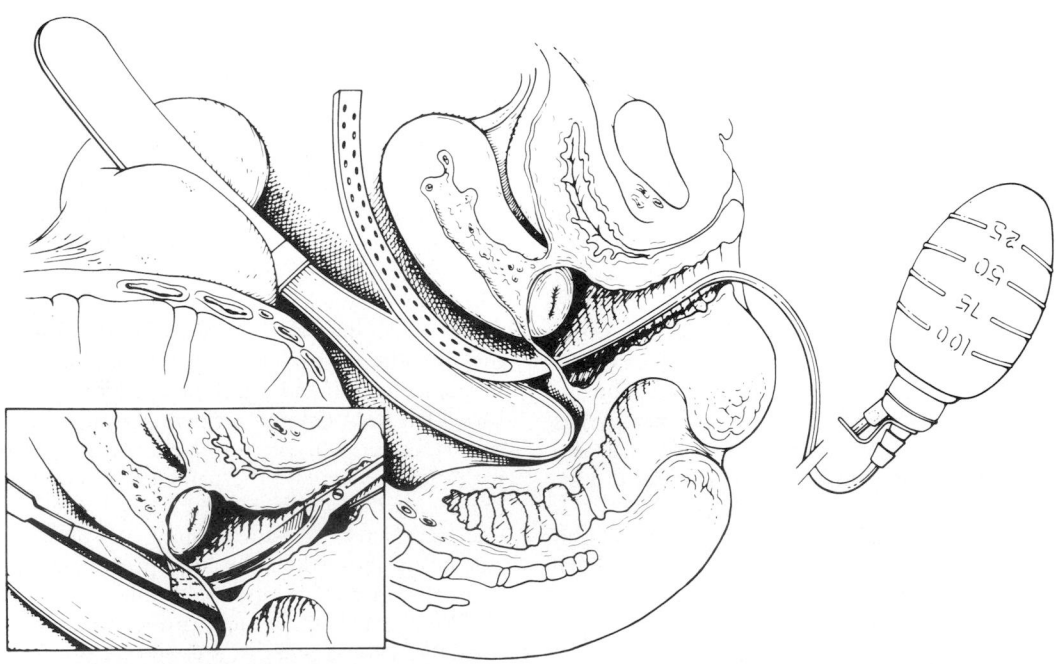

FIGURE 28.9. Drainage of pelvis through the cul-de-sac. A long Kelly clamp is inserted in the
vagina and opened slightly as the posterior vaginal fornix is pushed upward. The scalpel incises
between the jaws of the clamp. The drain is clamped and withdrawn through the vagina.

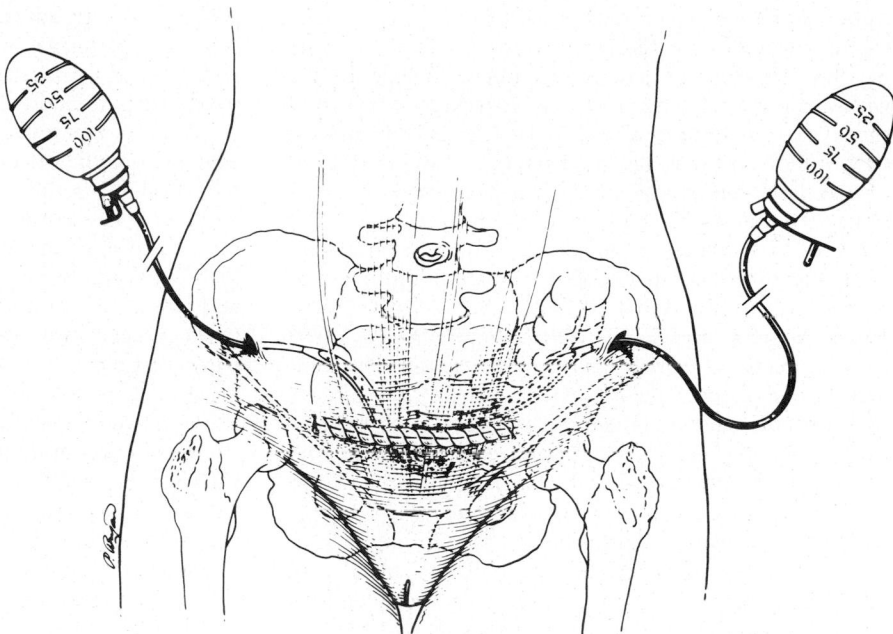

FIGURE 28.10. Bilateral trans-abdominal drainage through stab wounds. A closed suction drainage system is preferred.

tem can also be installed in the incision above the fascia with exit through a separate stab wound. This is especially important in diabetic and obese patients. Alternatively, the incision above the fascial closure can be packed open for a few days and closed secondarily to avoid incisional breakdown from infection.

PELVIC TUBERCULOSIS

Tuberculosis of the upper genital tract is a rare disease in the United States. However, it is a frequent cause of chronic PID and infertility in other parts of the world. For various reasons, the incidence of tuberculosis is again increasing in the United States. Therefore, cases of tuberculosis-associated PID may also become more evident. It should always be suspected in immigrants, especially those from Asia, the Middle East, and Latin America, and in patients with HIV. Pelvic tuberculosis is produced primarily by either *Mycobacterium tuberculosis* or *Mycobacterium bovis*. The primary site of infection for tuberculosis is usually the lung, with lymphatic spread from the Ghon complex to regional lymph nodes at the hilum usually occurring within 1 to 2 years. More rapid spread is due to hematogenous spread, which results in miliary disease often within the first year. The fallopian tubes are the predominant site of pelvic tuberculosis, but the bacilli also spread to the endometrium and occasionally the ovaries.

No location in the body is immune to the development of metastatic foci of infection. Tuberculosis of the bone, meninges, kidney, epididymis, fallopian tubes, and other sites can develop. At some sites of miliary spread, the lesions can remain quiescent for long periods before reactivation and further spread of the disease. Direct extension from one organ or system to an adjacent organ or system can also occur. Organs of the female reproductive tract are usually infected by hematogenous miliary spread from a primary pulmonary lesion, by hematogenous spread from a secondary miliary site, by lymphatic spread from a primary pulmonary site to intestinal lymph nodes and then to the pelvis, or by direct extension from adjacent abdominal organs (small intestines, appendix, rectum, bladder) that are the site of tuberculous infection. Fistulas between the intestinal tract and the fallopian tubes have been reported with pelvic tuberculosis.

A venereal transmission of the disease has been reported, with primary genital infection in the woman occurring after coitus with a sexual partner who had tuberculosis of the genitourinary tract. According to Sutherland and MacFarlane, it is not possible to prove conclusively that genitourinary tuberculosis in the male can be transmitted to the female through sexual intercourse. Because it has been shown that *M. tuberculosis* is present in the sperm of men with urogenital tuberculosis, the possibility of transmission to the pelvic organs of the female through intercourse must be accepted. Sutherland presents five cases in which sexual transmission of genitourinary tuberculosis from male to female presumably occurred. However, of 128 husbands of women with genital tuberculosis, only five (3.9%) were found to have active genitourinary tuberculosis. When tuberculosis of the vulva, vagina, and cervix is present without evidence of tuberculosis elsewhere in the body, venereal transmission should be suspected.

Pathology of Pelvic Tuberculosis

Both fallopian tubes are involved in almost all patients with pelvic tuberculosis. About one half of patients with tuberculous salpingitis have tuberculous endometritis.

Tuberculosis of the cervix is present in 5% of cases. The vagina and vulva are rarely involved. At operation, one may find evidence of generalized tuberculous peritonitis with small, grayish white tubercles covering all peritoneal surfaces of the abdominal and pelvic organs. The mucosa of the fallopian tubes may not be involved in generalized serosal tuberculous infection. At a later stage of infection, tuberculous salpingitis may grossly resemble other forms of PID involving the adnexa. Unless tubercles are seen, the diagnosis may not be apparent until microscopic sections are examined by the pathologist. A large pyosalpinx may contain the caseous material of a tuberculous infection but may also contain the purulent exudate of a secondary infection with other common organisms. Tubercles form in the lining of the tube. Some have caseation at the center, with giant cells and epithelioid cells. A proliferation of the mucosal lining of the fallopian tube may resemble a primary tubal carcinoma microscopically and may be confusing to the pathologist.

Tuberculous peritonitis is commonly associated with tuberculosis of the pelvis. Clinically, tuberculous peritonitis can be divided into two groups. In "wet" peritonitis there is an outpouring of straw-colored fluid into the peritoneal cavity, producing ascites. The peritoneum of the parietal wall and viscera is covered with innumerable small tubercles (Fig. 28.11). The tubes, in addition to being covered with miliary tubercles on the serosal surface, are usually slightly enlarged and distended. In contrast to other forms of salpingitis, the fimbriae may be patent. Within the tubal wall and tubal mucosa, the histology is typical of tuberculosis, with tubercle formation, multinucleated giant cells, and epithelioid reaction

(Fig. 28.12). In advanced cases, frank caseation is present. This pattern is usually associated with hematogenous spread of the tuberculous organism to the peritoneal surfaces and the pelvic organs.

Another type of tuberculous peritonitis encountered in women is the "dry" or adhesive type. Bowel adheres to bowel by innumerable dense adhesions that blend with the musculature. The muscle of the bowel is often invaded to some degree by the tuberculous process. Separation of these adhesions is extremely difficult surgically, and accidental injury to the bowel is common. The pelvic organs show evidence of tuberculous salpingitis with enlargement of the tubes, and occasionally pyosalpinges and even tuboovarian abscess formation.

Tuberculous involvement of the myometrium is rare. Tuberculous endometritis, however, is common, occurring in 60% to 70% of women with pelvic tuberculosis. Microscopically, tubercles are seen scattered throughout the endometrium, but they may be scanty. Tubercles are often seen in the endometrium removed by curettage in the premenstrual phase and are usually located in the endometrium adjacent to the tubal ostia. Apparently, the uterine cavity is protected from advanced tuberculous infection by the cyclic shedding of endometrial tissue in the reproductive years. Even in advanced pelvic tuberculous infections, evidence of caseation, fibrosis, and calcification are rarely seen in the uterine cavity. Occasionally, the endometrial cavity is obliterated by extensive adhesions. Total destruction of the endometrium can result in amenorrhea. Tuberculous pyometra can also develop, especially in postmenopausal women with an occluded internal cervical os.

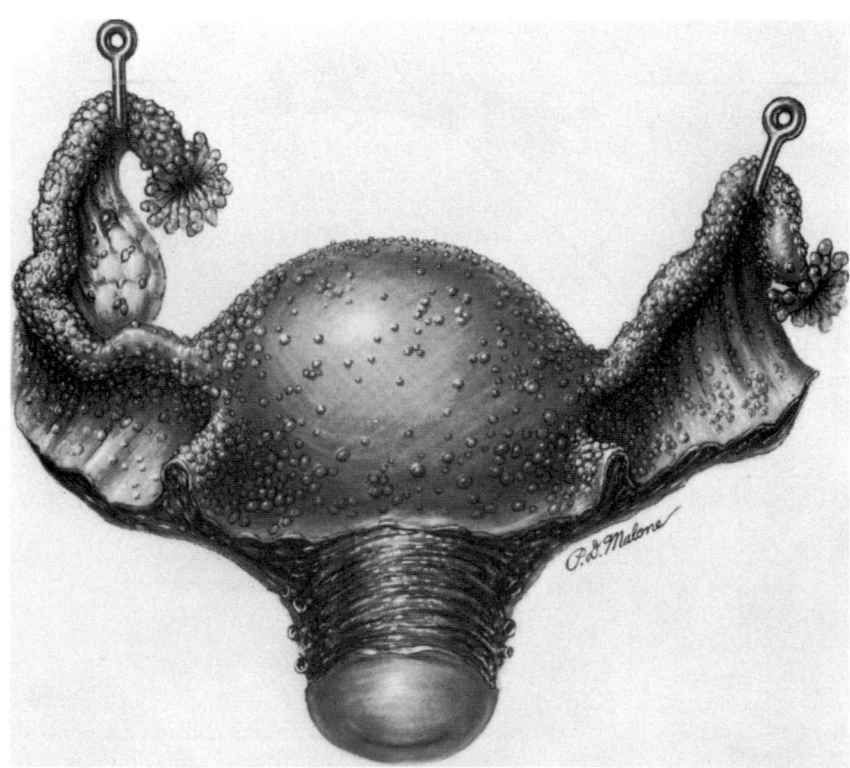

FIGURE 28.11. Typical specimen of tuberculosis of the reproductive organs as part of generalized tuberculous peritonitis.

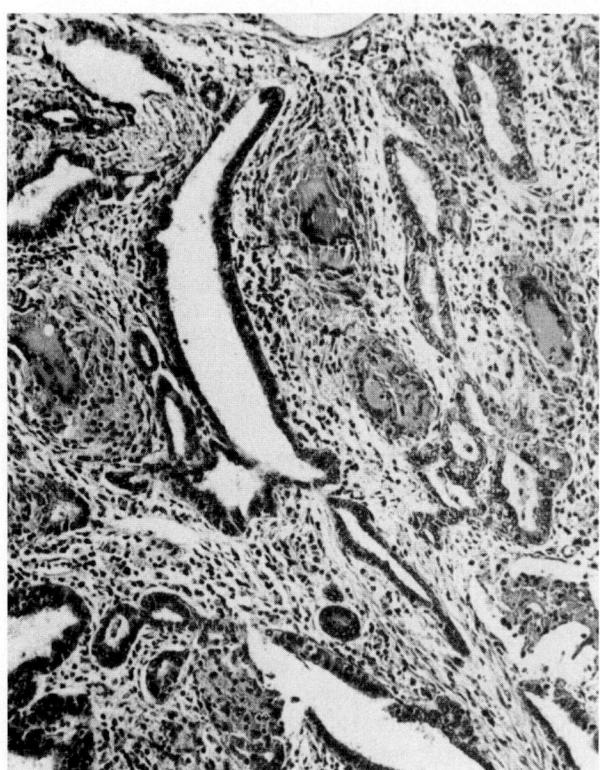

FIGURE 28.12. Tuberculosis of the fallopian tube. Note the multinucleated giant cells.

Tuberculous lesions of the cervix are rare. They can be either ulcerative or exophytic and can resemble a primary cervical malignancy or granuloma inguinale of the cervix. When there is a tuberculous lesion of the cervix, the cervical biopsy often reveals tubercles.

A tuberculous infection of the ovary usually involves only the surface of the ovary and represents simply an extension of infection from the peritoneal cavity and the adjacent fallopian tubes. The infection is usually limited to a perioophoritis. Extension of the tuberculous infection to the ovarian parenchyma can be prevented by the tunica albuginea. Tuberculous caseation can be found within the ovarian parenchyma, although this is uncommon. Presumably, it occurs as a result of hematogenous spread to the ovarian parenchyma rather than by direct extension through the ovarian capsule. However, a break in the tunica caused by ovulation may also allow the tubercular bacilli to gain access to the ovarian parenchyma. The ovaries are involved in about 25% of cases of pelvic tuberculosis.

It is uncommon for tuberculosis to involve the vulva and vagina. It is seen in only 2% of patients with pelvic tuberculosis. The gross appearance may be ulcerative with multiple sinuses, it may be hypertrophic with elephantiasis, or it may be similar to that of carcinoma.

Throughout the pelvic organs, the microscopic picture is similar, with tubercles of granulomatous inflammation, Langhans' giant cells, epithelioid cells, and central caseation associated with chronic inflammation.

With special stains, acid-fast bacilli can be demonstrated on careful microscopic examination of the tubercles.

Clinical Features of Pelvic Tuberculosis

Pelvic tuberculosis occurs most often in patients between the ages of 20 and 40 years. The age of patients with gynecologic tuberculosis has changed in recent years; the proportion of patients older than 40 years of age is now much higher than it was in the past. Falk and associates found that the incidence of pelvic tuberculosis in postmenopausal Swedish women is increasing. This was also the opinion of Sutherland, who reported an investigation from Glasgow in which 26 of 701 patients (3.7%) with proven gynecologic tuberculosis were postmenopausal.

The most common clinical symptoms of pelvic tuberculosis include pelvic pain, general malaise, menstrual irregularity, and infertility. Brown and associates found that menstrual irregularity occurred in nearly 50% of patients, whereas amenorrhea or oligomenorrhea was present in 27%. A low-grade fever that on occasion can produce a fulminating septic course is noted in most cases of active or subacute disease. The failure of fever to subside with high doses of broad-spectrum antibiotics is a classic feature of pelvic tuberculosis. A clinical course that is refractory to antibiotic therapy for the usual PID should always alert the clinician to the possibility of tuberculosis.

Among patients with pulmonary tuberculosis, the incidence of pelvic tuberculosis generally varies between 10% and 20%. Falk and associates noted that 38% of women with genital tuberculosis had previously had tuberculosis in other organs, usually the lungs. Often, the patient's clinical course is that of a chronic indolent illness.

Diagnosis of Pelvic Tuberculosis

The clinical symptoms and signs of pelvic tuberculosis should direct the clinician to the diagnosis. The disease is so uncommon that it is seldom encountered in the gynecologist's usual practice; therefore, the clinical index of suspicion is generally low. In many cases, the clinical presentation is obscure and the diagnosis is delayed. Howard Kelly once said that when competent gynecologists disagree about the diagnosis of an obscure pelvic condition, it usually is diagnosed as either an old ectopic pregnancy or pelvic tuberculosis.

More than two thirds of the cases are diagnosed at the time of laparotomy performed for some other indication, or at the time of investigation for infertility or abnormal uterine bleeding. The most common symptom is infertility, and the second most common symptom is lower abdominal and pelvic pain. Some patients are completely asymptomatic and are found to have pelvic tuberculosis during examination for other disorders such as infertility. A dilatation and curettage or endometrial biopsy is diagnostic in some cases, especially if performed in the late premenstrual phase of the menstrual cycle. In addition to standard microscopic sections, the specimen can be examined by fluorescent antibody technique. Acid-fast staining of tissue or culture of menstrual blood is effective in detecting the organism in about 10% of cases, according to Overbeck. Guinea pig inoculation with menstrual blood may be even more effective. The menstrual blood can be collected in a cervical cap. The culture or inoculation can be repeated many times before a positive result is obtained. Acid-fast stains of tissue suspected of tuberculous infection are important to confirm the diagnosis. Because some acid-fast bacilli are not tuberculous bacilli, it is important to obtain a positive culture whenever possible. A negative evaluation of the endometrium does not rule out pelvic tuberculosis, because the disease can be present in the fallopian tubes without tuberculous endometritis in 30% to 40% of cases.

On pelvic examination, bilateral adnexal tenderness is the rule. The tenderness is usually less marked than with acute gonococcal or streptococcal infections. Occasionally, a large tuberculous tuboovarian abscess is palpated on pelvic examination and even felt through the abdominal wall. The classic doughy feel of the broad ligament suggests a tuberculous inflammatory disease that is produced by a combination of thickening of the broad ligament, adherent bowel, and some ascitic fluid. On occasion, cul-de-sac nodules representing tubercles on the serosal surfaces of pelvic organs can be felt. The clinical detection of ascites is the strongest evidence obtainable in favor of pelvic tuberculosis. It was present in one fifth of the cases reported by Brown and associates. However, other causes of ascites must be considered, including ovarian carcinoma and cirrhosis of the liver. In differentiating tuberculous salpingitis from neisserial infections, the finding of a virginal outlet in the presence of obvious tubal inflammation should lend strength to the diagnosis of pelvic tuberculosis.

The diagnosis of tuberculosis cannot be made with certainty from a hysterosalpingogram, but it may be helpful. The radiographic criteria for a suspicion of pelvic tuberculosis by hysterosalpingogram have been described by Klein and associates as follows: calcified lymph nodes or smaller, irregular calcifications in the adnexal areas; obstruction of the fallopian tube in the zone of transition between the isthmus and the ampulla; multiple constrictions along the course of the fallopian tube; endometrial adhesions or deformity or obliteration of the endometrial cavity in the absence of a history of curettage or abortion; and vascular or lymphatic extravasation of contrast material. Although a conclusive diagnosis of pelvic tuberculosis can be made only from a positive culture, these authors conclude that hysterosalpingography is a useful aid, especially in patients who are asymptomatic except for infertility.

When the diagnosis of pelvic tuberculosis cannot be made in other ways, laparoscopy has been used. Because numerous adhesions may be present, making the introduction of the trocar hazardous, we believe that laparoscopy should be used with particular care. If possible, biopsy specimens of tubal fimbriae or other suspicious areas should be examined histologically or cultured to confirm the diagnosis. In addition to disclosing numerous adhesions, laparoscopy may reveal widespread miliary tubercles involving the omentum and peritoneal surfaces. Matted adnexal masses may be seen. Microscopic examination of peritoneal fluid shows a predominance of lymphocytes.

Vaginal cytology is of limited value in diagnosing tuberculosis. The cytologist must be familiar with the morphology of epithelioid cells in the vaginal smear. Only in cases of tuberculosis of the cervix may cytology be helpful. Patients with pelvic tuberculosis should also have an examination and special diagnostic procedures to rule out tuberculous infections in the upper genital tract. Chest radiograph, tuberculin skin test, pelvic ultrasonography, intravenous pyelogram, and urine, gastric, and sputum cultures for *M. tuberculosis* should be done. In some patients, exploratory laparotomy is needed to make the diagnosis.

Treatment of Pelvic Tuberculosis

Before the advent of antituberculous drug therapy, surgery was often used in the treatment of pelvic tuberculosis. Primary surgical treatment was technically difficult, sometimes ineffective, and associated with a high risk of fistula formation and persistent draining sinuses. With the advent of effective drug therapy, the surgical treatment for genital tuberculosis has been restricted to specific indications. Beginning with streptomycin more than 30 years ago, and later isoniazid and para-aminosalicylic acid, it became evident that many cases of pelvic tuberculosis could be cured or controlled with antituberculous drug therapy. There have been major advances in the antibiotic treatment of this disease, including the use of isoniazid with rifampin, with or without ethambutol, given sometimes for a period of 2 years or longer. Sutherland analyzed the results obtained with various drug schedules. The drugs that have been used to treat tuberculosis are isoniazid, rifampin, streptomycin, ethambutol, and pyrazinamide. Isoniazid and rifampin are the most effective and have the lowest toxicity. They should be the foundation of most drug regimens. The addition of ethambutol may not be of benefit, at least not in pulmonary tuberculosis. Severe and sometimes fatal hepatitis, which can develop even after months of treatment, has been associated with isoniazid therapy. The risk of developing hepatitis increases with age and with the daily consumption of alcohol. Liver function studies should be done before treatment is started, and patients should be carefully monitored with liver function studies throughout the course of therapy and later. The regimen options and dosage recommendations of the American Thoracic Society and the CDC from 1993 for the treatment of tuberculosis are given in Tables 28.5 and 28.6.

The therapeutic success of modern antituberculous drug treatment regimens is difficult to assess in view of the limited number of cases available in the literature. The cure rate varies in the literature from 65% to 95%. Kardos removed the fallopian tubes from 168 patients

TABLE 28.5.
Regimen Options for the Initial Treatment of Tuberculosis

Option 1	Option 2	Option 3
Administer daily INH, RIF, and PZA for 8 wk, followed by 16 wk of INH and RIF daily or two to three times per week.[a] In areas where the INH resistance rate is not documented as less than 4%, EMB or SM should be added to the initial regimen until susceptibility to INH and RIF is demonstrated. Continue treatment for at least 6 mo and 3 mo beyond culture conversion. Consult a tuberculosis medical expert if the patient is symptomatic or smear- or culture-positive after 3 mo.	Administer daily INH, RIF, PZA, and SM or EMB for 2 wk, then administer the same drugs two times per week[a] for 6 wk (by DOT). Next, administer INH and RIF two times per week for 16 wk (by DOT). Consult a tuberculosis medical expert if the patient is symptomatic or smear- or culture-positive after 3 mo.	Treat by DOT, three times per week[a] with M, RIF, PZA, and EMB or SM for 6 mo.[b] Consult a tuberculosis medical expert if the patient is symptomatic or smear- or culture-positive after 3 mo.

INH, isoniazid; RIF, rifampin; PZA, pyrazinamide; EMB, ethambutol hydrochloride; SM, streptomycin sulfate; DOT, directly observed therapy.
[a]All regimens administered two times a week or three times a week should be monitored by DOT for the duration of therapy.
[b]The strongest evidence from clinical trials is the effectiveness of all four drugs administered for the full 6 months. There is weaker evidence that SM can be discontinued after 4 months if the isolate is susceptible to all drugs. The evidence for stopping PZA before the end of 6 months is equivocal for the three times a week regimen, and there is no evidence on the effectiveness of this regimen with EMB for less than full 6 months.

TABLE 28.6.
Dosage Recommendations for the Initial Treatment of Tuberculosis

Drug	Dosage		
	Daily	Two Times a Week	Three Times a Week
Isoniazid	5 mg/kg Max 300 mg	15 mg/kg Max 900 mg	15 mg/kg Max 900 mg
Rifampin	10 mg/kg Max 600 mg	10 mg/kg Max 600 mg	10 mg/kg Max 600 mg
Pyrazinamide	15–30 mg/kg Max 2 g	50–70 mg/kg Max 4 g	50–70 mg/kg Max 3 g
Ethambutol hydrochloride	5–25 mg/kg Max 2.5 g	50 mg/kg Max 2.5 g	25–30 mg/kg Max 2.5 g
Streptomycin sulfate	15 mg/kg Max 1 g	25–30 mg/kg Max 1.5 g	25–30 mg/kg Max 1 g

after medical treatment for 10 months and found active tuberculosis in 35% of the surgical specimens. The experience of Sutherland suggests, however, that the results of treatment may be improved with newer drugs. The patients under treatment must be followed up closely for evidence of regression or remission of the pelvic tuberculosis. Only about 50% of patients with genital tuberculosis have the disease in the endometrial cavity; therefore, repeat endometrial biopsies and culture of menstrual egress provides only limited diagnostic information. The progress of the disease can be monitored closely by evaluating the size of adnexal masses with pelvic examinations and ultrasonography, as well as tracking the ESR, WBC count, and temperature response. Prolonged follow-up is probably indicated in all cases, because recurrence of the tuberculous pelvic lesion 5 years and even later after the end of drug treatment has occasionally been found.

Surgery in the management of patients with pelvic tuberculosis should be reserved for specific indications, as outlined by Schaefer and by Sutherland. In general, surgery is reserved for those patients who have failed to respond to an adequate trial of medical therapy. Our indications for the surgical treatment of pelvic tuberculosis include the following:

1. Persistence or enlargement of an adnexal mass after 4 to 6 months of antituberculous antibiotic therapy. The rare possibility of an ovarian tumor must always be considered, even though pelvic tuberculosis is also present. In a 1980 report by Sutherland, the persistence or development of substantial pelvic masses was the indication for surgery in 36 of 91 women with proven tuberculosis of the genital tract treated by surgery. Pelvic ultrasonography should be useful in following the response of adnexal masses to treatment.

2. Persistence of pelvic pain or recurrence of pelvic pain while on medical therapy. In Sutherland's report, 40 of 91 patients were operated on because of pain.
3. Primary unresponsiveness of the tuberculous infection to antibiotic therapy, as shown by persistent spiking temperature, leukocytosis, elevated ESR, and evidence on biopsy specimens of continued endometrial infection. Of the 91 women in Sutherland's report, 10 were operated on because of persistence of endometrial tuberculosis.
4. Difficulty in obtaining patient cooperation for continued long-term therapy. In these cases, we are accustomed to giving a brief course of streptomycin, 0.5 g every 12 hours intramuscularly for 1 week before surgery, to perform definitive surgery, and then we give 0.5 g every 24 hours in the postoperative period for 2 weeks. A persistent effort should be made to obtain the patient's cooperation for continued antituberculous therapy postoperatively. It is advisable to continue treatment for a year or longer. Isoniazid and rifampin should be used if possible. A common reason for failure of treatment is a tendency for the physician to discontinue drugs after only a few months because the patient appears well.

The preferred surgical treatment includes total abdominal hysterectomy and bilateral salpingo-oophorectomy. The nature of this inflammatory disease may make this operative procedure technically difficult, with an increased risk of injury to bowel and bladder. Consequently, in the event of a frozen pelvis from pelvic tuberculosis, it is occasionally necessary to perform only a subtotal abdominal hysterectomy and adnexectomy. Adhesions, which are invariably present and usually widespread, may make the dissection more difficult and injury more likely. However, it is usually possible to do this operation without a high incidence of bowel fistulas and other significant complications. Sutherland reported the results of surgery in 77 patients operated on while antituberculous therapy was administered. There were no deaths, no fistulas, and few late complications.

For young patients who are eager to attempt future childbearing, conservative adnexectomy should be carried out only if it is possible to do so after the extent of the adnexal disease is carefully evaluated and is found to be minimal. It is unwise for the surgeon to be committed to a specific operative procedure before the time of surgery, because conservative pelvic surgery for tuberculosis may constitute poor surgical judgment once the operative findings are known. The patient should be forewarned that conservative surgery will be performed only if the disease is minimal and such surgery is considered medically advisable.

Conservation of an ovary at the time of operation for pelvic tuberculosis is occasionally possible if the ovary is involved only on the surface. However, if one finds gross evidence of ovarian enlargement or other gross evidence of infection deep in the ovarian parenchyma, the ovary

should be removed. Bisection of ovaries to assess the presence of disease deep in the ovarian parenchyma is not advisable.

Reactivation of silent pelvic tuberculosis after tubal reconstructive surgery has been reported by Ballon and associates and by others. We believe that reconstructive tubal surgery has no place in the management of patients whose infertility is the result of bilateral tubal obstruction from tuberculous salpingitis.

Pregnancy After Pelvic Tuberculosis

It is evident from the literature, including the studies of both Schaefer and Sutherland, that only about 5% of patients with genital tuberculosis are capable of becoming pregnant, and only 2% carry a pregnancy to term. It is also evident that in the presence of tuberculous tuboovarian abscesses, pregnancy is extremely rare, and conservative surgery for the purpose of preserving fertility is unwarranted. Only when there is minimal pelvic disease without adnexal masses should conservative surgery be considered.

BIBLIOGRAPHY

Ballon SC, Clewell WH, Lamb EJ. Reactivation of silent pelvic tuberculosis by reconstructive tubal surgery. *Am J Obstet Gynecol* 1975;122:991.

Bell TA, Holmes KK. Age-specific risks of syphilis, gonorrhea, and hospitalized pelvic inflammatory disease in sexually experienced U.S. women. *Sex Transm Dis* 1989;11:291.

Brown AB, Gilbert RA, Te Linde RW. Pelvic tuberculosis. *Obstet Gynecol* 1953;2:476.

Centers for Disease Control and Prevention. Sexually transmitted diseases: treatment guidelines. *MMWR* 2002;51(RR-6):48–52.

Centers for Disease Control and Prevention. Initial therapy for tuberculosis in the era of multidrug resistance. *JAMA* 1993;270:694.

Chow AW, Pattern V, Marshall JR. The bacteriology of acute pelvic inflammatory disease. *Am J Obstet Gynecol* 1975;122:876.

Collins CG, Jansen FW. Management of tubo-ovarian abscess. *Clin Obstet Gynecol* 1959;2:512.

Eilard ET, Brorsson JE, Hanmark B, et al. Isolation of *Chlamydia* in acute salpingitis. *Scand J Infect Dis* 1976;9:82.

Eschenbach DA. Epidemiology and diagnosis of acute pelvic inflammatory disease. *Obstet Gynecol* 1980;55:142.

Eschenbach DA, Holmes KK. Acute PID: current concepts of pathogenesis, etiology and management. *Clin Obstet Gynecol* 1975;18:35.

Falk HC. Cornual resection for the treatment of recurrent salpingitis. *Am J Surg* 1951;81:595.

Fitz-Hugh T. Acute gonococcic peritonitis of the right upper quadrant in women. *JAMA* 1934;102:2084.

Franklin EW, et al. Management of pelvic abscess. *Clin Obstet Gynecol* 1973;16:66.

Ginsburg DS, Stern JL, Hamod KA, et al. Tubo-ovarian abscess: a retrospective review. *Am J Obstet Gynecol* 1980;138:1055.

Golde SH, Israel R, Ledger WJ. Unilateral tubo-ovarian abscess: a distinct entity. *Am J Obstet Gynecol* 1977;17:807.

Hager WD, Eschenbach DA, Spence MR, et al. Criteria for diagnosis and grading of salpingitis. *Obstet Gynecol* 1983;61:113.

Hager WD, Majmudar B. Pelvic actinomycosis in women using intrauterine contraceptive devices. *Am J Obstet Gynecol* 1979;133:60.

Heaton FC, Ledger WJ. Postmenopausal tubal ovarian abscess. *Obstet Gynecol* 1976;47:90.

Hemsel DL, Ledger WJ, Martens M, et al. Concerns regarding the Centers for Disease Control's published guidelines for pelvic inflammatory disease. *Clin Infect Dis* 2001;32:103–107.

Hemsell DL, Wendel GD, Hemsell PG, et al. Inpatient treatment for uncomplicated and complicated acute pelvic inflammatory disease: ampicillin/sulbactam vs. cefoxitin. *Infect Dis Obstet Gynecol* 1993;1:123.

Henry-Suchet, Soler A, Loffredo V. Laparoscopic treatment of tubo-ovarian abscesses. *J Reprod Med* 1984;29:579.

Jacobson L, Westrom L. Objectivized diagnosis of acute pelvic inflammatory disease. *Am J Obstet Gynecol* 1969;105:1088.

Kaplan AL, Jacobs WM, Ehresman JR. Aggressive management of pelvic abscess. *Am J Obstet Gynecol* 1967;98:982.

Kaplan RL, Sahn SA, Petty TL. Incidence and outcome of the respiratory distress syndrome in gram-negative sepsis. *Arch Intern Med* 1979;1939:867.

Kardos F. Late results in women with genital tuberculosis. *Obstet Gynecol* 1967;29:247.

Kelly H. *Operative gynecology*, vol II. New York: Appleton, 1898:199, 212, 374, 412, 432, 433.

Kirtley L, Benigno BB. The residual adnexa following surgery for pelvic inflammatory disease. Resident Research Day. Atlanta, Emory University School of Medicine, Gynecology and Obstetrics Department, 1979. Unpublished data.

Klein TA, Richmond JA, Mishell DR Jr. Pelvic tuberculosis. *Obstet Gynecol* 1976;48:99.

Landers DV, Sweet RL. Tubo-ovarian abscess: contemporary approach to management. *Rev Infect Dis* 1983;5:876.

Larsen B. Pelvic inflammatory disease in teenagers. *Clinical Advances in the Treatment of Infections* 1991:5.

Lemeke R, Lsonka GW. Antibodies against pleuropneumonia-like organisms in patients with salpingitis. *Br J Venereal Dis* 1962;38:212.

Loy RA, Gallup DG, Hill JA, et al. Pelvic abscess: examination and transvaginal drainage guided by real-time ultrasonography. *South Med J* 1989;82:788.

Martens MG, Faro S, Maccato M, et al. In-vitro susceptibility testing of clinical isolates of *Chlamydia trachomatis*. *Infect Dis Obstet Gynecol* 1993;1:40.

McNamara MT, Mead PB. Diagnosis and management of the pelvic abscess. *J Reprod Med* 1976;17:299.

Mickal A, Sellmann AH. Management of tubo-ovarian abscess. *Clin Obstet Gynecol* 1969;12:252.

Mickal A, Sellmann AH, Beebe JL. Ruptured tubo-ovarian abscesses. *Am J Obstet Gynecol* 1968:100:432.

Monif GR. Clinical staging of acute bacterial salpingitis and its therapeutic ramifications. *Am J Obstet Gynecol* 1982;143:489.

Monif GR. Significance of polymicrobial bacterial superinfection in the therapy of gonococcal endometritis-salpingitis-peritonitis. *Obstet Gynecol* 1980;55:1545.

Monif GR, Welkos SL, Baer H, et al. Cul-de-sac isolates from patients with endometritis-salpingitis-peritonitis and gonococcal endocervicitis. *Am J Obstet Gynecol* 1976;126:158.

Olak J, Christon NV, Stein LA, et al. Operative vs. percutaneous drainage of intra-abdominal abscesses. *Arch Surg* 1986;121:141.

Overbeck L. Is tuberculosis of the female urogenital tract an entity? *J Obstet Gynaecol Br Commonw* 1966;73:624.

Paavonen J, Kiviat N, Brunham RC, et al. Prevalence and manifestations of endometritis among women with cervicitis. *Am J Obstet Gynecol* 1985;152:280.

Pedowitz P, Bloomfield R. Ruptured adnexal abscess (tubo-ovarian) with generalized peritonitis. *Am J Obstet Gynecol* 1964;88:721.

Peterson IIB, et al. Pelvic inflammatory disease: key treatment issues and options. *JAMA* 1991:266:2605.

Phillips AJ, D'Abling G. Acute salpingitis subsequent to tubal ligation. *Obstet Gynecol* 1986;67:55.

Rivlin MR, Hunt JA. Ruptured tubo-ovarian abscess: is hysterectomy necessary? *Obstet Gynecol* 1983;61:169.

Schaefer G. Female genital tuberculosis. *Clin Obstet Gynecol* 1976;19:223.

Sutherland AM. Laparoscopy in diagnosis of pelvic tuberculosis. *Lancet* 1979;2:95.

Sutherland AM. The management of genital tuberculosis in women. *Gazzet San* 1970;19:180.

Sutherland AM. Postmenopausal tuberculosis of the female genital tract. *Obstet Gynecol* 1982;59:545.

Sutherland AM. Surgical treatment of tuberculosis of the female genital tract. *Br J Obstet Gynaecol* 1980;87:610.

Sutherland AM. The treatment of tuberculosis of the female genital tract with rifampicin, ethambutol, and isoniazid. *Arch Gynecol* 1981;230:315.

Sutherland AM. Twenty-five years' experience of the drug treatment of tuberculosis of the female genital tract. *Br J Obstet Gynaecol* 1977;84:881.

Sutherland AM, MacFarlane JR. Transmission of genitourinary tuberculosis. *Health Bull (Edinb)* 1982;40:87.

Svensson L, Westrom L, Ripa KT, et al. Differences in some clinical laboratory parameters in acute salpingitis related to culture and serologic findings. *Am J Obstet Gynecol* 1980;138:1017.

Svensson L, et al. Contraceptives and acute salpingitis. *JAMA* 1987;251:2553.

Sweet RL. PID and infertility in women. *Infect Dis Clin North Am* 1987;1:199.

Sweet RL, Gibbs RS. *Infectious diseases of the female genital tract*. Baltimore: Williams & Wilkins, 1990:241.

Sweet RL, Roy S, Faro S, et al. Piperacillin-tazobactam versus clindamycin and gentamicin in the treatment of hospitalized women with pelvic infection. *Obstet Gynecol* 1994;83:280.

Sweet RL, Schacter J, Robbie M. Failure of beta-lactam antibiotics to eradicate *Chlamydia trachomatis* in the endometrium despite clinical care of acute salpingitis. *JAMA* 1983;250:2641.

Sweet RL, Draper DL, Schacter J, et al. Microbiology and pathogenesis of acute salpingitis as determined by laparoscopy: what is the appropriate site to sample? *Am J Obstet Gynecol* 1980;138:985.

Tatum HJ, et al. The Dalkon shield controversy: structural and bacteriological studies of IUD trials. *JAMA* 1975;231:711.

Tyrrel RT, Murphy FB, Bernardino ME. Tubo-ovarian abscesses: CT-guided percutaneous drainage. *Radiology* 1990;175:87.

Vermeeren J, Te Linde RW. Intraabdominal rupture of pelvic abscesses. *Am J Obstet Gynecol* 1954;68:402.

Washington AE, et al. Hospitalization for PID: epidemiology and trends in the U.S., 1975 to 1981. *JAMA* 1984; 251:2529.

Weiner S, Wallach EE. Ovarian histology in pelvic inflammatory disease. *Obstet Gynecol* 1974;43:431.

Westrom L. Incidence, prevalence and trends of acute pelvic inflammatory disease and its consequences in industrialized countries. *Am J Obstet Gynecol* 1980;138:880.

Westrom L. Introductory address: treatment of pelvic inflammatory disease in view of etiology and risk factors. *Sex Transm Dis* 1984;11:437.

Wetchler SJ, Dunn LJ. Ovarian abscess: report of a case and a review of the literature. *Obstet Gynecol Surv* 1985;40:476.

Wharton LR. Pelvic abscess: a study based on a series of 716. *Arch Surg* 1921;2:246.

Willson JR, Black JR. Ovarian abscess. *Am J Obstet Gynecol* 1964;90:34.

Worthen NJ, Gunning JE. Percutaneous drainage of pelvic abscesses: management of the tubo-ovarian abscess. *J Ultrasound Med* 1986;5:551.

Te Linde's Operative Gynecology, ninth edition, edited by John A. Rock and Howard W. Jones, III. Lippincott Williams & Wilkins, Philadelphia © 2003.

CHAPTER

29

Surgery for Anomalies of the Müllerian Ducts

JOHN A. ROCK   LESLEY L. BREECH

Maldevelopment of the müllerian ducts occurs in a variety of forms, and each anomaly is distinctive. Nevertheless, some generalizations can be made. Classifications of vaginal anomalies based on certain anatomic findings are useful in organizing the type of malformation, but there usually are exceptions to each rule. Thus, what appears, after a preliminary diagnostic evaluation, to be an apparently isolated vaginal malformation may be found later to be associated with a uterine or renal anomaly. A comprehensive preoperative evaluation of patients with suspected malformations of the müllerian ducts is essential, but a clear understanding of the particular anomaly may not be established until the time of surgical correction. Reproductive surgeons must therefore be equally skilled in both uterine and vaginal reconstruction.

The patient with a uterovaginal anomaly often relies entirely on her physician to clarify the reproductive consequences associated with her diagnosis. The physician can help to allay her anxieties by making a prompt evaluation and giving a full and accurate description of the reproductive implications or the obstetric consequences of her particular uterovaginal anomaly.

CLASSIFICATION OF UTEROVAGINAL ANOMALIES

Classifications of uterovaginal anomalies originally were organized on the basis of clinical findings. Our improved understanding of the embryologic development of most uterovaginal anomalies has enabled categorization on this basis. The 1988 American Fertility Society (AFS) classification of müllerian anomalies (Table 29.1) offers an alternative based on the degree of failure of normal uterine development. Anomalies are grouped according to similarities of clinical manifestations, treatment, and prognosis for fetal salvage. The AFS classification system is weighted primarily toward disorders of lateral fusion and does not include associated vaginal anomalies, although the scheme does allow the user to describe anomalies involving the vagina, tubes, and urinary tract as associated malformations.

No classification of müllerian maldevelopment can focus entirely on the uterus, however. The vagina is often involved, and sometimes the tubes are involved as well. This discussion follows a suggested modification of the AFS classification of uterovaginal anomalies (Table

TABLE 29.1.
American Fertility Society Classification of Müllerian Anomalies[a]

Classification	Anomaly
Class I	Segmental, müllerian agenesis–hypoplasia
	A. Vaginal
	B. Cervical
	C. Fundal
	D. Tubal
	E. Combined anomalies
Class II	Unicornuate
	A. Communicating
	B. Noncommunicating
	C. No cavity
	D. No horn
Class III	Didelphus
Class IV	Bicornuate
	A. Complete (division down to internal os)
	B. Partial
Class V	Septate
	A. Complete (septum to internal os)
	B. Partial
Class VI	Arcuate
Class VII	Diethylstilbestrol related

[a]This classification allows the user to indicate the malformation type and provides additional findings to describe associated variations involving the vagina, cervix, tubes (right, left), and kidneys (right, left).
Adapted from the American Fertility Society. Classification of müllerian anomalies. *Fertil Steril* 1988;49:944.

TABLE 29.2.
American Fertility Society Classification of Uterovaginal Anomalies

CLASS I. DYSGENESIS OF THE MÜLLERIAN DUCTS

CLASS II. DISORDERS OF VERTICAL FUSION OF THE MÜLLERIAN DUCTS

A. *Transverse Vaginal Septum*
  1. Obstructed
  2. Unobstructed

B. *Cervical Agenesis or Dysgenesis*

CLASS III. DISORDERS OF LATERAL FUSION OF THE MÜLLERIAN DUCTS

A. *Asymmetric-Obstructed Disorder of Uterus or Vagina Usually Associated With Ipsilateral Renal Agenesis*
  1. Unicornuate uterus with a noncommunicating rudimentary anlage or horn
  2. Unilateral obstruction of a cavity of a double uterus
  3. Unilateral vaginal obstruction associated with double uterus

B. *Symmetric-Unobstructed*
  1. Didelphic uterus
    a. Complete longitudinal vaginal septum
    b. Partial longitudinal vaginal septum
    c. No longitudinal vaginal septum
  2. Septate uterus
    a. Complete
      1) Complete longitudinal vaginal septum
      2) Partial longitudinal vaginal septum
      3) No longitudinal vaginal septum
    b. Partial
      1) Complete longitudinal vaginal septum
      2) Partial longitudinal vaginal septum
      3) No longitudinal vaginal septum
  3. Bicornuate uterus
    a. Complete
      1) Complete longitudinal vaginal septum
      2) Partial longitudinal vaginal septum
      3) No longitudinal vaginal septum
    b. Partial
      1) Complete longitudinal vaginal septum
      2) Partial longitudinal vaginal septum
      3) No longitudinal vaginal septum
  4. T-shaped uterine cavity (diethylstilbestrol related)
  5. Unicornuate uterus
    a. With a rudimentary horn
      1) With endometrial cavity
        a) Communicating
        b) Noncommunicating
      2) Without endometrial cavity
    b. Without a rudimentary horn

CLASS IV. UNUSUAL CONFIGURATIONS OF VERTICAL-LATERAL FUSION DEFECTS

Modified from the American Fertility Society. Classification of müllerian anomalies. *Fertil Steril* 1988;49:944.

29.2) that comprises four groups based on embryologic considerations.

Class I. Dysgenesis of the Müllerian Ducts

Dysgenesis of the müllerian ducts, which includes agenesis of the uterus and vagina (the Mayer-Rokitansky-Küster-Hauser syndrome), is an impairment of the reproductive system characterized by no reproductive potential other than that achieved by *in vitro* fertilization in a host uterus.

Class II. Disorders of Vertical Fusion of the Müllerian Ducts

Disorders of vertical fusion can be considered to represent faults in the junction between the down-growing müllerian ducts (müllerian tubercle) and the up-growing derivative of the urogenital sinus. Typically, these disorders are characterized by an atretic portion of vagina that can be quite thick, extending through more than half the distance of the vagina, or it can be quite thin and limited to a small obstructing membrane.

Regardless of the length of the septum, a disorder of vertical fusion should be regarded as a transverse vaginal septum and classified as either obstructed or unobstructed. The so-called partial vaginal agenesis with uterus and cervix present is probably a misnomer for a large segment of atretic vagina. Cervical agenesis or dysgenesis is also included in the group of disorders of vertical fusion.

Class III. Disorders of Lateral Fusion of the Müllerian Ducts

Disorders of lateral fusion of the two müllerian ducts can be symmetric-unobstructed, as with the double vagina, or asymmetric-obstructed, as with unilateral vaginal obstruction. Obstructions associated with disorders of lateral fusion are particularly noteworthy in that they are observed clinically only as unilateral obstructions that almost invariably are associated with absence of the ipsilateral kidney. Bilateral obstruction is thought to be associated with bilateral kidney agenesis and subsequent nonviability of the developing embryo.

The three varieties of asymmetric obstruction with ipsilateral renal agenesis are as follows:

1. Unicornuate uterus with a noncommunicating horn that contains menstruating endometrium
2. Unilateral obstruction of a cavity of a double uterus
3. Unilateral vaginal obstruction

The five groups of symmetric-unobstructed disorders of lateral fusion are as follows:

1. The didelphic uterus
2. The septate uterus
3. The bicornuate uterus
4. The T-shaped uterine cavity, which may be hypoplastic and irregular, and which is associated with diethylstilbestrol (DES) exposure *in utero*
5. The unicornuate uterus with or without a rudimentary horn

The first three groups are types of double uteri; differentiation between a septate uterus (second group) and a bicornuate uterus (third group) requires visualization of the fundus. The septum within the septate uterus is complete or partial. When the septum is complete, there inevitably are two cervices with a longitudinal vaginal septum that can extend to the introitus or partially down the vagina. The bicornuate uterus also can have a partial or almost complete separation of the uterine cavities. The term *arcuate uterus* is used primarily by radiologists to refer to a slight septum in the uterine fundus that forms no clear separation of the uterine cavities. This type of uterus is usually included in the category of partial septate uterus.

The unicornuate uterus may have an attached horn with a cavity that communicates with the unicornuate uterus, or there may be no uterine horn or a uterine horn with no cavity. Some debate has focused on whether the unicornuate uterus with a communicating horn can represent a hypoplastic side of a bicornuate uterus.

Class IV. Unusual Configurations of Vertical-Lateral Fusion Defects

This final category includes combinations of uterovaginal anomalies and other disorders. Unusual uterovaginal configurations have been described that do not fit a particular category, and vertical and lateral fusion disorders can coexist.

Unusual configurations of vertical-lateral fusion defects can be seen with abnormalities of the lower urinary tract. Singh and co-workers have described a patient who was noted to have a persistent hymen and a longitudinal vaginal septum with a didelphic uterus. The patient was noted also to have a double urethra and bladder and left renal agenesis.

Obstructive lesions require immediate attention to relieve retrograde flow of trapped mucus and menstrual blood and increasing pressure on surrounding organs and structures. When no obstruction is present, attention may not be required immediately, but it will always be required eventually to establish or improve reproductive or coital function.

EMBRYOLOGY

The reproductive organs in the female (and in the male) consist of external genitalia, gonads, and an internal duct system between the two. These three components originate embryologically from different primordia and in close association with the urinary system and hindgut. Thus, the developmental history is complex (Figs. 29.1 and 29.2). Even in the 3.5- to 4-mm embryo, it is possible to recognize the bilateral thickenings of the coelomic epithelium known as the gonadal ridges medial to the mesonephros (primitive kidney) in the dorsum of the coelomic cavity. At about the sixth week of gestation, in the 17- to 20-mm embryo, the gonad can be distinguished as either a testis or an ovary.

In the female, the labia minora and majora develop from the labioscrotal folds, which are ectodermal in origin. The phallic portion of the urogenital sinus gives rise to the urethra. The müllerian (paramesonephric) duct system is stimulated to develop preferentially over the wolffian (mesonephric) duct system, which regresses in early female fetal life. The cranial parts of the wolffian ducts can persist as the epoöphoron of the ovarian hilum; the caudal parts can persist as Gartner's ducts. The müllerian ducts persist and attain complete development to form the fallopian tubes, the uterine corpus and cervix, and a portion of the vagina.

Origin of the Müllerian Ducts

About 37 days after fertilization, the müllerian ducts first appear lateral to each wolffian duct as invaginations of the dorsal coelomic epithelium. The site of origin of the invaginations remains open and ultimately forms the fimbriated ends of the fallopian tubes. At their point of origin, each of the müllerian ducts forms a solid bud. Each bud penetrates the mesenchyme lateral and parallel to each wolffian duct. As the solid buds elongate, a lumen appears in the cranial part, beginning at each coelomic opening. The lumina extend gradually to the caudal growing tips of the ducts.

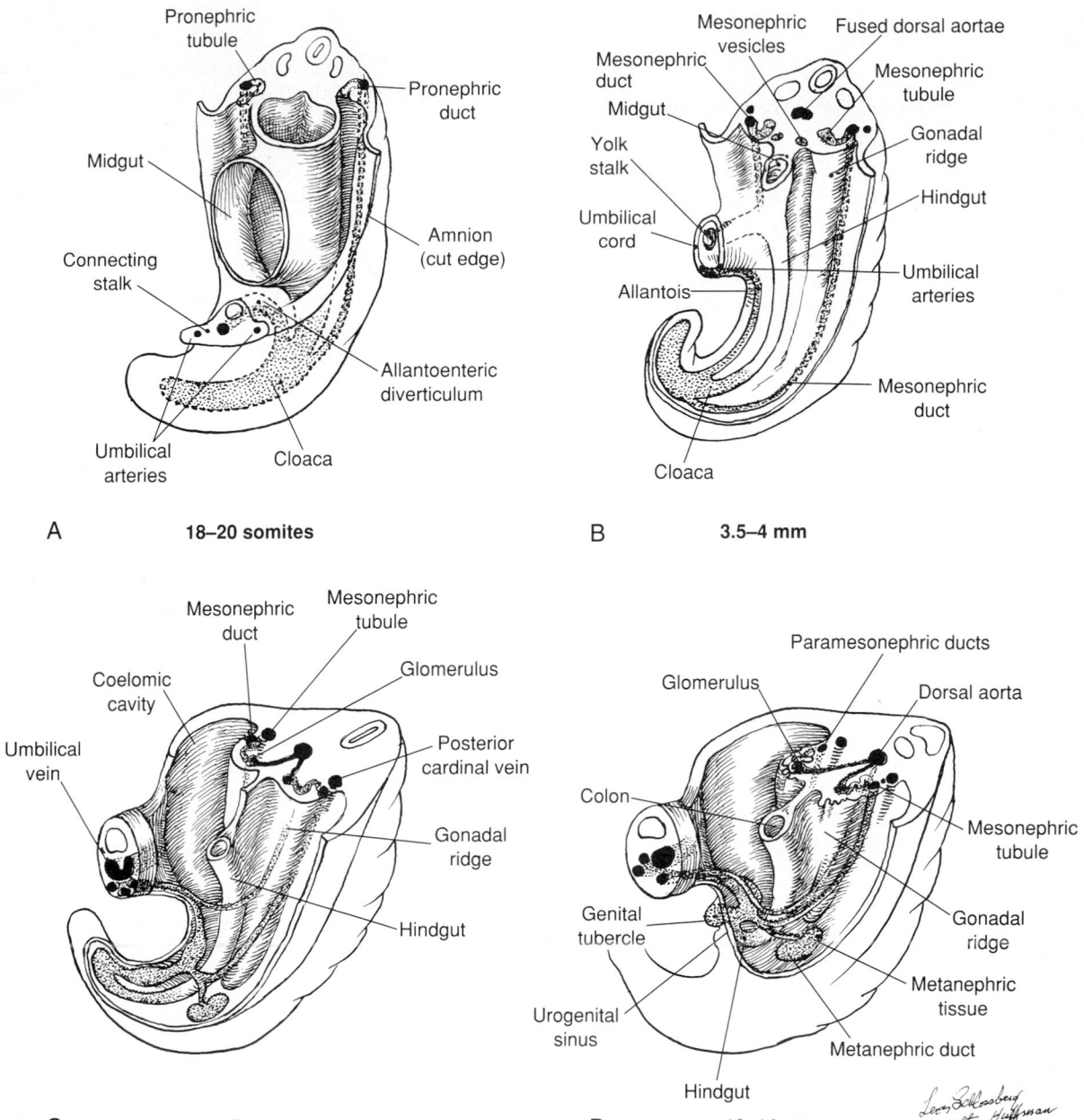

FIGURE 29.1. Diagrammatic representation of the development of the female reproductive organs and structures in early embryogenesis. **A:** At the 18- to 20-somite stage (fourth week), the gonadal ridges have not yet begun to form. **B:** In the 3.5- to 4-mm embryo (fifth week), the gonadal ridges can be recognized as thickenings of the coelomic cavity just medial to the mesonephric tubules. (Gonadal differentiation into either testis or ovary does not occur until the sixth week of development.) The allantoenteric diverticulum is joined caudally to the dilated cloaca. **C: and D:** The genital tubercle and labial folds form in the region just anterior to the cloaca. The cloaca later divides into the ventral urogenital sinus and the dorsal rectum. The development of the urinary system closely parallels that of the reproductive system. The nonfunctioning pronephric tubules shown in **(A)** develop to form the mesonephric ducts shown in **(B)** and **(C)**. The permanent kidneys eventually develop from the metanephric tissue, and the urinary collecting system develops from the metanephric ducts. The paramesonephric (müllerian) ducts are apparent by the 12- to 14-mm stage **(D).** (Their subsequent development is illustrated in Figure 29.2.)

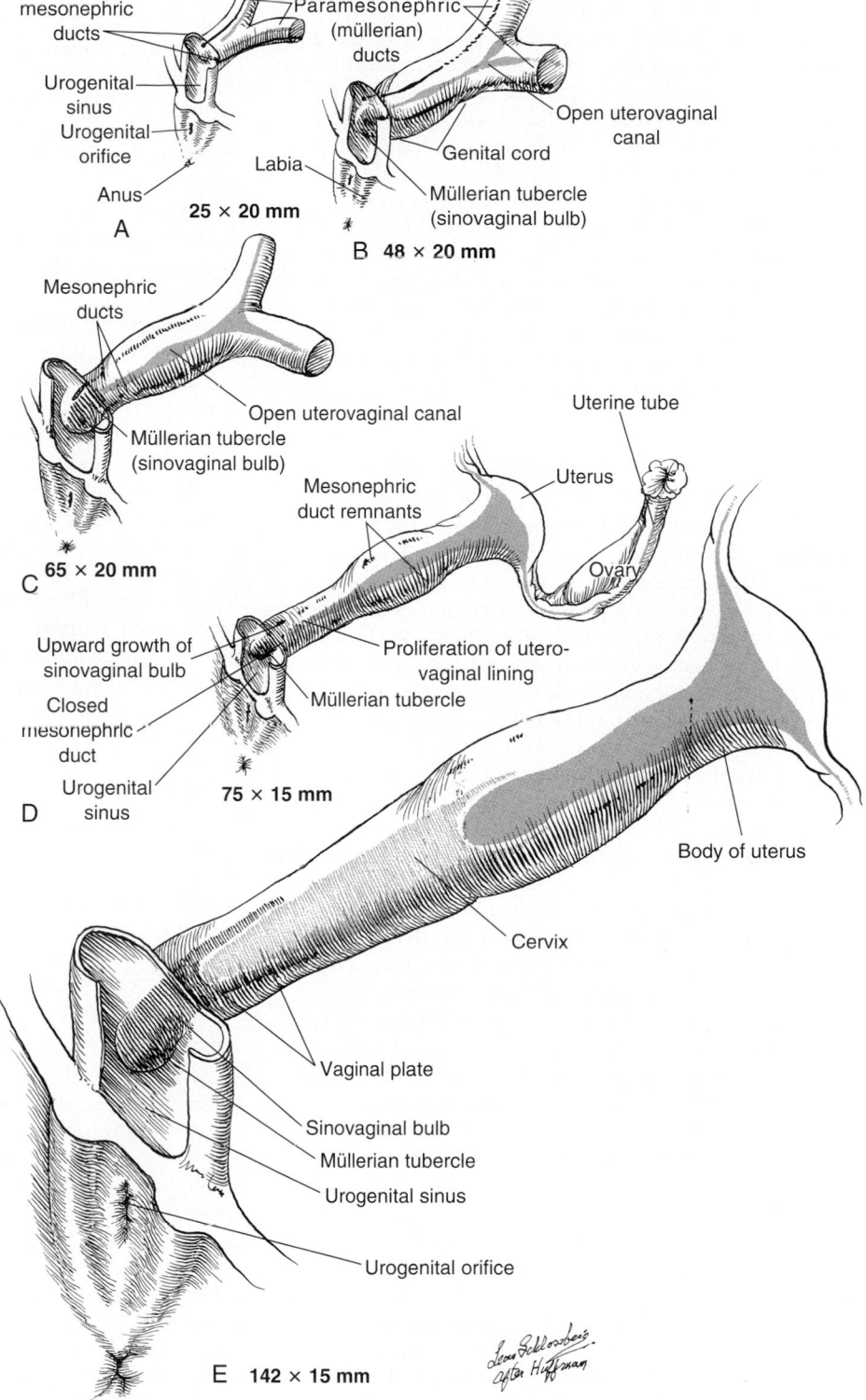

FIGURE 29.2. Further development of the paramesonephric (müllerian) ducts and the urogenital sinus. **A:** Early development of the paramesonephric ducts. The cranial ends of the paramesonephric ducts develop first. These ends remain open to form the fimbriated ends of the fallopian tubes. The paramesonephric ducts grow caudally and cross the mesonephric ducts ventrally. **B:** Eventually, they fuse together to form the uterovaginal canal. **C:** Further caudal development brings this structure into contact with the wall of the urogenital sinus, producing the müllerian tubercle. The caudal ends of the fused paramesonephric ducts form the uterine corpus and cervix. Together with the urogenital sinus, they also form the vagina. The cranial point of fusion of the paramesonephric ducts marks the location of the future uterine fundus. The fallopian tubes form from the unfused cranial parts of the paramesonephric (müllerian) ducts. The proliferation of the lining of the uterovaginal canal above the upward growth of the sinovaginal bulb from below (**D**) forms the vaginal plate (**E**), which later becomes canalized to leave an open vaginal canal. Thus, the vagina is of composite origin. The mesonephric ducts in the female degenerate but can persist into adult life as Gartner's ducts.

Eventually, the caudal end of each müllerian duct crosses the ventral aspect of the wolffian duct. The paired müllerian ducts continue to grow in a medial and caudal direction until they eventually meet in the midline and become fused together in the urogenital septum. A septum between the two müllerian ducts gradually disappears, leaving a single uterovaginal canal lined with cuboidal epithelium. Failure of reabsorption of this septum can result in a septate uterus. The most cranial parts of the müllerian ducts remain separate and form the fallopian tubes. The caudal segments of the müllerian ducts fuse to form the uterus and part of the vagina. The cranial point of fusion is the site of the future fundus of the uterus. Variations in this site of fusion can result in an arcuate or bicornuate uterus. Complete failure of fusion can result in a didelphic uterus.

Development of the Vagina

The vagina is formed from the lower end of the uterovaginal canal, which developed from the müllerian ducts and the urogenital sinus (Fig. 29.2). The point of contact between the two is the müllerian tubercle. A solid vaginal cord results from proliferation of the cells at the caudal tip of the fused müllerian ducts. The cord gradually elongates to meet the bilateral endodermal evaginations (sinovaginal bulbs) from the posterior aspect of the urogenital sinus below. These sinovaginal bulbs extend cranially to fuse with the caudal end of the vaginal cord, forming the vaginal plate. Subsequent canalization of the vaginal cord occurs, followed by epithelialization with cells derived mostly from endoderm of the urogenital sinus. Recent proposals hold that only the upper one third of the vagina is formed from the müllerian ducts and that the lower vagina develops from the vaginal plate of the urogenital sinus. Recent studies also suggest that the vaginal canal is actually open and connected to a patent uterus and tubes, even in early embryonic life, and that the vagina does not form and later become canalized from an epithelial cord of squamous cells growing upward from the urogenital sinus. Most investigators now suggest that the vagina develops under the influence of the müllerian ducts and estrogenic stimulation. There is general agreement that the vagina is a composite formed partly from the müllerian ducts and partly from the urogenital sinus.

At about the 20th week, the cervix takes form as a result of condensation of stromal cells at a specific site around the fused müllerian ducts. The mesenchyme surrounding the müllerian ducts becomes condensed early in embryonic development and eventually forms the musculature of the female genital tract. The hymen is the embryologic septum between the sinovaginal bulbs above and the urogenital sinus proper below. It is lined by an internal layer of vaginal epithelium and an external layer of epithelium derived from the urogenital sinus (both of endodermal origin), with mesoderm between the two. It is not derived from the müllerian ducts.

Anomalies in Organogenesis of the Vagina

Anomalies in the organogenesis of the vagina are easily understood. If there is failure in the development of the müllerian ducts at any time between their origin from the coelomic epithelium at 5 weeks of embryonic age and their fusion with the urogenital sinus at 8 weeks, the sinovaginal bulbs will fail to proliferate from the urogenital sinus and the uterus and vagina will fail to develop. Congenital absence of the uterus and the vagina, known as the Mayer-Rokitansky-Küster-Hauser syndrome, is the most common clinical example of this anomaly.

Transverse Vaginal Septum

A transverse vaginal septum can develop at any location in the vagina but is more common in the upper vagina at the point of junction between the vaginal plate and the caudal end of the fused müllerian ducts. This defect presumably is caused by failure of absorption of the tissue that separates the two or by failure of complete fusion of the two embryologic components of the vagina. A large segment of vagina can be atretic. In past reviews, this has been termed *partial vaginal agenesis with a uterus present*. Elucidation of the cause of a high transverse vaginal septum is more difficult. A local abnormality of the vaginal mesoderm or failure of canalization of the epithelial vaginal plate can provide the answer, but why the abnormality should occur at this particular site is not evident. The proportion of the vagina originating from the urogenital sinus can at times be considerably more than one fifth, and a high transverse vaginal septum thus may represent the junction of an abnormally long urogenital sinus contribution and a short müllerian portion. Alternatively, the high transverse septum could be the sequela of a local infection of the septum at the end of the vagina. Septa in other areas of the vagina are unexplained by this theory, which has not gained widespread acceptance.

Disorders of Ineffective Suppression of Müllerian Ducts

When abnormal gonadal development is caused by ineffective suppression of the müllerian ducts, ambiguous external genitalia frequently are accompanied by a small rudimentary uterus or a partially developed vagina. Additionally, when there is a genetic loss of cytoplasmic receptor proteins within androgenic target cells, such as occurs in the androgen insensitivity syndrome (formerly called testicular feminization syndrome), the vagina is incompletely developed because the existing male gonads suppress the development of the müllerian ducts. Because these genetically male patients are seen clinically as phenotypic XY females without a completely formed vagina, it is important that a vagina be surgically constructed so that these patients may have satisfactory sexual function in their female gender role.

Congenital rectovaginal fistula, imperforate (covered) anus, hypospadias, and other anatomic variants of cloacal dysgenesis also can occur. These anomalies can be associated with maldevelopment of the müllerian and mesonephric duct derivatives.

Müllerian Duct Abnormalities

Abnormalities in the formation or fusion of the müllerian ducts can result in a variety of anomalies of the uterus and vagina—single, multiple, combined, or separate. Just as the entirely separate origin of the ovaries from the gonadal ridges accounts for the infrequent association of uterovaginal anomalies with ovarian anomalies (see Chapter 26), so do the close developmental relationships of the müllerian and wolffian ducts explain the frequency with which anomalies of the female genital system and urinary tract are associated. Failure of development of a müllerian duct is likewise associated with failure of development of a ureteric bud from the caudal end of the wolffian duct. Thus, the entire kidney can be absent on the side ipsilateral to the agenesis of a müllerian duct.

Depending on the timing of the teratogenic influence, renal units can be absent, fused, or in unusual locations in the pelvis. Ureters can be duplicated or can open in unusual places such as the vagina or uterus. Jones and Rock have pointed out that failure of lateral fusion of the müllerian ducts with unilateral obstruction is associated consistently with absence of the kidney on the side with obstruction. Bilateral obstruction has not been observed clinically, presumably because it would be associated with bilateral renal agenesis, a condition that would not allow the embryo to develop. According to Thompson and Lynn, 40% of female patients with congenital absence of the kidney are found to have associated genital anomalies.

Much investigation has been undertaken to determine a genetic relationship in the development of disorders of the müllerian ducts. Familial aggregates of the most common disorders of the müllerian differentiation are best explained on the basis of polygenic or multifactorial inheritance. No information exists on the number and chromosomal location of responsible genes. Single mutant genes are responsible for the McKusick-Kaufman syndrome and the hand-foot-genital syndrome. Hand-foot-genital syndrome is a rare, dominantly inherited condition that affects both the distal limbs and the genitourinary tract. A nonsense mutation of the HOXA13 gene has been identified in several families. HOX gene mutations have been reported in several families with multiple müllerian abnormalities. Reproductive abnormalities involving the uterus and vagina may also be associated with other more complex malformation syndromes, in which the molecular basis of many of the syndromes remains unknown.

CONGENITAL ABSENCE OF THE MÜLLERIAN DUCTS

The disorders of müllerian agenesis include congenital absence of the vagina and uterus. Often referred to in the literature simply as congenital absence of the vagina

(vaginal agenesis), this condition is more accurately labeled aplasia (or dysplasia) of the müllerian ducts because the lower vagina generally is normal, but the middle and upper two thirds are missing. Despite the absence of the uterus, rudimentary uterine primordia are found that are comparable to each other in size and appearance. Tubes and ovaries in patients with congenital absence of the müllerian ducts generally are normal. The syndrome, usually referred to as the Mayer-Rokitansky-Küster-Hauser syndrome, is associated with a heterogeneous group of disorders that have a variety of genetic, endocrine, and metabolic manifestations and associated anomalies of other body systems.

Characteristics of Women with Müllerian Agenesis

- Congenital absence of the uterus and vagina (small rudimentary uterine bulbs are usually present with rudimentary fallopian tubes)
- Normal ovarian function, including ovulation
- Sex of rearing: female
- Phenotypic sex: female (normal development of breasts, body proportions, hair distribution, and external genitalia)
- Genetic sex: female (46,XX karyotype)
- Frequent association of other congenital anomalies (skeletal, urologic, and especially renal)

Partial agenesis of the vagina with the uterus present and a transverse vaginal septum both are categorized as disorders of vertical fusion. These two disorders have a low incidence of associated urinary tract anomalies, another circumstance that sets them apart from the Mayer-Rokitansky-Küster-Hauser syndrome.

Realdus Columbus first described congenital absence of the vagina in 1559. In 1829, Mayer described congenital absence of the vagina as one of the abnormalities found in stillborn infants with multiple birth defects. Rokitansky in 1838 and Küster in 1910 described an entity in which the vagina was absent, a small bipartite uterus was present, the ovaries were normal, and anomalies of other organ systems (renal and skeletal) were frequently observed. Hauser and associates emphasized the spectrum of associated anomalies. Pinsky suggested that congenital absence of the vagina is part of a symptom complex and not a true syndrome. Over the years, the disorder has come to be known as the Mayer-Rokitansky-Küster-Hauser syndrome, the Rokitansky-Küster-Hauser syndrome, or simply the Rokitansky syndrome (Fig. 29.3). Counseller found that the condition occurred once in 4,000 female admissions to the Mayo Clinic. Evans estimated that vaginal agenesis occurred once in 10,588 female births in Michigan from 1953 to 1957.

Individuals with an absent vagina and the classic Mayer-Rokitansky-Küster-Hauser syndrome usually are first seen by a gynecologist at age 14 to 15 years, when the absence of menses causes concern. Such young

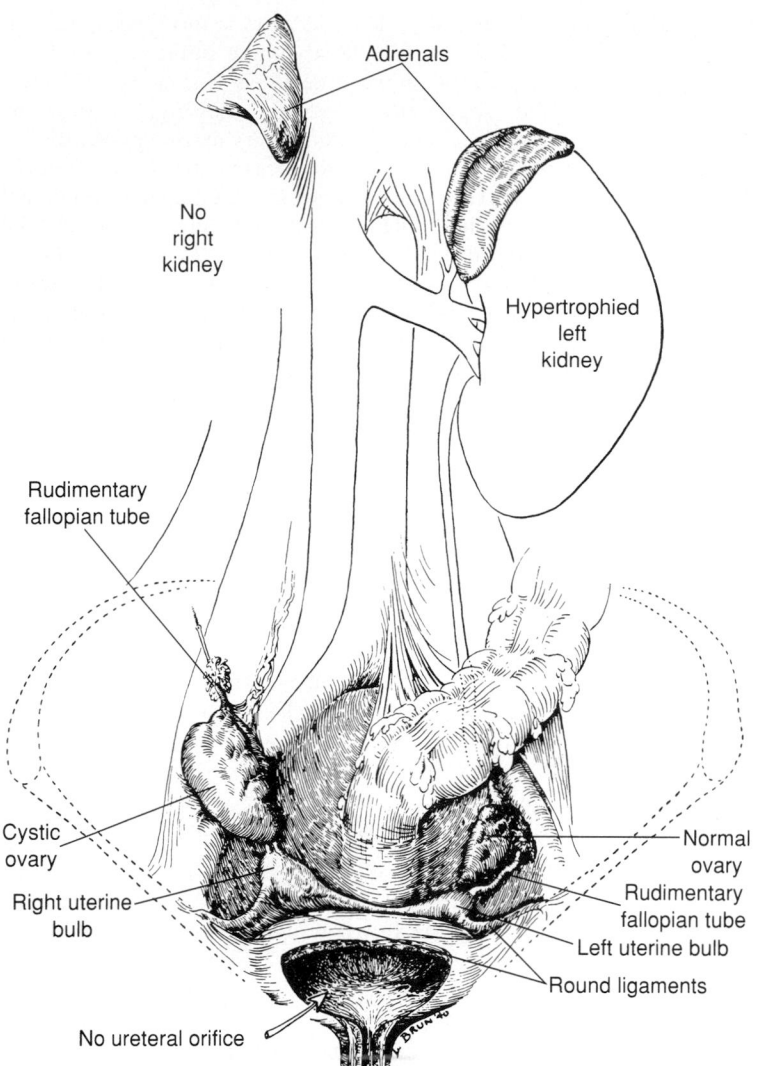

FIGURE 29.3. Typical findings in a patient with Mayer-Rokitansky-Küster-Hauser syndrome. Note the absence of the right kidney and right ureteral orifice. The uterus is represented by bilateral rudimentary uterine bulbs joined by a band behind the bladder. The ovaries appear normal although there is malposition of the right ovary.

women have a normal complement of chromosomes (46,XX) and usually have normal ovaries and secondary sex characteristics, including external genitalia. Menstruation does not appear at the usual age because the uterus is absent, but ovulation occurs regularly. There are some exceptions to the rule of normal ovaries. For example, polycystic ovaries and gonadal dysgenesis have been reported in patients with congenital absence of the vagina.

Etiologic Factors

An exclusively genetic etiology cannot be ascribed to vaginal agenesis because almost all patients have a normal karyotype (46,XX) and because the discordance of vaginal agenesis in three sets of monozygotic twins has been reported. The occurrence of complete vaginal agenesis in sisters with a 46,XX karyotype suggests an autosomal mode of inheritance for these patients. Shokeir investigated the families of 13 unrelated females with aplasia of müllerian duct derivatives. Similarly affected females were found in 10 families. Usually there was an affected female paternal relative, suggesting female-limited autosomal dominant inheritance of a mutant gene transmitted by male relatives.

Other investigators point to the variety of associated anomalies as support for the etiologic concept of variable expression of a genetic defect possibly precipitated by teratogenic exposure between the 37th and the 41st gestational day, the time during which the vagina is formed. Knab has suggested five possible etiologic factors of the Mayer-Rokitansky-Küster-Hauser syndrome:

1. Inappropriate production of müllerian regressive factor in the female embryonic gonad
2. Regional absence or deficiency of estrogen receptors limited to the lower müllerian duct
3. Arrest of müllerian duct development by a teratogenic agent
4. Mesenchymal inductive defect
5. Sporadic gene mutation

Knab believes that the teratogenic and the mutant gene etiologies are the most probable.

Anomalies Associated with Müllerian Agenesis

Many patients with müllerian agenesis have associated anomalies of the upper müllerian duct system together with associated anomalies of other organ systems. By gentle rectal examination, the physician can feel an absence of the midline müllerian structure that should represent the uterus. The physician instead feels a smooth band (possibly a remnant of the uterosacral ligaments) that extends from one side of the pelvis to the other. In Mayer Rokitansky-Küster-Hauser syndrome, the uterus is represented by bilateral rudimentary uterine bulbs that vary in size, are not usually palpable, are connected to small fallopian tubes, and are located on the lateral pelvic side wall adjacent to normal ovaries. Depending on their size, these rudimentary uterine bulbs may or may not contain a cavity lined by endometrial tissue (Fig. 29.4). If present, the endometrial tissue can appear immature or, rarely, can show evidence of cyclic response to ovarian hormones. The endometrial cavity does not communicate often with the peritoneal cavity because the tube may not be patent at the point of junction between the tube and the rudimentary uterine bulb. In rare instances, however, active endometrium can exist within the uterine anlagen and the endometrial cavity, enabling communication with the peritoneal cavity through patent fallopian tubes. Reports have described several patients with functioning endometrial tissue in one or both rudimentary uterine bulbs (Fig. 29.4B. The patient can develop a large hematometra due to cyclic accumulation of trapped blood. Cyclic abdominal pain is relieved by excision of the active uterine anlagen. A patient with Mayer-Rokitansky-Küster-Hauser syndrome was reported who had a 4-cm endometrioma removed from the left ovary by laparotomy at the time of operation to create a vagina. Myomas have been known to form in the muscular wall, and mild dysmenorrhea has been attributed to their presence. A small myoma has been found, in addition to the tube and ovary, in the inguinal canal and in the inguinal hernia sac.

Chakravarty and colleagues and Singh and Devi have demonstrated that the rudimentary bulbs have the potential for function. These authors used these rudimentary uterine bulbs to reconstruct a midline uterus. The reconstructed uterus was then connected to a newly constructed vagina. A surprising number of patients who have undergone this procedure have experienced cyclic menstruation, although recurrent stenosis and obstruction of the rudimentary horns are the most common results of such efforts. The authors of this chapter have had no experience with this technique and question its usefulness. However, these rudimentary uterine bulbs usually are insignificant structures that cause no problems.

Associated Urologic and Renal Anomalies

Fore and associates reported that 47% of patients in whom evaluation of the urinary tract was performed had associated urologic anomalies. In other studies, approximately one third of patients with complete vaginal agenesis were found to have significant urinary anomalies, including unilateral renal agenesis, unilateral or bilateral pelvic kidney, horseshoe kidney, hydronephrosis, hydroureter, and a variety of patterns of ureteral duplication. A significant number of patients with partial vaginal agenesis also have associated urinary tract anomalies.

Associated Skeletal and Other Anomalies

Associated skeletal anomalies have been recognized since congenital absence of the vagina was first described. In a review of 574 reported cases, Griffin and associates found a 12% incidence of skeletal abnormalities. Most of these abnormalities involve the spine (wedge vertebrae,

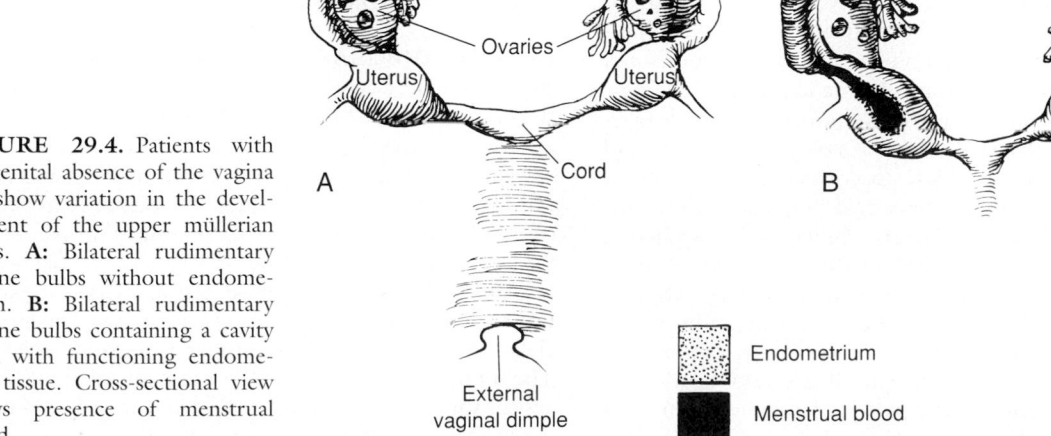

FIGURE 29.4. Patients with congenital absence of the vagina can show variation in the development of the upper müllerian ducts. **A:** Bilateral rudimentary uterine bulbs without endometrium. **B:** Bilateral rudimentary uterine bulbs containing a cavity lined with functioning endometrial tissue. Cross-sectional view shows presence of menstrual blood.

fusions, rudimentary vertebral bodies, and supernumerary vertebrae), but the limbs and ribs also can be involved. Other anomalies include syndactyly, absence of a digit, congenital heart disease, and inguinal hernias, although the latter are more often present in patients with androgen insensitivity syndrome than in patients with Mayer-Rokitansky-Küster-Hauser syndrome (Fig. 29.3).

Treatment for Disorders of Müllerian Agenesis

Preoperative Considerations

If functioning endometrial tissue is present with the anlagen, then symptoms from cryptomenorrhea will begin shortly after female secondary sex characteristics develop. Prompt removal of the active uterine bulbs affords complete relief of symptoms.

Occasionally, older patients with the classic Mayer-Rokitansky-Küster-Hauser syndrome consult a gynecologist because of difficult or painful intercourse. The indication for operation in these patients is obvious. Of all patients, they are the most satisfied with the operative results.

Most commonly, patients age 14 to 16 years are seen by a gynecologist because of primary amenorrhea. An examination may not have been done by a previous physician because the patient was "too young," but various hormonal medications may have been given with hope that menstruation would begin. An inaccurate examination may have led to the mistaken diagnosis of imperforate hymen. Futile attempts to incise the hymen may have resulted in scarring of the apex of the vaginal dimple before a correct diagnosis of congenital absence of the vagina was finally made. In the past it was customary to advise delaying surgery to create a vagina for these young patients until just before their marriage. This led to difficulties, particularly when complications developed that required a delay in marriage until the vagina healed completely. More recently, it has become usual to perform the procedure when patients are 17 to 20 years old and are emotionally mature and intellectually reliable enough to manage without difficulty the vaginal form that is used to maintain the neovaginal space.

PSYCHOLOGICAL PREPARATION OF THE PATIENT. Insufficient attention has been given to the psychological aspects of this problem. The patient with congenital absence of the vagina cannot be made into a whole person simply by creating a perineal pouch for intercourse. Establishment of sexual function is only one concern and may be the easiest problem to correct. Evans reported that 15% of his patients have real psychiatric difficulty. He and David and associates suggest that psychiatric help should be initiated before the operation. Weijenborg and others described the effect of a group program on women with Rokitansky syndrome. The authors held group sessions conducted by a gynecologist, a female social worker, and a woman with Rokitansky syndrome. Seventeen patients participated. Three women had elected not to create a vagina, six women created a vagina by dilatation or sexual activity, and eight women had undergone a vaginoplasty. Indices of psychological distress were measured before the program, at initiation of the program, and at the last group session. The results demonstrated that women with Rokitansky syndrome felt less anxious, less depressed, and less sensitive to interpersonal contact after participation in the semistructured program. These data support the value of group interaction in patients with Rokitansky syndrome.

Learning about this anomaly, especially at a young age, is a shock and is accompanied by diminished self-esteem. Such patients can be encouraged by having their gynecologist offer appropriate surgery to establish coital function. The gynecologist can point out that, functionally, the patient will be like thousands of young women who have had a hysterectomy because of serious pelvic disease, and who have satisfied their desire to be a parent through adoption or gestational surrogacy.

When counseling patients at the time of diagnosis, gestational surrogacy should definitely be included in the discussion. Until recently, the literature had provided only sparse evidence regarding the use of this modality in this population. Beski and others confirmed the use of gestational surrogacy in a small population. The treatment cycles resulted in six clinical pregnancies (42.9% pregnancy rate per embryo transfer and 54.5% per oocyte retrieval) and three live births (21.4% per embryo transfer, 27.3% per retrieval, and 50% per patient). Several authors have reported on the genetic offspring of patients with vaginal agenesis. Petrozza and others reported a retrospective study in 1997, describing a large number of treatment cycles for patients with Rokitansky syndrome. The authors attempted to determine an inheritance pattern of the syndrome through a questionnaire sent to all centers performing surrogacy treatment in the United States. A total of 162 *in vitro* fertilization/ surrogacy treatment cycles were reviewed for 58 patients with congenital agenesis of the uterus and vagina. The treatment resulted in 34 live births (17 females, 17 males). One child had a nonspecific middle ear defect and hearing loss. The authors concluded that congenital absence of the uterus and vagina was not commonly inherited in a dominant fashion. These findings suggest inheritance of this disorder in children of affected mothers is likely via a polygenic mechanism.

PATIENT COOPERATION. Regardless of which operative technique is chosen, the patient must cooperate if the operation is to be successful. When a McIndoe operation is performed, patients must understand the need to wear a form continuously for several months and intermittently for several years until the vagina is no longer subject to constriction and until regular intercourse is taking place. The operation should not be performed until preoperative interviews determine that the patient understands her essential role in its success. This is especially important when the patient is a young teenager. The single most important factor in determining the success of vaginoplasty is the psychosocial adjustment of the patient to her congenital vaginal anomaly.

Laboratory and Diagnostic Testing

A complete chromosomal analysis should be performed in all patients. If there is a suspicion of ovarian dysgenesis, androgen insensitivity syndrome, or some aberration of the classic Mayer-Rokitansky-Küster-Hauser syndrome, then a consideration of additional SRY analysis should be entertained to assess the possible presence of any Y chromosome. An intravenous pyelogram should be done preoperatively. This also provides an adequate survey for anomalies of the spine. If a pelvic mass is present, then additional special studies, including ultrasonography, should be performed to differentiate between hematometra, hematocolpos, endometrial and other ovarian cysts, and pelvic kidney.

Evaluation of Cyclic Pain

Some patients without a pelvic mass complain of cyclic pain. This pain can be ovulatory or possibly a result of dysmenorrhea originating in well-developed rudimentary uterine bulbs. The physician can differentiate between the two by asking the patient to keep a basal body temperature chart and to mark the days when pelvic pain is present. Occasionally there is a question about whether a patient has congenital absence of the vagina or an imperforate hymen with cryptomenorrhea. The diagnosis is clarified simply by placing a metal catheter or similar instrument in the urethra and a finger in the rectum. If the metal instrument in the urethra can be easily felt through the anterior rectal wall, then the vagina is probably absent. On the other hand, an intervening mass between the rectal finger and the instrument in the urethra can represent a hematocolpos behind an imperforate hymen. The hymen bulges from the force of accumulated blood in the vagina, especially when the hematocolpos is palpable suprapubically.

METHODS OF CREATING A VAGINA

There is no unanimity of opinion regarding the correct approach to the problem of vaginal agenesis (Table 29.3). With the development of the Ingram method for vaginal dilatation, fewer patients require surgical vaginoplasty. The role of tissue expanders in vaginoplasty has been reviewed by Patil and Hixon. Labial expansion with an expander having a capacity of 250 mL provides a flap 10 cm long and 8 cm wide with a 4-cm projection. Thus, well-vascularized flaps can be available to provide an outlet for stenosis-free vaginoplasty. This approach has been suggested to maximize the success of surgical vaginoplasty. A review of the methods devised for the formation of a vagina follows. The editors of this book have found the modified McIndoe technique to give the most consistently satisfactory results.

Nonsurgical Methods

In 1938, Frank described a method of creating an artificial vagina without operation. In 1940, he reported re-

TABLE 29.3.
Classification of Methods to Form a New Vagina

NONSURGICAL (INTERMITTENT PRESSURE ON THE PERINEUM)

Active Dilatation
Passive Dilatation

SURGICAL
Without Use of Abdominal Contents
Without cavity dissection
  Vulvovaginoplasty
  Constant pressure (Vecchietti)
No attempt to line cavity (now unacceptable)
Lining cavity with grafts
  Split-thickness skin grafts (McIndoe operation)
  Dermis grafts
  Amnion homografts
Lining cavity with flaps
  Musculocutaneous flaps
  Fasciocutaneous flaps
  Subcutaneous pedicled skin flaps
  Labial skin flaps (can be created with tissue expander)
  Penoplasty (transsexualism)
With Use of Abdominal Contents (Cavity Lining With)
Peritoneum
Free intestinal graft
Pedicled intestine

markably satisfactory results in eight patients treated with this method. His follow-up study showed that a vagina formed in this manner remained permanent in depth and caliber, even in patients who neglected dilatation for more than 1 year. It has been emphasized that the pelvic floor itself is embryologically deficient in some patients. Indeed, the ease with which some patients are able to create a vagina with intercourse alone or with other intermittent pressure techniques can be explained on this basis. Five patients were reported to have developed enteroceles, one after coitus alone, three after a Williams vulvovaginoplasty, and three after a McIndoe operation. This complication can develop when the vaginal mucosa is brought in close proximity to the pelvic peritoneum, but a relative embryologic weakness or an absence of endopelvic fascia can also contribute to this complication. Rock, Reeves, and associates at the Johns Hopkins Hospital reported that an initial trial of vaginal dilatation was successful in 9 of 21 patients.

Prompted by the rewarding results of Broadbent and Woolf, Ingram has described a passive dilatation technique of creating a new vagina. Instructing his patients in the insertion of dilators (Fig. 29.5) specially designed for use with a bicycle seat stool, Ingram was able to produce satisfactory vaginal depth and coital function in 10 of 12 cases of vaginal agenesis and 32 of 40 cases of various types of stenosis.

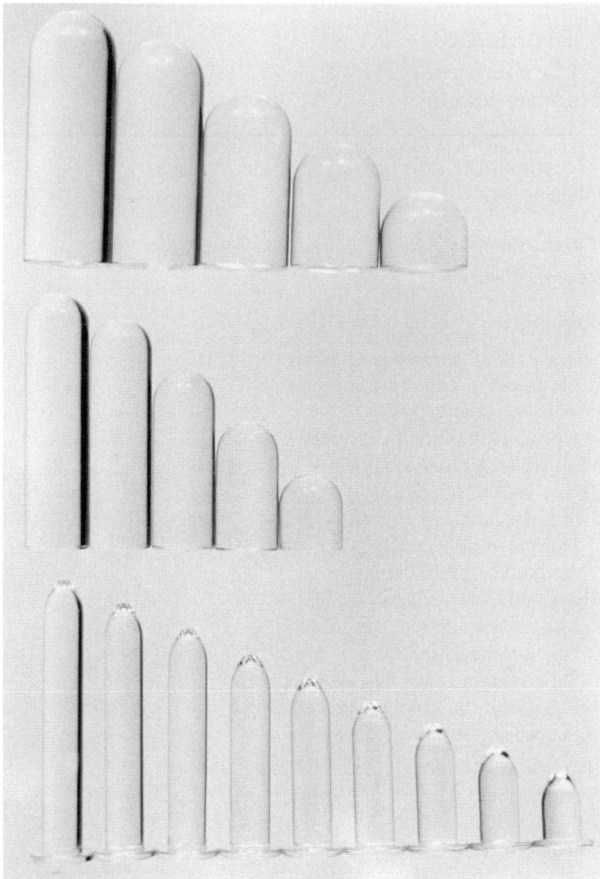

FIGURE 29.5. Vaginal dilators for use in Ingram passive dilatation technique to create a new vagina. The set consists of 19 dilators of increasing length and width. (Courtesy of Faulkner Plastics, Tampa, FL)

The Ingram technique for passive dilatation has several advantages. The patient is not required to press the dilator against the vaginal pouch. A series of graduated Lucite dilators slowly and evenly dilate the neovaginal space. The patient should be carefully instructed in the use of dilators, as recommended by Ingram, beginning with the smallest dilator. The patient is shown and instructed with the use of a mirror how to place a dilator against the introital dimple. The dilator may be held in place with a supportive undergarment and regular clothing worn over this.

The patient is shown how to sit on a racing type bicycle seat that is placed on a stool 24 inches above the floor. She is instructed to sit leaning slightly forward with the dilator in place for at least 2 hours per day at intervals of 15 to 30 minutes. Follow-up is usually at monthly intervals and the patient can expect to graduate to the next size larger dilator about every month. An attempt at sexual intercourse may be suggested after the use of the largest dilator for 1 or 2 months. Continued dilatation is recommended if intercourse is infrequent. In our experience, functional success rates are outstanding. Rock and Roberts reported the largest series of vaginal

agenesis patients who used the Ingram method of dilatation to create a neovagina. The records of 51 patients with müllerian agenesis were reviewed: 37 patients attempted vaginal dilatation and 14 young women underwent a surgical intervention. Functional success was defined as satisfactorily achieving intercourse or accepting the largest dilator without discomfort in the clinic visit. All patients were followed up for at least 2 years and for an average of 9.25 years. Functional success was achieved in 91.9% of those who attempted dilatation (Table 29.4). Thus, passive dilatation should be suggested as an initial therapy for vaginal creation. If dilatation is unsuccessful, operative vaginoplasty is indicated.

Surgical Methods

During the past 3 decades, experience has proved the Abbe-Wharton-McIndoe procedure (more popularly called the McIndoe operation) for dealing with complete absence of a vagina to be generally superior to others in most cases. In special circumstances, alternative methods of creation of a neovagina may be indicated.

Historical Development of Surgical Procedures

In 1907, Baldwin used a double loop of ileum to line a space dissected between the rectum and bladder, leaving the mesentery connected to the bowel. The continuity of the intestinal tract was reestablished by an end-to-end anastomosis. He reported that the new vagina was absolutely normal in every way. In 1910, Popaw constructed a vagina using a portion of the rectum that was moved anteriorly. This operation was modified by Schubert in 1911. The rectum was severed above the anal sphincter and moved anteriorly to serve as the vagina. The sigmoid was sutured to the anus to reestablish the continuity of the intestinal tract. Both operations had soberingly high morbidity and mortality rates, and their popularity declined. Today, segments of sigmoid are used most often to create a vaginal pouch or extend vaginal length in patients who have lost vaginal function as a result of extensive surgery or irradiation for pelvic malignancy. Some patients who are treated for multiple genitourinary or gastrointestinal abnormalities may be treated with a bowel vaginoplasty during a combined procedure.

TABLE 29.4.
Outcomes of Patients With Vaginal Agenesis Who Attempted Dilatation

Patients	Totals	Percent
Successful dilatation	34/37	91.9%[a]
Failed dilatation	3/37	8.1%

[a] $p < .001$.
Modified from Roberts CP, Haber MJ, Rock JA. Vaginal creation for müllerian agenesis. *Am J Obstet Gynecol* 2001;185:1349.

Less formidable procedures involving dissection of a space between the bladder and rectum and lining of this space with flaps of skin from the labia or inner thighs also were tried. Marked scarring resulted, and hair usually grew in the vagina. Extensive plastic procedures to construct a vagina are no longer necessary or desirable and have been discarded in favor of safer procedures unless there is the problem of maintaining a vaginal canal after an extensive exenterative operation for pelvic malignancy. In this case, the physician may want to consider using the gracilis myocutaneous flap technique described by McCraw and associates in 1976.

The Abbe-Wharton-McIndoe Operation

The operation most popular today for creating a new vagina began with simple surgical attempts to create a space between the bladder and the rectum. These early attempts were often made in patients with cryptomenorrhea. However, such a space usually would constrict because the surgeon would fail to recognize the importance of prolonged continuous dilatation until the constrictive phase of healing was complete.

At the Johns Hopkins Hospital in 1938, Wharton combined an adequate dissection of the vaginal space with continuous dilatation by a balsa form that was covered with a thin rubber sheath and was left in the space. He did not use a split-thickness skin graft. Instead, he based his operation on the principle that the vaginal epithelium has remarkable powers of proliferation and in a relatively short time will cover the raw surface. Recalling that a similar process occurs in the fetus when the epithelium of the sinovaginal bulbs and the urogenital sinus form the vaginal canal, Wharton merely applied this same principle in the adult. This simple procedure is entirely satisfactory as long as the space is kept dilated long enough to allow the epithelium to grow in. Occasionally, however, even after several years, the vault of the vagina remains without epithelial covering. Coital bleeding and leukorrhea result from the persistent granulation tissue, and there is a tendency for vaginas constructed by this method to be constricted by scarring in the upper portion. In Counseller's 1948 report from the Mayo Clinic of 100 operations to construct a new vagina, 14 were performed by Wharton's method, with excellent results in all 14 patients. It was stated that the disadvantages of persistent granulation tissue with bleeding and leukorrhea were of no consequence. This has not been the experience of the editors of this book.

When inlay skin grafts were first used to construct a new vagina, the results were poor because the necessity for dilatation of the new vagina again was not recognized. Severe contraction, uncontrolled by continuous or intermittent dilatation, almost invariably spoiled the results. Although Heppner, Abbe, and others preceded him by many years in using a skin-covered prosthesis in neovaginal construction, it was Sir Archibald McIndoe, at the Queen Victoria Hospital in England, who popularized the method and gave it substantial clinical trial. He emphasized the three important principles used today in successful operations for vaginal agenesis:

1. Dissection of an adequate space between the rectum and the bladder
2. Inlay split-thickness skin grafting
3. The cardinal principle of continuous and prolonged dilatation during the contractile phase of healing

Other tissues such as amnion and peritoneum have been used to line the new vaginal space, but they have not had substantial success. However, Tancer and associates reported good results with human amnion. Karjalainen and associates stated that a more physiologic result was achieved with an amnion graft than with a skin graft. Nevertheless, concerns about the transmission of human immunodeficiency virus with human amnion now limit this option.

TECHNIQUE OF ABBE-WHARTON-MCINDOE OPERATION

Taking the Graft. After a careful pelvic examination is performed under anesthesia to verify previous findings, the patient is positioned for taking a skin graft from the buttocks. For cosmetic reasons, the graft should not be taken from the thigh or hip unless for some reason it cannot be obtained from the buttocks. Patients may be asked to sunbathe in a brief bathing suit before coming to the hospital so that its outline can be seen; an attempt should be made to take the graft from both buttocks within these borders. The quality of the graft determines to a great extent the success of the operation. We have found the Padgett electrodermatome to be the most satisfactory instrument for taking the graft. With relatively little experience and practice, the gynecologic surgeon can successfully cut a graft of controlled width and thickness (Fig. 29.6). The instrument is set and checked for taking a graft approximately 0.018 inch thick and 8 to 9 cm wide. The total graft length should be 16 to 20 cm. If the entire graft cannot be taken from one buttock, then a graft 8 to 10 cm long is needed from each buttock.

The skin of the donor site is prepared with an antiseptic solution (povidone-iodine), which is then thoroughly washed away. The skin is then lubricated with mineral oil as assistants steady and stretch the skin tight.

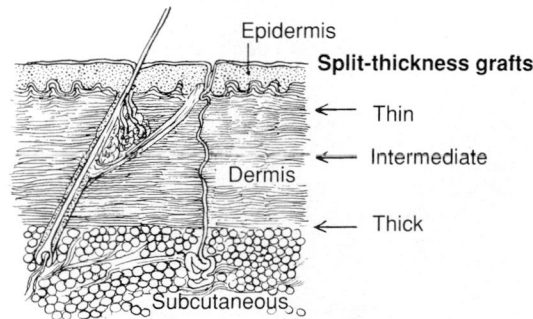

FIGURE 29.6. Section of split-thickness skin grafts. Grafts should be uniform in thickness. The Padgett electrodermatome is set to take a graft approximately 0.018 inch thick. A graft that is slightly thick is better than a thin graft.

Considerable pressure should be applied uniformly across the dermatome blade. The thickness of the graft must have minimal variation. A graft that is a little too thick is better than one that is a little too thin. There should be no breaks in the continuity of the graft. The graft is placed between two layers of moist gauze and the donor sites are dressed. The donor site is soaked with a dilute solution of epinephrine for hemostasis, and a sterile dressing is applied. A pressure dressing is then placed over the site; this dressing can be removed on the seventh postoperative day. The sterile dressing dries in place over the donor site and ultimately will fall off by itself. Moistened areas on the dressing can be dried with cool air. If there is separation and evidence of some superficial infection, then merbromin can be applied to these areas.

Creating the Neovaginal Space. The patient is placed in the lithotomy position and a transverse incision is made through the mucosa of the vaginal vestibule (Fig. 29.7A). The space between the urethra and bladder anteriorly and the rectum posteriorly is dissected until the undersurface of the peritoneum is reached. This step may be safer with a catheter in the urethra and sometimes a finger in the rectum to guide the dissection in the proper plane. After incising the mucosa of the vaginal vestibule transversely, the physician often is able to create a channel on each side of a median raphe (Fig. 29.7B), starting with blunt dissection and then dilating each channel with Hegar dilators or with finger dissection. In some instances, it may be necessary to develop the neovaginal space by dissecting laterally and bringing the fingers toward the midline. The median raphe is then divided, thus joining the two channels. This maneuver is helpful in dissecting an adequate space without causing injury to surrounding structures.

To avoid subsequent narrowing of the vagina at the level of the urogenital diaphragm, it may be helpful to incise the margin of the puborectalis muscles bilaterally along the midportion of the medial margin (Fig. 29.7C). Although useful in all circumstances, incision of the puborectalis muscle is more important in cases of androgen

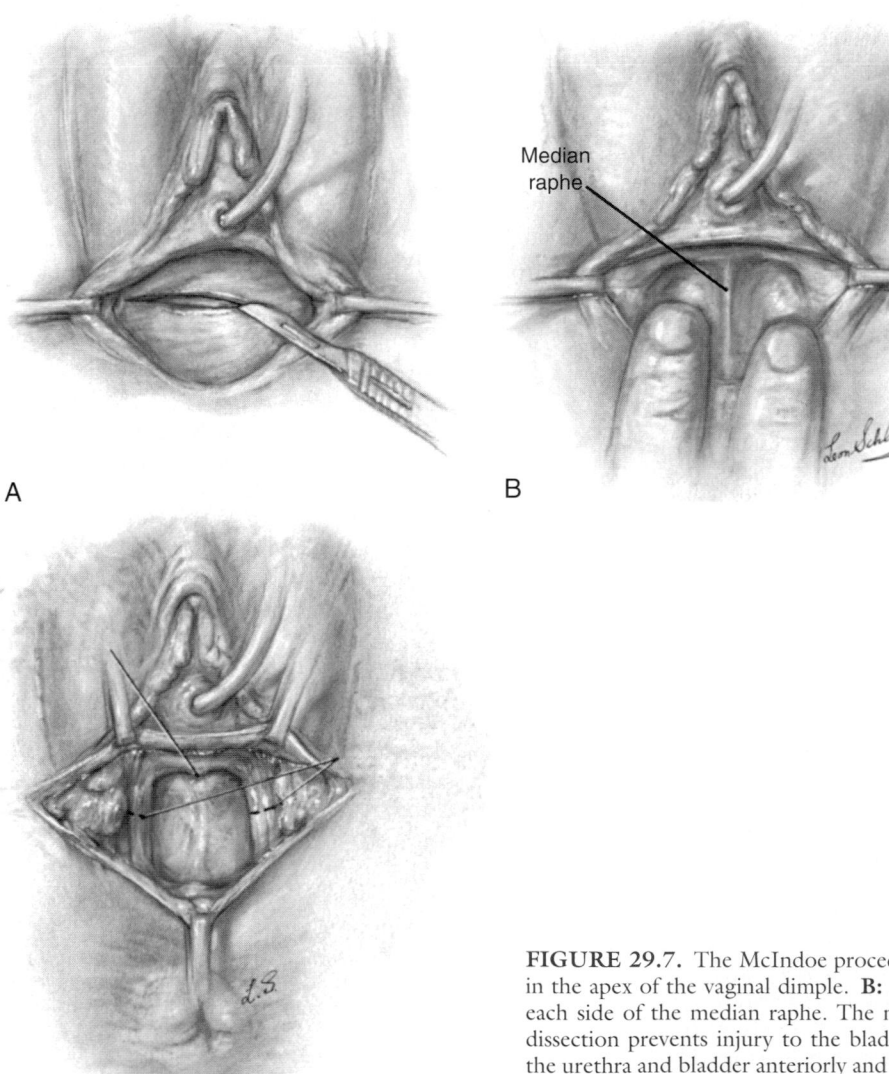

FIGURE 29.7. The McIndoe procedure. **A:** A transverse incision is made in the apex of the vaginal dimple. **B:** A channel can usually be dissected on each side of the median raphe. The median raphe is then divided. Careful dissection prevents injury to the bladder and rectum. **C:** A space between the urethra and bladder anteriorly and the rectum posteriorly is dissected until the undersurface of the peritoneum is reached. Incision of the medial margin of the puborectalis muscles will enlarge the vagina laterally.

insensitivity syndrome with android pelvis, in which the levator muscles are more taut against the pelvic diaphragm, than in cases of gynecoid pelvis. Incision of the puborectalis muscle causes no difficulty with fecal incontinence, significantly improves the ease with which the vaginal form can be inserted into the canal in the postoperative period, and has eliminated the problem of contracture of the upper vagina caused by a poorly applied form. The dissection should be carried as high as possible without entering the peritoneal cavity and without cleaning away all tissue beneath the peritoneum. A split-thickness skin graft will not take well when applied against a base of thin peritoneum. All bleeders should be ligated by clamping and tying them with very fine sutures. It is essential that the vaginal cavity be dry to prevent bleeding beneath the graft. Bleeding causes the graft to separate from its bed, resulting in the inevitable failure of the graft to implant in that area and in local graft necrosis.

Preparing the Vaginal Form. Early skin grafts were formed over balsa, which has the advantages of being an inexpensive, easily available, light wood that can be sterilized without difficulty. It also can be whittled easily in the operating room to a proper shape to fit the new vaginal space. However, uneven pressure from the form can cause a skin graft to slough in places, and pressure spots are associated with an increased risk of fistula formation. The Counseller-Flor modification of the McIndoe technique (Fig. 29.8) uses, instead of the rigid balsa form, a foam rubber mold shaped for the vaginal cavity from a foam rubber block and covered with a condom. The foam rubber is gas sterilized in blocks measuring approximately $10 \times 10 \times 20$ cm. The block is shaped with scissors to approximately twice the desired size, compressed into a condom, and placed into the neovagina (Fig. 29.8A through C). The form is left in place for 20 to 30 seconds with the condom open to allow the foam rubber to expand and conform to the neovaginal space (Fig. 29.8D). The condom is then closed and the form is withdrawn. The external end is tied with 2-0 silk, and an additional condom is placed over the form and tied securely (Fig. 29.8E and F).

Sewing the Graft Over the Vaginal Form. The skin graft is then placed over the form and its undersurface exteriorized and sewn over the form with interrupted vertical mattress 5-0 nonreactive sutures (Fig. 29.8G and H). Where the graft is approximated, the undersurfaces of the sutured edges are also exteriorized.

The graft should not be "meshed" to make it stretch farther, and the edges of the graft should be approximated meticulously around the form without gaps. Granulation tissue develops at any place where the form is not covered with skin. Contraction usually occurs where granulation tissue forms. After the form has been placed in the neovaginal space, the edges of the graft are sutured to the skin edge with 5-0 nonreactive absorbable sutures, with sufficient space left between sutures for drainage to occur. The physician must be careful not to have the form so large that it causes undue pressure on the urethra or rectum. A balsa form should have a groove to accommodate the urethra. With a foam rubber form, this is unnecessary. A suprapubic silicone catheter is placed in the bladder for drainage. If the labia are of sufficient length, then the form can be held in place by suturing the labia together with two or three nonreactive sutures.

Replacing with a New Form. After 7 to 10 days, the form is removed and the vaginal cavity is irrigated with warm saline solution and inspected. This is usually performed with mild sedation and without an anesthetic. The cavity should be inspected carefully to determine whether the graft has taken satisfactorily in all areas of the new vagina. Any undue pressure by the form should be noted and corrected. It is especially important that there not be too much pressure superiorly against the peritoneum of the cul-de-sac. Such a constant upward pressure could result in weakness with subsequent enterocele formation. The new vaginal cavity must be inspected frequently to detect and to prevent pressure necrosis of the skin graft.

The patient is given instructions on daily removal and reinsertion of the form and is taught how to administer a low-pressure douche of clear warm water. She is advised to remove the form at the time of urination and defecation, but otherwise to wear it continuously for 6 weeks. A neoprene form, which is much easier to remove and keep clean than a foam rubber form, is substituted for the original form in 6 weeks. A new form is molded with a sterile sheath cover (condom) to fit the size of the vaginal canal. The patient is instructed to use the form during the night for the following 12 months. If there has been no change in the caliber of the vagina by that time, then it is unlikely to occur later, and insertion of the form at night can be done intermittently until coitus is a frequent occurrence. However, if there is the slightest difficulty in inserting the form, then the patient should be advised to use the form continuously again. Most patients are able to maintain the form in place simply by wearing a panty girdle and perineal pad. Douches are advisable during residual vaginal healing and discharge.

RESULTS AND COMPLICATIONS

Results with the McIndoe operation have improved over the years. Recently reported percentages of satisfactory results have ranged from 80% to 100%. The serious complications formerly associated with the McIndoe operation have been significantly reduced by improvements in technique and greater experience. Serious complications do still occur, however, including a 4% postoperative fistula rate (urethrovaginal, vesicovaginal, and rectovaginal), postoperative infection, and intraoperative and postoperative hemorrhage. Failure of graft take is also still reported as an occasional complication. Failure of graft take often leads to the development of granulation tissue, which might require reoperation, curettement of the granulation tissue down to a healthy base, and even regrafting. Minor granulation can be treated with silver nitrate application. The functional result is more

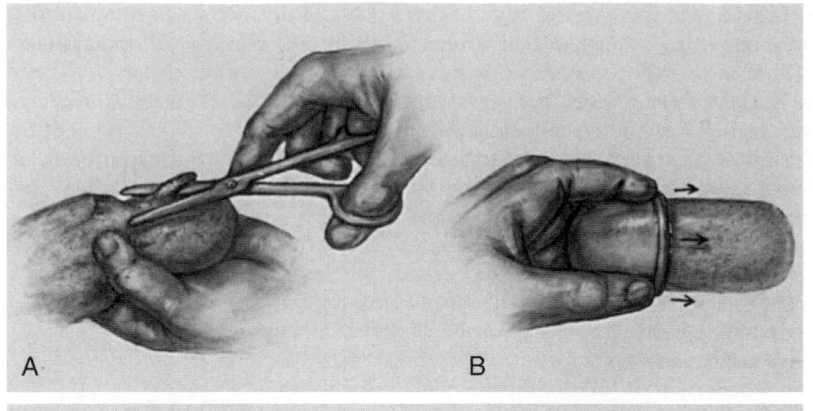

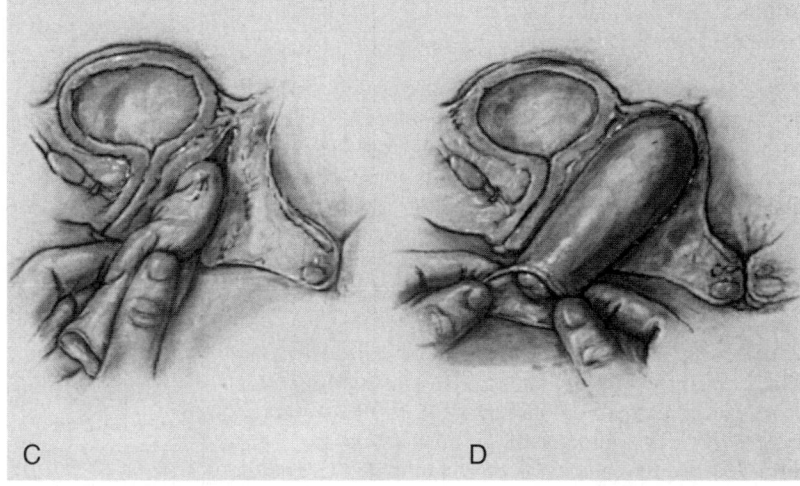

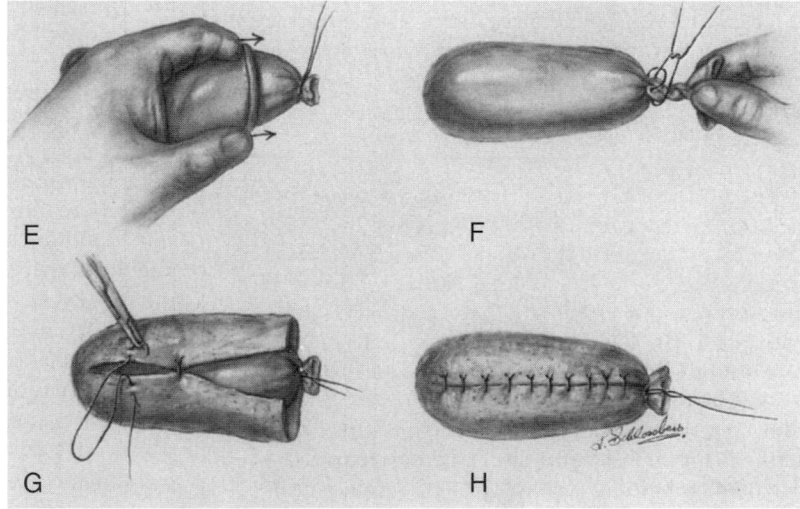

FIGURE 29.8. Counseller-Flor modification of the McIndoe technique. **A:** A form is cut from a foam rubber block. **B:** A condom is placed over the form. **C:** The form is compressed and placed into the vagina. **D:** Air is allowed to expand the foam rubber, which accommodates to the neovaginal space. The condom is closed and the form removed. A second condom is placed over the form (**E**) and tied securely (**F**). **G:** The graft is then sewn over the form with interrupted 5-0 nonreactive sutures. **H:** The undersurfaces of the sutured edges of the graft are exteriorized. The vaginal form is ready for insertion into the neovagina.

important than the anatomic result in evaluating the success of this operation. Although a vagina of only 4 cm is adequate for some couples, in most instances a vagina smaller than 4 cm causes major problems.

The postoperative results have improved significantly since the balsa vaginal form was replaced by the foam rubber form. Between 1950 and 1989, the McIndoe operation was performed on 94 patients at the Johns Hopkins Hospital. During these 39 years, 83% of the 94 pa-

tients had a 100% take of the graft; in only 3 cases was there a significant area over which the graft failed.

Urethrovaginal fistula has become even more infrequent since the introduction of the suprapubic catheter and the foam rubber form. The catheter is removed when the patient is voiding well and has no residual urine. In general, the patient is able to void without difficulty within the first few days of the procedure. Prophylactic broad-spectrum antibiotics started within 12 hours of surgery and continued for 7 days are of definite value in reducing the incidence of graft failures from infection in the operative site.

Because of the excellent results obtained after a modified McIndoe vaginoplasty, this operation is recommended as the procedure of choice for women unable or unwilling to obtain a neovagina with dilatation methods. Women with a flat perineum with no dimple or pouch have no alternative other than the McIndoe vaginoplasty to obtain a neovagina for comfortable sexual relations.

It is important that a McIndoe operation be performed correctly the first time. If the vagina becomes constricted because of granulation tissue formation, injury to adjacent structures, or failure to use the form properly, then subsequent attempts to create a satisfactory vagina are more difficult. The first operation has the best chance of success.

Ozek, like many other surgeons, modified the McIndoe procedure by describing an X-type perineal incision and the use of a perforated vaginal mold during the postoperative period. He postulated that this incision minimized stricture at the vaginal introitus and provided greater ease of dissection of the vaginal cavity. He reinforced that the overall procedure is simple with a generally uneventful postoperative course. Complications included infection, failure of skin graft take, stress urinary incontinence, partial graft loss, and vaginal stricture. All were treated satisfactorily except the patient with stress urinary incontinence.

Despite any minor modifications of the McIndoe vaginoplasty, the essential components of dissection of an adequate space, split-thickness skin grafting, and continuous dilatation during the contractile phase of healing remain unchanged. Recent reviews continue to support the safety and efficacy of the procedure. Hojsgaard and Villadsen reported 26 patients who underwent vaginoplasty, 18 of whom had Rokitansky syndrome. All patients were recorded as having a satisfactory result with complete graft take, adequate vaginal dimensions, and no strictures or fistulas giving symptoms. Complete take was achieved in 33% of patients within a week postoperatively, and after one further grafting procedure, an additional 38% had complete take. The intraoperative and early postoperative complications were perforation of the rectum in one patient (3.8%) and postoperative bleeding in three patients (11.5%). The late complications were vaginal stricture in three patients (11.5%), urethrovaginal fistula in two patients (7.7%), and rectovaginal fistula in one patient (3.8%). Alessandrescu and colleagues described the surgical management of 201 cases of Rokitansky syndrome. The surgeon substituted a modified transverse perineal incision and a perforated, rigid plastic mold. Intraoperative and postoperative complications consisted of two rectal perforations (1%), eight graft infections (4%), and 11 infections of graft site origin (5.5%). Sexual satisfaction was investigated with both objective and subjective criteria. Among the 201 cases, 83.6% had anatomic results evaluated as "good," 10% as "satisfactory," and 6.5% as "unsatisfactory." More than 71% of patients rated their sexual life as "good" or "sat-

isfactory" and reported that they had been able to experience orgasms related to vaginal intercourse. Twenty-three percent reported the ability to have sexual intercourse but had no ability to achieve orgasm and only 5% percent expressed dissatisfaction with their sexual performance. Strickland and colleagues reported on the coital satisfaction, perception of vaginal competence, and impact on lifestyle of adult women undergoing vaginoplasty as adolescents. Ten of 22 women responded to a questionnaire at a median of 18 years (range = 5–13 years) following surgical intervention with a McIndoe vaginoplasty. All of the women had sexual experience and 80% were sexually active at the time of evaluation. The most frequent difficulty reported was vaginal dryness and lack of lubrication with sexual intercourse. Ninety percent of the subjects expressed satisfaction that sexual ability was acceptable. This experience also supports the role of the McIndoe vaginoplasty in providing young women with vaginal agenesis long-term coital ability and minimal disabilities.

Development of Malignancies. At least 10 case reports exist of malignant disease developing in a vagina created by various techniques; these reports were reviewed by Gallup, Castle, and Stock. The authors reported a patient who was initially treated for intraepithelial malignancy by total vaginectomy combined with a split-thickness skin graft vaginoplasty to reconstruct a functional vagina. The authors noted a lesion in her vaginal apex 7 years later. These findings suggest that epithelium transplanted to the vagina can assume the oncogenic potential of the lower reproductive tract. It is therefore important that patients have long-term follow-up examinations after split-thickness skin graft vaginoplasty.

The Williams Vulvovaginoplasty

Construction of a perineal bridge to help contain the vaginal mold was a routine part of the operation described by McIndoe, but it was not adopted subsequently by others. However, Williams described a similar vulvovaginoplasty procedure in 1964 and advised that it could be used to create a vaginal canal. In 1976, he reported that the procedure was unsuccessful in only 1 of 52 patients. Feroze and co-workers reported that the anatomic results were good in 22 of 26 patients. According to these authors, the advantages of the Williams operation are its technical simplicity, its absence of serious local complications even when performed as a repeat procedure, the ease of postoperative care, the absence of postoperative pain, the speed of recovery, the possible elimination of dilators and consequent applicability to patients who do not intend to have regular intercourse in the near future, and the higher success rates of primary and repeat procedures. The technique is not applicable to patients with poorly developed labia. It does result in an unusual angle of the vaginal canal, which is reported to straighten to a more normal direction with intercourse. If a very high perineum is created, urine can momentarily collect in the pouch after urination, giving the impression of postvoid incontinence. Failure of the suture line to heal by primary intention results in a large area of granulation tissue and most likely an unsatisfactory result.

Williams believes that if the urethral meatus is patulous, a vulvovaginoplasty should not be performed because the urethra might be stretched further by coitus. He suggests that varying deficiencies in muscular and fascial tissue can explain why some patients with uterovaginal agenesis are able to develop a satisfactory vaginal canal with simple intermittent pressure with coitus, whereas others are prone to develop enteroceles.

The technique of vulvovaginoplasty described by Williams is as follows (Fig. 29.9). A horseshoe-shaped incision is made in the vulva to extend across the perineum and up the medial side of the labia to the level of the external urethral meatus. The success of the operation depends on the appropriation of sufficient skin to line the new vagina. For this reason, the initial mucosal incisions are made as close to the hairline as possible and approximately 4 cm from the midline. After complete mobilization, the inner skin margins are sutured together with knots tied inside the vaginal lumen. A second layer of sutures approximates subcutaneous fat and perineal muscles for support. Finally, the external skin margins are approximated with interrupted sutures. If the procedure is performed properly, it should be possible to insert two fingers into the pouch to a depth of 3 cm. An indwelling bladder catheter is used. The patient is confined to bed for 1 week to avoid tension on the suture line. Examinations are avoided for 6 weeks, at which time the patient is instructed in the use of dilators.

Capraro and Gallego have advised a modification of the Williams technique. They make the U-shaped incision in the skin of the labia majora at the level of the urethra or even lower, claiming that this modification results in a vulva more normal to sight and touch and still

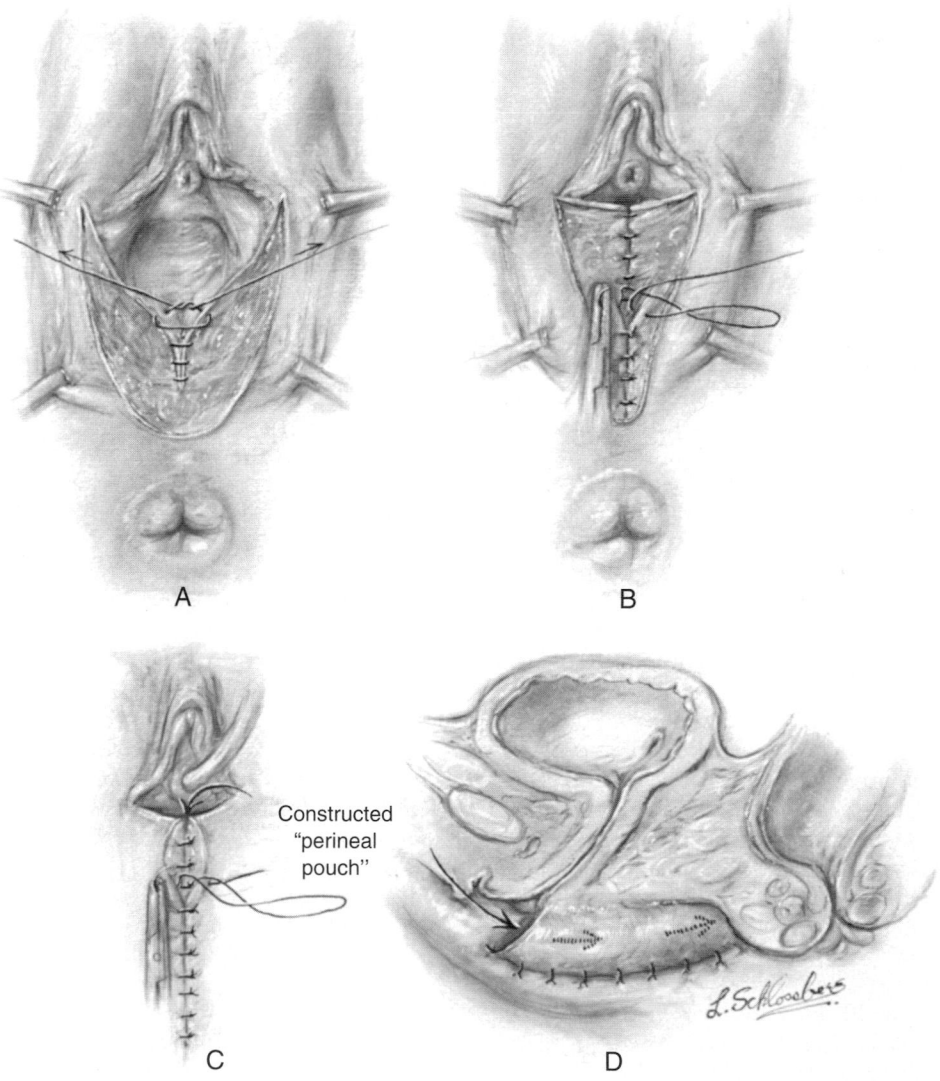

A   B

Constructed
"perineal
pouch"

C   D

FIGURE 29.9. The Williams vulvovaginoplasty. **A:** through **C:** No. 3-0 polyglycolic acid sutures can be used throughout to close both inner and outer skin margins and the tissue between. **D:** The entrance to the pouch should not cover the external urethral meatus.

satisfactory for intercourse, and that it avoids trapping stagnant urine in the vaginal pouch. Other modifications have been made by Feroze and associates and by Creatsas.

The Williams vulvovaginoplasty is a useful operation and should certainly be considered the operation of choice for patients needing a follow-up to an unsatisfactory McIndoe operation or a supplement to a small vagina resulting from extensive surgery or radiation therapy. Rarely does a patient with a solitary kidney low in the pelvis not have room for dissection of an adequate vaginal space.

Alternative Techniques

Several authors, including Adamyan and Soong and Templeman and colleagues, have described the laparoscopic use of the peritoneum to create a neovagina in patients with vaginal agenesis. Adamyan and Soong reported a group of 45 patients without significant postoperative complications. The most common postoperative problem involved the formation of granulation tissue at the vaginal vault. Templeman and others described the laparoscopic mobilization of peritoneum for the creation of a neovagina in only one patient. The peritoneum was grasped through a perineal dissection and sutured to the introitus. A pursestring closure was placed at the apex. Stenting of the neovagina was continued for 3 months postoperatively followed by rigid dilator use. At 9-month follow-up evaluation, an 8- by 2-cm vagina was described, with squamous epithelialization present. Both groups describe the technique as safe and efficient, producing a neovagina with apical granulation tissue as the only complication.

The Vecchietti operation was first described in 1965 by Giuseppe Vecchietti. He subsequently reported his cumulative 14-year experience in 1979 and 1980. Veronikus and colleagues reviewed the use of the technique and described a laparoscopic modification that uses cystoscopy to confirm bladder integrity. The Vecchietti procedure is a surgical technique for the treatment of vaginal agenesis that constructs a dilatation-type neovagina in 7 to 9 days. The procedure uses specialized equipment including a traction device, a ligature carrier, and an acrylic shaped olive. The process is in two steps, with essential operative and postoperative components. The operative phase involves positioning the olive at the perineum and the traction sutures extraperitoneally. Classically performed through a Pfannenstiel incision; the ligature carrier introduces the suture into a newly dissected vesicorectal space. The olive is threaded with suture at the perineum and the suture is reintroduced at the abdomen. The suture is then guided lateral to the rectus muscles bilaterally in a subperitoneal fashion and advanced along the sidewall. The traction device, which provides constant traction on the olive, is positioned on the abdomen. During the postoperative invagination phase, the neovagina is created by applying constant traction to the olive. The process reportedly occurs at a rate of 1.0 to 1.5 cm per day, developing a 10- to 12-cm vagina in 7 to 9 days. Patients are instructed on the use

of a vaginal obturator to be used as an outpatient. Borruto reported on Vecchietti's personal series of vaginal agenesis patients, comprising 522 consecutive patients. The surgical complications included one bladder and one rectal puncture with the ligature carrier and three cases of vaginal vault bleeding. At 100% follow-up at 1 month, dyspareunia was initially reported to be 12%, but resolved in all cases by 3 months. There were no reported failures of the neovaginal construction with 1- and 2-year follow-up of 70% and 30%, respectively.

Modifications of the Vecchietti approach include the use of laparoscopy and elimination of the dissection of the vesicorectal space. The first description of a laparoscopic modification was published by Gauwerky and colleagues. The vesicorectal space was dissected laparoscopically. The threads of the olive device were positioned using a probe introduced into the abdomen through the perineum. Six small abdominal incisions were used for laparoscopic instruments and the traction springs of the specialized device. In 1995, Laffarque and others described a laparoscopic intervention, creating a neovagina in three patients without dissection of the vesicorectal space. At completion of the procedure, cystoscopy was used to confirm bladder integrity. Some experts believe the theoretical risk of bladder or rectal perforation without the dissection of the vesicorectal space is unacceptably high. Fedele and others modified the approach to use a combined laparoscopic-ultrasonographic technique. The ultrasound assists in identifying the space of connective tissue between the bladder and rectum. The operating time for this modified procedure was only 40 minutes. After 10 days, the patient engaged in sexual intercourse. One-month evaluation confirmed a 12-cm vaginal length. Long-term follow-up outcomes are not available.

Bowel vaginoplasty is a well-known alternative for creation of a neovagina. The Ruge procedure and others are characterized by the formation of a neovagina using sigmoid colon grafts. Advocates propose that scar formation and vaginal stenosis occur less often than with other procedures; however, the disadvantage is the necessity of an abdominal laparotomy. Ota and colleagues reported a laparoscopic-assisted Ruge procedure. Mesenteric dissection and sigmoid resection were performed laparoscopically. A 3.5-cm incision was used for appropriate bowel suturing. The segment of sigmoid colon was mobilized and brought to the introitus. The serosal layer of the pediculate end was stabilized to pelvic peritoneum. The patient remained hospitalized for 14 days. The benefit of this modification is certainly the accomplishment of a difficult surgical procedure endoscopically. Other advantages include the functional, ample vaginal length (12 cm) without postoperative dilatation. Disadvantages include the extended postoperative hospitalization period and the small number of patients evaluated.

Makinoda and colleagues reported a nongrafting method of vaginal creation. This group reported 18 women who underwent a two-step protocol. The initial step used noninvasive dilatation using a vaginal mold based on the technique of Frank. The second step was a surgical procedure via a perineal approach. The apex of the dilated vaginal space was incised and further dissection between the bladder and rectum was carried to the peritoneal cavity. After peritoneal perforation, the uterine structures, when present, were pulled down and sutured to the newly created vaginal space. A firm vaginal mold was inserted and recommended for use for 6 months postoperatively. The authors propose a benefit of avoidance of grafting. The time course for success with the initial dilatation step may be unacceptably long in many patients (mean = 10.90 ± 9.8 months). No significant surgical complications were reported despite the theoretical risk of ureteral contortion and kinking when pulling the rudimentary uterine structures inferiorly. During the follow-up period, shrinkage of the vaginal length and diameter was noted in some patients who had been noncompliant with the mold or without coitus. The authors noted a minimal vaginal length of 5 cm in a patient who was noncompliant with the mold and nonsexually active. The authors dispute the necessity of any lining of the neovaginal space. In their experience, significant narrowing or contraction of the margins did not occur. They maintain that the vaginal space is maintained by suturing the muscular buds of the uterus to the pressure-created neovaginal space.

A spatial W-plasty technique using a full-thickness unilateral groin graft has been described in a limited number of patients by Chen and others. The authors advocate an earlier intervention with the premise that a full-thickness graft may grow as the patient grows. This is recommended to eliminate psychological issues in patients who would be treated during the late teens, when sexual identity may be forming.

Acquired Vaginal Insufficiency

Unusual types of infection and atrophy can rarely cause closure of part of the vagina, but acquired vaginal inadequacy most often is the result of treatment of various gynecologic malignancies with surgery or radiation, or a combination of both. Restoration and maintenance of vaginal function are important elements of the treatment plan for such malignancies, especially when the patient is young and otherwise healthy. The techniques of vaginal reconstruction in gynecologic oncology have been reviewed by Magrina and Masterson, by Pratt, and by McCraw and associates.

DISORDERS OF VERTICAL FUSION

The problems associated with vertical fusion include transverse vaginal septum with or without obstruction. Although imperforate hymen is a vertical fusion problem, the hymen is not a derivative of the müllerian ducts; therefore, this condition is discussed elsewhere (see Chapter 34).

Transverse Vaginal Septum

No reliable epidemiologic data exist regarding the incidence of transverse vaginal septum. Reported incidences vary from 1 in 2,100 to 1 in 72,000. It is probably less common than congenital absence of the vagina and uterus. It has been diagnosed in newborns, infants, and older adolescent girls. Its etiology is unknown, although McKusick has suggested that some and perhaps most cases are the result of a female sex-limited autosomal recessive transmission. There is a developmental defect in vaginal embryogenesis that leads to an incomplete fusion between the müllerian duct component and the urogenital sinus component of the vagina. The incomplete vertical fusion results in a transverse vaginal septum (AFS class IIA) that varies in thickness and can be located at almost any level in the vagina (Fig. 29.10). Lodi has reported that 46% occur in the upper vagina, 40% in the midvagina, and 14% in the lower vagina. Rock, Zacur, and associates have noted septa in the upper, middle, and lower thirds of the vagina in 46%, 35%, and 19% of patients, respectively. In general, the thicker septum is noted to be more common closer to the uterine cervix. In contrast to congenital absence of the müllerian ducts, the transverse vaginal septum is associated with few urologic or other anomalies. Imperforate anus and bicornuate uterus can be found, as reported by Mandell and colleagues. The lower surface of the transverse septum is always covered by squamous epithelium. The upper surface can be covered by glandular epithelium, which is likely to be transformed into squamous epithelium by a metaplastic process after correction of the obstruction.

In neonates and young infants, imperforate transverse vaginal septum with obstruction can lead to serious and life-threatening problems caused by the compression of surrounding organs by fluid that has collected above the septum. The fluid undoubtedly comes from endocervical glands and müllerian glandular epithelium in the upper vagina that have been stimulated by the placental transfer of maternal estrogen. Continued fluid collection in infants, even after the first year, has been reported; thus, the possibility of a fistula between the upper vagina and the urinary tract should be considered. The distended upper vagina creates a large pelvic and lower abdominal mass that can displace the bladder anteriorly, displace the ureters laterally with hydroureters and hydronephrosis, compress the rectum with associated obstipation and even intestinal obstruction, and limit diaphragmatic excursion to indirectly compress the vena cava and produce cardiorespiratory failure. Fatalities have been reported. The hydrocolpos develops along the axis of the upper vagina and therefore may not necessarily cause the outlet or perineum to bulge when there is compression of the mass from above. After careful preoperative radiologic and endoscopic investigations of the infant, the septum should be removed through a perineal approach. Bilateral Schuchardt incisions may be required to ensure that the septum has been removed. Because of the subsequent tendency for vaginal stenosis and reaccumulation of the fluid in the upper vagina, follow-up studies to assess the recurrence of urinary obstruction are important. Vaginal reconstruction may be required in later years to allow satisfactory menstruation and coitus.

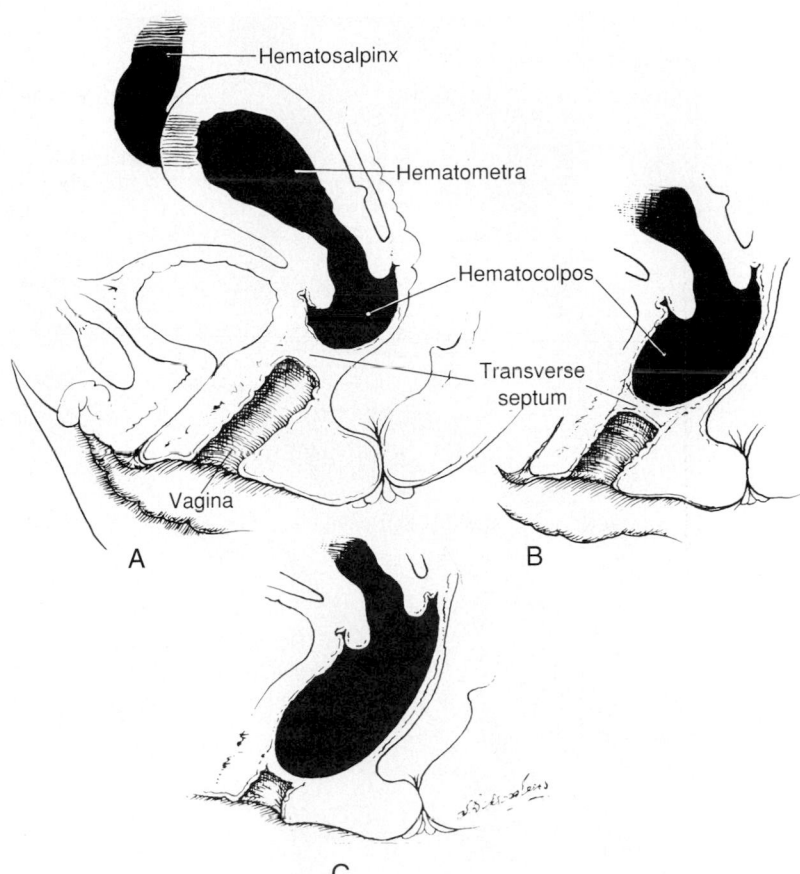

FIGURE 29.10. Positions of septum responsible for complete vaginal obstruction. High (**A**), mid (**B**)), and low (**C**) transverse vaginal septa. Note the position of the hematocolpos. Lower vaginal septa allow more blood to accumulate in the upper vagina. The vaginal mass shown in (**C**) is more accessible through rectovaginal examination.

A hematocolpos may not develop until puberty. Symptoms include cyclic lower abdominal pain, no visible menstrual discharge, and gradual development of a central lower abdominal and pelvic mass. Sometimes a small tract opens in the septum, some menstrual blood escapes periodically, and symptoms are variable. A septum large enough to allow pregnancy to occur can still cause dystocia during labor. Cyclic hematuria may be present if a communication between the bladder and upper vagina exists. The pelvic organs of a woman with a transverse vaginal septum are shown in Figure 29.11. The woman developed severe cyclic pain at the time of onset of menstruation, but there was no external bleeding until menstrual blood finally began to flow through the small sinus. Pelvic examination per rectum revealed a cervix and a normal-sized corpus. The ovaries were palpable but adherent, probably because of organized blood from hematosalpinx and hematoperitoneum. Remarkably, the woman had little dysmenorrhea after beginning to menstruate externally. Coitus was fairly satisfactory before surgical correction, but the shortness of the vagina was something of a handicap. The obstructing membrane was excised and an anastomosis of the upper and lower vagina was performed.

The findings of 26 patients with complete transverse vaginal septum reported from the Johns Hopkins Hospital by Rock, Zacur, and colleagues have shown that associated congenital anomalies include urinary tract anomalies, coarctation of the aorta, atrial septal defect, and malformations of the lumbar spine. Vaginal patency and coital function were successfully established in all patients, and 7 of 19 patients attempting pregnancy eventually had children. The incidence of endometriosis and spontaneous abortion was high. A lower pregnancy rate and more extensive endometriosis were present when the transverse septum was located high in the vagina, suggesting that retrograde flow through the uterus and fallopian tubes occurs earlier in these patients. More extensive dissection between the bladder and rectum was required to identify the upper vagina when the septum was thick and high. Exploratory laparotomy was necessary in five patients to guide a probe through the uterine fundus and cervix and to assist in locating a high hematocolpos.

Surgical Technique for a Transverse Vaginal Septum

A transverse incision is made through the vault of the short vagina (Fig. 29.11A). A probe is introduced through the septum after a portion of the barrier has been separated by sharp and blunt dissection. The physician usually finds some areolar tissue in dissecting the space between the vagina and the rectum. Palpation of a urethral catheter anteriorly and insertion of a double-gloved finger along the anterior wall of the rectum posteriorly provides the proper surgical guidelines so that

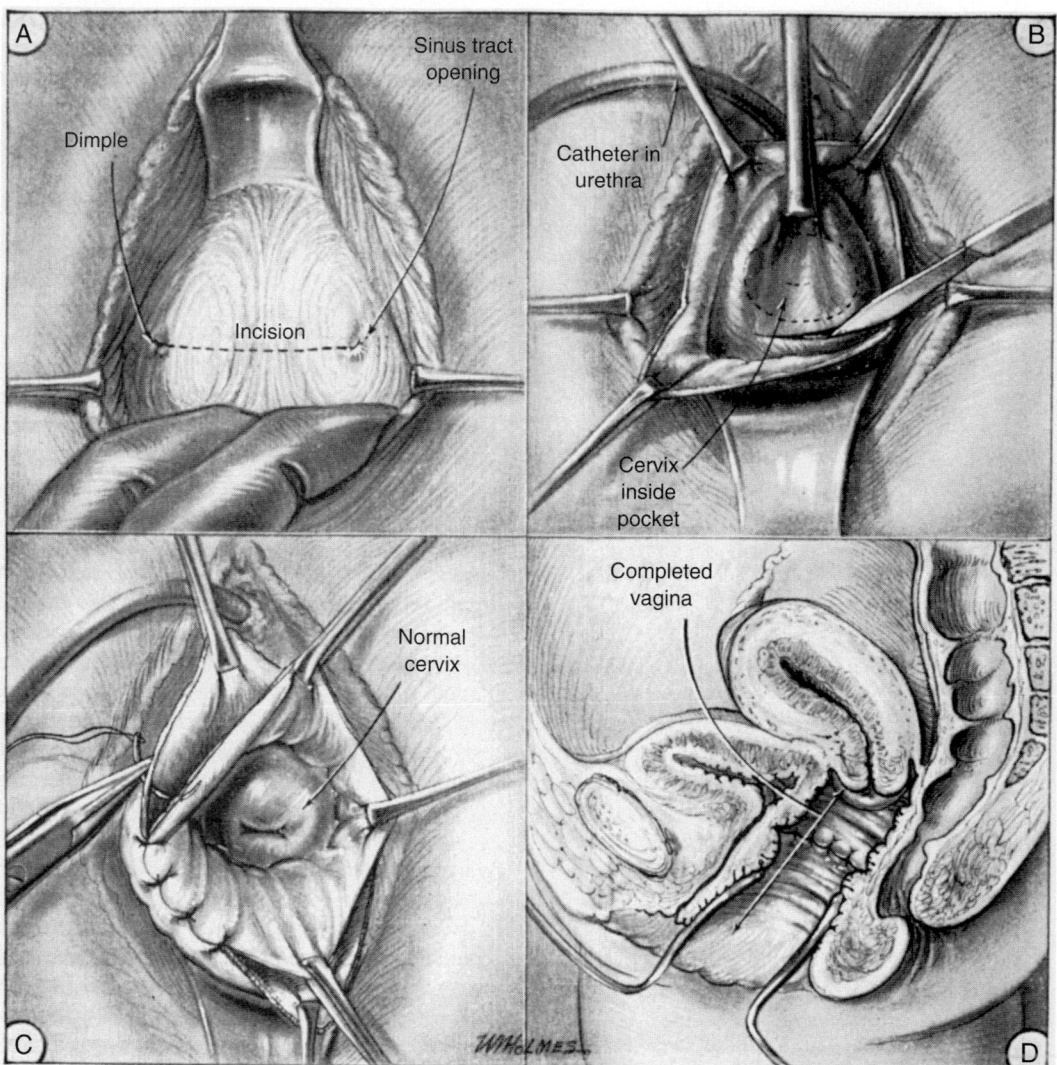

FIGURE 29.11. Surgical correction of transverse vaginal septum. **A:** The upper end of a short vagina. The small sinus tract opening, through which the patient menstruated, is shown. The line of incision is drawn through the mucous membrane between the vaginal dimple and the sinus. **B:** Areolar tissue is dissected through to the pocket of mucosa that covered the cervix. The mucosa is incised. **C:** An anastomosis is made between the lower vagina and the upper vagina. **D:** Completed vagina. It is slightly shorter than normal but of normal caliber.

the bladder and rectum can be avoided during this blind procedure. After the dissection is continued for a short distance, the cervix can usually be palpated, and continuity can be established with the upper segment of the vagina (Fig. 29.11B and C). The lateral margins of the excised septum are extended widely by sharp knife dissection to avoid postoperative stricture formation. The edges of the upper and the lower vaginal mucosa are undermined and mobilized enough to permit anastomosis with the use of interrupted delayed-absorbable sutures (Fig. 29.11C). Figure 29.11D shows the completed anastomosis with a vagina that is of normal caliber but has a length slightly shorter than average. A soft foam rubber vaginal form covered with a sterile latex sheath can be placed in the vagina and removed in 10 days for evaluation of the healing process. The form can be worn

for 4 to 6 weeks until complete healing has occurred. After this, coitus is permitted. If the patient is not sexually active, then vaginal dilatation may be necessary to maintain established patency. Alternatively, a silicone elastomer (Silastic) vaginal form can be inserted at night until the constrictive phase of healing is complete.

HIGH TRANSVERSE VAGINAL SEPTUM. If the length of the obstructing transverse vaginal septum is such that reanastomosis of the upper and lower vagina is impossible, as is the case with a high transverse vaginal septum, in which a significant portion of vagina is atretic, then a space is created between the rectum and bladder to permit identification of the obstructed vagina (Fig. 29.12). The mass that has resulted from accumulated menstrual blood must be distinguished from the bladder anteriorly

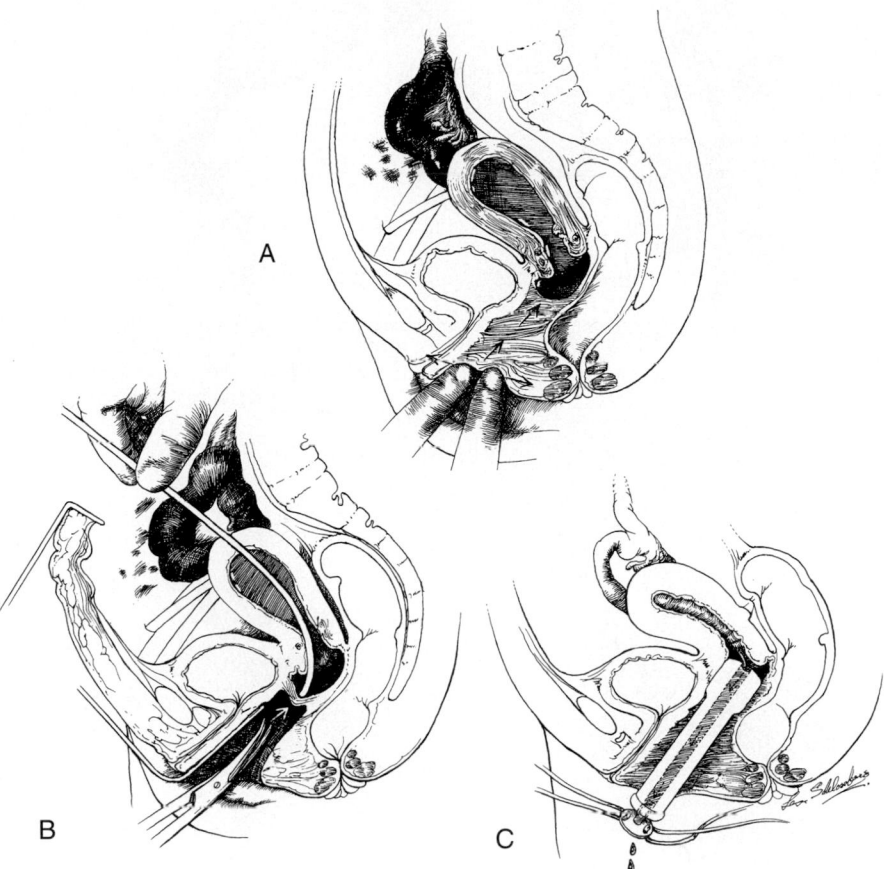

FIGURE 29.12. Correction of an atretic vagina. **A:** A large portion of atretic vagina is palpated with two fingers. Once the vaginal space is developed, it may be necessary to open the abdomen via laparotomy and pass a probe through to the uterine fundus **(B)** to tent out the septum, which may then be safely excised. **C:** An acrylic resin (Lucite) form is then placed into the vagina and secured with rubber straps.

and the rectum posteriorly, a process that is facilitated by the mass itself. When differentiation is impossible, however, exploratory laparotomy can be performed. During this procedure, a probe is passed through the fundus of the uterus to tent out the vaginal septum and enable the surgeon to excise it from below and resect it safely.

In most surgical procedures to remove the high transverse vaginal septum, the obstructing membrane can be readily identified (Fig. 29.13), after which the operator can probe the mass with an aspirating needle to identify old menstrual blood. The upper vagina is then opened and the septum excised. Because the distance between the septum and the upper vagina is too great to permit an anastomosis, an indwelling acrylic resin (Lucite) form, consisting of a bulbous end and a channel through which menstrual blood can drain, is placed into the vagina and anchored with a retaining harness. The bulbous end of the form, in most instances, is retained in the upper vagina and should be left in place for 4 to 6 months while epithelialization is accomplished. After its removal, vaginal dilatation should be practiced on a daily basis for 2 to 4 months to prevent contracture of the space. It is essential to the success of the operation that the new space not become constricted; to avoid constriction, the form must be worn for many months during the constrictive phase of healing. As an alternative to the Lucite form, the physician can consider using a split-thickness graft to bridge the gap. The graft is usually sutured *in situ* in the vagina rather than sutured to a form. An ingenious but rather complicated Z-plasty method of bridging the gap has been described by Garcia and by Musset. A simpler flap method was described by Brenner and associates.

A transverse vaginal septum diagnosed after the onset of puberty presents numerous problems. Often, a large segment of the vagina is absent, making anastomosis of the upper and lower segments difficult. Furthermore, postoperative vaginal dilatation is necessary to prevent stenosis at the anastomosis site. Poor compliance with dilatation in a poorly motivated pubertal patient is always a concern. However, rarely is the surgeon able to delay vaginoplasty until the patient is more mature because of increasingly severe cyclic abdominal pain caused by the hematocolpos. Thus, a difficult vaginoplasty can have less than optimal results.

Hurst and Rock have described an alternative approach to maximize surgical resection and anastomosis in women with a high transverse vaginal septum. Aspiration of the hematocolpos under ultrasound guidance was necessary to relieve the acute pain and delay surgery. Continuous oral contraceptives were used to delay recurrence of hematocolpos. Most important, vaginal dilatation was used to lengthen the lower vaginal segment to facilitate resection and reanastomosis (Fig. 29.14). In all three patients, the approach was successful.

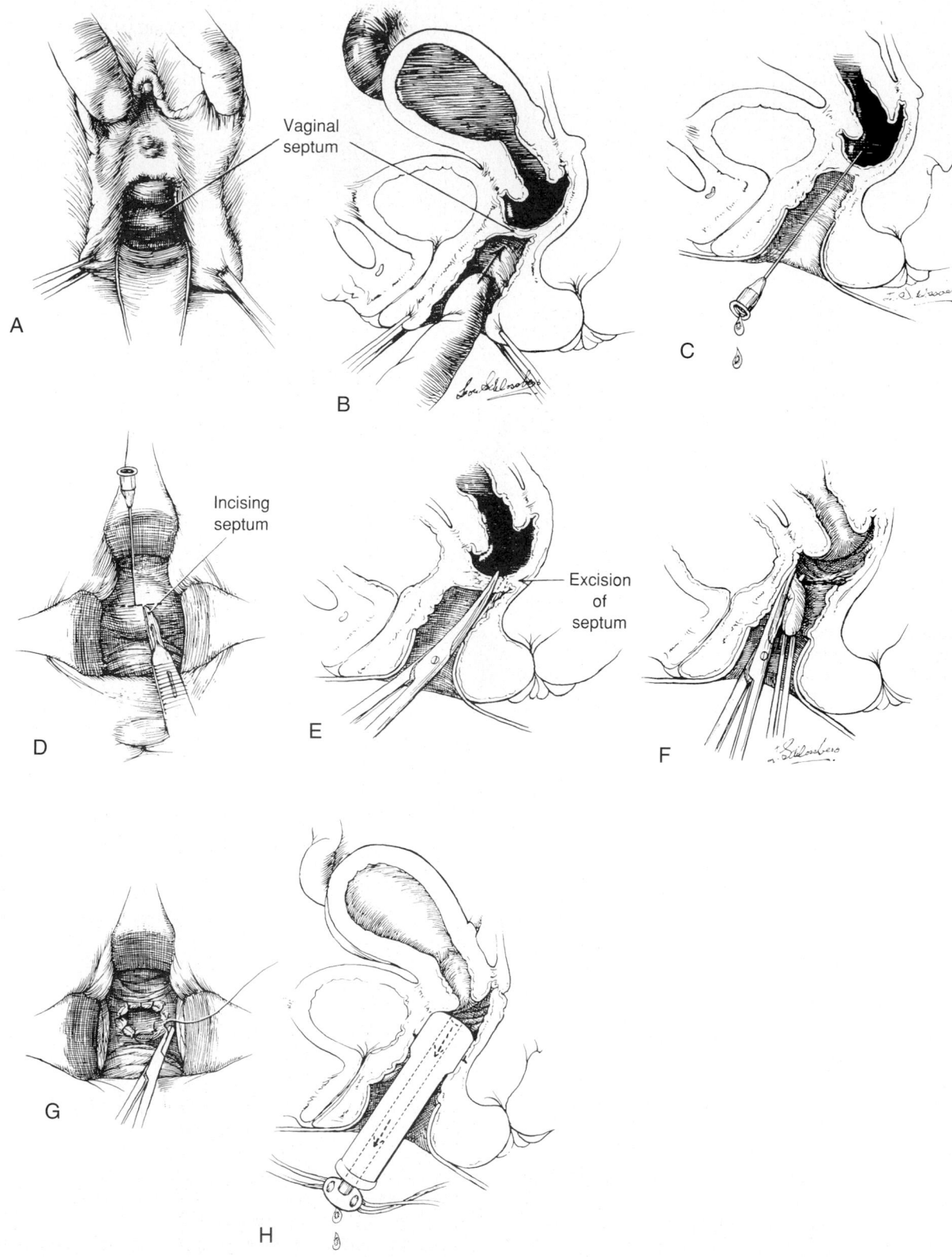

FIGURE 29.13. A high transverse vaginal septum. **A:** The neovaginal space is dissected, revealing a high obstructing vaginal membrane. **B:** This can be palpated with the middle finger. **C:** A needle is then placed into the mass. **D:** The incision is made with a sharp knife, and considerable bleeding can occur. **E:** The septum is excised. **F:** The septum is removed. **G:** After the septum is removed, the wall of the septum is oversewn with interrupted sutures of 2-0 chromic catgut. **H:** Because the distance between the septum and the upper vagina is too great to allow anastomosis, an acrylic resin (Lucite) form is placed in the vagina so that epithelialization can occur over the form while vaginal patency is maintained. The form, in place, is fitted with a plastic retainer. Rubber straps can be placed through the retainer and attached to a waist belt to allow constant upper pressure so that the form is retained in the upper vagina. Modification of this method includes a small adapter to allow drainage through the acrylic resin (Lucite) form, preventing the accumulation of old blood and mucus in the upper vagina. (From Rock J. Anomalous development of the vagina. *Semin Reprod Endocrinol* 1986;4:24, with permission.)

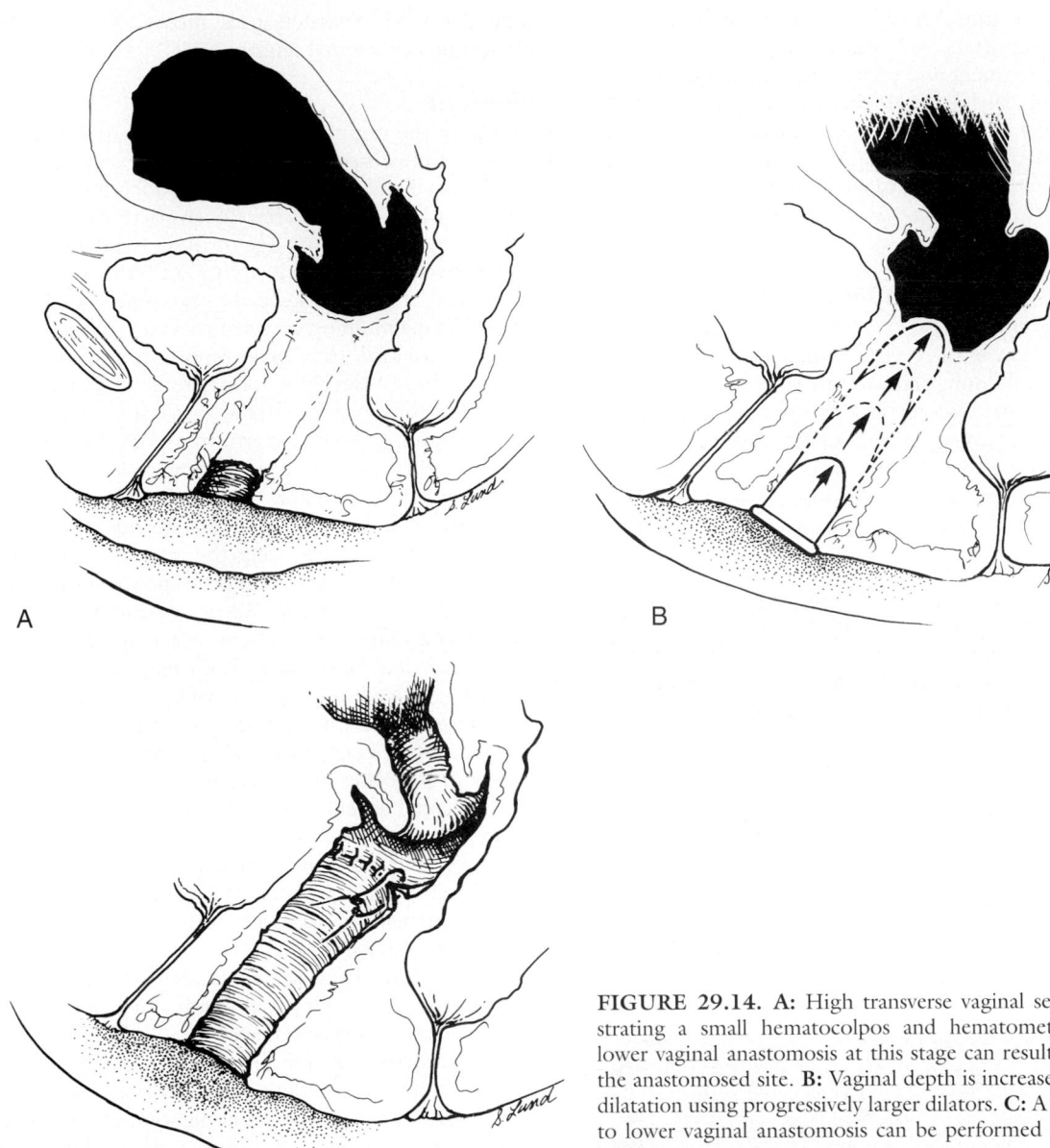

A

B

C

FIGURE 29.14. A: High transverse vaginal septum demonstrating a small hematocolpos and hematometra. Upper to lower vaginal anastomosis at this stage can result in stenosis at the anastomosed site. **B:** Vaginal depth is increased with passive dilatation using progressively larger dilators. **C:** A primary upper to lower vaginal anastomosis can be performed easily after dilatation.

Congenital Absence or Dysgenesis of the Cervix

Agenesis or atresia of the cervix (AFS class IIB) is a relatively infrequent müllerian anomaly. When this anomaly does occur, it is often in association with absence of a portion or all of the vagina. In many cases of cervical agenesis or atresia, retention of menstrual blood initiates symptoms of cyclic lower abdominal pain without menstrual flow, causing the patient to seek gynecologic evaluation and care. In past times, diagnosis was suspected on the basis of a history and physical findings but was not proved until the time of surgery. Today, diagnosis of cervical agenesis or atresia is still usually difficult before operation, but the possibility of making a correct diagnosis before surgery does exist, with the help of modern diagnostic tools. Early diagnosis offers significant advan-

tages in patient care, the most important of which is effective presurgical planning and preparation.

Diagnosis of Cervical Dysgenesis

Patients with congenital absence of the cervix present a diagnostic challenge. Patients with cervical aplasia with a functioning midline uterine corpus have aplasia of the lower two thirds of the vagina with an upper vaginal pouch. Similarly, some patients have a considerable atretic segment of vagina and an upper vaginal pouch with a properly developed uterine cervix and corpus above. Differentiation of these two müllerian anomalies is essential. Ultrasonography may be helpful. Valdes and associates have reported the use of preoperative ultrasonography in the evaluation of two patients with atresia of the vagina and cervix. Magnetic resonance imaging

(MRI) has been found to be helpful in confirming this diagnosis, as reported by Markham and associates. The lower uterine segment and cervical tissue can be carefully examined (Fig. 29.15). With cervical dysgenesis there is no vaginal dilatation with the accumulation of blood, as seen with a high transverse vaginal septum. Both ultrasonography and MRI are most helpful when they are correlated with the findings of a careful pelvic examination under anesthesia.

Anatomic Variations of Congenital Cervical Anomalies

Two basic categories of cervical anomalies have been observed in several configurations. Patients exhibiting the first type, cervical aplasia, lack a uterine cervix (Fig. 29.16A), and the lower uterine segment narrows to terminate in a peritoneal sleeve at a point well above the normal communication with the vaginal apex. The second type, cervical dysgenesis, can be described as four subtypes:

1. Intact cervical body with obstruction of the cervical os (the cervix is usually well formed, but a portion of the endocervical lumen is obliterated) (Fig. 29.16C)
2. Cervical body consisting of a fibrous band of variable length and diameter (endocervical glands may be noted on pathologic examination) (Fig. 29.16B)
3. Stricture of the midportion of the cervix (which is hypoplastic with a bulbous tip and no identifiable cervical lumen) (Fig. 29.16D)
4. Fragmentation of the cervix (with portions that can be palpated below the fundus and that are not connected to the lower uterine segment) (Fig. 29.16E)

Associated anomalies of the urinary tract are rare, but they do occur. Variable portions of the vagina can be

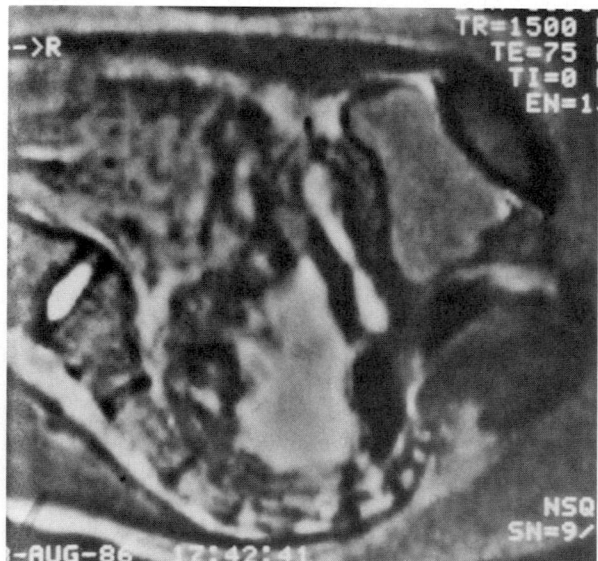

FIGURE 29.15. Magnetic resonance T1-weighted image showing atretic segment of distal cervix. The tip of an atretic cervix is shown. No vagina is noted.

atretic. Cervical obstruction is most often associated with a vagina of normal length.

Treatment

When both the vagina and cervix are absent and a functioning uterine corpus is present, it is difficult to obtain a satisfactory fistulous tract through which menstruation can occur. Many methods have been tried, most of them involving creation of a passage through the dense fibrous tissue between the uterine cavity and the vagina and placement of a stent to keep the tract open. Occasional successes in maintaining an open passageway and normal cyclic menstruation have been reported, but endocervical glands do not develop, and there is no way to compensate for the absence of the cervical mucus, which plays an important role in sperm transport. Even though cyclic ovulatory periods can be achieved in a few patients, pregnancy is unlikely. Eventually the uterovaginal tract closes from constriction by fibrous tissue. Endometriosis can develop along the tract. Endometriosis also can develop in ovaries and other pelvic sites because of retrograde menstruation. Recurrent and severe pelvic infection is a common problem and may require total hysterectomy and removal of both ovaries. As *in vitro* fertilization procedures began to offer the possibility for a host uterus to carry a pregnancy to term, procedures to establish a fistulous tract were abandoned. Nevertheless, Cukier and associates in 1986 reported treating a patient with congenital absence of the cervix by construction of a splint that extended into the neocervical canal such that a split-thickness skin graft could actually be placed within the endocervical canal. This patient has continued to menstruate without difficulty, although pregnancy has not been accomplished.

Many authors have recommended hysterectomy as an initial procedure for a patient with a functioning uterine corpus and congenital absence of the cervix and vagina. A hysterectomy eliminates much needless suffering from associated problems such as cryptomenorrhea, sepsis, endometriosis, and multiple operations. If the hysterectomy is performed soon enough, before the problems become great, it may be possible to conserve the ovaries and their useful functions. The reconstructive surgeon should be prepared to perform a vaginoplasty with use of a split-thickness graft if hysterectomy is performed, particularly if there has been a vaginal dissection. If the neovaginal space is allowed to close and scar, then future operations to develop an adequate neovagina are associated with increased risks of graft failure and fistula formation.

Despite the overall poor results from reconstruction for congenital absence of both the cervix and the vagina, clinical experience suggests that cannulization procedures can be worthwhile for a few carefully selected cases with adequate stroma to allow a cervicovaginal anastomosis. If a long segment of cervix is fibrous cord, a cervical grafting technique may be required. If a fragmented cervix is noted, then hysterectomy is usually warranted. Those few patients who have achieved a pregnancy after

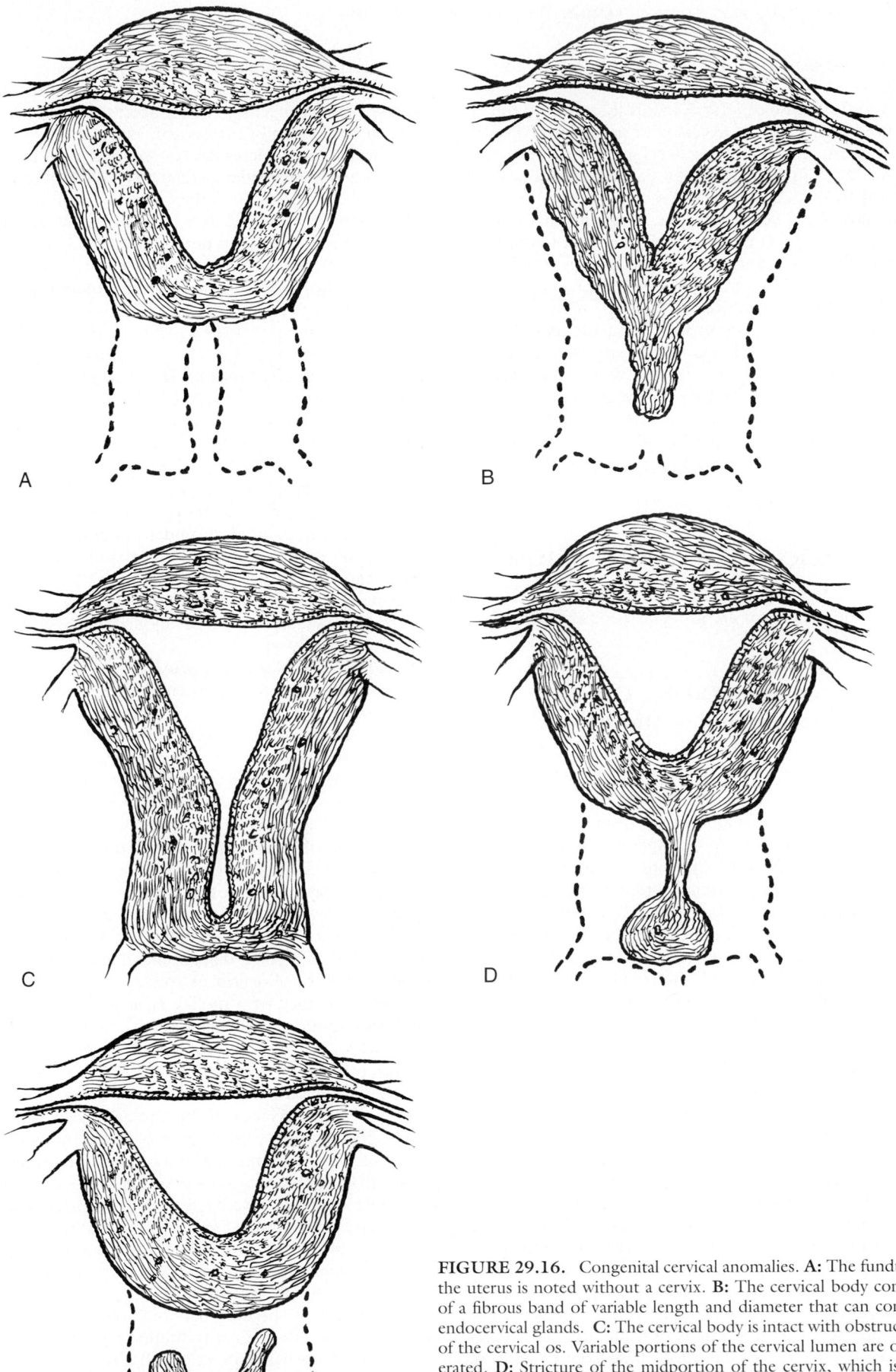

FIGURE 29.16. Congenital cervical anomalies. **A:** The fundus of the uterus is noted without a cervix. **B:** The cervical body consists of a fibrous band of variable length and diameter that can contain endocervical glands. **C:** The cervical body is intact with obstruction of the cervical os. Variable portions of the cervical lumen are obliterated. **D:** Stricture of the midportion of the cervix, which is hypoplastic with a bulbous tip. No cervical lumen is identified. **E:** Cervical fragmentation in which portions of the cervix are noted with no connection to the uterine body. Hypoplasia of the uterine cavity can be associated with cervical cord fragmentation.

cervical reconstruction have had a well-formed cervical body.

Anecdotal case reports occasionally appear in the literature confirming the necessity of palpable cervical tissue. Letterie described the development of a cervicovaginal tract in an adolescent patient with a core of cervical tissue. The tract has remained patent for menstrual flow for 2 years; however, pregnancy has not yet been attempted. Data published by the senior author regarding the long-term follow-up of 21 patients with abnormal cervical development support the success of cannulization in only selected patients with sufficient rudimentary cervical tissue. All of the patients with fragmentation of the cervix ($n = 4$) eventually underwent hysterectomy. Only those patients with a well-formed cervical body, with at least a palpable cord or only distal obstruction, achieved successful surgical outcomes (4/7 patients). Only one patient, with distal obstruction, treated with cannulization using a full-thickness skin graft, achieved pregnancy.

DISORDERS OF LATERAL FUSION

Failures of lateral fusion of the two müllerian ducts cause vaginal anomalies that are grouped as obstructed or unobstructed.

The Unobstructed Double Uterus (Bicornuate, Septate, or Didelphic Uterus)

Complete failure of medial fusion of the two müllerian ducts can result in complete duplication of the vagina, cervix, and uterus. Partial failure of fusion can result in a single vagina with a single or duplicate cervix and complete or partial duplication of the uterine corpus. A failure of absorption of the uterine septum between the two fused müllerian ducts causes the septum to persist inside the uterus to a variable extent while the external appearance remains that of a single uterus. The septum can be so complete that it divides both the uterine cavity and endocervical canal into two equal or unequal components. More often, incomplete disappearance of the septum leaves only the upper uterine cavities divided. Each of these and a variety of other forms of double uteri have their own individual features of clinical significance. When no obstruction is present, surgical reconstruction is performed primarily because of difficulties with reproduction.

Some aspects of lateral fusion disorders remain controversial because information is still inaccurate or incomplete. Many reports are based on small samples of selected patients, patients who have been diagnosed as having one anomaly or another based on incomplete data, and patients who have received unification operations without preliminary studies to rule out other causes of reproductive difficulty. A comparison of results from one series to the next is difficult because authors have used different classifications based on a variety of embryologic, anatomic, physiologic, functional, and ra-diologic considerations. Unknown numbers of uterine anomalies may have escaped detection because reproductive performance is generally acceptable and gynecologic difficulties do not necessarily occur.

The müllerian ducts undergo multiple steps in development including caudal, medial growth followed by fusion and later resorption of the remaining septum. Apoptosis has been proposed as a mechanism by which the septum regresses. Bcl-2, a protein involved in regulating apoptosis, was found to be absent from the septa of several uteri. The absence of this critical protein may play a pivotal role in the persistence of the septum and lateral fusion disorders.

Historical Development of Surgical Procedures

Ruge, in 1882, first reported excision of a uterine septum in a woman who had suffered two pregnancy losses. The woman subsequently carried a pregnancy to term. Paul Strassmann of Berlin and later Erwin Strassmann, his son, were strong advocates of uterine unification operations. The studies of Jones and Jones have contributed greatly to modern understanding of the management of uterine anomalies. Their studies began with a report in 1953 of a series that was started in 1936. Updates have been published from time to time. Wheeless, Rock, Andrews, and others have joined in these reports.

Diagnosis of Uterine Anomalies

If a uterine anomaly is associated with obstruction of menstrual flow, then it causes symptoms that will come to the attention of the gynecologist shortly after menarche. Unobstructed uterine anomalies are diagnosed later in a variety of circumstances. Young girls may notice difficulty in using tampons or later difficulty in coitus if a longitudinal vaginal septum is present. This can lead to the diagnosis of an associated uterine anomaly. A patient with an anomalous upper urinary tract on intravenous pyelogram may be found to have a uterine anomaly on gynecologic evaluation. A uterine anomaly is occasionally found when a patient complains of dysmenorrhea or menorrhagia or when a dilatation and curettage (D&C) is performed for abortion or some other indication. A palpable mass may be a uterine anomaly but should be confirmed as such by ultrasonography, hysterography, or laparoscopy. Woelfer and colleagues recently described the use of three-dimensional ultrasonography in screening for congenital uterine anomalies. During an investigation of the correlation of uterine anomalies with obstetric complications, the authors assessed the potential value of three-dimensional ultrasound for screening. More than 100 women with uterine anomalies were identified. Seventy-two arcuate uteri, 29 septate, and five bicornuate uteri were described. The authors emphasized how the three-dimensional ultrasound may overcome the limitations of conventional two-dimensional ultrasonography in providing a coronal view of the uterus, thus differentiating between arcuate, bicornuate, and subseptate uteri. This technique remains investigational. Semmens has pointed out that the diagnosis of a uterine anomaly can also be made from astute observation of an abnormal uterine contour during pregnancy, either in the antepartum period or at the time of abdominal or vaginal delivery. The abnormal contour is caused by a combination of fetal malpresentation and an anomalous uterus. An anomalous uterus can also be diagnosed when a pregnancy occurs despite the presence of an intrauterine contraceptive device. Persistent postmenopausal bleeding despite recent D&C can lead to a diagnosis of an anomalous uterus. Sometimes the diagnosis is made as an incidental finding at laparotomy. However, most uterine anomalies are diagnosed after hysterosalpingography to evaluate infertility or reproductive loss, usually from repeated spontaneous abortion.

Uterine Anomalies and Reproductive History
Although some uterine anomalies can cause infertility, most patients with uterine anomalies are able to conceive without difficulty. There is no question that uterine anomalies can be associated with perfectly normal reproductive performance. Overall, however, the incidences of spontaneous abortion, premature birth, fetal loss, malpresentation, and Caesarean section are clearly increased when a uterine anomaly is present. It is impossible to predict which patients with uterine anomalies will have these problems.

Etiology of Reproductive Failure
The etiology of reproductive failure in patients with uterine anomalies remains unclear. Mahgoub believes that the presence of a uterine septum can lead to abortion because of diminished intrauterine space for fetal growth or because of implantation of the placenta on a poorly vascularized septum. Mizuno and associates have attached importance to the inadequacy of vascularization of the uterine septum. Associated cervical incompetence, luteal phase insufficiency, and distortion of the uterine milieu have all been implicated in the etiology of increased reproductive loss. However, it is as yet unexplained why some patients with a uterine anomaly have normal reproductive function, whereas others abort early in pregnancy. Interestingly, it has been reported that the chance for a liveborn child increases with each pregnancy loss. It is unknown whether this apparent "conditioning" of the uterus is due to better vascularization, better myometrial stretching and accommodation, or some other factor.

A medical history of three or more episodes of spontaneous abortion or premature labor merits hysterosalpingography to determine whether structural abnormalities of the uterus are present. An abnormality is found in about 10% of such cases. Among chronic early second-trimester aborters, the incidence may be higher. The etiology of spontaneous abortion is complex, and a complete workup should be done even when an anomalous uterus has been found. A careful history should include a detailed discussion of each previous pregnancy loss and inquiry into DES exposure or other drug or chemical toxicity, specific medical illnesses, and exposure to contagious diseases. A family history should emphasize repro-

ductive failures among family members of both the patient and the husband. Specific medical diseases such as thyroid disease, diabetes mellitus, renal disease, and systemic lupus erythematosus should be ruled out. The possibility of infection by such agents as *Neisseria gonorrhoeae, Chlamydia, Mycoplasma, Toxoplasma,* and *Listeria* should be considered. Chromosome analyses should be done. Abnormalities in aborted tissue are found in more than 50% of spontaneous abortions, and abnormalities appear in up to one fourth of couples with a history of habitual abortion. Identifying such couples makes it possible to offer genetic counseling for subsequent pregnancies. Uterine leiomyomas, especially lower uterine segment and submucous leiomyomas, can cause spontaneous abortion. Basal body temperature charts, serum progesterone determinations, and endometrial biopsies timed in the luteal phase help determine the presence of luteal phase deficiency. The cervix should be studied for incompetence.

Couples with multiple etiologies for reproductive loss should have all other problems corrected before metroplasty is considered. Indeed, correcting other factors first may correct the problem of reproductive loss without metroplasty. In 1977, Rock and Jones reported on seven patients who had anomalous uterine development and extrauterine factors in the etiology of their reproductive loss. These patients had already had 16 pregnancies, 5 (29%) of which resulted in a liveborn child. After therapy to correct the extrauterine factor, the success rate increased to 71%. Stoot and Mastboom reported an impressive increase in reproductive performance among uterine anomaly patients by simple improvement of abnormal carbohydrate metabolism.

Hysterographic Studies
Proper technique during the performance of hysterosalpingography to diagnose uterine anomalies is important. The hysterogram must be taken at right angles to the axis of the uterus for a true assessment of the deformity to be made. The study is best done under fluoroscopy. A septate uterus cannot be distinguished from a bicornuate uterus by hysterogram alone (Fig. 29.17). The external uterine configuration also cannot usually be determined by pelvic examination alone, but some idea of the configuration can be obtained by ultrasonography. McDonough and Tho have suggested the use of double-contour pelvic pneumoperitoneum-hysterographic studies for precise identification of müllerian malformations. Of course, laparoscopy is even more certain. If the uterine corpus has not been previously visualized, the physician must be prepared to correct either anomaly (i.e., obstructed or unobstructed), depending on the findings at laparotomy.

Additional Testing
A complete investigation should also include an assessment of tubal patency and an intravenous pyelogram. A variety of upper urinary tract anomalies are seen, including absence of one kidney, horseshoe kidney, pelvic kidney, duplication of the collecting system, and ectopically

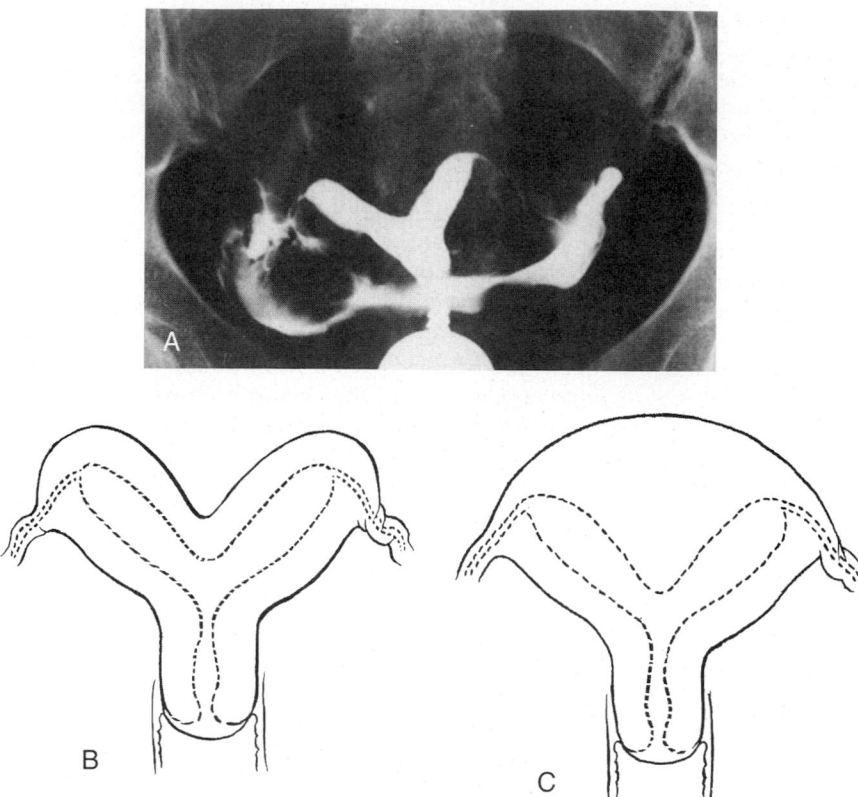

FIGURE 29.17. A: A hysterogram of a double uterus. A bicornuate uterus (**B**) and a septate uterus (**C**) are types of double uteri. Visualization of the fundus is required to determine the type of uterus.

located ureteral orifices. The lower urinary tract (bladder and urethra) is much less often anomalous.

The Double Uterus and Obstetric Outcome

The percentage of full-term pregnancies with various types of double uteri in an unselected series of women who have not been operated on is unknown. For all types combined, it is probably approximately 25%. In patients selected for operation, it probably increases from approximately 5% to 10% to approximately 80% to 90%. Because patients with uterine anomalies who have relatively normal obstetric histories cannot be identified, there is confusion in the literature about which anomalies are more often associated with obstetric difficulties and which are relatively benign in their effect. Special diagnostic procedures to detect uterine anomalies are not usually performed before reproductive performance is tested. A didelphic uterus is the exception. This anomaly can be diagnosed easily on routine pelvic examination by identification of two complete cervices and perhaps also a longitudinal vaginal septum. A study by Heinonen in Finland of 182 women with uterine anomalies indicated that pregnancies in the septate uterus had a better fetal survival rate (86%) than they did in the complete bicornuate uterus (50%) or in the unicornuate uterus (40%). These findings differ from prevailing opinions that the septate uterus is associated with the highest reproductive loss, as proposed by Jones and Jones. A recent report by Woefler and others supports Jones and Jones' opinions by noting that women with a septate uterus had a signif-

icantly higher proportion of first trimester loss than women with a normal uterus.

In 1968, Capraro and colleagues reported on 85 patients with uterine anomalies seen between 1962 and 1966. One uterine anomaly was seen for every 645 admissions (0.145%). Metroplasty was considered necessary in only 14 (16%) of these 85 cases. According to Jones and Jones, only one third of patients with a double uterus have important reproductive problems. In most instances, the presence of a double uterus is not in itself an indication for metroplasty.

In 1980, Jewelewicz and co-workers estimated the spontaneous abortion rate to be 33.8% in women with a bicornuate uterus, 22.2% in those with a septate uterus, and 34.6% in those with a unicornuate uterus. More recently, Ludmir and associates reported that high-risk obstetric intervention did not significantly increase the fetal survival rate for uncorrected uterine anomalies. Capraro and associates found a preoperative fetal salvage rate of 33.3% for the septate uterus, 10% for the bicornuate uterus, and 0% for the didelphic uterus. Postoperatively, the fetal salvage rate was 100% for the bicornuate uterus, 80% for the septate uterus, and 66% for the didelphic uterus. The report gives the improved salvage figures, compared with several previous studies, after abdominal metroplasty.

Ravasia and others described the incidence of uterine rupture in a cohort of women with müllerian duct anomalies who attempted vaginal birth after prior Caesarean delivery (VBAC). Of the 1,813 patients who attempted VBAC between 1992 and 1997, only 25 patients with known müllerian duct anomalies attempted a trial of labor. This included 14 patients with a bicornuate uterus, five with a septate uterus, four with a unicornuate uterus, and two with uterine didelphys. Uterine rupture was diagnosed in two patients with müllerian anomalies. The authors proposed several mechanisms for the greater incidence of uterine rupture in this population: abnormal development of the lower uterine segment, previous scar similar to a vertical or classic incision, and the possibility of abnormal traction on the uterine scar during labor.

THE DIDELPHIC UTERUS. A didelphic uterus with two hemicorpora is easily diagnosed because all patients have two hemicervices visible on speculum examination, and most, if not all, have a longitudinal sagittal vaginal septum. In the series reported by Heinonen and associates, all 21 patients with a didelphic uterus had a vaginal septum. Conversely, a patient with a longitudinal vaginal septum usually has a didelphic uterus. The indication for uterine unification is related to the role of this anomaly as an etiologic factor in reproductive loss. Of all the uterine anomalies (except arcuate uterus), the didelphic uterus is associated with the best possibility of a successful pregnancy. However, there is still some increase in perinatal mortality, premature birth, breech presentation, and Caesarean section for delivery. Heinonen and associates reported a fetal survival rate of 64% without metroplasty. Musich and Behrman stated that the didelphic uterus offers the best chance for a successful pregnancy (57%) and should not be considered an appropriate indication for metroplasty. However, W. S. Jones considered the didelphic uterus to give the worst obstetric outcome. In the opinion of the editors of this book, a unification operation for a didelphic uterus is not often indicated, and the results may be disappointing, especially when an attempt is made to unify the cervix. Not only is this procedure technically difficult in a complete didelphic anomaly, but it can also result in cervical incompetence or cervical stenosis.

THE SEPTATE UTERUS. Most patients who are evaluated for repeated abortion and who are found to have a uterine anomaly have a septate uterus. A few have other anomalies, mostly the bicornuate uterus. In our experience, fetal survival rates are higher after septate uterus repair than after other repairs. In 1977, Rock and Jones reported on 43 patients with septate uteri selected for Jones metroplasty at the Johns Hopkins Hospital. Of these 43 patients, 95% became pregnant postoperatively, 73% carried to term, and 77% delivered a liveborn child. Similarly, hysteroscopic metroplasty for the septate uterus provides a substantial improvement in obstetric outcome. Data obtained from retrospective studies suggest that hysteroscopic metroplasty is associated with favorable outcomes, with a pregnancy rate of approximately 80% and a miscarriage rate of only approximately 15%. Recently, the histologic features of the septum in this abnormal uterus have been described. Dabirashrafi

and colleagues noted less connective tissue in uterine septa. Poor decidualization and placentation were suggested as a cause.

Finally, the AFS class VA uterus (a double cervix and uterine cavity with a single fundus) can result from a rotation abnormality during the descent of the müllerian ducts. Among the reported cases of the septate uterus, the incidence of the complete septum involving the cervix varies from 4% to 29%. If the dextrorotating müllerian ducts overrotate, the senior author theorizes (J. A. Rock, personal observations, 1991) that the septum fails to absorb after fusion of the ducts. In virtually every patient with a complete septate uterus, the left cervix is higher than the right. In one patient, one cervix has been noted above the other (Fig. 29.18). This rotation abnormality may be a factor associated with lack of absorption of the uterine septum in these patients.

Uterine Anomalies and Menstrual Difficulties
Dysmenorrhea and abnormal and heavy menstrual bleeding have been reported to occur more frequently with any form of double uterus and to be relieved after unification operations. Capraro and associates reported several cases in which dysmenorrhea was cured by metroplasty. Erwin Strassmann also believed that all cases of dysmenorrhea and menorrhagia associated with uterine anomalies were relieved by unification of the two uterine cavities. Generally, however, dysmenorrhea and menorrhagia are inappropriate indications for uterine unification, and the operation should not be performed solely for these reasons.

Uterine Anomalies and Infertility
Opinions differ considerably in terms of whether infertility is a proper indication for metroplasty. Erwin Strassmann stated that primary infertility could be cured in 60% of patients with uterine anomaly if all other causes of

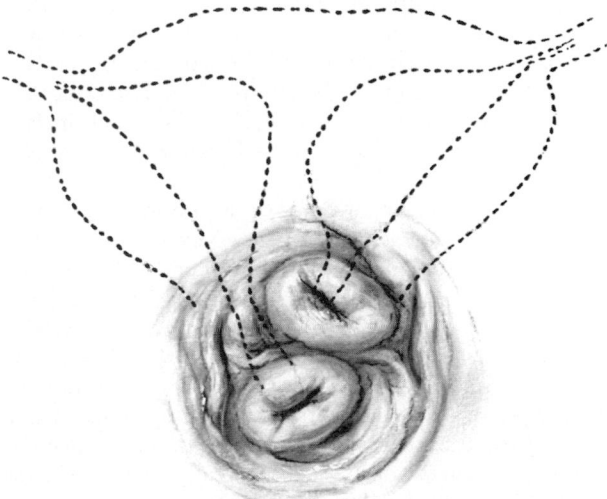

FIGURE 29.18. A double uterus with two cervices and a single fundus (class V). Note that the left cervix is positioned over the right cervix. This rotation abnormality may be a factor associated with a lack of absorption of the uterine septum.

infertility were excluded. Strassmann reported eight metroplasties for primary sterility that yielded nine pregnancies and seven liveborn children, although the number of patients who conceived was not given. Similar reports of small numbers of patients can be found throughout the literature. Heinonen and Pystynen indicated that uterine anomalies are rarely the reason for infertility. Nonuterine causes of infertility must be ruled out before metroplasty, as a last resort, is considered.

Certainly, a full infertility investigation to rule out other causes should be completed before the anomalous uterus is blamed. Even when no other cause for infertility is found, if the uterus is septate or bicornuate, then there may not be any proper indication for metroplasty. This question of when to perform metroplasty simply has not yet been answered. The decision is difficult, and becomes even more difficult, when the opportunity for metroplasty presents itself because a septate or bicornuate uterus requires laparotomy for some other reason, such as endometriosis or tubal occlusion.

Surgical Technique for Uterine Unification

Traditionally, the septate uterus has been unified with either the Jones or the Tompkins procedure. Clinical reports by Chervenak and Neuwirth, Daly, Walters, and co-workers, DeCherney and associates, and Israel and March have favorably compared hysteroscopic or resectoscopic incision of a uterine septum with the more traditional transabdominal approach. Term pregnancy rates after these procedures have approached 80% to 85%. Several attempts may be necessary to incise a wide septum, although the septum usually can be incised completely at the first operation.

TRANSCERVICAL LYSIS OF THE UTERINE SEPTUM. Abdominal metroplasty for transfundal incision or for excision of the septum associated with the septate uterus generally has been abandoned. With hysteroscopic scissors, the procedure can be tedious, especially with a large, broad septum. Although the hysteroscope and scissors are still used for cutting the septum, the resectoscope has been found to be comparable. The optics are excellent, and the septum can be electrosurgically incised with little difficulty. Laser-assisted procedures have also been described.

Before transcervical lysis of a uterine septum, a gonadotropin-releasing hormone agonist may be given for 2 months to reduce the amount of endometrium that can obscure the surgeon's view during the procedure. Many authors do not consider routine preoperative preparation of the endometrium essential and may only use medications in procedures involving exceptionally wide septa or complete septa that involve the lower one third of the uterine cavity or the cervical canal. If medical preparation is not used, surgical intervention should be scheduled during the early proliferative phase of the cycle to avoid bleeding and impaired visualization from a vascular endometrium associated with the secretory phase. Transcervical lysis is usually performed in conjunction with laparoscopy under general endotracheal anesthesia. The uterine cavity is distended with dextran 70 (Hyskon) by way of the resectoscope, which is inserted into the cervix. The septum is then electrosurgically incised by advancing the cutting loupe, using the trigger mechanism of the resectoscope. The uterine septum is incised until the tubal ostia are visualized and there is no appreciable evidence of the septum. The procedure is performed under simultaneous laparoscopy to limit the risks of uterine perforation. The laparoscopic light can be turned off so that the light from the hysteroscope can be clearly visualized through the fundus. Most patients can be discharged within 4 hours of the procedure. There is no role for placement of a postoperative intrauterine device. The benefit of routine procedure-related antibiotic therapy has not been well supported with evidence; however, it is recommended to administer antibiotics before the procedure and to continue for 5 days after surgery to limit the risks of infection. If excessive bleeding occurs after the procedure, a Foley catheter should be placed in the uterine cavity for tamponade and removed in 4 to 6 hours. Hormonal therapy is the most commonly used postoperative treatment regimen. The aim of the treatment is the promotion of rapid epithelialization. Dabirashrafi and colleagues reported that estrogen therapy did not appear to demonstrate a benefit. Further evidence is necessary before dismissing the current trend of postoperative estrogen therapy.

Transcervical lysis also can be performed to repair a complete septate uterus (i.e., a single fundus with two cavities and two cervices). In this instance, a no. 8 Foley catheter is inserted into one cervix and indigo carmine is injected into the cavity. The other cavity is distended with dextran 70 (Hyskon) by way of the resectoscope. The septum is electrosurgically incised at a point above the internal cervical os until the Foley catheter is visualized. The septum is then incised in a superior direction until the tubal ostium is visualized and there is no appreciable septum (Fig. 29.19).

After transcervical lysis of a uterine septum, a 2-month delay before attempting pregnancy is suggested to allow complete resorption of the septum. Delivery may be vaginal. The Jones procedure is used to repair a septate uterus when a particularly broad septum cannot be easily incised with the resectoscope. The Strassmann procedure is used for unification of a bicornuate uterus. The safety and efficacy of hysteroscopic resection of the uterine septum in patients with a class Va septate uterus has been demonstrated by the senior author. Historically, case reports such as that of Hundley and colleagues, was the only source of information about this interesting variant; however, one of the largest populations of patients with a complete septum was reported in 1999 by Roberts and Rock. The patients underwent hysteroscopic metroplasty with preservation of the cervical portion of the septum. With the exception of one case of pulmonary edema, no significant intraoperative or postoperative complications were reported. Postoperative hysteroscopy revealed only minor fundal septal remnants without clinical significance.

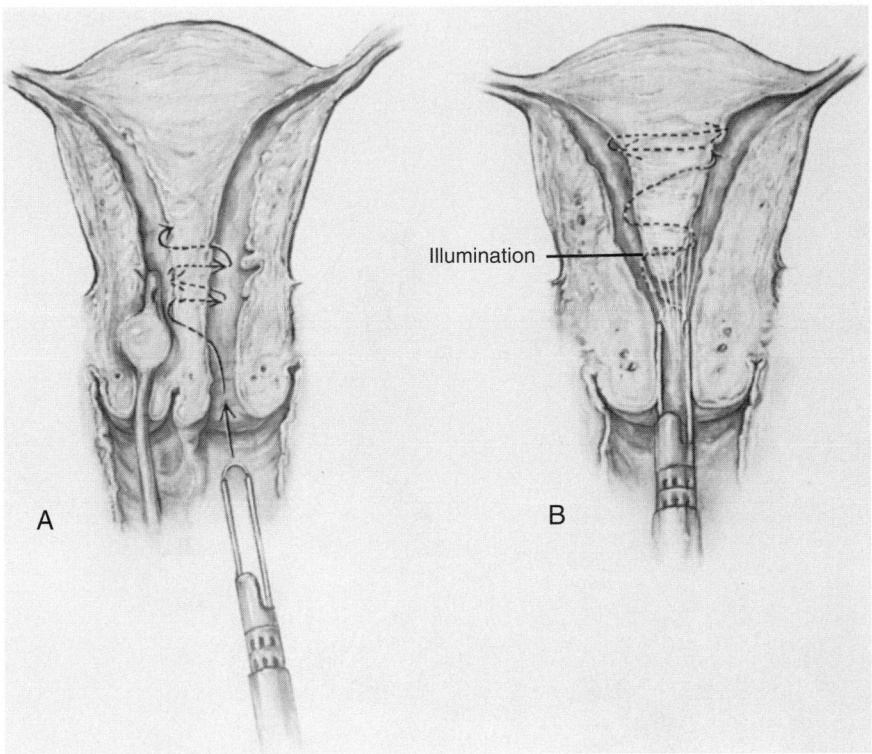

Illumination

FIGURE 29.19. Resectoscopic metroplasty. **A:** A Foley catheter is placed in one cavity of a complete septate uterus (American Fertility Society class VA uterus). The resectoscope is inserted in the opposite cavity, and the septum is incised until the Foley is visualized. The septum can be easily incised with the resectoscope until both internal os are visible. **B:** A septate uterus with a single cervix. The septum can be incised with the straight loupe of the resectoscope.

THE MODIFIED JONES METROPLASTY. In the modified Jones unification operation (Fig. 29.20), the abdomen is generally opened through a transverse incision. If only the unification operation is planned, then a Pfannenstiel incision is permissible. The pelvic viscera are inspected. The septate uterus may demonstrate a median raphe across the fundus, but it is surprising how often the corpus looks normal. To facilitate manipulation, a traction suture of heavy silk is placed through the top of the septum. This suture is removed from the site when the septum is excised.

No attempt is made to stain the uterine cavity with methylene blue. Normal unstained endometrial tissue can be easily differentiated from the myometrium.

There are essentially two methods to control bleeding during this procedure. In the first, a tourniquet is applied at the junction of the lower uterine segment and cervix by inserting a 0.5-inch Penrose drain through an avascular space in the broad ligaments just lateral to the uterine vessels on each side. The tourniquet is placed around the lower uterine segment and is tied anterior to the uterus. Because the uterine corpus receives a significant blood supply through the ovarian arteries, tourniquets should also be tied around the infundibulopelvic ligaments on each side, using the same hole in the broad ligament. All tourniquets must be tied tightly enough to occlude both the arterial supply to and the venous drainage from the uterus. If only the venous drainage is occluded, then the corpus becomes engorged and congested and bleeding is increased. If the arterial supply is occluded, then the uterus blanches and the bleeding is minimal. A sterile Doptone can be used to establish dis-

appearance of uterine artery pulsations. Hypotensive anesthetic techniques used in conjunction with the tourniquets allows a uterine unification operation to be accomplished with negligible blood loss.

The alternative method for hemostasis uses up to 20 units of vasopressin that is diluted in 20 mL of saline and injected into the anterior and posterior walls of the uterus before the incision is made.

The uterine septum should be surgically excised as a wedge (Fig. 29.20D). The incisions begin at the fundus of the uterus. The approach to the endometrial cavity should be handled carefully so that it is not transected (Fig. 29.20E). The original incisions at the top of the fundus are usually within 1 cm, and sometimes even less, of the insertion of the fallopian tubes. If the incision is directed toward the apex of the wedge, however, there seems to be little danger of transecting the tube across its interstitial transit in the myometrium.

After the wedge has been removed, the uterus is closed in three layers with interrupted stitches; 2-0 nonreactive suture on an atraumatic tapered needle is convenient. Two sizes of needles are needed: a half-inch needle for the inner and intermediate layers and a large needle (three fourths half-round) for the outer muscular layer. The inner layer of stitches must include about one third of the thickness of the myometrium, because the endometrium alone is too delicate to hold a suture and will be cut through. The inner sutures should be placed through the endometrium and the myometrium in such a way that the knot is tied within the endometrial cavity (Fig. 29.20G–H). While the suture is being tied, the two lateral halves of the uterus should be pressed together

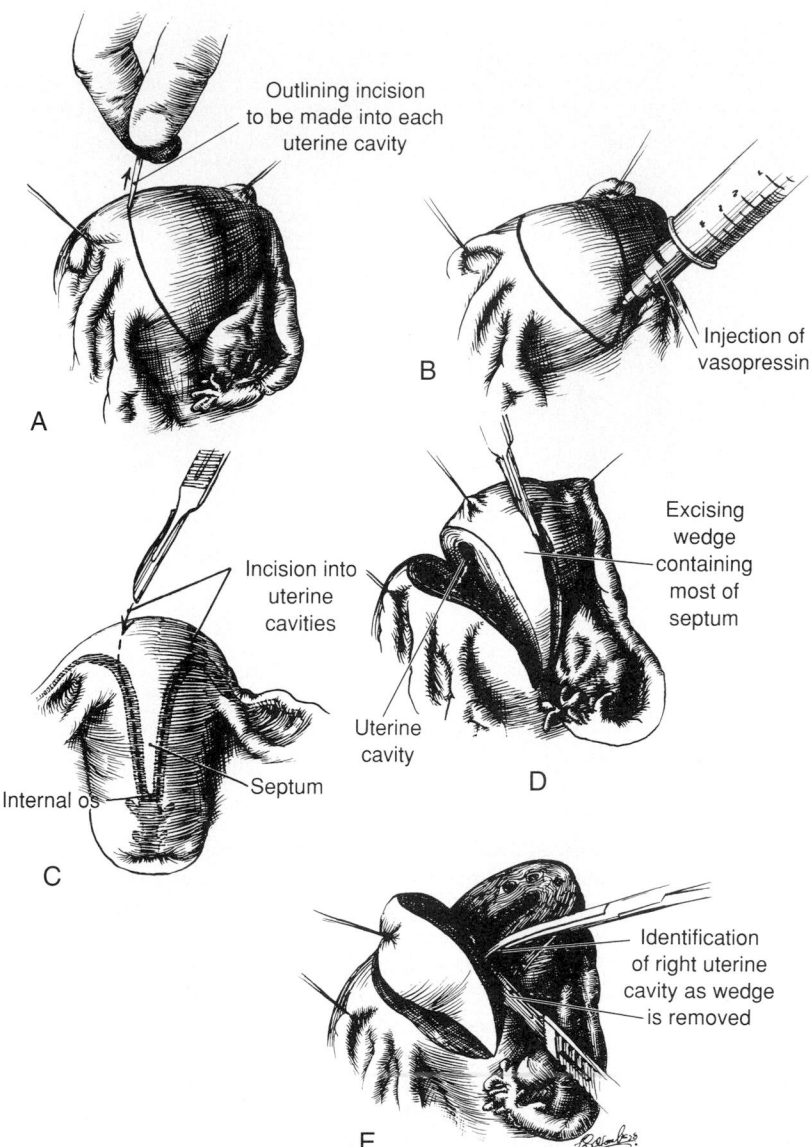

Outlining incision
to be made into each
uterine cavity

A

Injection of
vasopressin

B

Incision into
uterine
cavities

Internal os

Septum

C

Excising
wedge
containing
most of
septum

Uterine
cavity

D

Identification
of right uterine
cavity as wedge
is removed

E

FIGURE 29.20. The modified Jones metroplasty. See the text for a full description of the various steps in the operative repair of a septate uterus by excision of a wedge.

both manually and with the guy sutures to relieve tension on the suture line and to reduce the possibility of cutting through. These sutures are placed alternately, first anterior and then posterior. After the first few stitches are placed and before the first layer is completed, the second layer can be started to reduce tension.

As the operation proceeds, the third layer of stitches is begun in the serosa both anteriorly and posteriorly (Fig. 29.20I–K). Finer, nonreactive suture material can be used to approximate the serosal edges of the uterus more precisely to prevent adhesion formation to the suture line (Fig. 29.20K–L). By the conclusion of the operation, the uterus appears near normal in configuration. The striking feature is usually the proximity of the insertions of the fallopian tubes. Special care must be exercised not to obstruct the interstitial portions of the fallopian tubes while placing the fundal myometrial and serosal sutures.

The final size of the uterine cavity seems to be relatively unimportant to reproductive capability; uterine symmetry appears to be a more important factor. Often the constructed cavity is quite small compared with the normal uterus. Whether the surgeon removes the septum with the Jones procedure or lyses the septum transcervically, postoperative hysterogram films often show small dog-ears that are leftover tags from the original bifid condition of the uterus. Such dog-ears do not seem to interfere with function, although a postoperative roentgenogram cannot be considered normal in the sense that it does not have the appearance of a normal endometrial cavity after such an operation. If a double cervix is present, the physician should not attempt to unify the cervix because an incompetent cervical os will result. To allow the uterine incision the best possible opportunity to heal, a delay of 4 to 6 months in attempting pregnancy is advised after abdominal metroplasty.

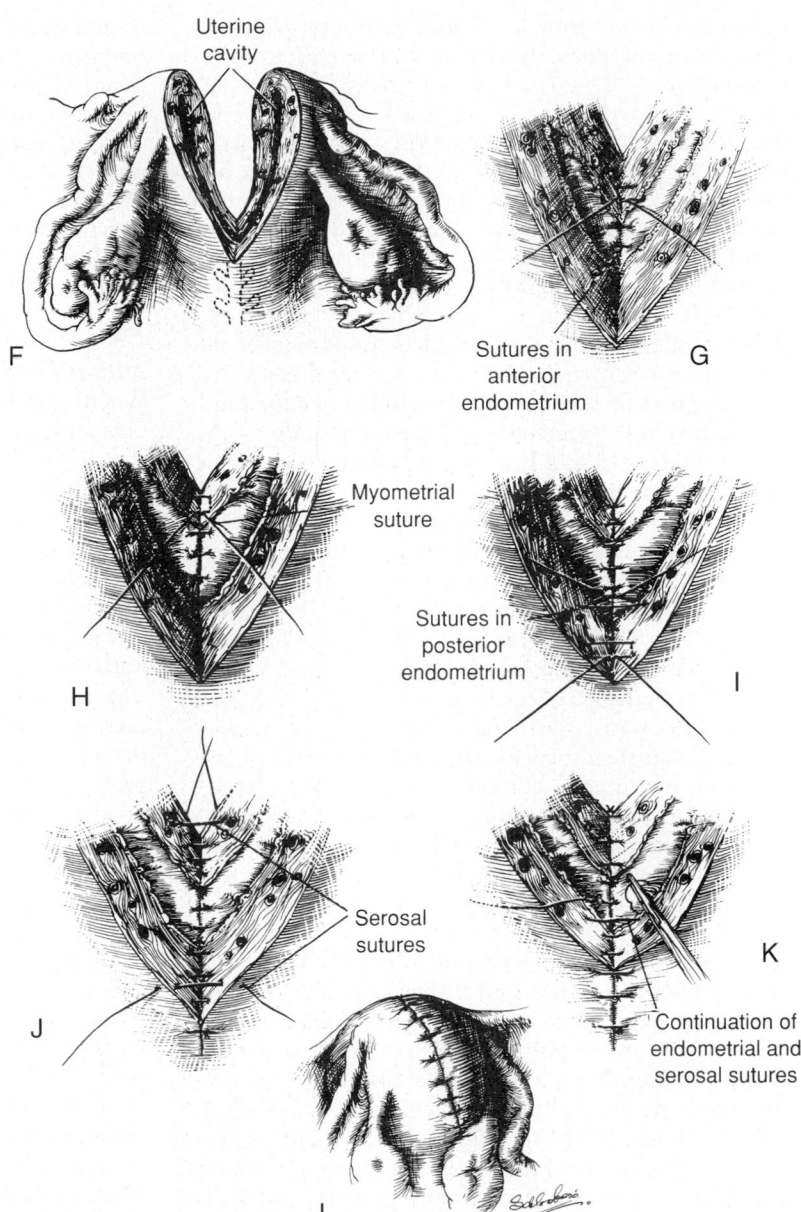

FIGURE 29.20. (continued) The modified Jones metroplasty. See the text for a full description of the various steps in the operative repair of a septate uterus by excision of a wedge.

THE JONES METROPLASTY VERSUS THE TOMPKINS PROCEDURE. The technique of modified Jones metroplasty is a compromise between the classic Jones metroplasty and the Tompkins metroplasty. In the Jones operation, the entire septum is removed. In the Tompkins operation, a single median incision divides the uterine corpus and septum in half. The incision is carried inferiorly until the endometrial cavity is reached. Each lateral septal half is then incised to within 1 cm of the tubes. No septal tissue is removed. The myometrium is reapproximated, taking care not to place sutures too close to the interstitial portion of the tubes. Proponents of the Tompkins technique suggest that it is simpler than the classic Jones procedure, that it conserves all myometrial tissue and leaves the uterotubal junction in a more nor-

mal and lateral position, and that it provides better results than the Jones metroplasty. Good results with the Tompkins technique have been reported by McShane, Reilly, and Schiff.

THE WEDGE METROPLASTY VERSUS TRANSCERVICAL LYSIS. There are obvious advantages to a transcervical incision of a uterine septum for patients with a septate uterus. Morbidity is decreased after the procedure and delivery can be vaginal. Term pregnancy rates are comparable to those after abdominal metroplasty for repeated pregnancy wastage.

Most of the septa associated with a septate uterus can be cut through the cervix by way of the hysteroscope or the resectoscope. Nevertheless, cases of broad uterine septum can benefit from the wedge metroplasty, and reconstructive surgeons should be knowledgeable in its performance.

THE STRASSMANN METROPLASTY. The Strassmann procedure is not easily adapted to the septate uterus, but it is the procedure of choice for unification of the two endometrial cavities of an externally divided uterus, both bicornuate and didelphic (Fig. 29.21). A bicornuate uterus cannot be repaired through transcervical lysis because perforation will result. When there has been failure of fusion of the two müllerian ducts, inspection of the pelvic cavity often reveals a broad peritoneal band that lies in the middle between the two lateral hemicorpora. This rectovesical ligament is attached anteriorly to the bladder, folds over and is attached between the uterine cornua, continues posteriorly in the cul-de-sac, and ends with its attachment to the anterior wall of the sigmoid and rectum. It is not invariably present, but when it is, its potential significance in the etiology of the anomaly, possibly by preventing the two müllerian ducts from joining, must be considered. This rectovesical ligament must be removed before a unification procedure can be performed (Fig. 29.21A).

For hemostasis, tourniquets are used in a manner similar to that described for the modified Jones procedure. The two uterine cornua are incised on their median sides in their longitudinal axes, deeply enough to expose the uterine cavities (Fig. 29.21B). Superiorly, the incision must not be too close to the interstitial portion of the fallopian tubes. Inferiorly, the incision is carried far enough to join the two sides into a single endocervical canal. If it appears that a deeper incision will compromise the competence of the cervix, then a double cervical canal can be left. If the cervix is already duplex, then it should not be joined. As the incision in the myometrium releases the internal stresses in the walls of the hemicorpora, each one everts and is perfectly positioned for apposition, almost as if the original intention in embryologic development is finally to be realized. The suture technique for joining the two sides (Fig. 29.21C–E) is exactly the same as for the modified Jones procedure. The suture line in the uterine corpus should be observed for several minutes to determine the adequacy of hemostasis. Occasionally it is necessary to place one or two extra sutures to control bleeding.

A uterine suspension can be performed as necessary. However, in the event of pregnancy, the shortened round ligaments can produce symptoms from an enlarging uterus. Presacral neurectomy in association with uterine unification should be considered only in patients with severe midline dysmenorrhea.

The cervix should be dilated to ensure proper drainage from the uterine cavity. This can be accomplished transvaginally after the abdominal procedure or from above by inserting a dilator through the cervical canal into the vagina to be removed later.

The operative technique should always be consistent with the goal of maintaining or enhancing fertility and possibly achieving a successful pregnancy. Tissue surfaces should be kept moist throughout the procedure, and instruments should be selected and used in such a way that tissue damage is minimized. Abdominal packs should be placed in plastic bags to avoid adhesions, or no-lint laparotomy pads can be used. Talc should be carefully washed from gloves, and meticulous aseptic technique should be used. The appendix should not be removed. Lactated Ringer solution containing heparin and corticosteroid can be used for peritoneal lavage throughout the procedure.

Cervical Incompetence Associated with a Double Uterus

When a patient with an anomalous uterus, with or without unification, becomes pregnant, she must be watched closely for evidence of cervical incompetence, especially if a history of previous reproductive loss suggests cervical incompetence. Heinonen and associates improved fetal survival rate from 57% to 92% by cervical cerclage. Cerclage was used mostly in patients with a partial bicornuate uterus. In these patients, the fetal salvage rate was improved from 53% before cerclage to 100% afterward. Prematurity also was decreased, from 53% to 3%. The authors stress that cervical incompetence, not the uterine anomaly, is the proper indication for cerclage in these patients. However, the frequency with which these problems are found together suggests the importance of doing a careful evaluation for both problems. Some reproductive losses from a uterine anomaly might be prevented by cerclage of an incompetent cervix during metroplasty. However, routine cerclage at the time of metroplasty is not recommended.

Attempts to unify a double cervix or a septate cervix also are not recommended because of the possibility of causing cervical incompetence. However, a double or septate cervix can adversely affect the outcome of delivery if vaginal delivery is attempted, and delivery should be by Caesarean section if it appears that the cervix will cause dystocia.

Mode of Delivery After Metroplasty

The scar formed in the myometrium after unification is as strong as, if not stronger than, the scar formed after Caesarean section. The biologic conditions under which healing occurs are entirely different in these two situations. Endomyometritis is a common complication after Caesarean section but is not a complication of uterine unification. Of 71 known pregnancies in Strassmann's collected series reported in 1952, 61 were delivered vaginally. There were no cases of uterine rupture during pregnancy or delivery. Despite evidence that the uterine scar heals securely after unification operations, our policy is to recommend delivery by elective Caesarean section in all patients who have undergone abdominal metroplasty. Patients can deliver vaginally after a metroplasty by hysteroscope or resectoscope.

Diethylstilbestrol-Related Uterine Anomalies

Exposure of the female fetus to DES can cause significant anomalous development of the uterus, as reported

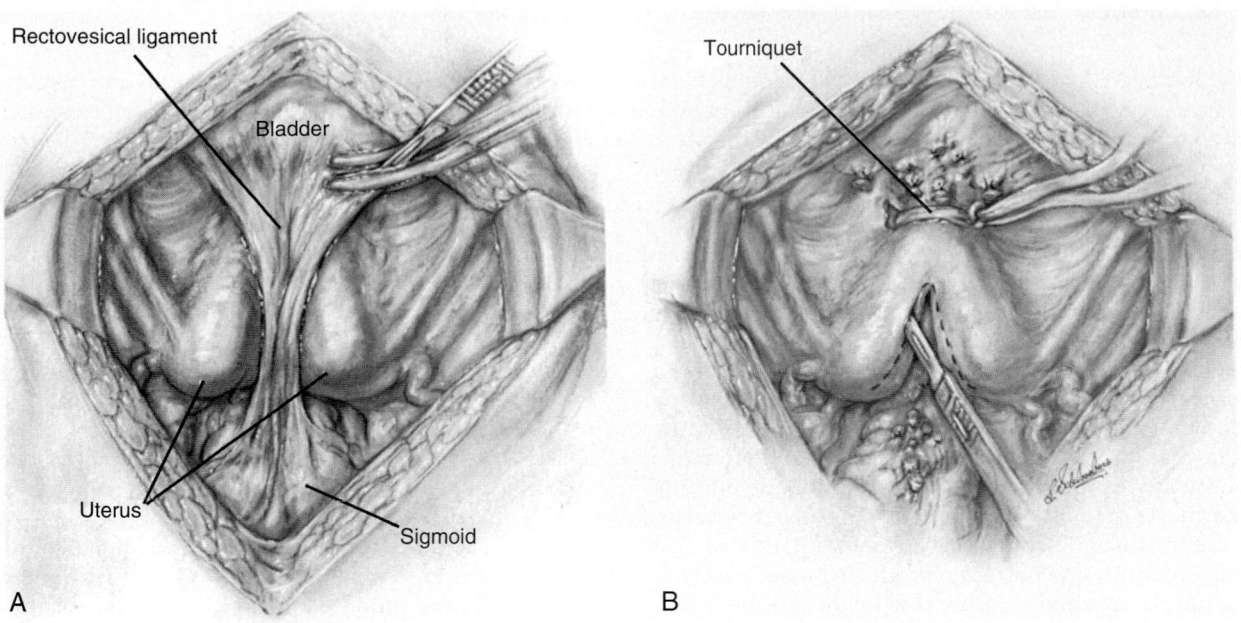

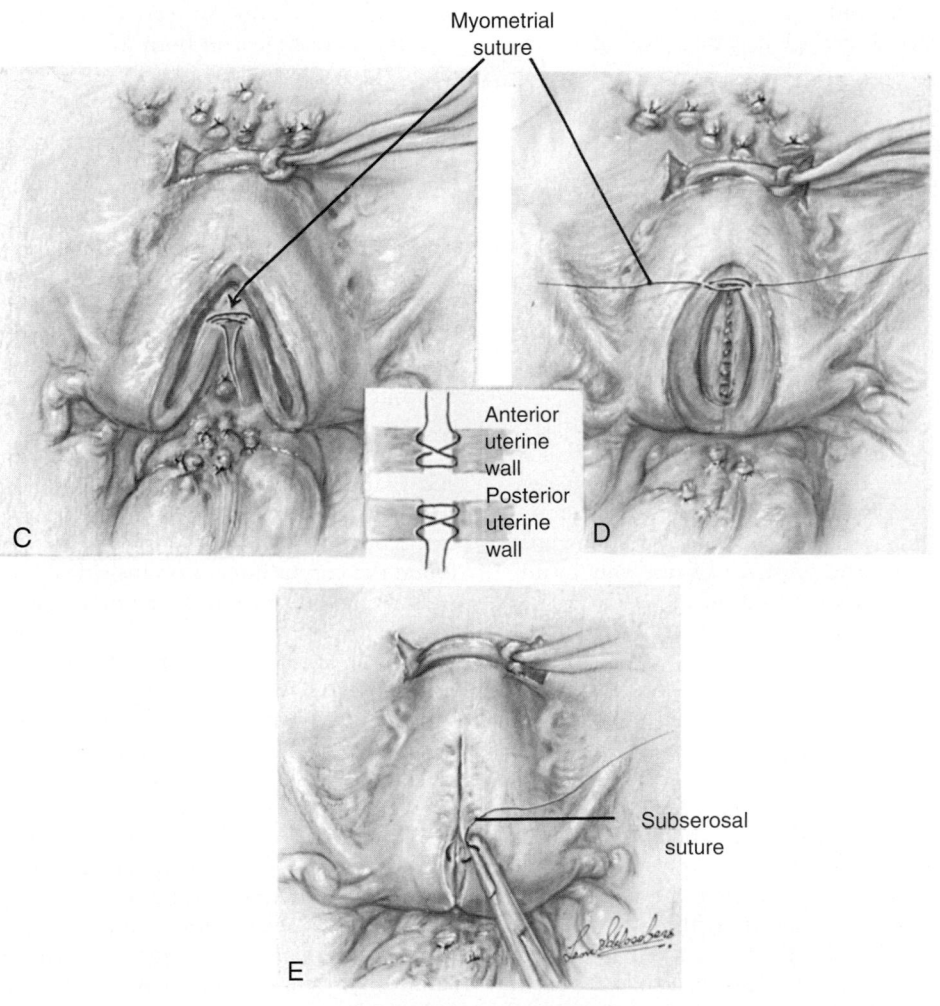

FIGURE 29.21. The Strassmann metroplasty with modification. **A:** If a rectovesical ligament is found, it should be removed. **B:** An incision is made on the medial side of each hemicorpus and carried deep enough to enter the uterine cavity. The edges of the myometrium will evert to face the opposite side. **C:** and **D:** The myometrium is approximated by use of interrupted vertical figure-of-eight 3-0 polyglycolic acid sutures. One should avoid placing sutures too close to the interstitial portion of the fallopian tubes. **E:** A continuous 5-0 polyglycolic acid subserosal suture is used as a final layer. Tourniquets are removed, and defects in the broad ligament are closed.

by Kaufman and associates and by Haney and colleagues. The T-shaped uterus is the variant most commonly seen. It is associated with an increased rate of spontaneous abortions, preterm deliveries, and ectopic pregnancies.

Nagel and Malo determined the feasibility of correcting the uterine malformations seen in DES-exposed women by incising constriction rings and septa. Their goal was to incise the irregular uterine walls until the cavity assumed a smooth, straight line from the lower uterine cavity to the uterine tubal ostium. Their results suggested that metroplasty can decrease pregnancy loss but does not enhance fertility. The editors of this book suggest that the rare patient can benefit from a uterine reconstructive procedure, but that most will not. Surgeons may never develop a large series to document efficacy of surgical outcomes because patients with this anomaly will eventually age beyond reproductive years, and some latitude is required in cases that might possibly benefit from metroplasty.

DES-exposed patients must be monitored closely for evidence of dilatation and effacement of the cervix early in pregnancy. Cervical cerclage may be indicated in some patients.

Unicornuate Uterus

A unicornuate uterus can be present alone or with a rudimentary horn or bulb on the opposite side. In a series reported by Heinonen and associates, 11 of 13 patients with a unicornuate uterus had a rudimentary horn, and two did not. The rudimentary anlage (uterine muscle bundle or bulb) can communicate directly with the unicornuate uterus. In some instances, there is no cavity within the anlage or there is no rudimentary horn. Most rudimentary horns are noncommunicating (90% according to O'Leary and O'Leary). The two sides may be connected by a fibromuscular band, or there may be no connection and no communication between the two uterine cavities. Fedele and associates have found sonography useful in determining the presence of not only a rudimentary horn but also a cavity within.

Associated Anomalies

Urinary tract anomalies are often associated with a unicornuate uterus. On the side opposite the unicornuate uterus there may be a horseshoe or a pelvic kidney, or the kidney may be hypoplastic or absent. This is especially true if there is associated müllerian duct obstruction. When all müllerian duct derivatives and the kidney are absent on one side, this implies failure of development of the entire urogenital ridge, including the genital ridge where the ovary forms. In addition, the ovary may be malpositioned (Fig. 29.22). Rock, Parmley, and associates reported a unilateral ovary located above the pelvic brim in four cases of uterine anomalies. The orifice of the müllerian duct develops at about the level of the fourth thoracic vertebra (T4) in the embryo. The tip subsequently migrates along the course of the müllerian duct into the pelvis. The orifice of the duct or the fimbriated end of the tube comes to lie in the pelvis as a result of differential growth of the fetus. The subsequent differential growth is retarded so that the portion of the urogenital ridge that gives rise to both the gonad and tube does not displace into the pelvis. Malpositions of the ovary and tube are the result.

Reproductive Performance

According to Heinonen and associates, the unicornuate uterus carries the poorest fetal survival rate (40%) of all uterine anomalies. In 1957, Jones reported similar findings. The abnormal shape, the insufficient muscular mass of the uterus, and the reduced uterine volume and inability to expand may explain the poor obstetric outcome.

Moutos and colleagues compared the reproductive performance of the unicornuate uterus with that of the didelphic uterus. Twenty of the 29 women with a unicornuate uterus produced a total of 40 pregnancies, whereas 13 women with a didelphic uterus produced a total of 28 pregnancies. The percentages of pregnancies resulting in preterm delivery, term delivery, and living children were similar in both groups. The authors concluded that reproductive performance of the unicornuate uterus was not different from that of the didelphic uterus, that it is uncommon for either malformation to be a primary cause of infertility, and that there is insufficient information to support recommendation of placement of a cervical cerclage in the absence of cervical incompetence. Thus, there is no evidence that uterine reconstruction should be performed for patients with a unicornuate (or a didelphic) uterus.

Because most cases of unicornuate uterus have a noncommunicating rudimentary uterine horn on the opposite side, there is danger of pregnancy in the rudimentary horn from transperitoneal migration of sperm or ovum from the opposite side. According to Holden and Hart, approximately 350 cases of pregnancy in a rudimentary horn have been reported since the original case report by Mauriceau in 1669. O'Leary and O'Leary found the corpus luteum on the side contralateral to the rudimentary horn containing a pregnancy in 8% of cases. Signs and symptoms of an ectopic pregnancy develop with eventual rupture of the horn if the pregnancy is not detected early. Rupture through the wall of the vascular rudimentary horn is associated with sudden and severe intraperitoneal hemorrhage and shock. Death can occur in a few minutes. It is surprising that the current mortality rate has decreased to 5%.

Very little, if anything, can be done to improve the reproductive performance of patients with a unicornuate uterus. The physician should observe closely for cervical incompetence and perform cerclage as indicated. Andrews and Jones have suggested that removal of the rudimentary uterine horn may improve the chances of a successful pregnancy, but the experience is too small to support a definite recommendation. Cases of asymmetric development of the unicornuate uterus with an opposing rudimentary uterine horn are not amenable to unification.

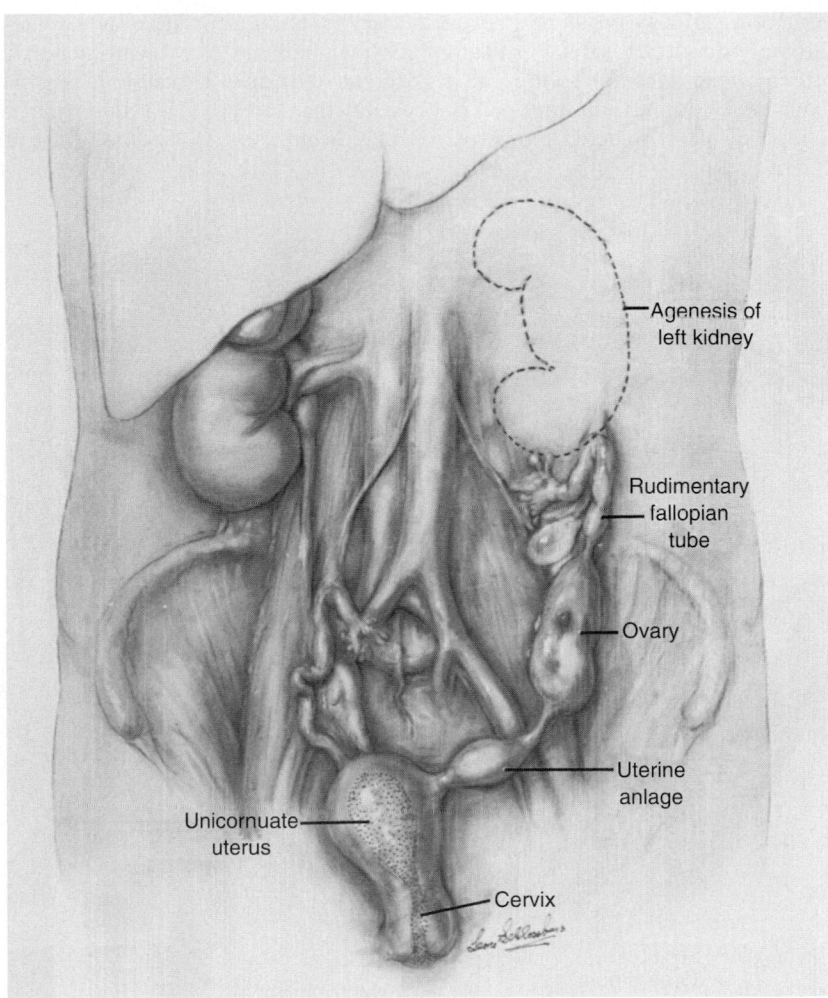

FIGURE 29.22. A unicornuate uterus associated with ovarian malposition on the left. Note that the ovary and the tube are slightly above the pelvic brim. In this instance, the ovary measured 6 inches long.

Labels on figure: Agenesis of left kidney; Rudimentary fallopian tube; Ovary; Uterine anlage; Unicornuate uterus; Cervix

Longitudinal Vaginal Septum

Failure of fusion of the lower müllerian ducts that form the vagina can result in a vagina with a longitudinal septum. The septum can be partial or complete. Young patients have difficulty using tampons. In cases of didelphic uterus with a longitudinal vaginal septum, one uterine hemicorpus is usually better developed than the other. If intercourse consistently occurs on the vaginal side connected to the uterine hemicorpus that is less well developed, then infertility or repeated abortion could result. For these reasons, the septum should be removed (when the patient is not pregnant) unless there is a contraindication. This can usually be accomplished easily with reasonable precautions against injury to the urethra, bladder, and rectum.

Haddad and colleagues reported their experience over a 24-year period with management of the longitudinal vaginal septum. The retrospective review of 202 patient charts described a complete septum (extending from cervix to introitus) in 45.6% of patients, high partial in 36.1%, and a medium or low partial, involving only the distal vagina, in 18.3%. Uterine malformations were noted in 87.8% of cases. The frequency of uterine malformations was 99.4% in cases of complete or partial

high septum and 30.3% in cases of partial medium or low septum. The most common malformation was class Va complete septate uterus in 59.5% of malformations, followed by class III didelphys uterus (24.3%) and class Vb partial septate uterus (15%). Section or resection was performed in 201 cases. Bladder injury in one patient was the only reported complication. As highlighted by the high prevalence of associated uterine malformations in this review, management should always include an assessment of uterine anatomy.

Asymmetric Obstruction of the Uterus or Vagina

Unicornuate Uterus and Noncommunicating Uterine Anlage Containing Functional Endometrium

If one müllerian duct develops normally while the opposite müllerian duct fails to develop or develops incompletely, then a relatively normal unicornuate uterus is found on one side and the cervix, musculature, uterine cavity, endometrium, fallopian tube, blood supply, and ligamentous attachments are absent or hypoplastic to a varying degree on the other side. Obstruction to menstruation can also occur to varying degrees on the improperly developed side. For example, if a rudimentary uterine horn does not communicate externally but does have an endometrium-lined uterine cavity, then clear symptoms of obstructed menstruation may begin soon after menarche, and severe dysmenorrhea will be present. Cryptomenorrhea can be overlooked as the diagnosis because there is cyclic menstruation from the opposite side. It is important to make the diagnosis as soon as possible, because if the lumen of the tube communicates with the

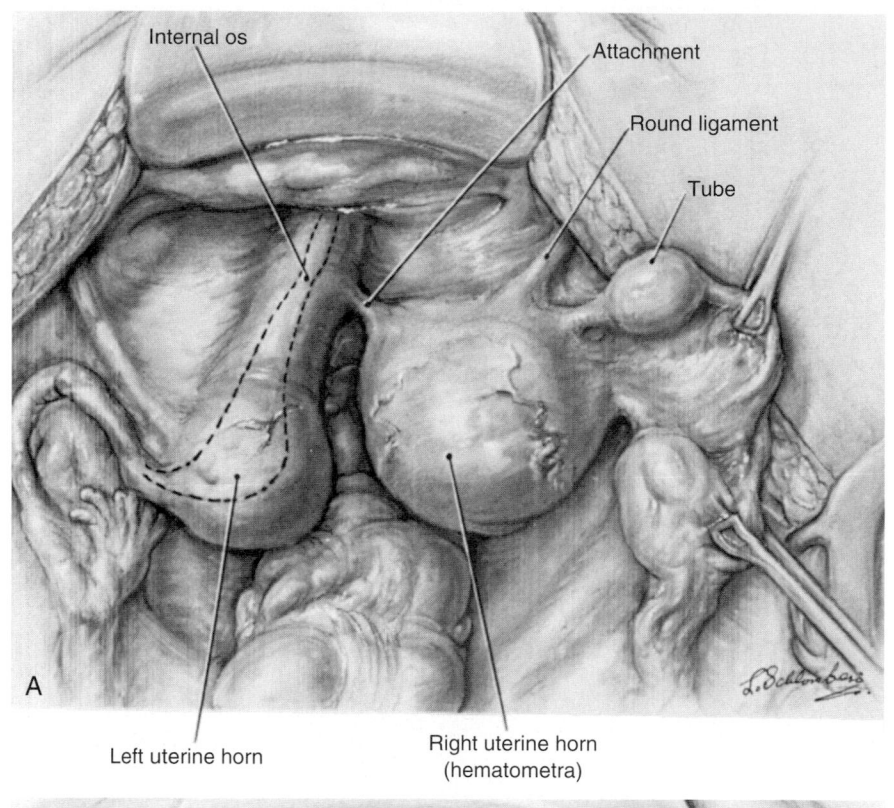

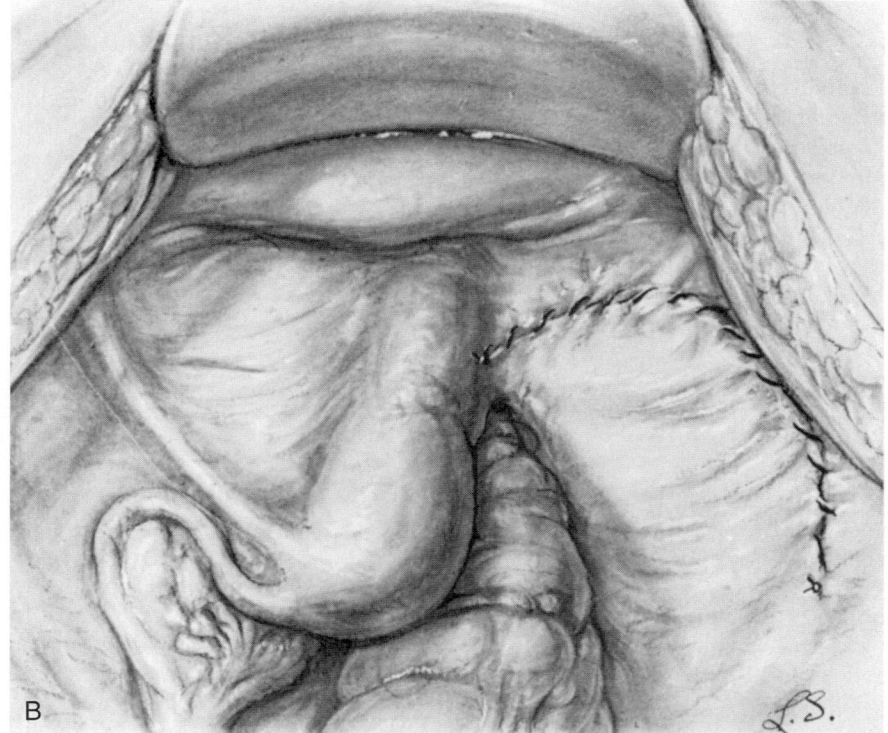

FIGURE 29.23. A: A noncommunicating rudimentary horn with functional endometrium that contains menstrual blood under pressure. Note the congenital abnormality of the fallopian tube, which prevented retrograde menstruation. **B:** The same patient after excision of the rudimentary horn.

endometrial cavity of the rudimentary uterus, then retrograde menstruation and pelvic endometriosis will develop, and reproductive potential can be destroyed. During the operation illustrated in Figure 29.23, which was performed to remove an obstructed rudimentary uterine horn, the fallopian tube was obstructed and retrograde menstruation was impossible. Occasionally, the fallopian tube connected to the rudimentary uterine horn may not be patent because of incomplete development.

Unilateral Obstruction of a Cavity of a Double Uterus

Another example of a rare obstructed lateral fusion problem is the complete septum between two uterine cavities illustrated in Figure 29.24. One cavity communicated with a cervix and the other did not. This could represent an example of unilateral failure of cervical development. The patient complained of incapacitating dysmenorrhea that appeared shortly after the menarche and lasted 5 days. A tense, cystic mass was palpable in the right half of the pelvis. The operation, described originally by Jones

in the second edition of this book, consisted of making an incision through the anterior wall of the cystic right portion of the uterus. It was found to contain old menstrual blood. The entire septum was excised and the uterus was reconstructed by anastomosis of the two cavities. A continuous lock-stitch was reinforced by interrupted myometrial sutures, and the plastic reconstruction of the uterus was completed by a third layer of interrupted sutures uniting myometrium and serosa.

Sanders and colleagues described several cases in which the role of interventional radiology was crucial in the management of obstructive anomalies. The report described the drainage of a noncommunicating right uterine cavity distended with blood in a unicornuate uterus in a 14-year-old patient. Adequate access was established by using ultrasound-guided needle aspiration followed by a hysteroscopic excision. The assistance of interventional radiologic procedures, including percutaneous drainage and dilatation of small maldeveloped areas, may allow access to areas otherwise inaccessible by conventional mechanisms and assist in preserving reproductive function.

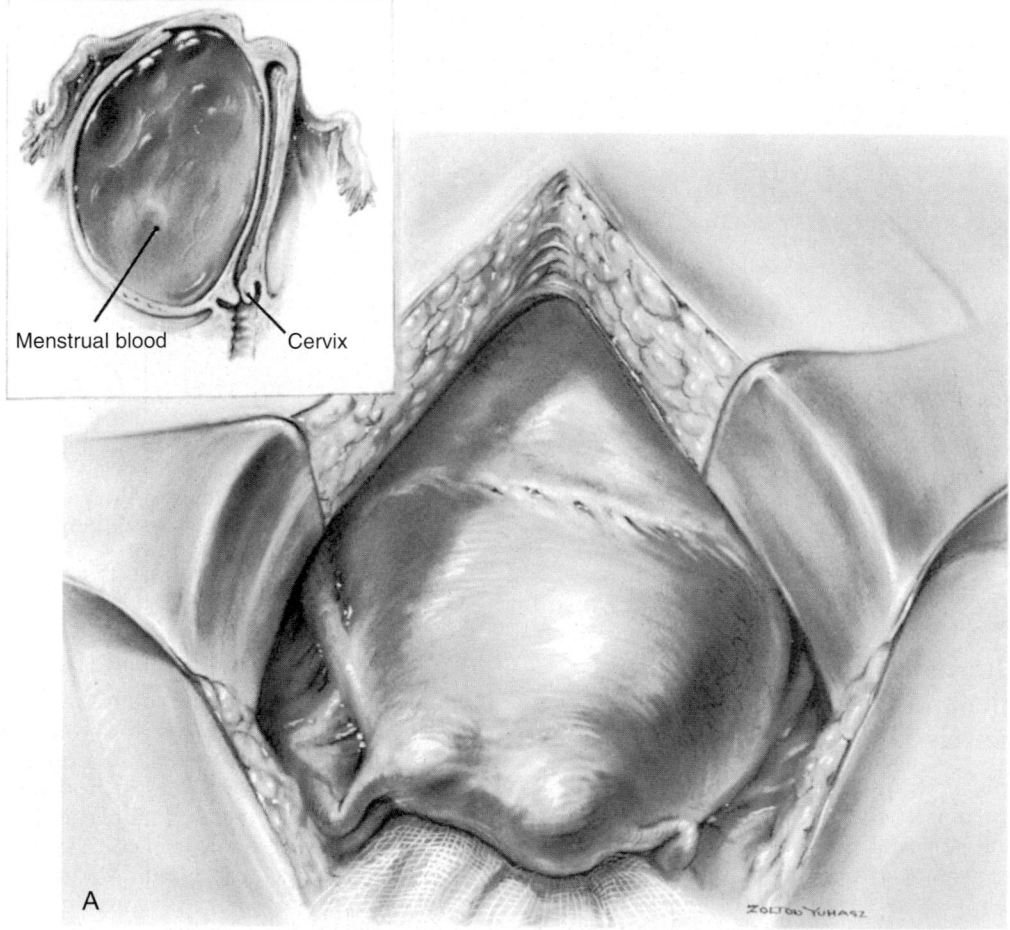

FIGURE 29.24. A: A double uterus seen at operation. Hematometra in the right uterine cavity (*inset*), which does not communicate with the other cavity or the cervical canal. *(continued)*

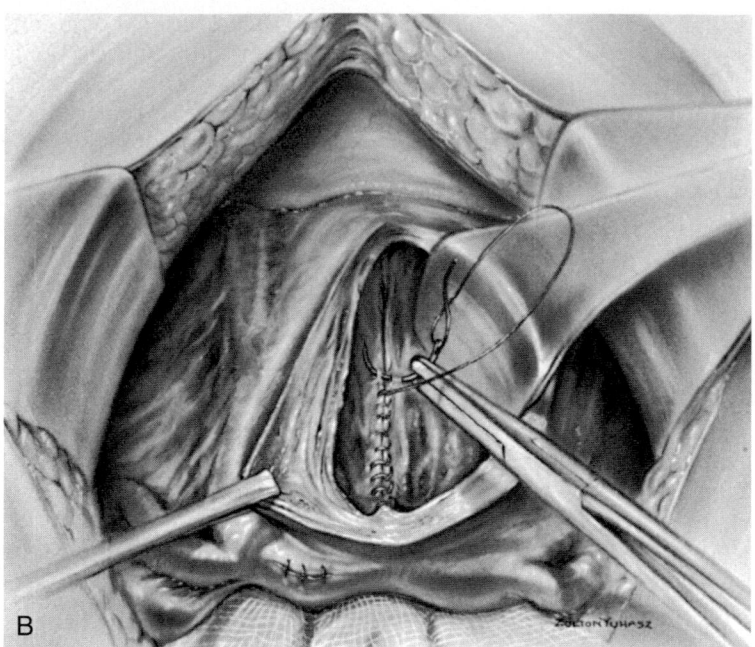

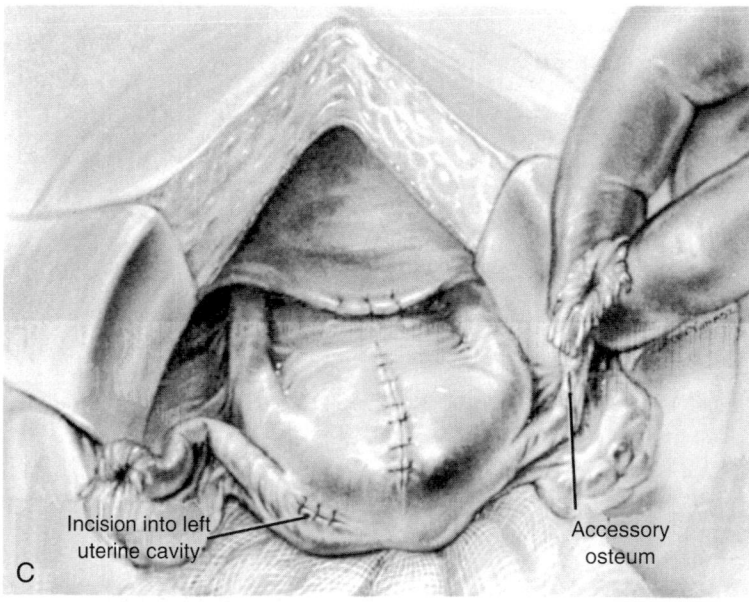

FIGURE 29.24. *(Continued)* **B:** The septum of the double uterus has been excised and anastomosis is performed to unite the two cavities. **C:** Anastomosis is completed. The small incision in the left uterine cavity was made before the septum was removed for the purpose of orientation.

Double Uterus with Obstructed Hemivagina and Ipsilateral Renal Agenesis

The unique clinical syndrome consisting of a double uterus, obstruction of the vagina (unilateral, partial, or complete), and ipsilateral renal agenesis is rare. The renal agenesis (mesonephric involution) on the side of the obstructed vagina associated with a double uterus and double cervix is suggestive of an embryologic arrest at 8 weeks of pregnancy that simultaneously affects the müllerian and metanephric ducts. The exact cause is unknown.

Diagnostic Groups

Clinical symptoms vary depending on the uterovaginal relations in individual cases, but the syndrome can be described generally in three groups. Group 1 patients have complete unilateral vaginal obstruction without uterine communication, resulting in a paravaginal mass and symptoms of severe dysmenorrhea and lower abdominal pain. Menses are regular. Group 2 patients have an incomplete unilateral vaginal obstruction without uterine communication. The presenting symptoms are lower abdominal pain, severe dysmenorrhea, excessive foul mucopurulent discharge, and, in some instances, intermenstrual bleeding. Group 3 patients have complete vaginal obstruction with a laterally communicating double uterus. They have a paravaginal mass, lower abdominal pain, and dysmenorrhea. Menses are regular. A 10-year review of patients with this anomaly was published by Phupong and colleagues. Most patients presented with dysmenorrhea (73%), or a pelvic or paravaginal mass (71%). The right uterus and vagina were affected in 63.5% of patients.

Because menses in patients with this syndrome are rarely irregular, the possibility of this syndrome as a diagnosis can easily be overlooked. A careful pelvic examination is necessary to make the correct diagnosis. MRI can identify the obstructed vagina, double uterus, and absence of a kidney on the side of the obstruction (Fig. 29.25), but it may not be helpful if there is incomplete vaginal obstruction or a uterine communication.

Complete unilateral vaginal obstruction (group 1) can go unrecognized for a number of years after the onset of menses. The vagina is quite distensible and can accommodate a large amount of accumulated blood in the obstructed side. There is sufficient absorption of menstrual blood between periods so that each subsequent flow can add to the increments of accumulated blood without pain. Nevertheless, once retrograde menstruation occurs, endometriosis invariably is the result.

Surgical Treatment

Careful excision of the vaginal septum is the treatment of choice for a unilateral vaginal obstruction. Prophylactic antibiotics should be administered before surgery. After opening the vaginal pouch, the surgeon should use suction and lavage to remove the pooled blood and mucus. Phupong and colleagues' review also confirms the suc-

cessful use of this primary therapy in 84.3% of patients. Haddad and colleagues reported a similar experience in a report describing patient management over a 27-year period. Excision of the vaginal septum was successful in 88% of patients with complete excision in one procedure in 92% of those patients. In cases of pyocolpos or hematocolpos, distention and stretching of the septal tissue may increase the risk of inadequate resection and possible postoperative stenosis; the authors found the use of a two-step graduated resection advantageous to ensure adequate resection. A limited resection (3 cm) was performed to allow adequate drainage, followed by a return to the operating room in approximately 1 month to remove any remaining septum.

Because the obstructing septum is usually thick, removal can be difficult. Clamps should be used to isolate a generous vaginal pedicle while the suture is being tied in place to prevent slippage of tissue. Such pedicles generally retract during healing, and formation of a vaginal stenosis is avoided. In most instances, surgery is restricted to excision of the septum, and abdominal exploration is unnecessary. Uterine reconstruction is not indicated for cases of lateral communication of the uterine horns. Some authors have reported the use of hemi-hysterectomy in patients with a high, thick-walled obstruction, massive ovarian involvement, endometriosis, or adenomyosis; however, this is generally not recommended in young patients.

Reproductive Performance

Reproductive performance for patients with this disorder is usually consistent with that of patients with a double uterus unless the delay in diagnosis and resection of the obstructing septum has been sufficient to destroy tubal function or to cause the development of endometriosis.

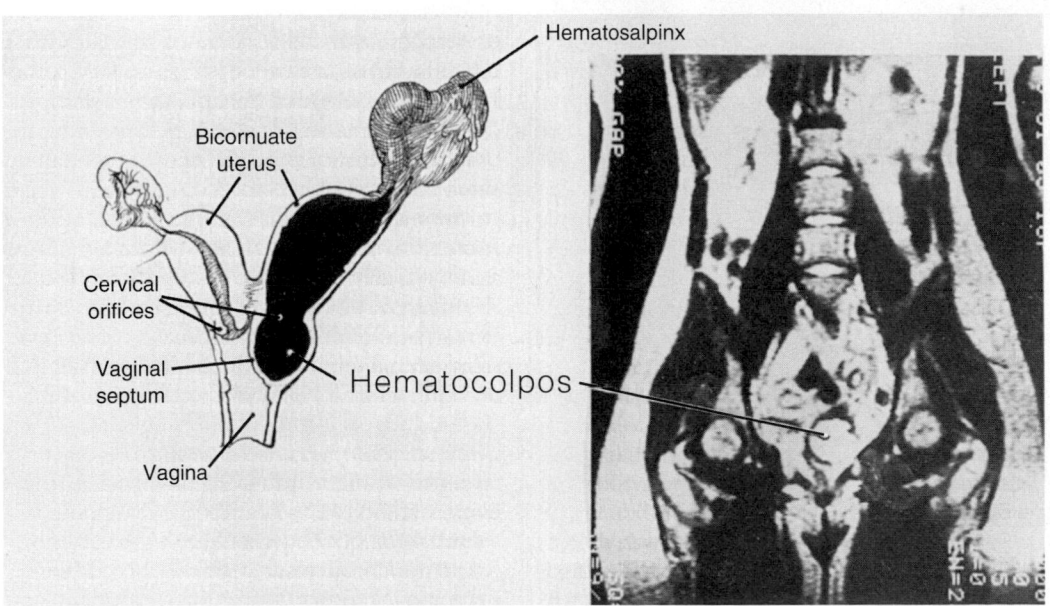

FIGURE 29.25. A double uterus with unilateral complete vaginal obstruction and ipsilateral renal agenesis. Magnetic resonance imaging reveals the left hematocolpos, both uteri, and absence of the left kidney on the side of the vaginal obstruction.

Haddad and colleagues' review was notable for a predominance of pregnancies (80%) in the contralateral endometrial cavity.

UNUSUAL CONFIGURATIONS OF VERTICAL-LATERAL FUSION DEFECTS

Unusual configurations of both vertical and lateral fusion defects may occur simultaneously. Figure 29.26 depicts the radiographic evaluation (MRI) of a young woman in whom cryptomenorrhea developed above a transverse

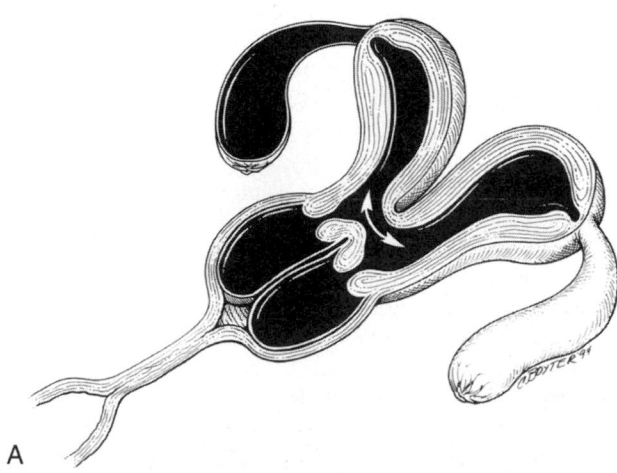

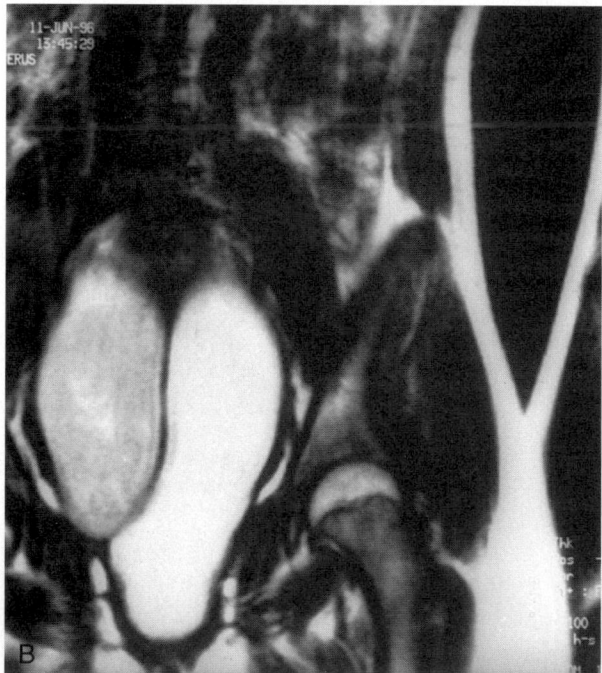

FIGURE 29.26. An unusual combination of both vertical and lateral fusion defects. **A:** A didelphys uterus with an intrauterine communication and a longitudinal vaginal septum are present proximal to a transverse vaginal septum. **B:** The magnetic resonance image demonstrates the presence of both septa.

vaginal septum. The MRI study depicting the hematocolpos also suggests the longitudinal vaginal septum. Incision, drainage, and resection of the transverse vaginal septum allowed appropriate evaluation of the more proximal müllerian anatomy. The artist's depiction in Figure 29.26 demonstrates the unusual constellation of a didelphys uterus with an intrauterine communication of the cavities and a longitudinal vaginal septum. This type of atypical combination occurs frequently enough to emphasize the importance of proper delineation of individual anatomy preoperatively for proper surgical preparation.

Müllerian duct anomalies can occur in association with a variety of other problems. For example, Stanton reported that in a series of 70 patients with bladder exstrophy, 30 (43%) had reproductive tract abnormalities. He suggested that the true figures were actually higher. Müllerian abnormalities included absence of the vagina; septate vagina; unicornuate, bicornuate, and didelphic uterus; and absent uterus. Fewer müllerian anomalies are seen with epispadias. Jones investigated anomalies of the external genitalia and vagina in 30 patients with bladder exstrophy seen at the Johns Hopkins Hospital and suggested operative techniques for correction of these anomalies. Techniques for the management of other gynecologic and obstetric problems (especially uterine prolapse) also have been discussed by Weed and McKee and by Blakeley and Mills. A number of other rare combinations of congenital malformations of the vagina and perineum have been found in association with uterine anomalies. Their surgical correction, especially in children, is reported by Hendren and Donahoe and by others. Several authors have considered the uterovaginal anomalies that occur in association with multiple other gastrointestinal and genitourinary abnormalities. Goh described an infant girl with complete duplication of the bladder, urethra, uterus, and vagina associated with a urogenital sinus and an anterior ectopic anus. Gastol and Magalhaes also described children with complete duplication of the bladder, urethra, vagina, and uterus. These complex anomalies include significantly more defects than lateral fusion concerns in the müllerian ducts. These cases emphasize the variable anatomy in this rare group of anomalies and that a substantial effort should be placed on defining anatomy before surgical exploration and management. Sheldon and others reviewed 13 consecutive cases of vaginal reconstruction in pediatric patients with multisystem anomalies. The review emphasized several important principles involved in the surgical management: (1) all anticipated perineal reconstruction should be performed in a single stage, (2) urethral catheterization has an important role, (3) urinary reconstruction is often intimately involved in the vaginal reconstruction, (4) avoidance of overlapping suture lines is essential for optimal healing, (5) maximum growth potential of the neovagina should be considered, and (6) meticulous follow-up of proper routine dilatation of the neovagina should be expected. Coordinated reconstruction of all organ systems is especially important in these complex cases.

Müllerian duct anomalies are seen with the McKusick-Kaufman syndrome, an autosomal recessive disorder. Other clinical findings reported with this syndrome include hydrometrocolpos, postaxial polydactyly, syndactyly, congenital heart disease, intravaginal displacement of the urethral meatus, and anorectal anomalies. In 1982, Jabs and co-workers added the most recent unusual case to the few cases previously reported in the literature.

Müllerian duct anomalies may also affect the development of the fallopian tube. Although extremely rare, episodes of unilateral or bilateral absence of the fallopian tube have been reported. Of the less than 10 cases in the literature, Eustace reported two of the described cases. He hypothesized that compromise of the local blood supply to the caudal aspect of the Müllerian duct was a more likely cause than a fusion disorder. This situation could affect fallopian tube development to a variable extent with even some effect on ovarian development.

BIBLIOGRAPHY

Abbe R. New method of creating a vagina in a case of congenital absence. *Med Rec* 1898;54:836.

Adamian LV, Maurvatov KD, Sorour YA, et al. Medicogenetic features and surgical treatment of patients with congenital malformations of the uterus and vagina. *Int J Fertil* 1996,41:293.

Adamian LV. Laparoscopic management of vaginal aplasia with or without functional noncommunicating rudimentary uterus. In: Arrequi ME, Fitzgibbons RJ, Katkhouda N, et al, eds. *Principles of laparoscopic surgery.* New York: Springer-Verlag, 1995:646.

Alessandrescu D, Peltecu GC, Buhimschi CS, et al. Neocolpopoiesis with split-thickness skin graft as a surgical treatment of vaginal agenesis: retrospective review of 201 cases. *Am J Obstet Gynecol* 1996;175:131.

American Fertility Society classification of müllerian anomalies. *Fertil Steril* 1988;49:952.

Andrews MC, Jones HW. Impaired reproductive performance of the unicornuate uterus: intrauterine growth retardation, infertility, and recurrent abortion in five cases. *Am J Obstet Gynecol* 1982;144:173.

Baldwin JF. The formation of an artificial vagina by intestinal transplantation. *Ann Surg* 1984;40:398.

Blakeley CR, Mills WG. The obstetric and gynaecological complications of bladder exstrophy and epispadias. *Br J Obstet Gynaecol* 1981;88:167.

Beski S, Gorgy A, Venkat G, et al. Gestational surrogacy: a feasible option for patients with Rokitansky syndrome. *Hum Reprod* 2000;15:2326.

Borruto F. Mayer-Rokitansky-Küster Syndrome: Vecchietti's personal series. *Clin Exp Obstet Gynecol* 1992;19:273.

Brenner P, Sedlis A, Cooperman H. Complete imperforate transverse vaginal septum. *Obstet Gynecol* 1965;25:135.

Broadbent TR, Woolf RM. Congenital absence of the vagina: reconstruction without operation. *Br J Plast Surg* 1977;30:118.

Busacca M, Perino A, Venezia R. Laparoscopic-ultrasonographic combined technique for the creation of a neovagina in Mayer-Rokitansky-Küster-Hauser syndrome. *Fertil Steril* 1996;66:1039.

Buttram VC Jr. Müllerian anomalies and their management. *Fertil Steril* 1983;40:159.

Buttram VC Jr, Gibbons WE. Müllerian anomalies: a proposed classification (an analysis of 144 cases). *Fertil Steril* 1979;32:40.

Capraro VJ, Chuang JT, Randall CL. Improved fetal salvage after metroplasty. *Obstet Gynecol* 1968;29:97.

Capraro VJ, Gallego MB. Vaginal agenesis. *Am J Obstet Gynecol* 1976;124:98.

Chakravarty BN. Congenital absence of the vagina and uterus—simultaneous vaginoplasty and hysteroplasty. *J Obstet Gynecol (India)* 1977;27:627.

Chakravarty BN, Gun KM, Sarkar K. Congenital absence of vagina: anatomico-physiological consideration. *J Obstet Gynecol (India)* 1977;27:621.

Chen YI, Cheng T, Lin H, et al. Spatial W-plasty full thickness skin graft for neovaginal reconstruction. *Plast Reconstr Surg* 1994;94:727.

Chervenak FA, Neuwirth RS. Hysteroscopic resection of the uterine septum. *Am J Obstet Gynecol* 1981;141:351.

Counseller VS. Congenital absence of the vagina. *JAMA* 1948;136:861.

Counseller VS, Davis CE. Atresia of the vagina. *Obstet Gynecol* 1968;32:528.

Counseller VS, Flor FS. Congenital absence of the vagina. *Surg Clin North Am* 1957;37:1107.

Creatsas GC. Creatsas modification of Williams vaginoplasty. *J Gynecol Surg* 1991;7:219.

Cukier J, Batzofin JH, Conners JS, et al. Genital tract reconstruction in a patient with congenital absence of a vagina and hypoplasia of the cervix. *Obstet Gynecol* 1986;68:325.

Dabirashrafi H, Bahadori M, Mohammad K, et al. Septate uterus: new idea on the histologic features of the septum in the abnormal uterus. *Am J Obstet Gynecol* 1995;172:105.

Daly DC, Tohan N, Walters C, et al. Hysteroscopic resection of the uterine septum in the presence of a septate cervix. *Fertil Steril* 1983;39:560.

Daly DC, Walters CA, Soto-Albors CE, et al. Hysteroscopic metroplasty: surgical technique and obstetrical outcome. *Fertil Steril* 1983;39:623.

David A, Carvil D, Bar-David E, et al. Congenital absence of the vagina: clinical and psychological aspects. *Obstet Gynecol* 1975;46:407.

Davydov SN. Colpopoiesis from the peritoneum of the uterorectal space. In: *Proceedings of the Ninth World Congress of Obstetrics and Gynecology, Tokyo, 1979.* Amsterdam, Excerpta Medica, 1980:793.

DeCherney A, Polan ML. Hysteroscopic management of intrauterine lesions and intractable uterine bleeding. *Obstet Gynecol* 1983;61:392.

DeCherney AH, Russell JB, Graebe RA, et al. Resectoscopic management of müllerian fusion defects. *Fertil Steril* 1986;45:726.

Dillon WP, Mudaliar NA, Wingate NB. Congenital atresia of the cervix. *Obstet Gynecol* 1979;54:126.

Eustace DL. Congenital absence of fallopian tube and ovary. *Eur J Obstet Gynecol Reprod Biol* 1992;46:157.

Evans TN. The artificial vagina. *Am J Obstet Gynecol* 1967;99:944.

Evans TN, Poland ML, Boving RL. Vaginal malformations. *Am J Obstet Gynecol* 1981;141:910.

Farber M, Marchant DJ. Reconstructive surgery for congenital atresia of the uterine cervix. *Fertil Steril* 1976;27:1277.

Farber M, Mitchell GW. Bicornuate uterus and partial atresia of the fallopian tube. *Am J Obstet Gynecol* 1979;134:881.

Farber M, Mitchell GW. Surgery for congenital absence of the vagina. *Obstet Gynecol* 1978;51:364.

Farber M, Mitchell GW. Surgery for congenital anomalies of müllerian ducts. *Contemp Obstet Gynecol* 1977;9:63.

Fayez JA. Comparison between abdominal and hysteroscopic metroplasty. *Obstet Gynecol* 1986;68:399.

Fedele L, Doeta M, Vercellini P, et al. Ultrasound in the diagnosis of subclasses of unicornuate uterus. *Obstet Gynecol* 1988;71:274.

Fedele L, Borruto F, Bianchi S, et al. A new laparoscopic procedure for creation of a neovagina in Mayer-Rokitansky-Küster-Hauser syndrome. *Fertil Steril* 1996;66:854.

Feroze RM, Dewhurst CJ, Welply G. Vaginoplasty at the Chelsea Hospital for women: a comparison of two techniques. *Br J Obstet Gynaecol* 1975;82:536.

Fore SR, Hammond CB, Parker RT, et al. Urologic and genital anomalies in patients with congenital absence of the vagina. *Obstet Gynecol* 1975;46:410.

Frank RT. The formation of an artificial vagina without operation. *Am J Obstet Gynecol* 1938;35:1053.

Frank RT. The formation of an artificial vagina without operation. *NY State J Med* 1940;40:1669.

Frank RT, Geist SH. The formation of an artificial vagina by a new plastic technic. *Am J Obstet Gynecol* 1927;14:712.

Gallup DG, Castle CA, Stock RJ. Recurrent carcinoma in situ of the vagina following split thickness skin graft vaginoplasty. *Gynecol Oncol* 1987;26:98.

Garcia J, Jones HW. The split thickness graft technic for vaginal agenesis. *Obstet Gynecol* 1977;49:328.

Garcia RF. Z-plasty for correction of congenital transverse vaginal septum. *Am J Obstet Gynecol* 1967;99:1164.

Gastol P, Baka-Jakubiak L, Skobejko-Wlodarska L, et al. Complete duplication of the bladder, urethra, vagina, and uterus in girls. *Urology* 2000;55:578.

Gauwerky JFH, Wallwiener D, Bastert G. An endoscopically assisted technique for reconstruction of a neovagina. *Arch Gynecol Obstet* 1992;252:59.

Geary WL, Weed JC. Congenital atresia of the uterine cervix. *Obstet Gynecol* 1973;42:213.

Genest D, Farber M, Mitchell GW, et al. Partial vaginal agenesis with a urinary-vaginal fistula. *Obstet Gynecol* 1981;58:130.

Goh DW, Davey RB, Dewan PA. Bladder, urethral, and vaginal duplication. *J Pediatr Surg* 1995;30:125.

Goodman FR, Bacchelli C, Brady AF, et al. Novel HOXA13 mutations and the phenotypic spectrum of hand-foot-genital syndrome. *Am J Hum Genet* 2000;67:197.

Goodman FR, Scambler PJ. Human HOX gene mutations. *Clin Genet* 2001;59:1.

Graves WP. Method of constructing an artificial vagina. *Surg Clin North Am* 1921;1:611.

Griffin JE, Edwards C, Madden JD, et al. Congenital absence of the vagina. *Ann Intern Med* 1976;85:224.

Haddad B, Louis-Sylvestre C, Poitout P, et al. Longitudinal vaginal septum: a retrospective study of 202 cases. *Eur J Obstet Gynecol Reprod Biol* 1997;74:197.

Haddad B, Barranger E, Paniel BJ. Blind hemivagina: long-term follow-up and reproductive performance in 42 cases. *Hum Reprod* 1999;14:1962.

Haney AF, Hammond CB, Soules MR, et al. Diethylstilbestrol-induced upper genital tract abnormalities. *Fertil Steril* 1979;29:142.

Hauser GA, Keller M, Koller T. Das Rokitansky-Küster Syndrom. Uterus bipartitus solidus rudimentarius cum vagina solida. *Gynecologia* 1961;151:111.

Hauser GA, Schreiner WE. Das Mayer-Rokitansky-Küster Syndrom. *Schweiz Med Wochenschr* 1961;91:381.

Heinonen PK. Longitudinal vaginal septum. *Eur J Obstet Gynecol Reprod Biol* 1982;13:253.

Heinonen PK, Pystynen PP. Primary infertility and uterine anomalies. *Fertil Steril* 1983;40:291.

Heinonen PK, Saarikoski S, Pystynen P. Reproductive performance of women with uterine anomalies. *Acta Obstet Gynecol Scand* 1982;61:157.

Hendren WH, Donahue PK. Correction of congenital abnormalities of the vagina and perineum. *J Pediatr Surg* 1980;15:751.

Hickok LR. Hysteroscopic treatment of the uterine septum: a clinician's experience. *Am J Obstet Gynecol* 2000;182:1414.

Hojsgaard A, Villadsen I. McIndoe procedure for congenital vaginal agenesis: complications and results. *Br J Plast Surg* 1995;48:97.

Holden R, Hart P. First-trimester rudimentary horn pregnancy: preruptureultrasounddiagnosis. *Obstet Gynecol* 1983;61[Suppl]:56.

Homer HA, Li T, Cooke ID. The septate uterus: a review of management and reproductive outcome. *Fertil Steril* 2000;73:1.

Hucke J, Pelzer V, Bruyne FD, et al. Laparoscopic modification of the Vecchietti-operation for creation of a neovagina. *J Pelvic Surg* 1995;1:191.

Hundley AF, Fielding JR, Hoyte l. Double cervix and vagina with septate uterus: an uncommon müllerian malformation. *Obstet Gynecol* 2001;98:982.

Hurst BS, Rock JA. Preoperative dilatation to facilitate repair of high transverse vaginal septum. *Fertil Steril* 1992;57:1351.

Ingram JM. The bicycle seat stool in the treatment of vaginal agenesis and stenosis: a preliminary report. *Am J Obstet Gynecol* 1981;140:867.

Israel R, March CM. Hysteroscopic incision of the septate uterus. *Am J Obstet Gynecol* 1984;149:66.

Jabs EW, Leonard CO, Phillips JA. New features of the McKusick-Kaufman syndrome. *Birth Defects* 1982;18:161.

Jacob JH, Griffin WT. Surgical reconstruction of congenital atresia of the cervix. *Am J Obstet Gynecol* 1961;82:923.

Jacobsen LJ, DeCherney A. Shall we operate on Müllerian defects? Results of conventional and hysteroscopic surgery. *Fertil Steril* 2000;73:1376.

Jeffcoate TNA. Advancement of the upper vagina in the treatment of haematocolpos and haematometra caused by vaginal aplasia. Pregnancy following the construction of an artificial vagina. *J Obstet Gynaecol Br Comm* 1969;76:961.

Jewelewicz R, Husami N, Wallach EE. When uterine factors cause infertility. *Contemp Obstet Gynecol* 1980;16:95.

Jones HW. An anomaly of the external genitalia in female patients with exstrophy of the bladder. *Am J Obstet Gynecol* 1973;117:748.

Jones HW. Reproductive impairment and the malformed uterus. *Fertil Steril* 1981;36:137.

Jones HW, Delfs E, Jones GE. Reproductive difficulties in double uterus: the place of plastic reconstruction. *Am J Obstet Gynecol* 1956;72:865.

Jones HW, Jones GE. Double uterus as an etiological factor in repeated abortion: indications for surgical repair. *Am J Obstet Gynecol* 1953;65:325.

Jones HW, Mermut S. Familial occurrence of congenital absence of the vagina. *Am J Obstet Gynecol* 1972;114:1100.

Jones HW, Rock JA. *Reparative and constructive surgery of the female generative tract.* Baltimore: Williams & Wilkins, 1983.

Jones HW, Wheeless CR. Salvage of the reproductive potential of women with anomalous development of the müllerian ducts: 1868-1968-2068. *Am J Obstet Gynecol* 1969; 104:348.

Jones TB, Fleischer AC, Daniell JF, et al. Sonographic characteristics of congenital uterine abnormalities and associated pregnancy. *J Clin Ultrasound* 1980;8:435.

Jones WS. Obstetric significance of female genital anomalies. *Obstet Gynecol* 1957;10:113.

Karjalainen O, Myllynenl O, Kajanoja P, et al. Management of vaginal agenesis. *Ann Chir Gynaecol* 1980;69:37.

Kaufman RH, Binder GL, Gray PM, et al. Upper genital tract changes associated with exposure in utero to diethylstilbestrol. *Am J Obstet Gynecol* 1977;128:51.

Knab DR. *Müllerian agenesis: a review.* Bethesda, MD: Department of Gynecology/Obstetrics, Uniformed Services University School of Medicine and Naval Hospital, 1983.

Kusuda M. Infertility and metroplasty. *Acta Obstet Gynecol Scand* 1982;61:407.

Laffarque F, Giacalone PL, Boulot P, et al. A laparoscopic procedure for the treatment of vaginal aplasia. *Br J Obstet Gynaecol* 1995;102:565.

Lees DH, Singer A. Vaginal surgery for congenital abnormalities and acquired constructions. *Clin Obstet Gynecol* 1982;25:883.

Letterie GS. Combined congenital absence of the vagina and cervix. *Gynecol Obstet Invest* 1998;46:65.

Lodi A. Contributo clinico statistico sulle malformazion della vagina osservate nella clinica Obstetrica e Ginecologica di Milano dal 1906 al 1950. *Ann Ostet Ginecol Med Perinat* 1951;73:1246.

Ludmir J, Samuels P, Brooks S, et al. Pregnancy outcome of patients with uncorrected uterine anomalies managed in a high risk obstetric setting. *Obstet Gynecol* 1990;75:907.

Maciulla GJ, Heine MW, Christian CD. Functional endometrial tissue with vaginal agenesis. *J Reprod Med* 1978;21:373.

Magalhaes ML, Campos LA, Souza LC, et al. A case of association of duplication of the urogenital and intestinal tracts. *J Pediatr Adolesc Gynecol* 1999;12:165.

Magrina JF, Masterson BJ. Vaginal reconstruction in gynecological oncology: a review of techniques. *Obstet Gynecol Surv* 1981;36:1.

Mahgoub SE. Unification of a septate uterus: Mahgoub's operation. *Int J Gynecol Obstet* 1978;15:400.

Makinoda S, Nishiya M, Sogame M, et al. Non-grafting method of vaginal construction for patients of vaginal agenesis without functioning uterus (Mayer-Rokitansky-Küster Syndrome). *Int Surg* 1996;81:385.

Mandell J, Stevens PS, Lucey DT. Diagnosis and management of hydrometrocolpos in infancy. *J Urol* 1978;120:262.

Markham SM, Parmley TH, Murphy AA, et al. Cervical agenesis combined with vaginal agenesis diagnosed by magnetic resonance imaging. *Fertil Steril* 1987;48:143.

Matsui H, Seki K, Sekiya S. Prolapse of the neovagina in Mayer-Rokitansky-Küster-Hauser Syndrome. *J Reprod Med* 1999;44:548.

McCraw JB, Massey FM, Shanklin KD, et al. Vaginal reconstruction with gracilis myocutaneous flaps. *Plast Reconstr Surg* 1976;58:176.

McDonough PG, Tho PT. Use of pelvic pneumoperitoneum: a critical assessment of 12 years experience. *South Med J* 1974;67:517.

McIndoe AH. The treatment of congenital absence and obliterative conditions of the vagina. *Br J Plast Surg* 1950;2:254.

McIndoe AH, Banister JB. An operation for the cure of congenital absence of the vagina. *J Obstet Gynaecol Br Emp* 1938;45:490.

McKusick VA. Transverse vaginal septum (hydrometrocolpos). *Birth Defects* 1971;7:326.

McKusick VA, Bauer RL, Koop CE, et al. Hydrometrocolpos as a simply inherited malformation. *JAMA* 1964;189:119.

McKusick VA, Weilbaccher RG, Gragg GW. Recessive inheritance of a congenital malformation syndrome. *JAMA* 1968;204:111.

McShane PM, Reilly RJ, Schiff I. Pregnancy outcomes following Tompkins metroplasty. *Fertil Steril* 1983;40:190.

Mizuno K, Koike K, Ando K, et al. Significance of Jones-Jones operation on double uterus: vascularity and dating of endometrium in uterine septum. *Jpn J Fertil Steril* 1978;23:9.

Moutos DM, Damewood MD, Schlaff WD, et al. A comparison of the reproductive outcome between women with a unicornuate uterus and women with a didelphic uterus. *Fertil Steril* 1992;58:88.

Murphy AA, Krall A, Rock JA. Bilateral functioning uterine anlagen with the Rokitansky-Mayer-Küster-Hauser syndrome. *Int J Fertil* 1987;32:296.

Musich JR, Behrman SJ. Obstetric outcome before and after metroplasty in women with uterine anomalies. *Obstet Gynecol* 1978;52:63.

Musset R. Traitement chirurgical des cloisans transversales due vagin d'origine congenitale par la plastie en "Z" a l'Hopital Lariboisiere. *Gynec et Obstet* 1956;55:382.

Nagel TC, Malo JW. Hysteroscopic metroplasty in diethylstilbestrol-exposed uterus and similar fusion anomalies. *Fertil Steril* 1993;59:502.

Niver DH, Barrette G, Jewelewicz R. Congenital atresia of the uterine cervix and vagina-three cases. *Fertil Steril* 1980;33:25.

Nunley WC, Kitchin JD. Congenital atresia of the uterine cervix with pelvic endometriosis. *Arch Surg* 1980;115:757.

O'Leary JL, O'Leary JA. Rudimentary horn pregnancy. *Obstet Gynecol* 1963;22:371.

Ota H, Tanaka J, Murakami M, et al. Laparoscopy-assisted Ruge procedure for the creation of a neovagina in a patient with Mayer-Rokitansky-Küster-Hauser syndrome. *Fertil Steril* 2000;73:641.

Ozek C, Gurler T, Alper M, et al. Modified McIndoe procedure for vaginal agenesis. *Ann Plast Surg* 1999;43:393.

Patil V, Hixon FP. The role of tissue expanders in vaginoplasty for congenital malformations of the vagina. *Br J Urol* 1992;70:554.

Petrozza JC, Gray MR, Davis AJ, et al. Congenital absence of the uterus and vagina is not commonly transmitted as a dominant genetic trait: outcomes of surrogate pregnancies. *Fertil Steril* 1997;67:387.

Phupong V, Pruksananonda K, Taneepanichskul S, et al. Double uterus with unilaterally obstructed hemivagina and ipsilateral renal agenesis: a variety presentation and a ten-year review of the literature. *J Med Assoc Thai* 2000;83:569.

Pinsky L. A community of human malformation syndromes involving the müllerian ducts, distal extremities, urinary tract, and ears. *Teratology* 1974;9:65.

Popaw DD. Utilization of the rectum in construction of a functional vagina. *Russk Virach St Peter* 1910;43:1512.

Pratt JH. Vaginal atresia corrected by use of small and large bowel. *Clin Obstet Gynecol* 1972;15:639.

Ravasia DJ, Brain PH, Pollard JK. Incidence of uterine rupture among women with müllerian duct anomalies who attempt vaginal birth after cesarean delivery. *Am J Obstet Gynecol* 1999;181:877.

Roberts CP, Haber MJ, Rock JA. Vaginal creation for müllerian agenesis. *Am J Obstet Gynecol* 2001;185:1349.

Rock JA, Baramki TA, Parmley TH, et al. A unilateral functioning uterine anlage with müllerian duct agenesis. *Int J Gynecol Obstet* 1980;18:99.

Rock JA, Carpenter SE, Wheeless CR, et al. The clinical management of maldevelopment of the uterine cervix. *J Pelvic Surg* 1995;1:129.

Rock JA, Jones HW. The clinical management of the double uterus. *Fertil Steril* 1977;28:798.

Rock JA, Jones HW. The double uterus associated with an obstructed hemivagina and ipsilateral renal agenesis. *Am J Obstet Gynecol* 1980;138:339.

Rock JA, Jones HW Jr. Vaginal forms for dilatation and/or to maintain vaginal patency. *Fertil Steril* 1984;42:187.

Rock JA, Parmley T, Murphy AA, et al. Malposition of the ovary associated with uterine anomalies. *Fertil Steril* 1986;45:561.

Rock JA, Reeves LA, Retto H, et al. Success following vaginal creation for müllerian agenesis. *Fertil Steril* 1983;39:809.

Rock JA, Roberts CP, Hesla JS. Hysteroscopic metroplasty of the class Va uterus with preservation of the cervical septum. *Fertil Steril* 1999;72:942.

Rock JA, Schlaff WD. The obstetrical consequences of uterovaginal anomalies. *Fertil Steril* 1985;43:681.

Rock JA, Schlaff WD, Zacur HA, et al. The clinical management of congenital absence of the uterine cervix. *Int J Gynecol Obstet* 1984;22:229.

Rock JA, Zacur HA. The clinical management of repeated early pregnancy wastage. *Fertil Steril* 1983;39:123.

Rock JA, Zacur HA, Dlugi AM, et al. Pregnancy success following surgical correction of imperforate hymen and complete transverse vaginal septum. *Obstet Gynecol* 1982;59:448.

Rotmensch J, Rosensheim N, Dillon M, et al. Carcinoma arising in the neovagina: case report and review of the literature. *Obstet Gynecol* 1983;61:534.

RugeE. Ersatz der durch die flexur mittels laparotomie. *Dtsch Med Wochenschr* 1914;40:120.

Sanders BH, Machan LS, Gomel V. Complex uterine surgery: a cooperative role for interventional radiology with hysteroscopic surgery. *Fertil Steril* 1998;70:952.

Schubert G. Uber Scheidenbildung bei angeborenem Vaginaldefekt. *Zentralbl Gynaekol* 1911;45:1017.

Semmens JP. Abdominal contour in the third trimester: an aid to diagnosis of uterine anomalies. *Obstet Gynecol* 1965;25:779.

Sheldon CA, Gilbert A, Lewis AG. Vaginal reconstruction: critical technical principles. *J Urol* 1994;152:190.

Shokeir MHK. Aplasia of the müllerian system: evidence for probably sex-limited autosomal dominant inheritance. *Birth Defects* 1978;14:147.

Simpson JL. Genetics of the female reproductive ducts. *Am J Med Genet* 1999;89:224.

Singh KJ, Devi L. Hysteroplasty and vaginoplasty for reconstruction of the uterus. *Int J Gynecol Obstet* 1980;17:457.

Singh M, Gearheart JP, Rock JA. Double urethra, double bladder, left renal agenesis, persistent hymen, double vagina and uterus didelphys. *Adolesc Pediatr Gynecol* 1993;6:99.

Soong YK, Chang FH, Lai YM, et al. Results of modified laparoscopically assisted neovaginoplasty in 18 patients with congenital absence of the vagina. *Hum Reprod* 1996;11:200.

Stanton SL. Gynecologic complications of epispadias and bladder exstrophy. *Am J Obstet Gynecol* 1974;119:749.

Stoot JE, Mastboom JL. Restriction on the indications for metroplasty. *Acta Eur Fertil* 1977;8:79.

Strassmann EO. Operations for double uterus and endometrial atresia. *Clin Obstet Gynecol* 1961;4:240.

Strassmann EO. Plastic unification of double uterus. *Am J Obstet Gynecol* 1952;64:25.

Strassmann P. Die operative vereinigung eines doppelten uterus. *Zentralbl Gynakol* 1907;29:1322.

Strickland JL, Cameron WJ, Krantz KE. Long-term satisfaction of adults undergoing McIndoe vaginoplasty as adolescents. *Adolesc Pediatr Gynecol* 1993;6:135.

Tancer ML, Katz M, Veridiano NP. Vaginal epithelialization with human amnion. *Obstet Gynecol* 1979;54:345.

Templeman CL, Hertweck SP, Levine RL, et al. Use of laparoscopically mobilized peritoneum in the creation of a neovagina. *Fertil Steril* 2000;74:589.

Thompson DP, Lynn HB. Genital anomalies associated with solitary kidney. *Mayo Clin Proc* 1966;41:538.

Thompson JD, Wharton LR, Te Linde RW. Congenital absence of the vagina. *Am J Obstet Gynecol* 1957;74:397.

Tompkins P. Comments on the bicornuate uterus and twinning. *Surg Clin North Am* 1962;42:1049.

Ulfelder H, Robboy SJ. The embryologic development of the human vagina. *Am J Obstet Gynecol* 1976;126:769.

Valdes C, Malini S, Malinak L. Sonography in the surgical management of vaginal and cervical atresia. *Fertil Steril* 1983;40:263.

Vecchietti G. Neovagina nella sindrome di Rokitansky-Küster-Hauser. *Attual Ostet Ginecol* 1965;11:129.

Vecchietti G, Ardillo L. *La sindrome di Rokitansky-Küster-Hauser. Fisiopatologia e clinica dell-aplasia vaginale con corni uterini rudimentali.* Roma: Societa Editrice Universo, 1970.

Vecchietti G. Le neo-vagin dans le syndrome de Rokitansky-Küster-Hauser. *Rev Med Suisse Romande*1979;99:593.

Vecchietti G. Die neovagina beim Rokitansky-Küster-Hauser-Syndrom. *Gynäkologe* 1980;13:112.

Veronikus DK, McClure GB, Nichols DH. The Vecchietti operation for constructing a neovagina: indications, instrumentation, and techniques. *Obstet Gynecol* 1997;90:301.

Weed JC, McKee DM. Vulvoplasty in cases of exstrophy of the bladder. *Obstet Gynecol* 1974;43:512.

Weijenborg PT, terKuile MM. The effect of a group programme on women with the Mayer-Rokitansky-Küster-Hauser-Syndrome. *Br J Obstet Gynaecol* 2000;107:365.

Wharton LR. Congenital malformations associated with developmental defects of the female reproductive organs. *Am J Obstet Gynecol* 1947;53:37.

Wharton LR. Further experiences in construction of the vagina. *Ann Surg* 1940;111:1010.

Wharton LR. A simple method of constructing a vagina. *Ann Surg* 1938;107:842.

Williams EA. Congenital absence of the vagina, a simple operation for its relief. *J Obstet Gynaecol Br Comm* 1964;71:511.

Williams EA. Uterovaginal agenesis. *Ann R Coll Surg Engl* 1976;58:266.

Williams EA. Vulvo-vaginoplasty. *Proc R Soc Med* 1970;63:40.

Woelfer B, Salim R, Banerjee S. Reproductive outcomes in women with congenital uterine anomalies detected by three-dimensional ultrasound screening. *Obstet Gynecol* 2001:98;1099.

Te Linde's Operative Gynecology, ninth edition, edited by John A. Rock and Howard W. Jones, III. Lippincott Williams & Wilkins, Philadelphia © 2003.

CHAPTER

30

Leiomyomata Uteri and Myomectomy

LESLEY L. BREECH   JOHN A. ROCK

Leiomyomata are the most common tumors of the uterus and the female pelvis. This chapter discusses the pathologic and clinical features of uterine leiomyomata, the choice of treatment, and the indications and techniques for myomectomy.

Hysterectomy is sometimes required for the management of leiomyomata. It is also performed for many other indications, but leiomyomata uteri is the most common indication for hysterectomy. Refer to Chapter 31 for a complete discussion of hysterectomy.

Advances in gynecologic surgery just 100 years ago finally brought this common and sometimes fatal disease of women under reasonable control. Before the 20th century, no effective treatment was available. Uterine leiomyomata often grew to enormous size and caused great suffering from bleeding, pain, and emaciation (Fig. 30.1). Death from this benign disease was not uncommon. Progress in gynecologic surgery and anesthesia finally allowed the safe removal of these tumors by skilled gynecologic surgeons.

No one played a more important role in this endeavor than Drs. Kelly and Cullen. Working together at the Johns Hopkins Hospital, they gradually developed surgical techniques that were successful in preventing and controlling intraoperative hemorrhage. Several illustrations from their magnificent treatise, *Myomata of the*

Uterus, published in 1907, are included in this chapter. In the preface, Cullen wrote:

> It was my good fortune to come to Baltimore in 1891, shortly after the hospital opened. At that time many cases of myoma were considered inoperable, and even when hysterectomy was undertaken it was only in the cases in which a stout rubber ligature could be temporarily tied around the cervix and when, as happened in some cases, this ligature slipped, alarming hemorrhage followed. Then came the systematic controlling of each of the cardinal vessels; later the bisection, and finally the transverse severance of the cervix as a preliminary feature of the operation in exceptionally difficult cases, until at present a myomatous uterus that cannot be removed is almost unheard of. I have watched the gradual simplication of the surgical procedures with the greatest interest. Many American surgeons have had much to do with the wonderful advance in this direction, but I know of no other man, either here or abroad, who has done as much toward this advancement as Howard A. Kelly.

The mortality rate for 1,373 operations performed for uterine leiomyomata at the Johns Hopkins Hospital between 1889 and 1906 was 5.75%; it was less than 1% for 238 operations performed between 1906 and 1909. In 55 patients, no operation was attempted because of

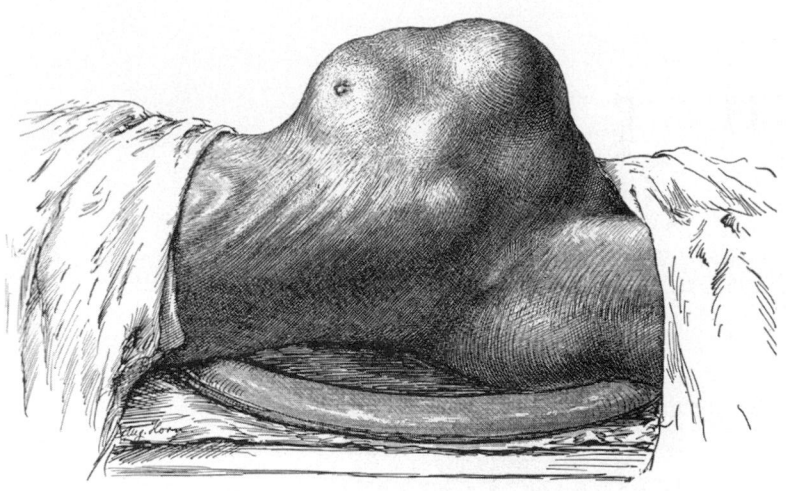

FIGURE 30.1. The patient is thin and emaciated, the outline of the ribs being prominent. Such advanced and neglected cases of multiple uterine leiomyomata are rarely seen today.

refusal or the patient's weakened condition. Among these patients, 21 deaths occurred in the hospital. Death from uterine leiomyomata is a rare occurrence today. The almost total elimination of mortality caused by this tumor represents a major milestone in the health care of women.

During the past century, hysterectomy and myomectomy by the traditional and classic techniques have been the main treatment for women with uterine leiomyomata and significant symptoms, and they continue to be so today. Each year in the United States, about 175,000 hysterectomies are performed with uterine leiomyomata as the primary indication. However, this traditional management will change in the future, for several reasons:

1. Concern regarding the increasing costs of health care has focused on the need to use effective but less expensive methods of management of uterine leiomyomata.

2. Advances in surgical technology now allow certain patients to be treated with new, minimally invasive techniques, including laparoscopic hysterectomy, laparoscopic-assisted vaginal hysterectomy, laparoscopic myomectomy, laparoscopic myoma coagulation (myolysis), and hysteroscopic resection of submucous myomata. Under proper circumstances, these procedures can be safe, effective, and less costly, but more time is needed before they will be available to a greater number of patients in need.

3. Interest in nonsurgical management also appears to be increasing with more data available regarding minimally invasive procedures including uterine artery embolization. This procedure is emerging from an investigational realm to common clinical practice. As more long-term data become available, outcomes and prognosis may be more clearly delineated.

4. A medical approach to the management of patients with leiomyomata is now available. Gonadotropin-releasing hormone (GnRH) analogs, administered for 4 to 6 months, cause most uterine leiomyomata to shrink. However, the myomata regain their original size several months after the GnRH analog is discontinued. This medical regimen has been useful as an adjunct to surgical management. Women who become symptomatic with leiomyomata just before menopause can be treated temporarily with GnRH analogs and can possibly avoid surgical therapy.

5. Uterine leiomyoma is a major public health and women's health care problem. Society has a legitimate reason for interest and concern and has questioned the advisability of hysterectomy for the management of most cases of uterine leiomyomata. Many women insist on the preservation of uterine function for future childbearing, and sometimes even when future childbearing is not desired or not likely to occur. There will probably be a greater emphasis on expectant management, medical management, minimally invasive surgical procedures, and conservational management of uterine leiomyomata in the future.

In the future, the traditional and classic techniques of hysterectomy and myomectomy will be required less often for patients with symptomatic leiomyomata. At present, however, these operations are still appropriate in many situations.

ETIOLOGY, PATHOLOGY, AND GROWTH CHARACTERISTICS OF UTERINE LEIOMYOMATA

A leiomyoma is a benign tumor composed mainly of smooth muscle cells but containing varying amounts of fibrous connective tissue. The tumor is well circumscribed but not encapsulated. Various terms are used to refer to the tumor, such as *fibromyoma, myofibroma, leiomyofibroma, fibroleiomyoma, myoma, fibroma,* and *fibroid.* The latter designation is the one most commonly used, but it is the least accurate and acceptable. The term *leiomyoma* is a reasonably accurate one that emphasizes the origin of this tumor from smooth muscle cells and the predominance of the smooth muscle component.

The tissue culture work of Miller and Ludovici suggested an origin from smooth muscle cells. The studies of Townsend and associates suggest a unicellular origin for leiomyomata.

Leiomyomata are the most common tumors of the uterus and female pelvis. It is impossible to determine their true incidence accurately, although the frequently quoted incidence of 50% found at postmortem examinations seems reasonable. Leiomyomata are responsible for about one third of all hospital admissions to gynecology services. It is well recognized that the incidence is much higher in black women than in white. In a careful study of leiomyomata among women in Augusta, GA, Torpin and associates found the incidence among black women to be three and one third times that among white women. There is no explanation for this racial difference. Leiomyomata also are larger and occur at a younger age in black women. In our institution, a large degenerating intramural leiomyoma was removed from a 1-year-old black girl; the tumor had enlarged the uterus to the level of the umbilicus. In black women, leiomyomata are not uncommon before 30 years of age. However, they are uncommon in either race before 20 years of age. Patients with uterine leiomyomata often have a positive family history of uterine leiomyomata. This suggests the presence of a gene encoding for their development.

About 40% to 50% of leiomyomas show karyotypically detectable chromosomal abnormalities that are both nonrandom and tumor-specific. Identified chromosomal abnormalities include t(12;14)(q15;q23-24), del(7)(q22q32), rearrangements involving 6p21, 10q, trisomy 12, and deletions of 3q. Interestingly, a recent study of 217 myomas found a positive correlation between the presence of a cytogenetic abnormality and the anatomic location of the myoma. In this study by Brosens and colleagues, submucous myomas were consistently shown to have fewer cytogenetic abnormalities when compared with intramural and subserous lesions (12% versus 35% and 29%, respectively). An increased prevalence in certain races, twin studies indicating higher correlation with hysterectomy in monozygotic twins, and increased incidence in first-degree relatives all seem to support an inherited predisposition. The true genetic contribution to the development of uterine leiomyoma remains to be defined.

Most of the data concerning the incidence of uterine leiomyomata are based on gross examination of the uterus, routine pathology reports, or the clinical diagnosis of uterine leiomyomata. Cramer and Patel subjected 100 uteri to gross serial sectioning at 2-mm intervals. They found 649 leiomyomata, roughly threefold the number identified by routine pathologic examination. Admittedly, some were only a few millimeters in diameter, but all were grossly visible. In 48 uteri with no mention of leiomyomata in the routine report, 27 were found to have small tumors. The incidence of leiomyomata was the same in premenopausal and postmenopausal uteri, although the average number of leiomyomata and the average size of the largest leiomyoma were greater in the premenopausal women. This

work has important implications for future epidemiologic studies. It also suggests that it is almost never possible to surgically remove all leiomyomata when a myomectomy is performed.

The growth of leiomyomata is dependent on estrogen production. The tumors thrive during the years of greatest ovarian activity. Continuous estrogen secretion, especially when uninterrupted by pregnancy and lactation, is thought to be the most important underlying risk factor in the development of myomata. After menopause, with regression of ovarian estrogen secretion, growth of leiomyomata usually ceases. Actual regression in the tumor size may occur. There are rare instances, however, of postmenopausal growth of benign leiomyomata, suggesting the possibility of postmenopausal estrogen production either in the ovary or elsewhere. Postmenopausal ovarian cortical stromal hyperplasia may be associated with an increase in estrogen secretion by the ovary. The postmenopausal ovarian stroma in a variety of presumably inactive ovarian tumors, including mucinous cysts and Brenner tumors, can also produce estrogen. When a central pelvic tumor presumed to be uterine leiomyomata enlarges after menopause, one should think of the possibility of malignant change in the leiomyoma itself or in the adjacent myometrium, or of the growth of a new pelvic tumor of extrauterine origin.

Older nulliparous women have an increased risk of developing leiomyomata. However, in multiparous women, the relative risk decreases with each pregnancy. A woman who has had five term pregnancies has only one fifth the risk of a nulliparous woman of developing myomata. The risk is reduced in women who smoke and is increased in obese women; this is possibly related to the conversion of androgens to estrogen by fat aromatase.

The observation that leiomyomata may show significant enlargement during pregnancy provides further clinical evidence of the relation of estrogen and progesterone to the growth of these tumors. However, a better blood supply during pregnancy might also encourage their growth. In a prospective ultrasonographic study of 29 pregnant patients with uterine leiomyomata, Aharoni and associates found no evidence of enlargement of the myomata in 78%. Lev-Toaff and colleagues also confirmed that some leiomyomata do enlarge during pregnancy in response to estrogen and progesterone.

In the initial two decades following the introduction of oral contraceptives containing high-dose estrogen, there was a striking increase in the occurrence of large leiomyomata among young women of all racial backgrounds who took these pills. Although the growth of uterine leiomyomata is not invariably stimulated, oral contraceptives containing high-dose estrogen should not be prescribed for women with these tumors. Oral contraceptives with low-dose estrogen are less likely to stimulate growth. According to Parazzini and associates, there is no significant relation between the occurrence or growth of leiomyomata and the newer oral contraceptives that contain much smaller amounts of estrogens and progestins, and some believe that the risk of developing myomata is reduced with these low-dose pills.

Scientific investigators have been intrigued by the observation that leiomyomata develop during the reproductive years, sometimes grow during pregnancy, and regress after menopause. Nelson, Lipschutz, and others have produced multiple leiomyomata artificially on the serosal surface of the uterus and other peritoneal surfaces in guinea pigs given prolonged estrogen injections. Spellacy and co-workers found that levels of plasma estradiol were the same in patients with and without leiomyomata. However, Wilson and associates found a significantly higher concentration of estrogen receptors in leiomyomata than in myometrium. Farber and colleagues reported that these tumors bind about 20% more estradiol per milligram of cytoplasmic protein than does the normal myometrium of the same organ. This observation was not uniformly true for all leiomyomata, suggesting that different cellular components with a leiomyoma may be associated with different biologic activity. Otubu and co-workers found the concentration of estradiol to be significantly higher in leiomyomata than in normal myometrium, especially in the proliferative phase of the menstrual cycle. Soules and McCarty reported that leiomyomata had more estrogen receptors than did normal uterine tissues in the first phase (days 1 through 9) and in the second phase (days 10 through 18) of the menstrual cycle. Gabb and Stone found that the ability to convert estradiol to estrone was similar in leiomyomata and myometrium. However, Pollow and associates found the conversion of estradiol into estrone to be significantly lower in leiomyomata than in myometrium. This difference in conversion rate could result in a relative accumulation of estrogen in a leiomyoma, causing a hyperestrogenic state within the tumor and surrounding tissues. The enzyme 17β-hydroxy dehydrogenase accelerates the conversion of estradiol to estrone. Leiomyomata have a low concentration of 17β-hydroxy dehydrogenase, which results in a relative accumulation of estradiol in leiomyomatous tissue. These findings may explain the myometrial hypertrophy that is invariably present with leiomyomata.

Other abnormalities in endocrine function have also been suggested. Ylikorkala and colleagues found that pituitary function may be abnormal in women with leiomyomata. Patients with leiomyomata had a low follicle-stimulating hormone level and a diminished follicle-stimulating hormone response to pituitary GnRH. There was an excessive prolactin response to thyrotropin-releasing hormone. Spellacy found that the peak levels of human growth hormone reached during a hypoglycemic test were twice as high in patients with leiomyomata as in the control group. Reddy and Rose suggested the possibility that 5α-reduced androgens may play a role in the pathophysiology of uterine leiomyomata, because a significant increase in 5α-reductase has been found in leiomyoma tissue as compared with myometrium and endometrium. Influenced by the experimental investigations of Lipschutz and associates, Goodman in 1946 treated patients with uterine leiomy-

omata with progesterone and noted a decrease in tumor size in all patients. However, Segaloff and colleagues reported no effect in their study. Goldzieher and co-workers produced histologic evidence of extensive degenerative changes in leiomyomata by administering high-dose progestin therapy (medrogestone in high doses for 21 days). Filiceri and associates have reported the regression of a uterine leiomyoma after long-term administration of a long-acting luteinizing hormone-releasing hormone agonist given to suppress ovarian estrogen secretion. Coutinho successfully used a potent 19-norsteroid antiestrogen–antiprogesterone to treat excessive uterine bleeding in 16 patients with uterine leiomyomata. A reduction in the size of the tumors was noted.

Although the exact etiology of uterine leiomyomata is not known, the puzzle may be solved bit by bit by the research of Kornyei and colleagues, Wilson and co-workers, Tamaya and associates, Buchi and Keller, Sadan and colleagues, and others who continue to investigate estrogen and progesterone as possible growth factors. Although some data are conflicting, evidence suggests that both estrogen and progesterone are involved in the growth of uterine leiomyomata. The possibility that progesterone may play a role in the growth of leiomyomata is suggested by the work of Kawaguchi and co-workers, who found a higher mitotic count in leiomyomata obtained in the proliferative phase of the menstrual cycle.

Anderson and associates have shown that medroxyprogesterone acetate, a progestin, causes a decrease in connexin-43 messenger ribonucleic acid levels in primary cultures of human myometrium and leiomyoma. Connexin-43 is a gap junction protein whose formation is stimulated by 17β-estradiol.

According to the research data of Brandon and colleagues, progesterone receptor messenger ribonucleic acid is overexpressed in uterine leiomyomata, compared with normal adjacent myometrium, suggesting that amplified progesterone-mediated signaling is instrumental in the abnormal growth of these tumors. It is possible that the increased amount of progesterone receptor is caused by an alteration of estrogen or estrogen receptors in leiomyomata. The work of Kastner and co-workers and Nardulli and associates has demonstrated that progesterone receptor expression is regulated by estrogen.

Research in recent years has also focused on polypeptide growth factors in the stimulation of growth of leiomyomata. Polypeptide growth factors that have been investigated include epidermal growth factor, transforming growth factor-alpha, insulin-like growth factor (IGF), and fibroblast growth factor. Other growth factors may also be involved. Polypeptide growth factor research has been performed by Goustin and colleagues, by Hoffmann and co-workers, by Lumsden and associates, and by others. A brief review of this research has been written by Vollenhoven and associates, who have been involved in the study of IGFs in uterine leiomyomata.

Results from a study by Strawn and colleagues demonstrate that IGF-I stimulates leiomyoma growth in a dose-related manner over that of normal myometrial tissue in monolayer culture. This stimulatory effect, in the absence of sex steroid hormones or other growth factors, provides additional support that IGF-I may play an important direct role in the pathogenesis of these tumors, possibly by modulating the response of these tumors to various levels of sex steroids. Dawood and Kahn-Dawood were unable to find any significant elevation in peripheral levels of serum IGF-I in nonpregnant premenopausal women with uterine leiomyomata of 14 weeks' gestational size. The authors state, "Nevertheless, the finding does not detract from the potential paracrine or autocrine role that IGF-I produced by leiomyoma cells may have either on the growth of its own or adjacent myomas or on the vascular supply and blood flow of the uterus and myomas."

Rein and co-workers have proposed a hypothesis to explain the pathogenesis of myomata. This hypothesis suggests a critical role for progesterone in their growth. They state:

> The initiation and growth of myomas likely involves a multistep cascade of separate tumor initiators and promotors. The initial neoplastic transformation of the normal myocyte involves somatic mutations. Although the initiators of the somatic mutations remain unclear, the mitogenic effect of progesterone may enhance the propagation of somatic mutations. Myoma proliferation is the result of clonal expansion and likely involves the complex interactions of estrogen, progesterone, and local growth factors. Estrogen and progesterone appear equally important as promotors of myoma growth.

To treat patients with uterine leiomyomata properly, the gynecologic surgeon must be familiar with their pathology, growth characteristics, and clinical features. Leiomyomata may be single, but most are multiple. They develop most commonly in the uterine corpus and much less often in the cervix. They may develop in the round ligaments, but this is rare. Because they arise in the myometrium, they are all interstitial or intramural in the beginning. As they enlarge, they can remain intramural, but growth often extends in an internal or external direction. Thus, the tumor can eventually become subserous or submucous in location. A subserous tumor can become pedunculated and occasionally parasitic, receiving its blood supply from another source, usually the omentum. A submucous tumor can also become pedunculated and may gradually dilate the endocervical canal and protrude through the cervical os. Indeed, a submucous myoma may descend through the vagina. Rarely, chronic uterine inversion results if the prolapsing submucous leiomyoma is attached to the top of the endometrial cavity and pulls the uterine fundus downward through the cervix.

In general, subserous leiomyomata contain more fibrous tissue than submucous leiomyomata. However, submucous leiomyomata contain more smooth muscle tissue than subserous leiomyomata. Sarcomatous change is more common in submucous tumors.

The typical uterine leiomyoma is a firm multinodular structure of variable size. The largest tumor, reported by Hunt in 1888, weighed more than 65 kg. Tumors of 4 to 5 kg are not rare, but most are smaller. At the operating table, leiomyomata appear as nodular tumors of different sizes that distort the uterus in various ways, depending on their size, location, and direction of growth. Growth between the leaves of the broad ligament and origin from the cervix may make surgical removal difficult. Subserous and subserous pedunculated tumors, as well as intraligamentous tumors, may create problems in diagnosis because they are difficult to distinguish from tumors arising from the adnexal organs (Fig. 30.2). When tumors cause symmetric enlargement of the uterus, they may be mistaken for a pregnant uterus on bimanual examination.

The "normal" intramural leiomyoma on section protrudes from the surrounding compressed myometrium. Ordinarily there is a clear distinction between the myoma and the myometrium so that dissection between the

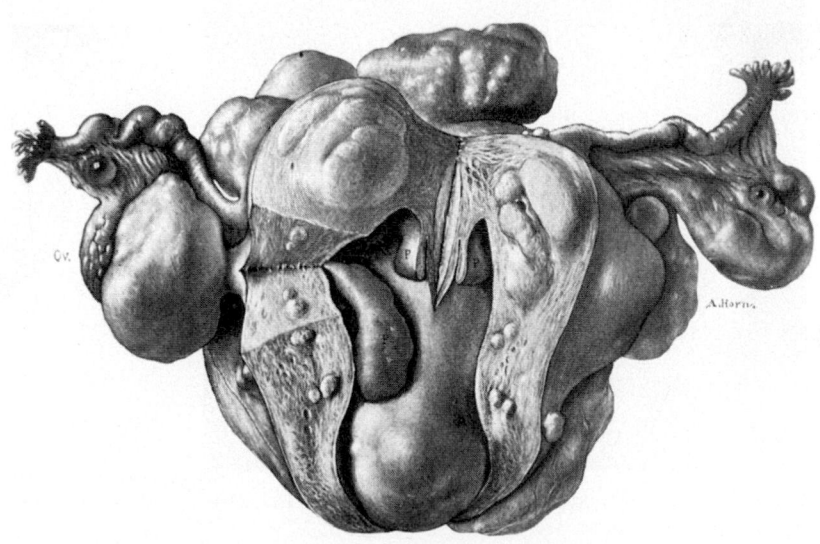

FIGURE 30.2. The uterine corpus is almost completely replaced by small and large myomas in intramural, subserous, and submucous positions. Some are pedunculated. A pedunculated submucous myoma is dilating the endocervical canal. A pedunculated subserous myoma is adjacent to the left ovary and will interfere with its palpation.

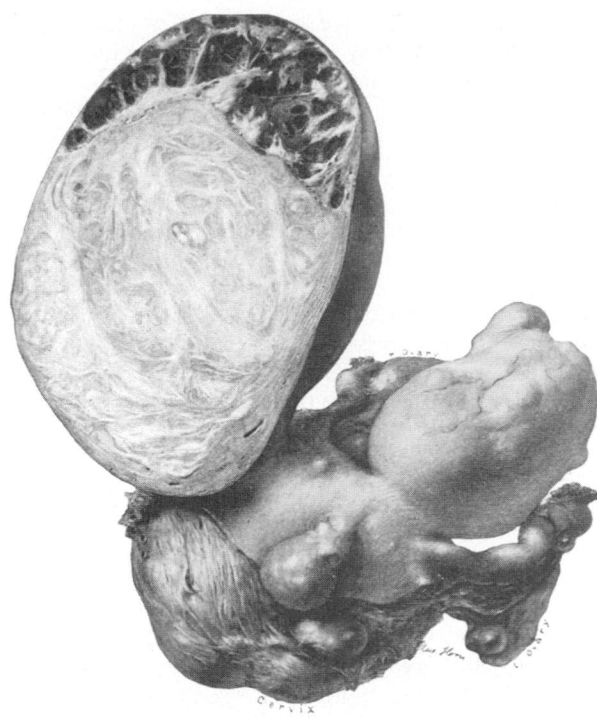

FIGURE 30.3. Multiple leiomyomata are present. A large subserous myoma has undergone partial cystic degeneration.

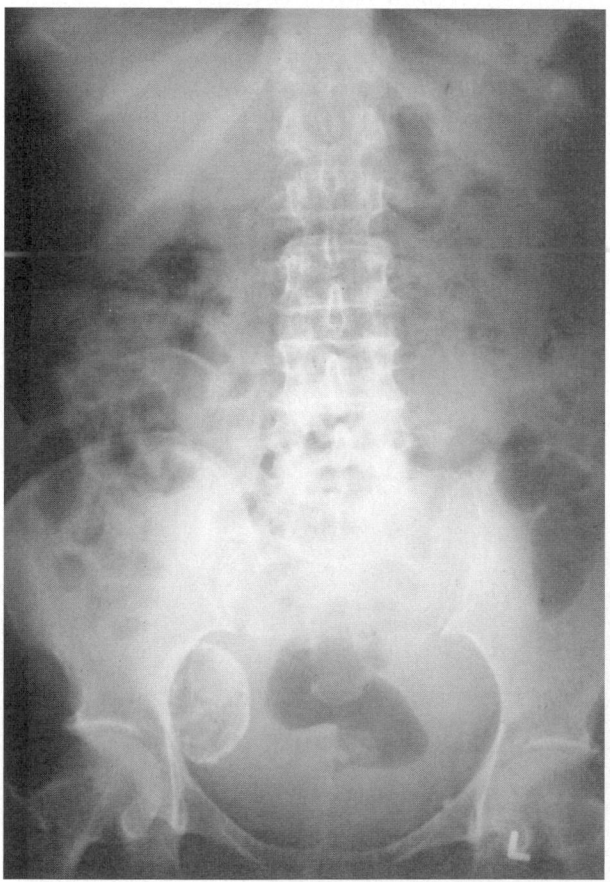

FIGURE 30.4. An abdominal radiograph shows typical calcification in a leiomyoma.

two is easy to accomplish. Myomata usually can be removed from surrounding myometrium with ease. Although these tumors are not encapsulated, a clear distinction can usually be made between a myoma and the myometrium that surrounds it. The cut surface appears as glistening pinkish white and gray. It is firm, and there is a whorl-like arrangement of the muscle and the fibrous tissue. In contrast to this typical appearance, the myometrium may be thickened by a diffuse, ill-defined nodularity of smooth muscle. This so-called diffuse leiomyomatosis usually involves all parts of the myometrium and causes symmetric enlargement of the uterine corpus. The nodules of smooth muscle are not distinct, contain little collagen, and merge with one another and the surrounding hypertrophied myometrium.

The extracellular matrix of leiomyomata is composed mostly of collagen but also contains proteoglycans and fibronectin. According to Fujita, myomata contain 50% more collagen than does normal myometrium, and the ratio of collagen type I to collagen type III is increased in myomata. Proteoglycans provide hydrated spaces between myoma cells. Fibronectin is a glycoprotein that mediates adhesion between myoma cells and extracellular matrix.

The most common change in leiomyomata is hyaline degeneration. The cut surface of a hyalinized area is smooth and homogeneous and does not show the whorl-like arrangement of the rest of the leiomyoma. Almost all leiomyomata, except the smallest, have scattered areas of hyaline degeneration. Eventually these may become liquefied and form cystic cavities filled with clear liquid or gelatinous material (Fig. 30.3). Sometimes the

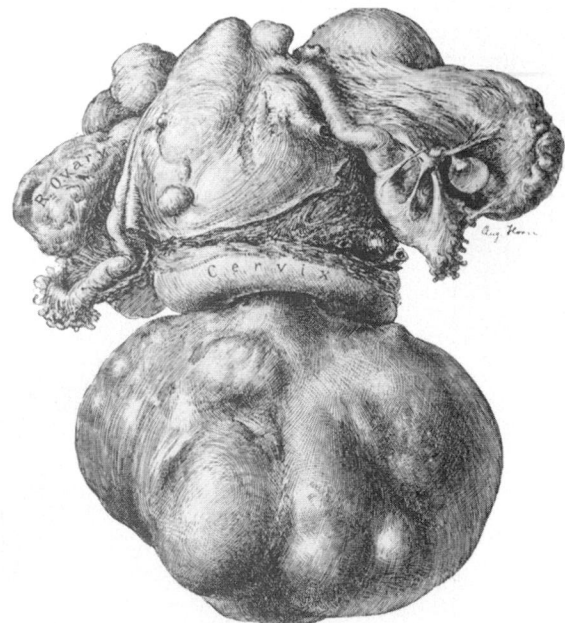

FIGURE 30.5. A large submucous pedunculated myoma has dilated the cervix and is now located in the vagina. Its pedicle is attached inside the uterine cavity. Morcellation of the myoma performed transvaginally allows clamping and ligation of the pedicle.

cystic change is so great that the leiomyoma becomes a mere shell and is truly a cystic tumor. Softness of a tumor does not necessarily indicate cystic degeneration. Fleshy leiomyomata may be equally soft.

Over time, with continued diminished blood supply and ischemic necrosis of tissue, calcium phosphates and carbonates are deposited in myomata. Their presence is evidence of a continuum of degenerative changes. The calcium may be deposited in varying amounts. If it is deposited at the periphery of the tumor, the leiomyoma may resemble a calcified cyst. Other calcified leiomyomata may show an irregular or diffuse distribution throughout with a honeycomb or mulberry appearance. When the degenerative change is advanced, the leiomyoma may become solidly calcified. Such calcified tumors have been called "wombstones." Calcified leiomyomata are seen most often in elderly women, in black women, and in women who have pedunculated subserous tumors. They are easily seen radiographically (Fig. 30.4).

Leiomyomata may undergo changes as a result of infection. Submucous leiomyomata are most commonly infected when they protrude into the uterine cavity, or especially into the vagina (Fig. 30.5). The pedunculated submucous leiomyoma thins out the endometrium as it grows inward, and eventually the surface becomes ulcerated and infected (Fig. 30.6). An intramural leiomyoma in an involuting puerperal uterus can also become infected when endometritis is present. Microscopic abscesses can be found, and gross abscesses occasionally occur, particularly if the leiomyoma descends as low as the cervical canal. Such infections are usually streptococcal and may be virulent. *Bacteroides fragilis* infections also occur. Parametritis, peritonitis, and even septicemia may result.

Necrosis of a leiomyoma is caused by interference with its blood supply. Occasionally a pedunculated subserous leiomyoma twists, and if an operation is not done immediately, infarction results. Necrosis sometimes occurs in the center of a large tumor simply as a result of poor circulation. Necrotic leiomyomata are dark and hemorrhagic in the interior. Eventually the tissue breaks down completely. So-called red or carneous degeneration is seen occasionally, especially in association with pregnancy. This condition is thought to result from poor

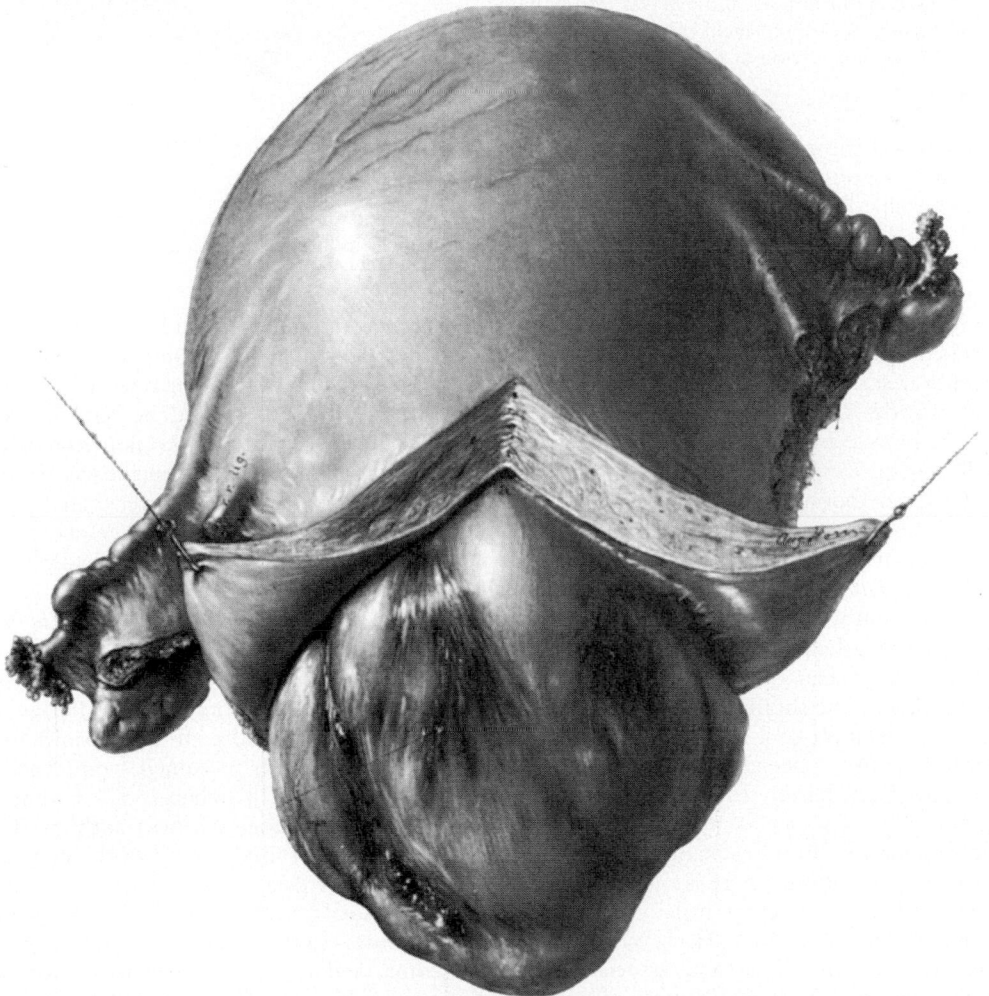

FIGURE 30.6. Pedunculated submucous myoma showing necrosis and ulceration.

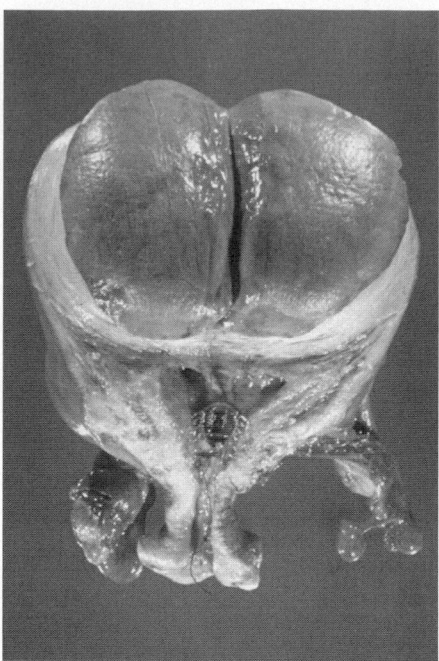

FIGURE 30.7. Degenerating leiomyoma showing carneous discoloration caused by thrombosis and extravasation of blood into the myoma tissue. A Dalkon shield can be seen in the endometrial cavity. See color version of figure.

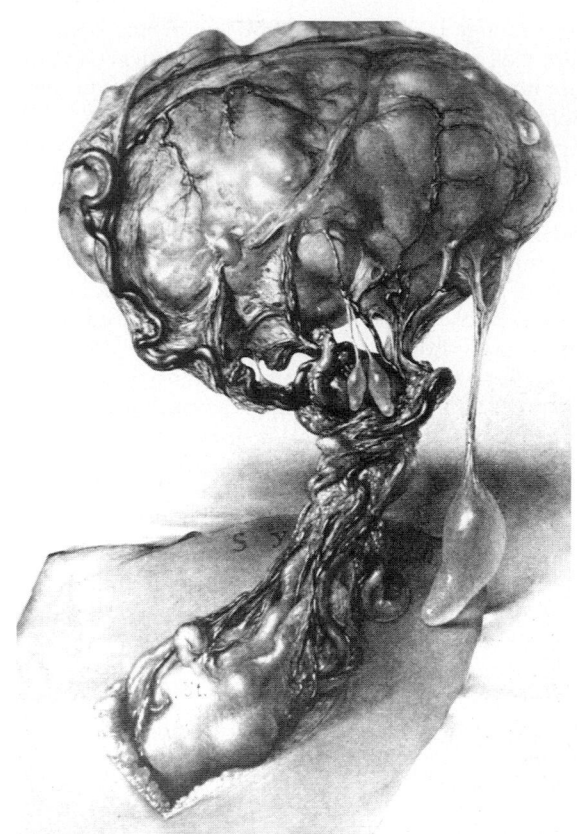

FIGURE 30.8. A subserous pedunculated myoma receives tenuous blood supply through its uterine pedicle. Such a myoma may wander in the upper abdomen and eventually receive its blood supply from other sources. It may also twist on its pedicle and undergo infarction.

circulation of blood through a rapidly growing tumor. Thrombosis and extravasation of blood into the myoma tissue are responsible for the reddish discoloration (Fig. 30.7).

A subserous and especially a subserous pedunculated myoma may gradually outgrow its blood supply (Fig. 30.8). To keep the myoma tissue from undergoing complete ischemic necrosis, the omentum becomes adherent to the peritoneal surface of a pedunculated subserous myoma and provides whatever blood supply is needed. Eventually, the pedicle may disappear or twist, and the myoma will become completely free from the uterus, wander in the upper abdomen, and receive its "parasitic" blood supply from the omentum and other sources.

On occasion, fat occurs in leiomyomata as true fatty degeneration. The cut surface may have a yellowish discoloration. Infrequently, a deposit of true fat may form a fibrolipoma; however, the presence of fat in a leiomyoma is rare. Indeed, if fat is seen grossly or microscopically in a curettage specimen, one should not assume that it represents fatty degeneration of a leiomyoma. One should assume that the uterus has been perforated and that fragments of fat have been curetted from the mesentery or omentum.

The most important, but rare, change in a leiomyoma is sarcomatous degeneration. There is much variation in the reported incidence of sarcoma in leiomyomata. The incidence given by Novak is 0.7%. However, a review of 13,000 myomata by Montague and associates at the Johns Hopkins Hospital revealed 38 cases of malignant change, the incidence of sarcoma thus being 0.29%.

Corscaden and Singh indicated by their study that the true incidence of sarcoma developing within uterine leiomyomata is no higher than 0.13% and is probably as low as 0.04%. It should be remembered that because most women with uterine leiomyomata do not undergo surgical removal, the true incidence of sarcoma in leiomyomata is probably much lower than 1 per 1,000 (0.1%).

After hysterectomy in 1,429 patients with presumed benign leiomyomata, the histologic diagnosis of leiomyosarcoma was made in seven (0.49%), according to a study by Leibsohn and co-workers. There was no evidence of malignancy in the endometrial sampling of any of these seven patients, and the diagnosis was suspected intraoperatively in only three. Uterine weights ranged from 120 to 1,100 g. In a woman between 41 and 50 years of age with presumed symptomatic leiomyomata, there is a 1 in 112 chance of a leiomyosarcoma being present, according to these authors. This information has important implications in the consideration of conservative or delayed treatment for these women. Parker and associates found that the total incidence of uterine sarcomas (leiomyosarcoma, endometrial stromal sarcoma, and mixed mesodermal tumor) among patients operated on for presumed benign uterine leiomyoma is lower (0.23%) than the 0.49% reported by Leibsohn.

The difficulty in defining the true incidence of sarcomatous change is understandable if one is familiar with the histology of leiomyomata. Abundantly cellular leiomyomata are relatively common, and at first glance they suggest sarcoma; however, they lack a significant number of mitotic figures, and patients from whom such tumors are removed all remain well. Misinterpretation of the histologic picture of this type of cellular leiomyoma undoubtedly accounts for the increased incidence of leiomyosarcoma reported by some. When cutting leiomyomata in the operating room, the surgeon finds that sarcomatous areas have a somewhat characteristic appearance, although the histologic diagnosis certainly cannot be made by gross examination. A sarcoma is likely to occur in a rather large leiomyoma and toward the center of the tumor, where the blood supply is poorest. Instead of being firm fibrous tissue that grates when scraped with a knife blade, the tissue is soft and homogeneous, and is described as resembling raw pork. Later, as necrosis of the malignant tissue occurs, it becomes more friable and hemorrhagic.

It has been difficult to understand uterine leiomyosarcoma because pathologists do not agree on the criteria necessary for diagnosis. Some pathologists rely on the mitotic count. All tumors with less than five mitotic figures per 10 high-power fields are considered benign. All tumors with more than 10 mitotic figures per 10 high-power fields are called malignant. Those in between can be called "smooth muscle tumors of uncertain malignant potential."

Other pathologists believe the mitotic count may have some significance but choose to rely instead on the presence of nuclear hyperchromatism, nuclear pleomorphism, or giant cells and other bizarre cell forms to make the diagnosis. Corscaden and Singh believe that no combination of histologic features is reliable and that only smooth muscle tumors that metastasize or recur are definitely malignant. We believe that all of these features should be taken into consideration for diagnosis and prognosis. When the tumor is confined to the uterus, both mitotic grade and histologic grade are important in the diagnosis and prognosis. A poor prognosis is associated with high mitotic counts and extremely atypical and anaplastic cytologic features. Bell and colleagues at Stanford University Medical Center assessed a variety of histopathologic features of 213 problematic smooth muscle neoplasms for which there were at least 2 years of clinical follow-up data. From the wide variety of light-microscopic features assessed, the important predictors that emerged were mitotic index, the degree of cytologic atypia, and the presence or absence of coagulative tumor cell necrosis. Previously, the mitotic index was relied on exclusively to determine whether a uterine smooth muscle tumor was benign or malignant, but currently an approach is used that incorporates additional histopathologic features.

A normal chromosome complement (46,XX) was observed by Meloni and co-workers in about 50% of leiomyoma cases. About 50% showed clonal abnormalities, such as those of chromosomes 1, 7, and 13, and t(12;14). Interstitial deletions of chromosome 7 were the ones most often involved, suggesting that this abnormality may be of primary importance in the cellular proliferation of leiomyomata. A relation between more aggressive histology and chromosomal abnormalities was also suggested.

Tumors that show obvious evidence of blood vessel invasion or spread to contiguous organs are rarely cured. The extent of the disease at the time of initial diagnosis is of even greater significance. In other words, when the diagnosis is suspected for the first time by the pathologist when he examines routine sections from a uterine leiomyoma, the patient almost always survives. However, if the diagnosis is made preoperatively by the gynecologist or is suspected during the operative procedure because of invasion of surrounding organs, the prognosis is grave. The management of leiomyosarcoma is discussed in Chapter 47.

An unusual atypical smooth muscle tumor was first described in the stomach by Martin and associates in 1960. Variously called *bizarre leiomyoma, leiomyoblastoma, clear-cell leiomyoma,* and *plexiform tumorlet,* these atypical smooth tumors probably all belong together. The term *epithelioid leiomyoma* was adopted by the World Health Organization. Kurman and Norris have proposed that this term be used for all atypical leiomyomata. Histologically, the characteristic feature is the mixture of rounded polygonal cells and multinucleated giant cells present in epithelioid clear-cell and plexiform patterns. Clinically, in the uterus most of these tumors are benign. They may rarely exhibit malignant potential. Malignancy is difficult to predict from histologic criteria because some metastases occurred from tumors that demonstrated very few mitoses. Kurman and Norris have suggested, however, that epithelioid neoplasms having more than five mitotic figures per 10 high-power fields should be called *epithelioid leiomyosarcomas* and that the term *epithelioid leiomyoma* should be applied when there is a lower level of mitotic activity. Although combination therapy (surgery plus radiation therapy or chemotherapy) may not be indicated for a patient with an epithelioid leiomyoma, follow-up should be considered essential, as emphasized by Klunder and colleagues.

An unusual benign form of leiomyomata uteri, *intravenous leiomyomatosis,* was first recognized at the turn of the century and has been reported sporadically since then. Before 1982, about 50 cases had been reported, according to Bahary and co-workers. Probably at least that many have been reported since then. Marshall and Morris presented the first detailed report of this entity in the American literature in 1959. The characteristic feature of this peculiar smooth muscle tumor is the extension of the polypoid intravascular projections into the veins of the parametrium and broad ligaments. Although there may be some difficulty in distinguishing such lesions from low-grade sarcoma, they are distinctly different histologically from stromatosis uteri because the intravenous plugs are mainly smooth muscle in origin. In 1966, Edwards and Peacock collected 32 cases of intravenous leiomyomatosis, including two cases of their own, and reviewed the clinical experience with this condition. In approximately 50% of the cases, the intravenous tumor was confined to the parametrium; in 75%, it extended no further than the veins of the broad ligament. The observations of Edwards and Peacock suggest that the severed intravenous extensions are probably incapable of independent parasitic existence and remain dormant after removal of the uterus. However, the cases presented by Bahary and associates tend to refute this idea. Total surgical excision of the tumor should be attempted for successful therapy. Some patients have survived for many years after incomplete resection of the tumor. A review of 14 cases of this rare uterine tumor from the file of the Armed Forces Institute of Pathology has been reported by Norris and Parmley. In this series, two of three patients with incomplete resection had a recurrence; the recurrent tumor was excised surgically, and the patients were alive and free of disease 5 and 11 years after operation. The authors concluded that this tumor behaves clinically like a benign neoplasm, although its wormlike extensions may involve uterine, vaginal, ovarian, and iliac veins. The uterine veins in the broad ligaments are the most common sites of extension. The mitotic index is quite low, with the most active lesions showing only one mitosis per 15 high-power fields. The material from the Armed Forces Institute of Pathology provides histologic evidence consistent with both theories of origin of intravenous leiomyomatosis, namely, that it may be the result of unusual vascular invasion from a leiomyoma or may arise *de novo* from the wall of veins within the myometrium.

Extension of benign leiomyomatosis up the vena cava and into the right atrium has been reported in several cases, with a fatal outcome in some. Before 1994, approximately 27 cases of intravenous leiomyomatosis extending to the heart were reported. Several recent cases requiring open-heart surgery to remove the intracardiac tumor thrombosis have been successful and without recurrence. All reported cases occurred in women. Tierney and colleagues reported that substantial quantities of cytoplasmic estradiol and progesterone receptors were found in the right atrial tumor removed from a patient with intravenous leiomyomatosis. Their patient was treated with the antiestrogen tamoxifen because of residual tumor in the vena cava that could be estrogen dependent. Irey and Norris have presented evidence that female reproductive steroids can produce intimal proliferation of veins in predisposed persons. Interestingly, of the 30 patients with leiomyomata and leiomyosarcomas of the vena cava reviewed by Wray and Dawkins, 80% were female. Both intravenous leiomyomatosis and benign metastasizing leiomyoma have been reported to metastasize to the lung. As suggested by Banner and co-workers, by Horstmann and associates, and by Evans and colleagues, oophorectomy may be indicated in patients with these conditions, again because of the possibility that these tumors may be estrogen dependent or that estrogens may have the ability to stimulate their development, whether in a uterine or extrauterine location and whether they appear to be endothelial or mesenchymal in origin.

The possibility of metastases from a histologically benign uterine leiomyoma has been discussed by Idelson and Davids and by Clark and Weed. When such a case occurs, it is usually settled by finding a sarcomatous component in the leiomyoma or by finding evidence of intravenous leiomyomatosis. However, more than 12 cases have now been reported in which a benign uterine leiomyoma metastasized. Idelson and Davids' case showed metastases to the aortic lymph nodes. The patient reported by Cramer and associates had metastatic tumor to the omentum, ovary, periaortic lymph node, and lung. In each location, the histology and estrogen receptor content of the tumor resembled those of a benign leiomyoma. The recommended treatment consists of surgical removal with castration and little or no estrogen replacement.

Leiomyomatosis peritonealis disseminata is sometimes confused with intravenous leiomyomatosis. However, only subperitoneal surfaces of the uterus and other pelvic and abdominal viscera are involved with leiomyomatosis peritonealis disseminata, and invasion of the lumen of blood vessels does not occur. Only about 15 cases have been reported, according to Pearce. All occurred in patients in the reproductive years who often had large uterine leiomyomata and were usually pregnant or taking oral contraceptives. The condition is likely to be confused with a disseminated intraabdominal malignancy, but it is entirely benign histologically and clinically. Parmley and colleagues have demonstrated the histologic similarities between this peritoneal lesion and the decidual change of the mesothelium in the pelvis, and they propose that the condition represents a benign reparative process in which fibroblasts replace soft peritoneal decidua. They suggest that this fibrocytic reaction occurs during pregnancy and especially in the postpartum period, resulting in nodules with a pseudoleiomyomatous pattern. Similar findings have been noted in patients with endometriosis treated with prolonged Enovid therapy. These findings indicate that prolonged and continuous stimulation of subperitoneal decidua by either endogenous or exogenous estrogen and progesterone is important in the pathogenesis of this condition. Parmley and co-workers suggest that the condition is more appropriately called disseminated fibrosing deciduosis. Goldberg and associates, on the other hand, on the basis of electron microscopy studies, believe that the tumors arise from smooth muscles of small blood vessels. This has been confirmed by Ceccacci and colleagues. It has been possible to show a continuum from fibroblastic cells through myofibroblasts to leiomyocytes. Although the cell of origin of this tumor is still controversial, the tumor is benign and the acceptable treatment to date is total abdominal hysterectomy and bilateral salpingo-oophorectomy. If this tumor occurs in the omentum, an omentectomy should also be performed to define more clearly the histologic nature of the lesion.

In attempting to distinguish between benign and malignant disease in a patient with uterine leiomyomata who also has unusual clinical findings, it is appropriate to keep the entities mentioned earlier (intravenous leiomyomatosis, atypical bizarre leiomyoma, benign metastasizing leiomyoma, and disseminated intraperitoneal leiomyomatosis) in mind. Although they all have features similar to those of malignant disease, they are almost always benign and amenable to treatment. One should also remember that benign uterine leiomyomata have been associated with pseudo-Meigs' syndrome in a few cases. Meigs reported five cases in 1954. In these cases, the ascites did not reappear after removal of the uterine leiomyomata.

There is a high frequency of endometrial hyperplasia when the uterus contains leiomyomata. Degligdish and Loewenthal reported that cystic glandular hyperplasia is often found in the endometrium at the margin of the leiomyoma. Yamamoto and co-workers have reported high concentrations of estrone and estrone sulfatase activity in the endometrium overlying a myoma. They suggest that the local hyperestrogenism in the endometrium overlying a leiomyoma may assist in the genesis or enlargement of these tumors.

Gynecologic surgeons are especially concerned about the vascularity of individual leiomyomata and about the blood flow to the uterus in the presence of multiple and sometimes very large leiomyomata. These considerations are pertinent when surgery, especially myomectomy, is contemplated.

According to Vollenhoven and associates, the vascularization of leiomyomata was studied by Vasserman and colleagues, and the findings were presented to the World Congress of Gynecology and Obstetrics in 1988. Using femoral arteriography, selective intraoperative angiography, radiography, and injection of surgical specimens, these investigators showed that leiomyomata have a rich vascular supply, including blood lakes within tumors. They found more than one nutrient vessel per myoma. Venous channels were predominantly peripheral, whereas the arterial supply was both internal and peripheral. Farrer-Brown and co-workers, using radiologic methods, demonstrated that myomata in various locations within the myometrium can cause congestion and dilatation of endometrial venous plexuses by obstructing venous return. These obstructions can result in ectasia of endometrial and myometrial venules (Fig. 30.9). The degree of vascularity of leiomyomata was also studied by Karlsson and Persson. Vascularity varied from many, to few, to no intrinsic vessels demonstrable. Generally, the sum of the width of the uterine arteries increases with the size of the uterus, but the diameter of the two sides sometimes differs markedly. A rich vascularity was found in 22 of 34 uteri with leiomyomata, but with increasing size there is a tendency to less vascularity. In none of five cases with very large (20 cm or more) leiomyomata uteri

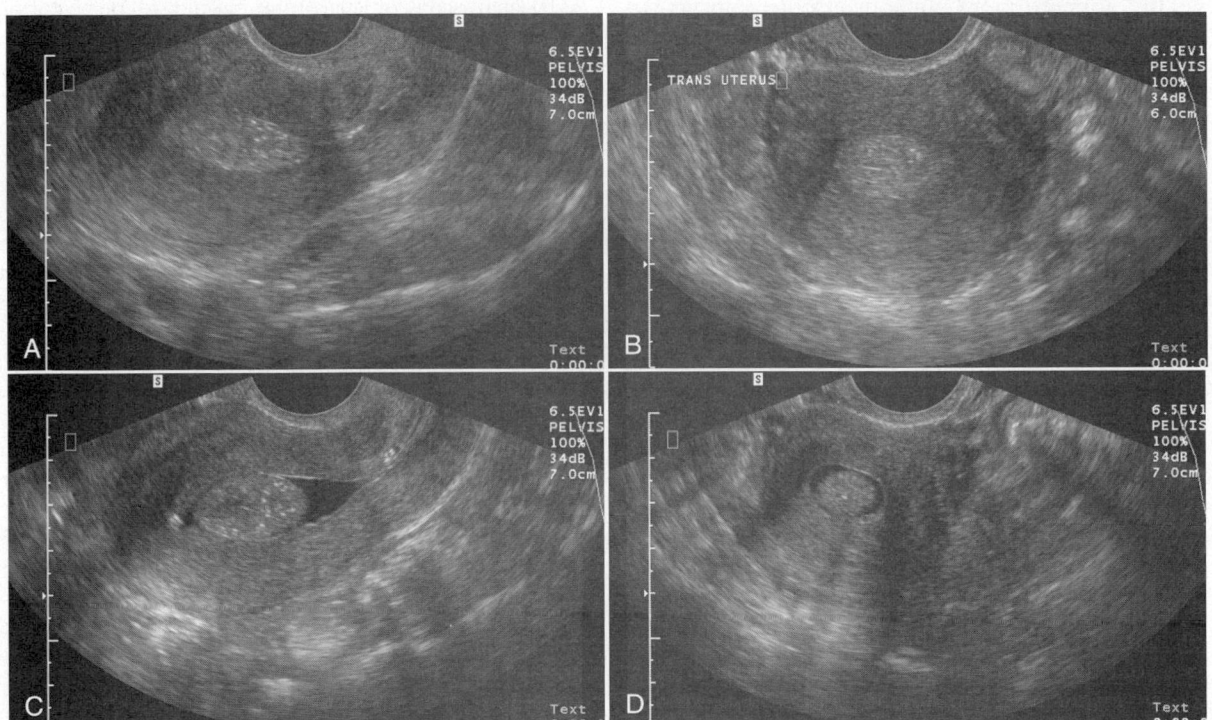

FIGURE 30.9. Sonographic images of a 48-year-old patient with a history of pelvic pain. Both transabdominal and transvaginal images were obtained on cycle day 8. Longitudinal (**A**) and transversely oriented (**B**) transvaginal images reveal a suspicious endometrial cavity, suggesting a thickened lining, endometrial polyp, or a submucosal myoma. **C** and **D:** Fluid-enhanced sonohysterographic studies clearly demonstrate a mass lesion and not generalized thickening of the endometrial lining. The patient underwent a hysteroscopy and uterine curettage, which revealed a histologically confirmed endometrial polyp. (Images courtesy of Jeff Dicke, M.D.)

was the vascularity rich. The intrinsic vessels were few in two cases and absent in three cases.

The total blood flow in a myomatous uterus is greater than the total blood flow in a normal uterus. Blood flow in a myomatous uterus, gram for gram, is less than blood flow in a normal uterus. Blood flow in myomata is reduced compared with blood flow in normal myometrium in the same uterus. Blood flow within a myoma varies from one location to another.

CLINICAL FEATURES OF UTERINE LEIOMYOMATA

Asymptomatic Leiomyomata

Most leiomyomata are asymptomatic. Untold numbers of such symptomless leiomyomata are removed surgically by either hysterectomy or myomectomy when they would have been better left undisturbed. The incidence of malignancy in leiomyomata is less than 0.1%, which is lower than the operative mortality rate of hysterectomy in the average hospital; therefore, unless there is some reason to suspect malignant change, the danger of the operation for asymptomatic leiomyomata may exceed the danger of malignancy. A history of rapid growth, however, particularly postmenopausal growth, does indicate removal, even when the tumor produces no symptoms. Signs of rapid enlargement are important in all patients but are even more ominous in older patients. In younger patients, the most common reason for rapid enlargement of a uterus with leiomyomata is pregnancy. If pregnancy can be ruled out, a leiomyosarcoma may be suspected but is rarely found.

Small leiomyomata that are asymptomatic need only to be observed from time to time, with pelvic examinations perhaps every 6 to 12 months and pelvic ultrasonography when indicated. In the beginning, frequent examination may be indicated to determine the growth rate. Such tumors may remain remarkably constant in size for years. If small leiomyomata are discovered late in menstrual life, it is unusual for symptoms to appear or for surgical treatment to be required. Larger tumors can also be watched safely, but if a policy of watchful waiting is adopted, one should be very sure of the nature of the tumors. If there is uncertainty of the uterine or ovarian origin of a tumor, as may well be the case when the tumor fills the whole pelvis or when a pedunculated tumor is felt in the adnexal region (Fig. 30.10), special diagnostic procedures may be indicated. Pelvic examination by an experienced gynecologist can usually clear up the uncertainty. In difficult cases, an examination under anesthesia may be necessary. Laparoscopy may be of great value in determining the nature of an adnexal mass. Before invasive techniques are used, however, noninvasive special diagnostic procedures should be done. These include radiographic studies of the abdomen and pelvis, ultrasonography (US), and computed tomography (CT). The characteristic calcification in a leiomyoma may be seen on radiographs. The US and CT features of uterine leiomyomata have been well described. However, mistakes in the interpretation can still be made. Tada and associates re-

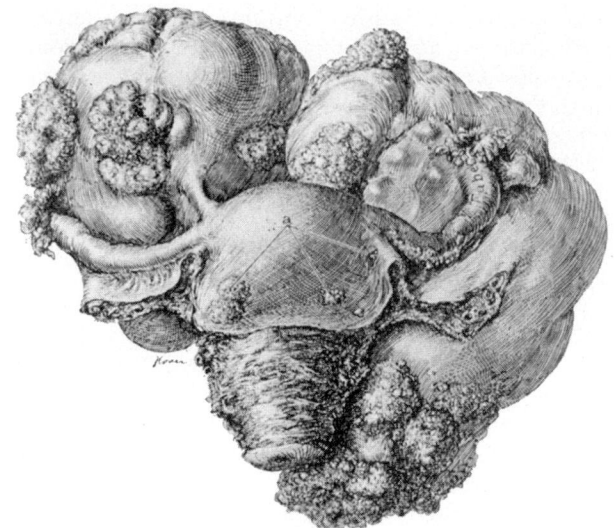

FIGURE 30.10. Although this central pelvic mass may feel like a multiple leiomyomatous uterus on bimanual pelvic examination, it is actually a bilateral ovarian malignancy. Differentiation between these two diagnoses may require special diagnostic procedures.

ported that 5% of patients given the diagnosis of uterine leiomyomata by CT actually had an ovarian tumor at operation. Therefore, if uncertainty about the diagnosis persists, laparoscopy or laparotomy should still be performed.

When large asymptomatic leiomyomata occur in premenopausal women who have had their families or in whom future childbearing is not important, a recommendation for removal may be made. It is impossible to predict which patients will become symptomatic in the remaining years before menopause. However, such tumors, with additional years to grow, are likely to require surgical removal eventually. Therefore, it is better to remove them when the patient is a good operative risk and when conservation of normal ovaries with a good blood supply can be easily accomplished. Such tumors should usually be 12 to 14 weeks in gestational size or larger. Depending on a variety of factors, either myomectomy or hysterectomy can be recommended to the patient. GnRH agonists may be useful in women approaching menopause to control symptoms or asymptomatic uterine myoma growth until menopause. The regrowth of tumors after the cessation of treatment limits the usefulness of these agents, however. Nakamura and Yoshimura reported their experience with GnRH agonists in the treatment of uterine leiomyomata in perimenopausal women. One third of patients reached menopause after 16 weeks of treatment, thus avoiding the need for surgery.

Reiter and colleagues studied 93 consecutive patients undergoing hysterectomy for leiomyomata. When the uterus was larger than 12 weeks' gestational size, there was no increased incidence of surgical complications compared with women with smaller uteri. On the basis of this small series, the authors concluded that hysterectomy need not be recommended to women with large asymptomatic uterine leiomyomata to avoid a possible increased risk of surgical complications.

There is no uniform size of an asymptomatic leiomyomatous uterus that can be used as an indication for hysterectomy or myomectomy. When size is the only significant indication for surgery in an asymptomatic patient, the location of the tumors is more important than the total uterine mass. When the leiomyomata are located in the cornual area or in the lateral wall of the uterus and obscure the anatomy of the adnexa and broad ligament, the risk of error in the early recognition of an ovarian tumor is greater. In such cases, one must carefully weigh the advantages and disadvantages of the conservative approach to the management of uterine leiomyomata. When adnexal tumors are present, it is critical that the origin of these tumors be confirmed. The diagnostic studies mentioned earlier should be performed to establish clearly that the tumors are of uterine origin before a decision is made to follow up the patient rather than operate. It is unacceptable to wait to see whether an adnexal tumor enlarges before identifying the site of origin of the mass as either uterine or ovarian. Ovarian carcinoma remains the most lethal disease of the female reproductive tract and the most difficult to diagnose early. Every diagnostic and therapeutic effort must be made to avoid errors in the clinical evaluation of pelvic neoplasms (Fig. 30.10). In women who are approaching menopause, relatively large uterine leiomyomata can be kept under observation with the knowledge that after menopause they will not increase in size and may actually regress somewhat. Still, one must be certain that the entire central pelvic mass is a leiomyomatous uterus. Patient management is largely dependent on knowledge of the exact location and size of leiomyomas. Imaging modalities play an important role in determining patient management, especially when differentiating a benign leiomyoma from other pathologic conditions that may require different therapies.

Uterine size as an indication for surgical intervention in women with leiomyomata has been thoughtfully discussed by Friedman and Haas. These authors point out that many gynecologists advocate surgical removal of leiomyomata when the uterus reaches 12 weeks' gestational size or greater, regardless of the presence or absence of significant symptoms. The reasons given for surgical intervention include the following:

- The inability to accurately assess the ovaries by examination
- The possible malignancy of the pelvic mass
- The potential for compromise of adjacent organ function if the mass continues to enlarge
- The greater risk of surgical complications if the mass grows to a larger size
- The potential for better fertility if myomectomy is performed when the uterus is smaller
- The possibility of continued growth of uterine leiomyomata if hormone replacement therapy is given after menopause

Friedman and Haas find very little in the literature to support these indications for surgical intervention and believe the availability of modern high-resolution US and magnetic resonance imaging (MRI) allows for expectant management in many patients with large asymptomatic uterine leiomyomata. They prefer to give primary consideration to the presence and severity of myoma-related symptoms in deciding whether surgical intervention is indicated. We believe that such a course of expectant management is appropriate only when there is certainty regarding the benignity of the central pelvic mass and all of its components, and when it is possible to get the patient to return for periodic assessment of gynecologic symptoms and findings on pelvic examination. Repeat MRI may also be required occasionally.

If one elects to observe a patient with a relatively large asymptomatic uterine leiomyoma, it is a good rule to obtain an excretory urogram or renal ultrasound. Everett and Sturgis showed many years ago that sometimes there is evidence of ureteral compression at the pelvic brim so that hydroureter and hydronephrosis develop (Fig. 30.11). It is usually the symmetrically enlarged uterus with intramural leiomyomata that extends near or above the umbilicus and rests on the pelvic brim that compresses the ureters, in the same way as a symmetrically enlarged gravid uterus. The process is usually slow and painless even when moderate to severe hydronephrosis has occurred. Pyelographic evidence of kidney damage may be the determining factor in a decision to operate on a patient with an entirely asymptomatic leiomyoma. The irregularly and asymmetrically enlarged uterus with subserous tumors usually does not produce pressure on the ureters.

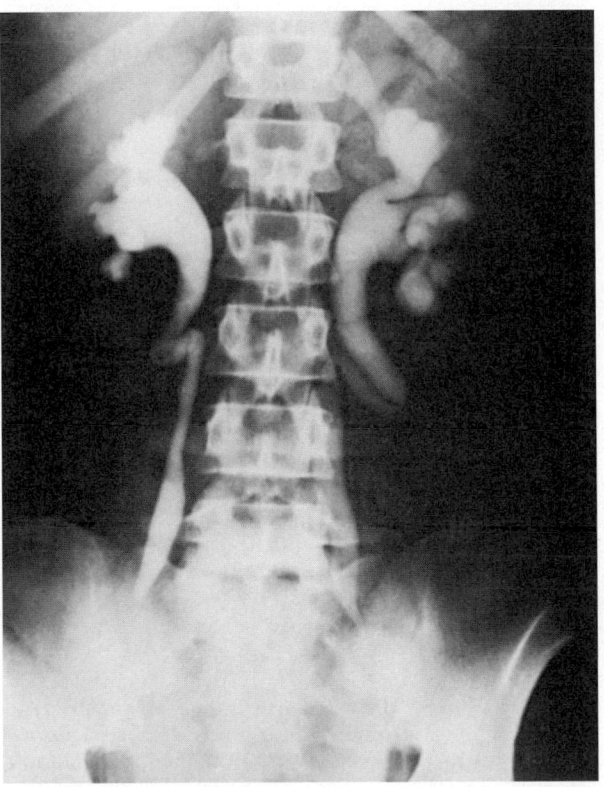

FIGURE 30.11. Bilateral ureteral obstruction and dilatation from pressure of large leiomyomata.

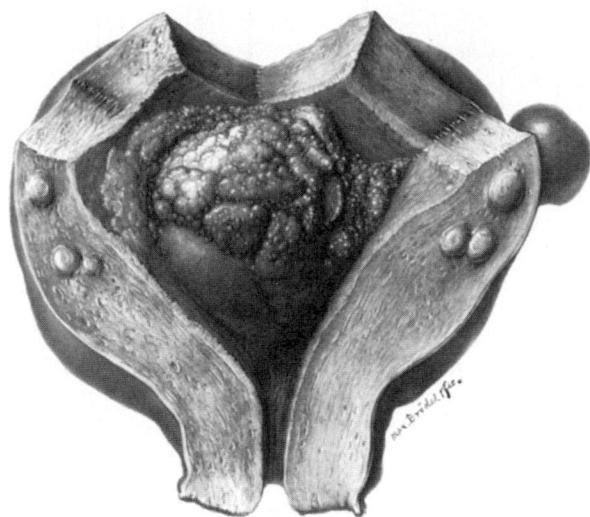

FIGURE 30.12. Adenocarcinoma of the endometrium is present in a symmetrically enlarged leiomyomatous uterus.

After menopause, asymptomatic leiomyomata generally should be left undisturbed. Again, the gynecologist must be absolutely certain that an ovarian neoplasm can be ruled out. In the postmenopausal years, shrinkage of myomata and the myometrium occurs. However, the myometrial shrinkage may be disproportionately greater than the myoma shrinkage. Therefore, a myoma in an intramural location before menopause may become a submucous myoma after menopause and then become

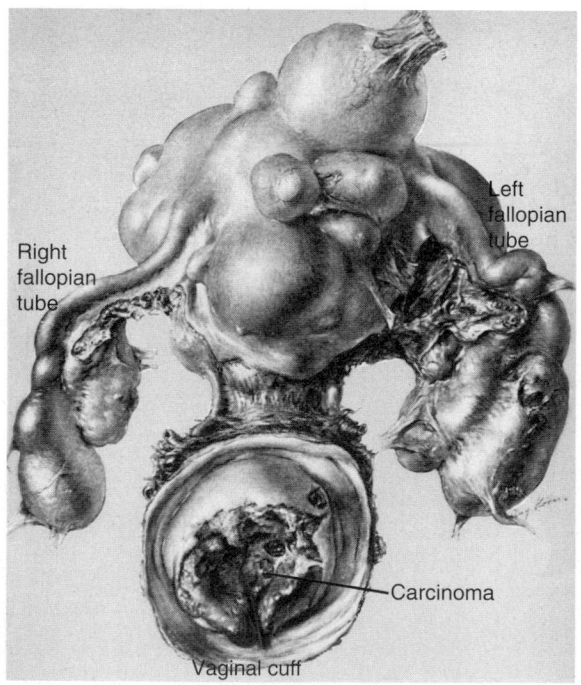

FIGURE 30.13. This specimen shows multiple uterine leiomyomata but also shows chronic pelvic inflammatory disease and cervical carcinoma. Patients with uterine leiomyomata may have abnormal bleeding, but a coexisting cervical carcinoma may also cause bleeding.

symptomatic for the first time, usually with postmenopausal bleeding.

In menopausal women, the appearance of even the slightest trace of vaginal bleeding should make one suspect cervical or endometrial malignancy or the possibility of sarcomatous change in the leiomyoma or elsewhere in the uterus (Figs. 30.12 and 30.13). Careful pelvic examination, Papanicolaou smear, and evaluation of the cervix by colposcopy or biopsy, pelvic US, fractional curettage, and perhaps hysteroscopy should be done. If the bleeding remains unexplained and the presence of atrophic vaginitis or the use of exogenous estrogens has been excluded, the leiomyomatous uterus should be removed because of the danger of sarcomatous change or other significant problems.

Transabdominal and endovaginal US are the standard imaging modalities for the detection of leiomyomas. Pelvic US by transvaginal and transabdominal techniques is most useful because of good patient tolerance, relatively low cost, availability, and accuracy when performed by well-trained and experienced ultrasonographers (Fig. 30.14). Ultrasonography is the most cost-effective screening mechanism for uterine masses suggestive of myomas. Sonographic criteria for diagnosis have been well described. Generally, abdominal US is unable to detect myomas less than 2 cm in diameter. Endovaginal probes have allowed for improved visualization of both the uterus and adnexa. With higher frequencies, sensitivity in the detection of small myomas has substantially increased. In a series evaluated by Fedele and colleagues using endovaginal ultrasound before hysterectomy, submucous leiomyomas were identified with a sensitivity of 100%. Difficulties may arise, however, if myomas are small or pedunculated, patients are obese, or the uterus is retroverted.

Transvaginal fluid-enhanced vaginal probe sonography (sonohysterography) is a useful technique to assess myomata that distort the endometrial cavity. This technique has little to no complications and is generally well tolerated with only mild cramping described by patients. The limitation of detection of leiomyomas with this modality is 0.5 cm diameter. In a study by Hoetzinger, the majority of intrauterine myomata (14 of 16, or 88%)

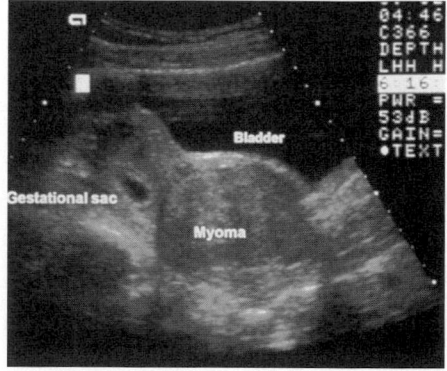

FIGURE 30.14. An ultrasonography study shows a cervical myoma and a very early intrauterine pregnancy. See color version of figure.

were detected by sonohysterography. Ultrasound transducing catheters have been suggested as a potential tool to supplement abdominal and endovaginal sonography. Three-dimensional data display has recently undergone development and application in sonography (Fig. 30.9).

There is no technique that reliably identifies a leiomyosarcoma. Plain abdominal or pelvic radiographs and hysterosalpingography are older, standard techniques that are still useful in assessing uterine size, calcification in myomata, intrauterine filling defects caused by submucous myomata, and tubal patency. These techniques, combined with US, are the most useful for assessing patients with a central pelvic mass thought to be a leiomyomatous uterus. CA-125 levels may be elevated in women with uterine leiomyomata, but the levels are generally lower than those in patients with ovarian cancer.

Symptomatic Leiomyomata

Less than 50% of patients with uterine leiomyomata have symptoms. Symptoms may be single or multiple and depend on the location, size, and number of tumors present. A clinical and pathologic study of 298 patients with uterine leiomyomata by Persaud and Arjoon revealed no significant relation between the presenting symptoms and the presence of degenerative changes in the tumors. Some form of degeneration was demonstrated in 65% of the specimens, with hyaline degeneration accounting for 63% of all types of degeneration. Hyaline degeneration produces no characteristic symptoms. Symptoms, especially pain and fever, may be present in some patients with red degeneration of a leiomyoma during pregnancy, with torsion and infarction of a subserous pedunculated leiomyoma, or with an infected leiomyoma. A discussion of the signs and symptoms caused by uterine leiomyomata follows.

Abnormal Bleeding

It is surprising but not unusual that even patients with large uterine leiomyomata may have a history of normal menstruation. Such patients should be questioned carefully about recent slight increases in the amount, duration, and frequency of menstruation. Some patients with a history of normal menstruation are found to have iron-deficiency anemia from a gradual increase in menstrual blood loss that even the patient has not recognized. If a case of uterine leiomyomata is to be followed, the patient should be asked to monitor her menstrual blood loss carefully and should be given instructions to keep a menstrual calendar and monthly record of the number of pads or tampons used each day. A more objective measurement of the amount of menstrual blood loss using the method of Hallberg and Nilsson may be helpful in doubtful cases. Iron depletion may not be evident by laboratory determination unless one performs an iron stain of the bone marrow or serum ferritin levels. In the early months of increased menstrual blood loss, the hemoglobin and hematocrit values are normal. Heavy menstruation does not cause anemia until iron stores are first depleted.

Abnormal bleeding occurs in about one third of patients with symptomatic uterine leiomyomata and commonly indicates that treatment is necessary. The menstrual flow is usually heavy (menorrhagia), but it can also be prolonged (metrorrhagia) or both heavy and prolonged (menometrorrhagia). Abnormal bleeding may be associated with submucous, intramural, and subserous tumors, but there is a distinct clinical impression that bleeding is more common and more severe in the presence of submucous tumors. The submucous leiomyoma bleeds freely at menstruation and may also bleed between periods as a result of passive congestion, necrosis, and ulceration of the endometrial surface over the tumor and ulceration of the contralateral uterine surface. If the submucous myoma is pedunculated, there is usually a constant, thin, blood-tinged discharge in addition to the menorrhagia. An intramural tumor that is just beginning to encroach on the uterine cavity can also be responsible for menorrhagia. Intramural leiomyomata near the serosal surface and pedunculated subserous tumors can also be associated with abnormal bleeding. When bleeding occurs with such tumors, however, one should search for some other lesion to account for it. The mere presence of leiomyomata in a woman who has abnormal uterine bleeding is not proof that the leiomyomata are causing the bleeding. This fact is important, particularly when there is intermenstrual bleeding. When a patient with leiomyomata has intermenstrual bleeding, it is a rule on our service to examine and study the cervix carefully with special diagnostic procedures and to sample and evaluate the uterine cavity before we proceed with treatment of the leiomyomata. If an endometrial or cervical malignancy is detected, the treatment of the leiomyomata will need to be altered.

There are several mechanisms by which leiomyomata can cause abnormal bleeding, although a single specific mechanism may not be apparent in a particular patient. According to Sehgal and Haskins the surface area of the endometrial cavity in a normal uterus is 15 cm^2. The surface area of the endometrial cavity in the presence of leiomyomata may exceed 200 cm^2. These authors demonstrated a correlation between the severity of the bleeding and the area of endometrial surface. In addition to an increased surface area from which to bleed, the endometrium may demonstrate local hyperestrogenism in areas immediately adjacent to submucous tumors, and endometrial hyperplasia and endometrial polyps are commonly found. Deligdish and Loewenthal noted a broad spectrum of histologic abnormalities in the endometrium associated with leiomyomata, ranging from atrophy to hyperplasia. Thinning and ulceration of the endometrial surface may be present over large submucous tumors; smaller ones may show slight thinning without ulceration. The presence of leiomyomata may interfere with myometrial contractility as well as contractility of the spiral arterioles in the basalis portion of the endometrium. Miller and Ludovici suggested that anovulation and dysfunctional uterine bleeding are more common in the presence of uterine leiomyomata.

Sampson in 1913 was the first to study the blood supply of uterine leiomyomata and its effect on uterine bleeding. More recent studies have been performed by Faulkner and by Farrer-Brown and associates. The most prominent and important change is the presence of endometrial venule ectasia. Tumors that are strategically located in the myometrium may cause obstruction and proximal congestion of veins in the myometrium and endometrium. Thrombosis and sloughing of these large dilated venous channels within the endometrium produce heavy bleeding (Fig. 30.15).

Makarainen and Ylikorkala have presented evidence that further supports the concept that prostanoids play a role in primary menorrhagia. They found that the production of 6-keto-prostaglandin F_1 alpha (6-keto-$PGF_{1\alpha}$), a metabolite of prostacyclin (PGI_2), and thromboxane B_2 (TXB_2), a metabolite of thromboxane A_2 (TXA_2), was normal in menorrhagic endometrium. However, the balance between TXA_2 and PGI_2 shifted to a relative TXA_2 deficiency and was negatively related to blood loss in patients with menorrhagia. Although ibuprofen decreased the blood loss in patients with primary menorrhagia, it failed to reduce myoma-associated menorrhagia. The authors suggest that uterine factors other than prostanoids are more important in causing menorrhagia associated with uterine leiomyomata.

In most cases, when bleeding occurs postmenopausally and leiomyomata are discovered on bimanual examination, the bleeding is due to some other factor, such as cervical or endometrial abnormalities, atrophic vaginitis, or exogenous estrogen, and the leiomyomata are purely incidental. However, the postmenopausal leiomyoma *can* be responsible for the bleeding. As stated

earlier, leiomyomata that do not bleed during the menstrual life of the patient have been found to migrate to a submucous position in later years. This occurs because after menopause the myometrium atrophies and the uterine wall becomes thinner. Leiomyomata also shrink somewhat, but not as much as the surrounding myometrium. Thus, a leiomyoma that was intramural before menopause may work itself into a submucous position after menopause, become ulcerated, and bleed. Postmenopausal growth of uterine leiomyomata may indicate malignant change, especially if associated with postmenopausal bleeding. We have rarely observed postmenopausal growth in a leiomyoma without finding malignancy in the tumor; whenever there is enlargement of the leiomyoma after menopause, one should seriously consider the possibility of sarcomatous change and remove the leiomyoma.

Patients with heavy menstruation and uterine leiomyomata should be evaluated for the presence of submucous myomata. Even patients without palpable evidence of uterine leiomyomata or uterine enlargement who have heavy menstruation should be evaluated for the presence of submucous myomata. When endometrial curettage is performed, irregularity of the uterine cavity may suggest the presence of a submucous myoma. However, a submucous myoma may not be detected with the curette. An accurate diagnosis is more likely to be made by hysterosalpingography, conventional transvaginal or transabdominal US, sonohysterography, MRI, or hysteroscopy. Cincinelli and colleagues reported their experience with transabdominal sonohysterography, a technique that involves transabdominal ultrasonographic scanning while 30 mL of sterile isotonic saline is slowly injected into the uterine cavity. According to these investigators, this technique provided the most accurate evaluation of the size of submucous myomata, intracavitary and intramural growth, and location within the uterine cavity, with sensitivity, specificity, and predictive values of 100%.

Pressure

Evidence of pressure on nearby pelvic viscera may be an indication for treatment. The urinary bladder suffers most often from such pressure, giving rise to urgency and frequency of urination and sometimes even urinary incontinence (Fig. 30.16). Although this symptom is common with large leiomyomata, one frequently finds the pelvis filled with leiomyomata when there is no urinary frequency. Occasionally, acute retention of urine or overflow incontinence results from a leiomyoma and necessitates surgical intervention. These effects can occur as a result of rapid interior growth of the leiomyoma with compression of the urethra and bladder neck against the pubic bone. More often, a tumor the size of a 3-month pregnancy may become incarcerated in the cul-de-sac, wedging the cervix forward against the urethra and obstructing the flow of urine through the urethra. A large pedunculated submucous tumor may fill and distend the vagina and press the urethra against the symphysis, causing urinary retention.

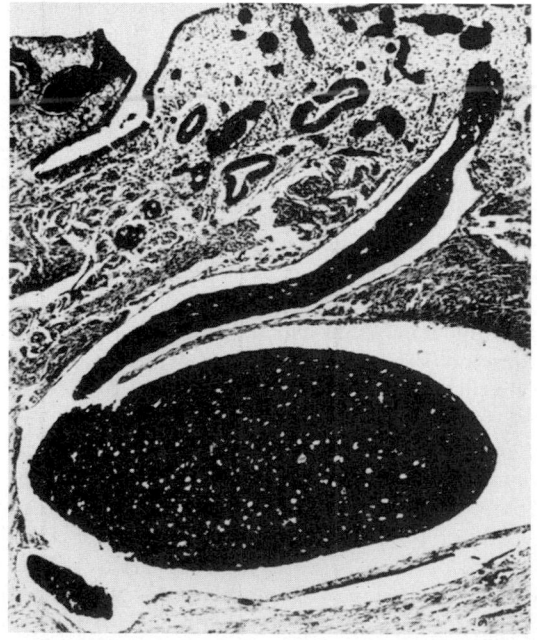

FIGURE 30.15. Dilated endometrial venous space communicating with a grossly enlarged vessel in the inner myometrium of a uterus with submucous leiomyomata. (From Farrer-Brown G, Beilby JO, Tarbit MH. Venous changes in the endometrium of myomatous uteri. *Obstet Gynecol* 1971;83:743.)

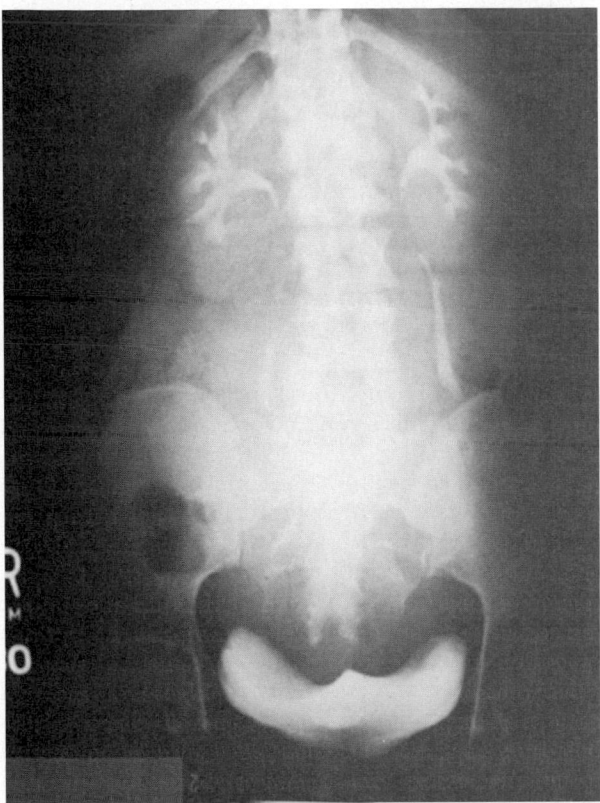

FIGURE 30.16. Cystogram and intravenous pyelogram showing distortion of the bladder by pressure from a leiomyoma.

As pointed out by Mattingly, one can expect to encounter women who have uterine leiomyomata of significant size and in addition have protrusion of the bladder base and posterior urethra through a widened levator muscle hiatus and a weakened urogenital diaphragm. Both conditions are relatively common. In addition to the usual symptoms produced by the leiomyomata, socially disabling stress urinary incontinence may be present. When the anterior wall of the uterus is greatly distorted by the presence of these tumors, pressure against the bladder can cause urinary frequency. If anatomic pressure equalization incontinence is also present, it may be aggravated by the increased intravesical pressure caused by the leiomyomata. However, the presence of anatomic stress urinary incontinence has no etiologic relation to the uterine enlargement caused by the leiomyomata.

Silent ureteral obstruction from pressure against the pelvic brim is an uncommon complication of uterine enlargement caused by multiple large leiomyomata. Such an asymptomatic anatomic change occurs more often with a symmetrically enlarged leiomyomatous uterus that becomes large enough to fill the pelvis and compress the ureter against the pelvic side walls (Fig. 30.11). Although an infrequent complication, the obstruction can occur in either ureter, depending on the location of the uterine tumors. If there has been no infection or parenchymal damage to the kidney, this anatomic alteration is completely reversible with removal of the uterus and relief of the pressure against the ureter. However, if urinary tract obstruction from leiomyomata has been neglected, uremia may result. Removal of the tumor and relief of obstruction are necessary to restore kidney function. Chronic bladder neck obstruction from uterine leiomyomata can be so severe as to cause a remarkable increase in the thickness of the bladder wall and enlargement of the bladder resembling that seen in men with urethral obstruction from prostatic enlargement. Indeed, in these neglected cases, the bladder may fill the entire lower abdominal wall so that an incision above the umbilicus is required to enter the peritoneal cavity to remove the tumor without injury to the bladder.

The bowel is less apt to show symptoms from pressure than is the bladder, but constipation can be caused and aggravated by pressure of leiomyomata against the rectum. The small intestines can become entwined with subserous pedunculated tumors, causing intermittent intestinal obstruction.

Pain

Abdominal and pelvic pain or discomfort, a feeling of heaviness in the pelvis, and dyspareunia are present in about one third of patients with symptomatic uterine leiomyomata and may be an appropriate reason for operative intervention. There are several causes of pain with leiomyomata. However, the usual hyaline or cystic degeneration of these tumors does not produce symptoms. In rare instances, pedunculated subserous leiomyomata twist and give rise to a clinical picture of acute abdominal pain, much like that seen with a twisted ovarian tumor. These pedunculated tumors twist more often during pregnancy and after menopause. Acute carneous or red degeneration of a leiomyoma can occur at any period of reproductive life, although pain from this form of degeneration is more common during pregnancy. Dysmenorrhea, acquired in the fourth or fifth decade, may be the outstanding symptom of the growth of leiomyomata. A common symptom complex resulting from leiomyomata at this time of life is menstrual pain coupled with increased menstrual flow. Diffuse adenomyosis can also cause these symptoms, and the differentiation of this condition from a symmetrically enlarged intramural leiomyoma may be extremely difficult and may require MRI. The differentiation is purely academic, for in either case surgery is indicated if the symptoms are of sufficient severity.

Patients who have uterine leiomyomata and pain may have concomitant pelvic disease such as ovarian pathology, pelvic inflammatory disease, tubal pregnancy, endometriosis, or urinary tract or intestinal pathology, including appendicitis. One must be careful to rule out other pathology that may be obscured by uterine leiomyomata.

Abdominal Distortion

Distortion of the normal abdominal wall contour due to large tumors may justify their removal. Tumors of such size often give rise to other symptoms also, so there is ample reason for surgical interference. However, when no other symptoms are present, one may recommend removal of the tumors if the abdominal distortion is of such a magnitude as to be embarrassing to the patient.

Rapid Growth

Evidence of rapid growth of uterine leiomyomata, as observed by the same examiner over time or as confirmed by US, is an indication for surgical intervention. Such rapid growth in a premenopausal patient is only rarely due to sarcoma. Parker and others reviewed the medical records of 1,332 women admitted for surgical management of uterine leiomyoma. They actually found no correlation between rapid growth and the presence of uterine sarcoma. It may be due to pregnancy or to the use of oral contraceptives containing large amounts of estrogens. In the latter case, these drugs should be discontinued and an alternative method of contraception prescribed. In the postmenopausal patient, however, growth of a uterine leiomyoma is highly suggestive of a malignancy. The malignancy may be a sarcomatous change in the leiomyoma itself, a sarcoma or carcinoma in the endometrium causing uterine enlargement, or an ovarian neoplasm whose estrogen secretion is stimulating enlargement of the leiomyoma or whose growth may be mistaken for rapid enlargement of uterine leiomyomata. Although malignancy is not invariably found, the chances in its favor are so great that one must proceed on the assumption that it exists and must perform dilatation and curettage followed by removal of the enlarged uterus.

Rapid growth of a leiomyomatous uterus is difficult to define in exact terms. Buttram and Reiter have arbitrarily defined it as a gain of 6 weeks or more in gestational size within a year or less. Although this definition could apply in premenopausal women, it might be disastrous to wait for this amount of growth in a postmenopausal woman. It is important to have a definite method of documenting uterine size at periodic intervals. Repeated sounding of the uterine cavity may be of some benefit, although leiomyomatous growth is not always accompanied by concomitant enlargement of the uterine cavity. It is important to document the size of specific leiomyomata or the total uterine size in terms of centimeters or grams of uterine weight rather than in terms of gestational size of the uterus, although the latter method has become quite popular. Changes in a patient's weight can make evaluation of growth more difficult. A uterine leiomyoma can erroneously appear to be growing in a patient who is dieting and losing weight when actually the tumor is just felt more easily. Conversely, in a patient who is gaining weight rapidly, the tumor will be more difficult to feel and may appear to be getting smaller. Ultrasonography is a much more objective way of establishing the size of a uterine leiomyoma in the beginning and, when indicated, of evaluating its rate of growth. There is a need for more information about the natural growth patterns of myomata before and after menopause.

Although leiomyomata can increase dramatically in size during pregnancy, usually there is no appreciable growth. Winer-Muram and co-workers studied 89 pregnant women with uterine leiomyomata documented by US examination. In 83 of the patients, there was no demonstrable increase in the size of the leiomyomata. In six patients there was an increase in size of up to 4 cm. Those myomata that increase in size during pregnancy will decrease in size a few weeks after the pregnancy is over.

Spontaneous Abortion and Other Pregnancy-Related Problems

Uterine leiomyomata are associated with a significantly increased risk of spontaneous abortion. In a collected series of patients undergoing myomectomy, Buttram and Reiter reported that 41% had spontaneous abortions. This rate was reduced to 19% after myomectomy. Various mechanisms have been proposed to explain the occurrence of spontaneous abortion from uteri with leiomyomata. These include disturbances in uterine blood flow, alterations in blood supply to the endometrium, uterine irritability, rapid growth or degeneration of leiomyomata during pregnancy, difficulty in enlargement of the uterine cavity to accommodate for the growth of the fetus and placenta, and interference with proper implantation and placental growth by poorly developed endometrium or by subjacent leiomyomata. Implantation in a thin, poorly vascularized endometrium over a submucous leiomyoma is doomed to failure, because proper growth and development of the embryo and placenta are impossible (Fig. 30.17). Matsunaga and Shiota found a twofold increase in the number of malformed embryos recovered from patients with uterine leiomyomata having artificial termination of pregnancy. Uterine leiomyomata may be associated with premature delivery, stillbirth, and interstitial pregnancy, as in the case reported by Starks, although we are unaware of good statistics regarding these associations. Muram and associates have followed patients with leiomyomata through pregnancy with US. When a leiomyoma was in close proximity to the placental site, an increased incidence of pregnancy-related complications was seen. These were mainly bleeding complications, but pain, premature delivery, and postpartum hemorrhage also occurred. Exacoustos and Rosati reviewed the US scans of 12,708 pregnant patients. Four hundred ninety-two patients had myomata. A statistically significant increased incidence of threatened abortion, threatened preterm delivery, abruptio placentae, and pelvic pain was observed in patients with myomata. Abruptio placentae was particularly evident in women with myoma volumes greater than 200 cm³, submucosal location, or superimposition of the placenta. The authors suggest that US findings make it possible to identify women at risk for myoma-related complications of pregnancy. Factors responsible for spontaneous abortion in patients without uterine leiomyomata may also be responsible for spontaneous abortion in patients with leiomyomata.

Occasionally, pregnancy causes a remarkable growth of leiomyomata in the same way that the myometrium

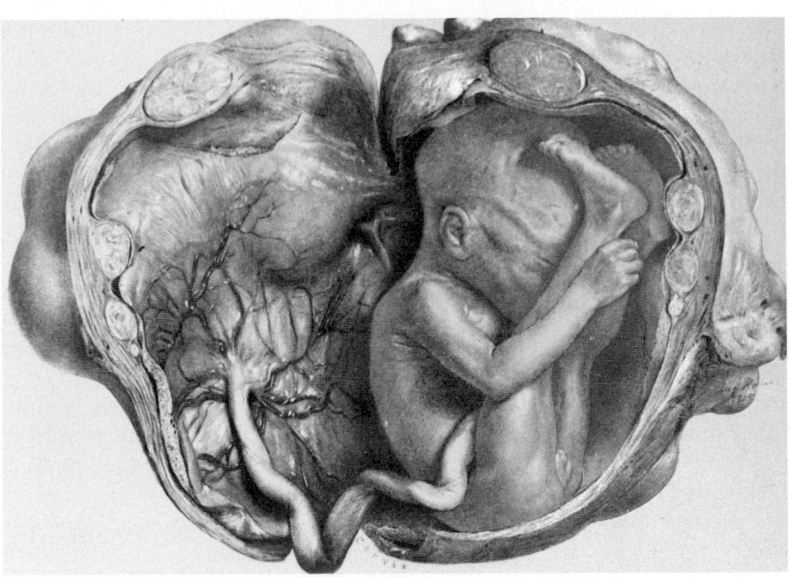

FIGURE 30.17. When the placenta is implanted over a myoma in the uterine wall, the blood supply to the fetus may be tenuous.

undergoes hypertrophy in pregnancy. Red or carneous degeneration of leiomyomata during pregnancy is associated with pain, tenderness over the tumor, low-grade fever, and leukocytosis. Management should be expectant with analgesic medications and bed rest. If premature uterine contractions occur, B mimetics can be given. Pain usually subsides within a few days. Operation is not indicated unless it is necessary to rule out other problems that require surgery for relief, because differentiation from appendicitis, placental abruption, twisted ovarian cyst, and other problems may be difficult. After delivery, leiomyomata involute and generally return to their prepregnancy size by the third postpartum month.

Torsion with infarction of subserous pedunculated leiomyomata is more common in pregnancy. A leiomyoma may interfere with labor and delivery by causing an abnormal presentation, by causing dysfunctional labor, or by obstructing the pelvis. A submucous leiomyoma in the lower uterine segment may entrap the placenta, necessitating manual removal. Indeed, furious postpartum hemorrhage can result if a submucous leiomyoma is disturbed at delivery or during exploration of the uterine cavity. Immediate hysterectomy may be necessary to control the bleeding.

Most patients with uterine leiomyomata have no difficulty conceiving and carry their pregnancies to term without complications. The only problem encountered may be a difficulty in estimating gestational age from uterine size because of the presence of leiomyomata.

Infertility

When asymptomatic leiomyomata are discovered in young women, the question of how these tumors relate to sterility and pregnancy usually arises. A number of factors may be responsible for infertility in a patient with uterine leiomyomata. Anovulatory cycles may occur more commonly. There may be interference with sperm transport caused by distortion and an increased surface area within the uterine cavity, impingement of leiomyomata on the endocervical canal or interstitial portion of the fallopian tube, or interference with prostaglandin-induced uterine contractions, which are thought to enhance sperm migration. Endometrial changes (atrophy, ulceration, focal hyperplasia, and polyps), vascular alterations (venous congestion, venule ectasia, impaired blood flow), and enlargement of the uterine cavity may be present. Because uterine leiomyomata occur in later reproductive years, relatively greater difficulty accomplishing conception can be expected in older couples.

The finding of small leiomyomata in sterile women is not an indication for immediate myomectomy. Quite often, an infertile patient with uterine leiomyomata is found to have some other cause of infertility. Tubal inflammatory disease with associated pelvic adhesions is especially common in patients with uterine leiomyomata. Both marital partners should have a complete infertility investigation, and the leiomyomata should be disregarded for a while. The ultimate decision regarding disposal of the tumors depends on their size and location. Usually, small subserous leiomyomata are not considered a factor in infertility. Even if the woman fails to become pregnant, removal of small subserous leiomyomata is not justified. When leiomyomata are intramural or submucous and of significant size, they may well be factors causing the infertility, and a myomectomy may be rewarded with a subsequent pregnancy.

When an unsuspected asymptomatic leiomyomatous uterus of significant size is found in a woman who is planning to become pregnant in the future, great tact is required in describing the problem to the patient. The best surgical and obstetric judgment is needed to make a proper recommendation. Should the patient be discouraged from attempting pregnancy because the risk of complications may be increased? Should a myomectomy be advised before pregnancy is attempted, with the knowledge that postmyomectomy adhesions may cause infertility? Such questions cannot be answered in a stereotypical manner. Each case presents its own problems, and the answers depend on the patient's age, her general physical health, her pelvic findings, and, most important, her own desires. All must be considered before a final recommendation can be made. In general terms, under these circumstances, an attempt to become pregnant will be rewarded with a satisfactory outcome in most cases. If pregnancy does not occur or is not successful, a myomectomy may be advised, but one must keep in mind that all causes of infertility, spontaneous abortion, and other pregnancy-related problems must also be investigated in patients with uterine leiomyomata; uterine leiomyomata represent an infrequent cause of infertility.

Eldar-Geva and colleagues performed a retrospective review of the treatment outcome of 106 assisted reproductive technology cycles in 88 patients with uterine myomata (subserosal, intramuscular without cavity distortion, and submucosal). Patients underwent controlled ovarian hyperstimulation and advanced reproductive technology. Not surprisingly, pregnancy (30.1%) and implantation (15.7%) rates were significantly lower in women with submucosal myomas; however, both pregnancy (16.4%) and implantation (6.4%) rates were also significantly lower in women with intramural myomas. In some advanced assisted reproductive technology patients, this information may influence the decision for surgical intervention regardless of menstrual pattern.

A review of information about infertility and uterine leiomyomata was published by Wallach and Vu, by Vercellini and colleagues, and by Verkauf.

Miscellaneous Signs and Symptoms

A variety of other unusual problems may be associated with uterine leiomyomata and may require treatment. Ascites and uterine inversion have already been mentioned. Sudden intraperitoneal hemorrhage can result from rupture of a dilated vein beneath the serosal surface of a subserous leiomyoma. Although leiomyomata are more often associated with iron-deficiency anemia from chronic uterine blood loss, occasionally patients present with polycythemia. Islands of extramedullary erythropoiesis have been found in leiomyomata. Arteriovenous shunts within the tumors have been found and may be etiologically important in polycythemia. If the tumor obstructs the ureters and causes back pressure on the renal parenchyma, erythropoiesis can be stimulated. Weiss and co-workers and other investigators have found marked erythropoietin activity within uterine leiomyomata. The polycythemia in these cases is cured by hysterectomy.

CHOICE OF TREATMENT FOR UTERINE LEIOMYOMATA

Six hundred fifty thousand hysterectomies are performed annually in the United States. About 175,000 are performed with uterine leiomyomata as the primary indication. Nearly 17,000 myomectomies are performed each year, and it is believed that this number is increasing substantially. There are no statistics to indicate the number of hysteroscopic and laparoscopic myomectomies performed each year. Effective medical therapies are available to use as adjuncts to surgical treatment. Abnormal bleeding from a leiomyomatous uterus can be controlled by ovarian irradiation if the patient is not a suitable surgical candidate. However, surgery is the preferred method of therapy for many reasons, especially because there are so few patients whose medical condition cannot be improved sufficiently to allow surgery.

Hysterectomy (abdominal, vaginal, and laparoscopy assisted) is discussed in Chapter 31. In this chapter, surgical techniques that allow conservation of uterine function are discussed, as are medical therapies that can be used as adjuncts to surgical therapy.

Medical Management of Uterine Leiomyomata

Most (70% to 80%) uterine leiomyomata are asymptomatic and are discovered initially during a routine pelvic examination. Such patients require an explanation and reassurance and reexamination at periodic intervals. An initial baseline pelvic US examination or MRI study may be indicated for comparison with future examinations and to evaluate the adnexa if the ovaries cannot be felt on pelvic examination. An experienced pelvic examiner can be fairly certain that a central pelvic mass is a leiomyomatous uterus. However, pelvic US examinations and repeat pelvic examinations can add to the certainty of the diagnosis. If the diagnosis remains doubtful, however, visualization of the mass, usually by laparoscopy, is indicated. Patients with an asymptomatic central pelvic mass should be followed up with periodic pelvic examination only when the mass is benign, usually a leiomyomatous uterus. Otherwise, expectant management is not appropriate.

Effective medical treatment that is likely to result in the permanent cure of uterine leiomyomata is not yet available. Surgical excision by a variety of techniques remains the most effective and widely used method of management for patients with significant symptoms. Medical therapies are available as an adjunct to surgical treatment or as a temporary substitute for definitive surgical treatment.

Hormonal therapy for the management of uterine leiomyomata has been the subject of investigation for many years. There is no support for the use of danazol or progestins in view of the disappointing results reported. Antiprogestin therapy with mifepristone (RU486) for 3 months has been shown by Murphy and colleagues to decrease leiomyoma volume by an average of 49%, with a variation of 0% to 87%. The immunoreactivity of progesterone but not estrogen receptors in the myoma and myometrial tissue was decreased significantly by RU486 treatment, suggesting that regression of these tumors may be attained through a direct antiprogesterone effect. All patients became amenorrheic. Side effects were mild, and bone density was not diminished. An effective dose to cause a clinically significant (50%) decrease in leiomyoma volume appears to be 25 mg daily. Additional experience is needed to further evaluate these promising results. Reinsch and associates have demonstrated that RU486 and leuprolide acetate are both effective in decreasing blood flow to the uterus. It is suggested that a decrease in uterine artery blood flow may provide a mechanism for a decrease in uterine size.

Gestrinone, a synthetic derivative of ethinyl-nortestosterone with antiestrogen and antiprogesterone properties, has been shown by Coutinho and associates to induce regression of leiomyomata. The treatment lasted 6 months to 1 year. The best results were obtained when the drug was administered intravaginally. Even the regression of large leiomyomata lasted up to a year after treatment. Side effects, though mildly androgenic, were well tolerated.

Many studies have been performed to investigate the treatment of patients with uterine leiomyomata with GnRH analogs. GnRH analogs bind to GnRH receptors, resulting in a biphasic response: a temporary increase in the levels of gonadotropins and gonadal steroids (agonist phase) is followed by chronic suppression of gonadotropin and gonadal steroid secretion (desensitization phase). In 1 to 3 weeks, a profound hypogonadotropic hypogonadal state begins and exists as long as the treatment lasts, but it is promptly reversed when treatment is discontinued. GnRH agonist treatment results in "medical oophorectomy" and "medical menopause" and is associated with the usual symptoms of a profound hypogonadal state (e.g., hot flashes, insomnia, mood lability, headaches, vaginal dryness, arthralgias, and myalgias). According to Friedman and associates, these adverse effects of treatment are self-limited and disappear within 3 to 6 months of cessation of GnRH agonist treatment. Dawood and colleagues describe a significant reduction in trabecular bone density after 24 weeks of GnRH agonist treatment that may not be completely reversible when treatment is discontinued. A mean reduction in trabecular bone density of 1% per month occurs in women treated for 6 months. Some of this bone loss may be permanent, but some is reversible.

Friedman and colleagues state that the average reduction in uterine and myoma volume is 40% to 50% after 3 to 6 months of GnRH agonist treatment; this is generally confirmed by others. Most of the response occurs in the first 12 weeks, and it is variable and unpredictable.

According to the analysis by these investigators, 4% of patients had an increase in uterine volume ranging from 0.1% to 25%; 24% had decreases in uterine volume ranging from 0.1% to 25%; 51% had decreases in uterine volume ranging from 25.1% to 50%; and 21% had decreases in uterine volume greater than 50%. No factors were found to predict the degree of uterine shrinkage. There were negative correlations with body weight, pretreatment uterine volume, age, height, and serum estradiol concentration.

It is commonly thought that GnRH analogs affect leiomyomata by reducing vascularity and the individual cell size within the tumor. The biochemical changes in leiomyomata obtained from women treated with the GnRH agonist leuprolide acetate depot for 3 months were studied by Rein and co-workers. The concentrations of amino acids contained in collagen were significantly greater in uterine myomata from treated patients than in myomata from placebo-treated controls. These investigators suggest that the reduction in uterine myoma volume associated with GnRH agonist therapy is due primarily to alterations in the extracellular matrix rather than to a reduction in the number or volume of cells in the myoma.

Because uterine leiomyomata are hormone-sensitive neoplasms that can be stimulated to grow by estrogen, some clinicians have been reluctant to prescribe oral contraceptive pills in patients with leiomyomata. However, Friedman and Thomas and others have demonstrated conclusively that oral contraceptives containing 30 to 35 μg of ethinyl estradiol do not cause uterine leiomyomata to increase in size. Therefore, low-dose contraceptives can be used to manage menorrhagia in patients with uterine leiomyomata. Friedman and Thomas demonstrated a significant decrease in the mean duration of menstrual flow and a significant increase in hematocrit values in response to low-dose oral contraceptives in patients with uterine leiomyomata.

When myoma-associated menorrhagia is more severe, GnRH agonist and iron treatment may be more effective than oral contraceptives. In about two thirds of patients, GnRH agonist treatment induces amenorrhea. Most of the remaining patients experience very light, irregular vaginal bleeding or spotting, according to Friedman. A combination of menstrual suppression and iron therapy allows correction of iron deficiency and iron-deficiency anemia during a 6-month treatment period. Ovulatory menses resume 3 to 24 weeks after the last depot GnRH agonist injection. Stovall and associates reported that a GnRH agonist plus iron was more effective than iron alone in treating anemia in patients with leiomyomata and in alleviating menorrhagia. With such effective treatment now available, there is rarely a need to use blood transfusions to correct anemia caused by myoma-associated menorrhagia. Only patients with significant symptoms from severe anemia may require transfusion.

Medical therapy may also be used transiently before surgery. By initiating the medication preoperatively, the maximum decrease in myoma volume may play a role in determining the route of surgery. If a hysterectomy is planned, the pharmacologic effect may facilitate a vaginal hysterectomy when the uterus is of borderline size. Vercellini and colleagues performed a multicenter, prospective, randomized, controlled study to assess if this shrinkage may increase the likelihood of a vaginal procedure. One hundred and twenty-seven premenopausal women with uterine volumes of 12 to 16 weeks were enrolled. After examination and disposition for an abdominal or vaginal hysterectomy, patients were randomized for GnRH therapy. Clinical assessment after the treatment course showed that abdominal hysterectomy was no longer indicated in 25 of 53 (47%) patients. No appreciable difference was found between the groups in postoperative complications. These findings are consistent with previously published studies, as well.

GnRH agonist treatment alone cannot be given for periods longer than 6 months. A prolonged hypoestrogenic state is undesirable for a number of reasons, the most important being the loss of trabecular bone. If there are circumstances that require that GnRH treatment be extended beyond 6 months, consideration should be given to adding low-dose steroids after 3 months of GnRH therapy. The usual postmenopausal estrogen-progestin replacement regimen can be prescribed without interfering with the reduction in uterine volume anticipated. Loss of trabecular bone may not be as great. By adding estrogen-progestin replacement to GnRH agonist therapy, the adverse effects of a prolonged hypoestrogenic state may be prevented, and treatment with GnRH agonists may be prolonged. Friedman and colleagues treated 51 premenopausal women with large, symptomatic myomata with leuprolide acetate depot for 104 weeks. After the first 12 weeks, 0.75 mg of estropiptate plus 0.7 mg of norethindrone were added on days 1 through 14 each month. Menorrhagia and other symptoms of uterine leiomyomata were controlled successfully. Hemoglobin and hematocrit levels increased. Symptoms of hypoestrogenism (hot flashes, vaginal dryness) were decreased significantly. Bone density decreased in the first 12 weeks, but only a small additional decrease occurred between weeks 12 and 52.

The use of GnRH analogs in the medical management of uterine leiomyomata is an emerging issue. How valuable it will be remains to be seen. Additional information and experience will define its use more exactly. For example, it may be possible for patients with symptomatic uterine leiomyomata who are approaching menopause to be managed medically through menopause without having a hysterectomy. It may be possible to improve fertility in some patients with uterine leiomyomata by treatment with GnRH analogs without myomectomy. With additional data, these and other questions can be answered.

Vaginal Myomectomy

In 1845, Atlee performed the first successful vaginal myomectomy on a patient with a submucous pedunculated myoma.

When a submucous myoma becomes pedunculated within the uterine cavity, there is a natural tendency for the uterus to try to expel it through the endocervical canal. Eventually, the cervix dilates. Even very large submucous pedunculated myomata can be delivered gradually through a markedly dilated cervix. Because adequate blood circulation through a long pedicle is difficult to maintain, the myoma becomes necrotic and infected (Figs. 30.5 and 30.6).

Patients complain of cramping lower abdominal pain; pressure and heaviness in the pelvis; a thin, bloody, foul discharge; difficulty with urination; and other symptoms. Episodes of profuse vaginal hemorrhage can occur. Such large submucous myomata may resemble a fetal head.

After satisfactory preoperative preparation, including broad-spectrum antibiotics and correction of anemia, vaginal myomectomy should be performed in the operating room. Morcellation may be required to remove very large tumors in many small pieces. Usually there is very little bleeding. One should avoid too much downward traction on the tumor because the uterine fundus may invert. Eventually, the pedicle is identified. It should be clamped and ligated as high as possible within the uterine cavity. If ligation of the pedicle is not possible, the clamps can be left in place and safely removed 48 hours later.

Smaller submucous pedunculated myomata can be diagnosed by hysteroscopy, by hysterosalpingography, by US, or at the time of dilation and curettage. They can also be felt on digital exploration through a slightly dilated external cervical os. If the myoma can be grasped with an instrument (ring forceps, Allis clamp, and so forth), it can be removed by twisting it free of its attachment. A tonsil snare can also be used. Bleeding is usually minimal. If brisk bleeding does occur, a 26-French, 30-mL Foley catheter can be inserted through the cervix and inflated for tamponade. If necessary, the cervix can be sutured around the catheter to hold it in place.

To gain access to submucous pedunculated myomata that are higher in the endocervical canal or uterine cavity, special procedures are required. An attempt at hysteroscopic removal may be successful. Alternatively, the cervix can be dilated with instruments or with *Laminaria japonica,* as described by Goldrath. Dührssen incisions can be made in the cervix. Also, the cervix can be incised by having the surgeon perform a vaginal hysterotomy (Fig. 30.18A and B). After the bladder is advanced, the cervix is dilated and an anterior midline incision is made in the cervix high enough to identify the myoma. The pedicle of the myoma is ligated as high as possible (Fig. 30.18C and D). The incision in the cervix is repaired with 2-0 interrupted delayed-absorbable sutures. The vaginal mucosa is reapproximated with 3-0 delayed-absorbable sutures (Fig. 30.18E and F).

A submucous pedunculated myoma may be solitary, and there may not be other myomata in the uterus. In fact, many patients exhibit no evidence of uterine enlargement. After a successful vaginal myomectomy, most patients are asymptomatic and menstruate normally. A few even become pregnant and deliver vaginally without difficulty. Cervical incompetence has been reported. Hysterectomy or myomectomy is required only for those few patients who have multiple leiomyomata and continue to have significant symptoms.

Excellent results of vaginal removal of submucous pedunculated myomata in 151 patients were reported by Goldrath. Ben-Baruch and co-workers also achieved excellent results in 43 of 46 women in whom vaginal myomectomy was attempted. Vaginal myomectomy is rec-

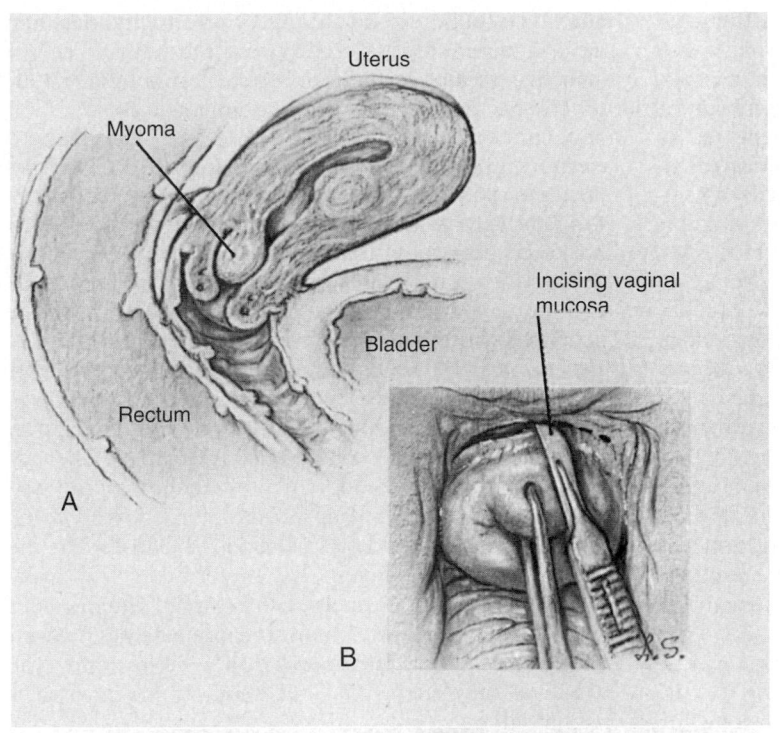

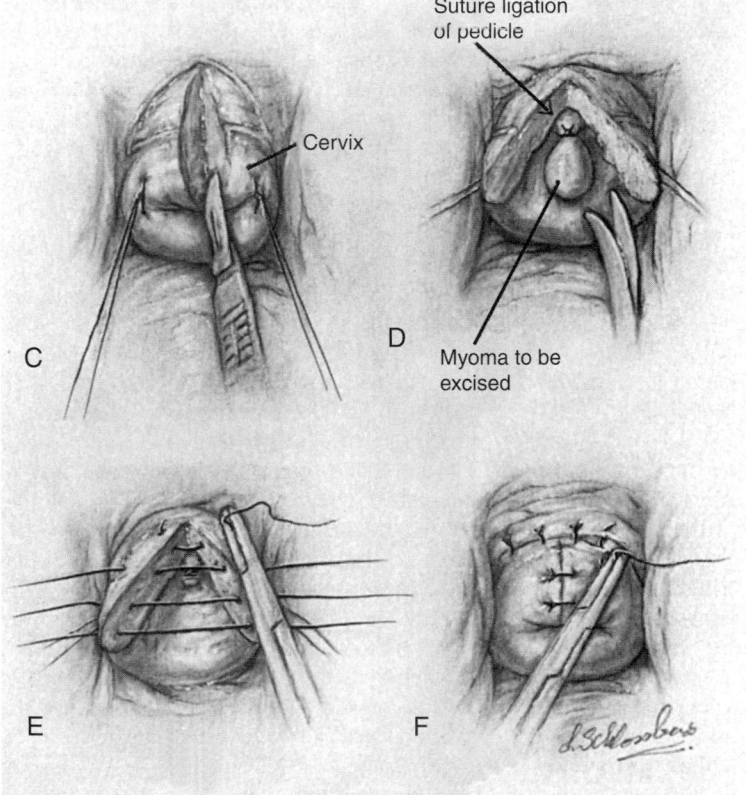

FIGURE 30.18. Transvaginal removal of a pedunculated submucous myoma that presents itself at the external cervical os. **A:** Sagittal view of uterus, demonstrating the location of the myoma originating on the posterior wall of the fundus just above the cervix. **B:** A transverse incision made anteriorly through the vaginal mucosa at the cervicovaginal junction. **C:** After the bladder is advanced bluntly, the cervix is incised anteriorly in the midline. **D:** The myoma and its pedicle are exposed, and the pedicle is suture ligated for hemostasis. **E:** After the myoma is excised, the cervix is reapproximated with interrupted 0-0 absorbable, nonreactive sutures. **F:** The overlying vaginal mucosa is sutured with interrupted 3-0 absorbable sutures.

ommended as the most appropriate initial treatment for pedunculated submucous myomata.

Vaginal myomectomy is traditionally used for submucosal myomas; however, it has been described for other myomas. Davies and colleagues reported a prospective study regarding the safety and efficacy of excision of intramural and subserosal leiomyoma by a vaginal route. Preoperative criteria included (1) uterine size less than or equal to 16 weeks' gestation, (2) good uterine mobility, (3) adequate vaginal access, (4) the presence of intramural or subserosal myomas, and (5) the absence of adnexal pathology. Essentially, an open abdominal myomectomy technique was performed through an anterior or posterior colpotomy. The uterus was manipulated to bring the myoma into the colpotomy. The management of 35 women was described. The mean number of myomas removed was 2.5 per patient with mean mass of 113.8 g. Three patients (8.6%) required conversion to a laparotomy. Neither mean blood loss nor length of hospital stay was improved. Additionally, four (11.4%) patients developed pelvic hematomas postoperatively. At this time this procedure does not seem to provide inherent benefits over an open abdominal myomectomy or a laparoscopic approach. With further review, better outcome data may demonstrate the advantages of this technique.

The tissue removed at vaginal myomectomy must be submitted for pathologic examination to rule out malignancy.

Hysteroscopic Resection of Submucous Myomata

Hysteroscopic resection of submucous myomata was first reported by Neuwirth and Amin in 1976 and was reported again by Neuwirth in 1978. A urologic resectoscope was used. In 1981, Goldrath and associates used "photocoagulation" of the endometrium with the neodymium:yttrium-aluminum-garnet (Nd:YAG) laser to treat patients with menorrhagia. Many subsequent reports by Derman and associates, Donnez and colleagues, Goldenberg and co-workers, Corson, Indman, Hallez, Baggish and associates, Wamsteker and colleagues, and others have confirmed the advantages of hysteroscopic treatment of menorrhagia in women with and without submucous leiomyomata. The menorrhagia associated with submucous myomata can sometimes be managed with oral contraceptives as long as the bleeding is not too severe. A favorable response can also be expected with GnRH analogs, but the menorrhagia usually reappears when the treatment is discontinued. Friedman has reported three cases of severe menorrhagia with resultant anemia requiring transfusions in women with submucous leiomyomata treated with leuprolide acetate. Both oral contraceptives and GnRH analogs are counterproductive in women who are seeking relief from infertility. The uterine cavity can be curetted several times, but the benefit of this procedure is temporary at best.

When hysteroscopic resection of submucous myomata is performed, menorrhagia can be controlled in more than 90% of patients. According to Indman, the mean number of pads used during the heaviest day of menses decreased from 17.8 before treatment to 6.8 after treatment in women undergoing myoma resection only, and from 21.4 to 1.7 pads per day in women whose treatment also included endometrial ablation. Dysmenorrhea was also reduced significantly. Forty-eight of 51 women (94%) with uterine leiomyomata who were seen with menorrhagia were able to avoid major gynecologic surgery for up to 5 years of follow-up. In the report of 156 patients by Derman and associates, 91.3% of patients did not require further surgery after 6 years of follow-up, and 83.9% did not require further surgery after 9 years of follow-up. Further review in recent papers supports Derman's results. Magos and colleagues performed a prospective observational study to identify factors that influence outcomes of hysteroscopic myomectomies by following up patients for almost 8 years. One hundred and twenty-two patients enrolled in the study, and results suggest that hysteroscopic myomectomy is successful in treating menstrual symptoms in four of five cases. In addition, statistical analysis demonstrated that outcome is significantly better when the uterus is only slightly enlarged and if the myoma is mainly submucous in nature.

If endometrial ablation is performed with myoma resection, pregnancy is not likely to occur subsequently. Without simultaneous endometrial ablation, 21 patients became pregnant after myoma resection only, with 18 infants delivered in the series reported by Derman and colleagues. The pregnancy rates among women who wished to conceive varied between 47% and 66% in several reports. These rates are comparable to those reported for abdominal myomectomy.

Donnez and co-workers used a biodegradable GnRH agonist (Zoladex Implant ICI) preoperatively in a series of 60 women with large submucous myomata. Submucous myomectomy by hysteroscopy and Nd:YAG laser was easily performed. In 12 patients, the procedure was accomplished in two stages. Perino and associates used GnRH agonists in 58 women with submucous leiomyomata diagnosed during investigation for infertility or menstrual disorder. There was a significant reduction in operating time, intraoperative bleeding, infusion volume, and failure rate in the treated group compared with the control subjects. Myoma size is reduced and hemoglobin concentration is restored to normal preoperatively.

When submucous myomata extend deeply into the myometrium, it may not be possible to perform a complete resection for obvious technical reasons. However, it should be possible to remove most irregularities in the uterine cavity and to restore the contour of the cavity to almost normal in most cases. According to Wamsteker and colleagues, hysteroscopic resection of submucous myomata with more than 50% intramural extension should be performed only in selected cases. Repeat procedures may be needed in cases of initial incomplete resection.

To avoid the possibility of inadvertent uterine perforation or to allow its prompt diagnosis if it occurs, hysteroscopic resection is usually performed under laparo-scopic guidance. However, as reported by Sullivan and co-workers, laparoscopy may be insufficient to evaluate fully the possible sequelae of uterine preformation. Laparotomy may be necessary to assess the pelvic viscera fully. Letterie and Kramer were able to safely substitute intraoperative transabdominal ultrasonographic guidance for laparoscopy. In their opinion, operative hysteroscopy with intraoperative ultrasonographic guidance provide an accurate and precise method to monitor intrauterine surgery, and it can be used to enhance the performance of hysteroscopic myomectomy and endometrial resection. Intraoperative US guidance provided sufficient details of the relation between the hysteroscope and the myoma and uterine walls to gauge the depth of resection and prevent uterine perforation.

The success and safety of the procedure depend on the experience and skill of the operator. During hysteroscopic resection, vascular spaces are opened in the endometrium and myometrium. Large volumes of fluid are instilled into the uterine cavity. Fluid balance must be monitored carefully by the surgeon and the anesthesiologist to avoid fluid overload.

All tissue must be submitted for pathologic examination. Among 92 patients undergoing hysteroscopic resection in the series reported by Corson and Brooks, two cases of leiomyosarcoma were diagnosed. Leiomyosarcoma is said to be more common in submucous leiomyomata than in intramural or subserous leiomyomata.

As time passes after hysteroscopic resection of submucous myomata, the possibility of recurrent problems increases because of regrowth of myomata. However, this is no more likely to occur than it is with standard abdominal myomectomy. The experience of many investigators has demonstrated that hysteroscopic management of menorrhagia in patients with submucous leiomyomata is a reasonable alternative to classic surgical hysterectomy or myomectomy. The occasional psychological problems and complications of hysterectomy are avoided. An abdominal incision is avoided, there is less discomfort, the procedure can often be performed in an outpatient setting, and the patient can usually resume normal activity after a very brief recovery period.

Hysteroscopic resection of a small submucous myoma is illustrated in Figure 30.19. Details of the indications, technique, complications, and results of hysteroscopic resection are also provided in Chapter 17.

Laparoscopic Myomectomy

When abdominal myomectomy is indicated, the laparoscopic approach can be offered as an alternative to the standard "open" abdominal myomectomy in selected patients. However, this procedure is appropriate in very few patients for several reasons. First, myomectomy is indicated in infertility patients only if there is significant distortion of the uterine wall or endometrial cavity or if there is obstruction or distortion of the fallopian tubes by myomata. Second, myomectomy is indicated in patients who wish to retain their uterus only if the myomata are large or are significantly symptomatic with menorrhagia. In both circumstances, the myomata are likely to be multiple and large, and laparoscopic myomectomy is rarely the most appropriate procedure for removal.

There are limitations to laparoscopic myomectomy, and these are mostly technical. Myomata in certain loca-

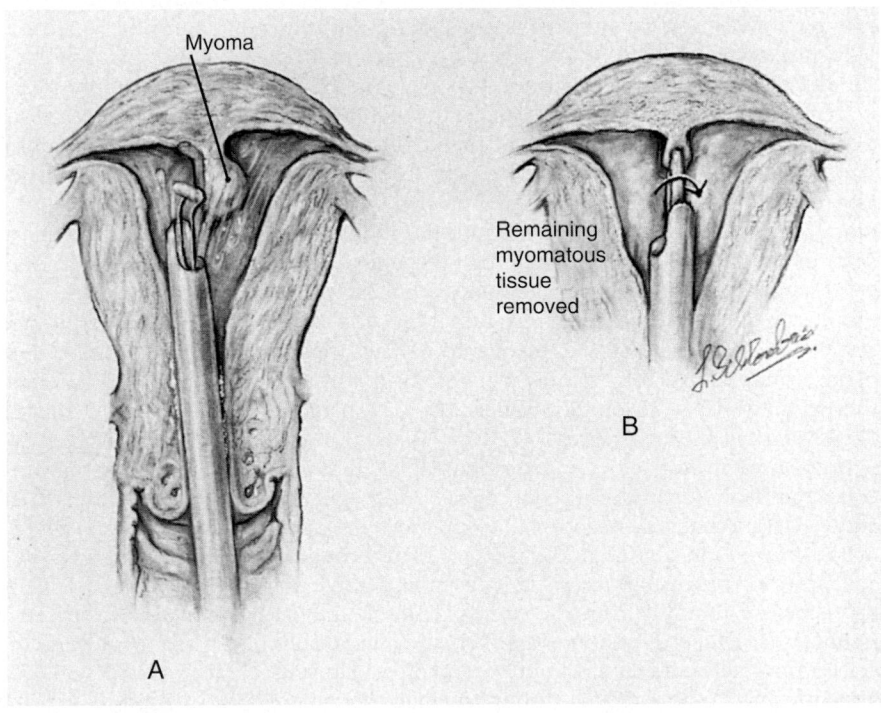
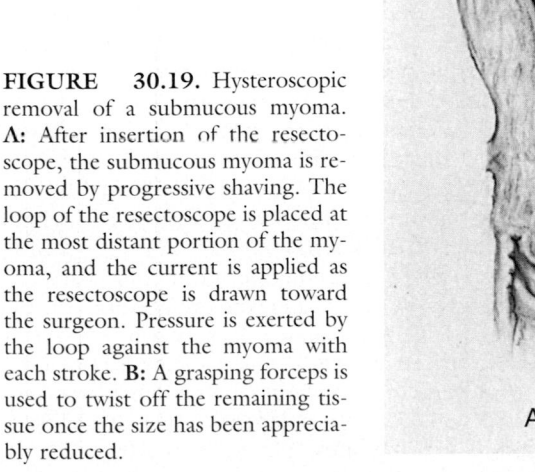

FIGURE 30.19. Hysteroscopic removal of a submucous myoma. **A:** After insertion of the resectoscope, the submucous myoma is removed by progressive shaving. The loop of the resectoscope is placed at the most distant portion of the myoma, and the current is applied as the resectoscope is drawn toward the surgeon. Pressure is exerted by the loop against the myoma with each stroke. **B:** A grasping forceps is used to twist off the remaining tissue once the size has been appreciably reduced.

tions are difficult to remove. When myomata are large or multiple, or both, operative time and blood loss may be unacceptable. When myomata are embedded deeply in the myometrium, proper repair of the uterine wall may be difficult or impossible, and uterine rupture may occur in a subsequent pregnancy. Retrieval of the resected myomata from the peritoneal cavity can also pose problems. Large myomata must be morcellated into smaller pieces for retrieval. Retrieval through the posterior vaginal fornix or though the abdominal wall requires separate additional incisions, which somewhat defeats the idea of a minimally invasive procedure. Only very skillful laparoscopists should attempt extensive myomectomy through the laparoscope. According to Mais and colleagues, operation time for myomectomy was significantly longer for laparoscopy than for laparotomy when more than four myomata had to be removed and the largest myoma was greater than 6 cm. Dubuisson and co-workers also reinforce the difficulty of the technique by reporting conversion to laparotomy at a rate of 7.5% (93.7% due to operative difficulties) and a complication rate of 3.8%. These authors echo similar intraoperative concerns: (1) the location of the hysterotomy, (2) the type of hysterotomy, (3) the uterine suture, and (4) removal of the myoma. In addition, they report that one third of patients developed adhesions at the uterine scar.

Several technical innovations have been developed to facilitate laparoscopic myomectomy. Electrosurgical and laser techniques are used in ingenious ways. Special traction devices, including corkscrews of various sizes, are required. The operator must be able to provide hemostasis using monopolar cutting current and bipolar forceps. Aquadissection can be used to establish planes for dissection between myomata and the surrounding myometrium. Special techniques of approximating myometrium with larger curved needles are used with extracorporeal suture tying. Autologous blood donation with intraoperative transfusion when necessary reduces the risk of homologous transfusion. Larger myomata can be removed vaginally with morcellation through a posterior colpotomy incision. In cases of myomas of extreme size, Pelosi and colleagues proposed the use of hand-assisted laparoscopy to avoid a laparotomy. This technique allows the insertion of a hand into the abdomen to assist in dissection. This is accomplished through a glove-sized incision at laparoscopy, while preserving the pneumoperitoneum. A cylindrical serrated morcellator can also be used to convert smaller myomata to small strips of tissue, which can then be removed abdominally through the trocar sleeve or through a minilaparotomy incision. Retrieval of all bits and pieces of myoma tissue from the peritoneal cavity can be a tedious challenge. Hirai and colleagues from Japan described a microwave coagulator and electromechanical tissue borer to minimize invasion of the myometrium and abdominal wall. The proposed advantage of this technique is that, by morcellating the tissue before removal from the uterus, less myometrial trauma is sustained. Horizontal and perpendicular blades at the tip rotate and hollow out the myoma, allowing large myomas to be removed through a small uterine in-

cision. The authors described the use in five patients with four of the five having myomas weighing less than 170 g. The blood loss and operating time were not substantially different than with conventional abdominal procedures. Long-term data regarding myometrial strength over time and pregnancy outcomes are not yet available. More experience with this procedure is necessary to determine its role in myomectomy.

Another technical innovation called *myolysis* has been described by Goldfarb and is based on earlier experience in Europe. Either Nd:YAG laser or bipolar needles are used laparoscopically to penetrate the myomata at multiple sites at a 90-degree angle to the uterus. In response to treatment, the myomata ultimately atrophy. The technique is based on the theory that the coagulating effects of lasers or the bipolar needle can necrose myometrial stroma, denature protein, destroy vascularity, and result in substantial shrinkage of myomas when deprived of their blood supply. Goldfarb advises treatment with GnRH agonists before surgery. The ideal candidates for myolysis are perimenopausal women who have symptomatic leiomyomata measuring 3 to 10 cm or uterine size less than 14 weeks' gestation. Goldfarb combines myolysis with endometrial ablation in patients with symptomatic myomas with persistent uterine bleeding. The addition of myolysis to endometrial ablation increased the rate of postsurgical amenorrhea from 36.5% to 57% and second procedures, including hysterectomy, were reduced from 38% to 12.5%. Goldfarb described significant adhesions at follow-up laparoscopy in patients treated with the Nd:YAG laser technique due to excessive serosal injury from multiple punctures. A circumferential technique was later developed to destroy vasculature instead of the myomatous tissue. The devascularized myoma becomes cyanotic, loses viability, and fibroses. Phillips and colleagues reported on women who underwent elective diagnostic laparoscopy to evaluate adhesions associated with previously performed myolysis. Mean adhesion score was only 1.15 ± 0.6 on a scale of 10.

Zreik and colleagues at Yale University modified the myolysis procedure to include cryotechnology to "freeze" uterine leiomyomas. The technique, *cryomyolysis*, was described in a prospective pilot study of 14 patients. All patients were pretreated with GnRH agonist therapy for 3 months. Thirteen of the 14 endoscopic procedures were performed by laparoscopy and the remaining one by hysteroscopic visualization. Cryoprobe placement was verified and freezing was performed at an internal probe temperature of $-180°C$ until the ice ball encompassed the entire fibroid or reached maximum size. A thaw cycle was then performed, followed by one more freeze-thaw cycle. A hollow track remained within the frozen myoma after removal of the cryoprobe. MRI studies were used to assess uterine and myoma size. The uterus enlarged by 22% after discontinuation of the GnRH therapy. Myoma volume decreased by 6% over 4 months postoperatively, with some patients having a decrease of more than 50%. Four of six women who underwent second-look office laparoscopy had adhesion formation at freezing sites. The authors attributed risk and severity of adhesion formation to the number of punctures with the cryoprobe. The role of this therapy in conservative treatment of uterine myomata remains to be defined.

Hysteroscopic myomectomy and endometrial resection can be performed simultaneously if submucous myomata are present. In more than 300 myolysis procedures, the author reported minimal morbidity with a 30% to 50% reduction in myoma size beyond the reduction achieved with GnRH agonist treatment. No regrowth occurred after several years of follow-up, even after estrogen replacement therapy. Bipolar coagulation myolysis may be less likely to cause damage to the uterine serosa and less likely to cause adhesion formation postoperatively. According to Goldfarb, "As a same-day procedure, myoma coagulation appears to be an extremely safe alternative to hysterectomy, allowing the patient to avoid major surgery and its subsequent recovery time, while providing an alternative solution for patients with symptomatic leiomyomas."

Nezhat and co-workers used a combination of laparoscopy and minilaparotomy to perform myomectomy in 57 women with uteri at 8 to 26 weeks in gestational size. In this laparoscopically assisted myomectomy procedure, the myomata were removed and the uterus repaired through the minilaparotomy incision. It was technically less difficult than laparoscopic myomectomy and allowed better closure of the uterine defects. This technique may be preferable in the case of large myomas in that it is easier to achieve conventional multilayer suturing and easier to extract myomas.

A significant disadvantage of myomectomy is the risk of postoperative pelvic adhesions. The adhesions may adversely affect fertility, give rise to pain, and increase the risk of ectopic pregnancy or even intestinal obstruction. Several studies have demonstrated that the risk of postoperative adhesions decreases when a laparoscopic approach is used in lieu of an open abdominal approach. Literature review demonstrates that the average rate of postoperative adhesions after laparoscopic myomectomy is 41% versus more than 90% after a myomectomy via laparotomy. Dubuisson and colleagues assessed adhesion formation after laparoscopic myomectomy in a prospective manner. Forty-five patients underwent a second look after laparoscopic myomectomy. Seventy-two sites were evaluated. The overall rate of postoperative adhesions was 35.6% per patient. The rate of adhesions per myomectomy site was 16.7%. The rate of adhesions on the adnexa was 24.4%. Associations with the occurrence of adnexal adhesions included an additional surgical procedure carried out at the same time, the existence of adhesions before the operation, and posterior location of the myoma. Several factors may increase the risk of postoperative adhesion formation after a laparoscopic myomectomy. Recognition of these factors may be helpful in limiting adhesion formation.

The use of uterine suture appears to increase the risk of uterine adhesions. In some studies, the frequency doubled after suturing. The suture induces local tissue ischemia with inflammatory changes, which slow the healing process and induce the formation of adhesions. Contradictory data have been published regarding adhesion formation and the use of bipolar coagulation during a laparoscopic procedure.

The location of the myoma also affects adhesion formation. Adhesions are more likely to form when the myomectomy site is located on the posterior uterine wall. During laparoscopy, a uterine incision must be made over each individual myoma. With laparotomy, a single anterior uterine incision may be used for polymyomectomy even when posterior myomas are present.

The prior existence of pelvic adhesions significantly increases the risk of postoperative adnexal adhesions, but has not been shown to affect adhesions at the myomectomy site.

Laparoscopic myomectomy is further discussed in Chapter 16.

Abdominal Myomectomy

The first successful abdominal myomectomy was performed in the United States by the Atlee brothers, Washington and John, in 1844.

The first abdominal multiple myomectomy was performed by W. Alexander of Liverpool in 1898. In the early part of the 20th century, the technique of abdominal myomectomy was refined by many notable gynecologic surgeons, including Kelly, Cullen, Mayo, Rubin, Bonney, and others. The procedure did not gain popularity until the middle of the 20th century. The incidence of complications, including hemorrhage, infection, and postoperative intestinal obstruction from adhesions, was considered to be too high. Advances in surgical techniques to control intraoperative bleeding during myomectomy, along with advances in anesthesia, blood transfusion therapy, and GnRH analogs, have made myomectomy a safe alternative to hysterectomy in women with symptomatic leiomyomata. The number of myomectomies performed in the United States is increasing.

Because myomectomy is rarely an emergency, time is available to prepare the patient for surgery. It is important that she be properly informed of the reasons myomectomy has been recommended. She should understand the nature of the procedure so she can know what to expect and what is expected of her. It is especially important that she be informed of the possibility that intraoperative findings may contraindicate myomectomy and require that hysterectomy be performed instead. For example, myomectomy may not be technically feasible if diffuse leiomyomatosis is found. The technical challenge of removing a large cervical myoma can also preclude myomectomy.

A preoperative hysterosalpingogram may indicate distortion of the fallopian tubes or uterine cavity, findings that are important in planning the technique of myomectomy. An assessment of fallopian tube patency is helpful in predicting fertility. If the tubes are occluded, however, myomectomy is not necessarily contraindicated. According to Seoud and associates, myomectomy does not interfere with *in vitro* fertilization performance

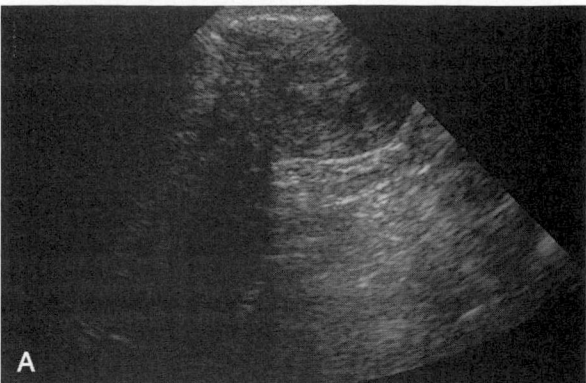

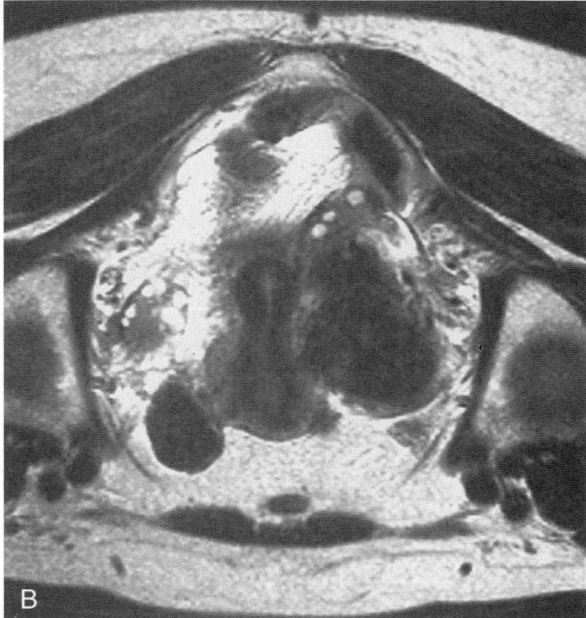

FIGURE 30.20. A: The ultrasound evaluation of this patient with a very large leiomyoma was not helpful in delineating the leiomyoma from the adnexa. B:The magnetic resonance imaging study demonstrated multiple leiomyomas distinctly separate from the adnexa bilaterally. The ovaries are seen bilaterally with multiple cysts. (Image courtesy of Deborah Baumgarten, M.D.)

in relation to overall and ongoing pregnancy rates. The patient whose tubes are occluded should understand that fertility may not be established by myomectomy, and assisted reproductive technologies may still be required after myomectomy. Tubal reconstruction procedures are uniformly unrewarding when performed at the same time multiple myomectomy is done. Indeed, tubal reconstruction may not always be necessary to establish tubal patency. In a report by Lev-Toaff and associates, nonfilling of the fallopian tubes was present on the preoperative hysterosalpingogram unilaterally in two patients and bilaterally in another two. In all four patients, tubal patency was shown after myomectomy. In the experience of these authors, hysterosalpingography before myomectomy can assist the gynecologic surgeon in planning the surgical approach by showing the presence, size,

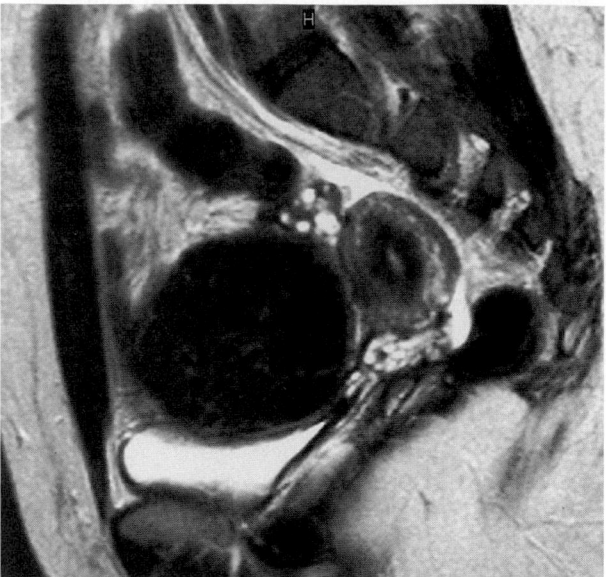

FIGURE 30.21. On magnetic resonance imaging, a large anterior, pedunculated leiomyoma is shown as a separate entity from the ovary in this patient. The ovary is displaced superiorly. (Image courtesy of Deborah Baumgarten, M.D.)

and location of submucous leiomyomata and concomitant tubal disease.

Imaging modalities such as transabdominal and transvaginal US and MRI play an important role in the management of patients with leiomyomata, especially those patients who are being prepared for myomectomy. As explained by Mayer and Shipilov, US is the preferred method for screening and initial evaluation of the pelvis. In many cases, it is the only imaging study necessary. There are special cases for which US cannot provide all the diagnostic information required. In a study by Schwartz and colleagues, US results were inconclusive in 20% of cases and did not yield a definitive diagnosis in 59% of cases. MRI was more definitive in all cases (Fig 30.20). The preoperative diagnosis of submucous leiomyomata by MRI may allow hysteroscopic resection and avoid abdominal myomectomy in some cases. Differentiation between uterine leiomyomata and adnexal pathology is more accurate with MRI and thus avoids the need for laparoscopy or laparotomy in some cases (Fig. 30.21). MRI studies can differentiate between uterine leiomyomata, diffuse and localized adenomyosis, and diffuse leiomyomatosis. MRI is the most accurate imaging technique for the detection and localization of leiomyomata (Fig 30.22). Hricak and co-workers were able to identify accurately by MRI all subserosal (9 of 9), all intramural (37), and 10 of 11 submucosal leiomyomata. Myomata as small as 0.3 cm can be detected. Various degrees of cellularity, degeneration, necrosis, and calcification can be identified by MRI, and sarcomatous change can be suspected. MRI provides imaging planes that are not available on transabdominal or transvaginal US, a feature that permits better visualization of the more lateral and posterior areas of the pelvis. MRI is the

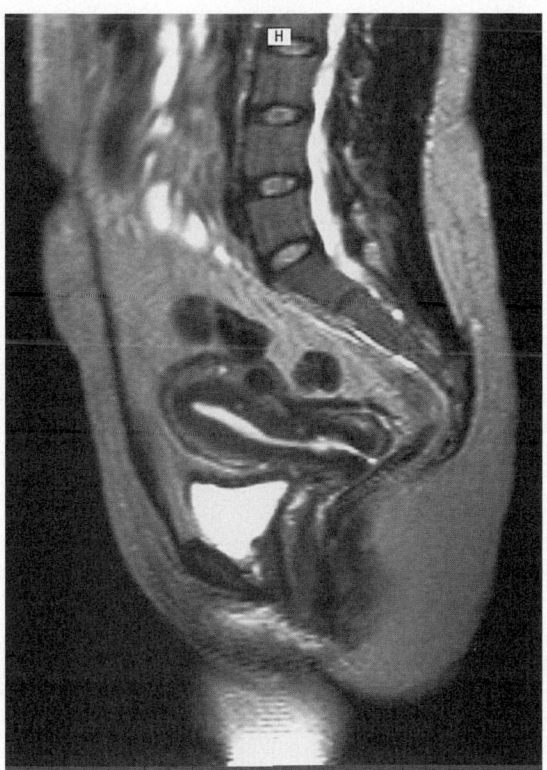

FIGURE 30.22. The location of this small posterior intramural leiomyoma is clearly delineated in this magnetic resonance image. The cervical canal is also easily visible. (Image courtesy of Deborah Baumgarten, M.D.)

most accurate method for preoperative localization of leiomyomata and surgical planning for myomectomy. Given the greater costs of MRI, it should be used judiciously. However, as noted by Mayer and Shipilov, the effective cost differential between MRI and US is decreasing.

As discussed by Wiskind and Thompson, one of the most serious risks of surgical bleeding during myomectomy is the risk associated with homologous blood transfusion. The first rule in reducing or eliminating the need for transfusion is to bring the patient to the operating room with the highest possible hemoglobin and hematocrit level. About 30% of myomectomy patients have associated menorrhagia. These small repeated menstrual hemorrhages deplete the body's iron stores over time and eventually result in iron-deficiency anemia of various degrees of severity. Patients scheduled for myomectomy benefit from oral iron supplementation. In a study by Thompson, the liberal use of oral iron therapy preoperatively was shown to decrease the number of blood transfusions on the gynecologic surgical service at the Johns Hopkins Hospital. A blood transfusion is seldom necessary to correct iron-deficiency anemia in a gynecologic patient. Blood transfusions should generally be reserved for patients with hypovolemic shock or aregenerative forms of anemia. In most other circumstances, elective surgery should be delayed until the anemia has been corrected by oral iron supplementation.

Occasionally, patients with a myomatous uterus have iron-deficiency anemia due to menstrual bleeding that is too heavy or too continuous to allow a response to oral iron therapy. In this situation, it may be beneficial to induce amenorrhea with hormonal therapy to allow the anemia to be corrected more expeditiously. Amenorrhea can be induced with progestational agents such as norethindrone or medroxyprogesterone acetate, with danazol, or with GnRH agonists. Several studies have demonstrated a significant increase in hemoglobin and hematocrit values in patients with leiomyomata treated preoperatively for 8 to 24 weeks with GnRH analogs compared with matched control groups. Friedman and colleagues also found a significant increase in serum iron and total iron-binding capacity in a study group treated with the GnRH agonist leuprolide acetate. In some patients, oral iron was also given. In an evaluation of 265 patients, GnRH agonists plus iron were more effective than iron alone in treating the anemia of patients with uterine leiomyomata, according to Stovall and co-workers. In a double-blind, placebo-controlled, multicenter study, Friedman and associates reported resolution of menorrhagia in 97% of uterine leiomyomata patients treated with GnRH agonists.

Preoperative treatment with GnRH analogs can actually reduce the operative blood loss during myomectomy, according to studies by Friedman and colleagues, Andreyko and co-workers, Moghissi, and others. In a prospective, randomized study of 50 patients undergoing hysterectomy for symptomatic leiomyomata, Stovall and colleagues found a significant decrease in operative blood loss between those patients who received 2 months of leuprolide acetate treatment preoperatively and matched control subjects. An elegant study by Friedman and associates demonstrated a significant decrease in operative blood loss during myomectomy between patients with pretreatment uterine volumes greater than 600 cm^3 who were treated with depot leuprolide acetate for 12 weeks preoperatively and a matched control group. However, there was no significant difference in blood loss between the two groups when patients with smaller uterine volumes (150 to 600 cm^3) were included in the analysis. It has been suggested that the hypoestrogenic environment caused by GnRH analog therapy reduces the vascular supply to uterine leiomyomata. However, even in patients not treated with GnRH agonists, blood flow has been observed to be lower in myomata and adjacent tissue.

The advantages and disadvantages of the preoperative collection of autologous blood are discussed in Chapter 18. Intraoperative autotransfusion and normovolemic hemodilution are also discussed. These techniques of reducing or avoiding the risk of homologous blood transfusion are discussed in detail by Wiskind and Thompson.

Perioperative antimicrobial prophylaxis is indicated with myomectomy. It is preferable to perform the operation in the follicular phase of the menstrual cycle. This avoids the chance of encountering an unknown or unsuspected pregnancy and reduces the problems encountered when a fresh corpus luteum is inadvertently traumatized.

After induction of anesthesia, the patient is placed in Allen universal stirrups, the bladder is emptied, and a careful pelvic examination, including a rectovaginal-abdominal bimanual examination, is performed under anesthesia. Preparation and draping are done to allow access to the vagina and cervix in case it is necessary to place an instrument through the cervix and into the endometrial cavity during the procedure. Cervical dilatation should be done to facilitate postoperative drainage from the endometrial cavity, especially for cases in which the endometrial cavity has been entered during the myomectomy.

Many of the general principles of pelvic surgery are applicable to myomectomy. Perhaps the most important of these is optimum exposure at the operative site. This is accomplished primarily by an adequate incision, but there must also be proper retraction, good lighting, and able assistants. Although a Pfannenstiel incision is considered adequate for myomectomy on a small uterus, we prefer the Maylard incision for larger uteri, even those that exceed a size equivalent to a 12-week pregnancy. A Maylard incision provides excellent exposure throughout the pelvis. Because it is a transverse incision, it is stronger and provides better cosmesis than a vertical midline incision. A Bookwalter retractor optimizes exposure of the operative site. A Pfannenstiel incision can be used for removal of a small solitary myoma.

The importance of adequate exposure cannot be overemphasized. With proper exposure, operative time can be shortened and surgical bleeding can be more easily identified and controlled. Limited exposure may lengthen operative time, increase the risk of inadvertent injury to other pelvic structures, and force abandonment of a myomectomy in favor of a hysterectomy in especially difficult cases.

After the peritoneal cavity is entered, the abdomen is explored as usual. Adhesions in the pelvis must be carefully released or excised so that the intestines can be placed in the upper abdomen and held there with packs. The operation is performed according to microsurgical techniques and principles. For example, the laparotomy packs that are used to hold the intestines in the upper abdomen are placed in plastic bags to reduce the microscopic trauma to peritoneal surfaces caused by regular laparotomy packs. Lintless laparotomy packs are preferred. Several laparotomy packs in plastic bags can be used to fill the cul-de-sac, thus elevating and stabilizing the uterus for easier access. Visualization of the operative site can be improved by the liberal use of suction to remove blood from the field. Suction should be used instead of sponges because it allows for a more accurate determination of blood loss and is less traumatic to tissues.

The operative field is kept moist and free of clots with a solution of lactated Ringer solution containing heparin. Very fine instruments and sutures are used when possible, and tissue is handled gently to avoid unnecessary trauma to serosal surfaces. Traumatic instrumentation (e.g., uterine elevators with teeth, Kocher clamps, or any instrument on the uterine serosa) must be avoided. Sutures on serosal surfaces should be of a fine absorbable nonreactive material. Running suture lines are preferable to avoid extra knot volume, which may contribute to adhesion formation. If pelvic adhesions develop after myomectomy, future fertility may be adversely affected. Performing the operation in a way that minimizes adhesion formation greatly improves the possibility of a successful result.

At this point in the operative procedure, one should pause and evaluate the size, location, and number of myomata present. Special note should be made of their proximity to the endocervical canal, uterine vessels, and fallopian tubes. One must decide if myomectomy is still feasible, how the leiomyomata will be removed (and in what sequence), and how the uterus will be reconstructed.

The conservation of uterine function with myomectomy requires control of bleeding from uterine incisions and myoma beds. Contrary to hysterectomy for leiomyomata, conservation of the uterus requires that the blood supply to the uterus through the uterine and ovarian vessels remain intact. Removing multiple myomata embedded deeply in a vascular myometrium can result in considerable blood loss. Proper application of special techniques to limit blood loss can allow multiple myomectomies even in uteri up to 20 weeks' pregnancy size if satisfactory reconstruction is possible.

Controlled hypotensive anesthesia has become a useful adjunct to decrease surgical bleeding in selected patients. The main mechanism in the control of operative field bleeding with hypotensive anesthesia is the reduction of venous tone. This can be accomplished by specific vasodilating agents, such as nitroglycerin or sodium nitroprusside, epidural or spinal anesthesia, some inhalation anesthetic agents, and ganglionic blockade, to achieve and maintain a target mean blood pressure of 60 mm Hg. Our experience with this technique has been favorable. Venous bleeding can be further reduced if the patient is placed in a moderate Trendelenburg position. This facilitates venous drainage from the lower extremities and pelvis by gravity and may further reduce the blood pressure at the operative site.

Induced hypotension is contraindicated in patients with cerebrovascular disease, myocardial ischemia, peripheral vascular disease, severe renal or hepatic disease, and hypovolemia. None of these contraindications is seen very often in myomectomy patients. An anesthesiologist experienced with the technique is an essential requirement. The decision to use hypotension should be made jointly by the surgeon and the anesthesiologist. It is essential that the blood pressure be returned to normal before closure of the incision to ensure that adequate surgical hemostasis has been established.

Early proponents of myomectomy focused on methods to temporarily occlude uterine blood flow to control hemorrhage and provide a bloodless operative field. One of the earliest methods was simply to have an assistant grasp the broad ligaments firmly with each hand during myomectomy to impede blood flow through the uterine vessels. In the 1920s, Victor Bonney introduced a specially designed clamp that was placed around the uterine vessels and the round ligaments. The ovarian vessels were occluded with ring forceps. Using this technique, he was able on one occasion to remove more than 200 myomata from a single uterus. Rubin, in 1938, was the first to use an elastic rubber tourniquet through the broad ligament, encircling the cervix and occluding the uterine vessels during myomectomy. Rubber-shod clamps applied to the broad ligaments have also been used to occlude the uterine vessels and control bleeding.

Gynecologic surgeons do not often have the opportunity to use tourniquets to control bleeding; however, a myomectomy is particularly suited to their use. We prefer to use tourniquets fashioned in the manner of a Rumel-type tourniquet, which is used by vascular, thoracic, and trauma surgeons to occlude major vessels. Initially, a small hole is made in an avascular space in the broad ligament on either side of the uterine isthmus just lateral to the uterine vessels. A 5-French pediatric feeding tube is looped around the upper cervix through the holes in the broad ligament, and the two ends of the tube are then threaded through a 4-inch length of 35-French Malecot catheter and held with a clamp. A loop tourniquet can then be placed around each infundibulopelvic ligament through the same holes in the broad ligaments (Fig. 30.23A).

As the tourniquets are being placed, controlled hypotension is induced by the anesthesiology staff. Before the tourniquets are tightened, the location of the uterine arterial blood flow is identified with a sterile Doptone. When everything is in readiness and the plan of opera-

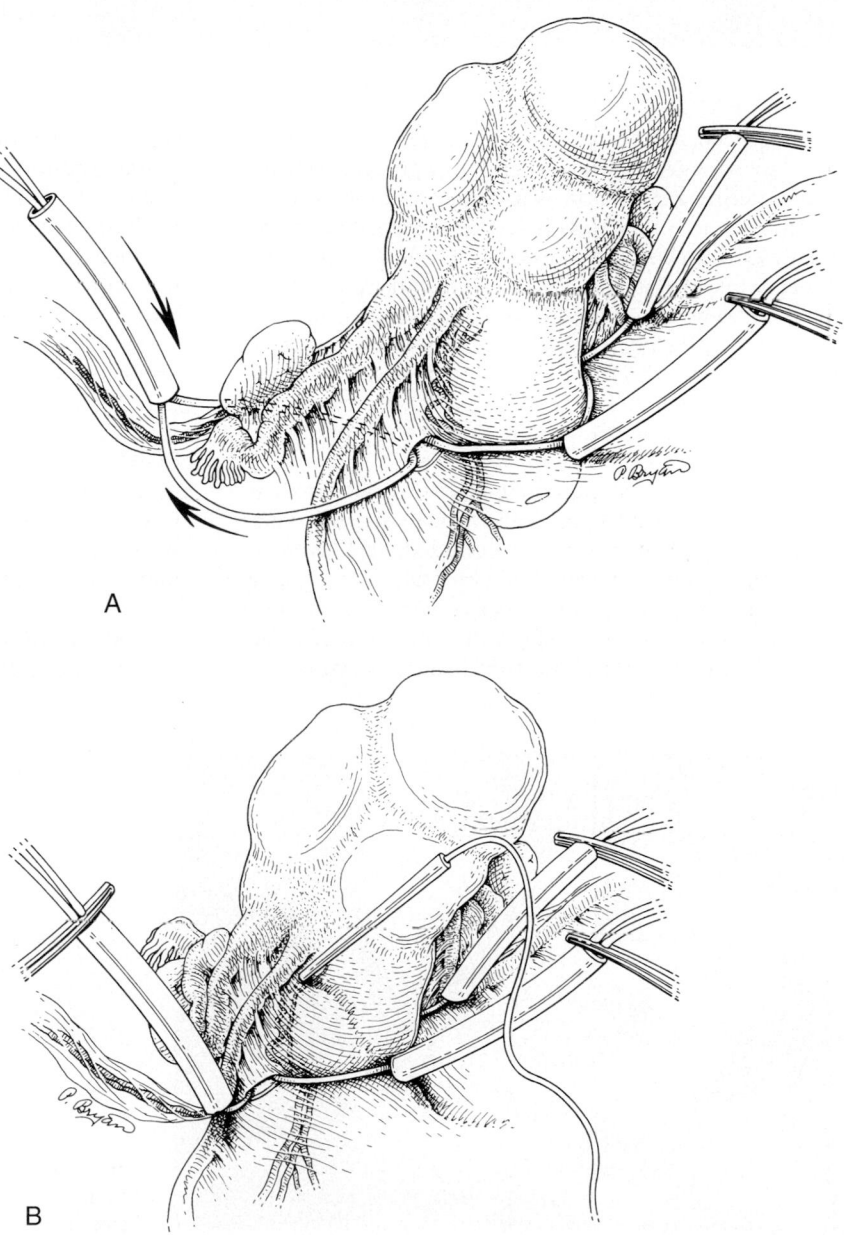

A

B

FIGURE 30.23. A: Through a small hole in the broad ligament on each side of the uterus, a Rumel tourniquet is placed around the lower uterus and around each infundibulopelvic ligament. **B:** When the tourniquets are tightened sufficiently, the blood flow to the uterus stops. The absence of arterial pulsations can be determined with the sterile Doptone.

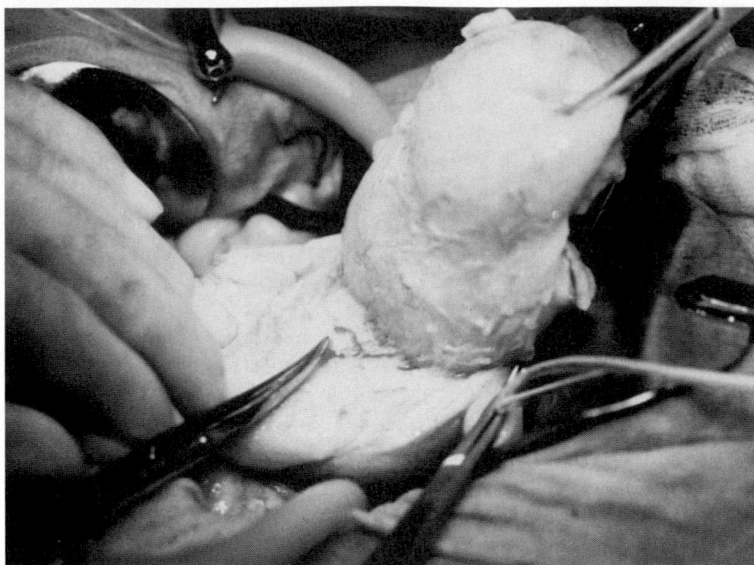

FIGURE 30.24. With tourniquets properly secured, myomectomy can be performed with minimal blood loss. See color version of figure.

tion has been selected by the surgical team, the tourniquets are snugged down and tightened progressively until the uterine arterial flow is no longer audible with the Doptone (Fig. 30.23B). It is very important that the arterial blood flow be occluded. If the venous flow is occluded while the arterial flow remains intact, blood loss could actually be increased with the tourniquets. The mean blood pressure should be reduced to the target hypotensive level (about 60 mm Hg) before the tourniquets are tightened. The higher the blood pressure, the tighter the tourniquets must be to occlude the uterine circulation.

With the combination of properly applied tourniquets and controlled hypotensive anesthesia, the entire circulation to the uterus can be occluded. The myomectomy can then be performed in a bloodless field, greatly facilitating complete removal of all tumors and a neat reconstruction of the uterus (Figs. 30.24 and 30.25). Occasionally, a large cervical or broad ligament myoma pre-

vents placement of the tourniquets. In this situation, the offending tumor should be removed first, the defects repaired when feasible, and the tourniquets applied for the remainder of the multiple myomectomy.

Once the tourniquets are tightened in place, the myomectomy should proceed expeditiously to prevent ischemic damage to the uterus, tubes, and ovaries. The length of time the pelvic structures can be without blood flow before irreversible damage occurs is unknown. We generally do not release the tourniquets until the myomectomy is complete (usually within an hour) and have not experienced any adverse events. Lock also agrees that intermittent release of the tourniquets is unnecessary. However, because the potential for injury does exist, tourniquet time should be monitored and kept to a minimum. The tourniquets should not be tightened until the surgical team is ready to perform the myomectomy. Intermittent release of the tourniquets should be considered if the operating time becomes excessive. We usu-

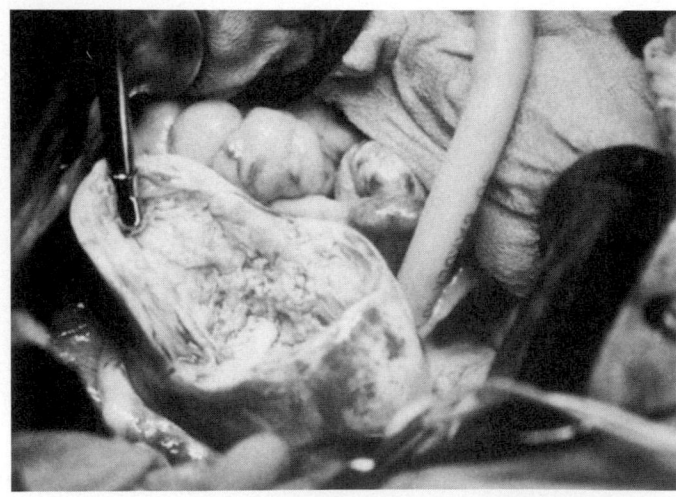

FIGURE 30.25. The use of tourniquets to control bleeding facilitates closure of the myoma bed and uterine incision. See color version of figure.

ally release the tourniquets around the ovarian vessels as the uterine serosa is being closed to restore circulation to the tubes and ovaries and to restore some collateral flow to the uterus. After reconstruction of the uterus is complete, the determination of adequate hemostasis in the uterus cannot be made until all the tourniquets are released and the blood pressure has returned to normal. Sometimes additional sutures are required for hemostasis. Before the abdomen is closed, the small holes in the broad ligament are repaired with figure-of-eight sutures.

Tourniquets are not necessary for every myomectomy, especially when the tumors are small or pedunculated. However, they are safe and inexpensive to use and can be of great benefit when large or multiple intramural myomata must be removed. A criticism of uterine tourniquets is that they are traumatic to pelvic structures. Our experience, to the contrary, is that soft plastic tubes used as tourniquets are quite atraumatic. No injuries attributable to these tourniquets have occurred in several hundred cases.

An alternative to the use of tourniquets to control bleeding during myomectomy is the local injection of vasoconstrictive agents. Perhaps the most commonly used agent is vasopressin, a synthetic derivative of the antidiuretic hormone from the posterior lobe of the pituitary gland. In addition to this antidiuretic effect, vasopressin induces smooth muscle contraction of the gastrointestinal tract and the vascular bed. In particular, it has been found to have a potent vasoconstrictor effect on the nonpregnant uterus when injected locally. It has a plasma half-life of 10 to 20 minutes and has been used effectively as a hemostatic agent during myomectomy. Pharmacologic vasoconstriction can be accomplished with vasopressin (antidiuretic hormone), 20 U (Pitressin). Twenty units of vasopressin are diluted in 20 mL of normal saline and injected into the superficial myometrium and serosa overlying the myoma. The effect usually lasts for 30 minutes.

Dillon reported that with the use of vasopressin, 72% of patients requiring myomectomy did not need blood replacement, compared with control subjects. Frederick and co-workers noted significantly less blood loss compared with an untreated group. Ginsburg and associates compared vasopressin with mechanical vascular occlusion and found that there were no demonstrable differences in blood loss, morbidity, or transfusion requirements between the two techniques. A favorable experience with vasopressin has also been reported by Semm and Mettler.

The weight of evidence in current clinical investigation indicates that vasopressin is as effective as mechanical vascular occlusion in controlling blood loss with myomectomy. Nevertheless, careful dissection around myomata and prompt suturing with exertion of direct pressure to bleeding vessels by the operative assistant are necessary to minimize blood loss. Care should be taken to avoid injecting the solution directly into a vascular channel, and no more than 30 mL per patient is recommended because of potential side effects. Vasopressin should not be used in patients with vascular disease, es-

pecially disease of the coronary arteries. Inadvertent intravascular injection can cause anginal pain; larger doses can cause myocardial infarction. Water intoxication can also occur as a result of the antidiuretic effect of vasopressin. This effect is potentiated in patients taking tricyclic antidepressants.

Although late postoperative bleeding does occur with the use of vasopressin, it is not a common complication. Arterial bleeding masked by vasopressin still requires suture ligation. Because of the short half-life of vasopressin, the hemostatic effect is observed only for 20 to 30 minutes and should be over before the incisional closure is started. However, some do claim that vasopressin simply delays bleeding, gives a false sense of security, and is not particularly effective for larger myomata and very extensive myomectomies.

For a variety of reasons, epinephrine as a vasoconstrictive agent is not recommended for use in gynecologic surgery.

Since its introduction into clinical practice in 1972, the CO_2 laser has been touted as a tool that increases surgical precision and decreases bleeding, tissue injury, and adhesion formation. The laser can be used to make a single uterine incision through which multiple myomata are removed. An elliptical incision can also be made around the base of larger myomata to facilitate their removal. Myomata less than 1 cm in diameter can be vaporized directly with the laser, which destroys tissue by vaporizing cellular water. Despite the favorable results reported by Weather, Reyniak and Corenthal, McLaughlin, and Starks, we believe that there is no clear advantage in using the CO_2 laser for abdominal myomectomy, especially considering the added cost to the patient.

Although the methods described earlier to control bleeding during myomectomy are helpful, they cannot substitute for good surgical techniques. Adherence to basic principles is essential for good results. Perhaps the most important of these is careful planning of the uterine incisions. Only a minimal number of incisions should be made. If possible, removal of all leiomyomata should be accomplished through a single incision in the anterior uterine corpus, and in the midline when feasible to avoid the vascular areas of the uterus and broad ligaments laterally. Even intramural leiomyomata in the posterior uterine wall can be removed through anterior incisions. Incisions in the posterior uterine wall may be necessary, however, if posterior subserous tumors are being removed. If posterior uterine incisions are made, adhesions are more likely to develop and will likely involve the tubes and ovaries as well.

As many tumors as possible should be removed through a single incision. Methods of removing myomata through a single anterior incision have been described by Bonney. The linear or elliptic incision should usually be over the largest myoma. It should be carried through the superficial myometrium directly into the underlying myoma. The myoma is then grasped with a double-tooth tenaculum or a large Lahey thyroid clamp for traction. The plane of cleavage between the myoma and the surrounding myometrium is easily identified. Sometimes in

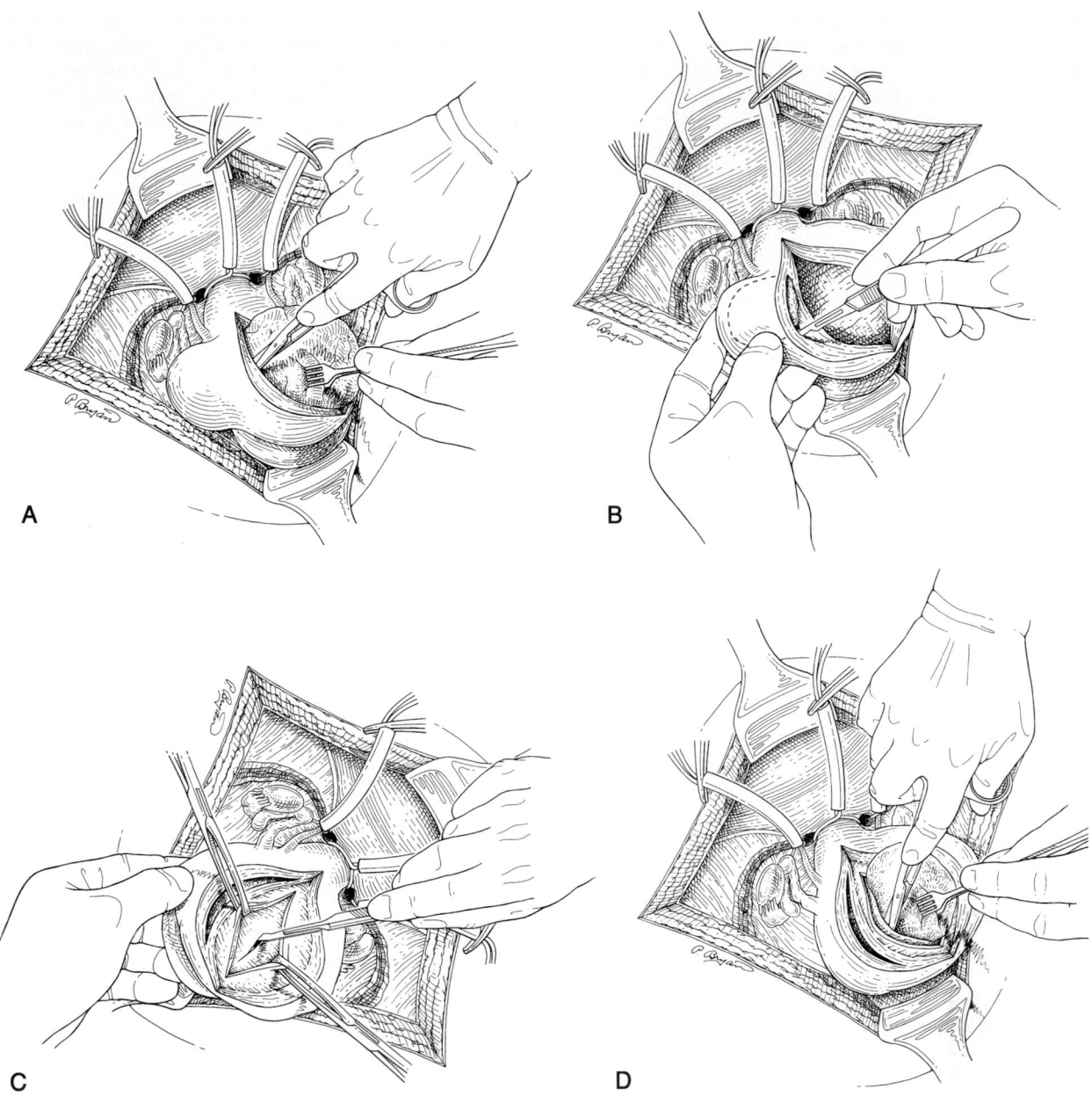

FIGURE 30.26. The sequence of steps in a multiple myomectomy is shown in these illustrations. **A:** Through a transverse Maylard incision, tourniquets are placed to occlude the uterine and ovarian artery flow. Through a single incision in the anterior myometrium, a large anterior myoma is removed first. All other myomas are removed through this incision. **B:** A smaller intramural myoma is removed through the same incision. **C:** To avoid making a separate incision in the posterior uterine wall, a large posterior myoma is removed through the uterine cavity. After an incision has been made through the anterior endometrium, an incision is made in the posterior endometrium directly over the posterior myoma. **D:** The myoma in the posterior uterine wall is dissected from its bed and removed through the uterine cavity. An incision in the posterior uterine serosa is thus avoided.

patients who have been treated with GnRH analogs, the plane of cleavage may seem less distinct. Sharp dissection with the scalpel or Metzenbaum scissors, or blunt dissection with the finger or knife handle, is required to enucleate the myoma from its bed. Sometimes the myoma is larger than expected. It may then be necessary to enlarge the incision or to remove the tumor by morcellation. Other adjacent tumors should be removed through the same incision. Any entry in the endometrial cavity should be noted, and a special attempt should be made to close it with sutures placed in the underlying supporting myometrium. Examples of the step-by-step planning and

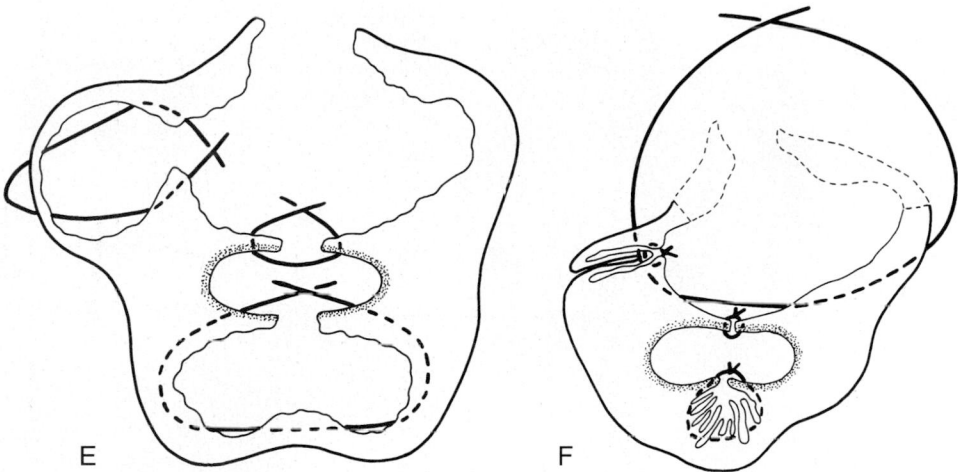

FIGURE 30.26. *Continued* **E:** Multiple sutures (2-0 delayed-absorbable) are used to close the defect in the posterior uterine wall first. Incisions in the uterine cavity are closed. Then the defects in the anterior uterine wall are closed. **F:** Trimming excess myometrium from the anterior uterine wall allows a better approximation of the myometrium. The edges of the serosa are closed with a continuous "baseball" stitch with 4-0 delayed-absorbable sutures.

performance of a multiple myomectomy are illustrated in Figures 30.26 and 30.27.

The muscle fibers and blood vessels surrounding a myoma are compressed by its growth. This compression of surrounding tissue forms a pseudocapsule around the myoma. No large blood vessels enter the myoma, and there is no vascular pedicle. If the dissection can be carried out between the myoma and the pseudocapsule, blood loss can be minimized. If blood vessels are cut or left on the surface of the myoma, it usually means that the dissection has been carried out in an improper plane. Dissection in the proper plane may be more difficult if the patient received GnRH analog therapy preoperatively.

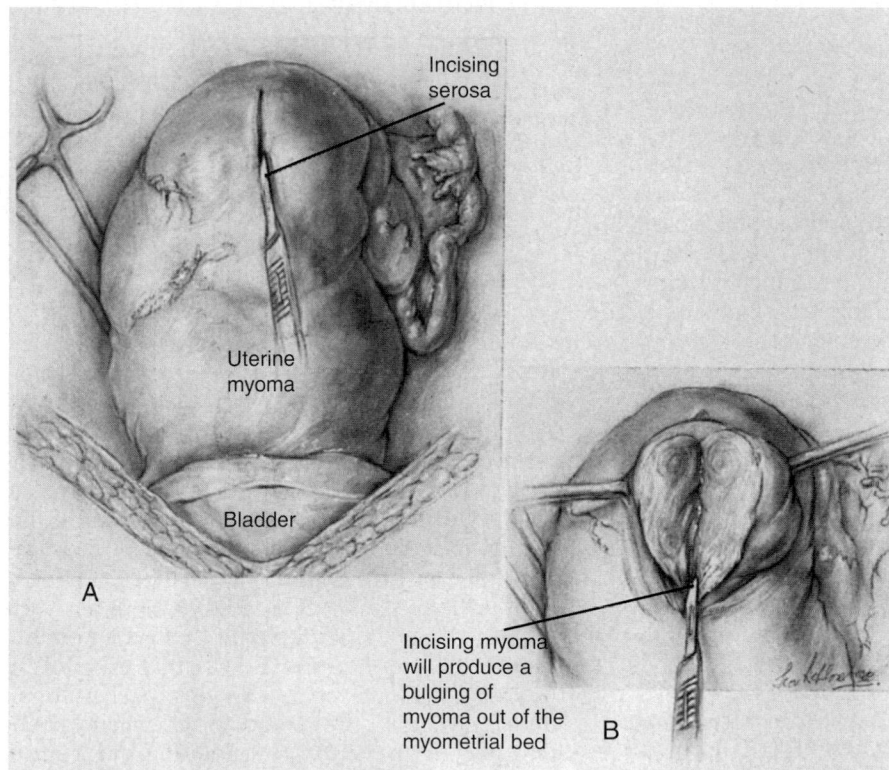

FIGURE 30.27. Techniques of multiple myomectomy. **A:** A vertical incision is made over a myoma on the anterior surface of the fundus as close to the midline as possible. Many myomas can be removed through this single incision. **B:** The incision is extended into the substance of the myoma. *Continued*

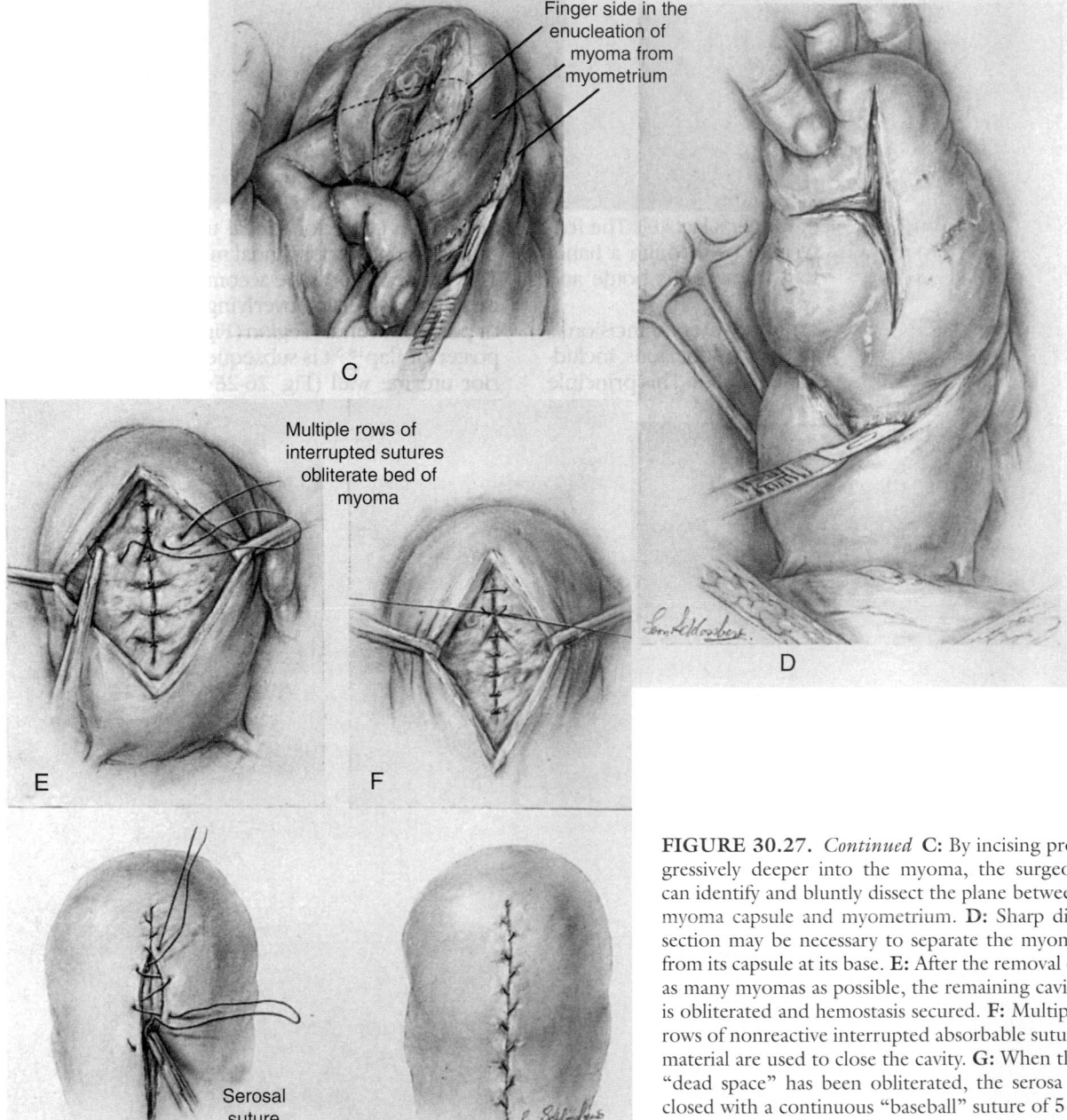

Finger side in the enucleation of myoma from myometrium

Multiple rows of interrupted sutures obliterate bed of myoma

Serosal suture

C

D

E

F

G

H

FIGURE 30.27. *Continued* **C:** By incising progressively deeper into the myoma, the surgeon can identify and bluntly dissect the plane between myoma capsule and myometrium. **D:** Sharp dissection may be necessary to separate the myoma from its capsule at its base. **E:** After the removal of as many myomas as possible, the remaining cavity is obliterated and hemostasis secured. **F:** Multiple rows of nonreactive interrupted absorbable suture material are used to close the cavity. **G:** When the "dead space" has been obliterated, the serosa is closed with a continuous "baseball" suture of 5-0 or 6-0 nonreactive absorbable material. **H:** This type of closure approximates the serosal edges.

Several ingenious techniques for removing leiomyomata and for repairing defects have been described. For example, Bonney's hood can be used to remove a large leiomyoma in the uterine fundus. The myoma is first exposed through an elliptic incision made transversely across the anterior fundus, taking care to avoid the interstitial portion of the fallopian tube on each side (Fig. 30.28A and B). After the primary tumor is removed (Fig. 30.28C), other leiomyomata can also be removed through the same incision. Excess myometrium can be trimmed away (30.28D). Interrupted sutures obliterate the dead space, approximate the myometrium, and accomplish satisfactory hemostasis. The sutures are placed in such a way that the posterior flap of myometrium is folded over the anterior uterine wall and sutured in place, thus fashioning Bonney's hood (Fig. 30.28D).

Meticulous closure of defects from the enucleated myomata is essential to maintain hemostasis postoperatively, but this should be deferred until all the tumors are removed. Hypertrophy of the normal myometrium is always present with uterine leiomyomata. Some of this hypertrophied myometrium is considered excess and can be trimmed to facilitate a more normal reconstruction of the uterus. Involution of the myometrial hypertrophy is expected to occur in the first few months after myomectomy. Therefore, only a small amount of normal my-

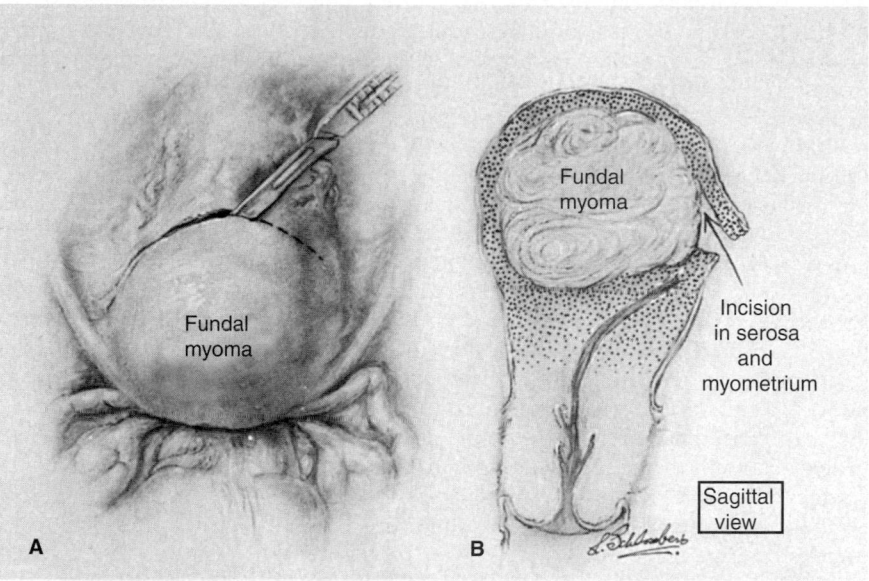

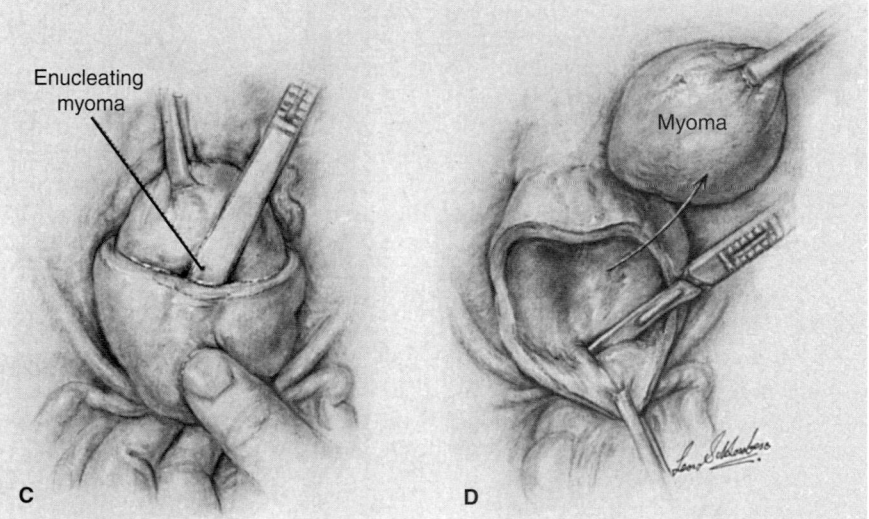

FIGURE 30.28. Technique of myomectomy using an anterior hood incision as described by Bonney. **A:** A transverse incision is made in the anterior fundal wall over the myoma. **B:** Sagittal view of the location of the incision. **C** and **D:** Using blunt and sharp dissection, the surgeon enucleates the myoma from its bed. Excess hypertrophied myometrium may be trimmed and removed before closure of myometrium and serosa.

ometrial tissue should be removed. In reconstructing the uterus, the surgeon should refer to fixed points such as the attachments of the round ligaments and fallopian tubes on each side of the corpus. Symmetric reconstruction is preferred but is not always possible. The myoma beds are usually closed with interrupted figure-of-eight or mattress 2-0 delayed-absorbable sutures. Large defects can be closed initially with a pursestring suture to obliterate the dead space. Several layers of sutures may be required. One must be careful to avoid occlusion of the uterine vessels, the endocervical canal, or the interstitial portion of the fallopian tubes. Transfundal or transcervical chromotubation to test fallopian tube patency after uterine reconstruction is complete is not usually possible because of leakage of the dye through the myometrial incisions.

In closing a myomectomy incision, the security of the closure comes from sutures placed in the myometrium. If possible, these sutures and knots must not

be exposed. In Figure 30.26E and F, several techniques of closing myometrial defects are illustrated. The serosal edge of the uterine incision should be carefully approximated with a continuous 5-0 or 4-0 delayed-absorbable "baseball" stitch.

The tourniquets are removed, the hypotensive anesthesia is reversed, and the uterus is carefully inspected for evidence of bleeding. Additional sutures are sometimes required. If a uterine suspension is needed, a modified Coffey or modified Gilliam technique along with uterosacral ligament plication is used.

Adhesion prevention can also be achieved by the use of absorbable or nonabsorbable barriers. The absorbable barrier Interceed (oxidized regenerated cellulose) can be placed over the uterine corpus to protect the tubes and ovaries from denuded peritoneal surfaces and uterine incision. Alternatively, a nonabsorbable barrier, Gore-Tex (polytetrafluoroethylene surgical membrane), can be sutured over the uterine incisions with 7-0 absorbable minimal reactive sutures. The use of Gore-Tex has been associated with a reduction in new adhesion formation. Diamond and the Seprafilm Adhesion Study Group assessed the efficacy of Seprafilm (HAL-F) Bioresorbable Membrane (sodium hyaluronate and carboxymethylcellulose) in reducing the incidence, severity, extent, and area of uterine adhesions after myomectomy. This prospective, randomized, blinded, multicenter study involved an independent gynecologic surgeon's review of each patient's second-look laparoscopy. One hundred and twenty-seven women undergoing uterine myomectomy with at least one posterior uterine incision were randomized to treatment with Seprafilm or no treatment at the completion of the myomectomy. All indices, including incidence, severity, and extent of adhesions, were decreased in the treatment group. This suggests that newer barriers may also have a role in adhesion prevention. Free grafts of peritoneum or omentum should not be used to cover uterine incisions.

Second-look laparoscopy may be indicated in patients with multiple incisions or in those with posteriorly located incisions adjacent to the adnexa. Early adhesions can be easily lysed, and an additional barrier membrane can be placed. The role of second-look laparoscopy is not well defined, and conflicting studies can be found in the literature regarding the efficacy of this procedure.

A comprehensive review of methods to prevent adhesion formation in gynecologic surgery has been published by Damario and Rock and by diZerega.

Results of Myomectomy

An extensive multiple myomectomy is a major operation with the potential for a higher morbidity than that found with hysterectomy. The major immediate postoperative complications after myomectomy are febrile morbidity and intraperitoneal bleeding.

Postoperative febrile morbidity may be related to extensive tissue trauma or to infection for a variety of reasons. Perioperative antibiotics are routinely given, but antibiotics are not usually continued beyond the day of operation. Any evidence of infection in the recovery period should be treated vigorously and promptly because infection in the operative site may be adhesiogenic and may have devastating effects on future fertility. Unfortunately, subclinical infection in the operative site may not be recognized and therefore may not be treated, but it can also have adverse effects on fertility because of de novo adhesion formation. For these reasons, meticulous and sterile surgical technique during myomectomy must be impeccable.

Intraperitoneal bleeding after myomectomy is usually due to failure to achieve hemostasis of the myometrial vessels during closure of the myoma beds and uterine incisions. Although we do use a heparin solution (5,000 U of heparin per 1,000 mL of lactated Ringer solution) for irrigation during myomectomy, there is no evidence to suggest that this contributes to occult intraperitoneal bleeding.

The diagnosis of intraperitoneal bleeding in the postoperative patient may be difficult. The vital signs can remain stable for several hours before rapidly deteriorating. Peritoneal signs are often subtle and may be masked by incisional pain and analgesic medications. In addition, the peritoneal cavity has an enormous capacity for accommodating occult blood loss. Indeed, as much as 3,000 mL of blood can be shed into the peritoneal cavity with only a 1-cm increase in the abdominal radius.

Therefore, patients must be carefully monitored for the first 24 hours after myomectomy. Vital signs are routinely checked every 15 minutes for the first 2 hours after surgery, then every 30 minutes until stable. Subsequently, they are monitored every 2 to 4 hours for the first 24 hours postoperatively. A hematocrit is usually performed 6 hours after the operation is completed and again on the first postoperative morning. It can also be performed whenever there is a suspicion of intraperitoneal bleeding, anemia, or hypovolemia. Any sign of restlessness, tachycardia, or tachypnea may be an indication of blood loss, especially when associated with hypotension.

When occult postoperative intraperitoneal bleeding is suspected, peritoneal lavage can be a valuable diagnostic tool. If the lavage solution yields a red blood cell count of $100,000/mm^3$, intraperitoneal bleeding is likely and reexploration is indicated without delay. Lavage is unnecessary when the diagnosis of intraperitoneal bleeding is unequivocal and associated with definite hypovolemia. In this situation, immediate return to the operating room for reexploration is indicated.

Postoperative bleeding after myomectomy can be devastating. Intraoperative control of bleeding during an extensive multiple myomectomy often requires that the uterine blood flow be impeded with tourniquets, clamps, or the local injection of vasoconstrictive agents. However, the demonstration of adequate surgical hemostasis in the uterus cannot be made until the uterine circulation has been fully restored. Assiduous attention to this principle intraoperatively prevents postmyomectomy bleeding in almost all cases.

Reports by Smith and Uhlir, Rosenfield, and LaMorte and associates indicate that the morbidity of myomectomy is no greater than the morbidity of hysterectomy. Verkauf reviewed current published reports and found that the operative risk of myomectomy does not exceed that of hysterectomy. One case of disseminated intravascular coagulation, hemolytic anemia, and acute renal failure associated with extensive multiple myomectomy was reported by Sacks and Hoyne.

Myomectomy has an excellent record in reducing heavy menstruation in patients with a complaint of menorrhagia. In more than 80% of patients, menorrhagia is cured or significantly improved. Pelvic pain and discomfort and dysmenorrhea can also be relieved, but the results are not as dramatic because leiomyomata are often associated with other gynecologic diseases (e.g., endometriosis and pelvic inflammatory disease) that can also cause pelvic pain.

The impact of abdominal myomectomy on infertility is difficult to assess. Other factors besides leiomyomata may be present to a varying degree. The extent to which the uterine cavity or the fallopian tubes are distorted also varies. The percentage of patients in each series who wish to conceive after myomectomy is not the same. There is also considerable variation in the surgical technique and skill of the gynecologic surgeon. Prospective, randomized, controlled studies are lacking. These and other factors make it difficult to assess the impact of abdominal myomectomy on infertility.

There are a number of published reports regarding women who experience recurrent pregnancy wastage or prior infertility with another cause, and who undergo myomectomy. According to Verkauf's review, conception occurs in more than half of such women who were not previously pregnant. A review of nine abdominal myomectomy reports by Vercellini and colleagues indicates similar results. Two hundred thirty-four women similarly evaluated and treated by myomectomy were included in Verkauf's review. Of patients with leiomyoma-associated infertility without other apparent cause, 59.5% conceived. Among patients who had additional treated infertility factors, 50% conceived after myomectomy. Eighty-six percent of pregnancies occurred within 2 years of the operation. The conception rate among women older than age 35 may not be as good. Also, the postmyomectomy conception rate may be lower when the uterus is greater than 12 weeks' gestational size and when more than four myomata are removed. When abdominal myomectomy includes removal of submucous myomata, Garcia and Tureck report that 53% of patients attempting to establish a pregnancy conceive. Both Li and colleagues and Vercellini and co-workers published retrospective reviews supporting excellent conception and pregnancy rates following abdominal myomectomies. Vercellini's work suggests that certainly age at the time of the procedure is important as it was one of three independent variables (age, duration of infertility before surgery, and the presence of other infertility factors) associated with postoperative cumulative conception rate.

Buttram and Reiter reviewed 1,914 cases of myomectomy and compared preoperative and postoperative abortion rates. The reduction in abortion rate after myomectomy from 41% to 19% suggests improvement in reproductive salvage through the use of this procedure. According to Verkauf's review, 69.2% of women with previous recurrent pregnancy wastage conceived after myomectomy and had a reduction in fetal loss.

An ultrasonographic study of uterine remodeling after conservative myomectomy was reported by Beyth and associates. There was a gradual decrease in uterine volume in all patients during the 6 months after myomectomy, with the most remarkable decrease occurring in the first 2 to 3 months. Presumably, this represents an involution of myometrial hypertrophy and postoperative healing of uterine incisions. We recommend that all patients use local methods of contraception (diaphragm, condoms, and spermicidal jelly or foam) for at least 3 months to avoid conception until the myomectomy incisions are healed.

Finally, there is the matter of recurrence of myomata after myomectomy. In Verkauf's review, leiomyomata recurred in 7.5% of patients, and 6.8% required reoperation. Most recurrences appeared more than 3 years after myomectomy, thus allowing sufficient time for conception to occur before recurrence. Friedman and associates investigated a concern that GnRH agonist–induced myoma shrinkage would make some small intramural and submucosal tumors "invisible" at myomectomy, causing early "recurrence" of leiomyomata once gonadal suppression ceased and estrogen production returned. In their study, there was no difference in myoma recurrence between women pretreated with GnRH agonists (67%) and those treated with placebo (56%) 27 to 38 months after myomectomy. Their myoma recurrence rate of 61% is much higher than that previously reported in combined myomectomy series. The authors believe that this discrepancy is most likely due to the use of high-resolution US to diagnose small myomata that would otherwise be missed on bimanual examination.

Matta and colleagues reported that after GnRH analog treatment, the US outline of some myomata was lost or obscured. Such myomata are probably more difficult to identify and remove with myomectomy and may be more likely to reappear when GnRH analog treatment is discontinued after myomectomy.

Embolotherapy

With current technology progressing toward less invasive therapies, the minimally invasive procedure of uterine artery embolization (UAE) is gaining popularity. This procedure can potentially obviate the need for surgical procedures in patients who suffer from symptomatic leiomyomas.

In the female genital tract, embolotherapy for control of hemorrhage from malignancy was first reported in the late 1970s. In 1980, Pais and colleagues described successful embolization for postpartum hemorrhage. Many more reports followed in the mid 1980s. In the early 1990s, Ravina and co-workers began utilizing embolotherapy as a preoperative maneuver to decrease intraoperative blood loss during surgery for myomas. The protocol generally included embolization about 24 hours before the surgery; however, some occurred a few days or weeks before surgery. Such an improvement in symptoms occurred that many surgeries were canceled altogether. This serendipitous discovery led to the performance of UAE as a primary procedure. UAE for leiomyomas was first performed in the United States by Goodwin and colleagues in 1995. Since then, several large series have been reported and experience continues to grow.

UAE is appropriate for patients with symptomatic leiomyomas and preference for other medical or surgical treatment. Clinical findings, therapeutic goals, and overall medical conditions factor into the decision making. Several concerns have developed in treating patients who may desire future conception. Hypotheses include reduced fertility as a consequence of injury to the uterus or ovaries, placental insufficiency resulting from inadequate blood flow through the uterus, or uterine rupture during pregnancy from UAE induced myoma necrosis. In practice, there have been no reports of decreased fertility after occlusion of the major uterine vessels either by surgical or radiologic technique. In addition, there are numerous reports of successful pregnancies after these procedures. Amenorrhea has been reported in 1% to 2% of patients after UAE; however, some authors have attributed this to the coincidental onset of menopause.

Contraindications to this procedure include pregnancy, active pelvic infection, severe contrast medium allergy, arteriovenous malformations, desire for future pregnancy, and undiagnosed pelvic mass. The technique is generally preceded by preprocedural testing and patients are pretreated with intravenous antibiotics. Many perform preliminary arteriographic mapping of the pelvis. A review by Hutchins and Worthington-Kirsch provides an excellent description of the procedure.

The technical success rate is consistently reported in the 96% to 98% range with experienced teams. Eighty percent to 90% of embolized patients have reported improvements in menorrhagia, bulk related symptoms, or both. Reduction in overall uterine volume peaks at more than 60% by 6 to 9 months after the procedure. Individual myomas show average volume reductions of 60% to 65%.

Forty percent of patients develop a syndrome of fever and malaise in the first 10 to 14 days after UAE. This is also associated with leukocytosis. This entity is well described as postembolization syndrome. It is typically self-limited and resolves in 3 to 5 days and rarely requires treatment except antipyretics. Other complications include those that may be attributed to the angiographic component and target or nontarget organ embolization. Groin infections, groin bleeding or hematoma, contrast-induced renal damage, and vascular damage may be attributed to the angiographic component. Uterine infection or perforation, sexual dysfunction, and myoma sloughing may be attributed to the target organ effects. Reported nontarget organ embolization complications include ovarian sequelae, sciatic nerve effects, and gluteal muscle pain. Current experience confirms a major complication rate of less than 1%.

BIBLIOGRAPHY

Adamson G. Myomectomy. GnRH analogs and adhesions. *Prog Clin Biol Res* 1993;381:155.

Aharoni A, Reiter A, Golan D, et al. Patterns of growth of uterine leiomyomata during pregnancy: a prospective longitudinal study. *Br J Obstet Gynaecol* 1988;95:510.

Amussat JZ, quoted by Rubin IC. Progress in myomectomy. *Am J Obstet Gynecol* 1942;44:197.

Anderson J, Grine E, Eng CLY, et al. Expression of connexin-43 in human myometrium and leiomyoma. *Am J Obstet Gynecol* 1993;169:1266.

Andreyko J, Blumenfeld Z, Marshall L. Use of an agonistic analog of gonadotropin-releasing hormone (nafarelin) to treat leiomyomas: assessment by magnetic resonance imaging. *Am J Obstet Gynecol* 1988;158:903.

Ariel IM, Trinidad S. Pulmonary metastases from a uterine "leiomyoma." *Am J Obstet Gynecol* 1966;94:110.

Babaknia A, Rock JA, Jones HW Jr. Pregnancy success following abdominal myomectomy for infertility. *Fertil Steril* 1978;30:644.

Baggish MS, Sze EH, Morgan G. Hysteroscopic treatment of symptomatic submucous myomata uteri with the Nd:YAG laser. *J Gynecol Surg* 1989;5:27.

Bahary CM, Gorodeski IG, Nilly M, et al. Intravascular leiomyomatosis. *Obstet Gynecol* 1982;59:735.

Baines RE. Problems associated with myomectomy in Cape Town. *S Afr Med J* 1971;45:668.

Baird DT, Bramley TA, Hawkins TA, et al. Effect of treatment with LHRH analog Zoladex on binding of oestradiol, progesterone and epidermal growth factor to uterine fibromyomata. *Horm Res* 1989;32:154.

Banner AS, Carrington CB, Emory WB, et al. Efficacy of oophorectomy in lymphangio-leiomyomatosis and benign metastasizing leiomyoma. *N Engl J Med* 1981;305:204.

Beacham WD, Webster HD, Lawson EH, et al. Uterine and/or ovarian tumors weighing 25 pounds or more. *Am J Obstet Gynecol* 1971;109:1153.

Bell SW, Kempson RL, Hendrickson MR. Problematic uterine smooth muscle neoplasm. *Am J Surg Pathol* 1994;18:535.

Ben-Baruch G, Schiff E, Menashe Y, et al. Immediate and late outcome of vaginal myomectomy for prolapsed pedunculated submucous myoma. *Obstet Gynecol* 1988;72:858.

Berkeley AS, DeCherney AH, Polan ML. Abdominal myomectomy and subsequent fertility. *Surg Gynecol Obstet* 1983;156:319.

Beyth Y, Jaffe R, Goldberger S. Uterine remodelling following conservative myomectomy: ultrasonographic evaluation. *Acta Obstet Gynecol Scand* 1992;71:632.

Bonney V. Abdominal myomectomy. In: Berkeley AS, Bonney V, eds. *A textbook of gynaecological surgery*, fifth ed. New York: Paul B. Hoeber, 1948.

Bonney V. The technique and results of myomectomy. *Lancet* 1931;220:171.

Brandon DD, Bethea CL, Strawn EY, et al. Progesterone receptor messenger ribonucleic acid and protein are overexpressed in human leiomyomas. *Am J Obstet Gynecol* 1993;169:78.

Brosens I, Deprest J, Dal Cin P, et al. Clinical significance of cytogenetic abnormalities in uterine myomas. *Fertil Steril* 1998;69:232.

Brown AB, Chamberlain R, TeLinde RW. Myomectomy. *Am J Obstet Gynecol* 1956;71:759.

Brown JM, Malkasian GD, Symmonds RE. Abdominal myomectomy. *Am J Obstet Gynecol* 1967;99:126.

Buchi KA, Keller PJ. Cytoplasmic progestin receptors in myomal and myometrial tissues. *Acta Obstet Gynecol Scand* 1983;62:487.

Buchi KA, Keller PJ. Estrogen receptors in normal and myomatous human uteri. *Gynecol Obstet Invest* 1980;11:59.

Buttram VC, Reiter RC. Uterine leiomyomata: etiology, symptomatology, and management. *Fertil Steril* 1981;36:433.

Ceccacci L, Jacobs J, Powell A. Leiomyomatosis peritonealis disseminata: report of a case in a non pregnant woman. *Am J Obstet Gynecol* 1982;144:105.

Cincinelli E, Romano F, Anastasio PS, et al. Transabdominal sonohysterography, transvaginal sonography, and hysteroscopy in evaluation of submucous myomas. *Obstet Gynecol* 1995;85:42.

Clark DH, Weed JC. Metastasizing leiomyoma: a case report. *Am J Obstet Gynecol* 1977;127:672.

Cohen LS, Valle RF. Role of vaginal sonography and hysterosonography in the endoscopic treatment of uterine myomas. *Fertil Steril* 2000;73:197.

Cole P, Berlin J. Elective hysterectomy. *Obstet Gynecol* 1977; 129:117.

Colgan T, Pendergast S, LeBlanc M. The histopathology of uterine leiomyomas following treatment with gonadotropin-releasing hormone analogs. *Hum Pathol* 1993;24:1073.

Corscaden JA, Singh BP. Leiomyosarcoma of the uterus. *Am J Obstet Gynecol* 1958;75:149.

Corson SL. Hysteroscopic diagnosis and operative therapy of submucous myoma. *Obstet Gynecol Clin North Am* 1995; 22:739.

Corson SL, Brooks PG. Resectoscopic myomectomy. *Fertil Steril* 1991;55:1041.

Coutinho E. Treatment of large fibroid with high doses of gestrinone. *Gynecol Obstet Invest* 1990;30:44.

Coutinho E, Boulanger G, Goncalves M. Regression of uterine leiomyomas after treatment with gestrinone, an antiestrogen, antiprogesterone. *Am J Obstet Gynecol* 1986;155:761.

Cramer SF, Meyer JS, Kraner JF, et al. Metastasizing leiomyoma of the uterus: S-phase fraction, estrogen receptor, and ultrastructure. *Cancer* 1980;45:932.

Cramer SF, Patel A. The frequency of uterine leiomyomas. *Am J Clin Pathol* 1990;94:435.

Damario M, Rock J. Methods to prevent postoperative adhesion formation in gynecologic surgery. *J Gynecol Techniques* 1995;1:1.

Daniell J, Gurley L. Laparoscopic treatment of clinically significant symptomatic uterine fibroids. *J Gynecol Surg* 1991;7: 37.

Darai E, Dechaud H, Benifla JL, et al. Fertility after laparoscopic myomectomy: preliminary results. *Hum Reprod* 1997;12:1931.

Davids A. Myomectomy: surgical techniques and results in a series of 1,150 cases. *Am J Obstet Gynecol* 1952;63:592.

Davies A, Hart R, Magos AL. The excision of uterine fibroids by vaginal myomectomy: a prospective study. *Fertil Steril* 1999;71:961.

Dawood MY, Khan-Dawood FS. Plasma insulin-like growth factor-I, CA-125 estrogen and progesterone in women with leiomyomas. *Fertil Steril* 1994;61:217.

Dawood M, Lewis V, Ramos J. Cortical and trabecular bone mineral content in women with endometriosis: effect of gonadotropin releasing hormone agonist and danazol. *Fertil Steril* 1989;52:21.

DeCherney A, Maheux R, Polan M. A medical treatment for myomata uteri. *Fertil Steril* 1983;39:429.

Degligdish L, Loewenthal M. Endometrial changes associated with myomata of the uterus. *J Clin Pathol* 1970;23:677.

Derman SG, Rehustrom J, Neuwirth RS. The long-term effectiveness of hysteroscopic treatment of menorrhagia and leiomyomas. *Obstet Gynecol* 1991;77:591.

Diamond MP. Reduction of adhesions after uterine myomectomy by Seprafilm membrane (HAL-F): a blinded, prospective, randomized, multicenter clinical study. *Fertil Steril* 1996;66:904.

Dillon T. Control of blood loss during gynecologic surgery. *Obstet Gynecol* 1962;19:428.

diZerega G. Contemporary adhesion prevention. *Fertil Steril* 1994;61:219.

Donnez J, Gillerot S, Bourgoujon D, et al. Neodymium:YAG laser hysteroscopy in large submucous fibroids. *Fertil Steril* 1990;54:999.

Dubuisson JB, Chapron C, Fauconnier A. Laparoscopic myomectomy: operative technique and results. *Ann N Y Acad Sc* 1997;828:326.

Dubuisson JB, Chapron C, Fauconnier A, et al. Laparoscopic myomectomy and myolysis. *Curr Opin Obstet Gynecol* 1997;9:233.

Dubuisson JB, Lecuru F, Foulot H, et al. Myomectomy by laparoscopy: preliminary report of 43 cases. *Fertil Steril* 1991;56:828.

Dubuisson JB, Fauconnier A, Chapron C, et al. Second look after laparoscopic myomectomy. *Hum Reprod* 1998;13:2102.

Edwards DR, Peacock JF. Intravenous leiomyomatosis of the uterus: report of 2 cases. *Obstet Gynecol* 1966;27:176.

Eldar-Geva T, Meagher S, Healy DL, et al. Effect of intramural, subserosal, and submucosal uterine fibroids on the outcome of assisted reproductive technology treatment. *Fertil Steril* 1998;70:687.

Evans AT, Symmonds RE, Gaffey TA. Recurrent pelvic intravenous leiomyomatosis. *Obstet Gynecol* 1981;57:260.

Everett HS, Sturgis WJ. The effect of some common gynecological disorders upon the urinary tract. *Urol Cutan Rev* 1940;44:638.

Exacoustos C, Rosati P. Ultrasound diagnosis of uterine myomas and complications in pregnancy. *Obstet Gynecol* 1993;82:97.

Farber M, Conrad S, Heinrichs WL, et al. Estradiol binding by fibroid tumors and normal myometrium. *Obstet Gynecol* 1972;40:479.

Farquhar C, Vandekerckhove P, Watson A, et al. Barrier agents for preventing adhesions after surgery for subfertility. *Cochrane Database of Systematic Reviews* 2000;1.

Farrer-Brown G, Beilby JO, Tarbit MH. The vascular patterns in myomatous uteri. *J Obstet Gynaecol Br Commonw* 1970; 77:967.

Farrer-Brown G, Beilby JO, Tarbit MH. Venous changes in the endometrium of myomatous uteri. *Obstet Gynecol* 1971;38: 743.

Faulkner RL. The blood vessels of the myomatous uterus. *Am J Obstet Gynecol* 1944;47:185.

Fedele L, Bianchi S, Dorta M, et al. Transvaginal sonography versus hysteroscopy in the diagnosis of uterine submucous myomas. *Obstet Gynecol* 1991;77:745.

Feeney JG, Basu SB. *Bacteroides* infection in fibroids during the puerperium. *BMJ* 1979;2:1038.

Filiceri M, Hall D, Loughlin J, et al. A conservative approach to the management of uterine leiomyoma. Pituitary desensitization by a luteinizing hormone releasing hormone analog. *Am J Obstet Gynecol* 1983;147:726.

Frederick J, Fletcher A, Simeon D, et al. Intramyometrial vasopressin as a hemostatic agent. *Br J Obstet Gynaecol* 1994; 101:435.

Friedman A. Acute urinary retention after gonadotropin-releasing hormone agonist treatment for leiomyomata uteri. *Fertil Steril* 1993;59:677.

Friedman A. The biochemistry, physiology and pharmacology of gonadotropin releasing hormone (GnRH) and GnRH analogs. In: Barbieri RL, Friedman F, eds. *Gonadotropin releasing hormone analogs: applications in gynecology*. New York: Elsevier, 1991:10.

Friedman A. Use of gonadotropin-releasing hormone agonists before myomectomy. *Clin Obstet Gynecol* 1993;36: 650.

Friedman AJ. Vaginal hemorrhage associated with degenerating submucous leiomyomata during leuprolide acetate treatment. *Fertil Steril* 1989;52:152.

Friedman A, Barbieri R, Benacerraf B, et al. Treatment of leiomyomata with intranasal or subcutaneous leuprolide, a gonadotropin-releasing leuprolide, a gonadotropin-releasing hormone agonist. *Fertil Steril* 1987;48:56.

Friedman A, Barbieri R, Doubilet P, et al. A randomized double-blind trial of a gonadotropin-releasing hormone agonist (leuprolide) with or without medroxy progesterone acetate in the treatment of leiomyomata uteri. *Fertil Steril* 1988;49:404.

Friedman A, Daly M, Juneau-Norcross M, et al. Predictors of uterine volume reduction in women with myomas treated with a gonadotropin-releasing hormone agonist. *Fertil Steril* 1992;58:413.

Friedman A, Daly M, Juneau-Norcross M, et al. A prospective randomized trial of gonadotropin-releasing hormone agonist plus estrogen-progestin or progestin "add-back" regimens for women with leiomyomata uteri. *J Clin Endocrinol Metab* 1993;76:1439.

Friedman A, Daly M, Juneau-Norcross M, et al. Recurrence of myomas after myomectomy in women pretreated with leuprolide acetate depot or placebo. *Fertil Steril* 1992;58:205.

Friedman AJ, Haas ST. Should uterine size be an indication for surgical intervention in women with myomas? *Am J Obstet Gynecol* 1993;168:751.

Friedman A, Harrison-Atlas D, Barbieri R, et al. A randomized, placebo-controlled, double-blind study evaluating the efficacy of leuprolide acetate depot in the treatment of uterine leiomyomata. *Fertil Steril* 1989;51:251.

Friedman A, Hoffman D, Canite F, et al, for the Leuprolide Study Group. Treatment of leiomyomata uteri with leuprolide acetate depot: a double-blind, placebo-controlled, multicenter study. *Obstet Gynecol* 1991;77:720.

Friedman A, Juneau-Norcross M, Rein M. Adverse effects of leuprolide acetate depot treatment. *Fertil Steril* 1993;59:448.

Friedman A, Lobel S, Rein M, et al. Efficacy and safety considerations in women with uterine leiomyomas treated with gonadotropin-releasing hormone agonist: the estrogen threshold hypothesis. *Am J Obstet Gynecol* 1990;163:111.

Friedman A, Rein M, Harrison-Atlas D, et al. A randomized, placebo-controlled, double-blind study evaluating leuprolide acetate depot treatment before myomectomy. *Fertil Steril* 1989;52:728.

Friedman A, Thomas P. Does low-dose combination oral contraceptive use affect uterine size or menstrual flow in premenopausal women with leiomyomas. *Obstet Gynecol* 1995;85:631.

Fujita M. Histological and biochemical studies of collagen in human leiomyomas. *Hokkaido Igaku Zasshi* 1985;60:602.

Gabb RG, Stone GM. Uptake and metabolism of tritiated oestradiol and oestrone by human endometrial and myometrial tissue *in vitro*. *J Endocrinol* 1974;62:109.

Gal D, Buchsbaum HJ, Voet R, et al. Massive ascites with uterine leiomyomas and ovarian vein thrombosis. *Am J Obstet Gynecol* 1982;144:729.

Garcia CR, Tureck RW. Submucosal leiomyomas and infertility. *Fertil Steril* 1984;42:16.

Gehlback D, Sousa R, Carpenter S, et al. Abdominal myomectomy in the treatment of infertility. *Int J Obstet Gynecol* 1993;40:45.

Gilbert HA, Kagan AR, Lagasse L. The value of radiation therapy in uterine sarcoma. *Obstet Gynecol* 1975;45:84.

Ginsberg E, Benson C, Garfield J, et al. The effect of operative technique and uterine size on blood loss during myomectomy: a prospective randomized study. *Fertil Steril* 1993;60:956.

Golan A, Bukovsky I, Pansky M, et al. Pre-operative gonadotropin-releasing hormone agonist treatment in surgery for uterine leiomyomata. *Hum Reprod* 1993;8:450.

Goldberg MF, Hurt G, Frable WJ. Leiomyomatosis peritonealis disseminata. *Obstet Gynecol* 1977;49:46s.

Goldenberg M, Sivan E, Sharabi Z, et al. Outcome of hysteroscopic resection of submucous myomas for infertility. *Fertil Steril* 1995;64:714.

Goldfarb H. Laparoscopic coagulation of myoma (myolysis). *Obstet Gynecol Clin North Am* 1995;22:807.

Goldfarb HA. Nd:YAG laser laparoscopic coagulation of symptomatic myomas. *J Reprod Med* 1992;37:636.

Goldfarb HA. Removing uterine fibroids laparoscopically. *Contemp Obstet Gynecol* 1994;39:50.

Goldfarb HA. Myoma coagulation (myolysis). *Obstet Gynecol Clin North Am* 2000;27:421.

Goldrath MH. Vaginal removal of the pedunculated submucous myoma: historical observations and development of a new procedure. *J Reprod Med* 1990;35:921.

Goldrath MH, Fuller TA, Segal S. Laser photovaporization of endometrium for the treatment of menorrhagia. *Am J Obstet Gynecol* 1981;140:14.

Goldzieher JW, Maqueo M, Ricaud L, et al. Induction of degenerative changes in uterine myomas by high-dosage progestin therapy. *Am J Obstet Gynecol* 1966;96:1078.

Gomel V. From microsurgery to laparoscopic surgery: a progress. *Fertil Steril* 1995;63:464.

Goodman AL: Progesterone therapy in uterine fibromyoma. *J Clin Endocrinol Metab* 1946;6:402.

Goodwin SC, Vedantham S, McLucas B, et al. Uterine artery embolization for uterine fibroids: Results of a pilot study. *J Vasc Interv Radiol* 1997;8:517.

Goustin AS, Leof EB, Shipley GD, et al. Growth factors and cancer. *Cancer Res* 1986;46:1015.

Gutmann J, Thornton K, Diamond M, et al. Evaluation of leuprolide acetate treatment on histopathology of uterine myomata. *Fertil Steril* 1994;61:622.

Hallberg L, Nilsson L. Determination of menstrual blood loss. *Scand J Clin Lab Invest* 1964;43:352.

Hallez JP. Single-stage hysteroscopic myomectomies: indications, techniques, and results. *Fertil Steril* 1995;63:703.

Hanson H, Rotman C, Rana N, et al. Laparoscopic myomectomy. *Obstet Gynecol* 1992;80:885.

Harris W. Uterine dehiscence following laparoscopic myomectomy. *Obstet Gynecol* 1992;80:545.

Hart R, Molnar BG, Magos A. Long term follow-up of hysteroscopic myomectomy assessed by survival analysis. *Br J Obstet Gynaecol* 1999;106:700.

Healy D, Frazer H, Lawson S. Shrinkage of a uterine fibroid after subcutaneous infusion of a LHRH agonist. *BMJ* 1984;289:1267.

Healy D, Lawson S, Abbott M, et al. Toward removing uterine fibroids without surgery: subcutaneous infusion of a luteinizing hormone-releasing hormone agonist commencing in the luteal phase. *J Clin Endocrinol Metab* 1986;63:619.

Hirai K, Kanaoka Y, Isshiko O, et al. A novel technique for myomectomy: intranodal surgery with an elctromechanical tissue borer. *J Reprod Med* 2000;45:813.

Hoetzinger H. Hysterosonography and hysterography in benign and malignant diseases of the uterus. A comparative *in vitro* study. *J Ultrasound Med* 1991;10:259.

Hoffmann GE, Rao V, Barrows GH, et al. Binding sites for epidermal growth factors in human uterine tissues and leiomyomas. *J Clin Endocrinol Metab* 1984;17:44.

Horstmann JP, Pietra GG, Harman JA, et al. Spontaneous regression of pulmonary leiomyomas during pregnancy. *Cancer* 1977;39:314.

Hricak H, Tscholakoff D, Heinrichs L. Uterine leiomyomas: correlation of MR, histopathological findings, and symptoms. *Radiology* 1986;158:385.

Hunt SH. Fibroid weighing one hundred and forty pounds. *Am J Obstet* 1888;21:62.

Hutchins F. Myomectomy after selective preoperative treatment with a gonadotropin-releasing hormone analog. *J Reprod Med* 1992;37:699.

Hutchins FL. Uterine fibroids: diagnosis and indications for treatment. *Obstet Gynecol* 1992;80:545.

Hutchins FL, Worthington-Kirsch R. Embolotherapy for myoma-induced menorrhagia. *Obstet Gynecol Clin N Am* 2000;27:397.

Idelson MG, Davids AM. Metastasis of uterine fibroleiomyomata. *Obstet Gynecol* 1963;21:78.

Indman PD. Hysteroscopic treatment of menorrhagia associated with uterine leiomyomas. *Obstet Gynecol* 1993;81:716.

Ingersoll FM, Malone LJ. Myomectomy: an alternative to hysterectomy. *Arch Surg* 1970;100:557.

Interceed (TC7) Adhesion Barrier Study Group. Prevention of postsurgical adhesions by Interceed (TC7), an absorbable adhesion barrier: a prospective, randomized multicenter clinical study. *Fertil Steril* 1989;51:933.

Irey NS, Norris HJ. Intimal vascular lesions associated with female reproductive steroids. *Arch Pathol* 1973;96:227.

Jones HW Jr, Andrew MC. Congenital anomalies and infertility. In: Ridley JH, ed. *Gynecologic surgery*, second ed. Baltimore: Williams & Wilkins, 1981.

Karlsson S, Persson P. Angiography in uterine and adnexal tumors. *Acta Radiologica Diagnostica* 1980;21:11.

Kastner P, Krust A, Turcotte B, et al. Two distinct estrogen-regulated promotors generate transcripts encoding the two functionally different human progesterone receptor forms A and B. *EMBO J* 1990;9:1603.

Kawaguchi J, Fujii S, Konishi I, et al. Mitotic activity in uterine leiomyomas during the menstrual cycle. *Am J Obstet Gynecol* 1989;160:637.

Kelly HA, Cullen TS. *Myomata of the uterus*. Philadelphia: WB Saunders, 1907.

Kettel L, Murphy A, Morales A, et al. Rapid regression of uterine leiomyomas in response to daily administration of gonadotropin-releasing hormone antagonist. *Fertil Steril* 1993;60:642.

Kiltz R, Rutgers J, Phillips J, et al. Absence of a dose-response effect of leuprolide acetate on leiomyomata uteri size. *Fertil Steril* 1994;61:1021.

Klunder KB, Svanholm H, Frimodt-Moller PC. Uterine bizarre leiomyoma. *Acta Obstet Gynecol Scand* 1982;61:121.

Kornyei J, Csermely T, Szekely JA, et al. Two types of nuclear Ez binding sites in human myometrium and leiomyoma during the menstrual cycle. *Exp Clin Endocrinol* 1986;87:256.

Kurman RJ, Norris HJ. Mesenchymal tumors of the uterus. VI. Epithelioid smooth muscle tumors including leiomyoblastoma and clear cell leiomyoma. *Cancer* 1976;37:1853.

LaMorte A, Lalwani S, Diamond M. Morbidity associated with myomectomy. *Obstet Gynecol* 1993;82:897.

Lapan B, Solomon L. Diffuse leiomyomatosis of the uterus precluding myomectomy. *Obstet Gynecol* 1979;53:825.

Leibsohn S, D'Ablaing G, Mishell DR, et al. Leiomyosarcoma in a series of hysterectomies performed for presumed uterine leiomyomas. *Am J Obstet Gynecol* 1990;162:968.

Letterie GS, Kramer DJ. Intraoperative ultrasound guidance for intrauterine endoscopic surgery. *Fertil Steril* 1994;62:654.

Lev-Toaff AS, Coleman BG, Arger PH, et al. Leiomyomas in pregnancy: sonographic study. *Radiology* 1987;164:375.

Lev-Toaff A, Karasick S, Toaff M. Hysterosalpingography before and after myomectomy: clinical value and imaging findings. *Am J Radiol* 1993;160:803.

Li TC, Mortimer R, Cooke ID. Myomectomy: a retrospective study to examine reproductive performance before and after surgery. *Hum Reprod* 1999;14:1735.

Ligon AH, Morton CC. Genetics of uterine leiomyomata. *Genes Chromosomes Cancer* 2000;28:235.

Lipschutz A. Experimental fibroids and the antifibromatogenic action of steroid hormones. *JAMA* 1942;120:171.

Lipschutz A, Murillo R, Vargas L. Antitumorigenic action of progesterone. *Lancet* 1939;2:420.

Lock FR. Multiple myomectomy. *Am J Obstet Gynecol* 1969;104:642.

Loeffler FE, Noble AD. Myomectomy at the Chelsea Hospital for Women. *J Obstet Gynaecol Br Commonw* 1970;77:167.

Lumsden MA, West CP, Bromley J, et al. The binding of epidermal growth factor to the human uterus and leiomyomata in women rendered hypo-oestrogenic by continuous administration of an LHRH-agonist. *Br J Obstet Gynaecol* 1988;95:1299.

Magos AL, Bournas N, Sinha R, et al. Vaginal myomectomy. *Br J Obstet Gynaecol* 1994;101:1092.

Maheux R, Guilloteau C, Lemay A, et al. Luteinizing hormone-releasing hormone agonist and uterine leiomyomata: a pilot study. *Am J Obstet Gynecol* 1985;152:1034.

Maheux R, Guilloteau C, Lemay A, et al. Regression of leiomyomata uteri following hypo-oestrogenism induced by repetitive luteinizing hormone-releasing hormone agonist treatment: preliminary report. *Fertil Steril* 1984;42:644.

Mais V, Ajossa S, Guerriero S, et al. Laparoscopic versus abdominal myomectomy: a prospective, randomized trial to evaluate benefits in early outcome. *Am J Obstet Gynecol* 1996;174:654.

Makarainen L, Ylikorkala O. Primary and myoma-associated menorrhagia: role of prostaglandins and effects of ibuprofen. *Br J Obstet Gynaecol* 1986;93:974.

Malone LJ, Ingersoll FM. Myomectomy in infertility. In: Bermen SG, Kistner RW, eds. *Progress in infertility*. Boston, Little, Brown, 1975.

Marshall JF, Morris DS. Intravenous leiomyomatosis of the uterus and pelvis: case report. *Ann Surg* 1959;149:126.

Martin JF, Bazin P, Feroldi J, et al. Tumeurs myoides intramurales de l'estomac. Considerations microscopiques apropos de 6 cas. *Ann Anat Pathol* 1960;5:484.

Matsunaga E, Shiota K. Ectopic pregnancy and myoma uteri: teratogenic effects and maternal characteristics. *Teratology* 1980;21:61.

Matta W, Shaw R, Hesp R, et al. Reversible trabecular bone density loss following induced hypo-estrogenism with GnRH analog buserelin in premenopausal women. *Clin Endocrinol* 1988;29:45.

Matta W, Stabile I, Shaw RW, et al. Doppler assessment of uterine blood flow changes in patients with fibroids receiving the gonadotropin-releasing hormone agonist buserelin. *Fertil Steril* 1988;49:1083.

Mattingly RF. Large myomata uteri and stress urinary incontinence. In: Nichols DH, ed. *Clinical problems, injuries, and complications of gynecologic surgery.* Baltimore: Williams & Wilkins, 1983.

Mayer D, Shipilov V. Ultrasonography and magnetic resonance imaging of uterine fibroids. *Obstet Gynecol Clin North Am* 1995;22:667.

Mayo WJ. Some observations on the operation of abdominal myomectomy for myomata of the uterus. *Surg Gynecol Obstet* 1911;12:97.

McLaughlin D. Metroplasty and myomectomy with CO_2 laser for maximizing the preservation of normal tissue and minimizing blood loss. *J Reprod Med* 1985;30:1.

Meigs JV. Pelvic tumors other than fibromas of the ovary with ascites and hydrothorax. *Obstet Gynecol* 1954;3:471.

Meloni AM, Surti U, Contento AM, et al. Uterine leiomyomas: cytogenetic and histologic profile. *Obstet Gynecol* 1992;80:209.

Meyer W, Mayer A, Diamond M, et al. Unsuspected leiomyosarcoma: treatment with a gonadotropin-releasing hormone analog. *Obstet Gynecol* 1990;75:529.

Miller NF, Ludovici PP. On the origin and development of uterine fibroids. *Am J Obstet Gynecol* 1955;70:720.

Mixson W, Hammond D. Response of fibromyomas to a progestin. *Am J Obstet Gynecol* 1961;82:754.

Moghissi K. Hormonal therapy before surgical treatment for uterine leiomyomas. *Surg Gynecol Obstet* 1991;172:497.

Montague A, Swartz DP, Woodruff JD. Sarcoma arising in leiomyoma of uterus: factors influencing prognosis. *Am J Obstet Gynecol* 1965;92:421.

Muram D, Gillieson MS, Walters JH. Myomas of the uterus in pregnancy: ultrasonographic follow-up. *Am J Obstet Gynecol* 1980;138:16.

Murphy A, Kettel L, Morales A, et al. Regression of uterine leiomyomata in response to the anti-progesterone RU486. *J Clin Endocrinol Metab* 1993;76:513.

Murphy A, Morales A, Kettel L, et al. Regression of uterine leiomyomata to the antiprogesterone RU486: dose-response effect. *Fertil Steril* 1995;64:187.

Nakamura Y, Yoshimura Y. Treatment of uterine leiomyomas in perimenopausal women with gonadotropin-releasing hormone agonists. *Clin Obstet Gynecol* 1993;36:660.

Nardulli AM, Greene GL, O'Malley BW, et al. Regulation of progesterone receptor messenger ribonucleic acid and protein levels in MCF-cells by estradiol: analysis of estrogen's effect on progesterone receptor synthesis and degradation. *Endocrinology* 1988;122:935.

Nelson WO. Endometrial and myometrial changes including fibromyomatous nodules, induced in the uterus of the guinea pig by the prolonged administration of oestrogenic hormone. *Anat Rec* 1937;68:99.

Neuwirth RS. Hysteroscopic management of symptomatic submucous fibroids. *Obstet Gynecol* 1983;62:509.

Neuwirth RS. A new technique for and additional experience with hysteroscopic resection of submucous fibroids. *Am J Obstet Gynecol* 1978;131:91.

Neuwirth RS, Amin HK. Excision of submucous fibroids with hysteroscopic control. *Am J Obstet Gynecol* 1976;126:95.

Nezhat C, Nezhat F, Bess O, et al. Laparoscopically assisted myomectomy: a report of a new technique in 57 cases. *Int J Fertil* 1994;39:39.

Nisolle M, Smets M, Malvaux V, et al. Laparoscopic myolysis with the Nd:YAG laser. *J Gynecol Surg* 1993;9:95.

Nordic Adhesion Prevention Study Group. The efficacy of Interceed (TC7) for prevention of reformation of postoperative adhesions on ovaries, fallopian tubes, and fimbriae in microsurgical operations for fertility: a multicenter study. *Fertil Steril* 1995;63:709.

Norris HJ, Parmley T. Mesenchymal tumors of the uterus versus intravenous leiomyomatosis: a clinical and pathologic study of 14 cases. *Cancer* 1975;36:2164.

Novak ER. Benign and malignant changes in uterine myomas. *Clin Obstet Gynecol* 1958;1:421.

Otubu JA, Buttram VC, Besch NF, et al. Unconjugated steroids in leiomyomas and tumor bearing myometrium. *Am J Obstet Gynecol* 1982;143:130.

Pais SO, Glickman M, Schwartz PE, et al. Embolization of pelvic arteries for control of postpartum hemorrhage. *Obstet Gynecol* 1980;55:741.

Parazzini F, Negri E, La Vecchia C, et al. Oral contraceptive use and risk of uterine fibroids. *Obstet Gynecol* 1992;79:430.

Parker W. Myomectomy: laparoscopy or laparotomy? *Clin Obstet Gynecol* 1995;38:392.

Parker WH, Fu YS, Berek JS. Uterine sarcomas in patients operated on for presumed leiomyoma and rapidly growing leiomyoma. *Obstet Gynecol* 1994;83:414.

Parmley TH, Woodruff JD, Winn K. Histogenesis of leiomyomatosis peritonealis disseminata (disseminated fibrosing deciduosis). *Obstet Gynecol* 1975;46:511.

Pearce PH. Leiomyomatosis peritonealis disseminata. *Am J Obstet Gynecol* 1982;144:133.

Pelosi MA, Pelosi MA, Eim J. Hand assisted laparoscopy for megamyomectomy. *J Reprod Med* 2000;45:519.

Perino A, Chianchiano N, Petronio M, et al. Role of leuprolide acetate depot in hysteroscopic surgery: a controlled study. *Fertil Steril* 1993;59:507.

Persaud V, Arjoon PD. Uterine leiomyoma: incidence of degenerative change and a correlation of associated symptoms. *Obstet Gynecol* 1970;135:432.

Phillips D. Laparoscopic leiomyoma coagulation (myolysis). *Gynecol Endosc* 1995;4:5.

Pollow K, Geilfub J, Boquoi E, et al. Estrogen and progesterone binding proteins in normal human myometrium. *J Clin Chem Clin Biochem* 1978;16:503.

Prayson RA, Hart W. Pathologic considerations of uterine smooth muscle tumors. *Obstet Gynecol Clin North Am* 1995;22:637.

Ranney B, Frederick I. The occasional need for myomectomy. *Obstet Gynecol* 1979;53:437.

Ravina JH, Aymard A, Ciraru-Vigneron N, et al. Value of preoperative embolization of uterine fibroma: report of a multicenter series of 31 cases. *Contracept Fertil Sex* 1995;23:45.

Reddy VV, Rose LI. Δ^4-3-Ketosteroid 5 α-oxidoreductase in human uterine leiomyoma. *Am J Obstet Gynecol* 1979;135:415.

Reich H. Laparoscopic myomectomy. *Obstet Gynecol Clin North Am* 1995;22:757.

Rein MS, Barbieri RL, Friedman AJ. Progesterone: a critical role in the pathogenesis of uterine myomas. *Am J Obstet Gynecol* 1995;172:14.

Rein MS, Powell WL, Walters FC, et al. Cytogenetic abnormalities in uterine myomas are associated with myoma size. *Mol Hum Reprod* 1998;4:83.

Rein MS, Barbieri RL, Welch W, et al. The concentrations of collagen-associated amino acids are higher in GnRH agonist treated uterine myomas. *Obstet Gynecol* 1993;82:901.

Reinsch R, Murphy A, Morales A, et al. The effects of RU486 and leuprolide acetate on uterine artery blood flow in the fibroid uterus: a prospective, randomized study. *Am J Obstet Gynecol* 1994;170:1623.

Reiter RC, Wagner PL, Gambone JC. Routine hysterectomy for large asymptomatic uterine leiomyomata: a reappraisal. *Obstet Gynecol* 1992;79:481.

Reyniak J, Corenthal L. Microsurgical laser techniques for abdominal myomectomy. *Microsurgery* 1987;8:92.

Riley P. Treatment of prolapsed submucous fibroids. *S Afr Med J* 1982;62:22.

Rosenfield DC. Abdominal myomectomy for otherwise unexplained infertility. *Fertil Steril* 1986;46:328.

Ross R, Pike M, Vessey M, et al. Risk factor for uterine fibroids: reduced risk associated with oral contraceptives. *BMJ* 1986;293:359.

Rubin I. Progress in myomectomy. Surgical measures and diagnostic aids favoring lower morbidity and mortality. *Am J Obstet Gynecol* 1942;44:196.

Rubin I. Uterine fibromyomas and sterility. *Clin Obstet Gynecol* 1958;1:501.

Sacks P, Hoyne P. Disseminated intravascular coagulation, hemolytic anemia, and acute renal failure associated with multiple myomectomy. *Obstet Gynecol* 1992;79:835.

Sadan O, Vauiddekinge B, Van Gelderen CJ, et al. Oestrogen and progesterone receptor concentrations in leiomyoma and normal myometrium. *Am Clin Biochem* 1987;24:263.

Sampson JA. The influence of myomata on the blood supply of the uterus with special reference to abnormal uterine bleeding. *Surg Gynecol Obstet* 1913;16:144.

Schlaff WD, Zerhoun E, Huth J, et al. A placebo-controlled trial of a depot gonadotropin-releasing hormone analog (leuprolide) in the treatment of uterine leiomyomata. *Obstet Gynecol* 1989;74:856.

Schwartz L, Panageas E, Lange R, et al. Female pelvis: impact of MR imaging on treatment decisions and net cost analysis. *Radiology* 1994;192:55.

Segaloff A, Weed JC, Sternberg WH, et al. The progesterone therapy of human uterine leiomyomas. *J Clin Endocrinol Metab* 1919;9:1273.

Sehgal N, Haskins AL. The mechanism of uterine bleeding in the presence of fibromyomas. *Am J Surg* 1960;26:21.

Semm K, Mettler L. Local infiltration of ornithine 8-vasopressin (POR8) as a vasoconstrictive agent in surgical pelviscopy. *Endoscopy* 1988;20:298.

Seoud M, Patterson R, Muasher S, et al. Effects of myomas or prior myomectomy on *in vitro* fertilization (IVF) performance. *J Assist Reprod Genet* 1992;9:217.

Singhabhandhu B, Akin JJ Jr, Ridley JH, et al. Giant leiomyoma of the uterus: report of a case and review of the literature. *Am Surg* 1973;39:391.

Smith DC, Uhlir J. Myomectomy as a reproductive procedure. *Am J Obstet Gynecol* 1990;162:1476.

Soules MR, McCarty KS Jr. Leiomyomas: steroid receptor content: variations within normal menstrual cycles. *Am J Obstet Gynecol* 1982;143:6.

Spellacy WN, LeMaire WJ, Buhi WC, et al. Plasma growth hormone and estradiol levels in women with uterine myomas. *Obstet Gynecol* 1972;40:829.

Starks GC. CO_2 laser myomectomy in an infertile population. *J Reprod Med* 1988;33:184.

Starks GC. Unilateral twin interstitial ectopic pregnancy, a case report. *J Reprod Med* 1980;25:79.

Stovall T. Gonadotropin-releasing hormone agonists: utilization before hysterectomy. *Clin Obstet Gynecol* 1993;36:642.

Stovall T, Ling F, Henry L, et al. A randomized trial evaluating leuprolide acetate before hysterectomy as treatment for leiomyomas. *Am J Obstet Gynecol* 1991;164:1420.

Stovall TG, Summit RL, Washburn SA, Ling FW. Gonadotropin-releasing hormone agonist before hysterectomy for leiomyomas: results of a multicentre, randomised controlled trial. *Br J Obstet Gynaecol* 1998;105:1148.

Stovall T, Muneyyirei-Delale O, Summitt R, et al, for the Leuprolide Acetate Study Group. GnRH agonist and iron versus placebo and iron in the anemic patient before surgery for leiomyomas: a randomized controlled trial. *Obstet Gynecol* 1995;86:65.

Strawn EY, Novy MF, Burry KA, et al. Insulin-like growth factor I promotes leiomyoma cell growth *in vitro*. *Am J Obstet Gynecol* 1995;172:1837.

Sullivan B, Kenney P, Seibel M. Hysteroscopic resection of fibroid with thermal injury to sigmoid. *Obstet Gynecol* 1992;80:546.

Tada S, Tsukioka M, Ishii C, et al. Computed tomographic features of uterine myoma. *J Comput Assist Tomogr* 1981;5:866.

Tamaya T, Fujimoto J, Okada H. Comparison of cellular levels of steroid receptors in uterine leiomyomata and myometrium. *Acta Obstet Gynecol Scand* 1985;64:307.

Thompson J. Anemia due to gynecologic disease. *South Med J* 1957;50:679.

Tierney WN, Ehrlich CE, Bailey JC, et al. Intravenous leiomyomatosis of the uterus with extension into the heart. *Am J Med* 1980;69:471.

Torpin R, Pond E, Peoples WJ. The etiologic and pathologic factors in a series of 1,741 fibromyomas of the uterus. *Am J Obstet Gynecol* 1942;44:569.

Townsend DE, Sparkes RS, Baluda MC, et al. Unicellular histogenesis of uterine leiomyomas as determined by electrophoresis of glucose-6-phosphate dehydrogenase. *Am J Obstet Gynecol* 1970;107:1168.

Tulandi T, Murray C, Guralneck M. Adhesion formation and reproductive outcome after myomectomy and second-look laparoscopy. *Obstet Gynecol* 1993;82:213.

Upadhyaya N, Doddy M, Googe P. Histopathologic changes in leiomyomata treated with leuprolide acetate. *Fertil Steril* 1990;54:811.

Vasserman J, Baracat E, Bondu KC, et al. Vascularization of uterine myomata. *Abstracts of the 12th World Congress of Obstetrics and Gynecology* 1988:108.

Vercellini P, Maddalena S, De Giorgi O, et al. Determinants of reproductive outcome after abdominal myomectomy for infertility. *Fertil Steril* 1999;72:109.

Vercellini P, Bocciolone L, Rognoni M, et al. Fibroids and infertility. *Adv Reprod Endocrinol* 1992;4:47.

Vercellini P, Zaina B, Yaylayan L, et al. Hysteroscopic myomectomy: long term effects on menstrual pattern and fertility. *Obstet Gynecol* 1999;94:341.

Vercellini P, Crosignani PG, Mangioni C, et al. Treatment with a gonadotrophin releasing hormone agonist before hysterectomy for leiomyomas: results of a multicentre randomised controlled trial. *Br J Obstet Gynaecol* 1998;105:1148.

Verkauf B. Changing trends in treatment of leiomyomata uteri. *Curr Opin Obstet Gynecol* 1993;5:301.

Verkauf B. Myomectomy for fertility enhancement and preservation. *Fertil Steril* 1992;58:1.

Vollenhoven BJ, Lawrence AS, Healy DL. Uterine fibroids: a clinical review. *Br J Obstet Gynaecol* 1990;97:285.

Wallach E, Vu K. Myomata uteri and infertility. *Obstet Gynecol Clin North Am* 1995;22:791.

Wamsteker K, Emanuel MH, deKruif JH. Transcervical hysteroscopic resection of submucous fibroids for abnormal uterine bleeding: results regarding the degree of intramural extension. *Obstet Gynecol* 1993;82:736.

Watanabe Y, Nakamura G. Effects of two different doses of leuprolide acetate depot on uterine cavity area in patients with uterine leiomyomata. *Fertil Steril* 1995;63:487.

Weather L. Cardon dioxide laser myomectomy. *J Natl Med Assoc* 1986;78:933.

Weiss DB, Aldor A, Aboulafia Y. Erythrocytosis due to erythropoietin-producing uterine fibromyoma. *Am J Obstet Gynecol* 1975;122:358.

West C, Lumsden M, Lawson S, et al. Shrinkage of uterine fibroids during therapy with goserelin (Zoladex): a luteinizing hormone-releasing hormone agonist administered as a monthly subcutaneous depot. *Fertil Steril* 1987;48:45.

Wilson EA, Yang F, Rees ED. Estradiol and progesterone binding in uterine leiomyomata and in normal uterine tissues. *Obstet Gynecol* 1980;55:20.

Winer-Muram HT, Muram D, Gillieson MS, et al. Uterine myomas in pregnancy. *Can Med Assoc J* 1983;128:949.

Wiskind A, Thompson J. Abdominal myomectomy: reducing the risk of hemorrhage. *Semin Reprod Endocrinol* 1992;10:358.

Wong GC, Muir SJ, Lai AP, et al. Uterine artery embolization: a minimally invasive technique for the treatment of uterine fibroids. *J Women's Health and Gender-Based Medicine* 2000;9:357.

Wray RC Jr, Dawkins H. Primary smooth muscle tumors of the inferior vena cava. *Ann Surg* 1971;174:1009.

Yamamoto T, Urabe M, Naitoh K, et al. Estrone sulfatase activity in human leiomyoma. *Gynecol Oncol* 1990;37:315.

Ylikorkala O, Kauppila A, Rajala T. Pituitary gonadotrophins and prolactin in patients with endometrial cancer, fibroids or ovarian tumours. *Br J Obstet Gynaecol* 1979;86:901.

Zawin M, McCarthy S, Scoutt LM, et al. High-field MRI and US evaluation of the pelvis in women with leiomyomas. *Magn Reson Imaging* 1990;8:371.

Zreik TG, Rutherford TJ, Palter SF, et al. Cryomyolysis, a new procedure for the conservative treatment of uterine fibroids. *J Am Assoc Gynecol Laparosc* 1998;5:33.

Te Linde's Operative Gynecology, ninth edition, edited by John A. Rock and Howard W. Jones, III. Lippincott Williams & Wilkins, Philadelphia: © 2003.

CHAPTER

31

▼

Hysterectomy

HOWARD W. JONES, III

Hysterectomy is the most common operation performed by the gynecologist, and it is the second most common major surgical procedure done in the United States. Only cesarean section is more common. There are many indications for hysterectomy and the uterus can be removed using any of a variety of techniques and approaches, including abdominal, vaginal, or laparoscopic. The gynecologic surgeon should be not only technically adept at these various procedures, but also should use history, physical examination, and discussion with the patient to match the surgical procedure to the patient in order to obtain the most satisfactory outcome.

HISTORY

The history of hysterectomy is long and varied. Although significant advances in the technique of hysterectomy did not occur until the 19th century, earlier attempts are known. Some references to hysterectomy even date to the 5th century BC, in the time of Hippocrates. The earliest attempts at removal of the uterus were made vaginally for indications of uterine prolapse or uterine inversion. By the 16th century AD, a number of hysterectomies already had been done in Europe, including Italy, Germany, and Spain. In 1600, Schenck of Grabenberg cataloged 26 cases of vaginal hysterectomy.

Vaginal hysterectomies were done sporadically through the 17th and 18th centuries. In 1810, Wrisberg

presented a paper to the Vienna Royal Academy of Medicine recommending vaginal hysterectomy for uterine cancer. Three years later, the German surgeon, Langenbeck, successfully performed a vaginal hysterectomy for uterine cancer. The first vaginal hysterectomy performed in the United States was in 1829 by John Collins Warren at Harvard University; however, the patient expired on the fourth postoperative day. Three years following Warren's attempt in Pittsburgh, Herman and Werneberg successfully performed a vaginal hysterectomy for uterine cancer. By the late 19th century, techniques for vaginal hysterectomy were systematically studied and developed by Czerny, Billroth, Mikulicz, Schroeder, Kocher, Teuffel, and Spencer Wells.

The earliest abdominal hysterectomy attempts usually involved uterine leiomyomas that had been misdiagnosed as ovarian cysts. In early 19th century, laparotomy for ovarian cysts still was considered dangerous, despite initial successes by McDowell in the United States and Emiliami in Europe in 1815. Abdominal hysterectomy for any reason was considered impossible to accomplish successfully. Many of the earliest myomectomies involved pedunculated tumors. Washington L. Atlee of Lancaster, PA performed the first successful abdominal myomectomy in 1844; although in a series of 125 surgeries, he did not attempt to remove the uterus.

The first abdominal hysterectomy was attempted by Langenbeck in 1825. The 7-minute operation for advanced cervical cancer resulted in the patient's demise several hours later. Abdominal section was commonly complicated by postoperative hemorrhage that was often lethal. In the mid-19th century, Manchester, England surgeon, A.M. Heath, was the first to ligate the uterine arteries, but it would be nearly 50 years before his practice became more common.

Successful surgery depends on control of bleeding, infection, and pain. Ligatures were known to be used to clamp bleeding vessels as early as 1090 and artery forceps were invented in the mid-16th century by Ambroise Pare. However, information regarding the pathophysiology of hemorrhage, shock, and blood transfusions was not available until the 20th century. The importance of infection control was first recognized by Austrian Ignaz Semmelweiss in his work with childbed fever. His 1840s work was furthered by Joseph Lister in the 1860s, and aided by notable discoveries by Louis Pasteur and Robert Koch. American Crawford W. Long first used ether as anesthesia in 1842, and Scotsman Sir James Y. Simpson initiated use of chloroform in his obstetric practice.

Although the mentioned advances were made to decrease surgical and postoperative bleeding, it was not until 1864 that much success in this area was achieved. Frenchman Koeberle introduced his method of securing the large vascular pedicle of the lower uterus with his tool, the serrenoeud. This ligature en masse around the lower uterus with the corpus amputated above was the usual technique of controlling bleeding with hysterectomy in the earliest years. The stump thus formed was such a large mass of tissue that it could not always be safely returned to the peritoneal cavity owing to risk of intraperitoneal bleeding; often the stump was fixed extraperitoneally in the incision so that it could be clamped later if necessary.

W.A. Freund of Germany further refined hysterectomy techniques in 1878 using anesthesia, antiseptic technique, Trendelenburg position, and ligature around ligaments and major vessels. The bladder was dissected from the uterus and the cardinal and uterosacral ligaments were detached; the pelvic peritoneum then was closed. Late in the 19th century, further refinements were made to abdominal hysterectomy by the Johns Hopkins Hospital, where they reduced their mortality to 5.9%.

In the early decades of the 20th century, hysterectomy became more commonly used as treatment for gynecologic disease and symptoms. Gynecology as a specialty was developing and little else but surgery was available to gynecologists to help their patients. Major discoveries and concepts of reproductive organ physiology and pathology were just beginning. As surgery became safer, gynecologists concentrated on developing newer surgical procedures. Estrogen and progesterone were not discovered until the late 1920s and early 1930s.

As gynecology matured as a specialty in medicine, knowledge of reproductive organ function and disease became more complete; special and more accurate diagnostic techniques were developed (e.g., the excretory urogram was developed in 1923); and effective nonsurgical methods of therapy were discovered. In the modern practice of gynecology, appropriate use of this knowledge and advanced modern diagnostic technologies allow more correct choices of treatment for complicated medical diseases. With proper use of blood transfusions and antibiotics, and with improvements in anesthetic techniques, a hysterectomy can be done fairly safely by the skillful gynecologic surgeon. Mortality from hysterectomy in most medical centers is one to two per 1,000. It is possible to report no mortalities in a series of several thousand hysterectomies. However, morbidity continues to plague the procedure. Complications may occur in as many as 25% of patients undergoing vaginal hysterectomy and 50% of those undergoing abdominal hysterectomy. Some complications may be serious (e.g., infection, hemorrhage, urinary tract and intestinal tract injury, and pulmonary embolus). It should be emphasized that the ability to perform several hundred hysterectomies with a low mortality and morbidity rate, although extremely desirable, is not ipso facto evidence that gynecologic surgery is being practiced correctly. Along with low morbidity and mortality rates, the physician also must be certain that only patients with proper indications are chosen for surgical treatment.

To formulate proper indications for hysterectomy, the surgeon must have a thorough understanding of the physiology and pathology of the female reproductive organs, clinical manifestations of pelvic disease, and normal and abnormal psychosocial-sexual development. This knowledge and understanding is the absolute foundation on which the pyramid of successful practice of gynecologic surgery is built. The surgeon must use this knowledge and his or her own wisdom to determine if a patient is a candidate for surgical therapy, remembering that it is only the occasional gynecologic patient who requires surgery for relief. If the patient requires surgical intervention, she must be properly prepared for surgery, and the surgeon must properly perform the surgery and provide proper postoperative care. In the practice of gynecologic surgery, most mistakes are made by those physicians who may know how, but may not understand when and why. Referring to this point, the late Richard W. Te Linde, professor of gynecology at the Johns Hopkins University and the original author of this text, said:

> The ease with which the average hysterectomy may be done has proven both a blessing and a curse to womankind. There is no doubt that a hysterectomy done with proper indications may restore a woman to health and even save her life. However, in the practice of gynecology, one has ample opportunity to observe countless women who have been advised to have hysterectomies without proper indications. . . . I am inclined to believe that the greatest single factor in promoting unnecessary hysterectomies is a lack of understanding of gynecologic pathology. The greatest need today among those who are performing pelvic surgery is a better knowledge of gynecologic pathology.

As Te Linde stated, many women have benefited from hysterectomy. However, considerable concern has been expressed that this same operation is overused and not always performed for proper indications. The medical profession has a strong tradition of accountability for the quality of patient care, evident in daily rounds and conferences, chart reviews, audits, hospital tissue and credential committees, specialty and subspecialty board certification and recertification, specialty society activities, rules and regulations of the Joint Commission on Accreditation of Hospitals, licensure, continuing medical education requirements, and so forth. Nevertheless, accusations of unnecessary operations, including unnecessary hysterectomies, still arise from unions, insurance companies, consumer groups, media, state and federal agencies, the US Congress, and members of the medical professions.

A review by the Centers for Disease Control and Prevention (CDC) estimated that from 1988 to 1990, 1.7 million US women had a hysterectomy, an overall rate of 56.8 procedures per 10,000 women 15 years old and older. Strongly linked to age, the rate peaked at 100.5 hysterectomies per 10,000 women 30 to 54 years old. The 30- to 54-year-old age range accounted for 74% of all hysterectomies performed in the US. Approximately 20% of women 40 years old had had a hysterectomy, and 37% of women 65 years old. These numbers have declined since the 1970s. Authors of the CDC paper, Wilcox and colleagues, account for the shift in numbers with second opinions for surgery, quality assurance programs, higher levels of education, media campaigns, and alternatives to hysterectomy, such as medical therapies and more conservative surgical procedures.

As we have seen in this brief historical review, hysterectomy has developed and evolved in the past 150 years from an extremely dangerous and infrequently performed operation that was almost abandoned to an important and major therapeutic modality that can save life and improve health assuming that proper patient selection, preparation, and skillful performance are employed. Nevertheless, because of significant rates of mortality and morbidity in all age and diagnosis groups, hysterectomy cannot be considered a low-risk operation to be used for treating relatively minor gynecologic symptoms or disease. However, as demonstrated by Carlson and colleagues in the Maine Women Health Study, hysterectomy is highly effective for relief of symptoms associated with common nonmalignant gynecologic conditions. In this study, symptom relief following hysterectomy is associated with a marked improvement in the quality of life. A study by Clarke and associates yielded similar findings.

INDICATIONS FOR HYSTERECTOMY

Because hysterectomy is the second most common surgical procedure performed in the United States, regulatory agencies, insurance companies, and the general public have studied its appropriate indications very extensively. In some cases, a pathologically normal uterus may be removed as part of an operation to treat stress urinary incontinence with pelvic relaxation, whereas in other instances hysterectomy is done as part of the surgery for endometriosis or in association with ovarian

cancer. Many times, there is no histopathologic or anatomic abnormality of the uterus; some critics have been quick to label these procedures "unnecessary hysterectomies."

Although it is undoubtedly true that some hysterectomies are done that are not indicated and others are performed for marginal indications, most are done for sound indications to relieve present symptoms, prevent future symptoms, or save life. Surgeons need to constantly review their practices to be sure that they conform to currently accepted guidelines for hysterectomy. Although some tried and true indications such as endometrial cancer have been unwavering, other indications, such as sterilization or even menorrhagia and dysmenorrhea, remain highly controversial. The more common indications for hysterectomy are listed in Table 31.1; these and others are discussed in detail on the following pages.

Abnormal Uterine Bleeding

Abnormal uterine bleeding can be caused by anatomic or pathologic abnormalities such as leiomyomas; polyps or cervical cancer; or hormonal imbalances leading to heavy, prolonged, or irregular uterine bleeding. In the absence of tumor, infection, pregnancy, or endometriosis, this type of bleeding generally is referred to as dysfunctional uterine bleeding. Although it was a common indication for hysterectomy in the past, today these symptoms usually can be managed by hormonal manipulation. The cause of bleeding can be evaluated by careful history, pelvic examination, endometrial biopsy, hysteroscopy, dilatation and curettage, and pelvic ultrasound. In women more than 40 years old or those with persistent bleeding, an endometrial biopsy or D&C is necessary to rule out endometrial hyperplasia or cancer.

Pinion and colleagues conducted a randomized trial of hysterectomy, endometrial laser ablation, and transcervical endometrial resection for dysfunctional uterine bleeding. Hysteroscopic endometrial ablation was superior to hysterectomy in terms of operative complications and postoperative recovery. Satisfaction after hysterec-

TABLE 31.1.
Indications for Hysterectomy

Benign Disease	Malignant Disease
Abnormal bleeding	Cervical intraepithelial neoplasm
Leiomyoma	
Adenomyosis	Invasive cervical cancer
Endometriosis	Atypical endometrial hyperplasia
Pelvic organ prolapse	Endometrial cancer
Pelvic inflammatory disease	Ovarian cancer
	Fallopian tube cancer
Chronic pelvic pain	Gestational trophoblastic tumors
Pregnancy related conditions	
Miscellaneous	

tomy was significantly higher, but between 70% and 90% of women were satisfied with the outcome of hysteroscopic surgery. According to these authors, hysteroscopic surgery can be recommended as an alternative to hysterectomy for dysfunctional uterine bleeding. According to Brooks and associates, greater familiarity with the technique of resectoscopic endometrial ablation, improved patient selection for the procedure, and the use of appropriate pharmacotherapy for suppressing endometrial growth prior to ablation probably substantially improve the rate of success, reduce procedural costs, and further enhance the cost advantage of this procedure over hysterectomy.

Transvaginal endometrial resection requires advanced hysteroscopic training and experience, but hysteroscopic rollerball ablation and, more recently, microwave and thermal endometrial ablation techniques have been introduced that require less technical skill. In a prospective, randomized trial from Denmark, Boujida et al. found similar and significantly reduced bleeding at both 2- and 5-year follow-up in women treated with either endometrial resection or rollerball ablation. In this series, 15 of the patients required a second treatment for persistent bleeding, and 15% had undergone hysterectomy for bleeding and/or pain. Bain et al. compared the results of endometrial resection with microwave endometrial ablation in a prospective, randomized group of 249 women followed for 2 years. Average age was 42 years, and approximately 45% reported complete amenorrhea, whereas another 45% had decreased bleeding. About 20% reported similar or increased dysmenorrhea, and 12% of the women in each group underwent hysterectomy within 2 years of initial treatment. In this and other similar studies, persistent bleeding, dysmenorrhea, and pelvic pain resulted in diminished quality of life scores compared to the general, age-matched population. Alexander et al. reported higher levels of satisfaction and a better overall quality of life in women managed by hysterectomy compared to those treated by ablation or resection in the follow-up of Pinion's randomized study.

Approximately 20% to 30% of hysterectomies are performed with dysfunctional uterine bleeding as the primary indication. Hysterectomy is not indicated unless the bleeding is recurrent, severe, and unresponsive to hormonal therapy and endometrial curettage on several occasions. Endometrial resection or ablation should be considered, especially for the patient 40 to 50 years of age. When hysterectomy is necessary, usually it can be done vaginally unless contraindicated. Recalcitrant dysfunctional uterine bleeding is not an indication for bilateral oophorectomy at the time of hysterectomy. Hysterectomy is very rarely required to treat dysfunctional uterine bleeding in young women.

Uterine Leiomyomas

Uterine leiomyomas are the most common reason for hysterectomy, accounting for approximately 30% of the indication for this procedure. Abdominal or vaginal hysterectomy may be indicated if the myomas are associated with discomfort, urinary frequency or obstruction, menorrhagia, metrorrhagia, or if they are significantly increasing in size. Uterine leiomyomas are common benign tumors of the myometrium that usually do not cause symptoms or require removal. The patient with small, asymptomatic uterine leiomyomas may be followed with periodic pelvic examinations. If the uterus is not too large, then a conservative approach with uterine curettage rather than hysterectomy should be tried first. If a submucous myoma is found by hysterography, hysteroscopy, or uterine curettage, then it is unlikely that conservative measures will relieve the patient's bleeding. Depending on the circumstances, a submucous myoma may be removed with the hysteroscope, by myomectomy, or with hysterectomy. If symptoms do not appear before menopause, then it is unlikely that a hysterectomy will be needed after menopause. No new myomas appear after menopause, and myomas already present cease to grow and usually become smaller.

Management of uterine leiomyomas is not always surgical. Hormonal management with gonadotropin-releasing hormone (GnRH) analogs can be used alone or in conjunction with conservative surgery or even hysterectomy. Transcervical hysteroscopic myomectomy has been used for small submucosal myomas that cause abnormal bleeding. Recently, electrosurgical ablation and arterial embolization have been reported to provide good results in patients with larger intramural myomas. These techniques are discussed in Chapter 30.

It is possible for a leiomyomatous uterus to be rather large and still cause no symptoms. When it reaches the size of a 12- to 14-week pregnant uterus, a recommendation for removal may be made based on size alone. However, Reiter and colleagues stated that hysterectomy need not be recommended to asymptomatic women with larger uteri. Yet, Hillis and associates present clear evidence that when the uterine weight exceeds 500 g, there is an increased risk of complications from abdominal hysterectomy. When deciding not to operate but to follow such a patient, the physician must be extremely careful that all components of the pelvic mass indeed are benign. There is always the possibility that one or more of the components of the mass is an ovarian tumor, the removal of which should not be delayed. Some idea of the various components of the mass may be obtained from pelvic ultrasound or computed tomography (CT). Although an abdominal approach usually is preferred when hysterectomy is indicated for large leiomyomas, many gynecologists still prefer vaginal hysterectomy with morcellation.

Rapid enlargement of a leiomyomatous uterus may indicate sarcomatous change. However, according to Parker and associates, of 371 women operated on for rapid growth of the uterus, only one patient was found to have sarcoma. Among 198 patients who met a definition of rapid growth (an increase by 6 weeks gestational size over 1 year), two were diagnosed with endometrial stromal sarcoma. The incidence of leiomyosarcoma in patients presumed to have benign leiomyomata is approximately 0.2% to 0.7%. Leibsohn and colleagues, reviewed 1,429 patients who underwent hysterectomy for presumed benign leiomyomata. A histologic diagnosis of leiomyosarcoma was made in seven (0.49%). The possibility that a benign leiomyoma may at some time undergo sarcomatous change is not an indication for hysterectomy. In young women, rapid growth of a leiomyomatous uterus is more commonly an indication of associated pregnancy. In this situation, a pregnancy test is indicated before hysterectomy is recommended.

A pedunculated myoma protruding through the cervical os always is infected and should be removed by vaginal myomectomy to prevent unavoidable bacterial contamination of the peritoneal cavity with abdominal removal. This may be done by passing a pretied laparoscopic Endoloop around the pedunculated myoma and cinching it down before cutting the pedicle. Several weeks later, hysterectomy may be done with less risk of infection.

Adenomyosis

Adenomyosis is an uncommon indication for hysterectomy. Dysmenorrhea, menorrhagia, uterine enlargement, and tenderness may indicate adenomyosis. Depending on the severity of symptoms, hysterectomy may be indicated after failure of response to more conservative measures, such as hormonal therapy and uterine curettage. The diagnosis may be suggested by magnetic resonance imaging, ultrasound, or CT scan, and core needle biopsy can be done with guidance under local anesthesia to confirm the diagnosis preoperatively. In many cases, a preoperative diagnosis of adenomyosis may not be confirmed by pathologic study of the removed uterus, and minimal adenomyosis found by careful pathologic study is probably of no clinical significance. In a study of validation of hysterectomy indications by Gambone and colleagues, adenomyosis represented the least verified indication, with only 38% of pathology reports providing confirmation. These authors stated that adenomyosis should no longer be considered a reliable indication for hysterectomy and recommended that patients suspected of having adenomyosis should be considered under other categories (i.e., chronic pelvic pain or recurrent uterine bleeding). We do not agree that adenomyosis should no longer be mentioned as an appropriate indication for hysterectomy, but do agree that it should be an uncommon indication.

Patients with dysmenorrhea, heavy, prolonged menstrual flow and an enlarged, tender uterus will experience a dramatic relief of symptoms from hysterectomy. Most should probably undergo attempts at hormonal management and D&C prior to hysterectomy. Ultrasound-directed core needle biopsy of the myometrium often provides a tissue diagnosis prior to hysterectomy.

Symptomatic Vaginal Relaxation, Uterine Descensus, and Prolapse

Symptomatic descent or prolapse of the uterus, usually associated with symptomatic vaginal wall relaxation (i.e., cystourethrocele, enterocele, and rectocele), with or without stress urinary incontinence, is a common indication for vaginal hysterectomy with restoration of normal anatomy and proper support to the vaginal outlet, vaginal walls, and vaginal vault, accounting for approximately 15% of hysterectomies. It should be emphasized that this operation is indicated only if symptoms are severe enough to justify the risk involved; if conservative measures, such as Kegel exercises or vaginal estrogen, have failed to give sufficient relief of symptoms; and, most of all, if the patient is asking for relief. The use of pessaries to manage pelvic relaxation is discussed in Chapter 35. An operation to correct asymptomatic and mild to moderate anatomic relaxation of the vaginal walls and uterine descensus rarely is indicated. Too many surgeries are performed for this indication in asymptomatic patients.

Hysterectomy is not a necessary part of surgical procedures to correct stress urinary incontinence. For example, if a suprapubic colpourethropexy is indicated to correct stress urinary incontinence, then hysterectomy is not indicated unless other conditions are present. Vaginal repair of a large symptomatic cystocele and enterocele usually is more successful if vaginal hysterectomy also is done at the same time.

Obstetric Problems

Hysterectomy in obstetric practice is discussed in Chapter 32. Uncontrollable postpartum hemorrhage; uterine rupture; uterine inversion; placenta accreta; and interstitial, abdominal, or cervical pregnancy are obstetric catastrophes that may require abdominal hysterectomy to prevent death from hemorrhage.

Septic abortion usually is treated successfully with antibiotics and evacuation of retained infected placental and fetal parts. Few patients are unresponsive to medical therapy and curettage. However, occasionally, the physician also may need to do an abdominal hysterectomy when there is severe infectious septic shock, peritonitis, and impairment of renal function perhaps associated with infection with clostridia microorganisms.

Associated Pelvic Conditions

In the circumstances discussed in the sections that follow, the uterus may be excised as part of an operation to remove the diseased adnexa even though there is no pathology in the uterus itself. In the past, hysterectomy was recommended if the tubes or ovaries were irreparably damaged or required removal, rendering conception impossible. However, modern assisted reproductive technology has changed our thinking in this area, and the possibilities, risks, benefits, and costs should be discussed with these patients and their partners before surgery so they may make an informed decision about hysterectomy at the time of adnexal surgery for inflammatory disease, ectopic pregnancy, or neoplasm.

Pelvic Inflammatory Disease

As discussed in Chapter 28, an acute exacerbation of chronic pelvic inflammatory disease (PID) with bilateral tuboovarian abscesses usually can be treated successfully with conservative medical management, including antibiotics for polymicrobial infection and drainage of pus when this is indicated by either posterior colpotomy or CT-guided needle aspiration. In our experience, at least 80% of patients respond to this management. Surgery may be recommended for those patients who do not respond, patients with a ruptured tuboovarian abscess, or patients with significant symptoms of chronic PID. Usually, a bilateral salpingo-oophorectomy is necessary because extensive adnexal disease is found bilaterally. Occasionally, it is possible to conserve the function of one ovary. Hysterectomy usually is recommended in women who are not interested in taking advantage of the new reproductive technologies for achieving pregnancy. For those who are, the uterus may be left in place, even though both tubes and ovaries have been removed. Chronic pelvic pain often occurs in women with PID, and this may be more likely if an ovary or the uterus is left behind.

Pelvic Endometriosis

Extensive pelvic endometriosis unresponsive to hormonal therapy may require surgery for relief. Young women who have not completed childbearing should have conservative surgery, including removal of all visible and palpable endometriosis, possible presacral neurectomy, and possible uterine suspension. For older women with no desire for pregnancy or for patients whose symptoms and pelvic findings of endometriosis have recurred following a previous conservative operation (or operations), a more extensive operation usually is indicated. Under these circumstances, abdominal hysterectomy with bilateral salpingo-oophorectomy is the procedure of choice unless the patient insists on the uterus remaining for the purpose of using new reproductive technologies to achieve conception. The management of pelvic endometriosis is discussed in Chapter 25.

Ectopic Pregnancy

Certain ectopic pregnancies may require hysterectomy. A hysterectomy may be required for cervical pregnancies, interstitial pregnancies, or abdominal pregnancies when the placenta cannot be removed without removing the uterus. It also may be permissible to perform a hysterectomy in a patient who has had repeated tubal pregnancies that have completely destroyed both fallopian tubes to the point that their function cannot be restored and whose condition during surgery is completely stable. Again, it is necessary for the patient to give specific permission for hysterectomy after being fully informed of all options for future reproduction. The surgical management of ectopic pregnancies is discussed in Chapter 22.

Neoplastic Diseases

Cervical Intraepithelial Neoplasia

Under most circumstances, cervical intraepithelial neoplasia may be adequately treated by a loop electrode excision procedure (LEEP), cryosurgery, laser surgery, or cervical conization (see Chapter 45). Sometimes hysterectomy is recommended for patients who do not desire more children and have other indications for hysterectomy. Vaginal hysterectomy is preferred unless contraindicated by adnexal disease, uterine enlargement, or other circumstances. A vaginal cuff should be removed with the uterus when the carcinoma *in situ* extends close to or on to the adjacent vaginal fornix.

Early Invasive Cervical Cancer

A simple, total hysterectomy is an adequate operation for early invasive cervical cancer if an adequate cervical conization examination shows superficial, microscopic stromal invasion limited to a depth of ≤3 mm or a lateral spread of <7 mm. There should be no confluence of tumor in the stroma and no evidence of vascular or lymphatic space invasion. Either abdominal or vaginal hysterectomy is satisfactory in this situation.

Most patients with stage IB1 and IIA carcinoma of the cervix may be treated with radical hysterectomy, bilateral pelvic lymphadenectomy, and partial vaginectomy, as discussed in Chapter 46. Treatment with primary surgery rather than irradiation is especially indicated in premenopausal women in whom ovarian conservation is an added bonus.

Endometrial Hyperplasia, Adenocarcinoma, and Sarcoma of the Uterus

Atypical endometrial hyperplasia is considered, by most authorities, to be a precursor to endometrial adenocarcinoma and, therefore, an appropriate indication for hysterectomy. Less severe forms of hyperplasia usually are reversible with progestational therapy and thus do not require hysterectomy.

Total abdominal hysterectomy is an important part of the management of endometrial adenocarcinoma and uterine sarcomas. Even though various combinations of adjuvant irradiation and chemotherapy also may be used, the most important part of the treatment is hysterectomy. Paraaortic and pelvic lymph nodes should be sampled in selected cases and enlarged nodes should be removed, but therapeutic pelvic lymphadenectomy usually is not required. Peritoneal washings should be sent for cytologic examination. A complete discussion can be found in Chapter 47.

Ovarian and Fallopian Tube Neoplasms

Malignant neoplasms of the ovaries and fallopian tubes are diagnosed, staged, and debulked surgically. In addition to bilateral salpingo-oophorectomy, a total abdominal hysterectomy is done almost always because of the frequent serosal tumor involvement. A subtotal rather than total hysterectomy may be done when extensive disease is spread throughout the abdomen, the cervix is encased in tumor, and removal of the cervix does not help with efforts to decrease the bulk of the tumor. These patients are almost always treated with adjuvant chemotherapy. In some patients with limited disease, conservation of the uterus and the opposite ovary may be indicated when fertility is desired. The treatment of ovarian malignancies is discussed in Chapter 48.

Trophoblastic Disease

Trophoblastic disease of the uterus usually is treated successfully with chemotherapeutic agents. Hysterectomy is rarely necessary, but it may be done in patients with a persistent disease involving the uterus that is resistant to chemotherapy. Hysterectomy is the treatment of choice in patients with a diagnosis of placental site trophoblastic tumor.

Malignant Disease of Other Adjacent Pelvic Organs

When malignant disease of other adjacent organs is treated surgically, a hysterectomy may be done for the operation to be technically adequate or to provide better exposure for radical pelvic resection. This is frequently true of carcinoma of the rectum, but also may be true of carcinomas of the cecum, sigmoid, or bladder that may be adherent to the uterus. Hysterectomy also may be required in operations for retroperitoneal tumors.

Miscellaneous and Unusual Indications

Cervical Problems

Cervical stenosis with recurring hematometra or pyometra despite one or more unsuccessful attempts to keep the cervix open may require abdominal hysterectomy for final solution. This situation almost always occurs in a postmenopausal patient and, not infrequently, malignancy is found in the uterine cavity or endocervical canal.

Rarely, an anomalous development of the müllerian duct system may leave the adolescent patient with a uterine cavity lined with functioning endometrium, but with congenital absence of the cervix and vagina. It is almost impossible to create a suitable endocervical canal and functional vagina at menarche to allow a permanently patent external exit for the menstrual flow. Hysterectomy is necessary to prevent recurrent hematometra and endometriosis from retrograde menstrual flow.

Chronic Pelvic Pain

Chronic pelvic pain often presents a difficult problem for the gynecologic surgeon. Women with chronic pain are miserable and may have an unsympathetic personality. In these women, it is unclear whether their long-standing discomfort has resulted in their dependent, helpless, pain medication–seeking behavior or whether their symptom of pain is another manifestation of their personalities. Many of these women do not have an identifiable cause of pain, such as endometriosis; thus, surgery is of questionable benefit. However, in many cases, the frustrated surgeon may be tempted to proceed with hysterectomy and often oophorectomy in an attempt to alleviate the patient's symptoms. If this fails, the surgeon is able to say, "I have done all I can do" forward her to another doctor, and eliminate the almost daily phone calls and office visits. It is important to remember that even when a specific organic cause of pain is identified and treated—surgically or otherwise—women with a long-standing history of pain often require counseling to correct the secondary emotional problems that result from chronic pain. The complexities of this topic are covered in Chapter 27.

Hysterectomy is rarely indicated for nonspecific pelvic pain. These women should be thoroughly evaluated as outlined in the preceding, and surgery should be reserved for those in whom specific organic pathology is demonstrated. Diagnostic laparoscopy may by helpful in these patients. Successful management of chronic pelvic pain usually is the result of a multidisciplinary team effort.

The Pelvic Congestion Syndrome and the Allen-Masters Universal Joint Syndrome

Patients with "pelvic congestion syndrome" complain of backache, pelvic heaviness, dysmenorrhea, and heavy menstrual flow. They often also have dyspareunia and chronic fatigue that may be out of proportion to any anemia. Careful inspection of the pelvis at laparotomy or laparoscopy shows dilated pelvic veins.

Allen and Masters described a series of women with symptoms similar to pelvic congestion syndrome but whose pelvic discomfort began after vaginal delivery and their pelvic examination is characterized by a tender, retroverted uterus and a cervix that can be easily moved in any direction. This mobility led to the nickname of the universal joint syndrome. Women with this syndrome, which is more formally know as the Allen-Masters syndrome, have unilateral or bilateral pelvic fascial defects and/or visible defects in the broad ligaments.

These syndromes have been controversial since they were first described. It has never been clear if the vascular congestion or pelvic fascial defects are a cause of pelvic pain and whether or not hysterectomy is the appropriate management.

Surgical Sterilization

When requested and indicated, surgical sterilization usually should be accomplished by tubal ligation instead of hysterectomy. Hysterectomy for sterilization is associated with more complications, a longer period of recovery, and more costs than tubal ligation. Therefore, hysterectomy is inappropriate for sterilization except in selected patients with other gynecologic disease or symptoms that, in all likelihood, will require hysterectomy in the near future. For example, a 30-year-old patient with a 10-week-sized myomatous uterus and menorrhagia who requests sterilization may be advised to have a total hysterectomy rather than tubal ligation and myomectomy. A 40-year-old patient with severe cervical dysplasia who requests surgical sterilization may be advised to have a hysterectomy rather than tubal ligation and cervical conization. A 35-year-old patient with symptomatic uterine descensus and vaginal relaxation who requests surgical sterilization may be advised to have a vaginal hysterectomy and repair rather than a tubal ligation.

PREOPERATIVE COUNSELING

The gynecologist needs to talk with the patient while trying to decide whether a hysterectomy is indicated. Fortunately for the patient and the gynecologist, time for talking is available in almost every instance. A hysterectomy is rarely an emergency. Unfortunately, the time may not be used properly. In a survey of women who underwent hysterectomy, Neefus and Taylor found that there is an urgent need for patient education on the physical, psychological, and sexual aspects of hysterectomy.

Often, the need for hysterectomy is obvious. There is a complete prolapse, or a large and symptomatic leiomyomatous uterus, or an endometrial cancer. Under these and other obvious circumstances, the patient should be told that a hysterectomy is recommended and why. The indication for surgery should be explained clearly and in language that the patient can understand. Treatment alternatives should be mentioned and the reason to prefer hysterectomy should be explained. The risks, benefits, and side effects must be reviewed, but in such a way that the patient is not unduly alarmed. Then the patient and the physician should spend the time necessary to discuss any questions that the patient may have. Additionally, the patient should be encouraged to discuss details about the operation and how long it will take, the recuperation period in the hospital and at home, whether or not ovarian function should be conserved, and possible hormone replacement therapy. Patient information pamphlets and videos also are useful for preoperative education.

Because the uterus is the main organ associated with reproduction, it is an important part of a woman's self-image, and, in some cultures, a woman's sexuality and reproductive potential are viewed as important parts of her value or status in her family or society as a whole. For these reasons, it is absolutely necessary for the gynecologic surgeons to understand and help patients cope with the emotional turmoil that accompanies hysterectomy. For some women who have had their children and need a hysterectomy for prolonged heavy bleeding and cramping associated with uterine fibroids or those with a diagnosis of endometrial cancer, the indications are clear, the benefits are obvious, and the loss of reproductive capacity often is not of great concern. The emotional stress of hysterectomy on these women is usually minimal and psychological adjustment often is rapid and complete. However, the young woman needing a hysterectomy for cervical cancer or a ruptured cornual pregnancy may have considerable difficulty adjusting to the loss of her uterus. Even the 32-year-old woman with three children and severe uterovaginal prolapse may not be comfortable with the idea of hysterectomy. The gynecologist must be sensitive to these possible concerns and anxiety. Even when the patient does not express any emotional distress, the gynecologist can provide an opening for the patient to discuss her feelings by statements such as, "Most studies have shown no change in sexuality and sexual function after hysterectomy, but I know many patients have concerns about this. Do you have any questions?" The support of the patient's husband or partner and her family and friends are very useful elements to prevent and manage depression and the emotional stress of hysterectomy. The wise surgeon includes members of this support group in preoperative discussions and encourages them to ask questions or express opinions that may be actually questions or opinions of the patient that she is hesitant to express.

Despite improvements in preoperative counseling in recent years, some women are depressed after hysterectomy. In most counseling, this depression is short-lived and self-limiting but the gynecologist should be alert for severe or prolonged symptoms of continued lack of energy, inability to return to normal activities of daily living, sleep difficulties, or other indicators of depression following surgery. Occasionally, antidepressants and/or psychiatric consultation may be necessary. The psychological aspects of pelvic surgery are extensively reviewed in Chapter 3.

Management of Normal Ovaries

Should normal ovaries be removed at the time of hysterectomy for benign disease? Although there are a few general guidelines, each patient must be approached individually. *Bilateral oophorectomy is recommended for postmenopausal women* because there is no evidence for persistent hormonal function or other metabolic activity. There is no doubt that bilateral oophorectomy removes the risk of ovarian cancer.

Four case-control studies that found a lower risk of ovarian cancer among women who had a history of previous hysterectomy have been analyzed by Weiss and Harlow. They believe the difference is explained by incidental screening for visible ovarian malignancy at the time of hysterectomy in those women in whom the ovaries are not removed. Those women with grossly normal ovaries have a reduced risk of developing symptomatic ovarian cancer over the next few years.

An analysis of the Cancer and Steroid Hormone Study by Irwin and colleagues from the CDC, including women 20 to 54 years old, found a relative risk (RR) of ovarian cancer of 0.6 in women who had a hysterectomy with ovarian conservation, unilateral or bilateral. The inverse association between hysterectomy and ovarian cancer risk was still present 10 years after surgery (RR = 0.6) but disappeared after two decades. The reason(s) for this risk reduction is unknown, but may be related to the opportunity to examine the ovaries at the time of hysterectomy with removal of those that are abnormal and conservation of those that are grossly normal. Other possible mechanisms include reduction in ovarian blood flow and steroidogenesis after hysterectomy, a higher frequency of previous oral contraceptive use among women who undergo hysterectomy, and protection of ovaries from transtubal migration of potential vaginal carcinogens.

Recent studies also have shown a decrease in the risk of breast cancer in women who have undergone bilateral oophorectomy. This is of particular importance in women from families with a history of ovarian or breast cancer and those with known BRCA gene mutations. In a series of 177 women with BRCA1 or BRCA2 mutations who were enrolled prospectively and followed for up to 6 years, Kauff et al., reported a 4% incidence of breast cancer among the 69 women who underwent prophylactic oophorectomy compared to a 13% incidence among those who elected follow-up surveillance only. In a similar retrospective review of 259 women compared with matched controls, the risk of breast cancer was reduced by 50% in the women who had bilateral oophorectomy. In both series, the risk of peritoneal or ovarian cancer was decreased by 95%.

Clearly, there are some significant potential benefits to oophorectomy at the time of any pelvic surgery in women with a strong family history of ovarian or breast cancer. However, in other premenopausal women, the advantages and disadvantages of "incidental" or "prophylactic" oophorectomy are not so clear-cut.

Traditionally, many gynecologists have recommended against oophorectomy in women under the age of 40 and offered oophorectomy to those between 40 and 50 years old. There are no data to support this approach.

In a study of 165 premenopausal women who were prescribed estrogen replacement therapy following bilateral oophorectomy, Castelo-Branco et al., found that only one third continued their medication for 5 years. Fear of cancer was the most common reason for discontinuation. Thus, the anticipated protection from osteoporosis and results of premature menopause that result from oophorectomy may not be effectively prevented by oral hormone replacement therapy because many patients stop or do not take estrogen as prescribed.

The average age of natural menopause in the United States is about 51 years. It seems reasonable to discuss the possibility of oophorectomy prior to planned hysterectomy for benign disease in women over age 45. However, it should be made clear to those women that there are some definite disadvantages to oophorectomy, especially if they do not or cannot use estrogen replacement therapy postoperatively. Each patient brings her own ideas and experiences to this discussion and the surgeon should try to counsel her and her family so she will be happy with her decision about oophorectomy.

Subtotal Versus Total Hysterectomy for Benign Conditions

In the United States, and throughout most of the world, hysterectomy—whether done transvaginally or through an abdominal incision—usually includes removal of the cervix. Over the past 50 years, subtotal, or supracervical, hysterectomy has come to be viewed as a suboptimal procedure reserved for those rare instances where concern over blood loss or anatomic distortion dictates limiting the extent of dissection. Recently, there have been some concerns about a reduced quality of orgasmic function and bladder dysfunction after the cervix has been removed. Much has been written about this in the lay media, and there are undoubtedly some women who develop problems after hysterectomy. However, almost all controlled studies have shown no difference in sexual or bladder function after simple hysterectomy for benign disease. My own clinical experience over 30 years also confirms this impression.

Nonetheless, the routine practice of removing the cervix at the time of hysterectomy for benign disease is now being challenged as many traditional surgical procedures are being modified to accommodate minimally invasive techniques. A new technique of total laparoscopic hysterectomy (as initially described by Semm) involves coring out the endocervical tissue and presumably the squamocolumnar junction area, which should practically eliminate the risk of cervical cancer. More recently, a laparoscopic tissue morcellator has been used to perform a supracervical hysterectomy. Experience with these newer, minimally invasive techniques is still inadequate to evaluate their effectiveness and morbidity rates or to develop indications and contraindications for their use.

PREPARATION FOR HYSTERECTOMY

A complete history and physical examination is indicated prior to any operative procedure. This evaluation is detailed in Chapter 6, but a few points deserve emphasis. Although it is appropriate to ensure all gynecologic symptoms have been evaluated carefully and a pelvic examination performed, a complete physical evaluation is necessary to be sure the patient can safely tolerate anesthesia and major surgery. Appropriate consultation should be sought where indicated to assure safe anesthesia administration and anticipation of any perioperative medical problems. In addition to a preoperative hematocrit or hemoglobin and other laboratory tests as indicated by the patient's medical condition, it is important to have a recent Pap smear to rule out cervical neoplasia and a recent pregnancy test in reproductive-age women prior to hysterectomy.

Preoperative chest x-rays are no longer routinely recommended but may be indicated in women with cardiorespiratory disease or malignancy. An intravenous pyelogram or CT scan of the abdomen and pelvis may be useful in women with uterine or extrauterine pelvic masses, but these are not indicated routinely.

Although the value of a bowel preparation prior to simple hysterectomy has been questioned in recent years, we prefer to have the colon evacuated prior to pelvic surgery in order to facilitate exposure and reduce trauma to the bowel caused by retraction and packing. We recommend a clear liquid diet on the day prior to surgery and usually one or two Fleet enemas the evening prior to surgery. A Dulcolax suppository (Boehringer Ingelheim, Germany) immediately on arising on the morning of surgery will evacuate any residual feces in the sigmoid and prevent contamination of the field during surgery. A complete mechanical or antibiotic bowel preparation is indicated only when intestinal surgery is a possibility.

Infection risk is decreased by routine use of intravenous antibiotics given immediately prior to induction of anesthesia. Second generation cephalosporins such as cefoxitin are commonly used. Prospective, randomized trials have shown a significant reduction in the risk of febrile morbidity and infection in both abdominal and vaginal hysterectomy. Some have suggested that bacterial vaginosis increases the risk of postoperative infections after vaginal hysterectomy, but preoperative evaluation and treatment remains controversial. Although povidone-iodine douches and antibiotic scrubs prior to surgery have been widely used in the past, no added benefit is apparent when perioperative intravenous antibiotics are employed.

If necessary, the pubic and/or vulvar hair should be clipped with an electric clipper or even scissors rather than shaved. The patient should be instructed not to shave the operative site prior to surgery because it has been shown to increase the risk of wound infection and cellulitis.

THE CHOICE OF APPROACH: ABDOMINAL, VAGINAL, OR LAPAROSCOPIC

With the introduction of laparoscopically assisted hysterectomy, there has been a resurgence of interest in vaginal hysterectomy. Transvaginal surgery is the special province of the gynecologic surgeon and vaginal hysterectomy is the showcase operation. It has many advantages over abdominal hysterectomy, but there are certain patients in whom the abdominal approach is indicated and still others for whom a laparoscopically assisted vaginal hysterectomy (LAVH) should be the procedure of choice.

The diagnosis may make the choice of approach obvious in some patients, whereas in others the decision to proceed with hysterectomy or not depends on the promise of low morbidity and a rapid return to functionality offered by a vaginal hysterectomy. For example, women with extensive, painful endometriosis, very large uterine fibroids or cancer usually are best managed by an abdominal hysterectomy, which provides better exposure and the opportunity to visualize and operate on the adnexal structures, the ureter and even the upper abdominal contents. Conversely, a woman in her forties with dysmenorrhea and menorrhagia may choose vaginal hysterectomy over endometrial ablation, but would not accept abdominal hysterectomy because the longer recovery time would interfere too much with her work and family life. An LAVH may be the right compromise for a 42-year-old woman with a 6-cm complex adnexal mass and heavy periods with dysmenorrhea. After careful inspection of the adnexal mass shows no signs of malignancy, the infundibulopelvic ligament can be divided laparoscopically, and the hysterectomy initiated from above and completed vaginally. By definition, if the uterine vessels are ligated transvaginally, the procedure is described as a *laparoscopically assisted vaginal hysterectomy*. If the uterine vessels are ligated, coagulated, or stapled through the laparoscope, the operation is a *laparoscopic hysterectomy*. Many gynecologists who have had limited experience with vaginal hysterectomy during their training may use the laparoscopically assisted technique to gain experience and confidence in performing vaginal hysterectomy. Several techniques for laparoscopic hys-

terectomy have been described. These involve a supracervical hysterectomy and one of the alleged advantages to this approach is cervical preservation. There is little evidence that orgasmic function is better preserved or enhanced when the cervix is retained at the time of hysterectomy or that posthysterectomy vaginal vault prolapse is less common; the marketing appeal appears to be removing the uterus through three or four small "keyhole" abdominal incisions. This method does not appear to offer any advantage over vaginal hysterectomy.

There have been several large reviews of the results and complications of abdominal, vaginal, and laparoscopic hysterectomy techniques. One of the largest was a comparison of 2,563 hysterectomies done by 37 private practice gynecologists at a large suburban general hospital. This retrospective review by Johns et al., was not randomized or controlled, but it does provide a good view of outcomes and complications (Table 31.2). When the study was initiated in 1991, 65% of hysterectomies were done abdominally, but 3 years later only 36% were still being done through an abdominal incision. The incidence of vaginal hysterectomy remained unchanged at about 20% during the course of the study, whereas the use of LAVH increased from 12% to 45%. Operating time was shortest for vaginal hysterectomy (63 minutes) but interestingly, the longest operative time was for LAVH (102 minutes). Abdominal hysterectomy averaged about 82 minutes. The length of hospital stay was similar for both vaginal hysterectomy and LAVH. Intraoperative and postoperative complications were more common with abdominal hysterectomy. Total hospital charges were somewhat lower for the vaginal hysterectomy patients. Although experience with laparoscopy undoubtedly has decreased operative time and the risk of complications, and decreased use of disposable laparoscopic instruments has lowered costs, more recent stud-

---

TABLE 31.2.
Characteristics of Hysterectomy by Different Approaches

	Abdominal	Vaginal	LAVH
Number of patients	1,184	530	839
Uterine wt. (Ave.)	216 g	113 g	129 g
Operative time (Ave.)	82 min	63 min	102 min
Blood loss[a] (Ave.)	5.35%	5.19%	6.0%
Complications			
Fever >101°F	9.1%	3.2%	2.0%
Transfused	2.5%	0.9%	0.6%
Bowel, bladder or ureteral injury	1.0%	0.9%	0.7%
Death	0	1 pt.	0
Hospital stay	60 h	40 h	40 h
Hospital charges	$6,552	$5,879	$6,431

[a] Blood loss is percent change in preoperative versus postoperative hematocrit.

From: Johns DA, Carrera B, Jones J, et al. *Am J Obstet Gynecol* 1995;172:1709, with permission.

ies confirm the higher morbidity and greater cost of the laparoscopically assisted approach compared with simple vaginal hysterectomy.

Maresh et al. reviewed the histories and outcomes of some 37,298 women who underwent hysterectomy for nonmalignant indications in the United Kingdom during 1994 and 1995. The most common indication was abnormal uterine bleeding (46%). Sixty-seven percent of the patients had an abdominal hysterectomy, 30% a vaginal hysterectomy, and only 3% were treated by LAVH. Intraoperative and severe postoperative complication rates were highest for the LAVH group.

The push toward shorter hospital stays, led by insurance companies in the United States, has resulted in early ambulation, rapid progression of diet, and an average hospital stay of only 3 to 4 days associated with abdominal hysterectomy. The traditional indications for abdominal hysterectomy, including malignant disease and large uterine size, continue to be tested by new concepts and aggressive approaches using vaginal surgery. Vaginal hysterectomy with laparoscopic lymphadenectomy is now a recognized option for the management of endometrial cancer and vaginal hysterectomy is being increasingly recommended for women with enlarged uteri. In a prospective, randomized study, Darai et al. compared vaginal hysterectomy to LAVH in 80 women who met the following criteria: a uterus >280 g and at least one other relative contraindication to vaginal surgery—previous pelvic surgery, history of PID, moderate or severe endometriosis, concomitant adnexal masses indication for adnexectomy and/or nulliparity without uterine descent. The operative times were long in both groups, indicating the complexity of the surgery, but the vaginal hysterectomy group was significantly shorter (108 minutes versus 160 minutes $p < 0.001$). The average uterine weight was slightly greater in the LAVH group (513 g versus 424 g), and three women had to be converted to abdominal hysterectomy in this group. Vaginal morcellation of the uterus was done in all women in both groups. Serious morbidity was minimal, and the authors concluded that vaginal hysterectomy could be done safely in many patients with traditional indications for the abdominal approach, and that laparoscopy did not seem to increase successful operability or decrease morbidity.

Thus, the indications and relative contraindications for abdominal, vaginal, or laparoscopic hysterectomy are constantly evolving. The individual gynecologic surgeon needs to use his or her experience, knowledge, and judgment to counsel the patient so that together they may decide on the approach that best suits the patient's need and the surgeon's skills.

TOTAL ABDOMINAL HYSTERECTOMY: SURGICAL TECHNIQUE

Previous editions of Te Linde's text have described gradually evolving modifications of Edward H. Richardson's technique for abdominal hysterectomy with which thousands of gynecologic surgeons have been trained over the years. The operative technique was first published in 1929, and because Te Linde felt it was a classic, he quoted it word-for-word in the fourth edition of this textbook with two added "modifications." This was the edition on my bedside table when I was a resident. I have had the good fortune to operate with many fine surgeons, including E. Stewart Taylor and Felix Rutledge, and have been challenged by many young residents over the years. These experiences have been further enhanced by discussions of surgical technique with gynecologists from around the world, who have suggested changes or ideas that I have tried and sometimes incorporated into my basic technique for abdominal hysterectomy. Although it is important to learn a basic technique for standard abdominal hysterectomy, every surgeon should be interested in observing new and different techniques or modifications to be tried from time to time when appropriate. As a resident, you should try each different technique used by each different attending physician, always asking why this clamp is used, that suture or needle is selected, or the cuff is left open or closed. Having tried many different ideas, each gynecologic surgeon gradually evolves his or her own basic techniques that feel comfortable, work for him or her, and make sense. Because each patient is unique, it also is useful to have experience with different techniques and various modifications of the basic operation so that when the occasion calls for it, an alternative technique that is more suitable for the particular situation can be employed. Our basic technique for abdominal hysterectomy and several modifications are described in the following.

On the day of surgery, the surgeon always attempts to see the patient and her family and supporters before she is brought into the operating room. Although surgery may be routine to the gynecologist, major surgery is often a once-in-a-lifetime, frightening experience for the patient. The calm reassurance of the surgeon and the professional and caring nature of the entire operative team is very helpful to the patient and her family at this point. The focus of attention should be on the patient and her surgery. A certain amount of relaxed chatter about someone's birthday or hospital gossip is reasonable, but the patient should feel that the concentration of the surgical team is focused on the surgery at hand. Remarks about how fat the previous patient was or how the surgeon had to stay up all night with a difficult patient in labor are not appropriate. An equipment problem or technical difficulties that affect the operation certainly should be discussed with the surgeon prior to starting the procedure; however, it is inappropriate to talk about these in front of the patient. Remarks such as, "The table is broken and won't go down" or "We weren't able to get your favorite retractor today" may not affect the performance of the operation, but such statements just before a patient is ready to be anesthetized may raise serious doubts as to whether the operative team is optimally prepared for this operation, and may raise uncomfortable questions later if complications or unexpected results occur.

Positioning

The patient is brought into the operating room and placed in the supine position on the operating table. It is nice to place a warm blanket on the bed immediately prior to the patient's arrival and to cover the patient with a blanket from the warmer when she is positioned because most operating rooms are somewhat cool and the patient is only lightly clothed.

When the patient has been anesthetized, a careful examination under anesthesia is done. At this point, the surgeon should concentrate on potential problems affecting resectability. Is there nodularity from endometriosis in the cul-de-sac that may make dissection of the rectum off of the posterior cervix difficult? Is the myoma in the broad ligament really wedged into the pelvic sidewall or can it be mobilized? The mobility and descent of the uterus under anesthesia is particularly important when a vaginal hysterectomy is being considered. These potential problems and possible solutions should be considered and possibly discussed with the operative team while the surgeon scrubs.

The vagina and perineum are prepped with antiseptic solutions and a Foley catheter is inserted. I prefer to position the patient supine on the operative table with a soft pillow under her knees to provide gentle flexion. The patient's legs provide a table on which instruments can be placed. Some surgeons prefer the patient to be positioned in the low Allen stirrups with her legs slightly apart. This allows an assistant to stand between the legs and ready access to the vagina for examination or manipulation, or the urethra for cystoscopy.

The abdomen then is prepped from the anterior thighs to the xiphoid and sterile drapes applied. In most instances, abdominal hysterectomy for benign disease can be done through a low transverse incision; most gynecologists prefer a Pfannenstiel incision, which is cosmetically appealing and strong. If more exposure is required, a Cherney or Maylard incision can be used, but a midline incision generally is done if malignant disease is present or exposure to the upper abdomen may be required. The choice of abdominal incision is discussed in Chapter 12.

Once the abdomen is opened, the pelvic pathology is carefully evaluated and the abdomen explored. The operating surgeon should examine the appendix and palpate the upper abdominal organs, including the kidneys, liver, gallbladder, stomach, spleen, diaphragm, and omentum. The retroperitoneal nodes in the pelvic and paraaortic area should be palpated and the area of the pancreas gently examined to identify any abnormalities. The status of these organs should be recorded in the operative note and an intraoperative consultation may be indicated if abnormalities are identified.

After the abdomen has been explored, a slight Trendelenburg position should be requested, a self-retaining retractor placed, and the bowel packed superiorly to afford good exposure of the pelvis. Any adhesions of the small bowel or rectosigmoid may need to be divided at this time so that the bowel can be mobilized out of the operative field. In relatively thin patients with benign disease, I prefer to use a Kirschner retractor, which is light and simple and provides a choice of several fairly wide, shallow blades that fit on a square frame, allowing adjustable retraction laterally, inferiorly, and superiorly. The cecum and sigmoid are packed first with separate packs and a third rolled or folded pack is placed in the center behind the superior retractor blade to hold back the small bowel. In larger patients, or patients with a longer midline incision, a Bookwalter retractor with its many options of blades and variable positioning is invaluable.

Hysterectomy

When the bowel has been packed away and exposure to the pelvis is satisfactory, the round ligaments and uteroovarian ligaments are grasped on each side with a Kocher clamp, elevating the uterus out of the pelvis. In some cases of extensive inflammatory disease, endometriosis, or very large fibroids, uterine mobility is limited; but in most benign conditions uterine mobility is satisfactory. The operator is generally on the patient's left side so that the right-handed surgeon can use his or her dominant hand to extend down into the pelvis. The first assistant is on the opposite side. The uterus is retracted to the patient's right side and the left round ligament is stretched taut. A 0 delayed absorbable suture is placed under the round ligament approximately halfway between the uterus and the pelvic sidewall (Fig. 31.1). The small artery of Sampson runs just under the round ligament and, in many cases, transilluminating this area allows the surgeon to easily visualize the artery and be sure that the suture is passed under it so that the ar-

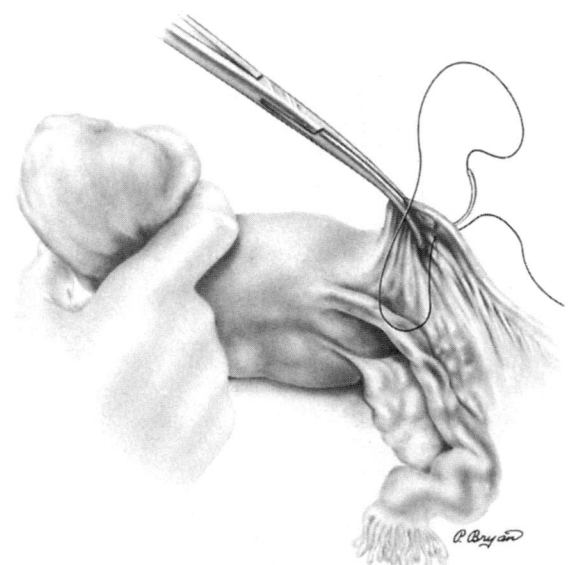

FIGURE 31.1. The technique of abdominal hysterectomy begins with the round ligament. The ligament is clamped, ligated with a transfixion suture, and cut. The broad ligament is opened.

tery will be ligated. A second suture is placed approximately 1 cm medial to the first suture; these two sutures are now tied simultaneously by the surgeon and first assistant.

With traction on these sutures, the round ligament is held taunt and divided with Metzenbaum scissors between the two suture ligatures. This opens the retroperitoneal space, which is almost always a free space for blunt dissection, even in the patient with extensive tumor, inflammatory disease, or endometriosis. If the ovaries are to be removed at the time of hysterectomy, the peritoneal incision then is extended superiorly, lateral to the ovary and parallel with the infundibulopelvic ligament. The peritoneal incision also can be extended anteriorly around to the bladder reflection, but the peritoneum over the anterior cervix does not need to be divided at this time because it may bleed, and exposure of this area is not yet required. With the index finger and the tip of the suction or the back of a tissue forceps, the surgeon gently divides the loose areolar tissue of the retroperitoneum, identifying the external iliac artery on the medial surface of the psoas muscle. In most cases, the artery can be identified very easily and blunt dissection is used to expose it superiorly to the level of the bifurcation of the common iliac artery. The ureter always crosses the pelvic brim at this location and should be identified easily on the medial leaf of the peritoneum at this point. The internal iliac or hypogastric artery dives into the pelvis at this location parallel to the ureter, and it should be identified also. This retroperitoneal exploration may seem awkward at first, but with practice the external and internal iliac arteries and ureter can be visualized easily in 10 to 20 seconds.

If the ovary is to be removed, a hole in the peritoneum between the ureter and the ovarian vessels superior to the ovary can be made under direct vision. We use a fairly fine sharp-pointed 9-in. clamp that can be passed gently through the peritoneum from lateral to medial against and between two fingers supporting the

medial side of the peritoneum. Alternatively, the peritoneum may be divided sharply or with the Bovie. We prefer to use a fairly delicate clamp on the infundibulopelvic ligament because it reminds us to isolate the vessels and take a fairly small pedicle. If there is significant inflammation or edema, a larger clamp such as a Heaney clamp may be used on the infundibulopelvic ligament pedicle (Fig. 31.2). A second, back clamp then is placed and the ovarian vessels divided between the two clamps. This pedicle then is ligated with a free-tie and then a second transfection suture ligature is placed for safety between the free-tie and the clamp. Zero-gauge delayed absorbable sutures and ties are used throughout. The suture ligature is placed distal to the free-tie so that if the needle happens to puncture one of the ovarian vessels, the vessel has already been ligated by the more proximal free-tie. The back clamp is ligated with a single free-tie and the posterior peritoneum then is torn or cut above the ureter toward the back of the uterus, mobilizing the ovary which is then tied to the clamp on the left tube and round ligament to keep it from flopping around and obscuring the operative field. The sutures on the round ligaments and infundibulopelvic ligament then are cut. The procedure is repeated on the patient's right side.

If the ovary and tube are to be left at the time of hysterectomy, a window in the peritoneum beneath the fallopian tube between the uterus and ovary is made sharply or bluntly and a heavy clamp such as a Heaney, Kocher, or similar clamp is used to clamp the uteroovarian pedicle (Fig. 31.3). The round ligament should not be included in this clamp. The clamp that was initially placed on the round ligament and fallopian tube just lateral to the uterine fundus at the beginning of the procedure serves as the back clamp for this pedicle. The tube and uteroovarian ligament are divided and the pedicle ligated as previously noted with a free-tie followed by a suture ligature. The ovary and tube may be left in the posterior pelvis if exposure is adequate or gently packed

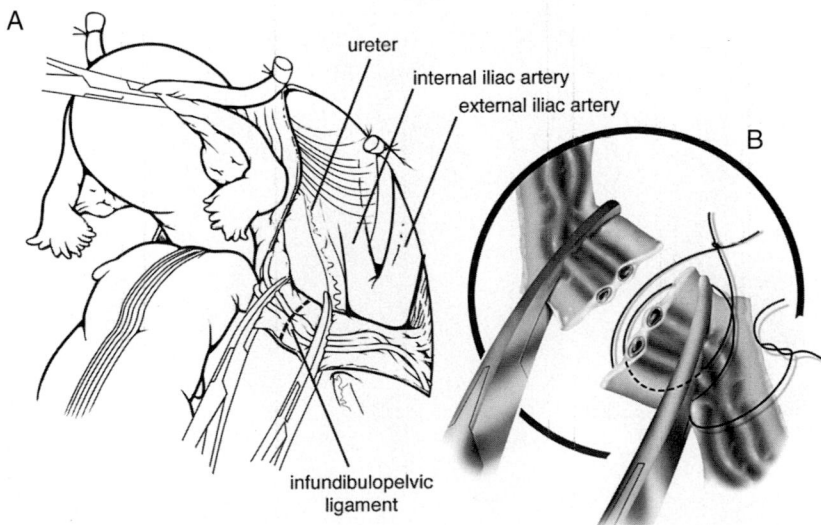

FIGURE 31.2. A: The infundibulopelvic ligament is doubly clamped and the ovarian vessels are cut between the clamps. Care is taken to be sure the ureter is clear as the clamps are applied. **B:** The proximal pedicle is ligated with a free tie followed by a transfixion suture ligature.

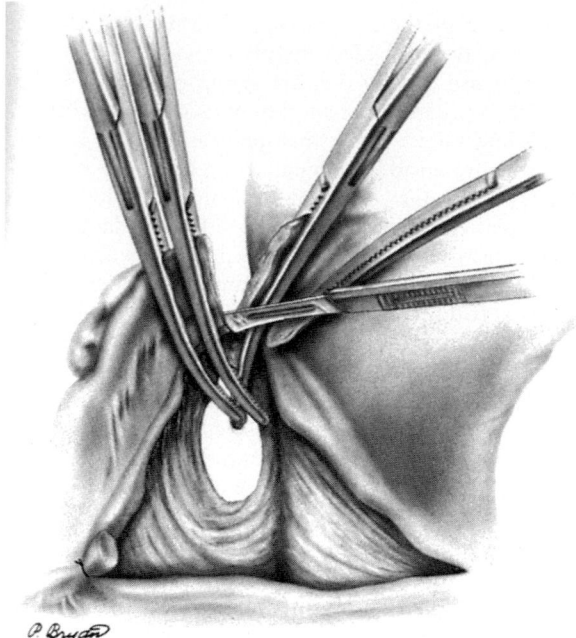

FIGURE 31.3. When the ovary is to be conserved, a peritoneal window is made above the ureter and one or two clamps used to clamp the tube and uteroovarian ligament. This is divided and doubly ligated.

in the paracolic gutter, with care being taken to ensure that the blood supply is not compromised.

The next step is the dissection of the bladder from the anterior cervix. At this point, the peritoneum is divided just inferior to its attachment to the lower uterine

segment. If the peritoneum is divided just inferior to its attachment, it is usually mobile and an avascular plane of loose areolar tissue usually can be identified between the posterior bladder wall and the anterior cervix. We begin this dissection sharply using the Metzenbaum scissors. With upward traction on the bladder peritoneum and the uterine fundus stretched tightly out of the pelvis, the tips of the Metzenbaum scissors should rest lightly on the fascia overlying the cervix and small bites used to develop this tissue plane, dissecting the bladder from the anterior cervix (Fig. 31.4). This dissection should take place over the cervix, because if is carried too far laterally, bleeding may be encountered and the ureters could be injured. Except in patients with a previous Caesarean section or an adherent bladder for other reasons, this bladder dissection often can be done bluntly, but it is good practice to do it sharply from time to time so that in those patients where sharp dissection is required, the procedure will be familiar. Blunt dissection of the bladder can be accomplished easily by grasping the uterus and lower uterine segment between both hands and gently using the first one or two fingers to advance the bladder, as illustrated in Richardson's classic paper (Fig. 31.5). It also is possible to use your right hand, placing the thumb in front on the anterior cervix and the fingers behind the uterus. The thumb is gently pushed toward the cervix and inferiorly toward the vagina, gently dissecting the bladder off of the cervix and lower uterine segment. With this technique, the pressure is against the cervix rather than against the bladder, which should minimize the risk of bladder injury. Excessive force should not be used. As the bladder is dissected below the cervix, the thumb in front and the fingers behind come into

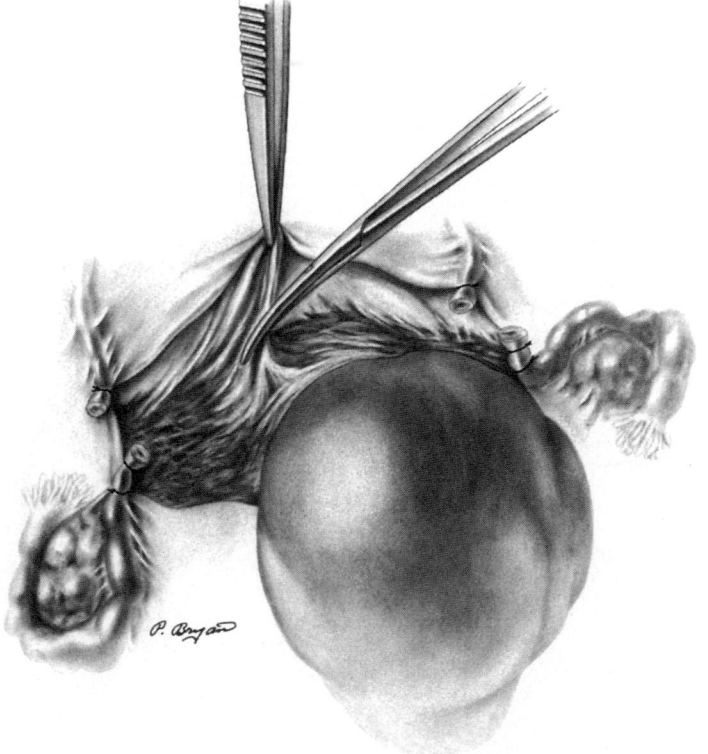

FIGURE 31.4. The bladder is mobilized inferiorly by sharp dissection away from the cervix. To avoid unnecessary bleeding, this step may be done in stages as necessary.

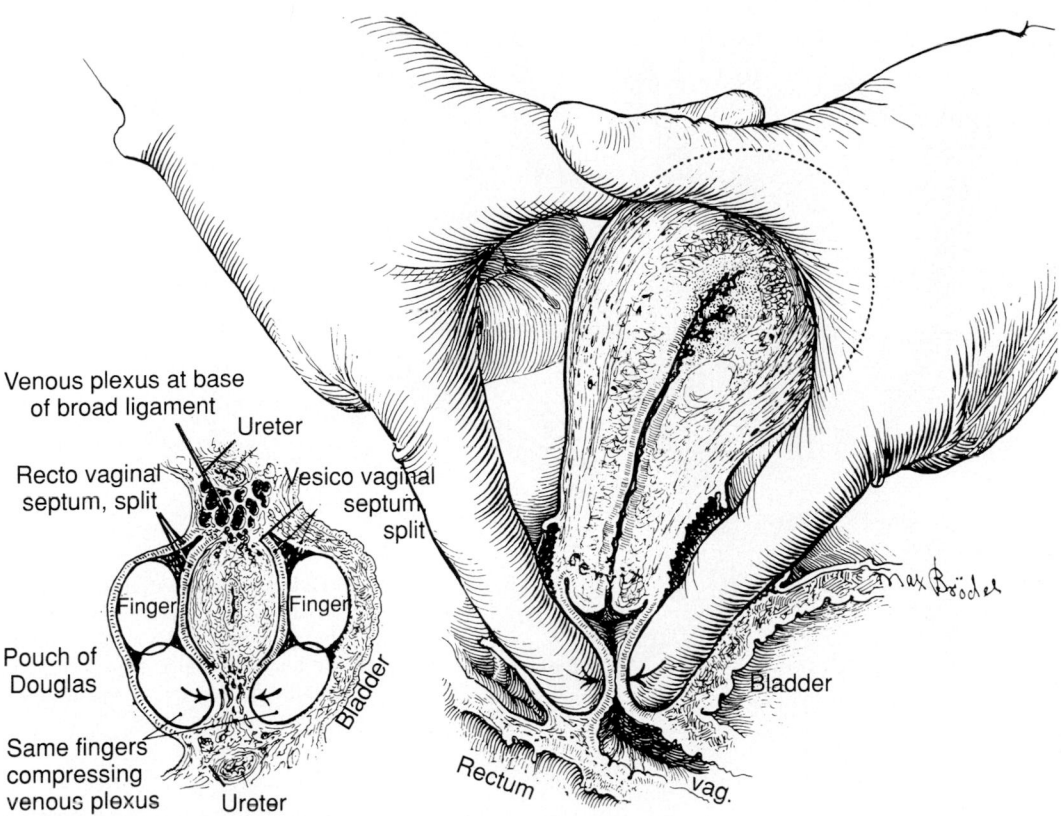

Venous plexus at base
of broad ligament

Ureter

Recto vaginal
septum, split

Vesico vaginal
septum,
split

Finger   Finger

Pouch of
Douglas

Bladder

Same fingers
compressing
venous plexus

Ureter

Rectum   vag.

Bladder

FIGURE 31.5. The bladder and, if necessary, the rectum can be gently advanced with blunt dissection. The depth of this dissection can be checked by squeezing the anterior and posterior fingers together below the cervix. (From: Richardson EH. A simplified technique for abdominal panhysterectomy. *Surg Gynecol Obstet* 1929;48:248, with permission.)

closer opposition because they now have only the vaginal wall between them. The dissection is extended laterally to encompass the full cervix. Usually, it is not necessary to dissect the rectum off of the posterior cul-de-sac; but if adherent rectum prevents good posterior exposure, it should be dissected free after the uterine vessels have been divided.

Once the bladder has been freed from the anterior cervix the uterine artery and vein are skeletonized. The uterus is pulled sharply to the patient's right side, and the surgeon gently dissects the loose fatty tissue adjacent to the lateral lower uterine segment on the left. The uterine artery is usually found immediately adjacent to the uterus at the level of the internal cervical os. In most patients, the uterine artery is easily exposed by holding the tissue laterally and gently "raking" with the Metzenbaum scissors slightly opened from medial to lateral. When the vessels are exposed, a fairly heavy, slightly curved clamp then is used to clamp the vessels just adjacent to the uterus (Fig. 31.6). We prefer to use a Heaney, Zepplin, or Masterson clamp for these pedicles. The tip of the clamp should be around the vessels and the clamp should come across the pedicle as close to a right angle as possible rather than at the diagonal so that the least amount of tissue will be incorporated in the pedicle. The tip of the clamp should not include too much cervical or uterine

tissue because this makes application of subsequent clamps more difficult. A second clamp can be placed above the first for added safety, if desired and a third, or back clamp used to prevent annoying back bleeding from the uterus after the vessels have been cut.

If exposure is satisfactory, we skeletonize the uterine vessels on the patient's right side and place a clamp on these vessels as well. If the uterus is small, no back clamp is required because the four major vessels supplying the uterus have now been clamped or ligated. Next, the uterine vessels are cut with scissors or a knife and the pedicle doubly ligated with zero delayed absorbed sutures. We prefer to use a CT-2 (Ethicon) or similar small tapered point needle for these pedicles because we feel that large needles are more difficult to place in the small confines of the deep pelvis. If a back clamp has been used, it is now ligated and removed so that the field is not obscured by an excessive number of clamps.

Hemostasis should be good at this point. The bladder is again checked to ensure it is well below the cervix. If the rectum needs to be dissected from the posterior cervix, this should be done now. The peritoneum of the posterior cul-de-sac between the uterosacral ligaments can be divided easily, and blunt dissection of the posterior vaginal wall from the anterior rectum usually is easy, although the rectosigmoid occasionally may be densely

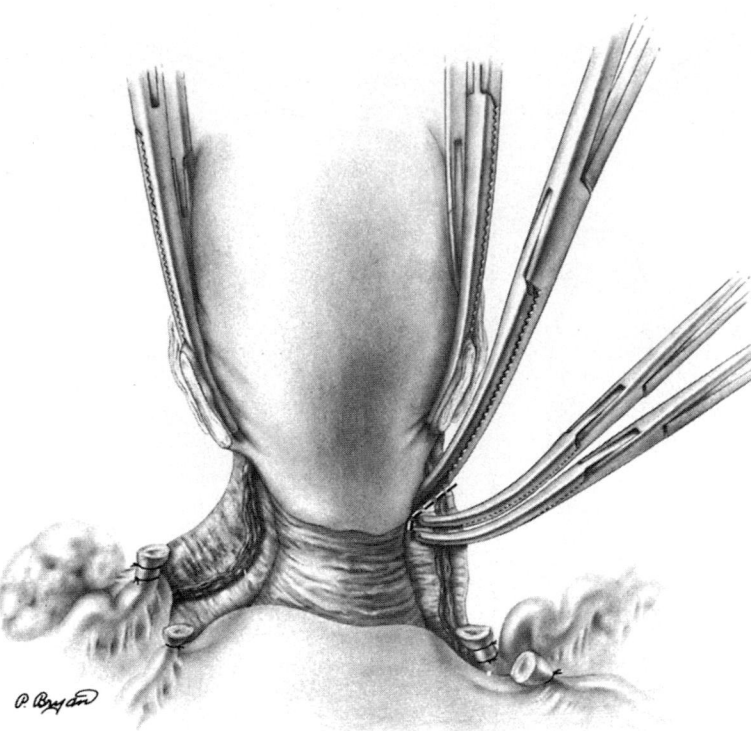

FIGURE 31.6. After the uterine vessels are skeletonized, they are clamped and cut along the dotted lines. To avoid clamping the ureter, the lowest clamp is placed first, at the level of the internal cervical os and at right angles to the lower uterine isthmus.

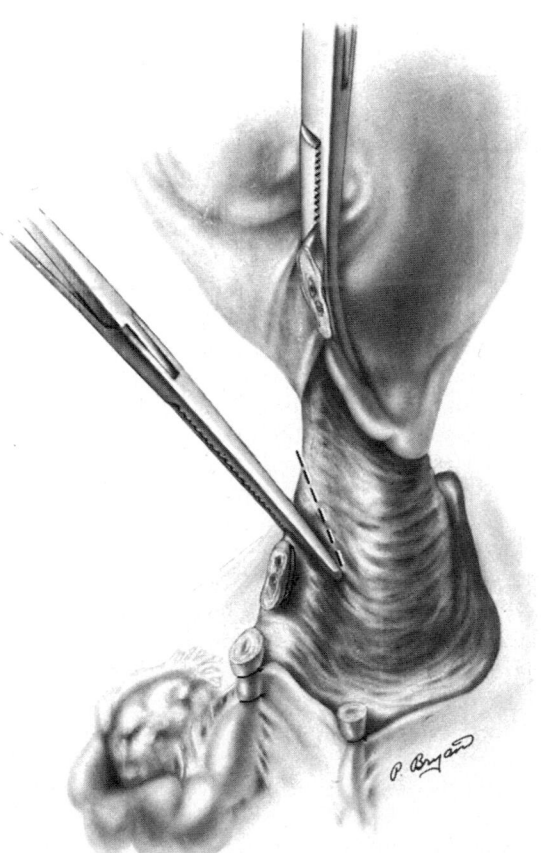

FIGURE 31.7. After the uterine artery and vein have been ligated, the remaining lower portion of the broad ligament is clamped with a series of straight clamps. The tips are placed on the edge of the cervix and the back of the jaw immediately adjacent to the previous pedicle.

adherent to the posterior uterine segment or cervix by endometriosis or PID. If the bladder and/or rectum is too densely adherent and there is concern that further attempts at dissection may damage them or cause troublesome bleeding, a supracervical hysterectomy should be considered at this point.

Once the bladder anteriorly and the rectum posteriorly have been freed from the cervix, the uterus is placed on tension, exposing the deeper portions of the broad ligament and pulling the lower uterine segment away from the ureter. In most cases, a series of straight Heaney or Zepplin clamps can be used to successfully clamp this remaining portion of the broad ligament (Fig. 31.7). The tips of the clamps should be placed on the lateral portion of the cervix and the upper portion of the jaw should lie immediately adjacent to the previous pedicle. As the clamp is gently squeezed closed, the tip slides off of the firm cervix. By staying close to the cervix in this way, the risk of damaging the ureter, which is not too far away laterally, is minimized. The pedicle then is cut with heavy scissors or a knife. A millimeter or two of tissue may be left medial to the clamp as insurance, but this is not necessary. The tip of the transfixion suture needle is placed at the lateral tip of the clamp jaw; if the pedicle is longer than 1 cm, we recommend using a Heaney suture ligature so that the upper end of the pedicle is secondarily transfixed to prevent it from slipping out of the ligature. While good exposure is maintained, one or two pedicles are tied on each side and then the procedure is repeated on the opposite side until the level of the cervical–vaginal junction has been reached. Once again, the bladder and rectum are checked and advanced if necessary to be sure that they are well clear and the vaginal walls exposed.

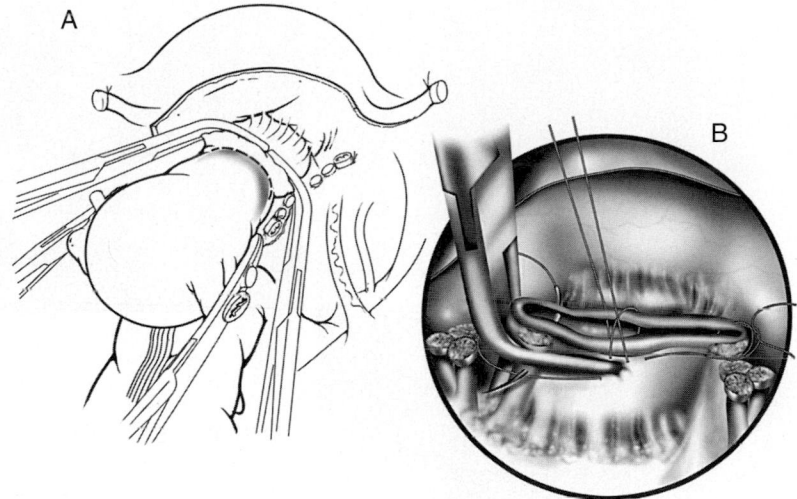

FIGURE 31.8. A: After checking to be sure the bladder and rectum are clear, the vagina is cross clamped with long, sharply curved Zepplin clamps just below the cervix *(dotted line)*. The vagina is divided just above the clamps with a knife or angled scissors. B: The vaginal cuff then is closed with a figure-of-eight in the middle and Heaney suture ligatures on the angles including the uterosacral and cardinal ligaments for support.

Sharply angled large Zepplin clamps are used to clamp across the vagina below the cervix. These clamps include the base of the cardinal ligaments laterally, the uterosacral ligament posteriorly, and the vaginal wall anteriorly and posteriorly. A clamp is applied from each side; in most cases, the tips of these clamps meet in the middle just below the cervix (Fig. 31.8). A knife or heavy, sharply angled Harrington scissors are used to divide the vagina above these clamps and below the cervix. The uterus is removed and placed in a pan on the back table for later examination. A single figure-of-eight suture is placed between the tips of the two clamps to close the midportion of the vagina. The ends of this suture are held initially and not tied. A Heaney suture ligature is placed on each of the lateral clamps with the second bite going through the uterosacral ligament posteriorly. Inclusion of the uterosacral and cardinal ligament in this pedicle provides excellent support of the vaginal apex. When these lateral sutures have been tied, the figure-of-eight suture in the middle then is tied also. The lateral sutures are cut and the figure-of-eight in the middle of the cuff is held to provide traction on the vaginal apex.

In the classic Richardson technique, the peritoneum over the posterior cervix is divided, the peritoneum is dissected off the cul-de-sac, and the rectovaginal septum entered to reflect the rectum posteriorly. In our experience, this has not been necessary in the vast majority of patients with benign disease. In contrast to the anterior bladder dissection, this posterior peritoneum is much more adherent. There is usually some bleeding associated with this dissection, making it both bloody and time consuming. The uterosacral ligaments also are clamped separately and subsequently attached to the vaginal cuff for support. In the technique described above, this is accomplished in a single step.

Finally, the vagina usually is entered sharply in most hysterectomy techniques. If the anatomy is distorted by a cervical myoma or any other reason, it may be advantageous to enter the vagina sharply and circumscribe the cervix starting from the point of normal anatomy and proceeding carefully to the abnormal area. With the approach described, the vagina is never opened to the pelvic cavity, minimizing contamination from vaginal bacteria. The vaginal cuff obviously is closed with our technique, but most surgeons today close the vagina at the time of hysterectomy because infection is uncommon with the use of prophylactic antibiotics.

Closure

After the pelvis has been copiously irrigated with warm saline, the pedicles are inspected carefully to be sure that hemostasis is present. Electrocautery or suture ligatures with 3-0 absorbable sutures on fine needles are used to control small bleeders. The location of the ureters, bladder, and major vessels should be known when placing these sutures. The pelvis is not reperitonealized, but the rectosigmoid colon is gently laid over the vaginal cuff to cover this raw surface and minimize the risk of adhesions. The packs and retractor are removed, the abdomen checked again for hemostasis, and the omentum placed anteriorly to minimize the risk of small bowel adhesions to the abdominal incision. The peritoneum is closed with delayed absorbable suture, although some surgeons today feel that it is unnecessary to close the anterior abdominal peritoneum. The fascial closure should be commensurate with the patient's risk of infection and hernia. Generally, a running monofilament delayed absorbably suture such as PDS (Ethicon) on a CT-1 needle can be used. If there is a significant risk of dehiscence secondary to infection, obesity, or other medical problems, interrupted sutures, or a mass closure technique may be used. Closure techniques are illustrated in Chapter 12. Because patients are often discharged by the third or fourth postoperative day, we generally prefer to close the skin with a subcuticular absorbable suture, which eliminates the necessity for a return to the office for suture or staple removal.

After the patient has been taken to the recovery room, the surgeon should speak with the family to assure them that the patient is doing well and to review the operative findings with them. A careful operative note

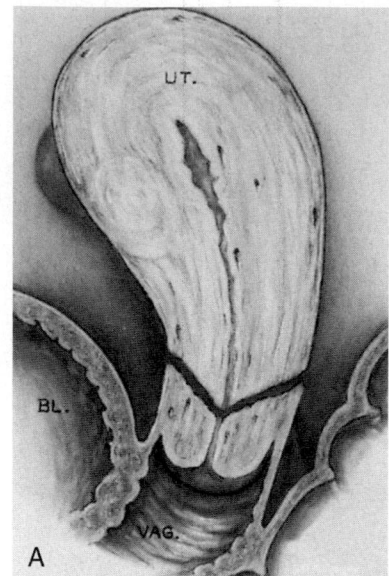

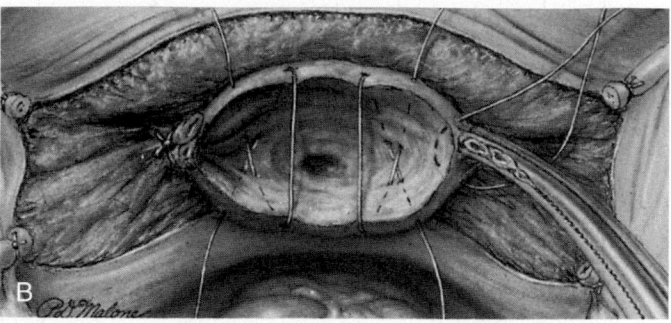

FIGURE 31.9. Subtotal or supercervical hysterectomy. **A:** After the uterine vessels have been ligated, the fundus is amputated using the electrocautery in a shallow cone-shaped technique. **B:** The cervix or lower uterine segment then is closed with several large figure-of-eight sutures. We do not recommend the lateral suture shown here because of the risk of ureteral injury.

should be dictated with emphasis on any unusual findings or variations from standard techniques.

SUBTOTAL ABDOMINAL HYSTERECTOMY

The technique of subtotal or supracervical abdominal hysterectomy is similar to the technique for abdominal hysterectomy as described, until after the uterine vessels have been clamped and ligated. At this point, care should be taken to be sure that the bladder and rectum have been advanced at least far enough so that the cervix can be clearly visualized both anteriorly and posteriorly. The uterus is stretched out of the pelvis and electrocautery is used to cut the cervix anteriorly just above the level of the ligated uterine vessels (Fig. 31.9). A shallow v-shaped incision is used both anteriorly and posteriorly until the uterine fundus is excised. The "coagulate" mode of the electrocautery is used and homeostasis usually is excellent. Several generous figure-of-eight sutures on a large needle then are used to close the upper endocervix in a hemostatic fashion. The top of the cervix is checked for bleeding and the bladder peritoneum may be used to cover this cervical stump to minimize the risk of adhesions.

VAGINAL HYSTERECTOMY

The patient is placed in the dorsal lithotomy position using either the Allen stirrups or the "candy cane" hanging stirrups. Although the Allen stirrups provide better support for the patient's legs during the course of the operation, they may render it more difficult for the surgical assistants to position themselves comfortably. The examination under anesthesia is crucial to ensure that the vaginal approach to hysterectomy is reasonable and that

exposure will be satisfactory. The lower abdomen, inner thighs, vulva, vagina, peritoneum, and buttocks are carefully prepped and draped as a sterile field. I prefer to sit during a vaginal hysterectomy, but it is important that the operator's stool be high enough so that the surgical assistants do not hurt their backs bending over. In some situations, it may be preferable for the entire operating team to stand during the course of a vaginal hysterectomy.

A weighted speculum is placed in the posterior vagina and a narrow Deaver retractor placed anteriorly under the bladder. The cervix is grasped with the tenaculum, although in some cases, if there is significant prolapse, a short-handled Leahey thyroid clamp will serve very well and its shorter length is less unwieldy. The vaginal mucosa around the cervix where the vaginal incision is to be made is injected with approximately 10 cc of Lidocaine with 1/100,000 epinephrine (Fig. 31.10). This causes vasoconstriction minimizing annoying oozing from the vaginal mucosa during the course of the procedure. This solution is readily available and is used for convenience, but a dilute solution of pitressin or even normal saline will suffice if the epinephrine is unavailable or the patient's medical condition contraindicates its use. Prior to injection, the cervix is gently manipulated in and out of the pelvis to visualize the bladder and rectal reflection.

With continuing traction on the tenaculum pulling the cervix down the vagina, the vaginal mucosa over the anterior cervix at the junction between the cervix and vaginal fornix is incised. This may be done with a knife or electrocautery (Fig. 31.11). The anterior vaginal retractor should push upward while the cervix is retracted downward so that the incision separates as the operator divides the mucosa. This incision is developed until the operator detects entry into the plane between the cervix and bladder. The assistant now holds the cervical tenaculum while the surgeon holds the paravesical

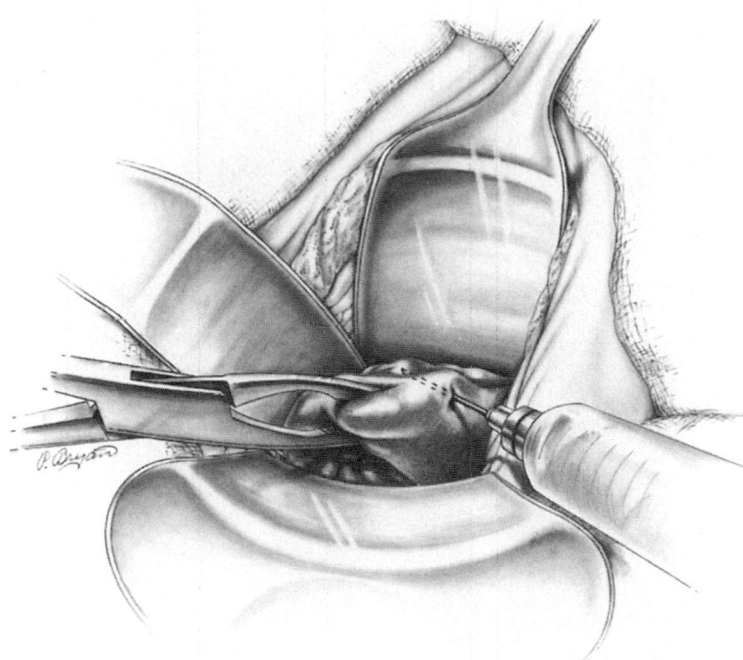

FIGURE 31.10. The cervix is grasped with a tenaculum and a hemostatic agent is injected beneath the vaginal mucosa around the cervix.

tissue anteriorly and with Metzenbaum scissors gently develops the plane between the anterior cervix and posterior bladder (Fig. 31.12A,B). As with abdominal hysterectomy, once this plane has been entered, the bladder usually is separated easily with blunt dissection. However, this is more difficult to do from below than abdominally and considerable experience is necessary before this plane can be found confidently. If problems are encountered with the anterior dissection of the bladder, the surgeon should place a small sponge in the area and begin the posterior dissection. Once the bladder has been separated off of the anterior cervix using a combination of sharp and blunt dissection, the Dever

retractor is placed anteriorly and the bladder gently retracted. This should expose the peritoneum, which attaches the bladder to the anterior uterine wall. The anterior uterine wall then can be grasped with tissue forceps and divided with Metzenbaum scissors (Fig. 31.13A,B). A small gush of peritoneal fluid is encountered occasionally, which may be disconcerting to the surgeon as he may think the bladder has been entered. With this small incision under direct vision, a finger or the retractor blade should be carefully placed and the uterine fundus and bowel identified. If there is still concern about injury to the bladder, a Foley catheter may be inserted and the bladder irrigated.

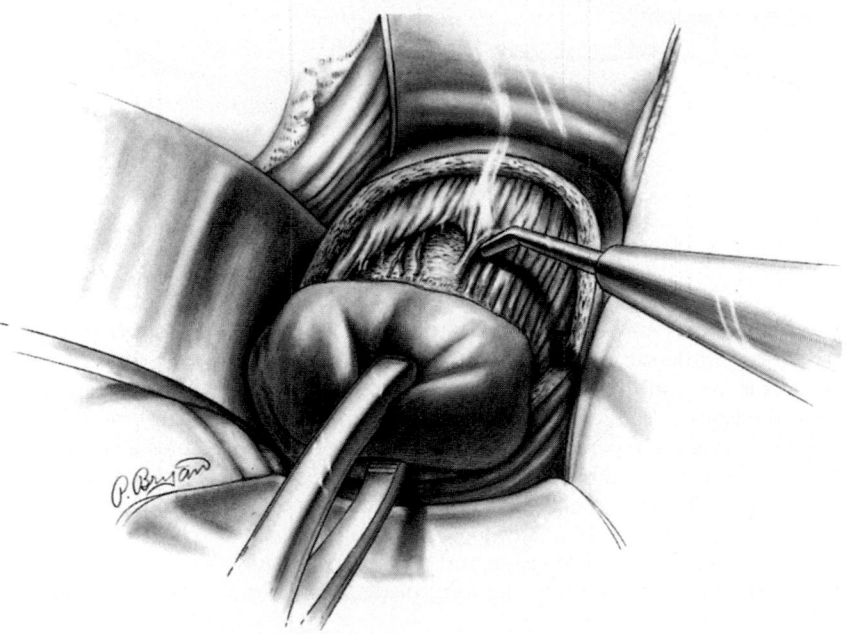

FIGURE 31.11. The incision in the vaginal mucosa is extended anterior to the cervix. The blade tip of the Bovie unit or Metzenbaum scissors are used to dissect the bladder away from the cervix and lower anterior uterine segment.

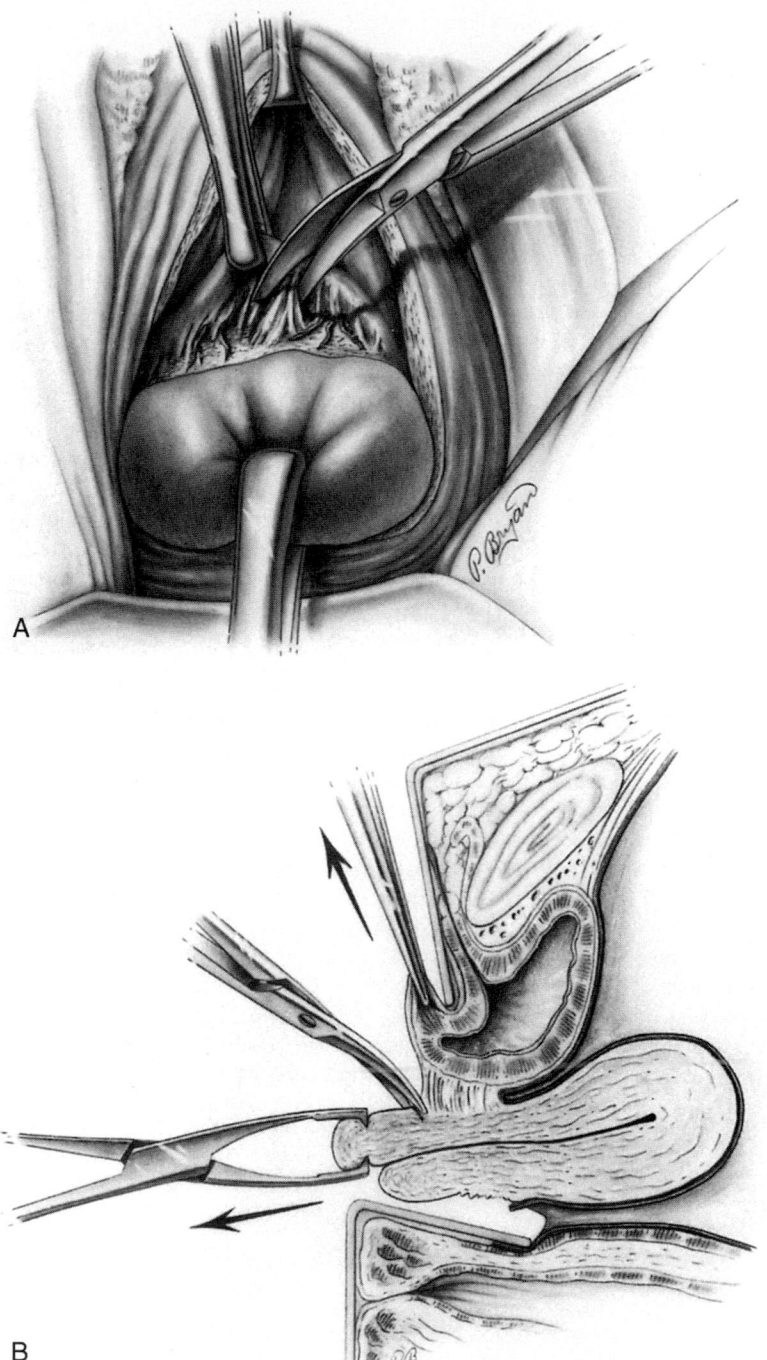

FIGURE 31.12. A: Scissors dissection is used to separate the bladder from the anterior cervix. **B:** The handle of the scissors should be elevated and the points directed downward against the uterus. Strong traction and countertraction facilitate the dissection.

The cervix then is retracted anteriorly exposing the posterior cul-de-sac. An elliptical incision from 8 to 4 o'clock is made in the posterior cervix where the mucosa joins the vagina. Metzenbaum scissors are used to dissect this mucosa and the peritoneum of the cul-de-sac is identified. This also is entered sharply with the Metzenbaum scissors and divided laterally to the uterosacral ligaments on each side (Fig. 31.14). Although many surgeons insert two fingers into this incision and tear it laterally until it is large enough to insert the long-bladed speculum,

I prefer to use a narrow Heaney retractor in the cul-de-sac and clamp the uterosacral ligament on each side, divide it, and ligate the ligament with a Heaney suture ligature of 0 delayed absorbable suture. These may be tied and held to facilitate closure of the cuff at the end of the procedure. At this point, the posterior incision is usually wide enough to insert the long-billed weighted speculum.

A finger is next placed in the posterior incision and the back wall of the uterus and broad ligaments palpated.

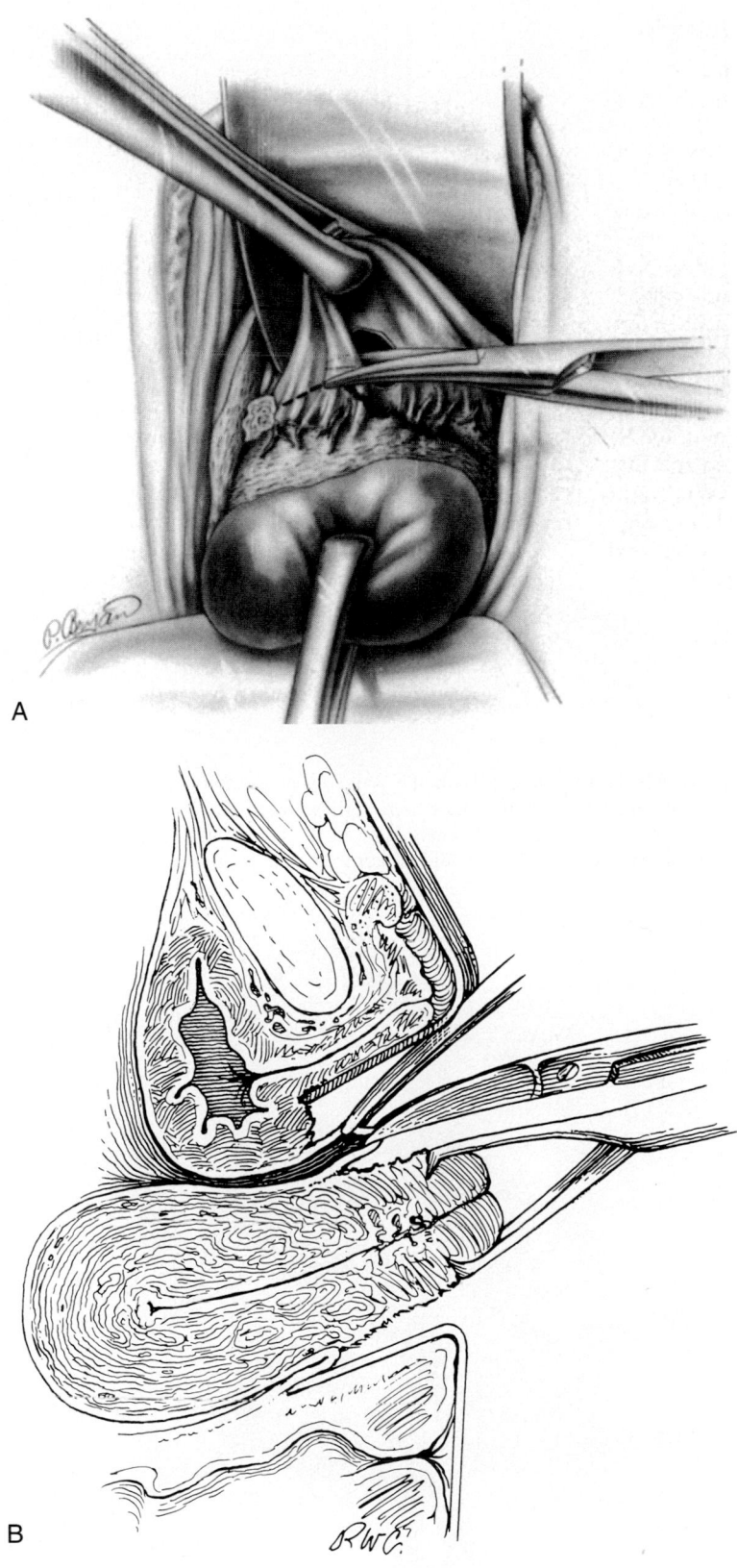

A

B

FIGURE 31.13. A: The peritoneum is incised sharply and the incision enlarged so that a retractor can be easily placed. If entering the peritoneal cavity anteriorly is difficult, it can be delayed until later but should be done before the uterine vessels are clamped and ligated. **B:** A small incision is made in the peritoneal reflection between the bladder and the uterus.

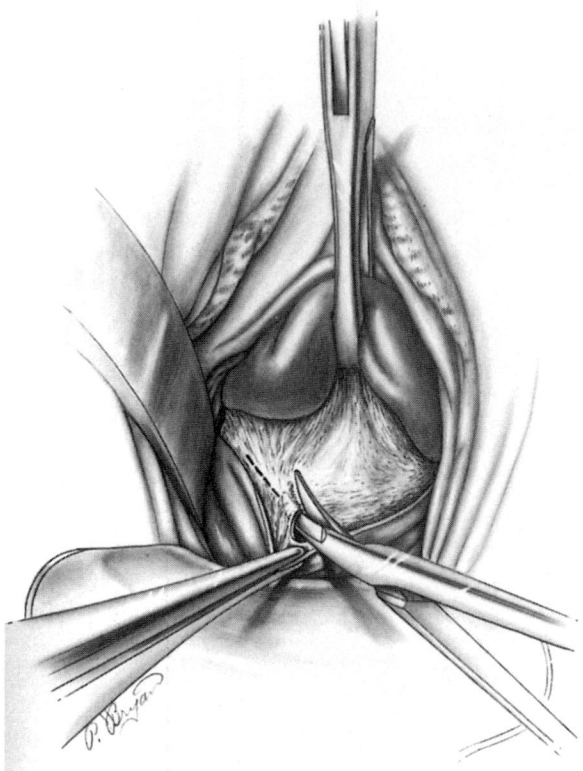

FIGURE 31.14. Dissection in the proper plane leads to the peritoneum, which should be incised with scissors. The peritoneal incision is extended laterally as far as the uterosacral ligaments. The cuff bleeding should be controlled at this point.

The right-handed surgeon next places a Heaney clamp on the left uterosacral ligament as it joins the uterus (Fig. 31.15). Care must be used to ensure that the tip of the Heaney clamp is pushed up against the side of the cervix. The pedicle is cut and sutured with a Heaney stitch. This stitch is held long for later manipulation. A second clamp is now placed on the cardinal ligament. Once again, the tip is placed on the edge of the cervix squeezing it out as the clamp is closed. The other end of the jaw is immediately adjacent to the uterosacral ligament pedicle. Placing the tip against the cervix is important to avoid wandering laterally with the clamp away from the cervix where the ureter might be injured. Placing the other end of the jaw adjacent to the previous pedicle avoids leaving gaps in the clamped and ligated tissue, which may lead to troublesome bleeding. After this clamp has been placed, the cardinal ligament is divided with curved scissors and a Heaney suture ligature is placed. Many surgeons prefer to leave a tag on this suture as well, but I generally cut these ligatures to avoid loosening them with prolonged traction during the course of the surgical procedure. The uterosacral and cardinal ligament on the patient's right side then are clamped, ligated, and divided as described.

At this point, it is important to be sure that the anterior cul-de-sac has been entered, and, if not, this is the time to get in anteriorly. Because the uterosacral and cardinal support has now been divided, usually it is possible to pull the uterus well down into the vagina, affording better exposure so that the bladder peritoneum can be identified and divided. The tip of the curved Dever re-

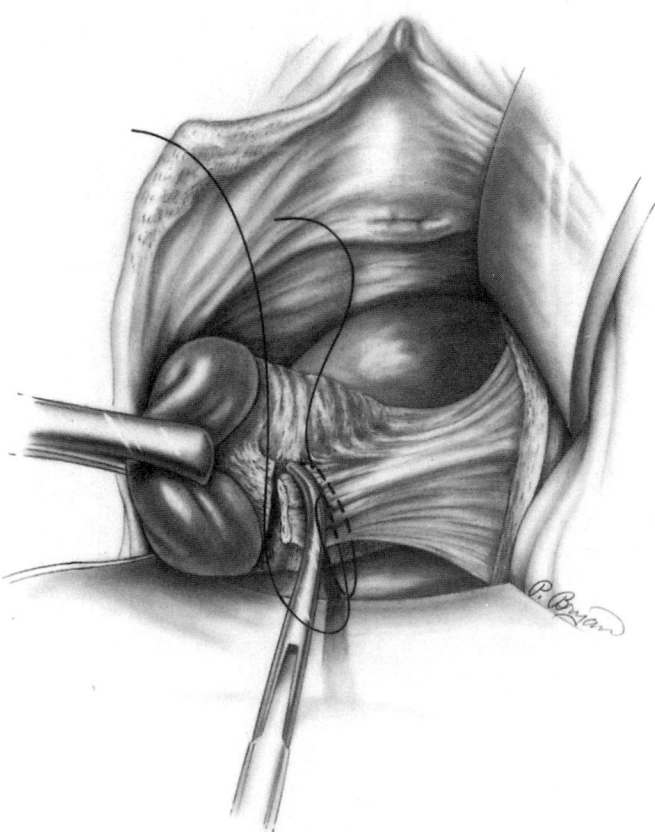

FIGURE 31.15. Staying as close to the uterus as possible, the paracervical uterosacral and cardinal ligament tissue is successively clamped, cut, and ligated with a Heaney clamp and a Heaney transfixion stitch.

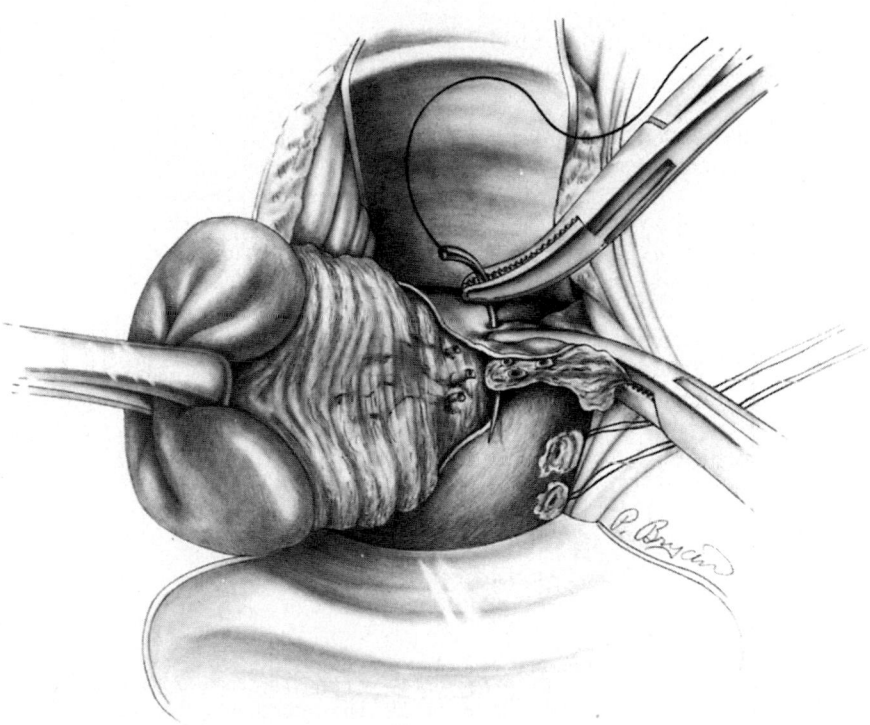

FIGURE 31.16. The uterine vessels are clamped with a single Heaney clamp, which also includes the anterior and posterior peritoneum. This vascular pedicle is doubly ligated with simple suture ligatures.

tractor is placed in the anterior cul-de-sac and the bladder retracted anteriorly. Downward traction is applied to the cervix and a curved Heaney clamp is used to clamp the uterine vessels on each side. Peritoneum should be included in the clamp tip both anteriorly and posteriorly on this bite. Tissue forceps may be used to pull the anterior peritoneum into the clamp jaws, if necessary. The pedicle is divided and the stump of the uterine vessels identified. This pedicle is ligated twice with 0 delayed absorbable sutures (Fig. 31.16).

After the uterine vessels have been secured on both sides, the surgeon places a forefinger behind the uterus and, with the cervix on traction, gently palpates the remaining portion of the broad ligament on each side. If a sharp band of tissue is palpable, it is advisable to place one or more clamps on the remaining broad ligament before attempting to invert the fundus posteriorly. However, if there is no palpable band of tissue, the uterine fundus can be retroverted through the posterior cul-de-sac and curved Heaney clamps used to clamp the upper portion of the broad ligament, including the round ligament and fallopian tube and uteroovarian ligaments. One clamp occasionally can be placed across the structures, but two clamps are required most often, with one being placed through the posterior cul-de-sac, including the fallopian tube and uteroovarian ligament while a second clamp is placed through the anterior cul-de-sac encompassing the upper portion of the broad ligament and round ligaments. The tips of these clamps should meet. A single suture ligature is satisfactory for the round ligament pedicle, but the uteroovarian ligament contains significant blood supply and double ligation with a free-tie followed by a suture ligature is advisable. In some

cases, clamps can be placed on these pedicles on both sides before the uterus is removed, whereas better exposure is obtained in other cases by placing clamps on one side and dividing these pedicles before placing the clamps on the opposite side. After the uterus has been removed, the exposure usually is better and the ties and suture ligatures can be placed more precisely.

At this point, the ovaries should be carefully inspected and the pedicles examined for hemostasis. The bowel can be pushed gently out of the way with a sponge on a ring forceps and the ovaries brought down into the fields for examination. If it is desired to remove the ovaries as part of the operation, the ovaries or fallopian tubes should be grasped with Babcock clamps and brought into the field one at a time. If mobility is a problem, the round ligament pedicle should be clamped separately from the uteroovarian pedicle (Fig. 31.17). Ligating these two separately should improve mobility. With long retractors laterally and anteriorly and the weighted speculum posteriorly, the ovaries and infundibulopelvic ligament should be visualized and a long curved clamp, such as a Zepplin or kidney pedicle clamp, can be used to clamp the infundibulopelvic ligament just above the ovary. A large tissue bundle should not be grasped because the ureter is not far away. The ovaries and fallopian tube are excised and the infundibulopelvic ligament pedicle doubly ligated with a free-tie followed by a suture ligature. The procedure then is repeated on the opposite side.

The cuff and pedicles then are inspected for hemostasis. Bleeding is sometimes found to occur between pedicles where traction has torn the tissue between clamps. These bleeding points may be grasped with an

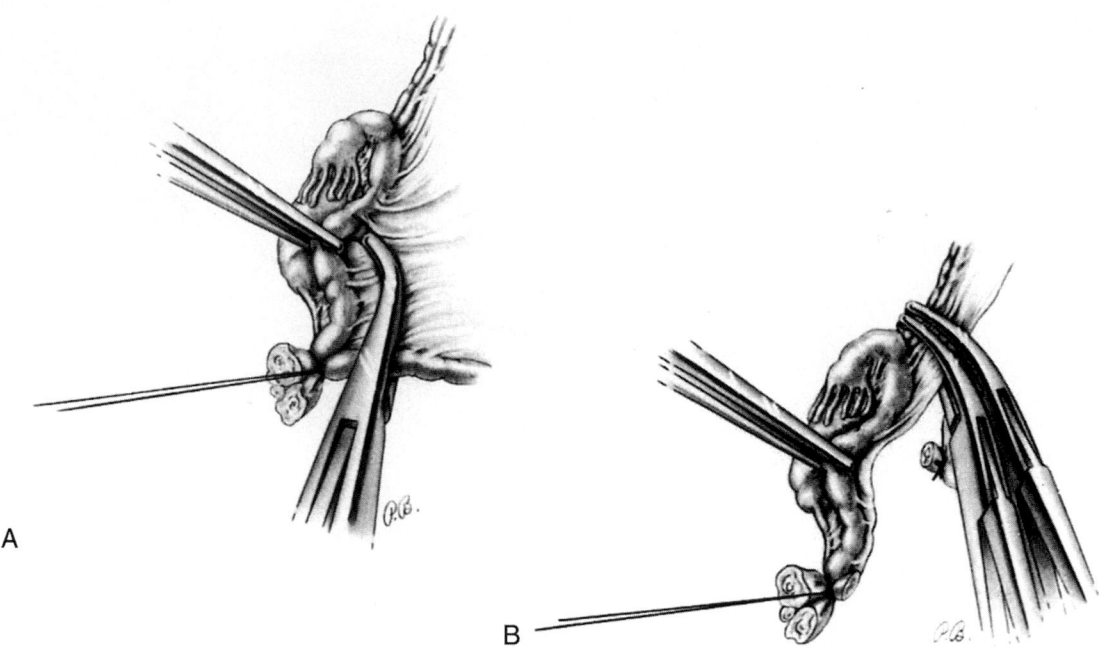

FIGURE 31.17. A: If the ovaries are to be removed, separate clamps are placed on the round ligament and uteroovarian ligament. **B:** The infundibulopelvic ligament must be securely clamped and ligated.

Allis clamp and a mattress suture used to ligate these annoying bleeders. Once again, care should be used to avoid clamping or suturing large pedicles because the ureter may be ligated or kinked.

After the uterus has been removed and hemostasis has been achieved, a careful assessment of the pelvic support should be done. The previously placed sutures on the uterosacral ligaments that have been held long are used to place the uterosacral ligament pedicles on tension and a finger is placed in the posterior cul-de-sac to feel for a potential enterocele. If this finger can be hooked in a pouch of cul-de-sac, a wedge of posterior vaginal mucosa and cul-de-sac should be excised and the uterosacral ligament plicated together in a McCall's culdoplasty to eliminate posthysterectomy enterocele, as described in Chapter 35.

Although some prefer not to close the pelvic peritoneum, I believe it is a good practice because it extraperitonealizes the pedicles, so that if bleeding occurs it will be seen vaginally and any infection of the pedicles is less likely to produce an intrapelvic abscess. A sponge or ring forceps is introduced into the cavity, and the bladder peritoneum gently raked down until its edge can be visualized through the vagina. It is grasped with tissue forceps and a running suture of 2-0 delayed absorbable material is used for a peritoneal purse string closure. The suture is started at 12 o'clock and several bites of peritoneum are taken around the pelvis in a clockwise fashion. Care is taken to avoid suturing vascular pedicles to minimize the risk of hematoma above the previous ligature. After the circular peritoneal pursestring suture has been placed, the pedicles are once again examined before the pursestring is tied down, finally closing the pelvis.

The vaginal cuff then is supported by plicating the uterosacral ligaments and cardinal ligaments together with the vaginal mucosa at the apex of the vagina. Although some surgeons simply tie the ligatures, holding each pedicle together in the midline, we prefer a separate stitch. A suture is passed through the vaginal mucosa lateral to the left uterosacral ligament, then through the ligament, across to the opposite side, through the right uterosacral ligament and then out through the lateral vaginal mucosa. A similar stitch is placed through the cardinal ligament and vaginal mucosa and both sutures then are tied, incorporating the cardinal and uterosacral ligaments into the cuff for support. The posterior vaginal mucosa then is closed with a series of interrupted sutures or, if bleeding on the vaginal cuff has been a problem, a series of figure-of-eight sutures can be used. In most cases, this mucosa is closed vertically, although if it seems to lie in a horizontal fashion, it can be closed horizontally just as well. We generally leave 1 to 2 cm of anterior vaginal mucosa under the bladder open for drainage if there is no bleeding from the vaginal mucosa.

The bladder is emptied with the red rubber catheter. No packing is used in the vagina if only a simple vaginal hysterectomy without repair has been done.

Laparoscopically Assisted Vaginal Hysterectomy

In an LAVH, the uterine artery and vein are ligated transvaginally as would normally be done in a vaginal hysterectomy. In a laparoscopic hysterectomy, the uterine vessels are ligated, coagulated, or stapled via the laparoscope. Several different techniques for total laparoscopic hysterectomy have been described in the literature, but we feel that indications for this procedure are either nonexistent or extremely limited. The procedure requires an extremely experienced laparoscopist and achieves results that are inferior to those of standard abdominal or vaginal hysterectomy with no less morbidity.

LAVH may be indicated when there is suspicious adnexal pathology that can be evaluated laparoscopically. When the benign nature of the situation is identified, the oophorectomy and hysterectomy can be initiated laparoscopically and completed vaginally.

The abdominal laparoscopic approach follows the same sequence as an abdominal hysterectomy. The vaginal portion of the operation is identical to a simple vaginal hysterectomy.

An examination under anesthesia is performed with the patient in the Allen stirrups, and the vagina and perineum as well as the abdomen are prepared and draped. The bladder is catheterized with a Foley catheter, and the cervix grasped with the tenaculum. An intrauterine manipulating device is inserted so that the uterus can be manipulated to facilitate laparoscopy. A small 5-mm incision is made through the umbilicus and the abdomen inflated and distended with carbon dioxide. A 5-mm laparoscopic trocar is introduced, and the laparoscope used to visualize the pelvis and abdomen. If there is an adnexal mass present, it is carefully evaluated for adhesions, external excrescences, or the presence of ascites or metastatic disease. Two lateral trocars are inserted in the lower quadrants, and washings are obtained for cytology, if appropriate.

The uterus is elevated and deviated to one side, and the round ligament on the opposite side is grasped with a bipolar cautery and cauterized. We have used bipolar cautery for hemostasis because it is rapid and inexpensive, but sutures, staples, or clips also can be used. The round ligament is divided with the laparoscopic scissors (Fig. 31.18), and the peritoneum divided cephalad toward the infundibulopelvic ligament. The retroperitoneal space is opened gently with traction on both sides, and the ureter is visualized either transperitoneally or retroperitoneally. The infundibulopelvic ligament is placed on traction and a bipolar cautery used to cauterize the ovarian artery and vein. This should be done as far away from the pelvic sidewall as possible to minimize the risk of injury to the ureter and iliac vessels. When satisfactory desiccation of the tissue has been obtained with cautery, the scissors are used to divide the infundibulopelvic ligament. In many cases, the ligament is only partially transected before additional cautery is required to achieve complete hemostasis. Again, the ovarian vessels also may be sutured, stapled, or clipped. When the infundibulopelvic ligament has been divided completely, the ovary is retracted anteriorly and the posterior peritoneum under the fallopian tube is either torn or divided sharply with the ureter in direct view. This procedure then is repeated on the opposite side. After both ovaries have been freed, the peritoneum over the anterior broad ligament and bladder is divided sharply with the scissors. Hydrodissection can be used to develop the space be-

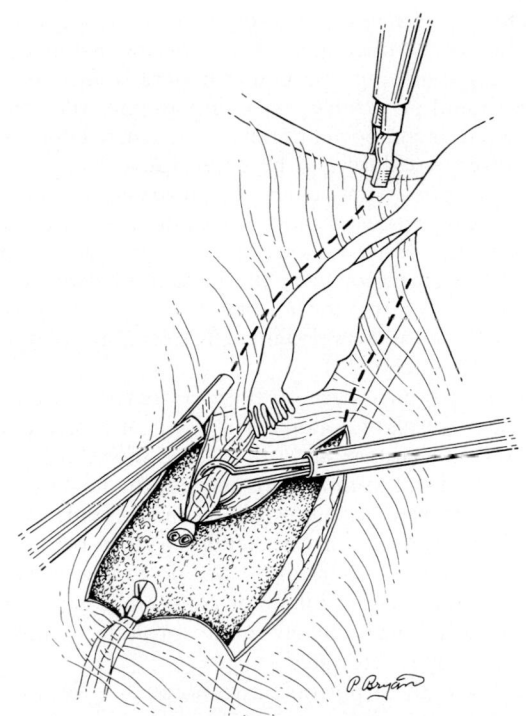

FIGURE 31.18. The round ligament is electrocoagulated and the infundibulopelvic ligament is ligated or coagulated and the peritoneum is divided laterally.

tween the bladder and anterior cervix, but this is not required. At this point, the laparoscopic procedure is completed, and the remainder of the operation is done vaginally, exactly as one would perform a standard vaginal hysterectomy. Because the infundibulopelvic ligaments and round ligaments have already been divided via the laparoscope once the uterine vessels have been ligated from below, there is only minimally fatty, relatively avascular, parametrial tissue to be divided before the uterus can be removed.

Coagulation or stapling of the uterine vessels from above, through the laparoscope, has been associated with a relatively high incidence of ureteral injury; therefore, we recommend vaginal ligation of the uterine vessels.

Once the vaginal hysterectomy has been completed and the peritoneum closed, the laparoscope is used to check the pelvis for hemostasis, and the laparoscopic instruments are removed, the pneumoperitoneum evacuated and the trocar incisions closed.

POSTOPERATIVE CARE

Although routine postoperative care is thoroughly reviewed in Chapter 7, there are several facets that should be emphasized following hysterectomy.

Several studies over the past few years have indicated that early feeding after hysterectomy is safe and actually results in earlier discharge. After vaginal hysterectomy, patients are immediately given a regular diet as soon as postanesthesia nausea resolves. In many cases, patients are also able to tolerate solid food on the first postoperative day following abdominal hysterectomy. The surgeon should nevertheless take into account the amount of dissection and bowel trauma that occurred during the operative procedure and be conservative with the diet orders if a postoperative ileus is anticipated. Patients and their caregivers always should be cautioned not to eat or drink if they feel nauseous or are vomiting. Having a bowel movement or even the passage of flatus are no longer requirements for hospital discharge as long as the patient has good bowel sounds, is tolerating solid food, and is not distended.

Most patients have a Foley catheter for bladder drainage overnight following abdominal hysterectomy, although Richardson and others have shown it is possible to avoid this in most patients with the help of good, enthusiastic anesthesiologists and nursing staff. In most situations, however, a catheter is inserted before hysterectomy and removed on the first postoperative day. In patients with bladder injury or continuous epidural for postoperative pain relief, more prolonged catheter drainage may be indicated.

The length of postoperative hospitalization has decreased dramatically in the last 20 years. Although it was common in the past for women to remain in the hospital for 7 to 10 days after abdominal hysterectomy, most patients are now discharged home in 3 or 4 days. After vaginal hysterectomy, 2- or 3-day hospitalization is the norm; Stovall and others have shown it is possible to discharge many patients less than 24 hours after vaginal hysterectomy. This trend toward a shorter hospital stay requires better patient education and a reasonable home environment to which the patient can be safely and comfortably discharged. The surgeon must also carefully evaluate the patient prior to discharge and resist pressure from insurance companies and hospital administrators when the patient's condition indicates that she is not suitable for an early discharge. The patient and her family must be instructed on proper care. Can she take a bath? Can she go up and down the stairs? Can she pick up her grandchild? How soon can she drive a car? A printed set of instructions for home care as well as answers to frequently asked questions are good ideas. Liberal use of home visiting nurses is also recommended, especially in older or more debilitated patients or in those whose home situation may be less than ideal.

COMPLICATIONS

Complications from hysterectomy can be diagnosed intraoperatively or postoperatively. In a thorough review, Harris found an overall complication rate of up to 50% but serious complications requiring reoperation or long-term disability are relatively uncommon. Reoperation rates of 4% to 4.3% have been reported by Gambone et al. and Brown and Frazer. The most common complications include infection, hemorrhage, and injuries to adjacent organs (Table 31.3). In general, the lowest rates

TABLE 31.3.
Complications of Hysterectomy

Complication	Abdominal	Vaginal	LAVH
Bleeding	1%	0.7%	
Hemorrhage	1%–2%	1%–5%	1%
Transfusion	2%–12%	2%–8.3%	1.58%
Infection			
Unexplained fever	10%–20%	5%–8%	2.14%
Operative site	6.6%–24.7%	3.9%–10%	0.54%
Wound	4%–8%	NA	NA
Pelvic	3.2%–10%	3.9%–10%	1.27%
Urinary tract	1.1%–5%	1.7%–5%	0.81%
Pneumonia	0.4%–2.6%	0.29%–2%	0.11%
Injuries			
Bladder	1%–2%	0.5%–1.5%	1%
Bowel	0.1%–1%	0.1%–0.8%	0.1%–1%
Ureter	0.1%–0.5%	0.05%–0.1%	0.19%
Vesicovaginal fistula	0.1%–0.2%	0.1%–0.2%	0.22%
Trocar injuries	—	—	0.5%

From: Harris WJ. *Obstet Gynecol Surv* 1995;50:795, with permission.

of complication are associated with vaginal hysterectomy. Laparoscopic procedures have their own sets of unique complications related to insertion of the trocars. Prevention and management of hemorrhage, infection, and operative injury complications are extensively discussed in several chapters of this text.

Several factors have been consistently shown to be associated with an increased risk of complications related to hysterectomy. These are increasing age, medical illness, obesity, and malignancy. These conditions are beyond the control of the gynecologic surgeon but they should be considered in the risk:benefit ratio when considering surgery and every effort should be made to have the patient in the best possible condition at the time of surgery.

BIBLIOGRAPHY

ACOG technical bulletin. *Chronic pelvic pain*. 1996;223.

Allen WM, Masters WH. Traumatic laceration of uterine support: the clinical syndrome and the operative treatment. *Am J Obstet Gynecol* 1955;70:500.

Aravantinos DJ. Keeping or removing the ovaries at the time of hysterectomy. *Eur J Obstet Gynecol Reprod Biol* 1988;28:146.

Atkinson SM, Chappell SM. Vaginal hysterectomy for sterilization. *Obstet Gynecol* 1972;39:759.

Atlee WL. Case of successful extirpation of a fibrous tumor of the peritoneal surface of the uterus by the peritoneal section. *Am J Med Sci* 1845;9:26.

Ballard CA. Therapeutic abortion and sterilization by vaginal hysterectomy. *Am J Obstet Gynecol* 1974;118:891.

Barillot I, Horoiot JC, Cuisenier J, et al. Carcinoma of the cervical stump: a review of 213 cases. *Eur J Cancer* 1993;29A:1231.

Berman M, Grosen E. A new method of continuous vaginal cuff closure at abdominal hysterectomy. *Obstet Gynecol* 1994;84:478.

Bernstein S, McGlynn E, Siu A, et al., for the Health Maintenance Organization Quality of Care Consortium. The appropriateness of hysterectomy: a comparison of care in seven health plans. *JAMA* 1993;269:2398.

Black N, Clarke A, Rowe P, et al. A prospective cohort study of the clinical management of total abdominal hysterectomy for benign disease. *J Obstet Gynaecol* 1995;15:394.

Boike G, Elfstrand E, Del Priore G, et al. Laparoscopically assisted vaginal hysterectomy in a university hospital: report of 82 cases and comparison with abdominal and vaginal hysterectomy. *Am J Obstet Gynecol* 1993;168:1690.

Bradham D, Stovall T, Thompson C. Use of GnRH agonist before hysterectomy: a cost simulation. *Obstet Gynecol* 1995; 85:401.

Broder MS, Kanouse DE, Mittman BS, et al. The appropriateness of recommendations for hysterectomy. *Obstet Gynecol* 2000;95:199.

Brook R, for the Health Maintenance Organization Quality of Care Consortium. The appropriateness of hysterectomy: a comparison of care in seven health plans. *JAMA* 1993; 269:2398.

Brooks P, Clouse J, Morris L. Hysterectomy vs. resectoscopic endometrial ablation for the control of abnormal uterine bleeding: a cost-comparative study. *J Reprod Med* 1994;39: 755.

Browne DS, Frazer MI. Hysterectomy revisited. *Aust NZ J Obstet Gynaecol* 1992;31:148.

Bukovsky I, Liftshitz Y, Langer R, et al. Ovarian residual syndrome. *Surg Gynecol Obstet* 1988;167:132.

Burkhart FL, Daly JW. Sciatic and peroneal nerve injury: a complication of vaginal operations. *Obstet Gynecol* 1966;28:99.

Cardosi RJ, Hoffman MS. Determining the best route for hysterectomy. *OBG Mgmt* 2002;July:24.

Carenza L. Keeping or removing the ovaries at the time of hysterectomy. *Eur J Obstet Gynaecol Reprod Biol* 1988;28:155.

Carlson K, Miller B, Flowler F. The Maine Women's Health Study: I. Outcomes of hysterectomy. *Obstet Gynecol* 1994;83:556.

Carlson K, Miller B, Flowler F. The Maine Women's Health Study: II. Outcomes of non-surgical management of leiomyomas, abnormal bleeding, and chronic pelvic pain. *Obstet Gynecol* 1994;83:566.

Carlson K, Nichols D, Schiff I. Indications for hysterectomy. *N Engl J Med* 1993;328:856.

Clarke A, Black N, Rowe P, et al. Indications for and outcome of total abdominal hysterectomy for benign disease: a prospective cohort study. *Br J Obstet Gynaecol* 1995;102: 611.

Cohen MM. Long term risk of hysterectomy after tubal sterilization. *Am J Epidemiol* 1987;125:410.

Copenhaver EH. Vaginal hysterectomy, past, present and future. *Surg Clin North Am* 1980;60:437.

Cruikshank SH. Avoiding ureteral injury during total vaginal hysterectomy. *South Med J* 1985;78:1447.

Cruikshank S, Kovac S. Anterior vaginal wall culdoplasty at vaginal hysterectomy to prevent posthysterectomy anterior vaginal wall prolapse. *Am J Obstet Gynecol* 1996;174:1863.

Dao AH, Cartwright PS. Fallopian tube prolapse following abdominal hysterectomy. *J Tenn Med Assoc* 1987;80:141.

Darai E, Soriano D, Kimata P, et al. Vaginal hysterectomy for enlarged uteri, with or without laparoscopic assistance: randomized study. *Obstet Gynecol* 2001;97:712.

Dexeus S, Munos A, Tusquets JM. Preservation of the ovaries: a controversial subject. *Eur J Obstet Gynaecol Reprod Biol* 1988;28:146.

Domenighetti G, Luraschi P, Gutzwiller F, et al. Effect of information campaign by mass media on hysterectomy rates. *Lancet* 1988;2:1470.

Domengihetti G, Luraschi P, Marazzi A. Hysterectomy and the sex of the gynecologist. *N Engl J Med* 1985;313: 1482.

Dorsey J, Steinberg E, Holtz P. Clinical indications for hysterectomy route: patient characteristics or physician preference? *Am J Obstet Gynecol* 1995;173:1452.

Drife J. Conserving the cervix at hysterectomy. *Br J Obstet Gynaecol* 1994;101:563.

Dunnihoo D, Huddleston H, North S. Femoral nerve palsy as a complication of vaginal hysterectomy: review of the world literature. *J Gynecol Surg* 1994;10:1.

Elkins T, Hopper J, Goodfellow K, et al. Initial report of anatomic and clinical comparison of the sacrospinous ligament fixation to the high McCall culdoplasty for vaginal cuff fixation at hysterectomy for uterine prolapse. *J Pelvic Surg* 1995;1:12.

Ewen S, Sutton C. Initial experience with supracervical laparoscopic hysterectomy and removal of the cervical transformation zone. *Br J Obstet Gynaecol* 1994;101:225.

Fernstrom I. The normal anatomy of the uterine artery. *Acta Radiol* 1955;122(Suppl):21.

Finazzo MS, Hoffman MS, Roberts WS, et al. Previous pelvic surgery in patients with ovarian cancer. *South Med J* 1988;81:1518.

Funt MI, Benigno BB, Thompson JD. The residual adnexa: asset or liability? *Am J Obstet Gynecol* 1977;129:251.

Gambone JC, Lench JB, Slesinski MJ, et al. Validation of hysterectomy indications and the quality assurance process. *Obstet Gynecol* 1989;75:1045.

Gambone JC, Reiter RC, Lench JB. Quality assurance indicators and short-term outcome of hysterectomy. *Obstet Gynecol* 1990;76:841.

Gambone J, Reiter R, Lench JB, et al. The impact of a quality assurance process on the frequency and confirmation rate of hysterectomy. *Am J Obstet Gynecol* 1990;163:545.

Garry R. Initial experience with laparoscopic-assisted Doderlein hysterectomy. *Br J Obstet Gynaecol* 1995;102:307.

Goldman JA, Feldberg D, Dicker D, et al. Femoral neuropathy subsequent to abdominal hysterectomy: a comparative study. *Eur J Obstet Gynaecol Reprod Biol* 1985;20: 385.

Gray LA. Indications, techniques, and complications in vaginal hysterectomy. *Obstet Gynecol* 1966;28:714.

Gray LA. Open cuff method of abdominal hysterectomy. *Obstet Gynecol* 1975;46:42.

Gray LA. *Vaginal hysterectomy.* Springfield, IL: Charles C Thomas, 1963.

Griffith-Jones MD, Jarvis GJ, McNamara HM. Adverse urinary symptoms after total abdominal hysterectomy: fact or fiction. *Br J Urol* 1991;67:295.

Grody M. Vaginal hysterectomy: the large uterus. *J Gynecol Surg* 1989;5:301.

Haas S, Acker D, Donahue C, et al. Variation in hysterectomy rates across small geographic areas of Massachusetts. *Am J Obstet Gynecol* 1993;169:150.

Hacker NF, Charles EH, Savage EW. Postcoital posthysterectomy vaginal vault disruption with hemorrhagic shock. *Aust NZ J Obstet Gynaecol* 1980;20:182.

Hankinson S, Hunter D, Colditz G, et al. Tubal ligation, hysterectomy, and risk of ovarian cancer: a prospective study. *JAMA* 1993;270:2813.

Harris W. Early complications of abdominal and vaginal hysterectomy. *Obstet Gynecol Surv* 1995;50:795.

Harris M, Olive D. Changing hysterectomy patterns after introduction of laparoscopically assisted vaginal hysterectomy. *Am J Obstet Gynecol* 1994;171:340.

Hasson HM. Cervical removal at hysterectomy for benign disease: risks and benefits. *J Reprod Med* 1993;38:781.

Heaney NS. A report of 565 vaginal hysterectomies performed for benign pelvic disease. *Am J Obstet Gynecol* 1934;28:751.

Helstrom L, Lundberg PO, Sorbom D, et al. Sexuality after hysterectomy: a factor analysis of women's sexual lives before and after subtotal hysterectomy. *Obstet Gynecol* 1993;81:357.

Hemsell DL, Johnson ER, Hemsell PG, et al. Cefazolin for hysterectomy prophylaxis. *Obstet Gynecol* 1990;76:603.

Hendricks-Mathews M. The importance of assessing a woman's history of sexual abuse before hysterectomy. *J Fam Prac* 1991;32:631.

Henrotin F. Vaginal hysterectomy. In: Kelly HA, Noble CP, eds. *Gynecology and abdominal surgery.* Philadelphia: WB Saunders, 1910:759.

Hillis S, Marchbanks P, Peterson H. The effectiveness of hysterectomy for chronic pelvic pain. *Obstet Gynecol* 1995;86:941.

Hillis S, Marchbanks P, Peterson H. Uterine size and risks of complications among women undergoing abdominal hysterectomy for leiomyomas. *Obstet Gynecol* 1996;87:539.

Hoffmann M, DeCesare S, Kalter C. Abdominal hysterectomy versus transvaginal morcellation for the removal of enlarged uteri. *Am J Obstet Gynecol* 1994;171:309.

Howard F. The role of laparoscopy in chronic pelvic pain: promise and pitfalls. *Obstet Gynecol Surv* 1993;48:357.

Irwin KL, Lee NC, Peterson HB, et al. Hysterectomy, tubal sterilization, and the risk of breast cancer. *Am J Epidemiol* 1988;127:1192.

Irwin KL, Weiss NS, Lee NC, et al. Tubal sterilization, hysterectomy, and the subsequent occurrence of epithelial ovarian cancer. *Am J Epidemiol* 1991;134:362.

Isaacs JH. Vaginal hysterectomy and vaginal repair. In: Breen JL, Osofsky HJ, eds. *Current concepts in gynecologic surgery.* Baltimore: Williams & Wilkins, 1987:81.

Jacobs I, Oram D. Prevention of ovarian cancer: a survey of the practice of prophylactic oophorectomy by fellows and members of the Royal College of Obstetricians and Gynaecologists. *Br J Obstet Gynaecol* 1989;96:510.

Jaszczak SE, Evans TN. Intrafascial abdominal and vaginal hysterectomy: a reappraisal. *Obstet Gynecol* 1982;59:435.

Jelen I, Bachmann G. An anatomical approach to oophorectomy during vaginal hysterectomy. *Obstet Gynecol* 1996;87:137.

Johns D. Laparoscopically assisted vaginal hysterectomy: a cost-effective approach. *Female Patient* 1994;19:46.

Johns D, Carrera B, Jones J, et al. The medical and economic impact of laparoscopically assisted vaginal hysterectomy in a large, metropolitan, not-for-profit hospital. *Am J Obstet Gynecol* 1995;172:1709.

Kauf ND, Satagopan JM, Robson ME, et al. Risk-reducing salpingo-oophorectomy in women with a BRCA1 or BRCA2 mutation. *NEJM* 2002;356:1609.

Kelly HA. Ligature of the trunks of the uterine and ovarian arteries as a means of checking hemorrhage from the uterus and broad ligaments in abdominal operations. *Johns Hopkins Hospital Rep* 1891;2:220.

Kelly HA. *Operative gynecology.* New York: Appleton, 1896.

Kelly HA. *Operative gynecology,* vol 2. New York: Appleton & Company, 1901.

Kelly HA, Cullen TS. *Myomata of the uterus.* Philadelphia: WB Saunders, 1909.

Kelly HA, Noble CP. *Gynecology and abdominal surgery,* vol 1. Philadelphia: WB Saunders, 1907.

Kerlikourske K, Brown J, Grady D. Should women with familial ovarian cancer undergo prophylactic oophorectomy? *Obstet Gynecol* 1992;80:700.

Kohli N, Mallipeddi PK, Neff JM, et al. Routine hematocrit after elective gynecologic surgery. *Obstet Gynecol* 2000;95:847.

Kovac S. Guidelines to determine the route of hysterectomy. *Obstet Gynecol* 1995;85:18.

Kovac SR. Hysterectomy outcomes in patients with similar indications. *Obstet Gynecol* 2000;95:787.

Kovac SR. Intramyometrial coring as an adjunct to vaginal hysterectomy. *Obstet Gynecol* 1986;67:131.

Kovac SR, Cruikshank SH, Retto HF. Laparoscopy assisted vaginal hysterectomy. *J Gynecol Surg* 1990;6:185.

Lalinec-Michaud M, Englesmann F. Depression and hysterectomy: a prospective study. *Psychosomatics* 1984;25:550.

Lalinec-Michaud M, Engelsmann F, Marino J. Depression after hysterectomy: a comparative study. *Psychosomatics* 1988;29:307.

Langer R, Neuman M, Ron-el R, et al. The effect of total abdominal hysterectomy on bladder function in asymptomatic women. *Obstet Gynecol* 1989;74:205.

Lash AF, Stepto RC. Chicago technique for vaginal hysterectomy at the Cook County Hospital. *Clin Obstet Gynecol* 1972;15:755.

Lazarus ML, Levanthol ML. Total abdominal and vaginal hysterectomy: a comparison. *Am J Obstet Gynecol* 1985;61:2.

Lipscomb G, Ling F, Stovall T, et al. Peritoneal closure at vaginal hysterectomy: a reassessment. *Obstet Gynecol* 1996;87:40.

Luoto R, Kaprio J, Reunanen A, et al. Cardiovascular morbidity in relation to ovarian function after hysterectomy. *Obstet Gynecol* 1995;85:515.

Lynch HT, Harris RE, Guirgis HA, et al. Familial association of breast/ovarian carcinoma. *Cancer* 1978;41:1543.

Lynch HT, Lynch PM. Tumor variation in the cancer family syndrome: ovarian cancer. *Am J Surg* 1979;138:439.

Lyons TL. Laparoscopic supracervical hysterectomy. *Obstet Gynecol Clin North Am* 2000;27:441.

Magos A, Bournas N, Sinha R, et al. Vaginal hysterectomy for the large uterus. *Br J Obstet Gynaecol* 1996;103:246.

Manyonda IT, Welch CR, McWhinney NA, et al. The influence of suture material on vaginal vault granulations following abdominal hysterectomy. *Br J Obstet Gynaecol* 1990;97:608.

Mathieu A. History of hysterectomy. *West J Surg Obstet Gynecol* 1934;42:2.

Mazdisnian F, Kurzel R, Coe S, et al. Vaginal hysterectomy by uterine morcellation: an efficient, non-morbid procedure. *Obstet Gynecol* 1995;86:60.

McCall ML. Posterior culdoplasty. *Obstet Gynecol* 1957;10:595.

Mead PB, Eschenbach DA, Ledger WJ, et al. Reconsidering bacterial vaginosis. *Contemp Obstet Gynecol* 1989;34:76.

Morgan K, Thomas E. Nerve injury at abdominal hysterectomy. *Br J Obstet Gynaecol* 1995;102:665.

Moschowitz AV. The pathogenesis, anatomy, and cure of prolapse of the rectum. *Surg Gynecol Obstet* 1912;15:7.

Munro M, Deprest J. Laparoscopic hysterectomy: does it work? A bicontinental review of the literature and clinical commentary. *Clin Obstet Gynecol* 1995;38:401.

Muntz HG, Falkenberry S, Fuller AF. Fallopian tube prolapse after hysterectomy: a report of two cases. *J Reprod Med* 1988;33:467.

Nathorst-Boos J, Fuchs T, von Schoultz B. Consumer's attitude to hysterectomy: the experience of 678 women. *Acta Obstet Gynecol Scand* 1992;71:230.

Nehra PC, Loginsky SJ. Pregnancy after vaginal hysterectomy. *Obstet Gynecol* 1984;64:735.

Neuman M, Beller U, Chetrit A, et al. Prophylactic effect of the open vaginal vault method in reducing febrile morbidity in abdominal hysterectomy. *Surg Gynecol Obstet* 1993;176:591.

Nezhat C, Bess O, Admon D, et al. Hospital cost comparison between abdominal, vaginal, and laparoscopy-assisted vaginal hysterectomies. *Obstet Gynecol* 1994;83:713.

Nezhat F, Nezhat C, Gordon S, et al. Laparoscopic versus abdominal hysterectomy. *J Reprod Med* 1992;37:247.

Nezhat C, Nezhat F, Seidman D, et al. Vaginal vault evisceration after total laparoscopic hysterectomy. *Obstet Gynecol* 1996;87:868.

Nichols DH, Randall CL. *Vaginal surgery,* third ed. Baltimore: Williams & Wilkins, 1989.

Nichols DH, Willey PS, Randall CL. Significance of restoration of normal vaginal depth and axis. *Obstet Gynecol* 1970; 36:251.

Olsson J, Ellstrom M, Hahlin M. A randomized prospective trial comparing laparoscopic and abdominal hysterectomy. *Br J Obstet Gynaecol* 1996;103:345.

Ostrzenski A. A new, simplified posterior culdoplasty and vaginal vault suspension during abdominal hysterectomy. *Int J Obstet Gynecol* 1995;49:25.

Papanicolaou GN, Traut HF. The diagnostic value of vaginal smears in carcinoma of the uterus. *Am J Obstet Gynecol* 1941;42:193.

Parazzini F, Negri E, Vecchia C, et al. Hysterectomy, oophorectomy, and subsequent ovarian cancer risk. *Obstet Gynecol* 1993;81.363.

Parker WH. Total laparoscopic hysterectomy. *Obstet Gynecol Clin North Am* 2000;27:431.

Parker W, Fu Y, Berek J. Uterine sarcoma in patients operated on for presumed leiomyoma and rapidly growing leiomyoma. *Obstet Gynecol* 1994;83:414.

Parys BT, Haylen BT, Hutton JL, et al. The effects of simple hysterectomy on vesicourethral function. *Br J Urol* 1989; 64:594.

Pelosi M, Kadar N. Laparoscopically assisted hysterectomy for uteri weighing 500 g or more. *J Am Assoc Gynecol Laparosc* 1994;1:405.

Pelosi M, Pelosi M III. Laparoscopic supracervical hysterectomy using a single-umbilical puncture (mini-laparoscopy). *J Reprod Med* 1992;37:777.

Pelosi M, Pelosi M III. Randomized comparison of laparoscopy-assisted vaginal hysterectomy with standard vaginal hysterectomy in an outpatient setting. *Obstet Gynecol* 1993;81:800.

Pinion S, Parkin D, Abramovich D, et al. Randomized trial of hysterectomy, endometrial ablation, and transcervical endometrial resection for dysfunctional uterine bleeding. *Br Med J* 1994;309:979.

Piscitelli J, Bastian L, Wilkes A, et al. Cytologic screening after hysterectomy for benign disease. *Am J Obstet Gynecol* 1995;173:24.

Piver MS. Hereditary ovarian cancer. *Gynecol Oncol* 2002;85:9.

Pratt JH. Vaginal hysterectomy by morcellation. *Mayo Clin Proc* 1978;43:374.

Prior A, Stanley K, Smith ARB, et al. Effect of hysterectomy on anorectal and urethrovesical physiology. *Gut* 1992;33:264.

Raju K. A randomized prospective study of laparoscopic vaginal hysterectomy versus abdominal hysterectomy each with bilateral salpingo-oophorectomy. *Br J Obstet Gynaecol* 1994;101:1068.

Randall CL, Hall DW, Armenia CS. Pathology in the preserved ovary after unilateral oophorectomy. *Am J Obstet Gynecol* 1962;84:1233.

Ramirez PT, Klemer DP. Vaginal evisceration after hysterectomy: a literature review. *Obstet Gynecol Surv* 2002;57:462.

Ranney B. Multiple diagnoses and procedures during hysterectomy. *Int J Gynecol Obstet* 1990;33:325.

Rebbeck TR, Lynch HT, Neuhausen SL, et al. Prophylactic oophorectomy in carriers of BRCA1 or BRCA2 mutations. *NEJM* 2002;346:1616.

Redeimeier D, Rozin P, Kahneman D. Understanding patients' decisions: cognitive and emotional perspectives. *JAMA* 1993;270:72.

Reich H, McGlynn F, Sekel L. Total laparoscopic hysterectomy. *Gynaecol Endosc* 1993;2:59.

Reiter R, Gambone J, Lench J. Appropriateness of hysterectomies performed for multiple preoperative indications. *Obstet Gynecol* 1992;80:902.

Reiter R, Wagner P, Gambone J. Routine hysterectomy for large asymptomatic uterine leiomyomata: a reappraisal. *Obstet Gynecol* 1992;79:481.

Richards DH. A post-hysterectomy syndrome. *Lancet* 1974;2: 983.

Richardson AC, Lyon JB, Graham EE. Abdominal hysterectomy: relationship between morbidity and surgical technique. *Am J Obstet Gynecol* 1973;115:514.

Richardson EH. A simplified technique for abdominal panhysterectomy. *Surg Obstet Gynecol* 1929;48:248.

Richardson R, Bournas N, Magos A. Is laparoscopic hysterectomy a waste of time? *Lancet* 1995;345:36.

Riedel H-H, Leihmann-Willenbrock E, Semm K. Ovarian failure phenomena after hysterectomy. *J Reprod Med* 1986;31:597.

Roman L, Morris M, Eifel P, et al. Reasons for inappropriate simple hysterectomy in the presence of invasive cancer of the cervix. *Obstet Gynecol* 1992;79:485.

Rudy D, Bush I. Sexual dysfunction after hysterectomy. *Contemp Obstet Gynecol* 1993;38:39.

Schilling J, Wyss P, Faisst K, et al. Swiss consensus guidelines for hysterectomy. *Int J Gynecol Obstet* 1999;64:297.

Senior CC, Steigrad SJ. Are preoperative antibiotics helpful in abdominal hysterectomy? *Am J Obstet Gynecol* 1986;154:1004.

Sheth S. The place of oophorectomy at vaginal hysterectomy. *Br J Obstet Gynaecol* 1991;98:662.

Siddle-N, Sarrel P, Whithead M. The effect of hysterectomy on the age at ovarian failure: identification of a subgroup of women with premature loss of ovarian function and literature review. *Fertil Steril* 1987;47:94.

Sightler S, Boike G, Estape R, et al. Ovarian cancer in women with prior hysterectomy: a 14-year experience at the University of Miami. *Obstet Gynecol* 1991;78:681.

Simel D, Matchar DB, Piscitelli JT. Routine intravenous pyelograms before hysterectomy in cases of benign disease: possibly effective, definitely expensive. *Am J Obstet Gynecol* 1988;159:1049.

Smith HO, Thompson JD. Indications and technique for vaginal hysterectomy. *Contemp Obstet Gynecol* 1986:28:125.

Souza AZ, Fonseca AM, Izzo VM, et al. Ovarian histology and function after total abdominal hysterectomy. *Obstet Gynecol* 1986;68:847.

Speroff T, Dawson NV, Speroff L, et al. A risk-benefit analysis of elective bilateral oophorectomy: effect of changes in compliance with estrogen therapy on outcome. *Am J Obstet Gynecol* 1991;164:165.

Stergachis A, Kirkwood KS, Grothaus LC, et al. Tubal sterilization and the long-term risk of hysterectomy. *JAMA* 1990;264:2893.

Storm HH, Clemmenson IH, Manders T, et al. Supravaginal uterine amputation in Denmark 1978-1988 and risk of cancer. *Gynecol Oncol* 1992;45:198.

Stovall TG, Ling F, Crawford D. Hysterectomy for chronic pelvic pain of presumed uterine etiology. *Obstet Gynecol* 1990;75:676.

Stovall T, Muneyyirci-Delale O, Summitt R, et al., for the Leuprolide Acetate Study Group. GnRH agonist and iron versus placebo and iron in the anemic patient before surgery for leiomyomas: a randomized controlled trial. *Obstet Gynecol* 1995;86:65.

Stovall T, Summitt R, Bran D, et al. Outpatient vaginal hysterectomy: a pilot study. *Obstet Gynecol* 1992;80:145.

Stovall T, Summit R, Lipscomb G, et al. Vaginal cuff closure at abdominal hysterectomy: comparing sutures with absorbable staples. *Obstet Gynecol* 1991;78:415.

Summitt R, Stovall T, Bran D. Prospective comparison of indwelling bladder catheter after vaginal hysterectomy. *Am J Obstet Gynecol* 1994;170:1815.

Summitt RL Jr, Stovall TG, Lipscomb GH, et al. Randomized comparison of laparoscopy assisted vaginal hysterectomy with standard vaginal hysterectomy in an outpatient setting. *Obstet Gynecol* 1992;80:895.

Summitt R, Stovall T, Lipscomb G, et al. Outpatient hysterectomy: determinants of discharge and rehospitalization in 133 patients. *Am J Obstet Gynecol* 1994;171:1480.

Sutton C. Treatment of large uterine fibroids. *Br J Obstet Gynaecol* 1996;103:494.

Symmonds RE, Pettit PDM. Ovarian remnant syndrome. *Obstet Gynecol* 1979;54:174.

Taylor HC Jr. Vascular congestion and hyperemia. Part II. The clinical aspects of the congestion fibrosis syndrome. *Am J Obstet Gynecol* 1949;57:637.

Taylor HC Jr. Vascular congestion and hyperemia. Part III. Etiology and therapy. *Am J Obstet Gynecol* 1949;57:654.

Thompson JD, Birch HW. Indications for hysterectomy. *Clin Obstet Gynecol* 1981;24:1245.

Vessy M, Villard-MacKintosh L, McPherson K, et al. The epidemiology of hysterectomy: findings in a large cohort study. *Br J Obstet Gynaecol* 1992;99:402.

Vietz P, Ahn S. A new approach to hysterectomy without colpotomy: pelviscopic intrafascial hysterectomy. *Am J Obstet Gynecol* 1994;170:609.

Wall L. A technique for modified McCall culdoplasty at the time of abdominal hysterectomy. *J Am Coll Surg* 1994;178:507.

Watson T. Vaginal cuff closure with abdominal hysterectomy: a new approach. *J Reprod Med* 1994;39:903.

Weiss NS, Harlow BL. Why does hysterectomy without bilateral oophorectomy influence the subsequent incidence of ovarian cancer? *Am J Epidemiol* 1986;124:856.

Wilcox L, Koonin L, Pokras R, et al. Hysterectomy in the United States, 1988–1990. *Obstet Gynecol* 1994;83:549.

Wingo PA, Huezo CM, Rubin GL, et al. The mortality risk associated with hysterectomy. *Am J Obstet Gynecol* 1985;152:803.

Wuest JH, Dry TJ, Edwards JE. The degree of coronary atherosclerosis in bilaterally oophorectomized women. *Circulation* 1950;1:1345.

Zakut H, Lotan M, Bracha Y. Vaginal preparation with povidone-iodine before abdominal hysterectomy: a comparison with antibiotic prophylaxis. *Clin Exp Obstet Gynecol* 1987;14:1.

Te Linde's Operative Gynecology, ninth edition, edited by John A. Rock and Howard W. Jones, III. Lippincott Williams & Wilkins, Philadelphia: © 2003.

CHAPTER

32

▼

Gynecologic Surgery for Obstetric Patients

LYNN P. PARKER   JOSEPH BRUNER

A

▼

Obstetric Problems

LYNN P. PARKER

HYSTERECTOMY FOR OBSTETRIC PROBLEMS

Horatio Storer performed the first caesarean hysterectomy in 1869. Initially the procedure was performed only for emergency situations, but in the early 20th century it became an accepted means of sterilization. As other forms of sterilization such as tubal ligation became accepted, the procedure once again has become limited to treatment of hemorrhage and a few other specific indications.

Peripartum hysterectomy can be performed in conjunction with a caesarean delivery (e.g., caesarean hysterectomy) or after a vaginal delivery for complications such as postpartum hemorrhage. The procedure also can be performed for either elective or emergency reasons. Although classified as elective, these procedures are most often performed for specific indications, such as uterine

leiomyomata. The term elective is used in this chapter in the context of indicated but nonemergency reasons.

Although there is little controversy regarding peripartum hysterectomy for emergency conditions, there is significant debate in modern obstetrics regarding an elective hysterectomy performed at the time of caesarean delivery. There has been legitimate concern about increased morbidity from peripartum hysterectomy, including damage to surrounding structures and possible reoperation. However, Plauché has pointed out that morbidity often is associated with the conditions leading to the hysterectomy and not necessarily the procedure itself. Lower morbidities have been reported for elective caesarean hysterectomies when compared with emergency hysterectomies. However, there is inherent bias in these retrospective reviews. Emergent surgery for life-saving maternal indications would be expected to have higher morbidities, such as blood loss and injury to sur-

829

rounding structures. Unfortunately, there are no randomized prospective studies of elective caesarean hysterectomy, and it is unlikely that such a study ever will be done in modern obstetrics.

Emergency Peripartum Hysterectomy

There are several indications for emergency peripartum hysterectomy. The three most common reasons are uterine rupture, abnormal placentation, and uterine atony. Although the exact incidence of emergency peripartum hysterectomy is not known, several authors have reported a rate of 0.004 to 1.5 per 1,000.

Obstetric hemorrhage secondary to a variety of etiologies is a common indication reported for peripartum emergency hysterectomy. Clark and associates reviewed 70 cases of emergency hysterectomy for obstetric hemorrhage. Sixty (86%) of these procedures were performed after caesarean delivery and 10 (14%) were performed after vaginal delivery. Uterine atony and placenta accreta accounted for almost three fourths of the cases. Other indications were uterine rupture, extension of the uterine incision, and fibroids precluding closure of the uterine incision.

Chestnut and associates reported that in 44 women undergoing emergency hysterectomy, 20 (45%) procedures were performed for uterine rupture, seven (16%) were performed for uterine atony, and four (9%) were performed for placenta accreta. Other indications included broad ligament hematoma, placenta previa, and chorioamnionitis. Twenty-nine of the cases in this series were emergency caesarean hysterectomies, and 15 were postpartum hysterectomies.

Zelop and colleagues reported that in 117 cases of peripartum hysterectomy, uterine atony accounted for 25 (21%) of the cases, and most (75, or 64%) were secondary to abnormally adherent placentation. The rate of emergent hysterectomy increased with increasing parity, placenta previa, and history of previous caesarean section.

It is clear from the recent literature that abnormal adherent placentation or placenta accreta (with or without hemorrhage) is emerging as the most common condition leading to an emergency hysterectomy. In four studies from 1993 to the present, 190 (47.7%) of the 398 emergent peripartum hysterectomies were performed owing to placenta accreta. Four of these studies are outlined in Table 32A.1. The increase in placenta accreta is no doubt related to the high caesarean delivery rate in this country, which has quadrupled over the last 25 years. Placenta previa also is significantly associated with placenta accreta. Zelop et al. reported the risk of peripartum hysterectomy in women with placenta previa increases from seven per 1,000 deliveries in nulliparous women to one in four deliveries in women with four or more live births. Clark and colleagues also reported that with placenta previa and one previous caesarean delivery, the risk of a placenta accreta was 24%, a risk that increased as the number of caesarean deliveries increased.

Zorlu et al., evaluated the indications for emergent hysterectomy in two distinct time periods. Forty-three patients underwent emergent hysterectomy between 1985 and 1989. The incidence of hysterectomy was one in 2,495 deliveries and the indications for hysterectomy included uterine atony (42%), placenta accreta (25.5%), and uterine rupture (21%). Between 1990 and 1994, the incidence of hysterectomy decreased to one in 4,228 deliveries. In this group, the indications for hysterectomy were placenta accreta (41.7%), uterine atony (29.2%), and uterine rupture (20.8%). The authors felt the increase in placenta accreta as an indication for emergent hysterectomy most likely reflected an increase in the caesarean section rate nationwide.

Elective Caesarean Hysterectomy

Numerous conditions have been reported as indications for elective caesarean hysterectomy. Some of the more common ones include uterine leiomyomata, cervical intraepithelial neoplasia or microinvasive cervical cancer, and menstrual abnormalities. In retrospective reviews that go back to the 1950s and 1960s, sterilization is listed as an indication, but it is also the most controversial. Many of the women who undergo elective hysterectomy also have one or more other indications for the procedure. Chronic pelvic pain, menstrual abnormalities, chorioamnionitis, and perhaps placenta previa without accreta are indications that probably engender significant

TABLE 32A.1.
Indications for Emergency Hysterectomy for Obstetric Hemorrhage

Indication	Clark et al., 1984 (*n* = 70)	Bakshi et al., 2000 (*n* = 39)	Stanco et al., 1993 (*n* = 123)	Zelop et al., 1993 (*n* = 117)
Uterine atony/hemorrhage	30 (43%)	11 (28%)	44 (35.9%)	25 (21.3%)
Placenta accrete/percreta	21 (30%)	20 (51%)	61 (49%)	75 (64.1%)
Uterine rupture	9 (13%)	5 (15%)	14 (11.5%)	—
Extension of uterine incision	7 (10%)	—	—	—
Leiomyomas	3 (4%)	2 (5%)	3 (2.4%)	—
Uterine infection	—	—	—	17 (14.5%)
Other	—	1(1%)	1(1.2%)	—

TABLE 32A.2.
Surgical Complications of Caesarean Hysterectomy: Literature Review 1951 to 1984 ($n = 5,220$)

Indication	Number	Percentage
Postoperative hemorrhage	172	3.3
Bladder laceration	144	2.8
Ureteral injury	23	0.44
Fistula		
Vesicovaginal	24	0.46
Uterovaginal	5	0.1
Rectovaginal	1	0.02
Total	30	0.57
Thromboembolic events	27	0.52
Puerperal morbidity	35.3	
(mean of 10 studies reporting)		
Maternal mortality	38	0.73

From: Plauché WC. Cesarean hysterectomy: indications, technique, and complications. *Clin Obstet Gynecol* 1986;29:318, with permission.

controversy. A good case either for or against each of these indications can be made depending on the surgeon's training, experience, and philosophy. In general, however, as these indications increase in number, the issue becomes less controversial.

Morbidity and Mortality of Hysterectomy

As stated, the condition leading to emergency hysterectomy also is responsible for much of the morbidity reported with the procedure. Two other important factors associated with morbidity, both of which are difficult to quantify, are training and experience (or surgical skill) of the surgeon. Chestnut and associates reported statistically significant reductions in operative time, estimated blood loss, intraoperative and total blood replacement, and length of hospital stay if the patient was in the care of an experienced surgeon. It seems reasonable, however, to conclude that morbidity and complications are higher in women undergoing emergency versus elective

procedures despite the skill of the surgeon. Plauché's summary of the operative and postoperative complications of caesarean hysterectomy from a literature review of over 5,000 such procedures is presented in Table 32A.2.

Morbidity of Emergency Hysterectomy

Zelop and associates (1993) reported 102 (87%) of the patients in their series required transfusion of blood products. Complications of four series, totaling 349 cases of emergency peripartum hysterectomy, are summarized in Table 32A.3. Maternal mortality rates in these studies varied between 0% and 4.5%. As with morbidity, mortality is better correlated with the specific complication than with the hysterectomy per se.

Morbidity of Elective Caesarean Hysterectomy

In a review of 80 women undergoing elective caesarean hysterectomy, McNulty reported that only five (6%) experienced febrile morbidity, and 15 (19%) received blood transfusion. Four (5%) women sustained bladder injuries and four (5%) women developed broad ligament hematomas. However, Strickland et al. also reviewed 188 patients who had undergone elective caesarean hysterectomy. In their study, 40% of patients undergoing elective hysterectomy had estimated blood loss greater than 1,000 cc, 21% risk of infection, and four patients (2%) needed cystotomy. Yancey and colleagues compared the outcomes in 43 women undergoing scheduled caesarean hysterectomy with those in 86 women who underwent caesarean delivery and subsequent scheduled hysterectomy. Although women in the caesarean hysterectomy group were more likely to need a blood transfusion than were women in the subsequent hysterectomy group (odds ratio 3.4; 95% confidence interval of 1.4 to 8.4), they were less likely to have other complications, such as infection (odds ratio 0.34; 95% confidence interval of 0.25 to 0.45). The overall postoperative complication rate was the same in both groups (51%). Thus, it is likely that elective caesarean hysterectomy is not associated

TABLE 32A.3.
Complications of 349 Cases of Emergency Peripartum Hysterectomy

Complication Incidence (%)

	Clark et al. ($n = 70$)	Bakshi et al. ($n = 39$)	Stanco et al. ($n = 123$)	Zelop et al. ($n = 117$)
Infection	50	20.5	9	50
Wound infection	12	—	9	3.4
Blood transfusion	96	80	82	87
Coagulopathy	6	2.5	5.7	27
Urologic injury	4	7.7	13	10.2
Death	1	0	0	0

with an increased risk of complications or morbidity compared with a caesarean delivery followed by an elective hysterectomy at a later time. However, in a healthy population, one must weigh the infectious risk of blood transfusion versus the benefit of the combined procedure. As pointed out by Baker and D'Alton, there is little doubt that elective caesarean hysterectomy does result in increased morbidity when compared with a caesarean delivery and a tubal ligation.

Emergency Versus Elective Hysterectomy

In two studies comparing emergency with elective peripartum hysterectomy, morbidity was greater when associated with the emergency procedure. Estimated blood loss, number of women transfused, and operating time were all higher in the emergency group (Table 32A.4).

Caesarean Hysterectomy Technique

Elective caesarean hysterectomy can be accomplished through either a midline or low transverse (Pfannenstiel) skin incision. Often it is more prudent to use a midline skin incision in cases of emergency peripartum hysterectomy if one anticipates that a hypogastric artery ligation may be required.

After the caesarean delivery, the placenta is quickly removed unless there is a contraindication to do so. No attempt is made to remove the placenta in cases of placenta accreta because significant life-threatening hemorrhage can ensue. In cases of placenta percreta involving the posterior wall of the bladder, a partial cystectomy may be required. In these cases, the bladder trigone and ureteral orifices must be carefully identified and urologic consultation may be needed. In cases of anterior placenta previa and suspected placenta accreta, it is prudent to arrange for urologic support preoperatively. In cases of suspected accreta, interventional Radiology may preoperatively place hypogastric artery balloons bilaterally. These inflated balloons may significantly decrease blood loss during the procedure, thus avoiding the need for embolization.

The uterine incision can be closed with a running no. 1 suture in a locking fashion. The bladder flap should be dissected well down before the start of the hysterectomy, and accomplished best at the time of the caesarean delivery. The bladder should be dissected off the anterior, lower uterine segment with sharp dissection if firm adhesions are encountered. Firm adhesions often are present in patients who have undergone multiple caesarean deliveries. If bleeding is a problem, further dissection of the bladder from the lower uterine segment can be accomplished after ligation of the uterine artery.

The actual hysterectomy is begun by double ligating the round ligament close to the uterus and ligating the distal stump with a 0-Vicryl suture ligature. The vesicouterine serosa where the bladder was attached before its dissection then is extended laterally to the severed round ligaments.

The peritoneal incision should be extended superiorly. Because the ureters are dilated in pregnancy, they should be identified quickly to avoid injury. The ureter can be seen crossing the iliac artery at the level of the bifurcation in the medial leaf of the broad ligament and is most easily identified at this location. The uteroovarian ligaments can be secured by first making a "window" through the posterior leaf of the broad ligament and then doubly clamping, cutting, and ligating the uteroovarian ligament bilaterally (Fig. 32A.1). The uterine vessels are skeletonized as in the nonpuerperal hysterectomy. These vessels are large and easy to identify. Dissection is made easier with continuous upward traction of the uterus. The uterine vessels are clamped bilaterally (usually with a Heaney or Zepllin clamp). Next, this pedicle on each side is cut and doubly ligated (Fig. 32A.2). A clamp placed above this pedicle and next to the uterus helps prevent back-bleeding, which can be significant in a pregnant uterus. Because the vascular pedicle may be large, a second straight clamp may be placed on each side to further secure the pedicle. This pedicle is formed with scissors or a scalpel, and secured using a 0-Vicryl suture. As with all hysterectomies, care must be exercised in identifying and avoiding the ureter. The next pedicles encountered should be the broad ligament, the base of which is the cardinal ligament. A

TABLE 32A.4.
Comparison of Emergency Versus Elective Peripartum Hysterectomy

	Chestnut et al., 1985		Gonsoulin et al., 1991	
	Emergency	Elective	Emergency	Elective
Mean operating time (min)	150[a]	126	105[b]	83
Estimated blood loss (mL)	3,003[a]	1,102	1,495[b]	875
Blood transfusion (% of patients)	100[a]	66	68[b]	15
Febrile morbidity (% of patients)	61[a]	27	18	11
Urologic injury (% of patients)	4.6	0	0	1

[a] $p < .05$.
[b] $p < .05$.

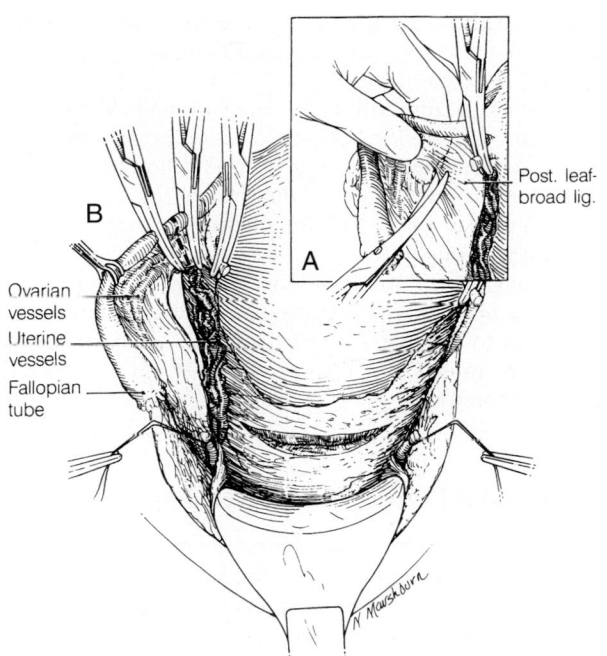

FIGURE 32A.1. A: The posterior leaf of the broad ligament adjacent to the uterus is perforated just beneath the fallopian tube, uteroovarian ligaments, and ovarian vessels. **B:** These are then doubly clamped close to the uterus and severed. (From: Cunningham FG, MacDonald PC, Gant NF, et al. Caesarean section and caesarean hysterectomy. In: *Williams obstetrics,* 19th ed. Norwalk, CT: Appleton & Lange, 1993:591, with permission.)

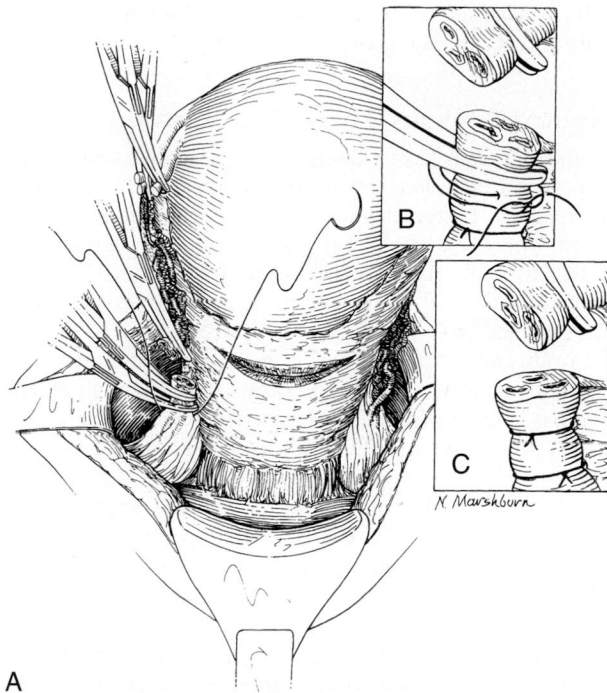

A

FIGURE 32A.2. A: The uterine artery and veins on either side are doubly clamped immediately adjacent to the uterus and divided. **B,C:** The vascular pedicle is doubly suture ligated. (From: Cunningham FG, MacDonald PC, Gant NF, et al. Caesarean section and caesarean hysterectomy. In: *Williams obstetrics,* 19th ed. Norwalk, CT: Appleton & Lange, 1993b:591, with permission.)

straight clamp, such as a Heany or Zeppllin, can be used for these ligaments. It is better to take several small pedicles instead of one large pedicle because an excessively large pedicle can slide out of a part of the clamp. This is especially true with the edematous tissues associated with pregnancy. Once the cardinal and uterosacral ligaments have been clamped, cut, and tied at a level below the cervix, the specimen can be removed by clamping across the vagina on each side and incising the vaginal mucosa (Fig. 32A.3). Then the cervix should be inspected to ensure that it has been removed completely.

After removal of the uterus and cervix, each of the angles of the lateral vaginal fornix is secured to the cardinal and uterosacral ligaments with a figure-of-eight 0-Vicryl or equivalent suture. There is no unanimity of opinion regarding whether the vaginal cuff should be run (with a locking 0-Vicryl or equivalent suture) and left open or closed. The vaginal cuff can be closed with interrupted figure-of-eight sutures. If there is continuous oozing, as with a coagulopathy or in the presence of purulent fluid, then the vaginal cuff is left open to allow for adequate drainage. Hemostatic agents such as Gelfoam, with or without topical thrombin, or Surgicel can be considered. An intraperitoneal suction drain can prove helpful in monitoring patients who are at high risk of developing hematoma or abscess.

There is no consensus of opinion regarding reperitonization of the pelvis. It is not necessary in most cases.

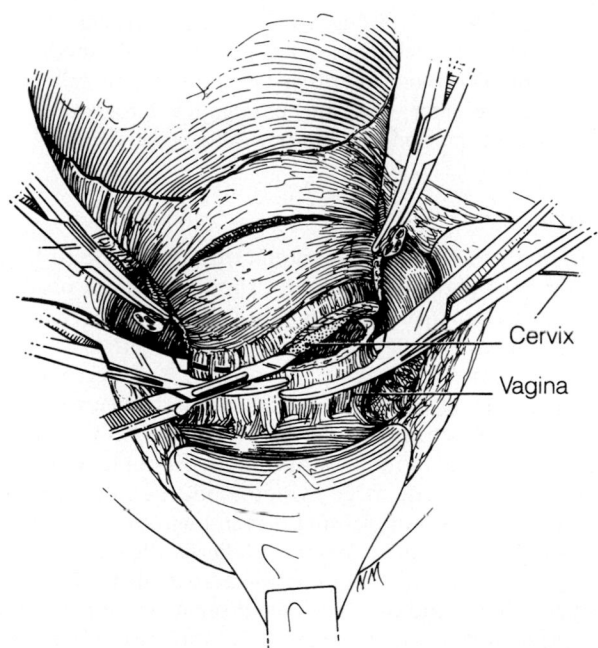

FIGURE 32A.3. A curved clamp is swung in across the lateral vaginal fornix below the level of the cervix, and the tissue is incised medially to the point of the clamp. (From: Cunningham FG, MacDonald PC, Gant NF, et al. Caesarean section and caesarean hysterectomy. In: *Williams obstetrics,* 19th ed. Norwalk, CT: Appleton & Lange, 1993b:591, with permission.)

All pedicles should be closely inspected for bleeding before the abdominal incision is closed.

Subtotal Versus Total Hysterectomy

Some clinicians have a tendency to perform a subtotal or supracervical hysterectomy in most cases of emergency peripartum hysterectomy. There is a general belief that both operating time and blood loss are significantly lower with the subtotal technique. In addition, it is said that the risk of bladder or ureteral injury is less. There is no question that in the select patient who has been or is hemodynamically unstable, it may be prudent to perform a supracervical hysterectomy, especially if all bleeding has been controlled to that point. However, it is necessary to remove the cervix in cases of placenta previa or placenta accreta involving the lower uterine segment.

Despite the reputed advantages of a supracervical hysterectomy, there is evidence that performance of a complete hysterectomy with removal of the cervix adds little to either operating time or blood loss. Clark and associates reported no significant differences in mean values for blood loss and operating time in obstetric patients undergoing emergency total hysterectomy versus supracervical hysterectomy. Mean hospital stay also was not significantly different. However, the women in this study were not randomized to supracervical versus total hysterectomy. In 1998, Zorlu and associates also reported no significant difference between total and supracervical hysterectomy in operative time, blood transfusion, and mean hospital stay. It is important to separate emergency caesarean hysterectomy for hemorrhage, and so on from elective peripartum hysterectomy for indications such as microinvasive cervical cancer because the blood loss and other morbidity is generally significantly greater for the emergency procedure. A prospective, randomized study would be very helpful.

Summary

Although there has been significant concern regarding the role of peripartum hysterectomy in modern obstetrics, it is clear that this operation is indeed important in the armamentarium of the practicing obstetrician. First and foremost, emergency peripartum hysterectomy is unavoidable by its very nature. Second, elective caesarean hysterectomy should be performed only for certain indications in modern obstetrics. Examples of these indications include large symptomatic uterine leiomyomas, some cases of placenta previa, microinvasive cervical carcinoma, some patients with cervical carcinoma *in situ*, and severe debilitating menstrual aberrations or other pelvic pathology (e.g., symptomatic endometriosis or pelvic inflammatory disease). Routine use of elective caesarean hysterectomy for the sole purpose of sterilization is not justified.

The most significant complications or morbidities associated with emergency peripartum hysterectomy are infection, urologic injury, and blood loss with the need for transfusion. Importantly, much of the morbidity is related to the need for the hysterectomy (e.g., uterine atony related or unrelated to chorioamnionitis, placenta accreta, placenta previa).

The risk of morbidity associated with an elective hysterectomy for specific indications is not greater than the risk associated with caesarean section followed by interval hysterectomy, except for the relative risk of requiring a blood transfusion, which is higher in the caesarean hysterectomy group.

Finally, it is critically important that the techniques and skills necessary to perform peripartum hysterectomy be taught to residents in obstetrics. This often life-saving procedure must be among the skills of any completely trained obstetrician-gynecologist.

POSTPARTUM HEMORRHAGE

Postpartum hemorrhage is poorly defined by estimation of blood loss. It is difficult, if not impossible, to determine actual blood loss or a percentage of blood loss. Additionally, blood volume expansion is variable during pregnancy and can be affected be several factors, including hypertension, renal disease, maternal size, and the presence of multifetal gestations. The potential effects of blood loss largely depend on the degree of blood volume expansion. For example, the average blood loss from a caesarean delivery is 1,000 to 1,100 mL. This degree of blood loss is generally well tolerated by the normal pregnant woman. A blood loss of 500 to 750 mL, however, may not be tolerated in a woman with poor to no blood volume expansion, or one who is hemoconcentrated secondary to severe preeclampsia or eclampsia. Gilstrap and Ramin have defined clinically significant hemorrhage as that amount of bleeding "that produces signs and symptoms of hemodynamic instability or that is likely to produce such if left unabated."

Incidence and Etiology

Although the exact incidence of hemorrhage associated with pregnancy is unknown, it remains one of the leading causes of maternal mortality in this country. Kaunitz and associates reported that 13% of more than 2,000 maternal deaths were secondary to hemorrhage, and one third of these occurred postpartum. Rochat and colleagues reported a similar incidence of 11% of maternal deaths owing to hemorrhage.

Uterine causes account for 90% of postpartum hemorrhage and are more severe than nonuterine causes. Uterine causes of postpartum hemorrhage include uterine atony, abnormal placentation, retained placental products, uterine inversion, or rupture. Nonuterine causes include vaginal lacerations, hematoma, or coagulopathy. The potential for postpartum hemorrhage exists whenever there is overdistention of the uterus, as occurs with multifetal gestations, hydramnios, and macrosomic fetuses. Dysfunctional labor (e.g., protracted active phase and prolonged second stage of labor) also places patients at risk. The extended use of oxytocin, grand multiparity, and chorioamnionitis also appear to be associated with this complication.

Although prophylactic use of uterotonics has become routine in the management of the third stage of labor, the types of drugs used have varied. Van Selm and associates performed a double-blind randomized control trial evaluating the efficacy of prophylactic use of oxytocin plus ergometrine versus sulprostone (a prostaglandin E_2 analog) plus placebo in women at high risk for atonic postpartum hemorrhage. In this study, women were included who had a history of postpartum hemorrhage greater than 1,000 cc. Sixty-nine women were enrolled, but no statistically significant difference was seen in the two groups in terms of blood loss or need for transfusion.

Amant and associates compared use of misoprostol and methylergometrine for prevention of postpartum hemorrhage. Postpartum hemorrhage occurred in 4.3% of the methylergometrine group and 8.3% of the misoprostol group. However, patients receiving misoprostol had a higher incidence of fever related to the medication than patients in the methylergometrine group.

Management

The most important aspects in the management of postpartum hemorrhage are prompt recognition of the condition and ascertainment of its etiology. Recognition is no problem with external bleeding, and such bleeding almost always can be controlled with medical or minor surgical means. Hypotension without obvious external blood loss always should serve as a sign of potential internal bleeding, and virtually all such hemorrhage requires a major surgical procedure to arrest the hemorrhage. If the etiology of the hemorrhage is not determined quickly, coagulopathy may complicate the clinical presentation, thereby making diagnosis difficult.

Medical Management

Uterine atony is obvious and easy to diagnose by palpation of the uterus. If atony it not present, the cervix and vagina should be carefully inspected for lacerations. The placenta also should be inspected for missing fragments, and careful palpation of the uterine cavity should be performed. If the source of bleeding still is not obvious or if bleeding is seen around venipuncture or catheter sites, then the patient should be evaluated for a coagulopathy. A thrombin-clot (clot retraction test) tube will reveal gross disruption in coagulation within minutes. Useful laboratory tests include prothrombin time, partial thromboplastin time, platelets, fibrinogen, and fibrin degradation product levels. Before surgical intervention, an ultrasound examination of the uterine cavity may prove useful for the identification of an accessory placental lobe or fragment.

Except in cases of profuse bleeding, medical management of hemorrhage generally is a good place to start. The hallmarks of medical management consist of volume replacement and oxytocic agents, including intravenous oxytocin and parenteral methylergonovine and prostaglandins. Volume can be maintained with crystalloid and blood or blood products. Invasive monitoring, such as with a pulmonary artery catheter, generally is not necessary and may be dangerous in the presence of a coagulopathy. Monitoring of urine output, vital signs, and oxygen saturation may be more helpful. Volume replacement generally is adequate when the blood pressure is maintained at 90 to 100 mm Hg systolic, the pulse is less than 100 beats per minute, and the urine output is at least 25 to 30 mL per hour. When a patient has required transfusion of significant amounts of packed red blood cells, transfusion of coagulation products should be performed to replace those lost in the hemorrhage and no delay should occur in doing so. Calcium also should be replaced in these patients, because of risk of complications related to hypocalcemia in patients who receive massive transfusions. Coagulation factors also should be replaced in patients who receive extensive transfusions with packed red blood cells. Fluid overload generally can be detected with a stethoscope and an oxygen monitor in conjunction with clinical signs and symptoms. Diuretics only should be used to remove excess fluid if the patient becomes hypoxic related to volume overload. A medical management protocol is summarized in Table 32A.5.

Surgical Management

Lower genital tract lacerations usually are best managed by suturing. The rare case of uterine rupture also is managed surgically. Other techniques to control hemorrhage include uterine and uteroovarian artery ligation, hypogastric or internal iliac artery ligation, hysterectomy, or uterine or hypogastric artery embolization.

TABLE 32A.5.
Medical Management Protocol for Postpartum Hemorrhage

GENERAL

Large-bore intravenous line
Foley catheter

DRUGS

Oxytocin, dilute solution of 20 U in 1,000 mL of normal saline or Ringers solution, given as i.v. infusion
Methylergonovine, 0.2 mg i.m.
15-methyl $PGF_{2\alpha}$, 0.25 mg i.m. or intramyometrially every 15 to 60 min as indicated

VOLUME REPLACEMENT

Crystalloid, 3 mL/mL of estimated blood loss (maintain urine output $\geq$30 mL/h)
Packed red blood cells
Fresh frozen plasma, platelets, or cryoprecipitate, as indicated

---

From: American College of Obstetricians and Gynecologists. *Diagnosis and management of postpartum hemorrhage.* ACOG Technical Bulletin No. 143, 1990, with permission.

Uterine packing, which until recently was abandoned by most clinicians, may allow adequate time for blood and fluid replacement before surgical intervention. Maier described the use of a packing device called a Torpin packer. The device uses a plunger to place several yards of 4-inch-wide gauze into the uterine cavity. It has been used successfully to control postpartum hemorrhage in nine women. Not only does this technique allow for volume replacement, but also it can slow bleeding enough to allow for surgical techniques short of hysterectomy, or actually stop the bleeding so that no further treatment is necessary. Other methods of uterine tamponade reported in the literature have included the use of a Foley catheter with a 30- to 50-cc balloon or a Sengstaken-Blakemore tube with the esophageal balloon inflated with 50 cc of normal saline.

The choice of a specific surgical technique to control bleeding depends on several factors, such as the degree of hemorrhage, the condition of the patient, parity, and the desire for future childbearing, although probably the single most important factor is the experience of the surgeon.

ARTERIAL EMBOLIZATION

Angiographically directed arterial embolization has been described for the successful control of obstetric and gynecologic bleeding. Gelfoam, polyvinyl alcohol dehydrated particles, and other substances have been used for such embolizations. Pelage and associates, in two separate reports, describe use of arterial embolization in patients with primary or secondary postpartum hemorrhage. They define primary postpartum hemorrhage as that which occurs within 24 hours after delivery. Twenty-seven women were identified in this group, and two of these patients had already undergone hysterectomy in an unsuccessful attempt to control the hemor-

rhage. Immediate decrease or cessation of bleeding occurred in all patients. Two patients required repeat embolization the next day with no further complications. Fourteen women were diagnosed with secondary postpartum hemorrhage after the first 24 hours following delivery. All the women had complete resolution of bleeding with embolization with no further complications. Arterial embolization can be performed quickly and safely, in many cases more quickly than an operating room can be readied. Therefore, it should be considered in patients with postpartum hemorrhage. There have been reports of successful pregnancies following embolization, rendering it an attractive alternative to hysterectomy in the patient who desires preservation of fertility.

UTERINE ARTERY LIGATION

Uterine artery ligation is a relatively safe procedure that can be performed by most obstetricians and allows for future childbearing. The technique consists of ligating the uterine artery and vein at the lower uterine segment 2 to 3 cm below the level of the uterine incision. An absorbable ligature is placed 2 to 3 cm medial to the uterine vessels through the myometrium (in order to obliterate any intramyometrial ascending branches) and then lateral to the vessels through the broad ligament. It is imperative that the bladder be advanced prior to placement of the suture to prevent bladder injury. Because of collateral flow from the ovarian artery, some recommend that a second ligature be placed at the junction of the uteroovarian ligament and uterus. The technique of uterine artery ligation is shown in Figs. 32A.4 and 32A.5.

O'Leary and O'Leary, in a review of 90 women who underwent uterine artery ligation (30 were for uterine atony), reported that only six (7%) procedures resulted

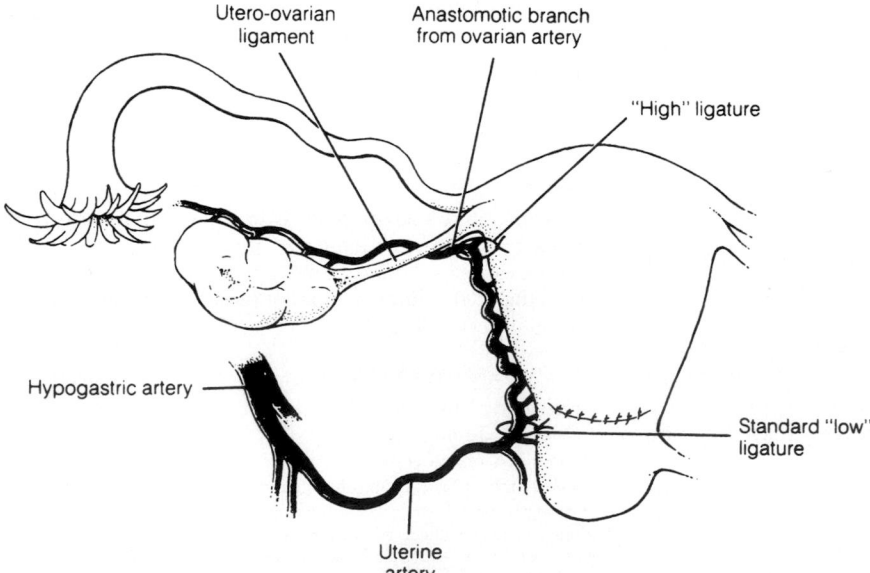

FIGURE 32A.4. Uterine artery ligation. (From: Clark SC, Phelan JP. Surgical control of obstetric hemorrhage. *Contemp Obstet Gynecol* 1984;24:70, with permission.)

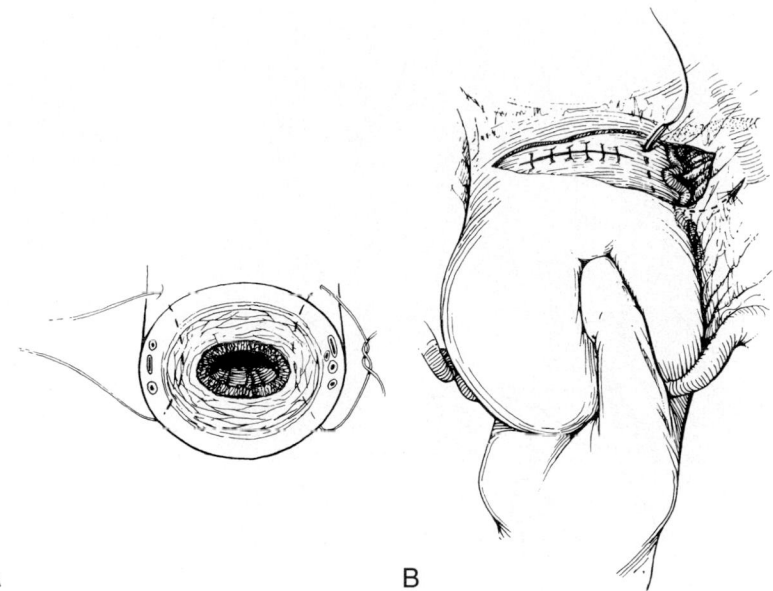

FIGURE 32A.5. Uterine artery ligation. **A:** Lateral view demonstrating ligature placement. **B:** Anatomic relation of ligature to uterine wall and vessels. (From: Floyd RC, Morrison JC. Postpartum hemorrhage. In: Plauche WC, Morrison JC, O'Sullivan MJ, eds. *Surgical obstetrics.* Philadelphia: WB Saunders, 1992:272, with permission.)

A   B

in failure. There were no major complications from the procedure itself. O'Leary reported a greater than 95% success rate in a follow-up review of 265 women who underwent uterine artery ligation.

This technique is most useful (and successful) when hemorrhage is of a moderate degree or less and originates from the lower uterine segment. Such an example is bleeding from a low placental implantation site. A uterine artery ligation also can prove beneficial for lower segment extensions or lacerations, as well as for a uterine artery laceration itself. Philippe et al., reported a vaginal approach to ligation of the uterine arteries in two patients after vaginal delivery, but a larger case series would have to be performed to determine the feasibility of this approach.

B-Lynch also described five cases in which hemorrhage was controlled by placing an absorbable suture vertically from 3 cm below the uterine incision to 3 cm above the uterine incision on the right side of the uterus. The stitch is then taken vertically over the fundus and placed horizontally in the posterior uterus at the same level as the anterior suture. The suture is threaded over the left side of the uterus to place another stitch on the left from 3 cm above the uterine incision to 3 cm below the uterine incision. The long suture is tied compressing the fundus. The uterine incision is closed in the usual fashion. Although this technique has successfully controlled uterine hemorrhage and has not been reported to cause any complications, too few cases have been reported for satisfactory evaluation.

HYPOGASTRIC ARTERY LIGATION

The major blood supply to the uterus and pelvis comes from the internal iliac artery, commonly called the hypogastric artery. Bilateral ligation of this artery can ef-

fectively control significant bleeding and thus prevent the need for hysterectomy and permanent sterilization. Burchell has aptly described the physiology of internal iliac artery ligation. It appears that ligation of this artery controls bleeding by converting an arterial system into a venous system, which decreases the pulse pressure by as much as 85%. This allows pressure and packing to produce clotting. Hypogastric artery ligation probably interferes little, if at all, with subsequent pregnancies. Mengert and colleagues reported successful pregnancies in five women who had undergone internal iliac artery ligation. This technique also may prove useful for controlling bleeding in patients with large hematomas of the broad ligament or for a lacerated artery that has retracted into the broad ligament. Such vessels or active bleeding sites often are difficult to identify. If the bleeding is from the hypogastric vein, ligation of the hypogastric artery decreases outgoing flow as well as allows exposure to the vein.

The technique of hypogastric artery ligation is illustrated in Fig. 32A.6. The peritoneum overlying the common iliac artery is opened by directly cutting on the surface of the artery. The ureter should be identified and retracted medially if necessary. The sheath covering the internal iliac (hypogastric) artery then can be opened longitudinally. A right-angle clamp then is gently passed under the artery with blunt dissection. Great care must be taken not to perforate the internal iliac vein. The ligation should be performed about 2 cm distal to the bifurcation to avoid disrupting the posterior division of the hypogastric, which can lead to ischemia and necrosis of the skin and subcutaneous tissue of the gluteus. Two nonabsorbable sutures of 2-0 silk should be used for ligation. It is important that hypogastric artery ligation be performed bilaterally to adequately decrease pressure to the uterus. Clark and associates reported on the successful control of bleeding in eight (42%) of 19 women who

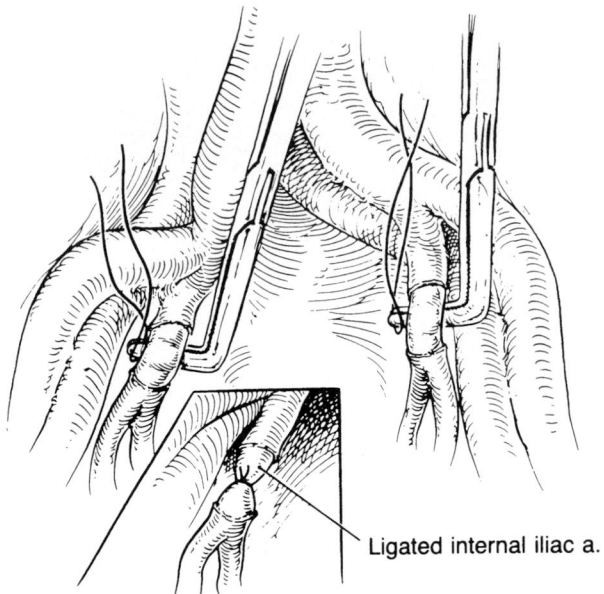

Ligated internal iliac a.

FIGURE 32A.6. Ligation of both hypogastric arteries. (From: Cunningham FG, MacDonald PC, Gant NF, et al. Caesarean section and caesarean hysterectomy. In: *Williams obstetrics,* 19th ed. Norwalk, CT: Appleton & Lange, 1993d:543, with permission.)

underwent hypogastric artery ligation. In a review of hypogastric artery ligation from three series, Clark reported that this procedure prevented hysterectomy in about half of the cases associated with uterine atony and placenta accreta. Interestingly, in the series by Clark and associates, the success of this procedure did not appear to be related directly to the conditions for which it was performed. It must be noted, however, that the number of patients in each category is small.

Although this procedure is successful in about 50% of the cases and does not interfere with subsequent fertility, it is not technically easy to perform and requires special expertise and skill. Many obstetricians have little, if any, experience with this procedure. Moreover, potential complications of hypogastric artery ligation include laceration of the iliac vein, ligation of the external iliac artery, ureteral injury, and death.

HYSTERECTOMY

Because of the lack of experience and skill with the technique of hypogastric artery ligation, many clinicians prefer to do a hysterectomy to control postpartum hemorrhage. Peripartum hysterectomy has been discussed in a previous section. Hysterectomy usually is the safest procedure and also the quickest that can be performed for refractory bleeding. For example, Clark and associates report that patients undergoing hypogastric artery ligation who subsequently required hysterectomy had an increased incidence of cardiac arrest secondary to blood loss. The increased morbidity associated with hypogastric artery ligation followed by

hysterectomy may be secondary to a delay in attempting conservative management short of hysterectomy. Hypogastric artery ligation was attempted before hysterectomy 64% of the time in nulliparous women, compared with 10% of the time for parous patients. Lack of experience with hypogastric artery ligation adds to the overall time required to attempt the procedure and therefore overall blood loss.

In a review of 70 women who underwent emergency hysterectomy, Clark and colleagues (1984) reported that almost all required blood transfusion, and 50% had postoperative febrile morbidity. The most common indication for hysterectomy in this series was uterine atony, followed by placenta accreta. Of the 70 procedures, 60 were performed after caesarean delivery. Mean operating time was 3.1 hours, and mean blood loss was 3,575 mL.

LATE POSTPARTUM HEMORRHAGE

Late postpartum hemorrhage is that which occurs more than 24 hours after delivery. The etiology of such bleeding includes placental site subinvolution, infection, coagulopathy, and retained products of conception. Initial therapy for this complication is the same as for early hemorrhage. If infection is present, antibiotics should be used. Endometrial curettage may be necessary for retained placental fragments. Angiographic embolization may prove especially useful in the case of late postpartum hemorrhage. Uterine artery ligation, hypogastric artery ligation, and hysterectomy are rarely required for control of late postpartum hemorrhage.

Summary

Puerperal hemorrhage is unpredictable in onset, duration, severity, and etiology. Such hemorrhage remains a major life-threatening possibility of any delivery. All physicians caring for pregnant women must remain alert and prepared for such a possibility at any hour of the day or night. Such preparation includes the provision of adequately trained nursing support and medical and laboratory facilities to meet such a need. The physician caring for such women should be trained in the appropriate choice and application of the medical and surgical principles and techniques described in this chapter. The choice of a specific surgical procedure is dependent on several factors, the most important of which is the experience and skill of the surgeon. Finally, although it is important to attempt to preserve fertility in some women, especially nulliparous women, procrastination in the face of profuse hemorrhage can increase the risk of both mortality and morbidity.

EPISIOTOMY

An episiotomy is a surgical incision into the perineal body for the purpose of either aiding the actual delivery process or preventing tears and lacerations.

Incidence

The incidence or frequency of episiotomy varies according to parity, patient population, indication, and the health care provider practicing obstetrics. In 1983, Thacker and Banta reported that about two thirds of all vaginal deliveries in the United States were associated with the performance of an episiotomy. Thorpe et al. reported that episiotomy was performed in 62% of patients in their series. In 1996, Bansal and associates reported a decrease in the use of episiotomy from 86.8% to 10.4% between 1976 and 1994 at their institution. In a review of 20,000 women who delivered vaginally, Owen and Hauth reported that approximately two thirds of primiparous and one third of multiparous women had episiotomies. Among medical professionals there is extreme variability in the use of episiotomy. Robinson and associates evaluated 1,576 consecutive spontaneous vaginal deliveries and revealed that midwives had a lower incidence of episiotomy use (21%) followed by medical school faculty (33%). Private practice providers had the highest rate of episiotomy (55%). Other predictors of episiotomy were prolonged second stage of labor, fetal macrosomia, and epidural anesthesia. Hueston reported that nulliparity, use of forceps, or vacuum extraction also were predictors of episiotomy.

Indications

Both the performance of and need for routine episiotomy with every vaginal delivery have been challenged. Although there is little justification for the routine performance of episiotomy for all vaginal deliveries, appropriate indications for this procedure do exist. Probably the two most common indications are to prevent third- or fourth-degree lacerations and to provide more room for vaginal delivery (e.g., with operative vaginal delivery). This argument is countered by the experience of Bansal et al., who report a reduction in the incidence of third- and fourth-degree lacerations with a decrease in the episiotomy rate. Other common indications are summarized in Table 32A.6. There is not a unanimous opinion regarding the prophylactic use of episiotomy for all

---

TABLE 32A.6.
Some Common Indications for Episiotomy

Significant risk of major perineal laceration
Operative vaginal delivery
    Forceps application
    Vacuum application
Breech delivery
Twin delivery
Fetal macrosomia
Shoulder dystocia
Preterm delivery

From: Cunningham FG, MacDonald PC, Gant NF, et al. Conduct of normal labor. In: *Williams obstetrics*, 19th ed. Norwalk, CT: Appleton & Lange, 1993c:371, with permission.

---

preterm births. It is reasonable to conclude, however, that episiotomy is not indicated if the perineum is already appropriately relaxed, as is often the case with the multiparous patient.

It has been clinically taught that routine episiotomy prevents vaginal and perineal damage associated with subsequent pelvic relaxation. However, few published data support the premise that "prophylactic" episiotomy prevents cystocele, rectocele, enterocele, uterine, or vaginal prolapse, or stress urinary incontinence. Rockner and associates evaluated pelvic floor muscle strength using vaginal cones, and revealed women with episiotomies had less strength than those with spontaneous vaginal deliveries. Neural testing of the perineal musculature in other studies showed that the amount of denervation was associated with weight of the baby, length of second stage of labor, and was unrelated to episiotomy. Sleep and Grant looked at deliveries in those who restricted use of episiotomy and those reported liberal use of episiotomy. Over 3 years of follow-up, there was little difference between the two groups in severity of incontinence or the reported incidence of incontinence. These studies indicate that episiotomy does not appear to be beneficial in preventing pelvic relaxation.

In addition, few data support prophylactic episiotomy for the prevention of "trauma" to the fetus, especially the preterm fetus. Thus, it appears that the major indication for episiotomy in modern obstetrics is to provide more room when deemed necessary for operative delivery or when the failure to do so might result in significant perineal lacerations.

Technique: Midline Versus Mediolateral Episiotomy

There is little question that the midline perineal incision is easier to perform and repair and is associated with less postoperative pain than the mediolateral episiotomy. In general, it is also associated with less blood loss and better anatomic results. Midline perineal incisions are used more frequently in the United States, whereas mediolateral episiotomy is used more commonly in Europe. The major disadvantage of midline episiotomy is an increased risk of third- and fourth-degree lacerations. Owen and Hauth report that 20% of primiparous women with a midline episiotomy had a third- or fourth-degree laceration, compared with 9% of women with a mediolateral incision, and only 1% when no episiotomy was performed. Of interest, multiparous women with a midline episiotomy had fewer third- and fourth-degree lacerations than those with a mediolateral episiotomy. Although these data appear to favor performing either a mediolateral episiotomy or no episiotomy at all, caution must be exercised when interpreting the data because this was not a randomized, prospective study and does not control for possible confounding factors. For example, patients who underwent episiotomy may have had larger babies, a higher incidence of forceps assistance, or other characteristics resulting in an increased risk of laceration.

Although the mediolateral episiotomy may be associated with fewer third- and fourth-degree lacerations (at

TABLE 32A.7.

Relation of Lacerations to Type of Episiotomy in 7,675 Primiparous Women

Laceration	Type of Episiotomy		
	Midline (n = 4,822)	Mediolateral (n = 79)	None (n = 2,774)
Second-degree	1425 (30%)	26 (33%)	375 (14%)
Third- or fourth-degree	968 (20%)	7 (9%)	52 (1%)
Other	295 (6%)	7 (9%)	274 (10%)
Totals	2688 (56%)	40 (51%)	701 (25%)

From: Owen J, Hauth JC. Episiotomy infection and dehiscence. In: Gilstrap LC III, Faro S, eds. *Infections in pregnancy.* New York: Alan R. Liss, 1990:61, with permission.

TABLE 32A.8.

Complications of Episiotomy

Infection
Hematoma
Third- and fourth-degree extensions
Cellulitis
Dehiscence
Abscess formation
Incontinence of flatus
Incontinence of stool
Rectovaginal fistula
Impaired pudendal nerve conduction
Poor sphincter tone
Necrotizing fasciitis
Death

From: Ramin SM, Gilstrap LC III. Episiotomy and early repair of dehiscence. *Clin Obstet Gynecol* 1994;37:816, with permission.

least in the primiparous patient) (Table 32A.7), there are several disadvantages to this technique. Blood loss is greater, mediolateral episiotomies are more difficult to repair, and anatomic results may be faulty. Postoperative pain also is more common, and can be very troublesome. The decision to perform a mediolateral or midline episiotomy must be based on clinical judgment and experience.

Episiotomy Repair

An episiotomy can be repaired in numerous ways. One popular method is to close the vaginal mucosa and submucosa with a continuous locking suture of chromic catgut 2-0 or Vicryl, followed by closure of the fascia and muscle of the perineal body with three or four interrupted sutures of 2-0 chromic catgut or Vicryl. The skin of the perineum can then be closed with a continuous subcuticular stitch (2-0 or 3-0 chromic or Vicryl) or by interrupted sutures of 3-0 or 4-0 chromic or Vicryl through the subcutaneous tissue and skin. Others have recommended the use of polyglactin sutures instead of chromic. Mackrodt and associates reported decreased perineal pain when polyglactin was used compared to chromic. In cases of fourth-degree lacerations, it is important to approximate the edges of the rectal mucosa with a running submucosal 3-0 or 4-0 chromic or polyglactin suture, followed by a second, reinforcement layer of the rectovaginal septal tissue. If the external anal sphincter is severed, it should be carefully reapproximated with several interrupted 2-0 chromic or polyglactin sutures through the muscle and fibrous capsule. The technique for primary episiotomy closure is shown in the section on secondary repair.

Complications of Episiotomy
Extensions and Fistula Formation
The major complications of episiotomy are summarized in Table 32A.8. Probably the single most common complication is extension (i.e., third- or fourth-degree lacer-

ation). Extensions in turn can lead to incontinence of flatus and stool, rectovaginal fistula, and infection. The association of extensions with the type of episiotomy has been discussed already. In the report by Harris, 11.6% of the more than 7,000 women with midline episiotomies had a third- or fourth-degree laceration. In the women with these lacerations, 2% had poor sphincter tone and 0.1% developed a rectovaginal fistula. Signorello and colleagues performed a retrospective cohort study to evaluate the relationship between midline episiotomy and anal incontinence postpartum. Women with episiotomies had a higher risk of fecal incontinence 3 months and 6 months postpartum. Episiotomy tripled the risk of fecal incontinence at 3 months and 6 months postpartum and doubled the risk of flatus incontinence compared with women with spontaneous lacerations. In a prospective evaluation of 16,583 deliveries, Walsh et al. found that 0.56% of deliveries were complicated by third-degree lacerations. Lacerations were not prevented by episiotomy, but were associated with forceps delivery. Of the 81 patients followed, 30 had abnormal anorectal examination; 7% were incontinent of stool, and 12% were incontinent of flatus.

Fistula is fortunately an uncommon complication of episiotomy. Causes include unrecognized lacerations in the rectovaginal septum at the time of episiotomy repair or infected hematoma. Risk factors for fistula formation include obesity, poor hygiene, malnutrition, anemia, history of inflammatory bowel disease, connective tissue disease, or prior exposure to radiation therapy. Half of these fistulae spontaneously heal, but repair should be considered if the patient is very symptomatic.

Infection
Infection is relatively uncommon after episiotomy. Harris reported an episiotomy infection rate of only 0.1% associated with a third- or fourth-degree laceration. In the series of more than 20,000 women reported by

Owen and Hauth, only 10 (0.05%) women developed infected episiotomies.

Dehiscence

The exact incidence of episiotomy dehiscence is unknown, but it appears to occur infrequently. In a review of 390 women with fourth-degree perineal lacerations, 18 (4.6%) experienced a dehiscence, and 11 of these were associated with infection.

Several predisposing factors have been reported to be associated with episiotomy dehiscence, including infection, human papilloma virus, cigarette smoking, hematoma, or trauma. Infection is probably the most common factor. In the study by Ramin and associates, 86% of patients with midline episiotomy dehiscence and 69% of patients with mediolateral episiotomy dehiscence had evidence of infection that was based on the presence of fever or purulent discharge. Infection with human papillomavirus also has been reported by some to be associated with dehiscence. In the report by Snyder and associates, active lesions, history thereof, or subsequent development of infection with human papilloma virus (HPV) was found in 29.8% of patients with episiotomy breakdown compared to 13.8% of patients in the control group ($p < 0.023$). Herpes simplex and other sexually transmitted diseases were not significantly associated with episiotomy dehiscence. Although inadequate or "faulty" repair has been reported to be associated with dehiscence, this is a rare cause.

Diagnosis

The diagnosis of obvious dehiscence is relatively easy. In women with incomplete dehiscence and infection, however, the diagnosis may not be so obvious. Pain, fever, induration, and purulent discharge are common symptoms. For example, in the series of 34 women reported by Ramin and colleagues, pain and purulent discharge were present in two thirds of the women, and fever was present in almost half (44%). The women with actual or impending dehiscence also may complain of passing flatus or stool from the vagina. In Arona's study, the most common presenting symptoms were pain, incontinence of flatus or feces, and discharge.

Early Repair of Dehiscence

In the past, it has been taught that repair of episiotomy dehiscence should be delayed for several months to allow for revascularization and healing. Few data support this opinion. Moreover, not only is delayed repair an inconvenience for the woman, but it is also associated with fecal incontinence and loss of sexual function. Delay also can increase the hospital stay, cost, and increase risk of litigation.

There are many advantages to early repair of episiotomy dehiscence. Hauth and colleagues reported on the efficacy and safety of early repair in eight women who had a dehiscence of a fourth-degree midline episiotomy. Early repair was successful in seven of the eight women.

One woman developed a pinpoint rectovaginal fistula 4 days after early repair. This was fixed with a 1-cm rectal flap 4 months later.

Monberg and Hammen reported on the successful resuturing of episiotomy breakdown in 20 women with infection, dehiscence, or both. Although four of the women had superficial reseparation, all subsequently healed spontaneously.

Hankins and associates updated the initial report by Hauth and colleagues to include 22 women with dehiscence of an initial fourth-degree repair, four with dehiscence of a third-degree repair, and five with breakdown of a mediolateral repair. Initial success of early repair was achieved in 29 (94%) of 31 women. Two women with a pinpoint rectovaginal fistula were subsequently repaired with a rectal flap procedure. Of the 27 women with a follow-up of 1 year or greater, all were continent and had resumption of normal coital activity. The follow-up of the 22 women with early repair of episiotomy dehiscence revealed no complications in 18 patients. Occasional incontinence of flatus and stool, dyspareunia, dyschezia, and numbness occurred in the remaining patients. All of the symptoms resolved by 9 months except for two patients who had persistent dyspareunia.

Ramin and coworkers reported on the early repair of 34 women with episiotomy dehiscence, most of whom were infected (Table 32A.9). These women received care from a large urban hospital serving primarily an indigent population. The timing of repair for dehiscence ranged from 3 to 13 days. Two women with initial third-degree episiotomy dehiscence had unsuccessful repairs. Thus, successful repairs were accomplished in 32 (94%) of the women. The average time from delivery to subsequent discharge after repair of the dehiscence was 15.5 days. This is similar to the time reported by Hankins and colleagues. This time probably can be shortened significantly with outpatient management of the wound and

---

TABLE 32A.9.

Characteristics of 34 Patients with Episiotomy Dehiscence and Subsequent Early Repair

Characteristic	Midline	Mediolateral
Total number of patients	21	13
Type of delivery		
Spontaneous	11	0
Outlet forceps	3	3
Low forceps	7	10
Extension		
None	1	5
Third-degree	9	6
Fourth-degree	11	2
Evidence of infection	18 (86%)	9 (69%)
Early repair failures	1	1

From: Ramin SM, Ramus RM, Little BB, et al. Early repair of episiotomy dehiscence associated with infection. *Am J Obstet Gynecol* 1992;167:1104, with permission.

repair in ambulatory care units. Arona and associates reported on 23 patients who underwent early repair of episiotomy dehiscence with an outpatient debridement procedure. All repairs were successful with no subsequent breakdown.

Secondary Repair Technique

Before attempting a closure, it is important to prepare the wound for repair. The first step is cleaning and debridement of the episiotomy site. This can be accomplished either on the ward with intravenous sedation or local anesthesia or in the operating room under regional anesthesia. All necrotic tissue and suture fragments should be removed and the wound irrigated with a diluted povidone-iodine solution or half-strength Dakin's solution. Broad-spectrum antibiotics are indicated for overt infection or significant cellulitis. After initial debridement, the wound should be scrubbed and cleaned at least twice daily. Scrub brushes impregnated with povidone-iodine or gauze dressing pads can be used. A 1% lidocaine jelly is applied to the wound several minutes before cleansing, and analgesics should be used as necessary. The liberal use of sitz baths helps keep the wound clean.

Secondary repair of the episiotomy is not attempted until the wound is free of exudate and covered by granulation tissue. A mechanical bowel preparation with an oral electrolyte solution should be administered the evening before surgery for fourth-degree breakdowns. Prophylactic antibiotics are recommended for all repairs. One to three doses of a first-generation cephalosporin generally proves satisfactory.

The first step in the surgical repair of dehiscence is debridement of granulation tissue and dissection to ensure good tissue mobility. If the anal sphincter muscle has been severed, extensive retraction usually has occurred. It is important to identify the fibrous capsule and mobilize the muscle and capsule for successful reapprox-

imation. If the rectal mucosa has been lacerated, it should be reapproximated as described in this chapter. In a prospective, randomized trial, Fitzpatrick et al., compared 55 women who underwent a sphincter overlap procedure compared to 57 women who underwent staple approximation repair of third-degree lacerations. In this study, there were no significant differences in anal manometry or endoanal ultrasound in the two groups. Therefore, either approach is acceptable. The rest of the closure is the same as for a secondary episiotomy repair. The secondary repair of a fourth-degree episiotomy breakdown is shown in Figs. 32A.7 through 32A.10.

Postoperatively, women can be placed on a regular diet if the rectal mucosa is not involved. If the rectal mucosa is involved, a low-residue diet should be used for several days and advanced to a regular diet. Stool softeners may prove useful, but diarrhea should be avoided because of the increased likelihood of infection. Postoperative care should also include sitz baths and a heat lamp.

The care and repair of a mediolateral episiotomy dehiscence are the same as for a midline repair. More extensive tissue mobilization may be required with the repair of a mediolateral episiotomy dehiscence.

Prevention of Dehiscence

Even with good surgical technique and meticulous attention to closure of the rectal mucosa and control of bleeding, not all cases of episiotomy dehiscence can be prevented. The role of prophylactic antibiotics, if any, in preventing dehiscence is unclear. In a study by Goldaber and associates, however, the authors reported that dehiscence, as well as infection, "was not associated with any readily preventable antepartum or intrapartum factors."

Hematoma

The most common cause of hematoma formation is an unligated bleeding vessel in the episiotomy incision, but can include an acquired or congenital coagulopathy, fail-

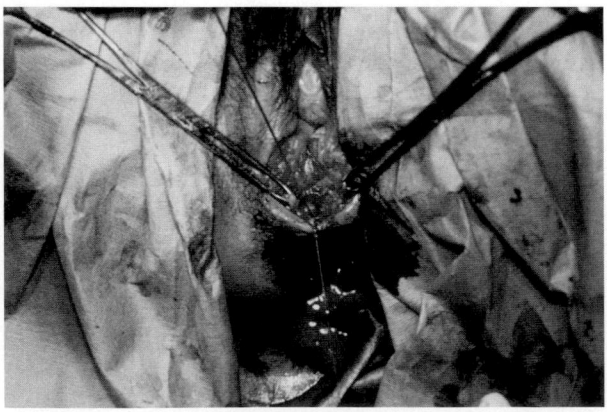

FIGURE 32A.7. Secondary closure of fourth-degree episiotomy breakdown. Rectal mucosa has been closed with 4-0 running chromic submucosal suture and reinforced with a second layer of 3-0 chromic suture through the rectovaginal septum. (Courtesy of Larry Gilstrap, University of Texas, Dallas.)

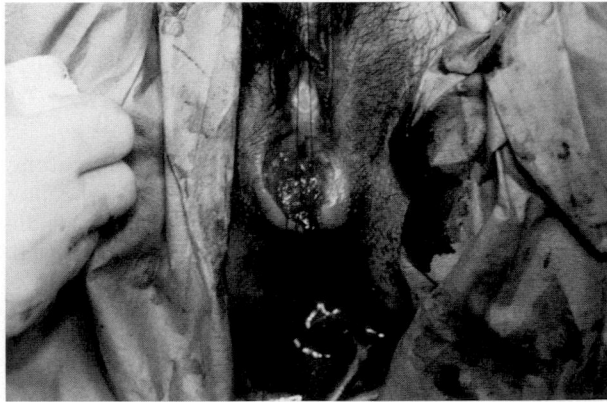

FIGURE32A.8. The anal sphincter muscle has been reapproximated end to end with several interrupted 2-0 chromic sutures through the muscle and capsule. (Courtesy of Larry Gilstrap, University of Texas, Dallas.)

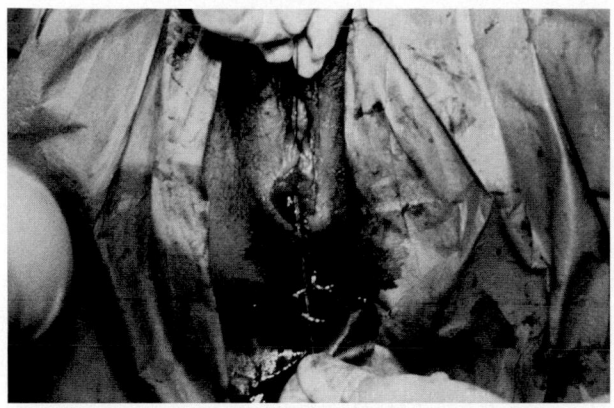

FIGURE 32A.9. The vaginal mucosa and bulbocavernous muscle have been closed with 2-0 chromic suture. (Courtesy of Susan Ramin, University of Texas, Dallas.)

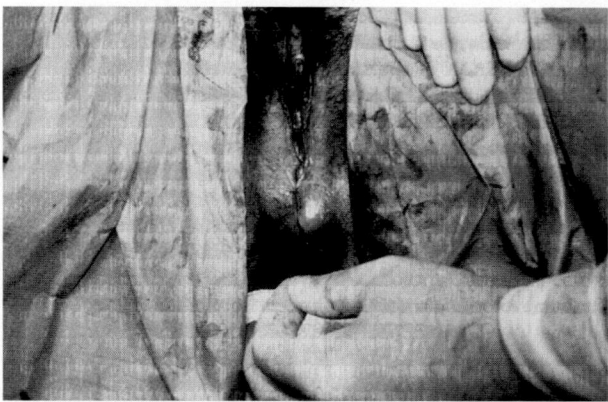

FIGURE 32A.10. Secondary repair of fourth-degree episiotomy dehiscence is completed. (Courtesy of Susan Ramin, University of Texas, Dallas.)

ure to obliterate the soft-tissue dead space, or poor approximation of the wound. Treatment consists of observation if the hematoma site is not expanding and is not infected. If expanding or infected, the episiotomy probably should be opened. An actual bleeding vessel is identified rarely. Coagulation studies, antibiotics, and blood products should be used as indicated.

Necrotizing Fasciitis

Fortunately, this is a rare complication of episiotomy. These infections, which involve the myofascial planes adjacent to the wound, are associated with risk factors including diabetes, intravenous drug use, malnutrition, obesity, steroid use, and an immunocompromised state. Anaerobic bacteria such as *Clostridium perfringens* or *Bacteroides fragilis* are common etiologic agents of fasciitis. However, aerobic Gram-positive cocci such as hemolytic streptococci also can be involved. Quick recognition of the problem is imperative to patient survival. Treatment consists of mandatory extensive debridement of all involved fascial layers, along with appropriate broad-spectrum antibiotics. Mortality is high and can approach 50%.

Summary

Although there are appropriate indications for performing an episiotomy, the routine performance of episiotomy for all deliveries cannot be justified. The most common complications of episiotomy are extension, infection, and dehiscence. Episiotomy dehiscence can result in significant discomfort and morbidity, especially if repair is delayed. Although classically it has been espoused that repair of episiotomy dehiscence should be delayed for several months, most experts now recommend early repair. Published data support the recommendation for early repair of episiotomy dehiscences (Table 32A.9). Such repairs have a 95% success rate. Before attempting repair, however, the wound must be clean and free of infection.

ACKNOWLEDGMENT

The current authors appreciate and acknowledge contributions made to this chapter by the preceding authors, Dr. Larry C. Gilstrap III and Dr. Norman F. Grant.

BIBLIOGRAPHY

Alamia Jr V, Meyer BA. Peripartum hemorrhage. *Obstet Gynecol Clin North Am* 1999;26:385.

Allen RE, Hoster GL, Smith ARB, et al. Pelvic floor damage and childbirth: a neurophysiologic study. *Br J Obstet Gynaecol* 1990;97:770.

Amant F, Spitz B, et al. Misoprostol compared with methylergometrine for the prevention of postpartum haemorrhage: a double-blind randomised trial. *Br J Obstet Gynaecol* 1999; 106:1066.

American College of Obstetricians and Gynecologists. *Diagnosis and management of postpartum hemorrhage*. ACOG Technical Bulletin No. 143, 1990.

Angioli R, Gomez-Marin O, et al. Severe perineal lacerations during vaginal delivery: the University of Miami experience. *Am J Obstet Gynecol* 2000;182:1083.

Arona AJ, Al-Marayati L, et al. Early secondary repair of third- and fourth-degree perineal lacerations after outpatient wound preparation. *Obstet Gynecol* 1995;86:294.

Argentine Episiotomy Trial Collaborative Group. Routine vs selective episiotomy: a randomised controlled trial. *Lancet* 1993;342:1517.

Baker ER, D'Alton ME. Caesarean section and caesarean hysterectomy. *Clin Obstet Gynecol* 1994;37:806.

Bamigboye AA, Hofmeyr GJ, Merrell DA. Rectal misoprostol in the prevention of postpartum hemorrhage: a placebo-controlled trial. *Am J Obstet Gynecol* 1998;179:1043.

Bansai RK, Tan WM, Ecker J, et al. Is there a benefit to episiotomy at spontaneous vaginal delivery? A natural experiment. *Am J Obstet Gynecol* 1996;175:897.

B-Lynch C, Coker A, Lawai A, et al. The B-Lynch surgical technique for the control of massive postpartum haemorrhage: an alternative to hysterectomy? Five cases reported. *Br J Obstet Gynaecol* 1997;104:372.

Burchell RC. Physiology of internal iliac artery ligation. *J Obstet Gynaecol Br Commonw* 1968;75:642.

Casele HL, Laifer SA. Successful pregnancy after bilateral hypogastric artery ligation: a case report. *J Reprod Med* 1997;42:306.

Castaneda S, Karrison T, Cibilis LA. Peripartum hysterectomy. *J Perinat Med* 2000;28:472.

Chan C, Razvi K, et al. The use of a Sengstaken-Blakemore tube to control post-partum hemorrhage. *Int J Gynecol Obstet* 1997;58:251.

Chestnut DH, Eden RD, Gall SA, et al. Peripartum hysterectomy: a review of caesarean and postpartum hysterectomy. *Obstet Gynecol* 1985;65:365.

Clark SL. Uterine and hypogastric artery ligation. In: Phelan JP, Clark SL, eds. *Caesarean delivery.* New York: Elsevier, 1988:238.

Clark SL, Phelan JP, Yeh SY, et al. Hypogastric artery ligation for obstetric hemorrhage. *Obstet Gynecol* 1985b;66:353.

Clark SL, Yeh SY, Phelan JP, et al. Emergency hysterectomy for obstetric hemorrhage. *Obstet Gynecol* 1984;64:376.

Connolly AM, Thorp, Jr JM. Childbirth-related perineal trauma: clinical significance and prevention. *Clin Obstet Gynecol* 1999;42:820.

Craig S, Chau H, Cho H. Treatment of severe postpartum hemorrhage by rectally administered gemeprost pessaries. *J Perinat Med* 1999;27:231.

Cunningham FG, MacDonald PC, Gant NF, et al., eds. Abnormalities of the third stage of labor. In: *Williams obstetrics,* 19th ed. Norwalk, CT: Appleton & Lange, 1993a:615.

Cunningham FG, MacDonald PC, Gant NF, et al., eds. Caesarean section and caesarean hysterectomy. In: *Williams obstetrics,* 19th ed. Norwalk, CT: Appleton & Lange, 1993b:591.

Cunningham FG, MacDonald PC, Gant NF, et al., eds. Conduct of normal labor. In: *Williams obstetrics,* 19th ed. Norwalk, CT: Appleton & Lange, 1993c:371.

Cunningham FG, MacDonald PC, Gant NF, et al., eds. Injuries to the birth canal. In: *Williams obstetrics,* 19th ed. Norwalk, CT: Appleton & Lange, 1993d:543.

De Loor JA, van Dam PA. Foley catheters for uncontrollable obstetric or gynecologic hemorrhage. *Obstet Gynecol* 1996;88:737.

Dildy GA, Scott JR, et al. Pelvic pressure pack for catastrophic postpartum hemorrhage. *Obstet Gynecol* 2000;95:7S.

Eason E, Feldman P. Much ado about a little cut: is episiotomy worthwhile? *Obstet Gynecol* 2000;95:616.

Eason E, Labrecque M, et al. Preventing perineal trauma during childbirth: a systematic review. *Obstet Gynecol* 2000;95:464.

Ferguson II JE, Bourgeois FJ, Underwood, Jr PB. B-Lynch suture for postpartum hemorrhage. *Obstet Gynecol* 2000;95:1020.

Fitzpatrick M, Behan M, O'Connell PR, et al. A randomized clinical trial comparing primary overlap with approximation repair of third-degree obstetric tears. *Am J Obstet Gynecol* 2000;183:1220.

Floyd RC, Morrison JC. Postpartum hemorrhage. In: Plauché WC, Morrison JC, O'Sullivan MJ, eds. *Surgical obstetrics.* Philadelphia: WB Saunders, 1992:272.

Gilstrap LC, Hauth JC, Hankins GDV, et al. Effect of type of anesthesia on blood loss at caesarean section. *Obstet Gynecol* 1987;69:328.

Gilstrap LC, Ramin SM. Postpartum hemorrhage. *Clin Obstet Gynecol* 1994;37:824.

Goldaber KG, Wendel PJ, McIntire D, et al. Postpartum perineal morbidity after fourth-degree perineal repair. *Am J Obstet Gynecol* 1993;168:489.

Gonsoulin W, Kennedy RT, Guidry KH. Elective versus emergency caesarean hysterectomy cases in a residency program setting: a review of 129 cases from 1984 to 1988. *Am J Obstet Gynecol* 1991;165:91.

Handa VL, Harris TA, Ostergard DR. Protecting the pelvic floor: obstetric management to prevent incontinence and pelvic organ prolapse. *Obstet Gynecol* 1996;88:470.

Hankins GDV, Hauth JC, Gilstrap LC III, et al. Early repair of episiotomy dehiscence. *Obstet Gynecol* 1990;75:48.

Hansch E, Chitkara U, McAlpine J, et al. Pelvic arterial embolization for control of obstetric hemorrhage: a five year experience. *Am J Obstet Gynecol* 1999;180:1454.

Hauth JC, Gilstrap LC III, Ward SC, et al. Early repair of an external sphincter ani muscle and rectal mucosal dehiscence. *Obstet Gynecol* 1986;67:806.

Henriksen T, Bek KM, Hedegaard M, et al. Episiotomy and perineal lesions in spontaneous vaginal deliveries. *Br J Obstet Gynaecol* 1992;99:950.

Homsi R, Daikoku NH, Littlejohn J, et al. Episiotomy: risks of dehiscence and rectovaginal fistula. *Obstet Gynecol Surv* 1994;49:803.

Hsu YR, Wan YL. Successful management of intractable puerperal hematoma and severe postpartum hemorrhage with DIC through transcatheter arterial embolization-two cases. *Acta Obstet Gynecol Scand* 1998;77:129.

Hueston WJ. Factors associated with the use of episiotomy during vaginal delivery. *Obstet Gynecol* 1996;87:1001.

Klein MC, Gauthier RJ, Jorgensen SH, et al. Does episiotomy prevent perineal trauma and pelvic floor relaxation. Online. *J Curr Clin Trials* 1992;2 (Document No. 10).

Klein MC, Gauthier RJ, Robbins JM, et al. Relationship of episiotomy to perineal trauma and morbidity, sexual dysfunction, and pelvic floor relaxation. *Am J Obstet Gynecol* 1994;171:591.

Klein MC, Janssen PA, MacWilliam L, et al. Determinants of vaginal-perineal integrity and pelvic floor functioning in childbirth. *Am J Obstet Gynecol* 1997;176:403.

Larsson PG, Platz-Christensen JJ, Bergman B, et al. Advantage or disadvantage of episiotomy compared with spontaneous perineal laceration. *Gynecol Obstet Invest* 1991;31:213.

Lede RL, Belizan JM, Carroli G. Is routine use of episiotomy justified? *Am J Obstet Gynecol* 1996;174:1399.

Liu CM, Hsu JJ, Hsieh TT, et al. Postpartum hemorrhage of the uterine artery rupture. *Acta Obstet Gynecol Scand* 1998;77:695.

Maier RC. Control of postpartum hemorrhage with uterine packing. *Am J Obstet Gynecol* 1993;169:317.

Marcovici I, Scoccia B. Postpartum hemorrhage and intrauterine balloon tamponade: a report of three cases. *J Reprod Med* 1999;44:122.

McNulty JV. Elective caesarean hysterectomy revisited. *Am J Obstet Gynecol* 1984;149:29.

Monberg J, Hammen S. Ruptured episiotomies resutured primarily. *Acta Obstet Gynecol Scand* 1987;66:163.

Myers-Helfgott MG, Helfgott AW. Routine use of episiotomy in modern obstetrics: should it be performed. *Obstet Gynecol Clin N Amer* 1999;26:305.

Oei PL, Chua S, Tan L, et al. Arterial embolization for bleeding following hysterectomy for intractable postpartum hemorrhage. *Int J Gynecol Obstet* 1998;62:83.

O'Leary JA. Stop OB hemorrhage with uterine artery ligation. *Contemp Obstet Gynecol* 1986;28:13.

O'Leary JA. Uterine artery ligation in the control of postcesarean hemorrhage. *J Reprod Med* 1995;40:189.

Owen J, Andrews WW. Wound complications after caesarean sections. *Clin Obstet Gynecol* 1994;37:842.

Owen J, Hauth JC. Episiotomy infection and dehiscence. In: Gilstrap LC III, Faro S, eds. *Infections in pregnancy.* New York: Alan R. Liss, 1990:61.

Patino JF, Castro D. Necrotizing lesions of the soft tissue: a review. *World J Surg* 1991;15:235.

Payne TN, Carey JC, Rayburn WF. Prior third- or fourth-degree perineal tears and recurrence risks. *Int J Gynaecol Obstet* 1999;64:55.

Pelage JP, Le Dref, O, Mateo J, et al. Life-threatening primary postpartum hemorrhage: treatment with emergency selective arterial embolization. *Radiology* 1999;208:359.

Pelage JP, Soyer P, Repiquet D, et al. Secondary postpartum hemorrhage: treatment with selective arterial embolization. *Radiology* 1999;212:385.

Philippe HJ, d'Oreye D, Lewin D. Vaginal ligature of uterine arteries during postpartum hemorrhage. *Int J Gynecol Obstet* 1997;56:267.

Plauche WC. Caesarean hysterectomy: indications, technique, and complications. *Clin Obstet Gynecol* 1986;29:318.

Plauche WC. Peripartal hysterectomy. In: Plauche WC, Morrison JC, O'Sullivan MJ, eds. *Surgical obstetrics.* Philadelphia: WB Saunders, 1992:447.

Ramin SM, Gilstrap LC III. Episiotomy and early repair of dehiscence. *Clin Obstet Gynecol* 1994;37:816.

Ramin SM, Ramus RM, Little BB, et al. Early repair of episiotomy dehiscence associated with infection. *Am J Obstet Gynecol* 1992;167:1104.

Roberts WE. Emergent obstetric management of postpartum hemorrhage. *Obstet Gynecol Clin N Amer* 1995;22:283.

Robinson JN, Norwitz ER, Cohen AP, et al. Episiotomy, operative vaginal delivery, and significant perineal trauma in nulliparous women. *Am J Obstet Gynecol* 1999;181: 1180.

Robinson JN, Norwitz ER, Cohen AP, et al. Predictors of episiotomy use at first spontaneous vaginal delivery. *Obstet Gynecol* 2000;96:214.

Rochat RW, Koonin LM, Atrash HK, et al. Maternal mortality in the United States: report from the Maternal Mortality Collaborative. *Obstet Gynecol* 1988;72:91.

Selo-Ojeme DO, Okonofua FE. Risk factors for primary postpartum haemorrhage. *Arch Gynecal Obstet* 1997;259:179.

Signorello LB, Harlow BL, Chekos AK, et al. Midline episiotomy and anal incontinence: retrospective cohort study [comment]. *BMJ* 2000;320:86–90.

Sleep J, Grant A. West Berkshire perineal management trial: three years follow-up. *BMJ* 1987;295:749.

Snyder RR, Hammond TL, Hankins GDV. Human papillomavirus associated with poor healing of episiotomy repairs. *Obstet Gynecol* 1990;76:664.

Stanco LM, Schrimmer DB, Paul RH, et al. Emergency peripartum hysterectomy and associated risk factors. *Am J Obstet Gynecol* 1993;168:879.

Strickland JL, Griffen WT, Llorens AS, et al. Caesarean hysterectomy: a procedure for modern obstetrics? *So Med J* 1989;82:1245.

Sturdee DW, Rushton DI. Caesarean and post-partum hysterectomy 1968–1983. *Br J Obstet Gynaecol* 1986;93:270.

Thacker SB, Banta HD. Benefits and risks of episiotomy: an interpretive review of the English language literature, 1860–1980. *Obstet Gynecol Surg* 1983;38:322.

Thorp JM Jr, Bowes WA Jr. Episiotomy: can its routine use be defended? *Am J Obstet Gynecol* 1989;160:1027.

Thorp JM Jr, Bowes WA Jr, Brame RG, et al. Selected use of midline episiotomy: effect on perineal trauma. *Obstet Gynecol* 1987;70:260.

Van Selm M, Kanhai HH, Keirse MJ. Preventing the recurrence of atonic postpartum hemorrhage: a double-blind trial. *Acta Obstet Gynecol Scand* 1995;74:270.

Varma A, Gunn J, Lindow SW, et al. Do routinely measured delivery variables predict anal sphincter outcome? *Dis Colon Rectum* 1999;42:1261.

Varmi A, Gunn J, Gardiner A, et al. Obstetric anal sphincter injury: prospective evaluation of incidence. *Dis Colon Rectum* 1999;42:1537.

Vedantham S, Goodwin SC, McLucas B, et al. Uterine artery embolization: an underused method of controlling pelvic hemorrhage. *Am J Obstet Gynecol* 1997;176:938.

Viktrup L, Lose G, Rolff M, et al. The symptom of stress incontinence caused by pregnancy or delivery in primiparas. *Obstet Gynecol* 1992;79:945.

Wagaarachchi PT, Fernando L. Fertility following ligation of internal iliac arteries for life-threatening obstetric haemorrhage. *Human Reprod* 2000;15:1311.

Walsh CJ, Mooney EF, Upton GJ, et al. Incidence of third-degree perineal tears in labour and outcome after primary repair. *Br J Surg* 1996;83:218.

Woolley RJ. Benefits and risks of episiotomy: a review of the English-language literature since 1980. Part I. *Obstet Gynecol Surv* 1995;50:806.

Woolley RJ. Benefits and risks of episiotomy: a review of the English language literature since 1980. Part II. *Obstet Gynecol Surv* 1995;50:821.

Yancey MK, Harlass FE, Benson W, et al. The perioperative morbidity of scheduled caesarean hysterectomy. *Obstet Gynecol* 1993;81:206.

Zelop CM, Harlow BL, Frigoletto FD, et al. Emergency peripartum hysterectomy. *Am J Obstet Gynecol* 1993;168:1443.

Zorlu CG, Turan C, Isik AZ, et al. Emergency hysterectomy in modern obstetric practice: changing clinical perspective in time. *Acta Obstet Gynecol Scand* 1998;77:186.

B
▼
Ovarian Tumors Complicating Pregnancy

LYNN P. PARKER

The coexistence of an ovarian tumor with pregnancy presents problems to both the clinician and the patient, the most serious being that of malignancy. This possibility must be discussed with the patient when obtaining informed consent before surgery. The therapeutic implications of possible hysterectomy with loss of current pregnancy and loss of future fertility result in an emotionally charged environment, because of the young age of the patient, the desire to preserve the pregnancy, as well as her reproductive capacity, and ovarian function.

INCIDENCE

Cancer complicates 1:1,000 pregnancies in the United States. The most common malignancies seen in pregnancy include malignant melanoma (2.6:1,000), Hodgkin's disease (1:1,000 to 6000), breast cancer (1:3,000 to 10,000), cervical cancer (1.2:10,000), ovarian cancer (1:10,000 to 100,000), colorectal cancer (1:13,000), and leukemias (1:75,000 to 100,000).

Benign ovarian tumors complicating pregnancy are more common. The exact incidence, however, depends on whether one considers simple cysts noted on ultrasound examination (one in 50 live births) or during pelvic examination (one in 80 live births), or those that ultimately require laparotomy (one in 1,000 to one in 1,500 live births). Ueda and Ueki reported 106 patients who required ovarian surgery during pregnancy. Of these cases, 29.2% were physiologic, 66% were benign, and 4.7% were malignant. In this study, the incidence of benign tumor was 1:112 deliveries, and 1:1,684 deliveries were malignant tumors.

Koonings and colleagues noted the incidence of ovarian tumors complicating caesarean section to be about one in 200 caesarean births, and Ballard observed that ovarian tumors complicated termination of pregnancy in one of 594 procedures. Hill and colleagues reported that ovarian cysts were diagnosed in 4.1% of second- or third-trimester ultrasounds. Most of these cysts were less than 3 cm and resolved spontaneously. Eighteen of the 7,996 patients had an exploratory laparotomy, which was equivalent to one surgery in 444 deliveries. All of these lesions were benign on pathologic examination.

DIAGNOSIS

The appropriate diagnosis of ovarian tumors complicating pregnancy depends on the use of certain windows of opportunity, namely, the initial pelvic examination in the first trimester, the initial ultrasound, and careful evaluation at the time of operative intervention. This includes thorough pelvic examination at the time of termination of pregnancy and careful examination of the ovaries at the time of caesarean section or postpartum tubal ligation.

The increasing (nearly routine) use of ultrasound examination affords an excellent opportunity for the diagnosis of coexistent ovarian pathology; it is for this reason that such an examination should always include the adnexa.

Perkins and coworkers evaluated 1,001 patients with first-trimester ultrasound and determined that a simple ovarian cyst was seen in 29% of these patients. Incidence of ovarian cyst decreased after 8 weeks, and absence of a cyst was more often associated with blighted ovum.

Resta and coworkers have reported that the upper limits of normal size for the corpus luteum of pregnancy is 2 cm. Most studies evaluating ovarian cysts in pregnancy rely on second trimester ultrasound characteristics or persistence of a cyst to try to eliminate false-positive results caused by the corpus luteum.

Lavery and colleagues, in a review of 3,918 ultrasound examinations at 20 weeks' gestation, noted cyst formation greater than 2 cm in 2.4% of examinations. Only nine patients (0.23%) required surgical intervention. Hogston and Lifford, in a review of 26,000 patients who received routine ultrasound, noted an incidence of cyst formation of 0.52%. All complex cysts and those greater than 6 cm were operated on primarily (10%). Eighty-five percent of the remaining patients who were followed conservatively showed a spontaneous resolution, with the exception of five patients who ultimately required laparotomy.

Bromley and coworkers evaluated the accuracy of sonographic diagnosis of adnexal masses during pregnancy. They evaluated all patients with an adnexal mass measuring 4 cm or greater noted beyond 12 weeks' gestation. One hundred and thirty-one lesions were noted; of these 89.3% were accurately diagnosed as benign. Of the 10.7% of lesions with sonographic characteristics of malignancy, one of 14 (7%) of these patients had ovarian cancer, for a 0.8% malignancy rate in this study.

Doppler sonography also has been evaluated for use in complex adnexal masses in pregnancy. Wheeler and Fleischer evaluated 34 pregnant patients with complex adnexal masses. Diagnosis made by color Doppler sonography was compared to actual histopathologic diagnosis. Three malignant and five low malignant potential tumors were correctly identified with a sensitivity of 0.89 and a mean pulsatility index (PI) of 0.71. The mean PI for benign lesions was >1, and the negative predictive value for PI > 1 was 0.93. The positive predictive value for PI < 1 was 0.42, indicating that some benign lesions were incorrectly classified as malignant when a PI < 1 is used as a cutoff for possibly malignant tumors. However, color Doppler appears to be highly predictive of a benign lesion when the PI is >1.

From a treatment standpoint, the first trimester is clearly the best time to diagnose an adnexal mass complicating pregnancy. Because tumors are rarely symptomatic during this period, most such tumors are discovered by ultrasound examination (or later, as an incidental finding at caesarean section). With the increasing incidence of ultrasound evaluation and use of caesarean section, recent articles suggest that only about 50% of ovarian tumors complicating pregnancy are symptomatic. When symptomatic, the patient typically presents with abdominal pain, abdominal distention, and vague gastrointestinal complaints. All these symptoms can be directly attributable to pregnancy itself; therefore, it is not surprising that most pregnant women with these symptoms are not evaluated for an ovarian tumor.

Ovarian tumors complicating pregnancy can be divided into three groups, depending on the severity of presentation.

- Those who are asymptomatic
- Those with symptoms compatible with torsion
- Those with catastrophic presentations consistent with hemorrhage, rupture, and shock

A successful outcome for both mother and fetus depends on a high index of suspicion with early diagnosis. One should consider an ovarian mass in any woman who experiences abdominal pain in pregnancy. Furthermore, torsion, rupture, infection, or hemorrhage of an ovarian tumor should be included in the differential diagnosis of any catastrophic abdominal obstetric event. This is particularly true during times of rapid change in uterine size or position (e.g., 8 to 16 weeks), during termination of pregnancy, during labor and delivery, or in the immediate postpartum period.

The incidence of torsion complicating ovarian tumor in the nonpregnant state is about 2%. Torsion complicating ovarian tumor during pregnancy is much higher, varying from 11% to 50%. Ueda and Ueki report a 21.8% rate of torsion in ovarian tumors in pregnancy. Other recent studies in which there is a high incidence of incidental asymptomatic tumors report much lower incidences of torsion, rupture, and dystocia. Nevertheless, it is clear that the unrecognized symptomatic ovarian tumor complicating pregnancy can become catastrophic, accompanied by hemorrhage, shock, peritonitis, or

death. Wang et al., retrospectively evaluated 174 patients who underwent surgery for ovarian masses during pregnancy. These patients were divided into two groups: those with emergency surgery (32 patients) and those with elective surgery (142 patients). They found in the emergency surgery group that half of the surgeries occurred in the first trimester; they contributed to 75% of total fetal wastage and 87% of spontaneous fetal loss; and tumor sizes were significantly larger. In their experience, tumors <5 cm in size never caused symptoms requiring surgery. Therefore, size of tumor, ultrasound characteristics, color Doppler flow, as well as symptoms are important in determining the management of pregnant patients with adnexal masses.

PATHOLOGY

Benign neoplasms complicating pregnancy include two tumorlike conditions with which every gynecologist should be familiar. Hyperreactio luteinalis (first described by Burger in 1938 as a grossly multicystic, usually bilateral ovarian enlargement, often 15 to 20 cm in size) is a term used to describe numerous luteinized follicular cysts of the ovary complicating pregnancy (Fig. 32B.1). Microscopically, one notes extensive luteinization of the theca and granulosa cell layers. Bradshaw et al. suggest the hyperandogenicity seen in this condition is related to increased ovarian sensitivity to human chorionic gonadotropin (hCG). Therefore, it is seen in conditions where the hCG is elevated, such as hydatidiform mole, multiple gestations, choriocarcinoma, and erythroblastosis fetalis. Hyperreactio luteinalis also has been associated with normal pregnancy, and there has not been an association with fetal virilization. These tumors spontaneously regress after delivery, but may take up to 6 months to resolve. Hyperreactio luteinalis also may occur in subsequent pregnancies.

Luteoma of pregnancy is a specific benign, usually unilateral, solid lutein cell tumor of the ovary found in late pregnancy, often noted at caesarean section (Fig. 32B.2). First described by Sternberg in 1963, this tumor is grossly bosselated, soft, fleshy, yellow, or hemorrhagic. Microscopically, it exhibits an acidophilic granular cytoplasm with sparse lipid formation and a distinctive reticular pattern. It is likely the most common cause of maternal virilization during pregnancy. The etiology is unknown, but theories have included luteinized stromal cells present prior to pregnancy that respond to hCG or "hyperluteinized" theca cells, granulosa cells, or a combination of the two. Fifty percent of female infants born to virilized mothers with pregnancy luteoma exhibit signs of virilization.

The important clinical implication with both of these lesions is that if they are recognized or suspected, simple biopsy without further surgery is adequate therapy, because both invariably resolve spontaneously.

The most common benign neoplasm of the ovary in pregnancy is the benign cystic teratoma, which occurs in about 36% of such cases (Fig. 32B.3). The second most

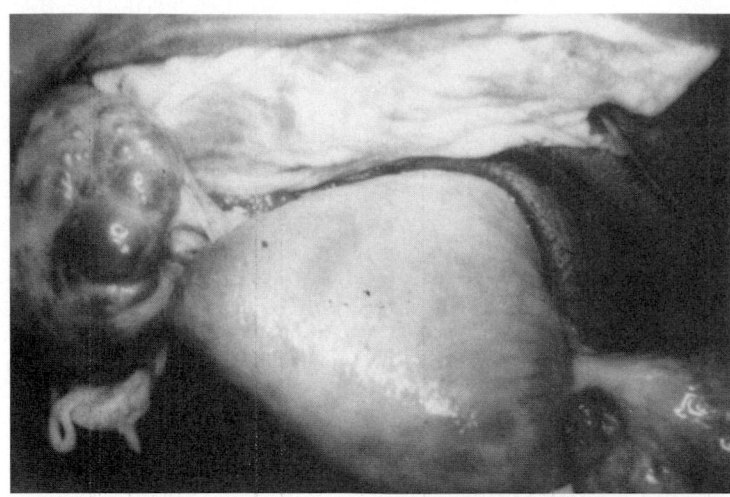

FIGURE 32B.1. Hyperreactio luteinalis (multiple theca luteal cysts) is a tumorlike condition complicating pregnancy. Usually, it is bilateral and resolves spontaneously. (Courtesy of David Barclay, Little Rock, AR.)

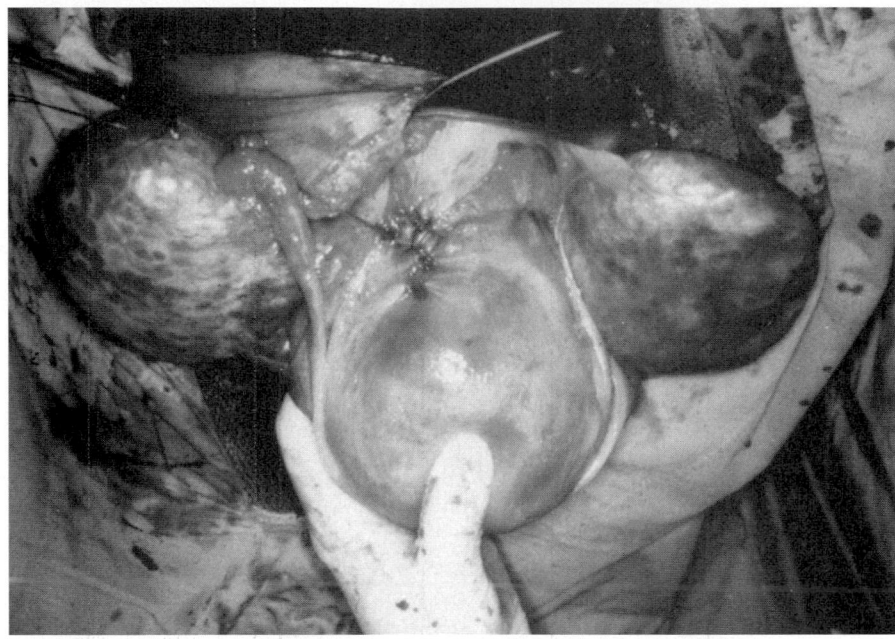

FIGURE 32B.2. Luteoma of pregnancy. Typically occurring late in normal pregnancies and usually unilateral and solid, this lesion resolves spontaneously. (Courtesy of David Barclay, Little Rock, AR.)

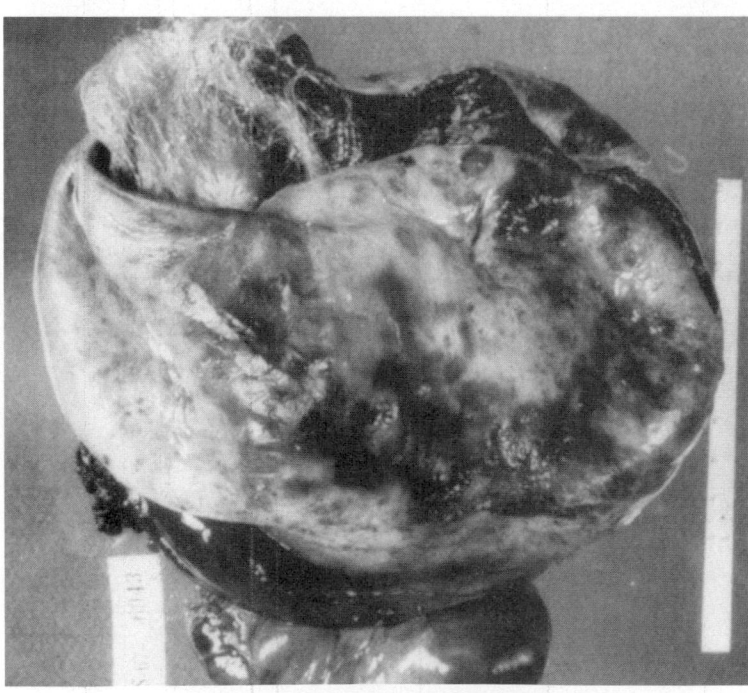

FIGURE 32B.3. The benign cystic teratoma is the most common benign neoplasm of the ovary complicating pregnancy. This tumor has undergone torsion and infarction.

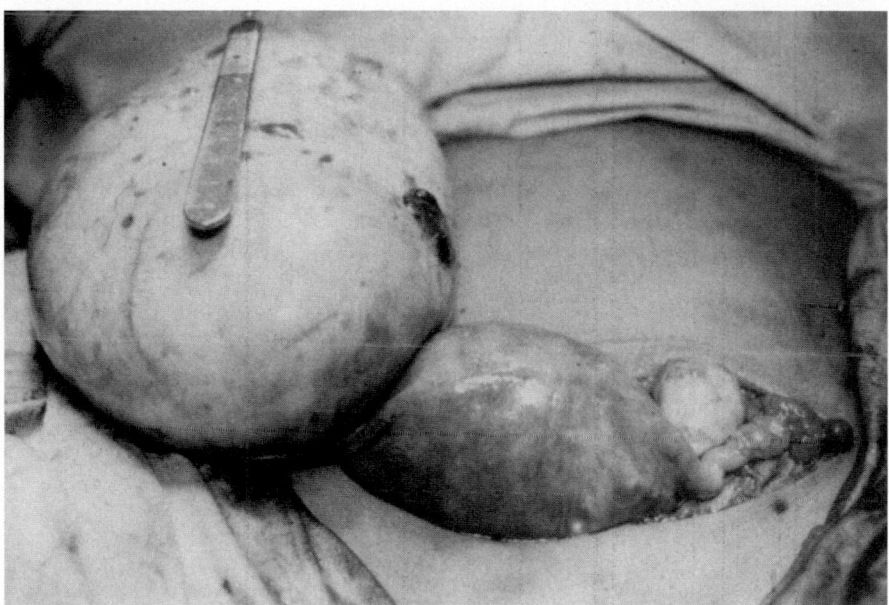

FIGURE 32B.4. A mucinous cystadenoma complicating pregnancy. Tumors of epithelial origin are the second most common benign neoplasm of the ovary complicating pregnancy. Mucinous tumors are relatively more common in pregnancy.

common group of ovarian tumors complicating pregnancy is that of cystadenomas. These represent about 15% of tumors (Fig. 32B.4). Endometriomas, simple cysts, corpus luteal cysts, tubal cysts, myomas, and other miscellaneous tumors constitute the remaining types of tumors seen in pregnancy (Table 32B.1).

Malignant ovarian tumors constitute about 1% to 2% of all adnexal masses that complicate pregnancy and require surgical exploration. The single most common malignant ovarian tumor complicating pregnancy probably is dysgerminoma. Malignant tumors of epithelial origin as a group, however, are more common; tumors of low

TABLE 32B.1.
Pathology of Pelvic Masses Complicating Pregnancy

	Bromley n = 131	Hill n = 19	Wheeler n = 34	Ueder n = 106	Total 290
Dermoid	40	8	8	48	104 (36%)
Endometrioma	15	1	2	10	28 (9.7%)
Functional cysts	14	1	0	6	21 (7.2%)
Cystadenomas	13	4	10	18	45 (15.5%)
Tubal cyst	9	2	0	0	11 (3.8%)
Fibroids	4	0	2	0	6 (2.1%)
Adenocarcinoma of the ovary	1	0	1	2	4 (1.4%)
Corpus luteum	0	2	2	15	19 (6.6%)
Serous cystadenoma/endometrioma	1	0	0	0	1 (0.3%)
Cystadenofibroma	2	0	0	0	2 (0.6%)
Fibrothecoma	1	0	0	0	1 (0.3%)
Serous cystadenofibroma	1	0	0	0	1 (0.3%)
Dermoid/fibrothecoma	1	0	0	0	1 (0.3%)
Fibroma	0	1	0	4	5 (1.7%)
Tavlov cyst	1	0	0	0	1 (0.3%)
Struma ovarii	2	0	0	0	2 (0.6%)
Luteoma of pregnancy	1	0	1	0	2 (0.6%)
Echinococcal cyst	1	0	0	0	1 (0.3%)
Dysgerminoma	0	0	1	1	2 (0.6%)
Lymphoma	0	0	1	0	1 (0.3%)
Low malignant potential tumors	0	0	6	1	7 (2.4%)
Embryonal carcinoma	0	0	0	1	1 (0.3%)
Twenty-four normal ovaries at follow-up in the Bromley study					24 (8.3%)

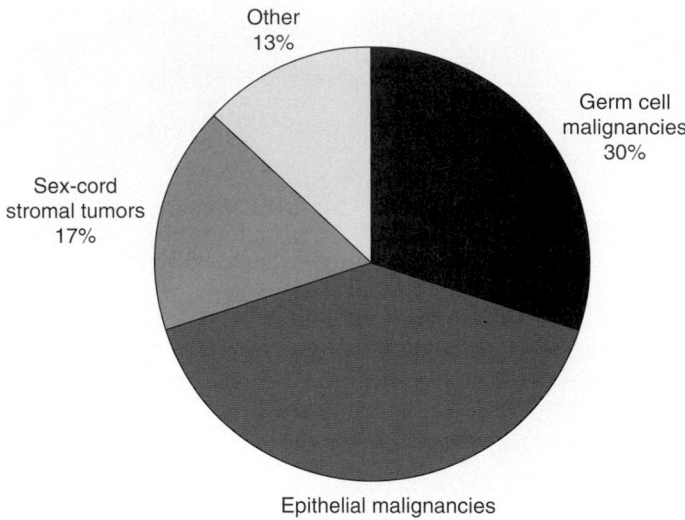

FIGURE 32B.5. The approximate relative frequency of the most common malignant ovarian tumors.

malignant potential occur most frequently (Fig. 32B.5). Sex cord stromal tumors are the third most common primary malignant ovarian neoplasms, representing about 17% to 20% of such tumors. Krukenberg and other metastatic tumors represent about 12% to 13% of malignant ovarian neoplasms complicating pregnancy.

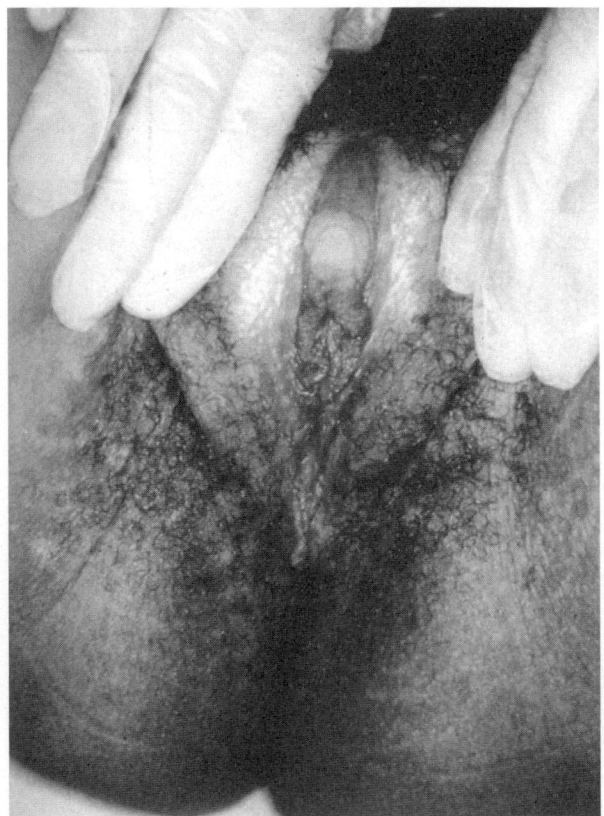

FIGURE 32B.6. Virilization occurring in late pregnancy secondary to a pregnancy luteoma. Note clitoral hypertrophy and hirsutism. (Courtesy of David Barclay, Little Rock, AR.)

Whether malignant or benign, most ovarian tumors complicating pregnancy are unilateral. Karlen and associates reported 90% of dysgerminomas in pregnancy to be unilateral, and Young and colleagues reported 35 of 36 sex cord stromal tumors to be unilateral when complicating pregnancy. Even malignant tumors of epithelial origin noted during pregnancy are unilateral in 90% of cases. The rarer germ cell tumors, such as endodermal sinus tumors, virtually always are unilateral as well. It is also interesting that most bilateral tumors occurring in pregnancy are not malignant; these include benign cystic teratoma, endometriosis, and hyperreactio luteinalis. The most common bilateral malignant ovarian tumors are the metastatic Krukenberg types. Somewhat less common are primary malignant tumors of epithelial origin.

Virilization secondary to an ovarian tumor sometimes complicates pregnancy (Fig. 32B.6). The classic painting entitled *Magdalena Ventura with Husband and Son,* painted in 1631 by Ribera, documents such a problem (Fig. 32B.7). Magdalena, after having several children, became virilized at age 37, with apparent infertility thereafter. However, when she was 52, a son was born. One would speculate that she probably had an ovarian Sertoli-Leydig cell tumor. Young and colleagues, however, pointed out that although about 50% of Sertoli-Leydig cell tumors in the nonpregnant state are functional, only about 15% of those complicating pregnancy result in maternal virilization. They proposed two possible explanations for this apparent decrease in virilization. The first is that the most active of such tumors result in anovulation; therefore, women with virilizing tumors rarely become pregnant. The second is that the placenta may aromatize the tumor-produced androgens into estrogens. In any event, Sertoli-Leydig cell tumors are not the most common tumors in pregnancy associated with virilization. This distinction falls to those tumors associated with a functioning ovarian stroma. The most common virilizing ovarian tumor that complicates pregnancy is the luteoma, followed by Krukenberg tumors and mucinous epithelial tumors (Table 32B.2).

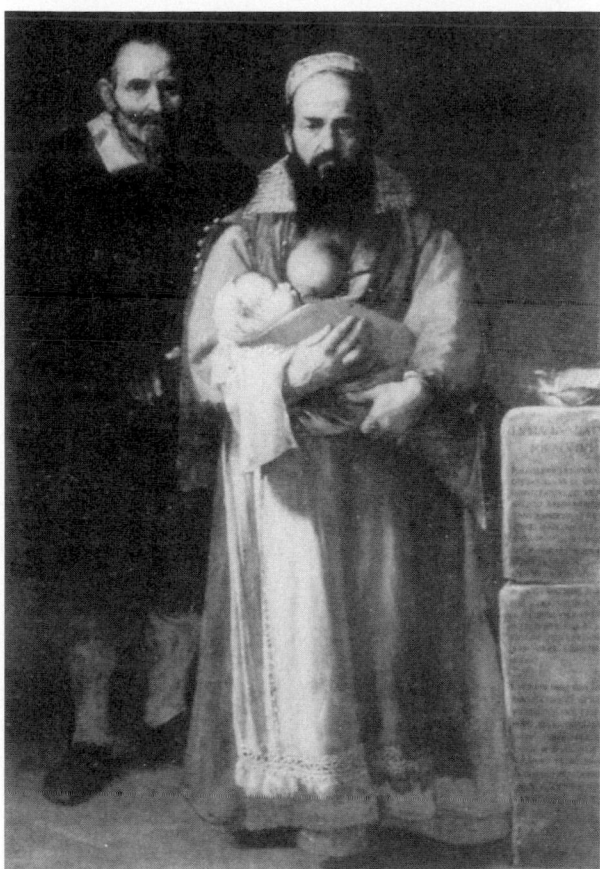

FIGURE 32B.7. The painting by Ribera entitled *Magdalena Ventura with Husband and Son*. The most common virilizing tumors of the ovary complicating pregnancy are those with functioning stroma. (Reprinted with permission.)

TABLE 32B.2.
Differential Diagnosis of Virilizing Ovarian Tumors Associated with Pregnancy[a]

HISTOLOGIC DIAGNOSIS

Luteoma
Hyperreactio luteinalis
Sex cord disorders
    Granulosa theca
    Thecomas
    Theca-lutein cyst
    Sertoli-Leydig
    Hilar cell tumor
    Hilar cell hyperplasia
    Stromal luteomas
    Stromal hyperthecosis
    Unclassified sex cord stromal tumors
Other ovarian tumors
    Krukenberg tumors
    Mucinous cystadenocarcinoma
    Dermoid
    Brenner tumor

From: XX, with permission.

The clinical implications of virilizing tumors complicating pregnancy are somewhat different from those of such tumors in the nonpregnant state. Virilization usually occurs late in pregnancy, is of short duration, and usually is reversible. The majority of such cases, as mentioned, are secondary to luteoma; therefore, they resolve spontaneously. If sex cord stromal or epithelial tumors are present, the ultimate outcome remains quite good. However, patients with Krukenberg lesions have a poor outcome.

Malignancies also can be metastatic to the placenta or products of conception. Although this is an uncommon occurrence, tumors that may metastasize to the placenta include malignant melanoma, leukemias and lymphomas, breast carcinoma, lung carcinoma, and some sarcomas.

THERAPY

Surgery

The first successful oophorectomy for an ovarian tumor complicating pregnancy was performed in 1846 by Bund. Although the woman survived, the fetus aborted

at 12 weeks' gestation. At about the same time, J. Marion Sims was the first to successfully remove an ovarian tumor in a pregnant woman and to have both the woman and fetus survive. As late as 1906, McKerran reported a 21% maternal mortality rate and a 50% fetal mortality rate with surgical management of ovarian tumors in pregnancy.

In general, one should avoid elective surgery in the first trimester, because many lesions represent the cystic corpus luteum of pregnancy and resolve spontaneously. Therefore, ultrasound should be repeated in 6 weeks to determine if the mass is persistent before considering surgical intervention. Buttery and colleagues noted an abortion rate of about 30% in those patients operated on in the first trimester, so first trimester procedures are high risk. Nevertheless, symptomatic, complex, bilateral, and solid tumors should be operated on immediately (Fig. 32B.8). Preoperative evaluation should be limited to careful clinical evaluation and pelvic ultrasound examination. Barium enema, computed tomography, and other such studies are best avoided. Magnetic resonance imaging can be used safely in pregnancy, but has not been helpful in evaluation of adnexal masses.

Tumor markers such as CA-125 are not helpful in pregnancy, because they can be elevated owing to the pregnancy and not the mass. Alpha fetoprotein is heterogenous and the yolk sac variant can be separated by affinity chromatography to determine if the elevation is owing to the yolk sac or liver variant. Lactate dehydrogenase (LDH) can be produced by dysgerminomas. Except for preeclampsia, LDH levels should remain within normal limits in pregnancy.

Wang et al., in their evaluation of surgical management of ovarian masses in pregnancy, found that elective

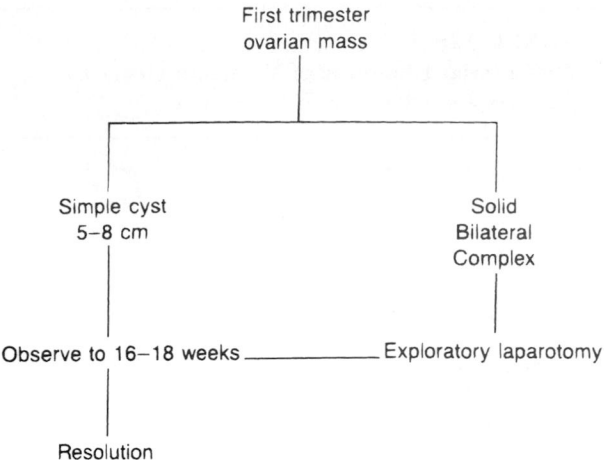

FIGURE 32B.8. Algorithm for the surgical management of ovarian tumors complicating pregnancy in the first trimester. Symptomatic, solid, bilateral, and complex lesions should be operated on when discovered.

surgery had a much lower rate of fetal wastage and was more likely to occur in the second trimester. Therefore, elective management of adnexal masses in pregnancy appears to be safer than awaiting symptoms or emergency intervention.

The optimum time for surgical intervention is 16 to 18 weeks. In general, the first trimester should be avoided if possible because of the naturally occurring high rate of spontaneous abortion. It is difficult to avoid the conclusion that any pregnancy loss occurring within a short time of surgery is related to the surgery, so that if it is possible to wait until the second trimester, the risk of an unrelated spontaneous abortion is decreased. Patients in whom the asymptomatic mass is noted at or near term, may be considered for delivery by caesarean section with careful surgical evaluation of the adnexa. Vaginal delivery in this situation has been associated with torsion, rupture, and hemorrhage that can occur during labor or immediately postpartum. The size and ultrasound characteristics of the mass will help to guide the clinician's decision concerning the best route of delivery. Caspi et al. described conservative management of 63 patients who had dermoid cysts <6 cm. None of these patients had an increase in size of the dermoid during pregnancy. In this study, 55 patients had normal vaginal deliveries and none had complications related to the cyst. They also evaluated the use of ultrasound guided cyst aspiration in patients with persistent simple cysts into the second trimester. In this study, 50% of the patients avoided surgical intervention with this procedure. Every case of an adnexal mass should be independently evaluated to determine the best management.

General anesthesia is the anesthesia of choice, although a combination of epidural and general anesthesia can be considered. One should remember that delayed gastric emptying and esophageal reflux can occur in pregnancy; therefore, appropriate precautions are necessary. One also should be aware of and prevent vena caval and aortic compression.

The next consideration is laparoscopy versus laparotomy as primary surgical management. Several case series have evaluated the safety and efficacy of laparoscopic management of adnexal masses in pregnancy. These studies have shown that laparoscopic surgery can be used without increased risk to mother or fetus. Moore et al. evaluated 14 patients with adnexal masses treated with laparoscopy. The average gestational age was 16 weeks, with average operating time of 84 minutes. The tumors included three mucinous cystadenomas, three mature teratomas, three functional cysts, and one endometrioma. Three patients had tumors greater than 10 cm; the remainder were >7 cm in size. There were no postoperative complications except for one case of mild peritonitis that spontaneously resolved. Laparoscopy should be considered early in the second trimester if the mass is mobile, accessible, and does not have characteristics of malignancy such as ascites or carcinomatosis.

If laparotomy is the chosen surgical approach, a vertical incision is preferred, because after 16 weeks' gestation the ovary is an abdominal rather than pelvic structure. The incision should be placed higher than usual. Thorough gross examination of the lesion, with frozen section, as well as evaluation of the upper abdomen, omentum, and paraaortic nodes, should be performed, along with pelvic washings. The involved ovary should be sent for frozen section to establish a preliminary diagnosis. The contralateral ovary should be carefully inspected. However, biopsy or wedge resection of the contralateral ovary should be avoided if no gross evidence of involvement is present. One possible exception is if the primary tumor is a dysgerminoma, because these tumors can involve the contralateral ovary in a clinically undetectable, microscopic manner. If the patient has a malignant germ cell tumor or low malignant potential tumor, staging should be performed to include omentectomy, peritoneal biopsies, and pelvic and paraaortic lymph node biopsies on the side of the mass. If the tumor is mucinous, either cystadenoma or low malignant potential tumor, an appendectomy should be performed.

The uterus should be handled gently in any case, and frequent irrigation should be used to prevent the tissue from drying. When ovarian cystectomy is required, a closure with use of a 5-0 suture internal closure is recommended. Alternatively, one can decide to perform no closure. The traditional Buxton-type closure should be avoided.

Before the decision is made to perform oophorectomy, one must always consciously exclude hyperreactio luteinalis and luteoma of pregnancy. Furthermore, because most malignant ovarian tumors are unilateral, total abdominal hysterectomy and bilateral salpingectomy are rarely indicated (Fig. 32B.9). Total hysterectomy and removal of ovaries should never be performed on the basis of a frozen section diagnosis of borderline or low-grade malignancy, unless the patient has clearly expressed a desire to abort this pregnancy and does not wish to preserve fertility and ovarian function.

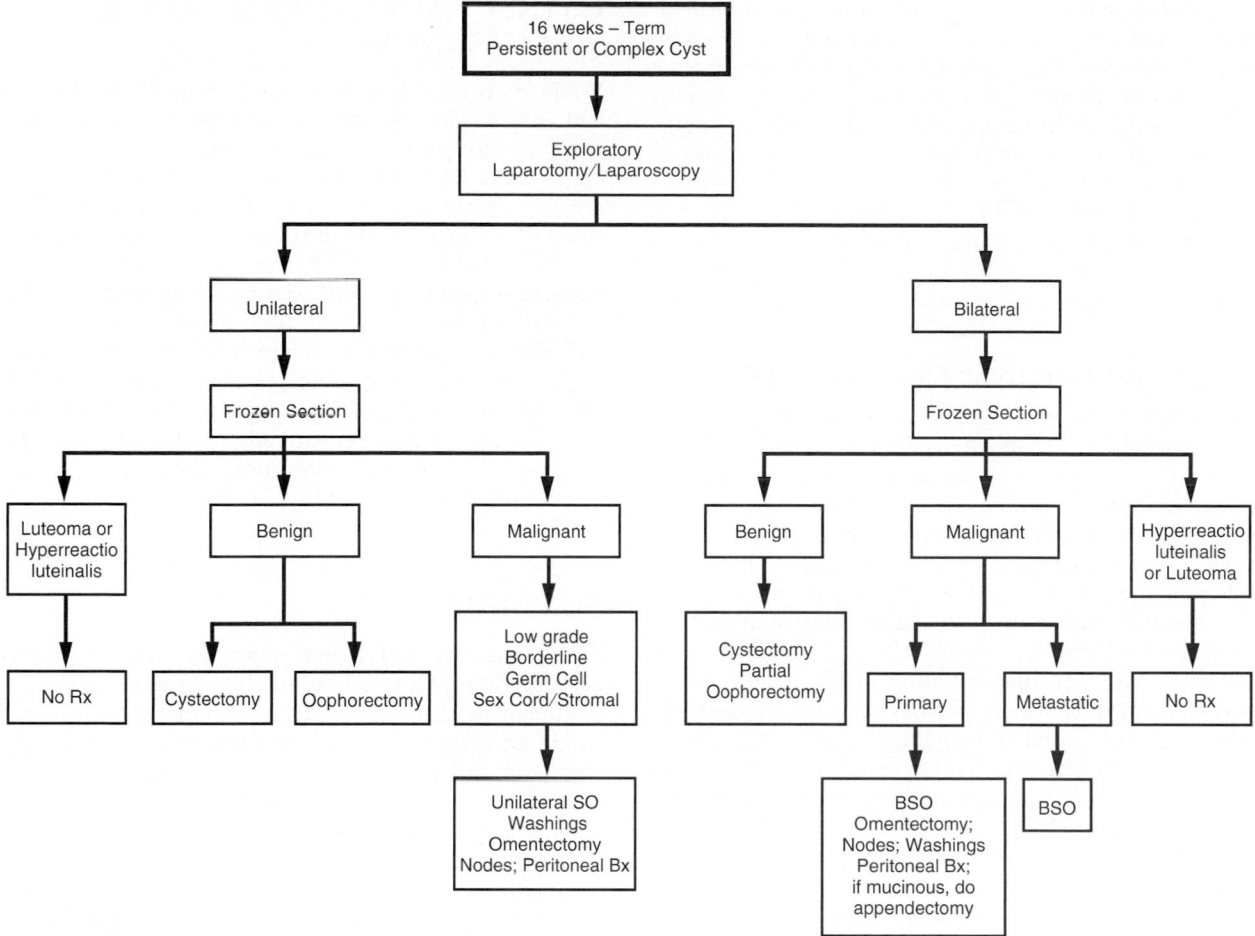

FIGURE 32B.9. Algorithm for the surgical management of ovarian tumors occurring after 16 weeks' gestation. BSO, bilateral salpingo-oophorectomy; SO, salpingo-oophorectomy, TAH, total abdominal hysterectomy.

When faced with a clearly malignant bilateral tumor, one usually treats the patient as if she were nonpregnant, with total hysterectomy, bilateral salpingo-oophorectomy, pelvic and abdominal washings, omentectomy, and pelvic and paraaortic node biopsies. Even with bilateral malignant disease, one can consider omitting hysterectomy if the uterus is not grossly involved, thus allowing preservation of the existing pregnancy, especially because platinum based chemotherapy can safely be given during pregnancy. Although other tumors are known to metastasize rarely to either the placenta or fetus, primary ovarian tumors almost never do so.

All the possible findings at surgery and possible surgical management options should be carefully discussed with the patient, and a good understanding of the planned therapy should be agreed on by all. A careful preoperative note about the discussion should be made in the patient's chart. The family should be informed of the findings and plans during the course of surgery and consultation should be obtained if necessary.

The role of progesterone to prevent labor in the postoperative period is unclear, but should be considered if the surgery occurs in the first trimester. The patient should be monitored for contractions and fetal heart tones checked in the postoperative period. If contractions occur these can be treated with hydration, sedation, indomethacin (if before 32 weeks), or standard tocolytic therapy.

Treatment Outcome

Conservative surgical treatment outcome for benign disease should be excellent. With malignant disease, the overall 5-year survival rate depends on stage and cell type. In the largest series of malignant ovarian tumors, Novak and colleagues reported a 5-year survival rate of 75%. Karlen and associates, in a review of 27 dysgerminomas, reported a tendency toward local recurrence with conservative treatment but an overall 5-year survival rate of 90%. Young and coworkers, in a review of 36 sex cord stromal tumors, noted a 5-year survival rate of 100%, although they cautioned that granulosa cell tumors are prone to late recurrence. However, patients with Krukenberg tumors or metastatic disease have a poor prognosis.

Fetal mortality also should be minimal with early diagnosis and appropriate surgical intervention. Although Karlen and associates reported a fetal mortality rate of 25%, two of the five deaths were secondary to hysterotomy. Young and colleagues reported three fetal deaths in 36 cases, two of which resulted from hysterectomy. Ueda et al. reported on 106 surgeries with a spontaneous abortion rate of 10%. Two patients desired termination of pregnancy in the second trimester owing to ovarian diagnosis, and one fetus died despite intensive efforts.

Adjunctive Cytotoxic Chemotherapy

At no time is the treatment of cancer during pregnancy more complicated than when adjunctive therapy is indicated. Can such therapy be given safely during pregnancy? Although single-agent or combination chemotherapy may be teratogenic in the first trimester, it is now apparent that cytotoxic chemotherapy can be used safely in the second and third trimesters. Antimetabolite therapy, including both aminopterin and methotrexate, has been reported to be associated with an increased rate of congenital abnormalities. The aminopterin syndrome, which consists of cranial dysostosis, hypertelorism, anomalies of the external ear, micrognathia, and cleft palate, has occurred in the fetuses of about 20% of patients treated in the first trimester. The risk decreases if the drugs are given in the second or third trimester. The alkylating agent chlorambucil has been associated with congenital abnormalities, namely, renal aplasia, cleft palate, and skeletal anomalies, but only with first-trimester exposure. Cisplatin also has been used in a limited number of patients in the second and third trimesters without apparent problems. Antitumor antibiotics such as bleomycin, doxorubicin, and daunorubicin have shown no adverse fetal outcomes. Vincristine and vinblastine cause malformations in animals, but have not been reported in humans exposed. Taxol is very effective in treatment of epithelial ovarian malignancies, but its safety in pregnancy is unknown.

Besides such congenital abnormalities and spontaneous abortions, other concerns with the use of chemotherapy in pregnancy include sterility, low birth weight, pancytopenia, delayed cognitive development, and carcinogenesis. The risk and benefits to the fetus and mother must be considered prior to beginning therapy. Of course, cytotoxic chemotherapy has other effects, including hematopoietic depression and infection. For this reason, the timing of chemotherapy in relation to anticipated delivery must be assessed carefully so that delivery does not occur when the patient is pancytopenic.

Reports in the literature describe safe treatment of germ cell tumors of the ovary with bleomycin, etoposide, and cis-platinum (BEP), vincristine, actinomycin D, and cyclophosphamide (VAC), or vinblastine, bleomycin, and cis-platinum (VPB). In epithelial malignancies, cis-platinum alone versus cis-platinum and cyclophosphamide have been used.

OTHER ISSUES SURROUNDING MALIGNANCY

Symptom control is very important in pregnant patients with malignancy. Symptoms commonly seen in malignancy include pain, nausea, vomiting, anorexia, dyspnea, fatigue and depression. Oxycodone, hydrocodone, with acetaminophen can be used safely for pain. Codeine should be avoided in the first trimester because of possible fetal malformation. Opiates can be used, but the neonate should be monitored for withdrawal after delivery. For nausea, options include chlorpromazine, prochlorperazine, prednisone, metoclopramide, and ondansetron. Morphine and albuterol have been successfully used to control dyspnea in patients with malignancy. Forty percent of patients with advanced cancer have depression. Fluoxetine has been used safely in pregnancy, and should be considered in these patients.

SUMMARY

The evaluation and management of ovarian tumors complicating pregnancy must be different from the treatment of such tumors in the nonpregnant woman. Although many tumors are asymptomatic, torsion, rupture, and hemorrhage are more common during pregnancy and can adversely affect maternal and fetal outcome if not appropriately diagnosed.

However, the outlook for malignant ovarian tumors complicating pregnancy is much better than it is for these tumors occurring in nonpregnant women. An increased incidence of tumors of borderline malignancy and early-stage epithelial tumors, as well as an increased incidence of germ-cell tumors, allows more conservative therapy. Consequently, in many patients, the pregnancy and future ovarian and reproductive function can be preserved. Furthermore, pregnancy does not preclude adjunctive cytotoxic chemotherapy, which can be initiated safely in the second and third trimesters.

In the final analysis, under optimum circumstances, achieving the therapeutic goal of both a healthy mother and child should be the rule rather than the exception when ovarian tumors complicate pregnancy.

BIBLIOGRAPHY

Aiman J. Virilizing ovarian tumors. *Clin J Obstet Gynecol* 1991;34:835.

Boulay R, Podczaski E. Ovarian cancer complicating pregnancy. *Obstet Gynecol Clin North Am* 1998;25:385.

Bradshaw KD, Santos-Ramos R, Rawlins SC, et al. Endocrine studies in a pregnancy complicated by ovarian theca lutein cysts and hyperreactio luteinalis. *Obstet Gynecol* 1986;67:66S.

Bromley B, Benacerraf B. Adnexal masses during pregnancy: accuracy of sonographic diagnosis and outcome. *J Ultrasound Med* 1997;16:447.

Buller RE, Darrow V, Manetta A, et al. Conservative surgical management of dysgerminoma concomitant with pregnancy. *Obstet Gynecol* 1992;79:887.

Caspi B, Ben-Arie A, Appelman Z, et al. Aspiration of simple pelvic cysts during pregnancy. *Gynecol Obstet Invest* 2000; 49:102.

Caspi B, Levi R, Appelman Z, et al. Conservative management of ovarian cystic teratoma during pregnancy and labor. *Am J Obstet Gynecol* 2000;182:503.

Check JH, Choe JK, Nazari A. Hyperreactio luteinalis despite absence of a corpus luteum and suppressed serum follicle stimulating concentrations in a triplet pregnancy. *Hum Reprod* 2000;15:1043.

De Palma P, Wronski M, Bifernino V, et al. Krukenberg tumor in pregnancy with virilization. *Eur J Gynaecol Oncol* 1995;16:59.

Dgani R, Soham Z, Atar OE, et al. Ovarian carcinoma during pregnancy. *Gynecol Oncol* 1989;33:326.

Dildy GA, Moise KJ, Carpenter RJ, et al. Maternal malignancy metastatic to the products of conception: a review. *Obstet Gynecol Surv* 1989;44:535.

Ebert U, Loffler H, Kirch W. Cytotoxic therapy and pregnancy. *Pharmacol Ther* 1997;74:207.

Elerding SC. Laparoscopic surgery in pregnancy. *Am J Surg* 1993;165:625.

Farahmand SM, Marchetti DL, Asirwatham JE, et al. Ovarian endodermal sinus tumor associated with pregnancy: a review of the literature. *Gynecol Oncol* 1991;41:156.

Fleischer AC, Shah DM, Entman SS. Sonographic evaluation of maternal disorders during pregnancy. *Radiol Clin North Am* 1990;28:51.

Frederiksen MC, Casanova L, Schink JC. An elevated maternal serum alpha-fetoprotein leading to the diagnosis of an immature teratoma. *Int J Gynecol Oncol* 1991;35:343.

Garcia-Bunuel RG, Berek JS, Woodruff JD. Luteomas of pregnancy. *Obstet Gynecol* 1975;45:407.

Greskovich Jr JF, Macklis RM. Radiation therapy in pregnancy: risk calculation and risk minimization. *Semin Oncol* 2000;27:633.

Henderson CE, Giovanni E, Garfinkel D, et al. Platinum chemotherapy during pregnancy for serous cystadenocarcinoma of the ovary. *Gynecol Oncol* 1993;49:92.

Hill LM, Connors-Beatty DJ, Nowak A, et al. The role of ultrasonography in the detection and management of adnexal masses during the second and third trimesters of pregnancy. *Am J Obstet Gynecol* 1998;179:703.

Hogston P, Lifford RJ. Ultrasound study of ovarian cysts in pregnancy: prevalence and significance. *Br J Obstet Gynaecol* 1986;93:625.

Hopkins MP, Duchon MA. Adnexal surgery in pregnancy. *J Reprod Med* 1986;31:1035.

Illingworth PJ, Johnstone FD, Steel J, et al. Luteoma of pregnancy: masculinisation of a female fetus prevented by placental aromatisation. *Br J Obstet Gynaecol* 1992;99:1019.

Karlen JR, Akbari A, Cook WA. Dysgerminoma associated with pregnancy. *Obstet Gynecol* 1979;53:330.

Kier R, McCarthy SM, Scoutt LM, et al. Pelvic masses in pregnancy: MR imaging. *Radiology* 1990;176:709.

King LA, Nevin PC, Williams PP, et al. Treatment of advanced epithelial ovarian carcinoma in pregnancy with cisplatin-based chemotherapy. *Gynecol Oncol* 1991;41:78.

Kobayashi H, Yoshida A, Kobayashi M, et al. Changes in size of the functional cyst on ultrasonography during early pregnancy. *Am J Perinatol* 1997;14:1.

Koonings PP, Platt LD, Wallace R. Incidental adnexal neoplasms at caesarean section. *Obstet Gynecol* 1988;72:767.

MacDougall M, LeGrand SB, Walsh D. Symptom control in the pregnant cancer patient. *Semin Oncol* 2000;27:704.

Malfetano JH, Goldkrand JW. Cisplatinum combination chemotherapy during pregnancy for advanced epithelial ovarian carcinoma. *Obstet Gynecol* 1990;75:545.

Manganiello PD, Adams LV, Harris RD, et al. *Obstet Gynecol Surv* 1995;50:404.

Matsuyma T, Tsukamoto N, Matsukuma K, et al. Malignant ovarian tumors associated with pregnancy. *Int J Gynecol Oncol* 1989;28:61.

Metz SA, Day TG, Pursell SH. Adjuvant chemotherapy in a pregnancy patient with endodermal sinus tumor of the ovary. *Gynecol Oncol* 1989;32:371.

Mooney J, Silva E, Tornos C, et al. Unusual features of serous neoplasms of low malignant potential during pregnancy. *Gynecol Oncol* 1997;65:30.

Moore RD, Smith WG. Laparoscopic management of adnexal masses in pregnant women. *J Reprod Med* 1999;44:97.

Nezhat F, Nezhat C, Silfen SL, et al. Laparoscopic ovarian cystectomy during pregnancy. *J Laparoendosc Surg* 1991; 1:161.

Nicklas AH, Baker ME. Imaging strategies in the pregnant cancer patient. *Semin Oncol* 2000;27:623.

Novak ER, Lambrose CD, Woodruff JD. Ovarian tumors in pregnancy. *Obstet Gynecol* 1975;46:401.

Pavlidis NA. Cancer and pregnancy. *Ann Oncol* 2000;11(Suppl 3):247.

Perkins KY, Johnson JL, Kay HH. Simple ovarian cysts: clinical features on a first-trimester ultrasound scan. *J Reprod Med* 1997;42:440.

Piana S, Nogales FF, Corrado S, et al. Pregnancy luteoma with granulosa cell proliferation: an unusual hyperplastic lesion arising in pregnancy and mimicking an ovarian neoplasia. *Pathol Res Pract* 1999;195:859.

Rodriguez M, Harrison TA, Nowazki MR, et al. Luteoma of pregnancy presenting with massive ascites and markedly elevated CA-125. *Obstet Gynecol* 1999;94:854.

Sandmeier D, Lobrinus JA, Vial Y, et al. Bilateral Krukenberg tumor of the ovary during pregnancy. *Eur J Gynaec Oncol* 2000;21:58.

Sasa H, Komatsu Y, Kobayashi M. Ovarian carcinoma in the first trimester. *Int J Gynecol Obstet* 1998;60:283.

Schapira DV, Chudley AE. Successful pregnancy following continuous treatment with combination chemotherapy before conception and throughout pregnancy. *Cancer* 1984;54: 800.

Schover L. Psychosocial issues associated with cancer in pregnancy. *Semin Oncol* 2000;27:699.

Schwartzberg BS, Conyers JA, Moore JA. First trimester of pregnancy laparoscopic procedures. *Surg Endosc* 1997;11:1216.

Shibahara H, Wakimoto E, Mitsuo M, et al. A case of a patient diagnosed with malignant mixed mullerian tumor of the ovary who conceived after conservative surgery and adjuvant chemotherapy. *Gynecol Oncol* 1997;65:363.

Silva PD, Proto M, Moyer DL, et al. Clinical and ultrastructural findings of an androgenizing Krukenberg tumor in pregnancy. *Obstet Gynecol* 1988;71:432.

Stedman CM, Kline RC. Intraoperative complications and unexpected pathology at the time of c-section. *Obstet Gynecol Clin North Am* 1988;15:745.

Sternberg WH, Barclay DL. Luteoma of pregnancy. *Am J Obstet Gynecol* 1966;95:195.

Tawan K, Baker TH. Ovarian tumors in pregnancy. *J Int Coll Surg* 1964;41:60.

Tewari K, Brewer C, Cappuccini F, et al. Advanced-stage small cell carcinoma of the ovary in pregnancy: long-term survival after surgical debulking and multiagent chemotherapy. *Gynecol Oncol* 1997;66:531.

Tewari K, Cappuccini F, Disaia PJ, et al. Malignant germ cell tumors of the ovary. *Obstet Gynecol* 2000;95:128.

Thornton JF, Wells M. Ovarian cysts in pregnancy: does ultrasound make traditional management inappropriate? *Obstet Gynecol* 1987;69:717.

Ueda M, Ueki M. Ovarian tumors associated with pregnancy. *Int J Gynecol Obstet* 1996;55:59.

Van der Zee AG, deBruijn HW, Bouma J, et al. Endodermal sinus tumor of the ovary during pregnancy. *Am J Obstet Gynecol* 1991;164:504.

Wang PH, Chao HT, Yuan CC, et al. Ovarian tumors complicating pregnancy: emergency and elective surgery. *J Reprod Med* 1999;44:279.

Weinreb JC, Brown CE, Lowe TW, et al. Pelvic masses in pregnant patients: MR and US imaging. *Radiology* 1986;159:717.

Wheeler TC, Fleischer AC. Complex adnexal mass in pregnancy: predictive value of color doppler sonography. *J Ultrasound Med* 1997;16:425.

Williams SF, Schilsky RL. Antineoplastic drugs administered during pregnancy. *Semin Oncol* 2000;27:618.

Young RH, Dudley AG, Scully RE. Granulosa cell, Sertoli-Leydig cell, and unclassified sex cord stromal tumors associated with pregnancy: a clinicopathological analysis of thirty-six cases. *Gynecol Oncol* 1984;18:181.

Yuen PM, Chang AMZ. Laparoscopic management of adnexal mass during pregnancy. *Acta Obstet Gynecol Scand* 1997;76:173.

Zanotti KM, Belinson JL, Kennedy AW. Treatment of gynecologic cancers in pregnancy. *Semin Oncol* 2000;27:686.

Fetal Surgery

JOSEPH P. BRUNER

The emerging subspecialty of fetal diagnosis and therapy is rapidly expanding, incorporating aspects of obstetrics, perinatology, radiology, genetics, pediatric surgery, neonatology, reproductive medicine, and clinical ethics. The purpose of this section is to provide an overview of the newer operative techniques of surgery on the fetus. This review is not meant to be definitive, but to acquaint the reader with the many *in utero* operative interventions available for the treatment of fetal anomalies.

NEEDLE PROCEDURES

Fluid-filled spaces in the fetus can be aspirated with a fine needle to prevent abnormal development. In congenital cystic adenomatoid malformation of the lung, type I (CCAM I), one or several large fluid-filled cysts can occupy a large volume of the closed intrathoracic space, preventing normal lung growth and leading to pulmonary hypoplasia; cause mediastinal shift, disrupting normal cardiovascular hemodynamics and leading to development of nonimmune hydrops; or compress the esophagus, impeding fetal swallowing and causing polyhydramnios. All of these complications may be relieved by aspiration of one or more cysts. Similar complications may result from primary fetal hydrothorax (PFHT) or pleural effusion. In both cases, a single thoracentesis may provide definitive antepartum therapy, although fluid reaccumulation is the rule. Depending on the rate of reaccumulation and the gestational age

of the fetus, a few simple aspirations may be preferable to a more invasive needle-catheter procedure for placement of a shunt for continuous drainage (see the following). Decompression immediately prior to delivery may aid in neonatal resuscitation. Most simple aspirations can be performed in the outpatient setting, and fetal paralysis rarely is necessary. Biochemical testing of the aspirated fluid provides no clinically useful information.

Vesicocentesis for decompression of the fetal bladder is both therapeutic and diagnostic in cases of distal urinary tract obstruction owing to posterior urethral valves. The initial drainage procedure will yield urine that may have been present for weeks, and determination of urinary electrolytes and proteins may not reflect current function. Refilling of the bladder is encouraging, but repeat aspiration 2 or 3 days after the first procedure will collect urine that has drained from the upper tracts. Improvement in electrolyte measurements may indicate improving function with decompression, but this specimen still may not be diagnostic. A third procedure after another 2- to 3-day interval will result in a fresh specimen for analysis. Hypotonic values of electrolytes and microproteins identify a fetus that is a good candidate for more invasive suprapubic shunt placement for continuous bladder drainage (Table 32C.1) (see Needle-Catheter Techniques).

Massive fetal ascites may cause obstructed labor and delivery if the abdominal girth is significantly enlarged. Paracentesis often allows vaginal delivery and may aid neonatal resuscitative efforts.

TABLE 32C.1.
Urine Values to Predict Absence of Significant Underlying Renal Damage

Sodium	≤100 mg/dL
Chloride	≤90 mg/dL
Osmolality	≤200 mOsm/L
β_2-Microglobulin	≤4 mg/L
Total protein	≤20 mg/dL

From: Johnson MP, Corsi P, Bradfield W, et al. Sequential urinalysis improves evaluation of fetal renal function in obstructive uropathy. *Am J Obstet Gynecol* 1995;173:59.

NEEDLE-CATHETER TECHNIQUES

Fine needle aspiration of a fluid-filled space in the fetus may not provide definitive therapy. Cysts in the lung or other locations, a pleural effusion, or an obstructed bladder may reaccumulate rapidly in a fetus remote from term, making continuous drainage desirable. In carefully selected cases, placement of a small lumen shunt for continuous decompression into the amniotic fluid may prevent further organ damage until delivery can be accomplished.

When indicated, shunts usually are placed after 18 weeks' gestation. Each case should be carefully evaluated, and the procedure attempted only when significant progressive loss of fetal organ function is anticipated without intervention. Specific contraindications to placement of a shunt for continuous decompression are operator inexperience, the presence of other severe congenital anomalies that make fetal survival unlikely, an abnormal fetal karyotype, or evidence of severe, irreversible end organ injury as described in the preceding section. Other risks include membrane rupture, preterm labor, chorioamnionitis, and iatrogenic injury to the uterus or fetal organs, including bleeding. The procedure may be unsuccessful, or the successfully implanted shunt may become dislodged or obstructed, making repeated procedures necessary. Even after successful shunt placement, progressive loss of organ function may occur, which may not be evident until after delivery. Potential candidates must be thoroughly counseled regarding the potential risks and benefits of the procedure and any alternative therapies.

After selection of an appropriate candidate, procedures usually are performed in an operating room to allow for maintenance of a sterile field and adequate maternal analgesia. The trocar set (Rocket of London or the Harrison catheter, San Francisco) should be examined to ensure that the appropriate introducer, sharp trocar, double pigtail catheter, and pusher are available. Short-acting tocolytics are commonly used, as are systemic or intraamniotic antibiotics. Careful ultrasonographic examination of the uterine contents must be performed to confirm that placental location, fetal lie, and amniotic fluid volume are adequate to accomplish successful shunt placement. The maternal abdomen is sterilely prepped, and a small skin incision is made with a no. 11 scalpel blade at the optimal insertion site for the trocar and introducer. The assembled apparatus is advanced into the uterine cavity under direct ultrasonographic guidance (Fig. 32C.1). The instruments should be as perpendicular as possible to the uterine wall and fetal skin surface to reduce the amount of manipulation required. The fetal bladder should be entered suprapubically, and the pleural space entered laterally. The trocar assembly is inserted several centimeters into the fluid-filled space, and the utmost care must be exercised to avoid laceration of internal fetal organs; this risk in minimized by withdrawing the sharp trocar tip into the introducer sleeve after fetal entry is achieved. When the introducer is properly positioned, confirmed by ultrasonographic visualization in at least two scanning planes, the sharp trocar is removed and the shunt is fed completely into the lumen of the hollow introducer. It is important that excessive fluid not be allowed to escape, or the target space may become too small for successful completion of the procedure; sterile saline may be reinstilled through the trocar as needed. The pusher is used to advance the distal end of the double pigtail catheter into the fluid-filled space. The pusher is used to hold the shunt in position while the in-

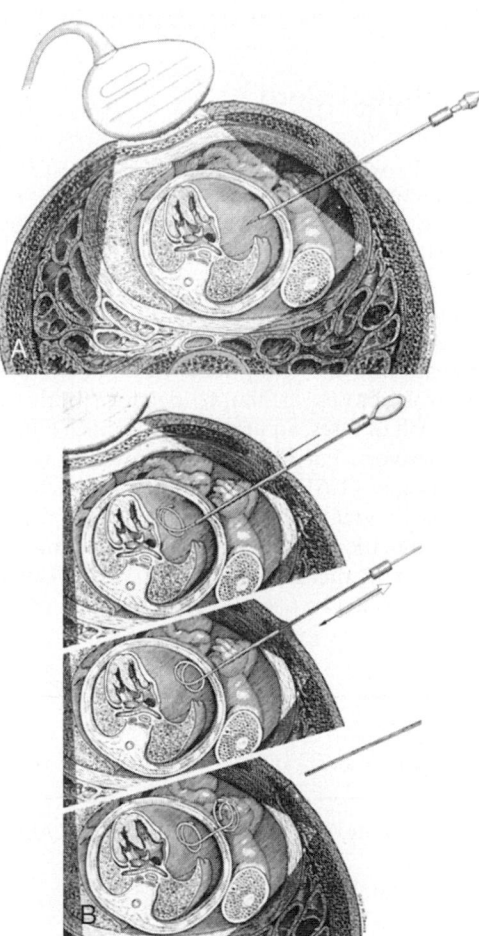

FIGURE 32C.1. A, B: A properly positioned double pigtail shunt has the proximal coil within the fluid-filled fetal organ, and the distal coil in the amniotic cavity. (Montemagnor R, Soothill P. Invasive procedures. In: Fisk NM, Moise KJ, eds. *Fetal therapy: invasive and transplacental.* New York: Cambridge University Press, 1997:22.)

troducer is withdrawn from the fetus, leaving the proximal coil of the catheter in the amniotic space. The introducer must not be withdrawn through the uterine wall until the proximal coil has completely exited the instrument tip, or the proximal end of the shunt may become embedded in the uterine wall. Successful placement of the shunt will result in rapid decompression of the fluid-filled space. Fetal well-being and uterine quiescence are confirmed by electronic monitoring, and serial ultrasonographic follow-up is scheduled.

ENDOSCOPIC TECHNIQUES

Endoscopic fetal surgery has been performed to interrupt umbilical cord blood flow for selective termination of monochorionic twins, especially the twin reversed arterial perfusion syndrome (TRAPS); for interruption of interfetal vascular placental anastomoses in the twin-to-twin transfusion syndrome (TTTS); to release trapped limbs in the amniotic band syndrome; and for direct fetal therapy of congenital diaphragmatic hernia (CDH), spina bifida, and sacrococcygeal teratoma (SCT).

The Umbilical Cord

Termination of one of multiple fetuses is most commonly performed by lethal injection into the heart or thorax of the target fetus. This should not be performed in monochorionic twin gestations, however, because of the presence of patent interfetal placental vascular anastomoses. In these cases, any toxic substance injected into one twin may be inadvertently shunted to the normal cotwin. Even if the injection is successful, the normal cotwin may exsanguinate into the dying fetus through the placental vascular anastomoses, leading to death of both twins in up to one half of cases, and neurologic injury in up to one third of survivors. Further, this technique is not possible in most cases of TRAPS, in which the parasitic twin does not possess an identifiable thorax or heart. In these instances, termination is best accomplished by interruption of blood flow in the umbilical cord. This is often most easily accomplished by occlusion of a segment of cord us-

ing a bipolar forceps. Using this technique, a 3- to 5-mm port is placed under ultrasonographic guidance. A small camera may be introduced for direct visualization of the umbilical cord, but this is usually unnecessary. A bipolar forceps is then introduced and used to grasp the umbilical cord of the anomalous fetus. Capture of the correct cord can be confirmed by compression of the cord vessels with the forceps, which results in deceleration of the heart rate of the attached fetus. A low-energy current (40 to 50 W) is passed through the forceps until cessation of blood flow is seen with color Doppler ultrasonography. During this process, ultrasonic microbubbles may be seen rising from the fulguration site, and an audible "pop" may be heard. A second occlusion should be performed in an adjacent cord site. An agonal fetal heart rate may persist for several minutes after complete cessation of blood flow in the umbilical cord. In a report of 10 cases of endoscopic umbilical cord occlusion performed for TTTS and TRAPS, Deprest and Ville were successful in every attempt, usually in less than 15 minutes. Two cases were complicated by iatrogenic rupture of the membranes, and pregnancy termination was elected. In the remaining eight cases, healthy babies were delivered at a mean gestational age of 35 weeks, more than 15 weeks after the procedure.

The Placenta

The most common contemporary indication for fetal endoscopy is treatment of TTTS by selective laser photocoagulation of placental interfetal vascular anastomoses. For many years, poor understanding of the underlying pathophysiology of this disease led to much confusion about appropriate diagnostic criteria, indications for treatment, and effective therapeutic options. In retrospect, overdiagnosis was common, and many cases of true TTTS were probably undertreated. The recent introduction of a staging system has greatly simplified diagnostic criteria, and clarified indications for the most appropriate treatment based on the level of disease. The staging of TTTS, introduced by Quintero (1999), is based on ultrasonographic findings and is summarized in Table 32C.2. Stage I is characterized by the twin oligo-

TABLE 32C.2.
Staging of Twin Transfusion Syndrome Based on Sonographic and Doppler Findings

Stage	Poly/Oligohydramnios[a]	Absent Bladder in Donor	CADs[b]	Hydrops	Demise
I	+1	−2	−2	−2	−2
II	+1	+1	−2	−2	−2
III	+1	+1	+1	−2	−2
IV	+1	+1	+1	+1	−2
V	+1	+1	+1	+1	+1

[a] Polyhydramnios, MVP of <8 cm; oligohydramnios, MVP of <2 cm.
[b] CADs, defined as the presence of at least one of the following: (a) UA AED/REDV; (b) REFD; or (c) pulsatile umbilical venous flow (PUVF).
From: Quintero RA, Morales WJ, Allen MH, et al. Staging of twin-twin transfusion syndrome. *J Perinatol* 1999;19(8):551, with permission.

hydramnios-polyhydramnios sequence (TOPS), and is further defined as a maximum vertical pocket of amniotic fluid less than 2 cm in the "stuck" twin, and greater than 8 cm in the polyhydramnic sac. Because the accuracy of diagnosis is most uncertain at this stage, treatment is more conservative. After 26 weeks' gestation, massive polyhydramnios may cause maternal discomfort or an overdistended uterus. Amnioreduction may be useful in relieving maternal symptoms, and decompression of the uterus may aid in prolonging the pregnancy. At earlier gestational ages, close observation for progression of disease is warranted. Amnioreduction is associated with a complication rate of 6% per procedure, or 15% per pregnancy. The most common catastrophic complications are spontaneous delivery (3.1%), placental abruption (1.3%), and chorioamnionitis (0.9%). Even if the pregnancy continues, membrane disruption (6.2%) or bleeding into the amniotic fluid may frustrate more invasive treatment in the likelihood of disease progression. Stage II is defined by the absence of an identifiable bladder in the "stuck" twin after prolonged ultrasonographic examination. Stage III is characterized by critically abnormal Doppler measurements in one or both twins, including absent or reversed end diastolic velocities (AEDV/REDV) in the umbilical artery, reverse flow in the ductus venosus, or pulsatile umbilical venous flow. Progression to more advanced stages of the disease leaves little doubt as to the diagnosis of true TTTS, and fetal mortality approaches 100% in the absence of treatment. Furthermore, although amnioreduction is associated with a 95.5% perinatal survival rate in Stage I TTTS, survival decreases to 81% in Stage II disease, and 46.2% in Stage III. Among survivors, respiratory distress occurs in 41.3%, periventricular leukomalacia in 24.5%, renal failure in 3.0%, necrotizing enterocolitis in 4.1%, and cranial ultrasound is abnormal in 24.5% at 4 weeks of life. Neurologic sequelae include cerebral palsy in up to 22.5% after treatment with amnioreduction. Because of increased mortality and morbidity with progressive disease, more definitive treatment by selective laser photocoagulation of placental anastomoses is indicated in Stage II and III TTTS. In Stage IV TTTS, nonimmune hydrops is seen in one or both twins. Laser photocoagulation of placental vessels is indicated for treatment unless the death of one twin seems imminent. Because the risk of neurologic sequelae and even death of the unaffected cotwin are so great when one monochorionic twin dies *in utero,* umbilical cord occlusion of the hydropic fetus, as described, may be preferable. Stage V TTTS is characterized by intrauterine fetal demise. Careful examination of the surviving cotwin should be performed for evidence of neurologic injury.

Selective laser photocoagulation of placental vessels is performed in the United States under general endotracheal anesthesia. The use of general anesthesia provides maternal comfort during the procedure, which may last as long as 1 to 2 hours. Maximum uterine relaxation is also achieved, and the possibility of fetal movement is minimized. After a detailed ultrasonographic assessment of the uterine contents, a small stab wound is created in the maternal abdomen and a 3- to 5-mm operating endoscope is inserted into the polyhydramnic sac, taking care to avoid the placenta. In cases with anterior placental implantation, use of a flexible endoscope or insertion of a side-firing laser through a second port have been described by Quintero. Color Doppler ultrasonography of the uterine wall may help to avoid maternal vessels during trocar placement. If bloody amniotic fluid is encountered, owing to bleeding during trocar placement or after a previous amnioreduction, poor visualization may make further progress impossible unless a large volume amnioexchange is performed with an irrigator-aspirator. Even if the fluid is clear, amnioreduction often is required at this point in order to bring the placental surface into the focal zone of the operating endoscope. Examination of the vascular equator of the monochorionic placenta is performed then, and all interfetal vascular anastomoses are identified. It is important to note that the unequal amniotic fluid volumes characteristic of TTTS displace the membranous equator, so that it no longer coincides with the vascular equator. In the placenta, arteries pass over veins. Normally, an artery from one fetus enters a cotyledon, and a paired vein is seen exiting the cotyledon within a few millimeters and returning to the cord insertion site. Arteriovenous (av) anastomoses are identified when an artery from one fetus is seen entering the placenta, and an unpaired vein exits within a few millimeters and courses to the opposite cord insertion. Arterioarterial (aa) anastomoses and venovenous (vv) anastomoses traverse the vascular equator in an unbroken line. Although the overwhelming majority of TTTS cases are caused by av anastomoses, all patent anastomoses should be occluded in order to achieve the therapeutic goal of creating functional dichorionic twins. The advantage of doing so is prevention of serious sequelae in the event of intrauterine demise of one twin, as described. On the other hand, a cotyledon is lost every time a vessel is occluded. Photocoagulation sites should be carefully planned, therefore, to occlude the minimal number of vessels possible, because the "stuck" twin may already be struggling to survive with a minimal number of cotyledons available for exchange. Once a photocoagulation site is selected, a 400-u YAG laser fiber is passed through the operating channel of the endoscope and advanced to within 5 to 10 mm of the vessel. The laser is activated at a low energy level (20 to 60 W), and photocoagulation performed until the placental surface blanches, usually several seconds. On average, 3.1 vascular anastomoses are occluded per procedure. On completion of photocoagulation, further amnioreduction is performed as needed to normalize the amniotic fluid volume in the polyhydramnic sac. Postoperative tocolysis and pain relief is provided as indicated, and discharge usually occurs within 1 to 2 days. Serial ultrasonographic examinations are scheduled until delivery.

When the severity of TTTS is corrected by stage, and perinatal survival compared between amnioreduction and selective laser photocoagulation of placental vessels, it becomes clear that the more invasive laser therapy does not improve survival in early stage disease. Perinatal mortality increases significantly with increasing severity of disease treated with amnioreduction; however, in contrast to the stable mortality rate seen with laser treatment. In stages III and IV, survival is clearly superior with selective laser photocoagulation of placental vessels. Moreover, neurologic morbidity among survivors is reduced to 4% to 6% after laser therapy.

The Membranes

The amniotic band syndrome (ABS) is widely believed to result from disruption of the amnion prior to 18 weeks' gestation. Although the sequelae of early membrane disruption can be devastating, occasionally only the umbilical cord or a single limb are encircled by a constricting membrane. In this situation, endoscopic release of the amniotic band may prevent severe disfigurement or amputation of a limb, or even death owing to umbilical cord strangulation. Selection of appropriate candidates, timing of the procedure, and long-term outcomes of treated fetuses are still unknown. Color Doppler ultrasonography has been used to monitor arterial blood flow velocities in the affected limb presurgery and postsurgery.

The Fetus

Congenital diaphragmatic hernia (CDH) is a developmental defect in the fetus that allows extrusion of abdominal contents into the thoracic cavity. The biological sequelae are similar to those seen with other space-occupying lesions of the thorax, such as CCAM and pleural effusion, described in the preceding, including pulmonary hypoplasia, hydrops, and polyhydramnios. Early attempts to treat CDH *in utero* were based on the techniques established for neonatal repair, and required open hysterotomy with partial delivery of the fetus. Perinatal mortality and maternal morbidity were unacceptably high, and continuous attempts to improve outcomes led to a gradual evolution in patient selection and operative approaches. In spite of the progression of technological innovations that have spurred the evolution of intrauterine treatment of CDH to its current state, contemporaneous advances in neonatal care also have improved outcomes in those newborns receiving standard therapy. At the present time, intrauterine treatment of CDH has not been demonstrated to improve survival compared to standard neonatal care, and disease-related morbidity among survivors is still prohibitive.

Attempts to manage congenital cystic adenomatoid malformation (CCAM), sacrococcygeal teratoma (SCT), and spina bifida endoscopically have been reported, but a variety of diagnostic and technical obstacles have prevented development of acceptable techniques. Because 15% of CCAM lesions resolve spontaneously, minimally invasive treatment prior to the onset of hydrops depends on the development of early markers for identification of aggressive tumors. The blood vessels feeding SCTs can be coagulated by application of an external energy source, but iatrogenic injury of the adjacent fetus has not been prevented. Spina bifida has defied attempts at endoscopic repair because of insurmountable technical difficulties, but these may soon be overcome with the aid of robotic technology (see the following).

HYSTEROTOMY
Lethal Malformations

Open fetal surgery was first performed in New York in 1963 for direct transfusion of fetuses severely affected by erythrocyte isoimmunization. These attempts preceded the introduction of clinical ultrasonography and much of the anesthetic and laboratory support taken for granted today. The results were not encouraging, and efforts were quickly abandoned. Modern techniques of open fetal repair through a hysterotomy were developed in the 1980s to treat lethal malformations such as CDH, CCAM, and SCT, already described. Although most of the specialized operative procedures and instruments still used today grew out of these efforts, lethal fetal anomalies are uncommon, and intrauterine intervention rarely is indicated. In any given year, only a handful of open fetal procedures were performed. With the advent of intrauterine repair for nonlethal anomalies, the number of open fetal surgical procedures has increased markedly, resulting in improved techniques, lower morbidity, and wider applications.

Nonlethal Malformations

Open fetal repair of a nonlethal anomaly was first performed for spina bifida (myelomeningocele) in 1997. Nonlethal fetal malformations are relatively common compared to lethal anomalies, and the annual number of cases immediately increased from a few to dozens. For the first time, surgical outcomes became rapidly available. Instead of waiting months for the opportunity to implement new devices and techniques, innovations could be tested as quickly as a week. Because fetal surgery for treatment of nonlethal malformations is elective, the fetuses are healthy except for the anomaly being treated, and the mothers are likewise free of serious surgical and medical risks. Therefore, fetal and maternal effects of surgical procedures could be assessed independently of the systemic disease common in life-saving procedures.

When performing open fetal repair of a nonlethal malformation, a combination of general and epidural anesthesia is used as evidence suggests this combination is superior to either individually in preventing uterine contractions. The indwelling epidural catheter also enables administration of continuous postoperative analgesics. The gravid uterus is exposed via a low transverse laparotomy incision and exteriorized. A vertical skin incision is used in obese patients or those with a previous vertical incision. The fetus and placenta are then localized with a sterile ultrasound transducer and the hysterotomy location chosen. Initial uterine entry is accomplished through a 1- to 2-cm hysterotomy. The foot plate of a US Surgical CS-57 autostapling device is passed into the uterine cavity. The stapler is examined manually and with color Doppler ultrasonography to exclude the presence of fetal tissue, and then used to create a 6- to 8-cm uterine incision (Fig. 32C.2). The fetus is directly visualized and manually positioned within the uterus such that the myelomeningocele sac is in the cen-

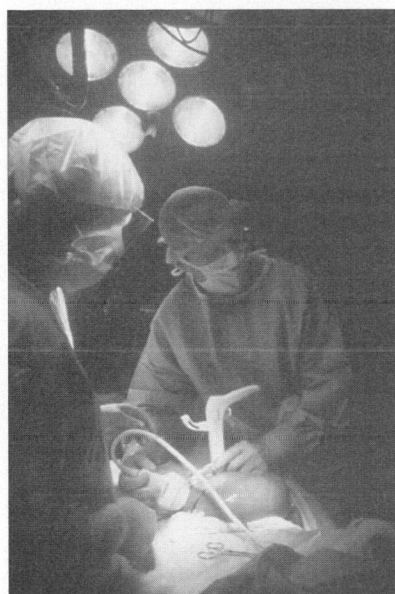

FIGURE 32C.2. The uterine autostapler is positioned in the uterine wall, ready to be engaged to create a hysterotomy.

ter of the hysterotomy (Fig. 32C.3). During the procedure the fetal heartbeat is monitored by ultrasound, by continuous electronic fetal monitoring (EFM), or by continuous fetal oxygen saturation monitoring. The myelomeningocele is closed in standard multilayered fashion under magnification regardless of the gestational age. The uterus is closed in two layers. The first layer incorporates the absorbable polyglycolic acid staples left by the autostapling device. As the last stitches of this layer are placed, warmed Ringer's lactate, mixed with 500 mg of Nafcillin or vancomycin, is added to the uterus until the amniotic fluid index is normal. Finally, an imbricating layer of suture is placed. The abdominal fascial layer and dermis are closed in routine fashion. Patients receive 24 hours of broad spectrum intravenous antibiotics. Intravenous magnesium sulfate is continued until the next

morning. A subcutaneous terbutaline pump is initiated on the first postoperative day. Indomethacin is administered preoperatively, and continued for 48 hours. Patients stay in the hospital until they tolerate a regular diet, have return of bowel function, are able to ambulate without assistance, demonstrate good tocolytic control, and have good postoperative pain management with oral medications. The average time of hospital discharge is the third postoperative day.

The most notable outcome of intrauterine myelomeningocele repair is a marked reduction in the need for ventriculoperitoneal shunt placement after delivery (59% versus 91%; $p = 0.01$). In cases with upper level of the lesion ≤L4 and repaired ≤25 weeks' gestation, the shunt rate at one year of age was 17%. The median age at shunt placement was also older among study infants (50 versus 5 days; $p = 0.006$). These results may be explained by the reduced incidence of hindbrain herniation among study infants (38% versus 95%; $p < 0.001$) (Fig. 32C.4). Follow-up of leg and bladder function is frustrated by the young age of the children treated *in utero* so far. Following hysterotomy, study patients experienced an increased risk of oligohydramnios (48% versus

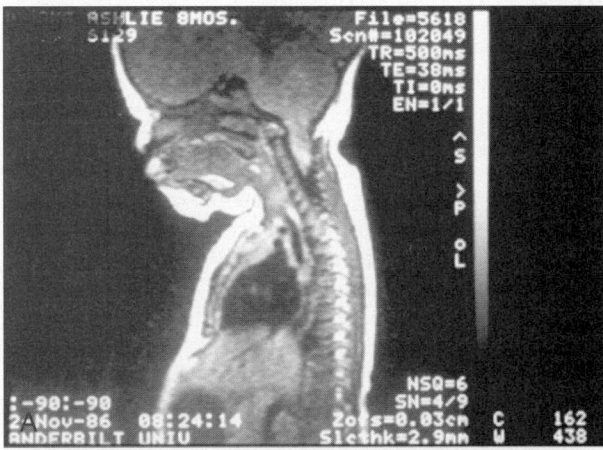

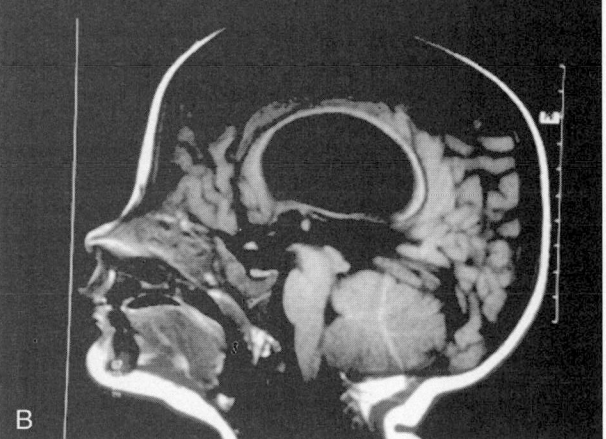

FIGURE 32C.4. Hindbrain herniation into the top of the spinal canal (**A**) is reversed by repair of the lesion *in utero* (**B**).

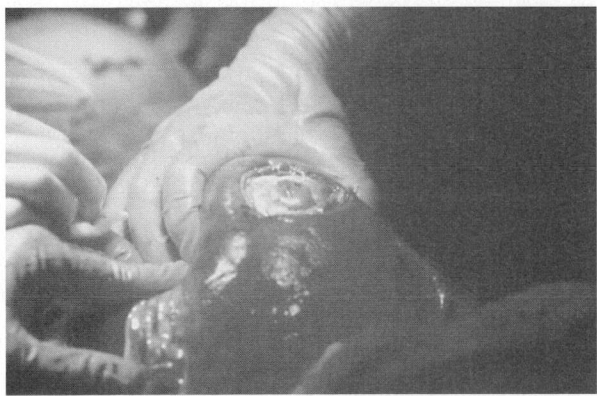

FIGURE 32C.3. The fetal myelomeningocele is centered in the hysterotomy. The uterine wall is extremely compliant with adequate anesthesia. Polyglycolic acid staples line the hysterotomy edge with negligible blood loss.

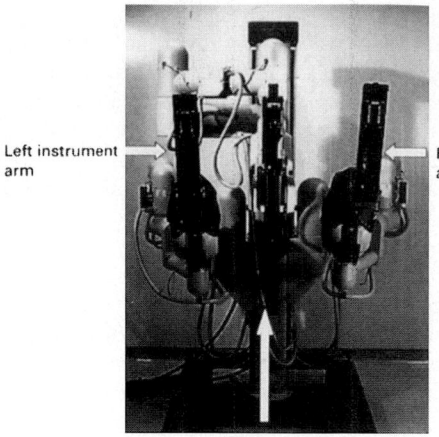

FIGURE 32C.5. The first-generation robotic endoscopic operating system interposes computer technology between the surgeon and the patient, improving performance.

4%; $p = 0.001$) and hospital admission for preterm uterine contractions (50% versus 9%; $p = 0.002$). The estimated gestational age at delivery was earlier for study patients (33.5 weeks versus 37.0 weeks; $p < 0.001$).

ROBOTICS

After intrauterine repair of spina bifida through a hysterotomy, all babies are delivered preterm by caesarean section, not only in the index pregnancy, but in all future pregnancies as well. Efforts to reduce maternal and fetal morbidity and fetal mortality by use of an endoscopic approach were unsuccessful owing to insurmountable technical difficulties (see the preceding). Although the endoscopic approach to myelomeningocele repair was abandoned, investigators continue to hope that a technological breakthrough will allow a return to minimally invasive fetal neurosurgery. Recently, Aaronson and coworkers reported repair of a spina bifida–like lesion in six fetal lambs using a robotic endoscopic operating system (Fig. 32C.5). In contrast to the earlier experience with standard laparoscopic techniques, the

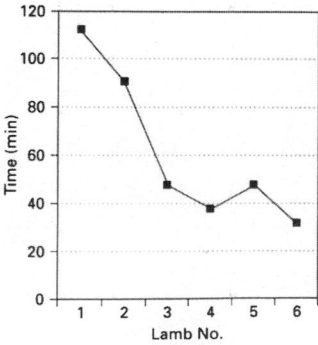

FIGURE 32C.6. After attaching the robot to the operating ports, surgery time is remarkably brief, reflecting high efficiency, and the learning curve is extremely short.

average operating time was only 30 minutes by the third case (Fig. 32C.6). If further refinement of robotic systems occurs, with development of smaller and more specialized instruments, human applications for fetal repair will soon follow. Return to minimally invasive myelomeningocele repair potentially will allow vaginal delivery of most patients at term. The risk:benefit ratio of fetal surgery thus may be expected to shift dramatically, enlarging the list of ethically acceptable indications for prenatal intervention.

BIBLIOGRAPHY

Aaronson OS, Tulipan N, Cywes R, et al. Robot-assisted endoscopic intrauterine myelomeningocele repair: a feasibility study. *Pediatr Neurosurg* 2002;36:85.

Adzick NS, Harrison MR, Crombleholme TM, et al. Fetal lung lesions: management and outcome. *Am J Obstet Gynecol* 1998;179:884.

Albanese CT, Lopoo J, Goldstein RB, et al. Fetal liver position and perinatal outcome for congenital diaphragmatic hernia. *Prenat Diagn* 1998;18:1138.

Bruner JP, Jarnagin BK, Reinisch L. Percutaneous laser ablation of fetal congenital cystic adenomatoid malformation: too little, too late? *Fetal Diagn Ther* 2000;15:359.

Bruner JP, Richards WO, Tulipan NB, et al. Endoscopic coverage of fetal myelomeningocele in utero. *Am J Obstet Gynecol* 1999;180:153.

Bruner JP, Tulipan N, Paschall RL, et al. Fetal surgery for myelomeningocele and the incidence of shunt-dependent hydrocephalus. *JAMA* 1999;282:1819.

Bruner JP, Tulipan N, Richards WO, et al. In utero repair of myelomeningocele: A comparison of endoscopy and hysterotomy. *Fetal Diagn Ther* 2000;15:83.

DeLia JE, Kuhlmann RS, Harstad TW, et al. Fetoscopic laser ablation of placental vessels in severe previable twin-twin transfusion syndrome. *Am J Obstet Gynecol* 1995;172:1202.

Deprest JAM, Ville Y. Obstetric endoscopy. In: Harrison MR, Evans MI, Adzick NS, et al., eds. *The unborn patient*, 3rd ed. Philadelphia: WB Saunders, 2001:213.

Freda VJ, Adamsons K. Exchange transfusion in utero: report of a case. *Am J Obstet Gynecol* 1964;89:817.

Graf JL, Albanese CT, Jennings RW, et al. Successful fetal sacrococcygeal teratoma resection in a hydropic fetus. *J Pediatr Surg* 2000;35:1489.

Harrison MR, Adzick NS, Flake AW, et al. Correction of congenital diaphragmatic hernia in utero. VI. Hard-earned lessons. *J Pediatr Surg* 1993;28:1411.

Harrison MR, Adzick NS, Bullard KM, et al. Correction of congenital diaphragmatic hernia in utero. VII: a prospective trial. *J Pediatr Surg* 1997;32:1637.

Haverkamp F, Lex C, Hanisch C, et al. Neurodevelopmental risks in twin-to-twin transfusion syndrome: preliminary findings. *Eur J Pediatr Neurol* 2001;5:21.

Hecher K, Plath H, Bregenzer T, et al. Endoscopic laser surgery versus serial amniocenteses in the treatment of severe twin-twin transfusion syndrome. *Am J Obstet Gynecol* 1999;180:717.

Hedrick HH, Estes JM, Sullivan KM, et al. Plug the lung until it grows (PLUG): a new method to treat congenital diaphragmatic hernia in utero. *J Pediatr Surg* 1994;29:612.

Hedrick MH, Ferro MM, Filly RA, et al. Congenital high airway obstruction syndrome (CHAOS): a potential for perinatal intervention. *J Pediatr Surg* 1994;29:271.

Holzbeierlein J, Pope JC IV, Adams MC, et al. The urodynamic profile of myelodysplasia in childhood with spinal closure during gestation. *J Urol* 2000;164:1336.

Johnson MP, Corsi P, Bradfield W, et al. Sequential urinalysis improves evaluation of fetal renal function in obstructive uropathy. *Am J Obstet Gynecol* 1995;173:59.

Mari G, Roberts A, Detti L, et al. Perinatal morbidity and mortality rates in severe twin-twin transfusion syndrome: results of the International Amnioreduction Registry. *Am J Obstet Gynecol* 2001;185:708.

Mychalishka GB, Bealor JF, Graf JL, et al. Operating on placental support: the ex utero intrapartum treatment (EXIT) procedure. *J Pediatr Surg* 1997;32:227.

Paek BW, Jennings RW, Harrison MR, et al. Radiofrequency ablation of human fetal sacrococcygeal teratoma. *Am J Obstet Gynecol* 2001;184:503.

Quintero RA. Treatment of previable premature ruptured membranes. In: Quintero RA, ed. *Diagnostic and operative fetoscopy.* London: Parthenon, 2002.

Quintero RA, Bornick PW, Allen MH, et al. Selective laser photocoagulation of communicating vessels in severe twin-twin transfusion syndrome in women with an anterior placenta. *Obstet Gynecol* 2001;97:477.

Quintero R, Morales W, Allen M, et al. Staging of twin-twin transfusion syndrome. *J Perinatol* 1999;19:550.

Quintero RA, Morales WJ, Bornick MH. et al. Minimally invasive intraluminal tracheal occlusion in a human fetus with left congenital diaphragmatic hernia at 27 weeks' gestation via direct fetal laryngoscopy. *Prenat Neonat Med* 2000;5:134.

Quintero RA, Morales WJ, Mendoza G, et al. Selective photocoagulation of placental vessels in twin-twin transfusion syndrome: evolution of a surgical technique. *Obstet Gynecol Surv* 1998;53:S97.

Quintero RA, Morales WJ, Phillips J, et al. In utero lysis of amniotic bands. *Ultrasound Obstet Gynecol* 1997;10:316.

Tulipan N, Bruner JP. Myelomeningocele repair in utero: a report of three cases. *Pediatr Neurosurg* 1998;28:177.

Tulipan N, Bruner JP, Hernanz-Schulman M, et al. The effect of intrauterine myelomeningocele repair on central nervous system structure and neurologic function. *Pediatr Neurosurg* 1999;31:183.

Tulipan N, Hernanz-Schulman M, Bruner JP. Intrauterine myelomeningocele repair reverses preexisting hindbrain herniation. *Pediatr Neurosurg* 1999;31:137.

VanderWall KJ, Bruch SW, Kohl T, et al. Fetoscopic tracheal clip occlusion for the treatment of congenital diaphragmatic hernia. *J Pediatr Surg* 1996;31:1101.

Ville Y, Hecher K, Gagnon A, et al. Endoscopic laser coagulation in the management of severe twin-to-twin transfusion syndrome. *Obstet Gynecol Surv* 1998;53:597.

Te Linde's Operative Gynecology, ninth edition, edited by John A. Rock and Howard W. Jones, III. Lippincott Williams & Wilkins, Philadelphia © 2003.

CHAPTER
33

▼

Surgical Conditions of the Vulva

IRA R. HOROWITZ   JOSEPH BUSCEMA

BHAGIRATH MAJMUDAR

The vulva and the adjacent perianal skin are desig nated the anogenital area. These tissues are derived from ectoderm and are considered separately from the vagina and cervix, which are of mesodermal origin. Multifocal diseases, particularly human papillomavirus (HPV), can affect all of the aforementioned epithelia. A complete vulvar examination should, therefore, include the vulva, perineum, anal area, urethral meatus, buttocks, and thighs. It is difficult to appreciate subtle skin changes in patients with dark skin; therefore, an adequate light source is necessary.

VULVAR DERMATOSIS

In 1987, the International Society for the Study of Vulvovaginal Diseases (ISSVD) revised the terminology initially established by that organization in 1976 to describe the nonneoplastic epithelial disorders which include psoriasis, lichen planus, lichen simplex chronicus, candidiasis, and condyloma acuminata. In their 1976 classification, the ISSVD categorized hyperplastic dystrophy with and without atypia. In the classification of 1987, squamous cell hyperplasia is without atypia and lesions with atypia are considered vulvar intraepithelial neoplasia (VIN).

Treatment of Vulvar Pruritus

Before any therapy for vulvar lesions caused by chronic irritation is begun, an accurate tissue diagnosis must be established. The epidermis may be thickened and the skin markings accentuated (lichenification), but the extent of the epithelial proliferation cannot be assessed without biopsy. Usually a 3- or 4-mm Keyes punch biopsy is used to obtain a small biopsy in the office under local anesthesia. The specimen is oriented with the epithelial surface up on a square of filter paper or Telfa before being placed in fixative. This allows correct orientation of the tissue so that a full-thickness, nontangential, microscopic section can be prepared (Fig. 33.1). Occasionally, experienced clinicians make a tentative diagnosis based on history and physical examination. A trial of topical therapy may be used for 6 to 8 weeks to evaluate the response, but if the response is less than satisfactory or if there is any suspicion of invasion, a biopsy must be done. All patients should be given detailed instructions to eliminate local irritants. Associated vaginitis should be treated vigorously. Topical medications for control of the symptoms must be given a satisfactory trial. Vulvectomy should *not* be performed for chronic dermatitis or for the benign dystrophies, including lichen sclerosus, before careful histologic evaluation is done. Systemic etiologies such as diabetes, anxiety, Sjögren's syndrome, hepatic or renal diseases, or drug reactions

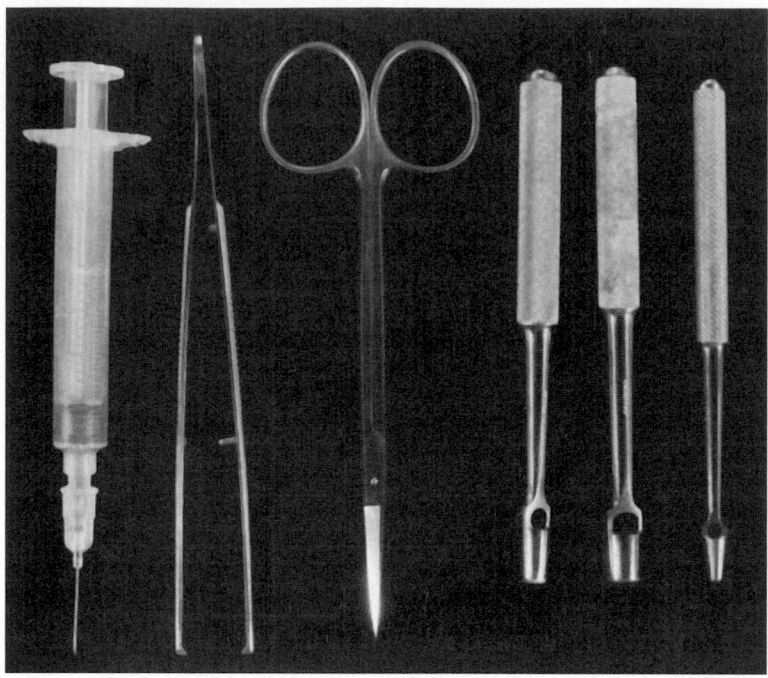

FIGURE 33.1. Biopsy instruments (dermatologic punch).

may exist. Cutaneous etiologies such as candidiasis, vaginitis, and contact or atopic dermatitis can also occur.

Topical Agents

Topical agents have been effective in treating vulvar pruritus and should be tried initially. When they are ineffective, often it is secondary to their inability to penetrate the thickened hyperkeratotic surface. Initially, treatment for a specific disease should be instituted. For example, topical steroids should be used for psoriasis, antifungals for candidiasis, and appropriate ablative therapy for molluscum contagiosum and condylomata acuminata. Vulvar dermatoses such as lichen simplex chronicus, lichen planus, seborrheic dermatitis, lichen sclerosus, and plasma cell vulvitis can be effectively treated with high-potency topical steroids such as betamethasone. Many of these patients also present with vulvar dysesthesia (vulvar burning) and can be treated with tricyclic medications such as amitriptyline and nortriptyline.

For historic purposes, no chapter on vulvar pruritus would be complete without mentioning alcohol injection and the Mering procedure. Before treatment with amitriptyline became popular, patients with recalcitrant pruritus and vulvar dysesthesia were treated with local alcohol injection. The anogenital area was prepped and draped in a sterile manner after the induction of general or regional anesthesia. The region was then divided into 1-cm squares with a marking pen of brilliant green. Absolute alcohol, 0.2 mL, was then injected subcutaneously at the intersection of these lines (Fig. 33.2). Postoperatively, the patients were treated with cold packs and cool sitz baths for 1 week.

Mering Procedure

The Mering procedure requires hospitalization and careful surgical technique (Fig. 33.3). The skin is shaved, thoroughly cleaned, and the incision is outlined with a marking pencil. The incision is made on the outer surface of the labium majus. It extends to the fascia of the urogenital diaphragm from the level of the clitoris to slightly beyond the fourchette, and may continue inferiorly to the level of the anal orifice, depending on the extent of the pruritus. The nerves in the adjacent tissue are severed with a finger placed on each side, moving from the lateral aspect of the clitoris toward the midline, over the clitoris, where the fingers meet. The procedure interrupts branches of the ilioinguinal and genitofemoral nerves (Fig. 33.4). Blunt dissection extends posteriorly to the lateral side of the rectum, outside the external anal sphincter. If the perianal area is involved, blunt dissection may extend to the posterior limit of the anal orifice, where the two fingers meet behind the anus in the midline breaking up the branches of the pudendal nerve.

It is important that hemostasis be meticulously maintained because the accumulation of blood and fluid could produce local cellulitis, which delays recovery. A small, flat Jackson-Pratt drain should be placed under the flap on each side. The underlying tissue is approximated with absorbable sutures, and the skin is sutured with polyglycolic acid or polyglactin 910 material. The area must be packed tightly for 24 hours, and the patient should use ice packs or cool tub baths. Domeboro sitz baths (Burow's solution) may help to relieve edema.

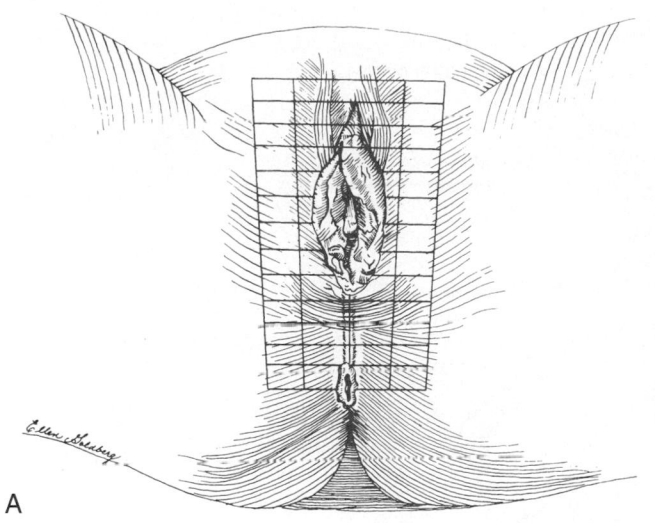

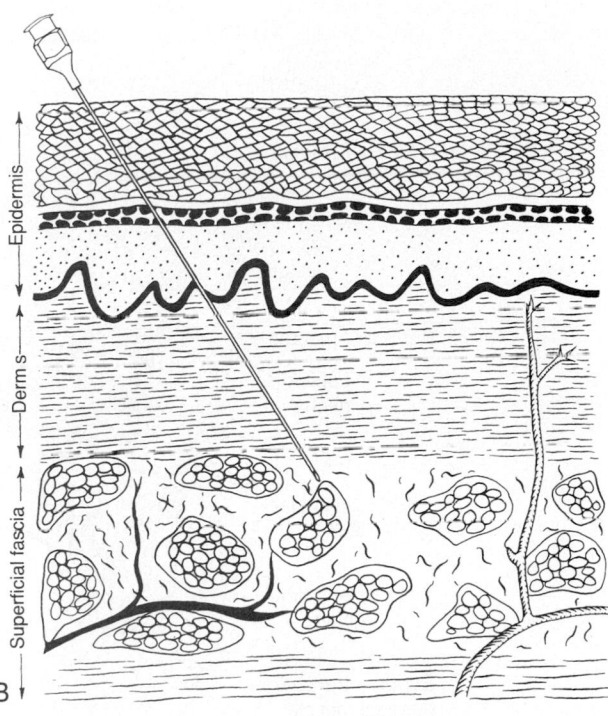

FIGURE 33.2. A: Marking of external genitalia into 1-cm squares in preparation for alcohol injection. **B:** Depth of penetration of 25-gauge needle into the subcutaneous tissue. (From Woodruff JD, Thompson B. Local alcohol injection in the treatment of vulvar pruritus. *Obstet Gynecol* 1972;40:18, with permission.)

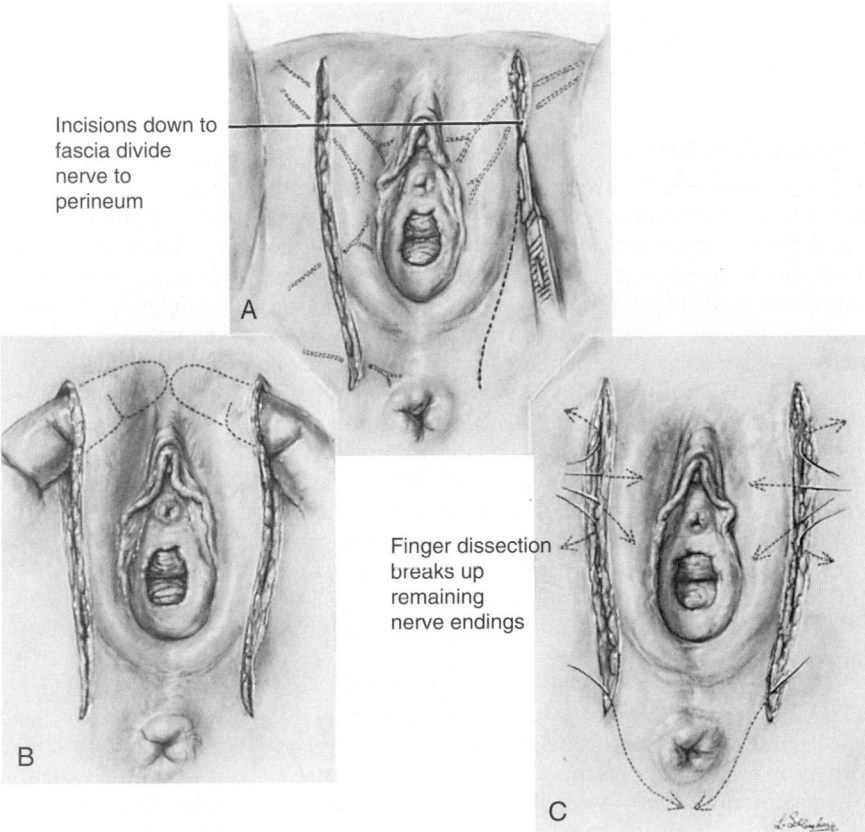

Incisions down to fascia divide nerve to perineum

Finger dissection breaks up remaining nerve endings

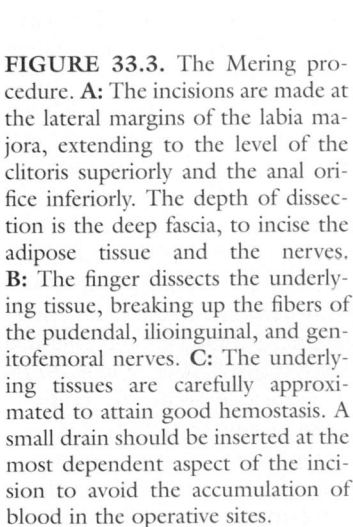

FIGURE 33.3. The Mering procedure. **A:** The incisions are made at the lateral margins of the labia majora, extending to the level of the clitoris superiorly and the anal orifice inferiorly. The depth of dissection is the deep fascia, to incise the adipose tissue and the nerves. **B:** The finger dissects the underlying tissue, breaking up the fibers of the pudendal, ilioinguinal, and genitofemoral nerves. **C:** The underlying tissues are carefully approximated to attain good hemostasis. A small drain should be inserted at the most dependent aspect of the incision to avoid the accumulation of blood in the operative sites.

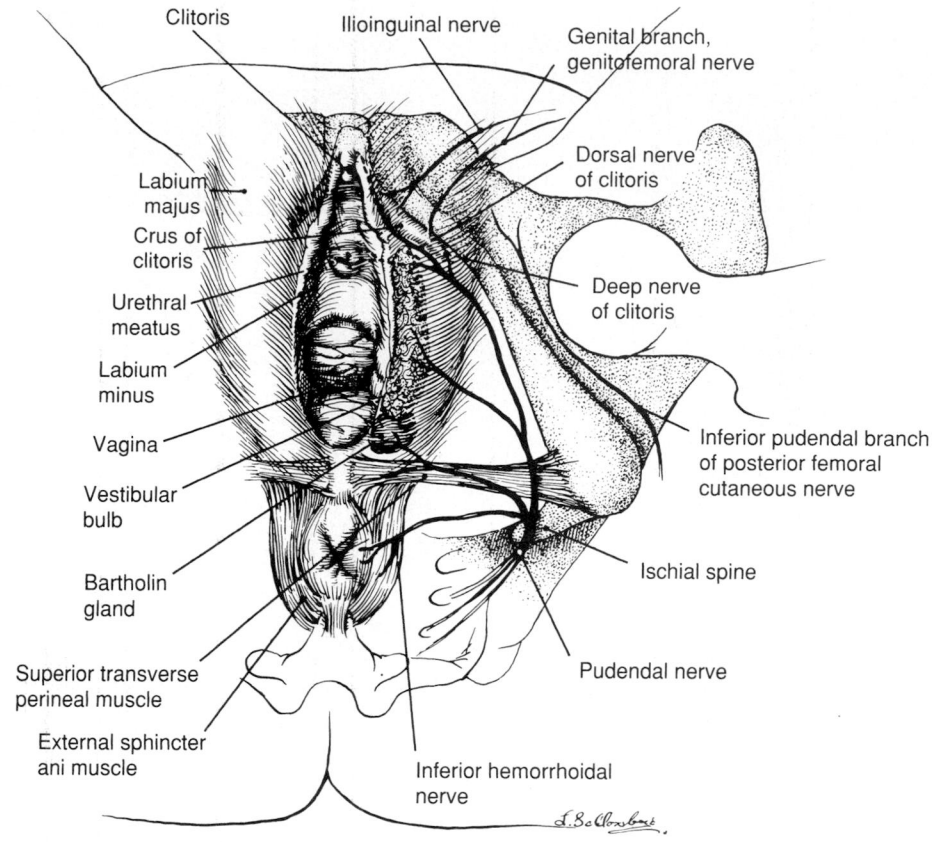

FIGURE 33.4. Nerve supply to anogenital region. (From Woodruff JD, Julian CG. In: Ridley JH, ed. *Gynecologic surgery: errors, safeguards and salvage.* Baltimore: Williams & Wilkins, 1974, with permission.)

Specific Infections

Although infections involving the vulva are treated with antibiotics rather than surgery, their appearance may resemble carcinoma in situ or even invasive cancer of the vulva. An accurate diagnosis may require cultures, viral testing, or even biopsy. Appropriate therapy is based on a correct diagnosis. Treatment of vulvitis secondary to an infectious process varies depending on the infection present. Viral infections such as HPV (condylomata) are strongly associated with intraepithelial neoplasia and carcinoma. These lesions are discussed later in this chapter. Molluscum contagiosum, a member of the pox family, requires accurate identification and resection of the umbilicated lesions with a dermal curette. These lesions are usually circular and umbilicated. Molluscum contagiosum in an adult may be an indicator of underlying HIV infection. Therefore, the patient's background should be appropriately discussed.

Herpes genitalis is caused by the herpes simplex virus (HSV). Fifteen percent of patients present with HSV type 1, and 85% present with HSV type 2. The patients with primary herpes present with high fevers, malaise, myalgias, painful vulvovaginal lesions, and inguinal adenopathy. The ulcers are small but coalesce into larger ulcers. The primary treatment of these sexually transmit-

ted diseases is presented in Table 33.1. Rarely, herpes genitalis can also cause meningitis, encephalitis, and hepatitis. If a pregnant patient has HSV, the newborn should be evaluated for this possibility.

Granuloma inguinale is caused by *Calymmatobacterium granulomatis* and presents as painless papular nodules or ulcerations. These lesions can occur in the genital, perianal, oral, and inguinal regions. When large and destructive, it may clinically simulate malignancy. Cytology and biopsy accompanied with Warthin Starry stains may establish the true diagnosis. The condition should be considered in all cases in which clinically malignant lesions are repetitively negative by biopsies. Lymphogranuloma venereum (LGV) is caused by *Chlamydia trachomatis* types L1, L2, and L3. LGV presents with papular or vesicular lesions on the vulva that can also ulcerate. LGV lesions are usually painless and heal spontaneously. As with herpes, these patients present with headaches, myalgias, arthralgias, and inguinal adenopathy. Chancroid is caused by *Haemophilus ducreyi*. The chancroid lesions present as multiple papules that become pustular and ulcerate. These lesions are very tender and have a ragged edge sitting on an erythematous base (halo). More than 50% of these patients present with large inguinal lymph nodes called buboes. These lymph nodes may become suppurative. Lymph

TABLE 33.1.
Treatment of Sexually Transmitted Diseases

Disease	Primary Treatment	Alternative Treatment
Syphilis	Benzathine penicillin, 2.4 million U IM × 1 dose	Tetracycline or erythromycin, 500 mg q.i.d. × 15 days
Herpes		
Primary	Acyclovir, 5 mg/kg q8h IV × 7–10 days	Acyclovir, 200 mg 5 × daily PO × 7–10 days
Disseminated	(inpatient)	(outpatient)
Encephalitis		
Hepatitis	Acyclovir, 10 mg/kg q8H IV	
Meningitis		
Frequent	Acyclovir, 200 mg 5 × daily PO × 5 days	Acyclovir, 800 mg PO b.i.d. × 5 days
recurrence		
Chronic	Acyclovir, 200 mg PO 2–5 × daily	Acyclovir, 400 mg PO b.i.d.
suppression		
LGV	Doxycycline, 100 mg × 3 weeks, and aspiration of fluctuant nodes; do not incise and drain lymphnodes	Tetracycline or erythromycin, 500 mg PO q.i.d. × 3 weeks
GI	Tetracycline, 500 mg PO q.i.d. × 3 weeks or until all lesions have healed	
Chancroid	Ceftriaxone, 250 mg IM q.i.d. × 7 days	Erythromycin, 500 mg PO q.i.d., or Bactrim, 2 tablets PO b.i.d. × 7 days

LGV, lymphogranuloma venereum; GI, granuloma inguinale.
Modified from Horowitz IR, Gomella LG, eds. *Obstetrics and gynecology on call,* first ed. East Norwalk, CT: Appleton & Lange, 1992:167.

nodes and soft tissue in the inguinal area can also be involved secondary to LGV and granuloma inguinale.

Syphilis is caused by the spirochete *Treponema pallidum.* The primary lesions usually have a painless, coin-shaped ulcer with a raised border and an indurated base. They can present 10 to 90 days after exposure and resolve in 2 to 6 weeks. Untreated syphilis results in a secondary phase characterized by skin rash, generalized adenopathy, and moist, papular anogenital lesions called condyloma latum. This is followed by a latent phase leading to tertiary syphilis. The latter can involve the cardiovascular, musculoskeletal, or central nervous system. *T. pallidum* can also cross the placenta and result in syphilis in the newborn infant. More than one STD can be seen in the same patient and can combine with AIDS.

Hidradenitis

An infectious process commonly demanding extensive local surgery is suppurative hidradenitis. This pustular disease begins as an infection in the apocrine sweat glands. The early manifestations often are cyclic, because the secretory activity of the apocrine glands corresponds to the progestational phase of the menstrual cycle. Consequently, in the early stages of the disease or in the chronic pruritic phase (Fox-Fordyce disease), the use of hormonal therapy, such as oral contraceptives, may help to modify the secretory activity of the glands. Once the disease extensively involves the deeper tissues, local and systemic agents usually are ineffective. Isotretinoin (Accutane) has been effective in some cases, but care must be taken in prescribing this agent because it is a powerful teratogen. Culturing exudates and treating with appropriate antibiotics may provide palliation and further delay surgery. The pustules often infect the entire area, so that pressure at one point may produce exudation of purulent material from sinus tracts (Fig. 33.5A). Because the entire anogenital area is honeycombed by the underlying infection, simple incision into a few of the pustules is useless. Extensive debridement must be performed to allow healing from the base.

The incision extends into the underlying fat, and the involved skin is removed in segments, leaving bridges of normal skin between the excised pustules. Loose approximation of the skin edges can be performed with polyglycolic acid or polyglactin 910 suture material; more commonly, the entire area is left open and treated locally to promote granulation (Fig. 33.5B). Results of therapy are rewarding in most cases, and skin grafting usually is unnecessary. The patient must be treated with antibiotics both before and after surgery. Ampicillin usually is recommended, but cultures should be obtained from the draining sinuses to check for organisms that are resistant. Vulvectomy has been used with success in some cases, but it is more traumatic to the patient both physically and psychologically. It is imperative that a thorough histologic evaluation be performed by the pathologist. Squamous cell carcinoma has been reported to arise in diffuse perineal suppurative hidradenitis.

Crohn's Disease

Crohn's disease, a chronic granulomatous inflammatory disease of the bowel, affects the vulva and perianal area in about 25% to 30% of the cases in which there is

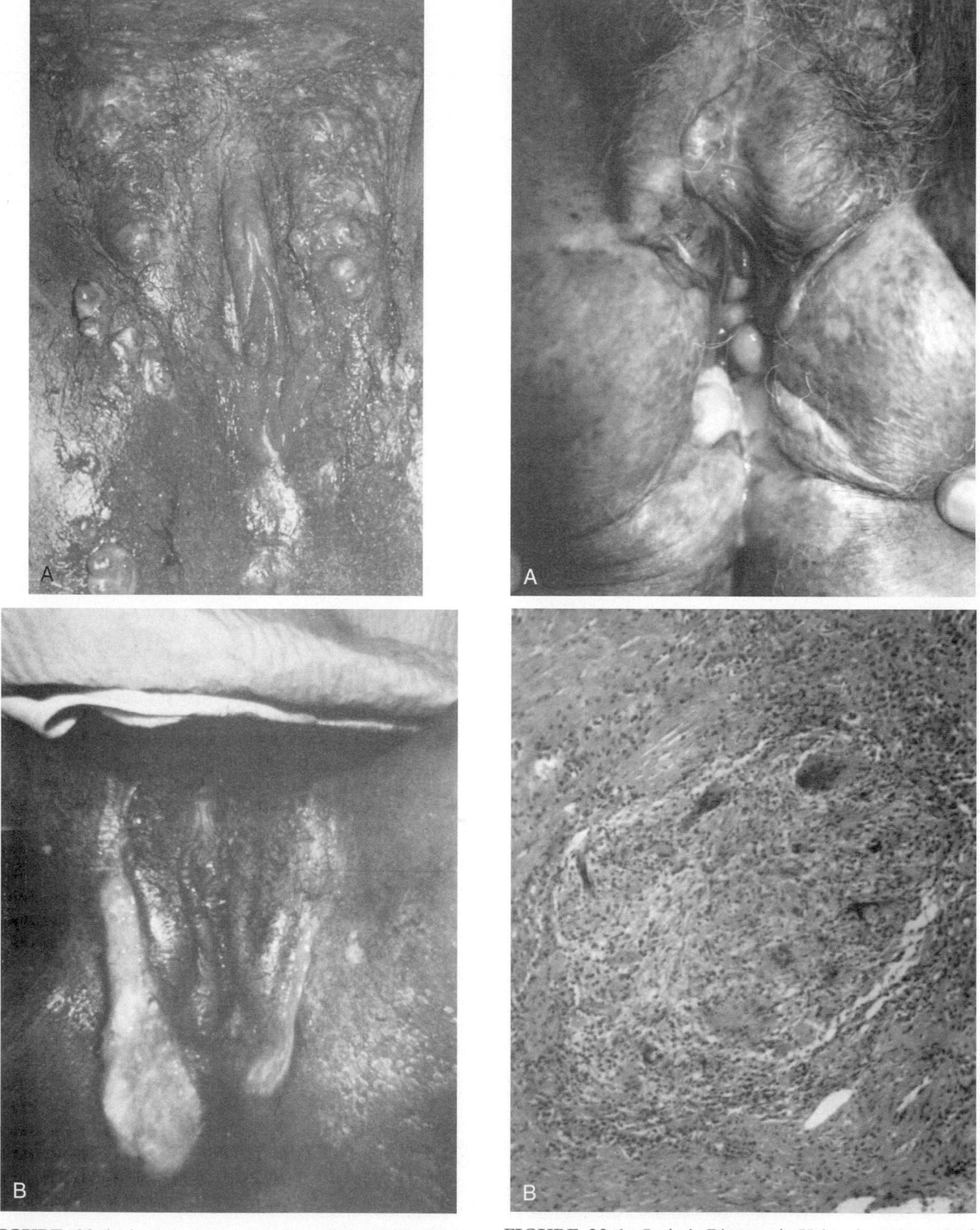

FIGURE 33.5. A: Extensive suppurative hidradenitis with numerous communicating sinuses. **B:** Same vulva 4 weeks after debridement with exuberant granulations (complete healing in 2 months).

FIGURE 33.6. Crohn's Disease. **A:** Vulva showing multiple fistulae and fibrosis causing tissue contraction and distortion. **B:** Microscopic section to show noncaseating granuloma. No microorganisms were seen by special stains.

classic intestinal involvement. The draining sinuses often communicate with the vagina or the rectum, thus resulting in the formation of fistulous tracts (Fig. 33.6A). On rare occasions, the vulva may be primarily involved, even though the small and large bowel apparently are not affected or affected subsequently. Crohn's disease can also present as unilateral labial hypertrophy.

Before any surgical therapy is begun, the diagnosis can be confirmed by studying the bowel or by obtaining a biopsy specimen of the affected tissues in the perineum. The presence of noncaseating granuloma without demonstrable organisms is characteristic of Crohn's disease (Fig. 33.6B). Further deterioration of the tissue may result from attempts to excise a draining sinus produced by Crohn's disease. Rectal incontinence can result from destruction of the anal sphincter or the development of a rectovaginal fistula.

Immunocytochemistry of Crohn's lesions has documented *Escherichia coli* and streptococcal antigens. In addition to short-term metronidazole, patients have responded to prolonged treatment (3 to 6 months) with broad-spectrum antibiotics such as ciprofloxacin. Methotrexate therapy is effective in reducing the requirement for prednisone in patients with chronically active Crohn's disease. Other drugs used in the medical management of Crohn's disease include 5-aminosalicylic acid, cyclosporine, azathioprine, 6-mercaptopurine, and mesalamine.

In addition to pharmacotherapy, a submucosal anal pull-through procedure may bring relief. Layered surgical repair of a fistula caused by Crohn's disease usually is unsuccessful, particularly without appropriate medical management. However, after appropriate medical therapy, surgical excision of the tract is usually effective (see Chapter 39). Results are difficult to predict because multiple areas of the terminal colon and small intestine may be affected, and any affected area may involve the vagina or perineum. Medical therapy should always be given during this type of surgical procedure and should be continued postoperatively for at least 2 months.

Trauma

Major trauma to the vulva most often occurs when young girls experience injuries as a result of sledding or bicycling accidents. Hematomas and occasionally lacerations can develop when the vaginal area forcefully comes in contact with the crossbar of a bicycle (as during a fall from a bicycle seat), or when the girl is thrown from a sled against an obstacle such as a tree or fence (Fig. 33.7). Trauma also can result from sexual assault, and the gynecologist must be sensitive to this possibility even when the initial history suggests another etiology. Women or girls who are victims of sexual assault should receive testing for pregnancy and sexually transmitted diseases as well as counseling.

Most traumatic injuries do not require surgical attention. Patients should be treated conservatively with

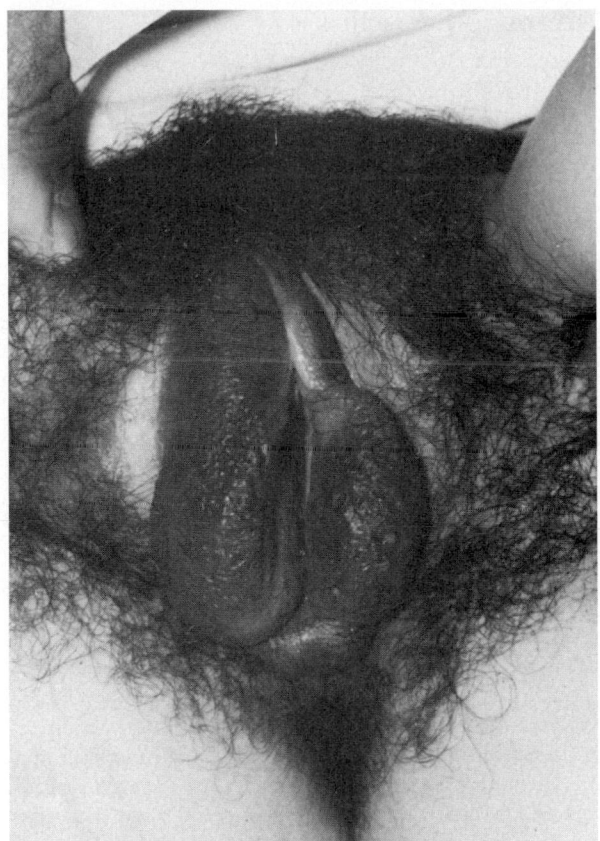

FIGURE 33.7. Hematoma of the vulva. (From Woodruff JD, Julian CG. In: Ridley JH, ed. *Gynecologic surgery: errors, safeguards and salvage.* Baltimore, Williams & Wilkins, 1974, with permission.)

activity restriction and with the immediate and continued use of Burow's solution (aluminum sulfate, calcium acetate; available as Domeboro tablets or powder) added to the sitz bath to reduce edema. Antibiotics may be used as prophylaxis against superinfection in damaged tissues. If a hematoma increases in size and extends well into the perineum or over the lower abdominal wall, incising the vulvar skin, evacuating the hematoma and ligating the bleeding vessels may reduce the period of convalescence. Goldman and co-workers reported 30% of patients with genital trauma not associated with parturition have a urologic injury. When a hematoma produces urethral obstruction, evacuation may reduce the time an indwelling urethral catheter is needed. If the hematoma is not expanding, it should be followed conservatively. Most vulvar hematomas resolve spontaneously; surgical intervention, on the other hand, can result in significant morbidity, including infection. Frequently, a distinct bleeding site is not identified. If, however, the clot becomes secondarily infected, it requires prompt evacuation and drainage. Lacerations into the rectum or urethra should be repaired expeditiously.

Necrotizing Fasciitis

Necrotizing fasciitis of the vulva is an uncommon invasive infection characterized by rapid progression and a high mortality rate ranging from 12% to 60%. Multiple bacterial pathogens are implicated, including staphylococci, streptococci, and gram-negative bacilli. Associated vascular thrombosis leads to skin and subcutaneous tissue necrosis. Fisher's criteria have been emphasized in the diagnosis and help to exclude clostridial infections. Diabetes mellitus is the most common predisposing condition, although other factors, such as radiation, have been identified.

Devascularization of the skin proceeds with sparing of underlying muscle and bone. Early skin changes include hemorrhagic bullous formation. Typically, the underlying fascial necrosis exceeds the boundaries of visible skin involvement. Inflammatory alterations and edema usually are present. Most patients present with fever, tachycardia, and signs of systemic toxic reaction. Prompt diagnosis is important because this disorder progresses rapidly.

Treatment combines expeditious surgery, antibiotics, and maintenance of circulation and tissue oxygenation. Surgical treatment should include aggressive excision of nonviable skin, subcutaneous tissue, and avascular fascia. Extensive debridement down to and including the fascia must be performed until viable, well-vascularized tissue margins are identified. Wounds are packed, not primarily closed. Broad-spectrum antibiotic coverage is advisable, and, when applicable, control of diabetes is advantageous.

Fournier's gangrene presents in a manner similar to that of necrotizing fasciitis and nonclostridial myonecrosis. Infections develop in the labia and spread to the perineum, buttocks, and abdominal wall. Treatment consists of a combination of surgery, broad-spectrum antibiotics, and hyperbaric oxygen.

Nodular Fasciitis

Nodular fasciitis is composed of fibroblasts and myofibroblasts in the subcutaneous tissues and are usually found on the extremities. There have been 11 cases reported in the English literature. Microscopically, the lesions consist of fibroblasts and myofibroblasts and have histologic similarities to a myogenic sarcoma. Wide local excision, as previously described, is adequate therapy for these patients.

CYSTS OF THE VULVA

Bartholin Duct Cysts

Obstruction of the Bartholin duct, usually near the orifice, is common. Although such obstructions can result from gonococcal infection, other infections and trauma more commonly explain the occlusion. During a mediolateral episiotomy or a posterior colporrhaphy, for example, sutures can easily injure or even ligate the duct. The lining of the main cyst is transitional epithelium. The mucus-se-

creting glands are not affected by the obstruction but may be distorted by the infectious process. During the acute infection, which may precede the actual cyst formation, an abscess often develops with symptoms of tenderness, swelling, and erythema. Depending on the cause, secretion from the cyst may be mucoid or cloudy.

Incision and drainage bring almost immediate relief to the patient and can be accomplished under local anesthesia. A small wick can be left in the cavity to maintain adequate drainage. A small incision (2 cm) is made in the cyst wall in the area of the normal duct orifice and a culture is obtained for *Neisseria gonorrhoeae*, Chlamydia, and aerobic and anaerobic bacteria. A Word catheter (Fig. 33.8) is inserted and the catheter bulb inflated with 2 to 3 mL of saline. If the catheter remains in place for 3 to 4 weeks, the tract becomes epithelialized and the catheter can be removed. Broad-spectrum antibiotics are given before surgery.

Marsupialization seldom can be accomplished during the acute stage, but the procedure is useful for chronic or recurrent abscesses. Injection of an antibiotic into the abscess has been tried as treatment for the acute infection but has proved to be less effective than systemic antibiotic therapy.

Most Bartholin duct cysts are uninfected and asymptomatic. They are usually found during routine pelvic examinations. Patients may even be unaware of large cysts. When symptoms do occur, most patients complain of discomfort during coitus or pain while sitting or walking. These require marsupialization only if they are symptomatic.

Technique of Excision

It is seldom necessary to excise a Bartholin duct cyst, particularly in the younger patient, unless there is induration at the base. The latter may signify deep-seated

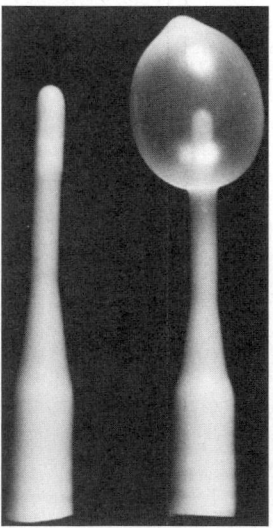

FIGURE 33.8. The Word catheter (*left*) is inserted into the Bartholin duct cyst through a vaginal incision. The bulb is inflated with saline solution (*right*), and the end of the catheter is placed in the vagina.

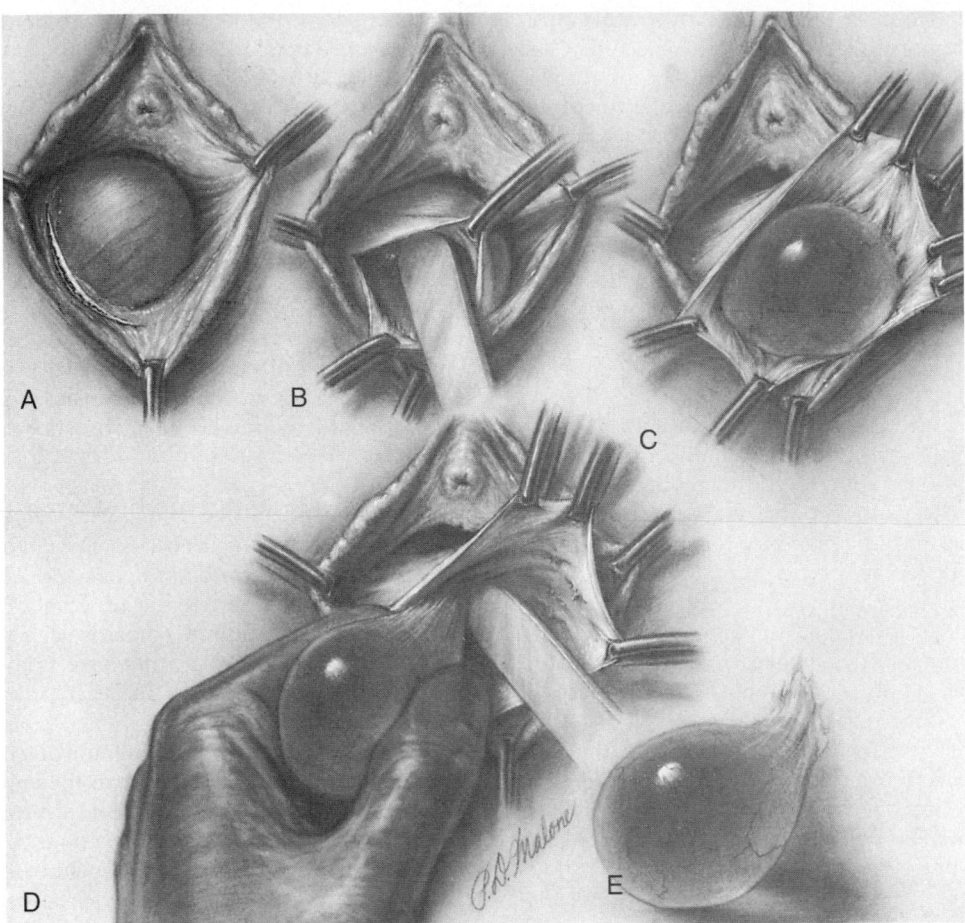

FIGURE 33.9. Excision of a Bartholin gland cyst. **A:** An incision is made in the mucosa over the cyst. **B:** Dissection is begun, using the handle of the scalpel. **C:** Dissection has been continued by sharp and blunt dissection. **D:** Dissection is almost complete. **E:** Intact cyst after removal.

infection that is inaccessible by marsupialization. Conversely, this may represent neoplasm in the base of the gland, an issue of greater concern in the patient older than 40 years of age or in patients with coexisting Paget's disease. An elliptical incision in the vaginal mucosa is made as close as possible to the site of the gland orifice (Fig. 33.9). An incision on the mucosal side is preferable because an incision through the vulvar skin makes it difficult to dissect the cyst wall from the skin without incising or tearing the skin. If an opening is accidentally made through the skin, a permanent fenestration may result. Difficulty is not usually encountered during dissection of the cyst from the inner surface of the vulvar skin when the incision is made on the mucosal side. Excising a small ellipse of mucosa with the cyst allows the surgeon to have a site for traction and reduces the risk of rupturing the cyst. Because cyst formation usually is preceded by inflammation, the wall is adherent and cannot be easily enucleated with blunt dissection only. The blunt-pointed Mayo scissors serve admirably for sharp dissection of the cyst from its bed (Fig. 33.9C). The cyst can be mobilized further with the handle of the scalpel. A large cyst may develop posteriorly and may approximate the rectum.

The rectal wall can easily be distinguished from the cyst by inserting a finger into the rectum during dissection.

Complete removal of the gland tissue adherent to the cyst wall is essential because residual glandular tissue may result in the formation of a tender nodule or recurrent cyst. If the margins of the cyst have become obscured, the cyst can be opened and the wall dissected from the surrounding tissue.

Directly beneath the Bartholin duct is the vestibular bulb, which is composed of anastomosing venous channels. In the dissection of the gland from the vestibular bulb, additional care must be taken to avoid troublesome bleeding. To ensure permanent hemostasis, the entire cavity must be obliterated by approximating the walls with fine delayed-absorbable suture material after excision of the cyst.

Approximation of the vaginal mucosa is best accomplished with a continuous or interrupted mucosal suture of 3-0 delayed-absorbable material. Persistent bleeding from the labia or vestibular bulb may cause a postoperative hematoma of the labia, which can progress to include the mons pubis and the abdominal wall beneath the Scarpa fascia. Bed rest, ice packs, and a pressure dressing on the vulva are the methods of treatment for a hematoma; attempts to ligate the venous bleeding points are futile. Although the blood usually reabsorbs with time, sometimes evacuation and drainage are necessary. If the bleeding deep in the bed of the gland seems uncontrollable, deep mattress sutures can be placed from the skin through the bleeding bed into the vagina. The sutures should not be tied too tightly because necrosis may result, with fenestration of the vaginal outlet. A small drain should be stitched into the bed with fine absorbable sutures to avoid the accumulation of blood and serous fluid.

Technique of Marsupialization

Drainage of a Bartholin duct cyst by marsupialization is not as technically involved as excision and eliminates many complications. The procedure makes it possible to avoid excising the gland with the cyst and to preserve the secretory function of the gland for lubrication.

The procedure can be performed under local, regional, or general anesthesia. A wedged-shaped, vertical incision is made in the vaginal mucosa over the center of the cyst, just outside the hymenal ring (Fig. 33.10A). The incision should be as wide as possible to enhance the postoperative patency of the stoma. After the cyst wall is opened and the cyst is drained of its contents, the lining of the cyst is everted and approximated to the vaginal mucosa with interrupted sutures of 2-0 delayed-absorbable material (Fig. 33.10B). Drains and packs are not necessary, but the patient's postoperative care should

include daily sitz baths beginning on the third or fourth postoperative day.

As a result of closure and secondary fibrosis of the orifice after marsupialization, 10% to 15% of cysts recur. Abscess formation is another occasional sequela of marsupialization.

Marsupialization has had limited use since the Word catheter was introduced. The catheter accomplishes the same result as surgery with minimal or no trauma. The nipple of the catheter can be inserted into the vagina. There is essentially no discomfort with the procedure, and coitus can be resumed normally. Because this procedure can be performed with local analgesia in the office setting and yields results comparable to those of marsupialization, its use should be encouraged.

Hydrocele or Cyst of the Canal of Nuck

Hydrocele is an uncommon vulvar cyst. The cyst appears as a dilatation in the labium majus and adjacent labium minus and must be differentiated from a Bartholin duct cyst. Figure 33.11 shows a hydrocele. The patient underwent two procedures for drainage of a Bartholin duct cyst, but the mass recurred after each procedure.

A hydrocele is a cystic, fluid-filled hernia of the peritoneum that accompanies the round ligament and extends from the inguinal canal into the vulva. When this sac extends into the inguinal canal, it is known as a cyst of the canal of Nuck. On rare occasions, a loop of intestine may follow the pathway of the round ligament,

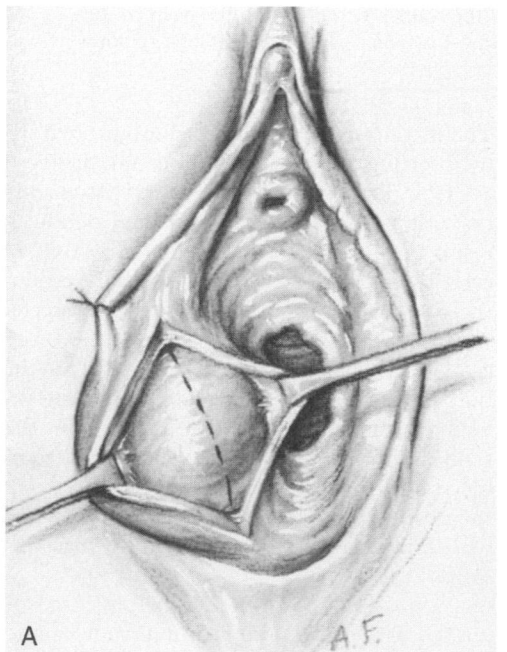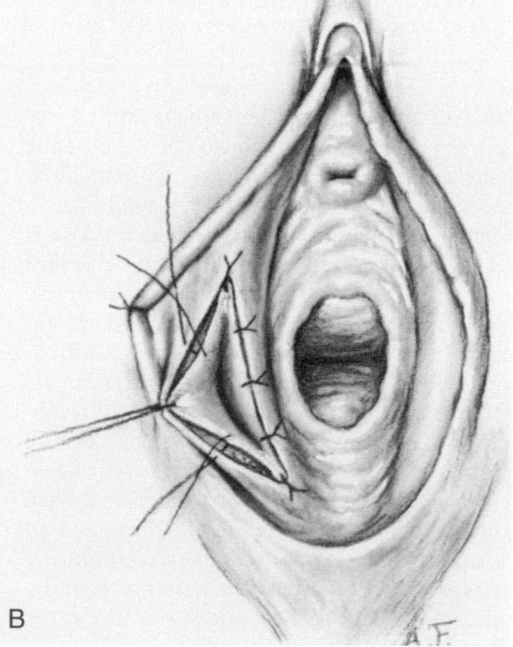

FIGURE 33.10. A: Incision for marsupialization. **B:** Marsupialization. (From Tancer ML, Rosenberg M, Fernandez D. Cysts of the vulvovaginal [Bartholin's] gland. *Obstet Gynecol* 1956;7:609).

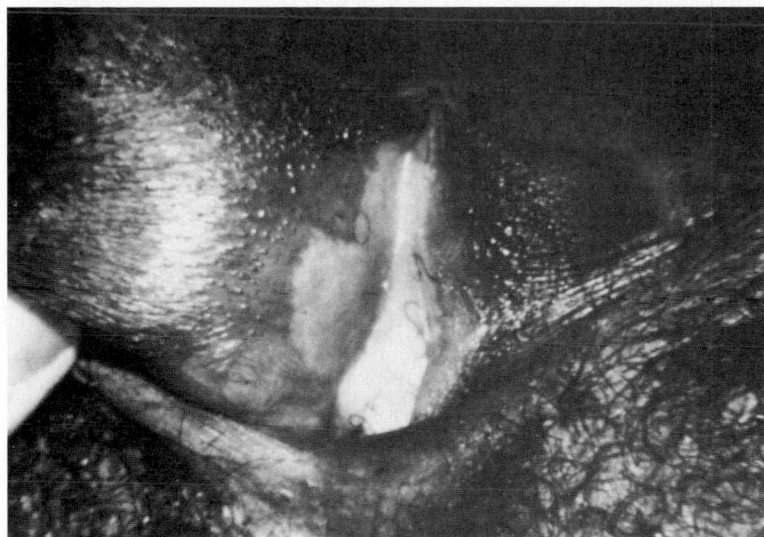

FIGURE 33.11. A hydrocele is caused by the extension of a peritoneal sac with the round ligament from the inguinal canal into the vulva.

forming a hernia in the vulva. When a hydrocele is treated as a Bartholin duct cyst by incision and drainage, peritoneal fluid may reaccumulate above the drainage site and the hydrocele recurs.

Kizer and colleagues reported a rare case of meconium hydrocele in a female newborn. The hydrocele was filled with meconium from a perforation of the bowel and spillage of meconium into the infant's peritoneal cavity and into the vulvar hydrocele. Although this has been reported in male infants, it seems to be the first reported case of a meconium hydrocele in a female infant.

Surgical treatment for a hydrocele begins with an incision into the cystic mass. The external inguinal ring is identified by inserting a finger in the cyst anteriorly to the inguinal canal. The peritoneal lining is excised from the cavity, and the external inguinal ring is closed along with the subjacent tissue in the anterior vulva. If a hernia is present, inguinal herniorrhaphy should be performed along with excision of the peritoneal covering of the round ligament.

VULVAR VESTIBULITIS SYNDROME

Vulvar vestibulitis is a clinical syndrome consisting of three characteristics as defined by the ISSVD in 1991: (1) severe pain on vestibular touch or attempted vaginal entry, (2) tenderness to pressure localized within the vulvar vestibule, and (3) physical findings confined to vestibular erythema of varying degrees. This syndrome is chronic and multifactorial. Etiologies include chronic or recurrent candidiasis, HPV infections, recurrent bacterial vaginosis, trauma, chemical and surgical destructive techniques, alterations of vaginal pH, irritants (soaps, detergents, douches, deodorants), and idiopathic causes. Wilkinson and colleagues found

HPV in only 3 of 31 cases evaluated for subtypes 6, 11, 16, and 18. However, Bornstein and associates identified a significant number of their patients with HPV 16/18.

Medical Treatment

A careful diagnostic evaluation is essential because of the apparent multifactorial etiology of vulvar vestibulitis. If an infectious etiology is present, it is imperative to treat it. Recombinant α-interferon is efficacious in treating vulvar vestibulitis syndrome (VVS) with a history of condylomata acuminata or subclinical HPV.

Chronic recurrent candidiasis is treated with prolonged oral administration of ketoconazole or fluconazole. Topical anticandidal regimens should be prescribed when oral antifungal medications are discontinued.

In addition to being treated for the infectious etiology, all patients should be started on a course of topical steroids. Horowitz treats all patients with VVS with hydrocortisone acetate 1% or 2.5% with 1% pramoxine HCl ointment (Pramosone) for 2 to 3 months. After 3 months of this therapy, the patients are placed on desoximetasone 0.25% ointment (Topicort). Only after failing topical steroids are the patients considered for surgical treatment. Amitriptyline has been used successfully in some patients. Doses of 25 to 75 mg taken 3 hours before bedtime is prescribed. Patients with vulva dysesthesia or interstitial cystitis benefit most from medical therapy with amitriptyline.

Surgical Treatment

Carbon dioxide laser ablation of the vestibular glands has not been shown to be optimal and has resulted in scarring and increased dyspareunia in some patients. In 1995, Reid and associates reported long-term results with the flashlamp-excited dye laser in nonresponders to

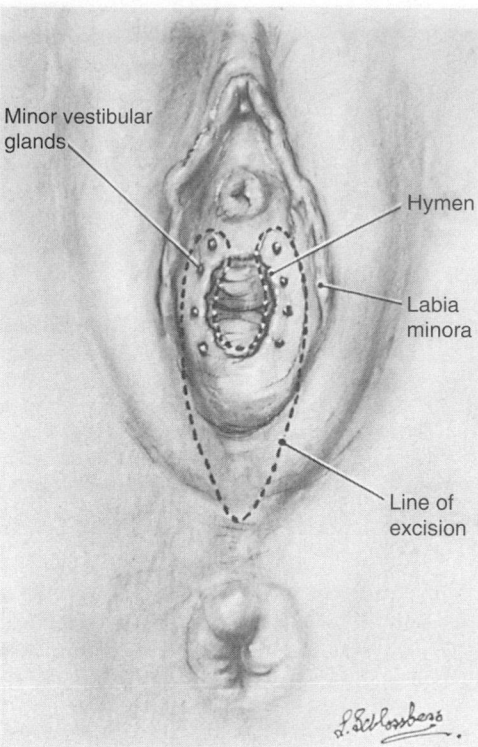

FIGURE 33.12. The minor vestibular glands exit lateral to the hymenal ring. They are very superficial and thus seldom produce definable "nodules," even when chronically infected.

medical therapy. Those with poor responses to laser vaporization were then treated with gland resection. Overall response rates were 62% to 80%, depending on the distribution of tenderness.

Primary surgical therapy has produced relief of symptoms in 75% to 90% of patients. This technique was initially described by Woodruff and associates in 1981 and

Friedrich in 1987, and was modified by Marinoff and Turner in 1991 to include the periurethral Skene gland openings. The outer incision extends circumferentially from the periurethral glands along Hart's line to the contralateral glands. The proximal vaginal margin is just inside the hymenal ring. This horseshoe-shaped epithelium is superficially excised and sent for histologic diagnosis. In almost all cases, the histology consists of nonspecific periglandular chronic inflammation, much less impressive than might be expected based on the severe symptoms described. As in a perineoplasty, the vaginal mucosa is undermined and the vagina advanced to approximate edges. The wound is closed in two interrupted layers of 3-0 polyglactin 910 (Vicryl) or polyglycolic acid (Dexon) sutures (Fig. 33.12). Postoperative treatment is the same as for perineoplasty. Coitus should be avoided for 2 to 3 months after surgery.

Several of Horowitz's patients (unpublished report) had severe levator spasm secondary to anticipation of vulvodynia. This learned response has been treated successfully with biofeedback in several patients. Glazer and colleagues were the first to report the treatment of VVS with electromyographic biofeedback of pelvic floor musculature. Seventy-eight percent (22 of 28) resumed coitus by the end of the treatment period.

SOLID TUMORS

The incidence of solid, benign tumors in the vulva is low; but a variety of benign tumors, including fibromas, fibromyomas, lipomas, hemangiomas, neurofibromas, and endometriomas have all been reported. These tumors can originate from any of the three germinal layers that constitute the anogenital area. One occasionally sees a solid vulvar tumor composed of benign breast tissue or a benign fibroadenoma arising therefrom (Fig. 33.13). Lactational changes can be seen in this tissue. Such an

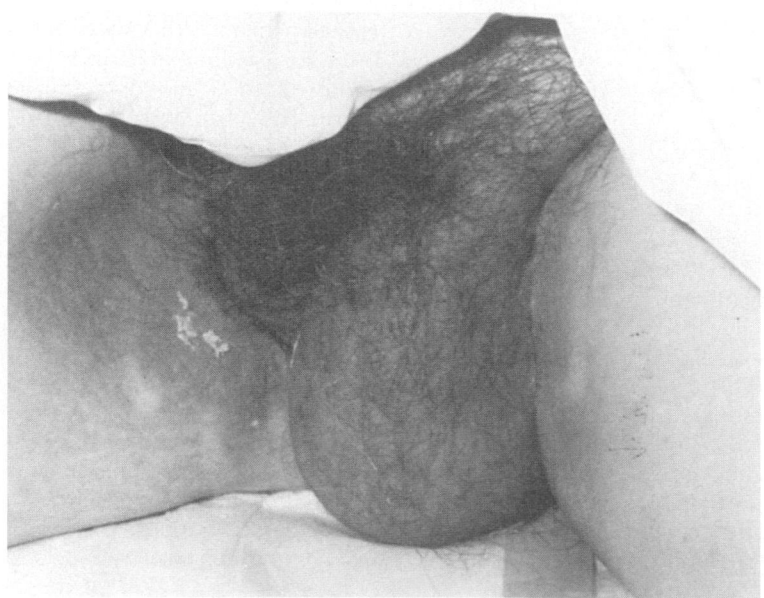

FIGURE 33.13. Fibroadenoma of the vulva arising from the embryonic breast tissue, the caudal end of the milk line.

event is accounted for by the embryologic milk line caudally ending in the vulvar area. Degenerative changes and necrosis often occur in the larger tumors and should not be confused with malignancy. Lipomas often are mistaken for cystic lesions because of their consistency, whereas hernias and hydroceles of the canal of Nuck must be differentiated from neoplastic growths because they require different surgical approaches.

Most solid tumors should be excised, both to ascertain the diagnosis and to relieve the patient's discomfort. Small, pedunculated tumors can be removed by simple ligation of the stalk; the deeply situated lesions require more extensive local dissection. All nevi showing hemorrhage, sudden enlargement, and pruritus should be suspected to be melanomas and excised widely.

The boundaries of such mesodermal tumors are difficult to delineate, but most of the tumors are benign. Even recurrence does not signify malignant alteration; the fibromyoma may recur if incompletely excised, even when the original specimen had no histologic evidence of malignancy. Although a sarcoma rarely arises in the vulva, histologic studies must be carefully made because degenerating atypical multinucleated cells of a benign or reactive tissue can be confused as indicative of malignancy.

As in any vulvar surgery, hemostasis is important because compression is difficult to obtain in these soft tissues. Extravasation of blood can dissect the fascial planes well out to the vulva, thigh, flanks, and abdominal wall. Closed suction drains should be used in the wounds if hemostasis is not complete.

Condyloma Acuminatum

Condyloma acuminatum is one morphologic manifestation of HPV infection in the lower genital tract. These lesions have an incubation period ranging from several weeks to 8 months; however, clinical infection usually is apparent in 6 to 8 weeks after exposure. Transmission of the virus is attributed to coitus, and the process is efficient, because most sexual partners are affected subclinically if not clinically. The disease process continues increasing in prevalence. Interestingly, clinically apparent condyloma constitute only a fraction of HPV infections. Most are undetected in asymptomatic patients with no clinical findings.

Numerous HPV subtypes have been identified. HPV subtypes 6, 11, 16, 18, and 31 account for most genital tract infections. Careful histopathologic and virologic study of vulvar lesions has demonstrated an association of HPV 6 and HPV 11 with most exophytic condylomata, as well as flat cervical condylomas and low-grade cervical dysplasias. HPV 16 and HPV 18 are only infrequently identified in benign lesions. Reid and associates demonstrated that these are the typical viral types found in association with high-grade dysplasia and invasive carcinomas. In 1988, Buscema and colleagues and others reported on vulvar lesions, including condylomata, VIN, and invasive cancers in patients at Johns Hopkins Hospital. HPV 16 was identified in only 12% of condylomata

but 81% of VIN III; this study supported the concept of HPV 16 as the dominant oncogenic virus in vulvar neoplasms.

Condylomata acuminata that manifest on the vulva are frequently associated with cervical, vaginal, and anal HPV infection. Careful clinical evaluation mandates vaginal/cervical cytology and colposcopy in patients who present with vulvar warts. This is appropriate not only to exclude cervical and vaginal dysplasia but also to define the extent of condylomatous involvement and permit appropriate tailoring of regional therapy.

Condylomata acuminata are small and usually multifocal lesions. They may be accompanied by pruritic discomfort or irritation. Warts initially may be reddish brown because of parakeratosis; however, with time and exposure to local trauma, they become gray or white. The latter appears to be associated with hyperkeratosis and the generalized keratin disturbance associated with viral infection (Fig. 33.14). Unless they are traumatized, bleeding is not a typical feature. In pregnancy, however, because of marked vascular alterations, condyloma of the vagina and perineum can be a source of abundant bleeding if laceration occurs. Massive vulvar and perianal condylomata may occur in certain circumstances, preventing identification of the introitus and anal orifice; conditions that foster this growth potential include immunosuppression and, less frequently, pregnancy (Fig. 33.15). Those lesions that were previously called giant condyloma are now regarded as verrucous carcinoma. In the spectrum of condylomatous growths, the dividing line between condyloma and verrucous carcinoma is indistinct because of the structural benignancy of both.

Various treatment approaches are available and are characterized by their inability to eliminate the offending agent—the virus. Interferon offers a nonspecific antiviral therapy, and research is currently progressing on the development of HPV vaccines. α-Interferon has been used intralesionally for refractory condylomata. Studies have cited its use two to three times weekly. Flulike effects should be anticipated for at least several weeks. Efficacy has been demonstrated with this technique, although treatment is cumbersome, can be costly, and remains investigational. Its primary role has not been defined.

At the present time, only a variety of ablative approaches are available for management of condyloma. These should be individualized with consideration of prior treatment, volume and location of disease, the presence or absence of associated dysplasia, and other idiosyncratic patient factors. The most common approach to vulvar condylomata is the local application of 25% podophyllum resin, often prepared in benzoin. This method, although reasonably well tolerated in the office setting, often requires numerous applications. Burning discomfort ensues after sustained contact, which is necessary for efficacy. Most recommend that the agent be left in place for 6 hours before tub baths, so compliance may be problematic. Podophyllum appears to be more effective on exophytic, rather than flat, condylomata. Use is restricted to the vulva in nonpregnant patients; vaginal application may lead to undesirable absorption

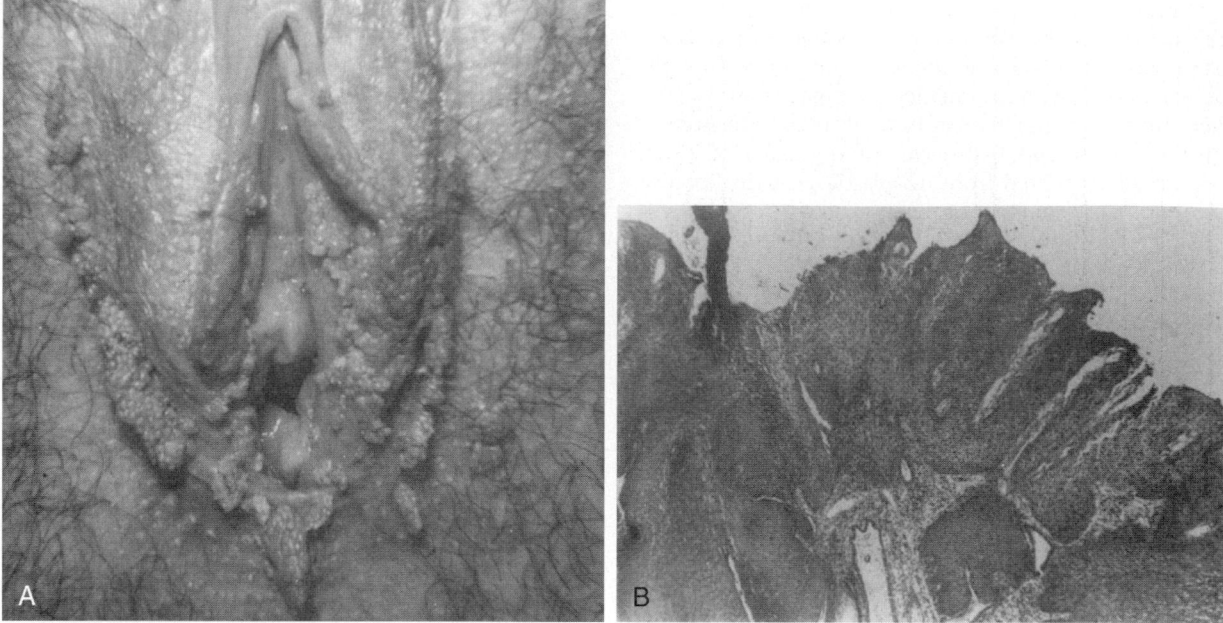

FIGURE 33.14. A: Condylomata acuminata, gross. Condylomata acuminata involving labia majora and minora. Note exophytic quality and lack of pigmentation. **B:** Condylomata acuminata, microscopic. Epidermal hyperplasia featuring acanthosis and elongated, distorted rete pegs is evident. Keratin disturbances are present.

and neurotoxicity. An alternative is halogenated acetic acid, either bichloroacetic or trichloroacetic (TCA). Our preference is 90% TCA. This agent quickly interacts with cellular proteins, inducing a coagulative effect, and rapidly turns lesions a brilliant white. Advantages include its

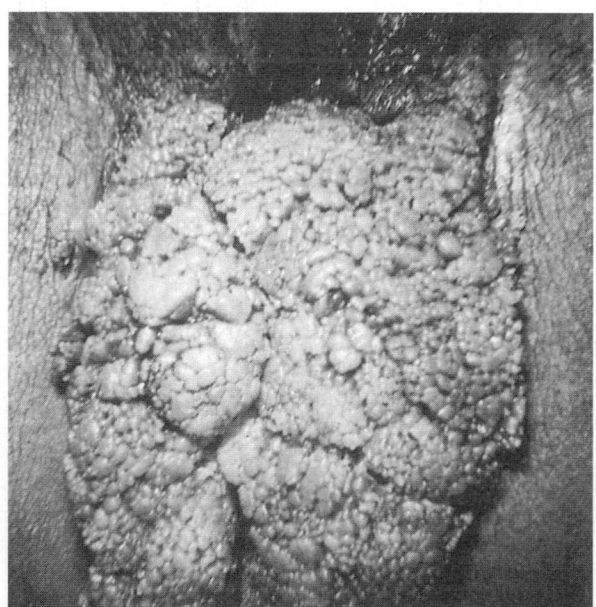

FIGURE 33.15. Massive condylomata acuminata now considered as verrucous carcinoma.. Note abundant exophytic lesions producing confluent, cauliflower-like growth. Lesion is present on perineum and totally obscures anal orifice. Patient is 23 years old and is maintained on prednisone because of neurosarcoidosis.

ability to sustain a prompt chemical effect on the condyloma, its availability for intravaginal use and use during pregnancy, and the fact that is can be rapidly neutralized with sodium bicarbonate, which may be dissolved in water and applied as a cooling paste.

Surgical excision, cautery, destruction, and laser ablation are reserved for certain patients. Criteria for selection may include the following:

- Extensive volume of condylomata exceeding what may be resolved with chemical agents
- Multicentric HPV infections, particularly with involvement of the vagina, urethra, or anus
- Failure of concerted office therapy with topical chemical agents
- Additional presence of significant intraepithelial neoplasia
- Immunocompromised state in some hosts

One should certainly use biopsy liberally to evaluate presumed condylomata that are refractory to topical treatment or that have an atypical appearance. This helps prevent sustained, ineffective chemical treatment of high-grade VIN, often presenting as a flat and pigmented verrucous lesion in the younger patient, and helps exclude a frank cancer with warty features. Large, sessile condylomata or those that grow rapidly, bleed abnormally, or become necrotic or invasive should arouse the suspicion of malignancy.

Cryotherapy has been used on the vulva to eradicate warts. The freezing induces localized tissue necrosis. Although healing usually is satisfactory, and numbing effects induce analgesia, application is limited by delivery systems and probe-tip sizes. Larger condylomatous masses are more difficult to treat, as are vaginal lesions. Depth of apparent tissue destruction can be difficult to assess.

Electrocautery with a loop has been used effectively, particularly with massive lesions. Analgesic needs are definitely a factor in this approach. Smaller lesions may be fulgurated. Buildup of charred tissue can be removed by abrasion to identify residual warty tissue. The precision and depth of tissue injury can be problematic.

Colposcopically directed laser ablation performed by trained personnel in appropriately selected cases may afford effective treatment. Condylomatous lesions may be vaporized; starting at the center of the lesion causes the wart to collapse inward toward the beam. The level of the adjacent normal skin should be selected as a landmark. In treating condylomata, there is no need for deep laser vaporization into the dermis, exceeding the so-called first laser surgical plane. Issues of appropriate power density may be debated; however, the inexperienced laser surgeon should use lower-power densities (larger spot size or lower laser output) to protect against unnecessarily deep laser injury. In experienced hands, higher laser output may be feasible, which speeds the procedure. Power densities of 500 to 800 W/cm^2 normally are used for vaporization. Lower power densities are associated with undesirable thermal injury to adjacent tissues. Sites of laser vaporization should be wiped with moistened gauze sponges to remove carbon and thermally coagulated tissue and to permit accurate assessment of depth and remaining disease. Large lesions can be dealt with by laser excision followed by vaporization at the base (see Chapter 15). Clinicians are advised to use protective eyewear during vaporization to prevent possible conjunctival condyloma.

Brush laser vaporization of the normal epithelium surrounding warty lesions is commonly done to destroy subclinical HPV and reduce the risk of clinical recurrence. This technique uses lower power densities (200 to 300 W/cm^2) to superficially denude 1 to 2 cm of adjacent epidermis. The rationale for this approach is the presence of HPV in tissue proximal to the condyloma, as demonstrated by Ferenczy and colleagues. Brush vaporization and laser treatment of so-called subclinical HPV infection that may be appreciated with the colposcope have been proposed to lessen the viral reservoir and reduce recurrence rates.

Nevertheless, recurrences must be anticipated in 25% to 50% of patients with extensive disease treated with the laser, particularly if immunocompromised. These patients require further treatment with either laser or chemical approaches, such as 5-FU topically. If disease is minimal, they can be observed.

Patients subjected to extensive laser treatment require considerable local care while healing proceeds. Cool tub or sitz baths with Burow's solution followed by the application of silver sulfadiazine (Silvadene) cream and 5% lidocaine (Xylocaine) ointment often afford relief and protect against bacterial superinfection. Narcotics for pain management are appropriate short-term drugs. Prophylactic systemic antibiotics do not appear to be indicated. Weekly office follow-up is advised for 2 to 3 weeks to assess tissue healing, prevent undesirable areas of tissue

agglutination, and allow potential early identification of recurrences, which can be managed with chemical ablation. Patients should be followed up carefully for several months after treatment to monitor for recurrences.

The Ultrasonic Surgical Aspirator has also been efficacious in treating condyloma. Tissue cell damage is 25 to 30 μm, which is similar to that caused by a cold scalpel. This contrasts with electrocautery at 75 to 100 μm. The tip vibrates at 23,000 cycles per second. Tissue is fragmented and aspirated, providing a specimen for histologic evaluation. The Ultrasonic Surgical Aspirator is discussed in Chapter 14.

Regardless of the selected approach to therapy, all patients should be advised to have their consorts examined to lessen the risk of reexposure to lesions with a large viral burden. This theoretically helps diminish treatment failures. Patients with HIV or other types of immunosuppression need to be more closely followed up.

Hidradenoma (Sweat Gland Tumor) of the Vulva

A rare benign tumor of the vulva, hidradenoma, was first described by Schickele in 1902. The tumor is characterized by its intricate papillary adenomatous pattern, which may be readily mistaken for cancer.

Clinically, a hidradenoma is small, rarely more than 1 cm in diameter (Fig. 33.16A). Its consistency can range from firm to as soft as a sebaceous cyst, with which it is often confused. Most of these lesions are found in the interlabial folds, in the labia majora, or in the perineum. Because these tumors are apocrine in origin, the labia minora location is unusual. The occasional occurrence of reddish brown pulpy material on the surface results when the tumor is evulsed through the duct of the sweat gland.

These lesions have been carefully studied in numerous laboratories, and the complex microscopic patterns have been repeatedly stressed (Fig. 33.16B). The superficial papillary adenomatous pattern appears aggressive, but careful inspection shows that the glandular structures are lined by a single layer of well-organized cuboidal cells. In some parts of the tumor, the pink-staining secretory elements can be identified superficial to the basal layer. Beneath the epithelium is an indefinite layer of flattened myoepithelial cells. When the clear cell variant of the myoepithelium proliferates, an ominous picture is created, yet this clear cell hidradenoma also behaves in a benign manner. Although hidradenocarcinoma occasionally does occur, a finding of distinct adenocarcinoma in the vulva should initiate a search to rule out a metastatic lesion from another primary site.

Hidradenomas are classically asymptomatic, and most lesions are discovered during a routine pelvic examination. Curative treatment consists of local excision; recurrences result only from incomplete excision.

Hemangioma

Hemangiomas are common vulvar lesions that usually do not require treatment. The lesions normally are small, are often multiple, and may bleed with trauma. On occasion,

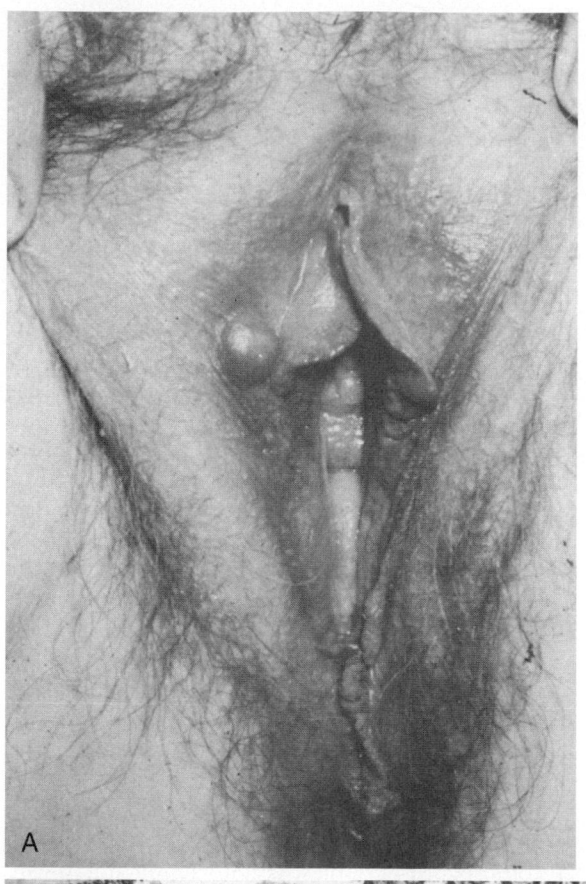

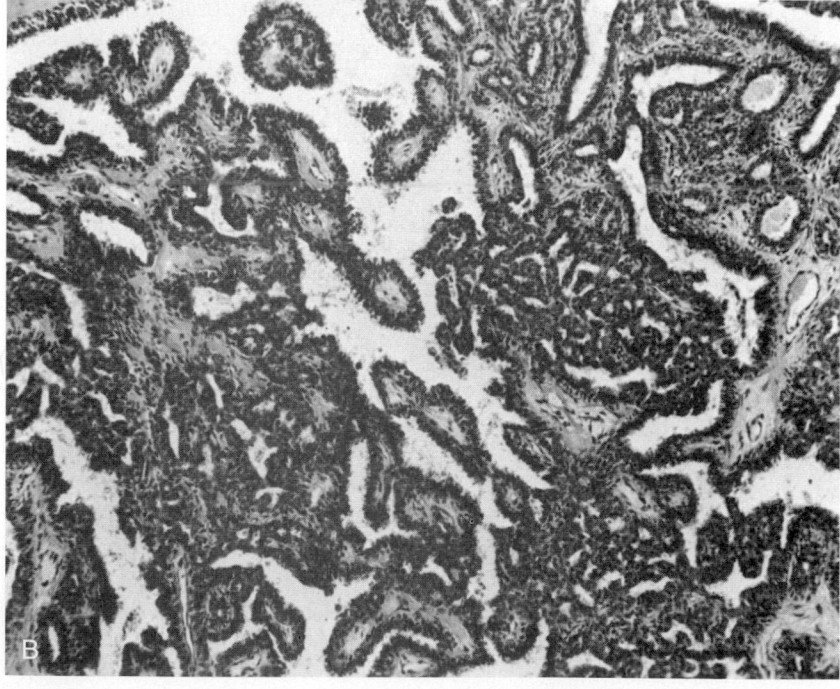

FIGURE 33.16. A: Hidradenoma of the vulva. **B:** Low-power magnification section of hidradenoma of the vulva. (**A:** From Novak E, Woodruff JD. *Obstetric and gynecologic pathology*, seventh ed. Philadelphia: WB Saunders, 1974.)

keratinization causes the superficial surface to appear white or gray-white (angiokeratoma). Hemangiomas should be differentiated from small varicosities, which commonly are seen in the postmenopausal patient.

An accurate diagnosis is imperative because a malignant melanoma can be misinterpreted as a hemangioma.

The abrupt appearance of any pigmented lesion demands biopsy. In 2 of 11 melanomas seen in our clinic, the lesions were diagnosed as hematoma or angioma, and a correct diagnosis was provided only by histologic study. Angiokeratoma, a benign tumor, is a distinct clinicopathologic entity. Aggressive angiomyxoma, although

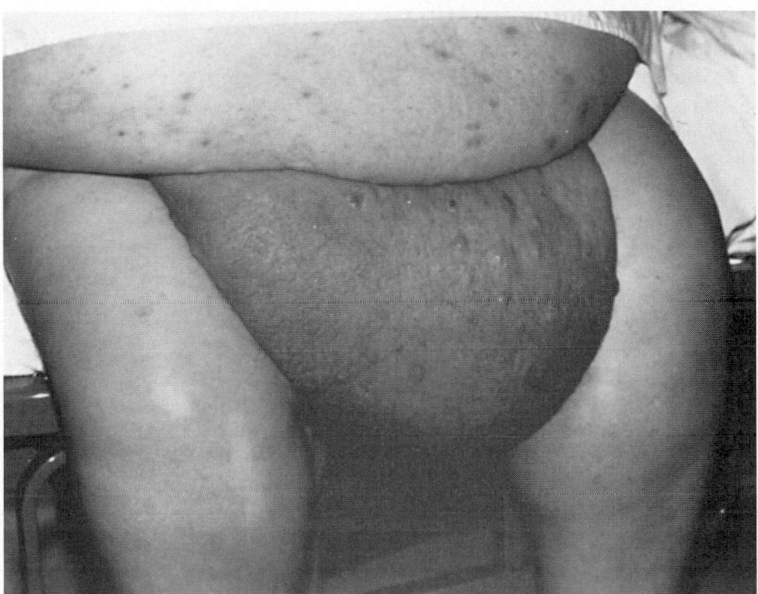

FIGURE 33.17. A benign angiolipoma noted for its massive size.

structurally benign, is known for its large size and local recurrences. Some tumors, although benign, can be massive in size and thereby pose operative problems (Fig. 33.17).

The best treatment for congenital hemangioma is careful observation. The lesions regress spontaneously in almost all cases, and attempts at excision may be mutilating. If bleeding is a problem, the troublesome vascular channels can be treated by surgical ligation or embolization.

VARICOCELE AND VARICES

Varices are common on the vulva, and the larger lesions are almost routinely unilateral. As with most varicosities, treatment depends on size and symptoms. Whereas varicoceles in the scrotum arise from dilatation of the veins in the pampiniform plexus of the inguinal canal, the lesions on the vulva arise from the pudendal veins (Fig. 33.18). Careful evaluation usually demonstrates more extensive involvement of the tributaries of the hypogastric vein with varicosities of the gluteal vessels over the buttock.

If the patient experiences discomfort from the engorgement that follows exercise or standing for long periods, ligation is indicated with excision of the segment of vulvar skin that contains the varices. Knowledge of the intricate vascular system that supplies the external genitalia is necessary to ensure that surgery will result in long-term success and will prevent recurrences. Horowitz has treated several patients using selective embolization with success.

Granular Cell Tumors

Granular cell tumors (GCTs) were first described by Weber in 1854. It wasn't until 1926 that Abrikossoff coined the term *myoblastoma*. Later the tumor was termed *granular cell schwannoma*. The current nomenclature recognizes the term *granular cell tumor*. Although frequently benign, GCTs can present as a malignant form that is multicentric and metastatic in vital organs. Horowitz and associates reported on 20 patients presenting with GCTs of the vulva over a 31-year period at the Emory University Teaching Hospitals. Seventy percent of the patients were African-American, and the mean age was 50 years. Ninety percent of the lesions were on the labia majora, with lesion size ranging from 0.4 × 0.4 cm to 7 × 8 × 12 cm. Nineteen of 20 patients were treated with a wide local excision. The twentieth patient required radical excision because of the size of the lesion. This patient eventually died of pulmonary metastasis. Only two patients presented with multiple le-

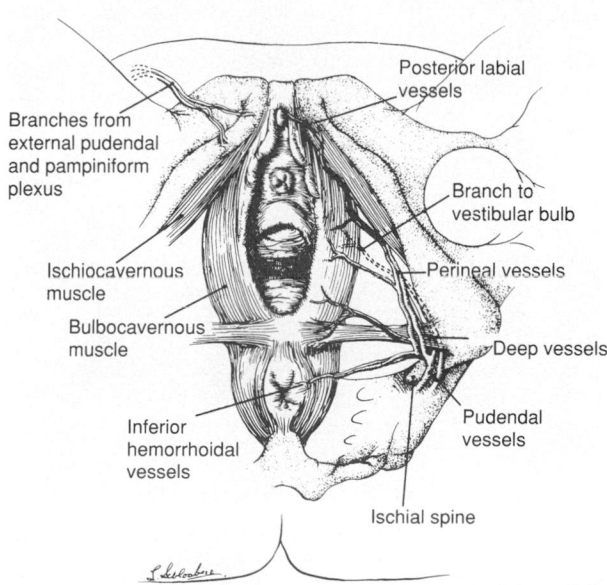

FIGURE 33.18. Vascular supply of the vulva.

sions. Twelve lesions were stained for S-100. All were positive, which suggests a neural Schwann cell origin.

Sometimes the overlying pseudoepitheliomatous changes are misinterpreted as carcinoma in situ (CIS) or early invasive cancer (Fig. 33.19). Identification is possible with recognition of the granular cells dispersed within the underlying stroma or within the tumor. In a few patients, GCT has behaved in a malignant fashion, but an appearance of a second lesion at a site outside the vulva usually indicates multiple primary lesions rather than metastasis.

WHITE LESIONS OF THE VULVA

The terms *kraurosis* and *leukoplakia* have been overused in the past. In 1877, Schwimmer reported that leukoplakia on the buccal surfaces of the mouth was a premalignant lesion, and Beisky later described kraurosis as an atrophic lesion similar to lichen sclerosus. Because of these early reports, every lesion on the vulva that appeared white and constricted the vaginal outlet was called kraurosis. Moreover, conditions as varied as leukoderma and invasive cancer have been called leukoplakia. Other terms, such as *primary senile atrophy* and *atrophic*

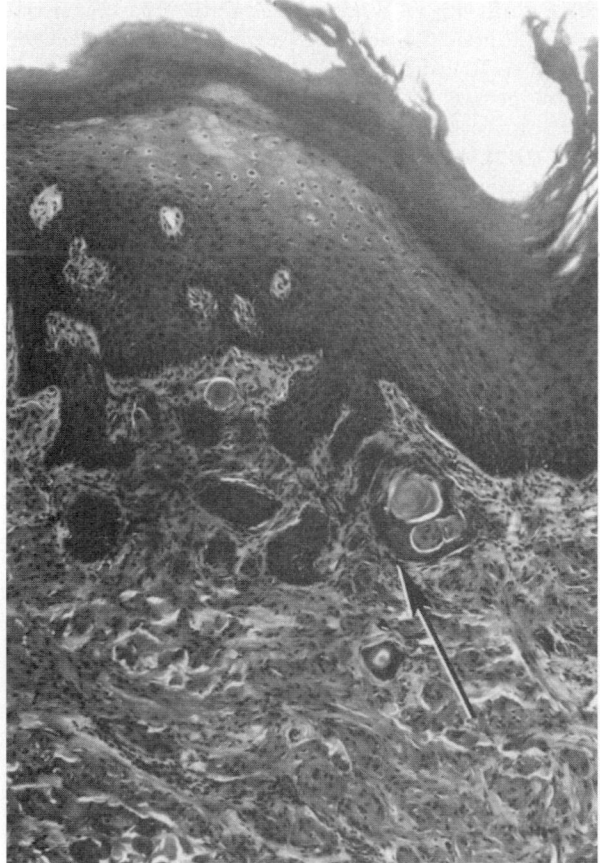

FIGURE 33.19. Granular cell tumor. Note the pseudoepitheliomatous hyperplasia, nests of large, pale "granular cells" beneath the epithelium.

leukoplakia, have been used interchangeably. They are nonspecific and should be eliminated.

Although some physicians have suggested that lichen sclerosus and kraurosis have different histopathologies, their microscopic appearance is similar. A safe approach would be for surgeons to describe the anatomic appearance (i.e., whether the vulva is shrunken and constricted or thickened and leathery), leaving it up to the pathologist, who is familiar with both histology and anatomy, to define the cellular and histologic abnormalities.

Depigmentation Lesions

Leukoderma and *vitiligo* are terms that are used interchangeably. Treatment is not required unless the symptoms of the commonly associated chronic dermatitis cannot be controlled by local medications. The hyperkeratotic lesions comprise a number of diverse entities that share a white to grayish white epithelial appearance in a moist environment. Biopsy is the only reliable criterion for accurate assessment.

Hyperkeratosis

Both chronic infections and benign tumors, most commonly condylomata acuminata, appear white because keratin absorbs moisture, which reflects light back to the observer.

To avoid the ambiguous term *leukoplakia*, Jeffcoate, in 1966, introduced the term *dystrophy* into the nomenclature of benign epithelial lesions of the vulva. Predictions about the malignant potential of vulvar dystrophy vary; of all the types of dystrophy, the one most often benign is lichen sclerosus. As noted earlier, the terminology for vulvar dystrophies has been altered. Vulvar dystrophy has been classified in three categories: squamous hyperplasia, lichen sclerosus, and VIN. Typical squamous cell hyperplasia is characterized by a thickened, hyperkeratotic squamous epithelium, elongated rete pegs, and often an infiltration of the underlying tissue with chronic inflammatory cells. Typical hyperplasia is a benign form of chronic dermatitis with hyperkeratosis and acanthosis; thus, the designation "dystrophy" should be eliminated.

Lichen Sclerosus

Lichen sclerosus is characterized by hyperkeratosis, thinning of the epidermis, loss of rete peg architecture, collagenization of the underlying tissue, and associated middermal inflammatory infiltrate (Fig. 33.20). It can occur at any age. The disease has been noted in the prepubertal child, and it occurs during the menstrual years. Nevertheless, it is seen most often in the postmenopausal woman when the lesions more commonly are symptomatic, perhaps because of the additional epithelial compromise caused by atrophy. The genetic aspects of lichen sclerosus have not been clearly identified, but the finding of lesions in both mother and child has been documented.

If biopsy specimens reveal lichen sclerosus, the patient should be treated with ultrapotent corticosteroids.

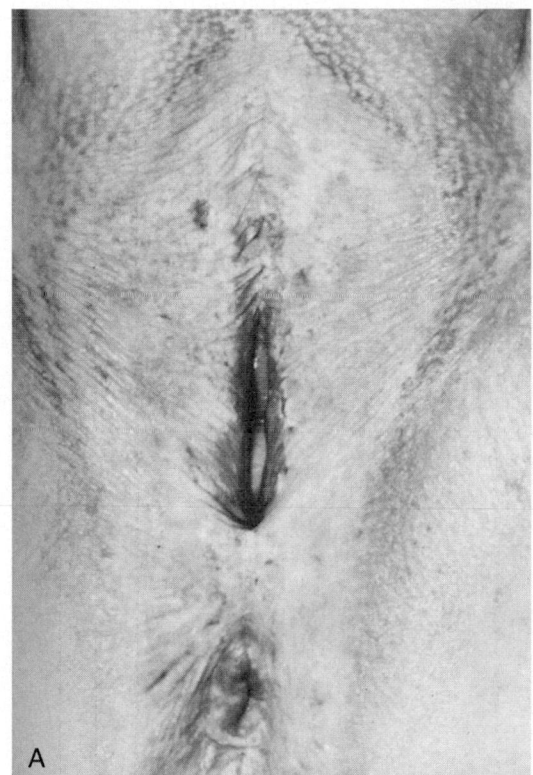

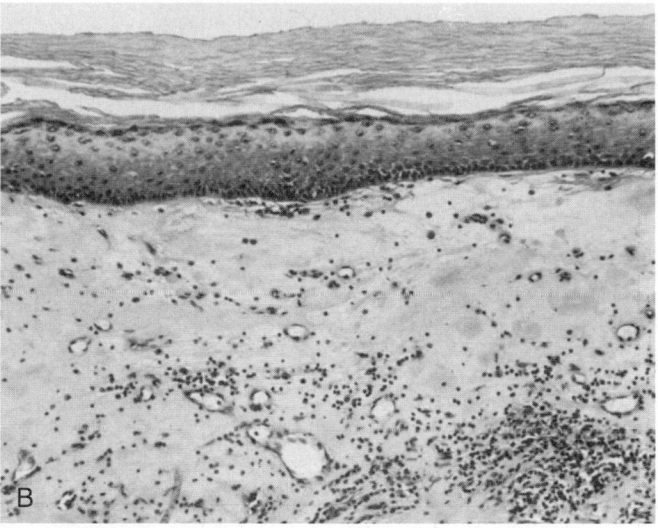

FIGURE 33.20. Vulvar dystrophy, lichen sclerosus. **A:** Distorted vulva with superficial ulcerations and extensive hyperkeratosis and loss of normal architecture. **B:** Microscopic picture of lichen sclerosus composed of epidermal diminution, subepidermal collagenization, and mid-dermal lymphocytic infiltrate.

Many series over the past few years have shown an excellent clinical response to 0.05% clobetasol proportionate topical ointment or cream. In a series of 81 women with biopsy-proven lichen sclerosus, Lorenz and co-workers reported that 77% had complete remission of symptoms and another 18% experienced significant improvement. Patients were treated with topical application of clobetasol cream twice daily for 1 month, at bedtime for another month, and, finally, twice a week for 3 months. They continued to use the cream on an "as needed" basis once or twice a week. Many patients continue to require occasional, episodic therapy for symptomatic flare-ups, but the long-term effects of these ultrapotent steroids on the vulva has not been well studied. Some experts recommend maintenance therapy with lower potency corticosteroids such as triamcinolone or 0.1% betamethasone. Topical testosterone has been recommended in the past, but Borentein and associates compared the results of 2% testosterone propionate to 0.05% clobetasol dipropionate; at 1 year follow-up, 80% of the clobetasol treated patients reported symptomatic improvement compared with 40% of those treated with testosterone.

Many patients with chronic vulvar dermatitis, stenosis of the outlet specifically related to lichen sclerosus, and vestibulitis have an associated constriction of the vaginal outlet with resultant dyspareunia. Local intravaginal or vulvar applications of estrogen do not improve this condition. Plastic surgery to the outlet (Fig. 33.21) may be helpful. By excising a triangular area of skin beneath the fourchette, the surgeon can undermine and evert the adjacent vaginal epithelium, incise the transverse perineal

muscle and fascia, and cover the denuded area with a flap of vaginal mucosa. The procedure is simple, and the use of delayed-absorbable suture material lessens the incidence of wound breakdown, which commonly occurs when absorbable suture is used. The results of this procedure have been most satisfactory; about 95% of patients are greatly relieved of dyspareunia. Breech and Laufer have reported good results in a few patients by suturing a protective covering of oxidized regenerated cellulose gauze (Surgicel, Johnson and Johnson, Arlington, TX) to the raw surfaces of the inner labia and clitoris after division of intracoital adhesions to prevent recurrence.

Vulvar Intraepithelial Neoplasm

The first two cases of CIS of the skin were described by Bowen in 1912. Bowen also stated that although stromal invasion had not developed in patients observed over periods of 12 to 16 years, curettage and cauterization did not eliminate recurrence of the lesions.

In 1958, Woodruff and Hildebrandt reported 13 cases of VIN. They suggested that because the histology varied from one area to another in the same section, the general term *carcinoma in situ* should be used to designate the lesion. Today, the term *vulvar intraepithelial neoplasia* is commonly used, and intraepithelial lesions are subdivided into VIN I, corresponding to mild dysplasia, VIN II, similar to moderate dysplasia and VIN III, which corresponds to severe dysplasia or CIS.

An increase in the incidence of VIN III was first noted by Woodruff and associates in 1973. Whereas only

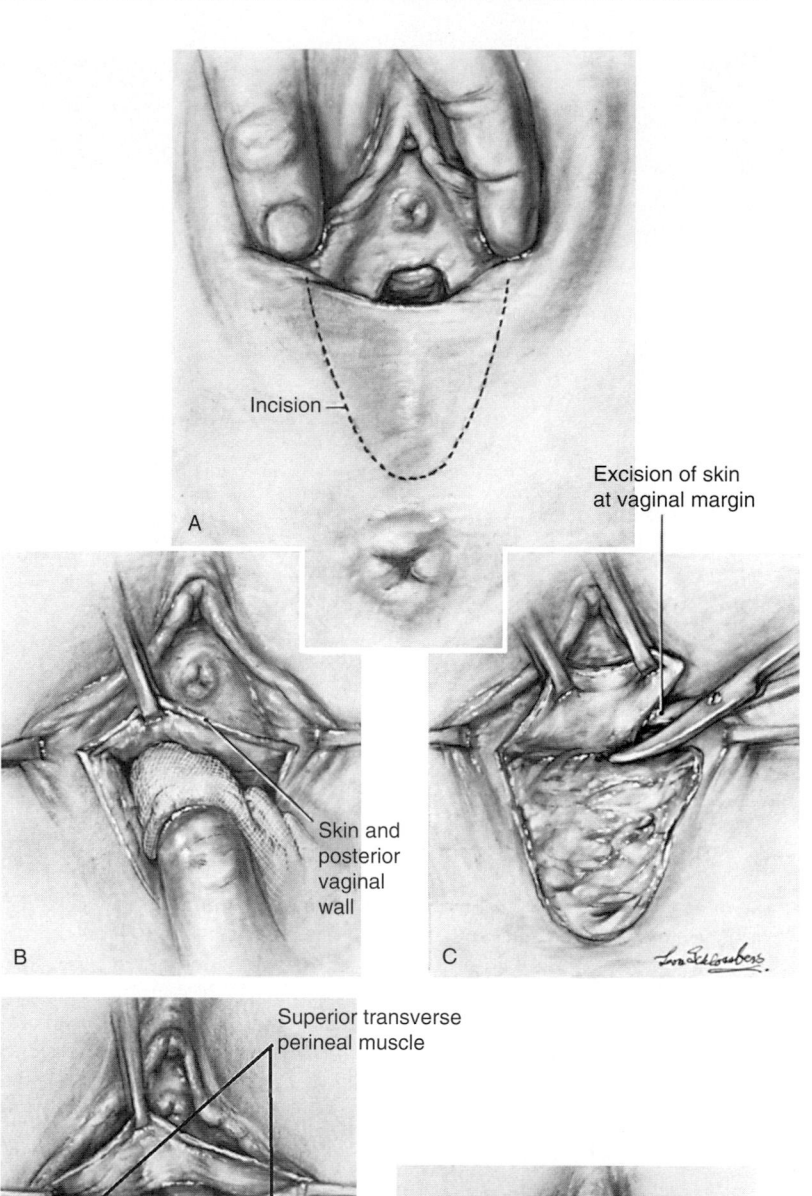

Incision

Excision of skin
at vaginal margin

Skin and
posterior
vaginal
wall

A

B

C

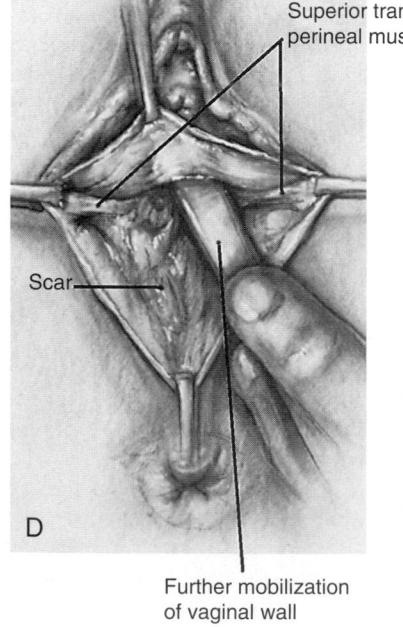

Superior transverse
perineal muscle

Scar

D

Further mobilization
of vaginal wall

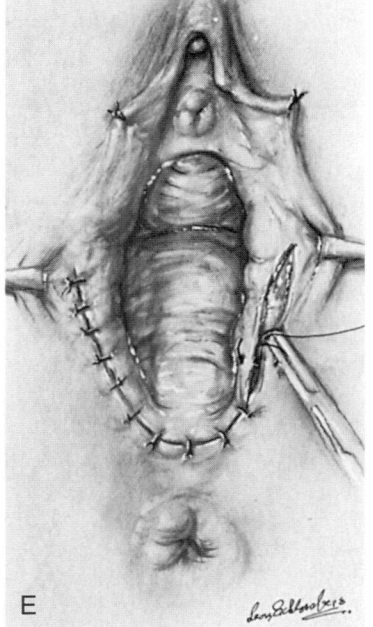

E

FIGURE 33.21. Perineoplasty. **A:** The incisional line is identified. The incision must be sufficiently extensive to allow for postoperative retraction and subsequent constriction of the outlet. **B:** The vagina is undermined to allow for exteriorization without tension. **C:** The scarred skin of the fourchette is excised. The vaginal epithelium is preserved for exteriorization. The vaginal epithelium is sufficiently undermined for the margins to be approximated to the skin (**D**) without tension (**E**). Occasionally, a small incision is made into the midline of the exteriorized mucosa to allow for an adequate outlet without tension.

13 cases of CIS were recorded in 1958 at our clinic, representing less than 20% of all vulvar neoplasia, the current incidence of VIN III has markedly surpassed that of invasive cancer. The upward trend is due to a real increased incidence of the disease process as well as an increased frequency of diagnosis as a result of increased awareness by patients, clinicians, and pathologists. Intraepithelial squamous lesions involving the whole lower genital tract, including the vulva, vagina, and cervix (Fig. 33.22), are associated with HPV. The increased frequency with which these lesions have been diagnosed may correlate with the increased sexual freedom that resulted from the introduction of oral contraceptives. VIN in younger women is strongly associated with HPV. In our clinic, 81% of VIN III lesions were positive for HPV 16 and also E-6 and E-7 transcripts have been detected in HPV-16 positive VIN lesions. However, HPV is much less frequently identified in VIN lesions of older women, perhaps suggesting another etiology.

Clinical Features

Symptoms

Pruritus is the predominant symptom of most vulvar disease, including cancer, yet itching was the primary symptom in only 50% of patients with in situ cancer in a series reported by Buscema and associates. Other presenting complaints were the presence of a lump, bleeding, and pain. In a small percentage of the cases, the lesion was discovered on routine examination; but, in others, the diagnosis commonly was made in patients seen during follow-up of cervical neoplasia.

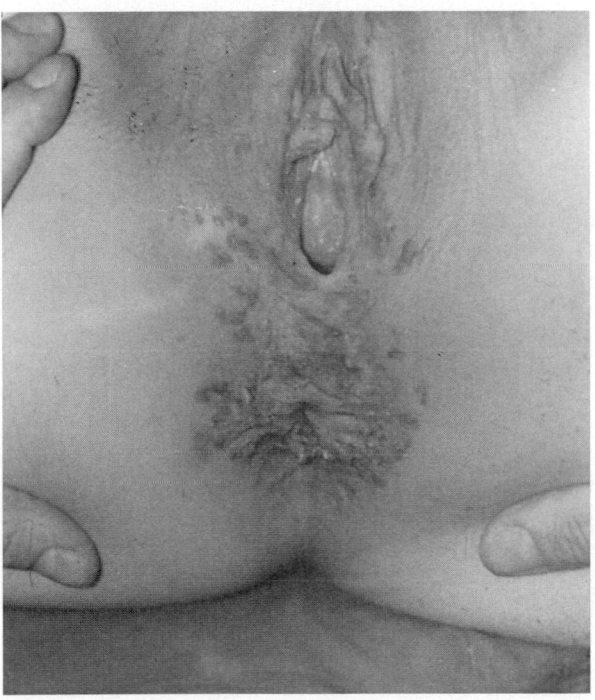

FIGURE 33.22. Multiple foci of carcinoma in situ in a young patient. Note the vulvar and perianal involvement.

Diagnosis

The best technique for early diagnosis is careful inspection of the external genitalia including perianal areas, thighs, and buttocks under a bright light. If suspicion is aroused either by history or preexisting neoplasia in the lower genital canal or by the suggestion of an abnormal configuration, magnification should be used. An experienced colposcopist can describe white lesions and areas of abnormal vasculature. As a screening procedure, however, colposcopy has not contributed to the early detection of vulvar neoplasia. The use of nuclear staining, specifically 1% toluidine blue and tetracycline fluorescence, has delineated foci of increased metabolic activity, but the false-negative and false-positive rates are high enough to make the results unpredictable.

Careful visual evaluation of the vulvar region should be directed at the focally white, hyperkeratotic areas, and at the more important, slightly elevated, papillary areas of skin. Atypical pigmentation, most significantly gray-white areas that are even minimally ulcerated or slightly elevated above the surrounding skin, should be viewed with suspicion (Fig. 33.23A). Biopsy provides the final diagnosis.

Pathologic Diagnosis

Biopsy with a Keyes punch can be performed in the office with the use of local anesthesia. Knife biopsies often are tangential and contain only the superficial layers, which results in a less than accurate histologic interpretation. Correct orientation of the tissue in the fixative is mandatory if accurate evaluation of the specimen is to be rendered. Such orientation can be obtained by placing the biopsy specimen on filter paper and toweling with the epithelial surface exposed, so that the pathologist can embed the specimen accurately. Tangential cutting may result in the erroneous diagnosis of invasive disease. Cytology has not proved to be a satisfactory screening technique in the evaluation of the precursory cellular atypias in vulvar neoplasia.

The classic bowenoid changes vary from one microscopic section to another, but typical sections show loss of polarity, hyperchromasia, anaplasia, individual cell keratinization, corps ronds, and mitotic activity on the surface (Fig 33.24B). Abnormal mitosis may abound. Other gross variations include the erythroplastic lesion (erythroplasia of Queyrat) with immature cells extending from base to surface, and lesions that appear almost normal, being marked only by intraepithelial pearl formation at the rete tips in a background of marked dysplasia. Papillary lesions showing changes of high-grade dysplasia were previously designated as *bowenoid papulosis*, a term discontinued by ISSVD.

Multicentricity

Multifocal areas of neoplasia that involve the external genitalia, perineum, and the epithelium of the lower genital canal are common; in fact, more than half the patients with intraepithelial disease in the lower genital

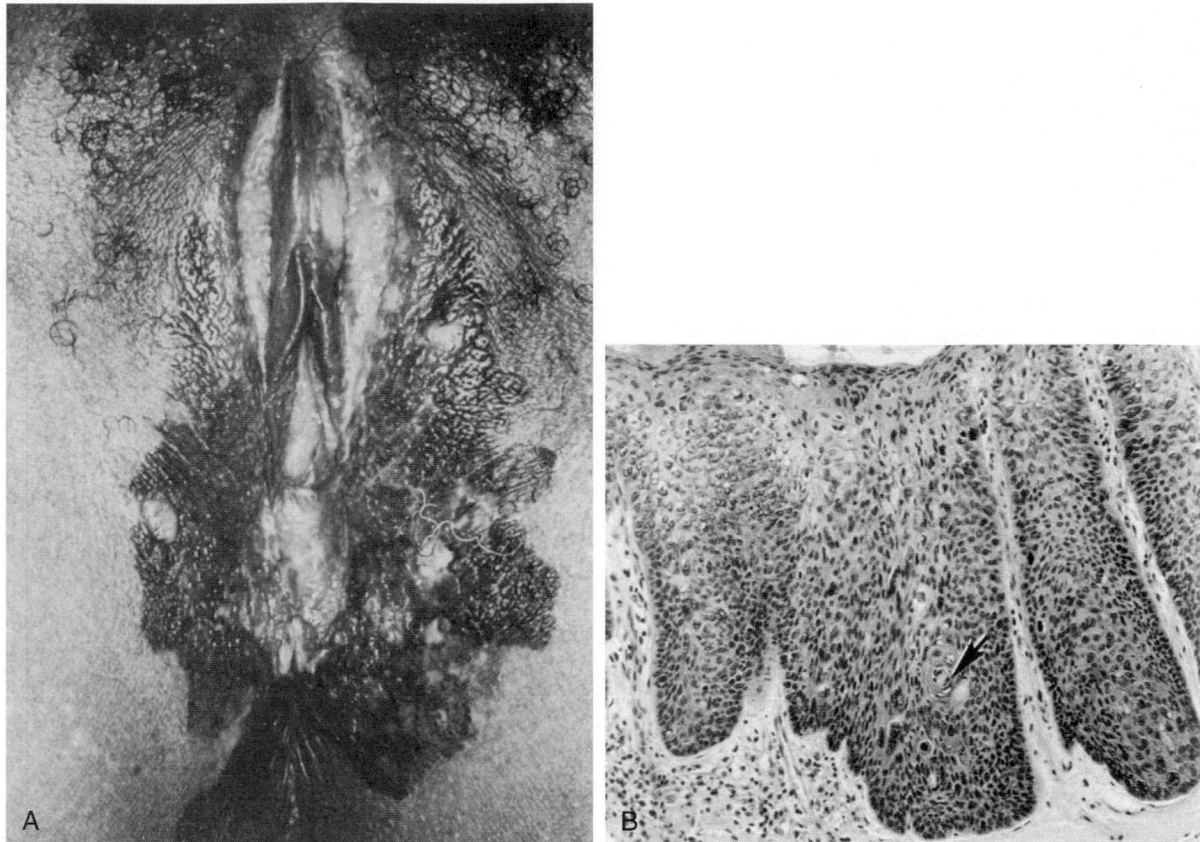

FIGURE 33.23. A: Carcinoma in situ of vulva showing multiple patterns, particularly atypical pigmentation. **B:** Carcinoma in situ of the vulva. There is full-thickness alteration in the architecture with elongation and distortion of the rete pegs. At *arrow*, there is intraepithelial pearl formation. (×160).

tract have multifocal lesions. These lesions suggest an infectious, possibly viral origin for the neoplasia. In contrast, patients older than 60 years of age with invasive or in situ cancer more commonly have unifocal disease. When the vulva is the primary site of the lesion, the cervix, vagina, and perianal areas are frequent sites for associated neoplastic alterations. The combination of vulvar and cervical cancer makes up about 20% of all multicentric neoplasia in the lower genital tract.

The most pressing question about multifocal disease is whether invasive disease that develops from in situ lesions will arise in many foci or in only one focus. Only two of our patients with in situ neoplasia younger than 40 years of age have developed invasive cancer, and both cases appeared as solitary perianal lesions. Because the vulva and the cervix are of different embryologic origins, the tendency to correlate the histopathology of one area with that of the other may be unrewarding. For example, the full-thickness changes that signal cervical intraepithelial neoplasia are not as comparable when they occur on the vulva. Keratinization at the rete tips with intraepithelial pearl formation may indicate on the other hand, a preinvasive disease in the anogenital area anywhere (Fig. 33.23B).

Treatment and Results

Although surgical excision of vulvar intraepithelial neoplasia is favored, patients typically do not require total vulvectomy. Modesitt and colleagues found invasive cancer in 22% of patients with biopsies consistent with VIN III. Vulvectomy may be appropriate for selected patients who are elderly, particularly if they have extensive disease, or for patients with Paget's disease. Wide local excision usually is successful, but an attempt should be made to obtain clear margins. The adjacent loose skin of the vulva provides sufficient extra skin to cover minor defects without a skin graft and without significant deformity. The incidence of recurrence is no greater with local excision than with total vulvectomy, but it still approaches 30% to 40%. Positive margins have been indicative of an increased risk of recurrence in some series. Unless invasive cancer is suspected in the area of the positive margins, immediate reexcision is usually not indicated, but careful follow-up is necessary because recurrence is common.

A skinning vulvectomy, in which the epidermis and underlying dermis of the vulva and often the perineal area are removed and replaced by a skin graft, has been used for the treatment of extensive or multifocal vulvar

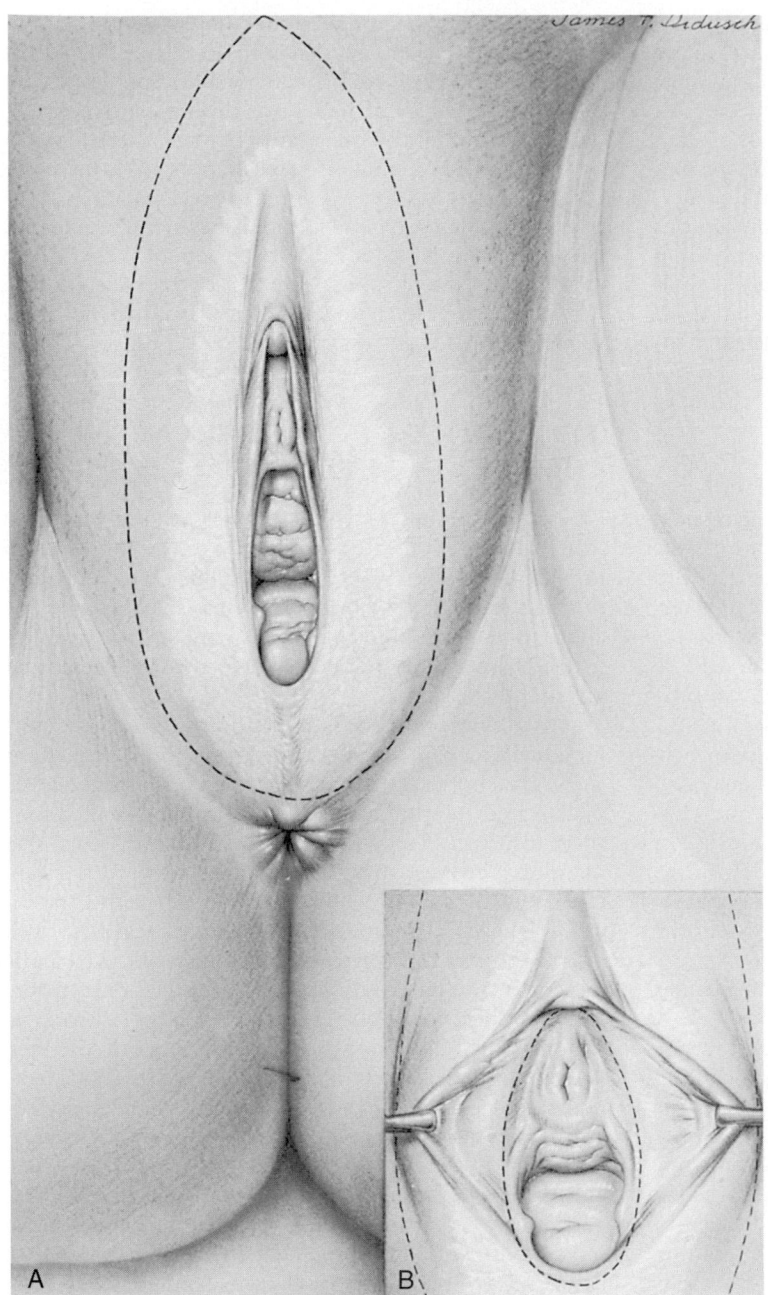

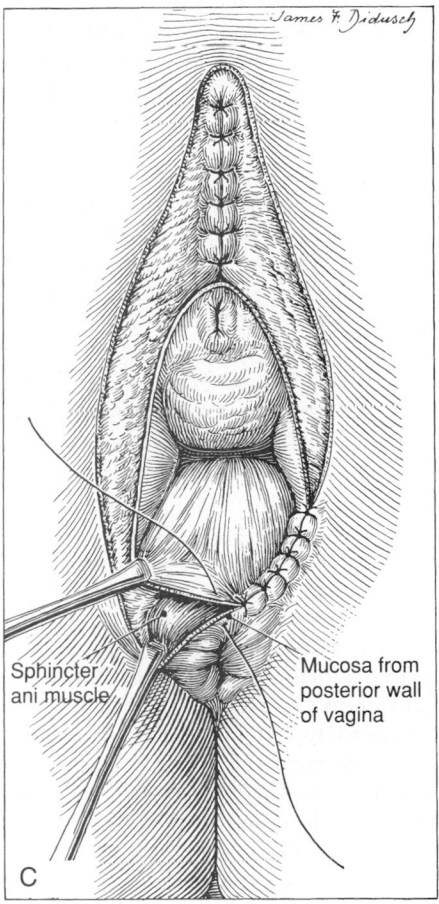

Sphincter ani muscle

Mucosa from posterior wall of vagina

FIGURE 33.24. Conservative vulvectomy for vulvar carcinoma in situ.

in situ disease. This procedure is usually recommended in younger women with extensive lesions in an attempt to restore normal anatomy and sexual function. However, the technique requires surgery at a donor site, which produces an additional scar in a patient who usually is young. Furthermore, it imposes prolonged bed rest, near complete immobilization of the lower extremities, and indwelling bladder catheterization for 5 to 6 days while the skin graft heals.

The carbon dioxide laser has been successfully used in the treatment of in situ vulvar neoplasia. This approach is of particular appeal for the younger patient with multifocal, viral proliferative disease. This subset of patients with VIN is undoubtedly at lower risk for occult invasion. Emphasis in therapy should be directed toward preservation of maximum tissue and vulvar function. Given these considerations and the reality of recurrences, laser ablation provides an effective medium. Pretreatment requirements include careful examination of the lower genital tract and the liberal use of biopsies to identify areas of possible invasion and multicentric disease. The risk of invasive cancer is greater in the older patient. The desire for cosmetic results is less, so that the use of surgical excision is favored in older women.

The laser itself is directed colposcopically after examination of tissues prepared by the application of dilute acetic acid. The latter may enhance detection of minimal viral changes not readily seen with the naked eye. Although benign condylomata can be adequately treated by superficial vaporization (so-called first and second plane), laser treatment of VIN must address the extension of disease into the hair follicles (pilosebaceous ducts). This mandates deeper laser vaporization beyond the papillary dermis and into the upper reticular dermis (third plane). The colposcope permits recognition of landmarks that characterize these levels. Baggish and co-workers identified skin appendage involvement in 36% of cases of vulvar in situ carcinoma and predicted that laser vaporization to a depth of 2.5 mm would effectively treat involved appendages in 95% of cases. Shatz and associates advocated ablation of VIN to a depth of 1 to 2 mm in nonhairy and hairy skin to achieve similar success. In laser treatment of VIN, the use of appropriate power densities should be emphasized. Low-power densities lead to thermal conduction injury in adjacent and underlying normal tissue. The latter increases the risk of scarring. Power densities of greater than 750 W/cm^2 are recommended. However, the deeper extent of vaporization required for VIN III, particularly in hair-bearing areas of the vulva, results in considerably greater postoperative pain, a longer period of healing, and an increased risk of scarring and subsequent chronic pain and dyspareunia so that many experts have abandoned the use of the laser in favor of surgical excision for VIN III. Bornstein and Kaufman have proposed combining laser ablation with surgical excision in the treatment of selected patients with VIN. Laser is used particularly in areas where excision hampers preservation of anatomy, such as in the clitoral region.

The Ultrasonic Surgical Aspirator can assist the surgeon in ablating to depths comparable to those achieved with the CO$_2$ laser. The advantage of this instrument is its ability to obtain additional tissue that might identify an occult cancer. Ultrasonic Surgical Aspirator and laser ablation also may be used to treat perianal intraepithelial neoplasia. In this setting, two concerns should be kept in mind. This location appears to be associated with a greater risk for the development of invasive squamous cancer, and the likelihood of fibrosis, scarring, and stricture is heightened. As with all treatments for VIN, the potential for recurrence and the need for further follow-up must be appreciated. With ablative approaches such as laser, diligence must be exercised to exclude invasion.

Topical agents have been used in the treatment of VIN with inconsistent results. Most notable among these topical treatments has been 5-FU (Efudex 5%). Efudex is not recommended by the manufacturer for this use, and they specifically recommend against its use in the vagina. The mechanism of action appears to be related to the inhibition of DNA and RNA synthesis; the latter is not specific to dysplastic or HPV-infected cells. Normal epithelium is susceptible to the agent, and a component of hypersensitivity reaction appears operative in its mode of action. For cases in which treatment is effective, denudation of the epithelium is a requisite finding. This understandably leads to localized discomfort and pain, often reported as intense burning. Treatment regimens with topical 5-FU are diverse, and no standardized administration protocol has been widely adopted. One technique is topical application on an alternate-night basis for as long as 6 weeks; patient compliance problems typically lead to earlier curtailment. Among young patients with erythroplastic VIN, a 50% to 60% complete response rate has been reported. The hyperkeratotic VIN lesion has not proved to be as responsive to 5-FU.

TECHNIQUE OF CONSERVATIVE (SIMPLE) VULVECTOMY

Conservative (simple) vulvectomy is recommended in many patients with extensive Paget's disease of the vulva or widespread VIN where it is difficult to rule out invasive cancer, even with multiple biopsies. It may also be appropriate when premalignant lesions, such as granulomatous diseases, do not respond to medical therapy or wide local excision.

An outline of the surgical margins is made with a surgical marking pen. The initial incision should be made at the vaginal outlet so that the urethral borders can be well demarcated and the vaginal epithelium undermined for a short distance. If the incision is begun at the lateral skin margins, bleeding can mask the area, making the incision at the outlet more difficult to define. When the first incision is made at the outlet, a small pack can be placed into the vagina to control the bleeding while the elliptic incision at the outer skin margins of the lesion is made. The skin incision usually encompasses most of the labia majora, depending on the extent of the lesion. The incision through the skin is made with a knife to avoid tissue necrosis that occurs at the skin margins when an electrosurgical instrument is used. Minor vessels can be coagulated.

Major bleeding concerns may arise at the clitoris, particularly from the dorsal vein. Hemostatic sutures must be used to control the bleeding. A second point of concern is the pudendal vessels, which enter at the lower one third of the vulva close to the opening of the Bartholin duct. Branches of the pudendal vessels extend down to the anus as the inferior hemorrhoidals, and bleeding may be rather profuse in this area (Fig. 33.18).

Because the lesions for which conservative vulvectomy is performed are superficial, dissection does not need to extend down to the deep fascia or to the muscles of the urogenital diaphragm. Although it is unnecessary to remove the bulbocavernous and ischiocavernous muscles, they may be difficult to avoid when the vulva is quite atrophic. Removal of some of the adipose tissue, particularly in the obese patient, allows for better approximation of the skin edges to the vaginal mucosa. The incision can be carried almost to the anal orifice; careful dissection here is important, so that the external anal sphincter is not damaged. If the disease extends onto the anal mucosa or the protruding hemorrhoidal tissue, the mucosa should first be carefully dissected from the underlying external sphincter, excised with the tumor-free margins, and sutured to the perianal skin with 3-0 delayed-absorbable material. In the remaining vulva, the underlying tissues are approximated in layers with absorbable sutures, and the skin edges are approximated with interrupted absorbable sutures (Fig. 33.24C). If bleeding is a problem, a small drain can be placed at the lower end of the incision, but it is much better to achieve meticulous hemostasis and use a firm pack against the area for 24 hours.

During closure of the perineal defect above the anal orifice and posterior vaginal introitus, the surgeon should evert the vaginal epithelium over the perineum in approximation to the anal orifice rather than suture the lateral skin edges snugly across the perineum and fourchette. Everting the vaginal mucosa allows for satisfactory coitus, whereas tightly approximated skin across the posterior fourchette may constrict the vaginal introitus and predispose to pain, dyspareunia, and fissuring.

When the firm packing has been removed after 24 hours, the entire area should be exposed. Initial application of ice packs to the operative site for 24 to 48 hours seems to provide more comfort to the patient than heat. Later, warm air blown across the perineum is both comforting and therapeutic because it helps to keep the operative site dry and stimulates blood flow, enhancing the healing process. An indwelling urethral catheter or a suprapubic catheter is used while the suture line undergoes initial healing of the skin edges. The suprapubic catheter can be maintained for 4 to 5 days, if desired. A single dose of a cephalosporin such as Cefazolin (1 g) intravenously is recommended immediately before surgery. Infrequently, a local cellulitis may develop, necessitating antibiotic therapy; extended-spectrum cephalosporins and semisynthetic penicillins have proved effective.

Vulvar Reconstruction

Procedures performed for extensive VIN 3 or Paget's disease include total or partial vulvectomy, skinning vulvectomy, and multiple wide excisions. These may occasionally result in large denuded areas, creating challenges for reconstruction. With the advent of laser ablation and the Ultrasonic Surgical Aspirator, fewer procedures such as skinning vulvectomy are performed for VIN.

Reconstructive efforts for superficial excisions typically require split-thickness grafts. Such grafts are ill-suited for reconstruction after radical excision because the depth of tissue defect is too great, and poor cosmetic and functional results ensue. A buttock donor site is preferred. Perioperative antibiotics are used. Bowel preparation and slow postoperative feeding minimize contamination of the graft site.

Split-thickness skin grafts can be procured with an air-driven dermatome. The size of the vulvar defect helps to determine donor site excision. Meticulous hemostasis should be sought before application of the graft. Fine absorbable sutures are used to secure the skin edges of the

graft. The donor site should be covered with an occlusive dressing, such as Op-Site or Tegaderm, until significant healing occurs. A soft pressure dressing is tied over the graft site and kept in place for 5 days, accompanied by an indwelling catheter for urinary drainage.

ACKNOWLEDGEMENTS

The authors want to recognize Dr. J. Donald Woodruff who has been a coauthor of this chapter for several editions and who has served as a mentor to the current authors.

BIBLIOGRAPHY

Abramov Y, Elchalal U, Abramov D, et al. Surgical treatment of vulvar lichen sclerosus: a review. CME review article. *Obstet Gynecol* 1996;51:3.

Adelson MD. Ultrasonic surgical aspiration in the treatment of vulvar disease [Letter, Comment]. *Obstet Gynecol* 1991;78(3 Pt 1):477.

Aranda FI, Laforga JB. Nodular fasciitis of the vulva. Report of a case with immunohistochemical study. *Pathol Res Pract* 1998;194(11):805.

Baggish MS, Sze EH, Adelson MD, et al. Quantitative evaluation of the skin and accessory appendages in vulvar carcinoma in situ. *Obstet Gynecol* 1989;74:169.

Barbero M, Micheletti L, Preti M, et al. Biologic behavior of vulvar intraepithelial neoplasia: source, logic and clinical parameters. *J Reprod Med* 1993;38:108.

Bloss JD. The use of electrosurgical techniques in the management of premalignant diseases of the vulva, vagina, and cervix: an excisional rather than an ablative approach. *Am J Obstet Gynecol* 1993;169:1081.

Bornstein J, Heifetz S, Kellner Y, et al. Clobetasol dipropionate 0.05% versus testosterone propionate 2% topical application for severe vulvar lichen sclerosus. *Am J Obstet Gynecol* 1998;178:80.

Bornstein J, Kaufman RH. Combination of surgical excision and carbon dioxide laser vaporization for multifocal vulvar intraepithelial neoplasia. *Am J Obstet Gynecol* 1988;158:459.

Bornstein J, Lahat N, Sharon A, et al. Telomerase activity in HPV-associated vulvar vestibulitis. *J Reprod Med* 2000;45(8):643.

Bornstein J, Pascal B, Abramovici H. Intramuscular beta-interferon treatment for severe vulvar vestibulitis. *J Reprod Med* 1993;38:117.

Bornstein J, Sova Y, Atad J, et al. Development of vaginal adenosis following combined 5-fluorouracil and carbon dioxide laser treatments for diffuse vaginal condylomatosis. *Obstet Gynecol* 1993;81:896.

Bornstein J, Zarfati D, Fruchter O, et al. A repetitive DNA sequence that characterizes human papillomavirus integration site into the human genome is present in vulvar vestibulitis. *Eur J Obstet Gynaecol Reprod Biol* 2000;89:173.

Bouchard S, Yazbech S, Lallier M. Perineal hemangioma, anorectal malformation, and genital anomaly: a new association? *J Pediatr Surg* 1999;34:1133.

Bowen JD. Precancerous dermatoses. *J Cutan Dis* 1912;30:241.

Breech LL, Laufer MR. Surgicel in the management of labial and clitoral hood adhesions in adolescents with lichen sclerosus. *J Pediatr Adolesc Gynecol* 2000;13:21.

Bresci G, Parisi G, Banti S. Long term therapy with 5-aminosalicylic acid in Crohn's disease: is it useful? Our four years' experience. *Int J Clin Pharmacol Res* 1994;14:133.

Buscema J, Naghashfar Z, Sawada E, et al. The predominance of human papillomavirus type 16 in vulvar neoplasia. *Obstet Gynecol* 1988;71:601.

Buscema J, Stern J, Woodruff JD. The significance of histologic alterations adjacent to invasive vulvar carcinoma. *Am J Obstet Gynecol* 1980;137:902.

Buscema J, Woodruff JD, Parmley TH, et al. Carcinoma in situ of the vulva. *Obstet Gynecol* 1980;55:225.

Collins CG, Hansen LH, Theriot EA. Clinical stain for use in selecting biopsy sites in patients with vulvar disease. *Obstet Gynecol* 1966;28:158.

Coppelson M. Colposcopic features of papillomaviral infection and premalignancy in the female lower genital tract. *Dermatol Clin* 1991;9:251.

Crum CP, McLachlin CM, Tate JE, et al. Pathobiology of vulvar squamous neoplasia. *Curr Opin Obstet Gynecol* 1997 (Feb);9:63.

Dalziel KL, Millard R, Wojnarowska F. The treatment of vulval lichen-sclerosus with a very potent topical steroid (clobetasol propionate 0.05%) cream. *Br J Dermatol* 1991;124:461.

Davis BL, Robinson DG. Diverticula of the female urethra: assay of 120 cases. *J Urol* 1970;104:850.

DiBonito L, Falconieri G, Bonifacio-Gori. Multicentric papillomavirus infection of the female genital tract: a study of morphologic pattern, possible risk and viral prevalence. *Pathol Res Pract* 1993;189:1023.

DiPaola GR, Gomez-Rueda N, Arrighi L. Relevance of microinvasion in carcinoma of the vulva. *Obstet Gynecol* 1975;45:647.

Ersan Y, Ozgultelxin R, Cetinkale O, et al. Fournier-gangran. *Langenbecks Arch Chir* 1995;380:139.

Farley DE, Katz VL, Dotters DT. Toxic shock syndrome associated with vulvar necrotizing fasciitis. *Obstet Gynecol* 1993;82:4:660.

Feagan BG, Rochon J, Fedorak RN, et al. Methotrexate for the treatment of Crohn's disease: the North American Crohn's Study Group Investigators. *N Engl J Med* 1995;332:292.

Ferenczy A, Mitao M, Nagai N, et al. Latent papillomavirus and recurring genital warts. *N Engl J Med* 1985;313:784.

Fisher JR, Conway MJ, Takeshita RT, et al. Necrotizing fasciitis: importance of roentgenographic studies for soft-tissue gas. *JAMA* 1979;241:803.

Frega A, di Renzi F, Stentella P, et al. Management of human papillomavirus vulvoperineal infection with systemic β-interferon and thymostimulin in HIV-positive patients. *Int J Gynecol Obstet* 1994;44:255.

Friedman-Kien AE, Eron LJ, Conaut M, et al. Natural interferon alpha for treatment of condylomata acuminata. *JAMA* 1988;259:533.

Friedrich EG Jr. International Society for the Study of Vulvovaginal Disease. New nomenclature for vulvar disease: report of the Committee on Terminology. *Obstet Gynecol* 1976;47:122.

Friedrich EG Jr. Topical testosterone for benign vulvar dystrophy. *Obstet Gynecol* 1971;37:677.

Friedrich EG Jr. *Vulvar disease: diagnosis and management*, second ed. Philadelphia: WB Saunders, 1983:488.

Friedrich EG Jr, Kalra PS. Serum levels of sex hormones in vulvar lichen sclerosus and the effect of topical testosterone. *N Engl J Med* 1984;310:488.

Friedrich EG Jr, Wilkinson EJ. Mucous cyst of the vulvar vestibule. *Obstet Gynecol* 1973;42:407.

Friedrich EG, Wilkinson EJ, Steingraeber PH, et al. Paget's disease of the vulva and carcinoma of the breast. *Obstet Gynecol* 1975;46:130.

Furlonge CB, Thin RN, Evans BE, et al. Vulvar vestibulitis syndrome: a clinicopathological study. *Br J Obstet Gynaecol* 1991;98:703.

Glazer HI, Radke G, Swencionis C, et al. Treatment of vulvar vestibulitis syndrome with electromyographic biofeedback of pelvic floor musculature. *J Reprod Med* 1995;40:283.

Goldman HB, Idom CB, Dmochowski RR. Traumatic injuries of the female external genitalia and their association with urological injuries. *J Urol* 1998;159(3):956.

Haefner HK, Tate JE, McLachlin CM, Crum CP. Vulvar intraepithelial neoplasia: age, morphological phenotype, papillomavirus DNA, and coexisting invasive carcinoma. *Hum Pathol* 1995;26:147.

Haley JC, Mirowski GW, Hood AF. Benign vulvar tumors. *Semin Cutan Med Surg.* 1998;17:196.

Hatch K. Colposcopy of vaginal and vulvar human papillomavirus and adjacent sites. *Obstet Gynecol Clin North Am* 1993;20:203.

Hatch KD. Vulvovaginal human papillomavirus infections: clinical implications and management. *Am J Obstet Gynecol* 1991;165:1183.

Herzog TJ, Rader JS. The Ultrasonic Surgical Aspirator in the gynecologic oncology patient. *Adv Obstet Gynecol* 1994;1:325.

Hoffman MS, Pinelli DM, Finan M, et al. Laser vaporization for vulvar intraepithelial neoplasia III. *J Reprod Med* 1992;37:135.

Hoffman MS, Roberts WS, LaPolla JP, et al. Laser vaporization of grade 3 vaginal intraepithelial neoplasia. *Am J Obstet Gynecol* 1991;165:1342.

Horowitz BJ. Interferon therapy for condylomatous vulvitis. *Obstet Gynecol* 1989;73:446.

Horowitz IR, Copas P, Majmudar B. Granular cell tumors of the vulva. *Am J Obstet Gynecol* 1995;173:1710.

Horowitz IR, Gomella LG, eds. *Obstetrics and gynecology on call*, first ed. East Norwalk, CT: Appleton & Lange, 1992:167.

International Society for the Study of Vulvar Disease, Committee on Terminology. New nomenclature for vulvar disease. *Obstet Gynecol* 1989;160:769.

Japaze H, Dinh T, Woodruff JD. Verrucous carcinoma of the vulva: study of 24 cases. *Obstet Gynecol* 1982;60:462.

Jeffries DJ. Acyclovir update. *BMJ* 1986;293:1523.

Julian CG, Callison J, Woodruff JD. Plastic management of extensive vulvar defects. *Obstet Gynecol* 1971;38:193.

Kent HL, Wisniewski PM. Interferon for vulvar vestibulitis. *J Reprod Med* 1990;35:1138.

Kizer JR, Bellah RD, Schnaufer L, et al. Meconium hydrocele in a female newborn: an unusual case of a labial mass. *J Urol* 1995;153:188.

Kornbluth A, Marion JF, Solomon P, et al. How effective is current medical therapy for severe ulcerative and Crohn's colitis? An analytic review of selected trials. *J Clin Gastroenterol* 1995;20:280.

Lijnen RL, Blindeman LA. VIN III (bowenoid type) and HPV infection. *Br J Dermatol* 1994;131:728.

Lorenz B, Kaufman RH, Kutzner S. Lichen sclerosus–therapy with clobetasol propionate. *J Reprod Med* 1998;43:790–794.

Majmudar B. Tumors of the vulva, Section 15. In: *Conn's current therapy 2000*. Philadelphia: WB Saunders, 2000.

Majmudar B, Castellano PZ, Wilson RW, et al. Granular cell tumors of the vulva. *J Reprod Med* 1990;35:1008.

Mann MS, Kaufman RH, Brown D Jr, et al. Vulvar vestibulitis: significant clinical variables and treatment outcome. *Obstet Gynecol* 1992;79:122.

Marinoff SC, Turner ML. Vulvar vestibulitis syndrome: an overview. *Am J Obstet Gynecol* 1991:165:2:1228.

Marinoff SC, Turner ML, Hirsch RP, et al. Intralesional alpha interferon: cost-effective therapy for vulvar vestibulitis syndrome. *J Reprod Med* 1993;38:19.

Matthews D. Marsupialization in the treatment of Bartholin's cyst and abscesses. *Obstet Gynaecol Br Commonw* 1966;73:1010.

McKay M. Dysesthetic (essential) vulvodynia treatment with amitriptyline. *J Reprod Med* 1993;38:9.

McKay M. Subsets of vulvodynia. *J Reprod Med* 1988;3308:695.

McKay M. Vulvodynia: diagnostic patterns. *Dermatol Clin* 1992;10:423.

McKay M, Frankman O, Horowitz BJ, et al. Vulvar vestibulitis and vestibular papillomatosis: report of the ISSVD Committee on Vulvodynia. *J Reprod Med* 1991;36:413.

Mering JH. A surgical approach to intractable pruritus vulvae. *Am J Obstet Gynecol* 1952;64:619.

Modesitt SC, Waters AB, Walton L, et al. Vulvar intraepithelial neoplasia III: occult cancer and the impact of margin status on recurrence. *Obstet Gynecol* 1998;92(6):962.

Morin C, Bouchard C, Brisson J, et al. Human papillomaviruses and vulvar vestibulitis. *Obstet Gynecol* 2000;95(5):683.

Moscicki A, Palefsky JM, Gonzales J, et al. Colposcopic and histologic findings and human papillomavirus (HPV) DNA test variability in young women positive for HPV DNA. *J Infect Dis* 1992;166:951.

Novak ER, Woodruff JD. *Gynecologic and obstetric pathology,* eighth ed. Philadelphia: WB Saunders, 1979.

O'Connell JX, Young RH, Nielsen GP, et al. Nodular fasciitis of the vulva: a study of six cases and literature review. *Int J Gynecol Pathol* 1997;16:117.

Paavonen J. Vulvodynia: a complex syndrome of vulvar pain. *Acta Obstet Gynecol Scand* 1995;74:2343.

Parks JS, Jones RW, McLean MR, et al. Possible etiologic heterogeneity of vulvar intraepithelial neoplasia: a correlation of pathologic characteristics with human papillomavirus detection by in situ hybridization and polymerase chain reaction. *Cancer* 1991;67:1599.

Patsner B. Treatment of vaginal dysplasia with loop excision: report of five cases. *Am J Obstet Gynecol* 1993;169:179.

Pincus SH. Vulvar dermatoses and pruritus vulvae. *Dermatol Clin* 1992;10:297.

Price LM, Mendolsohn SS, Youngs GR, et al. Unilateral vulvar hypertrophy and Crohn's disease. *Int J STD AIDS* 1995;6:146.

Rader JS, Leake JF, Dillon MB, et al. Ultrasonic surgical aspiration in the treatment of vulvar disease. *Obstet Gynecol* 1991;77:573.

Reid R, Greenberg M, Jenson AB, et al. Sexually transmitted papillomaviral infections. I. The anatomic distribution and pathologic grade of neoplastic lesions associated with different viral types. *Am J Obstet Gynecol* 1987;156:212.

Reid R, Greenberg MD, Lorincz AT, et al. Superficial laser vulvectomy. IV. Extended laser vaporization and adjunctive 5-fluorouracil therapy of human papillomavirus–associated vulvar disease. *Obstet Gynecol* 1990;76:439.

Reid R, Greenberg MD, Pizzuti DJ, et al. Superficial laser vulvectomy. *Am J Obstet Gynecol* 1992;166:815.

Reid R, Omoto KH, Precop SL, et al. Flashlamp-excited dye laser therapy of idiopathic vulvodynia is safe and efficacious. *Am J Obstet Gynecol* 1995;172:1684.

Santos JV, Baudet JA, Lasellas FJ, et al. Intravenous cyclosporine for steroid-refractory attacks of Crohn's disease: short and long term results. *J Clin Gastroenterol* 1995;20:207.

Schover L, Youngs DD, Cannata NW. Psychosexual aspects of the evaluation and management of vulvar vestibulitis. *Am J Obstet Gynecol* 1992;167:630.

Shakla VK, Hughes LE. A case of squamous cell carcinoma complicating hidradenitis suppurativa. *Eur J Surg Oncol* 1995;21:106.

Shatz P, Bergeron C, Wilkinson EJ, et al. Vulvar intraepithelial neoplasia and skin appendage involvement. *Obstet Gynecol* 1989;74:769.

Sherman KJ, Daling JR, Chu J, et al. Genital warts, other sexually transmitted diseases, and vulvar cancer. *Epidemiology* 1991;2:257.

Sobel JD. Management of recurrent vulvovaginal candidiasis with intermittent ketoconazole prophylaxis. *Obstet Gynecol* 1985;65:435.

Taussig FJ. *Diseases of the vulva.* New York: Appleton Century-Crofts, 1931.

Theusen B, Andreasson B, Bock JE. Sexual function and somatopsychic reactions after local excision of vulvar intraepithelial neoplasia. *Acta Obstet Gynecol Obstet Gynecol Scand* 1992;71:126.

Turner ML, Marinoff SC. General principles in the diagnosis and treatment of vulvar diseases. *Dermatol Clin* 1992;10:275.

Umpierre SA, Kaufman RH, Adam E, et al. Human papillomavirus DNA in tissue biopsy specimens of vulvar vestibulitis patients treated with interferon. *Obstet Gynecol* 1991;78:693.

van Beurden M, ten Kale FJ, Smits HL, et al. Multifocal vulvar intraepithelial neoplasia grade III and multicentric lower genital tract neoplasia associated with transcriptionally active human papillomavirus. *Cancer* 1995;75:2879.

Vuopala S, Pollanen R, Kaappila A, et al. Detection and typing of human papillomavirus infection affecting the cervix, vagina, and vulva: comparison of DNA hybridization with cytological, colposcopic and histological examination. *Arch Gynecol Obstet* 1993;253:75.

Welsh DA, Powers JS. Elevated parathyroid hormone-related protein and hypercalcemia in a patient with cutaneous squamous cell carcinoma complicating hidradenitis suppurativa. *South Med J* 1993;86:1403.

Wharton LR Jr, Everett HS. Primary malignant Bartholin gland tumors. *Obstet Gynecol Surv* 1951;6:1.

Wilkinson EJ, Guerrero E, Daniel R, et al. Vulvar vestibulitis is rarely associated with human papillomavirus infection types 6, 11, 16, or 18. *Int J Gynecol Pathol* 1993;12:344.

Woodruff JD, Genadry R, Poliakoff S. Treatment of dyspareunia and vaginal outlet distortions by perineoplasty. *Obstet Gynecol* 1981;57:750.

Woodruff JD, Hildebrandt EE. Carcinoma in situ of the vulva. *Obstet Gynecol* 1958;12:414.

Woodruff JD, Julian C, Paray T, et al. The contemporary challenge of carcinoma in situ of the vulva. *Am J Obstet Gynecol* 1973;115:677.

Woodruff JD, Richardson EH Jr. Malignant vulvar Paget's disease. *Obstet Gynecol* 1957;10:10.

Woodruff JD, Sussman J, Shakfeh S. Vulvitis circumscripta plasmacellularis. *J Reprod Med* 1989;34:369.

Woodruff JD, Thompson B. Local alcohol injection in the treatment of vulvar pruritus. *Obstet Gynecol* 1972;40:18.

Wu AY, Sherman ME, Rosenshein NB, et al. Pathologic evaluation of gynecologic specimens obtained with the Cavitron ultrasonic surgical aspirator (CUSA). *Gynecol Oncol* 1992;44:28.

Wysoki RS, Majmudar B, Willis D. Granuloma inguinale (donovanosis) in women. *J Repro Med* 1988;33:709.

Te Linde's Operative Gynecology, ninth edition, edited by John A. Rock and Howard W. Jones, III. Lippincott Williams & Wilkins, Philadelphia © 2003.

CHAPTER
34

▼

Surgical Conditions of the Vagina and Urethra

JOHN A. ROCK   IRA R. HOROWITZ

CELIA E. DOMINGUEZ

THE VAGINA

The Imperforate Hymen and Its Complications

The hymen, the junction of the sinovaginal bulbs with the urogenital sinus, is a thin mucous membrane, sometimes cribriform in appearance, which is composed of endoderm from the urogenital sinus epithelium. The müllerian ducts meet the sinovaginal bulbs at the most cephalad tip of the invaginating urogenital sinus. The vaginal plate elongates and canalizes to form the vagina. If the vaginal plate does not canalize, a transverse vaginal septum is the result. Canalization of the most caudal portion of the vaginal plate at the urogenital sinus establishes a patent hymen. The hymen usually is perforated during embryonic life to establish a connection between the lumen of the vaginal canal and the vaginal vestibule, and it usually is torn early in the prepubertal years. If canalization fails and there are no perforations, the hymen is called *imperforate.*

Although variations in hymen development occur, complete blockage by the hymen of the vaginal orifice is rare, occurring in approximately 0.05% to 0.1% of newborn females. In 1986, Mor and colleagues described the types of hymenal shape in the newborn infant from examination performed within the first 24 hours of life. In 53.5%, a smooth hymen with a central orifice was observed; a folded hymen with a central orifice was seen in 27%; a folded hymen with an eccentric orifice occurred in 4.5%; an anterior opening of the hymen was in 10.8%; a posterior opening was found in 0.6%. The researchers found that 3% had hymenal bands and 0.3% of the newborns had an almost imperforate hymen. Pokorny and Kozinetz described the various configurations and anatomic details of the prepubertal hymen. In a case series of 265 children with known genital problems, three main hymenal configurations were observed: fimbriated, circumferential, and posterior rim. Interestingly, bleeding without a history of trauma was associated with hymenal bumps or breaks suggestive of trauma (31%) or with other hemorrhagic vulvar lesions (40%).

Stelling and colleagues have recently evaluated the genetic transmission of imperforate hymen and reported that the occurrence of imperforate hymen in two consecutive generations of a family is consistent with a dominant mode of transmission, either sex-linked or autosomal. It has also been reported that transmission may be recessively inherited. Taken together they concluded that imperforate hymen is caused by mutations of several genes and emphasize the importance of evaluation of all family members of affected patients.

Symptoms

If an imperforate hymen is noticed before puberty, the condition can be treated when the condition is entirely asymptomatic. Cases, which are recognized at birth, present with a thin bulging membrane between the labia, which represents a mucocolpos. When the hymen is incised, the vagina is found to contain mucoid fluid that is the result of accumulated cervical secretion. This is caused by the stimulation of the infant's cervical mucous glands by maternal estrogen in the presence of an intact hymen. Prenatal diagnosis of imperforate hymen and mucocolpos has been described with second trimester antenatal sonography demonstrating a thin membrane that distended the vagina and spread the labia majora.

Most commonly, imperforate hymen is not detected until puberty with girls presenting at 13 to 15 years of age, when symptoms begin to appear but menstruation appears not to have begun. The symptoms after the onset of puberty are due to the accumulation of menstrual blood within the vaginal outlet tract. The blood of the first cycle period or two is collected in the vagina, which can hold a large volume of blood without undue stretching and with no other symptoms. This accumulated menstrual blood in the vagina is called *hematocolpos*. The patient may feel a slight fatigue and have cramping discomfort suggesting menstruation, but she has no history of any passage of menstrual blood through the vaginal outlet. Figure 34.1A shows bulging of the imperforate hymen, which may be dark in color because of occult blood showing through the stretched mucous membrane; Figure 34.1B shows extrusion of accumulated blood after the hymen is incised.

As menstruation continues to occur, however, the vagina becomes greatly overdistended, and the cervical canal also begins to dilate. Accumulation of menstrual

blood in the uterine cavity, with subsequent *hematometra*, may occur. When the intrauterine pressure reaches a certain point, retrograde passage of blood into the tubes causes hematosalpinx. Associated or other adhesion formation within or at the fimbriated ends of the tubes may seal them, so that little or no blood enters the peritoneal cavity. In some cases, however, blood passes freely into the peritoneal cavity, forming hematoperitoneum (Fig. 34.2). A tender mass often is palpable suprapubically, the result of uterine enlargement and upward displacement, bladder distention, or both. If hematoperitoneum occurs, the irritation of the free blood may cause all the symptoms and signs of peritonitis.

The most common symptoms of vaginal overdistention are lower abdominal pain, discomfort in the pelvis, and pain in the lower back. Hematocolpos should be included in the differential diagnosis of amenorrheic girls presenting with persistent lower back pain. Irritation of the sacral plexus is believed to be the etiology of this referred pain pattern. The lower abdominal discomfort often is aggravated on defecation and if extensive blood accumulation occurs in the vagina, constipation may result from pressure and obstruction of the underlying rectum. Urination can be difficult as a result of pressure of the distended vagina, which can compress the urethra and prevent emptying of the bladder; urinary obstruction can ensue. Bladder symptoms can present as cramplike pains in the suprapubic region, along with symptoms of dysuria, frequency, and urgency; overflow incontinence may eventually develop and hydronephrosis is a rare complication. Girls presenting with severe dysmenorrhea and duplicate vagina and didelphic uterus should be evaluated for unilateral imperforate hymen.

Rock and colleagues followed pregnancy success subsequent to the surgical correction of imperforate hymen between 1945 and 1981 at the Johns Hopkins Hospital. Twenty-two patients of mean age 14.7 years were admitted for surgical correction of imperforate hymens. As-

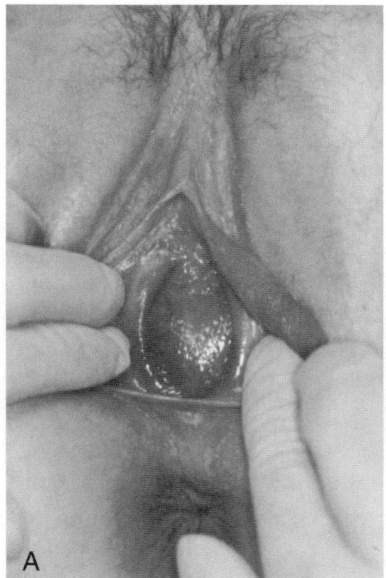 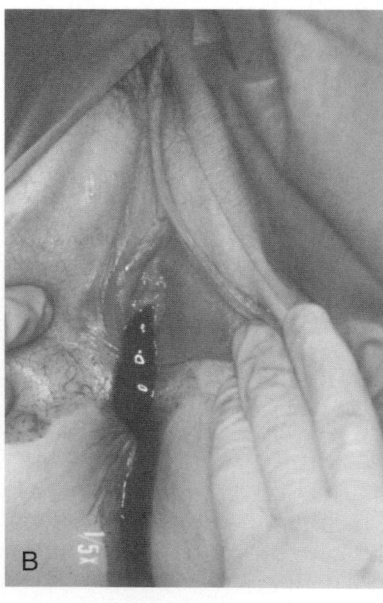

FIGURE 34.1. A: An imperforate hymen, membrane protrusion with a dark tinge posterior representing a hematocolpos **B:** Extrusion of accumulated blood at time of incision into membrane. See color version of figure.

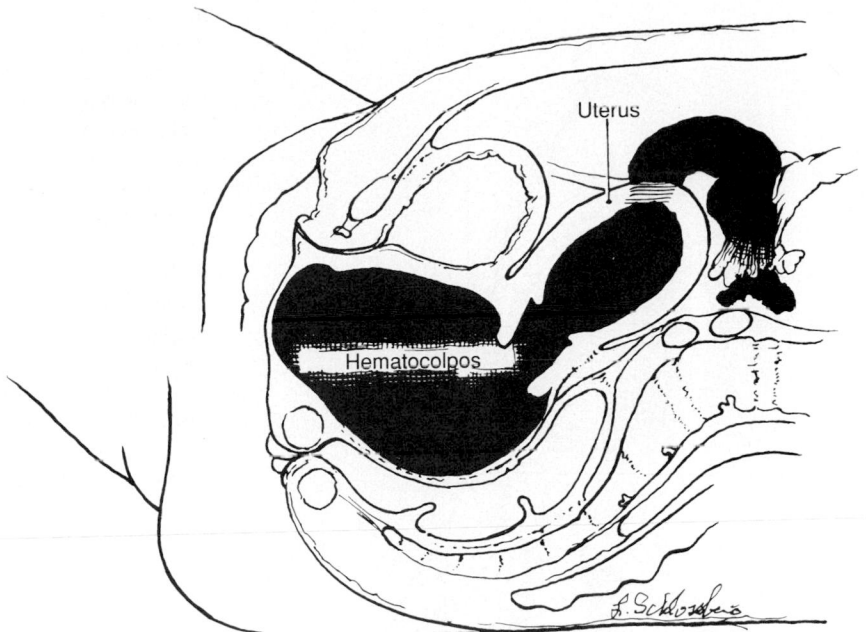

FIGURE 34.2. Hematocolpos, hematometra, hematosalpinx, and hematoperitoneum consequent to an imperforate hymen.

sociated anomalies, including urinary tract anomalies, were rare. Thirteen patients subsequently conceived, and 10 patients were observed to have living children. The great distensibility of the vagina probably protects the adolescent patient with an imperforate hymen from abnormal retrograde menstruation, and the possible subsequent development of pelvic endometriosis with imperforate hymen as the cause is unlikely as long as the diagnosis is made reasonably early.

Treatment

When an imperforate hymen is discovered before puberty, the hymenal membrane can simply be incised, preferably at the 2-, 4-, 8-, and 10-o'clock positions. The quadrants of the hymen are then excised, and the mucosal margins are approximated with fine delayed-absorbable suture (Fig. 34.3). To prevent scarring and stenosis, which could result in dyspareunia, the hymenal tissue should not be excised too close to the vaginal mucosa. All unnecessary intrauterine instrumentation should be avoided because, if hematocolpos has already developed (Fig. 34.2), there is the risk of perforating the thin, overstretched uterine wall.

No further surgical intervention is generally needed. If the uterine mass does not regress within 2 to 3 weeks, however, inspection and dilatation of the cervix should be performed to make certain that drainage from the uterus is satisfactory.

Anomalies of the External Genitalia and Vagina

Construction of Female External Genitalia

Sexually ambiguous external genitalia defects of the urogenital sinus are remarkably constant in appearance, regardless of the etiology of the anomaly. Such genitalia differ only in their degree of malformation and occupy a range of positions somewhere intermediate to the genitalia of a normal female and that of a normal male. These anomalies can be anatomically identical to each other whether their etiologic factor is congenital adrenal hyperplasia (CAH), male hermaphrodism, true hermaphroditism, or some other intersex syndrome. External genitalia proceeds along the female lines except in the presence of some virilizing influence acting on the developing embryo (i.e., androgens). The conversion of testosterone to dihydrotestosterone by 5α-reductase activity occurs in the skin of the external genitalia and urogenital sinus in early gestation. Masculinization of the external genitalia ensues in the presence of functional androgens regardless of genetic sex. In the case of female pseudohermaphrodism, XX chromosomes in the presence of a virilizing influence, fusion of the scrotolabial folds may be sufficient to obscure or conceal the vagina from the outside or even to entirely suppress its formation. The urethra can be formed for varying distances or along the entire length of the phallus. Therefore, the operative procedure for reconstruction of ambiguous genitalia into feminine genitalia does not vary in its essential elements, regardless of the cause of the intersexuality. The common goals for the female reconstruction of ambiguous genitalia include reduction of clitoral size, creation of labia minora, and exteriorization of the vagina.

Any reconstruction of the external genitalia with the objective of producing normal female appearance and function requires a full understanding of the surgical anatomy. It is essential to accurately identify the site of communication of the vagina with the urogenital sinus (UGS). In their classic paper in 1969, Hendren and Crawford recognized the variability of the communica-

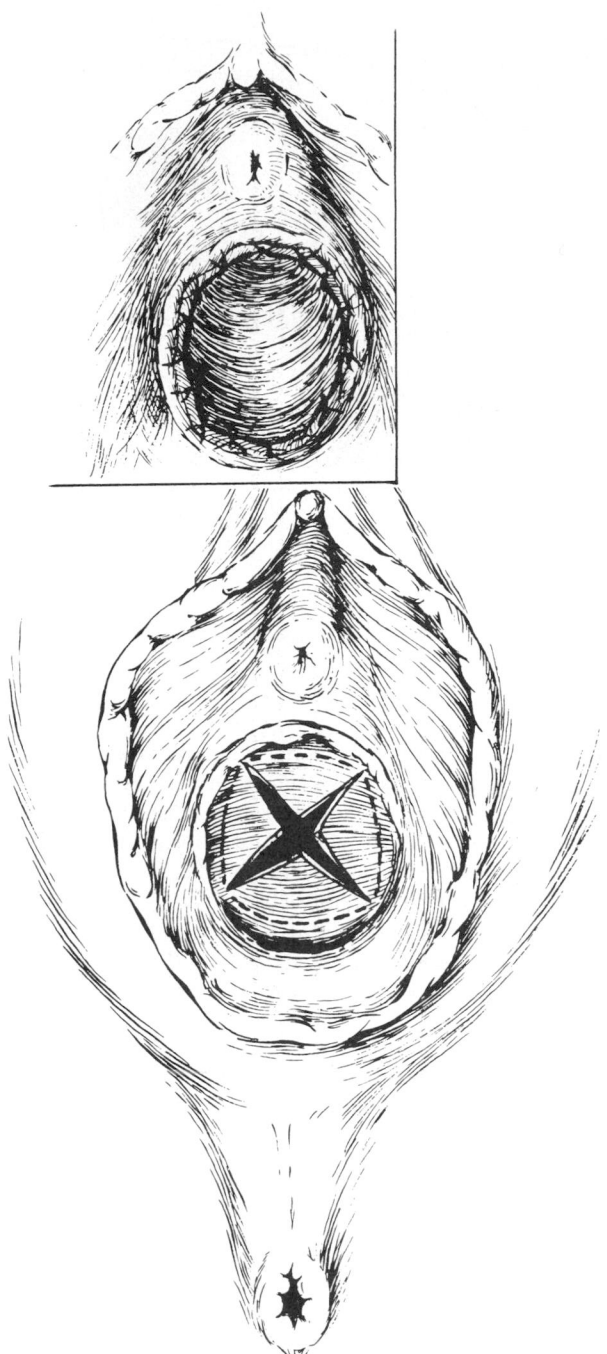

FIGURE 34.3. Excision of imperforate hymen. Stellate incisions are made through the hymenal membrane at the 2-, 4-, 8-, and 10-o'clock positions. The individual quadrants are excised along the lateral wall of the vagina, avoiding excision of the vagina. (*Inset*) Margins of vaginal mucosa are approximated with fine delayed-absorbable suture.

tion of the vaginal insertion into the UGS. Figure 34.4 illustrates the spectrum of vaginal communication with the urethra; with Figure 34.4A representative of a low distal communication (infrasphincteric) and Figure 34.4B representative of a high proximal communication (suprasphincteric). In 95% of cases, the vaginal commu-

nication is in relation to the caudal UGS derivatives (infrasphincteric) with the vagina communicating with that portion of the UGS that in a male gives rise to the membranous portion of the male urethra and that in the female becomes the vaginal vestibule. If this usual relation is confirmed at surgery, the persistent, anomalous urogenital sinus may be incised to the vaginal communication without fear of disturbing the urinary sphincter. In less than 5% of cases, the vagina communicates high, with the portion of the UGS that becomes the prostatic urethra in the male or the entire urethra in the female (suprasphincteric). Knowledge of the possible variants in communication of the vagina with the UGS is critical before entertaining surgical correction. Preoperatively genitography showing the relationship of the UGS, urethra, vagina, and bladder may be helpful. Contrast is injected retrogradely through the perineal meatus of the UGS. Delineation of this anatomy can be elucidated at the time of surgery with the use of endoscopy to evaluate where the vagina communicates with the UGS. In 1989, Bargy and colleagues described the anatomic lesions in the intersexual states based on clinical and anatomic observations.

One objective of the reconstruction procedure for external genitalia is to delay the procedure until the anomalous structures are of a size to permit easy identification of all structures, yet to complete the procedure before the anomalies may prove embarrassing or alarming to either the patient or the patient's family. There are many psychological advantages to proceeding as early as possible. As observed by Azziz and coworkers, however, vaginal repair may be delayed until menarche, when maturity and the desire for sexual activity are usually well established.

Most hermaphrodites reared as girls have a vagina or vaginal pouch, although in some instances it is rudimentary. Only rarely is there no vagina, despite ambiguity of the external genitalia. The choice of operative procedure must conform to the observed anatomy. Thus, these choices are considered in the context of several categories based on anatomic structure of the anomaly.

WHEN THE VAGINA IS PRESENT AND THE VAGINO-SINUS COMMUNICATION IS LOW. The basic operation is, in essence, a modification of one described at length by Young that was previously performed successfully by various surgeons, notably in Europe. Patients with adrenal hyperplasia usually require only reconstruction of the external genitalia. However, when exploratory laparotomy is necessary to remove contradictory sex structures in other types of intersexuality or to establish the diagnosis, reconstruction of the genitalia may be accomplished at the same operation.

When the operation is performed at the ideal age, the structures are so small that it is impossible to introduce a finger into the urogenital sinus, and all tissues must be grasped throughout the operation with fine delicate tissue forceps. Operating loupes (2.5 ×) are of great benefit to the surgeon. Small bipolar forceps and microscissors are also useful. Fine, 5-0 or 6-0 synthetic absorbable

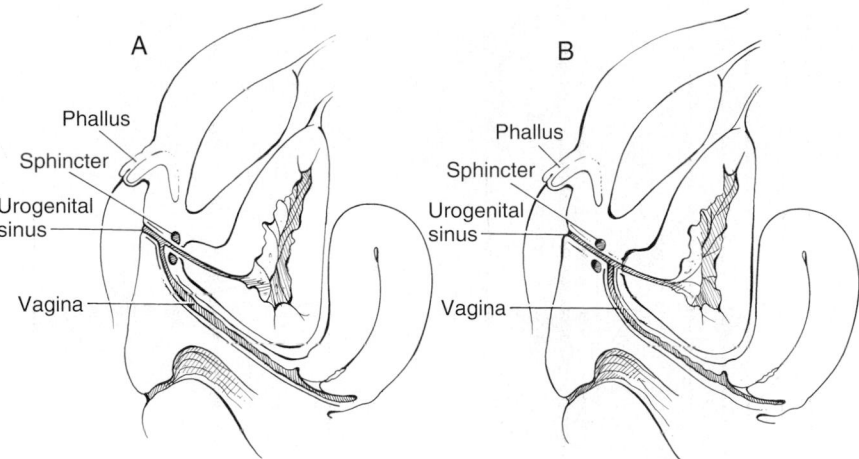

FIGURE 34.4. Illustration of the spectrum of vaginal communication with the urethra. **A:** Representative of a low distal communication (infrasphincteric). **B:** Representative of a high proximal communication (suprasphincteric).

suture material on an atraumatic needle is used throughout the procedure.

In cases of simple labial fusion, a cutback vaginoplasty (Fig. 34.5) would be sufficient to restore "normal" female genital anatomy. In cases of low vaginal confluence with the UGS (Fig. 34.4A), reconstruction may be done either by freeing the posterior vaginal wall and suturing up to the perineal external opening (Fig. 34.6) or, if a patient has copious subcutaneous fat and difficulty exists in approximating the vagina to the perineal skin, use of a posterior flap technique, as used by Fortunoff and co-workers, should be considered (Fig. 34.7).

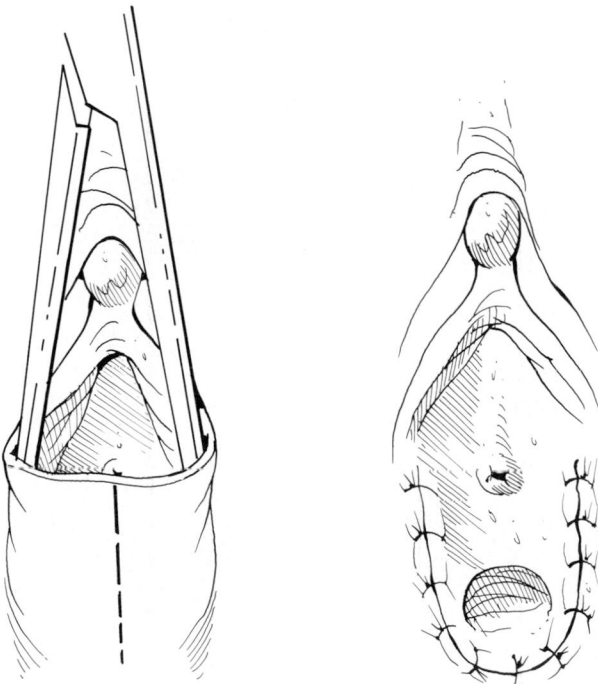

FIGURE 34.5. In cases of simple labial fusion, a cutback vaginoplasty is sufficient to restore "normal" female genital anatomy.

Initially, the UGS may be thoroughly investigated with a small McCarthy panendoscope to determine accurately the position and size of the vaginal communication. If a sound or catheter can be easily introduced into the meatus of the urogenital sinus and into the vagina, use of the endoscope may be omitted. Special care is needed not to introduce the sound into the urethra. A sound accidentally introduced into the urethra poses the danger of incising the distal urethral meatus. After the UGS is incised (to within 2 or 3 cm of the anus), the urethral orifice may be identified (Fig. 34.6A and B). A small Foley catheter may then be introduced through the urinary meatus for purposes of identification throughout the remainder of the operation. To attach the edges of the vagina to the skin, it is usually necessary to free the vagina posteriorly and laterally to secure sufficient mobilization to have these structures meet without tension. It is unnecessary to free the vagina anteriorly, because this requires its separation from the urethra. Sufficient mobilization can ordinarily be obtained by lateral and posterior dissection. When sufficient freedom has been attained, the edges of the vagina may be secured to the skin with interrupted 5-0 sutures on an atraumatic reserve-cutting needle. In the infant, four or five sutures around the edge of the vagina are usually sufficient. The edges of the incised sinus membrane may then be sutured to the skin anteriorly (Fig. 34.6D–G). A small sponge impregnated with petroleum jelly may be introduced into the vagina to maintain its patency during the healing process. The indwelling catheter may be left in place for a few days until edema of the surrounding structures has subsided. An indwelling catheter is particularly useful in children with metabolic disorders that require accurate urine collection. A pressure dressing for 24 hours reduces the incidence of incisional hematoma.

Figure 34.7 illustrates vaginoplasty with a posterior flap as advocated by Fortunoff and is useful in cases with anticipated difficulty in bringing the vaginal orifice to the outside. Briefly, a posterior based U-flap is drawn with corners on either side of the perineal body near the rectum (Fig. 34.7A–C). This flap must be wide enough for tension-free anastomosis. This posterior flap is dissected

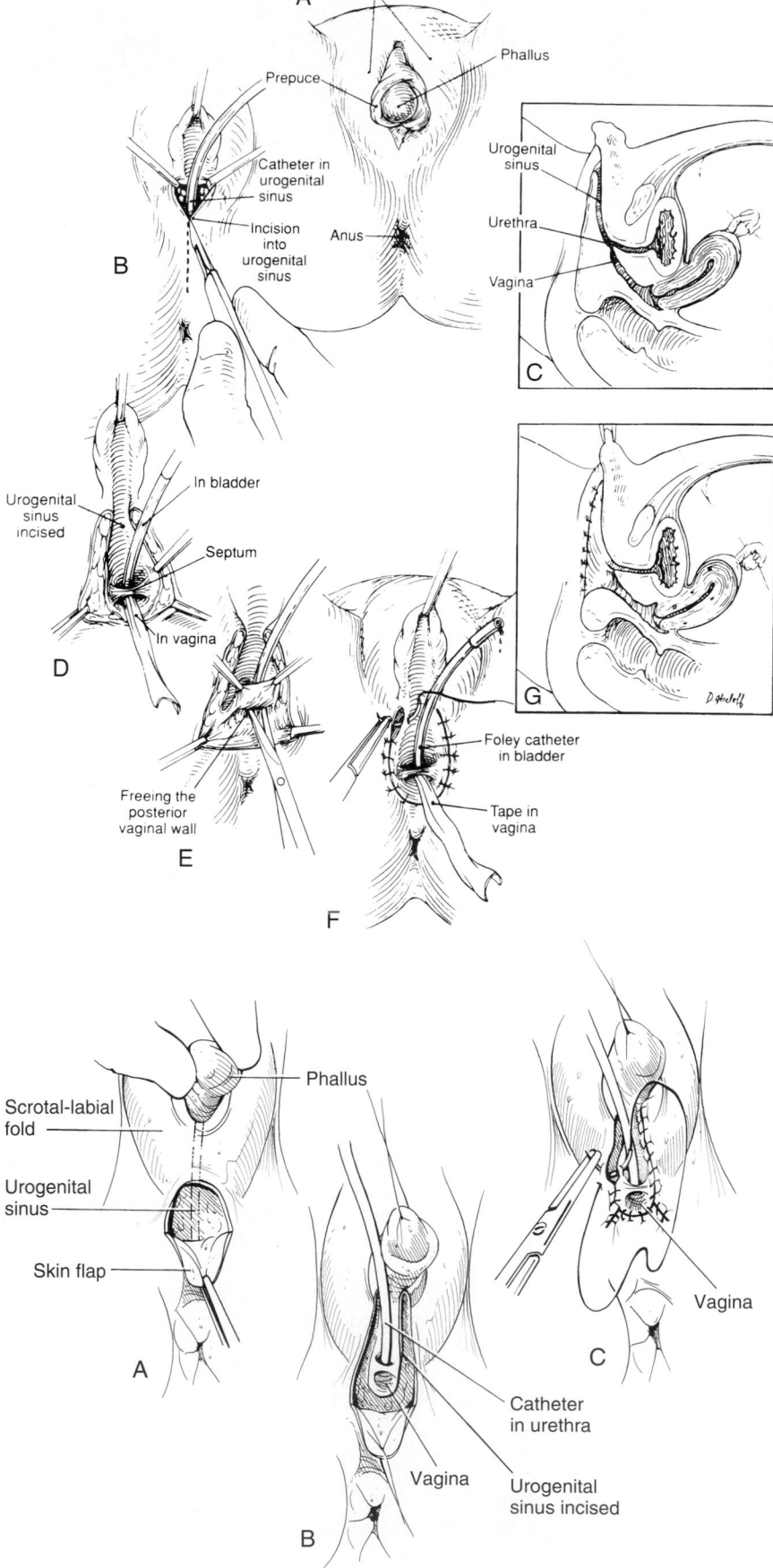

FIGURE 34.6. A: The external genitalia of an 18-month-old female with congenital adrenal hyperplasia. The operation is the same, regardless of the etiology of the "virilizing" deformity. **B:** Beginning of the operation. Incision into the urogenital sinus. If the external meatus is large enough and the urogenital sinus will accommodate it, it is sometimes possible to introduce a catheter into the bladder through the urethra and introduce a sound into the vagina beside this. When the structures are large enough, this maneuver greatly facilitates the operative procedure by ensuring their identification. **C:** Lateral view showing the relations among the various structures. **D:** Situation after incision of the urogenital sinus. **E:** With the glass catheter in the bladder, the posterior vaginal wall is freed to make it possible to bring it to the skin edge without undue tension. **F:** The operative situation after the edges of the vagina are sutured to the skin and after the edges of the mucous membrane of the urogenital sinus are also sutured to the skin along the line of incision. **G:** Lateral view at the completion of the operation.

FIGURE 34.7. A posterior flap technique for when there is difficulty bringing the vaginal orifice to the outside.

in the midline and is carried out between the rectum and UGS.

Sutures are individually placed through the posterior based flap and into the split posterior vagina. Sutures are tied after all have been placed. Because the anterior wall is not disturbed, no anterior flap is required. Finally, the phallic skin is divided in the midline and moved inferiorly to create the labia minora.

Surgical reconstruction of an enlarged clitoris has undergone significant evolution. Traditionally, the clitoris was simply amputated and a nonfunctioning cosmetic clitoris was fashioned. Although several children so treated now have normal adult sexual function, the literature is lacking in follow-up data on large patient groups. Surgical efforts now focus on concealment, plication, resection, and reduction, with an attempt to provide a normal cosmesis without sacrificing sensation or vascularity of the glans.

The clitoral flap technique has provided a somewhat better cosmetic result than simple amputation. This procedure attempts to preserve a shell of the glans on a pedicle flap. The shaft of the clitoris is subtotally resected and the stumps are reanastomosed (Fig. 34.8). The nerve supply to the glans is severed during this procedure, with the result that sensation in the glans is diminished. Sexual function, however, seems to be satisfactory.

Rajfer and colleagues have suggested a dorsal approach to the subtotal resection of the corpora (Fig. 34.9), which has the advantage of preserving the ventral nerve supply. and which should preserve sensation in the glans. This approach is theoretically desirable and can be recommended for suitable cases. As mentioned earlier, however, lack of clitoral sensation does not seem to significantly affect the later sexual behavior of patients treated by procedures that sever the dorsal nerves to the glans.

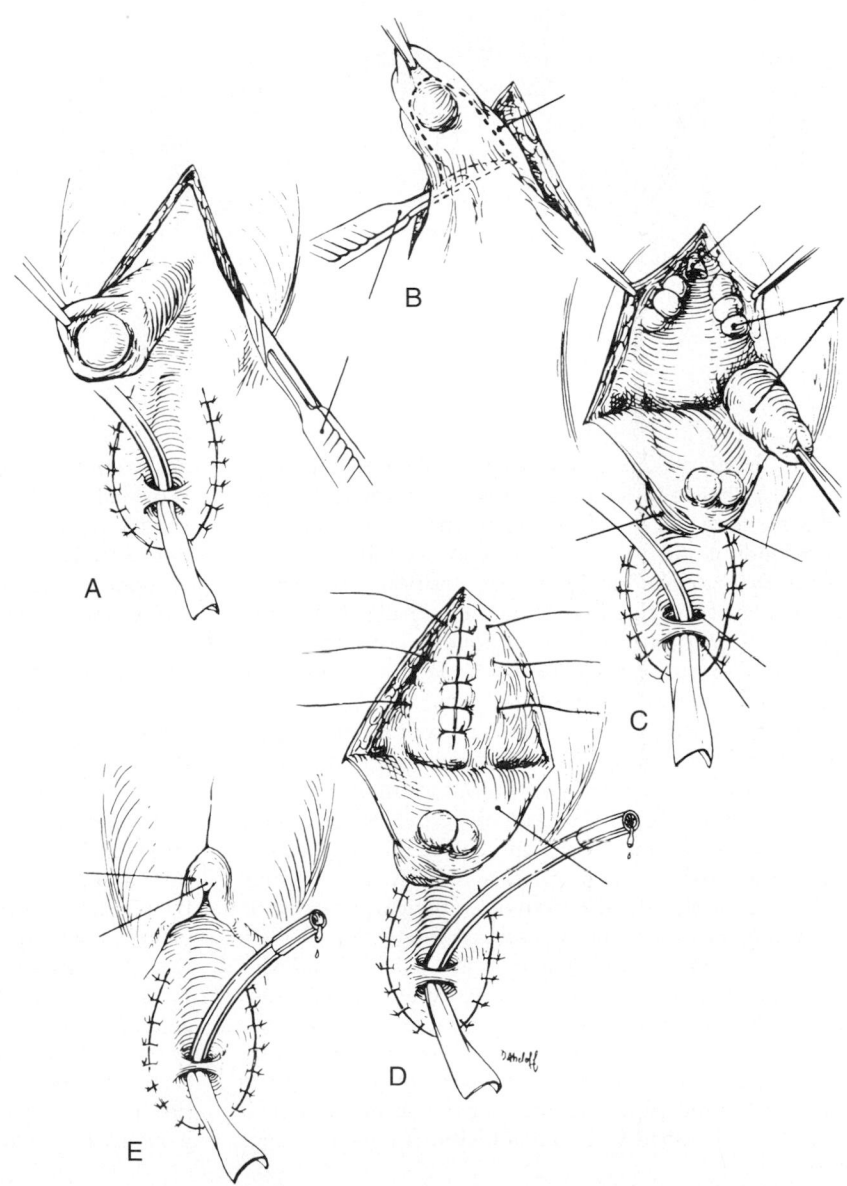

FIGURE 34.8. Clitoral reduction via the clitoral flap technique. A: The initial incision. B: The flap must be as wide as possible at the base to preserve the circulation for the glans. The glans cannot be preserved completely because the blood supply will be insufficient to maintain it. It must be as thin a shell of the glans as possible. C: The shaft of the phallus has been removed. D: There has been some closure of the space from which the corpora were removed. E: The flap has been sutured into place.

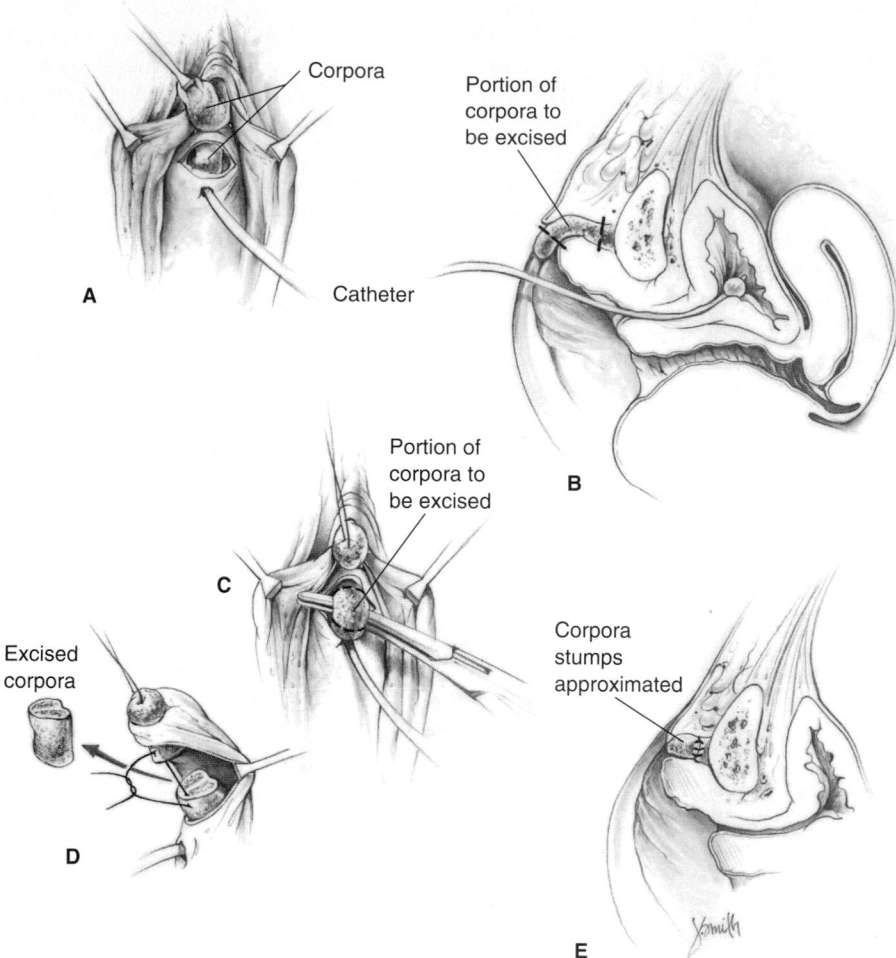

FIGURE 34.9. Clitoral reduction with the corpora exposed through a dorsal incision (operation of Rajfer and colleagues). **A** through **C:** Corpora are approached and removed through a posterior incision in the phallus. **D:** Diagram of the excised portion of the corpora. **E:** The corpora are removed and stumps approximated.

In 1999, Baskin and colleagues described the anatomic studies of the human clitoris. As in the human penis, the nerves in the clitoris form an extensive network surrounding the tunica of the corporeal body with a nerve-free zone at the 12-o'clock position. The normal clitoris has corporeal bodies that are smaller but analogous to those of the penis. Their function should be considered if extensive resection is considered with care to preserve the dorsal aspect of the glans.

Rink and Adams reviewed the present state of the art of feminizing genitoplasty. They advocated clitoral reduction without sacrificing sensation or vascularity of the glans, recommending a subtunical reduction of erectile tissue as described by Kogan and colleagues. The glans is preserved with its neurovascular supply intact along Buck's fascia and the dorsal tunic of the corpora, yet the cavernous erectile tissue is excised. Figure 34.10 illustrates this surgical management; additionally, the phallus is degloved and this skin is used to create the labia minora. An incision is made around the corona of the phallus and continued inferiorly around the urethral meatus. Preservation of this meatal plate improves cosmesis and increases blood supply to the glans. The neurovascular bundle is identified with lateral incisions into the tunica

of the corpora along the phallus from the glans backward proximal to the corporal bifurcation. The cavernous erectile tissue is dissected from the inferior aspect of the dorsal tunic and excised, and the proximal and dorsal corpora are suture-ligated. The glans is secured to the inferior aspect of the pubis or to the corporal stumps.

WHEN THE VAGINAL ORIFICE IS OBSCURED. As mentioned previously, preoperative identification and catheterization or sounding of the vaginal orifice is key to the performance of a successful, one-stage procedure. When the vagina cannot be located by sounding, it sometimes can be seen by endoscopy. When sounding and vision both fail, an attempt before surgery to introduce a small (no. 4 or 5) ureteral catheter into the vagina by blindly probing through the endoscope along the posterior wall of the urogenital sinus may assist in the identification of the vagina. Sometimes this catheter finds the orifice. If so, it may be left within the vagina as a guide during surgical exposure of the area (Fig. 34.11). If the vaginal orifice cannot be located, a planned two-stage operation may be indicated. The objective of the first stage is to obtain cosmetically satisfactory female genitalia by removing the clitoris and partially excising

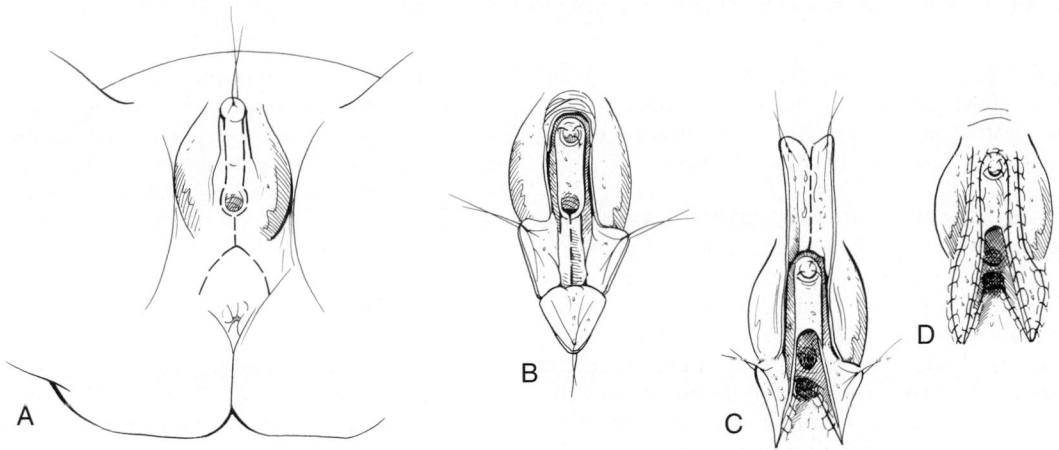

FIGURE 34.10. Surgical management of the clitoris with creation of labia minora and a posterior flap technique for vaginoplasty. **A:** Incision around the corona of the phallus continued inferiorly around the urethral meatus. **B:** Proposed incision into the posterior wall of the urogenital sinus. **C:** Degloving of the phallus. Sutures are individually placed through the posterior based flap and into the split posterior vagina. **D:** The phallic skin is divided in the midline and moved inferiorly to create the labia minora. (From Rink RC, Adams MC. Feminizing genitoplasty: state of the art. *World J Urol* 1998;16:212, with permission.)

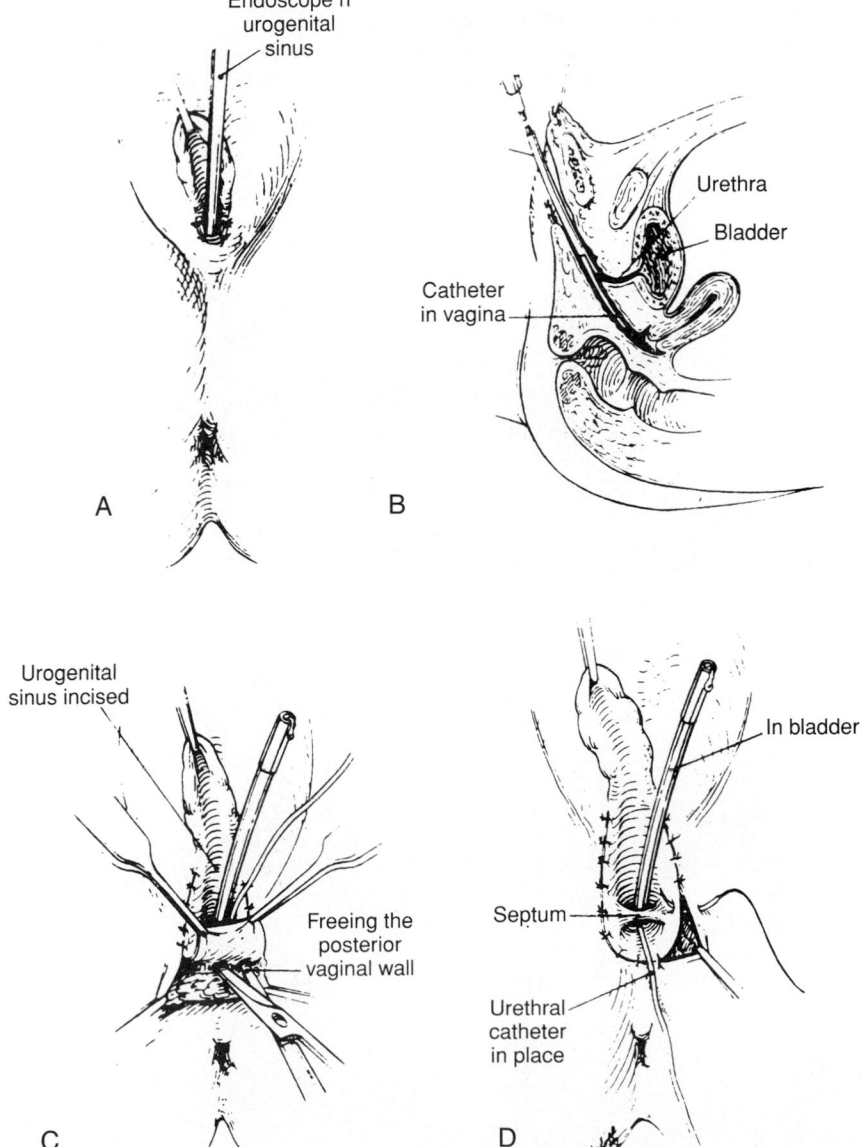

FIGURE 34.11. Operative procedure when it is difficult to locate vaginal orifice by sounding. An operative endoscope can be used to probe with a small ureteral catheter. **A:** The orifice is enlarged to accommodate the endoscope. **B:** The tip of the catheter has found the vaginal opening and entered the vagina. **C:** Freeing the posterior vaginal wall with the ureteral catheter in the vagina and a stiff catheter in the urethra. **D:** The vaginal portion of the operation is complete.

the urogenital sinus without exteriorizing the vagina. The second stage, exteriorization of the vagina, may be postponed until a later date, when identification of the vaginal orifice by sounding becomes possible.

WHEN THE VAGINOSINUS COMMUNICATION IS BLOCKED. Rarely does the vagina not communicate with the UGS. The vagina with the UGS is homologous with the hymenal area, and the hymen rarely is imperforate in an otherwise normal female. For such a circumstance, we have found it helpful to pass a uterine sound downward through the fundus via hysterotomy into the vagina, thus forming a protrusion on the perineum. With such a guide, the edges of the vaginal epithelium can be located and sutured to the skin (Fig. 34.12). Until the uterus enlarges somewhat from its infantile state, the cavity is not large enough to accommodate even a uterine sound. Therefore, if such an operation is contemplated, it should not be done until there is a palpable enlargement of the uterus at the onset of puberty. Evaluation of uterine volume sonographically as a predictor of uterine size adequacy may be helpful.

WHEN THE VAGINOSINUS COMMUNICATION IS HIGH. Hendren has been especially interested in patients whose vaginosinus communication involves the proximal urethra (suprasphincteric). He has advocated an operation that disconnects the vagina from the urethra and repositions the vaginal orifice in the perineum, the "pull-through" vaginoplasty. In his hands, this procedure seems to have been satisfactory for some patients. The procedure requires positioning the new vaginal orifice in the perineum (Fig. 34.13). The vast majority of patients with ambiguous external genitalia and a vagina have a vaginosinus communication well distal to the proximal urethra (infrasphincteric), and consideration of the procedure advocated by Hendren is not necessary. In patients in whom the vagina enters the UGS proximal to the external sphincter, the pull-through vaginoplasty of Hendren and Crawford or the method described by Passerini-Glazel can be used to prevent incontinence. Hendren and Crawford's vaginal pull-through remains the basis for reconstruction today. Modification to this procedure has evolved in an attempt to decrease the complexity and decrease the tendency of an isolated vagina toward stenosis. Rink and co-workers have favored a one-stage procedure using a perineal prone approach with no division of the rectum.

RESULTS OF REVISION OF EXTERNAL GENITALIA. Among 28 patients with adrenogenital syndrome and good follow-up treated at the Johns Hopkins Hospital,

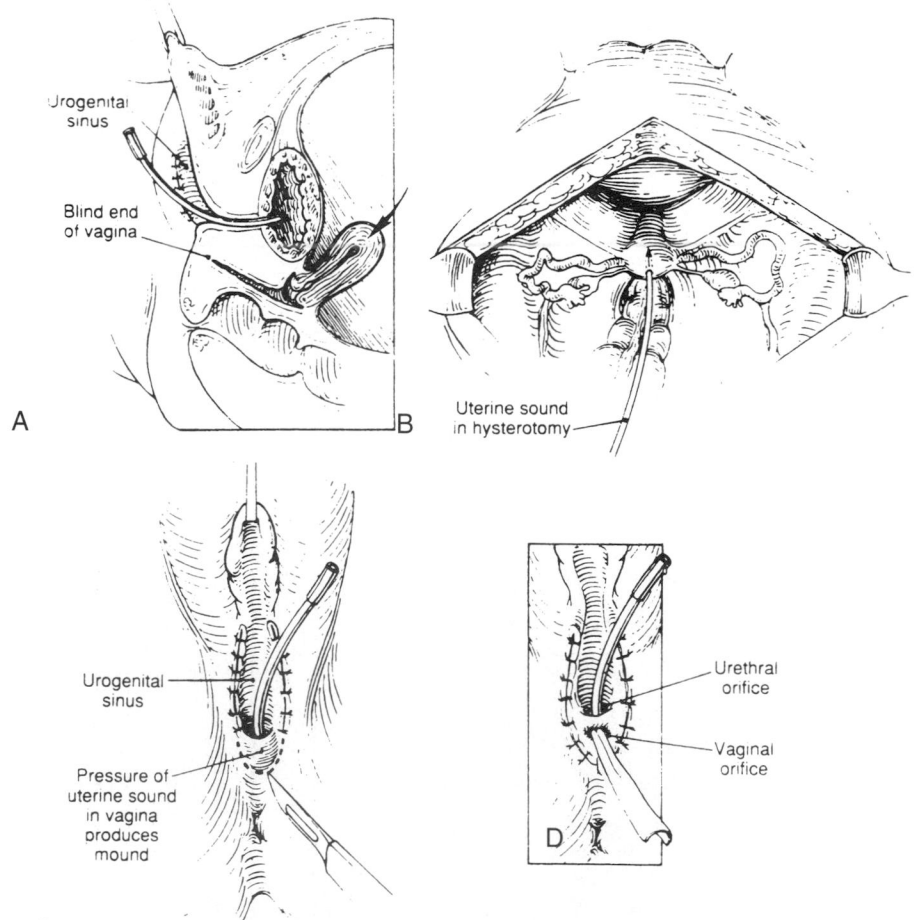

FIGURE 34.12. A: A situation in which the vaginal orifice is imperforate. **B:** A uterine sound has been passed through the fundus into the vagina. **C:** The tip of the sound can be palpated in the perineum. **D:** The completed procedure.

22 (87.6%) needed further vaginal reconstructive surgery to achieve an adequate vaginal size to allow comfortable intercourse. Of the 22 patients, five had undergone more than one surgical attempt at reconstruction. The mean age of patients undergoing repeat procedures was 7.1 years. The mean age at first surgery for the whole group was 23.6 months. Vaginal reconstructive surgery was performed on 18 of these patients and was successful in 13 (72%) of the procedures. It generally is recommended that exteriorization of the vagina be postponed until near puberty, when feminization occurs and the young woman is sufficiently mature to comply with a postoperative dilatation program. The results of exteriorization performed during infancy must be followed up carefully for evidence of narrowing. In 2000, Krege and colleagues reported on the long-term follow-up of female patients with CAH from 21-hydroxylase deficiency, with special emphasis on the results of vaginoplasty. They reported that the main problem during the long-term

follow-up was intravaginal stenosis, with all those affected 9 of 25 (36%) having undergone a single-stage procedure early in life to correct ambiguous genitalia (mean age, 4.7 years; range, 2 to 9 years). They suggested that vaginoplasty should be undertaken at the beginning of puberty, because higher estrogen levels may prevent stenosis and dilatation may be performed. In addition, 16 patients answered questionnaires that included psychological profile and the researchers found that 14 had problems with their overall body image. Patients with correction of vaginal stenosis were particularly anxious about sexual intercourse and had problems with orgasm.

Costa and colleagues have evaluated the vaginal size and sexual activity after different techniques of feminization of external genitalia in patients with pseudohermaphrodism. All patients who underwent clitoroplasty reported orgasms and 29% of the patients who had clitoridectomy reported no orgasm. Fifty percent of the pa-

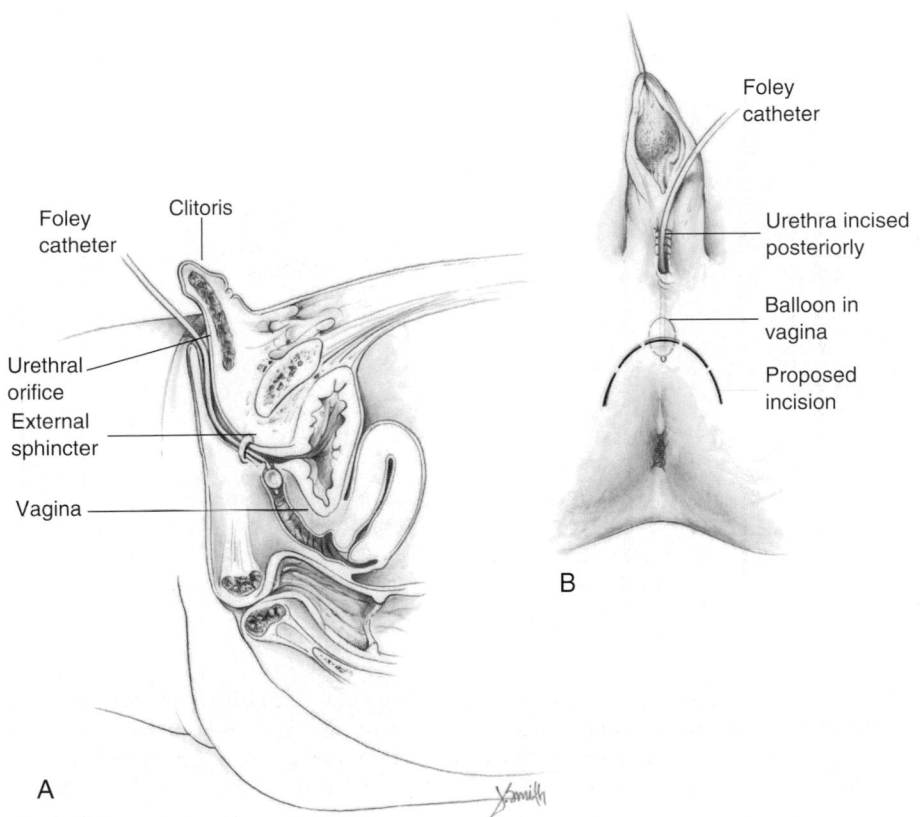

FIGURE 34.13. A perineal pull-through vaginoplasty according to Hendren. **A:** Sagittal view in diagram of high suprasphincteric vaginal communication to the urogenital sinus. A small Foley catheter is placed in the vagina to aid in its manipulation and localization. **B:** The location of the initial incision in relation to the balloon in the vagina.

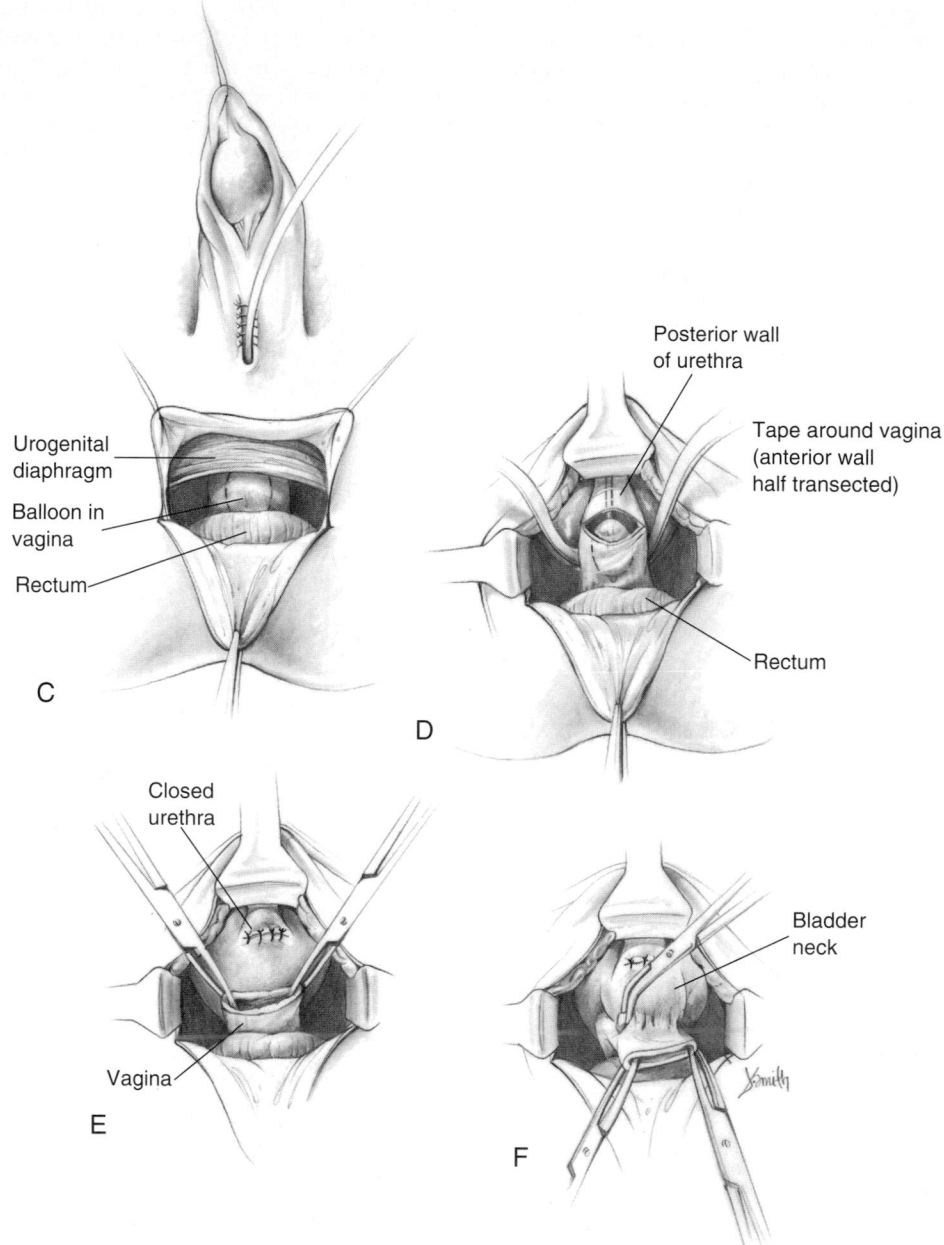

FIGURE 34.13. *(Continued)* **C:** The flap is retracted posteriorly, and the dissection is carried along the anterior wall of the rectum until the vagina (as identified by the balloon) is approached. **D:** The vagina is identified by the Foley balloon catheter. The vagina is open. Care should be taken to pull a flap of vagina distal so that there will be no problem in closing the urethra. **E:** The urethra is closed. Clips are placed on the vagina to bring it down to the perineum. **F:** The vagina is further mobilized.

tients who submitted to neovaginoplasty reported pain or bleeding during sexual intercourse. Satisfactory sexual intercourse was reported after vaginal dilation with acrylic molds by 87%. The clinicians concluded that surgical correction of external genitalia performed in childhood and vaginal dilation with acrylic molds performed when they wished to start having sexual intercourse resulted in best outcome.

Historically it has been assumed that psychosexual development of infants with intersex disorders is mostly due to rearing rather than being intrinsic. Over the past decade, the role of testosterone imprinting of the fetal brain has been studied to evaluate the role of this hormone in determining male sexual orientation. Studies in the 1990s of girls with CAH have confirmed that such children engage in more rough-and-tumble play than

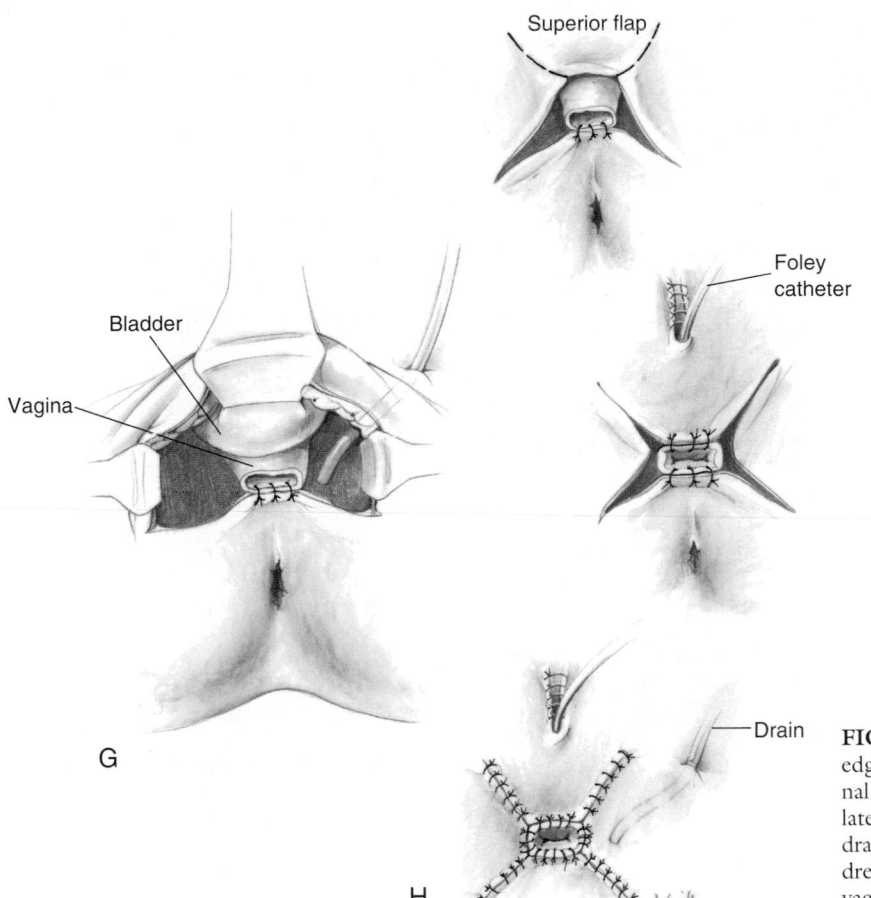

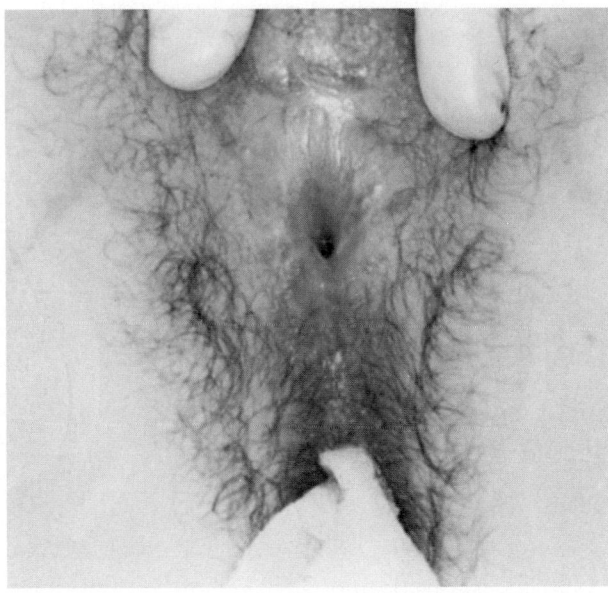

FIGURE 34.13. *(Continued)* **G:** The edge of the vagina is attached to the original flap of perineal skin. **H:** Anterior and lateral flaps are attached. Note the use of a drain in the perivaginal space. (From Hendren WH. Reconstructive problems of the vagina and the female urethra. *Clin Plast Surg* 1980;7:207, with permission.)

their affected peers and that difficulties with adjustment to their assigned gender may exist. Nonetheless, few studies have been conducted to address the social, psychological, and sexual outcomes for affected adolescents and adults, although it appears that most function in the normal range and are well adjusted. The majority of girls appear not to overtly demonstrate sexual identity problems.

SECONDARY OPERATIONS. A secondary operation on the vaginal outlet may be required. This is generally the case if the basic operation is deliberately accomplished in two stages, whatever the reason. A secondary operation may be indicated, for example, when an infant's vaginal orifice is not readily identifiable, yet it seems desirable to construct cosmetically acceptable female genitalia at a very early age. In this circumstance, the clitoroplasty can be done in the newborn, and the vagina may be exteriorized at puberty.

When the complete operation is attempted at an early age, the vagina is sometimes not satisfactorily exteriorized. Vaginal stenosis may require reconstruction at the time of puberty (Fig. 34.14). In this circumstance, there usually has been a failure to carry the midline incision far enough posteriorly, and a second procedure is re-

FIGURE 34.14. External genitalia of a 15-year-old patient with vaginal stenosis. Revision of the external genitalia, including an exteriorization of the vagina, had been performed in infancy.

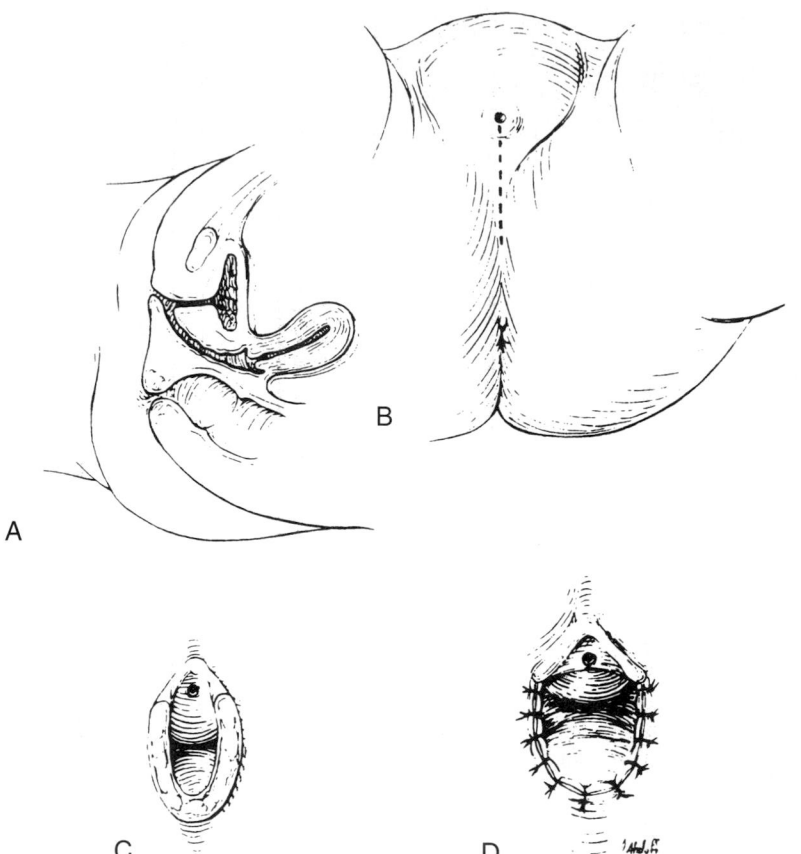

FIGURE 34.15. A: Repeated operation on the vaginal outlet when the operation was not completed at the first procedure. **B:** The posterior incision. **C:** The vagina is exposed. **D:** The closure.

quired to complete the first one by continuing the midline incision far enough posteriorly.

In other cases, contraction at the vaginal outlet may occur even if the operation is adequately performed. A minor revision of the vaginal orifice is required to enlarge

the vaginal orifice by making an incision in the midline and closing it at 90 degrees to the original axis of the incision (Fig. 34.15). In some instances, it may be necessary to create flaps to enlarge the vaginal orifice (Fig. 34.16).

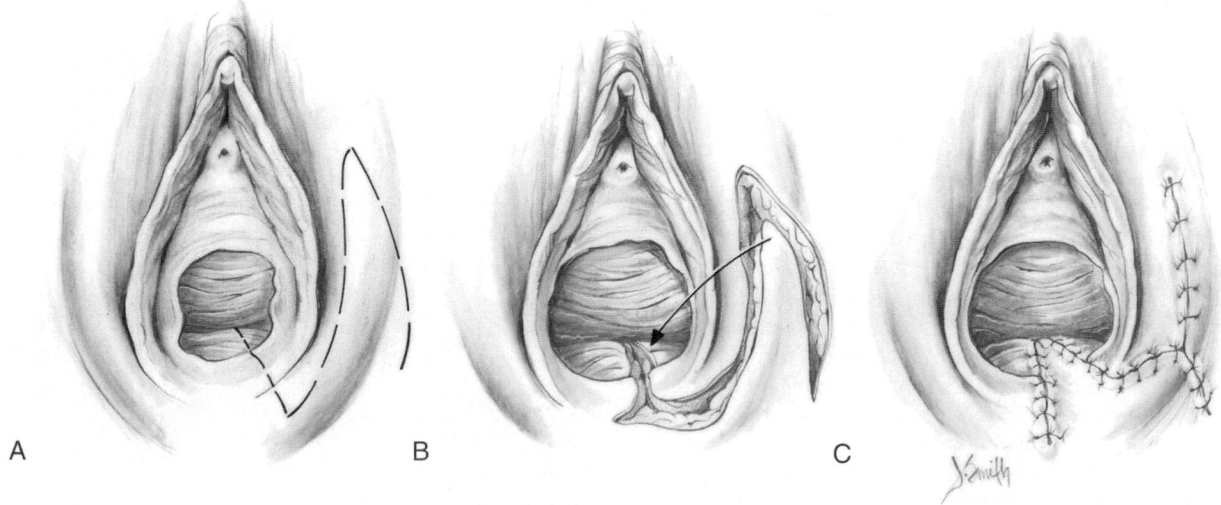

FIGURE 34.16. Labial cutaneous flap. **A:** An incision is made through the labia skin and subcutaneous fat. **B:** The flap is rotated into the perineotomy incision. **C:** The flap is sutured in place by interrupted 3-0 delayed-absorbable sutures. This may be repeated on the other side if required.

Bladder Exstrophy

Exstrophy of the bladder is a rare, congenital anomaly occurring in live births in a 1:25,000 to 1:40,000 ratio. There is a male predominance over females in a ratio of about 2:1. Classic bladder exstrophy is characterized by (1) absence of the lower anterior abdominal wall, (2) absence of the anterior wall of the bladder so that the posterior bladder wall and the ureteric orifices are exposed, (3) a poorly defined bladder neck and urethra, and (4) wide separation of the pubic symphysis. A genital abnormality typically present in females with bladder exstrophy is anterior displacement and narrowing of the vagina (Fig. 34.17) and separation of the clitoris into two distinct bodies (Fig. 34.18).

Bladder exstrophy, cloacal exstrophy, and epispadias are variants of the exstrophy epispadias complex. These defects have been attributed to failure of the normal process of ingrowth of mesoderm and the consequent lack of reinforcement of the cloacal membrane. The normal cloacal membrane is bilaminar and occupies the caudal end of the germinal disc. An ingrowth of mesenchyme between the ectodermal and endodermal layers of the cloacal membrane forms the lower abdominal wall musculature and the pelvic bones. After mesenchymal ingrowth occurs, descent of the urorectal septum divides the cloacal membrane into the bladder anteriorly and the rectum posteriorly. The urorectal septum eventually meets with the posterior remnant of the cloacal membrane, which perforates to form the anal and UGS openings. The paired genital tubercles migrate medially and fuse in the midline anterior to the cloacal membrane before perforation. Without its normal support from mesenchymal derivatives, the cloacal membrane is subject to premature rupture. Depending on the extent of the infraumbilical defect and the stage of development when rupture occurs, bladder exstrophy, cloacal exstrophy, or epispadias develops (Fig. 34.19).

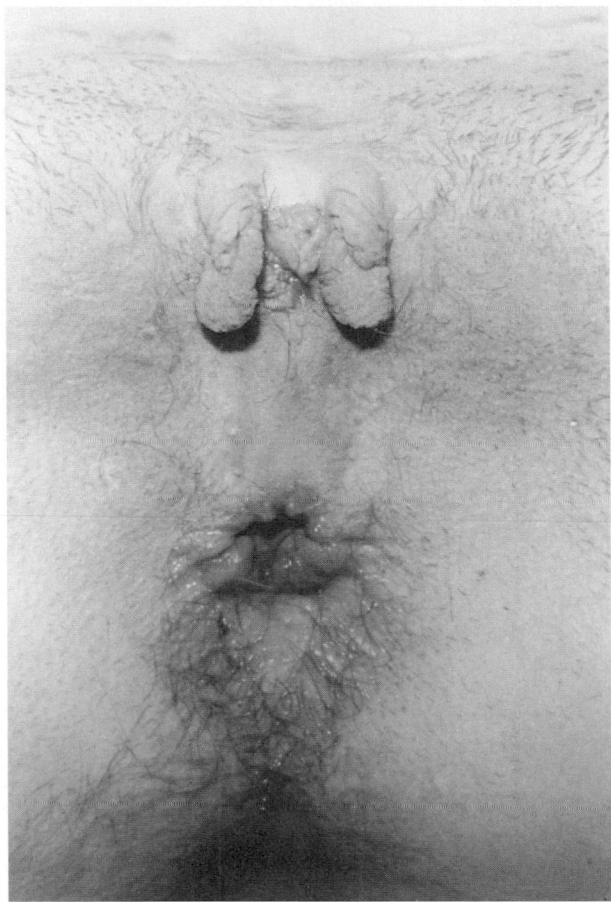

FIGURE 34.18. Preoperative photograph of a patient undergoing reconstruction of the external genitalia. Note the bifid clitoris and small anterior vaginal orifice.

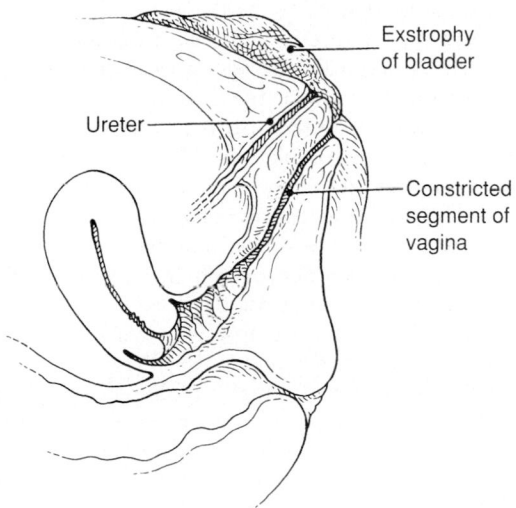

FIGURE 34.17. Common gynecologic anomaly seen in females with bladder exstrophy. The vagina is rotated anteriorly and constricted over its distal portion.

TREATMENT. Our understanding of appropriate urologic management of bladder exstrophy has evolved greatly over the past few decades, and improved management has markedly increased the life expectancy and quality of life of patients with this anomaly. Historical methods of treatment involved bladder excision and a urinary diversion procedure such as ureterosigmoidostomy. These techniques are complicated by serious sequelae including pyelonephritis, hyperchloremic acidosis, rectal incontinence, ureteral obstruction, and later development of malignancy.

Modern urologic management of bladder exstrophy relies on a staged approach to functional bladder closure. The initial procedure consists of primary bladder closure with or without iliac osteotomies to aid closure of the pelvic ring and growth and improvement of bladder capacity. The second-stage procedures usually involve bladder neck reconstruction to improve continence and bilateral ureteral reimplantations to prevent reflux. Both failures and primary reconstruction have also been performed using continence urostomies such as the Mainz II pouch. Mingen and co-workers and Gerharz and colleagues have reported their success using this technique.

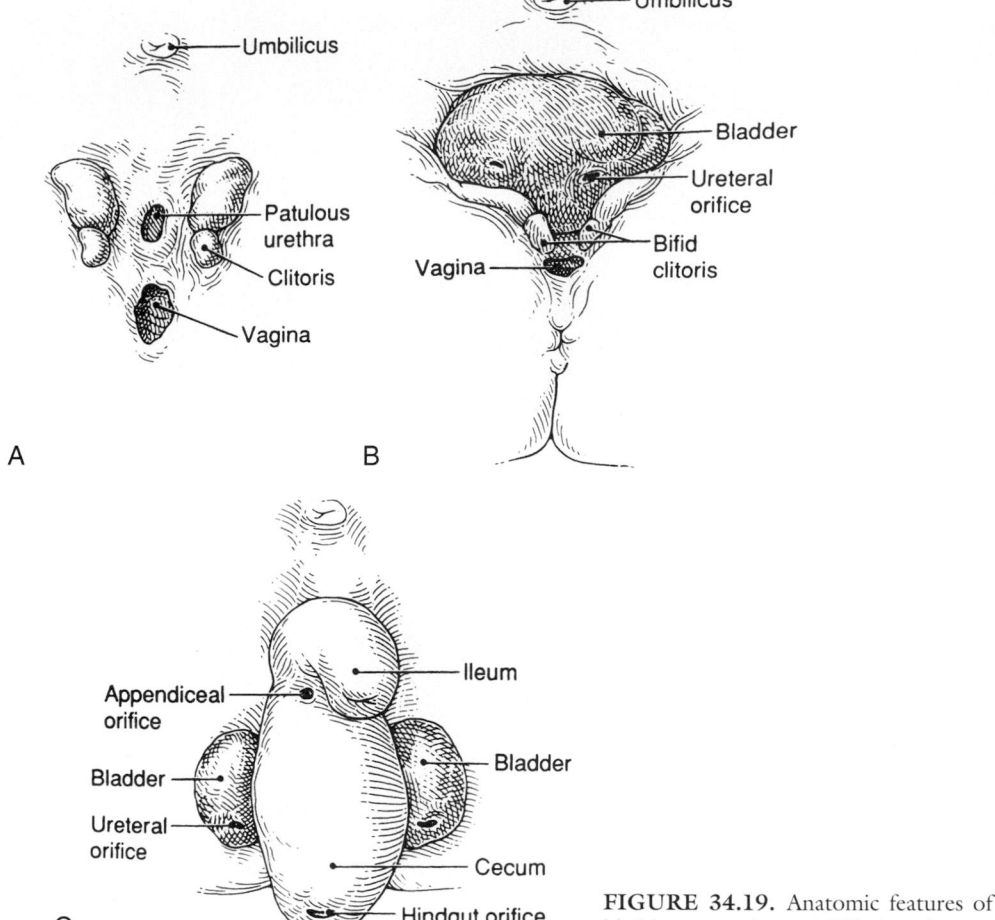

FIGURE 34.19. Anatomic features of (**A**) epispadias, (**B**) classic bladder exstrophy, and (**C**) cloacal exstrophy in females.

The prognosis using modern-day procedures is good. Although deficiency of the pelvic floor and a predisposition for pelvic organ prolapse are not unusual with bladder exstrophy, the condition of bladder exstrophy itself can often be corrected and associated genital anomalies can be managed to allow comfortable sexual activity and possibly even pregnancy.

The adjunctive procedures that may be important with surgical correction of bladder exstrophy are those that address the correction of anterior displacement and narrowing of the vagina and separation of the clitoris into two distinct bodies that are so typically associated with bladder exstrophy.

The procedure for correcting the external genitalia has evolved from one that was first described by Howard Jones, Jr., in 1973. Particular emphasis is placed on attainment of an adequate vaginal diameter without further predisposing to subsequent prolapse. The first step is vertical incision into the posterior raphe of what resembles fused scrotolabial folds; next, Allis clamps are placed laterally for traction. Fine-needle point electrocautery is then used to further open the incision, with special care taken not to take this incision too far posteriorly. The lateral portions of the incision are secured

with 3-0 nonreactive absorbable sutures for further traction. The posterior vaginal edges are undermined to allow their mobilization to the exterior. The vaginal mucosa is then approximated to the perineal surface with interrupted and figure-of-eight sutures, incorporating the superficial perineal muscles into the closure. In the more posterior portion of the closure, 2-0 nonreactive absorbable suture is used, because this is the area of greatest tension. At completion, there is a significant increase in the diameter of the vagina, and the vaginal orifice usually accommodates two fingers.

Postoperative active dilatation therapy has recently been advocated. Experience with management of ambiguous genitalia has shown a decrease in the incidence of postoperative vaginal stenosis if dilatation therapy is employed during the constrictive phase (the first 6 weeks) of healing. For this reason, following reconstruction of the external genitalia and exteriorization of the vagina, appropriately sized Lucite dilators are used once or twice a day for this 6-week period or until healing is complete.

Reapproximation of the bifid clitoris (Fig. 34.20) is primarily cosmetic and is not always performed. The technique involves excising a diamond-shaped area of

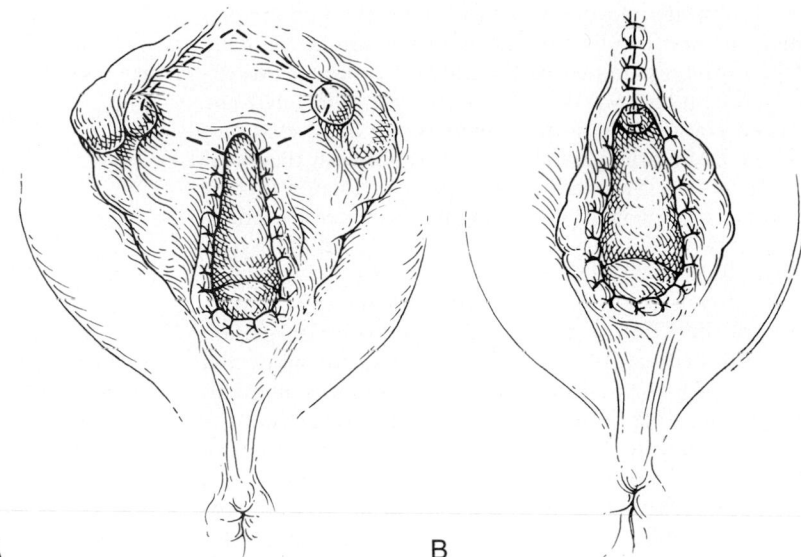

FIGURE 34.20. Schematic depiction of procedure to reapproximate the clitoris. A vulvovaginoplasty has already been performed to exteriorize the vagina. **A:** A diamond-shaped piece of skin and subcutaneous tissue between the clitoral bodies is excised. **B:** The clitoral bodies are then undermined and mobilized to the center for a side-to-side reapproximation.

skin and subcutaneous tissue between the clitoral bodies. The medial aspect of each side of the clitoris is then denuded and undermined to allow a central reapproximation with a side-to-side closure.

ADJUNCTIVE TREATMENTS. Stanton mentioned that perineotomy was performed in six patients with bladder exstrophy in which the labia and clitoris were reapproximated by a Z-plasty technique. Still others have described rather extraordinary efforts to restore the mons pubis and female escutcheon with skin flaps of hair-bearing areas. These latter reports, however, fail to mention correction of the vaginal anomaly.

Other series have described a wide range of both genital and extragenital abnormalities in association with bladder exstrophy. Stanton reviewed 70 patients with bladder exstrophy and observed an increased incidence of various müllerian anomalies. Eleven patients were also observed to have associated rectal prolapse. Blakely and Mills observed various extragenital abnormalities in their series including rectal prolapse, imperforate anus, exophthalmos, renal agenesis, and spina bifida.

RESULTS. Jones reviewed the records of all female patients diagnosed with bladder exstrophy at Johns Hopkins Hospital over a 20-year time span. Of 18 patients with adequately described external genitalia, 13 had small, anteriorly displaced vaginal orifices, and the remaining five patients had vaginal orifices of normal size and location. Therefore, while demonstrating phenomena very typical of bladder exstrophy, all female patients do not demonstrate the defect of narrowing of the vagina. Damario and colleagues have recently updated the Hopkins series, documenting continuing excellent long-term results.

Several series have reviewed subsequent pregnancy outcomes in patients with bladder exstrophy. Clemetson extensively reviewed the literature in 1958 and found 45 patients who underwent 64 pregnancies. A very high in-

cidence of uterine prolapse was observed both before and after pregnancy. In addition, there was a higher incidence of premature labor and malpresentations (24%). Krisiloff and colleagues also reported a high incidence of uterine prolapse related to pregnancy, which occurred in 6 of 7 women. Burbige and co-workers reported on 14 pregnancies in patients with a history of bladder exstrophy. Uterine prolapse occurred in 7 of 11 patients, all of whom had undergone a previous urinary diversion procedure.

The mode of delivery in patients with prior urinary diversion procedures has primarily been spontaneous vaginal delivery. The increased incidence of premature labor and malpresentation, however, has warranted an increased rate of Caesarean sections for obstetric indications. In patients with a prior bladder reconstruction, most surgeons advocate an elective Caesarean section to eliminate stress on the pelvic floor and to avoid trauma to the delicate urinary sphincter mechanism.

MANAGEMENT OF UTERINE PROLAPSE WITH BLADDER EXSTROPHY. Several mechanisms have been proposed to explain the high incidence of uterine prolapse in patients with bladder exstrophy. These mechanisms include (1) a deficiency of the pelvic floor due to the wide separation of the pubic symphysis, (2) an inherent deficiency of the cardinal ligament complex, and (3) the abnormal axis and short length of the vagina.

Because wide separation of the pubic symphysis results in an enlarged genital hiatus and deficiency of the pelvic floor, it is possible that iliac osteotomy may be helpful in deterring pelvic organ prolapse by closer approximation of the levator ani and puborectal muscles. Although Gearhart and Jeffs suggest that iliac osteotomies may not be necessary if primary bladder closure is performed in the first 72 hours of life, perhaps the procedure should be given increased consideration in female patients who present such a high risk for uterine prolapse later in life.

It appears important not to extend the midline perineal incision too far posteriorly in revision of the genitalia in these patients. As the incision proceeds posteriorly, the midline septum thickens to approximately 2 cm. At this point, the levator ani muscles may be severed, further enlarging the genital hiatus. It is prudent, therefore, to be more conservative; postoperative dilator therapy may aid in achieving further vaginal diameter if needed.

A case referred to us illustrated this point. A 16-year-old nulliparous patient with bladder exstrophy and a history of staged bladder reconstruction underwent revision of the external genitalia. A large posterior incision into the perineal body had left a gaping introitus, and uterine prolapse had occurred several months after this procedure. Our initial approach was to reconstruct the perineal body to help contain the uterus and improve support to the pelvic floor. This reconstruction has been successful, without further prolapse 5 years after the procedure. A similar case was reported by Blakely and Mills, who observed uterine prolapse occurring very soon after enlargement of the vaginal introitus.

Management of uterine prolapse associated with bladder exstrophy may be difficult. The patient frequently desires preservation of her child-bearing capacity. Sacrospinous fixation of the cervix may be considered, although an abnormally short vagina may produce difficulty in obtaining the suspension without significant suture bridges. An abdominal sacrocervicopexy may also be considered. Dewhurst and coworkers described this approach in 1980. They suspended the uterus to the sacrum using Ivalon sponge in a patient with procidentia following repair of bladder exstrophy.

The high historical incidence of uterine prolapse and the potential difficulties managing this problem highlight the need for the reconstructive surgeon to give extra thought and care to revision of the external genitalia in females with bladder exstrophy. Inappropriate reconstruction may actually accelerate genital prolapse. In addition, elective Caesarean section may be the most judicious mode of delivery for limiting traumatic insults to the pelvic floor that could further increase the propensity for prolapse. Ricci and co-workers evaluated 17 patients (15 children, 2 young adults) with bladder exstrophy for latex allergy. Twelve shared latex sensitization with five demonstrating symptoms. The multiple operative and cystoscope procedures performed on this group of patients has resulted in significant latex exposure and sensitization similar to that seen in health care workers.

Carcinoma of the Vagina

Carcinoma of the vagina is uncommon, occurring in less than 2% of patients with gynecologic malignancies. The average age at presentation is 60 years. Vaginal carcinoma is most frequently secondary to metastases from tumors of the cervix and vulva rather than originating in the vagina. Lesions that encroach on the outer vagina from the vulva must be separated from lesions that originate in the vaginal canal to be considered a vaginal primary.

The International Federation of Obstetrics and Gynecology (FIGO) has agreed on the following exclusionary criteria for the classification of vaginal cancer:

1. A vaginal growth extending to the portio of the cervix and reaching the area of the external os should always be considered a carcinoma of the cervix.
2. A vulvar growth that has extended to the vagina should be classified as carcinoma of the vulva.
3. A vaginal growth that is limited to the urethra should be classified separately as carcinoma of the urethra.

Clinicians now satisfy the staging criteria for the diagnosis of primary carcinoma of the vagina by showing a histologically negative cervix, urethra, vulva, and endometrium.

The criteria for the definition of primary carcinoma of the vagina were established after many clinicians reported the recurrence of vaginal lesions after treatment of carcinoma in situ of the cervix. Tumors recurred in 1% to 6% of cases. Today, extension of carcinoma in situ and invasive carcinoma of the cervix to the vaginal fornices or upper vagina can be easily identified with the use of colposcopy.

The clinical stages of carcinoma of the vagina agreed on by FIGO are listed in Table 34.1. In 1973, Perez and coworkers proposed that stage II be divided into stage IIa and IIb to provide a more accurate definition of the extent of the lesion. In the proposed modified FIGO classification, stage IIa includes subvaginal infiltration not extending into the parametrial regions, whereas stage IIb includes parametrial or paravaginal infiltration not extending to the pelvic wall. This classification has not been accepted by FIGO. Creasman and colleagues queried the National Cancer Data Base (NCDB), a central registry of hospital case data for 1985 through 1994. Of the 4,885 cases, 75% were invasive and 90% epithe-

TABLE 34.1.
International Federation of Obstetrics and Gynecology Classification of Vaginal Carcinoma

PREINVASIVE CARCINOMA

Stage 0   Carcinoma in situ, intraepithelial carcinoma.

INVASIVE CARCINOMA

Stage I   Carcinoma limited to the vaginal wall.
Stage II   Carcinoma involving the subvaginal tissue, but not extending onto the pelvic wall.
Stage III Carcinoma extending onto the pelvic wall.
Stage IV   Carcinoma extending beyond the true pelvis or involving the mucosa of the bladder or rectum. Bullous edema that does not permit a case to be allotted to stage IV.
Stage IVa Spread of the growth to adjacent organs.
Stage IVb Spread to distant organs.

From Pettersson F, ed. *Annual report on the results of treatment in gynecologic cancer.* Stockholm: FIGO, 1988:174.

lial. Survival at 5 years was as follows: stage 0, 96%; stage I, 73%; stage II, 58%; stage III-IV, 36%. The overall 5-year survival rate with melanoma was 14%.

Symptoms

The diagnosis of vaginal tumors frequently is delayed because of the lack of early symptoms. Progressive vaginal discharge and postmenopausal bleeding are the most frequent symptoms. Postcoital bleeding can also herald the presence of a vaginal or cervical carcinoma. More than 10% of patients are asymptomatic at the time of diagnosis.

Women with a history of vaginal, vulvar, and cervical intraepithelial neoplasia have an increased risk of vaginal carcinoma. These patients should receive annual Papanicolaou smears even if they have undergone a hysterectomy. Having a hysterectomy for other than preneoplastic or neoplastic conditions does not increase the risk for developing vaginal carcinoma.

The symptoms of vaginal carcinoma resemble those of cervical carcinoma, except that obvious bleeding occurs later than with neoplasms on the cervix. The overt bleeding eventually forces the patient to see her physician for diagnosis. The type of pelvic pain is frequently indicative of lesion location. The posterior vagina, the most common location of vaginal carcinomas, presents with tenesmus and other bowel symptoms. Anterior tumors, on the other hand, result in urethral and bladder symptoms.

Histopathology

The most common histologic type of primary vaginal tumor is squamous carcinoma, which accounts for 84% to 90% of all vaginal cancers (Table 34.2). Adenocarcinoma, including diethylstilbestrol (DES)-related cases, represents about 4% to 9% of vaginal cancers. Sarcomas, including leiomyosarcoma and sarcoma botryoides, account for 2% to 3% of vaginal lesions, and melanomas account for 1% to 2% of malignant neoplasms of the vagina. Rare tumors such as endodermal sinus tumors or neoplasms originating in embryologic cloacal remnants may form a transitional cell neoplasm that involves the vagina.

Squamous carcinoma of the vagina is discovered in 10% to 15% of cases after the finding of squamous cancer in other parts of the lower genital tract, such as the vulva or cervix. This has led to the theory of multicentric origin of squamous cancer in the lower genital tract. Woodruff and Parmley and others emphasize this correlation and have recommended that patients with squamous cancer in one area be categorized as high risk for the development of squamous carcinoma in other sites of the lower genital tract. A viral etiology such as the human papilloma virus is most likely responsible for these findings.

Carcinoma may arise in the neovagina lined with a split-thickness skin graft from the buttock or lateral thigh. Carcinoma of the neovagina is a rare cancer; only nine cases have been reported. The primary carcinoma seems to be related to the transplanted tissue. In three cases, adenocarcinoma was associated with the use of a large or small bowel intestinal graft for vaginal reconstruction. Five cases of squamous cell cancer arising from the graft have been documented. The transplanted epithelium in the vagina may be exposed to an unidentified carcinogen or mutagen, as has been documented with the vulva, and can undergo malignant transformation in this environment. These observations underscore the need for regular pelvic examinations after operative vaginoplasty with either a bowel graft or a split-thickness skin graft.

DES, a nonsteroidal estrogenic hormone thought to enhance embryo implantation and placental development, was introduced into clinical obstetrics in 1944 in Boston and became popular and widely used during the next two decades. Women with a history of previous spontaneous abortions or other risk factors for early pregnancy loss of multiple gestations were given DES. It is known now that DES use during the first trimester of pregnancy may cause vaginal neoplasia. It was not until the late 1960s, however, when a cluster of cases of adenocarcinoma appeared in young women younger than age 25 years (all offspring of DES-treated women) that Herbst and colleagues connected the result with the unusual cause.

From 1944 to 1970, about 1.5 to 2 million female offspring were exposed to DES. Fortunately, the incidence of vaginal adenocarcinoma in these young women has been quite low, ranging from 0.14 to 1.4 in 1,000 exposed women. More than 500 documented cases have been reported to the DES registry to date.

Observations of the development of vaginal adenosis and adenocarcinoma in teenage girls whose mothers were given DES before the 18th week of pregnancy brought new insights to the study of squamous tumor cells in the lower genital tract and greatly increased our understanding of the embryologic development of the vagina. The effect of the DES drug provided an indisputable histologic foundation for the development of an uncommon vaginal adenocarcinoma in women younger than 29 years of age. Twenty-five percent of women exposed in utero have anatomic cervical, vaginal, and urinary tract abnormalities.

The DES-associated adenocarcinoma originally was thought to arise from mesonephric remnants in the

---

TABLE 34.2.
Histologic Types of Vaginal Cancer and Frequency of Occurrence

Type	Frequency (%)
Squamous carcinoma	84–90
Adenocarcinoma (including DES-related)	4–9
Sarcoma	2–3
Melanoma	1–2
Other	1–2

DES, diethylstilbestrol.

vagina, and the disease consequently was mislabeled as a clear cell carcinoma. However, electron microscopic analysis of the ultrastructure of both the adenocarcinoma and the vaginal adenosis allowed Fenoglio and colleagues to clearly define these lesions as composed of columnar epithelium, similar in all respects to endocervical epithelium, and of paramesonephric (müllerian) origin. The colposcopic studies of Stafl and Mattingly and of others confirm these observations.

Vaginal adenosis has been found by colposcopic examination to occur in 34% to 90% of exposed offspring and vaginal adenocarcinoma in 50%. Although the hypothesis is still unproven, there is a strong possibility that the benign vaginal lesion is the cell of origin for vaginal adenocarcinoma. The risk of development of clear cell adenocarcinoma in an exposed female between birth and age 34 is 1 in 1,000.

Etiology

During embryologic development, the vagina is formed from the columnar epithelium of the müllerian ducts and UGS. The tissue then transforms into squamous epithelium, so that the vaginal and cervical epithelium have a common embryologic origin. Squamous metaplasia within the vaginal adenosis has been observed with a colposcope, and transformation of the metaplastic tissue also has been demonstrated in the development of intraepithelial neoplasia. Although many agents have been postulated as carcinogenic factors, none have been positively demonstrated. It is quite possible that squamous carcinoma arises from the effects of an oncogenic agent on the transformation zone within the foci of vaginal adenosis. The studies now being done on the effects of DES may find some interesting causative factors that influence vaginal carcinoma.

Carcinoma of the vagina also may share a common causative denominator with cervical carcinoma. Because slightly more than 50% of the cases occur in the posterior wall of the upper third of the vagina, which is the end point of vaginal coitus, vaginal carcinoma could be venereally induced. As with cervical carcinoma, primary carcinoma of the vagina usually occurs in sexually active women. Except for the cases of adenocarcinoma in young women exposed to DES, squamous carcinoma of the vagina is unquestionably associated with sexual activity. As with cervical intraepithelial neoplasia and carcinoma, the human papilloma virus is probably responsible for the majority of vaginal carcinomas.

Site of Lesion

Plentl and Friedman found that 51% of vaginal carcinoma lesions occur in the upper third of the vagina, 30% in the lower third, and 19% in the middle third. In the lower third, lesions most often occur in the anterior wall, whereas in the upper third, lesions most often appear in the posterior vaginal wall. Although the location is observed on diagnosis, the precise site of origin is difficult to pinpoint because the tumors usually have spread to various parts of the vagina by that time.

Pathways of Spread

The lymphatic drainage of the vagina takes place through different pathways. The upper third drains by way of the cervical lymphatics, the lower third passes by way of the vulvar lymphatics, and the middle third communicates with both the upper and the lower lymphatic channels. The vaginal vault and the anterior wall of the upper vagina drain to the interiliac pelvic lymph nodes, where they communicate with the external iliac, the hypogastric, and the common iliac nodes. The lymphatic drainage of the posterior vagina communicates directly with the deep pelvic nodes, including the inferior gluteal, sacral, and rectal nodes.

Because the major pathways of lymphatic drainage are to the superior and inferior gluteal muscles and the common iliac lymph nodes, the potential for extrapelvic spread of vaginal carcinoma is great. When extrapelvic spread occurs, prognosis usually is poor. The primary site of origin of the tumor is an important indicator of lymph node metastases, whether the tumor will metastasize to the inguinal-femoral chain or to the deep pelvic lymph nodes. When the disease involves the lower third of the vagina, 6% to 7% of patients have metastases to the inguinal-femoral lymph nodes.

Diagnosis

In general, invasive carcinoma of the vagina appears as either a raised exophytic lesion or an ulcerative, depressed lesion in the vaginal wall. Biopsy can be performed on both types of lesions easily, and diagnosis can be established without difficulty. Vaginal cytology usually is positive if an adequate cell sample is obtained from the exfoliated lesion, although, as often happens with cervical carcinoma, many cases of false-negative cytology occur even when an invasive lesion is present. Colposcopy, Lugol solution, or both can be used to demarcate the areas for biopsy, although iodine staining usually is unnecessary if the lesion is clearly visible.

Identifying vaginal carcinoma at an early stage can be a major problem because the first lesions appear within the epithelial cells, frequently indistinguishable from the remainder of the vaginal epithelium. Only by colposcopic examination or with iodine staining can alterations in the surface epithelium of the vagina be identified. Ng and associates have achieved an accuracy of 88% to 90% in detecting dysplastic lesions in DES-exposed patients with adenosis, but their technique requires separate, four-quadrant vaginal smears from the walls of the vagina to increase the sensitivity of the Papanicolaou smear. Herbst and co-workers emphasize the advantage of iodine staining of the vagina to reveal occult lesions that may be associated with adenosis. Stafl and Mattingly reported an accuracy of 96% in detecting abnormal epithelial lesions of the vagina in DES-exposed females by careful examination and colposcopy.

Because the vaginal speculum can obscure surface lesions and delay early diagnosis, the instrument should be rotated during the examination, so that the entire canal can be inspected. With iodine staining, the clinician can detect multifocal lesions, but the entire vagina also should be cytologically tested. A thorough colposcopic examination can be used to detect vaginal carcinoma, if the clinician has that expertise.

Treatment

Primary vaginal carcinoma is treated either with surgery or with radiotherapy. The choice of treatment depends on three factors: the size of the lesion, the location of the tumor in the vagina, and the clinical stage of the disease.

STAGE 0 LESIONS. Easiest to treat by far is vaginal intraepithelial neoplasia III (VAIN III), and it offers the most hopeful prognosis. Either surgery or radiotherapy can be used, depending on the location of the lesion. If the disease is located in the upper vagina and the margins of the disease are distinct, a partial vaginectomy, with or without hysterectomy, is a practical and successful method of treatment.

The carbon dioxide laser has proved to be a simple, effective means of treating noninvasive vaginal carcinoma. Laser therapy offers conservative treatment for both focal and multicentric lesions without impairment of normal coital function. Because there is a risk of residual disease in 10% of laser-treated patients, careful colposcopic and cytologic follow-up are critical. Histologic study is difficult after the treated lesions are vaporized by the carbon dioxide laser. An alternative ablative technique is the ultrasonic surgical aspirator, the tip of which vibrates 23,000 times per second, fragmenting and aspirating the tissue in contact with it. This technique permits histologic evaluation of the collected tissue fragments. The operative site also heals faster secondary to decreased thermal damage. Robinson and colleagues reported their experience in treating 46 patients with VAIN. Sixty- six percent (29) of those initially treated with ultrasonic surgical aspiration did not have recurrence. Fifty-two percent of patients treated for recurrent disease (17) did not experience a recurrence. The mean duration of follow-up was 21 months.

Nonsurgical methods such as administration of 5-fluorouracil vaginal cream have also proved efficacious in treating VAIN.

Radiation therapy is rarely used to treat VAIN. However, radiation is an excellent modality for suspected invasion when the medical risk for further evaluation by surgery is too great.

A vaginal cylinder, such as the Bloedorn applicator, can be used for radiotherapeutic treatment to deliver 70 Gy to the vaginal surface over a period of about 72 hours. If the lesion is confined to the vaginal fornices, vaginal colpostats can be used to deliver a similar dosage. Lesions in the lower third of the vagina may be treated by partial vaginectomy or by intravaginal irradiation using a variety of brachytherapy techniques.

STAGE I LESIONS. Surgery, radiation, or both are the primary modalities for treating vaginal carcinomas. Lesions in the vaginal fornix can be treated with a radical Wertheim hysterectomy, partial vaginectomy, and bilateral pelvic lymphadenectomy. Treatment for this lesion is similar to that for stage Ib cervical carcinoma. If pelvic lymph nodes are histologically positive or if paraaortic lymph nodes look suspicious, a paraaortic lymphadenectomy should be performed. If the lymph nodes are histologically positive for carcinoma, pelvic radiation with or without paraaortic radiation should be administered. As with cervical carcinoma, the size of the lesion is prognostic of our ability to adequately treat these patients with primary surgery. Large lesions not permitting clear surgical margins (e.g., proximity to the bladder or rectum) should be treated with primary radiation therapy. Radical surgery also may require the replacement of the upper vagina with a split-thickness skin graft to reestablish normal vaginal length for a sexually active woman. Irradiation therapy is an alternative treatment for this stage of disease.

The radical Wertheim hysterectomy has been quite successful in treating stage I adenocarcinoma in young women who were exposed to DES in utero. More than 75% of patients are cured. Magrina and associates treated a patient with stage I disease at their institution with laparoscopic radical parametrectomy and pelvic and aortic lymphadenectomy. The role of laparoscopy in the treatment of vaginal carcinoma will continue to expand. Although its role in parametrectomy may be debated, laparoscopy to excise the pelvic and periaortic nodes before radiation may be beneficial to patients with advanced disease.

Radiation therapy is the preferable treatment for large proximal lesions or middle or distal vaginal tumors. A combination of teletherapy (external beam) and interstitial or intracavity therapy is used.

STAGE II AND STAGE III LESIONS. More extensive lesions of the vagina pose an extremely difficult therapeutic problem for the gynecologist. Because the vagina is surrounded by the levator ani muscles of the pelvic diaphragm, penetration of the lateral wall of the vagina by the invasive tumor frequently is associated with fixation of the disease to the adjacent pelvic musculature. Even radical surgery cannot effectively control the disease when it extends beyond the confines of the vagina into the paravaginal tissues. Instead, the major method of treatment for stage II and stage III lesions is radiotherapy.

When stage II lesions involve the anterior or posterior wall of the vaginal septum, an anterior or posterior exenteration with pelvic node dissection may be required. When the disease includes the lower third of the vagina, a groin dissection is necessary also. Because surgery must be so extensive, its usefulness is limited when the disease affects the paravaginal region (stage IIb) or the lateral vaginal wall (stage III).

STAGE IV LESIONS. When advanced lesions involve only the bladder or the rectum, exenteration may be required to control the disease effectively. Unfortunately, pelvic exenteration, either anterior or posterior, can be used only when there is no other extension of the disease, and it is rare for the bladder and rectum to be involved without involvement of the adjacent paravaginal tissues. If the patient is not an acceptable surgical risk for exenteration, external beam megavoltage irradiation therapy followed by intravaginal or interstitial irradiation can be used to control the local disease and to offer palliation. If the tumor does not respond after 5,000 cGY of irradiation treatment to the whole pelvis, an exenteration may be required to control the disease in properly selected patients. Exenteration is also recommended for central recurrences without lymph node metastasis.

Irradiation Therapy

Irradiation treatment of vaginal carcinoma is easily divided between lesions in the upper and middle thirds and the lower third of the vagina.

UPPER AND MIDDLE THIRDS OF THE VAGINA. Because the lymphatic drainage of the upper and middle vagina extends through the hypogastric and pelvic nodes, full pelvic irradiation is necessary. Treatment usually includes a combination of techniques.

External beam megavoltage therapy using 4,500 to 5,000 cGY focused on the midplane of the pelvis is used to treat the full pelvis and to encompass the vagina. A vaginal implant of radium, cesium, or iridium follows, delivering an additional 3,000 to 4,000 cGY to a depth of 0.5 to 1.0 cm or more, depending on the thickness of the lesion.

At the M.D. Anderson Hospital, Brown and coworkers demonstrated the efficacy of using a radium needle implant for localized lesions. When the implant is used, high doses of radiation to the entire vagina, bladder, and rectum are avoided. Interstitial needles and iridium wires have been used as a primary treatment for localized vaginal lesions, and they can be used for persistent disease.

LOWER THIRD OF THE VAGINA. Lesions in the lower third of the vagina frequently metastasize to the inguinal-femoral lymphatics and must be treated with full external and intravaginal irradiation followed by external beam irradiation treatment to the inguinal-femoral lymph nodes. The inguinal-femoral regions require either a surgical groin dissection or the application of 5,000 to 6,000 cGY of electron beam teletherapy in addition to full pelvic irradiation. When vaginal lesions have metastasized to the groin lymph nodes, the cure rate is equally poor for both methods. In general, the presence of tumor in the groin nodes is a poor prognostic sign, suggesting that the deep pelvic nodes also may be involved in about 6% to 7% of cases. Because the incidence of vaginal cancer is so low, the exact frequency with which the deep pelvic nodes are involved has not been documented.

Chemoradiation for large bulky lesions may play a role in vaginal carcinoma, just as it does in cervical or vulvar lesions. Agents such as cisplatin, 5-fluorouracil, and hydroxyurea have been successfully used.

The number of patients with vaginal carcinoma reported to the FIGO registry by international clinics between 1979 and 1981 totals 547. Seventy-eight percent of these patients were treated by radiation. Only 38.6% of these patients were alive at 5 years. Results from other institutions that primarily have followed radiation therapy show that only stage I lesions have an adequate 5-year survival rate (Table 34.3).

In a retrospective analysis of 134 patients with carcinoma of the vagina treated at Washington University, Perez and Camel report an actuarial disease-free, 5-year survival rate of 85% for stage I lesions, 51% for stage IIa

---

TABLE 34.3.
Absolute 5-Year Survival After Irradiation Therapy for Carcinoma of the Vagina

	Proportion Surviving			
FIGO Stage	M.D. Anderson Hospital[a] 1948–1967	University of Maryland[a] 1957–1970	Washington University[b] 1950–1977	Vienna University[c] 1950–1977
I	11/16 (69%)	5/6 (83%)	33/39 (85%)	45/60 (75%)
II	13/19 (68%)	20/31 (64%)	28/60 (47%)	43/95 (45%)
IIa		13/20 (65%)	21/39 (51%)	
IIb		7/11 (63%)	7/21 (33%)	
III	4/15 (27%)	8/20 (40%)	4/12 (33%)	44/145 (30%)
IV	0/11 (0%)	0/7 (0%)	1/8 (19%)	12/62 (19%)
I–IV	28/61 (46%)	33/64 (52%)	66/119[d] (53%)	144/362 (40%)

[a] Data from Hilgers RD. Squamous cell carcinoma of the vagina. *Surg Clin North Am* 1978;58:25.

[b] Data from Perez CA, Camel HM. Long-term follow-up in radiation therapy of carcinoma of the vagina. *Cancer* 1982;49:1308.

[c] Data from Kucera H, Langer M, Smekal G, et al. Radiotherapy of primary carcinoma of the vagina: management and results of different therapy schemes. *Gynecik Ibcik* 1985;21:87.

[d] Not included in the figure 119 are 15 patients of the total patient group of 134 who were stage 0.

TABLE 34.4.
Carcinoma of the Vagina: Comparison of Survival

| Investigators | Years Studied | Stage | | | | |
		I	II	III	IV	Total
Puthawala et al., 1983	1976–1979	1/1 (100%)	12/16 (75%)	2/9 (22%)	0/1 (0%)	15/27 (56%)
Gallup et al., 1987	1971–1984	4/4 (100%)	6/12 (50%)	0/4 (0%)	2/8 (25%)	12/28 (43%)
Brown et al., 1971	1948–1967	11/16 (69%)	13/19 (68%)	4/15 (27%)	0/11 (0%)	28/61 (46%)
Nori et al., 1983	1950–1974	10/14 (71%)	4/6 (61%)	1/3 (33%)	0/13 (0%)	15/36 (42%)
Perez, 1981	1965–1981	26/32 (81%)	22/52 (42%)	3/10 (30%)	1/11 (9%)	52/105 (50%)
Prempree, 1982	1957–1975	7/9 (78%)	21/37 (57%)	10/26 (39%)	0/8 (0%)	38/80 (48%)
Benedet et al., 1983	1950–1980	20/28 (71%)	12/24 (50%)	2/13 (15%)	0/10 (0%)	34/75 (45%)
Manetta et al., 1988	1976–1986	5/7 (71%)	7/15 (47%)	1/3 (33%)	1/4 (33%)	14/29 (48%)

Adapted from Manetta A, Perito JL, Larson JE, et al. Primary invasive carcinoma of the vagina. *Obstet Gynecol* 1988;72:77.

lesions, 33% for stage IIb lesions, 33% for stage III lesions, and 19% for stage IV lesions. The actuarial study demonstrated that beyond stage I of the disease, control is poor. For stage IIa lesions, local control of the disease was achieved in only 65% of cases at the University of Maryland because external irradiation was not used in all cases. Pelvic control was achieved in 48% of stage IIb and stage III lesions, but in none of the seven patients (0%) with stage IV disease.

Overall survival rates for stages I through IV from published reports are outlined in Table 34.4. The highest survival rates are observed in stage I disease, whereas few patients survive for 5 years after the diagnosis of stage IV disease.

THE URETHRA

The female urethra develops from the caudal end of the UGS after it separates from the vaginal canal between the 8th and 12th week of embryologic life. Because the vagina and urethra are so closely integrated, the urethra shares many common disease processes and anatomic defects with the vagina. Bacteria in the lower genital tract frequently colonize in the outer urethra, harbor in the paraurethral glands, and enter the bladder to produce acute infections. A bacterial infection in the lower genital tract may not become clinically manifest for several years, until a Skene duct cyst or a urethral diverticulum develops.

Estrogen deficiency causes atrophic changes of the vaginal mucosa and can have a similar effect on the urethral mucosa. Thinning of the epithelium and irritation of the sensory nerve fibers can cause urinary frequency and dysuria. Prolapse at the external meatus also may result from atrophic changes of the urethra.

Diverticulum of the Urethra

Despite the many documented cases of urethral diverticula, the condition has not been well recognized by the medical profession. Anderson observed a urethral diverticulum in 3% of 300 cases undergoing treatment for cervical carcinoma. The condition probably occurs more frequently than it is diagnosed; whenever an article reporting on urethral diverticulum appears in the literature, there is a coincident upsurge in the number of cases diagnosed.

Etiology

In 1941, Parmenter suggested several congenital factors that could develop into a urethral diverticulum, including Gartner duct, a faulty union of primal folds, cell nets, and wolffian ducts or vaginal cysts that rupture into the urethra. Additional possible causes include trauma at childbirth, surgical trauma, urethral stone, urethral stricture, and infection of the urethral glands.

Of the many possible causes of urethral diverticula that have been considered, none have been proved. Two of the most probable causes are *Gonococcus neisseria* infection (although gonococci are seldom cultured) and infection of the suburethral tissue by vaginal flora. Huffman's experiments support the notion that a suburethral infection can develop into an abscess that becomes lined with epithelium. Huffman demonstrated periurethral openings by constructing wax models of infected urethras. The usual organisms cultured are *Escherichia coli, Aerobacter aerogenes,* and other gram-negative bacilli, *Staphylococcus aureus,* and *Streptococcus faecalis.*

Symptoms

Dysuria, urgency, frequency, and hematuria occurred together in 85% to 90% of 32 cases reviewed by Peters and Vaughn. Other frequently occurring symptoms are a lump in the vagina caused by protrusion of the diverticulum sac into the vagina, dyspareunia (intermittent discharge from the urethra), and pain on walking. Pyuria and cystitis also occur, depending on the location of the diverticular orifice. If the opening is sufficiently close to the outer end of the urethra, there may be no leakage of purulent exudate back into the bladder, which may explain the absence of symptoms of cystitis in 5% of cases.

If the diverticulum is located in the posterior urethra near the urethrovesical junction, stress urinary incontinence may be a significant symptom. In a review of 70 cases from the Johns Hopkins Hospital, Ginsberg and Genadry found that 17% of the diverticula were located in the proximal (outer) urethra, 43% in the midurethra, and 31% in the distal (posterior) urethra; in the remaining cases, the site was not specifically identified.

Not only are urinary tract symptoms the most common clinical expression of the urethral lesion, but a history of recurrent refractory cystitis is a clue that a diverticulum is the source of the infection.

Diagnosis

Urethral diverticula usually are small, varying from 3 mm to 3 cm in diameter. Some of the larger sacs cover the entire length of the urethra. On palpation of a suburethral mass, tenderness commonly is found. Pressure on the mass may cause the escape of urine or exudate from the urethral meatus.

An examination of the floor of the urethra through the water cystoscope while suburethral pressure is being applied reveals an opening in 50% to 70% of cases. The pressure may force contents of the diverticulum into the

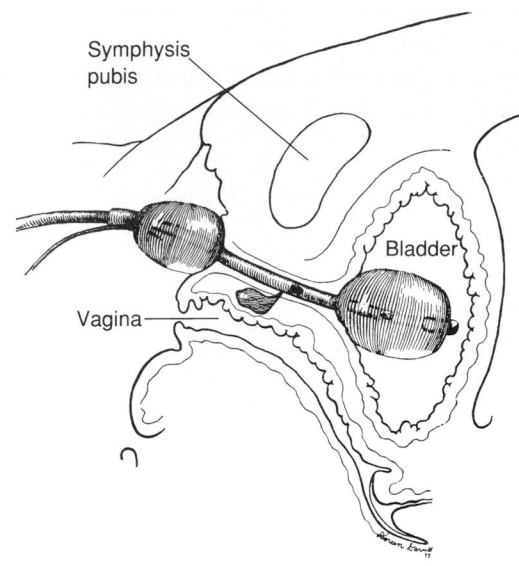

FIGURE 34.22. Double-ballooned catheter inserted for positive-pressure urethrography. (From Davis JH, Cian L. Positive-pressure urethrography: a new diagnostic method. *J Urol* 1958;80:34, with permission.)

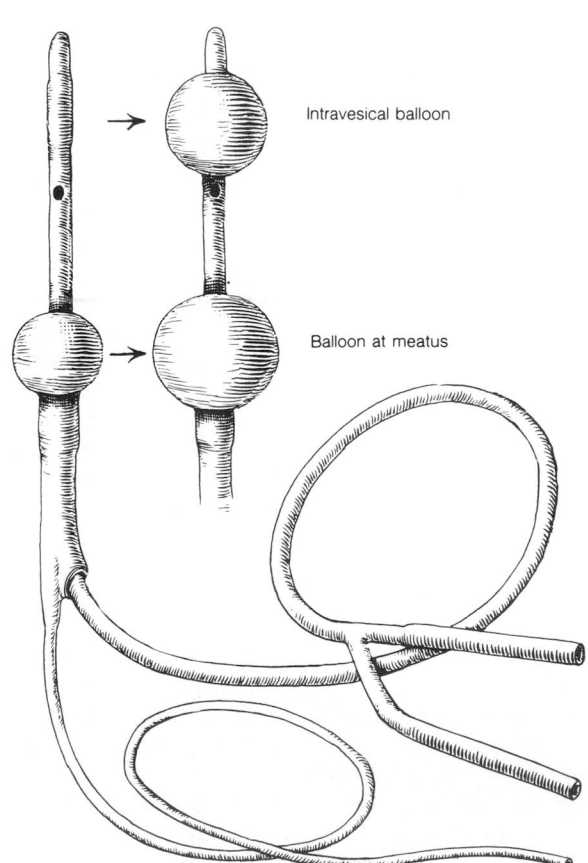

FIGURE 34.21. Double-ballooned catheter for positive-pressure urethrography. (From Davis JH, Cian L. Positive-pressure urethrography: a new diagnostic method. *J Urol* 1958;80:34, with permission.)

urethra while it is being viewed. Some of the openings are extremely small and may be missed. Inflammatory swelling can result in edema of the orifice, which makes visualization difficult or impossible.

The diagnosis of urethral diverticulum is firmly established by means of positive-pressure urethrography (PPUG). A special catheter is used to block the urethra at both ends and to fill it and the diverticulum under pressure with water-soluble contrast medium (Figs. 34.21 through 34.23). If the urethral orifice to the diverticulum is quite large, a voiding cystourethrogram together with a positive pelvic film may demonstrate the diverticulum. Although not as sensitive as PPUG, VCUG (voiding cystourethrography) may assist in identifying a urethral diverticulum. Wang compared VCUG and PPUG in evaluating 120 women. Twenty of 120 women demonstrated diverticulum. Thirteen were positive on PPUG and 10 with VCUG. If the surgeon's suspicion is high for urethral diverticulum, magnetic resonance imaging should be considered if both the PPUG and VCUG studies are negative.

Occasionally a diverticulum occurs with no clinical evidence of inflammation. If the diverticulum is diagnosed during a careful pelvic examination, and if the patient is completely asymptomatic except for a previous history of urinary tract problems, surgery is not necessary. With a complication rate of 15% to 20%, diverticulectomy should not be considered a quick and easy procedure. Removal of an asymptomatic urethral diverticulum may create more problems than it prevents, particularly if the sac is small or located in the floor of the posterior urethra. Only if a patient experiences acute or recurrent symptoms should urethral surgery be performed. Leng and McGuire classify urethral diverticulum as true versus pseudodiverticulum (Table 34.5).

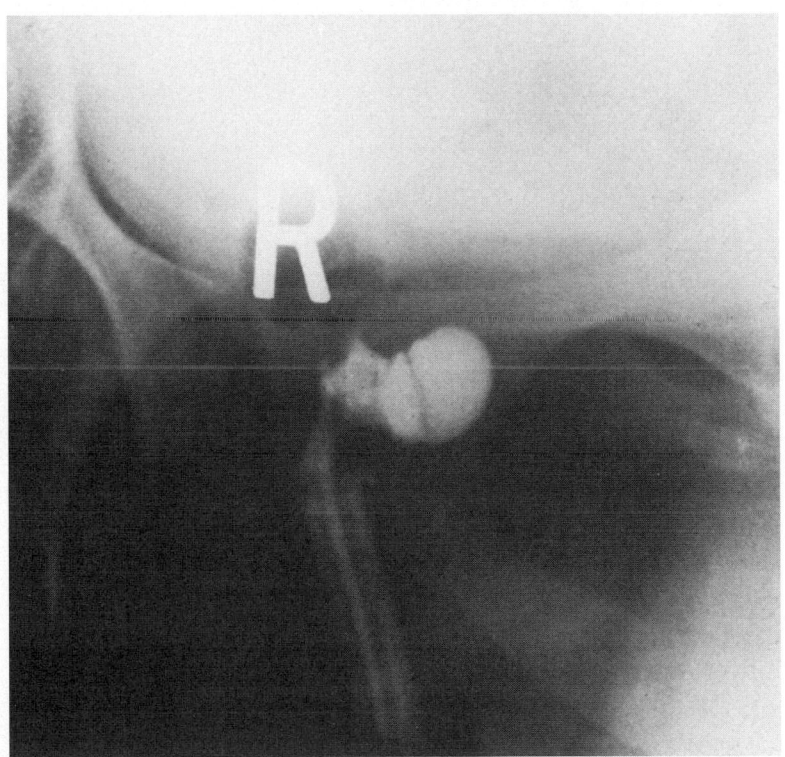

FIGURE 34.23. A large urethral diverticulum filled with contrast medium.

Treatment

A diverticulum that requires treatment must be completely excised before the defect in the urethra can be closed. Failure to remove the entire diverticulum results only in recurrence of the problem. Many techniques have been used to identify the anatomic boundaries of the diverticulum. One popular method is to pass a sound into the diverticulum through the urethral orifice. Another method is to distend the diverticulum by injecting it with fibrinogen and thrombin mixed in a syringe to form a firm fibrin clot. However, direct anatomic dissection of the diverticulum from the paraurethral fascia and vaginal wall without visual enhancement of the anatomic boundaries offers a better success rate. The smooth covering of a diverticulum protruding into the vagina can be easily distinguished from the rugal folds of the vaginal mucosa.

If the wall of the diverticulum is left unopened until the dissection has reached the base of the diverticulum sac, its neck can be visualized directly while it is removed. Inadvertent removal of a portion of the urethral floor along the base of the diverticulum is too common an error; if the mucosa is closed with too much tension, a urethral stricture or a postoperative fistula may result.

EXCISION AND LAYERED CLOSURE. A midline incision is made through the vaginal mucosa, which is then separated from the wall of the diverticulum (Fig. 34.24A). The wall of the diverticulum also is dissected from the paraurethral fascia in as wide a circumference as can be developed.

The diverticulum is opened and the interior of the cavity is inspected. If the orifice of the diverticulum is large, the opening of the urethra can easily be seen, especially if a catheter has been placed in the urethra and bladder (Fig. 34.24B). The rest of the thin, friable mucosa of the diverticulum is separated from the vaginal mucosa and fascia before the neck of the diverticulum is trimmed near the urethral orifice. The lining of the diverticulum is friable because of inflammatory changes and the thin layer fragments during the dissection. Meticulous sharp dissection is required to separate the

TABLE 34.5.
Urethral Diverticulum

True Diverticulum	Pseudodiverticulum
No prior urethral surgery	History of urethral surgery
Chronic recurring symptoms of urgency, dysuria, dyspareunia, dribbling	Relatively few voiding symptoms
Chronic lower urinary tract infections	Cystoscopy demonstrates broad-mouthed ostium to diverticulum
Narrow necked ostium not readily apparent on radiography or cystoscopy	More likely to have stress incontinence

From Leng WW, McGuire EJ. Management of female urethral diverticula: a new classification. *J Urol* 1998;160(4)1297–1300.

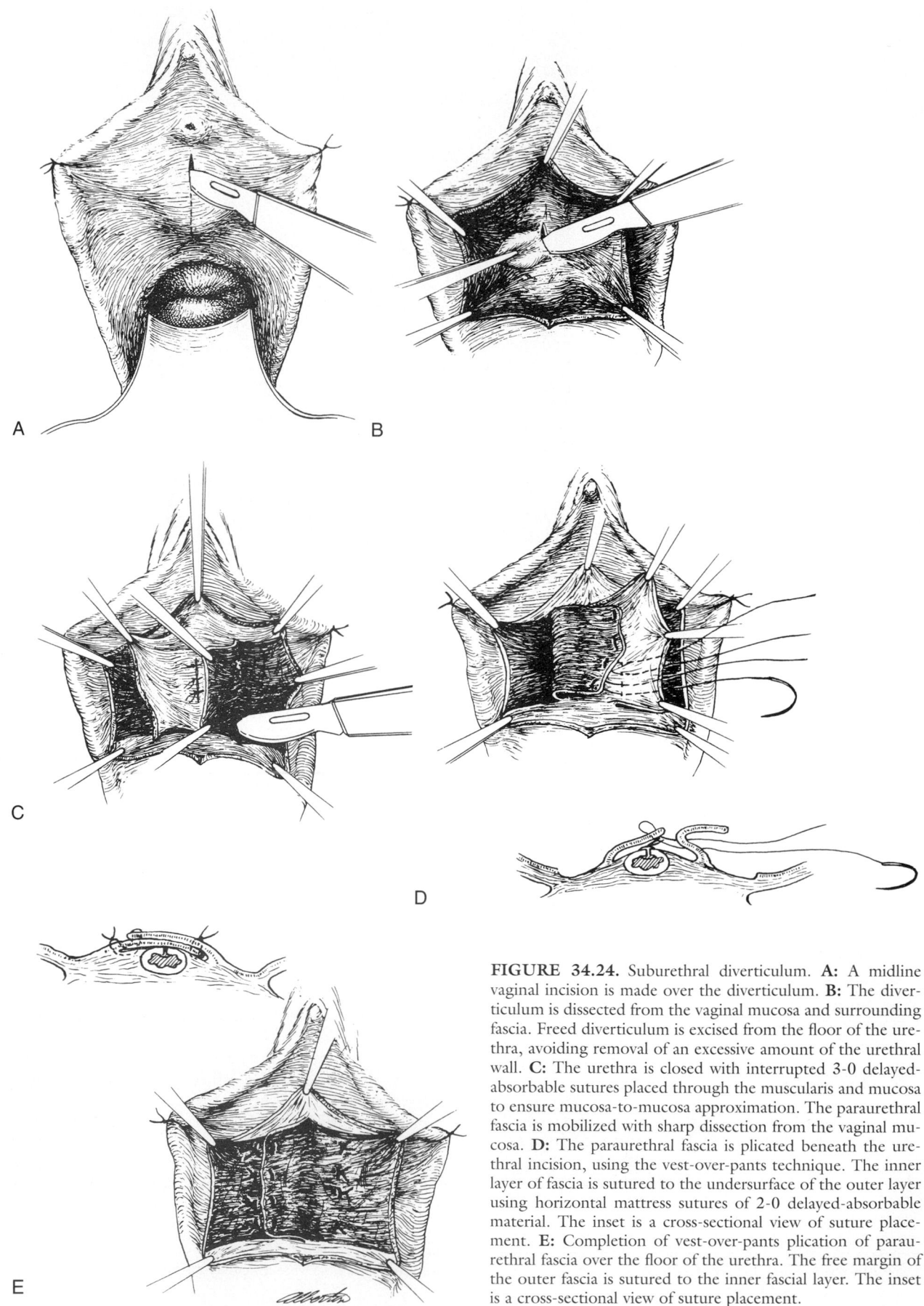

FIGURE 34.24. Suburethral diverticulum. **A:** A midline vaginal incision is made over the diverticulum. **B:** The diverticulum is dissected from the vaginal mucosa and surrounding fascia. Freed diverticulum is excised from the floor of the urethra, avoiding removal of an excessive amount of the urethral wall. **C:** The urethra is closed with interrupted 3-0 delayed-absorbable sutures placed through the muscularis and mucosa to ensure mucosa-to-mucosa approximation. The paraurethral fascia is mobilized with sharp dissection from the vaginal mucosa. **D:** The paraurethral fascia is plicated beneath the urethral incision, using the vest-over-pants technique. The inner layer of fascia is sutured to the undersurface of the outer layer using horizontal mattress sutures of 2-0 delayed-absorbable material. The inset is a cross-sectional view of suture placement. **E:** Completion of vest-over-pants plication of paraurethral fascia over the floor of the urethra. The free margin of the outer fascia is sutured to the inner fascial layer. The inset is a cross-sectional view of suture placement.

lining completely from the vagina and from the floor of the urethra. We repeat, in caution, that the neck of the diverticulum should be carefully resected to avoid eversion and to prevent the removal of mucosa from the urethral floor.

The urethral defect is closed with 3-0 delayed-absorbable sutures interrupted so that the edges can be inverted (Fig. 34.24C). After the interrupted sutures are tied, the paraurethral fascia is closed in a double-layer "vest-over-pants" technique in which the layer of fascia from one side of the urethra is sutured beneath the opposite and overlapping fascia and fastened to the urethral wall on that opposite side. The top layer of fascia is then sutured at its edge to the underlying fascial layer. The fascial margins are sutured by more durable 2-0 delayed-absorbable sutures (Fig. 34.23D and E), and the vaginal mucosa finally is trimmed and closed, also with interrupted 2-0 delayed-absorbable sutures. Faerber as well as Leng and McGuire have advocated diverticulectomy and placement of pubovaginal slings. Faerber uses the sling for intrinsic sphincter deficiency whereas Leng and McGuire have recommended fascial slings to close the defect if it is too large for reinforcement.

The bladder is filled with 300 mL of distilled water, and a suprapubic Silastic catheter is inserted and left in place until the morning of the fifth postoperative day. A suprapubic catheter is used in preference to a urethral catheter for three major reasons: to avoid trauma to the operative site, to avoid the necessity for transurethral catheterization during attempts to initiate voiding, and to avoid the discomfort of a urethral catheter. On the fifth day after surgery, the patient should attempt to void with the three-way stopcock of the suprapubic catheter closed to allow the bladder to fill.

URETHROTOMY. Urethrotomy has been used by Edwards and Beebe and by Kropp to treat diverticula. Splitting the floor of the urethra from the meatus down its full length to the site of the orifice of the diverticulum allows the sac to be well visualized during excision. As a rule, however, cases of urethral diverticula can be successfully repaired without such an extensive incision that requires the floor of the urethra to heal along its entire length. Healing is particularly a problem if there has been recent infection in the diverticulum.

MARSUPIALIZATION. In 1970, Spence and Duckett recommended marsupialization of the diverticulum to prevent recurrence, to minimize operating time, and to reduce blood loss. This procedure has been endorsed by Lichtman and Robertson and by Ginsberg and Genadry. Stress urinary incontinence has not been reported as a complication, but only, we suspect, because marsupialization is not used to treat lesions in the posterior urethra near the bladder base. Marsupialization is a useful procedure when diverticula occur in the outer third of the urethra, where a permanent opening in the outer floor of the urethra would not adversely influence intraurethral pressure.

Complications of Diverticulectomy

Complications arise in about 20% of cases treated for diverticula of the urethra. Urethral stricture can occur when too much urethral mucosa is removed, but strictures usually can be resolved by urethral dilatations. Urethral fistula, a serious and troublesome complication of diverticulectomy, occurs in about 5% of treated patients.

Postoperative fistulas frequently develop when acute or subacute infection in the walls of the diverticulum causes the urethral mucosa to become friable; the urinary incontinence that develops from urethral fistulas is far more troublesome than the initial symptoms of the diverticulum.

Closure of a urethral fistula is difficult because the blood supply to the floor of the urethra is delicate, and scarring and infection often develop with repeated efforts to close the urethra. A fistula in the outer part of the urethra may be asymptomatic and may not need to be repaired, but there normally are complaints with an outer fistula of spraying of urine when voiding.

Urethral Prolapse

Although there have been few recent reports of urethral prolapse, nearly 400 cases have been published in the English literature since 1732. More than half these cases occurred in infants and children; the remainder occurred in elderly patients.

Urethral prolapse is characterized by a sliding outward of the urethral mucosa around the entire urethral meatus. The urethra may become cyanotic, edematous, and infarcted (Fig. 34.25). Symptoms vary greatly. Prolapse may cause no discomfort, in which case it is detected only by bloody discharge of congested tissues that are breaking down, but more often there are complaints of severe and continuous pain, urinary frequency, and tenesmus. Occasionally, in a small child, tissue reaction and edema of the outer urethra produces urinary retention rather than the more usual urinary frequency.

Urethral prolapse is thought to be the result of poor development of or atrophic changes in the collagen and

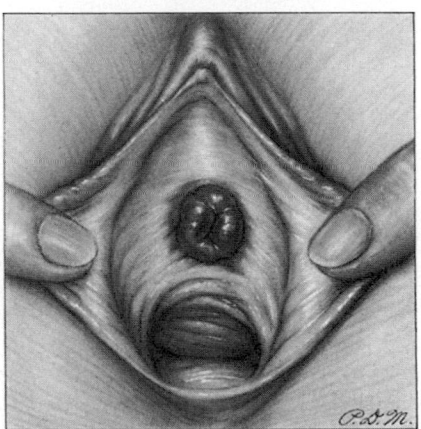

FIGURE 34.25. Prolapsed urethra.

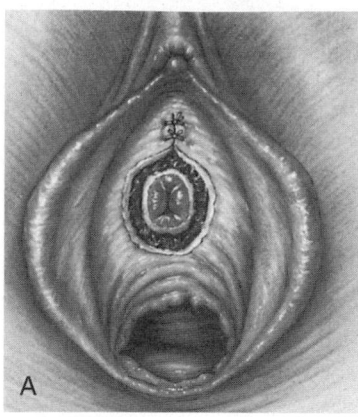
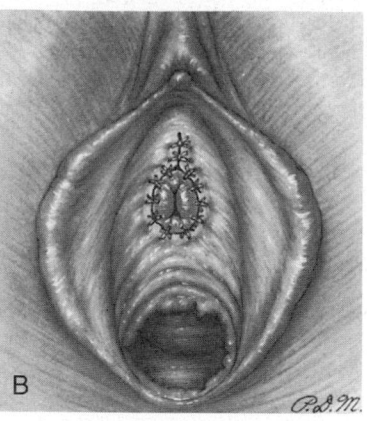

FIGURE 34.26. Operation for urethral prolapse. **A:** The prolapsed mucosa has been excised. **B:** Completed operation. Cut edges of urethral and vaginal mucosa are sutured with 3-0 delayed-absorbable sutures.

elastic tissues of the submucosa. In infants, prolapse usually follows a severe coughing or crying spell. In some older patients, too, prolapse has followed paroxysms of coughing. In older patients, diminished tone and elasticity of tissue alone may be sufficient to cause some cases of urethral prolapse.

Treatment of urethral prolapse may be palliative or surgical. Hot, moist compresses provide temporary comfort. A small mass of tissue can be reduced, but recurrence is common.

Surgical Techniques

Several surgical procedures have been suggested, including the one advocated by Kelly and Burnam in which the prolapsed mucosa is excised by a circular incision (Fig. 34.26A). The cut edges are then sutured with 3-0 delayed-absorbable suture material, avoiding an excessive number of stitches, which can result in stricture of the urethral meatus (Fig. 34.26B). In most cases this circumcision technique has proved to be the preferred method of correction.

Cryosurgery also has been used to treat urethral prolapse. The method is extremely effective in producing complete annular necrosis and healing of the prolapsed tissue (Fig. 34.27). The cryosurgery procedure can be performed without anesthesia, although for a young child a local anesthetic is advisable. A suprapubic Silastic catheter is inserted and is left in postopera-

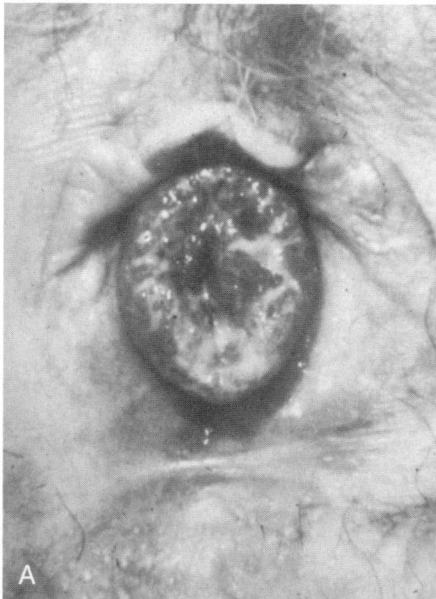
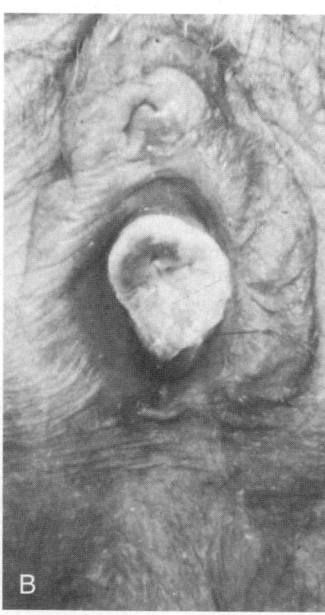
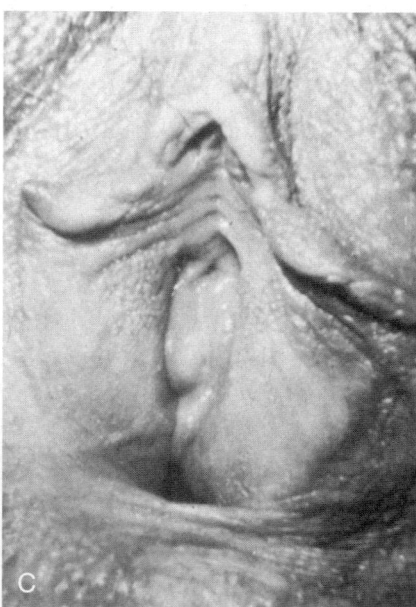

FIGURE 34.27. Cryosurgery in the treatment of urethral prolapse. **A:** Urethral prolapse in an elderly woman. **B:** Regression of urethral prolapse after cryosurgery. **C:** Repeated cryosurgery of urethral prolapse resulted in complete regression and healing of the urethral meatus within 8 weeks.

tively to permit bladder drainage until complete, spontaneous voiding can occur. The catheter also helps to prevent postoperative trauma at the suture line around the meatus.

BIBLIOGRAPHY

Al-Kurdi M, Monaghan JM. Thirty two years experience in management of primary tumors of the vagina. *Br J Obstet Gynaecol* 1981;88:1145.

Anderson MJ. The incidence of diverticula of the female urethra. *J Urol* 1967;98:96.

Azziz R, Mulaikal RM, Migeon CJ, et al. Congenital adrenal hyperplasia: long-term results following vaginal reconstruction. *Fertil Steril* 1986;46:1011.

Bailez MM, Gearhart JP, Migeon C, et al. Vaginal reconstruction after initial construction of the external genitalia in girls with salt-wasting adrenal hyperplasia. *J Urol* 1992;148:680.

Ball HG, Berman ML. Management of primary vaginal carcinoma. *Gynecol Oncol* 1982;14:154.

Bargy F, Laude F, Barbet JP, et al. The anatomy of intersexuality. *Surg Radiol Anat* 1989;11:103.

Baskin LS, Erol A, Li YW, et al. Anatomical studies of the human clitoris. *J Urol* 1999;162:1015.

Benedet JL, Murphy KJ, Fairey RN, et al. Primary invasive carcinoma of the vagina. *Obstet Gynecol* 1983;62:715.

Benjamin J, Elliott L, Cooper JF, et al. Urethral diverticulum in the adult female: clinical aspects, operative procedure, and pathology. *Urology* 1974;3:1.

Blaikley JB, Dewhurst CJ, Ferreira HP, et al. Vaginal adenosis: clinical and pathological features with special reference to malignant change. *J Obstet Gynaecol Br Commonw* 1971;78:1115.

Blakely CR, Mills WG. The obstetric and gynaecological complications of bladder exstrophy and epispadias. *Br J Obstet Gynaecol* 1981;88:167.

Breslow A. Thickness, cross-sectional areas, and depths of invasion in the prognosis of cutaneous melanoma. *Ann Surg* 1970;172:902.

Brown GR, Fletcher GH, Rutledge FN. Irradiation of in situ and invasive squamous cell carcinoma of the vagina. *Cancer* 1971;28:1278.

Burbige KA, Hensle TW, Chambers WJ, et al. Pregnancy and sexual function in women with bladder exstrophy. *Urology* 1986;28:120.

Choo YC, Anderson DG. Neoplasms of the vagina following cervical carcinoma. *Gynecol Oncol* 1982;14:125.

Chung AF, Casey MJ, Flanner JT, et al. Malignant melanoma of the vagina: report of 19 cases. *Obstet Gynecol* 1980;55:720.

Clemetson CA. Ectopia vesicae and split pelvis: an account of pregnancy in a woman with treated ectopia vesicae and split pelvis, including a review of the literature. *J Obstet Gynecol Br Emp* 1958;65:973.

Committee on Genetics, 1999–2000, Kaye CI, Cunniff C, et al. Evaluation of the newborn with developmental anomalies of the external genitalia. *Pediatrics* 2000;106:138.

Costa EM, Mendonca BB, Inacio M, et al. Management of ambiguous genitalia in pseudohermaphrodites: new perspectives on vaginal dilation. *Fertil Steril* 1997;67:229.

Creasman WT, Phillips JL, Menck HR. The National Cancer Data Base report on cancer of the vagina. *Cancer* 1998;83:1033.

Curra QJ, Rendtorff RC, Chandler RW, et al. Female gonorrhea: its relationship to abnormal uterine bleeding, urinary tract symptoms and cervicitis. *Obstet Gynecol* 1975;45:195.

Damario MA, Carpenter SE, Jones HW Jr, et al. Reconstruction of the external genitalia in females with bladder exstrophy. *Int J Gynaecol Obstet* 1994;44:245.

Davis BL, Robinson DG. Diverticula of the female urethra: assay of 120 cases. *J Urol* 1970;104:850.

Davis HJ, Cian LG. Positive pressure urethrography: a new diagnostic method. *J Urol* 1958;80:34.

Davis IIJ, Te Linde RW. Urethral diverticula: an assay of 121 cases. *J Urol* 1956;75:753.

Dewhurst J, Topliss PH, Shepherd JH. Ivalon sponge hysterosacropexy for genital prolapse in patients with bladder exstrophy. *Br J Obstet Gynaecol* 1980;87:67.

DiSaia PJ, Morrow CP, Townsend DE. *Synopsis of gynecologic oncology.* New York: John Wiley & Sons, 1975.

Eddy GL, Marks RD, Miler MC III, et al. Primary invasive vaginal carcinoma. *Am J Obstet Gynecol* 1991;165:282.

Edwards E, Beebe RA. Diverticula of female urethra. Review: new procedure for treatment: report of 5 cases. *Obstet Gynecol* 1955;5:729.

Faerber GJ. Urethral diverticulectomy and pubovaginal sling for simultaneous treatment of urethral diverticulum and intrinsic sphincter deficiency. *Techniques in Urology* 1998;4:192.

Fenoglio C, Ferenczy A, Richard RM, et al. Scanning and transmission electron microscopic studies of vaginal adenosis and the cervical transformation zone in progeny exposed in utero to diethyl-stilbestrol. *Am J Obstet Gynecol* 1976;126:170.

Fortunoff FS, Latimer JK, Edson M. Vaginoplasty technique for female pseudohermaphrodites. *Surg Gynecol Obstet* 1964;118:545.

Frick HC. Primary carcinoma of the vagina. *Am J Obstet Gynecol* 1968;101:695.

Frick HC, Jacox HW, Taylor HC. Primary carcinoma of the vagina. *Am J Obstet Gynecol* 1968;101:695.

Gallup DG, Morley GW. Carcinoma in situ of the vagina: a study and review. *Obstet Gynecol* 1975;46:334.

Gallup DG, Talledo OE, Shah KJ, et al. Invasive squamous cell carcinoma of the vagina: a 14-year-old study. *Obstet Gynecol* 1987;69:782.

Gearhart JP, Jeffs RD. State-of-the-art reconstructive surgery for bladder exstrophy at the Johns Hopkins Hospital. *Am J Dis Child* 1989;143:1475.

Gerharz EW, Hohl UN, Weingartner K, et al. Experience with the Mainz modification of ureterosigmoidostomy. *Br J Surg* 1998;86:427.

Ginsberg DS, Genadry R. Suburethral diverticulum: classification and therapeutic considerations. *Obstet Gynecol* 1983;61:685.

Hamilton W, Boyd JD, Mossman HW. *Human embryology,* third ed. Cambridge: W Heffer & Sons, 1962.

Hendren WH. Surgical management of urogenital sinus abnormalities. *J Pediatr Surg* 1977;12:339.

Hendren WH. Reconstructive problems of the vagina and the female urethra. *Clin Plast Surg* 1980;7:207.

Hendren WH, Crawford JD. Adrenogenital syndrome: the anatomy of the anomaly and its repair. *J Pediatr Surg* 1969;4:49.

Herbst AL, Cole P, Norusis MJ, et al. Epidemiologic aspects and factors related to survival in 384 registry cases of clear cell adenocarcinoma of the vagina and cervix. *Am J Obstet Gynecol* 1979;153:876.

Herbst AL, Scully RE, Robbo SJ. The significance of adenosis and clear-cell adenocarcinoma of the genital tract in young females. *J Reprod Med* 1975;14:5.

Herbst AL, Ulfelder H, Poskanzer EC. Adenocarcinoma of the vagina: association of maternal stilbestrol therapy with tumor appearing in young women. *N Engl J Med* 1971;284:878.

Herman JM, Homesley HD, Dignan MB. Is hysterectomy a risk factor for vaginal cancer? *JAMA* 1986;256:601.

Herzog TJ, Rader JS. The ultrasonic surgical aspirator in the gynecologic oncology patient. In: Rock JA, Faro S, Gant NF Jr, et al, eds. *Advances in obstetrics and gynecology,* vol 1. St Louis: Mosby–Year Book, 1994:325.

Hilgers RD. Pelvic exenteration for vaginal embryonal rhabdomyosarcoma: a review. *Obstet Gynecol* 1975;45:175.

Hilgers RD. Squamous cell carcinoma of the vagina. *Surg Clin North Am* 1978;58:25.

Hines M. Abnormal sexual development and psychosexual issues. *Baillieres Clin Endocrinol Metabol* 1998;12:173.

Hines M, Kaufman FR. Androgen and the development of human sex-typical behavior: rough-and-tumble play and sex preferred playmates in children with congenital adrenal hyperplasia (CAH). *Child Dev* 1994;65:1042.

Hoffman MJ, Adams WE. Recognition and repair of urethral diverticula. *Am J Obstet Gynecol* 1965;92:106.

Hopkins MP, Morley GW. Squamous cell carcinoma of the neovagina. *Obstet Gynecol* 1987;69:525.

Houghton CRS, Iversen T. Squamous cell carcinoma of the vagina: a clinical study of the location of the tumor. *Gynecol Oncol* 1982;13:365.

Huffman JW. The detailed anatomy of the paraurethral ducts in the adult human female. *Am J Obstet Gynecol* 1948;55:86.

Hutch JA. *Anatomy and physiology of the bladder, trigone and urethra.* New York: Appleton-Century-Crofts, 1972.

International Federation of Obstetrics and Gynecology. *Annual report on the results of treatment of carcinoma of the uterus, vagina and ovary,* vol 18. Stockholm: Norestedt, 1982.

Jones HW Jr. An anomaly of the external genitalia in female patients with exstrophy of the bladder. *Am J Obstet Gynecol* 1973;117(6):748.

Jones HW Jr, Verkauf BS. Surgical treatment in congenital adrenal hyperplasia: age at operation and other prognostic factors. *Obstet Gynecol* 1970;36:1.

Kamat MH, DelGaiso A, Seebode D. Urethral prolapse in female children. *Am J Dis Child* 1969;118:691.

Kanbour AE, Klionsky BK, Murphy AL. Carcinoma of the vagina following cervical cancer. *Cancer* 1974;34:1838.

Kelly HA, Burnam CF. Malfunctions of the urethra. In: Kelly HA, ed. *Diseases of the kidneys, ureters, and bladder.* New York: D Appleton, 1922:564.

Klaus H, Stein RT. Urethral prolapse in young girls. *Pediatrics* 1973;52:645.

Klobe JM. Pathologische Anatomieder weiblichen sexual Organe. *Vien* 1864.

Kogan SJ, Smey P, Levitt SB. Subtunical total reduction clitoroplasty: a safe modification of existing techniques. *J Urol* 1983:746.

Krege S, Walz KH, Hauffa BP, et al. Long-term follow-up of female patients with congenital adrenal hyperplasia from 21-hydroxylase deficiency, with special emphasis on the results of vaginoplasty. *Br J Urol Int* 2000;86:253.

Krisiloff M, Puchner PJ, Tretter W, et al. Pregnancy in women with bladder exstrophy. *J Urol* 1978;119:478.

Kropp KA. The female urethra. In: Glenn JF, ed. *Urologic surgery.* Hagerstown, MD: Harper & Row, 1975.

Kucera H, Langer M, Smekal G, et al. Radiotherapy of primary carcinoma of the vagina: management and results of different therapy schemes. *Gynecik Ibcik* 1985;21:87.

Latourette HB. End results of treatment of cancer of vagina. *Ann N Y Acad Sci* 1964;114:1020.

Lee RA, Symmonds RE. Recurrent carcinoma in situ of the vagina in patients previously treated for in situ carcinoma of the cervix. *Obstet Gynecol* 1976;48:61.

Lee RA. Diverticulum of the urethra: clinical presentation, diagnosis and management. *Clin Obstet Gynecol* 1984;27:490.

Leng WW, McGuire EJ. Management of female urethral diverticula: a new classification. *J Urol* 1998;160:1297.

Lichtman A, Robertson J. Suburethral diverticula treated by marsupialization. *Obstet Gynecol* 1976;47:203.

Lintgen C, Herbert P. Clinical-pathological study of 100 female urethras. *J Urol* 1946;55:298.

Livermore GR. Treatment of prolapse of the urethra. *Surg Gynecol Obstet* 1921;32:557.

Magrina JF, Walter AJ, Schild SE. Laparoscopic radical parametrectomy and pelvic and aortic lymphadenectomy for vaginal carcinoma: A case report. *Gynecol Oncol* 1999;75:514.

Manetta A, Gutrecht EL, Berman ML, et al. Primary invasive carcinoma of the vagina. *Obstet Gynecol* 1990;76:639.

Manetta A, Perito JL, Larson JE, et al. Primary invasive carcinoma of the vagina. *Obstet Gynecol* 1988;72:77.

Marcus R Jr, Million RR, Daly JW. Carcinoma of the vagina. *Cancer* 1978;42:2507.

Marcus SL. Multiple squamous cell carcinoma involving the cervix, vagina and vulva: the theory of multicentric origin. *Am J Obstet Gynecol* 1960;80:802.

Melneck S, Cole P, Anderson D, et al. Rates and risks of DES-related clear cell adenocarcinoma of the vagina and cervix. *N Engl J Med* 1987;316:514.

Merino MJ. Vaginal cancer: the role of infectious and environmental factors [Review]. *Am J Obstet Gynecol* 1991;165:1255.

Mingin GC, Stock JA, Hanna MK. The Mainz II pouch: experience in 5 patients with bladder exstrophy. *J Urol* 1999;162:846.

Mor N, Merlob P, Reisner SH. Types of hymen in the newborn infant. *Eur J Obstet Gynecol Reprod Biol* 1986;22:225.

Murad TM, et al. The pathologic behavior of primary vaginal carcinoma and its relationship to cervical cancer. *Cancer* 1975;35:787.

Ng AB, Reagan JW, Hawliczek S, et al. Cellular detection of vaginal adenosis. *Obstet Gynecol* 1975;46:323.

Nori D, Hilaris B, Stanimir G, et al. Radiation therapy of primary vaginal carcinoma. *Int J Radiat Oncol Biol Phys* 1983;8:1471.

Nori D, Hilaris BS, Shu F. Radiation therapy of primary vaginal carcinoma. *Int J Radiat Oncol Biol Phys* 1981;70:20.

Parmenter FJ. Diverticulum of the urethra. *J Urol* 1941;45:749.

Passerini-Glazel G. A new 1-stage procedure for clitorovaginoplasty in severely masculinized female pseudohermaphrodites. *J Urol* 1989; 142:565.

Pathak UN, House MJ. Diverticulum of the female urethra. *Obstet Gynecol* 1970;36:789.

Perez CA. Definitive radiotherapy for carcinoma of the vagina. *Int J Radiat Oncol Biol Phys* 1981;7:20.

Perez CA, Arneson AN, Dehner LP, et al. Radiation therapy in carcinoma of the vagina. *Obstet Gynecol* 1974;44:862.

Perez CA, Arneson AN, Galakatos A, et al. Malignant tumors of the vagina. *Cancer* 1973;31:36.

Perez CA, Camel HM. Long-term follow-up in radiation therapy of carcinoma of the vagina. *Cancer* 1982;49:1308.

Peters WA III, Kumar NB, Morley GW. Carcinoma of the vagina. *Cancer* 1985;55:892.

Peters WA, Vaughn EJ Jr. Urethral diverticula in the female: etiologic factors and postoperative results. *Obstet Gynecol* 1976;47:549.

Pettersson F. *Annual report on the results of treatment in gynecological cancer.* Stockholm: FIGO, 1988:174.

Pirtoli L, Santoni R. Radiation therapy of the primary vaginal carcinoma. *Acta Radiol Oncol Radiat Phys Biol* 1980;19:353.

Plentl AA, Friedman EA. *Lymphatic system of the female genital tract.* Philadelphia: WB Saunders, 1971.

Pokorny SF, Kozinetz CA. Configuration and other anatomic details of the prepubertal hymen. *Adolesc Pediatr Gynecol* 1988;1:97.

Prempree T. Role of radiation therapy in the management of primary carcinoma of the vagina. *Acta Radiol [Oncol]* 1982;21:195.

Prempree T, Vlravathana T, Slawson RG, et al. Radiation management of primary carcinoma of the vagina. *Cancer* 1977;40:101.

Pride GL, Bucher DA. Carcinoma of vagina 10 or more years following pelvic irradiation therapy. *Am J Obstet Gynecol* 1977;127:513.

Pride GL, Schultz AE, Chuprevich TW, et al. Primary invasive carcinoma of the vagina. *Obstet Gynecol* 1979;53:218.

Puthawala A, Sved AM, Nalick R, et al. Integrated external and interstitial radiation therapy for primary carcinoma of the vagina. *Obstet Gynecol* 1983;62:367.

Rajfer J, Ehrlich RM, Goodwin WE. Reduction clitoroplasty via ventral approach. *J Urol* 1982;128:341.

Rastogi BL, Bergman B, Angawall L. Primary leiomyosarcoma of the vagina: a study of five cases. *Gynecol Oncol* 1984;18:77.

Reddy S, Lee MS, Graham JE, et al. Radiation therapy in primary carcinoma of the vagina. *Gynecol Oncol* 1987;26:19.

Reid GC, Schmidt RW, Roberts JA, et al. Primary melanoma of the vagina: a clinicopathologic analysis. *Obstet Gynecol* 1989;764:190.

Reiner WG. Sex assignment in the neonate with intersex or inadequate genitalia. *Arch Pediatr Adolesc Med* 1997;151:1044.

Reuben SC, Young J, Mikuta JJ. Squamous carcinoma of the vagina: treatment, complications, and long-term follow-up. *Gynecol Oncol* 1985;20:346.

Ricci G, Gentili A, Di Lorenzo F, et al. Latex allergy in subjects who had undergone multiple surgical procedures for bladder exstrophy: relationship with clinical intervention and atopic diseases. *BJU Int* 1999;84:1058.

Ries J, Ludwig H. Zur therapie des primaren karzinoms der vagina. *Strahlentherapie* 1962;118:92.

Rink RC, Adams MC. Feminizing genitoplasty: state of the art. *World J Urol* 1998;16:212.

Rink RC, Pope JC, Kropp BP, et al. Reconstruction of the high urogenital sinus: early perineal prone approach without division of the rectum. *J Urol* 1997;158:1293.

Robinson JB, Sun CC, Bodurka-Bevers D, et al. Cavitational ultrasonic surgical aspiration for the treatment of vaginal intraepithelial neoplasia. *Gynecol Oncol* 2000;78:235.

Rock JA, Katz E. Ambiguous genitalia. *Semin Reprod Endocr* 1987;5:327.

Rock JA, Schlaff WD. Congenital adrenal hyperplasia: the surgical treatment of vaginal stenosis. *Int J Gynaecol Obstet* 1986;24:417.

Rock JA, Zacur HA, Dlugi AM, et al. Pregnancy success following the surgical correction of imperforate hymen as compared to the complete transverse vaginal septum. *Obstet Gynecol* 1982;59:448.

Rubin SC, Young J, Mikuta JJ. Squamous carcinoma of the vagina: treatment, complications, and long-term follow-up. *Gynecol Oncol* 1985;20:346.

Rutledge FN. Cancer of the vagina. *Am J Obstet Gynecol* 1967;97:635.

Rutledge FN, Boronow RC, Wharton JT. *Gynecologic oncology.* New York: John Wiley & Sons, 1976.

Sander R, Nuss RC, Rhadgan RM. DES-associated vaginal adenosis followed by clear-cell adenocarcinoma. *Int J Gynecol Pathol* 1986;5:362.

Schubert G. Uber scheidenbildung bei angeborenem vaginaldefekt. *Zbl Gynak* 1911;45:1017.

Sholem SL, Wechsler M, Roberts M. Management of the urethral diverticulum in women: a modified operative technique. *J Urol* 1974;112:485.

Smith FR. Clinical management of cancer of the vagina. *Ann N Y Acad Sci* 1964;114.1012.

Smith WG. Invasive carcinoma of the vagina. *Clin Obstet Gynecol* 1981;24:503.

Spence H, Duckett J. Diverticulum of the female urethra: clinical aspects and presentation of simple operative technique for cure. *J Urol* 1970;104:432.

Spirtos IM, Doshi BP, Kapp DS, et al. Radiation therapy for primary squamous cell carcinoma of the vagina: the Stanford University experience. *Gynecol Oncol* 1989;35:20.

Stafl A, Mattingly RF. Vaginal adenosis: a precancerous lesion? *Am J Obstet Gynecol* 1974;120:666.

Stanton SL. Gynecologic complications of epispadias and bladder exstrophy. *Am J Obstet Gynecol* 1974;119:749.

Stelling JR, Gray MR, Davis AJ, et al. Dominant transmission of imperforate hymen. *Fertil Steril* 2000;74:1241.

Stern A, Patel S. Diverticulum of the female urethra: value of the postvoid bladder film during excretory urography. *Radiology* 1976;121:22.

Stock RG, Chen AS, Seski J. A 30-year experience in the management of primary carcinoma of the vagina: analysis of prognostic factors and treatment modalities. *Gynecol Oncol* 1995;56:45.

Stuart GC, Allen HH, Anderson RJ. Squamous cell carcinoma of the vagina following hysterectomy. *Am J Obstet Gynecol* 1981;139:311.

Tait L. Sacular dilatation of the urethra: removal, cure. *Lancet* 1875;2:625.

Thigpen JT, et al. A phase II trial of cisplatin in advanced recurrent cancer of the vagina: a GOG study. *Gynecol Oncol* 1986;23:101.

Underwood PB, Smith RT. Carcinoma of the vagina. *JAMA* 1971;217:46.

Usherwood MM. Management of vaginal carcinoma after hysterectomy. *Am J Obstet Gynecol* 1975;122:352.

Wang AC, Wang CR. Radiologic diagnosis and surgical treatment of urethral diverticulum in women. A reappraisal of voiding cystourethrography and positive pressure urethrography. *J Reprod Med* 2000;45:377.

Weed JC, Lozier C, Daniel SJ. Human papilloma virus in multifocal, invasive female tract malignancy. *Obstet Gynecol* 1983;62:832.

Wharton JT. Carcinoma of the vagina and urethra. In: Rovinsky D, ed. *Obstetrics and gynecology.* Hagerstown, MD: Harper & Row, 1972.

Wharton JT. Carcinoma of the vagina. In: Rutledge F, Boronow RC, Wharton JT, eds. *Gynecologic oncology.* New York: John Wiley & Sons, 1976:259.

Wharton JT, Kearns W. Diverticulum of the female urethra. *J Urol* 1950;63:1063.

Wheeless CR Jr, McGibbon B, Dorsey JH, et al. Gracilis myocutaneous flap in reconstruction of the vulva and female perineum. *Obstet Gynecol* 1979;54:97.

Whelton JA, Kottmeier HL. Primary carcinoma of the vagina. *Acta Obstet Gynecol Scand* 1962;41:22.

Winderl LM, Silverman RK. Prenatal diagnosis of congenital imperforate hymen. *Obstet Gynecol* 1995; 85(5 pt 2):857.

Woodruff JD, Parmley TH. Epidermoid carcinoma of the vagina. In: Hafez EC, Evans TN, eds. *The human vagina*. New York: Elsevier North Holland, 1979.

Young HH. *Genital abnormalities, hermaphroditism and related adrenal diseases*. Baltimore: Williams & Wilkins, 1937.

Young RH, Scully RE. Endodermal sinus tumor of the vagina: a report of nine cases and review of the literature. *Gynecol Oncol* 1984;18:380.

SURGERY FOR CORRECTION OF DEFECTS IN PELVIC SUPPORT AND PELVIC FISTULAS

Te Linde's Operative Gynecology, ninth edition, edited by John A. Rock and Howard W. Jones, III. Lippincott Williams & Wilkins, Philadelphia © 2003.

CHAPTER

35

Surgical Correction of Defects in Pelvic Support

A

Pelvic Organ Prolapse

CARL W. ZIMMERMAN

The judgment as to surgical correction should depend upon a correlation of the history and physical findings. Even marked prolapse in the absence of complaint should rarely be corrected. The patient should ask the gynecologist for relief; the gynecologist should not urge the patient to have corrective surgery if she does not feel sufficiently uncomfortable to request it.

Te Linde, 1966

BASIC CONCEPTS

Pelvic organ prolapse is the downward displacement of structures that are normally located adjacent to the vaginal vault. Because these displacements are each associated with a defect in support structures, they may each be considered hernias. These conditions are common, affecting a progressively larger percentage of women as age advances. Whereas mortality is negligible,

significant morbidity is associated with prolapse. Women in developed countries who have access to modern health care can benefit from the advances that have been made in treating prolapse. If the problem is viewed from a worldwide perspective, however, the scope of suffering is much greater. In areas of high parity and little or no access to health care, countless women suffer from problems associated with pelvic organ prolapse with no real possibility of resolution. The direct effect that these conditions have on urinary, gastrointestinal, and sexual functions can only be appreciated by those women burdened with these problems on a daily basis.

Treatment of pelvic organ prolapse and the associated symptoms constitutes a major subject in gynecology. Especially in the advanced state, treatment of these conditions is one of the most challenging problems pelvic surgeons can face. Indeed, success in treating prolapse is frequently used to judge the skill of those surgeons. Providing permanent relief from this classic malady, by restoring normal anatomy and maximum physiologic function, always tests the ingenuity of gynecologists. As medical sophistication has progressed, so has the ability to understand more completely and better treat pelvic organ prolapse.

A brief review of the history of treatment of prolapse is helpful in understanding modern treatments and current concepts of these conditions. Because it was mentioned in the writings of Hippocrates and Galen, prolapse was clearly known to the ancients. Early treatments may seem quaint by today's standards. Yet, some of these interventions continue to be used today. Fortunately, others have not survived. Vaginal packing, tampons, massages, and exercises were used with some success. Other patients were suspended from their feet for a period of 24 hours to treat prolapse. Rodericus A. Castro advised that prolapse should be attacked with a red hot iron as if to burn it, "when fright would cause it to recede into the vagina." Various caustics were used, including silver nitrate, nitric acid, acid nitrate of mercury, hot metal, and sulfuric acid.

Perhaps the first real advance in treatment was the development of pessaries. These devices functioned as trusses. Their fitting and placement became an art form. They continue to bring relief to a large number of women without doing serious harm. They were especially popular in the middle of the 19th century. Some were held in place by waistbands. In some cases, pessaries were deliberately left in place until erosions occurred. The subsequent healing was expected to reduce the caliber of the vagina with scarification adding to support, but serious complications could occur. Reports exist of neglected pessaries being retrieved from the peritoneal cavity.

The earliest surgical attempts to relieve prolapse were relatively simple. These procedures included labial suturing and removing portions of the vaginal epithelium to reduce the caliber of the vaginal vault. Although Heming operated on the anterior vaginal wall in 1831, surgery for uterovaginal prolapse was not common until the advent of anesthesia and antisepsis in the middle of the nineteenth century. The first vaginal hysterectomy for prolapse was performed by Samuel Choppin of New Orleans in 1861. Many years passed before this surgical application became common. By the beginning of the 20th century, European and American reports of hysterectomy, colporrhaphy, cervical amputation, transposition/interposition operations (Manchester-Fothergill), cervical ligament plications, colpocleisis (LeFort), ventral fixation of the uterus to the abdominal wall, and trachelorrhaphy for procidentia were being published. The timing of this ingenious variety of operations is certainly consistent with the development of surgical procedures in all fields of medicine.

During the 20th century, advances in understanding and treatment of prolapse have progressed at an ever-increasing rate. In 1909, George R. White of Georgia published an account of cystocele repair using a transvaginal paravaginal approach. This report appears seminal and modern when viewed from today's perspective. His correct perspective on the importance of lateral vaginal support took nearly 50 years to be rediscovered by mainstream gynecologic surgeons. The paravaginal repair was not widely known and accepted at the time because it was overshadowed by the work of Howard A. Kelly of Johns Hopkins. This great and influential surgeon popularized the concept of fascial attenuation. Midline anterior and posterior plications were touted as the correct surgical approach to the problem of prolapse. The Kelly-Kennedy anterior plication and levator ani plication of the posterior vaginal wall remain as commonly performed procedures today.

In the 1950s, Milton L. McCall of Louisiana developed a culdoplasty technique that emphasized the importance of the uterosacral ligament. He believed this operation prevented enteroceles and posthysterectomy vaginal vault prolapse when it was performed at the time of hysterectomy. Currently, the restitution of vaginal vault support at the time of any type of hysterectomy is considered a very important step in prevention of future prolapse.

In the 1960s, Baden and Walker of Texas began to systemize a new defect-specific approach to pelvic organ prolapse repair. Page 1 of their 1992 book stated, "In a sense, the defect approach reverses the prior evolution toward 'compensatory' reparative techniques—our goal is to return all vaginal supports to their original anatomic status." Many other surgeons have contributed to this powerful concept of pelvic reconstructive surgery. A. Cullen Richardson of Georgia developed the concept of classifying fascial defects as proximal, distal, central, and lateral. This observation and the teaching of such master surgeons as David H. Nichols of Rhode Island and Massachusetts encouraged gynecologists to not only identify and repair each vaginal defect but to return support attachments to their original anatomic location. Emphasis was focused on the hernial nature of prolapse, which led to the abandonment of absorbable suture in favor of permanent suture in repairs. In the 1990s, pelvic anatomist John O. L. DeLancey of Michigan published a biomechanical analysis of normal vaginal anatomy. His observations have the precision of an engineer's work and identify specific surgical goals for each of three vaginal levels of support. Proximal vaginal suspension, mid-vaginal lateral attachment, and distal vaginal fusion to the perineum and urogenital fascia are the basic concepts modern pelvic surgeons must satisfy to complete a prolapse surgery.

A fusion of anatomic, physiologic, and biomechanical principles has allowed surgeons to offer their patients better treatments for prolapse than have historically been available. This brief and incomplete historical discussion outlines the evolution of the current understanding of a complex topic. Historically ineffective treatments of the presurgical era gave way to surgical approaches for advanced cases. In surgery, anatomically distorting operations have been replaced by anatomically restoring procedures.

There are many interesting aspects of the historical development of this subject; refer to previous editions of this book and to the bibliographic selections at the end of this section for additional material.

A better understanding of a problem always leads to more questions that deserve answers. For example, the process of childbirth is regarded as an important cause of vaginal prolapse. Little or no effort has been made to analyze the forces of childbirth as they relate to specific patterns of damage to the deep endopelvic connective tissue. Delineation of these patterns would assist the surgeon in recognizing defects and undoubtedly improving operative outcome. A better understanding of the effects of labor and delivery might also lead to techniques designed to reduce the potentially damaging effects of these obstetric events. Prolapse prevention is underused in the practice of gynecology. Teaching patients about physical therapy of the pelvic floor, better lifestyle, and proper evacuation habits should be part of the gynecologist's job. The long-term benefits of an organized program of prolapse prevention have never been evaluated.

Controversy exists as to the best surgical management for specific cases of female pelvic organ prolapse. In fact, now that reparative options are no longer limited to midline plications, more procedures are available than ever before. Vaginal, abdominal, laparoscopic, minimally invasive devices, and combined approaches have their advocates. The necessary randomized trials with matched controls will likely never be done to generate evidence-based outcomes, especially because two of the most powerful variables are surgical skill and experience. Surgical techniques for prolapse must be carefully evaluated so that anatomic and functional results will continue to improve.

The authors in the various sections of this chapter describe operations that gynecologic surgeons should consider when repairing pelvic organ prolapse. Each of these surgeons possesses a combination of operative skill, experience, and special interest in their topics that have led to their selection. The operative techniques presented should be combined with appropriate clinical evaluation and skillful technical performance to obtain maximum benefit for the patients.

ANATOMIC CONSIDERATIONS

The normal position and support of the uterus, vagina, bladder, and rectum rely on an interdependent system of bony, muscular, and connective tissue elements. This entire system of support is three-dimensional, and even subtle alterations in one part may lead to stresses in other parts that eventually lead to failure of normal anatomy. An understanding of normal applied pelvic anatomy is imperative in the repair of pelvic organ prolapse.

The bony pelvis has a central opening that is necessary for reproductive function. During evolutional transition to upright bipedal posture, the potential for prolapse became more likely because of gravitational stress. In the human female, a lordosis of the lumbosacral portion of the spine places the pelvic inlet in a position rem-

iniscent of the posture of a quadruped. The physical result of this shift is that the posterior aspect of the pelvic inlet is approximately 60 degrees above the anterior aspect (Fig. 35A.1). The more vertical orientation of the pelvic inlet deflects force onto the superior symphysis pubis rather than the pelvic outlet and urogenital hiatus. Consequently, the pelvic outlet is shielded from downward stresses in the anatomically normal woman.

The muscles of the pelvic diaphragm primarily provide pelvic support. These muscles form a basin or covering of the pelvic outlet and are often grouped together as the levator ani or levator sling (Fig. 35A.2). Within this diaphragm is the urogenital hiatus, which is large enough to allow childbirth. This potentially large defect explains why prolapse is such a significant problem. The most medial portion of the pelvic diaphragm is formed by the puborectalis, the muscular boundary of the urogenital hiatus. The obstetric axis of the pelvis passes through the urogenital hiatus medial to the puborectalis muscle. In the standing patient, the puborectalis muscle is horizontal and is palpable as a 2- to 2.5-cm band of voluntary muscle on each lateral side of the distal one-third of the vagina. When well innervated and contracted, the puborectalis muscle closes the distal vagina and displaces the posterior rectum anteriorly. Forming

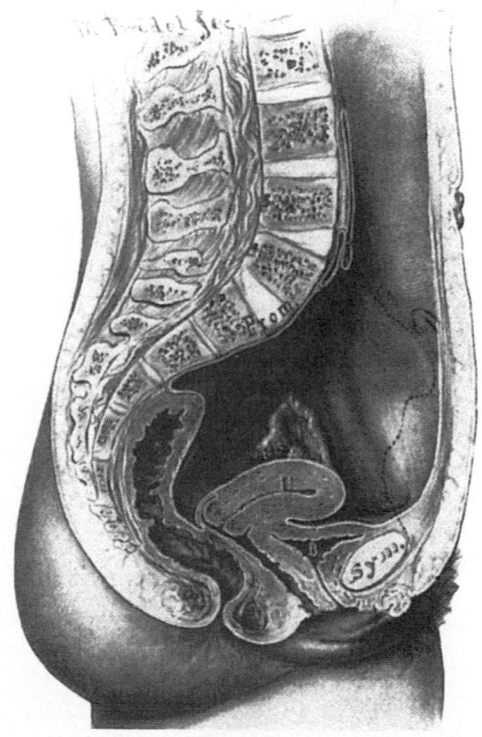

FIGURE 35A.1. The relationship between the pelvic floor and the abdominal cavity. Notice the lordosis of the lumbosacral spine and the almost vertical orientation of the pelvic inlet. (From Kelly HA. *Gynecology.* New York: D. Appleton & Co., 1928:2. Used with permission of the Department of Art as Applied to Medicine, Johns Hopkins Medical School.)

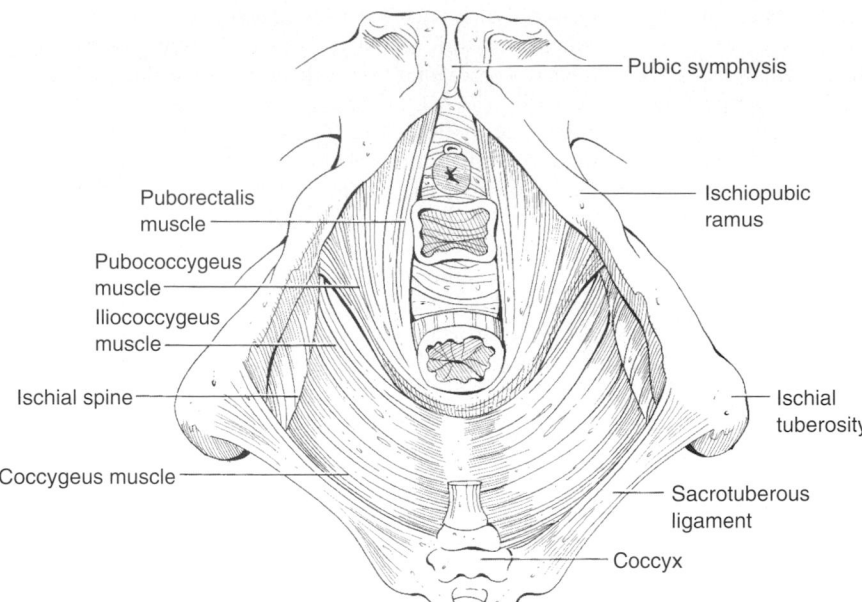

FIGURE 35A.2. The pelvic diaphragm viewed from below.

the bulk of the pelvic diaphragm, the pubococcygeus and iliococcygeus muscles cover the posterior and lateral portions of the pelvic outlet (Fig. 35A.3). The superior insertion of the ileococcygeus is an important landmark in pelvic support anatomy. The insertion of the ileococcygeus is a thickening of the pelvic sidewall parietal fascia that extends from the ischial spine posteriorly to a point on the pubic bone known as the pubic tubercle. This line of insertion is known as the arcus tendineus levator ani or muscular arch (Figs. 35A.4 and 35A.5). Immediately inferior to the muscular arch is a thickening of the parietal fascia of the belly of the ileococcygeus muscle known as the arcus tendineus fascia pelvis (fascial

arch) or white line. This structure is the lateral attachment point for the pubocervical fascia and proximal rectovaginal septum. The white line serves the function of midvaginal lateral support. Paravaginal and proximal pararectal defects are located immediately medial to the white line. In the standing patient, the white line is nearly horizontal; in the lithotomy position, it is nearly vertical.

During paravaginal repair, the white lines are palpable as stringlike structures between the ischial spines and the pubic arch. Recently, another fascial thickening has been described that runs posteriorly from the white line and serves as lateral support for the distal rectovaginal

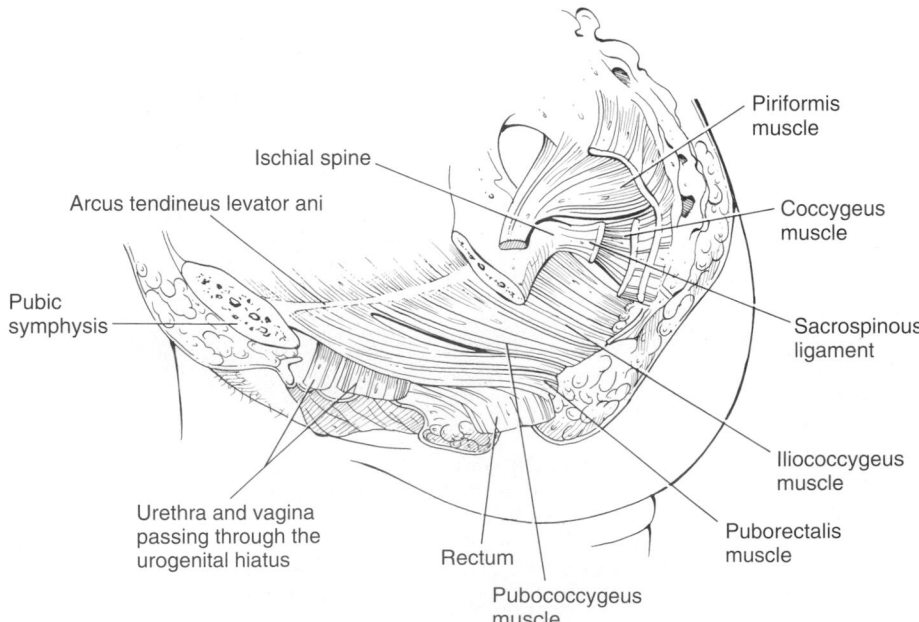

FIGURE 35A.3. Muscles of the pelvic floor, lateral view.

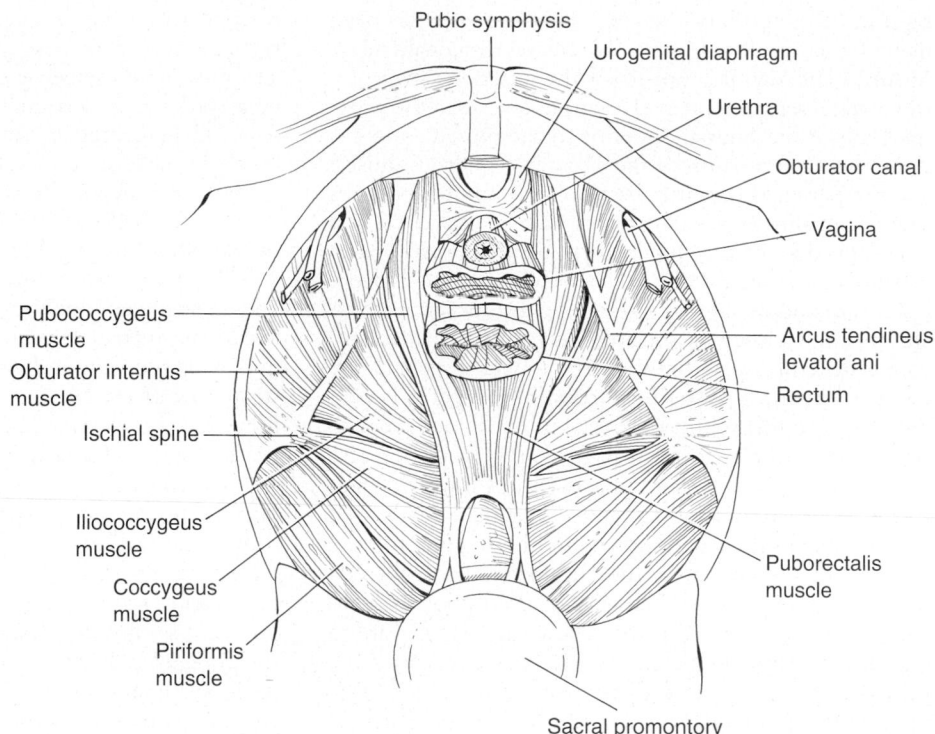

Pubic symphysis

Urogenital diaphragm

Urethra

Obturator canal

Vagina

Pubococcygeus muscle

Obturator internus muscle

Ischial spine

Iliococcygeus muscle

Coccygeus muscle

Piriformis muscle

Arcus tendineus levator ani

Rectum

Puborectalis muscle

Sacral promontory

FIGURE 35A.4. The pelvic diaphragm viewed from above.

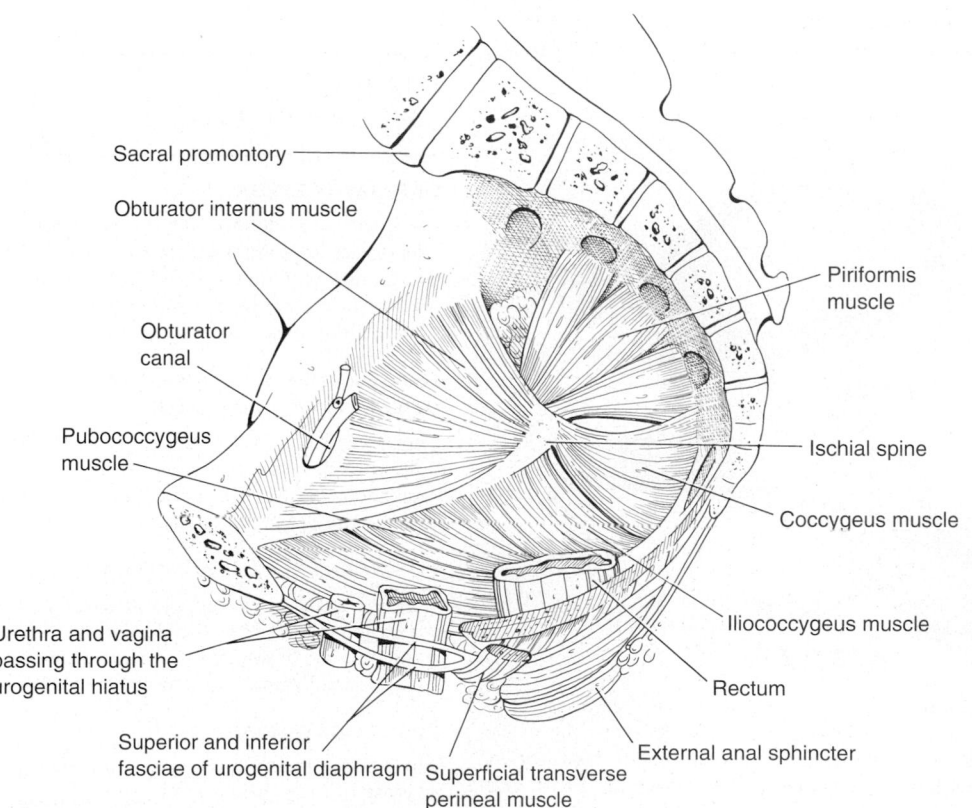

Sacral promontory

Obturator internus muscle

Obturator canal

Pubococcygeus muscle

Urethra and vagina passing through the urogenital hiatus

Superior and inferior fasciae of urogenital diaphragm

Superficial transverse perineal muscle

Piriformis muscle

Ischial spine

Coccygeus muscle

Iliococcygeus muscle

Rectum

External anal sphincter

FIGURE 35A.5. Sagittal view of the pelvis.

septum of the posterior vagina. This structure has been named the arcus tendineus fasciae rectovaginalis (Fig. 35A.6). The lateral supports of the anterior and posterior vaginal septa merge and are not separate in the proximal half of the vagina. Superior to the muscular arch is the uppermost portion of the obturator internus muscle and the parietal obturator fascia. The obturator internus muscles qualify as pelvic muscles because they form the lateral borders of the upper portion of the pelvic basin inferior to the linea terminalis. Posterior to the iliococcygeus, the pelvic floor is covered by the coccygeus muscle and the closely associated sacrospinous ligament. These structures pass between the ischial spine and the coccyx. The most posterior portion of the pelvis is covered by the piriformis muscle. The midline confluence of the levator muscles forms a particularly strong band of connective tissue between the coccyx and anus known as the levator plate or median raphe. This plate is oriented horizontally in the standing patient. The vagina and the rectum are suspended by the endopelvic fascia directly over the levator plate. Weakness of the pubococcygeus and iliococcygeus muscles may allow the levator plate to sag and descend permanently. This descent causes the genital hiatus to open as it does during defecation. This increased opening changes the normal horizontal axis of the proximal vagina to a vertical orientation and predisposes it to prolapse.

The pudendal nerve is an important motor and sensory nerve of the pelvic floor and perineum. It descends from the area posterior to the ischial spine under the sacrospinous ligament into Alcock's canal. Alcock's canal is located in the ischiorectal fossa immediately adjacent to the inferior fascia of the pelvic diaphragm. In this location,

the pudendal nerve is subjected to significant stretch and pressure during the descent of a fetus through the pelvis. The muscles of the pelvic diaphragm are also subjected to great pressure and stretch during labor. Magnetic resonance imaging studies have demonstrated myopathy and breaks in the levator muscles of parous women. Neuropathy of the pudendal nerve and myopathy of the levator muscles are believed to be active contributing factors in the development of pelvic organ prolapse.

The connective tissues of the pelvis are collectively known as the endopelvic fascia. This fibroelastic connective tissue matrix contains varying amounts of smooth muscle. It supports and invests all the midline organs and structures of the pelvis. Only the ovaries and fallopian tubes lie outside this investment. At various locations, the endopelvic fascia manifests different characteristics. These forms include loose areolar tissue capable of distention, neurovascular sheaths, septa and ligaments that support and separate the pelvic organs, and dense skeletal muscle investments. In the central pelvis, the visceral peritoneum drapes over the midline structures, dipping into recesses but not descending into direct contact with the muscular pelvic floor. The irregular space between the pelvic diaphragm, the muscular pelvic sidewall, and the visceral peritoneum is the location of the endopelvic fascia (Tables 35A.1–35A.8). The endopelvic fascia may be divided into three parts: parietal fasciae, visceral fasciae, and deep endopelvic connective tissue.

The parietal fasciae of the endopelvic fascia are relatively dense membranes investing the pelvic surface of

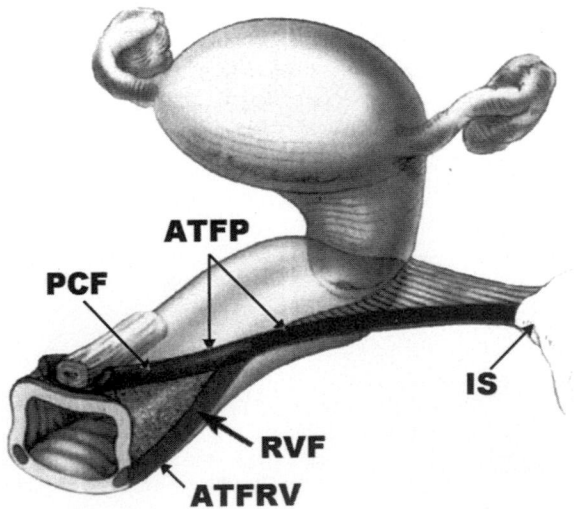

FIGURE 35A.6. The lateral attachments of the pubocervical fascia (PCF) and the rectovaginal fascia (RVF) to the pelvic sidewall. Also shown are the arcus tendineus fascia pelvis (ATFP), arcus tendineus fasciae rectovaginalis (ATFRV), and ischial spine (IS).

TABLE 35A.1.
Parietal Pelvic Fasciae

OBTURATOR FASCIA

Particularly well-defined in the area superior to the arcus tendineus levator ani and below the linea terminalis. This fascia may represent a vestigial portion of the levator ani whose origin has been lowered through evolution to the level of the muscular arch.

LEVATOR ANI FASCIA (SUPERIOR FASCIA OF THE PELVIC DIAPHRAGM)

This fascia is continuous across the pelvic floor, blending laterally with the obturator fascia at the arcus tendineus levator ani and centrally with the levator plate and the visceral fasciae at the urogenital hiatus.

COCCYGEUS FASCIA (SACROSPINOUS LIGAMENT)

This important pelvic support structure extends from the ischial spine laterally to the sacrum medially and is an important alternative source of proximal support when the uterosacral ligament is unavailable or insufficient.

PIRIFORMIS FASCIA

This fascia is the thinnest and most posterior of the parietal fasciae of the pelvis.

---

the skeletal muscles of the pelvic sidewall (Table 35A.1). They are similar in structure, form, and function to other parietal fasciae of the body, such as the rectus abdominis fasciae. At muscular margins, they blend with the various periostea of the bony pelvis.

The visceral pelvic fasciae are loose, highly elastic, and relatively ill-defined encasements of the central pelvic organs, taking the form of sheaths and sleeves (Table 35A.2). These structures allow for the high degree of physiologic distention necessitated by the function of the pelvic organs. The visceral fasciae blend intimately with the organs that they encase.

The deep endopelvic connective tissue is of central importance in the applied anatomy of the pelvis and is especially significant to the pelvic reconstructive surgeon. This structure is part of a continuum of retroperitoneal connective tissue that extends from the respiratory diaphragm in the upper abdomen to the pelvic diaphragm. Included in this continuum of structures are the mesenteries and ligaments of the upper abdomen. Anatomists debate whether the condensations of this connective tissue should be considered as true ligaments and fasciae. Part of this debate stems from the fact that some of these structures contain a significant muscular component and others serve as neurovascular conduits. Certainly, from a functional standpoint in the pelvis, they meet criteria for being so named. The endopelvic connective tissue is continuous from one part to the other. Separate portions serve different functions, take various forms, and therefore are given different names. The named structures of the deep endopelvic connective tissue include six ligaments, two septa, and one ring. Important anatomic details of these elements are summarized in the following tables.

The six pericervical ligaments form the paracolpium (Tables 35A.3, 35A.4, and 35A.5). The net effect of these structures is the suspension of the cervix in the posterior pelvis and the consequent placement of the vagina directly over the levator plate and away from direct exposure to the urogenital hiatus. In the normal anatomic position, pressure from above tends to close

TABLE 35A.2.
Visceral Pelvic Fasciae

PELVIC ORGANS AND STRUCTURES INVESTED BY VISCERAL FASCIAE

Vagina
Uterus
Bladder
Rectum

PELVIC ORGANS AND STRUCTURES NOT INVESTED BY VISCERAL FASCIAE

Fallopian tubes
Ovaries

TABLE 35A.3.
Components of the Deep Endopelvic Connective Tissue: Uterosacral Ligaments

ORIGIN
Periosteum of sacral vertebra 2, 3, and 4.

INSERTION
The points of insertion are on the posterior and lateral supravaginal cervix at the 5-o'clock and 7-o'clock positions. The ligaments are continuous with and form part of the pericervical ring.

NEUROLOGIC CONTENT
Uterosacral plexus of autonomic nerves.

VASCULAR CONTENT
Minimal.

MUSCULAR CONTENT
Rectouterine muscle.

FUNCTION
These structures are the primary proximal suspensory elements of the uterovaginal complex. They hold the cervix in the posterior pelvis at the level of the ischial spines with the uterus in anteflexion and the vagina suspended over the levator plate.

SYNONYM
Rectal pillar.
The uterosacral ligaments blend as continuous structures superiorly and laterally with the cardinal ligaments and distally with the proximal rectovaginal septum.

the vaginal vault and results in no tendency toward prolapse.

Two septa or fasciae (Tables 35A.6 and 35A.7) are located within the deep endopelvic connective tissue. These condensations of fibroelastic connective tissue are in close contact with the vaginal epithelium and visceral fasciae of the adjacent organs. Clinically, they are separate from their adjacent structures. When the septa and their supports are intact, the vaginal and rectal axes have a posterior angle of 130 degrees at the anterior point of their suspension over the levator plate. Distal to the puborectalis muscle, the vagina is nearly vertical as it passes through the urogenital hiatus. The proximal two-thirds of the vagina is nearly horizontal and is suspended over the levator plate. The normal vaginal axis is oriented posteriorly toward a point just above the center of the fourth sacral vertebra. This area is the level of the origin of the uterosacral ligaments.

The pericervical ring (Table 35A.8) is the single location where all deep endopelvic connective tissue support structures converge. Simply stated, the goal of the defect-specific pelvic reconstructive surgeon is the resti-

TABLE 35A.4.
Components of the Deep Endopelvic Connective Tissue: Cardinal Ligaments

ORIGIN

The hypogastric root with fibrous connections to the lateral abdominal and pelvic walls.

INSERTION

The points of insertion are on the lateral supravaginal cervix at the 3-o'clock and 9-o'clock positions. This insertion is continuous with and forms part of the pericervical ring.

NEUROLOGIC CONTENT

Portions of the uterosacral plexus.

VASCULAR CONTENT

Uterine artery and veins.

MUSCULAR CONTENT

Minimal smooth muscle content with no named component.

URINARY

The distal ureter passes under the uterine artery within the superior portion of the cardinal ligament.

FUNCTION

These ligaments are the primary vascular conduits of the uterus and vagina, providing lateral stabilization to the cervix at the level of the ischial spines.

SYNONYMS

Mackenrodt's ligament, lateral cervical ligament, and proper cervical ligament.

TABLE 35A.5.
Components of the Deep Endopelvic Connective Tissue: Pubocervical Ligaments

ORIGIN

Inferior surface of the superior pubic ramus medially and the arcus tendineus fascia pelvis laterally.

INSERTION

The points of insertion are on the anterior and lateral supravaginal cervix at the 11-o'clock and 1-o'clock positions. This insertion is continuous with and forms part of the pericervical ring.

VASCULAR COMPONENT

Artery and veins of the bladder pillar.

FUNCTION

These ligaments are the least well-developed of the pericervical ligaments, serving as a vascular conduit and for minimal cervical stabilization.

SYNONYM

Bladder pillar.

TABLE 35A.6.
Components of the Deep Endopelvic Connective Tissue: Pubocervical Septum or Fascia

SHAPE

Trapezoidal with the narrow end located distally.

CONTENTS

Fibroelastic connective tissue and smooth muscle.

FUNCTION

Anterior vaginal support including suspension of the bladder.

SYNONYMS

Vesicovaginal septum or fascia, pubovesicocervical septum or fascia.

BOUNDARIES

Distal: Pubic tubercles laterally and the pubic arch centrally fusing with the urogenital diaphragm.
Lateral: Arcus tendineus fascia pelvis or white line.
Proximal: Pericervical ring centrally and both pubocervical and cardinal ligaments laterally.
Superior: Visceral fascia of the bladder.
Inferior: Epithelium of the vagina.

TABLE 35A.7.
Components of the Deep Endopelvic Connective Tissue: Rectovaginal Septum or Fascia

SHAPE

Trapezoidal with the narrow end located distally.

CONTENTS:

Fibroelastic connective tissue and smooth muscle.

FUNCTION:

Posterior vaginal support, stabilization of the rectum, and perineal suspension.

SYNONYM:

Denonvilliers' fascia.

BOUNDARIES

Distal: Fusion with the proximal perineal body at the central tendon of the perineum.
Lateral: In the distal half of the vagina, the lateral boundary is the arcus tendineus fasciae rectovaginalis; in the proximal half of the vagina, the lateral boundary is the arcus tendineus fascia pelvis.
Proximal: Uterosacral ligaments laterally and the pericervical ring centrally.
Superior: Epithelium of the vagina.
Inferior: Visceral fascia of the rectum.

TABLE 35.8.
Components of the Deep Endopelvic
Connective Tissue: Pericervical Ring

SHAPE

Collar of connective tissue encircling the supravaginal cervix.

CONTENTS

Fibroclastic connective tissue.

FUNCTION

Cervical stabilization within the interspinous diameter by connecting with all other named components of the deep endopelvic connective tissue.

SYNONYM

Supravaginal septum.

CONNECTIONS

Anterior: The pericervical ring is located between the base of the bladder and the anterior cervix where it connects with the pubocervical ligaments at the 11-o'clock and 1-o'clock positions and the proximal pubocervical septum centrally.
Lateral: Cardinal ligaments at the 3-o'clock and 9-o'clock positions.
Posterior: The pericervical ring is located between the rectum and the posterior cervix where it connects with the uterosacral ligaments at the 5-o'clock and 7-o'clock positions and the proximal rectovaginal septum centrally.

TABLE 35A.9.
Avascular Spaces of the Pelvis

Prevesical
Paravesical
Vesicovaginal
Vesicocervical
Rectovaginal
Pararectal
Retrorectal

tution of the anatomy of the pericervical ring. If the dissection and reconstructive efforts during such a surgery do not extend proximally to the interspinous diameter, the surgery is likely to fail. Because the cervix is located on the anterior vaginal wall, the pubocervical septum is shorter than the rectovaginal septum by a length equal to the diameter of the pericervical ring. If one carries this line of reasoning further, an inherent structural problem is present in the posthysterectomy prolapse patient. If the cervix and its surrounding support tissues are absent, no completely anatomic method to reconstruct the proximal anterior vaginal support exists. Some form of anatomic distortion (e.g., shortening of the vagina or plication) is necessary to compensate for this defect. Likely, this dilemma is the reason that the dominant support defect in the posthysterectomy patient is most frequently in this location.

The three-dimensional structure of the endopelvic fascia has another distinguishing anatomic characteristic that is of interest to the pelvic surgeon. Outside the confines of the named condensations of this tissue are avascular potential spaces (Table 35A.9). When properly used, these spaces give the surgeon access to vital support structures deep within the pelvis. Gynecologic oncologists base their surgical training around mastering the surgical manipulation of these spaces, usually from the abdominal approach. These spaces are not only avail-

able to the vaginal reconstructive surgeon, but they are also critical in identification of pelvic support landmarks.

DeLancey's biomechanical analysis of normal uterovaginal support by the deep endopelvic connective tissue helps to unify the anatomic principles pertinent to pelvic organ prolapse (Fig. 35A.7). These concepts of support also help to define a set of goals for the reconstructive surgeon. Each goal must be satisfied for long-term success of a prolapse surgery. DeLancey divided vaginal support into three levels (Fig. 35A.8). Proximal vaginal level I support is attributed to suspension by the ligaments of the paracolpium. Damage to level I support results in uterovaginal prolapse, posthysterectomy vaginal prolapse, and enterocele. The cause for level I support problems is necessarily at or above the level of the ischial spines. The primary load-bearing elements are the uterosacral ligaments and to a lesser extent the cardinal ligaments. This fact is consistent with cadaver observations made many years ago by Mengert showing that prolapse occurred only after 85% of the integrity of the paracolpium was severed. Mid-vaginal level II support is due to lateral attachment of the fascial septa to the pelvic sidewalls. The septa attach to the arcus tendineus fascia pelvis and the arcus tendineus fasciae rectovaginalis. Damage at this level results in paravaginal and pararectal defects. Level III support is attributed to fusion to the urogenital diaphragm anteriorly and to the proximal perineum posteriorly. Damage at these sites results in urinary incontinence anteriorly and in perineal body deficits posteriorly. Cystocele and rectocele are central defects within the fabric of the pubocervical and rectovaginal septa.

ETIOLOGY AND PREVENTION

In the vast majority of women who will develop pelvic organ prolapse, the process begins with their first **vaginal delivery.** Each subsequent vaginal delivery contributes to the likelihood that a clinical prolapse will occur. Labor and delivery are certainly desired, necessary, and important physiologic events. Nonetheless, it does have a destructive aspect contributing to the development of pelvic organ prolapse. Commonly, many years pass and other factors contribute to the progression of prolapse before such patients present for evaluation.

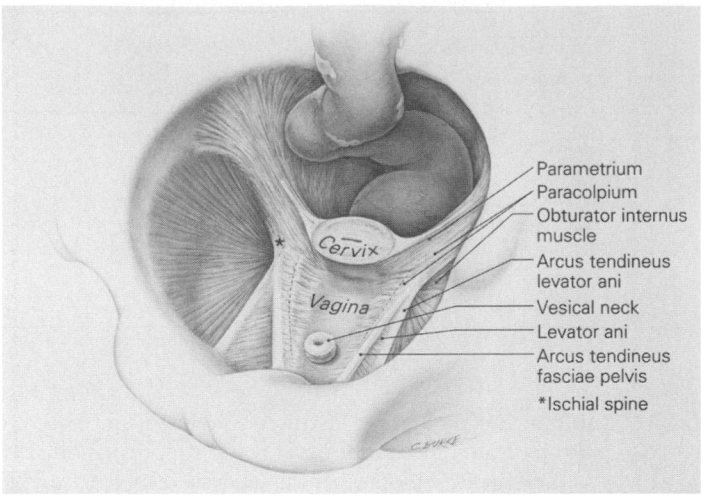

FIGURE 35A.7. Three-dimensional view of the endopelvic fascia. Notice the location of the cervix in the proximal anterior vaginal segment. (From DeLancey JO. Anatomic aspects of vaginal eversion after hysterectomy. *Am J Obstet Gynecol* 1992;166:1717–1728.)

During labor, the fetal presenting part (about 95% are vertex) must overcome a significant amount of soft tissue resistance presented by the lower uterine segment and cervix, the endopelvic fascia, and the muscular pelvic floor. Because of the lordosis of the lumbosacral spine, the obstetric axis of the pelvis is noticeably angled, differing by 90 degrees between the inlet and outlet. This angle occurs at the level of the ischial spine and causes the baby's head to extend sharply beginning at the level of the interspinous diameter. Thus, the fetus is driven by

strong uterine contractions through a low-velocity, high-pressure, arcing transit through the pelvis. Labor aided by maternal pushing and, at times, by physician traction has a damaging effect on the intricately constructed support structures of the pelvis.

In the initial phase of a nulliparous labor, the fetal head engages, flexes, and descends to a point immediately proximal to the interspinous diameter. Clinical examination at this stage commonly finds the cervix held in a far posterior position as a result of the strength and suspensory function of the uterosacral ligaments. In this situation, great pressure is placed on the anterior vaginal segment. The most common fetal presentation is the left occipitoanterior position, which places the rotating arc of the fetal head on the maternal right. As the fetal head overcomes the resistance of the pubocervical septum, significant downward pressure is placed on the maternal right pelvic sidewall. This event likely explains the preponderance of full-length right paravaginal defects as the most common fascial defect in anterior vaginal relaxation. As further descent occurs, the cervix rotates anteriorly, representing uterosacral damage proximal to the ischial spines. The fetus then rotates into the occipitoanterior position as it encounters the interspinous diameter. This diameter is the narrowest in the pelvis and therefore is the plane of greatest pressure during labor and delivery. The anterior sacrococcygeal curvature is concave. As the fetus passes under the pubic arch, this concavity makes it necessary for the fetal head to extend to complete labor. This change in orientation places intense pressure on the posterior pericervical ring. The usual result is further uterosacral stress and a transverse proximal detachment of the rectovaginal septum at its junction with the pericervical ring. As extension of the head progresses, the rectovaginal septum is displaced distally, resulting in the creation of a nidus for proximal vaginal enterocele and mid-vaginal rectocele formation. If the rectovaginal septum is displaced far enough distally, pararectal defects form as the septum is sheared away from its lateral attachments. The process of rectovaginal

FIGURE 35A.8. The endopelvic fascia of a posthysterectomy patient divided into DeLancey's biomechanical levels: level I—proximal suspension; level II—lateral attachment; level III—distal fusion. (From DeLancey JO. Anatomic aspects of vaginal eversion after hysterectomy. *Am J Obstet Gynecol* 1992;166:1717–1728.)

detachment and displacement weakens proximal support for the perineal body and predisposes to perineal descent. Subsequent deliveries progressively contribute damage to the endopelvic fascia. During descent and extension, the fetus passes through the urogenital hiatus. During this process, pressure is transmitted to the levator muscles and the pudendal nerve. If a patient dilates completely, pushes in an attempt to deliver, and then receives a cesarean section, she may have much of the same fascial damage as a woman with a successful vaginal delivery. A nulliparous patient with prolapse would likely suffer from isolated failure of the paracolpium, with the pericervical ring and fascial septa remaining intact.

A major shortcoming of the profession is that the effect of labor and delivery on the female pelvis has not been more completely objectified. Only recently has the study of pudendal neuropathy and levator myopathy been brought under scientific scrutiny. Even less has been done to determine the most common overall patterns of fascial and ligament damage during parturition. The pattern described in the previous paragraph is simply the most common one encountered. Other fetal presentations would result in different patterns of damage. Any experienced prolapse surgeon recognizes the variations in pattern of herniation, leading to the adage that no two patients are exactly alike. However, knowledge of the common pattern does help the surgeon who is new to the defect-specific approach know where to look to identify fascial edges and visually discriminate between the various tissues in the dissection field.

Fortunately, most women who bear children will not suffer a significant, symptomatic degree of prolapse. Parturition then is a necessary cause but not a sufficient cause for the vast majority of prolapse cases. Other factors work over time and in combination with the damage caused by childbirth to convert incipient prolapse into a clinically apparent problem.

Prolapse becomes more common with advancing age. The likely cause is general weakening of tissues including the pelvic floor muscles. Passage of time increases the cumulative effect of contributing causes on the pelvic floor. Most cases of prolapse become evident after the age of menopause. Virtually all the tissues of the pelvis possess estrogen receptors, and the atrophic changes that occur in the absence of estrogen are a contributing cause for prolapse. With age and a prolonged hypoestrogenic state, osteoporosis may develop. The kyphotic changes in the spine that result from osteoporosis displace the pelvic inlet into a more horizontal plane. This change in the pelvic inlet allows the weight of the abdominal contents to act more directly on the pelvic floor and on the urogenital hiatus.

Lifestyle may contribute to prolapse. Lifting objects heavy enough to require a Valsalva maneuver or fixation of the respiratory diaphragm displaces stress directly down on the pelvic floor. This process may be aided by shoulder, back, and extremity weakness. Defecation or micturition are commonly assisted with straining. This straining occurs when the pelvic diaphragm is intentionally relaxed. This action places substantial force on a passive pelvic floor and open urogenital hiatus several times a day. Straining has essentially the same effect as heavy lifting. Obesity, which is epidemic in the United States, directly increases the load on the pelvic floor and decreases mobility, as well as the ability to do muscle strengthening exercises.

Medical conditions and their complications may contribute to the development of prolapse. A few examples suffice to illustrate how a chronic medical condition or the treatments for medical problems may affect the pelvic floor. The natural history of diabetes mellitus includes neuropathy and obesity, both of which contribute to the tendency to prolapse. Chronic cough accompanying asthma, bronchitis, or smoking places repeated stresses on the pelvic floor. The effects of repeated or paroxysmal coughing help to convert incipient prolapse into a clinical problem. Smoking also has antiestrogenic properties, contributes to vascular disease, and creates a chronic hypoxic state. Corticosteroid therapy is used in many chronic medical conditions. The weakening effect of these medications on connective tissue is well known. People with constitutional connective tissue disorders have been shown to be at increased risk for prolapse. Ehlers-Danlos syndrome, for example, is characterized by generalized fascial and connective tissue weaknesses. The pelvic floor is also affected by these deficits. More subtle connective tissue weakness, such as joint hypermobility, has been shown to increase the long-term risk for prolapse. This list is by no means complete. Any condition that affects the physical load on the pelvic floor or the integrity of the muscular and connective tissues of the pelvis will increase the likelihood that symptomatic prolapse will develop.

Some medical conditions may reduce the tendency to develop prolapse. This is the case for any condition that causes an inflammatory reaction in the paracervical or parametrial tissues with subsequent tissue fibrosis. Pelvic inflammatory disease, puerperal or postabortal sepsis, endometriosis, and pelvic radiation therapy are conditions that could lead to such a circumstance. Pelvic adhesions, regardless of the cause, might be dense and numerous enough to suspend a prolapse. Large uterine leiomyomata can mechanically prevent the development and descent of prolapse.

The list of contributing causes to pelvic organ prolapse is varied. Prevention should begin early in a woman's life and be continued into the later years. Many of the measures discussed as preventions also have a positive effect on a woman's general health. Any discussion of pelvic organ prolapse prevention must include the obstetric management of childbirth. Vaginal delivery undoubtedly has a primary and profound effect on pelvic support anatomy. Debates have occurred for decades about the wisdom of operative vaginal deliveries, optimal length for the second stage of labor, management of macrosomia, utility of episiotomy, and multiple other obstetric practices. In truth, little evidence-based information exists regarding these concepts as they relate to the subsequent development of prolapse. The most likely major contributing factor is simply vaginal delivery. The pelvis is contoured so that even in a normal labor and delivery, substantial forces are applied to the endopelvic fascia, muscular floor of the pelvis, and pudendal nerve. The greatest forces generated are at the level of the interspinous diameter. This plane is the location of the singularly important pericervical ring and its junction with every other septa and ligament associated with normal vaginal support. For example, an episiotomy may shorten the second stage of labor but is unlikely to have any effect on the stresses generated in the interspinous diameter. Does prophylactic cesarean section represent the ultimate in prolapse prevention? This tactic certainly has attained popularity in some parts of the world. One might argue that if vaginal delivery is a necessary cause for prolapse, then this strategy would be preventative. This topic has generated an active and emerging debate in obstetrics and gynecology. Evidence-based resolutions to these questions are unlikely to ever be available. In my opinion, prophylactic cesarean section will never be widely applied. Replacing a desired physiologic process with a major surgery is illogical when the consequence to be prevented is relatively uncommon and not life threatening. However, occasional patients may present convincing arguments in favor of prophylactic cesarean section. The individual practitioner and patient must resolve the course of action in the privacy of the consultation room.

In the adult parous woman, strategies to prevent the development of prolapse center on efforts that decrease physical stress on the urogenital hiatus and strengthen the pelvic floor. Physical therapists have known for years that protection of the lower back is improved by strengthening the shoulder girdle, quadriceps, and abdominal muscles, as well as the muscles of the low back. This same concept is valid for protection of the pelvic floor. A program of exercise that develops strength in all these muscle groups allows women to accomplish the activities they desire without straining or using a Valsalva maneuver. Care must be taken to respect the urogenital hiatus so that during such training, undue stress is not repeatedly placed on the pelvic floor. Likewise, in daily activity, the proper techniques to lift, push, and pull objects should be learned and practiced. The control of obesity must be considered part of the effort to reduce the load placed on the pelvic floor. Osteoporotic spinal changes cause a gradual kyphosis, replacing the normal lumbosacral lordosis. The net effect is to rotate the pelvic brim into a more horizontal position. This shift places more stress on the pelvic floor. Estrogen therapy not only prevents osteoporosis but also has positive effects on the various estrogen-sensitive tissues of the pelvis.

Pelvic floor strengthening by voluntary contraction of the muscles innervated by the pudendal nerve was popularized by Arnold Kegel. The associated exercises have been known by his name ever since. Many women know this term because it is used frequently in postpartum instructions. Several different strategies help to remind patients to do their Kegel exercises. One of the most effective is briefly outlined below. The Kegel contraction is confirmed during the pelvic examination to ensure that the patient understands the correct muscles to contract. Frequently, patients will either perform a Valsalva maneuver or tighten the gluteus maximus muscle instead of the external anal sphincter and levator ani muscles. The proper time to Kegel is after micturition. After the bladder is emptied, the patient is instructed to lean as far forward as her stability allows. While leaning forward, she performs three isometric Kegel exercises by tightening the muscles until they voluntarily relax on their own. The dependent portion of a cystocele is below the level of the internal urethral orifice. The forward tilt physically elevates the bladder floor and allows for more complete emptying. The muscular action of the Kegel contractions also aids the process of emptying. Coupling this activity with voiding habituates the patient to perform the exercises several times a day. The result is the combination of more complete emptying and a strengthened pelvic floor, both of which are advantageous for the patient. The patient may then be able to recruit the Kegel contraction to prevent incontinence or to protect against sudden increases in abdominal pressure. If the patient knows how to use Kegel muscles that are strong and easily controlled, they become an asset in her daily life.

Splinting is particularly effective in alleviating the dysfunctional defecation related to symptomatic rectoceles. If a significant rectocele/enterocele herniation is present, patients frequently experience entrapment of the leading edge of the descending bowel movement. Entrapment leads to straining, which further enhances the entrapment. Often patients in this circumstance will strain until the bowel movement fragments, which allows partial defecation and descent of another segment of stool into the rectal pocket. Several trips to the toilet and a large segment of the day may be required to complete this process. This unfortunate problem may be avoided if the patient simply places upward pressure with her finger tips against the perineum or the area lateral to the perineum during the initial urge to defecate. Occasionally, the patient needs to place one or two fingers against the posterior vaginal wall. These maneuvers effectively reduce the rectocele pocket allowing the stool to evacuate while bypassing the rectocele. This "digital defecation" or splinting technique may avoid surgery and certainly empowers the patient to be in better control of her daily activities. I encourage the use of this technique postoperatively to protect the suspended posterior vaginal segment against undue strain. This protective maneuver is particularly important while acute healing is underway.

Control of chronic diseases and habits are helpful preventative strategies. Effective treatment of persistent cough may decrease incontinence and prevent progression of prolapse. Cessation of smoking certainly may be considered part of the preventative effort. Diabetic complications such as obesity, myopathy, and neuropathy are prevented by modern management strategies.

The prevention of pelvic organ prolapse involves care of the entire body. A healthy, fit, and well nourished patient who is aware of ways to actively protect her pelvic floor is less likely to experience this potentially disabling problem. Many of the strategies outlined in this section should be part of the care of patients from their obstetric years onward. Prevention is always preferable to intervention in the operating room.

CLINICAL EVALUATION

The correct management of pelvic organ prolapse depends on a careful evaluation of each patient. Only after a thorough history and physical examination is the practitioner able to develop an effective treatment plan for the individual patient.

The history should begin with the patient's perception of the problem. This information helps to determine what specific goals the patient may have. The patient might be afraid that the prolapse could rupture or that it may be caused by a malignant growth. Reassurance may suffice if such ideas are the major concern. Patients may or may not be interested in coital function, further childbearing, or simply knowing that the vagina is present if social circumstances change. Some women have grown accustomed to advanced prolapse and may describe very little inconvenience related to the herniation. These people may simply want to know if the prolapse represents any threat to their longevity. Other women are very conscious of an anatomically minor prolapse or may have pain unrelated to the prolapse. The patient may have unrealistic expectations or may be ready for intervention before the physician's operative criteria are met. In this situation, the pelvic reconstructive surgeon needs to be honest and forthright in discussing what will or will not improve after a surgery. A careful micturition, defecation, and sexual history may be invaluable in developing a treatment plan. Patients must be placed at ease and reassured during the evaluation before a full history concerning the details of pelvic functions can be obtained. Stress, urge, and neurogenic urinary incontinence may be differentiated by history. Obviously, the evaluations and treatments differ for each of these conditions. The complex topic of urinary incontinence is covered in detail elsewhere in this book. The mechanics involved in defecation are important. Determine the number of trips to the toilet and the compensatory measures necessary to complete evacuation. Fecal incontinence is a condition that patients are notoriously reluctant to discuss. This condition may or may not be due to physical damage to the anal continence control mechanism. The patient may be continent or incontinent of gas, liquid, or solids. Each patient may safely be presumed to desire urinary and bowel continence. Marked variation exists in patients' sexual goals. The practitioner should learn about these goals in a respectful and nonjudgmental way. Collecting sexual function information is an art, critical to the development of a management plan.

The past surgical history helps the surgeon assess the status of the patient in general and of the pelvis in particular. Specific interest should be placed on previous attempts to correct pelvic organ prolapse. Before her visit, the patient may be asked to prepare a list of previous surgeries so that none are overlooked. The route of hysterectomy and the indications for the procedure may be helpful. If previous prolapse surgery has been performed, the physician should try to obtain the operative notes. The anatomic details, type of suture used, and other details of the operative technique may help predict problems such as the likely location of anatomic distortion (previous plications) or the location of previously placed foreign bodies (e.g., meshes). Multiple previous attempts at repair necessitate a combination of caution and experience in order to achieve a successful outcome.

The medical history should be used to determine whether medical conditions exist that would likely interact with surgery or recovery. A complete pelvic reconstructive surgery may last several hours, involve significant blood loss, and require combined vaginal and abdominal approaches. Obviously, the patient needs the physical reserve to withstand this degree of stress. Patients with morbid obesity, limited pulmonary and cardiac function, thromboembolic risks, entrenched tobacco addiction, or limited mobility are not ideal candidates for this type of surgery. A complete list of current medications, including herbals and over-the-counter preparations, and treating physicians is also helpful.

The proper physical examination of the prolapse patient requires that the examining physician have a working knowledge of normal pelvic anatomy. Older systems for recording physical findings related to prolapse relied on subjective terms such as mild, moderate, and severe. These terms have limited utility in accurately describing prolapse and in effective communication between examiners. Two systems are currently in use that encourage a complete examination and that more objectively record anatomic detail. Each of these systems has strengths and weaknesses. The Baden-Walker Halfway System is user friendly, easy to record, and maximizes the amount of detail that can be recorded in a very brief space. Proponents of this system maintain that the essence of the prolapse examination is recorded after writing six numbers and some editorial notes. Critics note that the abbreviation of detail means that some compromises are made along the way. The second system is the **P**elvic **O**rgan **P**rolapse—**Q**uantification or **POP-Q** system. This is a more complex system incorporating more specific detail of the physical findings. Even for those clinicians accustomed to its use, the number of measurements needed requires additional time to acquire. The beauty of this system is that, theoretically, physician-to-physician variation is minimized. The POP-Q is currently used in many serious papers on the subject of prolapse. Interested physicians should become familiar with both of these systems. More important than any system is an accurate and anatomically based assessment of the patient at the time of examination.

Baden-Walker Halfway System

The extent of prolapse is recorded using a number (0 to 4) at each of six sites in the vagina. There are two sites on the anterior, superior, and posterior walls of the

TABLE 35A.10.
Primary and Secondary Symptoms at Each Site Used in the Baden-Walker Halfway System

Anatomic Site	Primary Symptoms	Secondary Symptoms
Urethral	Urinary incontinence	Falling out
Vesical	Voiding difficulties	Falling out
Uterine	Falling out	Heaviness and so forth
Cul-de-sac	Pelvic pressure (standing)	Falling out
Rectal	True bowel pocket	Falling out
Perineal	Anal incontinence (gas/feces)	Too loose

From: Baden WF, Walker T. *Surgical repair of vaginal defects.* Philadelphia: JB Lippincott, 1992:12.

vagina. Table 35A.10 lists the anatomic sites and the associated symptoms. The six numbers are recorded as a measure of descent. For all sites except the perineum, the hymen is used as a fixed anatomic reference point. Zero indicates normal anatomic position for a site, whereas 4 represents maximum prolapse. Between these extremes, the intervening numbers grade descent using a halfway system as illustrated in Figure 35A.9. The examination is performed with the patient straining so that maximum descent is attained. The patient may wish to stand to demonstrate maximum descent.

The perineum is graded using the familiar perineal laceration system used in obstetrics (Fig. 35A.9). The patient is asked to hold or Kegel to evaluate the amount of muscular and fascial compensatory support. Editorial comments may include the site of dominant prolapse, lo-

cation of scars, palpable plications, and the type of efforts necessary to demonstrate maximum prolapse. Strength of the levator contraction may be recorded as 0 to 4.

Example: 12/44/32. A dominant complete proximal prolapse is noted with enterocele, significant cystocele and rectocele, and perineal attenuation to the level of the external anal sphincter. 2/4 levator strength is present.

Although this type of notation encodes much information in a small space, no specific location of fascial defects is indicated.

Pelvic Organ Prolapse—Quantification System (POP-Q)

This system was developed as an effort to introduce more objectivity into the quantification of pelvic organ prolapse. For example, measurements in centimeters are used instead of grades. Nine specific measurements are recorded as indicated in Figure 35A.10. Point Aa is defined as being 3 cm proximal to the external urethral meatus on the anterior vaginal wall. Point Ap is defined as being 3 cm proximal to the hymen on the posterior vaginal wall. Points Ba and Bp are defined as points of maximum prolapse excursion on the anterior and posterior vaginal walls respectively. Measurements are recorded as negative numbers when proximal to the hymen and positive numbers when distal to the hymen. POP-Q sites C and D are identical in location to Baden-Walker sites three and four in the proximal vagina. In addition, measurements of the total vaginal length, genital hiatus, and perineal body are taken. All measurements are recorded on a tic-tac-toe style grid (Fig. 35A.11). When combined with sagittal line drawings, a fairly complete picture of prolapse is attained (Fig.

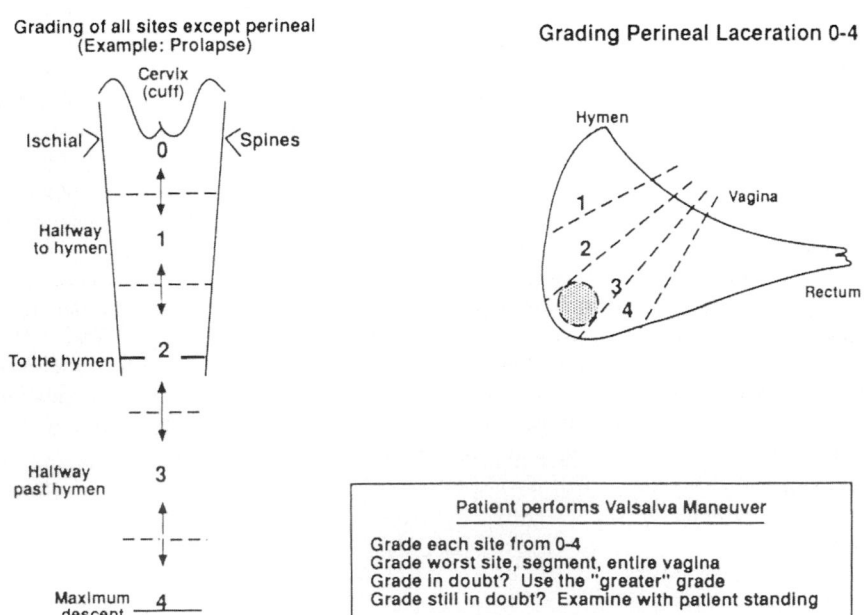

FIGURE 35A.9. Guidelines on how to assign grades in the Baden-Walker Halfway System. (From Baden WF, Walker T. *Surgical repair of vaginal defects.* Philadelphia: JB Lippincott, 1992.)

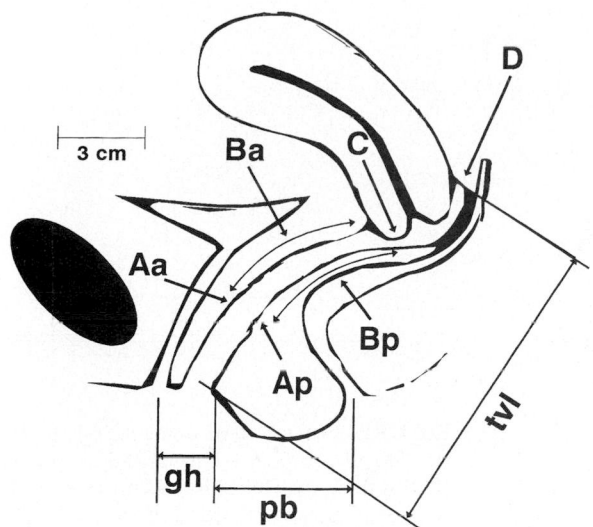

anterior wall	anterior wall	cervix or cuff
Aa	**Ba**	**C**
genital hiatus	perineal body	total vaginal length
gh	**pb**	**tvl**
posterior wall	posterior wall	posterior fornix
Ap	**Bp**	**D**

FIGURE 35A.10. The nine specific sites of measurement used in the Pelvic Organ Prolapse—Quantification System (POP-Q). gh, genital hiatus; pb, perineal body; tvl, total vaginal length. (From Bump RC, Mattiasson A, Bø K, et al. The standardization of terminology of female pelvic organ prolapse and pelvic floor dysfunction. *Am J Obstet Gynecol* 1996; 175:10.)

FIGURE 35A.11. The tic-tac-toe grid used to record measurements in the Pelvic Organ Prolapse—Quantification System (POP-Q) . (From Bump RC, Mattiasson A, Bø K, et al. The standardization of terminology of female pelvic organ prolapse and pelvic floor dysfunction. *Am J Obstet Gynecol* 1996; 175:10.)

35A.12). Ordinal stages of pelvic organ prolapse are then assigned from stage 0 (no prolapse) to stage V (complete prolapse) so that the outcome of cases of like magnitude may be compared.

This system is a physical examination tool and does not assign the specific location of fascial defects.

After a general physical examination is performed, the prolapse may be evaluated. Any surgical scars on the abdomen should be correlated with the surgical history. Patients frequently forget procedures that may have an impact on the treatment plan. The physician should pay particular attention to the suprapubic region where previous incontinence procedure incisions may be located.

The pelvic examination is initiated with the patient in the lithotomy position. Hip mobility should be evaluated because adequate abduction and flexion of the thighs is required for a vaginal procedure. Thigh and buttock obesity may also be limiting factors. If exposure is limited, an extended procedure performed vaginally is not in the patient's or surgeon's best interest.

The labia are opened for introital inspection. Prolapse may be internal (proximal to the hymen) or external (distal to the hymen) at rest. The extent of the prolapse may change considerably if the patient is asked to strain. This difference may be especially pronounced in patients with healthy pelvic floor muscles and an undescended levator plate. These two structures may help hold a prolapse in place. The patient may give a history of a prolapse that is not apparent on examination or not

as large as she describes. In such a case, the patient is examined while she is in the standing position; or she may be asked to perform the maneuvers necessary to demonstrate the full extent of the prolapse.

The dominant prolapse is considered to be the first hernia to descend or the most dependent part of a prolapse that has previously descended. Proper identification of the dominant prolapse provides key clues about where the most significant fascial damage is located. The dominant prolapse is located and replaced in order to examine the remainder of the vaginal vault. A large dominant prolapse often fills the urogenital hiatus and introitus, preventing incipient hernias from fully developing. Usually an anterior prolapse is easily replaced by placing a tongue blade or Ayre spatula in each anterior lateral sulcus. If a paravaginal defect is present, this maneuver replaces the anterior vaginal wall. If this maneuver does not reduce the hernia, a central anterior defect is likely present. A dominant posterior segment prolapse may be replaced with the posterior blade of a disjoined Sims' speculum. A dominant superior segment prolapse may be replaced with a large cotton swab, a sponge stick, or, in advanced cases, by attaching a tenaculum to the cervix. After replacement of the dominant prolapse, the secondary sites of prolapse become more apparent. An isolated single-site prolapse is rare. The location of the cervix or hysterectomy scar helps determine the location of the dominant prolapse. Frequently displaced, either anteriorly or posteriorly, these sites are often not at the most dependent part of the prolapse. The posthysterectomy scar is commonly a transverse fibrous band that

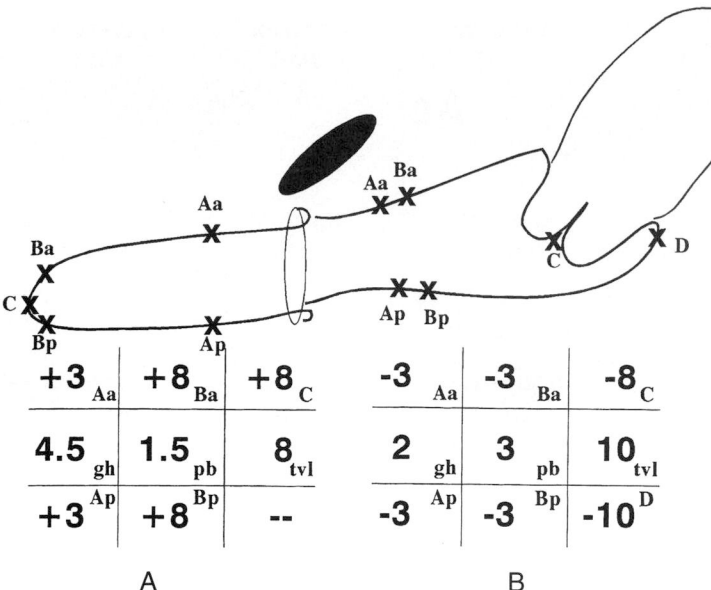

+3 Aa	+8 Ba	+8 C
4.5 gh	1.5 pb	8 tvl
+3 Ap	+8 Bp	--

A

-3 Aa	-3 Ba	-8 C
2 gh	3 pb	10 tvl
-3 Ap	-3 Bp	-10 D

B

FIGURE 35A.12. Two examples of the Pelvic Organ Prolapse—Quantification System (POP-Q). (From Bump RC, Mattiasson A, Bø K, et al. The standardization of terminology of female pelvic organ prolapse and pelvic floor dysfunction. *Am J Obstet Gynecol* 1996; 175:10.)

may be slightly retracted. To either side of the band are dimples in the epithelium corresponding to the location of the insertion of cardinal and uterosacral ligament remnants. Incomplete evaluation may lead to incomplete repair that results in recurrent prolapse and multiple trips to the operating room. The support structures of all vaginal segments and levels are interdependent. Complete restoration of all defects is necessary for a successful outcome.

Careful inspection of the vaginal epithelium reveals the location of rugae. The presence of these folds implies that endopelvic fascia is adherent to the epithelium in that location. The lateral vaginal sulci are the location of the junction of the pubocervical and rectovaginal septa to their respective lateral arcuate attachments. The pattern of rugae and the condition of the sulci should correlate with the pattern of fascial breaks found at surgery. The vaginal epithelium should also be inspected for atrophy created by the absence of the effects of estrogen. Local or systemic administration of estrogen before surgery assists in dissection and subsequent healing. Occasionally, an external prolapse may develop pressure ulcers as a result of entrapment when the patient is sitting. These lesions must be properly evaluated to rule out malignancy.

Rectovaginal examination assists in the evaluation of the posterior and superior vaginal segments. The uterosacral ligaments should be palpable immediately medial to each ischial spine. If the uterus is present, the uterosacrals may be more easily palpated with traction placed on the cervix. Anterior displacement of the rectal examining finger toward the vagina helps to distinguish between rectocele and enterocele. During the rectal examination, the patient is asked to strain. If an enterocele is present, it bulges down in the nonrugated vaginal epithelium proximal to the tip of the examining finger. Palpating the transversely detached proximal edge of the

rectovaginal septum is possible during this maneuver. This sharp border may retract distally all the way to the perineum. Perineal descent is also evaluated at the time of rectal examination. The levator plate is immediately posterior to the rectum and should be horizontal and immovable. The perineum is evaluated last. The perineum is triangular in the sagittal plane. The base is on the rectal side, and the apex, at the hymen. Perineal attenuation is very common in parous women. Apposition of the thumb of the examining hand while the index finger is in the rectum proximal to the anterior aspect of the external anal sphincter allows for evaluation of the integrity of this muscle. Voluntary contraction of the sphincter may be helpful. The S3 neurologic segment is necessary to contract this muscle. S3 also controls the ability to spread the toes if the integrity of that segment is in question.

The strength of the pelvic diaphragm is directly correlated with the ability to voluntarily contract these muscles. This ability is best tested clinically with light pressure placed on the posterior vaginal wall by the examining digits. The patient may need coaching in order to elicit a response. This time is an excellent opportunity to instruct the patient in the importance of postvoiding Kegel exercises and perineal support (splinting) during defecation.

If muscle activity is elicited, it may be subjectively graded from 0 to 4. If no muscle activity is detected, a more formal neurologic and medical workup should be considered. Pudendal nerve motor latency studies may reveal significant neuropathies. Magnetic resonance imaging of these patients has revealed the presence of advanced muscle atrophy and muscular detachments as well. The presence of such findings erodes the surgeon's ability to correct prolapse.

The presence of urinary incontinence should be noted during any part of the evaluation of prolapse. In an advanced prolapse, assessment of incontinence should be conducted with the prolapse in a reduced state. A pessary or loose vaginal packing may be helpful in accomplishing this goal. Incontinence may be masked by a hypotonic bladder or reverse kinking of the urethra if a cystocele is large. Repair of a large prolapse may be followed by the appearance of urinary incontinence if the preoperative evaluation is not performed with the prolapse reduced.

When a large prolapse is present, the trigone of the bladder is often located outside the vaginal introitus. In this degree of displacement, one may deduce the location of the trigone as being directly adjacent to the location of a Foley catheter bulb. The course of the ureter in a large prolapse is from the superior and lateral aspect of the anterior prolapse to the area of the trigone. The ureter may often be palpated in this location. If the prolapse is chronic and advanced, hydroureter and even hydronephrosis may be present. In this circumstance the ureters lose their cordlike consistency and are more difficult to palpate or recognize at the time of surgery. Dilation or prolapse makes the ureter more susceptible to injury. Intraoperative placement of ureteral catheters may be helpful in such a patient.

Occasionally, a patient presents with the cervix near the level of the hymen. If no other signs of prolapse are present, the alert examiner is aware of the possibility of

an elongated cervix. Sometimes surgery is not necessary in these patients. If surgery is performed, the technique of hysterectomy needs to take into consideration the elongation of the cervix. Often the paracolpium is properly placed in the interspinous diameter in these patients.

The examiner should not underestimate the value of an examination under anesthesia to supplement information that has been gathered preoperatively. With the patient and her pelvic diaphragm relaxed, the full extent of prolapse may become more apparent. Deep structures of importance, such as the ischial spines and uterosacral ligaments, may be more easily palpated. An examination under anesthesia should be performed before initiating a prolapse surgery.

A number of ways may be used to summarize the array of clinical findings discussed in this section. My preference is to use a pelvic organ prolapse map (Figs. 35A.13 and 35A.14). Key anatomic landmarks are schematically outlined. The three-dimensional structure of the vagina is reduced to two dimensions as if the vagina were divided at the 3-o'clock and 9-o'clock positions. A Baden-Walker profile can be recorded vertically on the map with numbers placed beside the appropriate anatomic location. As seen in Figure 35A.15, fascial defects can be sketched on the map at their suspected or known location. Editorial notes regarding the prolapse

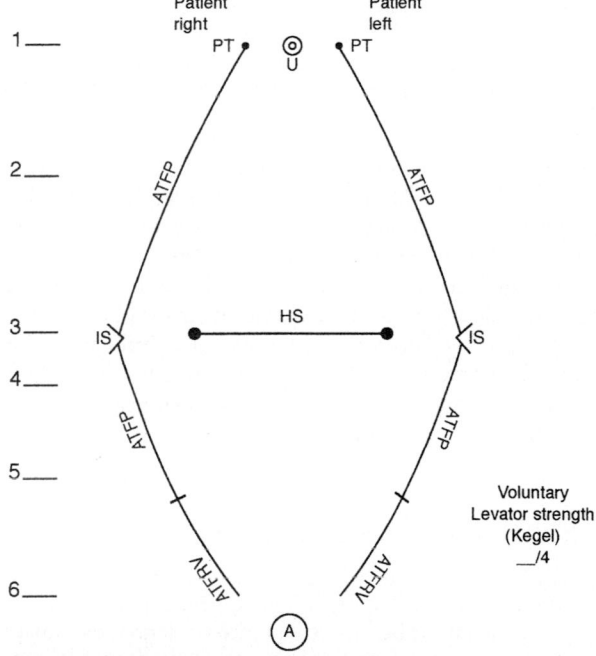

FIGURE 35A.13. Key elements of pelvic support anatomy. Three dimensions are reduced to two by dividing the vagina at the 3-o'clock and 9-o'clock positions. Baden-Walker vaginal support profile sites: 1, urethral; 2, vesical; 3, uterine; 4, cul-de-sac; 5, rectal; 6, perineal. PT, pubic tubercle; ATFP, arcus tendineus fascia pelvis; ATFRV, arcus tendineus fasciae rectovaginalis; IS, ischial spines; U, urethra; Cx, cervix; A, anus.

FIGURE 35A.14. Key elements of posthysterectomy pelvic support anatomy. Three dimensions are reduced to two by dividing the vagina at the 3-o'clock and 9-o'clock positions. Baden-Walker vaginal support profile sites: 1, urethral; 2, vesical; 3, uterine; 4, cul-de-sac; 5, rectal; 6, perineal. PT, pubic tubercle; ATFP, arcus tendineus fascia pelvis; ATFRV, arcus tendineus fasciae rectovaginalis; IS, ischial spines; U, urethra; HS, hysterectomy scar; A, anus.

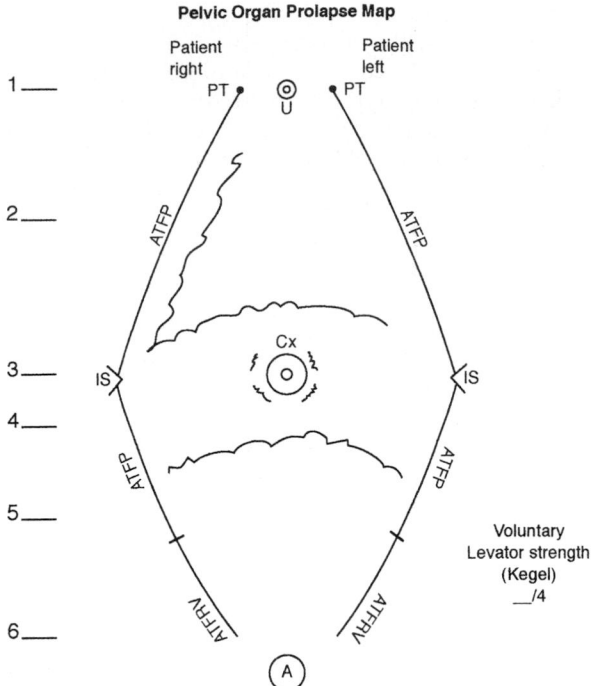

FIGURE 35A.15. The most frequently encountered pattern of fascial damage in pelvic organ prolapse: (1) full-length right paravaginal defect; (2) transverse proximal detachment of the pubocervical septum; (3) transverse proximal detachment of the rectovaginal septum. This pattern of damage is consistent with the mechanics of a left occipitoanterior delivery. Baden-Walker vaginal support profile sites: 1, urethral; 2, vesical; 3, uterine; 4, cul-de-sac; 5, rectal; 6, perineal. PT, pubic tubercle; ATFP, arcus tendineus fascia pelvis; ATFRV, arcus tendineus fasciae rectovaginalis; IS, ischial spines; U, urethra; Cx, cervix; A, anus.

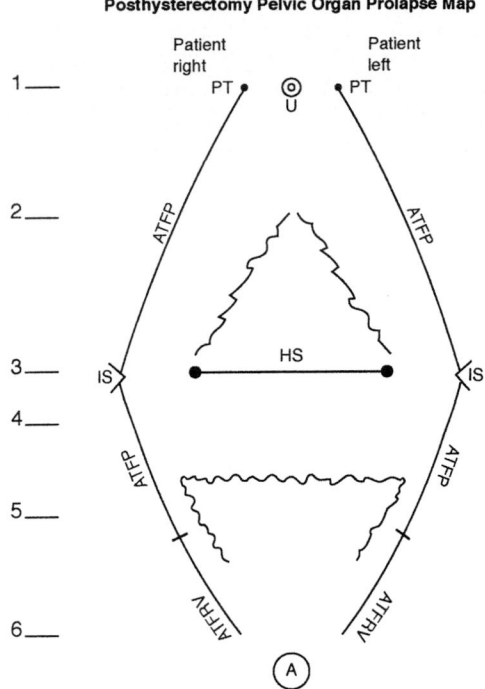

FIGURE 35A.16. An infrequently encountered inverted "V" anterior central fascial defect. Posteriorly, the proximal detachment of the rectovaginal septum has retracted toward the perineum, creating an enterocele and rectocele. Notice the bilateral pararectal defects. Baden-Walker vaginal support profile sites: 1, urethral; 2, vesical; 3, uterine; 4, cul-de-sac; 5, rectal; 6, perineal. PT, pubic tubercle; ATFP, arcus tendineus fascia pelvis; ATFRV, arcus tendineus fasciae rectovaginalis; IS, ischial spines; U, urethra; HS, hysterectomy scar; **A,** anus.

can be written in the space provided. The pattern that is noted in Figure 35A.15 is the one most commonly seen in pelvic organ prolapse surgery; however, many variations on this theme are encountered (Fig. 35A.16). Another diagram may be drawn to indicate the exact locations of fascial defects at the time of surgery.

A thorough history and physical examination improves the treatment of the prolapse patient. The physical findings must be recorded in an anatomically accurate and understandable way.

CHOICE OF TREATMENT

Vaginal reconstructive surgery is concerned with the return of abnormal organ relationships to a usual or normal state. There is no one site or degree of damage that must be repaired or restored; there are many and they occur in various combinations at various times of life, from different etiologic factors, in varying degrees, and with varying degrees of symptoms and disability.
Nichols and Randall, 1989.

Patients with pelvic organ prolapse have highly individualized perceptions of their situation. The single most important concept in the treatment of these conditions is to understand the patient's fears, concerns, and limitations related to the prolapse. The patient's expectations and her ability to tolerate surgery should be expertly evaluated. The physician's job is to educate the patient regarding options of treatment. After informed consent is given, the appropriate course of action is usually obvious to both the doctor and the patient. If the chosen course of action fails or becomes inappropriate over the course of time, the clinical evaluation and decision process can be revisited.

Nonsurgical Management

Regardless of the degree of prolapse, no surgery should be done unless the patient experiences a sufficient degree of morbidity. Most symptoms relate to quality of life issues. Generally, preventative measures should be the most widely applied techniques. Pelvic floor exercises, weight loss, treatment of chronic diseases, physical therapy, cessation of smoking, and estrogen therapy are all considerations in the conservative treatment of pelvic organ prolapse. These interventions have been discussed in the previous section of this chapter and should be employed regardless of whether expectant management or surgical intervention is the plan. During expectant management, periodic examinations should be done to determine the status of pelvic organ support and the degree of progression. Symptoms and the ability to participate in daily activities may be reviewed in order to reinforce the patient's motivation to continue preventative measures.

Pessaries are ingenious devices that have been used for a long period of time. They were originally the product of an age when surgery was not an option for the prolapse patient. They are available in a variety of shapes and sizes depending on the needs of the patient. In general, the greater the degree of prolapse and the more strenuous the daily activities of the patient, the less likely it is for a pessary to be a permanent solution. As the prolapse expands, occupies the urogenital hiatus, and dilates the introitus, the pressure of the prolapse tends to expel the pessary.

A pessary may be valuable for a patient to wear in order to feel more comfortable during a specific activity, such as exercise. If a patient of limited activity and acute onset advanced prolapse can be successfully fitted with a pessary, it may prevent progression and result in long-term improvement in intestinal and urinary function. Teaching patients to hold a pessary in place manually (splinting) during the process of defecation is helpful. In a patient with significant anterior segment prolapse, the insertion of a pessary elevates the bladder floor and can allow for more functional and complete voiding.

The utility of these devices is directly proportional to the efforts of the physician and the patient. If both parties are interested, pessaries can have a valuable place in the management of prolapse. Pessaries are more thoroughly discussed in Section F of this chapter.

Surgical Principles and Management

The management of advanced and symptomatic prolapse is primarily surgical. In 1997, 226,000 women underwent pelvic organ prolapse surgery in the United States. This condition is one of the most common indications for major surgery. Eleven percent of all women will experience some type of prolapse surgery during their lifetimes, and 30% of these women will undergo another operation for recurrence. Prolapse is a high-incidence problem that commands a substantial expenditure of health care dollars. Only those patients who request relief should be considered surgical candidates. Once the decision is made to operate, quality of life goals need to be established. If the patient can tolerate a lengthy operation and especially if she desires coital function, a reconstructive operation should be considered. The restoration of normal anatomy (form) maximizes the potential that symptoms and limitations (function) will be corrected or significantly improved. Restoration of normal anatomy automatically addresses the questions of vaginal axis, caliber, and depth. If the patient does not desire coital function, an occlusive procedure, such as colpocleisis, might be the best choice. Colpocleisis with vaginectomy has a very low failure rate, but the end does not justify the means in all patients.

Choosing the correct operation for prolapse is critical for success. The general plan for the procedures that will best correct the problems of the individual patient may be developed from details gathered during the preoperative examination and examination under anesthesia. Specific details become evident only during the intraoperative dissection. The goals of the operation are the restoration of normal form and function. Isolated areas of prolapse are uncommon. Childbirth places damaging pressure on all segments of support during the various phases of labor and delivery. Restricting an operative procedure to the repair of a single dominant or symptomatic site of prolapse simply transfers the stress to a different vaginal segment. An incomplete reconstruction may result in a secondary prolapse descending as a new dominant prolapse. Sometimes prolapse can return quickly. Perhaps the best known example of this phenomenon is the observation by Burch that many patients developed an enterocele after his anterior urethropexy procedure. An active search for potential and undeveloped defects must be done at the time of prolapse surgery. Site-specific repair of all segments and levels is the best insurance against failure.

The route of operation is a matter of debate. Vaginal surgery is the historical hallmark of the gynecologic surgeon. Although surgical training in vaginal techniques has eroded in recent years, a resurgence of interest in these operations is occurring. The vaginal approach requires either limited or no access to the peritoneal cavity and is surgically less stressful on the patient.

During the last three decades a significant change has occurred in the way prolapse surgery is conceptualized and performed. Anatomically distorting distal plications have been replaced by defect-specific anatomic restorations. Several aspects of the defect-specific method favor the vaginal approach. Fascial defects can be best identified when the full extent of the vaginal segment to be repaired is dissected and exposed. Such dissections are only possible vaginally. The detached fascial edge of a paravaginal defect may retract across the midline to the contralateral side of the body. This retraction leaves the fascial edge in a position that is impossible to reach from the abdominal or endoscopic approach. No one questions that a paravaginal defect can be identified from the abdominal/endoscopic operative approach. A question does remain about whether the retracted fascial edge can be accessed and reattached to the white line using the abdominal or laparoscopic approach. Likewise, a proximal rectovaginal septal defect that has retracted distally to the perineum would be very difficult to find and resuspend from above. All the major support anatomic landmarks and tissues are accessible vaginally. These points include the arcus tendineus fascia pelvis, arcus tendineus fasciae rectovaginalis, ischial spines, uterosacral ligaments, sacrospinous ligaments, and virtually all components of the deep endopelvic connective tissue. For most initial reconstructions, the vaginal operative route is superior to any other approach. The vaginal route is also preferred for patients with failures from previous operations. This approach is especially useful when a previous operation did not use the defect-specific approach and did not include the use of permanent suture for critical support sites.

The discussion and opinions in the previous paragraph do not preclude the use of abdominal and laparoscopic techniques for certain problems in pelvic reconstructive surgery. Procedures to correct stress urinary incontinence are discussed extensively in Chapter 36. Anterior urethropexy approached through the prevesical space with a suprapubic incision or laparoscopic technique has some advantages when compared with a suburethral sling urethropexy. No iatrogenic paravaginal defect is necessary during anterior urethropexy, for example. Such defects are made with pubovaginal sling procedures of all types. Some intentionally created defects are larger than others. To spend time and effort to reconstruct the pubocervical fascia anatomically from white line to white line and then to destroy part of the paravaginal support intentionally in order to allow passage of the sling material into the prevesical space does not make good sense. The primary prevesical space approach avoids this destructive necessity. Kelly-Kennedy plications and paravaginal repairs have been shown to be ineffective as incontinence procedures. Work continues to develop an effective totally vaginal operation to cure stress incontinence. A vaginal incontinence operation would avoid iatrogenic paravaginal damage and an abdominal or laparoscopic incision.

The abdominal approach is useful in some cases of prolapse in which one or more previous pelvic support operations have failed. Abdominal sacral colpopexy is an option to keep in mind in this situation. Colpopexy may be useful in a circumstance in which considerable scar is present from previous surgery. For example, consider a patient with a previous aggressive distal plication and a proximal support failure. Significant fibrolysis would be necessary to gain access to the proximal structures necessary to repair the prolapse. A rescue abdominal sacral colpopexy may more easily and effectively correct the prolapse. Occasional patients whose support has failed following a site-specific operation with permanent suture may also benefit from this operation. Abdominal sacral colpopexy is not a site-specific operation; however, it provides substantial proximal support and protects vaginal length.

During a prolapse surgery, the surgeon may determine that adequate support or repair is not attainable through the primary approach. No harm is done in using a combined approach. If support is not satisfactory after a vaginal procedure, an abdominal sacral colpopexy can be done at that time. Conversely, a vaginal examination should be performed after an abdominal sacral colpopexy to determine whether the vaginal axis, caliber, and depth are acceptable. The patient with proper informed consent would likely prefer a combined procedure to subsequent surgery.

Suture selection for pelvic reconstruction has changed with the realization that prolapse surgery is really a series of herniorrhaphies. No surgeon would consider performing repair of an inguinal hernia with rapidly absorbable suture. In the days of distal plications, the use of such suture was common. Today most experts recommend that fascial defects be repaired with permanent su-

ture. In an attempt to compromise, some surgeons use delayed absorbable sutures. They reason that the suture material is not needed after healing has been completed. Monofilament and polyfilament sutures are acceptable. Monofilament sutures occasionally erode and cause an unpleasant whisker effect in the vagina. If erosion occurs, the suture can be removed. My choice of suture is interwoven braided polyester for fascial repairs. This suture is affordable and easily tied, has no sharp end, and rarely causes a reaction or erosion.

All prolapse patients should be carefully evaluated for concomitant vaginal, uterine, adnexal, pelvic, or abdominal disease, which may change the operative approach selected for correction of prolapse. Orthopedic problems and obesity must be factored into the decision-making process because adequate vaginal access is also important.

Young patients with uterovaginal prolapse may request preservation of their fertility. Unless the problem is severe, these patients should be advised to complete their childbearing so that a definitive operation can be performed. Ring-type pessaries that permit intercourse may provide temporary relief. A unilateral sacrospinous ligament fixation with the uterus in place is beneficial and does not prohibit subsequent vaginal childbirth. Various abdominal or endoscopic uterine suspensions may also be considered. In general, retention of the uterus when a significant degree of prolapse is present compromises the long-term operative result. The cervix limits access to the structures of the paracolpium that are necessary to achieve proper proximal suspension of the vaginal vault. At the same time, removal of the cervix creates an inherent defect in the proximal anterior vaginal wall. The posthysterectomy vault prolapse is in many instances a result of this defect. Care must be taken to compensate for this weakness at the time of hysterectomy. This area is the location of the pericervical ring whose proper attachments are so important to normal vaginal support. No totally anatomic method to close this space exists. To achieve a satisfactory result is easier at hysterectomy than at subsequent posthysterectomy repair. Plication of the cardinal ligaments and McCall's culdoplasty are necessary components of hysterectomy cuff repair.

Various grafts and synthetic meshes can be valuable tools in prolapse surgery. For example, in a posthysterectomy prolapse, a small piece of foreign material used to bolster the area left by the absence of the cervix may decrease the amount of anatomic distortion needed to close such a defect. These materials are useful and necessary in abdominal sacral colpopexy. The overzealous use of grafts and meshes is unnecessary and may predispose to the annoying problem of erosion. Procedures that require the use of foreign materials to compensate for absent fasciae should be viewed with suspicion. Even in an advanced prolapse, the fascia is present in most cases. Fasciae, unlike muscles, do not atrophy. They may be retracted and scarred, but they are available for dissection and reattachment if the surgeon is trained in the proper techniques.

Complications occurred in 15.5% of prolapse surgeries in 1997 (Table 35A.11). The majority of these complications can be addressed in the operating room. Gynecologic surgeons have been well trained to irrigate

TABLE 35A.11.
Frequency and Percentage of Morbidity Associated with Pelvic Organ Prolapse Surgery, 1997

Morbidity	Frequency	Percent of All Surgeries*
Infections	14,824	5.4
Bleeding complications	13,945	5.4
Surgical injury	9,546	4.2
Pulmonary complications	3,024	1.3
Cardiovascular complications	2,407	1.1
Wound complications	1,368	0.6
Cerebrovascular complications	249	<0.1
Other complications	165	<0.1
Total morbidity	45,528	15.5

* $N = 225,964$ women undergoing prolapse surgery.

From: Brown JS, Waetjen LE, Subak LL, et al. Pelvic organ prolapse in the United States, 1997. *Am J Obstet Gynecol* 2001;186:712–716. Reprinted with permission.

inside the abdomen. The same principles are applicable when operating vaginally. In the operating room after the surgical prep and draping are completed, a vaginal lavage rinses the vagina of nonadherent bacteria. Intraoperative irrigation at frequent intervals also helps to prevent infection. Irrigation as described and prophylactic antibiotics greatly help reduce the incidence of postoperative infection. A vaginal pack may help initial adherence of the vaginal epithelium to the endopelvic fascia and may reduce hematoma formation. Packs should be removed the day after surgery.

The pelvis is a busy place anatomically. The deep dissections necessary for the correction of prolapse predispose the patient to injury to adjacent structures. Development of proper surgical planes helps to minimize the potential for such injuries. Vascular injuries are usually immediately apparent and can be corrected during the operation. Intestinal and urinary injuries are often more subtle. The surgeon should not conclude the operative procedure without some reassurance of the integrity of these structures. Cystoscopy is a valuable skill that should be used by the pelvic support surgeon. A high rectal examination may suffice for intestinal reassurance unless damage is suspected higher than the examination extends.

Preoperative and postoperative care is discussed elsewhere in this text. Early ambulation and thrombosis prophylaxis are particularly important in the usual prolapse patient. The patient should be at sexual pelvic rest for approximately 6 weeks. The patient may be quite anxious about sexual activity. Sexual rehabilitation may require time, reassurance, and the helpful advice of the physician. Straining to void and defecate should be minimized. The act of perineal splinting postoperatively helps to protect the perineum from downward displacement during defecation. Lifting should be restricted to those things that can be accomplished with available strength in the shoulders, back, and legs.

The care of patients with pelvic organ prolapse can be equally challenging and rewarding. Attention to the details of anatomy, physical diagnosis, reconstructive surgical techniques, and good medical care will yield the best results.

BIBLIOGRAPHY

Baden WF, Walker T. *Surgical repair of vaginal defects.* Philadelphia: JB Lippincott, 1992.

Barber MD, Visco AG, Weidner AC, et al. Bilateral uterosacral ligament vaginal vault suspension with site-specific endopelvic fascia defect repair for treatment of pelvic organ prolapse. *Am J Obstet Gynecol* 2000;183:1402–1411.

Bonney V. An address on genital displacements. *BMJ* 1928;1:432.

Bonney V. The principles that should underlie all operations for prolapse. *J Obstet Gynaecol Br Emp* 1934;41:669.

Brown JS, Waetjen LE, Subak LL, et al. Pelvic organ prolapse in the United States, 1997. *Am J Obstet Gynecol* 2002;186:712–716.

Buller JL, Thompson JR, Cundiff GW. Uterosacral ligament: description of anatomic relationships to optimize surgical safety. *Obstet Gynecol* 2001;97:873–879.

Bump RC, Mattiasson A, Bø K, et al. The standardization of terminology of female pelvic organ prolapse and pelvic floor dysfunction. *Am J Obstet Gynecol* 1996;175:10–17.

Cunningham F, Gant N, Gilstrap L, et al. *Williams obstetrics,* twenty-first ed. New York: McGraw-Hill, 2001.

DeLancey JO. Anatomy and biomechanics of genital prolapse. *Clin Obstet Gynecol* 1993;36:897–909.

DeLancey JO. Structural anatomy of the posterior pelvic compartment as it relates to rectocele. *Am J Obstet Gynecol* 1999;180:815–823.

Emge LA, Durfee RB. Pelvic organ prolapse: four thousand years of treatment. *Clin Obstet Gynecol* 1966;9:997.

Francis CC. *The human pelvis.* St. Louis: CV Mosby, 1952.

Gershenson DM, ed. Reconstructive pelvic surgery. *Operative Techniques in Gynecologic Surgery* 1996;1:2.

Grody MH. *Benign postreproductive gynecologic surgery.* New York: McGraw-Hill, 1995.

Grody MH, Nyirjesy P, Kelley LM, et al. Paraurethral fascial sling urethropexy and vaginal paravaginal defects cystopexy in the correction of urethro-vesical prolapse. *Int Urogynecol J* 1995;6:80–85.

Hollinshead WH, Rosse C. *Textbook of anatomy,* fourth ed. Philadelphia: Harper & Row, 1985.

Hoyte L, Schierlitz L, Zou K. Two- and 3-dimensional MRI comparison of levator ani structure, volume, and integrity in women with stress incontinence and prolapse. *Am J Obstet Gynecol* 2001;185:11–19.

Jenkins II VR. Uterosacral ligament fixation for vaginal vault suspension in uterine and vaginal vault prolapse. *Am J Obstet Gynecol* 1997;177:1337–1344.

Kegel AH. Physiologic therapy for urinary stress incontinence. *JAMA* 1952;10:915.

Kovac SR. Guidelines to determine the route of hysterectomy. *Obstet Gynecol* 1995;85:18–23.

Leffler KS, Thompson JR, Cundiff GW. Attachment of the rectovaginal septum to the pelvic sidewall. *Am J Obstet Gynecol* 2001;185:41–43.

McCall ML. Posterior culdoplasty. *Obstet Gynecol* 1957;10:595–602.

Mengert WF. Mechanics of uterine support and position. *Am J Obstet Gynecol* 1936;31:775.

Nguyen JK, Lind LR, Choe JY, et al. Lumbosacral spine and pelvic inlet changes associated with pelvic organ prolapse. *Obstet Gynecol* 2000;95:332–336.

Nichols DH, Clarke-Pearson DL. *Gynecologic, obstetric, and related surgery,* second ed. St. Louis: CV Mosby, 2000.

Nichols DH, Milley PS, Randall CL. Significance of restoration of normal vaginal depth and axis. *Obstet Gynecol* 1970;36:251.

Nichols DH, Milley PS. Surgical significance of the rectovaginal septum. *Am J Obstet Gynecol* 1970;108:215–220.

Nichols DH, Randall CL. *Vaginal surgery,* fourth ed. Baltimore: Williams & Wilkins, 1996.

Reiffenstuhl G, Platzer W, Knapstein P-G. *Vaginal operations: surgical anatomy and technique,* second ed. Baltimore: Williams & Wilkins, 1994.

Retzy SS, Rogers RM, Richardson AC. Anatomy of female pelvic support. In: Brubaker LT, Saclarides TJ, eds. *The female pelvic floor: disorders of function and support.* Philadelphia: FA Davis, 1996:3–21.

Richardson AC, Lyon JB, Williams NL. A new look at pelvic relaxation. *Am J Obstet Gynecol* 1976;126:568–573.

Shull B. Clinical evaluation and physical examination of the incontinent woman. *J Pelvic Surgery* 2000;6:334–343.

Shull BL, Bachofen C, Coates KW, et al. A transvaginal approach to repair of apical and other associated sites of pelvic organ prolapse with uterosacral ligaments. *Am J Obstet Gynecol* 2000;183:1365–1374.

Singh K, Reid WM, Berger LA. Magnetic resonance imaging of normal levator ani anatomy and function. *Obstet Gynecol* 2002;99:433–438.

Subak LL, Quesenberry CP, Posner SF, et al. The effect of behavioral therapy on urinary incontinence: a randomized controlled trial. *Obstet Gynecol* 2002;100:72–78.

Sze EH, Karram MM. Transvaginal repair of vault prolapse: a review. *Obstet Gynecol* 1997;89:466–475.

Sze EH, Kohli N, Miklos JR. Comparative morbidity and charges associated with route of hysterectomy and concomitant Burch colposuspension. *Obstet Gynecol* 1997;90:42–45.

Te Linde RW. Prolapse of the uterus and allied conditions. *Am J Obstet Gynecol* 1966;94:444.

Toglia MR, DeLancey JO. Anal incontinence and the obstetrician-gynecologist. *Obstet Gynecol* 1994;84:731–740.

Uhlenhuth E. *Problems in the anatomy of the pelvis.* Philadelphia: JB Lippincott, 1953.

Uhlenhuth E, Nolley GW. Vaginal fascia, a myth? *Obstet Gynecol* 1957;10:349–358.

Ulfelder H. The mechanism of pelvic support in women: deductions from a study of the comparative anatomy and physiology of the structures involved. *Am J Obstet Gynecol* 1956;72:856–864.

Wall LL. Birth trauma and the pelvic floor: lessons from the developing world. *J Women's Health* 1999;8:149–155.

B

Correction of Anterior Compartment Defects

CARL W. ZIMMERMAN   BOBBY SHULL

SITE-SPECIFIC REPAIR OF CYSTOURETHROCELE

CARL W. ZIMMERMAN

The anterior compartment of the vagina extends from the pubic symphysis anteriorly to the posterior aspect of the cervix. The lateral boundaries are the white lines or arcus tendineus fasciae pelvis. The anterior compartment separates the bladder from the lumen of the vagina. Support of the bladder is the function of the pubocervical septum that is part of the deep endopelvic connective tissue. In the anatomically normal woman, the epithelium of the anterior vaginal wall firmly adheres to the pubocervical septum, creating rugae. Rugae are responsible for the finely ridged texture of the vaginal wall. The linear attachment of the pubocervical septum to the white line forms the anterior lateral sulci of the vagina. In the standing woman, the proximal two-thirds of the anterior vaginal segment is nearly horizontal. In the lithotomy position, the anterior vaginal wall is more nearly vertical. The cervix and its surrounding ring

and ligaments comprise the proximal portion of the anterior vaginal segment. As a result, the pubocervical septum is shorter than the rectovaginal septum by the diameter of the cervix. In the absence of the cervix, an inherent defect is present that cannot be repaired in a completely reconstructive fashion. Compensating for the absence of the cervix at the time of hysterectomy is possible by using careful techniques of cuff repair. The failure to correct anatomically for the absent cervix in the posthysterectomy prolapse patient leads to many problems.

Labor and delivery apply intense pressure to all components of vaginal support. During descent, flexion, internal rotation, and extension, specific stresses are focused on the pubocervical septum before external rotation and expulsion of the fetus. The damage that results from the passage of a baby through the obstetric axis of the pelvis is the nidus for symptomatic prolapse of the anterior vaginal segment. The anatomic components of anterior prolapse are cystocele, urethrocele, paravaginal defects, and uterine procidentia. Prolapse may occur without childbirth; however, this clinical circumstance is the exception rather than the rule. Other etiologic factors are normally required for the development of pelvic organ prolapse. These factors include time, age, repeated pelvic stresses, and lack of estrogen.

For most of the 20th century, the assumption was made that, during childbirth, gradual attenuation of the endopelvic fascial support structures occurred. Howard Kelly of Baltimore championed this concept. His influence was considerable, and, as a result, anatomically distorting midline anterior plications became the standard of care. The Kelly–Kennedy plication was used to correct the perceived attenuated and stretched support of the bladder and anterior vaginal wall. This method of prolapse correction has been shown to have an unacceptable failure rate and has not proven to be a satisfactory treatment for urinary incontinence. This procedure is seldom used today.

In 1909, George White of Georgia noted that the repair of lateral anterior vaginal wall support was sufficient to correct cystocele. His observation remained largely unknown to mainstream gynecologic surgeons until the 1960s. Beginning with observations by Burch and others, the significance and importance of the lateral support of the anterior vagina began to emerge. Burch initially performed his anterior urethropexy using the white line as the ventral attachment point. He quickly abandoned the white line in favor of the more substantial Cooper's ligament. Subsequently, the importance of paravaginal defects in anterior vaginal relaxation has gradually become more and more apparent. Paravaginal defects are created when the pubocervical septum is separated from the arcus tendineus fascia pelvis. A paravaginal defect is a connection between the vesicovaginal space and the paravesical space. A trampoline analogy is useful in illustrating the difference between central and paravaginal defects. A central defect would result from a tear in the fabric of the trampoline. A lateral or paravaginal defect is analogous to unhooking the fabric from the side frame of the trampoline. Either defect results in a failure of the support of the trampoline. The correction of lateral defects is now considered to be a necessary component of anterior vaginal reconstruction.

A Kelly–Kennedy plication procedure bunches connective tissue in the midline. This operation actually places more stress on paravaginal defects by pulling the detached edge of the pubocervical septum further away from the pelvic sidewall. Pelvic surgeons have learned how to identify fascial defects. To visually distinguish between the visceral fascia of the bladder wall and the pubocervical septum is possible. The bladder wall is red, distensible, and highly elastic. The pubocervical septum that is part of the deep endopelvic connective tissue is whiter in color, stands out as a separate layer, and, when closely examined, has a coarse fibrous texture. During dissection, if the surgeon irrigates with saline, the color distinction between the visceral fascia of the bladder wall and the pubocervical septum becomes even more apparent.

In the 1970s, A. Cullen Richardson of Georgia formally described specific breaks in the deep endopelvic connective tissue (Fig. 35B.1). His observations have been confirmed by others, and these defects are described by their location and direction. For location, the terms distal, proximal, central, and lateral are used. For direction, the terms transverse and longitudinal are used. Anatomically specific terms improved the description of

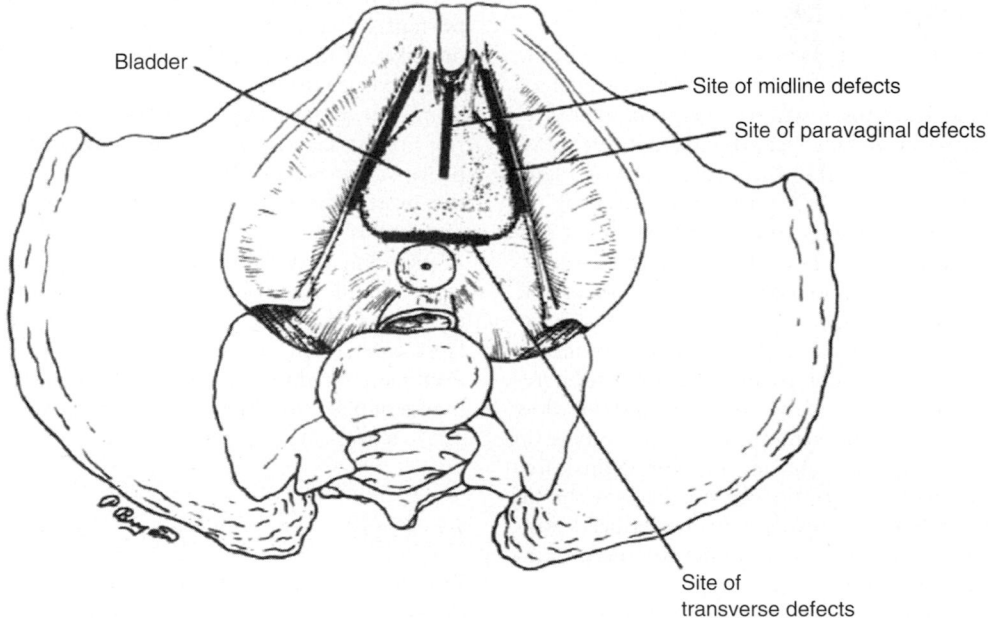

Bladder

Site of midline defects

Site of paravaginal defects

Site of
transverse defects

FIGURE 35B.1. The anterior vaginal segment from above. Potential sites of fascial defects are shown in bold lines. (Richardson AC. The rectovaginal septum revisited: its relationship to rectocele and its importance in rectocele repair. *Clin Onstet Gynecol* 36:976–983.)

fascial defects. In older literature, for example, lateral defects were termed displacement cystoceles, and central defects were termed distention cystoceles.

The next major conceptual step occurred after the biomechanical observations of DeLancey (Figs. 35A.7 and 35A.8). He recognized that each portion of the vagina relies on a different method of support to preserve normal anatomy. The proximal one-third of the vagina is suspended by the structures of the paracolpium, primarily the uterosacral ligaments (Fig. 35A.8). The middle one-third of the vagina is supported by lateral attachments to the pelvic sidewall at the arcus tendineus fasciae pelvis. The distal one-third of the anterior vagina fuses with the relatively immovable urogenital diaphragm. These concepts become very important in site-specific repairs. Any operation that does not account for the normal attachments at all three DeLancey levels is likely to fail. Specifically, the proximal extent of the operation should extend to the interspinous diameter and include proximal suspension of the pubocervical septum. The lateral extent of the operation should ensure bilateral attachments of the pubocervical septum to the parietal superior fasciae of the pelvic diaphragm. Each lateral attachment should include the entire length of the white line from the ischial spine to the pubic tubercle. Distally, the integrity of the connection between the pubocervical septum and the urogenital diaphragm should be assured. The only way to achieve these goals is a full-length and full-width dissection, followed by a meticulous correction of fascial defects. After the surgeon becomes practiced at detecting these separations, the reattachment becomes a relatively straightforward exercise in reconstruction.

EVALUATION OF THE PATIENT WITH A CYSTOCELE

Cystoceles are common in parous women, and most are asymptomatic. If they are large enough or accompanied by incontinence, the patient will seek surgical relief. Prevention and physical therapy were discussed in the previous section of this chapter. Incontinence is a major symptom in parous women. Cystocele and paravaginal repair may improve the symptoms; however, these surgeries do not represent a cure for incontinence. The correction of anterior vaginal defects does play a major role in the treatment of incontinence. Cystocele and paravaginal defects should be corrected at the time of incontinence procedures in order to improve long-term results. Reverse kinking of the urethra and outflow obstruction may hide the symptom of incontinence in the presence of a large and chronic anterior vaginal prolapse. Evaluation of the continence mechanism should be performed with a large prolapse in the reduced position in order to avoid the frustrating development of incontinence after prolapse repair.

Physical examination and surgical treatment of the patient with anterior vaginal prolapse should not be limited to the anterior vagina. Complete integrity of vaginal support depends on the normality of the support of each vaginal segment. Burch learned this lesson early in the course of developing his anterior urethropexy. Anterior displacement of the vaginal axis by placement of the urethropexy sutures led to the development of an enterocele in a significant portion of patients. This minor change in the axis of the vagina led to the conversion of an incipient defect into a symptomatic clinical problem.

The physical examination should be recorded in a way that is accurate and complete. Either the Baden–Walker Halfway System or the POP-Q system is recommended. Narrative notes can supplement either of these methods. Using a pelvic organ prolapse map to diagram the location of defects found on physical examination is helpful (Figs. 35A.13 and 35A.14). Another map may be created at the time of surgery when the defects are actually visualized. The pattern of the presence and absence of rugae is extremely important. Rugae indicate the presence of underlying fascia. In an advanced prolapse, rugae continue to be present even though they may be displaced by the distorted anatomy. Fascia does not atrophy. The most likely place to find rugae in an advanced or chronic prolapse is immediately proximal to the urethra. Both labor and prolapse displace anatomic structures from a proximal to distal direction.

Paravaginal defects may be detected by physical examination. A tongue blade or Ayre spatula may be used to replace the anterior lateral sulci. When a paravaginal defect is present, replacement of the sulci causes the anterior vaginal wall to retract into a normal anatomic position. If a central defect is present, a central bulge remains. Removing each of the bolsters in turn may help determine whether paravaginal defects are unilateral or bilateral. In most cases, a right paravaginal defect is present (Fig. 35A.15). Less commonly, a concomitant or isolated defect is diagnosed on the left. The findings in a defect analysis should correlate with the pattern of rugae.

The location of the cervix or hysterectomy scar is important in determining the location of the dominant prolapse. If the majority of the herniation is anterior to the cervix or hysterectomy scar, the anterior prolapse is dominant. Conversely, if the prolapse is primarily posterior to the cervix or hysterectomy scar, the dominant prolapse is posterior. If the cervix or hysterectomy scar is the most dependent part of the prolapse, the superior segment is dominant. Such observations are important in planning a successful surgery. A large dominant prolapse will fill the urogenital hiatus and prevent an incipient defect from developing. If only the dominant prolapse is repaired, incipient defects will probably become dominant rapidly. Restitution of all the normal attachments of pelvic organ support is the goal of the pelvic reconstructive surgeon.

SURGICAL TECHNIQUE

The site-specific correction of anterior vaginal defects depends on access to all normal support structures. Complete restoration of the pubocervical septum and the pericervical ring is the surgical goal. Normal anatomy of the pubocervical septum (Table 35A.6) and pericervical ring (Table 35A.8) has been described. Operative goals of anterior vaginal reconstruction are summarized in Table 35B.1. A full-length and full-width dissection of the anterior vaginal wall is necessary. If each operative goal is not satisfied, the long-term success of the surgery is jeopardized.

The patient's legs are carefully positioned in adjustable stirrups before the surgery to avoid peripheral neuropathy, joint stress, and femoral fracture. No rotational stress should be present at the hip or knee. Ideally, the angles of the hip and knee should be 90 degrees. If extended, a line connecting the foot and knee should intersect with the contralateral shoulder. Compromises in position may be needed in patients with obesity, limitations of motion, inadequate joint mobility, or other orthopedic problems. The vaginal operative approach may not be ideal in patients whose physical limitations prevent adequate operative exposure.

The procedure begins with a lavage of the vaginal vault to remove nonadherent bacteria. Irrigation at intervals throughout the procedure serves the same purpose as irrigation during abdominal surgery. An anterior midline vaginal incision begins the surgery. If a concomitant hysterectomy is performed, the anterior midline of the vaginal cuff may be used as the starting point for the anterior vaginal wall incision. This maneuver ensures adequate proximal surgical access. In the posthysterectomy patient, the initial incision is made immediately anterior to the hysterectomy scar (Fig. 35B.2). The hysterectomy scar is usually visible as a transverse fibrous band with lateral dimples that signify the location of the remnants of the uterosacral ligaments. The midline incision is extended distally to the plane where the pubocervical septum fuses with the urogenital diaphragm. The goal of the anterior vaginal incision is to allow separation of the epithelium from the underlying deep endopelvic connective tissue (Fig. 35B.3). The plane of separation is continued laterally in each direction to the pelvic sidewall. Separating the deep endopelvic connective tissue from the undersurface of the vaginal epithelium facilitates the dissection. This separation should begin immediately lateral to the line of incision. Once the correct dissection plane is es-

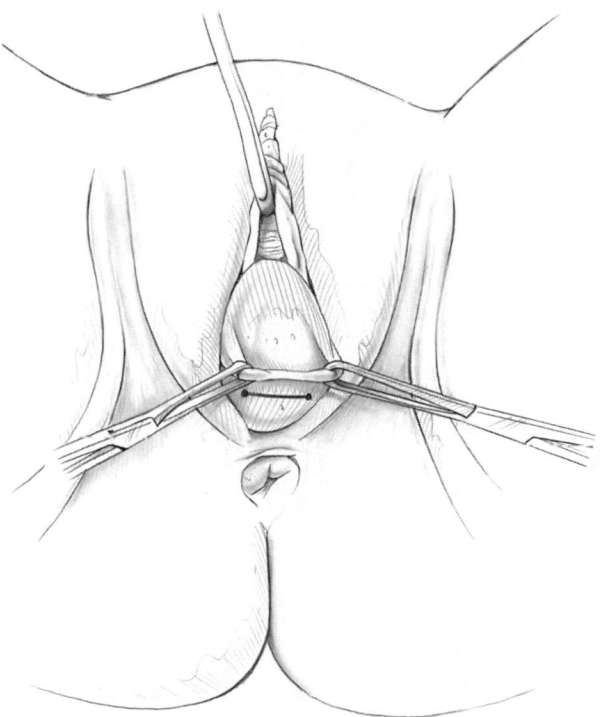

FIGURE 35B.2. A dominant anterior posthysterectomy prolapse is grasped with two Allis clamps. Notice the hysterectomy scar posterior to the clamps. The initial anterior incision will be made in the crease between the clamps.

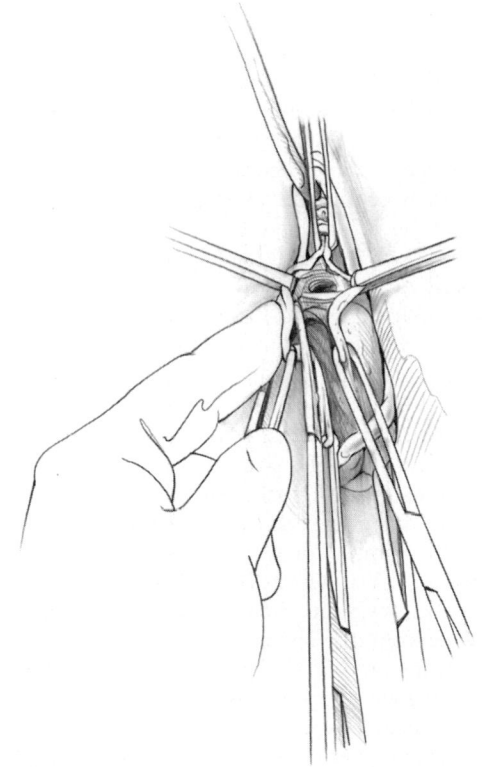

FIGURE 35B.3. The vesicovaginal space is developed by separating the endopelvic connective tissue from the vaginal epithelium.

TABLE 35B.1.
Operative Goals of Anterior Vaginal Reconstruction

Central: Reconstruct the pubocervical septum or repair of distention cystocele.
Proximal: Reattach the proximal pubocervical septum to the suspensory support of the paracolpium. Rebuild the pericervical ring and compensate for the defect left by the absence of the cervix (DeLancey Level I).
Lateral: Reattach the pubocervical septum to the arcus tendineus fasciae pelvis (white line) or paravaginal repair (DeLancey Level II).
Distal: Urethropexy (DeLancey Level III).

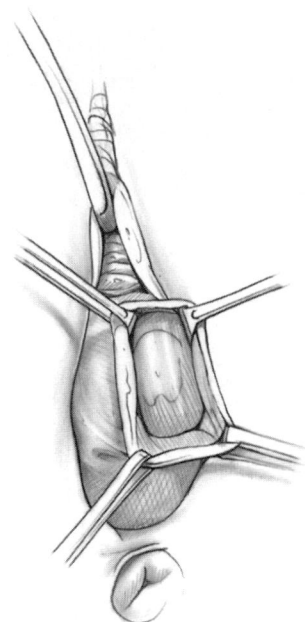

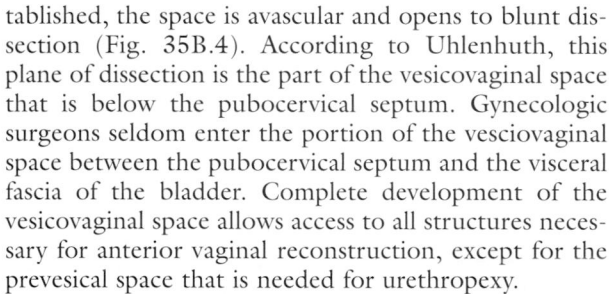

FIGURE 35B.4. Demonstration of the avascular vesicovaginal space.

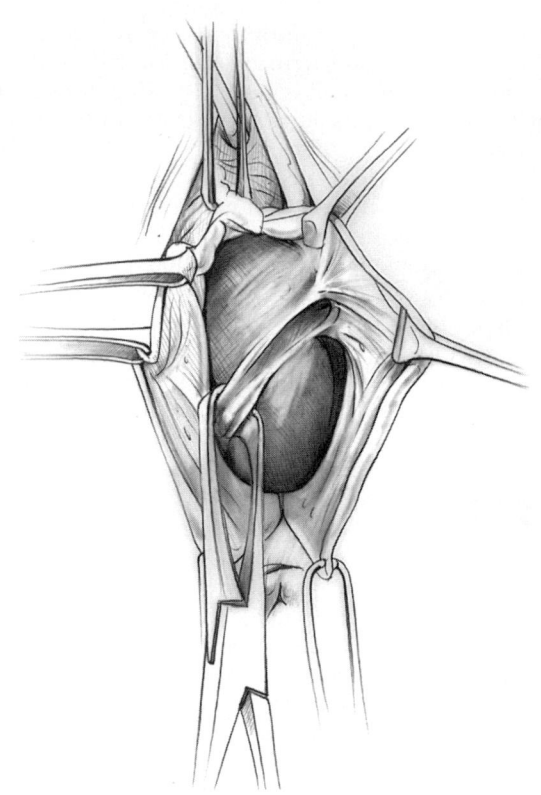

FIGURE 35B.5. Initial identification of the ragged edge of the pubocervical septum. The central Allis clamp is grasping the fascial edge. The right paravaginal defect can be seen in the upper left portion of the incision.

tablished, the space is avascular and opens to blunt dissection (Fig. 35B.4). According to Uhlenhuth, this plane of dissection is the part of the vesicovaginal space that is below the pubocervical septum. Gynecologic surgeons seldom enter the portion of the vesciovaginal space between the pubocervical septum and the visceral fascia of the bladder. Complete development of the vesicovaginal space allows access to all structures necessary for anterior vaginal reconstruction, except for the prevesical space that is needed for urethropexy.

The arcus tendineus fascia pelvis or white line extends from the ischial spine to the pubic tubercle. In the lithotomy position, the distal end of this structure is approximately 60 degrees above the horizontal plane. The white line may be visible to the surgeon. This structure is the fascial white line, not the arcus tendineus levator ani. The easiest place to palpate the white line is adjacent to its terminus at the ischial spine. Once a suture is placed around the white line and is under slight tension, the entire length of the structure is often palpable. Before initiating a paravaginal repair, the ischial spines must be palpable at the proximal extent of the dissection.

After the completion of dissection, an inspection may be started for fascial defects (Fig. 35B.5). The visceral fascia of the bladder is red, muscular, and distensible and has little tensile strength. The pubocervical septum is whitish, fibrous, strong, and in a different plane than the underlying visceral fascia. Irrigation with saline causes the subtle color difference between the visceral fascia of the bladder and the pubocervical fascia to become more obvious. Careful inspection reveals the presence of fascial edges. These edges are not smooth but are ragged and often

beveled or splayed. If the full thickness of the most obvious portion of the fascial edge is grasped with an Allis clamp, the entire length of the defect may become visible (Fig. 35B.6). The fascial edge may retract and create a wide paravaginal defect. In an advanced or chronic prolapse, the fascial edge may retract to the contralateral side of the midline.

The ability to recognize fascial defects is acquired during careful dissection and observation. The exact pattern of fascial damage cannot be determined until dissection is completed in the operating room. The most common pattern of anterior fascial damage is a full-length right paravaginal defect and a transverse proximal separation of the pubocervical septum from the pericervical ring (Fig. 35A.15). This pattern of fascial damage is consistent with the most common fetal presentation, left occipitoanterior position, at the time of delivery. The effects of the dynamics of a typical labor on pelvic support anatomy are described in Section A of this chapter. A left paravaginal defect or bilateral paravaginal defects may be encountered. The key to successful repair is the ability to visually distinguish between the visceral fascia of the bladder wall and the pubocervical septum.

After all the secondary adhesions are freed, the edge of the fully mobilized pubocervical septum should precisely extend to the desired reattachment point—the

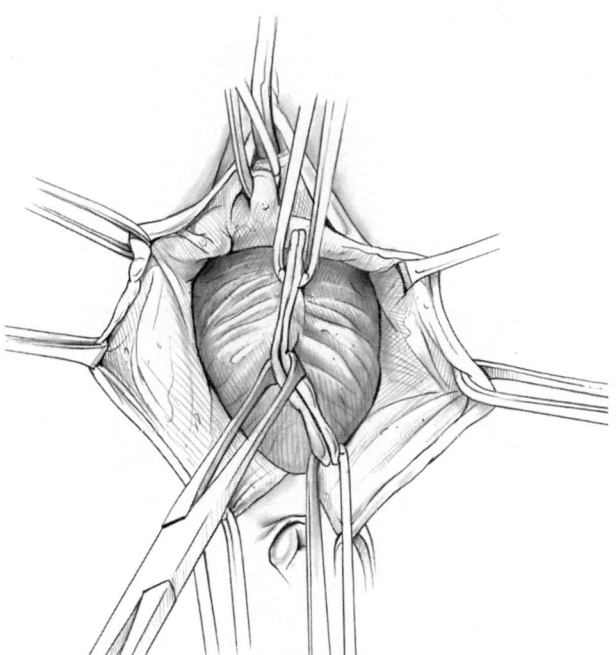

FIGURE 35B.6. After all secondary adhesions are released, the fascial edge is much more apparent when grasped by Allis clamps. A full-length right paravaginal defect is seen with the pubocervical edge retracted to the midline of the body.

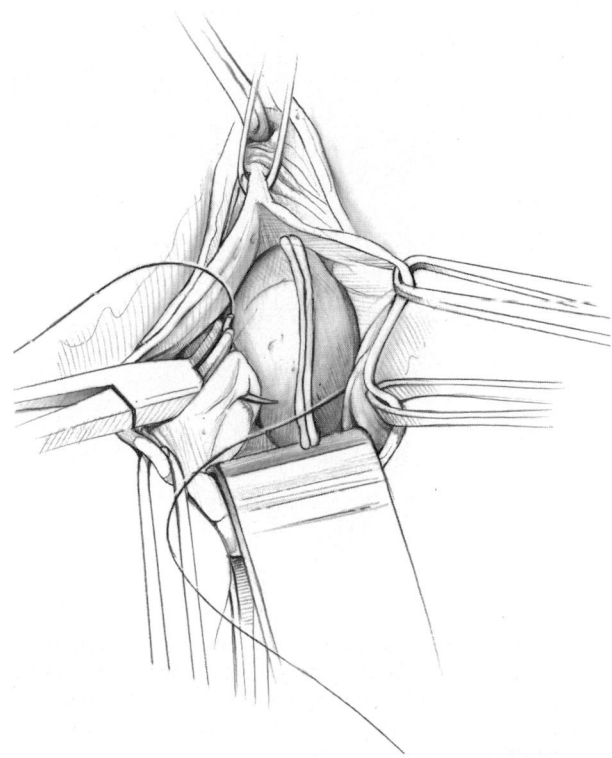

FIGURE 35B.7. A 0-gauge interwoven braided polyester suture is placed through the right white line adjacent to the ischial spine.

white line. Paravaginal sutures should connect the arcus tendineus fascia pelvis and lateral edge of the pubocervical septum. The placement of all sutures on a given side should precede tying. Commonly, between three and eight sutures are required for each paravaginal defect. Placement of the paravaginal sutures should begin proximally in the area adjacent to the ischial spine and proceed distally until the defect is completely closed (Figs. 35B.7, 35B.8, and 35B.9). If one accepts the premise that these defects are hernias, absorbable sutures have no place in their correction. Zero-gauge braided polyester is a useful suture; it is a soft and pliable product that is easily tied and not prone to erosion. Anatomic repairs restore the normal axis, caliber, and depth of the vagina and do not distort the anatomy of the vagina (Fig. 35B.10). The absence of anatomic distortion reduces the tension on the sutures and decreases the likelihood of suture erosion.

First, repair the largest lateral defect and then check the contralateral side to see whether the paravaginal attachment is intact. Checking the proximal portion of the contralateral paravaginal attachment is especially important because closure of the first lateral defect may allow a separation of the pubocervical fascia from the opposite pelvic sidewall to become apparent. After lateral reattachment has been completed, central defects should be repaired. The most common central defect is a proximal transverse separation of the pubocervical fascia from the cervix or hysterectomy scar. Occasionally, a central defect

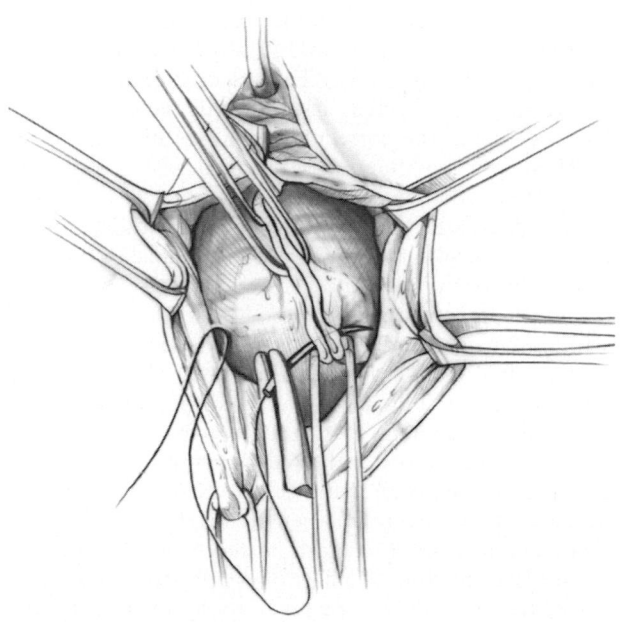

FIGURE 35B.8. The 0-gauge interwoven braided polyester suture from Fig. 35B.7 is passed through the detached edge of the pubocervical fascia to complete the most proximal paravaginal suture. The visceral fascia of the bladder wall is avoided to minimize the potential for urinary injury.

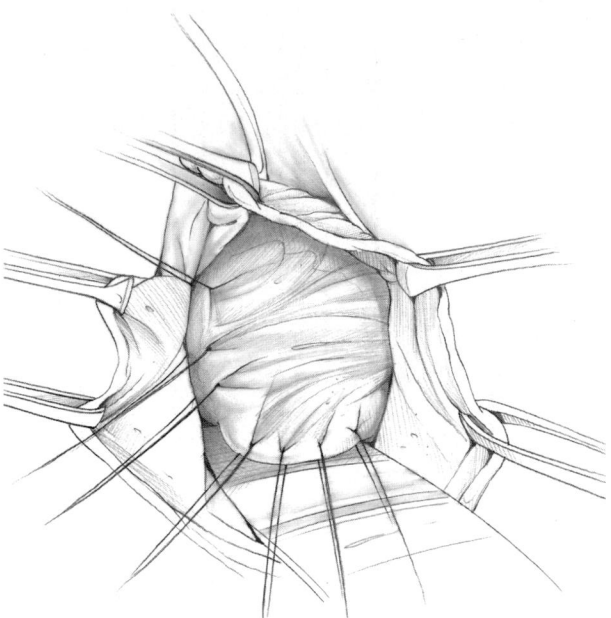

FIGURE 35B.9. Four paravaginal sutures have been placed to completely close the right paravaginal defect. Three sutures have been placed between the proximal edge of the pubocervical septum and the remnants of the hysterectomy scar to close the proximal transverse cystocele.

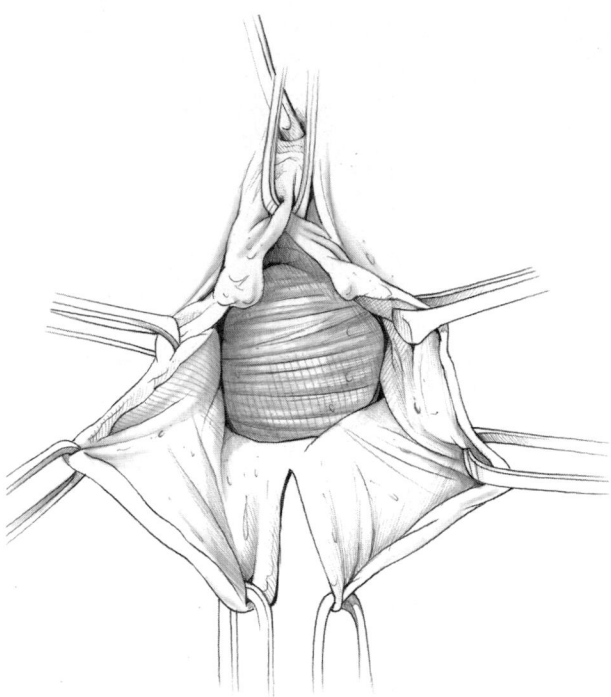

FIGURE 35B.10. After the sutures in Fig. 35B.9 are tied, the pubocervical septum is restored to its normal anatomic location.

may be encountered, which is in the configuration of an inverted "V" (Figure 35A.16). This type of central fascial defect is not commonly associated with paravaginal defects.

When all fascial defects are repaired, the pubocervical septum assumes its normal configuration with the distal end 60 degrees above the horizontal plane. The restoration of normal anatomy should always be in the mind of the site-specific surgeon. When fascial defects are properly identified, dissected, and repaired, the pubocervical fascia will be in the correct anatomic position as a hammock supporting the anterior vaginal wall and bladder with firm attachment to the pelvic sidewalls.

Proximal attachment of the pubocervical septum is the most difficult problem in anterior vaginal reconstruction. After paravaginal and central defects have been repaired, the transverse proximal edge of the pubocervical septum remains unattached. Normally, the proximal edge of the pubocervical septum connects with the pericervical ring, pubocervical ligaments, and the anterior portion of the cardinal ligaments. After hysterectomy, the normal proximal connections of the pubocervical septum are interrupted by removal of the cervix. No completely anatomic method exists to compensate for the absence of the cervix and to close the defect created by its absence.

If a hysterectomy is a part of the prolapse procedure, corrective measures can be taken to compensate for the absence of the cervix during the surgery. Plication of the cardinal ligaments across the midline and a McCall's culdoplasty with a permanent suture closes the cervical defect. Following this plication, the proximal edge of the pubocervical septum is attached in a site-specific fashion to the anterior aspect of the cardinal ligaments. Careful

attention to vaginal cuff support and closure is the most important part of a hysterectomy from the perspective of prolapse prevention.

In the posthysterectomy patient, the closure of the proximal anterior defect and the subsequent attachment of the proximal pubocervical septum are difficult. The cardinal ligaments and uterosacral ligaments are key anatomic landmarks that are difficult to identify or mobilize during a posthysterectomy anterior vaginal dissection. Attachment of the pubocervical septum to the hysterectomy scar with permanent suture may provide sufficient support. The hysterectomy scar can mimic the function of the pericervical ring, especially if a concomitant vaginal suspension or colpopexy is performed during the same surgery.

Placement of a bolster may be necessary when identifiable structures provide insufficient support. The surgeon may select from a variety of fascia or mesh products for this part of the reconstruction. I generally use cadaveric fascia or a permanent interlocked polyester fiber mesh for this portion of the operation. I do not recommend the use of an extruded polytetrafluoroethylene graft in this area because of its tendency to erode when placed in close proximity to the epithelium. A small piece of material, slightly larger than a commemorative postage stamp, adequately covers the defect caused by the absence of the cervix. The bolster should be attached by permanent sutures to both of the white lines in the fashion of a paravaginal repair (Figs. 35B.11 and 35B.12). The middle portion of the bolster may be secured to the underlying tissue to prevent rolling and gathering of the material. Bolsters may also be used to compensate for pubocervical

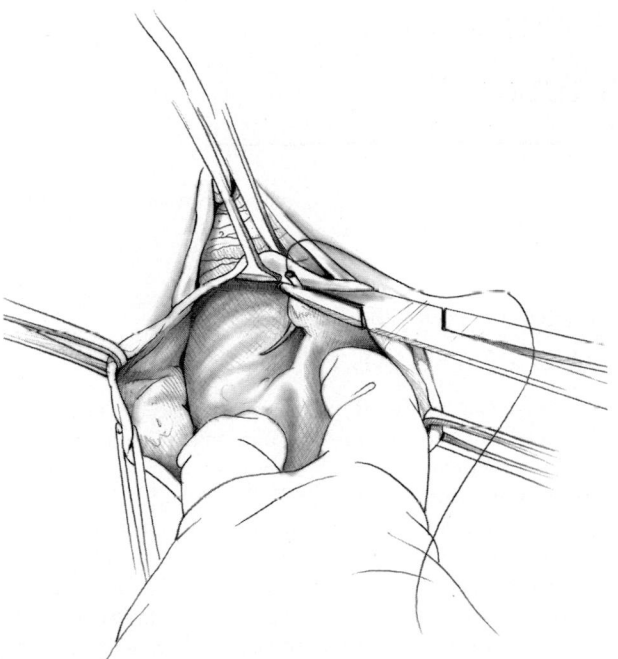

FIGURE 35B.11. A 0-gauge interwoven braided polyester suture is placed in the left white line. This suture will be one of the anchor sutures for the interlocked polyester fiber graft shown in Fig. 35B.12.

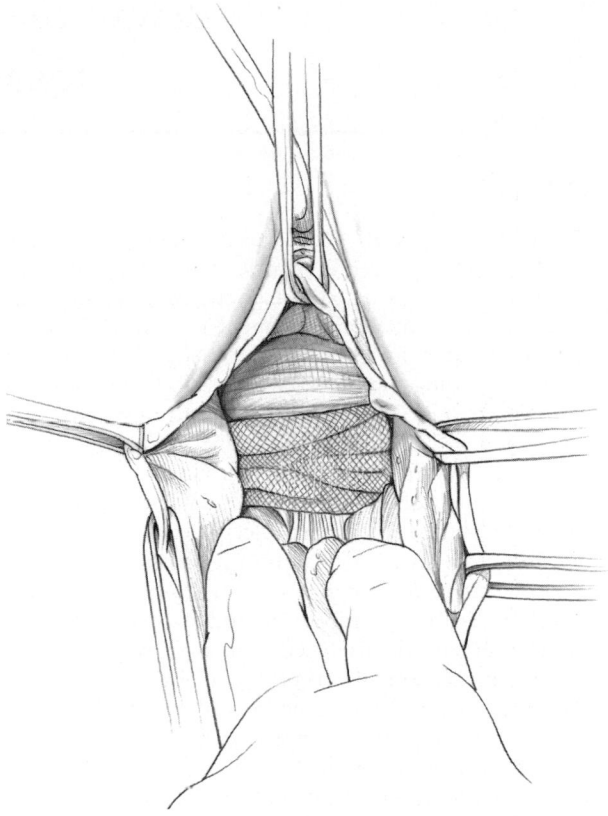

FIGURE 35B.12. The completed anterior vaginal reconstruction prior to closure of the incision. The interlocked polyester fiber graft is placed to reinforce the inherent area of weakness created by the absence of the cervix.

fascia that is significantly scarred or attenuated. Scarring is especially common in a patient who has had more than one previous pelvic support procedure. Scarring and retraction of the pubocervical septum may prevent adequate repair and require the use of a larger bolster.

Excessively distended vaginal epithelium may need to be trimmed. The amount of tissue removed should allow the epithelium to smoothly adhere to the underlying deep endopelvic connective tissue. The epithelium is not a support structure. Iatrogenic narrowing of the vaginal vault does not increase the likelihood of a successful operation. Absorbable suture is used for epithelial closure. During closure of the incision, attaching the proximal vaginal epithelium to the pubocervical septum near the level of the cuff is helpful.

After reconstruction of the pubocervical septum, both lateral anterior sulci should be visible (Fig. 35B.13). Permanent sutures and bolster material should not be exposed in the vaginal vault. The integrity of the rectum, bladder, and ureters should be confirmed.

The repair of anterior vaginal wall defects has undergone a recent conceptual revision. Anatomically distorting midline plications have been replaced by anatomically restoring operations that resemble herniorrhaphies. Anatomic landmarks define the extent of the components of the surgery. Permanent suture is used for support attachments. Anatomic restoration allows maximum potential for normal urinary, intestinal, and sexual function in the patient. To paraphrase the biological adage: function follows form.

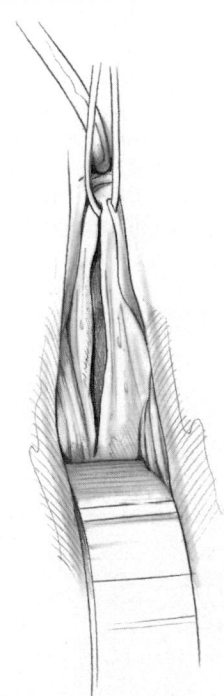

FIGURE 35B.13. Excessive vaginal epithelium has been trimmed. Notice the anterior lateral sulci, the normal orientation of the anterior vaginal plane, and normal vaginal depth as indicated by the Heaney retractor.

PARAVAGINAL DEFECT REPAIR

BOBBY SHULL

HISTORY

In 1909, George R. White quoted Ahlfelt, who said, "the only problem in plastic gynecology left unsolved by the gynecologist of the past century (the 19th century) is that of permanent cure of cystocele." Three years later, in 1912, White reviewed the current theories regarding the etiology of cystocele: overstretching and thinning of the vaginal wall and other supports of the bladder, which allow the bladder to descend in the form of a hernia; stretching of the firm attachment of the bladder to the uterus; and stretching of the ligamentous suspension of the bladder. He rejected each of these theories and also described his autopsy findings regarding the dissection of the anterior vaginal segment. One year before Howard Kelly's report on midline plication of the anterior segment, he discussed vaginal paravaginal repair for the management of certain types of cystocele; however, his theory and recommendation for surgical management did not gain widespread acceptance.

In 1923, Victor Bonney described the "periurethral wedge" that he found attached "to the subpubic angle, the rami of the pubes, and the edges of the levatores ani" and the association between this wedge and the mechanism of continence. Bonney suggested a retropubic repair of the loosened periurethral wedge in the treatment of incontinence. In 1961, Burch reported his experience with colposuspension. He attached the paravaginal fascia to the white line of the pelvis in his first seven patients. Subsequently, he chose Cooper's ligament as the point of fixation. The Burch procedure, as we have come to understand it, no longer uses the white line of the pelvis as a point of fixation. In the next decade, Richardson and colleagues published a "new"

and controversial look at pelvic relaxation and its relationship to fascial defects.

ANATOMIC CONCEPTS AND PHYSICAL FINDINGS

Stimulated by the work of Richardson and Baden, I have found it valuable to consider that isolated defects in the anterior compartment not only do occur but must be properly identified and specifically repaired to offer the best opportunity for cure of anatomic and functional complaints of the anterior vaginal segment. The pubocervical fascia is a trapezoid, part of which was described by Bonney more than 70 years ago. The fascia or fibromuscular tissue of the anterior vagina fuses with the perineal membrane distally, is attached to the arcus tendineus fasciae pelvis from a point just posterior to the pubic ramus to a point just anterior to the ischial spine bilaterally, and is attached to the cervix or to the vaginal cuff and base of the broad ligament and cardinal-uterosacral ligaments (Fig. 35B.14).

There are four clinically identifiable areas in which defects in this support are likely to occur:

- Laterally, where the pubocervical fascia attaches to arcus tendineus fascia pelvis (paravaginal defect)
- Transversely, in front of the cervix where the pubocervical fascia blends into the pericervical ring of fibromuscular tissue, or in the case of a woman who has had a hysterectomy, at the vaginal cuff (transverse defect)
- Centrally, in the area immediately anterior to the vaginal mucosa in between the lateral margins of the pubocervical fascia (midline or central defect)

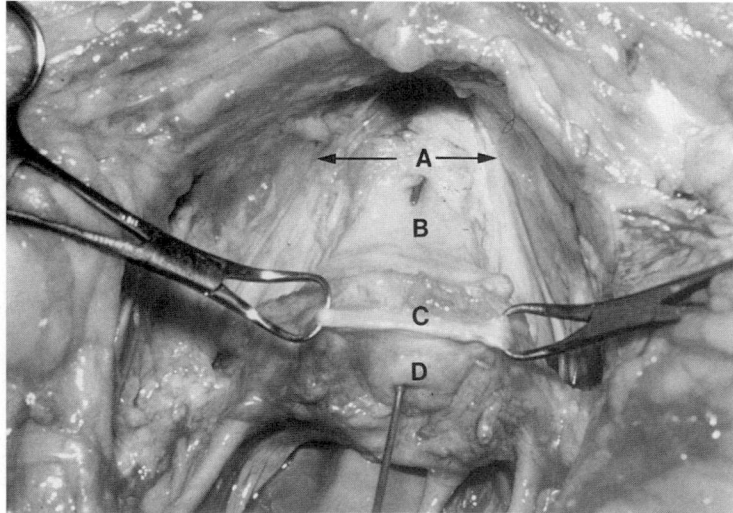

FIGURE 35B.14. An autopsy dissection of the pubocervical fascia. **A:** Arcus tendineus fasciae pelvis. **B:** Silver wire through the urethra. **C:** Towel clamps on the superior portion of the pubocervical fascia. **D:** Silver wire through the cervix. (From Shull BL. Clinical evaluation of women with pelvic support defects. *Clin Obstet Gynecol* 1993;36:939.)

• Distally, where the urethra perforates the urogenital diaphragm

These isolated defects may occur in combination, requiring the surgeon to identify and repair each defect individually. The clinical evaluation provides clues about the site of the fascial defect. The examination should be performed with the woman in the lithotomy position and the physician using only the posterior blade of the speculum. The patient is asked to strain or bear down maximally while the physician observes the landmarks of the anterior vagina. It is difficult to recognize an abnormal examination without having an understanding of normal. In a woman with normal support and no functional complaints, there is minimal descent of the urethra and urethrovesical junction on straining. There are lateral sulci in the anterior vagina at the site of attachment of the pubocervical fascia to the arcus tendineus fascia pelvis that extend from the back of the pubic bone to a point just anterior to the ischial spine (Fig. 35B.15). The anterior vaginal wall is normally about a centimeter shorter than the posterior vaginal wall. There are usually rugae in the epithelium overlying the urethra and bladder.

In a woman with paravaginal loss of support, one or both lateral sulci will be lost. Observations by DeLancey have shown that defects occur with equal frequency on the left and right sides and are associated with hypermo-

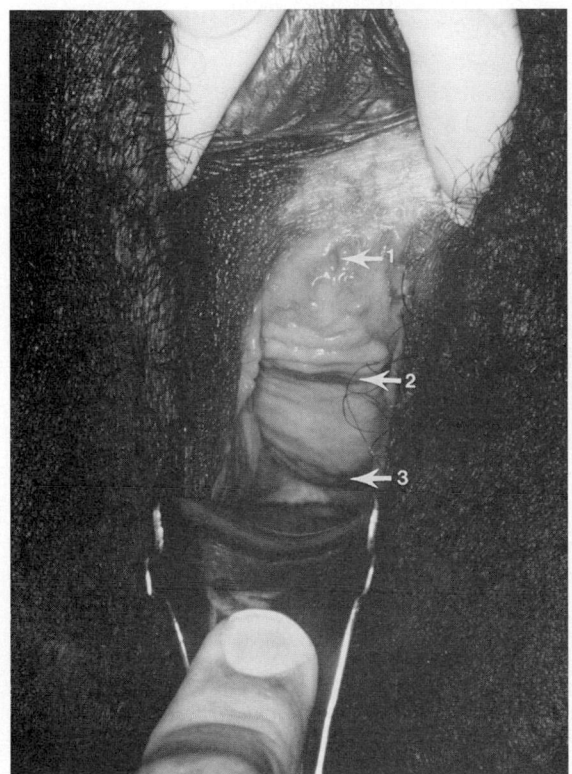

FIGURE 35B.15. Normal support for the urethra (1), urethrovesical junction (2), and bladder (3) in a woman with no functional complaints. (From Shull BL. Clinical evaluation of women with pelvic support defects. *Clin Obstet Gynecol* 1993;36:939.)

bility of the urethra and urethrovesical junction. When the support defect is predominantly paravesical, the support for the bladder is also poor. Loss of paravaginal support can also be detected during use of the bivalve speculum when the clinician finds that the sides of the vaginal walls collapse through the open sides of the bivalve speculum, obscuring view of the cervix or vaginal apex.

Baden and Walker have recommended the use of a curved ring forceps to elevate the lateral aspects of the anterior vagina to their normal points of attachment along the pelvic sidewall. The curved arms of the ring forceps are directed laterally and posteriorly toward the ischial spines as the patient bears down. When this lateral elevation corrects the support defect, the diagnosis of a paravaginal defect can be made (Fig. 35B.16). If the patient continues to have a bulge of tissue through the open arms of the forceps, she either has a midline loss of support or a combined midline and lateral loss of support. Imaging studies such as MRI and ultrasound provide details not only about connective tissue support in the pelvis but also about muscle integrity.

Women with complete eversion of the anterior vaginal segment must, by definition, have not only paravaginal loss of support for the urethra, urethrovesical junction, and bladder but also loss of support for the transverse portion of the pubocervical fascia. The eversion may occur in association with procidentia or posthysterectomy vaginal prolapse (Fig. 35B.17). In my own practice, management of the prolapsed anterior vaginal segment is technically the most challenging dilemma because it may require correction of a complex set of problems, including urinary incontinence; incomplete bladder emptying; impaired intravaginal intercourse; symptoms of prolapse, such as pressure, fullness, and a sense of things falling out; or any combination of these. Successful management of prolapse of the anterior vagina should ultimately result in correction of the poor support, maintenance or enhancement of the ability to have intravaginal intercourse, and maintenance or enhancement of urinary continence. A particularly difficult challenge is the patient with complete eversion of the vagina. Vaginal and abdominal operations for the treatment of vaginal vault prolapse are usually successful in suspension of the vaginal cuff. However, a 1992 study found a 15% to 25% incidence of postoperative urinary incontinence and a 15% incidence of persistent or recurrent cystocele.

OPEN RETROPUBIC TECHNIQUE

Paravaginal defects can be surgically repaired through an open retropubic incision, through a vaginal retropubic incision, or laparoscopically. I use the open retropubic repair primarily in the treatment of women who have genuine urinary incontinence associated with paravaginal defects. The operation can be performed with or without hysterectomy. If hysterectomy is performed, I prefer the intrafascial technique and incorporate the cardinal uterosacral ligaments into the angles and the pubocervical and rectovaginal fascia to minimize the occurrence of

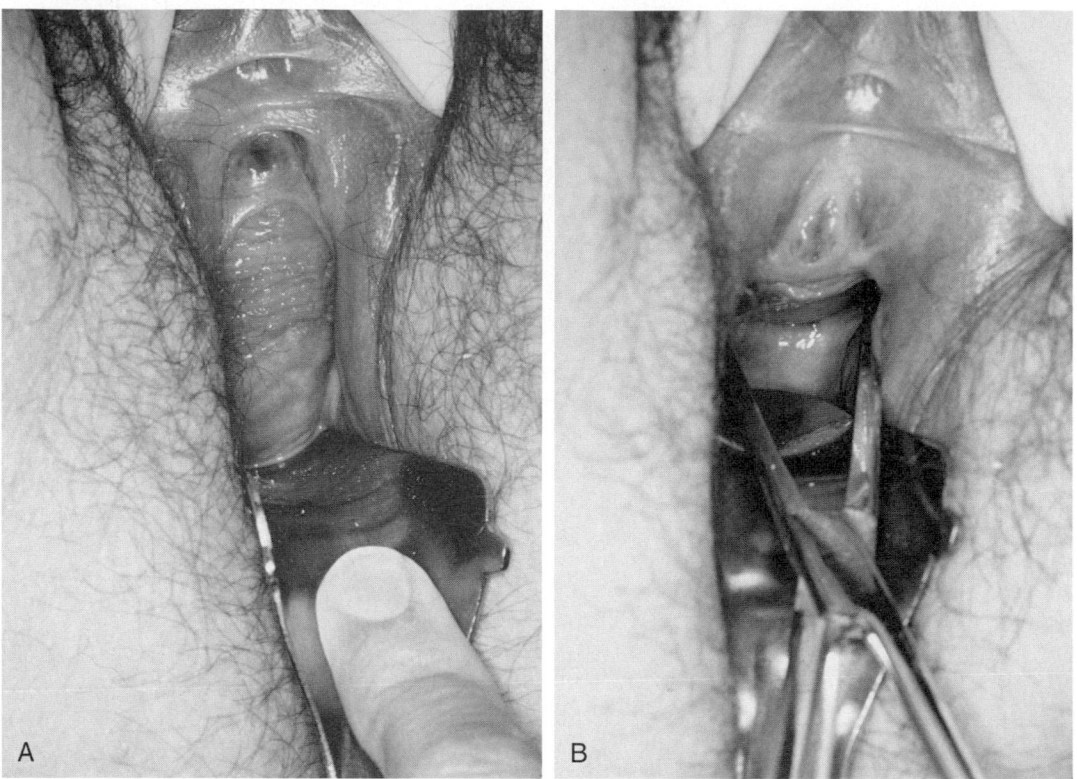

FIGURE 35B.16. A: Lateral loss of support with flattening of the urethrovesical junction. **B:** Lateral support with curved forceps restores normal support. (From Shull BL. Clinical evaluation of women with pelvic support defects. *Clin Obstet Gynecol* 1993;36:939.)

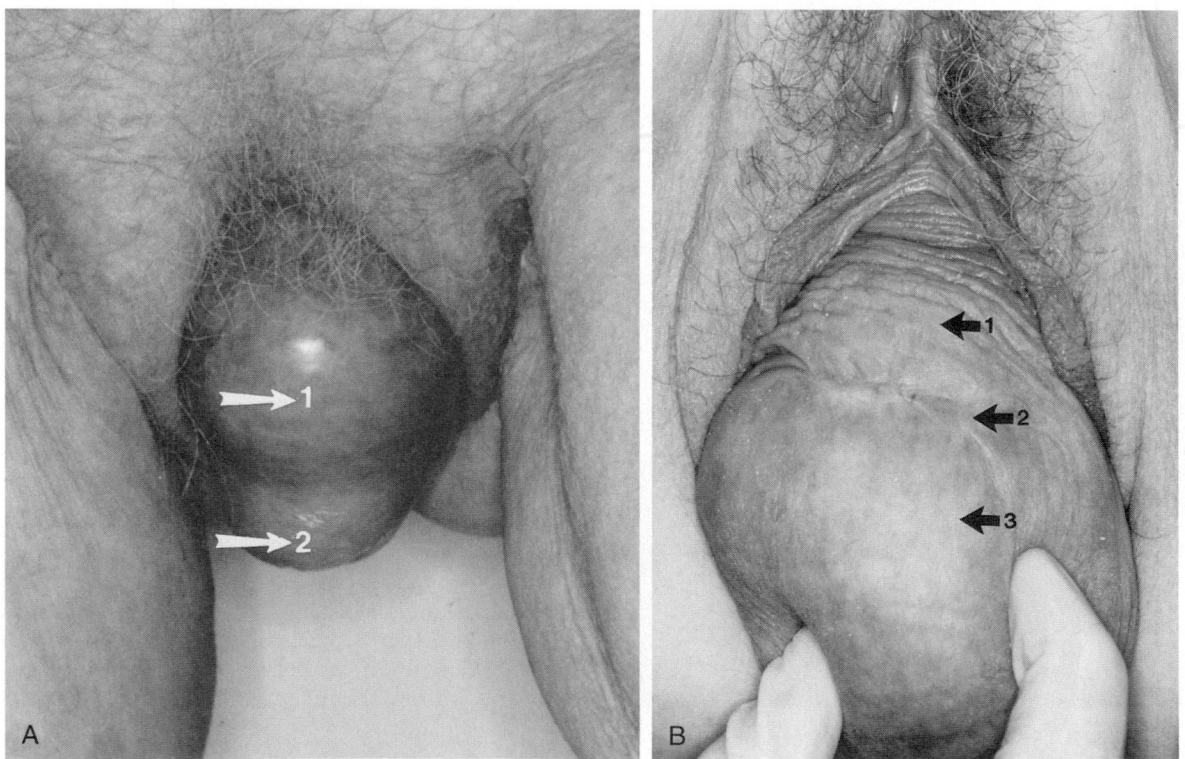

FIGURE 35B.17. *A:* Physical findings in the standing patient who has prolapse of the anterior segment (1) as well as uterine prolapse (2). **B:** Posthysterectomy prolapse of the anterior vaginal segment (1), vaginal cuff (2), and enterocele (3). (From Shull BL. Clinical evaluation of women with pelvic support defects. *Clin Obstet Gynecol* 1993;36:939.)

postoperative enterocele formation. In women with a preoperative enterocele and prior hysterectomy, I repair the enterocele in association with the paravaginal defect repair. The paravaginal repair is performed after completion of the hysterectomy or culdoplasty. The patient's legs are in low leg holders, and she is draped so that there is access to the abdomen as well as to the vaginal canal. A Foley catheter drains the urinary bladder. I prefer a low transverse abdominal incision made about one finger breadth cephalad to the symphysis pubis. The incision is carried to the anterior sheath of the rectus fascia, which is incised sharply. The rectus muscles are reflected laterally. The transversalis fascia is separated from the superior ramus of the pubic bone, and the space of Retzius is entered immediately medial to the superior ramus of pubis on each side. The loose areolar tissue can easily be dissected away from pubic bone by use of either the index finger or a pair of long tissue forceps. The bony landmarks in the pelvis are identified by palpation. The symphysis pubis, the midline landmark, is almost always convex. The pubic bone extends laterally and gently curves posteriorly. The next palpable landmark is the obturator neurovascular canal, which can be felt along the inferior border of the superior ramus of pubis about 7 to 10 cm lateral to the midline. The foramen feels like the buttonhole of a shirt or blouse. About 7 to 8 cm directly dorsal to the obturator canal is the ischial spine. The arcus tendineus fascia pelvis, more commonly known as the white line, extends from the back of the pubic bone to the ischial spine. The arcus is a condensation of the fascia of the obturator internus muscle and the levator ani muscles. The arcus tendineus musculi levator ani demarcates the origin of the pubococcygeal muscle from the inferior ramus of pubis and the condensation of the levator arcus (Fig. 35B.18).

After the bony landmarks have been identified by palpation, I use long tissue forceps to develop the space between the obturator internus fascia and the urethra and bladder. Veins coursing along the inner aspect of the superior ramus of pubis can be a source of troublesome bleeding. It is best not to traumatize them with a retractor or tissue forceps; however, when they bleed, electrocautery promptly controls the bleeding. A set of larger veins that course between the anterior surface of the urethra and the back of the pubic bone can also be the source of considerable bleeding. When they obstruct the dissection or interfere with the operative repair, they should be clipped with silver clips and divided sharply to fall out of the operative field. After the proper cleavage plane has been established, a fluffed up 4-in piece of gauze should be placed in the space to rest on the anterior surface of the vagina. Then a small or medium malleable ribbon retractor should be used to hold the bladder and urethra medially while the remaining landmarks are identified by direct visualization. To minimize bleeding, the bladder should never be reflected off of the anterior surface of the vagina. The vessels in the bladder generally course medially to laterally across the operative field. The vessels in the vagina generally course anteriorly to posteriorly. I dissect both the left and the right sides of the space of Retzius before beginning any of the operative repair. I find it helpful to use the long extension for the electrocautery in case it is necessary to cauterize bleeding points.

Because I am left-handed, it is easier for me to stand on the patient's right side and sew on her left side. The first assistant standing on the patient's left side can sew across the table on the patient's right-hand side. With this approach, a forehand stitch can be used to sew away from the bladder and urethra. If the surgeon chooses to stand on one side to do both sides of the repair, he or she will need to backhand the sutures when sewing on the side of the table on which he or she is standing. I prefer to use round tapered needles and 2-0 nonabsorbable suture for the repair. A long needle driver such as is used in chest surgery allows one to reach even the deepest portion of the retropubic space without having a hand directly in the operative field.

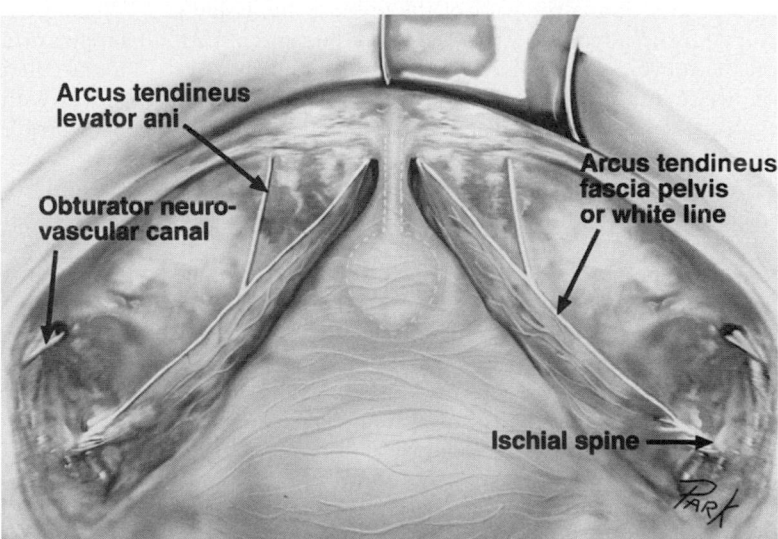

FIGURE 35B.18. The key anatomic landmarks in the space of Retzius in a woman with normal findings. (From Shull BL. How I do abdominal paravaginal repair. *J Pelvic Surg* 1995;1:43.)

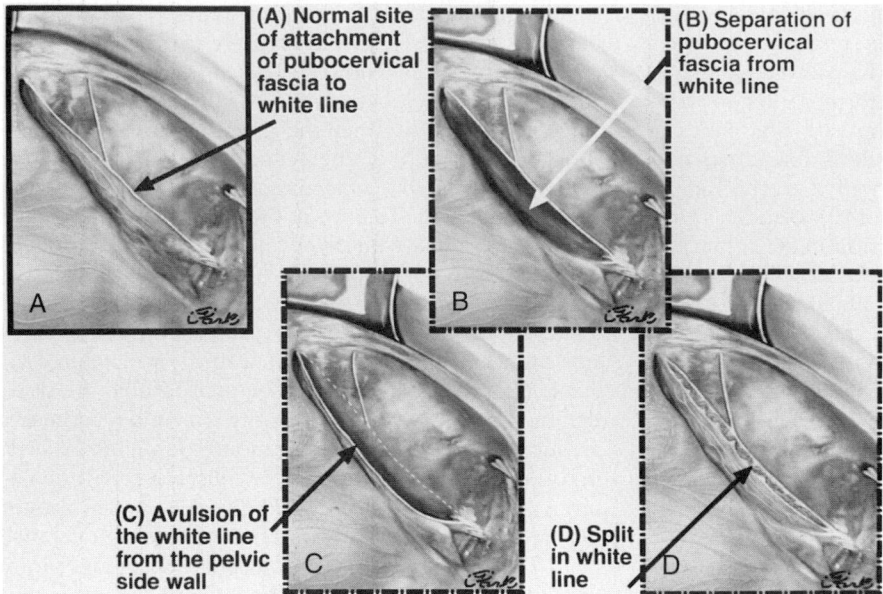

FIGURE 35B.19. Examples of the three types of paravaginal defects. **A:** Normal anatomy on the right side. **B:** Avulsion of the pubocervical fascia from the white line. **C:** Avulsion of the white line from the pelvic side wall. **D:** A split in the white line. (From Shull BL. How I do abdominal paravaginal repair. *J Pelvic Surg* 1995;1:43)

Paravaginal defects can occur in one of three different ways (Fig. 35B.19):

1. The entire arcus may remain attached to the pelvic sidewall with the pubocervical fascia breaking away from the arcus (Fig. 35B.19B).
2. The arcus may pull away from the side of the pelvis but remain attached to the pubocervical fascia (Fig. 35B.19C)
3. The arcus may split, with a portion of it remaining attached to the sidewall and a portion tearing away but remaining attached to pubocervical fascia (Fig. 35B.19D)

In any circumstance, the goal of the operative repair is to reattach the pubocervical fascia to the arcus tendineus fasciae pelvis as well as to the fascia overlying the obturator internus muscle.

The easiest point of identification of the white line is near its insertion at the back of the pubic bone. Using a pair of tissue forceps to grasp the white line and place it on tension makes it easier to identify the remainder of the white line as it courses toward the ischial spine. The smooth white fibromuscular tissue of the pubocervical fascia is always medial to the white line. The most dependent portion of the operative field is the perivesical space adjacent to the ischial spine. Any bleeding results in the collection of blood in that space; therefore, I prefer to initiate the repair near the vaginal apex while the field is quite dry.

I place my nondominant hand into the vaginal canal to elevate the periurethral and perivesical tissue to its site of normal attachment along the white line. The first suture is placed near the apex of the vagina through the perivesical portion of the pubocervical fascia. When permanent sutures are used, one should avoid penetration of the vaginal epithelium. If the needle is placed at a right angle to the fibromuscular tissue, it is easier to re-

trieve and place it through the white line and obturator internus fascia at a point 1 to 2 cm anterior to its origin at the ischial spine. The suture is securely tied with a series of four knots and the excess trimmed. I prefer to place the next suture at the opposite end of the repair through the pubocervical fascia near the distal portion of the urethra. The needle is regrasped and placed through the white line near its origin from the back of the pubic bone. The suture is similarly secured with four knots and the excess cut. At that point, the two extreme ends of the repair have been performed (Fig. 35B.20). The pubocervical fascia and white line stand out on relief, making it easier to determine the placement of subsequent sutures. I prefer to place the remaining sutures sequentially beginning proximal to the apical stitch. About four to six sutures are required on each side. In some patients, the vascular supply to the vagina is so generous that it is impossible to avoid suturing through or around a vessel. When each suture is tied as placed, significant bleeding is rarely a problem. Bleeding becomes a problem, however, if a needle is placed through a vein and the needle is removed without tying the suture down. Bleeding can also be a problem if one chooses to dissect the bladder or urethra off of the anterior surface of the vagina. When the sutures have all been placed on one side, the suture line adjacent to the urethra and urethrovesical junction is about horizontal to the floor (Fig. 35B.21). The suture line from the urethrovesical junction to the apex of the vagina angles gently posteriorly. The same sequence of sutures is repeated on the opposite side. I have used this repair for hundreds of patients over 14 years and have not left a drain in the space of Retzius in a single patient.

In patients who undergo a retropubic repair only, my goal is to dismiss them on the same day the procedure is performed. In these patients, I inject the incision site with a short-acting local anesthetic agent before making the incision and with a longer acting local anesthetic

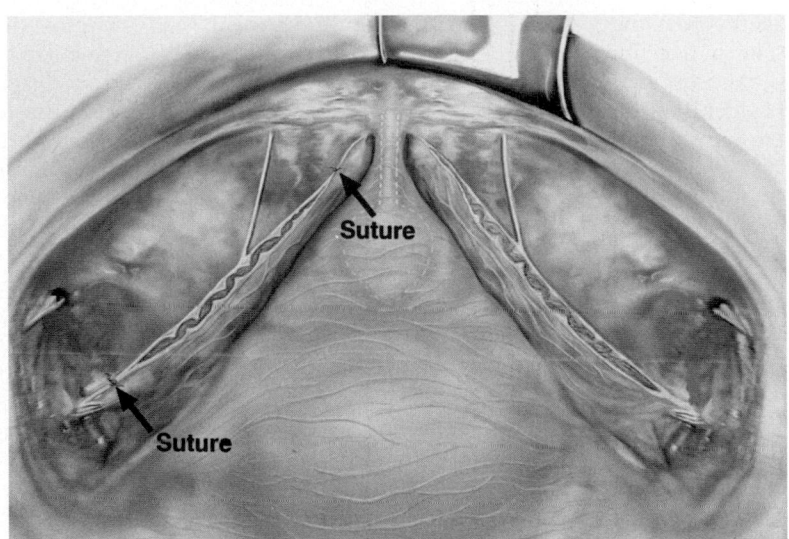

FIGURE 35B.20. A patient with bilateral paravaginal defects. The repair has been started on the left with sutures at the two extremes of the defect. (From Shull BL. How I do abdominal paravaginal repair. *J Pelvic Surg* 1995;1:43.)

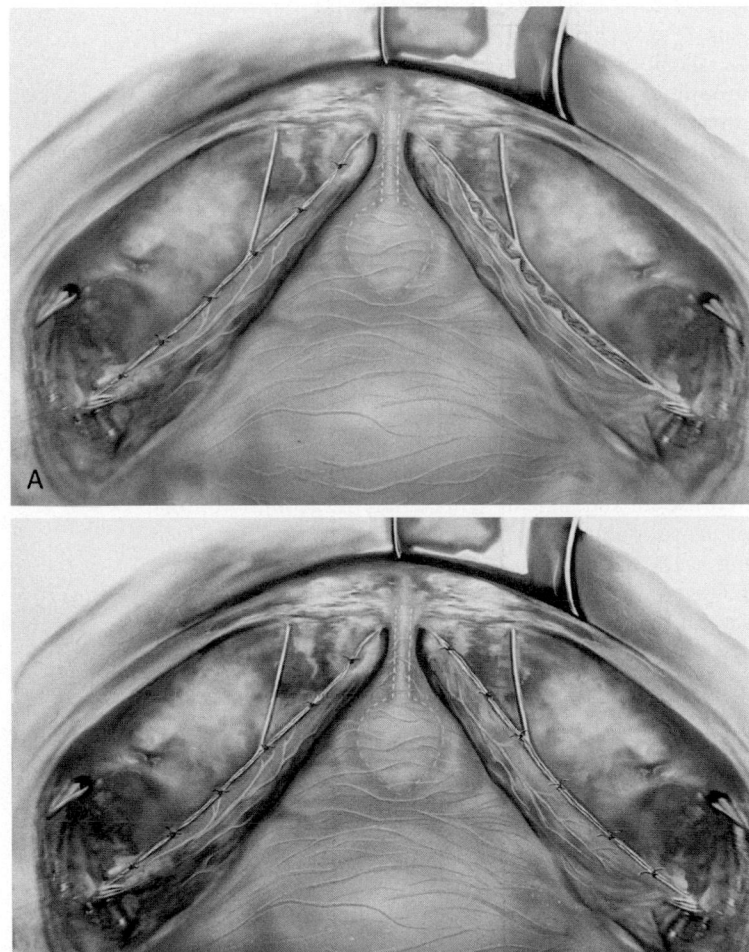

FIGURE 35B.21. A: The repair is complete on the left side. **B:** Both sides are repaired. (From Shull BL. How I do abdominal paravaginal repair. *J Pelvic Surg* 1995;1:43.)

agent when the wound is closed. When the patient is fully awake and can ambulate, the indwelling Foley catheter is used to empty the bladder fully. Next, the bladder is filled retrograde with 300 mL sterile saline and the catheter is removed. The patient is allowed to void. If she voids more than 150 mL, she is dismissed without a catheter; if not, she is dismissed doing intermittent clean self-catheterization (ICSC). For the last 4 years, all my patients with retropubic repair only have been dismissed on the same day of surgery.

In patients who have more extensive surgery and are admitted overnight, the same catheter management is employed the morning following surgery after the patient has breakfast.

In the exceptional patient who cannot perform ICSC, either a family member is taught to perform the catheterization or the patient is dismissed with a Foley catheter to closed drainage. A few days later, the patient returns for retrograde filling and a test of bladder function.

Some surgeons who treat vaginal eversion by sacral colpopexy have begun to incorporate the paravaginal repair as a part of the total vaginal reconstruction. After completion of the sacral colpopexy, the paravaginal repair is performed as previously described. Others perform a combined Burch procedure and paravaginal repair in association with a sacral colpopexy. After the sacral colpopexy is completed, the sutures adjacent to the urethra and the urethrovesical junction are placed through the Cooper ligament, as is done in the modified Burch colposuspension. The perivesical loss of support is then repaired with a series of paravaginal sutures.

VAGINAL RETROPUBIC TECHNIQUE

The vaginal approach to the paravaginal repair is particularly helpful in women whose primary complaint is pelvic organ prolapse without significant urinary incontinence. The vaginal approach requires greater technical skills than does the open retropubic repair. It has a limited use for the general gynecologic surgeon. The angle of the subpubic arch is the most important factor affecting access to the retropubic space. In a woman with a subpubic arch that admits three or more finger breadths, several retractors can easily be placed in the retropubic space, making the vaginal approach technically possible. In a woman with prolapse of the anterior segment and a narrow subpubic arch, I prefer a combination approach, managing the defects that can be handled appropriately through a vaginal incision and completing the retropubic repair through a transabdominal incision.

In the vaginal approach to paravaginal repair, the following steps are used. The patient's legs are placed in high leg holders and she is draped for vaginal surgery. The bladder is drained before the initiation of the surgical procedure. All segments of the vaginal canal area are thoroughly evaluated to confirm the fascial defects. The anterior vaginal segment is examined, specifically to ob-

serve loss of lateral sulci, lack of rugation of the epithelium along the base of the bladder, and elongation of the anterior vaginal wall (Fig. 35B.22). Marking sutures are placed through the vaginal epithelium at the level of the urethrovesical junction several millimeters lateral to the normal location of the lateral sulci (Fig. 35B.23). In women who have previously had a hysterectomy, marking sutures are placed at the vaginal apices. In a woman undergoing concomitant hysterectomy, a posterior colpotomy is performed. The anterior epithelium is sharply circumscribed and an anterior colpotomy is performed by sharp dissection. A retractor is placed to elevate the bladder ventrally. The ureters are identified by palpation. The cardinal-uterosacral ligament pedicles are clamped, divided, and tagged to be used later for support of the vaginal apices. A cross-clamp, cut, and tie technique is used to perform the hysterectomy. Salpingo-oophorectomy is performed if indicated. The cardinal-uterosacral ligament pedicles are sewn into the ipsilateral angles of the vaginal cuff, initiating the reconstructive procedure. At that point, tension can be placed on the cardinal-uterosacral ligament pedicle, and the ligament itself can be palpated as it courses posterior and medial to the ischial spine back to the sacrum. Nonabsorbable sutures are used to

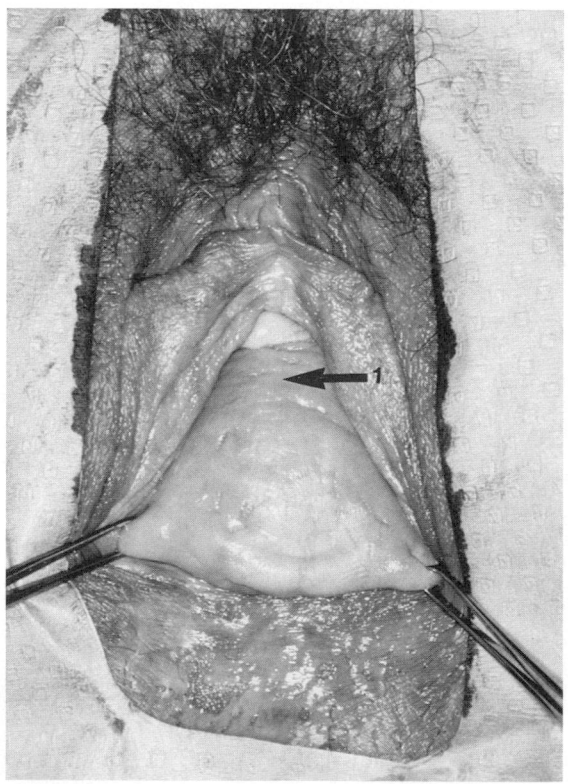

FIGURE 35B.22. A patient with loss of support laterally, centrally, and superiorly. A few rugae can be seen in the upper third of the pubocervical fascia closest to the urethrovesical junction. The remainder of the anterior segment is elongated and has lost its rugae. The apices prolapse less than 1 cm past the hymen. (From Shull BL. Clinical evaluation of women with pelvic support defects. *Clin Obstet Gynecol* 1993;36:939.)

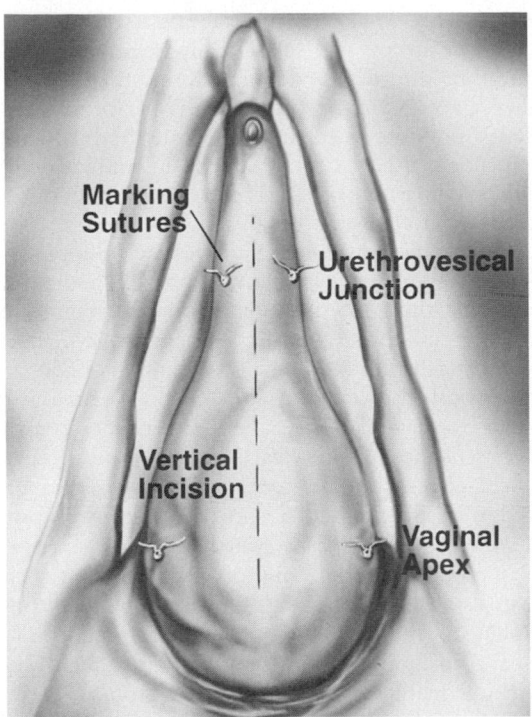

FIGURE 35B.23. A patient with prolapse of the anterior vagina. Marking sutures are at the urethrovesical junction and apices. The dotted line indicates the midline incision to be made. (From Shull BL, Benn SJ, Kuehl TJ. Surgical management of prolapse of the anterior vaginal segment: an analysis of support defects, operative morbidity, and anatomic outcome. *Am J Obstet Gynecol* 1994;171:1429.)

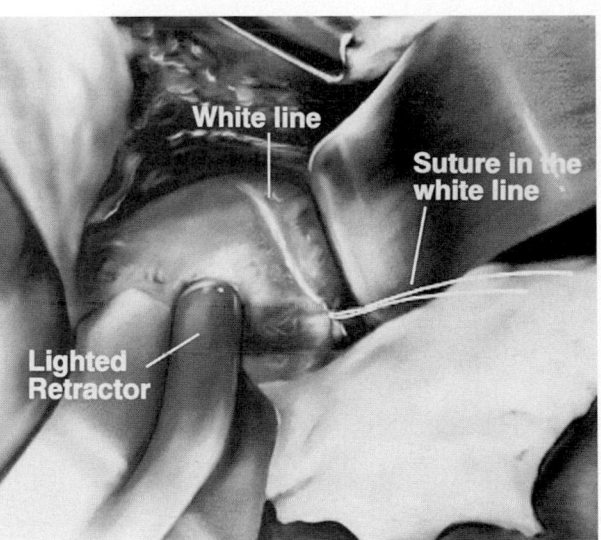

FIGURE 35B.24. A fiberoptic, right-angle retractor is in the retropubic space, retracting the bladder medially and providing illumination to the retropubic space. The suture is through the arcus tendineus fasciae pelvis (*white line*) about 2 cm ventral to the ischial spine. (From Shull BL, Benn SJ, Kuehl TJ. Surgical management of prolapse of the anterior vaginal segment: an analysis of support defects, operative morbidity, and anatomic outcome. *Am J Obstet Gynecol* 1994;171:1429.)

initiate the culdoplasty. Regardless of the technique of culdoplasty, the sutures are left untied until the paravaginal dissection and repair have been performed. Tying the culdoplasty sutures at this stage of the operation reduces the field of vision and makes subsequent dissection technically more difficult.

I initiate reconstruction of the anterior segment by placing Allis clamps along the cut edge of the epithelium at about the 3- and 9-o'clock positions. With sharp dissection, the pubocervical fascia is dissected off of the epithelium up to the urethrovesical junction, and the dissection is continued laterally until the index finger can be passed between the vaginal epithelium and the pubocervical fascia into the retropubic space just anterior to the ischial spine. With the index finger in the retropubic space, the dissection is continued anteriorly along the inferior ramus of pubis and medially to the symphysis pubis. Small individual veins may require isolation and ligation. A gauze sponge is placed into the retropubic space lateral to the bladder, and a long, lighted bayonet retractor is used to displace the empty bladder and urethra medially. A right-angle retractor with a fiberoptic light source is placed in the posterior aspect of the retropubic space, providing retraction and illumination. Another right-angle retractor is placed in the lateral aspect of the field, displacing the vaginal epithelium laterally. The obturator internus

fascia and the condensation of the arcus tendineus fasciae pelvis are identified first by palpation and next by visualization. With use of a long, straight needle driver and a small, round, tapered needle, the first suture is placed into the tendinous arch and obturator fascia 2 to 3 cm anterior to the ischial spine (Fig. 35B.24). The suture remains armed and is marked with a small clamp. I have found it handy to have a series of six clamps, each identified by one to six pieces of tape, so that sutures can be marked sequentially and can be remembered by the appropriately marked clamp. Traction is placed on the first suture, making it easier to visualize the tendinous arch and to facilitate placement of subsequent sutures. A series of four to six sutures is used from this point anterior to the spine to the attachment of the white line along the posterior aspect of the pubic bone (Fig. 35B.25).

Next, the suture that is placed closest to the posterior surface of the pubic bone is used to penetrate the lateral edge of the periurethral portion of the pubocervical fascia near the mid-portion of the urethra (Fig. 35B.26). The same suture is then used to penetrate the undersurface of the vaginal epithelium about halfway between the marking suture of the urethrovesical junction and the urethral meatus. The suture in the vaginal epithelium is placed several centimeters medial to the cut edge. The second suture penetrates the pubocervical fascia near the urethrovesical junction and the undersurface of the vaginal epithelium at the site of the previously placed marking suture. The third suture penetrates the perivesical fascia and the undersurface of the vaginal epithelium. This sequence is repeated until the suture placed closest

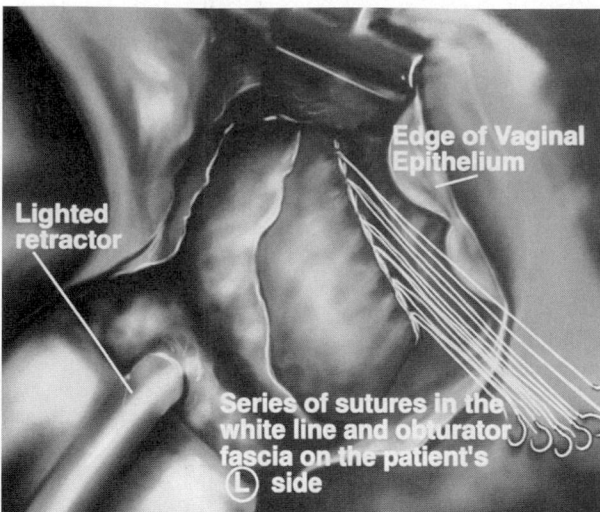

FIGURE 35B.25. A series of sutures has been placed in the arcus tendineus fasciae pelvis from a point ventral to the ischial spine to the back of the pubic bone. (From Shull BL, Benn SJ, Kuehl TJ. Surgical management of prolapse of the anterior vaginal segment: an analysis of support defects, operative morbidity, and anatomic outcome. *Am J Obstet Gynecol* 1994;171:1429.)

to the ischial spine is used to secure the most cephalad portion of the pubocervical fascia to the undersurface of the vaginal epithelium near the apex. It is necessary to pick up the lateral edge of the pubocervical fascia to avoid injury to the bladder and urethra as well as to avoid placing undue tension on the anterior segment. It is also necessary to place the sutures in the vaginal epithelium several centimeters away from the cut edges of the midline incision to allow adequate tissue for midline closure. When all sutures are placed with three points of penetra-

tion (the white line, pubocervical fascia, and vaginal epithelium), they are tied sequentially beginning with the periurethral suture and ending with the stitch nearest the vaginal apex. A similar procedure is performed on the patient's opposite side. At that point, the bilateral paravaginal defects have been repaired. If a midline defect in pubocervical fascia exists, it is closed with a series of 2-0 interrupted nonabsorbable sutures.

If a hysterectomy has been done, the culdoplasty and peritoneal sutures are tied next, providing depth and support to the posterior portion of the vaginal cuff. Once the culdoplasty sutures have been tied, they are used to attach the transverse or superior portion of the pubocervical fascia to the apex of the vagina. In this manner, the lateral, central, and superior or transverse portions of the pubocervical fascia have been repaired. The cut edges of the anterior epithelium are approximated with interrupted absorbable sutures. Most patients require a posterior colporrhaphy and perineorrhaphy in addition to the anterior vaginal reconstruction. The goals of the reconstructive procedure include establishment of normal support for all segments of the vagina, a posterior axis for the vaginal canal, and vaginal depth adequate for intravaginal intercourse. A gauze pack is placed in the vaginal canal, and a transurethral catheter is used to drain the bladder.

In the patient who has previously had a hysterectomy, the operation is begun by placing marking sutures at the site of the urethrovesical junction near the creation of the new lateral sulci and at the apex of the vagina near the expected approximation of the cuff anterior to the ischial spines. I prefer a vertical incision in the anterior vagina extending from the urethrovesical junction to the apex of the vaginal cuff. Other authors have described bilateral periurethral incisions extending from the urethrovesical junction to a point just anterior to the spine. With use of the single vertical incision, the dissection is continued laterally and superiorly to the vaginal cuff. When an enterocele is present, the sac is opened and an

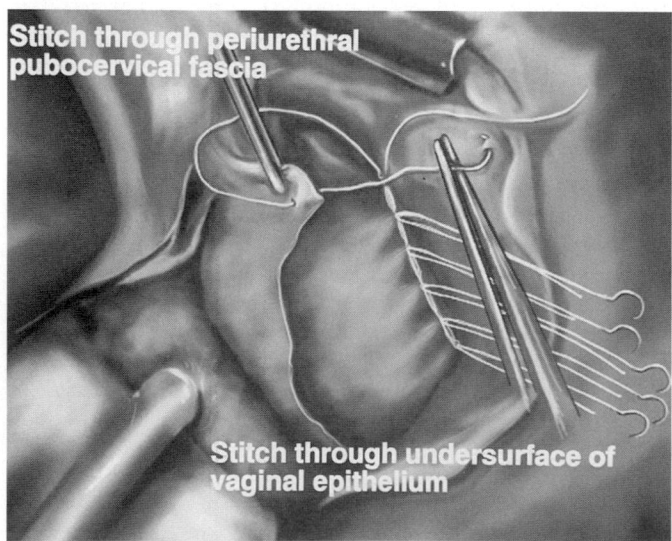

FIGURE 35B.26. The suture in the arcus tendineus fasciae pelvis near the pubic bone is also sewn into the lateral margin on the pubocervical fascia periurethrally and into the undersurface of the vaginal epithelium at the site of the marking suture at the urethrovesical junction. (From Shull BL, Benn SJ, Kuehl TJ. Surgical management of prolapse of the anterior vaginal segment: an analysis of support defects, operative morbidity, and anatomic outcome. *Am J Obstet Gynecol* 1994;171:1429.)

enterocele repair is performed. I identify the remnants of the uterosacral ligaments at the 4- and 8-o'clock positions and use them to suspend and support the transverse portion of the pubocervical and rectovaginal fascia, closing the space where an enterocele occurs. The sutures should be placed, but remain untied until the anterior dissection and repair have been completed. After the uterosacral sutures have been placed, or in cases where no enterocele is present, the dissection is continued laterally until the index finger can be placed into the retropubic space just anterior to the ischial spine. The vaginal paravaginal repair, midline and transverse repair, and posterior colporrhaphy and perineorrhaphy are performed as described in the preceding paragraphs.

The patients are ambulated and fed an oral diet on the afternoon or evening of the day of surgery. The transurethral catheter management is the same as for an abdominal repair. If the patient can void spontaneously with a residual volume of less than 150 mL, no further catheterization is required. If she cannot, she is taught ICSC and is dismissed with instructions to continue ICSC clean self-catheterization until she can spontaneously void 150 mL or more and has a postvoid residual volume of 150 mL or less.

SUMMARY

There are several ways to approach the management of paravaginal defects of the anterior compartment. In a woman with genuine urinary incontinence as a primary complaint, an open retropubic paravaginal repair may provide excellent relief. However, a valid criticism is that this procedure has not been subjected to the rigorous preoperative and postoperative urodynamic testing used for the Burch colposuspension and the Marshall-Marchetti-Krantz procedure. Reports by Richardson and associates and Shull suggest that paravaginal repair is efficacious in the management of genuine urinary incontinence in properly selected patients. My clinical impression, documented by longitudinal follow-up of my own patients, is that women with uncomplicated urinary incontinence, urethral hypermobility, a positive provoked full-bladder stress test, and lateral loss of support, as well as women with no incontinence but paravesical defects and cystocele, are candidates for paravaginal repair. Colombo and associates performed a randomized comparison of the Burch procedure and abdominal paravaginal defect repair for urinary incontinence and reported the Burch procedure was superior for the treatment of urinary incontinence. The patients who underwent a paravaginal repair resumed spontaneous voiding more quickly. Many surgeons now combine the principles of the Burch procedure and the paravaginal defect repair to offer superior results for cure of urinary incontinence as well as correction of anterior support loss.

In patients who have no significant urinary incontinence but who have prolapse of the anterior vaginal segment with paravaginal defects, the vaginal paravaginal repair is an effective method of management. The advantages include an opportunity for repair of isolated defects in the pubocervical fascia as well as repair of all other support defects with a single approach. The potential disadvantages include the greater technical difficulty of the repair and the unknown effects of extensive anterior dissection on bladder innervation. In my series of patients treated with vaginal paravaginal repair, all have had support defects in one or more additional sites. The transvaginal approach to paravaginal repair is particularly attractive because the coexisting anterior support defects as well as defects in all other sites can be repaired vaginally, thereby providing the patient with the advantages of vaginal surgery: less manipulation of the bowel, avoidance of an abdominal incision, and decreased adverse effects on pulmonary function.

BIBLIOGRAPHY

Addison WA, Timmons MC. Abdominal approach to vaginal eversion. *Clin Obstet Gynecol* 1993;36:995.

Aronson MP, ed. Reconstructive pelvic surgery. *Operative Techniques in Gynecologic Surgery* 1996;1:65–122.

Baden WF, Walker T. *Surgical repair of vaginal defects.* Philadelphia: JB Lippincott, 1992.

Bonney V. On diurnal incontinence of urine in women. *J Obstet Gynaecol Br Emp* 1923;30:358.

Burch JC. Cooper's ligament urethrovesical suspension for stress incontinence. Nine years' experience—results, complications, technique. *Am J Obstet Gynecol* 1968;100:764–774.

Burch JC. Urethrovaginal fixation to Cooper's ligament for correction of stress incontinence, cystocele, and prolapse. *Am J Obstet Gynecol* 1961;81:281–290.

Colombo M, Milani R, Vitobello D, et al. A randomized comparison of Burch colposuspension and abdominal paravaginal defect repair for female stress urinary incontinence. *Am J Obstet Gynecol* 1996;175:78–84.

DeLancey JO. Pelvic organ prolapse: clinical management and scientific foundations. *Clin Obstet Gynecol* 1993;36:895–995.

DeLancey JO. Structural support of the urethra as it relates to stress urinary incontinence: the hammock hypothesis. *Am J Obstet Gynecol* 1994;170:1713.

DeLancey JO. Fascial and muscular abnormalities in women with urethral hypermobility and anterior vaginal wall prolapse. *Am J Obstet Gynecol* 2002;187:93–98.

Grody MH. *Benign postreproductive gynecologic surgery.* New York: McGraw-Hill, 1994.

Horbach NS, ed. Surgery for stress urinary incontinence. 1997;2:1–55.

Kelly HA. Incontinence of urine in women. *Urol Cutan Rev* 1913;17:291–293.

Kovac SR, Cruikshank SH. Pubic bone suburethral stabilization sling: an anatomic approach to urinary stress incontinence. *Contemp Obstet Gynecol* 1998; 43:52–76.

Kovac SR. Follow-up of the pubic bone suburethral stabilization sling operation for recurrent urinary incontinence. (Kovac procedure). *J Pelvic Surg* 1999;5:156–160.

Pillai-Allen A, Benson JT. Cystocele. In: Brubaker LT, Saclarides TJ, eds. *The female pelvic floor: disorders of function and support.* Philadelphia: FA Davis, 1996:269–277.

Richardson AC, Edmonds PB, Williams NL. Treatment of stress urinary incontinence due to paravaginal fascial defect. *Obstet Gynecol* 1981;57:357.

Richardson AC, Lyon JB, Williams NL. A new look at pelvic relaxation. *Am J Obstet Gynecol* 1976;126:568.

Shull BL. How I do abdominal paravaginal repair. *J Pelvic Surg* 1995;1:43.

Shull BL, Baden WF. A six-year experience with paravaginal defect repair for stress urinary incontinence. *Am J Obstet Gynecol* 1989;160:1432.

Shull BL, Benn SJ, Kuehl TJ. Surgical management of prolapse of the anterior vaginal segment: an analysis of support defects, operative morbidity, and anatomic outcome. *Am J Obstet Gynecol* 1994;171:1429.

Shull BL, Capen CV, Riggs MW, et al. Preoperative and postoperative analysis of site-specific pelvic support defects in 81 women treated with sacrospinous ligament suspension and pelvic reconstruction. *Am J Obstet Gynecol* 1992;166:1764.

Uhlenhuth E. *Problems in the anatomy of the pelvis.* Philadelphia: JB Lippincott, 1953.

Weber AM, Walters MD. Anterior vaginal prolapse: review of anatomy and techniques of surgical repair. *Obstet Gynecol* 1997;89:311–318.

White GR. An anatomic operation for the cure of cystocele. *Am J Obstet Dis Women Child* 1912;65:286.

White GR. Cystocele. A radical cure by suturing lateral sulci of vagina to white line of pelvic fascia. *JAMA* 1909:53:1707–1710.

Zimmerman CW. New concepts in restoration of the anterior vaginal compartment. *Operative Techniques in Gynecologic Surgery* 2001;6:116–120.

C

Posterior Compartment Defects

MARVIN H. TERRY GRODY

Over the past decade, our increased understanding of pelvic support defects and the associated anatomy of the pelvic fascia and ligaments has provided pelvic surgeons with new concepts that encourage anatomically restorative methods of effecting repair of the posterior pelvic compartment. A defective perineal body or an inadequately unified rectovaginal septum (RVS) can lead to progressive deterioration throughout the pelvic connective tissue network. Posterior repair was once widely regarded as a simple tail end, an inconsequential sequel to a large procedure that usually included a vaginal hysterectomy and anterior compartment repair. Viewed all too often by the operator as nothing more than a glorified episiotomy, together with his or her desire to be done as quickly as possible, the colpoperineorrhaphy (if it truly could be labeled as such in most cases) has often consisted of merely an excision of perhaps too much mucosa followed by a few hastily thrown, small-caliber, rapidly absorbable stitches.

Perhaps this low perception of posterior repair, as well as the lack of attention paid to it, compared with other seemingly more important and complicated pelvic surgical procedures, has led us to the dilemma of universal dissatisfaction with the results of this phase of surgical repair. As always, the primary operative goal has been and should be the elimination of symptoms that have brought the patient to the operating table in the first place. So what good have we accomplished if we correct the presenting complaint of vaginal protrusion and substitute instead permanent coital dysfunction? The widely revered English gynecologist Victor Bonney steadfastly proclaimed the impossibility of correcting vaginal deformities without some subsequent significant coital limitation. In the United States, Joseph Pratt contended that a loss

of 25% to 45% of vaginal depth could almost inevitably be anticipated in secondary pelvic reconstructive procedures, despite one's best efforts to retain satisfactory vaginal sexual function. Such a stance by these two giants unfortunately reflects the general opinion and experience, including that of highly renowned practitioners in our specialty, from the very beginning of pelvic corrective surgery to the present time. Such a situation is no longer acceptable. Our greater comprehension of pelvic anatomy, our improved surgical skills, and our willingness to accept the role to be played in achieving success at all levels by a tediously and meticulously conducted repair of posterior pelvic lesions should and must lead to markedly more positive results for patient and surgeon alike. There is no excuse today for coital compromise and current techniques should lengthen, not shorten, the vagina.

To enhance any discussion of pelvic reparative procedures, an understanding of the nature of the tissues can be most beneficial. In the pelvis, we colloquially speak of fascia, ligaments, septa, pillars, and diaphragms. This terminology is nothing more than convenient identification of the same continuous pelvic connective tissue network (with variations in thickness, width, length, strength, and, to some degree, cellular composition). A perfect example is the term *endopelvic fascia*, which is used freely as a substitute for connective tissue located anywhere from the pelvic brim down to the perineum. The innuendo of such nomenclature spawns exaggeration. Thus, the pelvic surgeon should understand the anatomic vagaries so that he or she does not ascribe more strength to a particular tissue than it really has. Also, despite quality differences in the various areas of pelvic connective tissue, the surgeon must not forget that strength is meaningless if weakness in any site is omitted from repair because of the delicate interdependent nature of this tissue. Enterocele can develop after isolated anterior repair, and anterior compartment breakdown can occur secondary to a lack of attention to "silent" weakness when only posterior compartment correction is made.

THE VAGINAL AXIS

Only in recent years has the concept of the *normal vaginal axis* appeared in the gynecologic literature. It is highly unlikely that successful pelvic repair of any kind will occur without full comprehension by the surgeon of the structural importance of the normal vaginal axis. Without restoration of this balance of suspension and support, which I regard as the central core of the entire delicate interdependent network of pelvic connective tissue, complete integrity of pelvic anatomy cannot be achieved, including that of the mid-pelvis and the anterior pelvic compartment, as well as the posterior division.

A vagina with a normal vaginal axis has an almost vertical distal one third and an almost horizontal upper two thirds, the latter projecting into the sacrococcygeal bony curve. The posterior vaginal fornix is, therefore, located deep in the posterior pelvis, well behind an imaginary vertical line that is drawn through the anus. Early in the gynecologist's career, from repetitive experience in the examination of healthy nulliparous pelves, such an anatomic mindset should be established regarding the constancy of the normal, firmly supported and suspended vagina, with emphasis on its morphologic relation to its neighboring organs and the tissues that hold it so. Nothing could be more straightforward, but seldom does such a mental etching develop. Yet how else will the surgeon who may have no difficulty recognizing a rectocele bulging into the vagina comprehend the associated roles played by a disintegrated perineal body, the various possible sites and extents of rifts in the fascia of Denonvilliers, and the defective levator musculature and its accompanying fallen levator plate? Without initially understanding the varied tissue complex vital to the sound composition of the normal vaginal supports, the anatomically naive operator performs the same abbreviated tenuous operation on every patient who has a bulging posterior wall. Precise recognition of the peculiar defects and their extent in each patient gives the surgeon the opportunity to tailor an operation that will suit only that patient.

The basic elements that ensure a healthy axis are, from top to bottom, the cardinal-uterosacral complex, the RVS (fascia of Denonvilliers), the perineal body, and the levator plate (Fig. 35C.1). The cardinal-uterosacral fibers (the upper paracolpium) suspend the proximal vagina posterosuperiorly by their extensions, which attach to the posterolateral pelvic walls and sacrum. Ligamentous strands also project downward to help form the anterior wall of the cul-de-sac and then blend securely into the next vital part of axis maintenance, the RVS. This relation is important to understand because separation of this connection transversely is the cause of the uppermost type of rectocele. Only if the surgeon is aware

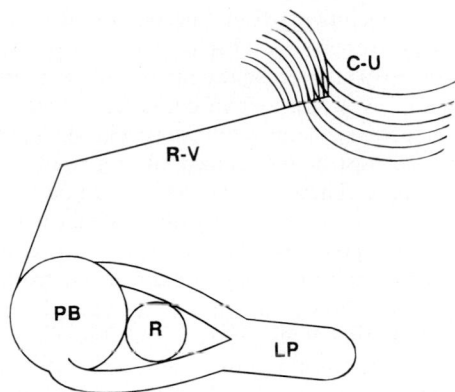

FIGURE 35C.1. Mainstays of vaginal axis integrity. C-U, cardinal–uterosacral ligament complex; LP, levator plate with connecting arms on either side around the rectum; PB, perineal body; R, rectum; R-V, rectovaginal septum. (From Grody MHT, ed. *Benign postreproductive gynecologic surgery.* New York: McGraw-Hill, 1994)

of such dissociation can appropriate repair at this level occur.

THE RECTOVAGINAL SEPTUM

The establishment of the RVS as a distinct anatomic entity with precise boundaries and function is attributed to Denonvilliers. It is the most important finite constituent of normal posterior pelvic integrity. Beginning superiorly at the cul-de-sac, this thin but strong tissue sheet runs downward to integrate distally into the perineal body. Laterally, this trapezoidal layer fuses into the iliococcygeal fascial coverings. In the normal female, it lies directly in contact with the posterior vaginal wall, accounting for its previous inclusion as part of the vagina. However, it can be bluntly separated and demonstrated to form the anterior limit of the rectovaginal space. It probably should be considered, together with the fibromuscular bands that extend bilaterally from the vaginal wall to the pelvic diaphragm at the sides, as part of the mid-paracolpium.

This remarkably strong, thin tissue layer consists of dense collagen fibers (mostly lateral), some smooth muscle (mostly in the midline, contributing to its resiliency), and what is probably its most important component, dense elastin distributed throughout the entire structure. Nowhere else in the entire pelvis are the elastic fibers as dense as they are in this unique cellular composition. This is understandable because of the need for physiologic expansion without destruction during the descent of the presenting part in childbirth. Yet, it is tearing and separation within the RVS, occurring during childbirth because of overdistention, which is thought to play the primary role as a cause of rectocele in most cases. According to A. Cullen Richardson, it has been shown that this process can cause horizontal detachments from the perineal body, which itself can be damaged extensively in the process of labor, and detachments from the deep endopelvic connective tissue superiorly. This type of transverse injury seems unquestionably to be the major predecessor of rectocele; it can exist alone or in conjunction with vertical defects, as further delineated more specifically in the next few pages. It must be recognized and repaired for a successful outcome. These specific defects can be fairly well-delineated preoperatively by way of bidigital examination, especially in the erect posture with an accompanying Valsalva maneuver, with the index finger of one hand in the rectum and the index and middle fingers of the other hand in the vagina (Figs. 35C. 2 and 35C.3). Use of a single hand, with thumb in the vagina and index finger in the rectum, is too limited to be adequately informative. Most certainly these specific defects in the RVS can and should be identified at surgery after the operative wound has been opened to its fullest extent.

The correct appraisal of points of injury cannot be emphasized enough. Only with this knowledge can the surgeon specifically address each defect. Too often I have seen the ignorantly conceived sequence of inadequate and limited dissection, excessive mucosal excision, and routine midline suture placement bringing together inconsequential perirectal fibers from each side, creating an unsupported narrow vagina in association with total disregard for discovery of specific defects and their magnitude. The operator mistakenly thinks a good job has been done only to be confronted weeks or months later with a recurrence of the same objectively visible deformity. Sometimes, to the surprise and dismay of the surgeon, a previously small and unrecognized enterocele suddenly pops boldly into view concomitantly with the other lesions.

Traditionally, RVS defects have been thought most commonly to be linear in nature, primarily as the result of many years of attenuation subsequent to the initial trauma of vaginal childbirth. Erroneously the feeling prevailed, for more than a century, that the RVS fibers

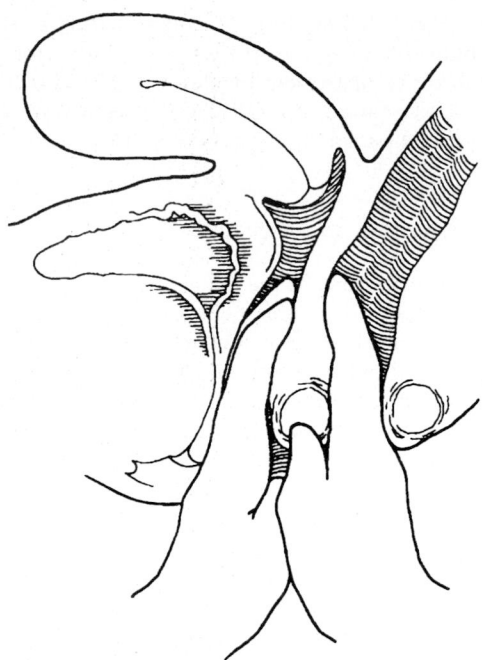

FIGURE 35C.3. Sketch of examiner's fingers (both hands) in the standing patient. Not only does digital opposition from separate hands allow deep posterior compartment assessment, but the two vaginal fingers can be rotated 180 degrees to judge anterior compartment defects under Valsalva conditions. (From Grody MHT, ed. *Benign postreproductive gynecologic surgery.* New York: McGraw-Hill, 1994.)

simply disappeared, thereby allowing the rectum to bulge through the length of the posterior vaginal wall, more or less in the midline. From this evolved a standard method of repair, described in one textbook after another, and taught and employed for multiple decades (including my own textbook and videos and teaching instructions, sorry to say) that essentially, in almost every case, resorted to a linear longitudinal repair. This technique has involved a series of side-to-side stitches, beginning, when presumably performed correctly, just posterior to the level of the ischial spines and extending down to the area of the perineal body. The tissues united from each side were a combination of residual connective tissue, areolar tissue, segments of lateral wall fascia, and too often, bites into levator muscle. If true elements of RVS happened to be included, it was usually by sheer accident. Nothing could be more unanatomic, less reliable, or unnecessarily constrictive. Even though we know better, this incorrect, truly archaic approach persists in a significant number of major medical institutions despite the revolutionary anatomic disclosures that have been exposed in the past decade.

In the early 1990s, after prolonged and intensive anatomic investigation, A. Cullen Richardson declared unequivocally that the primary reason for connective tissue defects in the female pelvis was tears, not attenuation. Such a monumental conclusion, stunningly contradictory to all traditional concepts up to that time, even

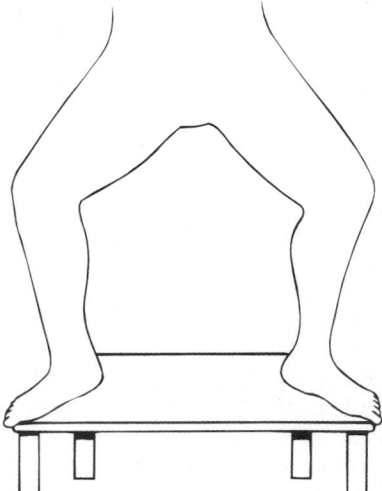

FIGURE 35C.2. Sketch demonstrating stance for examination of the erect patient. (From Grody MHT, ed. *Benign postreproductive gynecologic surgery.* New York: McGraw-Hill, 1994.)

though presented by a gynecologic surgeon of recognized high stature who arguably additionally was our finest clinical anatomist of the female pelvis at that time, was not readily understood or accepted. The major thrust of Richardson's argument embraced the concept of evolution of rectoceles primarily from detachment in the RVS that could, in almost every case, be clearly identified if one only looked for the torn separations, although nobody was doing that at that time. Reluctant at first to accept this radical revelation, we slowly broke through our confusion and, as a logical sequence, as instructed by Richardson, we began repairing rectoceles simply by reuniting the torn edges appropriately with the standard surgical stitches. Thus, we were finally restoring the original anatomy, quite obviously and easily demonstrated at the operating table just before vaginal mucosal dissection, after full dissection and exposure of the operative field, and finally after full unification of the septum. The vehicle for such convincing display of anatomic logic and gratifying accomplishment became the rectal examining index finger. How good it feels that we now have a good unifying anatomic concept that provides us with clear surgical principles to use when reconstructing defects which produce a rectocele.

Although the best opportunity for full comprehension of locating and repairing the torn defects is by observation and participation in the operating room, sketches can also be illustrative. Figure 35C.4A reveals a

transverse RVS tear at the vaginal vault with the separated segment, retracted into the perineal area, being drawn with clamps upward to be repositioned in its normal environment preparatory to surgical reunification. The edges of the torn fascia are then sutured together with a series of interrupted, delayed absorbable sutures as shown in Figure 35C.4B. Figure 35C.5 displays exactly the opposite type of tear, that is, RVS transversely torn as its fibers enter into their perineal body attachment. Here the clamps are shown drawing the RVS segment that has retracted upward being drawn down to the perineal area for operative realignment. In each case, a rectally inserted index finger can demonstrate that, except for scraps of areolar tissue, the anorectal mucosal wall is the only layer that prevents the finger from falling into the operative field as it produces rectocele simulation with forward pressure. When the clamps draw the long torn RVS segments into normal anatomic position, the anorectal finger cannot advance at all, despite strong effort, because of the natural strong barrier effect of the replaced RVS. Although these two types of transverse detachment seem to be the most common, others that are either U-shaped at the bottom (Fig. 35C.6) or inverted U-shapes at the top of the posterior compartment are not that unusual. The same is true for more or less linear (longitudinal) tears near one side or the other directly adjacent to the pelvic sidewalls, rarely in the midline. Occasionally a hockey-stick type of lesion, combin-

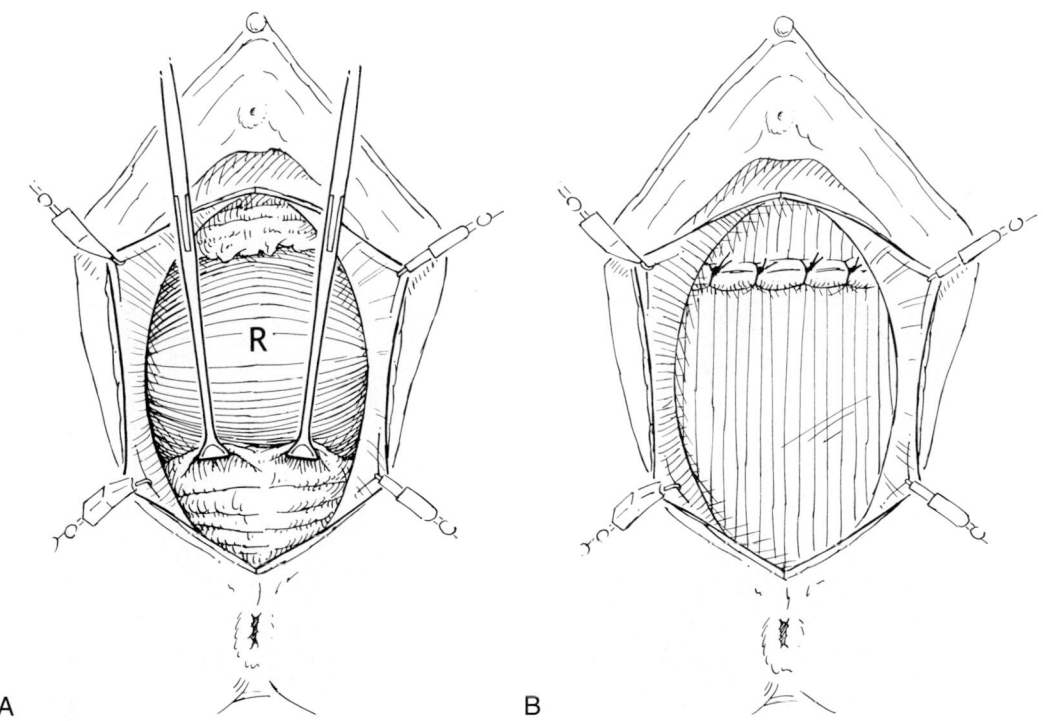

A   B

FIGURE 35C.4. A: The rectovaginal septum (fascia of Denonvilliers) has been detached transversely at the vaginal vault. Clamps are drawing the retracted edge upward for reunion with its upper segment over the bulging rectum that forms the rectocele (R). The flaps of longitudinally incised vaginal mucosa are drawn laterally, framing the operative wound. **B:** The site-specific restoration of the torn defect of the rectovaginal septum (RVS) at the vault has been performed. The reunited well-preserved fascial sheet is flat; the bulging rectocele has been eliminated.

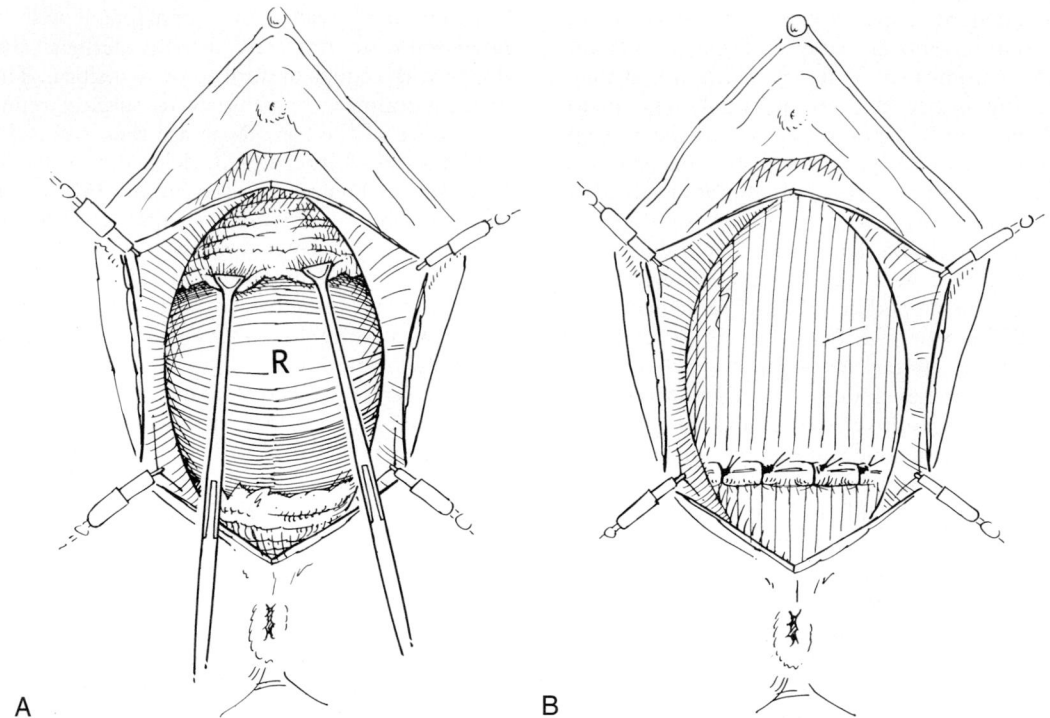

FIGURE 35C.5. A: In a similar setting to that of Figure 35C.4, a rectocele (R) is denoted bulging through a defect created by a distal tear of the RVS at its juncture with the perineal body. The upwardly retracted segment is being drawn downward. **B:** Defect-directed restitution of the separation has been completed. The rectocele has been obliterated.

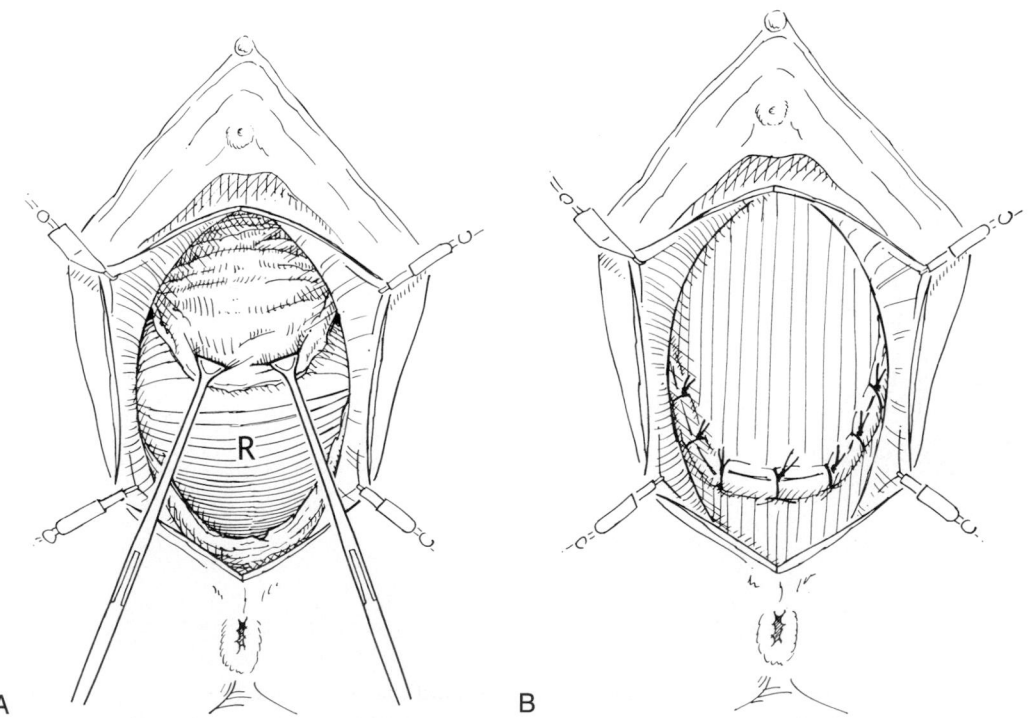

FIGURE 35C.6. A: This sketch reveals a distal U-shaped lesion that has allowed a rectocele (R) to form through the gap in the RVS. **B:** RVS integrity has been restored by appropriately placed sutures reuniting the torn edges denoted in Fig. 8 with simultaneous disappearance of the rectocele.

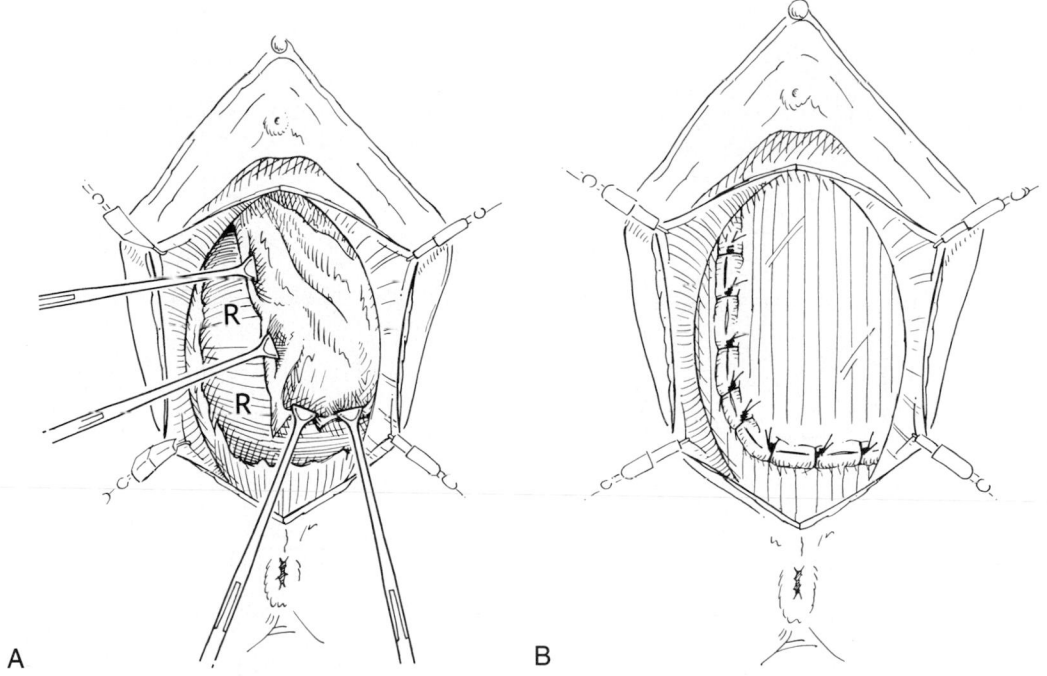

A   B

FIGURE 35C.7. A: A right-sided hockey stick defect has opened to a forward-thrusting rectal wall. The deflected RVS flap is seen being pulled back to normal position. **B:** The RVS has been reconstituted in the same manner as seen in the previous figures. With this combined longitudinal-transverse repair, the rectal distortion is gone.

ing a longitudinal tear and a transverse tear in continuity, as shown in Figure 35C.7, is discovered. A rare type of combined or double defect in which the Denonvilliers fascia has been torn transversely both at the vault and at the perineal body but retaining strong attachments bilaterally is diagrammatically shown in Figure 35C.8. The major conceptual breakthrough discussed in this chapter is that tears in Denonvilliers fascia, not attenuation, is the cause of a rectocele. These tears, transverse, longitudinal, hockey stick, or even occasionally stellate, can be identified without difficulty. The repair itself is much easier and more confidence-inspiring than the traditional method of fishing around to find scraps of muscle to plicate in the midline.

Over many years of observation, one gains the distinct impression that most rectoceles are progressive, particularly when subject to unfavorable circumstances such as smoking, chronic pulmonary disease, occupational heavy lifting, and menopausal atrophy, especially in the absence of estrogen replacement. The rectovaginal tear becomes more manifest, and the bulge enlarges, advancing from a small asymptomatic lesion to one annoying enough to evoke a subjective request for relief. In addition, it is not uncommon for a patient to appear for the first time with full-blown rectovaginal separation and an accompanying large, protruding rectocele that she states began as a small ball and simply grew larger with time. However, many women reveal early defects that never change over time. Certainly, there is no justification for operating on these patients "prophylactically" unless the patient requires surgery for other distinctly disabling sit-

uations in the anterior or mid-pelvis. Not to repair this "silent" posterior defect at the same time under these circumstances is poor practice and a disservice to the patient.

On other occasions, a large cystocele (almost certainly temporally preceding the development of posterior defects) can dominate the situation and, simply by compression, prevent the appearance of a rectocele despite the coexistence of a clearly definable rectovaginal septal separation. This impairment can even run the full posterior vaginal length with no rectocele becoming apparent because of cystocele domination. Recognition and repair of this asymptomatic lesion at the time of anterior correction is imperative. Otherwise, with the opposing force removed, a rectocele can seem to burst forth suddenly through the disparate rectovaginal fibers and necessitate a return trip to the operating room at a future date. A generally accepted corollary observation, all too often ignored, warns that anterior lesions do not often exist alone and that some form of posterior repair, even if only a perineorrhaphy, should be included in the operative plan.

A very dramatic, though rare, type of rectocele is the invaginating mid-third lesion (Fig. 35C.9). It is delineated best by a rectal finger and is easily cured by a series of closure sutures while the rectum is digitally depressed. Long-term cures are usually ensured when the stitches are carried slightly beyond both extents of this limited type of defect.

In a last definitive statement about rectocele, I feel it is singularly important to stress that, despite their origi-

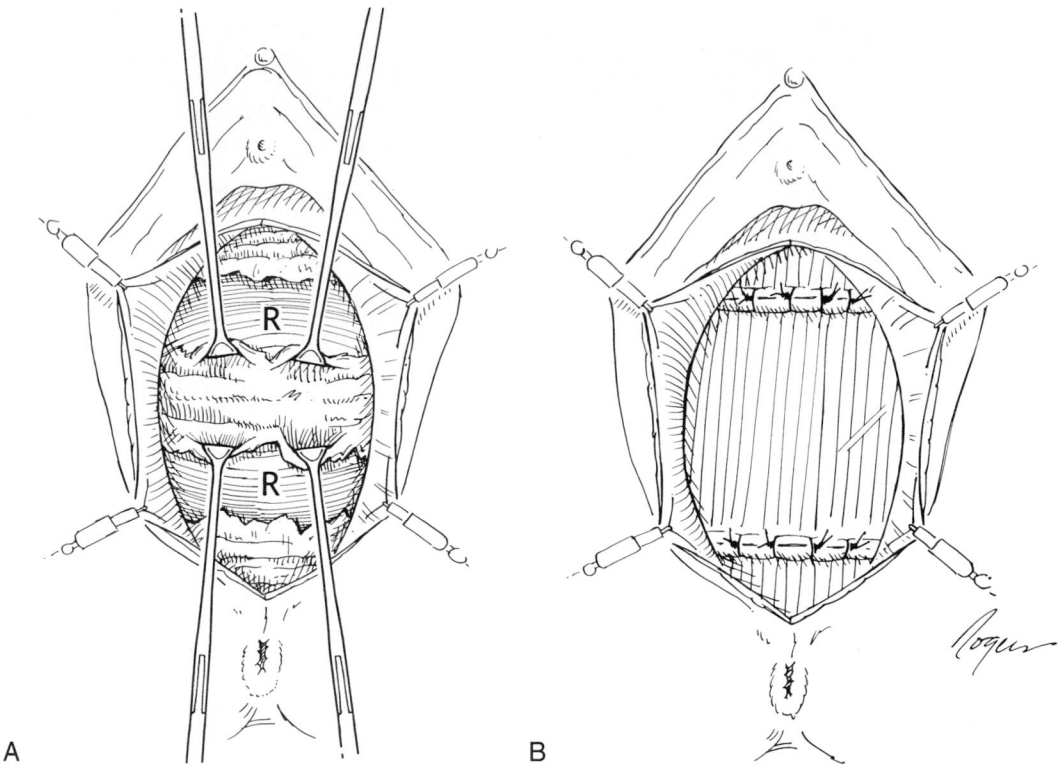

FIGURE 35C.8. **A:** In emphasis of possible tears of wide variance in the RVS, even stellate patterns, this sketch reveals a double defect, one at the top and one at the bottom, with intact lateral attachments of the RVS. Thus we define a "double rectocele" (R and R). **B:** Rectification is effected in standard fashion proximally and distally. Anatomic reestablishment of the RVS with full rectocele suppression is assured.

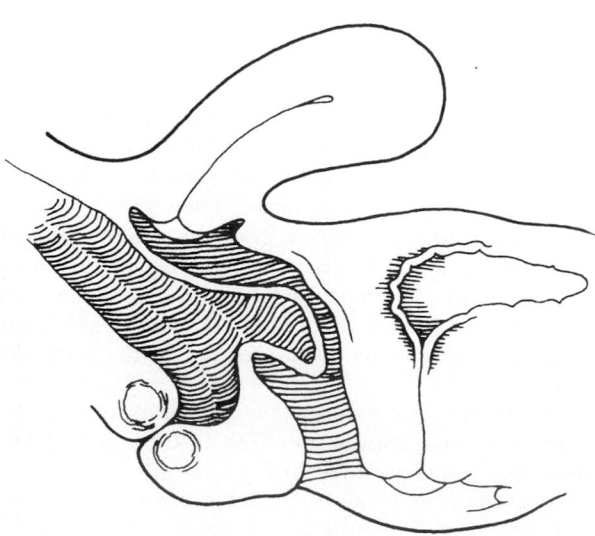

FIGURE 35C.9. Mid-vaginal rectocele as an isolated lesion. Vaginal axis is fairly normal. (From Grody MHT, ed. *Benign postreproductive gynecologic surgery.* New York: McGraw-Hill, 1994.)

nal distinctly different normal compositions, rectocele and its disordered anatomic neighbor, perineal body defects, almost always go together and must be linked invariably in the process of repair. Figures 35C.10 and 35C.11 illustrate these combined lesions in the area of the pelvic floor, always with associated loss of normal vaginal axis.

THE PERINEAL BODY

This solid, almost pyramidal structure should be regarded as a central core of posterior pelvic support. In its strategic position between the vagina in front and the anus and distal rectum behind, it acts as a hub with important connective tissue fibers and striated muscle strands feeding into it from every angle, much as the hub of a wheel grasps its spokes. Averaging 3.5 to 4 cm in depth (height) over a 4- × 4-cm base, figuratively speaking, it forms a dense, solid structure, when undamaged, that is totally different from the RVS that stretches above it. When its integrity has been compromised through structural tearing at vaginal delivery in earlier years and by aging, constipation, and chronic lung disease, its importance as a core of support may well be realized as its deterioration sets off a domino effect of supportive and suspensory failure. Weakened connective tissues of the

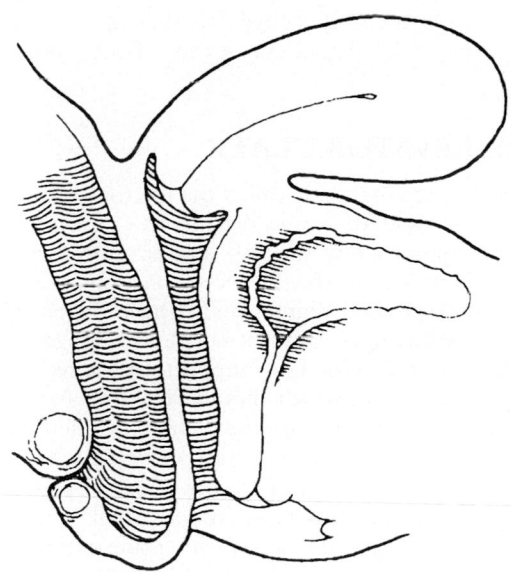

FIGURE 35C.10. Coexisting defective perineal body and low rectocele with associated vertical vagina. (From Grody MHT, ed. *Benign postreproductive gynecologic surgery.* New York: Mc-Graw-Hill, 1994.)

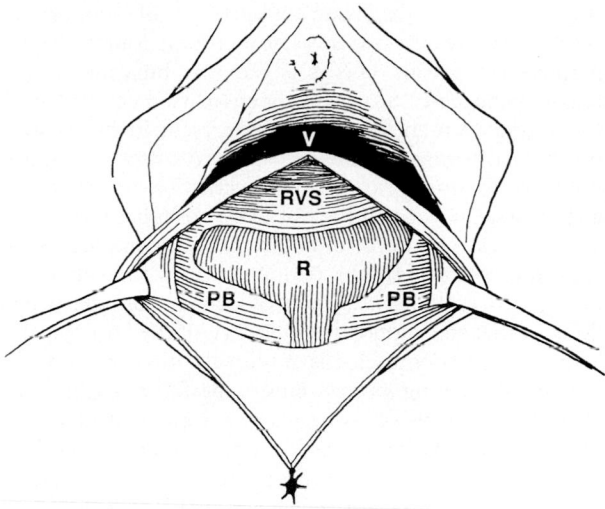

FIGURE 35C.11. Transverse separation of rectovaginal septum (RVS) from disrupted perineal body (PB) in low rectocele. R, rectum; V, vagina. (From Grody MHT, ed. *Benign postreproductive gynecologic surgery.* New York: McGraw-Hill, 1994.)

anterior and mid-pelvic compartments, as well as those of the posterior pelvis, can suddenly progress to produce disabling symptoms as this vital element of the vaginal axis falls apart.

Like other objectively detectable pelvic lesions that are asymptomatic, at least to the particular patient, a grossly damaged perineum can also be asymptomatic. In view of its key role of control, this seems strange and can only be explained, if the patient is not hiding her symptoms out of fear, by strong compensation from other pelvic muscles and connective tissue. However, because of its powerful pivotal role, if any major surgery is contemplated for other pelvic compartments, concomitant perineal body restitution becomes imperative if it is in any way deviant from acceptable normal bulks. A prime example occurs when patients undergo anterior pelvic compartment reconstruction, especially something like a suprapubic urethral suspension. If the vaginal axis already is less than it should be secondary to some perineal defects with or without an accompanying low rectovaginal separation, it is only further distorted by the periurethral surgery. In effect, the suprapubic urethral suspension pulls the anterior vaginal wall forward, opening up the vagina and setting the stage for development of pulsion enterocele, with or without rectocele. In 1961 and 1968, Burch reported a 15% chance of this occurring under these conditions, but many of us think the incidence today may be closer to 40% to 50% when simultaneous low colpoperineorrhaphy is not performed to maintain the normal axis. Thus, almost always, some form of perineal body restoration, at the least, is mandatory with any form of anterior repair. Much apprehension in this regard should exist today in association with the prolific frequency of the performance of the isolated

tension-free transvaginal tape employed for incontinence cure.

Also consider the silent perineal body defect that coexists in the multiparous woman in her late 30s or 40s who is undergoing a vaginal hysterectomy for symptomatic relief of one kind or another. Knowing that healthy perimenopausal women are likely to live well into old age, we have already accepted the dictum of obliterating the cul-de-sac at the time of hysterectomy to help prevent the future development of enterocele. Why, then, have we not similarly acknowledged the value of restoring the vaginal axis by what may be only a relatively minor procedure, a perineorrhaphy, at the same time as hysterectomy? For women who live long lives, this may well be considerably more protective than culdoplasty against a wider range of future pelvic breakdown. In actual practice, this presents a different selling proposition than the cul-de-sac closure; the patient is essentially unaware of a cul-de-sac closure, but a perineal repair hurts and may prolong the recovery period, at least from the patient's point of view. It has always been my custom, when vaginal hysterectomy is planned in the presence of a widely disrupted but as yet asymptomatic vaginal axis, principally because of perineal body disintegration, to make every effort to convince the patient to allow us to fix the perineum at the same time. Our arguments are rarely successful; the patient usually states that she would rather take her chances and see what happens later. Nonetheless, the argument for low posterior repair when pelvic surgery of another nature is to be performed (principally anterior compartment restitution or hysterectomy) should be pursued if one is to offer the best health care.

In attempting to justify the critical role of the perineal body in the chain of pelvic support, the skeptical resident or student may well challenge such a proposition by raising the issue of absence of supportive-suspensory breakdown in cases of chronic fourth-degree perineal laceration. This is a paradox, but one that is readily explicable. Strong compensatory mechanisms in the young woman, not generally present in the postreproductive woman, come into play to offset a negative influence for many years. Such a situation usually arises after a first delivery and is not likely to inflict significant lasting stress on the cardinal-uterosacral complex. Also, the rupture through the perineum takes the otherwise distributed stretch and strain of delivery off the pelvic floor so that the supportive influence of the levator plate and the levator muscles is minimally disturbed. Additionally, the young woman enjoys the full estrogen benefits of high levels of tissue texture, tone, collagen content, and vascularity, which are not present in the older woman. A major factor in most cases is the rapid neurogenic recovery after a first delivery, which is sometimes so effective that it offers compensatory resistance to involuntary fecal loss for many years. The older woman is not as fortunate. The decimated perineum has undergone years of wear and tear, the denervation of multiple deliveries has been compounded by the denervation of aging, and the atrophy of hypoestrinism has often set in. Tissues may have become further attenuated and inflexible through negative elements such as poor nutrition, constipation, indolence, and chronic coughing, which are not usually present in the premenopausal woman. Thus, the loss of perineal integrity in the postmenopausal woman presents a picture entirely different from that of the still reproductive woman.

Although of lesser interest to the reconstructive surgeon than the gross structural anatomy and its interrelations with adjacent tissues, a knowledge of the histologic composition of the perineal body is necessary to understand its function fully. It basically consists of a mixture of fibrous, elastic, muscular, and nerve cells. Because of its concentration of elastin and smooth muscle, it is flexible and mobilizes coordinately with activity in the vagina anteriorly and the anus and rectum posteriorly; it is attached at both places. A large number of ganglia and nerve fibers control this mobility and compliance, which extends to a rhythmic coordination with the musculoelastic rectovaginal septal activity above and the levator complex posterolaterally. Fibromuscular blending with the sphincter ani (behind), Colles fascia (above), and urogenital diaphragm (front) illustrates even further why widespread pelvic problems in both anatomy and function develop as the aging perineal body steadily dissolves. Problems are compounded by the greater extent and number of previously inflicted lacerations, poor operative repairs, poor healing capabilities, and hypoestrinism. The importance of surgically reestablishing a strong connection between the perineal body and the RVS has already been stressed. The impact of this restorative maneuver on correction of levator plate descensus cannot be emphasized enough because of the intimate association between the levator plate and the normal vaginal axis through its extensions into the perineal body. This leads to the last element of vaginal axis structure, the levator plate, a principal component of pelvic floor support.

THE LEVATOR PLATE

The structure commonly called the levator plate consists of a thick band of connective tissue representing the midline confluence of the two levator ani muscle complexes. It runs from the anorectal junction back to the lowermost vertebral segments. In the erect posture in the normal anatomic status, it lies almost horizontally as the fundamental pelvic floor support for the rectum and the vagina, both of which should lie almost flat also, in parallel, beyond the rectal verge. The cervix and the cul-de-sac also are situated above the levator plate, a very important feature in the prevention of pelvic prolapse as long as the levator plate remains horizontal. The levator plate fibers extend anteriorly on either side of the anorectal area to blend into the perineal body.

A precise definition of the status of the levator plate is not common in the evaluation of conditions of defective pelvic support, but it should be. If considered at all, it is by implication rather than by direct examination, which, in fact, can be easily accomplished. Except in marked obesity, the inferior borders of the levator musculature, medial to the inferior rami of the pubic bones, can be traced as they angle medially to meet behind the rectum to form their dense collagenous union so crucial to pelvic floor integrity. Assessment is made by lateral pressure of two fingers just inside the introitus against opposing pressure by the thumb of the same hand on the perineum. Analysis is best achieved in the erect patient, as above, when the index finger of the alternate hand is placed in the rectum and pressed downward and backward directly against the levator confluence. Levator attenuation, if it exists, can then be easily appreciated as the confluence is felt to be tilting downward, enlarging the rectogenitourinary hiatus. Pelvic structures can easily prolapse down this incline (Fig. 35C.12), much as a child might slide down a playground chute. In the presence of associated cardinal-uterosacral complex weakness, the downward prolapse can be accelerated.

The descent of the levator plate is a reflection of both inherent loss of levator muscle tone and overstretching of the fibers from pulsion effects from above. Additionally, as we are slowly discovering in explorations before repair of paravaginal defects in the anterior compartment from the vaginal approach, often one or the other, or both, of the levator muscle sets are shorn from its attachments to the arcus tendineus levator ani. When such a situation is discovered, it is imperative that the operator reattach the levator muscles to their origins at the same time as the paravaginal repair during anterior compartment restitution.

In view of current attitudes about rectovaginal septal tears, it is quite probable, in some cases, that we have falsely attributed weakness, deterioration, and attenuation within the levator plate as its cause of descent when,

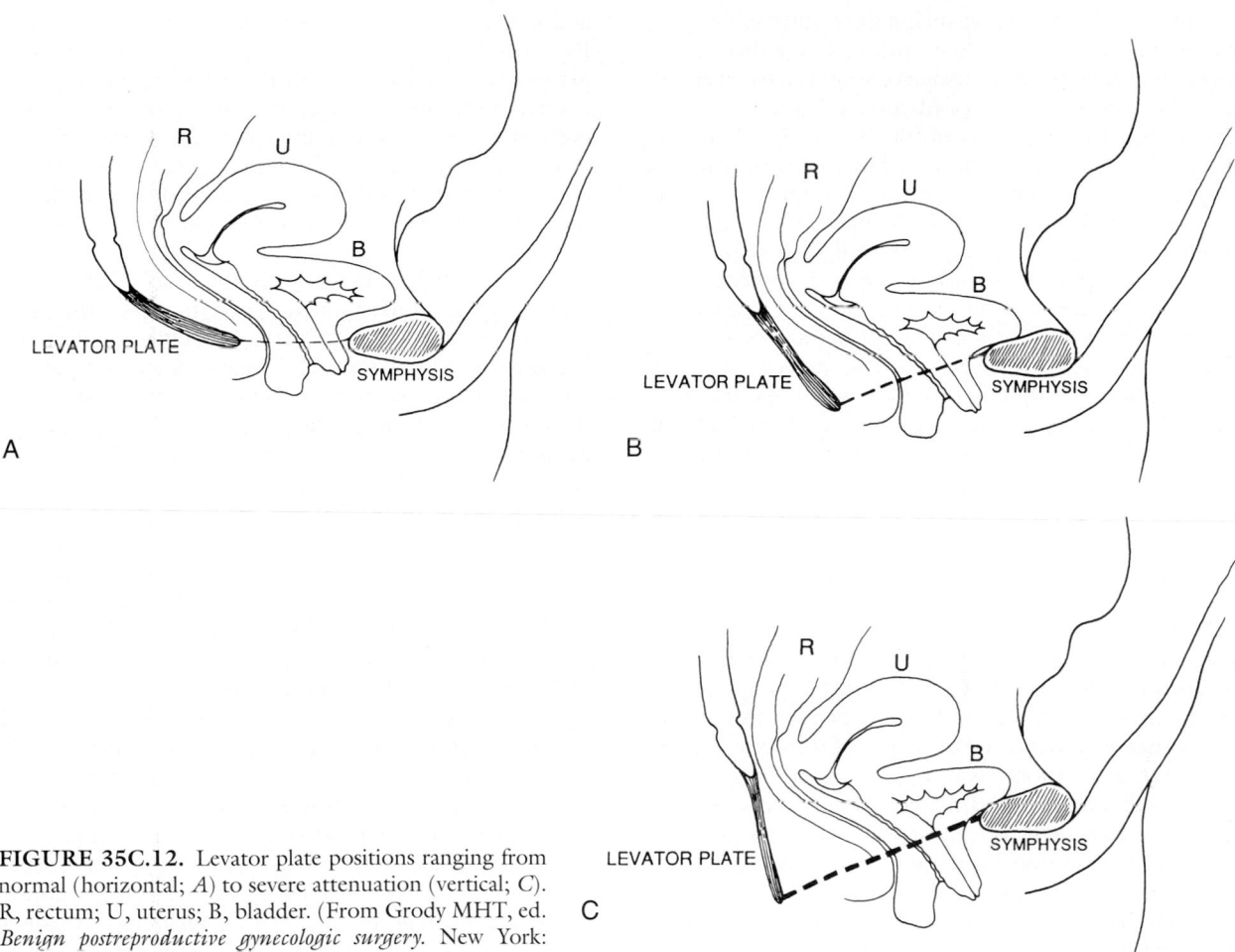

FIGURE 35C.12. Levator plate positions ranging from normal (horizontal; *A*) to severe attenuation (vertical; *C*). R, rectum; U, uterus; B, bladder. (From Grody MHT, ed. *Benign postreproductive gynecologic surgery.* New York: McGraw-Hill, 1994.)

in truth, it might be intrinsically strong and essentially unimpaired. If such is the case, and it certainly can be so in many instances, then the levator plate rotational descent in association with a progressively widened introitus may simply be the result of transverse RVS tears accompanied by perineal body destruction. Because it is accepted that all the female pelvic connective tissue is joined in an interdependent network, such a concept is most likely. Thus, restitution of the levator plate to its original horizontal anatomic position could be entirely dependent on full restoration of the RVS and the perineal body.

Recent discoveries at the Cleveland Clinic and Duke University introduce a new probability for levator plate descensus. Researchers there, using sophisticated electromyographic studies, have demonstrated concrete evidence of denervation injury involving the levator ani muscles specifically. They claim that this muscular complex is not innervated by the pudendal nerve but instead by a nerve traveling on its pelvic surface originating at levels S3 to S5 (the levator ani nerve). This must be considered a possible additional cause for rotational descent of the levator plate. This is best discovered clinically by testing the patient, preferably erect, with a finger in the rectum. When levator muscle capability is diminished or absent, whatever the cause, but especially by denervation, the valve-flap mechanism stressed for so many years by Robert Porges of New York University disappears. Translating this statement, when the patient is asked to cough or perform a Valsalva maneuver, normally the levator plate is snapped upward as part of the immediate resistance to increased abdominal pressure. In essence, this is truly a normal reflex action in which the pelvic floor shuts off the pelvis by an opposition response that is automatic. The impaired condition cannot do this.

Final commentary regarding anatomic distortions directly pertinent to both subjective complaints and corrective surgery in the posterior pelvic compartment is directed toward discovery of defects in the levator muscles themselves through relatively innovative techniques. Magnetic resonance imaging (MRI) has been well established as a useful adjunct in diagnosing and locating external anal disruption. Using similar MRI techniques, specific tears involving the levator muscles, either intrinsically or at the sites of their normal attachments, are being demonstrated at various major medical institutions. Additionally, patches of total muscle attrition can be located, and these are assumed to be neurogenic in origin.

In 2002, studies revealing such lesions, almost always attributable to previous trauma (obstetric), either directly to the musculature or to its nerve supply, have been presented by the University of Michigan, Loyola University of Chicago, the University of Illinois, the Royal Free and University College Medical School of London, and Brigham and Women's Hospital of Boston.

The clinical value of this information, it is currently thought, lies in the possible predictable degree of success or failure in pelvic floor reconstruction depending on the type, extent, and location of these levator defects, which seem to figure most seriously in the pubococcygeus and the puborectalis. How much these defect revelations may lead to any surgical correction is unexplored as yet, but much will depend on technical accessibility and the amount of associated nerve damage in any further assessments.

COLPOPERINEORRHAPHY

Dissection

Posterior repair is a colloquial term and probably should be discarded completely. Colporrhaphy is an appropriate particular designation, and when expressed as posterior colporrhaphy it indicates correction of rectocele. Further adjectival description, such as low posterior colporrhaphy or full-length posterior colporrhaphy, discloses the planned extent of the operation. Although this may seem minor in preparation for surgery, it can remind one of the degree of the lesion and it gives a clue to the time that may be necessary for the operation. Perhaps most importantly, it might divert surgeons from doing the same operation on everybody, stimulating them to find the precise lesions, either high, mid, or low, vertical or transverse, or combinations of these disruptions.

Similarly, perineorrhaphy, as a separate operation from colporrhaphy (although some form of it should almost always be performed in conjunction with colporrhaphy), deserves a listing apart from posterior repair. The extent of the dissolution of the perineal body to be repaired can be indicated by adding words in parentheses, such as mild, moderate, or severe. Certainly such detailing is impractical in an operating room schedule but not in a patient's chart, where it can serve as a distinguishing reminder, separating the particular patient from others.

The correct, combined terminology is posterior colpoperineorrhaphy. In most cases, some form of each is done concomitantly, as might be expected, considering the adjacent locations and the similar causes of injury.

Before the actual sharp invasion begins, reassessment under anesthesia, before "prepping" the field, is always prudent, using an index finger of one hand in the rectum and the first two fingers of the other hand in the vagina, as previously explained. The visual and tactile information perceived is invaluable, especially to neophytes, not only in highlighting up-to-the-moment precise areas for repair but also in clearly designating potential danger points in dissection that come from scarred distortion and closely adherent vaginal and rectal mucosal layers. Especially important is a true picture of dispersion of perineal body substance and the amount, if any, of disruption in all three levels of the external sphincter. However, one must correctly interpret and account for the distorted view interposed by the muscle relaxation inherent in anesthesia that is not present in the awake patient in whom muscle tone, such as it may be, exerts its influence.

Surgery should begin with the placement of Allis clamps at the mucocutaneous junction on either side, well out lateral to the fourchette, actually just outside the junction of the posterolateral vaginal sulci with perineal skin. Then the entire mucocutaneous junction, across the fourchette, between the two clamps should be either excised by scissors (my preference) or incised with a scalpel. Because of this large width, too many surgeons worry that this maneuver may lead ultimately to an introitus too narrow for coital comfort. This is a false concern at this point; the introitus, in most cases, at the outset, usually admits 8 to 12 fingers and the only objective at this time is attaining a wide and deep exposure of the full posterior pelvic compartment behind the posterior vaginal wall and at the vaginal vault. Such a goal can easily be achieved through appropriate dissection only if one begins in this manner. One cannot forget that the best pathway to good surgery is adequate exposure of the full operative field; this is especially true in the posterior pelvis. Avoiding an inadequate coital entry and instead aiming for a four-finger partially funnel-shaped coital portal can be guaranteed by the surgical adjustment described under the closure technique, which is used as the operation is terminated and is described later in this chapter. Therefore, ending with distal vaginal constriction should not be a problem.

Many gynecologists begin the posterior repair with Allis clamp placement well inside the area of the fourchette, actually at the lateral areas of the hymeneal ring. Such a maneuver is unquestionably restrictive and can forestall sufficient "work space" in obtaining comfortable access to the deep areas of cardinal-uterosacral ligament stumps, lateral vault connective tissue tears, and sacrospinous ligaments, not to mention encroachment on reaching far enough laterally to allow for satisfactory and substantial tissue involvement in the perineal body restitution that is so crucial in restoring the normal vaginal axis.

In association with the initial transverse incision, many gynecologic services routinely remove an inverted isosceles triangle of perineal skin in every case, as shown in Figure 35C.13. My colleagues and I feel this is often a very helpful technique, especially when the distance from fourchette to anus measures 3.0 to 4.5 cm, and the perineal body substance is split so that only vaginal mucosa and skin can be palpated against each other by pinching them together, sometimes for as much as 4 cm with only the external anal sphincter remaining intact. However, when the fourchette to anus distance is 2.5 cm or less, or when the perineal body defects are minor, removing perineal skin makes no sense.

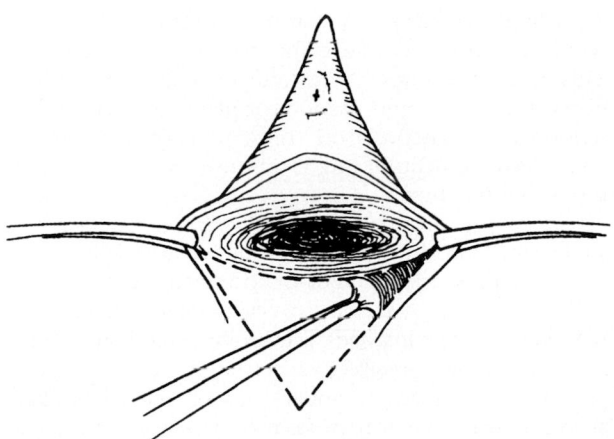

FIGURE 35C.13. Inverted isosceles triangle of skin being denuded from perineum in perineorrhaphy. (From Grody MHT, ed. *Benign postreproductive gynecologic surgery.* New York: McGraw-Hill, 1994)

The dissection then can be performed in standard fashion upward and laterally with concomitant midline vaginal wall incision completely up to the posterior vaginal vault. The dissection off the inner surface of the vaginal wall must be precisely meticulous to make certain that segments of rectovaginal fascia or any elements of connective tissue at all are not left behind, still attached to the vagina. This clearing process must be carried out bilaterally to the sidewall limits but not inadvertently beyond, for this could weaken the levator muscles and might enter the ischiorectal fossa. The landmarks for the lateral dissection boundaries are the posterior vaginal sulci on each side.

Correct technique in the dissection involves the use of T-clamps on the incised vaginal wall edges to create tension so as to allow curved Mayo scissors to do the clean stripping, pressing the concave side of the scissors against the convex curve of the nondominant index finger lying on the opposite vaginal epithelial surface in the vagina. Blunt dissection can be useful but only above the usually scarred perineal area and only where there is a clear plan of separation off the vaginal wall. Correct dissection techniques can be best learned and assessed from any of several operative videos in the American College of Obstetricians and Gynecologists (ACOG) audiovisual library in Washington, D.C.; precise tissue clearing cannot be emphasized enough. This can become especially difficult when the patient has undergone previous posterior repairs that present dense cicatrix between vaginal wall and anorectal mucosa, particularly in cases of indentations toward the rectum. Keeping the dissecting scissors always parallel to the vaginal wall is essential in prevention of inadvertent rectal entry.

Dissection depth can be regarded as complete once the level of the ischial spines has been reached, and they can easily be identified by palpation. Thus access to either cardinal-uterosacral stumps and/or sacrospinous ligaments can be assured if their involvement is deemed necessary for vault support insurance in the judgment of the surgeon in a particular case.

Repair

The surgeon has now arrived at the crux of the colporrhaphy, namely, discovery and labeling with Allis clamps all the torn edges of the RVS so that this fascia of Denonvilliers can be restored completely to original anatomic configuration. This maneuver is precisely what differentiates our current approved site-specific identification and defect-directed repair from the hopefully discarded traditional approach frequently used in the past.

Once the detached RVS edges have all been labeled, it is time for the second rectal examination. The examining index finger so placed must be pressed forward to simulate the rectocele, revealing the rectal wall bulging anteriorly in unrestricted fashion. Absolute verification of the preexisting absence of any form of connective tissue existing between the vaginal wall and the anorectal mucosa can then be verified by the placement of an opposing index finger in the operative wound. The two fingers all but touch each other, confirming that only the thin layer of lower intestinal wall separates them. Then, in dramatic fashion, as assistants draw the retracted rectovaginal segments together by approximating clasped opposite torn edges, temporarily restoring the natural RVS, the rectal finger can no longer be moved anteriorly because of the strong resistance of this natural barrier; implications of this demonstration are shown in Figures 35C.4, 35C.6, 35C.8, 35C.10, and 35C.12.

The balance of the operation then becomes much simpler and more reassuring than the traditional method of repair. All that is required is a sequential placement of interrupted stitches in appropriate points of reunion to create restitution of the normal RVS (Figs. 35C.5, 35C.7, 35C.9, 35C.11, and 35C.13). A continuous or running stitch is anathema; the potential for bunching, almost inevitable when this is done, and undue tension can ruin the operation. At the least, delayed absorbable suture material of sufficient caliber, at least 0, must be used. A good example is the popular polydioxanone (PDS, Ethicon, Wayne, NJ), which is monofilament. Monofilament suture is distinctly preferable to polyfilament or braided strands because of greater resistance to infection, especially in incompletely sterile areas such as the vaginal operative fields. There are many advocates pressing for nonabsorbable monofilament suture usage because a rectocele is unquestionably a herniation and should be treated as a hernia, and because there is considerably less risk of suture penetration into the rectum with the site-specific repair than with the old traditional method. A caution: almost all nonabsorbable sutures are stiff and the inflexible ends of the stitch knots not infrequently protrude through the vaginal mucosa in later months, causing no harm to the patient but inducing discouraging effects on an anticipatory penis. Polytetrafluorethylene suture (Gore-Tex, Gore, Inc., Flagstaff, AZ) is very soft and flexible and does not have the same effect.

Because of this remarkable alteration in the solution of the rectocele problem, it is strongly suggested, especially to the querulous or doubting reader, that a review of the solid evidence favoring this change be undertaken. If one did not hear directly any of Richardson's many lectures on the subject during the 1990s, good starting points are a viewing through the ACOG AudioVisual Library (AVL) of his video, "Anatomical Approach to Rectocele Repair," first presented in May 1993, with Paul Edmonds, and reading his cogent monograph published in 1995 (see bibliography). In 1997, Richardson and colleague William Saye made a graphic relevant presentation of posterior defect-specific correction at the annual meeting of the Society of Gynecologic Surgeons (SGS). Recent insights have been provided by Duke University (Cundiff et al, 1998) and an ACOG AVL video presentation dated May 2001. My colleagues and I at the Robert Wood Johnson Medical School–Camden (University of Medicine and Dentistry of New Jersey and Cooper Hospital, or UMDNJ) will have performed more than 200 of these site-specific repairs, including associated enterocele correction, sacrospinous ligament fixation, modified McCall suspension, and porcine derma and cadaveric grafts, by the end of 2003. Although still short-term postoperatively, our outcomes have been overwhelmingly rewarding both subjectively and objectively. As a direct outgrowth of this surgical activity, we are producing two new incisive educational videos scheduled for presentation at multiple scientific conferences, including those of SGS and ACOG, over the years 2003 and 2004.

Perineorrhaphy

Perineorrhaphy, although secondary to colporrhaphy in the total posterior pelvic correction, nonetheless plays a key role in the lasting endurance of an appropriate colporrhaphy, as described earlier. Briefly stated, an inadequately restored perineal body or, worse, ignored perineal body defects, present a major bottleneck to the success not only of posterior pelvic repair but also to any of the restorative measures, no matter how well executed, in the mid-pelvis (vaginal vault) and anterior pelvic compartment. Curiously, one of the foremost later consequences of such a surgical error is the occurrence or reappearance of an enterocele. The persistent perineal body defect is the "weak link in the chain," based on the precept that, as stated earlier, the integrity of normal pelvic anatomy depends on the unbroken continuity of its interdependent connective tissue network of which the perineal body is a crucial station (Fig. 35C.1).

Finally, a normal perineal body configuration inevitably restores the normal vaginal axis without which the entire reconstruction is threatened. A good long-term outcome is doomed without it, and this bodes poorly in a population with a steadily increasing life expectancy.

The bidigital examination, conducted initially on an outpatient basis and again at the operating table, easily imparts the degree of perineal body disintegration and accordingly signals the operator regarding the extent of required reparative effort for appropriate restitution. This means the surgery must ensure anchorage of RVS fibers from above and the levator plate connection posteriorly. Simultaneously one must remember that over-enthusiastic restitution might seriously interfere with future coital function.

Actual repair of the disrupted perineal body is rather straightforward. In various texts and monographs, often precise midline realignment of torn transverse perineal, bulbocavernosus, and pubococcygeal muscle fibers is described or at least implied. Truthfully, such tissue identification is rarely possible, especially in the aging postmenopausal woman, secondary to obliteration of exact anatomy from old cicatrix formation, years of wear and tear, neurologic and vascular attrition, and absence of estrogenic stimulation. The goal of repair is symmetrical restoration, as much as possible, by employing judiciously placed solid tissue bites into each side, using adequately reassuring interrupted stitches. Suture material can be either delayed absorbable synthetics of 0 caliber or, as many experts are currently advising, nonabsorbable strands of 0 bore. The preference for the former over the latter lies with the ready availability of delayed absorbable monofilament suture structure as opposed to the absence of practical nonabsorbable monofilaments other than polytetrafluoroethylene, as explained earlier in the colporrhaphy repair.

An anatomically correct fixed vaginal vault posterosuperiorly helps immeasurably in the enduring success of a colpoperineorrhaphy. Mid-pelvic vaginal cephalad suspension is discussed as a separate surgical entity elsewhere in this text. If the natural suspensory mechanism is intact and the surgeon deems tissue strength at that level is also sound, then nothing needs to be done. However, if there is even a minimal suggestion of vault prolapse, especially if an incipient enterocele is detected, then a procedure to correct this deficiency becomes imperative. Whether this is brought about by a sacrospinous ligament fixation, either unilateral or bilateral, or by a modified McCall procedure, or by some combination of the two, is unimportant because both have been shown to work well in the hands of skilled operators. It is strongly suggested that these techniques be considered for prophylaxis in cases of one or more disasters from previous failed corrective surgery and in situations in which inherent collagen deficiency is a marked probability. The surgeon is cautioned to make certain that no midline vault weakness or separation is left uncorrected in association with these suspensory techniques. Equally important is the vital necessity for direct tissue continuity with the uppermost extent of the RVS.

We always strive to achieve a vaginal length of at least 10 cm and often reach 11 to 12 cm. This can happen only when adequate vaginal wall remains. With the exception of large eversions, we rarely take off more than minimal amounts of vaginal mucosa, and this mucosa is taken only near the termination of the procedure to round off the right angles at the original fourchette. This is in sharp contrast to the earlier customary mucosal excision of many operators, especially those who still continue to excise at the outset. Our exception to these tactics occurs in very large eversions, whether anterior, posterior, central, or combined. In such instances, we remove truly excess vaginal wall, but this is done judiciously so as not to compromise the goals outlined above. One can always take off more, if necessary, when the final portion of the posterior closure ensues. We have experienced criticism by those who say 7 to 9 cm is an adequate vaginal depth and that we go too far. Our reason for this is our desire for overcorrection, when possible, to place a posterior vaginal vault as far behind the anterior edge of the levator plate as possible for the best prophylaxis against future enterocele, as long as we do not compromise functional vaginal diameter. In my 55 years of experience, this principle has paid off well, keeping later posterior breakdown to a bare minimum. This has proved to be especially true when judgment has dictated the need to combine a colpoperineorrhaphy with a vault fixation. Additionally, postreparative situations are capable of significant scarring regardless of how the surgery is conducted. Thus, when surgery is completed, what you have is what you get; the resiliency of the premenopausal resting vagina, capable of considerable stretching during coitus while still maintaining adequate support, is a luxury long gone. Fortunately, appropriate supplemental estrogen partially ameliorates any postoperative tendency for fixed or contracted dimensions.

Closure

One of the most common misconceptions of gynecologic surgeons is that excess vaginal mucosa should be removed. This is undoubtedly the greatest single factor in the undesirable development of an inadequate postrepair dysfunctional vagina. This concept, reinforced by the phrase that still echoes from one operating room to the next, "We must remove generous portions of mucosa," can and often does lead to regrettable impairment. Such a poor course, in the average case, beyond the obvious disability, interferes with restoration of a normal vaginal axis. Also, the inevitability of a shortened vagina increases markedly the potential for a later vault eversion. There is a false postulation that if something protrudes and should be inside, it must be in excess; therefore, some of it should be chopped off. Simple mathematics is ignored; no excess develops until what sticks out becomes larger than what originally was stuck in. Generally what we are dealing with, even in marked eversion (except for the extreme cases), is a single conical or ovoid expanse of vaginal wall protruding outside the introitus. We should dissect this freely enough for readjustment to form a functionally dimensional cylinder (Fig. 35C.14), bent appropriately to allow for apex placement deeply posterior toward the sacral hollow. The bend shapes naturally in association with appropriate reestablishment of a reunited RVS and a full perineal body, as the vaginal axis resumes its normal shape. It can happen that, despite all good intentions and seemingly accurate calculation, too much mucosa is removed. A

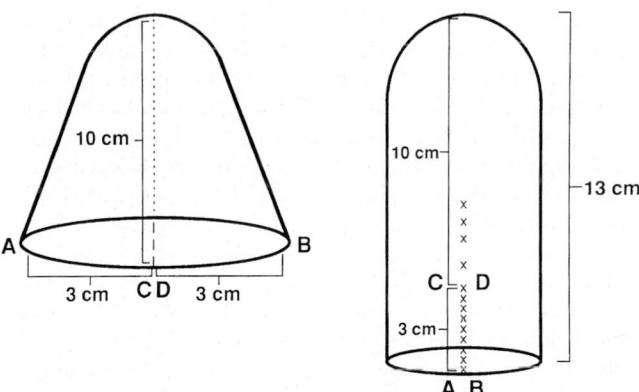

FIGURE 35C.14. Simple transformation. The cone, whether everted or still inverted, must be transformed into a cylindrical shape. Points A and B represent the lateral corners at the outset of surgery; C and D designate either side of the original fourchette as the posterior vaginal wall is bisected toward the vault. After thorough dissection, the reparative process moves C and D inward as the vagina is reshaped and lengthened, while A and B meet at the new fourchette. (Grody MHT, ed. *Benign postreproductive gynecologic surgery*. New York: McGraw-Hill, 1994.)

simple solution is to resuture back to the deficient area a measured segment of what was removed earlier. Therefore, do not discard any removed vaginal wall; keep it between moist gauze packs until the operation is over. The reattachment heals well.

Vaginal wall closure, as the operation progresses toward completion, is routinely accomplished by starting at the top of the opened posterior wall and then moving toward the perineum with a running (continuous) locking 2-0 rapidly absorbable suture. If colporrhaphy is performed as instructed in this chapter and vaginal mucosal excision has not been overzealous, then rarely is the vagina ever constricted so as to challenge future coital function using this simple method of reuniting the posterior wall. Nonetheless, it is still considered wise, and it certainly is harmless, to check the amplitude digitally arbitrarily after every two bites. If the vaginal depth is particularly deep, it is wise to start closing the mucosa immediately after completing the colporrhaphy and before perineorrhaphy is begun. Otherwise it may be a struggle to begin the mucosal reunion after the full repair itself is completed underneath.

Although the surgeon may have been very attentive to ensure adequate vaginal capacity for coital function throughout the posterior reparative process until the very end of the operation, it is possible to ruin all positive effects, from the patient's viewpoint, with the last few closure stitches in the area of the new fourchette. This happens when the vertical midline closure is continued, without interruption, from its starting point deep in the vagina down to the end in the perineal skin anterior to the anus. Initially, the operator is advised to create a wide horizontal entry across the fourchette to render full surgical exposure and to ignore functional introital room at that time. At this point, having avoided constriction so far by having already placed appropriate perineal body sutures, the operator will certainly create such an undesirable result if he or she unites the far reaches of either side to fashion the new fourchette. This is very simply averted by placing two to three interrupted 2-0 rapidly absorbable horizontal stitches on each side transversely, close to the "corners" (Fig. 35C.15). Corner sutures thus sited bring together juxtaposing edges of vaginal mucosa and perineal skin as shown in this sketch. These stitches should be placed when the vaginal longitudinal running stitch has closed to 2 cm from perineal skin where delay is made while the corner stitches are effected. This maneuver thereby produces a comfortable funnel-shaped vaginal entry and does not compromise the reestablished normal anatomy. This type of surgical consideration is especially critical with relevance to older couples in whom the reliable penile rigidity of youth has long disappeared.

Surgical Complications

If the rectal lumen is invaded and opened during the dissection, there is no cause for alarm. The most important factor is recognition. Once discovered, closure of the rent should not be effected at that time but should be postponed until the total dissection is completed. With the bowel lesion open, there is an available reference for

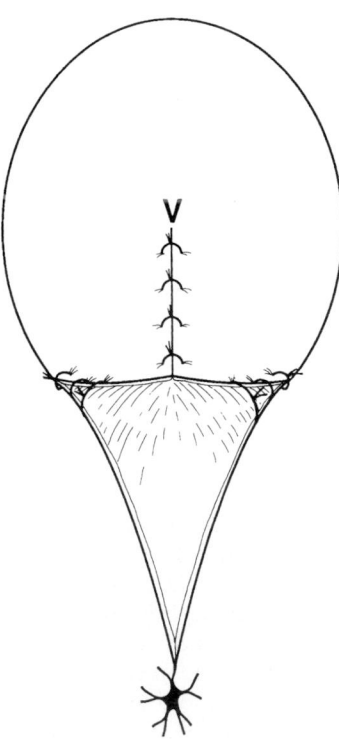

FIGURE 35C.15. Prevention of introital constriction by the placement of interrupted transverse closure sutures at the corners before completion of the longitudinal midline closure over the new fourchette. (From Grody MHT, ed. *Benign postreproductive gynecologic surgery.* New York: McGraw-Hill, 1994.)

the balance of the dissection. This reference would disappear if closure were performed immediately, placing the operator back to where he or she started with potential for reopening, especially in heavily scarred cases. If the bowel is empty preoperatively, as it should be, and jet-propelled lavage with Vital-Vue (American Cyanamid, Wayne, NJ) is maintained periodically throughout the procedure, no increased incidence of postoperative infection is noted. We do not use an intensive bowel preparation for any vaginal surgery because our long experience indicates no need for it. Very simply, the patient is instructed to eat a light lunch and to take liquids only at supper followed by a Fleet enema at bedtime the day before surgery. In view of the natural tissue resistance to traditional regional bacteria in this area in healthy women, the key elements in the prevention of subsequent trouble are appropriate preoperative antibiotic coverage, adequate lavage, and satisfactory surgical closure of the rectal lesion. Additional antibiotics are unnecessary, and the patient requires no special post-operative care and enemas should be used cautiously or not at all.

Using the modern method of defect-specific repair of the RVS, the risk of sutures being passed unintentionally through the anorectal mucosa is markedly diminished as compared to the old traditional method of posterior correction. Nonetheless, it can happen, especially in cases of dense scarring or distortion. For decades the universal admonition was, "After the operation is completed, the last thing to do is a rectal examination. If a stitch is felt, you must cut it through the anus by either palpation or small speculum exposure." This idea is incorrect. The time for recognition is during the procedure when the operative wound is still open and the target, found by rectal finger, can be removed easily and directly without the difficulty attendant to later stitch destruction rectally. In addition, cutting a suture after the operation is completed may jeopardize an otherwise effective repair by creating a weak area. While the wound is still open, a replacement stitch, this time without bowel penetration, can be positioned correctly. The surgeon's anxiety may be decreased by remembering that Edgar Poth, in 1968, showed that a stitch through the bowel, tied securely, led to no untoward consequences. He observed that an undisturbed benign course occurs, despite the errant intrusion, because of the forced penetration of the invading strand through the mucosa by the effects of adjacent progressive reactive edema. The suture, within a few hours, now buried beneath the mucosa, is covered by healing epithelial cells across the small defect. Again reassurance regarding absence of increased incidence of infection is emphasized without need for further antibiotic coverage if this protection was administered properly before the outset of the operation. Again, natural bacterial resistance of involved tissue is protective.

In extensive posterior repairs, particularly when a modified McCall procedure or correction of an enterocele is included, cystoscopy is necessary to reveal, hopefully, absence of untoward ureteral interference. Intravenously administered indigo carmine, as is customary, is used in this exercise, which should be performed before closure of the posterior vaginal wall.

Postoperative vaginal packing with an antibiotic-soaked gauze strip is considered compulsory at most major institutions. I believe that this pack should remain in position for 2 days (not 1, as in most other facilities). My experience reveals no negative effects. We believe this discourages serosanguineous fluid collections and protects the many delicately placed stitches against the undesirable pressure effects of postanesthetic retching and coughing that so commonly occur during this most vulnerable stage of healing.

A postoperative regimen for posterior compartment repair is always subservient to rules relevant to other procedures performed simultaneously. The specific course the patient should follow after colpoperineorrhaphy is relatively simple and can easily be incorporated with other instructions for accompanying operations, especially because the rules for recovery from any vaginal surgery mostly overlap anyhow. Mobility restrictions are minimal in the usual case. Immediately after leaving the hospital, the patient should begin walking about her house, even going up and down stairs, albeit slowly, and then outside ambulation as soon as is feasible. Too many gynecologic surgeons harbor the gross misconception that, after pelvic reconstructive surgery, the patient heals best by avoiding the erect posture "to keep the strain of upper body weight off the pelvis" that could interfere with the healing process. In my 55 years in the business of gynecology, my observations lie firmly in the opposite contention; early ambulation promotes good healing and potentiates better long-term results. Certainly it helps immeasurably in reducing serious lower extremity and pelvic vascular accidents that could lead to embolization. Also, increased activity, especially away from one's home, stimulates both appetite and psyche, obvious positive factors in good recovery. Constant caution, however, against heavy lifting and athletic jumping exercise, remains a lifetime warning from the outset.

Family support is unquestionably positive, although not necessary for the otherwise healthy and well-motivated woman who lives alone. However, in situations of adverse physical and/or mental capacity, family support is critical toward good recovery for all kinds of reasons; encouragement by the surgeon for family participation in the recovery phase is mandatory, especially with the elderly patient. I emphasize this point because, more and more, physicians are regarded by lay people as technologists lacking in the warmth, compassion, empathy, and even commiseration, that they would like to associate with health care.

Constipation, especially if it extends to impaction, can become the single greatest threat toward destroying even the best surgery. In my many years as a consultant of last resort in the area of recurrent pelvic floor breakdown, I can recite case after case of failed surgery where I am convinced that severe immediate postoperative constipation or chronic uncontrolled habitual constipation was a major factor of failure. Certainly the alert and responsible surgeon can and must order a prophylactic dietary regimen and has for ready disposal, both for prevention and cure, a vast armamentarium of benign medications, suppositories, and soft enemas that can obliterate this potentially catastrophic phenomenon.

The restorative influence of estrogen replacement on all the pelvic tissues cannot be emphasized enough. Estrogen receptors have been identified in tissues and organs throughout the pelvis, including urethra, bladder neck, anus, and uterosacral ligaments. Although their number diminishes with aging, the response to exogenous estrogen in previously atrophic hormone-deprived mucosal, muscular, and connective tissue in the pelvis can often be spectacular. This is thought to be due to the survival of a significant number of estrogen receptors. Clinically, many of us have long been aware of the crucial role played by estrogen in the rejuvenation and maintenance of tissue quality in the pelvis, particularly with reference to increased failure rates in its absence and better long-term outcomes in its continued presence. It is considered good advice not to perform any reconstructive or urogynecologic procedures until the patient has been under hormone replacement for at least 6 to 8 weeks and has a stated commitment for lifetime supplementation. In view of the well-publicized, astounding disclaimer of the National Institutes of Health in 2002 indicting oral combinations of estrogen and progesterone, many women have become fearful of taking estrogen at all in any form. It is essential for the surgeon to explain to the patient that the bad news was referable only to the combination of female hormones and not to estrogen administered alone through any route within safe but still effective limits.

In view of the recent awareness that conditions of connective tissue weakness are more common than we used to think, the ill effects of collagen deficiency states (usually of a congenital nature) on pelvic supportive and suspensory relations, particularly in the posterior compartment, must be recognized. Extensive clinical studies over the past several years have enlightened us immeasurably on the profound effects of this problem. If one adds to this the adverse effects on connective tissue of chronic cigarette smoking, particularly in the postmenopausal female (even after cessation of smoking for several years), the odds for long-term success in pelvic repair are certainly reduced. So the pelvic reconstructive surgeon should beware when the double-jointed, dislocation- and hernia-prone cigarette-smoking female presents herself for help! Certainly those so deprived require something extra, like a little overcorrection or an earlier and more liberal resort to graft materials.

Despite the best judgment, technique, material, and circumstances, occasionally the surgery breaks down in time, leading to recurrent lesions. Most likely this occurs secondary to previously existing or surgically induced pelvic denervation and subsequent atrophy despite adequate estrogen replacement therapy. Nerve damage and deterioration have been studied extensively in recent years in consideration of the roles they play in physiologic and anatomic disruption. It is generally concluded that, in some cases, it is difficult or impossible to overcome surgically the problems arising from long-standing denervation and its consequent destructive effects on muscle and connective tissue, especially in association with the wear and tear of aging. Can strategically placed grafts overcome this dilemma, at least partially?

Grafts, now in relatively common use in anterior pelvic correction, often in primary cases, are being applied in selective cases in the posterior pelvis. My colleagues and I are resorting to grafts at UMDNJ–Camden more than the average because, as an established referral center with a fellowship program, we experience a preponderantly heavier influx of patients with difficult and previously failed posterior pelvic defect repairs. The guidelines for the decision to include a graft as an addendum to our site-specific major repair depends almost entirely on our assessment of the quality of the available connective tissue, including the RVS itself, plus the ligamentous elements at the posterior vaginal vault. All the areas to be reunited or united into the repair itself are tested by a tugging maneuver, using an Allis clamp, before each stitch is placed at each particular point. When the connective tissue tears readily with only minimal or moderate tugging effort, it is judged to be inadequate and a graft as the appropriate substitute is considered expedient. In the uncommon situation (1 in 25 cases in our experience) in which exact delineation cannot be determined with confidence and we feel true attenuation has occurred, as in situations recording previous postoperative infection or those with a history of multiple recurrent and failed surgeries, we employ grafts without hesitation. Certainly, we regard any case that smacks of congenital collagen deficiency syndrome with great suspicion. In these instances, when our inner feelings create trepidation, we again apply a graft; even if we know it may be just prophylactic, we hope to prevent future breakdown. We have the same worries when we think denervation has contributed to connective tissue and muscle weakness, in which cases we sew in grafts and hope for good luck.

A graft should always be anchored into the resurrected RVS at the vault, sometimes including bites fixing it also to the cardinal-uterosacral ligament stumps or to the sacrospinous ligaments. On each side, the graft is attached by individual stitches to levator fascia and the same bind is made to the previously restored perineal body at the bottom.

Autologous fascia lata and rectus muscle fascia are not applicable to posterior repair augmentation because wide enough patches cannot be taken practically. I have used synthetic mesh with great success and I would not discourage its use in the future. However, a distinct trend toward the use of acellular collagen matrix has developed and it is popular in several major centers. The sources for this type of substitute support are most usually porcine derma and human cadaveric skin, both of which have been processed and reduced to matrix framework. The basic reasoning for using these materials is the presumption that, over several months, native fibroblasts will affix into this foreign tissue mesh, thereby producing a brand new effective barrier of connective tissue, really scar tissue. Because these substances have been in use

widely for only a few years, we require considerably more time to judge their true effectiveness.

Although I would like to omit entirely any reference to defecography, I cannot do so because of its progressively increasing appearance in diagnostic advisories affecting posterior pelvic surgery. This subject has provoked controversy and antagonism, even disdain, among gynecologists, who generally regard it as a worthless procedure, despite espousal from two groups, while conversely our operating neighbors, the colorectal surgeons, have embraced it with passion. The topic is covered in depth in Chapter 39 on Anal Incontinence. Simply, this particular diagnostic imaging technique seems to have become the major method for colorectal surgeons for discovery of a rectocele. The specific literature that covers colorectal surgery, plus several publications in radiology journals, is replete with monographs and studies on the apparent virtues of defecography in identifying rectoceles. Except for two U.S. medical centers in Chicago and Indianapolis, where reconstructive gynecologists employ this type of radiography primarily for sleuthing out what they have termed *sigmoidocele* (which carries its own inherent symptoms) that they claim escapes discovery by ordinary means of examination, gynecologic surgeons in general and pelvic reconstructive surgeons in particular, especially those who work primarily through the vaginal approach, ignore defecography completely and consider it a vehicle of no adjunctive contributing value. Most of us feel that the identification of a rectocele, together with attendant recognition of perineal body defects, is easily made from the patient's history and a thorough bidigital and bimanual examination, especially with the patient in the erect posture (Figs. 35C.2 and 35C.3).

From the outpatient examination as described, plus bimanual/bidigital examination on the operating room table just before initial incision, again as soon as the operative field is completely exposed, and finally after identification of the torn RVS edges, we know all that is necessary to perform not only just a proper rectocele repair but also a good vault suspension and a perineorrhaphy. If there really is such a separate diagnosis as sigmoidocele, then it will automatically be corrected at the upper end of the weakness causing enterocele under the direct vision afforded by appropriate enterocele exposure. In 55 years of practice and through multiple conversations with skilled pelvic surgeons, we collectively feel the concept of sigmoidocele is unacceptable.

In a relatively small but significant number of cases, there is also need for repair of the external anal sphincter. A history of fecal incontinence and a corroborative physical examination indicate the need for addition of sphincterpexy as discussed in Chapter 39. However, the necessity to discover any history of fecal incontinence, including its impending development (fecal staining), during the initial interview must be emphasized. The doctor must press the question because women who readily volunteer urinary incontinence are often too embarrassed to mention fecal incontinence. Knowing about this symptom in advance of surgery allows for sphincterpexy to be included simultaneously with perineorrhaphy. Sphincterpexy is generally not time-consuming under these circumstances. Finally, the surgeon is reminded that external anal sphincter defects, primarily in the upper and middle loops, are best evaluated during the surgery with a finger in the rectum when the dissection has been completed.

Figures 35C.16 and 35C.17 illustrate the changes that should occur in a correctly engineered posterior colpoperineorrhaphy performed under the best conditions with the best tissue available. The role of a good perineal body restitution in producing a normal vaginal axis is obvious. Also implied by these two sketches is the reason why we at Cooper Hospital/UMDNJ–Camden rarely consider any vaginal mucosa to be in excess, usually trimming, at the most, the square corners at the introitus. Our persistence in dissecting cleanly and widely to the side walls and almost to the depth of peritoneum affords us the architectural privilege of effecting a deep posterior vault. This allows shifting of the vaginal wall, none of which is removed except in extreme eversion, to suit our surgical goals, which is to reestablish a normal vaginal axis. Without this restored axis and its accompanying depth, penile penetration may be too limited for enjoyable copulation.

One often hears that there is no need to worry whether the vagina seems somewhat foreshortened because repetitive coital activity will lengthen it. In view of the current anatomic revelations, such thinking is archaic and silly. Most of these repairs are done in postmenopausal women who are married to or having rela-

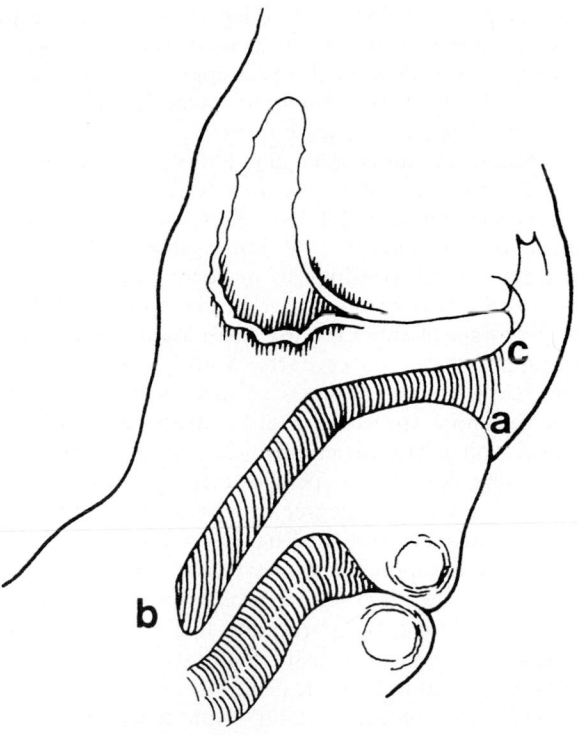

FIGURE 35C.17. Posthysterectomy, postperineorrhaphy illustration revealing restored curved cylindrical vagina, marked by a, b, and c, with functional measurements and normal axis after repair. (From Grody MHT, ed. *Benign postreproductive gynecologic surgery*. New York: McGraw-Hill, 1994.)

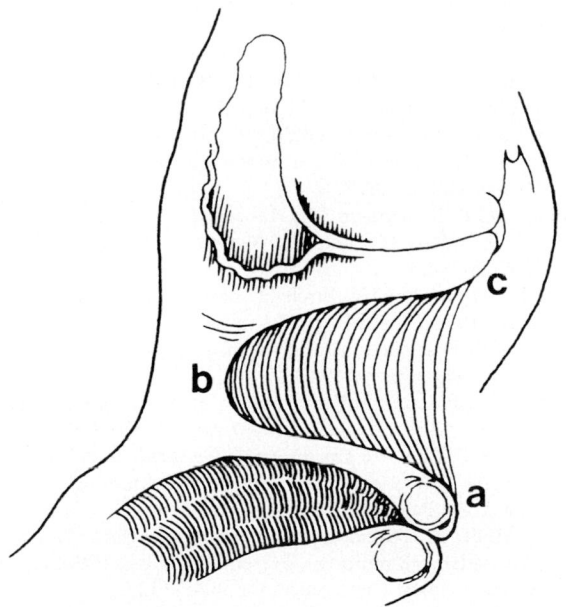

FIGURE 35C.16. Posthysterectomy case with severe perineal defects exaggerating an abnormally shaped conical vagina marked by points a, b, and c. (From Grody MHT, ed. *Benign postreproductive gynecologic surgery*. New York: McGraw-Hill, 1994.)

tionships with men of equal age. Because these men have lost their youthful sexual proclivities, they do not function as human dilators. Even if extension of length by coitus could occur, because deep surgical support is usually absent in such deficient vaginas, the stretched vault will simply begin telescoping outward, setting the stage for an enterocele.

One of the most common errors in mucosal closure is the compulsion to eliminate the "dead space" underneath. Spaces between organs are natural in the pelvis, thereby allowing one organ to function without disturbing adjacent structures. During coitus, problems will ensue if the vagina is bound tightly anteriorly or posteriorly to even a partially full bladder or rectum, respectively. The original design calls for sliding action, so that surgery should not fix the vagina to the rectum or bladder.

Because so many of our young gynecologists are enamored with the laparoscope, and because of some scattered attempts to suggest its possible use in posterior colporrhaphy, I am compelled to vehement exhortation against its use in this scenario. Although I must acknowledge that laparoscopists can skillfully restore satisfactory vaginal vault support by an assortment of methods via the abdomen, it seems ridiculous, even foolhardy, to conceive even for a moment an alternative approach to any further surgical restoration of an area so easily and rapidly accessible to direct exposure vaginally. Can you just imagine a ludicrous attempt at perineorrhaphy through an abdominally placed laparoscope? Believe me, it has been tried. Our current defect-specific methods, as described, provide a much easier approach to the surgical site. So, close the book on colporrhaphy by laparoscopy. There is no excuse for it.

Despite all the current new and exciting evidence-based knowledge about posterior pelvic defects and the logical surgical sequel I have described, a significant horde of nonbelievers and immovable traditionalists wish to and will continue to perform colporrhaphy in the old method that we have hoped to discard. I am deeply aware of an all too prevalent status countrywide through my various contacts. Some argue that they have had such a high degree of success in the past that they find no reason to change. In truth, all of us who consider ourselves meticulous precision-directed operators, using non–defect-specific techniques in the past, did achieve a certain degree of success. Why is this so? I believe this has happened because we re-created substantial vault support and reestablished a normal vaginal axis by returning the perineal body to normal, and because there was the pure good luck of a satisfactory natural response of scar tissue filling in between the top and the bottom. However, I cannot find any intelligent rationale to continue doing something in a non-anatomic way when we have learned the truth and can now reinvent the natural configuration. Most likely, our results of the past have not been as good as we would like to boast, and we cannot help but look forward to substantially greater success now that we know how to do it right.

In conclusion, I feel strongly that the supportive keystone for a sustained total pelvic outcome resides in the posterior pelvic compartment. Without its intact strength and stability, the balance of pelvic integrity is doomed to collapse. As a crucial segment in the ideal concept of pelvic reconstruction, a well-conceived, well-tooled posterior colpoperineorrhaphy can well be the cornerstone to long-term success beyond anything we have known before.

BIBLIOGRAPHY

Aldridge A, Watson P. Analysis of end results of labor in primiparas after spontaneous versus prophylactic methods of delivery. *Am J Obstet Gynecol* 1935;30:554.

Allen RE, Hosker GL, Smith ARB, et al. Pelvic floor damage and childbirth: a neurophysiological study. *Br J Obstet Gynaecol* 1990;97:770.

Barber MD, Bremer RE, Thor KB, et al. Innervation of the female levator ani muscles. *Am J Obstet Gynecol* 2002; 187:64.

Barber MD. Neurology becomes bigger focus in the study of pelvic floor disorders. *Cleveland Clinic Foundation Perspectives* 2002 (Sept).

Barbieri RL, York CM, Cherry ML, et al. The effects of nicotine, cotinine, and anabasine on rat adrenal 11 B-hydroxylase and 21-hydroxylase. *J Steroid Biochem* 1987;24:1.

Baron JA, LaVecchia C, Levi F. The centiestrogenic effect of cigarette smoking in women. *Am J Obstet Gynecol* 1990; 162:502.

Batra SC, Iosif CS. Effect of estrogen treatment on the peroxidase activity and estrogen receptors in the female rabbit urogenital tissues. *J Urol* 1992;148:935.

Benson JT. Pelvic floor neuropathy. In: *Female pelvic floor disorders*. New York: WW Norton, 1992:142.

Berglas B, Rubin IC. Study of the supportive structures of the uterus by levator myography. *Surg Gynecol Obstet* 1953; 97:677.

Berkley C, Bonney V. *Textbook of gynaecological surgery,* ed 5. London: Cassel, 1947.

Bradley CS, Beshara MN, Mikuta JJ, et al: An anatomic reconstruction of the pelvic floor and perineum. *J Pelv Surg* 2002;8:207.

Caraballo R, Maccarone JL, Holzberg A, et al: *New concepts in reconstructive pelvic surgery: slings, collagen matrix grafts, triggered sutures.* Video in production—publication date: March 6, 2003.

Chou Q, Kearny R, DeLancey JOL. *Location of defects in the levator ani muscle on magnetic resonance imaging using a structured system.* American Urogynecology Society presentation; paper 23. San Francisco: October 1, 2002.

Connell EB, Grody MHT. Estrogen: major factor in pelvic reconstructive and urogynecologic surgery. In: Grody MHT, ed. *Benign postreproductive gynecologic surgery.* New York: McGraw-Hill, 1994:8.

Cundiff GW. *Defect directed rectocele repairs: restorative and compensatory techniques* (video, 19 minutes). ACOG Audio-Visual Library, 2001, AVL 150.

Cundiff GW, Weidner AC, Visco AG, et al: An anatomic and functional assessment of the discrete defect rectocele repair. *Am J Obstet Gynecol* 1998;179:1451.

Damaser MS, Parikh M, Rasmussen ML, et al: *Three dimensional model of the normal female pelvic floor.* American Urogynecology Society presentation; paper 12. San Francisco: October 18, 2002.

Damaser MS, Parikh M, Rasmussen ML, et al. *Virtual reality model of the normal female pelvic floor.* American Urogynecology Society presentation; paper 15. San Francisco: October 18, 2002.

DeLancey JOL. Anatomic aspects of vaginal eversion after hysterectomy. *Am J Obstet Gynecol* 1992;166:1717.

DeLancey JOL. Anatomy and biomechanics of genital prolapse. *Clin Obstet Gynecol* 1993;36:897.

Dickinson RL. Studies of levator ani muscle. *Am J Obstet Dis Women* 1889;22:897.

Edmonds PB, Richardson AC. *Anatomical approach to rectocele repair* (video, 23 minutes). ACOG Audio-Visual Library, 1993, SGS 03.

Funt M, Thompson JD, Birch H. Normal vaginal axis. *South Med J* 1978;71:1534.

Gainey HL. Post-partum observation of pelvic tissue damage. *Am J Obstet Gynecol* 1943;45:457.

Gainey HL. Post-partum observation of pelvic tissue damage: further studies. *Am J Obstet Gynecol* 1955;70:800.

Grody MHT. *Complex procedures and methods in pelvic reconstructive and urogynecologic surgery.* Cassette II (video). New York: Parthenon, 1994.

Grody MHT. *Posterior colpoperineorrhaphy: bulwark of pelvic repair* (video, 38 minutes). Presented in May, 1994, ACOG Annual Clinical Conference, Orlando, FL.

Grody MHT. Posterior pelvis. III. Rectocele and perineal defects. In: *Benign postreproductive gynecologic surgery.* New York: McGraw-Hill, 1994:247.

Grody MHT. *Surgical repair in massive posthysterectomy posterior vaginal eversion* (video, 27 minutes). ACOG Audio-Visual Library, 1993, AVL 96.

Grody MHT. Wound healing and suture selection. In: Grody MHT, ed. *Benign postreproductive gynecologic surgery*. New York: McGraw-Hill, 1994:375.

Haadem K, Lennart L, Marten F, et al. Estrogen receptors in the external and sphincter. *Am J Obstet Gynecol* 1991; 164:609.

Halban J, Tandler J. *Anatomic and Atiologic der Genital prolapse beim Weibe*. Leipzig: Wilhelm Braumuller, 1907.

Handa VL, Harris TA, Ostergard. Protecting the pelvic floor: obstetric management to prevent incontinence and pelvic organ prolapse. *Obstet Gynecol* 1996;88:470.

Kearney R, DeLancey JOL, Chou Q. *The severity of defects seen in the levator ani muscle on MR imaging correlate with obstetric history*. American Urogynecology Society presentation; paper 14. San Francisco: October 18, 2002.

Longcope C, Johnson CC Jr. Androgen and estrogen dynamics in pre- and postmenopausal women: a comparison between smokers and non-smokers. *J Clin Endocrinol Metab* 1988;67:379.

Maccarone JL, Caraballo R, Holzberg A, et al. *Innovative defect-specific posterior pelvic surgery: triggered ligament sutures and collagen graft*. Video in production—publication date: May 1, 2003.

McCall ML. Posterior culdoplasty. *Obstet Gynecol* 1957;10:595.

Nichols DH. Posterior colporrhaphy and perineorrhaphy: separate and distinct operations. *Am J Obstet Gynecol* 1991;164:714.

Nichols DH, Milley PS, Randall CL. Significance of restoration of normal vaginal depth and axis. *Obstet Gynecol* 1970; 36:251.

Nichols DH, Randall CL. *Vaginal surgery*, third ed. Baltimore. Williams & Wilkins, 1989;21.

Norton PA, Boyd C, Deah S. Abnormal collagen ratios in women with genitourinary prolapse. *Neuro Urodyn* 1992; 11:2.

Norton PA. Histological and biochemical studies. In: Benson JT, ed. *Female pelvic floor disorders*. New York: WW Norton, 1992:166.

Norton PA. Pelvic floor disorders: the role of fascia and ligaments. *Clin Obstet Gynecol* 1993;36:926.

Poth EJ. Intestinal anastomosis; a unique technique. *Am J Surg* 1968;116:643.

Richardson AC. Personal communication: March 1995 and May 2001.

Richardson AC. The rectovaginal septum revisited: its relationship to rectocele and its importance to rectocele repair. *Clin Obstet Gynecol* 1993;36:976

Richardson AC. The anatomic defects in rectocele and enterocele. *J Pelv Surg* 1995;1:214.

Rogers RM Jr, Julian TM. Vaginal vault prolapse and interocele: prophylaxis and anatomic restitution during transvaginal surgery. *Oper Tech Gynecol Surg* 2001;6(3): 127.

Shull BL, Bachhofer C, Coates KW, et al. A transvaginal approach to repair of apical and other associated sites of pelvic organ prolapse with uterosacral ligaments. *Am J Obstet Gynecol* 2000;183:1365.

Shull BL, Capen CV, Riggs MW, et al. Pre- and post-operative analysis of site specific pelvic support defects in 81 women treated by sacrospinous ligament suspension and pelvic reconstruction. *Am J Obstet Gynecol* 1992;166:1764.

Singh K, Jakab M, Reid WMN et al. *Three-dimensional assessment of levator ani morphology in different grades of prolapse*. American Urogynecology Society presentation; paper 13. San Francisco: October 18, 2002.

Smith ARB, Hosker GL, Warrell DW. The role of partial denervation of the pelvic floor in the etiology of genitourinary prolapse and stress incontinence: a neurophysiologic study. *Br J Obstet Gynaecol* 1989;96:24.

Smith P, Heimer G, Norgren A, et al. Steroid hormone receptors in pelvic muscles and ligaments in women. *Gynecol Obstet Invest* 1990;30:27.

Snooks SJ, Swash M, Mathers SE, et al. Effect of vaginal delivery on the pelvic floor: a five year followup. *Br J Surg* 1990;77;1258.

Tobin CE, Benjamin JA. Anatomical and surgical restudy of Denonvilliers' fascia. *Surg Gynecol Obstet* 1945;80:373.

Warrell DW. Pelvic floor neuropathy: partial denervation in pelvic floor prolapse. In: Bensen JT, ed. *Female pelvic floor disorders*. New York: WW Norton, 1992:153.

Weinstein S. Vault prolapse. *Clin Pract Sexuality* 1991;7:17.

Wiskind AK, Thompson JD. Should cystoscopy be performed at every gynecological operation to diagnose unsuspected ureteral injury? *J Pelv Surg* 1995;1:134.

D

Vaginal Hysterectomy with Repair of Enterocele, Cystocele, and Rectocele

COMBINED COMPARTMENT DEFECTS

RAYMOND A. LEE

As noted in the previous sections, the supporting ligaments and fascia of the pelvis are closely related, one to another, so that prolapse of the uterus is often accompanied by relaxation of the anterior and posterior vaginal wall

Satisfactory, long-lasting surgical correction of uterine prolapse must, therefore, include correction of any and all pelvic support defects and the restoration of a normal, functional anatomy. To accomplish this, the attenuated uterosacral and cardinal ligaments must be shortened in a symmetrical fashion, the peritoneum of the posterior cul-de-sac must be appropriately excised, and the pararectal fascia must be approximated (obliteration of the cul-de-sac of Douglas). The levator hiatus also must be reduced and the levator plate repositioned to a normal inclination, the upper vagina restored over the levator plate, and the endopelvic (and levator) fascial attachments of the vagina reconstructed.

OPERATIVE TECHNIQUE

A well-planned and accomplished vaginal hysterectomy is a fundamental step to provide access to the supporting structures necessary for reconstruction of the pelvis. The degree of pelvic relaxation varies, but Figure 35D.1 illustrates a representative case of true uterine procidentia. A preliminary dilatation and curettage is done, and a frozen-section study of the endometrium is performed. With an assistant on either side, the surgeon grasps the tenacula, applying traction with the left hand, and delivers the cervix down and, in this case, completely out of

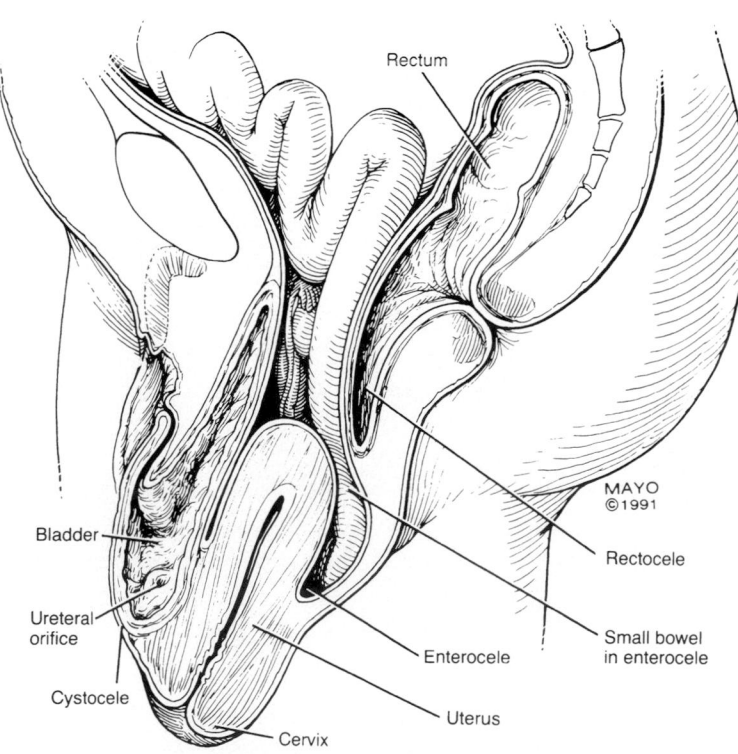

FIGURE 35D.1. Complete uterine procidentia with cystocele, enterocele, and rectocele. (From Lee RA. *Atlas of gynecologic surgery.* Philadelphia: WB Saunders, 1992. Reprinted with permission from the Mayo Foundation.)

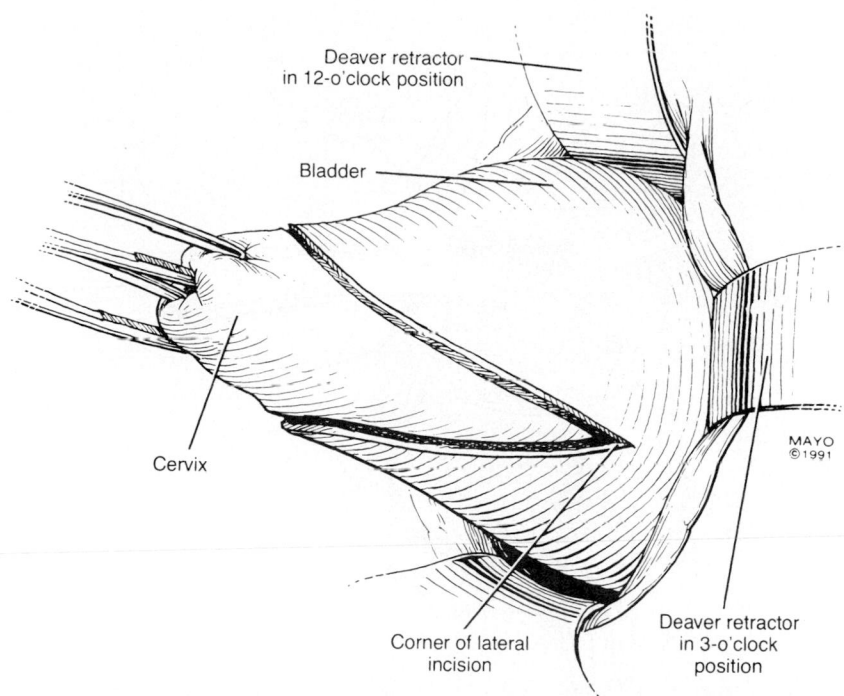

FIGURE 35D.2. With traction applied to the cervix, the lateral extent of the incision through the vaginal mucosa is assessed. (From Lee RA. *Atlas of gynecologic surgery*. Philadelphia: WB Saunders, 1992. Reprinted with permission from the Mayo Foundation.)

the vagina. This incision is continued (Fig. 35D.2) through the pubocervical fascia from the 9-o'clock (anterior) position to the 12-o'clock position, to the 3-o'-clock position. A similar incision is made posteriorly, where one can see the cervicopubic fascia pull away from the posterior aspects of the cervix. The anteriorly placed Deaver retractor is then inserted under the cut edge of

the anterior vaginal wall and bladder and is lifted superiorly; this maneuver opens the incision to permit direct visualization of the fold of the peritoneum, which can be incised accurately and safely. The vesicouterine fold of the peritoneum marks the anterior cul-de-sac and is identified as a concave line against the uterine wall (Fig. 35D.3A). The two layers of the peritoneum frequently

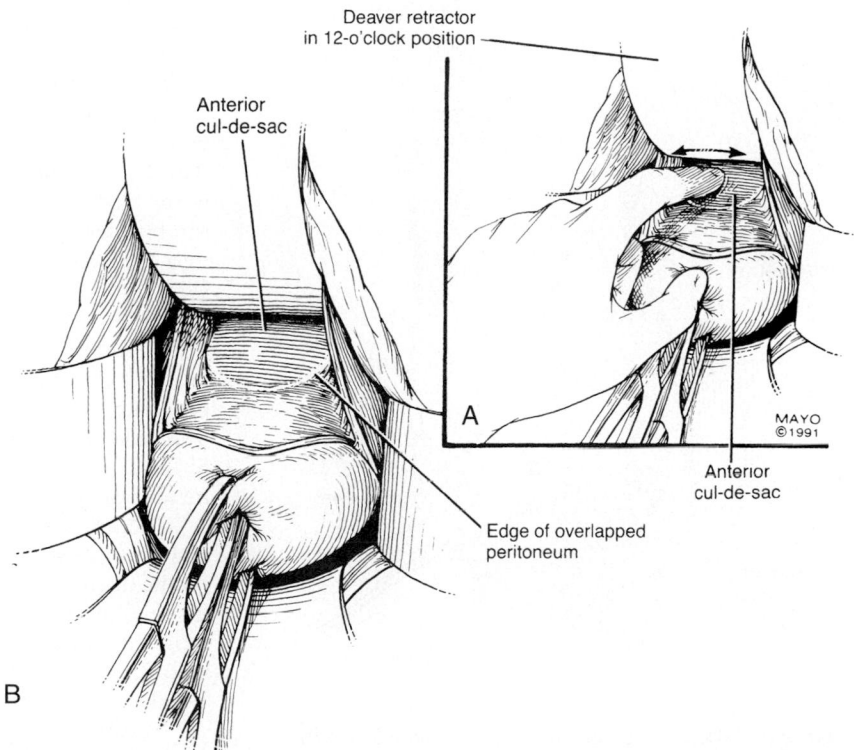

FIGURE 35D.3. A: The index finger of the surgeon's left hand feels the typically silky, smooth fold of the peritoneum of the anterior cul-de-sac. **B:** Concave line identifying the anterior cul-de-sac. (From Lee RA. *Atlas of gynecologic surgery*. Philadelphia: WB Saunders, 1992. Reprinted with permission from the Mayo Foundation.)

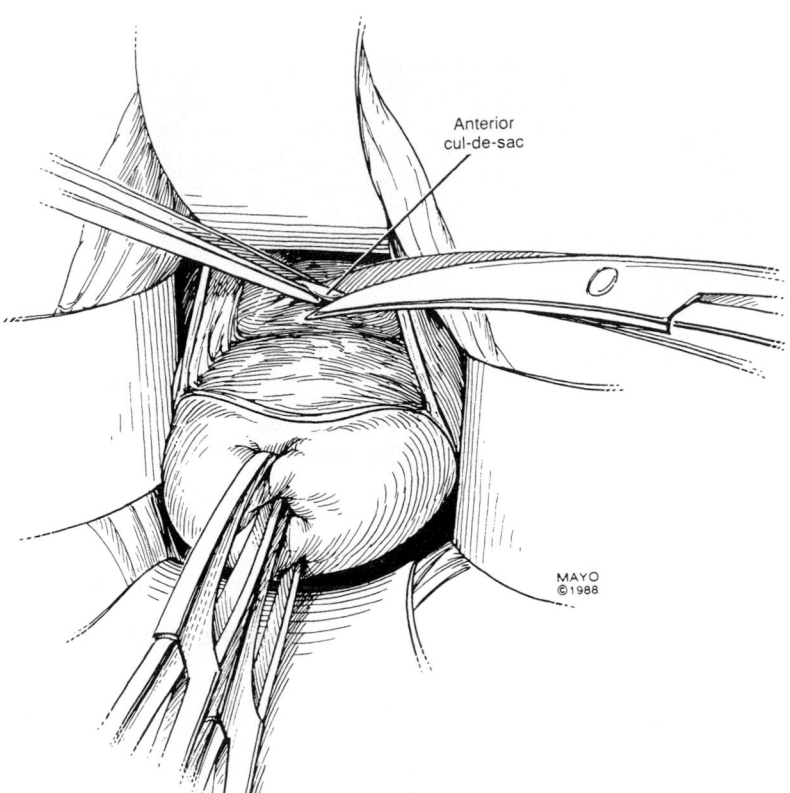

FIGURE 35D.4. Incision of the peritoneum of the anterior cul-de-sac. (From Lee RA. *Atlas of gynecologic surgery*. Philadelphia: WB Saunders, 1992. Reprinted with permission from the Mayo Foundation.)

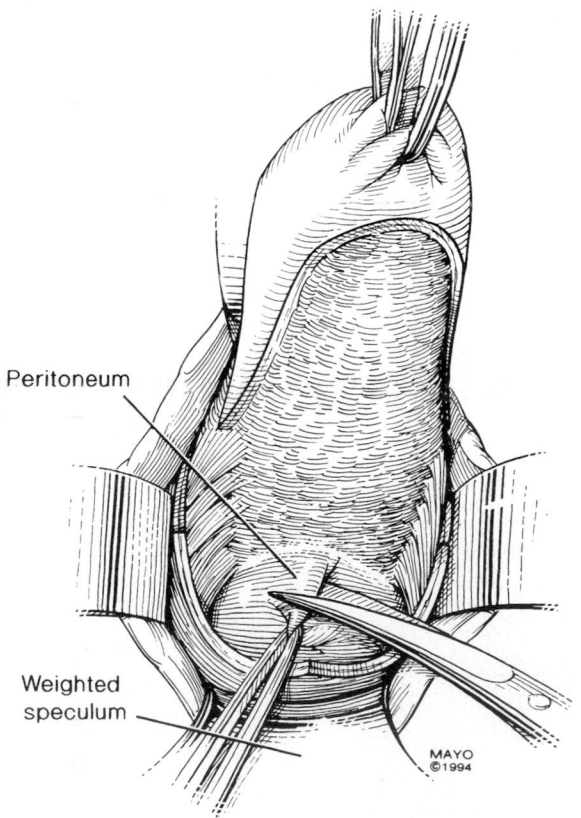

FIGURE 35D.5. Posterior cul-de-sac is incised. (From Lee RA. *Atlas of gynecologic surgery*. Philadelphia: WB Saunders, 1992. Reprinted with permission from the Mayo Foundation.)

move over each other (Fig. 35D.3B) to aid in further identification of the vesicouterine fold. The peritoneum is picked up with toothed forceps, and a Mayo scissors, with the points directed toward the uterus, is used to incise between the forceps and the uterine wall (Fig. 35D.4). The tips of the scissors are inserted into the peritoneal cavity and spread (a Russian forceps can be inserted through this opening and the fundus pushed down to detect the epiploic tags or bowel and to ensure that the peritoneal cavity has been entered). If urine was in the bladder, a gush of fluid would obviously be seen if the bladder was entered. A Deaver retractor is inserted into the anterior cul-de-sac in the 12-o'clock position. With upward traction of the Deaver retractor, there is an elevation of the base of the bladder and both ureters. With a similar technique, the posterior vaginal wall is detached from the cervix and posterior uterine wall. Appropriate traction with the forceps permits sharp dissection and incision of the posterior cul-de-sac (Fig. 35D.5). The posterior cul-de-sac is examined for any adhesions or bowel.

The left lateral vaginal wall is mobilized with sharp and blunt dissection, superior to the cervix (depending on the degree of the descent, 6 to 9 cm from the incision on the anterior vaginal wall). It therefore includes the most substantial supportive tissue of the uterosacral ligament (Fig. 35D.6). The ligament is cut and ligated with 1-0 delayed-absorbable suture.

Because of the extreme degree of prolapse, it is imperative to identify the ureter, which frequently is outside the vagina just cephalad to the uterosacral ligament

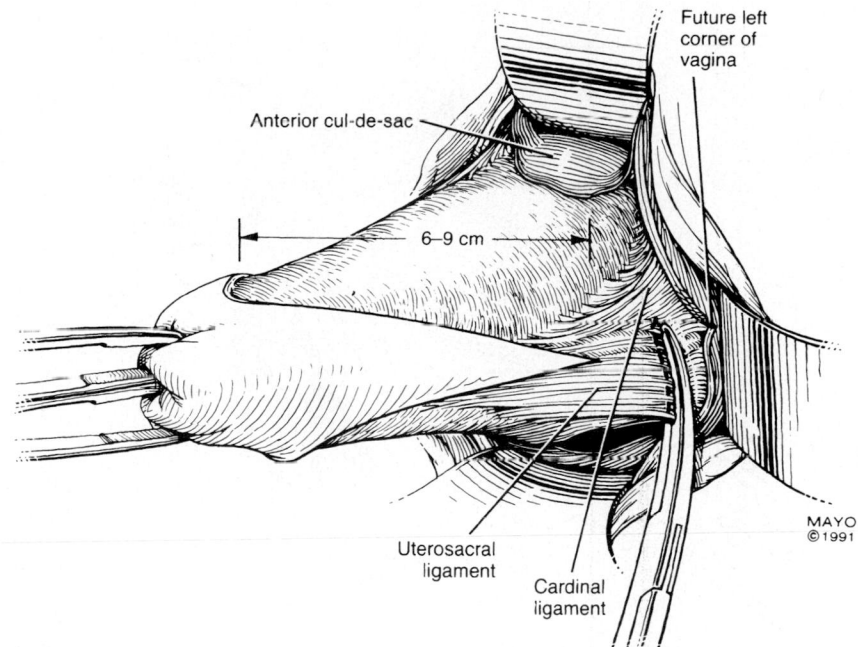

FIGURE 35D.6. A Heaney forceps is used to grasp the uterosacral ligament far superior (6 to 9 cm) to the incision on the anterior vaginal wall, thus capturing the most substantial supportive tissue available in this ligament. (From Lee RA. *Atlas of gynecologic surgery.* Philadelphia: WB Saunders, 1992. Reprinted with permission from the Mayo Foundation.)

tie. To identify the ureter, the surgeon inserts the left index finger into the anterior cul-de-sac and then palpates the exact location of the ureter between the index finger and the Deaver retractor in the 3-o'clock position (Fig. 35D.7A). The cardinal ligament is cut distal to the clamp

with an adequate cuff and is ligated with 1-0 delayed-absorbable suture (Fig. 35D.7B). The remainder of the cardinal ligament and its enclosed uterine vessel are clamped and tied in a similar fashion, including the anterior and posterior peritoneum (Fig. 35D.8). The right

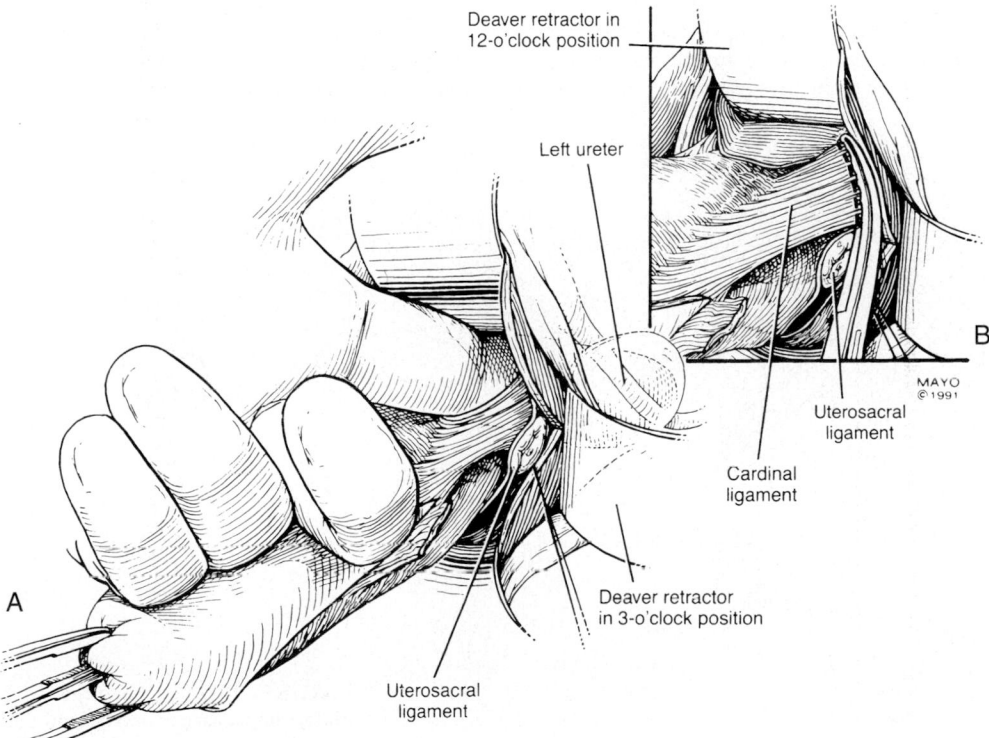

FIGURE 35D.7. A: The surgeon's left index finger is inserted through the anterior cul-de-sac, palpating the left ureter between the finger and the Deaver retractor in the 3-o'clock position. **B:** Portion of the cardinal ligament to be clamped after palpation of the ureter. (From Lee RA. *Atlas of gynecologic surgery.* Philadelphia: WB Saunders, 1992. Reprinted with permission from the Mayo Foundation.)

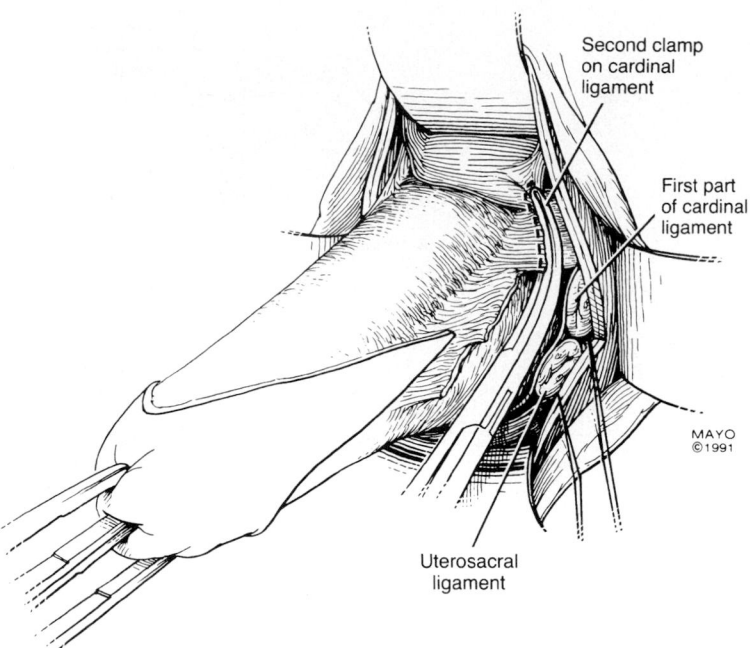

FIGURE 35D.8. The second portion of the cardinal ligament (including the uterine artery and vein) and the anterior and posterior peritoneum are included in the Heaney clamp. (From Lee RA. *Atlas of gynecologic surgery.* Philadelphia: WB Saunders, 1992. Reprinted with permission from the Mayo Foundation.)

uterosacral and cardinal ligaments are dealt with in the same way as those on the patient's left side. When tying a ligament stump, the surgeon must be careful to tie the knots far enough back on the stump to include all of the vessels and not allow any of them to slip out of the grasp of the knot. Each pedicle should be immediately adjacent to the next pedicle, such that there will not be a space between them sufficient to allow postoperative bleeding.

The surgeon then delivers the fundus through the posterior cul-de-sac by applying traction anteriorly on the tenacula. With a Heaney clamp across the right uteroovarian and round ligaments, the surgeon sharply divides the ligaments medial to the clamp (Fig. 35D.9). The left uteroovarian and round ligaments are divided in a similar fashion (Fig. 35D.10). The uterus is sent for immediate frozen-section histologic study. The uteroovarian and round ligaments then are ligated, and the operative area is inspected to ensure that hemostasis is complete. Occasionally, there will be sufficient space between either of the ligament stumps (uterosacral, car-

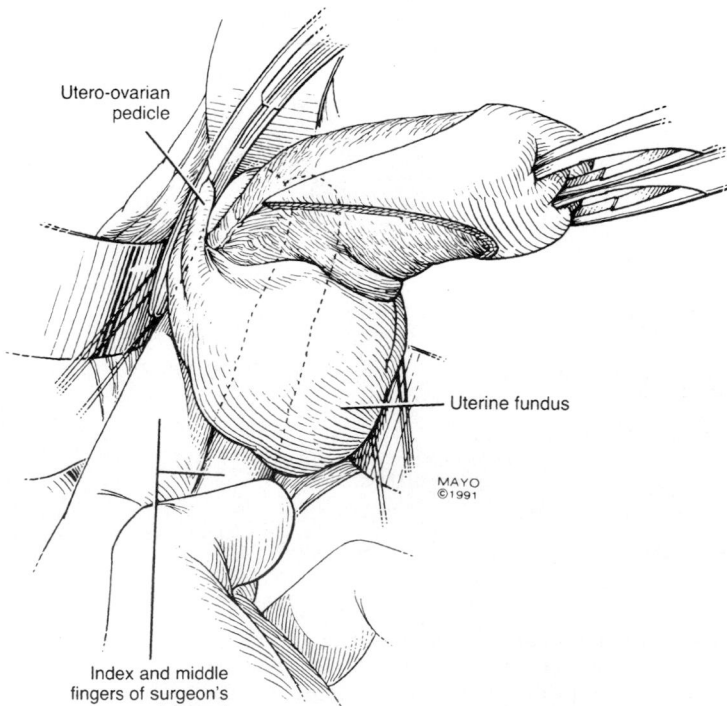

FIGURE 35D.9. The surgeon's left index and middle fingers are placed behind the uterus to protect any prolapsing bowel, after which the Heaney clamp is placed across the uteroovarian pedicle. (From Lee RA. *Atlas of gynecologic surgery.* Philadelphia: WB Saunders, 1992. Reprinted with permission from the Mayo Foundation.)

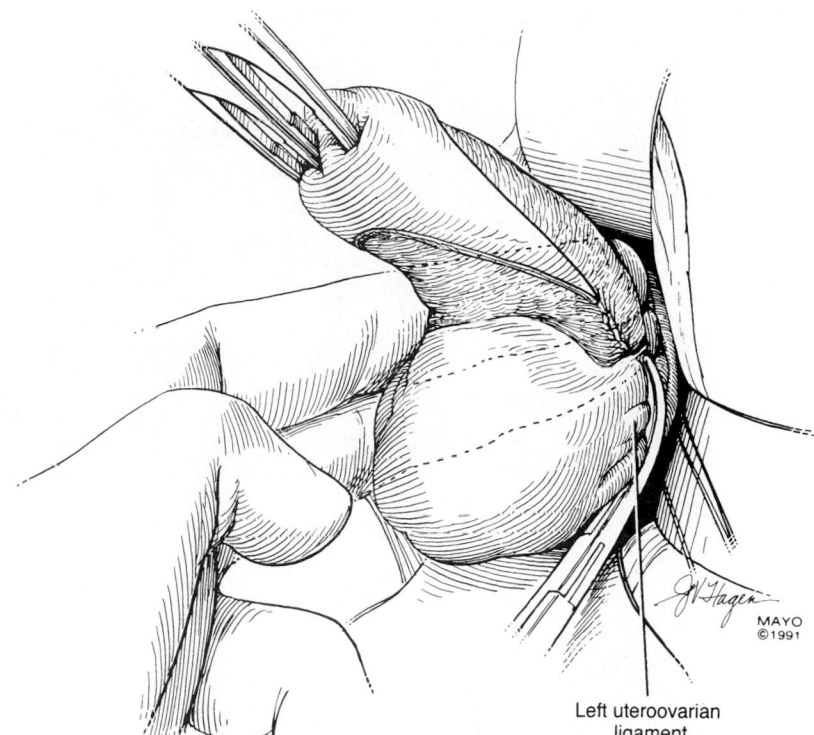

Left uteroovarian
ligament

FIGURE 35D.10. On the patient's left side, the fingers of the surgeon's left hand are placed behind the uterus to protect it, and the clamp is placed across the uteroovarian pedicle. (From Lee RA. *Atlas of gynecologic surgery.* Philadelphia: WB Saunders, 1992. Reprinted with permission from the Mayo Foundation.)

dinal, or uteroovarian) that a suture ligature should be placed to obtain perfect hemostasis. A salpingo-oophorectomy, if indicated, can be performed at this time. With Deaver retractors in the 9-o'clock and 12-o'-clock positions, Russian forceps are used to deliver the right tube and ovary. A Heaney clamp is placed proximal to the tube and ovary (Fig. 35D.11), incorporating the infundibulopelvic ligament. The clamp is placed to ensure that the entire tube and ovary have been excised but that the ureter, which is just cephalad to the clamp, is not in the clamp or included in the tie. After resection, the stump is ligated with a 1-0 delayed-absorbable suture

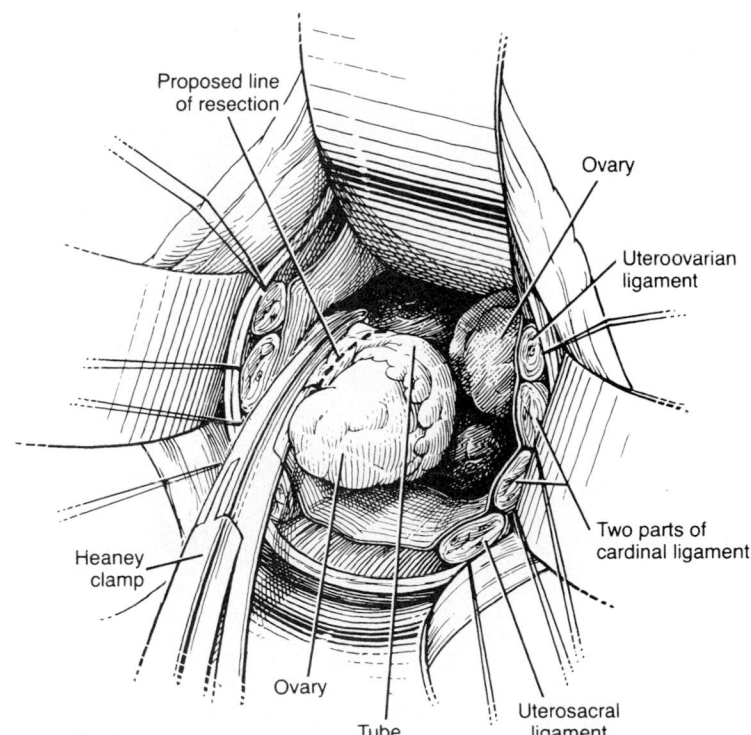

Proposed line
of resection

Ovary

Uteroovarian
ligament

Two parts of
cardinal ligament

Heaney
clamp

Ovary

Tube

Uterosacral
ligament

FIGURE 35D.11. The Heaney clamp is placed in a position proximal to the tube and ovary on the right side, incorporating the infundibulopelvic ligament. (From Lee RA. *Atlas of gynecologic surgery.* Philadelphia: WB Saunders, 1992. Reprinted with permission from the Mayo Foundation.)

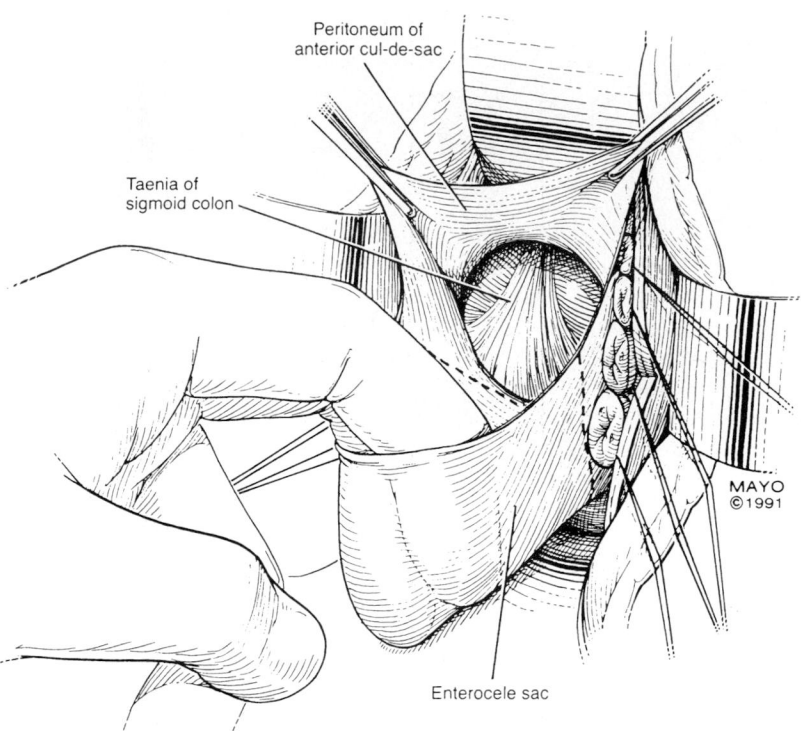

Peritoneum of anterior cul-de-sac

Taenia of sigmoid colon

Enterocele sac

MAYO ©1991

FIGURE 35D.12. Mobilized peritoneum of the posterior cul-de-sac with the line of proposed resection. (From Lee RA. *Atlas of gynecologic surgery*. Philadelphia: WB Saunders, 1992. Reprinted with permission from the Mayo Foundation.)

and permitted to retract into the abdomen. The left tube and ovary are removed in a similar manner.

The degree of enterocele varies, but there is always some enterocele present in cases of true procidentia. To aid in correction of the enterocele, a small abdominal pack is placed through the incision, and the table is placed in the slight Trendelenburg position to prevent the intestines from prolapsing into the operative field.

The peritoneum of the posterior cul-de-sac is sharply mobilized off the anterior surface of the rectum and lower sigmoid (Fig. 35D.12) and excised (Fig. 35D.13). At this point, the redundancy of the posterior vaginal wall is assessed, and an appropriately sized wedge of the posterior vagina is reflected inferiorly and placed under the tongue of the weighted speculum. Depending on the size of the enterocele, between one and three internal

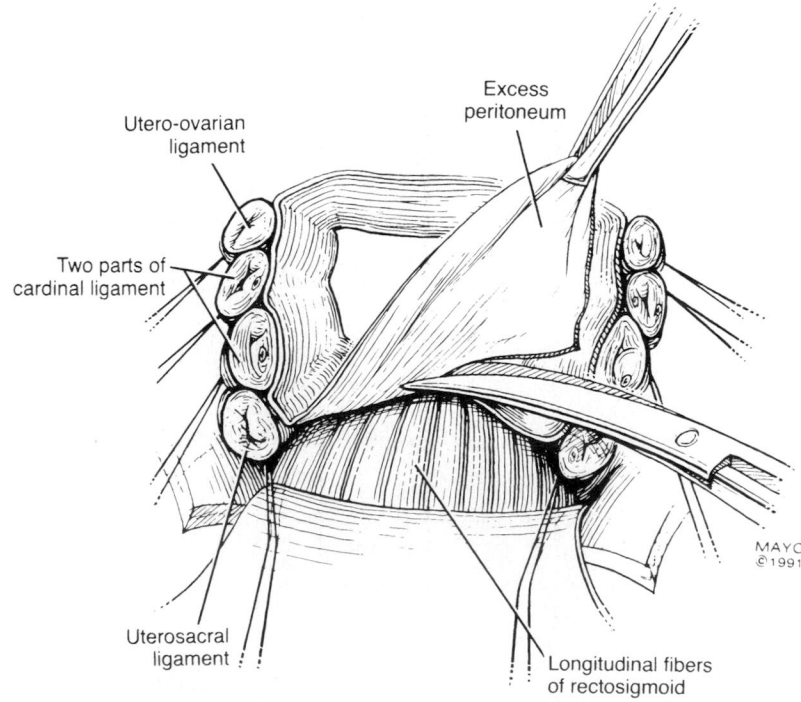

Utero-ovarian ligament

Two parts of cardinal ligament

Excess peritoneum

Uterosacral ligament

Longitudinal fibers of rectosigmoid

MAYO ©1991

FIGURE 35D.13. Mobilized and redundant peritoneum of the anterior sigmoid is excised flush with the rectal muscularis. (From Lee RA. *Atlas of gynecologic surgery*. Philadelphia: WB Saunders, 1992. Reprinted with permission from the Mayo Foundation.)

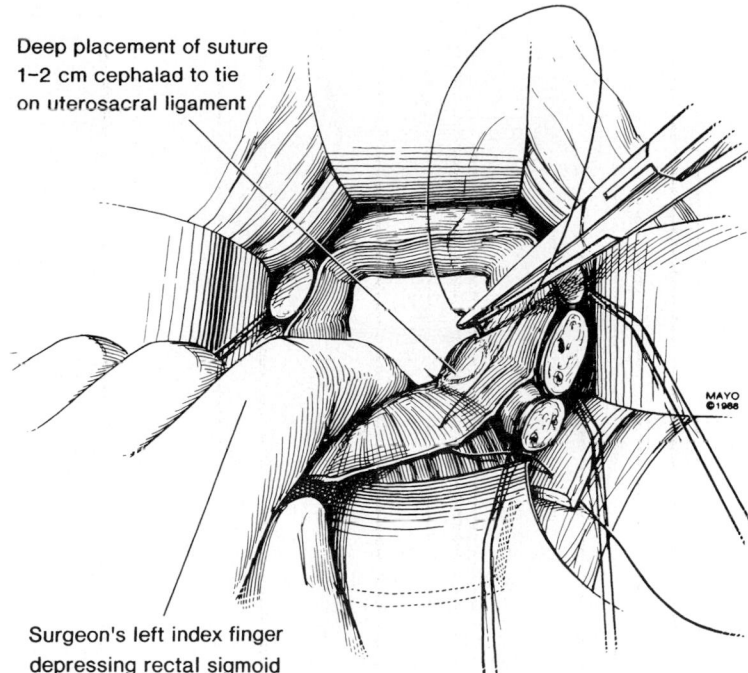

Deep placement of suture
1–2 cm cephalad to tie
on uterosacral ligament

Surgeon's left index finger
depressing rectal sigmoid

FIGURE 35D.14. The sigmoid is pressed down and to the patient's right side to place a suture deeply into the pararectal fascia. (Modified from Lee RA. *Atlas of gynecologic surgery*. Philadelphia: WB Saunders, 1992. Reprinted with permission from the Mayo Foundation.)

McCall sutures are placed. To place the internal McCall suture, the surgeon uses the left index and middle fingers to depress the sigmoid colon down and to the patient's right side (Fig. 35D.14). The monofilament zero suture is placed deeply into the left pararectal fascia, after which the suture is continued across the front of the sigmoid colon, where the surgeon presses the sigmoid down and to the patient's left side for a similar deep placement of the suture on the right pararectal fascia (Fig. 35D.15). This suture is tagged, after which additional internal McCall sutures may be placed (these sutures are tied after completion of the anterior colporrhaphy).

One to two external McCall sutures then are made with the following technique: the 1-0 delayed-absorbable suture is passed through the posterior vaginal wall and peritoneum to the same pararectal fascia used to make an internal McCall suture. The external suture, however, is made in a more cephalad position than is the internal one (Fig. 35D.16). The suture continues across the front of the sigmoid to the right pararectal fascia and is brought out through the vagina, where it is tagged to be tied at a later time.

The reperitonealizing suture (most cephalad to all sutures) is made in the following manner. A broad Allis forceps is used to grasp the anterior peritoneum, and the bladder is gently separated from the peritoneum to give adequate clearance for the later reperitonealizing suture. The peritonealizing suture passes through the peritoneum cephalad to the previously placed internal and external McCall sutures, picking up the peritoneum over the uterosacral and cardinal ligaments. The pursestring suture is tied, and the surgeon continues to reperitonealize the pelvis, moving the ligamentous stumps to the exterior. Thus, the reperitonealizing section is cepha-

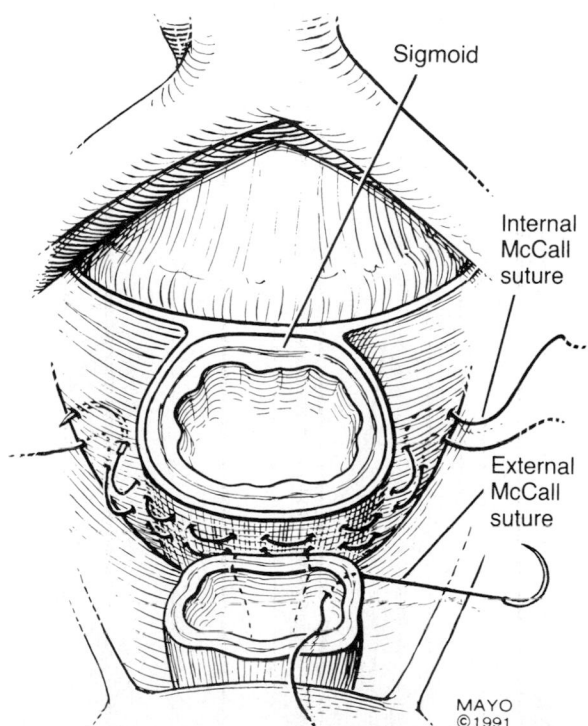

Sigmoid

Internal
McCall
suture

External
McCall
suture

FIGURE 35D.15. Previously made, internal McCall sutures are in place. An external McCall suture has been inserted through the vaginal mucosa to prepare the mucosa to be sutured into the pararectal fascia just superior to the internal McCall sutures. (From Lee RA. *Atlas of gynecologic surgery*. Philadelphia: WB Saunders, 1992. Reprinted with permission from the Mayo Foundation.)

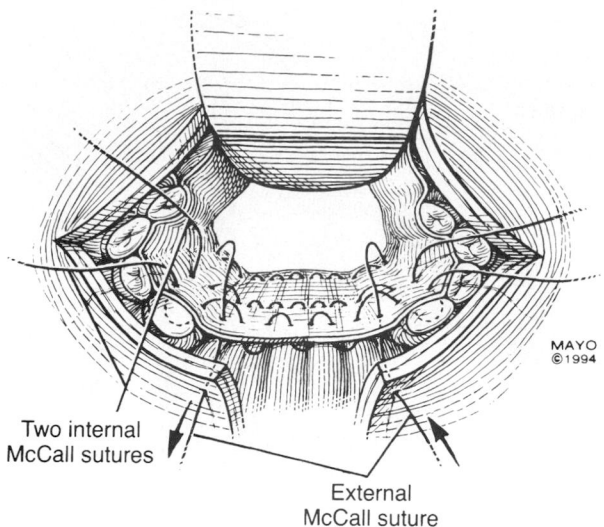

FIGURE 35D.16. Relative position of two previously placed, internal McCall sutures with an external McCall suture now placed in a more cephalad position. (Modified from Lee RA. *Atlas of gynecologic surgery.* Philadelphia, WB Saunders, 1992. Reprinted with permission from the Mayo Foundation)

lad to the external McCall sutures, which are cephalad to the internal McCall sutures (Fig. 35D.17).

After the surgeon is satisfied that the hemostasis has been completed, the vaginal vault closure may begin. In the posterior rectovaginal septum, the proximal (cephalad) edge of the endopelvic fascia is identified, and anteriorly the cervicopubic fascia is identified. At the left vaginal corner, a simple suture is placed starting through the posterior vaginal wall, including the endopelvic fas-

cia, and passing through and proximal to the tie of the uterosacral ligament but distal to the tie on the two portions of the cardinal ligament and the uteroovarian pedicle. It is continued through the anterior vaginal wall and endopelvic fascia (Fig. 35D.18A). This suture is tied and cut along with the previously tagged ligament stump ties on the left side. A second stitch is placed medial to the original suture, thus incorporating the very distal ends of the ligament stumps and the vaginal wall (Fig. 35D.18B).

ANTERIOR COLPORRHAPHY

To begin an anterior colporrhaphy, the surgeon places two straight clamps on the corners of the anterior vaginal wall and a third clamp just beneath the external urethral meatus. The surgeon then separates the anterior vaginal wall from the underlying cervicopubic fascia (Fig. 35D.19). With Allis forceps on the cut edge of the vagina, sharp dissection is used to free the vaginal wall from its underlying fascia, covering the base of the bladder (Fig. 35D.20A). The dissection is continued in a direction laterally and superiorly adjacent to the left descending pubic ramus (Fig. 35D.20B). A similar dissection is carried out on the patient's right side (Fig. 35D.21).

Although we have plicated the anterior cervicopubic fascia under the bladder and urethra in the traditional Kelly technique for many years with good success, newer anatomic concepts of pelvic support suggest that the cervicopubic fascia becomes detached, torn, or both, and reattachment or repair may serve to better correct anterior vaginal wall prolapse. These techniques are illustrated earlier in this chapter (Section B.)

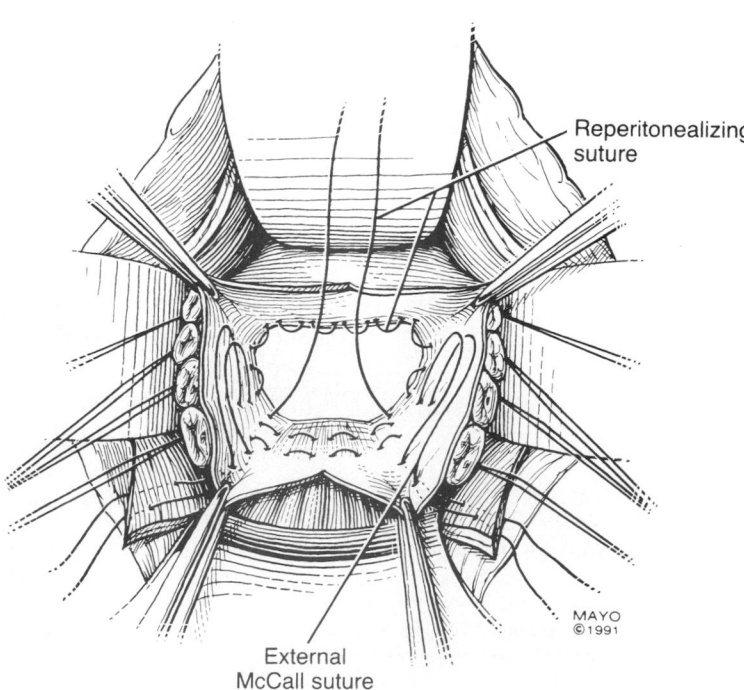

FIGURE 35D.17. Reperitonealizing suture placed cephalad to the previously placed internal and external McCall sutures. (From Lee RA. *Atlas of gynecologic surgery.* Philadelphia: WB Saunders, 1992. Reprinted with permission from the Mayo Foundation.)

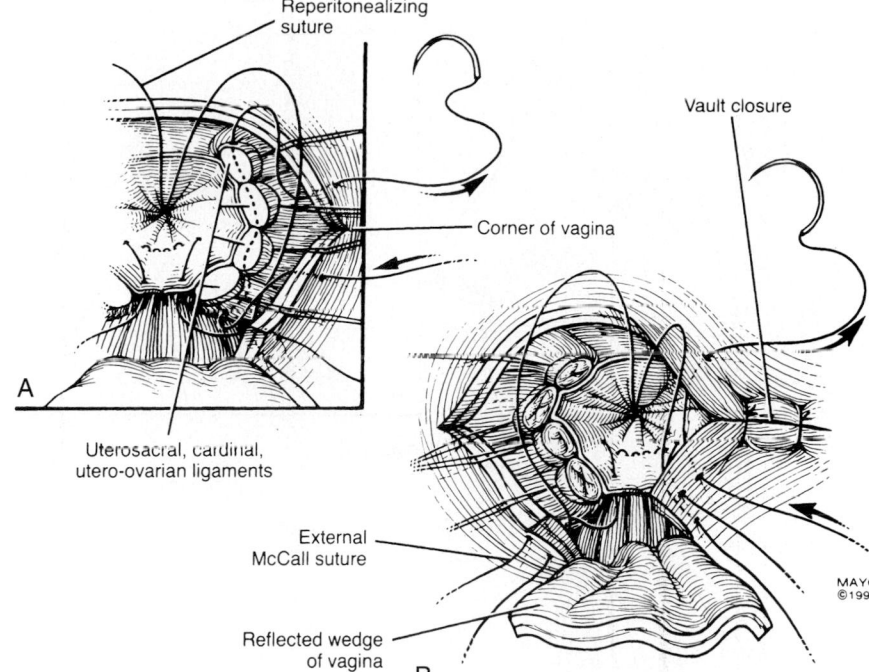

FIGURE 35D.18. A: Beginning on the patient's left vaginal fornix, the suture is passed through the vagina and then through the uterosacral ligament and two portions of the cardinal and uteroovarian pedicles. The suture is brought out at a position cephalad to its origin, where it is tied. **B:** As sutures are tied lateral to medial, care is taken that careful hemostasis is attained. (From Lee RA. *Atlas of gynecologic surgery*. Philadelphia: WB Saunders, 1992. Reprinted with permission from the Mayo Foundation.)

If a traditional colporrhaphy is used, adequate mobilization is important to ensure the surgeon has the freedom to plicate the bladder neck and urethra adequately, thereby providing a proper angular relation between the urethra and the base of the bladder, which ensures urinary control. We prefer to use interrupted 2-0 delayed-absorbable sutures, starting in a position immediately adjacent to the external urethral meatus. The first suture is made deeply in a position parallel and adjacent to the external urethral meatus on each side, sufficiently cephalad to incorporate the inferior aspects of the base of the posterior pubourethral ligament (Fig. 35D.22A). The sutures are tied, and each suture is appropriately placed (each succeeding suture is placed more laterally than the previously placed suture) in the lateral position so that sufficient support is created beneath the urethra, bladder neck, and base of the bladder. Additional sutures may be placed in the area of the proximal urethra and bladder neck to provide further plication and support of the tissues beneath the bladder (Fig. 35D.22B).

The redundant anterior vaginal wall is assessed and appropriately resected to ensure that the resultant suture line can be closed without tension. The vaginal walls are approximated with 3-0 delayed-absorbable suture in an interrupted fashion. As each edge of the vaginal wall is approximated, a small amount of the underlying cervicopubic fascia is incorporated to pull the vaginal wall to the level of the cervicopubic fascia and avoid potential empty space. At this point, we prefer to tie the internal and external McCall sutures. If these sutures are tied earlier in the procedure, it so elevates the apex and posterior vaginal wall that completion of the anterior repair is complicated.

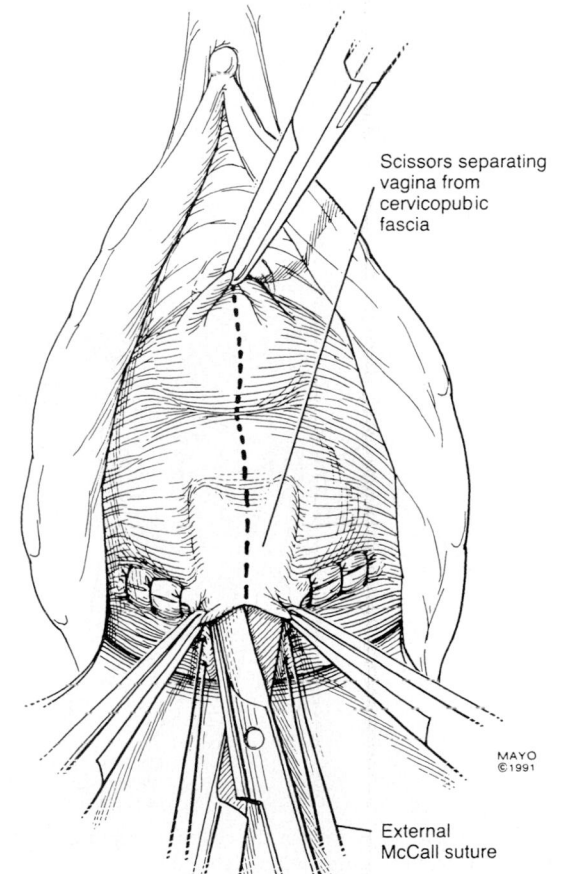

FIGURE 35D.19. After the vaginal mucosa is separated from the underlying cervicopubic fascia, the vaginal wall is incised vertically. (From Lee RA. *Atlas of gynecologic surgery*. Philadelphia: WB Saunders, 1992. Reprinted with permission from the Mayo Foundation.)

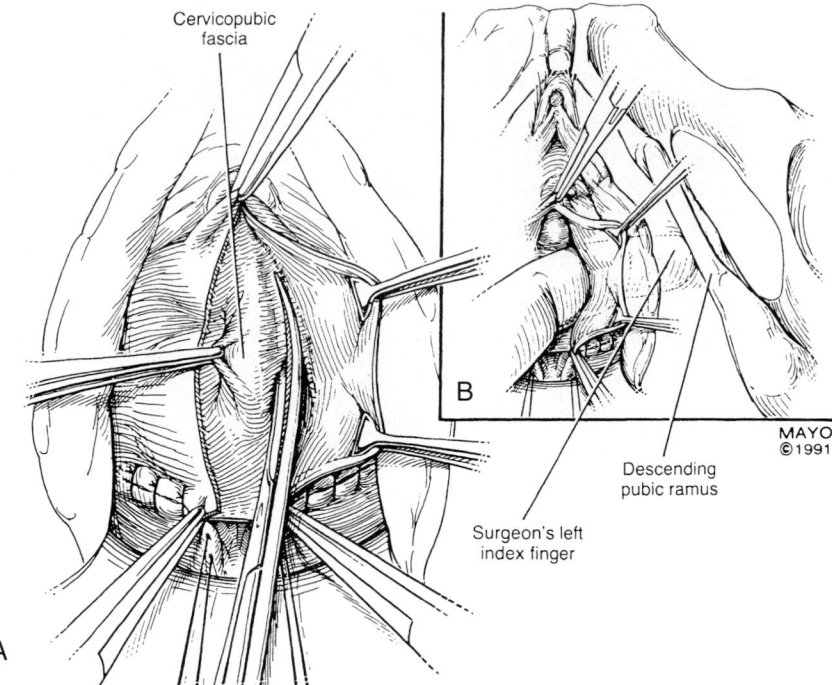

FIGURE 35D.20. A: As the assistant applies spreading traction on the clamps of the anterior vaginal wall, the surgeon, with two forceps in the left hand, applies countertraction on the bladder and, using Mayo scissors, sharply dissects the bladder with its cervicopubic fascia from the inferior surface of the vagina. **B:** The dissection is continued in a direction laterally and superiorly back to the left descending pubic ramus. (From Lee RA. *Atlas of gynecologic surgery*. Philadelphia: WB Saunders, 1992. Reprinted with permission from the Mayo Foundation.)

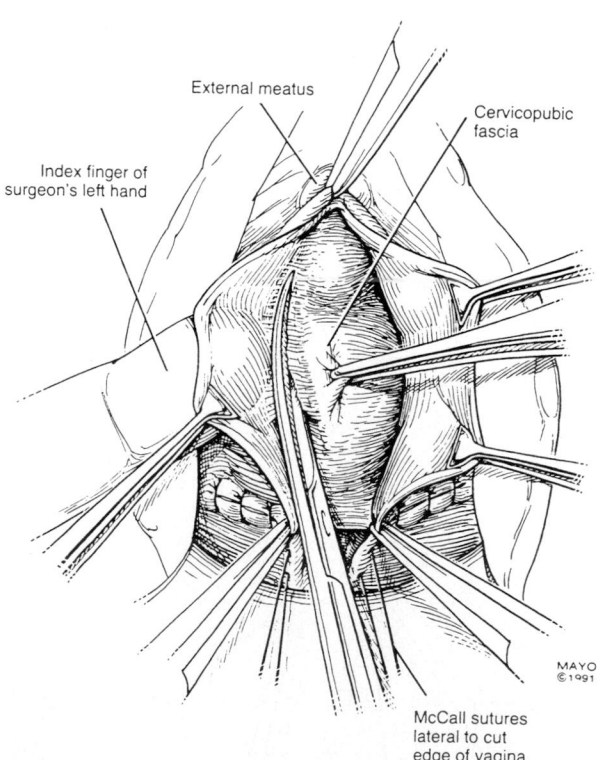

FIGURE 35D.21. A similar dissection is repeated on the right side, where the surgeon holds the Allis forceps in the left hand and may place the fingers on the outside of the vaginal wall; the assistant applies traction on the bladder to facilitate sharp, accurate, and wide dissection. (From Lee RA. *Atlas of gynecologic surgery*. Philadelphia: WB Saunders, 1992. Reprinted with permission from the Mayo Foundation.)

POSTERIOR COLPOPERINEORRHAPHY

As noted earlier, current concepts of vaginal support favor identification of the endopelvic fascia in the posterior rectovaginal septum and reattachment of the edges of this fascial sheet to the uterosacral ligaments superiorly and the pelvic sidewalls laterally. This posterior vaginal reconstruction is described in the previous segment of this chapter.

The traditional posterior colpoperineorrhaphy with plication of the fascia is not widely used currently, but is presented here for completeness. The repair is started by placing two Allis clamps on the right and left perineum, approximately where the marks remain from the weighted speculum that was just removed. A V-shaped incision is made between the tenacula (and tailored to the size of the patient's perineal body) (Fig. 35D.23A) and continued with scissors to dissect the appropriate wedge of redundant posterior vaginal wall and its underlying fascia, which is flush with the anterior wall of the rectum (Fig. 35D.23B). The width of the wedge of the vagina to be removed is determined by the degree of relaxation of the posterior vaginal wall and the need to preserve a functional vagina. The incision is continued superiorly until it meets the reflected upper triangular wedge of posterior vaginal wall that initially was placed under the weighted speculum. With 3-0 delayed absorbable suture, the surgeon closes the edges of the vaginal wall and the underlying rectovaginal fascia in a single layer (Fig. 35D.24). As each suture is tied in the midline, the diameter of the vagina is evaluated to ensure that there will be adequate room for vaginal function. At the appropriate level, the medial borders of the underlying

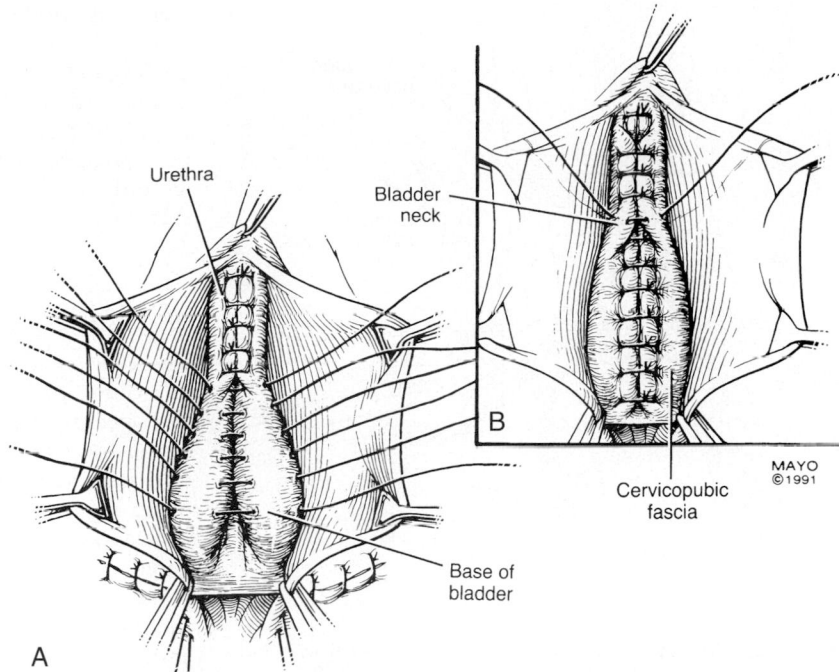

FIGURE 35D.22. A: Each suture is placed somewhat more laterally than the previously placed suture. **B:** Additional sutures may be placed in the area of the proximal urethra and bladder neck to provide further plication support of the tissues. (From Lee RA. *Atlas of gynecologic surgery*. Philadelphia: WB Saunders, 1992. Reprinted with permission from the Mayo Foundation.)

levator fascia are approximated in a single layer, after which the overlying vaginal mucosa is closed with interrupted sutures. Again, the diameter of the vagina is evaluated to ensure that appropriate support has been created without adversely compromising the vaginal diameter. The perineorrhaphy is completed by approximating the perineal muscles and the subcuticular closure of the skin.

The suture lines are inspected carefully to ensure that complete hemostasis has been obtained. The transverse suture line at the apex of the vagina is superior and is pulled posteriorly toward the hollow of the sacrum. The anterior suture line reveals the urethra and bladder neck to be tucked up under the symphysis pubic with a gentle curve representing the base of the bladder (Fig. 35D.25). The apex of the posterior suture line points di-

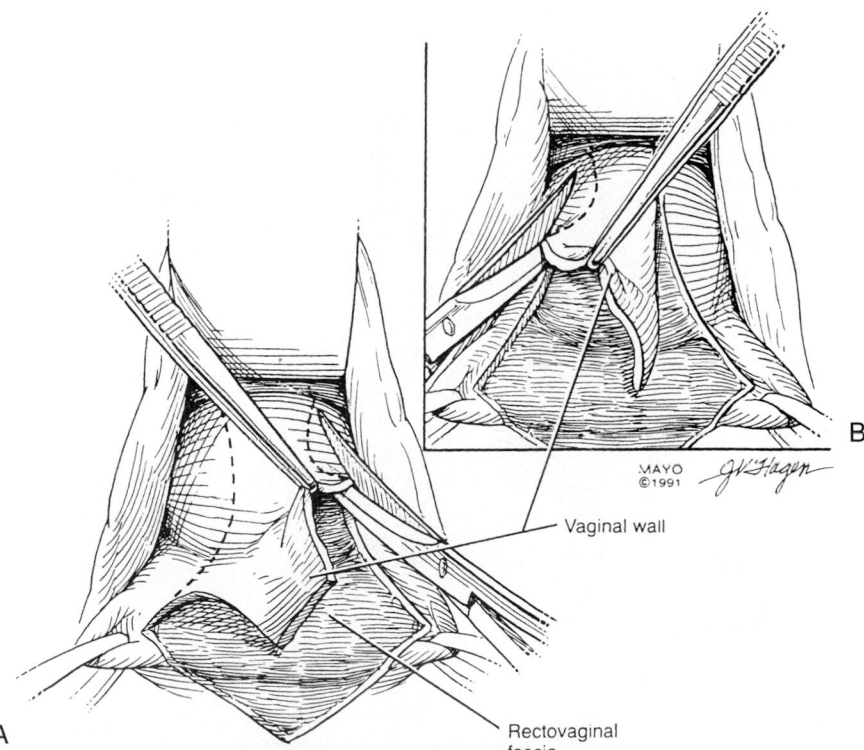

FIGURE 35D.23. Beginning at the introitus, the vaginal mucosa is incised flush with the underlying rectal muscularis. (From Lee RA. *Atlas of gynecologic surgery.* Philadelphia: WB Saunders, 1992. Reprinted with permission from the Mayo Foundation.)

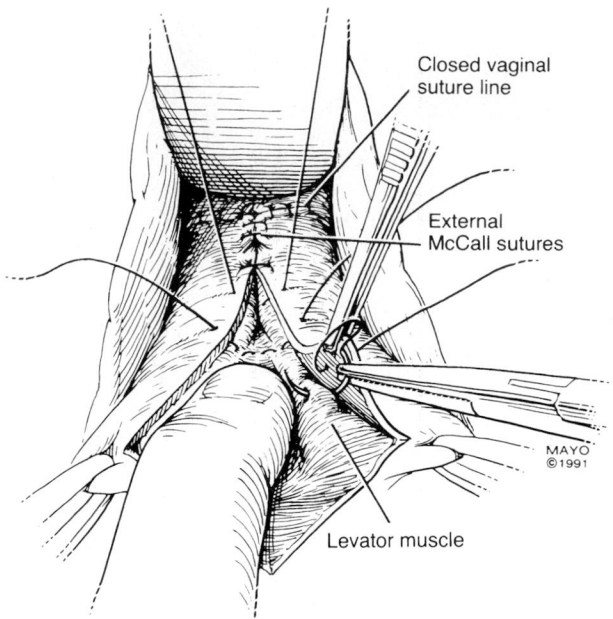

FIGURE 35D.24. High in the vagina, the vaginal wall and underlying rectovaginal fascia are approximated in a single layer. Care should be taken to avoid the development of a bar of approximated tissue that could be a source of dyspareunia. (From Lee RA. *Atlas of gynecologic surgery.* Philadelphia: WB Saunders, 1992. Reprinted with permission from the Mayo Foundation.)

rectly posteriorly toward the hollow of the sacrum, with a gradual elevation over the area of the lower portion of the levators. This positioning of the sutures ensures that the normal depth and diameter of the vagina are retained, so that when the patient is in the standing position the upper third of the vagina is approximately parallel to the floor. A small pack is placed in the vagina, and a 16-French catheter is placed in the bladder.

SUMMARY

There are several equally effective but different operative procedures to correct uterine procidentia; the technique and operative approach must be chosen according to the specific needs of the patient. The surgeon must be able to dissect, identify, resect, and approximate the appropriate supporting structures. To preserve a functional vagina in a patient with complete procidentia, the surgeon must have a full understanding of the principles of pelvic support. If a functional vagina is unimportant, then a tight, coned-down vagina (one finger in depth and diameter) offers the best long-term results.

ACKNOWLEDGMENT

This chapter is based on material from Lee RA. Atlas of gynecologic surgery. *Philadelphia, WB Saunders, 1992. Copyright 1994, the Mayo Foundation.*

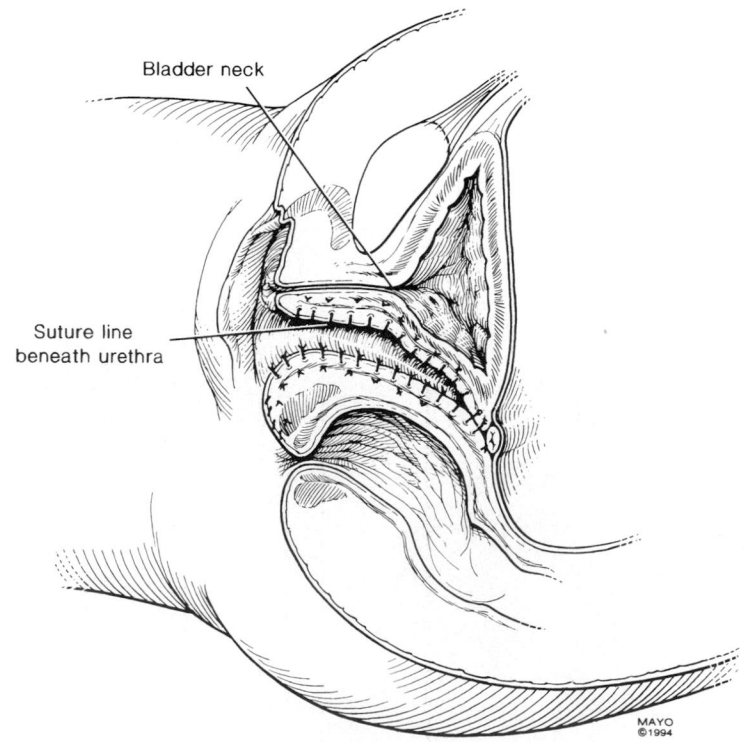

FIGURE 35D.25. Lateral view revealing the angular relation of the lower anterior vaginal wall and the apex of the vagina beneath the urethra and bladder neck as it meets the continued suture line beneath the base of the bladder. The upper portion of the posterior repair points back toward the hollow of the sacrum and continues with the gentle curve over the repair of the lower posterior vaginal wall. (From Lee RA. *Atlas of gynecologic surgery.* Philadelphia: WB Saunders, 1992. Reprinted with permission from the Mayo Foundation.)

BIBLIOGRAPHY

Brown JS, Waetijen LE, Subak LL, et al. Pelvic organ prolapse surgery in the United States, 1997. *Am J Obstet Gynecol* 2002;186:712–716.

Delancy JO. Fascial and muscular abnormalities in women with urethral hypermobility and anterior vaginal wall prolapse. *Am J Obstet Gynecol* 2002;187:93–98.

Hullfish KL, Bovbjerg VE, Gibson J, et al. Patient-centered goals for pelvic floor dysfunction surgery: what is success, and is it achieved? *Am J Obstet Gynecol* 2002;187:88–92.

Lee RA. *Atlas of gynecologic surgery.* Philadelphia, WB Saunders, 1992.

Lee RA. Vaginal hysterectomy with repair of enterocele, cystocele, and rectocele. *Clin Obstet Gynecol* 1993;36:967–975.

O'Boyle AL, Woodman PJ, O'Boyle JD, et al. Pelvic organ support in nulliparous pregnant and nonpregnant women: a case control study. *Am J Obstet Gyencol* 2002;187:99–102.

Thakar R, Stanton S. Management of genital prolapse. *BMJ* 2002;324:1258–1262.

Vineyard DD, Kuehl TJ, Coates KW, et al. A comparison of preoperative and intraoperative evaluations for patients who undergo site-specific operation for the correction of pelvic organ prolapse. *Am J Obstet Gynecol* 2002;186:1155–1159.

Webb MJ, Aronson MP, Ferguson KL, et al. Posthysterectomy vaginal vault prolapse: primary repair in 693 patients. *Obstet Gynecol* 1998;92:281–285.

E

Vaginal Vault Prolapse

MICKEY M. KARRAM   STEVEN D. KLEEMAN

As women live longer and healthier lives, pelvic floor disorders continue to become even more prevalent and an important health and social issue. It is estimated that by 2030, sixty-three million women will be 45 years of age or older and by 2050, thirty-three percent of the population will be postmenopausal. The lifetime risk of surgery for pelvic prolapse or incontinence has been estimated at 11% with a reoperation rate for failure at 29%. The management of pelvic organ prolapse can be difficult because different support defects often coexist. The pelvic surgeon must be adept in the thorough evaluation and management of these issues. An understanding of the anatomy and the relationship of the vagina to surrounding structures is imperative.

Our understanding of pelvic prolapse and the treatment thereof has changed in recent years. It was formerly taught that prolapse resulted from attenuation or stretching of endopelvic fascia. Richardson challenged this theory by introducing the concept of discrete breaks in endopelvic fascia. More recently, Richardson described apical enterocele as a separation of pubocervical fascia from rectovaginal fascia. This allows peritoneum of an enterocele sac to be in direct contact with vaginal epithelium. This is most common in the posthysterectomy patient. In women with a uterus and an enterocele, the defect results from a separation in the superior or transverse portion of the rectovaginal fascia. Thus, in patients undergoing hysterectomy, it is important to reattach the rectovaginal fascia to the pubocervical fascia and to provide good support to the vaginal

apex by reattaching the vaginal cuff to the uterosacral cardinal ligament complex.

DeLancey divided the support of the vagina into three levels. This concept is helpful in understanding normal anatomic relationships and helping to appreciate why certain repairs may work in some patients and not in others. Level I support defects are apical defects caused by loss of support of the uterosacral ligaments, paracolpium, and parametrium. Level II support defects result from disruption of the normal lateral attachment of the mid-vagina. Level III support defects result from defects in the perineal body or fusion of the distal urethra to the pubic bone (Fig. 35E.1).

The true incidence of vaginal vault prolapse is unknown. However, there is an overall perception that the number of procedures being performed for vaginal vault prolapse is increasing. The main goal of any procedure aimed at suspending the vaginal vault should be to suspend the vaginal vault as near as possible to its normal anatomic position. This should reapproximate the upper vagina in the midline over the levator plate. Distortion of the vaginal vault, whether in an anterior or posterior direction, can lead to a recurrent prolapse opposite the vaginal vault in a significant number of patients.

The ultimate goal of pelvic reconstructive surgery is "to restore anatomy, maintain or restore visceral function, and maintain or restore normal sexual function." It is extremely important to determine preoperatively whether lower urinary tract dysfunction, sexual dysfunction, and defecatory dysfunction exist. Urinary dysfunc-

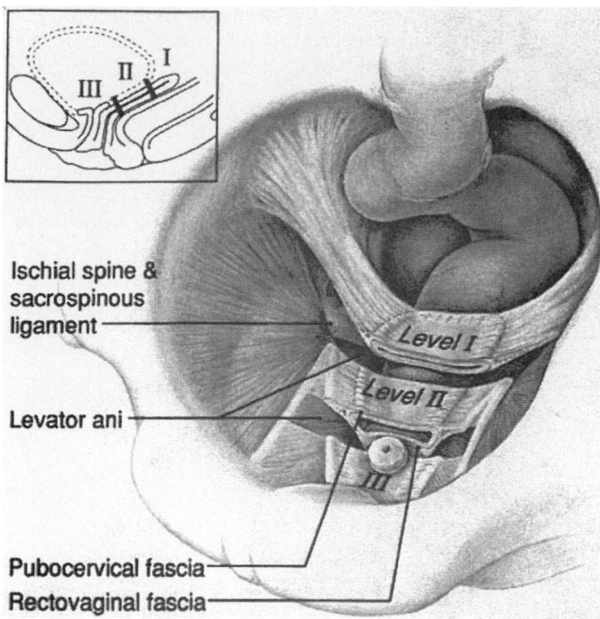

Ischial spine &
sacrospinous
ligament

Levator ani

Pubocervical fascia
Rectovaginal fascia

FIGURE 35E.1. Levels of support. DeLancey's biomechanical levels: level I —proximal suspension; level II—lateral attachment; level III—distal fusion. (From DeLancey JOL. Anatomic aspects of vaginal eversion after hysterectomy. *Am J Obstet Gynecol* 1992;166:1717–1728.)

tion may be masked in patients with advanced pelvic organ prolapse by obstructing or kinking the urethra. Thus, reductive maneuvers aimed at simulating what surgery will accomplish should be employed in the hope of identifying those patients who will require an antiincontinence procedure in conjunction with their pelvic reconstructive surgery. It is also important to initiate local estrogen therapy preoperatively in patients who have urogenital atrophy.

Many operations have been described for suspending the prolapsed vaginal vault. There is no general consensus on what is the best procedure. The procedure that the surgeon ultimately chooses is influenced by many factors, including the comfort and skill of the surgeon performing the operation, whether the prolapse is primary or recurrent, the patient's age, state of health, anticipated outcome, sexual activity, and overall state of the tissues. We believe it is important for the surgeon to have a variety of operative approaches available for the individual patient. We prefer to approach most cases transvaginally, reserving abdominal sacral colpopexy for patients who have failed a previous vaginal approach, have a foreshortened vagina, or in whom a compensatory procedure with the insertion of mesh is necessary to obtain a long-term durable repair. We believe the vaginal approach to pelvic prolapse has the advantage of decreased operative time, decreased incidence of adhesion formation, and quicker recovery time. Obliterative procedures including partial LeForte colpocleisis and colpectomy and colpocleisis can be used in elderly fragile patients who are no longer sexually active.

VAGINAL PROCEDURES TO SUSPEND THE VAGINAL APEX
McCall Culdoplasty

Several operations have been described and used by surgeons for vaginal vault suspension with correction of concurrent enterocele. McCall (in 1957) described his technique of surgical correction of enterocele at the time of vaginal hysterectomy. He used several nonabsorbable sutures to obliterate the enterocele (internal McCall sutures) by approximating both uterosacral ligaments and several bites of posterior peritoneum together. Delayed absorbable sutures were then inserted through the full thickness of the posterior vagina just lateral to the midline, passed through each uterosacral ligament and then back out the posterior vaginal wall. Additional external sutures are placed as required by the amount of prolapse. The internal sutures are then tied, and the external sutures are tied after the vaginal cuff is closed. This simple procedure obliterates the cul-de-sac, supports the vaginal apex, and lengthens the posterior vaginal wall (Fig. 35E.2). McCall originally reported on 45 cases and stated there was no evidence of enterocele recurrence.

Several modifications of McCall's technique have been described, most notably, the modified endopelvic fascia repair, which was popularized and reported on from the Mayo Clinic. A wedge of vaginal mucosa is removed from the anterior and posterior vaginal wall. This narrows the vault when closed and allows easier access to lateral supports of the vagina (i.e., cardinal and uterosacral ligaments and perirectal fascia). The enterocele sac is then dissected free and excised at the neck. The ureters are identified by palpation bilaterally. One to three internal McCall's sutures are placed as described above. After these sutures are placed and tagged, modified external McCall sutures are placed by passing delayed absorbable sutures through the posterior vaginal wall and peritoneum, through remnants of uterosacral and cardinal ligaments on the patient's left. Several bites of peritoneum overlying the rectosigmoid are taken, and then the right perirectal fascia and uterosacral are incorporated into the suture. Last, the suture is passed back out through the posterior vaginal wall. The number of internal and external sutures placed depends on the size of enterocele and redundancy of the upper vagina (Figs. 35E.3 and 35E.4). Two groups of investigators between 1952 and 1987 performed a total of 1,027 operations. The 1998 article by Webb reported on 660 women who underwent primary repair of vaginal vault prolapse. Follow-up was available on 514 of the 660 women. Eighty patients (11.5%) complained of a "bulge" or "protrusion" at the time of questioning. Eighty-two percent (385 patients) responded that they were very satisfied or somewhat satisfied with the operation. The most common operative complication was laceration of bowel or rectum in 16 patients (2.3%). Four patients (0.6%) suffered ureteral complication. Three of these were from obstruction and one developed a ureterovaginal fistula. Nine patients (1.3%) had a vault hematoma and four

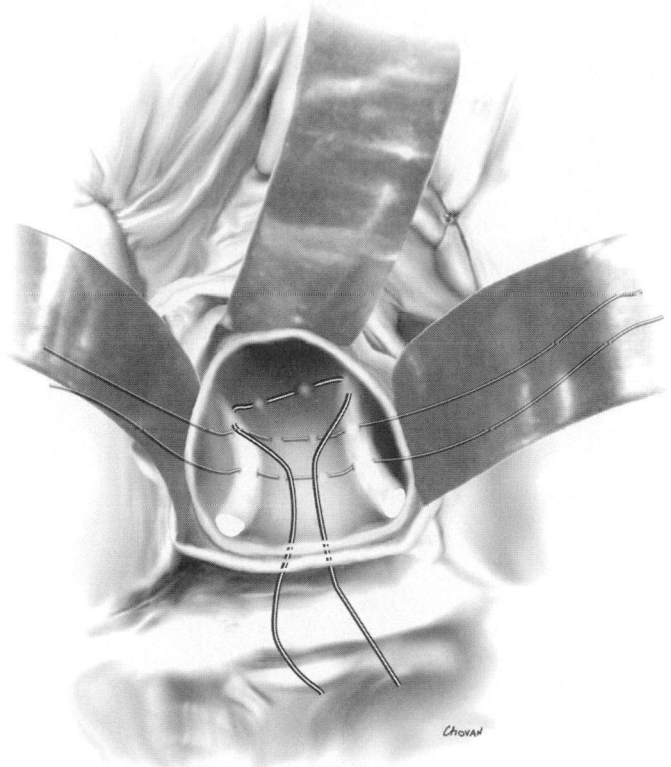

FIGURE 35E.2. McCall culdoplasty. Two internal sutures (permanent) and one external suture (delayed absorbable) have been placed. (From Baggish MS, Karram MM. *Atlas of pelvic anatomy and gynecologic surgery.* New York: Saunders, 2001.)

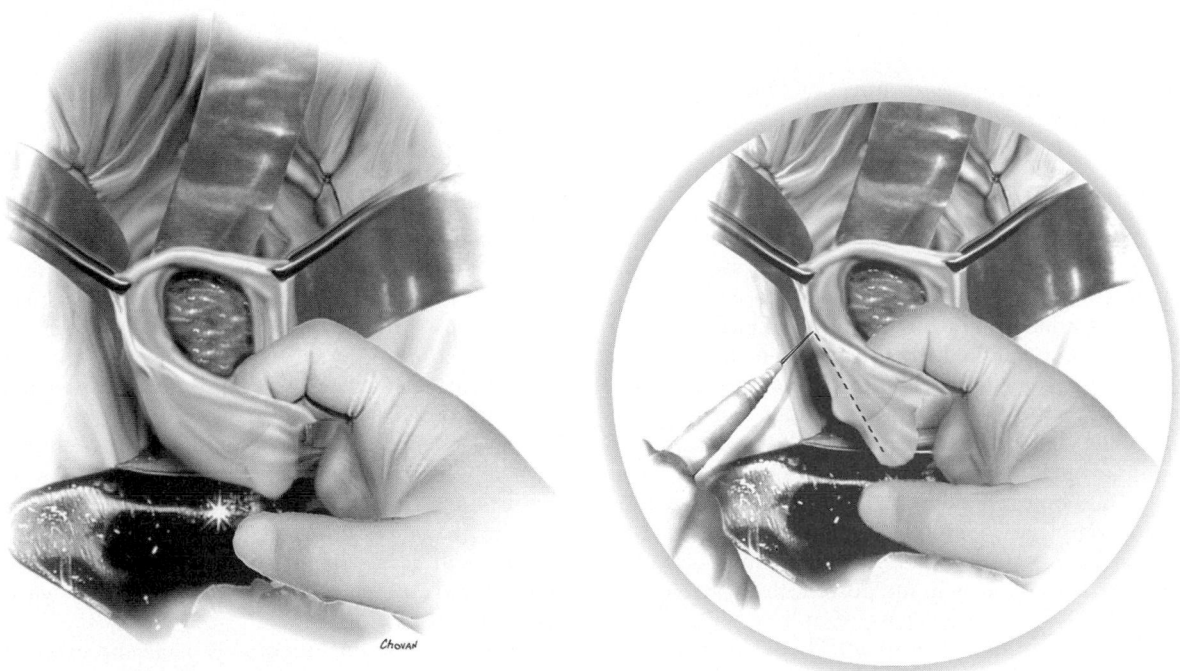

FIGURE 35E.3. Digital palpation of the posterior cul-de-sac and enterocele. **Inset:** The technique of removal of the redundant wedge of posterior vaginal wall and peritoneum. (From Baggish MS, Karram MM. *Atlas of pelvic anatomy and gynecologic surgery.* New York: Saunders, 2001.)

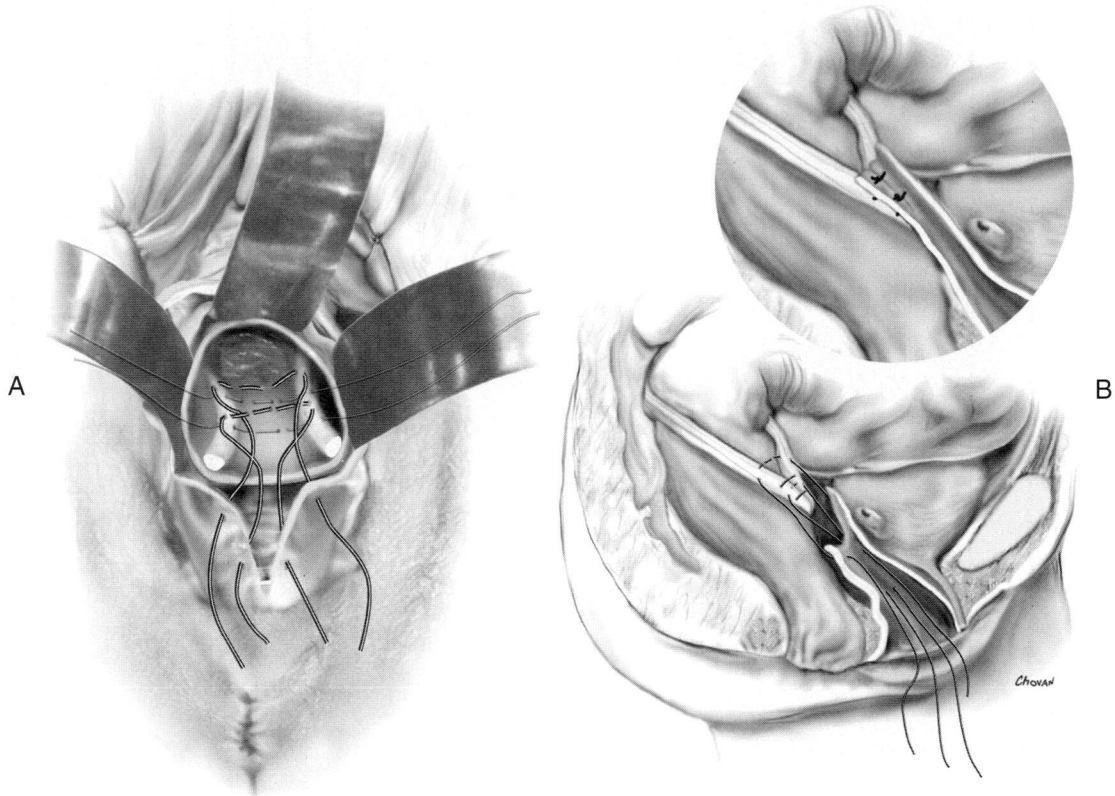

FIGURE 35E.4. A: Placement of internal and external McCall sutures after a wedge of posterior vaginal wall has been removed. **B:** Cross section of the upper vagina and vaginal vault before and after tying of sutures. (From Baggish MS, Karram MM. *Atlas of pelvic anatomy and gynecologic surgery.* New York: Saunders, 2001.)

(0.6%) had a cuff abscess or infection. Fifteen patients (2.2%) required blood transfusions.

Sacrospinous Ligament Fixation

To perform this operation, it is imperative that the surgeon be familiar with the anatomy of the sacrospinous ligament complex and of the pararectal space. Obtaining adequate exposure can be difficult and vascular complications, when encountered, may be life-threatening. The sacrospinous ligament is a cordlike structure that exists within the body of the coccygeus muscle. The sacrospinous ligament attaches medially to the sacrum and coccyx and attaches laterally to the ischial spine. The complex is collectively called the coccygeus-sacrospinous ligament complex (CSSL). The CSSL is best identified by palpating the ischial spine and tracing the finger-like ligamentous structure medially and posteriorly to the sacrum (Fig. 35E.5). The pudendal nerve and vessels pass directly posterior to the ischial spine. The sciatic nerve lies superior and lateral to the sacrospinous ligament. Superior to the ligament lies the inferior gluteal vessels and the hypogastric venous plexus (Fig. 35E.6). To avoid trauma to these structures it is important to place the fixation sutures two fingers medial to the ischial spine.

The apex of the vagina is grasped with two Allis clamps so the extent of the prolapse can be assessed. The vagina is then reduced to the sacrospinous ligament. Most surgeons prefer to use the sacrospinous ligament opposite their dominant hand; that is, the right-handed surgeon uses the right sacrospinous ligament, although some surgeons prefer to perform a bilateral fixation. Marking sutures can be used to identify the intended vaginal apex throughout the operation. It may be necessary to choose a different fixation point than the original vaginal cuff scar. This is best illustrated in a patient with a foreshortened anterior segment and a large enterocele. In this case, the new fixation point would be moved to an area over the enterocele. It is equally important to access the anterior and posterior segments of the vagina and the genital hiatus. If the patient requires an anterior vaginal wall repair or an anti-incontinence procedure, this should be performed in conjunction with the sacrospinous fixation.

A posterior vaginal incision is made and extended to the vaginal apex. Almost always an enterocele sac is present. The enterocele sac should be mobilized off the posterior vaginal wall up to its neck; the sac is then opened and the peritoneum excised. The defect is then closed with pursestring sutures.

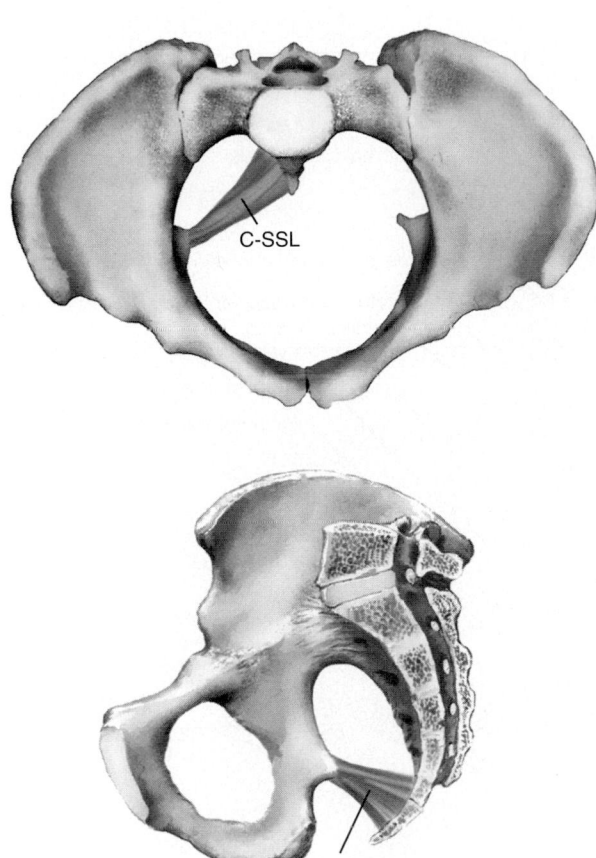

FIGURE 35E.5. The coccygeus-sacrospinous ligament complex (CSSL). Note that the sacrospinous ligament lies within the coccygeus muscle. (From Baggish MS, Karram MM. *Atlas of pelvic anatomy and gynecologic surgery.* New York: Saunders, 2001.)

The next step is entry into the perirectal space. The rectal pillar separates the rectovaginal space from the perirectal space. A window must be created through the rectal pillar, which is best accomplished by blunt dissection just lateral to the enterocele sac over the ischial spine. The window can also be created with the tips of scissors, a tonsil clamp, or a hemostat. The window should be gently enlarged to accommodate the vagina. The sacrospinous ligament can then be palpated by palpating the spine and moving the fingers dorsal and medial. It may be necessary to use blunt dissection to remove excess tissue from the CSSL.

Once the window has been created and the ligament is identified, a retractor (Briesky-Navratil, or Heaney) is used to displace the rectum medially. Great care must be taken to avoid raking the retractor over the anterior surface of the sacrum and causing damage to presacral nerves and vessels. When using the right sacrospinous ligament, the middle and index finger of the left hand are placed on the medial surface of the ischial spine. Then, under direct vision, the tip of the long-handled ligature carrier (Fig. 35E.7) penetrates the sacrospinous ligament two fingers medial to the ischial spine. There should be

considerable resistance as the carrier is pushed through the body of the ligament. If no resistance is felt, then the carrier either passed in front of or around the ligament. The ligament can be grasped with an Allis clamp or Babcock in order to isolate the tissue away from vessels and nerves. After the suture has been passed, the fingers of the left hand are withdrawn. The suture is then grasped with a nerve hook. A second suture is placed in a similar fashion approximately 1 cm medial to the first. If the surgeon doesn't desire a second passage, the suture can be cut in the midline and each end of the cut loop can be paired with its respective free suture. If a good purchase of tissue has been taken, the surgeon should be able to gently move the patient with traction of the suture.

In 1982, Miyazaki described a new technique for passing a suture through the sacrospinous ligament using a specially designed ligature carrier (Miya hook) (Fig. 35E.8). The proposed advantage of this technique is that it is safer and easier because the ligature carrier penetrates the sacrospinous ligament under direct palpation and is then passed downward into the safe perirectal space.

To use the Miya hook, the right middle finger tip is placed on the sacrospinous ligament, two finger breadths medial to the ischial spine and just below the superior margin. The Miya hook is held closed in the left hand and slid along the palmar surface of the right hand. The point of the hook then comes to rest just beneath the tip of the right middle finger. The handles are opened then lowered to a near horizontal position. The hook point should be at about a 45-degree angle. The tip of the right middle finger then confirms the hook point is placed two finger breadths medial to the ischial spine. The middle and index fingers then apply firm pressure downward just behind the hook hump so the hook penetrates the ligament. One can also place traction with the back of the thumb on the handle to help penetrate the ligament. The surgeon then closes and elevates the handles of the Miya hook and, with the index and middle fingers, clears the tissue from the point so as to make the suture visible. If there is too much tissue in the hook, the surgeon simply backs it out and takes a smaller bite. An assistant can then hold the handle elevated in a closed position. The rectum is held medially by a retractor and a notched speculum is inserted by palpation underneath the hook point. A nerve hook is then used to retrieve the suture.

Several other instruments have been designed to pass the suture through the ligament. These include the Laurus needle driver and Nichols-Veronikis ligature carrier (Fig. 35E.9).

Once the surgeon has the two sutures through the sacrospinous ligament, the vaginal vault can then be suspended. There are two ways for the surgeon to attach the sutures to the vagina. The first is to use a pulley stitch. Here the free end of the suture is threaded through a free needle, sewn into the full-thickness of the fibromuscular layer on the undersurface of the vagina, (excluding the epethelium) and then tied by a half hitch. Traction on the free end of the suture pulls the vagina directly

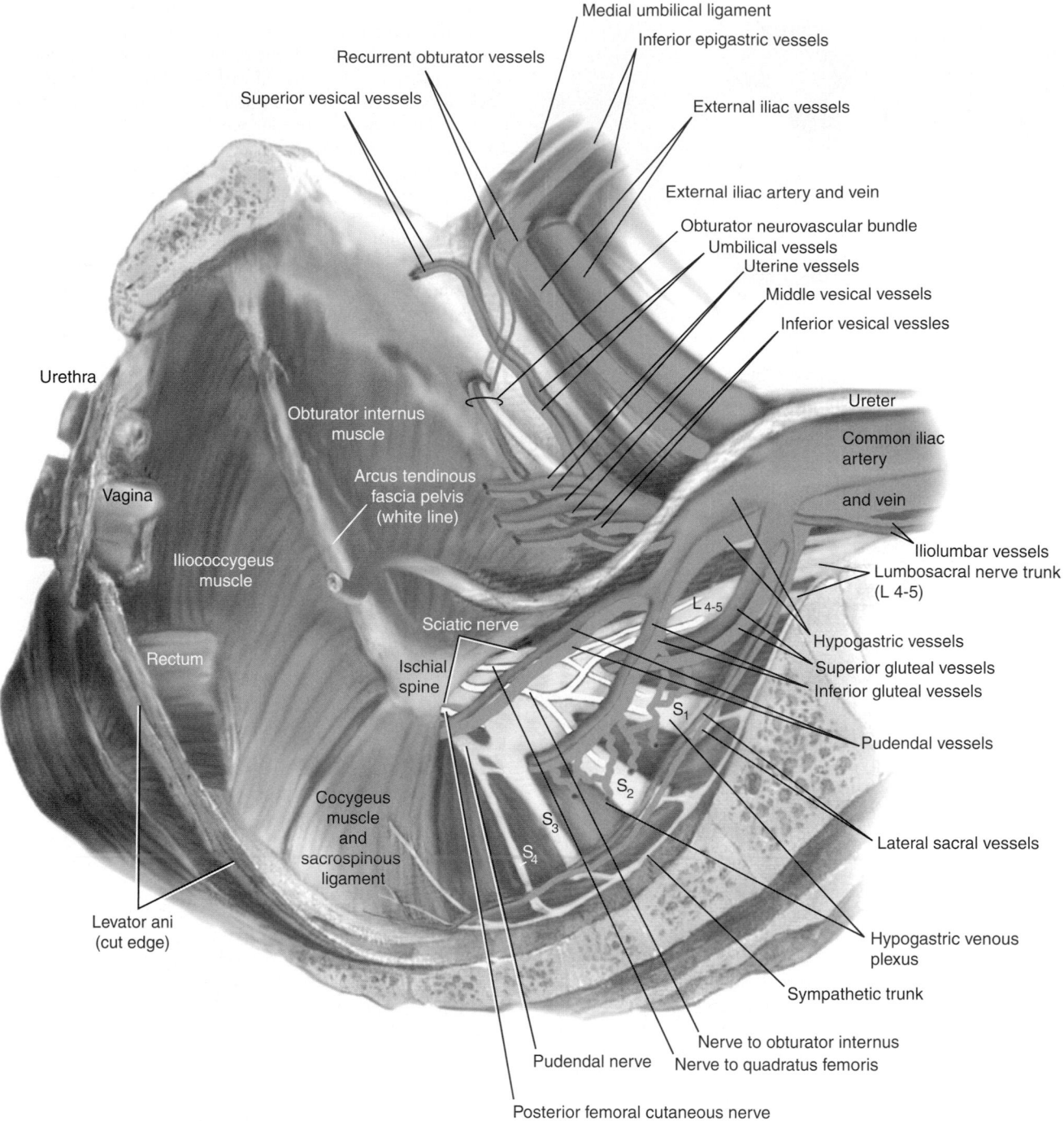

FIGURE 35E.6. Coccygeus-sacrospinous ligament anatomy. (From Baggish MS, Karram MM. *Atlas of pelvic anatomy and gynecologic surgery*. New York: Saunders, 2001.)

onto the ligament. A square knot is then used to fix the suture in place. Generally, when using this technique, permanent suture should be used.

The second technique can be used if the vagina is thin or if greater vaginal length is desired. This technique involves passing each end of the sutures through the full thickness of the vagina using 1-0 or 2-0 absorbable suture. The upper portion of the posterior vaginal wall should be closed with interrupted or running 3-0 absorbable sutures before tying the colpopexy sutures (Fig. 35E.10). If the colpopexy sutures are tied before the posterior wall is closed, the visibility of the vault is reduced and the colporrhaphy sutures are much more difficult to place. The vagina should come into contact with the sacrospinous ligament, especially if absorbable sutures are used. A suture bridge can predispose to recur-

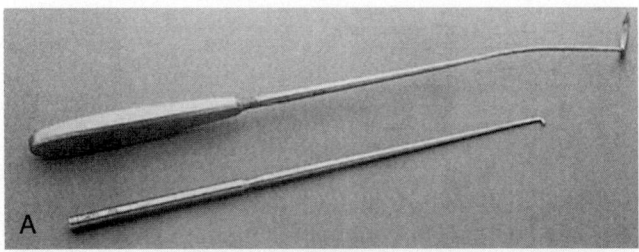
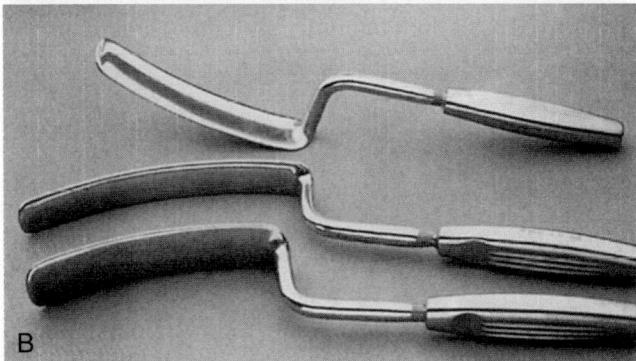

FIGURE 35E.7. A: Long-handled Deschamps ligature carrier and nerve hook. Note slight bend near the tip to facilitate suture placement into the coccygeus-sacrospinous ligament complex. **B:** Briesky-Navratil retractors, various sizes. (From Walters MD, Karram MM. *Urogynecology and reconstructive pelvic surgery,* 2nd ed. St. Louis: CV Mosby, 1999.)

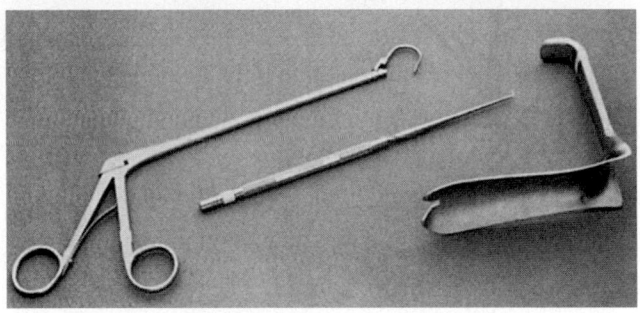

FIGURE 35E.8. Miya hook, notched speculum, and suture hook for use during sacrospinous ligament fixation. (From Walters MD, Karram MM. *Urogynecology and reconstructive pelvic surgery,* 2nd ed. St. Louis: CV Mosby, 1999.)

rent prolapse because a strong scar will not form before suture absorption.

After the colpopexy sutures are tied, a posterior colporrhaphy and perineorrhaphy is done. The vagina is then packed with moist gauze for 24 hours.

The overall results from sacrospinous fixation have been good. In 1997, Sze and Karram reviewed the literature on sacrospinous suspension and of the 1,137 patients available for follow-up, 36 (3%) had recurrent vault prolapse. Ninety-six (8%) had anterior wall prolapse and 25 (2%) had posterior wall prolapse. Some authors (Sze in 1997 and Shull in 1992) have reported a high incidence of anterior wall prolapse following sacrospinous fixation; others have not. Smilen and colleagues in 1998 compared patients with anterior vaginal wall defects undergoing anterior colporrhaphy with and without sacrospinous fixation to patients with a well supported anterior vaginal wall who were undergoing pelvic reconstructive procedures with and without sacrospinous fixation. They found no difference between the groups for subsequent anterior wall prolapse during the follow-up period. It has been our experience

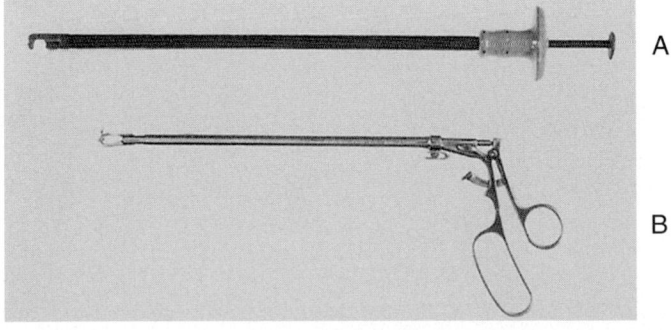

FIGURE 35E.9. Two specially designed instruments to facilitate passage of sutures through the sacrospinous ligament. **A:** Laurus needle driver (Microvasive-Boston Scientific Corporation, Watertown, MA). **B:** Nichols-Voronikis ligature carrier (BEI Medical Systems, Chatsworth, CA). (From Walters MD, Karram MM. *Urogynecology and reconstructive pelvic surgery,* 2nd ed. St. Louis: CV Mosby, 1999.)

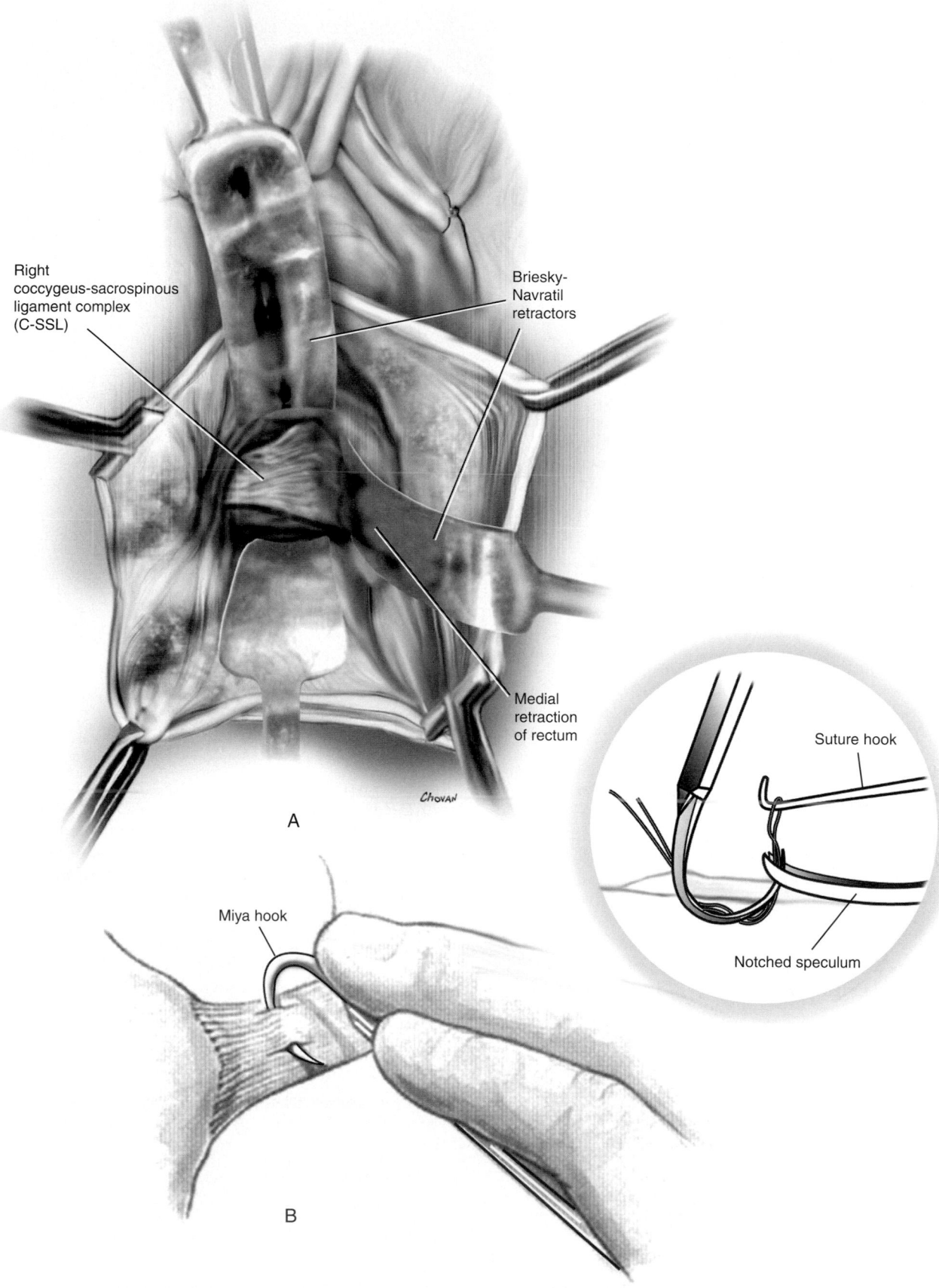

FIGURE 35E.10. A: Briesky-Navratil retractors are used to retract the rectum medially and bladder superiorly and depress the peritoneum. **B:** Technique of passage of a Miya hook through the ligament. **Inset:** Technique of retrieval of the suture.

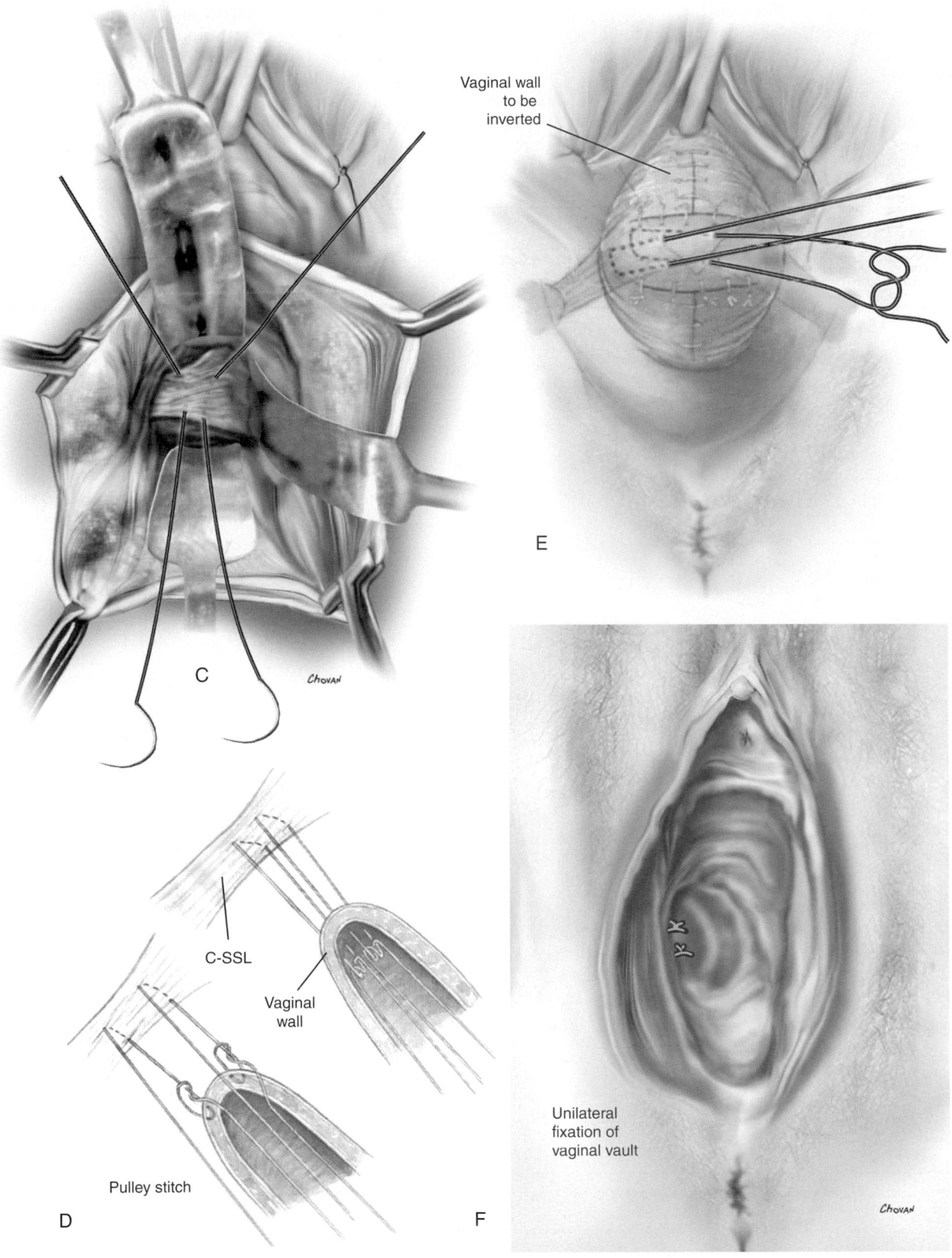

C

D

C-SSL

Vaginal
wall

Pulley stitch

Vaginal wall
to be
inverted

E

Unilateral
fixation of
vaginal vault

F

FIGURE 35E.10.   *(Continued)*: Two sutures have been passed through the complex. **D:** Technique of fixing the vaginal apex to the CSSL. If a pulley stitch is performed, then permanent sutures should be used. If the sutures are passed through the vaginal epithelium and tied in the vaginal lumen, then delayed absorbable sutures should be used. **E:** The vagina is closed before tying the suspension sutures. **F:** Tied sacrospinous sutures. (From Baggish MS, Karram MM. *Atlas of pelvic anatomy and gynecologic surgery.* New York: Saunders, 2001.)

that this operation does distort the vagina posteriorly and leaves the anterior segment vulnerable to recurrent prolapse. Table 35E.1 reviews published results of sacrospinous ligament suspension.

Complications can occur and the more common complications are discussed here. It is important to do frequent rectal examinations during this procedure to make sure that no inadvertent proctotomy has occurred. If evidence of suture penetration is evident, the offending suture should be removed and replaced. Lacerations should be closed in a standard two-layer fashion.

Hemorrhage can result from injury to the hypogastric venous plexus, inferior gluteal vessels, and internal pudendal vessels. Injury can occur from overzealous dis-

TABLE 35E.1.

Long-Term Complications, Follow-Up, and Recurrence of Prolapse After Sacrospinous Ligament Suspension

Investigation	Duration of Follow-Up	No. Available for Follow-Up	Vault	Anterior Wall	Posterior Wall	Unspecified/ Multiple Sites	No. Cured (%)	Cure Assessment[a]
Richter and Albright (1981)and Richter (1982)	1–10 yr	81	2/2	0/12	0/10		57 (70)	Objective
Nichols (1982)	≥2 yr	163	5/5				158 (97)[b]	
Morley and Delancey (1988)	1 mo–11 yr	92	3/3	2/11	0/0	0/3	75 (82)	Subjective/ Objective
Brown et al. (1989)	8–21 mo	11	1/1	0/0	0/0		10 (91)	Objective
Keetel and Herbertson (1989)	—	31	2/6				25 (81)	Objective
Cruikshank and Cox (1990)	8 mo–3.2 yr	48	0/1	0/5	0/2		40 (83)	Objective
Monk et al. (1991)	1 mo–8.6 yr	61	1/1	0/6	0/2		52 (85)	Objective
Backer (1992)		51	0/0	0/3	0/0		48 (94)	Objective
Heinonen (1992)	6 mo–5.6 yr	22	0/0	0/1	0/2		19 (86)	Objective
Imparato et al. (1992)	—	155	0/4			0/11	140 (90)	Objective
Shull et al. (1992)	2–5 yr	81	0/1	4/20	0/1	0/6	53 (65)	Objective
Kaminski et al. (1993)	—	23	2/2	0/1	0/0		20 (87)	Objective
Carey and Slack (1994)	2 mo–1 yr	63[d]	1/1	0/16	0/0		46 (73)	Objective
Porges and Smilen (1994)	—	76		?/1		0/2	—	Objective
Holley et al. (1995)	15–79 mo	36				0/33[e]	3 (8)	Objective
Sauer and Klutke (1995)	4–26 mo	24	3/5	1/3	0/1		15 (63)	Objective
Peters and Christenson (1995)	Median = 48 mo	30	0/0	0/0	4/6	0/1	23 (77)	Subjective/ Objective
Elkins et al. (1995)	3–6 mo	14		0/2			12 (86)	Objective
Sze et al. (1997)	7–72 mo	75	?/4	?/16	?/1	?/1	53 (71)	Objective
Ozcan et al. (1997)	4–54 mos	54	2/2	3/?	6/?		43 (80)	Objective
Hewson and Hon (1998)	8 mo–5 yr	114	2/2	6/6	?		(80)	Subjective
Meschia et al. (1999) TOTAL	1 mo–11 yr	1137	20/36	7/96	4/25	0/57		

[a] Subjective assessment, based on telephone interview or questionnaire; objective assessment, based on findings from pelvic examination.

[b] Cure rate applies to vaginal vault support only; does not include support defect at other site.

[c] Extrapolated from text.

[d] I ncludes 11 patients whose uteri were preserved.

[e] Includes 33 patients with anterior vaginal wall defects, 3 vaginal vault prolapses, and 8 posterior vaginal wall relaxations.

From Sze EHM, Karram MM. Vaginal operations to correct vaginal vault prolapse: a review. *Obstet Gynecol* 1997;89:466.

section or inappropriate needle passage through the sacrospinous ligament. If bleeding does occur initially, pressure should be applied to the bleeding area. Continued bleeding should be addressed with suture ligation and hemoclips. Because this area is difficult to approach transabdominally, every effort should be made to control bleeding transvaginally. An improperly placed retractor or inattentive assistance can cause damage to the presacral vessels by raking the tip over the bony sacrum.

Stress urinary incontinence may occur postoperatively and is probably the result of straightening of the posterior urethrovesical junction. It is important that all patients have adequate evaluation for potential stress incontinence. This is best done by preoperatively performing a stress test in the standing position with reduction of the prolapse.

A patient who complains of severe postoperative gluteal pain that runs down the posterior surface of the affected leg most likely has a pudendal nerve injury. Sutures that are placed too close to the ischial spine risk injury to the pudendal nerves and the sciatic nerve. If the patient has evidence of nerve injury, she should immediately undergo reoperation with removal of those sutures impinging on the nerve. New colpopexy sutures should be placed either more medial on the same side or the opposite sacrospinous ligament can be used.

In our experience, approximately 10% to 15% of patients have transient moderate to severe buttock pain on the side of the sacrospinous suspension. It is usually self-limiting and resolves by 6 weeks postoperatively. Reassurance and antiinflammatory agents are all that are necessary.

Vaginal stenosis can occur if too much vaginal tissue is removed before closing the vaginal incision. An aggressive posterior repair can also cause a constriction ring. If a constriction ring is present while the patient is still under anesthesia, it should be addressed at that time. The colporrhaphy sutures can be removed or lateral-relaxing incisions can be made in the vagina.

High Uterosacral Ligament Suspension with Fascial Reconstruction

In 1995, Richardson introduced a new approach to the management of enterocele and vault prolapse. The concept maintains that the endopelvic fascia that surrounds the vagina does not attenuate but breaks at specific points. The reconstruction aims to eliminate the enterocele by using principles of abdominal hernia surgery. This involves identifying the fascial defect, reduction of the enterocele sac, and closure of the fascial defect. In addition, the vagina is resuspended to its original level 1 support (the uterosacral ligaments).

Two Allis clamps are used to grasp the vaginal apex. With traction on the Allis clamps, the vaginal epithilium overlying the enterocele is incised. The enterocele sac is then dissected up to the neck of the hernia. The sac is opened and the cul-de-sac is palpated for adhesions and any unsuspected pathology. If adhesions are present, they should be carefully taken down. The excess peritoneum is excised. A Heaney retractor or Deaver is then placed anteriorly. The abdominal contents are carefully packed away with moist laparotomy sponges. The retractor is withdrawn and then replaced so as to elevate the sponges and abdominal contents out of the pelvis exposing the cul-de-sac (Fig. 35E.11).

Two Allis clamps are then placed where the remnants of uterosacral ligaments are believed to be, usually the 5-o'clock and 7-o'clock positions. It is sometimes necessary to trim excess vaginal mucosa to facilitate good traction on the uterosacral ligament. With tension on the Allis clamp directed outward, the pelvic sidewalls are palpated. The ischial spine is palpated transperitoneally and an attempt is made to palpate the ureter. If the uterosacral ligament is difficult to find, the Allis clamp can be repositioned. The ureter is usually found 2 to 5 cm ventral and lateral to the ischial spine. The ureter is best found by applying pressure to the pelvic sidewall with the tip of the index or middle finger and sweeping from an anterior superior to a posterior inferior position.

The uterosacral ligament remnants are then tagged with 0 permanent suture. The nondominant hand is used to displace the rectum medial and inferior. The needle is then passed through the remnant of the left uterosacral ligament from lateral to medial (for the right-handed surgeon). An assistant can place traction on the first suture throw and thereby allow the surgeon to place a better bite through the ligament, which should be slightly more medial and higher in the pelvis.. This "walking up" of the ligament allows both a better "purchase" of the ligament and helps identify the proximal part of the ligament. The same procedure is repeated on the patient's opposite side and these two sutures are then tagged.

The permanent sutures are then passed to the opposite side while taking successive bites through the peritoneum of the posterior cul-de-sac until the opposite uterosacral ligament is reached. The needle is then passed through the opposite uterosacral ligament. The suture should be passed from lateral to medial to avoid the ureter. Tying of these sutures obliterates the cul-de-sac and creates a firm ridge of tissue high up in the hollow of the sacrum. If an anterior colporrhaphy or sling procedure is indicated, it is done at this time.

Number 0 delayed absorbable suspension sutures are taken through the ridge of uterosacral ligament and then used to suspend the anterior and posterior vaginal walls and to reapproximate the pubocervical and rectovaginal fascia. One suture end is placed through the lateral aspect of posterior vaginal wall and the other end is passed out the lateral aspect of the anterior vaginal wall. This process is repeated for all suspension sutures. Cystoscopy is then performed to ensure that there is no ureteral compromise. Tying of these sutures suspends the vagina into the hollow of the sacrum and restores the continuity of the endopelvic fascia of the anterior and posterior vaginal walls.

There are three reports to date on the results of high uterosacral ligament suspension. In 2000, Shull and colleagues reported on their experience with 298 patients.

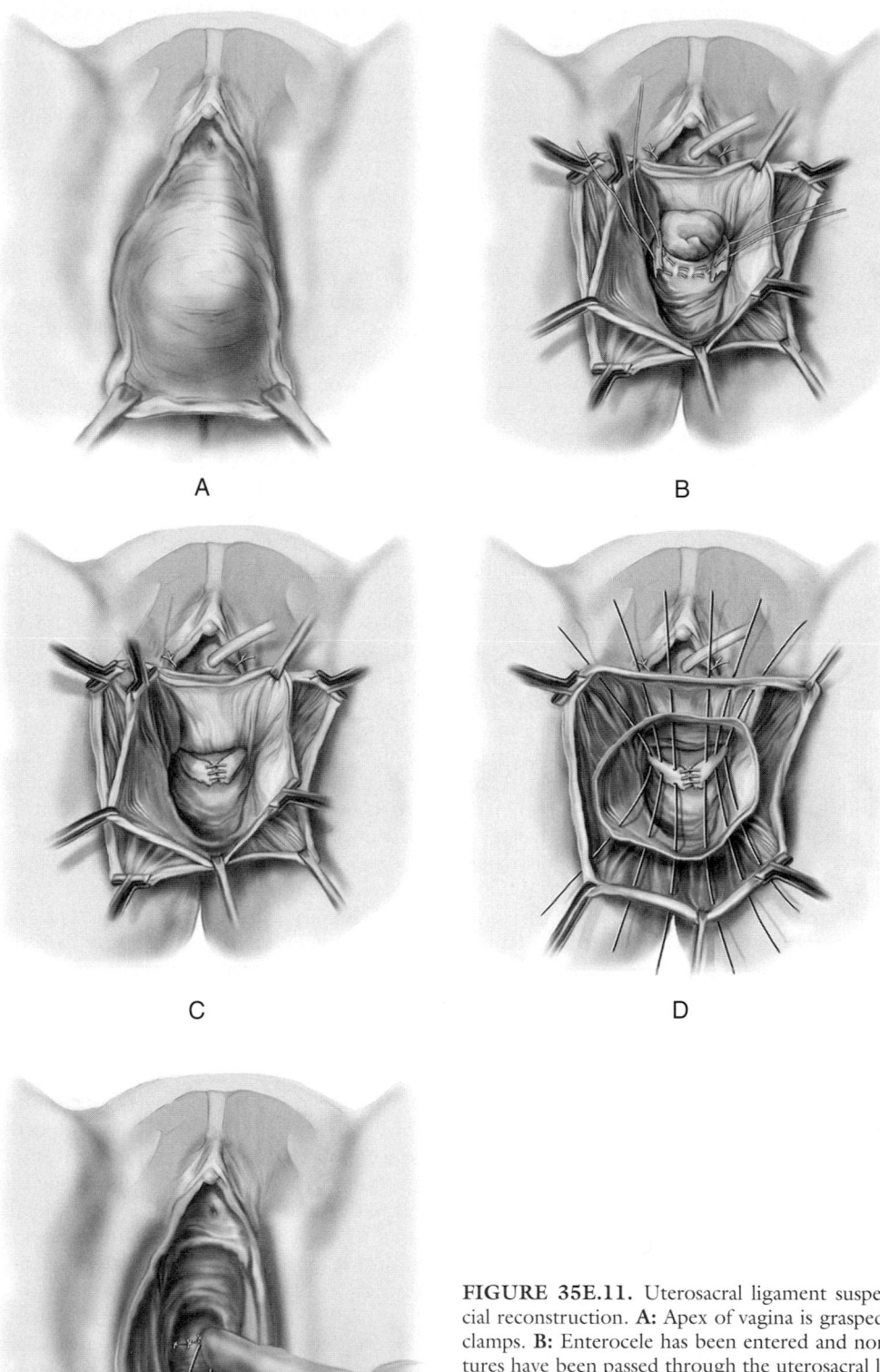

A

B

C

D

E

FIGURE 35E.11. Uterosacral ligament suspension with fascial reconstruction. **A:** Apex of vagina is grasped with two Allis clamps. **B:** Enterocele has been entered and nonabsorbable sutures have been passed through the uterosacral ligaments at the level of the ischial spines. **C:** Sutures have been tied across midline, creating a firm ridge to which the vagina will be anchored. **D:** Absorbable sutures are used to suspend anterior and posterior vaginal walls with their fascia to uterosacral ligaments. **E:** Tying of these sutures suspends the vagina into the hollow of the sacrum and restores the continuity of the endopelvic fascia of the anterior and posterior vaginal walls. (From Walters MD, Karram MM. *Urogynecology and reconstructive pelvic surgery,* 2nd ed. St. Louis: CV Mosby, 1999.)

TABLE 35E.2.

Investigator	Length of Follow-Up	No. Available for Follow-Up	Vault	Anterior Wall	Posterior Wall	No. of Reoperations
Shull (2000)	Up to 5 yrs	289	4 (1.3%)	35 (12%)	11 (4%)	2
Barber (2000)	3.5 mo–3.4 yr	39	7 (18%)	26 (67%)	21 (54%)	3
Karram (2001)	Up to 3.5 yr	168	14 (8%)	30 (18%)	46 (27%)	10 (6%)
TOTAL		496	25 (5%)	91 (18%)	78 (16%)	15 (3%)

Thirty-five (12%) had evidence of an anterior wall defect in the form of cystocele or urethrocele. However, 25 of these defects were noted to be only grade 1. Eleven (4%) patients developed posterior wall defects. In all, 38 patients (13%) had development of one or more support defects; however, 24 of these were grade 1 only. Two patients required another surgery for recurrent prolapse.

In 2000, Barber and colleagues reported their series of 46 patients, of whom 39 were available for long-term follow-up. Of note is that 19/26 anterior wall, 5/7 apical, and 13/21 posterior wall defects were designated as stage I. Three patients required another surgery for recurrent prolapse.

Karram and colleagues reported on 202 patients. One hundred and sixty-eight patients were available for follow-up either by phone or office visit. Eighty-nine percent of patients indicated that they were happy or satisfied with the procedure. The reoperation rate was 5.5%. These results are summarized in Table 35E.2.

Complications included hemorrhage with subsequent transfusion or bowel and bladder injury. The most common complication of this procedure, however, is ureteral injury or kinking. Karram and colleagues reported a 2.4% risk, Barber and colleagues reported an 11%, risk and Shull and colleagues reported a 1% risk. It is imperative that intraoperative cystoscopy be done to ensure ureteral patency. If ureteral spill is not observed, then the suspension sutures on that side should be cut and removed and the ureter reevaluated. Often, the suture can be replaced using a more medial placement into the uterosacral ligament complex.

Iliococcygeus Fascia Suspension

In 1963, Inmon described bilateral fixation of prolapsed vaginal vault to iliococcygeal fascia on three patients with inadequate uterosacral ligaments. In 1993, Shull and colleagues reported using this technique to treat 42 women. Their approach was to identify all fascial defects preoperatively. Before iliococcygeus suspension, any anterior compartment defects are fixed. A cul-de-sac repair may be undertaken to shorten and approximate the uterosacral ligaments.

Cuff suspension and posterior colporrhaphy are approached by excising a diamond-shaped section of tissue from the perineum and introitus. The vaginal epithelium is then freed from the rectum and rectovaginal fascia, and the dissection is carried laterally to the levators and cephalad to the cuff. The iliococcygeus muscle is identified lateral to the rectum and anterior to the ischial spine. The surgeon then uses the nondominant hand to press the rectum down and medially. A suture is placed just anterior to the ischial spine. Both ends of the suture are then passed through the ipsilateral vaginal apex. The same procedure is repeated on the patient's opposite side. If delayed absorbable suture is used, it should be passed through the full thickness of the vagina. If nonabsorbable suture is used, a pulley stitch similar to that described for sacrospinous fixation should be used. The sutures are then held to be tied after posterior colporrhaphy is finished (Fig. 35E.12).

A total of 152 patients were treated with this technique by Shull and colleagues and by Meeks and colleagues. A total of 13 patients (8%) developed recurrent pelvic prolapse at various sites. Two developed vault prolapses, eight developed anterior vaginal wall relaxation, and three developed posterior wall defects. They reported one rectal and one bladder laceration and two cases of hemorrhage requiring transfusion. Postoperative follow-up ranged from 6 weeks to 5 years.

Abdominal Sacral Colpopexy

Suspension of the vagina to the sacral promontory or into the hollow of the sacrum with an intervening mesh has been shown to be an effective treatment for vault prolapse. The patient is placed in Allen stirrups and is prepped and draped. Alternatively, the patient could be placed in the frog leg position. Either position allows access to the vagina during the operation. We generally use an EEA sizer for manipulation, although a sponge stick may also be used. A three-way Foley catheter is used to drain the bladder.

A laparotomy incision is made via a low transverse or vertical midline approach. Moist laparotomy sponges are then used to pack the bowel into the upper abdomen. Any adhesions should be carefully taken down. The course of the ureters and the cul-de-sac should be inspected and palpated. If the patient has a uterus, a hysterectomy should be done first and the cuff closed.

The vagina is then elevated using an EEA sizer (Fig. 35E.13). The peritoneum is then dissected off the anterior vaginal wall. The peritoneum on the posterior aspect

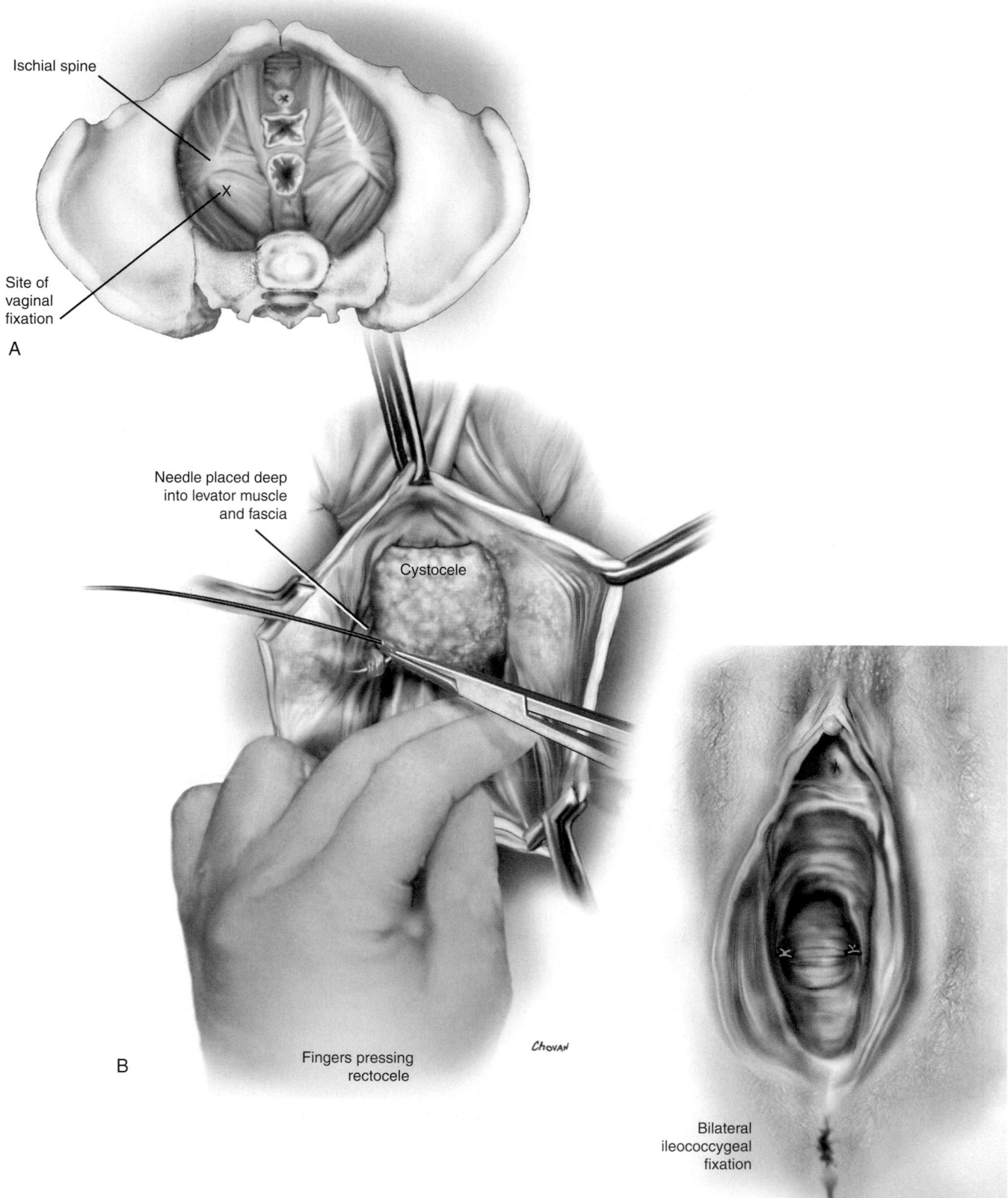

FIGURE 35E.12. Ileococcygeus fascia suspension. **A:** With the surgeon's finger pressing the rectum downward, the right ileococcygeus fascia suture is placed. **Inset:** Approximate location of the ileococcygeus fascia sutures. **B:** Bilateral ileococcygeus fascia suspension. (From Baggish MS, Karram MM. *Atlas of pelvic anatomy and gynecologic surgery.* New York: Saunders, 2001.)

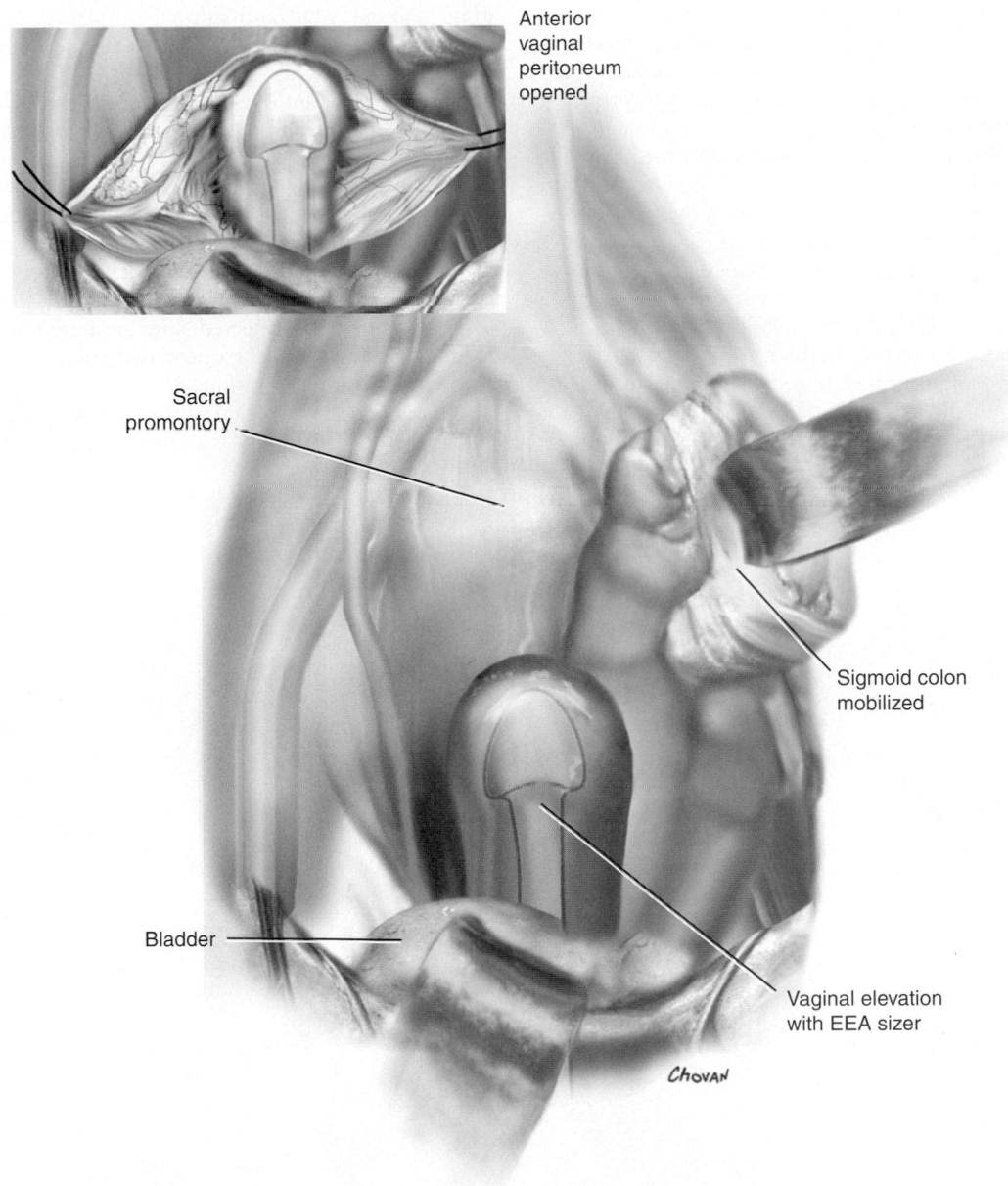

Anterior
vaginal
peritoneum
opened

Sacral
promontory

Sigmoid colon
mobilized

Bladder

Vaginal elevation
with EEA sizer

CHOVAN

FIGURE 35E.13. The vagina is elevated with an EEA sizer. The peritoneum over the vagina is opened, exposing the muscular portion of the vaginal wall (**inset**). (From Baggish MS, Karram MM. *Atlas of pelvic anatomy and gynecologic surgery.* New York: Saunders, 2001.)

of the vagina is incised in the midline and carried down into the cul-de-sac. The peritoneum is then dissected free laterally. Three to five pairs of 0 nonabsorbable suture are placed on the posterior aspect of the vagina about 1.5 to 2 cm apart. The suture should incorporate the full thickness of the vagina without entering the vaginal lumen. If the vagina is thin, imbricating sutures can be used to increase its thickness. The benefit of the EEA sizer is that penetration into the vagina is easily detected by the tactile sensation of the needle on the metal sizer.

The sutures are then placed through the mesh and tied down. In 1997, Cundiff recommended extending the mesh to the perineum. We generally extend the mesh approximately halfway down the posterior wall. We also place two to four pairs of 0 nonabsorbable suture on the anterior aspect of the vagina and attach a separate piece of mesh. This anterior mesh is sewn to the posterior mesh just proximal to the vaginal apex. Other potential configurations have also been described.

A Moschowitz or Halban procedure is then done to obliterate the cul-de-sac. To expose the presacral area, the rectosigmoid is then reflected to the left. The bifurcation of the aorta is palpated and again the right ureter is identified and retracted laterally. The peritoneum over the sacral promontory is opened and carried down over the anterior surface of the sacrum. With the peritoneum reflected, the middle sacral artery and vein are identified. The left common iliac vein and artery are also prone to injury and should be identified.

A subperitoneal tunnel can be created into the cul-de-sac by blunt and sharp dissection. The graft can then be placed retroperitoneally. Alternatively, the graft can be placed over the previous culdoplasty and can then be extraperitonealized by sewing the serosa of the sigmoid to the lateral peritoneum of the cul-de-sac.

The sacral promontory and the anterior longitudinal ligament are then exposed by blunt and delicate dissection. Two to four sutures of 0 nonabsorbable sutures are placed through the longitudinal ligament over the sacral promontory (Fig. 35E.14). The appropriate amount of

graft material is cut and sutures are placed through the graft and tied (Fig. 35E.15). There should be no tension on the graft material.

The peritoneum over the sacrum is then closed with a 2-0 or 3-0 absorbable suture. The peritoneum over the anterior vaginal wall is closed, thereby covering the mesh. Generally, a paravaginal repair is done and, when indicated, a retropubic urethropexy. Suprapubic telescopy or cystoscopy is preformed and a suprapubic catheter can be placed if desired. The abdomen is then closed.

The vagina is inspected and evaluated for any remaining defects. Usually a posterior colporrhaphy and a perineoplasty are also required.

It has been shown by multiple investigators that abdominal sacral colpopexy is a durable and strong surgical

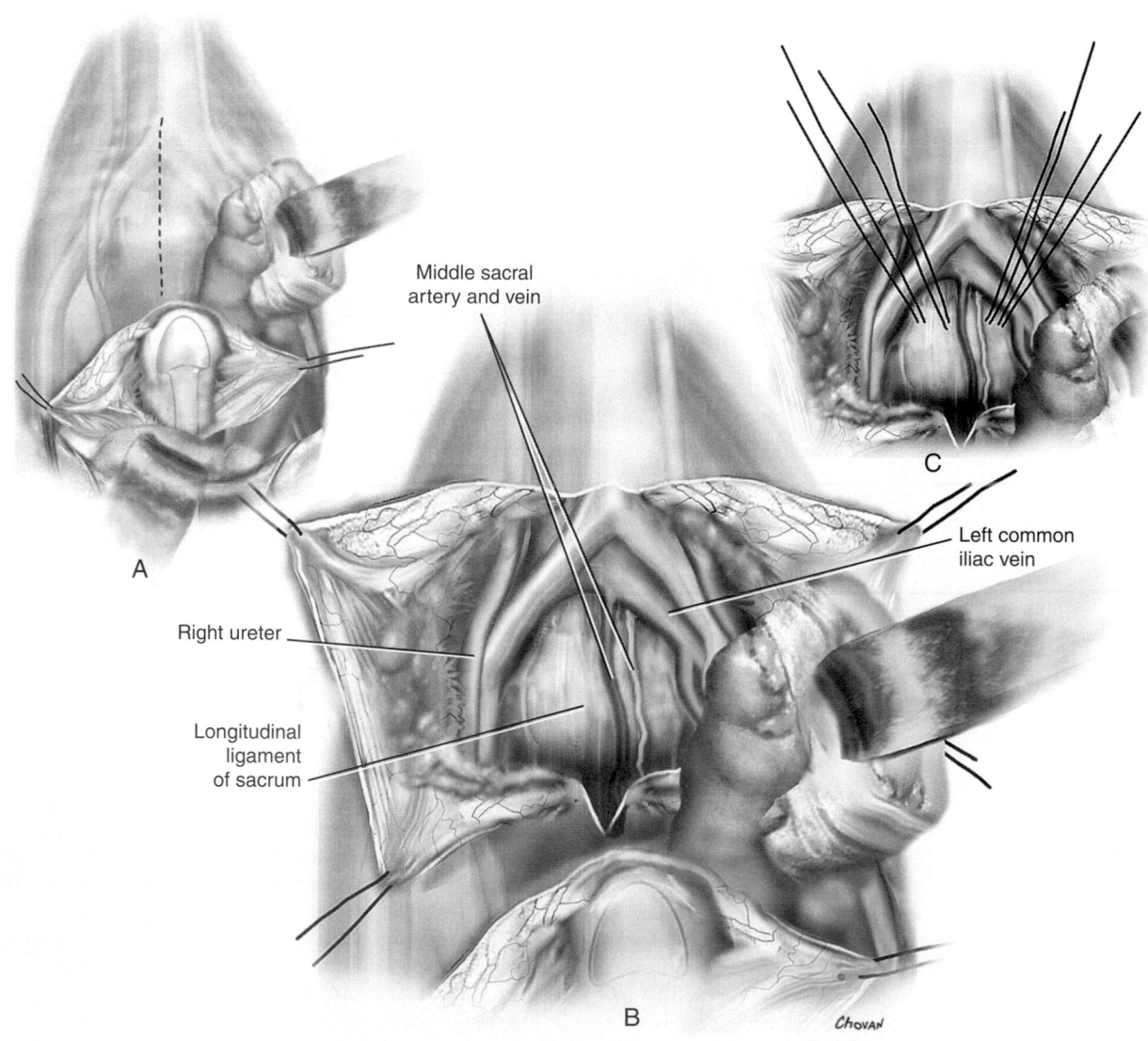

FIGURE 35E.14. Anatomy of the sacral promontory. **A:** Incision into the peritoneum. **B:** Dissection to the longitudinal ligament of the promontory. Note the vascularity of this area. **C:** Placement of permanent sutures through the longitudinal ligament of sacrum. (From Baggish MS, Karram MM. *Atlas of pelvic anatomy and gynecologic surgery.* New York: Saunders, 2001.)

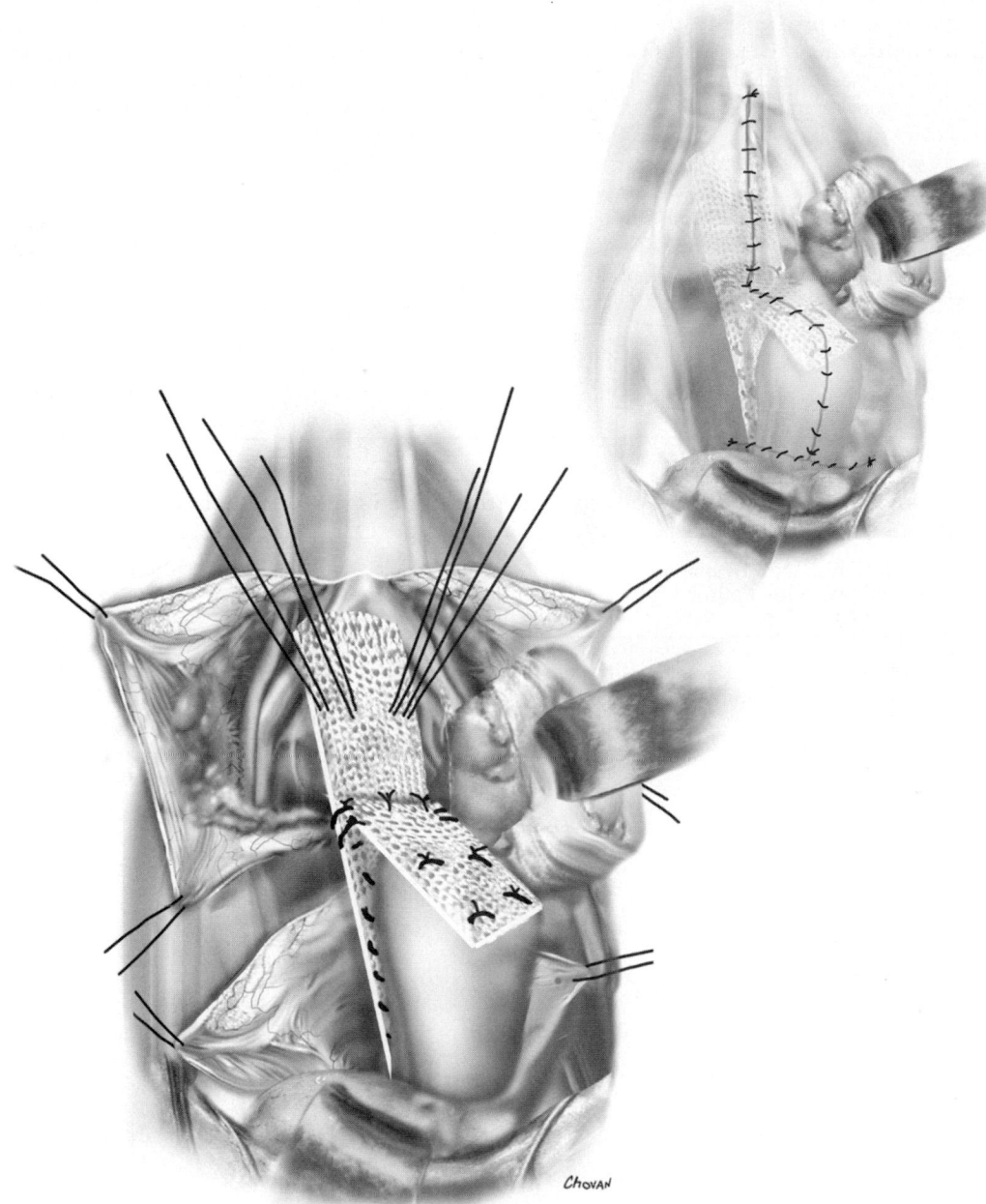

FIGURE 35E.15. Attachment of the mesh to the sacrum. Closure of the peritoneum over the mesh is shown in the inset. (From Baggish MS, Karram MM. *Atlas of pelvic anatomy and gynecologic surgery.* New York: Saunders, 2001.)

correction for vaginal vault prolapse. Benson and colleagues randomized patients with prolapse to abdominal sacral colpopexy versus bilateral sacrospinous ligament fixation. They found superior results with abdominal sacral colpopexy. The reoperation rate in the vaginal group was 33% and in the abdominal group 16%. Optimal results were obtained in only 29% of the vaginal group and 58% of the abdominal group. The time of operation was longer for the abdominal group.

Although the exact indications for abdominal sacral colpopexy are controversial, many surgeons use it as their primary surgery for all cases of posthysterectomy vault prolapse. Because of the increased operative time and longer time to recover, we generally use the abdominal approach for young patients with advanced prolapse, patients who have previously failed a vaginal approach, have a foreshortened vagina, or who have other coexisting conditions that predispose to continued marked increases in intraabdominal pressure and therefore possible subsequent failure.

Overall, the long-term results from sacral colpopexy have been very good. Addison and colleagues reported three recurrent prolapses after sacral colpopexy. In two patients the synthetic mesh had separated from the vaginal wall and in the third patient the posterior vaginal wall ruptured distal to the attachment of the mesh. The authors believed that failures can be minimized by performing meticulous culdoplasty and securing the mesh to the culdoplasty with permanent sutures to prevent the dissection of an enterocele. They also recommended attaching the mesh to the vagina at multiple sites. Long-term follow-up is summarized in Table 35E.3.

Intraoperative complications are unusual, and injury to bowel, bladder, ureter, and infection, as with all abdominal surgery, has been described. Hemorrhage, especially from presacral vessels, can be life threatening. Hemostasis can be difficult because damaged presacral vessels tend to retract beneath the bony surface. Sutures, hemoclips, and bone wax should be used initially. If these measures fail, then sterile thumbtacks can be employed. These stainless steel thumbtacks should be placed on the retracted bleeding vessel.

The most common long-term complication has been erosion of synthetic mesh. Kohli and colleagues in 1998 reported an incidence of 7%. Removal of the eroded mesh can be done via an abdominal or vaginal route. We have

TABLE 35E.3.
Long-Term Follow-Up and Recurrence of Prolapse After Abdominal Sacral Colpopexy

Investigator	Duration of Follow-Up (mo)	No. Available for Follow-Up	Vault[a]	Anterior Wall[a]	Posterior Wall[a]	Unspecified/ Multiple Sites	No. Cured (%)	Cure Assessment
Rust et al. (1976)	9–40	12	0/0	0/1	0/0	0/0	12/12 (100)	Objective[b]
Todd (1978)	NA	93	½	0/0	0/1	0/1	91/93 (98)	Objective[b]
Feldman and Birnbaum (1979)	1–48	21	0/1	0/2	0/1	0/1	20/21 (95)	Objective[b]
Cowan and Morgan (1980)	≤60	39	0/1	NA	NA	NA	38/39 (97)	Objective[b]
Addison et al. (1985)	6–126	56	2/2	0/0	0/0	0/0	54/56 (96)	NA
Drutz and Cha (1987)	3–93	15	1/1	0/0	0/2	0/0	14/15 (93)	Objective[b]
Angulo and Ligman (1989)	2–36	18	0/0	NA	NA	NA	18/18 (100)	Objective
Baker et al. (1990)	1–45	59	0/0	0/6	0/4	0/0	51/51 (100)	Subjective/ Objective
Maloney et al. (1990)	12–60	10	0/1	0/0	0/0	0/0	9/10 (90)	NA
Creighton and Stanton (1991)	3–35	23	2/2	0/0	0/0	0/0	21/23 (91)	Objective[b]
Synder and Krantz (1991)	≥6	116	?/8	NA	NA	?/24	108/116 (93)	Objective
Timmons et al. (1992)	9–216	162	0/1	0/0	3/3	0/0	161/162 (99)	Objective[b]
Imparato et al. (1992)	NA	63	?/4	0/0	0/0	?/10	59/63 (94)	Objective[b]
Traiman et al. (1992)	6–60	11	0/1	NA	NA	NA	10/11 (91)	NA
Iosif (1993)	12–120	40	1/1	0/1	0/2	0/0	39/40 (96)	Objective
Grunberger et al. (1994)	12–240	48	0/3	0/0	0/0	6/6	45/48 (94)	Objective
Vitranen et al. (1994)	12–96	27	0/1	0/1	0/0	0/1	23/27 (85)	Objective
Valaitis and Stanton (1994)	3–91	38	3/3	0/0	0/1	0/0	38/41 (93)	Objective
Van Lindert et al. (1996)	15–63	61	0/0	0/0	0/0	0/2	61/61 (100)	Objective[b]

[a] Denotes the number of patients with recurrent prolapse who underwent surgical repair/number of patients with recurrent prolapse.
[b] Extrapolated from text.
NA, Not available.

had good success removing the mesh via the vaginal route. With the patient prepped and draped, as much of the mesh as possible is exposed. The mesh is cut as high as possible and removed. The vaginal edges are then trimmed and closed in layers.

HIGH UTEROSACRAL LIGAMENT SUSPENSION

The vaginal approach of vaginal suspension to the uterosacral ligaments is discussed previously. The same concept can also be used in an abdominal approach.

After the abdominal wall has been opened and the bowel has been packed away, the remnants of the uterosacral ligaments are identified and tagged with suture near the ischial spine. The ureters are identified bilaterally. The enterocele is then addressed by obliteration of the cul-de-sac. The peritoneum over the vaginal apex is then opened and the endopelvic fascia is identified and reapproximated to form a continuos covering of endopelvic fascia over the vaginal epithelium. Nonabsorbable sutures are then used to suspend the vagina with the now intact endopelvic fascia to the uterosacral ligaments (Figs. 35E.16 and 35E.17).

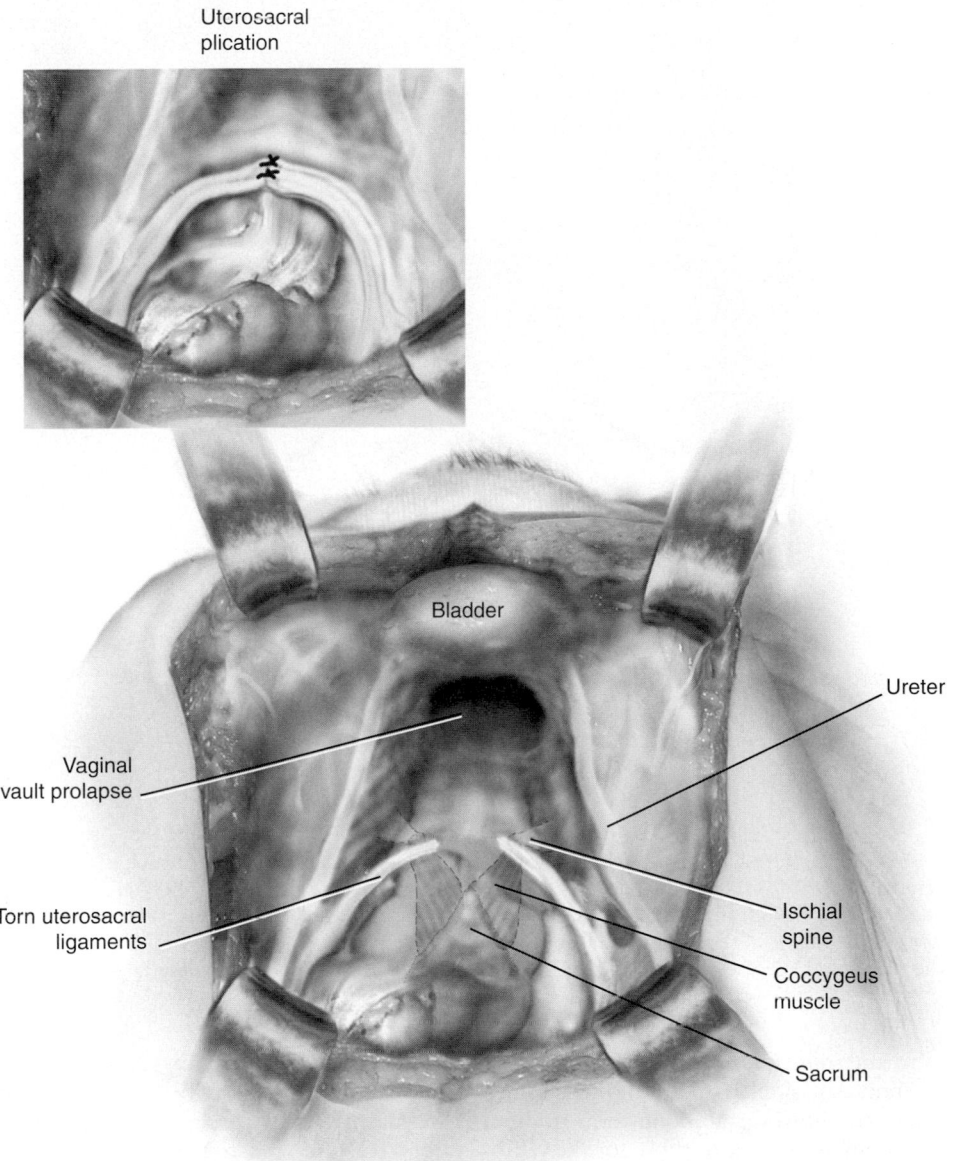

FIGURE 35E.16. Abdominal view of an enterocele and vaginal vault prolapse. Note the broken ends of the uterosacral ligaments at the level of the ischial spine. The inset demonstrates plication of ligaments, creating a firm durable ridge in the hollow of the sacrum to which the vaginal vault will be suspended. (From Baggish MS, Karram MM. *Atlas of pelvic anatomy and gynecologic surgery*. New York: Saunders, 2001.)

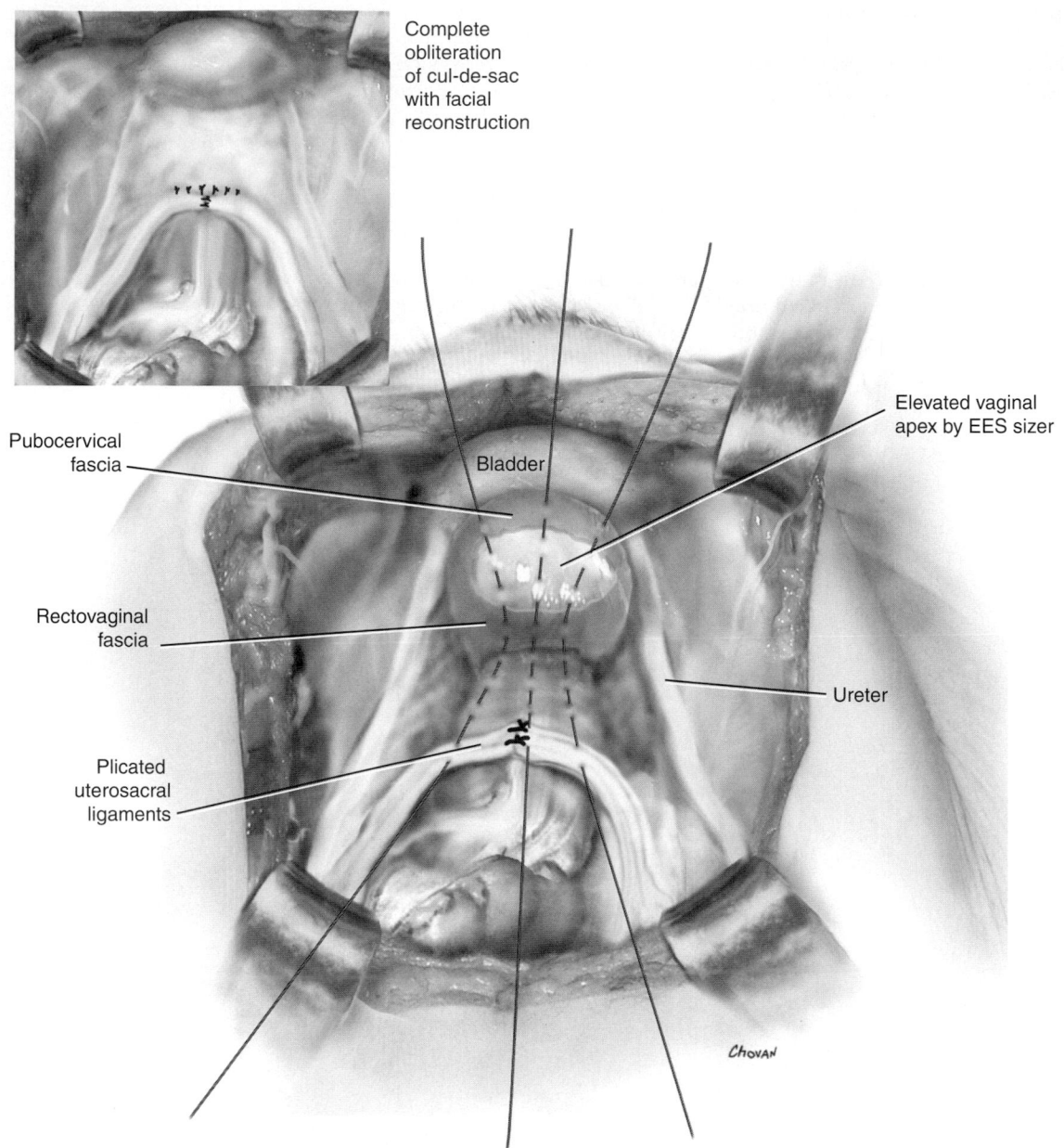

FIGURE 35E.17. Longitudinally placed nonabsorbable sutures are passed through the ridge of uterosacral ligaments, down the cul-de-sac to the edge of the rectovaginal fascia, into the vaginal vault, and finally, through the edge of pubocervical fascia. Tying of the sutures (**inset**) elevates the apex of the vagina to the uterosacral ligaments and reapproximates the pubocervical fascia with the rectovaginal fascia. (From Baggish MS, Karram MM. *Atlas of pelvic anatomy and gynecologic surgery.* New York: Saunders, 2001.)

Results for the abdominal approach to high uterosacral suspension should be similar to those for the vaginal approach. There are, however, no long-term studies available. Complications are similar to those for the vaginal approach.

Laparoscopic Approach

The techniques and concepts described earlier can also be approached via laparoscopy. The laparoscopic approach to the patient for positioning, port placement, and equipment is described elsewhere. The laparoscopic approach to these procedures requires patience, attention to detail, and the realization that there is a steep learning curve. It is our belief that the operation and subsequent outcomes should not be compromised for the purpose of having achieved the operation by this approach. Therefore, the surgical measures taken to achieve the underlying concepts should not be significantly altered or changed.

OBLITERATIVE PROCEDURES

Le Fort Partial Colpocleisis

At times, a patient may be sufficiently bothered by uterovaginal or vault prolapse but they medically are unable to undergo major reconstructive surgery. An obliterative procedure may then be undertaken. A Le Fort procedure is an option if the patient has her uterus and is no longer sexually active. The rate of postoperative urinary stress incontinence has been reported to be as high as 30% after this procedure, and, because the uterus is retained, it will be difficult to evaluate any future uterine bleeding or cervical pathology. Therefore endometrial biopsy and Papanicolaou smear must be done before surgery.

The procedure is started by placing the cervix on traction to evert the vagina. The vaginal mucosa is injected with 0.025% Marcaine with 1:200,000 epinephrine just below the epithelium. A Foley catheter with a 30-cc balloon is placed in the bladder for identification of the bladder neck.

A marking pen or scalpel is used to mark out the areas that are to be denuded both anteriorly and posteriorly. The area should extend 2 cm proximal to the tip of the cervix to 4 to 5 cm below the external meatus. A mirror image on the posterior aspect of the cervix should also be marked out.

The previously marked areas are removed by sharp dissection. The surgeon should leave the maximum amount of fascia behind on the bladder and rectum. Hemostasis is an absolute must.

The cut edges of the anterior and posterior vaginal wall are sewn together with interrupted delayed absorbable sutures. The knot should be turned into the epithelium-lined tunnels that were created bilaterally. The uterus and vaginal apex are gradually turned inward. After the vagina has been inverted, the superior and inferior margins of the rectangle can be sutured. A plication of the bladder neck should be routinely performed because of the high incidence of postoperative stress incontinence (Fig. 35E.18). Also, because there is no real support to the repair, an aggressive perineorrhaphy should be done to narrow the introitus.

In general, about 90% of patients have relief of symptoms and have good anatomic results. Complete breakdown and recurrence can be expected in 2% to 5% of patients. Results are summarized in Table 35E.4.

Early postoperative complications include hematoma and infection. These patients typically have other medical problems that may need to be addressed. Goldman and colleagues in 1985 reported on late postoperative complications from a modified Le Fort procedure in 118 patients. Ninety percent of patients had good anatomic results, whereas 85% had relief of symptoms. Two percent

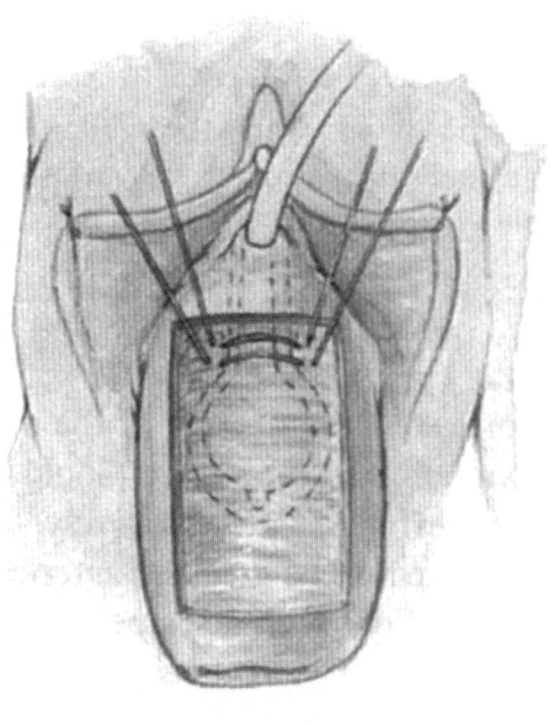

A

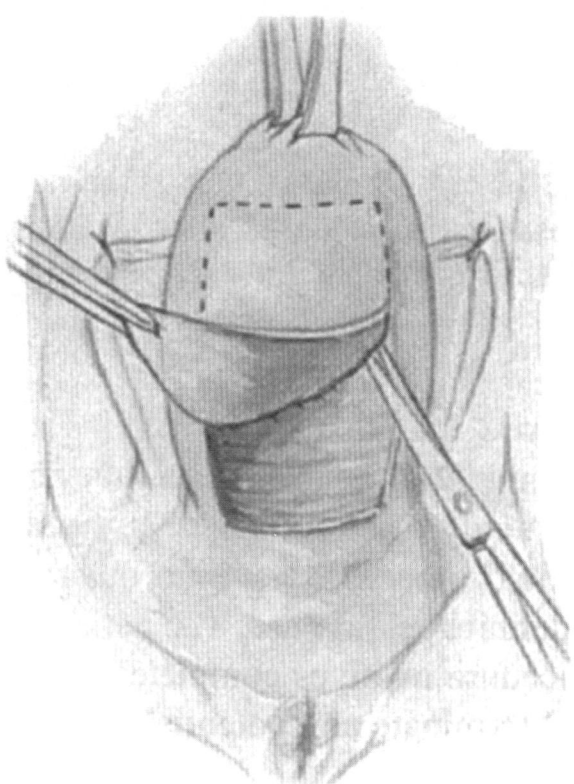

B

FIGURE 35E.18. Le Fort partial colpocleisis. **A:** The anterior vaginal wall has been removed and a plication stitch is placed at the bladder neck. **B:** The posterior vaginal wall is removed.

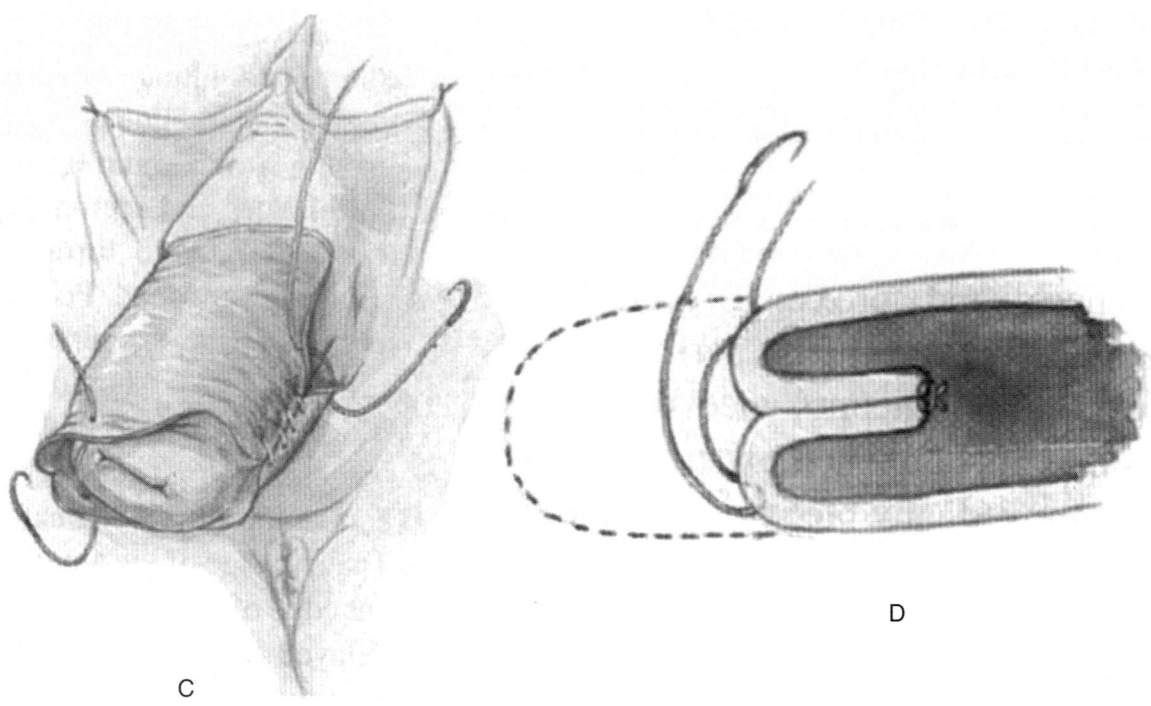

C

D

FIGURE 35E.18. *(Conrinued)* **C and D:** The cut edge of the anterior vaginal wall is sewn in the cut edge of the posterior vaginal wall in such a way that the uterus and vagina are inverted. (From Baggish MS, Karram MM. *Atlas of pelvic anatomy and gynecologic surgery.* New York: Saunders, 2001.)

to 5% had recurrence of their prolapse, 10.2% developed incontinence or worsening of their incontinence, and 1.8% had late vaginal bleeding.

Colpectomy and Colpocleisis

For patients with posthysterectomy vault prolapse who do not desire coital function and operative time is to be kept at a minimum, a colpectomy and colpocleisis can be done to treat the prolapse.

To perform this operation, the vaginal mucosa is completely excised from the underlying endopelvic fascia. A series of pursestring sutures are used to invert the prolapse and endopelvic fascia (Fig. 35E.19). Once the prolapse is reduced, a posterior colpoperineorrhaphy and levator plasty is done. Results are listed in Table 35E.4.

CONCLUSION

Our understanding and concepts of pelvic organ prolapse and its treatments are constantly evolving. This evolution will and must continue to facilitate our understanding of the complex and varied etiologies of pelvic organ prolapse. Surgical treatments must restore both anatomic and functional derangements. This evolution will also provide insight into preventive measures for women at risk for pelvic organ prolapse and pelvic floor dysfunction. We, as pelvic surgeons, must continue to evaluate and apply new principles and techniques to established surgical dictums. There must be continued research, education, and a thoughtful, honest comparison of long-term surgical outcomes if we are going to continue to improve our care to a growing number of afflicted but active patients.

TABLE 35E.4.
Long-Term Follow-Up and Recurrence of Prolapse After Le Fort Colpocleisis, Partial Colpectomy, and Total Colpectomy

Investigator	Duration of Follow-Up (mo)	No. Available for Follow-Up	Vault[a]	Anterior Wall[a]	Posterior Wall[a]	Unspecified/ Multiple Sites[a]	No. Cured/ Total (%)	Cure Assessment
LEFORT COLPOCLEISIS								
Phaneuf (1935)	NA	20	?/2	0/1	0/0	0/0	17/20 (85)	NA
Adair and DaSef (1936)	3–> 36	38	0/0	0/2	0/0	1/1	35/38 (92)	Objective[b]
Collins and Lock (1941)	1–48	31	0/2	0/0	0/0	0/0	29/31 (94)	Objective[b]
Mazer and Israel (1948)	24–132	38	1/1	0/0	0/0	0/0	37/38 (97)	NA
Wolf (1952)	NA	13	0/0	0/0	0/0	?/1	12/13 (92)	Objective
Falk and Kaufman (1955)	>24	100	0/0	0/2	0/2	0/0	96/100 (96)	Objective
Hanson and Keettel (1969)	≥60	216	3/3	0/1	1/1	0/8	203/216 (94)	Subjective/ Objective
Ridley (1972)	6–60	17	2/3	0/0	0/0	0/0	14/17 (82)	Subjective/ Objective
Ubachs et al. (1973)	≥36	93	2/3	0/0	0/0	0/5	85/93 (91)	Objective
Denehy et al. (1995)	4–40	20	0/0	0/0	0/0	1/1	19/20 (95)	Objective
PARTIAL COLPECTOMY								
Langmade and Oliver (1986)	12–144	102	0/0	0/0	0/0	0/0	102/102 (100)	NA
TOTAL COLPECTOMY								
Phaneuf (1935)	NA	5	0/0	0/0	0/0	0/0	5/5 (100)	NA
Adams (1951)	12–408	30	0/0	0/0	0/0	0/0	30/30 (100)	NA
Anderson and Deasy (1960)	6–12	18	0/0	0/1	0/1	0/0	16/18 (89)	Objective[b]
Ridley (1972)	6–60	41	0/0	0/0	0/0	0/0	41/41 (100)	Subjective/ Objective
Delancey and Morley (1997)	Mean = 35	33	1/1	0/0	0/0	0/0	32/33 (97)	Subjective/ Objective

[a] Number of patients with recurrent prolapse who underwent surgical repair/number of patients with recurrent prolapse.

[b] Extrapolated from text.

NA, Not available.

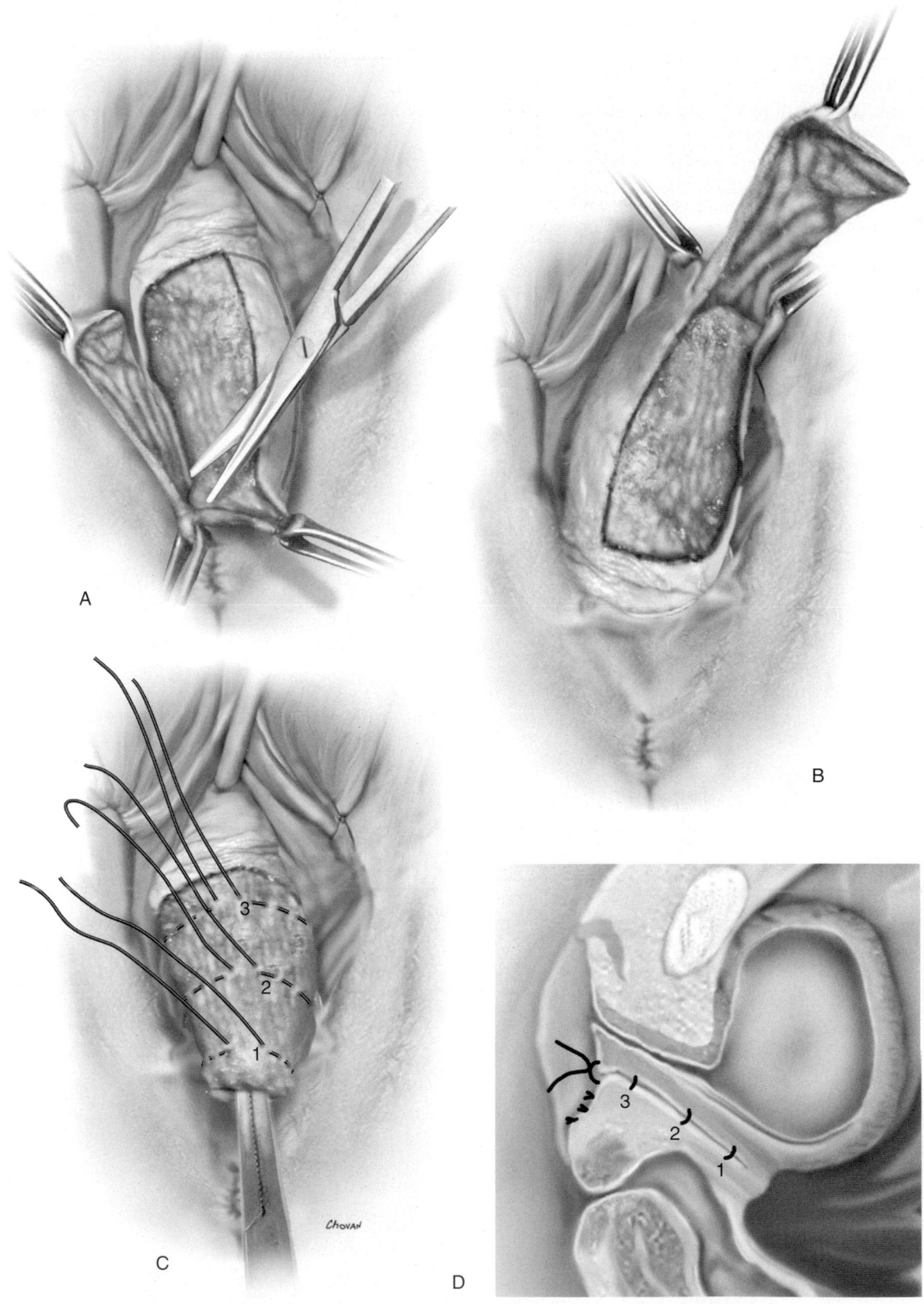

FIGURE 35E.19. Colpectomy and complete colpocleisis. **A and B:** After subcutaneous infiltration with lidocaine or bupivacaine hydrochloride in 1/200,000 epinephrine solution, the vagina is circumscribed by an incision at the site of the hymen and marked into quadrants. Each quadrant is removed by sharp dissection. **C:** Pursestring delayed absorbable sutures are placed. The leading edge of the soft tissue is inverted by the tip of a forceps. Pursestring sutures are tied 1 before 2 and 2 before 3, with progressive inversion of the soft tissue before the tying of each suture. **D:** The final relationship is shown in cross section. A perineorrhaphy is also usually performed. (From Baggish MS, Karram MM. *Atlas of pelvic anatomy and gynecologic surgery.* New York: Saunders, 2001.)

BIBLIOGRAPHY

Adair FL, DaSef L. The LeFort colpocleisis. *Am J Obstet Gynecol* 1936;32:334.

Adams HD. Total colpocleisis for pelvic eventration. *Surg Gynecol Obstet* 1951;2:321.

Addison WA, Livengood CH, Sutton GP, et al. Abdominal sacral colpopexy with Mersilene mesh in the retroperitoneal position in the management of posthysterectomy vaginal vault prolapse and enterocele. *Am J Obstet Gynecol* 1985;153:140–146.

Addison WA, Timmons MC, Wall LL, et al. Failed abdominal sacral colpopexy: observations and recommendations. *Obstet Gynecol* 1989;74(3 Pt 2):480–483.

Alevizon SJ, Finan MA. Sacrospinous colpopexy: management of postoperative pudendal nerve entrapment. *Obstet Gynecol* 1996;88(4 Pt 2):713–715.

Alsultan H, Suzanne F, Mansoor A, et al. Sacral colpopexy by the abdominal route: possible! *J Gynecol Obstet Biol Reprod (Paris)* 1995;24(4):452–453. French.

Anderson GV, Deasy PP. Hysterocolpectomy. *Obstet Gynecol* 1960;16:344.

Backer MH. Success with sacrospinous suspension of the prolapsed vaginal vault. *Surg Gynecol Obstet* 1992;174(5):419–420.

Barksdale PA, Elkins TE, Sanders CK, et al. An anatomic approach to pelvic hemorrhage during sacrospinous ligament fixation of the vaginal vault. *Obstet Gynecol* 1998;91(5 Pt 1):715–718.

Barksdale PA, Gasser RF, Gauthier CM, et al. Intraligamentous nerves as a potential source of pain after sacrospinous ligament fixation of the vaginal apex. *Int Urogynecol J Pelvic Floor Dysfunct* 1997;8(3):121–125.

Bissell D. Fascia lapping as applied to the tissues of the vaginal wall—a misnomer. *Surg Gynecol Obstet* 1929;48:549–550.

Bump RC, Hurt WG, Theofrastous JP, et al. Randomized prospective comparison of needle colposuspension versus endopelvic fascia plication for potential stress incontinence prophylaxis in women undergoing vaginal reconstruction for stage III or IV pelvic organ prolapse. The Continence Program for Women Research Group. *Am J Obstet Gynecol* 1996;175(2):326–333; discussion 333–335.

Cabrera JA, Szekely SJ. Sacrospinous ligament fixation. *Am J Obstet Gynecol* 1990;162(1):295–296.

Cespedes RD. Anterior approach bilateral sacrospinous ligament fixation for vaginal vault prolapse. *Urology* 2000;56(6 Suppl 1):70–75.

Collins CG, Lock FR. The LeFort colpocleisis. *Am J Surg* 1941;53:202.

Colombo M, Milani R. Sacrospinous ligament fixation and modified McCall culdoplasty during vaginal hysterectomy for advanced uterovaginal prolapse. *Am J Obstet Gynecol* 1998;179(1):13–20.

Costantini E, Lombi R, Micheli C, et al. Colposacropexy with Gore-Tex mesh in marked vaginal and uterovaginal prolapse. *Eur Urol* 1998;34(2):111–117.

Cowan W, Morgan HR. Abdominal sacral colpopexy. *Am J Obstet Gynecol* 1980;138(3):348–350.

Cruikshank SH, Cox DW. Sacrospinous ligament fixation at the time of transvaginal hysterectomy. *Am J Obstet Gynecol* 1990;162(6):1611–1615; discussion 1615–1619.

Cundiff GW, Harris RL, Coates K, et al. Abdominal sacral colpoperineopexy: a new approach for correction of posterior compartment defects and perineal descent associated with vaginal vault prolapse. *Am J Obstet Gynecol* 1997;177(6):1345–1353; discussion 1353–1355.

Delaere K, Moonen W, Debruyne F, et al. Hydronephrosis caused by cystocele. Treatment by colpopexy to sacral promontory. *Urology* 1984;24(4):364–365.

DeLancey JOL. Anatomic aspects of vaginal eversion after hysterectomy. *Am J Obstet Gynecol* 1992;166:1717–1728.

DeLancey JOL, Morley GW. Total colpocleisis for vaginal eversion. *Am J Obstet Gynecol* 1997;176:1228.

DeLancey JOL, Starr RA. Histology of the connection between the vagina and levator ani muscles; implications for urinary tract function. *J Reprod Med* 1990;35:765–771.

Delest A, Cosson M, Doutrelant C, et al. Enterocele. Retrospective study of 134 cases: risk factors and comparison between abdominal and perineal routes. *J Gynecol Obstet Biol Reprod (Paris)* 1996;25(5):464–470. French.

Denehy TR, Choe JY, Gregori CA, et al. Modified LeFort partial colpocleisis with Kelly urethral plication and posterior colpoperineoplasty in the medically compromised elderly: a comparison with vaginal hysterectomy, anterior colporrhaphy, and posterior colpoperineoplasty. *Am J Obstet Gynecol* 1995;173:1697.

Derry DE. On the real nature of the so-called "pelvic fascia." *J Anat* 1907;42:7–11.

Diana M, Schettini M. Treatment of vaginal vault prolapse with abdominal sacral colpopexy using Prolene mesh. *Minerva Gynecol* 1999;51(9):349–353.

Diana M, Zoppe C, Mastrangeli B. Treatment of vaginal vault prolapse with abdominal sacral colpopexy using Prolene mesh. *Am J Surg* 2000;179(2):126–128.

Dominguez Vazquez RH, Albarran de Regil CA. Sacrocolpopexy using Mersilene: report of 12 cases at the General Hospital Zone 7, Monclova, Coahuila. *Ginecol Obstet Mex* 1999;67:13–17. Spanish.

Dorsey JH, Sharp HT. Laparoscopic sacral colpopexy and other procedures for prolapse. *Baillieres Clin Obstet Gynaecol* 1995;9(4):749–756.

Falk HC, Kaufman SA. Partial colpocleisis: the LeFort procedure. *Obstet Gynecol* 1955;5:617.

Farrell SA, Scotti RJ, Ostergard DR, et al. Massive evisceration: a complication following sacrospinous vaginal vault fixation. *Obstet Gynecol* 1991;78(3 Pt 2):560–562.

Febbraro W, Beucher G, Von Theobald P, et al. Feasibility of bilateral sacrospinous ligament vaginal suspension with a stapler. Prospective studies with the 34 first cases. *J Gynecol Obstet Biol Reprod (Paris)*.1997;26(8):815–821. French.

Fothergill WE. The supports of the pelvic viscera: a review of some recent contributions to pelvic anatomy, with a clinical introduction. *J Obstet Gynaecol Br Emp* 1908;13:18–28.

Fox SD, Stanton SL. Vault prolapse and rectocele: assessment of repair using sacrocolpopexy with mesh interposition. *Br J Obstet Gynaecol* 2000;107(11):1371–1375.

Funt MI, Thompson JD, Birch H. Normal vaginal axis. *South Med J* 1978;71:1534.

Geomini PM, Brolmann HA, van Binsbergen NJ, et al. Vaginal vault suspension by abdominal sacral colpopexy for prolapse: a follow up study of 40 patients. *Eur J Obstet Gynaecol Reprod Biol* 2001;94(2):234–238.

Given FT, Muhlendorf IK, Browning GM. Vaginal length and sexual function after colpopexy for complete uterovaginal eversion. *Am J Obstet Gynecol* 1993;169(2 Pt 1):284–287; discussion 287–288. Review.

Goff BH. An histological study of the perivaginal fascia in a nullipara. *Surg Gynecol Obstet* 1931;52:32–42.

Goff BH. The surgical anatomy of cystocele and urethrocele with special reference to the pubocervical fascia. *Surg Gynecol Obstet* 1948;87:725–734.

Goldman J, Ovadia J, Feldberg D. The Neugebauer-LeFort operation: a review of 118 partial colpocleises. *Eur J Obstet Gynaecol Reprod Biol* 1985;12:31.

Hale DS, Rogers RM. Abdominal sacrospinous ligament colposuspension. *Obstet Gynecol* 1999;94(6):1039–1041.

Hanson GE, Keettel WC. The Neugebauer-LeFort operation: a review of 288 colpocleisis. *Obstet Gynecol* 1979;34:352.

Harer WB. Round ligament synthetic graft colpopexy. *Obstet Gynecol* 1994;83(6):1064–1066.

Heinonen PK. Transvaginal sacrospinous colpopexy for vaginal vault and complete genital prolapse in aged women. *Acta Obstet Gynecol Scand* 1992;71(5):377–381.

Hemelt BA, Finan MA. Abdominal sacral colpopexy resulting in a retained sponge. A case report. *J Reprod Med* 1999;44(11):983–985.

Hewson AD. Transvaginal sacrospinous colpopexy for posthysterectomy vault prolapse. *Aust N Z J Obstet Gynaecol* 1998;38(3):318–324.

Holley RL, Varner RE, Gleason BP, et al. Recurrent pelvic support defects after sacrospinous ligament fixation for vaginal vault prolapse. *J Am Coll Surg* 1995;180(4):444–448.

Holley RL, Varner RE, Gleason BP, et al. Sexual function after sacrospinous ligament fixation for vaginal vault prolapse. *J Reprod Med* 1996;41(5):355–358.

Hughes GW, Freeman RM. A modification of the technique of sacrospinous ligament fixation. *Br J Obstet Gynaecol* 1995;102(8):669–670.

Iosif CS. Abdominal sacral colpopexy with use of synthetic mesh. *Acta Obstet Gynecol Scand* 1993;72(3):214–217.

Kettel LM, Hebertson RM. An anatomic evaluation of the sacrospinous ligament colpopexy. *Surg Gynecol Obstet* 1989;168(4):318–322.

Kholi N, Sze E, Karram MM. Incidence of recurrent cystocele after transvaginal needle suspension procedures with and without comcomitant anterior colporrhaphy. *Am J Obstet Gynecol* 1996;175(6):1476.

Koster H. On the supports of the uterus. *Am J Obstet Gynecol* 1933;25:67–74.

Kulkarni S. Surgery for post-hysterectomy vaginal prolapse. *West Indian Med J* 1993;52(2):65–67.

Lahr SJ, Lahr CJ, Srinivasan A, et al. Operative management of severe constipation. *Am Surg* 1999;65(12):1117–1121; discussion 1122–1123.

Langmade CF, Oliver JA. Partial colpocleisis. *Am J Obstet Gynecol* 1986;154:1200.

Lansman HH. Posthysterectomy vault prolapse: sacral colpopexy with dura mater graft. *Obstet Gynecol* 1984;63(4):577–582.

Lecuru F, Taurelle R, Clouard C, et al. Surgical treatment of genito-urinary prolapses by abdominal approach. Results in a continuous series of 203 operations. *Ann Chir* 1994;48(11):1013–1019. French.

Lee RA, Symmonds RE. Surgical repair of posthysterectomy vault prolapse. *Am J Obstet Gynecol* 1972;112:953.

Lind LR, Choe J, Bhatia NN. An in-line suturing device to simplify sacrospinous vaginal vault suspension. *Obstet Gynecol* 1997;89(1):129–132.

Mattox TF, Kelly T, Bhatia NN. Modification of the Miya hook in vaginal colpopexy. *J Reprod Med* 1995;40(10):681–683.

Mazor C, Israel SL. The Le Fort colpocleisis: an analysis of 43 operations. *Am J Obstet Gynecol* 1948;56:944.

McCall ML. Posterior culdeplasty. *Obstet Gynecol* 1957;10:595.

Miyazaki FS. Miya hook ligature carrier for sacrospinous ligament suspension. *Obstet Gynecol* 1987;70(2):286–288.

Morley GW. Treatment of uterine and vaginal prolapse. *Clin Obstet Gynecol* 1996;39(4):959–969. Review.

Morley GW, DeLancey JO. Sacrospinous ligament fixation for eversion of the vagina. *Am J Obstet Gynecol* 1988;158(4):872–881.

Nichols DH, Randall CL. *Vaginal surgery,* third ed. Baltimore: Williams & Wilkins, 1989.

Nichols DH. Sacrospinous fixation for massive eversion of the vagina. *Am J Obstet Gynecol* 1982;152:901.

Norton PA. Pelvic floor disorders: the role of fascia and ligaments. *Clin Obstet Gynecol* 1993;36:926–938.

Olsen AL, Smith VJ, Bergstrom JO, et al. Epidemiology of surgically managed pelvic organ prolapse and urinary incontinence. *Obstet Gynecol* 1997;89:501–506.

Ostrzenski A. Laparoscopic colposuspension for total vaginal prolapse. *Int J Gynaecol Obstet* 1996;55(2):147–152.

Ozcan U, Gungor T, Ekin M, et al. Sacrospinous fixation for the prolapsed vaginal vault. *Gynecol Obstet Invest* 1999;47(1):65–68.

Papasakelariou C. Sacrospinous ligament fixation simplified with a new endoscopic suturing device. *J Am Assoc Gynecol Laparosc* 1996;3[Suppl 4]:S38.

Paraiso MF, Ballard LA, Walters MD, et al. Pelvic support defects and visceral and sexual function in woman treated with sacrospinous ligament suspension and pelvic reconstruction. *Am J Obstet Gynecol* 1996;175(6):1523–1530; discussion 1430–1431.

Patsner B. Abdominal sacral colpopexy in patients with gynecologic cancer: report of 25 cases with long-term follow-up and literative review. *Gynecol Oncol* 1999;75(3):504–508.

Patsner B. Mesh erosion into the bladder after abdominal sacral colpopexy. *Obstet Gynecol* 2000;95(6 Pt 2):1029.

Peters WA, Christenson ML. Fixation of the vaginal apex to the coccygeus fascia during repair of vaginal vault eversion with enterocele. *Am J Obstet Gynecol* 1995;172(6):1894–1900; discussion 1900–1902.

Phaneuf LE. The place of colpectomy in the treatment of uterine and vaginal prolapse. *Am J Obstet Gynecol* 1935;30:544.

Pohl JF, Frattarelli JL. Bilateral transvaginal sacrospinous colpopexy: preliminary experience. *Am J Obstet Gynecol* 1997;177(6):1356–1361; discussion 1361–1362.

Porges RF, Smilen SW. Long-term analysis of the surgical management of pelvic support defects. *Am J Obstet Gynecol* 1994;171(6):1518–1526; discussion 1526–1528.

Powell JL, Joseph DB. Abdominal sacral colpopexy for massive genital prolapse. *Prim Care Update Ob Gyns* 1998;5(4):201.

Powell JL, Joseph DB. Abdominal sacral colpopexy in patients with gynecologic cancer and "Burch" not "Birch." *Gynecol Oncol* 2000;77(3):483–484.

Randall C, Nichols D. Surgical treatment of vaginal inversion. *Obstet Gynecol* 1971;38:327.

Raz S, Nitti VW, Bregg KJ. Transvaginal repair of enterocele. *J Urol* 1993;149(4):724–730.

Ricci JV, Lisa JR, Thom CH, et al. The relationship of the vagina to adjacent organs in reconstructive surgery; a histologic study. *Am J Surg* 1947;74:387–410.

Ricci JV, Thom CH. The myth of a surgically useful fascia in vaginal plastic reconstruction. *Q Rev Surg Obstet Gynecol* 1954;2:253–261.

Richardson AC, Edmonds PB, Williams NL. Treatment of stress urinary incontinence due to paravaginal fascial defect. *Obstet Gynecol* 1982;57:357–362.

Richardson AC, Lyon JB, Williams NL. A new look at pelvic relaxation. *Am J Obstet Gynecol* 1976;126:568–573.

Ridley JG. Evaluation of the colpocleisis: a report of fifty-eight cases. *Am J Obstet Gynecol* 1972;113:1114.

Rodau SK, Thomason JL. Vaginal eversion repair. Sacrospinous ligament fixation procedure. *AORN J* 1988;47(2):539, 542–549, 552.

Rose CH, Rowe TF, Cox SM, et al. Uterine prolapse associated with bladder exstrophy: surgical management and subsequent pregnancy. *J Matern Fetal Med* 2000;9(2): 150–152.

Rust JA, Botte JM, Howlett RJ. Prolapse of the vaginal vault. Improved techniques for management of the abdominal approach or vaginal approach. *Am J Obstet Gynecol* 1976;125(6):768–776.

Salvat J, Slamani L, Vincent-Genod A, et al. Sacrospinous ligament fixation by palpation: variation of the Richter procedure. *Eur J Obstet Gynaecol Reprod Biol* 1996;68(1-2):1999–1203.

Sauer HA, Klutke CG. Transvaginal sacrospinous ligament fixation for treatment of vaginal prolapse. *J Urol* 1995; 154(3):1008–1012.

Schettini M, Fortunato P, Gallucci M. Abdominal sacral colpopexy with Prolene mesh. *Int Urogynecol J Pelvic Floor Dysfunct* 1999;10(5):295–299.

Schlesinger RE. Vaginal sacrospinous ligament fixation with the Autosuture Endostitch device. *Am J Obstet Gynecol* 1997;176(6):1358–1362.

Scotti RJ. Repair of genitourinary prolapse in women. *Curr Opin Obstet Gynecol* 1991;3(3):404–412. Review.

Shafik A, el-Sherif M, Youssef A, et al. Surgical anatomy of the pudendal nerve and its clinical implications. *Clin Anat* 1995;8(2):110–115.

Sharp TR. Sacrospinous suspension made easy. *Obstet Gynecol* 1993;82(5):873–875.

Shull BL, Baden WF. A six-year experience with paravaginal defect repair for stress urinary incontinence. *Am J Obstet Gynecol* 1989;160:1432–1435.

Shull BL, Benn SJ, Kuehl TJ. Surgical management of prolapse of the anterior vaginal segment: an analysis of support defects, operative morbidity, and anatomic outcome. *Am J Obstet Gynecol* 1994;171:1429–1439.

Shull BL, Capen CV, Riggs MW, et al. Preoperative and postoperative analysis of site-specific pelvic support defects in 81 women treated with sacrospinous ligament suspension and pelvic reconstruction. *Am J Obstet Gynecol* 1992;166(6 Pt 1):1764–1768; discussion 1768–1771.

Smilen SW, Saini J, Wallach SJ, et al.. The risk of cystocele after sacrospinous ligament fixation. *Am J Obstet Gynecol* 1998;179(6 Pt 1):1465–1471; discussion 1471–1472.

Snyder TE, Krantz KE. Abdominal-retroperitoneal sacral colpopexy for the correction of vaginal prolapse. *Obstet Gynecol* 1991;77(6):944–949.

Steiner RA, Healy JC. Patterns of prolapse in women with symptoms of pelvic floor weakness: magnetic resonance imaging and laparoscopic treatment. *Curr Opin Obstet Gynecol* 1998;10(4):295–301. Review.

Symmonds RE, Pratt JH. Vaginal prolapse following hysterectomy. *Am J Obstet Gynecol* 1960;79:899.

Symmonds RE, Williams TJ, Lee RA, et al: Posthysterectomy enterocele and vaginal vault prolapse. *Am J Obstet Gynecol* 1981;140:852, 2981.

Sze E, Karram MM. Vaginal operation to correct vaginal vault prolapse: a review. *Obstet Gynecol* 1997;89:466–475.

Sze E, Miklos J, Partoll L, Karram MM. Sacrospinous ligament fixation with transvaginal needle suspension for advanced pelvic organ prolapse and stress incontinence. *Obstet Gynecol* 1997;89:94–96.

Sze EH, Miklos JR, Partoll L, et al. Sacrospinous ligament fixation with transvaginal needle suspension for advanced pelvic organ prolapse ans stress incontinence. *Obstet Gynecol* 1997;89(1):94–96.

Thompson JD, Rock JA, eds. *Te Linde's operative gynecology,* seventh ed. Philadelphia: JB Lippincott, 1992: 904–914.

Thompson JR, Gibb JS, Genadry R, et al. Anatomy of pelvic arteries adjacent to the sacrospinous ligament: importance of the coccygeal branch of the inferior gluteal artery. *Obstet Gynecol* 1999;94(6):973–977.

Timmons MC, Addison WA, Addison SB, et al. Abdominal sacral colpopexy in 163 women with posthysterectomy vaginal vault prolapse and enterocele. Evolution of operative techniques. *J Reprod Med* 1992;37(4): 323–327.

Traiman P, De Luca LA, Silva AA, et al. Abdominal colpopexy for complete prolapse of the vagina. *Int Surg* 1992;77(2):91–95.

Ubachs JMH, Van Sante TJ, Schellekens LA. Partial colpocleisis by a modification of Le Fort's operation. *Obstet Gynecol* 1973;42:415.

Uhlenhuth E, Day EC, Smith RD, et al. The visceral endopelvic fascia and hypogastric sheath. *Surg Gynecol Obstet* 1948;86:9–28.

Unger JB. A persistent sinus tract from the vagina to the sacrum after treatment of mesh erosion by partial removal of a Gore-Tex soft tissue patch. *Am J Obstet Gynecol* 1999;181(3):762–763.

Van Lindert AC, Groenendijk AG, Scholten PC, et al. Surgical support and suspension of genital prolapse, including preservation of the uterus, using the Gore-Tex soft tissue patch (a preliminary report). *Eur J Obstet Gynaecol Reprod Biol* 1993;50(2):133–139.

Verdeja AM, Elkins TE, Odoi A, et al. Transvaginal sacrospinous colpopexy: anatomic landmarks to be aware of to minimize complications. *Am J Obstet Gynecol* 1995; 173(5):1468–1469.

Veronikis DK, Nichols DH. Ligature carrier specifically designed for transvaginal sacrospinous colpopexy. *Obstet Gynecol* 1997;89(3):478–481.

Virtanen H, Hirvonen T, Makinen J, et al. Outcome of thirty patients who underwent repair of posthysterectomy prolapse of the vaginal vault with abdominal sacral colpopexy. *J Am Coll Surg* 1994;178(3):283–287.

Wall LL. Abdominal-retroperitoneal sacral colpopexy for the correction of vaginal prolapse. *Obstet Gynecol* 1991;78(4): 724–726.

Wall LL, Hewitt JK. Voiding function after Burch colposuspension for stress incontinence. *J Reprod Med* 1996;41(3):161–165.

Watson JD. Sacrospinous ligament colpopexy: new instrumentation applied to a standard gynecologic procedure. *Obstet Gynecol* 1996;88(5):883–885.

Welgoss JA, Vogt VY, McClellan EJ, et al. Relationship between surgically induced neuropathy and outcome of pelvic organ prolapse surgery. *Int Urogynecol J Pelvic Floor Dysfunct* 1999;10(1):11–14.

White GR. Cystocele: A radical cure by suturing lateral sulci of vagina to white line of pelvic fascia. *JAMA* 1909;21: 1707–1710.

Winters JC, Cespedes RD, Vanlangendonck R. Abdominal sacral colpopexy and abdominal enterocele repair in the management of vaginal vault prolapse. *Urology* 2000;56[Suppl 6]:55–63.

F

The Nonsurgical Management of Pelvic Organ Prolapse: The Use of Vaginal Pessaries

RONY A. ADAM

The surgeon who treats patients with pelvic floor defects should also be familiar with the nonsurgical management of these disorders. Although pelvic organ prolapse prevalence has been and continues to rise steadily, pessary use has previously fallen out of favor, with renewed interest having been noted only recently. Various shapes and sizes allow a variety of pelvic floor defects to be adequately managed without the need for surgery. Vaginal pessaries have been used for the treatment of not only genital prolapse but also urinary incontinence, uterine retroversion, cervical incompetence, and more recently local administration of estrogen. Although both pessaries and pelvic floor muscle exercises have been used for a very long time with an abundance of expert opinion and case reports in the literature, rigorous investigations of these modalities is severely limited. This chapter reviews the primary indications for pessary use, some of the more commonly used pessary types and their proper fitting, subsequent follow-up, and potential complications.

HISTORY

References to female genital prolapse and its treatment can be found as early as 1550 BC in ancient Egyptian writings. Hippocrates (400 BC) prescribed succussion therapy where the patient was hung upside down by her feet and bounced up and down to reduce the prolapsed womb. Hippocrates also advocated inserting half a pomegranate soaked in wine into the vagina. Soranus (98 AD) described using pleasant fumigation around the patient's head to entice the prolapse to ascend, and foul odors near the vagina to force the organ upward. He also described the use of an astringent solution, manual reduction of the prolapse, and insertion of half a pomegranate dipped in vinegar, if succussion therapy failed. Soranos declared that a surgical procedure be undertaken only if the prolapsed uterus was gangrenous.

By the end of the 16th century, various pessaries of brass and waxed cork were used for uterine prolapse. The late 17th century saw a considerable number of medical therapies and pharmaceutical concoctions promoted for the treatment of genital prolapse, which persisted even into the 18th century. In the mid-19th century, the American Medical Association documented 123 differ-

ent pessaries. As the safety of surgical procedures has improved and concerns of adverse consequences of pessaries reported, there has been a tendency during the mid-20th century to use pessaries less in favor of corrective surgery. Modern pessaries are primarily made of silicone and rarely of latex rubber or acrylic. These materials have completely replaced the old Bakelite and hard rubber types used previously. Silicone is advantageous because it is inert, does not absorb secretions or odors, is flexible yet sturdy, and can be autoclaved for resterilization.

INDICATIONS AND CLINICAL CONSIDERATIONS

Cundiff and colleagues reported that 77% of responding members of the American Urogynecologic Society (AUGS) offer pessaries as first-line therapy for pelvic organ prolapse; 12% offer them only to women who are not considered good surgical candidates or to those who refuse surgery. This is in contrast to the distinct impression derived from reading the prevailing expert opinion found in the literature.

Most authors in the literature limit the use of pessaries for pelvic support defects to the patient who is considered a poor surgical candidate or to the elderly. Some advocate pessaries in patients who have prolapse-related vaginal and/or cervical ulcerations and for mucosal hypertrophy. In the AUGS survey, those who described themselves as gynecologists or urologists (as opposed to urogynecologists or obstetrician-gynecologists) were more likely to offer pessaries only to patients who were poor surgical candidates. Those in practice for more than 20 years were found to be less likely to use pessaries as a first-line management option, preferring to limit their use to nonsurgical patients.

Sulak and colleagues, in a retrospective study, reported their experience with 101 patients fitted with pessaries who were available for follow-up. Overall, 50 patients continued pessary use, four were deceased, 26 discontinued pessary and had surgery performed, and 21 had discontinued pessary use but no surgery performed. They found that among patients who were poor surgical candidates and patients who initially refused surgery, those with greater loss of pelvic support tended to continue pessary use, compared with women with milder pelvic support loss. Primary reasons for pessary discontinuation include inconvenience or inadequate relief of symptoms (40%), difficulty in removal (23%), discomfort (13%), patient requesting surgery (13%), pessary fell out (6%), and inability to urinate (5%). Of the 101 patients, 96 were fitted with a Gellhorn pessary. The remainder could not retain the pessary reportedly because of poor perineal support.

Wu and colleagues presented three therapeutic options to patients with symptomatic prolapse: expectant management, surgery, and pessary use. One hundred and ten women opted for and were fitted for pessaries as first-line therapy and were followed up prospectively. Initial fitting was successful in 81 (74%) of these women. These patients tended to be significantly older than those who were not fitted successfully (mean age 66 vs. 59 years of age). Mean parity of those who were successfully fitted initially was lower than for those whose fittings were unsuccessful. A history of pelvic surgery reduced the likelihood of successful initial pessary fitting as did a complaint of stress incontinence. The degree of pelvic organ prolapse did not predict failure of initial fitting, and neither did hormone replacement or the adequacy of the perineal body. In this study, the initial pessary used was a ring or a ring with support in the vast majority of cases (95%), with a cube pessary used for the remaining six patients. No differences were noted in efficacy between the ring with or without support. Following initial successful fitting ($n = 81$), the most common reasons for discontinuation include failure of sustaining pelvic support, urinary incontinence, vaginal discharge, pelvic pain, and vaginal abrasions and erosions. This occurred in 13 (16%) patients with an additional 6 (7.4%) patients lost to follow-up.

Given this information and the lack of additional objective data, the decision to use a pessary as first-line therapy rests with the physician and a well-informed patient. This requires frank discussion with the patient regarding potential risks and benefits of all the proposed management options before making a decision. Evidence suggests that most patients who wish to proceed with pessary use as initial management can be successfully fitted.

CLINICAL EVALUATION

The patient with pelvic floor dysfunction requires careful evaluation by history and physical examination as outlined elsewhere in this text. Important historical considerations include symptoms attributable to prolapse, including pelvic pressure, a sensation that something is falling out or protruding, and voiding and defecatory complaints. The clinical evaluation should be aimed at investigating and quantifying the specific pelvic support defects present in terms of anterior, posterior, and apical compartments. The Pelvic Organ Prolapse—Quantification (POP-Q) is a validated and accepted measure of the degree of pelvic organ prolapse. Testing for occult stress urinary incontinence by provocative ma-

neuvers with the prolapse reduced, using a Sims (or half) speculum, may help identify patients who will suffer from urinary leakage associated with pessary use. This may be helpful in the counseling of such a patient and perhaps in choosing a pessary with better support of the bladder neck to prevent such an undesirable outcome.

Evaluation for the estrogen status of the vaginal mucosa is necessary. The concern for pessary-associated erosion and ulceration in the atrophic vagina leads the vast majority of surveyed AUGS members (94%) to recommend concurrent estrogen replacement therapy in the absence of contraindications. Wu and colleagues reported that the incidence of vaginal abrasions increased as the vaginal epithelium exhibited more atrophy. Furthermore, those who experienced vaginal abrasions were more likely to discontinue pessary use.

TYPES OF PESSARIES

There have been hundreds of pessaries described throughout the ages. Currently, however, less than 20 pessary types are used for prolapse. Some types have been further modified for the nonsurgical management of stress urinary incontinence by increasing support to the bladder neck (Fig. 35F.1).

Of responding AUGS members, 78% tailored their choice of pessary type to the specific pelvic support defect. Of the members who reported using the same pessary for all types of prolapse, the ring was the most commonly used. Most respondents (59%) considered a weak pelvic diaphragm and only 44% considered a prior hysterectomy as important in the choice of pessary—generally favoring a space-occupying, rather than a supportive pessary in each of these circumstances. The supportive pessaries were defined as those that were derived by a spring mechanism (ring, Gehrung, lever-type pessaries) and reportedly supported by the symphysis pubis. The space-filling pessaries were defined as supported by the creation of suction between the pessary and the vaginal walls (e.g., cube) or by providing a diameter larger than the genital hiatus (donut, InflatoBall, Shaatz), or by both mechanisms (Gellhorn). Although these categories clearly simplify the analysis of data, such a functional classification has not been studied. It is unclear whether the mechanistic differences inferred by such a classification are indeed valid.

The AUGS survey shows that the ring pessary is the most commonly used, both among physicians who tailor their pessary choice based on the support defects present and those who use the same pessary for all types of prolapse (Table 35F.1). It is unclear whether this choice is related to perceived efficacy or to issues related to ease of management, patient acceptability, the patient's ability to remove the pessary, or other considerations.

Ring Pessary

The hinged spring circumference of the silicone-coated ring pessary allows for its compression in one direction,

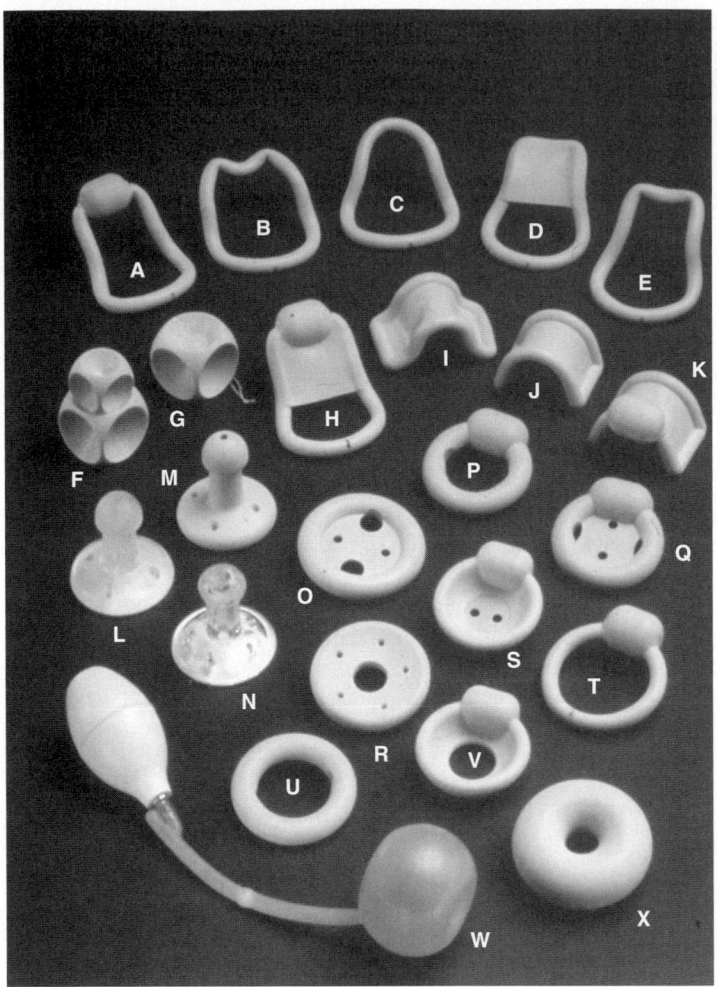

FIGURE 35F.1. Types of pessaries. A, Hodge with knob (silicone); B, Risser (silicone); C, Smith (silicone); D, Hodge with support; E, Hodge (silicone); F, Tandem-Cube (silicone); G, Cube (silicone); H, Hodge with support plus knob (silicone); I, Regula (silicone); J, Gehrung (silicone); K, Gehrung with knob (silicone); L, Gelhorn 95% rigid (silicone); M, Gelhorn flexible (silicone); N, Gellhorn rigid (silicone); O, Ring with support (silicone); P, Ring with knob (silicone); Q, Ring with support plus knob (silicone); R, Shaatz (silicone); S, Incontinence dish with support (silicone); T, Ring incontinence (silicone); U, Ring (silicone); V, Incontinence dish (silicone); W, InflatoBall (latex); X, Donut (silicone).

which makes for ease of insertion. These pessaries are similar in appearance to the contraceptive diaphragm, and may thus be more familiar and therefore acceptable to patients. It is recommended that once inserted behind the symphysis pubis, the ring be turned 90 degrees. The

TABLE 35F.1.
Vaginal Support Devices

Type	Sizes Available	Most Common Sizes	Number of Sizes
Gellhorn	1½–3½ in	2¼–3 in	9
Shaatz	1½–3½ in	2¼–3 in	9
Donut	2–3¾ in	2½–3¼	8
Inflatoball	S to XL	M, L	4
Ring and Ring with Support	0–13	3–6	14
Cube	0–7	2–4	8
Gehrung	0–9	3–5	10
Hodge	0–9	2–4	10
Smith	0–8	2–4	9
Risser	0–9	2–4	10

S, small; M, medium; L, Large; XL, extra large.

ring with support may provide additional support to a mild anterior vaginal defect, and it prevents the rare complication of an incarcerated herniated cervix through the open ring. The ring pessary is amenable for self-removal and insertion by the patient. It may be worn during coitus.

Donut Pessary

The silicone donut-shaped pessary may be used for higher degrees of prolapse. It is supported by the levator muscles and fills the upper vagina completely. It is, therefore, considered appropriate for the management of uterovaginal and vaginal vault prolapse. Insertion through the introitus is in the vertical plane, and the pessary is turned to a horizontal plane when inserted beyond the levator plate. It tends to be difficult for patients to remove this type of pessary by themselves. Coitus is not usually possible with this type of pessary.

The InflatoBall is a variant of the donut pessary. Made of latex rubber, it can be easily inserted and removed when deflated. When inflated, by use of a manual pump, it sits above the levator plate much like the donut pessary, with the valve stem tucked in the vagina (Fig. 35F.2). Because it is made of latex and therefore absorbs

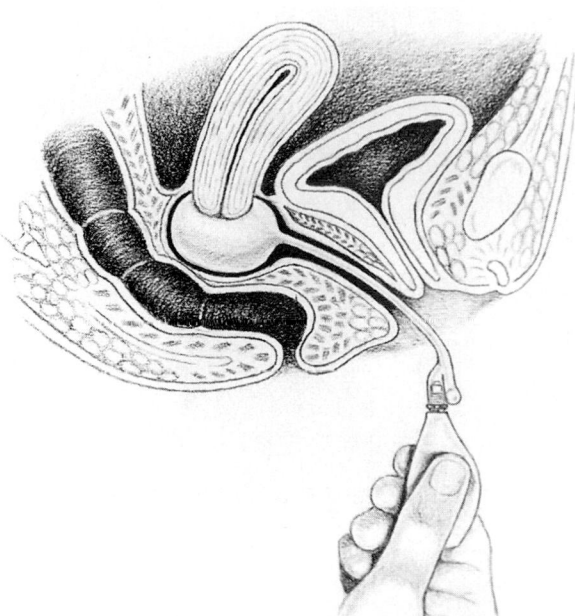

FIGURE 35F.2. InflatoBall pessary being inflated.

secretions and odors, the InflatoBall should be removed and cleaned every 1 to 2 nights and reinserted in the morning.

Gellhorn Pessary

The Gellhorn is useful in patients with severe degrees of uterovaginal or vaginal vault prolapse. Support derives from the base that sits above the levator plate and the stem that rests upon the distal posterior vagina and perineum (Fig. 35F.3). An adequate perineal body is considered by some to be important for the effectiveness of this pessary, whereas others believe that suction from the concave base contributes to its support. This pessary is somewhat difficult for patients to manage themselves. The Gellhorn pessary does not allow comfortable coitus because of its shape.

Shaatz Pessary

The Shaatz has a shape similar to that of the Gellhorn but has no stem. This may facilitate coitus in some patients. Self-management of this pessary is possible.

Cube Pessary

The concave walls of the cube pessary create suction and therefore adhere to the vaginal sidewalls. This results in effective support for severe uterovaginal or vaginal vault prolapse, but can potentially cause ulceration and erosion of the vaginal mucosa. It is therefore necessary to remove this pessary nightly. This is achieved by inserting fingers between the pessary and the vaginal walls to release the suction and grasp the pessary itself before pulling it out of the vagina.

Gehrung Pessary

The arch-shaped Gehrung pessary has a pliable metal frame that allows the pessary to be shaped to the patient's dimensions. The heels of the pessary rest upon the lateral aspects of the posterior vagina with the distal arch positioned behind the symphysis pubis (Fig. 35F.4). This underutilized pessary is effective in managing anterior and mild posterior compartment defects. Its shape makes this pessary somewhat difficult to insert, but also allows for intercourse.

Lever Pessaries

All lever pessaries in use today are modifications of the original Hodge pessary. The Smith modification is designed to fit a narrow pubic arch, whereas the Risser fits the wider pubic arch. The major function of these pessaries is the management of a retrodisplaced uterus. It has been proposed in the treatment of mild anterior and/or posterior compartment defects, as well as cervical incompetence during pregnancy. It is also useful in the management and workup of urinary incontinence. When placing a lever pessary in a patient with uterine retrodisplacement, the uterus must be first manually anteverted (Fig. 35F.5). Lever pessaries can be worn during intercourse and may be self-managed.

Incontinence Pessaries

Many of the previously described pessaries have undergone additional modification to manage concurrent stress urinary incontinence. This usually involves the addition of a knob that is positioned under the urethra to help prevent its descent. These pessaries and the Introl device, which is solely designed for treatment of stress incontinence, may be somewhat uncomfortable and occasionally cause voiding dysfunction. These issues are discussed in Chapter 36.

INITIAL FITTING

Pessary fittings are by trial and error. It is possible to achieve a good approximation regarding proper fit by digital measurement of the genital hiatus (width) and vaginal length (depth). Several sizes and pessary types should be available to facilitate a proper fit (Table 35F.1). A small amount of water-soluble lubricant on the leading edge of the pessary facilitates insertion. A well-fitting pessary should be comfortable to wear and should be retained despite ambulation and straining. Digital palpation around the periphery ensures that a finger can be easily inserted in between the pessary and vagina. The distal portion of the pessary rests behind the symphysis, or on the perineal body, depending on the pessary type. It should also allow for adequate emptying of the bladder, which can be assessed by measurement of spontaneous voided volume (with or without uroflowmetry) followed by a postvoid residual measurement (by catheterization or ultrasound).

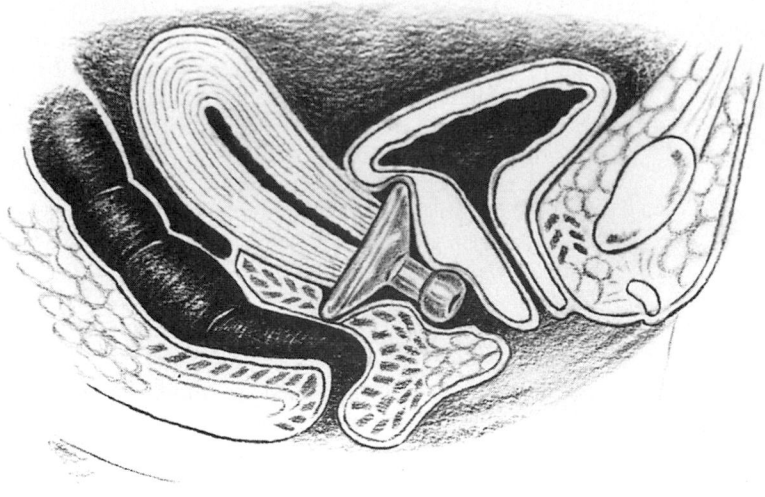

FIGURE 35F.3. Gellhorn placement.

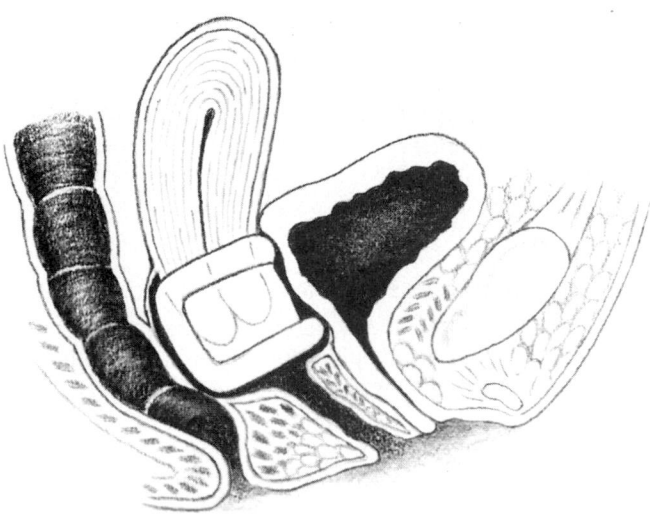

FIGURE 35F.4. Gehrung pessary in place.

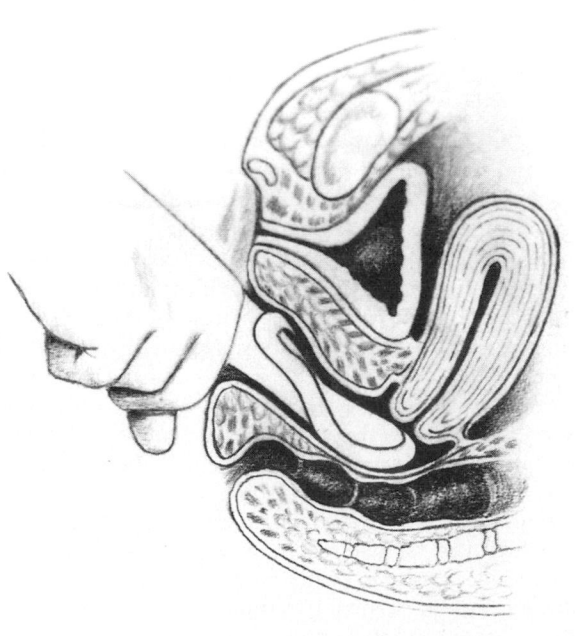

FIGURE 35F.5. Finger guiding the posterior bar of the lever pessary behind the cervix into the posterior fornix. Note the anteverted position of the uterus.

FOLLOW-UP

Although adequate follow up is essential given the nature of pessaries, there is considerable difference of opinion regarding optimal intervals. In the AUGS survey, there appeared to be no consistent trend in the regimens used. This is mostly likely due to the survey's failure to ask questions regarding specific pessaries and their follow-up. Similarly, a majority of those surveyed reported teaching all their patients how to change their pessaries themselves. However, these data were also not type specific. With the exception of the cube and InflatoBall pessaries, it appears possible to safely monitor patients by pessary removal and vaginal inspection by the physician (or well-trained nurse) at 3-month intervals, perhaps longer if the patient is adept at managing her own pessary and removes it regularly. Patients should be instructed to call or come in for a checkup if any warning symptoms or signs occur.

At each follow-up visit the patient should be asked about symptoms such as vaginal bleeding, malodorous discharge, pain, and discomfort. Any voiding difficulty with the pessary in place should be elicited, as should any symptoms or signs of urinary tract infection. Appropriate diagnostic tests should be performed if any abnormal symptoms are present.

At the set intervals determined by the patient and her care provider, the pessary is palpated to verify proper positioning. It is then gently removed with the aid of a water-soluble lubricant, and the vaginal and cervical surfaces are carefully inspected for any signs of erosion or abrasion. Suspicious lesions should be carefully inspected and biopsy considered. If the patient is satisfied with her pessary, it is reinserted if the inspection is negative. Voiding function can be assessed with the pessary in place if there is a concern regarding voiding function or urinary tract infection has occurred since the last follow-up visit.

A newly noted vaginal erosion may present a clinical dilemma in that prolapse-associated erosion is considered by some an indication for pessary use rather than a contraindication. If, however, such an erosion or serious abrasion is diagnosed after pessary insertion, but was not present before, relief of the mechanical pressures exerted by the pessary is indicated by withholding its use for 2 to 3 weeks. Use of local estrogen during this period facilitates further healing. This can be given as $\frac{1}{4}$ to $\frac{1}{2}$ applicator of estrogen cream applied intravaginally two to three times a week. If infectious vaginitis is noted, appropriate antibiotics should be prescribed. Following mucosal healing, replacement with the same or a slightly smaller pessary, or trying a different type altogether is a reasonable management option. Suspicious vaginal lesions should always be biopsied.

COMPLICATIONS

Most commonly, a discharge and odor develop with continued wearing of a vaginal pessary. In a preliminary study by Alnaif and Drutz, bacterial vaginosis was found more commonly in pessary users, with an odds ratio of 4.37.

Mucosal erosion and abrasions of the vagina and/or cervix are more common with cube and Gellhorn pessaries. They are also more likely in patients who do not remove and reinsert their own pessary, as well as in women with untreated vaginal atrophy. Recurrent erosions despite multiple attempts at pessary fitting with an adequately estrogenized vagina should prompt discontinuation of this mode of therapy. Pessary incarceration within the vagina with formation of vaginal adhesions has been described. Removal is facilitated by application of estrogen cream for several days.

Although rare, serious complications have been reported, mainly with the pessary that has been neglected, sometimes for many years. These include infections, fistulas, and even complete erosion with transmigration of the pessary into the bladder or the rectum. Herniation and incarceration of the cervix, and even small bowel, through neglected ring pessaries have been described. Unilateral and bilateral hydronephrosis with urosepsis and even uremia have also been reported.

Chronic irritation associated with prolonged, uninterrupted pessary use has been associated with vaginal cancer. The literature is comprised of case reports that do not allow concluding a causal relationship between pessary use and vaginal cancer. It appears to be more likely in the patient with a neglected pessary for many years, and perhaps with older pessaries made of rubber. Pessaries used in practice today are mostly made of inert medical grade silicone, which may reduce the risk of vaginal cancer further.

CONCLUSION

Although vaginal pessaries have been used throughout the millennia, their use has not been intensely studied. They remain a useful alternative either as initial management or reserved for those patients who are otherwise not candidates or desirous of surgery. Pessary types may, at the discretion of the physician, be chosen for specific pelvic support defects. Although follow-up regimens may be individualized, adequate follow-up and treatment of vaginal atrophy are important to prevent the minor and major complications that can be associated with pessary use.

BIBLIOGRAPHY

Alnaif B, Drutz HP. Bacterial vaginosis increases in pessary users. *Int Urogynecol J* 2000;11:219.

Bash KL. Review of vaginal pessaries. *Obstet Gynecol Surv* 2000;55:455.

Benson RC. *Pessaries: past and present.* Presented at the Postgraduate Course in Obstetrics and Gynecology. Iowa City, Iowa, 1959.

Bhatia NN, Bergman A, Gunning JE. Urodynamic effects of a vaginal pessary in women with stress urinary incontinence. *Am J Obstet Gynecol* 1983;147:876.

Chow SH, LaSalle MD, Rosenberg GS. Urinary incontinence secondary to vaginal pessary. *Urology* 1997;49:458.

Christ ML, Haja J. Cytologic changes associated with vaginal pessary use. With special reference to the presence of actinomyces. *Acta Cytol* 1978;22:146.

Cundiff GW, Weidner AC, Visco AG, et al. A survey of pessary use by members of the American Urogynecologic Society. *Obstet Gynecol* 2000;95:931.

Dasgupta P, Booth CM. Uraemia due to ureteric obstruction of a solitary kidney by a vaginal ring pessary. *Scand J Urol Nephrol* 1996;30:493.

Davila GW. Vaginal prolapse: management with nonsurgical techniques. *Postgrad Med* 1996;99:171.

Duncan LE, Foltzer M, O'Hearn M. Unilateral hydronephrosis, pyelonephritis and bacteremia caused by a neglected vaginal ring pessary. *J Am Geriatr Soc* 1997;45:1413.

Emge LA, Durfee RB. Pelvic organ prolapse: four thousand years of treatment. *Clin Obstet Gynecol* 1966;9:997.

Fritzinger KB, Newman DK, Dinkin E. Use of a pessary for the management of pelvic organ prolapse. *Lippincotts Prim Care Pract* 1997;1:431.

Goldstein I, Wise GJ, Tancer ML. A vesicovaginal fistula and intravesical foreign body. A rare case of the neglected pessary. *Am J Obstet Gynecol* 1990;163:589.

Greenhill JP. The non-surgical management of vaginal relation. *Clin Obstet Gynecol* 1972;4:1083.

Jay GD, Kinkead T, Hopkins T, et al. Obstructive uropathy from uterine prolapse: a preventable problem in the elderly. *J Am Geriatr Soc* 1992;40:1156.

Meinhardt W, Schuitemaker NWE, Smeets MJGH, et al. Bilateral hydronephrosis with urosepsis due to neglected pessary. *Scand J Urol Nephrol* 1993;27:419.

Merino MJ. Vaginal cancer: the role of infectious and environmental factors. *Am J Obstet Gynecol* 1991;165:1255.

Morley GW. Treatment of uterine and vaginal prolapse. *Clin Obstet Gynecol* 1996;39:959.

Ott R, Richter H, Behr J, et al. Small bowel prolapse and incarceration caused by a vaginal ring pessary. *Br J Surg* 1993;80:1157.

Poma PA. Management of incarcerated vaginal pessaries. *J Am Geriatr Soc* 1981;29:325.

Poma PA. Nonsurgical management of genital prolapse: a review and recommendations for clinical practice. *J Reprod Med* 2000;45:789.

Rachagan SP, Sinnathurary TA. The neglected ring pessary. *Asia-Oceania J Obstet Gynecol* 1986;12:75.

Roberge RJ, McCandlish MM, Dorfsman ML. Urosepsis associated with vaginal pessary use. *Ann Emerg Med* 1999;33:58.

Russell JK. The dangerous vaginal pessary. *BMJ* 1961;2:1595.

Schraub S, Sun XS, Maingon P, et al. Cervical and vaginal cancer associated with pessary use. *Cancer* 1992;69:2505.

Sulak PJ, Kuehl TJ, Shull BL. Vaginal pessaries and their use in pelvic relaxation. *J Reprod Med* 1993;38:

Wu V, Farrell SA, Baskett TF, et al. A simplified protocol for pessary management. *Obstet Gynecol* 1997;90:990.

Zeitlin MP, Lebherz TB. Pessaries in the geriatric patient. *J Am Geriatr Soc* 1992;40:635.

Te Linde's Operative Gynecology, ninth edition, edited by John A. Rock and Howard W. Jones, III. Lippincott Williams & Wilkins, Philadelphia © 2003.

CHAPTER
36

▼

Urinary Stress Incontinence

L. LEWIS WALL

Urinary incontinence has been defined by the International Continence Society as a condition in which involuntary loss of urine is a social or hygienic problem that is objectively demonstrable. Urinary incontinence is a particular medical problem for women because it is twice as prevalent among them as it is among men. Although involuntary urine loss is not a normal part of aging, it often becomes a clinical problem for the aging woman as the trauma of childbirth, the development of acute and chronic illnesses, and the loss of estrogenic stimulation at menopause weaken pelvic support and diminish the amount of normal homeostatic reserve available to cope with stresses placed on the bladder. At the consensus development conference on adult urinary incontinence in October 1988, the National Institutes of Health conservatively estimated the monetary costs of managing adult incontinence at $10.3 billion per year. By 1995, researchers estimated that the annual direct cost of urinary incontinence had reached $16.3 billion, with female incontinence accounting for $12.4 billion of this amount. The total societal cost of urinary incontinence was estimated by Wagner and Hu at $26.3 billion dollars for individuals over the age of 65. As our population grows older, and particularly as the women of the postwar "Baby Boom" generation reach menopause, the problem of urinary incontinence will occupy an increasingly larger place in gynecologic practice. Olsen and colleagues have demonstrated that an American woman has an 11.1% lifetime risk of requiring surgery for incontinence or prolapse by the age of 80, and nearly one third

of those women will require a second operation. Based on Census Bureau data and current levels of demand, Luber and coworkers have projected that the need for care for pelvic floor disorders (of which urinary incontinence is a major component) will increase twice as fast as the increase in population over the next 30 years. We do not yet have the resources in place to meet these needs. We must be ready to meet the medical and surgical challenges that this will present.

Urinary incontinence can be divided into two broad categories based on the route of urine loss (Table 36.1). *Extraurethral incontinence* refers to urine loss that occurs through an abnormal opening between the urinary tract and the outside, such as through a congenital defect or fistula. However, urinary incontinence occurs through the urethral lumen more typically. The most common form of *transurethral urinary incontinence* in women is stress incontinence. In this condition, urine loss occurs during periods of increased intraabdominal pressure, such as sneezing, coughing, or exercise, and results from incompetent closure of the urethra and bladder neck. A community survey of 1,060 randomly selected women more than 18 years of age in South Wales found that 22% of women had this complaint. In a survey of 144 collegiate female varsity athletes, Nygaard found that 27% complained of stress incontinence while participating in their sports. The activities most likely to produce urinary loss were jumping, high-impact landings, and running. Even in otherwise fit and vigorous women, the continence mechanism is particularly susceptible to stress incontinence.

TABLE 36.1.
Causes of Female Urinary Incontinence

EXTRAURETHRAL INCONTINENCE

Congenital
    Ectopic ureter
    Bladder exstrophy
Acquired (fistula)
    Ureteral
    Vesical
    Urethral
    Complex combinations

TRANSURETHRAL INCONTINENCE

Urethral sphincter incompetence (genuine stress incontinence)
    Incontinence caused by anatomic urethral hypermobility and loss of support
    Incontinence caused by intrinsic sphincteric deficiency
    Combination
Detrusor overactivity
    Idiopathic detrusor instability
    Neuropathic detrusor overactivity
    Detrusor hyperreflexia
    Reflex incontinence
Mixed incontinence (urethral sphincter incompetence and detrusor overactivity)
Urinary retention with bladder distention and overflow incontinence
    Genuine stress incontinence
    Detrusor hyperactivity with impaired contractility
    Combinations
Urethral diverticulum
Congenital urethral abnormalities (e.g., epispadias)
Uninhibited urethral relaxation (urethral instability)
Functional and transient incontinence

Urine loss in women also can occur for many reasons other than stress-related sphincteric failure. The most common of these other causes is uninhibited contractions of the bladder muscle (detrusor overactivity). When these detrusor contractions are caused by a neurologic lesion, such as multiple sclerosis or a cerebrovascular accident, the condition is called *detrusor hyperreflexia*. The term *reflex incontinence* is used to refer to hyperreflexia that occurs in spinal cord–injured patients, in whom involuntary urine loss occurring without urgency or a conscious need to urinate is precipitated by abnormal reflex activity. It is called idiopathic detrusor overactivity when no obvious neurologic reason for detrusor overactivity can be found.

A variety of other conditions also can cause transurethral urinary incontinence, including uninhibited urethral relaxation (urethral instability), overflow incontinence, urethral diverticula, congenital abnormalities, and functional disorders of urinary control. Patients who have acontractile or poorly functioning bladders can become incontinent when the bladder is overdistended. This is referred to often as *overflow incontinence*. In this situation, urine loss can occur for a variety of reasons. If the bladder is stretched to its physiologic limits, it loses its distensibility and develops increasing pressure owing to lowered compliance. This can increase intravesical pressure enough to overcome bladder outlet resistance, particularly if the patient coughs. In this situation, urine loss results from a combination of stress incontinence and low bladder compliance. Alternatively, the increasing bladder volume can trigger a detrusor contraction, which results in urine loss. In some patients, the detrusor contractions generated under these conditions are enough to cause incontinence but not enough to allow complete bladder emptying. These patients have increased residual urine in the presence of detrusor overactivity, a condition that has been called *detrusor hyperactivity with impaired contractility*. These conditions explain why measurement of the postvoid residual is an important part of the evaluation of any patient with urinary incontinence.

Urethral diverticula can cause incontinence by trapping urine during normal micturition and releasing it unexpectedly during other activities. Congenital abnormalities of the urethra, such as epispadias, can result in incontinence from sphincteric incompetence. Functional urinary incontinence can occur in patients with decreased mobility or debilitating diseases, such as arthritis; for example, if the patient is unable to walk quickly enough to a toilet and undo her clothing when the need to urinate arises. Changes in the living conditions and social environments of these patients may restore continence without significant medical or surgical intervention. Other miscellaneous conditions, such as untreated urinary tract infections, drugs, or the acute confusion associated with delirium, can cause transient urinary incontinence that may be cured by appropriate medical treatment. This is particularly important in elderly patients, in whom decreased physiologic reserve accounts for a greater risk for incontinence from such insults.

In summary, urinary incontinence is a *symptom*, not a diagnosis; the incontinent patient deserves an appropriate investigation before the start of treatment.

FUNDAMENTAL INVESTIGATIONS

A complete evaluation of the incontinent patient has six basic components.

1. A complete urinalysis and urine culture
2. A thorough history
3. A careful physical examination
4. Measurement of the residual urine volume after voiding
5. A frequency–volume bladder chart
6. Urodynamic testing

Although urinalysis serves as a screening test for many relevant metabolic and urinary tract disorders, a urine culture is essential to rule out infection in any patient with urinary tract symptoms. Failure to rule out infection can lead the clinician down the wrong track. Not to perform a urine culture on an incontinent patient before embarking on a series of sophisticated urodynamic investigations is akin to starting a workup for amenorrhea without checking to see if the patient is pregnant! When possible, infection should be eliminated before proceeding further with the evaluation of incontinence. The presence of unusual organisms, infections that persist after appropriate treatment, "sterile" pyuria, or other microscopic abnormalities provides reason to pursue a more extensive investigation of the upper urinary tract.

History

A careful review of the patient's history of incontinence allows the physician to determine the nature of the patient's complaint and its severity, helping to guide further investigations in appropriate directions. An adequate history should include the chief complaint (e.g., urine loss with coughing), its duration (e.g., since the birth of the patient's last child 5 years ago), any special circumstances or precipitating causes (e.g., associated change in medication, association with an acute illness such as bronchitis or stroke), and its progression (e.g., worsening rapidly during the past 3 months). Previous attempts at therapy, either medical or surgical, should be elicited, and some idea of the severity of the complaint obtained. The emotional distress reported by the patient does not correlate well with the amount of urine loss that can be demonstrated. Some women are distraught at a tiny amount of urinary leakage occurring during vigorous exercise, such as playing tennis; others tolerate wearing two or three incontinence pads per day with only minor complaints. Many patients feel that urinary incontinence is shameful and avoid seeking help because of their embarrassment. This can result in years of needless suffering. A solicitous inquiry about the presence of urinary incontinence during routine care may allow the patient to discuss this problem and avoid unnecessary delay in treatment.

Although the physiology of bladder function is still incompletely understood, in practical terms, the bladder has only two functions: to store urine and then to empty it completely at a socially acceptable time and place. This process involves a complex interplay of afferent sensory messages and efferent motor discharges modulated and directed by an intact nervous system. The bladder is an involuntary organ that is nonetheless under voluntary control; therefore, it is a unique entity, and the complex interplay between the cerebral cortex and bladder makes symptoms difficult to evaluate. This is not only because symptoms can have multiple causes but also because the patient frequently presents an interpretation of her symptoms in the guise of the symptoms themselves. However, these symptoms generally are referable to one of four major problems: (a) incontinence or problems with urine storage; (b) voiding difficulty or problems emptying the bladder; (c) problems with bladder sensation, such as pain or lack of bladder sensation; or (d) disorders of bladder contents, such as stones or hematuria (Table 36.2).

TABLE 36.2.
Classification of Lower Urinary Tract Symptoms

SYMPTOMS OF STORAGE DISORDERS

Stress incontinence
Urge incontinence
Mixed incontinence
Frequency
Nocturia
Nocturnal enuresis

SYMPTOMS OF ABNORMAL EMPTYING

Hesitancy
Straining to void
Incomplete emptying
Poor flow
Intermittent stream
Incomplete emptying
Postmicturition dribbling
Acute urinary retention

SYMPTOMS OF ABNORMAL BLADDER SENSATION

Urgency
Dysuria
Pain
Pressure
Decreased sensation

ABNORMAL BLADDER CONTENTS

Abnormal color
Abnormal smell
Hematuria
Pneumaturia
Stones
Foreign bodies
Miscellaneous

Failure to store urine leads to incontinence. Urinary frequency is the number of times per day that the patient voids. By convention, more than seven voids per day suggests a problem with frequency, but this is highly dependent on habit and fluid intake. Patients are notoriously inaccurate in estimating urinary frequency and should be encouraged to keep a frequency–volume bladder chart, or "urinary diary," for several days as part of their initial evaluation. The volume of each void should be measured and recorded, along with the time at which voiding occurred. The time and amount of all fluid intake also can be noted if desired. It is especially useful to have the patient record any episodes of incontinence and the circumstances under which these occurred (e.g., with sneezing, with urgency, while washing dishes). Patients often are surprised at the patterns revealed by their bladder charts, and the process of such record keeping plays a useful role in later bladder retraining programs. Approximate normal values for urine output are provided in Table 36.3. Frequency and urgency accompanied by high urine output, for example, may represent compul-

TABLE 36.3.
Approximate Normal Values for Daily Urine Output in Women

Parameter	Value
Total urine output in 24 h	1,500–2,500 mL
Daytime frequency of urination	7–8 voids
Nocturia	0–1 void
Average voided volume	250 mL
Largest voided volume (functional bladder capacity)	400–600 mL

sive water drinking rather than a basic fault with bladder physiology. Nocturia is defined as awakening from sleep with the need to urinate. If this occurs more than once per night, it may represent an abnormality, although nocturia is highly dependent on patient age and normally increases with advancing age. Urge incontinence refers to urine loss accompanied by a powerful desire to urinate (urgency). Urgency can result from detrusor overactivity (motor urgency), but it also can be associated with inflammatory bladder disorders and other causes of sensory urgency. It is important to differentiate urgency owing to urinary leakage or fear of leakage from urgency owing to pain or fear of pain. The former is more likely caused by detrusor overactivity; the latter is more likely caused by a sensory disorder. The symptom of stress incontinence refers to urine loss under conditions of increased intraabdominal pressure. This can be caused by urethral and bladder neck incompetence, but urine loss during physical exertion is sometimes also produced by detrusor contractions triggered by movement or changes of position.

Voiding difficulty in women has many causes, but only rarely is it caused by true outflow obstruction. Trouble starting the stream of urine (hesitancy), straining to void, and poor or intermittent flow can all reflect either urethral or detrusor dysfunction. Postmicturition dribbling can be a clue to the presence of a urethral diverticulum. Acute urinary retention is manifested as an inability to void that requires catheterization and results in the drainage of a large volume of urine. Although this can be psychological in origin, it also may represent serious underlying pathology. In such cases, a thorough diagnostic evaluation should be carried out before any woman is given the diagnosis of "hysterical" urinary retention.

Symptoms of disordered bladder sensation are the most difficult to evaluate because they are entirely subjective. Urgency, dysuria, and bladder pain all can accompany acute urinary tract infection, inflammatory bladder disorders such as interstitial cystitis, psychosomatic reactions to stress, or neoplasia. Feelings of pressure in the lower pelvis may represent the effects of a large prolapse or other gynecologic pathology, such as a large ovarian tumor or fibroid uterus. Often, such symptoms have no obvious explanation. A lack of bladder sensation or unconscious and unnoticed urine loss is worrisome because it may represent underlying neurologic disease.

Complaints of unusual urine are common and often are difficult to interpret. The patient may notice an unexpected change in the color or smell of her urine, for example. Such changes can be the result of recent dietary indiscretion or the normal mechanism of urine concentration at work in the kidneys, but they also can represent underlying metabolic disease, infection, or something more sinister. Hematuria in particular requires careful evaluation by urinary cytology, culture, cystoscopy, and urography, particularly if it is not related to an acute infection that clears promptly with appropriate antibiotic therapy. Gross hematuria is related to urinary tract malignancy in 22% of patients, and persistent microscopic hematuria also is associated with a neoplasm or other significant urologic lesion in more than 20% of cases. Urinary tract stones and foreign bodies that have been introduced into the bladder also can present in a myriad of ways. Therefore, it is clear that, although symptoms provide clues to the diagnostic possibilities and help point further investigations in certain directions, symptoms need some kind of objective confirmation before embarking on a course of therapy (e.g., surgery) that poses potentially significant risks for the patient. Nearly 30 years ago, Hodgkinson and colleagues estimated that between one third and one half of all "failures" in surgery for stress incontinence were caused by preoperative misdiagnosis. Surgical failure caused by an inadequate preoperative evaluation should not be tolerated.

An appropriate history also must include a review of previous attempts at therapy, including surgical procedures and their results, and any medications used in treating bladder disorders. Many medical conditions can affect bladder function, and a neurologic history is especially important in this regard. For example, diabetes and diseases requiring long-term corticosteroid use can impair wound healing if surgery is undertaken. Medications taken for apparently unrelated conditions can have a significant impact on bladder function. Tricyclic antidepressants, for example, have anticholinergic side effects that can precipitate voiding difficulty. Antihypertensive medications can create the opposite problem. The α-blockers (e.g., prazosin) that often are used in treating hypertension can cause drug-induced stress incontinence by relaxing the urethra and bladder neck; ACE-inhibitors sometimes produce a drug-induced cough that can cause stress incontinence.

Physical Examination

Physical examination of the incontinent patient encompasses three areas: a general physical examination, a neurologic screening examination with special emphasis on the lower extremities and perineal area, and the urogynecologic examination. The general physical condition of the patient should be evaluated, with special regard to her mobility, mental status, general level of activity, and potential fitness to undergo an operative procedure. The healthy 40-year-old woman with an active life style and mild stress incontinence requires a different management strategy from the 85-year-old, demented, bedridden nursing home patient with continuous urinary leakage. Transient urinary incontinence is a particular problem among elderly patients, for example, and correlates with increasing age and frailty. Because elderly patients have a diminished physiologic reserve owing to the aging process, are more likely to undergo a pathologic or pharmacologic insult to their systems, and are more prone to disorientation, sound medical management alone may cure their incontinence without resort to more drastic measures. Resnick has elegantly summarized these factors under the mnemonic DIAPPERS.

*D*elerium
*I*nfection
*A*trophic urethritis or vaginitis
*P*harmacologic causes
*P*sychological causes
*E*xcessive urinary production (e.g., diabetes, hypercalcemia)
*R*estricted mobility
*S*tool impaction

The neurologic examination is of particular importance for the incontinent patient because significant neurologic conditions can present initially as isolated disorders of bladder function. Although it is true that patients without an obvious neurologic deficit rarely have an occult neurologic problem, the incidence of neuropathology is higher among patients with bladder disorders than among the general population. Even though our understanding of the neurophysiology of lower urinary tract function is far from complete, it is clinically obvious that normal urinary control requires an intact neurourologic axis, extending from the cerebral cortex down through the pons and midbrain, then through the spinal cord to the peripheral nerves innervating the bladder. Table 36.4 summarizes the neuropathology that may impact bladder function. Although many authors have devoted extensive space to the description of multiple neurophysiologic loops and inhibitory and facilitative micturition reflexes, these remain areas of controversy even among neuroscientists. Until the neurophysiology of bladder function is more clearly understood, detailed descriptions of the processes involved belong in specialty texts that can devote appropriate space to the controversies in this area. Table 36.5 demonstrates the incidence of vesical dysfunction in various neuropathic conditions.

The neurologic examination of the incontinent patient does not have to be extensive. A general screening examination can be done in only a few minutes. If evidence of a previously unsuspected neurologic deficit is uncovered, then the patient may be referred for a more extensive neurologic evaluation. Particular importance should be given to the examination of the lower extremities and lumbosacral spine because of the importance of the micturition center in the sacral spinal cord. Lower-extremity reflexes and movement of the hip, knee, ankle, and foot should be evaluated. In addition, several sacral

TABLE 36.4.
Neurologic Causes of Bladder Dysfunction

DIFFUSE CEREBRAL CAUSES

Alzheimer's disease
Huntington's chorea
Pick's disease
Myxedema

FOCAL OR MULTIFOCAL CEREBRAL CAUSES

Parkinson's disease
Head injury
Multiple sclerosis
Cerebrovascular disease
Frontal tumor
Hydrocephalus

SPINAL CORD CAUSES

Trauma
Multiple sclerosis
Transverse myelitis
Vitamin B_{12} deficiency
Cervical spondylotic myelopathy

CAUDA EQUINA CAUSES

Central lumbar disk prolapse
Trauma
Spina bifida
Herpes zoster
Sacral agenesis

PERIPHERAL NERVE CAUSES

Diabetes mellitus neuropathy
Pelvic surgery or irradiation
Autonomic degenerations
Familial amyloid neuropathy
Alcoholic neuropathy
Guillain-Barré syndrome
Drug and heavy-metal toxic neuropathy
Familiar dysautonomia (Riley-Dray syndrome)

OTHER CONGENITAL DISORDERS

Porphyric neuropathy
Peroneal muscular atrophy
Friedrich's ataxia
Hereditary sensorimotor and autonomic neuropathies

OTHER DISEASES

Uremic neuropathy
Vasculitic neuropathy
Chaga's disease
Leprous neuritis

Rushton DN. In: Bradley WG, et al., eds. *Neurology in clinical practice.* Boston: Butterworth-Heinemann, 1991:665.

reflexes can easily be elicited on physical examination. These include the anal "wink," bulbocavernosus, and cough reflexes. Lightly stroking the buttocks lateral to the anal sphincter should elicit a rapid reflex contraction, or wink, of the external anal sphincter. Gently tapping or stroking the clitoris elicits a similar response (bulbocav-

TABLE 36.5.
Incidence of Neuropathic Bladder Dysfunction in Neurologic Diseases

Condition	Incidence (%)
Abdominoperineal resection	1–44
Radical hysterectomy	7–80
Polio (almost always recovers)	4–42
Diabetic neuropathy	2–83
Lumbar disk disease	6–18
Multiple sclerosis	
Presenting symptom	2–12
Overall incidence	33–78
Parkinsonism	37–70
Stroke	34–53
Meningomyelocele	97

Torrens MJ. In: Jordan, Stanton, eds. *The incontinent woman.* London: Royal College of Obstetricians and Gynaecologists, 1982.

ernosus reflex). A reflex contraction of the pelvic floor and perineum normally is elicited by a cough. The presence of these reflexes provides reassurance that the sacral spinal cord is intact; failure to elicit them, however, does not confirm the presence of a neuropathy, and such findings should be evaluated within the context of the overall picture presented by the patient. The skin overlying the perineum, buttocks, and medial thighs is innervated by the sacral spinal cord (dermatomes S-2 through S-4). Testing the sensitivity of this area to pinprick and light touch provides another means of evaluating the integrity of the sacral spinal cord.

Gynecologic examination of the incontinent patient differs only in degree from that of the continent patient. No patient complaining of stress urinary incontinence should undergo an operative procedure to correct this condition until her stress incontinence has been demonstrated repetitively on physical examination. Not only should she be proved to have stress incontinence, but also this should be confirmed with her as the problem for which she has been seeking help. Just because stress urinary incontinence can be demonstrated does not mean the patient needs an operation. Many multiparous women can be made to leak small amounts of urine if they cough during an examination with a full bladder. Some of these patients may have clinically significant stress incontinence, but many do not. The patient in whom stress incontinence can be demonstrated, for example, but who says that her real problem is that she cannot get to the toilet in time when she needs to urinate, is probably suffering from an overactive detrusor.

The condition of the external genitalia should be noted for signs of excoriation and atrophy. The condition, capacity, and mobility of the vagina should be noted because these can have significant implications for the choice of operation if surgical management is indicated. The presence and degree of any genitourinary prolapse should be noted, which may require simultaneous correction at the time of surgery.

URODYNAMIC TESTING

In the broadest sense, anything that provides objective information on lower urinary tract function can be considered a urodynamic study. A full discussion of the many complex and often controversial techniques that have been developed to look at bladder and urethral function lies beyond the scope of this chapter and can be found in a number of specialist monographs. The most important and useful of these techniques—the real workhorse of lower urinary tract investigation—remains the subtracted cystometrogram. Cystometry is the technique by which the pressure–volume relation of the bladder is measured, and it is used to assess bladder sensation, capacity, and compliance (change in pressure with change in volume), as well as detrusor activity. It is a way of attempting to reproduce the bladder cycle of filling and emptying in a clinical laboratory.

Because the bladder is a distensible organ that fills and empties regularly, much of its function can be understood using purely mechanical principles. Initially, the bladder accommodates a gradual increase in volume without a significant rise in detrusor pressure. At a volume of about 150 mL, the first sensation of fullness or first desire to void normally occurs, but this is followed by a period of voluntary cortical suppression of the micturition reflex until a socially acceptable time and place arises. At this time, the patient normally can generate a detrusor contraction and produce a concomitant rise in bladder pressure while relaxing the pelvic floor. This may appear as an isometric pressure rise if the detrusor contraction begins before the bladder neck is fully open. Normal voiding then is accomplished by a continuous detrusor contraction that is sustained until the bladder is empty, at which time the bladder relaxes and the pelvic floor resumes its normal tone (point 7). The cystometrogram is an attempt to reproduce these physiologic changes within the unphysiologic confines of a urodynamics laboratory.

To perform a cystometric study, pressure catheters, consisting of either fluid-filled lines or electronic microtip transducer pressure catheters, are placed in the bladder to measure bladder pressure. However, because the bladder is an intraabdominal organ measurement of bladder pressure alone is confounded by concurrent changes in abdominal pressure that can be mistaken for detrusor overactivity on a simple cystometrogram. Subtracted cystometry is used to correct this problem. Another catheter is placed in the vagina or rectum, and the pressure measured there is used as an approximation of intraabdominal pressure. The abdominal pressure (P_{abd}) then is subtracted from the intravesical pressure (P_{ves}) to arrive at the intrinsic bladder pressure or subtracted detrusor pressure (P_{det}), which represents the pressure in the bladder owing to the tone or contraction of the detrusor muscle ($P_{det} = P_{ves} - P_{abd}$). The bladder then

FILLING

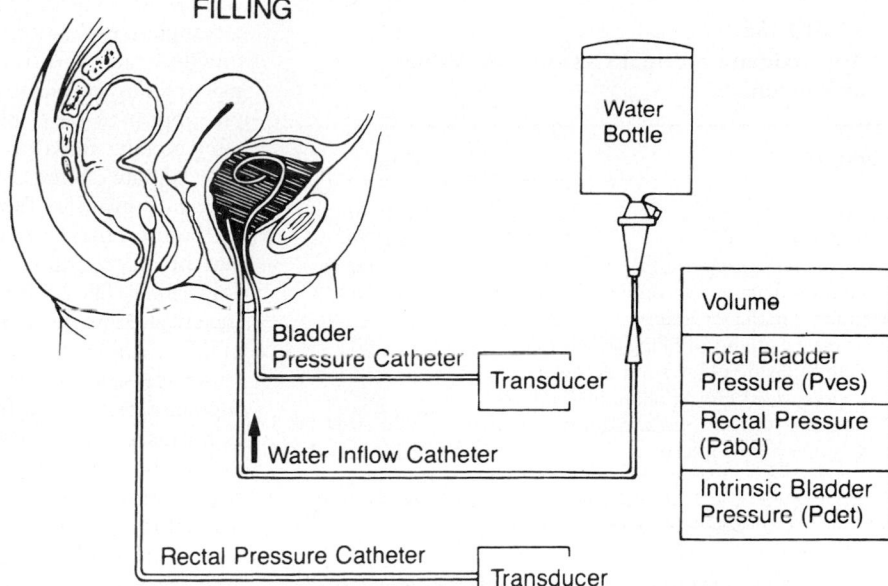

FIGURE 36.1. Filling cystometry. Pressure catheters are in place in the bladder and rectum. An additional filling catheter is placed in the bladder. Volume infused, total bladder pressure, rectal (abdominal) pressure, and subtracted detrusor pressure (intrinsic bladder pressure) are recorded. (From: Wall LL, Addison WA. Basic cystometry in gynecologic practice. *Postgrad Obstet Gynecol* 1988;8:1, with permission.)

is filled with sterile water (or radiocontrast dye, if fluoroscopy is being performed simultaneously) at a standard rate (usually 50 to 100 mL per minute), and the patient's sensations are recorded and correlated with the subtracted detrusor pressure (Fig. 36.1).

During filling, the subtracted detrusor pressure should remain stable, without phasic contractions. As her bladder is being filled, the patient should be asked to cough, change position, and perform various physical activities, such as heel bouncing, bending over, or standing up, in an attempt to provoke unstable detrusor activity. The use of such provocative maneuvers uncovers far more pathology than does supine filling alone. The patient should be asked to cough and strain in the erect position with her bladder full; every effort should be made to reproduce her leakage. The goal of cystometry is to reproduce the patient's symptoms in the urodynamics laboratory so that they can be correlated with measured bladder activity. For this reason, urodynamic studies are best done by a person, preferably the treating physician, who is thoroughly familiar with the patient's history and physical examination. Without this information, urodynamic studies are difficult to interpret accurately.

When the filling lines have been removed, the patient can be placed over a urine flowmeter and a study of the emptying phase of the bladder cycle begun (Fig. 36.2).

VOIDING

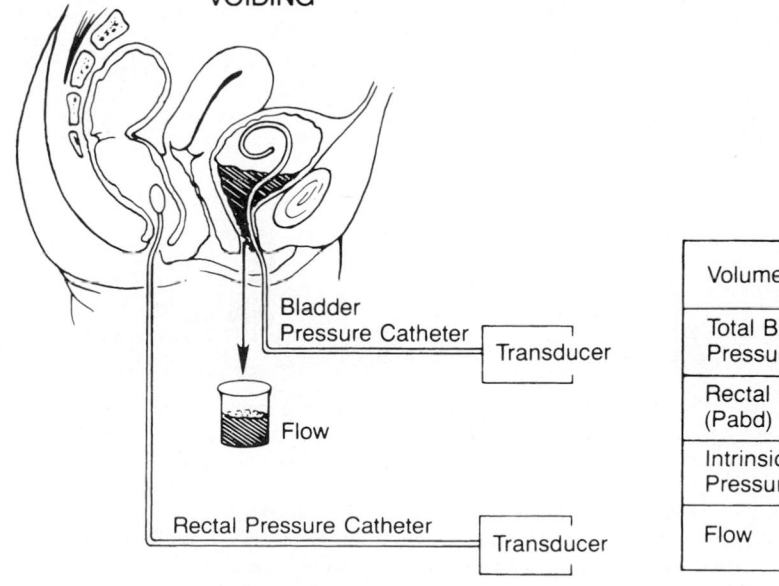

FIGURE 36.2. Voiding cystometry (pressure–flow voiding study). The filling catheter is removed. Volume voided, urine flow rate, total bladder pressure, rectal (abdominal) pressure, and subtracted detrusor pressure (intrinsic bladder pressure) are recorded. (From: Wall LL, Addison WA. Basic cystometry in gynecologic practice. *Postgrad Obstet Gynecol* 1988;8:1, with permission.)

TABLE 36.6.
Approximate Normal Cystometric Values in Women

Parameter	Value
Residue urine	<50 mL
First desire to void	150–250 mL
Cystometric capacity	400–600 mL
Maximum detrusor pressure during filling	<15 cmH$_2$O
Bladder compliance index	
(volume at end of filling in mL of fluid divided by resting detrusor pressure at end of filling in cmH$_2$O	20–100
Maximum detrusor pressure during voiding	<70 cmH$_2$O[a]
Peak urinary flow rate	>15 mL/s[a]

[a]A peak flow rate of <15 mL/s in conjunction with a detrusor pressure >50 cmH$_2$O is diagnostic of outflow obstruction.

This is called *voiding cystometry* or a *pressure–flow study*. Urine flow rate is measured and correlated with changes in bladder, abdominal, and subtracted detrusor pressures. The addition of pelvic floor or urethral sphincter electromyography and fluoroscopic visualization of a contrast-filled bladder may be necessary in some cases for a complete evaluation of bladder function. Patients with low flow rates and those who void primarily by abdominal straining or pelvic muscle relaxation only, for example, appear to be at higher risk for voiding dysfunction after certain kinds of antiincontinence operations. The approximate range of normal cystometric values in women is given in Table 36.6.

Figure 36.3 represents a stable cystometrogram in a patient with genuine stress incontinence. As the bladder is gradually filled with water, there is a slight rise in intravesical pressure. Abdominal pressure (rectal pressure in this example) remains constant, and the subtracted detrusor pressure is stable. The patient, who has been supine, rises to a standing position. The change in position causes a rise in both intravesical and rectal pressure as the abdominal contents shift, but the subtracted detrusor pressure remains stable. Sharp pressure spikes are generated by the patient coughing in the erect position with a full bladder. Because this patient is observed to leak urine under conditions in which increased intraabdominal pressure causes her intravesical pressure to rise beyond the limits that her urethra can hold, and because we know from the subtracted cystometrogram that there is no significant or sustained detrusor contraction, this

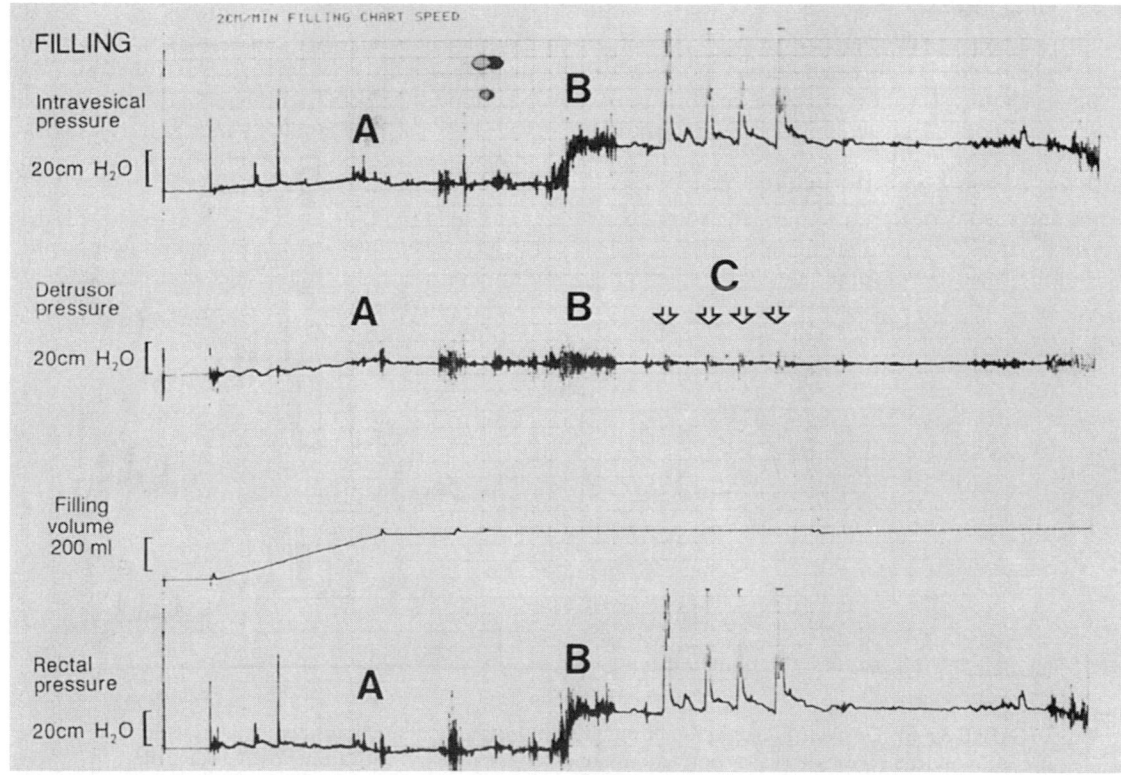

FIGURE 36.3. Stable filling cystometrogram showing genuine stress incontinence. During supine filling (**A**), there is no rise in detrusor pressure. When the patient stands up (**B**), there is a rise in intravesical and rectal pressure as the intraabdominal contents shift; however, the subtracted detrusor pressure remains stable. When the patient coughs in the erect position (**C, arrows**), the detrusor pressure remains stable. Coughs appear as sharp pressure spikes on the intravesical and rectal pressure tracings. Demonstration of urine leakage under these conditions gives the urodynamic diagnosis of genuine stress incontinence.

patient can be given the diagnosis of genuine stress incontinence.

Figure 36.4 is an example of an abnormal, unstable cystometrogram. During the filling phase, rectal pressure (abdominal pressure) remains low, whereas there are phasic pressure changes in both the intravesical and detrusor pressure tracings. This demonstrates unstable detrusor activity. Multiple sharp pressure spikes represent the patient coughing. In this case, coughing precipitates unstable detrusor activity. The significant and sustained increased detrusor pressure can be compared with the previous cystometrogram and indicate involuntary contraction of the detrusor muscles initiated in this case by coughing. These symptoms might have been misdiagnosed as simple stress incontinence and the patient subjected to an ineffectual and unnecessary operation if urodynamic studies had not been performed.

MANAGEMENT OF DETRUSOR OVERACTIVITY

The patient whose urinary incontinence is caused by uninhibited detrusor activity needs different treatment from the patient with simple stress incontinence. The therapeutic mainstays for patients with detrusor overactivity are behavioral modification and drug therapy.

Other, more complex therapies such as sacral nerve root stimulation or augmentation cystoplasty are sometimes indicated for complicated and refractory cases.

Behavioral modification, or bladder retraining for detrusor overactivity, is based on the premise that the basic problem with bladder function in these patients is that the bladder has escaped previously established cortical control. During normal development, the child goes through a period of automatic bladder emptying as soon as the urge arises. Gradually, the child is socialized to cultural norms and learns to suppress the emptying reflex and control bladder function. This results in the ability to postpone micturition until a socially acceptable time and place. The incontinent patient with an unstable detrusor has lost this ability and must regain it. Behavioral modification for the unstable bladder, therefore, is nothing more than a refresher course in toilet training for adults.

Bladder drill regimens attempt to reestablish cortical control over bladder function by gradually lengthening the time that micturition is postponed. Many studies have been done using both inpatient and outpatient training protocols, with excellent results. These regimens work well for patients with motor or sensory urgency, frequency, and urge incontinence, many of whom suffer from half-hourly or hourly urinary frequency and incontinence. The object of therapy is to break this vicious cycle and return them to a normal voiding pattern.

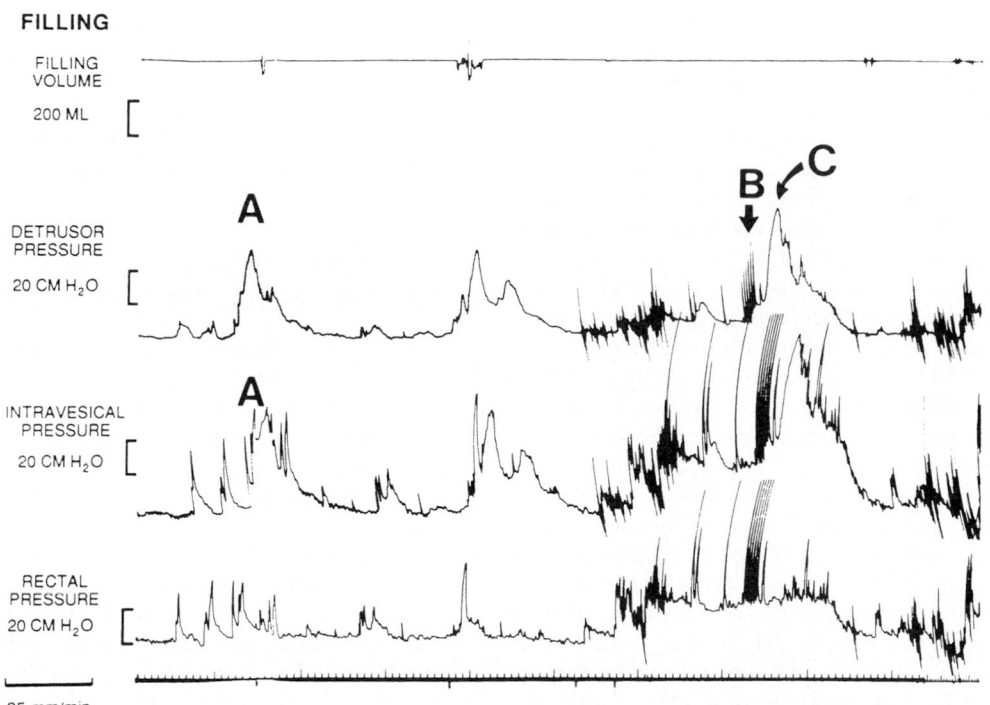

FIGURE 36.4. Unstable filling cystometrogram demonstrating detrusor instability. During filling, pronounced phasic detrusor contractions are demonstrated (**A**) with urine loss, making the diagnosis of motor urge incontinence owing to detrusor instability. Sharp pressure spikes (**B**) represent coughs, which in this case are followed immediately by an unstable detrusor contraction (**C**). Such patients can be misdiagnosed as having simple stress incontinence if urodynamic studies are not carried out.

To do this, the patient's baseline voiding pattern must first be established with a frequency–volume chart or urinary diary. Once this is done, the patient can be instructed to start a schedule that she can manage; for example, to void every 45 minutes during the day. The patient must then void by the clock, whether she needs to or not, on a rigid schedule throughout the day. At night, she voids only as the need arises and does not maintain a fixed schedule. Thus, when the patient gets up in the morning, she voids at 6:15, 7:00, 7:45, and so on. If it is 6:50 a.m. and she has a terrible urge to urinate, she must postpone it, even if this results in leakage. Similarly, if it is 7:45 a.m. and she does not feel the need to urinate, she must do so anyway. The object is to reestablish cortical control over bladder function and put the patient back in charge of her bladder. When she can complete this schedule successfully for 1 week, the interval is gradually increased by 15 minutes. Week by week, the voiding interval is increased by small amounts until the patient can control her bladder for 2 to 3 hours. These regimens are successful, but patient compliance is the absolute prerequisite for success. This can be enhanced by the unrelenting enthusiasm and support of her physician. The patient also must not try to do too much too soon. Gradual increases in the voiding interval are extremely important. As useful as this therapy is, however, some patients are unsuited to such an approach. Behavioral modification is an excellent tool for controlling idiopathic detrusor instability, but it works poorly for most patients with detrusor hyperreflexia caused by neurologic injury. These patients benefit from being placed on a timed voiding schedule, but they generally require drug therapy as well to control their detrusor contractions.

Drug therapy for detrusor overactivity is a reasonable and useful alternative to behavioral modification. All drug treatment for the unstable bladder is an attempt to interrupt the uncontrolled activity of the neuromuscular unit at some level, and because the main neurotransmitter in the bladder is acetylcholine, all drugs available for treating detrusor instability have anticholinergic properties and side effects to some extent. Typical anticholinergic side effects include a dry mouth from suppression of salivary and oropharyngeal secretions; constipation from decreased gastrointestinal motility; an increase in heart rate owing to vagal blockade; feelings of drowsiness; and transient blurring of the vision from blockade of the sphincter of the iris and the ciliary muscle of the lens of the eye. In general, these drugs are safe. The dosage usually is limited more by intolerance to their unpleasant side effects than by other, more serious, forms of toxicity. Extended-release preparations of some of these drugs are available (e.g., Ditropan XL, Detrol LA). Serum levels of these drugs are more tightly controlled than are the shorter-acting preparations; thus, the "peaks and troughs" are smoothed out, reducing the incidence of annoying side effects but without substantial compromise in therapeutic efficacy. Anticholinergic medications should be used cautiously in patients with significant cardiac arrhythmia or narrow-angle glaucoma, in whom they may cause a precipitous rise in intraocular pressure.

TABLE 36.7.
Drugs Useful in the Treatment of Detrusor Overactivity

Drug	Dose (mg PO)
Dicyclomine hydrochloride (Bentyl)	10–20 t.i.d. or q.i.d.
Hyoscyamine sulfate (Levsin)	0.125–0.25 q 4 h
Hyoscyamine sulfate, extended release (Levsinex)	0.375 mg–0.75 mg b.i.d.
Imipramine hydrochloride (Tofranil)	10 t.i.d.–50 b.i.d.
Oxybutynin chloride (Ditropan)	5–10 t.i.d. or q.i.d.
Oxybutynin chloride extended release (Ditropan XL)	5–15 mg q.d.
Propantheline bromide (ProBanthine)	15–30 q.i.d.
Tolterodine hydrochloride (Detrol)	2 mg b.i.d.
Tolterodine hydrochloride extended release (Detrol LA)	4 mg q.d.

The main drugs, and their usual dosages, that seem to be useful in treating detrusor overactivity are listed in Table 36.7. In addition to its anticholinergic effects, imipramine has both α-adrenergic effects that enhance urethral closure, as well as effects on the central nervous system that appear to be beneficial for patients with nocturnal enuresis. Some women appear to have perimenstrual exacerbation of their detrusor instability resulting from uterine prostaglandin synthesis and release. The addition of a prostaglandin synthetase inhibitor (e.g., mefenamic acid) around the time of menstruation can be of great benefit in selected cases. Older women with atrophic urethritis or vaginitis and detrusor instability also can benefit from appropriate hormone replacement therapy.

FACTORS CONTRIBUTING TO STRESS INCONTINENCE

As noted, stress incontinence is the most common form of urinary incontinence in women; however, the term *stress incontinence* is used to refer to three distinct entities: a symptom, a sign, and a condition. These three things are not the same, and their conceptual differences must be appreciated to understand which patients have clinically significant stress incontinence.

The *symptom* of stress incontinence refers only to the patient's complaint that she leaks urine when intraabdominal pressure is increased. Patients with this complaint may or may not have genuine stress incontinence as documented by urodynamic studies. The patient's report that she leaks urine when she engages in activities that raise her intraabdominal pressure should be taken seriously; but patients sometimes interpret what is happening and make their own diagnosis, which they then present to the physician as their symptom, rather than describing accurately what is occurring. Some patients may think that all female urinary incontinence is stress incontinence; therefore, they believe that they have this diagnosis if they leak. Other patients may not understand that the urgency that habitually accompanies the urinary leakage is a critically important part of their histories. Still others may have uncontrolled detrusor activity precipitated by physical exertion, which they describe as stress incontinence. The physician's task is that of a historian: to piece together and make sense of the patient's history. Failure to take a thorough history and analyze it carefully is one of the major sources of misdiagnosis in urogynecology. No patient should undergo a surgical operation for stress incontinence solely on the basis of her symptoms; the history must be confirmed by objective means.

The *sign* of stress incontinence is the physical demonstration and observation of urine loss during conditions of increased intraabdominal pressure (such as coughing) while the patient is being examined. The mere demonstration of the phenomenon of stress urinary leakage during a physical examination does *not* mean that the patient has a clinical problem with stress incontinence. As noted, stress incontinence is common among women. Hodgkinson emphasized that the relatively short and unprotected female urethra makes *all* women relatively susceptible to this form of urine loss. Indeed, several surveys of otherwise healthy, young nulliparous women have shown that half have experienced this symptom, and a significant number have experienced it frequently. According to the International Continence Society, incontinence exists when urine loss becomes a social or hygienic problem. Many women experience occasional stress urinary leakage that is only an annoyance or occasional inconvenience. They would not label themselves as incontinent, and these women do not need surgery; but studies also have shown that there is little relation between the volume of urine lost and the distress that this causes to an incontinent patient.

Which patients have the clinical *condition* or *diagnosis* of stress urinary incontinence? What factors push the mild, relatively common occurrence of female stress urinary leakage into the realm of a clinical problem? The clinical condition of stress incontinence exists along a spectrum and is influenced by the interaction of three separate factors. At one end of the spectrum is the young female athlete who leaks only drops of urine during violent physical activity; at the other end of the spectrum is the frail, elderly woman who leaks large amounts of urine if she merely changes position or reaches down to pick up a lightweight object. The degree to which either woman is bothered by the leakage is influenced by the cultural values and expectations she carries regarding urinary continence and incontinence, that is, the psychosocial milieu in which she lives. A biobehavioral model of stress incontinence thus can be created by looking at the interaction of these three determinants: the biologic strength or resiliency of the sphincteric mechanism; the level of physical stress placed on the continence mechanism; and the woman's personal and cultural expectations about urinary control (Fig. 36.5). This model explains the enormous variations found in symptoms, the

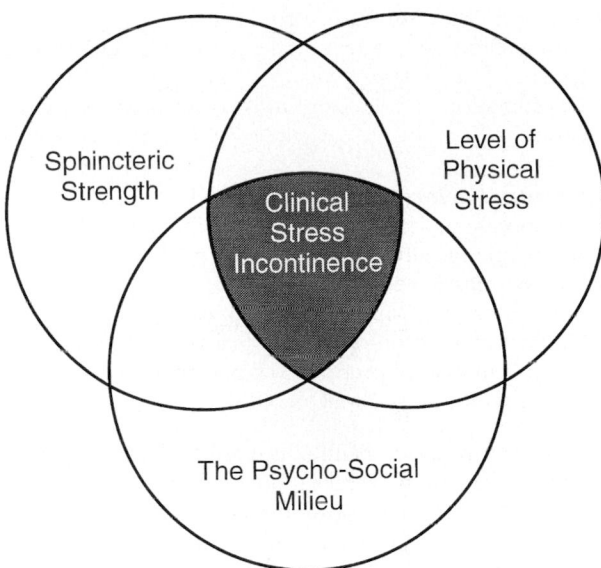

FIGURE 36.5. A biobehavioral model of stress incontinence. Clinical stress urinary incontinence results from the interaction of three distinct components: the inherent biologic strength of the urinary sphincter, the level of physical stress placed on the sphincter, and the psychosocial milieu in which the patient lives (i.e., her personal and cultural expectations concerning urinary control and urinary incontinence).

degree of leakage that can be demonstrated during physical examination, and patient's response to the stress incontinence. Modification of any one of these factors can influence the patient's clinical condition. For example, many patients give up certain physical activities when they start to cause stress incontinence (e.g., dancing, running, aerobic exercise). This may eliminate the incontinence problem, but it does so at a cost to quality of life. Other women manage to cope with stress incontinence by adopting new body postures during activities that cause them to leak, or they learn to strengthen the sphincteric mechanism through pelvic muscle exercises. Still other women are profoundly relieved to find out that the small amount of leakage they experience from time to time is not abnormal. In any case, the interaction of these three factors opens up a variety of management strategies for the stress incontinent woman. Surgical intervention is only one of these management strategies, and a surgical operation is designed primarily to influence the biologic competence of the sphincteric mechanism rather than either of the other factors that interact to produce the clinical problem.

What factors contribute to the structural and functional integrity of the sphincteric unit? Effective urethral closure is maintained by a variety of extrinsic and intrinsic factors.

Extrinsic Factors
- Endopelvic fascia and integrity of its lateral attachments to the pelvic sidewall
- Levator ani muscles

- Strength of levator muscle complex
- Connections of levator muscle complex to endopelvic fascia
- Coordination of levator muscle contraction with coughing

Intrinsic Factors

- Autonomic (sympathetic) innervation and tone (α-adrenergic receptors)
- Striated muscle of urethral wall
- Mucosal coaptation of urothelium
- Vascular congestion of submucosal venous plexus
- Smooth muscle of urethral wall and blood vessels
- Elasticity of urethral wall

The extrinsic factors influence urethral function indirectly by affecting urethral support, whereas the intrinsic factors affect urethral closure directly.

Stress continence is maintained by urethral support in a woman with a normal urethra. The urethra normally is supported by the endopelvic fascia, which attaches to the pelvic side walls along the arcus tendineus fasciae pelvis. The endopelvic fascia, when normally attached, permits the urethra to be compressed closed during episodes of increased intraabdominal pressure. The levator ani muscles are attached to the endopelvic fascia along the urethra and provide a muscular component to urethral support. This muscular component includes both *slow-twitch* muscle fibers (which help maintain effective closure over time), and *fast-twitch* muscle fibers (which respond quickly during coughing or other activity to maintain effective closure during periods of increased physical stress). This method of construction results in springy, resilient, and responsive support, much like that provided by a trampoline. It works remarkably effectively unless the lateral fascial supports are detached or the neuromuscular component is damaged. Damaged urethral support is manifested clinically by urethral hypermobility, which often results in incompetent urethral closure during physical activity and presents as stress urinary incontinence.

Intrinsic urethral functioning is more complicated and is not understood nearly as well as is urethral support. At least six (and probably more) factors are involved in normal urethral functioning, irrespective of the nature of urethral support. Important among these factors is the autonomic (sympathetic) innervation of the urethra, mediated principally by α-adrenergic receptors in the urethra and bladder neck. The degree of stimulation of these receptors has a direct influence on urethral closure. α-Stimulus produces an increase in urethral tone and enhances urethral closure, whereas α-blockade produces urethral relaxation and worsens urethral closure. This is why drugs such as phenylpropanolamine and pseudoephedrine are useful in treating stress incontinence, whereas antihypertensive medications such as prazosin can create stress incontinence as a side effect. The urethra also contains both smooth and striated muscle, the latter being under voluntary control at the level of the external urethral sphincter. The external sphincter serves mainly as a back-up mechanism for urinary control; the bladder neck and proximal urethra are the first line of defense against leakage. Proper closure of the urethra depends on the coordination of the muscular components as well as appropriate elasticity of the urethral wall, vascular congestion of the submucosal and periurethral venous plexuses, and coaptation of the urothelial folds, which is influenced at least in part by estrogen. Effective sphincteric dysfunction can be disrupted in many ways, including congenital developmental defects (epispadias, spina bifida), trauma, surgical denervation (radical hysterectomy), complete or partial urethrectomy (radical vulvectomy), urethral scarring from anterior colporrhaphy or bladder neck suspension surgery, and so forth. Restoration of normal urethral function in a patient who has developed intrinsic sphincteric failure is more complicated than is restoration of normal urethral support.

As these factors have become more clearly understood, it has become apparent that stress incontinence results from the interaction of the state of the intrinsic and extrinsic factors that normally result in continence. Patients fall along a continuum where both loss of urethral support and loss of urethral function interact with

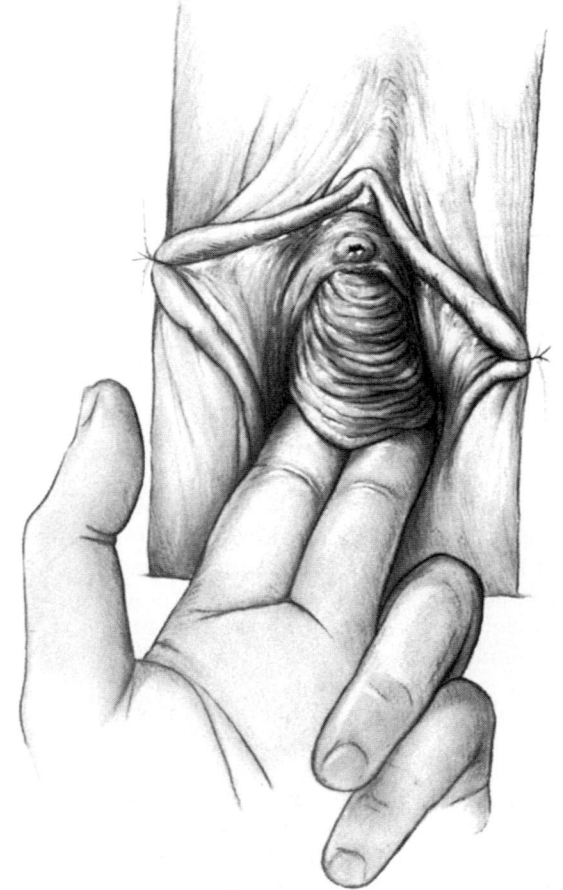

FIGURE 36.6. Loss of support of the urethra and bladder base manifested during straining.

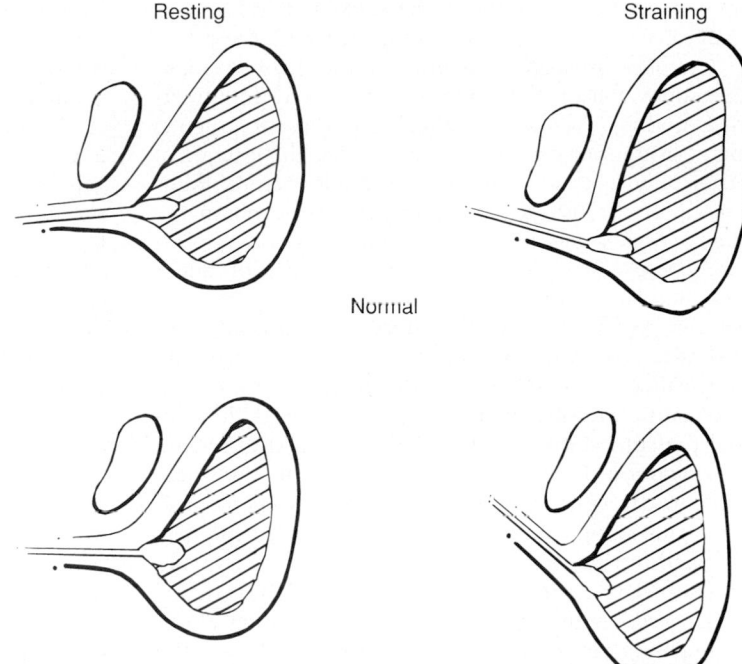

Resting   Straining

Normal

Hypermobile

FIGURE 36.7. The Q-tip test. A sterile cotton-tipped swab is inserted into the urethra to the level of the bladder neck. The patient then is asked to strain down. In the patient with normal urethral support, there is little change in the angle of the cotton-tipped swab with straining. In the patient with poor urethral support, there is a marked upward excursion of the cotton-tipped swab with straining. This is indicative only of urethral hypermobility; it is not a diagnosis of stress incontinence.

one another. Loss of urethral support is probably more common clinically than complete urethral failure, but elements of each condition probably are present in most women with stress incontinence.

Urethral support can be evaluated in several ways. The easiest way is simply by inspecting the urethra and bladder neck when the patient is at rest, and then when she is straining maximally (Fig. 36.6). Significant rotational descent of the urethra and bladder neck generally is easy to spot; however, this method of assessment is imprecise and highly subjective. Therefore, it is subject to tremendous individual variation and hence potential error. More precise ways of evaluating urethral support include lateral bead–chain cystourethrography (which is somewhat cumbersome and involves exposure to radiation), ultrasonography, and the "Q-tip test," which was originally introduced as an inexpensive way of evaluating urethral axial mobility as a substitute for radiographic studies. Current research is under way to investigate the utility of magnetic resonance imaging of the pelvic floor and urethra in evaluating these factors.

The simplest technique for evaluating urethral axial mobility involves placement of a lubricated sterile cotton-tipped swab into the urethra to the level of the bladder neck (the "Q-tip test"). The resting angle of the urethral axis is measured using a standard orthopedic goniometer oriented horizontally (usually with a line-level or similar standardized instrument). The patient then is asked to strain down using a Valsalva maneuver, and the maximum angle of excursion of the cotton-tipped swab is measured. A maximum straining angle greater than 30 degrees is conventionally taken to represent the presence of urethral hypermobility (Fig. 36.7).

The patient with hypermobility and stress incontinence usually is cured of leakage if the hypermobility is corrected; however, it is important to understand that a certain degree of urethral hypermobility can be present in normal multiparous women. Having urethral hypermobility and having clinical stress incontinence is *not* the same thing. Many women with severe stress incontinence have no urethral mobility at all, and many women with incontinence owing to other causes (e.g., detrusor instability) also have urethral hypermobility as a coincidental finding that is irrelevant to their main problem. No single bladder neck position is uniformly associated with continence or with incontinence. Similarly, there is no reason to believe that a patient with normal urethral support and no anatomic hypermobility can have her stress incontinence cured by an operation that is designed to reposition the urethra and restore urethral support. Patients who have stress incontinence in the presence of normal urethral support are different.

Evidence to suggest that the patient's problem primarily is caused by sphincteric weakness rather than loss of support can be obtained in several ways. During examination of the patient, an open ring forceps can be placed in the vagina with one arm in each lateral vaginal fornix, and used to support (not elevate) the urethra in its normal anatomic position. It is always possible to prevent stress incontinence if the examiner obstructs the bladder neck. The main usefulness of this test is not to find those patients who remain dry when it is performed, but rather those who continue to leak even though normal anatomic support has been restored. It would not be expected that these patients would become dry after undergoing a surgical operation to restore normal urethral support; such patients should be suspected of having a significant element of intrinsic sphincteric weakness.

Cystourethroscopic examination also can help identify patients with poorly functioning, scarred, foreshortened urethras. In many instances, the urethral lumen is open throughout its entire length so that the interior of the bladder can be seen from the distal urethra. Fluoroscopy of the bladder identifies patients in whom the bladder neck is gaping open at rest in the standing position. These women seem to be at higher risk of failure from standard bladder neck suspension operations. In addition to these somewhat subjective assessments of urethral function, attempts have been made to quantitate the effectiveness of the urethral closure mechanism using urodynamic measurement techniques, such as the urethral pressure closure profile or the leak-point pressure determination. In all cases, clinical judgment still is necessary to determine where a patient with stress incontinence falls along the continuum of anatomic hypermobility and intrinsic sphincteric dysfunction.

The urethral pressure profile (Fig. 36.8) was developed based on the idea that useful information about urethral function could be obtained by measuring the pressure along the length of the urethra. The idea behind this test was that there would be a direct relation between the pressure measurements obtained and the patient's continence status. The test is performed using a special catheter (usually one with two electronic microtip pressure transducers placed 6 cm apart), which is pulled from the bladder through the urethra to the outside environment at a fixed rate. As this catheter is pulled along, the transducer measures intravesical pressure until it enters the urethra, at which time the pressure rises to reflect the higher urethral pressure, peaking at the point of maximum urethral pressure. When the transducer finally exits the urethral lumen, the pressure drops precipitously to atmospheric pressure. This test generates a curve called the *urethral pressure profile*. The difference between the maximum urethral pressure and the intravesical pressure is called the *maximum urethral closure pressure*. This test is appealing because there is an intu-

itive sense that it must provide useful information about urethral strength; after all, for continence to exist, the pressure in the urethra must be higher than the pressure in the bladder.

Unfortunately, the urethral pressure profile has not lived up to the promise with which it began. First of all, the test does not actually measure pressure, but rather the unidirectional force exerted on the transducer surface as it is pulled through the urethra (Miyazaki's rule). The pressure reading that is obtained varies with the orientation of the transducer, rate of withdrawal, position of the patient, and bladder volume at which the test is done. Although it is true that women with stress incontinence have lower urethral pressures as a group than women without stress incontinence, there is a tremendous overlap between the two groups. Urethral pressure appears to fall normally with advancing age, and there does not appear to be any good correlation between urethral pressure and the severity of a patient's incontinence. It has been suggested that a low maximum urethral closure pressure (<20 cmH$_2$O, measured in a patient with a full bladder in the sitting position) is a risk factor for poor outcome in surgery for stress incontinence if a standard suspension procedure is performed, but this has not been a universal finding. Some of the differences in outcome may be related more to surgical technique among various authors than to significant differences in patients' sphincters. More important is the observation that urethral pressures do not change appreciably in patients who undergo successful surgery for stress incontinence. Achievement of continence is not associated with a significant rise in maximum urethral pressure. This finding is not what one would expect if the urethral pressure profile were actually a useful measurement of the closure strength or stress competence of the urethral sphincter mechanism. At best, the urethral pressure profile measures an indirect factor related to stress continence, but it is not a direct measurement of urethral sphincteric competence.

A potentially more useful test is the leak-point pressure determination. Whereas the urethral pressure profile

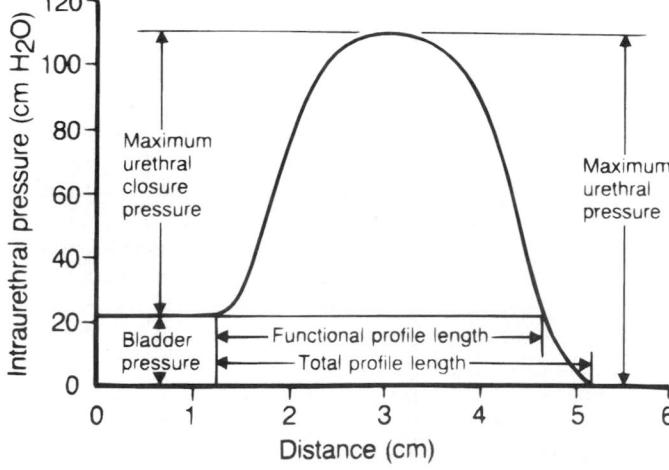

FIGURE 36.8. Component parts of the urethral pressure profile. (International Continence Society)

is a static test, the leak-point pressure measurement is a dynamic assessment of sphincteric integrity. Simply stated, the *leak-point pressure* is the total intravesical pressure needed to produce stress incontinence in a given patient. Work by McGuire has demonstrated that patients with lower leak-point pressures tend to complain of more severe incontinence and that leak-point pressures rise after successful treatment of stress incontinence. These are the results that one would expect to find if a test had a direct relation to sphincteric competence.

The technique for measuring leak-point pressures has not yet been standardized. Each laboratory must develop its own range of normal values. The volume of bladder filling and the size of the pressure measurement catheter both appear to be significant factors in the final determination of a leak-point pressure. McGuire obtains his readings using a 10F triple-lumen urethral catheter perfused through a constant pressure reservoir (275 cmH$_2$O) at a rate of 1 mL per minute, connected to a P23 Statham pressure transducer located at the level of the pubic symphysis with a frequency response of 0.2 seconds per 100 cmH$_2$O. Patients' bladders are filled with 20% iodinated contrast at a rate of 60 mL per minute through one of the ports of the triple-lumen catheter until a volume of 150 mL is reached, at which time the leak-point pressure is determined. The stress leak-point pressure as described by McGuire is the total intravesical pressure at which leakage is recorded radiographically during the fluoroscopic video urodynamic study. Patients are asked to strain slowly until they reach a pressure at which urine loss occurs (Valsalva leak-point pressure); if leakage does not occur, then they are asked to cough progressively with increasing vigor until leakage does occur (cough leak-point pressure). The lowest pressure at which leakage is seen to occur is taken as the true leak-point pressure. If leakage does not occur, the maximum pressure obtained can be recorded as an indicator of sphincteric strength (e.g., no leakage to 192 cmH$_2$O). In McGuire's experience, patients with leak-point pressures of less than 60 cmH$_2$O have severe incontinence owing to intrinsic sphincteric deficiency.

NONSURGICAL MANAGEMENT OF STRESS INCONTINENCE

Pelvic surgeons naturally tend to regard the solution to the problem of stress incontinence as surgical; however, surgery for urinary incontinence is almost always an elective procedure, never an emergency. It is a mistake of major proportions to persuade a patient to have incontinence surgery before she is ready. An operation should be carried out only when the problem has become severe enough for the patient to want to have it corrected, and when she understands the risks as well as the potential benefits of the procedure. Some women may not be bothered enough by the degree of their leakage to wish to undergo the expense and convalescence of surgery. Others may not have finished childbearing, and, although bothered by their leakage, they may be reluctant

to undergo an operation that may be damaged or undone by subsequent pregnancy, labor, and delivery. Still other incontinent women are frail and elderly and are reluctant to undergo an operation because of their general health. For all of these reasons, if nonsurgical approaches to restoring bladder neck support and urethral tone could be developed, such women could benefit greatly.

It remains unclear precisely how urethral tone, bladder neck and urethral mobility, and the state of pelvic floor innervation all interact to produce urinary continence. Recent work on the anatomy of this region suggests that the continence mechanism is more sophisticated and elaborate than heretofore recognized; clearly, however, much of the support of this region comes from the pelvic musculature. The musculature of the levator ani complex provides substantial support for the urethra, vagina, and rectum as they descend through the pelvic floor, by its connection with the endopelvic fascia.

The periurethral levator ani muscles contain both type I (slow-twitch) and type II (fast-twitch) muscle fibers, which allow them to maintain tone over a long period and increase tone suddenly to compensate for the increased abdominal pressure that occurs with coughing, sneezing, and straining. Rehabilitation of these muscle groups through exercise and physical therapy may serve to improve the continence mechanism in two ways. First, strengthening the striated urogenital sphincter could enhance its ability to constrict the urethral lumen. This may yield a stronger closure force in the urethra at rest or increase the forces of urethral closure generated during a cough or other stressful situations. Second, because the levator ani muscles are important to pelvic and urethral support, an exercise program could improve the support of the proximal urethra. Because these muscles can be activated during a cough, continence may be improved without a noticeable rise in resting urethral pressure measurements.

Arnold Kegel was the first person to investigate pelvic floor muscle strengthening in a systematic fashion. His method consists of developing the patient's awareness of the pubococcygeus muscle and then instructing her in exercises to strengthen this muscle with a crude pneumatic biofeedback device called a perineometer. Kegel originally stressed the importance of supervised instruction and encouragement in performing these exercises and reported good success rates in relieving symptomatic stress incontinence by his program. Although nearly all gynecologists are familiar with these exercises, they rarely are taught and used as Kegel did originally, and this form of therapy has often degenerated into a few brief words of oral instruction in which the patient is told to stop and start her urine stream a few times each day while voiding. Not only are programs based on this approach disappointing in their results, they can train women to become dysfunctional voiders.

For muscular rehabilitation of the pelvic floor to work, it must be supervised, done regularly, and aided by some form of feedback so that the patient can judge her progress. Bo and coworkers have clearly shown that enthusiastic supervision makes a dramatic difference in the degree of success that can be obtained by programs of pelvic muscle rehabilitation. Adjunct therapy, such as the use of electrical or magnetic stimulation of the pelvic muscles, weight training using intravaginal cones, and biofeedback devices, may help improve the results of these programs. Continuation of regular pelvic muscle exercise after the initial period of instruction is mandatory in order to maintain muscle tone and control over time.

This is not to suggest that physical therapy can cure or improve all cases of stress incontinence, but there is evidence to suggest that properly supervised and rigorously performed techniques for pelvic muscular rehabilitation can play a significant role in the treatment of genuine stress incontinence. Patients can expect improvement in their symptoms by tensing the musculature of the pelvic floor and holding these contractions for 5 seconds each, 15 to 20 times per session, three sessions per day. This strengthens the slow-twitch muscle fibers. Patients should also practice a similar number of rapid contractions to strengthen the fast-twitch muscle fibers. Pelvic muscle exercises should be taught to patients one-on-one during a pelvic examination because many patients contract the wrong muscles, and teaching *Kegel exercises* to large groups in classrooms is nearly worthless. Because pelvic muscle rehabilitation is virtually without side effects, involves the patient in her own care, and may prevent the development of subsequent pelvic relaxation if used regularly, gynecologists should make more use of it and should be encouraged to incorporate pelvic muscle exercises into routine health maintenance programs for women.

The tone of the urethra and bladder neck is maintained in large part by α-adrenergic activity from the sympathetic nervous system. For this reason, many pharmacologic agents have been used to treat stress incontinence, with varying degrees of success (Table 36.8). These drugs include imipramine (which has a concomitant relaxing effect on the detrusor), ephedrine, norephedrine, and phenylpropanolamine. Unfortunately, many of these compounds also increase vascular tone and therefore can lead to problems with hypertension, a condition that afflicts many postmenopausal women with stress incontinence. In 2000, a case-control study found that phenylpropanolamine-containing ap-

petite suppressants, and cough and cold remedies, were an independent risk factor in the development of hemorrhagic stroke in women between the ages of 18 and 49. These findings have led to a markedly diminished enthusiasm for the use of α-agonists in the treatment of stress incontinence.

Although the therapeutic role of α-agonists appears to be diminishing in the treatment of stress incontinence, the role of blockers, such as prazosin, in the creation of stress incontinence should not be overlooked. Such drugs commonly are used in treating hypertension because of their relaxing effects on vascular smooth muscle. The α-blockers also may relax the bladder neck and urethra to the point at which incontinence develops. Patients who present with complaints of stress incontinence while taking these drugs should have their antihypertensive medication changed before surgery is considered because their incontinence may resolve spontaneously with a change of medication.

Postmenopausal women with urogenital atrophy owing to estrogen deprivation and concurrent urinary incontinence should be placed on hormone replacement therapy as part of their therapeutic regimen, unless such therapy is contraindicated for other reasons. Not only do many complaints of urgency, frequency, and irritation often disappear, but evidence also suggests that estrogen replacement enhances the effectiveness of α-adrenergic receptors in the urethra.

Besides physical therapy and selected pharmacologic agents, electrical stimulation therapy has been used to treat stress incontinence. Passage of an electrical current through the muscles of the pelvic floor causes them to contract and simultaneously causes a reflex inhibition of detrusor activity. The stimulus can be applied transvaginally or transrectally in either continuous or intermittent fashion. Although many authors have reported good success rates using these devices, patient acceptance of the technique often is poor, and device failure sometimes occurs because of mechanical problems. Although this mode of therapy remains an option for the patient with stress incontinence, it is unlikely to be used extensively outside of a research setting. Recently, devices have been developed using pulsed magnetic technology to promote strengthening of the muscles of the pelvic floor. This technology is much less invasive than previous electrical stimulation devices, using a therapy chair instead of an intravaginal or intraanal device, and is better tolerated by patients. Although the initial results are somewhat encouraging, particularly for patients with mild incontinence, the long-term utility of this therapy has yet to be determined.

SELECTION OF OPERATIONS FOR STRESS INCONTINENCE

When a patient presents as a candidate for operative management of genuine stress incontinence, the surgeon faces an enormous array of potential procedures from which to choose. The world medical literature produces

---

TABLE 36.8.
Drugs Useful in the Treatment of Stress Incontinence

Drug	Dose (mg PO)
Pseudoephedrine	30–60 t.i.d. or q.i.d.
Ephedrine	15–30 t.i.d. or q.i.d.
Norephedrine	100 b.i.d.
Phenylpropanolamine	50–75 b.i.d.
Imipramine	10–25 t.i.d.

more than one article per week on stress incontinence, and probably more than 200 operations have been suggested as surgical cures for this condition. This alone should alert the surgeon to the fact that the ideal operation has yet to be devised. The major operations for stress incontinence can be grouped into seven categories (Table 36.9). Which of these many operations is the best?

Selection of the proper operation for a given patient depends on a variety of factors. The surgeon must first answer the question of what technical goals are to be achieved: Is the objective to correct urethral hypermobility? Is it to compensate for intrinsic sphincteric deficiency? Is it to do both? The surgeon must be clear about what is needed before embarking on an operative procedure. What other factors come into play in the case of a particular patient? A vigorous, active patient may need more durable urethral support than an elderly recluse. A morbidly obese patient with chronic respiratory problems who is a heavy smoker is different from a thin woman with normal lungs and sedentary habits. Are there reasons to avoid extensive intraabdominal surgery, or does the patient need a laparotomy for reasons other than stress incontinence? All of these factors must be

weighed when choosing a surgical procedure. One operation cannot fit the needs of every patient.

A review of the literature on the surgical treatment of genuine stress incontinence immediately reveals many problems. Many series are plagued by poor preoperative evaluation of patients, contain no urodynamic data, have short or shoddy follow-up, and use no objective criteria to define outcomes. Most published series represent the retrospective personal experience of one surgeon doing one procedure, and conclude (not surprisingly) that "my patients do pretty well." The history of the development of surgical treatments for stress incontinence is depressing, and tends to follow the seven stages in the career of medical innovation outlined by McKinlay:

1. The initial "promising report" of a new surgical procedure
2. Adoption of the technique by large groups of practitioners based on case reports and short case series
3. Public acceptance of the new procedure and payment for it by third-party insurance carriers–all without rigorous formal critical evaluation of the merits of the operation
4. Enshrinement of the innovation as a "standard procedure"
5. Gradual arousal of scientific curiosity (after several years and the performance of thousands of these operations) as to whether or not the procedure really works with the eventual organization of a randomized, controlled clinical trial to evaluate its efficacy
6. Discovery that the results of the operation are not what people thought they were, with the beginnings of professional denunciation of the procedure
7. Abandonment of the discredited operation

Unfortunately, this last step usually occurs only when a "replacement" operation is available. The replacement operation is inevitably early in its life cycle; thus, it is without any critical evaluation. The process is driven more by commercial interests and the egos of prominent surgeons who are invested in new operations than by any scientific foundation. This deplorable state of affairs should be replaced by a process that determines the best operation through prospective, randomized studies in which similar patients with urodynamically proven diagnoses are randomized to one of several operations done by one of several surgeons, who are also chosen randomly. The patients should be followed for several years postoperatively and evaluated by standardized criteria. Out of the vast literature on stress incontinence, only a few studies begin to approach these criteria.

Review of these studies shows that anterior colporrhaphy produces results consistently inferior to the Burch colposuspension or sling operations for the objective cure of genuine stress incontinence. Although it is obvious that anterior vaginal repair can produce a clinical cure in some patients that may be sustained over time, the available evidence strongly suggests that this operation should be used rarely today. Surgeons who routinely use anterior vaginal repair as their primary op-

---

TABLE 36.9.
Classification of Operations for Stress Incontinence

ANTERIOR COLPORRHAPHY WITH KELLY BLADDER NECK PLICATION

ABDOMINAL BLADDER NECK SUSPENSION PROCEDURES DESIGNED TO CORRECT INCONTINENCE CAUSED BY URETHRAL HYPERMOBILITY

Retropubic bladder neck suspension
    Marshall-Marchetti-Krantz procedure
    Burch colposuspension
Paravaginal bladder neck suspension
    Paravaginal defect repair
    Vaginal-obturator shelf procedure
Needle suspension procedures
    Pereyra procedure
    Modifications

OPERATIONS TO CORRECT INCONTINENCE CAUSED BY INTRINSIC SPHINCTERIC DEFICIENCY

Sling operations
    Organic materials
        Autologous materials (e.g., rectus fascia, fascia lata)
        Heterologous materials (e.g., porcine dermis, ox dura mater)
    Synthetic materials
Periurethral injections
    Teflon paste
    Collagen
    Carbon-coated zirconium oxide particles
    Fat
Artificial urinary sphincter

eration for genuine stress incontinence are doing their patients a disservice.

The other surgical alternatives can be divided into two broad groups: (a) those for most patients whose stress incontinence is primarily owing to hypermobility of the proximal urethra and bladder neck; and (b) the minority of patients whose incontinence is owing to insufficiency of the sphincteric unit itself. The former group should be cured of their incontinence if the anatomic hypermobility is corrected. The operations that do this best appear to be the retropubic bladder neck suspensions, such as the Burch colposuspension, or a "loose" sling operation. Needle-suspension procedures, such as the Pereyra procedure or one of its many modifications, appear to be much less successful over time in correcting stress incontinence, but perhaps slightly better than anterior colporrhaphy. In the practices of most gynecologists, patients with complex stress incontinence and intrinsic sphincteric failure rarely present as candidates for primary surgery. The patient with sphincteric damage almost always brings along some other baggage, such as a congenital abnormality of the lower urinary tract, previous failed incontinence surgery (often with multiple prior attempts at cure), incontinence developing after other pelvic surgery (e.g., a radical hysterectomy or radical vulvectomy), incontinence with a large enterocele or eversion of the vaginal vault, or significant pelvic trauma. Evaluation of these patients requires special care, particularly in the face of previous failed incontinence surgery. If residual hypermobility is present, all that may be required for cure is adequate repositioning of the bladder neck. This situation commonly occurs in patients who have had a failed anterior colporrhaphy, patients who have had a retropubic urethropexy performed with catgut instead of delayed-absorbable or permanent sutures, or patients who have had a needle-suspension procedure that failed because the permanent guy wire sutures broke or pulled through the supporting fascia. If the urethra and bladder neck are well supported and without excess mobility, however, further attempts to elevate them are unlikely to cure the patient's incontinence. These patients require operations that compensate for sphincteric damage by supporting and partially occluding the urethra and bladder neck (slings, periurethral injections, or an artificial urinary sphincter).

MANAGEMENT OF MIXED INCONTINENCE

Many patients present with both urinary incontinence caused by detrusor instability and genuine stress incontinence. Although there is nearly universal agreement that a bladder neck suspension operation is contraindicated in patients whose sole cause of incontinence is detrusor overactivity, the role of surgery in patients with mixed incontinence is more controversial. In general, the presence of preoperative detrusor instability is an unfavorable prognostic sign for the achievement of continence after an operation to cure coexistent genuine stress incontinence. Although the detrusor instability disappears in some patients postoperatively, some patients with previously stable cystometrograms develop new-onset instability after surgery. Karram and Bhatia carried out a retrospective review of 52 patients with mixed incontinence, 27 of whom were treated with primary surgery (Burch colposuspension) and 25 of whom were treated with various pharmacologic regimens. There was no statistically significant difference in outcome between the two groups, and all the surgical failures were caused by persistent detrusor instability rather than genuine stress incontinence. Therefore, the prudent course of treatment appears to be an initial trial of behavioral or pharmacologic therapy, or both, for detrusor instability before surgery. If the patient remains unhappy with her situation after a trial of conservative management, then she may be offered an attempt at surgical cure of her stress incontinence with the understanding that the outcome is unpredictable and the chances of complete success probably are diminished.

TECHNIQUES FOR RETROPUBIC BLADDER NECK SUSPENSION

The first retropubic bladder neck operation for stress incontinence was described in 1949 by Drs. Marshall, Marchetti, and Krantz of the Cornell University Medical Center. Since that time, a number of modifications of this basic operation have been described, but all of them share the common feature of correcting bladder neck displacement and urethral hypermobility by surgically resuspending these structures with an operation performed in the space of Retzius. The differences among these techniques owe largely to the different points to which portions of the endopelvic fascia are attached during the course of each operation (Fig. 36.9). Therefore, it seems logical to discuss retropubic bladder neck suspension operations as a group, describing the variations in surgical technique along the way.

These operations all attempt to prevent urethral hypermobility and the stress incontinence that results by stabilizing the endopelvic fascia from above. They do this by attaching the endopelvic fascia to various fixed points in the retropubic space. All of these operations successfully cure stress incontinence caused by anatomic hypermobility of the bladder outlet; they are less successful treating stress incontinence caused by intrinsic sphincteric dysfunction. Some of these techniques pull the bladder neck and urethra higher and tighter than do others. As pointed out in the following, the higher the point of fixation of the endopelvic fascia and the tighter the repair, the greater is the likelihood of developing both postoperative voiding difficulty and subsequent enterocele formation. The goal of surgery for stress incontinence should be to restore normal bladder function as far as is possible for each patient. Curing stress incontinence only to replace it with a vaginal vault eversion, chronic voiding difficulty, or intractable urge incontinence is not a surgical success for the patient. Each op-

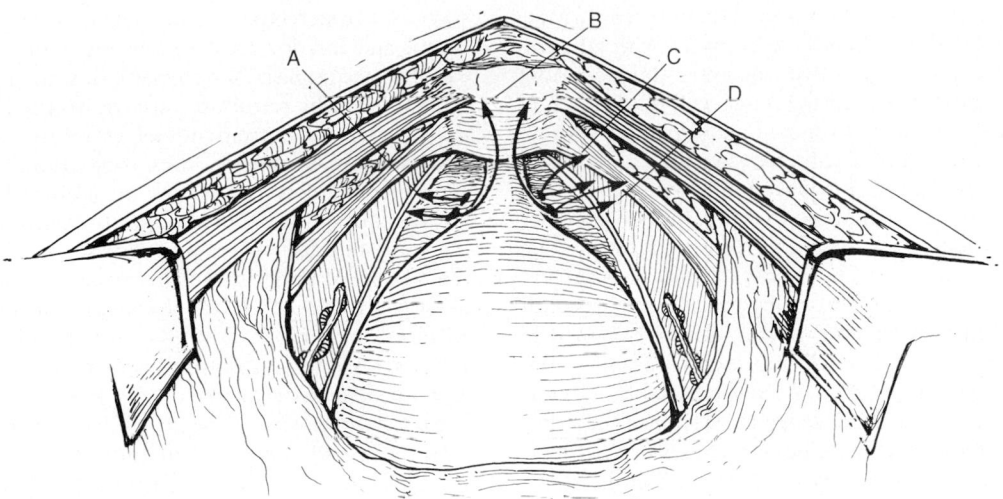

FIGURE 36.9. Points of reattachment of the endopelvic fascia during retropubic bladder neck suspension operations. **A:** Arcus tendineus fascia pelvis. **B:** Periosteum of the pubic symphysis. **C:** Iliopectineal ligament (Cooper ligament). **D:** Obturator internus fascia.

eration presents special challenges and the opportunity for special complications.

As in all other operations, having adequate access to and exposure of the operative field is a primary requirement for successful retropubic surgery. Generally speaking, these operations are easiest to perform when the surgeon has simultaneous access to the vagina as well as the abdominal operative field. This means that the patient is best positioned for this surgery in a modified lithotomy position. This can be done with traditional "candy cane" lithotomy stirrups, but use of Allen universal stirrups (Allen Medical Systems, Cleveland, OH) allows the patient to be positioned comfortably in a lithotomy position that keeps her knees and thighs away from the abdominal field (Fig. 36.10). We prefer to equip the patient with knee-high pneumatic compression boots during pelvic surgery to reduce the risk of venous thromboembolism. The boots should be used during surgery and also for the first few days postoperatively.

Both the vagina and abdomen should be prepared with povidone-iodine or an equivalent antiseptic solution, and draped as sterile operative fields. After the patient has been prepared and draped, a 14F or 16F Foley catheter is inserted through the sterile field into the urinary bladder and fixed to the drapes with a sterile clamp. Inserting the catheter as a sterile procedure after the patient has been draped allows the surgeon to manipulate the catheter and its balloon during the operation without becoming contaminated. Although some surgeons like to use a catheter with a 30-mL balloon, it is not necessary to use a balloon this large; a 5-mL balloon should be adequate. Prolonged bladder drainage with a large-volume balloon can cause irreversible damage to the bladder neck, and this should be avoided at all costs.

One of the irritations of doing retropubic surgery using both the vagina and abdomen is the need to change gloves frequently as the hand is moved from one field to the other. This nuisance can be avoided by using a dis-

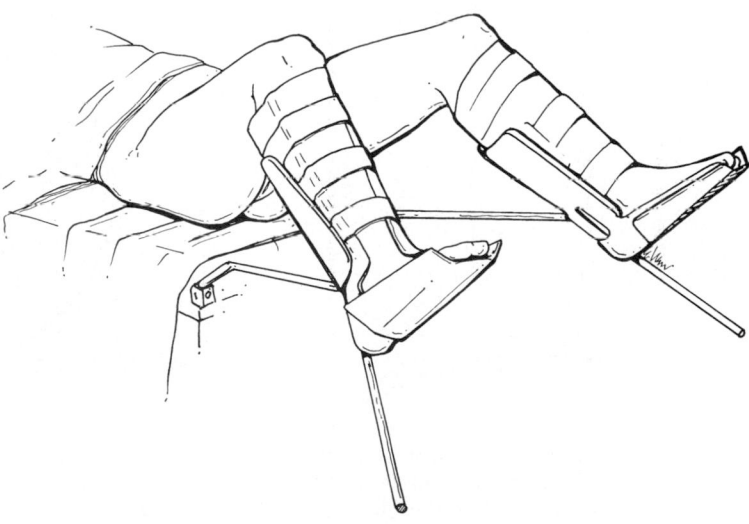

FIGURE 36.10. Positioning the patient for retropubic bladder neck surgery using Allen universal lithotomy stirrups. This allows the surgeon to have simultaneous access to both the vagina and the space of Retzius.

posable prostatectomy drape over the vagina (3M, Minneapolis, MN). These drapes are designed with an anterior slit that normally goes over the penis and a condom drape that is normally used for transrectal manipulation. The drape can be affixed over a woman's perineum to allow insertion of a Foley catheter through the anterior slit, whereas the condom is placed into the vagina. This effectively drapes the vagina so that the surgeon can continue to use one glove throughout the procedure (Fig. 36.11).

The type of incision chosen by the surgeon has a direct impact on how much exposure can be obtained in the retropubic space. The incision used for these operations should be as low and close to the back of the pubic symphysis as possible. A Cherney incision made one finger-breadth above the pubic bone provides excellent exposure of the retropubic space. Once the skin has been incised, the subcutaneous tissue can be divided with Bovie electrocautery. The incision should go down through the fascia directly to the rectus muscles, which are then cut free from their insertion onto the pubic bone, allowing the fascia and muscles to swing cranially as one unit, exposing the operative field. An incision this low does not hinder performance of other pelvic surgery,

such as a hysterectomy, and makes surgery in the deep lateral and inferior areas of the retropubic space much easier to accomplish. If necessary, this incision can be extended from the retropubic area up to the level of the iliac crests, giving tremendous exposure of the entire pelvic cavity. Of course, these operations can be done through a midline incision or a traditional Pfannenstiel incision made two or three finger-breadths above the pubic bone, but deep exposure in the space of Retzius is often a struggle under these circumstances. Such incisions do not provide good lateral exposure in the pelvis and require considerable additional retraction from a surgical assistant. A muscle-splitting incision, such as a Maylard incision, is a better alternative if the surgeon does not like a Cherney incision. Many different retractors can be used to provide exposure in the retroperitoneal space. We prefer to use a circular Turner-Warwick urology retractor, an extremely versatile instrument that allows traction to be placed from all angles using a variety of retractor blades of different sizes and shapes (Fig. 36.12).

At this point in the operation, the surgeon must decide if it is necessary to enter the peritoneal cavity or if the entire operation will be done in the retropubic space. Avoiding peritoneal entry theoretically decreases postop-

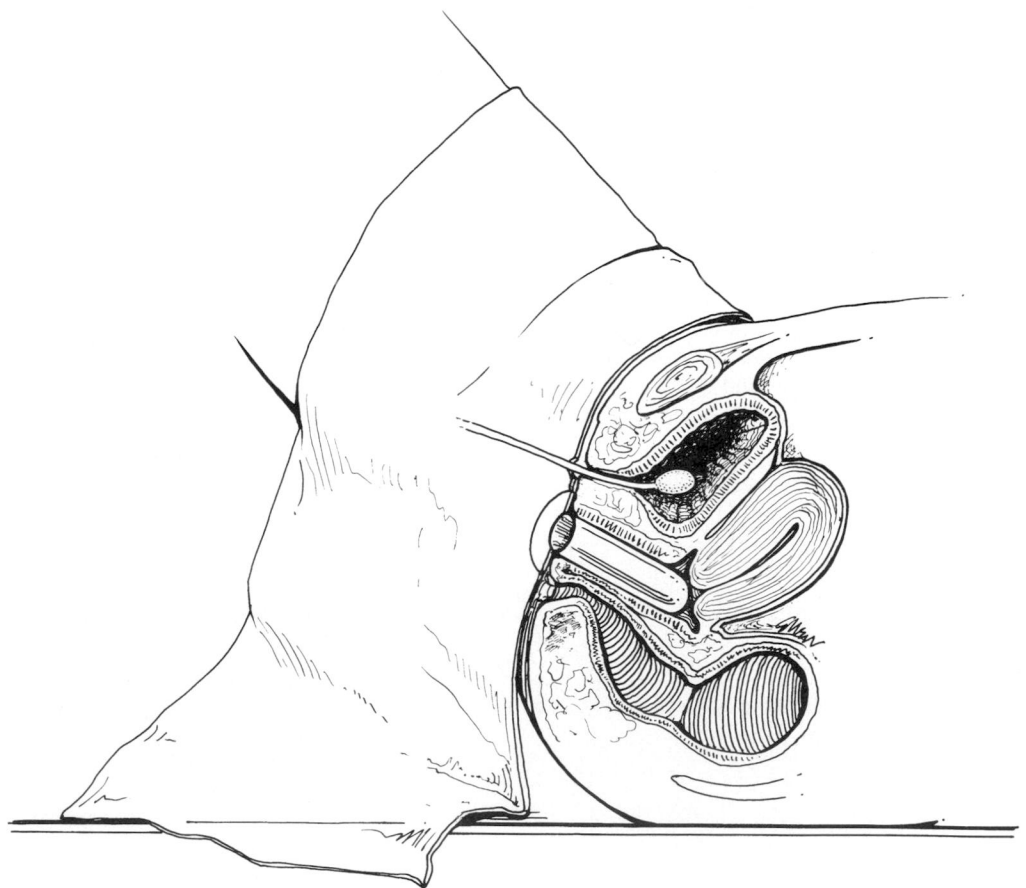

FIGURE 36.11. Use of a disposable prostatectomy drape in retropubic bladder neck suspension surgery. The transurethral Foley catheter is inserted through the anterior slit, and the sterile condom attached to the drape is placed inside the vagina.

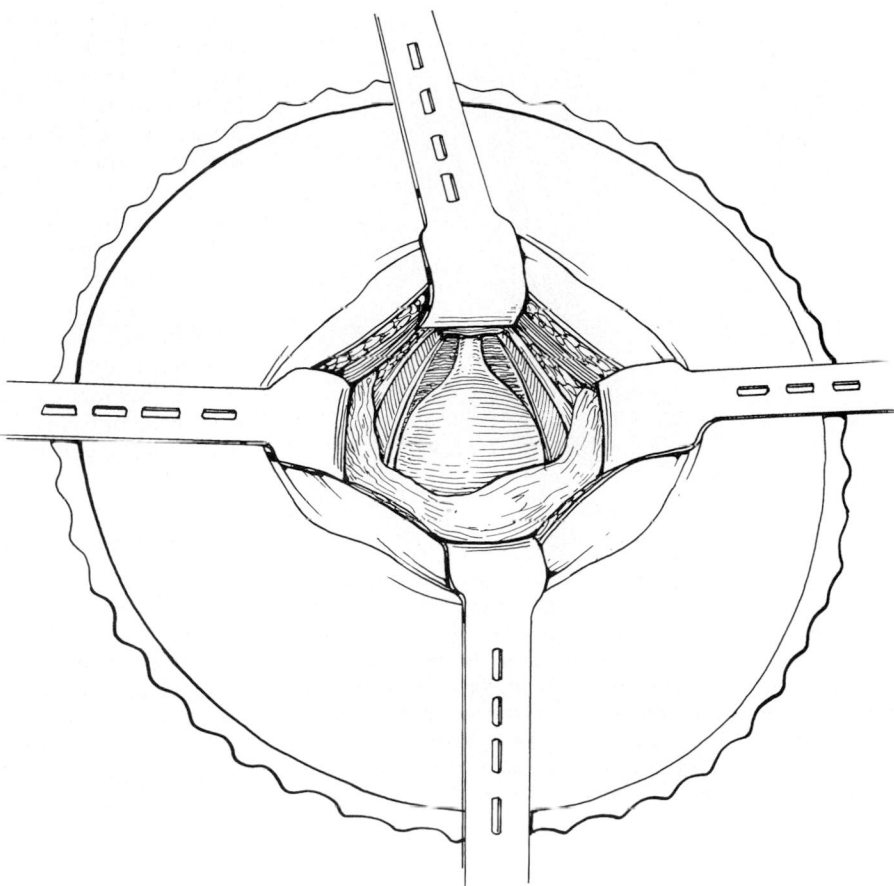

FIGURE 36.12. Use of a Turner-Warwick ring retractor, which allows positioning of multiple blades at different locations for enhanced surgical exposure.

erative morbidity and reduces the chance of the patient developing an ileus. If other pelvic surgery will be done at the same time, such as a total abdominal hysterectomy or removal of the patient's ovaries, then the abdomen must be entered of course. We generally prefer to open the peritoneal cavity for several reasons. First, it allows the surgeon to explore the abdomen and ensure that no unexpected pathology is present. Second, packing the intestines into the upper abdomen takes significant pressure off the space of Retzius from below. This makes operating in the deep lateral spaces of the pelvis significantly easier. Third, opening the peritoneal cavity allows the surgeon to perform a culdoplasty at the time of the operation to prevent the development of a future enterocele. This is a critical step that should not be neglected without good reason.

Virtually all of the operations that resuspend the urethra and bladder neck from above—the Marshall–Marchetti–Krantz (MMK), Burch, vaginal-obturator shelf, and needle-suspension operations—pull these structures anteriorly. Because the vagina is a circular tube, pulling the anterior vagina upward also pulls the posterior vagina upward and away from its normal position on the levator plate. This widens and opens the posterior cul-de-sac of Douglas, creating a potential space for enterocele formation. If the patient already has a degree of uterine prolapse, or if she has had a previous hys-

terectomy and has already started to develop an enterocele, then failure to close and support this space can create a rapidly progressing prolapse that may require corrective surgery within a few weeks of the operation. Case series of women who have undergone surgery for correction of posthysterectomy vaginal vault prolapse, for example, reveal that a large percentage of these patients have undergone retropubic bladder neck suspensions that clearly predisposed them to vault eversion. Wiskind and colleagues found that 27% of 131 women who underwent a Burch colposuspension for stress incontinence required subsequent surgery to correct a prolapse within 40 months of their initial operations (range, 9 to 70 months). Dr. Burch noticed this problem in his own patients and made a special point of performing a culdoplasty whenever he did this operation. Failure to appreciate such interrelations of support among the various pelvic compartments is a common problem in surgical practice, especially among urologists who are not accustomed to dealing with other pelvic support defects.

A variety of techniques of cul-de-sac closure exist. If a hysterectomy is being performed, then it is easy to identify the uterosacral ligaments at the time of surgery and tag them with permanent sutures (Fig. 36.13). Once the uterus has been removed, the cuff can be left open and a McCall culdoplasty performed from above (Fig. 36.14). This accomplishes closure and support of the

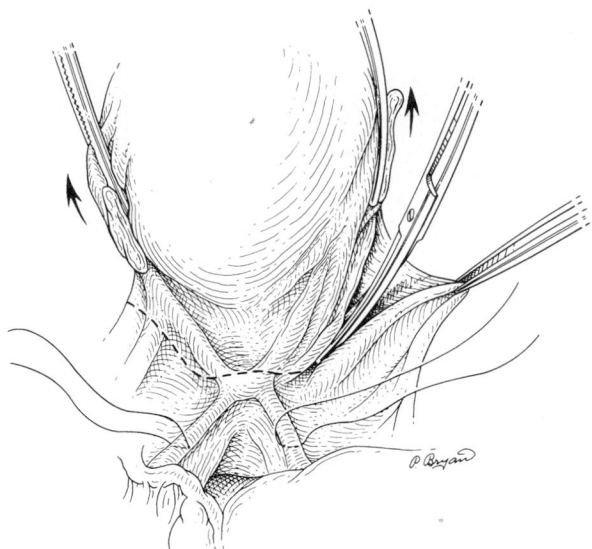

FIGURE 36.13. Modified McCall culdoplasty at the time of abdominal hysterectomy. The uterosacral ligaments are identified early in the course of the hysterectomy, before the uterus has been removed. This is aided by upward traction of the specimen through the use of Kocher clamps *(arrows)*. Permanent tag sutures are placed through each uterosacral ligament approximately 2 cm from the pelvic sidewall. (From: Wall LL. A technique for modified McCall culdoplasty at the time of abdominal hysterectomy. *J Am Coll Surg* 1994;178:507, with permission.)

cul-de-sac in a fashion similar to that obtained during a transvaginal McCall culdoplasty done at the time of a vaginal hysterectomy. If the patient has had a previous hysterectomy, the cul-de-sac can be closed using a single Moschowitz culdoplasty (which does, however, place the ureters at some risk) or a hemi-Moschcowitz culdoplasty on each side of the pelvis (Fig. 36.15). A Halban culdoplasty, which closes the cul-de-sac from front to back rather than side to side, is equally effective and poses less risk of inadvertently trapping or kinking a ureter along the pelvic sidewall.

With the intraabdominal portion of the operation completed, the surgeon's attention can be directed to the retropubic space. The space of Retzius is a potential space lying outside of the peritoneal cavity and inside the bony anterior pelvis. It is full of loose areolar connective tissue and, depending on the size of the patient, a varying amount of fat. To operate in this space, it must first be opened. Some surgeons do this by poking a finger behind the pubic symphysis and then sweeping their hands boldly along each side, pushing the bladder posteriorly as they go. Although this opens the space quickly in a patient who has not had previous retropubic surgery, the surgeon should remember that this is a highly vascular area, often with many large veins running in unexpected places along the edges of the bladder and vagina, the pelvic side walls, and the pubic symphysis. It is better to open this space gently and slowly, observing the variations in individual anatomy as this is done, using a malleable retractor, a sponge stick, and the blunt upper end of a pair of tissue forceps. If this is done systematically,

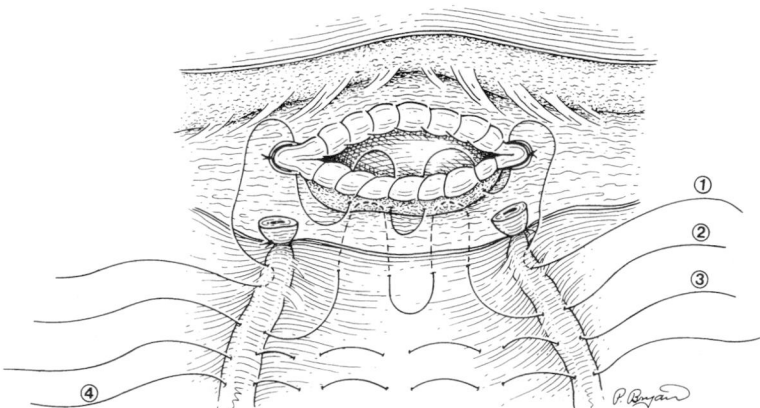

FIGURE 36.14. Modified McCall culdoplasty at the time of abdominal hysterectomy. Placement of the culdoplasty sutures. **1:** The initial delayed-absorbable suture is brought through the uterosacral ligament and the edge of the vaginal cuff and then is reefed through the vagina and posterior peritoneum before being brought out in a similar manner on the contralateral side. **2:** A second suture of delayed-absorbable material is placed in a similar manner, posterior to the first suture. **3 and 4:** The permanent tag sutures, which were placed through the uterosacral ligaments early in the hysterectomy, are reefed through the posterior peritoneum and brought through the uterosacral ligament on the contralateral side. When tied, these sutures obliterate the cul-de-sac and provide further support to the vaginal cuff. If desired, these sutures can be used to complete a full Moschcowitz culdoplasty. (From: Wall LL. A technique for modified McCall culdoplasty at the time of abdominal hysterectomy. *J Am Coll Surg* 1994;178:507, with permission.)

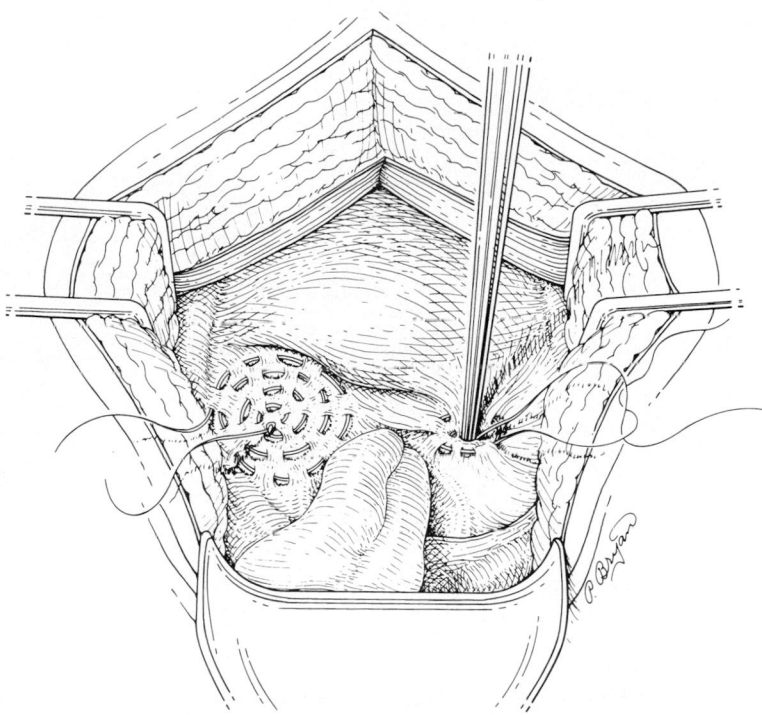

FIGURE 36.15. Hemi-Moschcowitz culdoplasty. A continuous circular suture is used to obliterate the cul-de-sac on each side. This can be reinforced over the top by interrupted sutures from front to back that plicate the uterosacral ligaments in the midline behind the vagina.

the entire space can be dissected out to expose the back of the pubic symphysis, iliopectineal ligament (Cooper ligament), urethra and anterior bladder, vagina, endopelvic fascia, attachments of the fascia along the arcus tendineus fasciae pelvis, obturator internus muscle, and obturator neurovascular bundle. These are the critical landmarks for surgeons operating in this space (Fig. 36.16).

The anatomy generally is different if the patient had previous surgery in the space of Retzius. Once opened, this space can scar down with remarkable tenacity. Reoperative surgery in this area often is difficult, with no good landmarks to guide the surgeon. In such cases, the first priority is always to establish normal anatomic relations. The space can be opened slowly and carefully by dissecting sharply with a pair of scissors directly down and along the back of the pubic symphysis. Often, the scarring that is encountered is worse directly behind the pubic bone (particularly if the patient had a previous MMK procedure). In such cases, the more lateral areas of the space of Retzius may be almost free of adhesions, and the work of surgical exposure can be started in these areas. As noted, the vascularity in the retropubic space may be remarkable and irregular in terms of the size of veins and their locations. Under these circumstances, careful dissection pays large dividends. Hemostasis, especially when dissection is taking place deep in the pelvis, is often aided by a monopolar cautery forceps operated by a foot pedal, with which aberrant veins can be grasped and cauterized. If bleeding does occur, often it can be controlled by upward compression from one of the surgeon's fingers in the vagina applied against a sponge forceps pressed down from above. This compresses the veins and allows them

to be cauterized, clamped with surgical clips, or ligated with sutures.

Once the space of Retzius is open, the endopelvic fascia must be identified. The bladder can be seen in the midline as a somewhat rounded structure, slightly humped along the edges. Immediately lateral to the bladder edge is the anterior vagina, which typically is marked by a rather exuberant venous plexus. Just lateral to this lies the exposed endopelvic fascia. It is into this sturdy, avascular connective tissue that the surgeon wants to place the supporting sutures. Failure to identify this tissue correctly means either a surgical failure or a surgical complication. Many MMK procedures have failed because the surgeon sutured the anterior bladder wall to the pubic symphysis, which does nothing to stabilize the endopelvic fascia and support the urethra. Moving the Foley catheter balloon within the bladder often helps identify the location of the bladder edge. If the landmarks are uncertain, the surgeon can use a sponge stick to dissect the bladder and vagina medially, exposing the underlying fascia (Fig. 36.17). If the veins running along the vaginal edge are sheared off during this process, significant hemorrhage can occur; the surgeon should be ready to deal with this problem. If the anatomy is uncertain, it is better to open the bladder and locate its edges directly than to place sutures in uncertainty. The dome of the bladder can be opened longitudinally along its anterior surface using a Bovie cautery for better hemostasis, left open during the procedure, and closed at the end of the case using a double layer of continuous 2-0 or 3-0 absorbable sutures, such as Vicryl. Many surgeons open the bladder routinely in performing these operations, although we do not. The bladder is a forgiving or-

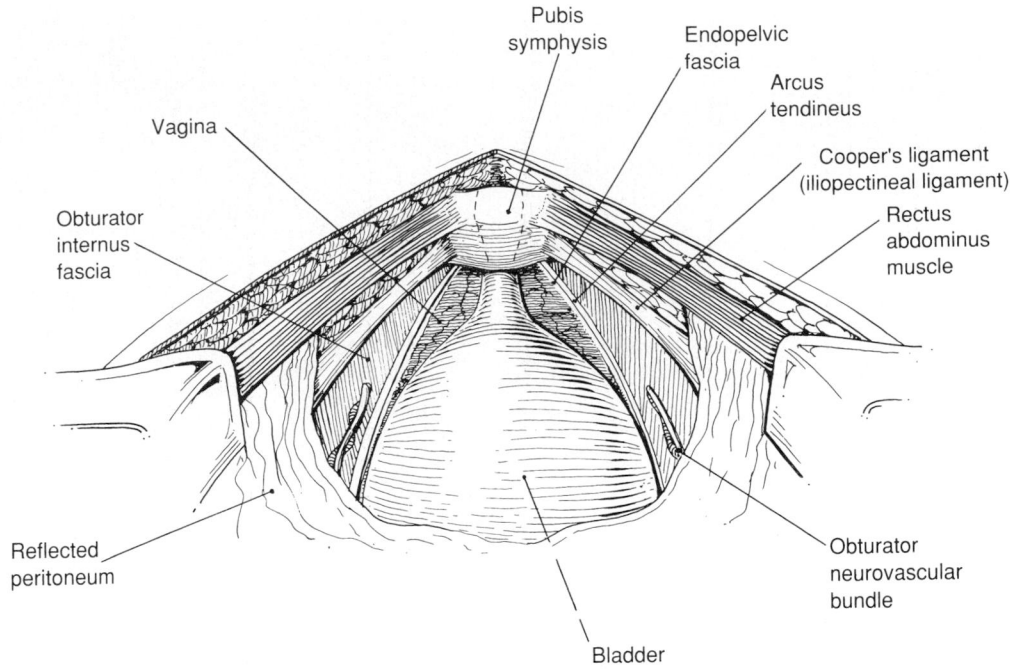

FIGURE 36.16. Anatomic landmarks in the space of Retzius.

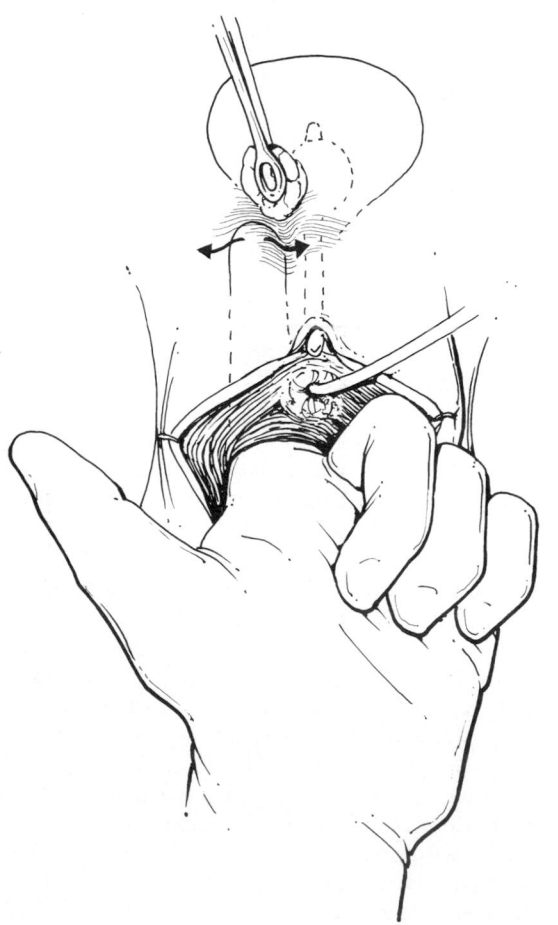

FIGURE 36.17. Medial dissection of the bladder edge to help expose the endopelvic fascia. The surgeon's left hand is in the vagina, elevating and stabilizing the endopelvic fascia, while the right hand moves the bladder medially with a sponge forceps.

gan and heals well after such trauma provided it is drained freely for a week after surgery and is not allowed to become overdistended.

Permanent (or at least delayed-absorbable) sutures should be used to fix the endopelvic fascia to the chosen points of attachment. The surgeon is repairing a support defect, much like a hernia. The use of catgut sutures for this type of surgery results in a significantly higher failure rate than more durable sutures. Nothing is more devastating to a patient with stress incontinence than to be dry in the immediate postoperative period, but to have her incontinence return by the time of her 6-week postoperative visit because her sutures dissolved before scar tissue could cement the results of the operation. We prefer to use 2-0 braided polybutilate-coated polyester (Ethibond). Full-thickness bites of tissue should be taken with the needle to ensure that the stitch is anchored well. It does not matter if the suture traverses the vagina; these sutures invariably reepithelialize without complication. However, it is important to make sure that the suture does not enter the bladder because this can cause stone formation, recurrent infection, and hematuria.

The sutures generally are placed by the surgeon operating with one hand in the vagina to stabilize the endopelvic fascia, while the other hand drives the needle (Fig. 36.18). Care should be taken to drive the needle carefully into the fascia, but not into the surgeon's finger! This can be accomplished by using the intravaginal finger to elevate and expose the fascia. This done, the surgeon's finger is withdrawn a little, and the suture is placed just proximal to the fingertip. Some surgeons perform this part of the operation using a sterilized sewing thimble on their intravaginal finger; other surgeons use an intravaginal retractor to elevate the endopelvic fascia. The stitches are placed along the edge of the bladder,

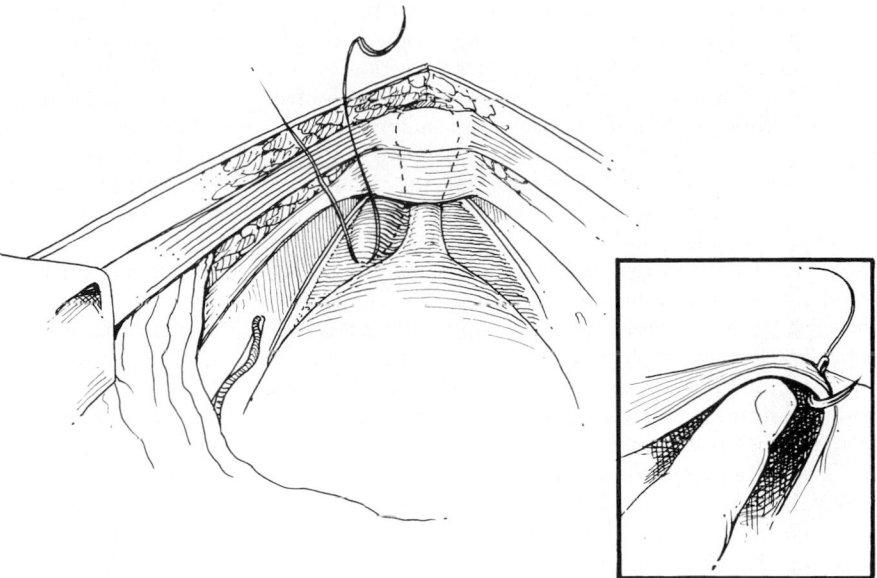

FIGURE 36.18. Placement of sutures through the endopelvic fascia. The surgeon tents the endopelvic fascia upward with a finger while the suture is placed *(inset)*.

beginning cranially and moving down progressively toward the bladder neck and distal urethra with each successive stitch. If a disposable prostatectomy drape is used as an intravaginal drape, care must be taken to withdraw the condom before placing the stitch to avoid suturing the drape into the vagina. Once the suture has been placed, it should be tied down against the endopelvic fascia. This prevents the suture from cutting through the vaginal tissues as it is pulled and manipulated during the remainder of the operation.

To this point, all of the retropubic bladder neck suspension operations are essentially the same; they differ primarily in where the sutures are placed into the endopelvic fascia and in where they are then attached. The MMK operation is performed by placing a series of sutures along the urethra to the level of the bladder neck and then driving the needle directly into the periosteum of the symphysis pubis (Fig. 36.19). This corrects stress incontinence by elevating the urethra into a fixed position behind the pubic symphysis from which it cannot descend; however, it often kinks the urethra into an unnatural position and also can be associated with significant postoperative voiding difficulty. The fact that the sutures are placed directly into the periosteum also puts patients at risk for developing osteitis pubis, a painful inflammatory condition that can totally disable an otherwise healthy woman for months. Placement of sutures too near or even into the urethra can lead to chronic irritative voiding symptoms. Because the supportive sutures are placed only along the urethra, only the urethra is supported; a traditional MMK operation does not correct a coexistent cystocele. At the same time, however, urethral elevation pulls the vagina forward and can predispose the patient to enterocele formation. The MMK procedure has been used by many surgeons for many years, and the published success rates are relatively consistent throughout the literature; however, consideration of the complications of this operation has led to the development of alternative techniques, and the operation

as originally described is falling out of favor among knowledgeable surgeons.

In 1961, John Burch of Nashville described a modification of the original MMK procedure. Burch thought that ". . . the Marshall-Marchetti-Krantz operation is not always easy to perform, the field is often deep and bloody, the edges of the urethra are difficult to define, and the periosteum on the posterior aspect of the symphysis is far from ideal as a holding structure." Based on these concerns, Burch looked for a different point of suture placement. Initially, he considered the fascia over the obturator internus muscle but abandoned this site in favor of the iliopectineal ligament of Cooper. Since the original description of this operation by Burch, it has been called by a number of names, including the Burch procedure, the Cooper ligament fixation, and the colposuspension. A number of modifications of technique have been described, ranging from extensive dissection

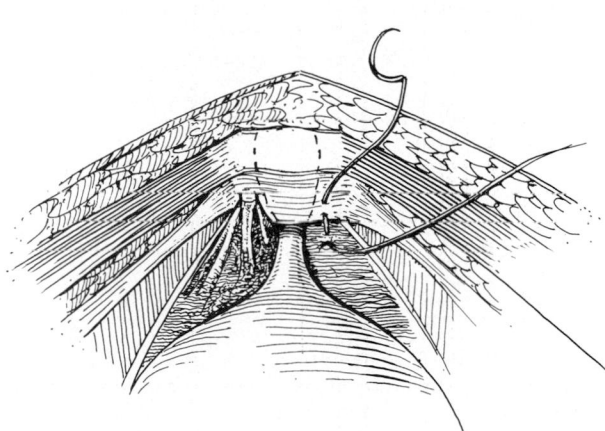

FIGURE 36.19. Placement of sutures for a Marshall-Marchetti-Krantz operation. Sutures are placed into the endopelvic fascia along the urethra and then into the periosteum along the back of the pubic symphysis.

and mobilization of the bladder neck so that the vagina comes into actual apposition with the Cooper ligament when the sutures are tied, to minimal dissection of the endopelvic fascia with tying of sutures under minimal tension. Either technique stabilizes the suburethral endopelvic fascia and prevents excessive urethral mobility. The more aggressive the dissection and the tighter the sutures are tied, the more the endopelvic fascia beneath the urethra is pulled up like a sling, and the greater is the opportunity for postoperative voiding difficulty as well as for enterocele formation. Complete apposition of the endopelvic fascia and vagina to the Cooper ligament is not necessary for success, particularly if permanent sutures are used; however, bridging or "bow-stringing" of absorbable sutures can lead to failure if scar tissue formation does not occur faster than suture dissolution.

Two to four permanent sutures are placed into the endopelvic fascia at the level of the bladder neck and along the bladder edge proximal to the bladder neck (Fig. 36.20). Most authors who have described their experiences with this operation prefer not to place sutures along the urethra, for fear of creating complications similar to those experienced with the MMK procedure. This leaves one to two finger-breadths of free space between the urethra and the back of the pubic symphysis, which is thought to prevent some of the postoperative voiding difficulty that can be experienced after the MMK operation. The sutures are tied down to prevent them cutting through the tissues as they are tied. The end of the needle then is passed at right angles through the thick portion of the Cooper ligament. The sutures are tied down, elevating the bladder neck and supporting the urethra.

Compared with the MMK operation, the Burch operation has some advantages. It can correct a coexistent cystocele, it does not produce osteitis pubis, and it has a

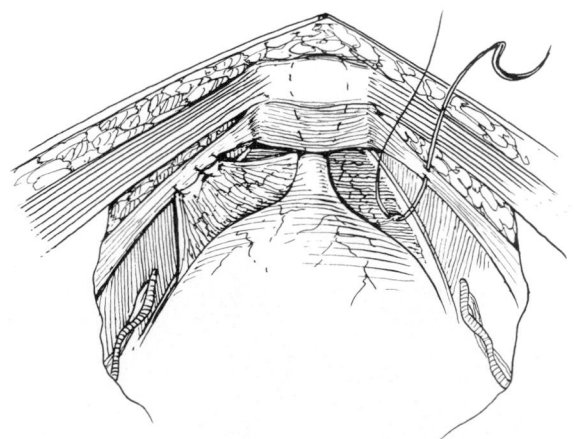

FIGURE 36.20. Placement of sutures for a Burch colposuspension operation. Sutures are placed into the endopelvic fascia along the bladder edge down to the level of the bladder neck and tied. The ends of the sutures are then passed through Cooper ligament. When tied, the bladder neck is elevated, but free space remains between the bladder neck and the back of the pubic symphysis.

firmer point of fixation along the Cooper ligament. Like the MMK operation, it is direct, reliable, and straightforward and does not depend on indirect attachments for success. There is widespread experience with this operation throughout the world, and it has been subjected to more rigorous investigation than any other operation for stress incontinence, including the MMK procedure. The published success rates are consistently high, and in comparative surgical studies, the Burch procedure consistently has the highest objective cure rates for stress incontinence of any standard operation.

As with any operation, there are complications with the Burch procedure, and most of these are related to the degree to which the bladder neck is elevated. The surgeon should remember that the object of this type of operation is primarily to correct urethral hypermobility, or abnormal urethral descent. Higher and tighter does not necessarily provide better support, but a higher and tighter suspension certainly can lead to problems, including outflow obstruction, voiding difficulty, detrusor instability, and enterocele formation.

Our expanding knowledge of retropubic anatomy has led to the realization that much of the hypermobility of the urethra and bladder neck that leads to prolapse and stress incontinence is caused by detachments of the endopelvic fascia from its normal connections to the pelvic sidewall. These defects can be corrected by reattaching the endopelvic fascia to the arcus tendineus, a procedure known as paravaginal repair (Fig. 36.21). Although it is theoretically possible to cure stress incontinence by identifying a defect only on one side and repairing it only on that side, virtually all surgeons who perform this operation reattach the endopelvic fascia bilaterally. After the space of Retzius has been dissected, the arcus can be identified running as a thin, white, wiry band along the pelvic sidewall from the pubic symphysis to the ischial spine. The vagina is placed on stretch, and an anchor stitch is placed into the endopelvic fascia, tied down, and then placed around the arcus on the pelvic sidewall (Fig. 36.22). This creates a small groove of tissue running along the arcus, and the endopelvic fascia and arcus then can be sutured together and the defect closed along its length. Again, owing to the similarities to hernia repair, it is better to use permanent sutures for this kind of surgery. Care should be taken to avoid injuring the obturator neurovascular bundle, which runs anterior to the arcus tendineus.

Early experience with this procedure suggests that it is durable, physiologic, and results in less voiding difficulty postoperatively than do other forms of retropubic bladder neck suspension surgery. In Shull and Baden's early series, 97% of patients undergoing this procedure had excellent functional results. A more recent randomized trial comparing the abdominal paravaginal defect repair with the Burch colposuspension conducted by Colombo and colleagues (1996) found that spontaneous voiding function returned more rapidly among patients undergoing paravaginal repair, but that both subjective (71%) and objective (61%) cure rates were much lower for these women than those patients who underwent a

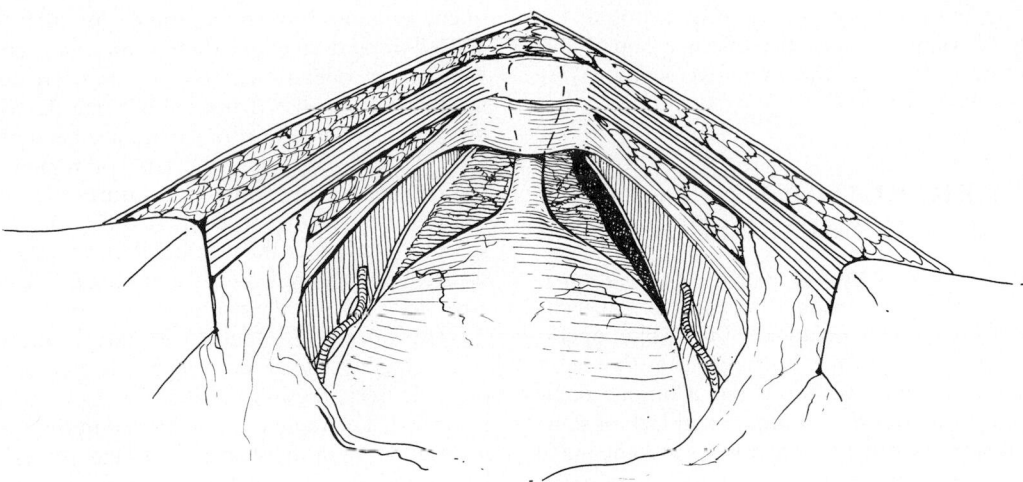

FIGURE 36.21. Detachment of endopelvic fascia from its normal attachment along the right side of the patient's pelvis. Fascial detachment leads to loss of support and the development of urethral hypermobility, which may cause stress incontinence.

Burch procedure (100% subjective and 100% objective cure).

The vagino-obturator shelf procedure represents a surgical procedure intermediate between the classic Burch operation and the paravaginal repair. Originally described by Turner-Warwick, it was an attempt to create a more physiologic and less obstructive retropubic bladder neck suspension operation than either the colposuspension or the MMK procedure. In this operative variation, the endopelvic fascia is sutured to the fascia covering the obturator internus muscle (Fig. 36.23). In Turner-Warwick's original description of the procedure, the endopelvic fascia is incised and sutures are placed directly into the underlying vagina, approximating the

vagina to the obturator fascia. This fascia generally is strong enough to hold sutures well, but sometimes the fascia is attenuated and an alternate point of attachment (usually Cooper ligament) must be used.

With the suspension procedure completed and hemostasis secured, any packs can be removed, and the peritoneum can be closed (if it was opened). A closed-suction drain (such as a Jackson-Pratt drain) can be placed in the space of Retzius and brought out through a separate stab incision through the fascia and anterior abdominal wall before closure of the main incision. If good hemostasis has been achieved, then drainage of this kind is not necessary, although some authors place such drains as a matter of routine. These drains can be re-

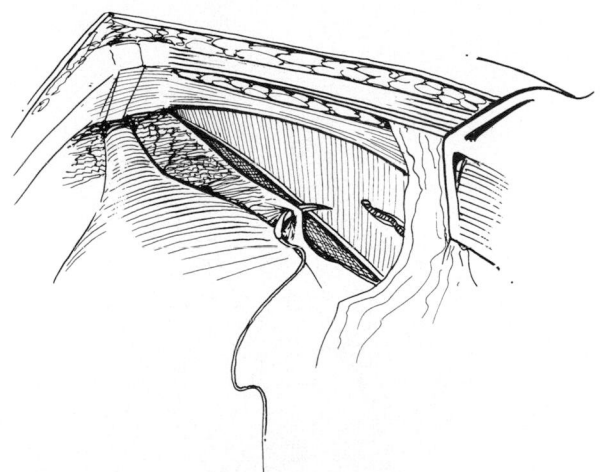

FIGURE 36.22. Reattachment of the endopelvic fascia to its normal location along the arcus tendineus fasciae pelvis. The first or key stitch should be placed to put the endopelvic fascia on stretch. Once this has been done, the line detachment can be resutured along its entire length from the pubic bone to the ischial ligament, if necessary.

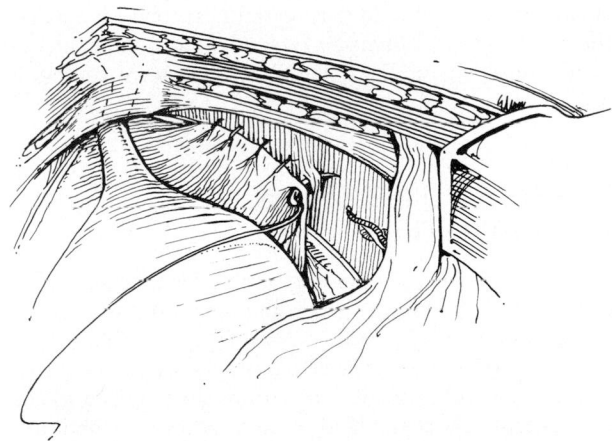

FIGURE 36.23. Vaginal-obturator shelf procedure. The endopelvic fascia is sutured to the fascia overlying the obturator internus muscle. The procedure is similar to a Burch colposuspension, but sutures are fixed at a level lower than the Cooper ligament, which runs above the obturator internus fascia.

moved on the first postoperative day if their output has been minimal. Many authors also place a suprapubic catheter before closure of the operative incision (see Postoperative Bladder Care).

RETROPUBIC BLADDER NECK SUSPENSION BY LAPAROSCOPY

Laparoscopic surgeons continue to advance their capabilities, and a number of authors have developed techniques to perform Burch (or, at least, Burch-like) operations for stress incontinence. Nearly every author who has written about these operations has a unique technique, and the variations in technique, and lack of standardized evaluations or measurements of outcome make the comparative evaluation of the laparoscopic approach problematic. Some surgeons have attempted to replicate the original Burch procedure laparoscopically, passing sutures through both the endopelvic fascia and the iliopectineal ligament of Cooper. Other surgeons have "modified" the technique, using hernia staples and synthetic mesh to accomplish bladder neck elevation. Definitive comparative studies have not been performed yet. The surgical studies that do exist are, for the most part, of questionable quality and cannot be said to have convinced the critical reader of the superiority of this approach to the treatment of stress incontinence. In view of the degree of scarring that usually occurs in the space of Retzius after bladder neck suspension surgery, laparoscopic techniques of bladder neck suspension seem feasible only in patients who have not previously undergone retropubic surgery. Because the goal of bladder neck suspension surgery is correction of the patient's stress incontinence rather than the demonstration of laparoscopic showmanship (or the generation of increased surgical fees), surgeons who perform laparoscopic Burch procedures should have previously acquired considerable operative experience performing these procedures using laparotomy, and should keep careful prospective data on their outcomes. Patients who are offered such procedures should be advised that their long-term success is unknown.

NEEDLE-SUSPENSION PROCEDURES

An alternative to the open retropubic bladder neck procedures described in the preceding is urethral suspension by a combined vaginal and abdominal approach in which the space of Retzius is traversed using a long needle that carries the suture with it. The suture then is fixed to the perivesical fascia at the bladder neck and to the abdominal fascia, suspending the bladder neck on a "swing" between the two sets of sutures. This class of operation was first described by Armand Pereyra in 1959, and he spent much of his career modifying, refining, and experimenting with this technique. The long-needle suspension procedures have proved to be popular, and many subse-

quent surgeons have made minor modifications to this procedure and attached their names to them as if they were unique operations; however, there are essentially no modifications in use that were not first described by the inventor. The modifications that have been proposed fall into five categories: (a) the type of vaginal dissection; (b) the method by which the sutures are anchored on the vaginal side of the field; (c) the way in which the space of Retzius is traversed; (d) the method by which sutures are anchored on the abdominal side of the operative field; (e) and the use of endoscopy.

The operation generally is started like an anterior colporrhaphy. The anterior vagina is incised and the endopelvic fascia around the bladder neck and urethra are identified. The vagina can be incised in the midline, as an inverted U, or in the shape of a T (Fig. 36.24). Once this has been done, an extensive bilateral dissection is carried out to mobilize the tissues up to the inferolateral edge of the pubic ramus. The endopelvic fascia then is perforated, either bluntly or by using a dissecting scissors, always with the instrument hugging the edge of the pubic bone to prevent injury to the bladder. Then, a finger can be inserted into the space to widen it further and to detach and mobilize the endopelvic fascia on each side before suture placement (Fig. 36.25).

At this point, a small suprapubic incision is made about two finger-breadths above the pubic symphysis. This incision is carried down through the subcutaneous fat to the level of the anterior rectus fascia. A special long needle threaded with suture then is punched through the fascia. Although several blind techniques have been described for doing this, it seems best to advance the needle through the space of Retzius by direct guidance from below. One of the surgeon's index fingers is inserted through the vaginal incision up into the space of Retzius. The needle can be popped through the abdominal fascia against the surgeon's finger, which can then

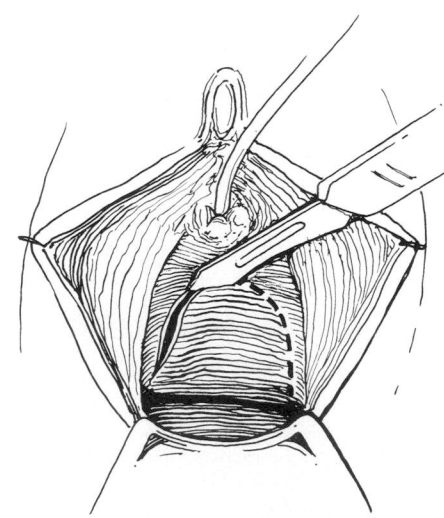

FIGURE 36.24. Opening the anterior vagina to expose the bladder neck using a U-shaped incision.

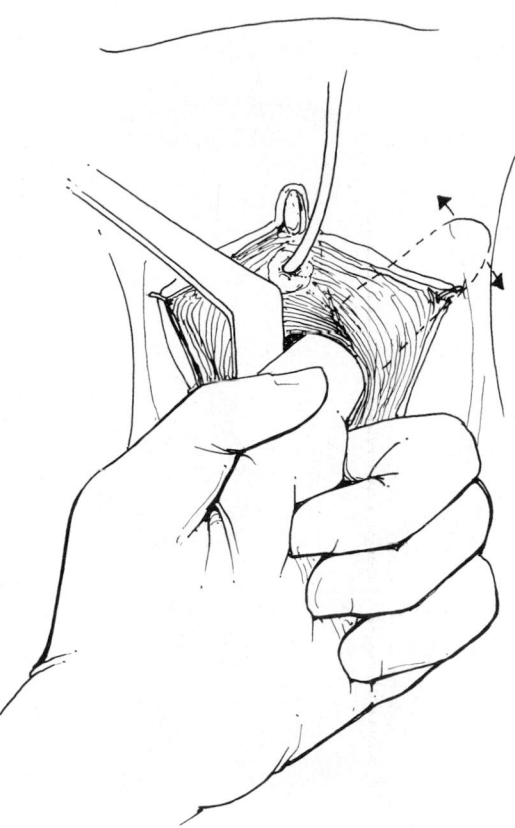

FIGURE 36.25. Perforation of the endopelvic fascia to open the space of Retzius and mobilize the periurethral tissues.

guide the needle safely through the retropubic space. The needle should exit the vaginal incision at the level of the bladder neck (Fig. 36.26). Mundy advocates a different technique, passing the needles transvaginally, starting from below and moving upward through the abdominal fascia. In either case, the suspensory suture should be fixed to the endopelvic fascia at the level of the bladder neck. After this is done, the needle is passed once more through the space of Retzius, and the other end of the suture is threaded through it. The needle then is pulled back up through the abdominal fascia, and the two ends of the suture are tied into the fascia.

Because this operation depends almost entirely on the integrity of the suture material and the way it is attached (rather than scarring), the type of suture used and the method by which it is affixed to the endopelvic fascia are of crucial importance. Heavy permanent sutures (0, 1, or 2) are preferable; absorbable sutures give inferior long-term success rates. Many types of suture fixation to the endopelvic fascia have been described, and these variations account for many of the new operations for stress incontinence that have been developed using long-needle techniques. In patients with poor connective tissue or weak fascia, there is a tendency for sutures to pull out or cut through like a cheese-wire. When this occurs, the support is lost, and the stress incontinence recurs. In the Stamey technique of needle suspension, a

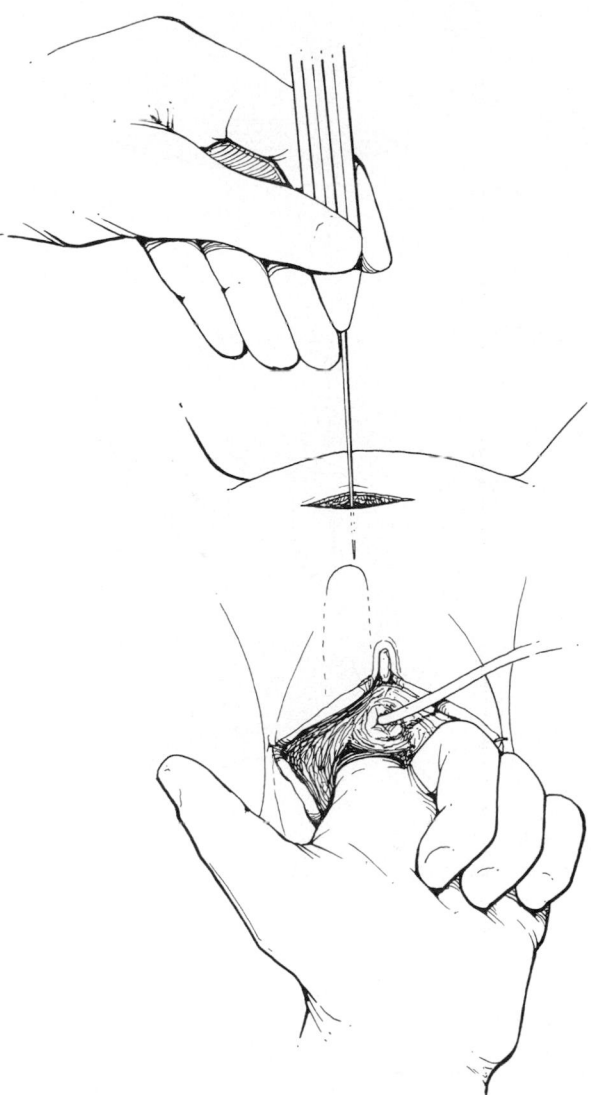

FIGURE 36.26. Guidance of the long needle through the space of Retzius using the surgeon's index finger.

small (1-cm) Dacron bolster is threaded over the suspending suture like a bead on a string to act as a stopper (Fig. 36.27). This buttress originally was thought to provide firmer support than the suture alone, but this method of anchoring tissue seems particularly vulnerable to pull-through. A more secure way of fastening the sutures is by passing the stitch through the tissue several times, incorporating wide helical bites of endopelvic fascia (with or without the vagina itself) before withdrawing the suture back through the space of Retzius (Fig. 36.28). Gittes and Loughlin recommend a no-incision technique in which the needles are passed blindly through the space of Retzius and anchored using helical bites of suture, incorporating the full thickness of the vagina at the bladder neck. The long-term results of this modification remain to be seen.

Pereyra designed a double-pronged needle for this operation, and several surgeons have modified this nee-

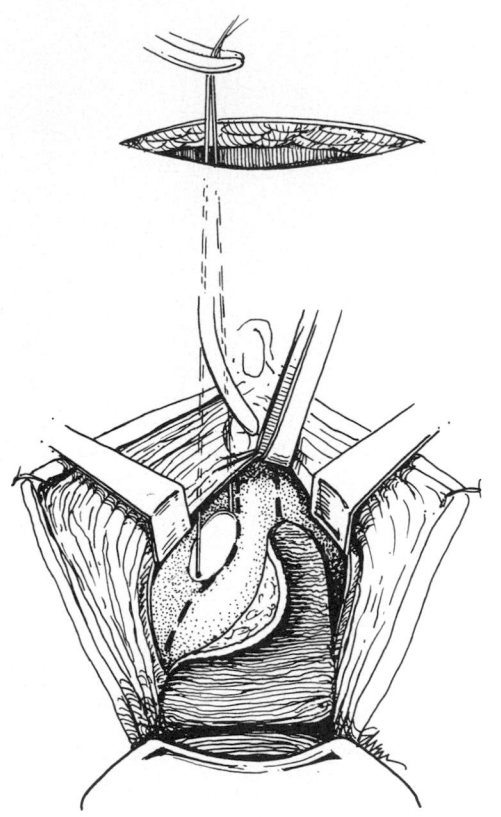

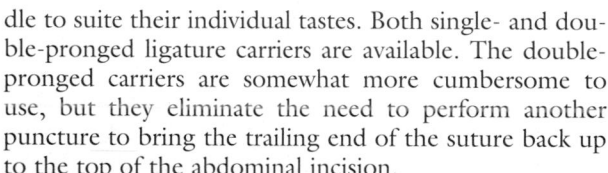

FIGURE 36.27. Stamey technique. Suture fixation using Dacron bolsters at the level of the bladder neck.

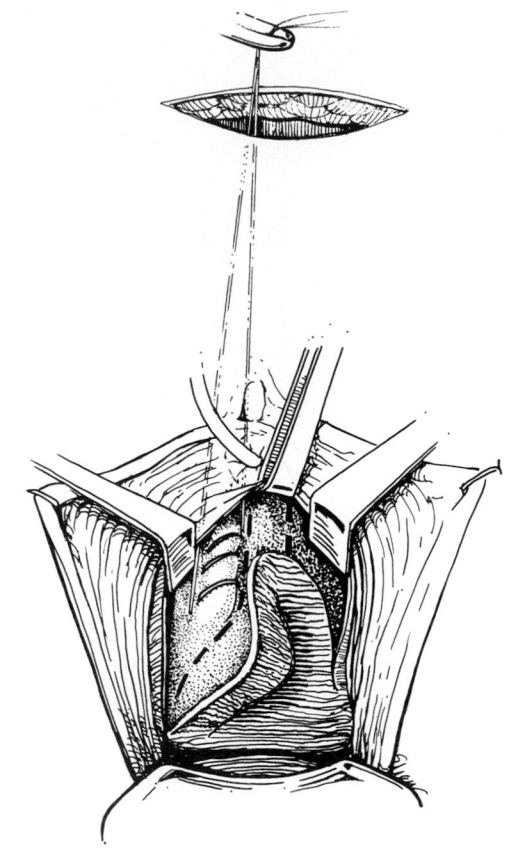

FIGURE 36.28. Fixation technique using helical sutures at the level of the bladder neck.

dle to suite their individual tastes. Both single- and double-pronged ligature carriers are available. The double-pronged carriers are somewhat more cumbersome to use, but they eliminate the need to perform another puncture to bring the trailing end of the suture back up to the top of the abdominal incision.

Abdominal fixation of the suspensory sutures can be done using several techniques. They can be tied down on each side of one long abdominal incision; they can be tied down in separate stab incisions on each side; or they can be tied together in the middle. Some surgeons tie the abdominal sutures down over buttresses; others do not. Leach advocates exposing the back of the pubic symphysis and fixing the suture to the periosteum of the pubic tubercle.

Undoubtedly the most important innovation in needle-suspension operations has been the use of intraoperative cystourethroscopy. Although viewing the urethra and bladder neck has not proved to be particularly helpful in determining how tight the sutures should be tied, it is invaluable in identifying injury to the bladder and urethra during the passage of the long needles. The most prudent way of performing intraoperative cystoscopy is to do it after each needle passage but before the needle is removed. The bulky needle is easy to see if it has penetrated the bladder, and moving the needle during cystoscopy allows the surgeon to see if the sutures have

been placed appropriately at the bladder neck. If cystoscopy is done at the end of the case, with suture but no needles *in situ*, a penetrating injury to the lower urinary tract can be missed because the sutures can be hidden by folds in the urothelium. Ureteral patency can be checked if 5 mL of indigo carmine dye is given intravenously at the end of the case and is observed to efflux from each ureteric orifice. This is advisable at the conclusion of any suspensory procedure for stress incontinence, not just in the case of needle-suspension operations.

At the end of the procedure, the surgeon must close the vaginal incision. This must be done before the suspensory sutures are elevated and tied. If the sutures are pulled up and tied down beforehand, it may be impossible to close the anterior vaginal incision because it will recede into an inaccessible retropubic position. It is exceptionally annoying when this happens; most surgeons only make this mistake once. When tying down the suspensory sutures, it should be remembered that needle-suspension operations are an attempt to cure stress incontinence caused by anatomic hypermobility. These operations work by preventing excessive urethral descent; therefore, it is only necessary to support the urethra at the lower border of the pubic symphysis. Pulling the sutures high and tight causes the same complications seen with open retropubic suspensions: voiding difficulty and a marked predisposition to develop pelvic prolapse.

Needle-suspension operations have many advantages over open retropubic bladder neck surgery. Usually, they can be performed quickly; many can be done in less than 30 minutes. They are relatively easy to perform, even in obese patients, and (when done properly) the morbidity is low. It is also easy to incorporate these procedures into other forms of vaginal surgery, such as transvaginal hysterectomy or anterior colporrhaphy.

Despite these advantages, there are many distinct disadvantages to needle-suspension procedures. The success of these operations in curing stress incontinence depends on the integrity of a single suture on each side—not tissue healing—and on a single point of anchoring on each side. The chance of the patient developing recurrent incontinence is high if either one of these components fails. There is no defined endpoint for suture elevation, and the results of the operation can range from complete failure to achieve the surgical goals by tying the sutures too loosely, to chronic urinary retention if the sutures are tied too tightly. The sutures pull through easily in patients with poor tissue. The use of buttresses can lead to infection, erosion, dyspareunia, chronic draining sinuses, and exuberant formation of granulation tissue with persistent vaginal bleeding. Many patients who undergo needle-suspension operations complain of a chronic pulling pain in the groin when they assume certain positions. This is caused by pulling or twisting of the permanent sutures that act as guy wires supporting the bladder neck. If performed carelessly, passage of the long needles can cause significant bleeding from the veins in the space of Retzius as well as major lacerations of the bladder and urethra. Overall, the success of needle-suspension operations is substantially lower than that obtained with open retropubic suspensions or sling operations. As the long-term results of these operations are becoming better known, fewer surgeons are performing them. Needle-suspension procedures are poor choices for young, otherwise healthy, active women with significant stress incontinence for whom long-term incontinence cure is desired.

SLING PROCEDURES

Sling operations work by providing both urethral support and partial urethral compression. In times past, sling operations were reserved primarily for complicated patients with special risk factors, such as patients who had undergone previous operations for stress incontinence that had failed, patients who developed stress incontinence after pelvic fractures or pelvic trauma, patients with stress incontinence and chronic obstructive pulmonary disease or other conditions characterized by chronically elevated intraabdominal pressure, patients with massive genital prolapse and stress incontinence, or patients with congenital urethral abnormalities (e.g., epispadias). Classically, sling operations were used for patients who had stress incontinence in the presence of normal urethral support, such as a patient who had previously undergone bladder neck suspension surgery that restored urethral support but was not successful in curing her stress incontinence. These patients continue to have stress incontinence because the sphincteric closure mechanism is deficient rather than because the urethra is poorly supported. Recently, many surgeons have begun to use slings as primary operations for stress incontinence. This trend has advantages as well as disadvantages.

Sling operations have a long history. The first reported operation was carried out by Giordano in 1907 using a gracilis muscle flap in a patient with epispadias. Since that time, many different sling procedures have been devised, but all of them use the principle of supporting the urethra and bladder neck in a hammock, which provides both elevation and partial compression of the urethra (Fig. 36.29). Many different synthetic and natural organic materials have been used in making the sling.

Organic Materials
- Autologous materials
  - Fascia lata
  - Rectus fascia

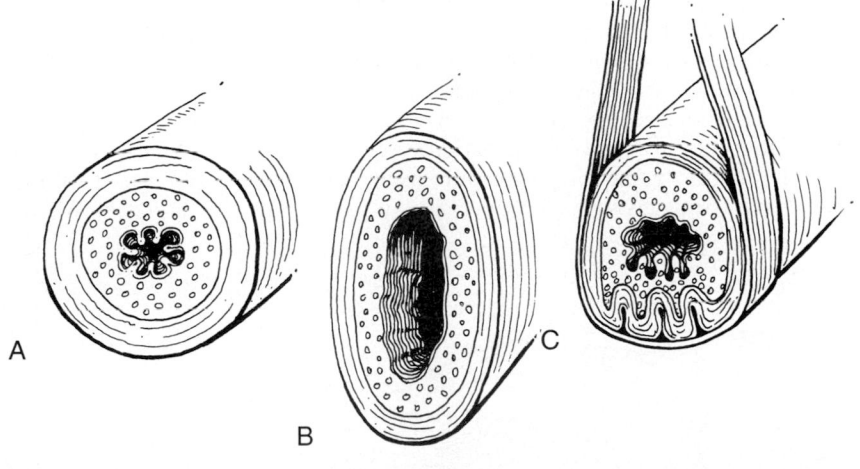

FIGURE 36.29. Mechanism of action of sling procedures for stress incontinence. **A:** Normal urethra. **B:** Incompetent urethra with intrinsic sphincteric deficiency. The lumen is gaping, scarred, and has lost its normal coaptation and pliability. **C:** Correction of intrinsic sphincteric deficiency using a sling operation. The urethra is supported and the urethral lumen is partially compressed by the sling.

—Vaginal patch
—Gracilis muscle
—Round ligaments
—Pyramidalis muscle
—Rectus muscle
- Heterologous materials
  —Lyophilized ox dura mater
  —Porcine dermis

Synthetic Materials
- Nylon
- Marlex mesh
- Mersilene mesh
- Silastic
- Gore-Tex
- Other synthetic materials

The use of "prepackaged" materials, either organic or synthetic, is appealing because it diminishes the amount of time that the operation takes as well as the need to harvest tissue from the patient. The materials used for synthetic slings are uniformly processed and are of consistent strength; however, almost all of the synthetic materials have been plagued by significant problems with infection and erosion. As consumer awareness of the problem of incontinence has increased, manufacturing companies have attempted to capitalize on the increasing demand for services by introducing new products, often in the form of handy surgical "kits." The US Food and Drug Administration regulations covering "devices" do not require testing as extensively as new drugs, only that they are shown to be "equivalent" to products already approved in the existing marketplace. Thus, "new and improved" products (such as the disastrous Protegen sling) may be used in large numbers of patients before the problems associated with them are apparent. In some series, one third of patients who underwent insertion of a synthetic sling had to have the sling removed; this is clearly an unacceptably high rate of complications. The patient, as well as the surgeon, should be wary of such products until data on long-term outcomes are available. Such problems are by no means limited to synthetic substances. Many commercial allografts (e.g., processed cadaveric fascia lata from tissue banks) appear to be plagued by inconsistent tissue strength, a propensity for autolysis, and occasional graft erosion—which seriously compromise their usefulness. Surgeons who elect to use these materials should be aware that they, too, have potential problems.

The urethrovesical sling procedure using autologous fascia lata is the "classic" sling operation in gynecology;

however, several variations of the operation have been developed and are increasing in popularity.

The fascia lata sling procedure (sometimes also known as the Goebel-Stoeckel-Frangenheim operation, after the German surgeons who pioneered many of the sling operations early in the last century) has four main components: (a) harvesting the fascia lata; (b) dissecting the bladder neck; (c) placing the sling in the proper position; and (d) fixing the sling to the anterior rectus fascia through a low abdominal incision.

The fascia lata is a broad, thick band of fascia lying along the middle third of the lateral thigh (Fig. 36.30). Harvesting this fascia requires a small, separate incision in the thigh and the use of a special instrument called a Masson fascial stripper. The patient should be positioned in a right lateral decubitus position on the operating room table, with her leg supported by pillows so that the left lateral thigh is parallel to the floor (Fig. 36.31). This area is prepared and draped as a sterile field. A small 3- to 4-cm incision is made longitudinally (or transversely) along the middle portion of the thigh, beginning about two finger-breadths above the lateral femoral epicondyle. This incision is carried down to the level of the fascia lata. The fascia is exposed broadly by undermining the overlying fatty tissues laterally and cranially for several centimeters. Two longitudinal incisions are made through the full thickness of the fascia lata about 2 cm apart, and the end is cut (Fig. 36.32). The small flap of fascia, thus raised, is grasped with two Kocher clamps, tagged with suture, and passed through the open end of the Masson fascial stripper (Fig. 36.33). The two Kocher clamps are held firmly in the surgeon's left hand to provide countertraction, while the right hand slides the stripper rapidly in one smooth motion as far as it can go along the fascia lata parallel to the underlying muscle (Fig. 36.34). When the instrument has been pushed as far as it can go, the inner cylinder of the fascial stripper is pulled back sharply, cutting the cranial end of the fascial strap. Then the instrument is removed, bringing the fascia out along with it. The tag sutures on its proximal end can be used to retrieve the fascial strap should it inadvertently become dislodged during the harvesting procedure.

Done properly, harvesting fascia lata is a nearly bloodless operation. Some surgeons like to place a small suprafascial Penrose drain or small flat suction drain in the incision for a few days, but this is not necessary generally. The fascial edges do not have to be reapproximated; the defect scars in naturally. The skin incision can be closed with interrupted sutures or stainless steel surgical clips. Many surgeons wrap the thigh loosely with an

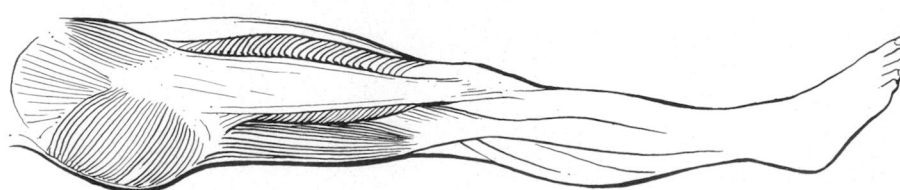

FIGURE 36.30. Location of the fascia lata.

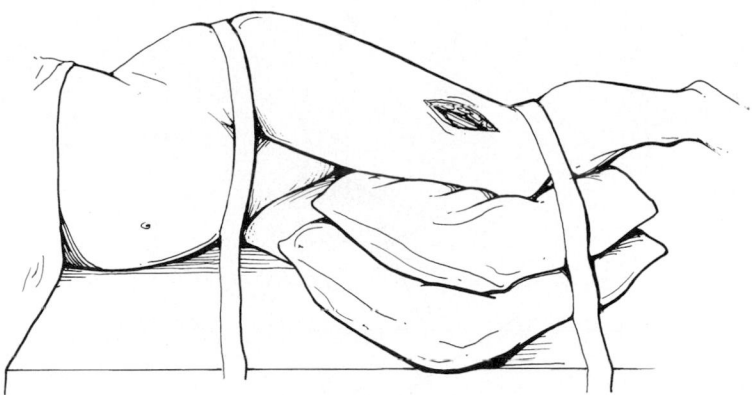

FIGURE 36.31. Proper positioning of the patient for harvesting a strip of fascia lata. A small longitudinal incision is made in the lateral thigh, through which the Masson fascial stripper is inserted.

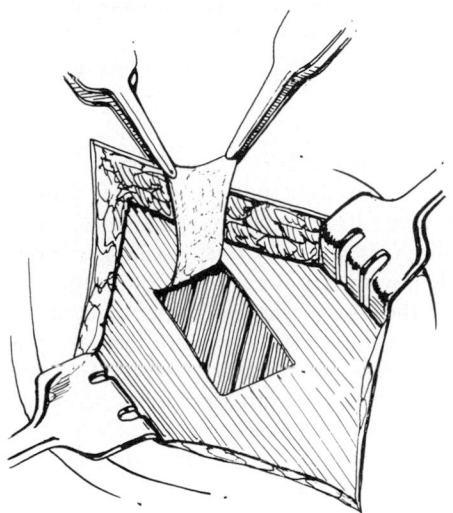

FIGURE 36.32. Harvesting the strip of fascia lata. Once the fascia lata is exposed, two longitudinal incisions are made through the full thickness of the fascia about 2 cm apart. The end is cut, and a small flap of fascia is raised.

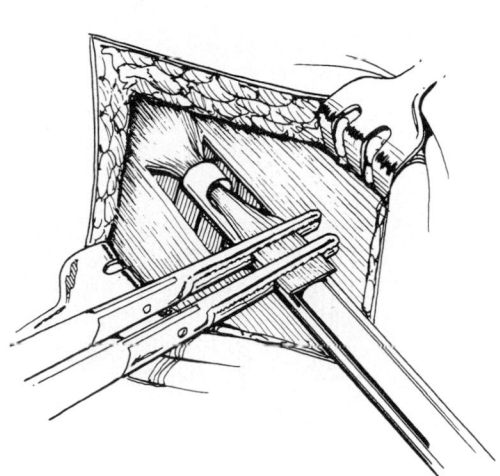

FIGURE 36.33. Harvesting the strip of fascia lata. The end of the fascial strip is passed through the Masson fascial stripper and grasped with two Kocher clamps.

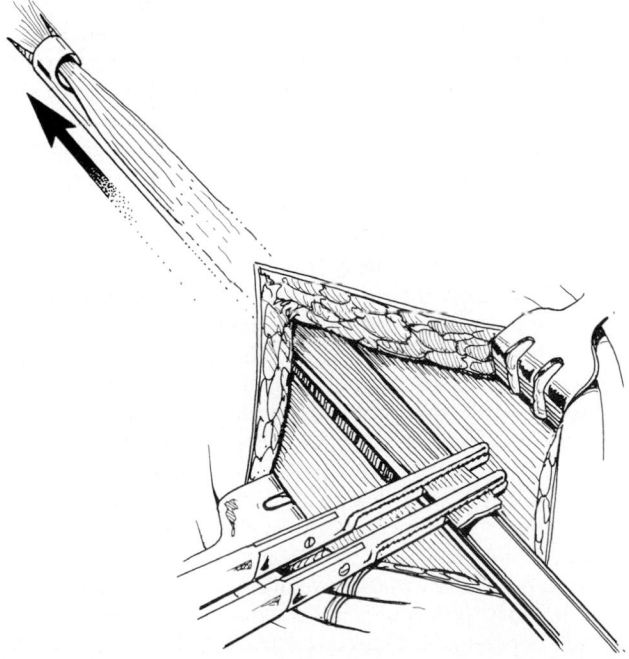

FIGURE 36.34. Harvesting the strip of fascia lata. With the strip of fascia held firmly by two clamps in the surgeon's left hand, the Masson fascial stripper is advanced rapidly up the thigh parallel to the underlying muscle, shearing off a long strip of fascia lata.

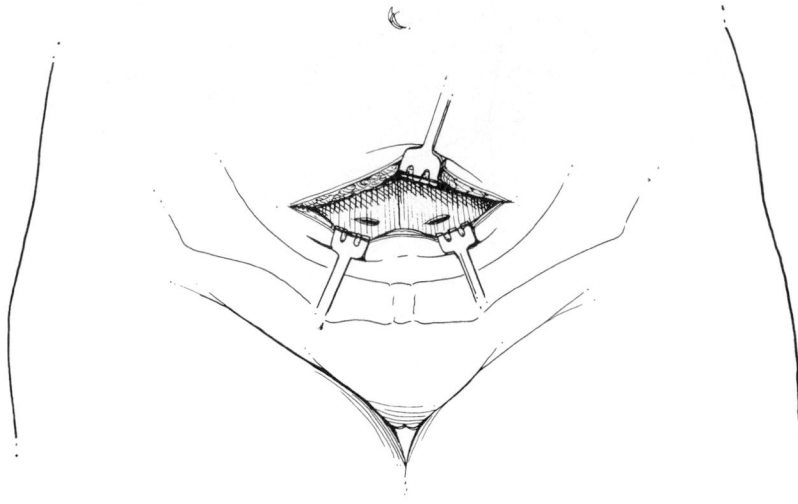

FIGURE 36.35. Abdominal incision for a fascia lata sling procedure. The anterior abdomen is opened with a transverse incision down to the level of the rectus fascia. Two small transverse incisions are then made in this fascia, through which the sling is passed.

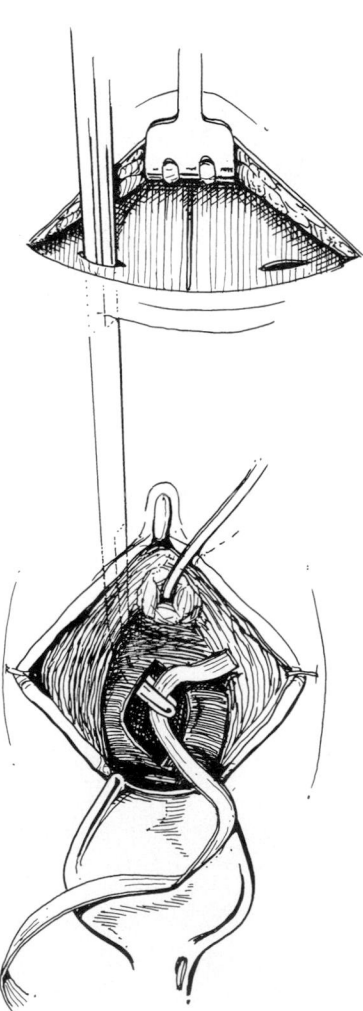

FIGURE 36.36. Passage of the fascia lata strap through the space of Retzius. A long clamp is passed down through the incision in the rectus fascia and through the space of Retzius under direct guidance from the surgeon's finger. The end of the fascial strap is grasped, and the end is pulled back up through the retropubic space through the incision in the rectus fascia on each side.

elasticized bandage for a few days to decrease any swelling that develops and stop any slow venous oozing. Most patients have some muscle tenderness along the lateral thigh for several days after the operation, but this generally resolves rapidly and without difficulty.

Once the fascial strap has been obtained, the patient is placed in a standard dorsal lithotomy position. A weighted vaginal speculum can be used to give greater vaginal exposure. The anterior vagina is opened to expose the endopelvic fascia under the bladder neck in exactly the same manner as if performing an anterior colporrhaphy or a needle suspension (see Fig. 36.24). Some surgeons prefer to perform a Kelly bladder neck plication at this point in the procedure, but this is not a universal practice. The endopelvic fascia is perforated lateral to the bladder neck, and the retropubic space is entered and dissected, just as would be done in a needle-suspension operation (see Fig. 36.25). A transverse suprapubic incision is made about two finger-breadths above the pubic symphysis, and the rectus fascia is exposed and incised (Fig. 36.35). A long Kelly clamp is passed down through the space of Retzius under direct guidance from the surgeon's finger, similar to the passage of a long needle during a Pereyra procedure. The strap of fascia is grasped at one end, and the clamp is pulled up through the space of Retzius close behind the pubic symphysis (Fig. 36.36). The end of the fascia lata strap is pulled through the abdominal incision in the rectus fascia and sewn into place. The procedure then is repeated on the opposite side as the sling is placed underneath the bladder neck.

The most crucial part of a sling procedure is placing the correct tension on the sling. The sling is always tighter when the patient is awake, with active muscle tone, and standing up than it is in the operating room when she is anesthetized, paralyzed, and lying in a dorsal lithotomy position. The most common mistake made by surgeons beginning to perform sling operations is making the sling too tight. This point cannot be overemphasized, particularly in the case of slings that are being used as primary procedures rather than secondary or "salvage" operations. It takes relatively little tension to obstruct the urethra, and the desire to make the patient dry often leads the surgeon to be overly zealous in tightening the sling. There should be just enough slack so that the tip of the surgeon's index finger can slide easily between the sling and the bladder neck (Fig. 36.37). The sling should be placed just at the level of the bladder neck, which is the major point of control for restoring continence in these patients (Fig. 36.38). Placement of the sling over the midurethra increases the likelihood of obstructed voiding. Once the sling has been placed correctly, it may be helpful to suture it into place with two to four small sutures that anchor it against the underlying endopelvic fascia. This prevents the strap from shifting its location once the vagina has been closed.

If the strip of fascia lata is not long enough to reach from the abdominal wall around the bladder neck and back up to the rectus fascia, several options are available

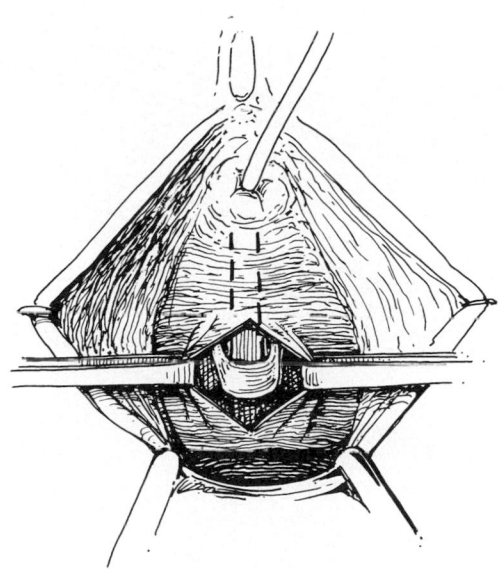

FIGURE 36.38. Placement of the sling at the level of the bladder neck.

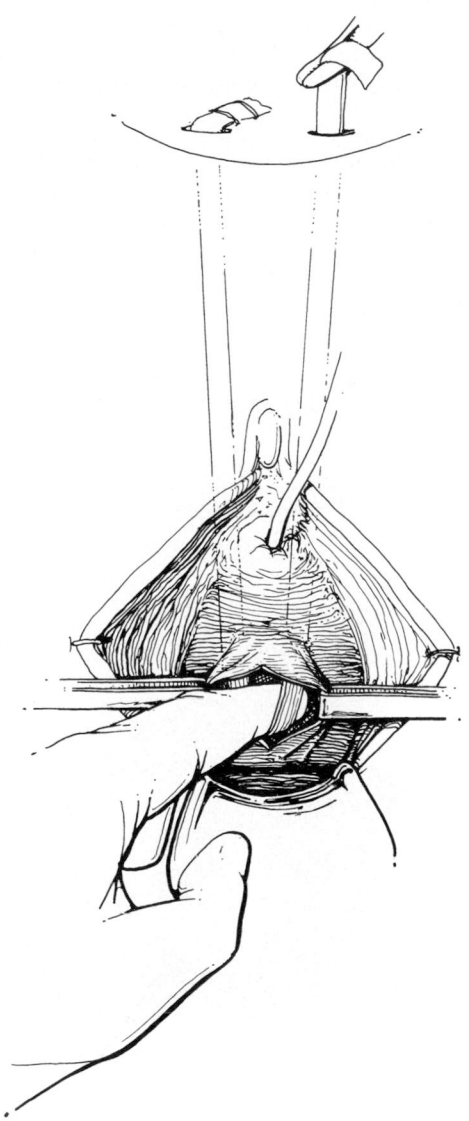

FIGURE 36.37. Adjusting tension on the fascia lata sling. There should be just enough slack so that the tip of the surgeon's index finger can slip between the sling and the bladder neck.

for lengthening it (Fig. 36.39). Wheeless recommends splitting the fascial strip down the middle and sewing the end back on itself to create a pair of pants appearance, thus doubling the length of the fascia. Ridley recommends splitting the fascial strip to lengthen it, but in such a manner that it is not narrowed in the middle. A piece of Mersilene mesh or tape can be sewn onto the end of the fascia lata to provide extra length, or long permanent sutures can be sewn to the ends of the fascial strip and the procedure completed as in a needle suspension of the bladder neck. This technique is similar to that used in the McGuire pubovaginal sling.

In 1942, Aldridge described a modified sling technique using rectus fascia instead of fascia lata. Using rectus fascia avoids the need to make a separate incision in the lower extremity and eliminates the repositioning of the patient that is required if fascia lata is harvested for use as a sling. In the Aldridge technique, rectus fascia is harvested through a transverse abdominal incision. A strip of fascia is raised on each side but left attached in the midline just above the pubic symphysis (Fig. 36.40). The anterior vagina is opened to expose the bladder neck, as in the other operations described. The ends of the rectus fascia are passed down from the abdominal field through the space of Retzius and crossed underneath the bladder neck (Fig. 36.41). Small permanent sutures are used to fix the strips of rectus fascia to the endopelvic fascia. The two fascial strips then are sutured to one another using permanent sutures, and the vagina is closed. Careful suturing of the fascial strips to each other is a crucial step in this operation. The integrity of the Aldridge sling depends on secure fastening of these fascial bands to one another; if these sutures break loose, the entire operation can fail. In addition, it is also more difficult to adjust the tension on the sling using the Aldridge technique because tension must be adjusted on two strips, each of which is fixed in place at one end. The

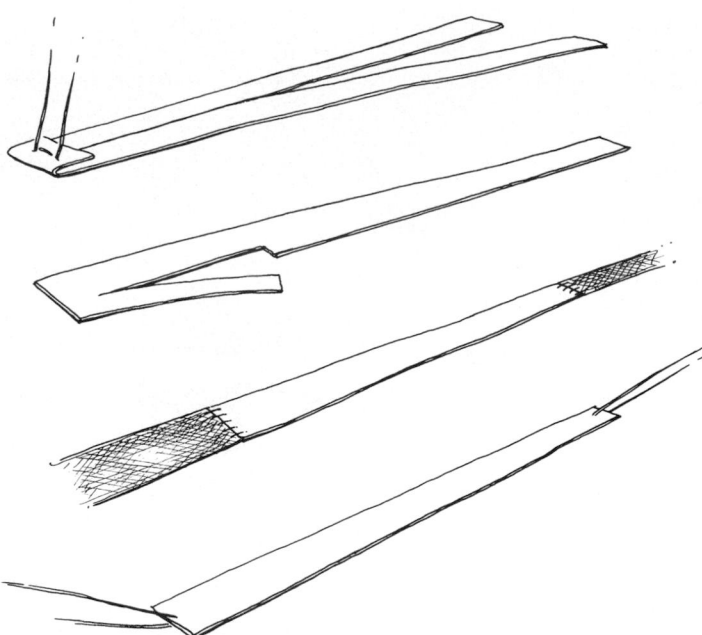

FIGURE 36.39. Options for lengthening a sling that is too short. **Top to bottom:** Splitting the fascial strap lengthwise and sewing the end over on itself for increased support; splitting off part of the sling as a lengthening mechanism; sewing artificial (e.g., Mersilene) mesh onto each end of the sling; sling lengthening using permanent sutures.

incision in the rectus fascia should be closed carefully with permanent sutures to diminish the risk of hernia formation when the Aldridge technique is used.

Rectus fascia harvested through a midline incision can be used as an alternative to the Aldridge sling procedure (Fig. 36.42). This technique is useful in patients who require both a sling and a laparotomy. A lengthy strip of fascia about 2 cm wide is obtained from the edge of the midline abdominal incision. As in the Aldridge procedure, the lower attachments of the fascia are left intact along the pubic symphysis. Because the abdomen is already open in most cases of this type, the space of Retzius can be completely exposed, and the fascial strap

passed through it under direct vision. A surgical assistant operating below opens the anterior vagina and exposes the bladder neck. The vaginal surgeon then perforates the endopelvic fascia lateral to the bladder neck under the guidance of the abdominal surgeon, and accepts the strip of rectus fascia that is passed down from above. The

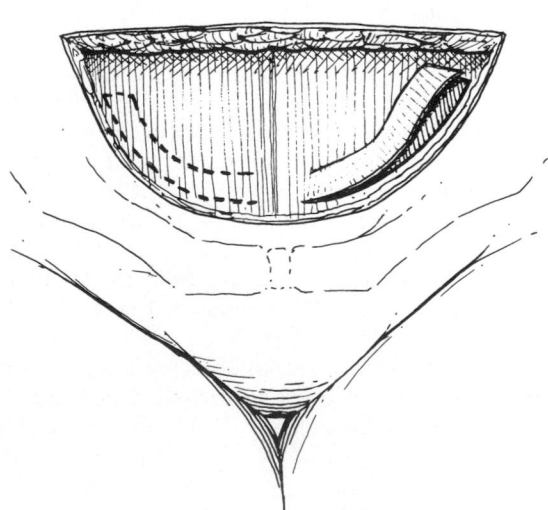

FIGURE 36.40. Aldridge modification of the sling procedure. Two strips of rectus fascia are developed, one on each side of the abdomen. The end of each strip of fascia is left attached in the midline just behind the pubic symphysis.

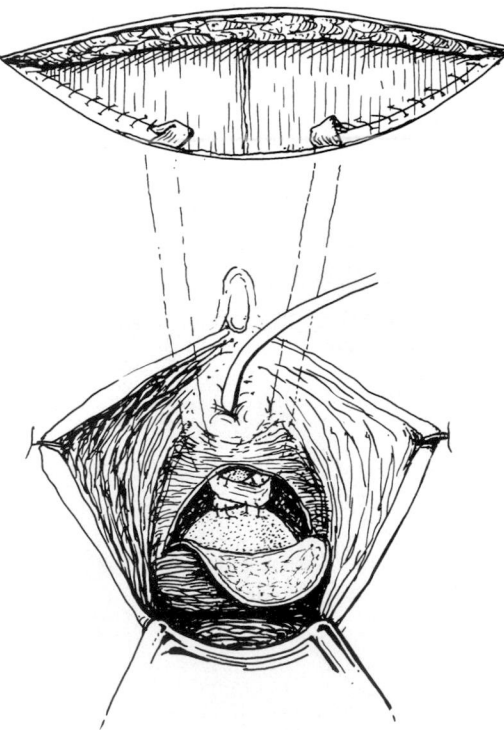

FIGURE 36.41. Aldridge modification of the sling procedure. The fascial strips are brought down through the space of Retzius on each side, crossed under the bladder neck, and sutured to each other.

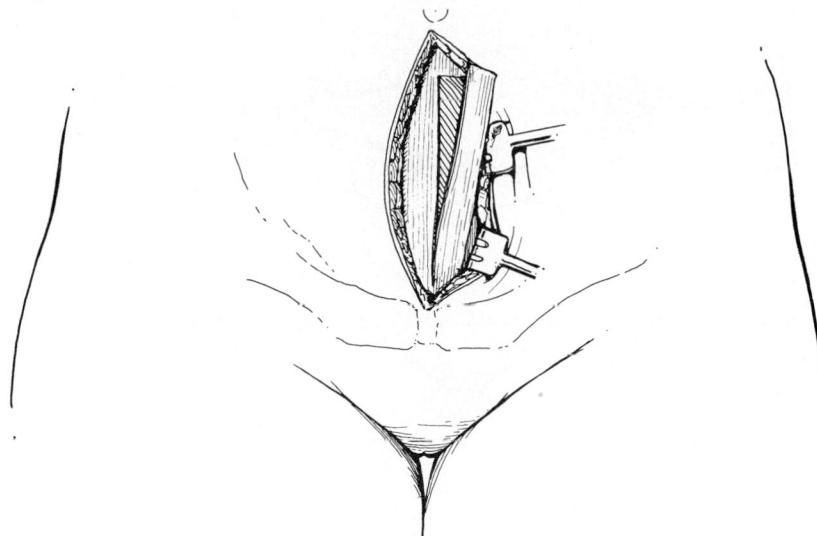

FIGURE 36.42. Harvesting a strip of rectus fascia through a midline incision for use in a sling procedure.

vaginal assistant pulls the strap across the bladder neck and passes it back up into the space of Retzius on the contralateral side. The abdominal surgeon adjusts the tension on the fascial strap according to the advice of the vaginal assistant. Depending on the amount of tension needed, the abdominal surgeon can sew the end of the fascial strap to the arcus tendineus, obturator internus fascia, or Cooper ligament, using permanent suture material (Fig. 36.43). Fine sutures can be placed to ensure proper positioning of the sling over the bladder neck. Once the sling has been fixed into position, the vaginal incision can be closed with absorbable sutures.

The McGuire pubovaginal sling operation is a modified needle-suspension procedure that uses a small piece of rectus fascia as the hammock in which the urethra rests. The patient should be placed in a modified lithotomy position for simultaneous abdominal and vaginal surgery. A transverse incision is made about two finger-breadths above the pubic symphysis to expose the un-

derlying rectus fascia. A transverse strip of this fascia about 15 cm long and 1.5 cm wide is harvested, taking the incision to the lateral edges of the rectus muscles (Fig. 36.44). A vaginal incision then is made to expose the bladder neck and endopelvic fascia, just as would be done in performing a needle-suspension procedure (see Figs. 39.24 and 39.25). A long clamp (or long needle) is passed down under direct finger guidance through the space of Retzius (see Fig. 36.26), grasping the end of the fascial strip, which has been prepared with permanent sutures affixed to each end. The ends of the sutures are grasped with the long clamp and pulled through the space of Retzius, leaving the fascial strap at the level of the bladder neck. The same procedure is repeated on the contralateral side (Fig. 36.45). The transverse incision in the rectus fascia should be closed before tying the sling sutures in place. One side can be tied down and anchored into position, using the other side to adjust the tension on the sling. These sutures can be tied down in-

FIGURE 36.43. Use of a longitudinal strip of rectus fascia as a sling procedure. The space of Retzius is opened completely. An assistant surgeon opens the anterior vagina from below. The fascial strap is passed down through an incision in the endopelvic fascia and back up from below into the space of Retzius on the other side of the bladder neck. The end of the fascial strap then is sewn into the obturator internus fascia or to the Cooper ligament, depending on the tension needed on the strap.

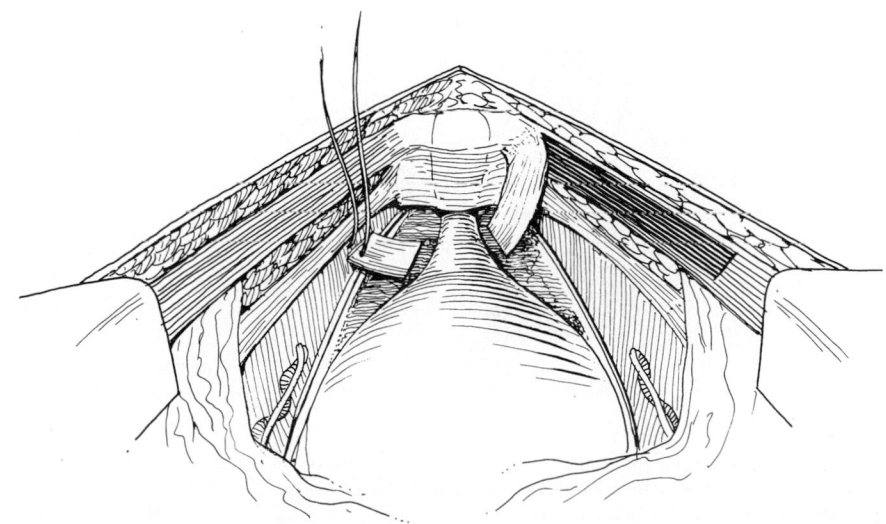

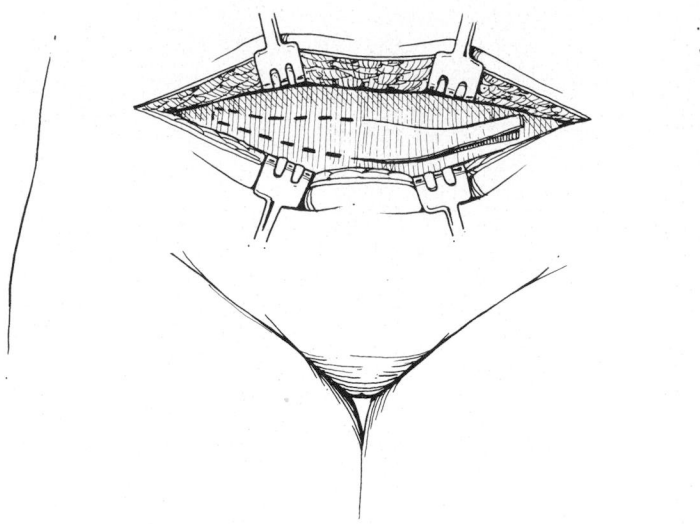

FIGURE 36.44. McGuire pubovaginal sling. Harvesting a transverse piece of rectus fascia.

dividually on each side, tied over a bolster, or tied down separately and then tied to one another in the midline, just as with a conventional needle-suspension operation.

Some surgeons have begun to use bone-anchors or bone-screws to which the slings are attached. Bone-anchors have been placed through abdominal incisions as

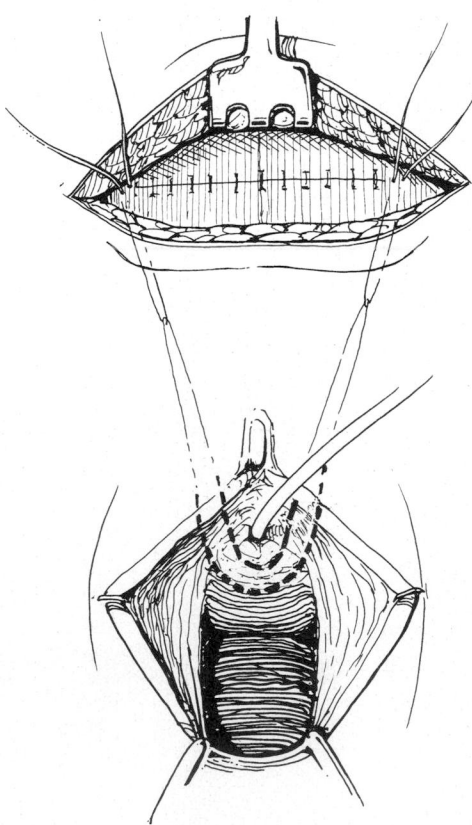

FIGURE 36.45. McGuire pubovaginal sling. Sutures are sewn into each end of the sling, passed through the space of Retzius, and tied down into the rectus fascia on each side, supporting the urethra in a "hammock."

well as transvaginally. In the transvaginal bone-anchor sling techniques, a vaginal incision is made through which the surgeon dissects and exposes the bladder neck. A "gun" then is introduced into the incision that shoots an anchor, a tack, or a screw into each side of the pubic symphysis to which the sling then is attached. In theory, such slings provide durable support without causing urethral obstruction. The procedure is quick and relatively easy to do; however, prospective, long-term studies of these operations have not yet been published and there are growing numbers of anecdotal reports of osteomyelitis, suture erosion, misapplied screws, dyspareunia, and operative failure that should give the thoughtful surgeon pause before uncritically abandoning older operations in favor of these techniques.

TENSION-FREE VAGINAL TAPE

In 1995, Ulmsten described an operation he called "intravaginal slingplasty" for the treatment of stress incontinence. This original operation has been modified and is now commonly known as the "tension-free vaginal tape" (or TVT) procedure (Ethicon Gynecare, Somerville, NJ). It represents the "next wave" of minimally invasive operations for the treatment of stress incontinence. The operation can be performed with conscious sedation under local anesthesia (as well as regional or general anesthesia) in an outpatient setting. The sling material is a knitted polypropylene mesh that is rapidly interpenetrated by fibroblasts, creating tough scar tissue that holds the sling in place, obviating the need for sutures.

In this operation, the skin, subcutaneous fat, and deep tissues behind the pubic symphysis in the space of Retzius are infiltrated with local anesthetic (e.g., 0.25% Marcaine). The surgeon then makes two small incisions just above and slightly lateral to the midline of the pubic bone. An additional incision approximately 1.5 cm in length is made with a scalpel 1 cm distal to the external urethral meatus. The incision then is opened slightly using sharp dissection with a scissors. The sling comes attached at each end to a curved trocar that is inserted along the urethra underneath the vaginal skin until the posterior border of the pubic bone is reached. The endopelvic fascia then is perforated by gentle leverage on the trocar with the aid of a detachable introducer. It is necessary to deviate the bladder neck away from the operative site on each side by the use of a rigid catheter guide inserted through an 18 Fr Foley catheter, which is affixed to the patient's ipsilateral thigh while the surgeon introduces the trocar on that side. The trocar then is rotated and forced up directly behind the pubic symphysis until it is pushed out through the abdominal incision on that side. Cystoscopy then is carried out to ensure the bladder has not been perforated by the trocar. The trocar introducer then is removed and the trocar is pulled through the abdominal incision. Next, an identical procedure is repeated on the contralateral side. The sling is placed loosely at the midurethra (not at the bladder neck, as is commonly the case for traditional sling operations), and does not appear to affect urethral mobility. This method seems to work by creating urethral compression during periods of increased intraabdominal pressure. The sling comes covered in a protective plastic sheath, which helps prevent contamination of the sling as it is passed through the vagina while permitting easy movement of the sling during insertion. Once the sheath has been removed, the polypropylene mesh grates against intervening fatty tissue and becomes difficult to manipulate, rapidly becoming incorporated into the surrounding tissue by fibroblasts. The three incisions then are closed.

The TVT operation is conceptually simple, technically straightforward, and can be performed quickly. In experienced hands, operative time is as little as 20 to 30 minutes. Long-term follow-up studies extending 3 years and beyond are becoming available from Europe and suggest that the operation is durable and has cure rates similar to those obtained by more traditional operations, such as the Burch colposuspension.

The TVT procedure is not without risk. As with any synthetic sling, the danger of mesh erosion is always present. At present, this risk appears to be lower than with many other synthetic materials; whether this impression will hold up over 5 to 10 years is not yet known. Because the mesh is rapidly incorporated into the patient's body, the sling is rapidly fixed into place. If the sling is too tight, intractable voiding difficulty can develop that requires transection of the tape. Should it become necessary to remove the tape completely, this appears to be a very challenging endeavor. Because the operative technique requires blind passage of a trocar through the space of Retzius, meticulous attention to the location of the trocar is imperative at all times. Some patients develop retropubic bleeding and hematoma formation that may require transfusion or surgical drainage. Most worrisome of all, there have been anecdotal case reports of bowel perforation, laceration of the great iliac vessels along the pelvic sidewall, and patient death from this procedure. A TVT operation should never be performed casually or by the inexperienced. It should only be performed by surgeons who are thoroughly familiar with the relevant anatomy and are experienced in the evaluation and treatment of urinary incontinence.

PERIURETHRAL INJECTIONS

Increasing attention has been devoted to the use of various kinds of paste that can be injected through a needle into the tissues around the bladder neck to restore continence. This concept is not new; it was first developed by Murless in 1938, but these techniques did not become popular until much later, owing to the lack of suitable materials for injection. Several different materials have been used for these procedures, and more are likely to be developed in the near future. The earliest substance used consisted of polytetrafluoroethylene micropolymer particles (Urethrin, Polytef' Mentor Corp., Santa Barbara, California). This was followed by glutaraldehyde cross-linked bovine collagen (Contigen; C. R. Bard, Inc., Covington, Georgia). More recently, a pyrolytic carbon-coated zirconium oxide bead paste (Durasphere; Carbon Medical Technologies, St. Paul, Minnesota) has been developed for this purpose. Some authors have even experimented with the periurethral injection of autologous fat. The materials can be injected transurethrally using a cystoscope, or periurethrally. In either case, the object of the injection is to improve coaptation of the urethra at the level of the bladder neck, thereby increasing the urethra's ability to remain closed during periods of increased intraabdominal pressure.

Polytetrafluoroethylene paste has been used for many years as an injectable material by otorhinolaryngologists in the treatment of a variety of vocal cord problems. Its use as an injectable for incontinence has been more recent. The paste is thick and rather difficult to inject, and requires a special power injector to use efficiently. Although reasonable success rates have been reported by some authors using this paste, the particles have been shown to migrate to other areas of the body, where they can set up a granulomatous reaction. This has diminished enthusiasm for the use of this material.

Contigen, on the other hand, does not have these problems. The material is a sterile, nonpyrogenic form of purified bovine dermal collagen that does not elicit a foreign-body reaction when injected into humans. The material is biodegradable and is replaced by the patient's own collagen over 3 to 4 months. Because it is biodegradable, more than one injection is necessary to achieve continence in some patients.

The carbon-coated zirconium oxide bead paste (Durasphere) appears to lie somewhere between the Teflon paste and the collagen in terms of ease of injection, requires less injectable material, and appears to have longer durability. Fat injection appears to have poor long-term success, and has never become popular as treatment.

The injection procedure can be done in an outpatient setting or in an ambulatory surgical center. The injection usually can be accomplished under local anesthesia. The periurethral tissues can be coated with 2%

lidocaine jelly 10 minutes before the procedure, and then 2 to 3 mL of 1% lidocaine can be injected periurethrally at the 5- and 7-o'clock positions. Patients generally are given a single dose of a cephalosporin antibiotic by mouth before the procedure.

Direct visualization of the bladder neck using a cystoscope equipped with a 0- or 30-degree lens is necessary to ensure proper placement of the collagen. The transurethral technique allows more accurate placement of the needle, but this can be offset by collagen oozing out of the urethral puncture site, bleeding into the operative field, or infection. Periurethral injection avoids penetration of the urothelium (unless the needle slips) and appears to be the preferred injection technique.

With the patient in a dorsal lithotomy position, prepared, draped, and given a local anesthetic as described earlier, a 22-gauge spinal needle is inserted into the periurethral tissues at the 4-o'clock position, with the bevel of the needle directed medially (Fig. 36.46). The needle is angled slightly toward the bladder neck and then is advanced under direct cystoscopic guidance until the tip of the needle can be seen causing the urethral mucosa to bulge inward at the level of the bladder neck. The collagen comes in a 3-mL Luer-Lok syringe injector, which attaches easily to the end of the needle. Durasphere is available in 1-mL syringes. The injection is made slowly under direct visualization; if the material is placed properly, the urethral lumen on that side gradually bulges out across the midline. The procedure should be repeated on the opposite side. One of the drawbacks to this procedure is that there is no sure way of knowing how much material to inject. The goal should be to get good coaptation of the urethral epithelium. Some patients require multiple injections to become dry; others require periodic injections to maintain continence.

Injection therapy appears to work by bulking up the tissues at the bladder neck so that the bladder neck is forced closed during coughing or sneezing (Fig. 36.47). There is no appreciable increase in passive urethral closure pressure when measurements are taken preoperatively and postoperatively, although leak-point pressures are increased after successful injection therapy.

Postoperatively, most patients are able to void before leaving the surgical center. Patients who cannot void are managed by clean intermittent self-catheterization, with a small catheter (14F or smaller). Indwelling catheters should be avoided so that the collagen around the urethral lumen is not distorted before it has had a chance to set up.

THE ARTIFICIAL URINARY SPHINCTER

The ultimate high-technology treatment of urinary incontinence owing to intrinsic sphincter deficiency is implantation of an artificial urinary sphincter. Many prototypes of these devices have been created; the AMS 800 (American Medical Systems, Minnetonka, MN) probably represents the final stage in the evolution of this concept. The artificial urinary sphincter is a small inflatable cuff that is placed around the bladder neck and proximal urethra. After allowing 6 weeks or so for healing to take place, this cuff then is inflated to compress the urethra. The device consists of a cuff, a pump (which usually is implanted within one of the labia majora), and a reservoir, which is placed in the abdomen beneath the fascia (Fig. 36.48). Once inflated, the cuff maintains urethral closure until the patient needs to void. The patient deflates the cuff by squeezing the labial pump with her fin-

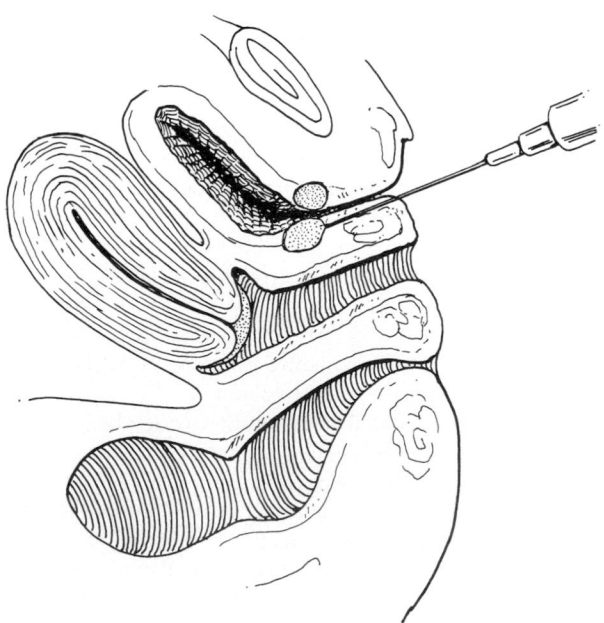

FIGURE 36.46. Periurethral injection of collagen around the bladder neck.

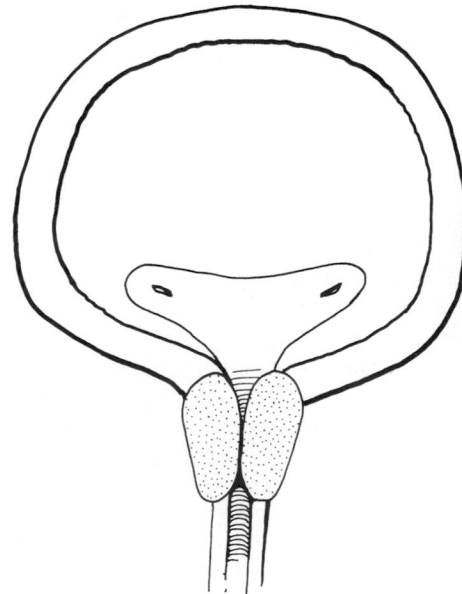

FIGURE 36.47. Bulking of the bladder neck and proximal urethra after successful collagen injection.

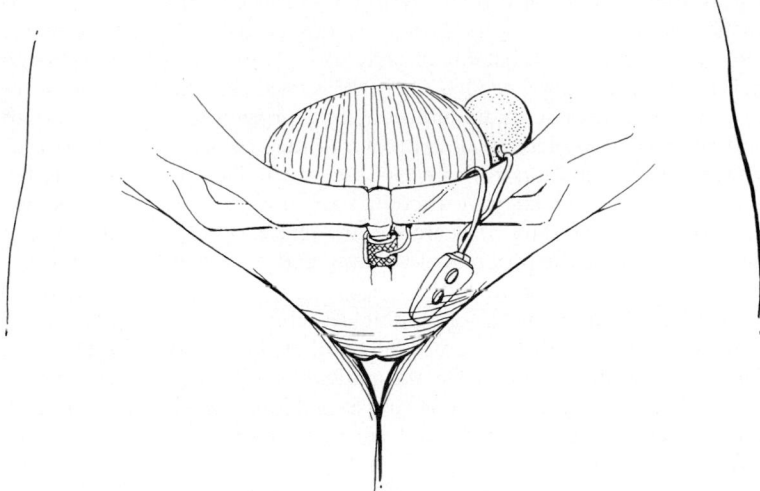

FIGURE 36.48. The artificial urinary sphincter in place.

gers, pumping fluid from the cuff into the reservoir. After voiding, the cuff automatically reinflates over 1 or 2 minutes and remains closed until the pump is reactivated.

There are several problems associated with artificial urinary sphincters, including erosion of the cuff, infection, and device failure. In general, artificial sphincters work better in men than women. Because the continuity of the male perineum is not broken by the presence of a vagina, when implanted in men, the artificial sphincter is protected from trauma by a thick cushion of tissue that carries with it an abundant blood supply. In women, the cuff of the artificial urinary sphincter must be placed into a relatively thin septum of tissue between the vagina and bladder neck, making it more susceptible to erosion and infection.

Artificial urinary sphincters are not an appropriate primary surgical treatment for stress incontinence, nor do they have any place in the primary, general practice of gynecologic surgery. Patients who are candidates for sphincter implantation represent only a tiny fraction of women with stress urinary incontinence. These patients should receive an artificial sphincter only after a full evaluation at a tertiary care medical center. The surgery should be done by an experienced surgical team that operates together on a regular basis and can provide specialized, life-long follow-up care for these patients.

POSTOPERATIVE BLADDER CARE

Management of the patient's bladder after surgery for stress incontinence is an extremely important, but often neglected, part of the overall operation. These patients have undergone surgery for abnormal bladder function, yet it is surprising how little attention is often paid to bladder function while they are recuperating in the postoperative period. There is often significant bleeding and edema in the perivesical tissues; sometimes there is direct trauma to the bladder. Alterations in bladder function

should be expected, and postoperative care should be planned accordingly.

The most important component of postoperative bladder care is making sure that the bladder is drained adequately and is not allowed to become overdistended. Overdistention of a traumatized bladder can result in serious long-term voiding dysfunction and can undo the results of a technically well-executed surgical procedure. In most cases, the bladder should be catheterized and the catheter left open to drain for at least 24 hours before voiding is attempted. Once voiding trials are begun, the technique of bladder management used varies according to the specifics of the individual patient. Whatever the method used, the object should be to provide regular, complete bladder emptying while avoiding overdistention of the bladder.

There is no one best method for postoperative bladder management. No matter what method is chosen, the surgeon must be aware that its implementation depends on effective nursing care. Nurses taking care of patients who have just undergone surgical procedures for stress incontinence must be impressed with the importance of the bladder management regimen because inattentive nursing care can have serious repercussions for these patients. For example, many clinicians put patients on a schedule whereby they are instructed to void every 4 hours once the catheter has been removed. In everyday life, there are few people who routinely wait 4 hours between voids; yet it is expected that a patient who has just had bladder neck suspension surgery and who is often receiving continuous intravenous fluid should wait this long. If the nurses are preoccupied, they may not check on such a patient until 6 hours have gone by, with the end result that the patient develops significant overdistention, which can cause irreparable damage to the bladder. A schedule whereby the patient voids every 2 hours is much more realistic and lessens the likelihood of postoperative overdistention.

Ideally, all patients undergoing stress incontinence surgery should be taught how to catheterize themselves.

Clean intermittent self-catheterization is well within the capabilities of most patients, if they are instructed properly. This involves the patient directly in her care, gives her a skill that may be needed for some weeks (as is the case with many patients undergoing sling procedures), and allows her an element of control that may compensate for lapses in nursing care on the ward. Patients should be encouraged to catheterize themselves after each void when voiding trials are begun. This allows the clinician to judge the progress of voiding, and the schedule can be modified as needed.

Catheterization with a suprapubic catheter also is an alternative. Such catheters can be inserted at the end of the operative procedure while the patient is still anesthetized. A variety of catheters are available commercially. They are easy to insert and are tolerated well by most patients. Alternatively, a silicone Foley catheter can be placed intraoperatively through a direct puncture into the bladder. The end of the catheter can be brought out through a separate stab incision through the fascia and the anterior abdominal wall, away from the operative incision. Suprapubic catheters should be placed into a bladder that has been distended by filling it with sterile water to a volume of about 400 mL. This makes the bladder easy to hit with a trocar or scalpel without the risk of injuring another structure. If a suprapubic catheter is inserted under direct vision during the operation, it is helpful to place a pursestring suture of 2-0 chromic catgut around the area in the distended bladder through which the incision will be made. Once the catheter has been inserted and its balloon has been inflated, the suture should be pulled tight and "snugged up" around the catheter to prevent leakage of urine from the cystotomy site. A catheter can be placed into an empty, nondistended bladder through a direct incision; however, when this is done, the bladder wall becomes thicker and more distensible at the catheter site when the bladder is subsequently filled. The seal obtained in such cases is not nearly as good as that obtained when the bladder has been distended before insertion of the catheter. Catheters placed with this technique often leak significantly through the abdominal incision in the postoperative period when they are clamped and the bladder starts to fill. This is unpopular both with patients and the nurses caring for them.

When voiding trials are to be begun, the suprapubic catheter should be clamped, and the patient should be instructed to void on a regular schedule. The patient should measure the amount of urine that she is able to pass, and the catheter should then be opened and allowed to drain for 20 minutes. The urine thus obtained should be recorded as the postvoid residual, and the catheter should then be reclamped. This catheter regimen allows both the volume voided and the residual urine to be checked regularly without the need for nursing personnel to insert and remove a transurethral catheter continually. When the voided volumes are large and the residuals are small (about 25% of the volume voided), the suprapubic catheter can be removed. If the patient is unable to void, the catheter can be opened every 2 hours to drain during the day. The catheter also can be left open to drain overnight, giving the patient a good night's sleep without the need to insert and remove a transurethral catheter.

Suprapubic catheters can be left in place for up to 6 weeks if needed. When they are left in place longer, they usually become encrusted and clogged. Sometimes this can be delayed by the use of ascorbic acid in large doses, 3 g by mouth three times per day. If suprapubic catheterization is needed for longer than 6 weeks, the catheter must be changed. If a small needle or trocar catheter has been used, this is difficult; however, if a silicone Foley catheter has been placed through an abdominal stab incision, the catheter tract usually remains open temporarily. The old catheter can be deflated and removed and a new catheter inserted through the tract left by the old one. When suprapubic catheters are removed, the clinician should make sure that the patient's bladder is empty. Failure to do this results in a geyser of urine spurting up from the hole, much to the dismay of all parties involved. This usually stops in less than 24 hours, but it can be unpleasant until the tract closes.

Long-term drainage of the bladder with a transurethral catheter should be discouraged. It is uncomfortable, irritating, and can lead to irreparable damage to the bladder neck, particularly if a large catheter balloon is used. There is no reason to place a catheter with a balloon larger than 5 mL. Suppressive antibiotics should not be used in catheterized patients. They do not reduce the incidence of urinary tract infections, but they do create resistant organisms that are more difficult to eradicate if an acute infection does occur. Establishment of normal bladder emptying and removal of the foreign body (i.e., the catheter) are the best defenses against infection. Patients who need long-term bladder drainage should be taught clean intermittent self-catheterization. If this is not possible, use of a suprapubic catheter is preferable.

Many patients develop transient urinary tract symptoms, such as urgency, frequency, and urge incontinence, in the first few weeks after bladder neck surgery. These patients should have a postvoid residual urine volume checked to make sure they are emptying completely, and they should be checked for the presence of an infection. Once these problems have been ruled out, it is best to wait a few weeks to let symptoms resolve before initiating any additional therapy. Treatment of such symptoms with anticholinergic medications in the immediate postoperative period often makes matters worse and can produce acute urinary retention. Most such symptoms resolve without the need for additional therapy. If they persist 3 months after surgery, further evaluation may be indicated.

A small percentage of patients develop intractable voiding difficulty followed antiincontinence surgery. If conservative approaches using anticholinergic medications and/or intermittent self-catheterization do not improve their symptoms, consideration can be give to either transvaginal or transabdominal urethrolysis to relieve the obstruction. In order to prevent rescarring, interposition of a bulbocavernosus or omental flap is useful. Some of these women develop recurrent stress incontinence; some continue to have voiding difficulty in spite of urethrolysis.

Clinicians who become adept at evaluating women with urinary incontinence and who become comfortable with all modalities of therapy for this condition—both nonsurgical and surgical treatment—find their practices enhanced and their clinical satisfaction increased. Patients who are cured of urinary incontinence are among the most grateful patients in gynecologic practice and are among the most rewarding to treat.

BIBLIOGRAPHY

Abrams P, Wein AJ (eds). The overactive bladder: from basic science to clinical management consensus conference. *Urology* 1997;50(Suppl 6A):1–114.

Addison WA, Livengood CH, Sutton GP, et al. Abdominal sacral colpopexy with Mersilene mesh in the retroperitoneal position in the management of posthysterectomy vaginal vault prolapse and enterocele. *Am J Obstet Gynecol* 1985; 153:140.

Amundsen CL, Visco AG, Ruiz H, et. al. Outcome in 104 pubovaginal slings using freeze-dried fascia lata from a single tissue bank. *Urology* 2000;56(6 Suppl 1):2–8.

Andersson KE, Chapple CR. Oxybutynin and the overactive bladder. *World J Urol* 2001;19:319–323.

Appell RA. Clinical efficacy and safety of tolterodine in the treatment of overactive bladder: a pooled analysis. *Urology* 1997;50(6A):90–96.

Appell RA. Periurethral collagen injection for female incontinence. *Prob Urol* 1991;8:208.

Appell RA, Sand P, Dmochowski R, et. al. Prospective randomized controlled trial of extended-release oxybutynin chloride and tolterodine tartrate in the treatment of overactive bladder: results of the OBJECT Study. *Mayo Clin Proc* 2001;76:358–363.

Azam U, Frazer M, Kozman E, et. al. The tension-free vaginal tape procedure in women with previous failed stress incontinence surgery. *J Urol* 2001;166:554–556.

Beck RP, Lai AR. Results in treating 88 cases of recurrent urinary stress incontinence with the Oxford fascia lata sling procedure. *Am J Obstet Gynecol* 1982;142:649.

Beck RP, McCormick S. Treatment of urinary stress incontinence with anterior colporrhaphy. *Obstet Gynecol* 1982;59:269.

Beck RP, McCormick S, Nordstrom L. A 25-year experience with 519 anterior colporrhaphy procedures. *Obstet Gynecol* 1991;78:1011.

Beck RP, McCormick S, Nordstrom L. The fascia lata sling procedure for treating recurrent genuine stress incontinence. *Obstet Gynecol* 1988;72:699.

Beckingham IJ, Wemyss-Holden, G, Lawrence WT. Long term follow-up of women treated with periurethral Teflon injections for stress incontinence. *Br J Urol* 1992;69:580.

Bennett D, Diokno A. Clean, intermittent self-catheterization in elderly patients. *Urology* 1984;24:43.

Berghmans LC, Hendriks HJ, Bo K, et al. Conservative treatment of stress urinary incontinence in women: a systematic review of randomized clinical trials. *Br J Urol* 1998;82: 181–191.

Bergman A, Ballard CA, Koonings PP. Comparison of three different surgical procedures for genuine stress incontinence: prospective randomized study. *Am J Obstet Gynecol* 1989a;161:1102.

Bergman A, Koonings PP, Ballard CA. Negative Q-tip test as a risk factor for failed incontinence surgery in women. *J Reprod Med* 1989b;34:193.

Bergman A, Koonings PP, Ballard CA. Primary stress urinary incontinence and pelvic relaxation: prospective randomized comparison of three different operations. *Am J Obstet Gynecol* 1989c;161:97.

Bergman A, McCarthy TA, Ballard CA. Role of the Q-tip test in evaluating stress urinary incontinence. *J Reprod Med* 1987;32:273.

Bidmead J, Cardozoa L, McLellan A, et. al. A comparison of the objective and subjective outcomes of colposuspension for stress incontinence. *BJOG* 2001;108:408–413.

Birhle W, Tarantino AF. Complications of retropubic bladder neck suspension. *Urology* 1990;35:213.

Black NA, Downs SH. The effectiveness of surgery for stress incontinence in women: a systematic review. *Br J Urol* 1996;78:497–510.

Black N, Griffiths J, Pope C, et. al. Impact of surgery for stress incontinence on morbidity: cohort study. *BMJ* 1997;3215; 1493–1498.

Black NA, Bowling A, Griffiths JM, et. al. Impact of surgery for stress incontinence on the social lives of women. *Br J Obstet Gynaecol* 1998;105:605–612.

Blaivas JG, Jacobs BZ. Pubovaginal fascial sling for the treatment of complicated stress urinary incontinence. *J Urol* 1991;145:1214.

Blakely CR, Mills WG. The obstetric and gynaecological complications of bladder exstrophy and epispadias. *Br J Obstet Gynaecol* 1981;88:167.

Blander DS, Zimmern PE. Cadaveric fascia lata sling: analysis of five recent adverse outcomes. *Urology* 2000;56:596–599.

Bo K, Hagan RR, Kvarsten B, et al. Pelvic floor muscle exercise for the treatment of female stress urinary incontinence III: effects of two different degrees of pelvic floor exercise. *Neurol Urodyn* 1990;9:489.

Bo K, Talseth T, Holme I. Single blind, randomised controlled trial of pelvic floor exercises, electrical stimulation, vaginal cones, and no treatment in management of genuine stress incontinence. *BMJ* 1999;318:487–493.

Bump RC. The mechanism of urinary continence in women with severe uterovaginal prolapse: results of barrier studies. *Obstet Gynecol* 1988;72:291.

Bump RC, Elser DM, Theofrastus JP, et al. Valsalva leak point pressures in women with genuine stress incontinence: reproducibility, effect of catheter caliber, and correlations with other measures of urethral resistance. *Am J Obstet Gynecol* 1995;173:551–557.

Burch JC. Cooper's ligament urethrovesical suspension for stress incontinence: nine years' experience-results, complications, technique. *Am J Obstet Gynecol* 1968;100:764.

Burch JC. Urethrovaginal fixation to Cooper's ligament for correction of stress incontinence, cystocele, and prolapse. *Am J Obstet Gynecol* 1961;81:281.

Cammu H, Van Nylen M, Amy JJ. A 10-year follow-up after Kegel pelvic floor muscle exercises for genuine stress incontinence. *BJU Int* 2000;85:655–658.

Carbone JM, Kavaler E, Hu JC, et. al. Pubovaginal sling using cadaveric bone anchors: disappointing early results. *J Urol* 2001;165:1605–1611.

Cardozo LD, Stanton SL, Williams JE. Detrusor instability following surgery for genuine stress incontinence. *Br J Urol* 1979;51:204.

Carr LK, Webster GD. Voiding dysfunction following incontinence surgery: diagnosis and treatment with retropubic or vaginal urethrolysis. *J Urol* 1997;157:821–823.

Chou Q, DeLancey JOL. A structured system to evaluate urethral support anatomy in magnetic resonance images. *Am J Obstet Gynecol* 2001;185:44–50.

Clemens JQ, DeLancy JOL, Faerber GJ, et. al. Urinary tract erosions after synthetic pubovaginal slings: diagnosis and management strategy. *Urology* 2000;56:589–595.

Colombo M, Milani R, Vitobello D, et al. A randomized comparison of Burch colposuspension and abdominal paravaginal defect repair for female stress urinary incontinence. *Am J Obstet Gynecol* 1996;175:78–84.

Colombo M, Vitobello D, Proietti FD, et. al. Randomised comparison of Burch colposuspension versus anterior colporrhaphy in women with stress urinary incontinence and anterior vaginal wall prolapse. *BJOG* 2000;107:544–551.

Constantinou CE. Determinants of cure by endoscopic suspension of the bladder neck in the incontinent female patient. *World J Urol* 1986;4:10.

Corcos J, Fournier C. Periurethral collagen injection for the treatment of female stress urinary incontinence: 4-year follow-up results. *Urology* 1999;54:815–818.

Cornella JA, Pereyra AJ. Historical vignette of Armand J. Pereyra, MD, and the modified Pereyra procedure: the needle suspension for stress incontinence in the female. *Int Urogynecol J* 1990;1:25.

Costa P, Mottet N, Rabut B, et. al. The use of an artificial urinary sphincter in women with type III incontinence and a negative Marshall test. *J Urol* 2001;165:1172–1176.

Cross CA, Cespedes RD, English SF, et. al. Transvaginal urethrolysis for urethral obstruction and after anti-incontinence surgery. *J Urol* 1998;159:1199–1201.

Crystle CD, Charme LS, Copeland WE. Q-tip test in stress urinary incontinence. *Obstet Gynecol* 1971;39:313.

Dainer M, Hall CD, Choe J, et al. The Burch procedure: a comprehensive review. *Obstet Gynecol Surv* 1999;54:49–60.

DeLancey JOL. Structural support of the urethra as it relates to stress urinary incontinence: the hammock hypothesis. *Am J Obstet Gynecol* 1995;173:1713–1723.

DeLancy JOL. The pathophysiology of stress urinary incontinence in women and its implications for surgical treatment. *World J Urol* 1997;15:268–274.

Demirci F, Petri E. Perioperative complications of Burch colposuspension. *Int Urogyn J* 2000;11:170–175.

Demirci F, Yucel N, Ozden S, et. al. A retrospective review of perioperative complications in 360 patients who had Burch colposuspension. *Aust NZ J Obstet Gynecol* 1999;39:472–475.

Demirci F, Yucel O, Eren S, et al. Long-term results of Burch colposuspension. *Gyn Obstet Invest* 2001;51:243–247.

Diokno A, Hollander J, Alderson T. Artificial urinary sphincter for recurrent female urinary incontinence: indications and results. *J Urol* 1987;138:778.

Donovan MG, Barrett DM, Furlow WL. Use of the artificial urinary sphincter in the management of severe incontinence in females. *Surg Gynecol Obstet* 1985;161:17.

Drutz HP, Shapiro BJ, Mandel F. Do static cystourethrograms have a role in the investigation of female incontinence. *Am J Obstet Gynecol* 1978;130:516.

El-Toukhy TA, Davies AE. The efficacy of laparoscopic mesh colposuspension: results of a prospective controlled study. *BJU Int* 2001;88:361–366.

Elkabir JJ, Mee AD. Long-term evaluation of the Gittes procedure for urinary stress incontinence. *J Urol* 1998;159:1203–1205.

Elliott DS, Boone TB. Is fascia lata allograft material trustworthy for pubovaginal sling repair. *Urology* 2000;56:772–776.

Enzelberger H, Helmer H, Schatten C. Comparison of Burch and Lyodura sling procedures for repair of unsuccessful incontinence surgery. *Obstet Gynecol* 1996;88:251–256.

Enzler M, Agins HJ, Kogan M, et. al. Osteomyelitis of the pubis following suspension of the neck of the bladder with the use of bone anchors. A report of four cases. *J Bone Joint Surg* 1999;81:1736–1740.

Evans JWH, Chapple CR, Ralph J, et al. Bladder calculus formation as a complication of the Stamey procedure. *Br J Urol* 1990;65:580.

Fantl JA, Bump RC, McClish DK. Mixed urinary incontinence. *Urology* 1990;36(Suppl):21SS.

Fantl JA, Hurt WG, Bump RC, et al. Urethral axis and sphincteric function. *Am J Obstet Gynecol* 1986;155:554.

Filbeck T, Ulrich T, Pichlmeier U, et. al. Correlation of persistent stress urinary incontinence with quality of life after suspension procedures: is continence the only decisive postoperative criterion of success? *Urology* 1999;54:247–251.

FitzGerald MP, Mollenhauer J, Bitterman P, et. al. Functional failure of fascia lata allografts. *Am J Obstet Gynecol* 1999;1339–1346.

FitzGerald MP, Mollenhauer J, Brubaker L. The face of rectus fascia suburethral slings. *Am J Obstet Gynecol* 2000;183:964–966.

Fleming GA. The FDA, regulation, and the risk of stroke. *N Engl J Med* 2000;343:1886–1887.

Francis W. The onset of stress incontinence. *J Obstet Gynaecol Br Commweal* 1960;67:899.

Franks ME, Lavelle JP, Yokoyama T, et. al. Metastatic osteomyelitis after pubovaginal sling using bone anchors. *Urology* 2000;56:330–331.

Galloway NTM, Davies N, Stephenson TP. The complications of colposuspension. *Br J Urol* 1987;60:122.

Galloway NTM, El-Galley RE, Sand PK et. al. Update on extracorporeal magnetic innervation (ExMI) therapy for stress urinary incontinence. *Urology* 2000;56(6 Suppl 1):82–86.

Gardy M, Kozminski M, DeLancey JOL, et al. Stress incontinence and cystoceles. *J Urol* 1991;145:1211.

German KA, Kynaston H, Weight S, et al. A prospective randomized trial comparing a modified needle suspension procedure with the vagina/obturator shelf procedure for genuine stress incontinence. *Br J Urol* 1994;74:188.

Gilja I, Pushkar D, Mlazuran B, et. al. Comparative analysis of bladder neck suspension using Raz, Burch, and transvaginal Burch procedures: a 3-year randomized prospective study. *Eur Urol* 1998;33:298–302.

Gittes RF, Loughlin KR. No-incision pubovaginal suspension for stress incontinence. *J Urol* 1987;138:568.

Glowacki CA, Wall LL. Bone anchors in urogynecology. *Clin Obstet Gynecol* 2000;43:659–669.

Goldman HB, Rackley RR, Appell RA. The efficacy of urethrolysis without re-suspension for iatrogenic urethral obstruction. *J Urol* 1999;161:196–199.

Gorton E, Stanton S, Monga A, et al. Periurethral collagen injection: a long-term follow-up study. *BJU Int* 1999;84:966–971.

Greenwald SW, Thornbury JR, Dunn LJ. Cystourethrography as a diagnostic aid in stress incontinence. *Obstet Gynecol* 1967;29:324.

Groutz A, Blaivas JG, Kesler SS, et. al. Outcome results of transurethral collagen injection for female stress incontinence: assessment by urinary incontinence score. *J Urol* 2000;164:2006–2009.

Haab F, Zimmern PE, Leach GE. Urinary stress incontinence due to intrinsic sphincter deficiency: experience with fat and collagen periurethral injections. *J Urol* 1997;157:1283–1286.

Handley-Ashken M, Abrams PH, Lawrence WT. Stamey endoscopic bladder neck suspension for stress incontinence. *Br J Urol* 1984;56:629.

Harris RL, Yancey CA, Wiser WL, et al. Comparison of anterior colporrhaphy with retropubic urethropexy for patients with genuine stress urinary incontinence. *Am J Obstet Gynecol* 1995;173:1671–1675.

Harvey MA, Baker K, Wells GA. Tolterodine versus oxybutynin in the treatment of urge urinary incontinence: a meta-analysis. *Am J Obstet Gynecol* 2001;185:56–61.

Haverkamp A, Steiner G, Muller SC, et al. Urethral erosion of tension-free vaginal tape. *J Urol* 2002;167:250.

Henalla SM, Hall V, Duckett JR, et al. A multicentre evaluation of a new surgical technique for urethral bulking in the treatment of genuine stress incontinence. *BJOG* 2000; 107:1035–1039.

Hertogs K, Stanton SL. Lateral bead-chain urethrocystography after successful and unsuccessful colposuspension. *Br J Obstet Gynaecol* 1985;92:1179.

Hertogs K, Stanton SL. Mechanism of urinary continence after colposuspension: barrier studies. *Br J Obstet Gynaecol* 1985;92:1184.

Hilton P. A clinical and urodynamic study comparing the Stamey bladder neck suspension and suburethral sling procedures in the treatment of genuine stress incontinence. *Br J Obstet Gynaecol* 1989;96:213.

Hodgkinson CP, Ayers MA, Drukker BH. Dyssynergic detrusor dysfunction in the apparently normal female. *Am J Obstet Gynecol* 1963;87:717.

Horbach NS, Blanco JS, Ostergard DR, et al. A suburethral sling procedure with polytetrafluoroethylene for the treatment of genuine stress incontinence in patients with low urethral closure pressure. *Obstet Gynecol* 1988;71:648.

Horton R. Surgical research or comic opera: questions, but few answers. *Lancet* 1996;347:984–985.

Huang YH, Lin AT, Chen PK, et al. High failure rate using allograft fascia lata in pubovaginal sling surgery for female stress urinary incontinence. *Urology* 2001;58:943–946.

Hunskaar S, Arnold EP, Burgio K, et al. Epidemiology and natural history of urinary incontinence. *Int Urogyn J* 2000;11:301–319.

Hutchings A, Black NA. Surgery for stress incontinence: a nonrandomized trial of colposuspension, needle suspension, and anterior colporrhaphy. *Eur Urol* 2001;39:375–382.

Jarvis JG, Fowlie A. Clinical and urodynamic assessment of the porcine dermis bladder sling in the treatment of genuine stress incontinence. *Br J Obstet Gynaecol* 1985;92: 1189.

Kammerer-Doak DN, Dorin MH, Rogers RG, et al. A randomized trial of Burch retropubic urethropexy and anterior colporrhaphy for stress urinary incontinence. *Obstet Gynecol* 1999;93:75–78.

Karram MM, Angel O, Koonings P, et al. The modified Pereyra procedure: a clinical and urodynamic review. *Br J Obstet Gynaecol* 1992;99:655.

Karram MM, Bhatia NN. Management of coexistent stress and urge urinary incontinence. *Obstet Gynecol* 1989;73:4.

Karram MM, Bhatia NN. Patch procedure: modified transvaginal fascia lata sling for recurrent or severe stress urinary incontinence. *Obstet Gynecol* 1990;75:461.

Karram MM, Bhatia NN. Transvaginal needle bladder neck suspension procedures for stress urinary incontinence: a comprehensive review. *Obstet Gynecol* 1989;73:906.

Kegel AN. Progressive resistance exercise in the functional restoration of the perineal muscle. Am J Gynecol 1948; 56:238.

Kelly HA, Dumm WM. Urinary incontinence in women without manifest injury to the bladder. *Surg Gynecol Obstet* 1914;18:444.

Kernan WN, Viscoli CM, Brass LM, et al. Phenylpropanolamine and the risk of hemorrhagic stroke. *N Engl J Med* 2000;343:1826–1932.

Kersey J. The gauze hammock sling operation in the treatment of stress incontinence. *Br J Obstet Gynaecol* 1983;90:945.

Kersey J, Martin MM, Mishra P. A further assessment of the gauze hammock sling operation in the treatment of stress incontinence. *Br J Obstet Gynaecol* 1988;95:382.

Kiewetter H, Fischer M, Wober L, et al. Endoscopic implantation of collagen (GAX) for the treatment of urinary incontinence. *Br J Urol* 1992;69:22.

Kobashi KC, Dmochowski R, Mee SL, et al. Erosion of woven polyester pubovaginal sling. *J Urol* 1999;162:2070–2072.

Koefoot RB, Webster GD. Urodynamic evaluation in women with frequency, urgency symptoms. *Urology* 1983;6:648.

Koelbl H, Stoerer S, Seliger G, et al. Transurethral penetration of a tension-free vaginal tape. *Br J Obstet Gynaecol* 2001;108:7653–7655.

Koelle D, Stenzl A, Koelbl H, et al. Treatment of postoperative urinary retention by elongation of tension-free vaginal tape. *Am J Obstet Gynecol* 2001;185:250–251.

Korn AP, Learman LA. Operations for stress urinary incontinence in the United States, 1988–1992. *Urology* 1996;48:609–612.

Kowalczyk JJ, Mulcahy JJ. Use of the artificial urinary sphincter in women. *Int Urogyn J* 2000;11:176–179.

Lamhut P, Jackson TW, Wall LL. The treatment of urinary incontinence with electrical stimulation in nursing home patients: a pilot study. *J Am Geriatr Soc* 1992;40:48.

Langer R, Ron-El R, Neuman M, et al. The value of simultaneous hysterectomy during Burch colposuspension for urinary stress incontinence. *Obstet Gynecol* 1988;72:866.

Langer R, Ron-El R, Newman M, et al. Detrusor instability following colposuspension for urinary stress incontinence. *Br J Obstet Gynaecol* 1988;95:607.

Langer R, Lipshitz Y, Halperin R, et al. Long-term (10–15 year) follow-up after Burch colposuspension for urinary stress incontinence. *Int Urogyn J* 2001;12:323–327.

Leach GE, Dmochowski R, Appell RA, et al. Female stress urinary incontinence clinical guidelines panel summary report on surgical management of female stress urinary incontinence. *J Urol* 1997;158:875–880.

Leach GE, Labasky RF. Bone fixation technique for transvaginal needle suspension. *Urol Clin North Am* 1989;16: 175.

Leach GE, Yip CM, Donovan BJ. Mechanism of continence after modified Pereyra bladder neck suspension. *Urology* 1987;29:328.

Lee PE, Kung RC, Drutz HP. Periurethral autologous fat injection as treatment for female stress urinary incontinence: a randomized double-blind controlled trial. *J Urol* 2001;165:153–158.

Lee RA, Symmonds RE. Repeat Marshall-Marchetti procedure for recurrent stress urinary incontinence. *Am J Obstet Gynecol* 1975;122:219.

Lee RA, Symmonds RE, Goldstein RA. Surgical complications and results of modified Marshall-Marchetti-Krantz procedure for urinary incontinence. *Obstet Gynecol* 1979; 53:447.

Liapis A, Pyrgiotis E, Kontoravdis A, et al. Genuine stress incontinence: prospective randomized comparison of two operative methods. *Eur J Obstet Gynecol Reprod Biol* 1996;64:69–72.

Lightner D, Calvosa C, Andersen R, et al. A new injectable bulking agent for treatment of stress urinary incontinence: results of a multicenter, randomized, controlled, double-blind study of Durasphere. *Urology* 2001;58:12–15.

Lose G, Jergenson L, Mortensen SO, et al. Voiding difficulties after colposuspension. *Obstet Gynecol* 1987;69:33.

Luber KM, Boero S, Choe JY. The demographics of pelvic floor disorders: current observations and future projections. *Am J Obstet Gynecol* 2001;184:1496–1503.

Mainprize TC, Drutz HP. The Marshall-Marchetti-Krantz procedure: a critical review. *Obstet Gynecol Surv* 1988;43:724.

Malizia AA, Reiman HM, Meyers RP, et al. Migration and granulomatous reaction after periurethral injection of Polytef (Teflon). *JAMA* 1984;251:3277.

Malone-Lee J, Shaffu B, Anand C, et al. Tolterodine: superior tolerability than and comparable efficacy to oxybutynin in individuals 50 years old or older with overactive bladder: a randomized controlled trial. *J Urol* 2001;165:1452–1456.

Marshall VF, Marchetti AA, Krantz KE. The correction of stress incontinence by simple vesicourethral suspension. *Surg Gynecol Obstet* 1949;88:509.

Marshall VF, Segaul RM. Experience with suprapubic vesicourethral suspension after previous failures to correct stress incontinence in women. *J Urol* 1968;100:647.

Massey JA, Anderson RS, Abrams P. Mechanisms of continence during raised intra-abdominal pressure. *Br J Urol* 1987;60:529.

McDuffie RW Jr, Litin RB, Blundon KE. Urethrovesical suspension (Marshall-Marchetti-Krantz): experience with 204 cases. *Am J Surg* 1981;141:297.

McGuire EJ. Bladder instability and stress incontinence. *Neurourol Urodyn* 1988;7:563.

McGuire EJ. Urodynamic findings in patients after failure of stress incontinence operations. In: Zinner NR, Sterling AM, eds. *Female incontinence.* New York: Alan R Liss, 1981:351 (*Proc Clin Biol Res* 78).

McGuire EJ, Bennett CJ, Konnak JA, et al. Experience with pubovaginal slings for urinary incontinence at the University of Michigan. *J Urol* 1987;138:525.

McGuire EJ, Fitzpatrick CC, Wan J, et al. Clinical assessment of urethral sphincter function. *J Urol* 1993;150:1452.

McGuire EJ, Lytton B. Pubovaginal sling procedure for stress incontinence. *J Urol* 1978;119:82.

McGuire EJ, Lytton B, Kohorn E, et al. The value of urodynamic testing in stress urinary incontinence. *J Urol* 1980;124:256.

McGuire EJ, Savastano JA. Stress incontinence and detrusor instability/urge incontinence. *Neurourol Urodyn* 1985;4:313.

McGuire EJ, Wang CC, Usitalo H, et al. Modified pubovaginal sling in girls with myelodysplasia. *J Urol* 1986;135:94.

McKinlay JB. From 'promising report' to 'standard procedure:' seven stages in the career of a medical innovation. *Milbank Mem Fund Q* 1981;59:374–411.

Menefee SA, Chesson RA, Wall LL. Stress urinary incontinence due to prescription medications: alpha-blockers and angiotensin converting enzyme inhibitors. *Obstet Gynecol* 1998;91:853–854.

Meschia M, Pifarotti P, Bernasconi F, et al. Tension-free vaginal tape: analysis of outcomes and complications in 404 stress incontinent women. *Int Urogyn J* 2001;(Suppl 2):S24–27.

Miklos JR, Sze EH, Karram MM. A critical appraisal of the methods of measuring leak-point pressures in women with stress incontinence. *Obstet Gynecol* 1995;86:349–352.

Miller JM, Perucchini D, Carchidi LT et al. Pelvic floor muscle contraction during a cough and decreased vesical mobility. *Obstet Gynecol* 2001;97:255–260.

Mittleman RE, Marraccinni JV. Pulmonary Teflon granulomas following periurethral Teflon injection for urinary incontinence. *Arch Pathol Lab Med* 1983;107:611.

Miyazaki FS. Misconceptions derived from the use of microtip catheters in tissue. *Neurourol Urodyn* 1996;15:672.

Miyazaki FS. The Bonney test: a reassessment. *Am J Obstet Gynecol* 1997;177:1322–1329.

Miyazaki F, Shook G. Ilioinguinal nerve entrapment during needle suspension for stress incontinence. *Obstet Gynecol* 1992;80:246.

Montz FJ, Stanton SL. Q-tip test in female urinary incontinence. *Obstet Gynecol* 1986;67:258.

Morgan JE, Farrow GA, Stewart FE. The Marlex sling operation for the treatment of recurrent stress urinary incontinence: a 16 year review. *Am J Obstet Gynecol* 1985;224.

Mundy AR. A trial comparing the Stamey bladder neck suspension procedure with colposuspension for the treatment of stress incontinence. *Br J Urol* 1983;55:687.

Murless BC. The injection treatment of stress incontinence. *J Obstet Gynaecol Br Emp* 1938;45:67.

Muzsnai D, Carrillo E, Dubin C, et al. Retropubic vaginopexy for correction of urinary stress incontinence. *Obstet Gynecol* 1982;59:113.

Norton PA, Baker JE. Postural changes can reduce leakage in women with stress urinary incontinence. *Obstet Gynecol* 1994;84:770.

Norton P, Karram M, Wall LL, et al. Randomized double-blind placebo-controlled trial of terodiline in women with idiopathic detrusor instability. *Obstet Gynecol* 1994;84:386.

Nygaard I, DeLancey J, Arnsdorf L, et al. Exercise and incontinence. *Obstet Gynecol* 1990;75:848.

Nygaard I, Thompson FL, Svengalis SL, et al. Urinary incontinence in elite nulliparous athletes. *Obstet Gynecol* 1994;84:183.

O'Leary JA. Osteitis pubis following vesicourethral suspension. *Obstet Gynecol* 1964;24:73.

Olsen AL, Smith VJ, Bergstron JO, et al. Epidemiology of surgically managed pelvic organ prolapse and urinary incontinence. *Obstet Gynecol* 1997;89:501–506.

Pages IH, Jahr S, Schaufele MK, et al. Comparative analysis of biofeedback and physical therapy for treatment of urinary stress incontinence in women. *Am J Phys Med Rehab* 2001;80:s494–502.

Parker RT, Addison WA, Wilson CJ. Fascia lata urethrovesical suspension for recurrent stress urinary incontinence. *Am J Obstet Gynecol* 1979;135:843.

Parnell JP, Marshall VF, Vaughan ED Jr. Management of recurrent urinary stress incontinence by the Marshall-Marchetti-Krantz urethropexy. *J Urol* 1984;132:912.

Peattie AB, Plevnik S, Stanton SL. Vaginal cones: a conservative method of treating genuine stress incontinence. *Br J Obstet Gynaecol* 1988;95:1049.

Peattie AB, Stanton SL. The Stamey operation for correction of genuine stress incontinence in elderly patients woman. *Br J Obstet Gynaecol* 1989;96:983.

Pereyra AJ. A simplified surgical procedure for the correction of stress incontinence in women. *West J Surg* 1959;67:223.

Pereyra AJ. Revised Pereyra procedure using collimated pubourethral supports. In: Slate WG, ed. *Disorders of the female urethra and urinary incontinence.* Baltimore: Williams & Wilkins, 1978:143.

Pereyra AJ, Lebherz TB. Combined urethral vesical suspension vaginal urethroplasty for correction of urinary stress incontinence. *Obstet Gynecol* 1967;30:537.

Pereyra AJ, Lebherz TB, Growdon WA, et al. Pubourethral supports in perspective: modified Pereyra procedure for urinary incontinence. *Obstet Gynecol* 1981;59:643.

Persson J, Bossmar T, Wolner-Hanssen P. Laparoscopic colposuspension: a short term urodynamic follow-up and a three-year questionnaire study. *Acta Obstet Gynecol Scand* 2000;79:414–420.

Peschers UM, Jundt K, Dimpfl T. Differences between cough and Valsalva leak-point pressure in stress incontinent women. *Neurourol Urodyn* 2000;19:677–681.

Peyrat L, Boutin JM, Bruyere F, et al. Intestinal perforation as a complication of tension-free vaginal tape procedure for urinary incontinence. *Eur Urol* 2001;39:603–605.

Ramon J, Mekras J, Webster GD. Transvaginal needle suspension procedures for recurrent stress incontinence. *Urology* 1991;38:519.

Raz S, Maggio AJ Jr, Kauman JJ. Why Marshall-Marchetti operation works . . . or does not. *Urology* 1979;14:154.

Reddy AP, DeLancey JOL, Zwica LM, et al. On-screen vector-based ultrasound assessment of vesical neck movement. *Am J Obstet Gynecol* 2001;185:65–70.

Reid GC, DeLancey JOL, Hopkins MP, et al. Urinary incontinence following radical vulvectomy. *Obstet Gynecol* 1990;75:852.

Resnick N. Noninvasive diagnosis of the patient with complex incontinence. *Gerontology* 1990;36 (Suppl Z):8.

Resnick N, Yalla S. Detrusor hyperactivity with impaired contractile function: an unrecognized but common cause of incontinence in elderly patients. *JAMA* 1987;257:3076.

Rezapour M, Ulmsten U. Tension-free vaginal tape (TVT) in women with recurrent stress urinary incontinence: a long-term follow-up. *Int Urogyn J* 2001;(Suppl 2):S9–11.

Richter HE, Varner RE, Sanders E, et al. Effects of pubovaginal sling procedure on patients with urethral hypermobility and intrinsic sphincteric deficiency: would they do it again? *Am J Obstet Gynecol* 2001;184:14–19.

Ridley JH. The Goebell-Stoeckel sling. In: Mattingly RF, Thompson JD, eds. *Te Linde's operative gynecology,* 6th ed. Philadelphia: JB Lippincott, 1985:623.

Ross J. Laparoscopy or open Burch colposuspension? *Curr Opin Obstet Gynecol* 19098;10:405–409.

Rottenberg RD, Weil A, Brioschi PA, et al. Urodynamic and clinical assessment of the Lyodura sling operation for urinary stress incontinence. *Br J Obstet Gynecol* 1985;92:829.

Seski JC. Iatrogenic intravesical foreign body following Marshall-Marchetti procedure for stress urinary incontinence. *Am J Obstet Gynecol* 1976;126:514.

Shapiro J, Hoffman J, Jersky J. A comparison of suprapubic and transurethral drainage for postoperative urinary retention in general surgical patients. *Acta Chir Scand* 1982;148:323.

Sharp HT, Doucette RC, Norton PA. Dyspareunia and recurrent stress urinary incontinence after laparoscopic colposuspension with mesh and staples: a case report. *J Reprod Med* 2000;45:947–949.

Shull BL, Baden WF. A six-year experience with paravaginal defect repair for stress urinary incontinence. *Am J Obstet Gynecol* 1989;160:1432–1440.

Sjoberg B. Hydrodynamics of micturition following Marshall-Marchetti-Krantz procedure for stress urinary incontinence. *Scand J Urol Nephrol* 1982;16:11.

Soergel TM, Shott S, Heit M. Poor surgical outcomes after fascia lata allograft slings. *Int Urogyn J* 2001;12:247–253.

Stamey TA. Endoscopic suspension of vesical neck for urinary incontinence. *Surg Gynecol Obstet* 1973;136:547.

Stamey TA. Endoscopic suspension of the vesical neck for urinary incontinence in females. *Ann Surg* 1980;192:465.

Stanton SL, Brindley GS, Holmes DA. Silastic sling for urethral sphincter incompetence in women. *Br J Obstet Gynaecol* 1985;92:747.

Stanton SL, Cardozo LD. A comparison of vaginal and suprapubic surgery in the correction of incontinence due to urethral sphincter incompetence. *Br J Urol* 1979;51:4978.

Stanton SL, Cardozo LD. Results of the colposuspension operation for incontinence and prolapse. *Br J Obstet Gynaecol* 1978;86:693.

Stanton SL, Cardozo LD, Chaudhury N. Spontaneous voiding after surgery for urinary incontinence. *Br J Obstet Gynaecol* 1978;85:149.

Stanton SL, Cardozo LD, Williams JE, et al. Clinical and urodynamic features of failed incontinence surgery in the female. *Obstet Gynecol* 1978;51:515.

Stanton SL, Norton C, Cardozo L. Clinical and urodynamic effects of anterior colporrhaphy and vaginal hysterectomy for prolapse with and without incontinence. *Br J Obstet Gynaecol* 1982;89:459.

Stanton SL, Williams JE, Ritchie D. The colposuspension operation for urinary incontinence. *Br J Obstet Gynaecol* 1976;83:890.

Steel SA, Cox C, Stanton SL. Long term follow-up of detrusor instability following colposuspension operation. *Br J Urol* 1986;58:138.

Stothers L, Goldenberg SL, Leone EF. Complications of periurethral collagen injection for stress urinary incontinence. *J Urol* 1998;159:806–807.

Sweat SD, Lightner DJ. Complications of sterile abscess formation and pulmonary embolism following periurethral bulking agents. *J Urol* 1999;161:93–96.

Swift SE, Ostergard DR. A comparison of stress leak-point pressure and maximal urethral closure pressure in patients with genuine stress incontinence. *Obstet Gynecol* 1995;85:704–708.

Tamussino KF, Hanzal E, Kolle D, et al. Tension-free vaginal tape operation: results of the Austrian registry. *Obstet Gynecol* 2001;98:732–736.

Tamussino KF, Zivkovic F, Pieber D, et al. Five-year results after anti-incontinence operations. *Am J Obstet Gynecol* 1999;181:1347–1352.

Theofrastus JP, Bump RC, Elser DM et al. Correlation of urodynamic measures of urethral resistance with clinical measures of incontinence severity in women with pure genuine stress incontinence. *Am J Obstet Gynecol* 1995;173:407–414.

Tschopp PJ, Wesley James T, Spekkens A., et al. Collagen injections for urinary stress incontinence in a small urban urology practice: time to failure analysis of 99 cases. *J Urol* 1999;162:779–783.

Turner-Warwick RT. Turner-Warwick vagino-obturator shelf urethral repositioning procedure. In: Gingell C, Abrams P, eds. *Controversies and innovations in urologic surgery.* New York: Springer-Verlag, 1988:195.

Ulmsten U, Henriksson L, Johnson P, et al. An ambulatory surgical procedure under local anesthesia for treatment of female urinary incontinence. *Int Urogyn J* 1996;7:81–86.

Ulmsten U, Johnson P, Rezapour M. A three-year follow up of tension free vaginal tape for surgical treatment of female stress urinary incontinence. *Br J Obstet Gynaecol* 1999;106:345–350.

Ulmsten U, Petros P. Intravaginal slingplast (IVS): an ambulatory surgical procedure for treatment of female urinary incontinence. *Scand J Urol Nephrol* 1995;29:75–82.

van Geelen JM, Theeues AGM, Eskes TKAB, et al. The clinical and urodynamic effects of anterior vaginal repair and Burch colposuspension. *Am J Obstet Gynecol* 1988;159:137.

Varner RE. Retropubic long-needle suspension procedures for stress urinary incontinence. *Am J Obstet Gynecol* 1990; 163:551.

Versi E, Apell R, Mobley D, et al. Dry mouth with conventional and controlled-release oxybutynin in urinary incontinence. The Ditropan XL Study Group. *Obstet Gynecol* 2000;95: 718–721.

Wagner TH, Hu TW. Economic costs of urinary incontinence in 1995. *Urology* 1998;51:355–361.

Wall LL. Diagnosis and management of urinary incontinence due to detrusor instability. *Obstet Gynecol Surv* 1990;45:1SS.

Wall LL. Innovation in surgery: caveat emptor. *Int Urogynecol J* 2001;12:353–354.

Wall LL. The muscles of the pelvic floor. *Clin Obstet Gynecol* 1993;36:910.

Wall LL. A technique for modified McCall culdeplasty at the time of abdominal hysterectomy. *J Am Coll Surg* 1994; 178:507.

Wall LL, Addison WA. Basic cystometry in gynecologic practice. *Postgrad Obstet Gynecol* 1988;9:1.

Diagnosis and management of urinary incontinence due to detrusor instability. *Obstet Gynecol Surv* 1990;45:1S–47S.

Wall LL, Addison WA. Prazosin-induced stress incontinence. *Obstet Gynecol* 1990;75:558.

Wall LL, Davidson TG. The role of muscular re-education by physical therapy in the treatment of genuine stress urinary incontinence. *Obstet Gynecol Surv* 1992;47:322.

Wall LL, DeLancey JOL. Observations on the diagnosis of stress urinary incontinence. *J Pelvic Surg* 1998;4:208–213.

Wall LL, DeLancey JOL. The politics of prolapse: a revisionist approach to disorders of the pelvic floor in women. *Perspect Biol Med* 1991;34:486.

Wall LL, Helms M, Peattie AB, et al. Bladder neck mobility and the outcome of surgery for genuine stress incontinence: a logistic regression analysis of lateral bead-chain cystourethrograms. *J Reprod Med* 1994;39:429.

Wall LL, Hewitt JK. Urodynamic characteristics of women with complete post-hysterectomy vaginal vault prolapse. *Urology* 1994;44:336.

Wall LL, Hewitt JK. Voiding function after the Burch colposuspension operation for stress incontinence. *J Reprod Med* 1996;41:161–165.

Wall LL, Hewitt JK, Helms MJ. Are vaginal and rectal pressures equivalent approximations of one another for the purpose of performing subtracted cystometry? *Obstet Gynecol* 1995; 85:488.

Wall LL, Norton PA, DeLancey JOL. *Practical urogynecology.* Baltimore: Williams & Wilkins, 1993.

Wall LL, Stanton SL. Transvesical phenolisation of pelvic nerve plexuses in female patients with refractory urge incontinence. *Br J Urol* 1989;63:465.

Wall LL, Warrell DW. Detrusor instability associated with menstruation: case report. *Br J Obstet Gynaecol* 1989;96:737.

Wall LL, Wiskind AK, Taylor PA. Simple bladder filling with a cough stress test compared to subtracted cystometry in the diagnosis of urinary incontinence. *Am J Obstet Gynecol* 1994;171:1472.

Walters MD, Diaz K. Q-tip test: a study of continent and incontinent women. *Obstet Gynecol* 1987;70:208.

Walters MD, Shields LE. The diagnostic value of history, physical examination, and the Q-tip cotton swab test in women with urinary incontinence. *Am J Obstet Gynecol* 1988; 159:145.

Wan J, McGuire EJ, Bloom DA, et al. Stress leak point pressure: a diagnostic tool for incontinent children. *J Urol* 1993;150:700.

Wan J, McGuire EJ, Bloom DA, et al. The treatment of urinary incontinence in children using glutaraldehyde cross-linked Contigen. *J Urol* 1992;148:127.

Weber AM. Is urethral pressure profilometry a useful diagnostic test for stress urinary incontinence. *Obstet Gynecol Surv* 2001;56:720–735.

Weber AM, Walters MD. Burch procedure compared with sling for stress urinary incontinence: a decision analysis. *Obstet Gynecol* 2000;96:867–873.

Webster GD, Sihelnik SA. Troubleshooting the malfunctioning Scott artificial urinary sphincter. *J Urol* 1984;131: 269.

Wefer J, Truss MC, Jonas U. Tolterodine: an overview. *World J Urol* 2001;19:312–318.

Weil A, Reyes H, Bischoff P, et al. Modifications of the urethral rest and stress profiles after different types of surgery for urinary stress incontinence. *Br J Obstet Gynaecol* 1984;91: 46.

Weiss RE, Cohen E. Erosion of buttress following bladder neck suspension. *Br J Urol* 1992;69:656.

Wheeless CR Jr. *Atlas of pelvic surgery,* 2nd ed. Philadelphia: Lea & Febiger, 1988.

Wilson L, Brown JS, Shin GP et al. Annual direct cost of urinary incontinence. *Obstet Gynecol* 2001;98:398–406.

Winters JC, Chiverton A, Scarpero HM, et al. Collagen injection therapy in elderly women: long-term results and patient satisfactions. *Urology* 2000;55:856–861.

Wiskind AK, Creighton SM, Stanton SL. The incidence of prolapse after the Burch colposuspension. *Am J Obstet Gynecol* 1992;167:399.

Wiskind AK, Miller KF, Wall LL. One hundred unstable bladders. *Obstet Gynecol* 1994;83:108.

Wolin LH. Stress incontinence in young healthy nulliparous female subjects. *J Urol* 1969;101:545.

Woodside JR. Pubovaginal sling procedure for the management of urinary incontinence after urethral trauma in women. *J Urol* 1987;138:527.

Yarnell JWG, Voyle GJ, Richards CJ, et al. The prevalence and severity of urinary incontinence in women. *J Epidemiol Community Health* 1981;35:71.

Zderic SA, Burros HM, Hanno PM, et al. Bladder calculi in women after urethrovesical suspension. *J Urol* 1988;139: 1047.

Zimmern PE, Hadley HR, Leach GE, et al. Female urethral obstruction after Marshall-Marchetti-Krantz operation. *J Urol* 1987;138:517.

Te Linde's Operative Gynecology, ninth edition, edited by John A. Rock and Howard W. Jones, III. Lippincott Williams & Wilkins, Philadelphia © 2003.

CHAPTER

37

▼

Operative Injuries to the Ureter

F.J. MONTZ   ROBERT E. BRISTOW

MARCELA G. DEL CARMEN

Ureteral injuries have been recognized as a potential complication of gynecologic surgical procedures since the inception of our discipline. Over the centuries, numerous unique surgical procedures or modifications thereof have been developed with the specific intent of decreasing the probability of ureteral injury. Despite these efforts, ureteral injury remains a very real complication of abdominal-pelvic surgery in the female patient, affecting as many as 1.5% of women taken to the operating theater. The risk of ureteral injury depends on the indication for and procedure performed, although an average incidence of about 0.4% is widely and consistently reported in case series. Therefore, it is evident that the gynecologic surgeon must be cognizant of ways to minimize the occurrence of these potentially disastrous complications as well as facile in the diagnosis and management of such an injury should it occur.

The goals of this chapter are to: (a) outline the functional anatomy of the ureter and illustrate how this leads to the ureter being in harm's way during gynecologic surgery; (b) summarize the basic principles of injury avoidance and, should injury occur, recognition and management; and (c) review the unique issues surrounding ureteral injury during the performance of specific groups of gynecologic surgical procedures.

FUNCTIONAL ANATOMY OF THE URETER

When viewed in cross section, the ureter can be divided into distinct layers: the lumen with transitional epithelium; the mucosa; the muscular layer, which is made up of longitudinal, circular, and spiral smooth muscle fibers; and the adventitia, which contains an intercommunicating network of blood vessels. The peritoneum lies over the ureter, making it a completely retroperitoneal structure (Fig. 37.1).

In normal adults, the ureter is between 25 and 30 cm in length from the renal pelvis to the trigone of the bladder. By convention, the ureter is divided into the abdominal and pelvic segments by the pelvic brim; each of these components is approximately 12 to 15 cm in length.

The abdominal ureter runs along the ventral surface of the psoas muscle and dorsal to the ovarian vessels to the level of the pelvic brim. The right ureter lies slightly lateral to the inferior vena cava and descends into the pelvis ventral to the common iliac artery at approximately the site of the latter's bifurcation. The left ureter runs lateral to the aorta and dorsal to the inferior mesenteric artery, ovarian vessels, and colon. The left ureter mirrors the right at the pelvic brim, entering the pelvis

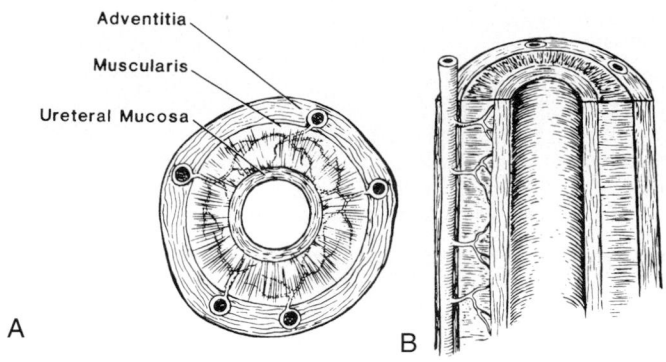

Adventitia

Muscularis

Ureteral Mucosa

A

B

FIGURE 37.1. Cross-sectional (**A**) and sagittal (**B**) views of the longitudinal arteries and veins in the adventitia. These arteries and veins provide the important collateral circulation along the course of the ureter.

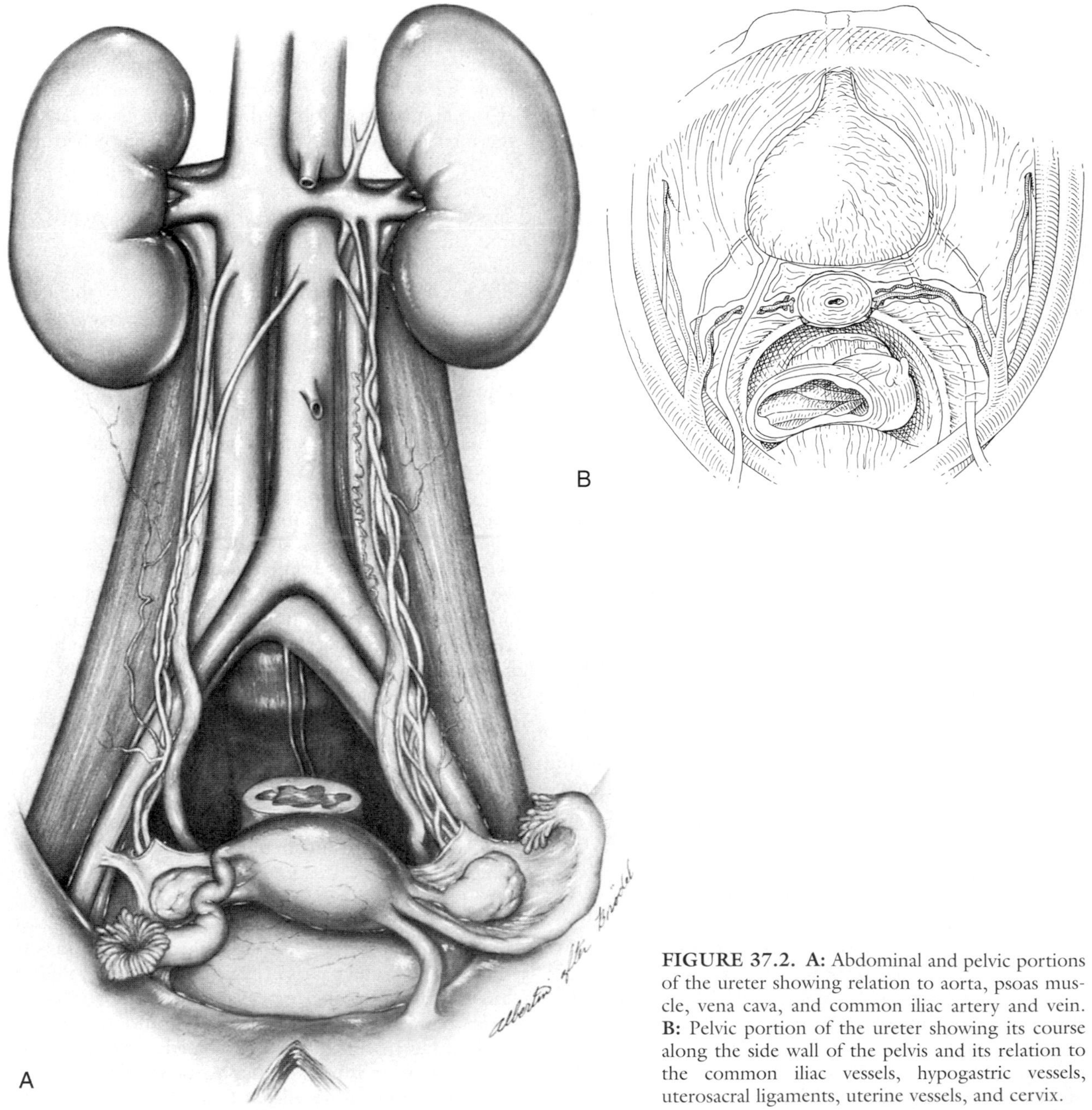

B

A

FIGURE 37.2. A: Abdominal and pelvic portions of the ureter showing relation to aorta, psoas muscle, vena cava, and common iliac artery and vein. **B:** Pelvic portion of the ureter showing its course along the side wall of the pelvis and its relation to the common iliac vessels, hypogastric vessels, uterosacral ligaments, uterine vessels, and cervix.

over the bifurcation of the left common iliac artery. The left ureter often is obscured by the sigmoid colon at the pelvic brim (Fig. 37.2).

There is little variance between the positions taken by the pelvic ureters. They descend into the posterior lateral pelvic sidewall lateral to the sacrum and next to the ventral border of the greater sciatic notch immediately ventral to internal iliac (hypogastric) artery. The ureters then deviate medially as they approach the ischial spine and lie medial to the internal iliac artery and the anterior branches thereof. The ureters subsequently course beneath the uterine artery (often referred to as water under the bridge). This passage occurs approximately 1.5 cm lateral to the internal cervical os and is the site of the ureteral entrance to the parametrial tissues. It is after this junction that the ureter passes into the tunnel of the cardinal ligament/anterior bladder pillar (often referred to as the web or the tunnel of Wertheim, named after an early champion of radical hysterectomy as treatment for cervical cancer). Once through the tunnel of Wertheim, the ureter travels medially and anteriorly over the vaginal fornix to enter the trigone of the bladder.

In those instances where there are not inflammatory or adhesive changes present and the anatomy has not been perverted, the ureters can be usually visualized through the peritoneum from above the pelvic brim to the tunnel of Wertheim. Once the ureters have entered the tunnel, they cannot be easily seen or palpated and, if identification is desired, they must be mobilized out of the parametrial tissue. Although the peristalsis that occurs in the normal ureter may be helpful in its identification, it is not uncommon that the ureter, following any degree of trauma, will have a degree of transient paralysis. Therefore, skill at definitively identifying the ureter based on its anatomy, not its motion, is essential for the pelvic surgeon.

Having defined the general anatomy of the ureter, it is valuable to appreciate that there is a significant degree of interpatient variability even in the pelvis that is free of inflammatory, infectious, neoplastic, congenital, or postsurgical changes.

The blood supply to the ureter is rich and the origin of such easily remembered: The ureter obtains part of its blood supply from every vessel that it transverses (Fig. 37.3). The small vessels that nourish the ureter are interconnected by a lush network of anastomosing arcades within the adventitial sheath. It is this vigorous and multiorigin blood supply that helps to make the ureter resistant to devascularization, even when it has been stripped of the surrounding ureteral sheath. Yet, although the ureter may be relatively difficult to devascularize, such injuries can occur and are more likely to happen if one fails to remember the origin of the blood supply, as illustrated in Fig. 37.3. Cephalad to the pelvic brim, the blood supply enters from the medial side; therefore, dissection and mobilization should be carried out from the lateral aspect of the ureter. The inverse is true below the pelvic brim.

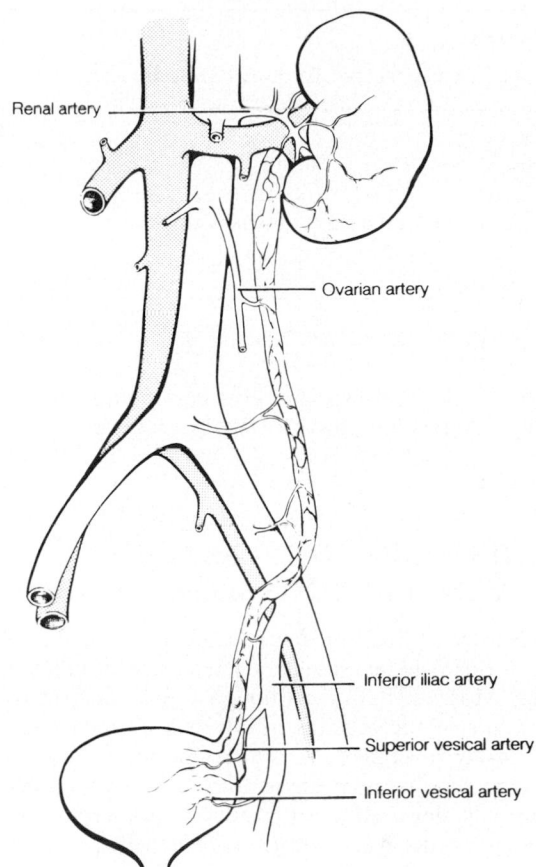

FIGURE 37.3. Blood supply of the ureter.

URETERAL INJURY

Thompson, in the preceding edition of this text, listed six types of operative ureteral injuries, which are shown in Table 37.1. Other authors have proposed that avulsion and stretch injuries also be listed as separate types, although we feel that these two categories are included (generally) under "transection" and "ischemia," respectively.

All of these injuries can and do occur, although relatively infrequently, during the performance of gynecologic surgical procedures. Additionally, angulation and ischemia can be the sequelae of nonsurgical processes (e.g., cervical myomas and radiation therapy, respectively). The specifics as to how these injuries occur and, more importantly, how they can be best avoided are discussed in subsequent sections of this chapter. Ureteral injuries most commonly occur at one of five different locales, as illustrated in Table 37.2.

Traditionally and in prior editions of this text it has been claimed that gynecologic surgery is the most common venue for iatrogenic ureteral injuries. However, modern single institutional reviews have reported that urological surgical procedures are most frequently associated with ureteral injury (42%) followed by gynecologic procedures (34%) and general surgical procedures

---

TABLE 37.1.
Types of Operative Ureteral Injuries

Crushing
Ligation
Transection
Angulation (with secondary obstruction)
Ischemia
Resection

(24%). Table 37.3 lists the most common elements regarding ureteral injuries associated with gynecologic surgery.

GENERAL PRINCIPLES OF PREVENTION AND MANAGEMENT

Forewarned is forearmed, or so the saying goes. However, is this true regarding the prevention of ureteral injuries? Most likely not. Although it is important to be cognizant of the settings in which a ureteral injury is more likely to occur (e.g., surgery performed for a malignancy, repeat caesarean section, large adnexal masses or fibroids, dense adhesions, severe endometriosis, etc.), there are no data supporting the belief that preoperative intravenous pyelogram, computed tomography, or prophylactic ureteral stint placement decreases the probability of a ureteral injury.

There are only a few truisms about the general prevention of ureteral injuries that the gynecologic pelvic surgeon can control. The most important is that the surgeon must constantly and unequivocally know where the ureter is. Not only is this supported by all of the references in this chapter, but also by our large personal experience. Often when we are called to assist a colleague who has induced a ureteral injury, it is evident that the surgeon did not know where the ureter was and therefore, ligated, incised, or transected it. The next truism is that staying outside of the adventitial sheath when performing ureteral dissection decreases the probability of devascularization and subsequent ischemia. This cannot always be accomplished, particularly in those settings

---

TABLE 37.2.
Common Sites of Ureteral Injuries

Cardinal ligament where the ureter crosses under the uterine artery
Tunnel of Wertheim
Intramural portion of the ureter
Dorsal to the infundibulopelvic ligament near or at the pelvic brim
Lateral pelvic sidewall above the uterosacral ligament

TABLE 37.3.
Ureteral Injury Associated with Gynecologic Surgery: "Most Commons"

Most common site: Pelvic brim near the infundibulopelvic ligament
Most common procedure: Simple abdominal hysterectomy
Most common type of injury: Obstruction
Most common "activity" leading to injury: Attempts to obtain hemostasis
Most common time of diagnosis: None: 50–50 split between intraoperative and postoperative
Most common long-term sequelae: None

---

where there is malignancy or significant scarring and fibrosis that accompany endometriosis or prior pelvic radiation (see following discussions). Finally, when using instruments that transmit energy to the tissues (e.g., electrocoagulation, whether monopolar or bipolar; argon beam coagulator; laser), the surgeon must know exactly how broad the zone of thermal injury is for that instrument at that power setting. Although the mean distance of thermal damage with most of these instruments is approximately 2 mm, it may be as much as 5 mm; therefore, use of these energy sources within this zone has the potential for delayed necrosis. The zone of thermal injury from the argon beam coagulator is much smaller, at 3 to 7 μ, but even this can be significant and must be considered when using this instrument.

Management of Ureteral Injury

It is an oversimplification to state that every specific type of ureteral injury can be managed in a specific and universally applicable way. Patient-unique variables play an important role in deciding what is best in a given setting. Regardless of this, general guidelines and techniques may be helpful. Our general recommendations for the management of ureteral injuries identified at the time of surgery are outlined in Table 37.4. Our preferences for these therapies are supported in the specifics and illustrations of each of these recommendations.

Management of Specific Injury Types
Ureteral Ligation
Complete ureteral ligation is an uncommon event. It is much more common that the ureter will be angulated or kinked by the placement of a suture that is either within the para-ureteral tissue or partially placed through the ureter. In the first instance, which is probably much more common than has been recognized, simple ureterolysis, making sure that one stays out of the adventitial sheath, is all that is necessary. In those instances where the ureter has been either partially or totally ligated, management begins by removing the suture. The surgeon must be completely confident that the ureter is

TABLE 37.4.
KGOS General Guidelines for Management of Ureteral Injuries Identified at Time of Surgery

Ureteral ligation: Deligation, assessment of viability, stint placement
Partial transection: Primary repair over ureteral stint
Total transection
> *Uncomplicated upper and middle thirds:* Uretero-ureterostomy over ureteral stint
> *Complicated upper and middle thirds:* Uretero-ileal interposition
> *Lower third:* Uretero-neocystotomy with Psoas hitch over ureteral stint

Thermal injury: Resection with management as per a transection

viable. There is no perfect way to guarantee this. Blanching and blood flow through the vessels in the adventitial sheath, ureteral peristalsis, and lack of discoloration are all valuable, although imperfect measures. If there is any question about viability, the segment of the ureter about which there is concern must be resected and handled as outlined in the following. A ureteral stint is placed once deligation has been effected. Theoretically, this can be done one of three ways: via ureterostomy, cystoscopy, or cystostomy. We strongly favor the last approach. Performing a ureterostomy when one is not necessary provides an unnecessary site for stenosis or a leak. Cystoscopy requires additional instrumentation, repositioning, and prepping of the patient if she has not been placed in the dorsal low-lithotomy position from the beginning of the case. Opening the dome of the bladder in an extraperitoneal (preperitoneal via the space of Retzius) fashion is easy, safe, and efficient. The negative aspects of this method of ureteral catheterization are the need for a short time interval of bladder rest (we prefer 3 days in the nonirradiated setting, and longer if pelvic radiation has been administered previously), and the potential difficulty of identifying the ureteral orifices if there has been internal bladder/trigonal injury. We have found that use of a no. 7 French double J ureteral stint and a right angle clamp to manipulate the stint make placement quite easy. The cystotomy is closed with two layers of suture: (a) a 2-0 chromic closing the urothelium; and (b) a 2-0 polyglycolic acid suture approximating the detrusor muscle in a running Lembert technique.

Partial Ureteral Transection

Repair of a partial transection is probably the easiest and fastest of all the ureteral injuries to manage. Because the ureterotomy already has occurred (although inadvertently), the ureteral stint is placed up and down through the ureterotomy. The ureter is repaired using 5-0 PGA suture over the ureteral stint. Excessive suture placement should be avoided because it is uncommon that more than three individual sutures are needed. Further additional suture placement does not increase the probability

of adequate watertight closure and simply increases the probability of infection, ischemia, and scar formation. A closed suction drain should be placed at the base of the repair.

Total Transection

UNCOMPLICATED UPPER AND MIDDLE THIRDS

A transection of the ureter in the upper and middle thirds is not an uncommon locale of transection in association with the performance of a paraaortic lymph node dissection or colonic resection. When this type of injury occurs, a ureteroureterostomy over ureteral stint is the recommended method of repair. The rules regarding performance of the ureteroureterostomy are the same as for the repair of the primary subtotal transection: a limited number of sutures using small-gauge PGA suture are placed over a ureteral stint, and the site of the repair is drained using a closed suction drain.

There are only two major modifications that we recommend. First, the surgeon should be assured that the ureteroureterostomy is completely tension free. In those instances where we have convinced ourselves (naively) that the repair was tension free when it was not, we have come to regret such a self-delusion. First, extra length of the proximal segment of ureter can be obtained by mobilizing the kidney, although care always must be taken to assure that the renal blood supply and drainage are not compromised. Second, we recommend that both ends (upstream and downstream) of the ureteroureterostomy site be spatulated. When the spatulating incision is made, care must be taken to assure that the blood vessels running in the ureteral sheath are not transected. If this occurs, the advantages of increasing the lumen at the site of the ureteroureterostomy are probably offset by the probability of a devascularization injury and subsequent sloughing of the site of repair. Although the vessels in the ureteral adventitial sheath usually can be visualized, such is not always the case. Of course, the spatulation should be done on opposing sides of the proximal and distal ureter so as to facilitate a watertight seal (Fig. 37.4).

COMPLICATED UPPER AND MIDDLE THIRDS

By convention, complicated upper and middle third ureteral injuries are those where one has resected a segment of the ureter and it can not be brought together in a tension-free fashion using either proximal or distal mobilization techniques as described. Although there are really two ways to effect repair (transureterureterotomy and ureteroenteroneocystomy), we strongly argue against the performance of the first technique. By definition, it doubles the number of urinary drainage systems that have been injured and, therefore, are at risk. For this reason, transurethroureterotomy has generally been abandoned and remains of historical interest only. Therefore, it is ureteroenteroneocystomy, in the form of an ureteroileal interposition, that is our standard for management of these injuries.

Ureteroileal interposition is a relatively easy procedure to perform. A healthy and mobile segment of the

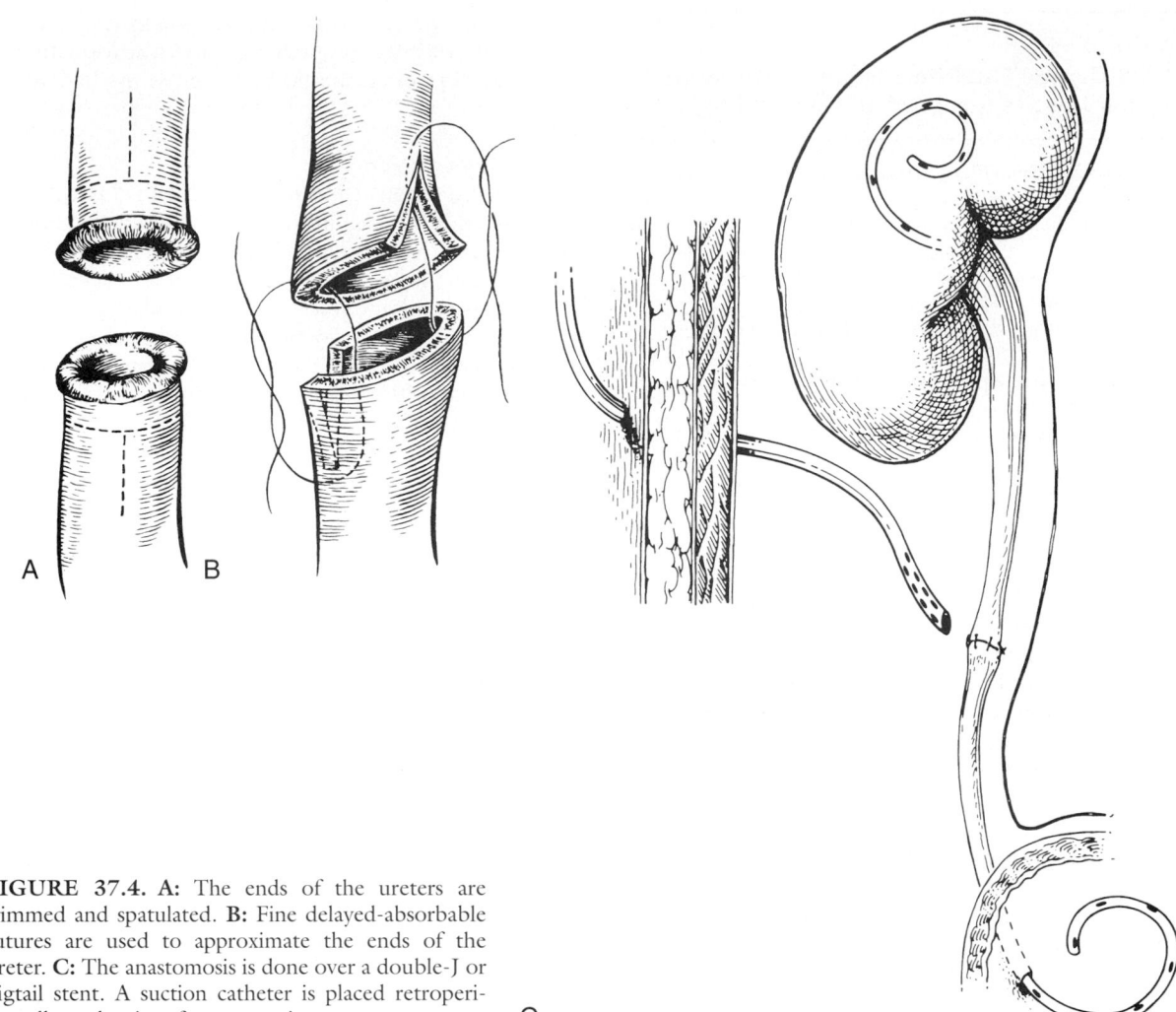

FIGURE 37.4. A: The ends of the ureters are trimmed and spatulated. **B:** Fine delayed-absorbable sutures are used to approximate the ends of the ureter. **C:** The anastomosis is done over a double-J or pigtail stent. A suction catheter is placed retroperitoneally at the site of anastomosis.

distal ileum is identified, and the vascular arcades assured to be adequate for viability. We prefer to perform this resection using linear stapling devices. The ileoileostomy is complete before the performance of the ureteroileoureteral repair. Thereafter, the proximal end of the loop of ileum is opened, a ureteral-ileal end-to-side anastomosis is performed over a ureteral stint. The same spatulating technique that was described in the preceding is used; however, we prefer to bring the ureter through the full thickness of the antimesenteric wall of the ileal segment. The full thickness ureter is splayed open inside of the ileal segment using a small-gauge PGA suture. In addition, the seromuscular portion of the ureter is attached to the serosa of the ileal segment so that the intra ileal anastomosis is completely tension free. After the proximal ureteroileal anastomosis is completed, the patent lumen of the proximal end of the ileal segment is closed. Either PGA staples (our preference) or a two-layer hand-sewn technique can be used. Closing the ileum with metal staples is not an acceptable option because of the potential for stone for-

mation on the permanent foreign body that is exposed to urine. The distal end of the ileal segment is opened with the staple line removed and the ureteroileal anastomosis to the distal segment completed over the ureteral stint, which has now been passed into the bladder via an antegrade technique. We secure the interposed ileal segment to the psoas muscle fascia so as to minimize tension on that bowel segment mesentery and potential tension on the proximal ureteroileal anastomosis that may be a result of the effect of gravity when the patient is in an upright position. The ureteral stint should remain *in vivo* for at least 6 weeks. A ureterogram to identify any persistent occult leaks is recommended prior to removing the stint via a transurethral cystoscopy. An illustration of the end result of a ureteroenteroneocystostomy is shown in Fig. 37.5. Even although this illustration does not show the ureteroileoureteral anastomosis described in the preceding, it does demonstrate the more commonly performed and similar procedure used for massive distal ureteral injuries.

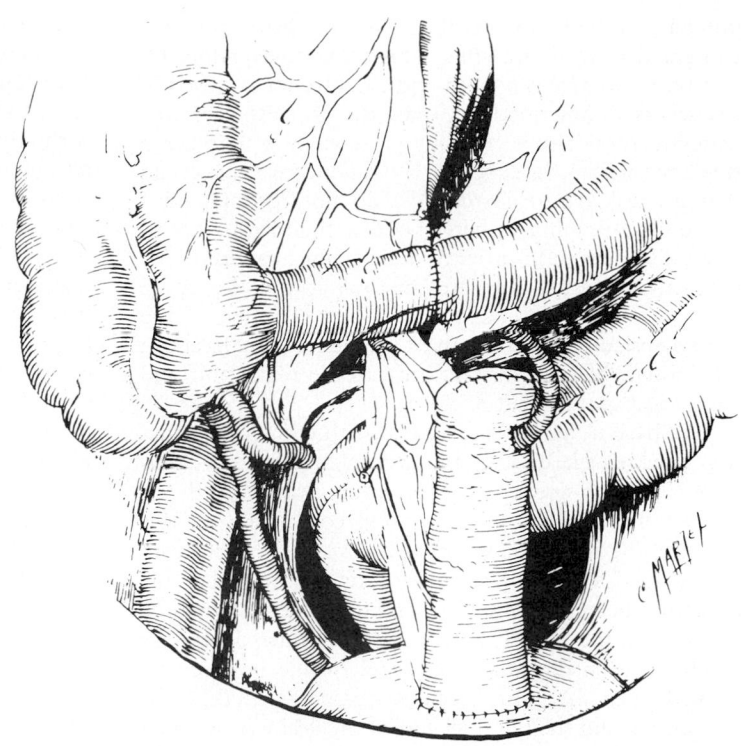

FIGURE 37.5. A segment of terminal ileum is substituted for the lower ureter. (From: Krupp P, Hoffman M, Roeling W. Terminal ileum as ureteral muscle: relationship to intubated ureterostomy. *J Urol* 1955;73:47, with permission.)

LOWER THIRD OF URETER

Following a ureteral transection within 6 cm of the ureterovesical junction or at the time of any resection of the lower third of the ureter, there must be a serious concern that vascularity of the distal remaining ureteral segment has been seriously compromised. Therefore, a ureteroureterostomy could not be performed safely. The standard for repair in these situations has become the ureteral-neocystostomy with psoas hitch over a ureteral stint. As with the performance of the ileal interposition, this is not a technically difficult procedure; it has a very high probability of a successful outcome if a meticulous focus on surgical technique is maintained. The first step in performing the ureteroneocystostomy is to tie off the distal segment of the ureter that is still attached to the bladder. Our preference is to double ligate the distal ureteral segment as close to the tunnel of Wertheim as possible in those instances where the ureteral damage has occurred proximal to the tunnel or, if the injury has occurred to the segment of the ureter that traverses the tunnel, as near the trigone as possible. Because the lumen of the remaining distal ureter is not in contact with the sutures, a permanent material can be used for the ligation. Silk (2-0) is our preference because of its handling characteristics; however, any of the synthetic, nonwoven suture materials is equally acceptable. After the distal ureter has been ligated, the bladder must be freed from its areolar attachment in the retropubic space. We perform this extensively using electrocautery, basically freeing the entire ventral surface of the bladder for almost 270 degrees in all planes. This helps to facilitate mobilization of the bladder toward the proximal ureter and can be done with no functional risk so long as the dorsal lateral blood supply is left intact. Once the bladder has been fully mobilized, we perform a cystotomy on the ventral aspect of the bladder dome. Our preference is that the cystotomy incision not run parallel to the longitudinal axis of the bladder, but deviate off toward the side of the proposed ureteroneocystostomy at a 15- to 30-degree angle. This angulation helps to "elongate" the bladder so that there is maximal length toward the side of implantation to allow for tension free attachment of the ureter. The ureteroneocystostomy is performed using the same technique for anastomosis, as described in the discussion of the ileal interposition procedure. The site where the ureter should be drawn into the bladder usually is self-evident. We attempt to place this attachment on the dorsal aspect of the bladder dome, some distance from the trigone so as to minimize any potential stenosis or injury to the contralateral ureteral orifice. Using direct tactile and visual guidance, with the primary surgeon's finger in the bladder, the ventral-lateral aspect of the bladder is attached to the psoas muscle tendon. We prefer to attach the bladder directly to the tendon using a pulley technique of two separate sutures of 3-0 nylon. The sutures are attached to the bladder wall without entering the bladder lumen. The sutures are tied down against the subtotal purchase of the bladder wall prior to placing the needle through the psoas muscle tendon. We place both sutures into the bladder wall before placing either suture through the psoas tendon. The sutures are placed through the tendon and using the actual tissue purchase in the tendon as the pulley, the bladder is then elongated toward and approximated to the tendon. Of course, the ureter is stinted and the bladder is closed in two layers, as described. We drain the site of the ureteroneocystostomy; however, our preference is to remove this drain within the first 2 to 3 days once we are certain that no leak has occurred. We do not recommend a suprapubic draining catheter because the bladder has to distend somewhat in order to drain against gravity. Many inexperienced surgeons are amazed at the degree of elongation that can be obtained and the size of the ureterovesicular gap that can be bridged if there has been a thorough bladder mobilization in the retropubic and paravesical spaces (Fig. 37.6).

We have never been presented with the clinical situation in which a large segment of distal ureter has been resected and an ureteroileoneocystomy was needed, although theoretically, such a setting could arise. In this instance, the ureteroileoneocystomy would be performed as described for the ureteroenterouréterostomy, the only difference being that the distal end of the ileum would be attached to the ventral aspect of the bladder dome. We would envision that this anastomosis would best be performed much like an ureteroneocystostomy with the bladder opened and the full thickness of the ileal wall attached to the vesicular lumen with a ureteral stint *in vivo*. We have not found a situation in which a Boari bladder flap (a flap of bladder wall fashioned into a tube to replace a missing ureteral segment) has been necessary in light of the availability of the other described surgical techniques.

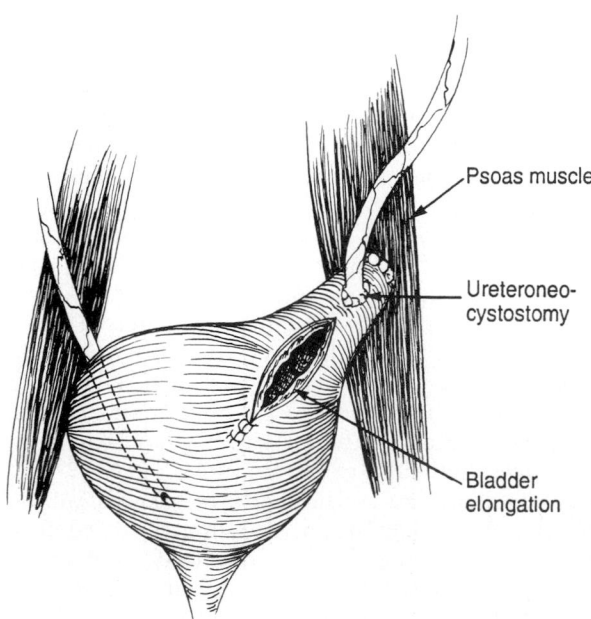

FIGURE 37.6. Bladder elongation performed to allow a tension-free ureteroneocystostomy. The bladder is anchored to the psoas muscle to avoid tension.

UNIQUE ISSUES ASSOCIATED WITH POSTOPERATIVE IDENTIFICATION OR APPRECIATION OF THE URETERAL INJURY

In most instances, the symptoms and findings associated with an intraoperative ureteral injury that were not appreciated at the time of surgery are subtle and may be overlooked easily. Signs and symptoms such as flank pain, temperature elevation, retroperitoneal fluid collection, and delay in return of bowel function (ileus) may or may not stimulate an investigation into the integrity and function of the ureter, depending on the degree of suspicion of the surgeon. From a laboratory perspective, even relatively inconsequential rises in serum creatinine (as little as 0.8 mg/dL) may be related to unilateral ureteral ligation. In contrast, it is unlikely that specific urinary tract symptomatology, such as the frank draining of urine from a drain or vaginal or abdominal incision will be ignored.

If there is any significant degree of suspicion that a ureteral injury has occurred, further evaluation must be undertaken expeditiously. Traditionally, unless there was concern that there was a ureteral fistula, these investigations began with the performance of an intravenous pyelogram (IVP). However, in the modern era, the investigation is more likely to begin with the performance of a computed tomography (CT) scan. The CT scan can give the same information regarding the integrity and function of the renal collecting system while offering the advantage of identifying urinomas and the postoperative anatomy of the surrounding structures. When there is excessive concern that high-grade or total ureteral obstruction is present and that intrinsic renal damage may result from intravenous contrast medium administration, a renal/proximal ureter ultrasound can be performed first. However, renal ultrasound has a false-negative rate of up to 25%; if ureteral dilation is not identified, obstruction cannot be ruled out completely.

A ureteral fistula may be suspected if there is urine leakage from the vagina. However, a bladder or urethral fistula also is possible, depending on the type of surgery. A simple test to differentiate between a ureteral and bladder fistula is the combination Pyridium (Parke-Davis, Morris Plains, NJ)-methylene blue test. The patient is asked to place the largest size tampon that she can comfortably wear into the vagina. She is given oral Pyridium and oral liquids for about 30 min. Orange-stained urine on the tampon indicates the presence of a ureteral or a cephalad bladder fistula. A fresh tampon then is inserted into the vagina, and a total of about 300 mL of methylene blue–stained sterile water is instilled transurethrally via catheter into the bladder. If there is no blue on the second tampon, the injury is ureteral except in the very smallest of vesicular fistulas. A cystoscopy may be performed to evaluate the intravesicular anatomy.

One of the most controversial issues regarding the management of ureteral injuries diagnosed in the postoperative period is how long one should wait before attempting repair. Our opinion is that some form of immediate intervention must be undertaken no matter what type of injury has occurred. If there is an obstruction without intraperitoneal or retroperitoneal leakage of urine, an immediate (same-day) attempt at ureteral stint placement should be undertaken. It is important to appreciate that the higher the grade of obstruction, the less likely that a retrograde stint can be placed successfully. In those instances where a retrograde stint cannot be placed, unless the patient is going to be taken to the operating room for an attempt at surgical correction of the obstruction within a very short time, an antegrade stint or drainage (tube nephrostomy) should be performed. A percutaneous nephrostomy usually can be done under fluoroscopic guidance by the interventional radiologist without too much difficulty. Any delay in relieving the obstruction can translate into further loss of renal parenchyma.

If there is no obstruction of the ureter but there is leakage of urine, whether the leakage is draining extracorporally or not, we similarly recommend that a ureteral stint be placed. Once drainage of urine has been (re)established and a ureteral stint is in place, the next decision is when surgical intervention should be undertaken. The information necessary to answer this question is multifactorial. For those women with high-grade obstructions, an attempt at surgical deligation (which is unlikely to be successful) or performance of the appropriate repair as described in the preceding, should be undertaken as soon as can be scheduled electively, unless the patient is critically ill and at a significant risk for suffering a life-threatening or fatal complication of a major surgical intervention. This is not a life-threatening emergency; the workup to localize the site of obstruction or leakage should be completed, the patient stabilized, the surgeons rested, and any appropriate consultation obtained. However, the best chance of healing with primary repair is when reoperation occurs within the first 48 hours. The longer the delay, the more edema, necrosis, and tissue damage reduce the possibility of successful primary repair.

In those instances where there is no major degree of obstruction and the obstruction is not the result of a "permanent" agent (metal clip or suture) or when only a ureteral leak occurs, a period of watchful waiting may be tried in the hope of avoiding surgical intervention entirely. If there is a ureteral leak, delay is advised only if a ureteral stint can be placed that stops the leakage. If there is persistent leakage despite these measures, there is probably little value in deferring a surgical attempt at repair unless the patient's general medical or psychiatric condition makes surgery unduly high risk.

SPECIFIC PROCEDURES

Laparoscopy-Associated Ureteral Injuries

Ureteral injuries at the time of laparoscopy are very uncommon, occurring in approximately 0.3% to 0.4% of all cases. Laparoscopic ureteral injuries are unique when compared to open injuries from two potentially complicating realities. First, these injuries are more likely to result from a thermal injury than incision, transection, or encroachment/ligation. Second, ureteral injuries in association with laparoscopy are more likely to be diagnosed

within a significant time interval (days or more) after the surgery. These two phenomena appear to decrease the probability of a successful primary repair and increase the risk of a long-term or even fatal complication. Prevention, recognition, and management are no different for laparoscopic-associated injuries than for those associated with any other setting. Although there have been reports of laparoscopic repair of ureteral injuries, experience is limited; the burden of proof that a laparoscopic repair is as good as an open repair rests on the surgeon who attempts it.

Complex Adnexectomy

Ureteral injury at time of complex adnexectomy is worthy of specific comment because: (a) it is in this setting that the ureter is commonly injured during gynecologic surgery; and (b) these injuries often can be avoided by using a retroperitoneal approach.

Every gynecologic or obstetric surgeon must be able to quickly and safely enter the retroperitoneum. This general skill is necessary in order to: (a) access the pelvic vessels for the purpose of establishing hemostasis; and (b) use the retroperitoneum as an adhesion and pathology free "space" in which to operate. Access is obtained most commonly for the latter purpose. Entrance into the retroperitoneum in the pelvis between the round ligament and infundibulopelvic ligament is safe, easy, and extremely useful. First, the round ligament is identified and transected (Fig. 37.7). We prefer to transect the round ligament at approximately its midpoint; thereby avoiding the major pelvic vessels (which lay laterally) as well as any inadvertent injury to the ovarian or uterine vessels (which sit medially). An incision in the lateral leaf of the broad ligament is made after the round ligament has been clamped, transected, and tied. This incision must be carried in a caudal-medial to cephalad-lateral fashion in order to avoid injury to the infundibulopelvic ligament. The incision should be generously carried above the pelvic brim and lateral to the cecum (on the patient's right side) or the sigmoid colon (on the patient's left side). Next, the potential space that exists between the medial leaf of the broad ligament and pelvic side wall is developed. We prefer to do this using the blunt end of DeBakey's forceps or special flattened Haney's retractors (so-called home boys). The separating action must be medial-to lateral/lateral-to-medial, with the instrument angulation toward the coccyx and not toward the sacral hollow. We actively avoid opening this space by finger dissection. We feel that this technique has limited capacity for visualization during the actual space development. Once this retroperitoneal space (which continues deep into the pelvis as the pararectal space) has been developed, the ureter is visible on the medial leaf of the broad ligament. If the surgeon cannot easily identify the ureter on the medial leaf of the broad ligament, its location can be identified by tracing the external iliac arteries cephalad to the common iliac artery. Invariably, the ureter crosses over the common iliac artery and enters into the pelvis where the common iliac artery bifurcates into the external and internal iliac arteries. We are not satisfied with

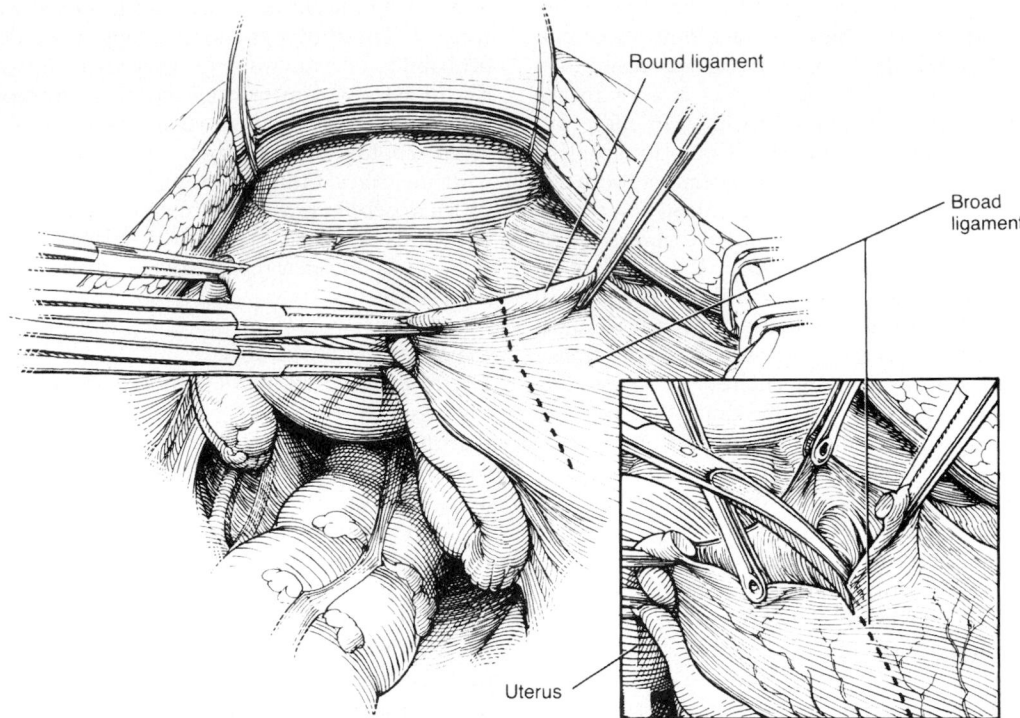

FIGURE 37.7. The initial step for ureteral identification is clamping and cutting of the round ligament. The loose areolar tissue is dissected and the ureter identified on the medial leaf of the broad ligament peritoneum.

simply "plucking" the ureter as some of our mentors did to assure themselves that they had identified this vital structure. We want to see it.

If a pelvic or adnexal mass is adherent to the medial leaf of the broad ligament or pelvic peritoneum overlying the ureter, we prefer to mobilize the ureter with its adventitial sheath under direct vision. Once the ureter has been mobilized, a simple atraumatic vessel loop is passed around it to facilitate positioning. It is always safest to mobilize the ureter off of the medial leaf of the broad ligament and out of harm's way prior to transecting the infundibulopelvic ligament or attempting resection of inflamed, scarred, or fibrotic peritoneum (Fig. 37.8). There are instances in the performance of gynecologic surgery for the management of malignant diseases when it is impossible to mobilize pathology off of the peritoneum or even the underlying ureter, even though the adventitial sheath has been entered. Occasionally, this occurs in benign conditions such as endometriosis. In this setting, the surgeon must decide whether to leave a little tumor or endometriosis on the ureter, risking subsequent obstruction, or resect a segment of ureter and repair accordingly.

Abdominal Hysterectomy for Benign Disease

Ureteral injury during resection of an adnexal mass focuses on surgical trauma to the ureter from the level of the pelvic brim to the tunnel of Wertheim. When discussing ureteral injuries associated with the performance

of an abdominal hysterectomy, the focus of our attention is where the ureter enters the tunnel of Wertheim, lateral to the uterosacral ligaments, until the ureter terminates in the bladder.

The essential, general caveats regarding how to avoid ureteral injury that we outline in this chapter apply to the prevention of these misadventures during the performance of an abdominal hysterectomy for benign disease. There are two additional techniques that can be employed to keep the ureter out of harm's way: (a) the performance of a partial intrafascial hysterectomy; and (b) the dissection of the ureter as if one were completing an MD Anderson type II radical hysterectomy.

Although intrafascial hysterectomy was a commonly performed surgical procedure before blood products and antibiotics became readily available, now it is generally relegated to surgical antiquity and is not part of the technical armamentarium of the modern gynecologic surgeon. In our opinion, there remains a place for this technique in those settings where: (a) it is certain that neither a cervical nor endometrial precancerous or cancerous process exists; or (b) skeletonization of the uterine vessels and mobilization of the ureter off of the medial leaf of the broad ligament leave the ureter in close proximity to the lateral edge of the cervix. Intrafascial hysterectomies can be performed easily using the Elkins' technique illustrated in Figs. 37.9 and 37.10.

In the era of gynecologic and obstetric subspecialization, it is unlikely that gynecologic surgeons who were not formally trained as radical pelvic surgeons will have

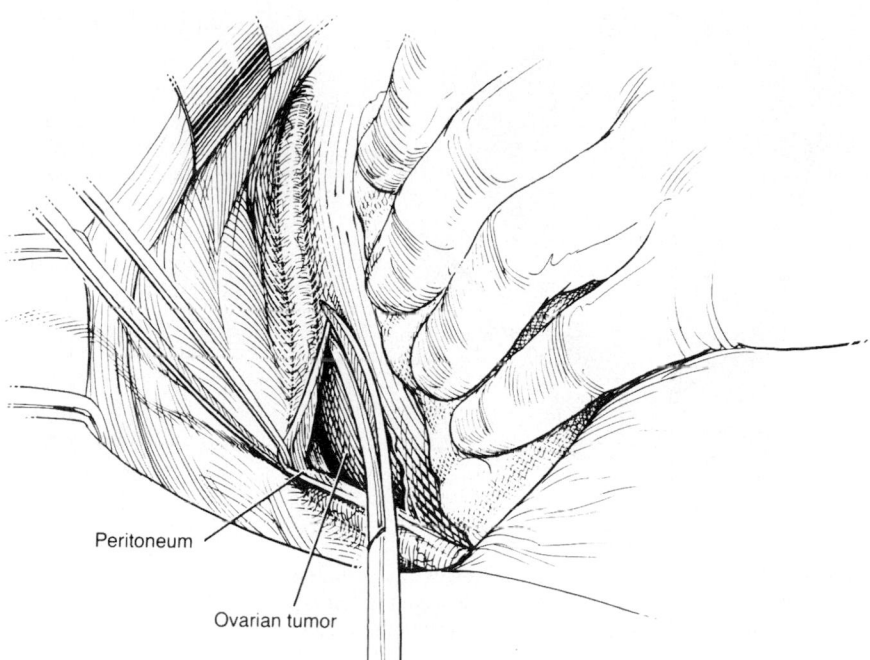

FIGURE 37.8. The ureter is dissected away from the peritoneum to be resected and ovarian mass/remnant.

mastered the performance of uterine artery ligation and ureteral dissection as is done in a type II radical abdominal hysterectomy. This is unfortunate because we have found this simple and safe technique, described elsewhere in this text, to be immensely helpful in the mobilization of the distal ureter when performing a hysterectomy on a woman with a lower uterine segment leiomyoma or severe endometriosis involving the uterosacral ligament.

Caesarean Hysterectomy

We feel this special situation is worthy of comment, even though numerically the procedure is of little significance as a source of operative ureteral injuries because of its relative rarity. Nevertheless, it is a common source of intraoperative consultations to advanced pelvic surgeons. An easy way to avoid ureteral injuries is to simply perform a supracervical hysterectomy; however, some surgeons

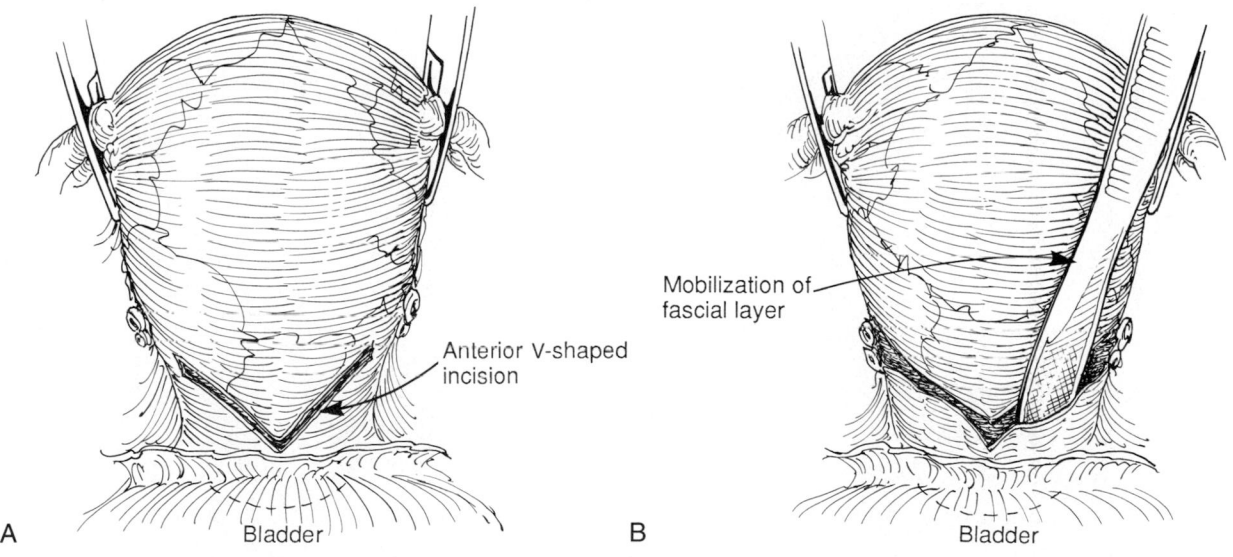

FIGURE 37.9. Partial intrafascial hysterectomy technique. **A:** Anterior V-shaped incision on the cervix of approximately 0.2 cm in depth after sharp and blunt dissection of the bladder flap has been completed and uterine vessel pedicles have been secured. **B:** Mobilization of a fascial layer with blunt end grasping forceps.

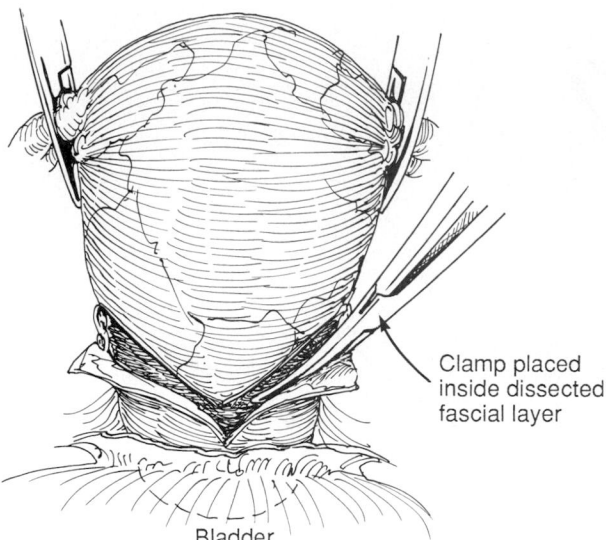

FIGURE 37.10. Partial intrafascial hysterectomy technique. Placement of all future clamps inside the dissected fascial layer provides an additional tissue layer between ureter and cervix.

find this a suboptimal choice. Therefore, in addition to the techniques outlined to this point, there may be value in either extending the hysterotomy incision caudally toward the cervix (Fig. 37.11) or making a similar incision into the cervix if a supracervical hysterectomy has been performed. This allows for the relatively easy placement of the forefinger of the nondominant hand into the endocervical canal and upper vagina, allowing tactile as well as visual guidance in the terminal parts of the procedure.

Vaginal Hysterectomy

Ureteral injury at the time of performance of a vaginal hysterectomy is a remarkably uncommon event, as discussed. However, because vaginal hysterectomies are performed often, a culdoplasty frequently is part of the reconstructive phase of the procedure, and this places the ureter at risk. There are few special maneuvers that can be taken to minimize the probability of injuring a ureter. Ureteral identification via the vaginal approach should be one of the most useful steps. Direct palpatory localization of the ureter, frequently presented as a straightforward endeavor, has proven to be much more problematic for us (Fig. 37.12).

There are ways to decrease the chance of injuring the ureter when performing a vaginal salpingo-oophorectomy. For obvious reasons, we are uncomfortable performing an oophorectomy and leaving the tubes *in vivo*. Our preference is to separate the "triple pedicle" into two parts: (a) containing the remnant of the uteroovarian ligament and fallopian tube; and (b) consisting simply of the round ligament. This allows for a "retrograde" approach to the infundibulopelvic ligament, assuring that the entire tube and ovary are removed as well as facilitating descent of the adnexa from of the pelvic brim and away from the ureter (Fig. 37.13).

Bladder Neck Suspension and Pelvic Organ Prolapse

One would anticipate that, by the very nature of the procedures being performed and the individual(s) performing them, ureteral injury in association with bladder neck suspension and pelvic organ prolapse would be a remarkably uncommon phenomenon. Apparently, there is

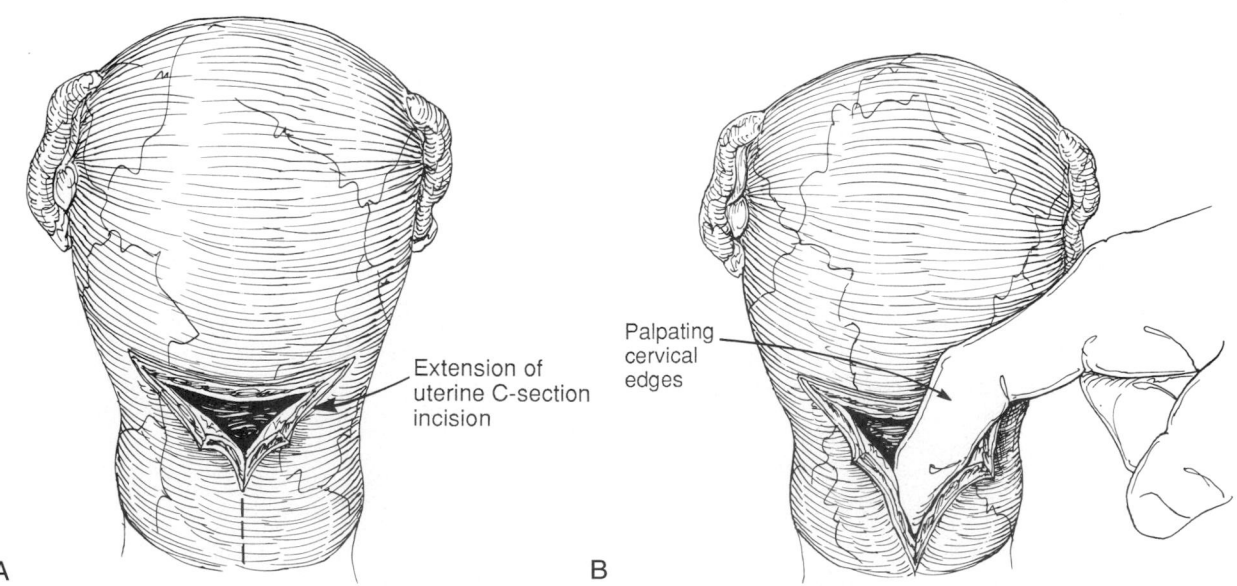

A   B

FIGURE 37.11. Avoiding ureteral injury with removal of the cervix at C-hysterectomy. **A:** Extension of uterine Caesarian section incision downward in the midline of the anterior cervix. **B:** Palpating cervical edges internally.

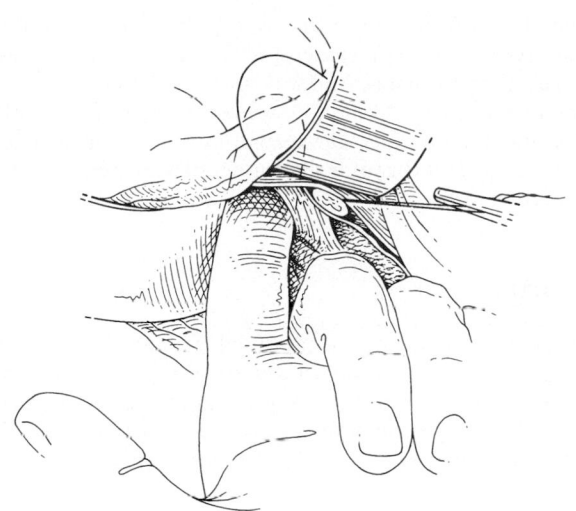

FIGURE 37.12. During vaginal hysterectomy, the ureter can be felt against a metal retractor placed in the paravesical space.

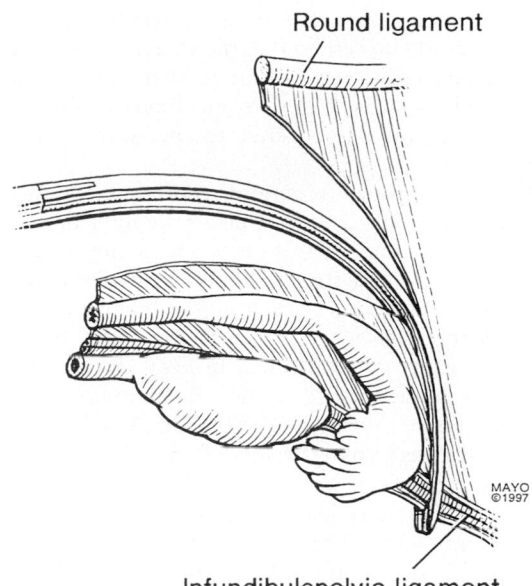

Round ligament

Infundibulopelvic ligament

FIGURE 37.13. The retrograde approach.

no protection granted by type of procedure or surgeon expertise. Although ureteral injury in association with the performance of bladder neck and pelvic organ prolapse surgery is less well studied than similar injuries associated with hysterectomy in the general field of gynecologic surgery, literature reviews report rates of about 0.1% when a Marshall-Marchetti-Krantz procedure is performed, and 0.4% and 1.3% when the Burch retropubic urethrovesical suspension procedure is employed. The data reporting on ureteral injury at time of transvaginal repair, as reviewed by Wiper and Walters, are even more scanty, without any legitimate percentages quoted. It has been proposed and reported that the risk of ureteral injury is less if the bladder neck suspension is performed using a laparoscopic, instead of an open technique; however, there are few retrospective series compared to historical reports to support this claim.

Ureteral injury during retropubic repair most often affects the distal ureter. As Wiper and Walters have stated, this injury can occur during three distinct parts of performance of the procedure: (a) vigorous dissection of the space of Retzius and the periurethral tissues; (b) high elevation of Burch colposuspension sutures; and (c) paravaginal defect repair performed in combination with the Burch procedure. We add an additional way that the ureters could be injured and (probably) occluded: If an excessive lateral mobilization of the bladder is performed, then the actual dorsal surface of the bladder in the vicinity of the trigone is exposed, and the ureter is brought into the operative field. If this has occurred and is not recognized by the operating surgeon, then the ureter could be either ensnared or kinked when the elevating sutures are placed.

Just as there are unique ways to injure the ureter at the time of retropubic urethropexy and paravaginal repair, there are specific steps that can be taken to avoid such injury. Dissection into and through the space of Retzius should be done under direct visualization, remaining as close to the symphysis pubis as possible. The amount of dissection that occurs over the paravaginal tissues should be kept to the minimal amount needed to guarantee accurate and appropriate placement of the sutures and not to mobilize the bladder off of the underlying vagina, thus potentially exposing the ureters. The urethrovesical junction (UVJ) must not routinely be elevated as high as possible. Unquestionably, this causes kinking not only of the urethra but also the ureters in certain patients. Repositioning of the UVJ into the intraabdominal pressure zone and to a zero angle at time of resting tension, performing the so-called Q-Tip (Johnson & Johnson, New Brunswick, NJ) test, is adequate.

Ureteral injury at time of transvaginal bladder neck suspension is a very uncommon sequela. However, ureteral injury at time of surgical correction of pelvic organ prolapse without bladder neck surgery is not uncommon. The method of ureteral injury may result from direct ligation or, more likely, from kinking as the redundant tissues are plicated. There is a significant degree of controversy as to whether or not a cystoscopy should be performed routinely in all patients undergoing retropubic urethropexies. Much of the controversy stems from whether or not the reporting authors have incidentally noted a bladder or ureteral injury simply at the time of a routine cystoscopy. It is our opinion that, in light of the minimal risk and cost of routine cystoscopy in this setting and the potential seriousness of an unrecognized ureteral injury, cystoscopy with concomitant administration of intravenous indigo carmine or methylene blue be performed routinely for documentation of vesicular integrity and ureteral patency.

Radical Pelvic Surgery

In the first edition of this text, Dr. TeLinde, while describing his performance of what is now known as an

MD Anderson type II radical hysterectomy, stated, ". . . one should be certain that the ureter is not included in the suture ligature, a likelihood that is not great although [it] can occur." This quote emphasizes that even a master surgeon was sensitive to the issue of ureteral injury.

Of all the groups of surgical procedures performed by practitioners of the art of pelvic surgery, those performed for the treatment of cancers affecting the female reproductive tract are the most likely to involve either intentional ureteral surgery or have the highest risk of an associated ureteral injury. It is very important to differentiate between an intentional ureteral disruption and one that is unintended or accidental. Intentional cutting of the waters or entry into the bladder may be an integral part of performing many of the most important operative procedures in the radical pelvic surgeon's armamentarium. The MD Anderson type IV radical hysterectomy—a total or anterior pelvic exenteration and resection of a fixed pelvic side wall mass that involves the ureter—should include ureteral surgery and some degree of reconstruction. As a result of the nature of gynecologic malignancies and the procedures performed to treat those diseases, intentional and sometimes unintentional ureteral injuries occur; although fortunately they are infrequent events. Additionally, the need to operate in a field that has been radiated or is acutely infected/inflamed, or in which multiple prior surgical procedures have been performed, compounds the cofactors that put the ureter at risk. It is evident that the radical pelvic surgeon must not only be a scholar of pelvic anatomy, but also a master of surgical handicraft in order to minimize the probability of inducing a ureteral injury.

How common are ureteral injuries in association with radical pelvic surgery? The largest volume of data addresses ureteral injuries at time of traditional Wertheim or MD Anderson type III radical hysterectomies. Angioli and Penalver, in their excellent recent review combining the major modern series, reported that there is an average rate of ureteral injury of just over 1% with a concomitant rate of bladder injury that is the same. Interestingly, as noted, these rates have been consistent over time and among different surgical groups during the last quarter century. There is a growing US and international experience with the performance of radical vaginal trachelectomy as fertility sparing treatment for women with FIGO stage I A 2 to I B 1 cervical cancer. The cumulative English-language data demonstrate that the rate of ureteral injuries in this setting is about the same as with radical abdominal hysterectomy, although rates of bladder injury are higher. In contradistinction to these relatively low rates of ureteral injury when a radical resection is performed in the nonirradiated field, the same procedure performed following therapeutic radiation therapy administered with curative intent as treatment of cervical cancer has an associated risk of a ureteral dysfunction of approximately 30%.

The incidence of ureteral injury at time of performance of simple extrafascial hysterectomy as part of treatment of endometrial cancer is low and similar to that when this procedure is performed for nonmalignant disease (see the preceding section). Ureteral injuries in association with lymph node dissections, sampling, or when performing "radical" oophorectomies are remarkably uncommon when those injuries that occur near the entrance to and through the tunnel of Wertheim are excluded from the data.

PREVENTION

In addition to all of the outlined caveats designed to minimize the probability of a ureteral injury during gynecologic surgery, are a few procedure-specific suggestions that may be helpful in avoiding these potentially lethal and often initially unrecognized events.

Radical Hysterectomy

Of all of the procedures performed by the radical pelvic surgeon, the radical hysterectomy requires the most specific attention to the paraurethral dissection to avoid an injury. Three steps are taken universally to minimize injury to the ureter as it enters and traverses the tunnel of Wertheim. First, we always free the ureter, leaving it inside its adventitial sheath and associated blood supply, from the medial leaf of the broad ligament. This separation is actually done approximately two-thirds of the way from the pelvic brim to the entrance into the tunnel. An atraumatic vessel loop is positioned around the ureter and placed under firm but gentle traction. Second, we develop the space of Morrow (Fig. 37.14). This, like the majority of spaces in the pelvis, is a potential space and a site medial to the ureter, cephalad to the entrance to the tunnel. By opening this space, we develop an easy entrance and route into the tunnel of Wertheim, progressively dissecting/tracking along the ventral-medial aspect of the ureter to avoid transection or inadvertent trigonal injury. Last, we fastidiously ensure that our ureteral dissection always stays outside of the ureteral sheath, whether it is in the tunnel of Wertheim or on the medial leaf of the broad ligament.

Although remaining outside of the ureteral sheath is relatively easy to assure while on the broad ligament, as the dissection is carried into the tunnel, it is easy to enter the sheath and thus devascularize a segment of the ureter. Such devascularization can be disastrous, particularly when radiation therapy has been administered. If the sheath is entered, it is important to recognize this fact, back out, and restart the dissection.

Radical Vaginal Trachelectomy

In our opinion, the real clue to performing a radical vaginal trachelectomy (RVT) without injuring the ureter is to be able to open the paravesical and pararectal spaces from their most inferior aspects. Numerous authors have described this technique; the explanation by Plante and Roy is the most useful for surgeons-in-training. Because there are few, if any, data that support the prophylactic

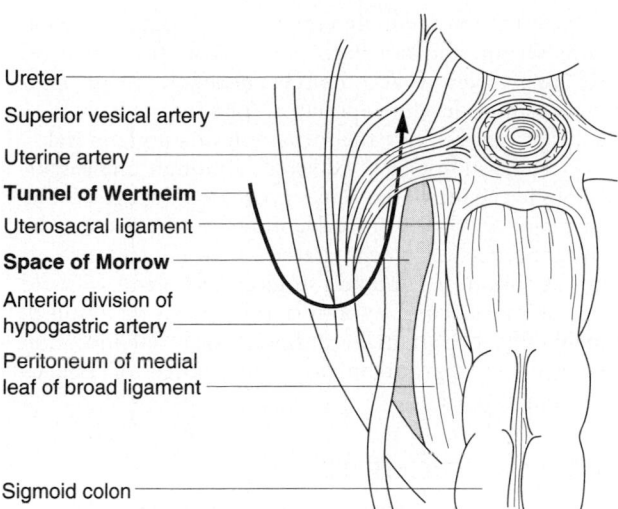

Ureter
Superior vesical artery
Uterine artery
Tunnel of Wertheim
Uterosacral ligament
Space of Morrow
Anterior division of
hypogastric artery
Peritoneum of medial
leaf of broad ligament
Sigmoid colon

FIGURE 37.14. The space of Morrow and the tunnel of Wertheim. (From: Greenfield. *Surgery,* 3rd ed. Philadelphia: Lippincott Williams & Wilkins, 2001:2189, with permission.)

placement of ureteral stints in an attempt to minimize ureteral injury, the performance of an RVT is the one procedure in which we would consider ureteral catheterization useful. Because the anatomy of the tunnel of Wertheim and the relationship of the ureter to the uterine arteries is literally upside down when performing an RVT, we have found that placement of ureteral stints is very helpful in localizing and following the course of the ureters.

Radical Oophorectomy

The successful performance of a difficult radical oophorectomy represents the mastering of most of the surgical procedures in which the radical pelvic surgeon should have become proficient. Therefore, all of the described steps are valuable to ensure that the ureter is not injured. The only additional specific point that we would like to make is that our preference, when performing a radical oophorectomy, is to immediately develop the paravesical spaces bilaterally at the very beginning of the dissection. This not only allows for the identification of the pelvic vessels and the mobilization of the involved pelvic peritoneum, but also makes it such that the ureter can be fully mobilized off of the pelvic peritoneum. This is actually the first maneuver that we perform once we have fully developed these spaces. We free the ureter from above the pelvic brim all the way to the tunnel of Wertheim, placing a vessel loop around the ureter near the midpoint of its descent through the pelvis. By having freed the ureter from the medial leaf of the broad ligament, that leaf can be employed as a "sheet" and pulled medially, literally peeling the extant tumor nodules off of the pelvic side walls and viscera until such point where the parietal peritoneum blends into the visceral peritoneum.

Lymph Node Dissection

Even experienced radical surgeons can injure a ureter at the time of an apparently easy and uncomplicated

paraaortic node dissection. What is the problem? Simply put, "get lost" and forget the essential rules of anatomy. When approaching the paraaortic nodes, the dissection often is carried in a caudal-cephalad fashion with imperfect visualization. Literally standing on one's head, it is not difficult to become disoriented and confuse the ureter for the ovarian vessels prior to their entrance into the infundibular pelvic ligaments. This problem serves to re-emphasize those three key words in avoidance of ureteral injuries by which even the most skilled and mature surgeons must live: anatomy, anatomy, anatomy.

MANAGEMENT

A few additional steps and techniques should be considered. First, if a ureteral leak has been identified postoperatively and the leak has developed in the setting of prior pelvic radiation, then an aggressive attempt at complete diversion via combined ureteral stint and tube nephrostomy should be undertaken. A period of many months should be allowed to pass before re-evaluating the patient radiographically to determine whether or not the leak has spontaneously healed. Although it is less likely that spontaneous closure will take place if the injury occurs in a radiated field because of the complex and risky nature of surgical correction in the radiated pelvis, it is in the patient's best interest to allow the maximal attempt for spontaneous healing prior to attempting a surgical repair. Second, if possible, the site of ureteral repair should incorporate, if not a new, at least an intact blood supply. Our threshold for performing an ureteroneocystostomy is very low when there is any concern regarding the integrity and functionality of the adventitial vascular arcade. It we elect to perform an ureteroureterostomy, we mobilize whatever residual omentum is available to wrap the site of repair, which has been stinted with an omental J flap. Although we employ drains at the site of ureteral injury, we only leave them *in vivo* for a few days and remove them after assuring that the creatinine of the drain effluent is the same as the patient's serum, and not her urine. Leaving the drains in over longer periods accomplishes nothing, in our opinion, except to develop a potential for a negative pressure tract that can facilitate the formation of a ureteral leak.

Ureteral injuries are expected, although unpleasant, realities in the life of the active gynecologic surgeon. The vast majority of these misadventures can be avoided by constant reflection on the ureteral anatomy and meticulous attention to optimal surgical technique. Should ureteral injury occur, an optimal outcome is the result of timely and preferentially intraoperative identification followed by appropriate site and source of injury–determined repair.

ACKNOWLEDGMENT

The authors are indebted to the contributors to a monograph edited by FJM on the same subject on which much of this material is based: Gershenson D, ed. Operative techniques in gynecologic surgery. In: Montz FJ, ed. Management of ureteral injuries. Philadelphia: WB Saunders, 1998:73, with permission.

BIBLIOGRAPHY

Angioli R, Penalver M. Ureteral injury at time of radical pelvic surgery. *Operat Tech Gynecol Surg* 1998;43:132.

Barber MD, Visco AG, Weider AC, et al. Bilateral uterosacral ligament vaginal vault suspension with site-specific endopelvic fascia defect repair for treatment of pelvic organ prolapse. *Am J Obstet Gynecol* 2000;183:1402.

Bristow RE, Smith-Sehdev AE, Kaufman HS, et al. Ablation of metastatic ovarian carcinoma with the argon beam coagulator: pathologic analysis of tumor destruction. *Gynecol Oncol* 2001;83:49.

Cornella JL, Lee RA. Management of ureteral injury at complex adnexectomy. *Operat Tech Gynecol Surg* 1998;3:97.

Cornella JL, Walter A. Prevention and early recognition of ureteral injuries at vaginal hysterectomy. *Operat Technol Gynecol Surg* 1998;3:115.

Covens A, Shaw P, Murphy J, et al. Is radical trachelectomy a safe alternative to radical hysterectomy for patients with stage I A-B carcinoma of the cervix? *Cancer* 1999;86:2273.

Daly JW, Higgins KA. Injury to the ureter during gynecologic surgical procedures. *Surg Gynecol Obstet* 1988;167:19.

Dargent D, Martin X, Sacchetoni A, et al. Laparoscopic vaginal radical trachelectomy. *Cancer* 2000;88:1877.

Drake MJ, Noble JG. Ureteric trauma in gynecologic surgery. *Int Urogynecol J Pelvic Floor Dysfunct* 1998;9:108.

Ehrlich RM, Skinner DG. Complications of transureteroureterostomy. *J Urol* 1975;113:467.

Elkins TE. Ureteral injury at time of abdominal hysterectomy for benign disease. *Operat Tech Gynecol Surg* 1998;3:108.

Eriksen BC, Hagen B, Kik-Nes SH, et al. Long term effectiveness of the Burch colposuspension in female urinary stress incontinence. *Acta Obstet Gynecol Scand* 1990;69:45.

Goldstein SL, Harold KL, Lentzner A, et al. Comparison of thermal spread after ureteral ligation with the Laparo-Sonic ultrasonic sheers and the Ligature system. *J Laparoendosc Adv Surg Tech A* 2002;12:61.

Gomel V, James C. Intraoperative management of ureteral injury during operative laparoscopy. *Fertil Steril* 1997; 55:416.

Goodno JA Jr, Powers TW, Harris VD. Ureteral injury in gynecologic surgery: a ten-year review in a community hospital. *Am J Obstet Gynecol* 1995;172:1817.

Haney NS. Technique of vaginal hysterectomy. *Surg Clin North Amer* 1942;22:73.

Harkk-Siren P, Kurki T. A nationwide analysis of laparoscopic complications. *Obstet Gynecol* 1997;89:108.

Harris RL, Cundiff GW, Theofrastous JP, et al. The value of intraoperative cystoscopy in urogynecologic and reconstructive surgery. *Am J Obstet Gynecol* 1997;177:1367.

Karram M, Goldwasser S, Kleeman S, et al. High ureteral sacral vaginal vault suspension with fascial reconstruction for vaginal repair of enterocele and vaginal vault prolapse. *Am J Obstet Gynecol* 2001;185:1339.

Klutke JJ, Klutke CG, Hsieh G. Bladder injury during the Burch retropubic urethropexy: is routine cystoscopy necessary? *Tech Urol* 1998;4:145.

Koelliker SL, Cronann JJ. Acute urinary tract obstruction. Imaging update. *Urol Clin North Am* 1997;24:571.

Kuno K, Menzin A, Kauder HH, et al. Prophylactic ureteral catheterization in gynecologic surgery. *Urology* 1998;52: 1004.

Liapis A, Bakas P, Giannopoulos V, et al. Ureteral injuries during gynecologic surgery. *Int Urogynecol J Pelvic Floor Dysfunct* 2001;12:391.

Mainprize TC, Drutz HP. The Marshall-Marchetti-Krantz procedure: critical review. *Obstet Gynecol Surv* 1988;43:724.

Mann WJ, Arato M, Patsner B, et al. Ureteral injuries in an obstetrics and gynecology training program: etiology and management. *Obstet Gynecol* 1988;72:82.

Mariotti G, Natale F, Trucchi A, et al. Ureteral injuries during gynecologic procedures. *Minerva Urol Nefrol* 1997;49:95.

Mattingly RF, Borkow HL. Acute operative injury to the lower urinary tract. *Clin Obstet Gynecol* 1978;5:123.

Meirow D, Moriel EZ, Zilberman M, et al. Evaluation and treatment of iatrogenic ureteral injuries during obstetrics and gynecologic operations for non-malignant conditions. *J Am Coll Surg* 1994;178:144.

Miklos JR, Kohli N. Laparoscopic paravaginal repair plus Burch colposuspension: review and descriptive technique. *Urology* 2000;56:64.

Monk BJ, Solkh S, Johnson MT, et al. Radical hysterectomy after pelvic irradiation in patients with high risk cervical cancer or uterine sarcoma: morbidity and outcome. *Eur J Gynaecol Oncol* 1993;14:506.

Munro M. Ureteral injury associated with gynecologic laparoscopy. *Operat Tech Gynecol Surg* 1998;3:84.

Neuman M, Eidelman A, Langer R, et al. Iatrogenic injuries to the ureter during gynecologic and obstetric operations. *Surg Gynecol Obstet* 1991;173:268.

Nezhat C, Nezhat F. Laparoscopic repair of ureter resected during operative laparoscopy. *Obstet Gynecol* 1992;80:543.

Oh BR, Kwon DD, Park KS, et al. Late presentation of ureteral injury after laparoscopic surgery. *Obstet Gynecol* 2000;95: 337.

Oh BR, Kwon DD, Park KS, et al. Late presentation of ureteral injury after laparoscopic surgery. *Obstet Gynecol* 2000;95: 337.

Piver M, Rutledge F, Smith J. Five classes of extended hysterectomy for women with cervical cancer. *Obstet Gynecol* 1974;44:265.

Plante M, Roy M. Radical trachelectomy. *Operat Tech Gynecol Surg* 1997;2:187.

Rosen DM, Korda AR, Waugh RC. Ureteric injury at Burch colposuspension: four case reports and literature review. *Aust NZ J Obstet Gynecol* 1996;36:354.

Saidi MH, Sadler RK, Vanvaillie TG, et al. Diagnosis and management of serious urinary complications after major operative laparoscopy. *Obstet Gynecol* 1996;87: 272.

Sandoz IL, Paul DP, MacFarlane CA. Complications of transureteroureterostomy. *J Urol* 1977;117:39.

Selzman AA, Spirnak JP. Iatrogenic ureteral injuries: a 20-year experience in treating 165 injuries. *J Urol* 1996; 155:878.

Speights SE, Moore RD, Miklos JR. Frequency of lower urinary tract injury at laparoscopic Burch and paravaginal repair. *J Am Assoc Gynecol Laparosc* 2000;7:515.

TeLinde RW. Cancer of the cervix uteri. *Operative gynecology.* Philadelphia: JB Lippincott, 1946:386.

Thompson JD. Operative injuries to the ureter: prevention, recognition, and management. In: Rock JA, Thompson JD, eds. *TeLinde's operative gynecology.* Philadelphia: JB Lippincott, 1997:1135 1173.

Webb JA. Ultrasonography and doppler studies in the diagnosis of renal obstruction. *BJU Int* 2000;86(Suppl 1):25.

Wiper DW, Walters MD. Ureteral injury at time of bladder neck suspension. *Operat Tech Gynecol Surg* 1998;3:126.

Woodland MB. Ureter injury during laparoscopy-assisted vaginal hysterectomy with the endoscopic linear stapler. *Am J Obstet Gynecol* 1992;167:756.

Yossepowitch O, Lifshitz DA, Dekel Y, et al. Predicting the success of retrograde stenting for managing ureteral obstruction. *J Urol* 2001;166:1746.

Te Linde's Operative Gynecology, ninth edition, edited by John A. Rock and Howard W. Jones, III. Lippincott Williams & Wilkins, Philadelphia © 2003.

CHAPTER
38

▼

Vesicovaginal
and Urethrovaginal Fistulas

G. RODNEY MEEKS   TED M. ROTH

Although it is difficult to accurately gauge the frequency with which genitourinary fistulae occur, the majority result from gynecologic surgery, specifically total abdominal hysterectomy. Prolonged obstructed labor remains a common cause of destruction of the urethra and base of the bladder in medically underprivileged countries, whereas elective vaginal and urogynecologic surgeries are the leading etiologies accounting for such fistulae in the United States. When a fistula becomes symptomatic depends on its cause, location, and size. Differences of opinion have developed regarding timing and route of repair; however, the final success of any fistula repair ultimately depends on a surgeon's experience, judgment, and appropriateness of technique.

HISTORICAL SURVEY

It is likely that vesicovaginal fistulae (VVF) have occurred since the beginning of recorded time. Professor Derry of the faculty of medicine of Fouad I University in Egypt, discovered a large vesicovaginal fistula in the mummy of Henhenit, a lady in the court of Mentuhotep of the Eleventh Dynasty who reigned about 2050 B.C. He found the pelvis was considerably contracted in the transverse diameter, and there was a through-and-through tear of the perineum. The Kahun papyrus,

which refers back to 2000 B.C. and generally is thought to contain the earliest gynecologic references, and the Eber's papyrus, from about 1500 B.C., make no mention of VVF. The Talmud, likewise, fails to give any evidence that ancient Hebrew physicians were cognizant of this malady. The first record of a VVF is found in the writings of ancient Hindu medicine, the Vedas and Upavedas. Avicenna, a Persian physician, was the first known writer to mention the occurrence of a VVF. He also recognized the association between such a lesion and labor. The delayed recognition of VVF as a clinical entity may be related to the prolonged influence of Arab physicians from 600 to 1600 A.D., who regarded postmortem examinations sinful, and, as men, were forbidden by their religion to practice obstetrics and gynecology.

In 1663, Hendrik Von Roonhuysen published his *Medico-Chirurgical Observations about the Infirmities of Women.* His innovations for the management of VVF included proper exposure with a speculum, marginal denudation of the fistula, and approximation of the denuded edges with "stitching needles made of stiff swan's quills." No figures or postoperative results were presented. Posthumously published in 1752, Johann Fatio described the first reported cures using Von Roonhuysen's technique.

A new era in the surgical treatment of VVF occurred in the 19th century. In 1834, de Lamballe was the first to emphasize tension-free closures. He also noted that newly acquired fistulae without evidence of induration at the edges might be cured by prolonged catheterization alone. De Lamballe also made attempts to cure VVF with pedicle flaps from labia, buttocks, and thigh. Simon of Darmstadt, a colleague of de Lamballe, suggested transverse colpocleisis in those cases that defied previous attempts at closure. Although this procedure was fraught with complications, partial colpocleisis was later espoused by Latzko to cure posthysterectomy fistulae.

In 1852, Marion Sims published his classic work, which formally established the technique of VVF repair. His contribution to this endeavor is recognized by the recent republication of his original paper. Although many of his innovations were not new, he attained greater success than anyone else, and his personality helped in bringing public attention to the treatment of women's diseases. Although Sims' only innovation was the use of silver wire suture, he standardized and defined the surgical principles of vesicovaginal repair that are used today.

As laparotomy became safer, many surgeons developed abdominal techniques for vesicovaginal fistula repair. Trendelenburg, in 1881 to 1890, described opening the bladder suprapubically, freeing the bladder wall, and closing the defect. Maisonneuve and Mackenrodt independently described separating the bladder from the vaginal mucosa, and suturing each as an individual layer. These principles are foundations for modern closure techniques.

In 1896, Kelly described a vaginal method of closing a large bladder defect. The bladder is freed away from the cervix to the level of the visceral peritoneum and closed. He also advocated the use of preoperative ureteral catheterization to minimize risk of ureteral injury, a technique first championed by Pawlik in 1882. By 1906, when Kelly described a suprapubic route for repair of vesicovaginal fistulae, at least 12 different surgical approaches had been detailed.

In 1942, Latzko described in detail the principles of his operation, based on the work by Simon, which is considered by some to be the gold standard for the surgical management of posthysterectomy VVF. He reported that 29 of 31 cases of vesicovaginal fistula treated by his method of partial colpocleisis were cured. The outcomes are impressive considering the majority of these patients had antecedent radical abdominal hysterectomy for cervix cancer.

ETIOLOGY/EPIDEMIOLOGY

The etiology of urogenital fistulae may be categorized as congenital or acquired, the latter being associated with childbirth, gynecologic surgery, malignancy, and radiation therapy. VVF in childhood usually occurs following penetrating trauma, foreign bodies, and genitourinary surgery. Congenital VVFs are extremely rare, and there are only nine cases described in the English and Japanese literature. Seven of nine were associated with other genitourinary malformations. This chapter focuses on acquired causes of VVF.

Much of the literature consists of retrospective case series and reflects the experience of a particular surgeon or fistula center. During a 15-year period of review, 303 women with genitourinary fistulae were seen at the Mayo Clinic (of whom 280 underwent surgical repair). Of the 190 patients with *vesicovaginal fistulae*, gynecologic surgery was responsible for 145 (82%) of the fistulae, 19 (11%) were from obstetric procedures, 13 (7%), followed treatment for malignant disease, and five (3%) were from trauma. Similarly, Goodwin found 74% of his cases to be of gynecologic origin, 14% of urologic origin, and 12% from radiation injury.

Culture and geography is reflected in the frequencies and etiologies of VVFs. In England, Kelly found that 95% of the vesicovaginal fistulae occurred with nonobstetric causes. In contradistinction, obstructed labor caused 98% of the vesicovaginal fistulae in Nigeria. The largest series of VVF details 1,443 cases in northern Nigeria between 1969 and 1980. Eighty-three percent resulted from prolonged obstructed labor and 13% resulted from "gishiri" cuts, a traditional tribal practice of cutting the anterior vagina with a razor blade to treat a variety of conditions, including obstructed labor, infertility, dyspareunia, backache, and goiter. Only 1% of fistulae in this study were associated with antecedent surgery.

In developing countries, obstetric trauma remains the leading cause of vesicovaginal fistulae. Most often the inciting event that leads to the formation of a VVF is prolonged and obstructed labor, which results in pressure necrosis. Introital stenosis secondary to female circumcision, cephalopelvic disproportion (from inadequate pelvic dimensions of early childbearing), an android pelvis, malnutrition, orthopedic disorders including rickets, and hydrocephalus contribute to dystocia. Fistulae may be caused by the misuse of forceps, destructive instruments used to deliver stillborn infants, or surgical abortion. Symphysiotomy and the postpartum use of intravaginal caustic agents also have a role.

The need to continue to implement health education programs in underdeveloped countries has been emphasized. So serious is the problem that a National Task Force on VVF was formed in Nigeria in 1990. The purpose of the task force is to prevent VVF through public awareness campaigns, education, and advocacy for women's medical and surgical services. In this population, there can be grave social consequences of VVF including divorce, poverty, and depression.

Premature childbearing as a result of early adolescent marriage continues to be epidemic in Africa. In sub-Saharan Africa, nearly 50% of the women are married by age 18, some by age 15 or younger. A recent case-control study from Onolemhemhen and Ekwempu in Katsina, Nigeria found that primiparous girls who married during early adolescence were more likely to experience vesicovaginal fistula than those who married at an older age. Uneducated women and those married to men who were unskilled laborers were 14 times more likely to sustain a vesicovaginal fistula than their cohorts. In contrast, Hilton and Ward in a review of 2,979 fistula repairs in 2,484 patients from southern Nigeria found that fistula patients were older and of higher parity; they appeared to have a higher literacy rate, and were more likely to remain in a married relationship despite being symptomatic with a VVF. Ibrahim and colleagues described 31 women treated over a 12-month period in a university teaching hospital in Sokoto, Nigeria. In contrast to previous reports, all cases were directly caused by obstructed labor, and none of the patients had undergone traditional surgical practices of gishiri or ritual circumcision. Because of variations in the populations studied, patient selection, and techniques employed, the rates of successful repair of VVF are difficult to compare.

In countries with more modern obstetric care, the most common cause of vesicovaginal fistula remains iatrogenic injury at the time of gynecologic or urological surgery. Predisposing risk factors for VVF include a history of pelvic irradiation, Caesarean section, endometriosis, prior pelvic surgery or pelvic inflammatory disease, diabetes mellitus, concurrent infection, vasculopathies, and tobacco abuse. Patients undergoing total abdominal hysterectomy are a particular risk. Although the incidence of VVF after hysterectomy is approximately one in 1,300 surgeries, there are only a few "large" series on which to base reliable estimates of risk. In a series of 17 cases of posthysterectomy fistulae reported over a 15-year period from Dublin, the risk of VVF was one in 605 for total abdominal hysterectomy, one in 571 for vaginal hysterectomy, and one in 81 for radical hysterectomy.

Using data from the National Patient Insurance Association in Finland, Harkki-Siren and associates reviewed the incidence of urinary tract injury on a national scale. During the study period, 62,379 hysterectomies were performed and 142 urinary tract injuries recorded. The incidence of bladder injury was 1.3 per 1,000 hysterectomies. The incidence of VVF was one in 1,200 procedures, one in 455 after laparoscopic hysterectomy, one in 958 after total abdominal hysterectomy, and one in 5,636 after vaginal hysterectomy. Risk of ureteral injury was greater with laparoscopic procedures than with open procedures. A recent series of 100 total laparoscopic hysterectomies included two VVF among the reported complications.

The underlying mechanism of posthysterectomy fistula formation is probably multifactorial. No single etiology seems to explain all fistulae, and multiple causes are likely. In some cases, a fistula may arise from avascular necrosis secondary to crush injury. Other times, there is an unrecognized cystotomy or partial tear of the bladder muscularis. Meeks and associates, in a rabbit model, demonstrated that suture material intentionally placed through the vaginal cuff and the bladder was not associated with the development of fistulae. Similar findings have been described in a canine model.

Bladder injury and urogenital fistulae are known complications of antiincontinence surgery. Urogenital fistulae also have been reported after such procedures. Synthetic sling materials are prone to infection and erosion. Kobashi reviewed cases in which sling removal was required after the use of a woven polyester sling treated with pressure-injected bovine collagen (ProteGen; Boston Scientific, Natick, MA). Thirty-four women, in a 2-year period, required sling removal and six had urethrovaginal fistulae. Although periurethral injectable materials are thought of as being relatively innocuous, two reports have linked the placement of periurethral collagen to the development of bladder neck fistulae in women with normal anatomy and following ileal bladder substitution.

Radiation-induced fistulae occasionally are associated with treatment for carcinoma of the cervix or other pelvic malignancies. However, fistulae are much less common today with modern close planning techniques. VVF formation does not always correlate with the absolute dose and distribution of radiation, or with the patient's weight or age; this suggests that some women are more sensitive to radiation therapy than others. Healthy tissues of the anterior vaginal wall tolerate radiation doses as high as 8,000 rads. Fistulae may appear during the course of radiotherapy (usually from necrosis of the tumor itself) or after treatment is completed. Late fistulae arise secondary to endarteritis obliterans within the first 2 years. In planning a repair, it is essential to rule out recurrent malignancy with biopsies of the fistula margins. Because of decreased vascularity of the adjacent tissue, healing is impaired and must be considered when planning repair of a radiation-induced fistula.

There are "fascinoma" case reports of vesicovaginal fistulae caused by vaginal foreign bodies, direct trauma from masturbation or automobile accidents, tuberculosis, schistosomiasis, bladder calculi, endometriosis, syphilis, lymphogranuloma venereum, and from idiopathic congenital causes.

Urethrovaginal fistulae are uncommon and usually occur after surgery for urethral diverticulum, anterior vaginal wall prolapse or urinary incontinence, and after radiation therapy. In these cases, the most common causes include tissue ischemia, problems related to healing, or radiation necrosis. Operative vaginal delivery also is a risk factor for the development of a urethrovaginal fistula. Pressure necrosis, resulting in a urethrovaginal fistula, can occur with a prolonged indwelling transurethral catheter. Urethrovaginal fistulae also may be congenital.

Vesicouterine and *vesicocervical fistulae* are rare. They are usually complications of gynecologic or obstetric surgery, occurring most frequently after Caesarean section. The clinical presentation may be similar to VVF, with urine egressing through the vagina. The examination fails to reveal a vaginal fistula, however, and rarely urine trickles down through the os. Cyclic hematuria (menouria) is common. An abdominal approach with interposition graft is favored for repair, using the techniques for VVF.

PREVENTION

Because the association of bladder injury at the time of hysterectomy and fistula formation seems intuitive, many of the techniques advocated to reduce the incidence of fistulae are directed toward protecting the bladder. The base of the bladder rests on the anterior lower uterine isthmus and the cervix, whereas the trigone is distal to the internal os. The bladder is subjected to trauma during dissection from the cervix and upper vagina. A fistula following injury in this area will be found in the posterior wall of the bladder superior to the interureteric ridge in almost all cases. Because the trigone overlies the upper one third of the anterior vagina, it is unlikely to be injured because dissection at this level is rarely needed during hysterectomy. Bladder injury associated with this procedure is rare because bladder dissection is minimal with supracervical hysterectomy. Harkki-Siren and colleagues reported 0 VVF after 1,000 supracervical hysterectomies in their review.

Tancer, in a retrospective study of 151 urogenital fistulae, found that 91% of the fistulae occurred after gynecologic procedures. Total hysterectomy was the most common antecedent procedure ($n = 110$), resulting in a vault fistula. Seventy percent occurred in the absence of factors that typically place the patient at risk. Tancer presented his suggestions and observations on avoiding injury to the bladder during total abdominal hysterectomy. These include the use of a two-way indwelling catheter, sharp dissection to isolate the bladder, an extraperitoneal cystotomy when the dissection is difficult, retrograde filling of the bladder when injury is suspected, and repair of an overt bladder injury only after mobilization of the injured area. Retrograde filling of the bladder also may help define the border of a bladder otherwise distorted or displaced by prior surgery or a lower uterine segment fibroid.

An intrafascial technique for removing the cervix at hysterectomy also may protect the bladder. The vesicocervical space must be completely developed, and the bladder must be thoroughly mobilized inferiorly and laterally. Before the cardinal ligament pedicles are developed and before the anterior vagina is incised, an inverted "T" or "V" incision is made in the pubocervical fascia. The fascia is separated from the cervix and upper anterior vagina. The exposed vaginal epithelium can be entered directly. In theory, the bladder has been mobilized from the site of entry into the vagina and is less likely to be compromised because it rests on the dissected fascia. Constant traction of the uterus cephalad and traction on the bladder caudad and inferiorly allows placement of clamps and sutures without injuring the bladder. In a recent review of 867 women who underwent intrafascial abdominal hysterectomy, there was a bladder injury incidence of 0.4%.

CYSTOTOMY AND REPAIR

The principles and technique of repairing a cystotomy are the same regardless of the inciting event. The margins of the wound should be delineated carefully to assess the extent of injury and prevent injury to the ureters. The closure is started slightly beyond the poles of the defect. The closure may be accomplished with interrupted or continuous sutures. The authors prefer to leave the sutures long at the poles to help with orientation and subsequent suture placement. Suture choice is physician dependent; usually natural or synthetic absorbable suture of 2-0 or 3-0 caliber. A point of contention is whether the bladder mucosa should be penetrated with the suture or if the sutures should be placed so as to entropion the edges of the wound. Benefits of the former include ease of suture placement and possibly improved hemostasis of the wound edges. The possibility of stone formation secondary to foreign body reaction is a drawback to "through-and-through" suture placement. Subsequent rows of continuous or interrupted sutures are placed in the musculo-fascial tissues to imbricate initial layers. If cystotomy occurs at the time of laparotomy in addition to the repair, a flap of peritoneum or omentum may be mobilized for further buttressing (Fig. 38.1). A watertight closure is assured by instilling 200 cc of sterile baby's formula or dilute methylene blue. Ureteral integrity and hemostasis of the repair may be assessed via cystoscopy. If the injury occurs extraperitoneally, the bladder may be drained for as little as 2 days. For repairs of injuries at the time of vaginal hysterectomy or intraperitoneal injuries, the bladder is drained for 7 to 10 days. Decisions regarding postoperative drainage of cystotomies depend on the extent of the injury, factors that may delay healing, and the security of the closure. Prior to removing the catheter, some advocate obtaining a cystogram to evaluate the integrity of the bladder.

Clinical Presentation of Fistulae

The most common presenting feature of vesicovaginal fistulae is continuous leakage of urine from the vagina. When vesicovaginal fistula follows gynecologic surgery, urinary leakage is most commonly recognized in the first 10 days after operation and less commonly, between the 10th and 20th postoperative days. Rarely does incontinence appear later. In the case of posthysterectomy VVF, onset of symptoms and early diagnosis may be delayed by postoperative vaginal cuff edema. In rare cases, it may be difficult to distinguish urine loss secondary to a VVF and other forms of urinary incontinence.

The size and location of the fistula determines the degree of leakage. Patients with small fistulae may void normal amounts of urine and notice only slight position-dependent drainage. Alternatively, they may experience leakage only at maximal bladder capacity. The patient may present with recurrent cystitis or pyelonephritis, unexplained fever, hematuria, flank, vaginal, or suprapubic pain, and abnormal urinary stream. Women with larger fistulae may not be able to collect enough urine intravesically in order to void normally. Irritation of the vagina, vulvar mucosa, and perineum follows and women complain of a foul ammoniacal odor. As urea is split by vaginal flora, the vaginal pH becomes alkaline, which precipitates greenish-gray phosphate crystals in the vagina and on the vulva. These crystals serve to further irritate what already may be compromised tissue. Large vaginal encrustations are seen with fistulae secondary to neglected vaginal foreign bodies. This constant leakage of urine may make the patient a social recluse; disrupt sexual re-

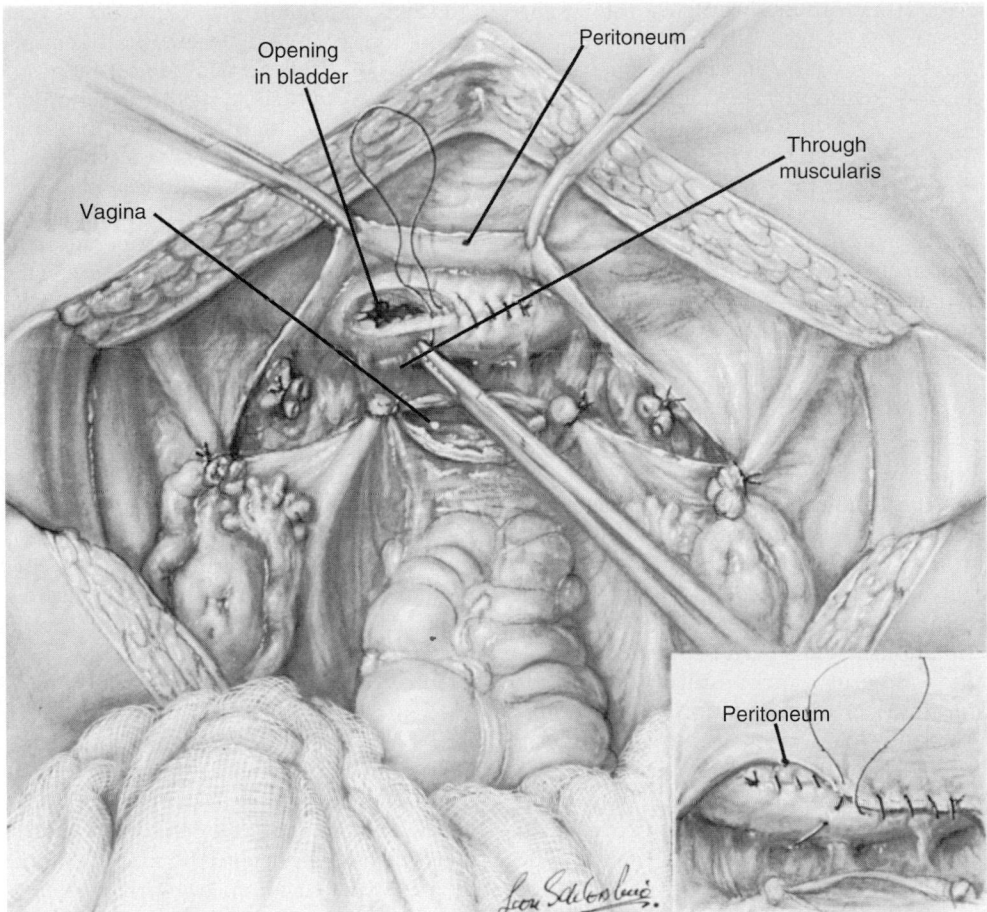

FIGURE 38.1. Closure of cystotomy associated with total abdominal hysterectomy. The bladder mucosa is closed with a continuous delayed-absorbable suture. The suture may invert the mucosa or may be through and through the mucosa. A second row of suture is placed in the musculofascial layer of the bladder to support the initial layer. The bladder peritoneum may be sutured over the operative site to protect it from postoperative pelvic cellulitis to further prevent leakage into the vagina. The edge of the bladder peritoneum also may be sutured to the anterior vaginal cuff.

lations; and lead to depression, low self-esteem, and insomnia. Steady incontinence of urine leads the majority of patients to use a variety of protective methods, including rubber sheets to protect her mattress, diapers or rubber pants to protect her clothing, and continence pad products.

Kursh and associates examined the records of 12 patients who had vesicovaginal fistula develop after total abdominal hysterectomy. Most of the patients had excessive postoperative abdominal pain, distention or paralytic ileus, or both. Hematuria and symptoms of irritability of the bladder were also noted in women who suffered a fistula. A prolonged, postoperative fever and increased white blood cell count occurred more often in the fistula group. The clinical features described are seen with an unrecognized bladder injury resulting in intraperitoneal extravasation of urine. Although in theory, with early recognition it may be possible to avert the formation of a vesicovaginal fistula, in Tancer's review more than 21%

of patients formed a VVF despite preventative maneuvers and repair of intraoperative bladder injury at the time of hysterectomy.

Urethrovaginal fistulae may present with a variety of complaints, depending on the location of the fistula. Patients with distal fistulae may be asymptomatic or complain of spraying of urine or an otherwise abnormal urinary stream. Midurethra fistulae may present with stress incontinence, recurrent cystitis, or no symptoms. Fistulae involving the proximal urethra and bladder neck present similarly to VVF.

Assessment

Even though a diagnosis is obvious in many patients, a thorough urologic investigation is mandatory, especially to rule out coexistent fistulae. In a series of 43 patients with VVF, Goodwin and Scardino found 12% to have associated ureterovaginal fistulae. Lee and associates found

10 of 53 patients (19%) with urethrovaginal fistulae also had a separate VVF.

An evaluation begins with a history and physical examination facilitated by use of a speculum, good lighting, and positioning. A history of large-volume vaginal leakage with no voided urine suggests a sizable vesicovaginal fistula, whereas lesser vaginal fluid drainage associated with regular voiding raises the possibility of a uterovaginal fistula or, perhaps, a very small or intermittent vesicovaginal fistula. Leakage from the vagina during and after voiding suggests a urethrovaginal fistula. Vaginal fluid may be collected for measurement of urea concentration, and a urinalysis and urine culture may identify the presence of a concomitant infection. Intravenous urography may aid in localizing the fistula and determining the adequacy of renal function. Urethrovaginal fistulae usually are easily distinguished on examination. Otherwise, the use of a Tratner catheter and contrast medium may aid in the diagnosis of a urethrovaginal fistula. Small fistulae can be identified more easily if a probe can be passed through the fistula from the vagina into the bladder.

Dye tests traditionally have been performed to evaluate the patients for a urinary tract fistula. With the patient in position for a pelvic examination on the examination table, a 16F Foley catheter is placed and a speculum is inserted into the vagina. In a patient with a larger vesicovaginal fistula, urine is easily seen in the vaginal vault; in some cases, the fistula itself is visualized. If not, the vaginal apex is sponged dry and 100 cc of a dilue solution of methylene blue or indigo carmine is instilled in the bladder via a Foley catheter. This is done with the speculum in place and the vaginal cuff or cervix and upper vagina in full view. The prompt appearance of blue dye indicates a vesicovaginal fistula. The vaginal apex should be carefully scrutinized to identify the site of the fistula. If no dye is seen, it is possible that the open speculum is occluding the fistula and it should be slowly rotated, partially closed, and slowly withdrawn to see if dye begins to leak into the vagina as the pressure from the speculum blades is changed. If dye is still not seen in the vagina, a tampon is inserted and the patient is asked to sit up and walk around for 15 or 20 minutes. With the patient on the examining table once again, the tampon is carefully removed. If blue dye stains the end near the vaginal apex, a small vesicovaginal fistula probably is present. If the tampon is wet with urine, but not blue, leakage from a ureterovaginal fistula is suspected. If the distal end of the tampon near the vaginal introitus is blue, urethral incontinence is present. The patient's symptoms of vaginal fluid leakage may result from leakage of urine from the ureter with pooling in the vagina and subsequent loss of this urine from the vagina when the patient changes position or moves about.

If the tampon has not yet been stained blue, further dye studies may be done to demonstrate a ureterovaginal fistula. The bladder is emptied and flushed with saline and 2 cc of sterile methylene blue or indigo carmine is injected intravenously (i.v.). A fresh tampon is inserted and left in place for 1 to 15 minutes. If the upper end of the new tampon is stained, a ureterovaginal fistula is probably present. The vagina apex is inspected carefully. Leakage of dye from one side of the postoperative vaginal apex strongly suggests the ureter on that side is most likely to be the site of the fistula, but this is not definitive. An i.v. urogram showing leakage, obstruction, or a retrograde pyelogram are indicated and not only show the side involved but the level of the fistula.

All patients should undergo cystourethroscopy. The exact location (in relation to the ureteral orifices), size, and underlying cause of the fistula should be determined. Additional fistulous communications need to be ruled out to reduce the opportunity for surgical failure. Careful attention should be paid to the bladder neck and urethra. Larger fistulae may prohibit or cause difficulty in performing liquid-based cystoscopy. In that case, the vagina may be packed with gauze; alternatively the bladder may be allowed to fill with air and dry cystoscopy performed with the patient in a jack-knife or knee-chest position. Carbon dioxide also may be used as a distention medium. At cystoscopy, urine fails to spurt through the orifice of the damaged or obstructed ureter, assuming that flow from the orifice was previously documented. On rare occasions, a compromised ureter continues to spurt urine from the ureteral orifice. With a previously ligated ureter or damaged kidney, the ureters may look atrophic and no urine flow is seen. Attempts to pass a catheter usually fail when the tip reaches the point of obstruction. A retrograde pyelogram sometimes is needed to fully evaluate the ureter. A ureterovaginal fistula is associated commonly with hydronephrosis and hydroureter because stenosis of the ureter occurs at the site of the injury. Scarring at the edges of a vesicovaginal fistula in the region of the ureteral orifice also may lead to ureteral stenosis and proximal dilatation. Further discussion of the differential diagnosis of urinary fistula is found in Chapter 37.

Although novel radiologic techniques are proving useful in other fields of medicine, their efficacy in the diagnosis of urogenital fistula does not surpass traditional methods. The use of computed tomography (CT) with intravaginal contrast has been reported with limited success. CT may be more helpful in evaluating for coexistent disease and the upper tracts prior to surgical correction. Recently, color Doppler ultrasound with contrast media has been described as a diagnostic tool. Sonography was positive in 11 of 12 (92%) patients with vesicovaginal fistula. (A jet phenomenon was demonstrated through the bladder wall, in the direction of the vagina, which was distinguishable from ureteral flow.)

All patients were known to have fistulae before enrollment into these studies and specificity of color Doppler for detection of VVF cannot be calculated. In fact, 100% were shown to have a fistula with dye tests. The benefits of color Doppler are that is it easy to learn, noninvasive, results in no radiation exposure, and can evaluate the distance from the fistula to the ureteral orifices. Abulafia and colleagues described the diagnostic use of transperineal ultrasound in a woman who was unable to undergo cystoscopy secondary to urethral obstruction. Ultrasonography and CT are unlikely to replace traditional diagnostic methods.

Preoperative urodynamic testing is defended by some authors. Hilton argues for its use before surgical repair of urogenital fistulae to establish the presence of abnormal lower urinary tract function. In this series, of the 38 patients evaluated, 47% had genuine stress incontinence, 40% showed detrusor instability, and 17% had impaired bladder compliance. The overall incidence of functional abnormality was highest in the patients with urethral or bladder neck fistulae. Most patients became continent after surgical treatment of the fistulae. Those who had urethral or bladder neck fistulae had more residual detrusor instability. Thomas and Williams argue that documenting abnormal urodynamic findings may protect the surgeon medico-legally and prepare patients for a less than perfect outcome. However, for the typical vaginal repair of a posthysterectomy VVF, *de novo* detrusor instability is rare.

Anatomic Considerations

Posthysterectomy fistulae are usually supratrigonal and medial to both ureteral orifices. Vaginally, this corresponds to the cuff. Fistulae from obstetric causes may be larger, more distal, and associated with urethral injury. Obstetric fistulae have been classified according to their anatomic location in relation to the cervix. They may have a single channel or multiple channels. There may be a single orifice on one side that tracts to multiple orifices on the other side, although this presentation is very unusual (Fig. 38.2).

Preoperative Care

Cystitis, vaginitis, and perineal dermatitis should be treated with the appropriate agent. Acute cystitis is uncommon in conjunction with a VVF; therefore, suppressive doses of antibiotics are unnecessary unless there is evidence for an upper tract infection. Perineal care is important and makes the patient more comfortable and tolerant of delayed closure. Frequent pad changes are required to minimize inflammation, edema, and vulvar irritation. Zinc oxide ointment or a cream containing lanolin may be especially helpful in the treatment of perineal and vulvar dermatitis. Inventive collection and drainage systems have been described for this purpose as well. Green and Philips described using dental prosthetic techniques to create a vaginal appliance to control urinary incontinence resulting from a VVF. Another system has been fashioned by gluing a Pezzer catheter to a fitted contraceptive diaphragm with rubber cement. This device traps urine in the vagina and diverts it to a collecting leg bag. It may be worn for the weeks or months before repair is carried out.

Every attempt should be made to divert the urinary stream to protect the perineum and allow the fistula margins to mature. In fact, small fistulae may close with catheter drainage alone. In a series of urogenital fistulae referred to a tertiary unit, 7% closed without the need for surgery (Hilton, unpublished data).

Medical therapy as an adjunct to surgery also is important. In the case of the malnourished patient, healing is improved if nutrition needs are optimized and anemia corrected prior to surgery. Some have described the preoperative use of steroids. Despite some success, there is

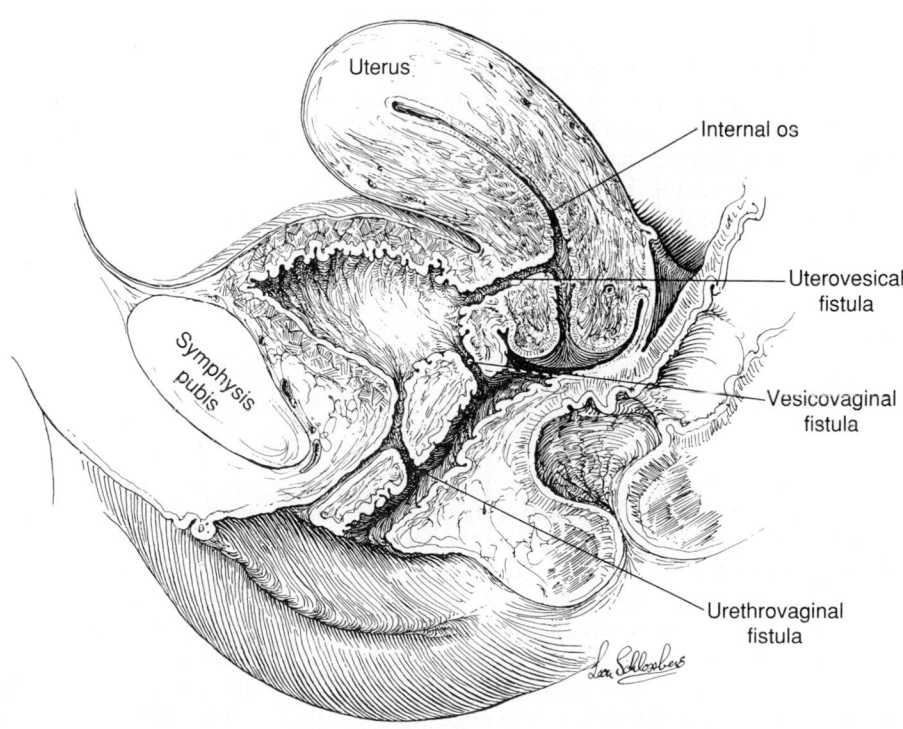

FIGURE 38.2. Sagittal section showing vesicocervical, vesicovaginal, and urethrovaginal fistulae.

no convincing evidence that steroids improve the tissues prior to closure, and they could interfere with healing when an early repair is attempted. Estrogen therapy may be used to improve tissue thickness and vascularity provided there are no contraindications. Hyperbaric oxygen has been described as an adjuvant to surgery for radiation-induced fistulae.

Surgical Technique

Surgery is the mainstay of therapy for urogenital fistulae. Following the tenets of Simms, Symmonds proposed several surgical principles to improve the success rate of fistula repair: (a) wide mobilization of the bladder; (b) excision of all scar tissue at the risk of increasing the size of the fistula in an attempt to create a "fresh bladder injury"; (c) a tension-free layer closure of the bladder and the vagina; (d) nontraumatizing technique; and (e) good hemostasis with complete bladder drainage postoperatively. These principles are the same for fistulae involving the urethra. Most authors agree that the best chance at closure of the fistula is the first attempt, although staged procedures have been described. Unfortunately, there are no controlled trials of route or timing of repair and the general view is for individualized management.

In general, the vaginal approach avoids the potential morbidity associated with abdominal surgery and is believed to provide a quicker recovery and a more cosmetic result. Because it does not require a laparotomy, it is considered to be easier, safer, and more comfortable for the patient. Success rates of 98% and 100% have been reported in two of the larger series. Although there are circumstances for which an abdominal approach has traditionally been favored, for example, larger fistulae, fistulae located high on the posterior wall, fistulae adjacent to the ureters, and concurrent intraabdominal pathology, the usual postsurgical fistula is low in the bladder and easily accessible in the anterior vaginal wall. The abdominal route of repair offers little benefit in this circumstance. However, an attempted vaginal repair of a fistula high in an immobile vaginal vault may be limited by visibility and lead to a less than satisfactory result.

Involvement of the ureter may require an abdominal approach to facilitate ureteral reimplantation or the placement of stents. Laparotomy is necessary in fistulae requiring bowel for augmentation cystoplasty. In certain circumstances, a combined vaginal and abdominal approach may be helpful. The authors have described a combined approach to the repair of a large fistula secondary to a vaginal foreign body that involved the trigone.

There is no consensus on the need to excise the fistulous tract. Some authors advocate its total removal, whereas others prefer to merely debride the margins, thereby avoiding an increase in the size of the defect. Iselin and associates advocate the excision of the fistula tract and vaginal cuff scar enabling the surgeon to suture viable tissues in every layer to promote wound healing obviating the need for interpositional flaps or grafts. They had a 100% cure rate on first attempt. In

his series of 65 transvaginal repairs, Raz did not excise the fistula tract in any patient and had no apparent adverse effects. Cruikshank did not excise the tract in a series of 11 patients and had a 100% cure rate. Zacharin warns that excision of the fistula scar markedly increases the risk of operative failure. Elkins and colleagues and Lawson also advised against excising the tract in large obstetric fistulae.

Suture preference for VVF repair is physician dependent. No data indicate any increased efficacy of synthetic over chromic suture in fistula repairs.

SURGICAL TECHNIQUE

Vesicovaginal Fistulae

Vaginal Repair

Patient positioning for greater visualization of the fistula edges is a matter of physician preference and some debate. Some prefer lithotomy position and others (e.g., Elkins) feel that adequate visualization, especially of the proximal urethra and bladder neck, can best be achieved by the knee-chest or Lawson position. Dropping the head of the table and elevating the buttocks may further facilitate exposure.

Technical difficulties encountered are likely to be resolved by improved exposure and accessibility of the fistula itself than a change in specific instrumentation. Because the vaginal walls normally are very pliable, retraction usually is sufficient for adequate exposure of the fistula. However, a narrow vaginal introitus, scarring of the vagina, a narrow subpubic arch, or a deep and fixed vaginal vault may limit exposure. An episiotomy or a Schuchardt's incision may allow access to the cuff, especially if the pubic arch is narrow, the vagina is deep or the introitus is constricted. In current practice, many surgeons avoid these incisions because of the increased morbidity. However, such incisions are invaluable and should be made without hesitation if exposure and accessibility are improved. In addition, the surgery may be facilitated by the placement of stay or traction sutures at the margins of the fistula or gentle traction on a Foley or Fogarty catheter placed through the fistula. These techniques help to identify the fistula's edges and may bring the tract closer to the surgeon. The Young prostatic retractor may be used in a similar fashion. Some fistula surgeons infiltrate the vaginal mucosa with saline or a dilution of epinephrine (1:200,000) to aid dissection and decrease oozing. This is not our current practice for repair of fistulae.

The two transvaginal repairs commonly performed are the flap splitting technique and the Latzko procedure. The *flap splitting technique* involves wide mobilization of the vaginal mucosa from the edge of the fistula. However, too much mobilization may lead to avascular necrosis of suture lines. The bladder is closed in two layers. A submucosal line of interrupted Lembert sutures is followed by a second layer to close the muscularis and reduce tension on the previous suture line (Fig. 38.3). Trigonal defects should be repaired in a transverse

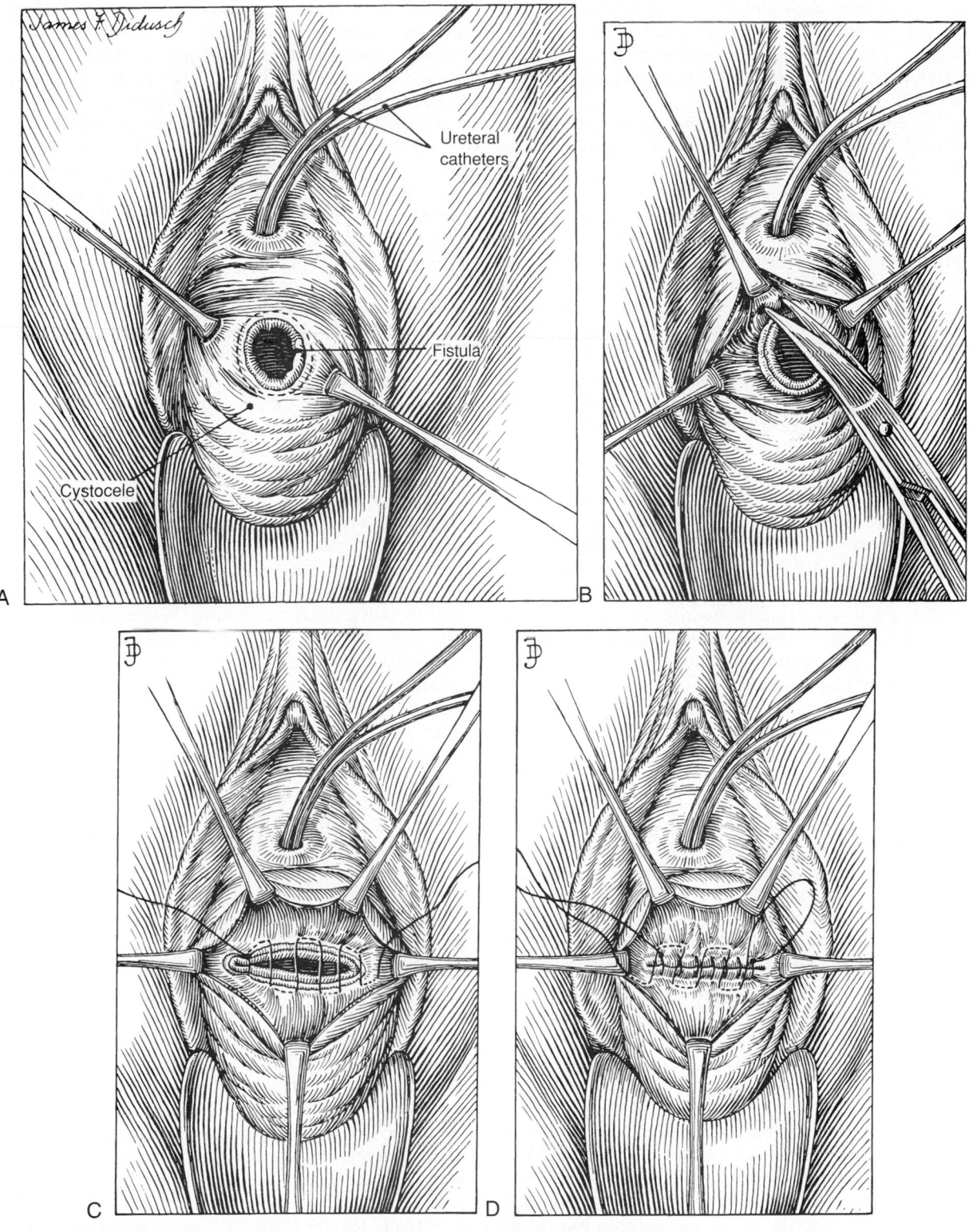

FIGURE 38.3. Flap-splitting closure of a simple vesicovaginal fistula. **A:** Ureters have been catheterized. An incision through the vaginal epithelium is made circumferentially around the fistula. **B:** The vaginal epithelium is widely mobilized from the bladder. The scarred fistula tract should be excised. **C:** A continuous (or interrupted) delayed-absorbable suture inverts the mucosa into the bladder. **D:** A second suture line is placed in the musculofascial layer to reinforce the first. Vaginal epithelium is trimmed and approximated.

direction. A vertical closure at the trigone may draw the ureters to the midline and lead to kinking or frank obstruction. This technique does not lead to vaginal foreshortening. Cure rates in some series approach those for the Latzko procedure.

The *Latzko procedure* is championed by many. It is an excellent procedure for correcting small posthysterectomy fistulae at the vaginal apex. It cannot be performed if the cervix remains *in situ*. The Latzko operation is a partial colpocleisis involving the upper 2 to 3 cm of vagina that surrounds the fistula (Fig. 38.4). An elliptical portion of vaginal epithelium is stripped from the anterior and posterior vaginal walls from around the fistula tract at least 2.5 cm in all directions. The walls have a natural tendency to fall together and are easily approximated without tension. The pubovesical fascia and vaginal mucosa are closed in layers using interrupted sutures. The vesical edges of the fistula are not denuded. The posterior vaginal wall becomes the posterior bladder wall and reepithelializes with urothelium. Theoretically because there are no sutures in the bladder wall with a Latzko repair, the bladder wall can fill without tension, obviating the need for prolonged catheterization.

Success rates for the Latzko partial colpocleisis are greater than 89% at the first attempt. Other advantages include short operating time, minimal blood loss, and low postoperative morbidity. Because posthysterectomy fistulae are almost always small and high in the vagina, the loss of vaginal depth and interference with sexual function should be minimal.

Interposition flaps or *grafts* may be used in large or recurrent fistulae, those involving the urethra or bladder neck, or fistulae requiring additional bulk. Pedicle flaps bring additional blood supply, improve the lymphatic drainage, and distance suture lines. In 1928, Martius first described the use of the labial fat pad as an interposition graft. The vascular supply to the graft inferiorly is from the internal pudendal artery and superiorly, the external pudendal artery. In mobilizing a labial fat pad pedicle, the surgeon must preserve one of these vascular bundles (Fig. 38.5). Birkhoff and colleagues reported a 100% success rate in six patients with transvaginal repairs of VVF using the Martius technique. In a series mostly of postobstetric injuries, Elkins and colleagues reported a success/closure rate of 96% (24 of 25 procedures).

Alternatively, a gracilis muscle flap may be used. First described by Ingelman-Sundberg in 1954, and later modified by Hamlin and Nicholson, the technique involves dissection of the gracilis muscle and separation of its attachment to the medial condyle of the femur. The blood supply, from the femoral artery, is preserved. The graft may be rotated or advanced directly and tunneled at the introitus up to the fistula. The gracilis muscle allows a bulky closure, when required, to urogenital fistulae. Fugiwara and associates have described the use of a gracilis myocutaneous graft in a patient with concurrent radiation-induced VVF and recto-vaginal fistulae.

A method using a pedicled flap of vaginal wall was presented recently as a case report by Hurley and Previte.

Although the results were good in this case, a subvaginal cyst may develop in the buried vaginal tissue.

Regardless of the route of repair for VVF, the closure should be watertight. The integrity of the repair may be tested during surgery with methylene blue or indigo carmine. The authors prefer to leave a pack in the vagina 24 hours postoperatively and continuously drain the bladder with a 16F Silastic suprapubic catheter for at least 3 weeks and discontinue the catheter after the patient successfully passes voiding trials. The patient is maintained on prophylactic antibiotics while the catheter is *in situ*.

Abdominal Repair

The patient should be in low, lithotomy position and the patient's legs should be placed in universal stirrups with the thighs flexed 15 degrees and abducted slightly. This allows vaginal access, the ability to elevate the fistula with the surgeon's hand, and the ability to perform cystoscopy.

O'Conor and coworkers pioneered an abdominal technique that can be performed extraperitoneally or intraperitoneally. The bladder is bisected with wide mobilization of the bladder and vagina. As much dissection as possible is performed to free the posterior wall of the bladder from the vagina. The fistula is excised with margins of viable tissue for closure. Stay sutures are placed on either side of the incision to facilitate exposure (Fig. 38.6). The bladder and vagina are finally closed in layers. Mondet and coworkers, in a recent review, evaluated the anatomic and functional results after transperitoneal-transvesical repair of VVF (after O'Conor). It is notable that in this series of 28 VVF, 33% required ureteral reimplantation. Overall success was 85% (24 of 28). The success rate was 87.5% for simple VVFs, 71% for complex VVFs, and 80% for fistulae requiring ureteral reimplantation. Ureteral reimplantation, although it makes the operation more complicated, does not worsen the prognosis. Nesrallah and associates had 100% success at correction of a series of 29 VVF, 34% of which had prior attempts using the O'Conor technique.

Modifications of O'Conor's technique to limit the amount of bladder dissection have been offered. Cetin and colleagues described a suprapubic transvesical repair that is extraperitoneal. Through a small vertical anterior cystotomy, the fistula tract is mobilized to the wound and circumferentially excised. The vagina and bladder are closed in separate layers. Success rates are comparable to the O'Conor and Latzko techniques. By performing the surgery extraperitoneally, perioperative morbidity may be reduced and recovery time shortened akin to vaginal repairs.

Ostad described an abdominal approach to repair with a free bladder mucosal graft in a series of six patients. Using a suprapubic cystotomy, the fistula tract was debrided and not excised. A free bladder mucosal graft was harvested from a healthy portion of the bladder and sutured in an interrupted fashion over the fistula. The donor site was allowed to reepithelialize and the bladder

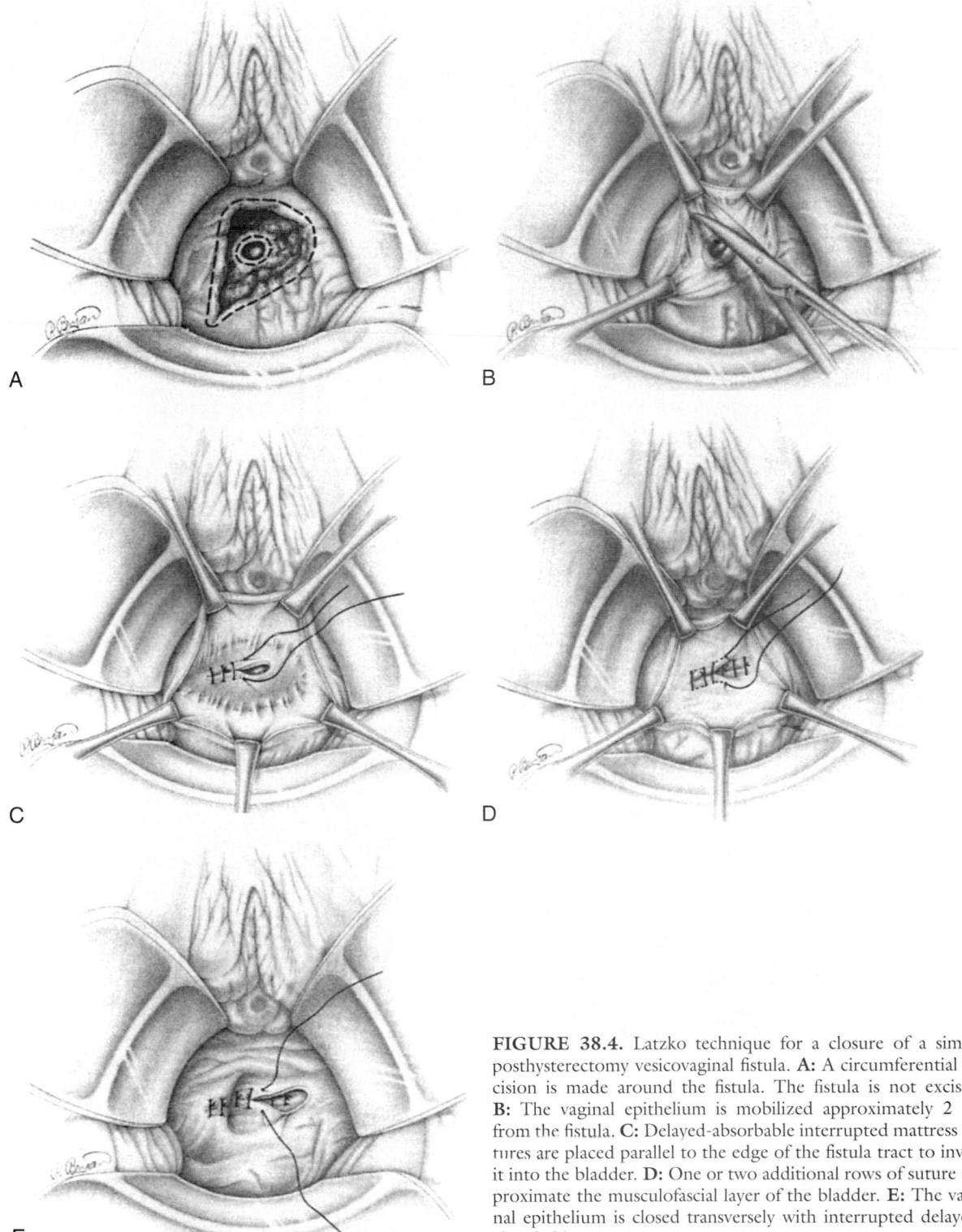

FIGURE 38.4. Latzko technique for a closure of a simple posthysterectomy vesicovaginal fistula. **A:** A circumferential incision is made around the fistula. The fistula is not excised. **B:** The vaginal epithelium is mobilized approximately 2 cm from the fistula. **C:** Delayed-absorbable interrupted mattress sutures are placed parallel to the edge of the fistula tract to invert it into the bladder. **D:** One or two additional rows of suture approximate the musculofascial layer of the bladder. **E:** The vaginal epithelium is closed transversely with interrupted delayed-absorbable sutures.

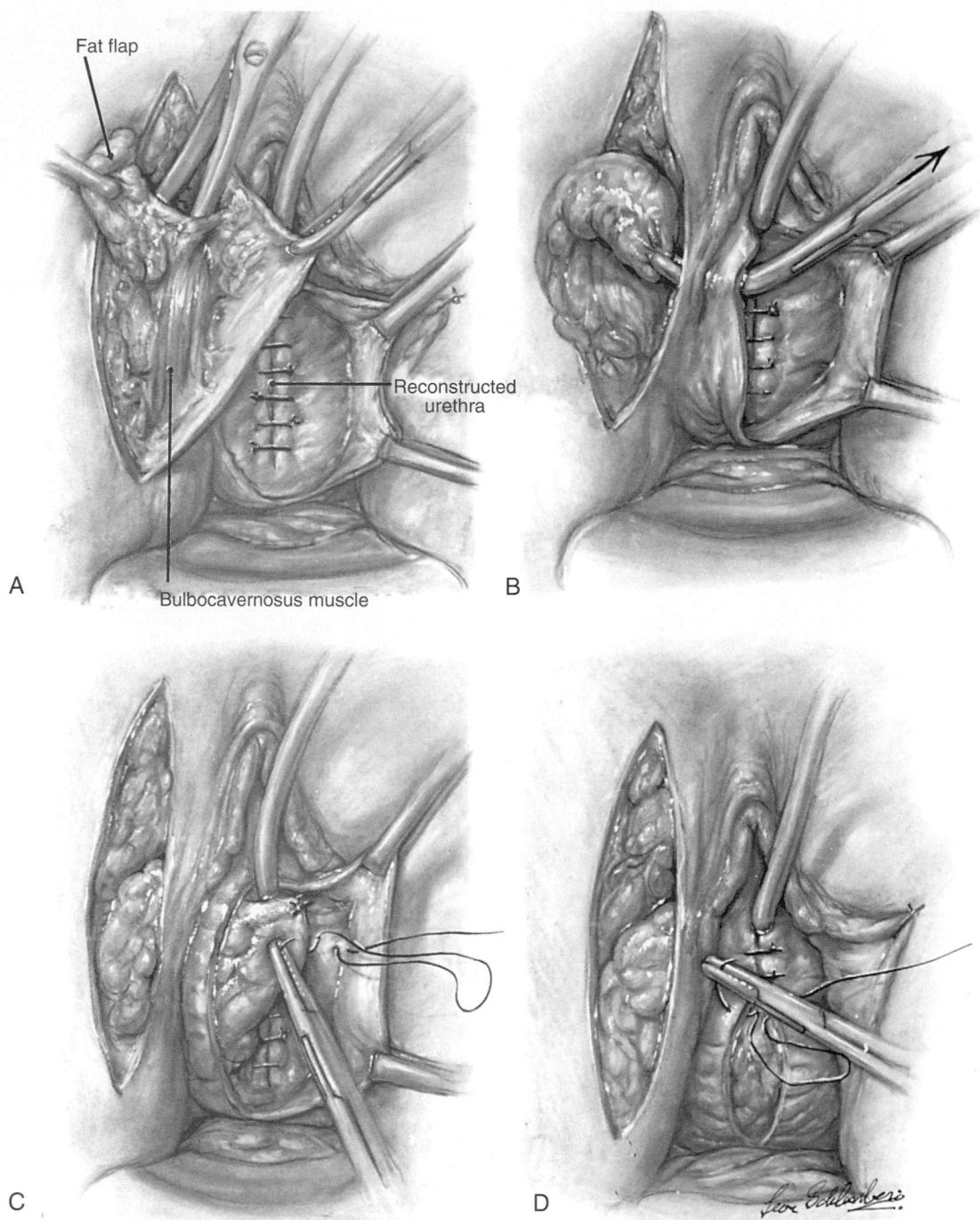

FIGURE 38.5. Martius bulbocavernosus fat pad graft for urethrovaginal or vesicovaginal fistula repair. **A:** The lateral margin of the labia majora is incised vertically. The fat pad adjacent to the bulbocavernosus muscle is mobilized, leaving a broad pedicle attached at the inferior pole. **B,C:** The fat pad is drawn through a tunnel beneath the labia minor and vaginal mucosa and sutured with delayed-absorbable sutures to the fascia of the urethra and bladder. **D:** The vaginal mucosa is mobilized widely to permit closure over the pedicle without tension. The vulvar incision is closed with interrupted delayed-absorbable sutures.

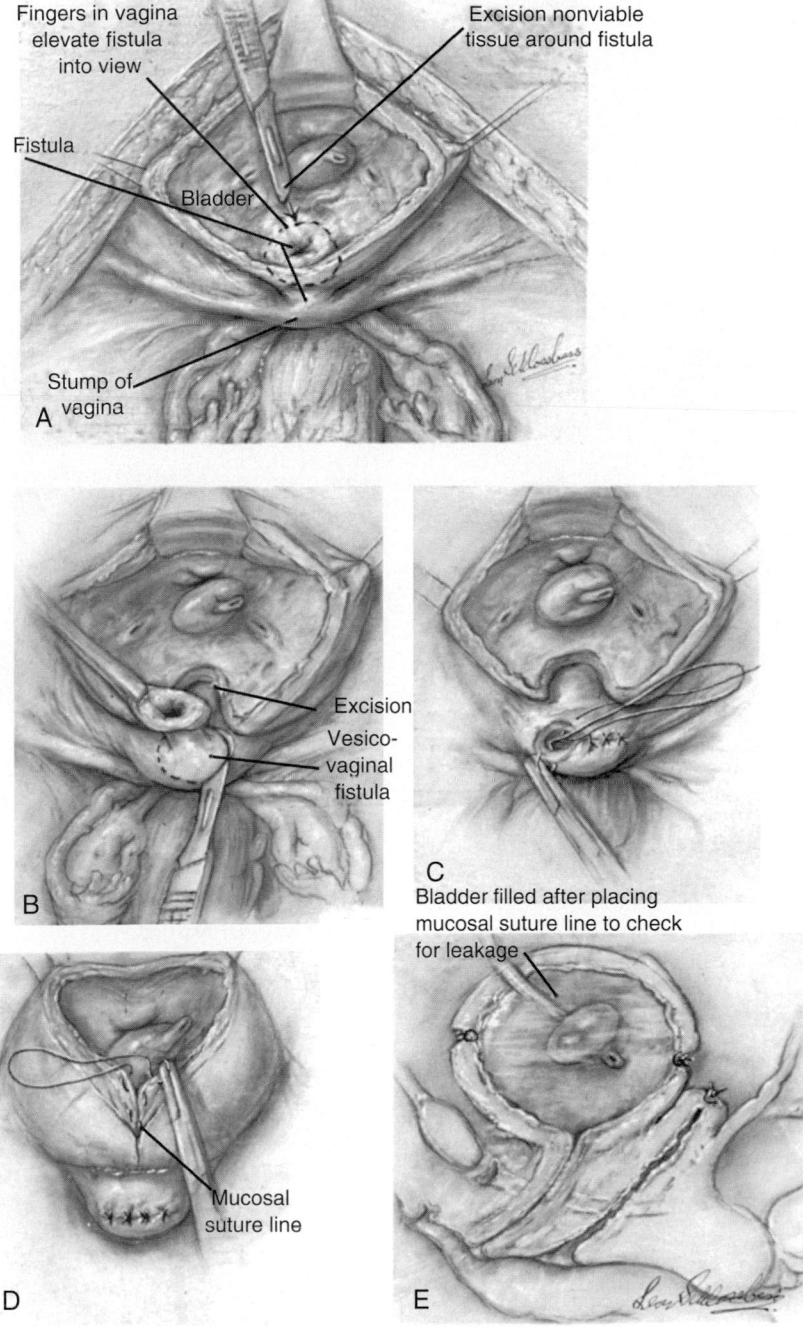

FIGURE 38.6. Transabdominal, transvesical closure of vesicovaginal fistula. **A:** A longitudinal incision is placed in the bladder dome. **B:** The incision is extended around the fistula. The fistulous tract and its vaginal orifice are completely excised. **C:** Interrupted delayed-absorbable sutures are used to close the vagina in one or two layers. **D:** Continuous delayed-absorbable suture closes the bladder mucosa longitudinally. **E:** A suprapubic catheter is placed into the bladder in an extraperitoneal location.   *(continued)*

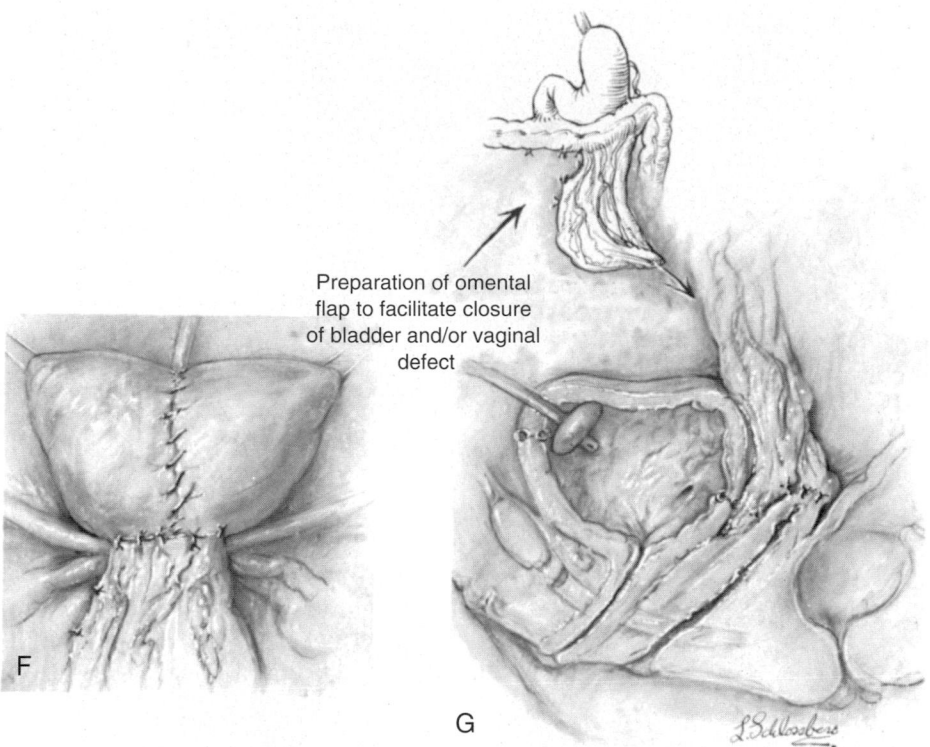

Preparation of omental flap to facilitate closure of bladder and/or vaginal defect

FIGURE 38.6. *(Continued)* **F:** The bladder muscularis is closed with delayed-absorbable continuous or interrupted sutures. **G:** An omental "J" flap can be interposed between the bladder closure and the vaginal closure.

drained for 3 weeks. Advantages include a reduced need for extensive dissection and the ability to tailor the graft to the patient's anatomy and proximity to the ureteral orifices.

The use of vascularized tissue grafts is helpful in assuring a successful abdominal repair. Omental flaps are excellent in this regard. In fact, one third of omental aprons may reach the deep pelvis without creating a flap. The omentum has a dual blood supply and may be mobilized based on either the right or left gastroepiploic arteries. A laparoscopic approach has even been described. Rectus muscles also have been used as grafts for abdominal repairs. A recent review by Evans and colleagues evaluated the use of interposition grafts for VVFs of benign and malignant etiologies. All repairs with grafts (12) were successful without regard to etiology, whereas only 16 of 25 (64%) of repairs without grafts were successful. The authors concluded that transabdominal VVF repairs should be performed with an interposition flap regardless of the appearance of healthy surrounding tissues and etiology.

Urethrovaginal Fistulae

The repair of urethrovaginal fistulae is more difficult than for VVF. Extensive urethral loss and lack of viable tissue may make conventional layered closures impractical. It is generally reported that the success rate of urethrovaginal fistula repair is 73% to 100%. The surgical principles of VVF repair also apply to the correction of urethrovaginal fistulae.

Urethral reconstruction begins by making a U-shaped flap of vaginal mucosa exposing the underside of the trigone and sphincter. The flap is rotated forward (Fig. 38.7). Two or three deep sutures are placed in the region of the sphincter and, when tied, will tighten the internal orifice. The flap of mucosa is drawn downward and an area 6 to 7 mm wide is denuded forward for a distance equal to the length of the flap.

The original flap is rotated forward so that the raw edges of the original flap may be sutured to the denuded area. When this step is repeated on the opposite side, an epithelial-lined tube is formed that serves as a urethra. Because the mucosal pedicles are relatively long, they are very susceptible to ischemia and subsequent necrosis. Thus, a layer of paraurethral fascia is plicated beneath the new urethral floor for support. The mucosal edges are approximated and this buries the newly constructed urethra and completely closes the wound.

Alternatively, Symmonds has described another technique for urethral reconstruction. The anterior vaginal wall is incised and extended around the margins of the urethral defect. The urethral margins are mobilized enough to provide a tension-free closure over a 12F catheter. This operation preserves the limited blood supply to the urethral margins by incising the vaginal mucosa at the lateral most margin of each side of the urethral remnant. No more than 2 mm of vaginal mucosa

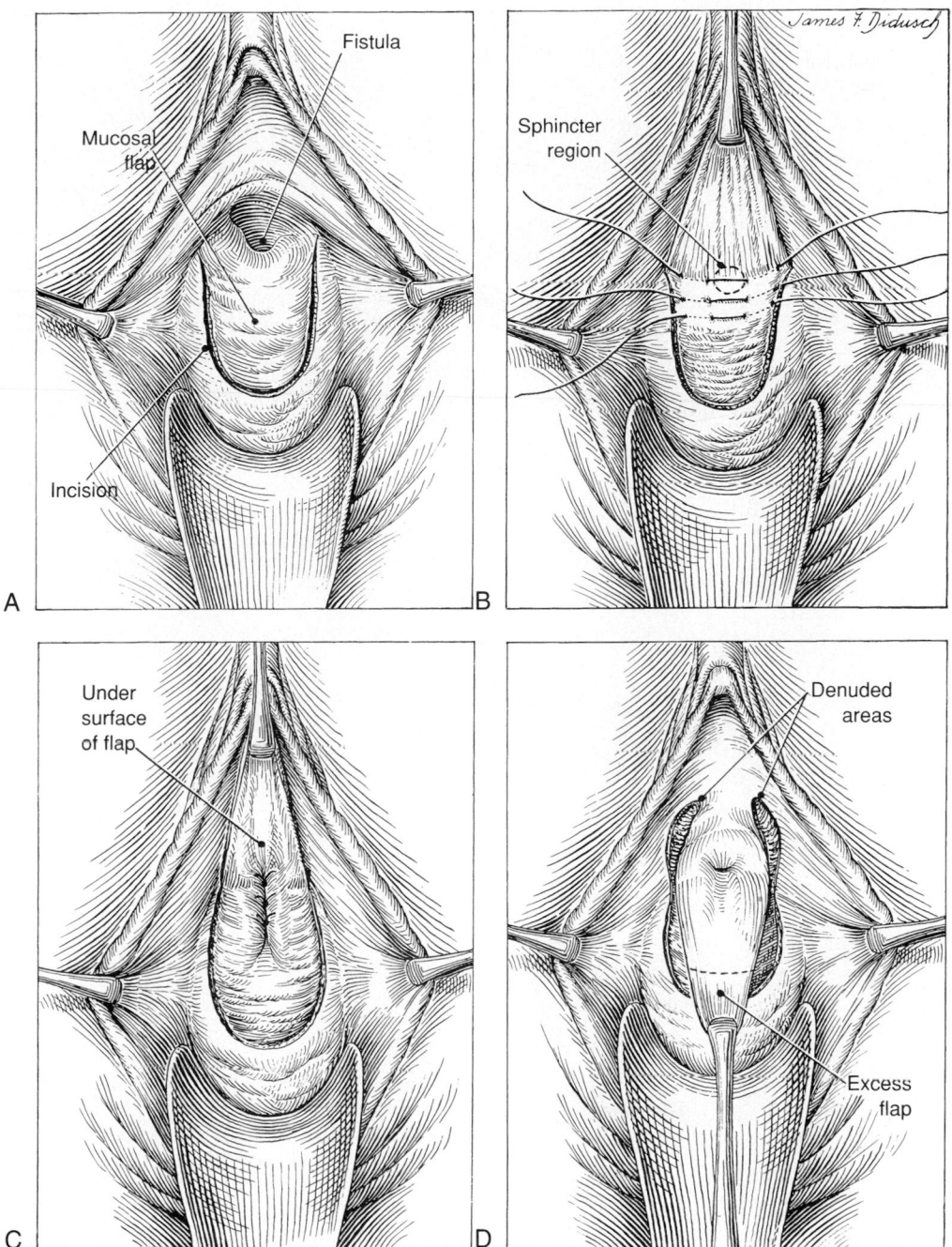

FIGURE 38.7. Reconstruction of urethra and repair of sphincter. **A:** A U-shaped incision is made through the vaginal epithelium. **B:** The flap is mobilized and rotated over the fistula. **C:** Three interrupted sutures of delayed-absorbable suture are placed in the sphincter region and the tissue inverted. **D:** The mucosal flap is pulled downward, and the incision is extended on both sides.   *(continued)*

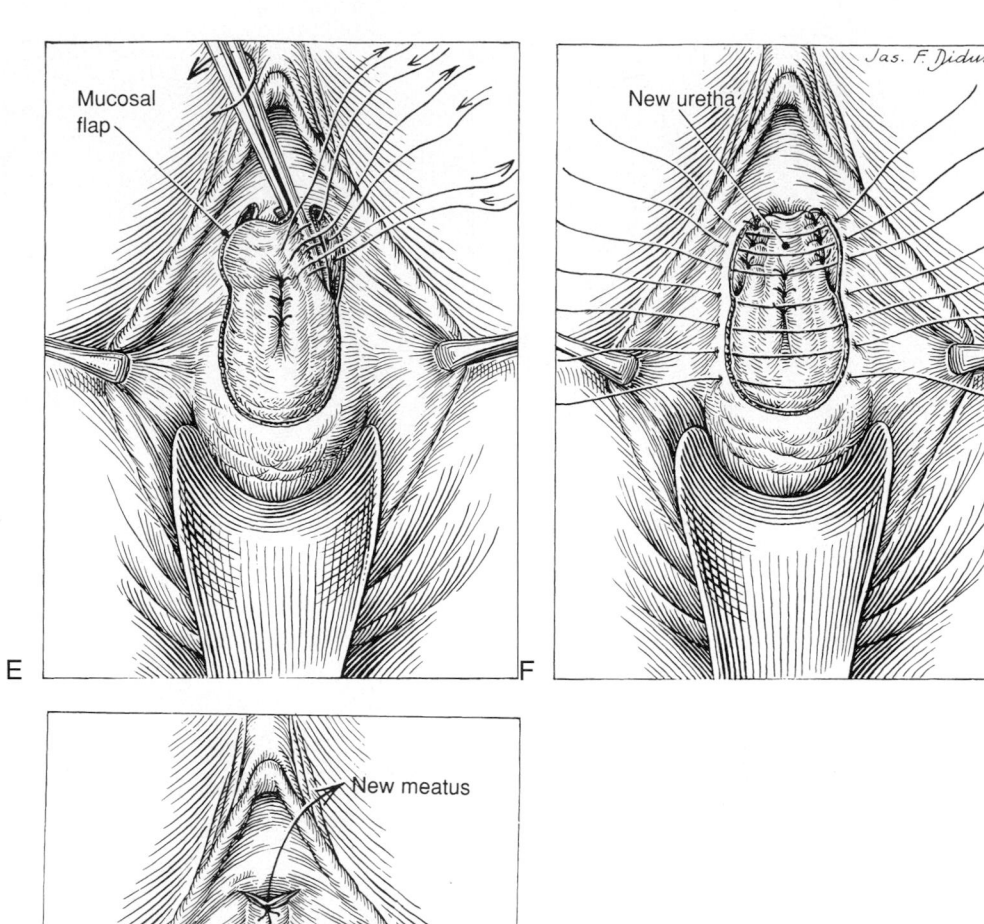

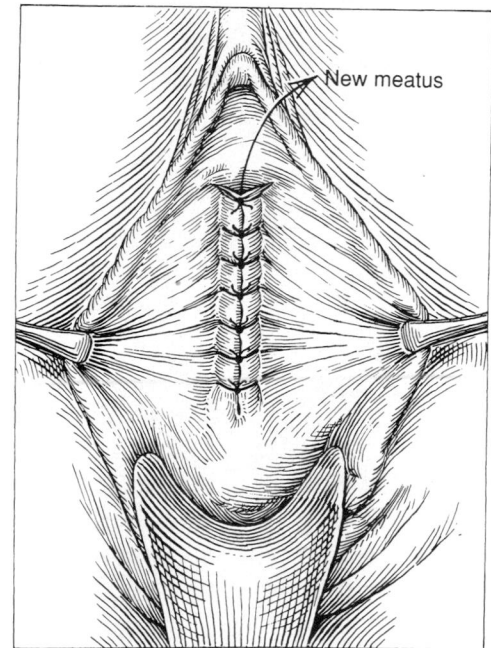

FIGURE 38.7. *(Continued)* **E:** The flap is rotated anteriorly and the incision edges approximated to form a tube. **F:** A layer of paraurethral fascia is plicated beneath the urethra. The vagina is approximated over the neourethra with interrupted delayed-absorbable sutures. **G:** Completion of the reconstruction, showing interrupted suture closure of suburethral mucosa.

remains attached to the urethral walls. Sharp dissection allows the edges of the retracted side walls to be freed while protecting the lateral paraurethral blood supply. Enough of the urethral tissue must be mobilized to permit approximation of the edges over a 12F catheter (Fig. 38.8). The small caliber urethra created by this technique may aid in establishing continence. The fascia adjacent to the newly created urethral tube is freed with sharp dissection avoiding deep lateral dissection that disrupts the blood supply.

Sutures are placed through the fascia and musculature of the urethral tube bilaterally. Each suture is held until placement of its counterpoint. The lower strand of the pair is tied across the urethral floor as are the upper strands. Alternatively, vertical mattress sutures may be used to approximate the fascia to support the urethral wall. The vaginal mucosa is closed without tension.

Interposition grafts may be used for either vaginal technique of urethral reconstruction and a suprapubic catheter is placed to allow continuous drainage for 12 to 14 days.

Using an abdominal approach, the urethra may be reconstructed using the bladder. Fernandes has reported tubularizing an anterior advancement flap of bladder to

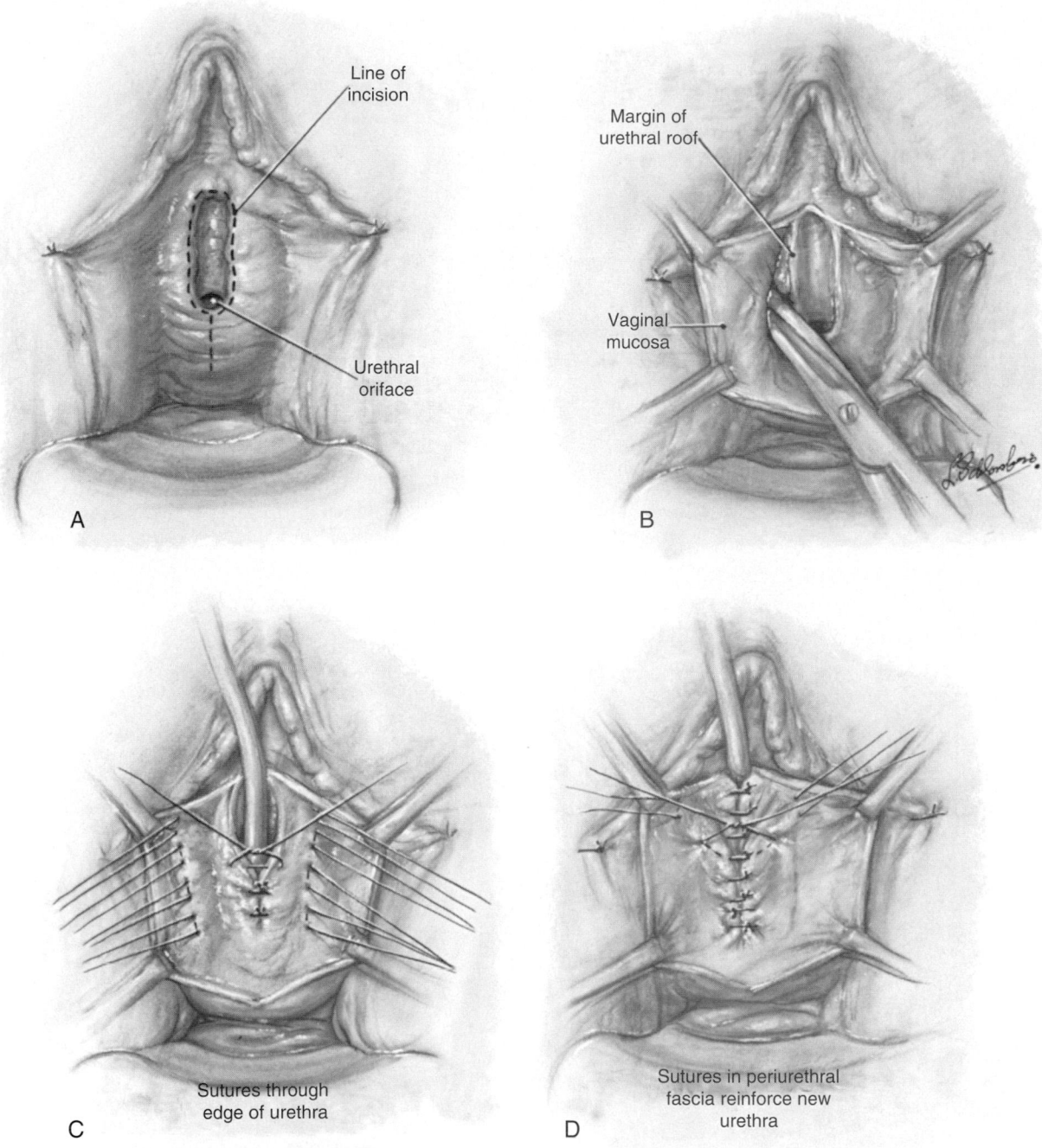

FIGURE 38.8. Reconstruction of total or partial loss of the urethral floor. **A:** A line of incision is made along the margins of the roof of the urethra and extended to the bladder base. **B:** The urethral margins and fascia are mobilized from the vagina to permit tension-free approximation of the urethral mucosa. **C:** Urethral edges are approximated over a 12F catheter with interrupted delayed-absorbable sutures. Mobilized urethral fascia is sutured on each side of the total length of the urethra. **D:** The lower strand of each suture is tied beneath the urethral floor, and the upper strands of the two sutures are used to pull the fascia beneath the urethra, where they are tied.

(continued)

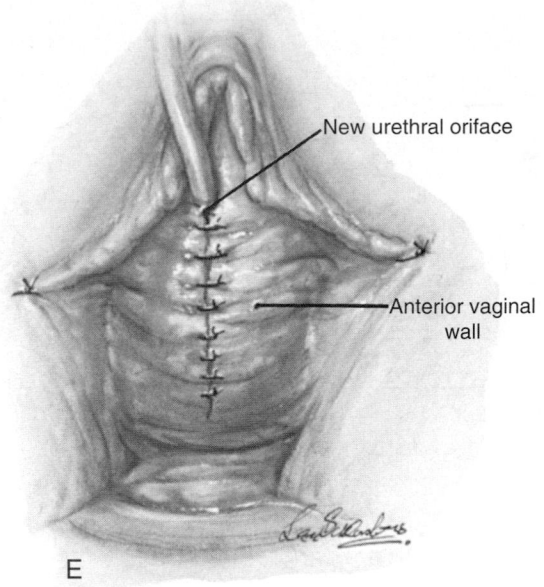

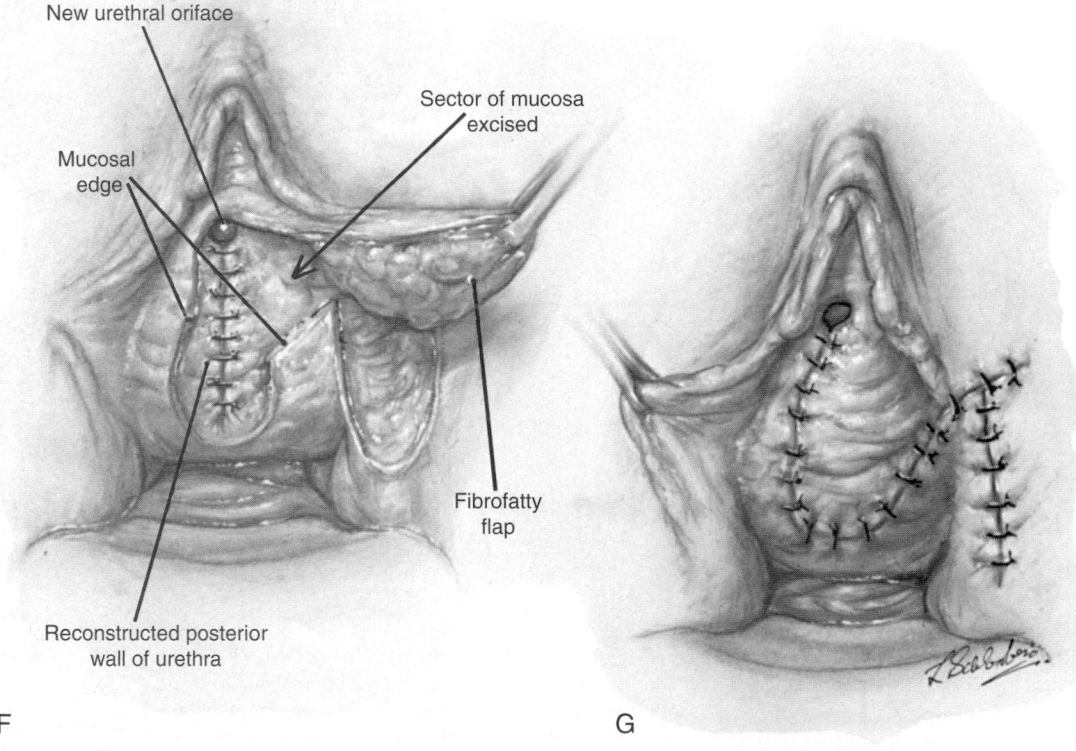

FIGURE 38.8. *(Continued)* **E:** The vaginal mucosa is closed without tension. **F:** For additional reinforcement, a U-shaped labial fat pad can be developed along the labia, leaving a broad pedicle superiorly. The vaginal mucosa between the urethral operative site and the labial graft is resected. **G:** The skin margins of the labial graft are sutured to the vaginal margins. The labial defect is closed.

reconstruct an entire urethra. Ome-Dare has used patch grafts of bladder mucosa for urethral reconstruction after gonococcal stricture with some success.

The use of a tubularized rectus abdominis muscle flap has also been described in a series of refractory urethrovaginal fistulae patients, all of whom had undergone at least one unsuccessful repair incorporating a Martius graft.

Minimally Invasive Management

Several minimally invasive approaches have been reported successful in closing small vesicovaginal fistulae. Fibrin occlusion of a vesicovaginal fistula was first reported by Pettersson and colleagues in 1979. The patient also had continuous bladder drainage for 8 weeks. Kanaoka and coworkers also reported the successful use of fibrin glue for a 1-mm complicated VVF for 4 years until the recurrence of an irreparable fistula requiring urinary diversion.

Fulguration of small VVF followed by continuous drainage also has been described by Stovsky and associates and Falk and Orkin with some success. Recently, Dogra and Nabi described the use of an endoscopic Nd-YAG laser to fulgurate a small 2- to 3-mm posthysterectomy VVF. They refer to the procedure as a "laser welding," but probably the denuded tract closes spontaneously after the 3-week period of continuous drainage.

McKay described successful transurethral suture repairs of two VVF using laparoscopic extracorporeal knot tying techniques. A 5-mm laparoscopic sleeve, for passage of the suture, is inserted along side a 17F cystourethroscope with a 30-degree lens.

Urinary Diversion and Reconstructive Techniques

In irreparable or recurrent VVF and cloacal defects following high-dose irradiation therapy for gynecologic malignancies, urinary diversion is the last resort to achieve a socially acceptable solution. Leissner and coworkers have reported the use of the Mainz III colon pouch for continent diversion. This group has also described the construction of a neovagina from redundant bladder or colon following urinary diversion.

An early technique of urinary diversion was implantation of the ureters into the sigmoid colon. Kidney failure, metabolic and electrolyte disturbance, and increased risk of colon cancer at the site of ureteral anastomosis led to its disfavor. Ureterosigmoid implantations are rarely performed in the United States, but continue to be used in developing countries. Ureteral implantation into an isolated ileal loop or into a continent colon or ileal pouch (see Chapter 50) is now the preferred method for fistulae that are irreparable.

Timing of Repair

The timing of repair remains controversial. The traditional belief is to wait a minimum of 3 to 6 months after the inciting event or the last attempt at repair, as inflammatory or necrotic fistula margins have been judged responsible for surgical failure and that the outcome of cancer therapy may be evaluated. This interim period of waiting is often very distressing for the patient. O'Conor has said, "a surgeon must stand firm in his conviction that an impatient patient is easier to manage than a surgical failure." Wein has attributed surgical failures to an inadequate delay until repair. Lee and Symmonds recommended delaying surgery to increase the success rate of the first attempt at repair. Symmonds recommends generally waiting 3 to 4 months for the tissues to "clean up," lose their edema, and obtain good vascularity and pliability.

Others propose that early intervention is safe. In 1960, Collins and associates reported on the use of oral steroids and early transvaginal repair of VVF. Patients received 100 mg of cortisone three times daily for 10 to 12 days preoperatively. Of 15 patients without a history of pelvic malignancy or radiation therapy, 13 (87%) had successful repairs. In this series, three of five (60%) patients with cervical cancer and irradiation induced fistulae had recurrences within a brief postoperative period. Eleven years later, these same authors reported a 28% failure rate in a series of 38 patients all of whom had a transvaginal repair and preoperative steroids within 60 days after diagnosis. The experience with steroids and early closure was again updated in 1984 with a series of 54 patients, 11% of whom required a second procedure for successful repair.

Reported series not using steroids are more favorable. Persky, also an advocate for early repair, reported a series of seven patients who all underwent successful transvesical repair using interposition grafts of peritoneum or omentum within 10 weeks of the antecedent surgery. Cruikshank also had success in 10 of 11 fistulae in his series repaired between 10 and 35 days after a hysterectomy. In a series from Duke University Medical Center, Iselin and colleagues had a 100% cure rate with an average time to repair of 16 weeks.

Treatment should be tailored to the individual patient. If the fistula is recognized within the first 48 hours postoperatively, the tissue should be more mobile, have less inflammation, and be amenable to early repair. Fistulae arising later usually are complicated by significant edema, inflammation, and induration. An interval of 3 months from injury to repair in obstetric and surgical fistulae allows inflammation and edema to resolve. Up to 1 year may be required for improvement in the tissues in radiation-induced fistulae prior to repair, that is, it is difficult to determine accurately when radiation necrosis has run its course. The outcome of prolonged catheterization alone for small fistulae is unpredictable. Large fistulae may be easier to repair once the tract is allowed to scar and edema resolves. On the other hand, the delay of closure may have a significant negative impact on a patient's quality of life.

The principles outlined for VVF repair also are applicable to urethrovaginal fistulae. Because the urethra has a minimum of redundant tissue with which to work, the tissues must be as near to normal as possible before a repair is undertaken. A delay of several months usually is recommended to allow tissues to completely heal and for inflammation to resolve.

Postoperative Care

How long to drain and whether to drain via transurethral or suprapubic routes are influenced by geography, culture, complexity of the fistula, and the technique used. Transurethral drainage for 10 to 14 days with an overall success rate of 70% was reported by Elkins in a series of 36 obstetrical fistulae. Tancer, in his series of Latzko closures, described removing the Foley catheter on the first or second postoperative day. All patients remained dry.

The surgeon should tailor the length of time to drain and route of drainage to the individual patient. Symmonds has recommended suprapubic catheters for distal fistulae involving the urethra or bladder neck. He argues that a transurethral catheter should not be used because of the proximity to the suture line and the risk of disrupting the wound. The authors prefer suprapubic catheters to facilitate voiding trials.

Excellent hydration will ensure irrigation of the bladder and prevent clots that could obstruct the catheter and lead to unwanted bladder distention and disruption of suture lines. As long as bladder drainage is adequate, prolonged bed rest and patient positioning in bed probably make little difference. Some surgeons advocate obtaining a cystogram to evaluate the integrity of the bladder prior to discontinuing bladder drainage, but this is not the authors' current practice.

Incontinence After the Repair

The occurrence of stress incontinence in patients after the successful repair of obstetric VVF has been long recognized and is estimated to occur in up to 10% to 12% of such patients. Waaldijk subjectively documented the occurrence of stress incontinence after repair of fistulae of varying types, describing 1% where there was no sphincter involvement in the fistula, 13% where there was sphincter involvement but with no tissue loss, and 16% where there was both sphincter involvement and tissue loss. In contrast, Hilton found that the incidence of urodynamically proven genuine stress incontinence associated with fistulae before repair was nine of 12 with sphincter involvement and five of 14 without such involvement. No patients complained of urge incontinence after surgery if they had stable bladders before repair, that is, there was no evidence of so-called *de novo* detrusor instability after surgery. In Hilton's series, all patients who complained of urgency after repair of their fistulae had abnormal cystometry preoperatively.

The extent of scarring in the area of the bladder neck and urethra may present a challenge to conventional techniques for surgical correction of stress incontinence. Successful anatomic restoration of the urethra is not synonymous with restoration of physiologic function, and incontinence may result. Birkhoff and colleagues and Hilton believe that the reestablishment of continence is facilitated by the use of the Martius interposition flap. In addition, Gray found that 50% of patients in his review were incontinent postoperatively without this added intervention. Authors have not advocated concomitant retropubic suspensions for fear of devascularizing or disrupting the suburethral repair. Preoperative urodynamics has not predicted which patients go on to suffer stress incontinence after fistula repair.

Periurethral injections traditionally have been appropriate in intrinsic sphincter deficiency with a relatively fixed or immobile bladder neck. This technique recently has been reported with initial short-term success in the stress incontinent, postfistula patient. Falandry has had some success with a modified needle suspension procedure in a group of 49 patients. Sixty-three percent were continent at a mean follow-up of 2 years.

CONCLUSION

The literature on urogenital fistulae is extensive, but largely based on small case series and a surgeon's or fistula center's experience with a particular technique. The principles of fistula surgery are well established: visualization of the tract, proper closure, assurance of adequate vascular supply to the repair, and appropriate bladder drainage. The diagnosis of the condition traditionally has been based on clinical methods and dye tests. Modern imaging techniques are increasingly being used in novel ways in other fields, but their utility in the detection of urogenital fistulae does not surpass conventional methods.

Appropriate management regarding timing of repair and surgical approach remains undecided. Minimally invasive approaches seem only appropriate for small, uncomplicated fistulae. Obstetric fistulae remain common in developing countries where access to adequate health care is limited, and fistulae in industrialized nations typically occur after surgery or radiation therapy for gynecologic malignancies.

The role of bladder injury antecedent to fistula formation seems obvious; thus, much of the effort in preventing VVF relies on protecting the bladder at the time of surgery or delivery. The risk of bladder injury is substantially higher at laparoscopic surgery and antiincontinence surgery. Despite preventative measures and good surgical technique, these injuries still occur. Even when recognized and repaired, fistulae may arise. It is likely that fistula formation is multifactorial.

Vesicovaginal and urethrovaginal fistulae represent particularly troublesome complications of obstetrics and gynecologic surgery, but they are no longer as Simpson said: "infirmaries beyond all relief and hope."

ACKNOWLEDGMENT

The authors wish to thank Dr. John D. Thompson for his enormous contribution to the previous editions of this text.

BIBLIOGRAPHY

Abulafia O, Cohen HL, Zinn DL, et al. Transperineal ultra-sonographic diagnosis of vesicovaginal fistula. *J Ultrasound Med* 1998;17:333–335.

Asanuma H, Nakai H, Shishido S, et al. Congenital vesicovaginal fistula. *Int J Urol* 2000; 7:195–198.

Billmeyer BR, Nygaard IE, Kreder KJ. Ureterouterine and vesicourethrovaginal fistulae as a complication of cesarean section. *J Urol* 2001;165:1212.

Birkhoff JD, Wechsler M, Romas NA. Urinary fistulae: vaginal repair using a labial fat pad. *J Urol* 1977;117:595.

Bruce R, El-Galley R, Galloway N. Use of rectus abdominis muscle flap for the treatment of complex and refractory urethrovaginal fistulae. *J Urol* 2000;163:1212–1215.

Carlin B, Klutke C. Development of urethrovaginal fistula following periurethral collagen injection. *J Urol* 2000; 164:124.

Cetin S, Yazicioglu A, Ozgur S, et al. Vesicovaginal fistula repair: a simple suprapubic transvesical approach. *Int Urol Nephrol* 1988;20:265–268.

Collins CG, Collins JH, Harrison BR, et al. Early repair of vesicovaginal fistula. *Am J Obstet Gynecol* 1971;111:524.

Conde-Agudelo A. Intrafascial abdominal hysterectomy: outcomes and complications of 867 operations. *Int J Gynaecol Obstet* 2000;68:233–239.

Cruikshank SH. Early closure of posthysterectomy vesicovaginal fistulae. *South Med J* 1988;81:1525.

De Lamballe J. *Traite des Fistules Vescio-uterines.* Paris: Bailliere, 1852.

Dogra PN, Nabi G. Laser welding of vesicovaginal fistula. *Int Urogynecol J Pelvic Floor Dys* 2001;12:69.

Dotters DJ, Droegemueller W. Diaphragm catheters for vesicovaginal fistula management. *Contemp Obstet Gynecol* 1992;36:45.

Elkins TE, DeLancey JOL, McGuire EJ. The use of modified martius graft as an adjunctive technique in vesicovaginal and rectovaginal fistula repair. *Obstet Gynecol* 1990;75:727.

Elkins TE, Drescher C, Martey JO, et al. Vesicovaginal fistula revisited. *Obstet Gynecol* 1988;72:307.

Evans DH, Madjar S, Politano VA, et al. Interposition flaps in transabdominal vesicovaginal fistula repairs: are they really necessary? *Urology* 2001;57:670.

Falandry L. Vaginal route treatment for residual incontinence after closing an obstetrical fistula: a series of 49 cases (French). *J Gynecol Obstet Biol Reprod* 2000;29:393–401.

Falk H, Orkin L. Nonsurgical closure of vesicovaginal fistulae. *Obstet Gynecol* 1957;9:538.

Falk HC, Tancer ML. After office hours: vesicovaginal fistula. *Obstet Gynecol* 1954;3:337–341.

Fatio J. *Helvetisch-vernunstige Wehenmutter.* (op. posthum.) Basel: 1752.

Fujiwara K, Koshima I, Tanaka K. Radiation-induced vesicovaginal fistula successfully repaired using a gracilis myocutaneous flap. *Int J Clin Oncol* 2000;5:338–344.

Goodwin WE, Scardino PT. Vesicovaginal and ureterovaginal fistulae: a summary of 25 years experience. *J Urol* 1980;123:370.

Gray LA. Urethrovaginal fistulae. *Am J Obstet Gynecol* 1968; 101:28.

Green DE, Philips GL. Case report: vaginal prosthesis for control of vesicovaginal fistula. *Gynecol Oncol* 1986;23:119.

Grody MH, Nyirjesy P, Chatwani A. Intravesical foreign body and vesicovaginal fistula: a rare complication of a neglected pessary. *Int Urogynecol J Pelvic Floor Dysfunc* 1999;10:407.

Hanai T, Miyatake R, Kato Y, et al. Vesicovaginal fistula due to a vaginal foreign body: a case report. *Acta Urol Jpn* 2000;46:141.

Harki-Siren P, Sjoberg J, Titinen A. Urinary tract injuries after hysterectomy. *Obstet Gynecol* 1998;92:113-118.

Hendren WH. Construction of female urethra from vaginal wall and a perineal flap. *J Urol* 1980;123:657.

Hilton P. Urodynamic findings in patients with urogenital fistulae. *Br J Urol* 1998;81:539.

Hilton P. Vesico-vaginal fistula: new perspectives. *Curr Opin Obstet Gynecol* 2001;13:513–520.

Hilton P, Ward A. Epidemiological and surgical aspects of urogenital fistulae: a review of 25 years experience in southeast Nigeria. *Int Urogynecol J Pelvic Floor Dysfunct* 1998; 9:189–194.

Hilton P, Ward A, Molloy M, et al. Periurethral injection of autologous fat for the treatment of post-fistula repair stress incontinence: a preliminary report. *Int Urogynecol J Pelvic Floor Dysfunct* 1998;9:118–121.

Huang S, Yao B, Chou C. Transvaginal ultrasonographic findings in vesicovaginal fistula. *J Clin Ultrasound* 1996; 24:209.

Hurley LJ, Previte SR. Vaginal pedicled flap for closure of vesicovaginal fistula. *Urology* 2000;56:856.

Ibrahim T, Sadiq A, Daniel S. Characteristics of VVF patients as seen at the specialist hospital Sokoto, Nigeria. *West Afr Med J* 2000;19:59–63.

Iselin CE, Aslan P, Webster GD. Transvaginal repair of vesicovaginal fistulae after hysterectomy by vaginal cuff excision. *J Urol* 1998;160:728.

Kelly J. Vesicovaginal and rectovaginal fistulae. *J R Soc Med* 1992;85:257.

Kobashi KC, Dmochowski R, Mee SL. Erosion of woven polyester pubovaginal sling. *J Urol* 1999;162:2070–2072.

Kuhlman JE, Fishman EK. CT evaluation of enterovaginal and vesicovaginal fistulae. *J Comput Assist Tomogr* 1990; 14:390.

Kursh ED, Morse RM, Resnick MI, et al. Prevention of the development of a vesicovaginal fistula. *Surg Gynecol Obstet* 1988;166(5):409.

Latzko W. Behandlung hochsitzender Blasen und Mastdarmscheiden Fisteln nach Uterus Extirpation mit hohom Scheidenverschluss. *Zentralbl Gynakol* 1914;38:906.

Latzko W. Postoperative vesicovaginal fistulae: genesis and therapy. *Am J Surg* 1942;58:211.

Leach GE. Urethrovaginal fistula repair with Martius labial fat pad graft. *Urol Clin North Am* 1991;18:409.

Lee RA, Symmonds RE, Williams TJ. Current status of genitourinary fistula. *Obstet Gynecol* 1988;72:313.

Leissner J, Black P, Filipas D, et al. Vaginal reconstruction using the bladder and/or rectal walls in patients with radiation-induced fistulae. *Gynecol Oncol* 2000;78:356–360.

Leissner J, Black P, Fisch M, et al. Colon pouch (Mainz pouch III) for continent urinary diversion after pelvic irradiation. *Urology* 2000;56:798–802.

Leng WW, Amundsen CL, McGuire EJ. Management of female genitourinary fistulae: transvesical or transvaginal approach? *J Urol* 1998;160:728–730.

Mackenrodt A. Die operative Heilung grosser Blasencheidenfisteln. *Zentralbl Gynak* 1894;18:180.

Madjar S, Gousse A. Postirradiation vesicovaginal fistula completely resolved with conservative treatment. *Int Urogynecol J Pelvic Floor Dysfunct* 2001;12:405–406.

Maisonneuve JG. *Clinique chirurgicale.* Paris: F Savy, 1863.

Marshall VF, Jeffs JD, Sarafyan WK. Urogenital sinus abnormalities in the female patient. *J Urol* 1979;122:508.

Martius H. Die operative Wiederherstellung der vollkommen fehlenden Harnrohre und des Schiessmuskels derselben. *Zentralbl Gynakol* 1928;52:480.

Martius H. *Gynecologic operations and their topographic-anatomic fundamentals.* Chicago: SB Debour, 1939.

McKay HA. Vesicovaginal and vesicocutaneous fistulae: transurethral suture cystorrhaphy as a new closure technique. *J Urol* 1997;158:1513.

Meeks GR, Sams JO, Field K, et al. Formation of vesicovaginal fistula: The role of suture placement into the bladder during closure of the vaginal cuff after transabdominal hysterectomy. *Am J Obstet Gynecol* 1997;177;1298.

Miklos JR, Sobolewski C, Lucente V. Laparoscopic management of recurrent vesciovaginal fistula. *Int Urogynecol J Pelvic Floor Dysfunct* 1999;10:116.

Moir JC. *The vesico-vaginal fistula.* London: Balliere, Tindall & Cox, 1961.

Moir JC. Vesicovaginal fistula as seen in Britain. *J Obstet Gynaecol Br Commonw* 1973;80:598.

Mondet F, Chartier-Kastler EJ, Conort P, et al. Anatomic and functional results of transperitoneal-transvesical vesicovaginal fistula repair. *Urology* 2001;58:882–886.

Morita T, Tokue A. Successful endoscopic closure of radiation induced vesciovaginal fistula with fibrin glue and bovine collagen. *J Urol* 1999;162:1689.

Mulvey S, Foley M, Kelly DG, et al. Urinary tract fistulae following gynaecological surgery. *J Obstet Gynecol* 1998; 18:369–372.

Nesrallah LJ, Srougi M, Gittes RF, et al. The O'Conor technique: the gold standard for supratrigonal vesicovaginal fistula repair. *J Urol* 1999;161:566.

O'Conor VJ Jr. Review of experience with vesicovaginal fistula repair. *J Urol* 1980;123:367.

O'Conor VJ Jr, Sokol JK, Bulkley GJ, et al. Suprapubic closure of vesicovaginal fistula. *J Urol* 1973;109:51.

Ojanuga D, Ekwempu CC. An investigation of sociomedical risk factors associated with vaginal fistula in northern Nigeria. *Women Health* 28:103;1999.

Omo-Dare P. Reconstruction of the urethra for stricture: description and evaluation of a technique. *J Urol* 1970; 103:69.

Ostad M, Uzzo RG, Coleman J, et al. Use of a free bladder mucosal graft for simple repair of vesicovaginal fistulae. *Urology* 1998;52:123.

Pawlik C. Ueberdie Operation der Blasenscheidenfisteln. *Ztschr F Gerburtsh U Gynakol* 1882;8:22.

Persky L, Forsythe WE, Herman G. Vesicovaginal fistulae in childhood. *Urology* 1980;15:36–39.

Pettersson S, Hedelin H, Jansson I, et al. Fibrin occlusion of a vesicovaginal fistula. *Lancet Apr* 1979;28:933.

Pruthi R, Petrus C, Bundrick WJ. New onset vesicovaginal fistula after transurethral collagen injection in women who underwent cystectomy and orthotopic neobladder creation: presentation and definitive treatment. *J Urol* 2000;164:1638–1639.

Ralph G, Tamussino K, Litchtenegger W, et al. Urological complications after radical hysterectomy with or without radiotherapy for cervical cancer. *Arch Gynecol Obstet* 1990;248:61.

Ramaiah KS, Kumar S. Vesicovaginal fistula following masturbation managed conservatively. *Aust NZ J Obstet Gynecol* 1998;38(4):475.

Raz S, Bregg KJ, Nitti VW, et al. Transvaginal repair of vesicovaginal fistula using a peritoneal flap. *J Urol* 1993;156:56.

Raz S. *Atlas of transvaginal surgery.* Philadelphia: WB Saunders, 1992:138–165.

Roth TM, Meeks GR, Blythe J, et al. Massive vesicovaginal fistula associated with a vaginal foreign body: a combined abdominal vaginal repair with gracilis muscle interposition flap. (case report). In press.

Rousseau T, Sapin E, Helardot PG. Congenital vesicovaginal fistula. *Br J Urol* 1996;77:760–761.

Schmidt JD, Buchsbaum HJ. Transverse colon conduit diversion. *Urol Clin North Am* 1986;13:233–239.

Schoenrock GJ, Cianci P. Treatment of radiation cystitis with hyperbaric oxygen. *Urology* 1986;27:271.

Sharma SK, Madhusudnan P, Kumar A, et al. Vesicovaginal fistulae of uncommon etiology. *J Urol* 1987;137:280.

Sims JM. On the treatment of vesico-vaginal fistula (classic articles in *Urogynecology*). *Int Urogynecol J Pelvic Floor Dysfunct* 1998;9:236–248.

Sims JM. On the treatment of vesicovaginal fistulae. *Am J Med Sci* 1852;23:59.

Stovsky MD, Ignatoff JM, Blum MD, et al. Use of electrocoagulation in the treatment of vesicovaginal fistulae. *J Urol* 1994;152:1443.

Symmonds RE, Hill LM. Loss of urethra: a report on 50 patients. *Am J Obstet Gynecol* 1978;130:130.

Tancer ML. Observations on prevention and management of vesicovaginal fistula after total hysterectomy. *Surg Gynecol Obstet* 1992;175:501.

Thomas K, Williams G. Medicolegal aspects of vesicovaginal fistulae. *Br J Urol Int* 2000;86:354–359.

Trendelenberg F. *Uber blasenscheidenfisteloperationen.* Leipzig: Samml Klin Vortrage, 1890.

Volkmer BG, Kuefer R, Nesslauer T, et al. Colour doppler ultrasound in vesicovaginal fistulae. *Ultrasound Med Biol* 2000;26:771.

Von Roonhuysen H. *Medico-chirurgical observations.* London: Moses Pitt at the Angel, 1676.

Waaldijk K. *The surgical management of bladder fistula in 775 women in Northern Nigeria.* Nymegen: Benda BV, 1989.

Wein AJ, Malloy TR, Carpiniello VL, et al. Repair of vesicovaginal and ureterovaginal fistulae by a suprapubic transvesical approach. *Surg Gynecol Obstet* 1980;150:57.

Te Linde's Operative Gynecology, ninth edition, edited by John A. Rock and Howard W. Jones, III. Lippincott Williams & Wilkins, Philadelphia © 2003.

CHAPTER
39

Anal Incontinence and Rectovaginal Fistulas

MICHAEL P. ARONSON   RAYMOND A. LEE

No symptom of pelvic floor dysfunction is more debilitating or has greater psychosocial impact on a woman than that of anal incontinence. The inability to control solid, liquid, or gaseous state stool can have a devastating effect on a woman's feelings of self-worth, her sexuality, and her ability to be an active social participant in her community. The evaluation and treatment of the anally incontinent patient is a challenging but rewarding task because relief of these symptoms can greatly improve the quality of a patient's life. Because the problem of anal incontinence is multifactorial, the approach to the problem often is multidisciplinary, involving health care providers from gynecology, colorectal surgery, and gastroenterology as well as nutrition and physical therapy. Anal incontinence is part of a spectrum of defecatory dysfunction that includes constipation, incomplete emptying of the bowels, urgency, frequency, and painful defecation. Outcomes for treatments should be understood in terms of impact on a patient's symptoms and her quality of life, not purely on anatomic result.

Although anal incontinence has a major impact on a patient's quality of life, most individuals are reticent to discuss this symptom with their health care providers. The prevalence and incidence of anal incontinence is difficult to establish because of underreporting. The lack of a uniform definition further confounds efforts. Fecal in-

continence is often thought of as the inability to control solid or liquid stool, whereas the term anal incontinence encompasses incontinence of gas as well. Nelson et al. reported an overall prevalence in a large, random sample of the general population in Wisconsin of 2.2%, with one third of these individuals being incontinent of solid stool. This figure may be low because their group interviewed only the head of each household and relied on that individual to know whom in their family was continent. In a questionnaire study designed to reflect the age and sex distribution of the adult population of Germany, Giebel et al. found a prevalence of 19.6%, with 4.8% being incontinent of solid stool. They found anal incontinence to be correlated with reduced social activities.

The incidence of anal incontinence is harder to estimate than the prevalence. There are no data regarding the incidence of anal incontinence in the community dwelling population, but Chassagne et al. reported on an elderly, long-term care facility population. They enrolled 1,186 individuals 60 years of age or older who did not have anal incontinence. After 10 months, 20% had developed anal incontinence. They identified five significant risk factors: history of urinary incontinence, neurologic disease, poor mobility, severe cognitive decline, and age older than 70 years.

It is well established that the presence of anal incontinence is associated with the presence of urinary incontinence as well as pelvic organ prolapse. The connective tissue, muscular, and neurologic elements of the pelvic floor function in concert with the organs they support as an interdependent unit to provide multiple functions simultaneously. In a cross-sectional community-based study involving 762 randomly selected women age 50 or older, Roberts et al. found 15.2% had anal incontinence, 48.4% had urinary incontinence, and 9.4% had both. Looked at another way, 59.6% of those with anal incontinence had concurrent urinary incontinence. Among patients presenting to a urogynecology clinic for evaluation of urinary incontinence, a high proportion have dual incontinence defined as concurrent urinary and anal incontinence. Leroi et al. (1999) found 28% of 409 patients in France, and Gordon et al. found 29% of 283 consecutive patients in Israel had dual incontinence. Clearly, the pelvic floor uses some common elements in maintaining continence of feces and urine; it follows that injury to one continent mechanism could also affect the other. An important development has been the beginning of an understanding of the relationship of vaginal birth to the problem of anal incontinence. In a review, Sultan et al. noted a reported 6.6-14% prevalence of anal incontinence in vaginally parous women. Because tools for treatment of this problem have limited success, it becomes important that future research should focus on the prevention of childbirth injuries that can contribute to anal incontinence.

In this chapter we examine the anal continence mechanism and try to understand how it can become damaged. Particular emphasis is placed on the effect of childbirth on the anatomic and neurologic aspects of that mechanism. We then review the evaluation of the anally incontinent patient and look at medical as well as surgical treatment options. Last, we review the etiology, evaluation, and techniques for surgical repair of extraanal incontinence of feces through a rectovaginal fistula.

ANAL CONTINENCE MECHANISM

Normal anal continence requires the coordinated control of multiple elements that act synergistically. They are summarized in Table 39.1. An anatomically and neurologically intact anal sphincter complex is necessary to keep the anal canal closed effectively. Intact anorectal sensation is necessary for the individual to perceive rectal filling and discriminate the nature of the rectal contents. Intact motor innervation is essential so that the sphincter mechanism can respond appropriately to the increased need for anal closure. The puborectalis muscle sling must be anatomically and neurologically intact to create an anorectal angle. The puborectalis muscle must be capable of willful contraction at the moment of need to increase that angle and move rectal contents off the sphincter complex into a capacious and distensible rectal reservoir. Last, gastrointestinal considerations such as colonic motility and stool consistency need to be reasonable for maintenance of continence. The complete interrelated mechanisms of defecation and anal control are

TABLE 39.1.
Mechanisms of Anal Continence

Anatomic
    Anal sphincter mechanisms
    Puborectalis sling/anorectal angle
Neurologic
    Intact pudendal enervation
    Anorectal reflex and sensory mechanisms
Functional
    Stool volume and consistency
    Colonic transit time
    Rectal capacity, distensibility and tone

more easily visualized once the principal elements of the anatomy related to continence are delineated.

Anatomy of the Anal Canal and Related Structures

The anal and rectal regions of the lower colon share a common embryologic origin—the posterior portion of the endoderm of the cloaca. During the development of these regions, the terminal end of the alimentary canal is surrounded by muscular sphincters of somatic origin. Thus, the anorectal region is composed of both visceral and somatic components. The visceral components include the rectum, internal anal sphincter, and lining of the upper part of the anal canal. The voluntary or somatic components are the epithelium of the lower part of the anal canal as well as the striated muscles of the pelvic floor and the external anal sphincter. The rectal mucosa consists of mucus-secreting columnar goblet cells, which invaginate to form tubular glands. The mucosa is surrounded by a muscularis mucosa and an inner circular layer of smooth muscle. This circular smooth muscle layer thickens distally to become the internal anal sphincter. An outer longitudinal layer of smooth muscle transitions distally into fibrous fascicles that travel between the internal and external anal sphincter and insert into the perianal skin, anchoring the sphincter complex and creating the puckering effect one sees on clinical examination.

The anal canal in the female is approximately 2.5 to 4 cm in length and normally remains completely collapsed because of the tonic contractions of the sphincters. Posterior to the anal canal is the coccyx, from which it is separated by intervening fibrofatty tissue. The levator ani muscles are posterior to the canal until it opens onto the perineal skin. The levator muscles also separate the lateral boundary of the anal canal from the ischiorectal fossa, through which pass the important nerves, lymphatics, and blood supply of the terminal rectum, anal canal, and perineum. The canal is fused anteriorly with the lower portion of the rectovaginal septum and perineal body (Fig. 39.1).

The lining of the anal canal is nonuniform. The proximal 1 cm is lined by rectal-type columnar mucosa, fol-

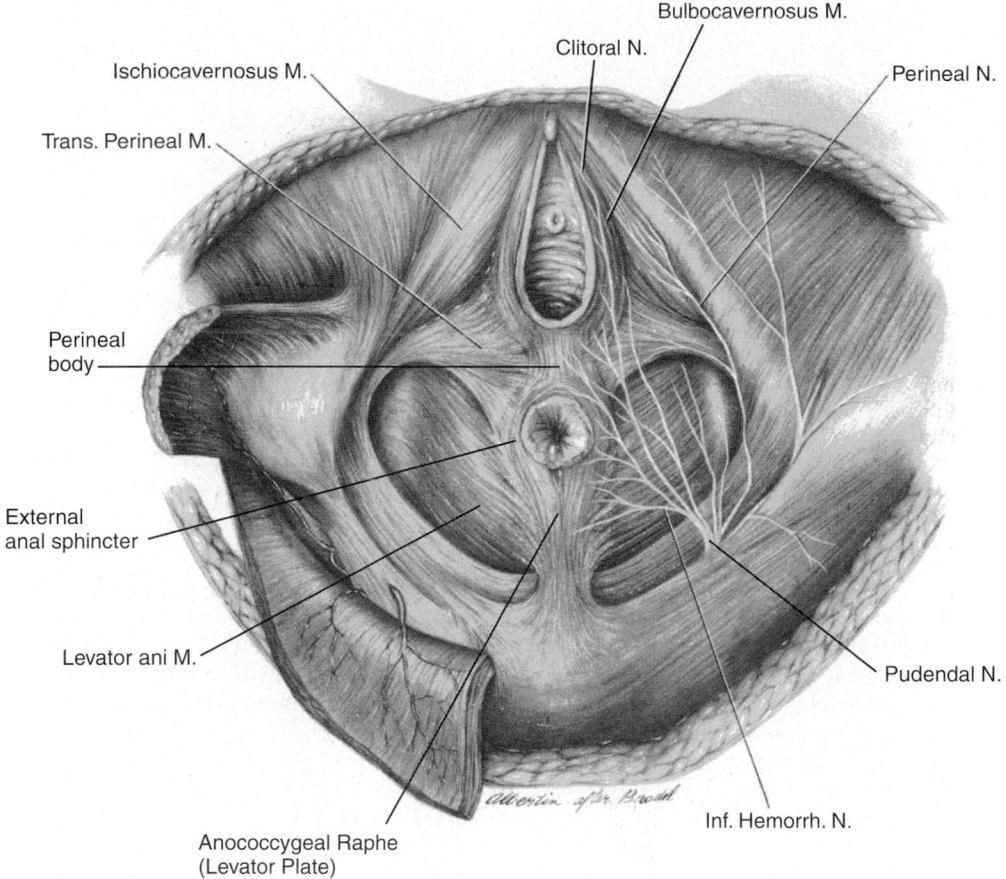

FIGURE 39.1. Location of the anal sphincter in relation to other structures of the female pelvic floor.

lowed by modified or stratified columnar epithelium for about 1.5 cm. The distal half of the anal canal is lined by squamous epithelium, which is richly supplied by branches of the inferior hemorrhoidal nerves and is exquisitely sensitive. As stated, the anal mucosa, like the rectum, also is surrounded by an inner circular layer of smooth muscle followed by an outer longitudinal layer. The longitudinal muscle layer of the anus forms fibrous bundles distally that fan out between the internal and external anal sphincters to gain attachment to the perineal skin. The main blood supply to the rectum and anal canal is from branches of the superior and inferior hemorrhoidal arteries.

The anatomic sphincter mechanism of the anal canal has been a matter of controversy since first described by Galen almost 2,000 years ago. It is most often thought of as consisting of three separate anatomic structures: the internal anal sphincter, the external anal sphincter, and the action of the most medial portion of the levator ani, the puborectalis muscle (Fig. 39.2). The circular smooth muscle layer of the rectal wall, under autonomic control, thickens at the proximal anal canal to form the internal anal sphincter. It can be identified on dissection or at the time of third- or fourth-degree obstetric laceration repair, as a thick fibrous white layer between the anal mu-

cosa and the external anal sphincter. The internal sphincter accounts for about 75% to 85% of the resting tone of the anal canal and is innervated by the autonomic nervous system, providing continuous involuntary muscle tone. The remainder of the resting tone of the anal canal is thought to be provided by the slow twitch fibers of the external sphincter.

The portions of the anal continence mechanism that are under voluntary control are the striated muscles of the external anal sphincter complex and the medial puborectalis portion of the pubococcygeus muscle. The fibers of the pubococcygeus that course behind the anorectum in a slinglike fashion are commonly referred to as the puborectalis muscle. Unlike most other striated muscles, the external anal sphincter and the puborectalis muscle maintain a constant muscular tone that is directly proportional to the volume of rectal contents. The tone of the puborectalis muscle wrapping around posterior to the junction of the rectum and the anal canal produces what is called the anorectal angle. The fibers of pubococcygeus that do not wrap around go on to form the fibrinous anococcygeal raphe, which inserts onto the last two segments of the coccyx. Gynecologists often refer to the anococcygeal raphe as the levator plate. Willful contraction of structurally and neurologically intact pu-

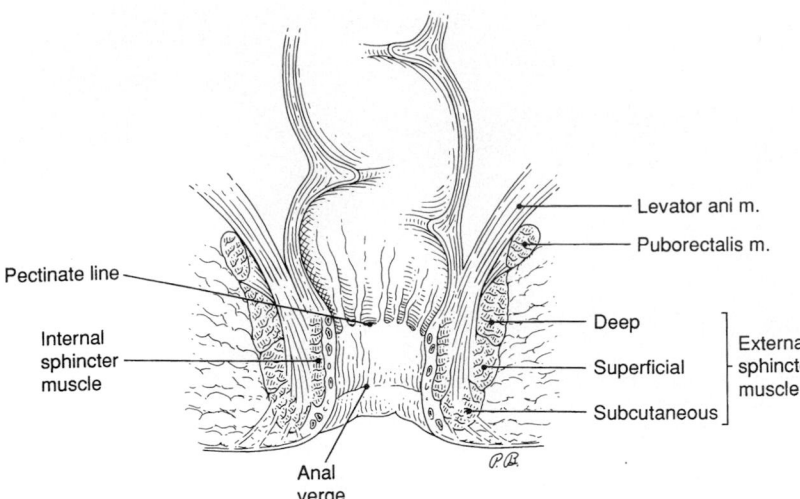

FIGURE 39.2. Diagrammatic illustration of the anal canal and sphincters.

borectalis and pubococcygeus muscles, along with the rest of the levator sling, can increase the anorectal angle and support the levator plate in a horizontal axis to aid in maintenance of continence.

The external anal sphincter complex is thought by different anatomists to be composed of one, two, or three parts. Most anatomists agree, however, that the entire external anal sphincter complex is innervated by perineal

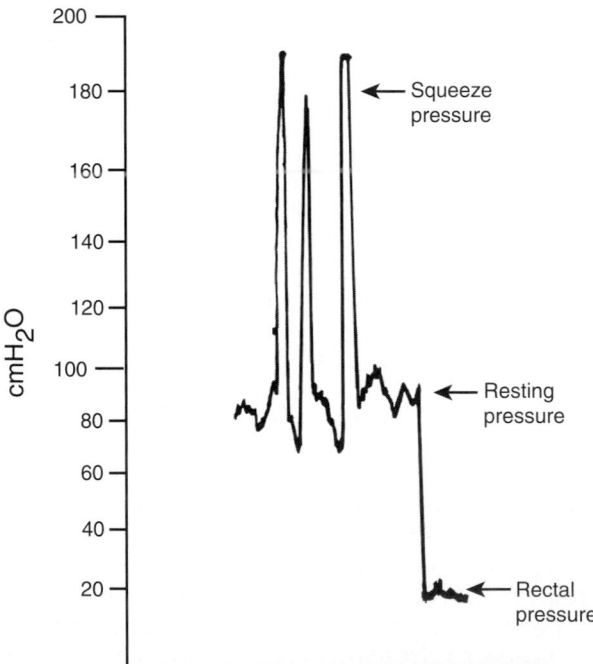

FIGURE 39.3. Anal manometry demonstrating pressures in the anal canal. Rectal pressure reflects intraabdominal baseline pressure recorded in the rectal reservoir. Resting pressure essentially reflects the effect of the involuntary, smooth muscle internal anal sphincter. Squeeze pressure largely reflects the transient contractile effort of the voluntary, striated external anal sphincter.

branches of the pudendal nerves emanating from S2-4. Although some authors refer to a three part sphincter as having superficial, medial, and deep portions (see Fig. 39.2), clinically the entire external sphincter responds to the same innervation and functions as a single unit. The subcutaneous part of the external sphincter is small and inserts on the perianal skin. The superficial part is more substantial and is attached posteriorly through the anococcygeal raphe to the coccyx. The deep portion is intimately related to the puborectalis muscle posteriorly, where its fibers loop around the anorectal junction. The external anal sphincter and puborectalis muscle are responsible for most of the voluntary squeeze pressure that is able to be exerted in the anal canal (Fig. 39.3).

To review, the puborectalis muscle originates from the pubic bone on either side of the midline, passes behind the vagina and rectum, and fuses posteriorly behind the anorectal junction to form a U-shaped sling around the rectum. Some fibers interdigitate with the walls of the anal canal (Fig. 39.4). The constant resting tone of the puborectalis muscle pulls the anorectal junction anteriorly to create an approximately 90-degree angle between the rectum and anal canal and maintains anorectal continence of solid stool by closing the rectal inlet. Both the puborectalis muscle and the external anal sphincter contain a majority of type I (slow twitch) muscle fibers that are ideally suited to maintaining constant tone over time. Each muscle also contains a smaller portion of type II (fast twitch) fibers, which allows them to respond quickly during sudden increases in intraabdominal pressure. The external anal sphincter is innervated by branches of the pudendal nerve (S2-4). The puborectalis muscle is innervated directly by the S3-4 pelvic nerves, as well as some collateral branches of the pudendal nerve.

Classically, the female anal sphincter complex has been thought of as being a broad band of tissue posteriorly but narrowing to a small tubular bundle of tissue anteriorly within the perineal body. The internal sphincter has most often been portrayed as a minor structure in the past. These concepts came from many centuries of anatomic study of cadavers augmented by observations in the delivery room of the transected ends of the anterior portion retracted into round holes in the perineal body at the time of third- and fourth-degree laceration repairs. In the recent past it has become possible to view this anatomy undisturbed in living, continent, nulliparous subjects with magnetic resonance imaging (MRI). In an early MRI study, Aronson et al. found the shape of the combined internal and external anal sphincter complex to be nearly cylindrical as it encircles the anal canal. Measured in the midline the anterior portion of the anal sphincter complex appeared as a broad band of tissue, not a narrow tube. The anterior sphincter complex averaged 1.8 cm in thickness and 2.8 cm in length. Fifty-four percent of the anterior thickness in this study was smooth muscle of the internal anal sphincter. Subsequent studies, including the cadaver studies of DeLancey et al. (1997), found a similar shape with a substantial contribution from the internal anal sphincter. This substantial anterior anal sphincter length and thickness, as well as the contribution from the internal sphincter, is important to keep in mind during primary repair of obstetric lacerations as well as in surgical correction of anal incontinence secondary to a chronic perineal laceration.

The tone of the levator ani muscle is stabilized by the skeletal muscles of the anterior compartment of the urogenital diaphragm, and the bulbocavernosus and transversus perinei muscles, which have a common insertion into the central perineal body between the anus and vaginal introitus. The perineal body is an important anatomic structure that is closely associated with the external anal sphincter and anal canal. The perineal body includes the insertion of two components of the transverse perineal muscles, a superficial and a deep muscle layer, both composed of striated muscle. The central raphe of the perineal body serves as a pivotal point tying in the transverse perineal musculature, the terminal end of the bulbocavernosus muscles, the external anal sphincter and, to an extent, the medial aspect of the levator ani or the puborectalis muscles (see Fig. 39.1). Trauma or separation of the perineal raphe causes relaxation of the perineal body, which is attached to the external anal sphincter. The resulting alteration of attachment may contribute to loss of control of both liquid stool and gas.

Physiology of Anal Continence

Anal continence is dependent on the complex interaction of many physiologic and anatomic factors. Often the focus is on the anatomic and neurologic aspects of continence that obstetricians see damaged in the labor room and try to repair. Many factors important to continence are actually quite distant from the pelvic floor. They can include problems with stool volume and consistency, colonic transit time, rectal capacity, and rectal distensibility. For example, a severe malabsorption syndrome delivering massive quantities of stool of a consistency that is difficult to manage can overwhelm even a normally adequate continent mechanism. The rectum needs to be capacious and distensible to serve as a storage vessel so that the timing of defecation may be consciously deferred. A patient with a radiation-damaged and fibrotic rectum may have lost that capacity. An individual must possess adequate mental faculties to recognize the need for evacuation, as well as sufficient mobility to transfer to an appropriate location for willful defecation, in order to remain continent. Although the relative importance of these factors has not been defined, it seems clear that for the normal patient with a normal consistency and quantity of stool and a capacious, compliant and evacuable rectal reservoir, three factors are crucial for continence—an anatomically and neurologically intact anal sphincter complex, an anorectal angle that can willfully be increased, and intact anorectal sensory and reflex mechanisms.

Function of anatomically intact external and internal anal sphincters is crucial for continence. The voluntarily controlled, striated muscle external sphincter, along with the puborectalis muscle, is responsible for continence at a moment of urgency. The involuntary, smooth muscle internal sphincter maintains continence in the anal canal on an ongoing basis. The relative role of both sphincters has long been a matter of controversy. Some authors believe that the internal anal sphincter primarily preserves continence at rest, whereas the external sphincter maintains continence in response to sudden increases in rectal pressure. To add to the confusion, patients with long-standing total disruption of both sphincters can sometimes maintain good control of solid stool purely with their puborectalis muscle and the use of constipating agents. The puborectalis muscle by itself can only maintain continence of solid feces; the internal and external sphincters in the anal canal maintain continence of liquid stool and flatus. The reader is referred to the excellent review of Dalley for further reading on the relative roles of the sphincters.

Anal continence and function depend on the constant vigilance of the anal sphincter muscles and puborectalis muscles. The maintenance of continuous tone is a quality of these voluntary muscles that is different from other muscles in the body. The level of tone depends on the volume of feces and gas in the rectum and is normally maintained even during sleep. Function of the muscles depends on normal innervation through the pudendal nerve and branches of the pelvic nerves arising from S3 and S4. These nerves may be damaged during vaginal birth, by constant straining with constipation, aging, and a variety of other factors. When anal incontinence is of neurogenic etiology, that is, caused by denervation injury of pelvic floor muscles including the external sphincter, rectal continence is exceedingly difficult to restore with surgery.

As intestinal contents fill the rectum, the constant resting tone of the puborectalis muscle holds the anorectal junction anteriorly to form a 90-degree angle (Fig. 39.4A). This angle is made more acute by the voluntary contraction of the pelvic floor muscles (Fig. 39.5A), and more obtuse by relaxation of these muscle and straining at defecation (Fig 39.5B). It had been suggested that

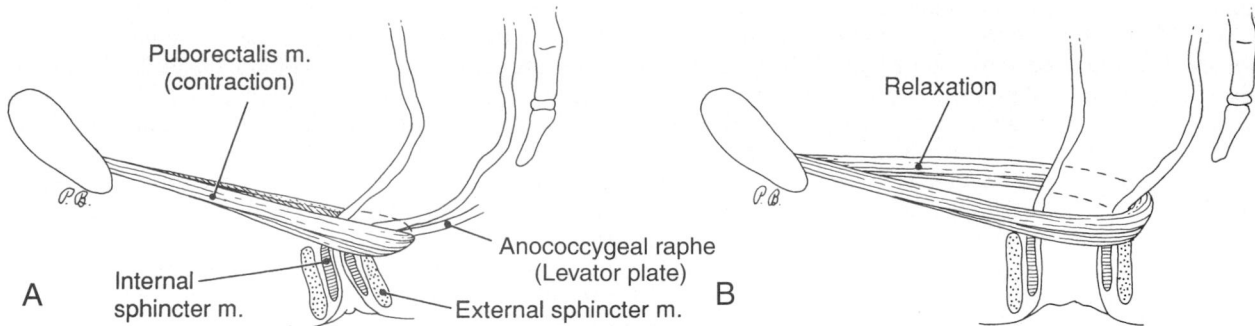

FIGURE 39.4. Function of the anal sphincter and puborectalis muscle. **A:** At rest, the constant tone of the puborectalis muscle pulls the anorectal junction anteriorly to create an approximately 90-degree angle between the rectum and anal canal, closing the rectal inlet and maintaining continence of solid stool. At moments of need this muscle can be contracted further, increasing the angle and supporting the stool bolus over the levator plate. **B:** During defecation, the puborectalis muscle relaxes, opening the rectal inlet, while intestinal peristalsis and the voluntary increase in intraabdominal pressure move stool into the anal canal. The anorectal angle is decreased and the stool bolus is lined up over the anal canal.

this acute angulation compresses the anorectum closed, creating a "flap-valve" effect that may contribute to the maintenance of anal continence. This theory has been questioned recently. Defecography studies have not confirmed the relation between the anorectal angle and anal continence, and the surgical restoration of the normal anorectal junction angle with a postanal repair, or retrorectal levatorplasty, has not been consistently associated with the return of continence.

For defecation to occur, the puborectalis muscle must voluntarily relax while intestinal peristalsis and a voluntary increase in intraabdominal pressure allows the stool to move downward into the anal canal (Figs. 39.4B and 39.5B). Of note is that when denervation of the pelvic floor musculature occurs, the muscles relax, lining up the rectum over the fatigable sphincter complex just as during an act of normal defecation. This relationship is unfavorable to continence and may contribute to in-

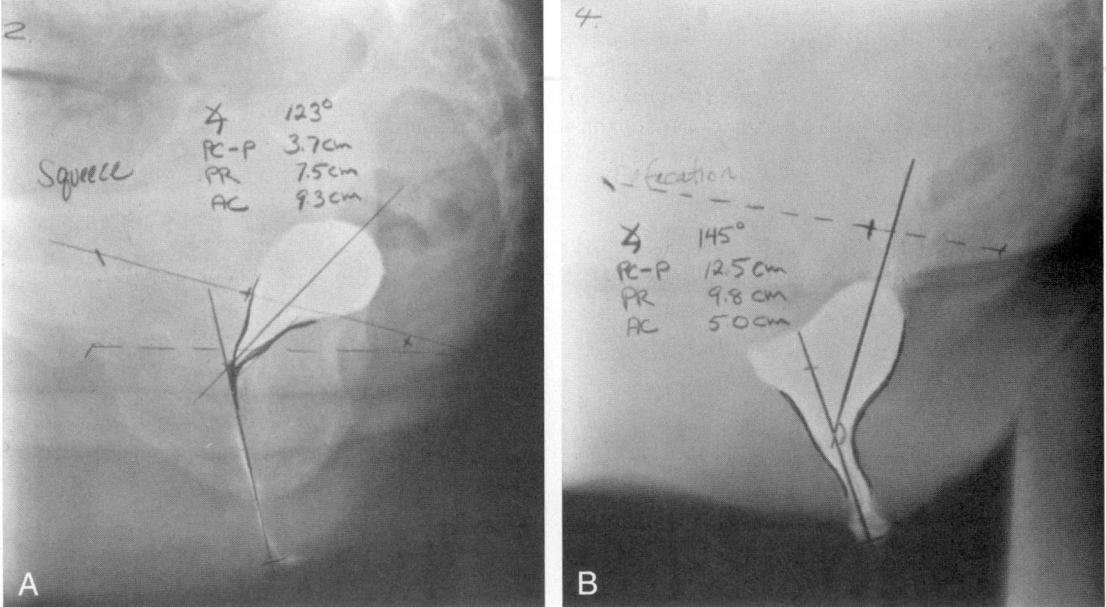

FIGURE 39.5. A: Lateral defecography of normal continent patient deferring defecation by contracting puborectalis sling, increasing anorectal angle, and exerting squeeze pressure in anal canal. Note how barium bolus is supported over levator plate and away from the fatigable anal sphincter complex. **B:** Lateral defecography of normal continent patient willfully defecating by relaxing puborectalis sling, decreasing anorectal angle, and decreasing pressure in the anal canal. Note how barium bolus becomes lined up over anal canal.

continence, especially in patients with compromised sphincter function.

The internal and external sphincters maintain continence below the level of the puborectalis muscle. As discussed, they are particularly important in the control of liquid stool and gas. At rest, the anal canal is kept closed by the baseline tone of the internal sphincter and the constant tonic activity of the external sphincter. When stool enters the rectum, the rectum accommodates or relaxes, allowing it to hold stool until defecation is socially convenient. Stool in the rectum also triggers relaxation of the internal anal sphincter, by the involuntary rectoanal inhibitory reflex, before distention is perceived (Fig. 39.6). This reflex relaxation of the internal sphincter allows the bolus to enter the proximal anal canal where discrimination of the solid, liquid, or gaseous nature of the bolus by the sensory-rich upper anal canal occurs. Subsequently, rectal distention and the presence of stool in the anal canal are consciously perceived, leading to voluntary contraction or relaxation of the pelvic floor muscles to maintain continence or permit defecation, respectively. These two sensory mechanisms, awareness of the degree of rectal distention and the ability to discriminate the nature of intestinal contents, are crucial to maintenance of continence.

As rectal filling continues, the internal sphincter contracts once again to facilitate rectal closure. If defecation or passage of gas is inconvenient, the external sphincter and puborectalis muscle can be firmly contracted. This helps force rectal contents back into a capacious and distensible rectal reservoir supported over the levator plate. Striated muscle such as the external sphincter and puborectalis can only be contracted maximally for approximately 1 minute, and by the end of 3 minutes most of the force of contraction is gone (Fig. 39.7). Injury to the internal sphincter that results in loss of tonicity of the anal canal can permit the involuntary passage of liquid stool and gas. Such an injury is particularly noticeable when the urge to defecate is persistent from a bolus of fecal material in the terminal rectum and when the voluntary contraction of the external sphincter and puborectalis muscle wanes.

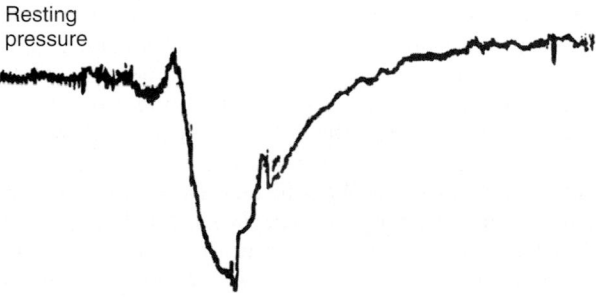

FIGURE 39.6. Rectoanal inhibitory reflex. Arrival of stool in the rectum triggers reflex relaxation of the internal anal sphincter allowing the bolus to enter the proximal anal canal where discrimination of the solid, liquid, or gaseous nature of the bolus by the sensory-rich upper anal canal occurs.

CAUSES OF ANAL INCONTINENCE
The Effects of Vaginal Birth

Although numerous causes are summarized in Table 39.2, in healthy adult women the most common cause of anal incontinence is obstetric injury to the pelvic floor. Vaginal birth may compromise the continence mechanism by direct anatomic injury to the anal sphincters, puborectalis sling, perineal muscles, and perineal fascia. It is now recognized that nerve injury occurs as well. Both of these injuries can lead to some degree of anal incontinence, either separately or in combination.

Damage to the anal sphincters is highly associated with the presence of anal incontinence. Thacker and Banta, in a 100-year review of the literature, reported an anal sphincter rupture rate of 0% to 24% at vaginal birth. Numerous authors have reported in case control studies that 6% to 44% of patients have some degree of anal incontinence after obstetric injury to the anal sphincter, despite immediate surgical repair. Sultan and colleagues (1993) prospectively studied 202 consecutive pregnant women with multiple modalities and found that 35% of

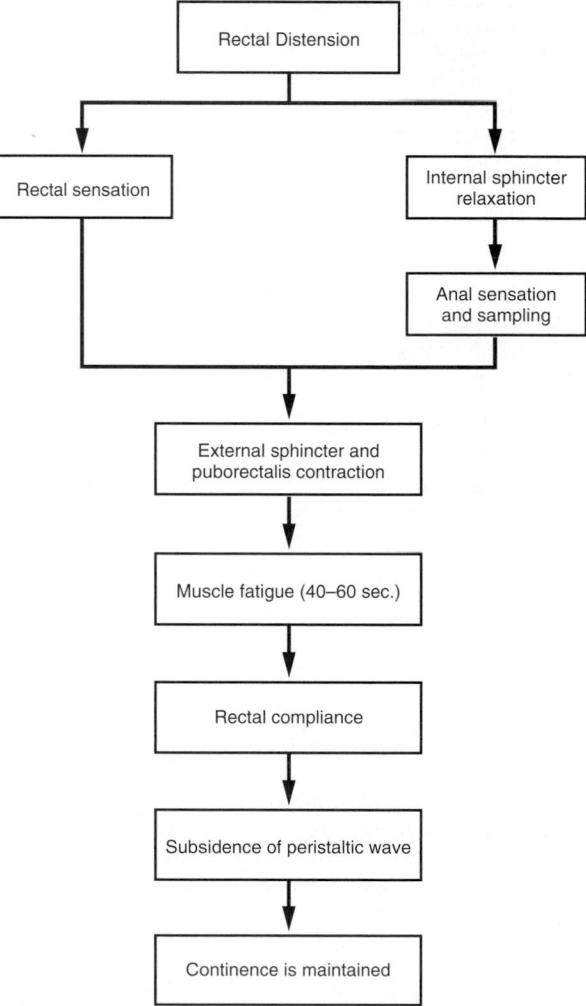

FIGURE 39.7. Algorithm for anal continence mechanism.

TABLE 39.2.
Causes of Anal Incontinence

ABNORMAL PELVIC FLOOR

Congenital anorectal malformations
Obstetric injury
    Third- or fourth-degree perineal lacerations
    Episiotomy breakdown
    Forceps delivery
Operative procedures
    Colpoperineorrhaphy
    Vulvectomy
    Difficult hysterectomy
    Colpotomy drainage of pelvic abscess
    Excision of Bartholin gland
    Hemorrhoidectomy
Trauma
    Impalement
    Pelvic fracture
    Foreign body
    Anal Intercourse
Inflammatory bowel disease
    Crohn's disease
    Tuberculosis
    Granulomatous venereal disease
    Ulcerative colitis
    Diverticulitis
    Perirectal abscess
Malignancy
    Carcinoma of the cervix
    Carcinoma of the vagina
    Carcinoma of the vulva
    Carcinoma of the rectum
Pelvic floor denervation
(idiopathic neurogenic incontinence)
    Vaginal delivery
    Chronic straining at stool
    Rectal prolapse
Aging

NORMAL PELVIC FLOOR

Diarrheal states
    Infectious diarrhea
    Inflammatory bowel disease
    Short-gut syndrome
    Laxative abuse
    Radiation enteritis
Overflow
    Impaction
    Encopresis
    Rectal neoplasms
Neurologic conditions
    Congenital anomalies (i.e., myelomeningocele)
    Multiple sclerosis
    Dementia, stroke, tabes dorsalis
    Neuropathy (i.e., diabetes)
    Neoplasms of brain, spinal cord, cauda equina
    Injuries to brain, spinal cord, cauda equina

---

primiparous women and 44% of multiparous women who delivered vaginally had an internal or external anal sphincter defect present postpartum. None of the nulliparas entering the study had a defect before delivery.

They found anal incontinence in their study population was significantly associated with the presence of a sphincter defect. Interestingly, a number of patients delivered over an apparently intact perineum had postpartum internal or external sphincter defects present on ultrasound, underscoring that the mechanism of these injuries is not completely understood.

Before the late 1980s there was little mention in the literature regarding anal incontinence as a sequela of sphincteric rupture. Hauth and associates reported that midline episiotomies extend to complete perineal lacerations in 4.6% to 8% of cases and state that appropriate repair can be expected to result in healing in 99% of cases with no subsequent problem with anal incontinence. It is now clear that sphincteric rupture occurs not infrequently and represents a serious injury that may have long-term consequences for the individual involved. In a study of 808 vaginally delivered women in Sweden, Zetterstrom et al. found sphincter tears detected at delivery to be associated with nulliparity (odds ratio [OR] 9.8: 95% confidence interval [CI] 3.6, 26.2), midline episiotomy (OR 5.5: 95% CI 1.4, 18.7), fundal pressure (OR 4.6: 95% CI 2.3, 7.9), postmaturity (OR 2.5: 95% CI 1.0, 6.2), and increased fetal weight (OR 1.3: 95% CI 1.1, 1.6). Of their subjects with primarily repaired sphincters, 54% reported at least "mild" anal incontinence at 5 months and 41% still had symptoms at 9 months postpartum.

The advantages and disadvantages of midline episiotomy have long been debated. Shiono and associates, using data from the Collaborative Perinatal Project, reported that midline episiotomy was associated with statistically significant 4.2-fold and 12.8-fold increases in the risk of third- and fourth-degree lacerations among primiparous and multiparous women, respectively. Studies by Green and Soohoo, Wilcox and associates, and Thorp and associates all suggest that midline episiotomy is associated with an increased risk of injury to the anal sphincter. Numerous authors have noted an association of the performance of midline episiotomy with third- or fourth-degree laceration even when other factors are controlled for. The suggested benefits of midline episiotomy include substitution of a routine straight surgical incision for an occasional ragged laceration; prevention of perineal, anal, and rectal trauma; prevention of pelvic relaxation; and reduction in the length of the second stage of labor. The Collaborative Perinatal Project data, however, indicated that 10% of women who had a midline episiotomy had a severe laceration. Shiono and associates believe that the risks and benefits of midline episiotomy as practiced in the United States should be reevaluated, especially because midline episiotomy may cause rather than prevent lacerations. Mediolateral episiotomy results in less risk of sphincter trauma but is not widely practiced in the United States. Data from Sultan (1993) and others suggest an association between sphincter rupture and the use of forceps, to a greater degree than with the use of vacuum, for assisted delivery.

The obstetric repair of a third- or fourth-degree laceration represents a primary surgical procedure that has significant implications for the patient's quality of life and can often leave a patient with some degree of incontinence; therefore, attention has begun to focus on the repair procedure itself. All who have attended at vaginal birth know that these lacerations often are repaired in the delivery room where conditions such as lighting, exposure, anesthesia, and asepsis are less than optimal. In addition, these injuries often are repaired by individuals of varying experience. The standard repair is taught most often as an end-to-end repair of a narrow tube of external anal sphincter with little attention being paid to possible internal sphincter damage. Evaluations of patients treated with current repair techniques have demonstrated unsatisfactory outcomes. Poen et al. reported on long-term clinical and functional results of standard primary repair of third-degree lacerations. They found significantly diminished squeeze pressures and increased first sensation of filling and anal mucosal electrosensitivity compared to controls. Forty percent of their study population had anal incontinence 5 years after repair. Eighty-eight percent of these subjects had a sphincter defect on anal endosonography. In a prospective cohort study of women after primary repair of anal sphincter laceration, Kammerer-Doak et al. found significantly decreased resting and squeeze pressures in study subjects versus controls. Forty percent of study subjects were found to have sphincter defects present on ultrasound despite primary repair, and a trend toward continued anorectal dysfunction was found in the laceration group.

The idea of a different repair using an overlapping technique for the external anal sphincter with a separate repair of the internal anal sphincter is the subject of some research interest at present. The internal sphincter can be identified as a band of white fibrous-appearing tissue between the anorectal mucosa and external sphincter. Sultan et al. (1999) published an initial experience with such a repair in 32 patients performed by two experienced surgeons with the patient moved to a well-lit operating room, given adequate anesthesia, and antibiotics. At follow-up all had apparent healing, 8% encountered incontinence of flatus, 15% had persistent external sphincter defects on ultrasound, and 44% had persistent internal sphincter defects. Fitzpatrick et al. prospectively randomized 112 primiparas who suffered a third-degree laceration to overlapping versus approximation repair. At 3 months they found no statistically significant difference in incontinence scores, anal manometry, or endoanal ultrasound. Interestingly, 66% of all subjects had a residual full-thickness defect present in their external anal sphincter regardless of type of primary repair. Further studies of these repair techniques are ongoing. In general, however, results may be improved in repair of obstetric sphincteric rupture by optimizing standard surgical considerations, including lighting, exposure, adequate anesthesia, use of antibiotics, and proper aseptic surgical technique.

Every effort should be made to perform a careful and complete repair of anal sphincter lacerations and to recognize and repair associated defects in both the internal and external anal sphincters and rectal mucosa. On occasion, the rectal mucosal repair breaks down, which can result in rectovaginal fistula. In Hibbard's series of 24 rectovaginal fistulae and 27 chronic perineal lacerations, 47 (92%) were caused by obstetric trauma. Additional studies by multiple authors support these high rates of obstetric trauma as an etiologic factor for anal incontinence. Even meticulously repaired lacerations occasionally completely break down, leaving the patient with an open cloacal deformity. Anal incontinence usually is a problem for these patients until the tissues are healed sufficiently to allow secondary repair. Even defects that do not completely break down and appear to have healed satisfactorily may have some persistent structural defects revealed by ultrasound. Most obstetric injuries are located in the anterior segment of the external anal sphincter. Even if the defect is properly repaired, ultrasound studies often demonstrate partial separation of the muscle fibers during healing. As noted by DeLancey et al. (1997), the resulting small defect may have a profound effect on the subsequent function of the anal sphincter, because there are no other muscles in this region that can compensate for the damage.

A second cause of persistent incontinence, even after successful anatomic repair of the anal sphincter, is denervation injury to the sphincter muscles. Snooks and colleagues (1984) demonstrated that there is physiologic evidence of denervation of the sphincter in 60% of patients with anal incontinence and an obstetric tear. In women who did not sustain any injury to the external sphincter during delivery, 42% had evidence of denervation. These denervation injuries were strongly associated with a prolonged second stage of labor, forceps delivery, and a large fetus, suggesting that the mode of injury of the pelvic nerves may be either from the stretching of the nerves during descent of the pelvic floor or from ischemic injury or the direct compression of the nerves. Most of these individuals reinnervate their pelvic floor over the first 6 months postpartum with improvement in their anal function, but many do not regain full neurologic function. At present there is no way to predict who will regain function. Much of what used to be termed idiopathic anal incontinence is now understood to be neurogenic anal incontinence.

Other Causes

In addition to obstetric trauma, anal incontinence may result from a number of other causes, as outlined in Table 39.2. These are common causes, but a promoter of incontinence over time is the fact that the normal process of aging results in decreased efficiency of the anal sphincter complex. Haadem et al. showed a natural decline with aging in resting and squeeze pressures in the anal canal in continent subjects. With increasing age, the internal sphincter generates a lower resting pressure and the proportion of fibrous tissue increases. The squeeze pressure able to be exerted by the external sphincter suffers a natural decline as well. Increasing age also is associated with prolonged pudendal nerve terminal motor latencies and elevated rectal and anal sensory thresholds. Because of this, many patients with damaged continent mechanisms may be able to compensate for this damage and remain continent until the natural decline of function with age unmasks their condition.

Functional problems of the bowel such as constipation or diarrhea can result in incontinence. Chronic constipation with its repeated straining at stools can cause stretch-induced injury to pudendal innervation. Overall, the most common cause of anal incontinence in the elderly, particularly those who are institutionalized, is fecal impaction with overflow incontinence. A diarrheal state can result in anal incontinence even in a patient with normal anorectal function, owing to the presence of large quantities of liquid stool that may overwhelm a normally functional mechanism. Neurologic disorders affecting sphincter control also may result in anal incontinence. Usually, the neurologic defect is widespread, and anal incontinence is but one manifestation.

Traumatic injury, more often a side-straddle injury in young girls, may result in simple or extensive laceration of the perineum. The extent of the injury may be difficult to determine because of pain, fear, edema, hemorrhage, and hematoma formation. Examination under anesthesia is advisable so that appropriate repair can be made, looking carefully for lacerations of the anal sphincter and rectum as well as other structures. Hematoma dissection above the levator muscles must be ruled out with pelvic ultrasound and with careful rectovaginal examination under anesthesia; above the levator muscles, there is nothing to impede the progression of a hematoma until the diaphragm is reached.

Rectal trauma from operative procedures can affect rectal capacity and compromise anal continence or perhaps lead to extraanal incontinence through a rectovaginal fistula. Entry into the rectum may occur during posterior colpoperineorrhaphy, especially when the anterior rectal wall and posterior vaginal walls are closely adherent with little, if any, septum between. Such an enterotomy should be repaired transversely if longitudinal closure would compromise rectal capacity. A difficult hysterectomy, either abdominal or vaginal, may result in injury to the rectum, especially when dissection behind the cervix is difficult because of dense adhesions, indurated tissue from infection, or involvement of the cul-de-sac and anterior rectal wall with endometriosis. If the rectal defect does not heal properly or is not closed properly, a high rectovaginal fistula may develop through the newly closed vaginal apex. Partial excision of anal sphincter and other muscles involved in maintaining anal continence may be required in extensive vulvectomy for cancer, and anal incontinence may result as reported by Berek and associates. Injury to the anterior rectal wall may occur during hemorrhoidectomy, excision of a Bartholin's gland, and colpotomy for pelvic abscess drainage.

Crohn's disease is the most important of the variety of inflammatory bowel diseases that may cause rectovaginal fistulae. Among 138 patients with rectovaginal fistulae seen at Duke University Medical Center, Bandy and associates reported that 15 (11%) were caused by Crohn's disease. The diagnosis, perioperative management, and surgical technique chosen for these patients constitute a special challenge for the gynecologic surgeon. Crohn's disease must be considered as a possible cause of rectovaginal fistula in any patient in whom other causes are not clear, particularly if the fistula orifice is tender to palpation. Crohn's disease also should be considered in the patient who has failed multiple attempts at fistula repair because the fistula tends to recur at the operative site in these individuals.

The role of diverticulitis as a cause of sigmoidovaginal fistulae has been highlighted by Tancer and Veridiano who report on 130 cases of sigmoidovaginal fistulae owing to diverticulitis. These fistulae usually present with a malodorous vaginal discharge in women older than 50 years of age, some years after a hysterectomy. Such fistulae commonly develop between the inflamed bowel segment and the apical vaginal scar from the previous hysterectomy, although they may infrequently occur through a retained cervix. Often, the diverticular disease is silent and is only discovered with further investigations of the fistula tract. A diverticular abscess may have formed and found drainage though the path of least resistance, which in this case is the thinned out scar of the vaginal cuff.

Malignant tumors may erode through the tissues between the vagina and the rectum. When a patient with tumor involvement of the rectovaginal wall receives radiation, sloughing of the tumor may result in a rectovaginal fistula. Radiation also may cause a rectovaginal fistula without tumor erosion.

Finally, anal incontinence may be idiopathic in about 10% of women. As stated, the mechanism of incontinence in these women is usually owing to pelvic floor denervation. This has been confirmed by studies demonstrating prolonged pudendal nerve terminal motor latencies in these patients. These individuals may present with a patulous anal sphincter, passive stretching of the puborectalis muscles, and a long history of straining with constipation. Forty percent to 60% of patients with rectal prolapse also have some degree of anal incontinence. Although this was originally thought to be secondary to a dilatation effect on the internal anal sphincter, there is evidence of associated neurogenic damage to the external sphincter muscles as well. Rarely, anal incontinence may be congenital, as seen in one of 5,000 newborn girls who have an imperforate anus with associated fecal incontinence through a congenital rectovaginal or rectoperineal fistula. Total rectal agenesis is rare. Paul and Lloyd reported hindgut duplication with a congenital rectovaginal fistula; however, most anal incontinence is acquired.

In summary, although an intact and functional anal sphincter complex and puborectalis sling are important in the maintenance of anal continence, it must be remembered that a variety of other factors are involved including intact anorectal sensation and reflexes, rectal capacity and distensibility, reasonable colonic transit time, appropriate stool volume and consistency, and adequate patient mental function and mobility.

EVALUATION OF ANAL INCONTINENCE

Over the past two decades, there have been several technologic advances in the development of objective radiologic and physiologic tests for the evaluation of anal incontinence. A careful history and physical examination are vital to eliciting the cause of, and guiding the management of, anal incontinence. Diagnostic tests such as anal endosonography, anal manometry, pelvic floor electromyography (EMG), and defecography can document the presence and severity of sphincter weakness. In addition, anal endosonography and defecography may uncover anatomic defects and gastrointestinal abnormalities not previously appreciated by physical examination alone. All of these objective studies are valuable as research tools and have done much to increase our understanding of anorectal anatomy and function; however, their clinical role still remains somewhat unclear. Ultrasound can be very useful in determining the presence of a segmental sphincter defect. Many of the above studies may prove most useful in patients with idiopathic anal incontinence or persistent incontinence after a failed surgical repair.

History and Physical Examination

Patients are reticent to discuss problems with anal incontinence. The gynecologist should enable the patient to overcome feelings of embarrassment by bringing the topic up in conversation during the taking of the history. Faltin et al. recently surveyed 666 patients in a general gynecologic outpatient clinic in Switzerland and found that 5.6% had anal incontinence. Of those individuals, only 20% had ever reported this symptom to a health care provider. For this reason, multiparous and elderly women should always be asked specifically about symptoms of anal incontinence in a nonthreatening way that invites discussion. The gynecologic examination always should include careful inspection of the posterior vaginal wall, perineum, anal sphincter, anal canal, and rectum, including assessment of the patient's function as well as her anatomy.

Once the history of defecatory dysfunction is elicited, the examiner should attempt to differentiate true incontinence from other conditions. Perianal leakage of material other than stool can occur because of prolapsing hemorrhoids, anorectal neoplasms, or sexually transmitted diseases. Poor hygienic practice can lead to patients noting fecal staining after bowel movements that does not truly represent anal incontinence. Anorectal frequency and urgency without the loss of bowel contents may occur in patients with inflammatory bowel disease, irritable bowel syndrome, and prior pelvic irradiation. In patients in whom the diagnosis is in doubt, the ability to retain an enema argues strongly against severe anal sphincter weakness.

The severity of the incontinence should be assessed by determining the frequency of leakage of gas, liquid stool, or solid stool, as well as the need for a perineal pad. The frequency and consistency of the stools also should be noted, preferably with a visual scale written form. Symptom diaries and questionnaires can be useful in helping to delineate a patient's problem. The effect of incontinence on quality of life can be ascertained by inquiring which activities patients have curtailed to avoid anal incontinence. Dietary habits should be discussed.

Screening for associated medical conditions such as diabetes mellitus, neurologic problems, and medication use should be included in the initial evaluation. Past surgical and obstetric history should be carefully reviewed for any prior gastrointestinal or anorectal surgery, number of vaginal deliveries, a history of prolonged labor, use of forceps, and significant perineal lacerations.

Physical examination should include a general screening neurologic examination in every patient to look for occult neurologic disease. Anal incontinence is rarely the presenting symptom in patients with spinal cord lesions. Pelvic examination should include a careful inspection of the perineal body and the posterior vaginal wall, along with palpation of the interdigitating perineal and levator muscles, anal sphincter, and rectum. A careful examination often reveals abnormalities. A gaping anus indicates a major loss of sphincter function and often is associated with rectal prolapse. Most obstetric injuries are associated with an anterior segmental defect in the external anal sphincter. This may appear as the loss of the perineal body and attenuation of the rectovaginal septum in some cases. In more subtle cases, the perineum was repaired and healed, but the anal sphincter beneath was either not repaired or did not heal when repaired. In such cases, in which the external sphincter is separated but the perineum is intact, there are no sphincter muscle fibers anteriorly; instead, there are only the dimples of the laterally retracted ends of the anal sphincter muscles. This produces a "dovetail" appearance, as described by Toglia and DeLancey, in which the normal radial distribution of the anal creases is absent anteriorly but is present laterally and inferiorly. If there is a question as to the presence of a segmental defect, endoanal or transperineal ultrasound can be useful in delineating the anatomy.

Next, a screening evaluation of the perineal reflexes to assess the integrity of the S2-4 dermatomes should be performed. Perception of pinpoint and light touch over the perineal skin and buttocks can be tested easily with the broken end of a wooden cotton swab or a safety pin. Light stroking of the inferolateral margin of the labia majora should cause a reflex contraction of the bulbocavernosus muscle within the labia. The anal wink reflex can be elicited by lightly stroking the perianal skin or touching it with a pin to cause a reflex contraction of the external anal sphincter. Asking the patient to cough also should elicit the reflex contraction of the external anal sphincter. With both of these maneuvers, the anal canal should constrict concentrically owing to contraction of the external sphincter, and the anus should be pulled inward secondary to the contraction of the puborectalis muscle. In women with separation of the external anal sphincter, voluntary contraction of the pelvic floor muscles causes an accentuation in the lateral perineal dimpling of the retracted ends. In patients with a denervated sphincter, there is no retraction of the anal skin during voluntary contraction. Patients who demonstrate abnormalities of these pelvic floor reflexes may require more in-depth neurologic evaluation.

Extraanal incontinence may come through a fistulous tract. A rectovaginal fistula is usually easily diagnosed by careful inspection of the posterior vaginal wall. By spreading the labia, a low fistula can be revealed, usually involving the area of a previous episiotomy or obstetric laceration. A high fistula can be seen using a bivalve speculum and often appears at the vaginal cuff scar. A straight-handled speculum can be useful because it can be rotated to allow full visualization of the anterior as well as posterior vaginal walls. The vaginal opening of a fistula may be localized by the presence of feces in the vagina or by the dark red rectal mucosa seen protruding at the fistulous opening, contrasting with the lighter vaginal mucosa. Colposcopic examination of the vagina sometimes assists in the identification of a small fistula orifice. When the fistula is small, it may be difficult to locate both the vaginal and rectal ends of the fistula, but both orifices must be located for complete care to be given. A small probe can be pushed gently from the vaginal side of the fistula and the tip felt on a rectally placed finger. Instillation of methylene blue through the vaginal orifice of the fistula may aid in the proctoscopic visualization of the rectal orifice. Carey describes the following examination technique to identify a suspected rectovaginal fistula. A Foley catheter with a 10-mL balloon is inserted into the anus while the posterior vaginal wall is painted with a concentrated solution of soap and water or, alternatively, the vagina can be filled with water. As the rectum is distended with air by a syringe attached to the Foley catheter, the vaginal orifice of the fistula may be localized by the presence of bubbles forming at the fistula site. A small probe may then be passed along the fistula tract.

Alternatively, when a rectovaginal fistula is suspected but cannot be identified, radiologic studies such as a vaginogram or fistulogram may identify a fistulous tract. These studies are superior to barium enema for identifying a fistula because they use a thin, water-soluble radioopaque medium rather than a thickened barium solution. Furthermore, although fistulae occasionally may be identified by barium enema, the intraluminal pressure of the bowel often is inadequate to force the barium solution through a small fistula opening. In addition, the presence of barium in the lower bowel may obscure a fistula tract.

When a rectovaginal fistula is diagnosed, it is important not to limit the evaluation to just identification of the fistulous tract but to complete a thorough assessment of the anal sphincter and pelvic floor because these patients may have multiple defects. If not properly evaluated preoperatively, the patient may undergo successful repair of her fistula only to become anally incontinent postoperatively. Her compromised sphincter function may have been adequate preoperatively when excess pressure was bypassing the sphincter through the fistula. After her fistula is repaired and the full force of rectal contents is delivered to the sphincter complex, there may not be adequate function to keep the patient continent. A full treatment of rectovaginal fistula management appears later in this chapter.

A thorough digital rectal examination should be performed after bimanual examination and careful inspection of the posterior vaginal wall. Any rectal mass must be noted and the stool consistency assessed. A gross assessment of the patient's resting and squeeze pressures within the anal canal, and her ability to contract her levator ani muscles should be included in every examination. Anal sphincter tone should be evaluated with the patient at rest and during sphincter contraction. An anterior sphincter defect may be easily detectable as the loss of the palpable muscular ring within the perineal body. Even in the absence of external anal sphincter muscle anteriorly, a scarified band of tissue can remain that completes the contractile ring and helps the patient maintain continence. Next, the anorectal axis can be assessed. On rectal examination, the puborectalis muscle is palpable posteriorly at the junction between the rectum and the anal canal. By directing the examining finger posteriorly, the angle between the anus and rectum can be estimated and should approximate 90 degrees in a normal woman. More important, when the patient is asked to squeeze the sphincter, the puborectalis muscle should pull the examiner's finger anteriorly toward the pubic bone.

The cause of anal incontinence can be identified in most cases by using these guidelines for careful evaluation of the perineum, posterior vaginal wall, pelvic floor muscles, external anal sphincter, and rectum. In the young parous patient, obstetric injury to the anterior anal sphincter complex is apparent most often on physical examination. One exception is that the integrity of the internal anal sphincter cannot be assessed adequately by physical examination alone but can be determined by radiologic and physiologic tests. A defect of the internal sphincter can be assumed, however, if there is significant thinning of the rectovaginal septum. In many of these cases, both the internal and external anal sphincters are injured. Certainly the patient with a cloacal deformity by definition has a segmental defect in both sphincters. From a practical and technical viewpoint, the internal anal sphincter cannot be repaired unless the external sphincter also is repaired, and surgery is rarely indicated for an isolated defect of the internal sphincter. When surgical repair of the external anal sphincter is indicated, however, one should consider repairing defects in the internal sphincter as well, although data regarding internal sphincter repair are, at present, scant and inconclusive.

Testing

After taking a history and performing a physical examination, there may be questions about a particular patient that thoughtful testing can answer. Is a segmental defect present in the internal or external anal sphincter? What is the functional status within the anal canal? Is rectal sensation normal? Is the innervation to the striated musculature of the continent mechanism intact? How does the patient actually defecate: Are rectoceles, enteroceles, or sigmoidoceles interfering? Is intussusception involved? Clearly many patients will have a diagnosis and be ready to proceed to treatment after their history and physical examination. For others, the picture will be less clear. Judicious use of testing based on the information needed to arrive at an accurate diagnosis and to plan successful treatment can be important.

Anal Imaging

Endoanal, transvaginal, and transperineal ultrasound techniques have made it easy and relatively inexpensive to identify defects in both the internal and external anal sphincters. These defects can go clinically unrecognized but may be amenable to surgical repair. Anal endosonography is a radiologic technique for assessing posttraumatic defects of the internal and external anal sphincters. High-resolution images of the separate sphincter muscles can be obtained using a rotating 7-MHz endoprobe. Anatomic defects can be identified as a loss of continuity of the muscle rings. Several studies have found that anal endosonography correlates well with needle EMG mapping of sphincter defects, manometric mapping of sphincter defects and with intraoperative findings. Ultrasound is less time consuming than EMG or manometry and much more comfortable for the patient. Other studies have established that transvaginal ultrasound is equally efficacious to endoanal ultrasound in identifying sphincter defects. Finally, Peschers et al. described normal sphincter and puborectalis anatomy as well as defects in both the internal and external sphincters using exoanal ultrasonography: a conventional 5-MHz convex transducer placed on the perineum. Ultrasound currently is the study of choice for establishing the presence or absence of a segmental anal sphincter defect. The approach chosen—endoanal, transvaginal, or transperineal—may depend on the equipment available and operator expertise.

Although endoanal ultrasound identifies anatomic defects or thinning of the internal anal sphincter, Heyer et al. showed that interpretation of external sphincter images is much more subjective and confounded by normal anatomic variations in the external anal sphincter. Indeed the external anal sphincter and perirectal fat are both echogenic and frequently indistinguishable; the external sphincter may be asymmetrical in the upper anal canal, particularly in women. A new imaging modality with better soft-tissue definition may be desirable. Magnetic resonance imaging (MRI) may prove to be superior to endoanal ultrasound because of high tissue contrast between the external anal sphincter and the perirectal fat. DeSouza et al. reported 100% concordance between MRI performed with an endoanal coil and surgical findings for presence, size, and location of anal sphincter tears in seven patients with obstetric trauma. Additionally, Lienemann et al. and Healy et al. have demonstrated that MRI also can define dynamic pelvic floor motion during defecation and squeeze. Rapid image acquisition is crucial for optimal visualization of dynamic motion, particularly because patients cannot maintain rectal expulsion or puborectalis contraction for more than 15 to 30 seconds. Prospective comparisons of endoanal MRI to endoanal ultrasound and barium defecography in anally incontinent subjects are in progress.

Although MRI is very effective at delineating the soft-tissue anatomy related to anal continence, whether it is performed with a body coil, phased array coil, endovaginal coil, or endoanal coil, the high cost of scanning, limited access to scanners, and the complexity of the examination itself keep MRI largely a research modality at present. This is especially true since ultrasound is now relatively inexpensive, widely available, and easy for the patient. MRI's exquisite soft-tissue differentiation and capability for multiplanar imaging makes it an excellent research modality for studying these structures undisturbed in living patients. Its clinical role in relation to anal incontinence is emerging.

Anal Manometry

Anal manometry provides information regarding function, sensation, compliance, and the presence of intact reflexes within the anal canal and distal rectum. The first part of this test is essentially a pressure profile of the anal canal, providing information on the functional status of the internal and external anal sphincters. Some computer-based, multichannel manometry equipment can provide graphic cross-sectional analysis of the anal canal to help detect the presence of segmental sphincter defects.

The test usually is performed with the patient in the left lateral decubitus position without any special bowel preparation. There are many different protocols for performing anal manometry. Most commonly, a fluid-filled pressure catheter with radial side ports located every 0.5 cm longitudinally and 90 degrees apart circumferentially connected to pressure transducers and a recording device is used to measure the anal canal pressures during rest and during voluntary contraction of the anal sphincter (Fig. 39.8). These pressures may be recorded either as the pressure catheter is slowly pulled continuously through the anal canal—a station pull-through technique—or at static points along the anal canal as the pressure catheter is pulled out in certain increments, usually every 0.5 cm. The average pressure measured at rest in the anal canal is the resting pressure and the highest pressure recorded along the anal canal with the patient at rest is the maximum resting pressure. The increase in

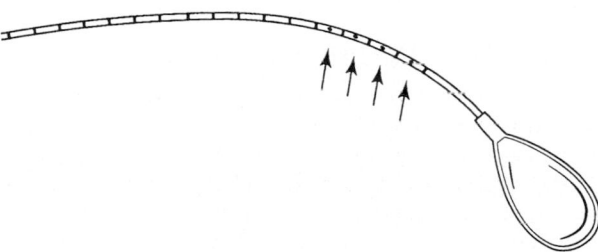

FIGURE 39.8. Anal manometry perfusion catheter. An open-tipped perfusion catheter with radial side ports located every 0.5 cm (*arrows*) records anorectal pressures. Distention of the balloon at the end of the catheter is used to determine rectal sensory thresholds and to elicit the rectoanal inhibitory reflex.

pressure over the basal canal pressure initiated by voluntary contraction of the anal sphincter is the squeeze pressure, and the highest such increment is the maximum squeeze pressure. The resting anal canal length is measured from the point at which the anal sphincter pressure continuously exceeds the average intrarectal pressure by 4 mm Hg. The resting pressure is largely a reflection of the internal anal sphincter function, whereas the squeeze pressure reflects the strength of the external anal sphincter voluntary contraction (Fig. 39.3).

A second part of anal manometry testing is the evaluation of rectal sensation. A balloon is placed in the rectum and incrementally distended. The minimum perceived volume, the volume causing the urge to defecate, and the maximum tolerable volume are recorded. Measurements of pressures within the balloon allow the calculation of rectal compliance. The presence of a reflex rectal contraction after a bolus of air is introduced into the balloon, followed by the return to normal baseline pressures as the rectum accommodates, also is noted. Most healthy patients have a minimal perceived volume of about 30 cc, and a maximum tolerable volume of about 300 to 350 cc, although this can be highly variable. When the rectal capacity is <200 cc, however, proctitis is often found.

"Normal" range for maximum resting pressure is 60 to 120 cmH_2O and for maximum squeeze pressure is 100 to 200 cmH_2O; however, there is tremendous overlap in values between patients who are continent and those who are incontinent. As a group, incontinent patients have lower values on anal manometry testing than continent patients, although there is no discriminatory level that can be used to predict incontinence. It has been suggested that patients with a maximum resting pressure of <20 cmH_2O and a maximum squeeze pressure of <40 cmH_2O are unlikely to be continent. Sentovich et al. found decreased resting and squeeze pressures in 90% of patients with a history of anal sphincter injury. Poen et al. found significantly decreased maximum squeeze pressures, and also found first sensation of filling to be significantly increased, in 40 subjects who had third-degree lacerations primarily repaired compared to controls. They also found that 35 (88% percent) of these subjects still had sphincter defects present on endoanal ultrasound despite apparently successful healing of their repair.

Pelvic Floor Electromyography

Pelvic floor EMG evaluates the pelvic floor muscles for evidence of nerve injury. The smallest functional neuromuscular unit is the motor unit, and injury to nerves or muscles produces characteristic changes recorded in the motor unit action potential. Concentric needle EMG involves placing a small needle with a recording electrode into the muscle being studied. The firing pattern of the motor units is assessed as the needle is being inserted, during spontaneous muscle activity, and during maximum voluntary contraction of the muscle. The characteristics of the recordings then can be evaluated. Single-fiber EMG allows the recording of action potentials from individual muscle fibers of a motor unit. When nerve injury occurs there is often reinnervation but with a change in fiber density. The reinnervation is more diffuse and results in less effective muscle contraction than the original active innervation. When these studies indicate nerve reinnervation, therefore, it reflects prior nerve damage that has healed. Needle EMG studies also can be used to map specific anatomic defects of the external anal sphincter but, as stated, this function currently is more often served by ultrasound studies.

Nerve conduction velocities, which are the actual speed of conduction of the action potential along the nerve, are another measure of nerve function. The nerve conduction velocity can be calculated by measuring the nerve latency, which is the delay between the stimulation of the nerve at a specific point and the response in the target muscle supplied by the nerve. Standardized latencies for most peripheral nerves have been established. Evaluation of pudendal nerve terminal motor latency (PNTML), as developed by Snooks and colleagues, is of interest in patients with anal incontinence. The pudendal nerve is stimulated as it courses behind the ischial spine into Alcock's canal and the time is measured until a response is detected in the external anal sphincter. Prolonged PNTMLs indicate nerve damage; however, this test only reflects the conduction time of the healthiest axon remaining in a nerve. Therefore, normal PNTMLs do not confirm a lack of damage to the whole nerve, only that at least one axon remains intact that can conduct a response normally. Cheong et al. found pudendal neuropathy in 36% (bilateral 21%, unilateral 15%) of 225 patients (174 women) presenting with anal incontinence. Osterberg et al. found a correlation between fiber density and clinical and manometric variables in 72 incontinent patients (63 women), but failed to find a correlation with PNTML. Vaccaro et al. found pudendal neuropathy to be an age-related phenomenon in patients with anal incontinence and constipation. A finding of prolonged PNTML may be of clinical significance; however, normal PNTMLs do not exclude the possibility of neurologic damage. Although PNTML testing is in use by many centers, it may lack sensitivity and specificity for detection of external anal sphincter weakness caused by pudendal nerve damage. The American Gastroenterological Association's (AGA) medical position statement on anorectal testing techniques of 1999 states that "although interesting from a research point of view, the clinical usefulness of this test is controversial. . . . The PNTML cannot be recommended for evaluation of patients with fecal incontinence."

Although suggestion of neurologic injury may be identified by careful physical examination, neither ultrasound nor anal manometry is helpful in identifying neuropathic patients. Identification of such patients is important. In the presence of neurologic damage patients are less likely to have a good functional response to operations designed to restore anal incontinence, even when the anatomic result appears completely successful. Knowledge of a patient's pelvic floor neurologic status can be particularly useful for counseling her on what to expect after surgical repair. Although the presence of pudendal neuropathy implies a poorer prognosis for the potential sphincteroplasty patient, it does not mean that many such patients could not derive significant improvement in their continence. Chen et al. found in a small group of patients undergoing sphincteroplasty that, based on continence scores, the one patient with no neuropathy had an excellent result; of seven patients with unilateral pudendal neuropathy 70% had a good to excellent result and 30% had a fair to poor result; whereas in four patients with bilateral neuropathy, half had a good to excellent result and the other half scored fair to poor.

Defecography

Defecography is a radiologic evaluation of the lower gastrointestinal tract. It was used initially in the evaluation of patients with defecation disorders, but more recently it has been used as part of the evaluation of anal incontinence. The rectum of the patient is filled with a barium-oatmeal or potato starch paste mixed to a consistency to approximate semisolid stool. The patient then is seated on a special commode chair and asked to defecate during fluoroscopy. Lateral radiographs usually are taken before, during, and after evacuation of the rectum (Fig. 39.5). Alternatively, cinedefecography can be performed, which is a videotaped dynamic fluoroscopic study.

The anorectal angle can be observed, as can the effect of willful contraction of the puborectalis muscle on this angle. It also provides information about rectal emptying and the mobility of the rectal wall. Anatomic abnormalities of the gastrointestinal tract not previously identified, such as intussusception, rectal prolapse, and rectal ulcers, can be detected by defecography. Now it is possible to perform a triple contrast study wherein the rectosigmoid, small bowel, and bladder are all opacified with contrast. These studies often reveal disturbances of dynamic pelvic floor motion and interaction of support defects in more than one compartment, for example, rectoceles, sigmoidoceles, enteroceles, and cystoceles.

In relation to anal incontinence, however, the clinical relevance of many of these findings is questionable because there are no findings that are specific for anorectal incontinence. Many of the anatomic abnormalities are also found in asymptomatic controls. Although the anorectal angle may be more obtuse in incontinent patients both at rest and during squeezing than in continent patients, recent studies have questioned the significance of the anorectal angle because of the wide overlap in measurements between the two groups. In addition, there is a significant intraobserver variation in the measurement of the anorectal angle from the same set of radiographic films among different radiologists. Last, surgical restoration of the angle with a postanal repair, or retrorectal levatorplasty, is poorly correlated with a return of continence. Therefore, the role of defecography in the evaluation of patients with anal incontinence is unclear.

In summary, because anal continence depends on multiple mechanisms, no one test is ideal for clinical evaluation of the incontinent patient. There is not a standard testing protocol for the anally incontinent patient. Testing should be individualized. Studies should be obtained only to gather specific information needed in the evaluation of an individual patient. Procedures thought by the AGA to be of value in selected patients follow: (a) symptom diary for diagnosis and monitoring of progress; (b) digital examination for basic qualitative assessment of resting and squeeze pressures; (c) anal ultrasound to assess anatomic integrity of the sphincters; (d) anorectal manometry to define sphincter weakness and predict response to biofeedback training; (e) rectal and anal sensory testing; and (f) testing of rectal compliance. Procedures of possible value for an individual patient might include: (a) surface EMG for evaluation of sphincter function and evacuation proctography; or (b) cinedefecography, when rectal prolapse is suspected. Testing procedures that are controversial for the clinical evaluation of anally incontinent individuals at present include: (a) pudendal nerve terminal motor latency testing for assessment of pudendal nerve function; and (b) MRI, because of its expense.

NONSURGICAL THERAPY OF ANAL INCONTINENCE

Although surgical therapy often is indicated in cases of anal incontinence, especially when there is a discrete anatomic defect in the neurologically intact anal sphincter mechanism, nonsurgical therapies also may be effective in these patients as well as in those with evidence of pelvic floor denervation. The goal of nonsurgical therapies is to minimize the threat to continence from intestinal contents by manipulating stool consistency and to maximize the patient's remaining sphincter function. Dietary manipulations and pharmacologic agents may reduce flatus and liquid stools, and pelvic floor exercises, biofeedback therapy, and transanal electrical stimulation facilitate maximization of anal sphincter function. Some early data imply a possible role for the use of sacral nerve stimulation as well.

To reduce the challenge to the sphincter mechanism, all conditions producing diarrheal states, such as inflammatory bowel disease and malabsorption syndromes, should be treated directly. For constipated patients, a high-fiber diet and the addition of an osmotic laxative (e.g., sorbitol 1 to 2 q.d. or b.i.d.), may produce soft, formed stools that are more easily managed by a compromised sphincter mechanism. Conversely, for patients with diarrhea, a low-residue diet to reduce stool bulk and constipating agents such as loperamide or diphenoxylate with atropine often are helpful. Patients should avoid foods that cause intestinal hypermotility as well as carbonated beverages and foods that tend to produce flatus. Many patients learn on their own that constipation helps them with continence and maintain themselves in a constipated state for many years before presenting to a health care practitioner. Santoro et al. studied amitriptyline for both its ability to slow colonic transit time resulting in a firmer stool that is passed less frequently, as well as improve pressure dynamics in the rectal reservoir. They found significant improvement in symptoms as well as manometric parameters in the study group. In some patients, a system of planned defecation with the use of glycerol suppositories or a daily tap water enema may leave the rectum clean between evacuations and decrease incontinence episodes.

Pelvic floor rehabilitation through physiotherapy with biofeedback, pelvic floor exercises, and transanal electrical stimulation may help improve anal sphincter function. These techniques are particularly helpful in patients with mild pelvic floor denervation to maximize the strength and function of the sphincter mechanism and levator sling. Rehabilitation techniques may be useful as an initial conservative measure in patients with recent obstetric trauma and evidence of pelvic floor nerve injury. Some reinnervation tends to occur over the first 6 months postpartum in these patients. Those who are not able to willfully contract their pelvic floor muscles immediately postpartum because of transient nerve injury may best benefit from electrical stimulation techniques. Pelvic floor rehabilitation may be useful preoperatively to try to maximize the outcome of a subsequent surgical repair. Patients who are improved but not totally continent after surgical repair also may benefit from these techniques to restore their margin of continence.

Pelvic floor exercises, similar to the Kegel exercises performed to improve urinary incontinence and pelvic support, may improve the functioning tone of the external anal sphincter. Biofeedback therapy using an anal balloon or plug electrode can facilitate the proper muscle contraction by measuring the strength of the sphincter contraction and by providing the patient with a visual demonstration of muscle function. Biofeedback therapy also has the advantage of being able to train patients to perceive decreasing volumes of air in the rectum and to coordinate this with the contraction of the external anal sphincter. Biofeedback therapy has been reported to improve anal incontinence in 50% to 90% of patients treated, with most studies showing improvement in about 80% of patients. Some effects of biofeedback training may be long-lasting in relation to anal incontinence. Enck et al. (1995) studied anally incontinent patients treated with biofeedback versus controls almost 10 years after treatment ended. They did not find a lasting difference in prevalence of anal incontinence but did find a significant difference in severity of incontinence measured in number and frequency of incontinent episodes. The success of biofeedback therapy seems primarily dependent on the improvement in rectal sensation; manometric studies have not consistently shown an increase in sphincter pressures after therapy. Suitable candidates for biofeedback therapy must have some degree of rectal sensation and be able to contract the anal sphincter voluntarily.

Transanal electrical stimulation can be used as an adjunct to pelvic floor exercises in patients who are unable to contract their pelvic floor muscles or who are unsuccessful with biofeedback therapy alone. An anal probe connected to a neuromuscular stimulation unit delivers a preset voltage to the external anal sphincter to induce contraction of the striated sphincter muscles. This technique causes minimal patient discomfort and has been associated with a significant increase in the MSP following therapy, with subsequent improvement in partial anal incontinence. It has not been successful in patients with major incontinence to solid stool. Transanal electrical stimulation also is unlikely to be successful in patients with a severely denervated anal sphincter because of the degree of irreparable end-organ damage. Such patients are likely to require surgical attention with an artificial anal sphincter, a gracilis muscle neoanal sphincter, or perhaps fecal diversion. In several recent reports, sacral neuromodulation has shown promise in treating urinary retention and urge urinary incontinence resistant to medical therapy. Two early reports of small groups of patients with anal incontinence by Matzel et al. and Malouf et al. have shown improvement in continence with sacral nerve stimulation.

SURGICAL THERAPY FOR ANAL INCONTINENCE

Most patients with anal incontinence who see an obstetrician-gynecologist present with a specific anatomic defect resulting from obstetric or postoperative trauma. These patients suffer from a long-standing disruption of the perineal body and anterior anal sphincter complex often called a chronic perineal laceration (Fig. 39.9). Approaches to the surgical repair of this problem are discussed at length in this chapter. The treatment of patients with idiopathic, neurogenic, or recurrent incontinence without an anatomic defect present requires more specialized care and more advanced procedures. These patients are most often referred to a colorectal surgeon or proctologist with a special interest in this area. Although a full discussion of these more difficult patients is beyond the scope of this chapter, some background is given for perspective. Papers that discuss surgical results for anal incontinence procedures most often use significant improvement on an incontinence scoring system scale as their criterion for success because total continence of solid, liquid, and gas occurs much less frequently. These procedures most often are measured on their impact on an individual's symptoms and quality of life.

In the mid-1970s, Sir Allan Parks proposed the postanal repair to treat idiopathic anal incontinence. The concept was to plicate the levator ani together behind the anorectal junction to increase the anorectal angle and augment what was proposed as a "flap valve" mechanism for continence involving the levator plate. Since that time, the idea of a flap valve mechanism has been discredited. Long-term results of the postanal repair have been disappointing. Keighley (1984) studied 105 patients who underwent this operation. With a follow-up

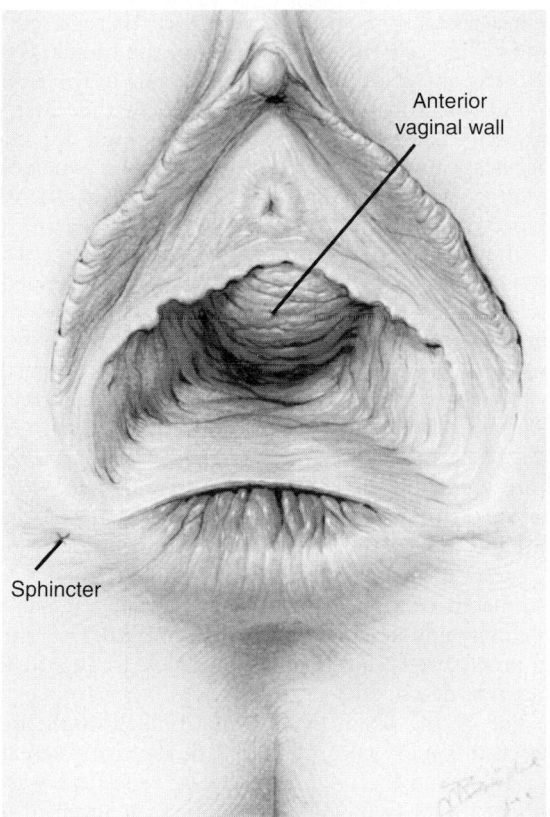

FIGURE 39.9. Chronic perineal laceration. Long-standing disruption of the perineal body and anterior anal sphincter complex usually secondary to obstetric trauma in the past. When the posterior vaginal wall heals directly to the anterior rectal wall above the hymenal ring, this is termed a cloacal deformity. Note the dimples on either side of the anal opening owing to the retraction of the ends of the torn external sphincter.

of at least 6 months he found that two thirds had regained continence. Studies with long-term follow-up are less encouraging. Based on a significant decrease in incontinence scores Matsuoka et al. (2000) found postanal repair successful in seven of 20 (35%) patients after a mean follow-up of 3 years. Setti Carraro et al. (1994) studied 34 postanal repair patients with a mean follow-up of 6.2 years. They found that only nine (26%) had continence of solid and liquids and five of the nine still leaked flatus. Recognizing that improvement, if not total continence, may be a significant goal, it is important to note that 28 of the 34 subjects assessed their outcome as improved, with the remainder relating no change.

A total pelvic floor repair has been proposed for these patients that involves a postanal repair, a plication of the levator muscles anterior to the rectum, as well as a sphincteroplasty. This operation was studied by Deen et al. (1993) in a prospective, randomized trial. A total pelvic repair was compared to anterior levator plication plus sphincteroplasty alone as well as to postanal repair alone. They found at 6 and 24 months a significantly better outcome for the total pelvic repair than for either of the other two procedures.

Muscle plasty procedures exist in which the gracilis muscle or gluteus muscle are swung as flaps to encircle the anal canal. Dynamic muscle plasty procedures involve stimulation of this muscle with an intramuscular neurostimulator to induce it to convert to the characteristics of normal external anal sphincter muscle. The muscle is continuously stimulated at a low frequency for 8 to 10 weeks until the transformation from a fast-twitch to a slow-twitch muscle has been achieved. At this point, the frequency of stimulation is increased so that the muscle contracts around the anal canal and occludes it continuously. When the patient wishes to defecate, the pulse generator can be turned off by a magnet. Once defecation is complete, the stimulator can be turned on again by the magnet. These are advanced procedures reserved for patients with difficult anal incontinence problems or multiple operative failures. In a series of 20 patients, reported by Hallan and associates, 12 have a functioning neoanal sphincter. Madoff et al. (1999) found a 70% reduction in solid stool incontinence in two thirds of patients undergoing a dynamic graciloplasty. However, one third of these patients experienced a major wound complication with their surgery.

Some investigators have used an artificial urinary sphincter around the anal canal in patients with severe anal incontinence. Although the initial results were good in a small series of patients, cuff erosion into the anal canal and infection have been significant problems that have caused a number of the sphincters to be removed. Last, for the patient with uncontrollable anal incontinence that cannot be addressed by any other procedure, a diverting colostomy may be a more manageable and preferable alternative to constant perineal soiling and the hygienic and social problems that it brings.

Chronic Perineal Laceration

In most cases of chronic perineal laceration with long-standing disruption of the anterior anal sphincter complex, classic symptoms include the progressive loss of control of gas and feces from the anus. The severity of symptoms generally varies with the degree of perineal laceration and sphincter loss. If the puborectalis muscle is left intact and is well innervated and functional, it can provide sufficient muscular contraction to permit control of feces when the patient is constipated or when the stool is of normal consistency. Such patients quickly learn this and maintain a constipated state in order to decrease their symptoms.

When the tear extends well above the external and internal anal sphincters, the high pressure zone of the anal canal is completely lost and gas and feces may escape at all times. A complete perineal laceration through the anal sphincter and possibly through the anorectal mucosa occurs not infrequently during vaginal delivery and must be recognized and adequately repaired at that time. If total anatomic reconstruction is not achieved, symptoms may develop within the first 7 to 10 days after delivery if not immediately. With injury to the internal or external anal sphincter, symptoms are usually those of incontinence of intestinal gas and liquid stool. Incontinence of solid stool occurs more commonly with complete breakdown of the perineal body, separation of the entire sphincter, and extension of the tear through the rectal mucosa (a fourth-degree perineal tear), particularly if the puborectalis muscle is compromised. If the entire perineal body is disrupted, including the internal and external anal sphincters, and the posterior vaginal wall heals directly to the anterior rectal wall above the level of the hymenal ring, then the patient is said to have a cloacal deformity (Fig. 39.9).

If repair at the time of delivery breaks down, it has been taught traditionally that a second attempt should be deferred for a minimum of 8 weeks to provide sufficient time for resolution of the inflammatory response, return of an adequate blood supply to the margins of the defect, and return of optimum viability of the perineal tissues. This delay also may allow time for some reinnervation to occur if the injury also was associated with pelvic floor denervation injury. A careful physical examination and perhaps a proctoscopic examination, should precede the second attempt so that the presence of an occult rectovaginal fistula can be excluded.

In order to avoid 2 months of uncomfortable symptoms, some surgeons have advocated an earlier repair. The results of early repair of an external anal sphincter and rectal mucosal dehiscence were first reported in 1986 by Hauth and associates. Each patient was seen within 10 days of delivery with dehiscence of a repaired fourth-degree laceration. Each patient underwent preoperative mechanical bowel preparation on admission, preoperative wound cleansing and debridement appropriate to the extent of superficial inflammation and necrosis, and preoperative intravenous antibiotic therapy. A range of 1 to 6 days elapsed to allow preparation of the wound area before a layered closure was performed. The bowel was rested for 10 days after the repair. Seven of eight cases were successfully repaired, with complete healing, normal external sphincter function, and no dyspareunia. Similar good results with early repair of dehiscence of fourth-degree episiotomy in 22 patients were reported by Hankins et al. The average hospital stay for debridement, intravenous antibiotic therapy, and repair was 15 days. Two patients developed pinpoint rectovaginal fistulae after early repair. Secondary repair in both cases was successful. The results of early repair of dehiscence after mediolateral episiotomies, as opposed to midline episiotomies, have been reported by Monberg and Hammen.

A number of techniques have been described over the past 100 years for reconstruction of a complete chronic perineal laceration, including the layered method of repair, the Warren flap procedure, and the Noble-Mengert-Fish operation. Today, some form of layered method of repair is performed most often. If the anorectal mucosa is intact and the injury is largely limited to the anal sphincter complex and perineal body, repair consists of anal sphincteroplasty with extensive perineorrhaphy. If the injury extends into the anal canal and involves the anorectal mucosa, this approach would essentially recreate a fresh fourth-degree perineal laceration, which would then be repaired in a standard layered fashion. Therefore, the initial layer of such a repair would include a suture line in the anorectal mucosa. Today in the antibiotic era this does not represent a significant problem, although infectious complications do occur. However, this was a major disadvantage to the layered approach in these patients in the preantibiotic era.

The Warren flap method, first described in 1882, avoids a mucosal incision in the anus, provides a pedicle graft of vaginal mucosa for enlargement of the perineal skin, and provides a more cosmetic result to the perineal body. However, the Warren technique offers no particular improvement in the results of the surgical correction of the muscular defect that produced the anal incontinence. The major advantage of the procedure is that a suture line is not created in the anal mucosa. With the Warren technique, the vaginal mucosa is turned backward and used as the new portion of the anterior wall at the end of the anal canal. The anal sphincter then is reapproximated over the inner portion of the vaginal flap, which remains attached to the anal mucosa. The Warren flap procedure is still used, although less frequently than when first described.

The Noble operation, or anal pull-through procedure as it is more commonly called, also avoids creating a suture line in the anal mucosa. The procedure was described originally in 1902 by Noble, but received little attention until described again independently by Mengert and Fish in 1955. Noble's original claims for the operation in the surgical era before the availability of antibiotics, blood banks, and modern advances in general anesthesia included: (a) elimination of the danger of infection or fecal matter from the rectum in the surgical wound; (b) avoidance of the tediousness of dissecting a vaginal flap; (c) minimal blood loss; and (d) uniformly good results. The most important advantage was the absence of a suture line in the anterior rectal wall. Although performed much less frequently than a layered approach today, interest in this operation remains, particularly for the treatment of rectovaginal fistula. Veronikas et al. reported a 94% anatomic success rate and 77% excellent functional success rate in 34 patients treated with this operation for primary and persistent rectovaginal fistulae.

Regardless of which approach is taken to repair of a chronic perineal laceration in the patient with anal incontinence, it is the sphincteroplasty itself that is the keystone to the repair. In the following we discuss techniques of anal sphincteroplasty as well as these three general approaches to overall repair of a chronic perineal laceration. The surgeon should keep in mind that the anal sphincteroplasty may be the most important part of the overall repair when transanal fecal incontinence is part of the indication for the operation.

Anal Sphincteroplasty

The anal sphincter complex is a surgical challenge to repair because both the internal and external sphincters have a constant tone that begins pulling against the healing area almost immediately. Functional results from this surgery are far from perfect. The overlapping repair was proposed for the external anal sphincter in the hopes that the scarified ends of the torn sphincter would bolster support for the reparative sutures and not allow them to pull through, resulting in a better anatomic result and, hopefully, better functional results. The advantage in terms of outcome seems to favor the overlapping approach over the end-to-end approximation method; however, more data clearly are needed in this area. Past studies of these operations are difficult to evaluate because the criteria for what constitutes success or cure often are poorly defined. Total continence of solid, liquid, and gaseous state stool often is not achieved. Again, improvement in continence and quality of life may represent the best outcome measure.

Blaisdell in an older report, and Arnaud in a more recent one reported success rates of approximately 60% using the end-to-end approach. Using the overlapping technique, Sitzler and Thompson reported a 74% success rate in 27 women, most of whom had obstetric sphincter injuries. The success rates for anal sphincter repair in patients with concurrent pudendal neuropathy are much lower than for those with intact innervation. Also, the continence rates after anal sphincteroplasty appear to diminish with time. Rothbarth et al. reported on 39 patients who had obstetric injuries and underwent overlapping sphincteroplasty. Their success rates were 77%, 67%, and 62% at 3, 9, and 12 months, respectively. They also found that patients with prolonged PNTMLs had significantly poorer outcomes.

The effect of pudendal neuropathy was striking in the study of Gilliland et al., who looked at a large group of patients who had undergone an overlapping sphincteroplasty with a median follow-up of 2.4 years. They found that 62% of 59 patients with normal pudendal function had a successful outcome, compared to only 17% of the 12 patients with unilateral or bilateral prolonged PNTMLs. A look at the degree and quality of long-term continence after sphincteroplasty was provided by the recent report from Malouf et al. from St. Mark's Hospital in the United Kingdom. They studied patients with a minimum of 5 years' follow-up (median 77 months) and found that 23 of 46 patients (50%) had a successful outcome with success being defined as no further surgery and episodes of urge fecal incontinence occurring once a month or less. Of the 23 patients judged to have a successful outcome, eight had no passive soiling, six had no fecal urgency, four were continent of solid and liquid stool, and none were fully continent of stool and flatus. Karoui et al. found success rates to deteriorate with time. They reported that poor results also were associated with the presence of an internal sphincter defect.

The importance of the internal anal sphincter to continence is a subject of recent interest. It has long been known that this structure contributes most of the resting tone in the anal canal and helps to maintain our day-to-day continence. Purposeful lateral disruption of the internal sphincter to aid with anal fissure healing has been shown to be associated with the development of at least transient incontinence. Vaizey et al. have identified primary degeneration of the internal sphincter as an independent cause of passive anal incontinence in some women with normal neurologic function and no obstetric trauma. It follows that repair of a disrupted internal sphincter should contribute to continence.

Little attention has been paid in the past to repair of the internal sphincter either at the time of initial obstetric injury or at the time of reconstruction of a long-standing injury. Repair of this smooth muscle structure that is tonically contracting against the suture line is more of a challenge in the healing phase than it is to actually accomplish in the operating room. Preliminary reports regarding this repair are mixed. Abou-Zeid reported on eight patients (two women) who had their ultrasonically established internal sphincter defects repaired end-to-end with 2-0 Vicryl. At a median follow-up of 15 months, all were improved and two achieved full continence. On the other hand, Leroi et al. (1997) reported on five patients with persistent incontinence after surgery that affected the internal sphincter. Three patients felt improved but none were fully continent. All had persistent defects on ultrasound postoperatively. Three had improvement of their resting pressure but only one was in the normal range. In a randomized trial addressing internal sphincter repair during total pelvic floor repair for anal incontinence, Deen et al. (1995) showed no differences in resting and squeeze pressures or in symptom relief.

Layered Method of Repair of Chronic Perineal Laceration

A transverse or crescent perineal incision is used at the junction of the posterior vaginal wall and anal mucosa. The lateral margins of the incision are extended to the region of the perineal dimple created by the retracted external sphincter, and a midline incision is made along the lower half of the posterior vaginal wall (Fig. 39.10A).

The edges of the vaginal and rectal mucosa are grasped separately with Allis clamps, and the anterior rectal wall is separated in the midline from the posterior vaginal wall with careful scissors dissection. The dissection is carried laterally by sharp dissection to the region of the external anal sphincter. The internal anal sphincter, which is the thickened distal condensation of the circular smooth muscle layer of the rectum, can be seen between the external anal sphincter and the anorectal mucosa as an area of white fibrous tissue (see Fig. 39.10B). Meticulous hemostasis and wide mobilization to allow closure without tension are crucial to success with this operation.

A fibrous scan that is retracted lateral to the wall of the anal canal (see Fig. 39.10B) often identifies the external sphincter. The exact anatomic margins of the external sphincter frequently are difficult to ascertain. A nerve stimulator can be used to identify contractile skeletal muscle. Alternatively, the Allis clamps containing the

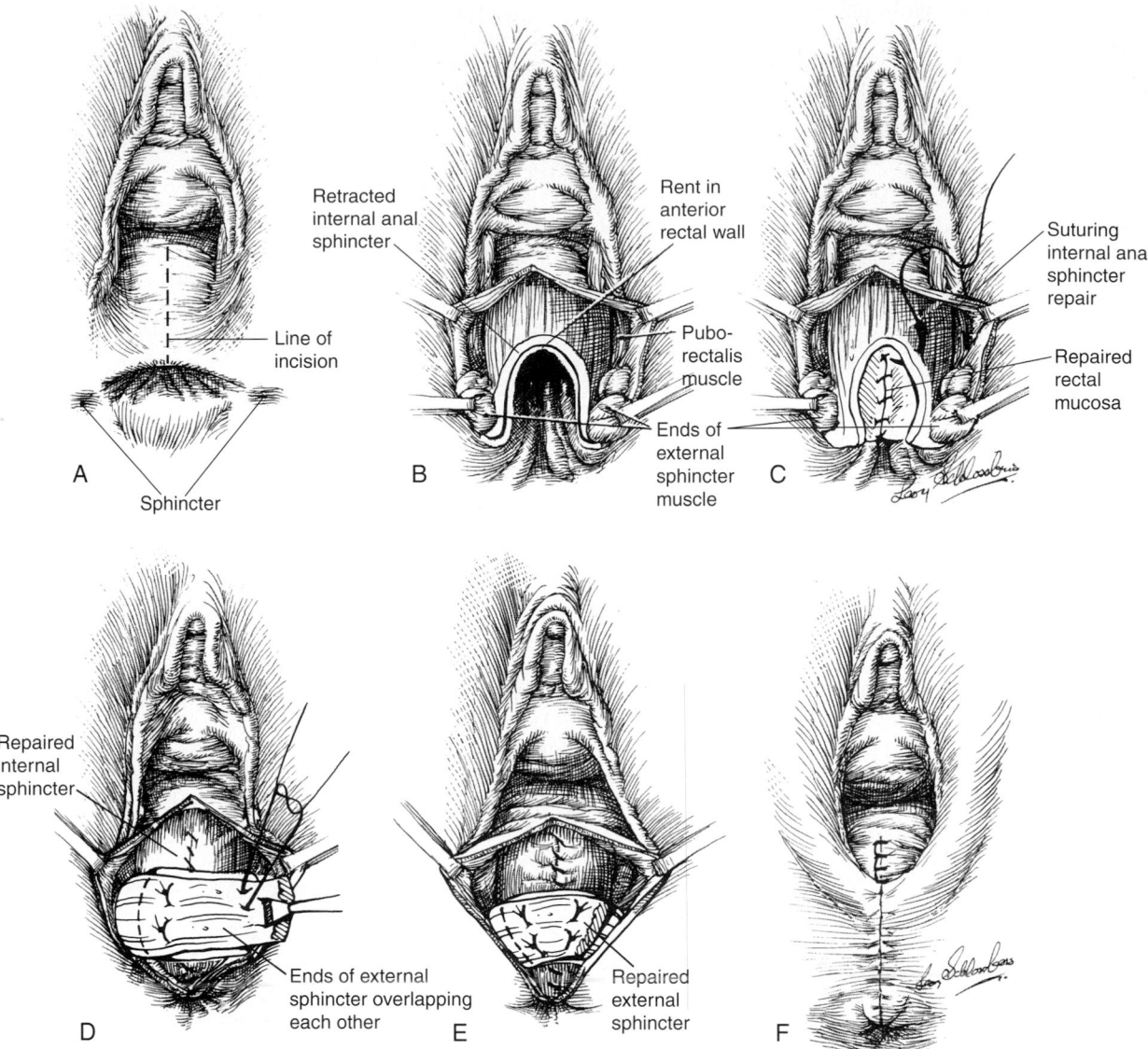

FIGURE 39.10. Layered closure of a chronic complete perineal laceration with overlapping sphincteroplasty. **A:** A transverse incision is made at the junction of the vaginal and rectal mucosa and extended up the midline of the posterior vaginal wall. **B:** The rectal wall has been separated from the posterior vaginal wall with careful sharp dissection. The ends of the external sphincter have been identified and grasped with Allis clamps. The internal anal sphincter can be seen between the external anal sphincter and the anorectal mucosa as an area of white fibrous tissue. **C:** The defect in the anal mucosa has been closed with a continuous 3-0 delayed-absorbable suture. The internal anal sphincter then is reapproximated over a length of 3 to 5 cm. This layer also serves to imbricate and isolate the mucosal layer and take tension off of it to help it heal and seal against infection. **D:** The ends of the external anal sphincter are widely mobilized with the scar tissue left on. Care should be taken to not to dissect beyond the 3- and 9-o'clock position as that is where the pudendal enervation to the sphincter enters laterally. The external sphincter then is brought together over the repaired internal sphincter with two rows of two horizontal mattress sutures of delayed-absorbable or permanent suture material. **E:** After the external sphincter has been repaired, the genital hiatus is narrowed by bringing the puborectalis muscles closer together with interrupted delayed-absorbable sutures placed in the fascia overlying them. **F:** The bulbocavernosus and superficial transverse perinei muscles have been reattached to the perineal body and the vaginal mucosa was closed with a continuous locking stitch of 3-0 delayed-absorbable suture that was continued subcuticularly to approximate the perineal skin.

ends of the external sphincter can be brought together in the midline and a circumferential sphincter tested for by inserting a double-gloved index finger into the rectum. If necessary, the clamps should be readjusted to incorporate more of the retracted muscle bundles until the constricted effect of the reapproximated sphincter can be demonstrated.

All scar tissue is excised from the margins of the anorectal mucosa, and the defect in the anal mucosa is closed using a continuous or interrupted suture of 3-0 delayed-absorbable material. A running suture may have the advantage of distributing tension along the entire suture line and helps prevent a gap in the closure that could occur from ischemia if an interrupted suture is tied too tight. A submucosally placed suture is ideal. Sometimes this tissue is quite friable and a full-thickness suturing of the mucosa is the safest method.

After the mucosal margins are approximated, a second supporting layer inverts the initial mucosal suture line. This layer often has been thought of in the past as "perirectal fascia," but in fact it is the thickened downward continuation of the circular smooth muscle layer of the rectum that is the internal anal sphincter. This appears as a white smooth layer of tissue between the anorectal mucosal closure and the external anal sphincter (see Fig. 39.10C). Great care should be taken in reapproximating this layer over a length of 3 to 5 cm because this muscle is responsible for most of the resting pressure in what is normally a 4-cm high pressure zone in the anal canal. This layer also serves to imbricate and isolate the mucosal layer and take tension off of it to help it heal and seal against infection.

In an approximation-type external anal sphincteroplasty, the external anal sphincter ends then are completely trimmed of scar tissue and united in the midline with interrupted number 0 or 2-0 delayed-absorbable sutures. Although some surgeons prefer a permanent suture, such as a braided silicone-treated polyester, a delayed-absorbable monofilament suture such as polydioxanone has the advantage of maintaining excellent tensile strength for an extended period of time while avoiding the presence of a permanent foreign body. This becomes particularly important in the event of wound infection. Four or five sutures are used to approximate the sphincter muscle. These can be placed 1 cm apart, full thickness with the nondominant index finger in the anal canal to aid in acquiring excellent purchase on both ends while assuring no penetration of the anal canal itself.

In an overlapping approach to the external anal sphincter, the scarified ends of the sphincter are important to the repair itself and are left in place. Because the external sphincter is a tonically contracted muscle, it pulls and adds tension to the closure site unavoidably. The concept of the overlapping sphincteroplasty is to use the scarred ends of the torn sphincter to help hold the sutures that reconstitute the circumferential sphincter. The ends are widely mobilized with the scar tissue left on. Care should be taken to try not to dissect beyond the 3- and 9-o'clock position because that is where the pudendal innervation to the sphincter enters laterally. The

external sphincter then is brought together over the repaired internal sphincter with two rows of two horizontal mattress sutures of delayed-absorbable or permanent suture material (see Fig. 39.10D).

An important part of the perineal reconstruction is the narrowing of the genital hiatus by bringing the puborectalis muscles closer together. One must remember that the bilateral arms of the puborectalis muscle do not normally come in contact with each other between the rectum and the vagina. Overzealous plication here can create posterior tissue banding that can lead to dyspareunia. Dissection should be carried out laterally to the fascia overlying the medial border of the puborectalis muscle. This fascia then should be brought together by a series of interrupted, delayed-absorbable sutures, taking care to not constrict the diameter of the vaginal canal. Plication of the puborectalis muscle itself can constrict the vagina. Each suture should be held tightly and the vagina tested before tying to assure that posterior banding is not created. If it is, that suture should be removed and another placed. Extending this procedure to the midportion of the vagina can produce excellent anatomic support for the underlying anal canal and rectal neck (see Fig. 39.10E).

Further support and elevation of the perineal body are provided by bringing together the disrupted ends of the superficial transverse perineal muscles and the bulbocavernosus muscles. These muscles normally insert on the perineal body, play a part in pelvic floor support, and should be included in perineal reconstruction, including obstetric repair, to re-establish and support the perineal body. After this step, the redundant vaginal mucosa is excised, and the remaining mucosa is approximated in the midline with a continuous 2 or 3-0 delayed-absorbable suture. This is followed by a subcuticular closure of the perineal skin (see Fig. 39.10F). Excessive narrowing of the vaginal introitus should be avoided because it can produce a painful midline scar and dyspareunia.

In 1937, Miller and Brown proposed making a paradoxic incision in the inferior portion of the anal sphincter at the 5- or 7-o'clock position to relax the tension on the suture line in patients undergoing sphincter repair. The procedure disrupts both the internal and external sphincters and is not without physiologic risk, such as poor healing and scarring of the sphincter with the potential for postoperative anal incontinence of gas and liquid feces. For these reasons, paradoxic incisions are not widely used at the present time. Nyam and Pemberton studied a similar procedure done for a different indication. They reported that although lateral internal sphincterotomy done for treatment of a chronic anal fissure led to fissure healing in 96% of 487 patients, anal incontinence occurred as a sequela in 53% of women treated. Although most of this incontinence was minor and transient, the incontinence was persistent in a small subgroup.

A preoperative mechanical bowel preparation is important. An oral bowel preparation should be given the evening before surgery is scheduled. If such a preparation is given the day of surgery, the patient may still be releasing stool during the operation. Although the patient may be given three doses of oral erythromycin, 500 mg, and neomycin, 1 g, the day before surgery, this may not be necessary in all patients.

The optimal postoperative diet for these patients is a matter of much controversy and little data. Decades ago these patients were given diverting colostomies to keep the fecal stream away from the repair until healing was complete. Patients would then have another procedure to close their colostomy. Most postoperative feeding regimens are based on the concept of keeping fecal material from the repair site for at least 4 to 5 days until the mucosal suture line has healed adequately and the reparative process is well established. A regimen of clear liquids for 3 to 5 days, with progression to a soft, low-residue diet for the next several weeks is a reasonable approach. Constipating agents can be useful immediately postoperatively but should not be used for a prolonged period of time because one wants the first bowel movement to be soft so as not to distend the repair. The use of an elemental liquid diet for 1 week postoperatively can be useful but is poorly tolerated by many patients and can lead to diarrhea in some. Stool softeners are advisable for 6 weeks postoperatively and after the first week or two of a clear liquid or low-residue diet, a high-fiber diet should be initiated.

Warren Flap Operation for Complete Third-Degree Tear

An inverted V-shaped incision is made in the posterior vaginal mucosa, outlining the flap that is to be turned down. The lower ends of the incision should be just lateral to the dimples caused by retracted sphincter ends (Fig. 39.11A). The length of the flap should measure a minimum of 3 cm to provide sufficient vaginal mucosa to be incorporated into the anal canal and cover the reconstructed perineal body.

Taking care to avoid injuring the bowel wall, the surgeon dissects the flap of mucosa free from the top downward (see Fig. 39.11B), stopping short of the margin between the vaginal and anal mucosa. If this margin is perforated, then the blood supply to the mucosal flap is compromised, thereby nullifying the advantage of the flap technique. The properly demarcated flap allows the areas overlying the sphincter ends to be denuded. The flap is grasped with two mucosal Allis clamps and is turned down to hang over the anus. The external anal sphincter ends then are dissected free, using Allis clamps for traction. An approximation- or overlapping-type external anal sphincteroplasty then is performed (see Fig. 39.11C). Although an approximation-type sphincteroplasty is pictured, an overlapping procedure could be incorporated into this procedure as described in the preceding (see Fig. 39-10D,E).

The fascia overlying the medial aspect of the puborectalis muscles is identified, and this tissue is brought together with a series of interrupted sutures for reinforcement in the manner described for the layered technique, using 0 or 2-0 delayed-absorbable sutures (see Fig. 39.11D). Each suture should be tested before tying to assure that the caliber of the vagina is not compromised.

Closure of the vaginal mucosa is carried out as in an ordinary perineal repair. Interrupted plication stitches of 2-0 delayed-absorbable suture are used to advance the fascia and shorten the muscle fibers of the perineal body, which strengthens the external sphincter as well. The margins of the vaginal mucosa and graft are approximated in the midline by a continuous locking stitch of 3-0 delayed-absorbable suture. The tip end of the vaginal mucosal flap should not be trimmed too closely, even though it protrudes somewhat from the repaired perineal body. It retracts as healing occurs (see Fig. 39.11E).

Noble Procedure for Complete Perineal Laceration

The torn perineal, anal, and rectal tissue in patients with a complete perineal laceration form a "butterfly" appearance across the perineum (Fig 39.12A). The "wings" of the butterfly are the lateral perineal dimples of the retracted ends of the external anal sphincter. The initial incision is outlined around the margins of this area following the margin of the anal mucosa along the anatomic defect in the rectovaginal septum. The perineal skin is left attached and held with Allis clamps to facilitate later dissection of the retracted ends of the external sphincter. A small margin of vaginal mucosa also is left attached to the anal wall for traction because the anal mucosa is so friable.

Atraumatic clamps are placed along the margin of the anal canal, and sharp dissection is used to carefully separate the anal wall from the overlying vaginal mucosa. The external anal sphincter remnants should be sharply mobilized and separated from the underlying anal wall (see Fig. 39.12B). The vaginal mucosa is widely mobilized from the anal canal and lower rectal wall laterally to the underlying levator muscles and proximally into the middle or upper one third. Adequate mobilization of the anterior anorectal wall allows it to be pulled outside the margin of the anal orifice without difficulty, thus avoiding sutures in the anorectal canal.

Once the ends of the external anal sphincter are mobilized to meet in the midline with traction on the Allis clamps, the overlying skin previously left attached is excised and the sphincter ends are approximated end-to-end in the midline (see Fig. 39.12C). Alternatively, one could perform an overlapping sphincteroplasty as described in the preceding (see Fig. 39-10D,E). Several of these sphincteroplasty sutures also should include the muscular layers of the anterior rectal wall to prevent it from retracting inward and to avoid tension on the suture line between the advanced anterior anorectal wall and the perineal skin. The genital hiatus should be narrowed by bringing the puborectalis muscles closer together as described in the preceding (see Fig. 39.12D). The transverse perineal muscles and the inferior margins of the bulbocavernosus muscles then are reapproxi-

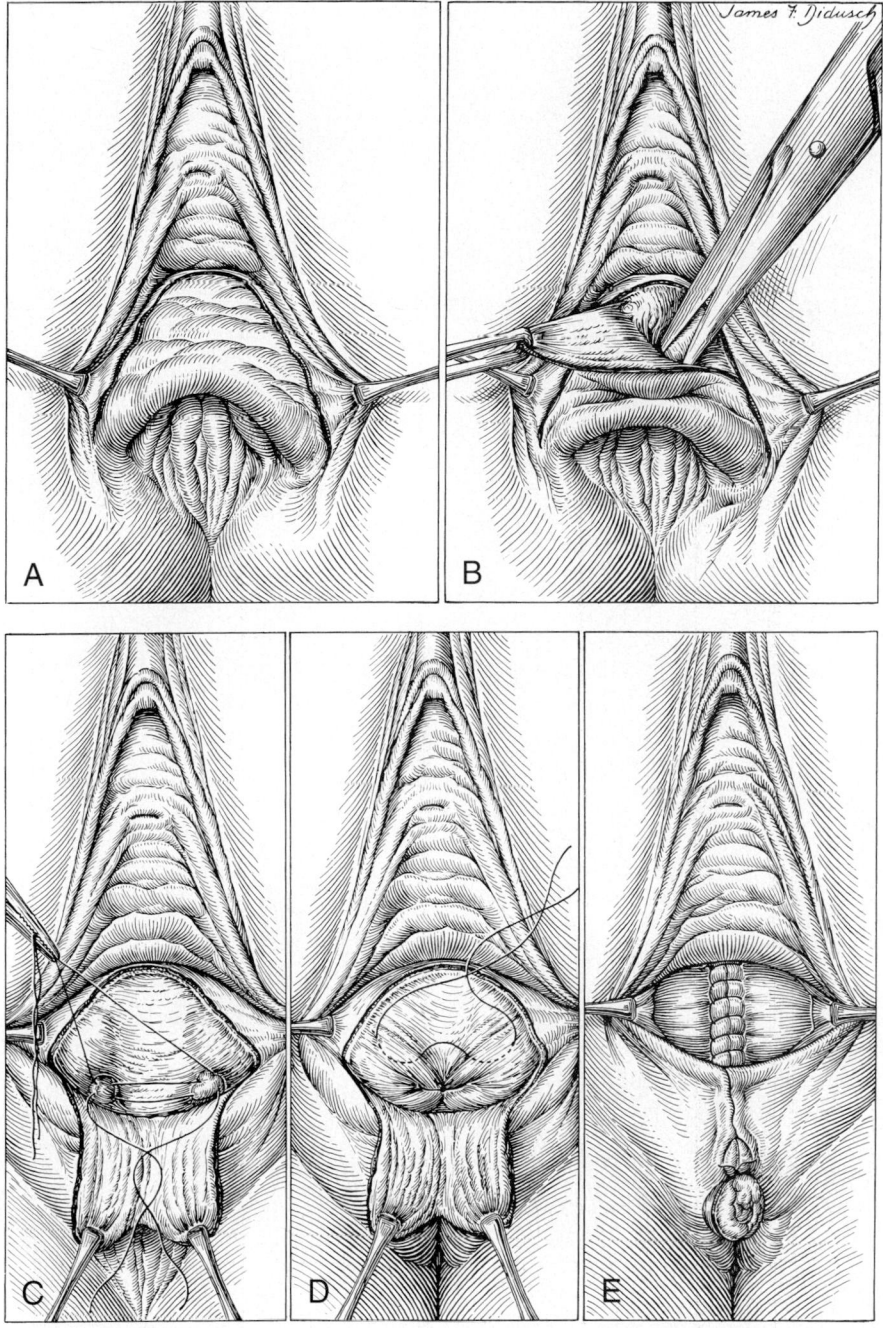

FIGURE 39.11. Warren flap operation for complete perineal laceration. **A:** The line of incision outlines the flap of vaginal mucosa. **B:** The flap is dissected free and turned back. **C:** The flap is retracted downward. The ends of the sphincter are delivered and are either sutured end to end as pictured or with an overlapping technique as described. **D:** The external sphincter has been re paired and the puborectalis muscles are then brought closer together taking care to not create a posterior band of tissue. **E:** The vaginal incision is closed with a continuous locking stitch that is continued subcuticularly over the perineum. The margins of the flap are included in the continuous suture, which may temporarily create a peaked appearance in the perineal skin. If the margins of the vaginal mucosal flap are redundant, it may be trimmed.

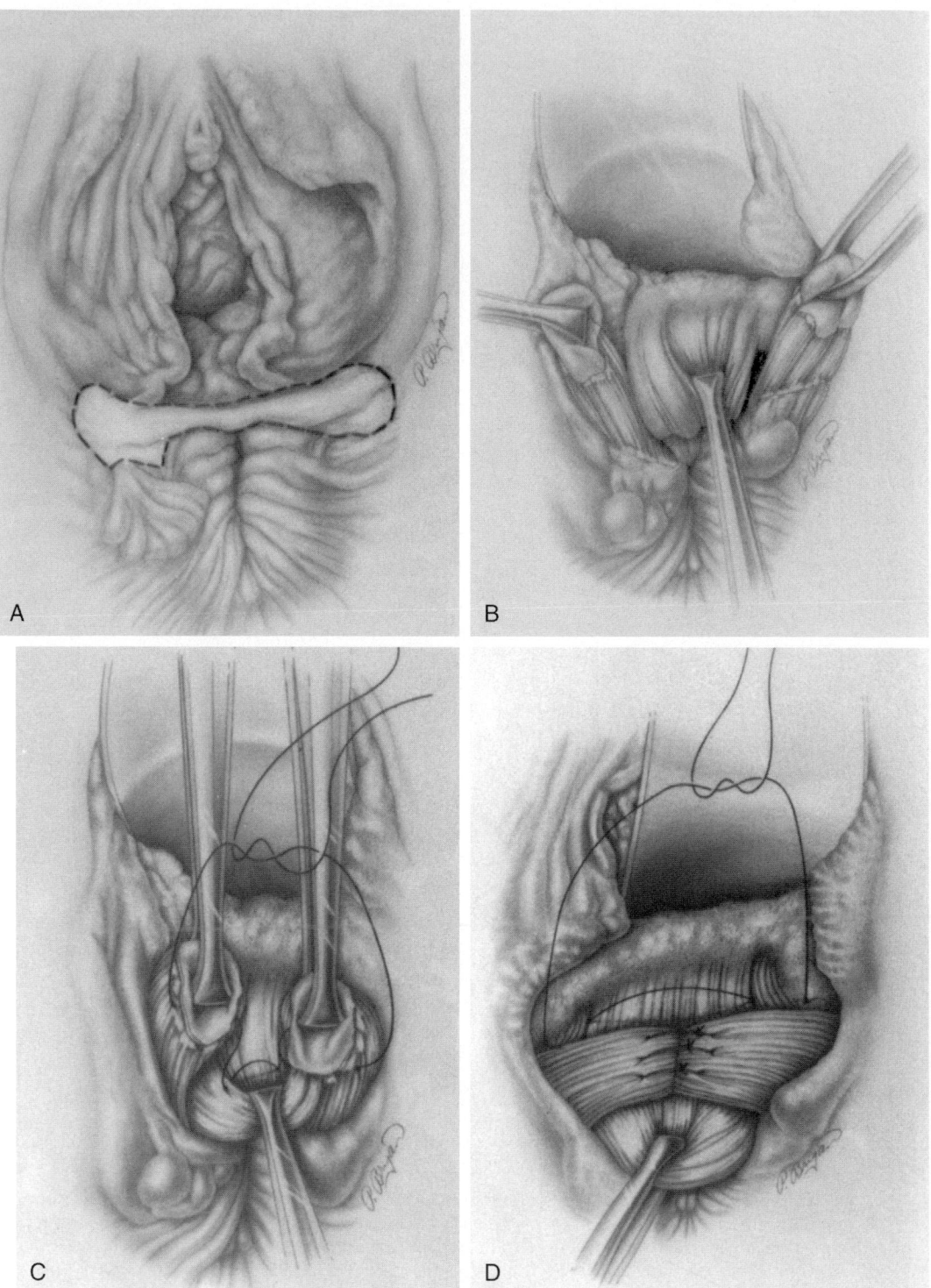

FIGURE 39.12. The Noble operation for complete perineal laceration. **A:** A "butterfly-shaped" scar is noted across the perineum where there is torn perineal, anal, and rectal tissues. The ends of the external anal sphincter can be recognized by lateral perineal dimpling. **B:** The anterior rectal wall is mobilized extensively from the posterior vaginal wall to allow it to be pulled down without tension. The wings of the butterfly are left attached to facilitate dissection of the retracted ends of the sphincter. **C:** Ends of the anal sphincter are trimmed and sutured together and to the pararectal fascia of the advanced anterior rectal wall. Several delayed-absorbable sutures are used. **D:** The levator muscles and pararectal fascia are brought closer together in the midline.

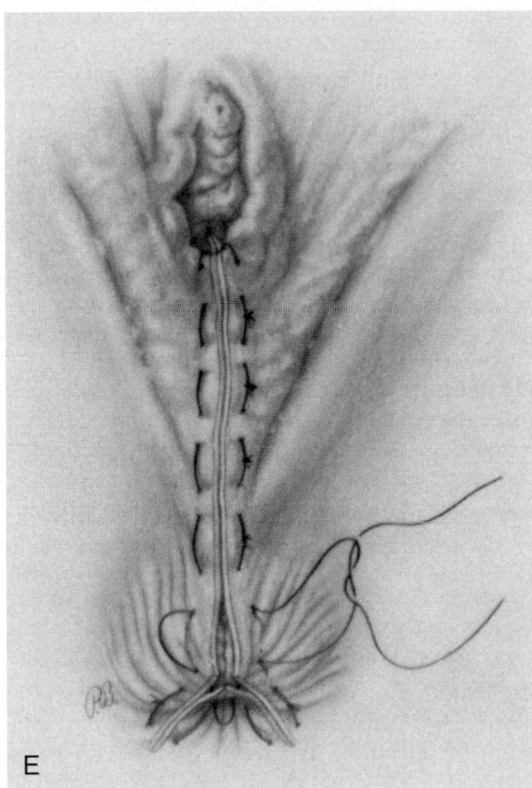

E

FIGURE 39.12. *(continued)* **E:** The transverse perineal muscles and the inferior margins of the bulbocavernosus muscles are brought together to reconstitute the perineal body and the vaginal mucosa and perineal skin are closed. The mobilized anterior wall of the anal canal is sutured without tension to the perineal skin.

mated, further reconstituting and supporting the perineal body.

The vaginal mucosa is trimmed, if necessary, and the margins of the posterior vaginal wall are approximated with a continuous locking stitch of 3-0 delayed-absorbable suture. The continuous suture closing the posterior vaginal mucosa is carried over the perineal body as a subcuticular stitch, and the perianal skin then is approximated at the midline. The mobilized anterior wall of the anal canal is drawn outside the reconstructed anal orifice and sutured without tension to the perianal skin (see Fig. 39.12E). The excess anal mucosa is trimmed. Care should be taken to remove as little of the distal anal canal as possible because this tissue contains the internal anal sphincter. Vertical mattress sutures of 3-0 delayed-absorbable suture are used to approximate the broad surface of the anal submucosa to the perianal skin. Any residual separation of the margins of the anal mucosa and perianal skin can be approximated with interrupted sutures.

RECTOVAGINAL FISTULAE

A rectovaginal fistula resulting in extraanal fecal incontinence is a distressing condition for the patient and her physician. Most fistulae actually arise in the anal canal beginning distal to the pectinate line (see Fig. 39.2) and should more accurately be considered anovaginal fistulae. The result of this condition often is the uncontrolled passage of flatus or stool from the anorectal canal through the fistulous tract into the vagina. It can be a socially disabling condition. Further, the difficulties of treatment leading to failure (contaminated operative site, high-pressure anal canal, usually without diversion), challenge both the patience of the affected individuals and the surgeon's skill.

There are several classifications systems for rectovaginal fistulae. We have favored that of low (vaginal opening near the posterior fourchette), mid (from the level of the cervix to just superior to the posterior fourchette), and high (the fistula is in the area of the posterior fornix).

Etiology

Although there are many different causes of rectovaginal fistulae (Table 39.3), numerous series report that obstetric trauma is the cause for the majority of them. Rectovaginal fistulae usually arise as a complication of a repaired fourth-degree perineal tear. Venkatesh et al. reported that even though this sequence of events may be the most common, only 0.1% of vaginal deliveries result in fistula formation. Risk factors for development of a rectovaginal fistula in association with vaginal deliveries include prolonged labor, difficult forceps delivery, shoulder dystocia, and a midline episiotomy.

A rectovaginal fistula may develop as a result of direct surgical injury to the rectum or vagina, ischemia, or postoperative infection. Other less common causes include blunt instrumentation or penetrating trauma caused by an accident. Occasionally, rectovaginal fistulae follow an infectious process such as a perianal abscess or an infected Bartholin duct cyst abscess. The most common cause of high rectovaginal fistulae is repeated bouts of diverticulitis with abscess formation followed by the formation of a sigmoidovaginal fistula or a combined sigmoidovesicovaginal fistula. Inflammatory bowel disease such as ulcerative colitis or Crohn's disease may result in complex rectovaginal fistulae. Crohn's disease is a transmural condition that often results in a rectovaginal fistula.

TABLE 39.3.
Causes of Rectovaginal Fistula

Congenital
Acquired
    Trauma
        Obstetric
        Operative
        Violent
    Infectious
    Inflammatory bowel disease
    Radiation
    Carcinoma

Radiation is a relatively infrequent cause of fistula formation, usually beginning as a proctitis with ulceration and fistula formation followed by a stricture. Fistulae may occur several years after completion of radiation therapy. Primary or metastatic disease in surrounding organs (rectum, cervix, uterus, or vagina) may result in rectovaginal fistulae. Because congenital rectovaginal fistula frequently is associated with other anomalies, its treatment is complex and beyond the scope of this chapter.

Clinical Evaluation

The most common symptoms are the passage of flatus and stool into the vagina. The severity of those symptoms may be affected by the size of the fistula and its number. There is usually a foul-smelling vaginal discharge with periodic, uncontrolled escape of gas. Occasionally, the fistula may develop immediately. More commonly, it appears 7 to 10 days after delivery. The breakdown of a primary repair, inadequate repair, or infection at the primary site may explain this delayed presentation. Because of the unpredictable condition and the desire to have more children, the patient may not seek medical attention for some time. Diarrhea, rectal bleeding, mucus discharge, and abdominal pain are caused by the underlying status of the bowel and do not result from the fistula per se.

The history frequently suggests the underlying cause of the fistula and may greatly influence the timing and route of repair. On physical examination, the location, size, and number of openings can be identified. The route of the fistula may be outlined by the passage of a thin probe from the vagina through the fistulous tract into the anal or rectal canal. Placing an examining finger in the rectum aids this process. Contraction of the puborectalis and external anal sphincter should be evaluated for competency. The perineal body is examined, and the tissues about the fistula are delineated to gain more insight into the cause of the underlying fistula. A proctosigmoidoscopic examination usually is done to ensure that the mucosa of the intestinal tract is normal.

In patients with a history compatible with a fistula but in whom no fistula opening can be identified, a simple office examination can be helpful. With the patient in a slight Trendelenburg position with a size 20 Foley urinary catheter, a 5-mL balloon is placed in the anal canal. Air is instilled through the catheter while the water-filled, or soap covered, vagina is observed for any escape of air bubbles originating from the anal canal. Contrast studies are necessary to define the sigmoidovaginal fistula or fistulae associated with primary bowel disease.

Surgical Management

Numerous operative procedures have been described for repair of rectovaginal fistula, including transvaginal, transanal, and abdominal approaches. Gynecologists usually use a transvaginal approach, whereas colon and rectal surgeons prefer the transanal technique. The determining factors to be considered include the cause of the fistula, its location and accessibility, and the status of the anal sphincter.

The most typical rectovaginal fistula is that following disruption of a primary repair of a fourth-degree laceration. It typically occurs low along the rectovaginal septum just inside the external anal sphincter. Generally, it presents 6 to 10 days after the initial repair with passage of air or stool through the vagina. Venkatesh et al. report that approximately 50% of these small fistulae may heal without operative intervention during the first 6 to 8 weeks postpartum.

Early Repair

As described, Hankins et al. recommended early repair of carefully selected rectovaginal fistulae and episiotomy breakdowns using a technique of early return to the operating room for debridement followed by daily cleansing of the wound area. After a 6- to 7-day interval, their patients were returned to the operating room for surgical repair of the fistula. With this approach, successful healing occurred in 90% of their patients. We prefer to wait 8 weeks to allow the surrounding inflammation to resolve before surgical intervention. Preoperative mechanical bowel preparation should be given. On the morning of operation, tap water enemas can be given until clear.

Appropriate treatment of a rectovaginal fistula requires consideration of the cause and location of the fistula and the condition of the involved tissues. For fistulae located in the lower portion of the anal canal, we prefer to use the lithotomy position to carry out the operative repair. For fistulae at the very apex of the vagina, an abdominal approach generally is required.

Low Rectovaginal Fistula: Technique of Repair

A technique for small rectovaginal fistulae involves a circular incision about the fistulous opening (Fig. 39.13), performed transvaginally. With traction on the vaginal wall and countertraction applied to the edge of the fistulous tract, the vagina is separated from the underlying rectal wall with sharp dissection, and this proceeds circumferentially (Fig. 39.14). This wide mobilization permits later approximation of the fresh injury free of tension. Once the vaginal walls are mobilized from the underlying rectum, the entire fistulous tract is excised to include a small rim of the rectal mucosa (Fig. 39.15) to convert the fistula to a fresh injury. With the surgeon's nondominant index finger lifting and supporting the anterior rectal wall, the initial sutures are placed extramucosally, including a portion of the muscularis and submucosa, with 3-0 delayed-absorbable sutures (Fig. 39.16). We frequently place all sutures throughout the length of the fistula, after which they are individually tied in the order in which they were placed. The initial suture line begins and is extended a full 5 to 8 mm above and below the site of the fistulous tract to assure complete closure. A second layer (Fig. 39.17) begins 5 mm above the previously closed suture line and

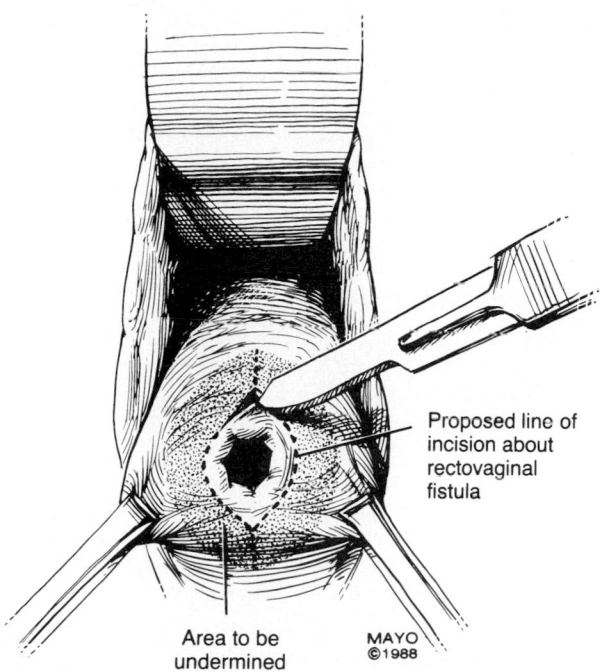

FIGURE 39.13. Small rectovaginal fistula with proposed line of initial incision.

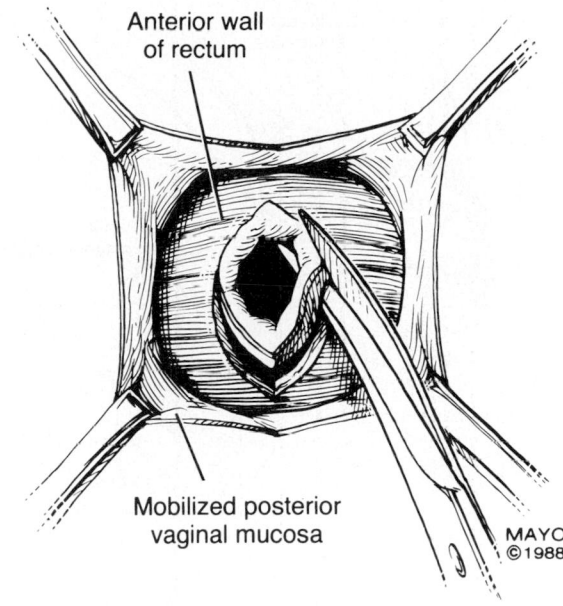

FIGURE 39.15. Excision of fistulous tract.

extends 5 mm distal to the fistulous closure, inverting the initial suture line into the rectum, and no sutures are located within the rectal lumen.

Once the wall of the rectum is reconstructed, the lower portions of the puborectalis muscle and the exter-

nal anal sphincter are approximated to add a third layer in the closure (Fig. 39.18 A), which helps to reconstitute the anterior rectal wall. Care should be taken that approximation is not carried so far superiorly that it results in a transverse bar across the posterior vaginal wall,

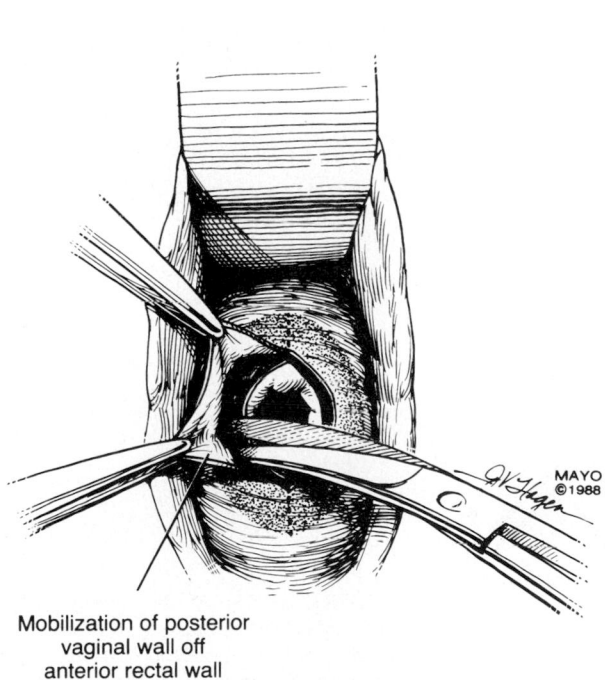

FIGURE 39.14. Incision of vaginal wall, mobilizing posterior vagina from underlying anterior anal canal.

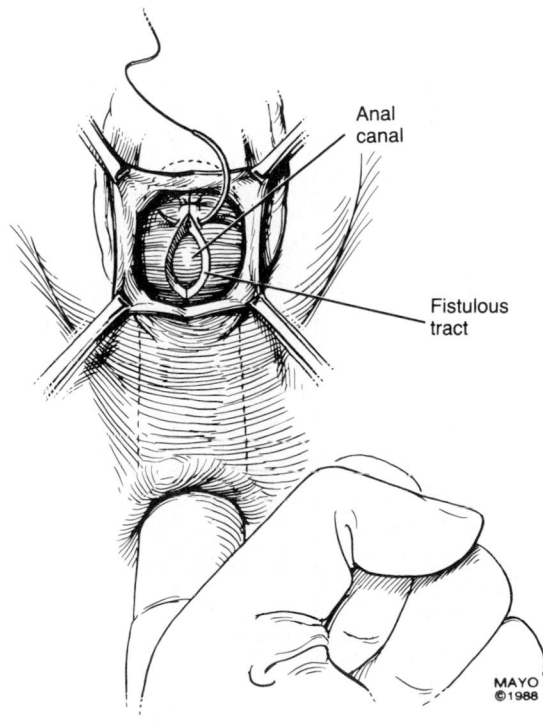

FIGURE 39.16. Extramucosal placement of sutures in wall of anterior anal canal.

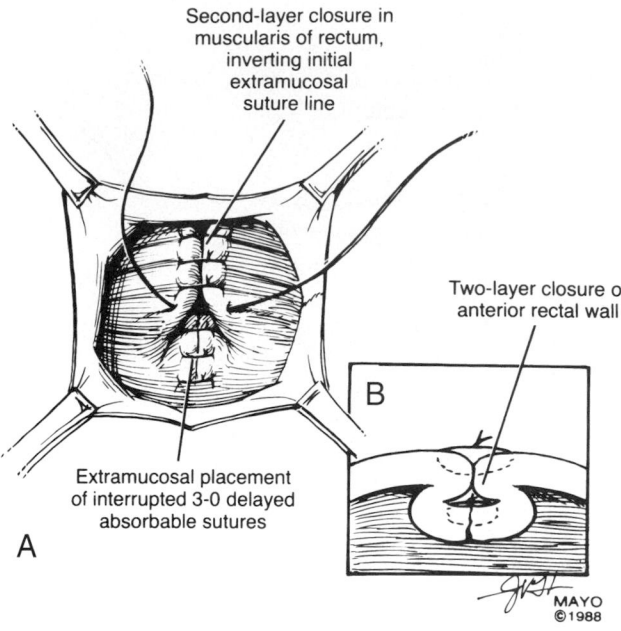

Second-layer closure in muscularis of rectum, inverting initial extramucosal suture line

Two-layer closure of anterior rectal wall

B

Extramucosal placement of interrupted 3-0 delayed absorbable sutures

A

MAYO
©1988

FIGURE 39.17. A: Inversion of initial suture line with approximation of muscularis of the anal canal. This thickened smooth muscle layer is the internal anal sphincter. **B:** Side view representing closure of the first and second layers in the anal canal.

which may lead to dyspareunia. Once the muscular walls are approximated, the vaginal wall is approximated with 3-0 delayed-absorbable sutures, accurately placed so as to promote primary apposition of the fresh edge of the vaginal wall (see Fig. 39.18B).

Occasionally, the fistulous tract is so close to the external anal sphincter that closure is difficult. In these conditions, the bridge of skin, sphincter, and perineal body are divided, and the fistula is thus converted to a fourth-degree tear (Fig. 39.19). The fistulous tract is excised, and the posterior vaginal wall is mobilized from the anterior anal wall (Fig. 39.20). The anal canal then is reconstructed with interrupted or running fine delayed-

absorbable sutures approximating the mucosa of the anal canal. This initial suture line then is inverted with a second layer of interrupted fine delayed-absorbable sutures approximating the retracted tissues of the internal anal sphincter, resulting in reconstruction of the anal canal (Fig. 39.21). The retracted ends of the external anal sphincter are approximated in the midline in an end-to-end fashion with fine delayed-absorbable sutures (Fig. 39.22). This results in a snug closure that is resistant to the passage of the surgeon's little finger. Alternatively, at this point one could perform an overlapping sphincteroplasty as described in the preceding (see Fig. 39.10D,E). The perineal body is reconstructed in such a fashion that

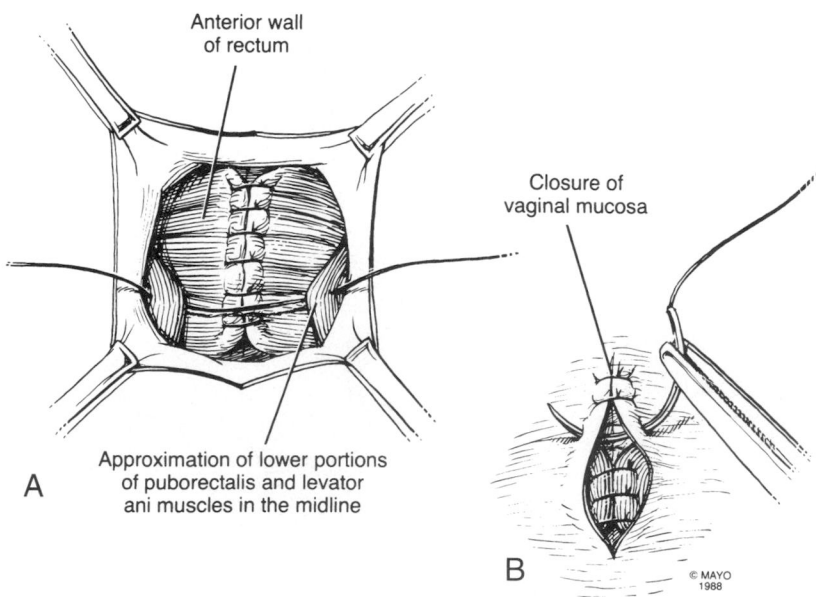

Anterior wall of rectum

Closure of vaginal mucosa

A

Approximation of lower portions of puborectalis and levator ani muscles in the midline

B

© MAYO 1988

FIGURE 39.18. A: Reconstruction of anal canal with approximation of portions of the puborectalis and external anal sphincter. **B:** Interrupted sutures approximating posterior vaginal wall.

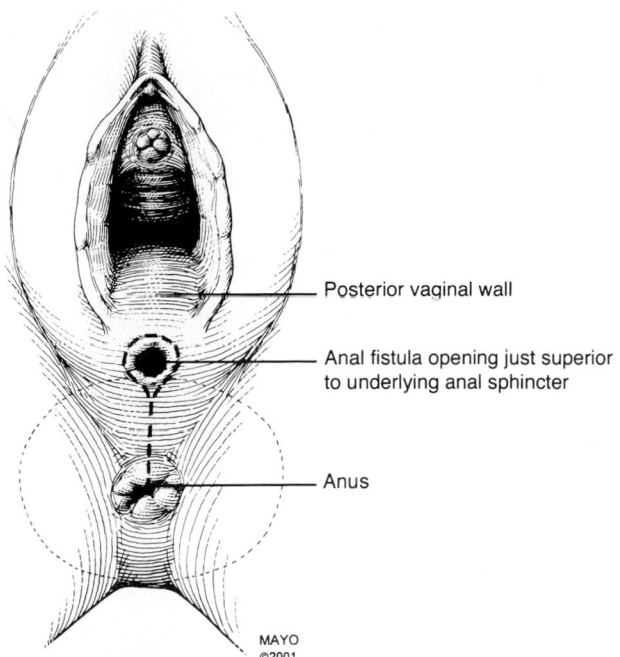

FIGURE 39.19. Proposed incision of perineal body and posterior vaginal wall with excision of fistulous tract.

there is significant support to the reconstructed anal sphincter and yet entrance to the vagina is not compromised Alternatively, one could perform an overlapping sphincteroplasty as described in the preceding (Fig. 39.23).

Considerable experience exists with the transanal flap approach to rectovaginal fistulae involving the lower portion of the rectovaginal septum. Rothenberger et al. reported on a technique that uses an endorectal flap consisting of mucosa, submucosa, and circular muscle fibers. The flap is twice as wide at the base as it is at the apex.

They achieved successful repair in 32 of 35 patients with rectovaginal fistulae. Hoexter et al. reported a similar high rate of fistula healing and improvement in anal continence, emphasizing several points for successful repair via endorectal flap: (a) elevating the rectal flap for at least 4 cm to the fistula; (b) excising the fistulous tract; (c) leaving the vaginal wound open for drainage; and (d) using an elliptic flap to avoid devascularization of the flap apex. Others have reported a high degree of efficacy of the endorectal flap for achieving both fistula healing and repair of any associated anal sphincter disruptions.

Repair of Radiation-Induced Fistula

Less commonly, a sizable rectovaginal fistula is located high in the posterior vaginal wall, frequently associated with a degree of stricture of the adjacent rectum and significant perirectal fibrosis and scarring. When this occurs, it is almost always after radiation therapy. Successful closure of the fistula requires aggressive excision of the surrounding tissues damaged by radiation. In selected patients, the fistula is best managed with a primary resection and anastomosis of the rectosigmoid through a lower midline incision. However, successful closure can be accomplished by means of a pedicled bulbocavernous muscle with an overlying labial fat pad (Martius procedure); this is performed vaginally.

Figure 39.24 depicts the usual location of the fistula, high in the posterior vaginal wall. Figure 39.25 outlines the potential sites from which the pedicled bulbocavernous Martius-type flap is obtained. Initially, an incision is made in the vagina to separate the scarred vagina from the underlying anterior wall of the rectum circumferentially. The edge of the scarred vaginal epithelium adjacent to the edge of the rectal mucosa is excised in anticipation of this being the site of the initial suture line approximating the squamous epithelium from the vulvar flap to the rectum in order to fill the defect in the rectum. With a

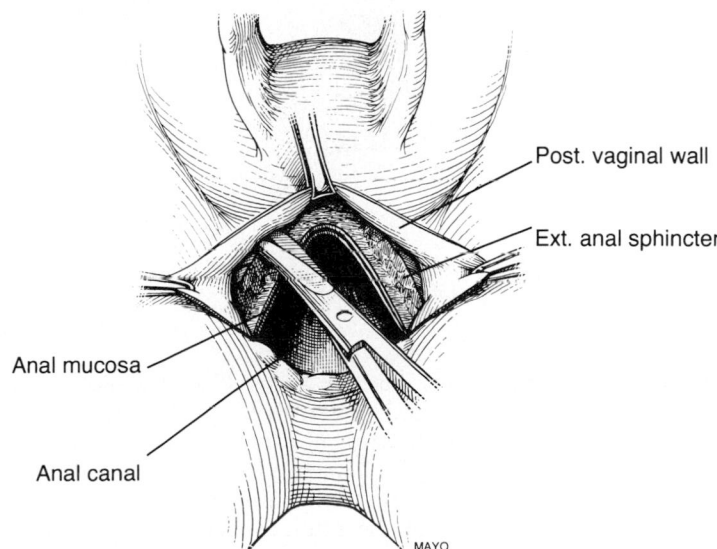

FIGURE 39.20. Mobilization of posterior vagina off anterior anal canal with conversion of rectovaginal fistula to fourth-degree injury.

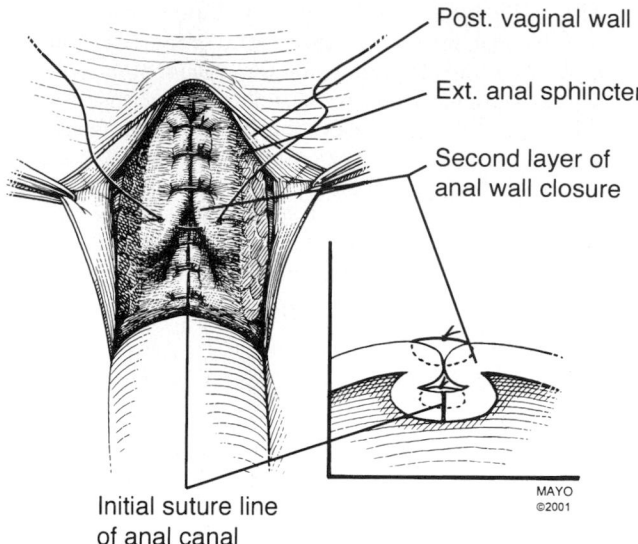

Post. vaginal wall

Ext. anal sphincter

Second layer of
anal wall closure

Initial suture line
of anal canal

MAYO
©2001

FIGURE 39.21. Two-layer reconstruction of anal canal.

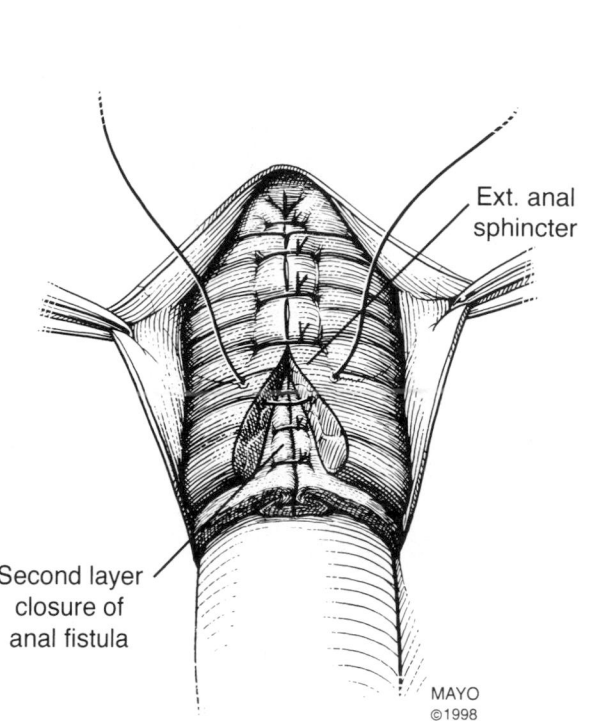

Ext. anal
sphincter

Second layer
closure of
anal fistula

MAYO
©1998

FIGURE 39.22. Reanastomosis of retracted external anal sphincter with surgeon's left index finger in the anal canal.

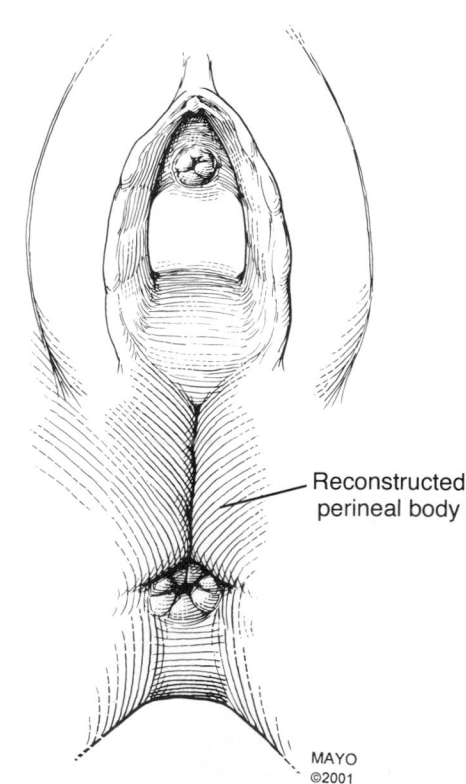

Reconstructed
perineal body

MAYO
©2001

FIGURE 39.23. Reconstructed perineal body with subcuticular approximation of skin of perineum.

Mayo scissors, a subcutaneous tunnel is made from the labium majus to the fistula under the labium and vaginal mucosa (Fig. 39.26). The free end of the muscle is guided through the subcutaneous tunnel with a single absorbable suture placed along its edge to assist in passage through the tunnel. The rectal defect is such that it cannot be closed primarily. Thus, the edge of the squamous epithelium from the vulvar graft is sutured to the edge of the rectal mucosa with 4-0 delayed-absorbable sutures. Occasionally, a Schuchardt incision is required in the vagina to obtain adequate exposure for the dissection.

The pedicled graft initially is closed, beginning at the 3-o'clock position, in a synchronous fashion such that the entire edge of the fistulous tract is in immediate proximity to the edge of the skin from the vulva (Fig. 39.27). Once in place, the muscle and subcutaneous tis-

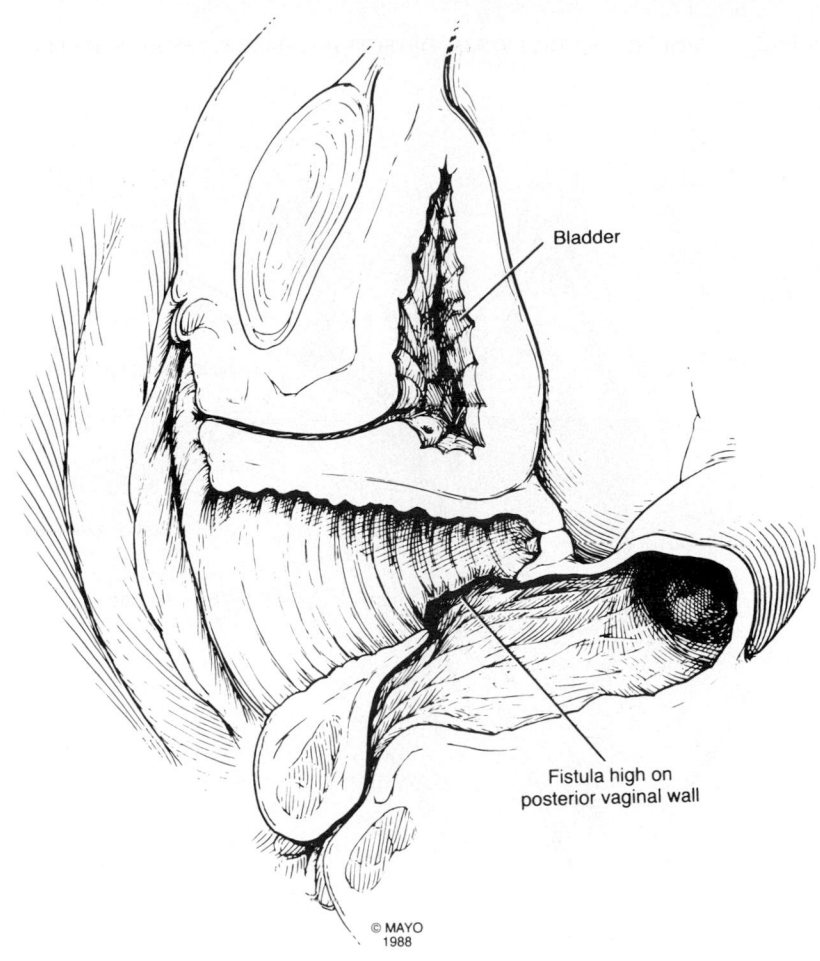

Bladder

Fistula high on
posterior vaginal wall

© MAYO
1988

FIGURE 39.24. Radiation-induced
fistula.

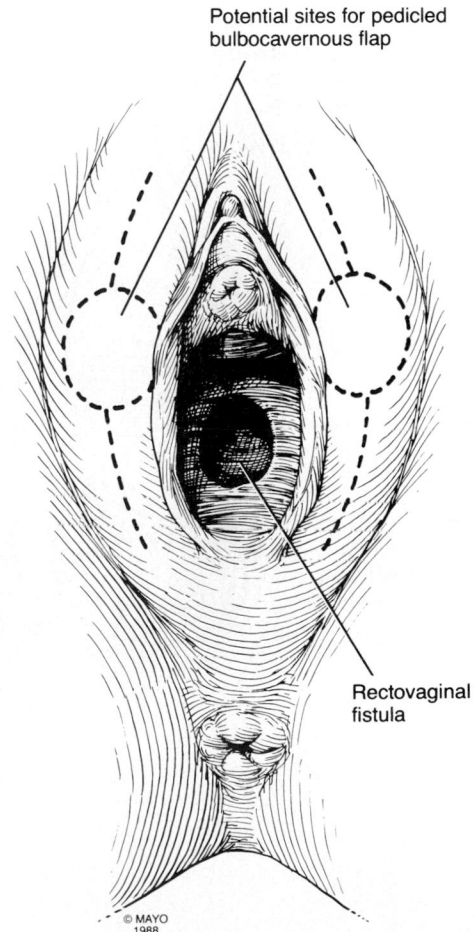

Potential sites for pedicled
bulbocavernous flap

Rectovaginal
fistula

© MAYO
1988

FIGURE 39.25. Proposed sites to harvest skin and subcutaneous tissue in
preparation to fill hole of rectovaginal fistula.

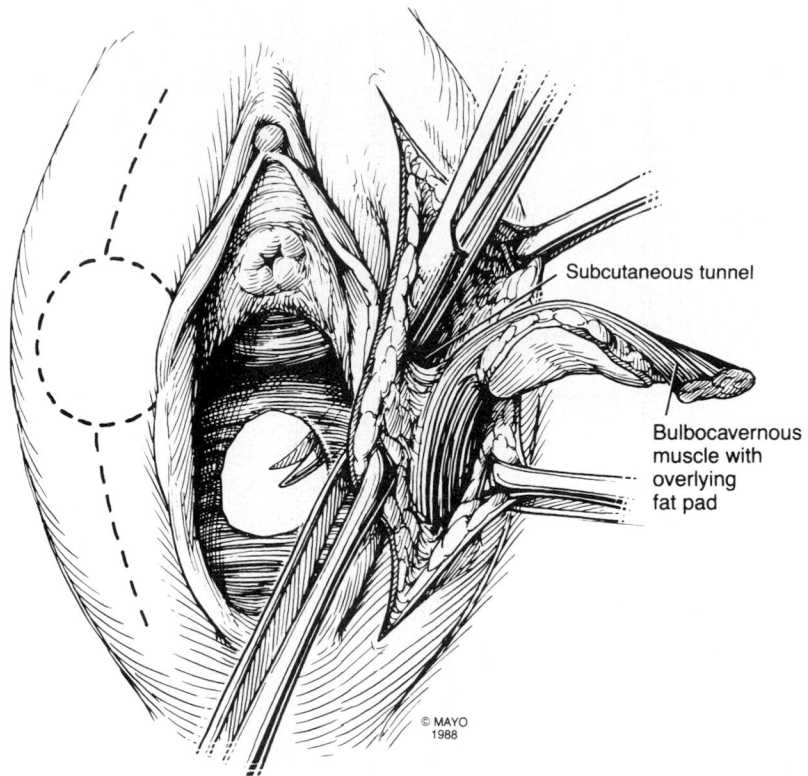

FIGURE 39.26. Mobilization of bulbocavernosus muscle with overlying fat pad.

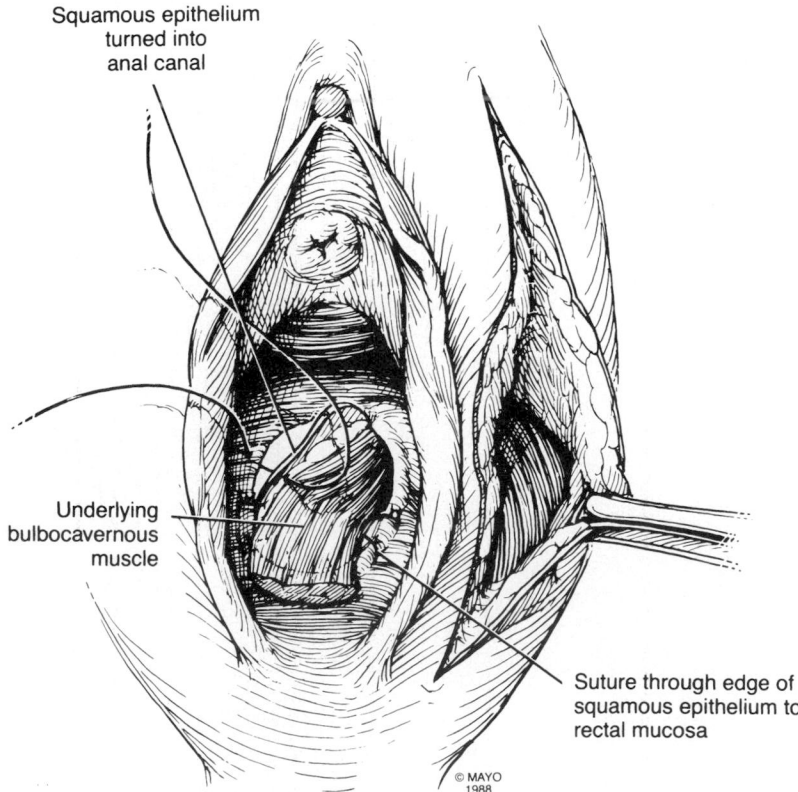

FIGURE 39.27. Suture fixation of pedicled skin to rectal mucosa.

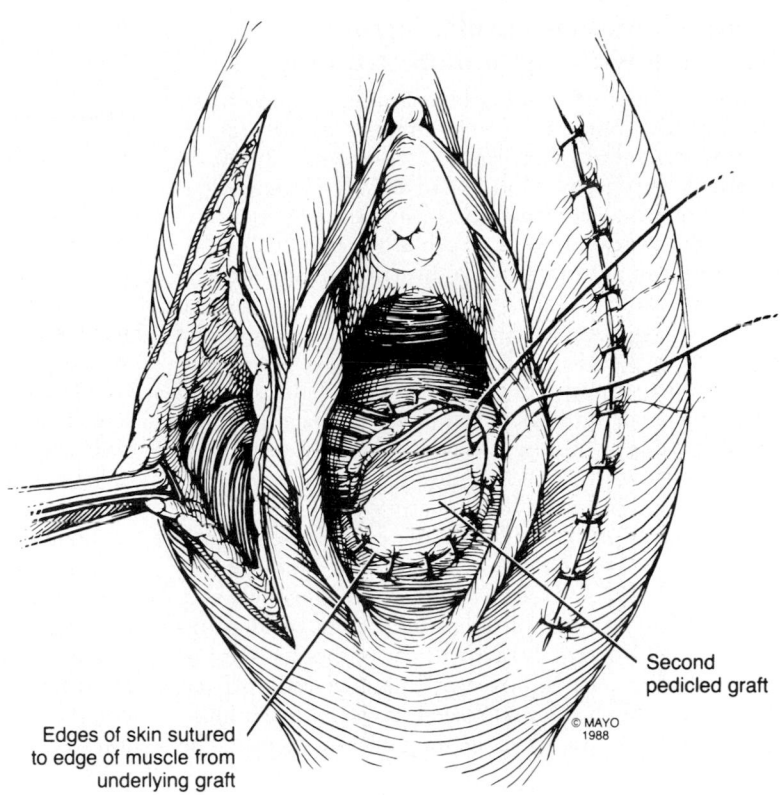

FIGURE 39.28. Approximation of the skin of the vulvar flap to the skin of the vaginal wall.

Edges of skin sutured to edge of muscle from underlying graft

Second pedicled graft

© MAYO 1988

sue of the graft are sutured to the surrounding connective tissue.

To provide coverage for the exposed Martius flap, which has been inserted as a plug into the rectum, a similar pedicled graft is developed from the patient's right side; this is placed such that the skin of the vulva is approximated to the skin of the vagina (Fig. 39.28). The edges are placed such that there is no exposed source for granulation tissue (Fig. 39.29).

A small suction catheter is placed between the two pedicled grafts and brought out through a stab wound lateral to the perineal incision. The vulvar incision is closed in layers with skin approximated with fine interrupted delayed-absorbable suture. In patients requiring a pedicled graft, the repair may result in a compromise of the vagina and a degree of colpocleisis. This results not only from the encroachment on the vaginal lumen with the pedicled grafts but also from the associated contracture caused by the underlying cause of the fistula—pelvic radiation. There is a tendency for further contracture and stenosis of the vagina, which may result in significant dyspareunia or apareunia.

Boronow has used bulbocavernosus-labial tissue graft to successfully treat radiation-induced rectovaginal fistulae. He reported on 25 radiation-induced vaginal fistulae in 22 patients. There were 16 rectovaginal fistulae, three vesicovaginal fistulae, and three combined vesicovaginal and rectovaginal fistulae. Successful closure was accomplished in 84% of the patients with rectovaginal fistulae.

Closed sites of harvest of bulbocavernous graft

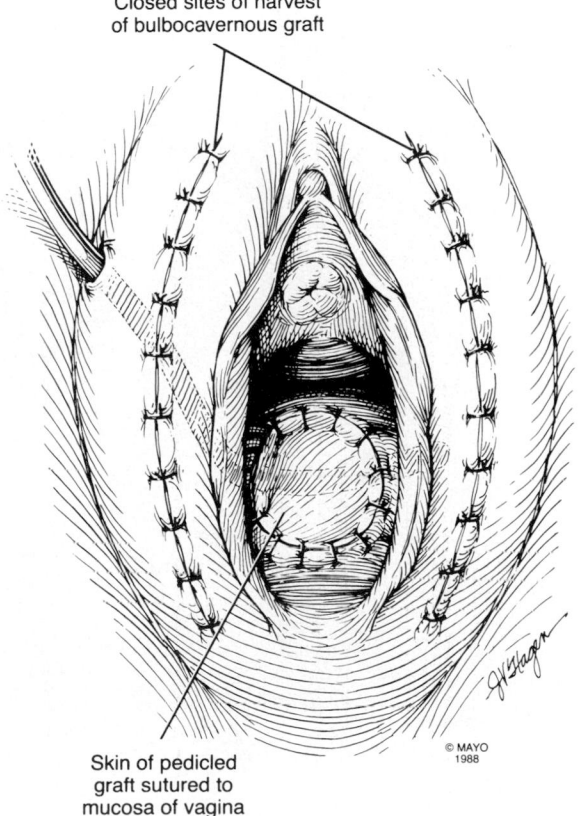

Skin of pedicled graft sutured to mucosa of vagina

© MAYO 1988

FIGURE 39.29. Reconstructed perineum in completed repair of fistula.

Sigmoidovaginal Fistula: Sigmoid Resection with Sigmoidorectostomy

Fistulae between the sigmoid colon and vagina occur infrequently, but the overwhelming majority result from diverticulitis of the sigmoid colon (Fig. 39.30) in a patient who has previously had a hysterectomy. Generally, the sequence of events consists of the patient experiencing repeated bouts of acute diverticulitis that finally result in perforation of a diverticulum and abscess formation with a fistulous tract communicating to the vagina. Passage of fecal material or gas through the vagina in the absence of a rectal communication should lead one to suspect a fistula arising from the sigmoid colon or small intestine. A proctoscopic examination should be done, although often it is impossible to visualize the fistulous orifice because of narrowing or fixation resulting from the inflammatory condition. Surgical intervention is indicated for a sigmoidovaginal fistula that is large enough to permit the passage of fecal material. In a few selected patients, a colostomy may be the only treatment, or the fistula may be divided and the sigmoidal defect closed with or without a temporary colostomy. In the overwhelming majority of patients, we prefer a sigmoid resection with primary anastomosis and closure of the opening into the vagina. The need for a temporary protective colostomy is determined on an individual basis.

Hartmann Procedure

Under some circumstances, the infected, inflammatory process is such that the sigmoid mass may be excised, but a primary anastomosis is ill advised. It may be more appropriate to excise the diseased colon, close the fistula in the vagina, and oversew the proximal end of the distal rectal stump. This procedure is accomplished with an inner layer of running 3-0 delayed-absorbable suture inverted with a second layer of interrupted 3-0 silk sutures. The tails on the tied silk sutures are left long to facilitate later identification of the rectal stump during reoperation (Fig. 39.31). The distal end of the descending colon is brought out as a colostomy, which is matured at that time. Later, usually after 2 to 3 months, reoperation can be done through the previous incision. The long ends of the silk ties facilitate identification of the proximal end of the distal rectal stump, which may be difficult to find otherwise. Placement of a gauze pack in the vagina with a large rectal tube in the anal stump also may help to identify these structures. Once identified, the descending colon is freed from the splenic flexure in a sufficient fashion to permit the primary descending colorectostomy in

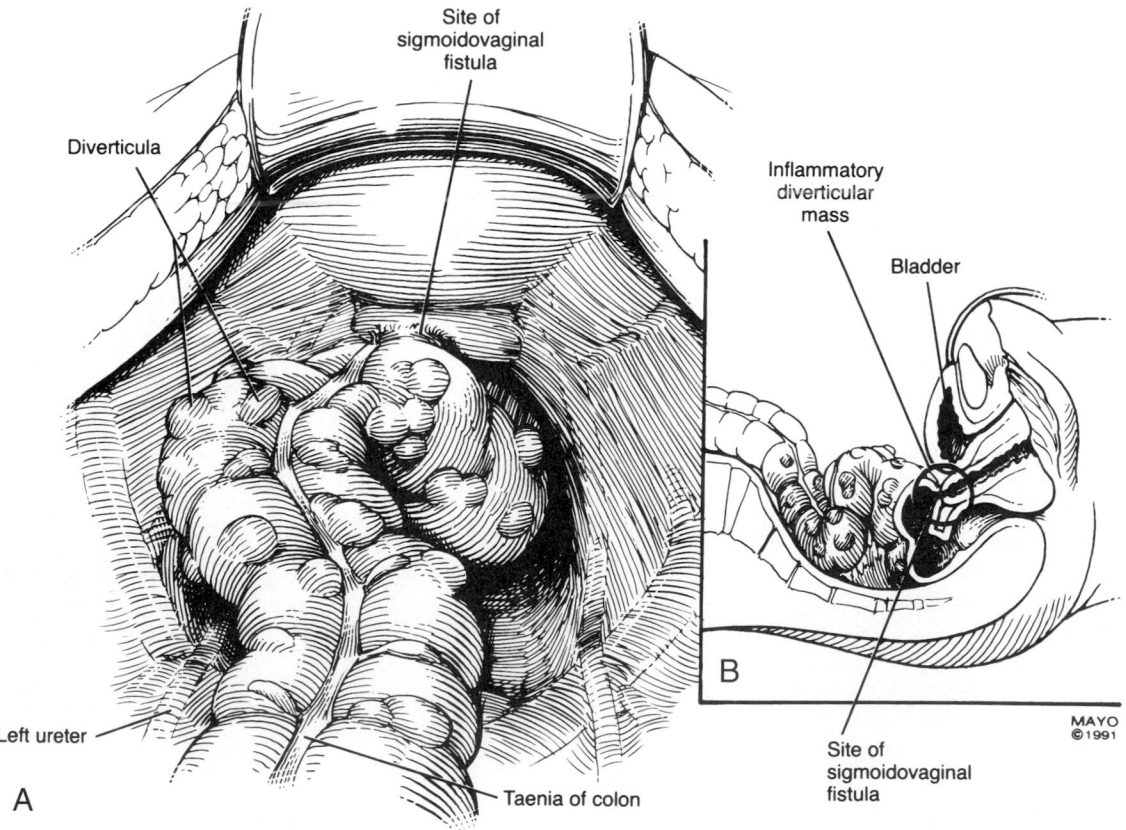

FIGURE 39.30. A: Sigmoid with multiple diverticula and site of sigmoidovaginal fistula. **B:** Site of sigmoidovaginal fistula at apex of vagina.

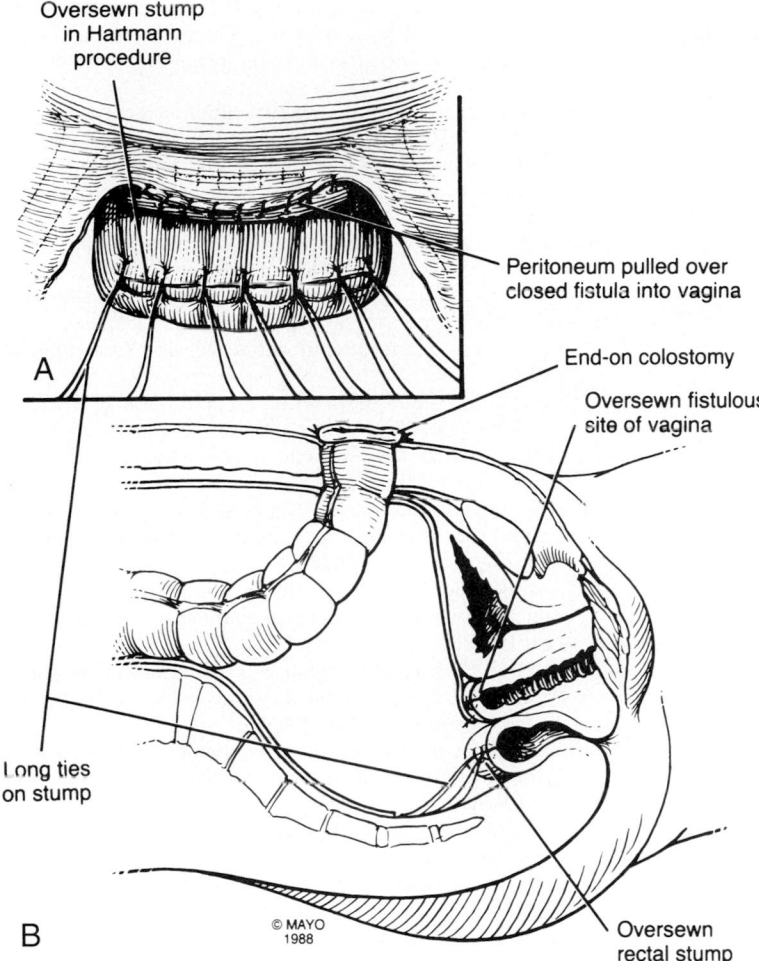

Oversewn stump
in Hartmann
procedure

Peritoneum pulled over
closed fistula into vagina

A

End-on colostomy

Oversewn fistulous
site of vagina

Long ties
on stump

B

© MAYO
1988

Oversewn
rectal stump

FIGURE 39.31. A: Separate closures of top of vagina and remnant of rectum. **B:** Matured colostomy and oversewn site of sigmoidovaginal fistula.

a noninfected field as a closing step in this two-stage procedure.

SUMMARY

The management of the anally incontinent patient is a complex undertaking whether that incontinence is transanal or extraanal through a rectovaginal fistula. Care must be taken in the assessment and diagnosis of these patients with testing judiciously used where it will provide clinically useful information. Because surgical results in anally incontinent patients are less than perfect, consideration should be given to initially trying nonsurgical management in appropriate patients. In those who fail conservative therapy, and in those who go directly to surgical therapy, a thoughtful preoperative work-up with extensive preoperative counseling regarding possible outcomes is crucial for the ultimate satisfaction of the patient. Surgery for anal incontinence and rectovaginal fistula repair requires thorough surgical planning, careful attention to detail, and a meticulous operative technique in order to provide the patient with optimal results.

BIBLIOGRAPHY

Aartsen EJ, Sindram IS. Repair of the radiation induced rectovaginal fistula without or with interposition of the bulbocavernosus muscle (Martius procedure). *Eur J Surg Oncol* 1988;14:171.

Abou-Zeid AA. Preliminary experience in management of fecal incontinence caused by internal anal sphincter injury. *Dis Colon Rectum* 2000;43(2):198.

Alexander AA, Liu J-B, Merton DA, et al. Fecal incontinence: transvaginal ultrasound evaluation of anatomic causes. *Radiology* 1996;199:529.

Allen RE, Hosker GL, Smith ARB, et al. Pelvic floor damage and childbirth: a neurophysiological study. *Br J Obstet Gynaecol* 1990;97:770.

Anthony S, Buitendijk SE, Zondervan KT, et al. Episiotomies and the occurrence of severe perineal lacerations. *Br J Obstet Gynaecol* 1994;101:1064.

American Gastroenterological Association Medical Position Statement on Anorectal Testing Techniques. *Gastroenterology* 1999;116:732.

Arnaud A, Sarles JC, Sielezneff I, et al. Sphincter repair without overlapping for fecal incontinence. *Dis Colon Rectum* 1991;34:744–747.

Aronson MP, Lee RA, Berquist TH. Anatomy of anal sphincters and related structures in continent women studied with magnetic resonance imaging. *Obstet Gynecol* 1990;76:846.

Ayoub SF. Anatomy of the external anal sphincter in man. *Acta Anat* 1979;105:25.

Bandy LC, Addison A, Parker RT. Surgical management of rectovaginal fistulas in Crohn's disease. *Am J Obstet Gynecol* 1983;147:359.

Bansal RK, Tan WM, Ecker JL, et al. Is there benefit to episiotomy at spontaneous vaginal delivery? A natural experiment. *Am J Obstet Gynecol* 1996;175:897.

Bartolo DCC, Roe AM, Locke-Edmunds JC, et al. Flap-valve theory of anorectal incontinence. *Br J Surg* 1986;73:1012.

Barton JR. A rectovaginal fistula cured. *Am J Med Sci* 1840;26:305.

Bartram CI, Sultan AH. Anal endosonography in faecal incontinence. *Gut* 1995;37:4.

Berek JS, Lagasse LD, Nacker NF, et al. Levator ani transposition for anal incompetence secondary to sphincter damage. *Obstet Gynecol* 1982;59:108.

Bielefeldt K, Enck P, Erckenbrecht JF. Sensory and motor function in the maintenance of anal continence. *Dis Colon Rectum* 1990;33:674.

Bielefeldt K, Enck P, Zamboglou N, et al. Anorectal manometry and defecography in the diagnosis of fecal incontinence. *J Clin Gastroenterol* 1991;13:661.

Birnhaum W. A method of repair for a common type of traumatic incontinence of the anal sphincter. *Surg Gynecol Obstet* 1948;87:716.

Blaisdell PC. Repair of the incontinent sphincter ani. *Surg Gynecol Obstet* 1940;70:692.

Boronow RC. Repair of the radiation-induced vaginal fistula using the Martius technique. *World J Surg* 1986;10:237.

Borrie MJ, Davidson HA. Incontinence in institutions: costs and contributing factors. *CMAJ* 1992;147:322.

Carey JC. A new method of diagnosing rectovaginal fistula: a case report. *J Reprod Med* 1988;33:789.

Chassagne P, Landrin I, Neveu C, et al. Fecal incontinence in the institutionalized elderly: incidence, risk factors, and prognosis. *J Urol* 1999;161(6):1813.

Chen AS, Luchtefeld MA, Senagore AJ, et al. Pudendal nerve latency. Does it predict outcome of anal sphincter repair? *J Clin Gastroenterol* 1998;27(2):108.

Cheong DM, Vaccaro CA, Salanga VD, et al. Electrodiagnostic evaluation of fecal incontinence [published erratum appears in *Muscle Nerve* 1995;18(11):1368]. *JAMA* 1995;274(7):559.

Christiansen J, Sparso B. Treatment of anal incontinence by an implantable prosthetic anal sphincter. *Ann Surg* 1992;215:383.

Cundiff GW, Nygaard I, Bland DR, et al. Proceedings of the American Urogynecologic Society Multidisciplinary Symposium on Defecatory Disorders. *Eur J Obstet Gynecol Reprod Biol* 2000;89(2):159.

Dalley AF II. The riddle of the sphincters: The morphophysiology of the anorectal mechanism reviewed. *Am J Surg* 1987;53:298. [Published erratum appears in *Am J Surg* 1987;53:398.]

Deen KI, Kumar D, Williams JG, et al. Randomized trial of internal anal sphincter plication with pelvic floor repair for neuropathic fecal incontinence. *Dis Colon Rectum* 1995;38:14.

Deen KI, Oya M, Ortiz J, et al. Randomized trial comparing three forms of pelvic floor repair for neuropathic faecal incontinence. *Br J Surg* 1993;80:794.

DeLancey JOL, Hurd WW. Size of the urogenital hiatus in the levator ani muscles in normal women and women with pelvic organ prolapse. *Obstet Gynecol* 1998;91:364.

DeLancey JOL, Toglia MR, Perucchini D. Internal and external anal sphincter anatomy as it relates to midline obstetric lacerations. *Obstet Gynecol* 1997;90:924.

Denny-Brown D, Robertson EG. An investigation of the nervous control of defecation. *Brain* 1935;58:256.

DeSouza NM, Puni R, Zbar A, et al. MR imaging of the anal sphincter in multiparous women using an endoanal coil: correlation with in vitro anatomy and appearances in fecal incontinence. *Am J Roentgenol* 1996;167:1465.

Elkins TE, DeLancey JOL, McGuire EJ. The use of modified Martius graft as an adjunctive technique in vesicovaginal and rectovaginal fistula repair. *Obstet Gynecol* 1990;75:727.

Emblem R, Dhaenens G, Ragnar S. The importance of anal endosonography in the evaluation of idiopathic fecal incontinence. *Dis Colon Rectum* 1994;37:42.

Enck P, Daublin G, Lubke HJ, et al. Long-term efficacy of biofeedback training for fecal incontinence. *Dis Colon Rectum* 1995;38(4):370.

Enck P, Kuhlbusch MTA, Lubke H. Age and sex and anorectal manometry in incontinence. *Dis Colon Rectum* 1989; 32:1026.

Faltin DL, Sangalli MR, Curtin F, et al. Prevalence of anal incontinence and other anorectal symptoms in women. *Int Urogynecol J* 2001;12:117.

Felt-Bersma RJF, Klinkenberg-Knol EC, Meuwissen SGM. Anorectal function investigations in incontinent and continent patients: differences and discriminatory value. *Dis Colon Rectum* 1990;33:479.

Felt-Bersma RJF, Luth WJ, Janssen JJWM. Defecography in patients with anorectal disorders: which findings are clinically relevant? *Dis Colon Rectum* 1990;33:277.

Ferrante SL, Perry RE, Schreiman JS. The reproducibility of measuring the anorectal angle in defecography. *Dis Colon Rectum* 1991;34:51.

Fitzpatrick M, Behan M, O'Connell PR, et al. A randomized clinical trial comparing primary overlap with approximation repair of third degree obstetric tears. *Am J Obstet Gynecol* 2000;183(5):1220.

Gaston EA. Physiology of faecal continence. *Surg Gynaecol Obstet* 1948;87:280.

Giebel GD, Lefering R, Troidl, et al. Prevalence of fecal incontinence: what can be expected? *Dis Colon Rectum* 1998;41(6):705.

Gilliland R, Altomare DF, Moreira H, et al. Pudendal neuropathy is predictive of failure following anterior overlapping sphincteroplasty. *Dis Colon Rectum* 1998;41(12):1516.

Goei R. Anorectal function in patients with defecation disorders and asymptomatic subjects: evaluation with defecography. *Radiology* 1990;174:121.

Goldaber KG, Wendel PJ, McIntire DD, et al. Postpartum perineal morbidity after fourth-degree perineal repair. *Am J Obstet Gynecol* 1993;168:489.

Goligher JC, Leacock AG, Brossy JJ. Surgical anatomy of anal canal. *Br J Surg* 1955;43:51.

Gordon D, Groutz A, Goldman G, et al. Anal incontinence: prevalence among female patients attending a urogynecologic clinic. *Am J Roentgenol* 1999;173(1):179.

Green JR, Soohoo SL. Factors associated with rectal injury in spontaneous deliveries. *Obstet Gynecol* 1989;73:732.

Haadem K, Dahlström JA, Ling L. Anal sphincter competence in healthy women: clinical implications of age and other factors. *Obstet Gynecol* 1991;78:823.

Hallan RI, George B, Williams NS. Anal sphincter function: fecal incontinence and its treatment. *Surg Annu* 1993;25:85.

Hankins GDV, Hauth JC, et al. Early repair of episiotomy dehiscence. *Obstet Gynecol* 1990;75:48.

Hauth JC, Gilstrap LC, Ward SC, et al. Early repair of an external sphincter ani muscle and rectal mucosal dehiscence. *Obstet Gynecol* 1986;67:806.

Healy JC, Halligan S, Reznek RH, et al. Dynamic MR imaging compared with evacuation proctography when evaluating anorectal configuration and pelvic floor movement. *AJR* 1997;169:775.

Heyer T, Enck P, Grantke B, et al. Anal endosonography: are morphometric measurements of the anal sphincter reproducible. *Gastroenterology* 1995;108:A613.

Henry MM, Swash M. *Coloproctology and the pelvic floor.* London: Butterworths, 1985.

Hibbard LT. Surgical management of rectovaginal fistulas and complete perineal tears. *Am J Obstet Gynecol* 1978;130:139.

Hoexter B, Labow SB, Moseson MD. Transanal rectovaginal fistula repair. *Dis Colon Rectum* 1985;28:572.

Ingleman-Sundberg A. Transplantation of the levator muscles in the repair of complete tear and rectovaginal fistula. *Acta Chir Scand* 1947;96:313.

Jackson SL, Weber AM, Hull TL, et al. Fecal incontinence in women with urinary incontinence and pelvic organ prolapse. *Obstet Gynecol* 1997;89:423.

Jacobs PPM, Scheuer M, Kuijpers JHC. Obstetric fecal incontinence: role of pelvic floor denervation and results of delayed sphincter repair. *Dis Colon Rectum* 1990;33:494.

Jorge JM, Wexner SD. Etiology and management of fecal incontinence. *Dis Colon Rectum* 1993;36:77.

Kamm MA. Obstetric damage and faecal incontinence. *Lancet* 1994;344:730.

Kammerer-Doak DN, Wesol AB, Rogers RG, et al. A prospective cohort study of women after primary repair of obstetric anal sphincter laceration. *Am J Obstet Gynecol* 1999; 181(6):1317.

Karoui S, Leroi AM, Koning E, et al. Results of sphincteroplasty in 86 patients with anal incontinence. *Ann Surg* 2000;232(1):143.

Keighley MR. Postanal repair for faecal incontinence. *J R Soc Med* 1984;77(4):285.

Keighley MRB. Faecal incontinence. In: Keighley MRB, Williams NS. *Surgery of the anus, rectum and colon.* Philadelphia: WB Saunders, 1993a:516.

Kodner IJ, Mazor A, Shemesh EI, et al. Endorectal advancement flap repair of rectovaginal and other complicated anorectal fistulas. *Surgery* 1993;114:682.

Kuhn RJP, Hollyock VE. Observations on the anatomy of the rectovaginal pouch and septum. *Obstet Gynecol* 1982;59: 445.

Kuijpers HC, Scheuer M. Disorders of impaired fecal control: a clinical and manometric study. *Dis Colon Rectum* 1990; 33:207.

Laurberg S, Swash M, Henry MM. Delayed external sphincter repair for obstetric tear. *Br J Surg* 1988;75:786.

Law PJ, Kamm MA, Bartram CI. A comparison between electromyography and anal endosonography in mapping external anal sphincter defects. *Dis Colon Rectum* 1990;33:370.

Law PJ, Kamm MA, Bartram CI. Anal endosonography in the investigation of faecal incontinence. *Br J Surg* 1991;78: 312.

Lee RA, ed. *Atlas of gynecologic surgery.* Philadelphia: WB Saunders, 1992.

Leroi AM, Kamm MA, Weber J, et al. Internal anal sphincter repair. *Int J Colorectal Dis* 1997;12(4):243.

Leroi AM, Weber J, Menard JF, et al. Prevalence of anal incontinence in 409 patients investigated for stress urinary incontinence. *Obstet Gynecol* 1999;94(5Pt1):689.

Levy E. Anorectal musculature. *Am J Surg* 1936;34:141.

Lienemann A, Anthuber C, Baron A, et al. Dynamic MR colpocystorectography assessing pelvic-floor descent. *Eur J Radiol* 1997;7:1309.

Lowry AC, Thorson AG, Rothenberger DA, et al. Repair of simple rectovaginal fistulas. Influence of previous repairs. *Dis Colon Rectum* 1988;31:676.

Madoff RD, Rosen HR, Baeten CG, et al. Safety and efficacy of dynamic muscle plasty for anal incontinence: lessons from a prospective, multicenter trial. *Eur J Radiol* 1999;9(3):436.

Madoff RD, Williams JG, Caushaj PF. Fecal incontinence. *N Engl J Med* 1992;326:1002.

Malouf AJ, Norton CS, Engel AF, et al. Long-term results of overlapping anterior anal-sphincter repair for obstetric trauma. *Lancet* 2000;355(9200):260.

Malouf AJ, Vaizey CJ, Nicholls RJ, et al. Permanent sacral nerve stimulation for fecal incontinence. *Dis Colon Rectum* 2000;43(8):1100.

Martius H. Die operative Wiederherstel-lung der vollkommen fehlenden. Harnrohare und des Schliessmuskels derselben. *Zentralb Gynakol* 1928;52:480.

Matsuoka H, Mavrantonis C, Wexner SD, et al. Postanal repair for fecal incontinence—is it worthwhile? *Dis Colon Rectum* 2000;43(11):1561.

Matzel KE, Stadelmaier U, Hohenfellner M, et al. Electrical stimulation of sacral spinal nerves for treatment of faecal incontinence [see comments]. *Int Urogynecol J Pelvic Floor Dysfunct* 1996;7(1):1.

Mazier WP, Senagore AJ, Schiesel EC. Operative repair of anovaginal and rectovaginal fistulas. *Dis Colon Rectum* 1995;38:4.

McIntosh LJ, Frahm JD, Mallett VT. Pelvic floor rehabilitation in the treatment of incontinence. *J Reprod Med* 1993;38:662.

Mengert WF, Fish SA. Anterior rectal wall advancement. *Obstet Gynecol* 1955;5:262.

Miller NF, Brown W. The surgical treatment of complete perineal tears in the female. *Am J Obstet Gynecol* 1937;34:196.

Milligan ETC, Morgan CN. Surgical anatomy of the anal canal, with special reference to anorectal fistulae. *Lancet* 1934;2:1150.

Miner PB, Donnelly TC, Read NW. Investigation of mode of action of biofeedback in treatment of fecal incontinence. *Dig Dis Sci* 1990;35:1291.

Monberg J, Hammen S. Ruptured episiotomies resutured primarily. *Acta Obstet Gynecol Scand* 1987;66:163.

Moore FA. Anal incontinence: a reappraisal. *Obstet Gynecol* 1973;41:483.

Nelson R, Norton N, Cautley E, et al. Community-based prevalence of anal incontinence. *JAMA* 1995;274(7):559.

Nielsen MB, Buron B, Christiansen J, et al. Defecographic findings in patients with anal incontinence and constipation and their relation to rectal emptying. *Dis Colon Rectum* 1993;36:806.

Nielsen MB, Hauge C, Pedersen JF, et al. Endosonographic evaluation of patients with anal incontinence: findings and influence on surgical management. *Am J Radiol* 1993;160:771.

Nivatvongs S, Stern HS, Fryd DS. The length of the anal canal. *Dis Colon Rectum* 1981;24:600.

Noble GH. A new technique for complete laceration of the perineum designed for the purpose of eliminating infection from the rectum. *Trans Am Gynecol Soc* 1902;27:357.

Nyam DC, Pemberton JH. Long-term results of lateral internal sphincterotomy for chronic anal fissure with particular reference to incidence of fecal incontinence. *Neurourol Urodyn* 1999;18(6):579.

Osterberg A, Graf W, Edebol Eeg-Olofsson K, et al. Results of neurophysiologic evaluation in fecal incontinence. *Dis Colon Rectum* 2000;43(9):1256.

Parks AG. Anorectal incontinence. *Proc R Soc Med* 1975;68:21.

Parks TG. The usefulness of tests in anorectal disease. *World J Surg* 1992;16:804.

Paul DJ, Lloyd TV. Hindgut duplication with rectovaginal fistula. *Obstet Gynecol* 1979;54:390.

Pemberton JH, Kelly KA. Achieving enteric continence: principles and applications. *Mayo Clin Proc* 1986;61:586.

Pescatori M, Pavesio R, Anastasio G, et al. Transanal electro-stimulation for fecal incontinence: clinical, psychologic, and manometric prospective study. *Dis Colon Rectum* 1991;34:540.

Peschers UM, DeLancey JO, Schaer GN, et al. Exoanal ultrasound of the anal sphincter: normal anatomy and sphincter defects. *Dis Colon Rectum* 1997;40(12):1430.

Poen AC, Felt-Bersma RJ, Strijers RL, et al. Third-degree obstetric perineal tear: long-term clinical and functional results after primary repair. *Br J Surg* 1998;85(10):1433.

Roberts PL, Coller JA, Schoetz DJ, et al. Manometric assessment of patients with obstetric injuries and fecal incontinence. *Dis Colon Rectum* 1990;33:16.

Roberts RO, Jacobsen SJ, Reilly WT, et al. Prevalence of combined fecal and urinary incontinence: a community-based study. *Dis Colon Rectum* 1999;42(7):857.

Rock JA, Woodruff JD. Surgical correction of a rectovaginal fistula. *Int J Gynecol Obstet* 1982;20:413.

Rockwood TH, Church JM, Fleshman JW, et al. Fecal Incontinence Quality of Life Scale: quality of life instrument for patients with fecal incontinence. *Dis Colon Rectum* 2000;43(6):813.

Rosenshein NB, Genadry RR, Woodruff JD. An anatomic classification of rectovaginal septal defects. *Am J Obstet Gynecol* 1980;137:439.

Rothbarth J, Bemelman WA, Mierjerink WJ, et al. Long-term results of anterior anal sphincteroplasty repair for fecal incontinence due to obstetric injury/with invited commentaries. *Dig Surg* 2000;17(4):390.

Rothenberger DA, Goldberg SM. The management of rectovaginal fistulae. *Surg Clin North Am* 1983;63:61.

Rothenberger DA, Christenson CE, Balcos EG, et al. Endorectal advancement flap for treatment of simple rectovaginal fistula. *Dis Colon Rectum* 1982;25:297.

Sandridge DA, Thorp JM. Vaginal endosonography in the assessment of the anorectum. *Obstet Gynecol* 1995;86:1007.

Sangwan YP, Coller JA. Fecal incontinence. *Surg Clin NA* 1994;74:1377.

Sangwan YP, Coller JA, Barrett RC, et al. Unilateral pudendal neuropathy. Impact on outcome of anal sphincter repair. *Dis Colon Rectum* 1996;39:686.

Santoro GA, Eitan BZ, Pryde A, et al. Open study of low-dose amitriptyline in the treatment of patients with idiopathic fecal incontinence. *Dis Colon Rectum* 2000;43(12):1676.

Sentovich SM, Blatchford GJ, Rivela LJ, et al. Diagnosing anal sphincter injury with transanal ultrasound and manometry. *Elder Care* 1997–1998;9(6 Suppl):3.

Setti Carraro P, Kamm MA, Nicholls RJ. Long-term results of postanal repair for neurogenic faecal incontinence. *Br J Surg* 1994;81:140.

Shafik A, Doss S. Surgical anatomy of the somatic terminal innervation to the anal and urethral sphincters: role in anal and urethral surgery. *J Urol* 1999;161(1):85.

Shiono P, Klehanoff MA, Carey JC. Midline episiotomies: more harm than good? *Obstet Gynecol* 1990;75:765.

Sitzler PJ, Thomson JP. Overlap repair of damaged anal sphincter. A single surgeon's series. *Dis Colon Rectum* 1996;13:56.

Snooks SJ, Henry MM. Faecal incontinence due to external anal sphincter division in childbirth is associated with damage to the innervation of the pelvic floor musculature: a double pathology. *Br J Obstet Gynaecol* 1985a;92:824.

Snooks SJ, Henry MM, Swash M. Anorectal incontinence and rectal prolapse: differential assessment of the innervation to puborectalis and external anal sphincter muscles. *Gut* 1985c;26:470.

Snooks SJ, Swash M, Setchell M, et al. Injury to innervation of pelvic floor sphincter musculature in childbirth. *Lancet* 1984;2:546.

Soffer EE, Hull T. Fecal incontinence: a practical approach to evaluation and treatment. *Am J Gastroenterol* 2000;95(8):1873.

Sorensen M, Tetzschner T, Rasmussen OO, et al. Sphincter rupture in childbirth. *Br J Surg* 1993;80:392.

Stewart LK, Wilson SR. Transvaginal sonography of the anal sphincter: reliable, or not? *J Am Geriatr Soc* 1999;47(7):837.

Strohbehn K, Ellis JH, Strohbehn JA, et al. MRI of the levator ani with anatomic correlation. *Obstet Gynecol* 1996a;87:277.

Sultan AH. Anal incontinence after childbirth. *Curr Opinion Obstet Gynecol* 1997;9:320.

Sultan AH, Kamm MA, Hudson CN, et al. Anal-sphincter disruption during vaginal delivery. *N Engl J Med* 1993;329:1905.

Sultan AH, Monga AK, Kumar D, et al. Primary repair of obstetric anal sphincter rupture using the overlap technique. *Br J Obstet Gynecol* 1999;106(4):318.

Sun WM, Donnelly TC, Read NW. Utility of a combined test of anorectal manometry, electromyography, and sensation in determining the mechanism of 'idiopathic' faecal incontinence. *Gut* 1992;33:807.

Swash M, Snooks SJ, Henry MM. A unifying concept of pelvic floor disorders and incontinence. *J R Soc Med* 1985b;78:906.

Tancer ML, Veridiano NP. Genital fistulas secondary to diverticular disease of the sigmoid colon. *Obstet Gynecol Surv* 1996;51:67.

Thacker SB, Banta HD. Benefits and risks of episiotomy: an interpretive review of the English language literature, 1860–1980. *Obstet Gynecol Surv* 1983;38:322.

Thomas TM, Egan M, Walgrove A, et al. The prevalence of faecal and double incontinence. *Commun Med* 1984;6:216.

Thorp JM, Bowes WA, Brame RG, et al. Selected use of midline episiotomy: effect on perineal trauma. *Obstet Gynecol* 1987;70:260.

Tjandra JJ, Milsom JW, Schroeder T, et al. Endoluminal ultrasound is preferable to electromyography in mapping anal sphincter defects. *Dis Colon Rectum* 1993;36:689.

Toglia MR, DeLancey JOL. Anal incontinence and the obstetrician-gynecologist. *Obstet Gynecol* 1994;84:731.

Uhlenhuth E, Wolfe WM, Smith EM, et al. The rectogenital septum. *Surg Gynecol Obstet* 1948;76:148.

Vaccaro CA, Cheong DM, Wexner SD, et al. Pudendal neuropathy in evacuatory disorders. *Dis Colon Rectum* 1995;38(2):166.

Vaizey CJ, Kamm MA, Bartram CI. Primary degeneration of the internal anal sphincter as a cause of passive faecal incontinence. *Lancet* 1997;349(9052):612.

Van Patter WN, Bargen JA, Dockerty MB, et al. Regional enteritis. *Gastroenterology* 1954;26:347.

Varma A, Gunn J, Gardiner A, et al. Obstetric anal sphincter injury: prospective evaluation of incidence. *Am J Obstet Gynecol* 2000;182(1 Pt 1):S1.

Venkatesh KS, Ramanujam PS, Larson DM, et al. Anorectal complications of vaginal delivery. *Dis Colon Rectum* 1989;32:1039.

Vernava AM III, Longo WE, Daniel GL. Pudendal neuropathy and the importance of EMG evaluation of fecal incontinence. *Dis Colon Rectum* 1993;36:23.

Veronikas DK, Nichols DH, Spino C. The Noble-Mengert-Fish operation revisited: a composite approach for persistent rectovaginal fistulas and complex perineal defects. *Am J Obstet Gynecol* 1998;179:1411.

Wall LL. The muscles of the pelvic floor. *Clin Obstet Gynecol* 1993;36;910.

Warren JC. A new method of operation for the relief of rupture of the perineum through the sphincter and rectum. *Trans Am Gynecol Soc* 1882;7:322.

Wilcox LS, Strobino DM, Baruffi G, et al. Episiotomy and its role in the incidence of perineal lacerations in a maternity center and a tertiary hospital obstetric service. *Am J Obstet Gynecol* 1989;160:1047.

Williams JG, Wong WD, Jensen L, et al. Incontinence and rectal prolapse: a prospective manometric study. *Dis Colon Rectum* 1991;34:209.

Wise WE, Aguilar PS, Padmanabhan A, et al. Surgical treatment of low rectovaginal fistulas. *Dis Colon Rectum* 1991;34:271.

Wiskind AK, Thompson MD. Transverse transperineal repair of rectovaginal fistulas in the lower vagina. *Am J Obstet Gynecol* 1992;167:694.

Zetterstrom J, Lopez A, Anzen B, et al. Anal sphincter tears at vaginal delivery: risk factors and clinical outcome of primary repair. *Obstet Gynecol* 1999;94(1):21.

RELATED SURGERY

CHAPTER

40

▼

Breast Diseases: Benign and Malignant

VICTORIA L. GREEN

The specialty of obstetrics and gynecology is devoted to the health care of women throughout their lifetime. Concerns about breast health are common to women from puberty to menopause and across all socioeconomic statuses. As the woman's primary care physician, obstetrician/gynecologists are becoming increasingly involved in not only the detection of breast masses but also the diagnosis, evaluation, and treatment of such lesions.

Although the etiology of most breast symptoms is a benign disorder, the fear of cancer is often the motivating factor for women seeking attention. Breast cancer remains the most common cancer in women, with the American Cancer Society (ACS) estimating nearly 183,000 cases in the United States in the year 2000. Cancer of the breast is second only to lung cancer in the number of cancer deaths in women, making it an especially dreadful adversary. Recent advances in hormonal treatment, genetic etiologies, and prophylactic prevention of breast cancer have thrust breast health issues into the forefront of the media and medical technology. The zeal to achieve the ideal cure or prevention strategy persists unabated in the medical profession and remains an ongoing challenge. A thorough understanding of the diagnosis and management of breast disease, as well as an appreciation of contemporary treatment options, are essential for the practicing gynecologist.

The purpose of this chapter is to review the anatomy, physiology, and pathology of the breast and to examine strategies for the diagnosis, management and treatment of benign breast conditions. A review of recent advances in breast cancer therapy is discussed, with emphasis on assessment of risk factors, breast cancer susceptibility testing and follow-up, mammographic screening recommendations, alternative imaging modalities, and tamoxifen chemoprevention in high-risk women. The woman in whom breast cancer develops requires a multidisciplinary team, including general surgeons, radiation oncologists, and medical oncologists. The gynecologist must be a knowledgeable participant in her treatment plan.

EMBRYOLOGY

The breasts, or mammary glands, are a distinguishing feature of mammals. In humans, embryologic differentiation of these paired glands begins at the fifth or sixth week of fetal development. Two ventral bands of thickened ectoderm (known as mammary ridges or "milk lines") develop and extend from the area of the future axilla at the base of the forelimb, to the future inguinal region of the hind limb (Fig. 40.1). With normal regression of the ridges (which occurs shortly after the sixth week of fetal development), only one gland persists on

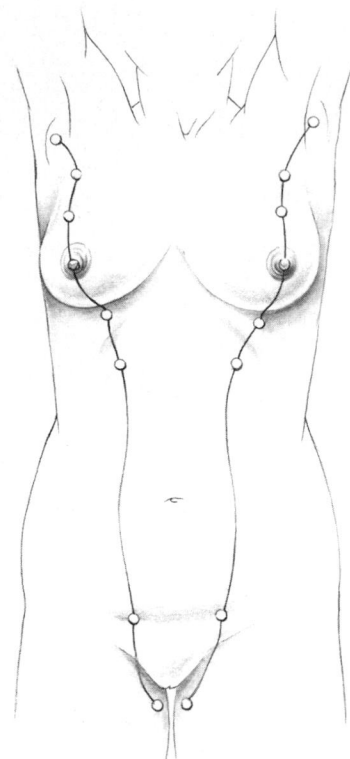

FIGURE 40.1. Mammary milk line.

each side, at the level of the thorax. This process is similar in both genders. Accessory mammary glands (polymastia) or accessory nipples (polythelia) may result along the original mammary ridge with failure of normal regression. This minor congenital anomaly may occur in both sexes with an estimated frequency of about 1%. One third of affected individuals may have multiple extra breasts or nipples.

Ingrowth of the remaining ectoderm into the underlying mesenchyme initiates the development of the primary bud of the mammary gland. As many as 15 to 20 secondary buds develop as outgrowths of each primary bud and extend into the surrounding connective tissues of the chest wall. Canalization of these epithelial cords (under the influence of placental sex steroids) during the third trimester marks the development of the lactiferous ductal system. Proliferation of basal mesenchymal cells initiates transformation into the fully formed nipple. Continued elevation is supported by both expansion of underlying connective tissue and smooth muscle development in the areolar gland. Failure of elevation of the nipple above the skin level occurs in 2% to 4% of the population, resulting in inverted nipples.

Anatomy

The breast, or mammary gland, is a highly modified sudoriferous gland situated between two layers of superficial fascia upon the pectoralis major, serratus anterior, and external oblique muscles. It is bordered by the sec-

ond rib superiorly, the sternum medially, the sixth intercostal space inferiorly, and the midaxillary line laterally. It is composed of 15 to 20 lobes, with the greatest volume of glandular tissue located in the upper outer quadrant. Fibrous septa, called *suspensory* or *Cooper's ligaments,* interdigitate between the parenchymal tissue to connect the two fascial planes. The ligaments permit mobility of the breast upon the anterior thoracic wall while also providing structural support (Fig. 40.2).

These anatomic landmarks gain importance in breast cancer development. Fixation of the breast to the underlying chest wall may result from cancer involving the area beneath the deep layer of superficial fascia and above the deep investing fascia of the pectoralis major muscle (retromammary bursa). Involvement of the Cooper's ligament in a malignant process may result in skin retraction or dimpling.

The breast lobes are arranged in a radial pattern and contain many lobules. Each lobule consists of 10 to 100 alveoli or tubulosaccular secretory units (Fig. 40.3). Breast cancer is thought to originate in these units, also called terminal duct lobular units. Each lobe terminates in a lactiferous duct, which opens onto the nipple. Beneath the areola, each lactiferous duct features a dilated portion called the lactiferous sinus. Inspissation of material in the lactiferous sinus may account for galactoceles.

The epidermis of the nipple and areola is highly pigmented. Additional increased pigmentation and size of the nipple–areolar complex is noted in pregnancy. The nipple contains the only muscle "within" the breast tissue. Smooth muscle fibers in the dense connective tissue of the nipple and the numerous sensory nerve cell endings account for erection of the nipple as a consequence of various sensory and thermal stimuli. This rich sensory innervation is also of great functional importance in the neurohumoral pathways necessary for "milk letdown" during suckling. The areola consists of many sweat, sebaceous, and accessory glands. During pregnancy, accessory glands called *Montgomery tubercles* become prominent.

The breast tissue is well supplied by an extensive arterial and venous system. The anterior perforating branches of the internal thoracic (internal mammary) artery supplies the medial and central aspect of the breast. The upper outer quadrant is supplied by the lateral thoracic artery, a branch of the axillary artery. The two vessels combined provide the major blood supply to the nipple. Other vessels supplying the breast include the anterior and lateral branches of the intercostals, other branches of the axillary artery (including the pectoral branch of the thoracoacromial artery), and the subscapular and thoracodorsal arteries.

Venous and lymphatic drainage of the breast follows the course of the superficial and deeper arteries. Principal venous drainage goes to the internal thoracic vein medially, to the axillary vein superolaterally, and by way of the intercostal veins to the vertebral and azygous veins posteriorly. This drainage pathway accounts for the frequent sites of metastases, because breast cancer enters the venous system and metastasizes to the lungs by way of the axillary or intercostal veins or to thoracic, abdom-

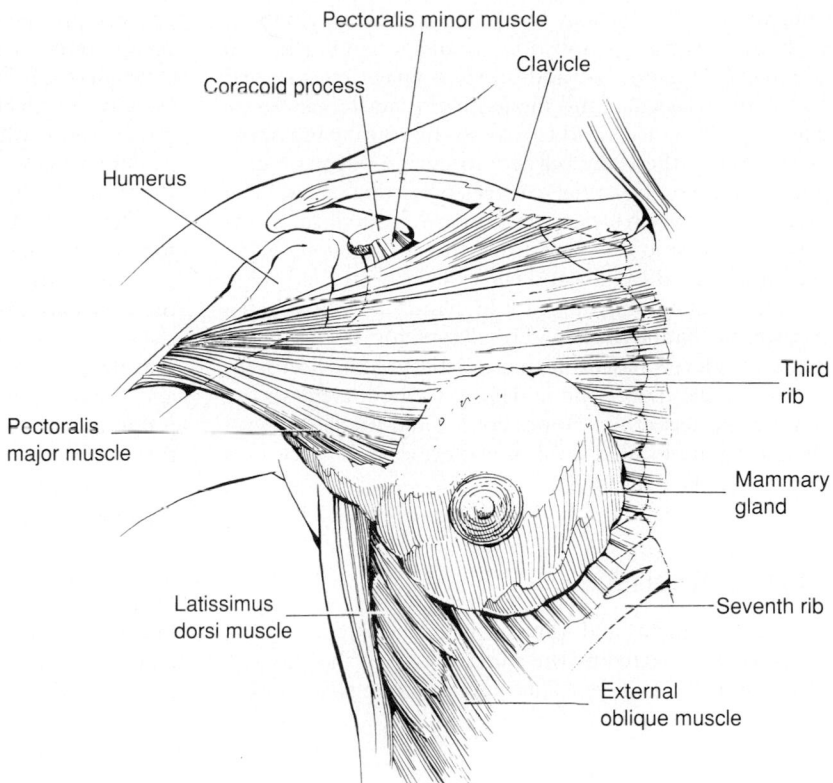

FIGURE 40.2. Topography of the breast. The breast lies approximately over the midportion of the hemithorax with the tail extending toward the axilla. Ramifications also penetrate the interstices of the underlying muscle. These extensions and the close adherence of the skin to subcutaneous breast tissue make complete subcutaneous mastectomy nearly impossible.

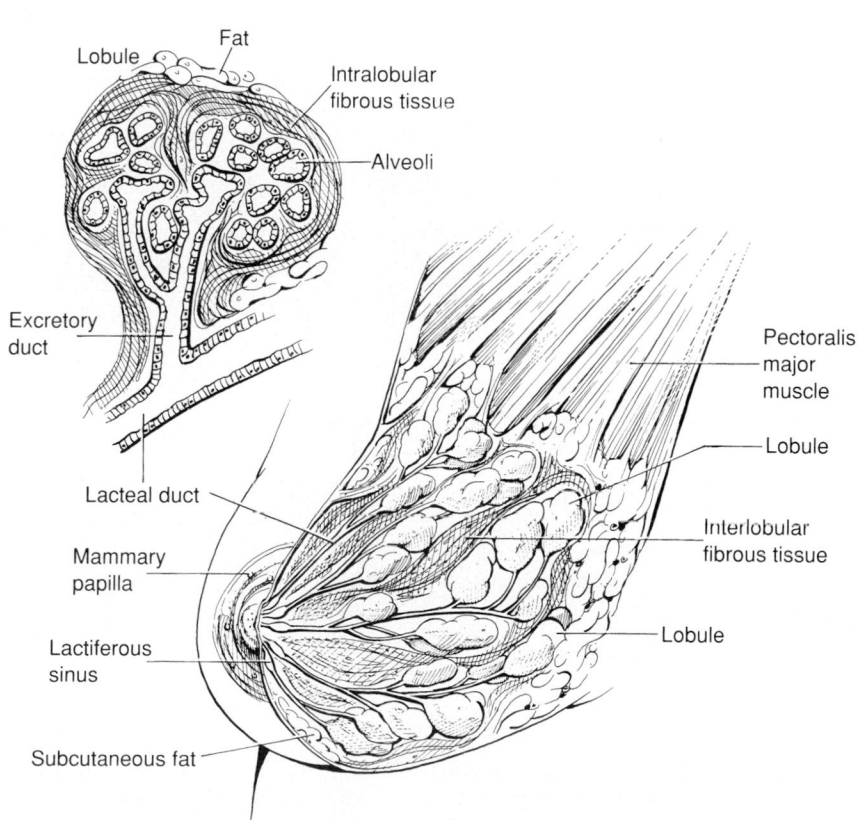

FIGURE 40.3. Internal structure of the breast. The breast is a large apocrine gland. The secreting parenchyma is composed of lobules containing acini, fat, and fibrous tissue. The ducts drain centrally toward large lacunae located directly beneath the nipple. These act as reservoirs until they receive the impetus for ejection.

inal, and pelvic organs by way of the vertebral vein. Similarly, the primary lymph node drainage is initially into the axillary region, but additional drainage can proceed to the infraclavicular and mediastinal (parasternal) areas, thus suggesting the need to extend the routine breast examination to the bony borders to ensure adequate coverage of these potential cancer-containing areas. The lymphatic plexus has deep and superficial drainage pathways. Lymphatic drainage from the deep lesions is directed toward the axilla and the axillary nodes, although all breast quadrants contribute lymph to the medial parasternal lymph nodes. This lymphatic plexus is divided into levels based on their relation to the pectoralis minor muscle. Level one nodes are located lateral to the muscle and level three nodes are located medially. Level two nodes are located deep or posterior to the pectoralis minor muscle (Fig. 40.4).

PHYSIOLOGY

The development and physiologic functioning of the breast is orchestrated by the anterior lobe of the pituitary gland and the ovaries. This development is a lifelong process that begins in utero. Transient enlargement of the breast bud and associated milklike nipple secretion ("witches milk") may occur in both newborn girls and boys as a result of transplacental transfer of maternal hormones (primarily estrogen). The fluid secretion may appear for a week postpartum, but subsequent involution of the tissue results by the third or fourth week postpartum.

Before the transformation that occurs at puberty, the function and histology of the human breast is identical in boys and girls. However, at puberty in girls, the rudimentary gland buds proliferate and increase in size, and the nipple and areola become pigmented. The ductal system develops as a consequence of estrogen stimulation and the lobular-alveolar system develops in response to progesterone secretion. The first *visible* manifestation of this hormonal response is a symmetric palpable enlargement beneath the nipple.

Menstruation, pregnancy, and menopause are additional sentinel events in the cycle of breast development. Before the onset of menstruation, breast transformation begins with ductal branching and proliferation of interductal stroma. With each menstrual cycle, ductal proliferation occurs under the influence of estrogen. Proliferation of the terminal duct structure and increased

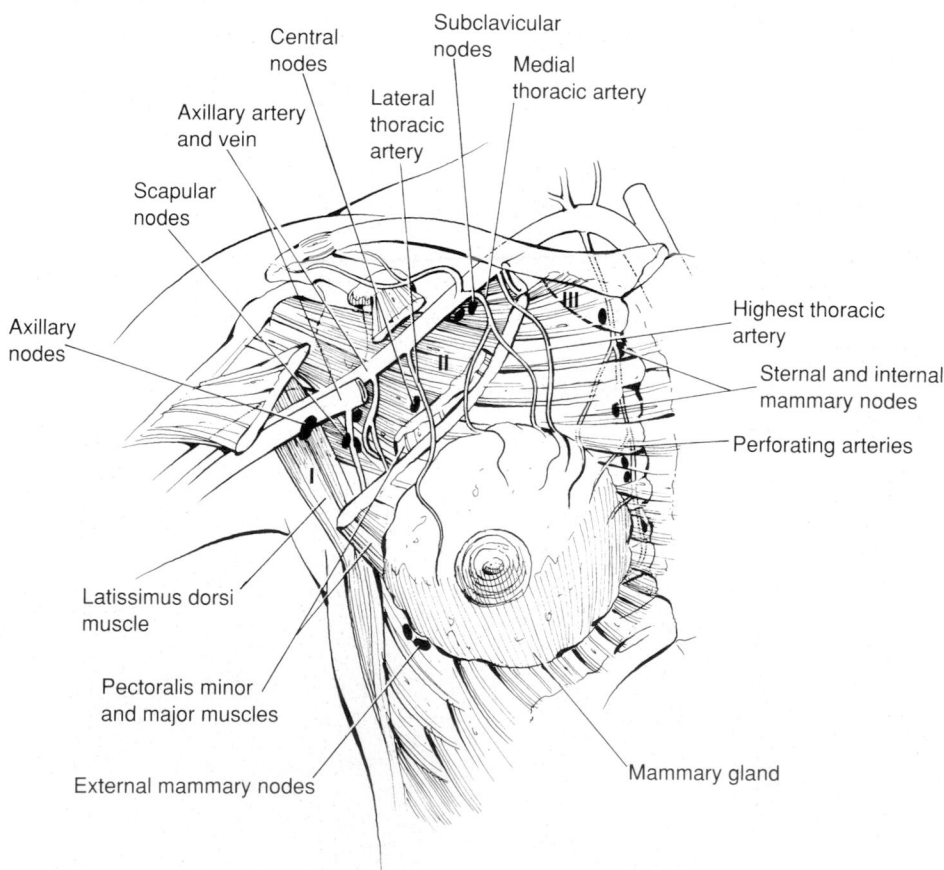

FIGURE 40.4. Lymphatics and blood supply of the breast. Lymphatic drainage from the outer half of the breast goes first to the axillary nodes, shown here at levels I, II, and III. Medial lesions are more likely to metastasize first to the internal mammary chain.

mitotic activity in the basal epithelial cells occur in the secretory phase under the influence of progesterone. Stromal proliferation and edema, in response to the hormonal milieu, accounts for the sense of fullness or tenderness experienced premenstrually. The decrease in hormones that occurs with menstruation signals disappearance of stromal edema, desquamation of epithelial cells, atrophy of intralobular connective tissue, and overall shrinkage in the size of the ducts.

Further maturation of the breast occurs with pregnancy. Significant development of glandular tissues and decrease in the surrounding stroma portends reversal of the stromal glandular relation seen before this stage. After pregnancy, these changes regress but do not return completely to their prepregnancy state. Menopause heralds a further reduction and shrinkage of the ducts, gland buds, and surrounding stroma.

Lactation

Hormonal and structural changes, which prime the breast for future milk production, occur during pregnancy. As previously occurred during puberty, increased estrogen and progesterone secretion in early pregnancy results in ductal development and maturation as well as enlargement of lobular size. During the latter half of pregnancy, glandular epithelium is transformed into secretory epithelium in response to insulin, thyroxine, growth hormone, and corticosteroids. Human placental lactogen and prolactin also play critical roles in breast development in pregnancy. Paradoxically, despite considerable increases in prolactin, its functioning is inhibited at the alveolar level by progesterone. Thus, lactation does not occur until the rapid decline of estrogen and progesterone that occurs with delivery.

Stimulation of the afferent neural arc suppresses prolactin inhibitory factor (PIF), allowing release of PRF and further elevation of the prolactin concentration. Breast suckling stimulates the neural arc as do auditory and visual stimuli. PIF is thought to be dopamine and PRF is thought to be thyroid-releasing hormone or thyrotropin-releasing hormone. Additionally, stimulation of the neural arc triggers release of oxytocin by involving the paraventricular and supraoptic nuclei of the hypothalamus. Oxytocin release from the posterior pituitary induces contraction of the myoepithelial cells surrounding the nipple ducts, resulting in milk letdown. Continued suckling induces additional prolactin secretion and replenishment of the milk supply. Discontinuation of suckling results in increased levels of PIF, which inhibit prolactin production. Ultimately, lactation ceases with resultant decrease in size of the alveoli.

PATHOLOGY

Table 40.1 lists the basic anatomic structures and the most commonly associated pathologic abnormalities. Most of the pathology of the breast involves the termi-

TABLE 40.1.
Breast Anatomic Structures and Associated Breast Lesions

Anatomic Structures	Lesions
Nipple	Paget's disease
	Nipple adenoma
Lactiferous duct	Papillomas
Adipose tissue	Traumatic fat necrosis
Terminal duct	Hyperplasia
Lobular unit (lobule, terminal duct, ductules)	Most carcinomas
	Fibroadenoma
	Cysts

Adapted from Cotran R, Kumar V, Robbins SL. *Pathologic basis of disease,* 5th ed. Philadelphia: WB Saunders, 1994.

nal duct lobular unit. A brief review of pathology of the breast follows.

Congenital Anomalies

Congenital abnormalities affecting the breast anlage include amastia, hypertrophy, asymmetry, and congenital inversion of the nipples. Additionally, supernumerary nipples or breasts may be seen—the result of persistence of epidermal thickenings along the milk line.

Inflammation

Acute mastitis or breast abscesses may develop during nursing or with other dermatologic conditions of the nipples. The breast is vulnerable to bacterial infection from tears or fissures in the nipples. The offending bacterium in puerperal mastitis is most commonly *Staphylococcus aureus* and *Streptococcus*. Treatment includes continued emptying of breast milk, either through nursing or pumping, and use of warm or cold compresses. The most effective broad-spectrum antibiotics are dicloxacillin or a first generation cephalosporin for 10 days. For those with penicillin allergies, erythromycin may be substituted.

Nonpuerperal mastitis is often associated with a sticky, multicolored discharge and is noted in individuals who are immunocompromised (e.g., diabetic patients), people who have undergone radiation treatment, and those who have an autoimmune disorder. Purulent discharges generally respond to antibiotics, but an abscess requires incision and drainage for complete resolution.

Duct ectasia is characterized by dilation of the ducts, inspissation of breast secretions, and marked periductal and interstitial chronic granulomatous inflammatory reaction. It is often association with a multicolored, sticky, spontaneous, bilateral nipple discharge coming from multiple ducts. It is most commonly seen in women in the fifth or sixth decade of life; however, the etiology is unknown. Periductal inflammation may result in nipple inversion, areolar thickening, and a breast mass that can mimic a cancer or nonpuerperal abscess. This condition is discussed further under the section on nipple discharge.

Galactocele occurs as a result of overdistention of lactiferous ducts with resultant inspissation of milk. It usually presents as a firm nontender mass in the outer quadrants of the breast, away from the areolar margin.

Fibrocystic Changes

Fibrocystic change (FCC) of the breast is the most frequently encountered benign breast disorder. It occurs most often in reproductive women between the ages of 30 and 50 years. It also occurs in approximately 10% of women younger than 21 years of age, so breast symptoms in a young population must not be ignored. Fibrocystic condition does not increase the risk of developing breast cancer but it does often make the physical examination of the patient more difficult (Fig. 40.5).

In 85% to 90% of cases of significant FCC, breast discomfort is the leading symptom. Women often present with a history of bilateral, menstrually related, painful, tender, and a nodular breasts, most often localized to the upper outer quadrants. Typically, the pain is most severe just before menses as a result of the normal physiologic stromal edema and ductal dilation.

The breast is normally an inhomogeneous appendage with uneven distribution of adipose and fibrous tissue. It is estimated that at least 50% of women have palpably irregular breasts. This "normal" anatomic asymmetry leads to physiologic inhomogeneity, irregularity, or lumpiness in some women. Nodularity, particularly as it waxes and wanes during the menstrual cycle, is a physiologic process. This nodularity and irregularity is often mistaken for a dominant breast mass. Evaluation of FCC, thus, creates a difficult dilemma for physicians. Providers must carefully decide whether their findings represent a dominant mass or an exaggeration of normal breast tissue associated with the "nodularity" of FCCs.

Dominant masses may represent a variety of benign and malignant processes, including fibroadenomas, macrocysts, prominent areas of FCC, fat necrosis, abscesses, or carcinoma. Dominant masses are distinguished by their persistence throughout the menstrual cycle and palpable difference on examination from the surrounding breast parenchyma. Often, evaluation of the contralateral breast assists in determination of whether an anatomic variation is a mass or normal breast tissue. However, any concern should be referred for evaluation or a repeat examination may be performed after a menstrual cycle to detect persistence. A delay of 1 to 2 months in a reproductive age woman is acceptable; however, a shorter-term follow-up is preferable in a menopausal woman because of the higher frequency of breast cancer in this age group. Breast masses are often easier to appreciate in postmenopausal women, because of atrophy of the surrounding nodular glandular elements. A *positive* mammogram is helpful. Conversely, a negative mammogram does not obviate the need to evaluate this mass by fine-needle aspiration (FNA) or a histologic method of biopsy because there is a 10% to 15% false-negative rate for mammography.

Fibrocystic change is a term proposed by the ACS. The terminology encompasses several histopathologic categories including macrocyst formation, hyperplasia of ductal epithelium, apocrine metaplasia, papillomatosis, duct ectasia, sclerosing adenosis, and stromal fibrosis, thus leading to significant confusion. Reporting criteria for pathologists may include all or only some of these groups. It is important to know whether *severe* ductal hyperplasia is included in the pathologist's category of FCC because this variant increases a patient's risk of subsequent development of breast carcinoma by three to five times that of the general population. Conversely, mild hyperplasia (which may also be included in the FCC categorization) does not increase a patient's risk of breast cancer development. Practitioners should attempt to describe exactly what they are feeling rather than use the undefined FCC term in the clinical arena. This term is not *clinically* meaningful in that it designates a heterogeneous group of processes, some pathologic and some physiologic.

In simple FCC, there is an increase in fibrous stroma associated with dilatation of ducts and cyst formation of various sizes. Occasionally, the cysts may be lined by epithelial proliferations of large cells with abundant cytoplasm. This variant is called apocrine metaplasia and is almost always benign. Epithelial hyperplasia occurs in the ducts and ductules. The more severe and atypical the hyperplasia, the greater the risk of breast cancer development. Sclerosing adenosis is characterized by intralobular fibrosis and proliferation of small ductules or acini. This variety is less common than cystic changes or epithelial hyperplasia. Treatment options for FCC-induced mastalgia are discussed later. Table 40.2 summarizes the various FCCs and their relative risks of breast cancer.

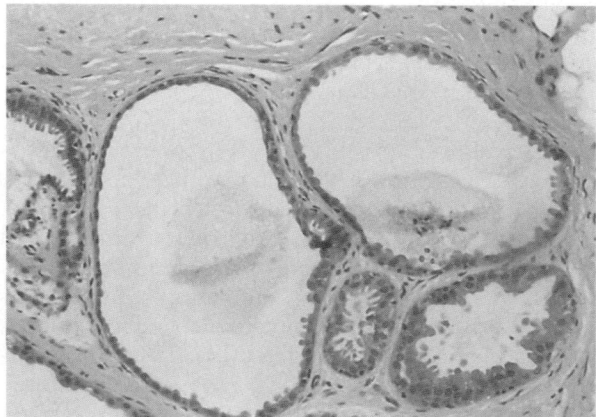

FIGURE 40.5. Histologic section of fibrocystic changes with cyst formation and at right lower corner apocrine metaplasia (H&E ×120) (Courtesy of Taalat Tadros, M.D., Emory University, School of Medicine, Atlanta, GA.)

TABLE 40.2.
Fibrocystic Changes and Relative Risk of Breast Carcinoma

Change	Risk
Fibrosis	No increased risk
Cystic changes	
Apocrine metaplasia	
Sclerosing adenosis	
Mild hyperplasia	
Hyperplasia–moderate to severe	1.5–2×
Marked ductal papillomatosis	
Atypical hyperplasia (ductal or lobular with duct involvement)	5×

Adapted from Cotran R, Kumar V, Robbins SL. *Pathologic basis of disease*, 5th ed. Philadelphia: WB Saunders, 1994.

Benign Tumors

Most women discover their own breast masses by chance or by periodic self-breast examination. Two thirds of the masses found during a woman's reproductive years are benign and include cystic changes, fibroadenomas, and papillomas. However, 50% of the palpable masses in perimenopausal women and the majority of lesions in postmenopausal patients are malignant. Once a lesion has been characterized as a mass or a lump, further evaluation is required. This may involve additional examinations at optimal times during the patient's menstrual cycle, radiologic imaging including mammography or ultrasound, FNA, or referral for excisional biopsy.

Because the incidence of breast cancer is extremely low in patients younger than 20 years of age, patients in this age group who have solid masses that appear to be benign when examined by ultrasonography can be monitored without biopsy at the discretion of the physician. However, the ability of the patient to follow up and other risk factors for breast cancer should be considered.

Gross cysts or macrocysts may be silent or painful. The consistency is a function of the pressure of the fluid within the cyst and the amount of normal breast tissue surrounding it. Cysts may be single or multiple and may be associated with a green-brown nipple discharge (although a thorough evaluation of the nipple discharge should occur despite the presumption of its origin). Of course, any dominant mass must be differentiated from a cancerous process.

Fibroadenomas are the most common benign tumors of the female breast and represent the most common breast tumor in women younger than 25 years of age. Fibroadenomas can occur at any age but are more common in women younger than 30 years of age. These tumors are clinically painless, well-circumscribed, freely movable with a rounded, lobulated, or discoid configuration. They are usually rubbery and firm, but when calcified, they may present as a stony hard mass. Multiple fibroadenomas may develop simultaneously or succes-

sively in one or both breasts in 10% to 15% of cases. Growth of the fibrous stromal and glandular tissue is thought to be the result of an unopposed estrogenic influence on susceptible tissue, aberrations of normal breast development, or the product of a hyperplastic processes, rather than a true neoplasm. These tumors often contain estrogen receptors, hence they may fluctuate in size with the menstrual cycle or increase in size during pregnancy. They routinely involute with menopause. Histologically, there are two proliferative patterns of epithelial and stromal elements. The stroma proliferates around tubular (pericanalicular) or compressed cleftlike (intracanalicular) ducts. In the pericanalicular pattern, there is a random or concentric proliferation of the stromal elements around the epithelial structures. The intracanalicular pattern is characterized by radial growth patterns of the stroma perpendicular to the epithelial components. The two patterns coexist in some lesions, but one pattern often dominates. They are uncommonly associated with carcinoma, but, rarely, in situ lobular or ductal carcinomas arise in or involve fibroadenomas (Fig 40.6).

Fibroadenomas infrequently grow to be very large (10 to 15 cm in diameter) although most are excised at 2 to 4 cm. The very large fibroadenomas are called *giant fibroadenomas*. When morphologic changes such as leaflike clefts and "slits" are present, these fibroadenomas are called *phyllodes tumors* (formerly known as cystosarcoma phyllodes). These can be benign or malignant lesions. Histologic examination reveals that these lesions have a more cellular stroma, rarely display a prominent pericanalicular growth pattern, and tend to occur in an older age group (Fig. 40.7).

Management of fibroadenomas is varied. The key to management in all clinical situations is individualization. In women younger than 25 years of age who have fibroadenomas diagnosed by concurring physical examination, sonography, and FNA, the risk of missing breast cancer is 1 in 229 to 1 in 700. This risk remains very low

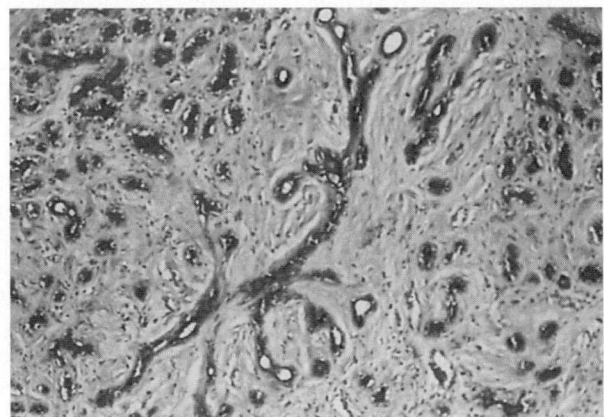

FIGURE 40.6. Histologic section of fibroadenoma with cellular stroma (in a pericanalicular pattern), ducts maintain patency (H&E ×240) (Courtesy of Taalat Tadros, M.D., Emory University, School of Medicine, Atlanta, GA.)

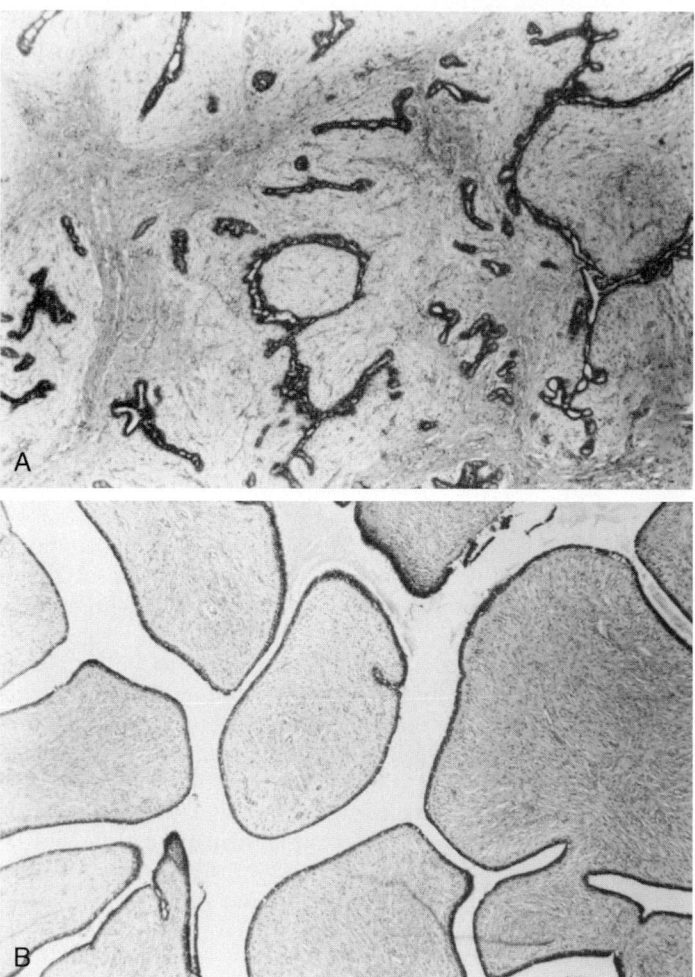

FIGURE 40.7. Benign tumors. **A:** A circumscribed breast tumor from a young patient illustrates fibroadenoma. A mixture of benign epithelial and stromal components is seen. **B:** Phyllodes tumor of the breast showing a pattern superficially similar to that of **(A)**. It is distinguished by its leaflike pattern of stromal growth in cystic spaces. The stroma is also markedly cellular. This tumor, although structurally benign, is capable of recurrence. (Courtesy of Bhagirath Majmudar, M.D., Emory University School of Medicine, Atlanta, GA.)

in women younger than 35 years who also have the battery of tests. Fibroadenomas do not regress spontaneously and tend to enlarge with time. Because of the low probability of cancer, conservatism is particularly acceptable in women younger than age 25 years if the fibroadenoma is not increasing in size or is not psychologically disturbing. If conservative management of fibroadenoma is to be advocated, physical examination, sonography, and FNA should be performed and all results should concur with a diagnosis of fibroadenoma. Mammography is an integral part of the evaluation in women older than 35 years (or younger depending on risk factors and clinical suspicion). Lesions greater than 3 cm should probably be evaluated for excision in a young woman.

Some authors promote excision of all fibroadenomas, regardless of histology, in women older than age 25 to 35 years. Clearly, if the FNA cytology reveals atypia or hyperplasia, excisional biopsy should be performed. Small, asymptomatic, mammographically detected fibroadenomas proven by FNA or core biopsy may be watched depending on clinical duration and patient risk factors. Although fibroadenomas may be suspected on the basis of their clinical presentation, a final diagnosis cannot be made without histologic or cytologic confirmation.

Intraductal papilloma is a papillary growth within a duct. These lesions are usually solitary and are found in the lactiferous ducts or sinuses. Clinically, they are rarely more than 1 cm in diameter and are associated with serous or bloody nipple discharge, or nipple retraction.

Breast cancer is discussed later in this chapter.

COMMON BREAST COMPLAINTS
Mastalgia

Breast pain, or mastalgia, is the primary presenting symptom for 28% to 40% of women presenting to the physician's office with a breast complaint. Because of the subjective nature of the problem, it was often ignored as a psychoneurotic disorder. Breast pain alone is rarely a presenting symptom of cancer; however, studies have indicated that nearly 10% of breast cancer patients had pain as the initial presenting symptom. The histologic cause of mastalgia is unknown.

Breast pain may be divided into cyclic, noncyclic, and nonbreast categories. A careful history should include the use of pain charts, documenting exactly when pain occurs during the month and the exact nature of the discomfort. In addition, a thorough physical examination and radiologic procedures (when appropriate) can assist in delineating these three groups. Research into the treatment of breast pain is difficult to interpret as a result of the heterogeneous nature of the pain, because breast pain is usually a symptom that resolves spontaneously within a short time and because one fifth of patients respond to placebo.

Cyclic mastalgia is often attributed to FCC, but scientific evidence concerning the etiology of cyclic breast pain has yet to be reported. The mechanism of pain is not understood, although there is some evidence that this could be related to a decreased progesterone:estrogen ratio during the luteal phase of the menstrual cycle or to an unusually high reactive state in the body's regulation of normal cyclic prolactin release. Because so many women experience asymmetric discomfort (i.e., more discomfort in one breast than in the other), it is unlikely that the sole basis of the monthly pain is hormonal.

Although mastalgia may be the presenting symptom, most patients are concerned with the possibility of cancer. Therefore, for 85% to 90% of patients without a dominant mass, reassurance is often sufficient without the need for medical intervention. Appropriate examination and testing should be performed, possibly including sonography, mammography (depending on age and risk factors), and frequent follow-up.

Those with severe and protracted symptoms merit treatment, particularly when symptoms interfere with lifestyle. A review of the literature reveals that nearly 60% to 80% of women experience regular premenstrual discomfort, although fewer than half consult their health care practitioner about the symptoms and even fewer (11% to 30%) describe their symptoms as being moderate-to-severe and necessitating treatment. Severe mastalgia may blanket a patient's everyday life, interfering with normal enjoyment and disrupting her daily routine. One study showed that mastalgia interferes with sexual activity in 48% of women, with physical recreation in 37%, and with social endeavors in 12%. Additionally, 8% to 15% of women list interference with work or school activity. Thus, breast pain impacts not only the individual sufferer but the patient's family and society at large.

Numerous treatments and therapies have been promoted to ameliorate cyclic breast pain. These have included decreasing caffeine intake, promoting weight loss, and taking diuretics (on the hypothesis that fluid retention is the basis of the pain), but scientific support for these methods is not available. Anecdotal evidence exists for the use of ginseng tea, vitamin A, vitamin B complex, and a supportive brassiere, but the extent to which these methods are effective is unclear. Depending on severity, acetaminophen or nonsteroidal anti-inflammatory medications may be helpful.

Several hormonal methods for treatment of cyclic breast pain have been advocated. No regimen is 100% ef-

fective, and some have a significant placebo response rate. Currently, danazol, an antigonadotropin, is considered the most effective and is the only medication approved by the Food and Drug Administration (FDA) for this problem. However, nearly 20% to 30% of patients experience the androgenic side effects of hirsutism, deepening voice, and amenorrhea, thereby limiting its widespread acceptance, even though response rates near 75% have been shown. Treatment should begin at 100 to 200 mg/day, although many patients may not experience relief until 400 mg/day is given. Recommendations on the length of treatment vary from 2 to 6 months. Upon discontinuation, the dose should be tapered to prevent rapid withdrawal. As with all hormonal medication, discontinuation may cause resumption of symptoms.

Because doses less than 400 mg/day do not ensure inhibition of ovulation, an effective method of contraception should be given to avert possible teratologic effects of the drug. Luteal phase-only danazol (200 mg/d) is an alternative treatment regimen that appears to be highly effective for the relief of premenstrual mastalgia. This regimen is associated with few side effects, but further study is necessary to ascertain whether such a regimen avoids potentially detrimental effects on lipid status.

Bromocriptine (Parlodel, Sandoz) is used to relieve galactorrhea but has also been effective for mastalgia in 40% to 78% of patients. Some investigators have used the TRH stimulation test (i.e., prolactin response 20 minutes after intravenous injection of 500 μg of TRH) to identify which patients affected with cyclic mastalgia are more likely to benefit from bromocriptine treatment. Patients with abnormal prolactin response to TRH had a statistically significant higher response to bromocriptine than those with a normal TRH response. The dosage of bromocriptine is similar to that discussed later in the section on nipple discharge. However, one third of patients experience side effects and 30% relapse once treatment is discontinued. Medication is usually discontinued after 2 months to review symptoms.

Gammalinolenic acid discovered in evening primrose oil at 3 to 4 g/day has been noted to have an overall useful response rate of 97% in some groups of women. Side effects were found in 12%, but all were insignificant. Other studies have revealed response rates of 44% and side effects of 2%. Gammalinolenic acid is a precursor of the unsaturated fatty acids and is essential for the production of beneficial prostaglandins in the body. Several hypotheses have been promoted to explain the effect. It appears to be due to modification of membrane fluidity and lipid-associated receptors, changes in the inositol cycle, or diminishing the response of the breasts to cyclic hormone activity. Yet, the delayed effectiveness (4 months) and the potential gastrointestinal and abortifacient side effects suggest caution in its use, especially in women desiring pregnancy.

Oral contraceptive pills (OCPs) may not be an alternative for all patients, but they may be a good option for patients seeking birth control in addition to relief of breast symptoms. Earlier studies used pills containing significantly higher progesterone contents than do present-day standard OCPs. Results indicate that symptoms of FCC are suppressed in 70% to 90% of patients who use the medication for 3 to 6 months. Maximum effects were noted after 2 years of use, but significant decreases in symptoms were noted after 1 year of use. Symptoms recur in up to 40% of patients when the high-dose OCP is discontinued. There is limited research on the effectiveness of the current low-dose formulations of OCPs in the treatment of mastalgia. However, in a recent study by Leonardi, 60% of patients with chronic mastalgia showed a reduction or improvement in symptoms while taking a *low-dose* OCP for 3 months. This study did not have a placebo group for comparison. The effectiveness appears to be due to the reduced ovarian estradiol production and the alteration of breast estrogen receptors caused by the progestin component of the pill. Although the older formulations appear to have some benefit, the new low-dose estrogen and the phased estrogen and progesterone dosage medications should be evaluated in a prospective trial to determine their effectiveness in the treatment of benign proliferative breast disease.

Tamoxifen (20 mg/day) has also been successful in the treatment of mastalgia. It has been heralded as the most effective and least toxic agent for the treatment of severe chronic breast pain. In one study comparing tamoxifen with danazol and placebo, tamoxifen had the greatest pain relief score, with nearly 75% of those receiving tamoxifen having significant pain relief compared with 65% with danazol and 38% with placebo. Twelve months after treatment was discontinued, 53% of women who received tamoxifen were still free of symptoms compared with 37% of the danazol-treated patients and none of the placebo-treated patients, suggesting that tamoxifen is highly efficacious and cost effective for the management of severe cyclical mastalgia. Lower dosages (10 mg/day) appear to have significantly fewer side effects and to be as effective in pain control as the higher dosages (20 mg/day). The metabolic effects on bone, mineral metabolism, and lipid profile were insignificant after 3 months of treatment. The effectiveness appears to be due to a reduction in nuclear volume and mitotic activity of the epithelium even when administered only in the luteal phase. However, lack of evidence of the long-term consequences of treatment portends caution in implementation of its use in benign breast disease.

Vitamin E has been beneficial in some studies for the relief of mastalgia. At dosages of 600 to 1,200 units/day, a 41% response rate with minimal side effects was found. The mechanism of action is unknown. Dietary flaxseed has also resulted in significant reduction in symptoms of severe cyclic mastalgia in a 3-month double-blind, randomized clinical trial. Women consuming a single daily muffin containing 25 g of ground flaxseed had improvement in symptoms. Flaxseed is a rich source of lignan precursors with antiestrogenic effects resulting in relief of breast pain. This nonpharmacologic alternative also has antiproliferative effects similar to tamoxifen in patients with breast cancer.

Recent studies support the effectiveness of gonadotropin-releasing hormone (GnRH) analogs for symptomatic treatment of fibrocystic mastalgia. When administered long-term, GnRH analogs result in marked reductions in blood levels of estrogen. Several investigations of depot GnRH treatment used for 3 to 6 months reported improvements in clinical mastalgia that was recurrent or refractory to other hormonal drugs. Monsonego and associates noted a 53% complete response rate in premenopausal patients with clinical, histologic, and ultrasonographic evidence of fibrocystic mastopathy and mastalgia after treatment with GnRH analogs. A statistically significant partial response was observed in 45% of patients. Further studies are required to determine the optimal length of treatment and the adverse effects on bone density and lipid metabolism generated by estrogen deficiency in premenopausal women.

Noncyclic mastalgia is seen less frequently than the cyclic variety. This form of mastalgia is usually anatomic in nature rather than hormonal. Although rare, it can be a sign of cancer and thus always demands an extensive breast examination and possible follow-up or consultation. Frequent causes include trauma, sports injury, and postsurgical biopsy. However, frequently the cause is unknown.

Exercise may result in excessive breast motion, leading to breast pain. Because the female breast contains minimal intrinsic structural support, breast motion is often difficult to reduce. It is suggested that the primary anatomic support for the breast is the Cooper's ligaments, but their true functional properties are unknown. Studies indicate a sports bra provides superior support for the breast in relation to the amplitude of movement, deceleration forces on the breast, and perceived pain when compared with fashion bras, crop tops, and bare-breasted motion.

Nipple pain or itching may be caused by local skin dryness, eczema, allergic reaction to clothing or clothes detergent, or, in pubescent girls, a physiologic result of anatomic growth. Symptomatic relief measures can include the use of antipruritis creams or ointments, such as calamine lotion, or other oils that enhance skin moisture such as vitamin E oil.

On the other hand, unilateral nipple itching must be viewed with suspicion so as not to miss the diagnosis of Paget's disease. Paget's disease often presents as a scaly pruritic nipple rash that is often mistakenly diagnosed as eczema. Nipple symptoms that do not resolve after 1 to 2 weeks of treatment requires biopsy to rule out Paget's disease. The skin presentation is often not associated with an underlying mass, so a heightened suspicion must always be present (Fig. 40.8).

Nonbreast sources that mimic breast pain include costochondritis, pleuritis, muscle pain including fibromyalgia, Tietze's syndrome, fractured rib, cervical radiculopathy, angina, cholecystitis or cholelithiasis, hiatal hernia, and peptic ulcer disease.

Nipple Discharge

Any breast complaint has the potential for creating an enormous amount of anxiety for patients. A thorough

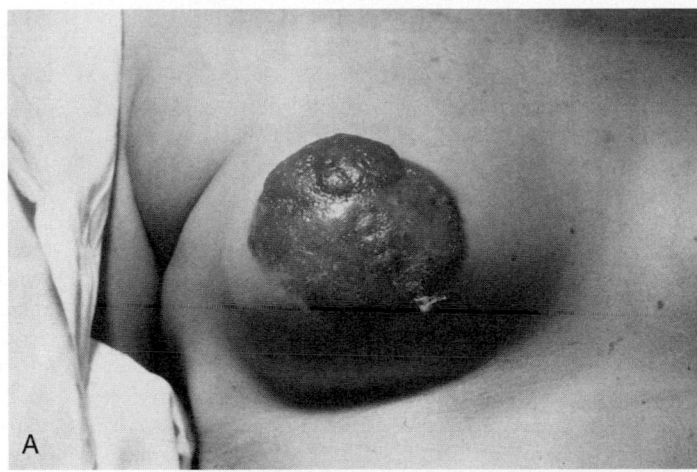

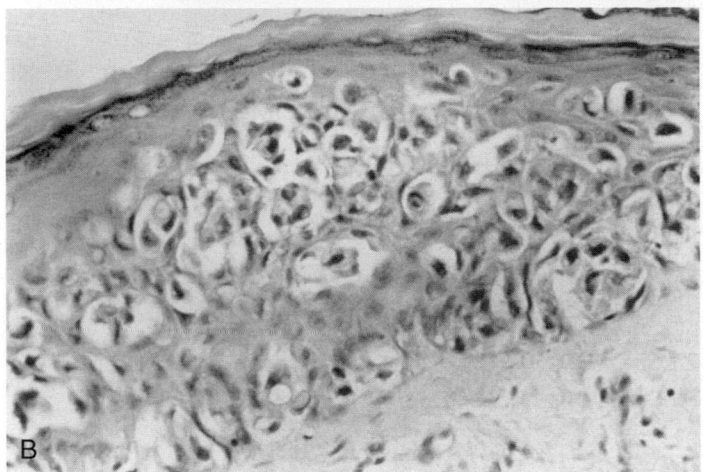

FIGURE 40.8. Paget's disease. **A:** Right breast showing an extensive area of erythema with a nodular surface suggesting Paget's disease. **B:** Skin biopsy specimen from a patient with Paget's disease shows intraepidermal collections of anaplastic cells (Paget cells) arranged singly and in microclusters. (Courtesy of Bhagirath Majmudar, M.D., Emory University School of Medicine, Atlanta, GA.)

understanding of the pathophysiology of common breast complaints, particularly those with low probability of association with cancer such as nipple discharge, is a necessary component of women's health care. This information can allay anxiety and prevent the emotional burden of unnecessary diagnostic evaluations. Nipple discharge is the third most common reason for women to consult their physicians regarding a breast problem. Complaints of nipple discharge not only account for 3% to 6% of office visits for women with breast complaints, but it also occurs in 10% to 50% of women with benign breast disease and in 10% to 15% of women with breast cancer, and it is responsible for 7% of breast operations.

Although *spontaneous* discharge from the nipples is uncommon, almost one half of women in their reproductive years can manually *express* one or more drops of nonpathologic liquid from the breast. The practice of squeezing the nipple either during breast self-examination (SBE), clinical breast examination (CBE), or sexual and physical activity can elicit fluid from almost all women of all ages. This outcome is the basis for suggesting that one should not attempt to elicit nipple discharge during an examination of an asymptomatic patient because pathologic discharge is likely to occur spontaneously without nipple manipulation. However, if nipple discharge is a complaint, the breast examination must include "milking" of the breast toward the nipple to delineate the exact ductal source of the problem.

Galactorrhea

Secretions from the breast may be divided into milky (galactorrhea) and nonmilky discharge with physiologic and pathologic causes in each category. Other investigators classify secretion from the nipples according to color, cellularity, and biology. Galactorrhea, which is the nonpuerperal secretion of breast milk, must be separated from other types of nipple discharge. This may be done by viewing a sample, under low-power magnification, for multiple fat droplets of various sizes. If the secretion does not contain fat droplets, it is not (by definition) galactorrhea and must be evaluated by other criteria. Galactorrhea usually results in bilateral nipple discharge from multiple ducts and is unassociated with a mass. On the contrary, pathologic sources of nipple discharge may be characterized by unilateral discharge from a single duct with an associated mass in some cases. Also, nipple discharge in women older than 50 years of age is of concern.

Although many hormones are involved in normal lactation and galactorrhea, prolactin is the most significant. Prolactin was isolated in 1971 and is secreted by the anterior pituitary, by chorion of pregnancy, and by decidual and endometrial tissue. In the nonpregnant state, the normal level is 0 to 20 ng/mL (in most laboratories). Prolactin (like luteinizing hormone) is secreted in a pulsatile fashion throughout the day with a circadian rhythm. It is greater during sleep, with a maximum between midnight and 6 AM, and it decreases during the day. It is increased by eating, physical and mental stress, exercise (poorly fitted bra resulting in breast stimulation), and sexual intercourse (excessive breast manipulation by the patient or her partner). However, these physiologic stimuli rarely cause prolactin to increase to more than 30 ng/mL. Pathologic sources of galactorrhea include medications, hypothalamic lesions or dysfunction, thyroid disorders, Forbes-Albright syndrome, chest lesion (chest trauma, burns, herpes zoster, lung cancer), renal disease, pituitary prolactin-secreting tumors, and nonpituitary prolactin-producing tumors (lung, kidney, craniopharyngioma). Not all patients with hyperprolactinemia display galactorrhea. The reported incidence is about 33 %.

The most common cause of physiologic nipple discharge is pregnancy. During pregnancy, prolactin values increase to 100 to 200 ng/mL, beginning as early as the 10th week of gestation. Lactation does not occur until after delivery because the peripheral action of prolactin is inhibited by estrogen and progesterone. During the process of suckling, prolactin increases to 300 to 600 ng/mL. After 6 months postpartum, there is no longer an increase from baseline associated with suckling. Therefore, amenorrhea, galactorrhea, or hyperprolactinemia more than 6 months after delivery is not physiologic. Any duration of galactorrhea demands evaluation in a nulliparous woman and, if at least 12 months have elapsed since the last pregnancy or weaning, in a parous woman.

The differential diagnosis of galactorrhea (excluding physiologic lactation) is a complex clinical challenge resulting from multiple factors involved in the control of prolactin release. A thorough and detailed history and physical examination are necessary to discern the cause. Prolactin itself, PIF, and prolactin releasing factors (PRFs), are the major substances involved in prolactin homeostasis. Thus, the pathologic cause of nipple discharge can be easily comprehended with an awareness of the release–inhibition pathway.

To be significant, a discharge should be true, spontaneous, persistent, and nonlactational. The most common source of galactorrhea is consumed medication; thus a thorough review of the patient's medication list is an essential part of the initial evaluation. Tranquilizers and antidepressant medications block the dopamine receptor, whereas antihypertensive agents, such as reserpine and methyldopa (Aldomet), inhibit the synthesis of dopamine. Opiates (including heroin), amphetamines, marijuana, phenothiazines, and anesthesia suppress dopamine release. OCPs may lead to milk secretion via hypothalamic suppression from excessive estrogen. This may result in reduction of PIF and release of pituitary prolactin by direct stimulation of pituitary lactotrophs.

In one study, about 40% of women taking low-dose OCPs had modest elevations of prolactin (20 to 40 ng/mL), although other research has yielded conflicting results.

Once medications and manual breast stimulation have been ruled out, the other sources of galactorrhea are less common. Stimulation of neurogenic reflexes result in hypothalamic reduction of PIF and hyperprolactinemia. This is the mechanism found to be operational with prolonged stimulation of the breast, thoracotomy scars, cervical spinal lesions, and herpes zoster. Hypothyroidism is the cause of hyperprolactinemia in 5% to 10% of cases. Hypothyroidism results in diminished circulating levels of thyroid hormone and consequently excess hypothalamic TRH. TRH acts as a PRF with resultant hyperprolactinemia. Because prolactin is predominantly excreted or cleared by the kidney, chronic renal failure results in hyperprolactinemia in 25% of affected patients. Lastly, Chiari-Frommel and Forbes-Albright syndromes result in amenorrhea after pregnancy and galactorrhea secondary to a pituitary tumor.

Hyperprolactinemia with normal thyroid and renal function studies, as well as a normal chest and breast examination may indicate a pituitary or hypothalamic problem. Prolactin-producing tumors, such as microadenomas and macroadenomas, account for a small percentage of cases. Evaluation of visual fields and a neurologic examination may be necessary. Imaging studies of the sella turcica, pituitary gland, and hypothalamic area are helpful to delineate problems. The coned-down view of the sella turcica, computed axial tomographic scans (CT), and magnetic resonance imaging (MRI) are the most common techniques to evaluate this area. Previous routine use of the coned-down view of the sella turcica and CT has been surpassed by MRI at some institutions. MRI provides better resolution, detects smaller lesions, and does not use radiation. It is much more costly than the sella turcica study. If the prolactin level is greater than 60 ng/mL, an imaging study should always be performed. However, with only mild elevation of the prolactin level (20 to 60 ng/mL), some investigators advise that imaging is unwarranted if there is more than a threefold (i.e., 200%) increase in prolactin after a TRH stimulation test. The reliability of this test is not supported in all circles; thus, many recommend a CT scan or MRI study for all patients who have persistently elevated prolactin levels.

Treatment of microadenomas (smaller than 1 cm) and macroadenomas (larger than 1 cm in diameter) is controversial. Depending on several factors, investigators promote surveillance, bromocriptine, or transsphenoidal resection. Prolactin-producing microadenomas rarely progress to macroadenoma size. Most are exceedingly slow growing or stable, which accounts for the recommendation for surveillance in most cases. Bromocriptine shrinks tumors and can prevent growth, although complete elimination of the tumor does not usually occur. Discontinuation of the drug usually leads to rapid regrowth. Transsphenoidal microsurgery is a safe procedure, but there is a high rate of recurrence.

If results of all tests are negative except for an elevated prolactin level, a provisional diagnosis of a dysfunction of the hypothalamus can be made. Small pituitary tumors may be missed; accordingly, a prolactin level should be obtained every 6 months. Repeat imaging, visual field, and neurologic examinations should be performed if an increase in the prolactin level is noted. However, a tumor may increase without a concomitant rise in the prolactin level.

If galactorrhea persists despite a normal prolactin level, normal examination, and negative imaging studies, the condition is called *idiopathic galactorrhea*. This may be caused by excessive sensitivity of the breasts to normal levels of circulating prolactin, intermittent elevations of prolactin, excess sleep-induced prolactin secretion, or elevated biologically active prolactin, which is not immunoreactive or detectable by current methods. Although androgens, danazol, and combined OCPs have been used for this purpose, the effectiveness of these drugs has been limited. The most common treatment for galactorrhea has been bromocriptine (Parlodel), a dopamine agonist. This drug has received negative publicity because there is an increased risk of hypertensive crises and strokes in postpartal women who use the medication. However, its use in women who are not recently pregnant or lactating continues to be recommended. Treatment begins with 1.25 mg orally twice daily and is increased to 2.5 mg orally twice daily once the patient is able to tolerate the side effects. Primary side effects include nausea and hypotension, which can be alleviated by administering the medication vaginally. Typical use of bromocriptine is for 2 years, followed by a period of cessation to determine whether symptoms return. It is prudent for the practitioner who prescribes bromocriptine to be aware of any government, manufacturer, or health advocate updates on the use of this drug.

Nonmilky Nipple discharge

Nonmilky nipple discharge is often divided into bloody and nonbloody categories (with physiologic and pathologic sources in each). Tests such as Hemoccult or urine dipstick may be helpful to discover occult blood in the secreted fluid but results should be scrutinized in the face of severe inflammation because this may lead to false-positive results. Additionally, although breast cancer presents as nipple discharge in 5% to 15% of cases, only 2% to 3% of *bloody* nipple discharges are associated with a malignancy. Breast cancer may also be associated with a watery or serous discharge, hence, no one piece of information can lead to a definitive diagnosis.

Physiologic causes of nonmilky, nonbloody nipple discharge include manual stimulation and poorly fitting brassiere as described earlier. Common causes of pathologic bloody nipple discharge include duct ectasia, mastitis, and intraductal papilloma.

Duct ectasia may present with a bloody nipple discharge, although more commonly a multicolored discharge is seen. Duct ectasia, without an associated mass, generally does not require more than symptomatic treatment, emphasizing gentle washing and application of moist packs. However, surgery may be appropriate in the presence of a mass, serosanguineous discharge, or excessive discomfort.

Mastitis, eczema, periareolar abscesses, and insect bites may present with purulent nipple discharge. Mastitis is discussed earlier under "Inflammation."

Unilateral or bilateral bloody nipple discharge may be elicited during and immediately after pregnancy in the absence of significant breast pathology. The phenomenon is likely due to the development of delicate, easily traumatized capillary networks within the ducts. If a breast mass is not found by physical examination or sonography, regular follow-up should be continued because the condition usually disappears shortly after delivery. If a mass is present, FNA or core needle biopsy should be performed.

Intraductal papilloma is the most common cause of bloody nipple discharge. It usually presents as a small, solitary, nonmalignant tumor of the dilated portion of the lactiferous duct that is found within a centimeter of the areola. Although it is not cancerous, an intraductal papilloma should be treated by excision through a circumareolar incision to rule out a malignancy. The surgical significance of nipple discharge rests on its frequency of association with cancer or precancerous mastopathy.

Physical examination, mammography, or galactography and sonography may be used to delineate the exact nature, location, and extent of the lesion preoperatively. Galactography involves the cannulation of the discharge-producing duct with a small catheter or needle and injection of a water-soluble contrast agent in the duct. Ductal orientated sonography uses modern high-resolution techniques to visualize the mammary ducts in detail. These procedures may be complementary, in that cases of ductal abnormalities have been missed by sonography yet visualized by galactography. However, researchers caution that modern galactography has a high false-negative rate, so it does not reliably exclude intraductal pathology and is, therefore, not a substitute for surgery in patients with pathologic discharge. Ultrasound may be used in pregnancy to delineate a mass. However, if there is a high suspicion for cancer, a shielded mammogram should be ordered.

Fiberoptic ductoscopy is an emerging technique allowing direct visualization of the ductal system of the breast through nipple orifice exploration. When this procedure was applied to women with nipple discharge, an 83% positive predictive value was noted. The positive predictive value was increased to 86% with the addition of ductal washings to obtain exfoliated cells for evaluation at the time of the ductoscopy. MRI has also been shown to be of diagnostic value, but it is not as informative as regular galactography. Both modalities may offer safe alternatives to galactography in guiding subsequent breast surgery in the treatment of nipple discharge.

If imaging studies were unable to preoperatively identify the specific ductal source of nipple discharge, surgical exploration may be required. Skin hooks are used to lift the skin flaps for easier visualization and exploration. The affected duct is identified and excised.

Hemostasis and closure techniques are similar to those used with excisional breast biopsies.

Papanicolaou and associates advocated cytologic analysis of breast secretions. Floria and associates concur, finding cytologic analysis in addition to galactography useful in identifying minimal breast cancer and in detecting premalignant lesions such as papillomatosis in patients with a nipple discharge but without a breast lump. Immunologic tests may also be performed on secreted fluid to detect high levels of carcinoembryonic antigen, indicating a latent malignancy. Conversely, Leis reported a false-negative rate for cytologic evaluation to be 16.4%. Because of the high false-negative rate, evaluation of a suspicious nipple discharge must continue despite negative cytology results.

Breast carcinoma and precancerous changes are thought to begin in the lining of the milk duct or terminal duct lobular unit, yet, until recently, we have not had direct access to this area for pathologic correlation other than by blindly removing tissue by core biopsy or FNA. Ductal lavage is a minimally invasive method of collecting ductal epithelial cells for cytologic evaluation. It is currently an investigational technique under review at several institutions. Dr. Rogsbert Phillips of Metro Surgical Associates in Atlanta, is a co-investigator and the expert consultant for the southeastern region. In a clinical trial of 507 high-risk women, cells collected through ductal lavage were shown to detect the presence of precancerous and cancerous changes in 20% of the women.

Each participant in the study had a normal mammogram or physical examination within 1 year of enrollment. The presence of these changes correlated with a fivefold to 18-fold increase in the risk of developing breast cancer depending on family history and the patient's risk of breast cancer development as determined by the Gail model. Ductal lavage may not only be a helpful adjunct to determine which high-risk women require closer, more active management, but it may also be used to track cell status in particular ducts over time. Because breast cancer is known to develop over time and to be present nearly 6 years before earliest detection on mammography, availability of this technique is surmised to provide practitioners with a tool to detect precancerous and cancerous breast cells *before* they become palpable cancers that can be imaged, thus allowing closer surveillance, surgical intervention, or chemoprevention. This procedure should be considered for (1) women with a prior history of breast cancer and (2) women at high risk for development of breast cancer as defined by Gail Index score, family history, BRCA mutation, or previous benign breast biopsies.

Ductal lavage involves placing a special suction cup over the nipple and applying negative pressure to collect the nipple aspirate fluid (NAF) (Fig. 40.9). A microcatheter is then inserted through the nipple orifice, into the identified fluid-yielding ducts. After saline infusion, the ductal fluid is withdrawn and sent for cytologic analysis. In preliminary trials, 79% of subjects yielded

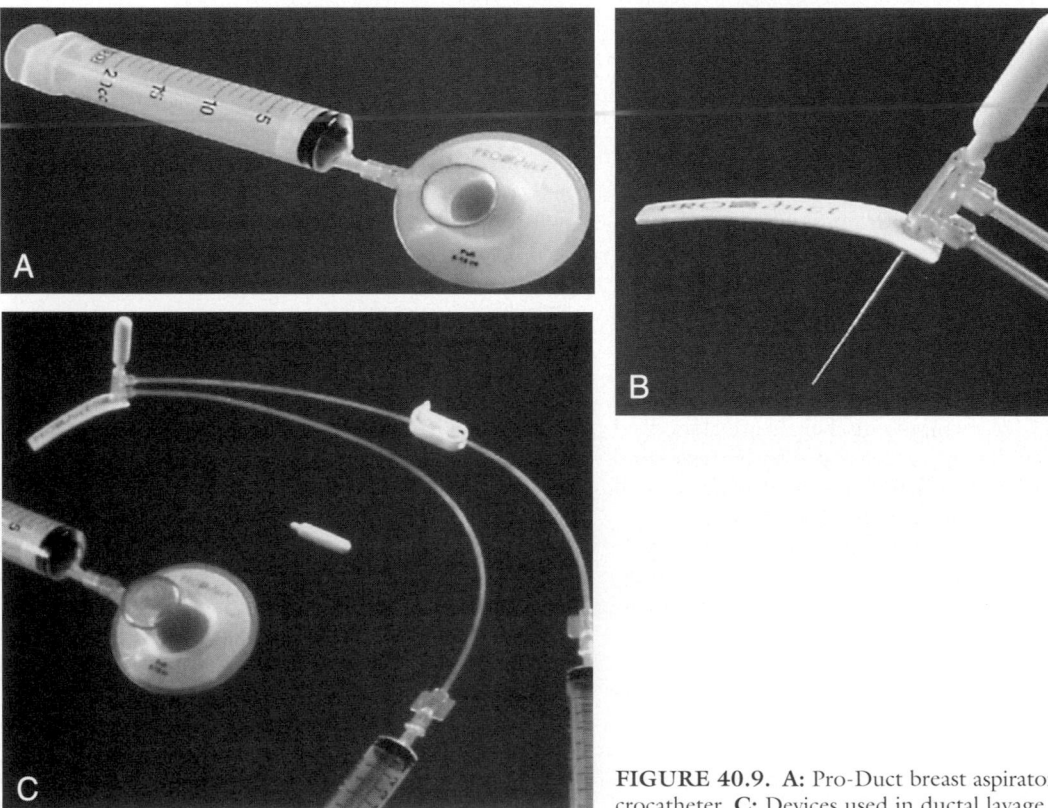

FIGURE 40.9. A: Pro-Duct breast aspirator. **B:** Breast microcatheter. **C:** Devices used in ductal lavage.

NAF, although this rate may be influenced by race and age, in that women older than 50 years, African-American, Mexican American, and Asian women typically yielded less NAF. The phase of the menstrual cycle, a history of pregnancy, or use of oral contraceptives did not significantly affect the availability of NAF. Hormone replacement therapy (HRT) in postmenopausal women tended to increase the amount of NAF obtained.

DIAGNOSIS

Breast cancer accounts for 30% of all cancers in women and 15% of death from cancer (second only to lung cancer). Gynecologists are in a crucial position for coordination of ongoing medical care for patients with breast problems. Breast symptoms are appropriately evaluated by a breast-oriented history, physical examination, cytology studies, and imaging techniques. If the diagnosis is in doubt, open surgical biopsy provides the definitive histologic diagnosis.

History

A thorough history is a vital aspect of the initial evaluation. However, breast cancer cannot be excluded by any single fact within the patient's history; rather, the history focuses attention on additional information. The practitioner should obtain detailed information about the patient's complaint and other pertinent positive and negative symptoms related to the complaint. The information necessary to assess breast health includes age, menstrual, gynecologic, sexual, reproductive, and lactation history, and any family history of breast disorders. In addition, a total body review of systems (e.g., headache, blurred vision for macroadenomas) should be focused on the patient's complaint. Of vital importance are the following:

- Menopause status
- Timing and specific nature of symptoms
- Cyclic changes
- Onset, duration, and growth pattern of any masses
- Presence of pain
- Attempted and successful relief measures
- Alleviating and aggravating factors
- Use of HRT or OCPs
- Presence or absence of risk factors for breast cancer

All previous breast diagnostic and surgical procedures should be documented. Past medical and surgical history, as well as current medications and social history (including smoking, alcohol, and educational level), should also be reviewed. Because most breast complaints in reproductive-aged women are due to a benign cause, reassurance may be an important aspect in reducing anxiety. However, the practitioner should notify the patient of any concerns regarding the history and examination to ensure that the patient understands the significance of follow-up and does not misconstrue the practitioner's reassurance to mean the diagnostic workup is completed.

Self-Breast Examination

Mammography remains the gold standard for early detection of breast carcinoma, but this technique it is not 100% effective. CBE and SBE are important facets of a breast screening program. Controversy exists regarding the utility of routine SBE for increasing the rate of breast cancer detection. Studies yield conflicting results. The research has been hampered by differing SBE education strategies, schedules of performance, and control groups. Although the results are often incongruous, some authors have found a 34% reduction in nodal involvement and increased survival in women performing SBE compared to women who do not. In addition, 70% to 90% of masses are first detected by the women themselves. These findings require assessment, but to negate SBE as an important component of overall personal health care seems inappropriate if there is any possibility that it will impact the survival rate in women. In breast disease wherein early detection is so clearly related to improved survival, the value of these relatively simple, economical, and minimally inconvenient techniques cannot be overemphasized. With this in mind, the American College of Obstetricians and Gynecologists (ACOG) and the ACS continue to recommend SBE be performed monthly beginning at age 20. Studies have shown that women who were more educated, more confident in performing SBE, and whose physicians recommended monthly SBE were more likely to perform SBE monthly. These results highlight the importance of physician recommendation of compliance with screening guidelines for early detection of breast cancer.

Effective instruction of patients in the technique of SBE incorporates description of the procedure while the patient views the health care provider's performance of the examination. Additionally, having the patient reiterate her understanding of what has been taught and then demonstrating her mastery of the technique using manufactured breast models further solidifies compliance. The patient should understand the significance of breast inspection in various positions as well as the utility of breast palpation in the standing as well as supine positions. The circular method of breast palpation is routinely the easiest to master, although for patients with pendulous breasts, positional changes to ensure positioning of the breast tissue upon the chest wall must be emphasized. The best time to perform the examination is usually the week after the menses, although menopausal women should pick a convenient time of the month such as their birth date or the first of each month. After hysterectomy, patients with continued estrogenic support of the ovaries should observe for breast fullness or tenderness. Breast examination should then be performed 7 to 10 days after maximal breast symptoms.

Clinical Breast Examination

As with SBE, the utility of routine CBE in asymptomatic women has been questioned. Query into its reliability and efficacy has been propagated; however, there is greater scientific support for CBE. The Canadian Health

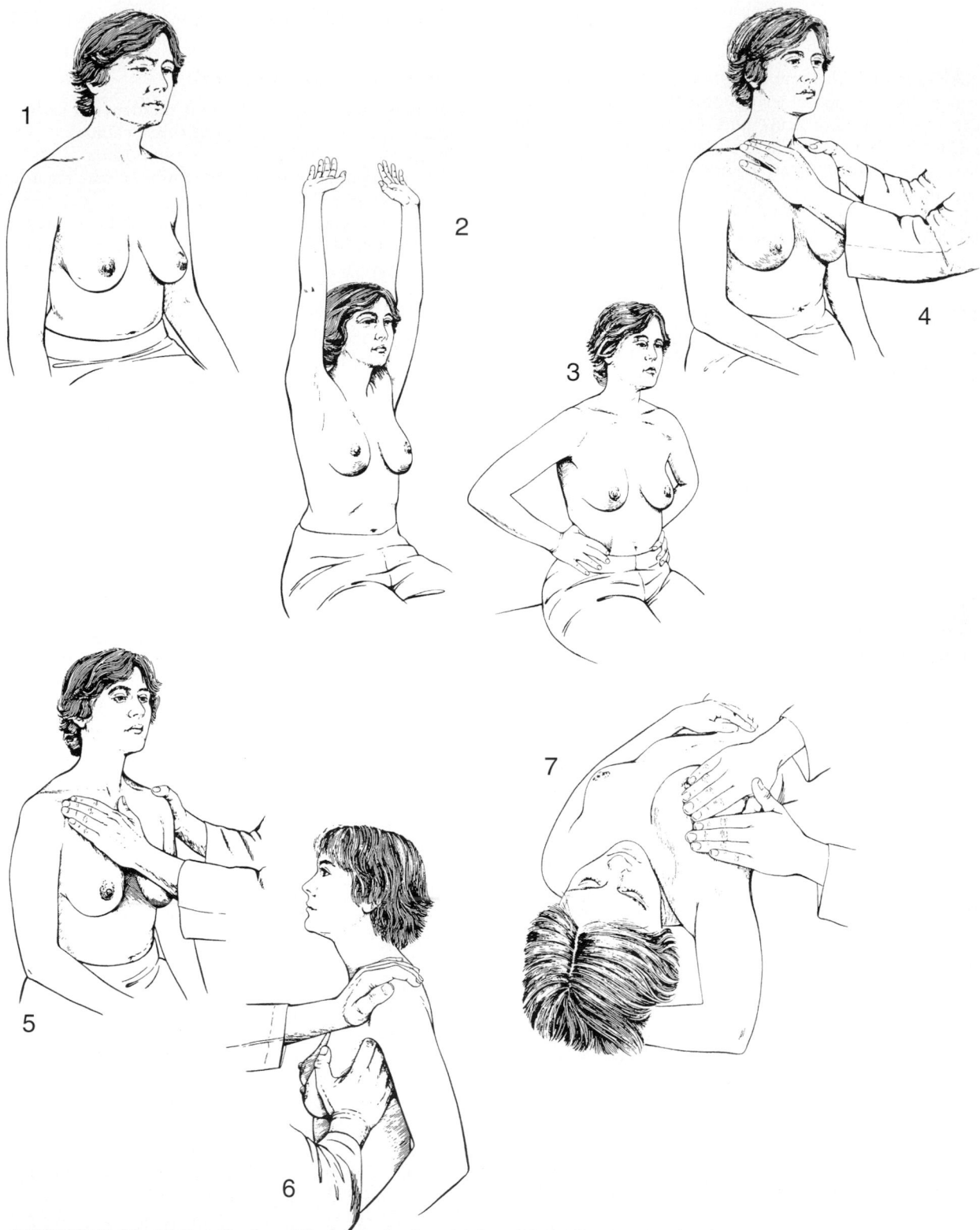

FIGURE 40.10. (*1*) Examination of the breasts begins with inspection. The patient is disrobed to the waist and comfortably seated facing the examiner. Asymmetry, prominent veins, and skin changes may be signs of disease. (*2*) The patient raises her arms above her head, thereby altering the position of the breasts. Immobility or abnormal cutaneous attachments may become evident. (*3*) Inward pressure on the hips tenses the pectoralis major muscle. Abnormal attachments to its overlying fascia and skin can produce retraction or dimpling of the skin. (*4*) Supraclavicular lymph nodes are examined by palpation. (*5*) The deltopectoral triangle is palpated for evidence of infraclavicular nodal enlargement. (*6*) Each axilla is examined for nodal enlargement. Proper placement of the examiner's hands and of the patient's arm is important. (*7*) Thorough palpatory examination of the entire breast for masses is performed with the patient in the supine position. A fine rotational movement of the hands is useful to appreciate the consistency of the underlying tissues. The examiner should check for nipple discharge by compressing the ducts in a clockwise manner toward the nipple. (From Scott JR, DiSaia PJ, Hammond CB, et al. *Danforth's obstetrics and gynecology,* 7th ed. Philadelphia: JB Lippincott, 1994:700)

Insurance Plan noted a 70% reduction in mortality from breast cancer as a result of physical examination. Although inferior to mammography, CBE has a sensitivity of 57% to 70% in detecting breast cancer. In addition, the ACS recommends annual CBE of women age 40 years and older and CBE every 3 years for women ages 20 to 39. Strategies to improve a practitioner's ability to detect a mass include increasing the time devoted to the examination, using a technique with variable degrees of pressure, and developing a systematic, consistent search mode. The size of the lesion, of course, is also correlated with the practitioner's ability to detect the mass.

To capture any benefit from early detection, CBE should be a routine part of the examination of gynecologic and obstetrics patients. Obstetrician/gynecologists should not abdicate their responsibilities by relying on previous examinations performed by other specialists. The practitioner must also be concerned with protecting himself or herself from future lawsuits due to errors of omission.

At least 3 to 5 minutes should be devoted to the CBE to improve mass detection. As with the SBE, CBE should be performed approximately 1 week after the end of the menstrual cycle to diminish the impact of luteal phase breast vascular or lymph congestion, which can obscure mass detection. Each portion of the breast examination should be performed with the patient in both the sitting and supine positions because positional changes often expose a lesion that was otherwise masked by the patient's normal anatomic variations.

The initial part of the examination should focus on breast inspection, viewing for symmetry, skin retraction, rashes, and nipple retraction or deviation (Fig. 40.10). Inspection should continue with the patient's arms raised overhead. Not only does this allow visualization of the lateral aspects of the breast (which are often obscured by excess arm girth), but also provides a complete view of the skin on the undersurface of the breast (inframammary ridge). Again, asymmetry and skin changes are sought. Inspection continues with placing the patient's hands behind her head with elbows retracted, or placing her hands on her hips while contracting the pectoralis muscles. In patients with rheumatoid arthritis or other conditions preventing pressure on the hip joint, other more comfortable options may be used. One may either have the patient grasp her fingertips at a level near the waistline, while pulling laterally or pressing her palms together while extended above the head. Because the breast lies upon the pectoralis muscle and Cooper's ligaments are attached to the muscle and the skin, tension on the muscle accentuates carcinoma invading these structures. The clinician should always survey the breast for nipple retraction or inversion, which can result from carcinomatous invasion of the tissue beneath the nipple (Fig. 40.11). Nipple inversion is significant only when developed secondarily and unilaterally. If gentle manual eversion may be accomplished, the inversion is a normal variation.

Another position for breast inspection that is especially helpful in women with pendulous breast is to have the woman lean forward while placing her hands on the practitioner's shoulders. Palpation of the breast in this position (while the breast tissue is away from the chest wall) is helpful to differentiate *chest wall* pain from true *breast* pain.

Next, the axilla is evaluated for masses. Several postures are helpful while the patient is in the seated position. (This part of the examination is repeated with the patient in the supine position.) The physician may hold the patient's elbow or wrist in his or her hand, with the patient's arm at a 90-degree angle and slightly abducted from her side (or gently across the front of the patient's torso). The opposite hand is then used to evaluate the axilla. Another position rests the patient's hand on the shoulder of the practitioner while asking the patient to relax her elbow. This allows the examiner to use both hands in evaluation of the axillary area. To allow proper assessment of the axilla for all positions, the patient's shoulder girdle must be relaxed.

Inspection of the breast is followed by palpation. The patient should be properly gowned with only the area being examined exposed. The patient must be positioned (by tilting her hips and torso) to allow the portion of the breast tissue being examined to lie directly upon the chest wall. For patients with pendulous breasts, this may require three to four positional changes for each breast. The pads of the fingers (and not the finger tips) are the most sensitive and should be used in examination. Three circular motions are made with three levels of pressure (superficial, medium, and firm) on each 1-cm

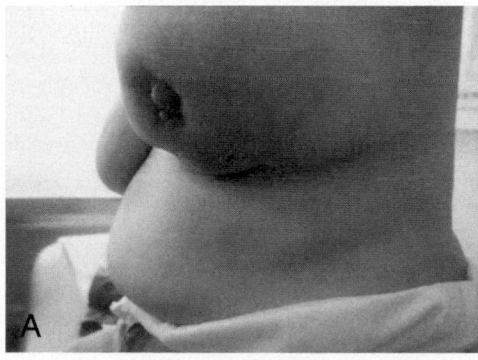
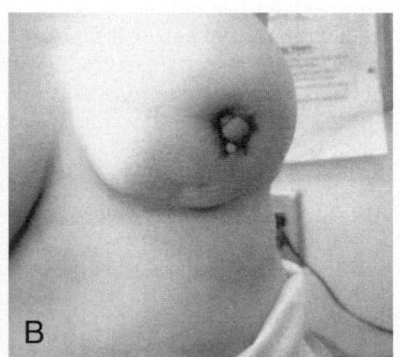

FIGURE 40.11. A 52-year-old patient with presentation to clinic for complaints of "hardening" in the lower part of her breast. **A:** Characteristic nipple retraction is seen. **B:** Also Peau d'orange changes are noted in the lower quadrants of the breast. (Courtesy of Jacqueline Foster, PA-C, Atlanta, GA.)

square area of the breast. Not only does this improve mass detection but also prevents masking a mass through excessive pressure.

Next, the patient should be placed in a comfortable supine position with her arm, on the same side as the breast being examined, raised above her head to evenly distribute the breast over the chest wall, thereby making its deeper regions accessible. The pattern of palpation is less important than the time spent on the examination. The circular pattern is the most frequently used. With the circular method of palpation, the breast tissue is examined with the pads of the fingers perpendicular to the rib cage. The examination proceeds clockwise around the full circumference of the breast at its perimeter and gradually moves inward toward the nipple. However, the "spoke and wheel" and "vertical strip" patterns should be mastered, because they may be helpful in certain clinical situations such as with patients with large breasts. Most practitioners use two hands to perform the breast examination, although a thorough and systematic use of a single hand is satisfactory. Use of the two-handed method uses the second hand to follow behind in the same pattern as the initial hand, thus providing dual evaluations of each area. The Mammocare method of breast examination uses a single hand for palpation in the vertical strip pattern. If the patient presents with breast complaints, it is advisable to palpate the unaffected breast first to a "tactile baseline" with which to compare the involved breast and prevent omitting lesions in the unaffected breast.

Palpation should extend beyond the actual breast tissue to encompass the supraclavicular and infraclavicular lymph nodes, the area adjacent to the sternum, approximately 1 to 2 cm below the inframammary ridge, and the axillary tail of Spence. The examination encompasses these areas to ensure nodal involvement along the sternum and inframammary ridge is discernible. Routine evaluation of the nipple for nipple discharge is controversial. Some authors do not recommend this as a routine portion of the breast examination in women without nipple discharge or complaints. It is well known that excessive breast manipulation can lead to a nipple discharge. If one does exclude this as a routine part of the examination, a *detailed* history should be obtained to rule out any nipple complaints. Patients often have such complaints but forget to relate this information to the practitioner, particularly if they have experienced the symptoms for an extended period of time. Squeezing the nipple may actually obstruct the ductal orifice and impede any discharge from coming to the surface. Using a milking technique improves the examiner's ability to elicit a nipple discharge. Each quadrant of the breast is "milked" by sliding the fingers from the outer quadrant in a clockwise fashion toward the nipple and documenting the location of any fluid accumulation.

To adequately evaluate the axilla in the supine position, the arm that has previously been raised and placed behind the head should be extended at a 90-degree angle from the chest wall. This maneuver relaxes the area to be examined for a more thorough evaluation. Continued placement of the patient's hand behind her head tenses the muscles in the area and hinders evaluation of the deeper regions of the axilla.

In this increasingly litigious society, breast assessment demands careful documentation of the history, examination, and disposition of the case. A clear and legible note should record all findings from the breast examination noting texture, size, consistency and a detailed description (including diagrams) of abnormal and suspicious features as well as the plan of action for follow-up. Although positive or abnormal findings are very important, it is important to list negative findings in the medical record as well.

Regardless of the pattern of breast examination used, the importance of using a consistent and methodical pattern of evaluation and allowing sufficient time for a thorough assessment should not be underemphasized as factors that increase detection capabilities.

Mammography

The etiology of breast cancer remains an enigma, and there is presently no known method of preventing breast cancer. Therefore, the major opportunity to alter the natural course of the disease is provided by diagnosing the disease at an early stage when the prognosis for cure is excellent. Mammography is the most effective screening method for detection of nonpalpable and minimally invasive breast cancer. The goal in clinical practice is to detect nonpalpable cancers by ordering screening mammography for all patients eligible by age, history, or both. Only mammographic imaging can detect small nonpalpable cancers, which, when treated, have an excellent 90% 10-year disease-free survival prognosis.

The value of mammography as a screening tool in the detection of breast cancer is well established. Although estimates vary, it has been suggested that a lesion must be 1.0 to 2.0 cm before it may be palpated. The kinetics of breast cancer growth are important for a full understanding of screening and detection. The average breast mass doubles volume every 100 days and doubles diameter every 300 days. A breast carcinoma grows for 6 to 8 years before reaching a diameter of 1 cm. In slightly less than another year, the carcinoma reaches 2 cm in diameter. It is estimated that, on the average, a mammogram detects a breast cancer 2 years before it is palpable.

Because mammography is a radiologic tool, accuracy depends on a number of factors, including expertise of the technician, size and density of the breast, and the location of the lesion. False-negative results occur even in the best installations (Table 40.3). Routinely, a false-negative rate of 10% to 15% is quoted; therefore, a normal mammographic examination does not rule out the presence of breast cancer. Thus, a palpable mass requires further evaluation despite a "negative" mammographic examination. Dense parenchymal tissue is the principal cause of false-negative mammograms. Other sources of error include misjudging a well-circumscribed carcinoma for a benign mass, misconstruing malignant calcifications for benign ones because they do not show the typical

TABLE 40.3.
Reasons for False-Negative Mammograms

Failure to image the region of interest
Poor image quality
Errors of perception
Breast cancer indistinguishable from normal breast tissue
Poor image quality due to overlying breast tissue

characteristics, not recognizing the indirect signs of malignancy such as asymmetry, and faulty radiographic technique. Guidelines promulgated by the American College of Radiology Mammography Accreditation Program have significantly reduced this latter problem. It is important to forewarn patients that adequate breast compression is essential to improved radiographic technique and to deliver a high-quality mammogram. Compression holds the breast motionless, decreasing artifact, separates tissues to disclose small lesions, improves image quality by decreasing radiation scatter, and reduces the radiation dose by decreasing breast thickness.

In some studies, HRT reduced the sensitivity of mammographic screening. In countries where HRT is widespread (as in the United States), the reduction in sensitivity may undermine the capacity of population-based mammographic screening programs to achieve their potential mortality benefit. For instance, in one research paper, among women who were diagnosed with cancer in the 2-year mammography screening interval, HRT users were more likely to have a false-negative result than nonusers (odds ratio, 1.60; 95% CI, 1.04 to 2.21). However, among women who did not have cancer diagnosed in the interval, HRT users were more likely to have a false-positive result (adjusted odds ratio, 1.12; 1.05 to 1.19).

Early detection by mammography reduces breast cancer mortality rate by approximately 18% to 30%, and widespread use of this imaging test, in conjunction with improved treatment, may be responsible for the recent decline in number of deaths due to breast cancer. Not only does mammographic imaging enable the detection of nonpalpable breast cancer, but early detection also permits breast conservation surgery (BCS). Moreover, it has been suggested that substantially greater reductions in mortality would have resulted if more rigorous screening guidelines were in place. These results have been achieved while maintaining acceptably low rates of recall for additional imaging after basic screening examination (10% for the initial prevalence screening and 5% for subsequent incidence screenings) as well as maintaining false-positive biopsy rates for nonpalpable lesions that are lower than those for lesions found at clinical examination. Positive predictive values for lesions for which biopsy is recommended on the basis of mammographic findings range from 25% for women in the fifth decade of life to 50% for women in the eighth decade of life, which are all within an acceptable range. This radiologic modality uses high-resolution techniques that enable

demonstration of fine spiculations and microcalcifications; high contrast, which allows visualization of subtle differences among soft-tissue densities; and high-luminance view boxes, which improve visualization of dense tissue (Fig. 40.12).

Mammography serves multiple purposes in the evaluation of women's breast health. Mammography is useful not only for screening but also in evaluating lesions identified by clinical symptoms (e.g., nipple discharge) or physical examination (e.g., a palpable mass or "suspicious" examination), called a *diagnostic mammogram*. Screening mammography is provided to an asymptomatic patient and may often be performed without the presence of a radiologist. On the other hand a diagnostic mammogram is administered to a patient with symptoms or a breast mass. The examination includes not only the craniocaudal and mediolateral view of the routine screening mammogram but also may include additional views as well as ultrasound and physical examination by the radiologist. Additionally, when a lesion is found in one breast, mammography is used to detect further lesions in the ipsilateral or contralateral breast, which ultimately may modify the treatment plan. Follow-up of breast cancer patients is also aided by the use of mammography. Finally, it is used as a baseline against which future mammograms can be compared.

In detection of breast cancer, there are several mammographic characteristics of malignancy, which include the presence of a mass, architectural distortion, asymmetrical density, and microcalcifications. Malignant lesions generally display more of these pathognomonic mammographic appearances than do benign lesions, but benign lesions may have similar features. Calcification in

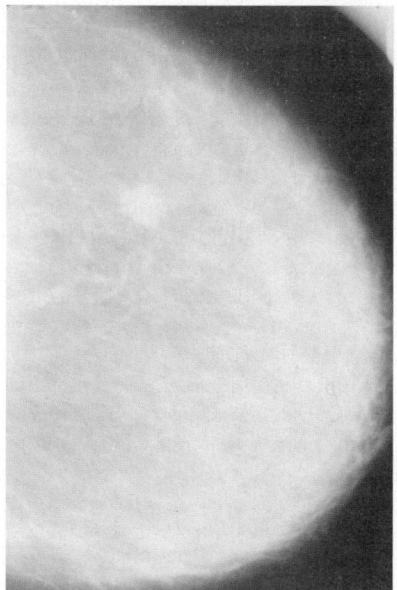

FIGURE 40.12. Mammogram of a 44-year-old woman with breast carcinoma in the upper quadrant. Characteristic features of spiculations interdigitating into the surrounding tissue and irregular margins are seen.

the breast can be benign or malignant. Round, smooth calcium deposits of uniform size generally tend to be associated with benign processes, whereas branching and polymorphic calcifications suggest the possibility of malignancy. The presence of clusters of microcalcifications in a small geographic area is also a suspicious finding. Microcalcifications play an important role in the early detection of breast cancer. However, calcifications occur in fewer than half of nonpalpable cases and fewer than half of these calcified lesions demonstrate the classic appearances suggestive of malignancy. The calcifications of FCCs often mimic those of malignancy, leading to unavoidable false-positive mammograms. Calcific-like deposits in the skin secondary to tattoos, deodorants, ointments, or sebaceous gland secretions can also be mistaken for malignancy. Therefore, clustered microcalcifications are a sensitive but not a specific sign of malignancy.

The radiation risks associated with x-ray mammography are considered negligible. Contemporary roentgenogram units, specifically designed for breast imaging, use the most advanced technology to obtain images of the highest quality with a considerable decrease in radiation dose to probably less than 0.2 to 0.3 rads (2 to 3 Cgy). Information from the Breast Cancer Detection Demonstration Project, sponsored by the ACS and the National Cancer Institute indicates an even lower average mid breast dose of 0.08 rads. A randomized, controlled study to determine the effect of such low doses of radiation on the incidence of breast cancer would be unfeasible because 20 million women would be required to offer enough statistical power for analysis. To put radiation risk in perspective, data presented by the National Council on Radiation Protection illustrate that mammographic examination of 100,000 women at age 45 years would *theoretically* result in the eventual loss of one life. This risk of death is tantamount to that incurred by a coast-to-coast round-trip airplane trip, a 660-mile trip by car, mountain climbing for about 15 minutes, or smoking about eight cigarettes. There have been no documented radiation-induced breast cancers from mammographic screening to date.

If new imaging techniques are to be effective in screening for early minimal breast cancer (defined as less than 5 mm in diameter) wherein the potential to reduce mortality is greatest, they must be able to detect lesions smaller than 5 mm and must help to accurately localize small abnormalities for surgical removal. They must also allow the simultaneous performance of procedures for procurement of the cytologic or histologic specimens necessary for accurate preoperative assessment, and they must provide some information regarding chemotherapeutic responses. To this end, ultrasound-guided biopsies, stereotactic needle biopsy, and MRI are being investigated and used.

Screening Guidelines

Mammography is known to reduce breast cancer mortality by up to 30%. Survival from breast cancer is influenced by tumor size, degree of invasion, and lymph node status at the time of diagnosis. The advantage of early detection and diagnosis is reduced mortality because of smaller-sized cancers, more localized lesions with a lower percent of positive nodes, and increased feasibility of breast conserving surgery. Clearly this fundamental tenet accentuates the importance of compliance with radiologic screening programs and knowledge of guidelines.

Women who have less than a high school education, who are a minority, who do not speak English as their primary language, and who are socioeconomically disadvantaged are less likely to report having had a mammogram in the previous year. According to data from the 1994 National Health Interview Survey, fewer than 60% of women age 50 years and older and 45% of women age 70 years and older reported having had a mammogram in the preceding 1 to 2 years. Only 38% of women aged 50 years and older with low income and 42% of those with less than a high school education had a recent mammogram. Clearly, efforts to increase screening should specifically target older women and socioeconomically disadvantaged women who are at the highest risk for underutilization of mammograms.

Multiple factors influence screening behavior, such as fear of the screening test, embarrassment, and lack of knowledge. Conversely, women with positive health behaviors, high social support, and positive mental health attributes are more likely to participate in mammographic screening programs. Physician recommendation of mammography was the strongest predictor of having obtained both a mammogram and CBE within the previous year. Even encouraging a single mammogram may develop a continued pattern of adherence to mammographic screening guidelines.

Randomized, controlled trials have clearly demonstrated a decreased mortality rate in women who received mammography at age 50 to 69. Even among this group of women, however, fewer than 40% have had a mammogram in the past year.

The controversy regarding screening in women younger than 50 years of age is multifold. Reduction of mortality rates as a result of screening is a subject of debate, the cost-effectiveness when compared with that in older women is unknown, and, finally, the frequency of screening intervals has become a point of disagreement among the committees that issue imaging guidelines. Authors have argued that mammograms performed in women younger than 50 years are not useful because younger women have more radiographically dense breast tissue that obscures abnormalities (Fig. 40.13). Some investigators have advocated yearly mammograms for all women 40 to 49 years old because breast cancer is often more aggressive and faster growing in younger women. The benefit of mammography in women age 40 to 49 years is less clear than for those age 50 and older. Moreover, the interpretation of the evidence for reduced mortality in women age 40 to 49 years has been the subject of much controversy. With increasing years of follow-up, evidence of a benefit for women in their 40s has increased and studies show that regular mammograms reduce the death rate from breast cancer in this age group

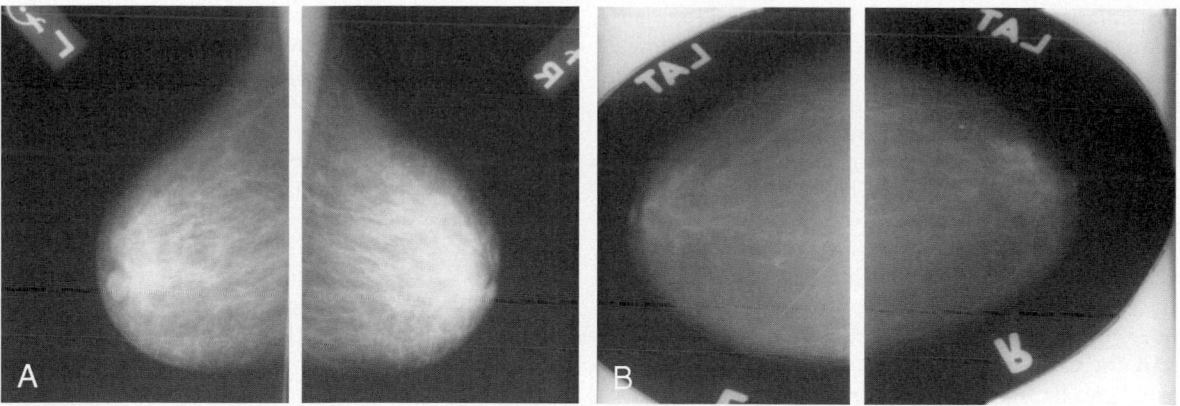

FIGURE 40.13. A: Mammogram of radiographically dense tissue of a 35-year-old patient with fibrocystic changes. **B:** Radiolucent tissue of an 87-year-old patient. Both mammograms are normal.

by about 17%. In 1993, the National Cancer Institute considered the evidence showing the benefits of screening mammography in women 40 to 49 years of age and, finding it equivocal, withdrew its recommendation for routine screening in women in this age group. In 1997, the National Institutes of Health (NIH) convened the Consensus Development Conference on "Breast Cancer Screening for Women Ages 40–49." The group declined to recommend routine screening in women age 40 to 49 years, instead advocating for a well-informed conversation between physician and patient regarding the present knowledge and the risks and benefits of screening for each woman. However, because of inadequate numbers of patients studied and a brief length of follow-up, ACOG continues to recommend offering screening mammography every 1 to 2 years for women 40 to 49 years of age and annually for women older than 50 years. Women who are at higher than average risk of breast cancer should seek expert medical advice about early screening and the frequency of screening (Table 40.4).

Although there are insufficient data regarding women age 70 years and older, the incidence of breast cancer does increase with age. Therefore, ACOG continues to recommend annual screening in this age group.

Digital Mammography

Many exciting developments are occurring in breast imaging. Although mammography still remains the gold standard for breast cancer screening and diagnosis, it often cannot differentiate benign from malignant disease and is less accurate in patients with dense glandular breasts, with diffuse involvement of the breast with tumor, and in those taking HRT. Ten percent to 20% of breast cancers detectable by physical examination are not visible radiographically. Furthermore, of the women who are referred for biopsy based on mammographic findings, only 20% to 40% of lesions actually prove to be malignant. Clearly, there is room for improvement in both breast cancer detection and lesion characterization.

Digital mammography is a rapidly evolving technology that has the potential to improve upon and ultimately replace or at least function as a complement to conventional film-screen mammography for the early detection of breast cancer. Digital mammography offers improved detection of early breast lesions secondary to improved efficiency of absorption of x-ray photons, as well as greater contrast resolution, especially in dense breast tissue. Systems are based on the absorption of x-rays by a phosphor material with subsequent conversion of the absorbed energy to electronic charge. The charge signal is then digitized and stored as a matrix in computer memory to represent the image.

Recent studies indicate digital systems may be superior to conventional film-screen mammography in detection of microcalcifications, which are the earliest evidence of minimal breast cancer. However, and thus room for caution, characterization of morphologic details is inferior with the digital system, presumably because of reduced spatial resolution. Furthermore, some lesions visualized on conventional film-screen mammography were not detected by digital detectors. Moreover, no statistically significant difference was found in the differentiation of benign from malignant lesions with this technique.

TABLE 40.4.
ACOG Breast Cancer Screening Guidelines

---

1. Annual clinical examination with a screening mammogram performed at 1- or 2-year intervals in women age 40 to 49 years, unless mammographic or physical findings suggest more frequent evaluation.
2. Annual screening and examination for women 50 years of age or older.

From American College of Obstetricians and Gynecologists. *Routine cancer screening. ACOG Committee Opinion 247.* Washington, DC: ACOG, 2000.

Digital mammography offers further technologic advancements that may continue to improve the accuracy of breast cancer diagnosis in the future. It holds the promise of computer aided diagnosis (CAD) and telemammography. Sophisticated computer techniques have been applied to the interpretation of radiologic images with ever-increasing success. CAD is the detection of a potential abnormality by means of computer analysis of the mammogram; that is, a second reading by a computer to increase the yield of screening mammography for the detection of early breast cancer or to decrease the number of biopsies performed for benign disease, thereby increasing diagnostic specificity. Information of this kind can be supplied to radiologists to help improve their diagnostic performance. Several investigators have demonstrated improved radiologist performance in lesion detection and characterization when a CAD system is used with digitized screen-film mammograms. Currently, in the absence of the advanced digital mammography technology, CAD requires the cumbersome and time-consuming initial step of digitizing film images to provide appropriate input for the computer. The CAD enhancement of digital mammography appears highly promising; however, further clinical studies are needed to evaluate the relative efficacy of different CAD methods. Moreover, the medicolegal status of CAD is uncertain at present and needs to be clarified.

Because digital images can be readily transmitted electronically for remote interpretation and consultation, digital mammography holds the promise of telemammography. In a study by Duding, image transmission time was approximately 1 minute per image and data loss was minimal even with adverse weather conditions.

Digital mammography also allows for combining several single images into a three-dimensional image called *tomosynthesis*. It has been proposed as a solution to the problem of false-negative conventional screen-film mammography due to masking from overlying structures, particularly in very dense breast tissue. Here, multiple images are acquired as the x-ray tube rotates in an arc above the breast and detector. By manipulating the digital image, any plane in the breast can be easily displayed. This pioneering technique permits blurring of the planes above and below the abnormal lesion, allowing more specific information about lesion surface characteristics and associated features. Ultimately such a system might substantially improve diagnostic accuracy.

Another potentially useful application of digital mammography is stereoradiography of the breast, also called *stereomammography*. With this technique, two images of the breast are taken at slightly different angles and later "fused" to provide greater perception of the relative depths of structures within the image. This approach may reduce obscuration by overlying structures, eliminate false-positive findings, and offer assistance with interventional procedures.

Dual-energy mammography is another technology that becomes practical once the image is digitized. This technique provides another approach to the problem of overlying breast tissue masking lesion detection. With this method, two exposures of the breast are made at substantially different x-ray spectra. Weighted subtraction of one image from the other provides additional information about breast tissue composition. Specifically, it may render calcifications more obvious in dense breast tissue.

Finally, expanding upon the advantages of breast MRI, which compares the differential blood flow of malignancies and normal tissue, digital mammography should be able to depict subtle differences in contrast uptake by tumors, compared with background tissue. Subtraction of a precontrast from a postcontrast image after the injection of intravenous contrast material should delineate a difference. Furthermore, because of its higher spatial resolution, this technology potentially allows for visualization of small arteries that may not be visible with MRI. Analogously, because even very small cancers develop an arterial supply through angiogenesis, it may be possible to detect cancers at a smaller size than those currently detected with conventional film-screen mammography as well as improve the accuracy of detection of the extent of cancer invasion.

Digital mammography offers other benefits including diagnostic signs that are identical for interpretation of screen-film mammography and digital mammography, which could facilitate the transition from one system to the other. Another variation, *mammoscintigraphy* may be helpful in identifying drug-resistant tumors before therapy. Although digital mammography may reduce some costs by eliminating film and film processing chemicals, decreasing film storage space, and reducing film library staff, immediate cost savings are unlikely. Substantial capital equipment costs are necessary in that the digital mammography systems cost four to five times the cost of conventional mammography units.

Despite its potential in the arena of breast cancer diagnosis, digital mammography is the only major imaging technique unavailable in the United States in digital form. There are currently four full-field digital mammography detectors undergoing testing for approval. They are manufactured by Fischer Imaging, Fuji Medical Systems, General Electric Medical Systems, and Trex Medical. The FDA has been unable to formulate a plan for manufacturers to demonstrate the safety and efficacy of this tool; thus, no system has been approved for marketing in the United States.

Major technical challenges remain, and further clinical studies are necessary to determine the actual clinical value of this modality as a probable adjunct to conventional mammography primarily in the area of dense breast tissue. The Diagnostic Mammography Trial, funded by the Office of Women's Health, will be of considerable assistance in determining the true efficacy of this evolving technology. Early analysis of data revealed approximately equal sensitivity of screen-film and digital mammography. However, digital mammography was shown to significantly lower the recall rate and offer a higher true-positive biopsy rate over conventional mammography in the population studied. As with all research studies, caution should be applied as preliminary results are based on only a limited amount of data.

Ultrasound

Ultrasound imaging of the breast has been an extremely valuable addition to the breast-imaging armamentarium. Ultrasound is currently used to guide aspirations and biopsies in mammographically detected nonpalpable lesions, thus likely preventing unnecessary open biopsy. The rate of inadequate samples in ultrasound-guided FNA was 0% for malignant lesions and 28.4% for benign (primarily due to the decreased cellularity of benign fibrous lesions) in a recent research study. It has also been invaluable in differentiating solid from cystic breast lesions where it has a 95% accuracy (Fig. 40.14). This procedure also has a high sensitivity of 96.9% and specificity of 98.4%. In younger women, an ultrasonically detected cyst may defer mammography and prevent unnecessary x-ray exposure. However, a normal sonogram at any age should not prevent further evaluation of an abnormal physical finding. Conversely, if a nonpalpable solid mass is detected by sonography but is not clearly seen on a mammogram, biopsy or needle localization must be performed during real time sonographic imaging (Fig. 40.15). The benefits of this diagnostic technique include the absence of radiation, noninvasive technique, lack of morbidity, and ease of repeated examinations.

Unfortunately, breast ultrasound in its current state, is extremely inefficient in detecting malignancy and is thus not suitable as a method of breast cancer screening (Fig. 40.16). In one study, only 44% of the mammographically detected nonpalpable lesions and 37% of the cancers could be visualized by high-frequency ultrasound. Ultrasound also has a low capacity for detecting small lesions or small aggregate groups of calcifications,

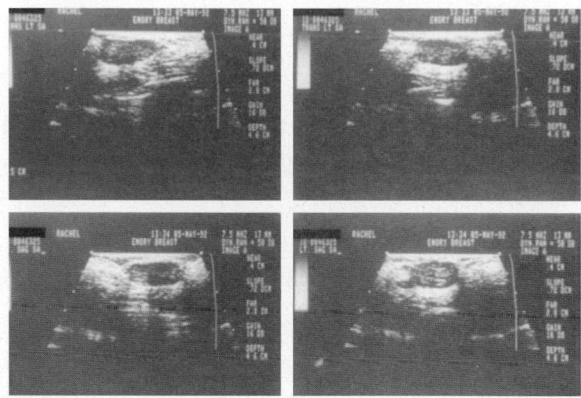

FIGURE 40.15. Ultrasound of a 27-year-old patient presenting with breast mass. Mammogram shows inhomogeneous internal structure, without through transmission, and indistinct margins on the lower border. Thus, if the typical features of a cyst are not met, ultrasound should not be used to delineate the mass further. Fine-needle aspiration showed fibroadenoma.

which may be evidence of early breast carcinoma. Because breast cancer control can be achieved only by early diagnosis of minimal breast cancer, diagnostic ultrasound in its present state of development is incapable of accomplishing this task. However, there is renewed interest in evaluating ultrasound as a potential adjunctive screening tool in women with radiographically dense breasts.

Blood flow in malignant breast lesions is considerably increased due to vascular proliferation. Doppler flow ultrasonography can detect increased blood flow and has the potential to distinguish benign from malignant lesions. As a rule, malignant lesions produce Doppler signals of higher frequency and amplitude during continuous flow through diastole. Presently, Doppler flow analysis is not sensitive enough to be used as a tool for

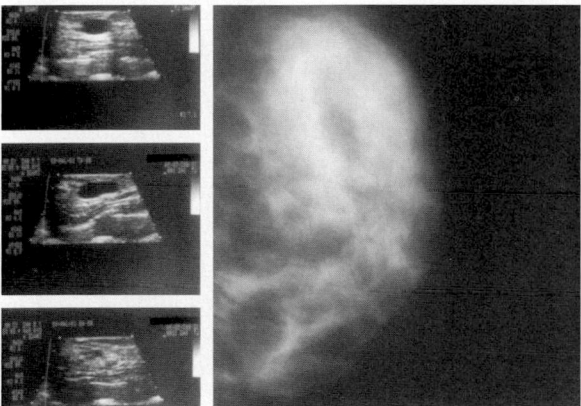

FIGURE 40.14. Ultrasound of a benign cyst in a patient with a "normal" mammogram. The mammogram did not detect the cyst due to the density of the tissue. The cyst shows the typical characteristics of through transmission, homogenous internal features without "debris," and smooth margins. The compressibility of the cyst can be seen in the second ultrasound screen.

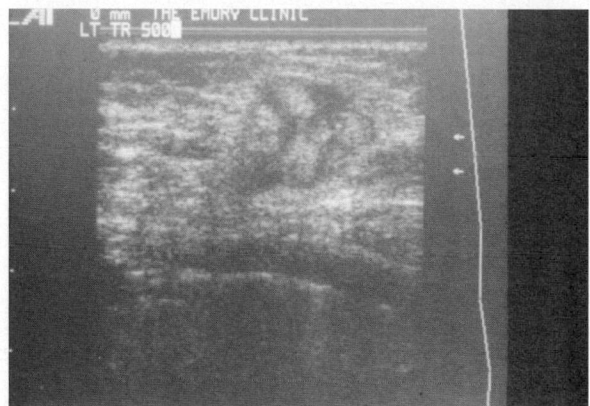

FIGURE 40.16. Ultrasound of a palpable mass in a 39-year-old patient that was not seen on mammography. Typical features of a cyst are not seen. Fine-needle aspiration showed invasive ductal carcinoma

distinguishing malignant from benign tissue, but it offers potential for advancement in the field.

Magnetic Resonance Imaging of the Breast

MRI is emerging as perhaps the most promising imaging modality as an adjunct for breast cancer detection to date (Fig. 40.17). Interventional MR machines have produced unique opportunities for image-guided surgery. MRI has excellent sensitivity in demonstrating breast cancer that is both mammographically and clinically occult, especially in dense breast tissue, but it has a low specificity. Nevertheless, contrast-enhanced MRI may be used more extensively in monitoring chemotherapeutic responses in breast cancer, in the preoperative evaluation of patients being considered for BCS, and intraoperatively to define the margins of the lesion and ensure complete excision.

Initial fervor over contrast-enhanced MRI of breast cancer and the ability to differentiate benign and malignant lesions with high specificity has been replaced by skepticism because of the significant overlap in contrast enhancement features in benign and malignant lesions and reported specificity ranging from only 37% to 97%. Published results, however, are from studies with relatively small numbers of patients. Further clinical investigation is needed to address the issue of cost effectiveness and to define the technical requirements for optimal imaging, interpretation criteria, and clinical indications for which MRI should be used as an adjunct to conventional imaging methods. One such trial, an international, multiinstitutional study funded by the National Cancer Institute, is currently underway.

This imaging modality has considerable benefits, including absence of ionizing radiation and lack of known radiobiologic hazards, but it is time consuming, expensive, and lacks sufficient resolution for the identification of small lesions. It is also especially deficient in detecting the aggregates of small calcifications that may be evidence of early carcinoma and appears limited due to the

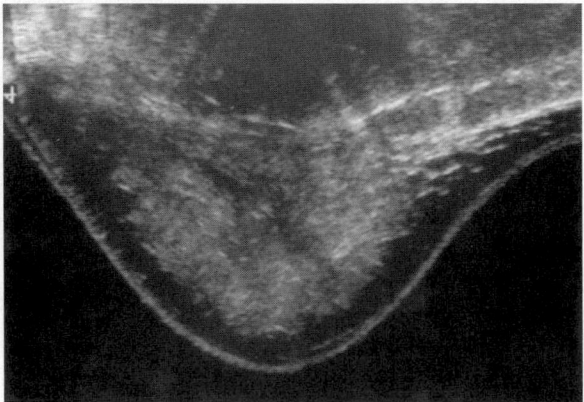

FIGURE 40.17. Magnetic resonance imaging (MRI) study of a 32-year-old patient with a normal examination. MRI results were normal. The patient was complaining of breast pain.

overlap in the enhancement kinetics and morphologic appearance of benign and malignant lesions, which severely limits its usefulness as a screening method. MRI, though, seems to be the most accurate method for detection of breast implant integrity.

Investigational Modalities

CT mammography requires a long and rigorous examination with delivery of a moderately high dose of radiation. The utility of CT mammography is that it can image the extreme medial and lateral portions of the breast at the points of attachment to the chest wall. It also may be useful for localizing those rare lesions that can be visualized only on the mediolateral mammographic view.

Xeromammography was introduced by Wolfe in 1972; however, xeroradiographic equipment is no longer manufactured and the vast majority of mammographic images are produced by the film-screen technique. The uniqueness of this technique revolves around edge enhancement and wide recording latitude. This allows detail of soft tissues of the breast, chest wall, and the thinner peripheral portions of the breast to be recorded in a single mediolateral view. This modality provides better detail of calcifications, but delivers about seven times more radiation to the midpoint of the breast than conventional film-screen mammography. Because the effects of radiation are cumulative, this technique is not recommended for screening purposes.

Thermography and transillumination have not demonstrated sensitivities specific enough for screening purposes.

Fine-Needle Aspiration

FNA or fine-needle aspiration biopsy (FNAB) was first reported by Martin and Ellis at Sloan-Kettering Cancer Center in 1930. Despite preliminary concerns and apprehension, the technique has gained acceptance and is currently regarded as the initial diagnostic procedure of choice for most palpable breast lesions. In response to the increasing frequency with which women are consulting their obstetrician-gynecologists about concerns related to their breasts, the American Board of Obstetrics and Gynecology (ABOG) has promulgated specific educational requirements for resident training in the various aspects of diagnosing and treating breast disease. Technical proficiency in this procedure is essential for the proper evaluation, treatment, and further definition of a palpable lesion.

FNA is recognized as highly accurate and cost effective when used in conjunction with clinical examination and imaging as part of the triple approach. Alone, this method is relatively accurate but has a false-negative rate as high as 20% according to the American Society of Cytology. The false-negative rate is highest in detection of lobular cancers and carcinoma in situ when one factors in the acellular aspirates. However, FNA has a sensitivity of 96% and specificity of 98% (similar to core biopsies), as

TABLE 40.5.
Advantages of Fine Needle Aspiration

Outpatient procedure
Minimal discomfort
Anesthesia not required
Negligible complication rate
Rapid diagnosis
Both diagnostic and therapeutic for breast cysts
Low false-negative rate

well as a 99% positive predictive value and 94% negative predictive value and an overall efficacy of 97%.

However, when FNA is combined with clinical examination and radiologic testing, the false-negative and false-positive rate of the triple test diagnosis approaches that of surgical biopsy and frozen section, respectively.

Morris and colleagues developed a triple test "score" by giving each component of the triple screen a 1,2, or 3 designation, depending on whether the mass was suspected to be benign, suspicious, or malignant by that method. Results indicate that masses with 6 points or higher should be considered malignant and should undergo definitive therapy. Whereas, masses with 4 points or lower were benign and should be clinically followed. Only those masses scoring 5 points required biopsy. Thus, the triple test "score" was able to decrease the number of patients needing surgical biopsy. The diagnostic accuracy and predictive value were 100%.

FNA provides a cytologic rather than histologic sample for review by the pathologist. It has multiple advantages (Table 40.5) over excisional biopsy and is helpful in confirming the clinical impression of both benign and malignant breast disease. Nevertheless, a negative cytologic report, as with a negative mammographic report,

must not be relied upon to rule out malignancy in a clinically suspicious lesion. A negative finding on FNA cytology may be unreliable and should not preclude further evaluation. Any clinically suspicious mass in a patient with negative FNA findings indicates that open excisional biopsy or other methods of detection including histologic evaluation should be performed. If breast cancer or a *specific* benign condition (e.g., apocrine metaplasia or fibroadenoma) is not detected by FNA, needle core biopsy or excisional biopsy is warranted. A positive finding of malignant cells expedites evaluation and allows early selection of appropriate therapy before further surgical intervention. The accuracy of aspiration cytology alone is good, ranging from 66% to 80% in palpable lesions later proved by biopsy to be carcinoma. When cyst aspiration is performed, the fluid may be discarded if it is clear (transparent and not bloody) and the mass disappears. If the cyst aspirate is bloody or the mass does not disappear, the patient should be considered a candidate for excisional biopsy. Additionally, if the cyst recurs after aspiration, excisional biopsy is warranted.

The recommendations of the National Cancer Institute Consensus Conference of 1997 include use of FNA for sufficiently defined palpable breast masses of clinical or patient concern, persistent or suspicious masses in patients with increased family risk factors, evaluation of nonpalpable mammographically suspicious breast lesions, or low risk for malignancy lesions when recommended follow-up with imaging is not feasible or accepted by the patient. FNA should not be used for investigation of microcalcifications but may be used under ultrasound or stereotactic guidance to investigate densities presumed to be nonmalignant. Doubtful densities are best assessed by core biopsy.

FNA is an easily mastered technique, but the adequacy of specimens is improved with experience and training (Fig. 40.18). Although there are no contraindi-

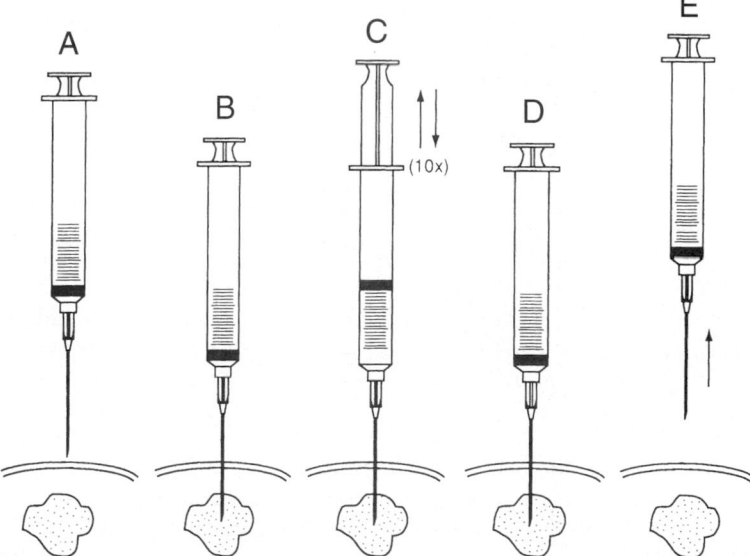

FIGURE 40.18. Overview of fine-needle aspiration. **A:** The mass is located. **B:** The needle is inserted into the mass without negative pressure. **C:** Negative pressure is applied while the needle is moved in a "jackhammer" fashion within the mass. **D:** Negative pressure is released. **E:** The needle is removed from the mass.

cations, the risks include infection, bleeding, and bruising at the site. Because the chest wall is immediately beneath the site, pneumothorax has been listed as a potential complication. The small size of the needle and assuring the mass is stabilized over a rib during the procedure significantly decrease this complication.

After the procedure is explained to the patient and consent has been obtained, the skin is cleaned with alcohol and wiped dry to prevent stinging when the needle is inserted. The lesion is identified and stabilized, preferably over a rib, between the fingers of the nondominant hand (Fig. 40.19). The table should be prepared for easy access because the nondominant hand should not be removed (once it has been placed alongside the mass) until the procedure is complete (Table 40.6). Stabilization of the hand throughout the procedure prevents frequent "loss" of the mass and repeated attempts to locate the targeted structure.

If anesthesia is desired, a small wheal is placed in the skin over the mass, assuring excess local anesthesia does not obscure the mass. Only the skin and immediate subcutaneous tissue need be anesthetized, because insertion directly into the mass is generally not painful. Only a very small amount of anesthesia is necessary because only that tissue immediately below the needle puncture site is involved, not the tissue "surrounding" the mass. Excess anesthesia may also interfere with cytologic interpretation. Whether to use anesthesia depends on the surgeon and patient preference. If the examiner is inexperienced, anesthesia may make subsequent attempts less worri-

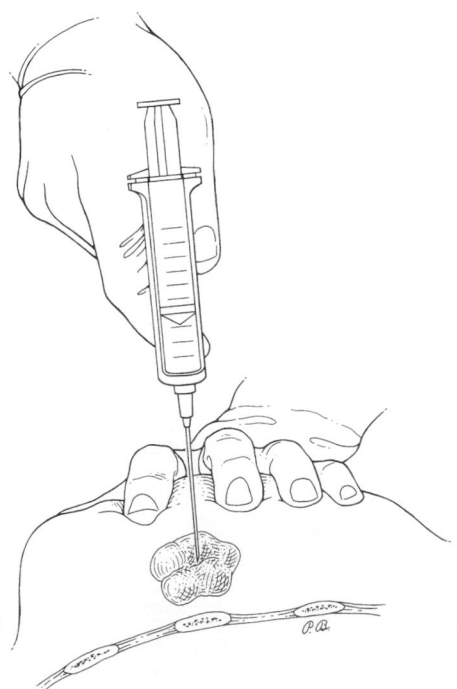

FIGURE 40.19. Technique of fine-needle aspiration. The mass is stabilized with the nondominant hand (preferably over a rib). After the needle is inserted into the mass, negative pressure is applied.

TABLE 40.6.
Equipment for Fine-Needle Aspiration

Fine-needle aspiration gun or 10-cc syringe
22 to 24 gauge needle with *clear* hub
Syringe holder (if desired)
Clear frosted-end glass slides
Alcohol or betadine pads
Fixative (if desired)
Gauze pads
Adhesive bandage
Toluidine blue if immediate microscopic examination desired
Local anesthesia if desired

some if the first attempt fails. Also, if the specimen is insufficient, a repeat procedure does not lead to additional apprehension in the patient.

A 22-gauge, 1.5-inch needle with a clear hub attached to a 10- to 20-mL syringe is then inserted into the central portion of the mass. Increasing the needle gauge does not increase the sample size. In fact, the larger the needle, the more blood aspirated and the greater the likelihood of hematoma formation. A pistol-grip holder may also be used, because the mechanics of hand motion are often easier with the holder. Mastery of both techniques (with the holder and without) is recommended because not all institutions have this equipment. If a holder is not used, two fingers are placed under the piston of the syringe and the thumb is used against the body of the syringe to pull the piston toward the examiner, applying negative pressure. With use of the holder, the grips of the holder are pulled together to apply negative pressure.

The lesion is sampled by moving the needle up and down within the mass several times. Several passes should be made into every portion of the mass to prevent false negative samples. Sampling only one axis of a mass could lead to sampling of the inflammatory reaction, which often surrounds a carcinoma, and failure to sample the malignant cells. If the lesion is cystic, liquid material is seen in the hub of the needle and possibly the body of the syringe. With a solid mass, one may not see evidence of cellular material in the hub; however, a thorough sampling should ensure an adequate specimen. About four to five passes along each axis increases the positive sampling rate. It is often helpful, in sampling very large masses, to release the suction before changing sampling axis. Thus, if the needle is inadvertently removed from the mass during a positional change, the specimen is not lost (by inadvertently aspirating into the syringe) as negative pressure was applied during the movement. When the examiner is in position for further sampling, he or she reapplies the negative pressure and continues the procedure along the new axis.

A subareolar lesion should not be approached through the nipple–areolar complex. This is very painful for the patient because the nipple and areola area is the site of the greatest sensory innervation. These lesions

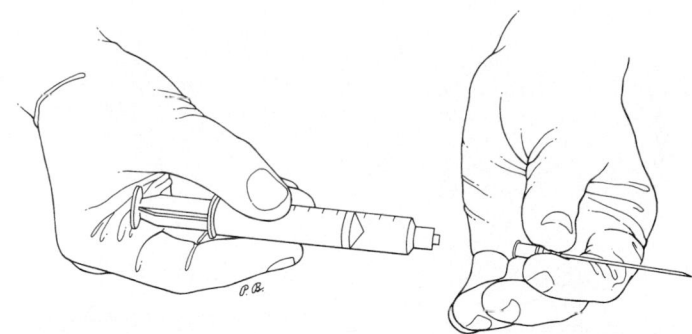

FIGURE 40.20. Technique of fine-needle aspiration—slide preparation. After the needle is removed from the mass, the needle is removed from the syringe and air is aspirated into the syringe. This avoids suctioning cellular material from the needle into the syringe; the cellular material should stay within the needle.

should be approached laterally through the parenchyma of the breast.

After about 10 to 15 seconds, or complete sampling along each axis of the mass, suction is released and the needle is removed from the lesion. Releasing the suction *before* removing the needle is a very important aspect of this procedure. Continued negative pressure upon removing the needle (without release of suction) forces aspiration of the specimen into the body of the syringe, from which it is difficult to retrieve. Once the needle is removed, pressure is applied to the puncture site (by an assistant or the patient) by holding pressure with a gauze pad for 1 to 2 minutes. Significant bleeding from the site of the needle puncture is often characteristic of carcinoma or an inflammatory lesion, although benign conditions and bleeding diathesis may also result in this complication. The patient usually does not require any dressing or bandage upon completion of the procedure.

Before sampling, it is often helpful to place 1 cc of air into the syringe. Upon release of negative pressure, the piston assumes its position at the 1-cc mark (it does not completely close). This approach is helpful in the process of expelling the cellular material onto the slide. Once the needle is removed from the mass, the material can be im-

mediately expressed onto the slide without removing the needle first. The tendency (without the initial aspiration of 1 cc of air) is to pull back on the piston while detaching the needle (and drawing in additional air), which inadvertently aspirates the material into the syringe. This tendency is even more prevalent when using the holder, wherein compressing the grips often accompanies needle detachment and essentially nullifies the procedure. The material should be expelled onto a glass slide (frosted ends facing up toward the practitioner) with the needle bevel down (Figs. 40.20 through 40.23). The bevel-down method prevents scatter of the specimen. Once the initial specimen is expelled onto the slide, the needle is *then* detached, air is drawn into the syringe, the needle is reattached, and any additional cellular material is placed onto the slide. The "detach, draw air, and reattach" portion is repeated until all the cellular material has been expelled.

If a large amount of fluid is obtained when aspirating a cyst (greater than 10 cc), one can detach the needle from the syringe while the needle remains in the mass. The fluid is processed or discarded, then the syringe is reattached to aspirate any additional fluid. Complete aspiration of a cystic mass should always be attempted.

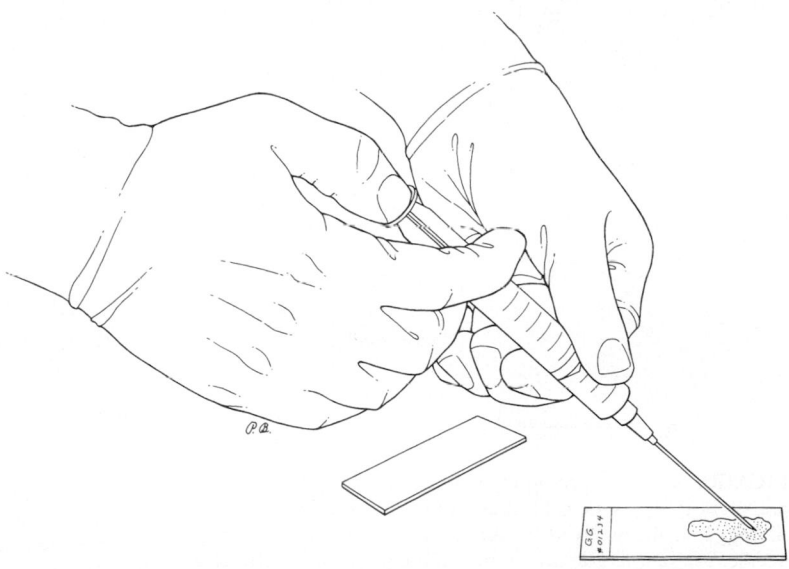

FIGURE 40.21. Technique of fine-needle aspiration—slide preparation. Cellular material is ejected onto a labeled slide.

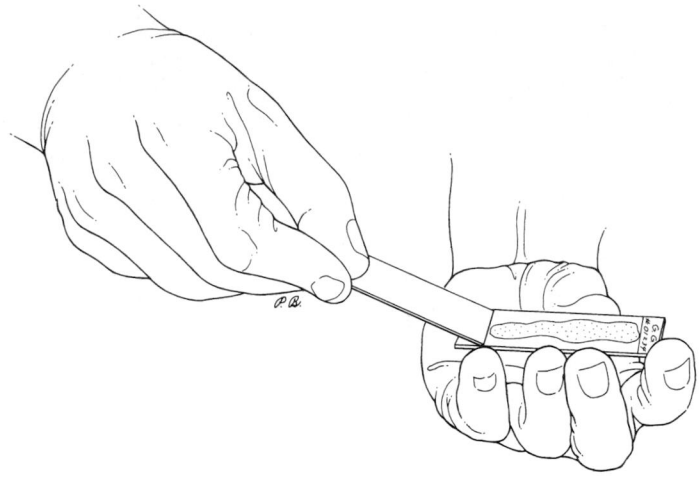

FIGURE 40.22. Technique of fine-needle aspiration—slide preparation. A smear is made using another glass slide at a 45-degree angle. Note the position of the hand stabilizing the slide, which allows the smear to be made.

One should not simply stop once clear fluid is obtained because at follow-up it will be difficult to determine whether the fluid has reaccumulated or is a remnant from the last procedure. This becomes important, because reaccumulated fluid in a cyst should be referred for excisional biopsy (Table 40.7).

Cells dry quickly, so it is crucial that immediate fixation with 95% ethanol or a spray fixative occur after smearing. Prompt fixation is not as vital when stains other than Papanicolaou are used such as Wright-Giemsa. To increase the adequacy of the sample, the first expulsion of material should be smeared and fixed immediately. Any additional material obtained upon drawing air and reattaching the needle can be placed on a separate slide with a minimal delay in fixation. The smear is made similar to a hematology smear. Hence, the examiner slides the edges of a second glass slide horizontally across the initial slide with the specimen. Another technique involves pressing the slides perpendicular to each other (like a cross). This technique decreases cellular crushing and improves the adequacy of the sample. Usually, one to three slides can be made from each aspirate.

Each slide may be immediately evaluated for adequacy. One or two drops of toluidine blue is applied to the cellular material and a cover slip is placed. The specimen is then examined microscopically to identify ductal cells or cellular material. Large breast lesions may require more than one aspiration to adequately evaluate the entire mass. The multidisciplinary team of the cytopathologist, obstetrician/gynecologist, and surgeon must work together in specimen interpretation. Special training is required for cytologic evaluation of specimens unlike for histologic samples. The examiner must provide the cytopathologist with an accurate clinical history, including age, clinical examination, and whether the patient is pregnant or lactating, because this information is crucial in interpretation of the sample. Figures 40.24 through 40.26 demonstrate examples of FNA cytology. FNA can produce bleeding into the breast tissue and a hematoma

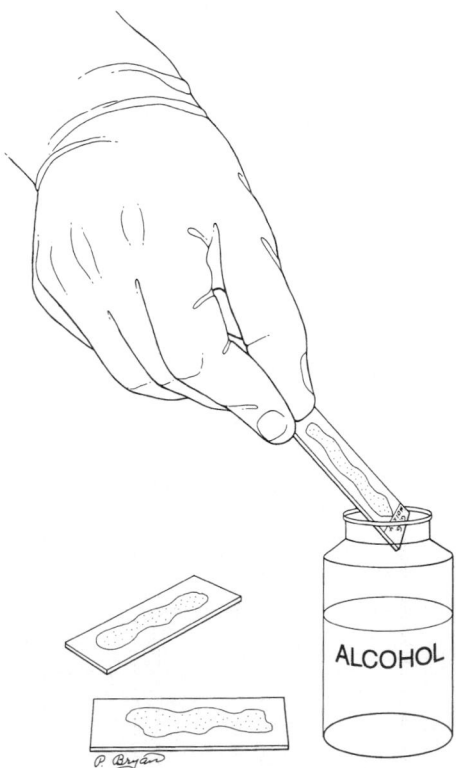

FIGURE 40.23. Technique of fine-needle aspiration—slide preparation. The slide is fixed as rapidly as possible to avoid air drying. Usually, two to three slides can be made from one fine-needle aspiration attempt. The technique chosen for slide preparation depends on the desire of the pathologist

TABLE 40.7.
Requires Open Biopsy

Bloody or serosanguineous fluid on aspiration
Failure of mass to disappear upon fluid aspiration
Recurrence of cyst after one or two aspirations
Bloody nipple discharge
Nipple excoriation
Skin edema and erythema suspicious of inflammatory breast carcinoma

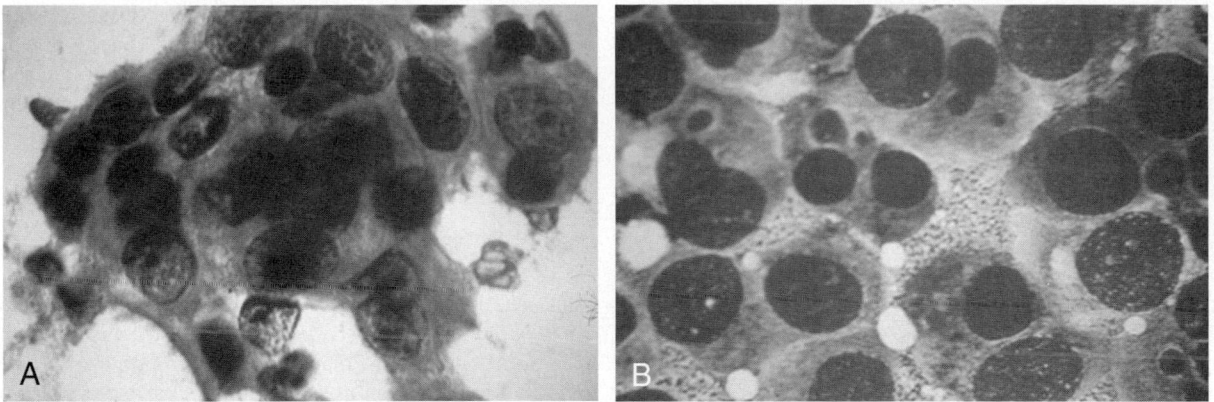

FIGURE 40.24. Fine-needle aspiration of ductal carcinoma. **A:** Smears are cellular with loosely cohesive cells arranged in a malignant cluster. Cells demonstrate clumping of chromatin and irregular nucleoli (Papanicolaou stain ×240). **B:** Single malignant cells with absence of myoepithelial cells are viewed using Diff-Quik stain (×400). Diff-Quik stains are air dried, thus the chromatin pattern is less demonstrative. (Courtesy of Taalat Tadros, M.D., Emory University, School of Medicine, Atlanta, GA.)

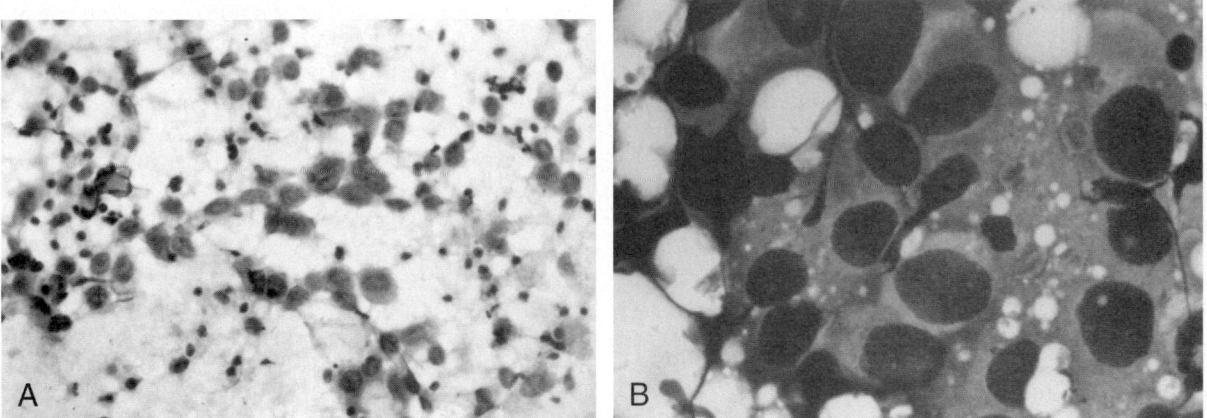

FIGURE 40.25. Fine-needle aspiration of medullary carcinoma. The smears are cellular. **A:** Loosely syncytial malignant aggregates (Papanicolaou stain ×240). **B:** Single malignant cells with benign lymphoid cells noted in the background (Diff-Quik ×400). (Courtesy of Taalat Tadros, M.D., Emory University, School of Medicine, Atlanta, GA.)

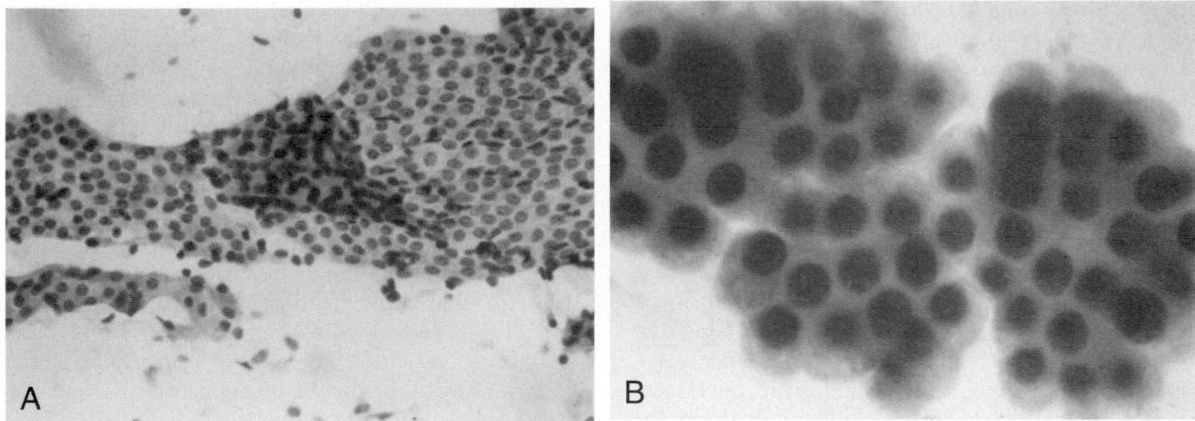

FIGURE 40.26. Fine-needle aspiration of fibrocystic change. **A:** View of uniform ductal cells in right upper quadrant with honeycomb pattern. Characteristic adherent bipolar naked nuclei of myoepithelial cells are noted. Stripped nuclei are seen in the background (Papanicolaou stain ×240). **B:** A flat sheet of apocrine cells are seen in this view. Cells have abundant granular cytoplasm and the nuclei have prominent nucleoli (Papanicolaou stain ×240). (Courtesy of Taalat Tadros, M.D., Emory University, School of Medicine, Atlanta, GA.)

formation beneath the surface, which can complicate mammographic interpretation. For this reason, mammograms (and probably ultrasounds) should be performed either before the FNA procedure or at least 2 weeks afterward.

Contemporary techniques for slide preparation have been developed to improve accuracy and decrease the number of inadequate specimens. Pathologists and cytotechnologists have traditionally been trained to stain cytologic smears with Papanicolaou stain. Diff-Quik, a nonalcohol-based preservative used for air-dried smears, has several advantages over the Papanicolaou stain that may improve both the false-positive and the false-negative smear rates. Smears naturally dry at the edges first. This is particularly true in cases of thin smears such as those obtained by FNA. Diff-Quik smears are air dried, which is technically easier for nonpathologists performing such aspirations. With the Papanicolaou stain method, cells are often lost during alcohol fixation, and background blood and cellular debris obscure details. Such problems have been noted to cause a large number of false-negative and false-positive smears. The Diff-Quik process eliminates cell loss, and background blood does not interfere with the staining of epithelial cells. Morphologic features with Diff-Quik are different from Papanicolaou and the Diff-Quik process accentuates distinct cell features. For instance, cytoplasmic structures and lactating cells are seen better with Diff-Quik versus nuclear processes that are viewed better with Papanicolaou stains. However, studies indicate that although Diff-Quik improves the speed of staining, no important quantifiable differences in nuclear morphology are detected.

Cytyc Thin Prep (TP) processing is being used as an alternative to the traditional method of preparing FNA (and Papanicolaou smear) samples. The TP uses a methanol-based medium in an automated processor that prepares monolayer slides from cells suspended in an alcohol-based preservative. The preparation of monolayered slides is intended to decrease cell loss, improve standardization of slides (fewer thick smears), and allow the preparation of several slides from a single aspirate for cases in which additional slides are required for special studies. A double blind study by Perez-Reyes and associates compared TP slides and conventional smears prepared from the same aspirate and showed only a 62% correlation in diagnosis. Fibroadenoma was particularly difficult to diagnose by the TP method, with a diagnostic correlation rate of only 19%. This great discrepancy may be due to TP's cell shrinkage and loss of background materials, such as stroma and adipose tissue, materials that are the sources of key cytologic criteria for differentiating fibroadenomas from FCC. Blood and cellular debris are often helpful in making a diagnosis of carcinoma as well. The authors also noted a decrease in cytologic detail, including size, shape, and nuclear texture, possibly as a result of components in the proprietary TP fixative or the manner in which the cells were transferred to the slide. The authors suggest that this novel preparatory procedure should be used only as an adjunctive method to conventional Papanicolaou and Diff-Quik smears unless further studies discern a much improved correlation rate. The fact that the TP method may be used to obtain several slides from the initial specimen should not be overlooked, however, and this may be one important reason for its occasional application in the future.

Core Needle Breast Biopsy

It is estimated that approximately 1 million breast biopsies will be performed this year to diagnose approximately 200,000 breast cancers. Percutaneous core needle biopsy may spare many of these women the need for a more deforming, invasive, and expensive surgical procedure. In the mid-1970s core biopsy was introduced to decrease the number of patients undergoing open biopsy for abnormal mammographic findings that ultimately resulted in benign results. With this procedure, a histopathologic diagnosis may be obtained compared with cytologic evaluation with FNA. Studies indicate a high degree of accuracy (98% positive predictive value and 80% negative predictive value), sensitivity of 89%, and specificity of 100% in confirming malignant invasion. False-negative results may occur, as with FNA, but false-positive results are rare except with radial scars. Increasing the number of core specimens by taking samples from several locations in the lesion may increase the representativeness of the specimens.

Percutaneous core breast biopsy may be performed under stereotactic (often called stereotactic needle biopsy) or ultrasound guidance. Both methods are highly accurate procedures that are faster, less invasive, and less expensive than surgical biopsy. Less tissue is removed during core needle biopsy, resulting in no deformity in the breast and minimal-to-no scarring on subsequent mammograms. Other advantages include the ability to distinguish between invasive and intraductal carcinoma. Because *any* pathologist can interpret the histologic material obtained from core needle biopsy, this obviates the need for the special skills of a cytopathologist. One disadvantage of core needle biopsy is that local anesthesia is needed because of the large size of the needle. A potential disadvantage of core needle biopsy is the risk of seeding the needle tract with tumor cells. Thus, placing the core needle biopsy tract within the future surgical excision field seems prudent in those patients undergoing BCS.

This biopsy procedure is most used in the assessment of BI-RADS category 4 lesions (Table 40.8). If core biopsy of a category 4 lesion yields a benign diagnosis, concordant with the imaging characteristics, the woman is usually spared the diagnostic surgical biopsy. Although most often performed for nonpalpable lesions, percutaneous imaging–guided core biopsy can also be helpful in the evaluation of palpable breast masses, particularly for those that are deep, mobile, or vaguely palpable. Performing the biopsy under imaging guidance can help ensure that the lesion has been sampled.

Stereotactic core needle biopsy may be used for all types of mammographic lesions (palpable lesions, non-

TABLE 40.8.
Breast Imaging Reporting and Data System (BI-RADS)

Category	Assessment Category	Follow-Up
1	Negative	Routine (annual)
2	Benign	
3	Probable benign	Short interval follow-up at 6 months for ipsilateral breast, followed by both breasts at 1, 2, 3 years after initial mammogram.
4	Suspicious for malignancy	Biopsy
5	Highly suggestive of malignancy	

palpable lesions, and calcifications), but requires dedicated equipment. Its sensitivity decreases with microcalcifications less than 1 cm in diameter, suggesting that mammographic lesions of this size and of high or intermediate suspicion should undergo excisional biopsy. It is also helpful in evaluating suspicious mammographic findings in cases of previous reduction mammoplasty because the mammographic appearance of a new cancer may be subtle and may simulate the benign changes that are expected of the mammoplasty procedure itself. On the other hand, ultrasound-guided core needle biopsy is used primarily for palpable lesions. It has several advantages, including real-time visualization of the needle, lack of ionizing radiation, accessibility to all parts of the breast and axilla, multipurpose use of equipment, and lower cost. However it is limited in detection of lesions less than 1 cm and has decreased sensitivity in detection of microcalcifications. The choice of stereotactic versus ultrasound guidance depends on several factors, including equipment availability, lesion visibility and accessibility, and preferences of the radiologist and the patient.

After administration of local anesthesia, the area is cleaned. As the core needle is introduced into the mass by the equipment, the tissue inside the core of the needle is cut from the surrounding tissue as the outer sheath is advanced. After removal of the sheath and core needle, a pressure dressing is applied. This procedure may obviate the need for needle localization surgical biopsy and studies indicate similar sensitivity and lower cost. The histologic core specimen may be used to determine hormone receptor status and to study other tumor markers using immunohistochemistry.

There are a number of new devices introduced for stereotactic biopsy of nonpalpable, mammographically detected lesions, including the vacuum-assisted core biopsy and the advanced breast biopsy instrumentation. Further data are necessary to evaluate the strengths and weaknesses of each technique.

Percutaneous core needle biopsy is a reasonable and accurate alternative to open surgical biopsy for the diagnosis of both palpable and nonpalpable breast lesions. Recent studies indicate this procedure can reduce the cost of diagnosing mammographically detected breast lesions by more than 50%. At a time when health care policy and re-imbursement decisions are influenced by cost consideration, increased use of this procedure is probable.

Open Surgical Biopsy

Open surgical biopsy includes excisional and incisional techniques. Incisional biopsy is a diagnostic procedure reserved for masses that are too large to be completely excised. There are currently few indications for the use of incisional biopsy because FNA and core needle biopsy usually provide sufficient tissue to make a diagnosis with less morbidity and lower cost. Conversely, excisional biopsy refers to the complete removal of a breast mass and is the definitive procedure for some benign breast masses. Excisional biopsy is usually an outpatient procedure performed under local anesthesia with intravenous sedation as needed.

Some authors recommend beginning the procedure by marking the incisional site with the patient in the sitting position. Conversely, others recommend locating the lesion with the patient in the same position in which the surgery is to be performed. This marking should be performed before injection of any anesthesia because the anesthetic may obliterate the outlines of the mass. Circumareolar incisions are the most ideal cosmetically and heal well. They are attempted for most benign masses despite having to tunnel a short distance to reach the lesion. This should not be done with suspected malignant lesions to prevent the spread of tumor cells along the tunnel, thus prohibiting breast-conserving therapy in the future. On the other hand, Langer or curvilinear lines (following the anatomic skin lines) may be used depending on the location of the lesion. Langer's lines may be defined by gently pinching the skin over the mass and noting the outline. Radial incisions are made over the axilla and inframammary portions of the breast but are ill-advised in the upper portions of the breast because of possible contracture and asymmetric cosmetic result. It is important to keep biopsy incisions within the boundaries of the future mastectomy or wide local excision site, which may be required for definitive treatment.

After marking the site of the lesion, the patient is placed supine with her arm extended comfortably on an arm board. In draping the patient, the nipple should be kept in view for orientation during surgery. Local anesthesia without epinephrine is infiltrated at the incision site and deeply around the mass with a 23-gauge needle. Very small masses may be obscured, however, by the use of large amounts of local anesthesia. The absence of epinephrine permits immediate visualization of blood loss, which helps in obtaining adequate hemostasis (rather than oozing later when the anesthetic has worn off, resulting in unsightly hematomas.) The incision is made with a no. 15 knife blade and carried through the skin and subcutaneous tissue to the lesion (Fig. 40.27).

Sharp dissection is used to develop the skin flaps to achieve better exposure. Blunt dissection increases adhesions and inflammation. The edges of the incision are retracted with skin hooks. Instruments that will crush the tissue are never used so as to prevent cutting the tumor into smaller pieces, thus making excision more difficult, or to prevent tumor seeding. The mass may be gently grasped with suture for traction while excision is performed with sharp dissection. Cautery should be used *only* for hemostasis, not for excision of the mass,

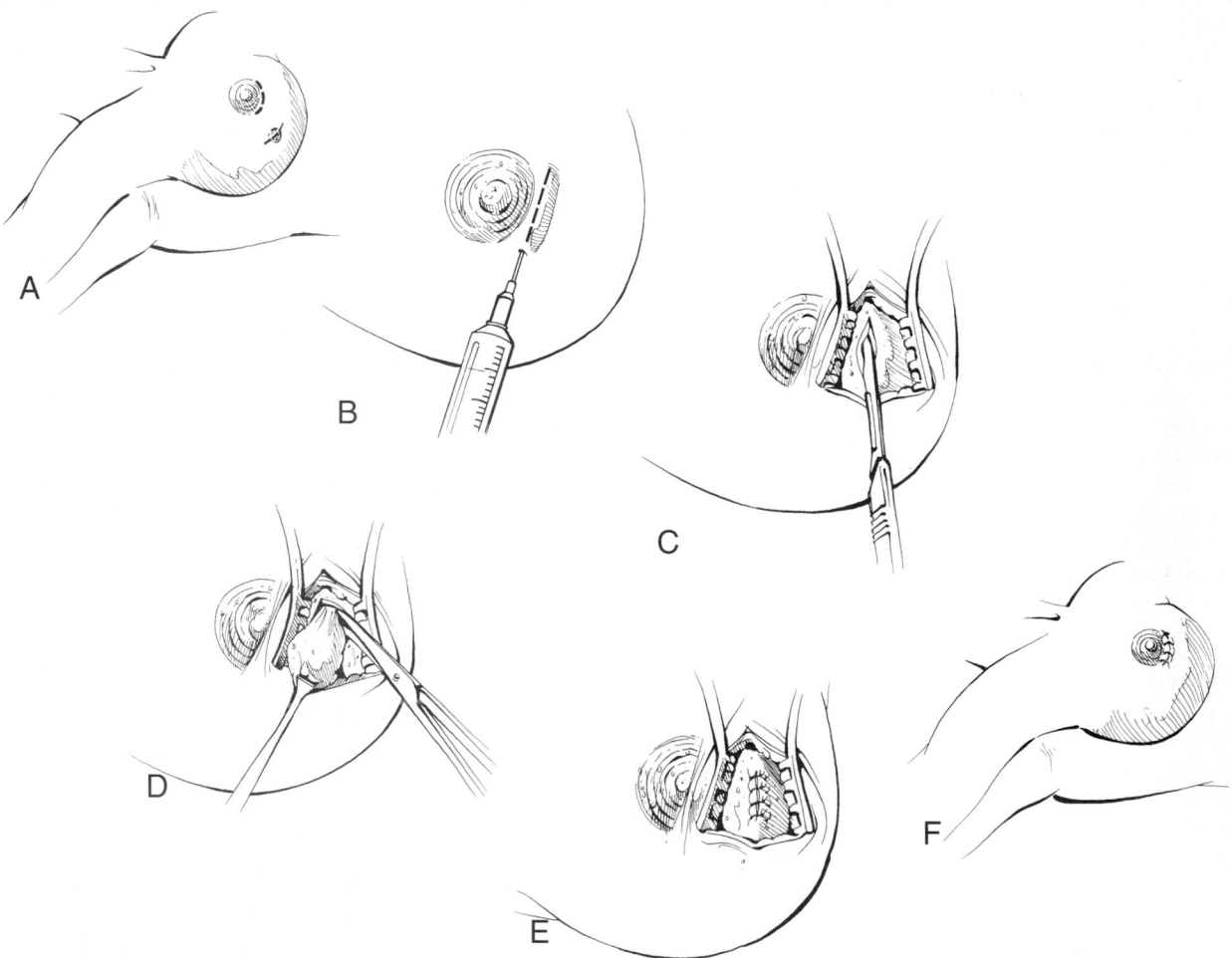

FIGURE 40.27. Technique of excisional biopsy. **A:** For cosmetic reasons, circumareolar incisions are preferable when the lesion is thought to be within 2 or 3 cm of the areola. Not more than one half of the areolar margin should be incised. A curved incision parallel to the areola is made over lesions further out from the center. When malignant disease is strongly suspected, the surgeon should attempt to avoid the probable path of the subsequent mastectomy incision. **B:** An intradermal wheal is raised along the path of the proposed incision using 1% lidocaine and a hypodermic (no. 25) needle. From the wheal, deeper injections of anesthetic are made around the circumference of the lesion and beneath it. **C:** The incision is carried down through the dense subcutaneous tissue and into the lobule containing the lesion. Self-retaining retractors are helpful when an assistant is not available. **D:** If the lesion is small or easily mobilized, it should be sharply dissected and excised with a thin margin of adjacent tissue. **E:** The lobular defect is sutured with fine absorbable suture material if the closure places no tension on the overlying skin. Bleeding is controlled with absorbable ligatures or electrocoagulation. Absolute hemostasis is essential. **F:** The skin is closed with interrupted 4-0 or 5-0 silk or nylon sutures. Drainage is seldom necessary. A pressure dressing for 24 to 48 hours is desirable if a significant amount of dead space has been left behind.

because heat may distort estrogen and progesterone receptor evaluation and margin delineation. If malignancy is suspected, the biopsy specimen should include a generous margin of normal tissue around the mass. Furthermore, estrogen and progesterone receptor status and human epidermal growth factor receptor 2 protein (HER2/neu) evaluation is critical. Ideally, the pathology department should receive the specimen on ice, because room temperature (heat) can damage the estrogen and progesterone receptors.

Closure of the defect left by the excised mass (dead space) is discouraged because of the increased risk of infection from suture placement and the potential for skin distortion. If a large defect is obtained, a minimum number of sutures should be used and drainage of the site bears additional significance. A subcuticular closure with 4-0 or 5-0 absorbable material using Steri-Strips is generally performed. Alternatively, nonabsorbable suture can be used and removed 1 or 2 weeks week postoperatively. To prevent hematoma formation, a snugly placed elastic dressing is applied for 24 to 48 hours. A bra should then be worn continuously for 3 to 7 days to minimize the risk of bleeding and discomfort. The patient should avoid heavy lifting with the affected arm and strenuous activity for 3 to 7 days.

Needle localization excisional biopsy is performed for suspicious nonpalpable abnormalities seen on mammography. In the radiology suite, under local anesthesia, the lesion is identified by fluoroscopy and a needle is placed near it. A hooked wire is inserted through the needle and located just beneath the lesion. After the needle is removed, the wire is stabilized on the skin, and the patient is transported to the operating suite for surgical excision. Incisions similar to those used for excisional biopsy are made, and the suspected abnormality and the wire are excised. Radiographic studies are performed on the specimen to ensure that the lesion originally noted on mammography has been excised in its entirety. This procedure can be done under local anesthesia in an outpatient setting. The complications are similar to those of excisional biopsies, including bleeding, hematoma formation, and infection (cellulitis, abscess). This procedure has been surpassed by percutaneous needle core biopsy (either stereotactic or ultrasound guided) and is used less often today.

BREAST CANCER

The risk of breast cancer has reached epidemic proportions, affecting one in eight women who live to the age of 85 years. Its incidence is more that two times that of all female pelvic cancers combined and is probably the most feared disease by women today. A millennium of scientific inquiry, theoretical investigation, and systematic experimentation has only now begun to provide the medical profession with prevention strategies for women at high risk.

Thus, breast cancer remains a leading cause of cancer-related mortality in women. Estimates by the ACS indicated nearly 183,000 women were expected to develop breast cancer and 40,800 women would die of the disease in the United States during the year 2000. Breast cancer is the most frequently diagnosed neoplasm in women and is second only to lung cancer in female deaths due to cancer. Men are not immune; 1,400 new cases of breast cancer were expected to be diagnosed in men in the year 2000. There is good news, though, in that the incidence rates appear to have leveled off in the 1990s after increasing about 4% per year in the 1980s. Additionally, mortality rates have declined since 1992, with the largest decreases noted in younger women (both black and white).

The increasing lifetime risk for development of breast cancer may be attributed to early detection of prevalent cases, primarily due to increased use of mammographic screening and lower mortality due to causes other than breast cancer. Terminating the lifetime risk calculation at age 85 years, however, assumes incorrectly that no women develop breast cancer after that age.

Risk Factors

The etiology of breast cancer is multifactorial and, although numerous risk factors have been identified, they only account for 21% of the risk of breast cancer in women age 30 to 54 years old and only 29% of that in women age 55 to 84 years. Furthermore, nearly three-fourths of women with breast cancer have no identifiable risk factors other than gender and age, thus all women should be considered at risk for breast cancer.

Previously identified risk factors for breast cancer include increasing age, nulliparity, delayed childbearing (childbirth before age 18 years portends one third the risk of breast cancer than in a woman delivering at age 35 years), personal or family history of breast cancer, oophorectomy, benign proliferative breast disease, obesity in postmenopausal women, a long menstrual history (menarche before age 12 and late menopause), and higher education and socioeconomic status. Other factors, such as fat intake, breast-feeding, previous abortions, smoking, and alcohol intake, have all been suggested to contribute to breast cancer risks, but the associations remain inconclusive, inconsistent, and controversial.

Breast cancer incidence and mortality rates vary among racial and ethnic groups. For all ages combined, white women are more likely to develop breast cancer, yet African-American women are more likely to die of breast cancer. Native Americans have the lowest incidence of breast cancer, nearly one third the risk of white women. In addition, Native American and Asian women have approximately one third the mortality of African-American women.

Family History

Family history is the most widely recognized breast cancer risk factor. First-degree female relatives of women with breast carcinoma have two to three times the general population risk of developing the disease. The risk increases even more if the affected relative was pre-menopausal with bilateral breast disease upon diagnosis (eightfold increased risk) compared with a post-menopausal affected relative with only unilateral disease (onefold to twofold increased risk). Centers for Disease Control and Prevention data indicate a 2.3 relative risk for patients with an affected mother or sister and a 1.5 relative risk for patients with an affected aunt or grandmother. The risk for patients with both an affected mother and sister has been listed between a twofold and 14-fold increase. First-degree relatives include the patient's mother, sister, or daughter. Second-degree relatives include grandmother, niece, and aunt.

Breast Cancer Susceptibility Genes

The past decade has witnessed an explosion of knowledge in the field of cancer genetics and inherited susceptibility to cancer syndromes. It has been estimated that approximately 5% to 10% of breast cancers are inherited in an autosomal dominant pattern. Breast cancer susceptibility genes, BRCA1 and BRCA2, were discovered in the early 1990s and mapped to chromosome 17q and 13q, respectively. In 1996, commercially available DNA-based carrier detection became available, opening up a quandary for women at risk for inherited forms of breast cancer. Because these tests are expensive, are often difficult to interpret, and are documented to have a significant psychologic impact for both positive and negative test results, as well as placing healthy individuals at risk for insurance and employment discrimination, the decision to undergo testing must be made after a thorough and informed discussion between the physician and the patient.

The only currently known BRCA genes are BRCA1 and BRCA2, thus the discussion herein is based only on these mutations. BRCA1 is a large protein, encoding for 1,863 amino acid pairs. Approximately 600 mutations have been found in the BRCA1 gene and nearly 500 in the BRCA2 gene. BRCA1 mutation is believed to account for nearly half of all inherited breast cancer cases and nearly 90% of the hereditary ovarian cancer cases. Similarly, BRCA2 mutations are responsible for approximately 40% of familial breast cancer and 5% to 10% of familial ovarian cancer. Li-Fraumeni syndrome, p53 mutations, Hras, and ataxia-telangiectasia appear to account for the other cases of inherited breast cancer.

Initial studies suggest that the lifetime risk of developing breast cancer in families with BRCA1 was approximately 80% to 90%, whereas the risk of ovarian cancer was approximately 30% to 60%. It is estimated, based on data from families linked to BRCA1, that 50% of female mutation carriers will develop breast cancer by age 50 years (compared with 1.7% in the general population at age 50 years) and 85% by age 70 years (compared with 11% in the general population at age 70 years). Pedigree analysis in BRCA2 carriers have identified a similar risk of development of female breast cancer to that seen with BRCA1 mutations. However, the risk of ovarian cancer for carriers of BRCA2 mutations is only 10%. The overall lifetime risk of developing breast *or* ovarian cancer is nearly 100%. BRCA mutation carriers not only have an increased overall risk of developing cancer, but commonly have a younger age of onset and a greater probability of second tumors. Accordingly, although the inherited mutations account for only 5% to 10% of all breast cancers, they account for nearly 25% of breast cancer cases diagnosed before the age of 30.

These initial studies have been questioned because penetrance (the percent of mutation carriers who develop disease) may be lower in women with a less strongly positive family history. Also, differences in penetrance have been noted among family members with identical BRCA1 mutations. It has been suggested that other genes may modify the penetrance of the suppressor gene. Alternatively, the gene–environment interaction may modify risk, including reproductive risk factors that affect breast and ovarian cancer incidence. Thus, population-based studies (versus studies based on specific families) suggest that the *actual* overall lifetime cancer risk of mutation carriers is closer to 56% for breast cancer and 16% for ovarian cancer. It is unclear whether these inconsistent results are related to the populations tested, to the size of the studies, or, perhaps, to differences in penetrance between different mutations. Further longitudinal studies may resolve this question.

Not only are the BRCA genes associated with increased risk of female malignancies, they have also been shown to be a marker for hereditary cancer syndromes in men. Male breast cancer is much more common in BRCA2 families than in the general population. Nearly 40% of male breast cancers are related to a BRCA2 mutation. In addition, other malignancies are increased in BRCA2 carriers, such as laryngeal, prostate, gallbladder, stomach, malignant melanoma, primary peritoneal carcinoma, and pancreatic cancer. Hence, the BRCA mutation may be transferred to a woman through a male relative. However, a male carrier of a BRCA1 mutation is much more likely to be cancer-free than is a woman who carries the same mutation. And, although a family history of breast cancer places a mutation carrier at increased risk not only for breast cancer but also for colon and ovarian cancer, similarly her brother will be at increased risk for colon cancer and potentially prostate cancer as well. It is therefore important to elicit a history of *all* related malignancies, not just a family history of breast and ovarian cancer. Patients are often unaware that the risk of transmission of a BRCA mutation is equally high from the paternal side and do not volunteer information about cancers from that side. Episodes of malignancies from both sides of the families must be elicited, including age of onset, bilaterality, and history of multiple primary cancers in an individual in the family.

Because of the large size of the gene and the number of different mutations, genetic testing has proven to be technically difficult. In some families, it may be impossible to distinguish disease-causing mutations from insignificant rare polymorphisms. Direct DNA sequencing and single-strand conformation polymorphism assay are the current methods used to map BRCA germline mutations. Because of the expense, labor intensity, sensitivity and specificity, testing is reserved for research settings and is not suited for wide-scale screening.

BRCA1 and BRCA2 are believed to be tumor suppressor genes. Although inheritance of familial cancer syndromes usually follows an autosomal dominant pattern of inheritance, as a tumor suppressor, BRCA mutations are recessive at the cellular level because inactivation of both gene copies is required for tumorigenesis. Mutations in both gene copies results in loss of the tumor suppressor function of the BRCA1 gene. Two hypotheses have been proposed for the key function of these genes. Loss of the tumor suppressor function may represent an initial event that facilitates the development of other genetic alterations, culminating in the development of a clinically recognizable cancer, or loss of function may increase the frequency of DNA strand breaks that lead to alterations in other cancer-causing genes. Inactivation of tumor suppressor genes is almost a universal step in the development of a wide range of cancers in humans and experimental animals. In individuals who are not genetically at increased risk for cancer, environmental mutagenesis with time can result in inactivation of both gene copies. In individuals who have inherited a mutation in one of these tumor suppressor genes, the probability of acquiring additional mutations to produce cancer is significantly increased.

Our knowledge regarding BRCA mutations is far from complete. Many incongruencies form the basis of our present information. It has been noted that various BRCA1 mutations may differ in the extent to which they predispose to breast or ovarian cancer depending on whether the mutation is located in the carboxyl terminus of the gene or proximal amino end of the gene. Penetrance also affects an individual patient's risk of development of the disease. Penetrance refers to phenotypic expression of the genetic mutation, here represented by development of breast or ovarian cancer. Routinely, most single gene forms of cancer (or mutations) are inherited in an autosomal dominant fashion with a high degree of penetrance. Studies have shown that inheritance of a single gene mutation is not sufficient to produce malignancy. Two or more mutations in a tumor suppressor gene must be acquired for a specific cell to make a malignant transformation.

Histologic differences in the hereditary breast cancers compared to the sporadic cancers may account for the earlier presentation of cancer in mutation carriers. It has been reported that BRCA1-associated breast cancers are characterized by higher-grade medullary features, overexpression of p53, aneuploidy, and high proliferation index relative to sporadic breast cancers. In fact, the presence of medullary cancer in a patient or a family member increases the suspicion of a BRCA1 mutation. Essinger and colleagues noted 19% of BRCA1 cancers were of the medullary variety, as compared with none in the sporadic cases, suggesting that medullary cancer alone may be an indication for susceptibility testing. Additionally, BRCA1-associated cancers are estrogen receptor negative 65% to 80% of the time, compared to a rate of 25% to 35% in sporadic cancers. In contrast, the excess of estrogen receptor–negative tumors is not demonstrated in the BRCA2-associated cancers. Moreover, the clinicopathologic characteristics of BRCA2-associated cancers are similar to sporadic breast cancers with the suggestion of higher grades. However, a number of studies have found no differences between prognosis in BRCA-associated cancers and sporadic cancers. Thus, the issue remains unresolved and suggests the need for longitudinal studies to ferret out this needed information.

The frequency of a BRCA1 mutation in the general population is estimated to be 1 in 500 to 1 in 1,000 (with BRCA2 mutations occurring somewhat less), although it appears to be higher in certain ethnic groups, such as Ashkenazi Jews in whom it is estimated to be 1%. In the Ashkenazi Jewish population (of eastern or central European origin), three different founder mutations have been identified: 185delAG and 5382insC in BRCA1, and 6174delT in BRCA2. Estimates indicate that 1 in 40 Ashkenazi individuals carry one of these founder mutations, and they are responsible for 25% of the early onset breast cancer in this population. Current investigations indicate the estimated gene frequency in the general population may be artificially high because of ascertainment bias in the initial studies of high-risk families.

BRCA Risk Assessment and Counseling

Genetic counseling is an essential element of breast cancer susceptibility testing. Recent policy statements of the American Society of Clinical Oncology (ASCO) and the American Society of Human Genetics mandates both genetic counseling and informed consent before any testing. Moreover, the State of New York has passed a law that stipulates the above requirements. The decision to proceed with genetic testing for BRCA1 or BRCA2 mutations is complex. Considerable caution must be used in counseling patients because definitive data are not available. The benefit of genetic testing remains hypothetical because there is no proof that testing would translate into a decrease in breast and ovarian cancer mortality. The ability to reassure those with negative tests is limited by the possible existence of other, as yet undiscovered, genes. Nonpenetrance of the gene may make pedigree interpretation difficult in that absence of cancer in a parent cannot necessarily be interpreted to mean that the children are not at risk.

The accuracy of screening tests is affected by the prior probability of having the condition and the sensitivity and specificity of the test. A history of multiple affected first-degree relatives, bilateral disease, early or premenopausal age of onset, and a family history of both ovarian and breast cancer increases the probability of having an inherited predisposition to breast cancer. Current protocols vary, but most recommend testing for women with a personal or family history of premenopausal breast cancer, personal or family history of ovarian cancer before age 70 years, family history of male breast cancer, or family history of known BRCA mutation carrier. The family history includes first-degree (mother, sister, daughter) and second-degree (grandmother, aunt, niece) relatives but, most importantly, includes relatives from both the maternal *and* paternal sides of the family. Given the current cost of testing ($2,400 to $2,500 at most institutions; 350$ for specific major mutations) and the fact that its benefits remain unproven, physicians should discourage individuals from undergoing testing in the absence of a strong family history or early disease.

It is preferable to test an *affected* family member to document the particular familial BRCA1 or BRCA2 mutation (there are more than 100 different BRCA1 mutations currently identified). A negative result is most meaningful in a situation in which the family member has previously tested positive. In the absence of the detectable mutation in the proband, the patient may be reassured that she does not have the high risk of cancer seen in her family. She should be counseled, however, that she still has the baseline risk of cancer seen in the general population (one in eight for women who live to age 85 years) and that she should continue usual care, such as mammography and breast examination. On the other hand, if the family member with cancer has not or cannot be tested, the interpretation of a negative result is more problematic. For such a woman, a negative BRCA test could have several possibilities: (1) a BRCA mutation is present but was not detected by the test (possibly due to the testing modality or polymorphisms); (2) there is no BRCA mutation, but another gene mutation exists (as yet unidentified or related to a regulatory gene); (3) the patient does not have inherited breast cancer predisposition. In the latter case, again, the woman still has a risk equal to the general population for sporadic forms of breast cancer. One study showed that one third of mutations detected involved deletions that are not currently detected by conventional techniques. In summary, present techniques do not identify all disease-causing mutations and patients need to be informed of the limitations of the present technology.

Several algorithms have been developed to estimate a woman's risk of developing breast cancer with the best known of these being the Gail and Claus models. The Gail Model Risk Assessment Tool (Fig. 40.28) incorporates the patient's race, current age, age at menarche and first live birth, number of first-degree relatives with

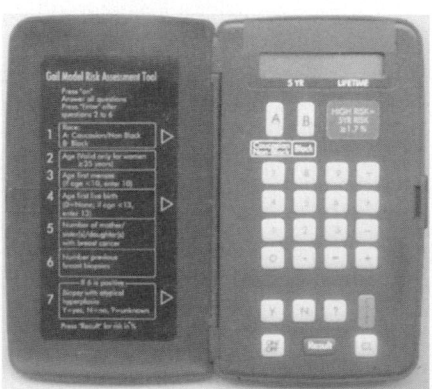

FIGURE 40.28. Gail model risk-assessment tool.

breast cancer, number of previous breast biopsies, and pathology results in generating an estimate of breast cancer risk. Conversely, the Claus model uses fewer categories including only the number of relatives with breast cancer, their relationship to the patient, and the relative's age of cancer diagnosis. Although helpful in diagnosis, models are often inapplicable to the proband. In particular, the Gail model cannot be used for women younger than 35 years of age and is less accurate in women who do not obtain annual mammograms. Counseling must stress these figures are estimates and not absolute risks, and thus balance the magnitude of risk for the individual patient.

A crucial question for women at increased risk for developing breast cancer is whether that risk can be modified. Although conceivably genetic testing and counseling may reduce both the incidence and mortality rate of cancer by identifying families with an inherited cancer predisposition, currently there are no definitive preventive measures available for cancers developing in patients with BRCA germline mutations. The field of molecular biology and genetics is growing exponentially, outpacing modern knowledge of how to apply susceptibility testing results to clinical care. Ongoing population-based longitudinal studies will greatly assist in decision making for patients at increased risk for disease.

Exogenous Hormones

No issue related to breast cancer risk has been fraught with as much controversy as has the use of exogenous hormones, specifically postmenopausal HRT and OCPs. The extensive research conducted to answer this question has expanded the debate rather than resolved it.

Hormonal Replacement Therapy

Currently, nearly 42 million American women are postmenopausal, and this number is predicted to increase to 62 million by 2020. Nearly 40% of postmenopausal women in the United States use HRT; thus, recent association of breast cancer with the use of HRT has received considerable attention in the medical and lay press.

Sufficient evidence exists to indicate the possibility of a slightly increased risk of breast cancer associated with long durations (10 or more years) of postmenopausal estrogen use. Nevertheless, we believe that patients must consider this possibility in their informed decision making.

Initial case control studies did not find an increased risk of breast cancer associated with the use of HRT, but these studies were limited by statistical power and methodologic problems. A review of the epidemiologic studies on postmenopausal hormone therapy and the risk of breast cancer also fails to provide definitive evidence regarding this issue because results are inconsistent. Categories of participants with increased risk are noted in some studies whereas other categories are refuted in the same study. The latest data from the Nurses Health Study and the Collaborative Group on Hormonal Factors in Breast Cancer refutes previous data and indicate that current users of HRT have a relative risk of 1.33 of developing breast cancer but note no increased risk with past use. The shear number of participants (more than 20,000 participants) warrants giving great credibility to these findings. In addition, four subsequent metaanalyses note a slight increased risk in long-term users of HRT (greater than 15 years), although here also there are conflicting results, affected by dosage and duration of HRT use. In contrast, the Four State Case Control Study and the Iowa Women's Health Study showed no change in the risk of breast cancer diagnosis with long-term current use. Note that metaanalyses have the same flaws in methodology and bias as the initial epidemiologic studies upon which they are based. Pooling several groups of data does not remove this problem, thus this information should be viewed with caution and the patient made aware of the lack of definitive information at this time. Nevertheless, the trend propels one to consider these findings in making recommendations to patients.

Two recent articles in *The Journal of the American Medical Association* and *The Journal of the National Cancer Institute* have joined the list of epidemiologic studies examining the potential risk for breast cancer associated with HRT. The key finding in both of these retrospective studies was the identification of an increased risk of being diagnosed with breast cancer associated with cyclic HRT, and with the duration of therapy. Importantly, continuous combined therapy, used by 80% of women on HRT, did not show an increased risk in either study. Again, differing dosages of estrogen and progesterone, regimens, and duration may flaw the results. Consequently, these results may reflect therapies that are different from the ones currently prescribed.

On the other hand, additional data are being compiled showing benefits to HRT when breast cancer is diagnosed. Survival data indicate that the risk of mortality from breast cancer was decreased among women who were using HRT at the time of diagnosis compared to age-matched nonusers. HRT user-associated cancers were more likely to be smaller, less likely to be associated with positive nodes, and more likely to be estrogen receptor positive. Possibly this information supports the idea that the increased risk of breast cancer diagnosis among users of HRT is likely to result from detection bias wherein participants were more likely to see a physician regularly, and have regular breast examination and mammography. In addition, a review of pathology data shows that HRT use is associated with an increased incidence of breast cancer with a favorable histology in an analysis of the Iowa Women's Health Study.

In summary, the studies over the preceding 25 years are contradictory and several studies lack statistical significance. Current information appears to suggest change in regimens for women on cyclic HRT. For women on the combined continuous regimen, the information is less definitive, thus investigators have attempted to provide credible data to assist in decision making. To project the impact of HRT on disease incidence and longevity in postmenopausal women with different risk factors for coronary heart disease (CHD) and breast cancer, Col and colleagues designed a mathematical decision-making analysis based on the Markov model. Their model indicated that use of HRT in newly postmenopausal women could result in gains in life expectancy, 3 years or more depending on their risk factor profiles. This is analogous to predicted life expectancy increases among 35-year-old women of 2.8 years for cessation of smoking, of 0.4 to 6.3 years for lowering serum cholesterol values, and of 0.9 to 5.7 years for lowering diastolic blood pressure. More importantly, for individuals with at least one risk factor for CHD, HRT should extend life expectancy, even for women having first-degree relatives with breast cancer. Even among women at high risk for breast cancer, the presence of even one risk factor for CHD tips the balance in favor of using HRT. The only category of women who would not benefit from HRT are women *without any* risk factors for CHD or hip fracture, but who have two first-degree relatives with breast cancer; these women should not receive HRT.

Although most women are fearful of the consequences of breast cancer, which claims 43,000 lives per year, more women die of CHD (230,000 per year) and nearly 65,000 women die each year of hip fractures. The lay population's perspectives of risk assessment is also unbalanced in that fewer than 3% of women age 50 to 59 have two or more first-degree relatives with breast cancer, but more than half of these same women have at least one risk factor for CHD (about 60% have hypertension, 50% have elevated serum cholesterol values, and 45% smoke). Despite the increased prevalence, nearly 100% of women are more concerned about the risk of breast cancer over the impact of CHD risk factors. Additionally, health care providers may be reluctant to prescribe HRT if more weight is placed on errors of commission (breast cancer) than on errors of omission (CHD or osteoporosis).

It is also worthwhile to counsel patients on other potential benefits of HRT, including prevention of osteoporosis, improved cognitive function, abatement of menopausal vasomotor symptoms, and decreased genitourinary symptoms as well as reduced risk of tooth loss and death of all causes before age 80 years. HRT has also been shown to have cardioprotective effects with improved lipid profiles, but in women with established CHD, an increased risk of second CHD event was noted in the first year of use. In the individual woman, the potential benefits of hormone use may outweigh the potential risk of cancer promotion. The use of hormonal therapy may be considered as long as such women are fully informed of the risks and benefits.

In summary, medical studies contain conflicting information regarding HRT use in postmenopausal women. In addition, the role these agents may play in the development of cancers in genetically predisposed women has not been evaluated. Caution should be applied in recommending the routine use of postmenopausal estrogen replacement in women with inherited breast cancer susceptibility until more information is known. HRT use increases longevity and can improve the quality of life for postmenopausal women. It should not be initiated solely for the purpose of secondary prevention of CHD events in women with established CHD, but it continues to show benefit in the majority of women without CHD risk factors. To make definitive recommendations, additional studies, especially prospective trials, are required. The Women's Health Initiative (funded by the NIH) may resolve these issues.

Oral Contraceptive Medications

OCPs are used by nearly 11 million women worldwide, and are the second most popular contraceptive method available (surpassed only by female sterilization). Since its approval by the FDA in 1960, OCPs have become one of the most extensively studied medications ever prescribed. Recent studies relating OCPs to breast cancer have yielded conflicting results, thus the issue continues to be controversial.

Case control studies including the Cancer and Steroid Hormone Study initially showed no overall association between OCP use and the development of breast cancer. However, the enrollees were not representative of the current OCP user who is younger, uses OCPs for longer duration, and delays initial versus subsequent pregnancies. Reanalysis of the data shows a correlation between certain subgroups and an increased risk of development of breast cancer, specifically among women using OCPs before their first full-term pregnancy, women age 25 to 34, and long-term users. Although incongruous, it may be that estrogen in OCPs stimulates breast cancer, promotes its growth, and makes it detectable, so that it is more likely to be diagnosed while the OCP user is younger, yet without conferring an increase in overall lifetime risk. Another possibility is that the increased risk seen in these analyses represents detection bias—that is, women taking OCPs are more likely to have breast examinations and they are more likely to have the diagnosis made while they are younger. In summary, there is a slightly increased risk of being diagnosed with breast cancer in OCP users younger than 35 years of age. By age 50 years, the cumulative risk is the same in users and nonusers, and there is no evidence of increased overall breast cancer risk even with prolonged duration of use. Furthermore, the Nurses Health Study, a prospective cohort study of more than 100,000 female nurses in the United States, showed no increased risk of breast cancer or breast cancer mortality in past users of OCPs.

Studies specifically of women at high risk for breast cancer have also generated contradictory results. In women with a family history of breast cancer and OCP use, a 1989 study by Murray (with more than 4,500 women) showed no association with subsequent development of breast cancer. Conversely, a study published in 2000 involving 426 families (3,300 women with a positive family history for breast or ovarian cancer) revealed a threefold increased risk of development of breast cancer in those with a family history compared to those without such history who also used OCPs. However, other authors belie the strength of the study and indicate they would continue to support use of low-dose formulations in women with a family history of breast cancer unless the cancer history was compelling.

The purported associations must be placed in perspective, though. It is evident that case control studies have inferior methodologic strength compared to the gold standard of randomized controlled trials. The conclusions may be imprecise because of the low numbers of participants in some studies. Also, studies have not included current low-dose formulations in wide scale, but have been based on previous high-dose OCPs, which clearly may confer higher risk. Also note, the categories associated with increased risk (use before pregnancy and women age 25 to 34) are at increased risk *without use of OCPs* because OCPs are purposely used to delay pregnancy. Finally, studies often include women with a family history of *both* ovarian and breast cancer, whereas there is evidence that OCPs actually decrease the risk of ovarian and endometrial cancer in the general population. Whether this decreased risk applies to women with an inherited predisposition to breast or ovarian cancer is unknown, especially because the risk of breast cancer is more common than ovarian cancer in these high-risk families.

Staging

Due to widespread adherence to mammographic screening, breast cancer is being detected at earlier stages. Nearly 56% of white women and 45% of African-American women are presenting with in situ or stage I disease. Breast cancer is staged clinically according to the status of the tumor, the regional lymph nodes, and distant metastasis (TNM system) (Table 40.9). Complete staging includes a through physical examination, mammography, pretreatment chest radiograph, and routine blood studies including hematology and liver panel. Routine bone scan is not cost effective in that only 0.6% of asymptomatic patients have a positive bone scan. Therefore, bone scans are indicated only in patients who are symptomatic or are at high risk for metastatic disease.

Mammography is essential to adequate staging, even in the most obvious cases. Synchronous cancer is present in 4% to 5% of patients, and multicentric disease may be discovered in the involved breast. The clinical nodal status is often incorrect, with a false-positive and false-negative rate of approximately 25%. The pathologic stage of the primary lesion based on histologic examination at the time of surgery is the main determinant of actuarial survival of the patient.

Staging is reflective of 5-year survival rates. The 5-year survival rate for localized breast cancer has increased from 72% in the 1940s to 96%. If the cancer has spread regionally, however, the rate is 77%. There is a significant decrease in survival to 21% for women with distant metastases. Seventy-one percent of women diagnosed with breast cancer survive 10 years, and 57% survive 15 years (Fig. 40.29).

Histology

Cancers of the mammary gland comprise a histologically heterogeneous group of tumors. More than 90% of breast cancers arise with the ducts. Infiltrating or invasive

TABLE 40.9.
TNM Staging System

DEFINITIONS

Primary Tumor (T)

Definitions for classifying the primary tumor (T) are the same for clinical and pathologic classification. The telescoping method of classification can be applied. If the measurement is made by physical examination, the examiner will use the major headings (T1, T2, or T3). If other measurements, such as mammographic or pathologic, are used, the examiner can use the telescoped subsets of T1.

TX	Primary tumor cannot be assessed	
T0	No evidence of primary tumor	
Tis	Carcinoma in situ: intraductal carcinoma, lobular carcinoma in situ, or Paget's disease of the nipple with no tumor	
T1	Tumor 2 cm or less in greatest dimension	
	T1a	0.5 cm or less in greatest dimension
	T1b	More than 0.5 cm but not more than 1 cm in greatest dimension
	T1c	More than 1 cm but not more than 2 cm in greatest dimension
T2	Tumor more than 2 cm but not more than 5 cm in greatest dimension	
T3	Tumor more than 5 cm in greatest dimension	
T4	Tumor of any size with direct extension to chest wall or skin	
	T4a	Extension to chest wall
	T4b	Edema (including peau d'orange) or ulceration of the skin of the breast or satellite skin nodules confined to the same breast
	T4c	Both (T4a and T4b)
	T4d	Inflammatory carcinoma

Note: Paget's disease associated with a tumor is classified according to the size of the tumor.

Regional Lymph Nodes (N)

NX	Regional lymph nodes cannot be assessed (e.g., previously removed)
N0	No regional lymph node metastasis
N1	Metastasis to movable ipsilateral axillary lymph nodes
N2	Metastasis to ipsilateral axillary lymph nodes fixed to one another or to other structures
N3	Metastasis to ipsilateral internal mammary lymph nodes

Pathologic Classification (pN)

pNX	Regional lymph nodes cannot be assessed (e.g., previously removed, or not removed for pathologic study)	
pN0	No regional lymph node metastasis	
pN1	Metastasis to movable ipsilateral axillary lymph nodes	
	pN1a	Only micrometastasis, none larger than 0.2 cm
	pN1b	Metastasis to lymph nodes, any larger than 0.2 cm
	pN1bi	Metastasis in one to three lymph nodes, any more than 0.2 cm and all less than 2 cm in greatest dimension
	pN1bii	Metastasis to four or more lymph nodes, any more than 0.2 cm and all less than 2 cm in greatest dimension
	pN1biii	Extension of tumor beyond the capsule of a lymph node metastasis less than 2 cm in greatest dimension
	pN1biv	Metastasis to a lymph node 2 cm or more in greatest dimension
pN2	Metastasis to ipsilateral axillary lymph nodes that are fixed to one another or to other structures	
pN3	Metastasis to ipsilateral internal mammary lymph nodes	

Distant Metastasis (M)

MX	Presence of distant metastasis cannot be assessed
M0	No distant metastasis
M1	Distant metastasis (includes metastasis to ipsilateral supraclavicular lymph nodes)

STAGE GROUPING

Stage 0	Tis	N0	M0
Stage I	T1	N0	M0
Stage IIA	T0	N1	M0
	T1	N1*	M0
	T2	N0	M0
Stage IIB	T2	N1	M0
	T3	N0	M0
Stage IIIA	T0	N2	M0
	T1	N2	M0
	T2	N2	M0
	T3	N1	M0
	T3	N2	M0
Stage IIIB	T4	Any N	M0
	Any T	N3	M0
Stage IV	Any T	Any N	M1

*Note: The prognosis of patients with N1a is similar to that of patients with pN0.

HISTOPATHOLOGIC TYPE

The histologic types are as follows:

Carcinoma, NOS (not otherwise specified)

Ductal
- Intraductal (in situ)
- Invasive with predominant intraductal component
- Invasive, NOS
- Comedo
- Inflammatory
- Medullary with lymphocytic infiltrate
- Mucinous (colloid)
- Papillary
- Scirrhous
- Tubular
- Other

Lobular
- In situ
- Invasive with predominant in situ component
- Invasive

Nipple
- Paget's disease, NOS
- Paget's disease with intraductal carcinoma
- Paget's disease with invasive ductal carcinoma
- Other
- Undifferentiated carcinoma

HISTOPATHOLOGIC GRADE (G)

GX	Grade cannot be assessed
G1	Well differentiated
G2	Moderately differentiated
G3	Poorly differentiated
G4	Undifferentiated

From American Joint Committee on Cancer. *Beahr's manual for staging of cancer,* 4th ed. Philadelphia: JB Lippincott, 1992.

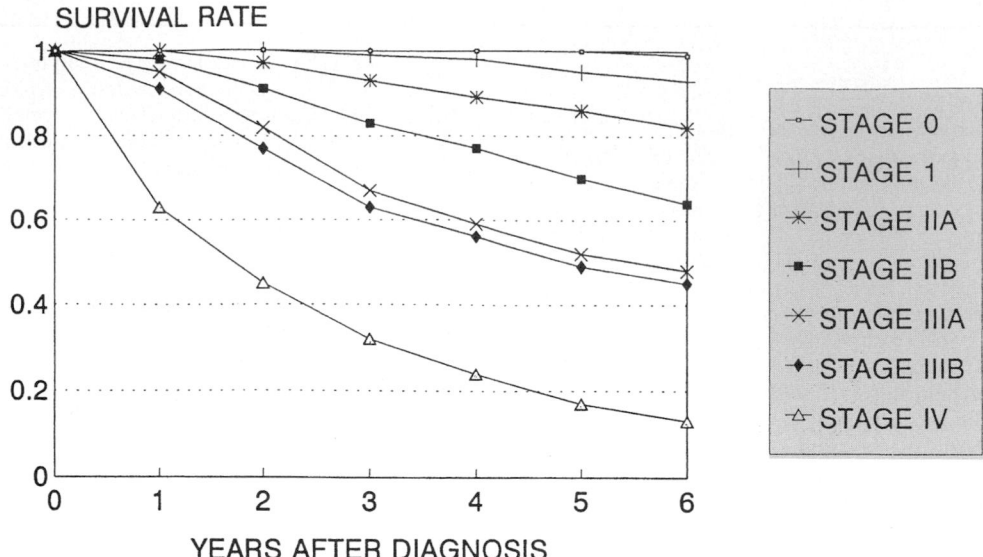

FIGURE 40.29. Relative survival rates according to stage of disease.

ductal carcinoma (IDC) is by far the most common histologic pattern of breast cancer seen, constituting 68% of cases (Fig. 40.30). Infiltrating lobular carcinoma (ILC) is the second most frequent cancer of the breast at 6.3% incidence. Other histologic subtypes include medullary carcinoma (2.8%), mucinous adenocarcinoma (2.2%), comedocarcinoma (1.4%), and Paget's disease (1.1%). Papillary carcinoma, tubular adenocarcinoma, and inflammatory carcinoma, each have an incidence of less than 1%. Inflammatory carcinoma is by far the most aggressive of the histologic types and has the poorest 5-year rate of 18%.

Terminology, however, has been confusing in that nearly three fourths of infiltrating carcinomas of the breast have been included in the imprecise category of *infiltrating ductal* or *adenocarcinoma, not otherwise specified.* Much of the terminology of breast cancer is divided

into lobular and ductal, based principally on historical perspectives. Initially, early classifications used the term *lobular* to refer to lobular carcinoma in situ and those without a lobular pattern were referred to as *ductal*, hence the term ductal has no specific meaning. In fact, the majority of breast cancers originate in the terminal duct lobular unit, but these terms have impelling familiarity and are thus the basis of much of the scientific literature. Some authors promote the histologic classification that recognized special types of mammary carcinoma defined in terms of specific histologic criteria (lobular, tubular, medullary, and mucinous carcinomas). Because of its familiarity and in order to judge against current literature, the earlier terminology is used herein.

IDC accounts for the majority of breast cancers. These lesions usually present as stony hard masses result-

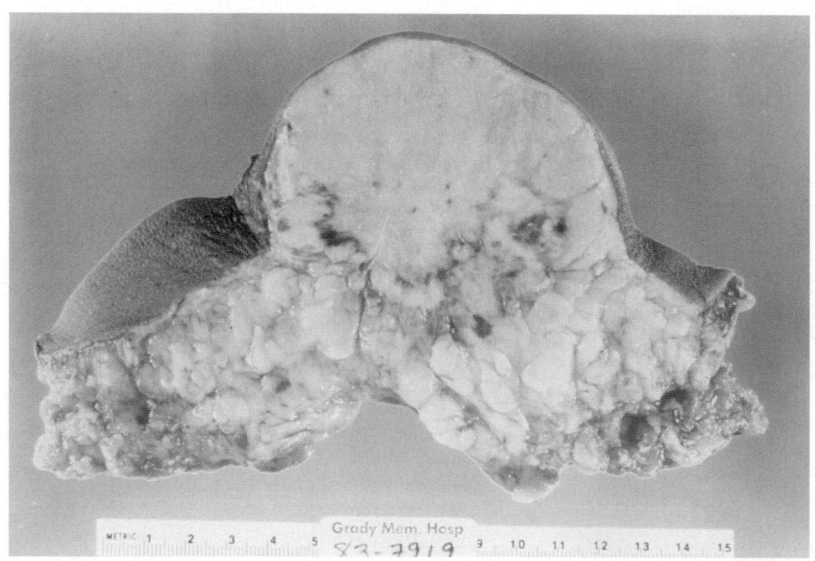

FIGURE 40.30. Invasive breast cancer. This mastectomy specimen shows a large tumor growing under the epidermis above and invading the soft tissue below. Foci of hemorrhage (*black areas*) are seen in the tumor.

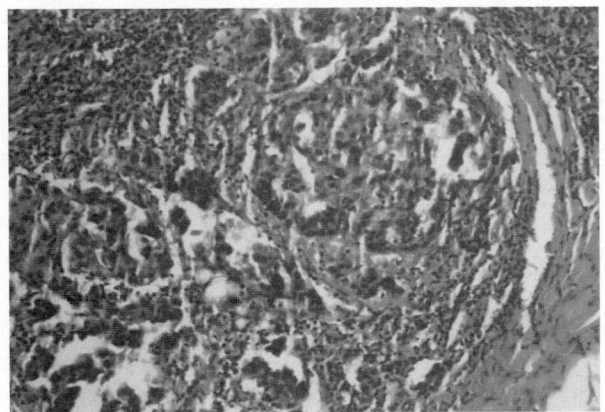

FIGURE 40.31. Histologic section of medullary carcinoma showing smooth margins, primitive malignant cells in syncytial growth surrounded by lymphoplasmacytic infiltrate (H&E ×240). (Courtesy of Taalat Tadros, M.D., Emory University, School of Medicine, Atlanta, GA.)

ing from the density of the fibrous tissue stroma. Tumors on average are approximately 2 cm and rarely exceed 4 to 5 cm. These are more often detected by mammography because of their increased frequency of calcifications compared to ILC. Additionally, this variant commonly metastasizes to the axillary lymph nodes.

Fleshy tumors are characteristic of medullary carcinoma, which can measure up to 5 to 10 cm in diameter.

The histopathologic appearance exhibits a predominance of syncytial cells, lymphocytic infiltrate, and a lack of microglandular structure (Fig. 40.31). As a group, these tumors tend to have a better prognosis than the other IDC variants.

Colloid carcinoma appears as a large, slow-growing, gelatinous mass usually found in older women. Pathologic review of the specimen reveals large lakes of mucin and isolated tumor groupings (Fig. 40.32).

Paget's disease is another form of IDC that originates in the excretory ducts of the breast. Involvement of the nipple–areolar complex may result in a firm consistency of the nipple, inflammation, ulceration, edema, and "weeping" of the skin. Characteristic Paget's cells appear in the epidermis as large anaplastic cells surrounded by a clear halo. Paget's may present solely with skin changes and the absence of an underlying mass. Thus, any nipple rash or skin changes that do not resolve with symptomatic treatment in a few weeks should be evaluated with dermatologic punch biopsy.

Finally, ILC arises from the terminal ductules of the breast and tends to be multifocal within the same breast as well as frequently bilateral. Involvement of the contralateral breast occurs in 20% of cases. Histologically, loosely, dispersed single-cell columns form strands of infiltrating tumor cells (Fig. 40.33).

In situ or noninvasive histologic variants of breast cancer also exist. Coincident with the widespread use of screening mammography, there has been a shift in the

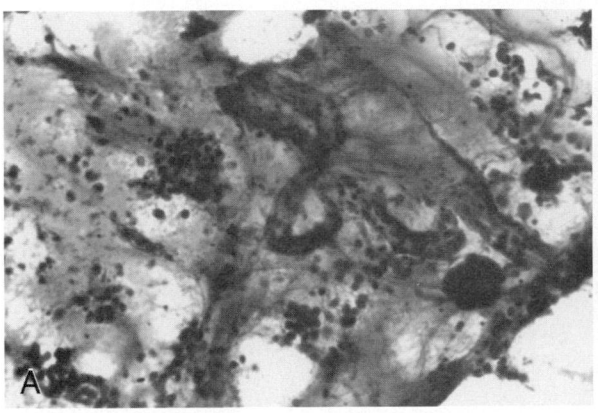

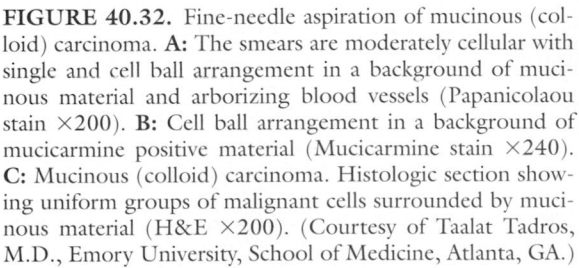

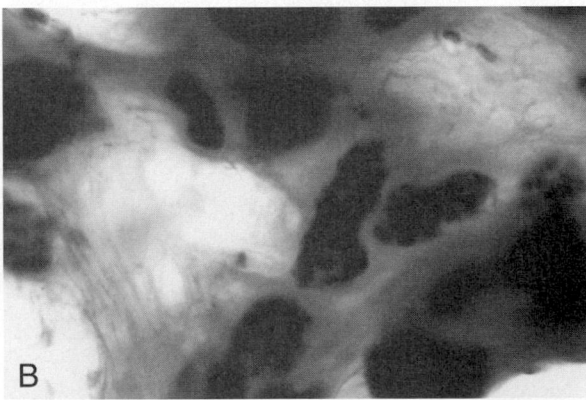

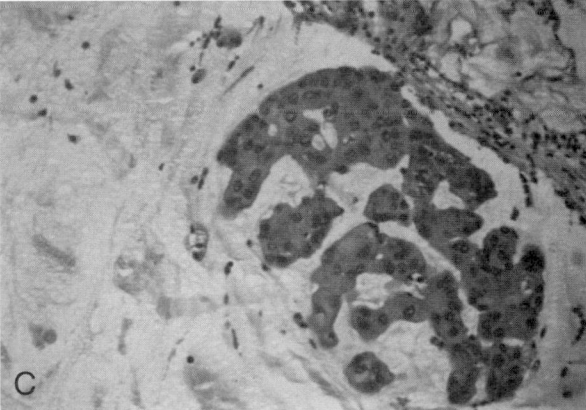

FIGURE 40.32. Fine-needle aspiration of mucinous (colloid) carcinoma. **A:** The smears are moderately cellular with single and cell ball arrangement in a background of mucinous material and arborizing blood vessels (Papanicolaou stain ×200). **B:** Cell ball arrangement in a background of mucicarmine positive material (Mucicarmine stain ×240). **C:** Mucinous (colloid) carcinoma. Histologic section showing uniform groups of malignant cells surrounded by mucinous material (H&E ×200). (Courtesy of Taalat Tadros, M.D., Emory University, School of Medicine, Atlanta, GA.)

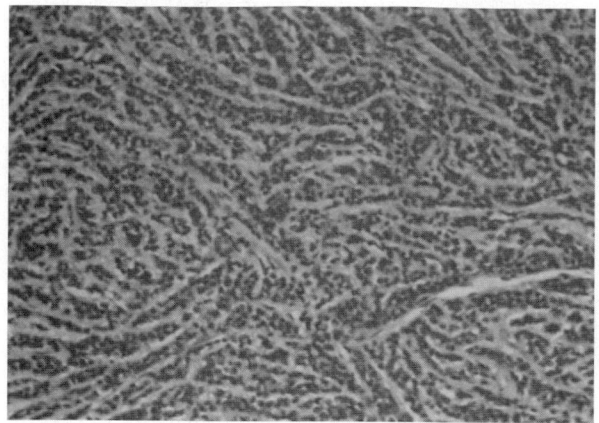

FIGURE 40.33. Histology of infiltrating lobular carcinoma, showing characteristic single small malignant cells in an Indian file pattern. Cells are diffusely infiltrating the stroma (H&E ×240). (Courtesy of Taalat Tadros, M.D., Emory University, School of Medicine, Atlanta, GA.)

stage at presentation of breast cancer toward earlier-stage disease, particularly for ductal carcinoma in situ (DCIS) (Fig. 40.34). Recent data from Surveillance, Epidemiology, and End Results shows nearly 300% change in incidence of DCIS in women age 50 years and older and greater than 100% increase in the incidence of stage I disease in the same group. The percentage of change was more pronounced in African-American women than in white women. DCIS is a nonobligatory precursor to IDC with variable rates of progression depending on histology, size, and margin status. DCIS refers to lesions with proliferation of malignant cells within the ductal system of the breast but without invasion of the stromal tissue (basement membrane). This category represents 20% of all newly diagnosed breast cancers with a 20-year survival rate of 97%. In at least 90% of patients, the diagnosis is made with mammography. Only about 10% of patients have a palpable mass. Because of the controversy as to the potential for progression of DCIS to IDC, optimal management is one of the biggest challenges in breast disease faced by clinicians. Although DCIS is a preinvasive form of breast cancer and is not life threatening, treatment options may include mastectomy, ra-

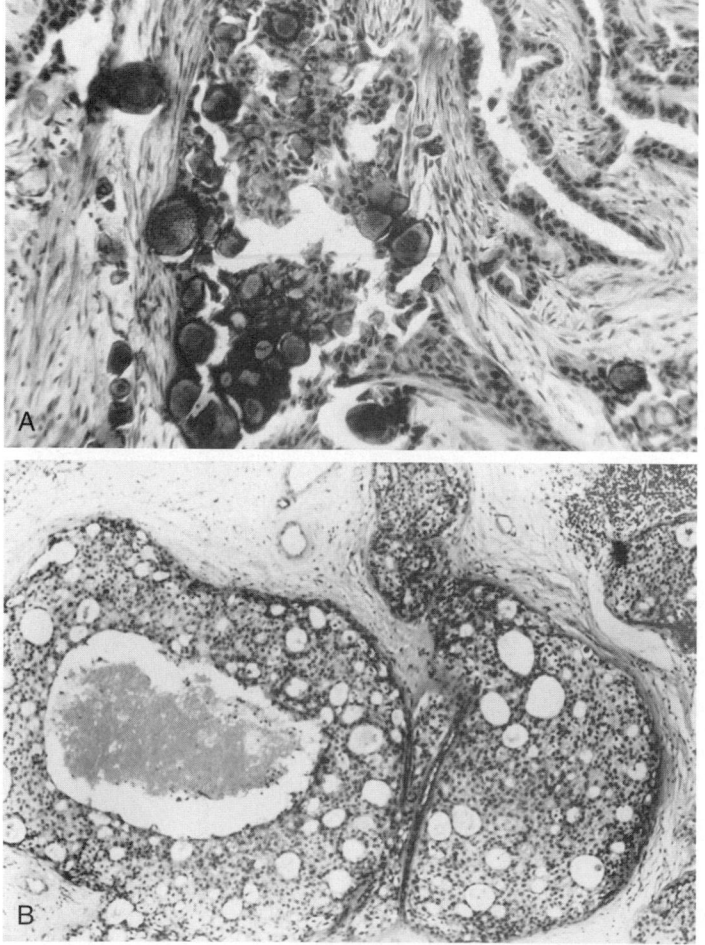

FIGURE 40.34. Ductal carcinoma in situ. **A:** A dilated duct is filled with proliferating atypical ductal cells interspersed with multiple microcalcifications. The microcalcifications were identified by mammogram. **B:** Ductal carcinoma in situ with central necrosis suggesting a comedo pattern.

diotherapy, or tamoxifen. Current treatment modalities may be overly aggressive because many cases of DCIS may not recur or progress to invasive cancer. Conservative contemporary treatments include lumpectomy with breast irradiation, excluding axillary dissection. Selected patients may be treated with only lumpectomy. Historically, multicentricity was used to justify mastectomy for DCIS. In the literature, estimates of multicentricity in DCIS range widely, from 2% to 78% depending on the definition and mode of detection. Until we are better able to identify those patients at low risk for progression, it is unlikely that current treatment will change.

Lobular carcinoma in situ (LCIS) refers to proliferation of cells within the breast lobules. LCIS is considered a predictive marker of future cancer rather than a cancer precursor. It is usually found *incidentally* by microscopy at the time of breast biopsy performed for another indication and does not present characteristic clinical or mammographic findings. It is typically multicentric and has a sevenfold to 10-fold increased risk of subsequent invasive breast cancer, which is typically ductal carcinoma. Studies of women with LCIS managed with biopsy alone demonstrate a risk of cancer development of approximately 1% per year.

Breast cancer may present with a firm consistency, fixed position (lack of mobility), dimpling or retraction of the overlying skin, nipple retraction, and irregular shape. Peau d'orange skin changes are associated with obstruction of the lymphatics and associated edema. This characteristic feature is not always associated with breast cancer and may be seen with mastitis. IDC frequently metastasizes to bone, lung, liver or brain, whereas ILC more often metastasizes to meningeal serosal surfaces. On the other hand, inflammatory cancer causes extensive swelling, redness, and tenderness, which is often mistaken for a hematoma or abscess.

In general, breast cancer is slightly more common in the left breast than in the right. In most women, the left breast is slightly larger than the right. The upper outer quadrant is more frequently involved in malignant changes (this is the site of the highest distribution of breast tissue), with the central and subareolar regions being second.

TREATMENT

Surgical Techniques

The first recorded operative treatment for breast cancer was in the Greco-Roman period 220 BC by a Greek physician names Leonides. A century ago, William Halsted published his first paper on the radical mastectomy for the control of breast cancer. This procedure was very extensive, including removal of the breast tissue en bloc, pectoralis muscles, and axillary lymph nodes to achieve superior local and regional control of disease in that day. Since the 1970s, the trend in surgery for breast cancer has been to employ more limited procedures. Taking into account the medical circumstances and the patient's preferences, treatment may involve lumpec-

tomy (local removal of the tumor) and removal of the lymph nodes under the arm, mastectomy (surgical removal of the breast) and removal of the lymph nodes under the arm, radiation therapy, chemotherapy, or hormone therapy. Currently, long-term updates of original prospective clinical trials have confirmed that BCS, which includes lumpectomy, axillary node dissection, and postoperative radiation therapy, is the appropriate primary therapy for most women with stage I and II breast cancer. The largest of the BCS trials, National Surgical Adjuvant Breast Project (NSABP) B-06, reviewed women over 15 years and proved the equivalence of the treatments. Other studies have shown congruent results demonstrating no statistically significant differences between rates of local and regional recurrences, distant metastasis, and overall survival between mastectomy and BCS. Tumor recurrence is 40% with BCS but decreased to 10% with the addition of radiation therapy, which is similar to treatment with modified radical mastectomy. Accordingly, the 1992 NIH Consensus Development Conference reported that "breast conservation treatment is an appropriate method of primary therapy for the majority of women with stage I and II breast cancer and is preferable because it provides survival equivalent to total mastectomy and axillary dissection while preserving the breast." However, the procedure remains underused, with studies indicating only 56% of women receiving the BCS compared to the modified mastectomy in some institutions. The appropriate candidate for mastectomy is primarily the patient in whom it is evident that BCS will not control the primary tumor. Cosmetic factors are important, but the primary concern is adequate removal of the primary tumor with pathologically negative margins. One other concern with respect to BCS is the necessity for radiation therapy and continued intense surveillance. For this reason, patients with certain medical conditions such as active or preexisting collagen vascular disease are not candidates for BCS, because these patients have been shown to have poor tolerance to radiation in the breast and chest wall areas (Tables 40.10 and 40.11). Axillary dissection continues to assume a position of diminishing importance in the treatment of breast carcinoma but remains controversial. As the role for systemic therapy even in patients with negative nodes expands, some investigators have stated that not all patients require an axillary dissection, but 30% of patients with no palpable lymph nodes (clinically negative axilla)

TABLE 40.10.
Absolute Contraindications to BCS

Pregnancy: first and second trimester
History of previous irradiation to the breast region
Multicentric Lesions
Diffuse, indeterminate or malignant-appearing microcalcifications
Patient's clear preference for mastectomy

TABLE 40.11.
Relative Contraindications to BCS

Large tumor/breast ratio (cosmetic result)
Large breast size (difficult to radiate)
Tumor location beneath the nipple
History of collagen vascular disease

have been found to have histologically positive lymph nodes. Because axillary nodal status is the best established indicator of their risk for systemic relapse, the potential of sentinel lymph node evaluation is evident.

The timing of surgery in relation to the menstrual cycle is a novel venue to understanding breast cancer biology. The effect of timing surgery during the menstrual cycle on breast cancer mortality has been debated since the first report by Hrushesky and colleagues in 1989. Recent metaanalysis of published data suggests a reduction in breast cancer mortality of 15% when breast cancer surgery is performed in the luteal phase of the menstrual cycle. There are two distinct postulates proposed to explain this phenomenon: (1) either the hormonal milieu in the host modulates the metastatic potential of breast cancer or (2) the events at the time of surgery can influence survival. It is well established that estrogen remains unopposed during the follicular phase of the menstrual cycle and is postulated to be the cause of the discrepancy in survival.

For patients with negative axillary involvement, the tumor size and histologic grade are the most useful prognostic factors. Among patients with invasive tumors of less than 1 cm in greatest diameter, the 5-year disease-free survival rate is more than 90%. Expression of the estrogen receptor or the progesterone receptor is associated with a better prognosis, primarily attributable to the responsiveness of these tumors to tamoxifen. The role of HER2/neu as a prognostic factor remains controversial. HER2 amplification has been associated with a poor prognosis primarily among patients with positive nodes. However, retrospective studies of node-negative patients have yielded conflicting results. A recent prospective study report showed a negative impact on disease-free survival for node-negative patients with overexpression of HER2. The role of HER2 as a predictor of response to chemotherapy is discussed in the section on Tumor-Specific Therapies.

Adjuvant Therapy

The role for adjuvant therapy is well accepted for most patients with early stage breast cancer. Recommendations for use of adjuvant systemic therapy for the treatment of patients with primary breast cancer were promulgated by the Sixth International Conference on Adjuvant Therapy of Primary Breast Cancer in 1998. This report recommends consideration of adjuvant chemotherapy regardless of age, menopausal status,

lymph node involvement, or hormone receptor status. The most frequently used chemotherapy regimens include CMF (cyclophosphamide, methotrexate, 5-fluorouracil); AC; FAC, fluorouracil, epirubicin (not available in the United States), tamoxifen, and cyclophosphamide. Omitting cyclophosphamide obviates the long-term risk for acute leukemia and substantially reduces the severity of alopecia and myelosuppression, thus it is a better tolerated regimen. Fifty percent to 80% of women have an objective response to FAC, and 40% to 60% have an objective response to CMF. Regimens containing anthracyclines (doxorubicin or epirubicin) were superior to CMF in the Early Breast Cancer Trialists' Collaborative Group overview. These chemotherapy regimens may cause short-term complications, including nausea, vomiting, myelosuppression, alopecia, and weight gain. Use of anthracycline-based chemotherapy has the long-term risks of cardiac dysfunction, premature menopause, and secondary malignancies. The risk of chemotherapy-induced ovarian ablation is approximately 70%, but is less common among women younger than 35 years of age and more common among women older than 45 years of age. Node-positive patients may benefit from the addition of paclitaxel to the AC regimen; therefore, until other studies are analyzed, treating node-positive patients with four cycles of AC (or CAF) followed by four cycles of paclitaxel is reasonable. In addition to chemotherapy, because estrogen receptor–positive tumors respond better to hormonal therapy (e.g., tamoxifen) than estrogen receptor–negative tumors, patients with estrogen receptive–positive tumors should receive tamoxifen for 5 years, regardless of age or menopausal status.

For postmenopausal patients with nodal involvement, tamoxifen is the standard adjuvant therapy.

Adjuvant therapy has also been proven to have added benefit for node-negative patients with breast cancer. Zambetti and colleagues found adjuvant chemotherapy increases disease-free survival in 85% of patients compared with 42% of untreated control subjects. Similar values have been verified in other studies. The goal is to determine which node-negative patients are at high risk for recurrence to avoid further unnecessary treatment in patients already cured of their disease. Several prognostic factors are currently used to predict recurrent disease, including the number of involved lymph nodes, tumor diameter, and receptor status. Other less well established prognosticators include S-phase fraction (an indicator of proliferative capacity), HER2/neu overexpression, histology, nuclear grade, and DNA aneuploidy. Thus, node-negative women with moderately or poorly differentiated invasive tumors of larger than 1 cm and negative hormone receptors should be offered chemotherapy. Because the risk for node-negative patients with well-differentiated tumors of less than 1 cm in size is 10% or less, adjuvant chemotherapy is not recommended. In addition to chemotherapy, patients who are premenopausal (or younger than 50 years of age) with negative nodes and estrogen receptor–positive tumors should be considered for a 5-year course of tamoxifen because even in node-negative patients, 30% of patients have a relapse in 5 years. The treatment of postmenopausal patients with negative nodes and hormone receptor–positive tumors is evolving. Randomized clinical trials showed that chemotherapy plus tamoxifen yields better survival rates than tamoxifen alone, but the absolute benefit is small and the use of chemotherapy in this setting should be individualized. However, the consensus panel recommends hormonal therapy as the treatment of choice for estrogen receptor–positive women with limited disease regardless of menopausal status, tumor size, or axillary involvement, especially for patients who are asymptomatic or are of advanced age. Hormone receptor status determines the likelihood that a patient will respond to hormonal therapy, with 75% to 80% of patients with estrogen receptor/progesterone receptor–positive tumors showing an objective response. Even patients with estrogen receptor/progesterone receptor–negative tumors had a 10% objective response rate. An assay for progesterone and estrogen receptors is important in all malignant specimens. One gram of tissue is necessary for the assay. Care must be taken to avoid heat and tissue ischemia, which will invalidate the assay. Therefore, patients with asymptomatic metastatic disease or progressive disease after receiving first- and second-line cytotoxic chemotherapy may still benefit from endocrine therapy.

The role of radiation therapy in breast cancer treatment has been more clearly defined in the last 2 decades. Radiation therapy is applied to DCIS, early stage invasive disease, locally advanced breast cancer, and as postmastectomy therapy. Because of the general acceptance of BCS (which is usually followed by radiation), radiation therapy has become an integral part of the treatment of early stage breast cancer. Whether radiation therapy is required for every patient with invasive breast cancer after BCS is still unresolved. Women who have undergone mastectomy and who have four or more positive lymph nodes or an advanced primary tumor benefit from postsurgical radiation. Radiotherapy should begin as soon as the wounds of surgery are healed. It is generally agreed that the breast should be treated with 180 to 200 cGy/day for 4.5 to 5.5 weeks for a total of 4,500 to 5,000 cGy. This is usually followed by a supplemental boost of 1,000 to 1,600 cGy, although this is also controversial. A total dose in excess of 5,000 cGy results in fibrosis, retraction, and an unacceptable cosmetic result.

Radiation is also useful in the palliative treatment of bone pain in advanced metastatic disease. Complications of radiation therapy include fatigue, development of dry skin, erythema or tanning, edema, and muscle stiffness within the tissues encompassed by the radiation beam. After completion of the irradiation treatment, most patients recover their normal skin color and texture within a few weeks. Edema can take much longer to resolve, especially in a large breast. Late complications from radiotherapy are unusual, including a very low incidence of rib fracture, radiation pneumonitis, brachyplexopathy, and pericarditis in cases of left-sided lesions. In the overwhelming majority of cases, a return to normal is the rule.

Ovarian ablation has been shown to reduce the risk of tumor recurrence and death in women younger than 50 years of age, at least in the absence of adjuvant chemotherapy. The combination of oophorectomy and chemotherapy was as effective as either treatment alone in premenopausal women, but the invasive nature of surgical feminine castration has limited its use in the United States. In addition, tamoxifen is effective in premenopausal women, and no randomized trial has shown the superiority of oophorectomy over tamoxifen.

Luteinizing hormone-releasing hormone analogs are an alternative to oophorectomy. These agents induce a "chemical castration" and are effective for premenopausal patients with metastatic breast cancer. Interest in the integration of the luteinizing hormone-releasing hormone agonist goserelin and leuprolide in the adjuvant setting is increasing, and large randomized trials are underway.

In the United States, primary breast cancer is the most common indication for high-dose chemotherapy (HDCT) with autologous peripheral blood (or bone marrow) stem cell transplantation (also called autologous bone marrow transplantation). With this technique, higher doses of chemotherapeutic agents are given, which has been shown to enhance cytotoxic effects, shorten the necessary duration of exposure to the chemotherapy, and decrease the development of tumor cell resistance. Some studies have shown a positive response in women with 10 or more positive lymph nodes or with recurrent or metastatic disease; however, the superiority of HDCT over full doses of standard chemotherapy has not been established. Nor have benefits been noted when HDCT follows conventional dose chemotherapy in women with complete or partial remission. Furthermore, this treatment requires extensive hospitalization and is accompanied by a mortality rate of 15% to 20%. Research in this area continues.

Sentinel Lymph Node Biopsy

Treatment of the axilla is an integral part of the management of patients with invasive breast cancer. In general, the standard treatment of the axilla involves level I and level II axillary lymph node dissection (ALND). Currently, there is no evidence that ALND improves survival, thus diminishing its importance, although the issue remains controversial. ALND, however, is an effective staging procedure and is essential for local control of disease in the axilla. The status of axillary nodes is one of the most well-established prognostic indicators for systemic relapse used to select patient subgroups for adjuvant chemotherapy. Patients with involvement of the lymph nodes have a 60% to 70% risk for relapse within 5 years, whereas 70% to 80% of patients with negative nodes are cured by local therapy.

The current standard of care for surgical management of invasive disease is complete excision of the tumor by either mastectomy or lumpectomy followed by ALND. It has been established that in melanoma, the first lymph node (the sentinel node) to receive drainage from the primary tumor can be used to predict the presence or absence of tumor in the remainder of the lymph nodes. Published and unpublished results in breast carcinoma surgery appear to support the same concept for axillary node breast metastases. Intraoperative lymphatic mapping and sentinel lymph node biopsy (SLNB) has emerged as a potential alternative to routine ALND in clinically node-negative early breast cancer and represents a major new opportunity obviating the need for more invasive surgical management of many tumors. Lymphatic mapping with selective lymphadenectomy is an attractive approach in breast cancer patients because it may lead to a substantial reduction in the need for axillary node dissection without compromising survival and regional control and without loss of prognostic staging information, thus translating into a significant reduction in patient morbidity and medical expenses. SLNB is highly accurate and sensitive in patients with small tumors, and no false-negative SLNB has been reported for a breast cancer smaller than 1.0 to 1.5 cm, resulting in a negative predictive value of 100%. In the future, axillary dissection might be avoided in patients who have no metastatic involvement of the SLN; however, the efficacy of SLNB in the setting of randomized, prospective trials must be tested first before abandoning ALND as the standard of care.

This procedure requires a concerted multidisciplinary approach encompassing the efforts of the nuclear radiologist, surgeon, and pathologist. It uses existing technology to exploit logical anatomic physiologic principles to identify occult regional lymph node metastases. The lymphatic flow is visualized and the first (sentinel) lymph node on a direct drainage pathway from the primary tumor is identified. This is the node at greatest risk of harboring metastatic deposits. Lymphoscintigraphy can indicate the number of sentinel nodes and their location.

The surgeon can use two techniques to find the node. Intraoperative SLN mapping is performed using a blue dye injected peritumorally, which stains the lymphatic duct (Fig. 40.35). This method was pioneered by Giuliano and associates. After 5 minutes, blue dye can be visualized traversing afferent lymphatics and collecting in an SLN through an axillary incision at the tumor site. There is a 93.5% success rate in identifying an axillary node as the sentinel node. The false-negative rate has been 0%. The main problems associated with the blue dye approach are the increased amount of dissection and tissue disruption required and the inability to localize possible sentinel nodes in the internal mammary or other nodal chain. Alternatively, a lymph node–seeking radioactive tracer (^{99m} Tc) migrates from the tumor site (when injected into the breast parenchyma) to the sentinel node and enables its retrieval with the use of a gamma detection probe. The drawbacks of this technique include a substantial learning curve, "shine-through" from the zone of diffusion around the injection site confusing and obscuring the activity in the

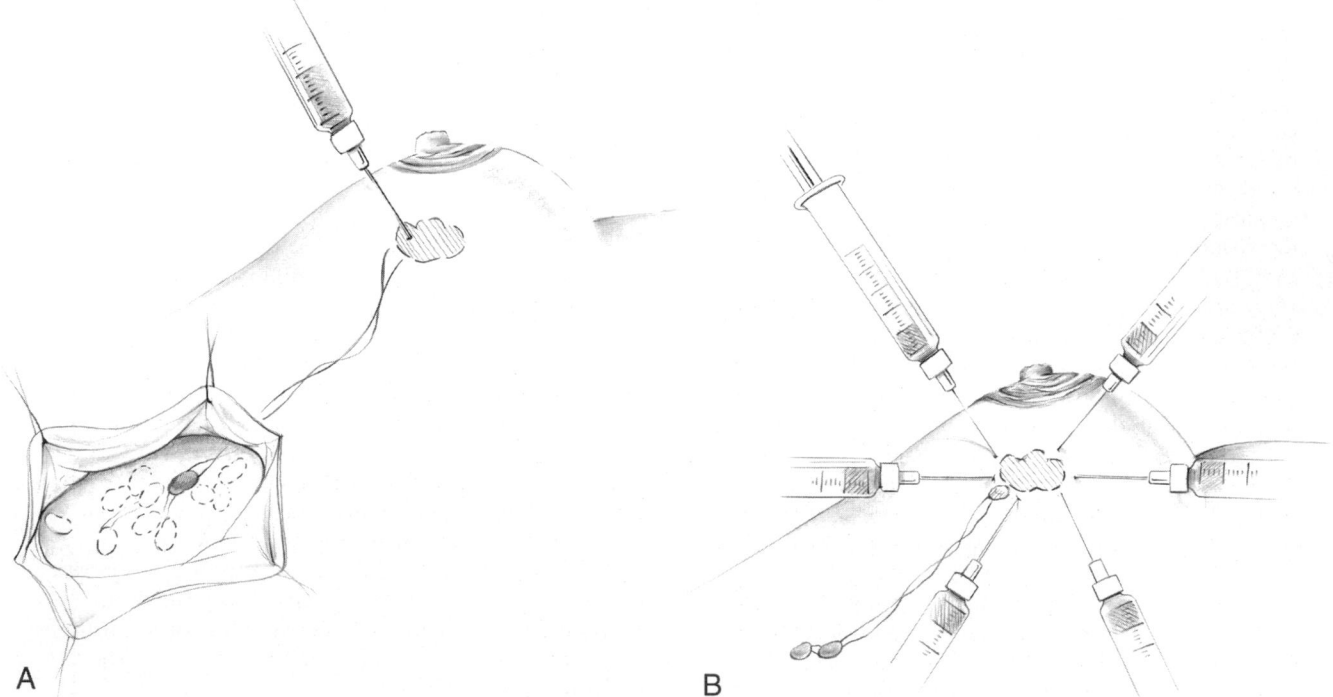

A   B

FIGURE 40.35. Sentinel lymph node mapping. A: Schematic diagram depicting the transit of blue dye, injected into the primary breast cancer, to the sentinel lymph node. B: Injection technique for lymphatic mapping and sentinel lymphadenectomy showing peritumoral injection. For a palpable lesion, dye is injected into the breast parenchyma around the tumor. If the tumor has previously been removed, dye is injected into the wall of the biopsy cavity.

axilla, and technical failure in 10% to 15% of cases. Blue dye and lymphoscintigraphy are complementary techniques, and optimal localization is achieved when the two methods are used together. Several authors have achieved greater than 95% success rate and quote a sensitivity of 98% when the procedures are used complementarily. The pathologist uses a number of techniques to identify tumor deposits in a lymph node, including serial sectioning and immunohistochemical techniques.

Other variations of the procedure have been espoused, including the addition of ultrasound to the protocol. Ultrasound locates the lymph node that has been identified through a radioactive tracer and located with the gamma camera. With the use of ultrasound, a localization wire can be placed, allowing easier access and less operative time for surgical dissection to the lymph node. Additionally, endoscopic axillary clearance after liposuction was promoted due to improved visualization and less traumatic surgery. Unfortunately this method is time-consuming, expensive, and shows no obvious advantage compared to the open SLNB. Until data regarding the long-term results of SLNB are available, these methods should be considered investigational.

Selective Estrogen Receptor Modulators

Selective estrogen receptor modulators (SERMs) were first evaluated in the 1960s as nonsteroidal antiestrogens. This group of drugs showed potent antifertility activity in rats, but paradoxically proved to be an inducer of ovulation in subfertile women. Clomiphene remains a vital part of the regimen for ovulation induction. Further study was commenced based on the compound's multifaceted actions on different types of receptors. Ancillary studies in this group of drugs focused upon treatments for advanced breast cancer; however, only tamoxifen was investigated further due to its high potency, efficacy, and modest side effects.

The strategic application of these medications was first noted in long-term adjuvant therapy for node-positive and node-negative, estrogen receptor–positive breast cancers. Additional benefits of tamoxifen treatment were later discovered in the laboratory followed by further elucidation in clinical studies into the prevention of bone loss. Tamoxifen is proven to exhibit selective estrogenic properties by conferring an overall lipid profile benefit and stabilization of bone mineral loss but with antiestrogenic actions in the breast. Tamoxifen decreases the serum levels of total cholesterol by 13% and those of low-density lipoprotein cholesterol by 19%. Therefore, tamoxifen has the added benefit of maintaining bone density and reducing the risk of myocardial infarction in postmenopausal women.

Tamoxifen citrate has been shown to be of immense significance in the battle against breast cancer. Tamoxifen has demonstrated benefit when used alone or in combination with chemotherapy in the treatment of advanced breast cancer and has proven efficacy in reducing tumor recurrence, prolonging disease-free survival, and lowering the incidence of contralateral breast cancer by 40% when administered as postoperative adjuvant therapy in stages I and II disease. The 1998 landmark report of the NSABP indicated tamoxifen (20 mg/day) reduced the risk of invasive breast cancer by 49% when used prophylactically in women 60 years of age and older, age 35 to 59 with a 5-year predicted risk for breast cancer of at least 1.66% by the Gail model algorithm or women with a history of lobular carcinoma in situ. Similar protection has also been shown in women with one, two, or even three first-degree relatives with breast cancer and in the subset of women with a 5 year predicted breast cancer risk greater than 5%. Tamoxifen administration in this randomized trial also reduced the risk of fractures; however, it did not alter the rate of ischemic heart disease. Tamoxifen has several side effects including development of menopausal vasomotor symptoms, a modest increase in the detection of endometrial cancer (risk ratio = 2.53), cataract formation, pulmonary embolism, stroke, and deep vein thrombosis. Recent studies also demonstrate that tamoxifen is a carcinogen in rat liver. Evaluation of these data by the International Agency for Research on Cancer resulted in classification of tamoxifen as a carcinogen; however, authors emphatically indicate that women should not discontinue therapy with tamoxifen based on concerns about endometrial cancer because the benefits outweigh its risks.

However, studies testing tamoxifen for primary prevention of breast cancer have not been as encouraging. Of note, two recently published reports of the European Breast Cancer Prevention Trials showed no significant reduction in breast cancer incidence with the tamoxifen. Several factors may account for the discrepancy, including dissimilar inclusion criteria, the length of treatment, and the length of follow-up. Nonetheless, these contradictory results have fueled controversy that may slow the use of tamoxifen for chemoprevention of breast cancer.

Raloxifene hydrochloride is a selective estrogen receptor modulator that has antiestrogenic effects on breast and endometrial tissue and estrogenic effects on bone, lipid metabolism, and blood clotting. This compound was first investigated for the prevention of osteoporosis, but beneficial "side effects" were seen in the prevention of breast and endometrial cancer. Raloxifene is approved for the prevention of osteoporosis because it increases bone mineral density in the spine and femoral neck and reduces risk of vertebral fracture. However, clinical experience with raloxifene in cancer management is insufficient to support its use for breast cancer treatment.

To date, the benefits of raloxifene make further study into this multifaceted agent compelling. Raloxifene binds to estrogen receptors to competitively block estrogen-induced DNA transcription in the breast and endometrium. SERMS have differing estrogenic activities due to individual structural deviations from 17β-estradiol. Studies indicate raloxifene preserves skeletal bone loss, confers a beneficial lipid profile, and does not lead to uterine bleeding or mastodynia, nor does it increase the risk of endometrial carcinoma. It has a convenient once-daily dosage and does not increase the risk of breast carcinoma. However, it predisposes women to deep vein thrombosis and leg cramps, and it has no effect on menopausal vasomotor symptoms.

Because of its absence of stimulation of the endometrium and breast, raloxifene is particularly attractive for prevention of osteoporosis in women with uteri in whom mastodynia, headaches, or dysphoric moods develop on HRT. Its most compelling use is in the treatment of women with benign but persistent bleeding on HRT, as well as in those at high risk for recurrent endometriosis or breast cancer on HRT. Because it has no effect on hot flashes or vaginal atrophy, it is not the method of choice for women with these as their primary symptoms.

Because more cases of breast cancer occur in women who are not at "increased" risk over the general population, prevention strategies focus on reduction of breast cancer in women at low to average risk for the disease. Results from the multicenter, randomized, double-blind Multiple Outcomes of Raloxifene Evaluation (MORE) trial revealed a 76% decreased risk of breast cancer among postmenopausal women with osteoporosis during 3 years of treatment with raloxifene; however, no objective tumor response was noted in patients with metastatic breast cancer in a phase II clinical trial. The Study of Tamoxifen and Raloxifene (STAR) trial is also underway and has enrolled 6,139 postmenopausal women at increased risk for breast cancer in the first year. The study is designed to determine whether raloxifene is as effective as tamoxifen in reducing breast cancer risk. In a one-to-one comparison, raloxifene (60 mg/day) appeared to effect about 50% of the change on bone turnover markers and bone density compared with 0.625 mg conjugated estrogens.

Several new SERMs are under investigation. Toremifene has shown efficacy similar to tamoxifen and may be a reasonable first-line alternative. Because of substantial cross-resistance between toremifene and tamoxifen, there is no role in patients who have tumors resistant to tamoxifen. Droloxifene and idoxifene have had minimal evaluation but show binding affinity to estrogen receptor–positive breast cancers and response rates of 0% to 70%.

Tumor-Specific Therapies

New, innovative treatment strategies are clearly needed to improve outcomes in breast cancer. Overexpression of HER2/neu in primary breast carcinomas induces cell transformation and has been shown to correlate with unfavorable tumor biology and a significantly worse clinical prognosis for patients with breast cancer. Amplification or overexpression of this protein is noted in 10% to 40% of human breast tumors and in 9% to 32% of ovarian cancer cases. In breast cancer patients, overexpression is linked to patient responsiveness or resistance to tamoxifen and chemotherapeutic regimens. In fact, overexpression of this gene product predicts *resistance* to tamoxifen therapy. Transtuzumab (Herceptin) is an FDA-approved monoclonal immunoglobulin G1 antibody with high affinity for the HER2/neu receptor.

Herceptin significantly inhibits the growth of breast tumors with high levels of the HER2 protein when administered alone or in combination with paclitaxel or carboplatin and has been shown to improve the overall response in women with metastatic breast cancer. Currently, Herceptin prolongs survival in metastatic breast cancer patients whose tumors overexpress the HER2/neu protein. Its effect on ovarian cancer is investigational at present. HER2/neu amplifications and Herceptin receptor response have the ability to predict disease outcome and therapy response in patients with breast cancer and have a potential to become a new modality for breast cancer treatment.

Herceptin has few additional side effects, apart from cardiac toxicity in patients concurrently receiving anthracyclines. It is thus reasonable for Herceptin to become a treatment option in metastatic breast cancer. Several institutions routinely incorporate HER2/neu status testing into the assessment of all patients with invasive breast disease. A number of approaches are being investigated as possible therapeutic strategies targeting HER2, including growth inhibitory antibodies, which can be used alone or in combination with standard chemotherapeutics; receptor inhibitors, developed to block receptor activity because phosphorylation is the key event leading to activation and initiation of the signaling pathway; and active immunotherapy, because the HER2 oncoprotein is immunogenic in some breast carcinoma patients.

Follow-up

Patients who have received definitive treatment for breast cancer have a 16% risk at 3 years of developing a second *primary* site of cancer including the contralateral breast, ovaries, endometrium, and large intestine. The risk of recurrent disease in the contralateral breast is estimated at 30% for patients with in situ carcinoma and 5% to 10% with invasive cancer. Follow-up visits should not only assess the patient's risk of additional disease but also respond to the patient's emotional needs. Some authors propose interval visits scheduled by the patient only when symptoms develop, because early detection of metastatic disease in the asymptomatic state does not improve disease-free or overall survival. Others, reviewing the psychosocial components of the visits, recommend scheduled visits.

Scheduled visits should occur every 3 months for 1 year then every 6 months thereafter in patients with previous mastectomy. Those with initial advanced disease should have regularly scheduled visits at 3-month intervals for their lifetime. BCS patients necessitate visits at an increased frequency for an extended period because early detection of recurrences may result in cure. Several regimens are proposed but all have basic similarities: visits at 3-month intervals for 1 year, every 6 months for 5 years, then annually with annual mammogram, chest radiograph, and alkaline phosphatase measurement. Most surgeons continue to recommend yearly complete blood counts and chemistry panels as well as chest radiograph, despite evidence of specificity in detection of metastatic disease. One series indicated less than 18% specificity for routine testing. Bone and liver scans are recommended only for symptomatic patients, in that no survival advantage is conferred by detecting asymptomatic disease. Others recommend visits every 3 months for 3 to 5 years, then every 6 months thereafter for patients with more advanced disease.

A review of systems should include frequent sites of recurrence such as nodal disease, lung, bone, liver, adrenal gland, and ovary. A focused history should include information on weight loss, local or distant skin changes (radiation effects or breast skin changes—ipsilateral and contralateral), mental status changes, headache or sensory deficits, pleuritic chest pain, shortness of breath, bone pain, changes in bowel function and melena or blood in the stools, and abnormal rectal or vaginal secretions. Physical examination should incorporate an evaluation of the remaining breast tissue and lymph node bearing areas, range of motion of the upper extremity, and increasing girth, which may indicate onset of lymphedema or axillary recurrence. Examinations of the chest and abdomen are performed to search for evidence of pleural effusions or hepatomegaly. Routine Papanicolaou smear, stool guaiac, and pelvic and rectovaginal examinations are also performed.

Estrogen Replacement in Breast Cancer Survivors

As more breast cancers are detected at an earlier stage, resulting in increased survival, there is a wealth of attention directed toward use of HRT in breast cancer survivors. There are no prospective trials providing conclusive evidence of a favorable risk-benefit ratio for estrogen use among breast cancer survivors. Authors have addressed the theoretical concerns of its use in patients through examinations of related studies. The possibility that a high estrogen environment might cause reemergence of neoplastic growth has been dispelled in studies of breast cancer survivors who subsequently chose to become pregnant. They found that pregnancy did not impact overall survival; in fact, in some reports, patients with breast cancer who became pregnant seemed to survive longer than patients who did not become pregnant. Furthermore, no consistent link has been noted between induced or spontaneous pregnancy termination and the development or outcome in breast cancer. Certainly, there is no consensus within the scientific literature to support withholding HRT for these cancer survivors.

Most authors recommend use of HRT for menopausal women who are disease-free and have symptomatic estrogen deficiency, especially after the first 2 years when the risk of recurrence is decreased. Furthermore, patients with localized node-negative breast cancers who are at low risk for recurrent disease may be excellent candidates for long-term replacement. ACOG recommends HRT use with a treatment plan that includes dietary control, exercise, smoking cessation, reduction of alcohol consumption, and weight reduction when appropri-

ate. Women with unexplained vaginal bleeding, acute vascular thrombosis, or significant liver function impairment would remain ineligible for use. All women should be carefully and completely counseled regarding the potential, albeit unproven, risks of disease recurrence balanced with the proven long-term benefits of HRT.

The Role of Lifestyle Modification, Tamoxifen Prophylaxis, and Prophylactic Surgery for Women with Predisposition to Cancer

Risk reduction in women at greatly increased risk for breast cancer because of hereditary mutations remains a dilemma. For this group, three management options are generally considered: cancer surveillance, prophylactic surgery (mastectomy or oophorectomy), and chemoprevention. In a consensus statement by the Cancer Genetics Study Consortium (CGSC), it is recommended that carriers of BRCA mutations have vigilant surveillance through monthly self-examination beginning in early adulthood (18 to 21 years), annual or semiannual CBE, and annual mammography starting at age 25 to 30 years.

Recommended breast cancer surveillance guidelines from ASCO include a thorough history and physical examination every 3 to 6 months for 3 years, followed by every 6 to 12 months for 2 years, then the patient may return to an annual schedule for examination. The CBE and BSE schedule is similar to that of CGSC. A routine pelvic examination should be performed annually. ASCO does not recommend routine chest radiograph, CT, or blood studies (alkaline phosphatase, complete blood count) although several institutional policies may include these routinely.

Even though self-examinations are free and of no real risk other than inducing anxiety, evidence to support its use is limited. A study from Shanghai of more than 250,000 women, who were randomized to no instruction or to intensive BSE instruction, failed to demonstrate any difference in the number of cancers detected or in the stage or size at which they were found. No reduction in mortality was seen, but more than twice as many benign lesions were found in the self-examination group.

The benefit of close follow-up alone for women at increased risk of breast cancer seems questionable from recent NSABP Study P-1 data, wherein, despite the close follow-up mandated by the trial, fully 25% of the cancers found were greater than 2 cm in diameter and 29% were node positive. Thus, it is not clear whether close clinical and yearly mammographic follow-up of women with a BRCA1 and BRCA2 mutation will reduce mortality from breast cancer.

Although the 1994 NIH Consensus Development Conference concluded that "there is no evidence available as yet that the current screening modalities of CA125 and transvaginal ultrasonography can be effectively used for widespread disease screening," these currently available screening tests may be applicable to patients at risk for hereditary ovarian cancer syndromes with appropriate counseling.

Although heredity may be the strongest risk for development of breast and ovarian cancer syndromes, reproductive risk factors may be modifiable. As with unaffected individuals, early age of first live birth and increased parity appear to lower the risk of breast cancer development. Use of fertility drugs and ovulation induction may need to be reevaluated. OCP use appears to increase the risk of breast cancer but decreases the risk of ovarian cancer. Modification of diet, alcohol consumption, exercise, or lactation are unlikely to have profound alterations on genetically determined breast cancer risk. There are few prospective, randomized, controlled studies that directly address breast cancer risk modification in women with hereditary breast cancer syndromes.

Prophylactic oophorectomy and mastectomy are attempts to remove at-risk healthy tissue before the onset of cancer. However, neither approach removes all the risk. Furthermore, there are undoubtedly modifying genes and environmental factors that play a role in the onset of carcinogenesis, but for BRCA1 and BRCA2 mutation carriers these remain unknown. Preliminary analysis of case control data from women with a BRCA mutation revealed a 64% reduction in breast cancer and 90% reduction in ovarian cancer risk with prophylactic oophorectomy, especially when performed at an early age. Delaying oophorectomy until age 40 years had minimal effect on the magnitude of risk reduction, suggesting that delaying surgery until after the completion of childbearing is a reasonable approach. At present, it can be stated that either tamoxifen or oophorectomy are valid options that may reduce the risk of breast cancer for women harboring BRCA1 or BRCA2 mutations. The costs (both emotional and financial) and benefits of these options must be carefully explained to the individual.

Prophylactic mastectomy has long been considered a potential approach to reducing the risk of breast cancer. Initially, subcutaneous mastectomy was performed wherein breast tissue is removed with preservation of the nipple–areolar complex; however, subsequent cases of breast cancer development were noted. This procedure has been largely abandoned because only 90% to 95% of the breast parenchyma is removed as residual ductal tissue remains adherent to the undersurface of the nipple–areolar complex and nipple sensation is not preserved. Conversely, simple or total mastectomy (skinsparing removal of the breast tissue) has supplanted the subcutaneous procedure, because the cosmetic result after this procedure is excellent. Total mastectomy reduces the amount of breast tissue remaining postoperatively; however, cases of breast cancer after this procedure have been reported. A recent retrospective study by the Mayo Clinic reviewed women who underwent bilateral prophylactic subcutaneous mastectomy due to a strong family history of breast cancer. The authors demonstrated a 90% reduction in the risk of breast cancer and decreased mortality during 14 years of follow-up. Of interest, unsuspected cancers were found in the prophylactic mastectomy specimens.

Although there is limited data regarding the efficacy of prophylactic surgery, statistical models suggest that certain woman at high risk for development of breast or ovarian cancer may gain 2.9 to 5.3 years of life expectancy by undergoing prophylactic mastectomies as well as 0.3 to 1.7 years in life expectancy with prophylactic oophorectomy. To place this gain in perspective, studies of mammography in normal risk women have life expectancy gains of less than 0.7 years. Whereas prophylactic surgery is not a panacea for women with a genetic predisposition for cancer, identification of the women at high risk and counseling of her options is an important aspect of her care. Prophylactic surgery may be a reasonable approach for women at substantially high risk for breast cancer who are willing to accept its irreversible consequence.

There is no clear evidence to suggest that women with breast cancer associated with a BRCA1 or BRCA2 mutation should be managed differently from those with sporadic cancers. BCS remains the standard of care for women with early stage sporadic breast cancer and is routinely offered to mutation carriers who have been diagnosed with breast cancer. BRCA mutation carriers are at increased risk for contralateral breast cancers; this risk may be as high as 60%. Thus, questions exist regarding optimal surgical management. Researchers question whether these patients may benefit from an ipsilateral mastectomy and contralateral prophylactic mastectomy

Breast Cancer and Pregnancy

Breast cancer is estimated to occur in 1 in 3,000 to 1 in 10,000 and have an incidence of 0.2% to 3.8% of pregnancies. Breast cancer in pregnancy has an overall worse prognosis due to the advanced stage at diagnosis; however, when patients are categorized according to stage at presentation and lymph node status, prognosis is similar in pregnant and nonpregnant patients. The normal pregnancy-associated changes in the breast make physical examination of the breast increasingly difficult as pregnancy advances. Physiologic edema and intensification of growth in the ductal and lobular system makes examination of the multinodular consistency of the breast challenging and may obscure early abnormalities. The intense hormonal milieu progressively causes greater breast volume and firmness. Benign masses also occur in pregnancy (Fig. 40.36).

Evaluation of a breast mass in a pregnant patient is unchanged from their nonpregnant counterparts. The conventional diagnostic modalities may be performed, including FNA, ultrasonography, core needle biopsy under local anesthesia, or excisional biopsy under local or general anesthesia without adverse sequelae. The finding of a thickness or a possible mass usually requires a short interval follow-up because the mass may feel similar to normal hypertrophic thickness as pregnancy advances. A mass that appears to "disappear" as pregnancy advances could actually be obscured by the normal changes in pregnancy and represent an ongoing developing breast carcinoma. For this reason, ultrasound may be used to evaluate an area that is "negative" on examination but was previously thought to harbor a mass lesion. Breast

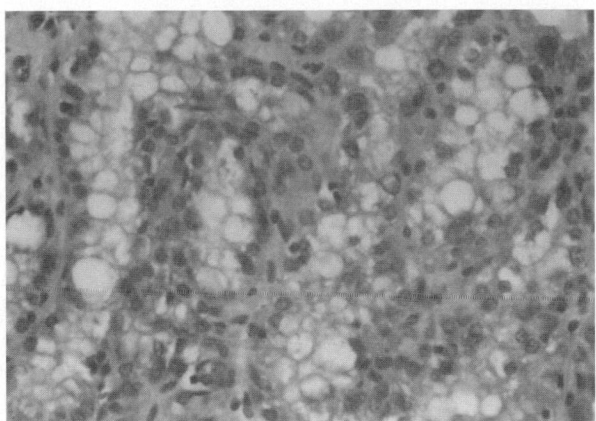

FIGURE 40.36. Lactating adenoma. Uniform cells have large nuclei and abundant vacuolated cytoplasm. Secretory material (milk) is present in the lumens (not seen in this figure).

ultrasonography during pregnancy is safe and helpful in differentiating between cystic and solid masses. However, ultrasound cannot distinguish benign solid masses from malignant masses. Little is known about the ultrasonographic appearance of normal breasts examined during pregnancy. Although no published data exist on MRI studies of the breasts of healthy pregnant or lactating women, MRI has been used in pregnancy and seems safe for fetuses because it does not expose them to ionizing radiation, although the safety committee indicates that the safety during pregnancy has not been proven. Recent reports on its use for fetal imaging in prenatal diagnosis contain limited follow-up of the infants, but no untoward effects have been reported. MRI may be particularly useful for the diagnosis or confirmation of bone metastases, liver metastases, or even brain metastases in the staging of patients, although head CT scans with abdominal shielding yield only small amounts of fetal exposure.

If an area is suspicious for malignancy, a shielded mammogram should be obtained during pregnancy; however, shielding cannot modify the internal radiation scatter dose from the breast to the fetus. If mammography is necessary in lactating women, it should be performed immediately after emptying the breast by nursing or pumping. One would expect mammography to be less sensitive during pregnancy because of increased density of breast tissue, but this has not been shown in practice. A recent study of 18 women revealed that few were noted to have an increased density category when comparing prepregnancy mammograms to those performed during pregnancy or lactation.

Any dominant mass should be evaluated as it would be in the nonpregnant patient to prevent diagnostic delay. Screening mammography may be deferred to limit fetal exposure but should be obtained without hesitation if the lesion requires additional evaluation. Radiation exposure to the fetus during mammography is estimated at less than 10 mrad depending on the gestational age, with increasing dose as the gravid fundus grows closer to the targeted breast tissue. If a palpable mass is felt, FNA is a

safe procedure in pregnancy. However, additional false-positive results may occur as a function of the increased cellularity and frequent mitosis that can occur normally during gestation. Thus, access to an experienced cytopathologist is vital. Core biopsies are more accurate, but milk fistulas, a complication seen in surgical biopsy, have been reported.

The risk for teratogenicity in subsequent fetal development may discourage the institution of therapy for cancer in pregnant women; however, established surgical and adjunctive therapies should be undertaken. Therapeutic termination does not appear to affect the survival in early stage breast carcinoma and is therefore not advocated. Modified radical mastectomy is the optimal treatment for local management of stage I and II. BCS is contraindicated in the first and second trimester due to the effect of the required adjunctive radiation on the fetus. Concerns continue to be raised about the future neurologic development and potential subsequent increased risk for childhood cancers among these newborns exposed to radiation; reliable long-term data are unavailable.

If the diagnosis is made during the third trimester, the patient may elect to be observed until delivery, when prompt treatment is initiated. Adjuvant therapy may also be delayed until delivery as long as the risks are exhaustively discussed with the patient. As in the nonpregnant patient, most recurrences occur within 2 years of treatment; therefore, patients with breast cancer are advised to delay pregnancy for 2 to 3 years and effective nonhormonal birth control should be administered. However, studies have not shown an adverse effect of subsequent pregnancy even in patients with positive axillary nodes or patients whose pregnancy occurred earlier than 2 years after completion of treatment. If nodal involvement is found, studies have indicated no adverse effects of the frequent forms of chemotherapy in the second or third trimesters, although long-term effects on the fetus are unknown. Methotrexate, taxanes, and tamoxifen should be avoided during pregnancy until further studies are available. Detailed studies of transplacental passage of chemotherapeutic agents to fetuses are also not available. The potential adverse effects of antineoplastic agents on fetuses and neonates include immediate effects, such as spontaneous abortion, teratogenesis, and organ damage, and delayed effects, such as growth retardation and gonadal dysfunction. Chemotherapy administration during the first trimester is associated with an increased incidence of stillbirths and congenital malformations. The risk of fetal malformation when chemotherapy is instituted in the first trimester is 12% compared with no increased risk with chemotherapeutic administration in the second and third trimester.

Staging procedures for breast cancer are often considered inappropriate in the gravid patient, but there are no contraindications for chest radiography performed with abdominal and pelvic shielding. In late pregnancy, the fetal shield may obscure the lower lung parenchyma; however, exposing third trimester fetuses to chest radiography presents no great concern. Alkaline phosphatase is elevated in normal pregnancy, making its use in evaluation of bone metastasis ineffectual. Conventional radiography, excluding the pelvis and abdomen (e.g., skull and long bones), can be performed. No adequate substitute for bone scanning exists, although articles have promoted certain modifications of the bone scanning technique for pregnant patients. Because the incidence of bone metastasis is very low in stage I and II disease, bone scanning can usually be avoided. On the other hand, in clinical stage III disease in which the possibility of bone metastasis is increased, treatment methods differ and may weigh in favor of provision of the test.

Whereas other human malignancies, including melanoma, hematopoietic malignancies, hepatoma, and choriocarcinoma, have been reported to cause fetal metastases, breast cancer has not. On the contrary, placental metastases from breast cancer and other solid tumors have been reported. Because half of these patients did not have visible lesions, microscopic examination of the placenta is warranted.

Rarely, breast fibroadenomas may infarct during pregnancy. These cases warrant close microscopic review because they may mimic carcinomas.

RISK MANAGEMENT AND PROFESSIONAL LIABILITY

Associated with the increased involvement in evaluation of diseases of the breast comes attached potential liability. Although medicolegal concerns should never alter method of practice, gynecologists must be cognizant of the legal environment. The special challenge of these cases derives from the emotionally charged nature of the cancer diagnosis, combined with high public expectations as to the current capability of breast cancer screening and treatment outcome. In this litigious society, nearly 80% of board-certified obstetricians/gynecologists in the United States have been sued for alleged malpractice. The most recent ACOG Professional Liability survey listed failure to diagnose breast cancer as the second leading primary allegation in claims against gynecologists (second only to surgical injury). Specifically, failure to diagnose breast cancer accounted for 53.7% of these claims with failure to diagnose cervical (18.1%) and ovarian cancers (5.9%) running a far second and third. According to the St. Paul Fire and Marine Insurance Company, the largest medical professional liability insurer, failure to diagnose cancer accounts for 46% of the total losses for insurers of the specialty of gynecology with a mean payment of $250,839.

Health care providers encounter a wide variety of legal issues with regard to patients with breast disorders, including liability for alleged misdiagnosis, delayed diagnosis of breast cancer, failure to obtain informed consent, and improper treatment of breast disease. Contextual legal issues other than medical malpractice often impact the care of breast disorders. For example, many state legislatures have mandated informed consent requirements for those treating patients with breast cancer.

Finally, legislation and litigation regarding insurance coverage for mammography screening, managed care policies, and new breast cancer treatments, such as HDCT and autologous bone marrow transplantation, are becoming increasingly common. The idea that physicians would not be brought into suits against Health Maintenance Organizations (HMO) and pharmaceutical companies has drastically changed, with more private doctors becoming involved in lawsuits against corporate entities.

The Physicians Insurers Association of America (PIAA) Breast Cancer Study, published in 1995, indicates that claims involving malignant neoplasms of the breast were the most common and the second most expensive condition resulting in physician malpractice claim payments. Analysis of the paid malpractice claims revealed women who were relatively young for the diagnosis of breast cancer (60% were younger than 50 years of age) and a high occurrence of false-negative mammogram results (nearly 80% of the claims had negative or equivocal mammogram results) were overrepresented. The average length of diagnostic delay was 14 months, with the average malpractice award or settlement increasing with longer periods of delay. The average indemnity payment increased by 36% over the 1990 study from $221,524 to $301,460 in 1995. Interestingly, radiologists have surpassed gynecologists as the most frequently sued practitioner, accounting for 24% of claims (gynecologists accounted for 23%). Specifically, this is a significant change from the previous study wherein gynecologists accounted for 39% of the claims and radiologists for 11%. In 1995, family practitioners accounted for 17%, surgical specialties for 14%, internal medicine for 4%, and pathologists for 2%.

Historically, U.S. jurisdictions used a "but for" test to establish legal, or proximate, causation. Causation in legal terminology signifies that the practitioner's action (e.g., delayed diagnosis) must have an association with the resultant injury (development of breast cancer) that is sufficiently close to hold the practitioner liable for damages. Under the "but for" test, malpractice damages are not awarded unless a better outcome was probable, better than even, or more likely than not, absent the actions of the practitioner. Under this test, only actions that possibly or with a likelihood of 50% *or greater* result in the alleged injury are deemed sufficient to make the practitioner liable for damages.

Historically, the "but for" standard was the most frequently used test of causation; however, this standard has been replaced in most states by causation theories that allow recovery in circumstances in which the probability that the negligent action led to patient injury is *less than* 50%. For instance, the "substantial factor" test permits recovery when the negligent behavior is a substantial factor in producing injury, even if the plaintiff's chance at a better outcome absent the actions of the practitioner was less than 50-50. A distinct, but related, alternative causation standard is the "loss of a chance" theory. Twenty-two states have adopted this theory as a standard. In those jurisdictions, a physician may be held liable for actions that deny the patient *some* chance or prospect of a better outcome. For instance, a delayed diagnosis that reduced a patient's chance of survival from 39% to 24% would preclude a verdict in favor of the physician in a "loss of a chance" state. Recovery would not be possible in a jurisdiction that followed the traditional "but for" causation analysis in which, as in this scenario, there was less than a probable impact on outcome. Hence the particular causation standard that a jurisdiction follows can have an enormous impact on the outcome of a medical malpractice liability case.

The most common reason underlying delay in diagnosis was physical examination findings that did not impress the physician (35%). Other reasons included failure to follow up in a timely fashion (31%), negative/misread mammogram (26%/23%), failure to perform a biopsy (23%), delayed/failure to consult (16%), failure to order/react to mammogram (11%/12%), communication failure (11%), and poor clinical examination (10%). Because mammography has a 15% to 20% false-negative rate, the practitioner should not rely on a "negative" mammogram in the face of a dominant lesion or suspicious examination. However, because mammography may not detect neoplastic changes in the breast until the cancer has been developing for 6 years, some lesions will not be seen on mammography in retrospect, some should be considered as subthreshold, and some are appropriately classified as missed.

The significance of medicolegal issues in the arena of breast cancer compels practitioners to develop risk management techniques that incorporate policies for reducing malpractice liability risk. The old adage "Good medicine is good law" is apropos as the guiding principles for care of women with breast disorders, which must be grounded in medical science and sound clinical judgment.

Patient education and effective communication are key components of good clinical care and effective risk management. One should not underemphasize significant diagnostic or therapeutic uncertainty in critical clinical decisions while maintaining an optimistic tenor in the doctor–patient relationship. This prevents the patient from misconstruing the importance or true implications of returning for follow-up examinations, repeat diagnostic tests, or other procedures. The clinician should allow the patient to participate in the decision-making process.

The best defense is an adequate record. For women with breast symptoms, the medical record should include a description and diagram of findings from the history and physical examination that will allow effective comparison during follow-up examinations. The chart notation "breasts okay" or "breasts normal" is not adequate chart documentation for a woman who presents with breast symptoms. The use of a printed encounter form designed specifically for breast complaints may facilitate suitable chart documentation. Documentation of a dominant mass, which may be measured or diagrammed, requires evaluation and resolution. Practitioners should make a record of each visit and any changes that occurred in the interval from the previous checkup. The re-

sults of any diagnostic tests should be documented, including patient notification and discussion. Clinicians should also record the rationale and factors of importance in their decision making in the medical record. If, ultimately, the patient's clinical course is unfavorable, prior documentation of the clinical reasoning may prove that the action taken was appropriate in light of the information available at the time.

The desired follow-up visits in women with breast complaints should be explicit and clear. Scheduled appointment dates are preferable to patient-initiated ("PRN") follow-up. Continuity of care for breast complaints must be carefully ensured, even when other medical problems or referred specialists become interposed. An extra effort to dispatch reminder telephone calls and letters are appropriate for patients with particularly suspicious clinical presentations who do not follow up for appointments. If a referral is made, follow-up is necessary to ensure the patient has seen the appropriate consultant and a copy of their recommendations should be made a part of the chart.

With the recent advancement in technology, medicolegal issues cannot be disregarded. The discovery of breast cancer susceptibility genes have prompted recent lawsuits charging physicians with failure to recommend monitoring or screening procedures for relatives of patients with hereditary forms of cancer.

Conclusion

The epidemic of breast cancer represents a significant public health problem affecting a large number of women. As obstetricians/gynecologists continue to care for women and expand their primary care function, we must remain knowledgeable of the changes in the field of breast disease. Advanced technology has improved the ability to define risk status and identify women with genetic predisposition to breast cancer development. Increased access to and use of screening mammography have been instrumental in decreasing the mortality rate associated with breast cancer by identifying earlier stage disease. Although changes in mammographic screening have occurred, a consensus on the evaluation of women younger than 50 years is controversial. Further radiologic technology in the arena of digital mammography may provide an alternative or adjunct to current conventional screen film. Although the impact of OCPs and HRT on the risk of breast cancer is unresolved, the information must be used to provide informed consent for patients while continuing to keep an eye on the horizon for supplementary information. Medicolegal concerns will continue to hover, but an accurate assessment and attention to testing and follow-up will decrease the delayed diagnosis in the future.

BIBLIOGRAPHY

Ad Hoc Committee on Genetic Testing/Insurance Issues. Genetic testing and insurance. *Am J Hum Genet* 1995;56: 327–331.

Adami HO, Persson I. Hormone replacement and breast cancer. *J Am Med Inform Assoc* 1995;274(2):178–179.

Ader DN, Browne MW. Prevalence and impact of cyclic mastalgia in a United States clinic-based sample. *Am J Obstet Gynecol* 1977;177(1):126–132.

Ader DN, Shriver CD. Cyclical mastalgia: prevalence and impact in an outpatient breast clinic sample. *J Am Coll Surg* 1997;185(5):466–70.

American Board of Obstetrics and Gynecology. An initiative for curriculum development and residency education. Presented at the Conference on Breast Disease, Chicago, May 1986.

American Cancer Society. *Cancer facts & figures 2000*. Atlanta, GA, 2000.

American College of Obstetrics and Gynecology. *ACOG Professional Liability Survey 1999*. Washington, DC: ACOG, 1999.

American College of Obstetricians and Gynecologists. *Breast-ovarian cancer screening. ACOG Committee Opinion 239*. Washington, DC: ACOG, 2000.

American College of Obstetricians and Gynecologists. *Carcinoma of the breast. ACOG Technical Bulletin 158*. Washington, DC: ACOG, 1991.

American College of Obstetricians and Gynecologists. *Guidelines for women's health care*. Washington, DC: ACOG, 1996.

American College of Obstetricians and Gynecologists. *Hormone replacement therapy in women with previously treated breast cancer. ACOG Committee Opinion 226*. Washington, DC: ACOG, 1999.

American College of Obstetricians and Gynecologists. *Nonmalignant conditions of the breast. ACOG Technical Bulletin 156*. Washington, DC: ACOG, 1991.

American College of Obstetricians and Gynecologists. *Professional liability and its effects: report of a 1999 survey of ACOG's membership*. Washington, DC: Conducted by Princeton Survey Research Associates. Princeton, NJ, December 1999.

American College of Obstetricians and Gynecologists. *Role of the obstetrician-gynecologist in the diagnosis and treatment of breast disease. ACOG Committee Opinion 186*. Washington, DC: ACOG, 1997.

American College of Obstetricians and Gynecologists. *Routine cancer screening. ACOG Committee Opinion 247*. Washington, DC: ACOG, 2000.

American College of Obstetricians and Gynecologists. *Tamoxifen and the prevention of breast cancer in high-risk women. ACOG Committee Opinion 224*. Washington, DC: ACOG, 1999.

Anderson I, Janzon L. Reduced breast cancer mortality in women under 50: updated results from Malmo Mammographic Screening Program. *Monogr Natl Cancer Inst* 1997;22:63–68.

Anonymous. Digital mammography. Why hasn't it been approved for U.S. hospitals? *Health Devices* 2000;29(1):14–21.

Anonymous. The management of ductal carcinoma in situ (DCIS). The steering committee on Clinical Practice Guidelines of the Care and Treatment of Breast Cancer. Canadian Association of Radiation Oncologists. *Can Med Assoc J* 1998;158[Suppl 3]:S27–S34.

Anonymous. The presentation and management of breast symptoms in general practice in South Wales. The BRIDGE Study Group. *Br J Gen Pract* 1999;49(447):811–812.

Arason A, Barkardottir RB, Egilsson V. Linkage analysis of chromosome 17q markers and breast-ovarian cancer in Icelandic families, and possible relationship to prostate cancer. *Am J Hum Genet* 1993; 52:711–717.

Armstrong BK. Estrogen therapy after the menopause—boon or bane? *Med J Aust* 1988;148:213–214.

Ayers JW, Gidwani GP. The "luteal breast": Hormonal and sonographic investigation of benign breast disease in patients with cyclic mastalgia. *Fertil Steril* 1983;40:779–784.

Badwe RA, Mittra I, Havaldar R. Timing of surgery with regard to the menstrual cycle in women with primary breast cancer. *Surg Clin North Am* 1999;79(5):1047–1059.

Bailar JC III. Mammography before age 50 years [Editorial]. *JAMA* 1988;259:1548–1549.

Baines CJ. Breast self-examination. *Cancer* 1992;69:1942.

Baines CJ. Changes in breast self-examination: behavior achieved by 89,835 participants in Canadian National Breast Screening Study. *Cancer* 1990;66:570.

Baines CJ. The Canadian National Breast Screening Study. Why: what next: and so what? *Cancer* 1995;76:2107–2112.

Baselga J, Seidman AD, Rosen PP, et al. Her2 overexpression and paclitaxel sensitivity in breast cancer; therapeutic implications. *Oncology (Huntington)* 1997;11[3 Suppl 2]:43–48.

Bassett LW, Manjikian V III, Gold RH. Mammography and breast cancer screening. *Surg Clin North Am*1990;70(4):775–800.

Bassett L. Winchester DP, Caplan RB, et al. Stereotactic core-needle biopsy of the breast: a report of the Joint Task Force of the American College of Radiology, American College of Surgeons, and College of American Pathologists. *CA Cancer J Clin* 1997;47(3):171–190.

Benjamin F. Normal lactation and galactorrhea. *Clin Obstet Gynecol* 1994;37(4):887–897.

Berchuck A, Carney M, Lancaster JM, et al. Familial breast-ovarian cancer syndromes: BRCA1 and BRCA2. *Clin Obstet Gynecol* 1998;41(1):157–166.

Bjurstam N, Bjorneld L, Duffy SW, et al. The Gothenburg Breast Screening Trial: first result on mortality, incidence, and mode of detection for women ages 39–49 years at randomization. *Cancer* 1997;80:2091–2099.

Bland breast book.

Blichert-Toft M, Anderson AN, Henriksen OB, et al. Treatment of mastalgia with bromocriptine: a double-blind cross-over study. *BMJ* 1979;1:237.

Bowers DG, Radlauer CB. Breast cancer after prophylactic subcutaneous mastectomies and reconstruction with silastic prostheses. *Plast Recontr Surg* 1969;44:541–544.

Branch LG. Breast health. In: Youngkin EQ, Davis MS, eds. *Women's health: a primary care clinical guide*. Norwalk, CT: Appleton and Lange, 1994.

Brody LC, Biesecker BB. Breast cancer susceptibility genes: BRCA1 and BRCA2. *Medicine* 1998;77(3):208–226.

Burke W. Oral contraceptives and breast cancer: a note of caution for high risk women [Editorial]. *JAMA* 2000;284(14):1837–1838.

Burke W, Daly M, Garber J, et al. Recommendations for follow-up care of individuals with an inherited predisposition to cancer. II. BRCA1 and BRCA2. *JAMA* 1997;277:120:997–1003.

Buzdar AU, Marcus C, Holmes F, et al. Phase II evaluation of LY156758 in metastatic breast cancer. *Oncology* 1988;45:344.

Cancer and Steroid Hormone Study of the Centers for Disease Control and the National Institute of Child Health and Human Development. Oral-contraceptive use and the risk of breast cancer. *N Engl J Med* 1986;315:405–411.

Cancer facts and figures 2000. American Cancer Society, 2000.

Cha CH, Kennedy GD, Niederhuber JE. Metastatic breast cancer. *Surg Clin North Am* 1999;79(5):1117–1143.

Chen LM, Karlan BY. Early detection and risk reduction for familial gynecologic cancers. *Clin Obstet Gynecol* 1998;41(1): 200–214.

Cheung KL. Management of cyclical mastalgia in oriental women: pioneer experience of using gamolenic acid (Efamast) in Asia. *Aust N Z Surg* 1999;69(7):494–494.

Chlebowski RT. Primary care: reducing the risk of breast cancer. *N Engl J Med* 2000;343(3):191–198.

Claus EB, Risch N, Thompson WD. Autosomal dominant inheritance of early-onset breast cancer: implications for risk prediction. *Cancer* 1994;73:643–651.

Col NF, Edkman MH, Karas RH, et al. Patient-specific decisions about hormone replacement therapy in postmenopausal women. *JAMA* 1997;277(14):1140–1147.

Colditz GA. Oral contraceptive use and mortality during 12 years of follow-up: the Nurses' Health Study. *Ann Intern Med* 1994;120:821–826.

Colditz GA, Hankinson SE, Hunter DJ, et al. The use of estrogens and progestins and the risk of breast cancer in postmenopausal women. *N Engl J Med* 1995;332:1589–1593.

Collaborative Group on Hormonal Factors in Breast Cancer. Breast cancer and hormonal contraceptives: further results. *Contraception* 1996;54[Suppl 3]:1S–106S.

Collins FS. BRCA1-Lots of mutations, lots of dilemmas. *N Engl J Med* 1996;334:186–188.

Controlled trial of tamoxifen as adjuvant agent in management of early breast cancer. Interim analysis at four years by Nolvadex Adjuvant Trial Organization. *Lancet* 1983;1: 257–261.

Controlled trial of tamoxifen as single adjuvant agent in management of early breast cancer. Analysis of six years by Nolvadex Adjuvant Trial Organization. *Lancet* 1985;1: 836–840.

Cooper DR, Butterfield J. Pregnancy subsequent to mastectomy for cancer of the breast. *Ann Surg* 1970;171: 429–433.

Cummings SR, Eckert S, Krueger KA, et al. The effect of raloxifene on risk of breast cancer in postmenopausal women: Results from the MORE randomized trial. *JAMA* 1999;281:2189–2197.

Data on file. Wyeth-Ayerst Laboratories, February 22, 2000.

Davies EL, Gateley CA, Miers M, et al. The long-term course of mastalgia. *J R Soc Med* 1998;91(9):464–464.

Dawes LG, Bowen C, Venta LA, et al. Ductography for nipple discharge: no replacement for ductal excision. *Surgery* 1998;124(4):685–691.

Delaloye JF, Antonescu C, Besseghir N, et al. Sentinel lymph node biopsy in breast cancer: the Lausanne experience. *Revue Medicale de la Suisse Romande* 2000;120(6):491–494.

Deliiski Y, Baichev G, Borchev G, et al. The treatment of cyclic mastalgia—a comparative study between the preparations bromocriptine and Geritamin. *Akusherstvo I Ginekologiia* 2000;39(1):27–29.

Delmas PD, Bjarnason NH, Mitlak BH, et al. Effects of raloxifene on bone mineral density, serum cholesterol concentrations and uterine endometrium in postmenopausal. *N Engl J Med* 1997;337(23):1641–1647.

DiSaia PJ, Creasman WT. *Clinical gynecologic oncology*, 5th ed. Mosby: St Louis, 1997.

Dooley W, Veronesi U, Phillips R, et al. Detection of pre-malignant and malignant breast cells by ductal lavage: results from a multicenter trial. Submitted for publication.

Dowlatshahi K. Yaremko ML, Kluskens LF, et al. Nonpalpable breast lesions: findings of stereotaxic needle-core biopsy and fine needle aspiration cytology. *Radiology* 1991;181: 745–750.

Duding KE, Abdel-Malek A, Barnett BG, et al. Data transmission integrity using satellite teleradiology testbed for digital mammography. In: Doi K, Giger ML, Nishikawa RM, et al, eds. *Digital mammography '96*. New York: Elsevier. 1996:177–182.

Dupont W, et al. Breast cancer risk associated with proliferative breast disease and atypical hyperplasia. *Cancer* 1993;71: 1258–1265.

Dupont WD, Page DL. Menopausal estrogen replacement therapy and breast cancer. *Arch Intern Med* 1991,151. 67–72.

Dupont W, Page D. Risk factors for breast cancer in women with proliferative breast disease. *N Engl J Med* 1985; 312:146–151.

Early Breast Cancer Trialists Collaborative Group. Tamoxifen for early breast cancer: an overview of the randomized trials. *Lancet* 1998;351:1452–1467.

Easton DF. Cancer risks in A-T heterozygotes. *Int J Radat Biol* 1994;66:S177–S182.

Easton DF. The inherited component of cancer. *Br Med Bull* 1994;50:527–535.

Easton DF, Bishop DT, Ford D, et al. Genetic linkage analysis of familial breast and ovarian cancer: results from 214 families. *Am J Hum Genet* 1993;52:678–701.

Easton DF, Ford D, Bishop DT. Breast Cancer Linkage Consortium. Breast and ovarian cancer incidence in BRCA1-mutation carriers. *Am J Hum Genet* 1995;56:265–271.

Edell SL, Eisen MD. Current imaging modalities for the diagnosis of breast cancer. *Del Med J* 1999;71(9):377–382.

Eeles RA, Stratton MR, Goldgar DE, et al. The genetics of familial breast cancer and their practical implications. *Eur J Cancer* 1994;30A:1383–1390.

Einstein AJ, Yang GC, Silberfarb JB, et al. Effect of ultrafast Papanicolaou staining on nuclear and textual features in breast cancer cytology. *Anal Quant Cytol Histol* 1997; 19(4):361–367.

Eisinger F, Jacquemier J, Charpin C, et al. Mutations in BRCA1: the medullary breast carcinoma revisited. *Cancer Res* 1998;58:1588–1592.

Ellis IO, Pinder SE. Fine needle aspiration (FNA) cytology of breast: refining the diagnosis. *Cytopathology* 1998; 9(5):289–290.

Eng C, Vijg J. Genetic testing: The problems and the promise. *Nat Biotechnol* 1997;15:422–426.

Esteva FJ, Hortobagyi GN. Adjuvant systemic therapy for primary breast cancer. *Surg Clin North Am* 1999;79(5): 1075–1090.

Ettinger B, Back DM, Mitlak BH, et al. Reduction of vertebral fracture risk in postmenopausal women with osteoporosis treated with raloxifene: results from a 3 year randomized clinical trial. *JAMA* 1999;282:637–645.

Fabian C, Kimler B, et al. Short-term breast cancer prediction by random periareolar fine-needle aspiration cytology and the Gail Risk Model. *J Natl Cancer Inst* 2000;92: 1217–1227.

Faiz O, Fentiman IS. Management of breast pain. *Int J Clin Pract* 2000;54(4):228–232.

Falun Meeting Committee and Collaborators. Falun meeting on breast cancer screening with mammography in women aged 40-49 years: report of the organizing committee and collaborators. *Int J Cancer* 1996;58:693–699.

Feig SA. Ductal carcinoma in situ: implications for screening mammography. *Radiol Clin North Am* 2000;38(4); 653–668.

Feig SA. Estimation of currently attainable benefit from mammography screening of women aged 40-49 years. *Cancer* 1995;75:2412–2419.

Feig SA. Increased benefit from shorter mammography screening intervals from women age 40-49 years. *Cancer* 1997; 80:2035–2039.

Feig SA, Yaffe MJ Digital mammography. *Radiographics* 1998;18(4):893–901.

Fernandez MA, Tortolero-Luna G, Told RS. Mammography and pap test screening among low-income foreign-born Hispanic women in USA. *Cadernos de Saude Publica* 1998;14[Suppl 3]:133–147.

Feuer EJ, Lap-Ming W, Boring CC, et al. The lifetime risk of developing breast cancer. *J Natl Cancer Inst* 1993; 85:892–897.

Feuer EJ, Wun LM, Boring CC, et al. The lifetime risk of developing breast cancer. *J Natl Cancer Inst* 1993;85(11): 892–897.

Fisher B, Anderson S. Conservative surgery for the management of invasive and noninvasive carcinoma of the breast: NSABP trials. National Surgical Adjuvant Breast and Bowel Project. *World J Surg* 1994;18:63–69.

Fisher B, Bauer M, Margolese R, et al. Five year results of a randomized clinical trial comparing total mastectomy and segmental mastectomy with or without radiation in the treatment of breast cancer. *N Engl J Med* 312:665, 1985.

Fisher B, Constantino J, Redmond C, et al. A randomized clinical trial evaluating tamoxifen in the treatment of positive tumors. *N Engl J Med* 1989;320320:479–484.

Fisher B, Costantino JP, Wickerham DL, et al. Tamoxifen for prevention of breast cancer: report of the National Surgical Adjuvant Breast and Bowel Project P-1 Study. *J Natl Cancer Inst* 1998;90:1371–1388.

Fisher B, Redmond C, Brown A, et al. Adjuvant chemotherapy with and without tamoxifen in the treatment of primary breast cancer: 5-year results from the National Surgical Adjuvant Breast and Bowel Project Trial. *J Clin Oncol* 1986;4:459–471.

Fisher B, Redmond C, Poisson R, et al. Eight year results of a randomized clinical trial comparing total mastectomy and lumpectomy with or without irradiation in the treatment of breast cancer. *N Engl J Med* 1989;320:822–828.

Fitzgibbons PL, Page DL, Weaver D, et al. Prognostic factors in breast cancer. College of American Pathologists Consensus Statement 1999. *Arch Pathol Lab Med* 2000;124(7): 966–978.

Fletcher SW, O'Malley MS, Bunce LA. Physicians' abilities to detect lumps in silicone breast models. *JAMA* 1985;253: 2224–2228.

Floria MG, Manganaro T, Pollicino A., et al. Surgical approach to nipple discharge: A ten-year experience. *J Surg Oncol* 1999;71(4):235–238.

Ford D, Easton DF. The genetics of breast and ovarian cancer. *Br J Cancer* 1995;72:805–812.

Ford D, Easton DF, Bishop DT, et al. Risk of cancer in BRCA1-mutation carriers. *Lancet* 1994;343:692–695.

Formenti S, Green G. An update on radiation therapy in breast cancer. *Hematol Oncol Clin North Am* 1999;13(2): 373–389.

Friedman LC, Moore A, Webb JA, et al. Breast cancer screening among ethnically diverse low-income women in a general hospital psychiatry clinic. *Gen Hosp Psychiatry* 1999;21(5):374–381.

Futreal A, Liu Q, Shuttuck-Eidens D, et al. BRCA1 mutations in primary breast and ovarian carcinomas. *Science* 1994;266:120–122.

Gail MH, Brinton LA, Byar DP, et al. Projection individualized probabilities of developing breast cancer for white females who are being examined annually. *J Natl Cancer Inst* 1989;81:1879–1996.

Gapstur SM, Morrow M, Sellers TA. Hormone replacement therapy and risk of breast cancer with a favorable histology. *JAMA* 1999;281(22):2091–2097.

Gemignani ML, Petrek JA, Borgen PI. Breast cancer and pregnancy. *Surg Clin North Am* 1999; 79(5):1157–1169.

Gisvold JJ, Goellner JR, Grant CS. Breast biopsy: a comparative study of stereotaxically guided core and excisional techniques. *AJR Am J Roentgenol* 1994;62:815–820.

Giuliano AE, Jones RC, Brennan M, et al. Sentinel lymphadenectomy in breast cancer. *J Clin Oncol* 1997;15: 2345–2350.

Goldenberg MM. Trastuzumab, a recombinant DNA-derived humanized monoclonal antibody, a novel agent for the treatment of metastatic breast cancer. *Clin Ther* 1999; 21(2):309–318.

Goldhirsch A, Glick JH, Gelber RD. et al. Meeting highlights: International consensus panel on the treatment of primary breast cancer. *J Natl Cancer Inst* 1998;90:1601–1608.

Goroll AH, May LA, Mulley AG. *Primary care medicine: office evaluation and management of the adult patient.* Philadelphia: JB Lippincott, 1995.

Gould SW, Lamb G, Lomax D, et al. Interventional MR-guided excisional biopsy of breast lesions. *J Magn Reson Imaging* 1998;8(1):26–30.

Grabrick DM, Hartmann LC. Cerhan JR, et al. Risk of breast cancer with oral contraceptive use in women with a family history of breast cancer. *JAMA* 2000;284(14):1791–1798.

Graves TA, Bland KI. Surgery for early and minimally invasive breast cancer. *Curr Opin Oncol* 1996;8:468–477.

Green VL. Advances in the treatment of breast diseases. In: Rock JA, Faro S., Gant NF, et al, eds. *Adv Obstet Gynecol* 1996;3:245–290.

Greenberg R. Skornick Y, Kaplan O. Management of breast fibroadenomas. *J Gen Intern Med* 1998;13(9):640–645.

Grumback Y. Fine needle cytology and core biopsy of nonpalpable breast lesions. When appropriate. *Archives D anatomie et de Cytologie Pathologiques* 1998;46(4): 219–221.

Halsted WS. The results of radical operations for the cure of carcinoma of the breast. *Ann Surg* 1907;56:1–19.

Hanna AK, Trapdoor J, Mira MK. Spectrum of benign breast disorders in a university hospital. *J Indian Med Assoc* 1997;95(1):5–8.

Hansen N, Morrow M. Breast disease. *Med Clin North Am* 1998;82(2):203–222.

Hartmann LC, Sellers TA, Schaid DJ, et al. Clinical options for women at high risk for breast cancer. *Surg Clin North Am* 1999;79(5):1189–1206.

Hartmann LC, Schaid DJ, Woods JE, et al. Efficacy of bilateral prophylactic mastectomy in women with a family history of breast cancer. *N Engl J Med* 1999;340:77–84.

Hatcher RA, Trussel J, Stewart F, et al, eds. *Contraceptive technology,* 17th ed. New York: Ardent Media, 1999.

Hawley W, Nuovo J, deNeef CP, et al. Do oral contraceptive agents affect the risk of breast cancer: a meta-analysis of the case-control reports. *J Am Board Fam Pract* 1993;6: 123–135.

Heland KV, Rutledge P. Medicolegal issues. *Obstet Gynecol Clin North Am* 1994;21:781–788.

Henderson IC, Hayes DF, Gelman R. Dose-response in the treatment of breast cancer: a critical review. *J Clin Oncol* 1988;6:1501–1515.

Hendrick RE, Smith RA, Rutledge JII III, et al. Benefit of screening mammography for women aged 40-49: a new meta-analysis for randomized controlled trials. *Monogr Natl Cancer Inst* 1997;22:87–92.

Hild F, Duda VF, Albert U, et al. Ductal orientated sonography improves the diagnosis of pathological nipple discharge of the female breast compared with galactography. *Eur J Cancer Prev* 1998;7[Suppl 1]:S57–S62.

Hindle WH. *Breast disease for gynecologists.* Norwalk, CT: Appleton & Lange, 1990.

Hogge JP, Artz DS, Freedman MT. Update in digital mammography. *Crit Rev Diagn Imaging* 1997;38(1): 89–113.

Hrushesky WJ, Bluming AZ, Gruber SA, et al. Menstrual influence on surgical cure for breast cancer. *Lancet* 1989;2:949–952.

Isaacs JH. Other nipple discharge. *Clin Obstet Gynecol* 1994;37(4):898–902.

Jackson IM, Litherland S, Wakeling AE. Tamoxifen and other antiestrogens. In: Powles TJ, Smith IE, eds. *Medical management of breast cancer.* London: Martin Dunitz, 1991.

Jacobs AJ, Gast MJ. Practical gynecology: clinical manual. Norwalk, CT: Appleton and Lange, 1994.

Jancin B. Dietary flaxseed may relieve cyclic mastalgia. *OB/GYN News* January 15, 2001.

Jordan VC, ed. *Tamoxifen for the treatment and prevention of breast cancer.* Melville, NY: PRR, Inc., 1999.

Jordan VC. Selective estrogen receptor modulation (SERM): an overview of strategies. In: Focus on postmenopausal health: current issues and new directions. Speaker Medical Education Meeting 1998. National Initiatives in Continuing Medical Education—Institute of Continuing Healthcare Education. Philadelphia, 1998.

Jordan VC. Tamoxifen: the herald of a new era of preventive therapeutics. *J Natl Cancer Inst* 1997;89(11):747–749.

Karp SE. Clinical management of BRCA1 and BRCA2 associated breast cancer. *Semin Surg Oncol* 2000;18:296–304.

Kavanagh AM, Mitchell H, Giles GG. Hormone replacement therapy and accuracy of mammographic screening. *Lancet* 2000;355(9200):270–274.

Keating NL, Cleary PD, Rossi AS, et al. Use of hormone replacement therapy by postmenopausal women in the United States. *Ann Intern Med* 1999;130:545–553.

Kline TS, Lash SR. Nipple secretion in pregnancy a cytologic and histologic study. *Am J Clin Pathol* 1962;37: 626–632.

Kochli OR. Development in minimally invasive breast surgery—overview and our own experience: new diagnostic and therapeutic challenges in breast cancer. *Gynakologisch-Geburtshilfliche Rundschau* 2000;40(1):3–12.

Kontostolis E, Stefanidis K, Navrozoglou I, et al. Comparison of tamoxifen with danazol for treatment of cyclical mastalgia. *Gynecol Endocrinol* 1997;11(6):393–397.

Krag DN, Meijer SJ, Weaver DL, et al. Minimal access surgery for staging of malignant melanoma. *Arch Surg* 1995;130: 654–660.

Kumar S, Mansel RE, Hugher LE, et al. Prolactin response to thyrotropin-releasing hormone stimulation and dopaminergic inhibition in benign breast disease. *Cancer* 1984;53:1311–1315.

Lando JF, Heck KE, Brett KM. Hormone replacement therapy and breast cancer risk in a nationally representative cohort. *Am J Prev Med* 1999;17(3):176–180.

Lawrence HC. History, physical examination, and education in breast self-examination. In: Seltzer V, ed. The role of the obstetrician-gynecologist in diagnosing and treating breast disease. *Clin Obstet Gynecol* 1994;37:881.

Letton AH, Mason EM, Rainshaw BJ. Twenty year review of a breast cancer screening project: ninety-five percent survival of patients with nonpalpable breast cancers. *Cancer* 1996;77:104–106.

Leis HP Jr, Cammarata A, LaRaja Rd. Nipple discharge: significance and treatment. *Breast* 1985;11:6.

Leis HP Jr. Management of nipple discharge. *World J Surg* 1989;13:736.

Leis HP, Dursi MD, Mersheimer ML. Nipple discharge: Significance and treatment. *N Y State J Med* 1967;67:3105–3110.

Lerman C, Croyle R. Psychological issues in genetic testing for breast cancer susceptibility. *Arch Intern Med* 1994;154: 609–616.

Lerman C, Marod S, Schulman K, et al. BRCA1 testing in families with hereditary breast-ovarian cancer: a prospective study of patient decision making and outcomes. *JAMA* 1996;275:1885–1892.

Li CP, Lee FY, Hwang SJ, et al. Treatment of mastalgia with tamoxifen in male patients with liver cirrhosis: a randomized crossover study. *Am J Gastroenterol* 2000;95(4):1051–1055.

Lieberman L. Clinical management issues in percutaneous core breast biopsy. *Radiol Clin North Am* 2000;38(4):791–808.

Lim VS, Kathpalice S, Frohman LA. Hyperprolactinemia and impaired pituitary response to suppression and stimulation in chronic renal failure: reversal after transplantation. *J Clin Endocrinol Metab* 1979;48:101–107.

Love RR, Barden HS, Mazess RB, et al. Effect of tamoxifen on lumbar spine bone mineral density in postmenopausal women after 5 years. *Arch Intern Med* 1994;154:2585–2588.

Love S, Lindsey K. *Dr. Susan Love's breast book,* 2nd ed. Addison-Wesley Publishing, 1995.

Love RR, Barden HS, Mazess RB, et al. Effect of tamoxifen on lumbar spine bone mineral density in postmenopausal women after 5 years. *Arch Intern Med* 1994;154: 2585–2588.

Love S, Schnitt S, Connolly J, et al. Benign breast diseases. In: Harris J, Hellman S, Henderson I, et al, eds. *Breast diseases.* Philadelphia: JB Lippincott, 1987.

Mahavni V, Buller RE. Estrogen replacement therapy in endometrial and breast cancer survivors. *Clin Obstet Gynecol* 1999;42(4):863.

Malkin D, Le FP, Strong LC, et al. Germ line p53 mutations in a familial syndrome of breast cancer, sarcomas, and other neoplasia. *Science* 1990;250:1233.

Marchant DL. Mammography. In: Sciarra JW, ed. *Gynecology and obstetrics.* Philadelphia: Harper & Row, 1993.

Martin HE, Ellis EB. Biopsy of needle puncture and aspiration. *Ann Surg* 1930;92:169–181.

Mason BR, Page KA, Fallon K. An analysis of movement and discomfort of the female breast during exercise and the effects of breast support in three cases. *J Sci Med Sport* 1999;2(2):134–144.

Maswell CJ, Kozak JF, Desjardins-Denault SD, et al. Factors important in promoting mammography screening among Canadian women. *Can J Public Health (Revue Canadienne de Sante Publique)* 1997;88(5):346–350.

Meden H, Kuhn W. Overexpression of oncogene c-erb-2 (HER2/neu) in ovarian cancer: a new prognostic factor. *Eur J Obstet Gynecol Reprod Biol* 1997;71(2):173–179.

Menard S, Tagliabue E, Campiglio M, et al. Role of HER2 gene overexpression in breast carcinoma. *J Cell Physiol* 2000;182(2):150–162.

Michels KV, Willett WC, Rosner BA, et al. Prospective assessment of breast feeding and breast cancer incidence among 89,997 women. *Lancet* 1996;347(8999):431–436.

Miki Y, Swenson J, Shuttuck-Eidens D, et al. A strong candidate for the breast and ovarian cancer susceptibility gene BRCA1. *Science* 1994;266:66–71.

Miller J. Benign breast disorders. In: Lemcke D, Pattison J, Marshall L, et al, eds. *Primary care of women.* Norwalk, CT: Appleton & Lange, 1995.

Mishell DR. Evaluating the benefits and risks of hormone replacement therapy. *ObGyn News* December 2000[Suppl].

Morris A, Pomier RF, Schmidt WA. Accurate evaluation of palpable breast masses by the triple test score. *Arch Surg* 1998;133(9):930–934.

Mouridsen H, Palshof T, Patterson J, et al. Tamoxifen in advanced breast cancer. *Cancer Treat Rev* 1978;5: 131–141.

Mulvihill JJ, Stadler MP. Breast cancer risk analysis and counseling. *Clin Obstet Gynecol* 1996;39(4):851–859.

Murray PP, Stadel BV, Schlesselman JJ. Oral contraceptive use in women with a family history of breast cancer. *Obstet Gynecol* 1989;73:977–983.

Mustafa IA, Bland KO. Physiologic effects of steroid hormones and postmenopausal hormone replacement on the female breast and breast cancer risk. *Ann Surg* 1998;228(5): 638–651.

National Cancer Institute Breast Cancer Screening Consortium. Screening mammography: a missed clinical opportunity: results of the NCI Breast Cancer Screening Consortium and National Health Interview Survey Studies. *JAMA* 1990;264:54–58.

National Cancer Institute—Consensus Conference. The uniform approach to breast fine needle aspiration biopsy. *Am J Surg* 1997; 174(4):371–385.

National Council on Radiation Protection and Measurements. *Mammography—a user's guide, NCRP report no 85.* Bethesda, MD: National Council on Radiation Protection and Measurements, 1986.

National Institutes of Health Consensus Development Conference Statement. Breast cancer screening for women ages 40-49. Bethesda, MD: NIH, January 21–23, 1997.

National Institutes of Health Consensus Development Conference Statement. Ovarian cancer: screening, treatment and follow-up. *Gynecol Oncol* 1994;55:S4–S14.

National Institutes of Health Consensus Development Conference. Consensus statement: treatment of early-stage breast cancer. *J Natl Cancer Inst Monogr* 1992;11:1–5.

Nettles-Carlson B. Problems of the breast. In: Fogel CI, Woods NF, eds. *Women's health care.* Thousand Oaks, CA: Sage Publications, 1995.

Newton KM, LaCroix AZ, Leveille SG, et al. Women's beliefs and decisions about hormone replacement therapy. *J Womens Health* 1997;6:459–465.

Nieweg OE, Jansen L, Valdes Olmos RA, et al. Lymphatic mapping sentinel lymph node biopsy in breast cancer. *Eur J Nucl Med* 1999;26[4 Suppl]:S11–S16.

Niklason LT, Christian BT, Niklason LE, et al. Digital tomosynthesis in breast imaging. *Radiology* 1997;205: 399–406.

Noguchi M, Tsugawa K, Miwa K, et al. Sentinel lymph node biopsy and axillary lymph node dissection. *Jpn J Cancer Chemother* 2000;27(7):961–966.

Nystrom L, Rutqvist LE, Wall S, et al. Breast cancer screening with mammography: overview of Swedish randomized trials. *Lancet* 1993;342:973–978.

O'Brien PM, Abukhalil IE. Randomized controlled trial of the management of premenstrual syndrome and premenstrual mastalgia using luteal phase-only danazol. *Am J Obstet Gynecol* 1999;180(1 pt 1):18–23.

Okazaki A, Hirata K, Okazaki M, et al. Nipple discharge disorders: current diagnostic management and the role of fiberductoscopy. *Eur Radiol* 1999;9(4):583–590.

O'Neil S, Castelli M, Gattuso P, et al. Fine needle aspiration of 697 palpable breast lesions with histopathologic correlation. *Surgery* 1997;122(4):824–828.

Orel S. MR imaging of the breast. *Radiol Clinics North Am* 2000;38(4):899–914.

Osborne MP. Chemoprevention of breast cancer. *Surg Clin North Am* 1999;79(5):1207–1222.

Page D, et al. Atypical hyperplastic lesions of the female breast. *Cancer* 1985;55:2698–2708.

Page KA, Steele JR. Breast motion and sports brassiere design. Implications for future research. *Sports Med* 1999;2(4): 205—211.

Papanicolaou GN, Holmquist DG, Batter GM, et al. Exfoliative cytology of the human mammary gland and its value in the diagnosis of cancer and other disease of the breast. *Cancer* 1958;11:377–409.

Parker SH, Dennis MA, Kaske TI. Identification of the sentinel node in patients with breast cancer. *Radiol Clin North Am* 2000;38(4):809–823.

Parker JD, Sabogal F, Gebretsadik T. Relationship between earlier and later mammography screening—California Medicare, 1992 through 1994. *West J Med* 1999;170(1): 25–27.

Pearson D. NWHN joins health research group in suit against dangerous lactation suppression drug: Parlodel withdrawn from market. *The Network News: National Women's Health Network* 1994;19:4.

Perlet C, Becker C, Sittel H, et al. A comparison of digital luminescence mammography and conventional film-screen system: preliminary results of clinical evaluation. *Eur J Med Res* 1998;3(3):165–171.

Petrakis ML, Mason L, Lee R. Association of race, age, menopausal status, and cerumen type with breast fluid secretion in nonlactating women, as determined by nipple aspiration. *J Natl Cancer Inst* 1975;54: 829–834.

Petrij-Bosch A, Peelen T, Van Vliet M, et al. BRCA1 genomic deletions are major founder mutations in Dutch breast cancer patients. *Nat Genet* 1997;17:341–345.

Physicians Insurers Association of America: Breast cancer study, June 1995. Washington, DC: Physician Insurers Association of American, 1995.

Physicians Insurers Association of America: Breast cancer study, March 1990. Lawrenceville, NJ: Physician Insurers Association of American, 1990.

Pisano ED, Yaffe MJ, Hemminger BM, et al. Current status of full-field digital mammography. *Acad Radiol* 2000;7(4): 266–280.

Plotkin D, Blankenship F. Breast cancer: biology and malpractice. *Am J Clin Oncol* 1991;14:254–266.

Powles T, Eeles R, Ashley S, et al. Interim analysis of the incidence of breast cancer in the Royal Marsden Hospital tamoxifen randomized chemoprevention trial. *Lancet* 1998;352:98–101.

Preece PE, Hughes LE, Mansel RE, et al. Clinical syndromes of mastalgia. *Lancet* 1976;2:670.

Preliminary data presented at the San Antonio Breast Conference. San Antonio, TX, December 2000.

Preliminary data presented by the American Society of Clinical Oncology Annual Meeting, May 2000, and the Second Annual Lynn Sage Breast Cancer Symposium, September 2000.

Presented by Drs. Barbara L. Weber, Steven A. Narod, and Andrea Eisen from Toronto at the American Society of Human Genetics, December 2000. As reported by Mitchel L. Zoler in *OB GYN News* 2000;35(23):1–2.

Pye J, Mansel R, Hugher L. Clinical experience of drug treatments for mastalgia. *Lancet* 1985;2:373.

Raffel L. Genetic counseling and genetic testing for cancer risk assessment. *Clin Obstet Gynecol* 1998;41(1):141–145.

Orel S. MR imaging of the breast. *Radiol Clin North Am* 2000;38(4):899–914.

Orel SG, Dougherty CS, Reynolds C, et al. MR imaging in patients with nipple discharge: initial experience. *Radiology* 2000;216(1):248–254.

Rea H, Bove F, Gentile A, et al. Prolactin response to thyrotropin-releasing hormone as a guideline for cyclical mastalgia treatment. *Minerva Medica* 1997;88(11):479–487.

Reference clinical report on file at PRO-Duct Health, Inc. Cyctyc Health Corporation, Boxborough, MA.

Reynolds HE. Advances in breast imaging. *Hematol Oncol Clin North Am* 1999;13(2):333–348.

Ribiero G, Jones DA, Jones M. Carcinoma of the breast associated with pregnancy. *Br J Surg* 1986;73(8):429–433.

Ries AG I, Fisner MP, Kosary CI, et al. SEER Cancer Statistics Review, 1973–1997. Bethesda, MD: National Cancer Institute, 2000.

Ries LA, Wingo PA, Miller DS, et al. The annual report to the nation on the status of cancer, 1973–1997, with a special section on colorectal cancer. *Cancer* 2000;88(10):2398–2424.

Romieu I, Willet WC, Colditz GA, et al. Prospective study of oral contraceptive use and risk of breast cancer in women. *J Natl Cancer Inst* 1989:81:1313–1321.

Romrell LJ, Bland KI. Anatomy of the breast, axilla, chest wall, and related metastatic sites. In: Bland KI, Copeland EM III, eds. *The breast: comprehensive management of benign and malignant diseases,* 2nd ed. Philadelphia: WB Saunders, 1998:19–37.

Ross RK, Paganni-Hill A, Wan PC, et al. Effect of hormone replacement therapy on breast cancer risk: estrogen versus estrogen plus progestin.

Rovno HD, Siegelman ES, Reynolds C, et al. Solitary intraductal papilloma: findings at MR imaging and MR galactography. *AJR Am J Roentgenol* 1999;172(1):151–155.

Runowiczz C. Hormone replacement therapy in cancer survivors: a con opinion. *CA Cancer J Clin* 1996;46(6): 365–373.

Rushton L, Jones DR. Oral contraceptive use and breast cancer risk: a meta-analysis of variations with age at diagnosis, parity, and total duration of oral contraceptive use. *Br J Obstet Gynaecol* 1992;99:239–246.

Sakorafas GH, Tsiotou AG, Sentinel lymph node biopsy in breast cancer. *Am Surg* 2000;66(7);667–674.

Sandrucci S, Casalegno PS, Percivale P, et al. Sentinel lymph node mapping biopsy for breast cancer: a review of the literature relative to 4791 procedures. *Tumori* 1999;85(6): 425–434.

Sands R, Studd J. Hormone replacement therapy for women after breast carcinoma. *Curr Opin Obstet Gynecol* 1996; 8:216–220.

Sangold GA, Kletzky OA, Marrs RP, et al. Hyperprolactinemia: comparison of thyrotropin-releasing hormone and tomography. *Obstet Gynecol* 1984;63:771–775.

Sattuck-Eidens D, Mcclure M, Simard J, et al. A collaborative survey of 80 mutations in the BRCA1 breast and ovarian cancer susceptibility gene. *JAMA* 1995;273:535–541.

Schilling RB, Cox JD, Sharma SR. Advanced digital mammography. *J Digital Imaging* 1998;11[3 Suppl 1]:163–165.

Schlesselman JJ. Net effect of oral contraceptive use on the risk of cancer in women in the United States. *Obstet Gynecol* 1995;85:793–801.

Schrag D, Kuntz KM, Garber JE, et al. Life expectancy gains from cancer prevention strategies for women with breast cancer and BRCA1 or BRCA2 mutations. *JAMA* 2000; 283(5):617 624.

Schwartz SI, Shires GT, Spencer FC, eds. *Principles of surgery,* 6th ed. New York: McGraw-Hill, 1994.

Scott S, Morrow M. Breast cancer: making the diagnosis. *Surg Clin North Am* 1999;79(5):991–1005.

Seidman H, Gelb SK, Silverberg E, et al. Survival experience in the Breast Cancer Detection Demonstration Project. *CA Cancer J Clin* 1987;37:258–290.

Seltzer MII, Perloff LJ, Kelley RI, et al. The significance of age in patients with nipple discharge. *Surg Gynecol Obstet* 1970;131:519.

Severin MJ. Hereditary cancer litigation: a status report. *Oncology* 1996;10:211–214.

Shen KW, Wu J, Lu JS, et al. Fiberoptic ductoscopy for patients with nipple discharge. *Cancer* 2000;89(7):1512–1519.

Sherrid P. Will boomer women defy the menopause? The drug industry is betting they will try. *US News & World Report* September 11, 2000.

Sherwin BB, Carlson LE. Estrogen and memory in women. *J SOGC* 1997;19(11)[Suppl]:7–13.

Sillero-Arenas M, Delgado-Rodriguez M, Rodigues-Canteras R, et al. Menopausal hormone replacement therapy and breast cancer: a meta-analysis. *Obstet Gynecol* 1992;79(2): 286–294.

Simpson JF, Wilkinson EJ. Malignant neoplasia of the breast: infiltrating carcinomas. In: Bland KI, Copeland EM III, eds. *The breast: comprehensive management of benign and malignant diseases,* 2nd ed. Philadelphia: WB Saunders, 1998:285–295.

Sitruk-Ware R, Sterkers N, Mauvais-Jarvis P. Benign breast disease: hormonal investigation. *Obstet Gynecol* 1979;53: 457–460.

Sneige N. Fine needle aspiration of the breast: a review of 1,995 cases with emphasis on diagnostic pitfalls. *Diagn Cytopathol* 1993;9(1):106–112.

Speroff L, ed. Oral contraceptives and the risk of breast cancer. *Obset Gynecol Clin Alert* 2000;17(8):60–61.

Speroff L. Postmenopausal hormone therapy and breast cancer. *Obstet Gynecol* 1996;87(2):44S–54S.

Speroff L, Glass R, Case N. *Clinical gynecologic endocrinology and infertility,* 5th ed. Baltimore, MD: Williams & Wilkins, 1994.

Stadmauer EA, O'Neill A, Goldstein LJ, et al. conventional dose chemotherapy compared with high dose chemotherapy plus autologous hematopoietic stem cell transplantation for metastatic breast cancer. *N Engl J Med* 2000;342(15):1069–1076.

Steinberg KK, Thacker SB, Smith SJ, et al. A meta-analysis of the effect of estrogen replacement therapy on the risk of breast cancer. *JAMA* 1991;265:1985–1990.

Strewing JP, Abeliovich D, Peretz T, et al. The carrier frequency of the BRCA1 185delAG mutation is approximately 1 percent in Ashkenazi Jewish individuals. *Nat Genet* 1995;11:198–200.

Swang ES, Esserman LJ. Management of ductal carcinoma in situ. *Surg Clin North Am* 1999;79(5):1007–1030.

Swift M, Reitnauer PJ, Morrell D, et al. Breast and other cancers in families with ataxia-telangiectasia. *N Engl J Med* 1987;316:1289–1294.

Swinford AE, Adler DD, Garver KA. Mammographic appearance of the breasts during pregnancy and lactation: false assumptions. *Acad Radiol* 1998;5:467.

Tabar L, Fagerberg G, Chen H-H, et al. Efficacy of breast cancer screening by age; new results from the Swedish Two-County trial. *Cancer* 1995;75:2507–2517.

Taghian AG, Powell SN. The role of radiation therapy for primary breast cancer. *Surg Clin North Am* 1999;79(5): 1091–1115.

Thomas DB, Gao DL, Self SG, et al. Randomized trial of breast self examination in Shanghai: methodology and preliminary results. *J Natl Cancer Inst* 1997;276:33–38.

Tsevat J, Weinstein MC, Williams LW, et al. Expected gains in life expectancy form various coronary heart disease risk factor modifications. *Circulation* 1991;83:1194–1201.

Uehara J, Mazario AC, Rodrigues de Lima G, et al. Effects of tamoxifen on the breast in luteal phase of the menstrual cycle. *Int J Gynecol Obstet* 1998;62(1):77–82.

Van Golan K, Milliron K, Davies S, et al. BRCA-associated cancer risk: molecular biology and clinical practice. *J Lab Clin Med* 1999;134(1):11–18.

Van Zee KJ, Ortega PG, Minnard E, et al. Preoperative galactography increases the diagnostic yield of major duct excision for nipple discharge. *Cancer* 1998;82(10): 1874–1880.

Varney H. *Varney's midwifery*, 3rd ed. Sudbury, MA: Jones and Bartlett Publishers, 1997.

Veronesi J, Luini A, Del Vecchio M. Radiotherapy after breast-preserving in women with localized cancer of the breast. *N Engl J Med* 1993;328:1587–1591.

Veronesi U, Mainsonneuve P, Costa A, et al. Prevention of breast cancer with tamoxifen: preliminary findings from the Italian randomized trial among hysterectomized women. *Lancet* 1998;352:93–97.

Veronesi U, Volterrani F, Luini A, et al. Quadrantectomy versus lumpectomy for small size breast cancer. *Eur J Cancer* 1990;26:671–673.

Walsh BW, Lewis HK, Wild RA, et al. Effect of raloxifene on serum lipids and coagulation factors in health postmenopausal women. *JAMA* 1998;279:1445–1451.

Warmuth MA, Sutton LM, Winer EP. A review of hereditary breast cancer: from screening to risk factor modification. *Am J Med* 1997;102(4):407–415.

Watt-Boolsen S, Eskildsen PC, Blaehr H. Release of prolactin, thyrotropin-releasing hormone stimulation and dopaminergic inhibition in benign breast disease. *Cancer* 1984;53:1311–1315.

Wertheimer MD, Costanza ME, Dodson TF, et al. Increasing the effort toward breast cancer detection. *JAMA* 1986;255:1311.

Wolfe S. The great mammogram debate. *Med Econ* 1997;60(8):41–44.

Wong AT, Salisbury E, Bilous M. Recent developments in stereotactic breast biopsy methodologies: an update for the surgical pathologist. *Adv Anat Pathol* 2000;7(1):26–35.

Wooster R, Bignell G, Lancaster J, et al. Identification of the breast cancer susceptibility gene BRCA2. *Nature* 1995;378:789–792.

Wooster R, Ford D, Mangion J, et al. Absence of linkage to the ataxia-telangiectasia locus in familial breast cancer. *Hum Genet* 1993;92:91–94.

Wrensch M, Petrakis H, et al. Breast Cancer incidence in women with abnormal cytology in nipple aspirates of breast fluid. *Am J Epidemiol* 1991;135:130–141.

Zylstra S. Office management of benign breast disease. *Clin Obstet Gynecol* 1999;42(2):234–248.

Te Linde's Operative Gynecology, ninth edition, edited by John A. Rock and Howard W. Jones, III. Lippincott Williams & Wilkins, Philadelphia © 2003.

CHAPTER

41

▼

The Vermiform Appendix in Relation to Gynecology

BARRY K. JARNAGIN

Appendectomy is the most common surgical procedure performed on an emergency basis and the most common cause of abdominal pain requiring surgery. The differential diagnosis of lower abdominal pain not only includes acute appendicitis, but many gynecologic problems, such as pelvic inflammatory disease, ectopic pregnancy, ovarian torsion, and ruptured ovarian cyst. Therefore, the differential diagnosis of lower abdominal pain is one of the most common and difficult diagnoses that the gynecologist is called on to make. It is a serious undertaking and one in which a mistake could be fatal.

Individuals have a 7% lifetime risk of developing appendicitis. In the United States, reports show that approximately 300,000 operations are done per year, with the greatest incidence in the second and third decade of life. Although the overall mortality rate with appropriate and timely treatment is much less than 1%, it remains approximately 5% to 15% in the elderly. The higher mortality and morbidity rate in the elderly is caused by the increased difficulty in diagnosing appendicitis in older people, which leads to a higher rate of perforation. The incidence of perforation in patients ranges from 17% to 40%, with a median of 20%. The perforation rate in the elderly patient is significantly higher, with rates as high as 60% to 70% reported. Several factors contribute to this, including significant delay in seeking care, nonspecificity

of the presenting symptoms and signs, diminished febrile response, and fewer abnormalities in laboratory parameters such as the white blood cell count. Although the mortality rate for acute appendicitis is less than 0.1%, the mortality rate for gangrenous appendicitis is about 0.6%, and the mortality rate for perforated appendicitis is 5%. Death usually is the result of uncontrollable sepsis with generalized peritonitis, intraabdominal abscesses, intestinal obstruction, pyelonephritis, and Gram-negative septicemia. The overall morbidity rate is about 15% to 20% in most reports of appendicitis, with wound infection from a gangrenous or perforated appendix being the most common complication. Preoperative antibiotic therapy has greatly improved the morbidity rate, but perforation of the appendix is not prevented by antibiotics. Nor has the incidence of perforation decreased in recent years. Acute inflammation of the appendix commonly extends to the right adnexa (Fig. 41.1) and can involve the left as well when a large periappendiceal abscess develops in the pelvis. When the appendix ruptures, bilateral tubal adhesions commonly occur that may result in sterility or tubal pregnancy as a sequela. Incidental appendectomy at the time of other pelvic surgery remains controversial, but proponents argue that appendectomy simplifies the differential diagnosis of lower abdominal pain and prevents the possibility of a ruptured appendix in the future. This controversy is discussed later in the chapter.

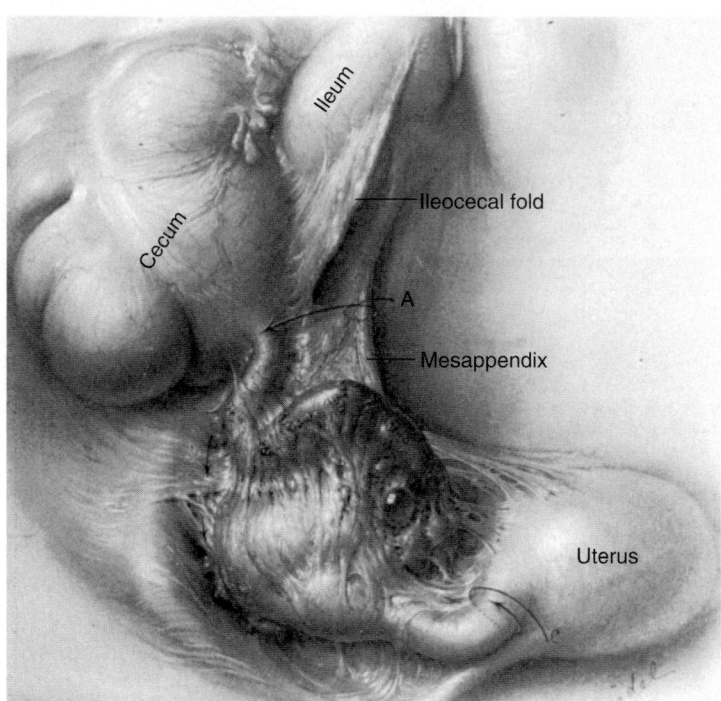

Cecum

Ileum

Ileocecal fold

A

Mesappendix

Uterus

FIGURE 41.1. As illustrated in this original Max Broedel drawing, inflammatory disease of the appendix can involve the fallopian tube or vice versa. Extensive adhesions can form. The tube and the appendix can be removed as a single mass.

HISTORY

The first known surgical removal of the appendix occurred in December of 1735 when Claudius Amyand operated on an 11-year-old boy with a longstanding scrotal hernia and fecal fistula. He found a perforated appendix in the hernia sac and removed it. The fistula closed and the boy recovered. The first known successful appendectomy for acute appendicitis was performed in 1880 by Lawson Tait, the renowned British abdominal and gynecologic surgeon who was also the first to operate successfully on a patient with a ruptured tubal pregnancy.

The recognition of appendicitis as a significant problem necessitating surgical removal was described by Fitz in 1886 and McBurney in 1889. Fitz described the sequence of appendiceal inflammation, perforation, abscess formation, and peritonitis.

In 1905, Kelly and Hudson coauthored a beautifully illustrated book entitled, *The Vermiform Appendix and Its Diseases.* The book is unexcelled in its definition of the pathology, clinical manifestations, and natural history of appendicitis and its complications. There have been numerous reviews through the years since that time.

ANATOMY AND FUNCTION OF THE APPENDIX

The base of the appendix arises from the inferior wall of the cecum about 2.5 cm from the ileocecal valve. The *taeniae coli* of the cecum form the outer longitudinal muscle of the appendix and, therefore, can be followed

inferiorly to help locate an appendix that is hidden. The appendiceal tip is found most commonly in a retrocecal position (65% of cases). Signs and symptoms of appendicitis may vary depending on the location of the appendix. The main blood supply to the appendix, the appendicular artery, is a branch of the ileocolic artery and is located in the mesoappendix. The base of the appendix is supplied by a branch of the posterior cecal artery.

The appendiceal wall is composed of smooth muscle; the narrow lumen is lined by colonic mucosa. A large number of submucosal lymphoid follicles are found in the appendix in teenagers and young adults. This number declines rapidly after 30 years of age. These lymphoid follicles function in the gut-associated lymphoid tissue secretory globulin immune system, but their function is not indispensable in the secretory immune system of the gut.

Anatomists have questioned the purpose of the appendix since its initial description. Leonardo DaVinci considered the appendix to serve and protect the cecum from rupture by too great an accumulation of "superfluous wind" because it had the ability to dilate and contract. Current belief is that the appendix is a vestigial organ with no function in humans. The appendix is absent in carnivores such as the dog, wolf, tiger, and lion. In herbivores, a long and well-developed cecum is noted. In omnivores, which include apes and humans, a portion of the cecum is smaller in diameter with a prominent lymphoid aggregation susceptible to inflammation or atrophy. The preserve of lymphoid aggregation has led to the hypothesis that the appendix has a role in immune surveillance of the gut. Others postulate an exocrine function to assist in the digestion of plants. In a 24-hour period, the adult human appendix produces a maximum of

2 mL of fluid containing mucin, amylase, and proteolytic enzymes. It is unlikely that this volume aids substantially in digestion. A pressure gradient normally exists along the long axis and prohibits the entrance of food or other intestinal contents into the lumen of the appendix.

ACUTE APPENDICITIS

Acute appendicitis is initiated by an obstruction of the appendiceal lumen. The obstruction can be caused by hyperplasia of lymphoid follicles of the appendix as part of a generalized response of lymphoid tissue to a systemic infectious disease, by bacterial enterocolitis, or by a fecalith, a foreign body, or intestinal parasites in the appendiceal lumen. An increase in intraluminal pressure distal to the obstruction from increased mucus secretion is followed by an increase in bacteria and, finally, the production of frank pus. The appendix becomes swollen and the appendiceal wall becomes edematous from obstruction of lymphatic and venous drainage. Ulceration of the mucosa allows invasion of the wall by bacteria. Further progression causes venous thrombosis and obstruction of blood flow through the appendiceal artery. Because this is an end-artery, no collateral circulation is available

to prevent ischemic necrosis and gangrene with eventual rupture of the wall. Escape of bacteria through the perforation causes peritonitis. Unless necrosis of the base of the appendix occurs, continued fecal contamination of the peritoneal cavity is prevented by the initial blockage of the appendiceal lumen. The infection in the right lower quadrant can be walled off efficiently in young, healthy patients. In females, this abscess usually involves the right adnexal organs to some extent. Generalized peritonitis may ensue in advanced age or in the presence of reduced host resistance from other illnesses or immunosuppression. A correlation between the clinical course and pathologic progress of appendicitis is illustrated in Figure 41.2.

Diagnosis of Acute Appendicitis

The diagnosis of acute appendicitis is based primarily on history and physical examination. Although all symptoms and signs should be listed, careful evaluation must be done with assignment of different weights to each as appropriate to the clinical setting. Pain is present in 95% of patients and is the most consistent symptom. The typical pain of acute appendicitis is diffuse and mild and initially located in the epigastrium and periumbilical region.

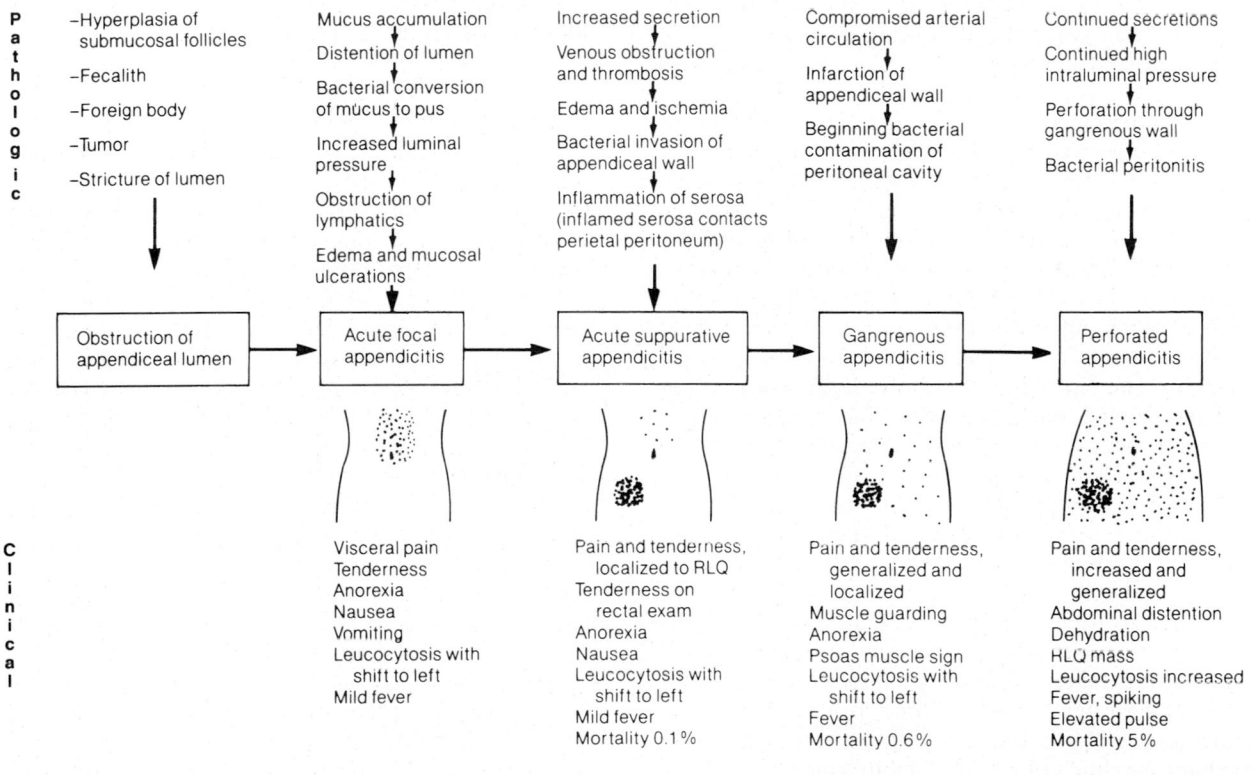

FIGURE 41.2. The clinical-pathologic correlations of appendicitis. (From: Sabiston DC Jr, ed. *Textbook of surgery.* Philadelphia: WB Saunders, 1991, with permission.)

Once local peritonitis occurs, the maximum tenderness usually is located in the region of the appendix. Anorexia, nausea, and occasional vomiting usually are present. (The diagnosis of appendicitis is in doubt if vomiting occurs first.) This classic sequence can be found in 50% of patients. However, it should be emphasized that the typical presentation is absent in the remaining 50%. Atypically, pain can be localized in the right lower quadrant in the beginning, or it can remain diffuse throughout the abdomen. Although the location of the cecum is constant, the inflamed appendiceal tip may be located in the right upper quadrant, in the cul-de-sac, or anywhere in between. The location and magnitude of the pain may vary with the position of the appendix and age of the patient. Elderly patients may have less severe pain and delayed localization in the right lower quadrant. Indeed, appendicitis in the elderly presents a real challenge to early diagnosis, because very few clinical findings may be present. This is the reason for the higher incidence of appendiceal perforation and, consequently, the higher morbidity and mortality in older patients, as confirmed in the 1986 report by Lau and associates.

In infants and children, the diagnosis is also more difficult and the incidence of appendiceal perforation higher. Improvement in the results for these two age groups depends on a higher index of suspicion and a lower threshold for intervention, which inevitably results in the removal of a larger number of normal appendixes. Improved diagnosis with ultrasound and computed tomography (CT) scanning may decrease the incidence of appendiceal rupture and also the frequency of exploratory laparotomy for what turns out to be a normal appendix. However, removal of a normal appendix in a symptomatic patient who is thought to have appendicitis, a potentially lethal disease, should not be considered an unnecessary operation. The number of elderly patients and children who die of appendicitis because of failure to operate early enough when the diagnosis is in doubt is much higher than the number of patients who die from a complication following removal of a normal appendix. The morbidity of negative laparotomy is minimal and is much more acceptable than the significantly higher morbidity of a perforated appendix. Unfortunately, after 60 years of age, about 50% of patients are found to have a ruptured appendix when the operation is finally done. The mortality rate in these patients is 5%; however, this represents more than 50% of all deaths from appendicitis.

Twelve to forty-eight hours usually elapse from the onset of symptoms until the patient consults her physician. On physical examination, patients with appendicitis classically have tenderness to direct palpation, rebound tenderness, and muscle guarding in the right lower quadrant over the point where the inflamed appendiceal serosa is in contact with the parietal peritoneum, often at McBurney's point, which is located at the junction of the middle and lateral thirds of a line drawn from the umbilicus to the right antero-superior spine. The Rovsing sign (pain in the right lower quadrant when pressure is applied in the left lower quadrant) as well as psoas and obturator muscle signs may be positive. A positive psoas sign is increased pain as the right leg is extended at the hip when the patient is in the left lateral decubitus position, indicating irritation of the psoas muscle by the inflamed appendix. A positive obturator sign is increased pain in the right lower abdomen when passively flexing the right hip and knee and internally rotating the leg at the hip, indicating irritation of the obturator muscle. Rectal and pelvic examinations always should be done and often reveal tenderness high on the right side of the pelvis. Pelvic inflammatory disease is almost always associated with bilateral adnexal tenderness. A pelvic mass from an inflamed appendix sometimes can be felt on pelvic examination. A tender, unilateral adnexal mass also may be found in a patient with ovarian torsion, but ultrasound should help make the diagnosis. As the disease progresses to gangrene and appendiceal rupture, a mass consisting of inflammatory adhesions, omentum, indurated bowel, mesentery, and pockets of purulent exudate usually can be felt in the right lower quadrant or right adnexa. Tenderness and muscle rigidity are more pronounced. If the infection fails to localize, generalized peritonitis ensues with diffuse tenderness, guarding, distention, ileus, dehydration, tachycardia, and spiking fever. All these signs may be less apparent in the elderly. Several studies over the past few decades have evaluated the clinical presentation of patients with acute appendicitis. A summary of the common history and physical findings is shown in Table 41.1.

Laboratory and Radiology Diagnosis

Minimal investigation is required when the history and physical examination are definitive. About two thirds of patients with appendicitis have an elevated white blood cell (WBC) count of greater than 10,000 WBC/mL. However, an elevated WBC is also found in acute pelvic inflammatory disease, diverticulitis, pyelonephritis, and in many patients with ovarian torsion. In elderly patients, however, the white cell count may be elevated only slightly or not at all, even though the differential count is abnormal. The erythrocyte sedimentation rate is elevated when the appendix is severely inflamed, but this is a very nonspecific test. Some white cells and red cells may be present in the urine of patients with appendicitis, although significant bacteriuria suggests a urinary tract infection is a more likely diagnosis.

Ultrasound is now a valuable adjunct to physical examination in young women with pelvic or lower quadrant pain. Graded abdominal compression is used to displace the cecum and ascending colon, exposing the retrocecal area and pelvis. A typical "target appearance" identifies the appendix by characteristic changes within its wall (Fig. 41.3). Findings associated with appendicitis include wall thickening beyond the normal 8 to 10 mm, luminal distention, lack of compressibility, and localized pain and tenderness at the site of the visualized appendix. Advanced cases are noted by asymmetric wall thickening, abscess formation, associated free intraperitoneal fluid, surrounding tissue edema, and decreased local ten-

TABLE 41.1.
Summary of Clinical Examination Operating Characteristics for Appendicitis

Procedure	Sensitivity	Specificity	LR+ (95% CI)	LR− (95% CI)
Right lower quadrant pain	0.81	0.53	7.31–8.46	0–0.28
Rigidity	0.27	0.83	3.76 (2.96–4.78)	0.82 (0.79–0.85)
Migration	0.64	0.82	3.18 (2.41–4.21)	0.50 (0.42–0.59)
Pain before vomiting	1.00	0.64	2.76 (1.94–3.94)	—
Psoas sign	0.16	0.95	2.38 (1.21–4.67)	0.90 (0.83–0.98)
Fever	0.67	0.79	1.94 (1.63–2.32)	0.58 (0.51–0.67)
Rebound tenderness test	0.63	0.69	1.10–6.30	0–0.86
Guarding	0.74	0.57	1.65–1.78	0–0.54
No similar pain previously	0.81	0.41	1.50 (1.36–1.66)	0.323 (0.246–0.424)
Rectal tenderness	0.41	0.77	0.83–5.34	0.36–1.15
Anorexia	0.68	0.36	1.27 (1.16–1.38)	0.64 (0.54–0.75)
Nausea	0.58	0.37	0.69–1.20	0.70–0.84
Vomiting	0.51	0.45	0.92 (0.82–1.04)	1.12 (0.95–1.33)

Source: Wagner JM, McKinney WP, Carpenter JL. Does this patient have appendicitis? *JAMA* 1996;276:1589–1594, with permission.

derness to compression. The sensitivity of ultrasound in the diagnosis of appendicitis from several centers has been reported to be as high as 80%, with a specificity as high as 90%.

CT is usually the initial imaging technique used in emergency departments in the United States today. CT imaging has a 90% sensitivity for detecting intraabdominal inflammation. A specific diagnosis can be made in 80% of these patients. A normal appendix may be difficult to locate on CT examination and may require extra scans at finer intervals. Appendicoliths are seen in one fourth of all people as a ringlike or homogenous calcified density on CT. Specific CT findings of appendicitis become more prominent with advanced diseases including

a distended, thick-walled, edematous appendix seen as a target structure (Fig. 41.4). Other findings include inflammatory streaking of surrounding fat and the presence of an appendicolith. CT findings suggestive of appendicitis include a pericecal phlegmon or abscess, and small amounts of right lower quadrant intraabdominal free air that signals perforation.

Standard abdominal radiography may show a calcified fecalith in the right lower quadrant along with a paucity of gas in the right lower quadrant of the abdomen. A loss of the right psoas shadow may be noted and represents late appendicitis with retroperitoneal inflammation. A perforated or gangrenous appendix may exhibit extraabdominal gas on radiographs, but this occurs in only 1% of cases. A sentinel loop ileus or a soft-tissue mass with or without gas bubbles also be may seen in advanced cases.

Barium contrast studies remain a simple, safe, and readily available test that may be helpful. However, ultrasound and CT examinations now are preferred. A barium study assures luminal patency of the appendix, colonic wall for mass effects or secondary effects of appendicitis, and right colonic or terminal ileal mucosal disease that may simulate appendicitis. When the barium contrast fills the appendix, a diagnosis of acute appendicitis is very unlikely but not impossible. Up to 10% to 20% of normal appendices do not fill during a barium study.

Laparoscopy can be both diagnostic and therapeutic for acute appendicitis. Some have advocated diagnostic laparoscopy in all women presenting with symptoms associated with acute appendicitis to reduce unnecessary appendectomy while also examining for gynecologic pathologies. The diagnostic error of presumed appendicitis in young, adult women in the reproductive years is 35% to 50%. According to Leape and Romanofsky, and Deutech and associates, about one third of patients who underwent laparoscopy for suspected appendicitis did not have appendicitis.

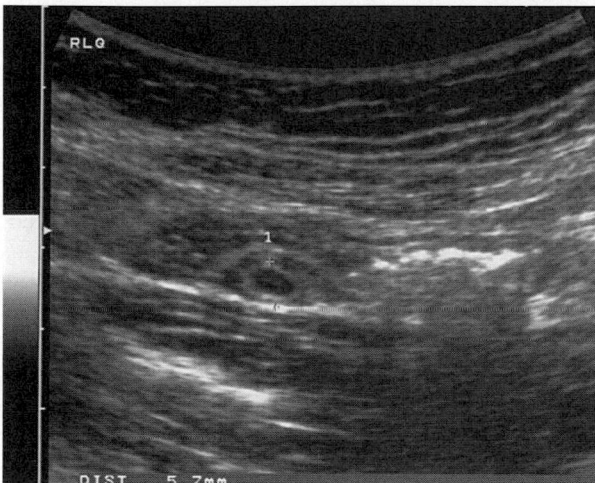

FIGURE 41.3. Transabdominal ultrasound of acute appendicitis. Note the "target-like" appearance produced by the thickened, inflamed wall of the appendix. (Courtesy of Arthur Fleischer, Vanderbilt University.)

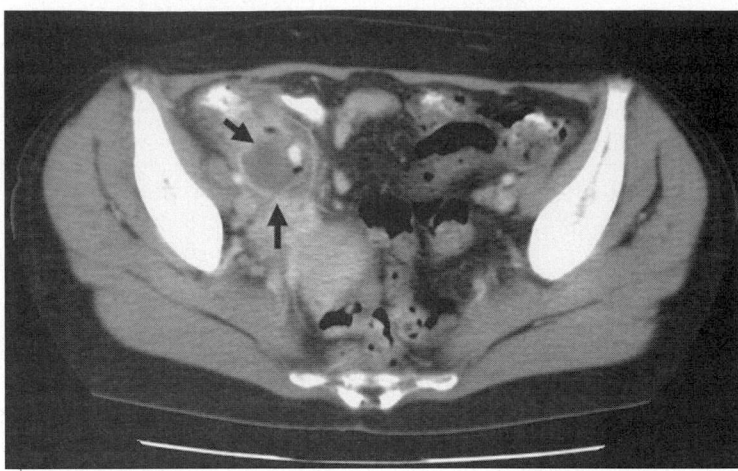

FIGURE 41.4. Computed tomography of appendiceal abscess. Note complex fluid mass with an enhancing rim in the right lower quadrant. (Courstey of Ronald Arildsen, Vanderbilt University.)

Because there is no single diagnostic test for acute appendicitis that is accurate and applicable to the general population, most physicians agree with Levine and associates that a decrease in the number of negative explorations is most likely to be achieved by sound clinical judgment supplemented by basic laboratory and radiologic studies. Using this standard classical approach assiduously, these authors reported negative laparotomy in only 7.4% of 282 patients with a preoperative diagnosis of suspected appendicitis. Most patients with the classic pattern of migratory abdominal pain, direct and rebound tenderness in the right lower abdominal quadrant, and increased metamyelocytes in the peripheral blood smear require prompt operation. However, when there is an atypical presentation in a young, adult women, close in-hospital observation may be indicated to allow progression of the clinical picture and complete the radiologic workup. Simultaneous evaluation by the general surgeon and gynecologist is also of benefit in improving diagnostic accuracy.

Laparoscopy may be indicated in problem patients. In almost all circumstances, a laparoscopy with negative findings is preferred to expectantly watching the appendix rupture or pelvic inflammatory disease progress untreated. An unnecessary delay increases the likelihood of perforation increasing morbidity and mortality In the younger patient, it also increases the risk of pelvic adhesions, infertility, and chronic pain. When surgery is performed within 24 hours of the onset of symptoms, less than 20% of appendixes are perforated, compared with over 70% when operation is delayed more than 48 hours after symptoms began. A delay in diagnosis in pregnant patients has especially devastating effects on the outcome. A proper evaluation of clinical presentation allows the index of suspicion to be set at the proper level so that a threshold for intervention can be reached before the appendix ruptures. According to Condon and Telford,

> The removal of a normal appendix in appropriate clinical circumstances never constitutes an unnecessary appendectomy. A policy of active surgical intervention on the basis of minimal clinical suspicion has been demonstrated to reduce both the morbidity and

mortality of appendicitis. Watching and waiting, however careful it may be, runs the risk of increasing both morbidity and mortality.

Treatment of Acute Appendicitis

There is general agreement that the treatment of acute appendicitis is appendectomy. Clinical experience and numerous reports on mortality clearly show the advantage of early operation. The current operative mortality without perforation is essentially nil, and only 3% of patients have postoperative complications. After perforation, the overall mortality rate is less than 5%, but more than 30% of patients have postoperative complications. These statistics have improved with the use of antibiotics and earlier intervention.

The patient with appendicitis should not be rushed to the operating room without adequate hydration and antibiotic treatment. Most surgeons use short-course (<24 hours) antimicrobial prophylaxis. One common combination is cefazolin and metronidazole to cover Gram-negative, -positive, and anaerobic bacteria. Recent studies have recommended monotherapy with a second-generation, broad-spectrum cephalosporin such as cefotetan for patients undergoing surgery. Antibiotics have been shown to be effective in reducing the incidence of postoperative wound infections if started preoperatively. Antibiotics can be discontinued immediately following surgery if the appendix is not gangrenous or perforated. However, if the appendix has ruptured, many surgeons switch to triple antibiotic therapy including ampicillin, metronidazole, and gentamicin to encompass a wide spectrum of enteric bacteria. Intravenous antibiotic therapy should be continued until the patient is well on the way to recovery, which is usually 3 to 5 days.

Postoperatively, if the appendix is not ruptured, the patient usually is discharged within 24 hours. However, if the appendix was ruptured or gangrenous, supportive treatment is continued in the ill patient. Food and fluid by mouth are restricted. Nasogastric suction is rarely used today. Wound infection is the most common complication after appendectomy. Other more serious complications include pelvic, subphrenic and intraabdominal abscess, fecal fistula, peritonitis, pyelonephritis, venous thrombosis, and intestinal obstruction. Septicemia, pneumonia, septic shock, renal failure, and pulmonary embolus can lead to death in the most advanced or neglected cases.

It is relatively safe to remove the appendix in virtually any patient. However, if there are significant medical contraindications to surgery in a nontoxic patient with a clear diagnosis of an appendiceal abscess, a nonoperative approach can be considered. If a distinct mass in the right iliac fossa is palpated and the patient has no systemic manifestations, the patient is kept nil per os (NPO) while intravenous fluids and broad-spectrum antibiotics are given to cover enteric organisms. The patient should be kept under close observation with the pulse closely followed because tachycardia is one of the first signs of sepsis. Other clinical parameters to follow include change in pain quality, white blood cell counts, differential counts, and serial radiologic evaluations including ultrasound and/or CT. Failure to respond to therapy after 24 to 48 hours indicates that operative intervention should be reconsidered. Patients with well-formed periappendiceal abscesses can undergo CT-guided placement of pigtail drainage catheters to help resolve the abscess more rapidly, rather than depending on the abscess to drain internally into the cecum. If the abscess is palpable, it is usually large and should be drained. Limitations of percutaneous drainage include the inadequacy of draining multiloculated abscesses, inaccessible location, and possible need for anesthesia. Periappendiceal abscesses usually resolve in 10 to 14 days without appendectomy or drainage. Most surgeons wait 6 to 12 weeks after nonoperative therapy to perform an interval appendectomy. Technical difficulties during interval appendectomy may be minimal but can be extreme depending on the nature of the initial abscess.

Open Technique

The standard management of appendicitis has been open appendectomy by way of a limited right lower quadrant incision. The surgeon should note the point of maximal tenderness prior to anesthesia and attempt to palpate masses after anesthesia. McBurney's point, at the junction of the middle and lateral thirds of a line drawn from the umbilicus to the right anterosuperior iliac spine, does not universally mark the tip of the appendix. In general, an inferior incision below the area of maximal tenderness helps in rotating the cecum into the wound. The McBurney incision is the classical oblique appendectomy incision through McBurney's point to the lateral edge of the rectus sheath; it can be extended into the lateral rectus sheath, if necessary. It is quite cosmetically acceptable when healed (Fig. 41.5). Alternatively, a skin line or transverse incision placed 1 to 2 cm medial to the anterosuperior iliac spine can be used. Both incisions generally are performed with a muscle-splitting technique through all layers lateral to the rectus abdominis muscle as entrance into the abdomen is gained. A low, horizontal skin incision also can be used and is possibly more

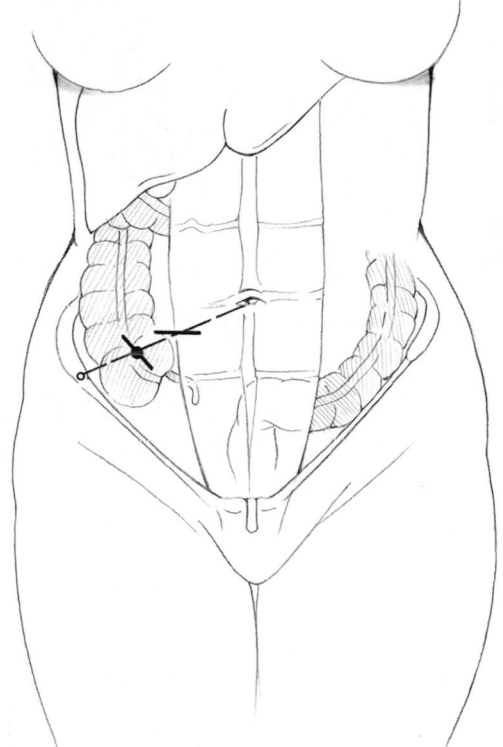

FIGURE 41.5. Common incisions for appendectomy. The classic McBurney incision over the cecum is not as easily extended to perform gynecologic procedures if needed.

cosmetic. The incision is continued through the superficial fascia until the external oblique muscle aponeurosis is exposed. The fibers of the aponeurosis are opened sharply, and the muscle fibers are bluntly separated, as are the fibers of the internal oblique and transverse abdominis muscles. The peritoneum is incised, and cultures can be obtained. The cecum is mobilized into the wound, and the appendix is mobilized as adhesions are bluntly and/or sharply dissected. The base of the appendix always lies at the confluence of the taeniae. When the appendix is mobile, the mesoappendix can be grasped near the tip of the appendix with a Kelly clamp and the appendix can be supported with a Babcock clamp near its base (Fig. 41.6). The mesoappendix can be ligated en masse with no. 3-0 absorbable suture if the pedicle is not too large or edematous. If this is not feasible, it is clamped and ligated with a succession of small bites with hemostats or Kelly clamps. Ligation of the mesoappendix usually is performed from the distal tip to the base of the appendix, but sometimes reversing the sequence can facilitate appendectomy. It may be appropriate to pass one suture into the musculature of the cecal wall and mesoappendix at the base of the appendix to ligate the accessory branch of the posterior cecal artery securely. Packs should be placed around the appendix to isolate it from the operative field. The appendix is double clamped with straight hemostats across the base, leaving sufficient space between clamps to permit passage of the cautery or

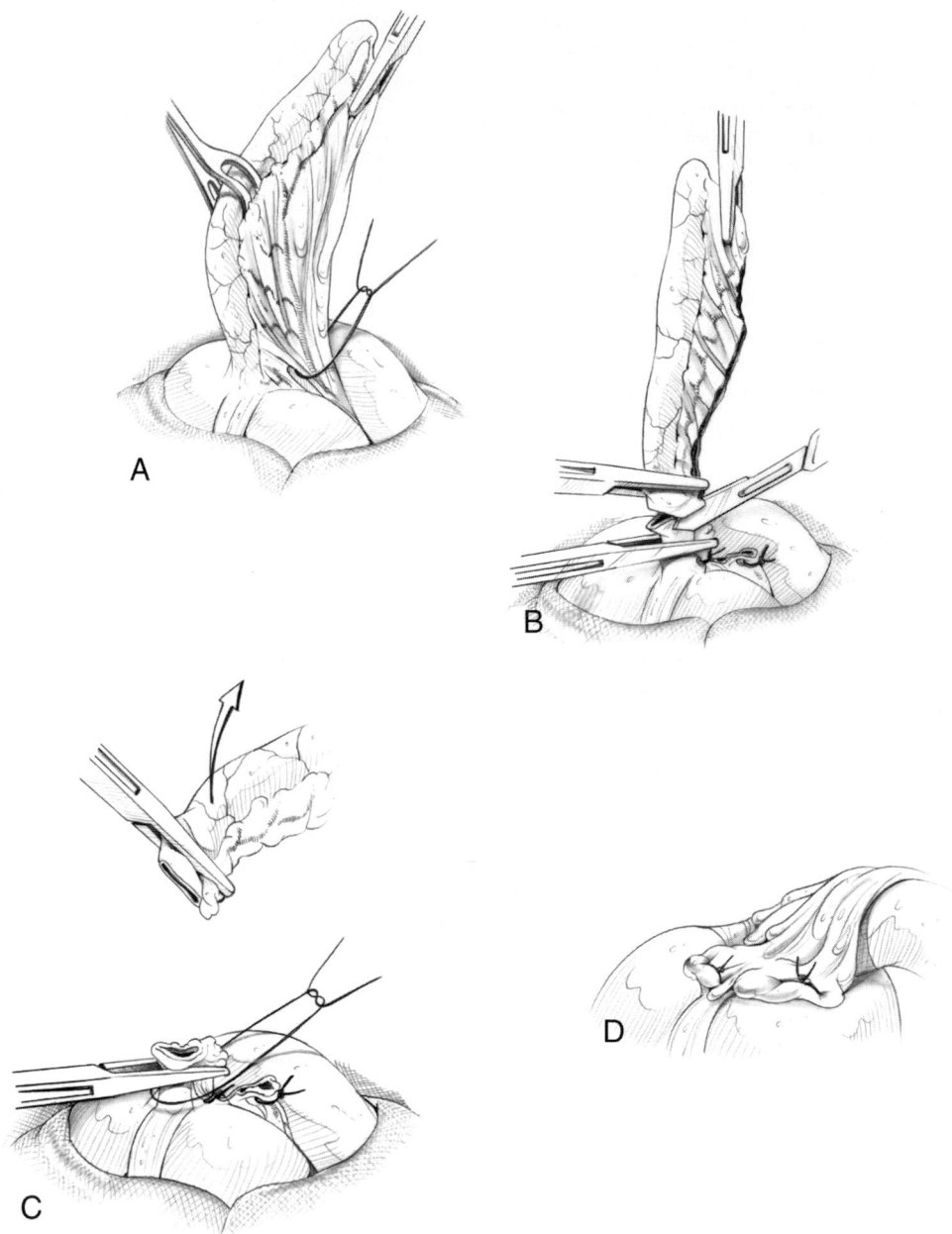

FIGURE 41.6. Technique of open appendectomy. **A:** The appendix is elevated by a Babcock clamp and the mesoappendix is ligated. Alternatively, small clamps may be used to clamp, cut and tie the mesoappendix. **B:** The operative field is isolated with gauze packs and the appendix is cross-clamped and divided between the two closely placed clamps. **C:** The stump of the appendix is ligated with a 2.0 absorbable ligature. **D:** The stump is usually cauterized and covered with the adjacent mesoappendix.

scalpel. The space between clamps can be crushed or milked prior to clamping to minimize contamination into the peritoneal cavity. The appendix is amputated with the scalpel or with cautery, and the appendix and the attached clamp are dropped into a small basin to avoid contamination. The appendiceal stump is then doubly ligated with 2-0 absorbable or delayed absorbable suture. The appendiceal stump may be cauterized to prevent mucocele formation or inverted with a

pursestring suture or Z-stitch in the cecum. If this is done, a purse-string suture of medium silk is placed around the base of the appendix. The circumference of the purse-string suture should be large enough to permit easy inversion of the stump. A half-knot is placed in the silk; after the appendix is amputated, the stump is inverted and the purse-string is drawn tight. The site of the inversion should be covered with mesoappendix or any convenient flap of fat. However, inversion of the stump is no longer considered necessary by many authors. It is not recommended when the appendix is inflamed. An abscess can form in the cecal wall or a space-occupying mass may be seen in the cecum on barium enema leading to diagnostic confusion. Copious irrigation with saline or antibiotic solution should be performed in cases of perforated appendicitis to reduce the risk of a pelvic or subhepatic abscess. The peritoneum and muscular fasciae are usually closed with a running absorbable suture. The skin can be closed in nonperforated cases of appendicitis, but delayed primary closure is routine in cases of ruptured appendicitis. Skin mattress sutures can be placed and left untied until the third to fifth postoperative day. If the wound is clean, the skin sutures are tied and adhesive strips placed. If the wound is not healthy, it should not be closed but packed with wet to dry dressings and allowed to granulate from the bottom until healing is complete, which may take approximately 1 month.

Laparoscopic Technique

Since it was first described by Semm in 1983, laparoscopic appendectomy has gained acceptance as both a diagnostic and treatment method for acute appendicitis. Many studies have demonstrated that a video-laparoscopic approach to acute appendicitis is safe and effective for the experienced endoscopist. The laparoscopic approach offers many potential advantages including less surgical tissue trauma, a better postoperative course, the ability to explore the entire abdominal cavity, assessment for the existence of associated pathologies, better cosmetic results, and a rapid return to normal activity. The ability to completely evaluate the pelvis and the entire peritoneal cavity when a healthy appendix is found is extremely important for the gynecologist in light of the other conditions that mimic appendicitis in women such as adnexitis, endometriosis, ovarian cysts, ectopic pregnancies, and even cholecystitis.

Removing a normal appendix during laparoscopic evaluation for suspected acute appendicitis can be performed with no added morbidity or increased length of hospitalization as compared to diagnostic laparoscopy. Initially, there were some concerns about an increased risk of intraabdominal abscess formation following laparoscopic surgery for acute appendicitis possibly secondary to peritoneal insufflation spreading local infection throughout the abdominal cavity and the carbon dioxide pneumoperitoneum creating a favorable environment for the survival of virulent anaerobic bacteria. However, many studies comparing open versus laparoscopic appendectomies have shown a lower morbidity rate with laparoscopy. The laparoscopic approach offers the advantage of shorter hospitalization and less morbidity, with a lower rate of abdominal wall infection. There is no significant difference in the rate of abscess formation in patients with perforated appendicitis. The interval until the patient may return to work is shortened and postoperative pain is decreased with the laparoscopic approach, and the quality of life appears to improve faster than when the traditional open approach is used. Obese patients may benefit substantially from the laparoscopic approach as it obviates the problems of a large incision, strong retraction, prolonged surgery, and wound infection that are associated with open surgery in the obese.

The disadvantages of the laparoscopic approach have been longer duration of surgery and higher costs. However, the length of surgery has been significantly reduced with improved surgical skills and experience. Also, the immediate cost difference appears to be diminished with the use of reusable laparoscopic equipment, and when the more rapid return to work and other activities is included, the laparoscopic approach turns out to be extremely cost effective. It is increasingly recommended as the procedure of choice for the diagnosis and treatment of suspected acute appendicitis.

The operation is conducted under general anesthesia with endotracheal intubation and muscle relaxation to allow controlled ventilation after the patient has been positioned in the modified dorsal lithotomy position with low stirrups. The position of the patient may be adjusted with Trendelenburg tilt or tilting the table to the left to optimize visualization of the appendix and better exposure to the structures on the right side of the pelvis and the right iliac fossa. The stomach and bladder are decompressed to minimize risk of injury during trocar insertion and allow optimal visualization of the operative field. Initially, an open or closed laparoscopic trocar insertion technique is utilized to place a 5- or 10-mm laparoscope. After viewing the location of the appendix, the accessory trocars can be placed in several different ways, again depending on the preference of the surgeon and anatomy of the appendix. We prefer placing the accessory trocars in the right and left lower quadrants and then one in the midline two finger breadths above the symphysis pubis. This places the trocars in positions familiar to the gynecologist and results in cosmetically appealing incisions. Atraumatic forceps are used through the lower right trocar to secure the tip of the appendix. If the appendix is markedly swollen, a pretied surgical loop can be placed at the tip and used for traction (Fig. 41.7). The appendix is elevated and retracted toward the pelvis, keeping the mesoappendix stretched. Adhesions can be separated from the appendix with sharp or blunt dissection. Dense and vascular adhesions require bipolar cautery, the harmonic scalpel, or clips. The appendix is skeletonized and isolated from the mesoappendix with bipolar cautery. (Metal clips, unipolar cautery, and the harmonic shears also may be used.) Special attention should be given to the appendicular artery that is located near the base of the appendix. The base of the appendix is secured by various methods: (a) three metal clips or three Endoloops with transection between them so that two ligatures remain at the base of the appendix; (b) the use of bipolar coagulation and resection; (c) the use of mechanical cutting and stapling devices; and (d) the use of endoloops with which self-locking extracorporeal slip-knots or normal surgical knots are made. Mechanical suturing devices can be used offering a secure and technically easy method, but this is an expensive option. We prefer the Endoloop technique using no. 1 chromic sutures. After isolating the appendix, two

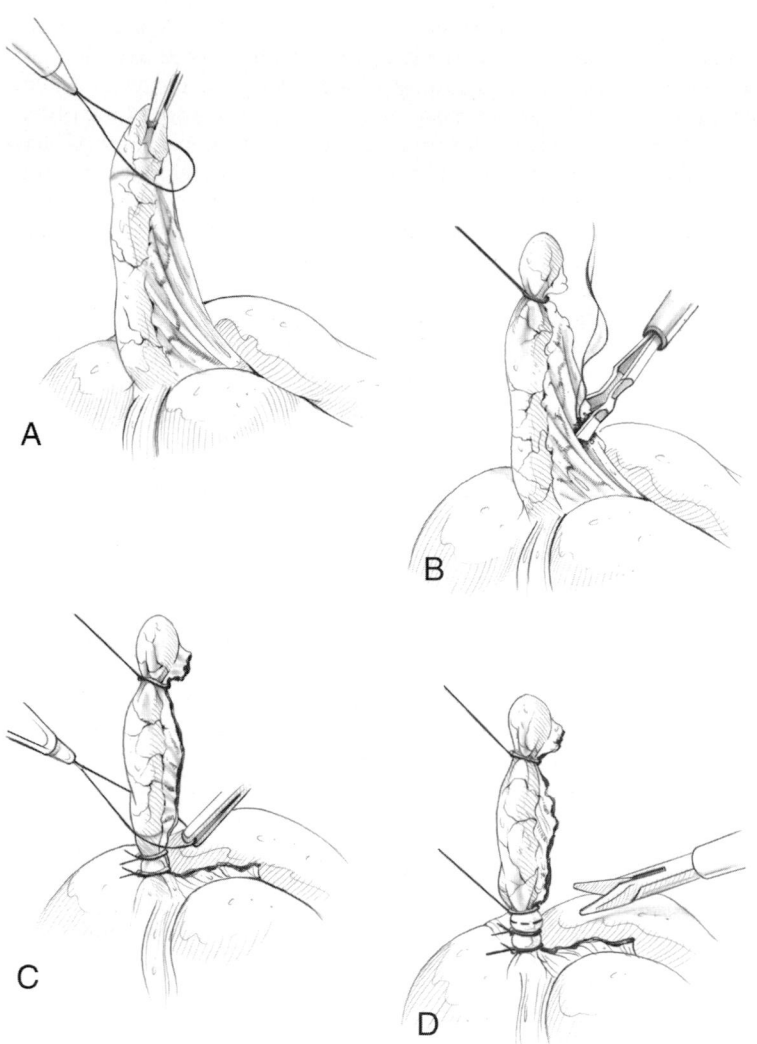

FIGURE 41.7. Laparoscopic appendectomy technique. **A:** The appendix is elevated with atraumatic forceps and a pretied suture loop is placed around the distal end to provide traction. **B:** The mesoappendix is divided using cautery. Clips or the harmonic scalpel also can be used. **C:** The skeletonized base of the appendix is then crushed with forceps to empty its contents and three ligatures are placed around the base. **D:** The appendix is divided, leaving two absorbable ligatures on the stump.

chromic Endoloop ties are placed securely at the base of the appendix. The area distal to the ties is then milked and the third Endoloop is placed 2 to 4 mm from the other ties. The appendix can be excised with scissors or harmonic scalpel, and removed through the larger trocar under direct visualization. The appendix can be placed in an endobag or surgical glove when there is the possibility of rupture. Some advocate cauterizing the stump; however, this can cause necrosis of the cecum at the site of the ligature on the appendicular stump and result in a subsequent cecal fistula. Care should be taken to remove the entire appendix because appendicitis of the appendicular stump has been reported. A total appendectomy can be achieved by ensuring that the mesoappendix is cleared off the base of the appendix until the three taenia on the cecum can be identified clearly. Stump invagination is not necessary and not performed routinely by this author because of the reasons previously discussed. If the surgeon desires to bury the stump, it is performed in a fashion similar to the open technique using no. 0 chromic catgut suture and one extracorporal knot. Careful irrigation and suction is performed after removal of the appendix.

The procedure is terminated in the usual laparoscopic fashion with the trocars removed and the scope skin incision closed with 4-0 delayed absorbable sutures or steri-strips. The fascia at the 10-mm incision must be closed with 0 or 2-0 delayed absorbable sutures. The postoperative course and hospital stay varies with the pathology and need for antibiotic coverage. Hospitalization generally is not required after uncomplicated laparoscopic appendectomy for an unruptured appendix. If the appendix is perforated at the base, the cecal strip would require suturing. If the appendix cannot be identified within an abscess cavity, the surgeon may place either a closed suction drain and plan an interval appendectomy, or convert to an open procedure.

APPENDICITIS IN PREGNANCY

In 1898, Hancock reported the first case of appendicitis complicating pregnancy. Appendectomy is the most common nonobstetrical operative intervention in the pregnant patient. The reported incidence of appendicitis in pregnancy varies from one in 355 to one in 11,479 deliveries. If ectopic pregnancy is excluded, appendicitis is responsible for about 75% of all cases of an acute abdomen during pregnancy. The incidence of acute appendicitis does not seem to be increased during pregnancy above that of the nonpregnant state, but the diagnosis often is delayed. Acute appendicitis occurs more often during the second trimester (50%) than during the first (10%) or third trimester (35%). Five percent of cases occur during labor or in puerperium. Although pregnancy does not appear to increase the incidence of appendicitis, it does increase the difficulty of diagnosis. This is because many abdominal symptoms are considered "normal" during pregnancy. Added to this are the anatomic changes in the location of the appendix. Baer and associates showed by repeat roentgenographic studies throughout pregnancy and the puerperium that the appendix rotated in a counterclockwise direction, with the tip displaced near the right kidney at term. The base of the appendix underwent upward and outward displacement after the third month, caused by the enlarging uterus, and reached the level of the iliac crest at the end of the sixth month. After the seventh month of pregnancy, in 88% of their cases, the appendix was found above the iliac crest. However, in interpreting these findings in relation to abdominal pain and tenderness, one must remember that in dealing with an abnormal appendix in which previous attacks of appendicitis may have occurred, adhesions can fix it in a low position and do not permit its upward displacement.

Ultrasound may be particularly useful in the diagnosis in pregnancy; but as noted, it may not be located in its normal, nonpregnant, right lower quadrant location. The most important step for the clinician is to consider the diagnosis of appendicitis in pregnancy.

The incidence of gangrenous and perforated appendix has been reported to be twice as high in pregnant patients as in women who are not pregnant and is highest in advanced pregnancy. In a pregnant patient, the omentum may not be able to reach the site of infection and perform its walling off function efficiently. If rupture is followed by abscess formation, the uterus is always a part of the abscess wall because of its proximity. Generalized peritonitis without abscess is more common in advanced pregnancy and is a serious threat to the expectant mother and her unborn child. The speed of onset and spread of peritonitis in pregnant patients can be insidious and strikingly rapid. The patient can become seriously ill and appear moribund within 24 hours. Peritonitis increases uterine irritability and the risk of preterm labor. Premature labor and delivery are the most serious fetal risks with up to 30% fetal mortality reported if perforation occurs. Maternal complications include wound infections, pelvic abscess, peritonitis, and pulmonary complications.

Treatment of Appendicitis in Pregnancy

Immediate operation is the treatment for acute appendicitis in pregnancy, regardless of the duration of pregnancy. Preoperative measures to improve the patient's condition should be brief and intensive. Although antibiotics may not be needed in simple acute appendicitis, antibiotic therapy should be initiated 30 minutes prior to surgery so that an adequate level can be present in the tissues when the incision is made. When a gangrenous or perforated appendix is found, antibiotics with broad-spectrum bacterial coverage should be continued or initiated immediately in both the pregnant and nonpregnant patient. One may choose to give cefoxitin and metronidazole. In the more serious cases, triple antibiotic therapy with ampicillin, gentamicin, and clindamycin should be used.

In this inflammatory environment, some suggest the use of nonsteroidal antiinflammatory drugs such as indomethacin or ibuprofen for tocolysis. Intravenous magnesium sulfate also can be used. Although the use of tocolytic agents to combat premature labor might seem reasonable, they should be used only in patients who are hemodynamically stable because they can increase pulmonary edema. As pointed out by deVeciana and associates, injudicious fluid management and tocolytic use can greatly increase the risk of pulmonary complications with antepartum appendicitis, especially in a third trimester patient with a perforated appendix. Spontaneous premature labor is more likely when the appendix has ruptured. Tocolytic agents are the most dangerous in the patients who need them the most.

Delay in operating also can stem from concern about what harm the operation will do to the pregnancy, with the consequent desire to operate only when acute appendicitis is definitely present. Such a delay only increases the risk of perforation with its attendant problems for both mother and fetus. Proper removal of a normal appendix found at operation for suspected appendicitis rarely is associated with preterm labor so the benefits clearly outweigh the minimal risks.

The anesthetic should be planned and administered to avoid hypotension and hypoxia. If the pregnancy is 3 months or less in duration, the appendix can be removed through the usual gridiron McBurney or Rockey-Davis incision. The more advanced the pregnancy, the higher should be the incision. If a midline incision is not used, it is important to center the incision over the point of maximum tenderness, which usually means using a high transverse muscle-cutting or a right paramedian incision. Tilting the patient to her left side minimizes displacement and handling of the uterus and relives the compression of the vena cava by the gravid uterus. The appendectomy should be done as quickly and atraumatically as possible, and the patient should be given intensive antibiotic therapy. In the case of appendiceal rupture with or without frank abscess formation, the patient should be treated immediately, in the same way as in the nonpregnant state, with the understanding that premature labor usually occurs as a result of the infection. Caesarean section should not be performed at that time of appendectomy with or without rupture to avoid infection in the newborn and postoperative endometritis and parametritis. Caesarean section in the third trimester patient with appendicitis is indicated only for strict obstetric reasons. Some authors have advised that a Caesarean section hysterectomy be performed to control the spread of infection into the uterus and broad ligaments.

Laparoscopic management of appendicitis now has been described with good results. The open laparoscopic technique is used, and all reports have shown success during all trimesters without complications. Some argue that the laparoscopic approach exposes the fetus to excessive risks from trocar placement and CO_2 insufflation. Others, however, note that laparoscopy expands the ability to explore the abdomen with less uterine manipulation and offers an increased ability for irrigation. Further, it increases the ability to locate the appendix and results in relatively small incisions compared to the open technique.

INCIDENTAL APPENDECTOMY IN GYNECOLOGIC AND OBSTETRIC SURGERY

Incidental appendectomy refers to the prophylactic removal of the normal-appearing appendix during surgery for another condition. In 1902, Howard Kelly of Johns Hopkins argued against incidental appendectomy because he felt it increased operative risk for the unproved benefit of reduction in the morbidity of acute appendicitis. He reported a survey of prominent surgeons of the day in which 37% said that they routinely performed incidental appendectomy. However, delayed diagnosis and a significant morbidity and even mortality associated with appendicitis in those days led Fischer in 1909 and Goldspohn in 1911 to endorse incidental appendectomy during other abdominal operations. However, the risk of morbidity and mortality have been substantially reduced in the past 50 years, and presently the use of incidental appendectomy at the time of gynecologic surgery is controversial. The decision to resect the appendix during routine gynecologic procedures depends on the risk: benefit ratio. It is estimated that at 60 years of age, about 125 incidental appendectomies need to be performed to prevent one case of appendicitis, 250 to prevent one ruptured appendix, and 5,000 to prevent one death. These benefits are greater in younger women in whom acute appendicitis is more common.

There are potential risks of the surgery. These include bleeding and hematoma formation, adhesion formation with subsequent intestinal obstruction, blowout of the appendiceal stump with abscess or fecal fistula or both, and others. However, in a careful review of the literature, Snyder and Selanders concluded that there was no statistically significant increase in morbidity or mortality when incidental appendectomy is performed at the time of routine abdominal hysterectomy, salpingectomy, tubal ligation, or Caesarean section. Good judgment must be exercised and good technique used in performance of the procedure, and circumstances should be favorable; including satisfactory condition of the patient during the operation, satisfactory tolerance of the anesthesia, and easy exposure of the appendix. If the patient has lost a great deal of blood or the operation has been unusually prolonged, appendectomy should be performed only when significant pathology of the appendix is found. Incidental appendectomy should not be performed in the presence of bowel obstruction or when severe postoperative ileus is likely.

One of the main advantages of incidental appendectomy is to eliminate the appendix from consideration when a patient presents subsequently with perplexing pelvic or abdominal pain. In addition to preventing appendicitis in future years, incidental appendectomy offers the advantage of removing unsuspected pathology. In a retrospective study of 260 women with pelvic or right iliac fossa pain, Lynch and coworkers reported that 90% of the women who had appendectomy in addition to hysterectomy, oophorectomy, or other gynecologic surgery reported relief of symptoms, compared to only 49% in the group who did not have an appendectomy. Quite probably all these appendices did not look grossly normal and this was not a prospective, randomized study; however, a significant incidence of "chronic obstructive appendicitis," endometriosis, and granuloma were found on microscopic examination of the removed appendices. Among the pathologic findings in clinically normal-appearing appendixes are acute, subacute, and chronic appendicitis, carcinoid tumors, and endometriosis. Others have reported about 10% of incidental appendectomy specimens show significant pathology. The incidence obviously depends on the definition of "incidental" and how carefully the appendix is examined by the pathologist.

Ectopic pregnancy and endometriosis have been reported in association with appendicitis. Panganiban and Cornog reported that four of 31 patients with endometriosis of the appendix had symptoms of appendicitis. The appendix is a common site of involvement in patients with pelvic endometriosis, although endometriosis is rarely confined only to the appendix. Pittaway found endometriosis in 13% of appendixes removed from patients with pelvic endometriosis at the Johns Hopkins Hospital. In 38%, the appendix was grossly normal when histologic evidence of endometriosis was found. The author concluded from the study that: (a) appendectomy is warranted in patients who are not interested in having children and are undergoing definitive surgery for endometriosis; and (b) appendectomy should be done when the appendix is abnormal, even in patients with endometriosis who are undergoing surgery to restore fertility.

The appendix is the most common site for carcinoid tumors, with an incidence of 0.03% of all appendixes removed. Almost all appendiceal carcinoids are benign. It is rare for the carcinoid syndrome to be present. In Waters' series of 830 patients in whom elective appendectomy was performed, six appendiceal carcinoid tumors were suspected or diagnosed on gross surgical appearance.

In summary, there are three main reasons to perform incidental appendectomy.

1. To reduce the risk of future mortality and morbidity from appendicitis, including possible infertility after a perforated appendix
2. To eliminate undiagnosed incidental pathology in the appendix

3. To eliminate the appendix from diagnostic consideration when the patient has abdominal or pelvic complaints in the immediate postoperative period and in future years

The incidence of appendicitis decreases with increasing age. The risk is greatest in girls 15 to 19 years old, and 70% of acute appendicitis occurs in patients under the age of 30. However, the rate of perforation increases with advancing age; in women over age 65, perforation occurs about 50% of the time. Using life table analysis, Snyder and Selanders estimated that for females 15 to 19 years old, 1000 incidental appendectomies would prevent 52 cases of appendicitis, five of which would be ruptured. For women 35 to 39 years old, 24 cases of appendicitis would be prevented by 1,000 incidental appendectomies; for patients 60 to 64 years old, only eight cases of acute appendicitis would be prevented, but four of these would rupture before diagnosis.

Studies show that incidental appendectomy is far more commonly done in women, probably because they more often have abdominal or pelvic surgical procedures such as hysterectomy, oophorectomy or cholecystectomy. It is also more commonly done in women 35 to 55 years old, probably for the same reason.

In a careful analysis of the potential cost savings of incidental appendectomy, Wang and Sax evaluated the impact of laparoscopy and managed care on this question. They reasoned that many of the primary procedures performed at the time of incidental appendectomy were now done via the laparoscope (laparoscopically-assisted vaginal hysterectomy and laparoscopic cholecystectomy). Taking into account long-term risk of appendicitis and complication, as well as various fee schedules and other surgical costs, they calculated that laparoscopic incidental appendectomy was not cost-effective at any age. Because there is very minimal cost associated with slightly increased operating time and a few sutures, with open appendectomy there are more cost savings for women under 30 years old when incidental appendectomy is done as part of an open abdominal procedure. With the frequent changes in managed care plans and strong pressure to minimize costs, they felt there was no incentive to spend money today (for incidental appendectomy) with the hope of saving money in the future (decreased risk of appendicitis at a later time).

Analyzing the various factors, it is easy to see why incidental appendectomy remains controversial. Many experts have suggested that it is most appropriate for women under 30 or 35 years old, especially if they have a history of pelvic pain, PID, or endometriosis. Because of the low risk of appendicitis, many experts do not recommend incidental appendectomy for women over 50 years old. In women between 35 and 50 years old who are undergoing gynecologic surgery, the status of the abdomen and pelvis, diagnosis, overall condition of the patient, and appearance of the appendix and surrounding structures all should be taken into account when deciding on the advisability of incidental appendectomy. The possibility of appendectomy should be discussed with the patient during the preoperative period and the benefits and risks ex-

plained. Informed consent should be documented in the chart. At the time of surgery, the appendix should be carefully examined; if abnormal or involved with the pelvic disease process, it should be removed. Women with mucinous ovarian tumor should have an appendectomy if possible to rule out an appendiceal primary.

BIBLIOGRAPHY

ACOG Committee Opinion. Incidental appendectomy. *Am Col Obstet Gynecol* 1995;164·1.

Affleck D, Handraham D, et al. The laparoscopic management of appendicitis and chololithiasis during pregnancy. *Am J Surg* 1999;178:523.

Aluarez C, Voitk A. The road to ambulatory laparoscopic management of perforated appendicitis. *Am J Surg* 2000; 179:63.

Anderson B, Niclen T. Appendicitis in pregnancy: diagnosis, management and complications. *Acta Obstet Gynecol Scand* 1999;78:758–762.

Attwood SA, Hifi AK, Murphy PG. A prospective randomized trial of laparoscopic versus open appendectomy. *Surgery* 1992;112:497.

Azaro E, Amaral P, Ettinger J, et al. Laparoscopic versus open appendectomy: a comparative study. *J Soc Laparoendoscop Surg* 1999;3:279.

Babaknia A, Parsa H, Woodruff JD. Appendicitis during pregnancy. *Obstet Gynecol* 1977;50:40.

Byrne DS, Bell G, Morrice JJ, et al. Technique for laparoscopic appendicectomy. *Br J Surg* 1992;79.574.

Chung R, Rowland D, et al. A meta-analysis of randomized controlled trials of laparoscopic versus conventional appendectomy. *Am J Surg* 1999;177:250.

Condon RE, Telford GL. Appendicitis. In: Sabiston DC Jr, ed. *Textbook of surgery.* Philadelphia: WB Saunders, 1991.

Deutsch AA, Zelikovsky A, Reiss R. Laparoscopy in the prevention of unnecessary appendectomies: a prospective study. *Dr J Surge* 1982;69:336.

deVeciana M, Towers CV, Major CA, et al. Pulmonary injury associated with appendicitis in pregnancy: who is at risk? *Am J Obstet Gynecol* 1994;171:1008.

DeVore GR. Acute abdominal pain in the pregnant patient due to pancreatitis, acute appendicitis, cholecystitis, or peptic ulcer disease. *Clin Perinatol* 1980;7:349.

El Ghoneimi A, Valla JS, Limmone B, et al. Laparoscopic appendectomy in children: report of 1,379 cases. *J Pediatr Surg* 1994;29:86.

Engstrom L, Fenyo G. Appendectomy: assessment of stump invagination versus simple ligation: a prospective randomized trial. *Br J Surg* 1985;72:971.

Farquharson RG. Acute appendicitis in pregnancy. *Scott Med J* 1980;25:36.

Fingerhut A, Millat B, Borne F. Laparoscopic versus open appendectomy: time to decide. *World J Surg* 1999;23:835.

Fitz RH. Perforating inflammation of the vermiform appendix, with special reference to its early diagnosis and treatment. *Trans Assoc Am Phys* 1886;1:107.

Flancbaum L, Nosher JL, Brolin RE. Percutaneous catheter drainage of abdominal abscesses associated with perforated viscus. *Ann Surg* 1990;56:52.

Fontanelli R, Paladini D, Raspagliesi F, et al. The role of appendectomy in surgical procedures of ovarian cancer. *Gynecol Oncol* 1992;46:42.

Forsell P, Pieper R. Infertility in young women due to perforated appendicitis? *Acta Chir Scand* 1986;5:30(suppl):53.

Frazee RC, Roberts JW, Symmonds RE, et al. A prospective randomized trial comparing open versus laparoscopic appendectomy. *Ann Surg* 1994;219:725.

Fritts LL, Orlando R III. Laparoscopy appendectomy: a safety and cost analysis. *Arch Surg* 1993;128:521.

Geerdsen JP. Sterility: a delayed complication after appendicitis acuta perforata in girls. *Nord Med* 1988;103:62.

Grubham J, Sutton C, Nicholson M. A case for the removal of the "normal" appendix at laparoscopy for suspected acute appendicitis. *Ann R Coll Surg Engl* 1999;81:279.

Halvorsen AC, Brandt B, Andreasen JJ. Acute appendicitis in pregnancy: complications and subsequent management. *Eur J Surg* 1992;158:603.

Halvorsen AC, Brandt B, Andreasen JJ, et al Pregnancy complicated by acute appendicitis: commentary. *Acta Obstet Gynecol Scand* 1991;70:183.

Herczeg J, Kovacs L, Kerseru T. Premature labour and coincident acute appendicitis not resolved by beta mimetic but surgical treatment. *Acta Obstet Gynecol Scand* 1983;62:373.

Horowitz MD, Gomez GA, Santiesteban R, et al. Acute appendicitis during pregnancy. *Arch Surg* 1985;120:1362.

Isaacs JH, Knaus JV. The detection of non-genital pelvic tumors mimicking gynecologic disease. *Surg Gynecol Obstet* 1981;153:74.

Jadallah FA, Abdul-Ghani AA, Tibblin S. Diagnostic laparoscopy reduces unnecessary appendectomy in fertile women. *Eur J Surg* 1994;160:41.

Kelly HA, Hurdon E. *The vermiform appendix and its diseases.* Philadelphia: WB Saunders, 1905.

Khalili T, Hiatt J, Savar A, et al. Perforated appendicitis is not contraindicated to laparoscopy. *Am Surg* 1999;65:965.

Kraemer M, Ohmann C, Leppert R, et al. Macroscopic assessment of the appendix at diagnostic laparoscopy is reliable. *Surg Endoscop* 2000;14:625.

Krukowski ZH, Irwin ST, Denholm S, et al. Preventing wound infection after appendicectomy: a review. *Br J Surg* 1988;75:1023.

Kum CK, Ngoi SS, Goh PY, et al. Randomized controlled trial comparing laparoscopic and open appendectomy. *Br J Surg* 1993;80:1599.

Kum CK, Sim EK, Goh PY, et al. Diagnostic laparoscopy: reducing the number of normal appendectomies. *Dis Colon Rect* 1993;36:763.

Langman J, Rowland R, Vernon-Roberts B. Endometriosis of the appendix. *Br J Surg* 1981;68:121.

Lau WY, Fan ST, Yiu TF, et al. Acute appendicitis in the elderly. In: Schwarts SI, ed. *The year book of surgery.* Chicago: Year Book, 1986.

Lechmann-Wfflenbrock E, Miecke H, Riedel HH. Sequelae of appendectomy, with special reference to intraabdominal adhesions, chronic abdominal pain, and infertility. *Gynecol Obstet Invest* 1990;29:241.

Lemieur T, Rodriguez J, Jacobs D, et al. Wound management in perforated appendicitis. *Am Surg* 1999;65:439.

Levine JS, Gomez GA, Dove DB, et al. Negative appendix with suspected appendicitis: an update. *South Med J* 1986;79:177.

Lim HK, Bae SH, Seo GS. Diagnosis of acute appendicitis in pregnant women: value of sonography. *AJR* 1992;159:539.

Lynch CB, Sinha P, Jalloh S. Incidental appendectomy during gynecological surgery. *Int J Gynecol Ostet* 1997;59:261.

Mahmoodian S. Appendicitis complicating pregnancy. *South Med J* 1992;85:19.

Mangi A, Berger D. Stump appendicitis. *Am Surg* 2000;66:739.

Mazze RI, Kallen B. Appendectomy during pregnancy: a Swedish registry study of 778 cases. *Obstet Gynecol* 1991;77:835.

McAnena OJ, Austin O, O'Connell PR, et al. Laparoscopic versus open appendicectomy: a prospective evaluation. *Br J Surg* 1992;79:818.

McBurney C. Experience with early operative interference in cases of disease of the vermiform appendix. *NY Med J* 1889;50:676.

McGee TM. Acute appendicitis in pregnancy. *Aust NZ J Obstet Gynecol* 1989;29:378.

Meynaud-Kraemer L, Cohn C, Vergnon P, et al. Wound infection in open versus laparoscopic appendectomy: a meta-analysis. *Int J Technol Assess Health Care* 1999;15:380.

Morrow CP. Is incidental appendectomy a safe practice? (editor's comments) In: Mishell DR, ed. *The year book of obstetrics and gynecology.* Chicago: Year Book, 1990.

Mueller BA, Daling JR, Moore DE, et al. Appendectomy and the risk of tubal infertility. *N Engl J Med* 1986;315:1506.

Nakhgevany KB, Clarke LE. Acute appendicitis in women of child-bearing age. *Arch Surg* 1986;121:1053.

Nase HW, Kovalcik PJ, Cross GH. The diagnosis of appendicitis. *Am Surg* 1980;46:504.

Nauta RJ, Magnant C. Observation versus operation for abdominal pain in the right lower quadrant. *Am J Surg* 1986;151:746.

Nezhat C, Nezhat F. Incidental appendectomy during video-laseroscopy. *Am J Obstet Gynecol* 1991;165:559.

Nguyen D, Silen W, Hodin R. Appendectomy in the pre-and post-laparoscopic eras. *J Gastroenterol Surg* 1999;3:67.

Nockers SR, Detmer DE, Fryback DG. Incidental appendectomy in the elderly? No. *Surgery* 1980;88:301–306.

Olsen JB, Myre CJ, Haahr PE. Randomized study of the value of laparoscopy before appendectomy. *Br J Surg* 1993;80:922.

Ozmen M, Zulfikaroglu B, et al. Laparoscopic versus open appendectomy: prospective randomized trials. *Surg Laparoscop Endoscop Percutan Technol* 1999;9:187.

Parsons AK, Sauer MV, Parsons MT, et al. Appendectomy at cesarean section: a prospective study. *Obstet Gynecol* 1986;68:479.

Paterson-Brown S, Thompson JN, Eckersley JRT, et al. Which patient with suspected appendicitis should undergo laparoscopy? *Br Med J* 1988;296:1363.

Pier A, Gotz F, Bacher C. Laparoscopic appendectomy in 625 cases: from innovation to routine. *Surg Laparos Endoscop* 1991;1:8.

Pittaway E D. Appendectomy in the surgical treatment of endometriosis. *Obstet Gynecol* 1983;61:421.

Pun P, McGuinness EPJ, Guiney EJ. Fertility following perforated appendicitis in girls. *J Pediatr Surg* 1989;24:547.

Rose PG, Reale FR, Fisher A, et al. Appendectomy in primary and secondary staging operations for ovarian malignancy. *Obstet Gynecol* 1991;77:116.

Schirmer BD, Schmieg RE Jr, Dix J, et al. Laparoscopic versus traditional appendectomy for suspected appendicitis. *Am J Surg* 1993;165:670.

Schreiber JH. Early experience with laparoscopic appendectomy in women. *Surg Endoscop* 1987;1:211.

Schreiber JH. Results of outpatient laparoscopic appendectomy in women. *Endoscopy* 1994;26:292.

Semm K. Endoscopic appendectomy. *Endoscopy* 1983;15:59.

Skoubo-Kristensen E, Hvid I. The appendiceal mass: results of conservative management. *Ann Surg* 1982;196:584.

Spirtos NM, Eisenkop SM, Spirtos TW, et al. Laparoscopy: a diagnostic aid in cases of suspected appendicitis. Its use in

women of reproductive age. *Am J Obstet Gynecol* 1987;
154:90.

Snyder TE, Selanders JR. Incidental appendectomy—yes or no?
A retrospective case study and review of the literature. *Infect Dis Obstet Gynecol* 1998;6:30.

Sugimoto T, Edwards D. Incidence and costs of incidental appendectomy as a preventive measure. *Am J Public Health* 1987;77:471.

Tamir IL, Bongard FS, Klein SR. Acute appendicitis in the pregnant patient. *Am J Surg* 1990;160:57

Temple L, Litwin D, McLeod R. A meta-analysis of laparoscopic versus open appendectomy in patients suspected of having acute appendicitis. *Can J Surg* 1999;42:377.

Wagner J, McKinney W, Carpenter J. Does this patient have appendicitis? *JAMA* 1996;276:1589.

Wang HT, Sax HC. Incidental appendectomy in the era of managed care and laparoscopy. *J Am Coll Surg* 2001;
192:182.

Wittich A, DeSantis R, Lockrow E. Appendectomy during pregnancy: a survey of two army medical activities. *Mil Med* 1999;164:671.

Udwadia T, Udwadia R. How we do it: laparoscopic appendicectomy. *Natl Med J India* 1999;12:281.

Yao C, Lin C, Yang C. Laparoscopic appendectomy for ruptured appendicitis. *Surg Laparoscop Endoscop Percutan Technol* 1999;9:271.

Te Linde's Operative Gynecology, ninth edition, edited by John A. Rock and Howard W. Jones, III. Lippincott Williams & Wilkins, Philadelphia © 2003.

CHAPTER
42

▼

Intestinal Tract in Gynecologic Surgery

KELLY L. MOLPUS

An indistinguishable overlap exists such that women may present with clinical signs and symptoms that are common to both primary gynecologic and digestive disorders. Intestinal disorders may be found intraoperatively at the time of gynecologic procedures. Additionally, gynecologic conditions may adversely affect the gastrointestinal tract. The gynecologic surgeon should have a basic understanding of the anatomy and physiology of the intestinal tract and should possess the fundamental skills necessary to recognize and correct common conditions affecting the digestive system. Meticulous dissection and cautious handling of tissues reduce the occurrence of intestinal injury and the risk of postoperative complications.

GASTROINTESTINAL DISORDERS THAT MIMIC GYNECOLOGIC PROBLEMS

Diverticulitis

Colonic diverticulitis may be confused with pelvic inflammatory disease (PID). These two processes generally do not occur in the same age group; however, rarely diverticulitis may occur in women younger than age 40 years. Patients with acute diverticulitis present with pain, altered bowel function, fever, and leukocytosis. Tenderness and guarding are usually localized to the left lower quadrant. One in five patients with acute diverticulitis also has signs and symptoms of colonic obstruction. Treatment for unruptured diverticulitis and PID are similar, and include intravenous fluid resuscitation, bowel rest, and broad-spectrum antibiotic coverage for anaerobes, gram-negative rods, and enterococci.

Diagnostic computed tomography (CT) scan clarifies whether a pericolonic abscess is present, and CT-directed drainage of an abscess expedites recovery and avoids surgical exploration in most cases. Nasogastric decompression is necessary in the setting of obstruction. If obstructive symptoms persist, or if bowel perforation has occurred, surgical exploration is warranted. If bowel perforation results in generalized peritonitis, consideration is given to diverting colostomy, with extensive irrigation and drainage of the peritoneal cavity.

Appendicitis

Perhaps one of the most frequently encountered diagnostic dilemmas is that of acute appendicitis versus PID. Appendicitis is most frequently seen during the second and third decades of life, which coincides with that of reproductive aged women at risk for PID. Whereas cervical motion tenderness is helpful in the diagnosis of PID and right-sided pain on rectal examination is helpful in the diagnosis of appendicitis, neither is pathognomonic. Peritoneal irritation from any source can be elicited by manipulation of the pelvic organs, so that manual manipulation of the cervix elicits an intensely painful response (cervical motion tenderness) in women with either PID or appendicitis. Similarly, rectal examination may illicit pain in a woman who has PID. Acute appendicitis will be overlooked by clinicians who assume the ailment is PID after finding cervical motion tenderness.

Historical information such as lateralization of pain (i.e., initial vague discomfort near the umbilicus that gravitates toward McBurney's point over time) with progressive anorexia raises suspicion for appendicitis. A history of prior PID, multiple sexual partners, recent acquisition of a new sexual partner, recent menses, and physical findings of a purulent cervical discharge suggest PID. Radiographic studies may be needed to clarify the diagnosis because acute appendicitis is a surgical emergency; PID, however, may be initially treated with broad-spectrum antibiotics and supportive care. Spiral CT scan has gained acceptance as an accurate determinant of the appendiceal anatomy. Contrasted CT imaging is also invaluable in the diagnosis of pelvic abscess. Bilateral pelvic abscesses are more characteristics of PID than an appendiceal process.

Meckel's Diverticulum

Meckel's diverticulum represents a residual portion of the vitelline (yolk) duct and is present in 1% of women. Diverticula average 5 cm in length and are located along the antimesenteric border of the ileum within 2 feet of the ileocecal valve. They are lined by ileal type mucosa, but at least one in five cases have ectopic pancreatic or gastric tissue. Acute symptoms result from inflammation, hemorrhage, or obstruction in approximately 5% of Meckel's diverticula. Inflammation and hemorrhage result from gastric acid secretion, and obstruction follows intussusception or torsion. Presenting signs and symptoms may mimic acute appendicitis or PID.

Most complications from Meckel's diverticula are during early childhood, and the likelihood of problems significantly decreases with advancing age. Accordingly, most surgeons believe resection of an asymptomatic Meckel's diverticulum in adulthood is unnecessary. Some recommend prophylactic removal if encountered during surgery, because morbidity associated with resection is low. It is generally agreed, however, that resection should be undertaken if the individual has previously been symptomatic, if the diverticulum is unusually long or has a narrow neck, or if thickening at the tip suggests ectopic gastric mucosa. Resection is accomplished by excising the base of the diverticulum with transverse closure of the enterotomy. Care is taken to avoid unnecessary resection of bowel wall to prevent luminal narrowing.

Volvulus

Sigmoid volvulus is an acute malrotation that presents with sudden onset of intense pain, similar to that of ovarian torsion. Volvulus is generally accompanied by obstipation, abdominal pain, and distention. Nausea and vomiting may occur. Volvulus is most commonly seen after the age of 60 years; however, cases in young individuals have been reported. Flatplate abdominal radiographic features are that of a markedly dilated, gas-filled sigmoid colon. Barium enema shows a tapered obstruction at the rectosigmoid junction with a typical bird's beak deformity. Sigmoid volvulus can usually be corrected nonoperatively with sigmoidoscopy or cautious barium enema. If volvulus is discovered at the time of surgery, initial management consists of untwisting the loop of bowel and observing for viability. Resection is infrequently necessary and should be reserved for devitalized bowel. Cecal volvulus is rare and tends to occur in the elderly population. This too is best managed by derotation, and resection is reserved for nonviability.

Pelvic Malignancies

Colorectal carcinomas may be difficult to distinguish from other pelvic malignancies. Advanced colorectal carcinoma may invade the vagina and/or bladder producing symptoms suggestive of a gynecologic or urologic problem. Advanced ovarian, cervical, and endometrial cancers may also invade surrounding organs leading to rectal bleeding. Resultant inflammation, tissue necrosis, and abscess formation contribute to the diagnostic dilemma. Historical information, thorough physical examination, colonoscopy or barium enema, cystoscopy, CT scan, and tissue biopsy can clarify the origin of pelvic malignancies in most cases.

Inflammatory Bowel Disease

Inflammatory bowel disease includes Crohn's disease (regional enteritis) and ulcerative colitis. Crohn's disease is an inflammatory process of uncertain etiology that usually involves the small bowel. It most frequently occurs in young adults with symptomatic onset during the late teens, but may occur at any age. Those affected have intermittent diarrhea, intestinal cramping, and weight loss. The extent of intestinal symptoms generally enables the clinician to distinguish inflammatory bowel disease from PID. Clinical findings, such as a functional ovarian cyst, may lead to overdiagnosis of a gynecologic disorder and result in unnecessary surgery. Gynecologic surgery is best avoided if possible in Crohn's patients because of the high risk of intestinal complications, even if the bowel is uninjured.

Medical management is the mainstay of treatment because there is a high recurrence rate that follows surgical resection. Therapy consists of bowel rest, nutritional support with total parenteral nutrition (TPN), and antiinflammatories such as sulfasalazine and corticosteroids. Surgery is reserved for patients whose disease is complicated by obstruction, perforation, fistula, or hemorrhage. Affected areas of the small intestine may be interspersed by normal segments of bowel. The appearance of Crohn's intestine is thickened walls with dull, purple-red discoloration, inflammatory exudate, and adherent mesenteric fat. If surgical resection is necessary, only the involved segments of bowel are removed.

Because of the high rate of anastomotic dehiscence following resections for Crohn's disease, some surgeons advocate stricturoplasty as an alternative to resection. Stricturoplasty is accomplished by opening the bowel longitudinally and closing transversely, creating a wider lumen. The appendix is eventually affected by Crohn's disease and ulcerative colitis in 25% and 50% of cases, respectively. Prophylactic appendectomy may be considered if the terminal ileum and cecum are not involved by active disease at the time of exploration. Fistulae (i.e., enterocutaneous, enterovaginal, enterovesical) are frequently associated with inflammatory bowel disease and its surgical management. Surgical correction is reserved for problematic fistulae that fail to respond to extended medical management. The intestinal defect, as the source of fistulous drainage, must be corrected for any chance of successful resolution.

Hemorrhoids

It has been said of hemorrhoids that few human afflictions cause greater distress without posing threat to life. Hemorrhoids are dilated perianal and rectal veins. Chronic pressure causes distention and loss of resistance in the venous wall, resulting in varices. The collection of blood further draws fluids into the dilated perianal skin. Internal hemorrhoids protrude into the rectal lumen and cause painless bleeding, which may be severe. Larger internal hemorrhoids can protrude through the anus, resulting in pain, itching, and burning. Spasm of the external sphincter may constrict the hemorrhoid, resulting in strangulation, necrosis, and extreme discomfort. This process is recognized clinically as thrombosed hemorrhoids, which are not actually thrombosed vessels but rather perianal hematomas. An understanding of the Bartholin's gland anatomy helps delineate a Bartholin's abscess from hemorrhoidal inflammation or a perirectal abscess.

If thrombosed hemorrhoids are recognized during the first 3 days of onset, incision and drainage or excision with primary closure are acceptable treatments. Excision is favored in most cases because excision reduces the chance of recurrence, has less postoperative bleeding, and avoids development of skin tags. Protruding symptomatic hemorrhoids can be excised by the radial hemorrhoidectomy technique. Removal of excessive anoderm predisposes to anal stricture and should be avoided. Regular postoperative bowel function and followup digital examinations are helpful in reducing stricture formation. Techniques of elastic ligation have also been developed and modified for selected use in the management of hemorrhoids. Symptomatic hemorrhoids persisting more than 72 hours may best be treated nonoperatively. Nonoperative intervention includes fiber laxatives, sitz baths, antiinflammatory medication, and topical steroids. Care is taken in the use of topical anesthetic ointments because these may worsen symptoms in some patients. Perianal lidocaine injection can alleviate sphincter spasm in markedly symptomatic individuals.

GYNECOLOGIC CONDITIONS THAT AFFECT THE GASTROINTESTINAL TRACT

Extensive endometriosis may involve the small or large intestine. Inflammation from small bowel endometriosis may result in adhesions, with painful peristalsis and intermittent or complete obstruction. Rectal implants and invasive endometriosis can manifest clinically as cyclic pain, intermittent diarrhea, bleeding, and pain associated with bowel movements. Rectovaginal endometriosis can cause perineal discomfort and a tender palpable mass on rectovaginal examination, which could mimic a perirectal abscess.

Pregnancy, either ectopic or intrauterine, must be considered in any symptomatic woman of reproductive age. Serum beta human chorionic gonadotropin (B-hCG) can be obtained rapidly in most hospital settings to rule out pregnancy. Tuboovarian abscess and adnexal torsion are often difficult to distinguish from inflammatory gastrointestinal conditions such as appendicitis or diverticulitis. All of these conditions may cause fever, nausea, anorexia, diarrhea, pain, and leukocytosis. Gynecologic infections may also adversely affect the intestinal tract, causing inflammation, adhesions, and obstruction. The fundamental history and physical examination help clarify the situation and separate gynecologic from gastrointestinal disorders in most cases.

PREOPERATIVE CONSIDERATIONS

Preoperative Bowel Prep

The surgical morbidity of gastrointestinal procedures is probably reduced in patients who undergo mechanical and antibiotic bowel preparation prior to surgery. The objectives of preoperative bowel prep are to reduce enteric volume and bacterial load. Potential benefits include better operative handling and exposure, reduced infectious complications, and enhanced anastomotic healing. A good mechanical bowel prep does eliminate stool and gas from the colon, thus improving exposure and making it easier to pack the bowel out of the operative field. Mechanical cleansing also allows for better visibility during intraoperative colonoscopy, if needed. The literature, however, is inconclusive as to whether or not bowel prep consistently reduces operative morbidity.

Various bowel preps have been proposed and used, including mechanical cleansing alone versus mechanical prep plus oral antibiotics, with or without parenteral antibiotics. In the past, such agents as castor oil, senna, bisacodyl, and magnesium citrate were used, but frequently resulted in inadequate bowel cleansing. Large volumes of isotonic solution and osmotic agents such as mannitol were more effective in bowel preparation; however, the prohibitive side effects included electrolyte and fluid abnormalities, nausea, vomiting, and abdominal distention.

Newer mechanical preparations usually consist of either polyethylene glycol or sodium phosphate. Polyethylene glycol is an effective, osmotically balanced solution that causes fewer electrolyte and fluid abnormalities. The major disadvantage is that 4 L must be consumed. Many patients are unable to complete this prep because of the large volume and the resultant gastrointestinal symptoms. Sodium phosphate has the advantage of being an effective cathartic while only requiring 90 cc of oral liquid. In randomized clinical trials comparing polyethylene glycol to sodium phosphate, patients who took sodium phosphate had significantly less trouble drinking the solution and reported less abdominal discomfort. Sodium phosphate provided a significantly better prep for colonoscopy. This trend was also observed in surgical patients, although not statistically significant. Polyethylene glycol and sodium phosphate should be used cautiously in debilitated patients and those with cirrhosis, renal impairment, electrolyte abnormalities, or ascites. They should not be used in patients with renal failure, congenital megacolon, bowel obstruction, or congestive heart failure.

Nonabsorbable or minimally absorbed oral antibiotics have traditionally been used in bowel preparation to reduce the intraluminal colonic flora. It is presumed that reduction in the bacterial load causes less peritoneal contamination and complications if the bowel is opened during surgery. Following colorectal surgery, cultures from wound infections and intraperitoneal abscesses most commonly reveal aerobic bacteria and other coliforms, such as *Escherichia coli, Streptococcus faecalis, Pseudomonas, Klebsiella,* and *Proteus,* and anaerobes, such as *Bacteroides* and *Clostridia.* In some randomized trials of oral preoperative neomycin and erythromycin compared with no oral antibiotics, the infection rate was significantly decreased. The patients studied had also been given a mechanical prep plus intravenous antibiotics. Other clinical studies have not shown an additional benefit to oral antibiotics when intravenous antibiotics are used. Similarly, oral antibiotics alone have not been proven to be superior to intravenous antibiotics alone for infection prophylaxis. Oral ciprofloxacin compared with no oral antibiotic has been noted to reduce postoperative infections. Metronidazole with either erythromycin or neomycin has also been effectively used. There are no data to support that one regimen is superior to another. In selected patients, the bowel prep regimen that we prefer is summarized in Table 42.1.

There are few randomized trials comparing mechanical bowel preparation with no preparation. The utility of bowel prep is called into question with collective retrospective data from trauma surgeries involving colonic injury and from emergent colorectal surgery for bowel obstruction. A recent review of 2,964 unprepped patients who underwent primary repair of colon injury reported an anastomotic leak rate of only 2.3%. Despite lack of consistent evidence supporting reduced morbidity, there is a general consensus regarding the potential benefit, such that the majority of gynecologic oncologists, surgical oncologists, and colorectal surgeons continue to recommend a preoperative bowel prep.

Positioning the Patient

Examination under anesthesia facilitates evaluation of anatomy and may clarify the likelihood of intestinal involvement by disease. Low dorsal lithotomy position is used if there is an expectation of possible rectosigmoid resection and anastomosis. Proper positioning reduces the risk of injury. The anesthetized patient is placed with

---

TABLE 42.1.
Bowel Preparation for Surgery

Your surgery is planned for:

Day _____ Date _____ Time _____

Follow these instructions on the day before surgery

Day _____ Date _____

6:00 a.m. - Only clear liquid foods today. Clear liquid foods would include beef or chicken broth, plain Jell-O, hot tea, popsicles, 7-Up, or clear fruit juices. Do not eat or drink any milk products. Do not eat or drink anything you cannot see through. Do not drink any alcoholic beverages.

10:00 a.m. - Take one Reglan 10-mg pill. This will help keep your stomach from being upset by the other medicines. You may repeat this every 4 hours, if needed for nausea.

11:00 a.m. - (1) Drink ½ of the 3-ounce bottle of Fleet Phospho-Soda. This is a strong laxative and will cause you to have diarrhea. (2) Take one of each of the antibiotic pills, Neomycin and E-mycin.

2:00 p.m. - Take one Reglan 10-mg pill.

3:00 p.m. - (1) Drink the second ½ of the bottle of Fleet Phospho-Soda. (2) Take the second dose of each of the antibiotic pills, Neomycin and E-mycin.

6:00 p.m. - Take one Reglan 10-mg pill.

7:00 p.m. - Take the third dose of each of the antibiotic pills, Neomycin and E-mycin.

12:00 Midnight - No eating, drinking, or smoking between now and surgery.

We understand this bowel prep may be difficult for you. However, we strongly encourage you to follow all of these steps as outlined. A proper bowel prep may help maximize your effective healing and minimize your chance of problems after surgery.

If you have any questions about these instruction, please call our office.

her hips at the end of the table and buttocks extending several centimeters beyond the table end. Padding is secured below the coccyx to avoid pressure point injury. Careful positioning ensures the thighs are slightly flexed and the weight of the legs is distributed evenly, with no pressure points from the stirrups. Lithotomy position also allows access for intraoperative pelvic examination and provides easy exposure to assess bladder or rectal integrity after pelvic dissection. Additionally, an assistant or surgeon can be positioned between the stirrups to elevate the vaginal apex or assist with a rectal anastomosis, or to enable dissection in the paraaortic and upper abdominal areas.

INTRAOPERATIVE CONSIDERATIONS

Lysis of Adhesions

Adhesions may be associated with prior surgical procedures, trauma, irradiation, infection, bleeding, or chemical irritants. Prior gynecologic surgery is the most frequently noted predisposing factor. After surgery, desiccated tissue surfaces in direct opposition are those at greatest risk for adhesion formation. History alone is not predictive, in that certain individuals have adhesions without identifiable predisposing factors. Others have a predilection for an exaggerated healing response and excessive adhesion formation.

Adhesiolysis may be necessary to mobilize the bowel, expose the surgical field, and circumvent obstruction. Constricting adhesive bands require transection. It is best to start with translucent adhesions that can be sharply lysed without difficulty. As adhesions become more dense, efforts are made to isolate a window such that an index finger and thumb can be placed behind and in front of the adhesion, respectively. Gentle blunt tissue dissection by rubbing the index finger and thumb back and forth helps to identify translucent adhesive bands that can be sharply lysed. There is often a recognizable white line between adhesions and their peritoneal attachment, which identifies a safe tissue plane for dissection (Fig. 42.1). Another plane ideal for sharp dissection is one followed in close parallel proximity to a recognizable structure, such as along a loop of small bowel. Inadvertent tissue injury is less likely with adhesiolysis close to the bowel wall than with cutting through the center of dense adhesions. Controlled traction and countertraction facilitates isolation and dissection, but excessive force is avoided. With dense adhesive bands, excessive force may literally tear a hole in the bowel wall, which may go unrecognized during surgery.

Intestinal Injury in Open Gynecologic Surgery

Most intestinal injuries in gynecologic surgery occur during abdominal procedures. One comprehensive clinical review estimated that 37% of injuries occurred during entrance into the peritoneal cavity, and 35% during lysis of

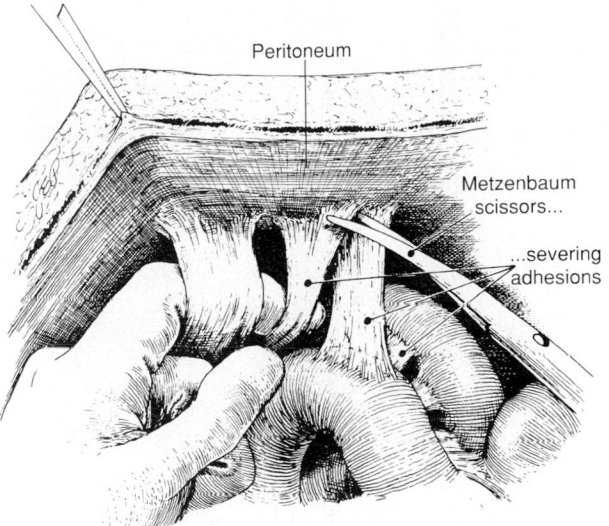

FIGURE 42.1. Traction-countertraction gives good exposure of an abdominal adhesion, which is lysed with scissors.

adhesions. Ten percent of injuries occurred during laparoscopic procedures, 9% during vaginal surgeries, and an additional 9% during dilatation and curettage as a consequence of uterine perforation. Enterotomy refers to a full-thickness opening in the bowel wall such that the lumen is entered. Enterotomy may be an incidental occurrence during dissection or an intentional orchestrated maneuver during gastrointestinal surgery. Unintentional enterotomies are best avoided by cautious entry into the peritoneal cavity and meticulous dissection of adhesions.

Adequate visualization and access are necessary for safe adhesiolysis. Ongoing visual and manual bowel inspection is advisable to ensure there is no compromise to wall integrity. If an inadvertent enterotomy occurs, the affected bowel must be mobilized from surrounding tissues to allow adequate exposure and a tension free repair. Although it is generally best to repair an enterotomy immediately, if the dissection is particularly difficult, it is advisable to finish the dissection so the extent of injuries can be assessed. The initial impression of a single enterotomy can be incorrect. Mobilization of tissues from the surrounding area may demonstrate multiple enterotomies within a single bowel segment or involvement of more than one loop of bowel (Fig. 42.2).

If an enterotomy is not immediately repaired, it should be marked with a suture of 3-0 silk tied loosely with the tails left long for easy identification. Eventual suture repair should be accomplished in a transverse direction to avoid excess narrowing of the lumen. This is most important in the small bowel. Staple repair is also acceptable if luminal diameter is not compromised. If multiple enterotomies occur within a localized segment of small bowel, the best plan may be to resect the damaged segment rather than individually repair three or four injuries. Resection of an affected bowel segment may also be necessary if the blood supply is compromised, if greater than 50% of the circumference is in-

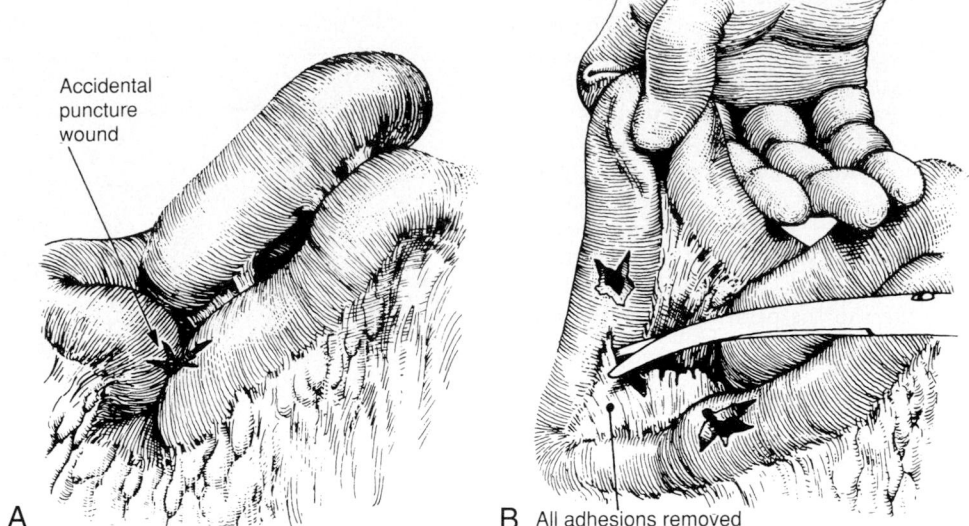

FIGURE 42.2. Sharp dissection of a loop of bowel containing an enterotomy is made to ascertain whether there is one enterotomy (**A**) or two enterotomies (**B**). Note that it appears that there is only one enterotomy (**A**); however, after dissection of adhesions (**B**), two enterotomies are apparent.

jured, if irregular edges preclude reapproximation, or if repair would result in excessive luminal narrowing.

In general, small bowel injury with intraperitoneal contamination by enteric content is associated with less morbidity than similar occurrence in the large bowel. Historically, large bowel injury (colotomy) with gross intraperitoneal contamination has been managed by diverting colostomy, with delayed surgical repair and colostomy closure after several months. Collective clinical experience from scheduled procedures and trauma surgeries have demonstrated that immediate repair without colostomy is associated with acceptably low morbidity. Suture and staple closure techniques, as well as segmental resection with anastomosis, have been successfully used. Furthermore, some studies suggest that immediate recognition and repair of intestinal injury is associated with less morbidity than the diversion techniques previously thought to be mandatory.

Aggressive peritoneal irrigation and administration of intravenous broad-spectrum antibiotics reduce bacterial count. Peritoneal drains should not be placed in the immediate vicinity of an anastomosis, because this can actually impede healing. However, there may be therapeutic benefit from suction drains in dependent regions, such as the pelvis and pericolic gutters, which prevent accumulation of fluid. A diverting colostomy is indicated when a full-thickness colonic injury occurs in those who have undergone irradiation, who are profoundly malnourished, or whose condition is unstable from shock or sepsis.

Intestinal Injury During Endoscopic Procedures

Gastrointestinal injury during laparoscopy can occur with introduction of the insufflating needle or trocar, and during cautery or sharp dissection. Good clinical judgment is necessary to determine which patients are appropriate candidates for laparoscopy. Previous surgeries, inflammatory conditions, and prior irradiation increase risk of injury from enteric adhesions, which fix intestine to the abdominal wall. Oxygenating the patient via bag-mask in preparation for intubation can distend the stomach below the level of the umbilicus, placing it at risk for injury. Nasogastric decompression before introduction of a Veress needle or trocar reduces this risk. In the presence of enteric adhesions, the laparoscopic trocar can be inadvertently placed into the stomach, transverse colon, or small intestine. Perforation is recognized by nonidentification of intraperitoneal structures, visual characteristics of intraluminal tissue, and reflux of enteric content. If perforation occurs, it is prudent to leave the trocar in position and convert to an open laparotomy. It is much easier to recognize injuries using the trocar to guide identification of the affected anatomy (Fig. 42.3).

Cautery or sharp dissection can result in enterotomy, which commonly occurs during adhesiolysis. The skill and comfort level of the laparoscopic surgeon determines whether the defect can be successfully repaired laparoscopically or whether laparotomy is required. The most serious laparoscopic intestinal injuries are those that go unrecognized at the time of surgery. Thermal injury from electrocautery or laser can have a potentially disastrous outcome. With electrosurgical injury, a progressive zone of tissue destruction extends well beyond the area of thermal contact, resulting in tissue necrosis and perforation 72 to 96 hours after surgery. Perforation may be signaled by high fever, leukocytosis, nausea, vomiting, and a generalized ill appearance. Signs of peritonitis are present on examination. Flat plate x-ray studies may be of limited benefit in the early postoperative period, because intraperitoneal air can persist for 7 days

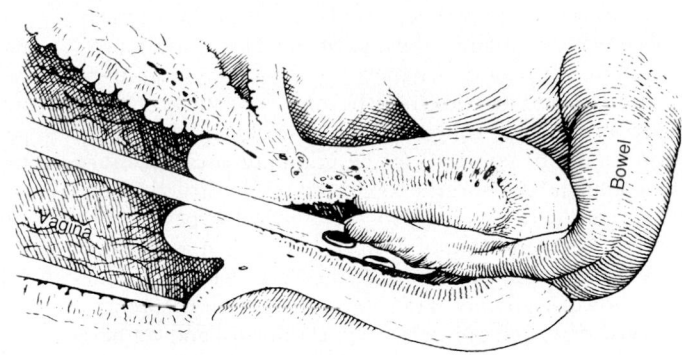

FIGURE 42.3. A suction cannula perforated the uterus during suction dilatation and curettage. With suction still on as curette is removed, the bowel is drawn through the uterus and vagina.

following surgery. CT scan using water-soluble contrast is better suited for this evaluation and should demonstrate extravasation of contrast material into the peritoneal cavity with possible abscess formation.

If perforation is suspected or confirmed, urgent re-exploration is warranted. Hypovolemia, electrolyte abnormalities, and anemia should be aggressively corrected. Broad-spectrum antibiotics are administered and nasogastric decompression is performed as the patient is prepared for surgery. At surgery, aggressive irrigation is necessary to enhance visibility. Copious enteric exudate causes a profound inflammatory response and generalized matting together of intraperitoneal content. Inspection of the small bowel is begun at the ileocecal junction and is done proximally in a hand over hand fashion. Careful examination of the bowel and mesentery is continued to the ligament of Treitz, followed by thorough inspection of the large intestine. The stomach and proximal small bowel are also inspected. In contrast to sharp enterotomy, which can be repaired primarily, significant thermal injury is best corrected by resection of affected bowel. At the very least, a wide margin of bowel wall is removed beyond any visible thermal injury. Because of enteric contamination, other necrotic tissues such as fulgurated endometriotic implants are at high risk for abscess formation and should be excised.

Intestinal Injury During Uterine Curettage

It is estimated that most uterine perforations go unrecognized; therefore, injury to pelvic viscera may also go unrecognized. If fundal perforation occurs during sharp or suction curettage, intestine and mesentery can be drawn into the uterine cavity by the curette. Evisceration as a consequence most commonly occurs during dilatation and curettage of the gravid uterus. Tactile feedback may suggest products of conception, when in fact what is felt is prolapsed abdominal viscera (Fig. 42.4). Recognition of this injury warrants immediate surgical exploration. With the abdomen open, the bowel is retrieved by gentle traction from above. The surgical objectives are to control hemorrhage from the uterine injury, thoroughly inspect the bowel, repair injuries, and complete the uterine evacuation. In women of reproductive age,

hysterectomy is avoided unless uterine preservation poses a significant threat to her health.

Radiation Injury

Radiation therapy for gynecologic cancers can cause intestinal injuries that require surgical correction. Also, damage from prior irradiation contributes to complications during other surgical procedures. The intestinal tract is adversely affected by radiation during treatment and soon thereafter (acute injury) or remote from treatment (late injury). The acute phase is associated with small bowel irritability, cramping, and diarrhea, with onset generally 2 to 3 weeks after initiation of therapy. Injury to the large bowel manifests acutely as proctosigmoiditis, with resultant pain, tenesmus, frequent bowel movements, and bleeding. Low residue diet, antispasmodics, and antiinflammatories are helpful in uncomplicated cases. In more severe cases, debilitating symptoms can adversely affect lifestyle. Intestinal adhesions, fibrosis, obstruction, perforation, abscess, and fistulae are potential late complications.

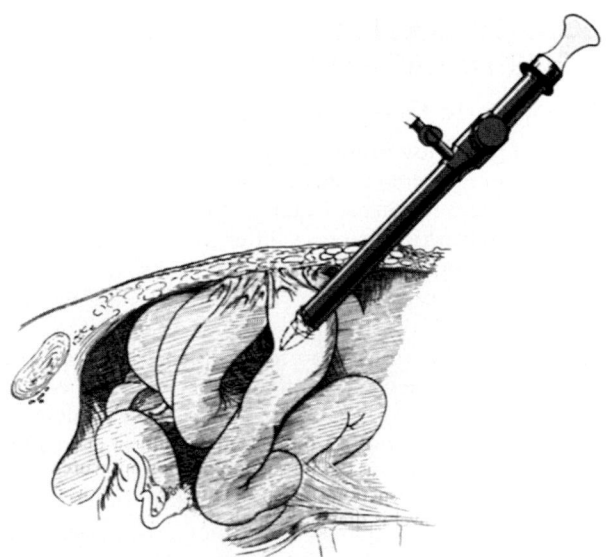

FIGURE 42.4. Perforation of trocar into small bowel.

Surgery in previously irradiated patients warrants special attention and is best performed by those experienced in this regard. Whenever possible, the surgical incision is made in a location beyond the radiation field. Extensive lysis of adhesions is best avoided, and dissection should be confined to the minimum area necessary to complete the surgical objectives. If obstruction occurs, consideration is given to intestinal bypass as opposed to extensive mobilization. Resection is avoided unless the anastomosis can be completed with nonirradiated bowel segments. This objective is often theoretical, because damaged bowel may appear normal and yet have significant microscopic endarteritis and vasculature obliteration. The characteristic pale, thickened bowel wall, telangiectatic vessels, and strictured lumen need not be present to indicate significant radiation injury. If resection is unavoidable, the suture line can be reinforced by wrapping the anastomosis with omentum, which elicits support of exogenous blood supply.

A vesicovaginal or rectovaginal fistula may develop if there is extensive damage to the intervening tissue. The time course of fistula occurrence is usually between 6 and 24 months after therapy, but it may present years after irradiation. The mechanism of late radiation injuries is believed to be obliterative vascular injury with compromised blood flow and tissue necrosis. Postirradiation rectovaginal fistulae are complex problems that rarely heal with simple excision, mobilization, and closure, such that they are probably best corrected using a three-staged approach. First, a diverting ileostomy or colostomy is performed to redirect the colonic content, reduce bacterial infiltration, and allow resolution of inflammation. Several months later, the objectives of the second surgery are complete resection of the fistulous tract and surrounding damaged tissue plus neovascularization via an omental flap or myocutaneous graft. The goal of the eventual third surgery is reversal of the diverting ostomy to reestablish normal intestinal continuity.

POSTOPERATIVE CONSIDERATIONS

Nasogastric Decompression

Some surgeons use routine postoperative nasogastric decompression to reduce nausea, vomiting, and abdominal distention and to enable healing of bowel anastomoses. These prophylactic objectives differ from the therapeutic goals of nasogastric decompression used to alleviate symptoms and expedite recovery from an existing ileus or small bowel obstruction. The literature, however, does not support routine postoperative use. Nasogastric tubes increase patient discomfort and increase the occurrence of sinus infections and epistaxis. A metaanalysis of selective versus routine nasogastric decompression after elective laparotomy included 26 trials and 3,964 patients. Routine postoperative decompression was associated with an increased incidence of pneumonia, atelectasis, and fever. Abdominal distention and vomiting were

increased in selectively treated patients who did not have nasogastric tubes, and eventual tube insertion was required in 5% to 7% of patients in this group. Nasogastric tube reinsertion was required in 2% of routinely decompressed patients. There was no significant difference in the occurrence of wound infections, wound dehiscence, or anastomotic leaks. The authors of this analysis concluded that, through the selective use of nasogastric decompression, only 1 in 20 patients require a nasogastric tube.

Early Postoperative Oral Feeding

There is a wide spectrum of practice patterns among surgeons regarding postoperative diet. For many decades, the conventional approach has been to wait for auscultation of bowel sounds before providing clear liquids and to wait for the occurrence of flatus before giving solid food. Inpatient managed care pressures and successful outpatient recovery following laparoscopic procedures have challenged clinicians to reevaluate traditional postoperative feeding regimens. Current trends are toward much more aggressive early postoperative feeding, even in the setting of bowel resection and anastomosis. Some randomized clinical trials have shown early feeding to be associated with increased frequency of nausea and vomiting, whereas others have shown no difference. The overall rates of ileus, anastomotic complications, and times required for return of bowel function are generally comparable. Early postoperative feeding, however, has not consistently resulted in shorter average length of hospital stay.

Supplemental Nutrition

Perioperative nutritional support is indicated in patients who have been without nutrition for more than 7 days, in patients who are malnourished (weight loss exceeds 15% of usual weight), and when expected duration of recovery is longer than 10 days. TPN has extended the lives of numerous surgical patients and enabled the resumption of normal lifestyle in many. Long-term parenteral nutrition, however, has morbidity that is not insignificant. The need for indwelling central venous access puts patients at risk for catheter sepsis and other catheter-related complications. Metabolic derangements and pancreatic or hepatic dysfunction are common. Intestinal mucosal atrophy results from nonuse in patients who are reliant solely upon parenteral nutrition.

Use of the gut for nutrition is advisable whenever possible. The advantages of enteral tube feeding over TPN include no requirement for venous access, enhanced intestinal lymphatic function, reversal of mucosal atrophy, decreased risk of bacterial translocation, and stimulation of intestinal adaptation. Adaptation is the process whereby the villous height and crypt depth increase, with gradual bowel dilation and lengthening, resulting in increased absorptive surface area. Enteral feeding is not indicated in patients with a nonfunctional intestinal tract or intestinal obstruction, or in those at high risk for aspiration.

Acute Gastric Distention

Acute gastric distention results from inhibition of gastric peristalsis. Postoperative gastric distention more commonly occurs after surgical manipulation in the vicinity of the stomach. Patients at increased risk are those who are diabetic, elderly, or medically debilitated. Short-term postoperative nasogastric decompression can prevent and manage this problem in those who are at high risk. Stimulatory agents such as metoclopramide may expedite gastric emptying in the nonobstructed patient.

Ileus

Postoperative ileus is a mechanical dysfunction in which the normal anterograde gastrointestinal peristalsis is disrupted. Ileus may involve any segment of the digestive tract, including the stomach, small bowel, or colon. In fact, ileus is most frequently a large bowel dysfunction, in that the colon is generally the last segment in the gastrointestinal tract to regain function after pelvic surgery. Postoperatively, the stomach and small intestine usually resume activity within 8 hours. At times, active small bowel peristalsis is noted at the conclusion of even complex abdominal procedures. In contrast, the colon may take 48 to 72 hours to regain function. Colonic dysfunction generally resolves from proximal to distal, such that rectosigmoid activity is the last to return.

Factors that predispose to ileus or worsen the severity of ileus include dehydration, electrolyte abnormalities, diabetes, long-term laxative use, bowel manipulation during surgery, extensive retroperitoneal dissection, general anesthetic agents, narcotic analgesics, immobility, urinary or gastrointestinal leak, peritonitis, abscess, and hematoma. Some degree of adynamic ileus results from all intraabdominal procedures. With return of bowel function, peristaltic pains are often severe, such that many patients describe them as being worse than surgical pain. Normal recovery of bowel function is evident by gradual increase in appetite, tolerance of oral nutrition, and flatus.

Significant delay in bowel function associated with worsening gas pains, nausea, and vomiting is suggestive of clinically significant ileus. Physical examination confirms abdominal distention with diffuse discomfort, hypoactive bowel sounds, and tympanic percussion. Correction of contributing factors and supportive care are the cornerstones of management. Therapeutic interventions include bowel rest, intravenous hydration, correction of electrolytes (i.e., potassium, sodium, and magnesium), physical activity, and judicious use of narcotic analgesia. If good bowel sounds for 24 hours or more suggest that colonic dysfunction is a predominant underlying factor, transrectal colonic stimulation (e.g., docusate sodium or stimulating enema) may be helpful. Patients with vomiting, those not responding to supportive

measures, and those with evidence of gastric or small bowel dilatations on x-ray study benefit from nasogastric decompression. Decompression is generally continued until flatus ensues and abdominal distention resolves.

Adynamic ileus must be distinguished from a mechanical small bowel obstruction. If the patient has not passed flatus within 4 to 5 days or does not respond to conservative measures, then the possibility of a mechanical small bowel obstruction should be considered. Early in the disease process, radiographs may provide little assistance in clarifying the diagnosis because the changes of postoperative ileus and early obstruction are similar. However, after 3 to 5 days, plain abdominal radiographs with supine, upright, and/or lateral recumbent views will help distinguish ileus from mechanical small bowel obstruction. The typical radiographic pattern of an ileus is that of intermittent air found throughout the gastrointestinal tract, including the colon and rectum. Upright views may show air-fluid levels within the small bowel and stomach, and, on occasion, the transverse colon (Fig. 42.5). In contrast, radiographic characteristics of mechanical small bowel obstruction include proximal distended loops with a paucity or absence of gas in the colon. The dilated small bowel loops with air-fluid levels may follow a stair-step pattern from the right lower quadrant to the left upper quadrant in parallel with the anatomic base of the small bowel mesentery.

With intermittent or partial small bowel obstruction, some gas is seen in the colon. Conversely, if the obstruction is in the proximal small bowel, there may be no distended loops at all. Radiographic studies can at times clarify the type of obstruction (mechanical vs. nonmechanical), the extent of obstruction (partial vs. complete), and the location of obstruction (stomach vs. small bowel vs. colon). If the diagnosis remains unclear, a water-soluble contrasted gastrointestinal study with small bowel follow-through can clarify the situation and local-

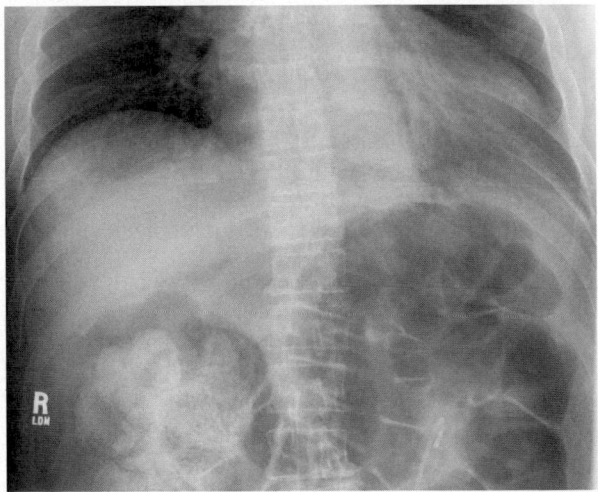

FIGURE 42.5. Kidney, ureter, bladder view of postoperative ileus.

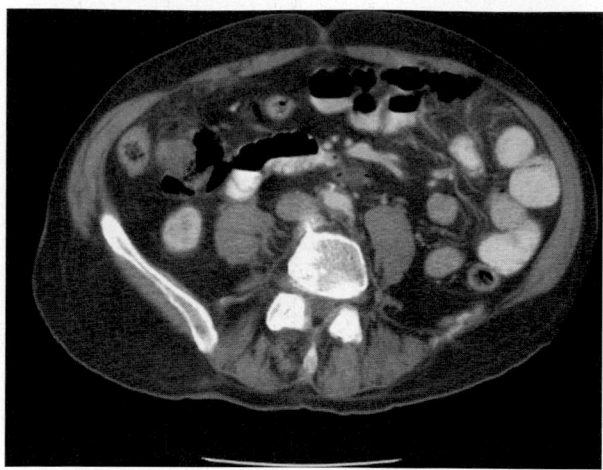

FIGURE 42.6. Computed tomography scan of small bowel obstruction; air-fluid levels in dilated small bowel.

ize the point of obstruction if present. Contrast material may also stimulate peristalsis and has been reportedly therapeutic in some cases of paralytic ileus.

Small Bowel Obstruction

Intraperitoneal adhesions are the most common etiology of intestinal obstruction. Malignancies and hernias are also frequent extrinsic causes. An estimated 85% of all small bowel obstructions are secondary to one of these three conditions. Intraluminal causes include tumors, polyps, gallstones, and bezoars. Obstructive intramural strictures can complicate irradiation or inflammatory bowel disease.

Early postoperative obstruction deserves a trial of nonsurgical management. Nasogastric decompression, supportive care, and correction of underlying contributing factors are as described for adynamic ileus. Supine position with legs flexed helps relax rectus abdominus muscles to facilitate examination. Early in the course of obstruction, there may be minimal to absent distention. Proximal obstruction may also manifest with minimal abdominal distention. High-pitched bowel sounds with metallic tones and rushes are suggestive of an obstructive process. Hypoactive or absent bowel sounds are more suggestive of paralytic ileus. Hypoactive bowel sounds may also occur with intestinal fatigue from long-standing obstruction, closed loop obstruction, or pseudoobstruction. Fewer than half of obstructed patients manifest the classic triad of rebound tenderness, guarding, and rigidity. Also, the physical findings of focal tenderness and guarding are neither sensitive nor specific in confirming underlying obstruction or ischemia.

The duration of asymptomatic intervals between peristaltic pains may suggest the level of obstruction. Peristaltic waves tend to be 3 to 5 minutes apart in high obstruction, whereas in distal obstruction, 10 to 15 minutes may lapse between episodes. Radiographically, small bowel distended by gas outlines the valvulae conniventes (plicae circulares), which traverse the entire diameter of the dilated bowel lumen. Valvulae conniventes are closely spaced and may appear to interdigitate. In contrast, distended colon highlights the haustra, which partially traverse the bowel lumen and are spaced more widely apart. The central abdomen is occupied by distended small bowel loops, whereas the abdominal periphery houses the colon. In the decompressed patient, character of gastric aspirate suggests the potential anatomic site of obstruction. Gastric outlet obstruction produces clear gastric secretions. Bilious output is suggestive of obstruction in the proximal to mid small bowel, or a colonic obstruction with a competent ileocecal valve. Feculent drainage is characteristic of a distal small bowel obstruction, or colonic obstruction with an incompetent ileocecal valve.

Intestinal obstruction leads to an accumulation of intraluminal fluid and gas with distention proximal to the occlusion (Fig 42.6). It is estimated that more than 70% of air in the gastrointestinal tract is from swallowing. Accordingly, distention is significantly worsened by swallowed air. With progressing distention comes tension and venous compression. Arterial inflow continues, resulting in blood accumulation within the bowel wall and lumen. Protein-rich fluid exudes from the capillaries, adding to tissue edema. Malabsorption combined with intestinal secretion further exacerbates intraluminal fluid collection. In the setting of complete obstruction, up to 7 to 8 L of fluid can accumulate, including 50% of plasma volume and 30% of circulating blood volume. Mucosal integrity is disrupted and enteric bacteria traverse the defective bowel wall, seeding the peritoneum. If the process goes uncorrected, intestinal viability is irreversibly damaged as tissue necrosis ensues.

If a decision is made for operative intervention, preparation concentrates on correction of hypovolemia, anemia, and electrolyte imbalances. Broad-spectrum antibiotics may suppress bacterial translocation and delay intestinal ischemia. Upon exploration, the point of obstruction is identified and corrected. All necrotic bowel must be resected. It is not always possible, however, to discern the viability of bowel in the setting of obstruction. Visible characteristics such as tissue color, extent of edema, and peristalsis are not consistently reliable. Active bleeding from the cut bowel edge is a more accurate indicator. Intraoperative Doppler testing of the antimesenteric border should provide characteristic arterial pulsations. Absent Doppler sounds do not necessarily indicate inadequate arterial blood flow. In this setting, viability can be confirmed by intravenous 10% fluorescein (15 mg/kg), followed in 10 minutes by Wood's lamp illumination. Observation of bowel wall fluorescence suggests adequate blood flow to support anastomotic healing. Bowel segments that are less than 2 cm in diameter with no fluorescence can be preserved, but should not be included in the anastomosis. Larger areas of nonfluorescence suggest ischemia and likely require resection.

Large Bowel Obstruction

The vast majority of large bowel obstructions are due to malignancy or inflammatory conditions. This is in contrast to small bowel obstructions for which adhesions are the principal etiology. The gynecologic surgeon may encounter large bowel obstruction from a primary colon or a gynecologic malignancy, ulcerative colitis, diverticular disease, pelvis abscess, or radiation injury. The onset of most colonic obstructions is insidious because of gradual luminal narrowing, which manifests clinically as decreased caliber stools, constipation, and bleeding. Progressive obstruction leads to obstipation, abdominal distention, colicky pain, nausea, and vomiting. Radiographic studies reveal a dilated colon proximal to the point of obstruction (Fig. 42.7). If the ileocecal valve is incompetent, the distention extends proximally into the small bowel as evident by dilated bowel loops with air-fluid levels. A more serious closed loop obstruction occurs when the ileocecal valve is competent. The cecum is commonly involved, and, as cecal dilation exceeds 10 to 12 cm, the risk of perforation increases significantly. Preoperative endoscopy or water-soluble contrast study can clarify the etiology and location of obstruction. Barium enema should not be performed in the setting of acute obstruction or suspected perforation to avoid barium peritonitis. If necessary, any viable segment of large bowel proximal to the point of obstruction can be exteriorized as a colostomy.

Ogilvie's syndrome (acute colonic pseudoobstruction) is a dysfunction of colonic peristalsis. Clinical presentation may be indistinguishable from a large bowel obstruction. The mechanism of colonic pseudoobstruction is theorized to be an imbalance between the proximal and distal colonic innervation. Parasympathetic innervation from the vagus nerve supplies the colon proximal to the splenic flexure. In contrast, the left colon receives parasympathetic innervation from the sacral plexus (S-2 to S-4). Most commonly, only the right colon is dilated. Ogilvie's syndrome is seen more commonly in elderly and debilitated patients and in those who are on narcotics and phenothiazine or tricyclic antidepressants. Supportive care includes hydration, correction of electrolyte abnormalities, and gastrointestinal decompression (nasogastric tube, rectal tube). Sequential radiographs are used to monitor cecal dilation to assess the risk of perforation. Endoscopic decompression or tube cecostomy are preferred alternatives to exploration, because surgical morbidity is significant. If necessary, intraoperative colonic decompression can be accomplished using an 18-gauge needle passed obliquely through the taenia coli and attached to suction. Decompression facilitates exteriorization of the bowel for diverting colostomy.

Fistulae

Postoperative intestinal fistulae are an especially challenging problem for patients and clinicians. An enterocutaneous or enterovaginal fistula may be difficult to confirm, even when clinical findings are strongly suggestive of a fistulous communication. The high-pressure bowel defect may be small with only intermittent drainage, thus obscuring localization. Oral administration of charcoal or of brilliant blue or carmine red dye confirms the diagnosis if characteristic color change is observed in the effluent. Clarification of the fistulous tract can be aided by a fistulogram. Contrast material is injected transcutaneously, and the pattern of flow is evaluated radiographically. Excessive force during injection is avoided to prevent dislodgment of the bowel from its adherence to the abdominal or vaginal wall.

Initial nonoperative management of fistulae in selected cases has gained wide acceptance. The fundamentals of conservative management include correction of underlying inflammatory processes and electrolyte abnormalities, nutritional support, and maintenance of adequate hydration. The more proximal the fistula, the greater the potential for physiologic derangements, and the less likely to close spontaneously with conservative management. Gastric, duodenal, and proximal jejunal fistulae can cause potentially fatal physiologic disturbances and thus require prompt intervention. Distal ilial or colonic fistulae are generally well tolerated and tend to close spontaneously if predisposing factors are circumvented. There must be no abscess, peritonitis, distal bowel obstruction, or foreign body within the fistulous tract. Prior irradiation is likely to preclude spontaneous healing.

Approximately two thirds of distal fistulae are expected to heal within 6 weeks if no complicating factors persist. A fistula that persists beyond 6 weeks is unlikely to heal without operative intervention. Depending on the clinical situation, it may be reasonable to wait an additional 1 to 2 months to optimize nutritional status and allow for resolution of inflammation. The appropriate time for surgical intervention must be individualized. The surgical objectives are to completely excise the fistulous tract and resect the affected bowel segment whenever possible. In certain circumstances, such as irradiated bowel or extensive adhesions, the fistula could be more aptly addressed by bypassing the diseased area. See Chapter 39 for a more extensive discussion of fistulae.

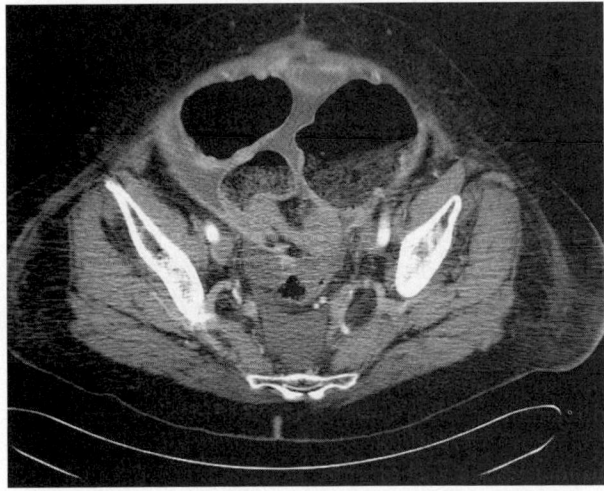

FIGURE 42.7. Computed tomography scan of colonic obstruction.

Dehiscence and Evisceration

Dehiscence implies postoperative wound separation and most commonly involves only the skin and subcutaneous tissue (superficial or incomplete dehiscence). Complete (deep) wound dehiscence refers to separation of the fascia and usually manifests with skin and subcutaneous disruption as well. Fascial disruption generally occurs between the fifth and tenth postoperative day, and is estimated to occur in approximately 1 in 200 high-risk patients. Complete dehiscence is most frequently associated with suture tearing through the tissue and is suspected in the setting of copious serous or serosanguineous drainage from the abdominal wound. The incision is explored with a sterile swab or gloved finger to assess for fascial defects. A small defect (1 to 2 cm) in an otherwise intact fascia with no associated bowel extrusion may be reapproximated with an interrupted fascial suture. Larger fascial defects and all defects with bowel herniation (evisceration) require immediate surgical attention.

Evisceration is an acute full-thickness wound disruption through which abdominal contents extrude and most commonly includes loops of distal small bowel and omentum. Evisceration is rare following laparoscopic procedures but should be suspected with a palpable or visible hernial defect and serosanguineous fluid drainage. Concomitant problems may include abnormal bowel function, nausea, vomiting, or evidence of bowel incarceration. CT and ultrasound imaging are useful if the diagnosis is uncertain. In preparing the eviscerated patient for surgery, she is kept in supine position and the exposed bowel is covered with towels moistened by sterile saline or povidone-iodine solution. If accomplished without difficulty, eviscerated organs should be cautiously replaced back into the abdomen. The protective towels can be secured using a sterile plastic drape and reinforced with an abdominal binder. Broad-spectrum antibiotics are administered, and steps are taken to correct fluid and electrolyte abnormalities. Sedatives and analgesics can reduce intraperitoneal pressure. Intraoperatively, all layers of the wound are inspected for infection, and devitalized abdominal wall tissue is sharply debrided. The bowel and mesentery are inspected for injury, viability, hemostasis, and obstruction, and the peritoneal contents are copiously irrigated. Bowel resection is generally not necessary, but it may be required if obstruction or ischemia is present. Dehiscence, evisceration, and closure techniques are discussed in more detail in Chapters 11 and 12.

Vaginal Evisceration

Protrusion of viscera through the vagina (Fig. 42.8) has been reported in association with surgery, enterocele, trauma, Valsalva maneuver, coitus, radiation, and foreign bodies. Small bowel and mesentery are most commonly involved, but evisceration may also include large bowel and omentum. Approximately two thirds of reported cases have occurred in patients with a history of prior surgery for pelvic relaxation or in the setting of symptomatic enterocele. Prior hysterectomy is a factor in only

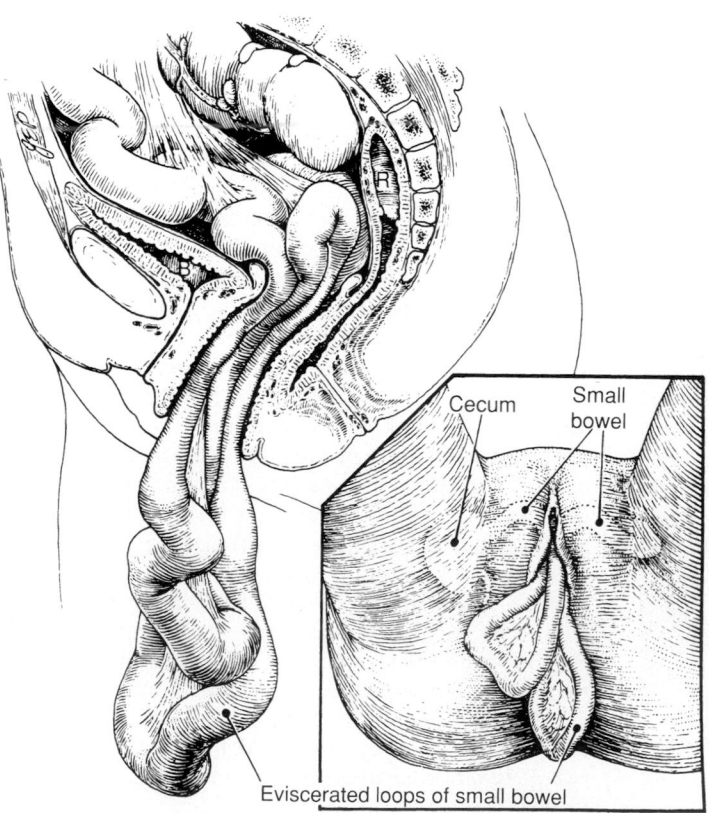

Cecum   Small bowel

Eviscerated loops of small bowel

FIGURE 42.8. Vaginal evisceration.

half of reported cases. This distressing situation tends to occur outside of the hospital setting and bacterial contamination is inevitable. Severe abdominal pain may indicate mesenteric compromise. Surgical preparation is similar to that for an abdominal evisceration, but in contrast, it is probably best to resist preoperative attempts at replacing the bowel transvaginally. Surgical management should be via exploratory laparotomy. During exploration, the eviscerated contents are replaced into the peritoneal cavity with a combination of gentle traction from above and guidance from below. Copious intraperitoneal irrigation and broad-spectrum antibiotics are used. Careful inspection of the bowel and mesentery are necessary to identify and repair injuries and to ensure viability. Severely damaged or obstructed bowel requires resection.

Short Bowel Syndrome

Short bowel syndrome results from loss of significant bowel length or inadequate function of normal length bowel. The net result is insufficient nutrient absorption necessary to meet the body's metabolic requirements. Causes include extensive surgical resection, regional enteritis (Crohn's disease), and radiation injury. In women, the average length of small bowel is approximately 600 cm (range 350 to 700 cm). In general, 50% of the small bowel can be resected without long-term impairment of nutritional status, as long as there is normal function in the remainder of the bowel. Severe nutritional deficiencies will likely result with loss of two thirds to three fourths of the small intestine. Malabsorption manifest as diarrhea, dehydration, weight loss, metabolic derangement, protein and nutrient deficiencies, and anemia (iron, folate, and B_{12} deficiencies). After undergoing an intestinal resection, the remaining small bowel has adaptation capacity that begins a few weeks postoperatively and maximizes by approximately 24 months.

Compensatory adaptation is via mucosal hypertrophy with increased villous height and crypt depth. Eventually, surface area and transit time are also increased through gradual dilation and lengthening of the bowel. Enteral feeding is an important stimulus for intestinal adaptation, and use of the gut for nutrition is encouraged whenever possible. Medical management of short bowel syndrome depends on the locations of abnormalities and the severity of resultant problems. Dehydration, electrolyte abnormalities, and specific nutrient deficiencies are corrected as needed. Therapy includes histamine (H2) blockers to reduce gastric secretions and antimotility agents, which improve absorption via increased transit time and reduced diarrhea. Broad-spectrum antibiotics may be beneficial in patients with enteric bacterial overgrowth and translocation.

Surgical therapy for short bowel syndrome begins with preemptive planning. A concerted effort is made to preserve as much small bowel and colon as possible at the time of any surgical resection. Whenever reasonable, therapeutic surgical procedures should be delayed until after the period of intestinal adaptation. Operative ma-neuvers designed to increase transit time and absorption include stricturoplasty, tapering, serosal patching, and interposing of a colonic segment or antiperistaltic small bowel segment. Additional long-term sequelae of short bowel syndrome include gallstones in 50% of patients. Accordingly, some surgeons advocate prophylactic cholecystectomy.

Hernias

Ventral or incisional hernias occur subsequent to 1% of gynecologic surgeries. Abdominal viscera are encased by a peritoneum-lined hernia sac, which protrudes through a fascial defect. The overlying skin and subcutaneous tissue remain intact. Patients tend to describe an insidious onset of abdominal fullness or pressure and often notice a focal area of distention. Symptoms generally worsen with prolonged standing and physical activity, and lessen at rest. Hernias that reduce spontaneously and those easily reduced manually can be managed without surgery. Any suspicion of bowel obstruction, incarceration, strangulation, or necrosis requires immediate surgical evaluation. The surgical objectives are to isolate and resect the hernia sac, reduce the sac contents, lyse pertinent adhesions, and inspect the viscera to ensure gastrointestinal integrity. Resection may be necessary to alleviate intestinal obstruction or remove severely damaged bowel. Before closure, steps are taken to acquire hemostasis, control infection, excise preexisting scar tissue, and mobilize the abdominal wall to enable a tension-free fascial approximation.

OPERATIVE TECHNIQUES

General Principles

Numerous variations exist on bowel resection and anastomotic techniques. Discussed in this text are some of the more commonly used methods, instruments, and materials. This review is by no means exhaustive given the vast array of reported options on this theme. Strict adherence to the fundamental principles of anastomosis is more important to successful healing than are the specific techniques or materials used (Table 42.2). Broad categories for consideration include whether to use open or closed technique and whether to use hand-sewn or staple closure. Anastomotic communication can be established via an end-to-end, side-to-side, or end-to-side alignment. Hand-sewn closure may be effectively accomplished using one or two layers of absorbable or permanent suture via continuous or interrupted methods. Additionally, specific suturing techniques (i.e., Lembert, Connell) can be selected (Fig. 42.9).

Staple anastomoses have largely replaced hand-sewn techniques. Technical ease and equivalent to superior results are among the potential advantages of stapling methods (Table 42.3). An overview of selected surgical procedures in this chapter includes hand-sewn and staple techniques, with a focus on modern surgical stapling. A more expansive discussion of hand-sewn maneuvers is

TABLE 42.2.
General Principles of Intestinal Anastomosis

INTESTINAL ANASTOMOSIS SHOULD

Be tension free
Avoid intraperitoneal spill of gastrointestinal content
Incorporate healthy tissue in the proximal and distal segments
Preserve adequate lumen
Be hemostatic and watertight/airtight
Be completed under optimal surgical exposure
Preserve maximum amount of normal bowel
Invert the tissue edges
Incorporate the submucosa, which is the strongest layer
Include bowel segments of the same diameter
Be performed in an infection free tissue bed
Not be done with an uncorrected obstruction or fistula

found in the seventh edition of *Te Linde's Operative Gynecology.*

Familiarity with open and closed anastomotic techniques provides the surgeon with a choice of repairs and facilitates intraoperative decision making. Open techniques (bowel lumens exposed) have gradually replaced closed techniques (lumens occluded) in most circumstances. Morbidity associated with open techniques is acceptably low. The extent of intraperitoneal spill can generally be controlled with aggressive preoperative bowel prep and atraumatic bowel clamps. Closed techniques are potentially advantageous in reducing complications from unprepped bowel or reanastomosis involving the colon.

Angiogenesis at the anastomotic margins begins within the first 72 hours of surgery if not impeded by infection or inflammation. The most important strength layer of the bowel wall is the submucosa, which must be incorporated into any anastomosis. Collagen is believed to be the single most important contributor to submucosal strength. The maximum anastomotic bursting pressure reflects the pressure required to disrupt an anastomosis and has been used experimentally to assess the strength of healing. The bursting pressure of an anastomosis increases rapidly during the early postoperative period. Sixty percent of the surrounding bowel wall strength is reached by postoperative day 3 to 4, and pressure tolerated by the anastomotic site approximates 100% of that tolerated by intact bowel wall by postoperative day 7. The ideal suture material should provide maximum strength during the lag phase of wound healing with minimal tissue reaction and inflammation. Although the perfect suture material is yet to be identified, modern monofilament and coated braided sutures represent progress toward this goal.

Double-layer intestinal closures have long been touted as more secure than single-layer closures. The traditional anastomosis includes a running inner layer of 3-0 chromic cat gut (absorbable) and an interrupted outer layer of 3-0 silk (nonabsorbable). Extensive clinical evidence, however, suggests single-layer closure to be equivalent and may offer some advantages over double layer anastomosis. Comparative animal studies have demonstrated more rapid vascularization and mucosal healing, and greater early anastomotic strength associated with single-layer repair. Double-layer closures, along with traditional sutures such as cat gut and silk, are associated with greater inflammation, reduced microneoangiogenesis, and less blood flow across the anastomosis. A single-layer reapproximation generally causes less narrowing of the intestinal lumen and can be accomplished in less time. When done properly, all hand-sewn techniques result in an inverted suture line.

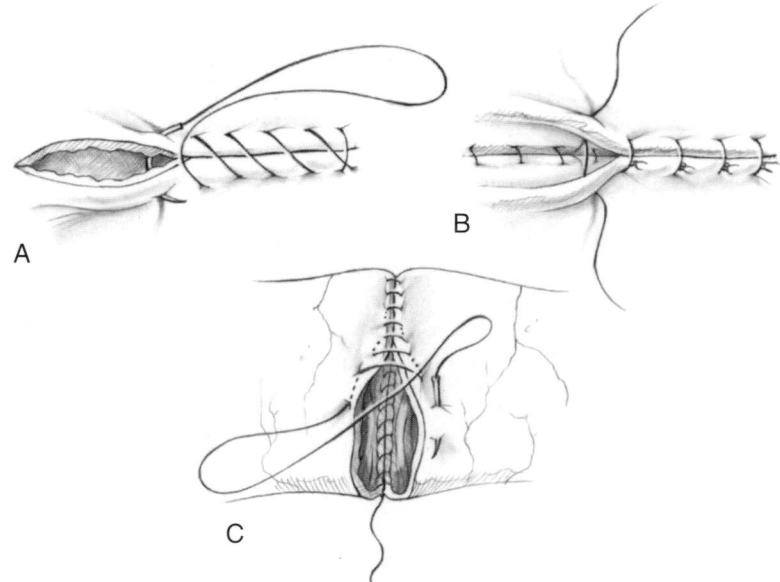

FIGURE 42.9. Commonly used suture techniques for intestinal anastomosis: continuous over-and-over suture (**A**), interrupted Lembert suture (**B**), and Connell continuous suture (**C**).

TABLE 42.3.
Staple Techniques

Advantages	Disadvantages
Better blood flow and oxygen delivery across the anastomotic line	Greater expense with stapling instruments
Less operative time required	Everted tissue edges using some techniques
Uniform staple placement is an inherent design of surgical staplers	Dependence on equipment that could malfunction
Less luminal narrowing	Staple lines may be less resistant to tension injury
Technically easier to learn and perform in most cases	Technically difficult to align the surgical staplers in some anatomic locations

Either continuous or interrupted closures can be used for intestinal anastomosis. Continuous technique is rapid and has the potential advantage of a more even tension distribution along the suture line. In comparison of running versus interrupted closure, animal studies have also shown reduced tissue oxygen tension, impaired collagen synthesis, and increased anastomotic complications using running closure. To date, however, randomized clinical trials are lacking, and retrospective studies show no consistent benefit of one technique over the other. Clinical and subclinical anastomotic leak rates, associated morbidity, and length of hospitalization are generally equivalent, even for high-risk patients (e.g., patients with prior radiation therapy, malnutrition, carcinomatosis).

SURGERY ON THE SMALL INTESTINE

Blood Supply to the Small Intestine

The small bowel receives its arterial blood supply from the superior mesenteric artery (SMA), which arises from the ventral surface of the abdominal aorta (Fig. 42.13). In addition to the small bowel, the SMA also gives rise to the middle and right colic arteries, which supply those regions of the colon. The most proximal small bowel is supported by the common inferior pancreaticoduodenal artery from the SMA. Arising from the left side of the SMA are a series of jejunal and ileal arteries that branch to form anastomotic arcades. Primary arcades terminate directly into the small bowel via vasa recta or extend to form secondary, tertiary, and quaternary arcades that eventually give rise to terminal vasa recta. Avascular spaces between the vasa recta are known as *windows of Deaver.* In general, up to 8 cm of small intestine can remain viable distal to the closest vasa recta because of intramural vascular communications.

The ileocolic artery arises from the right side of the SMA and traverses the base of the mesentery to form a loop anastomosis with the SMA in the region of the terminal ileum. This loop encircles an area devoid of vessels known as the *avascular space of Treves.* The arterial blood supply to the distal ileum is considered tenuous due to a decreased number of vasa recta from only primary vascular arcades. Because of the uncertain vascular status in

this area, it is recommended that 10 cm of terminal ileum also be removed during cecal resection to improve the anastomotic blood supply.

Small Bowel Resection

It is important to resect only the length of bowel necessary to adequately address the disease process, thereby sparing as much normal intestine as possible. For benign disease, bowel transection sites are located just proximal and distal to the abnormal segment. Moist laparotomy pads are positioned to isolate the surgical field from the remaining peritoneal contents. At the proposed transection sites, blunt dissection is used to make a small opening through the avascular mesenteric window adjacent to the bowel wall. The staple cartridge half of the gastrointestinal anastomotic (GIA) stapler is passed through the proximal mesenteric defect, perpendicular to the axis of the bowel. The anvil half is placed across the bowel and aligned with the cartridge. This effectively occludes the bowel as the GIA stapler is closed. Proper positioning is confirmed, and the stapler is fired by steady forward motion on the pusher-bar knife assembly. Upon release of the assembly and opening of the GIA handles, two double-staggered staple lines are noted with the intervening bowel transected. The same steps are carried out at the distal site for transection (Fig. 42.10).

For benign disease, the mesenteric resection can be carried out in close proximity to the bowel, with no need to remove an intervening wedge. The objective is to preserve as much intact mesenteric blood supply as possible. The peritoneum overlying the mesentery is opened with cautery. Visual inspection and transillumination help to identify mesenteric vessels, which are clamped, cut, and suture-ligated using 2-0 silk ligatures. Division of the mesentery completes the resection. In preparation for anastomosis, tissue attachments are cleared 5 mm from both stapled bowel edges to avoid incorporation of mesenteric fat.

Staple Anastomosis

Staple end-to-end anastomosis in the small bowel is rarely used because of excess narrowing of the lumen. More favorable are the staple side-to-side anastomotic techniques that are functionally likened to an end-to-end anastomo-

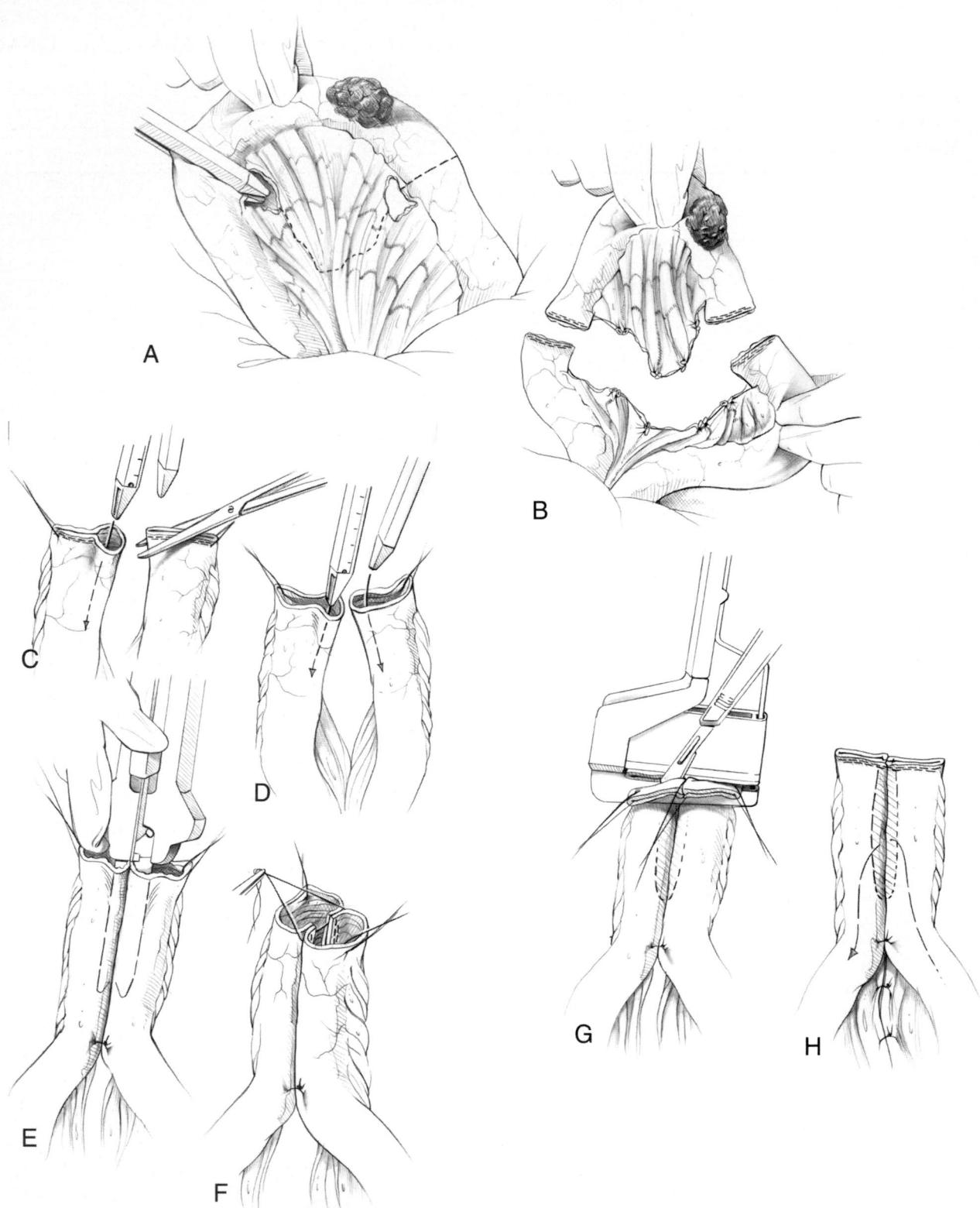

FIGURE 42.10. Small bowel resection with side-to-side (functional end-to-end) staple anastomosis. **A:** The two halves of the gastrointestinal anastomotic (GIA) stapler are passed through the mesenteric window and secured across the bowel. **B:** The GIA stapler has been fired proximal and distal to the abnormal bowel. Staggered double staple lines are noted to occlude each segment. Extent of mesenteric resection is tailored to the case-specific disease process. **C:** Full-thickness corners are sharply excised from the antimesenteric end of each bowel segment. The anvil and cartridge halves of the GIA stapler are inserted into each enterotomy. **D:** An open variation of this technique is such that the bowel segments are not occluded, and the GIA anvil and cartridge are introduced through each open lumen. **E:** Using either closed or open techniques, the GIA stapler is locked into position along the antimesenteric borders and fired by forward motion on the pusher-bar knife assembly. **F:** Firing the GIA stapler establishes a common enterotomy. **G:** The thoracoabdominal (TA) stapler is used to secure the open ends. Full-thickness bowel wall is circumferentially elevated above the staple line before firing. **H:** Shown is the resultant side-to-side functional end-to-end anastomosis. The mesenteric defect is closed with interrupted 3-0 silk sutures.

sis. Staple end-to-end techniques are more aptly used for anastomosing two segments of large bowel following transverse colectomy or rectosigmoid resection.

Side-to-Side (Functional End-to-End) Staple Anastomosis

The side-to-side functional end-to-end staple techniques have gained wide acceptance because of the technical ease, availability of reliable instruments, and capacity to join bowel lumens of different diameters. Following resection, the occluded bowel ends are juxtaposed with the antimesenteric edges aligned in parallel along a distance of approximately 8 cm. This alignment is secured by a seromuscular 3-0 silk suture placed at the proximal end. Mayo scissors are used to excise a full-thickness oblique segment from the antimesenteric corner of each staple-occluded bowel segment. The anvil half of the GIA stapler and the cartridge half are inserted into each enterotomy (Fig. 42.10). The stapler is secured into position by closing the lock lever such that the antimesenteric borders are aligned. Proper positioning is confirmed and the instrument is fired by sliding the pusher-bar knife assembly forward, and then returning it to the neutral position. This maneuver delivers two double-staggered staple rows and cuts the intervening bowel walls. The GIA instrument is disengaged and removed. The resultant enteroenterostomy is inspected to ensure patency, viability, and hemostasis.

The open bowel edges are grasped with Allis clamps, and a linear thoracoabdominal (TA) stapler is placed across the common lumen, ensuring that full-thickness bowel wall is circumferentially elevated above the staple line. After releasing the safety, the TA stapler is fired via steady closing grip on the handles. Excess tissue above the edge of the stapler is excised, and the instrument is released. Luminal capacity is evaluated by transmural palpation between the thumb and index finger, moving in a circular motion to outline the two layers of bowel wall (in contrast to the four palpable layers proximal to the common lumen). Oversewing the staple line is unnecessary unless there is concern regarding the anastomotic integrity.

An open variation of this technique is such that after resection, the ends of the in situ bowel are not occluded. Atraumatic bowel clamps, protective moist laparotomy pads, irrigation, and povidone-iodine–soaked gauze reduce enteric contamination. The antimesenteric borders are aligned and secured as described above. The anvil half of the GIA stapler is introduced through one open bowel lumen, and the cartridge half is introduced through the other. The GIA stapler is locked and fired along the antimesenteric borders, and the TA stapler is used to close the resultant common enterotomy. These staple techniques are also ideal for joining bowel segments of discordant diameters (i.e., ileocolonic anastomosis). The ileum and colon are aligned and secured in parallel along their antimesenteric borders. An enterotomy and colotomy are made through which the anvil

and cartridge halves of the GIA stapler are placed to initiate the anastomosis as described earlier. Proper alignment minimizes the residual large bowel segment that extends beyond the anastomosis, which is at risk for nonfunction and progressive symptomatic dilation (blind loop syndrome).

Side-to-Side Staple Anastomosis

Side-to-side techniques are less commonly used than they once were and have largely been replaced by end-to-end or functional end-to-end anastomoses. Nevertheless, side-to-side techniques are an effective means of reanastomosis, and they can be used to bypass an obstructed intestinal segment. Either hand-sewn or staple closure may be used. The antimesenteric borders are aligned, and the bowel segments are overlapped along 8 cm and secured into position such that the stapled bowel edges are at opposite ends of this alignment. Subsequent steps taken for the staple method are as previously described.

End-to-End Hand-Sewn Double-Layer Anastomosis

In performing an end-to-end anastomosis, it is desirable to have adequate and equivalent lumens in both the proximal and distal segments. The diameter of any lumen can be increased by transecting the bowel obliquely or via linear incision along the antimesenteric border (Cheatle slit). Noncrushing linen shod or rubber shod intestinal clamps are placed across the proximal and distal bowel to decrease intestinal spill. The bowel segments and mesenteries are aligned and secured by 3-0 silk seromuscular sutures placed midway between the mesenteric and antimesenteric borders. The traditional two-layer anastomosis includes a running inner layer of 3-0 chromic catgut and an outer layer of interrupted 3-0 silk sutures (Fig. 42.11).

The inner layer is closed first, starting on the mesenteric (posterior) bowel edges and continuing the closure around to incorporate the antimesenteric (anterior) edges. This is best accomplished with a double-arm needle, sewing in both directions. Suturing begins on the mucosal side, passing from in-to-out and then out-to-in, bringing the inverted bowel edges together. Full-thickness tissue bites are initiated approximately 3 mm from the edge and advanced approximately 3 mm between throws. After circumferential closure, the knot is tied toward the lumen and the bowel is rotated 180 degrees to expose the posterior wall. Rotation is facilitated by passing one stay suture through the mesenteric defect, with sustained counterclockwise rotational traction on both stay sutures. Interrupted seromuscular 3-0 silk sutures are placed to complete the mesenteric (posterior) outer layer. The bowel is rotated back 180 degrees into its normal anatomic position, and the anterior outer layer is lastly closed with interrupted silk Lembert sutures. If the bowel cannot be rotated, the mesenteric (posterior) outer segment must be sewn first.

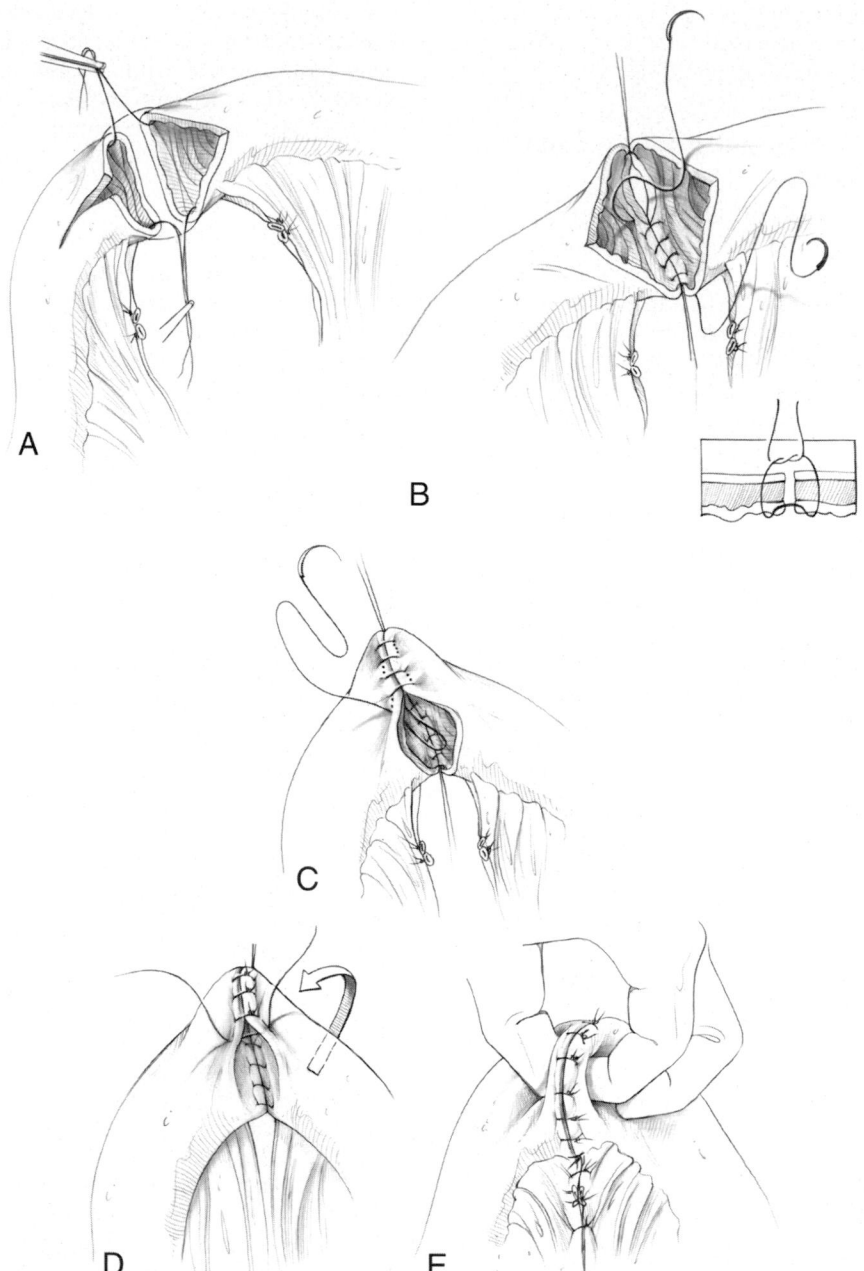

FIGURE 42.11. End-to-end hand-sewn double-layer small bowel anastomosis. **A:** The bowel segments are aligned end-to-end and secured by stay sutures placed midway between the mesenteric and antimesenteric borders. Each luminal diameter is increased via a linear incision along the antimesenteric border (Cheatle slit). **B:** The inner running layer is started on the mesenteric (posterior) bowel edges. A double-arm needle facilitates bidirectional sewing as the closure continues around the corners onto the antimesenteric (anterior) edges. **C:** The anterior inner layer is completed in a continuous over-and-over or Connell suture (shown). **D:** The bowel is rotated 180 degrees to expose the posterior wall. Interrupted seromuscular 3-0 silk sutures are placed to finish the posterior outer layer. **E:** The bowel is rotated back into its normal alignment, and the anterior outer layer is closed with interrupted silk sutures. The mesenteric defect is reapproximated and the adequacy of the lumen is assessed. **Inset:** Conventional inner layer inverting technique.

Side-to-Side Hand-Sewn Anastomosis

For hand-sewn technique, 5 cm length parallel linear enterotomies are made along the antimesenteric borders of each bowel segment. Elevation of the anterior bowel wall with gastrointestinal forceps, during either sharp or cautery incision, will reduce the likelihood of posterior wall injury. A row of interrupted 3-0 silk sutures are placed in Lembert fashion to join the posterior outer edges of the enterotomies. A running absorbable 3-0 suture is then used on the posterior inner layer sewing toward the surgeon and continuing around to the anterior edges of the enterotomies. A second posterior inner layer suture or a double-arm suture is continued away from the surgeon around the far end of the enterotomies. Suturing is continued along the anterior inner layer using the continuous over-and-over or Connell suture. The two suture ends are tied together across the anastomosis. The final anterior outer layer is placed using interrupted seromuscular sutures of 3-0 silk in Lembert fashion. Stay sutures are secured or removed, and the anastomosis is checked for integrity.

As a modification to the aforementioned procedure, the initial posterior layer of interrupted 3-0 silk Lembert sutures are placed before performing the enterotomies (Fig. 42.12). Silk sutures are placed such that the knots are secured on the outside. Parallel enterotomies are made approximately 4 mm above and below the edges of the suture line. The remaining steps in the anastomosis are completed as described previously.

SURGERY ON THE LARGE INTESTINE

Blood Supply to the Large Intestine

The SMA arises from the abdominal aorta and gives rise to the ileocolic, right colic, and middle colic arteries, which supply the right and transverse portions of the colon (Fig. 42.13). The inferior mesenteric artery (IMA) also arises from the abdominal aorta and gives off the left colic and sigmoid branches, which supply the descending and sigmoid colon. Each of these major vessels divide

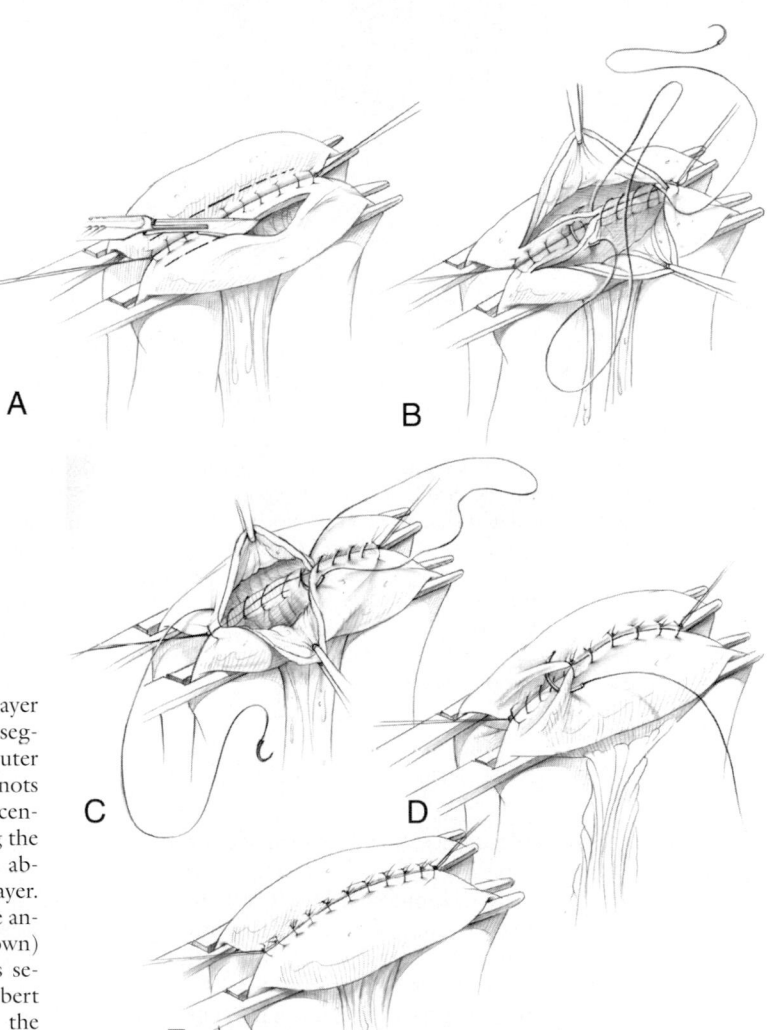

FIGURE 42.12. Side-to-side hand-sewn double-layer small bowel anastomosis. **A:** The occluded bowel segments are aligned in parallel, and the posterior outer layer is placed with interrupted 3-0 silk sutures. Knots are tied on the outside of the anastomosis. Five centimeter length parallel enterotomies are made along the antimesenteric borders. **B:** A double-arm, delayed absorbable 3-0 suture is used on the posterior inner layer. **C:** Sewing is continued around the corners onto the anterior edges using continuous over-and-over (shown) or Connell suture. **D:** The anterior outer layer is secured with interrupted seromuscular 3-0 silk Lembert sutures. **E:** Occluding clamps are released, and the completed anastomosis is checked for integrity.

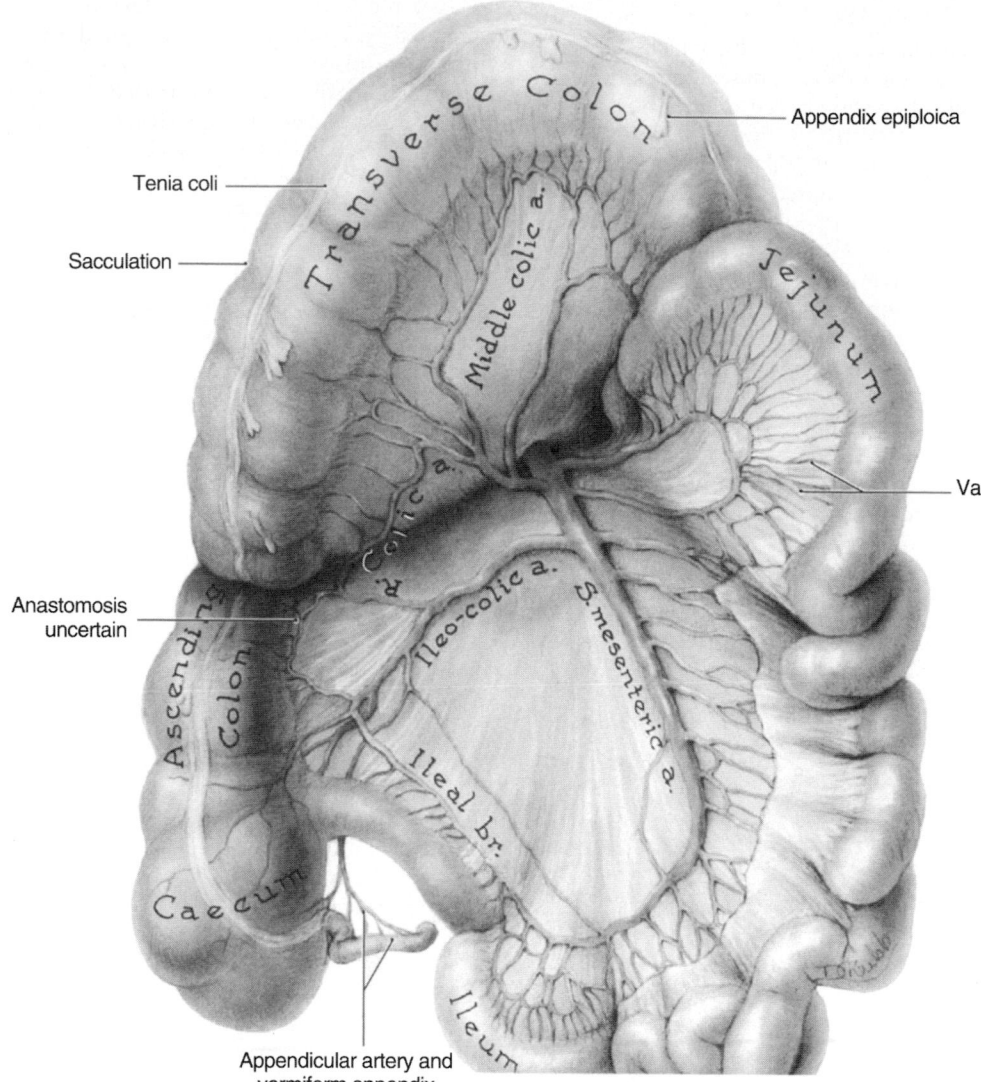

Tenia coli

Sacculation

Anastomosis
uncertain

Appendix epiploica

Va

Appendicular artery and
vermiform appendix

FIGURE 42.13. Intestinal blood supply—superior mesenteric artery. The peritoneum is in part stripped off. Observe the following: *(1)* The superior mesenteric artery, which ends by anastomosing with the ileal branch of the ileocolic artery. *(2)* Its branches: from its left side, *(a)* 12 or more jejunal and ileal branches. These anastomose to form arcades from which vasa recta pass to the small gut. From its right side, *(b)* the middle colic, the ileocolic, and commonly, but not here, an independent right colic artery. These anastomose to form a marginal artery (labeled in Fig. 42.14) from which vasa recta pass to the large gut. *(c)* The two inferior pancreaticoduodenal arteries (not in view) arise from the main artery either directly or in conjunction with the first jejunal branch. *(3)* Taeniae coli, sacculations, and appendices epiploicae distinguish the large gut from the smooth-walled small gut.

into numerous smaller branches, forming an anastomotic arcade that communicates from the cecum to the rectum via the marginal artery of Drummond. The marginal artery gives off numerous terminal vasa recta that directly supply the colon (Fig. 42.14). Arterial perfusion is thus preserved to any segment of the colon as long as the marginal artery is not disrupted. The marginal artery, however, is absent at the hepatic or splenic flexure in 1%

to 2% of the population. This anatomic inconsistency most often affects the left side, such that colon resection in this area should include removal of the splenic flexure. Again noted is the tenuous ileocolic blood supply, such that if the cecum is resected, 10 cm of terminal ileum should also be removed. The rectum derives its oxygenation from the IMA via the superior rectal artery and from the hypogastric artery via the middle and inferior

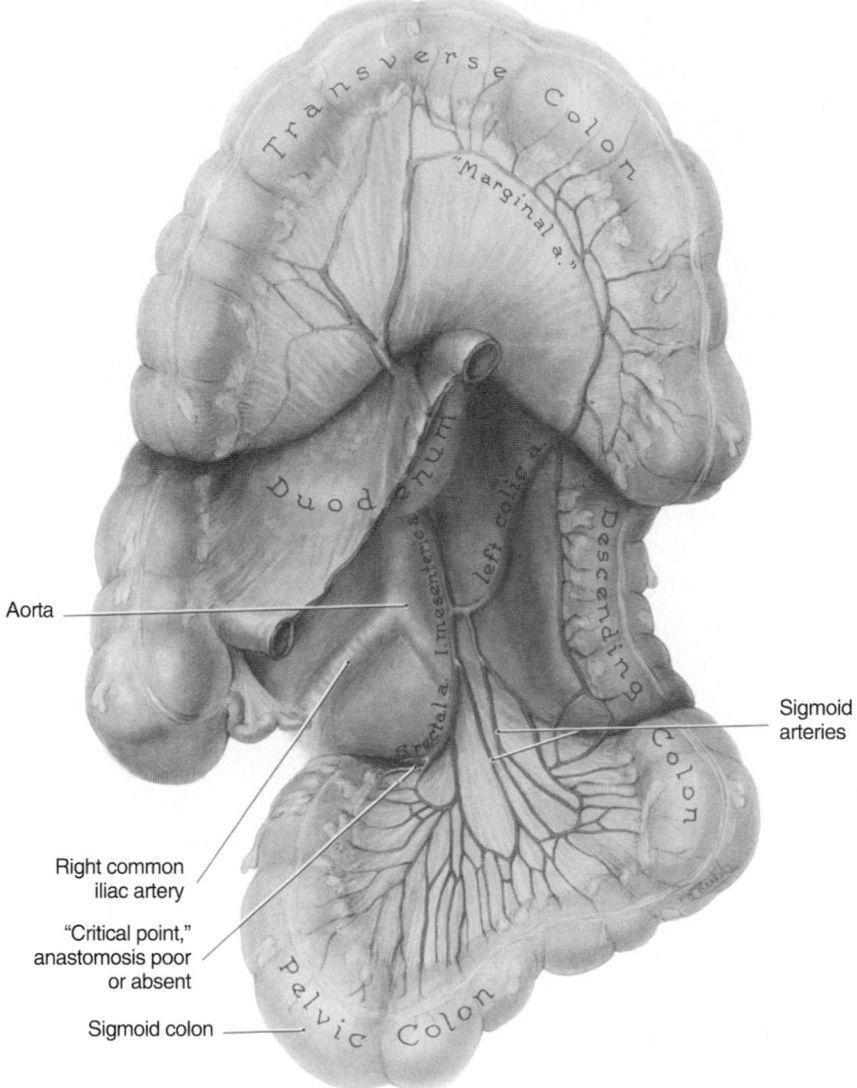

FIGURE 42.14. Intestinal blood supply—inferior mesenteric artery. The mesentery has been cut at its root and discarded with the jejunum and ileum. Observe the following: (1) The inferior mesenteric artery arising 1 to 1½ inches above the bifurcation of the aorta. On crossing the left common iliac artery, it becomes the superior rectal (haemorrhoidal) artery. (2) Its branches: (a) a single (superior) left colic artery and (b) several sigmoid arteries (inferior left colic arteries) springing from its left side. In this specimen, the two lowest sigmoid arteries spring from the superior rectal artery. The point at which the last sigmoid artery leaves the superior rectal artery is known as the critical point of Sudeck.

rectal arteries. An elaborate anastomotic lattice with other pelvic vessels encircles the rectum and anus.

Large Bowel Resection

The principles important in large bowel resection and anastomosis are essentially the same as those described previously for the small bowel. Segmental colon resection in gynecologic surgery is most commonly necessary because of malignancy or radiation injury. The gynecologic surgeon may also encounter benign conditions that require resection, such as severe endometriosis, diverticular disease, extensive adhesions, or nonreparable colonic injury. Large bowel resection for benign gynecologic conditions does not require segmental wedge resection of the mesentery. The integrity of the marginal artery is protected when the mesentery is transected close to the bowel wall through the vasa recta.

Mobilization of the Colon

The majority of large bowel resections require some degree of mobilization to ensure a tension-free anastomosis. The general objectives of colon mobilization are to gain retroperitoneal access and transect avascular attachments from the splenic and/or hepatic flexures. If needed, additional mobility is acquired via transecting the gastrocolic ligament. This also provides entry into the lesser omental sac, which facilitates resection of the gastrocolic ligament and infracolic omentum if necessary. Mobilization can be carried out before or after the segmental colon resection, depending on the clinical situation.

To free the right colon, retroperitoneal dissection is initiated at the base of the cecum and continued lateral and parallel to the ascending colon along the white line of Toldt. This is aided by medial traction on the ascending colon. The hepatocystocolic ligament is transected as

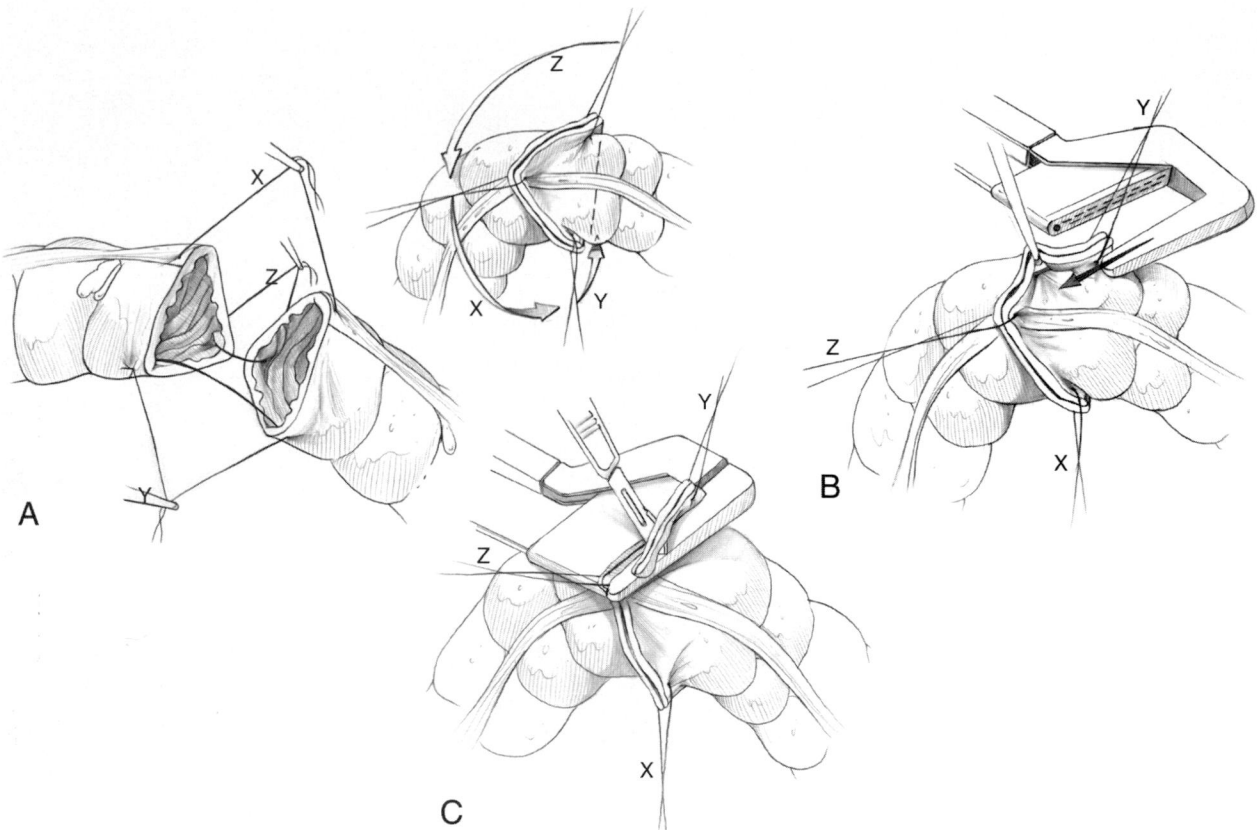

FIGURE 42.15. End-to-end colon staple anastomosis. **A:** The colon segments are aligned end-to-end, and 3-0 silk sutures are placed to divide the bowel circumference into equal one-third segments. **Inset:** The mesenteric (posterior) bowel edges are joined first. The bowel is rotated 180 degrees counterclockwise. This is done by passing stay suture *(y)* through the mesenteric defect, with continued counterclockwise rotational traction on sutures *(z)* and *(y)*. **B:** The thoracoabdominal (TA) stapler is used to close the posterior segments. Full-thickness bowel walls are lifted above the staple line with Allis clamps. **C:** After firing the stapler, excess tissue is sharply excised.

dissection is carried into Morison's pouch and along the proximal transverse colon. Mobilization of the left colon is initiated at the most distal site of retroperitonealized sigmoid colon, which is usually located at the pelvic brim. With medial retraction on the bowel, a peritoneal incision is made lateral and parallel to the descending colon. Dissection is continued around the splenic flexure as the lienocolic and phrenicocolic ligaments are transected. Excessive traction is avoided to prevent splenic capsule injury. The left lateral portion of the gastrocolic ligament is divided to access the lesser omental sac. This ligament can be completely transected along the transverse colon by dividing the omental vessels. If necessary, division of the gastrocolic ligament is accomplished along the greater curvature of the stomach by dividing the gastroepiploic and short gastric vessels.

End-to-End Staple Anastomosis

Transverse colon resection is used as an illustrative example of this technique. After completing the resection and mobilization of the left and right colon, the proximal and distal bowel edges are brought into close opposition. Their mesenteries are aligned, and seromuscular 3-0 silk sutures are placed, dividing the bowel circumference into equal one-third segments. The mesenteric (posterior) segment of the anastomosis is completed first. Bowel rotation of 180 degrees is facilitated by counterclockwise passage of one stay suture through the mesenteric defect, with continued counterclockwise rotational traction on the adjacent stay suture. Allis clamps are used to lift both full-thickness bowel walls into the noncutting TA stapler. The stapler is positioned such that the staple line extends just beyond the lateral edge of both stay sutures. Steady closing grip secures the device into position. After confirming proper placement, the safety latch is released, and firm closure of the handles fires the staple line. Excess tissue is sharply excised, and the stapler is released (Fig. 42.15).

The bowel is rotated back 180 degrees to its normal anatomic alignment. The two remaining equilateral segments are stapled from the serosal side in similar fashion. Alternatively, if the bowel is not easily rotated, the mesenteric (posterior) segment can be stapled first from

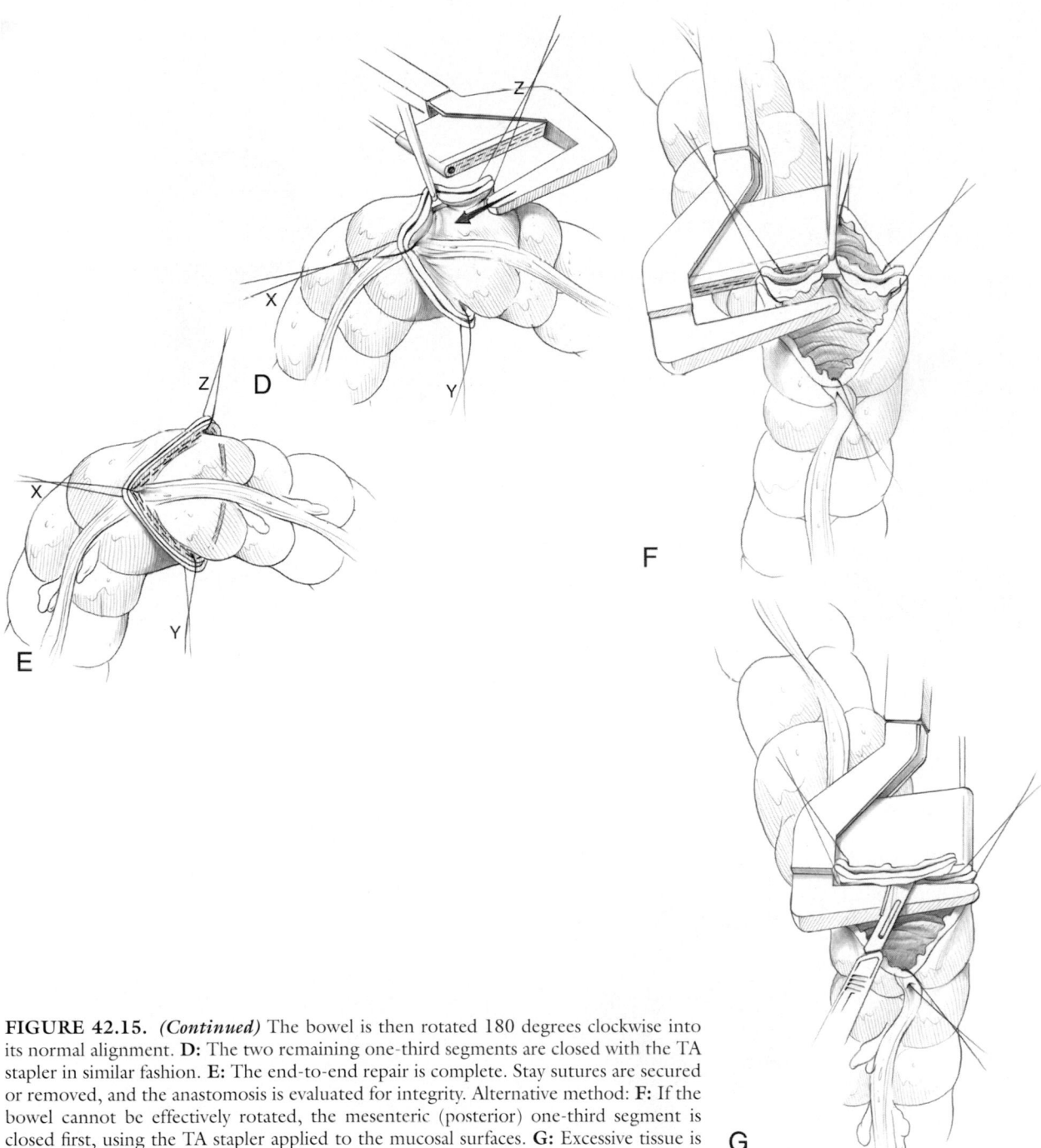

FIGURE 42.15. *(Continued)* The bowel is then rotated 180 degrees clockwise into its normal alignment. **D:** The two remaining one-third segments are closed with the TA stapler in similar fashion. **E:** The end-to-end repair is complete. Stay sutures are secured or removed, and the anastomosis is evaluated for integrity. Alternative method: **F:** If the bowel cannot be effectively rotated, the mesenteric (posterior) one-third segment is closed first, using the TA stapler applied to the mucosal surfaces. **G:** Excessive tissue is sharply excised. The two remaining one-third segments are closed from the serosal surfaces as described.

the mucosal side. The remaining segments are closed from the serosal side as described earlier. Slight overlap of adjoining staple lines ensures complete closure without hindering anastomotic healing. Adequacy of the lumen, integrity of repair, and hemostasis are confirmed before closing the mesenteric defect.

Sigmoid Resection

The appropriate site for sigmoid transection is identified proximal to the area of diseased bowel. A small mesen-

teric opening is made adjacent to the colon, through which the GIA cartridge is introduced. The GIA anvil is placed across the bowel, and the stapler is secured and fired, resulting in a transected sigmoid with occluded proximal and distal segments. Moist laparotomy towels are used to pack the proximal segment above the surgical field. The mesenteric peritoneum is opened adjacent to the bowel, and the incision is continued parallel to the sigmoid as the mesentery transitions from a medial to a posterior insertion (Fig. 42.16). Mesenteric vessels are clamped, cut, and secured with 2-0 silk ligatures. The

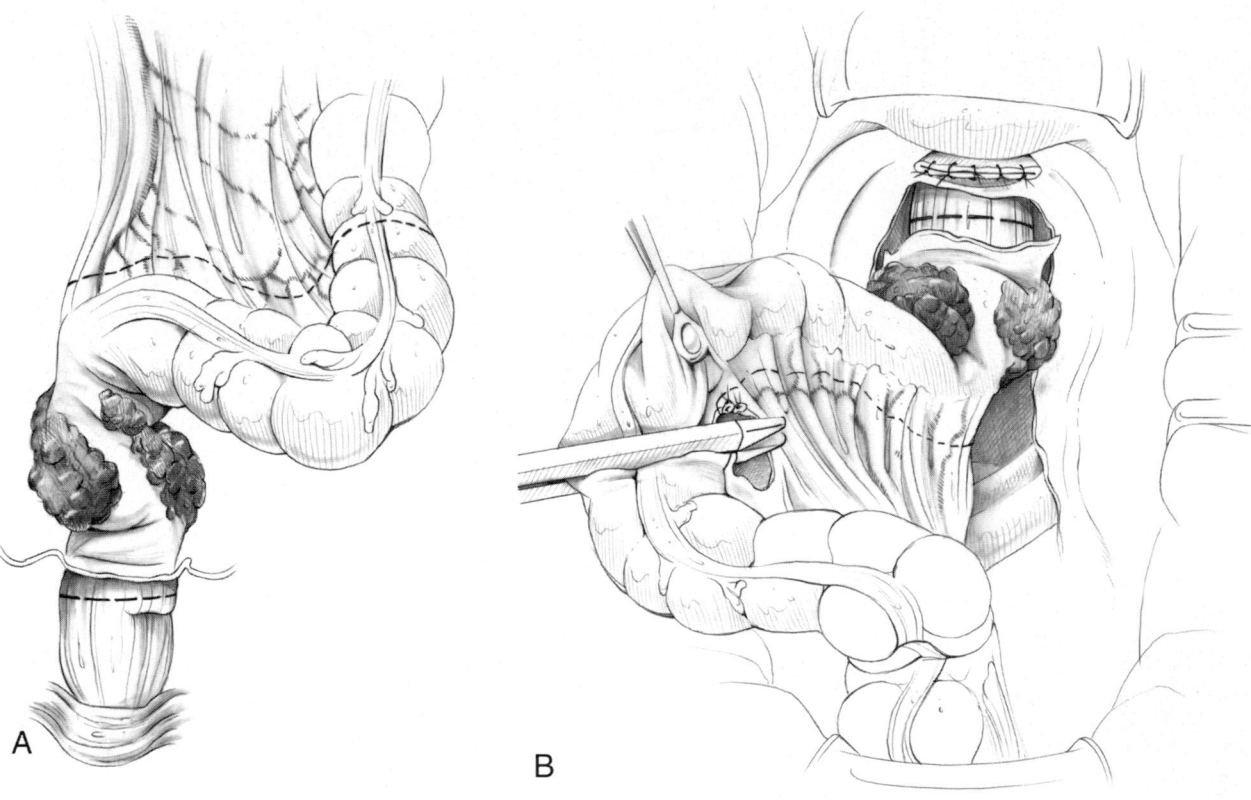

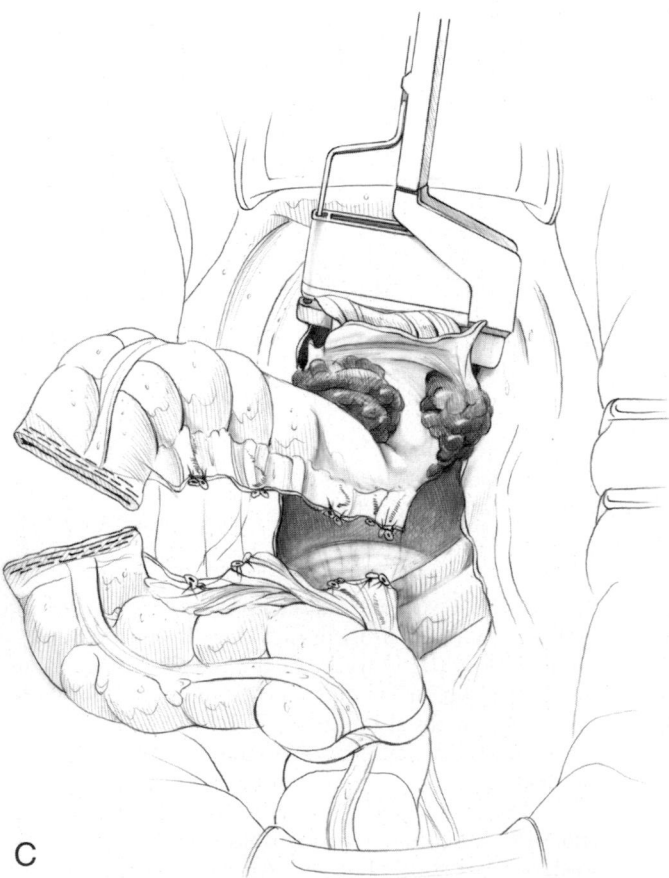

FIGURE 42.16. Sigmoid resection. **A:** An appropriate site for sigmoid transection is identified proximal to the area of diseased bowel. The amount of mesentery removed depends on the disease process. For most gynecologic conditions, an extensive mesenteric resection is not necessary. **B:** The gastrointestinal anastomosis stapler is used to divide the sigmoid colon. Sigmoid mesentery is transected by clamping, cutting, and securing the vessels with suture ligatures. **C:** The rectovaginal, retrorectal, and perirectal spaces are opened. Dissection is carried out until normal rectum is isolated below the diseased segment. The thoracoabdominal stapler is fired to occlude the rectum, which is then sharply excised to complete the resection.

rectovaginal space is opened between the uterosacral ligaments with cautery and sharp dissection. Blunt retroperitoneal dissection between the medial ureter and lateral hypogastric vessels exposes the perirectal space. Entry into the retrorectal space is aided by lifting the transected sigmoid. Retrorectal dissection is carried out to release the rectum from its attachments along the sacrum. Care is taken to avoid laceration of the presacral veins. The uterosacral ligaments are transected to gain exposure toward the distal rectum as the ureters are retracted laterally with a handheld malleable retractor. The rectal stalks are secured by dividing and ligating the posterior portion of the cardinal ligaments.

The extent of required dissection depends on the location and severity of disease. For nonmalignant pathology, dissection below the pelvic peritoneal reflection and levator ani is rarely necessary and may actually disrupt the blood supply. When normal rectum has been isolated below the diseased segment, the sigmoid resection can be finished. Pericolonic tissue attachments are cleared to expose smooth bowel wall. The TA stapler is guided across the rectum, ensuring the staple line incorporates only the rectum. The stapler is locked into position, checked for proper alignment, and fired by firm closure of the handles. Occluding clamps are placed across the bowel just above the staple line, and sharp dissection is used to transect the rectum and complete the resection.

Rectosigmoid End-to-End Staple Anastomosis

Before anastomosis, the descending colon is laid in the pelvis to ensure the colon and rectum can be approximated without tension. Redundant laxity of the colon should be observed. Any resistance or tension indicates the need for additional mobilization. The descending colonic lumen is occluded via an atraumatic clamp and the staple line is sharply excised. The appropriate diameter end-to-end anastomosis (EEA) stapler is selected based on the largest EEA sizer that can be placed into the lumen without undue stretch on the bowel wall. One milligram (one ampule) of intravenous glucagon causes relaxation of the muscularis and allows more accurate sizing.

Various designs of the EEA stapler exist, but generally the proximal portion consists of an anvil with a spike. An auto pursestring or hand-sewn pursestring is placed circumferentially around the open end of the descending colon. The anvil is positioned within the lumen, and the pursestring is secured around the base of the spike, the tip of which is directed toward the rectal stump. The anus is digitally dilated, and the lubricated shaft of the EEA stapler is introduced transanally. The shaft is visually and manually guided to the apex of the rectal stump. Clockwise rotation of the central wing nut advances the sharp trocar to pierce the apex of the rectal stump. The trocar is removed, leaving the hollow center shaft of the EEA in place through the rectum. The anvil spike from the descending colon is guided into the hollow center shaft of the rectal stump until it locks into place (Fig. 42.17). The central wing nut is further rotated clockwise until the indicator line is readily visible in the indicator window. This rotation draws the rectum and sigmoid colon into direct opposition. Normal anatomic alignment of the mesentery is confirmed. The safety is released, and steady, firm closure of the handles fires the instrument. The handles are released, and the central wing nut is rotated counterclockwise two complete turns. A gentle rocking motion back and forth frees the instrument tip from the anastomosis, as the EEA shaft is slowly withdrawn from the rectum.

The anastomotic integrity is confirmed through a series of checks. First, the staple line is visually and manually inspected. Second, the EEA instrument is inspected for two complete 360-degree tissue rings. This confirms circumferential stapling and resection of both the colonic and rectal segments. Third, the pelvis is filled with sterile crystalloid, and a rigid sigmoidoscope is used to insufflate the bowel. Manual occlusion of the proximal sigmoid ensures adequate testing pressure across the anastomosis. The anastomosis is observed while underwater, looking for air bubbles that would indicate an anastomotic leak (Fig. 42.18). Rigid sigmoidoscopy also allows direct internal inspection of the staple line, if necessary. If any of these methods suggest an incomplete anastomosis, the area in question is reinforced with interrupted 3-0 silk sutures, and the integrity is retested. Care is taken to avoid vascular compromise as the mesenteric defect is closed with interrupted sutures.

Postanastomotic morbidity and symptoms are largely related to the amount of residual rectum at the time of repair. Patients with a high colorectal anastomosis (11 cm or more above the anal verge) have relatively low morbidity and excellent functional results. Those who have undergone a low anastomosis (between 7 and 11 cm) have intermediate levels of morbidity, but generally have satisfactory functional results after several months of physiologic adaptation. In contrast, patients with a very low colorectal anastomosis (less than 7 cm from the anal verge) are at highest risk for complications, including anastomotic leak. These patients are also more likely to have chronic symptoms of gastrointestinal frequency, urgency, and incontinence. The sigmoid J-pouch for rectosigmoid anastomosis provides a reservoir that may decrease the frequency of stools and reduce the incidence of incontinence (Fig. 42.19). Accordingly, the J-pouch is considered if resection leaves less than 7 cm of rectum and if the colon is redundant enough to allow tension-free pouch construction. Postoperatively, some patients have a sense of incomplete evacuation and require suppositories or enemas.

Anastomotic leak is more common in colorectal anastomoses than in colon-to-colon anastomoses, in part because the rectum has no serosa. In ovarian cancer surgery, the estimated incidence of clinically significant anastomotic leak is 3% to 5%, but a wide range of this occurrence is reported in the literature. Traditionally, temporary diverting colostomies have been used to protect distal colonic anastomoses. Clinical studies do not support the notion that routine protective colostomies re-

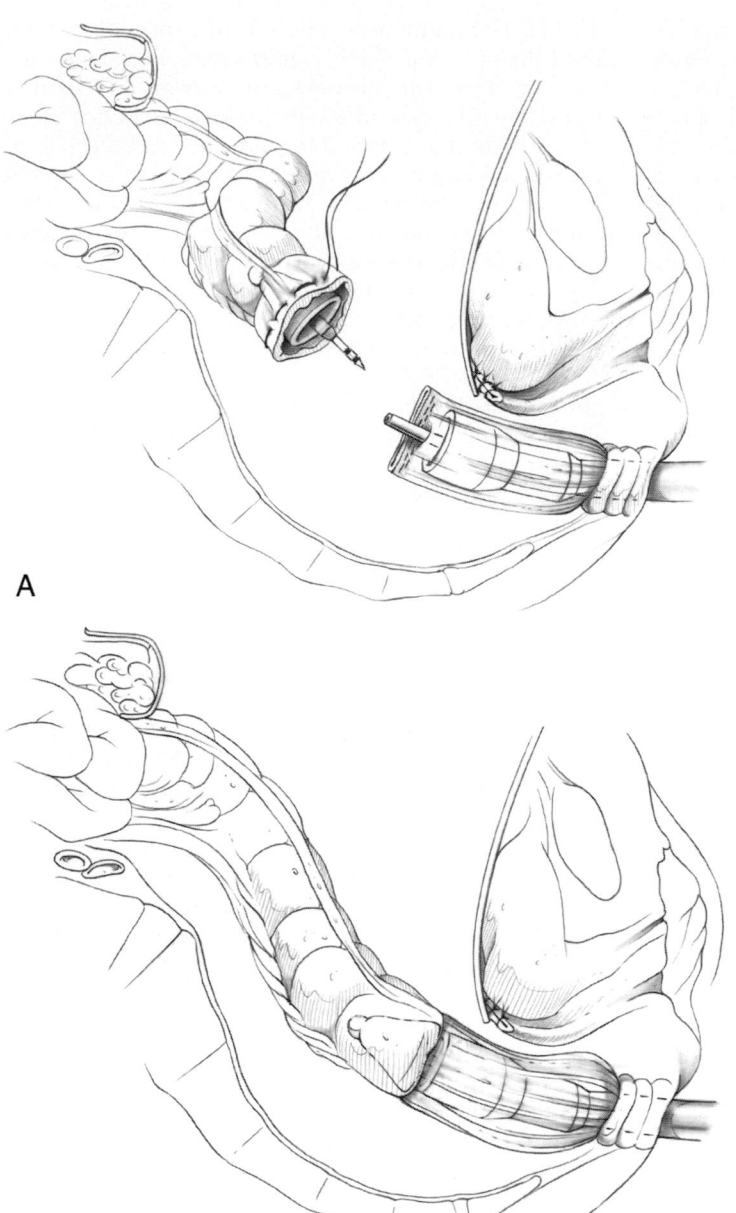

A

B

FIGURE 42.17. End-to-end rectosigmoid staple anastomosis. **A:** A pursestring suture holds the anvil and spike within the sigmoid lumen. The end-to-end anastomosis (EEA) stapler is inserted transanally. Clockwise rotation of the central wing nut advances the sharp trocar to pierce the apex of the rectal stump. In this illustration, the trocar has been removed and the hollow center shaft of the EEA remains in place. **B:** The spike and hollow center shaft are locked into position. Further rotation of the EEA central wing nut brings the sigmoid and rectum into direct opposition. The stapler is fired to deliver dual circular staple rows, as the knife transects the central tissue core to complete the anastomosis.

FIGURE 42.18. Testing the anastomotic integrity. The pelvis is filled with sterile crystalloid. The descending colon is manually occluded as air is insufflated via a rigid sigmoidoscope to create pressure across the anastomosis. Holding the anastomosis under water, it is examined for air bubbles that would suggest an anastomotic leak.

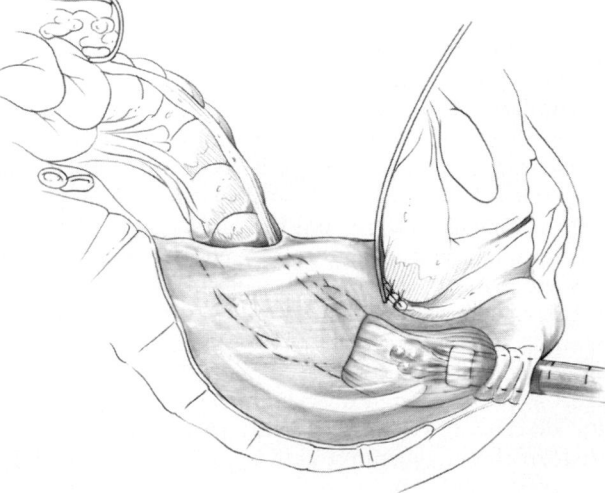

duce the risk of anastomotic breakdown. However, diversion of the fecal contents may reduce the severity of infectious complications if a leak occurs. Selective colonic diversion may be of benefit in cases of very low rectal anastomosis, prior radiation, unprepped bowel, and abscess or hematoma in the perianastomotic region.

End-to-Side Staple Anastomosis

End-to-side anastomotic techniques are advantageous for intestinal closure when the anorectal region is not readily accessible (e.g., supine position) or not necessary to complete the closure (e.g., ileocolonic or high rectosigmoid anastomosis). A high rectosigmoid repair is used for illustrative purposes. Following sigmoid resection, a small colotomy is made 3 to 4 cm from the end of the descending colon. The EEA instrument is introduced through the open lumen, and the hollow center shaft is advanced through the colotomy. The instrument is positioned such that the tip of the EEA rests perpendicular to bowel wall. A pursestring suture is used to secure the anvil spike within the rectal lumen. The end of the rectum is brought into close proximity with the side of the descending colon as the anvil spike is secured into

the EEA hollow center shaft. Clockwise rotation of the central wing nut brings the bowel edges into direct opposition. Rotation is continued until adequate closure is confirmed via the indicator window. The stapler is fired by closing the instrument grips. Counterclockwise rotation of the wing nut, followed by a subtle back and forth rocking motion, frees the instrument from the staple line. The open end of the descending colon is repaired using the TA stapler as previously described, and the integrity of the anastomosis is assessed.

End-to-End Hand-Sewn Single-Layer Colon Anastomosis

Before the common availability of surgical staplers, intestinal anastomoses were accomplished using hand-sewn techniques. Suture is still preferred over staple repair by some surgeons. Anastomosis can be accomplished using a single layer of delayed absorbable monofilament suture (small or large intestine) or nonabsorbable suture for large bowel (i.e., 4-0 polypropylene). The continuous closure has been proven efficacious in colon-to-colon repair and is used for this illustration. The bowel segments and mesenteric edges are aligned

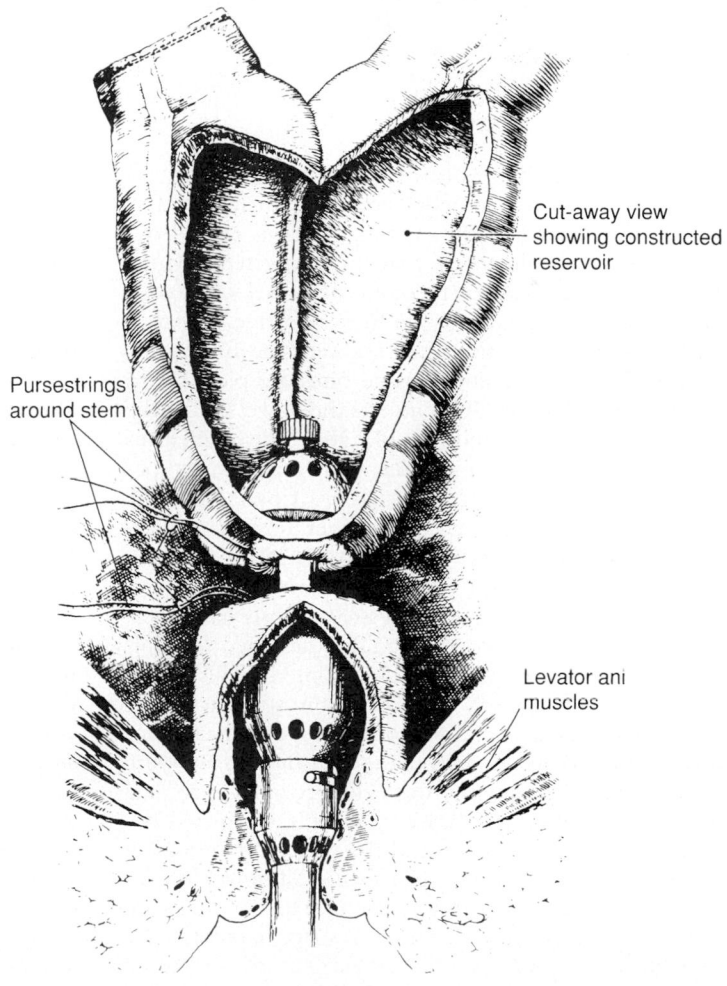

Cut-away view showing constructed reservoir

Pursestrings around stem

Levator ani muscles

FIGURE 42.19. Rectal J-pouch coloproctostomy.

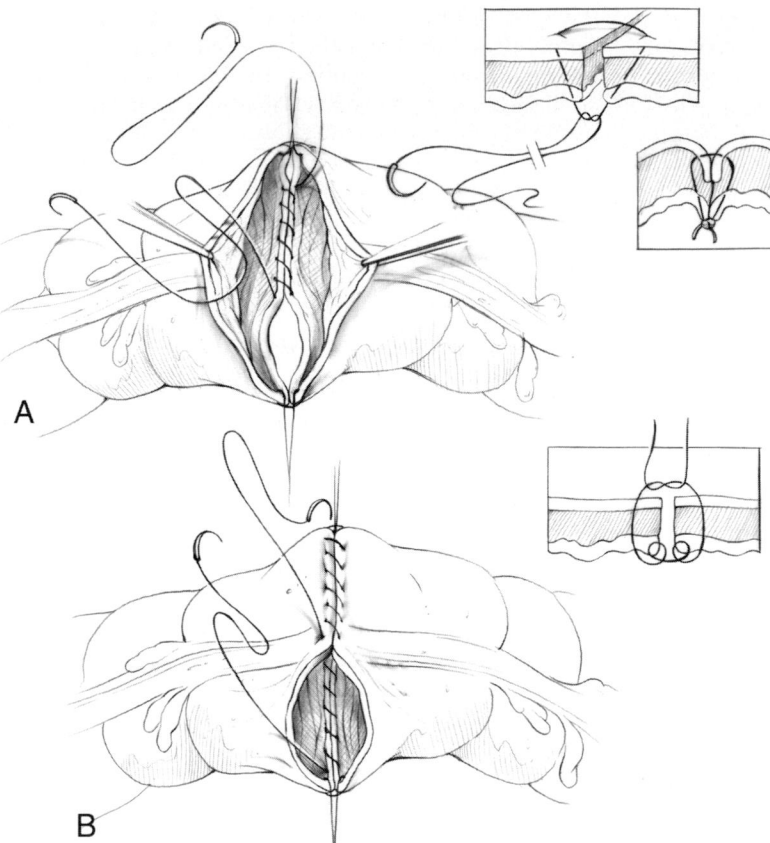

FIGURE 42.20. End-to-end hand-sewn single-layer colon anastomosis. **A:** The bowel edges are brought together and their alignment is stabilized with stay sutures. Sewing is started on the mucosal surfaces of the posterior bowel edges. A double-arm suture enables bidirectional sewing in a continuous fashion. **Insets:** The needle enters near the transected mucosal edge and passes obliquely through the bowel wall to exit 5 mm from the serosal edge. The needle is passed through the adjoining segment in the same oblique fashion, which inverts the tissue edges as the running suture is secured. **B:** Suturing is continued around the corners onto the anterior edges, which are closed from the serosal side. **Inset:** Alternative method of single-layer closure is the Gambee technique, which results in end-to-end opposition of the tissue edges without puckering the mucosa.

and secured with stay sutures. Suturing begins on the mesenteric (posterior) mucosal edges and is facilitated by a double-arm needle. The running stitch is carried out such that the needle enters near the transected mucosal edge and passes obliquely through the bowel wall to exit the serosa approximately 5 mm from the edge. The needle is passed through the adjoining segment in the same oblique fashion. Sequential tissue bites are placed 2 to 3 mm apart. This effectively inverts the bowel wall as the running suture is secured (Fig. 42.20). Bidirectional suturing is continued around the corners onto the antimesenteric (anterior) surfaces, which are closed from the serosal side. The Gambee single-layer technique is an equally effective method that results in end-to-end opposition of bowel edges without puckering the mucosa.

The interrupted single-layer anastomosis has generally been done as a closed technique designed to minimize intraoperative spill of enteric content. This closed technique is infrequently used today, but still plays a role in selected cases of unprepped bowel, especially those involving the colon. A pair of noncrushing clamps are placed across the lumen at both the proximal and distal sites for resection. The bowel is sharply transected between these paired clamps, and the mesenteric resection is completed as previously described. All bowel lumens remain occluded by a surgical clamp. The cut edges are held in close proximity with their respective mesenteries aligned. Interrupted 3-0 silk Lembert sutures are passed

full thickness through the bowel wall, being placed approximately 3 mm apart until they encompass the entire circumference. Some surgeons prefer to exclude the mucosa, because this adds no strength and may contribute to local tissue ischemia. Gentle traction and countertraction are applied along the untied sutures to guide the opposing bowel edges together. As the clamps are slowly removed, the sutures are tied. Patency of the lumen is assessed, and any insecure anastomotic areas are reinforced with additional sutures.

Colostomy

A colostomy should include tension-free bowel with noncompromised blood supply. The colon remains viable only about 2 cm beyond the closest intact vasa recta. The abdominal wall aperture must be generous enough to allow easy passage of the bowel with its intact mesentery, because even mild constriction may result in venous congestion, tissue edema, and necrosis. In gynecologic surgery, temporary colonic diversion may be necessary because of severe radiation injury (proctosigmoiditis), distal obstruction, perforation, or fistula. Permanent colostomy may be required if the rectum has been completely resected or is unacceptable for anastomosis. A diverting colostomy can also provide emergent decompression in the setting of complete large bowel obstruction at risk for perforation.

Perioperative Considerations

Preoperative consultation with an enterostomal therapist is very important in the perioperative planning and care. Counseling sessions, reading materials, support groups, and contact with other ostomy patients provide educational and emotional benefit. In nonemergent cases, the stoma appliance can be worn preoperatively to determine appropriate positioning and clarify postoperative expectations. The stoma should be located in an area that is easily seen and reached by the patient (Fig. 42.21). The tentative stoma site is marked preoperatively with indelible ink. As a general guide, a line is drawn connecting the anterior superior iliac spine to the umbilicus, and the colostomy is exteriorized through the rectus muscles at some point along this line. Placement is avoided within skin folds, surgical scars, and the umbilicus because the appliance will not seal securely with these skin irregularities.

Postoperatively, the enterostomal therapist can assist in teaching the patient independent ostomy care. Daily inspection is important to ensure tissue viability, adequate function, and nonretraction of the stoma. If tissue viability is in question, closer investigation under bright light is warranted. Insertion of a glass test tube or syringe with penlight transillumination allows for an easy bedside inspection of the internal bowel wall. If tissue viability remains uncertain, an anoscope or sigmoidoscope can be used. Focal ischemia is suggested if the mucosa is grey or dusky in appearance. Tissue necrosis distal to the skin edge may be safely observed and reevaluated after tissue sloughing and reepithelialization have occurred. Surgical correction is generally unnecessary in this setting. Deeper and more extensive necrosis indicates compromised blood flow and the need for colostomy revision. Excessive retraction, stricture, or peristomal herniation may also require surgical correction.

Some patients with an end sigmoid or descending colostomy prefer irrigation management over a collection appliance. Motivation, capacity for self-care, and relatively normal preoperative bowel function are requisite. Irrigation is started early in the postoperative period and is continued on a daily basis thereafter. The eventual goal is fecal continence between irrigations. Irrigation can also help reduce stoma odor and flatus, which can be further suppressed with a charcoal-based stoma cap. Some patients will develop predictable evacuation patterns such that irrigation is eventually not required. Others will be satisfied with the security of a continuous appliance.

End Colostomy Technique

Efforts are made to create the stoma at the site marked on the abdominal wall preoperatively. The bowel selected for use should be adequately mobilized so the distal end can be brought beyond the abdominal wall by several centimeters. To fashion the abdominal wall aperture, a 3-cm diameter circle is drawn on the skin at the marked site. Symmetry is aided by a circular guide such as the flat, round end of a 60-cc syringe plunger. Dissection is carried through the skin and subcutaneous tissue to the level of the rectus fascia. A core of subcutaneous adipose tissue is not necessarily removed. Cruciate incisions are made in the anterior rectus sheath, with each incision being approximately 4 cm in length. The rectus muscle fibers are bluntly separated until the posterior rectus sheath and peritoneum are reached, through which similar cruciate incisions are made. When separating the rectus abdominus muscle, care is taken to avoid injury of the inferior epigastric vessels. All layers of the abdominal aperture are manually dilated and should easily admit three fingers without stricture.

A Babcock clamp is inserted through the aperture to grasp the colon for exteriorization. The bowel is brought through the abdominal wall, such that the occluded end rests easily above the skin surface without tension. Large epiploic appendices can be removed with electrocautery if needed to ease exteriorization. Tissue viability is assessed to ensure noncompromised blood flow. Interrupted 3-0 silk seromuscular sutures are fixed to the posterior and anterior rectus sheaths to secure the alignment and reduce the chance of retraction or herniation. The lateral pericolic gutter is obliterated to prevent small bowel herniation. Maturation of the stoma is deferred until after the abdomen is closed.

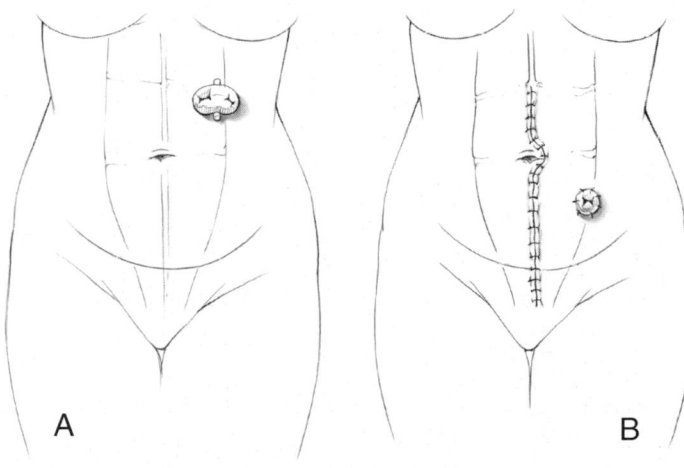

FIGURE 42.21. Positioning the stoma. **A:** Shown is a transverse loop colostomy positioned in the left upper abdomen. **B:** An end colostomy located in the left lower abdomen. As a guide, a line can be drawn to connect the umbilicus with the anterior-superior iliac spine, along which the end colostomy is positioned. The stoma is exteriorized through the rectus abdominus muscle and secured to skin that is devoid of folds or surgical scars.

A   B

Any remaining surgical objectives are completed, and the peritoneal cavity is irrigated and checked for hemostasis. The intraabdominal and extraabdominal bowel are again inspected before closing the surgical wound. After closure, the incision is protected with collodion or sterile towels. The exteriorized colon is opened, and the cut edges are observed for bleeding to ensure viability. Excessive bowel is trimmed such that approximately 2 to 3 cm remain above the skin surface. If viability is questionable, the edges are trimmed further until adequate blood flow is confirmed.

The stoma is matured using interrupted delayed absorbable sutures (3-0 polyglycolic acid). Stitches are initiated at the skin surface and carried in and out through the seromuscular bowel wall approximately 2 cm from the distal end and then full thickness through the cut bowel edge (Fig. 42.22). Sutures are placed circumferentially at about 5-mm intervals. As the sutures are tied,

the everted bowel wall is folded back on itself. The result is a slightly protruding stoma that enables a better appliance fit and is less prone to retraction. In patients with a thick abdominal wall, it may not be possible to have enough viable bowel for stomal eversion. In this scenario, a stoma flush with the skin surface is matured by securing the skin to full-thickness bowel edge using interrupted sutures. The appliance is fashioned and secured intraoperatively.

Diverting Loop Colostomy

A loop colostomy is technically less difficult to create and reverse than an end colostomy and can often be accomplished through a single incision. This is a good technique when a temporary diverting colostomy is needed. Readily mobile transverse or sigmoid colon is preferred. As a general rule, the loop colostomy is fashioned from

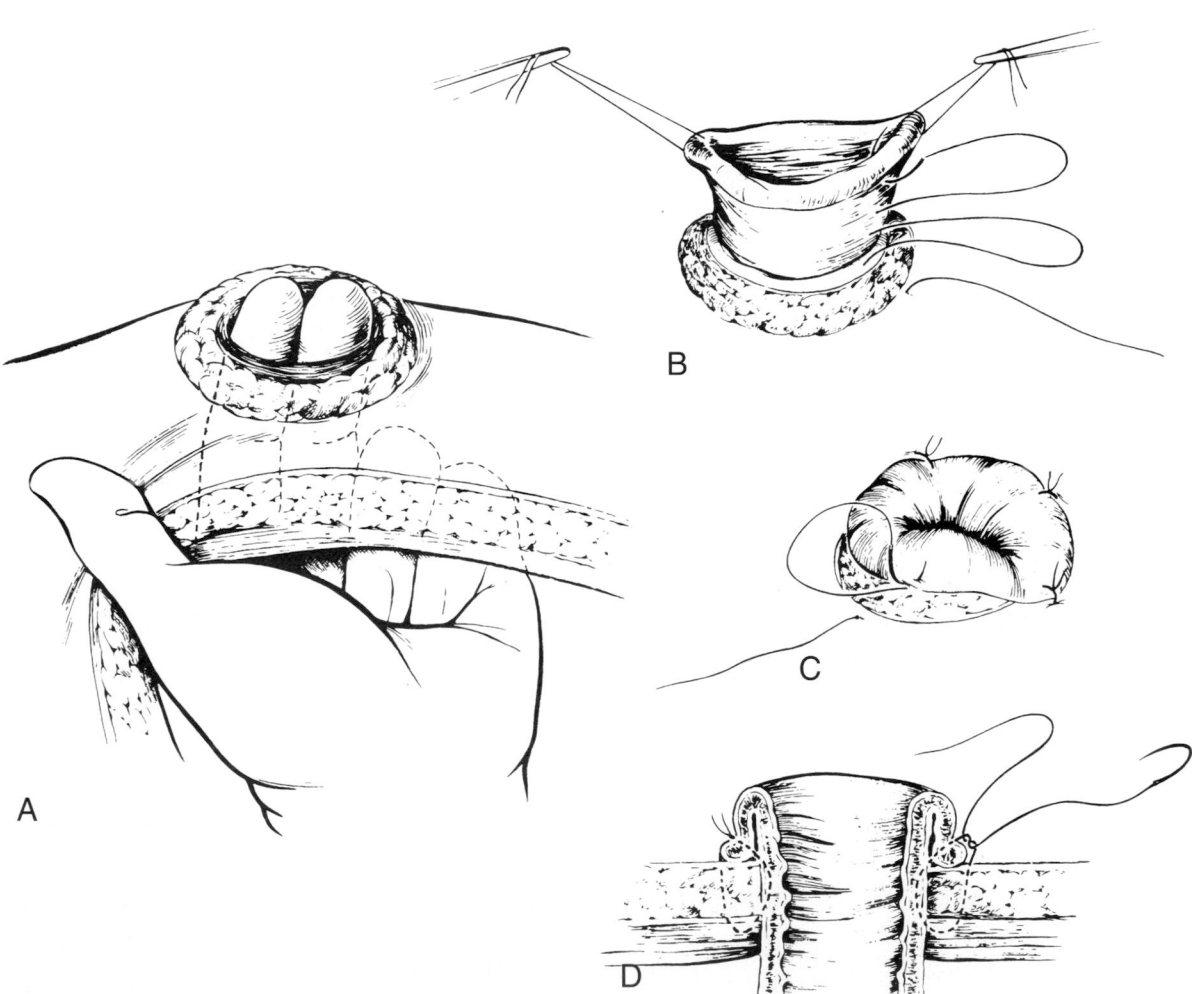

FIGURE 42.22. End colostomy. Technique for creating a bowel stoma that is elevated from the skin surface. This everted stoma is developed by excising a 3-cm circumferential segment of abdominal wall (**A**), anchoring the skin margin with the adjacent wall of the exteriorized bowel (**B**), and approximating the mucosal edge of the bowel to the skin (**C**). The cross-sectional view demonstrates how the bowel wall is anchored to the skin margin to prevent retraction (**D**).

the most distal site along the bowel that can be effectively used. Factors to consider are that the transverse colon is generally outside of the previous surgical or radiation field and the transverse colon has a lower bacterial count than the more distal colon. Alternatively, use of the sigmoid preserves a greater length of intact bowel. The traditional loop colostomy is described for illustrative purposes and uses the transverse colon with the stoma created in the left upper quadrant.

In comparison to an end colostomy, a larger aperture is required to bring two full segments of colon through the abdominal wall. A stoma site is selected overlying the rectus muscle, which avoids skin folds, surgical scars, and the umbilicus. A transverse incision is carried down through the anterior rectus fascia. Two evenly spaced, perpendicular fascial incisions can be used to increase the diameter of this aperture. The rectus muscle fibers are bluntly separated, and the posterior rectus sheath and peritoneum are incised in a manner similar to that of the anterior fascia. The opening is manually dilated and should easily admit four fingers without stricture.

The transverse colon is identified by the presence of tenia and the omental attachment. Once isolated, the bowel is followed in a hand-over-hand fashion until the most distal yet readily mobile segment is brought through the abdominal wall. Lifting the loop is simplified by using a half-inch diameter Penrose drain passed under the intestine. A bridge device is also passed through the adjacent mesenteric window and positioned onto the skin, thereby supporting the bowel loop above the skin surface. Fascial supporting sutures are generally not necessary as the normal healing process scars the stoma into position. Any extra length of the abdominal incision is closed. The stoma is matured by a sharp longitudinal incision through the tenia that is extended to within 1.0 cm of the skin edge at both ends. The stoma edges are everted and secured with interrupted skin to full-thickness bowel sutures using 3-0 delayed absorbable material (Fig. 42.23).

The traditional Hollister bridge frequently precludes a secure appliance fit. A number of various supporting devices have been used effectively. We prefer a supporting bridge fashioned from a 20-French thoracostomy tube. A segment of about 20 cm length is cut and passed through the mesenteric window underneath the bowel.

The ends are brought together over the bowel and sutured together to form a loop. This method requires no skin sutures, does not interfere with application of the collecting bag, and permits secure adherence between the stoma wafer and skin. After adequate healing (10 to 14 days), the bridge is easily removed by cutting the suture to open the loop and withdraw the tube.

Variations of the loop colostomy include the double-barrel colostomy in which the bowel is transected and both stomas are matured. An end colostomy with mucous fistula is used in the setting of distal obstruction, because the decompression provided by the mucous fistula avoids a closed loop obstruction. When the mucous fistula is placed immediately adjacent to the end colostomy, it is known as an end loop or terminal loop colostomy.

GASTRIC PROCEDURE
Open Gastrostomy

A gastrostomy tube avoids prolonged nasogastric intubation when long-term gastric decompression is needed. This access route can also be used for enteral hydration, nutrition, and medication administration in patients who have an intact intestinal tract. Gastrostomy is avoided in obtunded patients and those with massive ascites, esophageal varices, coagulopathy, or extensive tumor that precludes tension-free placement. Commercially available gastrostomy tubes generally have an inflatable balloon tip that secures the tube within the stomach. Other catheters such as a Foley, Robinson, or Malecot also suffice.

The technique of open gastrostomy begins with ensuring there is adequate mobilization to bring the stomach wall into direct opposition with the abdominal wall. An insertion site is chosen in the mid anterior gastric wall, away from the short gastric vessels. Cautery or sharp dissection is used to make a small puncture. Injury to the posterior gastric wall is avoided by making the gastrotomy directly over a nasogastric tube, which is secured into position with handheld traction. A stab incision is made through the skin of the left upper abdomen. A narrow clamp is passed from peritoneum through skin, and the tip of the gastrostomy tube is grasped and

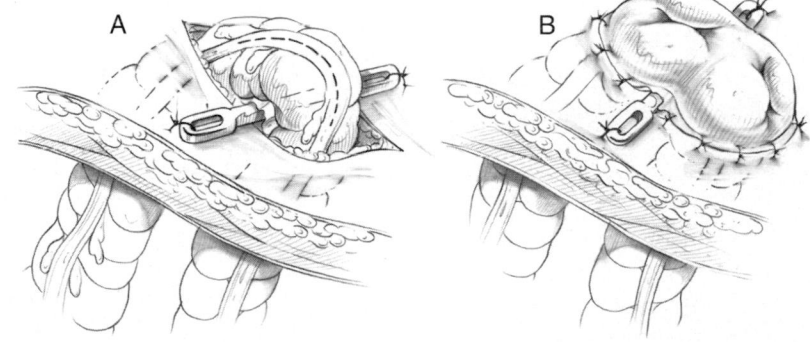

FIGURE 42.23. Transverse loop colostomy. **A:** An isolated loop of transverse colon is held above the skin surface by a supporting bridge. The bowel is opened via sharp incision through the tenia. **B:** The stoma is matured using interrupted 3-0 delayed absorbable sutures, which are placed from skin to full thickness bowel edge.

brought through the abdominal wall. The tube is guided into the stomach through the gastrotomy and secured in place with two pursestring sutures of 2-0 delayed absorbable or nonabsorbable material. The inner pursestring suture is first secured. The gastric wall is then elevated and held in position using Babcock clamps as the outer pursestring suture is tied securely around the tube in Stamm fashion. If a balloon apparatus is used, it is inflated with approximately 10 cc of fluid. Traction on the gastrostomy tube elevates the stomach to the abdominal wall peritoneum; these are then sutured together using interrupted 2-0 delayed absorbable sutures. The tube can be further secured at the skin surface using nonabsorbable suture. Similar techniques are also used to decompress the intestinal tract at other anatomic locations, such as via a tube jejunostomy.

This open technique can also be used for gastroduodenal tube insertion. Commercially available catheters (Moss gastrostomy tube, Moss Tubes, West Sand Lake, NY) have proximal ports for gastric decompression and distal ports to deliver enteral nutrition (Fig. 42.24). Intraoperatively, the tube is manually guided through the pylorus into the duodenum. Advantages of small bowel enteral nutrition include less gastroesophageal reflux and aspiration in comparison to gastric feedings. This also allows simultaneous enteral nutrition while decompressing the stomach. Such feedings are, however, more likely to cause cramping, abdominal distention, and rapid transit with diarrhea.

If a permanent gastrostomy is intended at the time of surgery, consideration is given to a gastric flap procedure. With this approach, a portion of the stomach wall is incorporated into the stoma. An inverted U-shaped flap is raised from the anterior stomach wall, with the base located near the greater curvature. An adequate flap reduces

gastric reflux onto the skin and should be 6 cm in width by 10 cm in length. The flap is closed around the gastrostomy catheter in continuum with the gastric closure, using two layers of delayed absorbable suture. The distal end of the flap is exteriorized and matured as a stoma.

Postoperatively, the gastrostomy tube is attached to low wall suction ($\leq$80 mm Hg) and irrigated frequently. The catheter is generally not removed before the fourth postoperative week to ensure adequate healing between the gastric wall and peritoneum. When the tube is discontinued, gastric leaking tends to persist for several days until the defect reepithelializes. Occasionally, a gastrocutaneous fistula persists which could require surgical closure. A long-term indwelling gastrostomy tube is replaced every 2 to 3 months to maintain adequate function. This is accomplished by decompressing the balloon and removing the old tube, with immediate replacement of a new tube through the mature tract.

Excessive tension can cause tissue ischemia and necrosis. Conversely, an inadequate seal can result in leakage of gastric content with resultant abscess and peritonitis. Surgical reexploration is necessary if the leak cannot be corrected by increasing balloon tension against the undersurface of the abdominal wall. Other potential gastrostomy complications include bleeding, tube malfunction, skin irritation, infection, and migration through the pylorus or gastroesophageal junction.

Endoscopic Gastric Procedures

Percutaneous procedures are currently available for patients in need of gastrostomy who are not undergoing laparotomy. Percutaneous endoscopic gastrostomy (PEG) and percutaneous endoscopic jejunostomy (PEJ) are performed under local anesthesia with intravenous sedation.

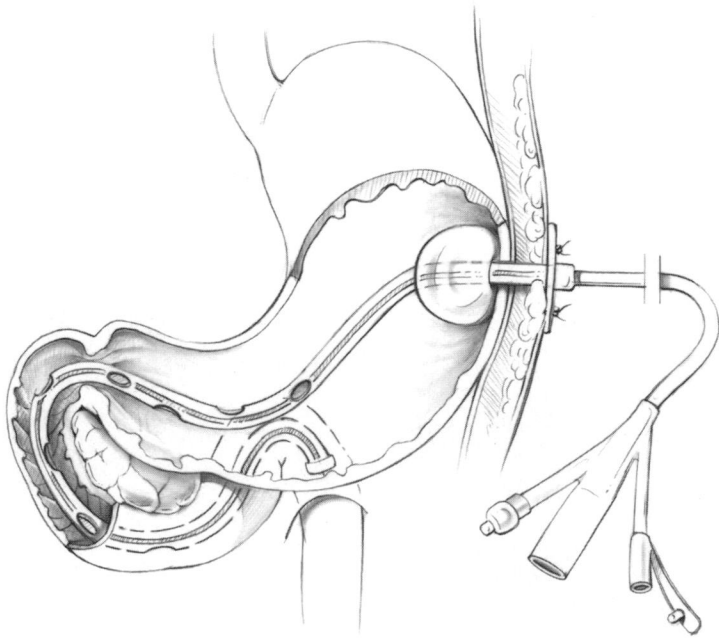

FIGURE 42.24. Gastrostomy tube. The gastric wall and abdominal wall are juxtaposed and held into position via balloon apparatus and suture fixation. Shown is a gastrostomy tube with proximal ports for gastric decompression, and distal ports for enteral nutrition (i.e., Moss gastrostomy tube, Moss Tubes, West Sand Lake, NY).

The PEG tube is placed via endoscopic gastric insufflation and transillumination to guide percutaneous needle and guide wire placement through the abdominal wall. An introducer is passed transcutaneously into the stomach over the guide wire. The introducer is withdrawn, leaving a sheath through which the gastrostomy tube is inserted. As the sheath is peeled away, traction on the tube draws the flange and stomach wall into juxtaposition with the abdominal wall. Another external flange or fixation suture is used to secure the apparatus into position. Using similar endoscopic techniques, a jejunostomy tube can be guided through the pylorus and duodenum, into the jejunum. Laparoscopic procedures have also been developed and are used by surgeons familiar with advanced laparoscopic techniques. Although less invasive than laparotomy, laparoscopic procedures usually also require general anesthesia.

BIBLIOGRAPHY

Adamson GD, Nelson HP. Surgical treatment of endometriosis. *Obstet Gynecol Clin North Am* 1997;24(2):375.

Beart RW, Kelly KA. Randomized prospective evaluation of the EEA stapler for colorectal anastomoses. *Am J Surg* 1981;141:143.

Bernard DK, Shaw MJ. Principles of nutrition therapy for short-bowel syndrome. *Nutr Clin Pract* 1993;8:153–160.

Brennan SS, Pickford IR, Evans M, et al. Staples or sutures for colonic anastomosis—a controlled clinical trial. *Br J Surg* 1982;69:722.

Burke P, Mealy K, Gillen P, et al. Requirement for bowel preparation in colorectal surgery. *Br J Surg* 1994;81:907–910.

Carey LC, Fabri PJ. The intestinal tract in relation to gynecology. In: Thompson JD, Rock JA, eds. *Te Linde's Operative Gynecology,* seventh ed. Philadelphia: JB Lippincott, 1992.

Cheatham ML, Chapman WC, Key SP, et al. A meta-analysis of selective versus routine nasogastric decompression after elective laparotomy. *Ann Surg* 1995;221(5):469; discussion 476–478.

Chung RS. Blood flow in colonic anastomoses: effect of stapling and suturing. *Ann Surg* 1987;206:335.

Clark JS, Condon RE, Barlett JG, et al. Preoperative oral antibiotics reduce septic complications of colon operations: results of prospective, randomized, double-blind clinical study. *Ann Surg* 1977;186:251–259.

Cohen Z, Sullivan B. Intestinal anastomosis. In: Wilmore DW, Cheung LY, Harken AM, et al, eds. *ACS surgery: principles and practice.* New York: WEBMD, 2002.

Coppa GF, Eng K. Factors involved in antibiotic selection in elective colon and rectal surgery. *Surgery* 1988;104:853 858.

Curran TJ, Borzotta AP. Complications of primary repair of colon injury: literature review of 2,964 cases. *Am J Surg* 1999;177:42–47.

Cutillo G, Maneschi F, Franchi M, et al. Early feeding compared with nasogastric decompression after major oncologic gynecologic surgery: a randomized study. *Obstet Gynecol* 1999;93(1):41–45.

Eskelinen M, Ikonen J, Lipponen P. Contributions of history-taking, physical examination and computer assistance to diagnose acute small bowel obstruction: a prospective study of 1333 patients with acute abdominal pain. *Scand J Gastroenterol* 1994;29:715.

Falcone RE, Wanamaker SR, Santanello SA, et al. Colorectal trauma: primary repair or anastomosis with intracolonic bypass vs. ostomy. *Dis Colon Rectum* 1992;35(10):957–963.

Fanning J, Andrews S. Early postoperative feeding after major gynecologic surgery: evidence-based scientific medicine. *Am J Obstet Gynecol* 2001;185(1):1–4.

Gambee LP, Garnojobst W, Harwick CE. Ten years experience with a single layer anastomosis in colon surgery. *Am J Surg* 1956;92:222.

Gillette-Cloven N, Burger RA, Monk BJ, et al. Bowel resection at the time of primary cytoreduction for epithelial ovarian cancer. *J Am Coll Surg* 2001;193:626.

Helton WS. Intestinal obstruction. In: Wilmore DW, Cheung LY, Harken Am, et al, eds. *ACS surgery: principles and practice.* New York, WEBMD, 2002.

Hesp F, Hendriks T, Lubbers EJ, et al. Wound healing in the intestinal wall: a comparison between experimental ileal and colonic anastomosis. *Dis Colon Rectum* 1984;24:99.

Jaeger W, Ackermann S, Kessler H, et al. The effect of bowel resection on survival in advanced epithelial ovarian cancer. *Gynecol Oncol* 2001;83:286.

Krebs HB. Intestinal injury in gynecologic surgery: a ten year experience. *Am J Obstet Gynecol* 1986;155(3):509–514.

Levine JH, Longo WE, Pruitt C, et al. Management of selected rectal injuries by primary repair. *Am J Surg* 1996;172(5):575–578; discussion 578–579.

MacMillan SL, Kammerer-Doak D, Rogers RG, et al. Early feeding and the incidence of gastrointestinal symptoms after major gynecologic surgery. *Obstet Gynecol* 2000;96(4):604–608.

Miettinen RP, Laitinen ST, Makela JT, et al. Bowel preparation with oral polyethylene glycol electrolyte solution vs. no preparation in elective open colorectal surgery: prospective, randomized study. *Dis Colon Rectum* 2000;43:669–677.

Mirhashemi R, Averette HE, Estape R, et al. Low colorectal anastomosis after radical pelvic surgery: a risk factor analysis. *Am J Obstet Gynecol* 2000;183:1375.

Mitchell GW Jr. Evisceration and repair of ventral hernias. In: Nichols DM, Ed. *Gynecologic and obstetrical surgery.* St. Louis, Mosby–Year Book, 1993.

Monk BJ, Berman ML, Montz FJ. Adhesions after extensive gynecologic surgery: clinical significance, etiology, and prevention. *Am J Obstet Gynecol* 1994;170:1396–1403.

Morrow CP, Curtin JP. Surgical anatomy. In: *Gynecologic cancer surgery.* Philadelphia: Churchill Livingstone, 1996.

Morrow CP, Curtin JP. Surgery on the intestinal tract. In: *Gynecologic cancer surgery.* Philadelphia: Churchill Livingstone, 1996.

Nichols RL, Smith JW, Garcia RY, et al. Current practices of preoperative bowel preparation among North American colorectal surgeons. *Clin Infect Dis* 1997;24:609.

Obermair A, Hagenauer S, Tamandl D, et al. Safety and efficacy of low anterior en bloc resection as part of cytoreductive surgery for patients with ovarian cancer. *Gynecol Oncol* 2001;83(1):115–120.

Oliveira L, Wexner SD, Daniel N, et al. Mechanical bowel preparation for elective colorectal surgery: a prospective, randomized, surgeon-blinded trial comparing sodium phosphate and polyethylene glycol-based oral lavage solutions. *Dis Colon Rectum* 1997;40:585–591.

Platell C, Hall J. What is the role of mechanical bowel preparation in patients undergoing colorectal surgery? *Dis Colon Rectum* 1998;41(7):875–882; discussion 882–883.

Pearl ML, Frandina M, Mahler L, et al. A randomized controlled trial of a regular diet as the first meal in gynecologic oncology patients undergoing intraabdominal surgery. *Obstet Gynecol* 2002;100:230–234.

Rex D. Should we colonoscope women with gynecologic cancer? *Am J Gastroenterol* 2000;95(3):812–813.

Santos JC Jr, Batista J, Sirimarco MT, et al. Prospective randomized trial of mechanical bowel preparation in patients undergoing elective colorectal surgery. *Br J Surg* 1994;81:1673–1676.

Schrock TR. Colorectal procedures. In: Wilmore DW, Cheung LY, Harken Am, et al., eds. *ACS surgery: principles and practice*. New York: WEBMD, 2002.

Schwartz SI. Small intestinal surgery incidental to gynecologic procedures. In: Nichols DH, ed. *Gynecologic and obstetric surgery*. St. Louis: Mosby–Year Book, 1993.

Schwartz SI. Surgery of the colon, incidental to gynecologic surgery. In: Nichols DH, ed. *Gynecologic and obstetric surgery*. St. Louis: Mosby–Year Book, 1993.

Stewart BT, Woods RJ, Collopy BT, et al. Early feeding after elective open colorectal resections: a prospective randomized trial. *Aust N Z J Surg* 1998;68(2):125–128.

Tamussino KF, Lim PC, Webb MJ, et al. Gastrointestinal surgery in patients with ovarian cancer. *Gynecol Oncol* 2001;80(1):79–84.

Taylor EW, Lindsay G. Selective decontamination of the colon before elective colorectal surgery. West of Scotland Surgical Infection Study Group. *World J Surg* 1994;18:926–931.

Van Der Krabben AA, Dijkstra FR, Nieuwenhuijzen M, et al. Morbidity and mortality of inadvertent enterotomy during adhesiotomy. *Br J Surg* 2000;87(4):467–471.

Wheeless Jr CR. The intestinal tract in gynecologic surgery. In: Rock JA, Thompson JD, eds. *Te Linde's operative gynecology,* eighth ed. Philadelphia: Lippincott-Raven, 1996.

Yoshioka K, Connolly AB, Ogunbiyi OA, et al. Randomized trial of oral sodium phosphate compared with oral sodium pico-sulphate (Picolax) for elective colorectal surgery and colonoscopy. *Dig Surg* 2000;17:66–70.

Zmora O, Pikarsky AJ, Wexner SD. Bowel preparation for colorectal surgery. *Dis Colon Rectum* 2001;44(10):1537–1549.

Te Linde's Operative Gynecology, ninth edition, edited by John A. Rock and Howard W. Jones, III. Lippincott Williams & Wilkins, Philadelphia: © 2003.

CHAPTER

43

▼

Nongynecologic Conditions Encountered by the Gynecologic Surgeon

KENNETH W. SHARP   V. SEENU REDDY

From time to time, the gynecologic surgeon may be faced with a surgical or even nonsurgical condition that arises in the gastrointestinal tract, urinary tract, or some other nongynecologic pelvic structure. Although careful preoperative evaluation should correctly identify most of these patients, occasionally women with symptoms of pelvic pain or findings of a pelvic mass may be thought to have pelvic inflammatory disease (PID), only to be found to have a ruptured appendix when the abdomen is opened; or an ovarian mass in a 35-year-old woman may be a metastasis from a primary cancer of the colon. In such patients, and on occasion when the gynecologic surgeon may be asked to consult or assist another pelvic surgeon, it is most helpful to understand the clinical presentation, workup, and management of some nongynecologic pelvic conditions. A discussion of these situations is presented in this chapter.

PREOPERATIVE DIAGNOSTIC EVALUATION

A careful history and physical examination combined with routine laboratory data remains the cornerstone of the preliminary evaluation. Although nongynecologic pelvic disorders that can be encountered by the gynecologic surgeon can occur at any age, they are most often found in the obese or elderly patient with an ill-defined pelvic mass. The symptoms often are vague and, particularly in the elderly patient, minimized. Additionally, most elderly patients often have a high threshold for pain.

Gastrointestinal Disease

Complaints such as pelvic pain, low-grade fever, altered bowel habits, hematochezia, or melena should arouse suspicions of intestinal disease. Although pelvic pain is frequent in patients with gynecologic conditions, it is also common in many rectal and urologic diseases. Pain extending outside the pelvis should heighten concern for nongynecologic disorders. Abdominal distention, nonspecific dyspeptic and postprandial pain, and unintentional weight loss may alert the clinician to evaluate the patient for nongynecologic conditions. In such instances, a gastrointestinal evaluation is essential before laparotomy.

A pelvic examination may reveal a right or left adnexal mass that may seem to be an inflammatory or neoplastic disorder of the tube or ovary or both, but this may not be the true situation. Line drawings and representative computed tomography (CT) scans depict various intestinal disorders that may be mistaken easily for ovarian or tubal conditions (Figs. 43.1 through 43.5). Digital rectal examination and testing of stool for the presence of occult blood should be a routine component of every physical examination. A positive test for occult blood is important in guiding further evaluation of the gastrointestinal tract, but a negative test does not reliably exclude the presence of a significant gastrointestinal lesion.

Appropriate preoperative evaluation of the patient with a suspected intestinal disorder may require a variety of studies. The workup of a patient with evidence of blood in her stool may involve a barium enema, colonoscopy, an upper gastrointestinal series, or even an upper tract endoscopy to look for ulcers, polyps, colon cancer, diverticular disease, or even inflammatory bowel disease. The patient with blood in the stool who has nor-

mal radiographic studies of the colon and stomach may need a small bowel series to look for Crohn's disease, distal small bowel tumors (carcinoids, lymphoma), or small bowel diverticula. In addition to being an invaluable aid in the detection of colon cancer and diverticulitis, a barium enema may detect appendicitis or an appendiceal abscess colonoscopy is considered to be an appropriate initial evaluation for a patient over the age of 50 who has blood in the stool because of the increasing incidence of colonic polyps and cancer in this age group. CT scans of the abdomen and pelvis are very useful in evaluating abdominal and pelvic masses and in delineating small bowel, colon, cecal, or appendiceal conditions. Figures 43.6 through 43.9 are examples of colonic conditions diagnosed by barium enema and CT studies.

Although the value of digital rectal examination and sigmoidoscopy in detecting lesions of the rectum and sigmoid cannot be overemphasized, the changing distri-

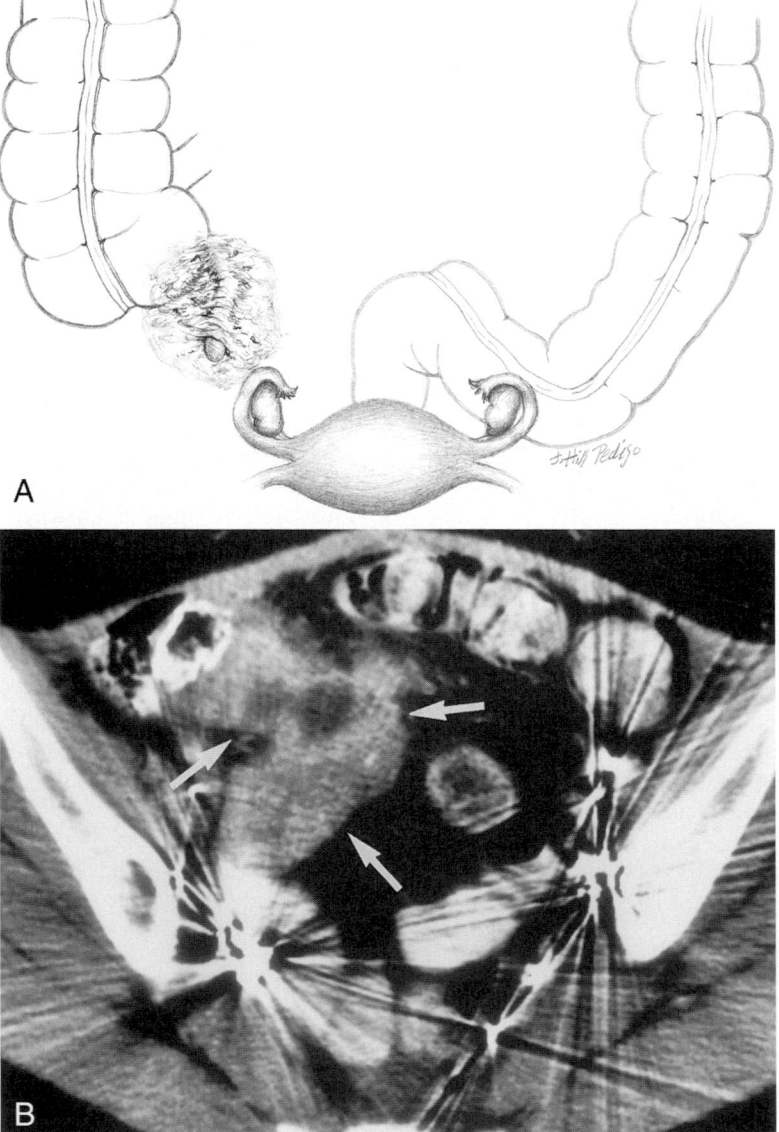

FIGURE 43.1. Appendiceal abscess. **A:** On bimanual examination, this abscess is felt to be slightly higher in the pelvis but can be mistaken for an adnexal condition. **B:** Computed tomography image shows inhomogeneous abscess *(arrows)* in the right side of the pelvis. Hemoclip artifact is also present. (Courtesy of T. Demos, Maywood, IL.)

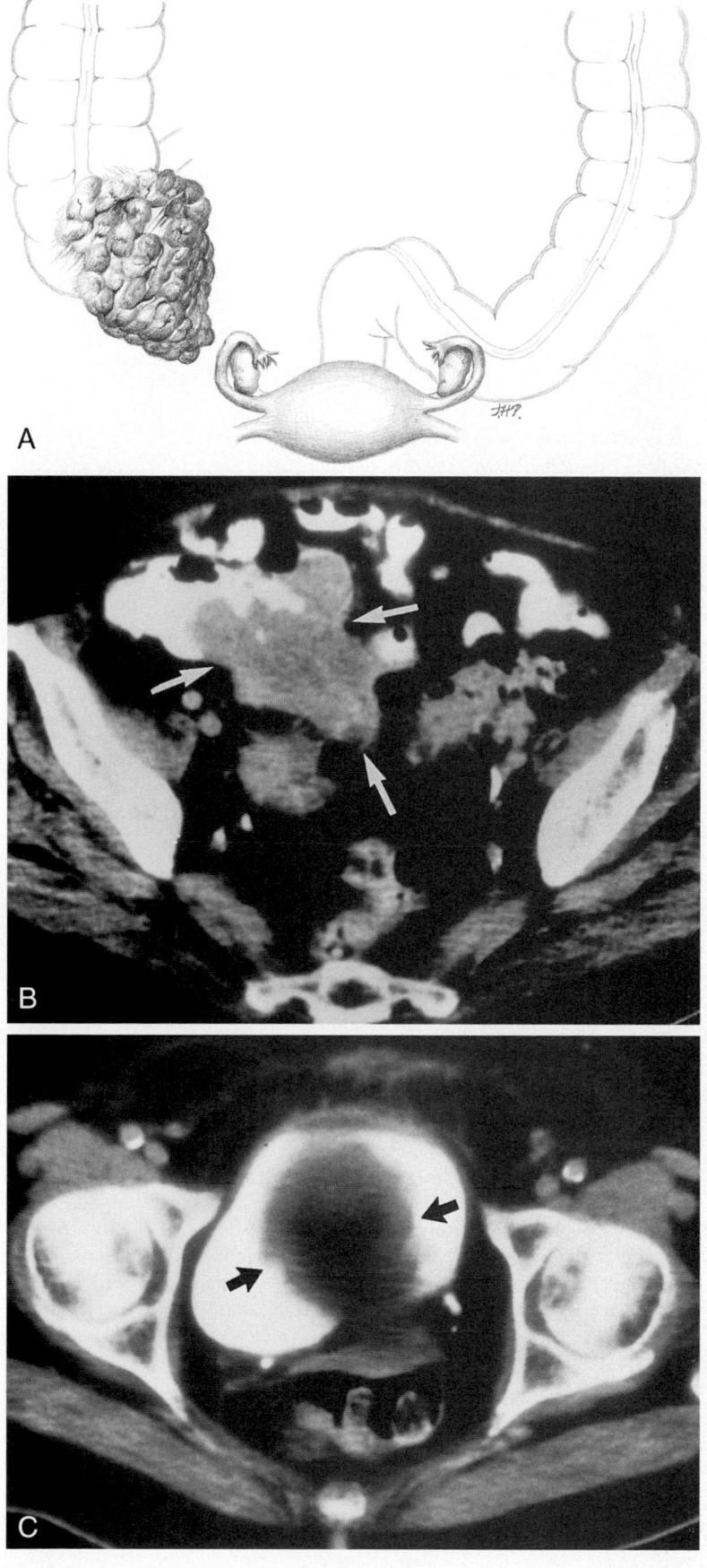

FIGURE 43.2. Cecal carcinoma. **A:** A cecal carcinoma encroaching on the right adnexa can be mistaken for an adnexal condition. **B:** Computed tomographic (CT) image shows a large neoplasm *(arrows)* extending from the cecum. **C:** CT image through the opacified urinary bladder shows invasions by the cecal neoplasm *(arrows)*. (Courtesy of T. Demos, Maywood, IL.)

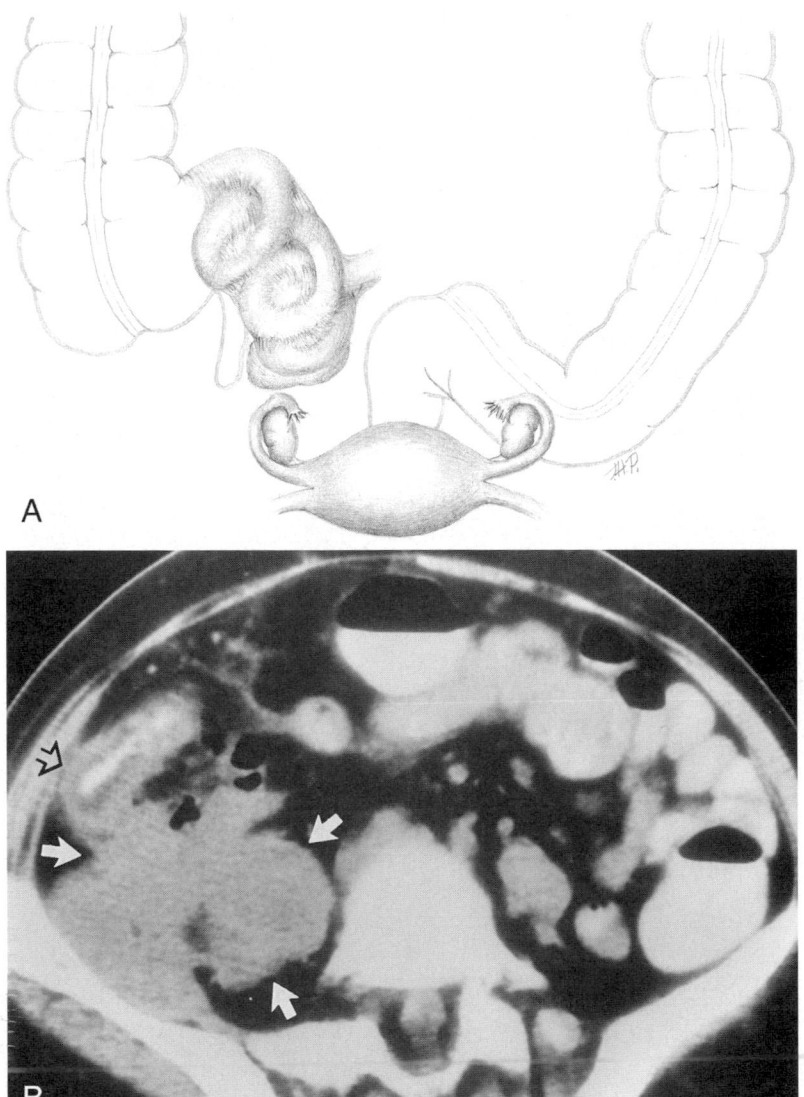

FIGURE 43.3. Crohn's disease with pelvic abscess. **A:** A conglutinant mass of small bowel adjacent to the right tube and ovary is Crohn's disease and can suggest inflammatory adnexal disease. **B:** Computed tomographic image shows a pelvic abscess *(closed arrows)* involving the iliacus and psoas muscles. The wall of the distal ileum *(open arrow)* is thickened because of Crohn's disease. (Courtesy of T. Demos, Maywood, IL.)

bution of colon cancer makes colonoscopy more important in the diagnostic workup. Cohn and Nance have noted that the incidence of left-sided colon and rectal cancer in their 1950 to 1954 series was 78.6% and right-sided colon was 21.4%. In their 1975 to 1979 series, the incidence of left-sided colon and rectal cancer had dropped to 68.4%, and the incidence of right-sided colon cancers had increased to 31.6%. A more recent report from McCallion suggests that proximal colon cancers increased in incidence from 23.5% in 1970 to 36.7% between 1990 and 1997. Because colon cancers that arise in the rectosigmoid or cecum may be palpable on pelvic examination, the gynecologist should not assume all palpable adnexal masses are ovary or tube. If the symptoms suggest colonic disease, even when the barium enema is reported to be normal, colonoscopy is indicated. Flexible sigmoidoscopy, which only evaluates the left colon, may be an inadequate examination in these patients because colon cancers are increasingly common in the proximal colon.

Unusual small bowel lesions may initially present as a pelvic mass; thus, small bowel barium contrast radiologic studies and CT scans often are helpful. CT scans are particularly useful in delineating mesenteric cysts (Fig. 43.10), volvulus of the small bowel, small bowel intussusception (Fig. 43.11), and Crohn's disease of the ileum (Fig. 43.12), any one of which may prolapse into the pelvis and be mistaken for a gynecologic condition. Gastrointestinal stromal tumors (previously termed leiomyomas or leiomyosarcomas) may occur in the small bowel and present as a solid pelvic mass, which easily could be diagnosed as a pedunculated uterine leiomyoma. They appear as solid masses adjacent to normal bowel on CT scan.

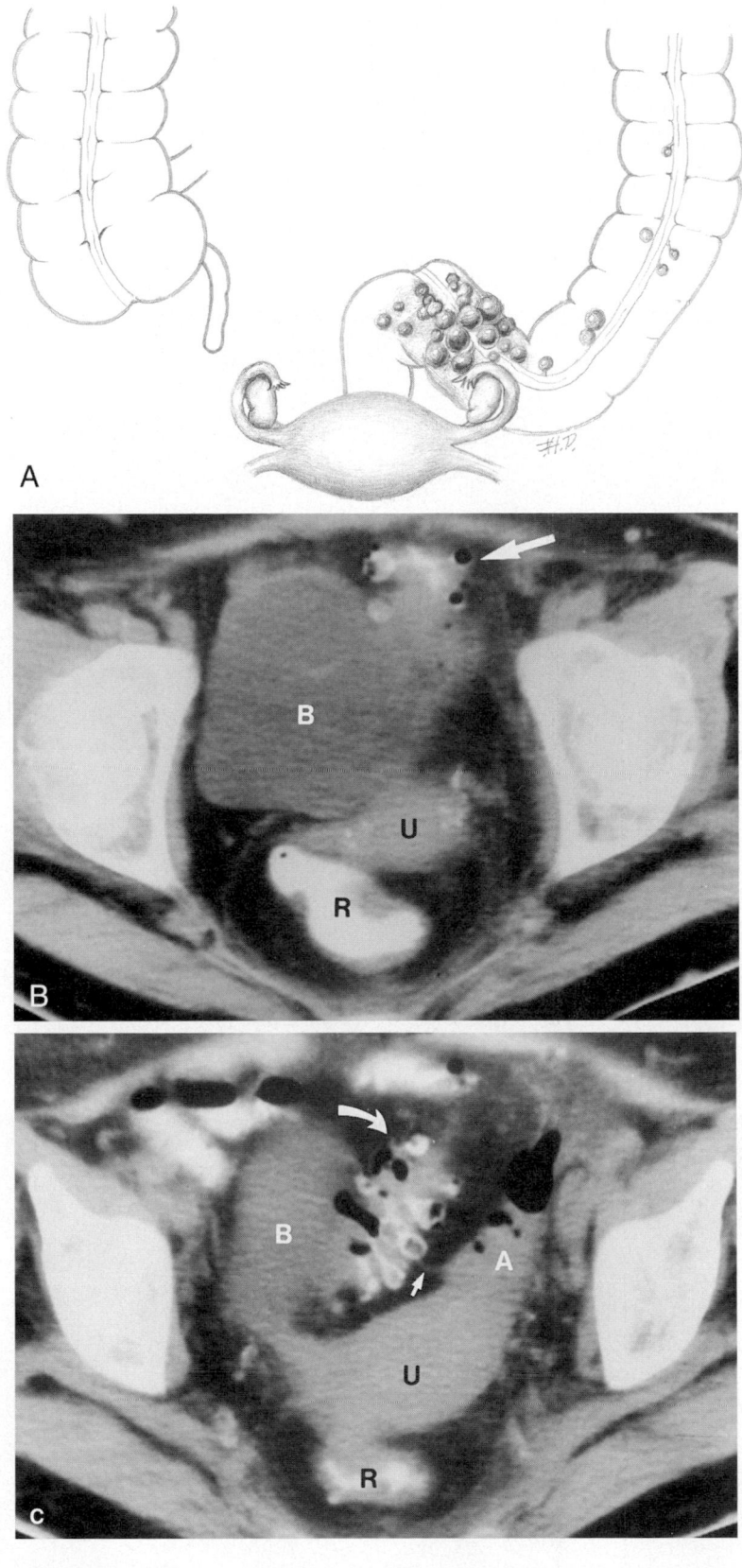

FIGURE 43.4. Sigmoid diverticulitis with abscess. **A:** This is easily confused with a left adnexal pathologic condition. **B:** Computed tomographic (CT) image low in pelvis shows sigmoid diverticula *(arrow)* with infiltration of adjacent fat. **C:** CT image at a higher level shows sigmoid diverticula *(arrow)* and a small sinus tract *(straight arrow)* leading to an abscess **(A),** which contains fluid and gas. The abscess is inseparable from the uterus (U). B, bladder; R, rectum. (Courtesy of T. Demos, Maywood, IL.)

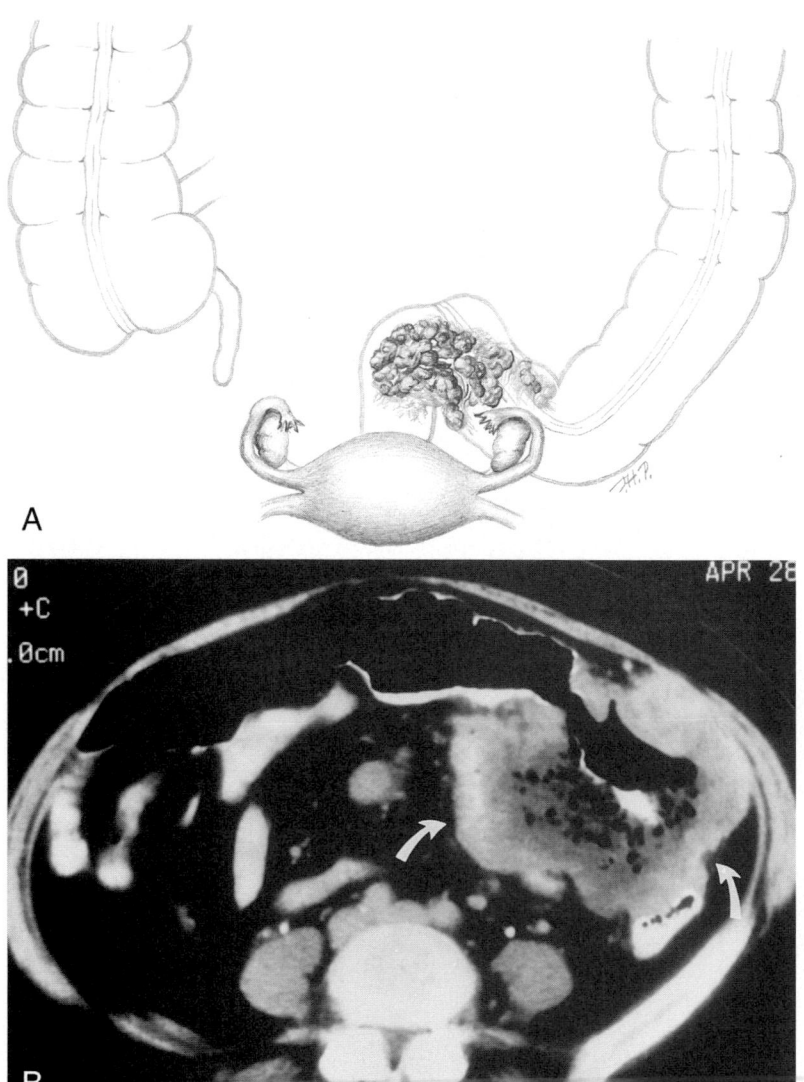

FIGURE 43.5. Rectosigmoid carcinoma. **A:** This tumor may encroach on the left adnexa and be mistaken for gynecologic disease. **B:** Computed tomographic (CT) image shows a large sigmoid carcinoma *(arrows)* containing a necrotic tumor and gas centrally. (Courtesy of T. Demos, Maywood, IL.)

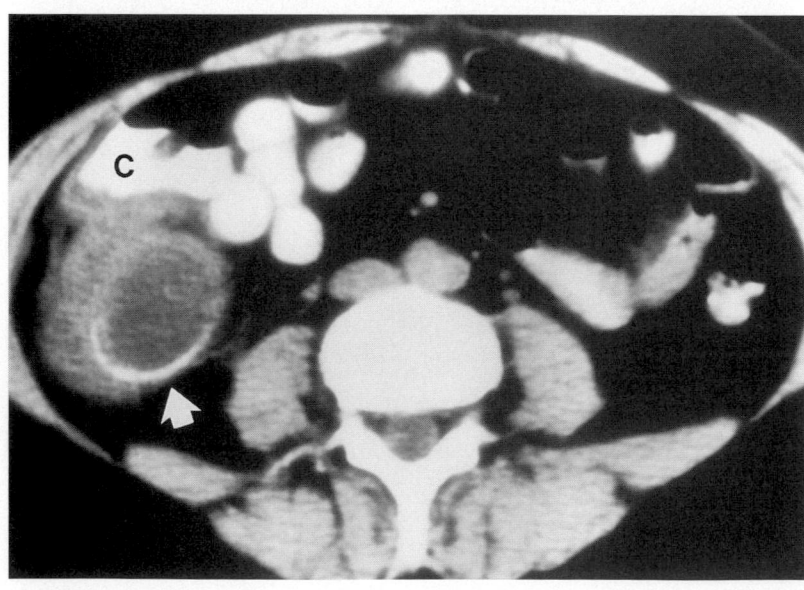

FIGURE 43.6. Infected mucocele of the appendix. Computed tomographic image shows a mucocele *(arrow)*, which has a thin rim of calcification and indents the cecum *(C)*. (Courtesy of T. Demos, Maywood, IL.)

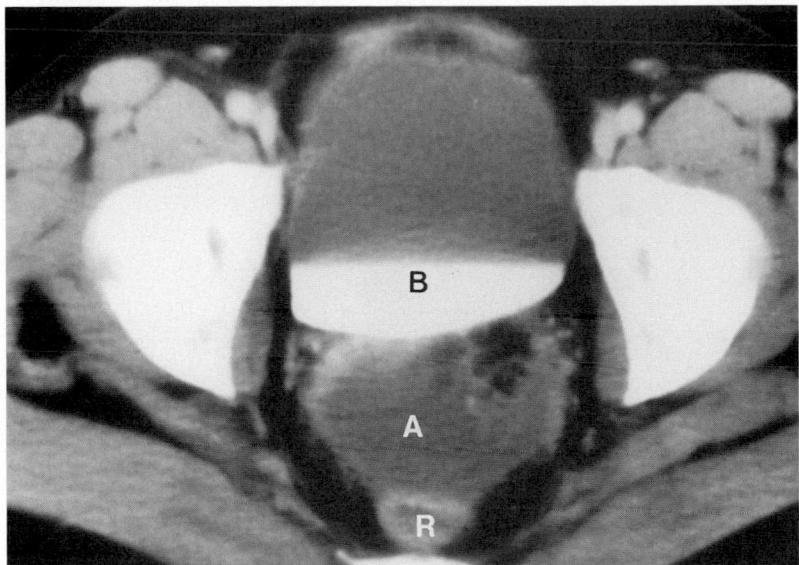

FIGURE 43.7. Appendicitis with pouch of Douglas abscess. Computed tomographic image shows a large abscess *(A)* between the rectum *(R)* and the bladder *(B)*. (Courtesy of T. Demos, Maywood, IL.)

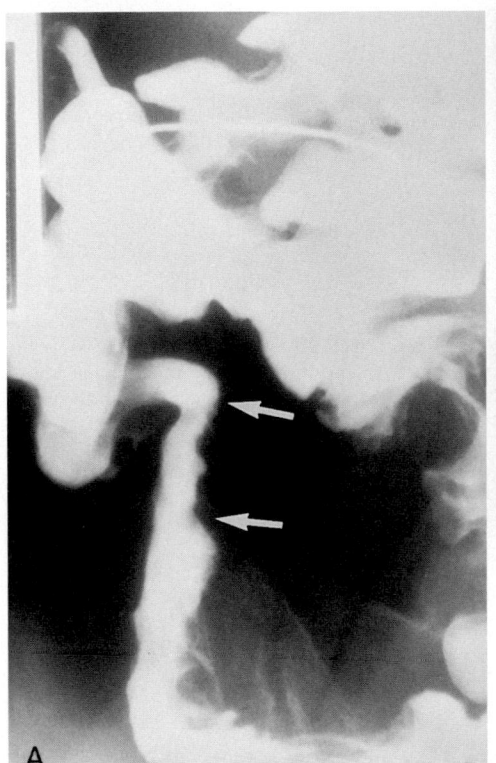

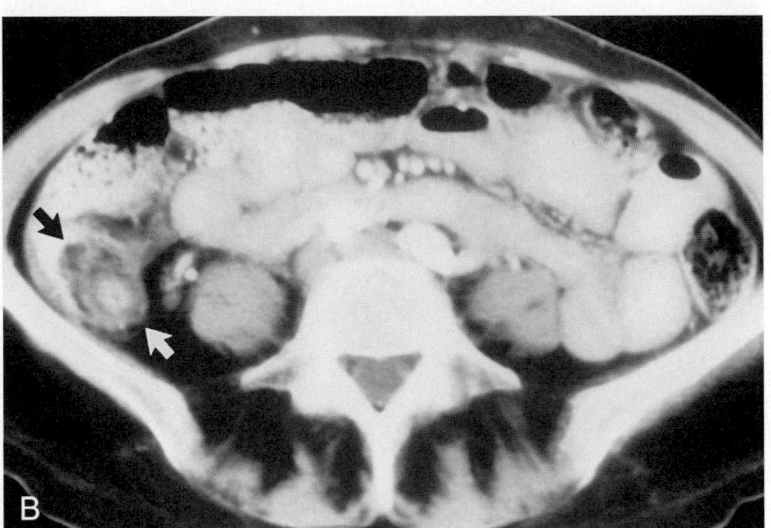

FIGURE 43.8. Non-Hodgkin's lymphoma of the terminal ileum. **A:** Barium enema shows irregular narrowing of the terminal ileum *(arrows)* and displacement of adjacent bowel loops. **B:** Computed tomographic image shows thickening of the wall of the terminal ileum *(arrows)*. (Courtesy of T. Demos, Maywood, IL.)

The role of laparoscopy in evaluation of unusual pelvic masses or pain cannot be ignored. Despite advances in endoscopy and imaging studies, we do not always get a clear idea of the nature of many unusual pelvic lesions. Diagnostic laparoscopy may be useful in these situations; this is covered in Chapter 16.

Urologic Tumors

Urinary conditions that occur concomitant with or mimic gynecologic disease include pelvic kidney, urachal cysts, carcinoma of the distal ureter, tumors of the bladder wall, hemangiopericytoma posterior to the bladder,

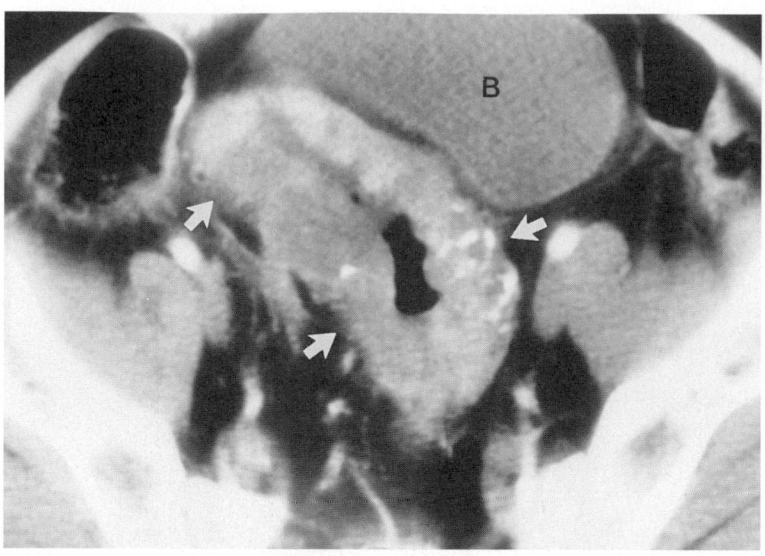

FIGURE 43.9. Ulcerative colitis with sigmoid carcinoma. Computed tomographic image shows circumferential sigmoid tumor *(arrows)*, which indents the bladder *(B)*. (Courtesy of T. Demos, Maywood, IL.)

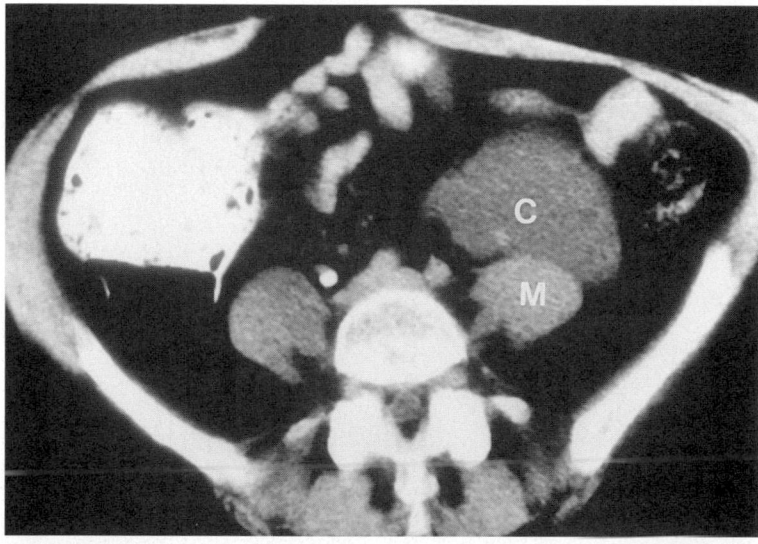

FIGURE 43.10. Mesenteric cyst (lymphangioma). Computed tomographic image shows the water density cyst *(C)*, which is indented by the psoas muscle *(M)*. (Courtesy of T. Demos, Maywood, IL.)

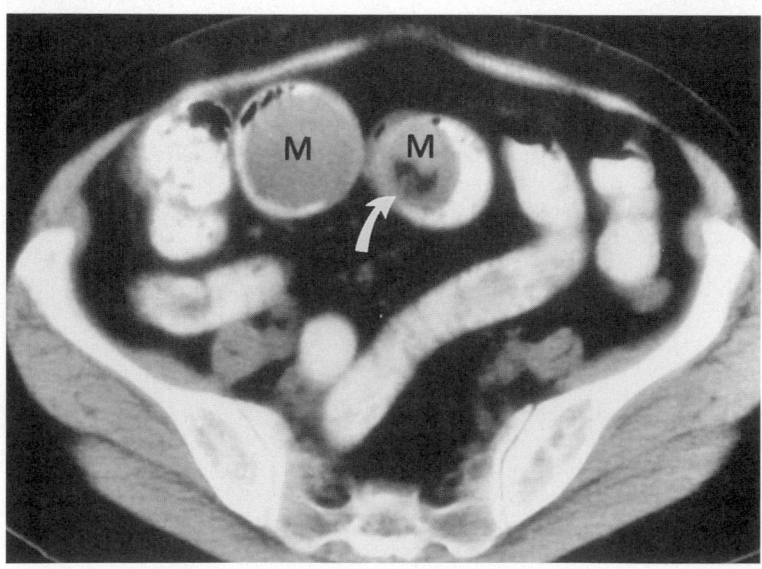

FIGURE 43.11. Small bowel polyp with ileoileal intussusception. Computed tomographic image shows intussuscept stetum *(M)* with associated mesenteric fat *(arrow)*. The intussusceptum is encircled by contrast material within the intussuscipiens. (Courtesy of T. Demos, Maywood, IL.)

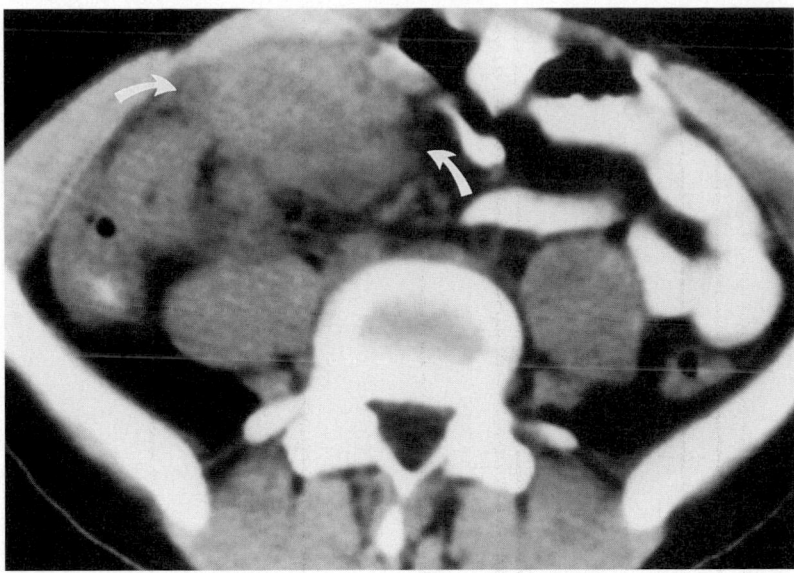

FIGURE 43.12. Crohn's disease with pelvic abscess. Computed tomographic image shows an inhomogeneous lesion *(arrows)* displacing the opacified intestine. This abscess cannot be differentiated from a phlegmon. (Courtesy of T. Demos, Maywood, IL.)

and bladder cancers, as shown in Figure 43.13. A routine urinalysis that reveals hematuria should raise suspicion of urinary tract disease. A urine culture should be obtained, and, if an infection is present, the hematuria should clear after a course of antibiotic therapy. For those patients without infection or with persistent hematuria after antibiotic therapy, an intravenous pyelogram and cystoscopy are warranted. CT is extremely useful in the evaluation of microscopic hematuria. Lang reported a 45% positive diagnosis rate for patients with previously undiagnosed urologic lesions who underwent careful multiphase helical CT with contrast.

A CT scan with intravenous contrast is extremely helpful in the preoperative evaluation of a pelvic mass prior to exploratory laparotomy, though an intravenous pyelogram (IVP) may be used if CT is unavailable. It establishes the function of the kidneys and determines the presence of a pelvic kidney or partially obstructed distal ureter. When a bimanual examination is performed, a large tumor of the distal ureter may be confused with an intraligamentous leiomyoma. Cystoscopy and retrograde pyelography are indicated in patients in whom suspicion of urinary tract disease is high and in patients who are allergic to the intravenous contrast media.

Retroperitoneal Tumors

Although gastrointestinal tract disease is the most frequent condition mistaken for gynecologic disease, retroperitoneal tumors occur often enough within the pelvis so that they should be considered, especially when dealing with vague or unusual pelvic symptoms and physical findings. Beck reported on seven collected series of retroperitoneal tumors and noted that the major

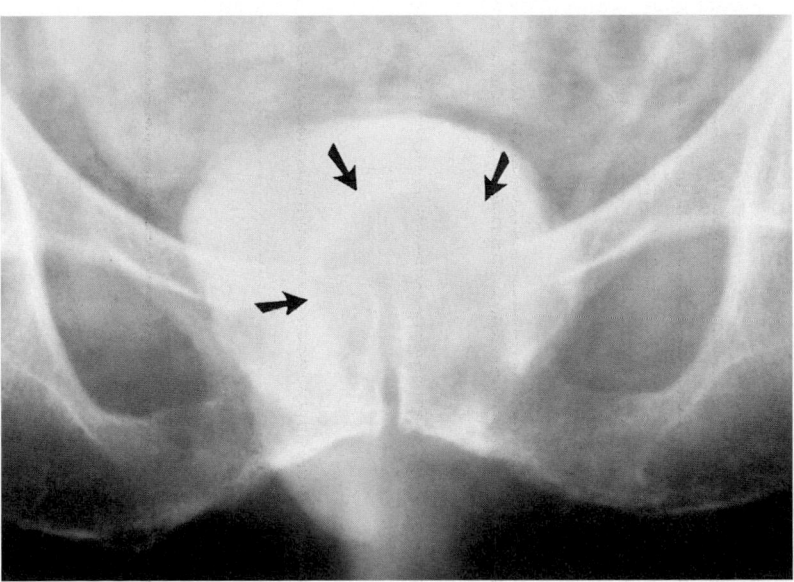

FIGURE 43.13. Urinary bladder carcinoma. Intravenous urogram shows inferior displacement of the bladder because of a cystocele. The bladder tumor produces a lobulated filling defect *(arrows)*. (Courtesy of T. Demos, Maywood, IL.)

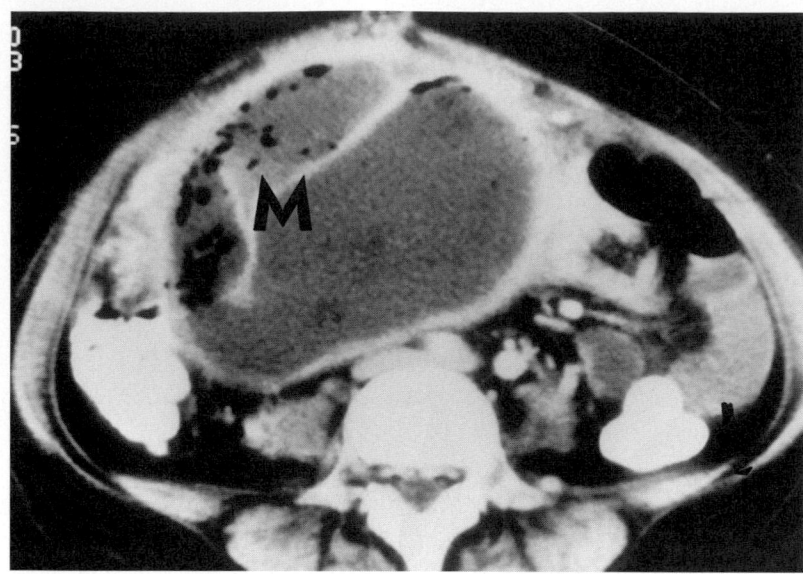

FIGURE 43.14. Necrotic retroperitoneal teratoma. Computed tomographic image shows a large septate mass *(M)*, which contains fluid and gas. Opacified intestine is draped around the lesion. (Courtesy of R. Benjoya, Libertyville, IL.)

symptoms include abdominal pain, abdominal mass or swelling, and weight loss, anorexia, or both. The symptoms depend on the location of the tumor in the retroperitoneal space. Retroperitoneal tumors in the pelvis may become manifest earlier than those in the abdomen because the bony confines of the pelvis cause pressure on adjacent organs earlier than in the upper abdomen.

Abnormal findings noted on an excretory urogram and upper and lower gastrointestinal radiologic studies may be secondary to extrinsic involvement rather than intrinsic pathology. The most reliable tools for diagnosing retroperitoneal tumors are CT and magnetic resonance imaging (MRI). Figures 43.14 through 43.16 demonstrate CT and MRI images of retroperitoneal conditions.

If the tumor is a lymphoma, a careful history may elicit complaints of fever, night sweats, pruritus, and weight loss. Patients with a lymphoma may have skin nodules, enlarged lymph nodes, liver and spleen enlargement, and areas of joint or bone tenderness, although this is usually representative of advanced disease. Figure 43.17 illustrates a CT image of a patient with an ileocecal lymphoma and mesenteric adenopathy. A biopsy of a peripheral lymph node or skin nodule may establish the diagnosis of lymphoma and provide enough tissue for proper characterization of the correct subtype. Additionally, a core needle biopsy of the bone marrow can be helpful as a staging procedure for a lymphoma. Staging and response to therapy of lymphomas is currently performed with positron emission tomography (PET) scans and CT. Historically, gallium scintigraphy and lymphan-

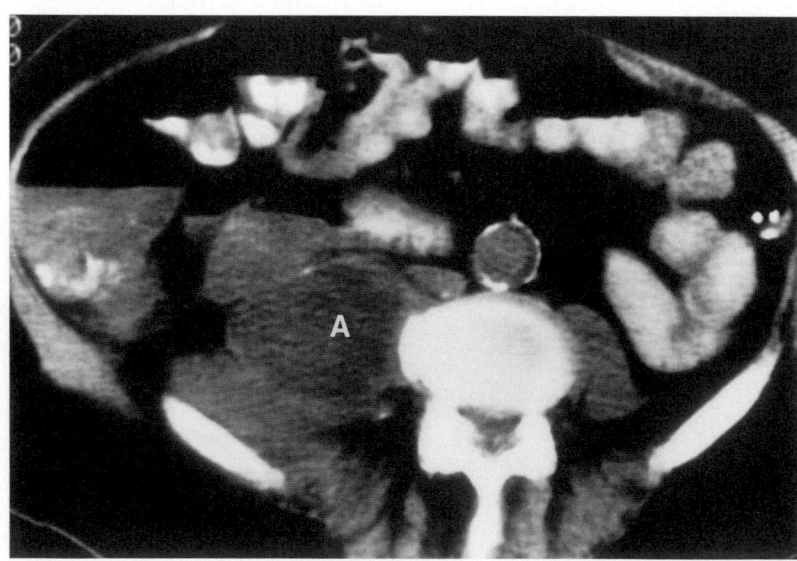

FIGURE 43.15. Large psoas abscess. Computed tomographic image shows a large low-density psoas abscess *(A)*. (Courtesy of T. Demos, Maywood, IL.)

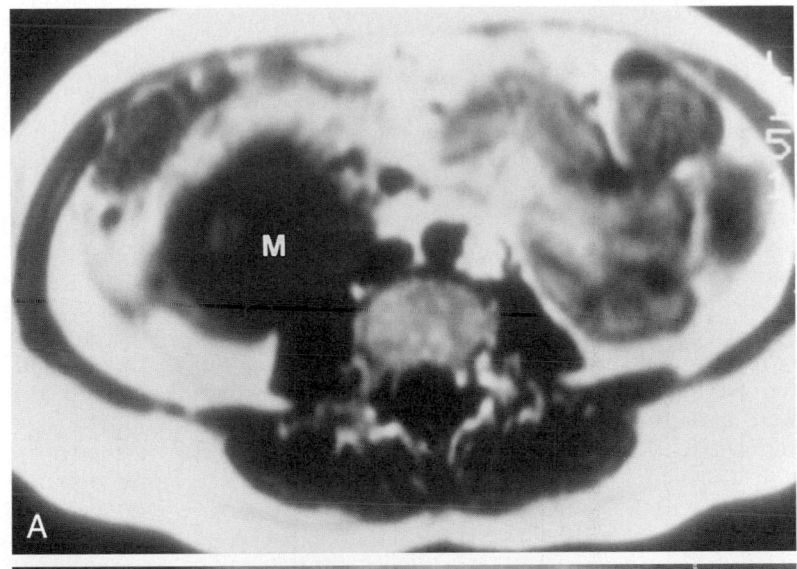

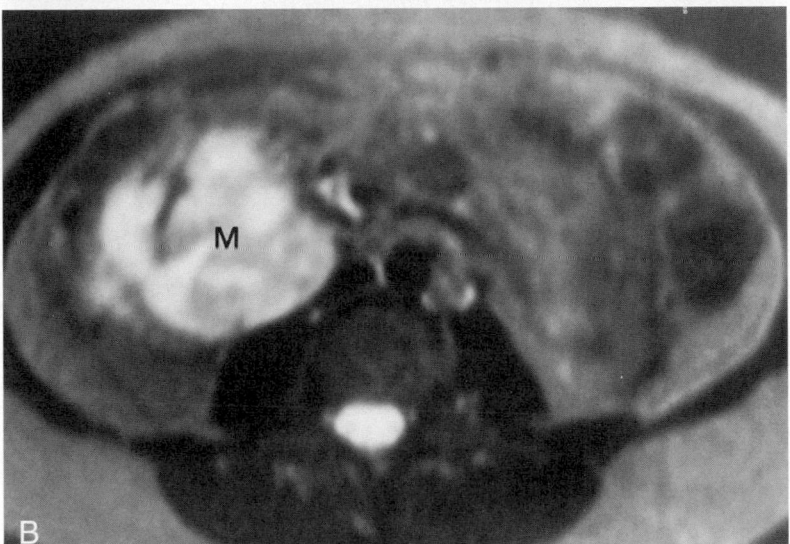

FIGURE 43.16. Retroperitoneal leiomyosarcoma. **A:** T1-weighted magnetic resonance image (MRI) shows a lobulated mass *(M)*, which has low signal. **B:** T2-weighted MRI shows the same mass *(M)*, which has heterogeneous high signal. (Courtesy of T. Demos, Maywood, IL.)

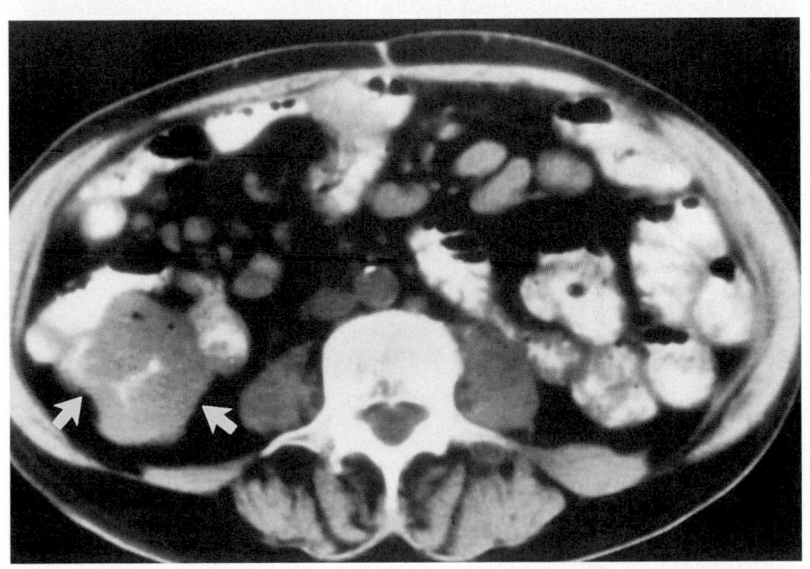

FIGURE 43.17. Ileocecal non-Hodgkin's lymphoma with mesenteric adenopathy. Computed tomographic image shows an ileocecal mass *(arrows)*. There are numerous oval, enlarged mesenteric lymph nodes between opacified loops of intestine. (Courtesy of T. Demos, Maywood, IL.)

giography have been used for staging, but are no longer widely employed.

There are rare neurogenic tumors that arise in the pelvis, in addition to very rare anterior meningoceles and arachnoid cysts (Fig. 43.18). The most common are those that arise from the nerve sheath of the obturator or sacral nerve complex, which are the neurofibromas (often associated with von Recklinghausen's disease) and the neurilemomas. Tumors also may develop from the sympathetic nervous system of the pelvis; these include ganglioneuroma, sympathicoblastoma, and neuroblastoma.

Soft-tissue sarcomas may occur anywhere in the retroperitoneal space. Lewis reported 500 patients with retroperitoneal sarcomas and found the most common were liposarcomas and leiomyosarcomas. Survival was inversely related to tumor size and complete surgical resection with a tumor-free margin offered the best survival. According to Adam and colleagues, these tumors are diagnosed most easily by CT scan, but ultrasonography, arteriography, and venography may be useful. Figure 43.19

demonstrates an intravenous urogram of a large pelvic neurofibroma with sarcomatous degeneration.

Orthopedic Disorders

Disorders that may arise from the bony pelvis include those that are congenital, iatrogenic, metabolic, or septic, as well as fractures and tumors. The congenital or developmental abnormalities include anterior sacral meningocele (discussed in the preceding), spondylolisthesis, and sacrococcygeal teratomas. Spondylolisthesis is a slow, forward displacement of the lumbar spine over the sacrum. The degree of slip usually is not severe enough to cause significant impairment. If the entire fifth lumbar vertebra is displaced forward of the sacrum (spondyloptosis), however, severe narrowing of the anteroposterior diameter of the pelvis and displacement of the pelvic viscera are noted. Pelvic examination is significantly abnormal. A pelvic radiograph defines the problem.

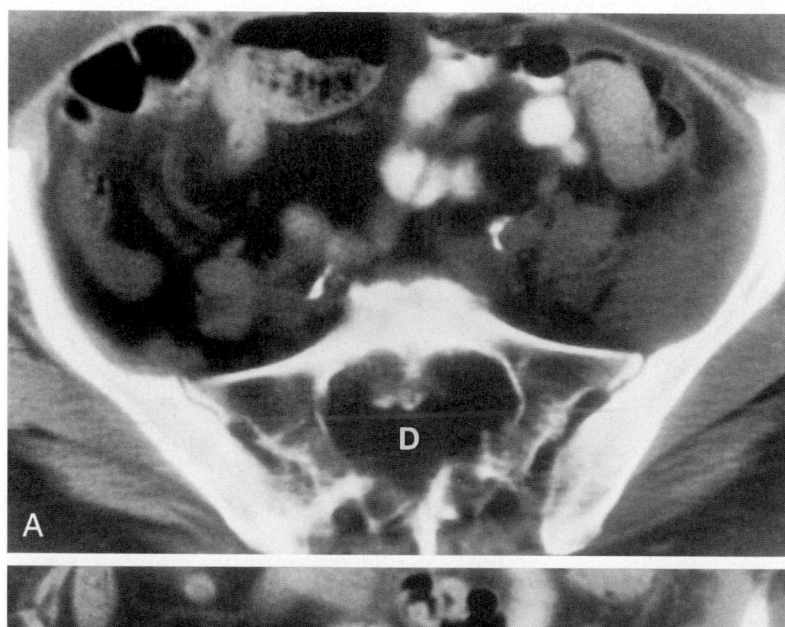
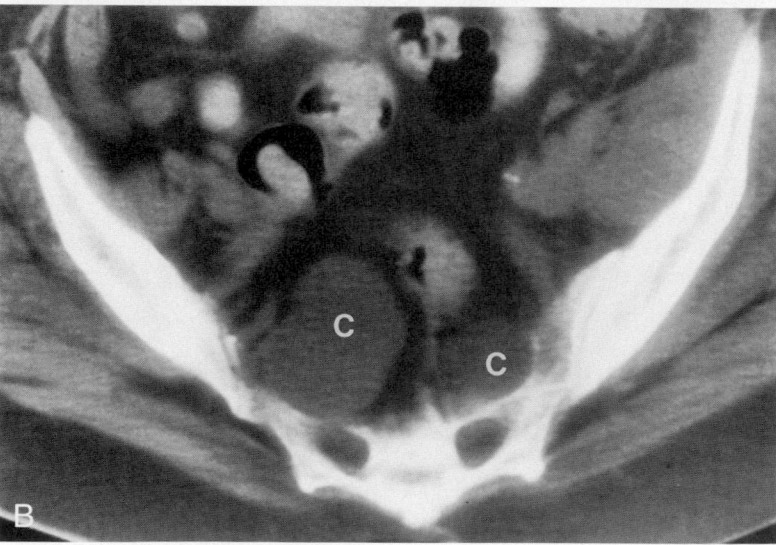

FIGURE 43.18. Arachnoid cysts. **A:** Computed tomographic (CT) image shows a central defect *(D)* of the sacrum. **B:** A more inferior CT image shows water density arachnoid cysts *(C)* bulging into the pelvis. (Courtesy of T. Demos, Maywood, IL.)

Sacrococcygeal teratomas usually are diagnosed by age 2 or 3 years; however, occasionally the dermoid forms are not discovered until early adulthood. These anomalies are four times more common in women, and malignant forms are more common in adults. Such lesions usually can be defined by ultrasonography and CT (Fig. 43.20).

Total hip arthroplasty has become commonplace since it was introduced in the 1960s. In some earlier cases, the inner wall of the acetabulum was penetrated, allowing the cement (methyl methacrylate) to flow into the pelvis to improve fixation. The cement produces a bony, hard mass fixed to the pelvic wall that varies in size, shape, and convolution. If such a mass is encountered on pelvic examination, it may represent a challenging diagnostic problem. Only a high degree of suspicion can warn the examining gynecologist that the hard, nodular fixed pelvic mass is a cementing substance that should not be disturbed.

Certain metabolic disorders of the skeletal system can cause gradual development of pelvic deformities that may be confusing on pelvic examination. With bone deficiency, sometimes there is inward protrusion of the femoral head through the inner acetabular wall (protrusio acetabuli). Other causes of protrusio acetabuli include Marfan's syndrome, Paget's disease of the bone, rheumatoid arthritis, and osteomalacia.

Fungal, parasitic, and pyogenic afflictions of the bony pelvis can cause the development of soft-tissue masses that may be difficult to diagnose. Most of these cases occur as acute, painful infectious processes, but some develop as subacute or chronic pyogenic infections. Pelvic examination may cause severe discomfort and produce findings suggestive of a deep fullness or masses on either pelvic side wall. Sometimes, such infections occur as a presacral abscess. There usually is associated tenderness over the sacroiliac joints and both buttocks. Figure 43.15 is a CT image of a large psoas abscess with perinephric extension.

A rather common cause of intrapelvic distortion is residual bony deformities caused by pelvic fractures that may occur in falls or automobile accidents. Radiologic examination of the pelvis reveals the cause of the unusual findings.

Primary bone tumors that involve the pelvis are rare except for those on the anterior sacrum. The sacrum is the primary site of more than 50% of chordomas (malignant) and 6% of giant cell tumors (benign). Pelvic and rectal pain, urinary frequency, and constipation are common symptoms. Radiologic studies of the pelvis usually are sufficient for diagnosis, and a technetium 99 bone scan may demonstrate bone destruction not apparent on the radiographic films. MRI gives far better detail to delineate bone and nerve involvement.

Vascular Considerations

Two significant vascular lesions are iliac aneurysms and arteriovenous fistulas. Isolated iliac aneurysms are rare, but many patients with abdominal aortic aneurysms have

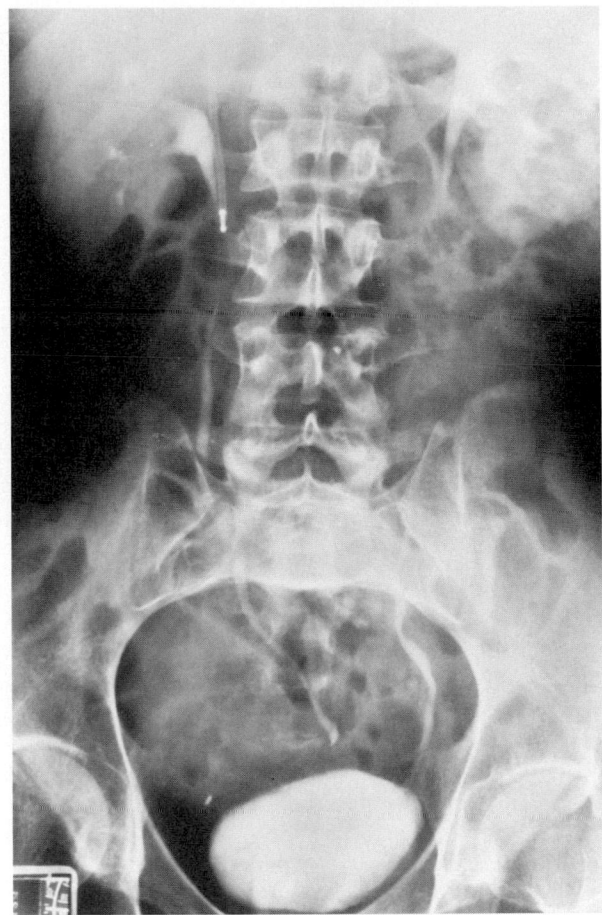

FIGURE 43.19. Neurofibromatosis with pelvic sarcoma. Intravenous urogram shows the distal right ureter displaced by a soft-tissue mass within the pelvis. (There is a ventriculoperitoneal shunt extending to the right upper quadrant.) (Courtesy of T. Demos, Maywood, IL.)

associated iliac aneurysms. This lesion is 10 times more common in men than women. They are more common on the common iliac and hypogastric arteries and are rare on the external iliac artery. Most iliac aneurysms remain asymptomatic until they rupture, unless they impinge on adjacent structures. Diagnosis of iliac artery aneurysms is difficult, but ultrasonography and CT may detect these aneurysms. Figure 43.21A shows a barium enema with extrinsic pressure on the colon by the iliac aneurysm. Figure 43.21B demonstrates an iliac arterial aneurysm on CT. Arteriovenous fistulae and malformations may be found in the rectum and colon—the presenting symptom is always hemorrhage, not pelvic pain. These lesions should not cause a palpable pelvic mass.

Nonsurgical Acute Abdomen

There are a number of nonsurgical causes of acute abdominal pain that may be mistaken for a gynecologic problem. Patients with sickle cell anemia may have attacks of bone and joint pain but also may suffer abdom-

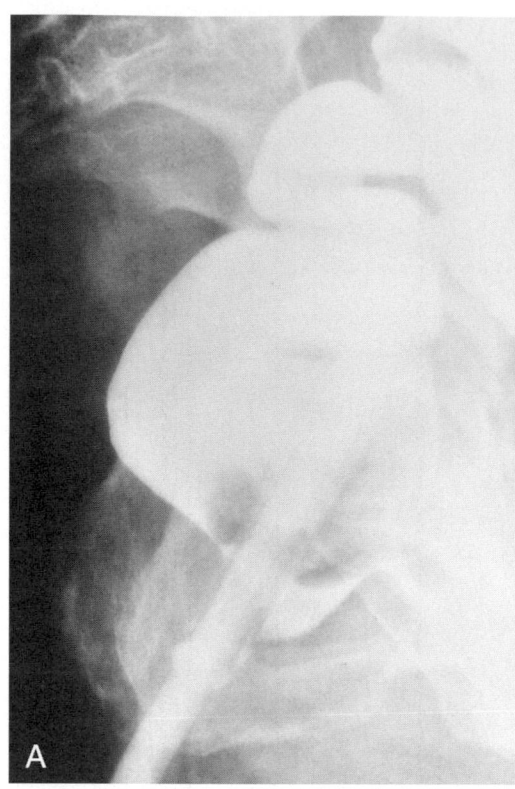

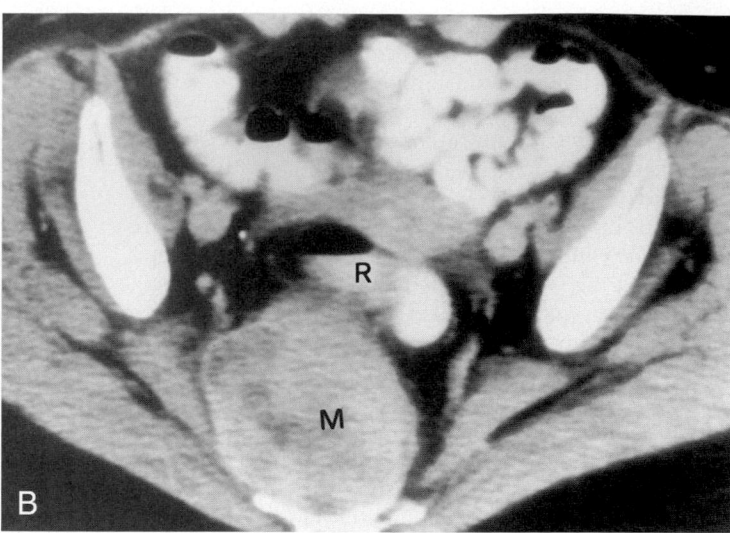

FIGURE 43.20. Presacral teratoma. **A:** Lateral view from a barium enema shows that the rectum is displaced anteriorly from the sacrum. **B:** Computed tomographic image shows a soft tissue mass *(M)*, which deforms the sacrum and displaces the rectum *(R)* anteriorly. (Courtesy of K. Baliga, Rockford, IL.)

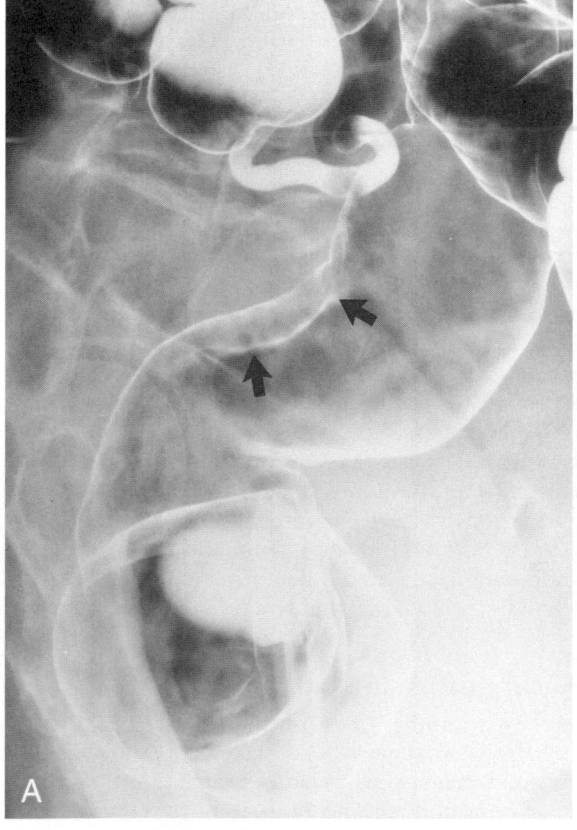

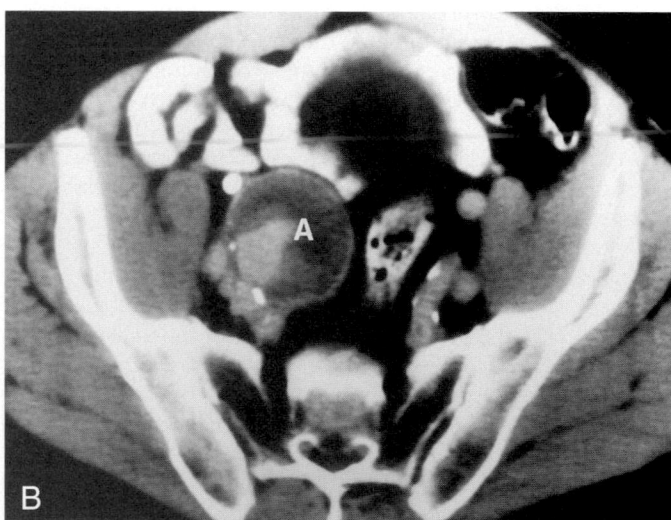

FIGURE 43.21. Iliac artery aneurysm. **A:** Barium enema shows extrinsic filling defect *(arrows)* of the rectosigmoid. **B:** Computed tomographic image shows an iliac artery aneurysm *(A)*, which contains a clot. Adjacent bowel is displaced. (Courtesy of T. Demos, Maywood, IL.)

inal pain. The major disabilities suffered by patients with sickle cell anemia are related to painful vasoocclusive crises and occlusion of the microvasculature by the sickling phenomenon. Precipitating factors are infection, hypoxia, dehydration, and acidosis. A careful family history and laboratory testing for sickle cells and hemoglobin S usually establish the diagnosis.

Recurrent attacks of abdominal pain occur with acute porphyria, an autosomal dominant condition most common in women in their third and fourth decades of life. Abdominal tenderness is less than expected for the severity of pain that is experienced. Activation of the disease is related to factors such as drugs, infection, low-calorie diets, and steroid hormones. Fever and leukocytosis may be present, and abdominal radiologic studies show distended loops of bowel. Diagnosis is made by determining a history of similar attacks and by the quantitative detection of excessive porphobilinogen and aminolevulinate in a 24-hour urine collection.

Other nonsurgical causes of abdominal pain include familial Mediterranean fever, lower-lobe pneumonia, rectus sheath hematoma (especially in anticoagulated patients), pyelonephritis, and acute viral gastroenteritis.

INTRAOPERATIVE MANAGEMENT OF NONGYNECOLOGIC PELVIC DISORDERS

Despite thorough preoperative history, physical examination, and proper imaging studies, the surgeon still encounters unexpected findings at abdominal exploration from time to time. Mechanical and antibiotic bowel preparation facilitates examination of the gastrointestinal tract, and—if the gynecologic surgeon is trained in bowel surgery—allow management of unexpected findings. Once the abdomen is opened, a thorough evaluation of the upper abdomen and then the pelvis should be made. If the upper abdomen is normal, then the upper abdominal contents should be packed away with laparotomy pads and the patient placed in the Trendelenburg position. Next, the pelvic findings should be assessed and the problem analyzed, with the tissues being put in as near an anatomically normal position as possible. If dense adhesions are present, these should be lysed by sharp dissection. If the disease involves the uterus or fallopian tubes and ovaries with extension into the surrounding organs, the appropriate surgery to remove the diseased organs should be undertaken. Depending on the pathology, this may be within the gynecologist's expertise; if not, however, another surgical specialist should be consulted.

The most common nongynecologic problems involve the gastrointestinal tract. If the colon and small bowel are normal, the gynecologic surgeon must consider retroperitoneal tumors or disease of the distal ureter or urinary bladder. If the patient has had an adequate bowel preparation and has been apprised of the various possible procedures that could be undertaken (i.e., colostomy, bowel resection, urinary diversion, ex-

cessive blood loss, and possibly, prolonged hospital stay), then definitive surgery should be carried out. If these precautions have not been taken preoperatively, the abdomen should be closed. Then the surgeon must explain to the patient and family the nature of the problem found at surgery and plans for future management, including referral and evaluation for possible additional surgery.

Gastrointestinal Disease
Appendicitis
Appendicitis frequently involves gynecologic conditions in the differential diagnosis. It is discussed in Chapter 41.

Cancer of the Colon and Rectum
Cancer of the colon is predominantly a disease of older people, but it can occur at any age. The incidence of right-sided colon cancer is steadily increasing so that discovery of a cecal mass in the pelvis is more common. Radical surgical removal of the primary lesion is the only acceptable curative therapy. If colon cancer is found unexpectedly and the bowel has had both mechanical and antibiotic preparation, an appropriate resection should be carried out by a surgeon experienced in colonic surgery. A sample of blood should be sent for carcinoembryonic antigen (CEA), because this may serve as a baseline value in long-term surveillance for recurrence or metastasis. The abdomen should be closed and definitive surgery performed at a later date if the patient has not had suitable bowel preparation or if a surgeon experienced in colorectal surgery is not available. The resection includes the entire segment of the involved portion of the colon and its associated lymphovascular pedicle. Resection of high rectal or distal sigmoid lesions often is difficult if the resection needs to extend below the peritoneal reflection. Primary resection of right colon lesions and anastomosis may be carried out even in the absence of prior bowel preparation with only a very low incidence of postoperative infection. Bilateral oophorectomy has been advocated for premenopausal patients with colorectal cancer to prevent metastases to the ovaries, but it is actually quite rare to develop isolated ovarian metastasis. (Fewer than 1% of women with colorectal cancer develop isolated ovarian metastasis that is potentially curable.) This strategy is unlikely to prolong survival. Routine prophylactic oophorectomy is not recommended.

Diverticulitis
The usual therapy for diverticulitis is medical. Most patients with mild uncomplicated diverticulitis are treated as outpatients with oral antibiotics. Patients with severe acute diverticulitis should be hospitalized for bowel rest and administration of intravenous fluids and broad-spectrum antibiotics. Repeated attacks of diverticulitis in the same area generally require surgical resection. Severe attacks with acute peritoneal signs, fistula formation, suspected abscess, or perforation require intravenous antibi-

otics directed against Gram-negative anaerobic bacteria, followed by surgical drainage or resection.

In operating on a patient for what was presumed to be recurring attacks of PID or an ovarian mass, however, the gynecologist may find a portion of the rectosigmoid involved with diverticulitis. If the patient has had repeated attacks of diverticulitis, the colon feels firm and there may be a significant mass effect, which is difficult to distinguish from a sigmoid carcinoma. If the patient is not symptomatic (obstruction, bleeding) the wisest course may be to simply close the patient and perform postoperative colonoscopy or barium enema. If the colon has been preoperatively prepared and cleansed, the patient may undergo elective resection of the involved segment of colon and a primary anastomosis with a very low operative risk. The surgeon may find more acute disease in the patient undergoing operation for acute pelvic pain or infection. A diverticular abscess may be uncovered or ruptured with manipulation of the diseased section. This should be treated with drainage and resection followed by a diverting colostomy, because many of these patients have not had adequate bowel preparation. Simple drainage of the diverticular abscess may suffice; however, the risk of an ongoing leak makes this a less optimal choice. Free perforation of the colon in diverticular disease is rare and must be treated by resection of the involved segment of colon. This obviously calls for significant experience in colonic surgery because these resections are done in the face of substantial edema and fibrosis in the colon mesentery, with a significant risk of hemorrhage or ureteral injury. Siting a colostomy on the abdominal wall in the emergency performance of a colostomy also is difficult if the surgeon is not experienced. The colostomy may be taken down at a later operation in 6 to 12 weeks after appropriate evaluation of the remaining colon with barium enema or colonoscopy.

Crohn's Disease

Crohn's disease (regional enteritis) is a chronic inflammatory disorder of the gastrointestinal tract of unknown cause. Because it most frequently involves the terminal ileum and proximal colon, it may be mistaken easily by history and pelvic examination as an inflammatory process of the appendix, fallopian tube, or ovary. The most common complaint is right lower quadrant pain that usually is associated with fever, diarrhea without blood, weight loss, fatigability, and a tender, palpable abdominal mass. The disease most commonly has its onset in young people, but occurs in all age groups. The complications of Crohn's disease are often local, resulting from intestinal inflammation and involvement of adjacent viscera. Intestinal obstruction, fistula formation, right ureteral obstruction and hydronephrosis, malabsorption, anorexia, and intestinal perforation with abscess formation are all possible manifestations and complications of this disease. Endoscopic examination of the colon and radiologic studies of the bowel (including CT scans demonstrating thickening of the bowel wall) are most important in establishing the diagnosis of inflammatory bowel disease. The operative finding of thickened mesentery with growth of mesenteric fat ("fat wrapping") around the circumference of leathery fibrotic bowel is almost always pathognomonic of Crohn's disease, although this can be seen with lymphomas or carcinoid tumors of the distal ileum.

Intraoperative management of incidentally discovered Crohn's disease depends on the indication for operation and the experience of the surgeon. Patients explored for PID found to have perforated Crohn's disease need resection, possibly including an ileostomy. Like complicated diverticular disease, these resections can be quite challenging and hazardous for the occasional surgeon. Patents explored for a mass and found to have diseased terminal ileum without perforation may be resected in some cases (if there is evidence of proximal obstruction) or the patient may be closed and further examinations carried out. Most patients with small bowel disease can have endoscopic biopsy to confirm the diagnosis and then are managed medically. Surgery is held in reserve until complications (stricture, obstruction, abscess) develop. Current surgical management of Crohn's disease involves very conservative resections preserving bowel length to avoid short bowel syndrome caused by repeated resections of progressively involved bowel. Crohn's disease is not cured surgically and recurs in over 75% of patients with ileocecal Crohn's disease, the most common site of the disease. Bypass procedures for obstructing Crohn's disease are of historical interest only; current surgical treatment involves resection or stricturoplasty.

Urologic Disease

The most common retroperitoneal urologic mass to be encountered is a pelvic or horseshoe kidney. Pelvic kidneys may be found anywhere in the pelvis and their ureters may take unusual courses, even crossing to the contralateral side. An important point to remember is that pelvic and horseshoe kidneys have an arterial supply that courses much more anteriorly than the normal kidney, and their collecting system lies anteriorly as well, exposing both to risk of injury. These anomalies should be identifiable readily if the patient has a CT scan with intravenous contrast or intravenous pyelogram preoperatively. An attempt should be made to identify a renal pelvis or ureter if the retroperitoneal pelvic mass appears to be a kidney at the time of surgery. Aspiration with a 22-gauge needle may reveal the presence of urine within the mass. Excretory urography can be performed during surgery by intravenously injecting 50 to 100 mL of contrast material and obtaining a 10- to 20-minute supine film. An alternative is to inject 5 to 10 mL of indigo carmine intravenously and obtain an aspirate from the suspected renal pelvis 5 to 10 minutes later. The presence of blue or green urine confirms that the mass is a functioning kidney. Palpation of the ipsilateral or contralateral side to ascertain that a kidney is present is not reliable. According to Schuster, "palpating the kidney" was done in almost all the reported cases of removal of a solitary pelvic kidney, and the surgeon thought a normal kidney was present in its usual proper position.

If the surgeon unwittingly attempts to remove a pelvic kidney, when the "tumor mass" is entered, bleeding becomes profuse. If the tumor mass is recognized as a kidney, the injured kidney usually can be repaired, but this should be performed by an experienced surgeon. Packing the wound stops some of the small bleeders and controls massive bleeding until the situation can be evaluated. If the vascular pedicle can be located, vascular or bulldog clamps can be placed across the vessels and left for about 30 minutes without harm to the kidney. The intrarenal blood vessels need to be individually ligated. Electrocautery does not stop parenchymal bleeding and may increase it. If defects in the collecting system are observed, these defects should be repaired with fine absorbable suture.

Tumors of the lower one third of the ureter are more frequent than tumors of the upper one third of the ureter. Although ureteral tumors normally are small, they can be large and infiltrate the surrounding tissue. When they infiltrate the surrounding tissues and are firm, theoretically they may be palpated on bimanual examination and mistaken for an adnexal or pelvic mass. The traditional treatment of ureteral tumors has been nephroureterectomy with removal of the entire renal unit and ureter. Current management is resection of the distal ureter with a cuff of bladder and reimplantation of the ureter into the bladder.

If an adequate preoperative workup has been carried out, it is unlikely that an unsuspected cancer of the bladder will be encountered. The surgeon may encounter a paraganglioma of the bladder wall invading adjacent loops of small bowel that had been mistaken for a leiomyoma or an adnexal mass. These tumors usually are benign and can be managed by resection of the involved portion of the bladder wall and small bowel. Hemangiopericytomas posterior to the bladder require total resection of the tumor mass.

Retroperitoneal Tumors

Although retroperitoneal tumors are relatively rare, the pelvic surgeon should be prepared to deal with them. Primary retroperitoneal tumors arise from retroperitoneal tissue that does not represent growth from another body organ in the retroperitoneum. Ackerman has compiled and classified all the possible retroperitoneal tumors. There is virtually no retroperitoneal tumor that should be resected if found unexpectedly at operation for other pelvic disease. Retroperitoneal sarcomas, teratomas, and sacral chordomas all need careful preresection imaging and very specialized surgical techniques. Even biopsy can cause severe bleeding and retroperitoneal masses should not be biopsied without intraoperative consultation with the appropriate consultant scrubbed in. These are never surgical emergencies and it is much more judicious to close the abdomen than venture into a difficult retroperitoneal tumor.

SUMMARY

A thorough history, physical examination, and appropriate laboratory and imaging procedures usually detect an unsuspected condition before laparotomy. Even if a comprehensive workup suggests gynecologic pathology, bowel preparation and a thorough discussion with the patient about problems that may be encountered will prevent many otherwise difficult, if not impossible, situations. Because gastrointestinal disease most often is the unexpected condition, the gynecologist should be aware of the correct management of these disorders. Urinary tract conditions and retroperitoneal tumors should be familiar to the gynecologic surgeon. However, in modern surgical practice, definitive management of nongynecologic conditions should be undertaken by the appropriate specialist and consultation should be requested for all but the most minor conditions.

BIBLIOGRAPHY

Andersson P, Sjodahl R. Controversies in surgical treatment of inflammatory bowel disease. *Eur J Surg Suppl* 2001;586: 73–77.

Bau A, Atri M. Acute female pelvic pain: ultrasound evaluation. *Semin Ultrasound CT MR* 2000;21(1):78–93.

Bauerfeind P. Colon tumors and colonoscopy. *Endoscopy* 2001;33(11):949–960.

Blumberg D, Ramanathan RK. Treatment of colon and rectal cancer. *J Clin Gastroenterol* 2002;34(1):15–26.

Cohn I, Nance JC. The colon and rectum. In: Sabiston DC Jr, ed. *Textbook of surgery.* Philadelphia: WB Saunders, 1986:1004.

Drennan DB. Orthopedic lesions. In: Isaacs JH, Byrne MP, eds. *Pelvic surgery: a multidisciplinary approach.* Mt Kisco, NY: Futura, 1987:173.

Elmas N, Killi RM, Sever A. Colorectal carcinoma: radiological diagnosis and staging. *Eur J Radiol* 2002;42(3):206–223.

Embury SH. Sickle cell anemia and associated hemoglobin pathology. In: Bennet JC, Plum F, eds. *Cecil textbook of medicine.* Philadelphia: WB Saunders, 1996.

Farrell RJ, Farrell JJ, Morrin MM. Diverticular disease in the elderly. *Gastroenterol Clin North Am* 2001;30(2): 475–496.

Farrell RJ, Peppercorn MA. Ulcerative colitis. *Lancet* 2002;359(9303):331–340.

Ferzoco LB, Raptopoulos V, Silen W. Acute diverticulitis. *N Engl J Med* 1998;338(21):1521–1526.

Gill SS, Heuman DM, Mihas AA. Small intestinal neoplasms. *J Clin Gastroenterol* 2001;33(4):267–282.

Hanauer SB. Inflammatory bowel disease. In: Bennet JC, Plum F, eds. *Cecil textbook of medicine.* Philadelphia: WB Saunders, 1996.

Horton KM, Corl FM, Fishman EK. CT of nonneoplastic diseases of the small bowel: spectrum of disease. *J Comput Assist Tomogr* 1999;23(3):417–428.

James MF, Hift RJ. Porphyrias. *Br J Anaesthesiol* 2000; 85(1):143–153.

Knaus JV, Barber HRK. Metastatic lesions presenting as pelvic mass. In: Isaacs JH, Byrne MP, eds. *Pelvic surgery: a multidisciplinary approach.* Mt Kisco, NY: Futura, 1987:69.

Kohler L, Sauerland S, Neugebauer E. Diagnosis and treatment of diverticular disease: results of a consensus development conference. The Scientific Committee of the European Association for Endoscopic Surgery. *Surg Endoscop* 1999; 13(4):430–436.

Lang EK, Macchia RJ, Thomas R, et al. Computerized tomography tailored for the assessment of microscopic hematuria. *J Urol* 2002;167:547–554.

Levin B. Neoplasms of the large and small intestines. In: Bennet JC, Plum F, eds. *Cecil textbook of medicine.* Philadelphia: WB Saunders, 1996.

Lewis JJ, Leung D, Woodruff JM, et al. Retroperitoneal soft-tissue sarcoma. Analysis of 500 patients treated and followed at a single institution. *Ann Surg* 1998;228:355–365.

McCallion K, Mitchell RMS, Wilson RH, et al. Flexible sigmoidoscopy and the changing distribution of colorectal cancer: implications for screening. *Gut* 2001;48:522–525.

O'Malley ME, Wilson SR. Ultrasonography and computed tomography of appendicitis and diverticulitis. *Semin Roentgenol* 2001;36(2):138–147.

Paulson DF. The urinary system. In: Sabiston DC Jr, ed. *Textbook of surgery.* Philadelphia: WB Saunders, 1986:1658.

Pignone M, Rich M, Teutsch SM, et al. Screening for colorectal cancer in adults at average risk: a summary of the evidence for the U.S. Preventive Services Task Force. *Ann Intern Med* 2002;137(2):132–141.

Rieber A, Nussle K, Reinshagen M, et al. MRI of the abdomen with positive oral contrast agents for the diagnosis of inflammatory small bowel disease. *Abdom Imag* 2002;27(4): 394–399.

Shanahan F. Crohn's disease. *Lancet* 2002;359(9300):62–69.

Smith RP. Lower gastrointestinal disease in women. *Obstet Gynecol Clin North Am* 2001;28(2):351–361, viii.

Stollman NH, Raskin JB. Diverticular disease of the colon. *J Clin Gastroenterol* 1999;29(3):241–252.

Thadani H, Deacon A, Peters T. Diagnosis and management of porphyria. *BMJ* 2000:320(7250):1647–1651.

Urban BA, Fishman EK. Targeted helical CT of the acute abdomen: appendicitis, diverticulitis, and small bowel obstruction. *Semin Ultrasound CT MR* 2000;21(1):20–39.

Urban BA, Fishman EK. Tailored helical CT evaluation of acute abdomen. *Radiographics* 2000;20(3):725–749.

Wolff BG, Devine RM. Surgical management of diverticulitis. *Am Surg* 2000;66(2):153–156.

Yahchouchy EK, Marano AF, Etienne JC, et al. Meckel's diverticulum. *J Am Coll Surg* 2001;192(5):658–662.

Young-Fadok TM, Roberts PL, Spencer MP, et al. Colonic diverticular disease. *Curr Probl Surg* 2000;37(7):457–514.

GYNECOLOGIC ONCOLOGY

Te Linde's Operative Gynecology, ninth edition, edited by John A. Rock and Howard W. Jones, III. Lippincott Williams & Wilkins, Philadelphia © 2003.

CHAPTER

44

▼

Malignancies of the Vulva

MITCHEL S. HOFFMAN

Carcinoma of the vulva is an uncommon malignancy accounting for 0.3% of all female cancers in the United States and 3% to 5% of all female genital malignancies. It is predominantly a disease of older women, with the median age being 67 years in a series of 415 patients reported by Cavanagh and associates in 1990. In this country as a whole, the steady increase in life expectancy has brought carcinoma of the vulva into a place of more importance among gynecologic malignancies. This is especially so in states with a large number of elderly citizens, such as Florida. The predominant histologic type is squamous cell carcinoma, which accounts for about 90% of the tumors in most series. This malignancy metastasizes primarily through the lymphatic system in an orderly manner through the superficial inguinal lymph nodes, the deep inguinal nodes, and the pelvic nodes. Just 50 years ago, the absolute 5-year survival rate for carcinoma of the vulva was 15%. However, a significant improvement in survival has occurred because of earlier diagnosis and a better understanding of the nature and modes of spread of this disease.

The survival of patients with invasive squamous cell carcinoma of the vulva is dependent on a number of histopathologic factors, but it most closely relates to the pathologic status of the inguinal lymph nodes. In the not too distant past, patients with invasive carcinoma of the vulva were routinely treated with radical vulvectomy and bilateral inguinofemoral and pelvic lymphadenectomy. Especially over the past decade, treatment of this malignancy has undergone a number of significant modifications that are applicable to most patients.

This chapter first reviews the epidemiology, clinical characteristics, staging, and prognostic factors for invasive carcinoma of the vulva. The broad spectrum of treatment of this disease is then reviewed with an emphasis on the surgical treatment. Finally, histologic variants of vulvar malignancy and their treatment are discussed individually.

EPIDEMIOLOGY

Invasive squamous cell carcinoma of the vulva is typically a disease of postmenopausal women, with a median age at diagnosis of about 65 years. However, the age range is wide, and some data suggest an increasing incidence in younger women. This has been attributed to some extent to the human papillomavirus or some other sexually transmitted factor, although the association is not nearly as strong as it is for cervical cancer. Furthermore, recent data have shown an association with coexistent vulvar intraepithelial neoplasia, basaloid or warty histology, and classic cervical cancer risk factors. Human papillomavirus does not appear to play a significant role in the epidemiology of invasive squamous cell carcinoma of the vulva in older women.

The other sexually transmitted factors that have been epidemiologically associated with vulvar cancer are the granulomatous venereal diseases, especially in countries where these are prevalent.

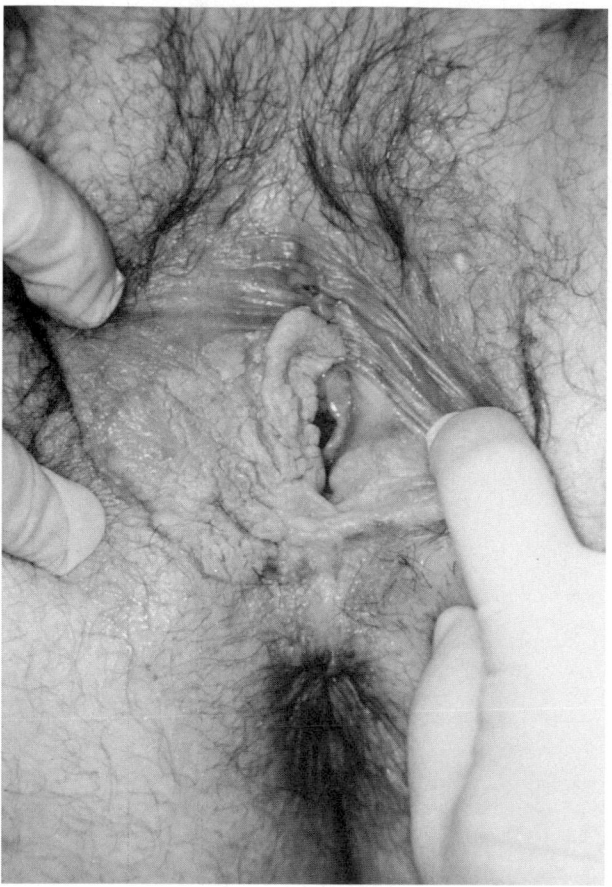

FIGURE 44.1. Carcinoma in situ of the vulva.

Vulvar carcinoma in situ (Fig. 44.1), like cervical carcinoma in situ, is considered a precursor to invasive disease, although the risk of progression appears to be lower. There are no substantial long-term natural history studies of untreated patients. Although Jones and Rowan found in seven of eight women with untreated vulvar intraepithelial neoplasia that invasive cancer developed within 8 years, three other studies found progression rates of 5% to 16%. Occult invasion has been discovered in 16% to 22% of patients undergoing excision of vulvar intraepithelial neoplasia III. The risk for invasive cancer may be greater with perianal location, increased age, and immunosuppression. Vulvar carcinoma in situ tends to be multifocal with a lower risk of invasive cancer in younger women, but it tends to be unifocal with a higher risk of invasive disease in older women. For this reason, as reported by Jones and Rowan in 1994, all patients should be treated, and long-term follow-up is mandatory. Although progression of vulvar intraepithelial neoplasia from grade 1 to grade 2 and grade 3 has been demonstrated, in the absence of atypical changes, other vulvar epithelial abnormalities do not appear to have significant precancerous potential. Patients who have cervical neoplasia are at increased risk for developing vulvar neoplasia, and vice versa. This so-called field phenomenon should heighten the physician's surveil-

lance for the development of other lesions once a lower genital tract neoplasm occurs.

Hypertension and diabetes mellitus are common in patients with invasive vulvar cancer, but this may simply be related to the elderly population affected. The associations of vulvar cancer with obesity and cigarette smoking are also unclear. There does not appear to be any significant association with parity or race. One group that does appear to be at increased risk for the development of invasive vulvar cancer is chronically immunosuppressed patients.

CLINICAL PRESENTATION

The most common initial symptom of vulvar cancer is pruritus vulvae, which may be of long duration. Vulvar pain, discharge, and bleeding are less commonly reported. The patient often becomes aware of a lesion on her vulva; but despite the superficial nature of the lesion, delay in seeking medical help is common. In a previous report by Cavanagh and associates in 1990, there was a patient delay of more than 12 months in 99 of 296 patients (33%). Rutledge and co-workers reported that 60% of their patients were aware of a vulvar mass or sore for an average period of 10 months before treatment. In 30% of their cases, there was a physician delay of 3

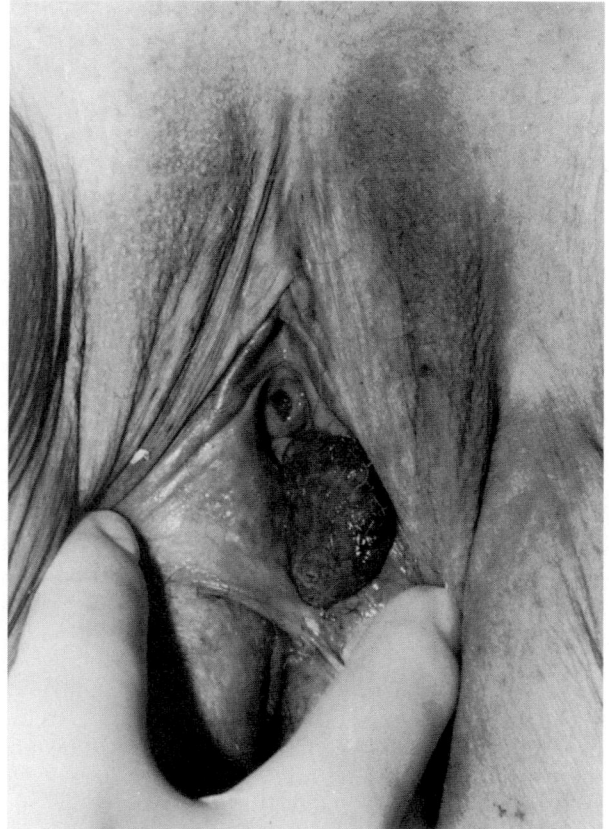

FIGURE 44.2. Exophytic vulvar cancer.

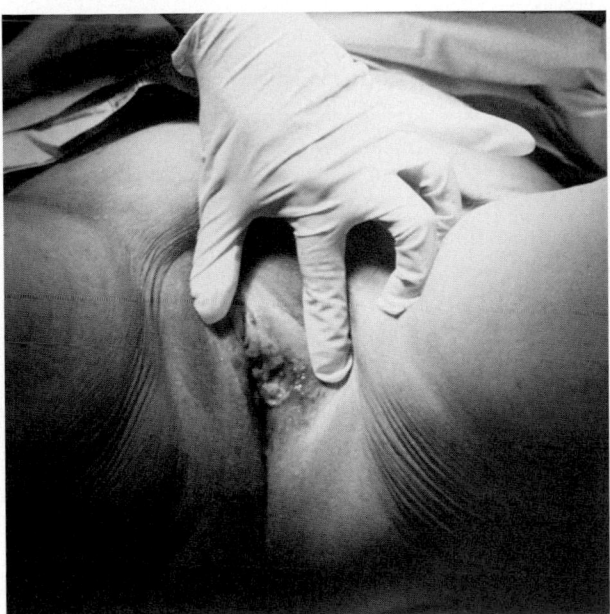

FIGURE 44.3. Ulcerating vulvar cancer.

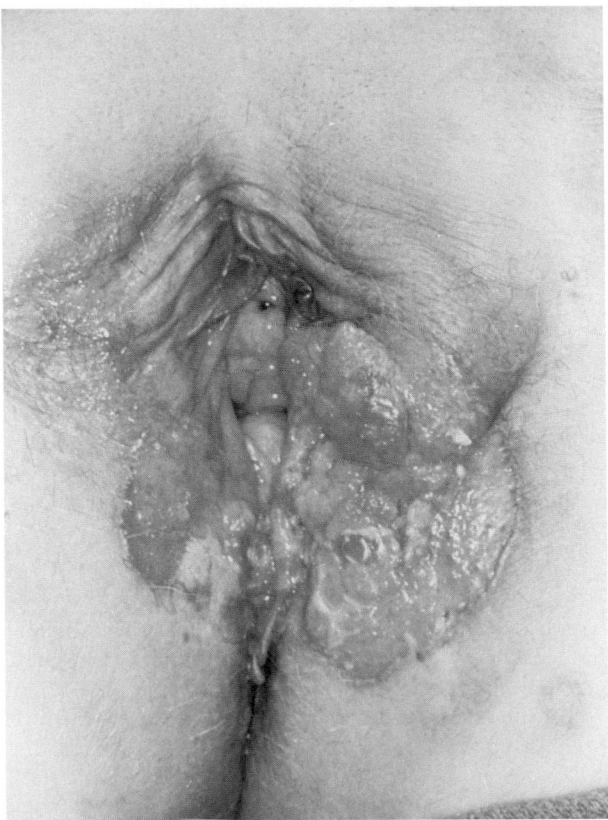

FIGURE 44.4. Flat vulvar cancer.

months or more, and 25% had been under medical treatment without having a biopsy. Boutselis reported a patient delay of 27% and a physician delay of 26% with an average delay of 3 to 9 months. In the series of Garcia and Boronow, patient delay ranged from 1 month to 8 years, and physician delay ranged from 2 to 12 months. Parker and co-workers reported that the duration of symptoms was 3 months or more in 70% of their patients, 6 months or more in 50%, and 12 months or more in 30%. These findings underscore the need for patient and physician education with regard to the early diagnosis of carcinoma of the vulva, and the importance of having a biopsy diagnosis before treating vulvar lesions. Biopsy of the vulva is a simple procedure that can be performed in the physician's office.

Invasive squamous cell carcinoma of the vulva involves the labia majora in about two thirds of patients. The remaining tumors involve the clitoris, labia minora or posterior fourchette, and perineum. These cancers can be exophytic, ulcerating, or flat (Figs. 44.2 through 44.4).

HISTOLOGY

Squamous cell carcinoma accounts for about 90% of the invasive vulvar malignancies in most large series. Melanoma is the second most common histologic type, accounting for 5% to 10% of vulvar cancers. Some of the less common vulvar malignancies include Bartholin's carcinoma (with most of these being adenocarcinoma or squamous carcinoma), basal cell carcinoma, verrucous carcinoma, adenocarcinoma, invasive Paget's disease, and sarcomas. This chapter mainly deals with invasive squamous cell carcinoma, followed by a discussion of the less common vulvar malignancies.

ROUTES OF SPREAD

Squamous cell carcinoma of the vulva can spread by local extension to involve the vagina, urethra, or anus. Spread from the primary site can occur by the lymphatic or the vascular system, but, by far, the most common is the lymphatic route. The lymphatics of the labia drain to the inguinal lymph nodes. The lymphatics of the perianal area drain in a similar manner, but lesions that extensively involve the anus or rectovaginal septum can drain directly into the pelvic lymph nodes. Although there are channels that drain the clitoris to the deep pelvic nodes, it appears that they are of minimal clinical significance. The lymphatics of the vulva are numerous and tend to cross the midline. The regional lymph nodes include the superficial inguinal lymph nodes, the deep inguinal lymph nodes, and the pelvic lymph nodes (external iliac, obturator, internal iliac, and common iliac lymph nodes). The superficial inguinal lymph nodes are the primary nodal group of the vulva and are located around the saphenous, superficial epigastric, and superficial circumflex iliac veins. These lymph nodes drain through the cribriform fascia to the deep femoral lymph nodes, which are mainly located medial to the femoral vein. Drainage from here is under the inguinal ligament into the pelvic lymph nodes. As is discussed later, the pelvic lymph nodes are virtually never positive in the absence of inguinofemoral lymph node metastases. In our own experience, of 122 patients with bilateral groin and pelvic

TABLE 44.1.
Clinical Staging of Invasive Cancer of the Vulva

Stage I	All lesions confined to vulva, with maximal diameter of 2 cm or less and no suspicious groin nodes
Stage II	All lesions confined to vulva, with diameter greater than 2 cm and no suspicious groin nodes
Stage III	Lesions extending beyond vulva but without grossly positive groin nodes
	Lesions of any size confined to vulva, with suspicious groin nodes
Stage IV	Lesions involving mucosa of rectum, bladder, or urethra, or involving bone
	All cases with distant or palpable deep pelvic metastases

TABLE 44.2.
FIGO Staging of Invasive Cancer of the Vulva

Stage 0	Carcinoma in situ, intraepithelial carcinoma
Stage I	Tumor confined to the vulva or perineum, or both; 2 cm or less in greatest dimension (no nodal metastasis)
Stage IA	Stromal invasion no greater than 1.0 mm*
Stage IB	Stromal invasion greater than 1.0 mm.
Stage II	Tumor confined to the vulva or perineum, or both; more than 2 cm in greatest dimension (no nodal metastasis)
Stage III	Tumor of any size with one or both of the following:
	Adjacent spread to the lower urethra, vagina, or anus.
	Unilateral regional lymph node metastasis
Stage IVA	Tumor invades any of the following: upper urethra, bladder mucosa, rectal mucosa, or pelvic bone, or bilateral regional node metastasis
Stage IVB, any T, any N, MI	Any distant metastasis including pelvic lymph nodes

* The depth of invasion is defined as the measurement of the tumor from the epithelial-stromal junction of the adjacent most superficial dermal papilla to the deepest point of invasion.

lymphadenectomy, not a single patient was found to have positive pelvic nodes in the presence of negative groin nodes. Overall, 20% to 40% of all patients with invasive squamous cell carcinoma of the vulva have lymph node metastases.

STAGING

In 1979, the International Federation of Gynecology and Obstetrics (FIGO) approved a clinical classification for invasive squamous cell carcinoma of the vulva (Table 44.1). This was based on an analysis of tumor (T) by size and location; node (N) status by palpation; distant metastases (M) as assessed by general and pelvic examination; evaluation of the bladder or rectum, or both; and radiologic investigation. Most patients with invasive carcinoma of the vulva are treated surgically, and it was recognized through a number of studies that there were substantial discrepancies between the clinical assessment of the inguinal lymph node status and the surgical pathologic findings. In 1988, FIGO approved a surgical staging system (Table 44.2). This system is based on well-established surgical-pathologic prognostic criteria. In 1995, stage I was divided into A and B based on a depth of invasion less or greater than 1 mm.

PROGNOSTIC FACTORS

Invasive squamous cell carcinoma of the vulva has a relatively low propensity for distant metastases. Recurrences tend to be local or regional, and even unremitting disease tends to remain locoregional for long periods of time. The dominant prognostic factor in this disease is the status of the inguinofemoral lymph nodes. Further definition of prognosis is done by evaluating a number of factors relating to the regional lymph nodes. In addition, several prognostic factors related to the primary tumor have been delineated. These primary tumor characteristics have been correlated with the likelihood of regional nodal involvement or risk of local recurrence.

Primary tumor factors that appear to have prognostic importance include depth of invasion or tumor thickness, tumor diameter, tumor differentiation, lymph-vascular space involvement, and margin status. Tumor involvement of the distal urethra, vagina, or perineum is also an adverse prognostic factor. Of less clear importance are cytologic grading, the local immunologic response to the tumor, tumor volume, tumor growth pattern, location, ulceration, amount of keratin, the presence of associated vulvar intraepithelial neoplasia or vulvar dystrophy, p53 overexpression, DNA ploidy, and proliferation index. Sedlis and colleagues reported on a Gynecologic Oncology Group (GOG) study of 272 patients with lesions less than or equal to 5 mm in tumor thickness. They found that histologic grade, capillary-like space involvement, tumor thickness, and clitoral or perineal location were all significant predictors of groin node metastases. A subsequent GOG study reported by Homesley and associates on 588 evaluable patients with invasive carcinoma found lymph-vascular space involvement, GOG tumor differentiation, age, and tumor thickness to be significant independent risk factors for groin node metastases. A few of the primary tumor characteristics, such as tumor diameter and lymph-vascular space involvement, may be significant independent predictors of survival. Other factors may be predictive of an increased risk of local recurrence, including margin status, large tumor size, and deep invasion.

The status of the groin nodes is clearly the most important prognostic factor for patients with invasive squamous cell carcinoma of the vulva. The overall 5-year survival rate for all treated patients is about 60%, with a corrected 5-year survival rate of about 70%. In the GOG study previously mentioned, 65.5% of the patients had negative groin nodes and 34.5% had positive nodes; this is consistent with our own experience and with other recent reports in the literature. In the GOG report, the survival rate for patients with negative lymph nodes was 90.9%, and with positive lymph nodes it was 57.7%, again consistent with the other recent reports in the literature. When the pelvic lymph nodes are known to be positive, the survival rate decreases to about 20%. Further definition of prognosis is achieved by examining a number of variables related to the lymph node metastases; the most significant of these is the number of nodes involved. Other factors that have been reported to be prognostically significant include bilateral involvement, extracapsular extension, clinical nodal status, size of the metastatic deposit inside the lymph node, percentage of nodal replacement, nodal immune response, and location of the metastases within the lymph nodes. Several studies have shown that when only one lymph node is involved, survival is still quite good, but survival rate decreases drastically with metastases to three or more nodes or with bilateral nodal involvement. In the 1991 GOG report, the relative survival rate was 75.2% when one or two nodes were involved and decreased to 36.1% when three or more nodes were involved. The survival rate was 70.7% with unilateral involvement versus 25.4% with bilateral involvement. On the basis of limited data from a few studies, it appears that large nodal diameter, extensive nodal replacement, and especially extracapsular extension of a lymph node metastasis are adverse prognostic factors. In a report by Origoni and colleagues in 1992, which was based on 53 vulvar cancer patients with groin node metastases, the survival rate varied from 90.9% when the diameter of the metastasis was less than 5 mm to 20% when it was larger than 15 mm, and from 85.7% to 25% when the metastases were intracapsular and extracapsular, respectively. Especially important are the data from the 19 patients in that study with a single positive node. For these patients, the 5-year cancer-related survival rate was 90% when the metastasis diameter was less than 5 mm versus 37.5% when it was 15 mm, and 85.7% when the metastasis was intracapsular versus 20% when it was extracapsular. Re-

sults from a study by Paladini and associates were similar; they reported that patients with intracapsular metastases tended to have recurrence at distant sites, whereas patients with extracapsular nodal disease were more likely to have local or groin recurrence. Both of the previously mentioned studies also revealed that a lack of active immune response within the lymph node metastases was an adverse prognostic factor. A 1995 study from the Netherlands (van der Velden and colleagues) found a predominantly distant failure pattern in a subgroup of patients with extranodal spread, multiple positive lymph nodes, and lymph nodes replaced greater than 50% by tumor. Hoffman and co-workers studied 48 patients with groin node metastases and reported prognostic significance for the size and number of the nodal metastases, but they found that the immune response and the location of the metastasis within the lymph node were much less important. Groin nodes that are both clinically and surgically positive may also portend a worse prognosis, which is probably a reflection of the factors mentioned earlier.

PRETREATMENT INVESTIGATION

Patients with carcinoma of the vulva are generally elderly and often have coexisting medical problems. A thorough preoperative evaluation by internal medicine and anesthesiology consultants is essential in the care of these patients. As previously discussed, these women have an increased incidence of cervical and vaginal neoplasia, which may be coexistent. Therefore, careful examination of these areas preoperatively is important. Beyond physical examination and a chest radiograph, routine studies to rule out metastatic disease are not indicated except in the presence of locally advanced disease. Cystoscopy, intravenous pyelography, or proctoscopy (or all three) is indicated if it appears that locally advanced cancer may be involving the bladder, bladder base, or rectum. Imaging the tumor with magnetic resonance imaging (MRI) or computed tomography (CT) may help to determine resectability and treatment planning. When a locally advanced tumor or obvious inguinal lymph node metastasis is noted, CT of the groins, pelvis, and abdomen is suggested. This aids in determining the resectability of the tumor and metastases, extension to the pelvic lymph nodes, and distant metastases (Fig. 44.5). Lymphography is rarely used and should be avoided because it can

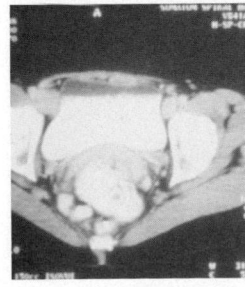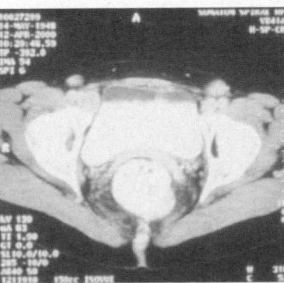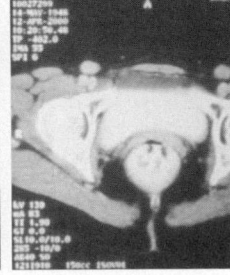

FIGURE 44.5. Patient had bilateral clinically positive inguinal lymph nodes. CT scan demonstrates their relationship to the femoral vessels and additional lymph node metastases above these.

increase the risk of cellulitis in a lymphedematous limb at a later date.

TREATMENT OF INVASIVE SQUAMOUS CELL CARCINOMA OF THE VULVA

Invasive squamous cell carcinomas of the vulva are a heterogeneous group of tumors requiring considerable flexibility in the approaches to treatment. Dating back to the favorable reports of Taussig in 1940 and Way in 1948, radical vulvectomy with bilateral inguinal lymphadenectomy performed by en bloc excision became the standard therapy applied to most patients with carcinoma of the vulva. This operation involves radical removal of the entire vulva, the mons pubis, the inguinofemoral lymph nodes, and often the pelvic lymph nodes. A large surgical defect is created that is generally closed under tension with a high subsequent breakdown rate and marked disfigurement of the genital area (Fig. 44.6). Important concerns with this approach for the treatment of vulvar cancer have led to a number of modifications, especially over the past 20 years (Fig. 44.7). Some of these concerns include the high rate and the severity of wound complications and the psychosexual effects of radical removal of the vulvar tissues. Other potential problems related to the standard approach include urinary or fecal incontinence and vaginal relaxation, the overtreatment of early cancer, the inadequate treatment of more advanced disease, and the lack of attention directed specifically at the local vulvar lesion to ensure an adequate margin of resection. What we wish to emphasize in this section are some treatment recommendations based on our own experience and on current literature on the subject.

Modifications in Regional Nodal Management

It should be kept in mind that certain vulvar cancers, by virtue of their anatomic extent, may have access to lymphatics that bypass the groins. These include tumors that extensively involve the anus (particularly the anal canal or its surrounding tissue), the rectovaginal septum, the vagina above the lower third, and the proximal urethra.

Separate Incisions

Although reported earlier by Kehrer, Taussig, Byron and associates, and Ballon and Lamb, it was only after later reports by Hacker and colleagues, DiSaia and associates, and others that separate incisions for the vulvar and inguinal phases of the operation came into increasing use (Fig. 44.7B). This has been one of the most important modifications of the classic en bloc excision. The separation of incisions results in a significant reduction in wound morbidity. Importantly, the separation allows for increased flexibility in the modification of the two aspects of the operation (regional and local). The report by Hacker and colleagues in 1981 consisted of 100 patients in whom three separate incisions were used to perform the bilateral inguinofemoral lymphadenectomy and radical vulvectomy, leaving a bridge of tissue between the incisions and sparing the mons pubis. Major groin wound breakdown occurred in 14 patients, which was a considerable reduction from the 50% or higher groin wound breakdown rate generally seen with the en bloc excision. In this report, there were no isolated recurrences in either the groin or the inguinal skin bridge. There were two recurrences in the inguinal skin bridge associated with other recurrence sites; both patients had originally had positive inguinal lymph nodes. In addition to these two patients, inguinal skin bridge recurrence has been reported in at least seven other patients. However, this

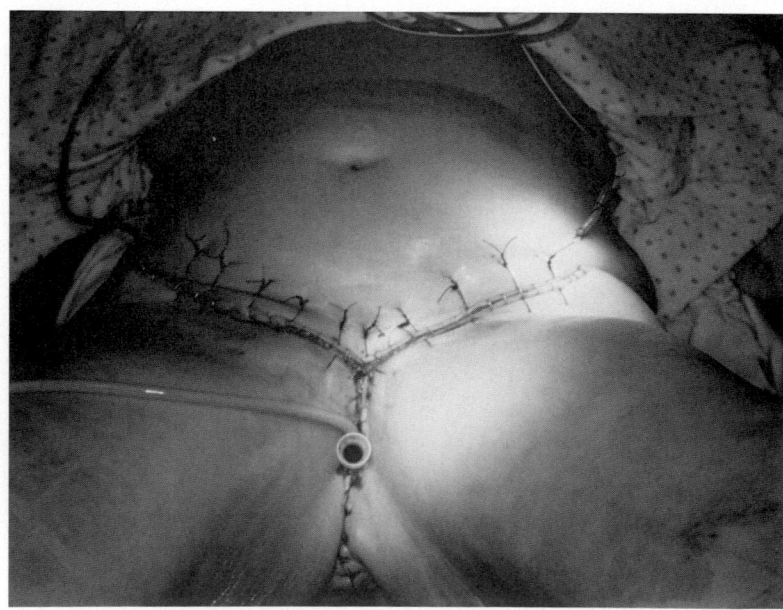

FIGURE 44.6. Closure of en bloc radical vulvectomy with bilateral inguinofemoral lymphadenectomy. Foley catheter and vaginal stent are in place.

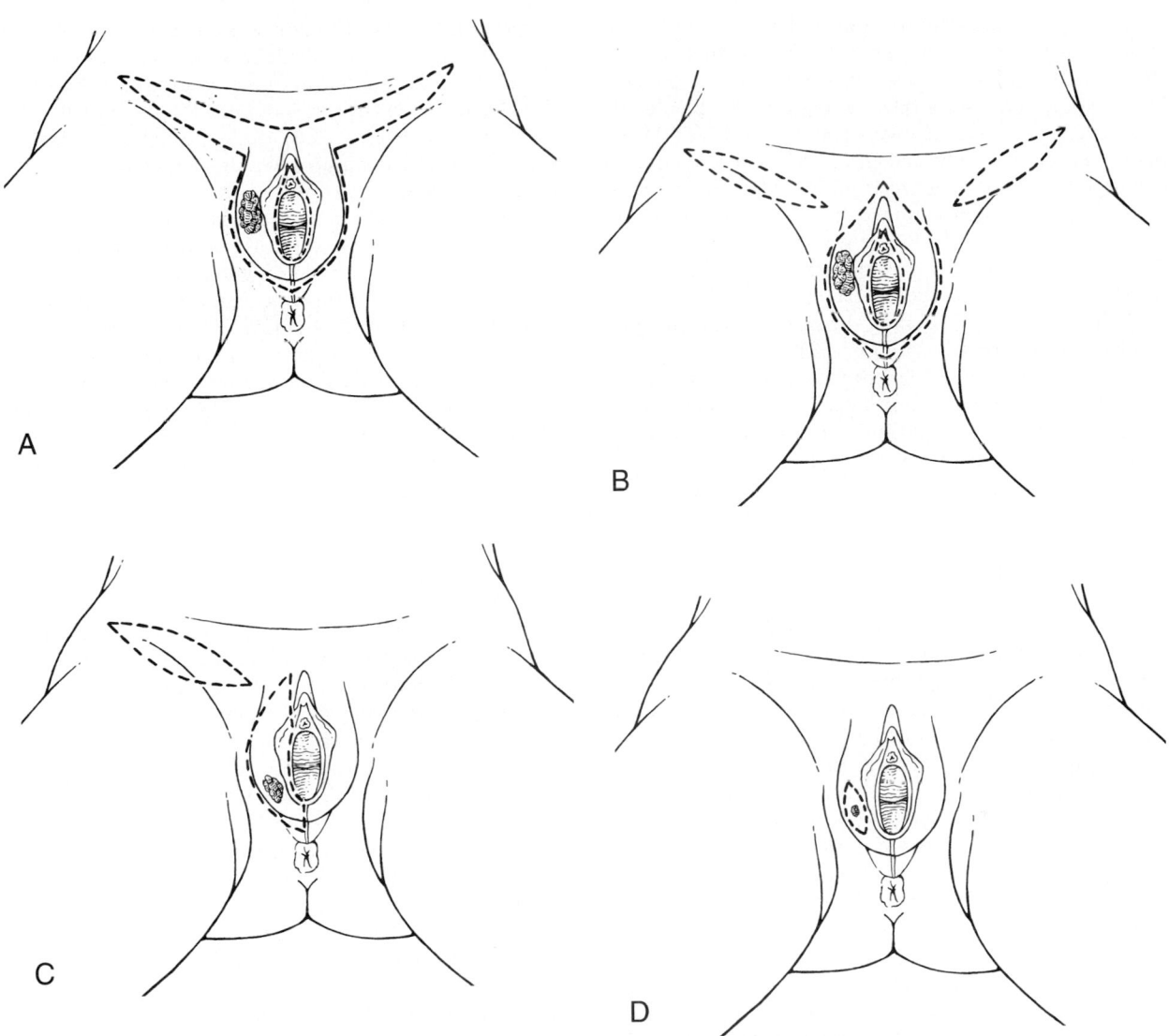

FIGURE 44.7. Modifications in regional nodal management. **A:** En bloc removal. **B:** Radical vulvectomy with bilateral inguinofemoral lymphadenectomy performed through three separate incisions. **C:** Unilateral lymphadenectomy for a well-lateralized lesion. **D:** Early lesion with lymphadenectomy omitted.

still appears to be a rare event. Some authors believe that in the presence of advanced disease or grossly positive inguinal lymph nodes, an en bloc excision of the tumor and the lymph nodes is still the best approach. En bloc excision is certainly warranted at times to obtain an adequate resection of the malignancy.

Transperineal Lymphadenectomy

Two studies have evaluated removal of the inguinal lymph nodes by mobilizing the vulvectomy incision. There is insufficient data to comment on the value of this approach, but it may be worth considering in particular situations.

Unilateral Groin Lymphadenectomy

Removing the inguinal lymph nodes only on the side of a unilateral tumor has been another proposed and stud-

ied modification (Fig. 44.7C). In 1981, Iversen reported on 53 patients with unilateral tumors and lymph node metastases. Eighty-three percent of these patients had only one positive ipsilateral node, 15% had bilateral positive nodes, and one patient had contralateral positive lymph nodes only. Other retrospective studies have confirmed these results. It has been stated by a number of authors, although without solid scientific data, that capillary or lymphatic space involvement by tumor may increase the risk of contralateral nodal metastases. Certainly, patients with tumors approaching the midline or involving more medial structures (perineum, clitoral hood or clitoris, vagina, and labia minora) are at increased risk for contralateral lymph node metastases. The issue of unilateral groin lymphadenectomy was studied to some extent in 1992 by Stehman and associates in a GOG study. Briefly, patients with early disease and negative ipsilateral superficial inguinal lymph nodes were treated with ipsilateral superficial inguinal lymphadenectomy and a modified radical vulvectomy. A few patients in this study did have a bilateral inguinal lymphadenectomy because of midline involvement. A total of 121 patients were in the study, and three experienced contralateral inguinal lymph node recurrences. The vulvar lesions of these three patients ranged from 0.6 to 2.5 mm in depth of invasion, and all were poorly differentiated. Although lesion location was not given for these three cases, a large percentage of patients included in this study had lesions approaching the midline, as defined by involvement of the labia minora. Tumors with capillary or lymphatic space involvement were excluded from this study. The role of unilateral inguinal lymphadenectomy in the management of invasive squamous cell carcinoma of the vulva requires further study; but, at present, it appears reasonable in a patient with a well-lateralized early tumor that is well differentiated, with no capillary or lymphatic space involvement, and with negative ipsilateral inguinal lymph nodes.

Superficial Inguinal Lymphadenectomy

A more limited resection of the inguinal lymph nodes in the management of superficially invasive vulvar cancer was reported by DiSaia and co-workers in 1979. The dissection he described is aimed at removal of the superficial lymph nodes above the cribriform fascia, mainly associated with the great saphenous and superficial epigastric veins. These lymph nodes are sent for frozen section analysis. If results are positive, a complete bilateral inguinofemoral lymphadenectomy is performed. In the 1979 study, DiSaia and colleagues also reported 79 cases of invasive squamous cell carcinoma of the vulva treated with radical vulvectomy and bilateral inguinal lymphadenectomy. In these cases, it was noted that the deep femoral lymph nodes were never positive in the absence of positive superficial inguinal lymph nodes. The

purpose of this modification was to reduce the morbidity of the inguinal lymphadenectomy. The dissection is less radical and resulted in only one groin breakdown in the 18 patients in the series of DiSaia and associates. The previously mentioned GOG study specifically studied the issue of superficial inguinal lymphadenectomy in patients with early carcinoma of the vulva. The study group included clinical stage I patients with tumor invasion of 5 mm or less and no capillary or lymphatic space involvement. A modified radical vulvectomy and ipsilateral superficial inguinal lymphadenectomy were performed, and 121 patients were evaluable. These were compared with a historical control group in the GOG registry who had undergone radical vulvectomy with bilateral inguinofemoral lymphadenectomy. Nine patients in this study, or 7.3%, experienced groin recurrences, versus no recurrence in the control group. Six of the groin recurrences were in the ipsilateral groin, and five of the nine patients died of the recurrent vulvar cancer. The interpretation from this study was that superficial inguinal lymphadenectomy may not be a valid treatment procedure even for early vulvar carcinoma. However, in a number of patients in this study, the tumors approached the midline, and there is valid concern that more medial tumors may have direct access to the deep inguinal lymph nodes. Another area of concern in this study is the high percentage of poorly differentiated tumors—almost twice as many as in the control group. Six of the nine groin recurrences in this study were from the poorly differentiated tumors. Whether poorly differentiated tumors are more likely to metastasize to deep inguinal or contralateral inguinal lymph nodes deserves further study. In addition, it is not clear whether the superficial inguinal lymphadenectomy described by DiSaia was universally applied to the patients in this study.

Table 44.3 summarizes the groin recurrences after superficial inguinal lymphadenectomy that have been reported in the literature. Because of the small numbers

TABLE 44.3.
Groin Recurrence After Superficial Lymphadenectomy

Investigator	Patient Age (y)	Tumor Size (cm)	Grade	Tumor Depth (mm)	Capillary or Lymphatic Space Involvement	Tumor Location	Months	Status (mo of follow-up)
Chu et al., 1981	45	1	2	3.5	NA	Periclitoral	0	NA
Burke et al., 1990	61	2	NA	4.0	(+)	Right labia major	27	AWD (3)
Podczaski, 1990	76	1	1	1.5	(−)	Left labia major	17	DOD
Kelley et al., 1992	52	NA	NA	<1	NA	Right labia major	31	A (27)
Stehman et al., 1992	72	1.5	2	3.2	(−)	NA	6.2	A(26)
	76	1.5	1	1.5	(−)	NA	16.5	DOD
	52	2	3	2.0	(−)	NA	2.9	DOD
	75	2	3	5.2	(−)	NA	4.6	A (19)
	75	2	3	3.0	(−)	NA	7.8	DOD
	84	1.5	2	2.0	(−)	NA	17.9	DOD

NA, not available; AWD, alive with disease; DOD, dead of disease; A, alive.

and lack of information in some of these patients, it is not possible to draw any definite conclusions. Again, factors worth studying with respect to the efficacy of superficial inguinal lymphadenectomy appear to be tumor grade, depth of invasion, the presence of capillary or lymphatic space involvement, and tumor location. If the status of superficial inguinal lymphadenectomy is to be further studied on the basis of its potential for reduced morbidity, then it will need to be done in carefully selected comparable groups of patients. The superficial lymph nodes removed should be reported as negative on frozen section during the course of the operation, and the patients should be those generally at low risk for lymph node metastases and should probably have tumors confined to the labia majora. Extending dissection to include removal of lymph nodes medial to the femoral vein may be considered in selected patients.

Sentinel Lymph Node Identification

A large number of reports have been published recently on sentinel lymph node detection. The concept relies on the presumption that the sentinel lymph node is the initial site of metastatic disease and that the histology of the sentinel lymph node reflects the histology of the rest of the nodes in the basin. Lymphatic mapping is considered by some authors to be the standard of care in the United States for the surgical treatment of the patient with melanoma and is coming into widespread use for breast cancer patients.

With lymphatic mapping, the pathologist has only a few lymph nodes to examine, allowing a more detailed examination. Techniques such as serial sectioning, immunohistochemical staining, and reverse transcriptase–polymerase chain reaction analysis can be applied, increasing the sensitivity of the examination and allowing the detection of micrometastases.

Sentinel lymph node detection is currently accomplished using two methods of lymphatic mapping, blue dye and radiocolloid. One to two milliliters of isosulfan blue dye (Lymphazurin) is injected around the periphery of the primary tumor, and the blue-dyed lymphatic channels are followed. An incision is made over the anticipated location, and the dyed lymph node or nodes are removed. Alternatively, the periphery of the tumor is injected with 400 mCi of technetium-labeled sulfur colloid 2 to 4 hours before surgery. An intraoperative gamma counter is used to identify one or more sentinel lymph nodes. The removed lymph nodes are checked with the gamma counter and complete removal is assured when the radioactivity in the inguinal area returns to background levels. Medical centers experienced in lymphatic mapping report that the two techniques are complementary.

In practice, lymphatic mapping is not always successful in identifying a sentinel lymph node. A formal lymph node dissection is reserved for those cases in which the sentinel node is positive or has not been successfully identified.

Experience with lymphatic mapping of vulvar cancer patients has increased substantially over the past 10 years. The technique is promising as a method to sub-

stantially reduce the morbidity of inguinal lymphadenectomy. Injection of radiocolloid is best done 2 to 4 hours before surgery, but this is painful. Unanswered questions include the incidence of "skip" metastases, the reliability of an isolated ipsilateral negative sentinel node with a midline lesion, the reliability of lymphatic mapping after prior excisional biopsy, and the optimal lymphatic mapping methodology for vulvar cancer patients.

Pelvic Lymph Nodes

During the late 1970s and early 1980s, several studies were published showing that carcinoma of the vulva metastasizes to the inguinofemoral lymph nodes before spreading to the pelvic lymph nodes. Extension of the groin lymphadenectomy to include removal of the pelvic lymph nodes continued to be performed in selected patients with positive inguinofemoral lymph nodes. A number of studies also showed that the 5-year survival rate of vulvar cancer patients with positive pelvic lymph nodes is less than 20%. A 1986 study by the GOG directed by Homesley compared pelvic lymph node dissection with groin and pelvic radiotherapy in patients with positive inguinofemoral lymph nodes. The study included 114 patients and showed no difference in morbidity between the two treatment arms and a better 2-year survival rate in the radiotherapy group (68% versus 54%). The improved survival was seen in those patients with suspicious or grossly positive lymph nodes or those with more than one positive groin lymph node. There was no evidence that groin radiation therapy was beneficial to those patients with occult metastases and only one positive groin node. Review of the pattern of recurrence in that study suggested that adjuvant radiation was more effective largely because groin recurrences were reduced. The value of removing positive pelvic lymph nodes before radiotherapy is unknown. In a patient with obvious inguinal lymph node metastases who is otherwise suitable, our practice is to extend the dissection and remove enlarged pelvic lymph nodes. Preoperative CT may help with such a decision (Fig. 44.5).

Primary Inguinal Radiotherapy

The use of elective radiotherapy to the groins in the place of bilateral inguinofemoral lymphadenectomy has been proposed as a modification with considerable potential for reducing morbidity. The method is believed to be appropriate only in the absence of clinically suspicious lymph nodes. Daly and Million reported on this method of treatment in six patients with minimum morbidity and no groin recurrences, but follow-up was short. Frischbier and Thomsen reported on this method for the treatment of 118 patients and reported a 70% survival rate for the N0, N1 group. Henderson and colleagues used the method for 91 N0, N1 patients with minimum morbidity. In that series, there were no groin recurrences in the radiotherapy field and two outside the field. In addition, there are extensive supporting data on elective nodal radiation for other sites, including the cervix, endometrium, vulva (pelvic), and head and neck. This issue was later addressed in another GOG study by Stehman and co-workers in 1992 in which there was a random-

TABLE 44.4.
Invasion of Less than 1 Millimeter: Nodal Disease

Investigator	Patients	Positive Nodes
Wilkinson, 1985	115	0
Hacker et al., 1984	34	0
Parker et al., 1975	19	0
Magrina et al., 1979	19	0
Struyk et al., 1989	11	0
Sedlis et al., 1987	32	1
Ross and Ehrmann, 1987	17	0
Kelley et al., 1992	24	1
Stehman et al., 1992	13	1
Magrina et al., 2000	40	0
TOTALS	324	3 (1%)

ization of patients with nonsuspicious groin lymph nodes to radical vulvectomy plus bilateral inguinofemoral lymphadenectomy, or radical vulvectomy plus radiation therapy to the groins bilaterally. This study was closed early because of a high incidence of recurrence in the radiated groins and reduced survival (in the first 49 evaluable patients, there were 5 groin recurrences in the irradiated patients and no groin failures in the operated group). Upon review, however, it was believed that the radiation program used in the study may not have provided an adequate dose to the depth where the lymph nodes were located. The role of elective primary groin radiotherapy in the management of invasive squamous cell carcinoma of the vulva, therefore, remains unclear.

Omitting Groin Dissection for Superficial Disease

Extensive data support the contention that a subset of early vulvar carcinomas (carefully studied pathologically) can be identified that have an extremely low risk of nodal involvement. This subset includes tumors confined to clinical stage I, which are unilateral, are well differentiated, have up to 5 mm of invasion, have no capillary or lymphatic space involvement, and have no confluence. The International Society for the Study of Vulvar Disease Task Force in 1981 believed that there was no appropriate definition for microinvasive carcinoma of the vulva. They suggested the classification of stage IA for tumors no more than 2 cm in diameter and no more than 1 mm in greatest depth. They also pointed out that there was a need for standardization of the definition of *depth of invasion*. In another GOG study reported by Sedlis and associates, a subgroup (63 of 272) of patients with early disease was identified as having a zero incidence of lymph node metastases. This subset included nonmidline tumors with no capillary or lymphatic space involvement that were well differentiated or were grade 2 and limited to 2 mm in thickness. Other factors that have been studied for the purpose of identifying a low-risk group include tumor volume (which does not appear to have received further attention since Wilkinson's report in 1985), tumors that are largely carcinoma in situ with very early stromal invasion and with a pushing rather than an infiltrative pattern, and factors such as tumor diameter, squamous cell type, the presence of an inflammatory response, and tumor ploidy.

There seems to be general agreement that the patients in whom it would be most reasonable to omit the lymphadenectomy are those with tumor invasion less than or equal to 1 mm. The risk of lymph node metastases in this group of patients is about 1% (Table 44.4). Based on this, FIGO stage I was recently divided into stages IA and IB. As reported in the literature, three of five patients with nodal disease or nodal recurrence in association with tumor invasion less than or equal to 1 mm had poorly differentiated cancers (Table 44.5). Thus, certain high-risk patients with superficially invasive tumors should still undergo a groin node dissection. These include women with suspicious lymph nodes, poorly differentiated tumors, tumors with capillary or lymphatic space involvement, and perhaps those with multiple foci

TABLE 44.5.
Invasion of Less than 1 Millimeter: Nodal Disease

Investigator	Patient Age (y)	Tumor Size (cm)	Grade	Tumor Depth (mm)	Capillary or Lymphatic Space Involvement	Months*	Status (mo of follow-up)
Sedlis et al., 1987	61	2.5	4†	1	(−)	0	NA
Atamede and Hoogerland, 1989	75	1.0	1	0.72	(−)	13	AWD
Van der Velden et al., 1992	84	1.0	3	0.3	(−)	20	DOD
Kelley et al., 1992	52	NA	NA	<1	NA	31	A (27)
Stehman et al., 1992	57	2.0	3	0.6	(−)	26	A (35)

NA, not available; AWD, alive with disease; DOD, dead of disease; A, alive.
* Months to diagnosis of nodal disease.

or broad areas of invasion, or aneuploidy. Meanwhile, in the report by Sedlis and colleagues on 272 patients with invasion of 5 mm or less, the groin nodes were positive in approximately 20%.

Modifications in Management of the Vulvar Phase of Treatment

The main type of morbidity relating to a radical vulvectomy is the subsequent sexual dysfunction and the sense of disfigurement that many patients suffer in silence. In some cases, there may also be compromised function of the anus or urethra. Additional types of morbidity are encountered in the treatment of locally advanced tumors because of the ultraradical therapy that may be required. If the local control and cure rate can be maintained, then the patient is likely to benefit from conservation of as much normal vulvar tissue as is feasible. In a 1979 study, DiSaia and colleagues reported complete preservation of sexual function in 17 of 18 patients who underwent wide local excision for early invasive tumors. They also reported that preservation of the mons pubis as well as the major portion of the superior aspect of the vulva resulted in an appreciably more satisfactory cosmetic result.

There is little additional information in the literature on sexual function as it relates to modifications of radical vulvectomy. It seems reasonable to assume, however, that the sparing of as much normal vulvar tissue as possible is less likely to produce sexual dysfunction and a sense of disfigurement than is radical vulvectomy. A modified radical vulvectomy is an ambiguously defined operation that generally refers to radical removal of the portion of the vulva containing the tumor (Fig. 44.8). Recommendations have included 1- to 3-cm skin margins in the treatment of well-localized, unifocal lesions, although most authors recommend a 2-cm margin.

The chief concern with a modified radical vulvectomy is the possibility of an increased risk of local recurrence, which centers around the issue of multicentricity (Fig. 44.9). Multicentricity has been reported to occur in 20% to 28% of invasive squamous cell carcinomas of the vulva. Ross and Ehrmann reported 15 of 64 stage I patients who had microscopic multifocal disease and 3 of 64 patients who had grossly multifocal disease. There may be an ongoing occult process within the vulva of patients with vulvar carcinoma, and biochemical abnormalities have been demonstrated in normal-appearing epithelium adjacent to malignancy. In the report by Ross and

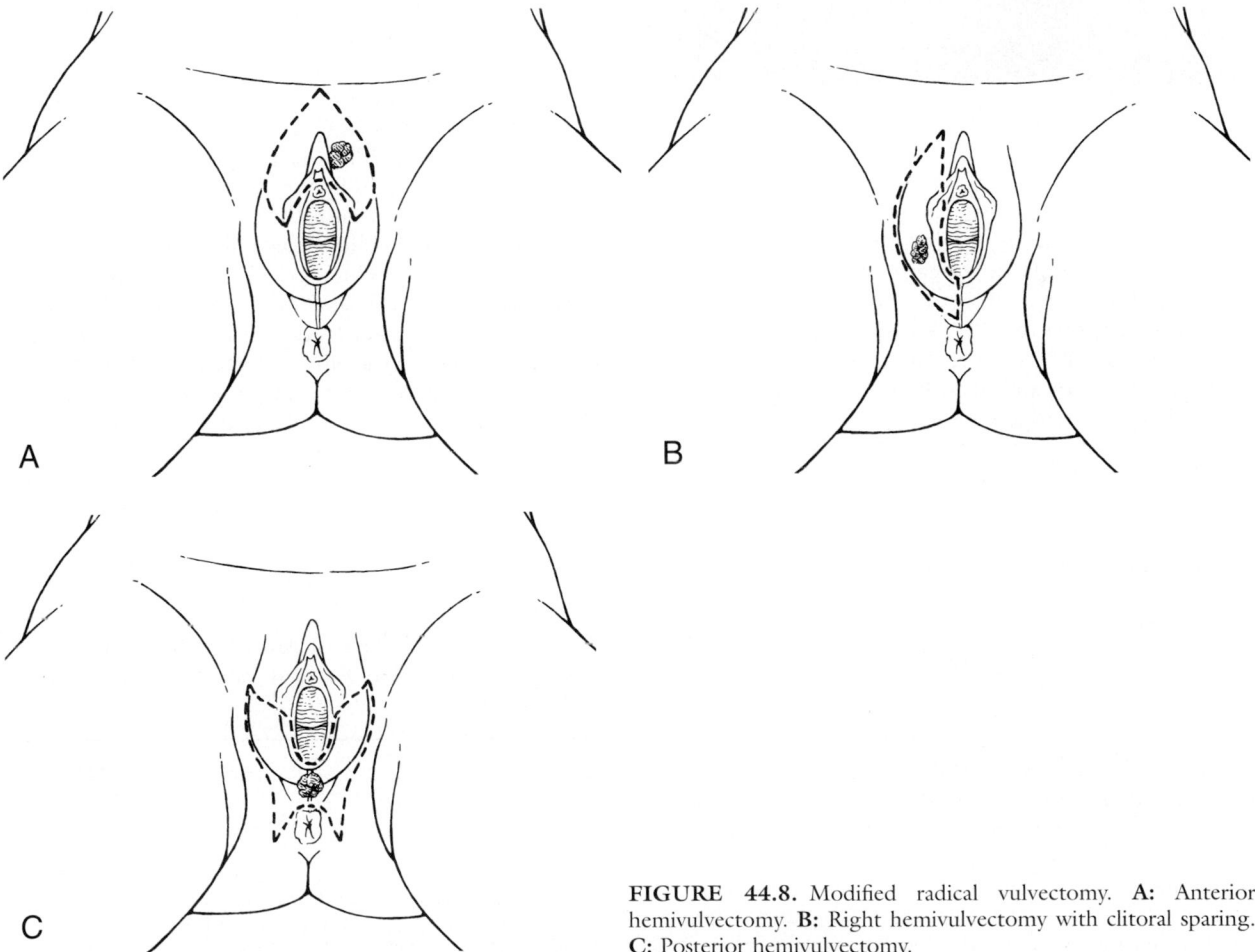

FIGURE 44.8. Modified radical vulvectomy. **A:** Anterior hemivulvectomy. **B:** Right hemivulvectomy with clitoral sparing. **C:** Posterior hemivulvectomy.

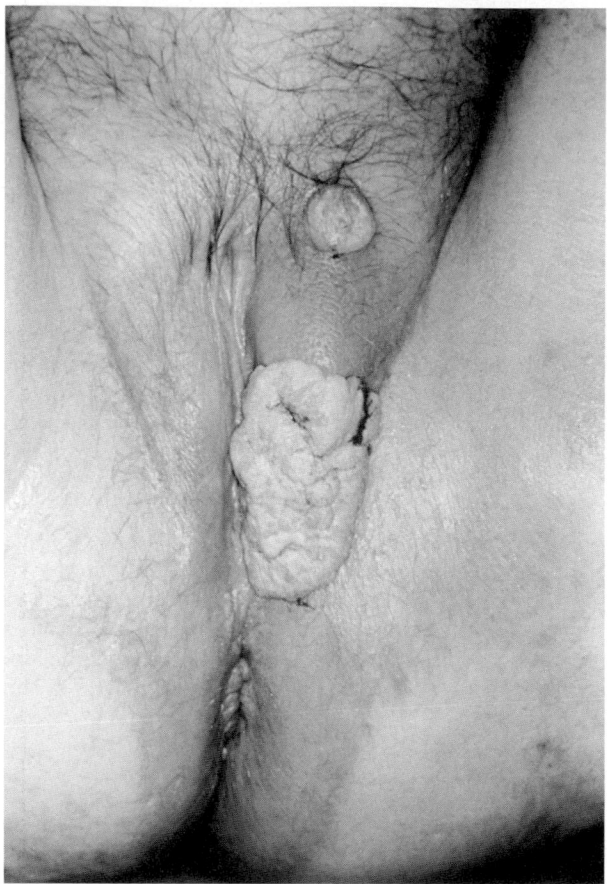

FIGURE 44.9. Multifocal carcinoma of the vulva.

Ehrmann, occult microscopic multifocal disease appeared in the immediate vicinity of the grossly evident tumor as surface noncontiguity of the primary lesion. Occult microscopic disease away from the primary tumor has not been reported, and the concern that microscopic multicentric foci might be left behind as a result of a modified operation does not appear to be valid. The potential for local microscopic noncontiguity of the tumor, however, would indicate the importance of an adequate tumor margin. In fact, two recent studies reported a higher local recurrence rate when the resected tumor-free margin was less than 1 cm. For most well-demarcated tumors, the gross and microscopic borders of the tumor correlate. One recent study found that ulcerative tumors with an infiltrative pattern of invasion involving mucosal epithelium may be more likely to extend beyond what is grossly apparent. Simonsen and colleagues noted that in many radical vulvectomies, margins are close. Iversen suggested that the goal in treating the primary tumor in vulvar squamous cell carcinoma of all stages should be adequate margins rather than removal of the entire vulva. Hacker and colleagues compared radical vulvectomy with wide local excision in the treatment of superficially invasive squamous cell carcinoma of the vulva. Fifty-six patients underwent radical vulvectomy and 28 patients underwent wide local excision. The local recurrence rate of 4%

TABLE 44.6.
Modified Radical Vulvectomy Literature: Local Recurrence

	Patients	Local Recurrence	Minimum Follow-Up (mo)
DiSaia et al., 1979	18	0	7
Hacker et al., 1984	28	1 (4%)	24
Burrell et al., 1988	28	0	16
Berman et al., 1989	50	4 (8%)	12
Sutton et al., 1991	56	7 (12%)	1
Stehman et al., 1992	121	10 (8%)	36
Hoffman et al., 1992	45	1 (2%)	12
Lin et al., 1992	12	2 (13%)	24
Andrews et al., 1994	28	2 (7%)	12
Burke et al., 1995	76	9 (12%)	NA
de Hullu et al., 2002	85	7 (8%)	NA
TOTALS	547	43 (8%)	

was identical in both groups. A later review by Hacker and van der Velden of literature regarding patients with vulvar cancer 2 cm or less in diameter showed a local invasive recurrence rate of 7.2% for 165 patients treated with radical local excision versus a local invasive recurrence rate of 6.3% for 365 patients treated with radical vulvectomy. In a comparative study at our institution, of 45 patients who underwent radical vulvectomy and 45 patients who underwent modified radical vulvectomy, the local recurrence rates were 2.2% and 4.4%, respectively. Several additional studies have reported excellent local control with the modified radical vulvectomy (Tables 44.6 and 44.7). In another GOG study, Stehman and colleagues analyzed recurrences following modified radical hemivulvectomy. The mean time to "relapse" on the vulva was 43.4 months and 11 of 18 patients had recurrence on the contralateral side from the primary lesion. A study by de Hullu et al. also reported a significant number of late recurrences following modified radical vulvectomy. From these results, it is apparent that women undergoing a modified vulvar operation for cancer are at high risk for later development of a new primary vulvar tumor and should have long-term close follow-up.

TABLE 44.7.
Comparative Studies of Modified Radical Vulvectomy Versus Radical Vulvectomy: Local Recurrence

	Patients	Recurrence
Modified Radical Vulvectomy	263	35 (13%)
Radical Vulvectomy	343	39 (11%)

Data from Hacker et al., 1984; Stehman et al., 1992; and Hoffman et al., 1992, de Hullu et al., 2002.

It appears reasonable to conclude that a modified radical vulvectomy is efficacious treatment for well-localized invasive squamous cell carcinoma of the vulva. Attention should be focused on obtaining a 2-cm skin margin around the tumor while sparing as much vulvar tissue beyond this as possible. Most patients with squamous cell carcinoma of the vulva are candidates for a modified radical vulvectomy performed separately from the groin lymphadenectomy. A few patients, however, by virtue of disease extent, require a radical vulvectomy. Whatever the vulvar phase of the operation is called, the aim should be to excise the tumor with a 2-cm margin.

Partial Urethral Resection

Because of tumor proximity, it is occasionally necessary to remove a portion of the urethra to obtain an adequate resection of a vulvar carcinoma. Although several authors have stated that removal of the outer urethra does not result in significant problems with incontinence, there are no substantial confirming data. In one small study, Reid and colleagues did find urinary incontinence to be a problem after resection of the distal urethra or even an excision close to the urethra. If a portion of the urethra is resected, a Foley catheter should be left in place (carefully taped to the leg) for about 1 week postoperatively to facilitate healing and splint the urethra. A surgical anti-incontinence procedure should also be strongly considered at the time of resection, especially if there is any preoperative stress urinary incontinence or if more than 1 cm of the urethra has to be removed.

Vulvar Cancer with Perianal Involvement

There is scant literature concerning the local management of vulvar cancer with perianal involvement (Figs. 44.9 and 44.10). However, we have noted that about one third of our patients who are referred for vulvar cancer have lesions with perianal or anal involvement, and we have reported on this aspect. The chief problems in the management of patients with these tumors are the difficulty in obtaining adequate surgical margins on the resection while attempting to preserve external anal sphincter function, and deciding which patients would be better treated either with a more radical excision and colostomy or with preoperative radiotherapy (Fig. 44.11). In our experience with vulvar carcinoma, partial resection of the external anal sphincter in combination with radical local resection of perianal tissue is associated with a significant rate of subsequent fecal incontinence. Careful sphincter reapproximation and levator muscle plication are important measures to minimize incontinence. Other important measures include good bowel preparation preoperatively, prophylactic antibiotics, and careful postoperative bowel management. In addition, we have had very good results with the use of cutaneous rhomboid flaps in the reconstruction of the perineum and perianal area. These flaps allow for reconstruction of a perineal body, they bring

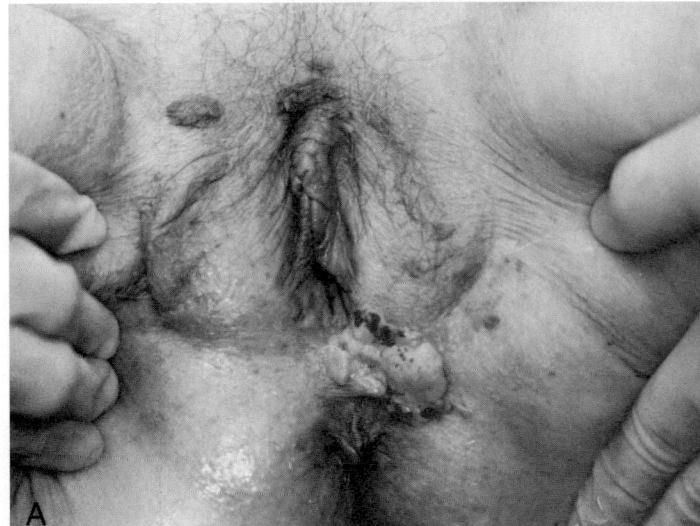
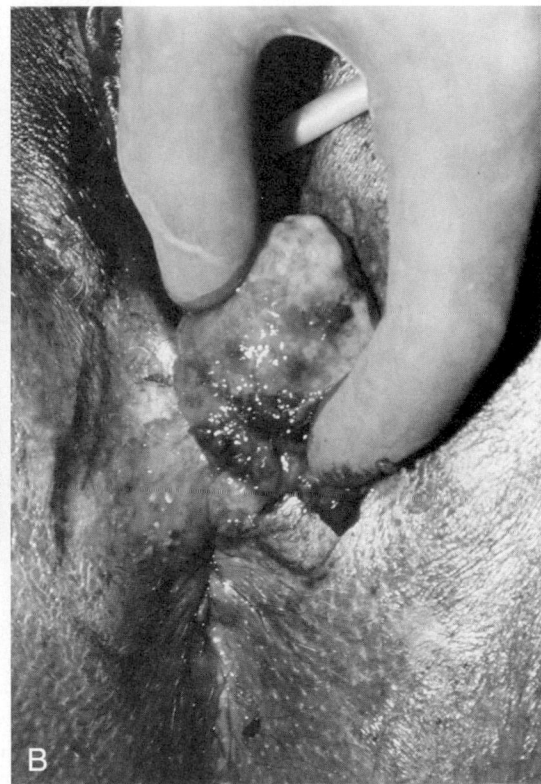

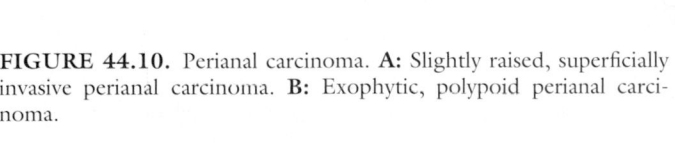

FIGURE 44.10. Perianal carcinoma. **A:** Slightly raised, superficially invasive perianal carcinoma. **B:** Exophytic, polypoid perianal carcinoma.

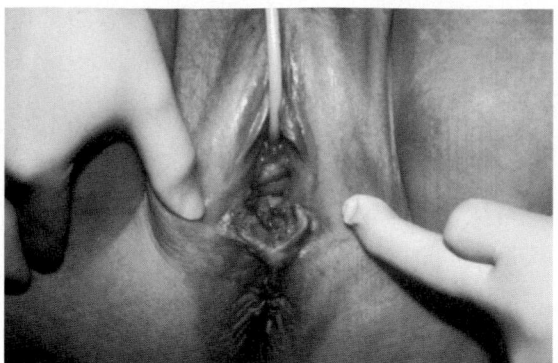

FIGURE 44.11. Perineal carcinoma encroaching upon the anus. See color version of figure.

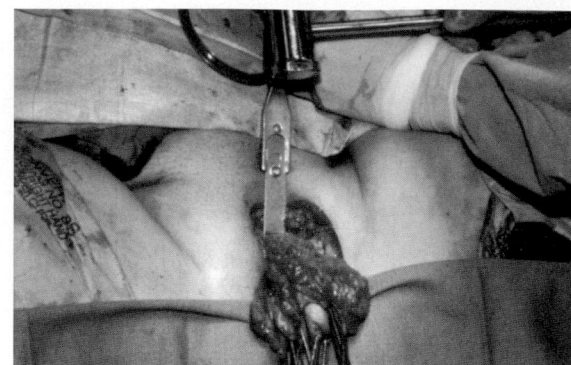

FIGURE 44.13. Locally advanced vulvar tumor fixed to the periosteum of the pubic bone. This portion of the bone is being removed with the tumor using a Richardson osteotome. See color version of figure.

tissue with a good blood supply into the area, which promotes healing, and they allow closure of the wound without tension on the anus.

LOCALLY ADVANCED DISEASE

About 30% to 40% of vulvar cancers have FIGO (clinical) stage III or IV disease. Although surgical staging was introduced by FIGO in 1988 and hard data on this system are still in relatively short supply, a review of our own patients suggests that this percentage probably still holds. We have considered carcinoma of the vulva to be locally advanced when the primary or recurring tumor cannot be locally managed by a radical vulvar resection (Fig.

44.12). Current approaches to the treatment of locally advanced vulvar cancer include ultraradical surgery, radiotherapy, and a combination of treatment modalities. This section reviews the current approaches to the treatment of locally advanced vulvar cancer.

Ultraradical Surgery

Ultraradical surgery has been used for patients with clinically resectable vulvar lesions and has generally consisted of a radical vulvar operation combined with a partial or total pelvic exenterative-type procedure. This has included resection of bone in a few reports (Fig. 44.13). Inguinofemoral and pelvic lymphadenectomies are usually performed as well (Fig. 44.14).

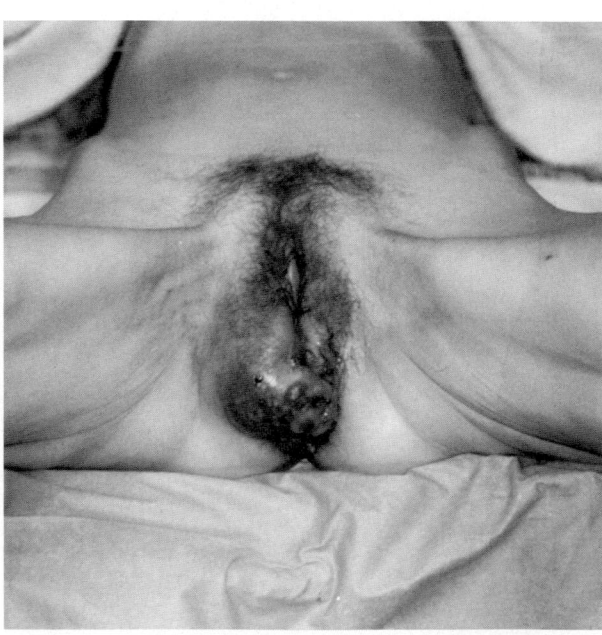

FIGURE 44.12. Locally advanced vulvar carcinoma. The lesion extensively involved the anus and lower rectovaginal septum but was mobile. There was no suspicious adenopathy.

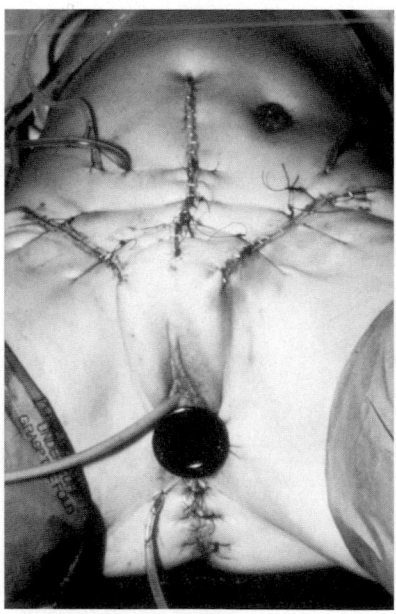

FIGURE 44.14. Completed posterior pelvic exenteration for a locally advanced vulvar cancer. Note the end-sigmoid colostomy, inguinal incisions, extended perineal incision, and a Youngs' dilator in the vagina. See color version of figure.

In some cases, resection can be limited to partial removal of the urethra or anus. Subsequent incontinence may occur, but this can be prevented to some degree by reconstructive efforts. Reid and associates reported problems with urinary incontinence in 4 of 4 patients who underwent resection of 1 to 1.5 cm of the distal urethra and in 2 of 14 patients who underwent resection within 1 cm of the urethra for carcinoma of the vulva. The value of urethral reconstruction in this setting is uncertain, but it seems worthwhile. Three recent studies have reported preservation of anal continence after partial sphincter resection and reconstruction for posteriorly located carcinoma of the vulva.

The cumulative literature from 1970 to 1995 includes 184 exenteration patients (Table 44.8). The postoperative mortality rate ranges from 0% to 20%, with a mean of about 4%. The cumulative disease-free survival rate for these patients is 46%. In those series that have included an analysis, the survival has correlated well with the status of the regional lymph nodes. Most studies have not differentiated inguinal and pelvic lymph nodes. There have been very few survivors with positive nodes, either in our series or elsewhere. Although not well addressed in the literature, there is also significant physical and psychological morbidity resulting from these operations as a result of the extensive nature of the surgery and the need for a permanent colostomy or urostomy, or both. It appears that the use of combined treatment modalities avoids the need for such extensive surgery in many of these patients (see later text). With these factors in mind, it may be reasonable to confine the use of ultraradical surgery to patients with clearly resectable lesions who have negative, or perhaps one or two microscopically positive, regional lymph nodes.

Radiotherapy

The use of primary radiotherapy for carcinoma of the vulva remains controversial but may be the only option available when the patient presents with unresectable disease. The literature concerning the use of radiotherapy for this disease consists of retrospective studies with small numbers of patients (many of whom were medically infirm or had locally advanced disease) who were treated with a variety of radiotherapy techniques (Table 44.9). Overall, this literature is difficult to interpret. The older literature is discouraging in terms of both low cure rates and vulvar skin intolerance. More recent literature describing the use of high-energy radiotherapy with its relative skin-sparing effects as well as the use of modern radiotherapy techniques has been encouraging. Whether normal bladder and bowel function is preserved with this type of treatment is difficult to determine.

We reported a series of 10 patients with locally advanced vulvovaginal malignancy treated mainly with teletherapy followed by interstitial needles to the local tumor bed for a tumor dose of 70 to 90 Gy. The therapy was highly morbid, with six patients developing severe radionecrosis (Fig. 44.15). However, seven patients remained alive with no evidence of recurrent disease at 1 to 3 years. The large volume of tissue that required implantation led to a fairly high degree of inhomogeneity across the implant, which we believe was the principal reason for the high morbidity rate.

The optimal techniques for radiotherapeutic treatment of carcinoma of the vulva have not been well defined. In the more recent literature, teletherapy has been administered to the whole pelvis, including the vulva and the groins, at a dose of 45 to 55 Gy. It is not uncommon for patients to require treatment interruption because of

TABLE 44.8.
Postoperative Mortality and Survival of Patients with Advanced Vulvar Cancer Treated by Ultraradical Surgery

Investigator	Patients	Postoperative Mortality	Disease-Free Survivors
Rutledge et al., 1970	13	0	10 (3 yr)
Thornton and Flanagan, 1973	12	1	4 (7 mo–9.5 yr)
Kaplan and Kaufman, 1975	9	1	4 (5 + y)
Krupp et al., 1975	13	2	3 (1.5–15 yr)
Adams and Daly, 1979	5	1	3 (10–41 mo)
Benedet et al., 1979	5	0	1 (>5 + yr)
Phillips et al., 1981	12	1	5 (52–153 mos)
Cavanagh and Shepherd, 1982	13	1	5 (>5 + yr)
King et al., 1989	7	0	3 (9 mo–18 yr)
Hopkins and Morley, 1992	19	0	10 (5 yr)
Grimshaw et al., 1991	23	0	15 (4–136 mo)
Miller and Morris, 1992	21	0	9 (5 year)
Hoffman et al., 1993	11	0	6 (30–84 mo)
Miller et al., 1995	21	0	7 (70% primary, 38% recurrent)
TOTALS	184	7 (3.8%)	85 (46%)

TABLE 44.9.
Radiation Alone for Vulvar Cancer, 1970 to Present

Investigator	Technique	Stage	Dose (Gy)	L/R Control (%)	Follow-Up (yr)	Serious Complication Rate (%)
Frischbier and Thomsen, 1971	MeV E	III-II	45–54	23/33 (70)	5	8
		III-IV		33/85 (39)		
Backstrom et al., 1972	60Co	IV	52–69	7/19 (36)	5	NA
Helgason et al., 1972	ORTH, 60Co + RI	I-IV Recurrence	15–58	16/29 (55)	2–5	—
			30	4/24 (17)	3	
Kuipers, 1975	MeV E	I-II	60–80	3/11 (27)	5	—
		III-IV		12/37 (32)		12
Jafari and Magalotti, 1981	60Co, t-Ces	II-IV	30–60	7/8 (88)	1–11	2
Pirtoli and Rottoli, 1982	ORTHO	I-IV	45–85	17/36 (47)	5	18
Miyazawa et al., 1983	Betatron + implant	III-IV Recurrence	40–50	2/12 (17)	2–11	—
			50–80	2/10 (20)		
Prempree and Amornmarn, 1984	60Co, MeV E + RI	Limited	40–60	8/8 (100)	>5	37
		Extensive	+ 15–55	0/13 (0)		
Carlino et al., 1984	Betatron + Ir I	I-IV	NG	2/8 (25)	<1	0
Fairey et al., 1985	60Co	I-II Local recurrence	50–55	3/6 (50)	>3	22
		Palliative		2/9 (22)		
			30	19/40 (48)		25
Pao et al., 1988	meg	III-IV	7.5–78	2/5 (40)	4	—
Slevin and Pointon, 1989	I ± meg	I-IV Recurrence	45–55	23/58 (40)	NA	5
		Palliative				
Hoffman et al., 1990	meg + Ir I	III-IV, Recurrence	44–90	8/10 (80)	1–4	60
Perez et al., 1993	meg ± Ir I	I-IV, Recurrence	50–70	NA/33	NA	25
Tewari et al., 1999	meg + Ir I	III-IV, Recurrence	24–55*	11/11 (100)	.75–6.5	18

L/R, local/regional; MeV, million electron volts; E, electrons; 60C, cobalt-60; ORTH, orthovoltage; RI, radium implant; t-Ces, teletherapy cesium; IrI, iridium implant; meg, megavoltage.
*Interstitial dose only.

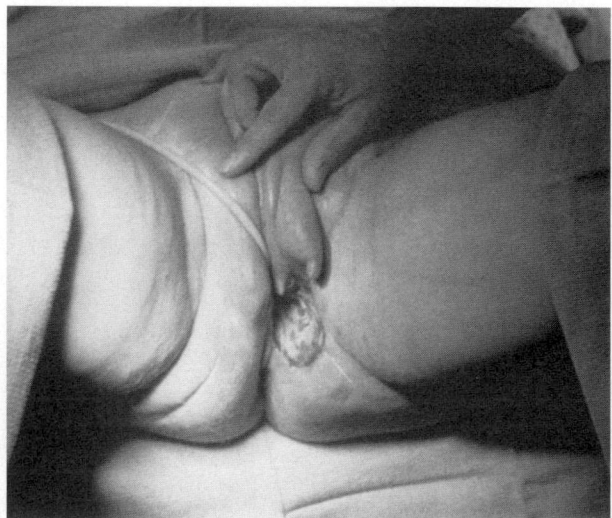

FIGURE 44.15. Radionecrosis with large ulcer.

vulvitis. The treatment regimen has been modified in some studies, with only brachytherapy or palliative treatment used. A few studies have described the use of a direct perineal portal. Treatment fields, the role of interstitial radiotherapy, the overall dose, and the integration of combination treatment with chemotherapy or surgery, or both, are among the issues to be studied. Preliminary results suggest that radiotherapy (possibly combined with chemotherapy) followed by a more limited resection is more efficacious than radiotherapy alone. These treatments are discussed in the next two sections.

Preoperative Radiotherapy

From the work of Boronow and others, data confirm that megavoltage radiotherapy can cause marked regression of even locally advanced vulvar carcinoma to the point where a more limited resection can be undertaken (often with an improved resection margin) with sparing of organ function and improved quality of life. In an update of his study in 1987, Boronow reported that, of 48 bladders and 48 rectums at risk, one bladder and two rectums were lost because of local failure, and one bladder and one rectum were lost because of radiation injury.

The report did not mention other types of bladder or bowel morbidity. Of 40 patients who underwent vulvectomy, 17 contained no identifiable residual cancer. There were no reported problems with wound healing. Similar results have been reported in other studies (Table 44.10). In these studies, survival with locally advanced disease so far has been comparable to that with ultraradical surgery. Again, the optimal radiotherapeutic techniques for such treatment are not well defined. Boronow's group has generally used a combination of external beam radiation and intracavitary brachytherapy, delivering a mean vaginal surface maximum dose of 86.26 Gy. His group and others have also used preoperative external beam therapy only, generally delivering a dose of about 50 Gy to the whole pelvis, including the vulva and groins. Surgery has generally been performed 2 to 6 weeks after completion of radiotherapy. Boronow and associates reported 42.5% of vulvectomy specimens and Hacker and colleagues reported 4 of 7 (57%) vulvectomy specimens to be negative for residual tumor.

Chemoradiotherapy

As with preoperative radiotherapy, combined chemoradiotherapy with or without resection has been used increasingly with promising results in squamous cell carcinomas of several different primary sites. This approach has been particularly successful in the treatment of squamous cell carcinoma of the anus. This type of carcinoma may be somewhat analogous to carcinoma of the vulva in terms of location and, in some instances, preservation of the anus. However, caution is warranted because the success experienced with squamous cell carcinoma of the anus may be a somewhat unusual phenomenon. Combination radiotherapy and chemotherapy at other sites, such as the cervix and the head and neck, has yielded less reliable clearance of tumor. There are few data on this type of treatment for carcinoma of the vulva, but in two of the more recent studies, the results were particularly promising.

The most commonly used chemotherapeutic agents are 5-fluorouracil, mitomycin-C, and cisplatin. Chemo-

therapy has been combined with external radiotherapy administered in a manner similar to that described in the previous sections. Most data have been accumulated over the past 15 years with the use of regimens similar to those used at other sites. Results suggest a high rate of local control for locally advanced or recurrent disease (Table 44.11). However, an increase in the degree of local morbidity is seen with this type of therapy. Most of these patients develop a moderate amount of mucositis in the vulvovaginal area (Fig. 44.16). This leads to dysuria and generalized pelvic and perineal discomfort. An indwelling catheter and the use of various perianal and rectal preparations help ease the discomfort, although treatment interruption is necessary at times. The GOG investigated the use of chemoradiotherapy for the treatment of advanced squamous cell carcinoma of the vulva (GOG 101, closed 2/94). Results from this study are included in Table 44.11 and confirm those reported by the other investigators.

Neoadjuvant Chemotherapy

A large number of pilot studies in the recent literature have reported on the use of neoadjuvant chemotherapy (NACT) in cervical cancer. The planned course of chemotherapy has been followed by surgery, radiotherapy, or both. Reported response rates have been high, and preliminary results with NACT followed by radical surgery are somewhat encouraging. However, in most of these reports, the lack of a control group and the short follow-up have not enabled clear conclusions to be drawn regarding the benefit of NACT in cervical cancer.

In 1993, Benedetti-Panici and colleagues reported the results of a pilot study using NACT followed by surgery in patients with locally advanced carcinoma of the vulva. Twenty-one patients with FIGO stage IVA (clinical) were treated. Chemotherapy consisted of cisplatin, 100 mg/m² intravenously on day 1, bleomycin, 15 mg intravenously on days 1 and 8, and methotrexate, 300 mg/m² intravenously plus citrovorum factor rescue dose on day 8, repeated every 21 days for two to three cycles. A partial response was observed in the primary tumor in

---

TABLE 44.10.
Preoperative Radiotherapy for Carcinoma of the Vulva

Investigator	Patients	Stage	Survival Rate (%)	Survival	Severe Complications (%)
Boronow et al., 1987 Boronow, 1973, 1982	48	III, IV, Recurrent	72	4–168 mo	23
Acosta et al., 1978	14	II-III	71	2 mo–8 yr	14
Jafari and Magalotti, 1981	4	II-III	100	4–5 yr	0
Hacker et al., 1984	8	IV	62.5	15 mo–10 yr	12
Carlino et al., 1984	6	II-III	66.6	15 mo	NA
Fairey et al., 1985	7	I-IV	86	13 mo–3 yr	14
Pao et al., 1988	2	I, III	100	1–2 yr	0
Rotmensch et al., 1990	16	III, IV	45	12–72 mo	4
TOTALS	105		69		19

TABLE 44.11.
Results of Chemoradiotherapy with and without Resection

Investigator	Radiotherapy (Gy)	Stage	Chemotherapy	Surgery	Proportion of Patients with Local Control	Severe Complications (%)
Kalra et al., 1981	^{60}Co (30)	III	Mit-C, 5FU	RV, GND (−)	1/1	0
Iversen, 1982	Meg (30–40)	Inoperable/Recurrent	Bleo	2 RV, GND	4/15 (26%) 1–4	40
Nori et al., 1983	Meg (34–58)	III–IV, Recurrent	Flagyl	1 vulv	5/6 (83%) 1–3	0
Levin et al., 1986	Meg (18–45)	T3N1–T4N0	Mit-C, 5FU	4RV	5/5 1–25 mo	17
Lovett et al., 1987	Meg (40 ± 1)	III, IV	DDP, 5FU	NA	1/2 10 mo	NA
Evans et al., 1988	Meg (20–64 ± 1)	NA	Mit-C, 5FU	NA	4/4 > 18 mo	NA
Thomas et al., 1989	Meg (40–64)	1.3–9 cm Recurrent 1.5–12 cm	5FU ± Mit-C	5 LE	7/9 (77%) 5–43 mo 8/12 (66%) 5–45 mo	9
Whitaker et al., 1990	Meg (25–45)	III, IV, Recurrent	Mit-C, 5FU	2 RV	3/12 6–9 mo	25
Carson et al., 1990	Meg (45–50)	III, IV, Recurrent	5FU, Mit-C DDP	4 RV, 3 LE	6/8 (75%)	12.5
Podczaski et al., 1990	Meg (51 + H)	IV	5FU, DDP	RV	1/1 8 mo	0
Berek et al., 1991	Meg (44–54)	III, IV	DDP, 5FU	3 RV, 1 PE	10/12 7–60 mo	0
Russel et al., 1992	Meg (46–78)	III, IV*	5FU ± DDP	1 RV	20/25 (80%) 2–52 mo	8
Scheistroen et al., 1993	Meg (9–45)	III, IV*	Bleo	4RV	6/20 (30%) 7–60 mo	30
Koh et al., 1993	Meg (34–70)	III, IV,* Recurrent	5FU	9LE, 2RV, 1PE	11/20 (55%) 14–75 mo	5
Sebag-Montefiore et al., 1994	Meg (45–50)	III, IV, Recurrent	Mit-C, 5FU	8RV	17/32 3–40 mo	11
Whalen et al., 1995	Meg (45–50 ± 1)	II, III†	Mit-C, 5FU	6 LE	14/19 11–72 mo	0
Eifel et al., 1995	Meg (40–50)	Recurrent-T4N3	DDP, 5FU	6LE, 1RV, 1PE, 3GND	4/12 (33%) 17–37mo	17
Lupi et al., 1996	Meg (NG)	Recurrent-T4N2	Mit-C, 5FU	18RV, 11LE, 29GND	25/31 (80%) 22–90 mo	20
Landoni et al., 1996	Meg (54)	II, III, IV,* Recurrent	Mit-C, 5FU	39RV, 30GND	47/58 (82%) 4–48 mo	20
Cunningham et al., 1997	Meg (50–65)	III, IV*	DDP, 5FU	NG	9/14 (64%) 7–81 mo	23
Moore et al., 1998	Meg (41–50)	III, IV*	DDP, 5FU	24LE, 24RV, 2PE	60/71 (84%) 22–72mo	21
Montana et al., 2000	Meg (47)	N2/N3 nodes	DDP, 5FU	34LE, 37GND	28/38 (74%) 56–89mo	47

Mit-C, mitomycin-C; 5FU, 5-fluorouracil; Bleo, bleomycin; DDP, cisplatin; RV, radical vulvectomy; GND, inguinal lymphadenectomy; Meg, megavoltage; vulv, vulvectomy; LE, local excision; PE, posterior exenteration; H, hyperthermia; I, implant; NG, not given.

*1988 staging.
†1992 staging.

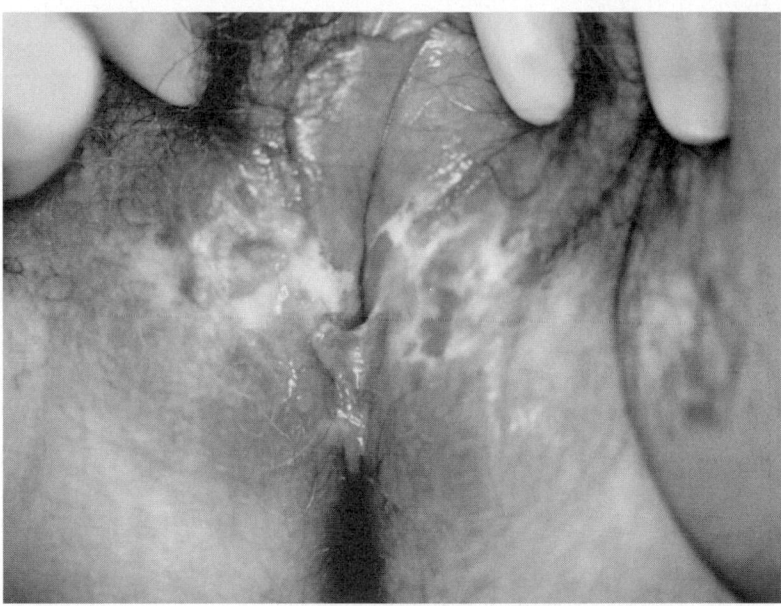

FIGURE 44.16. Desquamative vulvitis and mucositis during chemoradiotherapy.

two patients, and progression of disease was seen in two other patients. Eleven complete and three partial responses were noted in the patients with nodal disease. On pathologic examination of the 19 patients undergoing resection, 15 had inguinal lymph node metastases and nine of these had pelvic lymph node metastases. Local control was achieved in 12 of 21 (57%) of the patients (3 to 37 months), and the 3-year corrected survival rate was 24%.

The study just discussed does not suggest any benefit of NACT over the previously described treatment approaches, and the authors of that report state that they are studying the chemoradiotherapeutic approach.

Treatment of Locally Advanced Disease: Summary

Ultraradical surgery appears to be reasonable treatment for locally advanced but resectable carcinoma of the vulva, especially in the absence of nodal metastases. The role of radiotherapy in the treatment of this malignancy is still being defined. In our experience, teletherapy combined with interstitial needles for locally advanced carcinoma of the vulva appears to be effective but associated with extensive morbidity. With the use of more modern treatment techniques and better definition of the optimal delivery of radiotherapy to the vulva, the role of this modality may be expanded. A modified course of radiotherapy used in combination with other treatment modalities appears to be more efficacious than radiotherapy alone in the treatment of this disease. Combined treatment modalities for this disease present an important form of management. Especially in patients with locally unresectable disease, initial treatment with external radiation therapy possibly combined with chemotherapy appears to be the most reasonable approach. With the

use of radiologic techniques and perhaps random biopsies, an additional treatment course could be planned. Careful planning of how much surgery may be necessary or how much volume needs to be implanted may contribute to an overall decrease in morbidity in these patients.

Management of the regional lymph nodes in the context of combined treatment modalities has been variable and, by necessity, highly individualized.

The management of locally advanced vulvar cancer continues to evolve as reports of small series of these patients accumulate. Considering the relative paucity of data and the rarity and heterogeneity of these tumors, no clear-cut management guidelines can be constructed. It seems reasonable to individualize the management of these patients, carefully considering all of the various treatment modalities available.

RECURRENT SQUAMOUS CELL CARCINOMA OF THE VULVA

About 15% to 40% of patients with squamous cell carcinoma of the vulva develop recurrence after treatment. As discussed previously, the incidence of recurrence is influenced by a number of factors, including the original stage of the disease, the depth of invasion, and the regional lymph node status. About 70% of recurrences have a local component, and 55% to 90% of these are isolated local recurrences (Fig. 44.17). This is more likely to occur in the patient with negative lymph nodes at initial treatment. For patients with recurrent squamous cell carcinoma of the vulva, recurrence site is the strongest predictor of outcome. Only with an isolated local recurrence is there a reasonable expectation of successful salvage therapy (Table 44.12).

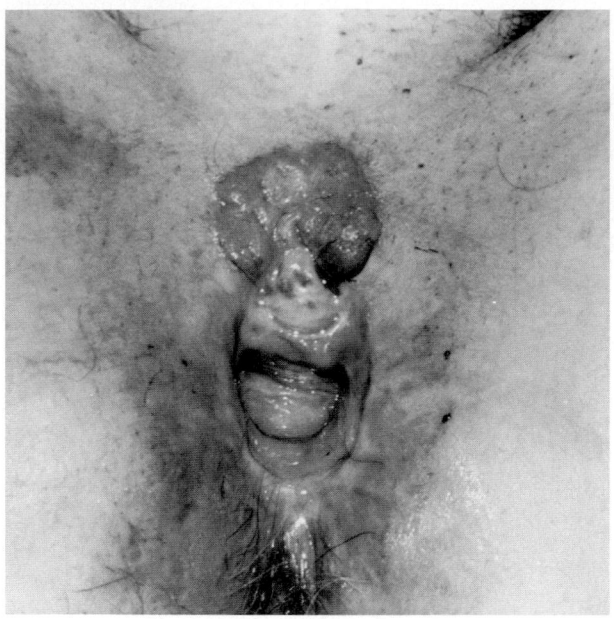

FIGURE 44.17. Local recurrence around urethral meatus.

The presence of inguinal nodal metastases, especially when multiple, bilateral, or extranodal, predisposes the patient to recurrence within the groin or pelvis and systemically. The prognosis for a patient with regional or systemic recurrence is poor. Regional recurrences do not lend themselves well to salvage resection, radiotherapy is not very effective against grossly recurrent disease, and there is no effective systemic therapy. A small percentage of patients with groin recurrence can be salvaged with resection followed by radiotherapy, and a few patients with regional recurrence may be candidates for combined resection and intraoperative radiotherapy.

Certain factors predispose the patient to develop local recurrence, including a close resection margin (less than 1 cm), deep invasion, and a large tumor size. When a patient develops an isolated local recurrence, the re-

ported salvage rate ranges from 40% to 80%. Treatment depends on the individual situation. When feasible, radical resection is performed. Otherwise, the best approach is probably preoperative radiotherapy with or without chemotherapy followed by resection.

OPERATIVE TECHNIQUES

Radical Vulvectomy with Bilateral Inguinofemoral Lymphadenectomy

The patient is placed in the "ski position" in adjustable stirrups so that the legs can be elevated to high lithotomy during the perineal phase of the operation.

The radical vulvectomy with bilateral inguinofemoral lymphadenectomy is performed with the use of two teams, and dissection of each groin is performed simultaneously. A crescent-shaped incision is made starting about 2 to 4 cm medial and about 2 cm caudal to the anterior superior iliac spine (Fig. 44.18). The incision gradually curves downward just above the superior border of the inguinal ligament medially to the inguinal ring or about 2 cm below and 2 cm medial to the pubic tubercle. Unless there is a large clitoral lesion or palpably suspicious nodes, the mons pubis is spared, and separate incisions with a skin bridge are made as illustrated. For anterior lesions such as those involving the clitoris, a portion of the mons pubis is included in the resection and the nodes on one or both sides may be done en bloc with the radical vulvectomy as illustrated in Figure 44.7A. From the lateral points, caudal incisions are carried medially so as to excise a strip of skin 2 to 4 cm in width. This incision is designed to extend from just below the fossa ovalis (this can generally be identified clinically as the area of femoral pulsation in the groin) to the top of the labiocrural fold above a point just medial to the external inguinal ring. In the presence of grossly positive inguinal lymph nodes, a wider resection of both the groin skin and fat is necessary to help ensure proper clearance. The separate skin incision may also be done

TABLE 44.12.
Vulvar Recurrence Site and Salvage Rate

Investigator	Patients	Local Recurrence Only (%)	Groin (± Local)	Pelvis (± Local)
Buchler et al., 1979	27	13/18 (72)	0/7	1/2
Podratz et al., 1982	59	15/30 (50)	NA	NA
Simonsen, 1984	41	11/29 (38)	1/12	—
Prempree and Amornmarn, 1984*	21	6/12 (50)	2/5	0/4
Hopkins et al., 1990	34	19/24 (79)	0/10	—
Tilmans et al., 1992	40	9/17 (53)	2/12	1/11
Piura et al., 1993	73	24/39 (61)	NA	NA
Stehman et al., 1996	37	13/21 (62)	0/12	—
Maggino et al., 2000	187	56/94 (60)	8/33	0/10
TOTALS	519	166/284 (58)	13/91	2/27

*All patients treated with radiotherapy only.

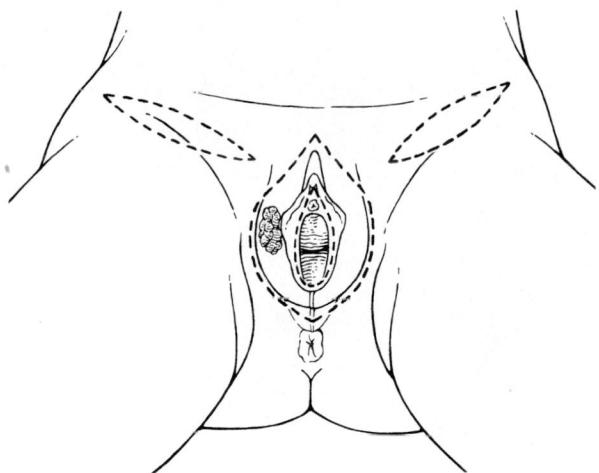

FIGURE 44.18. Incision for radical vulvectomy with separate incisions for bilateral inguinofemoral lymphadenectomy.

vertically (with the leg), centered across the fossa ovalis and about halfway between the femoral artery and pubic tubercle.

Leaving a layer of subcutaneous tissue with the skin, the superior incision is undermined so that the lymph node–bearing adipose tissue above the inguinal ligaments and around the superficial circumflex iliac, and superficial epigastric vessels is included with the resection. These vessels are ligated as they are encountered. The superior dissection over the groin area is carried down to the superior border of the inguinal ligament. The midline aspect of the superior flap can be mobilized off of

the pubic bone and rectus fascia at this point to facilitate later closure of the wound without tension. Dissection of the block of inguinal tissue is carried inferiorly off of the inguinal ligament. The lateral corners are dissected medially off of the sartorius fascia (Fig. 44.19). The inferior flap of the lower incision is also mobilized, especially medially, and the saphenous vein is identified as it enters the region of the femoral triangle (Figs. 44.20 through 44.22). Accessory saphenous veins can also be seen entering this area. The long saphenous vein is isolated and ligated with a free tie and a transfixion ligature of 2-0 polyglactin (Vicryl). The vein with its surrounding block of lymph node–bearing tissue is dissected superiorly off of the sartorius and adductor fascia. Dissection of the block of inguinal tissue is continued from the three sides toward the fossa ovalis. As this area is approached, the overlying cribriform fascia is recognized, and the femoral artery pulsation can be palpated in the lateral aspect. En bloc dissection continues and includes the contents of the fossa ovalis (Fig. 44.23). The area under the fascia lateral to the femoral artery should be left undisturbed. There are no lymph nodes of consequence here, and avoidance of this area prevents injury to the femoral nerve and possibly reduces subsequent lymphedema. Rather, resection of the cribriform fascia begins over the area of femoral pulsation, exposing the underlying femoral vessels. A few small branches of the femoral nerve are sacrificed during this dissection. The sheath of the femoral artery is incised along its anteromedial aspect from somewhere between the base of the fossa ovalis and the apex of the femoral triangle to its emergence from under the inguinal ligament. Branches, such as the external pudendal artery, are ligated as they are encoun-

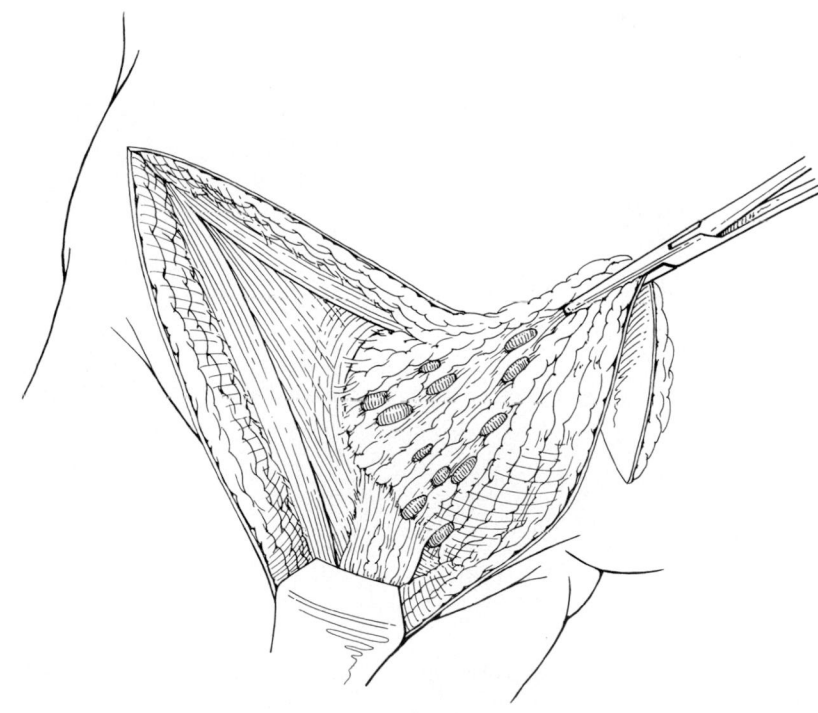

FIGURE 44.19. Corner of groin specimen dissected up medially off of sartorius muscle. Lateral portion of fossa ovalis and cribriform fascia are exposed.

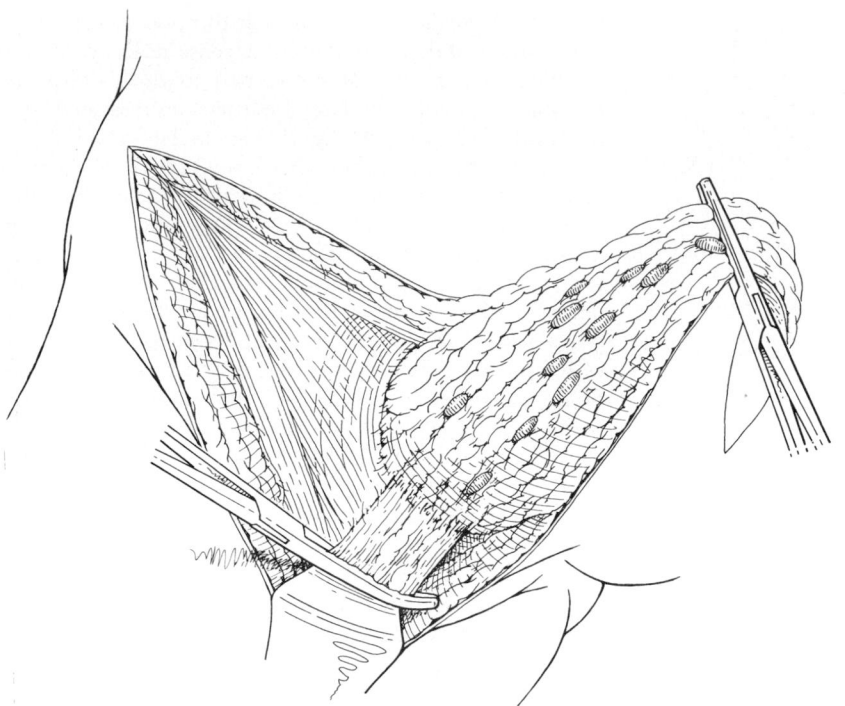

FIGURE 44.20. Block of lymph node bearing tissue overlying saphenous vein has been mobilized and clamped inferiorly.

tered. There is no purpose in dissecting under the artery or between the femoral artery and vein. Rather, the dissection that has been performed over the top of the artery is continued over the top of the vein, mobilizing the specimen to the medial aspect of the femoral vein. During this process, the saphenofemoral venous junction is identified, ligated with a 2-0 silk free-tie followed by a suture ligature for insurance, and transected, thus removing several centimeters of the saphenous vein with the specimen (Figs. 44.24 and 44.25).

An alternative method, as long as there are no adherent suspicious lymph nodes, is to dissect the saphenous vein free of the specimen so that it can be preserved, potentially reducing the risk of subsequent lymphedema. Complete dissection of the space medial to the vein is important because this is where most of the femoral groin nodes are located. The specimen is freed from the femoral vein medially, from the inguinal ligament superiorly, and from the underlying pectineal fascia. Dissection is continued toward and off of the

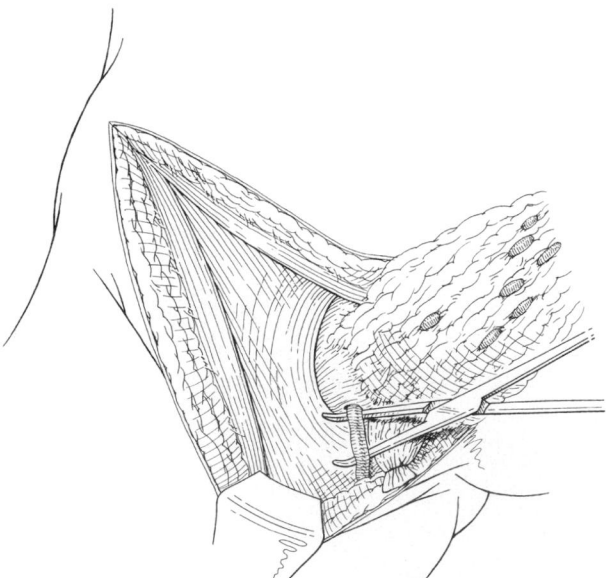

FIGURE 44.21. Segment of saphenous vein in groin is isolated.

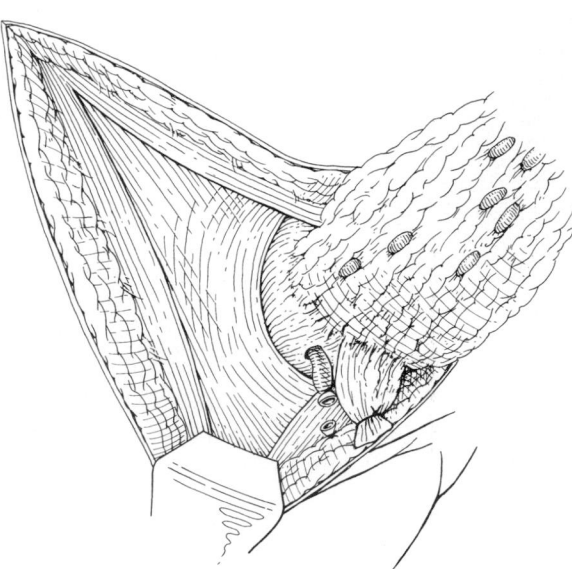

FIGURE 44.22. Saphenous vein has been transected and ligated near its entrance into the femoral triangle.

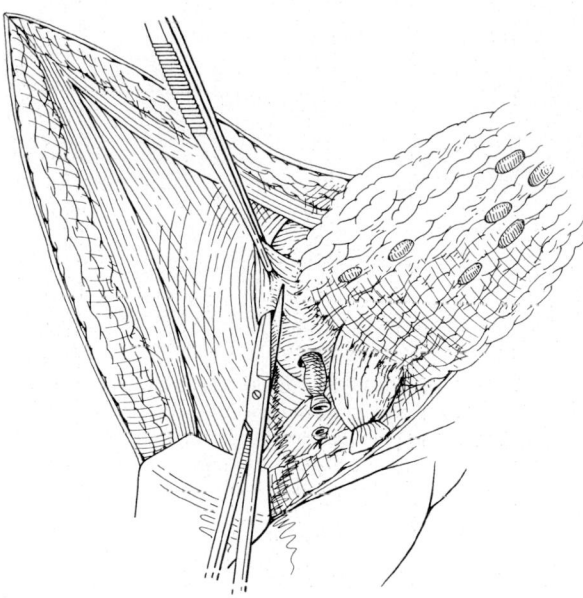

FIGURE 44.23. Dissection of the femoral lymph nodes beginning with separation of the cribriform fascia and contents of the fossa ovalis from the anterior aspect of the femoral artery.

adductor longus fascia until the labiocrural fold is reached.

To protect the femoral vessels in the event of subsequent wound breakdown, the sartorius muscle can be transposed over them at this point. We have largely discontinued the practice of transposing the sartorius muscles because of the improved healing of these wounds and less radical dissection. Alternatively, the vessels can be covered by a variety of other materials, and occasionally we use sartorius fascia. To do this, the muscle is divided with cautery at its tendinous attachment to the anterior superior iliac spine. The proximal end of the muscle is then mobilized and transposed so that it covers

the femoral vessels. It is sutured at this location to the inguinal ligament and pectineal fascia with 0 polyglactin (Fig. 44.26).

If a superficial inguinal lymphadenectomy has been chosen (also generally done through separate incisions), the same general dissection is done except that the cribriform fascia and underlying femoral lymph node–bearing tissue are left intact (Figs. 44.27 and 44.28). All lymph nodes around the saphenofemoral junction should be included, and any prominent deeper lymph nodes medial to the femoral vein should be removed.

If a prominent femoral lymph node can be identified at the most superior aspect of the dissection in the space just medial to the femoral vein (Cloquet node or node of Rosenmüller), this can be used as a sentinel lymph node when deciding on the risk of pelvic lymph node metastases. When such a lymph node is positive, a search should be made for further nodes above this by carrying the dissection up the femoral ring under the inguinal ligament.

A pelvic lymphadenectomy, when chosen, is done immediately after completion of the groin dissection. The pelvic lymphadenectomy is performed in a retroperitoneal manner through the same groin incisions, which can be extended laterally and superiorly (in a "J" or vertical manner), if necessary. About 2 cm above and parallel to the inguinal ligament, an incision is made through the external oblique, internal oblique, and transversalis musculofascial layers (Fig. 44.29). The retroperitoneal space is then opened bluntly, mobilizing the peritoneum and ureter medially. It is necessary to ligate and transect the inferior epigastric vessels and round ligament to fully develop this space. A self-retaining retractor or hand-held retractors can be used for adequate exposure of the retroperitoneal space. The pararectal and paravesical spaces are opened bluntly, fully exposing the iliac vessels and obturator fossa. All (or suspicious) lymph node–bearing tissue from the external iliac, internal iliac, and common iliac vessels, and in the obturator

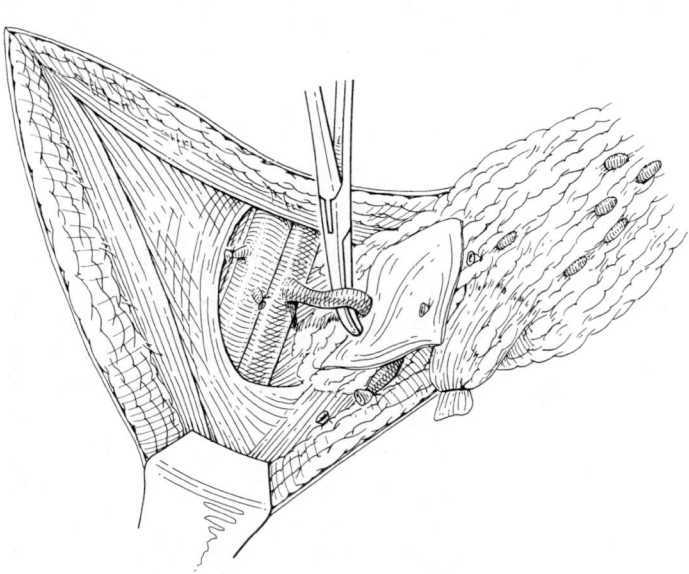

FIGURE 44.24. Groin specimen including cribriform fascia and femoral lymph nodes dissected to medial aspect of fossa ovalis and saphenous vein attachment. Termination of saphenous vein (saphenous bulb) is isolated.

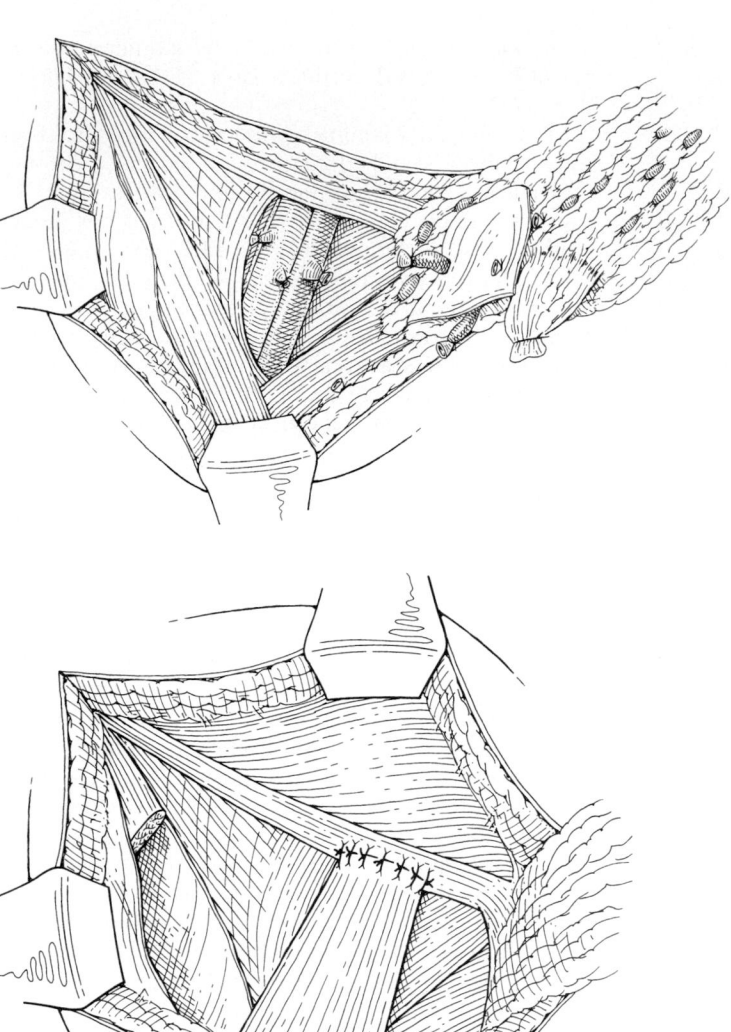

FIGURE 44.25. Saphenous bulb transected and ligated. Groin node dissection completed to beginning of planned vulvectomy incision. Fossa medial to femoral vein and overlying the pectineus muscle has been cleared of lymph node-bearing tissue.

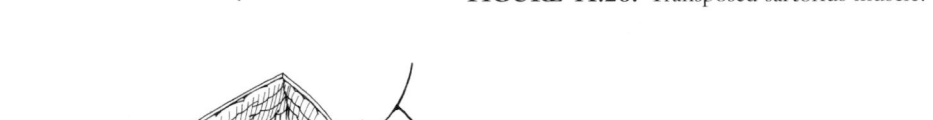

FIGURE 44.26. Transposed sartorius muscle.

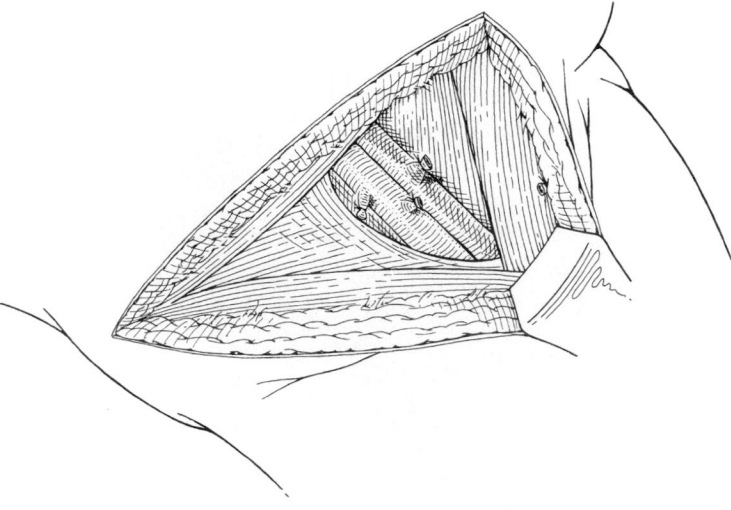

FIGURE 44.27. Inguinofemoral lymphadenectomy completed through a separate incision.

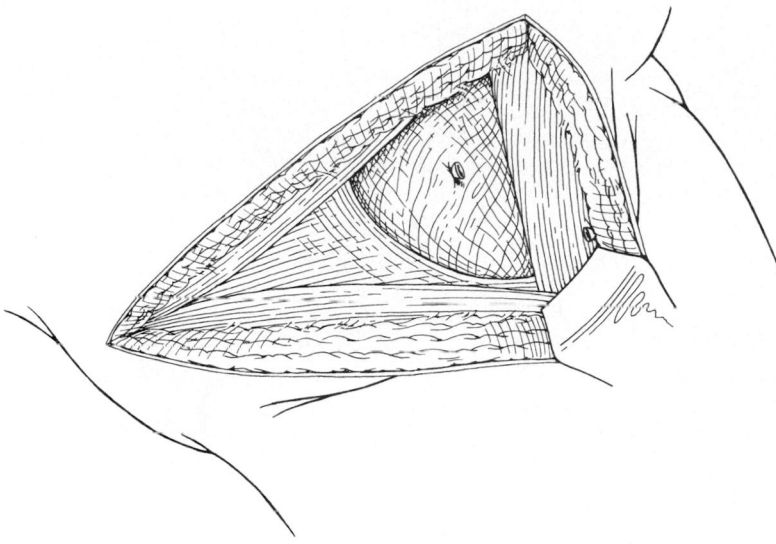

FIGURE 44.28. Completed superficial inguinal lymphadenectomy.

fossa above the obturator nerve, is removed by sharp dissection, with cautery, metal clips, and free-tie ligatures of 3-0 polyglactin used for hemostasis. Separate pelvic Jackson-Pratt drains can be placed at the discretion of the surgeon. The incised musculofascial tissues are closed in a single layer with no. 1 synthetic, absorbable, monofilament sutures. Special attention is paid to closure of the internal inguinal ring with 2-0 silk sutures. The wounds are copiously irrigated, and hemostasis is secured. When performed through separate incisions, the groin wounds are closed at this point.

Soft, active suction drains are placed in each groin and are brought out through separate stab wounds superolaterally. For groin wounds, we prefer to use a large mass closure with no. 2 polypropylene vertical mattress retention sutures (Fig. 44.30A). Three to five sutures are placed on each side. Each suture starts several centimeters from the edge of the superior flap with a bite then taken of the underlying inguinal ligament. This is designed to close the dead space under the superior flap. Under the inferior flap, a bite of sartorius, adductor, or pectineal fascia is taken (with care taken to avoid injury to the femoral vessels and nerve), followed by placement of the suture from inside to out through the inferior flap several centimeters from the edge. Again, this is designed to close the dead space of the inferior flap and, once pulled together, to close the dead space of the midline wound. Going back from inferior to superior, a small bite of each skin edge is then taken, which is designed to approximate these edges. The sutures are not tied until all have been placed. The sutures are tied somewhat loosely, with only enough tension to bring the wound together (Fig. 44.30B). The skin is further closed with stainless steel staples (Fig. 44.30C). En bloc groin incisions are closed in an identical manner, but this is delayed until completion of the entire resection. With separate incisions, the medial aspects of the groin wounds are under much less tension and are easily closed because of preservation of the inguinal skin bridge. These inci-

sions can probably be closed with simple sutures or staples. Separation of the groin and vulvar wounds and especially closure without tension are the factors thought to be largely responsible for the reduced wound complications seen with the three-incision technique.

After completion of the inguinofemoral lymphadenectomy, attention is turned to the radical vulvectomy. The surgeon may elect to change the position of the legs to high lithotomy; "high-low" Allen-Brown stirrups are useful for this purpose (for a difficult perineal dissection, high lithotomy with sling stirrups is preferred). With en bloc resection, the inguinal specimens are mobilized toward the vulva as just described (Fig. 44.31). From the point of completion of the inferior inguinal dissections, incisions are continued down along

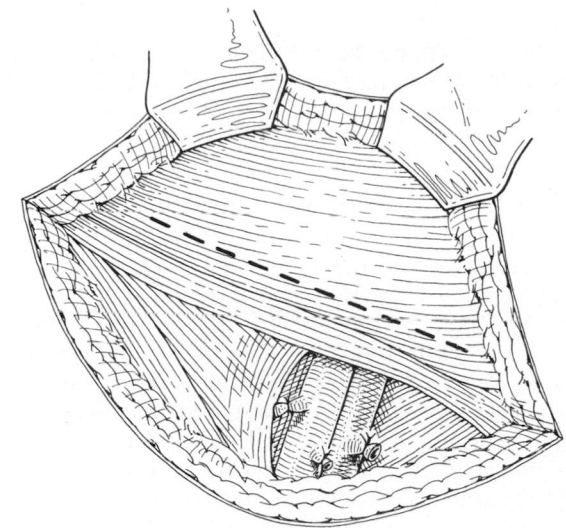

FIGURE 44.29. Incision for pelvic lymphadenectomy performed immediately after completion of the inguinofemoral lymphadenectomy.

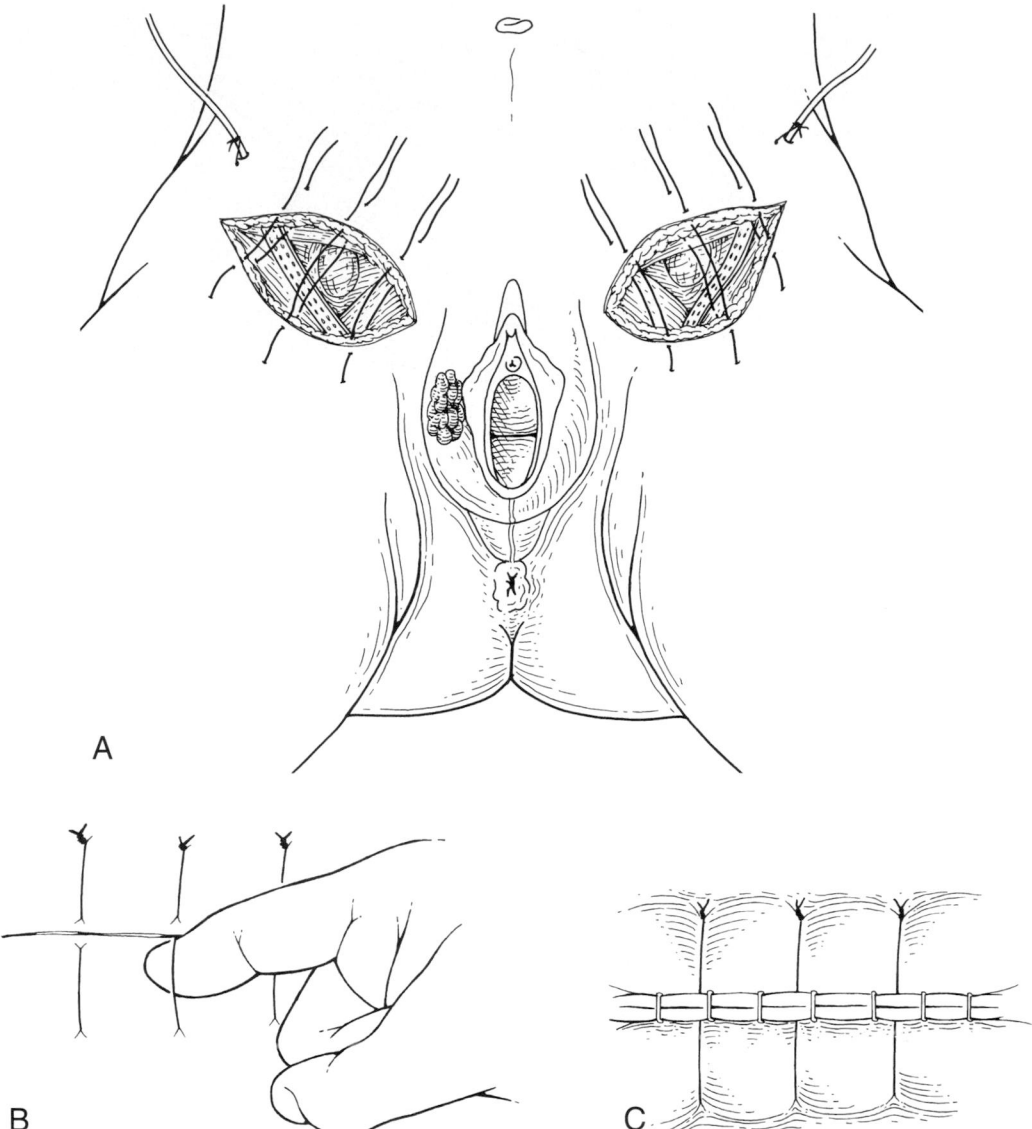

FIGURE 44.30. A: Large block closure of groin wounds (separate in this case) with vertical mattress retention sutures. Note drains in place. **B:** The groin closure sutures are tied somewhat loosely. **C:** Groin closure completed with stainless steel skin staples.

the labiocrural folds on each side and across the perineum, where they meet. A medial mucosal incision is made along the introitus extending through the anterior vestibule and around the urethral meatus.

When radical vulvectomy is performed through a separate vulvar incision, the same labiocrural, posterior, and mucosal incisions are used and the same vulvar tissue is excised (Fig. 44.32). The superior incision extends from the top of the labiocrural folds as an inverted V, with the point above the base of the clitoris. As previously discussed, a variable amount of superior tissue (i.e., mons pubis) is removed, depending on the location and size of the lesion.

The radical vulvectomy incisions may be modified somewhat depending on the location and extent of the tumor and the condition of the remaining vulvar skin. The surgeon should attempt to attain at least a 2-cm margin of normal-appearing skin or mucosa around the tumor. To accomplish this, it may be necessary to excise a portion of vagina, anus, or distal urethra. For an anterior lesion, it is reasonable to spare the perineal body; but for a posterior lesion, it is important to incorporate radical resection of this area. For a lesion (especially superficial) in proximity to the urethral meatus or anus, it is reasonable to limit the margin of resection to 1 cm to preserve these structures and their function.

The labiocrural incisions are extended to the lateral margins of the deep fascia of the urogenital diaphragm (Fig. 44.33). The internal pudendal vessels are ligated as they are encountered entering the vulva at about the 4-

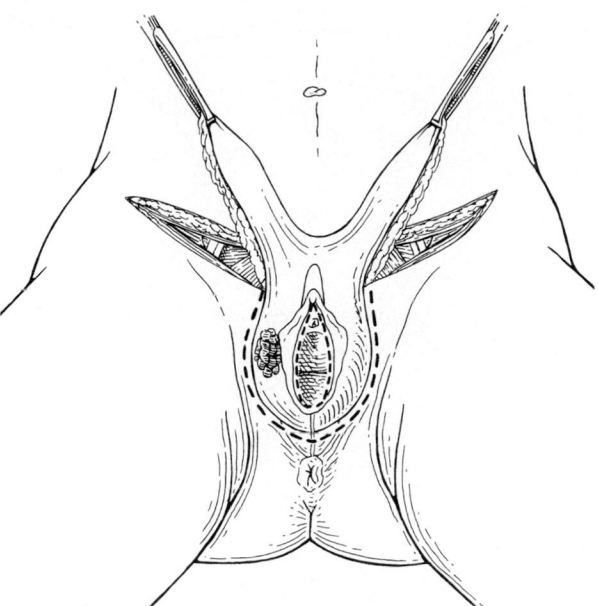

FIGURE 44.31. Bilateral inguinofemoral lymphadenectomy is complete. Planned incisions for the en bloc radical vulvectomy are shown.

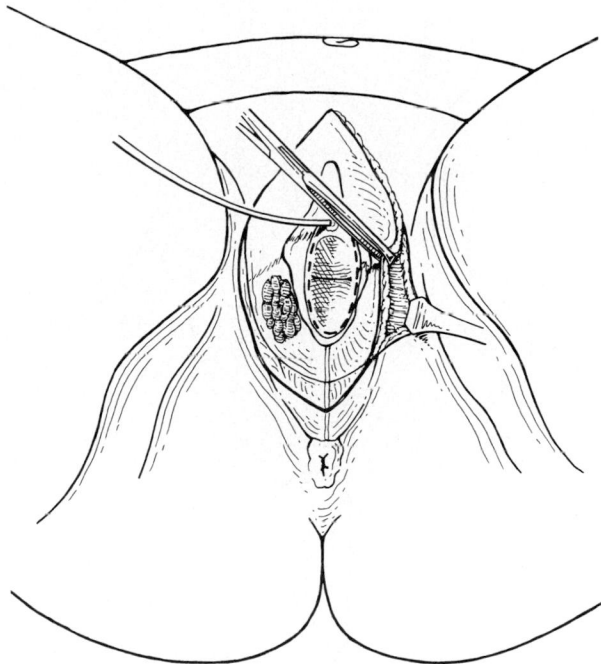

FIGURE 44.33. Labiocrural incisions extended to the deep fascia of the urogenital diaphragm.

o'clock and 8-o'clock positions. Superiorly, the specimen is dissected off the pubic periosteum and adductor fascia. The vascular base of the clitoris is clamped and transected, and a transfixion suture ligature is placed (Fig. 44.34). If deemed necessary, the attachment of the ischiocavernosus muscles can also be transected at this level. Dissection of the superior portion of the vulva off of the pubic bone and adductor fascia is completed and joined, in the midline, to the transvestibular mucosal in-

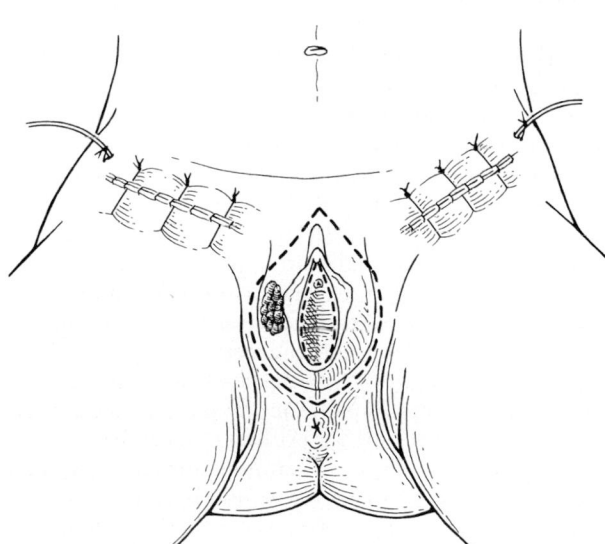

FIGURE 44.32. Bilateral inguinofemoral lymphadenectomy through separate incisions is completed and wounds are closed. Separate incisions for radical vulvectomy are marked.

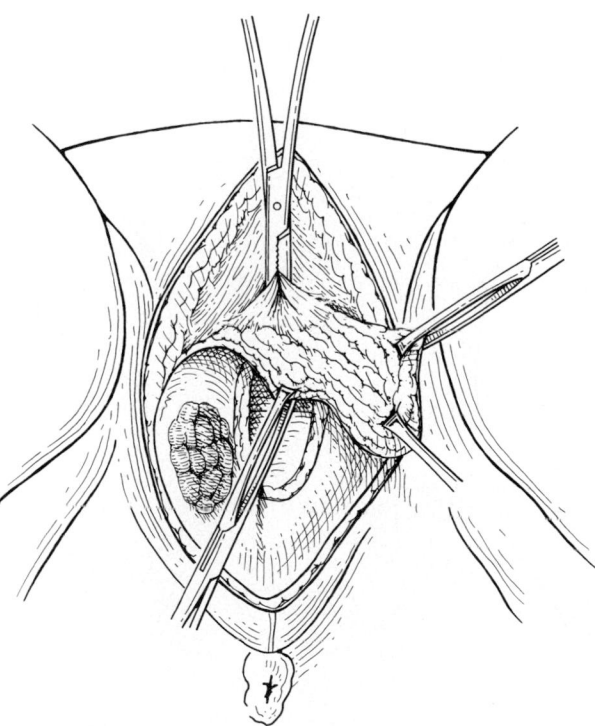

FIGURE 44.34. Dissection proceeds dorsally off of the pubic bone. The vascular base of the clitoris clamped, followed by transection and ligation.

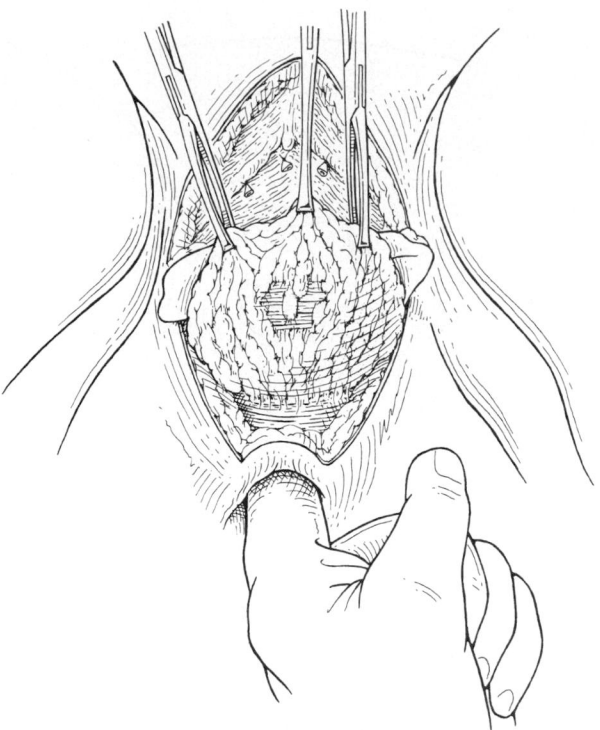

FIGURE 44.35. Perineal body and posterior vulvar tissues are dissected away from the anus.

cision above the urethra. Inferiorly, various portions of the perineum (and in some cases the anus) are dissected upward and cephalad toward the vaginal incision (Fig. 44.35). Care is taken as the vaginal incision is approached above the perineum to avoid injury to the anal canal. Using the index finger or a large Kelly clamp, the

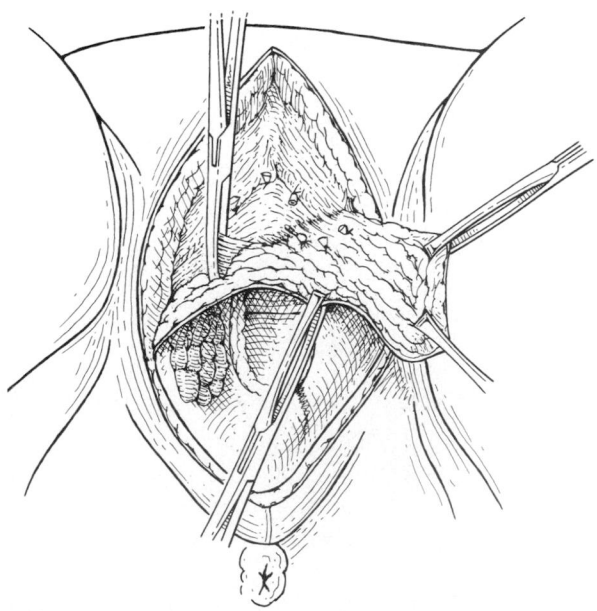

FIGURE 44.36. The vascular vestibular tissue along the sides of the vaginal tube is clamped. Transection and suture ligation follow.

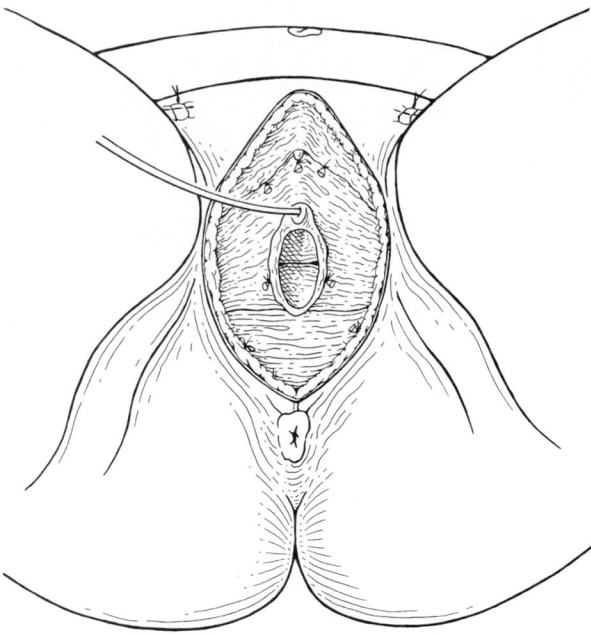

FIGURE 44.37. Radical vulvectomy resection is completed.

surgeon separates the vaginal tube bluntly from the vulvar tissues cephalad to the vestibular structures. The mucosal incision is then completed, separating the vagina (with the urethra) from the specimen. This dissection can be facilitated by splitting the specimen in the midline anteriorly or posteriorly. The remainder of the dissection off of the underlying deep fascia of the urogenital diaphragm is completed. Clamps and transfixion suture ligatures of no. 0 or 2-0 polyglactin are used during transection of the tissue along the side of the vaginal tube in the region of the vestibular bulbs (Fig. 44.36).

After removal of the specimen, the wounds are copiously irrigated with antibiotic solution and hemostasis is secured (Fig. 44.37). After en bloc resection, the superior abdominal wall flap and the groin and vulvar thigh flaps are further mobilized as necessary to achieve closure of the wounds without tension. Any ischemic-appearing skin is excised. It is very useful, especially if there is an element of vaginal relaxation, to mobilize the lower vagina to facilitate wound closure. Any pelvic relaxation defects (i.e., cystocele, rectocele, loss of the posterior urethrovesical angle) are repaired at this time. To the extent that it is necessary or possible, the perineal body is also reinforced or reconstructed at this time.

The vulvar wound and the perineal area are closed with vertical mattress 2-0 delayed-absorbable sutures (Fig. 44.38). Depending on the amount of tissue that has been removed, the superior portion of an en bloc wound may be difficult to close. When done through a separate incision, closure of the vulvar wound is under much less tension, again because of preservation of the inguinal skin bridges. Careful attention must be paid to closure of the periurethral area. The urethra should be secured on a straight course without tension. A hood of skin above the urethra is also avoided because this can obstruct the path of the urinary stream and cause spraying.

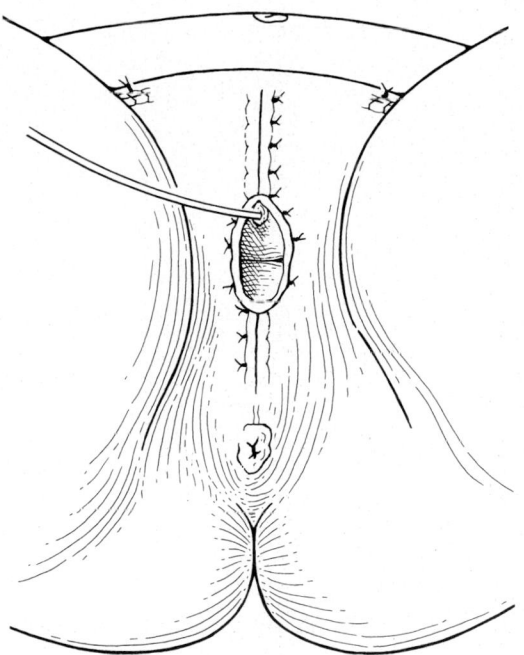

FIGURE 44.38. Closure of the vulvar wound is completed.

As previously discussed, it is reasonable in many patients to manage the vulvar lesion locally with a modified radical vulvectomy. This operation consists of radical removal of the portion of the vulva containing the tumor. It is performed with the techniques described earlier except that the excision is basically limited to removal of that particular part of the vulva. The lateral and deep tumor margins are not compromised by this operation. After the surgeon carefully demarcates a 2-cm radius of normal skin or mucosa around the tumor, an encompassing incision is designed that will readily close and be as cosmetically acceptable as possible (Fig. 44.8 and Figs. 44.39 and 44.40).

Postoperative Care

After closure, silver sulfadiazine (Silvadene, Hoechst Marion Roussel) cream is applied to the perineal wound and a light dressing is placed. In the recovery room, ice is applied to the vulvar wound, and this is continued off and on for 48 to 72 hours. On postoperative day 3 or 4, the patient is started on a regimen of cleansing the vulvar wound with a showerhead, followed immediately by complete drying of the area with a blow dryer using cool air. This is done three times a day, after each bowel movement, and is continued until the wounds are healed. If moisture in the wound is a problem despite this regimen, other useful measures include placing a roll of gauze between the legs and against the wound between washings, increasing the frequency of washings, and applying a heat lamp to the area three times a day between washings. All of these efforts are aimed at keeping this normally warm and moist area clean and dry, which reduces risk of infection and promotes healing. Intermittently leaving the legs slightly apart to air (the immodest position) is also beneficial.

Drains are removed on the second or third day. A compression dressing (rolled gauze and an abdominal binder) is maintained on the groins for an additional 24 to 48 hours to prevent lymphocyst formation. Compression boots may be continued during this time, and care is taken to avoid marked femoral vein compression.

A prophylactic antibiotic is continued for 24 hours, and Jobst compression boots (plus low-dose heparin in very high-risk patients) are used until the patient is ambulating. If the wounds are closed under tension, ambu-

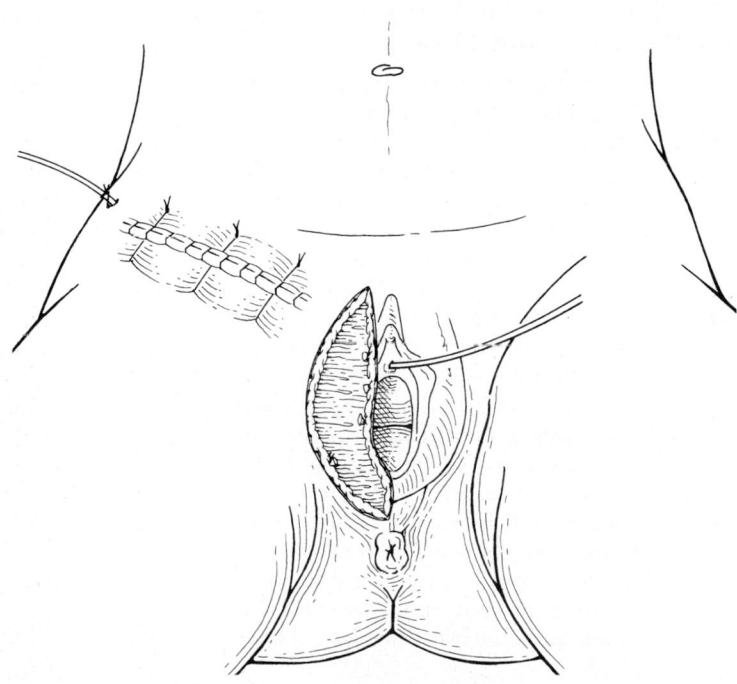

FIGURE 44.39. Radical hemivulvectomy.

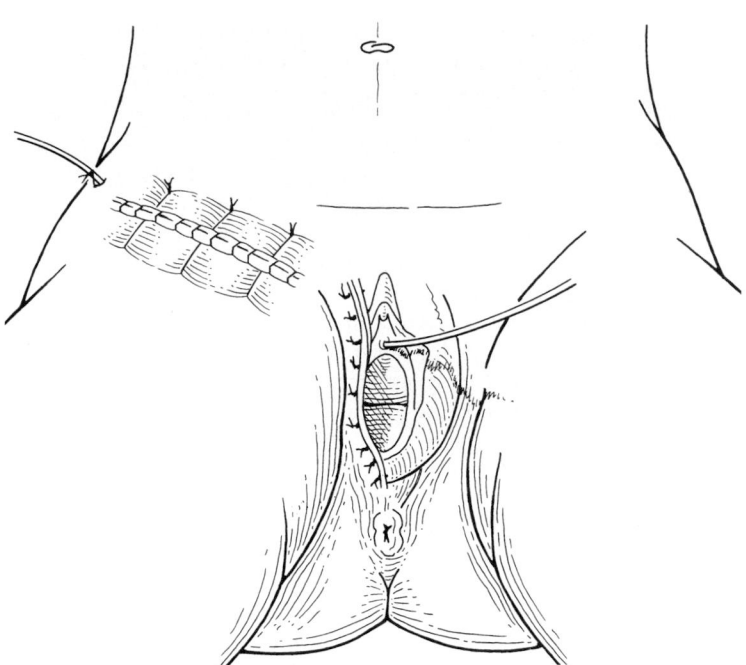

FIGURE 44.40. Closure of hemivulvectomy wound.

lation is restricted for 3 to 5 days, and the patient is instructed to avoid leg abduction when getting into and out of bed. A no. 18 Foley catheter is left in place for 3 to 5 days to act as a stent and divert urine while the urethra is healing. Depending on the degree of perineal or perianal resection, several days of bowel rest may be indicated, with or without constipating agents, followed by a stool softener.

Especially when lymph node dissection has been extensive or radiotherapy is planned, long-term use of fitted graduated compression stockings may be beneficial.

Reconstructive Techniques for the Vulva and Groin

After radical resection for carcinoma of the vulva, the wounds can generally be closed primarily. This is greatly facilitated when the incisions are modified somewhat (as with sparing of the mons pubis), and especially when separate incisions are used. When an extensive resection is necessary, it may not be possible to close the wound primarily, or at least not without considerable tension. This is often the case after resection of a recurrent tumor, where previous radical surgery has already left a paucity of tissue. If the area was treated previously with radiotherapy, then closure may be difficult because of the lack of elasticity of the fibrotic tissue and because of radiation-induced healing impairment. Under these various circumstances, closure of the incisions and healing can be greatly facilitated by a variety of reconstructive procedures. Other potential benefits of such reconstruction include maintenance of anal, urethral, and sexual function and a more cosmetically acceptable result.

Closure of groin and vulvar wounds using reconstructive techniques involves moving a block of expend-

able tissue (with its blood supply intact) from some nearby site into the deficient area. The mobilized block of tissue is commonly referred to as a flap. Flaps are classified according to what layers of tissue they include and according to their blood supply. The types of flaps that have been useful in reconstruction of the vulva and groin are full-thickness skin (random and arterial based), fasciocutaneous, and myocutaneous flaps. Some flaps remain completely attached at their base and are rotated into the defect, whereas others are partially separated from the base and are transposed as an island of tissue.

A full-thickness skin flap involves rotating an adjacent block of skin with its underlying subcutaneous tissue into the defect. The flap is mobilized from the donor site but remains attached at its base; through this base travels the arterial and venous circulation. The blood supply of the flap may be random, or it may depend on a specifically planned arterial source. A random flap relies on the many small musculocutaneous perforating vessels that are retained through the base. For this reason, the subcutaneous layer must be kept thick, and the length of the flap should not be much greater than the width of the base (1.0 to 1.5 times greater). This is the type of flap most commonly used for reconstruction of a radical vulvectomy wound.

A few specific arterial-based full-thickness skin flaps, sometimes called axial flaps, have been used for reconstruction in vulvar cancer patients. Arterial sources of these flaps have included the internal pudendal, circumflex iliac, superficial circumflex iliac, superficial inferior epigastric, superficial branch of the deep external pudendal, and superficial external pudendal arteries. With some of these arterial flaps, the deep fascia must be carefully mobilized with the subcutaneous tissue to maintain an adequate blood supply. The main advantage of an ar-

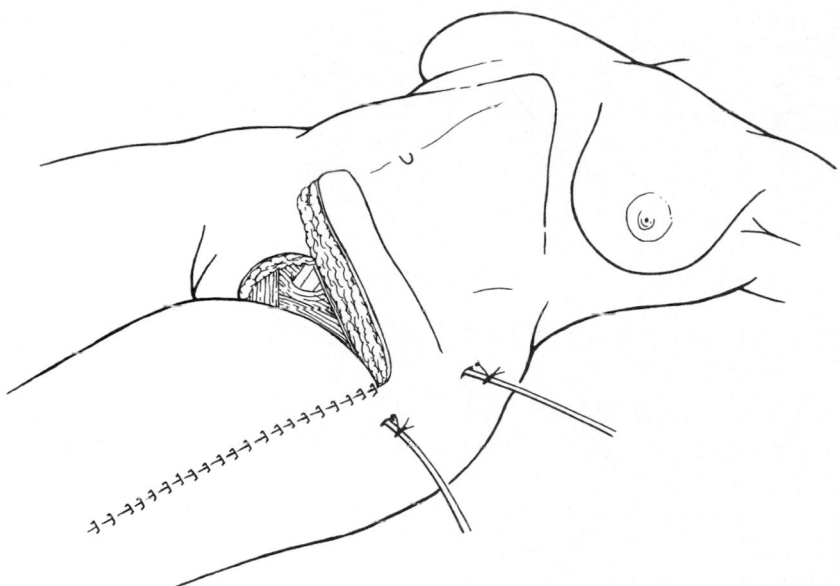

FIGURE 44.41. Tensor fascia lata flap being rotated to close a large groin wound.

terial flap, because of the good arterial blood supply, is that it can be considerably longer than a random flap. However, these flaps are technically more difficult to construct and have a low margin for error in terms of compromised blood supply.

As previously mentioned, some full-thickness skin flaps are designed to include the deep fascia taken off of the underlying muscle. These are known as fasciocutaneous flaps, and they are more reliable than random cutaneous flaps because the preserved fascial layer provides additional musculocutaneous perforators along its length. A fasciocutaneous flap can also be relatively long and is transposable as an island of tissue. Some fasciocutaneous flaps have a designated arterial blood supply. Locally useful fasciocutaneous flaps include the pudendal thigh, superior medial thigh, inferior gluteal, and island groin flaps.

A myocutaneous flap makes use of an expendable muscle with its intact overlying fascia and cutaneous tissue. The use of these flaps for vulvovaginal reconstruction began after the 1976 report by McCraw and colleagues. A substantial blood supply is preserved through a narrow pedicle connected to the muscle, which allows the flap to be transposed as an island with a wide arc of rotation. Another advantage of a myocutaneous flap is the capacity to bring tissue into the defect that has a blood supply separate and independent from that of the operative site. This makes these flaps particularly valuable in the reconstruction of heavily radiated tissues. These flaps are also somewhat bulky and have the ability to fill a large tissue defect. The main disadvantage of myocutaneous flaps is that they are technically demanding, and the survival ability of some of these flaps is somewhat tenuous.

The difficulties resulting from a large wound created by an extensive radical vulvectomy with bilateral inguinofemoral lymphadenectomy were previously discussed. Reconstruction of these wounds with bilateral

tensor fascia lata (TFL) myocutaneous flaps has been reported. The TFL originates from the anterior superior iliac spine. It inserts into the fascia lata and is supplied by the lateral femoral circumflex artery. The base is just lateral to the groin wound, into which the flap is directly rotated. The flaps are easily made long enough to reach and close the often large area created by resection of the mons pubis and anterior vulva. A TFL myocutaneous flap is also useful for reconstruction of the groin after extensive resection for recurrent disease (Fig. 44.41).

The rectus abdominis myocutaneous flap, based on the inferior epigastric artery, is also useful for reconstruction of a large groin defect. The block of tissue based on this muscle is taken from the abdominal wall, and the muscle is divided at the superior border of the flap. The island of cutaneous tissue is completely mobilized with its carefully preserved attachment to the muscle, and this is further mobilized inferiorly. This allows the island flap to rotate down easily into the groin (or vulva) through a generous subcutaneous tunnel. The rectus abdominis myocutaneous flap is also suitable for the reconstruction of large vulvar wounds (Fig. 44.42).

We commonly use flaps for vulvar wound reconstruction after radical resection of cancer involving the perineal or perianal tissues. Such a resection removes the entire perineal body as well as portions of the superficial muscles and leaves a large defect that is difficult to close (Fig. 44.43). Poor healing of this area may significantly compromise both anal and coital function. The use of flaps for such a defect allows closure without tension; brings tissue with a good blood supply into the area, which promotes healing, and helps recreate a perineal body. Preventing tension on the anal apparatus helps promote healing of its associated reconstructed musculature and helps preserve its function. Reconstruction of a perineal body separates the vagina from fecal contamination and helps create a smooth and less scarred platform

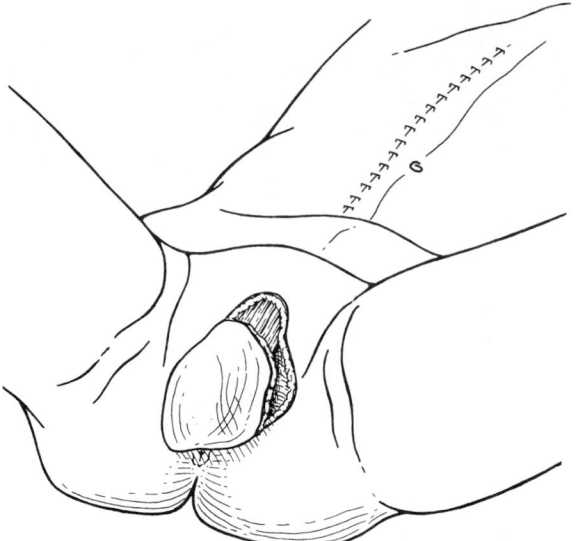

FIGURE 44.42. Rectus abdominis myocutaneous flap is brought through a subcutaneous tunnel to close a large perineal wound.

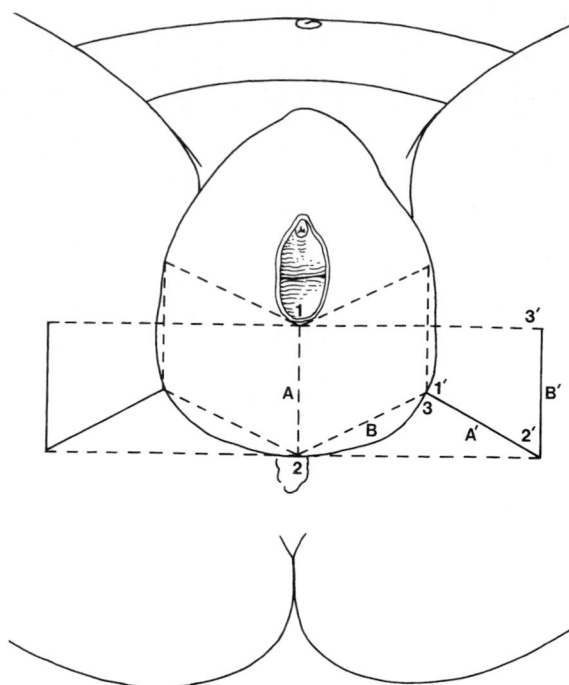

FIGURE 44.44. Planning rhomboid flap. Defect is divided into two rhomboids. Configuration and measurement of the flap are based on this rhomboid defect, as shown. Numbers and letters indicate proposed location of flap in reconstructed site.

for intercourse. For reconstruction of such defects, we prefer to use local, full-thickness rhomboid skin flaps (Figs. 44.44 through 44.47). Closure of a larger defect involving the perineal or perianal and vulvar areas may be better accomplished with gluteal thigh fasciocutaneous, gluteus maximus myocutaneous, or gracilis myocutaneous flaps.

Closure of a heavily radiated wound should be accomplished with a block of relatively unradiated tissue, the blood supply to which is unlikely to have been sig-

nificantly compromised by the prior treatment. In general, myocutaneous flaps are better for this purpose.

Many other flaps have been reported to be useful for groin and vulvar reconstruction and may be used depending on the individual situation and preference of the surgeon.

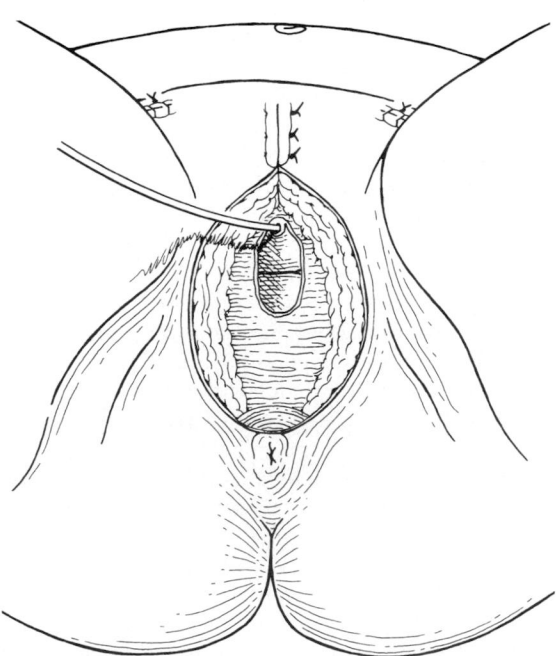

FIGURE 44.43. Extensive posterior vulvar resection leaves a large defect between the anus and the introitus.

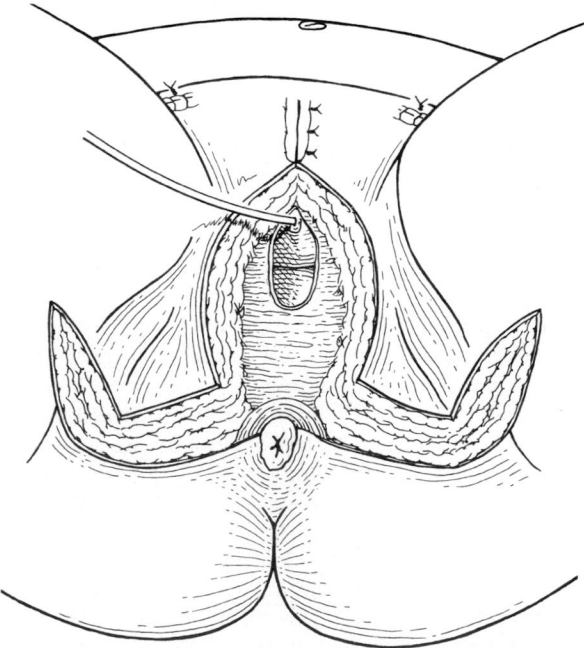

FIGURE 44.45. Bilateral rhomboid flaps are developed.

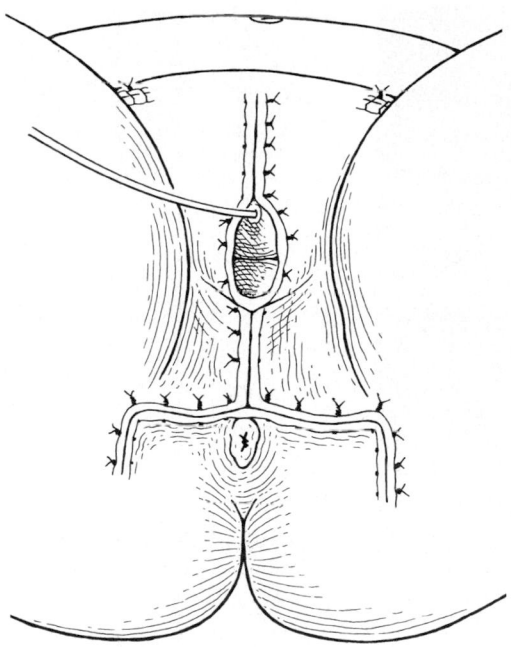

FIGURE 44.46. Posterior closure is accomplished with the rotated flaps.

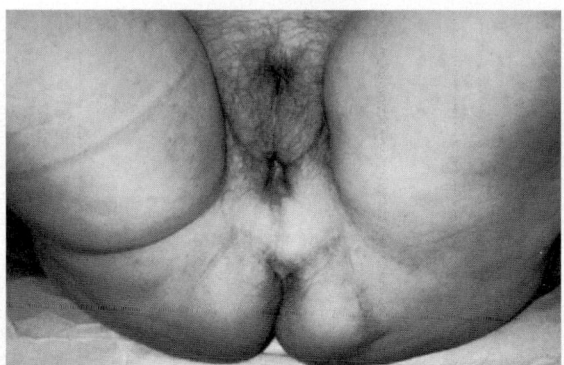

FIGURE 44.47. Healed rhomboid flaps. See color version of figure.

ADJUVANT THERAPY

This section deals with adjuvant therapy following radical or modified radical vulvectomy with inguinofemoral lymphadenectomy. The role of adjuvant therapy in the management of locally advanced vulvar cancer is discussed elsewhere in this chapter.

Other than with locally advanced disease, preoperative adjuvant therapy has generally not been used or recommended. An exception to this appeared in a report by Thomas and colleagues on a small number of patients treated primarily with chemoradiotherapy, with surgery used as salvage therapy. It was suggested by these authors that this type of therapy might be used as definitive management for those lesions encroaching on critical midline structures, such as the clitoris, urethra, vagina, and anal verge, where surgical removal is accompanied by major cosmetic and functional morbidity.

Postoperatively, the only adjuvant therapy that appears to be of value is radiotherapy. This can consist of radiotherapy to the local area of primary tumor resection, to the groins, or to the pelvic nodal areas, or to all three. Postoperative radiotherapy administered to the remaining vulvar tissues is rarely indicated but should be considered when an extensive tumor has been resected with positive or close margins that cannot be readily excised further. As discussed later, this type of therapy may be particularly indicated in some Bartholin cancers because they are sometimes difficult to resect widely as a result of their deep-seated location.

Postoperative adjuvant radiotherapy has been used primarily in patients with metastases to the groin lymph nodes. Substantial data now exists regarding the prognosis and recurrence pattern in these patients. Because

vulvar cancer has a recurrence pattern that tends to remain largely locoregional, its use for patients at high risk of recurrence is rational. There are further data to substantiate the benefit of radiotherapy in this setting. When a patient has metastases limited to microscopic involvement of one or perhaps two unilateral groin lymph nodes, the incidence of groin recurrence and pelvic lymph node metastases is very low, the overall prognosis is still reasonably good, and the benefit of postoperative radiotherapy is not great. If, however, there is gross replacement or extracapsular involvement of a lymph node, or involvement of three or more lymph nodes, the risk of groin recurrence and pelvic nodal metastases is substantial and the benefit of adjuvant postoperative radiotherapy is much more evident. In the GOG study previously discussed, the value of adjunctive radiation therapy was in the reduction of groin recurrences. When such treatment is anticipated, placement of metal clips to localize metastases may aid the radiation oncologist in treatment planning. Postoperative adjuvant chemotherapy, either alone or in combination with radiotherapy, has not been extensively studied, but it is unlikely to be of substantial benefit with use of the currently available agents.

MORTALITY AND MORBIDITY OF RADICAL VULVAR SURGERY

Even though most patients affected by invasive carcinoma of the vulva are elderly, radical vulvar surgery is generally well tolerated. This is attributed to the external nature of the operation, as well as to the intensive perioperative care that the patients receive. However, 2% to 4% of patients die in the first 4 weeks postoperatively, usually from cardiovascular or pulmonary complications. In addition, early groin wound complications are common, and long-term sexual dysfunction has generally been the rule. Treatment modifications over the past 2 decades undoubtedly have reduced the incidence and severity of these problems

Short-Term Complications

In published series of large numbers of patients undergoing en bloc radical vulvectomy with bilateral in-

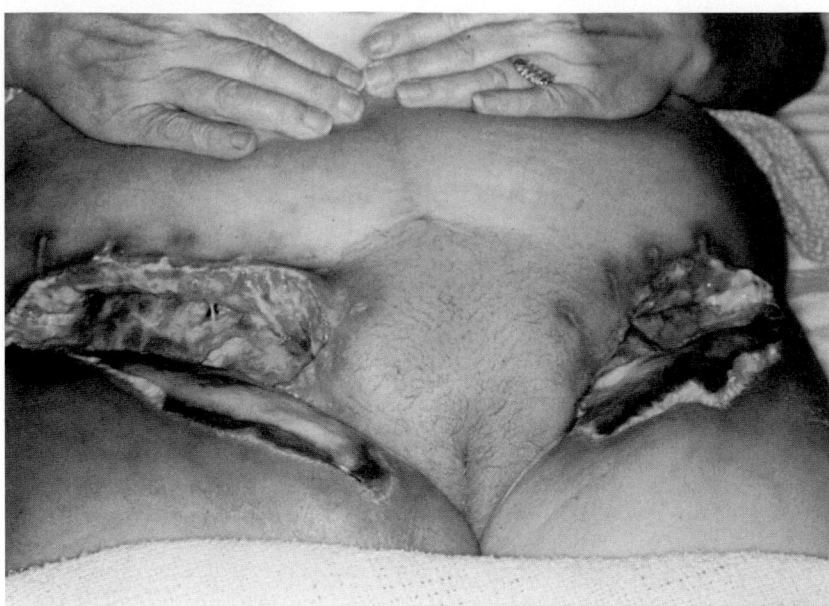

FIGURE 44.48. Bilateral groin wound breakdown (separate incisions in this case).

guinofemoral lymphadenectomy, a high percentage (overall about 50%) of significant wound breakdown in the inguinal sites has been reported (Fig. 44.48). Extensive undermining of skin, fluid collections in the wound, and infection are all contributing factors, but the main problem is the considerable tension placed on these wounds during closure. Suggested but unproven methods of prevention include prophylactic antibiotics, attempts to ligate lymphatics, and prophylactic suction drainage. Modifying the resection by preserving the mons pubis, minimizing undermining of skin, leaving a layer of fat with the skin, and excising any dark or dusky skin at the end of the operation reduce groin wound complications. With more extensive resection, plastic reconstruction (such as with TFL flaps) is also likely to be helpful. However, the single most effective method of reducing groin wound breakdown (to around 20%) has been the use of separate incisions, as previously discussed. Management of groin wound breakdown is similar to that of other wounds, with debridement and wet-to-dry dressings. During debridement, the surgeon must be cognizant of the femoral vessels. If infection has completely cleared, the wound is clean, and the tissues are pliable, secondary closure should be attempted.

About 10% to 20% of patients develop a clinically evident fluid collection (seroma or lymphocyst) in the groin. In recent years, we have seen a marked reduction in groin wound breakdown but an increased frequency of lymphocytes. When such fluid collections are small and asymptomatic, they should be left alone. The most commonly recommended treatment has been repeated aspirations until resolution. When there is infection, prompt hospitalization with drainage and intravenous antibiotics is necessary. For persistent collections, we prefer reinstitution of suction drainage combined with pressure.

Femoral nerve injury is a rare but potentially debilitating complication of inguinofemoral lymphadenectomy. Not uncommonly, a few sensory branches are sacrificed, resulting in numbness or paresthesia of the anterior thigh. However, surgical injury of a major portion of the nerve lateral to the artery results in significant and potentially permanent difficulty with ambulation. As previously discussed, this complication is prevented by avoiding dissection on the lateral side of the femoral artery.

Urinary tract infection is common in these patients and generally resolves with antibiotics or catheter removal. However, elderly patients sometimes tolerate urosepsis poorly and become profoundly ill. A diligent search for urinary tract infections, treatment of these infections, and removal of the Foley catheter as soon as is practical are important measures in these patients.

In the past, large series of patients undergoing en bloc radical vulvectomy with bilateral inguinofemoral lymphadenectomy reported a 1% to 2% incidence of severe postoperative hemorrhage from femoral vessel rupture. This was related to the extensive wound breakdown that occurred in a high percentage of these patients, with associated infection and necrosis involving the exposed and denuded femoral vessel walls. Coverage of the vessels by transposition of the sartorius muscle largely prevented this complication. With the use of separate incisions as well as other techniques that have reduced groin wound breakdown, and with avoidance of vessel skeletonization, postoperative femoral vessel rupture is now exceedingly rare. In our reported series of 415 surgically-treated patients, rupture occurred five times in the first 50 patients, but with routine transposition of the sartorius muscles and less skeletonization of vessels, no other patients had this complication. In current practice, transposition of the sartorius is rarely done.

Patients who have undergone radical vulvectomy with bilateral inguinofemoral lymphadenectomy are at high risk for thromboembolic complications because most are elderly and have coexisting medical problems, malignancy, and femoral vein trauma, and most have undergone prolonged surgery and prolonged bed rest. If prophylaxis fails, then treatment is promptly begun with intravenous heparin.

Rarely, a rectovaginal fistula develops days to weeks after radical vulvectomy. Prevention of this complication is based on preoperative evacuation of the colon, careful surgical dissection of this area, and prompt recognition of rectal entry. Surgical repair of the fistula is carried out once the area has healed and regained its elasticity.

Osteitis pubis and osteomyelitis are rare complications that may not become symptomatic until several weeks after radical vulvectomy. The patient complains of pain over the pubic bone and difficulty with ambulation, which may become chronic and debilitating. This complication is more likely to develop if the periosteum is traumatized, although this is not always avoidable. Extensive use of the cautery on the periosteum should be avoided. The mainstay of treatment is bed rest and nonsteroidal antiinflammatory drugs. Even more rarely, frank osteomyelitis of the pubic bone develops. This is a serious condition that requires debridement and drainage of the bone, along with prolonged antibiotic therapy.

Late Complications

After groin node dissection, it is not uncommon for a patient to develop some degree of lower extremity edema. It is most often transient or mild but persists chronically as a significant problem in about 10% of patients. Factors that have been implicated as contributing to this complication include the performance of a pelvic lymphadenectomy, groin radiotherapy, major groin wound breakdown, postoperative lower extremity lymphangitis, and preoperative lymphangiography. Suggested methods for reducing this problem include limiting the groin dissection to the superficial lymph nodes when feasible, confining femoral lymphadenectomy to the medial side of the femoral vein, avoiding pelvic lymphadenectomy, more tailored and selective use of adjuvant radiotherapy, sparing the saphenous vein, wearing fitted support stockings prophylactically for the first 6 months to 1 year after surgery, use of a low-dose prophylactic antibiotic to prevent lower extremity lymphangitis, and prompt antibiotic treatment of lymphangitis when it occurs. Management of lymphedema begins with patient education, avoidance of trauma to the affected leg, and meticulous skin and nail care. Constricting clothing or jewelry should be avoided. A treatment program with a physical therapist specifically trained in lymphedema management is particularly helpful. Components of management include intermittent leg elevation, manual lymphatic drainage (massage) combined with bandaging, a carefully tailored moderate exercise program, carefully fitted compression stockings, and a carefully fitted pneumatic compression device. There is no effective pharma-

cologic therapy and lymphangioplasty remains investigational. Some lymphedema patients occasionally develop lymphangitis, which presents with fever, pain, and redness of the involved extremity. This condition is treated promptly with an intravenous antibiotic, such as ampicillin-sulbactam (Unasyn), which covers streptococci.

A few good studies on sexual dysfunction after radical vulvectomy have been published. Generally, the capacity for intercourse remains. However, patients experience a marked sense of disfigurement and a reduction in genital sensitivity. Dyspareunia can occur as a result of stenosis or scar tissue (Fig. 44.49), but these problems are often surgically treatable. Some patients remain orgasmic. However, after surgery, 70% to 80% report the end of all sexual activity. There is increasing evidence to suggest that a modified radical vulvectomy, especially with preservation of the anterior vulvar structures, helps maintain sexual function. It does seem reasonable to assume that sparing of as much normal vulvar tissue as possible is less likely to produce sexual dysfunction and a sense of disfigurement than is radical resection.

During follow-up of radical vulvectomy patients, it is not uncommon to discover pelvic relaxation (cystocele or rectocele). This may be related to resection of the perineal body with the attendant loss of its support functions, or it may simply be a result of aging. If the patient's medical condition and extent of cancer surgery permit, any stress urinary incontinence or defects in vaginal support should be repaired at the time of radical vulvectomy because they are likely to worsen subsequently.

Spraying or misdirection of the urinary stream is related to poor alignment of the urethra, a hood of periclitoral tissue obstructing the path of the urinary stream (Fig. 44.49), or asymmetry created by a hemivulvectomy. Digital manipulation or the use of an applied collection or directing device is useful, but in some cases minor surgical revision is necessary.

Rarely, after inguinofemoral lymphadenectomy, a femoral or inguinal hernia develops. When a hernia or any apparent weakness of the femoral or inguinal canal is noted at the time of surgery, it should be repaired at that time. Avoiding incision of the inguinal ligament is also important in the prevention of this complication.

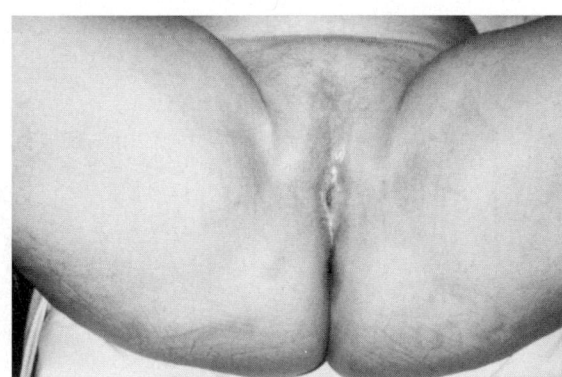

FIGURE 44.49. Marked introital stenosis following radical vulvectomy. See color version of figure.

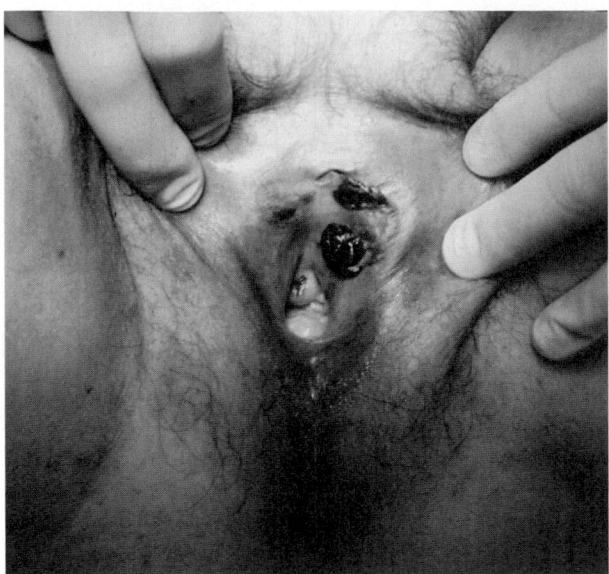

FIGURE 44.50. Melanoma of the vulva. Multifocal, darkly pigmented lesions are in the anterior vestibule.

VULVAR MELANOMA

Melanoma is the second most common histologic type of malignancy of the vulva but still accounts for only 5% to 10% of vulvar cancers (Fig. 44.50). This lesion occurs predominantly in white women in the seventh decade, and although the vulva covers only 1% to 2% of the body surface, vulvar melanoma accounts for 3% to 5% of malignant melanomas in women. The most common presenting symptoms are bleeding, a lump or changing mole, and pruritus or irritation. In a small percentage of patients, there is a family history of melanoma. Melanoma of the vulva is uncommon, so most of the literature on the subject consists of retrospective studies of small numbers of patients. For this reason, the behavior of this tumor is difficult to define, and a rationale for treatment has been slow to develop. However, it seems clear that the pattern of regional metastases is the same as that for squamous cell carcinoma; the behavior of the tumor is predicted best by a microstaging system. Importantly, the behavior of vulvar melanoma appears to be very similar to that of cutaneous melanomas in general.

As information has accumulated over the past 2 decades, it has become more reasonable to individualize treatment of vulvar melanoma based on clinical-pathologic factors, including microstaging, and to model overall treatment using experience derived from cutaneous melanomas in general.

What Do We Know about Cutaneous Melanoma?

Important areas of information that can be extrapolated from the general melanoma literature include individualization of management based primarily on microstaging, determination of what constitutes an adequate margin of

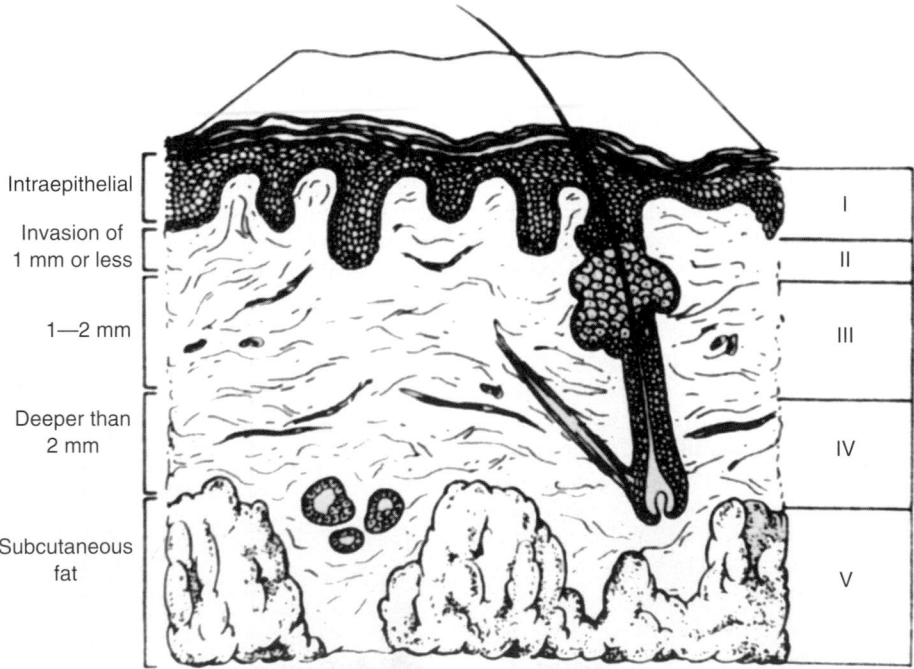

FIGURE 44.51. Levels of involvement of vulvar melanoma (Left, Chung; right, Clark). Level I (melanoma confined to the surface epithelium and pilar sheath) and level V (tumor extension into the underlying adipose tissue) are the same as Clark's levels I and V. Levels II, III, and IV are determined by measurements from the granular layer of the vulvar skin or the outermost epithelial layer of the squamous mucosa. (Chung AF, Woodruff JM, Lewis JL Jr. Malignant melanoma of the vulva: a report of 44 cases. *Obstet Gynecol* 1975;45:638).

resection, and definition of which groups of patients might benefit from an elective regional lymph node dissection.

Clark's classification has been used extensively for the microstaging of melanomas, with division into five levels of invasion (Fig. 44.51). Subsequently, Breslow's classification, based on millimeters of invasion from the upper granular layer of the epidermis to the deepest point of invasion, has become widely used. According to this method, tumor confined to a depth of 0.76 mm or less is generally within the epidermis and behaves as carcinoma in situ. In the recent literature, invasion of 0.76 to 1.49 mm is considered superficial; 1.5 to 4 mm, intermediate; and greater than 4 mm, deep. In 2002, the American Joint Committee on Cancer extensively revised the TNM staging system for cutaneous melanoma based on results of several large studies. (Table 44.13). Some tumors can be quite superficial in measurement and yet be deep melanomas according to Clark's classification.

TABLE 44.13.
TNM Staging System of the American Joint Committee on Cancer

---

pT	PRIMARY TUMOR
pTX	Primary tumor cannot be assessed*
pT0	No evidence of primary tumor
pTis	Melanoma in situ (Clark level I) (atypical melanocytic hyperplasia, severe melanocytic dysplasia, not an invasive malignant lesion)
pT1	**TUMOR 1 MM OR LESS IN THICKNESS**
pT1a	Clark level II or III, without ulceration
pT1b	Clark level IV or V, or with ulceration
pT2	Tumor more than 1 mm but not more than 2 mm in thickness
pT2a	Without ulceration
pT2b	With ulceration
pT3	Tumor more than 2 mm but not more than 4 mm in thickness
pT3a	Without ulceration
pT3b	With ulceration
pT4	Tumor more than 4 mm in thickness
pT4a	Without ulceration
pT4b	With ulceration
pN	**REGIONAL LYMPH NODES**
pN0	No regional lymph node metastatis
NX	Regional lymph nodes cannot be assessed
	Histologic examination of a regional lymphadenectomy specimen ordinarily includes six or more lymph nodes. If the lymph nodes are negative, but the number ordinarily examined is not met, classify as pN0. Classification based solely on sentinel node biopsy without subsequent axillary lymph node dissection is designated (sn) for sentinel node, e.g., pN1 (sn)
pN1	Metastasis in one regional lyph node
pN1a	Only microscopic metastasis (clinically occult)
pN1b	Macroscopic metastasis (clinically apparent)
pN2	Metastasis in two or three regional lymph nodes or intralymphatic regional metastasis
pN2a	Only microscopic nodal metastasis
pN2b	Macroscopic nodal metastasis
pN2c	Satellite or in-transit metastasis without regional nodal metastasis
pN3	Metastasis in four or more regional lymph nodes, or matted metastatic regional lymph nodes, or satellite or in-transit metastasis with metastasis in regional lymph node(s)
	Note: Satellites are tumor nests or nodules (macroscopic or microscopic) within 2 cm of the primary tumor. In-transit metastasis involves skin or subcutaneous tissue more than 2 cm from the primary tumor but not beyond the regional lymph nodes.
M	**DISTANT METASTASIS**
MX	Distant metastasis cannot be assessed
M0	No distant metastasis
M1	Distant metastasis
M1a	Skin, subcutaneous tissue, or lymph node(s) beyond the regional lymph nodes
M1b	Lung
M1c	Other sites, or any site with elevated serum lactic dyhydrogenase

Over the past 2 decades, the independent prognostic factors in cutaneous melanoma have been well defined. For the primary tumor, these include tumor thickness and ulceration. Clinical or microscopic satellites around the primary tumor are considered to be intransit lymphatic metastases. The dominant regional prognostic factors include the number or percentage of metastatic lymph nodes, macroscopic versus microscopic metastases, and the presence of clinical or microscopic satellites around a primary tumor. In patients with distant metastases, the site of metastases, the number of metastatic sites, and an elevated serum lactate dehydrogenase level were most predictive of poor survival. Based on the more precise delineation of prognostic factors, the American Joint Committee on Cancer (AJCC) revised the melanoma staging system in 2002.

The available literature suggests that adequate local treatment for a superficial cutaneous melanoma (less than 1.5 mm in thickness) consists of obtaining a 1-cm margin of skin and subcutaneous tissue. Current data support 2- to 3-cm margins for melanomas of intermediate thickness (1.5 to 4 mm). A study recently completed by the Intergroup Melanoma Trial supports a 2-cm margin for intermediate-thickness melanomas, and the World Health Organization is investigating this issue. Excision of underlying fascia continues to be controversial. The local management of deep (greater than 4 mm) melanomas is less clear. The risk of metastatic disease in these patients is high, which probably lessens the impact of local therapy.

It is generally agreed that melanomas less than 1 mm in thickness are associated with a very low risk of lymph node metastases, and elective regional lymph node dissection is not indicated in this group. Patients with melanomas greater than 4 mm in thickness have a high risk of both regional and systemic metastases, and they are less likely to benefit from elective lymph node dissection. There is significant controversy, however, about the benefit of prophylactic lymphadenectomy in patients with intermediate-thickness melanomas. The results of some retrospective studies have shown a beneficial effect of elective lymph node dissection on the survival of patients with intermediate-thickness melanomas. Two prospective studies, one from the Mayo Clinic and one multiinstitutional study directed by the World Health Organization, did not show any significant effect of elective lymph node dissection on survival. However, problems cited with these two studies have included the small numbers of intermediate-thickness melanomas and an imbalance of prognostic factors. In a recently completed Intergroup Melanoma Trial, patients with melanomas 1 to 4 mm thick on the trunk or proximal extremities were randomized to wide local excision with elective lymph node dissection versus wide local excision only. Overall survival was not significantly different. However, two subsets of patients had a significantly better overall 5-year survival rate with elective lymph node dissection. These subsets included patients age 60 years or younger and patients with a tumor thickness of 1.1 to 2.0 mm.

Intraoperative lymphatic mapping and sentinel lymph node biopsy are discussed earlier. Detection of occult melanoma cells by a more detailed examination of the sentinel nodes does correlate with recurrence and overall survival, and the information is potentially useful in the decision regarding adjuvant therapy. As these techniques come into more widespread use, recommendations regarding elective lymph node dissection are being reconsidered.

What Do We Know about Vulvar Melanoma?

As pointed out by Chung and colleagues, Clark's microstaging system for melanomas may be less suitable for vulvar tumors because of the lack of a well-defined papillary dermis in much of the vulvar skin and its virtual absence in the mucosal areas. Chung and associates proposed an alternative microstaging system (Fig. 44.51), which combines aspects of the Clark and Breslow systems. Because of the large percentage of vulvar melanomas that arise from or include mucosal membranes, caution is warranted in extrapolating data from squamous cell carcinoma of the vulva and from cutaneous melanomas in general. However, many of the tumors only superficially extend onto mucosal surfaces; until further data are available, it does appear reasonable to consider the available data on cutaneous melanomas in general and the data on squamous cell carcinoma of the vulva when managing a vulvar melanoma. Factors besides depth of invasion that seem to have an impact on the incidence of nodal metastases and survival include the AJCC stage, the presence of satellite lesions, tumor ulceration, central tumor location, tumor size, and capillary or lymphatic space involvement. The presence of any metastases indicates high-risk disease, although some studies report a few patients with positive groin nodes to be long-term survivors. In a recent retrospective report on 75 patients from the Norwegian Radium Institute, Scheistroen and associates identified nodal metastasis, angioinvasion, tumor thickness greater than 5 mm, clitoral or multifocal involvement, and aneuploidy as high-risk factors.

Diagnosis

When a vulvar melanoma is suspected, the diagnosis is best confirmed by an excisional biopsy. This allows pathologic evaluation of the entire lesion and, therefore, the most complete information on which to base definitive treatment. If the lesion is large, a generous incisional biopsy specimen is obtained from what appears to be the most significant portion of the lesion. Workup of the patient with a clinically localized vulvar melanoma beyond the superficial level need only consist of a careful history and physical examination, a chest radiograph, and a serum lactate dehydrogenase level. Depending on the results of these evaluations, further studies may be indicated.

Treatment

The traditional treatment for melanoma of the vulva has been radical vulvectomy with bilateral inguinofemoral and pelvic lymphadenectomy, the same treatment recommended for squamous cell carcinoma.

However, based on recent cutaneous melanoma literature, radical vulvectomy and the regional lymphadenectomy does not appear necessary in most cases.

As with squamous cell carcinoma, the main modification in the local management of vulvar melanomas has been to tailor the resection to the individual lesion. Accordingly, some patients still require radical vulvectomy or even more extensive surgery. For many patients, however, the local treatment consists of a wide or radical local excision. For apparently localized lesions amenable to local removal, margin size should probably be that which is appropriate for cutaneous melanomas in general, based on the depth of invasion of the melanoma as determined from the excisional biopsy. As with vulvar tumors in general, the excision is also tailored to the local vulvar anatomy. The frequent encroachment on midline vulvar structures by the melanoma creates difficulty in obtaining adequate margins while avoiding compromise of urinary or bowel function. The appropriate margin size of mucosally involved areas is much more difficult to define but should probably be at least the same as that for the cutaneous margin. The surgeon must frequently remove the clitoris, portions of the distal vagina, or part of the distal urethra, or all three. Because of the propensity for early hematogenous spread in patients with deeply invasive tumors, ultraradical resection is rarely, if ever, indicated. Trials are being carried out to determine the benefit of adjuvant systemic therapy (see later text).

Modifications of the regional nodal management of vulvar melanoma have also paralleled those for squamous cell carcinoma of the vulva and cutaneous melanomas. The same arguments regarding elective lymph node dissection for cutaneous melanomas apply to vulvar melanomas. Inguinal-femoral lymphadenectomy is not generally recommended for superficial or deeply invasive vulvar melanoma. Nodal metastases are rarely found in lesions with less than 1-mm invasion, and systemic disease is usually present in women with a depth of invasion greater than 4 mm. In patients with intermediate depth of invasion between 1 and 4 mm, the data are unclear, and many experts would continue to recommend regional lymphadenectomy in these patients. As with issues surrounding local tumor management, there is a small amount of literature supporting some of these concepts with site-specific vulvar melanoma data, including the possible benefit from elective lymph node dissection and removal of clinically positive lymph nodes. The overall incidence of lymph node metastases in vulvar melanoma patients is reported to be around 30%. As with squamous cell carcinoma, pelvic lymphadenectomy does not appear to be warranted for a melanoma confined to the vulva with negative inguinal lymph nodes. The role of pelvic lymphadenectomy in patients with positive inguinal lymph nodes is unclear, but considering the poor prognosis, the value would be of limited benefit at best. The value of elective radiotherapy to the regional nodes in melanoma patients is not known, so it should be used cautiously. If, during follow-up, isolated metastases appear in an undissected groin, they should be excised.

For patients in whom high-risk features have been identified after primary surgical therapy (e.g., positive lymph nodes, deep invasion), effective adjuvant treatment has not yet been identified. Radiotherapy may improve locoregional control of disease. One randomized study (mostly stage III resected cutaneous melanoma) demonstrated improved disease-free and overall survival with adjuvant interferon α-2b. Recurrent or metastatic disease carries a very poor prognosis in vulvar melanoma patients. Systemic therapy is of limited palliative benefit and most commonly consists of immunotherapy, chemotherapy (DTIC), hormonal therapy (tamoxifen), or all three.

Results

Overall, about one third of vulvar melanoma patients survive 5 years. This rate is lower than that reported for patients with squamous cell carcinoma of the vulva and with cutaneous melanomas in general. The worse prognosis has been attributed to an older age and a large percentage of deeply invasive and generally more advanced tumors at the time of diagnosis. According to several reports, survival of vulvar melanoma patients does correlate closely with depth of invasion. Other factors include the worse prognosis associated with mucosal melanomas in general and the difficulty in obtaining an adequate resection for the more centrally located tumors. Local recurrences are a common problem after removal of vulvar melanomas and tend to occur on the medial margin of resection. Local recurrences are reported to occur in about one third of patients, and the prognosis for these women is poor. Local tumor control and survival are reduced with more central and deeply invasive tumors. The presence of lymph node metastases also carries a poor prognosis, which has been correlated with the extent and number of lymph nodes involved. When the inguinal lymph nodes are positive, the reported survival rate is in the range of 10% to 31%. Vulvar melanomas have a propensity for late recurrence, and 5-year survival may not be an accurate predictor of cure in these patients.

BARTHOLIN GLAND CARCINOMA

A malignancy can arise from the Bartholin gland or duct, with most of the cancers being adenocarcinoma or squamous cell carcinoma. Other much rarer histologic types include transitional cell carcinoma, mixed carcinoma, and sarcoma. Bartholin carcinoma accounts for only 1% to 2% of vulvar malignancies, and, in some cases, a Bartholin origin is not clear-cut. Several criteria have been described to define a primary Bartholin malignancy, including anatomic position consistent with a Bartholin tumor, intact overlying skin, areas of apparent transition from normal to neoplastic elements, involvement of areas of the Bartholin gland with an origin histologically compatible with the gland, and no evidence of any other primary cancer. Although some of these criteria may not be met in an individual case, the tumor should at least be in a location consistent with a Bartholin tumor. As with the other rare types of vulvar malignancies, the available information on Bartholin malignancies is derived from retrospective studies of small series of patients.

Diagnosis

Bartholin carcinoma should be suspected when a tumor is noted in the region of Bartholin's gland, particularly in a woman older than 40 years of age (Fig. 44.52). The average age at diagnosis is about 50 years, but there is a wide age range. Many studies report a significant delay in diagnosis, attributed both to the deep-seated location of the tumor and to frequent misdiagnosis and treatment as a Bartholin abscess. When a woman presents with a Bartholin mass, biopsy or excision should be considered if she is older than 40 years of age, if the mass is suspicious, or when an apparently benign process does not resolve promptly with conservative therapy. Fine-needle aspiration for cytologic examination may be useful in some cases.

Treatment

Because of their deep location in the vulva, Bartholin malignancies tend to invade the ischiorectal fossa, close to the anorectum, or close to the pubic ramus, or all three, before they are diagnosed. These cancers also can erode through the overlying skin. Radical excision with an adequate margin tends to be more difficult with Bartholin malignancies. As with other vulvar cancers, surgical resection should be aimed less at a standard radical vulvectomy and more at adequate resection of the tumor. Depending on the tumor extent, local resection must consist of at least a radical hemivulvectomy; but it may need to include removal of portions of vagina, levator ani, ischiorectal fat, perineal body, anal sphincter, anorectum, or pubic bone, or all of these. In locally advanced but resectable cases, exenterative surgery or multimodality therapy may be necessary.

In relation to the difficulty in obtaining an adequate local resection, Copeland and associates reported improved local control with the administration of adjuvant

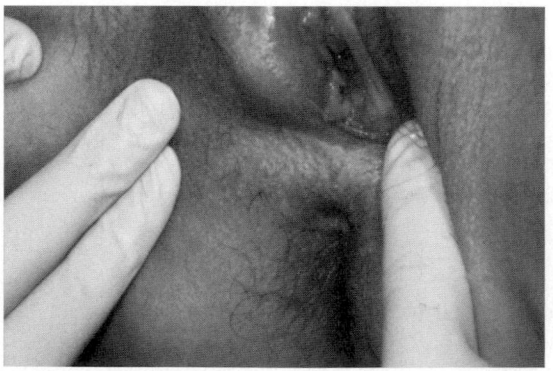

FIGURE 44.52. Right Bartholin gland carcinoma. See color version of figure.

postoperative radiotherapy. This is especially appropriate in the presence of close or positive margins. However, external radiotherapy alone should not be expected to control gross residual disease.

At the time of diagnosis, inguinal lymph node metastases are present in about half of patients with a Bartholin carcinoma. This propensity for lymphatic spread has been attributed to the frequent delay in diagnosis and the more advanced local extent of these tumors. The pattern of lymphatic spread is the same as that for other vulvar malignancies, primarily to the ipsilateral inguinofemoral lymph nodes. Unless a tumor is locally advanced, an ipsilateral inguinal lymphadenectomy is reasonable. As with other vulvar cancers, if positive nodes are found, dissection of the opposite groin or radiotherapy to the inguinal and pelvic nodal basins, or both, may be warranted. Inguinal lymphadenectomy in these patients appears to be both prognostic and therapeutic.

Local, regional, and distant recurrences are common with Bartholin malignancies, and overall survival rate is lower than that for carcinoma of the vulva in general. Copeland and associates reported on a series of 36 patients with this cancer. The local recurrence rate was 2 of 12 (17%) for patients treated with hemivulvectomy (with or without radiotherapy) and 5 of 24 (21%) for patients treated with radical vulvectomy.

Adenoid Cystic Carcinoma

Adenoid cystic carcinoma accounts for about 15% of Bartholin gland carcinomas. As seen with electron microscopy, the tumor contains glandlike lumens filled with eosinophilic material derived from basement membrane, so it is of squamous cell origin. The behavior of this rare malignancy appears to be different from that of other Bartholin and vulvar cancers and to be similar to that of adenoid cystic carcinomas arising from other sites, such as the salivary gland. These vulvar tumors have a high local recurrence rate and a propensity for hematogenous metastases usually developing subsequent to local recurrence. Both local recurrences and metastases can be slowly progressive over a period of years but are not very responsive to radiotherapy or chemotherapy. In view of the difficulty in obtaining adequate surgical margins with Bartholin malignancies in general, and the high local recurrence rate and uncertain sensitivity to radiotherapy with adenoid cystic carcinomas in particular, a concerted effort to obtain at least 2-cm margins should be made when resecting these tumors. Postoperative adjuvant radiotherapy for close or positive margins did appear to be of possible benefit in the 1986 report by Copeland and colleagues and in the report by Rosenberg and associates. From the scant information available, inguinal lymph node metastases occur less frequently with this tumor and have all been ipsilateral. The prognostic and therapeutic value of lymphadenectomy in these patients remains to be defined. The role of adjuvant postoperative chemotherapy for this malignancy also deserves further study.

BASAL CELL CARCINOMA

Although basal cell carcinoma is the most common malignancy of the skin, basal cell carcinoma of the vulva is a rarely reported tumor. Only 250 to 300 cases have been reported in the literature, although basal cell carcinoma constitutes 2% to 3% of vulvar cancers. The cause is unknown, but there is frequently a history of chronic vulvar irritation. This lesion shares many features with vulvar squamous cell carcinoma. The average age of patients at diagnosis is 65 years, and there is a predilection for white women. Common symptoms include chronic pruritus vulvae and the presence of a mass. Authors have repeatedly reported a delay in diagnosis. Most basal cell carcinomas occur on the labia majora and, less commonly, on the labia minora, urethral meatus, and prepuce of the clitoris. The gross appearance is variable. Tumor size has ranged from 0.2 to 10 cm in greatest diameter, averaging 1.5 to 2 cm. There are also reports of multifocal lesions.

Up to 20% of patients with vulvar basal cell carcinoma have a history of other primary cancers. These other cancers have infrequently included coexistent melanoma or squamous cell carcinoma. Keratinization and mature squamous differentiation are commonly found in basal cell carcinomas and do not alter the prognosis. These lesions must be carefully distinguished from the rarer basosquamous carcinoma, which contains a malignant squamous component. How often this occurs is uncertain, but it has been estimated to occur in 3% to 5% of basal cell carcinomas. Careful histologic evaluation of the biopsy material is necessary to rule out a malignant squamous component. With the exception of very large lesions, this is best accomplished by excisional biopsy.

One of the subtypes of basal cell carcinoma, adenoid basal cell carcinoma, must be differentiated from the more aggressive adenoid cystic carcinoma arising in a Bartholin gland or in the skin of the vulva. Merino and colleagues have suggested clinical and histologic criteria for this distinction.

In 1977, Safai and Good reviewed the literature and found 109 cases of basal cell carcinoma of the skin with metastases. These are rare cases, with an incidence of 0.028% to 0.1%. Basosquamous carcinoma of the skin, including the vulva, is a more aggressive neoplasm, with the squamous component metastasizing. Basal cell carcinoma of the vulva is also an indolent, locally invasive lesion that rarely metastasizes. There are only nine well-documented cases of metastatic basal cell carcinoma of the vulva in the literature. These have all been lymphatic metastases. When a patient with basal cell carcinoma has suspicious inguinal lymph nodes, these lymph nodes should probably be removed, especially if the vulvar tumor is large or locally advanced. If the inguinal lymph nodes are not suspicious, they can be removed if they become suspicious during follow-up.

Treatment

Most authorities agree that the treatment of choice for vulvar basal cell carcinoma is wide local excision including a generous amount of underlying subcutaneous tissue. For a multifocal lesion, complete vulvectomy may be appropriate. If a malignant squamous component is present, however, a radical or modified radical vulvectomy with inguinal lymphadenectomy should be performed. There is little information available on the use of radiotherapy or chemotherapy in the treatment of primary or metastatic basal cell carcinoma of the vulva, but there is one report of a locally advanced lesion that had a complete response to radiotherapy. Close follow-up is essential, because the local recurrence rate has been reported to be 10% to 21.5%.

Prognosis

The overall prognosis for patients with vulvar basal cell carcinoma is difficult to ascertain. In a review by Breen and colleagues, there was a 5-year survival rate of about 64%. However, they were unable to find documentation for a single death directly related to recurrent or residual basal cell carcinoma. Rather, they attributed the deaths to old age, attrition, and overzealous therapy.

The prognosis for the rare metastatic basal cell carcinoma of the vulva is even more difficult to predict. Sworn and co-workers concluded that the prognosis is similar to that for basal cell carcinoma at other skin sites. With basal cell carcinoma elsewhere on the skin, the mean survival after discovery of metastatic disease has been reported to be 10 to 14 months. However, Conway and Hugo reported prolonged survival if only regional lymph nodes are involved.

SARCOMA OF THE VULVA

Primary sarcoma constitutes 1% to 3% of all vulvar malignancies. The literature consists of case reports and small series of patients, often with very limited follow-up. In addition, this is a heterogeneous group because of the variety of histologic types and their associated differences in behavior. Hence, the natural history and appropriate treatment of these tumors have not been well defined.

Leiomyosarcoma

The most common histologic type of primary vulvar sarcoma is leiomyosarcoma. Most of these patients are in the age range of 40 to 50 years, but a few are younger (one patient was 17). At least three cases of pregnant patients with leiomyosarcoma have been reported. According to the descriptions, most patients present with an enlarging mass in the labia majora or Bartholin region. Like tumors at other sites, smooth muscle tumors of the vulva appear to have a range of appearances and behavior, from benign to malignant. Tavassoli and Norris reported 32 smooth muscle tumors of the vulva and attempted to delineate the histologic features that might relate to prognosis. They believed that their analysis was impeded by small numbers of patients in subgroups and by varied adequacy of excision. According to their results, prognosis was best predicted by three main determinants (size, tumor contour, and mitotic activity). Neoplasms greater than 5 cm that have infiltrating margins and five or more mitotic figures per 10 high-power fields are likely to recur unless controlled by total excision. It was also determined that lesions larger than 5 cm with infiltrative margins and prominent mitotic activity have a more aggressive behavior as the number of mitotic figures increases. The significance of mitotic activity could not be fully evaluated because of the small number of cases with intermediate grades of mitotic activity and because of other factors. The degree of cellular atypism did not correlate well with the mitotic activity or with recurrence. In 1996, Nielsen and colleagues proposed similar prognostic criteria, but included cytologic atypia. In keeping with a range of behaviors, according to the available reports, vulvar leiomyosarcomas may do well with adequate excision, may follow a slowly progressive course, or may rapidly progress to fatality. Local recurrences are common, and several authors have recommended early radical excision of these tumors to improve treatment results. As with the other genital tract sarcomas, there is a propensity for hematogenous metastases that may develop early. From the few studies reporting long-term follow-up, it appears that only about half of these patients are 5-year survivors. Information regarding the propensity of these tumors to metastasize to the regional lymph nodes, and the prognostic and therapeutic value of inguinal lymphadenectomy is scant. On the basis of general knowledge of the behavior of these types of sarcomas, the regional lymph nodes are probably at minimal risk with a low-grade tumor. In patients with high-grade tumors, removal of regional lymph nodes is probably of prognostic value only, although control of disease in the groin is a consideration. In a fit patient with a high-risk but apparently localized tumor, inguinal lymphadenectomy seems reasonable. Radiotherapy has been used in only a few cases with mixed results. Postoperative adjuvant radiotherapy to the pelvis (including the perineum) may be worthwhile in selected cases to improve local control. As with other genital tract leiomyosarcomas, chemotherapy has been of limited palliative benefit.

Other Sarcomas

According to our review, fourteen cases of *dermatofibrosarcoma protuberans* (DFSP) of the vulva have been reported. These patients ranged in age from 37 to 87 years and presented with a tumor characteristic of DFSP at other sites. The tumors range in maximum diameter from 1 to 8 cm and are multinodular, firm, seemingly well-circumscribed masses. The mass is reportedly mobile but fixed to the overlying skin from which it originated. The clinical impression of a mobile, well-circumscribed mass is apparently misleading, because fine microscopic projections of the tumor have been shown to extend well beyond the apparent mass. This explains the marked tendency of this tumor to recur locally and

the need for wide (3 cm has been recommended) surgical margins. Intraoperative frozen section analysis of margins has also been recommended. Despite this tendency for local recurrence, DFSP behaves like a low-grade sarcoma that rarely metastasizes. In the absence of suspicious lymph nodes, a lymphadenectomy is not warranted. Hematogenous metastases may be seen after multiple local recurrences. Local radiotherapy has not been useful for these tumors. With adequate resection, the overall prognosis for DFSP of the vulva should be good. Two cases of a fibrosarcoma arising in a vulvar DFSP have been reported, but the clinical behavior and prognosis for such tumors appear to be the same as those for DFSP alone.

Six cases of *malignant fibrous histiocytoma* of the vulva have been reported. The age range of these patients is 38 to 79 years. Five of the six tumors were on the labium majus, and the sixth was vulvovaginal. Based on these few reports and the more abundant literature on malignant fibrous histiocytoma at other sites, recommended treatment includes radical excision of the tumor with an inguinal lymphadenectomy. Adjuvant radiotherapy and chemotherapy may have a role, and the one vulvovaginal tumor reported was without evidence of recurrence 6 years after sequential chemotherapy and radiotherapy.

We found five reports of *pure fibrosarcoma* of the vulva. Two of these patients died with disseminated disease at 3 weeks and 16 months after diagnosis, and one patient had inguinal lymph node metastases but was without evidence of recurrence at 48 months. According to the general literature on fibrosarcomas, the malignant potential varies depending on the tissue of origin and the histologic pattern (cellularity, mitotic activity). Three of the four reported patients who were treated developed local recurrences (two of them repetitive), which is in agreement with the general behavior reported for these tumors. Again, the importance of wide excision at the time of primary treatment is emphasized. Fibrosarcomas are reported to only rarely metastasize to lymph nodes; however, as previously pointed out, one of the five described cases did have an isolated lymphatic metastasis.

Nineteen *primary epithelioid sarcomas* of the vulva have been reported. Nine of the women were 31 years of age or younger, and five of the lesions arose on the labium majus. Seven of the patients developed repetitive local recurrences (generally in the form of multiple subcutaneous nodules) and coincident or subsequent hematogenous or lymphatic metastases, or both, and died over the course of months to years. This tumor apparently penetrates along soft tissue planes, and there is reported difficulty in delineating tumor extent. Radical excision with wide, clear margins seems to be the most reasonable initial treatment. Regional lymphadenectomy should be considered on an individual basis.

A few malignant *rhabdoid tumors* of the vulva have also been reported. There is apparent difficulty distinguishing this malignancy histologically from epithelioid sarcoma. Both tumors present similarly as a benign-appearing labial mass in young women. Malignant rhabdoid tumors may follow an even more aggressive course.

Although sarcomas constitute only a small percentage of vulvar malignancies in general, they account for most vulvar cancers in children and young women. Overall, pediatric vulvovaginal *rhabdomyosarcomas* have a good prognosis and greatly reduced treatment morbidity because of the efficacy of combined treatment modalities (especially chemotherapy and brachytherapy). Rhabdomyosarcomas arising in older women and other histologic variants of rhabdomyosarcoma may not be so amenable to therapy.

At least 40 cases of *aggressive angiomyxoma* involving the female pelvis or perineum, or both, have been described, and at least 13 of these primarily involved the vulva. It is an unusual tumor derived from fibroblasts or myofibroblasts with nuclei that have no atypical features or mitotic activity. The tumor appears to be locally invasive and spreads by direct extension only. Local recurrences are common, although there have been no reported deaths attributable to this tumor. The mainstay of treatment is wide excision both primarily and for recurrences.

Isolated reports of a variety of other types of sarcomas arising in the vulva have been published. Treatment of these various sarcomas must be individualized according to the scant literature available, the potential aggressiveness of the malignancy as suggested by the pathologist, and the individual situation.

PAGET'S DISEASE OF THE VULVA

Paget's disease is classified, according to location, as mammary or extramammary disease. The original lesion described by Paget is a skin (nipple and areola) lesion related to an underlying invasive ductal adenocarcinoma. Extramammary Paget's disease most commonly involves the anogenital region, appearing as a patchy, reddish and whitish, velvety, and eczematous lesion (Fig. 44.53). Patients with Paget's disease of the vulva are usually white, postmenopausal women who complain of localized itching and burning.

Paget's disease of the vulva is of apocrine origin and is confined to the epithelium in most cases. However, invasive disease is present in about 15% to 25% of cases, either as a result of direct invasion through the basement membrane or, less commonly, because of the presence of an underlying apocrine gland adenocarcinoma. Histologically, intraepithelial Paget's disease appears as large, pale cells often in nests at the tips of the rete ridges (Figs. 44.54 and 44.55). The cells are often seen infiltrating upward in the epithelium, which is hyperkeratotic. The Paget's cells can be located within any of the skin adnexa.

Vulvar Paget's disease occurs with other malignancies in about 25% of patients; the most common of these is breast carcinoma. Other commonly associated malignancies are basal cell, rectal, and genitourinary carcinomas.

When Paget's disease involves the anus, there is a very high incidence of coexisting rectal cancer. Part of the preoperative workup should be directed at screening for these malignancies.

When a patient is diagnosed with Paget's disease of the vulva, the area of involvement should be carefully inspected and palpated to detect areas suspicious for invasive cancer. If the disease clinically appears to be intraepithelial, a wide local excision is performed, including a small amount of subcutaneous tissue. A well-known characteristic of intraepithelial Paget's disease is histologic extension far beyond that which is clinically apparent. Intraoperative assessment of margins with frozen sections is of questionable benefit. We have preferred to use the mapping technique described by Bergen and associates. Intraoperative mapping involves excising strips of tissue along the initially planned margins and sending them for frozen section analysis (Fig. 44.53B and C). While waiting for the frozen section reports, the central lesion is excised (Fig. 44.53D). Other methods that have been reported to be useful in ensuring clear margins include Mohs micrographic surgery and fluorescein dye with ultraviolet light. Colposcopy and toluidine blue staining are not helpful according to Friedrich and colleagues. An experimental technique reported to be potentially useful in evaluating histologically negative margins is the application of a panel of monoclonal antibodies that may detect occult Paget's cells.

When intraepithelial Paget's disease extends far beyond that which is clinically apparent, very extensive excision is necessary to obtain clear margins. Primary closure of vulvar wounds is desirable but may not be possible in such cases. Reported means of dealing with such cases include skin grafting and laser vaporization of the occult disease (guided by peripheral biopsies). There are a few reports of Paget's disease recurring within a skin graft. Topical 5-fluorouracil or bleomycin, administered either preoperatively or postoperatively, has also been used to treat the clinically negative disease. If it appears that excision of persistently positive margins may prevent primary closure, it is not unreasonable to close the wound and follow up the patient closely.

After excision of intraepithelial Paget's disease of the vulva, local recurrence develops in about one third of patients. This tends to take the form of multiple recurrences over a prolonged period of time. In some studies, recurrence risk has been correlated with excisional margin status, but it also has been pointed out that the initial disease in some cases is multifocal. Of particular concern are a few reports of patients whose recurrent lesions eventually became invasive. Whether such instances are preventable by diligently eradicating the full histologic extent of the disease remains unclear.

When vulvar Paget's disease is found to contain an invasive component, the treatment is radical surgery, as for squamous cell carcinoma. Overall, these patients have a high incidence of inguinal lymph node metastases with an associated poor prognosis. The role of adjuvant therapy in these patients is unclear.

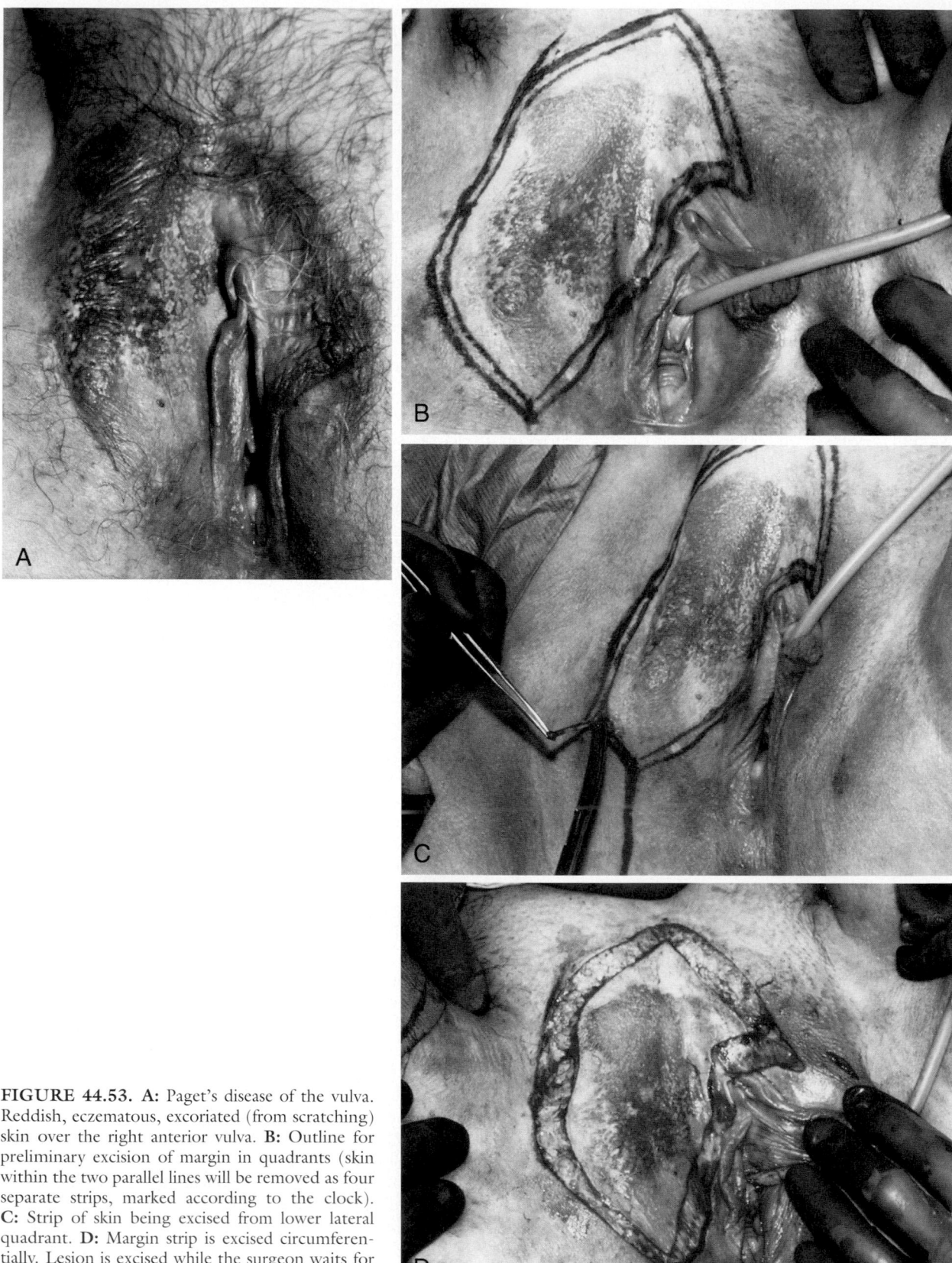

FIGURE 44.53. A: Paget's disease of the vulva. Reddish, eczematous, excoriated (from scratching) skin over the right anterior vulva. **B:** Outline for preliminary excision of margin in quadrants (skin within the two parallel lines will be removed as four separate strips, marked according to the clock). **C:** Strip of skin being excised from lower lateral quadrant. **D:** Margin strip is excised circumferentially. Lesion is excised while the surgeon waits for the frozen-section results.

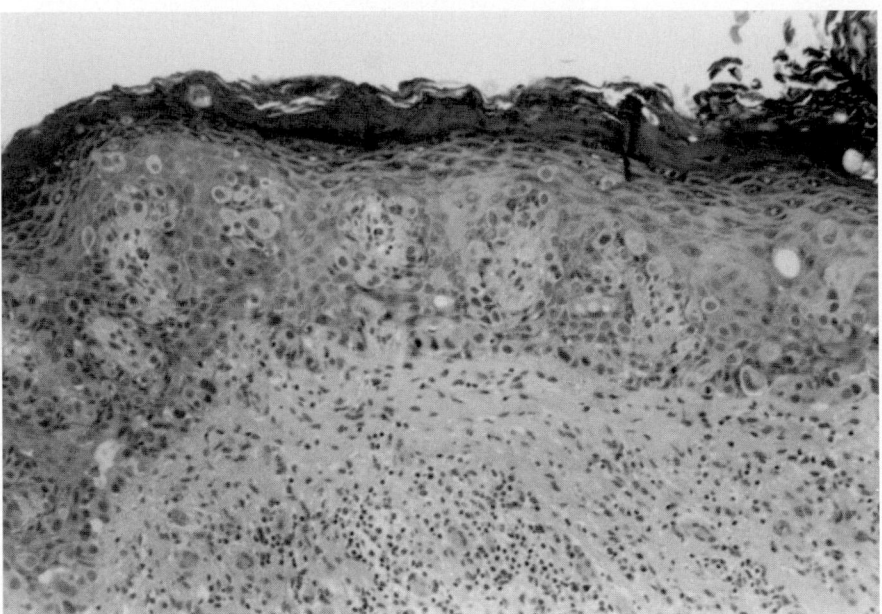

FIGURE 44.54. Microscopic section of intraepithelial Paget's disease of the vulva. Nests of large, pale cells infiltrate upward in the epithelium, which is hyperkeratotic.

Management of recurrent intraepithelial Paget's disease of the vulva is similar to that of the primary lesion, with excision of at least the clinically evident disease.

VERRUCOUS CARCINOMA OF THE VULVA

Verrucous carcinoma of the vulva is a rare variant of squamous cell carcinoma, with about 50 cases reported in the literature. This tumor was first described in the oral cavity by Ackerman in 1948 and most commonly occurs in the oral cavity, larynx, and anogenital region. The mean age of the women diagnosed with this malignancy of the vulva is about 50 years. The reported tumors have ranged from 1 to 10 cm in maximum diameter and appear as a slow-growing, cauliflower-like tumor (Fig. 44.56). Characteristically, verrucous cancers have well-demarcated borders that are pushing rather than infiltrating. Verrucous carcinoma can be confused with condyloma; when an apparent condyloma (especially when large and in an older woman) does not respond to the usual conservative measures, it should be excised. About one third of patients with vulvar verrucous carcinoma have a history of genital warts, and human papillomavirus (HPV) has been detected in some lesions, the most common type being HPV-6.

The diagnosis of verrucous carcinoma requires a large (preferably excisional) biopsy that must include the

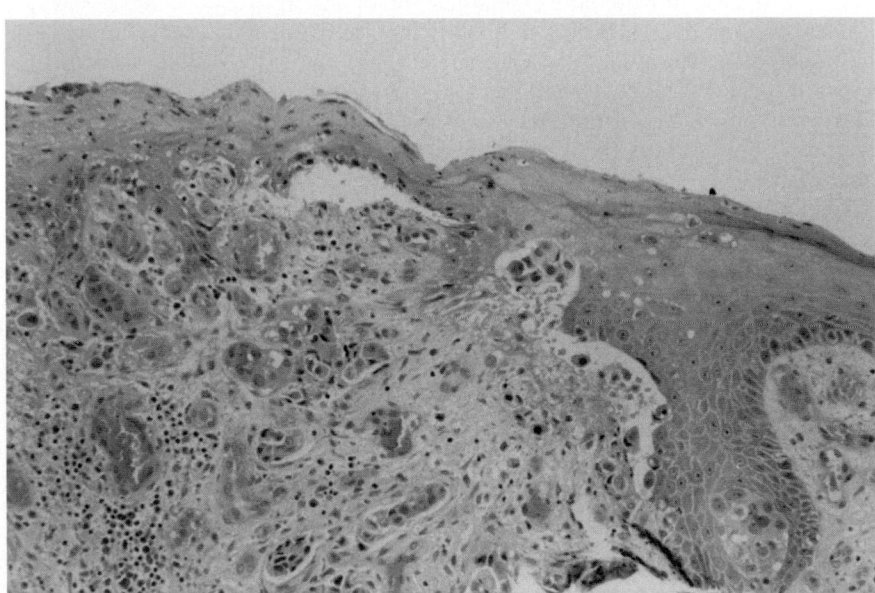

FIGURE 44.55. Microscopic section of invasive Paget's disease of the vulva. Nests of Paget's cells infiltrate the stroma.

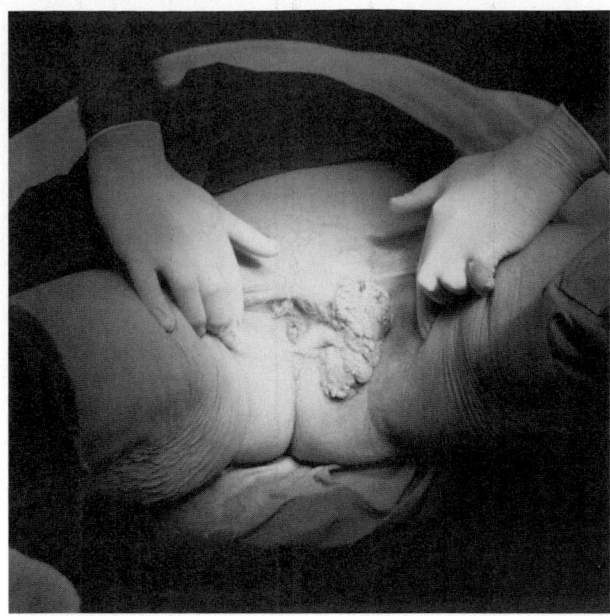

FIGURE 44.56. Verrucous carcinoma of the vulva. A large cauliflower-like tumor arising from the left labia majora.

base of the lesion. Verrucous carcinoma can also be confused with so-called warty carcinoma, another variant of well-differentiated squamous cell carcinoma that tends to remain in situ or superficially infiltrating. Differentiation of these two entities is not of great importance because both have a very low incidence of metastases and treatment is essentially the same.

Verrucous carcinoma is rarely associated with metastatic disease, and many of the reports of such spread have shown histologic evidence of nests of squamous cell carcinoma invading the stroma beneath the tumor. Some authors have suggested that if areas of distinct invasion are found beneath a verrucous lesion, the behavior may be more aggressive and treatment should be more radical. Inflammatory enlargement of the inguinal lymph nodes has been a frequently reported finding with verrucous carcinoma of the vulva.

It is generally agreed that the main treatment of verrucous carcinoma of the vulva is excision with free margins. How radical this resection should be is unclear, but local recurrences have not been uncommon. Local lesions have had a good initial response to radiation therapy but a high rate of subsequent recurrence and about a 30% incidence of anaplastic transformation with associated aggressive behavior. The few reported cases of metastatic verrucous carcinoma of the genital tract have followed radiotherapy. However, many tumors have been successfully treated with a combination of surgery and radiotherapy; when a tumor is locally advanced, this seems to be a reasonable treatment. Inguinal lymphadenectomy may be indicated in patients with large tumors, in patients with persistence or recurrence of disease, especially after radiotherapy, and in patients with infiltrating cancer beyond very early invasion below the verrucous tumor. Biopsy specimens may

be obtained of enlarged lymph nodes thought to be inflammatory.

Verrucous carcinoma of the vulva has been associated with second malignant tumors, most commonly of the cervix, breast, and anogenital skin. Although verrucous carcinoma of the genital tract is a slow-growing tumor that rarely metastasizes, a 1988 review by Andersen and Sorensen reported that 26.1% of the patients with this type of carcinoma had died of disease.

MERKEL CELL CARCINOMA OF THE VULVA

Merkel cell cancers are small cell (neuroendocrine) tumors of the skin that occur most commonly in sun-exposed areas (head, neck, and extremities) and behave in an aggressive manner. This malignancy was first described in 1972 by Toker, and about 500 cases have been reported since. At least 10 cases of vulvar origin have been reported. The ages of these ten patients ranged from 28 to 74 years, and the tumors occurred in all regions of the vulva (two in Bartholin glands). When originating from the vulva, Merkel cell carcinoma has behaved in a highly aggressive fashion (even more so than Merkel cell tumors in general), with nine patients having regional lymph node metastases. At least seven had distant metastases and died within 2.5 years of diagnosis. Surgery and radiotherapy appear to be of value for local control only, and as yet no effective systemic treatment exists. As in the treatment of small cell carcinoma of the lung, etoposide and cisplatin have been used for a few cases of Merkel cell carcinoma, with good responses. Three of the vulvar cases were treated with this regimen. Two progressed and one had a partial response of very short duration.

SUPERNUMERARY MAMMARY ADENOCARCINOMA

Ectopic breast tissue in the vulva is very rare, but at least nine cases of mammary-type adenocarcinoma arising in the vulva have been reported. These patients ranged in age from 49 to 71 years, and five of the nine presented with an asymptomatic vulvar nodule. Only one of the patients had evidence of primary breast cancer, but rather than representing metastatic disease, the vulvar lesion appeared to be primary from the vulva. The diagnosis of vulvar mammary adenocarcinoma is based primarily on the histologic pattern of the vulvar tumor. Other criteria can include the finding of adjacent normal mammary glandular elements (one case of adjacent in situ malignancy), the presence of estrogen or progesterone receptor positivity, positivity for common breast markers, and ruling out an origin from skin appendages.

One of the eight patients died of disease without treatment 1 month after diagnosis. The patient with coexistent primary breast carcinoma died of widespread metastatic (including cerebral) disease 22 months after the diagnosis. One patient had 2 of 10 positive ipsilateral inguinal lymph nodes and was placed on tamoxifen post-operatively; this patient remained without evidence of recurrence at 1 year. A fourth patient had extensive nodal metastases at the time of diagnosis, subsequently developed distant metastases, and died of disease 27 months after diagnosis despite chemotherapy. A fifth patient had 4 of 11 positive ipsilateral inguinal lymph nodes and was placed on tamoxifen postoperatively. After 2 years of disease-free survival, the patient stopped taking the tamoxifen and presented 4 months later with bony metastases. After radiotherapy and reinstitution of tamoxifen, she was disease free at 1 year of follow-up. A sixth patient had microscopic involvement in 1 of 14 ipsilateral lymph nodes. She received adjuvant chemotherapy with a plan for subsequent radiotherapy and tamoxifen. Follow-up was not available for the other three patients, but two of the three had undergone an inguinal lymphadenectomy, and in both cases there were positive lymph nodes.

Beyond surgical treatment, such a rare patient might be considered for adjuvant therapy (especially with metastatic disease) such as radiotherapy, tamoxifen (if estrogen receptor-positive), or chemotherapy.

OTHER REPORTED VULVAR MALIGNANCIES

There are scattered reports of a variety of adenocarcinomas arising in the vulva other than those previously discussed. Most of these have arisen from recognizable adenomatous sources, such as adnexal structures and endometriosis. There are five reports of malignancy arising in the vulva from isolated foci of extraovarian endometriosis; four were clear cell adenocarcinoma and the fifth was an endometrial stromal sarcoma. There are also rare reports of vulvar sebaceous carcinoma, mucinous carcinoma, lymphoma, and a peripheral primitive neuroectodermal tumor.

At least four endodermal sinus tumors of the vulva have been reported. The ages of these patients were 22 months, 2 years, 15 years, and 26 years, and all four presented with painless vulvar masses. Three of the four patients died of metastatic disease 6, 11, and 23 months after diagnosis. The 2-year-old patient remains without evidence of recurrence 5.5 years after local excision.

A variety of metastatic lesions to the vulva have been documented, most commonly from the gynecologic tract. Nongynecologic metastatic disease to the vulva is rare, with isolated reports of primary sites such as the urinary tract, the colorectum, the skin (melanoma), non-Hodgkin's lymphoma, and the breast.

BIBLIOGRAPHY

Abrao FS, Baracat EC, Marques AF, et al. Carcinoma of the vulva: clinicopathologic factors involved in inguinal and pelvic lymph node metastasis. *J Reprod Med* 1990;35:1113.

Achauer BM, Braly P, Berman ML, et al. Immediate vaginal reconstruction following resection for malignancy using the gluteal thigh flap. *Gynecol Oncol* 1984;19:79.

Ackerman LV. Verrucous carcinoma of the oral cavity. *Surgery* 1948;23:670.

Acosta AA, Given FT, Frazier AB, et al. Preoperative radiation therapy in the management of squamous cell carcinoma of the vulva: preliminary report. *Am J Obstet Gynecol* 1978;132:198.

Adams J, Daly JW. Proctectomy combined with vulvectomy for carcinoma of the vulva. *Obstet Gynecol* 1979;54:643.

Adelson MD, Miranda FR, Strumpf KB. Necrotizing fasciitis: a complication of squamous cell carcinoma of the vulva. *Gynecol Oncol* 1991;42:98.

Agarossi A, Vago I, Lazzarin A, et al. Vulvar Kaposi's sarcoma. A case report [Letter]. *Ann Oncol* 1991;2:609.

Agress R, Figge DC, Tamimi H, et al. Dermatofibrosarcoma protuberans of the vulva. *Gynecol Oncol* 1983;16:288.

Al-Ghamdi A, Freedman D, Miller D, et al. Vulvar squamous cell carcinoma in young women: a clinicopathologic study of 21 cases. *Gynecol Oncol* 2002;84:94.

Andersen ES, Sorensen IM. Verrucous carcinoma of the female genital tract: report of a case and review of the literature. *Gynecol Oncol* 1988;30:427.

Andersen WA, Franquemont DW, Williams J, et al. Vulvar squamous cell carcinoma and papillomaviruses: two separate entities? *Am J Obstet Gynecol* 1991;165:329.

Anderson BL. Sexual functioning complications in women with gynecologic cancer: outcomes and direction for prevention. *Cancer* 1987;60:2123.

Andreasson B, Moth J, Jensen SB, et al. Sexual function and somatopsychic reactions in vulvectomy operated women and their partners. *Acta Obstet Gynecol Scand* 1986;65:7.

Andreasson B, Nyboe J. Predictive factors with reference to low risk of metastases in squamous carcinoma of the vulva region. *Gynecol Oncol* 1985;21:196.

Andreasson B, Nyboe J. Value of prognostic parameters in squamous cell carcinoma of the vulva. *Gynecol Oncol* 1985;22:341.

Andreasson B, Visfeldt J, Bock JE, et al. Value of four models for selecting patients for local excision of invasive squamous cell carcinoma of the vulva. *J Reprod Med* 1990;35:1041.

Andrews SJ, Williams BT, DePriest PD, et al. Therapeutic implications of lymph nodal spread in lateral T1 and T2 squamous cell carcinoma of the vulva. *Gynecol Oncol* 1994;55:41.

Ansink AC, Sie-Go DMDS, van der Velden J, et al. Identification of sentinel lymph nodes in vulvar carcinoma patients with the aid of a patent blue V injection. *Cancer* 1999;86:652.

Anthony JP, Mathes SJ, Hoffman WY. Immediate flap coverage in the treatment of large surgical defects after tumor resection. *Surg Gynecol Obstet* 1993;176:355.

Atamdede F, Hoogerland D. Regional lymph node recurrence following local excision for microinvasive vulvar carcinoma. *Gynecol Oncol* 1989;34:125.

Atlante G, Lombardi A, Mariani L, et al. Carcinoma of the vulva (1981-85): analysis of a radio surgical approach. *Eur J Gynaecol Oncol* 1989;10:341.

Auger M, Colgan TJ. Detection of metastatic vulvar and cervical squamous carcinoma in regional lymph nodes by use of a polyclonal keratin antibody. *Int J Gynecol Pathol* 1990;9:337.

Ayhan A, Tuncer R, Tuncer ZS, et al. Risk factors for groin node metastasis in squamous carcinoma of the vulva: a multivariate analysis of 39 cases. *Eur J Obstet Gynecol Reprod Biol* 1993;48:33.

Baachi CE, Goldfogel GA, Greer BE, et al. Paget's disease and melanoma of the vulva. *Gynecol Oncol* 1992;46:216.

Bachrendtz H, Einhorn N, Pettersson F, et al. Paget's disease of the vulva: the Radiumhemmet series 1975–1990. *Int J Gynecol Cancer* 1994;4:1.

Backstrom A, Edsmyr F, Wicklund H. Radiotherapy of carcinoma of the vulva. *Acta Obstet Gynecol Scand* 1972; 51:109.

Bailey CL, Sankey HZ, Donovan JT, et al. Primary breast cancer of the vulva. *Gynecol Oncol* 1993;50:379.

Baird WL, Hester TR, Nahai F, et al. Management of perineal wounds following abdominoperineal resection with inferior gluteal flaps. *Arch Surg* 1990;125:1486.

Bakri YN, Akhtar M, El-Senoussi M, et al. Vulvar sarcoma: a report of four cases. *Gynecol Oncol* 1992;46:384.

Balch CM, Buzaid AC, Atkins MB. A new American Joint Committee on Cancer staging system for cutaneous melanoma. *Cancer* 2000;88:1484.

Balch CM, Buzaid AC, Soong SJ, et al. Final version of the American Joint Committee on cancer staging system for cutaneous melanoma. *J Clin Oncol* 2001;19:3635.

Balch CM, Soong SJ, Bartolucci AA, et al. Efficacy of an elective regional lymph node dissection of 1 to 4 mm thick melanomas for patients 60 years of age or younger. *Ann Surg* 1996;224:255.

Balch CM, Soong S-J, Milton GW, et al. A comparison of prognostic factors and surgical results in 1,786 patients with localized (stage 1) melanoma treated in Alabama, USA, and New South Wales, Australia. *Ann Surg* 1982;196:677.

Balch CM, Urist MM, Karakousis CP, et al. Efficacy of 2-cm surgical margins for intermediate-thickness melanomas (1 to 4 mm): results of a multi-institutional randomized surgical trial. *Ann Surg* 1993;218:262.

Ballon SC, Lamb EJ. Separate inguinal incisions in the treatment of carcinoma of the vulva. *Surg Gynecol Obstet* 1975;140:81.

Baltzer J, Kurzl RY, Lohe KJ, et al. Melanoma of the vulva. *J Reprod Med* 1986;31:825.

Barbero M, Micheletti L, Preti M, et al. Biologic behavior of vulvar intraepithelial neoplasia: histologic and clinical parameters. *J Reprod Med* 1993;38:108.

Barclay DL, Collins CG, Macey HB Jr. Cancer of the Bartholin gland: a review and report of 8 cases. *Obstet Gynecol* 1964;24:329.

Barnhill DR, Boling R, Nobles W, et al. Vulvar dermatofibrosarcoma protuberans. *Gynecol Oncol* 1988;30:149.

Barnhill DR, Hoskins WJ, Metz P. Use of the rhomboid flap after partial vulvectomy. *Obstet Gynecol* 1983;62:444.

Barton DPJ, Berman C, Cavanagh D, et al. Lymphoscintigraphy in vulvar cancer: a pilot study. *Gynecol Oncol* 1992; 46:341.

Barton DP, Hoffman MS, Roberts WS, et al. Use of local flaps in the preservation of fecal continence following resection of perianal neoplasias. *Int J Gynecol Cancer* 1992;3:318.

Benedet JL, Miller DM, Ehlen TG, et al. Basal cell carcinoma of the vulva: clinical features and treatment results in 28 patients. *Obstet Gynecol* 1997;90:765.

Benedet JL, Turlo M, Fairey RN, et al. Squamous carcinoma of the vulva: results of treatment, 1938 to 1976. *Am J Obstet Gynecol* 1979;134:201.

Benedetti-Panici P, Greggi S, Scambia G, et al. Cisplatin (P), bleomycin (B) and methotrexate (M) preoperative chemotherapy in locally advanced vulvar carcinoma. *Gynecol Oncol* 1993;50:49.

Ben-Izhak O, Levy R, Weill S, et al. Anorectal malignant melanoma. A clinicopathologic study, including immunohistochemistry and DNA flow cytometry. *Cancer* 1997;79:18.

Berek JS, Heaps JM, Fu YS, et al. Concurrent cisplatin and 5-FU chemotherapy and external radiation for primary treatment of advanced stage squamous carcinoma of the vulva. *Gynecol Oncol* 1991;40:171(abst).

Bergen S, DiSaia PJ, Liao SY, et al. Conservative management of extramammary Paget's disease of the vulva. *Gynecol Oncol* 1989;33:151.

Berman ML, Soper JT, Creasman WT, et al. Conservative surgical management of superficially invasive stage 1 vulvar carcinoma. *Gynecol Oncol* 1989;35:352.

Bertani A, Riccio M, Belligolli A. Vulval reconstruction after cancer excision: the island groin flap technique. *Br J Plast Surg* 1990;43:159.

Binder SW, Huang I, Fu YS, et al. Risk factors for the development of lymph node metastasis in vulvar squamous carcinoma. *Gynecol Oncol* 1990;37:9.

Bjerregaard B, Andreasson B, Visfeldt J, et al. The significance of histology and morphometry in predicting lymph node metastases in patients with squamous cell carcinoma of the vulva. *Gynecol Oncol* 1993;50:323.

Bock J, Andreasson B, Thorn A, et al. Dermatofibrosarcoma protuberans of the vulva. *Gynecol Oncol* 1985;20:129.

Borgno G, Micheletti L, Barbero M, et al. Topographic distribution of groin lymph nodes. *J Reprod Med* 1990;35:1127.

Boronow RC, Hickman BT, Reagan MT, et al. Combined therapy as an alternative to exenteration for locally advanced vulvovaginal cancer. II. Results, complications, and dosimetric and surgical considerations. *Am J Clin Oncol* 1987;10:171.

Bottles K, Lacey CG, Goldberg J, et al. Merkel cell carcinoma of the vulva. *Obstet Gynecol* 1984;63:61S.

Bouma J, Dankert J. Recurrent acute leg cellulitis in patients after radical vulvectomy. *Gynecol Oncol* 1988;29:50.

Boutselis JG. Radical vulvectomy for invasive squamous cell carcinoma of the vulva. *Obstet Gynecol* 1972;39:827.

Boyce J, Fruchter RG, Kasambilides E, et al. Prognostic factors in carcinoma of the vulva. *Gynecol Oncol* 1985;20:364.

Bradgate MG, Rollason TP, McConkey CC, et al. Malignant melanoma of the vulva: a clinico-pathological study of 50 women. *Br J Obstet Gynaecol* 1990;97:124.

Brand A, Covert A. Malignant rhabdoid tumor of the vulva: case report and review of the literature with emphasis on clinical management and outcome. *Gynecol Oncol* 2001;80:99.

Breen JL, Neubecker RD, Greenwald E, et al. Basal cell carcinoma of the vulva. *Obstet Gynecol* 1975;46:122.

Brennan MJ, Miller LT. Overview of treatment options and review of the current role and use of compression garments, intermittent pumps, and exercise in the management of lymphedema. *Cancer* 1998;83:2821.

Breslow A. Thickness, cross-sectional areas, and depth of invasion in the prognosis of cutaneous melanoma. *Ann Surg* 1970;172:902.

Breslow A, Macht SD. Optimal size of margins for thin cutaneous melanoma. *Surg Gynecol Obstet* 1977;145:691.

Brisigotti M, Moreno A, Murcia C, et al. Verrucous carcinoma of the vulva: a clinicopathologic and immunohistochemical study of five cases. *Int J Gynecol Pathol* 1989;8:1.

Brooks JJ, LiVolsi VA. Liposarcoma presenting on the vulva. *Am J Obstet Gynecol* 1987;156:73.

Brunschwig A, Brockunier A Jr. Surgical treatment of squamous cell carcinoma of the vulva. *Obstet Gynecol* 1967; 29:362.

Bryson SC, Dembo AJ, Colgan TJ, et al. Invasive squamous cell carcinoma of the vulva. Defining low and high risk groups for recurrence. *Int J Gynecol Cancer* 1991;1:25.

Buchler DA, Kline JC, Tunca JC, et al. Treatment of recurrent carcinoma of the vulva. *Gynecol Oncol* 1979;8:180.

Buhl A, Landow S, Lee YC, et al. Microcystic adnexal carcinoma of the vulva. *Gynecol Oncol* 2001;82:571.

Burger MPM, Hollema H, Emanuels AG, et al. The importance of the groin node status for the survival of T1 and T2 vulvar carcinoma patients. *Gynecol Oncol* 1995;57:327.

Burke TW, Levenback C, Coleman RL, et al. Surgical therapy of T1 and T2 vulvar carcinoma: further experience with radical wide excision and selective inguinal lymphadenectomy. *Gynecol Oncol* 1995;57:215.

Burke TW, Morris M, Levenback C, et al. Closure of complex vulvar defects using local rhomboid flaps. *Obstet Gynecol* 1994;84:1043.

Burke TW, Morris M, Roh RS, et al. Perineal reconstruction using single gracilis myocutaneous flaps. *Gynecol Oncol* 1995;57:221.

Burke TW, Stringer A, Gershenson DM, et al. Radical wide excision and selective inguinal node dissection for squamous cell carcinoma of the vulva. *Gynecol Oncol* 1990;38:328.

Burrell MO, Franklin EW III, Campion MJ, et al. The modified radical vulvectomy with groin dissection: an eight-year experience. *Am J Obstet Gynecol* 1988;159:715.

Buscema J, Naghashfar S, Sawada E, et al. The predominance of human papillomavirus type 16 in vulvar neoplasia. *Obstet Gynecol* 1988;71:601.

Buscema J, Stern J, Woodruff JD. The significance of histologic alterations adjacent to invasive vulvar carcinoma. *Am J Obstet Gynecol* 1980;137:902.

Buscema J, Woodruff JD. Progressive histobiologic alteration in the development of vulvar cancer. *Am J Obstet Gynecol* 1980;138:146.

Buzaid AC, Tinoco LA, Jendiroba D, et al. Prognostic value of size of lymph node metastases in patients with cutaneous melanoma. *J Clin Oncol* 1995;13:2361.

Byron RL, Lamb EJ, Yonemoto RH, et al. Radical inguinal node dissection in the treatment of cancer. *Surg Gynecol Obstet* 1962;114:401.

Calabro A, Singletary E, Balch CM. Patterns of relapse in 1001 consecutive patients with melanoma nodal metastases. *Arch Surg* 1989;124:1051.

Calame RJ. Pelvic relaxation as a complication of radical vulvectomy. *Obstet Gynecol* 1980;55:716.

Camacho-Martinez F, Moreno JC, Sanchez-Conejo MJ, et al. International dermatosurgery: advancement local flaps in the reconstructive treatment of vulvar carcinoma. *J Dermatol Surg Oncol* 1983;9:748.

Cardosi RJ, Speights A, Fiorica JV, et al. Bartholin's gland carcinoma: a 15-year experience. *Gynecol Oncol* 2001;82:247.

Carlino G, Parisi S, Montemaggi P, et al. Interstitial radiotherapy with Ir in vulvar cancer. *Eur J Gynaecol Oncol* 1984;3:183.

Carlson JW, McGlennen RC, Gomez R, et al. Sebaceous carcinoma of the vulva: a case report and review of the literature. *Gynecol Oncol* 1996;60:489.

Carson LF, Twiggs LB, Adcock LL, et al. Multimodality therapy for advanced and recurrent vulvar squamous cell carcinoma: a pilot project. *J Reprod Med* 1990;35:1029.

Carter J, Carlson J, Fowler J, et al. Invasive tumors in young women—a disease of the immunosuppressed? *Gynecol Oncol* 1993;51:307.

Castaldo TW, Petrilli ES, Ballon SC, et al. Endodermal sinus tumor of the clitoris. *Gynecol Oncol* 1980;9:376.

Cavanagh D, Beasley J, Ostapowicz F. Radical operation for carcinoma of the vulva: a new approach to wound healing. *J Obstet Gynaecol Br Commonw* 1970;77:1037.

Cavanagh D, Desai S. Invasive carcinoma of the vulva. *Aust N Z J Obstet Gynaecol* 1968;8:171.

Cavanagh D, Fiorica J, Hoffman MS, et al. Invasive carcinoma of the vulva: changing trends in surgical management. *Am J Obstet Gynecol* 1990;163:1007.

Cavanagh D, Hovadhanakul P, Taylor HB. Invasive carcinomas of the vulva: current view on diagnosis and treatment. *Mo Med* 1976;73:129.

Cavanagh D, Roberts WS, Bryson SCP, et al. Changing trends in the surgical treatment of invasive carcinoma of the vulva. *Surg Gynecol Obstet* 1986;162:164.

Cavanagh D, Shepherd JH. The place of pelvic exenteration in the primary management of advanced carcinoma of the vulva. *Gynecol Oncol* 1982;13:318.

Chafe W, Fowler WC, Walton LA, et al. Radical vulvectomy with use of tensor fascia lata myocutaneous flap. *Am J Obstet Gynecol* 1983;145:207.

Chafe W, Richards A, Morgan L, et al. Unrecognized invasive carcinoma in vulvar intraepithelial neoplasia (VIN). *Gynecol Oncol* 1988;31:154.

Chamlian DL, Taylor HB. Primary carcinoma of the Bartholin's gland. A report of 24 patients. *Obstet Gynecol* 1972;39:489.

Chandeying V, Sutthijumroon S, Tungphaisal S. Merkel cell carcinoma of the vulva: a case report. *Asia Oceania J Obstet Gynaecol* 1989;15:261.

Chapman GW Jr, Benda J, Lifshitz S. Adenoid cystic carcinoma of the vulva with lung metastases. A case report. *J Reprod Med* 1985;30:217.

Chen KTK. Merkel's cell (neuroendocrine) carcinoma of the vulva. *Cancer* 1994;73:2186.

Chen L, Schink JC, Panares BN, et al. Resection of a giant aggressive angiomyxoma in the Philippines. *Gynecol Oncol* 1998;70:435.

Cheung TH, Chan MK, Chang A. Aggressive angiomyxoma of the female perineum: case reports. *Aust N Z J Obstet Gynaecol* 1991;31:285.

Cho D, Buscema J, Rosenshein N, et al. Primary breast cancer of the vulva. *Obstet Gynecol* 1985;66[Suppl]:79.

Christophersen W, Buchsbaum HJ, Voet R, et al. Radical vulvectomy and bilateral groin lymphadenectomy utilizing separate groin incisions: report of a case with recurrence in the intervening skin bridge. *Gynecol Oncol* 1985;21:247.

Chu J, Tamimi HK, Figge DC. Femoral node metastases with negative superficial inguinal nodes in early vulvar cancer. *Am J Obstet Gynecol* 1981;140:337.

Chung AF, Woodruff JM, Lewis JL. Malignant melanoma of the vulva: a report of 44 cases. *Obstet Gynecol* 1975;45:638.

Clark WH, From L, Bernardino EA, et al. The histogenesis and biologic behavior of primary human melanomas of the skin. *Cancer Res* 1969;29:705.

Coates AS, Ingvar CL, Petersen-Schaefer K, et al. Elective lymph node dissection in patients with primary melanoma of the trunk and limbs treated at the Sydney Melanoma Unit from 1960 to 1991. *J Am Coll Surg* 1995;180:402.

Cohen R, Margolius KA, Guidozzi F. Non-gynaecological metastases to the vulva and vagina. *S Afr Med J* 1988;73:159.

Coldiron BM, Goldsmith BA, Robinson JK. Surgical treatment of extramammary Paget's disease: a report of six cases and a reexamination of Mohs micrographic surgery compared with conventional surgical excision. *Cancer* 1991;67:933.

Collins CG, Lee FYL, Roman-Lopez JJ. Invasive carcinoma of the vulva with lymph node metastases. *Am J Obstet Gynecol* 1971;109:446.

Committee on Gynecologic Oncology, International Federation of Obstetricians and Gynecologists. Changes in staging of cancer of the vulva and of the endometrium. *Int J Gynaecol Obstet* 1989;28:189.

Conway H, Hugo NE. Metastatic basal cell carcinoma. *Am J Surg* 1965;110:620.

Copas P, Dyer M, Comas FV, et al. Spindle cell carcinoma of the vulva. *Diagn Gynecol Obstet* 1982;4:235.

Copeland LJ, Cleary K, Sneige N, et al. Neuroendocrine (Merkel cell) carcinoma of the vulva: a case report and review of the literature. *Gynecol Oncol* 1985;22:367.

Copeland LJ, Sneige N, Gershenson DM, et al. Adenoid cystic carcinoma of Bartholin's gland. *Obstet Gynecol* 1986; 67:115.

Copeland LJ, Sneige N, Gershenson DM, et al. Bartholin gland carcinoma. *Obstet Gynecol* 1986b;67:794.

Corney RH, Everett H, Howells A, et al. Psychosocial adjustment following major gynaecological surgery for carcinoma of the cervix and vulva. *J Psychosom Res* 1992;36:561.

Creasman WT. New gynecologic cancer staging. *Obstet Gynecol* 1990;75:287.

Creasman WT. New gynecologic cancer staging. *Gynecol Oncol* 1995;58:157.

Creasman WT, Gallager HS, Rutledge F. Paget's disease of the vulva. *Gynecol Oncol* 1975;3:133.

Creasman WT, Phillips JL, Menck HR. A survey of hospital management practices for vulvar melanoma. *J Am Coll Surg* 1999;188:670.

Creasman WT, Phillips JL, Menck HR. The national cancer database report on early stage invasive vulvar carcinoma. *Cancer* 1997;80:505.

Crowley NJ, Seigler HF. The role of elective lymph node dissection in the management of patients with thick cutaneous melanoma. *Cancer* 1990;66:2522.

Crowther ME, Shepherd JH, Fisher C. Verrucous carcinoma of the vulva containing human papillomavirus-11: case report. *Br J Obstet Gynaecol* 1988;95:414.

Crum CP, Liskow A, Petras P, et al. Vulva intraepithelial neoplasia (severe atypia and carcinoma in situ). A clinicopathologic analysis of 41 cases. *Cancer* 1984;54:1429.

Crum CP. Carcinoma of the vulva: epidemiology and pathogenesis. *Obstet Gynecol* 1992;79:448.

Cruz-Jimenez PR, Abell MR. Cutaneous basal cell carcinoma of the vulva. *Cancer* 1975;36:1860.

Cunningham MJ, Goyer RP, Gibbons SK, et al. Primary radiation, cisplatin, and 5-fluororacil for advanced squamous carcinoma of the vulva. *Gynecol Oncol* 1997;66:258.

Curry SL, Wharton JT, Rutledge F. Positive lymph nodes in vulvar squamous carcinoma. *Gynecol Oncol* 1980;9:63.

Curtin JP, Rubin SC, Jones WB, et al. Paget's disease of the vulva. *Gynecol Oncol* 1990;39:374.

Curtin JP, Saigo P, Slucher B, et al. WJ. Soft-tissue sarcoma of the vagina and vulva: a clinicopathologic study. *Obstet Gynecol* 1995;86:269.

Daly JW, Million RR. Radical vulvectomy combined with elective node irradiation for TXNO squamous carcinoma of the vulva. *Cancer* 1974;34:161.

Davos I, Abell MR. Soft tissue sarcomas of the vulva. *Gynecol Oncol* 1976;4:70.

de Hullu JA, Hollema H, Piers DA, et al. Sentinel lymph node procedure is highly accurate in squamous cell carcinoma of the vulva. *J Clin Oncol* 2000:18;2811.

de Hullu JA, Hollema H, Lolkema S, et al. Vulvar carcinoma. The price of less radical surgery. *Cancer* 2002;95:2331.

de Hullu JA, Hollema H, Hoekstra HJ, et al. Vulvar melanoma. Is there a role for sentinel lymph node biopsy? *Cancer* 2002;94:486.

DeCesare SL, Fiorica JV, Roberts WS, et al. A pilot study utilizing intraoperative lymphoscintigraphy for identification of the sentinel lymph nodes in vulvar cancer. *Gynecol Oncol* 1997;66:425.

Dehner LP. Metastatic and secondary tumors of the vulva. *Obstet Gynecol* 1973;42:47.

Demian SDE, Bushkin FL, Echevarria RA. Perineural invasion and anaplastic transformation of verrucous carcinoma. *Cancer* 1973;32:395.

Deppe G, Cohen C, Bruckner H. Chemotherapy of squamous cell carcinoma of the vulva: a review. *Gynecol Oncol* 1979;7:345.

Deppe G, Malviya VK, Smith PE, et al. Limb salvage in recurrent vulvar carcinoma after rupture of femoral artery. *Gynecol Oncol* 1984;19:120.

Di Bonito L, Patriarca S, Falconieri G. Aggressive "breast-like" adenocarcinoma of vulva. *Pathol Res Pract* 1992;188: 211.

Diagnosis and treatment of peripheral lymphedema, consensus document of the International Society of Lymphology Executive Committee. *Lymphology* 1995;28:113.

DiSaia PJ. Management of superficially invasive vulvar carcinoma. *Clin Obstet Gynecol* 1985;28:196.

DiSaia PJ. The case against the surgical concept of en bloc dissection for certain malignancies of the reproductive tract. *Cancer* 1987;60:2025.

DiSaia PJ, Creasman WT, Rich WM. An alternative approach to early cancer of the vulva. *Am J Obstet Gynecol* 1979;133:825.

DiSaia PJ, Dorion GE, Cappuccini F, et al. A report of two cases of recurrent Paget's disease of the vulva in a split-thickness graft and its possible pathogenesis—labeled "retrodissemination." *Gynecol Oncol* 1995;57:109.

DiSaia PJ, Rutledge F, Smith JP. Sarcoma of the vulva: report of 12 patients. *Obstet Gynecol* 1971;38:180.

Dolan JR, McCall AR, Gooneratne S, et al. DNA ploidy, proliferation index, grade and stage as prognostic factors for vulvar squamous cell carcinomas. *Gynecol Oncol* 1993;48:232.

Donaldson ES, Powell DE, Hanson MB, et al. Prognostic parameters in invasive vulvar cancer. *Gynecol Oncol* 1981;11:184.

Dubreuilh W. Paget's disease of the vulva. *Br J Dermatol* 1901;13:1407.

Dudley AG, Young RH, Lawrence WD, et al. Endodermal sinus tumor of the vulva in an infant. *Obstet Gynecol* 1983;61:76S.

Dudzinski MR, Askin FB, Fowler WC. Giant basal cell carcinoma of the vulva. *Obstet Gynecol* 1984;63:57S.

Echt ML, Finan MA, Hoffman MS, et al. Detection of sentinel lymph nodes with Lymphazurin in cervical, uterine, and vulvar malignancies. *South Med J* 1999;92:204.

Egwuatu VE, Ejeckam GC, Okaro JM. Burkett's lymphoma of the vulva. Case report. *Br J Obstet Gynaecol* 1980;87:827.

Eifel PJ, Morris M, Burke TW, et al. Prolonged continuous infusion cisplatin and 5-fluorouracil with radiation for locally advanced carcinoma of the vulva. *Gynecol Oncol* 1995;59:51.

Elchalal U, Dgani R, Zosmer A, et al. Malignant fibrous histiocytoma of the vagina and vulva successfully treated by combined chemotherapy and radiotherapy. *Gynecol Oncol* 1991;42:91.

Elit L, Hancock G, Carey M, et al. Comparing the morbidity of single versus separate incision surgical approaches to vulvar cancer. *J Gynecol Tech* 1999;5:147.

Enker WE, Heilwell M, Janov AJ, et al. Improved survival in epidermoid carcinoma of the anus in association with preoperative multidisciplinary therapy. *Arch Surg* 1986;121: 1386.

Eriksson JE, Eldh J, Peterson LE. Surgical treatment of carcinoma of the clitoris. *Gynecol Oncol* 1984;17:291.

Evans LS, Kersh CR, Constable WC, et al. Concomitant 5-fluorouracil, mitomycin-C and radiotherapy for advanced gynecologic malignancies. *Int J Radiat Oncol Biol Phys* 1988;15:901.

Ewing TL. Paget's disease of the vulva treated by combined surgery and laser. *Gynecol Oncol* 1991;43:137.

Fairey RN, Mackay PA, Benedet JL, et al. Radiation treatment of carcinoma of the vulva: 1950–1980. *Am J Obstet Gynecol* 1985;151:591.

Fanning J, Lambert L, Hale T, et al. Paget's disease of the vulva: prevalence of associated vulvar adenocarcinoma, invasive Paget's disease, and recurrence after surgical excision. *Am J Obstet Gynecol* 1999;180:24.

Farias-Eisner R, Cirisano FD, Grouse D, et al. Conservative and individualized surgery for early squamous carcinoma of the vulva: the treatment of choice for stage 1 and II (T1-2, N0-1,M0) disease. *Gynecol Oncol* 1994;53:55.

Feuer GA, Shevchuk M, Calanog A. Vulvar Paget's disease: the need to exclude an invasive lesion. *Gynecol Oncol* 1990;38:81.

Figge DC, Tamimi HK, Greer BE. Lymphatic spread in carcinoma of the vulva. *Am J Obstet Gynecol* 1985;152:387.

Finon MA, Fiorica JV, Roberts WS, et al. Artificial dura film for femoral vessel coverage after inguinofemoral lymphadenectomy. *Gynecol Oncol* 1994;55:333.

Fioretti P, Gadducci A, Prato B, et al. The influence of some prognostic factors on the clinical outcome of patients with squamous cell carcinoma of the vulva. *Eur J Gynaecol Oncol* 1992;13:97.

Fiorica JV, Cavanagh D, Roberts WS, et al. Carcinoma-in-situ of the vulva: twenty-four years' experience. *South Med J* 1988;81:589.

Fiorica JV, Roberts WS, LaPolla JP, et al. Femoral vessel coverage with dura mater after inguinofemoral lymphadenectomy. *Gynecol Oncol* 1991;42:217.

Fishman DA, Chambers SK, Schwartz PE, et al. Extramammary Paget's disease of the vulva. *Gynecol Oncol* 1995;56:266.

Flamant F, Gerbaulte A, Nihoul-Fekete C, et al. Long-term sequelae of conservative treatment by surgery, brachytherapy, and chemotherapy for vulval and vaginal rhabdomyosarcoma in children. *J Clin Oncol* 1990;8:1847.

Flannelly GM, Foley ME, Lenehan PM, et al. En bloc radical vulvectomy and lymphadenectomy with modifications of separate groin incisions. *Obstet Gynecol* 1992;79:307.

Fletcher CD, Tsang WY, Fisher C, et al. Angiomyofibroblastoma of the vulva: a benign neoplasm distinct from aggressive angiomyxoma. *Am J Surg Pathol* 1992;16:373.

Franklin EW, Bostwick J III, Burrell MO, et al. Reconstructive techniques in radical pelvic surgery. *Am J Obstet Gynecol* 1977;129:285.

Frankman O. Stage III squamous cell carcinoma of the vulva. Results of a Swedish study. *J Reprod Med* 1991;36:108.

Frankman O, Kabulski Z, Nilsson B, et al. Prognostic factors in invasive squamous cell carcinoma of the vulva. *Int J Gynecol Obstet* 1991;36:219.

Friedrich E, Wilkinson E, Steingraeber P, et al. Paget's disease of the vulva and carcinoma of the breast. *Obstet Gynecol* 1975;46:130.

Friedrich EG, Wilkinson EJ, Fu YS. Carcinoma in situ of the vulva: a continuing challenge. *Am J Obstet Gynecol* 1980;136:830.

Frischbier HJ, Thomsen K. Treatment of cancer of the vulva with high-energy electrons. *Am J Obstet Gynecol* 1971;111:431.

Gadducci A, De Punzio C, Facchini V, et al. The therapy of verrucous carcinoma of the vulva: observations on three cases. *Eur J Gynaecol Oncol* 1989;10:284.

Gallousis S. Verrucous carcinoma: report of three vulvar cases and review of the literature. *Obstet Gynecol* 1972;40:502.

Ganjei P, Giraldo KA, Lampe B, et al. Vulvar Paget's disease: is immunocytochemistry helpful in assessing the surgical margins? *J Reprod Med* 1990;35:1002.

Garbe C, Buttner P, Bertz J, et al. Primary cutaneous melanoma. Identification of prognostic groups and estimation of individual prognosis for 5093 patients. *Cancer* 1995;75:2484.

Garcia C, Boronow RC. Carcinoma of the vulva-anatomic and histologic prognostic facts. *South Med J* 1972;65:237.

Genton CY, Maroni ES. Vulval liposarcoma. *Arch Gynecol* 1987;240:63.

George M, Durrant KR, Mangioni C, et al. Bleomycin (BLM), methotrexate (MTX) and CCNU as neoadjuvant treatment of carcinoma of the vulva. Second International Congress on Neo-Adjuvant Chemotherapy, February 19-21, Paris, 1988:67(abst).

Gershenwald JE, Thompson W, Mansfield PF, et al. Multi-institutional melanoma lymphatic mapping experience: the prognostic value of sentinel lymph node status in 612 stage 1 or II melanoma patients. *J Clin Oncol* 1999;17:976.

Ghamande SA, Kasznica J, Griffiths CT, et al. Mucinous adenocarcinomas of the vulva. *Gynecol Oncol* 1995;57:117.

Gil-Moreno A, Garcia-Jimenez A, Gonzalez-Bosquet J, et al. Merkel cell carcinoma of the vulva. *Gynecol Oncol* 1997;64:526.

Gleeson NC, Hoffman MS, Cavanagh D. Isolated skin bridge metastasis following modified radical vulvectomy and bilateral inguinofemoral lymphadenectomy. *Int J Gynecol Cancer* 1994;4:356.

Gleeson NC, Ruffolo EH, Hoffman MS, et al. Basal cell carcinoma of the vulva with groin node metastasis. *Gynecol Oncol* 1994;53:366.

Goldberg MI, Rothfleisch S. The tensor fascia lata myocutaneous flap in gynecologic oncology. *Gynecol Oncol* 1981;12:41.

Gordinier ME, Steinhoff MM, Hogan JW, et al. S-Phase fraction, p53, and HER-2/neu status as predictors of nodal metastasis in early vulvar cancer. *Gynecol Oncol* 1997;67:200.

Gould N, Kamelle S, Tillmanns T, et al. Predictors of complications after inguinal lymphadenectomy. *Gynecol Oncol* 2001;82:329.

Graziottin A, Maggino T, Francia G, et al. Non mutilant radical vulvectomy vs radical vulvectomy. *Eur J Gynaecol Oncol* 1983;4:128.

Green H. Adenocarcinoma of supernumerary breast of the labia majora in a case of epidermoid carcinoma of the vulva. *Am J Obstet Gynecol* 1936;32:660.

Green TH Jr, Ulfelder H, Meigs JV. Epidermoid carcinoma of the vulva: an analysis of 238 cases. Parts I and II. *Am J Obstet Gynecol* 1958;75:834.

Greenall MJ, Quan SHQ, Stearns MW, et al. Epidermoid cancer of the anal margin: pathologic features, treatment and clinical results. *Am J Surg* 1985;149:95.

Grimshaw RN, Aswad SG, Monaghan JM. The role of anovulvectomy in locally advanced carcinoma of the vulva. *Int Gynecol Cancer* 1991;1:15.

Grimshaw RN, Murdoch JB, Monaghan JM. Radical vulvectomy and bilateral inguino-femoral lymphadenectomy through separate incisions: experience with 100 cases. *Int J Gynecol Cancer* 1993;3:18.

Guerry R, Pratt-Thomas HR. Carcinoma of supernumerary breast of vulva with bilateral mammary cancer. *Cancer* 1976;38:2570.

Guidozzi F, Sadan O, Koller AB, et al. Combined chemotherapy and irradiation therapy after radical surgery for leiomyosarcoma of the vulva. *S Afr Med J* 1987;71:327.

Hacker NF, Berek JS, Juillard GJF, et al. Preoperative radiation therapy for locally advanced vulvar cancer. *Cancer* 1984;54:2056.

Hacker NF, Berek JS, Lagasse LD, et al. Individualization of treatment for stage 1 squamous cell vulvar carcinoma. *Obstet Gynecol* 1984;63:155.

Hacker NF, Berek JS, Lagasse LD, et al. Management of regional lymph nodes and their prognostic influence in vulvar cancer. *Obstet Gynecol* 1983;61:408.

Hacker NF, Leuchter RS, Berek JS, et al. Radical vulvectomy and bilateral inguinal lymphadenectomy through separate groin incisions. *Obstet Gynecol* 1981;58:574.

Hacker NF, Nieberg RK, Berek JS, et al. Superficially invasive vulvar cancer with nodal metastases. *Gynecol Oncol* 1983b;15:65.

Hacker NF, van der Velden J. Conservative management of early vulvar cancer. *Cancer* 1993;71:1673.

Hall DJ, Grimes MM, Coplerud DR. Epithelioid sarcoma of the vulva. Case report. *Gynecol Oncol* 1980;9:237.

Hall JSE, Amin UF. Fibrosarcoma of the vulva: case report and discussion. *Int Surg* 1981;66:185.

Har-Shai Y, Hirshowitz B, Marcovich A, et al. Blood supply and innervation of the supermedial thigh flap employed in one-stage reconstruction of the scrotum and vulva: an anatomical study. *Ann Plast Surg* 1984;13:504.

Hart WR, Millman RB. Progression of intraepithelial Paget's disease of the vulva to invasive carcinoma. *Cancer* 1977;40:2333.

Heaps JM, Fu YS, Montz FJ, et al. Surgical-pathologic variables predictive of local recurrence in squamous cell carcinoma of the vulva. *Gynecol Oncol* 1990;38:309.

Helgason NM, Haas AC, Latourette HB. Radiation therapy in carcinoma of the vulva: a review of 53 patients. *Cancer* 1972;30:997.

Helm CW, Hatch K, Austin JM, et al. A matched comparison of single and triple incision techniques for surgical treatment of carcinoma of the vulva. *Gynecol Oncol* 1992;46:150.

Helm CW, Hatch KD, Partridge EE, et al. The rhomboid transposition flap for repair of the perineal defect after radical vulvar surgery. *Gynecol Oncol* 1993;50:164.

Henderson RH, Parsons JT, Morgan L, et al. Elective ilioinguinal lymph node irradiation. *Int J Radiat Oncol Biol Phys* 1984;10:811.

Hendrix RC, Behrman SJ. Adenocarcinoma arising in a supernumerary mammary gland in the vulva. *Obstet Gynecol* 1956;8:238.

Hensley GT, Friedrich EG. Malignant fibroxanthoma: a sarcoma of the vulva. *Am J Obstet Gynecol* 1973;116:289.

Herod JJO, Shafi MI, Rollason TP, et al. Vulvar intraepithelial neoplasia with superficially invasive carcinoma of the vulva. *Br J Obstet Gynaecol* 1996;103:453.

Herod JJ, Shafi MI, Rollason TP, et al. Vulvar intraepithelial neoplasia: long term follow-up of treated and untreated women. *Br J Obstet Gynaecol* 1996;103:446.

Hilgers RD, Pai R, Bartow SA, et al. Aggressive angiomyxoma of the vulva. *Obstet Gynecol* 1986;68S:60.

Hitchcock CL, Bland KI, Laney RG III, et al. Neuroendocrine (Merkel cell) carcinoma of the skin: its natural history, diagnosis and treatment. *Ann Surg* 1988;207:201.

Hoffman JS, Kumar NB, Morley GW. Microinvasive squamous carcinoma of the vulva: search for a definition. *Obstet Gynecol* 1983;61:615.

Hoffman JS, Kumar NB, Morley GW. Prognostic significance of groin lymph node metastasis in squamous carcinoma of the vulva. *Obstet Gynecol* 1985;66:402.

Hoffman MS, Cavanagh D, Roberts WS, et al. Ultraradical surgery for advanced carcinoma of the vulva: an update. *Int J Gynecol Cancer* 1993;3:369.

Hoffman MS, Greenberg H, Roberts WS, et al. Management of locally advanced squamous cell carcinoma of the vulva. *J Gynecol Surg* 1991;7:175.

Hoffman MS, Greenberg S, Greenberg H, et al. The use of interstitial needles for the treatment of advanced or recurrent vulvar and distal vaginal malignancy. *Am J Obstet Gynecol* 1990;162:1278.

Hoffman MS, Gunasekaran S, Arango H, et al. Lateral microscopic extension of squamous cell carcinoma of the vulva. *Gynecol Oncol* 1999;73:72.

Hoffman MS, LaPolla JP, Roberts WS, et al. Use of local flaps for primary anal reconstruction following perianal resection for neoplasia. *Gynecol Oncol* 1990;36:348.

Hoffman MS, Mark JE, Cavanagh D. A management scheme for postoperative groin lymphocysts. *Gynecol Oncol* 1995;56:262.

Hoffman MS, Roberts WR, LaPolla JP, et al. Carcinoma of the vulva involving the perianal or anal skin. *Gynecol Oncol* 1989;35:215.

Hoffman MS, Roberts WS, Finan MA, et al. A comparative study of radical vulvectomy and modified radical vulvectomy for the treatment of invasive squamous cell carcinoma of the vulva. *Gynecol Oncol* 1992;45:192.

Hoffman MS, Roberts WS, LaPolla JP, et al. Recent modifications in the treatment of invasive squamous cell carcinoma of the vulva. *Obstet Gynecol Surv* 1989;44:227.

Hoffman MS, Roberts WS, Ruffolo EH. Basal cell carcinoma of the vulva with inguinal lymph node metastases. *Gynecol Oncol* 1988;29:113.

Homesley HD, Bundy BN, Sedlis A, et al. Assessment of current International Federation of Gynecology and Obstetrics staging of vulvar carcinoma relative to prognostic factors for survival (a Gynecologic Oncology Group study). *Am J Obstet Gynecol* 1991;164:997.

Homesley HD, Bundy BN, Sedlis A, et al. Prognostic factors for groin node metastasis in squamous cell carcinoma of the vulva (a Gynecologic Oncology Group study). *Gynecol Oncol* 1993;49:279.

Homesley HD, Bundy BN, Sedlis A, et al. Radiation therapy versus pelvic node resection for carcinoma of the vulva with positive groin nodes. *Obstet Gynecol* 1986;68:733.

Hopkins MP, Morley GW. Pelvic exenteration for the treatment of vulvar cancer. *Cancer* 1992;70:2835.

Hopkins MP, Reid GC, Johnston CM, et al. A comparison of staging systems for squamous cell carcinoma of the vulva. *Gynecol Oncol* 1992;47:34.

Hopkins MP, Reid GC, Morley GW. Radical vulvectomy. The decision for the incision. *Cancer* 1993;72:799.

Hopkins MP, Reid GC, Morley GW. The surgical management of recurrent squamous cell carcinoma of the vulva. *Obstet Gynecol* 1990;75:1001.

Hopkins MP, Reid GC, Vettrano I, et al. Squamous cell carcinoma of the vulva: prognostic factors influencing survival. *Gynecol Oncol* 1991;43:113.

Hording U, Junge J, Poulsen H, et al. Vulvar intraepithelial neoplasia III: a viral disease of undetermined potential. *Gynecol Oncol* 1995;56:276.

Hoyme UB, Tamimi HK, Eschenbach DA, et al. Osteomyelitis pubis after radical gynecologic operations. *Obstet Gynecol* 1984;63:47.

Husseinzadeh N, Recinto C. Frequency of invasive cancer in surgically excised vulvar lesions with intraepithelial neoplasia (VIN 3). *Gynecol Oncol* 1999;73:119.

Husseinzadeh N, Wesseler T, Newman N, et al. Neuroendocrine (Merkel cell) carcinoma of the vulva. *Gynecol Oncol* 1988;29:105.

Husseinzadeh N, Wesseler T, Schneider D, et al. Prognostic factors and the significance of cytologic grading in invasive squamous cell carcinoma of the vulva: a clinicopathologic study. *Gynecol Oncol* 1990;36:192.

Imachi M, Tsukamoto N, Kamura T, et al. Alveolar rhabdomyosarcoma of the vulva: report of two cases. *Acta Cytol* 1991;35:345.

Imachi M, Tsukamoto N, Shigematsu T, et al. Cytologic diagnosis of primary adenocarcinoma of Bartholin's gland: a case report. *Acta Cytol* 1992;36:167.

Irvin W, Pelkey T, Rice L, et al. Endometrial stromal sarcoma of the vulva arising in extraovarian endometriosis: a case report and literature review. *Gynecol Oncol* 1998;71:313.

Irvin WP, Cathro HP, Grosh WW, et al. Primary breast carcinoma of the vulva: a case report and literature review. *Gynecol Oncol* 1999;73:155.

Irvin Jr WP, Legallo RL, Stoler MH, et al. Vulvar melanoma: a retrospective analysis and literature review. *Gynecol Oncol* 2001;83:457.

Isaacs JH. Verrucous carcinoma of the female genital tract. *Gynecol Oncol* 1976;4:259.

Itala J, de Paola GR, Gomez-Rueda N, et al. Melanoma of the vulva: the experience of the University of Buenos Aires. *J Reprod Med* 1986;31:836.

Iversen T. Irradiation and bleomycin in the treatment of inoperable vulvar carcinoma. *Acta Obstet Gynecol Scand* 1982;61:195.

Iversen T. New approaches to the treatment of squamous cell carcinoma of the vulva. In: Pitkin RM, Scott JR, Kaufman RH, et al, eds. *Clinical obstetrics and gynecology*, vol 28. Philadelphia: Harper & Row, 1985:204.

Iversen T. Squamous cell carcinoma of the vulva: localization of the primary tumor and lymph node metastases. *Acta Obstet Gynecol Scand* 1981;60:211.

Iversen T. The value of groin palpation in epidermoid carcinoma of the vulva. *Gynecol Oncol* 1981;12:291.

Iversen T, Aalders JG, Christensen A, et al. Squamous cell carcinoma of the vulva: a review of 424 patients, 1956-1974. *Gynecol Oncol* 1983;9:271.

Iversen T, Aas M. Lymph drainage from the vulva. *Gynecol Oncol* 1983;16:179.

Iversen T, Abeler V, Aalders J. Individualized treatment of stage 1 carcinoma of the vulva. *Obstet Gynecol* 1981;57:85.

Jafari K, Magalotti M. Radiation therapy in carcinoma of the vulva. *Cancer* 1981;47:686.

Japaze H, Dinh TV, Woodruff JD. Verrucous carcinoma of the vulva: study of 24 cases. *Obstet Gynecol* 1982;60:462.

Jaramillo BA, Ganjei P, Averette HE, et al. Malignant melanoma of the vulva. *Obstet Gynecol* 1985;66:398.

Johnson TL, Kumar NB, White CD, et al. Prognostic features of vulvar melanoma: a clinicopathologic analysis. *Int J Gynecol Pathol* 1986;5:110.

Jones MA, Mann EW, Caldwell CL, et al. Small cell neuroendocrine carcinoma of Bartholin's gland. *Am J Clin Pathol* 1990;94:439.

Jones RW, Baranyai J, Stables S. Trends in squamous cell carcinoma of the vulva: the influence of vulvar intraepithelial neoplasia. *Obstet Gynecol* 1997;90:448.

Jones RW, Rowan DM. Vulvar intraepithelial neoplasia III: a clinical study of the outcome in 113 cases with relation to the later development of invasive vulvar carcinoma. *Obstet Gynecol* 1994;84:741.

Julian CG, Callison J, Woodruff JD. Plastic management of extensive vulvar defects. *Obstet Gynecol* 1971;38:193.

Kadar N, Nelson JH. Sling operation for total incontinence following radical vulvectomy. *Obstet Gynecol* 1984;64[Suppl]:85.

Kalra JK, Grossman AM, Krumholz BA, et al. Preoperative chemoradiotherapy for carcinoma of the vulva. *Gynecol Oncol* 1981;12:256.

Kaplan AL, Kaufman RH. Management of advanced carcinoma of the vulva. *Gynecol Oncol* 1975;3:220.

Karakousis CP, Emrich LJ. Tumor thickness and prognosis in clinical stage I malignant melanoma. *Cancer* 1989; 64:1432.

Kehrer E. Soll das vulvakarzinom operiert oder bestrahlt werden? *Geburtsch & Franuenk* 1918;48:346.

Kelley JL III, Burke TW, Tornos C, et al. Minimally invasive vulvar carcinoma: an indication for conservative surgical therapy. *Gynecol Oncol* 1992;44:240.

Kennedy JC, Majmuder B. Primary adenocarcinoma of the vulva, possibly cloacogenic: a report of two cases. *J Reprod Med* 1993;38:113.

Keys H. Gynecologic Oncology Group randomized trials of combined technique therapy for vulvar cancer. *Cancer* 1993;71:1691.

Khansur T, Sanders J, Das SK. Evaluation of staging workup in malignant melanoma. *Arch Surg* 1989;24:847.

Kim SH, Garcia C, Rodriguez J, et al. Prognosis of thick cutaneous melanoma. *J Am Coll Surg* 1999;188:241.

King LA, Downey GO, Savage JE, et al. Resection of the pubic bone as an adjunct to management of primary, recurrent and metastatic pelvic malignancies. *Obstet Gynecol* 1989;73:1022.

Kirkwood JM, Strawderman MH, Ernstoff MS, et al. Interferon alfa-2b adjuvant therapy of high risk resected cutaneous melanoma: the Eastern Cooperative Oncology Group Trial EST 1684. *J Clin Oncol* 1996;14:7.

Kirschner CV, Yordan EL, Geest KD, et al. Smoking, obesity, and survival in squamous cell carcinoma of the vulva. *Gynecol Oncol* 1995;56:79.

Knapstein PG. Reconstructive procedures following extended vulvectomy. In: Knapstein PG, diRe F, DiSaia P, et al, eds. *Malignancies of the vulva.* New York, Theime Medical Publishers, 1991.

Kneale BL. Microinvasive cancer of the vulva: report of the International Society for the Study of Vulvar Disease Task Force, VIIth Congress. *J Reprod Med* 1984;29:454.

Kodama S, Kaneko T, Saito M, et al. A clinicopathologic study of 30 patients with Paget's disease of the vulva. *Gynecol Oncol* 1995;56:63.

Koh W-J, Wallace III J, Greer BE, et al. Combined radiotherapy and chemotherapy in the management of local-regional advanced vulvar cancer. *Int J Rad Onc Biol Phys* 1993;26:809.

Konefka T, Senkus E, Emerich J, et al. Epithelial sarcoma of the Bartholin's gland primarily diagnosed as vulvar sarcoma. *Gynecol Oncol* 1994;54:393.

Krag Miller LB, Nygaard Nielsen M, Trolle C. Leiomyosarcoma vulvae. *Acta Obstet Gynecol Scand* 1990;69:187.

Krupp PJ, Bohm JW. Lymph gland metastases in invasive squamous cell cancer of the vulva. *Am J Obstet Gynecol* 1978;130:943.

Krupp PJ, Lee FY, Bohm JW, et al. Prognostic parameters and clinical staging criteria in epidermoid carcinoma of the vulva. *Obstet Gynecol* 1975;46:84.

Kuipers T. Carcinoma of the vulva. *Radiol Clin* 1975;44:475.

Kuller JA, Zucker PK, Peng TC. Vulvar leiomyosarcoma in pregnancy. *Am J Obstet Gynecol* 1990;162:164.

Kuppers V, Stiller M, Somville T, et al. Risk factors for recurrent VIN: Role of multifocality and grade of disease. *J Reprod Med* 1997;42:138.

Kurzl R, Messerer D. Prognostic factors in squamous cell carcinoma of the vulva: a multivariate analysis. *Gynecol Oncol* 1989;32:143.

Lambrou NC, Mirhashemi R, Wolfson A, et al. Malignant peripheral nerve sheath tumor of the vulva: a multimodal treatment approach. *Gynecol Oncol* 2002;85:365.

Landoni F, Maneo A, Zanetta G, et al. Concurrent preoperative chemotherapy with 5-fluororacil and mitomycin-C and radiotherapy (FUMIR) followed by limited surgery in locally advanced and recurrent vulvar carcinoma. *Gynecol Oncol* 1996;61:321.

Landoni F, Proserpio M, Maneo A, et al. Skin flap reconstruction of the perineal defect after radical vulvar surgery. *J Gynecol Surg* 1995;11:165.

Landthaler M, Braun-Falco O, Leitl A, et al. Excisional biopsy as the first therapeutic procedure versus primary wide excision of malignant melanoma. *Cancer* 1989;64:1612.

Lavie O, Comerci G, Daras V, et al. Thrombocytosis in women with vulvar carcinoma. *Gynecol Oncol* 1999;72:82.

Lawton FG, Hacker NF. Surgery for invasive gynecologic cancer in the elderly female population. *Obstet Gynecol* 1990;76:287.

Lawton G, Rasque H, Ariyan S. Preservation of muscle fascia to decrease lymphedema after complete axillary and ilioinguinofemoral lymphadenectomy for melanoma. *J Am Coll Surg* 2002;195:339.

Leake JF, Buscema J, Cho KR, et al. Dermatofibrosarcoma protuberans of the vulva. *Gynecol Oncol* 1991;41:245.

Leiserowitz GS, Russell AH, Kinney WK, et al. Prophylactic chemoradiation of inguinofemoral lymph nodes in patients with locally extensive vulvar cancer. *Gynecol Oncol* 1997; 66:509.

Lenaz MP, Nguyen TC, Hewett WJ. Leiomyosarcoma of the vulva. *Conn Med* 1987;51:705.

Lens MB, Dawes M, Goodacre T, et al. Elective lymph node dissection in patients with melanoma. Systemic review and meta-analysis of randomized controlled trials. *Arch Surg* 2002;137:458.

Lens MB, Dawes M, Goodacre T, et al. Excision margins in the treatment of primary cutaneous melanoma. A systematic review of randomized controlled trials comparing narrow vs. wide excision. *Arch Surg* 2002;137:1101.

Leuchter RS, Hacker NF, Voet RL, et al. Primary carcinoma of the Bartholin gland: a report of 14 cases and review of the literature. *Obstet Gynecol* 1982;60:361.

Levenback C, Coleman RL, Burke TW, et al. Intraoperative lymphatic mapping and sentinel node identification with blue dye in patients with vulvar cancer. *Gynecol Oncol* 2001;83:276.

Levenback C, Burke TW, Gershenson DM, et al. Intraoperative lymphatic mapping for vulvar cancer. *Obstet Gynecol* 1994;84:163.

Levenback C, Morris M, Burke TW, et al. Groin dissection practices among gynecologic oncologists treating early vulvar cancer. *Gynecol Oncol* 1996;62:73.

Levin M, Pakarakas RM, Chang HA, et al. Primary breast carcinoma of the vulva: a case report and review of the literature. *Gynecol Oncol* 1995;56:448.

Levin W, Rad FF, Goldberg G, et al. The use of concomitant chemotherapy and radiotherapy prior to surgery in advanced stage carcinoma of the vulva. *Gynecol Oncol* 1986;25:20.

Lewandowski G, O'Toole RV, Delgado G, et al. Carcinoma of the vulva. Significance of surgical margin involvement in assessing prognosis. *J Reprod Med* 1989;34:884.

Lin JY, DuBeshter B, Angel C, et al. Morbidity and recurrence with modifications of radical vulvectomy and groin dissection. *Gynecol Oncol* 1992;47:80.

Loree TR, Hempling RE, Eltabbakh GH, et al. The inferior gluteal flap in the difficult vulvar and perineal reconstruction. *Gynecol Oncol* 1997;66:429.

Loret de Mola Jr, Hudock PA, Steinetz C, et al. Merkel cell carcinoma of the vulva. *Gynecol Oncol* 1993;51:272.

Lotem M, Anteby S, Peretz T, et al. Mucosal melanoma of the female genital tract is a multifocal disorder. *Gynecol Oncol* 2003;88:45.

Lovett RD, Kuske RR, Perez CA, et al. Preliminary evaluation of toxicity and tumor response to radiotherapy with cisplatin and 5-fluorouracil for advanced or recurrent gynecologic malignancies. *Rad Oncol Biol Phys* 1987;13:129.

Lupi G, Raspagliesi F, Zucali R, et al. Combined preoperative chemoradiotherapy followed by radical surgery in locally advanced vulvar carcinoma. *Cancer* 1996;77:1472.

Mader MH, Friedrich EG Jr. Vulvar metastasis of breast carcinoma: a case report. *J Reprod Med* 1982;27:169.

Maggino T, Landoni F, Sartori E, et al. Patterns of recurrence in patients with squamous cell carcinoma of the vulva: a multicenter CTF study. *Cancer* 2000;89:116.

Magrina JF, Gonzalez-Bosquet J, Weaver AL, et al. Squamous cell carcinoma of the vulva stage 1A: long-term results. *Gynecol Oncol* 2000;76:24.

Magrina JF, Webb MJ, Gaffey TA, et al. Stage 1 squamous cell cancer of the vulva. *Am J Obstet Gynecol* 1979;134:453.

Malfetano J, Piver MS, Tsukada Y. Stage III and IV squamous cell carcinomas of the vulva. *Gynecol Oncol* 1986;23:192.

Malfetano JH, Piver MS, Tsukada Y, et al. Univariate and multivariate analyses of 5-year survival, recurrence, and inguinal node metastases in stage I and II vulvar carcinoma. *J Surg Oncol* 1985;30:124.

Mariani L, Conti L, Atlante G, et al. Vulvar squamous carcinoma: prognostic role of DNA context. *Gynecol Oncol* 1998;71:159.

Marsden DE, Hacker NF. Urinary problems following simple and radical vulvectomy. *J Gynecol Oncol* 2002;7:61.

Massad LS, DeGeest K. Multimodality therapy for carcinoma of the Bartholin Gland. *Gynecol Oncol* 1999;75:305.

Matias C, Nunes JF, Vicente LF, et al. Primary malignant rhabdoid tumour of the vulva. *Histopathology* 1990;17:576.

Mayer AR, Rodriguez RL. Vulvar reconstruction using a pedicle flap based on the superficial external pudendal artery. *Obstet Gynecol* 1991;78[Suppl]:964.

McCall AR, Olson MC, Potkui RK. The variation of inguinal lymph node depth in adult women and its importance in planning elective irradiation for vulvar cancer. *Cancer* 1995;75:2286.

McClay EF, Mastrangello MJ, Sprandio JD, et al. The importance of tamoxifen to a cisplatin-containing regimen in the treatment of metastatic melanoma. *Cancer* 1989;63:1292.

McClintock J, Hoffman MS, Fiorica JV, et al. Vulvar melanoma: a retrospective review of prognostic factors and outcome. *J Gynecol Surg* 1998;14:25.

McCraw JB, Massey FM, Shaklin KD, et al. Vaginal reconstruction with gracilis myocutaneous flaps. *Plast Reconstr Surg* 1976;58:176.

McKee PH, Hertogs KT. Endocervical adenocarcinoma and vulvar Paget's disease: a significant association. *Br J Dermatol* 1980;103:443.

Menzin AW, DeRisi D, Smilari TF, et al. Lobular breast carcinoma metastatic to the vulva: a case report and literature review. *Gynecol Oncol* 1998;69:84.

Merino MJ, LiVolsi VA, Schwartz PE, et al. Adenoid basal cell carcinoma of the vulva. *Int J Gynecol Pathol* 1982;1:299.

Mesko JD, Gates H, McDonald TW, et al. Clear cell ("mesonephroid") adenocarcinoma of the vulva arising in endometriosis: a case report. *Gynecol Oncol* 1988;29:385.

Messing MJ, Gallup DG. Carcinoma of the vulva in young women. *Obstet Gynecol* 1995;86:51.

Messing MJ, Richardson MS, Smith MT, et al. Metastatic clear-cell hidradenocarcinoma of the vulva. *Gynecol Oncol* 1994;48:264.

Micheletti L, Preti M, Zola P, et al. A proposed glossary of terminology related to the surgical treatment of vulvar carcinoma. *Cancer* 1998;83:1369.

Microinvasive cancer of the vulva: report of the ISSVD Task Force. *J Reprod Med* 1984;29:454.

Miller B, Morris M, Levenback C, et al. Pelvic exenteration for primary and recurrent vulvar cancer. *Gynecol Oncol* 1995; 58:202.

Misas JE, Cold CJ, Hall FW. Vulvar Paget's disease: fluorescein-aided visualization of margins. *Obstet Gynecol* 1991;97:156.

Misas JE, Larson JE, Podczaski E, et al. Recurrent Paget's disease of the vulva in a split-thickness graft. *Obstet Gynecol* 1990;76:543.

Mitchell MF, Prasad CJ, Silva EG, et al. Second genital primary squamous neoplasms in vulvar carcinoma. viral and histopathologic correlates. *Obstet Gynecol* 1993;81:13.

Miyazawa K, Nori D, Hilaris BS, et al. Role of radiation therapy in the treatment of advanced vulvar carcinoma. *J Reprod Med* 1983;28:539.

Modesitt SC, Waters AB, Walton L, et al. Vulvar intraepithelial neoplasia III: occult cancer and the impact of margin status on recurrence. *Obstet Gynecol* 1998;92:962.

Moller LBK, Nielsen MN, Trolle C. Leiomyosarcoma vulvae. *Acta Obstet Gynecol Scand* 1990;69:187.

Monaghan JM, Hammond IG. Pelvic node dissection in the treatment of vulval carcinoma: is it necessary? *Br J Obstet Gynaecol* 1984;91:270.

Monk BJ, Burger RA, Fritz L, et al. Prognostic significance of human papillomavirus DNA in vulvar carcinoma. *Obstet Gynecol* 1995;85:709.

Montana GS, Thomas GM, Moore DH, et al. Preoperative chemo-radiation for carcinoma of the vulva with N2/N3 nodes: a gynecologic oncology group study. *Int J Radiation Oncology Biol Phys* 2000;48:1007.

Moore RG, Steinhoff MM, Granai CO, et al. Vulvar Epithelioid sarcoma in pregnancy. *Gynecol Oncol* 2002;85:218.

Morley GW. Cancer of the vulva: a review. *Cancer* 1981; 48[Suppl 2]:597.

Morley GW. Infiltrative carcinoma of the vulva: results of surgical treatment. *Am J Obstet Gynecol* 1976;124:874.

Morrow CP, DiSaia PJ. Malignant melanoma of the female genitalia: a clinical analysis. *Obstet Gynecol Surv* 1976;31:233.

Mulayim N, Silver DF, Ocal IT, et al. Vulvar basal cell carcinoma: two unusual presentations and review of the literature. *Gynecol Oncol* 2002;85:532.

Nahai F. The tensor fascia lata flap. *Clin Plast Surg* 1980;7:51.

National Comprehensive Cancer Network (NCCN) melanoma practice guidelines. *Oncology* 1998;NCCN Proc 3:153.

National Institutes of Health Consensus Development Panel on Early Melanoma. Diagnosis and treatment of early melanoma. *JAMA* 1992;268:1314.

Ndubisi B, Kaminski PF, Olt G, et al. Staging and recurrence of disease in squamous cell carcinoma of the vulva. *Gynecol Oncol* 1995;59:34.

Newman PL, Fletcher CDM. Smooth muscle tumors of the external genitalia: clinicopathological analysis of a series. *Histopathology* 1991;18:523.

Nicklin JL, Hacker NF, Heintze SW, et al. An anatomical study of inguinal lymph node topography and clinical implications for the surgical management of vulvar cancer. *Int J Gynecol Cancer* 1995;5:128.

Nielsen GP, Rosenberg AE, Koerner FC, et al. Smooth-muscle tumors of the vulva. A clinicopathological study of 25 cases and review of the literature. *Am J Surg Path* 1996;20:779.

Nobler MP. Efficacy of a perineal teletherapy portal in the management of vulvar and vaginal cancer. *Ther Radiol* 1972;103:393.

Nori D, Cain JM, Hilaris BS, et al. Metronidazole as a radiosensitizer and high-dose radiation in advanced vulvovaginal malignancies: a pilot study. *Gynecol Oncol* 1983;16:117.

Odongo FN, Ojwang SB. Verrucous carcinoma of the vulva: report of two cases managed at Kenyetta National Hospital, and literature review. *East Afr Med J* 1990;67:830.

Ogino M, Sakamoto T, Inoue J, et al. Reconstruction of surgical defects using the gluteus maximus myocutaneous flap following radical vulvectomy. *Asia Oceania J Obstet Gynaecol* 1992;18:23.

Origoni M, Sideri M, Garsia S, et al. Prognostic value of pathological patterns of lymph node positivity in squamous cell carcinoma of the vulva stage III and IVA FIGO. *Gynecol Oncol* 1992;45:313.

Paget J. On disease of the mammary areola preceding cancer of the mammary gland. *St Barth Hosp Reports* 1874;10:87.

Paladini D, Cross O, Lopes A, et al. Prognostic significance of lymph node variables in squamous cell carcinoma of the vulva. *Cancer* 1994;74:2491.

Paley PJ, Johnson PR, Adcock LL, et al. The effect of sartorius transposition on wound morbidity following inguinal-femoral lymphadenectomy. *Gynecol Oncol* 1997;64:237.

Pao WM, Perez CA, Kuske RR, et al. Radiation therapy and conservation surgery for primary and recurrent carcinoma of the vulva: report of 40 patients and a review of the literature. *Int J Radiat Oncol Biol Phys* 1988;14:1123.

Parazzini F, Vecchia CL, Garsia S, et al. Determinants of invasive vulvar cancer risk: an Italian case-control study. *Gynecol Oncol* 1993;48:50.

Parker RT, Duncan I, Rampone J, et al. Operative management of early invasive epidermoid carcinoma of the vulva. *Am J Obstet Gynecol* 1975;123:349.

Parmley T, Woodruff J, Julian C. Invasive vulvar Paget's disease. *Obstet Gynecol* 1975;46:341.

Parry-Jones E. Lymphatics of the vulva. *J Obstet Gynaecol Br Commonw* 1963;70:751.

Partridge EE, Murad R, Shingleton HM, et al. Verrucous lesions of the female genitalia. II. Verrucous carcinoma. *Am J Obstet Gynecol* 1980;137:419.

Patsner B, Mann WJ Jr. Radical vulvectomy and "sneak" superficial inguinal lymphadenectomy with a single elliptic incision. *Am J Obstet Gynecol* 1988;158:464.

Patsner B, Hetzler P. Post-radical vulvectomy reconstruction using the inferiorly based transverse rectus abdominis (TRAM) flap: a preliminary experience. *Gynecol Oncol* 1994; 55:78.

Patsner B, Mann WJ. Serum squamous cell carcinoma antigen levels in patients with invasive squamous vulvar and vaginal cancer: a preliminary report. *Gynecol Oncol* 1989;33:323.

Pelosi G, Martignoni G, Bonetti F. Intraductal carcinoma of mammary-type apocrine epithelium arising within a papillary hydradenoma of the vulva: report of a case and review of the literature. *Arch Pathol Lab Med* 1991;115:1249.

Perez CA, Grigsby PW, Galakatos A, et al. Radiation therapy in management of carcinoma of the vulva with emphasis on conservation therapy. *Cancer* 1993;71:3707.

Perez CA, Kraus FT, Evans JC, et al. Anaplastic transformation in verrucous carcinoma of the oral cavity after radiation therapy. *Radiology* 1966;86:108.

Perrone T, Swanson PE, Twiggs L, et al. Malignant rhabdoid tumor of the vulva: is distinction from epithelioid sarcoma possible? *Am J Surg Pathol* 1989;13:848.

Perrone T, Twiggs LB, Adcock LL, et al. Vulvar basal cell carcinoma: an infrequently metastasizing neoplasm. *Int J Gynecol Pathol* 1987;6:152.

Petry KU, Kochel H, Bode U, et al. Human papillomavirus is associated with the frequent detection of warty and basaloid high-grade neoplasia of the vulva and cervical neoplasia among immunocompromised women. *Gynecol Oncol* 1996;60:30.

Phillips B, Buchsbaum HJ, Lifshitz S. Pelvic exenteration for vulvovaginal carcinoma. *Am J Obstet Gynecol* 1981;141:1038.

Phillips GL, Bundy BN, Okagaki T, et al. Malignant melanoma of the vulva treated by radical hemivulvectomy. *Cancer* 1994;73:2626.

Phillips GL, Twiggs LB, Okagaki T. Vulvar melanoma: a microstaging study. *Gynecol Oncol* 1982;14:80.

Pickel H. Early stromal invasion of the vulva. *Eur J Gynaecol Oncol* 1989;10:97.

Pinto AP, Signorello LB, Crum CP, et al. Squamous cell carcinoma of the vulva in Brazil: prognostic importance of host and viral variables. *Gynecol Oncol* 1999;74:61.

Pirtoli L, Rottoli ML. Results of radiation therapy for vulvar carcinoma. *Acta Radiol Oncol* 1982;21:45.

Piura B, Masotina A, Murdoch J, et al. Recurrent squamous cell carcinoma of the vulva: a study of 73 cases. *Gynecol Oncol* 1993;48:189.

Piver MS, Barlow JJ, Wang JJ, et al. Combined radical surgery, radiation therapy and chemotherapy in infants with vulvovaginal and embryonal rhabdomyosarcoma. *Obstet Gynecol* 1973;42:522.

Piver MS, Xynos FP. Pelvic lymphadenectomy in women with carcinoma of the clitoris. *Obstet Gynecol* 1977;49:592.

Plentl AA, Friedman EA. Clinical significance of vulvar lymphatics. Lymphatic system of the female genitalia: the morphologic basis of oncologic diagnosis and therapy. In: Plentl AA, Friedman EA. *Major problems in obstetrics and gynecology*, vol 2. Philadelphia, WB Saunders, 1971:27.

Plouffe K Jr, Tulandi T, Rosenberg A, et al. Non-Hodgkin's lymphoma in Bartholin's gland: case report and review of literature. *Am J Obstet Gynecol* 1984;148:608.

Podczaski E, Stryker J, Banducci D, et al. Multimodality approach to a massive carcinoma of the vulva. *Eur J Gynecol Oncol* 1990;11:415.

Podratz KC, Gaffey TA, Symmonds RE, et al. Melanoma of the vulva: an update. *Gynecol Oncol* 1983;16:153.

Podratz KC, Symmonds RE, Taylor WF, et al. Carcinoma of the vulva: analysis of treatment and survival. *Obstet Gynecol* 1983;61:63.

Podratz KC, Symmonds RE, Taylor WF. Carcinoma of the vulva: analysis of treatment failures. *Am J Obstet Gynecol* 1982;143:340.

Potkul RK, Barnes WA, Barter JF, et al. Vulvar reconstruction using a mons pubis pedicle flap. *Gynecol Oncol* 1994;55:21.

Powell JL, Donovan JT, Reed WP. Hip disarticulation for recurrent vulvar cancer in the groin. *Gynecol Oncol* 1992; 47:110.

Prempree T, Amornmarn R. Radiation treatment of recurrent carcinoma of the vulva. *Cancer* 1984;54:1943.

Preti M, Ronco G, Ghiringhello B, et al. Recurrent squamous cell carcinoma of the vulva. Clinicopathologic determinants identifying low risk patients. *Cancer* 2000;88:1869.

Proffitt SD, Spooner TR, Kosek JC. Origin of undifferentiated neoplasm from verrucous carcinoma of the oral cavity following irradiation. *Cancer* 1970;26:389.

Puig-Tintoré LM, Ordi J, Vidal-Sicart S, et al. Further data on the usefulness of sentinel lymph node identification and ultrastaging in vulvar squamous cell carcinoma. *Gynecol Oncol* 2003;88:29.

Raber G, Mempel V, Jackisch C, et al. Malignant melanoma of the vulva. Report of 89 patients. *Cancer* 1996;78:2353.

Ragnarsson-Olding B, Johansson H, Rutqvist L-E, et al. Malignant melanoma of the vulva and vagina: trends in incidence, age distribution, and long-term survival among 245 consecutive cases in Sweden 1960-1984. *Cancer* 1993; 71:1983.

Ragnarsson-Olding BK, Kanter-Lewensohn LR, Lagerlof B, et al. Malignant melanoma of the vulva in a nationwide, 25-year study of 219 Swedish females. Clinical observations and histopathologic features. *Cancer* 1999;86:1273.

Ragnarsson-Olding BK, Nilsson BR, Kanter-Lewensohn LR, et al. Malignant melanoma of the vulva in a nationwide, 25-year study of 219 Swedish females. Predictors of survival. *Cancer* 1999;86:1285.

Reid GC, Delancey JOL, Hopkins MP, et al. Urinary incontinence following radical vulvectomy. *Obstet Gynecol* 1990;75:852.

Reid R. Local and distant skin flaps in the reconstruction of vulvar deformities. *Am J Obstet Gynecol* 1997;177:1372.

Reintgen DS, Cox EB, McCarty KS, et al. Efficacy of elective lymph node dissection in patients with intermediate thickness primary melanoma. *Ann Surg* 1983;198:379.

Remmenga S, Barnhill D, Nash J, et al. Radical vulvectomy with partial rectal resection and temporary colostomy as primary therapy for selected patients with vulvar carcinoma. *Obstet Gynecol* 1991;77:577.

Roberts WS, Hoffman MS, LaPolla JP, et al. Management of radionecrosis of the vulva and distal vagina. *Am J Obstet Gynecol* 1991;164:1235.

Roberts WS, Kavanagh JJ, Greenberg H, et al. Concomitant radiation therapy and chemotherapy in the treatment of advanced squamous carcinoma of the lower female genital tract. *Gynecol Oncol* 1989;34:183.

Rockson SG, Miller LT, Senie R, et al. Workgroup III: diagnosis and management of lymphedema. *Cancer* 1998; 83:2882.

Rodriguez A, Isaac MA, Hidalgo E, et al. Villoglandular adenocarcinoma of the vulva. *Gynecol Oncol* 2001;83:409.

Rogo KO, Andersson R, Adbom G, et al. Conservative surgery for vulvovaginal melanoma. *Eur J Gynaecol Oncol* 1991;12:113.

Rose PG, Piver S, Tsukada Y, et al. Conservative therapy for melanoma of the vulva. *Am J Obstet Gynecol* 1988;159:52.

Rose PG, Roman LD, Reale FR, et al. Primary adenocarcinoma of the breast arising in the vulva. *Obstet Gynecol* 1990;76:537.

Rose PG, Tak WK, Reale FR, et al. Adenoid cystic carcinoma of the vulva: a radiosensitive tumor. *Gynecol Oncol* 1991;43:81.

Rosen C, Malmstrom H. Invasive cancer of the vulva. *Gynecol Oncol* 1997;65:213.

Rosenberg P, Simonsen E, Risberg B. Adenoid cystic carcinoma of Bartholin's gland: a report of five new cases treated with surgery and radiotherapy. *Gynecol Oncol* 1988;34:145.

Ross MJ, Ehrmann RL. Histologic prognosticators in stage I squamous cell carcinoma of the vulva. *Obstet Gynecol* 1987;70:774.

Rotmensch J, Rubin SJ, Sutton HG, et al. Preoperative radiotherapy followed by radical vulvectomy with inguinal lymphadenectomy for advanced vulvar carcinomas. *Gynecol Oncol* 1990;36:181.

Rouzier R, Haddad B, Dubernard G, et al. Inguinofemoral dissection for carcinoma of the vulva: effect of modifications of extent and technique on morbidity and survival. *J Am Coll Surg* 2003;196:442.

Rowley KC, Gallion HH, Donaldson ES, et al. Prognostic factors in early vulvar cancer. *Gynecol Oncol* 1988;31:43.

Russel AH, Mesic JB, Scudder SA, et al. Synchronous radiation and cytotoxic chemotherapy for locally advanced or recurrent squamous cancer of the vulva. *Gynecol Oncol* 1992;47:14.

Rutledge F, Smith JP, Franklin EW. Carcinoma of the vulva. *Am J Obstet Gynecol* 1970;106:1117.

Rutledge FN, Mitchell MF, Munsell MF, et al. Prognostic indicators for invasive carcinoma of the vulva. *Gynecol Oncol* 1991;42:239.

Safai B, Good RA. Basal cell carcinoma with metastasis. *Arch Pathol Lab Med* 1977;101:327.

Salti GI, Kansagra A, Warso MA, et al. Clinical node-negative thick melanoma. *Arch Surg* 2002;137:291.

Santala M, Suonio S, Syrjanen K, et al. Malignant fibrous histiocytoma of the vulva. *Gynecol Oncol* 1987;27:121.

Scheistroen M, Trope C, Kaern J, et al. Malignant melanoma of the vulva: evaluation of prognostic factors with emphasis on DNA ploidy in 75 patients. *Cancer* 1995;75:72.

Scheistroen M, Tropé C, Kaern J, et al. Malignant melanoma of the vulva FIGO stage 1: evaluation of prognostic factors in 43 patients with emphasis on DNA ploidy and surgical treatment. *Gynecol Oncol* 1996;61:253.

Scheistroen M, Tropé C. Combined bleomycin and irradiation in preoperative treatment of advanced squamous cell carcinoma of the vulva. *Acta Oncol* 1993;32:657.

Scherr GR, d'Ablaing G, Ouzounian JG. Peripheral primitive neuroectodermal tumor of the vulva. *Gynecol Oncol* 1994;54:254.

Schulz MJ, Penalver M. Recurrent vulvar carcinoma in the intervening tissue bridge in early invasive stage I disease treated by radical vulvectomy and bilateral groin dissection through separate incisions. *Gynecol Oncol* 1989;35:383.

Scurry J, Brand A, Planner R, et al. Vulvar Merkel cell tumor with glandular and squamous differentiation. *Gynecol Oncol* 1996;62:292.

Sebag Montefiore DJ, McLean C, Arnott SJ, et al. Treatment of advanced carcinoma of the vulva with chemoradiotherapy: can extensive surgery be avoided? *Int J Gynecol Cancer* 1994;4:150.

Sedlis A, Homesley H, Bundy BN, et al. Positive groin lymph nodes in superficial squamous cell vulvar cancer. *Am J Obstet Gynecol* 1987;156:1159.

Cady B. Sentinel lymph node procedure in squamous cell carcinoma of the vulva. *J Clin Oncol* 2000;18(15):2795.

Shanbour KA, Mannel RS, Morris PC, et al. Comparison of clinical versus surgical staging systems in vulvar cancer. *Obstet Gynecol* 1992;80:927.

Shen JT, D'ablaing G, Morrow CP. Alveolar soft part sarcoma of the vulva: report of first case and review of literature. *Gynecol Oncol* 1982;13:120.

Shepherd JH, Van Dam PA, Jobling TW, et al. The use of rectus abdominis myocutaneous flaps following excision of vulvar cancer. *Br J Obstet Gynaecol* 1990;97:1020.

Shivers SC, Wang X, Li W, et al. Molecular staging of malignant melanoma. Correlation with clinical outcome. *JAMA* 1998;280:1410.

Shutze WP, Gleysteen JJ. Perianal Paget's disease. Classification and review of management: report of two cases. *Dis Colon Rectum* 1990;33:502.

Siller BS, Alvarez RD, Conner WD, et al. T2/3 vulva cancer: a case-control study of triple incision versus en bloc radical vulvectomy and inguinal lymphadenectomy. *Gynecol Oncol* 1995;57:335.

Sim FH, Taylor WF, Ivins JC, et al. A prospective randomized study of the efficacy of routine elective lymphadenectomy in the management of malignant melanoma. *Cancer* 1978;41:948.

Simon KE, Dutcher JP, Runowicz CD, et al. Adenocarcinoma arising in vulvar breast tissue. *Cancer* 1988;62:2234.

Simonsen E. Invasive squamous cell carcinoma of the vulva. *Ann Chir Gynaecol* 1984;73:331.

Simonsen E. Treatment of recurrent squamous cell carcinoma of the vulva. *Acta Radiol Oncol* 1984b;23:345.

Simonsen E, Johnsson JE, Tropé C, et al. Stage I squamous cell carcinoma of the vulva. *Acta Radiol Oncol* 1984;23:443.

Singhal RM, Narayana A. Malignant melanoma of the vulva: response to radiation. *Br J Radiol* 1991;64:846.

Singletary SE, Shallenberger R, Guinee VF. Surgical management of groin nodal metastases from primary melanoma of the lower extremity. *Surg Gynecol Obstet* 1992;174:195.

Slevin NJ, Pointon RCS. Radical radiotherapy for carcinoma of the vulva. *Br J Radiol* 1989;62:145.

Sliutz G, Reinthaller A, Lantzsch T, et al. Lymphatic mapping of sentinel nodes in early vulvar cancer. *Gynecol Oncol* 2002;84:449.

Smith HO, Worrell RV, Smith AY, et al. Aggressive angiomyxoma of the female pelvis and perineum: review of the literature. *Gynecol Oncol* 1991;42:79.

Snijders-Keilholz T, Trimbos JB, Hermans J, et al. Management of vulvar carcinoma radiation toxicity, results and failure analysis in 44 patients (1980-1989). *Acta Obstet Gynecol Scand* 1993;72:668.

Soergel TM, Doering DL, O'Connor D. Metastatic dermatofibrosarcoma protuberans of the vulva. *Gynecol Oncol* 1998;71:320.

Soltan M. Dermatofibrosarcoma protuberans of the vulva. *Br J Obstet Gynaecol* 1981;88:203.

Soper JT, Elbendary AA, Hurteau JA, et al. Bulbocavernosus myocutaneous flap for perineal reconstruction. *J Gynecol Tech* 1996;2:141.

Stacy D, Burrell MO, Franklin EW III. Extramammary Paget's disease of the vulva and anus: use of intraoperative frozen-section margins. *Am J Obstet Gynecol* 1986;155:519.

Steeper TA, Rosai J. Aggressive angiomyxoma of the female pelvis and perineum: report of nine cases of a distinctive type of gynecologic soft-tissue neoplasm. *Am J Surg Pathol* 1983;7:463.

Stehman FB, Bundy BN, Ball H, et al. Sites of failure and times to failure in carcinoma of the vulva treated conservatively: a Gynecologic Oncology Group study. *Am J Obstet Gynecol* 1996;174:1128.

Stehman FB, Bundy BN, Dvoretsky PM, et al. Early stage I carcinoma of the vulva treated with ipsilateral superficial inguinal lymphadenectomy and modified radical hemivulvectomy: a prospective study of the Gynecologic Oncology Group. *Obstet Gynecol* 1992;79:490.

Stehman FB, Bundy BN, Thomas G, et al. Groin dissection versus groin radiation in carcinoma of the vulva: a Gynecologic Oncology Group study. *Int J Radiat Oncol Biol Phys* 1992;24:389.

Struyk APHB, Bouma JJ, van Lindert ACM, et al. Early stage cancer of the vulva: a pilot investigation on cancer of the Vulvain Gynecologic Oncology Centres in the Netherlands. Proceedings of the second meeting of the International Gynecologic Cancer Society, Toronto, 1989:303.

Sturgeon SR, Brinton LA, Devesa SS, et al. In situ and invasive vulvar cancer incidence trends (1973 to 1987). *Am J Obstet Gynecol* 1992;166:1482.

Sturgeon SR, Curtis RE, Johnson K, et al. Second primary cancers after vulvar and vaginal cancers. *Am J Obstet Gynecol* 1996;174:929.

Sutton GP, Miser MR, Stehman FB, et al. Trends in the operative management of invasive squamous carcinoma of the vulva at Indiana University, 1974 to 1988. *Am J Obstet Gynecol* 1991;164:1472.

Sworn MJ, Hammond GT, Buchanan R. Metastatic basal cell carcinoma of the vulva: a case report. *Br J Obstet Gynaecol* 1979;86:332.

Sykiotis C, Vitoratos N, Kalabokis D, et al. Dermatofibrosarcoma protuberans of the vulva. *J Gynecol Surg* 1999;15:149.

Tan GW, Lim-Tan SK, Salmon YM. Epithelioid sarcoma of the vulva. *Singapore Med J* 1989;30:308.

Tateo A, Tateo S, Bernasconi C, et al. Use of V-Y flap for vulvar reconstruction. *Gynecol Oncol* 1996;62:203.

Taussig FJ. Cancer of the vulva: an analysis of 155 cases. *Am J Obstet Gynecol* 1940;40:764.

Tavassoli FA, Norris HJ. Smooth muscle tumors of the vulva. *Obstet Gynecol* 1979;53:213.

Tawfik O, Huntrakoon M, Collins J, et al. Leiomyosarcoma of the vulva: report of a case. *Gynecol Oncol* 1994;54:242.

Taylor RN, Bottles K, Miller TR, et al. Malignant fibrous histiocytoma of the vulva. *Obstet Gynecol* 1985;66:145.

Terada KY, Coel M, Ko P, et al. Combined use of intraoperative lymphatic mapping and lymphoscintigraphy in the management of squamous cell cancer of the vulva. *Gynecol Oncol* 1998;70:65.

Terada KY, Shimizu DM, Wong JH. Sentinel node dissection and ultrastaging in squamous cell cancer of the vulva. *Gynecol Oncol* 2000;76:40.

Tewari K, Cappuccini F, Syed N, et al. Interstitial brachytherapy in the treatment of advanced and recurrent vulvar cancer. *Am J Obstet Gynecol* 1999;181:91.

Thomas G, Dembo A, DePetrillo A, et al. Concurrent radiation and chemotherapy in vulvar carcinoma. *Gynecol Oncol* 1989;34:263.

Thornton WN, Flanagan WC. Pelvic exenteration in the treatment of advanced malignancy of the vulva. *Am J Obstet Gynecol* 1973;117:774.

Tilmans AS, Sutton GP, Look KY, et al. Recurrent squamous carcinoma of the vulva. *Am J Obstet Gynecol* 1992;167:1383.

Tjalma WAA, Hauben EI, Deprez SME, et al. Epithelioid sarcoma of the vulva. *Gynecol Oncol* 1999;73:160.

Toker C. Trabecular carcinoma of the skin. *Arch Dermatol* 1972;105:107.

Trelford JD, Deer DA, Ordorica E, et al. Ten-year prospective study in a management change of vulvar carcinoma. *Am J Obstet Gynecol* 1984;150:288.

Trimble CL, Hildesheim A, Brinton LA, et al. Heterogeneous etiology of squamous carcinoma of the vulva. *Obstet Gynecol* 1996;87:59.

Trimble EL, Lewis JL Jr, Williams LL, et al. Management of vulvar melanoma. *Gynecol Oncol* 1992;45:254.

Ulbright TM, Brokaw SA, Stehman FB, et al. Epithelioid sarcoma of the vulva: evidence suggesting a more aggressive behavior than extra-genital epithelioid sarcoma. *Cancer* 1983;52:1462.

Ungerleider RS, Donaldson SS, Warnke RA, et al. Endodermal sinus tumor: the Stanford experience and the first reported case arising in the vulva. *Cancer* 1978;41:1627.

Valentine BH, Arena B, Green E. Laser ablation of recurrent Paget's disease of vulva and perineum. *J Gynecol Surg* 1992;8:21.

Van der Griend MD, Burda P, Ferrier AJ. Angiomyofibroblastoma of the vulva. *Gynecol Oncol* 1994;54:389.

van der Velden J, Kooyman CD, Van Lindert ACM, et al. A stage IA vulvar carcinoma with an inguinal lymph node recurrence after local excision: a case report and literature review. *Int J Gynecol Cancer* 1992;2:157.

van der Velden J, van Lindert ACM, Lammes FB, et al. Extracapsular growth of lymph node metastases in squamous cell carcinoma of the vulva. The impact on recurrence and survival. *Cancer* 1995;75:2885.

Veronesi U, Adamus J, Bandiera DC, et al. Inefficacy of immediate node dissection in stage I melanoma of the limbs. *N Engl J Med* 1977;297:627.

Veronesi U, Cascinelli N, Adamus J, et al. Thin stage I primary cutaneous malignant melanoma: comparison of excision with margins of 1 and 3 cm. *N Engl J Med* 1988;318:1159.

Veronesi U, Cascinelli N. Narrow excision (1-cm margin): a safe procedure for thin cutaneous melanoma. *Arch Surg* 1991;126:438.

Visco AG, Del Priore G. Postmenopausal Bartholin gland enlargement: a hospital-based cancer risk assessment. *Obstet Gynecol* 1996;87:286.

Waibel M, Richter K, Von Lengerken W, et al. Merkel cell carcinoma (neuro-endocrine carcinoma) in uncommon skin location, immunohistochemical and lectinhistochemical findings. *Zentralbl Pathol* 1991;137:140.

Watring WG, Roberts JA, Lagasse LD, et al. Treatment of recurrent Paget's disease of the vulva with topical bleomycin. *Cancer* 1978;41:10.

Way S, Benedet JL. Involvement of inguinal lymph nodes in carcinoma of the vulva. *Gynecol Oncol* 1973;1:119.

Way S. The anatomy of the lymphatic drainage of the vulva and its influence on the radical operation for carcinoma. *Ann R Coll Surg Engl* 1948;3:187.

Weissmann D, Amenta PS, Kantor GR. Vulvar epithelioid sarcoma metastatic to the scalp: a case report and review of the literature. *Am J Dermatopathol* 1990;12:462.

Whalen SA, Slater JD, Wagner RJ, et al. Concurrent radiation therapy and chemotherapy in the treatment of primary squamous cell carcinoma of the vulva. *Cancer* 1995;75:2289.

Wharton JT, Gallager S, Rutledge FN. Microinvasive carcinoma of the vulva. *Am J Obstet Gynecol* 1974;118:159.

Wheeless CR Jr, McGibbon B, Dorsey JH, et al. Gracilis myocutaneous flap in reconstruction of the vulva and female perineum. *Obstet Gynecol* 1979;54:97.

Wheelock JB, Goplerud DR, Dunn L, et al. Primary carcinoma of the Bartholin gland: a report of ten cases. *Obstet Gynecol* 1984;63:820.

Whitaker SJ, Kirkbride P, Arnott SJ, et al. A pilot study of chemoradiotherapy in advanced carcinoma of the vulva. *Br J Obstet Gynaecol* 1990;97:436.

Wick MR, Goellner JR, Wolfe JT, et al. Vulvar sweat gland carcinomas. *Arch Pathol Lab Med* 1985;109:43.

Wilkinson EJ, Kneale B, Lynch PJ. Report of the ISSVD Terminology Committee. *J Reprod Med* 1986;31:973.

Wilkinson EJ. Superficially invasive carcinoma of the vulva. *Clin Obstet Gynecol* 1985;28:188.

Winkelmann SE, Llorens AS. Case report: metastatic basal cell carcinoma of the vulva. *Gynecol Oncol* 1990;38:138.

Woolcott RJ, Henry RJ, Houghton CR. Malignant melanoma of the vulva: Australian experience. *J Reprod Med* 1988;33:699.

Zaidi SNH, Conner MG. Primary vulvar adenocarcinoma of cloacogenic origin. *S M J* 2001;94:744.

Zaino RJ, Husseinzadeh N, Nahhas W, et al. Epithelial alterations in proximity to invasive squamous carcinoma of the vulva. *Int J Gynecol Pathol* 1982;1:173.

Zerner J, Fenn ME. Basal cell carcinoma of the vulva. *Int J Gynaecol Obstet* 1979;17:203.

Zettersten E, Sagebiel RW, Miller III JR, et al. Prognostic Factors in patients with thick cutaneous melanoma (>4 mm). *Cancer* 2002;94:1049.

Zhang SH, Sood AK, Sorosky JI, et al. Preservation of the saphenous vein during inguinal lymphadenectomy decreases morbidity in patients with carcinoma of the vulva. *Cancer* 2000;89(7):1520.

Te Linde's Operative Gynecology, ninth edition, edited by John A. Rock and Howard W. Jones, III. Lippincott Williams & Wilkins, Philadelphia © 2003.

CHAPTER

45

▼

Cervical Cancer Precursors and Their Management

HOWARD W. JONES, III

Although cellular atypia adjacent to invasive squamous cell cancers of the cervix has long been recognized, it was not until the 1950s when carcinoma in situ of the cervix was characterized and its preinvasive potential became accepted. In their 1952 publication, Galvin, Jones, and Te Linde described their observations of the natural history of carcinoma in situ. Their report confirmed and advanced previous studies by Thomas Cullen and Pemberton and Smith. The concept of a clearly identifiable preinvasive neoplastic change in the cervical epithelium represented a major breakthrough in an understanding of the development and natural history of cervical cancer. However, it was the parallel development of cervical cytology that provided a technique that made this concept clinically useful. Because these preinvasive epithelial changes that have come to be known as *cervical intraepithelial neoplasia* (CIN) are asymptomatic and essentially unrecognizable on gross inspection or palpation, they were not particularly useful to the clinician until it was shown they could be diagnosed by cervical cytology. The introduction of practical cytology by Papanicolaou and Trout in 1943 and its later widespread adaptation into clinical practice represented the second major development that has led to the ability to screen asymptomatic women for invasive and then preinvasive cervical neoplasia. This had led to a dramatic 70% reduction in cervical cancer deaths in the United States over the past 50 years. In addition, those two developments provided the tools that have enabled us to understand the clinical development of cervical cancer.

This chapter discusses the cytologic, histologic, and molecular changes that occur in the cervix as cervical cancer develops and how CIN can be diagnosed and treated.

TERMINOLOGY

Although carcinoma in situ became well recognized as a full-thickness epithelial change without stromal invasion, the terminology and clinical significance of adjacent, less than full-thickness atypia was uncertain. In 1956, Reagan and Hamonic introduced the term *dysplasia* to designate these cervical epithelial abnormalities that were characterized by cytologic atypia, increased mitotic activity, and loss of polarity. If these basoid changes involved only the basal one third of the epithelium, they were referred to as mild *dysplasia*. Changes extending into the middle third of the cervical epithelium were classified as *moderate dysplasia*, and when more than two thirds of the epithelium was involved the lesion was designated *severe dysplasia*. At its first international meeting in 1961, the International Congress on Exfoliative Cytology accepted the following definition "only those cases should be classified as *carcinoma in situ* which, in the absence of invasion, show as surface lining epithelium in which, throughout its whole thickness, no differentiation takes place. The process may involve the lining of the cervical glands without thereby creating a new group. It is recognized that the cells of the uppermost layers may show some slight flattening." At this same meeting, dyplasia was defined as "all other disturbances of differentiation of the squamous epithelium of surface and glands. They may be characterized as of high or low degrees, terms that are preferable to 'suspicious' and 'nonsuspicious' as the proposed terms describe the histological appearance and do not express an opinion." It generally was assumed that these lesions represented a spectrum of disease and that the more severe abnormalities were more likely to progress to invasive cancer and to do so in a shorter period of time. However, it was not until the studies of Barron and Richart and later of Nasiell and her colleagues that the natural history of these preinvasive lesions became well understood.

The original cytologic classification introduced by Papanicolaou used a four- or five-step "class" designation, where "class 1" was normal, benign and "class 5" was suspicious of invasive cancer. This terminology was replaced gradually by the histologic terms of mild, moderate, or severe dysplasia and carcinoma in situ, although various modifications were formally or informally introduced and adopted in the United States and throughout the world. One of the most important values of an accurately defined and widely accepted terminology is that it allows investigators and clinicians to accurately observe and classify the natural history of a disease or lesion and the effect of various treatments on the outcome and to communicate these findings to others. Over time, it became clear that histopathologists and cytopathologists could not accurately and reproducibly differentiate between severe dysplasia and carcinoma in situ. In addition, clinicians managed these two lesions in a similar fashion. Therefore, in 1976 Richart proposed the terminology of *cervical intraepithelial neoplasia,* which combined the categories of severe dysplasia and carcinoma in situ into the term *CIN 3.* Cervical intraepithelial neoplasia, grade 1 (CIN 1) was essentially the same as mild dysplasia and CIN 2 was similar to moderate dysplasia. But CIN 3 combined severe dysplasia and carcinoma in situ, thus simplifying the classification from four categories to three (Table 45.1). This practical terminology was favored by clinicians and widely adopted throughout the world. It has been used for both cytologic and histologic diagnoses.

However, as the role of human papillomavirus (HPV) in cervical neoplasia became more evident and the difficulties of intraobserver variation with a lack of reproducibility of cytologic diagnoses became more well accepted, another change in terminology was undertaken. At a series of two large meetings held at the National Cancer Institute in Bethesda, MD, *The Bethesda System* was introduced and published in 1991 (Table 45.2). These conferences clarified a number of ill defined

TABLE 45.1.
The Changing Terminology of Cervical Cytology

Dysplasia	CIN	Bethesda*
Mild	Grade 1	Low-grade SIL
Moderate	Grade 2	High-grade SIL
Severe	Grade 3	High-grade SIL
Carcinoma in situ	Grade 3	High-grade SIL

* The Bethesda System classification of low-grade SIL includes both CIN 1 and HPV changes.

SIL, squamous intraepithelial lesion; CIN, cervical intraepithelial neoplasia; HPV, human papilloma virus.

or previously undefined problems with cytologic diagnoses, such as what constituted an adequate specimen for accurate interpretation. It tried to eliminate the term "atypia," which had become increasingly used to designate a wide range of nonspecific changes that were clinically confusing. The Bethesda System combined HPV cytopathologic effects, often referred to as *koilocytosis,* with mild dysplasia or CIN 1 into a category called *low-grade squamous intraepithelial lesion* (LSIL). More significant lesions including moderate and severe dysplasia and carcinoma in situ, or CIN 2 and 3, are combined into high-grade squamous intraepithelial lesion (HSIL). Pap tests with "cellular abnormalities that are more marked than those attributable to reactive changes but that quantitatively or qualitatively fall short of a definitive diagnosis of "squamous intraepithelial lesion" are placed in a category called *atypical squamous cells* (ASC). These specimens may be further categorized as *of undetermined significance* (ASC-US) or *cannot exclude high grade* (ASC-H). This latter category together with more specific diagnostic terminology for glandular abnormalities were new additions in the 2001 revision of the Bethesda System. Although the Bethesda System terminology for reporting the results of cervical cytology has been almost universally accepted in the United States and is used in many other countries, other terminology and definitions are used in Great Britain, Germany, Australia, and other countries, which creates some difficulty in publishing and understanding scientific studies from different countries.

In the United States, a typical laboratory that processes cervical cytology from an average, generally low-risk population reports epithelial cell abnormalities in about 5% to 6% of patients. Usually one half to two thirds of these abnormalities are ASC (2% to 4%), whereas 1% to 2% are LSIL and 0.5% to 1.0% are HSIL diagnoses, with occasional glandular cell abnormalities. The ratios of ASC to SIL diagnoses should be about 2:1 or, at most, 3:1 for most cytology laboratories.

The Bethesda System was designed and published to be used for cytologic diagnoses; however, it has been applied increasingly to histologic or tissue diagnoses. This is advantageous in that it provides uniformity between

TABLE 45.2.
Bethesda System of Cytologic Classification

THE 2001 BETHESDA SYSTEM (ABRIDGED)

SPECIMEN ADEQUACY
Satisfactory for evaluation (*note presence/absence of endocervical/transformation zone component*)
Unsatisfactory for evaluation . . . (*specify reason*)
    Specimen rejected/not processed (*specify reason*)
    Specimen processed and examined, but unsatisfactory for evaluation of epithelial abnormality because of (*specify reason*)

GENERAL CATEGORIZATION (OPTIONAL)
Negative for intraepithelial lesion or malignancy
Epithelial cell abnormality
Other

INTERPRETATION/RESULT
Negative for Intraepithelial Lesion or Malignancy
    Organisms
        Trichomonas vaginalis
        Fungal organisms morphologically consistent with *Candida* species
        Shift in flora suggestive of bacterial vaginosis
        Bacteria morphologically consistent with *Actinomyces* species
        Cellular changes consistent with herpes simplex virus
    Other nonneoplastic findings (*Optional to report; list not comprehensive*)
        Reactive cellular changes associated with inflammation (includes typical repair), radiation, intrauterine contraceptive device
        Glandular cells status posthysterectomy
        Atrophy
Epithelial Cell Abnormalities
    Squamous cell
        Atypical squamous cells (ASC)
            Of undetermined significance (ASC-US)
            Cannot exclude HSIL (ASC-H)
        Low-grade squamous intraepithelial lesion (LSIL)
            Encompassing human papillomavirus/mild dysplasia/cervical intraepithelial neoplasia (CIN) 1
        High-grade squamous intraepithelial lesion (HSIL)
            Encompassing moderate and severe dysplasia, carcinoma in situ, CIN 2 and CIN 3
        Squamous cell carcinoma
    Glandular cell
        Atypical glandular cells (AGC) (*specify endocervical, endometrial, or not otherwise specified*)
        Atypical glandular cells, favor neoplastic (*specify endocervical or not otherwise specified*)
        Endocervical adenocarcinoma in situ (AIS)
        Adenocarcinoma
Other (*List not comprehensive*)
    Endometrial cells in a woman ≥40 years of age

AUTOMATED REVIEW AND ANCILLARY TESTING (INCLUDE AS APPROPRIATE)

EDUCATIONAL NOTES AND SUGGESTIONS (OPTIONAL)

the diagnosis on the Papanicolaou test and the cervical biopsy. By combining moderate dysplasia, severe dysplasia, and carcinoma in situ, it lacks the imagined specificity that is occasionally helpful in clinical management decisions. The word "imagined" is used intentionally because many studies have shown that there is a significant lack of reproducibility in the diagnoses of various grades of dysplasia and even carcinoma in situ. There is no clear dividing line between the different cytologic or histologic grades of cervical epithelial atypias, lesions, or neoplasias and the diagnosis on the Papanicolaou or biopsy report is a general impression, not a precise predictor of the benign or malignant behavior of the cervical epithelium sampled.

EPIDEMIOLOGY

One of the earliest epidemiologic studies of any cancer was the observation of Rigoni-Stern published in 1842. This Italian noted that cervical cancer was found in married women but was virtually absent in celibate groups such as Catholic nuns. Others noted that cervical cancer was almost never found in virginal women and that a woman's risk of developing cervical cancer was directly related to the number of male sexual partners she had had. It was also reported that early age at first sexual intercourse, low socioeconomic status, cigarette smoking, and early age at first pregnancy increased a woman's risk of cervical neoplasia. More recently, it became obvious that immunosuppression from any cause, including infection with human immunodeficiency virus (HIV), substantially increased a woman's risk of cervical neoplasia. Oral contraceptive use has been reported to increase a woman's risk of cervical cancer as well, but the odds ratios are relatively low, and it is difficult to control for confounding factors.

Many epidemiologic studies have shown a pattern of cervical cancer that is typical for a sexually transmitted disease (STD). For this reason, investigators have focused on etiologic agents that might be passed venereally. Virtually every sexually transmitted agent has been studied for its relation to cervical neoplasia, including *Chlamydia*, gonorrhea, *Gardnerella*, *Mycoplasma*, *Trichomonas*, and herpes simplex virus (HSV). Although all STDs are associated with cervical neoplasia, the herpes simplex virus type 2 (HSV-2) received particular attention because it was reported that women whose blood contained antibodies to HSV-2 were at substantially higher risk of having cervical neoplasia compared with patients who were negative for such antibodies. These observations led investigators to conclude that HSV-2 may be of etiologic importance in the pathogenesis of cervical cancer. Although there is a relation between HSV-2 and virtually all other STDs and cervical neoplasia, it seems to be a casual rather than a causal relation.

As the epidemiologists studied the lifestyle characteristics of women with cervical cancer and the cytopathologist described the microscopic morphologic transition of the cervical epithelium, clinicians were observing certain abnormalities on the cervix in patients with the preinvasive changes of cervical dysplasia. First popularized by Hinsalmann in Germany, the colposcope is a magnifying instrument used to examine the cervix. With the colposcope, vascular changes and other epithelial patterns were recognized and correlated with the cytologic and histologic changes that were being described. These early neoplastic changes were most prominent adjacent to the squamo-columnar junction (SCJ) and this area was called the *transformation zone*. With time, colposcopic patterns associated with the developing stages of dysplasia and early invasive cancer were identified and described by Mestwerdt, Wespi, Kolstad, Stafl, Barghardt, Coupez, Coppelson, and others. In 1974, Stafl and Mattingly brilliantly synthesized these observations and the work of the epidemiologists and proposed a theory of the development of cervical cancer (Fig. 45.1). They did not know the identity of the environmental carcinogen that they presumed was sexually transmitted, but they proposed a framework that has been enormously useful for the clinician.

In 1976, Meisels and Fortin and, in 1977, Purola and Savia reported finding HPV in the nuclei of dysplastic squamous epithelial cells, particularly those that had koilocytotic features. These observations were confirmed by a number of other investigators, and it was suggested by zur Hausen that this virus may be important etiologically in cervical carcinogenesis. Using electron microscopy and antibodies to the HPV capsid protein, several investigators identified viral particles or HPV-related antigens in CIN. They were particularly prevalent in low-grade lesions and became less frequently observed as

the cells became less well differentiated. These observations strongly implicated HPV as a possible etiologic agent in cervical neoplasia and led to an explosion of molecular and clinical studies of HPV and its related lesions.

HUMAN PAPILLOMAVIRUSES

Human papillomaviruses are members of a large family of viruses known as the *Papovaviridae*. This includes another oncogenic DNA virus, the simian virus 40 (SV40), as well as the polyomavirus. All the viruses in this group are DNA tumor viruses. Although they have dissimilar DNA base pair sequences and dissimilar capsular antigens, they appear to produce neoplasms through similar mechanisms. The papillomaviruses have a tightly coiled, circular, double-stranded DNA molecule about 8,000 base pairs in length. The complete virion consists of a DNA core and a surrounding protein capsid that measures about 45 to 55 nm in diameter. The capsid has an icosahedral shape. Papillomaviruses are found throughout the animal kingdom and infect not only humans but cattle, rabbits, dogs, deer, monkeys, and birds. The viruses are highly species specific. Cross-infections between species have not been reported. Unlike many viruses that infect humans and that are classified by their surface antigens, the papillomaviruses are classified according to their DNA base pair sequence. The degree of relatedness is determined by the degree of hybridization homology.

Although in animals papillomaviruses can infect both epithelial cells and fibroblasts, the human papillomavirus

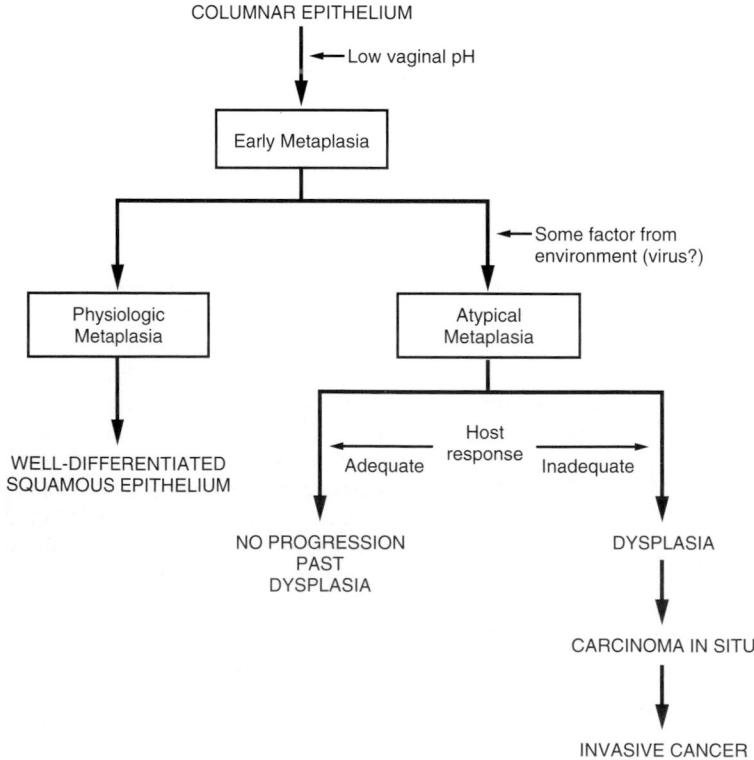

FIGURE 45.1. Diagrammatic illustration of the theory of development of cervical neoplasia proposed by Stafl and Mattingly. (From Stafl and Mattingly. Vaginal adenosis: a precancerous lesion? *Am J Obstet Gynecol* 1974:120:666.)

is an exclusively epitheliotropic organism that produces alterations in the supporting structures solely as a secondary effect related to infection of the epithelium. HPV infects virtually all surface epithelia, including the skin and mucous membranes. The infected epithelium is characterized by epithelial proliferation at the infected site, by various degrees of epithelial thickening, and by papillomatosis.

Many of the newly discovered HPV types were associated with cervical cancer and cancer precursors in the male and female anogenital tract. Because certain types were so consistently associated with neoplastic cervical lesions, attention was focused on these specific viral types in an effort to better understand their relation to the development of cervical neoplasia. HPV DNA was also found in many of the cervical cancer–related tissue culture cell lines that had been studied by investigators for many years for other purposes. These initial studies were expanded, and with increasing molecular sophistication came the discovery of more types, the sequencing of more types, and a better understanding of the relation between these types and cervical disease. At least 100 HPV types have been identified; about 25 of these affect the male and female anogenital tract.

The most prevalent anogenital HPVs can be divided into three groups that are predictive of their ability to produce neoplasia (Table 45.3). The group with a low oncogenic risk or no oncogenic risk includes HPV types 6, 11, 42, 43, and 44. Members of the low-oncogenic risk group are found in acuminate warts, in low-grade CIN lesions, and in the so-called flat condylomata. They are rarely found in high-grade CINs and are virtually never found in invasive squamous cell cancers of the cervix or in cervical adenocarcinoma. HPV types that are of intermediate oncogenic risk form the second group of anogenital HPV types. These viruses can be found in low-grade and high-grade CIN lesions but are infrequently seen in invasive carcinoma. The intermediate oncogenic risk group includes HPV types 31, 33, 35, 51, and 52. The anogenital HPV types with a high oncogenic risk are types 16, 18, 45, and 56. HPVs in this risk group are seen in low-grade lesions, are overrepresented in high-grade lesions, and are substantially overrepresented in invasive cancers. This overrepresentation is particularly striking with HPV type 18, which is found in less than 3% of high-grade CIN lesions but in 15% of invasive squamous cell carcinomas.

It was originally thought that there was a correlation between HPV type and a characteristic histologic pattern in the low-grade lesions. However, it has proved impossible at the light microscopic level to distinguish among histologically low-grade lesions that are induced by a virus with a low oncogenic risk, those that are induced by a virus with an intermediate oncogenic risk, and those that are induced by a virus with a high oncogenic risk. Morphologically, they all have a similar appearance, although there is widespread diversity in the histologic pattern of each type. In the high-grade CIN lesions in which differentiation is low, cell turnover is high, mitotic figures are frequent, and cytologic atypia is severe, infections with multiple different HPV types are uncommon, being found in only about 7% of cases. In addition, the distribution of viruses is more restricted among high-grade lesions, because the types with a low oncogenic risk or no oncogenic risk are almost never seen in such lesions when they are properly diagnosed, and the group with an intermediate oncogenic risk is much less common than the group with a high oncogenic risk. HPV type 16 is found in more than 70% of the high-grade lesions; the remaining 30% are caused by other members of the groups with a high or intermediate oncogenic risk.

Human Papillomavirus Genome

The viral genome of HPV can be divided into three regions: the upstream regulatory region (URR), the early region, and the late region. The URR is a noncoding region that has as its major functions the regulation of viral replication and the transcription of downstream sequences in the early region. The early and the late region both contain a series of open reading frames (ORFs), linear sequences that lack stop codons and hence are potentially transcribable into proteins. The early region transcribes proteins that are important in the early life cycle of the virus and interact with the cellular genome to program the host cell to produce new viral DNA. The late region, as the name implies, encodes for capsid proteins that surround the DNA core to produce the infectious unit—the complete virion.

The URR is not well understood but is known to be a regulatory region that contains binding sites for a number of transcription factors, including activator protein 1 (AP1) and keratinocytic specific transcription factor 1 (KRF1), as well as virally derived transcriptional factors.

TABLE 45.3.
Natural History of CIN—Literature Review

	Patients	Regress	Persist	Progress to CIN 3	Progress to Invasive Cancer
CIN 1	4,504	57%	32%	11%	1%
CIN 2	2,247	43%	35%	22%	5%
CIN 3	767	32%	>56%	—	>12%

CIN, cervical intraepithelial neoplasia.

These proteins and others are important in the transcription of the early region ORFs.

Six different ORFs have been identified in the early region of HPV. They are designated E_1, E_2, E_4, E_5, E_6, and E_7. These viral genes are extremely important because they control the process of viral replication, they encode for the maintenance of a high intracellular viral copy number, and they encode for the genes whose transcription produces the oncogenic proteins that transform the normal cervical cells into neoplastic cells. The E_6 and E_7 ORFs encode for two highly oncogenic proteins by which the oncogenic HPV types transform normal cervical cells into neoplastic cells.

The late-region ORFs, designated L_1 and L_2, are transcribed late in the replication cycle and encode for major and minor capsid proteins. The L_1-encoded protein predominates in the capsid, is highly conserved among papillomaviruses, and is similar in all HPV types. On the other hand, the L_2-encoded protein is highly variable between different HPV types, and largely accounts for the differences in antigenicity from one HPV type to another. All the proteins that are transcribed in the late region appear to be regulated by cell-derived transcriptional proteins that are produced only by squamous epithelial cells undergoing terminal maturation. The quantity of L_1- and L_2-encoded capsid proteins is highly correlated with terminal maturation of the epithelium. Well-differentiated HPV-induced lesions such as condylomata are generally rich in L_1- and L_2-encoded proteins, whereas high-grade CIN lesions, which tend to be highly undifferentiated, contain only small quantities of capsid proteins.

Natural History of Human Papillomavirus Infection

In recent epidemiologic studies that have used highly sensitive and specific HPV DNA detection techniques, it has been found, in contrast to the early studies, that almost all high-grade CIN lesions and invasive cancers contain HPV DNA. In addition, the covariables that have traditionally been associated with a high risk of developing cervical neoplasia are also highly correlated with the presence of HPV DNA. In a relatively large study of women attending a university health clinic, it was found that HPV DNA positivity was strongly correlated with an increasing number of sexual partners; the prevalence of HPV infection in women with 10 or more lifetime sexual partners was 69%, compared with 21% in women with only a single sexual partner. In Schiffman's studies, it was reported that women who are HPV DNA positive have a relative risk of 40 of having an abnormal Papanicolaou smear. He also reported that the attributable risk of HPV in such populations is greater than 90%. The only other covariable that was a significant contributor to risk was cigarette smoking. He also noted that "relative risks and attributable risks of this strength and consistency are so rare that the statistical association of HPV and cervical neoplasia is beyond question" and that "the epidemiological data support a central, causal role for genital HPV infection in the etiology of cervical neo-

plasia." Thus, the clinical, histologic, molecular, and epidemiologic data all support HPV as the causative agent for most, if not all, epithelial neoplasms of the cervix.

Through the "magic" of molecular biology, the natural history of HPV infections is becoming better understood. The papillomavirus requires access to basal or parabasal cells to infect the epithelium. In the cervix, this access occurs principally at the SCJ. Access also occurs in the thin, immature portions of the transformation zone (TZ), where the metaplastic squamous epithelium consists principally of immature basal- and parabasal-type cells. When a mitotically active epithelial cell is infected, the virus may remain in the cell in a latent form in which bare DNA resides in the nucleus and replication occurs only in synchrony with the normal cell cycle. This is termed a *latent infection*. These latently infected epithelial cells are morphologically normal, and because complete virion is not produced, patients who acquire and carry a latent infection are not infectious to others.

Latent infections can be detected only by molecular techniques such as HPV DNA hydridization. Patients who are latently infected cannot be identified clinically as having an HPV infection. Because latently infected individuals shed virus intermittently and in a nonpredictable fashion, there is substantial variation in HPV DNA detection in women who are screened sequentially over a period of time. In most women with an initial HPV infection, the infection appears to clear spontaneously, without therapeutic intervention, probably because of normal immunologic host defense mechanisms. In some individuals, however, for reasons that are not well understood, the latent papillomavirus begins to replicate independent of the host cell cycle, and large numbers of complete virions are produced. This is referred to as a *productive viral infection*. In a productively infected epithelium, viral replication takes place principally in intermediate and superficial cells, with the greatest number of viral particles found in the terminally differentiated epithelium. The control of viral replication is determined by the early genes, but as the epithelial cells mature and become differentiated, cell-derived, differentiation-specific transcriptional factors are produced by the host epithelial cells, and capsid proteins are synthesized to surround the viral DNA.

Since the importance of HPV in the etiology of cervical neoplasia has become more certain, various investigators have suggested that a vaccine against papillomavirus might prevent infection and perhaps even eliminate the virus in already infected individuals. This idea of immunization against HPV type 16 was recently tested in a clinical trial by Koutsky and colleagues, who prospectively randomized almost 2,400 young women who tested negative for HPV type 16 infection and immunized half with three doses of virus-like particle vaccine and treated the other half with placebo. The patients were then followed up for a median of 17 months, and the risk of developing a persistent HPV type 16 infection was 3.8 per 100 women-years in the placebo group compared with 0 in the vaccinated patients ($p > 0.001$). CIN developed in nine women in the placebo group, whereas there was no instance of CIN among the vaccinated women.

Cytologic and Colposcopic Changes

As viral replication takes place in the epithelium, it is accompanied by alterations that are often clinically evident and by changes in the cytology of the epithelial cells that allow such cells to be detected cytologically and histologically. Clinicians have observed that the earliest and most severe changes occur adjacent to the SCJ on the cervix. Anatomic studies have shown that the location of the SCJ is not fixed, but it changes during a woman's life. Under the influence of the vaginal pH, columnar cells on the exocervix are transformed into squamous cells by a process called *metaplasia*. There are three times in a woman's life that metaplasia is particularly active— in the embryologic development of the vagina and cervix, at puberty, and after the first pregnancy. During puberty and after pregnancy, the columnar epithelium of the endocervix is everted out onto the exocervix or portio of the cervix and metaplasia is stimulated. The columnar cells, starting with the epithelium on the tips of the glandular papillae, are changed into squamous epithelium. This process can be observed with the colposcope and the area of active metaplasia just lateral to the SCJ where this metaplastic change occurs is called the *transformation zone*—columnar epithelium is transformed into metaplastic squamous epithelia Figure 45.2. This epithelium can be recognized as a circumferential, pale white, translucent ring around the SCJ.

These metaplastic cells are very active and may be infected by HPV in the vagina. As described earlier, certain oncogenic HPV types may infect and transform the epithelial cells and the increased mitotic activity and DNA density can be identified as "white epithelium" following application of 3% to 5% acetic acid to the cervix. As CIN develops, vascular changes occur and these may be recognized as "punctation" or "mosaic." If the lesion progresses, bizarre vascular changes can be seen. These "atypical vessels" have grossly abnormal architecture and are colposcopic hallmarks of invasive cancer.

Women whose initial low-grade CIN lesions are caused by HPVs with a low oncogenic risk or no oncogenic risk either maintain an infected epithelium with persistent disease for long periods of time or, in most instances, seem to resolve the HPV infection over time without treatment. Lesions that are caused by HPV types with an intermediate or high oncogenic risk may undergo remission spontaneously, persist, or, in a minority of cases, progress. It is not well understood what influences a lesion to undergo remission, persist, or progress, but indirect clinical evidence suggests that HPV type, host immunologic factors, and cofactors such as other STDs may play a role.

Cellular Transformation

In patients whose lesions progress from a low-grade CIN to a high-grade CIN, the progression is accompanied by alterations in the virus-host interaction. These interactions appear to be critical to the transformation of nor-

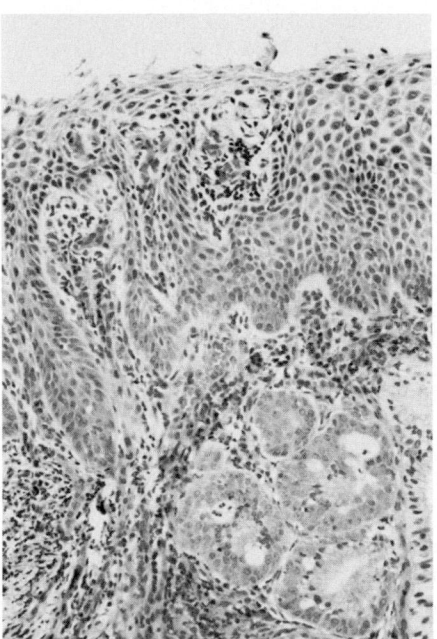

FIGURE 45.2. Histologic section of squamous metaplasia. Immature squamous metaplasia may be acetowhite colposcopically and may be confused with cervical intraepithelial neoplasia histologically. Although the metaplastic cells are immature, they are not pleomorphic or cytologically atypical. The growth pattern and cytology are regular, and there is a lack of the features that characterize human papillomavirus–related lesions. This section is typical of the epithelium from the immature transformation zone.

mal epithelial cells to neoplastic cells. The key alteration seems to be the integration of the viral DNA into host chromosomes. Because the episomal (nonchromosomal) virus that is found in latently or productively infected cells is in a circular form and because the DNA in the host chromosomes is linear, a change in the physical state of the virus must take place before the viral DNA can be integrated into the host chromosome. What initiates this change and the mechanism by which it occurs is not yet understood, but the circular strand of viral DNA is opened and the linear DNA can be spliced into the host DNA. It can then use the protein production apparatus of the transformed host cell.

Disruption of the viral genome at the E_1-E_2 ORFs appears to inactivate E_2 expression. Because the E_2-encoded proteins regulate the transcription of the early region and ORFs, the loss of E_2 control allows for the unregulated or overexpression of the E_6- and E_7-encoded proteins. The E_6 and E_7 proteins are highly oncogenic. They appear to disrupt the normal process of cellular replicative control by binding to key proteins that help regulate cell division. The E_6 protein binds to the p53 protein and causes its inactivation and more rapid degradation. The p53 protein is an important negative growth regulator that plays a key role in the control of cell division. The E_7 protein binds to cyclin A p107 and the retinoblastoma gene product, p105RB. The p105RB proteins are responsible for controlling the progression of cells from the G1 phase of the cell cycle to the S phase.

In tissue culture models, E_6- and E_7-encoded proteins have been shown to be capable of transforming normal epithelial cells to neoplastic cells, and it has further been reported that both E_6 and E_7 expression are necessary to maintain the transformed state. The oncogenic proteins encoded for by these viral genes appear to complement each other and are only weakly active when present alone. HPV viruses with a high oncogenic potential (e.g., HPV types 16 and 18) produce E_6- and E_7-encoded proteins that have a transforming potency greater than that of proteins produced by HPVs with an intermediate oncogenic risk. The E_6- and E_7-encoded protein produced by HPV types with little or no oncogenic risk (6 and 11) seem to be incapable of transforming cells *in vitro*. This feature probably accounts for the differences in risk rates between the viral subtypes (Table 45.3). The importance of E_6 and E_7 in maintaining the transformed cell state has been demonstrated by inserting an antisense message for these ORFs in tissue culture cells. Such insertion is capable of reversing the transformed phenotype.

Simple deregulation of the mitotic process appears to be insufficient for producing neoplastic transformation. Recent data suggest that mutations in other cellular genes whose proteins are important in regulating the mitotic process are required for transformation to occur. It is now evident that the process of malignant transformation usually involves five to six such mutations. The p53 antioncogene is responsible for ascertaining that the genome is intact after DNA replication before the cell is allowed to divide. If DNA coding errors are found, they are repaired and the cell is allowed to progress to and complete cell division, or, if repair is not possible, the cells are not allowed to divide and instead a process of programmed cell death (apoptosis) is initiated. E_6 and E_7 oncogenic proteins are produced, which bind to and inactivate p53 so that it can no longer carry out the function of surveillance and quality control over DNA replication. Thus, the epithelial cells, even with chromosomal mutations are able to complete repeated mitotic cycles. It is probably that the accumulation of mutated genes is required for the cervical epithelial cell to become fully transformed. These alterations that occur at the molecular level result in changes in the chromosome number, in mitotic abnormalities, and in morphologically identifiable abnormalities in the chromosomes and eventually result in the production of an aneuploid cell population. This process of malignant transformation probably starts at the point at which HPV is integrated into the host epithelial cell chromosomes.

The Role of Immunosuppression in HPV-Related Lesions

It is clear from multiple clinical observations that men and women who are immunosuppressed have a higher risk of developing HPV-related lesions of the anogenital tract. It is probably because of relative immunosuppression that some pregnant women develop vulvar condylomata that then undergo remission postpartum without any treatment having been administered. Similarly, women who undergo renal transplantation or women with chronic immunosuppression have a high risk of developing HPV-related lesions and a high risk of developing lower genital tract cancers. These data support the concept of HPV latency and argue for the strong role of an intact immune system in controlling HPV infections. More recent observations of men and women who are immunosuppressed secondary to infection with HIV confirm the importance of immunocompetence in suppressing latent HPV infection and in facilitating the acquisition of HPV infection. Not only are HPV-related lesions more common in immunosuppressed individuals, but they tend to be larger, more often multicentric, and more likely to recur after treatment.

A number of studies of women who have acquired immunodeficiency syndrome (AIDS) have confirmed that this group of individuals is at increased risk for developing HPV-related lesions. In one of the first studies of women with AIDS, it was reported that in a group enrolled in a methadone maintenance program in New York, 14 of 33 (42%) HIV-infected women with AIDS had abnormal Papanicolaou tests compared with 3 of 18 (17%) HIV-infected women without AIDS and 6 of 65 (13%) HIV seronegative women. In a more recent study, the prevalence of biopsy-proven CIN was five times higher in HIV seropositive women and increased progressively as the CD4 T-lymphocyte count decreased.

These observations support the model proposed earlier by Stafl and Mattingly in which the clinical development of invasive cervical cancer involves a struggle between the oncogenic effects of the HPV infection and the immunologic defense mechanisms of the woman.

SCREENING FOR CERVICAL NEOPLASIA

Cervical Cytology

After the introduction of cervical cytology for cervical cancer screening more than 50 years ago, multiple screening programs from all parts of the world have reported decreased rates of invasive cervical cancer and decreased death rates from a malignancy that had previously been the number one worldwide cause of cancer deaths in women. Yet, even today cervical cancer remains one of the leading causes of death for women in developing nations where Papanicolaou smear screening programs are nonexistent. The cervical screening program in the Province of British Columbia, Canada, is one of many examples of how effective cervical cytology screening can be. Since the implementation of a population-based Papanicolaou smear screening program in 1949, the incidence rate of invasive cervical cancer has decreased from more than 30 per 100,000 women to less than 5, and the mortality rate has decreased from 12 to about 3 per 100,000 (Fig. 45.3). These excellent results have been obtained through a combination of a population-based program with a central registry that notifies women every

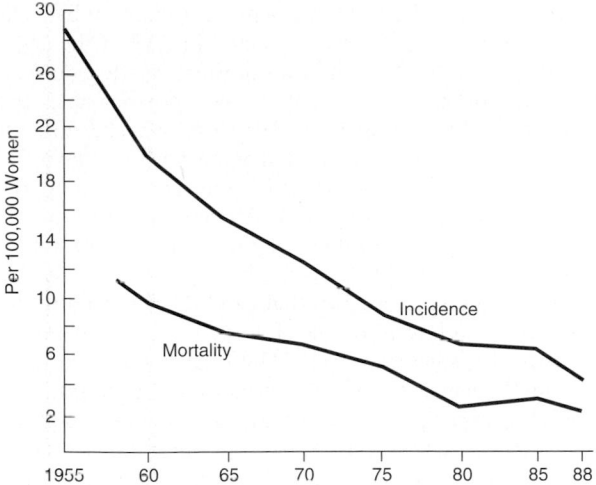

FIGURE 45.3. Incidence and mortality rate in women older than 20 years. British Columbia, 1988. (From Benedet JL, Anderson GH, Matisic JP. A comprehensive program for cervical cancer detection and management. *Am J Obstet Gynecol* 1992;166:1254–1259.)

3 years that their screening visit is due and follows up to be sure they do not default (a "call and recall" system), an excellent central cytology laboratory and well-trained clinicians to obtain the smears, and a network of colposcopy follow-up clinics where women with abnormal results are evaluated and treated. The program is well organized with quality control built in at every level and funding for this preventive health service and any follow up and treatment required is universally provided to all residents of the province. All of these elements are required to achieve excellent results from a screening program.

Despite the effectiveness of this and other cervical cytology screening programs, there are several limitations of Papanicolaou smear screening. A single Pap smear has a sensitivity of only about 50% to 60%. This means that a single test will not detect a cervical lesion in many women. However, even with this limited sensitivity, if three consecutive tests are negative, there is less than a 1% chance that the patient will have a cervical abnormality. A false-negative Papanicolaou smear may result from either screening or interpretation problems. Screening problems include lesions that do not shed cells or that are not sampled by the clinician. Or, sometimes, the diagnostic cells are not transferred from the spatula or collection device to the glass slide. Rarely, the slide preparation or staining is unsatisfactory. In other patients, problems with interpretation include failure to identify abnormal cells or misinterpretation of cells that are diagnosed as reactive or metaplastic when a dysplastic lesion exists. Various studies have shown that women who are diagnosed with invasive cervical cancer after a reportedly "negative" Papanicolaou smear most often have abnormal cells on review of their slides. The diagnostic cells may be few in number or obscured by blood or inflammatory changes. It is unfortunate that litigation over the

"missed diagnosis" of cervical neoplasia is such a common problem for cytology laboratories in the United States. The threat of a law suit may cause cytologists and cytopathologists to "overcall" a diagnosis and the gynecologist to recommend colposcopy and possibly cervical biopsy in a patient with any hint of abnormality. This not only increases the anxiety and morbidity associated with cervical cancer screening but it also increases the costs.

Liquid-Based, Thin-Layer Cytology

To decrease the false-negative rate of cervical cytology, attempts have been made to improve both specimen collection and quality and to reduce errors of interpretation. Over the past several years, several liquid-based techniques have been approved by the Food and Drug Administration in the United States. These techniques differ from the conventional method of Papanicolaou smear collection in several ways. Once the clinician obtains a scraping of the SCJ and transformation zone area of the exocervix, the spatula and brush are dipped and agitated in a small bottle of fixative solution to elute the cells rather than being smeared on a glass slide. The small bottle is labeled and sent to the cytology laboratory rather than sending a slide. Once in the lab, a machine prepares a slide containing about 40,000 representative epithelial cells in a thin layer. The slide is then stained with the conventional Papanicolaou stain and reviewed by the cytologists and cytopathologist. Several studies have shown that more diagnostic cervical cells are collected by this liquid-based technique and that the slides prepared from this sample provide a "cleaner" appearance with less clumping, blood, and inflammatory changes, thus providing a better specimen and hopefully a better interpretation. In a review, Dunton found that thin-layer, liquid-based cytology resulted in significantly fewer unsatisfactory and "satisfactory, but limited by" specimens and that more patients were diagnosed with both low- and high-grade lesion. The agency for Healthcare Research and Quality evaluated the literature available and concluded, "The relative true-positive rate for ThinPrep compared to conventional cytology is 1.13, suggesting a modestly higher sensitivity with ThinPrep, the relative false-positive rate is 1.12 suggesting a modestly lower specificity." This new technology costs more money than the conventional Papanicolaou smear, but theoretical analysis suggests that these costs are balanced by the possibility of less frequent screening intervals made possible by a more sensitive test. Liquid-based cytology reduces the rate of false-negative results from both screening and interpretation errors.

Computer-Assisted Diagnosis

It has long been believed that optical scanning by computer could be used for Papanicolaou smear interpretation but the differences in staining and the overlap of cells has made practical application very difficult. However, in the past several years, two different computer-based systems for cervical cytology use have been approved by the Food and Drug Administration. There are relatively few data published in the one system, which is commercially available in the United States. These techniques have been used mostly for quality control to identify slides that have been read as normal by cytotechnology screeners but that have cellular characteristics recognized by the computer as suspicious. In a primary screening trial, the AutoPap system was used to grade cervical cytology and the results compared with conventional screening. The computer "graded" each slide based on a number of characteristics and the 25% lowest scoring, "most normal" slides were diagnosed as within normal limits and received no further review. The other 75% were manually screened and the computer was used to identify 15% of the most suspicious for a second, manual rescreening. More than 25,000 slides were analyzed in this side-by-side comparison trial. Of the 70 cases of HSIL or greater, the computer-assisted arm identified 68 (including both invasive cancers) whereas the conventional screening arm identified 65 of the 70 patients with high-grade lesions. There was no statistically significant difference between these two arms. There is good evidence to suggest that computer-assisted diagnosis is even better when liquid-based, thin-layer slides are used because the background is much cleaner and there are fewer cell clumps with diagnostic cells obscuring one another. Although the initial cost of a computer-based system is large, considerable savings should be realized by the around-the-clock work and a reduced need for cytotechnologists who could concentrate on the diagnostic evaluation of high-risk slides identified by the computer on primary screening. More clinical experience with these computer techniques is needed but early results are promising.

Human Papillomavirus Testing

With the knowledge that cervical neoplasia is almost always (possibly always) associated with HPV, it was suggested that HPV testing could be used to screen women for cervical neoplasia. HPV testing in the past has been inaccurate and the complex laboratory techniques are not conducive to large volume clinical work. However, with the newer second-generation hybrid capture techniques, these problems seem to have been solved. Current technology uses DNA hybridization and quantification by a chemiluminescence reaction to identify the presence of any of 11 different, high- and intermediate-risk HPV. In a trial of 1,119 high-risk women in Costs Rica, Schiffman and colleagues demonstrated an 88% sensitivity to detect high-grade lesions compared with a Papanicolaou test sensitivity of 77.7%. Twelve percent of the women screened were HPV positive and were referred for colposcopy as compared with a 6.9% referral rate with the less sensitive Papanicolaou smear screening. In a similar trial from South Africa, Wright and colleagues instructed patients on self-collection of vaginal samples and were able to detect high-risk HPV DNA in 66% of the patients with high-grade lesions. This was almost identical to the 68% pickup rate of abnormal cytol-

ogy collected at the time of a pelvic examination by a clinician. High-risk HPV was detected in 84% of the specimens obtained by the clinician during a pelvic examination. In high-risk, sexually active populations, the problem of "false positive" HPV tests may be difficult because a certain number of women with a subclinical HPV infection clear the virus without cervical neoplasia ever developing. In the South African trial, 15% of the women who tested positive for HPV had no cervical lesion. Nevertheless, HPV testing is easy to perform and is a relatively inexpensive test that can be automated in the laboratory and requires no interpretation (a problem with the Papanicolaou test). These advantages must be weighted against its lack of specificity for high-grade lesions; however, it may be of particular benefit in resource-poor settings where cytology laboratories are not available. At the present time, HPV testing is being more widely used as a triage step in women with ASCs on Papanicolaou tests. This is discussed later in this chapter.

EVALUATION OF ABNORMAL CYTOLOGY

Following the announcement of the 2001 Bethesda System terminology for reporting the results of cervical cytology, the American Society of Colposcopy and Cervical Pathology sponsored a 3-day consensus conference to develop management guidelines. These are very detailed and carefully crafted to include almost all situations and were published by Wright and colleagues in 2002. It is important for the clinician to distinguish between cytologic or Papanicolaou smear abnormalities and biopsy or histologic abnormalities. In this section, the evaluation of cytologic abnormalities are discussed; in the following section, the management of patients with biopsy-proven abnormalities is presented. In both sections, high-grade abnormalities are discussed first because they are the least controversial and most important. Treatment rarely is initiated based on the results of cervical cytology alone. The Papanicolaou smear result, colposcopic impression, and biopsy diagnosis should all be in general agreement, although it is common that they may not agree precisely on the grade of abnormality.

High-Grade Squamous Intraepithelial Lesions

Approximately 0.5% of all Papanicolaou smears are diagnosed as HSIL (Fig. 45.4). When these patients are evaluated, more than 70% will have biopsy-proven moderate dysplasia (CIN 2) or worse, and 1% to 2% will have an invasive cancer. Because high-grade abnormalities may progress to invasive cancer or, indeed, be associated with an already existing invasive cancer, women with an HSIL Papanicolaou test should be referred for colposcopic evaluation.

In many cases, biopsy confirmation of the lesion will be done by loop electrode excision procedure (LEEP) of the whole transformation zone which serves as both a di-

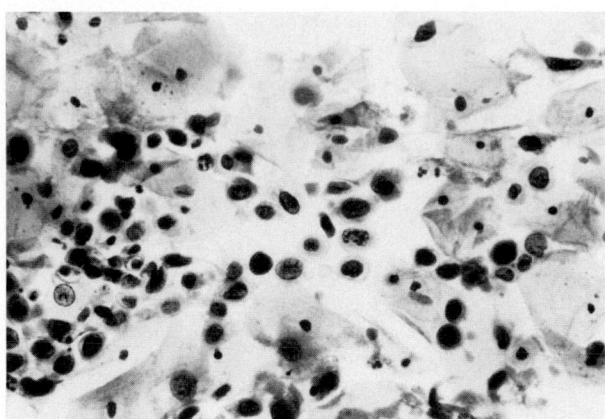

FIGURE 45.4. Papanicolaou smear showing high-grade cervical intraepithelial neoplasia. Normal superficial cells contain small, pyknotic, regular nuclei. Abnormal cells exfoliated from high-grade lesions are of the neoplastic basal and parabasal types, have an altered nuclear:cytoplasmic ratio, and contain very hyperchromatic, irregularly shaped, pleomorphic nuclei with a dense, abnormal chromatin pattern.

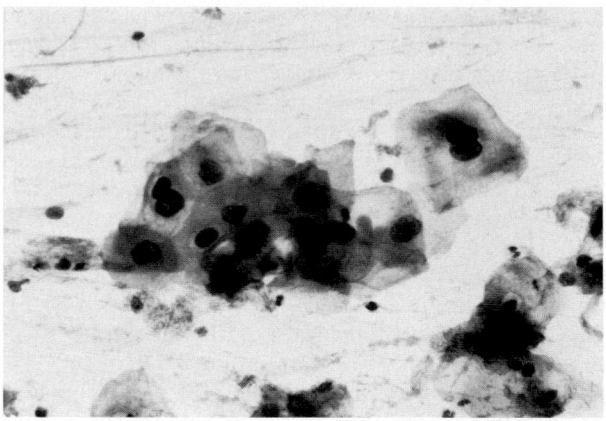

FIGURE 45.5. Papanicolaou smear showing low-grade cervical intraepithelial neoplasia. A cluster of superficial squamous cells containing hyperchromatic, atypical nuclei is seen. Several cells are binucleated. The cells with perinuclear clearing and nuclear atypia are referred to as koilocytes. These changes are characteristic of a productive human papillomavirus infection of the genital tract mucosa.

agnostic and a treatment procedure. This is particularly important in large, high-grade lesions because the colposcopic diagnosis of microinvasive cancer is difficult. Unless excision and histologic study of the whole transformation zone is done, microinvasive cancer may be missed.

If a woman with an HSIL Papanicolaou smear does not have a high-grade lesion identified on colposcopy, an endocervical curettage (ECC) should be done. If the origin of the HSIL Papanicolaou finding is still not identified, the clinician should request a review of the cytology, ECC, and any cervical biopsies. If the cytopathologist still believes that a high-grade lesion exists that has not been identified by biopsy, then the cervix and vagina should be reexamined and a LEEP or cone biopsy done, especially if the SCJ cannot be visualized.

Low-Grade Squamous Epithelial Lesion

Of all Papanicolaou smear diagnoses, about 1.5% to 2.0% are LSIL. Between 15% and 30% of these women have moderate dysplasia or worse, and 1 to 2 per 1,000 have invasive cancer (Fig. 45.5). Although the risk of a significant lesion is lower in these women, referral for colposcopic evaluation is still recommended.

There are many treatment options for women with mild dysplasia (CIN 1) on colposcopically directed biopsy. But because of the wide possibility of diagnosis in women with an LSIL Papanicolaou finding, colposcopic evaluation and biopsy confirmation of the diagnosis is indicated. In a patient with no visible lesion on the exocervix and vagina to explain the abnormal Pap test, an endocervical curettage is indicated.

When no lesion to explain the LSIL Papanicolaou finding can be found, the evaluation can be repeated in 4 to 6 months, a LEEP could be done, or consultation

with a more experienced colposcopist could be requested. In postmenopausal women, atrophy can cause minor cellular atypia, which can produce an LSIL Papanicolaou finding, so treatment with topical estrogen for 2 months may be helpful before repeating the cytologic study.

Atypical Squamous Cells

A diagnosis of ASC is the most common abnormal Papanicolaou diagnosis, occurring in 2.5% to 5.0% of all Papanicolaou smears. Although high-grade lesions are present in only 5% to 10% of these patients and because of the relatively large number of women with these ASC diagnoses, more women with a biopsy diagnosis of moderate dysplasia or worse present with an ASC Papanicolaou than any other Papanicolaou diagnosis, including HSIL. Even so, immediate referral to colposcopy for all these patients *is not cost effective* because there are so many women with no significant cervical abnormalities. Another option is to bring these patients back for *repeat Papanicolaou testing in 4 to 6 months*. This can lead to a delay in diagnosis, and it is not unusual for 20% or more of these patients to be lost to follow-up, producing an even greater delay. It is probably not of great importance if a progression from mild to severe dysplasia occurs during this follow-up or even lost to follow-up delay because treatment of various degrees of intraepithelial neoplasia is similar, but occasionally invasive cancer develops during this period. It has been estimated that there are about 1.25 million women each year in the United States with an ASC Papanicolaou finding. Even if the risk of cervical cancer is very low, with such a large number of women at risk, invasive cancer will already have developed or will develop during a follow-up management protocol.

The third management option for women with an ASC-US Papanicolaou finding is *triage by HPV testing*. Several large prospective studies have demonstrated the effectiveness of this approach. In a National Cancer Institute–sponsored randomized trial, Schiffman and colleagues randomized a group of 4,500 women with ASC-US Papanicolaou findings to immediate colposcopy, follow-up every 6 months until two consecutive ASC-US Paps, or HPV triage. All women were eventually colposcoped and treated by LEEP at 24 months if they had not already been diagnosed and treated for CIN earlier. In this study, HPV testing identified 95% of the patients with CIN 3 or greater and required colposcopy in only 55% of the patients. The follow-up arm was able to identify only 85% of the patients with a high-grade lesion and referred 60% for colposcopy. Even though the immediate colposcopy group should diagnose almost 100% of the CIN 3 lesions, it is very expensive in the United States where colposcopy charges are three to four times greater than an HPV test.

Patients with a Papanicolaou diagnosis of ASC-H should be referred for colposcopy because they have a 15% to 35% risk of having moderate dysplasia or worse. Even if colposcopic evaluation is negative, including an ECC, these patients need to be followed up carefully. The value of HPV testing in these patients is unproven; such patients usually test positive for high-risk HPV.

Glandular Abnormalities

In the 2001 Bethesda System, there are three categories plus adenocarcinoma under the classification of glandular cell abnormalities. These include atypical glandular cells (AGC), atypical glandular cells—favor neoplastic, and endocervical adenocarcinoma in situ (AIS). The cytologist should state if possible whether the glandular cells are endocervical, endometrial, or not otherwise specified. While it may be helpful for the clinician in the future, the experience with the different categories is still limited and it remains to be proven whether cytology can reliably differentiate between glandular dysplasia and AIS—and, indeed, between AIS and invasive adenocarcinoma.

Therefore, all patients with abnormal glandular cells of Papanicolaou smear should be referred for further evaluation. Follow-up studies show that 35% to 50% of these patients have a lesion and that most have squamous not glandular CIN (Fig. 45.6). A few have endocervical glandular dysplasia or AIS and a few have endometrial hyperplasia or adenocarcinoma. Endocervical glandular neoplasia is also HPV related so that it is often accompanied by a squamous dysplasia. For this reason, the diagnosis of moderate squamous dysplasia on the exocervix in a woman with an AGC Papanicolaou smear does not rule out an accompanying glandular lesion so that the workup for a possible glandular abnormality needs to be pursued. The association of HPV, especially type 18, suggests that HPV testing might also serve as a useful triage step in the evaluation of women with AGC findings, but this concept has not yet been proven clinically.

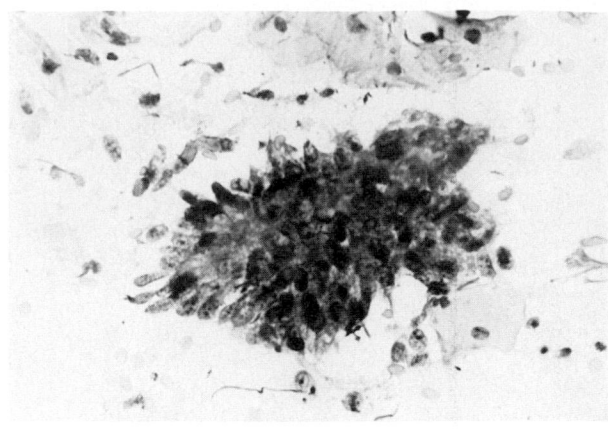

FIGURE 45.6. Papanicolaou smear showing adenocarcinoma in situ. A cluster of atypical endocervical cells with a feathered border and cytologically atypical nuclei characteristic of adenocarcinoma in situ is seen. Cells exfoliated from adenocarcinoma in situ tend to occur in clumps, which should raise the suspicion that a glandular neoplasm may be present.

Evaluation of the patient with an AGC Papanicolaou finding usually involves a colposcopic examination and an endocervical curettage, whether or not the SCJ can be visualized. If the ECC is positive for a glandular abnormality, a cone biopsy is indicated. Even though some experts are able to adequately evaluate endocervical glandular lesions with a LEEP specimen, we find that a LEEP often provides a specimen that is not deep enough and the deep endocervical margin is positive for glandular dysplasia or AIS. We recommend a traditional, deep, wide, cold knife cone biopsy under anesthesia in the operating room for the evaluation of glandular abnormalities. If the endocervical curettage is negative and the colposcopic examination is normal, the Papanicolaou diagnosis should be reviewed. Management options include a repeat Papanicolaou with or without colposcopy and ECC in 4 to 6 months or possible cone biopsy if suspicion of a cervical lesion is high.

These general guidelines should be helpful in most cases, but there are many special situations, including the evaluation of pregnant women, adolescents, and postmenopausal patients, in which alternative management plans may be more suitable. More extensive management guidelines are available in the *JAMA* article by Wright and colleagues or on the American Society for Colposcopy and Cervical Pathology Website: *www.asccp.org*.

Abnormal Papanicolaou Finding in Pregnancy

The pregnant woman with an abnormal Papanicolaou finding generally is evaluated by colposcopic examination and directed biopsy if a high-grade lesion is suspected. The goal of evaluation of the pregnant patient with CIN is to rule out invasive cancer. CIN is not treated in pregnancy but is followed up until the postpartum period when the patient usually is reevaluated and managed as indicated by the biopsy results and her social situation. During pregnancy, most clinicians do a cervical biopsy to confirm the diagnosis only if a high-grade lesion is suspected, although some recommend a confirming biopsy in all patients with a visible lesion. The pregnant cervix is very vascular especially in the later trimester, so a biopsy may bleed profusely and cervical trauma can initiate uterine contractions. An endocervical curettage is contraindicated in pregnancy. Rarely, a cone biopsy is required in pregnancy to rule out invasive cancer when colposcopy with directed biopsy does not eliminate that possibility. This can be a difficult and potentially bloody procedure and should be undertaken by an experienced gynecologist only after all other avenues to rule out invasion have been exhausted.

MANAGEMENT OF CERVICAL INTRAEPITHELIAL NEOPLASIA

The management of CIN or cervical dysplasia is almost always based on a colposcopically directed biopsy of the lesion rather than just the Papanicolaou or cytologic diagnosis or even the colposcopic impression. If there is a significant discrepancy between these diagnoses, the clinician should review the whole diagnostic evaluation to be sure cervical cancer is not being undertreated on the one hand or benign cervical inflammation or metaplasia is not being overtreated on the other hand. In addition to the biopsy diagnosis of the cervical lesion, the social situation of the patient often plays an important part in management decisions. For example, a 32-year-old mother of three with a three-quadrant CIN 1 lesion should probably be treated with LEEP or cryotherapy, whereas the same lesion in a 21-year-old unmarried student might well be watched for 12 months or so in hope that it will regress and no cervix will have to be removed or destroyed.

Treatment Indications

It is difficult, if not impossible, to write out a complete set of guidelines that encompasses every clinical situation. The preceding sections on the natural history of the transformation zone and CIN need to be applied to the specific patient and the various management options reviewed in order to select the best plan for that patient. In many cases, the patient may be helpful in the decision to treat or follow a lesion. Insurance coverage, school vacations, and equipment availability could all influence the choice or timing of treatment.

CIN 1—Mild Dysplasia

Reviews by Oster and more recently by Nuovo and colleagues have shown that regression occurs with no treatment in about 50% of women with a cervical biopsy showing CIN 1 during 12 to 24 months of follow-up (Table 45.3). Although good data do not exist, larger lesions and lesions that have persisted for a

longer time are probably less likely to regress spontaneously. Because the treatment options are the same and chance of complete cure approaches 100% for CIN 1 and CIN 2 or 3, the consequences of progression are minimal. It is, therefore, reasonable to manage a patient with CIN 1 by observation alone. Follow-up without biopsy-proven CIN 1 is not recommended because cytology and colposcopy are not sufficiently accurate to confidently rule out a more severe lesion (Fig. 45.7). The only two risks to this approach are that invasive cancer already exists and has been missed on the diagnostic evaluation of this patient or that the patient becomes lost to follow-up and does not reappear until her condition has progressed to invasive cancer. These risks are minimal, but in almost all series in which women with low-grade cervical abnormalities have been followed up with no treatment, invasive cancer has eventually been diagnosed in a few patients.

For this reason and because treatment is relatively easy with limited patient inconvenience, side effects, complications, and costs, CIN 1 lesions in women who have completed their families who have three- or four-quadrant lesions or who have had a lesion for 12 months or longer should be considered for treatment. These low-grade abnormalities have cure rates of 90% or better with LEEP, cryotherapy, or CO_2 laser vaporization. Traditional cold knife cone biopsy is probably associated with more morbidity and cost than is warranted by CIN 1.

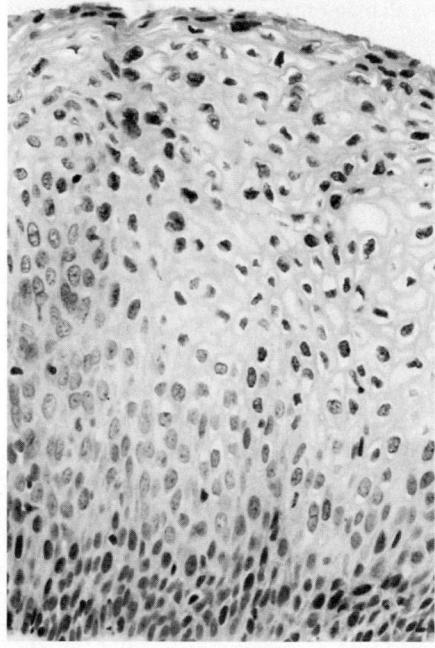

FIGURE 45.7. Histologic section of low-grade cervical intraepithelial neoplasia. A productive human papillomavirus infection in the cervical epithelium is characterized by cytologic atypia and hyperchromasia (heteroploidy), binucleated cells (lack of cytokinesis), and koilocytosis (binding of filaggrin). No other agent produces these changes, which are diagnostic.

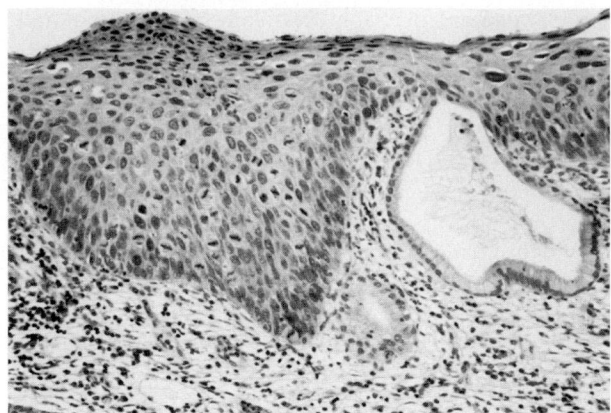

FIGURE 45.8. Histologic section of high-grade cervical intraepithelial neoplasia. This lesion has some features of low-grade cervical intraepithelial neoplasia but also contains abnormal mitotic figures—a diagnostic feature of an aneuploid, high-grade, human papillomavirus–related lesion.

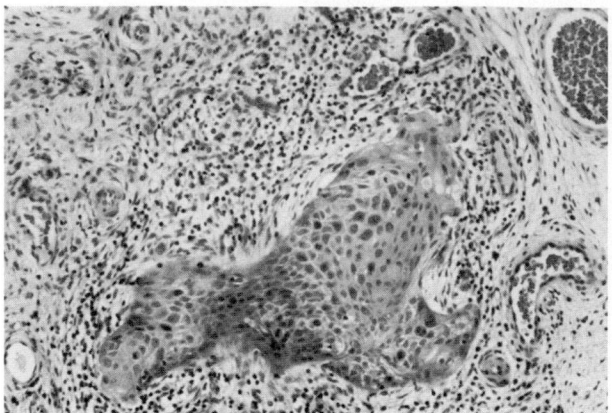

FIGURE 45.9. Histologic section of microinvasive squamous cell carcinoma. In microinvasive cancer, tongues of neoplastic epithelium extend through the plane of the basal lamina to split collagen bundles as they penetrate the cervical stroma, creating an irregular outline. Early invasion is commonly accompanied by a local inflammatory response.

Although patients with "atypical metaplasia" or chronic cervicitis have been treated with cautery or cryotherapy in the past, these are not generally indications for treatment under modern guidelines.

CIN 2 or 3—Moderate or Severe Dysplasia, Carcinoma in Situ

Patients with a biopsy diagnosis of CIN 2 or 3 have a less than 50% chance of regression and a significant chance of progression to carcinoma in situ (Fig. 45.8), so treatment is usually recommended. Pregnant women and, occasionally, very young women or those who wish to retain their fertility and have been previously treated for CIN may be followed up conservatively.

Although treatment of these lesions can be successful using either ablative or excisional techniques, high-grade lesions bordering on invasive cancer are best managed by excision, which makes a tissue specimen available for examination by the pathologist. In several large series of LEEP specimens, a few invasive cancers that had been unsuspected were diagnosed on histopathologic examination of the whole transformation zone. Cryotherapy or laser vaporization of such lesions would be inappropriate and could result in a deeply invasive cancer going untreated for several months or even several years.

A cold knife cone biopsy in the operating room under anesthesia is indicated when cytology, colposcopy, or directed punch biopsy suggests superficially invasive cancer. Negative margins and a large specimen in one piece that can be well oriented is essential for an accurate and complete diagnosis of microinvasive cervical cancer. A final diagnosis of microinvasive cervical cancer cannot be made on punch biopsy or endocervical curettage. It is necessary to examine tissue on all sides of the microinvasive focus to be sure more deeply invasive disease does not exist adjacent to the focal area sampled by punch biopsy or ECC (Fig. 45.9).

Adenocarcinoma in Situ or Glandular Dysplasia

These diagnoses also require a cone or large biopsy of the endocervical epithelium and stroma with negative margins for diagnosis. An endocervical curettage or punch biopsy are inadequate to rule out a more extensive, possibly invasive, lesion. As previously noted, I favor cold knife cone biopsy for the evaluation of glandular lesions.

The standard of care for AIS of the cervix in the United States is still simple hysterectomy, although there is some increasing interest in the use of cone biopsy alone for these patients. If cone biopsy is used as definitive management of AIS, the margins should be negative and enough sections of the cervix need to have been studied to be confident that an early invasive adenocarcinoma does not coexist. Glandular dysplasia can also be managed by cone biopsy if the margins are clear, but there are few data on this subject.

Treatment Techniques

In general, treatment techniques can be divided into ablative and excisional. Destructive methods such as cryotherapy, CO_2 laser ablation, and electrocautery rely on an accurate colposcopically directed biopsy diagnosis because no tissue specimen is provided by the treatment procedure. On the other hand, punch biopsy, LEEP, and cone biopsy all provide a specimen so these techniques are both diagnostic and therapeutic.

Punch Biopsy as Therapy

In most developed countries, women are highly screened; invasive cancers are uncommon, particularly in younger age groups; high-grade CIN is relatively uncommon; and most lesions that are detected are low-grade CINs found as incident cases. Because most of the cases of CIN are low-grade lesions that have developed between screening visits, the lesions tend to be small, to be located at the SCJ, and to occur in younger, often nulliparous women. For such patients, simple removal of the lesion with one or two punch biopsies or a small, segmental resection with an electrosurgical loop is adequate. Theoretically, the entire transformation zone should be destroyed or removed, but in some patients, these small biopsies clear the abnormalities.

Cryotherapy

Cryosurgery is a destructive technique that was introduced to gynecologists in the late 1960s to treat CIN. The cryosurgical instruments use nitrous oxide or carbon dioxide as a refrigerant to lower the temperature of the tissue below $-22°C$ and to produce cell death by intracellular and extracellular water crystallization. The refrigerant is applied to the cervix with a cryoprobe, which is placed in contact with the cervical epithelium. As the gas is circulated through the cryoprobe, it withdraws heat from the cervix until freezing temperatures occur. The cervix and cryoprobe generally reach a steady state after about 3 minutes of freezing, at which time the amount of heat brought to the cervix by the vascular supply balances the amount of heat withdrawn from the cervix by the evaporating cryogenic gas.

Tens of thousands of patients have been treated with cryotherapy, which has proved to be a predictable, reliable treatment technique with limited side effects and morbidity. Cryotherapy is used principally in patients whose lesions are confined to the exocervix because the depth of cryodestruction seldom exceeds 5 mm. The cure rates are dependent on the size of the lesion. They generally average about 90% for lesions involving one quadrant, but only 75% for lesions involving three or more quadrants. The cryocurability is not related to the histologic grade of the lesion, except as histologic grade influences lesional size and distribution. Opinions differ as to whether a single freeze-thaw cycle or a double freeze-thaw cycle is the optimal approach to cryotherapeutic treatment, but there appear to be no differences in cure rates between the two approaches.

The most important end point in cryotherapy is that the ice ball should extend well past the edge of the lesion. A minimum of 5 mm margin is recommended. The incidental, small CIN lesions can be treated adequately by cryotherapy with a single cryoprobe application. When multiple probe placements are required to cover the lesion, cryotherapy may not be the best treatment. It is generally useful to apply acetic acid and Lugol's to the cervix before cryotherapy to reestablish the size and distribution of the lesion.

Patients treated with cryotherapy may experience minor cramping during the procedure but otherwise the treatment is not painful. Thus, it is generally not necessary to anesthetize the cervix or give the patient premedication. After cryosurgery, about 20% of patients experience a profuse watery discharge that may require wearing a pad. Some patients experience light spotting,

particularly 12 to 15 days after cryotherapy when the eschar begins to separate from the treated areas.

Long-term complications of cryotherapy are minimal and consist principally of cervical stenosis or narrowing in 1% to 4% of patients. Several studies have reported that there is no change in fertility and that pregnancy complications seldom occur, except in patients who have excessive cervical fibrosis and in whom cervical dystocia may be a problem. Postcryotherapeutic healing is rapid (it is generally completed within 12 weeks) and usually restores the SCJ to be coincident with the external os. It is important, however, that the flat or shallow cone cryoprobe be used for treatment, because cryoprobes that have deep endocervical extensions may lead to cervical stenosis. In most patients, the SCJ will not be visible after the cervix has healed following cryotherapy. Cryosurgery is a safe, useful, inexpensive procedure that should be considered for any patient (particularly young and nulliparous patients) with a low-grade lesion confined to one or two quadrants of the exocervix.

Carbon Dioxide Laser

The CO_2 laser is another useful treatment modality for the management of CIN lesions. This laser is an instrument that produces a high-intensity columnar beam of light that can be concentrated to a small spot where it produces a small footprint and a high-power density. This concentration of energy vaporizes the tissue by rapidly boiling the intracellular water, causing the cells to explode. The CO_2 laser can be used to ablate tissue or to cut, depending on the spot size and the power density. When the energy is concentrated on an extremely small spot, the light beam penetrates the tissue deeply and rapidly. It can be used as a knife to excise a lesion, although this requires considerable skill and experience as well as an expensive laser. Surgical excision using the CO_2 laser is not often used for CIN these days. When the laser beam is defocused to spread the energy over a larger area but while it still retains sufficient power density to produce cellular destruction, it can be used to evaporate tissues fairly rapidly. The CO_2 laser is used to ablate CIN in patients whose lesion is confined to the portio and in whom invasive cancer has been ruled out by colposcopically directed biopsies and endocervical curettage.

The CO_2 laser has the following advantages: it can be used for either cutting or ablation; the healing after laser surgery is rapid; and there are minimal side effects, including limited vaginal discharge. Patients treated with the CO_2 laser generally have less cervical narrowing and a lower stenosis rate than those treated with cryotherapy. There is no diminution of fertility, and there are no obstetric complications after laser treatment. The major disadvantages of the laser are (1) its acquisition expense, (2) the time required to acquire and maintain laser skills, particularly for laser conization, and (3) the relatively high maintenance cost of the instrument. Use of the CO_2 laser for the management of CIN has decreased dramatically since the introduction of loop electrosurgical excision.

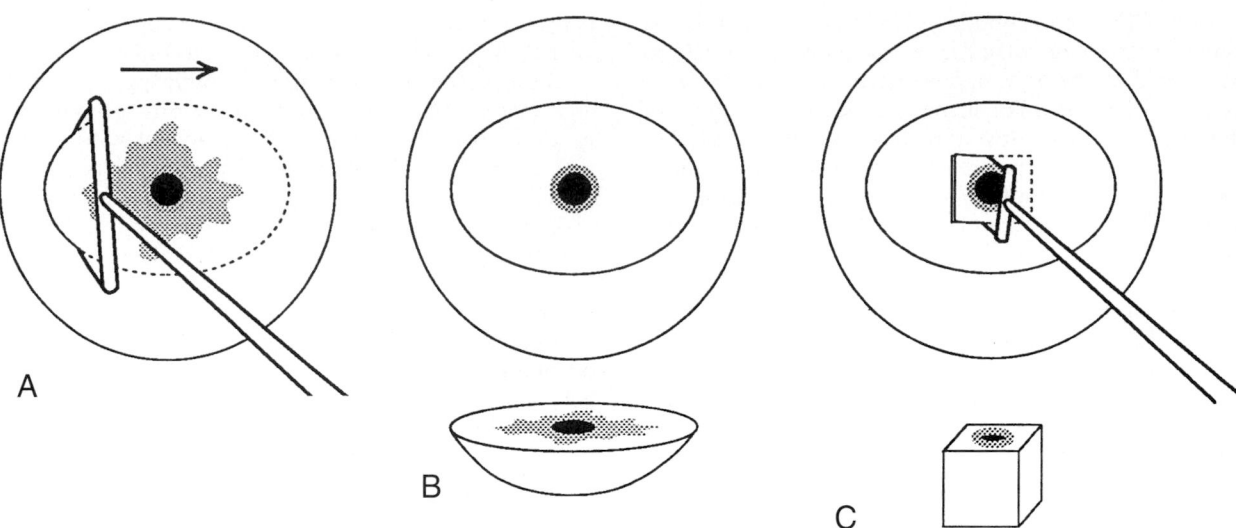

FIGURE 45.10. Diagram of approach to loop excision of small portio lesion, which can be removed by a single pass **(A)** of the 2-cm × 7-mm exoloop. **B:** Note the shallow dish configuration of the removed tissue. After the exocervical excision is completed, the canal is recolposcoped after additional acetic acid is applied. If residual disease is found in the canal, it can be removed by the endoloop **(C)**. (From Wright TC, Richart RM, Ferenczy A. Electrosurgery for HPV-related diseases of the anogenital tract. New York: ArthurVision, 1992.)

Loop Electrosurgical Excision

LEEP was introduced in the United Kingdom as large loop excision of the transformation zone after the modification of techniques originally developed in France. LEEP was introduced in North America in the early 1990s and, as in Europe, rapidly became the procedure of choice for the management of CIN.

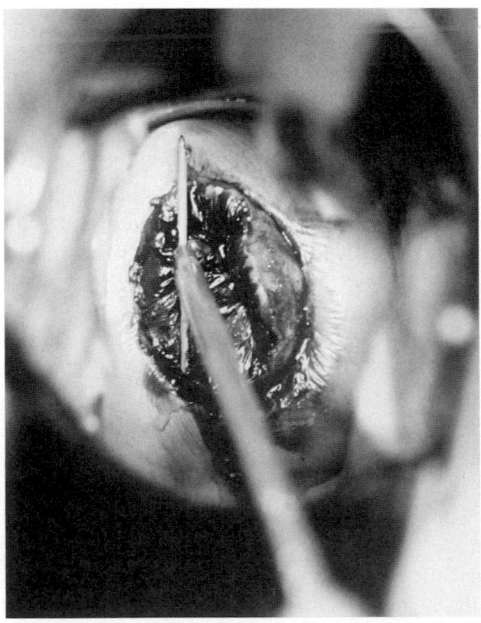

FIGURE 45.11. Loop electrosurgical excision procedure. Endosurgical loop is passed through a Lugol-stained cervix from right to left. Note cut surface of cervical stroma from the 12-o'clock to the 6-o'clock position. Also note lack of charring so commonly seen with laser ablation.

LEEP takes advantage of the properties of modern, solid-state, electrosurgical generators coupled with loop electrodes, made with a thin stainless steel or tungsten wire, to excise areas of CIN (Fig. 45.10). It is also possible to electrocoagulate tissue with a 5-mm ball electrode. LEEP is used under colposcopic control and has the advantage of being a diagnostic and therapeutic procedure at the same time. The fact that a tissue specimen is provided makes the procedure particularly useful in ruling out early invasive cancer and in identifying unsuspected AIS. Many authors have reported that 4 to 6 per 1,000 cases diagnosed by colposcopy, punch biopsies, and endocervical curettage as having CIN in fact have invasive cancer or AIS in the specimen removed by LEEP.

Because LEEP is easy to learn, easy to teach, and easy to apply, it can be used to treat patients with high-grade CIN without the disadvantages and great cost of cold knife conization (Fig. 45.11). The major advantage of LEEP over conventional cold knife conization is that the procedure can be performed under colposcopic control and the margins can be examined colposcopically after the initial excisions are completed. This gives the operator the opportunity to reexcise additional tissue if it is found colposcopically that residual CIN remains. For LEEP to be used effectively, the extent of excision and the choice of electrodes must be tailored to the size and distribution of the lesion. When disease extends into the canal, however, a loop endocervical excision procedure can be performed with use of a 1- ×1-cm loop electrode. If the lesion is present on both the portio and the canal, a "reverse cowboy hat" combined endocervical-portio excision is appropriate. The preferred electrode for the portio excision should not exceed 2.5 cm in width and 7 mm in depth. The use of extremely large electrodes may lead to inadvertent cervical amputations and significant reproductive and obstetric morbidity. The side effects and complications of LEEP are almost identical to those of the CO_2 laser.

Although low-grade lesions can readily be treated with cryotherapy, many gynecologists choose LEEP excision instead because of its ease of use, its limited morbidity, and the fact that it provides a specimen. Caution is advised in choosing LEEP for small lesions in women who have only small areas of CIN in a small, nulliparous cervix because it is possible to produce irreversible cervical damage. With few exceptions, all high-grade lesions should be removed with use of an excisional, rather than an ablative, procedure.

Cervical Conization

Traditional cold knife conization has been used successfully for generations to excise lesions that extend into the endocervical canal to rule out invasive cancer. The cone is generally planned to be both diagnostic and therapeutic, and the technique is widely understood and practiced (Fig. 45.12). We recommend cone biopsy for endocervical glandular lesions and for suspected microinvasion because accurate diagnosis of these lesions requires a large tissue specimen with negative margins. The cone usually is performed in an operating room under anesthesia and, thus, it is expensive. Because of the size of the specimen excised, bleeding and other sequelae such as cervical stenosis and infection are more common.

See and Treat

Because LEEP is a simple procedure that can be used for both diagnosis and treatment during a single office visit, its use has been recommended in the so called "see and treat" mode. With this application, patients who are detected as having an abnormal Papanicolaou smear are seen for colposcopy, and when a clear-cut colposcopically

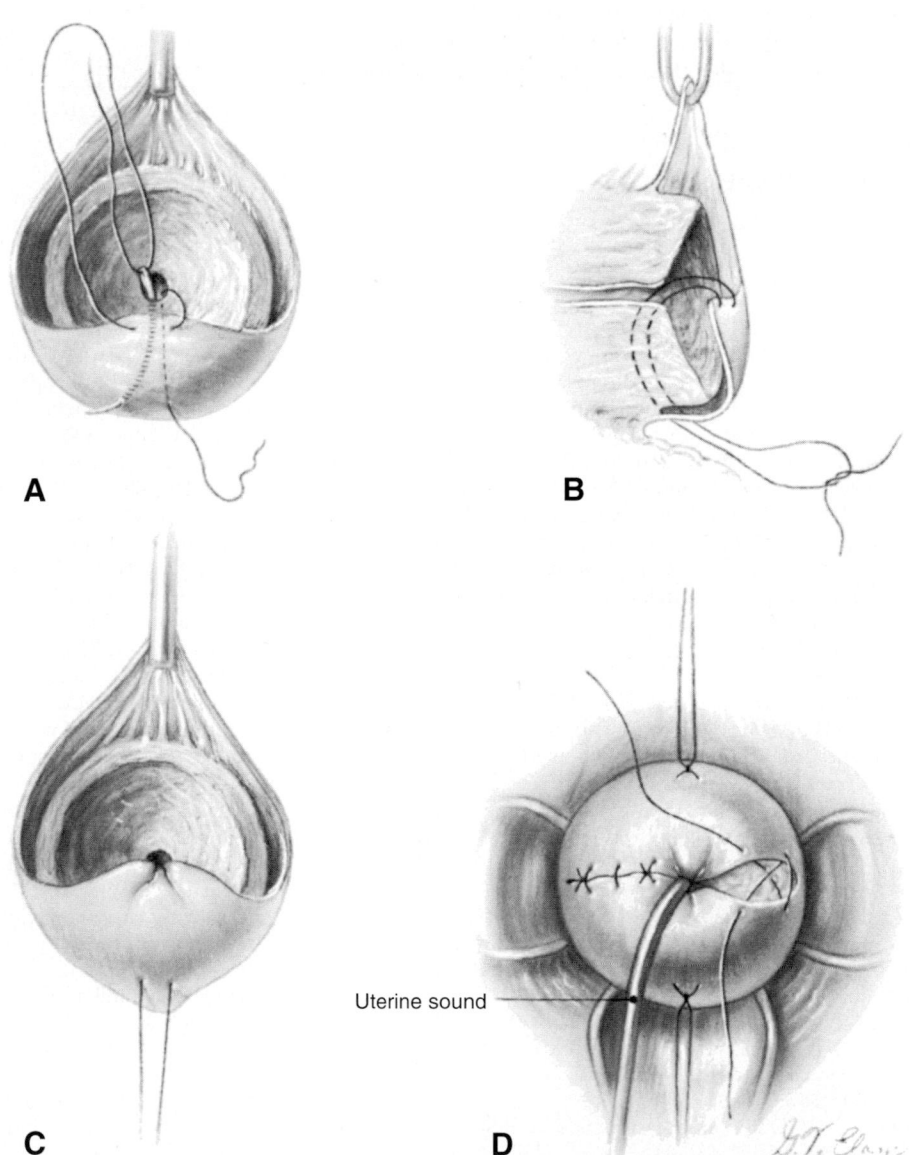

FIGURE 45.12. A: Mattress suture is placed as in Sturmdorf tracheloplasty. **B:** Method of action of suture in drawing the flap into the canal. **C:** The lower flap has been pulled into position. **D:** Anterior and posterior flaps have been drawn into the canal. Lateral mucosa wounds are being sutured.

Uterine sound

visible lesion is present, the lesion is removed in its entirety with use of the loop electrode. The patient does not first have to undergo cervical biopsies and an endocervical curettage.

The advantages to this approach are that the procedure is done in one office visit, thus reducing patient anxiety by eliminating the need to wait for a diagnosis to be rendered and to then return for additional treatment, and, if used appropriately, it may save time and money. The disadvantage to this approach is that the colposcopic appearance of squamous metaplasia, repair, or other non–HPV-related changes may mimic CIN, and some patients who do not have a CIN lesion may have benign epithelium excised inappropriately. For see-and-treat to be used effectively and appropriately, the colposcopist must be certain that the colposcopic changes that are seen are sufficiently characteristic that a diagnosis of an HPV-related lesion can be assured. Under these circumstances, see-and-treat may be the procedure of choice. Spitzer and colleagues have shown that in an inner-city clinic, the LEEP see-and-treat approach is highly beneficial and provides the opportunity to treat patients with significant lesions who might otherwise not return for their scheduled therapeutic follow-up visits.

BIBLIOGRAPHY

Agency for Health Care Policy and Research. Evaluation of Cervical Cytology. AHCPR Publication No. 99-E010, February, 1999.

American Cancer Society. Early Detection of Cervical Cancer. No. 52, 2002.

Anderson GH, Benedet JL, Le Riche JC, et al. Invasive cancer of the cervix in British Columbia: a review of the demography and screening histories of 427 cases seen from 1985–88. *Obstet Gynecol* 1992;80:1–4.

Barron BA, Richart RM. A statistical model of the natural history of cervical carcinoma based on a prospective study of 557 cases. *J Natl Cancer Inst* 1968;41:1343.

Barron BA, Richart RM. Statistical model of the natural history of cervical carcinoma, II: estimates of the transition time from dysplasia to carcinoma-in-situ. *J Natl Cancer Inst* 1971;45:1025.

Bedell MA, Jones KH, Laimins LA. The E_6-E_7 region of human papillomavirus type 18 is sufficient for transformation of NIH 3T3 and rat-1 cells. *J Virol* 1987;61:3635.

Benedet JL, Anderson GH, Matisic JP. A comprehensive program for cervical cancer detection and management. *Am J Obstet Gynecol* 1992;166:1254–1259.

Benedet JL, Anderson GH, Boyes DA. Colposcopic accuracy in the diagnosis of microinvasive and occult invasive carcinoma of the cervix. *Obstet Gynecol* 1985;65:557–562.

Bergeron C, Barrasso R, Beaudenon S, et al. Human papillomaviruses associated with cervical intraepithelial neoplasia: great diversity and distinct distribution in low- and high-grade lesions. *Am J Surg Pathol* 1992;16:641.

Berstein SJ, Sanchez-Ramos L, Ndubisi B. Liquid-based cervical cytologic smear study and conventional Papanicolaou smears: a metaanalysis of prospective studies comparing cytologic diagnosis and sample adequacy. *Am J Obstet Gynecol* 2001;185:308–317.

Brinton LA. Oral contraceptives and cervical neoplasia. *Contraception* 1991;43:581.

Brinton LA, Fraumeni JF. Epidemiology of uterine cervical cancer. *J Chronic Dis* 1986;39:1051.

Broker TR. Structure and genetic expression of papillomaviruses. *Obstet Gynecol Clin North Am* 1987;14:329.

Cordon-Cardo C. Mutation of cell cycle regulators: biological and clinical implications for human neoplasia. *Am J Pathol* 1995;147:545.

Cox JT, Schiffman MH, Winzelberg AJ, et al. An evaluation of human papillomavirus testing as part of referral to colposcopy clinics. *Obstet Gynecol* 1992;80:389.

Crum CP, Nuovo G, Friedman D, et al. Accumulation of RNA homologous to human papillomavirus type 16 open reading frames in genital precancers. *J Virol* 1988;62:84.

Cullen AP, Reid R, Campion M, et al. An analysis of the physical state of different human papillomavirus DNAs in intraepithelial and invasive cervical neoplasia. *J Virol* 1991;65:606.

Cullen TS. *Cancer of the uterus.* New York: Appleton and Company, 1900.

Dale GE, Coleman RM, Best JM, et al. Class-specific herpes simplex virus antibodies in sera and cervical secretions from patients with cervical neoplasia: a multi-group comparison. *Epidemiol Int* 1988;100:455.

Denny L, Kuhn L, Pollack A, et al. Evaluation of alternative methods of cervical cancer screening for resource-poor settings. *Cancer* 2000;89:826–833.

de Villiers EM. Heterogeneity of the human papillomavirus group. *J Virol* 1989;63:4898.

Doorbar J. An emerging function for E_4. *Papillomavirus Reports* 1991;2:145.

Doorbar J, Ely S, Steriling J, et al. Specific interaction between HPV 16 E_1-E_4 and cytokeratins results in collapse of the epithelial cell intermediate filament network. *Nature* 1991;352:824.

Dunton CJ. New technology in Papanicolaou smear processing. *Clin Obstet Gynecol* 2000;43:410–417.

Dyson N, Lowley PM, Munger K, et al. The human papillomavirus 16 E_7 oncoprotein is able to bind to the retinoblastoma gene product. *Science* 1989;243:934.

Finlay CA, Hinds PW, Levine AJ. The p53 protooncogene can act as a suppressor of transformation. *Cell* 1989;57:1083.

Firzlaff JM, Kiviat NB, Beckmann AM, et al. Detection of human papillomavirus capsid antigens in various squamous epithelial lesions using antibodies directed against the L_1 and L_2 open reading frames. *Virology* 1988;164:467.

Frazer IH, Tindle RW. Cell-mediated immunity to papillomaviruses. *Papillomavirus Reports* 1992;3:53.

Fu YS, Reagan J, Richart RM. Definition of precursors. *Gynecol Oncol* 1981;12:s220.

Fukushima M, Yamakawa Y, Shimano S, et al. The physical state of human papillomavirus 16 DNA in cervical carcinoma and cervical intraepithelial neoplasia. *Cancer* 1990;60:2155.

Galvin GA, Jones HW Jr, Te Linde RW. Clinical relationship of carcinoma in situ and invasive carcinoma of the cervix. *JAMA* 1952: 149: 744.

Gissman L, de Villiers EM, zur Hausen H. Analysis of human genital warts (condylomata acuminata) and other genital tumors for human papillomavirus type 6 DNA. *Int J Cancer* 1982;29:143.

Gissman L, Wolnik L, Ikenberg H, et al. Human papillomavirus types 6 and 11 DNA sequences in genital and laryngeal papillomas and in some cervical cancers. *Proc Natl Acad Sci USA* 1983;80:560.

Gissman L, zur Hausen H. Partial characterization of viral DNA from human genital warts (condylomata acuminata). *Int J Cancer* 1980;25:605.

Goldie JS, Kuhn L, Denny L, et al. Policy analysis of cervical cancer screening strategies in low-source settings: clinical benefits and cost-effectiveness. *JAMA* 2001; 285:3107–3115.

Gram IT, Austin H, Stalsberg H. Cigarette smoking and the incidence of cervical intraepithelial neoplasia grade 3 and cancer of the cervix. *Am J Epidemiol* 1992;135:341.

Gram IT, Macaluso M, Stalsberg H. Incidence of cervical intraepithelial neoplasia grade III, and cancer of the cervix uteri following a negative Pap-smear in an opportunistic screening. *Acta Obstet Gynecol Scand* 1998;77:228–232.

Grohs HK, Husain OAN, eds. *Automated cervical cancer screening.* New York: Igaku-Shoin, 1994.

Guijon FB, Paraskevas M, Brunham R. The association of sexually transmitted diseases with cervical intraepithelial neoplasia: a case control study. *Am J Obstet Gynecol* 1985;151:185.

Hallam NF, West J, Harper C, et al. Large loop excision of the transformation zone (LLETZ) as an alternative to both local ablative and cone biopsy treatment: a series of 1,000 patients. *J Gynecol Surg* 1993;9:77.

Ho GYF, Bierman R, Beardsley L. Natural history of cervicovaginal papillomavirus infection in young women. *N Engl J Med* 1998;338:423–428.

IARC Working Group on Evaluation of Cervical Cancer Screening Programmes. Screening for squamous cervical cancer: duration of low risk after negative results of cervical cytology and its implication for screening policies. *BMJ* 1986;293:659–664,

Jones HW III. Cervical intraepithelial neoplasia. In: *Bailliere's Clinical Obstetrics and Gynaecology,* vol 9(1). London: Bailliere Tindall, 1995.

Kiviat NB, Koutsky LA, Paavonen JA, et al. Prevalence of genital papillomavirus infection among women attending a college student health clinic or an STD clinic. *J Infect Dis* 1989;159:293, 302.

Kyaer SK, van den Brule AJ, Paull G, et al. Type specific persistence of high-risk human papillomavirus (HPV) as indicator of high grade cervical squamous intraepithelial lesions in young women: population based prospective follow up study. *BMJ* 2002;325:572–578.

Kolstad P, Klem V. Long-term follow-up of 1121 cases of carcinoma in situ. *Obstet Gynecol* 1979;48:125.

Koss LG. *Diagnostic cytology and its histopathologic basis.* Philadelphia: JB Lippincott, 1992.

Koss LG, Stewart FW, Foote FW, et al. Some histological aspects of behavior of epidermoid carcinoma in situ and related lesions of the uterine cervix. *Cancer* 1963;16:1160.

Koutsky L. Epidemiology of genital human papillomavirus infection. *Am J Med* 1997;102[Suppl]:3–8.

Koutsky LA, Ault KA, Wheeler CM, et al. A controlled trial of a human papillomavirus type 16 vaccine. *N Engl J Med* 2002;347:1645–1651.

Kottmeier HL. Evolution et traitment des epitheliomas. *Rev Fr Gynecol Obstet* 1961;56:821.

Kurman RJ, Jenson AB, Lancaster WD. Papillomavirus infection of the cervix. II: relationship to intraepithelial neoplasia based on the presence of specific viral structural proteins. *Am J Surg Pathol* 1983;7:39.

Kurman RJ, Sanz LE, Jenson AB, et al. Papillomavirus infection of the cervix. I: correlation of histology with viral structural antigens and DNA sequence. *Int J Gynecol Pathol* 1982;1:17.

Kurman RJ, Solomon D. *The Bethesda System for Reporting Cervical/Vaginal Cytologic Diagnoses.* New York: Springer-Verlag, 1994.

Lambert PF, Howley PM. Bovine papillomavirus type $1E_1$ replication-defective mutants are altered in their transcriptional regulation. *J Virol* 1988;62:4009.

Lancaster WD, Castellano C, Santos C, et al. Human papillomavirus deoxyribonucleic acid in cervical carcinoma from primary and metastatic sites. *Am J Obstet Gynecol* 1986; 154:115.

Lorincz AT. Human papillomavirus detection methods. In: Holmes KK, Mardh PA, Sparling PF, et al, eds. *Sexually transmitted diseases,* ed 2. New York: McGraw-Hill Information Service, 1990.

Lorincz AT, Reid R, Jenson AB, et al. Human papillomavirus infection of the cervix: relative risk associations of 15 common anogenital types. *Am J Obstet Gynecol* 1992;79:328.

Lucsley DM, Cullimore J, Redman CW, et al. Loop diathermy excision of the cervical transformation zone in patients with abnormal cervical smears. *BMJ* 1990;300:1690.

Lungu O, Sun XW, Felix J, et al. Relationship of human papillomavirus type to grade of cervical intraepithelial neoplasia. *JAMA* 1992;267:2493.

Mandelblatt JS, Lawrence WF, Womack SM, et al. Benefits and cost of using HPV testing to screen for cervical cancer. *JAMA* 2002; 287:2372–2381.

Manos MM, Ting Y, Wright KD, et al. Use of polymerase chain reaction amplification for the detection of genital human papillomaviruses. *Cancer Cells* 1989;7:209.

McIndoe WA, McLean MR, Jones RW, et al. The invasive potential of carcinoma in situ of the cervix. *Obstet Gynecol* 1984;64:451.

Meisels A, Fortin R. Condylomatous lesions of the cervix and vagina, I: cytologic pattern. *Acta Cytol* 1976;20:505.

Meisels A, Fortin R, Roy M. Condylomatous lesions of the cervix, II: cytologic, colposcopic, and histopathologic study. *Acta Cytol* 1977;21:379.

Meisels A, Roy M, Fortier M, et al. Condylomatous lesions of the cervix: morphologic and colposcopic diagnosis. *Am J Diagn Gynecol Obstet* 1979;1:109.

Montz FJ, Frederick KM, Farber L, et al. Impact of increasing Papanicolaou test sensitivity and compliance: a modeled cost and outcomes analysis. *Obstet Gynecol* 2001;97:781–788.

Morrison EA, Ho GY, Vermund SH, et al. Human papillomavirus infection and other risk factors for cervical neoplasia: a case control study. *Int J Cancer* 1991;49:6.

Moscicki A-B, Palefsky J, Gonzales J, et al. Colposcopic and histologic findings and human papillomavirus (HPV) DNA test variability in young women positive for HPV DNA. *J Infect Dis* 1992;166:951.

Moscicki A-B, Palefsky J, Gonzales J, et al. Human papillomavirus infection in sexually active adolescent females: prevalence and risk factors. *Pediatr Res* 1990;28:507.

Moscicki A-B, Shiboski S, Broering J, et al. The natural history of human papillomavirus infection as measured by repeated DNA testing in adolescent and young women. *J Pediatr* 1998;132:277–284.

Nanda K, McCrory D, Myers ER, et al. Accuracy of the Papanicolaou test in screening for and follow-up of cervical cytologic abnormalities: a systematic review. *Ann Int Med* 2000;132:810–819.

Nasiell K, Roger V, Nasiell M. Behavior of mild cervical dysplasia during long-term follow-up. *Obstet Gynecol* 1986;67:665–669.

Nasiell K, Nasiell M, Vaclavinkova V. Behavior of moderate cervical dysplasia during long-term follow-up. *Obstet Gynecol* 1983;61:609–614.

Nuovo J, Melnikow J, Willan AR, et al. Treatment outcomes for squamous intraepithelial lesions. *Int J Gynecol Obstet* 2000;68:25–33.

Orth G. Epidermodysplasia verruciformis: a model for understanding the oncogenicity of human papillomaviruses. In: Evered D, Clark S, eds. *Papillomaviruses.* New York: John Wiley & Sons, 1986:157.

Oster AC. Natural history of cervical intraepithelial neoplasia: a critical review. *Int J Gynecol Pathol* 1993;12:186.

Palefsky JM, Winkler B, Rabanus J-P, et al. Characterization of in vivo expression of the human papillomavirus type 16 E_4 protein in cervical biopsy tissues. *J Clin Invest* 1991; 87:2132.

Papanicolaou GN, Traut HF. *Diagnosis of uterine cancer by the vaginal smear.* New York: Commonwealth Fund, 1943.

Patnick J, Monsonego J, de Wolf C, et al. ESGO consensus document on cervical cancer screening. *Eur J Gynaecol Oncol* 2001;22:99–101.

Pemberton FA, Smith GV. The early diagnosis and prevention of carcinoma of the cervix: a clinical pathologic study of borderline cases treated at the Free Hospital for Women. *Am J Obstet Gynecol* 1929;17:165.

Pfister H. General introduction to papillomaviruses, properties of the virions, and classification. In: Pfister H, ed. *Papillomaviruses and human cancer.* Boca Raton, FL: CRC Press, 1990:2.

Purola E, Savia E. Cytology of gynecologic condyloma acuminatum. *Acta Cytol* 1997;21:26–31.

Reagan JW, Hamonic MJ. The cellular pathology in carcinoma in situ: a cytohistopathological correlation. *Cancer* 1956; 9:385.

Reid R. Colposcopy of cervical preinvasive neoplasia. In: Singer A, ed. *Premalignant lesions of the lower genital tract.* New York: Elsevier, 1990:87.

Reid R, Greenberg M, Jenson AB, et al. Sexually-transmitted papillomaviral infections. I: the anatomic distribution and pathologic grade of neoplastic lesions associated with different viral types. *Am J Obstet Gynecol* 1987;156:212.

Reid R, Greenberg MD, Lorincz AT, et al. Should cervical cytologic testing be augmented by cervicography or human papillomavirus DNA detection? *Am J Obstet Gynecol* 1991;164:1461.

Renshaw AA, Lezon KM, Wilbur DC. The human false-negative rate of rescreening Pap tests. Measure in a two-arm prospective clinical trial. *Cancer* 2001;93:106–110.

Richart RM. Cervical intraepithelial neoplasia: a review. In: Sommers SC, ed. *Pathology annual.* East Norwalk, CT: Appleton-Century-Crofts, 1973:301.

Richart RM. Colpomicroscopic studies of the distribution of dysplasia and carcinoma-in-situ on the exposed portion of the human uterine cervix. *Cancer* 1965;18:950.

Richart RM. A modified terminology for cervical intraepithelial neoplasia. *Obstet Gynecol* 1990;75:131.

Richart RM, Townsend DE. Outpatient therapy of cervical intraepithelial neoplasia with cryotherapy or CO_2 laser. In: Osofsky HJ, ed. *Advances in clinical obstetrics and gynecology,* vol 1. Baltimore: Williams & Wilkins, 1982:235.

Richart RM, Wright TC. Controversies in the management of low-grade cervical intraepithelial neoplasia. *Cancer* 1993;71:1413.

Richart RM, Wright TC. The histology of lower anogenital tract neoplasia. In: Singer A, Monaghan JM, eds. *Lower genital tract precancer: colposcopy, pathology, and treatment.* Oxford: Blackwell Scientific Publications, 1994:2.

Richart RM, Wright TC. The pathology of cervical neoplasia. In: Luesley D, Jordan J, Richart RM, eds. *Intraepithelial neoplasia of the lower genital tract.* New York: Churchill Livingstone, 1995:19.

Rigoni-Stern D. Fatti statistici relativi alle malattie cancerose. *Gior Serv Progr Pathol Terap* 1842;2:507.

Rollason TP. The normal anatomy and histology of the cervix, vagina, and vulva. In: Luesley D, Jordan J, Richart RM, eds. *Intraepithelial neoplasia of the lower genital tract.* Edinburgh: Churchill Livingstone, 1995:1.

Saslow D, Runowicz CD, Solomon D, et al. American Cancer Society guideline for the early detection of cervical neoplasia and cancer. *CA Cancer J Clin* 2002; 52:342–362.

Scheffner M, Werness BA, Huibregtse JM, et al. The E_6 oncoprotein encoded by human papillomavirus types 16 and 18 promotes the degradation of p53. *Cell* 1990;63:1129.

Schiffman MH. Recent progress in defining the epidemiology of human papillomavirus infection and cervical neoplasia. *J Natl Cancer Inst* 1992;84:394.

Schiffman MH, Bauer HM, Hoover RN, et al. Epidemiologic evidence that human papillomavirus infection causes most cervical intraepithelial neoplasia. *J Natl Cancer Inst* 1993;85:958.

Schiffman M, Herrero R, Hildesheim A, et al. HPV DNA testing in cervical cancer screening: results from women in a high-risk province of Costa Rica. *JAMA* 2000;283:87–93.

Sigurdsson K. Quality assurance in cervical cancer screening: the Icelandic experience 1964–1993. *Eur J Cancer* 1995;31A:728.

Sillman F, Stanek A, Sedlis A, et al. The relationship between human papillomavirus and lower genital intraepithelial neoplasia in immunosuppressed women. *Am J Obstet Gynecol* 1984;150:300.

Slattery ML, Overall JC, Abbott TM, et al. Sexual activity, contraception, genital infections, and cervical cancer: support for a sexually-transmitted disease hypothesis. *Am J Epidemiol* 1989;130:248.

Solomon D, Davey D, Kurman R, et al. The 2001 Bethesda System: terminology for reporting results of cervical cytology. *JAMA* 2002; 287: 2114–2119.

Spitzer M, Chernys AE, Seltzer VL. The use of large loop excision of the transformation zone in an inner city population. *Obstet Gynecol* 1993;82:731.

Stafl and Mattingly. Vaginal adenosis: a precancerous lesion? *Am J Obstet Gynecol* 1974:120:666.

Steller MA. Update on human papillomavirus vaccines for cervical cancer. *Curr Opin Invest Drugs* 2002; 3:37–47.

Street D, Delgado G. The role of p53 and HPV in cervical cancer. *Gynecol Oncol* 1995;58:287.

Sung H-Y, Kearney, KA, Miller M. Papanicolaou smear history and diagnosis of invasive cervical carcinoma among members of a large prepaid health plan. *Cancer* 2000;88: 2283–2289.

Teale G, Moffitt DD, Mann CH, et al. Management guidelines for women with normal colposcopy after low grade cervical abnormalities: population study. *BMJ* 2000;320:1693–1696.

Tjiong MY, Schegget JT, Burger MP, et al. Epidemiologic and mucosal immunologic aspects of HPV infection and HPV-related cervical neoplasia in the lower female genital tract: a review. *Intl J Gynecol Cancer* 2001;11:9–17.

Ursin G, Peters RK, Henderson BE, et al. Oral contraceptive use and adenocarcinoma of the cervix. *Lancet* 1994; 344:1390.

Van den Brule AJ, Walboomers JM, Maine M du, et al. Difference in prevalence of human papillomavirus genotypes in cytomorphologically normal smears is associated with a history of cervical intraepithelial neoplasia. *Int J Cancer* 1991;48:404.

Vermund SH, Kelley KF, Klein RS, et al. High risk of human papillomavirus infection and cervical squamous intraepithelial lesions among women with symptomatic human immunodeficiency virus infection. *Am J Obstet Gynecol* 1991;165:392.

Weid GL. *Proceedings of the First International Congress on Exfoliative Cytology.* Philadelphia: JB Lippincott, 1961.

Werness BA, Levine AJ, Howley PM. Association of human papillomavirus types 16 and 18 proteins with p53. *Science* 1990;248:76.

Wilbanks GD, Richart RM, Terner JY. DNA content of cervical intraepithelial neoplasia studied by two-wave-length Feulgen cytophotometry. *Am J Obstet Gynecol* 1967;98:792.

Wilbur DC, Norton MK. The primary screening clinical trials of the TriPath AutoPap system. *Epidemiology* 2002;13:S30–S33.

Wilbur DC, Prey Mu, Miller WM, et al. Detection of high grade squamous intraepithelial lesions and tumors using the AutoPap system: results of a primary screening clinical trial. *Cancer* 1999;87:354–358.

Willet GD, Kurman RJ, Reid R. Correlation of the histological appearance of intraepithelial neoplasia of the cervix with human papillomavirus types. *Int J Gynecol Pathol* 1989;8:18.

Wright TC Jr, Cox JT, Massad LW, et al. 2001 Consensus guidelines for the management of women with cervical cytological abnormalities. *JAMA* 2002;287:2120–2129.

Wright TC Jr, Denny L, Kuhn L, et al. HPV DNA testing of self-collected vaginal samples compared with cytologic screening to detect cervical cancer. *JAMA* 2000;283:81–86.

Wright TC, Ellerbrock TV, Chiasson MA, et al. Cervical intraepithelial neoplasia in women infected with human immunodeficiency virus: prevalence, risk factors, and validity of Papanicolaou smears. *Obstet Gynecol* 1994;84:591.

Wright TC, Koulos J, Schnoll F, et al. Cervical intraepithelial neoplasia in women infected with human immunodeficiency virus: outcome after loop electrosurgical excision. *Gynecol Oncol* 1994;55:253.

Wright TC, Richart RM, Ferenczy A. *Electrosurgery for HPV-related diseases of the anogenital tract.* New York: Arthur-Vision, 1992.

zur Hausen H. Human papillomaviruses in the pathogenesis of anogenital cancer. *Virology* 1991;184:9.

zur Hausen H. Human papillomaviruses and their possible role in squamous cell carcinomas. *Curr Top Microbiol Immunol* 1977;78:1.

zur Hausen H. Papillomaviruses in human cancer. *Cancer* 1987;59:1692.

Te Linde's Operative Gynecology, ninth edition, edited by John A. Rock and Howard W. Jones, III. Lippincott Williams & Wilkins, Philadelphia © 2003.

CHAPTER

46

▼

Cancer of the Cervix

DENNIS S. CHI   NADEEM R. ABU-RUSTUM

WILLIAM J. HOSKINS

In the first half of the 20th century, more women died from cervical cancer in the United States than from any other cancer. However, with the introduction of the Papanicolaou (Pap) smear in the 1940s, early detection and treatment of preinvasive disease became possible. Consequently, both the incidence and mortality rates owing to invasive cervical cancer in the United States declined approximately 75% by the end of the 20th century. The American Cancer Society estimates that in the year 2002, 13,000 women will be diagnosed with cervical cancer and 4,100 will succumb to the disease. Based on these figures, cervical cancer currently ranks as the third most common female genital tract malignancy in the United States (behind uterine corpus and ovarian cancer); it is the third most common cause of gynecologic cancer death.

Worldwide, however, over 370,000 cases are diagnosed annually, leading to approximately 190,000 deaths. This makes cervical cancer not only the most common gynecologic malignancy, but also the third most frequently diagnosed cancer in women (behind breast and colorectal cancer). In general terms, the disease is much more common in developing countries. Overall, 78% of cases occur in these areas. In developing countries, cervical cancer accounts for 15% of female malignancies, carrying a lifetime risk of about 3%. In contrast, in developed countries, cervical cancer accounts for only 4.4% of fe-

male malignancies, with a lifetime risk of 1.1%. The highest incidence rates are observed in Latin America, the Caribbean, sub-Saharan Africa, and Southern and Southeast Asia. In developed countries, the incidence rates generally are low, with age-standardized rates less than 14 per 100,000. Very low rates also are observed in China and Western Asia. This geographical disparity is felt to be related to the presence or absence of effective screening programs, because epidemiologic and biologic studies have not shown significant differences in tumor biology in countries with high rates of cervical cancer.

EPIDEMIOLOGY

In the United States, the peak age of developing cervical cancer is 47 years, but approximately 47% of women with invasive cervical cancer are less than 35 years old at diagnosis. Excluding childhood cancers and lymphomas, patients with cervical cancer die younger than women with any other type of cancer (average, 60 years). Older women (>65 years) account for 10% of patients with cervical cancer. Although these older patients represent only 10% of all cases, they are more likely to die of the disease owing to their more advanced stage at diagnosis.

Cervical cancer primarily affects women from lower socioeconomic classes and those with poor access to routine medical care. The incidence of cervical cancer in White women is about 7.6 per 100,000 women; for Black women, it is 12.0 per 100,000 women. Other ethnic groups in the United States also have higher incidence rates of invasive cervical cancer than White women. For example, Hispanic, Korean, and Alaskan native women have about twice the incidence rates of White women. Vietnamese women have five times the incidence of White women. On the other hand, Japanese and Chinese women residing in the United States have a slightly lower incidence than their White counterparts.

Although there are marked geographical variations in mortality rates for cervical cancer in the United States, sparse data on cervical cancer mortality rates exists by geographic region for Black women. For White women, elevated mortality rates are seen in the South, across Appalachia, in parts of the Midwestern states, and in the upper Northeast (Fig. 46.1). These high mortality rates may be attributed in part to rural and socioeconomic factors related to access to health care.

Black women with cervical cancer are approximately three times more likely to die from their disease as White women, with mortality rates of 5.7 and 2.2 per 100,000 women, respectively. This "mortality gap" persists when mortality is controlled for demographic characteristics, prognostic factors, and type of treatment. The most recent data on cervical cancer from the American Cancer Society report overall 5-year survivals of 72% for White women compared to 58% for Black women. The 5-year survivals for White women with localized, regional, and distant disease are 92%, 50%, and 15%, respectively. For Black women, the reported 5-year survivals are 86%, 37%, and 7%, respectively. These data suggest that improvements in screening alone may not close the mortality gap, and more data are needed to explain these survival differences between Black and White women. However, equal access to gynecologic oncologists recently has been shown to eliminate disparities in stage-adjusted survival among minority women treated at adjacent public and university hospitals.

FACTORS ASSOCIATED WITH CERVICAL CANCER DEVELOPMENT

A large number of epidemiologic studies have evaluated factors associated with the development of cervical cancer. Although the risk factors are similar for both invasive cervical cancer and its precursor lesions, the association of the risk factors generally is much stronger with invasive disease. The major risk factors found in most studies are markers of sexual behavior, such as number of sexual partners, age at first intercourse, and history of sexually transmitted disease. Corbett and Crompton reported on a patient who developed invasive squamous-cell carcinoma in only one cervix of a didelphic uterus. A longitudinal septum divided the vagina into two sides. The cancer was found on the side where the vagina was of normal caliber. No cancer was found on the side where

the vagina was too small to permit intercourse. This case and other studies, which demonstrated that the disease was much more frequent in married women than celibate women, that it was more common in prostitutes and incarcerated women than the general population, and that it was highly associated with a woman's lifetime number of male sexual partners, all argue for venereal transmission. The fact that a woman's risk was increased not only by her total number of sexual partners, but also by the total number of sexual partners that her male partner or partners had, further strengthens the epidemiologic evidence that cervical cancer behaves as a sexually transmitted disease.

With so much evidence suggesting that the development of cervical cancer is related to the sexual transmission of one or more agents, investigators have analyzed virtually every known sexually transmitted disease to determine the causative agent. The most popular candidates for almost a decade were the herpes simplex viruses. However, the most recent molecular research indicates that the human papillomavirus (HPV) is the probable causative agent.

Papillomaviruses are members of the A genus of the family Papovaviridae. This family of viruses includes the papillomaviruses, polyoma virus, and SV40 virus. They are all double-stranded DNA tumor viruses. More than 100 types of HPV have been characterized. Thirty-one types of HPV that infect the anogenital tract have been described. Studies that use sensitive molecular methods to detect and type HPV in cervical lesions now find that almost all cervical cancers and their precursors are associated with HPV DNA. Bosch and colleagues analyzed over 900 cervical cancer specimens collected from 32 hospitals in 22 countries. HPV DNA was detected in 93% of the tumors, with no significant variation in HPV positivity among countries. Either HPV type 16 or 18 was found in 64% of specimens. Subsequently, Walboomers et al. reanalyzed the HPV-negative cases from the former study. Of the 55 cases that were reanalyzed, 40 were found to have HPV DNA on more extensive testing. Combining these data with those reported by Bosch et al., and excluding inadequate specimens, the authors reported that 99.7% of the cervical carcinomas contained HPV DNA.

Numerous other studies have demonstrated the strong and consistent association between specific types of HPV DNA and invasive cervical cancer and that exposure to HPV precedes the development of cervical disease. Based on the wide body of evidence, the International Agency for Research on Cancer (IARC) of the World Health Organization (WHO) has classified HPV types 16 and 18 as carcinogens in humans. Discussion of the proposed mechanism by which HPV infection leads to cervical carcinoma is beyond the scope of this chapter; the interested reader is referred to excellent reviews of the topic.

The majority of women who are infected with HPV never develop cervical dysplasia or cervical cancer. Immunologic mechanisms are thought to clear the virus in these women. It is not known why some women are able to clear the virus, whereas others go on to develop cer-

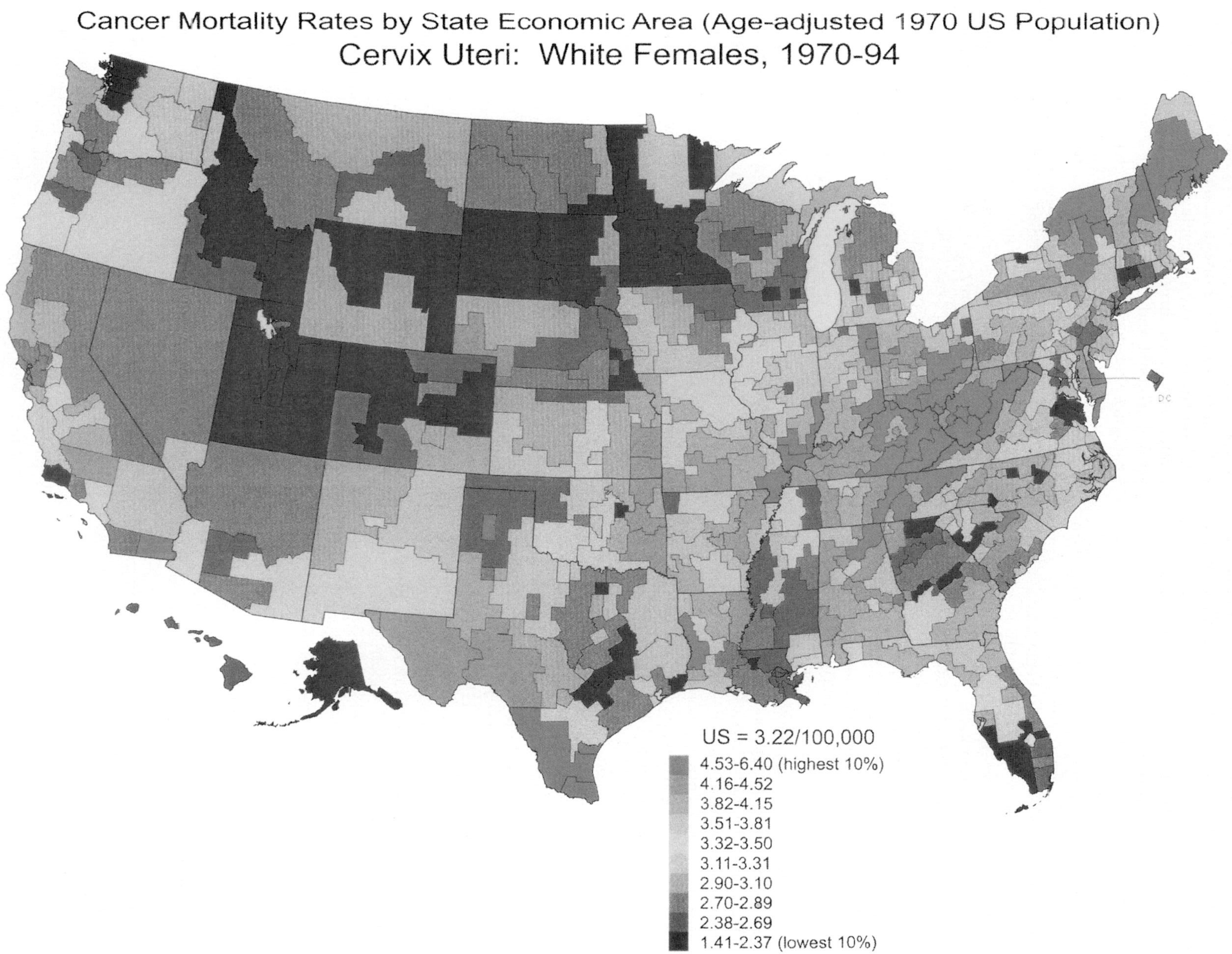

Cancer Mortality Rates by State Economic Area (Age-adjusted 1970 US Population)

Cervix Uteri: White Females, 1970-94

US = 3.22/100,000

4.53-6.40 (highest 10%)
4.16-4.52
3.82-4.15
3.51-3.81
3.32-3.50
3.11-3.31
2.90-3.10
2.70-2.89
2.38-2.69
1.41-2.37 (lowest 10%)

FIGURE 46.1. Cancer mortality rates by state economic area (age-adjusted 1970 US population) cervix uteri: white females, 1970–1994. (From: Devesa SS, Grauman DJ, Blot WJ, et al. *Atlas of cancer mortality in the United States, 1950–1994.* Bethesda, MD: National Institutes of Health, National Cancer Institute, 1999; NIH Publ No. 99-4564:217, with permission.)

vical cancer. Additional cofactors most likely contribute to the process; however, the exact mechanism is yet to be established. Risk factors for the development of cervical cancer, in addition to infection with the HPV virus, are listed in Table 46.1.

Population studies of women with invasive cervical carcinoma have demonstrated that early age of onset of sexual activity also plays a role in the later development of the disease. It is postulated that during the time of menarche in early reproductive life, the transformation zone of the cervix is more susceptible to oncogenic agents, such as HPV. Women who begin sexual activity before 16 years of age or who are sexually active within 1 year of beginning menses are at a particularly high risk of developing cervical carcinoma.

In a review of the literature, Szarewski and Cuzick concluded that a positive association between cigarette smoking and the development of cervical cancer had been reported by the majority of studies designed to address this question. Proposed mechanisms include diminished immune function secondary to a systemic effect of cigarette smoke and its byproducts or a local effect of tobacco-specific carcinogens.

The use of oral contraceptives also may play a role in the development of invasive cervical carcinoma, although this theory is more controversial. Because women who use oral contraceptives may be more sexually active than those who do not, this may represent a confounding factor rather than a true independent risk factor.

Immunosuppression has been demonstrated to be a risk factor for the development of cervical dysplasia and cancer. Porreco and colleagues reported a relative risk of 13.6 for the development of cervical carcinoma *in situ* for renal transplant recipients (who generally receive immunosuppressive agents) compared with women in the general population. Women who are infected with the human immunodeficiency virus (HIV) have an elevated prevalence of HPV infections, persistent HPV, and cervical dysplasia compared to women not infected with HIV. Although the exact magnitude of the increased risk of developing invasive cervical cancer among HIV-infected women compared to uninfected women is unclear, Maiman et al. have reported that cervical cancers that develop in HIV-infected women act aggressively, respond poorly to standard forms of therapy, and are associated with a poor prognosis. In 1993, the Centers for Disease Control and Prevention designated invasive cervical cancer as an AIDS case-defining illness.

However, the role of screening for HIV infection in women with newly diagnosed cervical cancer is not universally accepted and the yield may be extremely low, suggesting that decisions about screening for HIV in women with cervical cancer should be based on local prevalence rates. Such screening may be of benefit because the institution of highly active antiretroviral therapy yields longer survival and diminished morbidity, and improvement of immune status through antiretroviral therapy conceivably could improve cervical cancer outcome. The threshold prevalence of HIV infection among women with cervical cancer that justifies HIV screening is a clinical judgment that may be determined best in discussions between patients and treating physicians.

STAGING OF CERVICAL CANCER

In 1937, the Health Organization of the League of Nations adopted a clinical classification system for cervical cancer. Cervical cancer was the first cancer to be so classified. In 1950, this classification was modified to include preinvasive (*in situ*) cervical cancer, which was designated stage 0. New recommendations for the clinical classification of carcinoma of the cervix were adopted by the General Assembly of the International Federation of Gynecology and Obstetrics (FIGO) in 1961, and several other modifications have been made since then. The general use of this classification abroad and in the United States has been extremely helpful in reporting and comparing results of various modalities of therapy. Descriptions of the clinical stages in carcinoma of the cervix uteri as updated by FIGO in 1995 appear in Table 46.2. Although the TNM (tumor, regional nodes, and metastasis) staging system is included for completeness, most clinicians use the FIGO (International Federation of Gynecology and Obstetrics) staging.

Stages II, III, and IV have remained essentially unchanged through the various modifications (Fig. 46.2). The major redefinition and refinements have occurred in stage I disease. Microinvasive (stage IA) carcinoma has been subdivided into stage IA1 and IA2 based on the depth of cervical stromal invasion by carcinoma. Stage IB has been subdivided into stage IB1 and IB2 based on the size of the clinical lesion.

HISTOPATHOLOGY

The principal histologic type of invasive cervical cancer, occurring in about 80% to 90% of cases, is the squamous (epidermoid) lesion. In 1923, Martzloff classified these squamous tumors into three main histologic subtypes and grades. Grade 1 tumors contain well-differentiated spinal cells, keratin, and squamous pearls (Fig. 46.3A). Grade 2 tumors, the most common, are predominantly

---

TABLE 46.1.
Risk Factors for the Development of Cervical Cancer

Low socioeconomic status
Race (e.g., Black, Hispanic, Vietnamese)
Multiple sexual partners
Early age at first coitus
History of sexually transmitted disease
Infection with human papillomavirus
Cigarette smoking
Immunosuppression

TABLE 46.2.
Staging of Carcinoma of the Cervix Uteri (FIGO, 1995)

TNM Classification

Primary Tumor (T)	FIGO Classification	Definition
TX	C	Primary tumor cannot be assessed
T0	C	No evidence of primary tumor
Tis	0	Carcinoma *in situ*, intraepithelial carcinoma
T1	I	Cervical carcinoma confined to cervix (extension to the corpus should be disregarded)
T1a	IA	Invasive carcinoma, diagnosed microscopically only. All gross lesions, even with superficial invasion, are stage IB cancers. Invasion is limited to measured stromal invasion with maximum depth of 5 mm and maximum width of 7 mm.[a]
T1a1	IA1	Minimal microscopically evident stromal invasion. Measured stromal invasion with maximum depth of 3 mm and maximum width of 7 mm
T1a2	IA2	Measured stromal invasion with depth from 3B5 mm and maximum width of 7 mm
T1b	IB	Clinical lesions confined to the cervix or preclinical lesions >stage IA
	IB1	Clinical lesions no >4 cm in size
	IB2	Clinical lesions >4 cm in size
T2	II	Cervical carcinoma invades beyond the uterus but not to the pelvic wall or to the lower third of the vagina
T2a	IIA	No obvious parametrial invasion
T2b	IIB	Obvious parametrial invasion
T3	III	Extends to the pelvic wall or involves lower third of the vagina or causes hydronephrosis or nonfunctioning kidney
T3a	IIIA	Tumor involves the lower third of the vagina. No extension to the pelvic wall
T3b	IIIB	Tumor extends to the pelvic wall or causes hydronephrosis or nonfunctioning kidney
T4	IV	Carcinoma extends beyond the true pelvis or has clinically involved the mucosa of the bladder or rectum. A bullous edema as such does not permit a case to be alotted to stage IV
T4a	IVA	Spread of the growth to adjacent organs
T4b	IVB	Spread to distant organs

[a] The depth of invasion should not be more than 5 mm taken from the base of the epithelium, either surface or glandular, from which it originates. Vascular space involvement, either venous or lymphatic, should not alter the staging.
FIGO, International Federation of Gynecology and Obstetrics; TNM, tumor, regional nodes, and metastasis.

composed of transitional cells of the large-cell nonkeratinizing type (see Fig. 46.3B). Grade 3 tumors, the least common, are poorly differentiated small basal-cell-type tumors (see Fig. 46.3C). The classification of Martzloff did not prove to be clinically useful, mainly because biopsies taken from different areas of the same tumor often show different degrees of differentiation and different predominant cell types. Martzloff's work did stimulate Broders, Wentz and Reagan, and others to continue to categorize the histologic types and degree of differentiation of squamous-cell cervical tumors and to study their clinical behavior and response to treatment. The histologic classification of squamous-cell tumor types introduced in 1959 by Wentz and Reagan sometimes is used in pathology reports. However, Willen and coworkers were unable to confirm a predictive value for survival from the Wentz-Reagan classification. Similarly, most recent studies, including those by the Gynecologic Oncology Group (GOG), have shown the use of grading of squamous carcinomas to be of little predictive value.

A rare form of squamous-cell cancer of the cervix is a verrucous carcinoma. It is a very well-differentiated squamous-cell carcinoma with extensive keratinization that usually presents as a large bulky tumor of the cervix and often is confused with giant condylomas, such as those seen on the vulva. There is a sharp line between the tumor and underlying cervical stroma. Verrucous carcinoma has been shown to be associated with HPV infection. Although metastatic disease is rare, this tumor has been said to become more virulent if treated with irradiation. Goldberger and coworkers reported an unusually aggressive verrucous carcinoma of the cervix. According to deJesus and coworkers, at least 49 cases of this tumor have been reported in the female genital tract, sometimes as verrucous carcinoma and sometimes as squamous papillary tumor.

Adenocarcinomas of the cervix are becoming more common, especially in younger women. In a review of the Surveillance, Epidemiology, and End Results (SEER) Cancer Incidence Public-Use database from 1973 to 1996, Smith and colleagues reported that although the age-adjusted incidence rates per 100,000 for all invasive cervical cancers and squamous-cell cancers decreased by 37% and 42%, respectively, the rates for adenocarcinoma of the cervix actually increased 29% during the study pe-

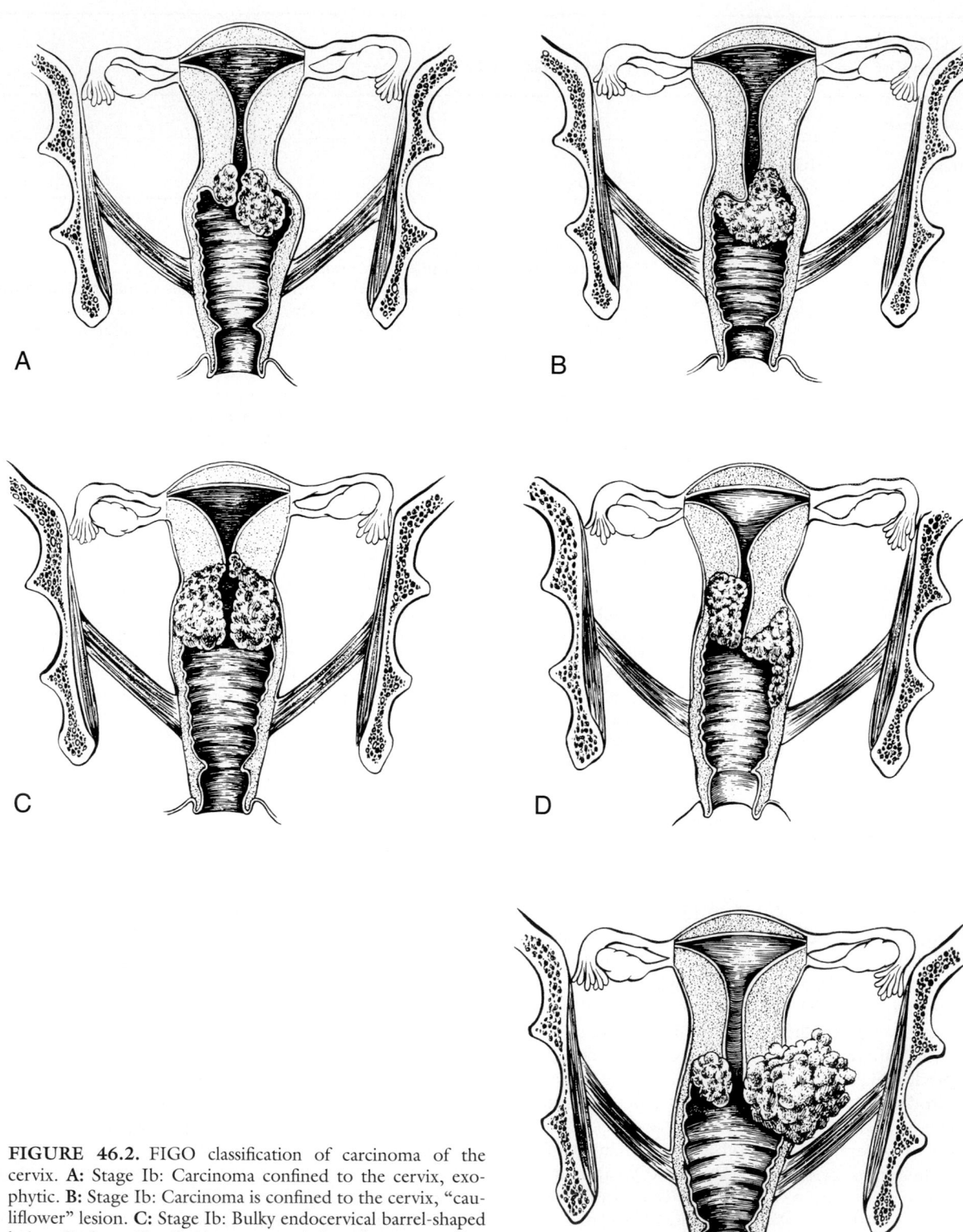

FIGURE 46.2. FIGO classification of carcinoma of the cervix. **A:** Stage Ib: Carcinoma confined to the cervix, exophytic. **B:** Stage Ib: Carcinoma is confined to the cervix, "cauliflower" lesion. **C:** Stage Ib: Bulky endocervical barrel-shaped lesion. **D:** Stage IIa: Carcinoma extends into the upper vagina or fornix. **E:** Stage IIb: Carcinoma extends into the parametrium but does not extend to pelvic wall.

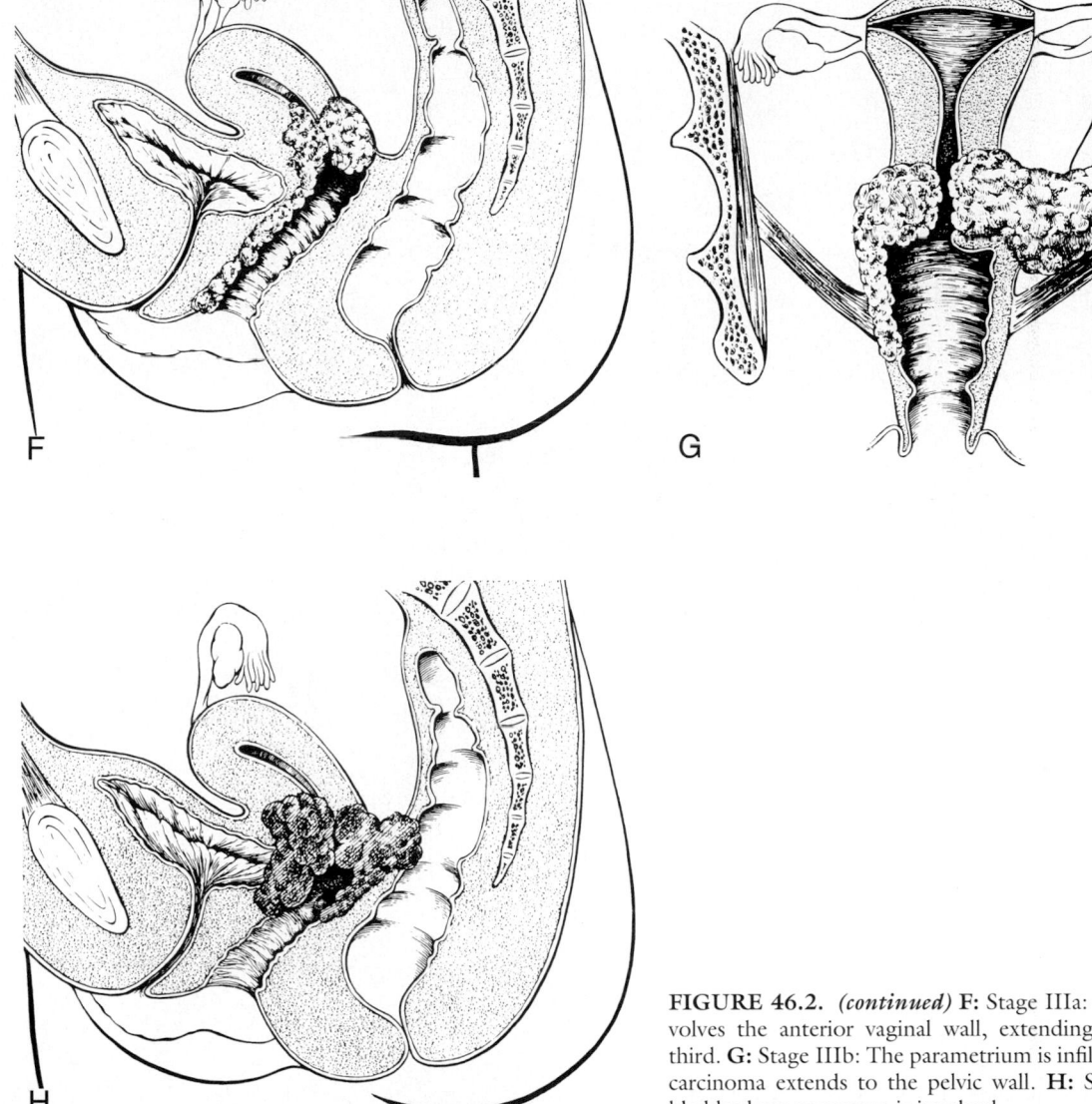

FIGURE 46.2. *(continued)* **F:** Stage IIIa: Carcinoma involves the anterior vaginal wall, extending to the lower third. **G:** Stage IIIb: The parametrium is infiltrated, and the carcinoma extends to the pelvic wall. **H:** Stage IVa: The bladder base or rectum is involved.

riod. These results suggest that current screening practices may be insufficient in detecting a significant proportion of adenocarcinoma precursor lesions.

About one-half of cervical adenocarcinomas are exophytic, usually polypoid or papillary; others diffusely enlarge or ulcerate the cervix. Approximately 15% of patients have no visible lesion because the carcinoma is within the endocervical canal. Even without visible signs or symptoms, the lesion may infiltrate deeply into the cervix. Drescher and colleagues reported a higher frequency of uterine corpus invasion, nodal metastasis, and ascites in 26 patients with cervical adenocarcinoma compared with 139 cases of squamous-cell carcinoma. More recent studies have reached contradictory conclusions regarding the prognostic significance of this histology.

In addition to pure (endocervical) adenocarcinoma (Fig. 46.4), cervical adenocarcinomas can exhibit a vari-

ety of patterns and can be composed of diverse cell types. Other histologic patterns include adenoma malignum, endometrioid, clear-cell, serous, and mesonephric. Different histologic patterns and cell types often appear in the same cervical tumor. Because mixtures are common, the designation of tumor type is based on the predominant component. If a second type composes 20% or more of the tumor, the lesion is designated as a "mixed-cell type." Not infrequently, an adenocarcinoma and squamous-cell carcinoma coexist in the same tumor and these lesions are referred to as adenosquamous carcinomas. The so-called glassy cell adenocarcinoma of the cervix is rare and considered a variant of poorly differentiated adenosquamous carcinoma. It is known to be especially aggressive, with frequent early distant metastasis. Clear-cell adenocarcinoma of the cervix can occur in the presence or absence of intrauterine exposure to diethyl-

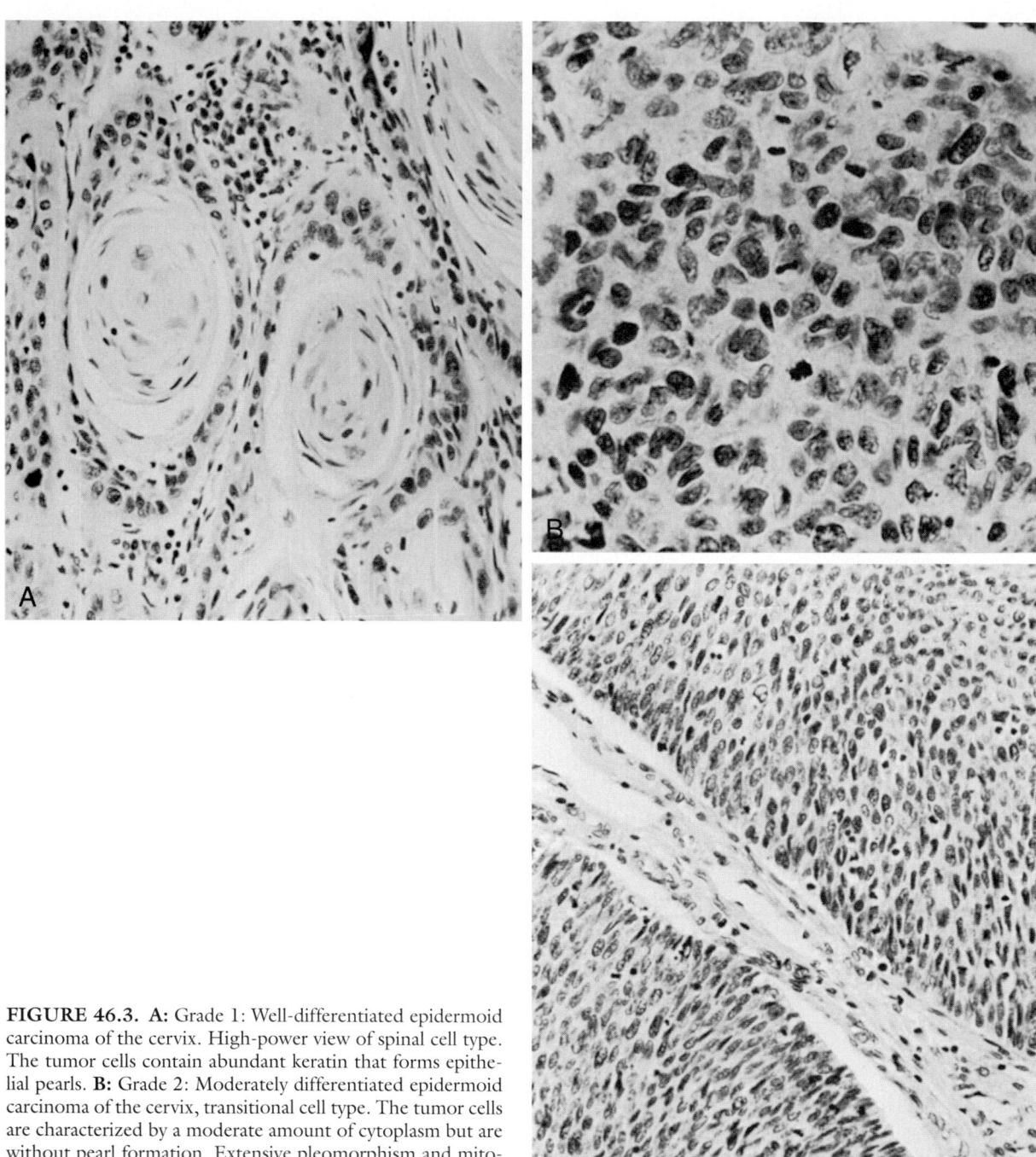

FIGURE 46.3. A: Grade 1: Well-differentiated epidermoid carcinoma of the cervix. High-power view of spinal cell type. The tumor cells contain abundant keratin that forms epithelial pearls. **B:** Grade 2: Moderately differentiated epidermoid carcinoma of the cervix, transitional cell type. The tumor cells are characterized by a moderate amount of cytoplasm but are without pearl formation. Extensive pleomorphism and mitosis are evident. The tumor is frequently classified as being of large cell, nonkeratinizing type. **C:** Grade 3: Poorly differentiated epidermoid carcinoma of the cervix, fat spindle or basal cell type. The tumor cells have little cytoplasm, numerous mitoses, and no keratin or epithelial pearls.

stilbestrol. Saigo and coworkers found that the endometrioid pattern was associated with a more favorable prognosis than any other histologic type of cervical adenocarcinoma; however, other authors believe that the subpatterns have no prognostic significance.

The early classifications of squamous-cell carcinoma of the cervix proposed by Martzloff and others divided these tumors into three categories: keratinizing squamous-cell carcinoma, large-cell nonkeratinizing squamous-cell carcinoma, and small-cell carcinoma. Over the years, however, it became apparent that the group designated as "small-cell carcinoma" was composed of a heterogeneous group of tumors, many of which displayed neuroendocrine differentiation. Recent changes in the nomenclature have led to the subdivision of these neuroendocrine tumors into typical carcinoid, atypical carcinoid, large-cell neuroendocrine carcinoma, and small-cell carcinoma. Typical carcinoid and atypical

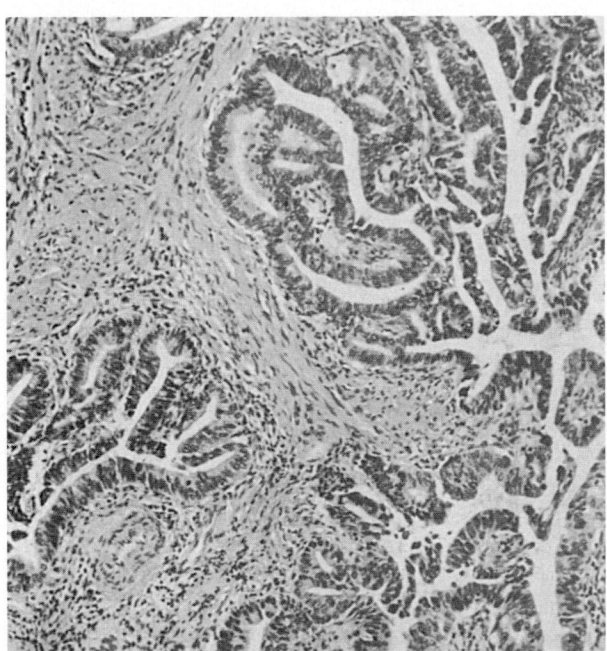

FIGURE 46.4. Adenocarcinoma of the cervix.

carcinoid tumors are rare in the cervix; therefore, their clinical and pathologic features have not been well characterized. Large-cell neuroendocrine and small-cell carcinomas are highly aggressive neoplasms, with a propensity to metastasize early and widely. Usual methods of therapy are not effective for these histologic types.

Various cervical sarcomas have been described by Rotmensch and coworkers. These tumors constitute less than 0.5% of all cervical cancers and include adenosarcomas, leiomyosarcomas, carcinosarcomas, and rhabdomyosarcomas. It is extremely rare for a lymphoma to develop primarily in the cervix, but lymphoma in the cervix is more likely to represent evidence of generalized lymphomatous disease.

CLINICAL PRESENTATION

Invasive cervical cancer is more likely than its intraepithelial precursors to cause symptoms such as abnormal vaginal bleeding (menorrhagia, metrorrhagia, postcoital bleeding, or postmenopausal bleeding). Many patients have a profuse and often malodorous discharge, especially when the disease is advanced. Thus, any patient with abnormal vaginal bleeding or discharge should have a complete pelvic examination, including a speculum examination with visualization of the cervix. Failure to examine the cervix in a patient with abnormal vaginal bleeding or discharge could result in failure to diagnose cervical cancer.

Pain is not a common complaint in patients with cervical cancer unless the disease is advanced. In more advanced stages, patients may complain of bladder and rectal symptoms. When the disease involves lumbosacral and sciatic nerve roots and the lateral pelvic sidewall, chronic boring pelvic bone pain radiating down the leg can be excruciating and indicative of advanced disease. Edema of the lower extremities likewise indicates tumor obstruction of lymphatic and/or venous drainage. Ascites is uncommon in cervical cancer.

Unfortunately, the physician cannot rely on the presence of symptoms to lead to a diagnosis of early carcinoma of the cervix. Many women remain without symptoms for many months. It is known that one third of patients with advanced stage III and IV disease have had symptoms for less than 3 months. The only way to diagnose cervical cancer in the earliest possible stages is to routinely apply special diagnostic procedures to large groups of women with and without gynecologic symptoms. This means screening the adult female population with Pap smears.

Invasive cervical lesions can be exophytic, infiltrative, ulcerative, or occult. The size of the visible lesion on the cervix may not correlate well with the extent or depth of invasion (Fig. 46.5).

An everted exophytic carcinomatous growth may be friable. Bits of tissue may break off on the examining fingers. On inspection, the friable exophytic cancer shows a

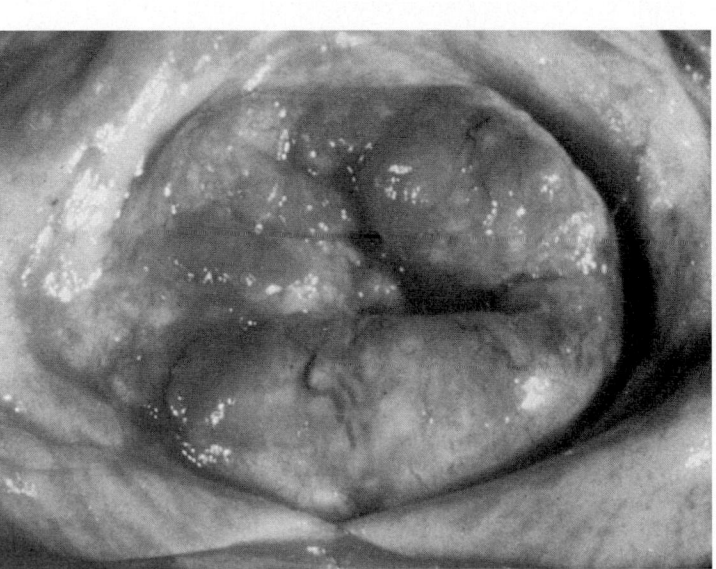

FIGURE 46.5. Squamous cell carcinoma, cervix uteri, FIGO stage IIA.

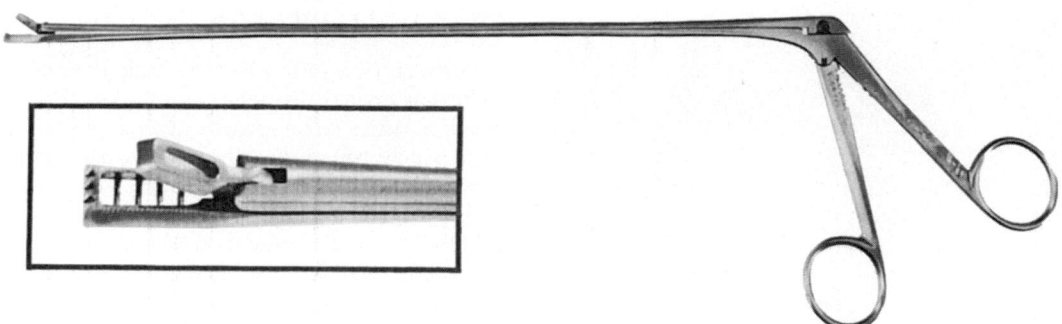

FIGURE 46.6. Kevorkian square-jawed cervical biopsy forceps.

rough, granular bleeding surface that can be sloughing and infected, with a foul-smelling discharge.

A tumor that develops beneath the mucosa of the exocervix and infiltrates the cervical stroma usually causes cervical enlargement. The surface of the cervix may feel smooth, but the cervical consistency to palpation is firm or nodular. It is characteristic of cervical cancers that develop in the endocervical canal to cause cervical enlargement and a firm cervical consistency before breaking through the mucosa of the exocervix to cause a lesion. This also is characteristic of many cervical cancers that develop in postmenopausal women. In fact, it is possible, although uncommon, for a cervical cancer that is developing high in the endocervical canal to invade the parametrial tissue and even obstruct the ureters before causing a visible cervical lesion. An ulcerative lesion can look like a fairly clean punched-out ulcer, but more commonly it is an irregular crater with a necrotic bleeding base and a foul-smelling discharge.

Any grossly visible lesion of the cervix should be considered suspicious for cancer, and biopsy should be performed. Good visualization with a speculum and adequate illumination are essential. A Pap smear should be taken even though it can be less accurate in the presence of a grossly visible cervical lesion.

Colposcopic examination is neither needed nor particularly effective for a gross cervical lesion, but can be helpful when there is a small surface lesion to identify the most abnormal area for directed biopsies. The primary benefit of colposcopy is in visualizing noninvasive, precursor, or minimally invasive lesions that cannot he visualized without magnification.

Cervical biopsy techniques are discussed in Chapter 45. Biopsies can be undertaken with any of a number of special instruments; the Kevorkian (Fig. 46.6), Younge, or Gaylor biopsy forceps are particularly functional for taking an adequate biopsy specimen. It is important to obtain a specimen where frank stromal invasion can be demonstrated, not from the exophytic portion where no benign stroma is present. Surgical conization under anesthesia is unnecessary when a grossly visible lesion is present; indeed, it is contraindicated in the presence of a gross lesion because it has the potential of delaying the initiation of definitive treatment. Iodine (Schiller) staining can be used to demarcate the vaginal margins of a neoplastic area from adjacent normal epithelium. All of these procedures, as well as the popular loop diathermy conizations, can be done in the outpatient setting. It is rarely necessary to take the patient to the operating room to diagnose cervical cancer. If an anesthetic is deemed necessary for some other reason, a careful pelvic examination under anesthesia, biopsy of any vaginal lesions, cervical and uterine sounding, cystoscopy and proctoscopy (if warranted), and even uterine curettage can be done. Useful information to plan treatment thus can be obtained.

PROGNOSTIC FACTORS

Several factors have been reported to affect prognosis in cervical cancer. However, the most important determinant of prognosis remains FIGO clinical stage. Based on studies by Piver, van Nagell, Delgado, and numerous others, which demonstrated the prognostic significance of depth of cervical stromal invasion and tumor size in early-stage disease, FIGO incorporated these factors into its current clinical staging system. The 5-year survival rates by stage as reported by FIGO in the most recent report are shown in Table 46.3.

TABLE 46.3.
5-Year Survival by FIGO Stage

Stage	Number of Patients	5-Year Survival Rate (%)
Ia1	787	94.6
Ia2	313	92.6
IB1	986	90.4
IB2	440	79.8
IIA	993	76.0
IIB	2,775	73.3
IIIA	131	50.5
IIIB	2,271	46.4
IVA	258	29.6
IVB	196	22.0

FIGO, International Federation of Gynecology and Obstetrics.

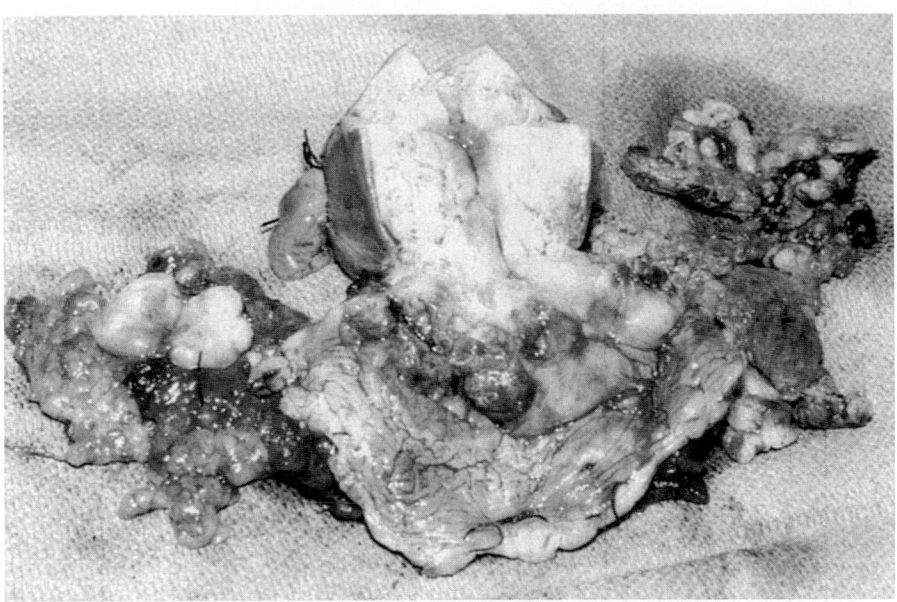

FIGURE 46.7. Squamous cell carcinoma, cervix uteri, FIGO stage IIa, with gross metastatic tumor in a right parametrial lymph node.

In addition to FIGO stage, other reported prognostic factors include endometrial cavity extension, regional (pelvic) and distant (paraaortic) lymph node metastases, histologic tumor grade, and lymphovascular space invasion (LVSI).

Uterine corpus and endometrial cavity extension from primary cervical cancer was originally thought to be a poor-prognosis factor. The original League of Nations classification of 1937 included such lesions in the stage II category. Over the years, classification of the disease based on extension to the uterine corpus or endometrial cavity has gradually been discounted. These lesions, classified as stage IC in 1950, were included in the broad category of stage IB in 1961. Despite the change in classification, we still have some concern about patients whose tumor extends into the corpus of the uterus. Evidence from Washington University reported by Perez and coworkers showed that tumor extension into the endometrial cavity lowers the 5-year survival rate of stage IB and IIA lesions by 10% to 20%. Lesions that involve the corpus also were found to have a twofold greater incidence of distant metastases when compared with lesions without corpus extension. Similar observations have been reported by Prempree and coworkers from 82 cases of stage I and II disease with endometrial extension. The absolute 5-year cure rates of 68% for stage I and 62% for II disease with endometrial extension reflects the higher risk of metastases: 20% for stage I cases and 24% for stage II cases. Such reports must be studied with consideration of the difficulty of establishing a diagnosis of endometrial extension by using microscopic study of endometrial curettage specimens. Frequently, the curettage specimen is contaminated by the cervical tumor, making it difficult to be certain about endometrial extension. Treatment planning is not altered by such observations, nor is a fractional curettage recommended as part of pretreatment evaluation.

Lymph node metastases, either regional (pelvic) or to higher level (common iliac and paraaortic) lymph nodes, have proved to be one of the most reliable prognostic factors for patients with cervical cancer (Fig. 46.7). The frequency of metastases to pelvic lymph nodes is about 0% to 0.5% for patients with stage IA1; 7% to 9% for stage IA2; 12% to 20% for stage IB; 20% to 38% for stage IIA; 16% to 36% for stage IIB; >35% for stage III; and >50% for stage IV. Preoperative detection of positive pelvic and paraaortic lymph nodes is unreliable, even with newer radiologic imaging techniques. Detection of positive lymph nodes is more accurately determined when lymphadenectomy is used in preoperative staging or treatment. Although Kolstad showed that when intraoperative lymphography is used, 15% to 25% more patients with stage IB disease are found to have positive regional lymph nodes, this technique is rarely used outside the research setting.

When patients with stage IB cervical cancer are primarily treated with radical hysterectomy and pelvic lymphadenectomy, the 5-year cure rate is about 90%, if there are no lymph node metastases. However, if metastatic disease to lymph nodes is found, the 5-year cure rate falls to about 65%. The number of positive nodes also influences prognosis. In a review of the literature, Hoskins reported an 83% survival rate for patients with stage IB and IIA disease who had negative lymph nodes at the time of radical hysterectomy and pelvic lymphadenectomy. The survival rate decreased to 57% in patients with one to two positive nodes and 31% in those with greater than three positive nodes.

Metastatic disease to paraaortic lymph nodes occurs in 4% to 7% of patients with stage I disease, 15% to 20% with stage II disease, 25% to 30% with stage III disease, and 30% to 50% with stage IVA disease. Most studies confirm that metastases to paraaortic nodes occur more frequently when positive pelvic nodes also are present.

The rarity of patients found to have positive paraaortic nodes when pelvic nodes are negative raises the question: How well sampled and/or sectioned were the pelvic nodes? Even with extended-field radiation therapy, the 5-year survival rate for patients with metastases to the paraaortic nodes is only about 25% to 35%.

Histologic tumor grade has been reported to affect prognosis. Early studies by Chung and coworkers and van Nagell and colleagues demonstrated a poorer prognosis among patients with poorly differentiated tumors. However, more recent studies by Zaino and the GOG have shown the grading of squamous tumors to be of little predictive value in cervical carcinoma. Shingleton and Orr reviewed nine publications that reported on 3,761 patients with predominantly squamous-cell carcinoma. Twenty-eight different factors were evaluated for prognostic significance. On multivariate analysis, tumor volume, lymph node metastasis, parametrial invasion, and LVSI were found to be significant independent prognostic factors but patient age and tumor grade were not.

On the other hand, tumor differentiation may have a significant prognostic role in adenocarcinoma of the cervix. Shingleton and Orr also reviewed eight studies containing 577 patients with adenocarcinoma of the cervix. As with squamous-cell carcinoma, the strongest independent prognostic variables were tumor size and nodal metastasis. However, unlike with squamous-cell carcinoma, tumor grade appeared to have prognostic significance.

Several investigators, including Swan and Roddick, Wheeless and Graham, and Julian and coworkers, have drawn attention to the fact that when there is a mixture of adenocarcinomatous and squamous elements—so-called adenosquamous tumors—the prognosis is poor and the incidence of pelvic lymph node metastases is high. Histologic combinations should be considered when comparing the prognoses of adenocarcinoma and squamous cancers of the cervix. The literature is mixed on the overall issue of whether adenocarcinoma in general and adenosquamous cancers in specific are more virulent and less curable than their squamous counterparts. Stehman and colleagues performed a multivariate analysis of prognostic variables for 626 patients with locally advanced cervical carcinoma treated with radiation therapy on three GOG protocols. Histologic cell type was not found to be a significant prognostic factor. A national pattern of care and evaluation study of the American College of Surgeons also failed to report statistically different 5-year survival rates for squamous and adenocarcinoma, regardless of type of therapy chosen.

In a GOG prospective study of 645 patients with stage IB squamous-cell carcinoma of the cervix treated with radical hysterectomy and pelvic lymphadenectomy, Delgado et al. identified three independent risk factors in relation to disease-free survival: the depth of invasion, the size of the tumor, and LVSI. The disease-free interval was 89% for those patients without LVSI compared to 77% for those found to have LVSI. Although not all studies have found LVSI to be an independent prognostic factor, as stated, in a review of nine studies (including the study by Delgado et al.) containing 3,761 patients,

Shingleton and Orr found LVSI to be a significant independent prognostic factor on multivariate analysis. The incidence of LVSI in early-stage lesions varies widely, depending on multiple factors, including the number of sections of the cervix prepared, the depth of stromal invasion, and the interest of the examining pathologist.

Observations from Austria and Germany indicate that there is considerable variation in the frequency with which LVSI is recognized by the pathologist. In a combined study of over 1,000 patients at three different reference centers (Graz, Munich, and Erlangen), Burghardt et al. reported the frequency with which LVSI was identified ranged from 9% in Munich, where only blood vessel involvement was so classified, to 43% in Graz, where it was classified as capillary-like space involvement. At the third center, Erlangen, the corresponding value was intermediate at 23%. Such variations in histopathologic criteria may well contribute to some of the controversy that exists regarding the prognostic significance of LVSI.

To this point, this discussion of prognostic factors has included only anatomic and morphologic factors. Peipert and associates emphasize that cancer, including cervical cancer, has both form and function. Accordingly, other clinical variables, such as patient's symptoms, symptom severity, and comorbidity, affect the survival rate of patients with invasive cervical cancer. Unless these variables are suitably included, prognostic estimates based on morphology alone are imprecise, and therapeutic evaluations can be misleading. According to Rutledge and associates, there is no consistent effect of age on survival rate in patients treated for cervical cancer. Younger patients with early-stage disease seemed to survive longer than older patients, but the tendency reversed when disease was advanced.

PRETREATMENT EVALUATION

When a diagnosis of invasive cervical cancer has been established histologically, the clinician should perform an evaluation of all pelvic organs to determine whether the tumor is confined to the cervix or has extended to the adjacent vagina, parametrium, endometrial cavity, bladder, ureters, or rectum. According to the FIGO guidelines for clinical staging, diagnostic studies may include intravenous urography (IVU), cystoscopic examination of the bladder and urethra, a proctosigmoidoscopic study, a barium enema (BE), and in the case of early-stage disease, a colposcopic study of the vagina and the vaginal fornices. Colposcopic findings may be used for assigning a stage to the tumor (for instance, FIGO stage IIA), but the results must be confirmed by biopsy. Chest radiographs and electrocardiographic studies are used to determine cardiopulmonary disease, particularly in the older patient. Pulmonary function studies can be important, especially for evaluating patients who are candidates for extensive surgery.

When studies detect ureteral obstruction, a tumor is classified as a stage IIIB lesion, regardless of the size of the primary lesion. Ureteral obstruction, either hydronephrosis or nonfunction of the kidney, is well established as an indicator of poor prognosis, as recognized in the FIGO classification. Retrograde pyelography can be performed after the ureteral obstruction is located for further evaluation; however, it is not routinely recommended. Kidney function studies such as serum creatinine and creatinine clearance provide important baseline information before treatment; complete urinalysis is useful for detecting the presence of albumin or white and red blood cells and renal tubular casts.

In women with bulky or advanced-stage tumors, the bladder mucosa also should be inspected cystoscopically for possible bullous edema, which indicates lymphatic obstruction within the bladder wall. Evidence of tumor in the bladder must be confirmed by biopsy before the lesion can be classified as stage IVA. Rectal mucosal lesions also require a biopsy via proctosigmoidoscopy, because they can be related to an inflammatory process rather than to the cervical tumor.

A pelvic examination must be performed as part of the staging process, and it may be necessary to have the patient completely relaxed by general anesthesia. In up to 20% of patients, the initial clinical classification of the disease has proved to be incorrect at the time of pelvic examination under anesthesia. Such an examination can reveal a more advanced stage of the disease than was originally found; additional biopsies (if indicated) or fractional curettage can be done as well as colposcopy, cystoscopy, and proctosigmoidoscopy. In today's health care climate, the cost of a separate examination under anesthesia should be reserved for only the most problematic cases.

Pretreatment pedal lymphangiography was used in the past to detect pelvic and paraaortic lymph node metastases, but the procedure is tedious and associated with many false-negative and -positive findings. When compared with lymphadenectomy, positive lymphangiograms have an accuracy rate of <75% and a false-negative rate as high as 50%. Furthermore, a lymphangiogram only detects metastatic lesions when the parenchyma of the lymph node has become distorted, by which time the lesions are macroscopic. The procedure thus is not recommended for routine use in the pretreatment evaluation of cervical cancer patients.

Surgical experience from pelvic lymphadenectomy has confirmed an error rate of 15% to 25% in the clinical staging of patients with stage IB or II lesions. In 10% to 30% of cases with stage II or III tumors, in addition to positive findings of occult pelvic lymph nodes, other metastases may be found in the paraaortic nodes. Unfortunately, pelvic examinations and clinical staging as defined by FIGO cannot detect such metastases. Consequently, there is a growing body of literature showing the superiority of cross-sectional imaging (computed tomography [CT] and magnetic resonance imaging [MRI]) over clinical staging in delineating the extent of disease in patients with cervical cancer. As stated earlier, official FIGO guidelines do not incorporate the use of either CT or MRI findings into the staging of cervical cancer. This is mainly owing to the belief that staging methods should be universally available and that staging should serve as a standardized means of communication between different institutions worldwide. However, as knowledge of prognostic factors and the value of cross-sectional imaging has accumulated, its use in treatment planning has increased without changing the official FIGO clinical staging guidelines.

In a Patterns of Care Study conducted between 1978 and 1988, Montana et al. reported a decrease in the use of IVU (86% to 42%) and BE (58% to 32%) in the staging of cervical cancer patients. During the same time period, the use of CT scan increased from 6% to 70%.

The value of CT scan in the pretreatment evaluation of patients with cervical cancer is in the assessment of advanced disease (stage IIB and greater) and in the detection and biopsy of suspected lymph node metastasis. The treatment plan for patients with locally advanced disease must be modified if upper abdominal tumor masses and/or distant metastasis are discovered. A metaanalysis by Schneidler et al. reported a positive predictive value of 61% for CT scan in the pretreatment evaluation of nodal disease in cervical cancer. Moreover, in experienced hands, fine-needle aspiration of retroperitoneal nodes with CT scan guidance has an accuracy rate of 80% to 95%. When the aspiration study unequivocally shows malignant cells, a surgical biopsy need not be performed. This information is most valuable in patients who have metastasis to the paraaortic nodes, because these patients would need the pelvic radiation fields extended to incorporate the involved region if there is no other evidence of distant metastasis.

The soft-tissue contrast resolution of CT scan does not allow for consistent tumor visualization at the primary cervical site; therefore, neither tumor size nor early parametrial invasion can be evaluated reliably. However, T2-weighted MR imaging allows consistent tumor visualization and has been reported to be 93% accurate in determining tumor size to within 5 mm of measurements of surgical specimens. The reported positive predictive value for MR imaging in detecting nodal disease and in identifying parametrial invasion (compared to surgical specimens) is 66% and 67%, respectively. Based on these promising results, the American College of Radiology Imaging Network (ACRIN) is performing a prospective trial in conjunction with the GOG evaluating the diagnostic performance of CT and MRI scan prior to radical hysterectomy and pelvic lymphadenectomy in patients with stage IB cervical cancer. The plan is to compare the diagnostic accuracy of the two scanning methods to each other and also to the clinical FIGO staging system. However, until the results of this and other similar studies have been reported, the clinician should not accept radiographic interpretations as definitive evaluations.

SURGICAL TREATMENT OF EARLY-STAGE CERVICAL CANCER

Based on the pretreatment evaluation of the patient, including the prognostic factors of tumor size, clinical stage of the disease, and risk of pelvic node metastases, a treatment schema can be developed for invasive cervical cancer as shown in Table 46.4. Almost all patients are

TABLE 46.4.
General Treatment Schema for Invasive Cervical Carcinoma[a]

Disease Stage	Treatment
Stage IA1	Simple hysterectomy, abdominal or vaginal, or cervical conization
Stages IA2,[b] IIA, IB1, and nonbulky IIA	Radical (class III)[c] hysterectomy, bilateral pelvic lymphadenectomy with postoperative irradiation, plus or minus concurrent chemotherapy in selected high-risk patients
Stages IB2 and bulky IIA[d]	Full external and intracavitary pelvic irradiation with concurrent chemotherapy followed by extrafascial abdominal hysterectomy
Stages IIB to IVA[e]	Full external and intracavitary pelvic irradiation with concurrent chemotherapy
Stage IVB	Palliative chemotherapy

[a] For individual patients, recommendations for treatment can vary, depending on the clinical circumstances.

[b] Some authorities recommend modified (class II) radical hysterectomy, bilateral pelvic lymphadenectomy for stage IA2 disease.

[c] Refer to Figure 46.8.

[d] Some authorities recommend radical (class III) hysterectomy, bilateral pelvic lymphadenectomy for stage IB2 and bulky stage IIA disease.

[e] A patient with a stage IVA lesion that extends only in the anterior or posterior direction may be a candidate for pelvic exenteration.

treated with either primary surgery or primary radiation therapy with concurrent chemotherapy. Some patients are appropriately treated with combinations of all three. The standard management of patients with early cervical carcinoma is surgical removal of the cervix. The extent of resection of the surrounding tissue depends on the size of the lesion and the depth of cervical stromal invasion.

Stage IA1 Disease

The exact definition of early-stage cervical cancer has been debated for several decades. This is illustrated by the fact that FIGO changed the definition of early-stage cervical cancer at least five times from 1960 to 1995. In 1985, FIGO defined stage IA cervical cancer as that which invaded the cervical stroma to a maximal depth of 5 mm with no greater than 7 mm of horizontal spread. Stage IA disease was further subdivided into stages IA1 and IA2. Stage IA1 was defined as minimal microscopic evidence of stromal invasion but with no exact measurement delineation. In general, these lesions were considered to be so superficial that they could not be measured accurately, with the invasive component usually measuring <1 mm in depth. All other stage IA cancers fell into the IA2 category.

Although many gynecologic oncologists believed that this was a step in the right direction, the feeling was that a more precise definition for stage IA1 was needed. Many physicians who used the FIGO staging system found it to be vague, with limited utility in the daily management of patients. Ideally, the clinical staging system for early cervical cancer should provide treatment options for individual patients within each stage grouping.

Specific criteria to define early invasive cancer of the cervix and possibly guide clinicians in the selection of less radical management of these lesions has been an area of investigation since Mestwerdt introduced the concept of microcarinoma of the cervix in 1947. In 1973, the Society of Gynecologic Oncologists (SGO) suggested a defi-

nition for microinvasive carcinoma of the cervix as being microscopic invasive cancer with a maximum depth of invasion of 3 mm. This definition gained many advocates, because it was felt that it could be used as a guide for therapy. Numerous reports showed that the frequency of nodal metastasis with ≤3 mm invasion was exceedingly rare. These studies suggested that patients with microinvasive cancers could be treated conservatively, possibly with a conization, whereas those who had >3 mm invasion or vascular lymphatic involvement might be considered for more radical therapy.

In an exhaustive review of the literature, Ostor identified 31 studies spanning the years 1976 to 1993 that reported on 3,598 patients with squamous-cell carcinoma of the cervix and ≤3 mm stromal invasion. Although not all patients had lymph nodes removed as part of their treatment, the calculated incidence of lymph node metastasis in this group of patients was <1%.

In 1995, FIGO made its most recent revision in the cervical cancer staging system. After an extensive evaluation of the data in the literature, as well as seeking advice from specialty societies and individuals worldwide, FIGO changed the definition of stage IA1 disease to lesions that invaded the cervical stroma ≤3 mm in depth and ≤7 mm in width.

Diagnosis

Because stage IA lesions in women without symptoms usually are detected by cytologically differential diagnosis is best made by an experienced colposcopist in conjunction with a colposcopically directed biopsy. If the question of microinvasion is raised from the colposcopic findings, the biopsy, or a curettage of the endocervical canal, then a conization of the cervix is mandatory to rule out the presence of frank or deeply invasive cancer. Colposcopic appearance alone is not sufficient to make a final diagnosis, but the colposcope is best used to identify the most suspect areas of the cervix, so that biopsy specimens can be obtained. When a suspicious lesion extends into the endocervical canal and cannot be entirely seen colposcopically, then the examination is considered inadequate or unsatisfactory and a cervical conization is required. Microinvasive carcinoma cannot be diagnosed from a punch biopsy because adjacent areas may contain more advanced tumor; conization is required for definitive diagnosis in this situation. The accuracy of the diagnosis depends on the adequacy of the cone and the adequacy of the pathologic examination of the cone. The entire cone should be blocked, so that an adequate number of histologic sections can be taken from each block. If the diagnosis is still not certain, more sections should be made. Excellent conization specimens are possible using loop diathermy equipment in the outpatient setting (local anesthesia). If small loops are selected, however, surgeons tend to remove multiple pieces of cervical tissue, which become difficult to orient in the pathology laboratory. Proper technique for large-loop excision is mandatory for best results.

Hysterectomy After Conization

To evaluate the extent of an early lesion, cervical conization occasionally is required. If simple extrafascial hysterectomy is subsequently chosen as the correct surgical treatment, the operation should be done within 48 hours of the conization or delayed until the cervix has healed, usually about 4 to 6 weeks later. If the hysterectomy is done after 48 hours and before the cervix has healed, the risk of serious postoperative infectious morbidity is increased. However, a radical abdominal hysterectomy and bilateral pelvic lymphadenectomy can be done at almost any time after cervical conization, even before the cervix is completely healed, without increasing the risk of serious postoperative infectious morbidity. The reason for this difference is not clear, but may be related to the fact that indurated and possibly infected paracervical and parametrial tissue is actually removed when an extensive hysterectomy is done. Whenever possible, the surgeon should avoid doing a diagnostic cervical conization in a patient with deeply invasive cervical cancer. Cervical conization is unavoidable in some patients to confirm a depth of invasion limited to the superficial 3 mm of cervical stroma, so that a more conservative extrafascial hysterectomy can be correctly chosen as adequate primary treatment.

Treatment

In 1996, the National Institutes of Health (NIH) invited an international panel of experts to develop a consensus conference statement on cervical cancer. After an extensive literature review and presentation of the scientific evidence, they concluded that patients who have squamous-cell carcinoma of the cervix with ≤3 mm stromal invasion and negative conization margins have virtually a 100% cure rate when treated with simple hysterectomy or conization alone. However, for patients treated by conization alone, both the internal conization margin and the postconization endocervical curettage must be negative for cancer and dysplasia, because the risk of

residual invasive cancer is significantly increased if either the margin or the curettage is positive. The choice of therapy should be influenced by the patient's desire to maintain fertility. Although LVSI generally is considered to be an adverse prognostic factor in cervical cancer, its prognostic significance in stage IA1 disease is uncertain. Because of this uncertainty, some clinicians suggested that the presence of LVSI in stage IA1 disease might be more appropriately treated with radical hysterectomy or radiation therapy.

Recurrence in the vaginal vault usually is the result of failing to accurately define the extent of the lesion and the presence of involvement of adjacent vaginal mucosa. This usually can be prevented with a careful colposcopic examination before hysterectomy. If vaginal fornices are involved, partial vaginectomy is easier to perform with hysterectomy if the operation is done vaginally (Fig. 46.8). Alternatively, if the woman is not a good surgical candidate, radiation therapy (usually in the form of brachytherapy alone) can be selected.

The surgeon might expect an increased morbidity with intracavitary irradiation of a recently coned cervix. The cervix must be allowed to heal completely before intracervical irradiation. The survival rates for microinvasive disease (all treatments) should reach 98% to 99% if patients are adequately studied and properly treated.

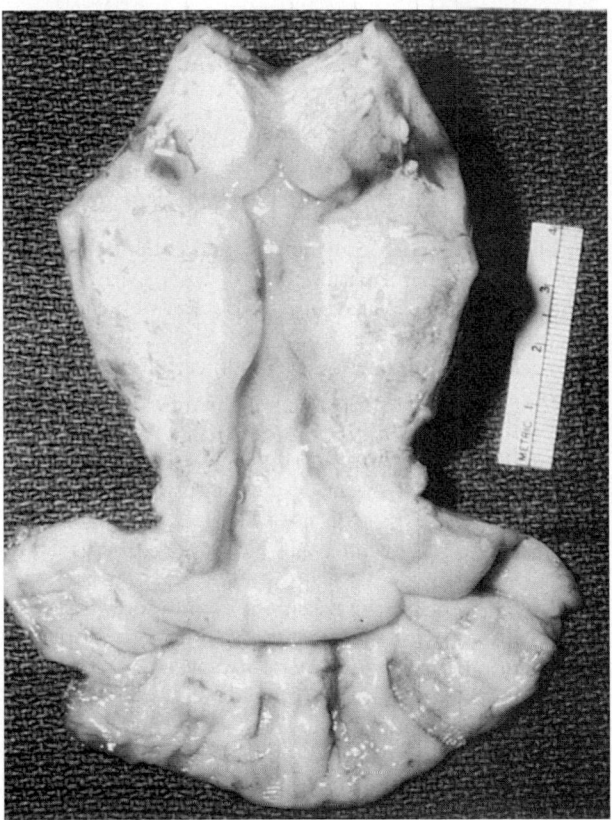

FIGURE 46.8. Vaginal hysterectomy and partial vaginectomy specimen from patient with squamous cell carcinoma, cervix uteri, FIGO stage IA1, with extension to adjacent vaginal fornix. Note uniform width of vaginal cuff.

Contrary to its squamous-cell counterpart, the currently accepted treatment for all early invasive adenocarcinomas of the cervix is radical surgery or radiation therapy. The reason for this disparity is that it is unclear if the FIGO definition and treatment of stage IA1 squamous-cell carcinoma of the cervix applies to glandular lesions. Only a few studies of microinvasive adenocarcinoma of the cervix have been done. Webb and colleagues recently reviewed the SEER Public-Use Database to identify 131 cases of cervical adenocarcinoma with 3 mm or less stromal invasion. Fifty patients had a radical hysterectomy and pelvic lymph node dissection and none were found to have lymph node metastasis. Furthermore, there were no deaths among the 54 patients treated with simple hysterectomy alone. Others have reported a 0% rate of lymph node metastasis with depths of stromal invasion of up to 5 and 12 mm. However, bilateral pelvic lymph node metastases have been reported with as little as 2.5 mm of stromal invasion. Furthermore, Elliot et al. reported a case of lymph node metastasis with cervical adenocarcinoma with <1 mm invasion and a second case of recurrence and death after radical hysterectomy and pelvic lymphadenectomy in a patient with 1.8 mm of stromal invasion. It appears that more information is needed before sound recommendations regarding conservative treatment options for microinvasive adenocarcinoma can be made.

Stages IA2, IB1, and Nonbulky IIA Disease

Owing to estimates of nodal involvement of 4% to 10%, the recommended treatment by the NIH Consensus Conference for patients with stage IA2 disease continued to be primary radical or modified radical hysterectomy with bilateral pelvic lymphadenectomy or primary radiation therapy. Again, the diagnosis of both stage IA1 and IA2 disease should be based on microscopic examination of removed tissue, preferably a conization or large-loop excision specimen, which must include the entire lesion. For stage IA2 disease, the depth of invasion should not be more than 5 mm taken from the base of the epithelium, either surface or glandular, from which it originates. The second dimension, the horizontal spread, must not exceed 7 mm. Vascular space involvement, either venous or lymphatic, should not alter the staging but should be specifically recorded because it can affect treatment decisions in the future. The remaining stage I cases should be allotted to stage IB.

For stage IA2 disease, standard treatment is class III radical hysterectomy with bilateral pelvic lymphadenectomy; however, some authors recommend a class II modified radical hysterectomy (Fig. 46.9). The class II hysterectomy removes the median half of the cardinal and uterosacral ligaments, ligating the uterine artery at the ureter. This more conservative operation has been used by some authors in the past three decades to excise small primary tumors while reducing the partial bladder denervation associated with the complete excision of the cardinal and uterosacral ligaments required for a class III

hysterectomy. Five-year survival rates of up to 97% to 98% have been reported for patients with small cervical lesions treated with class II hysterectomy. However, in a recent review of the data from the 1981 to 1984 GOG prospective protocol, Creasman and associates reported a 100% progression-free survival in 51 stage IA2 patients treated by class III radical hysterectomy and bilateral pelvic lymphadenectomy.

The role of the class II modified radical hysterectomy was recently evaluated in a randomized, prospective study reported by Landoni and colleagues. Two hundred forty-three patients with FIGO stages IB and IIA were randomized to either class II or III hysterectomy. The recurrence-free and overall survivals were similar between the two groups. Patients treated with Type II radical hysterectomy had a statistically significant reduction in operative time and postoperative morbidity, particularly bladder dysfunction. However, given the relatively high cure rate for early cervical cancer treated by radical hysterectomy, larger trials are necessary to prove equivalence in survival between the two types of hysterectomy. As stated by Rose, larger trials are required before we can accept these results as the new standard of care. The estimated extent of tissue resection in surgical procedures for early cervical cancer is summarized in Table 46.5.

Historical Points in the Development of Radical Surgery for Cervical Cancer

Although the first truly radical hysterectomy for cervical cancer was performed by John Clark while still a resident trainee at the Johns Hopkins Hospital in 1895, the pro-

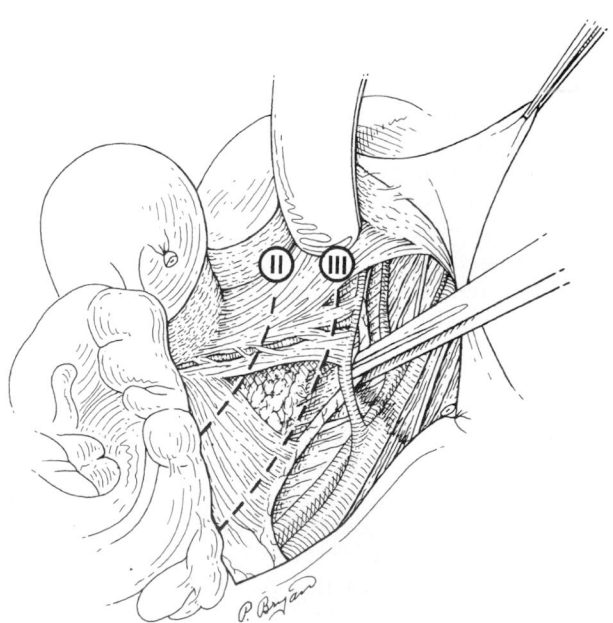

FIGURE 46.9. The cardinal ligament is excised medially in women with microscopic lesions (class II operation) or laterally in those with larger volume lesions (class III operation). (Modified from: Piver MS, Rutledge F, Smith JP. Five classes of extended hysterectomy for women with cervical cancer. *Obstet Gynecol* 1974;44:265, with permission.)

TABLE 46.5.
Comparison of Extent of Resection for Surgical Procedures to Treat Early-Stage Cervical Cancer

Tissue	Cervical Conization	Total Abdominal/ Vaginal Hysterectomy	Modified Radical Hysterectomy	Radical Abdominal Hysterectomy	Radical Vaginal Trachelectomy	Radical Vaginal Hysterectomy
Cervix uteri	Partially removed	Completely removed	Completely removed	Completely removed	Majority removed	Completely removed
Corpus uteri	Preserved	Completely removed	Completely removed	Completely removed	Preserved	Completely removed
Ovaries and tubes	Preserved	Preserved	Preserved	Preserved	Preserved	Preserved
Parametria and paracolpos	Preserved	Preserved	Removed at level of ureter	Removed lateral to ureter	Partially removed	Removed at level of ureter
Uterine vessels	Preserved	Ligated at level of cervical internal os	Ligated at level of ureter	Ligated at origin from hypogastric vessels	Descending cervicovaginal branch ligated	Ligated at level of ureter
Uterosacral ligaments	Preserved	Ligated at uterus	Divided midway to rectum	Divided near rectum	Partially removed	Partially removed
Vaginal cuff	Preserved	None removed	1–2 cm removed	≥2 cm removed	1–2 cm removed	≥2 cm removed

cedure is linked in perpetuity to Wertheim of Vienna, who reported his series of 500 cases of radical extended abdominal hysterectomy and partial lymphadenectomy performed from 1898 until 1911. Despite the enthusiasm of Wertheim, Schauta (who developed the vaginal radical hysterectomy), Okabayashi, and others, radical surgery was fraught with significant operative morbidity and mortality; the introduction of radium brought irradiation to the forefront of primary treatment for carcinoma of the cervix for the next several decades. In the United States, Joe V. Meigs reintroduced radical hysterectomy as a treatment of choice, publishing in 1944 a series of 344 cases. Until formalization of training fellowships in gynecologic oncology in the early 1970s, many outstanding gynecologic surgeons in the United States (Parsons, Ulfelder, Green, and many others) have made important contributions and modifications in the radical surgical approach that have markedly decreased complications while preserving the cure rate; today, superb performance of radical hysterectomy is the benchmark of the gynecologic oncology surgeon.

Patient Selection for Radical Hysterectomy

Simple hysterectomy is not adequate treatment for stage IB cervical cancer. In 1943, Jones and Jones reported a 5-year survival rate of only 41.6% in patients who had been treated for stage I cervical cancer with simple hysterectomy only. Such poor results also have been reported by Schmidt and others. When more than FIGO stage IA1 invasive cervical cancer is a surprise finding in a simple hysterectomy specimen, additional therapy, usually radiation therapy with or without chemotherapy should be given postoperatively. Suggested indications for radical abdominal hysterectomy are summarized in Table 46.6.

Although radical hysterectomy and pelvic lymphadenectomy occasionally are used to treat patients with adenocarcinoma of the endometrium with involvement of the cervical stroma (stage IIB) and, rarely, patients who have a small cervical cancer that persists or recurs in the cervix after primary radiation therapy, emphasis is given to the use of the operation as primary treatment for invasive cervical cancer in this chapter.

In most institutions, the majority of patients with stages IA2, IB1, and nonbulky IIA cervical cancer are of-

TABLE 46.6.
Indication for Radical Abdominal Hysterectomy

Indication	Extent of Disease
Invasive cervical cancer	Stage IA1 with lymphvascular invasion
	Stage IA2
	Stage IB1
	Stage IB2 (selected)
	Stage IIA (selected)
Invasive vaginal cancer	Stage I–II (limited to upper one third vagina, usually involving posterior vaginal fornix)
Endometrial carcinoma	Clinical stage IIB (gross cervical invasion)
Persistent of recurrent cervical cancer after radiotherapy	Clinically limited to cervix or proximal vaginal fornix

fered radical abdominal hysterectomy and bilateral pelvic lymphadenectomy as primary treatment.

Patients with bulky stage IB disease (currently FIGO stage IB2) have traditionally been treated with radical hysterectomy and bilateral pelvic lymphadenectomy or primary radiation therapy with equivalent survivals. However, patients with these larger lesions treated surgically have a very high risk of having an indication, such as lymph node metastasis, for postoperative pelvic radiation treatment. Landoni and colleagues performed a randomized trial of radical hysterectomy and pelvic lymphadenectomy versus pelvic radiation therapy for stage IB to IIA cervical cancer. Patients randomized to the surgery arm who had pathologic risk factors, such as lymph node metastasis, received adjuvant radiation therapy. Of the 55 patients with tumors >4 cm, 46 (84%) required postoperative irradiation. The disease-free and overall survival for these patients treated with surgery and radiation therapy was the same as that for patients with bulky tumors treated with radiation therapy alone; however, the combination therapy significantly increased morbidity. Subsequently, a randomized trial performed by the GOG demonstrated the benefit of the addition of cisplatin chemotherapy to pelvic radiation followed by extrafascial hysterectomy in this group of patients. Therefore, many experts feel that patients with FIGO stage IB2 and bulky IIA cervical cancer are best treated with concomitant cisplatin chemotherapy and radiation therapy followed by extrafascial hysterectomy.

In this country, patients with stage IIB invasive cervical cancer usually are excluded from primary treatment with surgery. They also are currently treated with concomitant radiation therapy and chemotherapy. Admittedly, in patients with large, friable tumors, it is somewhat difficult to be certain about extension of disease into the parametrium based on pelvic examination alone.

The clinical significance of parametrial involvement dates from the early studies of Kundrat and those of Sampson. Kundrat, working in Wertheim's clinic, in a careful study of more than 21,000 serial microscopic sections of the parametrium, found that the parametrium of one or both sides was involved in 44 of 80 patients. In a similar study at the Johns Hopkins Hospital, Sampson pointed out that the parametrium could feel indurated and yet show no evidence of cancer. Also, the parametrium can feel normal and yet contain cancer. Sampson emphasized that only by the microscope can the surgeon exclude cancer from the parametrium. More recently, Inoue and Okumura found parametrial extension in 7% of stage IB patients and in only 34% of stage IIB patients. Burghardt and Pickel found true parametrial involvement in only 19% of stage IIB patients. Matsuyama and coworkers found no parametrial cancer in 58% of stage IIB patients. These studies were based on careful examination of microscopic sections and reemphasize the difficulty of being certain about parametrial extension from pelvic examination alone. If there is suspicion of spread into the parametrial tissues by examination, CT scan, or MRI scan, it is reasonable to offer radiation therapy with concomitant chemotherapy as

primary treatment. When tumor has broken through the fibrous capsule within which it is contained in the cervix, the percentage of lymph nodes involved with metastatic disease more than doubles, and rates of persistent disease after surgery, with or without postoperative radiation, increase. Inoue and Okumura studied 628 operative specimens from patients treated with radical hysterectomy and lymphadenectomy and found that parametrial extension is an important factor in the number of positive lymph nodes found and in patient survival.

The major point to be emphasized is that the gynecologic surgeon should not attempt to treat a patient with a large cervical tumor with primary radical surgery unless there is reasonable assurance that the operation will result in the complete removal of the central tumor with an adequate margin of tumor-free tissue around it. The surgeon should not operate on patients with the idea that radiation therapy with or without chemotherapy can be used postoperatively to eliminate residual fragments of tumor tissue left behind after incomplete resection. Such patients usually are better treated with pelvic radiation therapy with or without chemotherapy from the beginning.

Primary radical surgical treatment is not contraindicated in any histologic type of cervical cancer. Shingleton and coworkers have suggested that the survival of patients with stage I adenocarcinoma of the cervix is better with surgery than with irradiation. Patients with stage I adenosquamous cancer, clear-cell cancer, and undifferentiated adenocarcinoma have a poorer prognosis, regardless of the method of treatment chosen, and are often considered for adjuvant radiation therapy and/or chemotherapy after primary surgery.

Patients considered for radical hysterectomy must be acceptable candidates for an operation and free of serious medical problems that contraindicate extensive surgery. In former years, some institutions limited radical surgery as primary treatment to premenopausal women so that ovarian function might be conserved. As experience has accumulated, it has become apparent that the operation is also well tolerated by older women. In a study of 45 women aged 65 years and older with cervical cancer, Fuchtner and associates concluded that age alone should not be a contraindication to extensive hysterectomy in the elderly patient with American Society of Anesthesiologists physical status I to III. Kinney and coworkers reported their experience with the Wertheim operation in a geriatric population. Thirty-eight selected women between 65 and 89 years of age (median age, 69 years) were compared with 320 patients younger than age 65. The survival rates were almost identical in the two groups. Perioperative morbidity was minimally increased in the geriatric group. Geisler recently compared the outcomes after radical hysterectomy and pelvic lymphadenectomy of 62 patients over age 65 to 124 matched controls age 50 or younger. Even using this relatively younger cohort for comparison, there were no significant differences in operative mortality or morbidity. However, to achieve such excellent results in older women, Kinney et al. pointed out that "meticulous sur-

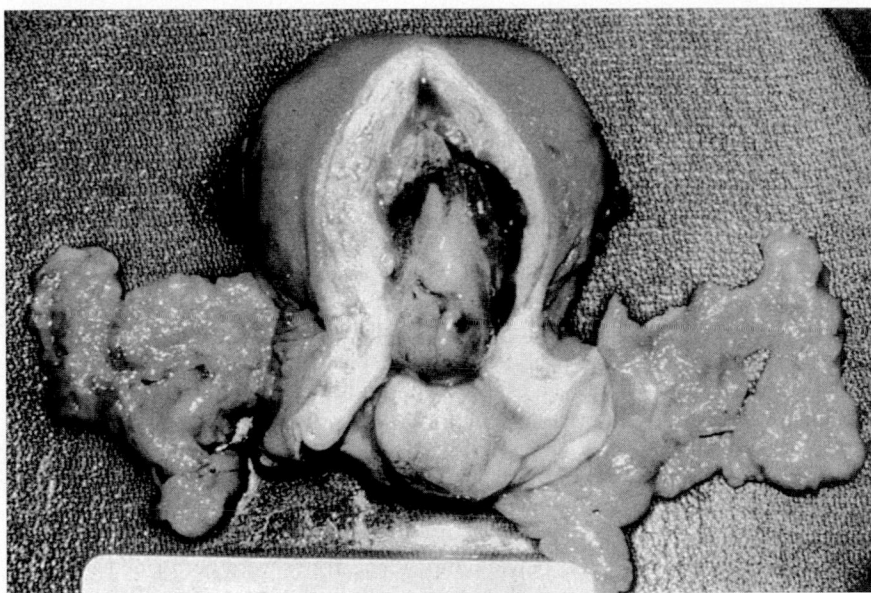

FIGURE 46.10. Squamous cell carcinoma, cervix uteri, FIGO stage Ib with intrauterine pregnancy, 16 weeks (lymphadenectomy specimen not included).

gical technique, high-quality ancillary services, and support from internal medicine and anesthesia services" are required. Such extended supportive care is not available in every hospital.

Extreme obesity (especially morbid obesity) presents especially difficult technical problems when radical surgery is chosen for primary treatment. Not only is the performance of the operation less satisfactory, but also there is an increased risk of wound dehiscence and evisceration, postoperative infection, intraoperative hemorrhage, pulmonary embolus, pulmonary atelectasis, and anesthesia-related and other problems. Unfortunately, primary treatment with radiation therapy with or without chemotherapy also is frequently less than satisfactory in extremely obese patients.

Studies by Soisson and Levrant have compared outcomes after radical hysterectomy for cervical cancer in obese versus nonobese women. They have found that survival is not compromised and the incidence of serious complications is not increased in obese patients. However, in obese women, the authors have reported that the operative technique is more difficult, the procedure lasts longer, and the surgery is associated with greater blood loss. Cohn et al. recently reported their results with radical hysterectomy for cervical cancer in 46 obese women. The median body mass index was 36 kg/m² and the median weight was 95 kg. Nine patients (20%) experienced postoperative morbidity, mostly related to wound complications. No patient developed a fistula. According to Massi and associates, the Schauta-Amreich vaginal hysterectomy can be used as an alternative to the radical abdominal hysterectomy in the presence of obesity or elevated surgical risks.

According to Shingleton, primary treatment with radical surgery paradoxically also can be riskier in very thin patients with a higher incidence of fistula. It may be speculated that easy exposure and lack of excess fatty tissue in these patients may result in removing essential vasculature around the ureters and bladder, and subsequently resulting in ischemic necrosis. A thin patient has less fat around the pelvic vessels and in the lymph fields; thus, the surgeon should be satisfied to remove less tissue in an operation that will still be adequate in a thin patient.

Once invasive carcinoma of the cervix is diagnosed in a pregnant patient, a decision must be made either to save the pregnancy or treat the cancer. Pregnancy is not a contraindication to primary treatment of stage IB or IIA carcinoma of the cervix with radical surgery (Fig. 46.10). In 1974, Sall and coworkers reported on 29 patients with stage IB carcinoma of the cervix in pregnancy treated with radical hysterectomy and pelvic lymphadenectomy. Twenty-eight patients were alive and well, and 23 patients had been followed for more than 5 years. There were no fistulas or major complications. Others have confirmed 5-year survival rates of 85% to 95% for patients treated with radical surgery for stage IB cervical cancer. Funnell and associates, operating on 17 pregnant patients suggested that the associated pregnancy changes facilitated the surgical dissection. Sood and colleagues performed a case-control study comparing the outcomes after radical hysterectomy and pelvic lymphadenectomy for 26 pregnant versus 26 nonpregnant patients. Operative times and postoperative complication rates were similar between the two groups. There was a statistically significant increase in blood loss at the time of surgery for pregnant patients; however, there was no difference in the frequency of blood transfusion. Eleven patients underwent surgical treatment in their third trimester of pregnancy with a mean planned delay in therapy of 16 weeks. None of the patients with the planned delay in therapy developed recurrent disease. The authors concluded that surgical management of early cervical cancer is safe during pregnancy. In select obstetric patients who desire to maintain their pregnancies, they agree with the conclusions of Greer and coworkers that planned delay in therapy to increase the likelihood of fetal maturity is safe for early stage I squamous-cell cancers diagnosed in the late second and early third trimester. All other patients should either be treated promptly in an attempt to cure the cancer.

Finally, based on data from Orr, Chapman, and others, extensive parametrectomy and pelvic lymphadenectomy appear to be appropriate management for selected patients found to have unexpected invasive cancer of the cervix on pathologic examination of a uterus removed for benign conditions. Low morbidity rates and acceptable rates of long-term disease-free survival have been reported.

Advantages of Radical Surgery as Primary Treatment for Invasive Cervical Cancer

The most important considerations in choosing a method of therapy for any cancer are, first, effectiveness of the treatment in curing the disease and, second, mortality and morbidity rates associated with the treatment plan. For the indications listed previously, the cure rates of primary radiation therapy and primary extensive surgery are about equal. The modern mortality rates also are about equal. Both modalities of therapy have a list of complications unique to each that seem about equal. There are, however, important major and minor advantages of primary radical surgery over irradiation for early-stage disease, some of which are discussed in the following.

ACCURATE EVALUATION OF EXTENT OF DISEASE

The findings at operation and from careful pathologic examination of the surgical specimen can be immensely helpful in selecting high-risk patients for adjuvant postoperative radiation therapy, chemotherapy, or both. Most patients with FIGO stages IA2, IB1, and nonbulky IIA disease are not found to have high-risk factors and thus are spared the potential morbidity associated with whole pelvic radiation therapy. Furthermore, the findings at operation and careful pathologic examination of the surgical specimen can be helpful in determining prognosis and in identifying patients at greatest risk for persistence or recurrence of disease. Such high-risk patients may require special diagnostic procedures and follow-up examinations at more frequent intervals.

In addition to an accurate assessment of the extent of the cervical cancer, primary surgical treatment allows for discovery of other intraabdominal incidental conditions and diseases entirely unrelated to the cancer. Ovarian malignancies, pelvic tuberculosis, sigmoid diverticulitis, cholelithiasis, and other diseases and conditions may be encountered at the time of operation.

PRESERVATION OF OVARIAN FUNCTION

When primary radiation therapy with or without chemotherapy is used to treat invasive cervical cancer in premenopausal women, premature loss of ovarian function is an unfortunate and inevitable result. When primary surgery is used instead, the function of normal ovaries can be conserved. Sutton and associates analyzed the incidence of ovarian metastasis for 991 patients with stage IB carcinoma of the cervix treated with radical hysterectomy and pelvic lymphadenectomy on a prospective GOG protocol. Ovarian spread was found in four of 770 patients (0.5%) with squamous-cell carcinoma and in two of 121 patients (1.7%) with adenocarcinoma. The difference was not statistically significant. All six patients with ovarian metastases had other evidence of extracervical disease. This study confirmed that ovarian metastasis is rare in patients with Stage IB cervical cancer and extremely rare in the absence of other evidence of extracervical disease.

Although the incidence of ovarian metastasis is slightly higher in women with *adenocarcinoma of the cervix* as compared with squamous-cell carcinoma, ovarian conservation should still be considered, especially in young women. Brand and Berek reported no ovarian metastases in more than 60 patients with adenocarcinoma of the cervix treated with extensive surgery. Angel and associates found no ovarian metastases in 41 patients with adenocarcinoma of the cervix who underwent oophorectomy. Greer and coworkers treated 55 patients with stage IB adenocarcinoma of the cervix with radical hysterectomy and pelvic lymphadenectomy. Ninety-one percent had ovarian preservation, and there was no evidence that this contributed to tumor recurrence. Hopkins and coworkers found that the best cumulative 5-year survival rate (93%) with cervical adenocarcinoma was in patients treated by radical hysterectomy without bilateral salpingo-oophorectomy, and concluded that "ovarian conservation seems to be an acceptable alternative to bilateral salpingo-oophorectomy" in young patients.

Some authors have advocated transposing the ovaries into the paracolic gutters at the time of radical hysterectomy in premenopausal women to protect the ovaries from radiation damage should postoperative pelvic radiation therapy be needed. The technique used for ovarian transposition was described by Husseinzadeh and coworkers. However, in the series reported by Chambers and coworkers there was a threefold increase in symptomatic benign ovarian cyst formation with lateral ovarian transposition compared to those that did not have their ovaries transposed. Furthermore, Anderson and coworkers reported that only four of 24 patients (17%) who had ovarian transposition retained ovarian function after postoperative radiation therapy. Moreover, after transposition, 17.6% of patients required surgical treatment for ovarian-associated pain or cysts. These data raise the question of whether paracolic gutter transposition actually achieves its goal of protecting the ovaries.

SEXUAL FUNCTION

Studies of the effect of surgical and radiation treatment for cervical carcinoma on sexual function have been published by Seibel and coworkers from Emory University and by others. Among patients treated with radiation, there are decreases in sexual enjoyment, ability to attain orgasm, frequency of intercourse, and desire for intercourse. Marked alterations can be seen and felt in the upper vagina and paravaginal tissues. The vagina usually is shorter from stenosis. The upper vagina is less pliable. Tissues are fixed and firm. The vaginal mucosa is thin, smooth, and dry with a tendency to split and bleed with slight trauma. Some of these changes are made more pronounced in young women because of hypoestrogenism from radiation-induced premature menopause. They are not completely reversed by intravaginal or oral administration of estrogen. Such functional and anatomic changes are not seen nearly as frequently in patients treated with primary extensive surgery. Even if the vagina has been surgically shortened by several centimeters with primary surgery, it remains soft, pliable, moist, and functional. Unfortunately, in those women who undergo postoperative adjuvant pelvic irradiation, some of this advantage is lost.

FEWER LATE RECURRENCES AND COMPLICATIONS

Late recurrences after treatment for cervical cancer are almost never seen after primary radical surgery. They occur more often when patients are treated with primary radiation therapy. The same can be said for complications of treatment. Because of the gradual and progressive obliterative endarteritis produced by irradiating tissue, complications resulting from ischemic changes (e.g., cystitis, proctitis, enteritis, colpocleisis, pyelonephritis) can be seen many years after radiation treatment. Late onset of complications after primary radical hysterectomy and pelvic lymphadenectomy are unusual. These points are especially important when selecting a method of primary treatment for young women.

PSYCHOLOGICAL BENEFITS

There are probably important psychological benefits of primary treatment with radical surgery, compared with radiation therapy. Most patients prefer to have the tumor removed and are especially encouraged when the surgeon can report that "the cancer is out" and that no evidence of metastatic disease was found at operation. Radiation therapy carries an unfortunate connotation in some patients who feel that it is the treatment of last resort, that the treatments are actually "cooking" the tissues in the pelvis, that the tumor is still there (albeit treated), or that irradiation can cause other cancers. All gynecologic surgeons have heard the disappointment patients express when they are told that they cannot be treated with an operation. Some patients continue to request an operation even after they have completed radiation therapy.

Justification for Pelvic Lymphadenectomy

For many years, there was competition between gynecologic surgeons who advocated radical vaginal hysterectomy without lymphadenectomy and those who advocated radical abdominal hysterectomy with lymphadenectomy. The advocates of extensive vaginal hysterectomy without lymphadenectomy (the Schauta-Amreich-Navratil operation) argued that their patients had fewer postoperative complications (especially urinary fistulas), a lower operative mortality rate, and a cure rate that was almost equal to that achieved by an abdominal operation that included lymphadenectomy. Furthermore, they pointed out that pelvic

lymphadenectomy is an incomplete operation at best, in that removal of all pelvic lymph nodes that can possibly be involved with metastatic tumor is technically impossible. This is especially true of those inferior gluteal nodes that are located in the region of the ischial spine, as pointed out by Reiffenstuhl. It also has been known since Henriksen's work that involvement of paraaortic lymph nodes can occur in a significant number of patients with metastasis to pelvic nodes, and paraaortic nodes cannot be completely removed and have not been routinely nor adequately sampled by gynecologic surgeons in abdominal operations for cervical cancer. However, even Navratil stated in 1965 that "indications for the Schauta operation must take the lymph node problem into account." Later he performed extraperitoneal pelvic lymphadenectomy with the Schauta operation in all cases of stage I and II that were locally advanced, as did Mitra.

In recent years, the operative mortality and complication rates in patients who have undergone radical abdominal hysterectomy and bilateral pelvic lymphadenectomy have significantly decreased. Operative mortality and fistulas occur in <1% and about 2% of patients, respectively. Therefore, one purported disadvantage of radical hysterectomy (high morbidity) has essentially been removed, and the surgeon can concentrate on the question of whether lymphadenectomy adds anything to the possibility of cure.

It is the opinion of some that pelvic lymphadenectomy is of no value in those 80% to 90% of patients who have negative lymph nodes. We disagree with this view. We believe that lymphadenectomy is helpful in achieving an adequate central dissection around the cervical tumor, the most important part of the operation. This is especially true of that part of the lymphadenectomy that involves removal of tissue from around the hypogastric vessels, from the obturator fossa, and from the lower presacral region. Admittedly, dissection of lymph nodes from the common iliac vessels and from the paraaortic region does not add to the completeness of the central dissection. Removal of these and other nodes, however, is helpful in prognosis and in identifying patients at greater risk for persistent disease who might receive adjuvant postoperative radiation therapy to the pelvis and perhaps to extended fields along the aorta. Although we seldom dissect and remove the highest paraaortic lymph nodes, we do remove the lowest paraaortic nodes around and just above the aortic bifurcation. If pelvic lymph nodes involved with tumor are found during the operation, a concerted effort is made to do a more complete paraaortic dissection. Although it is possible for paraaortic nodes to be directly involved without involvement of pelvic nodes, this is extremely rare. For the group of patients who usually would be chosen for treatment with primary radical surgery, routine extensive paraaortic lymph node dissection would not result in a therapeutic benefit very often. Podczaski and coworkers found positive paraaortic lymph nodes in seven of 52 patients (13.4%) with stage IB and IIA disease. Twenty-eight of the 52 patients, however, had bulky tumors >5 cm in greatest diameter. Currently, such patients are considered by many gynecologic oncologists not to be appropriate candidates for treatment with primary radical surgery. Patsner and coworkers performed paraaortic lymph node sampling in patients with small (tumor ≤3 cm) stage IB cervical cancer. Only two of the 125 patients who underwent radical hysterectomy, bilateral pelvic lymphadenectomy, and paraaortic node sampling had metastases to the paraaortic nodes. No patient had gross paraaortic nodal involvement, and both patients with microscopic paraaortic nodal metastases had grossly positive pelvic nodal involvement. These investigators recommended that paraaortic sampling in patients with small stage IB cervical tumors be restricted to patients with suspicious or positive pelvic or paraaortic nodes. The paraaortic region should be carefully palpated and any enlarged or firm nodes removed, but the gynecologic surgeon should be aware of the added morbidity associated with comprehensive paraaortic lymphadenectomy.

If a pelvic lymphadenectomy is not done in patients who have a radical hysterectomy for cervical cancer, at least 15% to 20% of patients (those with positive nodes) will be inadequately treated for their disease (unless perhaps all patients receive postoperative pelvic irradiation). In our judgment, it is better to do a pelvic lymphadenectomy in all patients and then give postoperative radiation therapy selectively than to avoid a lymphadenectomy and give postoperative radiation therapy to all patients.

A study reported by Downey and colleagues provides indirect evidence that postoperative pelvic irradiation is more effective in controlling disease after pelvic lymphadenectomy has removed clinically positive lymph nodes that contain metastatic tumor. The amount of irradiation required to eliminate tumor in lymph nodes is directly related to the volume of tumor present (Table 46.7). Thus, removing the larger nodes involved with tumor increases the probability of control of tumor with irradiation. Patients in this study who underwent resection of large positive pelvic nodes followed by postoperative extended-field irradiation had a surprisingly high 5-year recurrence-free survival rate of 51%. The advantages of surgical debulking of positive lymph nodes also was

TABLE 46.7.

Squamous Cell Carcinoma of the Cervix: Dose–Tumor–Volume Relation[a]

Tumor Volume (cm)	Dose (Gy)
<2	50
2	60
2–4	70
4–6	75–89
6	80–100

[a] Average radiation dose required to obtain 90% control in area treated.
From: Shingleton HM, Orr JW. *Cancer of the cervix: diagnosis and treatment.* New York: Churchill Livingstone, 1987:174, with permission.

discussed by Potish and coworkers in a later study from the same center. No patient with unresectable pelvic nodes survived 5 years. In 84% (49/58) of cases with grossly positive pelvic nodes, the nodes were able to be debulked. The 5-year actuarial relapse-free survival rates were the same for patients with only microscopically involved pelvic node metastases (56%) and for patients with grossly involved but surgically resected pelvic node metastases (57%). All patients with positive pelvic nodes received postoperative irradiation to the pelvis and paraaortic nodes. These authors believe that surgical debulking of grossly involved pelvic lymph nodes to microscopic residual disease can improve the chance of control with postoperative irradiation.

PERTINENT PELVIC ANATOMY

Arterial and Venous Anatomy

Although the lower portions of the aorta and vena cava are frequently incorporated into the operative field of the pelvic lymphadenectomy, the major operative dissection includes the common iliac, external iliac, and hypogastric (also known as the internal iliac) arteries and veins and their various branches and tributaries. The abdominal aorta emerges through the aortic hiatus of the diaphragm at the lower border of the last thoracic vertebra and descends along the ventral surface of the vertebral column, where it bifurcates into the left and right common iliac arteries at the fourth lumbar vertebra (Fig. 46.11). This is an important anatomic landmark because the bifurcation at L-4 lies directly beneath the umbilicus in most cases. Therefore, an abdominal midline incision that provides surgical exposure to the lower aorta needs to be extended somewhat above the umbilicus. The right common iliac artery crosses the upper portion of the left common iliac vein at the aortic bifurcation. This segment of the venous drainage of the left side of the pelvis joins with the right common iliac vein to form the vena cava, which lies directly along the right side of the aorta and on the right lateral side of the bodies of the lumbar vertebrae in its retroperitoneal course through the abdomen.

Both common iliac arteries continue along the medial border of the psoas muscle to the pelvic brim, where they divide into external iliac and hypogastric vessels. As shown in Fig. 46.11, this important vascular division marks the site where the ureters enter the pelvis from the abdomen, usually overlying the terminal end of the common iliac artery on the left and commonly crossing the actual bifurcation of the artery on the right. Both external iliac arteries pass beneath the inguinal ligament to proceed into the leg as the femoral artery. The external iliac artery makes no direct vascular contribution to the pelvis, although there is a fairly consistent arterial branch to the ureter from the midportion of the common iliac artery.

The external iliac vein emerges from beneath the inguinal ligament, where it courses along the lateral pelvic brim on the medial side of the artery until it reaches the proximal segment. Here, the vein passes directly beneath the artery at the bifurcation of the common iliac artery

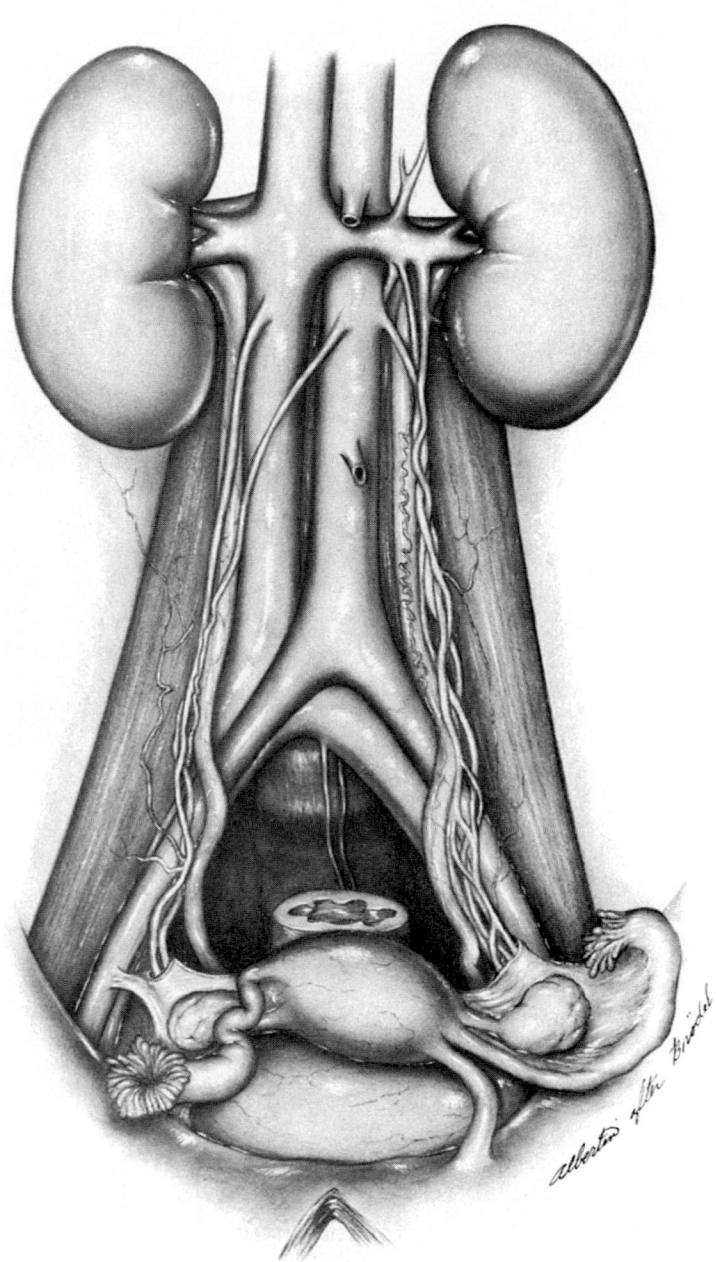

FIGURE 46.11. Abdominal and pelvic anatomy, showing the anatomic relations of the aorta, vena cava, iliac vessels, and ureters. Note the arteriovenous crossing of the right common iliac artery and the left iliac vein.

and then passes along the lateral side of the upper half of the artery. It then joins the left common iliac vein to become the inferior vena cava at the fifth lumbar vertebra. In dissecting the lymph nodes along the external iliac vessels, these anatomic landmarks are important to avoid trauma to the wall of the vein as it deviates from the medial to the lateral side of the arterial tree.

The hypogastric artery provides the major blood supply to the pelvic viscera. For descriptive purposes, it is conveniently divided into an anterior and a posterior division. The important branches of the hypogastric artery are shown in Figs. 46.12 and 46.13.

A fairly consistent arterial branch to the ureter arises from the hypogastric artery near the common iliac bifurcation. This vessel passes medially to the ureter and

should be preserved, if possible, during the dissection of the hypogastric vessels. The hypogastric artery continues beneath the coccygeus muscle through the ischiorectal fossa, where it becomes the internal pudendal artery to supply the perineum and vulva.

The major blood supply to the pelvic viscera is derived from the anterior division of the hypogastric artery. Figure 46.12 shows the anterior division which gives off the uterine artery before continuing along the posterolateral pelvic wall to supply the superior and inferior vesical branches to the bladder. The anterior division then continues as the obliterated umbilical artery as it passes cephalad along the inferior surface of the rectus muscle to the umbilicus. In dissecting along the hypogastric artery in a caudad direction, the uterine artery is the first vessel

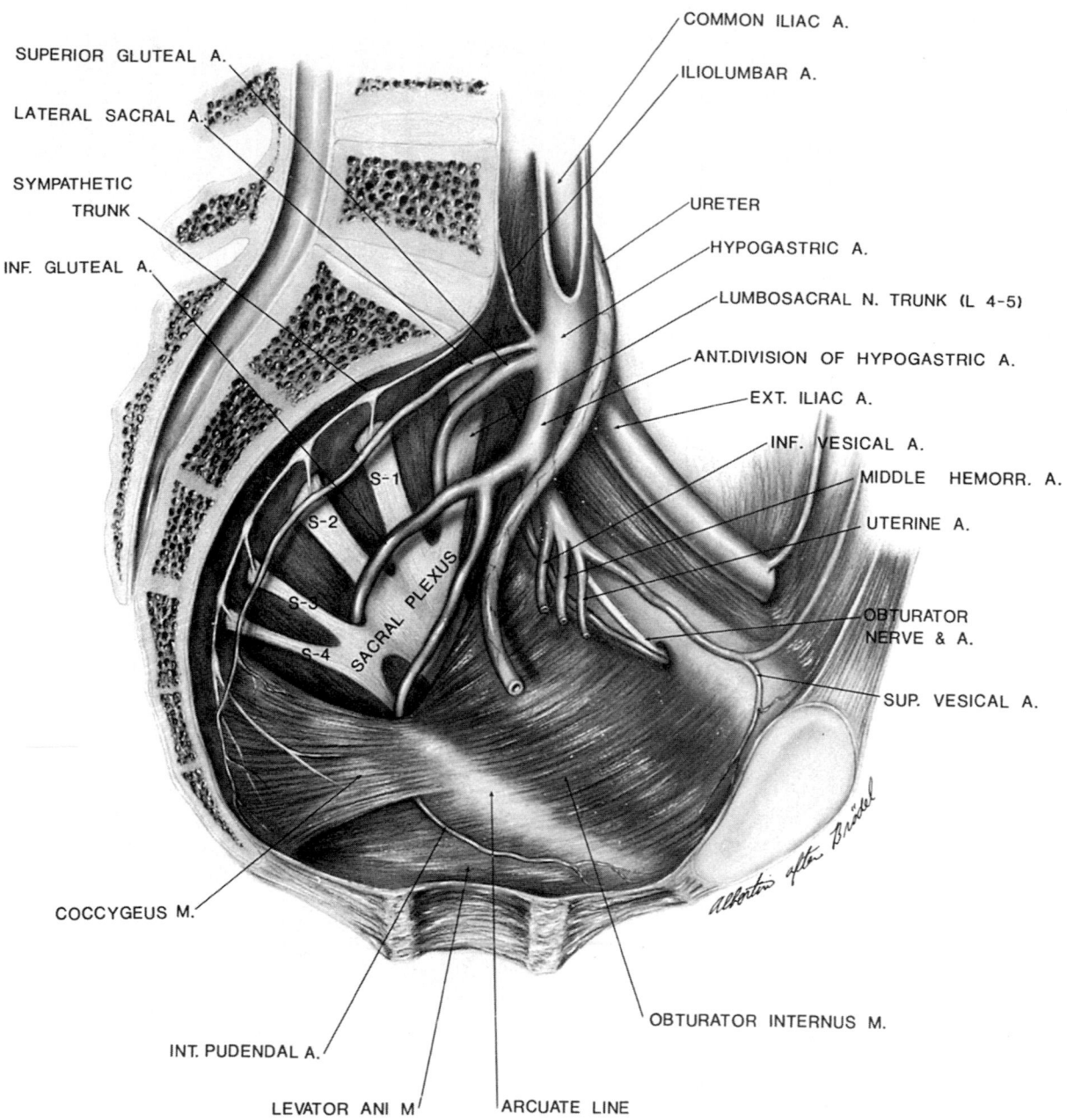

FIGURE 46.12. Anatomy of the arterial blood supply to the female pelvis showing relations of pelvic musculature, divisions of hypogastric artery, and lumbosacral and sacral nerve plexuses. Note that the anterior division of the hypogastric artery provides the blood supply to the pelvic viscera.

encountered; it emanates from the medial side of the vessel. Passing more inferiorly and medially is the middle hemorrhoidal artery, which supplies a major segment of the rectum and communicates with the superior hemorrhoidal (from the inferior mesenteric) and the inferior hemorrhoidal (from the internal pudendal) arteries.

The hypogastric vein and its tributaries course along the pelvic floor and medial side of the artery to drain the pelvis in close relation to the arterial blood supply. Its ex-

tensive anatomic variations and its location along the pelvic sidewall and floor place these tortuous, thin-walled veins in a precarious and vulnerable position for trauma during deep dissection of the pelvis. As shown in Fig. 46.13, the delicate tributaries of the trunk of the hypogastric vein extend into sacral foramina and pass beneath nerve fibers and muscles within the pelvis, so that their identity during the dissection of the pelvis frequently is obscured. The continuation of the hypogastric

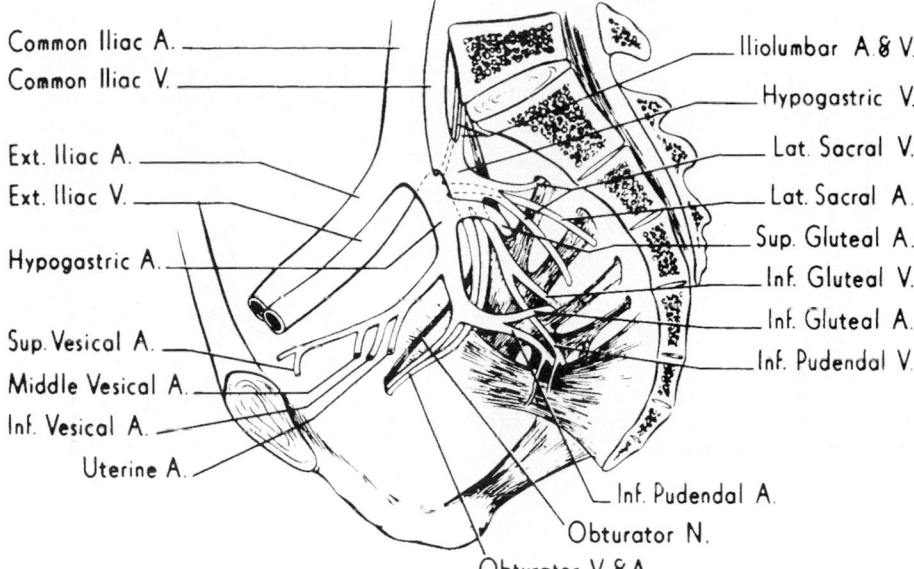

Common Iliac A.
Common Iliac V.

Ext. Iliac A.
Ext. Iliac V.

Hypogastric A.

Sup. Vesical A.
Middle Vesical A.
Inf. Vesical A.
Uterine A.

Iliolumbar A. & V.
Hypogastric V.
Lat. Sacral V.
Lat. Sacral A.
Sup. Gluteal A.
Inf. Gluteal V.
Inf. Gluteal A.
Inf. Pudendal V.

Inf. Pudendal A.
Obturator N.
Obturator V & A.

FIGURE 46.13. Anatomy of hypogastric vein. (From: Thompson JD. Extensive hysterectomy and bilateral pelvic lymphadenectomy. In: Coppleson M, ed. *Gynecologic oncology*, second ed. New York: Churchill Livingstone, 1992, with permission.)

vein, in association with the artery, beneath the coccygeus muscle is a frequent site of bleeding when dissection is undertaken along the pelvic floor. When this occurs, it is difficult to identify the vessel because it retracts beneath the margins of the muscle.

The profuse collateral blood supply to the ureter is an important anatomic safeguard that protects its pelvic segment from ischemic necrosis as a result of radical hysterectomy (Fig. 46.14). The ureter has the advantage of a multiple-source blood supply. This favorable collateral circulation permits interruption of small arteries and veins deep in the pelvis during extensive dissection of the base of the broad ligament without producing a significant incidence of ischemic necrosis and fistula formation. The freely anastomosing arterial and venous network that courses along the longitudinal surface of the ureter in its adventitial layer is supplied in its superior segment by branches from the renal and ovarian arteries. The middle segment of the ureter derives its blood supply directly from aortic branches and from a vessel from the common iliac artery. As the ureter enters the pelvis and courses along the lateral pelvic wall, it receives arterial branches from the uterine, vaginal, middle hemorrhoidal, and vesical arteries. As it approaches the trigone of the bladder, it has a rich arteriovenous collateral circulation from the arterial branches to the vagina and base of the bladder. Protection of this important vascular network is important for the integrity of the terminal ureter during extensive dissection of the cardinal ligament. Preservation of the lateral aspect of the posterior segment of the vesicouterine ligament has been recommended to ensure adequate vascularity to the terminal segment of the ureter, but we have encountered no difficulty in removing this tissue and have no hesitation in doing so to enhance the adequacy of the central dissection.

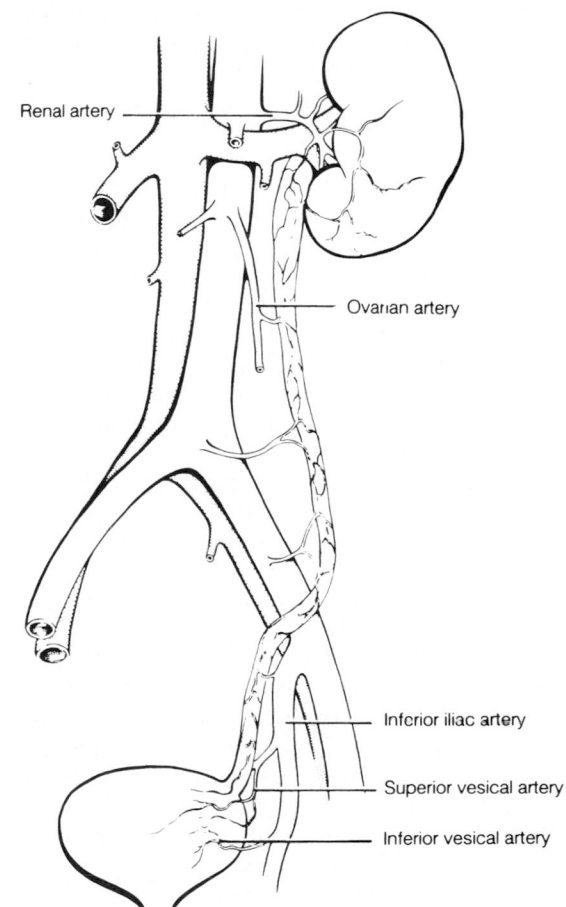

Renal artery

Ovarian artery

Inferior iliac artery

Superior vesical artery

Inferior vesical artery

FIGURE 46.14. Blood supply of the ureter showing multiple sources of collateral arterial circulation.

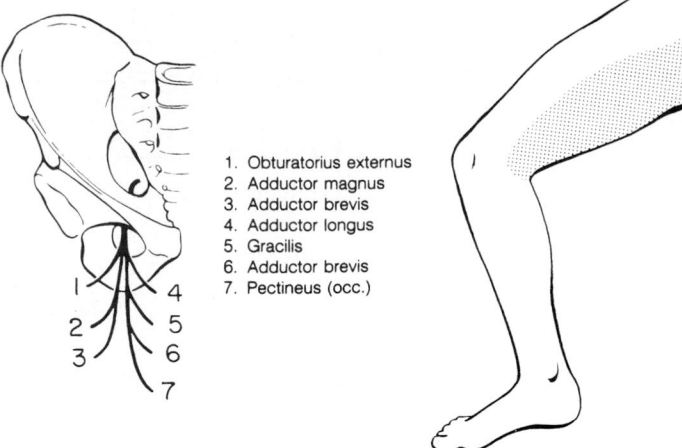

1. Obturatorius externus
2. Adductor magnus
3. Adductor brevis
4. Adductor longus
5. Gracilis
6. Adductor brevis
7. Pectineus (occ.)

FIGURE 46.15. Obturator nerve (L-2 through L-4): motor and sensory innervation.

Lymphatic Anatomy

The lymphatic drainage of the pelvis follows the course of the arterial and venous blood supply. Although there are multiple variations in the lymphatic anatomy of the pelvis, in general, lateral, superior, medial, and inferior lymph nodes and communicating lymphatic channels surround the common iliac, external iliac, and hypogastric vessels. One of the important pathways of the pelvic nodes and thin-walled lymphatics that drain the upper vagina, cervix, and uterus courses along the posterior aspect of the endopelvic fascia. Here, the pelvic nodes pass through the uterosacral ligament area and terminate in lymph nodes along the lateral aspect of the sacrum. These nodes communicate freely with lymphatic channels from the bifurcation of the common iliac artery near the lateral sacral and ischiosacral fossae. These can be difficult nodes to resect because they are closely attached to the thin-walled tributaries of the hypogastric vein. In dissecting the nodes from the bifurcation of the common iliac vessels, care must be taken to avoid injury to the hypogastric vein, which extends from beneath the artery on the medial side in this area.

The most direct lymphatic drainage of the cervix and upper vagina is through the lateral parametrium (cardinal ligament) to the hypogastric and obturator lymphatics. Because of the presence of obscure obturator veins and multiple venous tributaries from the hypogastric vein along the pelvic floor, the obturator dissection can be associated with troublesome venous bleeding. Injury also can occur to the obturator nerve, which arises from the anterior division of the second, third, and fourth lumbar nerves; enters the pelvis through the psoas muscle; and runs along the lateral pelvic wall in the obturator fossa to exit the pelvis through the obturator foramen along with the obturator vessels. It is a motor nerve to the adductor muscles of the thigh and is the only motor nerve that arises from the lumbar plexus without innervating any of the pelvic structures. Damage to the obturator nerve produces not only motor impairment to the adductor muscles but also sensory loss along the medial aspect of the thigh

(Fig. 46.15). Deep dissection posterior to the obturator nerve can be complicated by bleeding from the tributaries of the hypogastric and obturator veins so that dissection in this area, if necessary, must be done with great care, using clips on the small vessels and compression for troublesome venous bleeding.

Reiffenstuhl, in his classic study of the lymphatics of the female genital organs, describes efferent lymph channels from the cervix to the interiliac lymph nodes, the lateral and medial external iliac lymph nodes, the lateral and medial common iliac lymph nodes, the sacral lymph nodes, the subaortic lymph nodes, the aortic lymph nodes, the superior gluteal lymph nodes, the inferior gluteal lymph nodes, and the rectal lymph nodes. Of these, the inferior gluteal nodes are not technically possible to remove with the standard approach. This is because the nodes lie around the ischial spine in proximity to the inferior gluteal artery and pudendal artery and nerve. An imposing network of veins also surrounds the inferior gluteal nodes. They are thin-walled, easy to damage, difficult to expose, and difficult to control when damaged.

Reiffenstuhl's concepts of the lymphatic drainage of the cervix are partially shown in Figs. 46.16 through 46.19.

CONCEPT OF RADICAL ABDOMINAL HYSTERECTOMY AND BILATERAL PELVIC LYMPHADENECTOMY

There are several variations of hysterectomy used in the management of cervical carcinoma. The description of the five classes of hysterectomy by Piver and colleagues has found general acceptance. The first three classes are used in the primary treatment of cervical carcinoma, whereas the last two classes are generally reserved for patients with recurrent disease. The class I hysterectomy is a slight extension of the simple total hysterectomy, with removal of a small amount of parametrium. It is used as

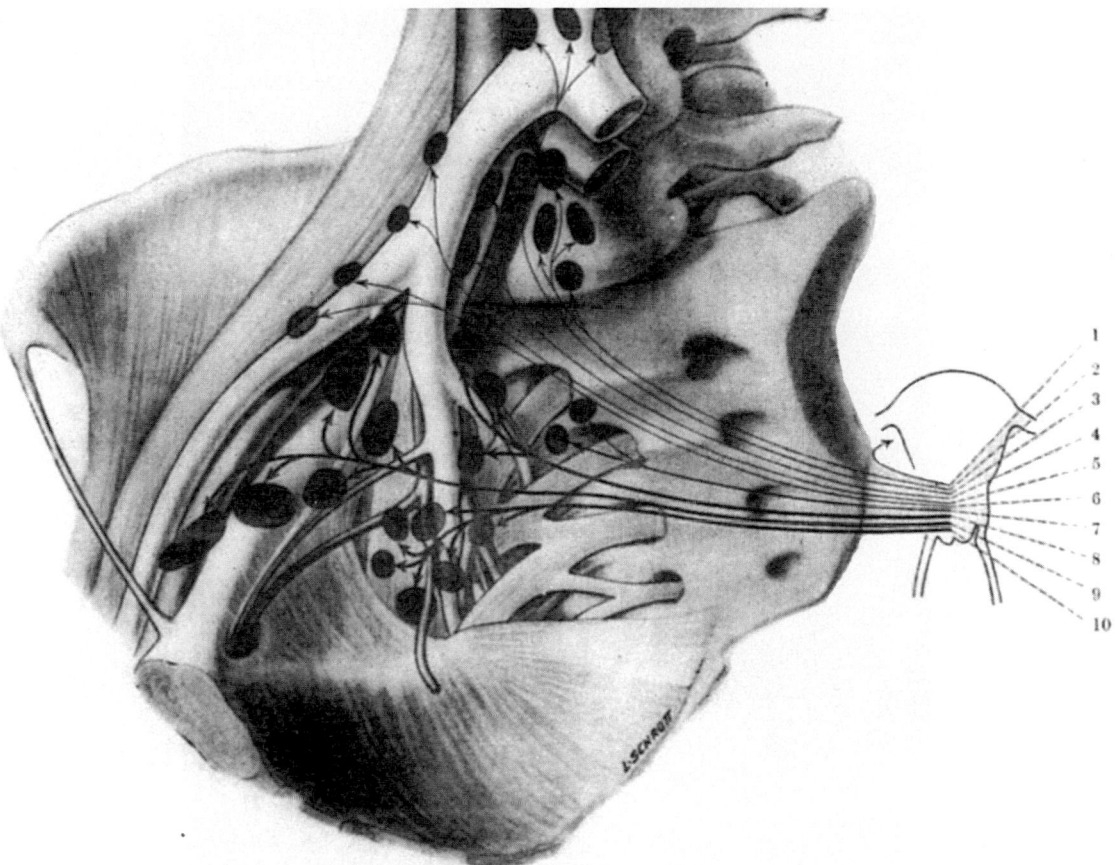

FIGURE 46.16. The regional lymph node stations of the uterine cervix. Channels 8, 9, and 10 (indicated by especially heavy lines) lead to those regional lymph node stations most frequently reached by the efferent lymph vessels of the cervix. Nonetheless, it is necessary to remember that carcinoma cells also can reach the pelvic lymph nodes by way of channels 1 through 7, without previous interruption, to: *(1)* rectal; *(2)* subaortic (promontorial); *(3)* aortic; *(4)* medial common iliac; *(5)* lateral common iliac; *(6)* lateral external iliac; *(7)* sacral; *(8)* superior gluteal; *(9)* interiliac; and *(10)* inferior gluteal lymph nodes. (From: Reiffenstuhl G. *The lymphatics of the female genital organs.* Philadelphia: JB Lippincott, 1964, with permission.)

primary treatment for stage IA1 disease and after concurrent chemotherapy and radiation therapy for stage IB2 and bulky stage IIA cervical carcinoma. The class II hysterectomy (see Fig. 46.9), also known as a modified radical hysterectomy, removes a more generous vaginal cuff, ligates the uterine artery on the medial side of the ureter (but does not dissect the ureter from the vesicouterine ligament), and removes the inner one third to one half of the cardinal ligament. As stated, some authors now recommend the performance of the class II hysterectomy for stage IA2 cervical carcinoma. The class III operation is the classic Meigs procedure, with removal of all of the parametrium and paravaginal tissue in addition to the pelvic lymph nodes (see Fig. 46.9). A more extensive procedure is performed in the class IV radical hysterectomy, in which the ureter is completely dissected from the cardinal and vesicouterine ligaments, the superior vesical artery is sacrificed, and three fourths of the vagina is removed as well as the uterus and para-

metria, along with a complete lymphadenectomy. A far more extensive procedure is done with the class V radical hysterectomy, in which the terminal ureter or a segment of the bladder or rectum is removed along with the uterus, parametria, adnexa, and pelvic lymph nodes.

Although many techniques emphasize a more or less extensive dissection in one phase of the operation or another, the management of the parametria and the dissection of the pelvic lymph nodes appear relatively uniform. Because the most serious complication of this procedure is related to ureteral fistulas and stenosis, many modifications have been undertaken to ensure an adequate blood supply to the terminal ureter. We agree that the terminal ureter must have a good blood supply and believe that this can be accomplished without jeopardizing the adequacy of the central dissection. The classic radical hysterectomy with wide resection of the parametrium, dissection of the terminal ureter from the vesicouterine ligament, and wide resection of the uterosacral ligaments,

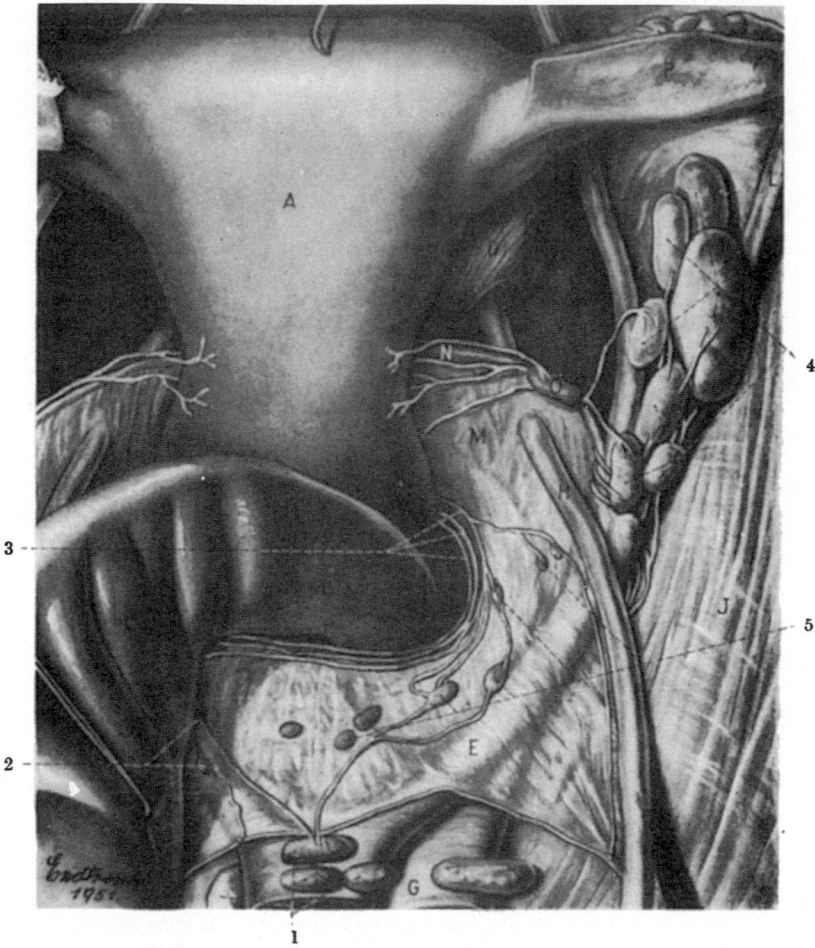

FIGURE 46.17. Lymphatic drainage of the cervix along the uterine artery and the sagittal rectal pillar (rectouterine ligament). The uterus is drawn markedly upward. **A:** View of the posterior surface of the uterus. Several lymph vessels from the cervix twine around the uterine artery *(N)*, pass the uterine Buretrol module *(O)*, which is located on the right side of the specimen at the lateral edge of the ureter *(H)*, and after crossing over the lateral umbilical ligament *(K)*, empty into the uppermost interiliac lymph nodes *(4)*. A few lymph channels from the cervix *(3)* run dorsally at the base of the Mackenrodt ligament *(M)* in the sagittal rectal pillar and reach the superior rectal lymph nodes *(2)* that lie along the like-named artery on the posterior surface of the rectum. The lymph vessels in the ureteral leaf, coming from the cervix, first run dorsally in the sagittal rectal pillar for some distance and, then before reaching the rectum, turn upward to the nodes in the ureteral leaf *(5)*. The ureteral leaf is a continuation of the sagittal rectal pillar cranially. The lymph channels then empty directly into the lowest aortic lymph nodes *(1)*. One lymph vessel from the cervix runs upward on the medial edge of the right ureter (variant). **A:** Uterus (intestinal surface); **B:** right ovary; **C:** rectum; **D:** urinary bladder (posterior surface); **E:** common external iliac artery; **F:** aorta; **G:** inferior vena cave; **H:** ureter; **J:** psoas muscle; **K:** lateral umbilical ligament; **L:** external iliac artery; **M:** Mackenrodt ligament; **N:** uterine artery; **O:** lymph node. **1:** Aortic lymph nodes; **2:** rectal lymph nodes; **3:** lymphatic vessels; **4:** interiliac lymph nodes; **5:** lymph nodes. (From: Reiffenstuhl G. *The lymphatics of the female genital organs.* Philadelphia: JB Lippincott, 1964, with permission.)

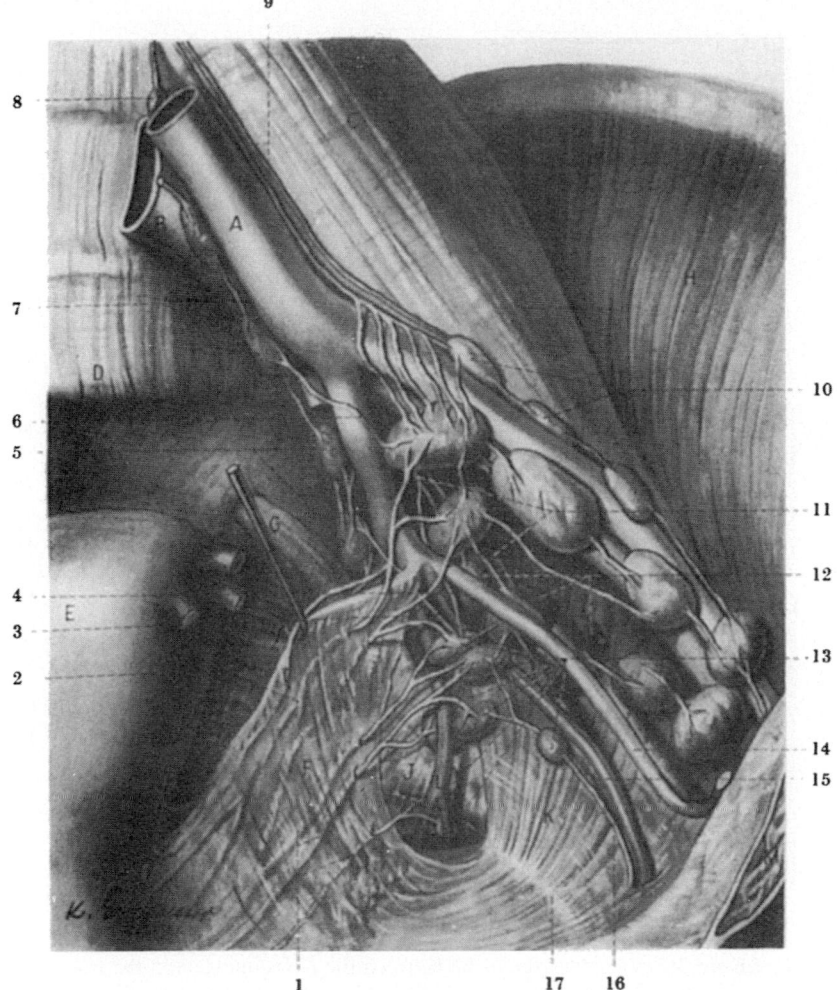

FIGURE 46.18. Inflow and outflow of the inferior gluteal lymph nodes. View of the anterior surface of Mackenrodt ligament (**F**). The uterine artery is drawn upward by means of a hook. The lateral portion of the pelvic origin Mackenrodt's ligament was removed to bring the deep nodes of the group in the sacral plexus (**J**) into view. The veins of the vesicouterovaginal plexus, which hide the nodes, were not drawn in. The lateral umbilical ligament *(14)* was left in place. Cervical lymphatic channels *(1)*, which run into the pelvic wall in the basal portions of the parametrium and then empty into the inferior gluteal lymph nodes *(13)*, predominate. These nodes extend along the inferior gluteal-internal pudendal artery down as far as the infrapiriforme foramen and, in part, lie behind the parietal blood vessels. From the inferior gluteal lymph nodes: (a), efferent vessels *(3)* run to the superior gluteal lymph nodes *(5)*; (b) vessels turn as deep channels *(4, then 11)* to the posterior side of the parietal blood vessels; and (c) connections run to those interiliac lymph nodes on the obturator artery *(12)*, which on their part, send their deep channels *(11)* upward to the deep lateral common iliac lymph nodes. From the uppermost interiliac lymph nodes lying in hypogastric angle, one lymph channel *(6)* reaches the medial common iliac lymph nodes *(7)* by crossing over the stem of the internal iliac artery. Note also the numerous efferent vessels of the uppermost interiliac nodes that cross over the initial portion of the external iliac artery and then run upward on the lateral edge of the common iliac artery as a cable *(9)*. **A:** Common iliac artery; **B:** common iliac vein; **C:** psoas muscle; **D:** promontory; **E:** uterus; **F:** Mackenrodt's ligament; **G:** first sacral nerve; **H:** iliac muscle; **J:** sacral plexus; **K:** internal obturator muscle; **L:** internal pudendal-inferior gluteal artery; **M:** internal oblique and transverse abdominal muscles. **1,2:** Cervical lymph vessels; **3,4:** efferent vessels; **5:** superior gluteal lymph nodes; **6:** efferent vessel; **7:** medial common iliac; and **8:** deep lateral common iliac lymph nodes; **9:** lymphatic vessels; **10:** lateral external iliac lymph nodes; **11:** efferent vessels; **12:** interiliac (obturator) and **13:** inferior gluteal efferent vessels; **14:** lateral umbilical ligament; **15:** obturator artery; **16:** lymphatic vessels; **17:** tendinous arch of the levator ani muscle. (From: Reiffenstuhl G. *The lymphatics of the female genital organs.* Philadelphia: JB Lippincott, 1964, with permission.)

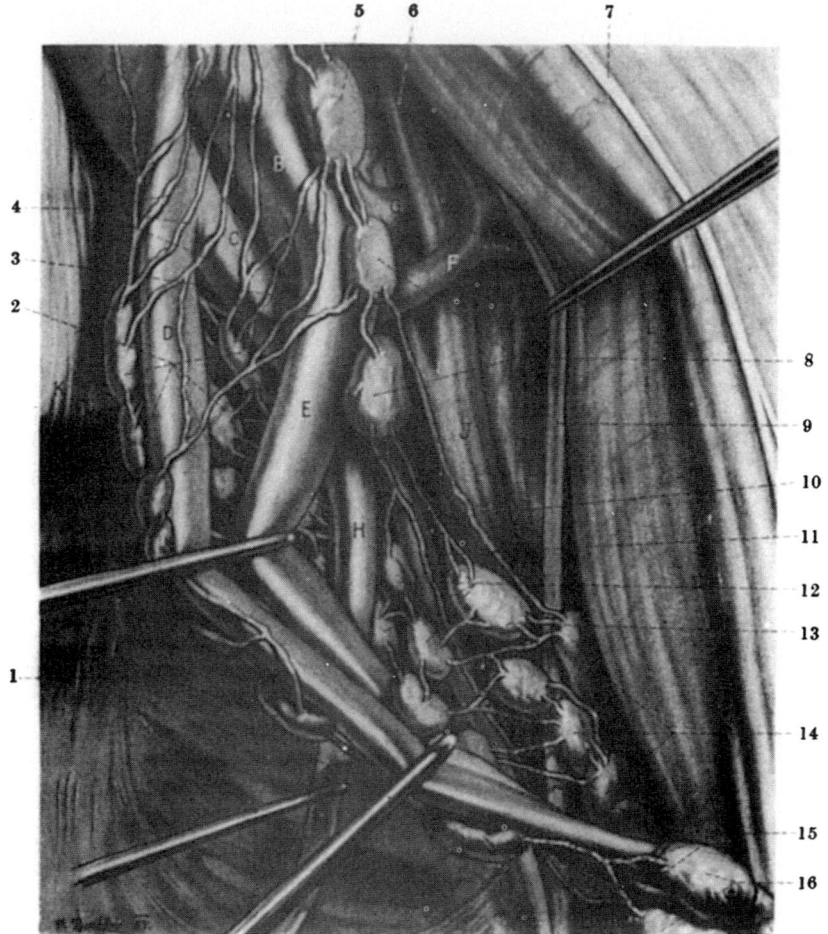

FIGURE 46.19. View into the niche between the psoas muscle and the external iliac vessels, down to the femoral ring. The blood vessels *(C,D,E,H)* were drawn medially by a hook (view of their posterior side!), and the psoas muscle **(L)** with the obturator nerve *(9)* was forced laterally. The lumbosacral trunk **(J)** appears at the bottom of the niche. The efferent channels of the uppermost interiliac lymph nodes climb over *(4)* the outer edge of the external and the common iliac arteries and reach the deep lateral common iliac lymph nodes. The deep efferent channels *(3)* of the uppermost interiliac lymph nodes; however, also open into the deep nodes located on the posterior side of the partial blood vessels, after crossing under the internal iliac artery **(C)**. The nodes *(12)* lying at the cranial edge of the obturator artery *(10)* and the nodes *(14)* of this group (interiliac lymph nodes) found lateral to the obturator nerve *(9)* send efferent vessels to the deep lateral external iliac lymph nodes *(8)*. From the great nodes on the femoral ring *(16)*, two primary lymphatic paths lead upward. One path *(15)* runs along the outer edge of the external iliac artery, where several superficial lateral external iliac lymph nodes *(1)* are located. The other, in the form of numerous lymph vessels, leads upward. **A:** Common iliac artery; **B:** common iliac vein; **C:** internal iliac artery (posterior aspect); **D:** external iliac artery (posterior aspect); **E:** external iliac vein (posterior aspect); **F:** iliolumbar artery; **G:** iliolumbar vein; **H:** lateral umbilical ligament; **J:** lumbosacral trunk; **K:** promontory; **L:** psoas muscle. **1:** Lateral external iliac; **2:** interiliac lymph nodes; **3:** deep efferent vessels; **4:** efferent vessels; **5:** deep lateral common iliac lymph node; **6:** half of fourth lumbar nerve; **7:** genitofemoral nerve; **8:** deep lateral external iliac lymph nodes; **9:** obturator nerve; **10,11:** efferent vessels; **12:** interiliac lymph nodes; **13:** obturator artery; **14:** interiliac lymph nodes; **15:** efferent vessels; **16:** femoral ring lymph nodes. (From: Reiffenstuhl G. *The lymphatics of the female genital organs.* Philadelphia: JB Lippincott, 1964, with permission.)

upper 2 to 3 cm of vagina, and paravaginal tissues, along with a thorough pelvic lymphadenectomy, constitute the traditional procedure that is used in our institution.

The major focus of the operation is the adequacy of the central dissection. The central cervical tumor must be removed with an adequate margin of uninvolved normal tissue around it. This is the most crucial point in the success of the operation and has been emphasized by many of the famous pelvic surgeons of former years, especially Parsons and Navratil. The central dissection can be facilitated by developing the pelvic spaces and using proper planes for dissection. Correct dissection along natural rather than artificial connective tissue planes and correct development of the pelvic spaces (paravesical, pararectal, vesicocervical, and rectovaginal) avoid unnecessary injury to pelvic vessels, keep blood loss to a minimum, and facilitate an adequate central dissection (Fig. 46.20). These connective tissue planes and pelvic spaces are beautifully described by Reiffenstuhl. The central dissection also is facilitated by a complete removal of the contents of the obturator fossa (except the obturator nerve), so that branches of the hypogastric artery and vein in the cardinal ligament are clearly visible and can be dissected away from their attachments to the lateral pelvic sidewall.

The importance of an adequate central dissection also was emphasized by Girardi and coworkers. By studying surgical specimens processed according to the giant-section technique of Burghardt and Pickel, parametrial lymph nodes were found in 280 (78%) of the 359 surgical specimens from radical hysterectomies. Metastatically involved parametrial nodes were found in 63 (22.5%) of these 280 specimens. The lymphatic drainage from the cervix to the pelvic lymph nodes runs through the parametrium, and deposits of tumor often are found there. An adequate central dissection must include removal of a wide margin of parametrial tissue around the central tumor and total removal of the parametria from the bladder, the rectum, and the lateral pelvic wall because positive lymph nodes can be found in the lateral as well as medial parametrium.

When a large vaginal cuff must be removed because of a bulky cervical tumor or involvement of adjacent vaginal mucosa, starting the operation from below may facilitate the central dissection. Sometimes, a bulky lesion is excised and fulgurated transvaginally. The formation of the vaginal cuff is done in a manner similar to that in the Schauta-Amreich procedure. The vaginal incision is made around the entire circumference of the vagina, mobilizing the vaginal cuff from paravaginal tissue. Further dissection into the paravesical space, vesicocervical space, and rectovaginal space from below may be easier than from above.

Superior to the midcommon iliac arteries and in the paraaortic region, lymph nodes are sampled in selected patients (usually stage IB1 and IIA). A special effort is made to remove any nodes that look or feel suspicious. The paraaortic lymph nodes then are sent for frozen section analysis. Approximately 5% to 10% of stage IB patients have paraaortic lymph node metastasis. Metastasis to the paraaortic lymph nodes is considered by many gynecologic oncologists as a contraindication to radical hysterectomy. These patients are currently being treated with extended-field radiation therapy with concurrent chemotherapy.

The pelvic component of the procedure is started by opening the paravesical and pararectal spaces bilaterally to assess resectability and exclude gross parametrial invasion. The bladder peritoneum and the posterior cul-de-sac peritoneum also may be opened to exclude gross extension of tumor in the anteroposterior plane. The pelvic lymphadenectomy can be performed prior to or after the radical hysterectomy depending on surgeon preference and anatomical considerations. A pelvic lymphadenectomy requires the bilateral removal of all visible nodal tissue with complete skeletonization of all the blood vessels from the midportion of the common iliac artery down to the point where the deep circumflex iliac vein

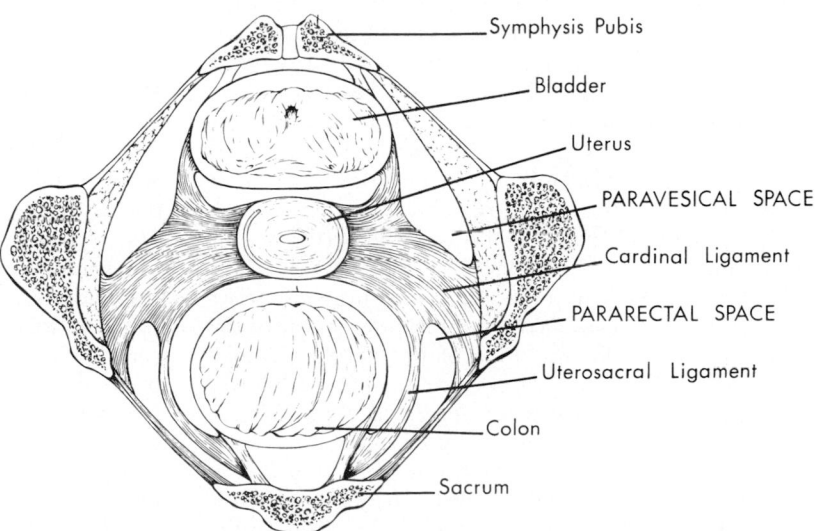

FIGURE 46.20. Cross section of pelvis showing paravesical and pararectal space. The base of the broad ligament (cardinal ligament) extends to the lateral pelvic wall and contains the major lymphatics draining the cervix.

crosses over the external iliac artery. Special attention is given to removal of lymph nodes that are located between the lower common iliac vessels and the psoas muscle (lateral common iliac nodes) at the point where the obturator nerve enters the obturator fossa through the belly of the psoas muscle. Complete removal of these nodes exposes the roots of the lumbosacral nerve plexus. The obturator nerve is dissected free from its entrance into the superior obturator fossa through the psoas muscle to its exit through the obturator foramen inferiorly. After removal of the hypogastric nodes, the uterine artery is transected at its origin from the hypogastric artery. The various vessels that compose the cardinal ligament are individually clipped or ligated at the lateral pelvic sidewall, and an attempt is made to remove as much of the cardinal ligament as possible. No attempt is made to do an en bloc removal of the nodes.

The ureters are left intact until the lymphadenectomy is completed if that order is chosen. The surgeon is cognizant of the closeness of the dissection to the central tumor throughout the remainder of the operation. The plane of dissection usually comes closest to the cervix in development of the vesicocervical space. The ureter is freed from its passage through the "tunnel," and the anterior and posterior parts of the vesicouterine ligament are ligated as close to the bladder as possible without injury. The periureteral sheath is carefully preserved, but the ureter usually is completely detached for a distance of 4 to 5 cm above its entrance into the bladder wall. The development of the posterior rectovaginal space allows identification of the posterior parametrium, including the uterosacral ligaments. This tissue is clamped and dissected away as close to the rectum as possible. The only remaining tissue to be clamped and removed is paravaginal, after which the specimen is removed by an incision in the vaginal wall at an appropriate distance from the cervix. Some authors recommend sending the distal vaginal margin of the specimen for frozen-section analysis to be certain that the inferior margin of the dissection has cleared the tumor.

Multiple approaches to performing a radical abdominal hysterectomy and bilateral pelvic lymphadenectomy have been described. The traditional transperitoneal approach has been used in our institution for many years with satisfactory results. The transverse Maylard or Cherney incisions are used by some, whereas others prefer midline incisions. Orr and Scribner have reported shorter hospital stays when a Pfannenstiel incision is used. Currie has presented and published a film using a transverse cosmetic incision with vertical fascial entry for selected patients.

After anesthesia is induced, some surgeons prefer that the patient is placed comfortably in stirrups with the buttocks brought to the edge of the "broken" table. Pneumatic compression devices are placed on both lower extremities and the knees are separated about 90 degrees. The thighs are elevated only 15 to 20 degrees relative to the abdomen. Care is taken to avoid pressure on the peroneal nerves in the legs. Proponents of this position claim several advantages. There is less strain on the

patient's lumbosacral spine when the thighs are slightly flexed. This is especially important for patients with lumbosacral back problems. It is possible to have a second assistant stand at the foot of the table between the patient's legs. His or her participation in the operation is greatly facilitated by being closer to the operative field. Finally, in this position, the urethral orifice, vaginal introitus, and anal orifice are all available for instrumentation in case this is necessary to clarify anatomy.

After the patient is positioned on the operating table, a careful rectovaginal-abdominal pelvic examination is done. This can be followed by cystoscopy or proctosigmoidoscopy if desired. It may be necessary to shave a small amount of the escutcheon, but vulvar hair is not shaved completely. The skin is prepared from the rib margin to the midthigh, with special attention given to the umbilicus, perineum, and vagina. The patient is draped, a transurethral Foley catheter is inserted into the bladder, and the operation is begun.

When operating abdominally, the exposure achieved depends on the choice of incision, the method of retracting, the placement and intensity of overhead lights, and the participation of willing and skillful assistants. Suction should be available to keep the field as dry as possible and is preferred over sponges for two reasons. First, sponges are more traumatic to delicate serosal surfaces and other tissues. Second, a determination of the amount of blood lost can be more accurate if the largest percentage has been suctioned from the operative field into a calibrated bottle and measured.

It usually is possible (and always desirable) to keep the number of clamps in the operative field to an absolute minimum. If the field is cluttered with clamps, the operator cannot see well to operate. There is an unfortunate tendency for gynecologic surgeons to use instruments that are too short. Pedicle clamps, tissue forceps, dissecting scissors, needle holders, and all other instruments must be longer when operating deep in the pelvis and when operating on obese patients. The handles of the instruments must come all the way out and above the level of the incision so that they do not interfere with the operator's vision.

SURGICAL TECHNIQUE

Preoperative Evaluation and Preparation

After the initial history and physical examination have indicated the possibility of primary treatment with radical hysterectomy and pelvic lymphadenectomy, the usual preoperative evaluation common before any extensive operation is indicated. We also recommend a chest x-ray to screen for cardiac or preliminary disease as well as the very low risk of pulmonary metastases. An intravenous pyelogram provides good visualization of the course and number of ureters. Many surgeons obtain a CT scan of the abdomen and pelvis that also shows the ureters and may provide additional information about nodal or other metastases. We believe the picture of the ureters and bladder is better on the IVP, and, for patients with clinical stage IB1 disease, enlarged nodes as CT scan would not make us cancel the surgical approach in favor of radiation therapy.

Contrary to the frequent practice of doing all possible tests on every patient, it is our practice to be selective and to do only those tests and procedures that are expected to yield useful information. It is not necessary (and indeed may be inappropriate) to subject every patient to a long list of preoperative procedures that are expensive and exhausting and have little, if any, expectation of providing useful information. Indeed, it is most unfortunate when a test or procedure yields questionable or suspicious findings that require one or more additional studies that, after delay, discomfort, and expense turn out to be negative or even perhaps nondiagnostic. Good judgment from an experienced clinician is usually the most helpful.

A young, healthy patient with a small cervical lesion requires an admission history and physical examination, chest radiograph and routine laboratory studies, and anesthesia consultation. If the patient is older, has medical complications, or has a larger or undifferentiated cervical lesion, the preoperative workup and preparation may be more involved and thorough. Larger lesions or those more likely to have metastases may be investigated by pelvic and abdominal CT scan or magnetic resonance scans, but we have rarely found those to be helpful in women with small cervical cancers. They may be most helpful when the clinician is on the fence trying to decide if surgery or radiation is the best management option—a clean, normal study may be reassuring that primary surgery is the way to go, whereas suspicious, enlarged nodes in a woman with a 4-cm cervical lesion helps make the decision to recommend radiation. Likewise, cystoscopy or proctoscopy are rarely indicated or helpful in the preoperative evaluation of early-stage cervical cancer. As much as possible should be done on an outpatient basis before admission to the hospital.

Bowel Preparation

In our institution, patients are asked to start a liquid diet 24 hours before surgery. They also are given a mechanical bowel preparation and sometimes oral antibiotics if significant peritoneal adhesions are anticipated or there is a history of previous pelvic surgery or radiation. An intestinal tube for suction is not necessary.

Evaluation at Laparotomy

As stated, the operation is initiated through a low transverse (Maylard, Cherney, Pfannenstiel) or a low midline incision. In most patients, the umbilicus identifies the location of the bifurcation of the aorta; therefore, extension of the incision about 2 to 3 cm above the umbilicus is recommended for adequate exposure of this area if a lower midline incision is used. The midline incision is protected by a moist pack beneath each arm of the self-retaining retractor to avoid excessive compression of the epigastric vessels that course beneath the rectus muscles. In case of a lengthy operative procedure, the mechanical retractors are released at periodic intervals to improve circulation through the abdominal musculature. The bladder is decompressed by an indwelling catheter throughout the procedure to facilitate exposure and maintain an accurate record of urine output.

Before initiating the pelvic procedure, the abdominal viscera and parietal peritoneum of the abdominal cavity are evaluated meticulously for possible evidence of metastatic tumor. The superior and inferior surfaces of the liver are carefully palpated, as is the region of the celiac plexus. The undersurface of the diaphragm is particularly vulnerable for metastases, especially the right hemidiaphragm, where the paraaortic lymphatics pass from the abdominal cavity into the mediastinum. The mesentery of the large and small bowel and the serosal surface of the bowel along with the omentum should be examined carefully for evidence of metastatic tumor. The kidneys are examined and the retroperitoneal space along the aorta and vena cava is palpated assiduously because these are the major sites of extrapelvic spread of cervical cancer. It is well known that 15% or more of paraaortic node metastases are occult; therefore, even the most unsuspecting node should be removed and evaluated histologically by frozen-section study for possible metastatic tumor. Therefore, it is our practice to sample any paracaval or paraaortic node that is identifiable before initiating the procedure and send it for frozen section analysis. If there is histopathologic evidence of unsuspected, metastatic tumor in a paraaortic lymph node, we generally do not proceed with a radical hysterectomy and the operation is abandoned. These patients are currently being treated with concurrent chemotherapy and extended-field radiation therapy.

Peritoneal washings for cytologic examination usually are not obtained because the yield is low and the prognostic significance is undetermined.

At this point in the procedure, any adhesions in the pelvis are lysed, and the intestines are placed in the upper abdomen and held there with packs. A suitable self-retaining retractor can be used. If Bookwalter, Turner-Warwick, or Balfour retractors are used in a lower midline incision, care must be taken to avoid compression of the femoral nerves by the lateral blades.

Evaluation of the extent of the pelvic tumor is carried out at this time by examining the course of the lymphatic drainage of the pelvis, which is carefully palpated along the pelvic vessels. When enlarged or clinically suspicious nodes are found, they are removed and immediately sent for frozen-section study while further evaluation of the pelvis is undertaken. The paravesical and pararectal spaces are important anatomic landmarks. When developed, they provide an opportunity for thorough exploration of the intervening base of the broad ligament (see Fig. 46.20). Tumor can extend into the base of the broad ligament without detection of anatomic evidence of disease before operation. This step, therefore, is a safeguard in determining the possible extension of tumor beyond the cervix and into the immediate paracervical tissues. When there is evidence of extracervical disease,

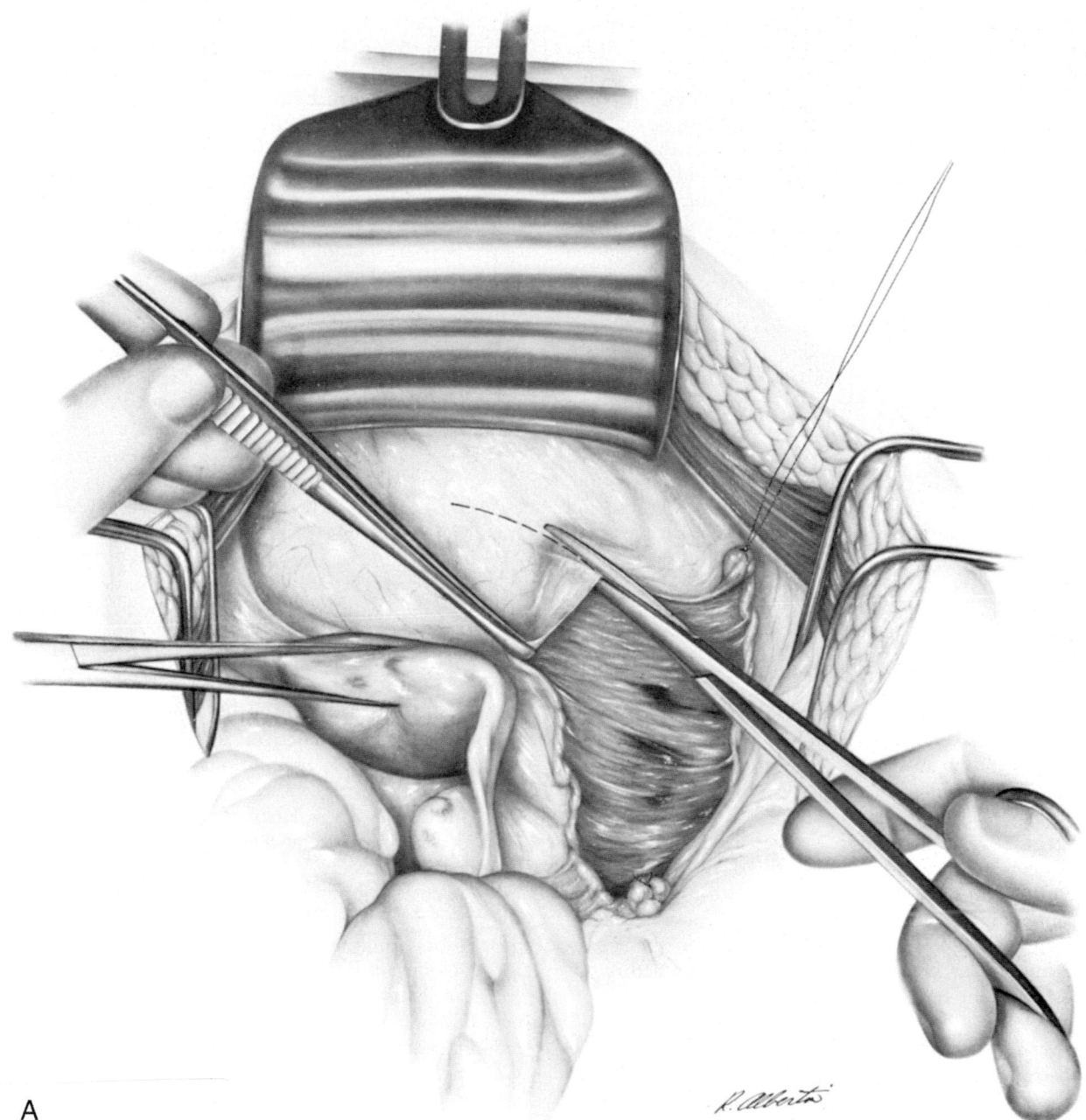

A

FIGURE 46.21. A: Opening the anterior leaf of the broad ligament after ligament, round ligament, and infundibulopelvic ligament.

we may abandon the surgical procedure unless there is clear evidence that the disease can be removed cleanly. In either case, full pelvic irradiation is indicated. Certainly, the lateral pelvic wall must be free of tumor. When the central tumor is clearly resectable, we do not hesitate to complete the operation, even if there is evidence of metastatic disease in the pelvic lymph nodes.

A decision must be made about conservation or removal of the tubes and ovaries before the pelvic planes and spaces are developed. If normal ovaries are conserved in premenopausal patients, the tubes usually also are left in. After the round ligaments are clamped, cut, and ligated, the uteroovarian ligaments and medial fal-

lopian tubes are clamped and doubly ligated. The infundibulopelvic ligaments are carefully mobilized, and the adnexal organs are packed out of the operative field with the intestines.

Development of Paravesical Space

The anterior leaf of the broad ligament forms the roof of the paravesical space and blends with the bladder peritoneum medially and the parietal peritoneum laterally. This deep fossa beneath the peritoneal covering is composed of loose connective tissue and fat. It occupies the area between the bladder and the retropubic space

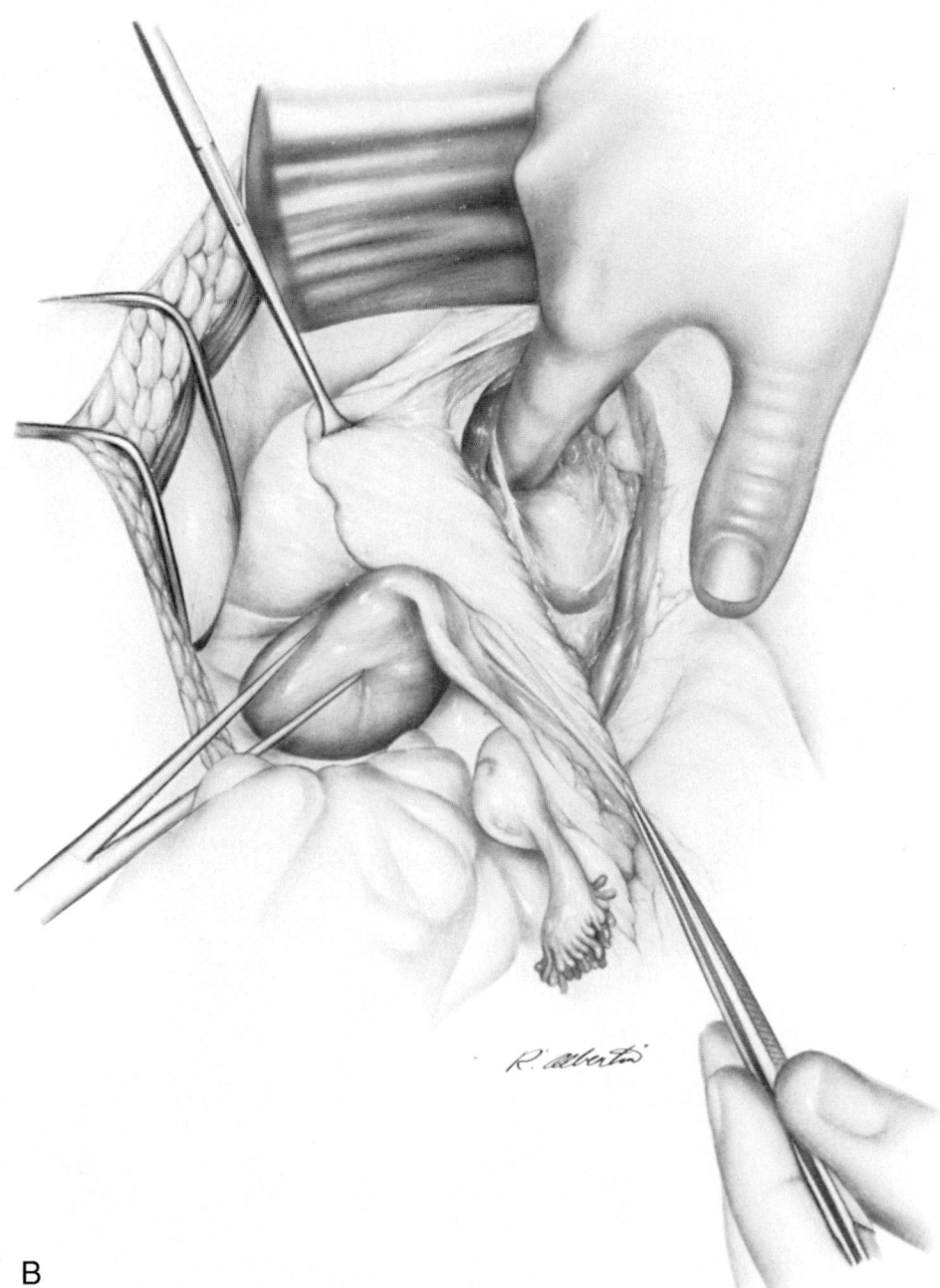

B

FIGURE 46.21. *(continued)* **B:** Development of paravesical space.

medially, with the pelvic sidewall and obturator muscle forming the lateral boundaries. The superior boundary is formed by the cardinal ligament, whereas the floor is composed of the levator ani muscle. After clamping and ligating the round ligament about midway along its course, the anterior leaf of the broad ligament is opened in an inferior direction, passing well into the pelvis before diverting the incision medially to reflect the bladder peritoneum from the lower uterine segment (Fig. 46.21A). The paravesical space can be entered without difficulty with gentle digital pressure, making certain that the dissection is initiated on the lateral side of the obliterated hypogastric artery (lateral umbilical ligament) and carried all the way down to the levator ani muscle (see Fig. 46.21B). The hypogastric artery gives off the superior vesical artery in this area and continues onto the undersurface of the rectus muscle, where it becomes the obliterated umbilical artery. There are no major blood vessels in this potential space, although occasionally an aberrant obturator vessel emerges from the inferior epigastric artery and courses along the posterior aspect of the pubic bone to the obturator space. With gentle digital dissection, the pelvic floor can be palpated and the posterior aspect of the space can be identified, including the anterior margin of the cardinal ligament.

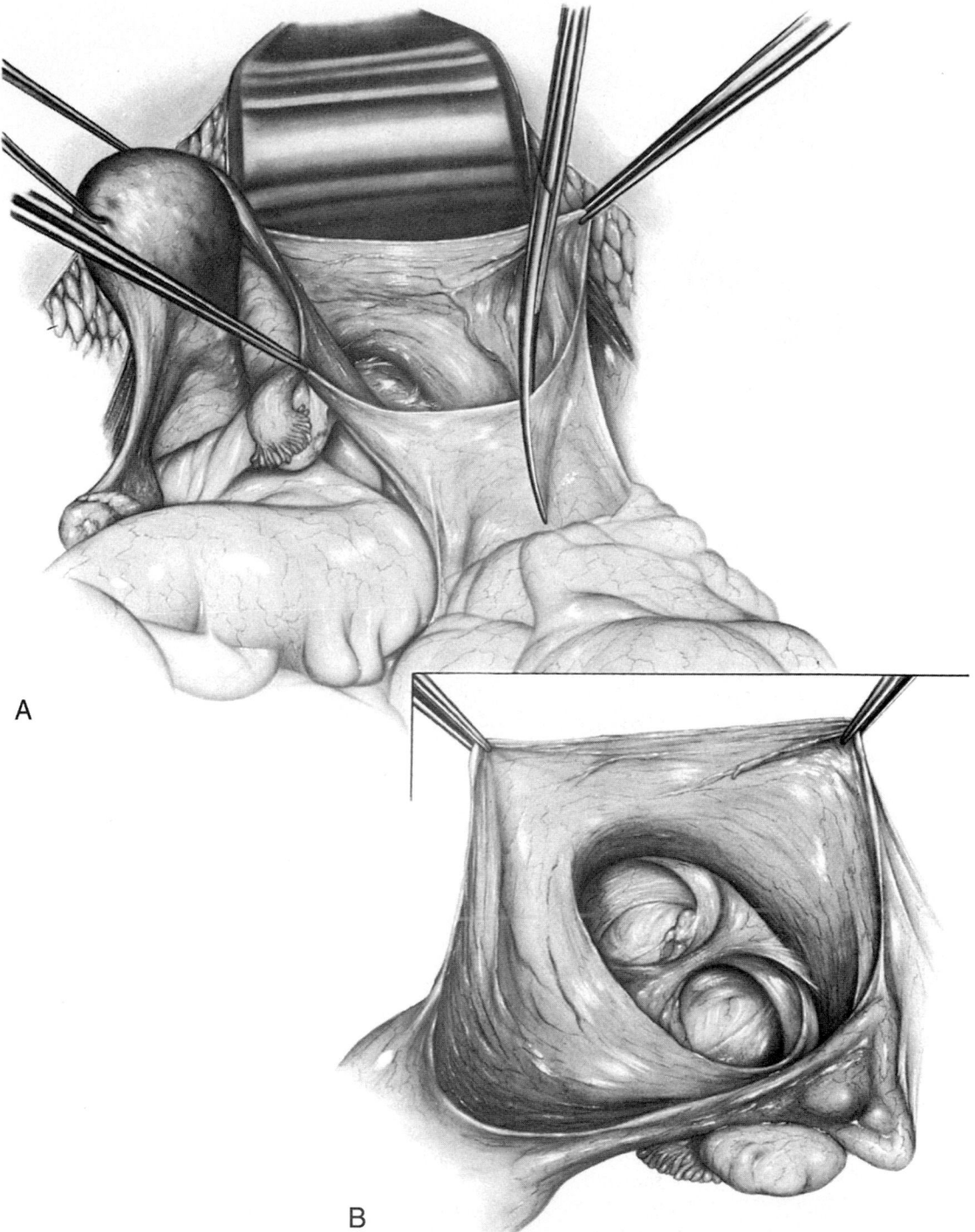

FIGURE 46.22. A: Extending the incision in the anterior leaf of the broad ligament in a cephalic direction along the lateral margin of the right infundibulopelvic ligament. **B:** Paravesical and pararectal fossae, with intervening base of broad ligament attached to pelvic floor and lateral pelvic wall.

Development of Pararectal Space

The pararectal space lies beneath the pelvic peritoneum and extends between the cardinal ligament laterally and the uterosacral ligament medially. It can be entered by extending the incision in the anterior leaf of the broad ligament in a cephalic direction along the lateral margin of the infundibulopelvic ligament (Fig. 46.22A). By retracting the infundibulopelvic ligament and displacing the uterus medially, the uterosacral ligament is placed on a stretch, and the pararectal space is widened. Dissection of this space is much more precarious than that of the paravesical space. Unskilled dissection in this area frequently is associated with troublesome bleeding. The medial border of the fossa is bounded by the uterosacral ligament and rectum, and the lateral border is formed superiorly by the piriformis muscle and inferiorly by the levator muscle. The sacrum forms the posterior margin of the space, and the ureter is attached to the peritoneum along the roof of the space before entering the medial aspect of the cardinal ligament. The hypogastric artery and vein are located in the deeper aspect of the pararectal space along the levator ani muscle. The cardinal ligament forms the caudal and lateral borders of this important area. Entry into the pararectal space must be made cautiously (see Fig. 46.22A) with medial displacement of the ureter and its attached peritoneum. A point between the ureter, which is attached to the medial leaf of peritoneum, and the hypogastric artery is selected. Blunt dissection should be used in this area, and careful handling of tissue is imperative to avoid unnecessary damage to small veins deep in this fossa. When the examining finger reaches the pelvic floor and levator ani muscle, the fossa narrows, and care must be taken to avoid damage to the lateral sacral and hemorrhoidal vessels. The dissection is carried vertically downward for a short distance. The further development of the space then changes to an inferior and caudad direction lateral to the rectum. If the development of the space is difficult, it should be delayed until a later time in the operation. When the paravesical and pararectal spaces have been dissected (Fig. 46.22B), the pelvic floor and cardinal ligament easily can be identified and palpated. In the absence of demonstrable tumor extension, the case is considered operable, and the lymph node dissection is initiated at this time.

Pelvic Lymphadenectomy

Dissection of the lymphatic tissue along the iliac vessels can begin in the region of the bifurcation of the common iliac artery and extend superiorly to the bifurcation of the aorta and inferiorly to the inguinal ligament and deep circumflex iliac vein, or it can begin at another point along the course of the iliac vessels. The opening of the posterior peritoneal leaf of the broad ligament must be extended to the area of the pelvic brim, where the ureter is easily identified as it enters the pelvis at the bifurcation of the common iliac artery. This dissection is made easier if the infundibulopelvic ligament has been ligated and divided; however, the ligament and ovarian vessels can be retracted medially if the adnexa are preserved. The ovary and tube also can be detached from the uterine corpus and gently tucked beneath the retractor above. In dissecting the presacral area in the angle of the bifurcation of the aorta, care must be taken to avoid bleeding from the middle sacral vessels as well as from the proximal part of the left external iliac vein, which courses through this retroperitoneal space. It is best to

occlude the middle sacral vessels with smaller vascular clips as they are identified, and if traumatized, the venous bleeding can be controlled with positive pressure against the sacrum and with vascular clips. The lymphatic tissue along the common iliac vessels is removed by sharp dissection with the points of the Metzenbaum scissors directed upward, while special care is taken to avoid trauma to the ureter (Fig. 46.23). The ureter is reflected medially during the dissection of the common iliac vessels and left attached to the parietal peritoneum to maintain its blood supply.

It is important to remove the loose areolar tissue and fascial sheath from the iliac vessels; however, to avoid trauma to the intima or wall of the vessels (particularly the veins), the surgeon should not attempt to skeletonize the pelvic vessels to the point of producing a pearl-white vascular tree. If there is tumor in the adventitia of the vessel wall, the patient probably will not be cured by this procedure; consequently, such compulsive surgical efforts produce far more complications than benefits. It is important to rotate the vessels medially and laterally with a vein retractor during the dissection of the common and external iliac trunks in order to obtain the posterior lymphatic chain behind the vessels along the psoas muscle. The genitofemoral nerve, which is seen lateral to the external iliac vessels, should be preserved, if possible, because damage to this peripheral nerve occasionally produces postoperative discomfort in the groin and medial aspect of the thigh.

The external iliac vessels are carefully dissected down to the point where the deep circumflex iliac vein crosses over the external iliac artery. At this point, care must be taken to avoid injury to the inferior epigastric artery and vein, which arise from the anterior and medial side of the iliac vessels and course along the anterior peritoneum onto the lower abdominal wall. The surgeon also must be cognizant of the anomalous obturator artery and vein, which can arise from the lower portion of the external iliac or inferior epigastric vessels and course over the pelvic sidewall into the obturator space. If accidentally traumatized, they should be ligated at their point of origin from the artery or vein. To avoid bleeding in the obturator space, these vessels are frequently occluded with small vascular clips as they pass through the obturator space, regardless of their origin. The clips also can be used to occlude the lymphatic channels coming into the pelvis from the leg.

The obturator space is entered by reflecting the external iliac vessels medially away from the psoas muscle and freeing the areolar tissue that lies directly between these vessels and the lateral pelvic wall (Fig. 46.24A), usually with blunt dissection. Once the space has been entered and the adjacent tissue cleaned from the external iliac vessels, the artery and vein are released and gently retracted laterally with a vein retractor, and the obturator space is clearly exposed. The lymphatic and areolar tissue are dissected from the obturator space to the region of the pelvic floor, with particular care taken to avoid trauma to the obturator nerve and vessels (Fig. 46.24B). The dissection is continued by removing all of

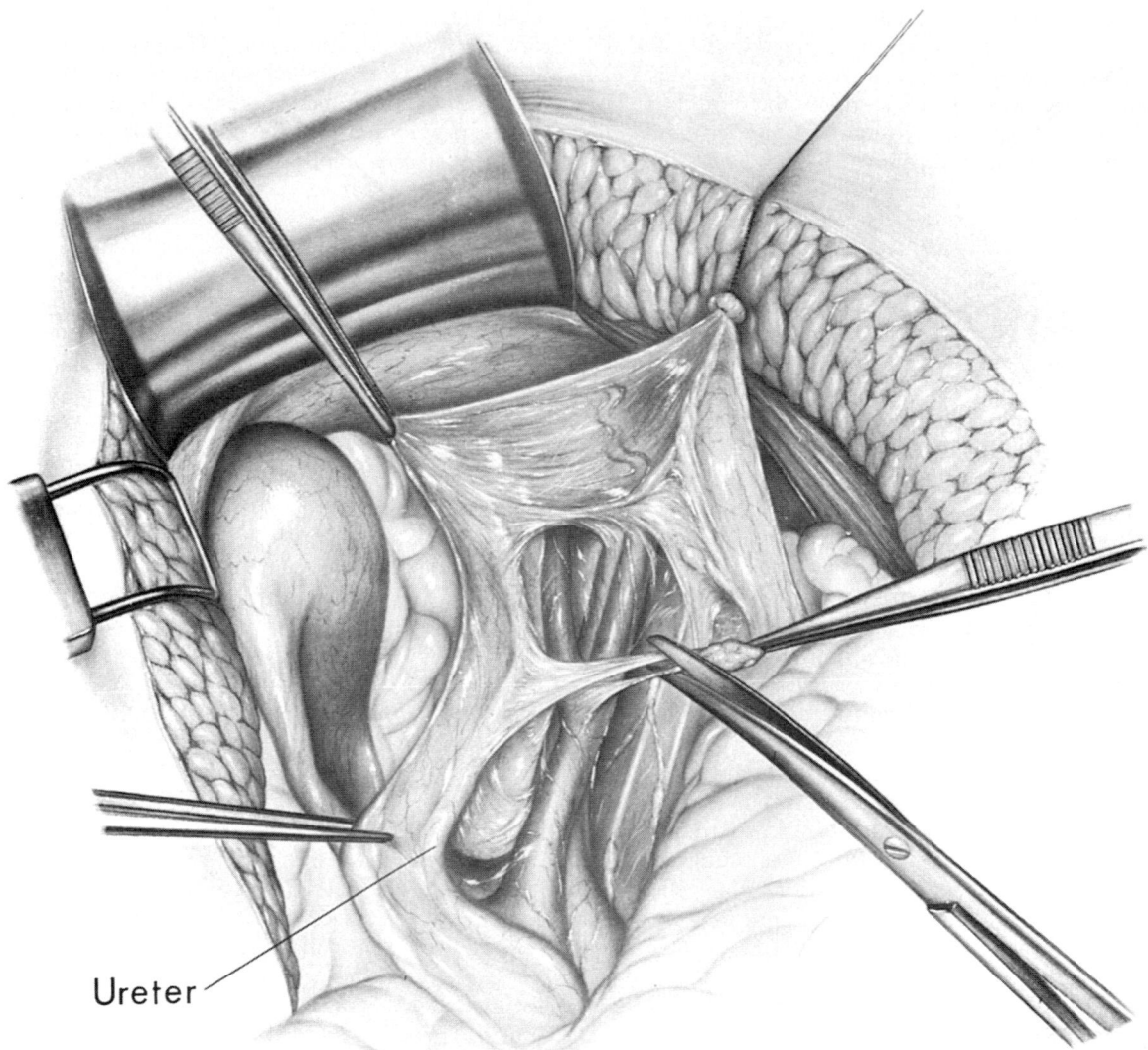

Ureter

FIGURE 46.23. Pelvic lymphadenectomy with dissection of right common iliac vessels and their branches, including the external iliac and hypogastric arteries and veins. Note attachment of ureter to parietal peritoneum. The genitofemoral nerve courses along the psoas muscle.

the nodes below the bifurcation of the iliac vessels, including the hypogastric nodes and the nodes in the obturator fossa. A lymph node may be encountered in the angle formed by the external iliac and hypogastric arteries and must be carefully dissected out, avoiding trauma to the adjacent hypogastric vein.

Retraction of the common iliac artery and vein medially exposes a group of lymph nodes that should be removed carefully. These lymph nodes are the lateral common iliac nodes. There is danger of venous bleeding in this area. When this area has been cleared, the surgeon can see the obturator nerve entering the obturator fossa through the body of the psoas muscle. The nerve roots of the lumbosacral plexus also are exposed. Particular care must be exercised in the dissection of the lateral sacral and sacroiliac plexus, just medial to the hypogastric artery and vein, near their origin. The rich arcade of small arteries and veins in-

creases the risk of bleeding in this area. When the vessels retract into the sacral foramen, control of bleeding becomes difficult.

The obturator artery can be identified as it courses along the lateral pelvic wall adjacent to the obturator nerve. The nerve, artery, and vein advance toward the obturator foramen, through which they leave the pelvis. Care must be taken to avoid trauma to all of the structures, particularly the obturator veins, which have a rich anastomotic network against the lateral pelvic wall and communicate freely with the adjacent hypogastric veins. It is best to ligate or clip the obturator vessels, but if uncontrolled bleeding occurs in this area, hemostasis is best obtained by packing the space tightly with a hot pack and providing adequate time for a fibrin clot to develop. If excessive bleeding occurs on one side of the pelvis, dissection can continue on the opposite side in the interim after pressure packing.

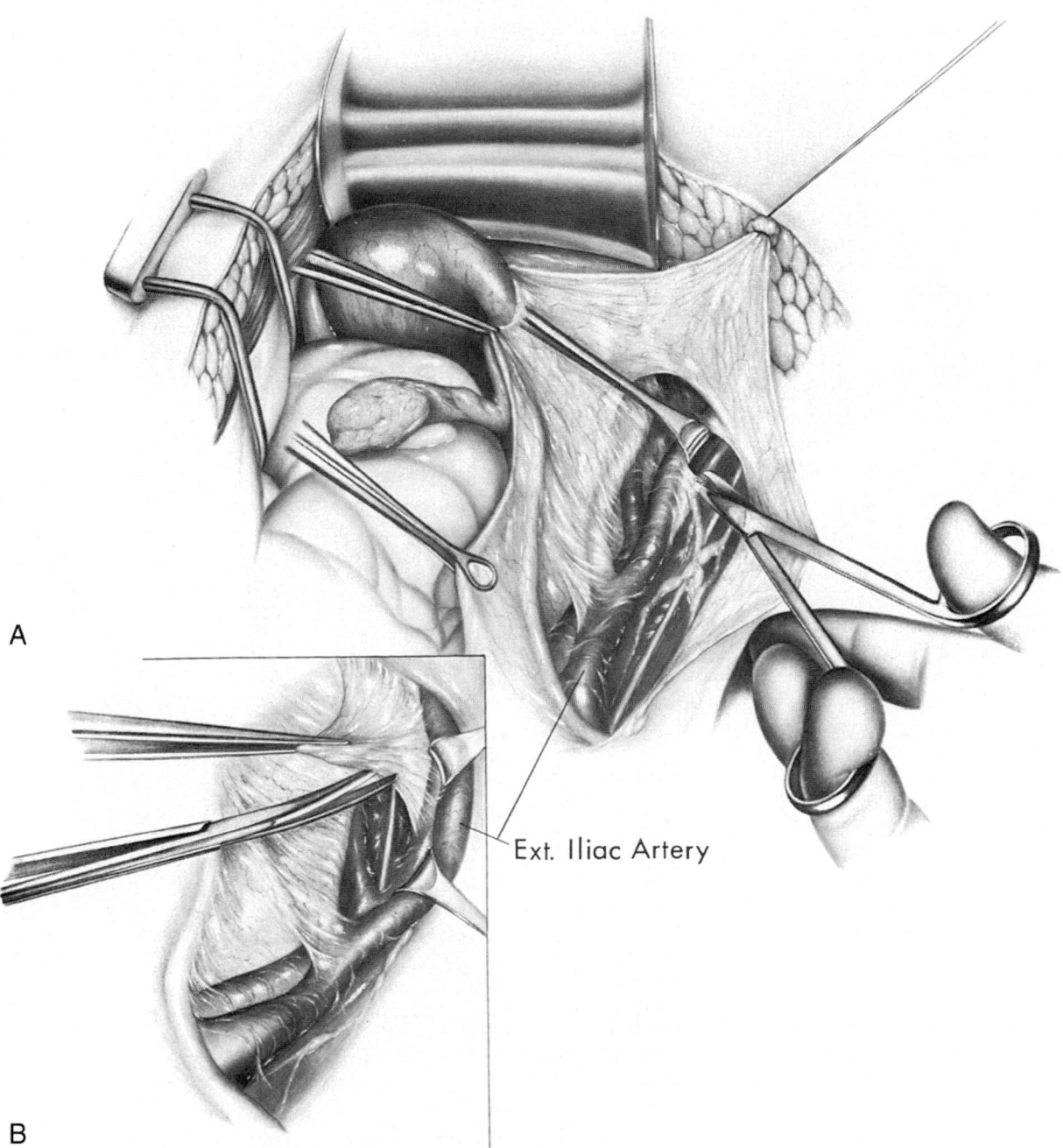

A

B

FIGURE 46.24. A: Entry into obturator space by medial reflection of external iliac vessels. **B:** Dissection of obturator fossa, demonstrating obturator nerve with areolar tissue attached superiorly to external iliac vessels.

Ext. Iliac Artery

Dissection of Hypogastric Artery, Uterine Artery, Bladder, and Ureter

The hypogastric artery is dissected with identification of the visceral branches of the anterior trunk, which include the uterine; superior, middle, and inferior vesical; vaginal; and middle hemorrhoidal arteries. The anterior division of the hypogastric artery continues along the paravesical fossa to become the obliterated lateral umbilical ligament beneath the anterior abdominal wall. If the su-

perior vesical artery is damaged, it can be ligated without serious compromise to the blood supply of the bladder. At this point, we ligate the uterine artery at its origin from the hypogastric artery. Some authors believe that a more adequate central dissection is achieved by ligating the anterior division of the hypogastric artery just distal to the point of origin of its posterior division rather than ligating the uterine artery individually. Whichever vessel is chosen, after double ligation, the distal branches traversing the cardinal ligament are removed with the spec-

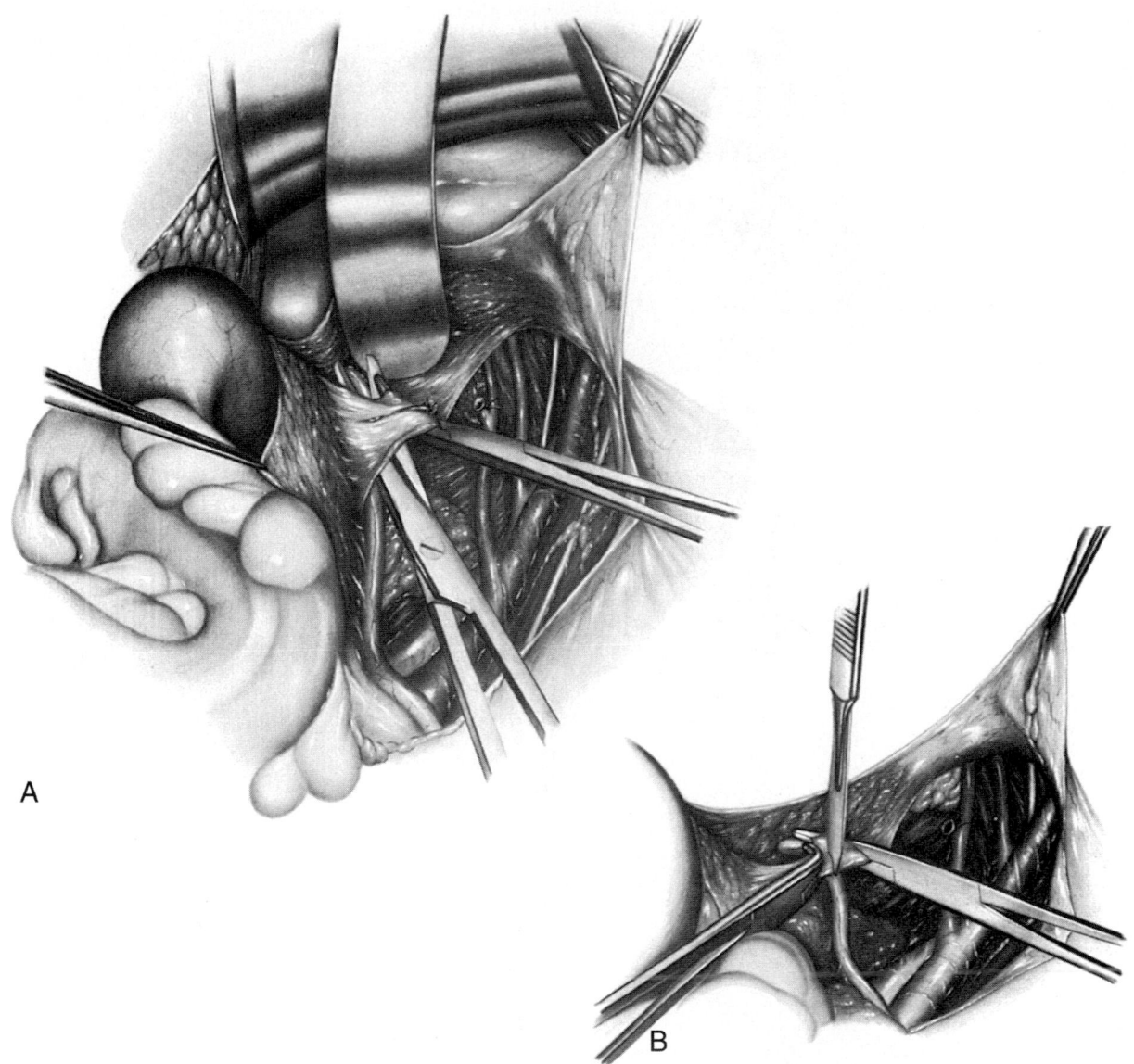

FIGURE 46.25. A: Metzenbaum scissors inserted above the ureter in the vesicouterine ligament or ureteral tunnel of the broad ligament. Note ligated uterine artery in anterior fascial sheath of tunnel. **B:** Roof of tunnel is opened between clamps.

imen. No attempt is made to remove the hypogastric vein. The other, adjacent veins should be ligated to avoid brisk bleeding in this area.

The bladder then is reflected off the lower uterine segment by incising the bladder peritoneum from its attachment to the uterus. The fascial adhesions of the base of the bladder are released from the cervix and upper vagina by electrocautery or sharp scissors dissection, and the vesicocervical space is developed inferiorly and laterally. The ureter tunnels between the anterior fascial bundles of the base of the broad ligament, commonly called the vesicouterine ligament. This fascial tunnel is carefully opened by sliding the Metzenbaum scissors or an Adson clamp, with concave surface pointed upward, along the anterior and medial surface of the ureter and by gently spreading the blades, as shown in Fig.

46.25A. The uterine artery and vein course along the fascial roof of this ligament. As shown in Fig. 46.25B, the anterior sheath of the vesicouterine ligament is opened by doubly clamping and incising this tissue. Each of the fascial bundles is suture ligated for control of bleeding, and the ureter is dissected free of its attachment to the posterior leaf of the vesicouterine ligament. Care must be taken to prevent damage to the adventitia and muscular wall of the ureter, which contain nutrient vessels from the collateral circulation. In the event that the blood supply to the ureter is compromised by thrombosis or trauma to the veins, fistula formation is a serious and frequent complication. The ureter is gently retracted with an umbilical tape or vein retractor. If forceps are used to handle the ureter, they should gently grasp only the adventitia.

Dissection of Cardinal Ligament

The base of the broad ligament (the cardinal ligament) then can be excised from its attachment at the lateral pelvic wall. The technique of clamping and ligating the vascular cardinal ligament varies, depending on the circumstances. Sometimes, part of the ligament can be in-cluded in a single clamp. Sometimes, it is better to ligate or clip individual vessels. The ligament is excised with sharp scissors dissection and ligated with 2-0 delayed ab-sorbable suture. A series of clamps are placed until the dissection is completed to the pelvic floor and along the paravaginal tissues (Fig. 46.26). If serious bleeding oc-curs in this region owing to trauma to the pelvic floor

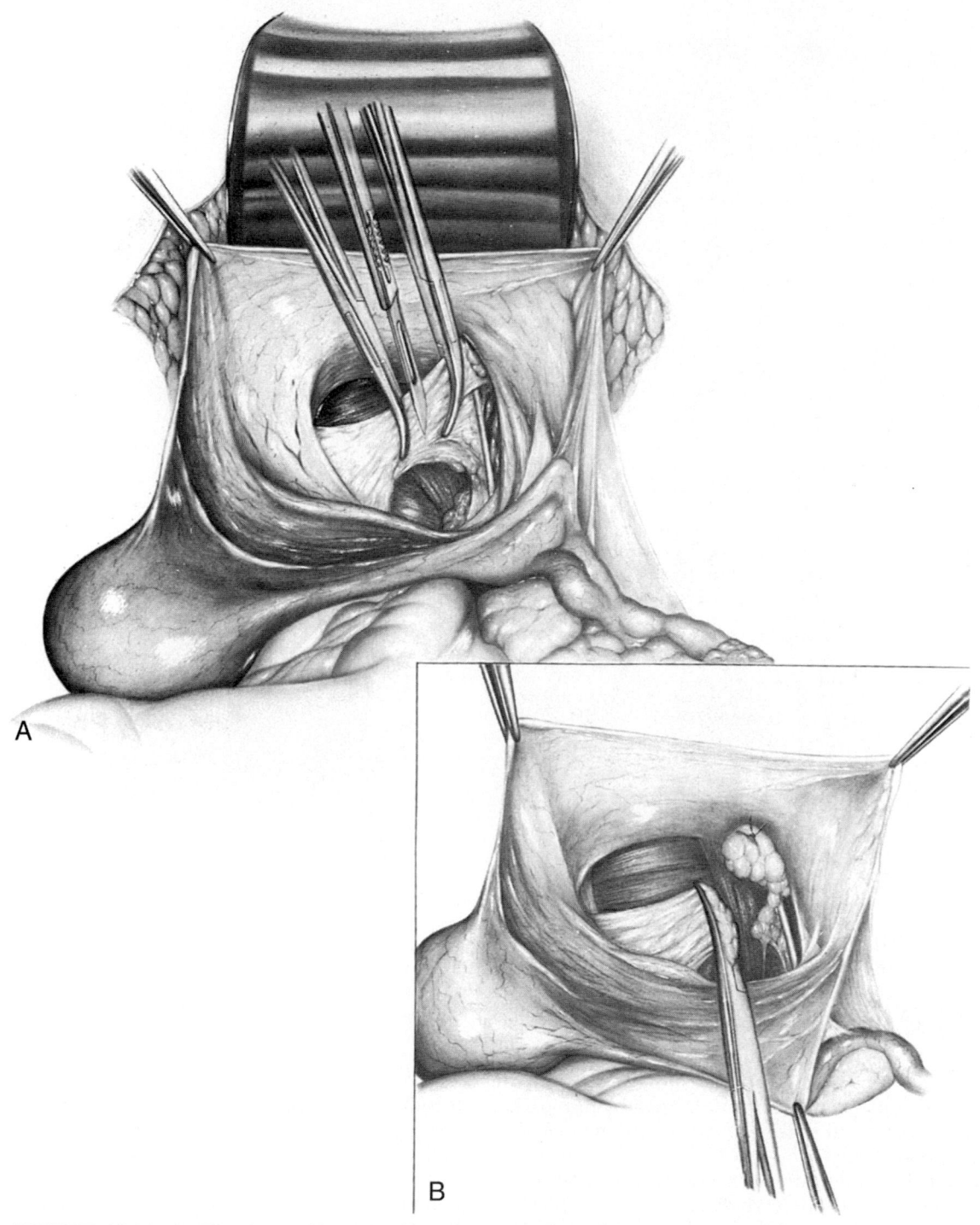

FIGURE 46.26. A: Clamping and incision of lateral portion of cardinal ligament adjacent to the lateral pelvic wall. **B:** Excised ligament showing pelvic floor and levator muscles. Dissected obturator nerve is seen in obturator space.

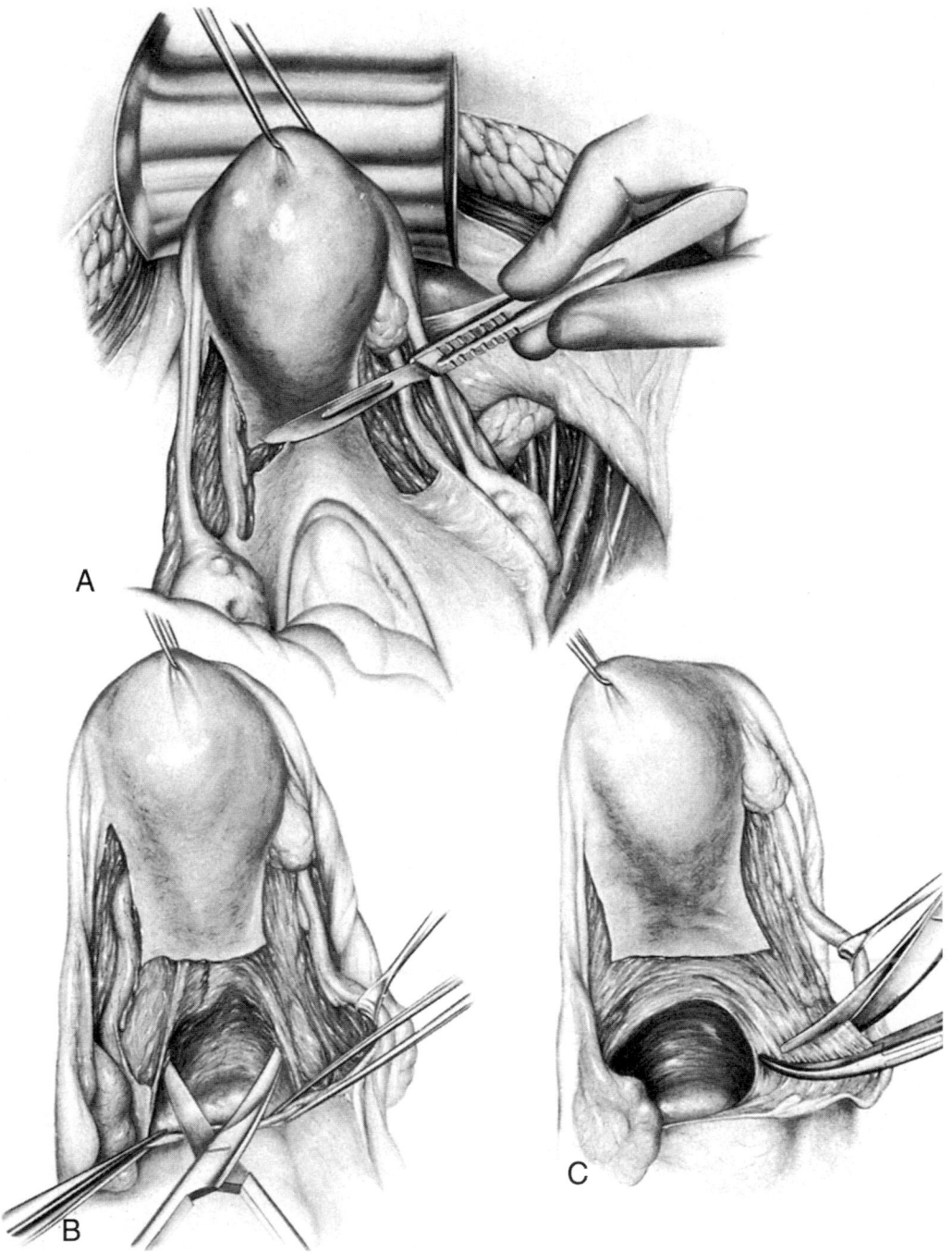

FIGURE 46.27. A: Cutting the cul-de-sac peritoneum as it reflects onto the rectum. Ureters course laterally, devoid of peritoneum. **B:** Dissection of the rectovaginal septum with development of rectal stalks (uterosacral ligaments). **C:** Clamping the uterosacral ligament. Ureter is gently retracted to avoid trauma.

veins, hemostatic control is best obtained by firm packing of the pelvis and shifting the dissection temporarily to the opposite side.

The uterosacral ligaments originate from a posterolateral position on the cervix where they are thickest and run posteriorly to the anterolateral aspect of the rectum. As the ligaments approach the rectum, they broaden so that they have a longer attachment to the rectum than to the cervix. Although these ligaments are called uterosacral, they actually originate on the cervix and terminate on the lateral rectosigmoid wall. Because of their almost in-line position relative to the rectal pillars, they are often considered the superior extensions of those structures. The uterosacral ligaments are

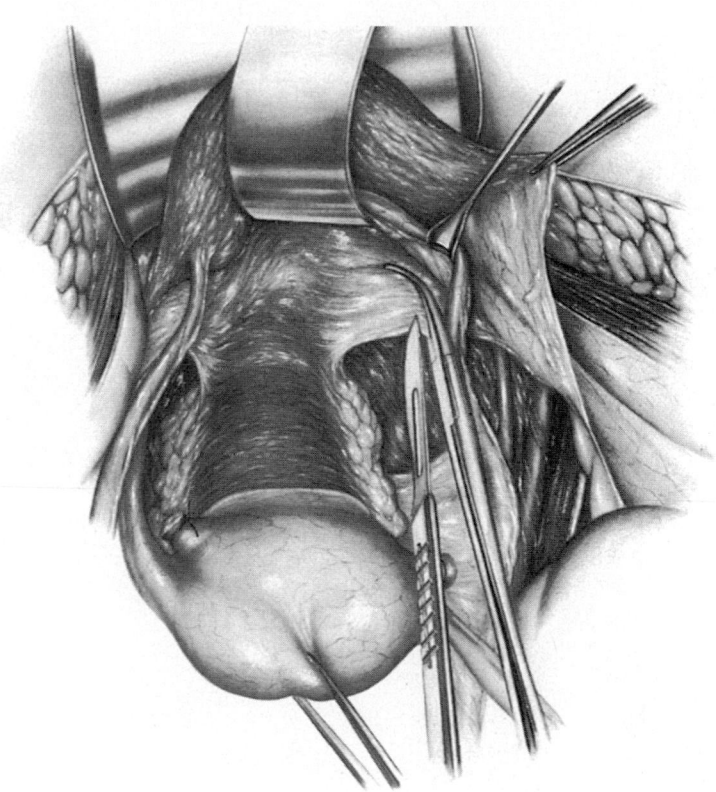

FIGURE 46.28. Dissection and retraction of bladder and terminal ureter from vagina and excision of the paravaginal fascia from the lateral pelvic wall.

stretched by sharply withdrawing the uterus forward. The peritoneal reflection of the cul-de-sac of Douglas then is incised, leaving a small segment of peritoneum attached to the anterior surface of the rectum. Care must be taken to avoid injury to the ureters, which are attached to the peritoneum just lateral to the uterosacral ligament (Fig. 46.27A). The rectovaginal space is opened by sharp scissors dissection and deepened by blunt and sharp dissection (Fig. 46.27B). This procedure separates the posterior reflection of the endopelvic fascia from the lateral wall of the rectum, which includes the more superficial uterosacral ligaments. The entire fascial bundle of the uterosacral ligament is identified, clamped as far posteriorly and close to the anterior rectal wall as possible, and cut and ligated (Fig. 46.27C). No attempt is made to divide the attachments to the sacrum. Using the endoscopic stapler to transect both the cardinal and uterosacral ligaments is advocated by some authors to significantly reduce operating time and blood loss without any adverse effects on complication or tumor recurrence rates. Continuation of this plane of dissection along the posterior endopelvic fascia frees the posterior aspect of the cervix from the pelvic floor.

It is important to dissect the paravaginal fascia to obtain all of the microlymphatic channels that communicate between the cervix and upper vagina (Fig. 46.28). The bladder then is dissected further from the upper portion of the vagina by sharp and blunt dissection, making certain to avoid trauma to the blood supply of this organ. It is important, therefore, that sharp dissection,

rather than blunt trauma, be used to free the base of the bladder from the anterior vagina to avoid forceful tearing of the blood vessels and musculature of the bladder. When the specimen is ready to be removed, a long right-angled Wertheim clamp is placed across the vagina below the cervix (not shown) to avoid gross spillage of tumor cells into the pelvis. The specimen then is removed by dividing the vagina above clamps placed on the lateral vaginal angles (Fig. 46.29).

Closure

The vaginal angles are suture ligated separately to secure hemostasis and then the remaining cuff is closed in an anterior to posterior direction using a continuous locking 2-0 delayed absorbable suture. No additional attempt is made to support the vaginal vault because all of the fascial support of the uterus and vagina has been removed. The remaining vagina, which has been shortened by about 2 to 3 cm, is well supported by its attachments to the levator ani muscles and urogenital diaphragm and mainly by the effects of postoperative fibrosis during the healing phase.

At the end of the procedure, some surgeons place suction catheters in the obturator fossae and along the lateral pelvic walls and bring them out through stab wounds in the lower abdomen. After the abdomen is closed, these catheters are connected to intermittent, low-suction drainage units. Traditionally, these drains were thought to be effective in preventing pelvic infection, and fistula and lymphocyst formation. However, re-

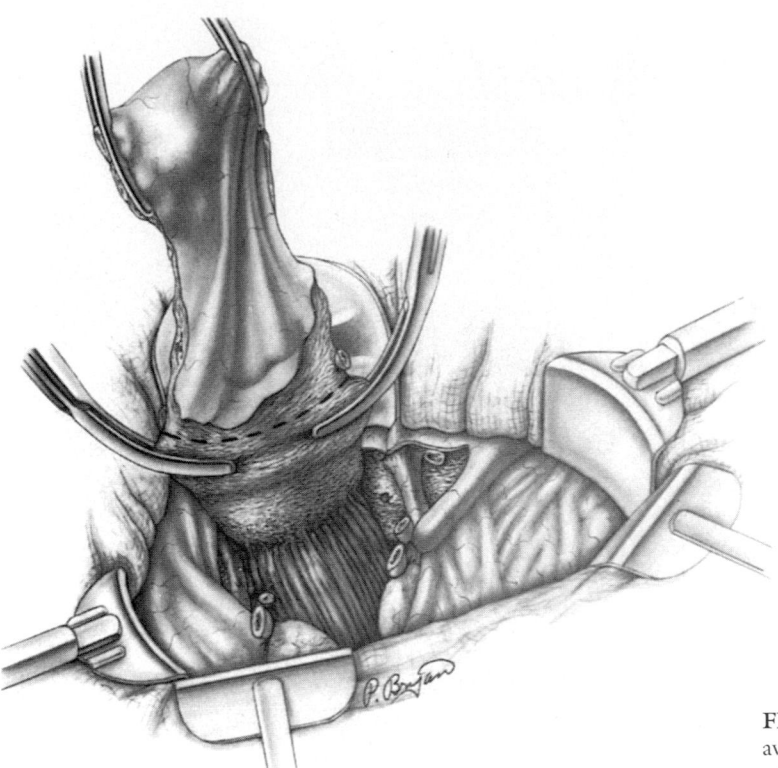

FIGURE 46.29. After clamping and ligating paravaginal tissue laterally, an incision is made in the vagina several centimeters below the cervix.

cent retrospective and prospective studies have demonstrated that the incidence of these complications is not decreased in patients who have retroperitoneal drains placed compared to those who do not. Furthermore, pelvic drains can adversely affect defense mechanisms leading to an increased risk of infection without benefit. Therefore, many gynecologic oncologists feel that the routine use of these retroperitoneal drains is unnecessary.

No attempt is made to suspend the ureters to the hypogastric artery, as suggested by Green and coworkers, or to place the terminal ureter on the inside of the peritoneal surface, as recommended by Novak. In view of the fact that the pelvis is well drained and the blood supply of the terminal ureter is preserved, we have had little difficulty with stenosis or fistula formation of the terminal ureter. Furthermore, there appears to be no benefit to reperitonizing the pelvis as described by Symmonds and Pratt.

If the tubes and ovaries are to be transposed out of the pelvis, a tunnel is dissected beneath the peritoneum laterally and superiorly toward each lateral gutter. An incision in the peritoneum is made as high as possible at the top of the tunnel. The adnexal structures are guided through the tunnel and through the incision at the top of the tunnel, making absolutely certain that the ovarian vessels in the infundibulopelvic ligament are not twisted. Permanent suture material is used to suture the tuboovarian pedicle as high as possible to the peritoneum and underlying muscle. Two large metal clips also are placed across the pedicle to identify later the location of

the ovaries with an abdominal radiograph. This ovarian suspension is done when there is a reasonable chance that a patient will need postoperative pelvic irradiation (see Figs. 46.30 and 46.31). In most operations, however, the tubes and ovaries can be left in their natural positions in the pelvis.

LAPAROSCOPICALLY ASSISTED RADICAL VAGINAL HYSTERECTOMY WITH PELVIC AND AORTIC LYMPHADENECTOMY

Over the last decade, laparoscopy has emerged as a new and exciting modality for the surgical management of cervical cancer. Currently, several surgical procedures are being performed completely by, or in combination with, the laparoscopic approach; in addition, laparoscopy has opened the door to new surgical approaches, and revived the utility of the radical vaginal hysterectomy (Schauta). It should be noted, however, that the data on laparoscopy in cervical cancer are largely from small retrospective or prospective studies, with a lack of randomized trials in humans, so far. Moreover, many initial reports combine a variety of gynecologic disease sites with a variety of surgical approaches. The four main laparoscopic procedures used in the management of primary cervical cancer include: (a) Laparoscopically as-

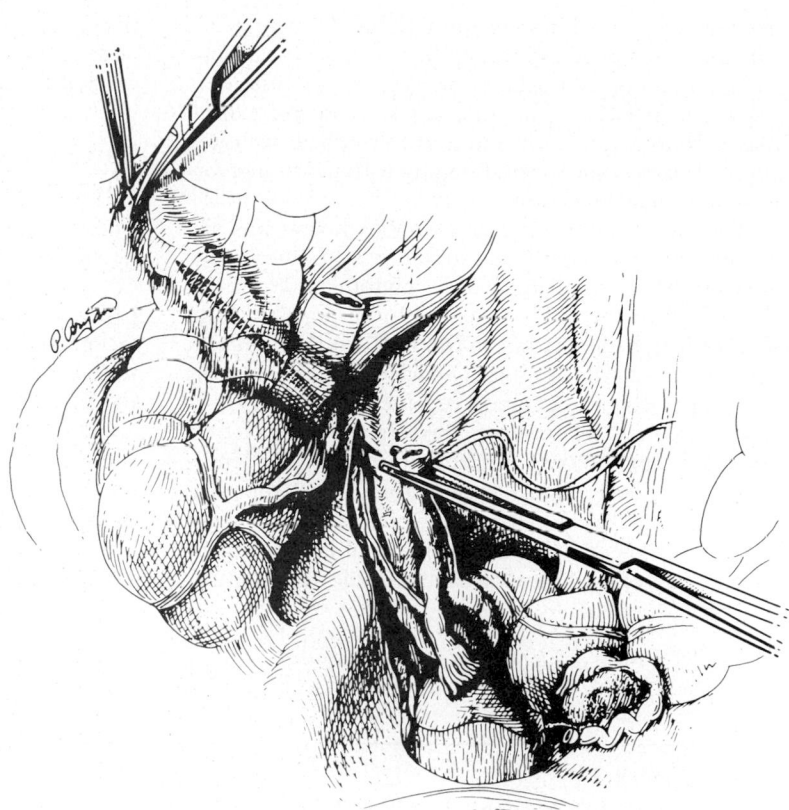

FIGURE 46.30. If the ovaries are to be suspended, a tunnel can be made under the peritoneum and the cecum on the right. The tube and ovary are guided through the tunnel to the new position in the right colic gutter above the pelvis.

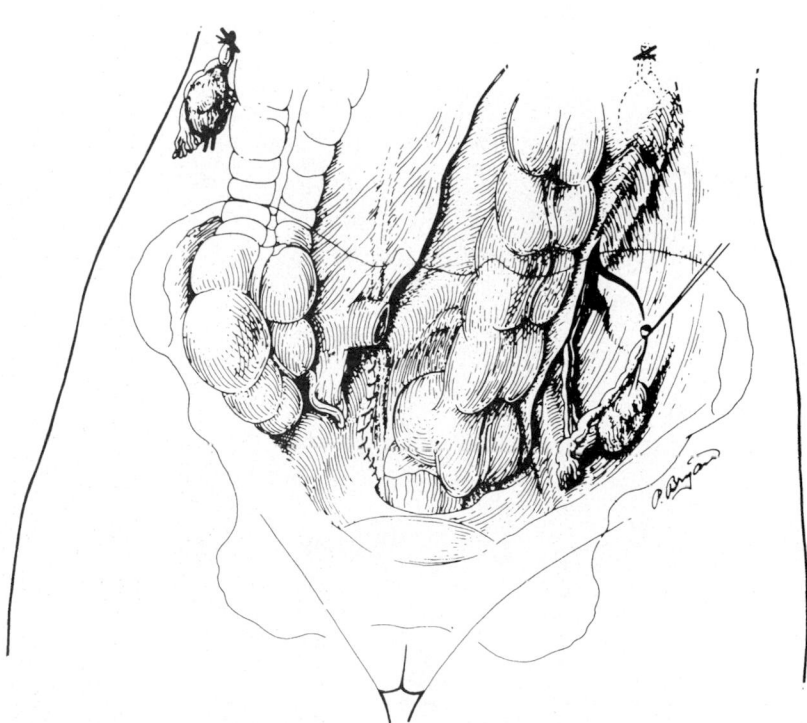

FIGURE 46.31. A similar procedure can be performed on the left. The ovarian vessels should not be twisted. Metal clips are placed on the pedicles to allow later identification with abdominal radiograph.

sisted radical vaginal hysterectomy (LARVH) with pelvic and aortic lymphadenectomy; (b) laparoscopically assisted radical vaginal trachelectomy (LARVT) with pelvic and aortic lymphadenectomy; (c) laparoscopic radical hysterectomy with pelvic and aortic lymphadenectomy; and (d) laparoscopic surgical staging with pelvic and aortic lymph node dissection.

The radical vaginal hysterectomy (Schauta) was historically associated with a reduction in postoperative mortality when compared to the abdominal Wertheim radical hysterectomy. However, with the popularization of pelvic lymphadenectomy in the 1940s as an important component in the surgical management of cervical cancer, the Schauta operation became less popular. Dargent is credited for reviving this operation through a combined laparoscopic retroperitoneal lymphadenectomy and radical vaginal hysterectomy. This approach became popular among gynecologic oncologists, and the LARVH is now available as another tool in the surgical management of early cervical cancer. Table 46.8 summa-

rizes reports on laparoscopic pelvic and aortic lymph node dissection with LARVH for stage IA2 to IIB cervical cancer.

Laparoscopically Assisted Radical Vaginal Hysterectomy Technique

The surgical technique for LARVH varies among surgeons. In general, for the treatment of early-stage cervical cancer, laparoscopy is used to perform a bilateral pelvic lymphadenectomy, transect the upper uterine attachments, and divide the uterine vessels. The procedure then is completed vaginally using a modified version of the Schauta radical vaginal hysterectomy.

However, the basic technique for LARVH may be summarized as follows: The gonadal vessels or utero-ovarian pedicles are divided (depending on desire for ovarian function) and the round ligaments are divided. The pararectal and paravesical spaces are opened (Fig. 46.32). A pelvic lymphadenectomy is performed to the

TABLE 46.8.

Summary of Laparoscopic Pelvic and Aortic Lymph Node Dissection with LARVH for Stage IA2–IIB Cervical Cancer

Author	n	LN	ORT	HD	Complications	Recurrence
Querleu, 1993	8	12.6	281	4.1	No major	2
Kadar, 1994	8	30.9	—	3	1 Reexploration	0
Garza, 1994	3	22	—	7	No major	0
Roy, 1996	25	27	270	7	1 Vascular 2 Cystotomy 1 Abscess 1 Hematoma	0
Primicero, 1996	17	14	—	—	No major	—
Schneider, 1996	33	27.2	295	11	1 Vascular 3 Cystotomy 1 Ureteral	1
Hatch, 1996	37	46	225	3	2 Cystotomy 2 UVF 11% Transfusion	—
Sardi, 1999	47	17	267	4	1 Ureteral 1 Abscess 1 Hematoma	4
Renaud, 2000	57	30	270	5	3 Cystotomy 1 Vascular 1 Abscess 1 Hematoma 4% Transfusion	2
9 Reports	235	27–28	270	4–5	4%–5% Cystotomy 1%–2% Ureteral 1%–2% Vascular 1%–2% Abscess 1%–2% Hematoma 6%–7% Transfusion	

HD, mean hospital stay in days; LARVH, laparoscopically assisted radical vaginal hysterectomy; LN, mean pelvic and aortic lymph nodes; n, number of patients; ORT, mean operating room time in minutes; UVF, ureterovaginal fistula.

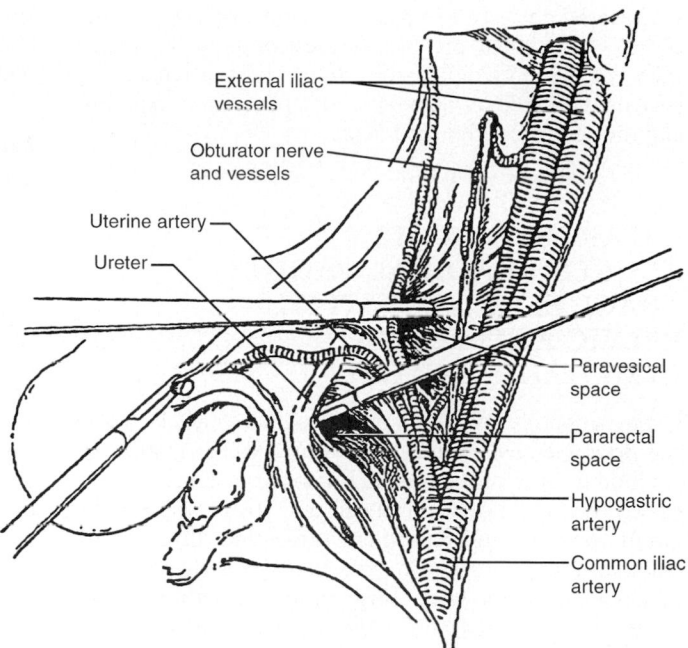

FIGURE 46.32. The paracervix as it appears after laparoscopic transperitoneal preparation. Both paravesical and pararectal spaces are developed. From Dargent D, Mathevet P. Shauta's vaginal hysterectomy combined with laparoscopic lymphadenectomy. *Bailleres Clin Obstet Gynecol* 1995;9:691, with permission.

same standards as the open approach, and the uterine artery is divided at its origin from the hypogastric artery with the endoscopic stapler or bipolar grasper (Fig. 46.33). The bladder peritoneum is incised and the ureter then is unroofed and reflected laterally with the medial stump of the uterine artery pulled medially with the uterus. The superior part of the vesicouterine ligament then is dissected and the ureter mobilized further later-

ally, then the vaginal component of the procedure is started. The vagina is incised 2 to 3 cm from the tumor margin, and a vaginal cuff is developed and approximated with Krobach (Marina Medical) or Allis clamps covering the tumor. The rectovaginal and vesicovaginal spaces are opened and the bladder pillars are dissected and divided after identifying the ureter. The posterior cul-de-sac is entered and the uterosacral ligaments are di-

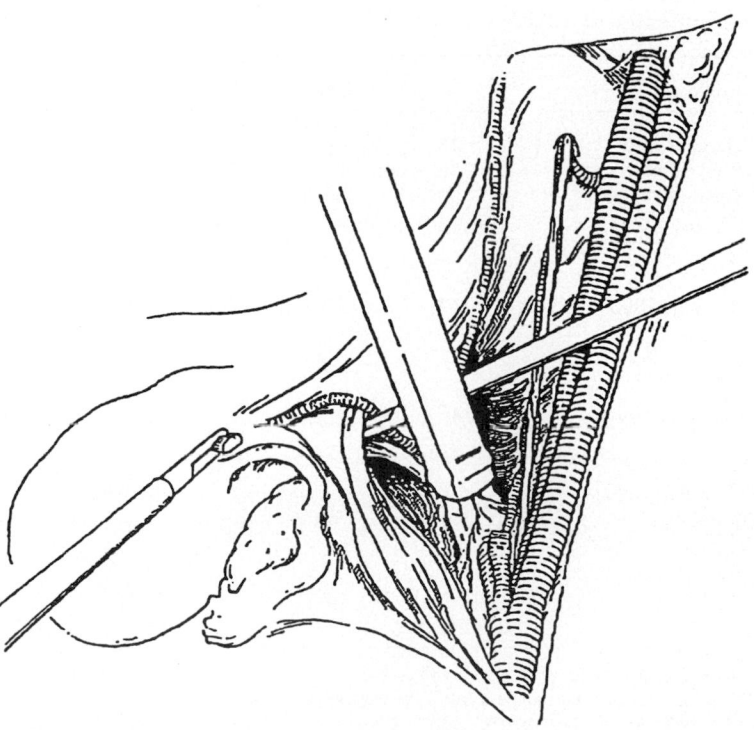

FIGURE 46.33. Division of the paracervix using the endo GIA stapler under laparoscopic guidance. (The anterior trunk of the hypogastric artery has been previously cut using the same device.) From Dargent D, Mathevet P. Shauta's vaginal hysterectomy combined with laparoscopic lymphadenectomy. *Bailleres Clin Obstet Gynecol* 1995;9:691, with permission.

vided approximately 2 to 3 cm from its insertion into the cervix. The caudal part of the vesicouterine ligament then is divided, avoiding the ureter and the remaining part of the cardinal ligaments, and parametria exposed and divided at the required level.

LAPAROSCOPICALLY ASSISTED RADICAL VAGINAL TRACHELECTOMY WITH PELVIC AND AORTIC LYMPHADENECTOMY

Laparoscopically assisted radical vaginal trachelectomy was developed by Daniel Dargent in 1987, in France. It is a modification of the LARVH with two main purposes, to: (a) treat early cervical cancer; and (b) preserve uterine morphology and reproductive function. One of the main advantages in learning the LARVH is that the experience gained allows the surgeon to offer radical trachelectomy to selected young women with early invasive cervical cancer who wish to preserve their fertility. So far, at least seven series are available in the English literature and more than 30 live births have been documented in women treated for early cervical cancer with this approach, including a case of pregnancy after radical trachelectomy and pelvic irradiation. The general eligibility criteria for radical vaginal trachelectomy include the following: desire for fertility, no clinical evidence of impaired fertility, lesion size <2 cm, FIGO stage IA2 to IB

lesions, no involvement of the upper endocervical canal by colposcopy, and negative regional lymph nodes. Table 46.9 summarizes the current literature on LARVT.

Laparoscopically Assisted Radical Vaginal Trachelectomy Technique

The technique for LARVT is described by Dargent, Plante, and Shepherd. In summary, the operation has two phases: the laparoscopic pelvic with, or without, aortic lymph node dissection, followed by the vaginal radical trachelectomy, if no malignancy is identified at laparoscopy. The laparoscopic approach is similar to the described technique for surgical staging and Schauta, and the vaginal component is summarized as follows. The cervical, vaginal, paracervical, and paravaginal tissue to be resected is outlined in Fig. 46.34. A vaginal cuff is delineated circumferentially approximately 1 to 2 cm from the cervicovaginal junction using eight straight Kocher clamps. The distance from the cervix where these clamps are placed determines the length of vaginal wall to be resected (Fig. 46.35). The vaginal mucosal ring elevated is infiltrated with 20 to 30 mL of Xylocaine 1% with adrenaline 1:200,000, or a similar solution to improve hemostasis and dissection. A circumferential mucosal incision then is made just above the Kocher clamps with care to stay superficial at the 3- and 9-o'clock positions, and the vaginal mucosa is separated. The vaginal edges created are grasped over the cervix with five or six Krobach clamps completely covering the cervix (Fig. 46.36). The vesicouterine space between the anterior as-

TABLE 46.9.
Summary of LARVT and Pelvic and Aortic Lymph Node Dissection

Author	n^a	LN	ORT	HD	Birth	Complications	Recurrence
Dargent, 1994	28	—	—	—	3	None	1 Aortic LN
Roy, 1998	30	—	285	4	4	4	1 Local
Shepherd, 1998	10	—	—	—	3	—	—
Covens, 1999	32	—	180	1	3	6% Transfusion 3% Infectious 3% Noninfectious	1 Local
Renaud, 2000	34	26	260	4	—	2 Vascular 1 Cystotomy 1 Hematoma 6% Transfusion	1 Local 1 Distant
Dargent, 2000	47	—	129	7	13	1 Cystotomy 5 Reexplored 6% Transfusion	1 Local 1 Distant
Shepherd, 2001	30	—	—	—	9	—	—
7 Reports	211	32	3–4	4	33	6% Transfusion 2%–3% Reoperation 1% Vascular 1% Cystotomy 1% Hematoma	2% Local 1%–2% Distant

^{a}Some patients may be reported more than once.

HD, mean hospital stay in days; LARVT, laparoscopically assisted radical vaginal trachelectomy; LN, mean pelvic and aortic lymph nodes; n, number of patients; ORT, mean operating room time in minutes.

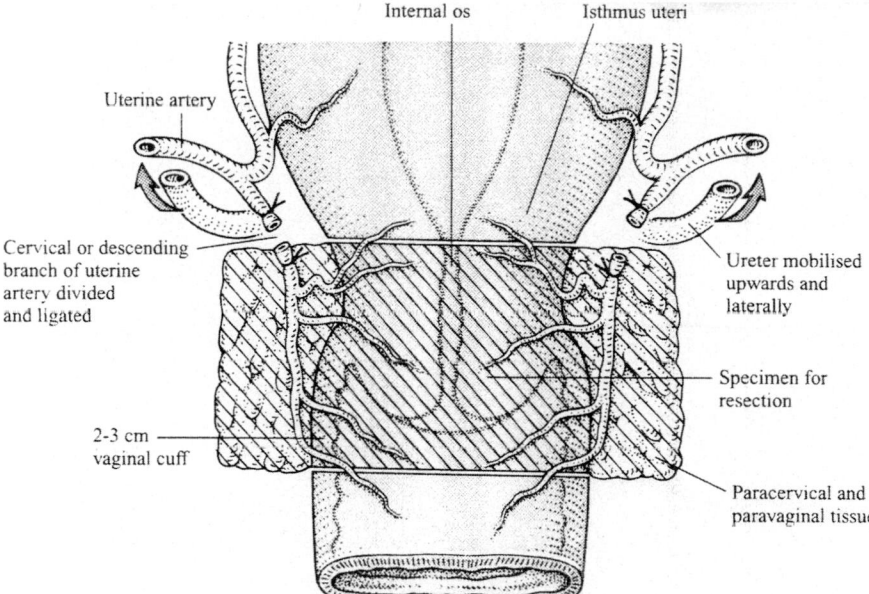

Internal os   Isthmus uteri

Uterine artery

Cervical or descending
branch of uterine
artery divided
and ligated

Ureter mobilised
upwards and
laterally

Specimen for
resection

2-3 cm
vaginal cuff

Paracervical and
paravaginal tissue

FIGURE 46.34. The cervical, vaginal, paracervical, and paravaginal tissue to be resected is outlined. Shepherd JH, Crawford RA, Oram DH. Radical trachelectomy: a way to preserve fertility in the treatment of early cervical cancer. *Br J Obstet Gynaecol* 1998;105:912, with permission.

pect of the isthmus and the posterior aspect of the bladder is developed sharply and the anterior aspect of the cervix and isthmus are palpated. The paravesical spaces then are developed by creating tension on the specimen with the Krobach clamps and countertraction with

Kocher clamps placed on the opposite vaginal mucosa at the 1- and 3-o'clock positions. Then the space is developed further, using Metzenbaum scissors bluntly and with gentle spreading. The knee of the ureter then can be identified as it turns to insert into the bladder (Fig. 46.37), and the surgeon's fingers are used to palpate and gently roll the distal ureter to hear the characteristic "click." Placement of temporary ureteral catheters pre-

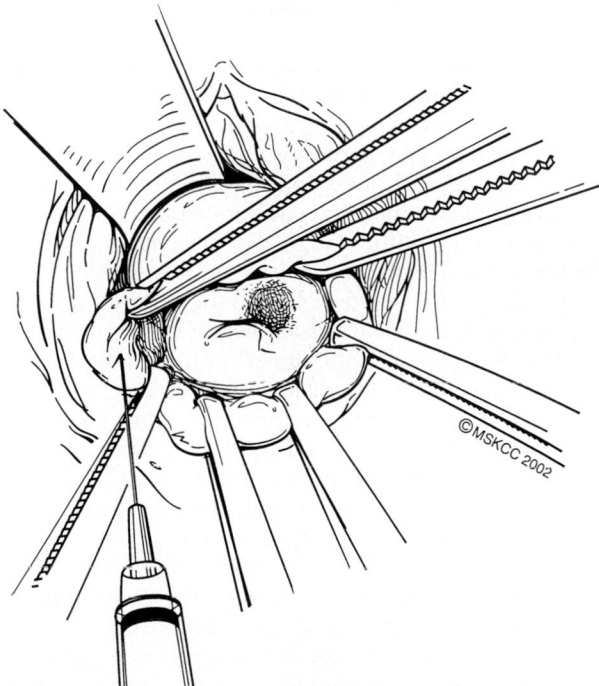

FIGURE 46.35. The vaginal-approach phase of a laparoscopically assisted radical vaginal trachelectomy. A vaginal cuff is delineated circumferentially approximately 1 to 2 cm from the cervicovaginal junction using eight straight Kocher clamps. The distance from the cervix where these clamps are placed will determine the length of vaginal wall to be resected.

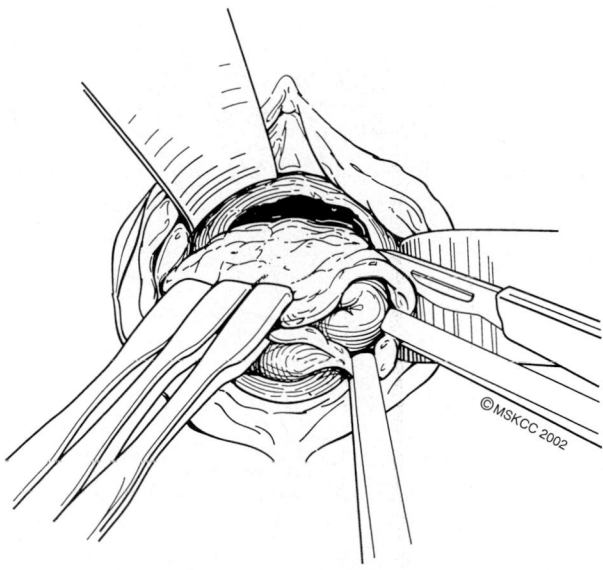

FIGURE 46.36. The vaginal-approach phase of a laparoscopically assisted radical vaginal trachelectomy. A circumferential mucosal incision is made just above the Kocher clamps, with care to stay superficial at the 3- and 9-o'clock positions, and the vaginal mucosa is separated. The vaginal edges created are grasped over the cervix with five to six Krobach clamps completely covering the cervix.

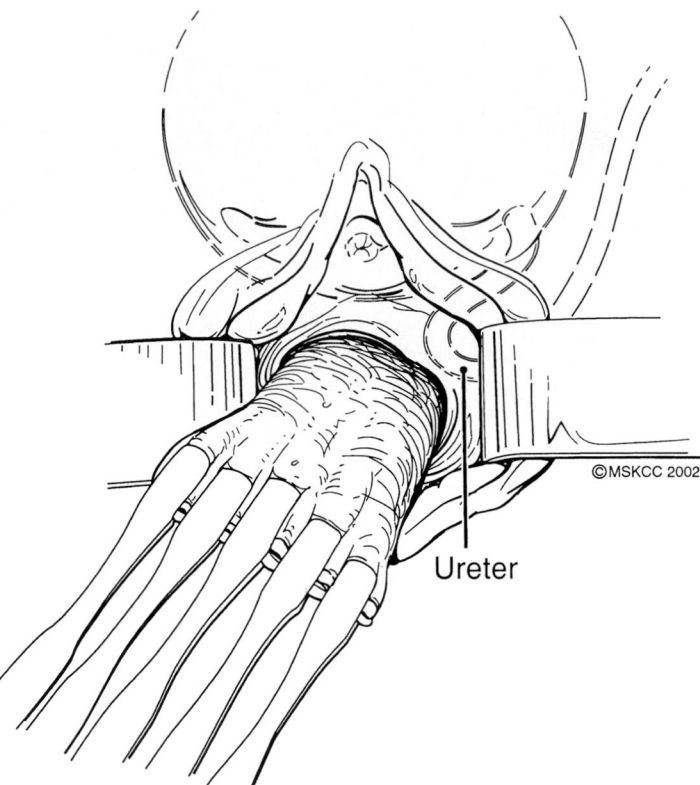

Ureter

FIGURE 46.37. The vaginal-approach phase of a laparoscopically assisted radical vaginal trachelectomy. The vesicouterine space between the anterior aspect of the isthmus and the posterior aspect of the bladder is developed sharply and the anterior aspect of the cervix and isthmus are palpated. The paravesical spaces then are developed by creating tension on the specimen with the Krobach clamps and counteraction with Kocher clamps placed on the opposite vaginal mucosa at 1 and 3 o'clock. Then, using Metzenbaum scissors bluntly and with gentle spreading the space is developed further. The knee of the ureter then can be identified as it turns to insert into the bladder.

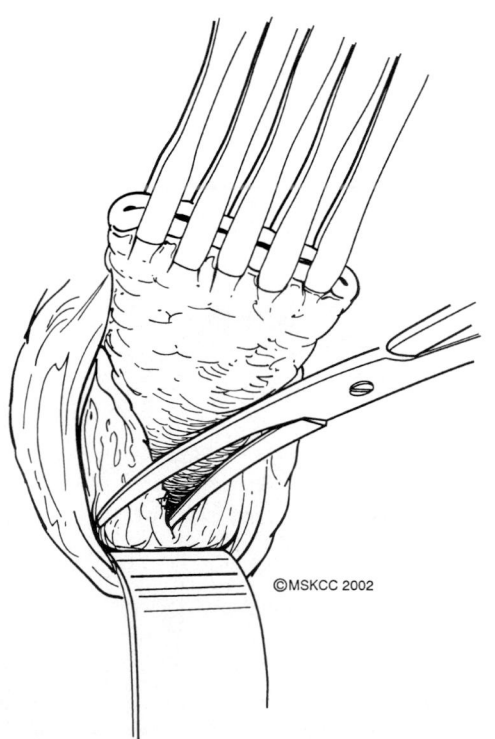

FIGURE 46.38. A posterior colpotomy then is performed in a similar fashion as for total vaginal hysterectomy, and the rectouterine/uterosacral ligaments are divided 1 to 2 cm from the cervix.

operatively may facilitate identification of the ureters and may be used at the surgeon's discretion.

The bladder pillars then are placed on tension and divided midway between the bladder base and anterior aspect of the specimen, keeping the ureter cephalad. A Babcock clamp may be placed at the knee of the ureter to facilitate identification and mobilization cephalad. A posterior colpotomy then is performed in a similar fashion to that of a total vaginal hysterectomy, and the rectouterine/uterosacral ligaments are divided 1 to 2 cm from the cervix (Fig. 46.38). With the knee of the ureter clearly identified, the necessary length of proximal parametria can be identified, clamped with a curved Heaney or Zeppelin clamp, and divided. The descending cervicovaginal branches of the uterine artery then are ligated and divided (Fig. 46.39). The specimen then is ready to be separated from the uterine corpus with a knife or diathermy (Fig. 46.40). Ideally, the resection is performed 10 mm above the tumor extent, with at least 5 to 10 mm of residual cervical canal. The resected cervical margins are evaluated by frozen section. In addition, an endocervical sample is obtained for analysis. If residual carcinoma is identified, the surgeon has to individualize the decision and feasibility of removing more cervical tissue versus proceeding with total hysterectomy. Ideally, the cervical specimen should be at least 1 cm long, with 1 cm of vaginal mucosa and 1 to 2 cm of parametrium. Hemostasis is secured, and a Foley catheter may be placed in the remaining os as a stent while the upper vagina heals around the newly formed

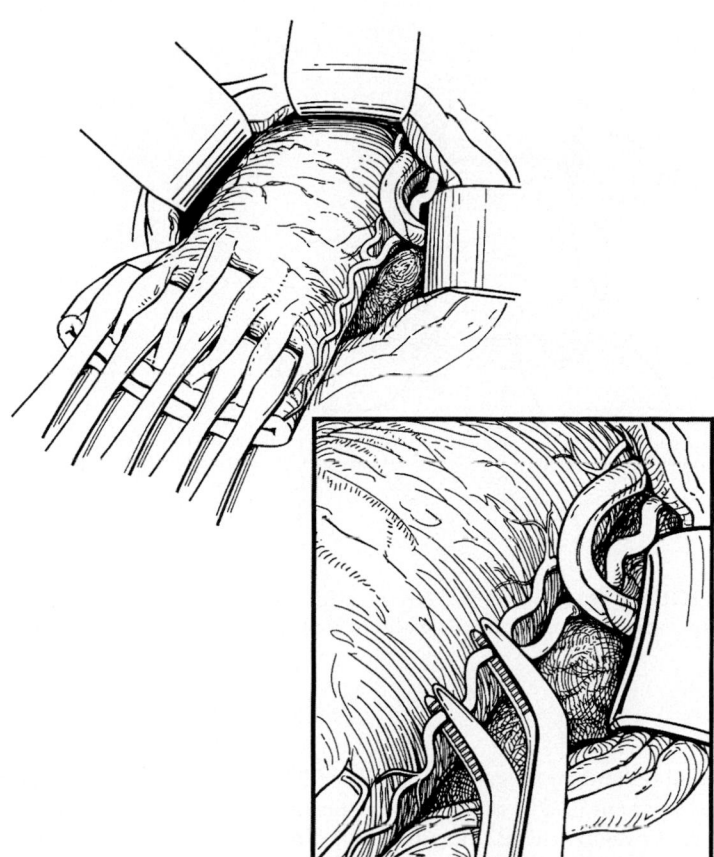

FIGURE 46.39. The vaginal-approach phase of a laparoscopically assisted radical vaginal trachelectomy. With the knee of the ureter clearly identified, the necessary length of proximal parametria can be identified, clamped with a curved Heaney or Zeppelin clamp, and divided. The descending cervicovaginal branches of the uterine artery then are ligated and divided. Figure © MSKCC, 2002.

cervix. A cervical cerclage with 0 Prolene or nylon is placed prophylactically with the knot tied posteriorly (Fig. 46.41), and the vaginal mucosa is sutured to the edges of the cervical stump with care not to occlude the os (Fig. 46.42). The patient is evaluated closely during the initial postoperative healing phase for any signs of cervical stenosis that may require dilatation.

LAPAROSCOPIC RADICAL HYSTERECTOMY WITH PELVIC AND AORTIC LYMPHADENECTOMY

Laparoscopic radical hysterectomy with pelvic and aortic lymph node dissection was first reported by Nezhat in 1992. This technically challenging procedure initially was received with caution by gynecologic oncologists who have used the abdominal radical hysterectomy as the traditional approach for decades. So far, no randomized trials are available for comparing these two surgical approaches; however, more than 150 patients have been reported with encouraging results. So far, the largest series reported has been by Spirtos et al., who describe 78 consecutive patients, all with early cervical cancer and a Quetelet body mass index <35, who underwent the procedure. In all, 94% of the procedures were completed laparoscopically with an average operative time of 205

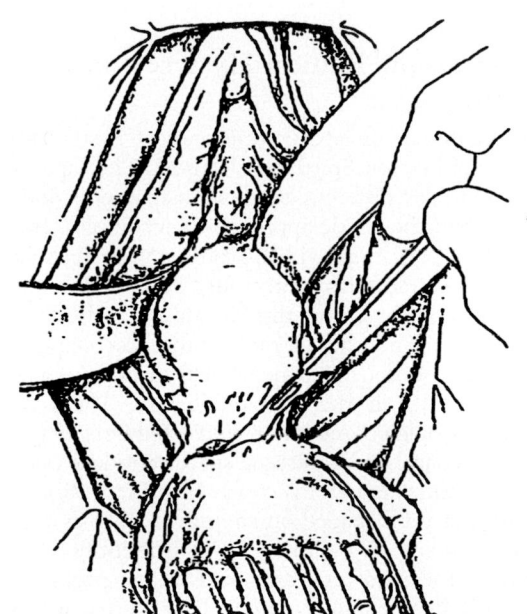

FIGURE 46.40. Dividing the uterus after preparation of the specimen. From Dargent D, Mathevet P. Shauta's vaginal hysterectomy combined with laparoscopic lymphadenectomy. *Bailleres Clin Obstet Gynecol* 1995;9:691, with permission.

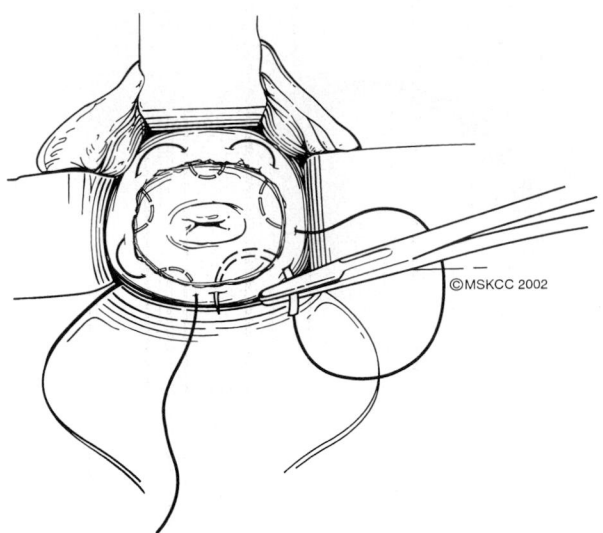

FIGURE 46.41. A cervical cerclage with no. 0 Prolene or nylon is placed prophylactically with the knot tied posteriorly.

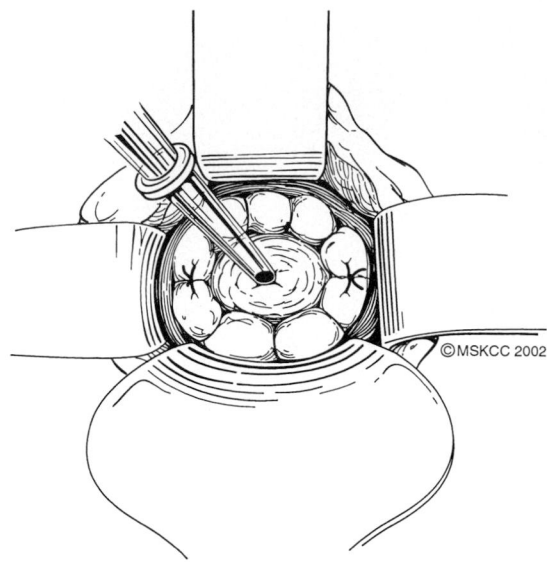

FIGURE 46.42. The vaginal-approach phase of a laparoscopically assisted radical vaginal trachelectomy. The vaginal mucosa is sutured to the edges of the cervical stump with care not to occlude the os.

minutes and an average blood loss of 225 mL, with only one patient (1.3%) requiring transfusion. There was one ureterovaginal fistula documented. The average lymph node count was 34, with 11.5% of patients having positive lymph nodes. Three patients (3.8%) had close or positive surgical margins, and 5.1% recurred with a minimum of 3-year follow-up. Table 46.10 summarizes reports on laparoscopic radical hysterectomy with pelvic and aortic lymphadenectomy.

Laparoscopic Radical Hysterectomy Technique

The technique of laparoscopic radical hysterectomy is well described by Spirtos and Chen. The laparoscopic approach uses different surgical instruments and techniques than the classic approach to accomplish the same procedure performed via laparotomy. The technique of laparoscopic radical hysterectomy described in this section relies on the use of the 10-mm argon beam coagulator (ABC) and the 12-mm endoscopic stapler. Four trocars are needed with the camera in the umbilical site and the ABC in the suprapubic site. The retroperitoneum is opened and the round ligaments coagulated. The paravesical and pararectal spaces are developed with the ABC and the ureter is clearly identified. Resection of the adnexa are managed on an individual basis as per the open approach. The uterine artery is identified after developing the pararectal and paravesical spaces and the umbilical ligament is isolated. The uterine artery and vein are stapled with the endoscopic stapler in one or two separate applications. The bladder flap then is developed. The posterior cul-de-sac peritoneum is incised and the rectouterine ligaments exposed. The ureter is then

unroofed from the parametria by placing medial traction on the stapled uterine artery stump and the bladder is dissected further inferiorly. The uterosacral/rectouterine ligaments are stapled or coagulated and the ureter is retracted laterally to resect the desired length of parametria with the stapler. Anterior colpotomy is performed at the desired vaginal length. A vaginal probe facilitates stretching the vagina for easier incision. The remaining parametria and paracolpos are resected with the ABC and staplers. The specimen is removed vaginally with a single tooth tenaculum, and the vaginal cuff is closed laparoscopically with endoscopic sutures or the endostich. The placement of ureteral catheters or stents to facilitate ureteric manipulation is optional. The pelvic and aortic lymphadenectomy is performed as described in the preceding. Pelvic drains usually are not necessary, and a suprapubic catheter is optional.

LAPAROSCOPIC SURGICAL STAGING

Currently available clinical staging methods and imaging studies are not 100% accurate in the detection of pelvic and aortic lymph node metastasis from cervical cancer, and pathologic evaluation of retroperitoneal lymph nodes remains the gold standard for establishing metastasis. In addition, identifying retroperitoneal nodal metastasis may alter the overall therapeutic approach and impact the patient's prognosis.

Laparoscopic surgical staging with pelvic and aortic lymph node dissection for cervical cancer was initially reported by Querleu, in France. Since this initial report, many investigators have adopted the laparoscopic pre-

TABLE 46.10.
Summary of Reports on Laparoscopic Radical Hysterectomy with Pelvic and Aortic Lymphadenectomy

Author	n^a	LN	ORT	HD	Complications	Recurrence
Nezhat, 1992–1993	7	28	315	2.1	None	None
Sedlacek, 1994–1995	14	16	420	5.5	1 VVF, 1 Ureteral injury	—
Ting, 1994	4	8	5–8	—	—	—
Osterzenski, 1996	6	—	280	2–6	1 Hydronephrosis	—
Spirtos, 1996	10	24.8	253	3.2	None	—
Kim, 1998	18	22	363	—	None	—
Hsieh, 1998	8	—	—	6.5	None	1 Distant
Spirtos, 2000	78	34	205	—	1.3% Transfusion, 3 Cystotomies, 1 UVF	4
8 Reports	146	28–29	300	4	3%–4% Conversion 2%–3% Cystotomy 2%–3% Ureteral injury 1%–2% Transfusion	3%–4%

^{a} Some patients may be reported more than once.

HD, mean hospital stay in days; LN, mean pelvic and aortic lymph nodes; *n,* number of patients; ORT, mean operating room time in minutes; UVF, ureterovaginal fistula; VVF, vesicovaginal fistula.

treatment surgical approach and continue to modify the technical details of the procedure. It is well established at this point that transperitoneal or extraperitoneal laparoscopic pelvic and aortic lymph node dissection for cervical cancer, in experienced hands, is feasible, yields similar results as the open approach, and is associated with low morbidity. Furthermore, this approach may provide valuable information that may not be available using clinical staging techniques. Computed tomography was able to detect retroperitoneal nodal metastasis in only 17% to 57% of cervical cancer patients staged laparoscopically. Table 46.11 summarizes selected reports on laparoscopic pelvic and aortic lymph node dissection in the management of stage I to IV cervical cancer.

Surgical Technique

The technique of laparoscopic surgical staging continues to evolve as experience with this minimally invasive approach increases. There are two main approaches: the transperitoneal approach (commonly used in the United States), and the extraperitoneal approach (popularized by Querleu and Dargent from France). For the transperitoneal approach, four laparoscopic trocars usually are needed (Fig. 46.43): 10-mm trocars in the umbilical and suprapubic regions, and 5-mm trocars just medial to the iliac crest on each side. For the aortic nodal dissection, the laparoscope is placed in the suprapubic region and the monitors are moved cephalad. For the pelvic lymphadenectomy, the laparoscope is placed in the umbilical region and the monitors are placed caudal. A variety of endoscopic tools may be used with similar results. The selection usually is based on the surgeon's preference and experience. Both monopolar and bipolar currents

are available and a wide variety of endoscopic dissecting instruments, clip appliers, and specimen retrieval devices are available. The 10-mm argon beam coagulator (ABC, Conmed, Utica, NY) is ideal in this setting. It works both as a dissector and a coagulator. A retroperitoneal nodal dissection may be satisfactorily completed in the majority of cases with the aid of a tissue grasper and an endoscopic clip applier. The right aortic nodal tissue is approached via a retroperitoneal incision over the right common iliac artery. The right ureter and gonadal vessels are identified, and the nodal tissue over the inferior vena cava is removed. The left aortic nodal tissue may be approached via the same incision. The inferior mesenteric artery, left ureter, and left gonadal vessels are identified, and the nodal tissue over the left aortic region is removed.

Dissection above the inferior mesenteric artery to include the infrarenal nodal regions may be accomplished through a similar approach, and a left-sided laparoscopic suprarenal retrocrural paraaortic lymphadenectomy in advanced cervical cancer has been described.

PATHOLOGIC EXAMINATION OF THE OPERATIVE SPECIMEN

Considerable useful information about the extent of the disease can be obtained by a careful pathologic examination of the operative specimen. This is helpful in determining prognosis but is also absolutely essential to the identification of patients at greater risk for persistent disease, so that additional therapy and close surveillance can be provided. Even though the operator may be fatigued at the end of the operation, he or she should

TABLE 46.11.

Summary of Pretreatment Laparoscopic Pelvic and Aortic Lymph Node Dissection in the Management of Stage I to IV Cervical Cancer

Author	n	Stage	PLN (% +)	PAN (% +)	ORT	HD	Complications
Querleu, 1991	39	IB–IIB	8.7 (12.8%)	—	90	1	3 Minor
Childers, 1993	18	IB–IVA	31.4 (both) (33.3%)	(6.2%)	75–175	1.5	Not significant
Fowler, 1993	12	IB	23.5 (16.7%)	6.5 (0%)	373 With laparotomy	7.4 With laparotomy	2 Minor
Su, 1995	38	—	15	—	77	—	1 Vascular 1 Ureteral
Recio, 1996	12	IB2	18 (25%)	7 (0%)	176	1	Not significant
Chu, 1997	67	IA2–IIIB	26.7 (12.8%)	8 (35.7%)	93	2	1 Vascular
Possover, 1998	26	IIB–IIIB	15.3 (11.5%)	6.8 (7.7%)	162	3.2	1 Vascular
Vidaurreta, 1999	84	IB2–IV	18.5 (45.2%)	—	108	1–2	1 Vascular
Schlaerth, 1999	40	IA–IIA	32.1	12.1	—	—	—
Querleu, 2000	53	≥IB2	With common iliac	20.7 (32%)	126	1–2	1 Ureteral
Altgassen, 2000	108	IA1–IVB	21–24.3	5.1–10.6	Aortic: 35–73 Pelvic: 61–70	—	3 Vascular
11 Reports	497	I–IV	9–32 (24%–25%)	6–21 (19%–20%)	120	1–2	1%–2% Vascular 0.4% Ureteral

HD, mean hospital stay in days; *n*, number of patients; ORT, mean operating room time in minutes; PAN, mean aortic lymph nodes; PLN, mean pelvic lymph nodes.

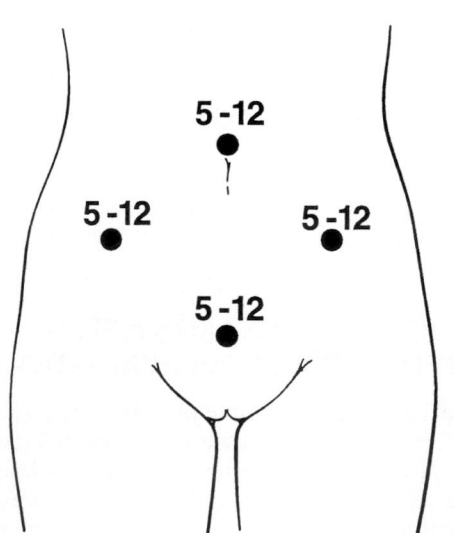

FIGURE 46.43. The transperitoneal minimally invasive approach for laparoscopic surgical staging. Four laparoscopic trocars usually are needed. Figure © MSKCC, 2002.

consider accompanying the specimen to the pathology laboratory, where it can be examined with the pathologist before it is placed in fixative and sectioned. The gynecologic surgeon then can point to worrisome parts of the specimen; such information assists the pathologist in taking sections. Critical margins of dissection can be pointed out and stained with India ink, so that they can be seen on microscopic slides. The primary cervical tumor should be measured as accurately as possible, so that at least an estimate of its size and volume can be recorded. Numerous microscopic sections of the cervix with adjacent vaginal cuff; lower uterine segment; and paravaginal, paracervical, and parametrial tissue should be examined to show the cell type, degree of differentiation, depth of stromal invasion, and presence or absence of invasion of lymphatic and vascular spaces. It is important to know not only the depth of invasion but also the thickness of the uninvolved fibromuscular stroma of the cervix, as pointed out by Kishi and coworkers. These authors found that the nodal metastasis and 5-year cancer death rates were 7% and 8%, respectively, in patients with uninvolved fibromuscular stroma thickness >3 mm, and 37% and 26%, respectively, in patients with the thickness <3 mm. Furthermore, the GOG has demonstrated that the percentage of invasion of tumor into the cervical stroma is an independent prognostic factor and is used to help determine the need for postoperative adjuvant treatment.

Unfortunately, the exquisite giant-section technique of pathologic examination used by Burghardt and coworkers is not available in any US pathology laboratory. These authors measured ratio of tumor size to the size of the cervix. The incidence of lymph node involvement increased with tumor size, reaching a maximum of 68.3% in the group with a ratio from 70% to 80% of cervical anatomic involvement. Surprisingly, direct spread into the parametrium seldom was found, even when large tumors were found to occupy the entire cervix. This finding is contrary to that of Bleker and coworkers, who found 16.8% unrecognized parametrial tumor involvement in patients with stage IB and IIA lesions. The 5-year survival rate fell with parametrial involvement.

Thorough examination of the lymphadenectomy specimens must be done. Tumor metastasis to lymph nodes affects patient survival adversely and would be an indication for postoperative adjuvant therapy. In patients with positive nodes, the pathologic examination should report whether the metastatic disease is microscopic or macroscopic, single or multiple, unilateral or bilateral. The location of lymph nodes positive for tumor also should be reported because the prognosis is especially poor in patients with positive common iliac or paraaortic nodes. The usual standard technique of pathologic examination of lymphadenectomy specimens involves removal of visible and palpable nodes from fatty tissue, with bisection of each node for microscopic examination. This standard technique may not be adequate for an accurate assessment of lymph node metastases. A significant increase in positive findings can be obtained if special pathologic examination techniques are used, as demonstrated by To and coworkers, Ahrens and Tschoke, and Wilkinson and Hause. With their technique of dissection of lymph nodes at multiple levels before paraffin embedding, To and coworkers showed that 9% of patients originally reported to have negative nodes actually had positive nodes.

An accurate assessment of the extent of disease by a careful pathology examination of the operative specimen is imperative in deciding whether additional treatment is needed. Indeed, it is such an important component in the surgical management of patients with cervical cancer that these patients should be operated on only in hospitals where such expert specimen evaluation is available.

POSTOPERATIVE COMPLICATIONS

Bladder

Neurogenic Dysfunction

A radical hysterectomy substantially denervates the bladder and upper urethra; the more extensive the dissection, the greater the degree of interference with their function. Parasympathetic and sympathetic nerve fibers to and from the bladder and urethra are removed, along with paracervical, paravaginal, cardinal ligament tissues, and pelvic lymph nodes. All patients have some degree of

bladder dysfunction; the incidence of significant bladder dysfunction can be as high as 50%.

Mundy and Sasaki and coworkers have suggested that the posterior part of the cardinal ligament (pars nervosa) contains the major part of the parasympathetic and sympathetic nerve supply to the bladder and urethra and that its removal is responsible for postoperative bladder dysfunction. Sasaki and coworkers demonstrated that removal of the anterior cardinal ligament (pars vasculosa) with preservation of the pars nervosa reduces the incidence of postoperative bladder dysfunction. The work of Kadar and coworkers and that of Asmussen and Ulmsten suggest that the nerve supply to the bladder and urethra can be spared without compromising the necessary extensive dissection and tissue removal around the central disease, thus sparing many patients the loss of urethrovesical function. Kuwabara and colleagues recently reported a decrease in bladder dysfunction by using a technique of intraoperative electrical stimulation to identify and preserve the vesical nerve branches These nerve-sparing modifications have not been widely adopted by gynecologic oncologists, presumably because of a concern that this same cardinal ligament tissue also carries lymphatic channels draining the cervix and should be removed in a complete central dissection. It seems, therefore, that some degree of bladder dysfunction is inevitable with a technique of radical hysterectomy that emphasizes adequacy of the central dissection and complete lymphadenectomy.

Studies have demonstrated that the bladder initially can be hypertonic, with decreased bladder capacity, increased resting pressure, and increased residual urine volume. Many patients have difficulty initiating micturition and experience a loss of sensation of bladder fullness. Using sensitive urodynamic instrumentation, Scotti and coworkers found a variety of abnormalities, including obstructive voiding patterns, immediate and delayed loss of compliance, sensory losses, and genuine stress incontinence. Some patients had complete absence of bladder contractions during voiding. Although these findings are quite compelling, Lin and associates recently reported normal preoperative urodynamic findings in only 17% of 210 patients with cervical cancer scheduled to undergo radical hysterectomy.

Techniques of managing the postoperative bladder have varied widely. Duration of catheter drainage, suprapubic versus transurethral drainage, the value of self-catheterization, and the value of cystometric studies have all been debated as described by Bandy and coworkers. These authors also found that patients receiving postoperative adjunctive pelvic radiation had significantly more contracted and unstable bladders than patients treated with surgery alone. Proper management of the bladder in the first several weeks after operation is essential to avoid overdistention. The duration of postoperative bladder catheterization has decreased in recent years. Chamberlin and investigators reported a contemporary median indwelling catheter duration of 6 days compared to 30 days in historical controls with no increase in complication rates.

Although some clinicians leave an indwelling catheter or suprapubic tube in place 2 to 3 weeks, we prefer continuous transurethral catheter drainage until the patient is ready for discharge, which is usually about 4 to 7 days after surgery. Early postoperative intravenous pyelography (IVP) in the absence of intraoperative urinary tract injury or clinical symptoms suggestive of injury is not indicated; moreover, an abnormal early IVP is not predictive of subsequent urinary tract dysfunction. When the patient is ready for discharge, the catheter is removed, and postvoid residuals are checked with a bladder scanner (transurethral catheterization also can be used). If the postvoid residual volume is below 50 to 75 mL and the volume of urine spontaneously voided is greater than the postvoid residual, then the patient is allowed to leave the hospital without an indwelling catheter. She must be thoroughly schooled in the importance of not allowing her bladder to become overdistended. Allowing the bladder to overdistend, especially in the early postoperative recovery period, can result in a flaccid bladder from stretching and decompensation of the detrusor muscle, prolongation of bladder dysfunction with high residual urine volumes, and the likelihood of urinary infections. Patients who have unacceptable postvoid residuals are best managed with prolonged indwelling catheter drainage for several weeks before attempting to remove it. If a serious episode of overdistention of the bladder ever occurs, continuous indwelling catheter drainage should be reinstituted, sometimes for several weeks, with the hope that permanent impairment of bladder function can be avoided. Urinary tract infections can occur in conjunction with bladder dysfunction and should be looked for with periodic urinalysis and culture and treated with appropriate antibiotics. Patients should be encouraged to maintain a urine output above 2,000 mL per day to avoid urinary tract infection.

In most patients, a satisfactory voiding pattern can be established within several months. Urodynamic studies, however, can show some evidence of slight and persistent chronic bladder dysfunction for several years. Fraser stated that 20% of his patients continued to report changes in bladder sensation as long as 5 to 15 years after operation. In many patients who have had properly performed radical hysterectomy and pelvic lymphadenectomy, it is inevitable that bladder function will never be completely normal again. With proper postoperative bladder care and rehabilitation, however, function should be satisfactory in most patients at the end of the first year. According to Fishman and coworkers, 35% of patients continued to express unhappiness at the extent and effect of their postoperative urinary dysfunction.

Fistula

In the absence of prior pelvic irradiation, bladder ischemia and vesicovaginal fistula are infrequent complications of this procedure. Vesicovaginal fistulas occur in less than 1% of patients (Table 46.12). Nearly one third

TABLE 46.12.
Urinary Fistulas in Nonirradiated Patients Treated by Radical Abdominal Hysterectomy

Investigators	Number of Patients	Ureteral Fistula (%)	Vesical Fistula (%)
Kaser et al., 1973	717	3.3	0.6
Park et al., 1973	156	0	0
Hoskins et al., 1976	224	1.3	0.45
Morley and Seski, 1976	208	4.8	0.5
Sall et al., 1979	349	2.0	0.8
Webb and Symmonds, 1979	423	1.4	0.7
Benedet et al., 1980	241	1.2	0.4
Langley et al., 1980	284	5.6	1.4
Lerner et al., 1980	108	0.9	0
Bostofte et al., 1981	479	3.8	1.4
Powell et al., 1981	135	1.5	0
Zander et al., 1981	1,092	1.4	0.3
Gitsch et al., 1984	187	0.5	NS
Shingleton, 1985	444	1.4	0.23
Artman et al., 1987	153	1.3	1.3
Larson et al., 1987	233	0.8	NS
Ralph et al., 1988	320	1.9	2.5
Lee et al., 1989	954	1.2	1.2
Kenter et al., 1989	213	3.3	3.3
Burghardt et al., 1989	325	2.5	2.8
Massi et al., 1993	228	0.9	0.4
TOTAL	7,473	2.0	0.9

NS, no sample.
From: Shingleton HM, Orr JW Jr, eds. *Cancer of the cervix.* Philadelphia: JB Lippincott, 1995, with permission.

of urinary tract fistulas following surgery heal spontaneously, as compared to none if adjuvant radiation therapy is given. The management of vesicovaginal fistulas is discussed in Chapter 38.

Ureter

Clark, working at the Johns Hopkins Hospital, published one of the first descriptions of radical hysterectomy for cervical cancer in 1895. Sampson, working in the same institution during the same time, recognized that injury to the ureter was the most serious problem associated with primary radical surgery for this disease. His publications on ureteral anatomy and blood supply and the relation between the ureter and gynecologic disease are classic and pertinent today. Devascularization and ischemic necrosis of the wall of the terminal ureter has proved to be one of the more serious complications of this operation. Wertheim found this complication to be one of the more serious sequelae. In Meigs' clinic, there was a 12.5% significant ureteral complication rate, including an 8.5% incidence of ureterovaginal fistulas and a 4% incidence of ureteral stricture. As recently as 1965, Talbert and coworkers reported that nine of 112 patients (8%) who had radical hysterectomy, usually preceded by radium, developed ureterovaginal fistulas, two of which were bilateral. Seven kidneys were lost. The incidence of ureteral stricture also was high. The high percentage of ureteral complications might have been related to a large number of patients with pelvic cellulitis and also a large number of patients (71%) who received preoperative radiation. It is well known that these two factors increase the risk of ureteral complications. In a report of 111 patients undergoing radical hysterectomy and lymphadenectomy for cervical cancer in the same institution, only two minor ureteral injuries and no fistulas occurred.

For many years, gynecologic surgeons have attempted to lower the rate of ureteral complications with special techniques. Novak, from Yugoslavia, reduced the incidence of ureteral fistulas to 2% after primary radical surgery by placing the dissected pelvic ureter on the inside (peritoneal surface) of the pelvic peritoneum and by preserving the lateral mesentery to the terminal ureter. Green and coworkers suggested that the terminal ureter should be lifted out of the accumulated fluid in the retroperitoneal space by suturing it to the obliterated hypogastric artery. Ohkawa developed a procedure that attempted to elevate and isolate the ureter from the infected retroperitoneal fluid and also to develop a new blood supply to the terminal ureter by placing it in a peritoneal envelope from the pelvic brim to the bladder. Blythe and coworkers compared this technique with simple retroperitoneal suction drainage first advised by Symmonds and Pratt. They found that ureteral obstruction and ureterovaginal fistulas occurred twice as often and that the operative time was extended 45 minutes to 1 hour with the Ohkawa technique. More recently, Patsner and others have recommended the routine use of the omental J-flap (omentopexy) at the conclusion of

radical hysterectomy and pelvic lymphadenectomy as an effective means of minimizing urinary tract fistulas.

Given a normal unirradiated ureter, we believe that the incidence of ureteral fistulas and permanent stenosis can be kept below 1% with meticulous intraoperative management of the ureter by a technically skillful operator who can prevent vascular trauma to the periureteral sheath and injury to the muscularis of the ureter.

Some temporary postoperative changes in ureteral function are an almost inevitable result of radical hysterectomy, as pointed out by Gal and Buchsbaum. Using special static and cinefluoroscopic intravenous pyelography techniques, these authors found ureteral dilation in 87% of patients in the first week after surgery. In most cases, by 6 weeks after surgery, the dilation had regressed and the pyelograms had returned to normal. Peristalsis was altered in the distal ureter, which appeared as a rigid conduit during the first postoperative week. Peristalsis had returned 1 month later. These changes may explain the increased frequency of urinary tract infections after radical hysterectomy and the possibility of permanent ureteral stenosis if radiation, serious infection, or lymphocyst formation is superimposed.

Table 46.12 shows the frequency of urinary fistulas in a collected series of 7,473 nonirradiated patients treated by radical hysterectomy as compiled by Shingleton and Orr. The management of ureterovaginal fistulas is discussed in Chapter 37.

Retroperitoneal Spaces

Traditionally, a closed system of constant suction was placed in the retroperitoneal spaces on each side at the end of the procedure. These drains were thought to be effective in preventing pelvic infection, fistula, and lymphocyst formation. However, recent retrospective and prospective studies have demonstrated that the incidence of these complications is not decreased in patients who have retroperitoneal drains placed compared to those who do not. Furthermore, the drains may actually increase infectious complications. Therefore, we do not routinely place drains in the retroperitoneal spaces.

Whether drains are placed or not a small percentage of patients develop lymphocysts. A lymphocyst becomes obvious by symptoms and examination in the weeks after radical hysterectomy and pelvic lymphadenectomy. It may be small and asymptomatic. Most patients with large lymphocysts complain of lower abdominal discomfort on the same side with radiation to the back, hip, or thigh. Some edema of the lower extremity on the same side may be present. Evidence of ureteral obstruction may be found on IVP.

Small lymphocysts that do not cause ureteral obstruction can be observed without treatment. Large symptomatic lymphocysts and those that cause ureteral obstruction should be aspirated either vaginally or abdominally with a needle. CT-directed needle aspiration can be done with local anesthesia and repeated as needed. The fluid should be submitted for cytologic examination. It is seldom necessary to perform open drainage of a lymphocyst. Mann and coworkers reported successful sclerosis of a recurrent lymphocyst by injection of a solution of tetracycline. Others have used povidone-iodine sclerosis.

Infection

Historically, patients were treated with antibiotics only if postoperative infection occurred. However, antibiotic prophylaxis has been associated with decreased febrile morbidity and decreased rates of serious infections in women undergoing radical abdominal hysterectomy. Furthermore, Orr and colleagues have demonstrated that a single dose of prophylactic antibiotic is as effective as a multiple-dose regimen and lessens patient exposure and cost. Thus, the prophylactic use of broad-spectrum antibiotics with both aerobic and anaerobic coverage has proved to be a useful addition to the surgical armamentarium.

We initiate single agent broad-spectrum antibiotic coverage immediately before surgery. The administration of the drug is timed to allow adequate distribution prior to incision. During an extended operation, if the antibiotic given has a short half-life, a second dose is administered.

When secondary infection occurs despite the use of prophylactic antibiotics, the appropriate cultures are obtained, and bacteria-specific, antibiotic therapy is chosen.

Venous Thrombosis and Pulmonary Embolus

Patients who undergo radical pelvic surgery fulfill the components of Virchow's triad and are at high risk for the development of venous thrombosis of the lower extremities and thromboembolic phenomena. Factors such as postoperative alteration of blood coagulation, trauma to the vein wall, and venous stasis are recognizable features of this type of surgery. In particular, pelvic lymphadenectomy invariably produces some trauma to the vein wall during the mobilization of the vessel and resection of the adherent lymphatic tissue. One of the biologic effects of radical surgery is the occurrence of local tissue necrosis during healing. This results in the release of tissue thromboplastin into the circulation, which contributes to venous thrombosis by acceleration of the clotting mechanism. The release of thromboplastin from the intima of the vein wall also provides an excellent nidus for the formation of fibrin, particularly in an area of the venous system where there is alteration in venous flow with stagnation of blood. This is frequently seen behind the valves of the veins of the lower extremity, where silent thrombosis is common. Prolonged immobilization of the lower extremities during a lengthy operative procedure is responsible for intraoperative venous stasis and clot formation. There is evidence to document that postoperative thrombosis of the lower extremity is a result of the surgical procedure in more than 50% of cases.

Efforts to decrease the frequency of this complication initially used prophylactic low-dose heparin, using 5,000 U subcutaneously, three times daily, beginning 2 hours before surgery, and given every 8 hours thereafter for the subsequent five postoperative days. By using perioperative heparin alone, the incidence of deep vein thrombosis in a study by Kakkar and associates was decreased from 24.6% in the untreated control group to 7.7% in the heparin-treated group of surgical cases. More impressive was the observation in a subsequent study by the same investigators that 16 patients in the control group, as compared with only two patients in the heparin-treated group, were found on autopsy study to have died of acute, massive pulmonary embolism.

Clarke-Pearson and coworkers have published numerous randomized trials on this subject. They have demonstrated that pneumatic calf compression is as effective as low-dose unfractionated heparin in the prevention of deep venous thrombosis after gynecologic oncology surgery. Moreover, patients receiving pneumatic calf compression have significantly less postoperative bleeding complications and retroperitoneal drainage. The recently developed low-molecular-weight heparins (LMWHs) have also been reported to be as effective as conventional, unfractionated heparin but the newer drugs are associated with fewer bleeding complications. Maxwell and colleagues performed a randomized trial comparing pneumatic calf compression to LMWH for deep vein thrombosis in gynecologic oncology patients undergoing major surgery. They found the two methods of prophylaxis were equally effective with no significant differences in bleeding complications.

We use intermittent pneumatic calf compression beginning in the operating room and continuing whenever the patient is in bed until she is discharged. These compression boots are used not only in our patients undergoing radical hysterectomy but in all our patients undergoing major gynecologic surgical procedures. In very high-risk patients, we add prophylactic LMWH.

Approximately 3% to 5% of patients with occult venous thrombosis of the lower extremities develop pulmonary emboli. Unfortunately, more than half of the cases of fatal pulmonary embolism occur in patients with silent venous thrombosis and without any clinical evidence of this complication before the acute pulmonary catastrophe. When evidence of venous thrombosis of the lower extremity is verified, full anticoagulation therapy is required for prevention of pulmonary embolism. In the rare case that a pulmonary embolus occurs after full anticoagulation has been achieved, it is necessary to prevent further migration of clot to the lung by either inferior vena cava ligation or the use of an intracaval Silastic umbrella. These complications are rare, but the sinister effects of thromboembolism must be carefully evaluated on a daily basis and a high index of suspicion needs to be maintained in this high-risk group of patients.

Hemorrhage

Intraoperative and postoperative pelvic hemorrhages also are discussed in Chapters 10 and 18.

Intraoperative Bleeding

Despite the surgeon's adequate technical skills and careful dissection, serious hemorrhage can suddenly appear, especially during retroperitoneal dissections on the lateral pelvic sidewalls and around the sacrum. When it happens, it is hoped that the operative field will not be cluttered with clamps; exposure, lighting, and suction will be adequate; the patient's condition will be stable; and anesthesia will be sufficient to maintain good relaxation. If the bleeding vessel cannot be clamped quickly, the simplest and most effective method of controlling the bleeding is provided by pressure applied by the index finger of the gloved hand. With cessation of bleeding, the operative site can be cleared of accumulated blood by suctioning, exposure of the area can be improved, and the surgeon can gain a few moments to evaluate the situation and choose the best possible course of action. Arterial bleeding is easy to identify and control with clips, clamps, or ligatures. The difficult problem with hemorrhage in the pelvis comes from lacerations of deep pelvic veins that are fragile, tortuous, distended, sometimes hidden or retracted from view, and sometimes held open by attachment of the vein wall to surrounding tissue. Blood returning through the lacerated vein can come from multiple sources unavailable for ligation. Placing clamps or sutures blindly is dangerous and can even make the problem worse. Sometimes, digital pressure for at least 7 minutes is the most effective procedure to control venous bleeding. Sometimes, additional careful dissection in the area is required to free the vessel above and below the bleeding point to allow more precise clipping or suture ligation. A cardinal rule in dissecting in the pelvis is to avoid creating a deep hole, the bottom of which cannot be exposed in case a deep vein is lacerated. This is the reason that dissection of the pararectal space, for instance, should not be forced if it does not develop easily.

Whenever an extensive pelvic dissection is anticipated, preparations should be made in advance in case severe intraoperative bleeding is suddenly encountered. Adequate quantities of blood should be available to replace lost volume. More blood should be requested in advance of its need, if possible. A responsible member of the operating team or anesthesia team should be assigned the task of monitoring blood loss, blood replacement, and urine output. When bleeding is profuse, in the excitement of the moment, it is possible to lose count of the number of units of whole blood, blood components, crystalloids, and other fluids that have been given and how much blood has been lost. A dependable route for administering blood must be maintained. Without it, rapid blood replacement is not possible. If massive hemorrhage occurs or if even a possibility of its occurrence exists, a Swan-Ganz or similar catheter should be placed for better monitoring of physiologic functions and blood replacement. In extreme cases in which no other vessels are available for rapid intraoperative blood volume replacement, transfusions can be given under pressure directly into the common iliac artery, with the needle pointed in the direction of the heart.

The most frequent site of troublesome intraoperative bleeding during radical hysterectomy occurs from the pelvic floor veins in the dissection of the cardinal ligament and the hypogastric vessels. The collateral venous circulation of the hypogastric veins is an ever-present source of potential hemorrhage owing to difficulty in identification of these vessels as they course among muscle bundles and fascial planes on the pelvic floor. The pararectal fossa, cardinal ligament, and presacral and paraaortic areas are frequent sites of venous bleeding. Therefore, meticulous dissection is important to avoid these complications. When venous bleeding does occur, it can be difficult to identify the site of the lacerated vein. In these circumstances, it is important to use compression of the pelvic floor veins by either a sponge stick or finger held in place for several minutes, or to use an abdominal pack placed firmly against the site of bleeding for a similar length of time. In these cases, it is advisable to keep pressure on the vein until full control of the bleeding has been established, in the meantime dissecting in other places in the pelvis. Only when the wall of a major pelvic vein has been severely traumatized and has retracted out of the operative field is there a serious problem in reestablishing hemostasis. In contrast to arterial bleeding, hemorrhage from deep pelvic veins is seldom improved by hypogastric artery ligation, owing to the extensive collateral venous circulation to the pelvis from the lower extremity and vena cava. It occasionally is beneficial to ligate the anterior division of both hypogastric arteries to determine whether interruption of the major arterial blood supply to the pelvis can reduce the venous bleeding. When more extensive trauma to the wall of the external or common iliac vein has occurred, it is necessary to place vascular clamps above and below the area of injury and to repair the defect with fine vascular sutures.

Postoperative Hemorrhage

This condition is a rare complication of radical pelvic surgery. Because all of the blood supply to the pelvis has been skeletonized as part of the operative procedure, it is exceedingly rare for secondary hemorrhage to occur unless there has been uncontrolled bleeding at the completion of the operation. In these cases, the pelvis usually is packed with multiple gauze packs, with one end exteriorized through the open vagina. Tamponade of the pelvis by means of an umbrella (Logothetopulos) gauze pack and external ring (see Chapter 18) has been advocated by some when there is persistent venous oozing in the pelvis at the completion of the operation. Pelvic packs should be advanced within 24 to 48 hours and removed shortly thereafter to avoid ascending infection from the vagina.

In certain cases of postoperative hemorrhage, selective embolization by invasive radiographic techniques can prevent reoperation.

Neuropathies

Nerve injury with radical hysterectomy was reviewed by Hoffman and coworkers, who reported its infrequent occurrence. The most important injuries are to the femoral, obturator, peroneal, sciatic, genitofemoral, ilioinguinal, iliohypogastric, lateral femoral cutaneous, and pudendal nerves. Awareness of the anatomic location of these nerves in the operative field, careful surgical technique in dissection and securing hemostasis, careful placement of self-retaining retractors, and careful positioning of patients in stirrups prevent most nerve injuries. Fortunately, most nerve injuries are not associated with serious or permanent disability.

However, injury to the obturator nerve can lead to difficulty with adduction of the lower extremity. Obturator nerve injuries are the most common neurologic injuries and they occur most frequently during the removal of the obturator lymph nodes from the obturator fossa. If the nerve is transected, it should be repaired as described by Vasilev and associates.

Rectum

Although much less frequent than bladder dysfunction, both acute and chronic rectal dysfunction may occur following radical hysterectomy. The rectal dysfunction is characterized by difficulty with defecation and loss of defecation urge. Barnes and associates reported that postoperative anorectal manometry studies were abnormal in all patients studied suggesting disruption of the spinal reflex arcs controlling rectal emptying, possibly secondary to partial denervation of the rectum. Dietary fiber modifications and rectal stimulation with suppositories over several weeks or months are effective in addressing these problems.

ADJUVANT THERAPY IN CONJUNCTION WITH RADICAL SURGERY

Postoperative Pelvic Irradiation

External-beam radiation therapy is used in the postoperative period as an adjunct to radical abdominal hysterectomy and bilateral pelvic lymphadenectomy in selected cases. It is given selectively to patients considered to be at high risk for persistent disease based on operative findings and careful study of the surgical specimens. Previously, if only one or two lymph nodes show micrometastases, postoperative irradiation may not be given. However, when several nodes are involved, the risk of persistent disease is greater, and postoperative irradiation is usually given, and can be extended as high as T-12 if proximal common iliac or paraaortic nodes are involved with metastatic disease. However, nodal metastasis is not the only risk factor for recurrence and other local tumor related factors may be indicators of high-risk tumors that may warrant adjuvant radiation therapy.

Sedlis et al., in a GOG randomized trial of pelvic radiation therapy versus no further therapy in selected patients with stage IB carcinoma of the cervix with negative lymph nodes after radical hysterectomy and pelvic lymphadenectomy, evaluated the benefits and risk of adjuvant pelvic radiation therapy aimed at reducing recurrence in this group of patients.

In this study, 277 eligible patients were entered with at least two of the following tumor-related risk factors: greater than one-third stromal invasion, capillary lymphatic space involvement, and large clinical tumor diameter. Table 46.13 summarizes the eligibility criteria: Of the 277 patients, 137 were randomized to pelvic radiation therapy and 140 to no further treatment. Twenty-one (15%) in the radiation therapy group and 39 (28%) in the no further treatment group had a cancer recurrence, 18 of whom were vaginal/pelvic in the radiation therapy, and 27 in the no further treatment group. Life table analysis indicated a statistically significant (47%) reduction in risk of recurrence (relative risk = 0.53, p = 0.008, one-tail) among the radiation therapy group, with recurrence-free rates at 2 years of 88% versus 79% for the radiation therapy and no further treatment groups, respectively. Toxicity was generally acceptable, with severe or life-threatening urologic adverse effects occurring in four (3.1%) in the radiation therapy group and two (1.4%) in the control group. The authors concluded that adjuvant pelvic radiation therapy following radical surgery in selected women with stage IB cervical cancer, reduces the number of recurrences at the cost of 6% grade 3 and 4 adverse events versus 2.1% in the control group.

Many physicians are currently using these data to identify node-negative patients with local risk factors following radical hysterectomy and pelvic lymphadenectomy to prescribe adjuvant radiation therapy.

Postoperative Adjuvant Chemoradiation

If invasive cervical cancer is unexpectedly found after a simple hysterectomy has been done, postoperative pelvic radiation therapy is recommended. Survival rates in these patients have improved with the advent of megavoltage irradiation, as reported by Andras and coworkers, Davy and coworkers, and Papavasilou and coworkers. Heller and coworkers reported 35 patients with invasive cervical carcinoma discovered in uteri removed for benign conditions. All patients received postoperative radiation

---

TABLE 46.13.

Eligibility Criteria for Radiation Therapy After Radical Hysterectomy in Node-Negative Patients

CLVI	Stromal Invasion	Tumor Size (cm)
+	Deep one third	Any
+	Middle one third	≥2
+	Superficial one third	≥5
−	Middle or Deep one third	≥4

From: Sedlis A, Bundy BN, Rotman MZ, et al. A randomized trial of pelvic radiation therapy versus no further therapy in selected patients with stage IB carcinoma of the cervix after radical hysterectomy and pelvic lymphadenectomy: a Gynecologic Oncology Group Study. *Gynecol Oncol* 1999;73:177–183, with permission.

therapy; patients with presumed stage IB disease had a corrected 5-year survival rate of 78%, and those with presumed stage IIB disease had a corrected 5-year survival rate of 67%. After radical surgery in high-risk, early-stage cancer of the cervix, Peters et al. reported a phase III trial of adjunctive concurrent chemotherapy and pelvic radiation therapy compared with pelvic radiation therapy alone. In all, 243 assessable patients with clinical stage IA (2), IB, and IIA carcinoma of the cervix, initially treated with radical hysterectomy and pelvic lymphadenectomy, and who had positive pelvic lymph nodes and/or positive margins and/or microscopic involvement of the parametrium were evaluated. Patients were randomized to receive platinum-based chemoradiation or radiation only. Patients in each group received 49.3 Gy radiation therapy in 29 fractions to a standard pelvic field. Chemotherapy consisted of cisplatin 70 mg/m^2 and a 96-hour infusion of fluorouracil 1,000 mg/m^2 day every 3 weeks for four cycles, with the first and second cycles given concurrent to radiation therapy.

Progression-free and overall survival are significantly better in women receiving chemoradiation. The projected progression-free survival at 4 years was 63% with radiation therapy alone, and 80% with chemoradiation. The projected overall survival rate at 4 years is 71% with adjuvant radiation therapy and 81% with adjuvant chemoradiation. However, grade 3 and 4 hematologic and gastrointestinal toxicity were more frequent in the chemoradiation group.

The authors concluded that the addition of concurrent cisplatin-based chemotherapy to radiation significantly improves progression-free and overall survival for high-risk, early-stage patients who undergo radical hysterectomy and pelvic lymphadenectomy for carcinoma of the cervix and are found to have positive pelvic lymph nodes and/or positive margins and/or microscopic involvement of the parametrium. Although the data from this study are compelling, use of this regimen should be undertaken only with understanding of the toxicities encountered.

The data from this randomized trial and the Sedlis trial currently provide practical guidelines for eligibility of patients for adjuvant postoperative radiation or chemoradiation following primary radical hysterectomy and pelvic lymphadenectomy.

Postoperative Extended-Field Irradiation or Chemoradiation

In selected cases, with multiple positive pelvic nodes, metastasis to common iliac nodes, or aortic nodal metastasis, patients are treated with pelvic and extended-field radiation to include the paraaortic lymph chain. To numerous previous studies can be added two studies from Japan that describe the results of paraaortic nodal irradiation in the treatment of cervical cancer. Inoue and Morita (1988) administered extended-field radiation after extensive surgery to 76 patients with aortic nodal metastases. Two patients developed severe intestinal complications that required reoperation. Postoperative

extended-field irradiation improved the survival rate of patients with four or more positive nodes from 39% to 69%, as well as the survival rate of patients with unresectable nodes from 0% to 44%. The authors concluded that postoperative extended-field irradiation can control the distant spread by way of lymphatic routes and can increase the survival time of patients. In addition, 86 patients with cervical cancer were treated with paraaortic nodal irradiation by Horii and coworkers (1988). None of the patients developed severe complications from the treatment. Based on their selection criteria for paraaortic nodal irradiation, the authors found a statistically significant improvement in the prognosis for the treated group.

In 1987, Jones reported on a collected series of 332 patients with paraaortic lymph node metastases who received extended-field radiation. Twenty-six percent were long-term survivors. Although it is true that most patients with positive paraaortic lymph nodes die of their disease (probably because systemic disease is already present), it also is clear that some patients are curable with extended-field radiation or chemoradiation, especially if the nodes are involved with only microscopic disease. The surgeon must anticipate a 10% incidence of enteric complications even with doses limited to 5,000 cGy. Again, micrometastatic disease is more likely to be eradicated by a dose of paraaortic radiation that can be tolerated by the patient. Patients with paraaortic nodes that contain a large volume of tumor are not likely to be cured even with a dose of paraaortic radiation that exceeds 5,000 cGy, unless the bulky nodes are excised before the irradiation.

Extended-field chemoradiation also may be used. The GOG reported on a multicenter trial of chemoradiation therapy to evaluate the feasibility of extended-field radiation therapy with 5-fluorouracil (5-FU) and cisplatin, and to determine the progression-free interval, overall survival, and recurrence sites in patients with biopsy-confirmed paraaortic node metastases from cervical carcinoma. In all, 86 evaluable stage I to IV patients with aortic metastases were reported. Radiation therapy doses were 4,500 cGy to paraaortic nodes, and concomitant chemotherapy consisted of 5-FU 1,000 mg/m^2 per day for 96 hours and cisplatin 50 mg/m^2 in weeks 1 and 5.

Initial sites of recurrence were pelvis alone, 20.9%; distant metastases only, 31.4%; and pelvic plus distant metastases, 10.5%. The 3-year overall and progression-free survival rates were 39% and 34%, respectively, for the entire group. Overall survival was stage I, 50%; stage II, 39%; and stage III/IVA, 38%.

GOG grade 3 and 4 acute toxicity was gastrointestinal (18.6%) and hematologic (15.1%). Late morbidity actuarial risk of 14% at 4 years primarily involved the rectum. The authors concluded that extended-field radiation therapy with 5-FU and cisplatin chemotherapy was feasible in a multicenter clinical trial, and that a progression-free survival of 33% at 3 years suggests that a proportion of patients achieve control of advanced pelvic disease and that not all patients with paraaortic metastases have systemic disease. This points to the importance of assessment and treatment of paraaortic metastases.

Adjuvant Postoperative Chemotherapy

Few studies of adjuvant chemotherapy following radical hysterectomy have been done. Wertheim et al. from Memorial Sloan-Kettering Cancer Center (MSKCC) in 1985 reported on a pilot study of adjuvant chemotherapy with cisplatin and bleomycin and pelvic radiation therapy in patients with cervical cancer at high risk of recurrence after radical hysterectomy and pelvic lymphadenectomy.

The continuous disease-free survival rate for the 32 evaluable patients was 84% at a median follow-up time of 28 months. In addition, the complications of this treatment program were not significantly greater than those observed in prior studies using the combination of surgery and adjuvant radiation therapy without chemotherapy. When compared with the results from historical controls in a large series of similar patients at the same institution, the results in this pilot study were encouraging and appeared to justify a randomized prospective clinical trial.

Two randomized trials have attempted to clarify the role of adjuvant postoperative chemotherapy. In 1992, Tattersall et al. reported a randomized trial comparing standard pelvic radiation therapy versus three cycles of combination chemotherapy with cisplatin, vinblastine, and bleomycin followed by pelvic radiation therapy. No difference in disease-free or overall survival emerged between the two treatment groups. Relapse was more common in patients with nonsquamous tumors (44%) and in those with metastases in several pelvic lymph nodes.

In 1996, Curtin et al. from MSKCC reported on a prospective multicenter randomized Phase III trial of adjuvant chemotherapy versus chemotherapy plus pelvic irradiation for high-risk stage IB to IIA cervical cancer patients after radical hysterectomy and pelvic lymphadenectomy. The objective was to compare the clinical efficacy of adjuvant chemotherapy alone versus chemotherapy plus whole pelvic radiation therapy on recurrence rates, patterns of recurrence, and survival of patients after radical hysterectomy and pelvic lymphadenectomy for cervical cancer at high risk for recurrence.

Risk factors included deep cervical invasion, tumor >4 cm, parametrial involvement, nonsquamous histology, and/or pelvic lymph node metastasis. Chemotherapy consisted of cisplatin and bleomycin alone or in combination with whole-pelvic radiation therapy. Eighty-nine patients were entered, 19 had recurrences, and 16 died. Nine of 44 (20%) patients receiving chemotherapy alone recurred compared to 10 of 45 (22%) patients receiving chemotherapy and radiation (p = NS). Patterns of recurrence were statistically similar between the two treatment arms, even among the subgroup of patients with more than three risk factors. In addition, both regimens were well tolerated. The authors concluded that recurrence rates and patterns of recurrences (local, regional, or distant) were not influenced by the addition of radiation therapy.

However, in view of the more recent randomized trial of adjuvant chemoradiation, most high-risk patients with nodal metastasis will probably be offered adjuvant platinum-based chemoradiation. Whether weekly cisplatin or other platinum-based regimes are the optimal choice remains to be determined.

FOLLOW-UP AFTER RADICAL SURGERY FOR CERVICAL CANCER

Despite carefully planned and executed radical surgery for early stage cervical cancer, 5% to 20% of patients in various series show evidence of recurrent or persistent tumor. About half occur in the first year after treatment. Almost all occur within the first 3 years. Few occur later. Recurrences many years later are extremely rare after primary surgical treatment and are more likely to be seen in patients treated with primary radiation therapy.

Persistent or recurrent disease after primary radical surgery may represent incomplete resection of the central tumor undetected at operation or by the pathologist's examination of the surgical specimen. Microscopic metastatic involvement of lymph nodes may be undetected by incomplete pathologic examination or these nodes may be left behind by incomplete lymphadenectomy. Viable tumor cells in small numbers may escape by way of lymphatics or vascular channels to distant sites and overcome host resistance. Probably in as many as 10% of patients with persistent disease, recurrence may result from continued growth of unrecognized intraperitoneal spread of tumor.

After the immediate postoperative recovery is completed, patients are scheduled for regular follow-up examinations, which vary depending on circumstances. Patients who are at greater risk for recurrence should be followed especially closely at frequent intervals. These usually are the same patients who have been given postoperative therapy, including patients with metastatic disease in lymph nodes and/or parametria, close surgical margins, large-volume cervical tumors, deep cervical stromal invasion, lymphatic and/or vascular channel involvement. The frequency of examination varies somewhat from patient to patient. Most patients are seen every 3 months during the first 3 years after primary treatment, every 6 months during the fourth and fifth years, and every 6 months to 1 year thereafter. Patients are instructed to report unusual signs or symptoms (e.g., vaginal bleeding or discharge, leg swelling, discomfort in the pelvis, discomfort or swelling in the legs, difficulty with urination or defecation, enlarged neck or groin nodes) at any time they appear. Krebs and coworkers, however, reported that 25% of their patients did not have symptoms when persistent disease was diagnosed. In the study reported by Larson and coworkers, 37% did not have symptoms.

A follow-up examination should include palpation of the neck for enlarged lymph nodes, abdominal and leg examination, and a speculum and bimanual rectovaginal pelvic examination. A vaginal cytology smear is performed with each visit. Computed tomography scan of the abdomen and pelvis, proctosigmoidoscopy, cystoscopy, IVP, and biopsy (needle, punch, or both) of any suspicious lesions may be required, depending on the patient's symptoms and examination findings. These special diagnostic procedures are not done routinely as part of postoperative follow-up surveillance in patients without symptoms. Positive findings are rare unless the patient has symptoms. For example, IVP seldom shows ureteral obstruction in a patient who does not also have symptoms of persistent pelvic side-wall disease, and is, therefore, not routinely done at specific intervals. It is in the patient's best interest to have follow-up examinations done in the same center in which her treatment was administered. Findings at each visit must be compared with previous information all the way back to her original presentation.

Soisson and coworkers reported a comparison of symptoms, physical examination, and vaginal cytology in the detection of recurrent cervical carcinoma after radical hysterectomy. The study group consisted of 203 women with stage IB and IIA cervical cancer followed at the Duke University Medical Center. Thirty-one (15%) patients developed recurrence. For the detection of recurrent tumor, vaginal cytology had a sensitivity and specificity of 13% and 100%, pelvic or general physical examination 58% and 96%, and the presence of suspicious symptoms 71% and 95%, respectively. Ninety-four percent of all patients with recurrent tumor had at least one abnormal surveillance index. Another Duke study by Weber and associates found that MRI correctly demonstrated the extent of recurrence in 18 of 21 cases.

Regular pelvic examinations and vaginal cytology smears may detect a central pelvic recurrence early. This can be a great advantage. Just as it is important to detect the original cancer in the earliest stage possible so that the patient can have the best possible chance of cure, it also is important to detect persistent disease at the earliest possible moment, for the same reason. For example, Jobsen and coworkers reported on the use of radiation therapy to treat locoregional recurrence of carcinoma of the cervix after primary surgery. The overall 5-year survival rate was 44%. Response to radiation therapy was strongly correlated with tumor volume, providing additional supportive evidence to the idea that persistent disease should be diagnosed as early as possible and, it is hoped, when the volume of persistent tumor is still small and responsive.

Patients with recurrent or persistent cancer of the uterine cervix after initial radiation therapy can have radical surgery provided the disease is limited and judged to be surgically resectable. Usually some type of pelvic exenteration is required to resect the recurrent tumor with negative margins. In carefully selected patients with centrally recurrent disease, 5-year survivals of 40% to 60% have been reported.

Tumor ulceration in the upper vagina can produce vaginal discharge and spotting, a palpable tumor mass, and induration and nodularity of tissue extending to the pelvic sidewalls. Pain may not be present unless the tumor involves nerve roots. Symptoms related to urination and defecation can result from pressure, infection, or tumor involvement of the bladder and rectum. Either unilateral or bilateral edema of the lower extremities or unilateral or bilateral hydroureter and hydronephrosis can

be an ominous sign of persistent disease, but these also can be the result of a combination of the effects of radical surgery and postoperative irradiation. When initially diagnosed, recurrences are central in about one fourth of patients, involve the pelvic sidewall in one fourth, and involve distant sites in one fourth; the remaining one fourth of patients have multiple sites of involvement.

About 20% to 25% of patients with recurrence after primary radical surgery still can be cured. The best chance of cure is in patients who had no postoperative radiation treatment and no metastatic disease to pelvic lymph nodes and in whom persistent disease is limited to the central pelvis. A combination of total pelvic irradiation plus vaginal brachytherapy can be effective in controlling the disease. The addition of concurrent platinum-based chemotherapy also should be considered. Chemotherapy can be given for palliation when there is evidence of unresectable persistent disease in the pelvis in patients who have already received postoperative pelvic radiation, or when there is persistent disease in distant sites.

Because recurrence or persistence of cervical cancer after treatment is difficult but important to detect as early as possible, attempts have been made to use a serum marker that would monitor the course of the disease. Kato and Torigoe isolated a squamous-cell carcinoma antigen from cervical carcinoma tissue. A squamous-cell carcinoma antigen radioimmunoassay kit, developed by Abbott Laboratories (Abbott Park, Illinois), has been tested but the role of this antigen in the follow-up of patients with cervical carcinoma is yet to be determined.

Although the early detection of persistence is the primary purpose of and justification for follow-up visits, assessment of urinary tract function also is important. Particular attention should be paid to bladder function and maintaining a satisfactory voiding pattern. Urinary tract infection should be diagnosed and treated promptly. If ureteral stenosis impairs renal function, early intervention can be successful in avoiding nephrectomy. This is more likely to be seen in patients who receive a combination of radical surgery and irradiation as primary treatment.

Rehabilitation of sexual function after surgical therapy for cervical cancer usually is easily done by the patient and her partner but is more difficult if the vagina and paravaginal tissues have received heavy doses of radiation or if the patient has lost ovarian function as a result of treatment. The gynecologic surgeon should inquire about sexual problems and should give advice and permission when needed. Counseling, including instruction in the technique of alternative means of sexual gratification (e.g., interfemoral intercourse) may be needed. If ovarian function has been lost as a result of treatment, estrogen replacement therapy should be provided, even though symptoms of hypoestrogenism are not present. If normal ovaries were conserved, their function should be monitored with periodic follicle-stimulating hormone and estrogen levels, so that estrogen replacement can be provided when ovaries cease functioning in future years. There may be other contraindications to estrogen replacement therapy in patients treated for cervical cancer, but a history of treatment for cervical cancer is not one of them.

And finally, patients who have been treated for cervical cancer are at greater risk for developing other primary cancers at different sites, especially if the treatment included irradiation. Detection of other primary cancers should be part of posttreatment follow-up. This subject has been studied by Hoffman and coworkers, Buchler, and others. Axelrod and coworkers reported that 3.9% of patients with invasive cervical cancer had second primaries. In 1987, Arneson and Kao reported that 61 new primary cancers were detected among 718 patients with invasive cervical cancer who had been studied from 1955 to 1979.

RADIATION THERAPY

Beginning in 1903, several methods of intracavitary therapy were developed, including the Stockholm technique from the Radiumhemmet; the Paris technique, designed at the Curie Foundation; and the Manchester technique from England. The Stockholm radium technique consisted of high-intensity central irradiation, repeated two or three times within 3 weeks, whereas the Paris technique used low-intensity central irradiation, continuously delivered over 1 week. The Manchester technique, derived from the Paris method, used low, hourly dosage rates that required at least two intracervical insertions of radiation sources. Other radioactive elements, including cesium and iridium, have to a large degree replaced radium in central brachytherapy.

With the establishment of the roentgen as a defined unit of radiation exposure (Stockholm, 1921), it became possible to measure the quantity of irradiation delivered to the tumor. Although many clinicians are most familiar with the dosing measure of rads, modern therapy is calculated in grays (Gy) [1 Gy = 100 rads; 1 centigray (1 cGy) = 1 rad]. High-energy, external-beam radiation sources, ranging to 25 mV for the betatron and linear accelerator, have significantly reduced the complication rates after radiation therapy and possibly improved the cure rates. An intracavitary pelvic dosage derived from the gamma rays of radium or cesium is complementary to the megavoltage external-beam irradiation to ensure tumoricidal dosages to the cervix, broad ligaments, and lateral pelvic walls. Extended fields of external radiation can deliver therapy to common iliac and aortic nodal tissues.

Survival rates of irradiation and primary surgery can be compared by analyzing the reports from patients treated for stage I cervical cancer. Patients treated by irradiation have an average 5-year survival rate essentially identical to the survival rate for those who undergo radical surgery (Table 46.14).

TABLE 46.14.
5-Year Survival Rates of Patients with Stage I Cancer of Cervix by Treatment Modality

Investigators	Number of Patients	5-Year Survival Rate (%)
SURGERY		
Morley and Seski, 1976	149	91.3
Zander et al., 1981	747	84.5
Noguchi, 1987	191	85.3
Barber, 1988	273	78.8
Carenza, 1988	105	85.7
Fuller et al., 1989	285	86.0
Kentler, 1989	178	87.0
Lee, 1989	237	86.1
Monaghan, 1990	494	83.0
Hopkins, 1991	213	89.0
Alvarez, 1991	401	85.0
Burghardt, 1992	443	83.4
Massi, 1993	211	75.8
TOTAL	3,526	84.2
RADIOTHERAPY		
Madowski et al., 1962	442	81.3
Kottmeier, 1964	611	89.5
Crawford et al., 1965	63	46.0
Masubuchi et al., 1969	152	88.2
Marcial, 1970	41	87.0
Neinminen and Pollanen, 1970	77	70.0
Fletcher, 1971	549	91.5
Newton, 1975	61	74.0
Einhorn, 1975	60	88.0
Petersson, 1987	160	76.9
TOTAL	2,196	85.1

The traditional brachytherapy systems for cervical cancer have been low-dose-rate systems delivering 0.4 to 2 Gy per hour, and typical implants have been of 24- to 72-hour durations. More recently, high-dose-rate systems have been employed, capable of delivering dose rates of more than 0.2 Gy per minute, thereby allowing treatments of only a few minutes' duration and adaptable to the outpatient, rather that the inpatient, setting. A comparison of 5-year survival rates of the two systems by clinical stage documents the usefulness of the newer system (Table 46.15).

In the United States, radical hysterectomy generally is recommended for women with stage IA2 and IB1 cervical cancer who are good operative risks, especially if they are premenopausal. Women with larger tumors and those who are at risk for surgical complications generally are referred for radiation therapy.

SUMMARY

Many improvements have been made in the operative technique of the radical hysterectomy and lymphadenectomy since its original description. The incidence of complications after this procedure has decreased during the past 75 years, and the survival rates have increased. The operation has achieved its peak of clinical usefulness during this period and is now considered to be the principal method of treatment of early invasive carcinoma of the cervix. Among the better surgical institutions, the meticulous execution of this operative procedure has reduced the incidence of complications to an acceptable and infrequent occurrence. The operation affords little additional surgical risk to the patient than a hysterectomy performed for benign disease. In medical centers in which the operation is performed well, the 5-year cure rate for stage IB1 carcinoma of the cervix is over 90%. Newer laparoscopic approaches are promising with comparable cure rates and the potential to retain fertility in carefully selected patients.

Comparative studies with primary radiation therapy have demonstrated an equal cure rate with primary radical surgery in the treatment of early-stage disease. However, the complications of irradiation are far more difficult to manage than are those of primary surgery. In young women, when preservation of ovarian function is important, primary surgery is a preferable choice of treatment.

The major limiting factor in the long-term surgical cure of cervical cancer is related to the spread of the disease at the time of initiation of treatment. Historically, in cases in which pelvic lymph nodes were positive for metastatic tumor, the 5-year cure rate was reduced to about 60%. However, numerous recently reported prospective, randomized trials have demonstrated the benefit of concurrent chemotherapy and radiation therapy in various settings. In the management of high-risk patients after radical hysterectomy and pelvic lymphadenectomy, including those with positive nodes, the reported 4-year disease-free survival is 80%.

It is important to understand that it is the individual surgical expertise that offers the highest cure rate and lowest incidence of complications to the patient with invasive carcinoma of the cervix. One of the greatest errors in clinical judgment is made by the gynecologist who attempts a radical hysterectomy and pelvic lymph node dissection without adequate surgical training and experience. Unless the pelvic surgeon is performing this type of surgery regularly in a well-staffed medical center with trained assistants, he or she would be well advised to refer the patient to an established cancer center. From the patient's point of view, the initial treatment, whether primary surgery or irradiation, provides the best chance for long-term cure of this disease. It would be to her advantage to have the treatment conducted in the most expert hands because secondary treatment for recurrent disease offers only limited potential long-term cure.

The gynecologic surgeon who becomes thoroughly familiar with the pathology and natural history of cervical cancer, who appreciates the history of the development of radical hysterectomy and pelvic lymphadenectomy as primary treatment of the disease, and who then thoroughly masters the technical details of performing the operation can feel enormous pride in his or her achievement because there is no greater challenge in gynecologic surgery and no greater personal satisfaction than that which comes to those who are able to perform the operation correctly and save a woman from the intense suffering and undignified death that cervical cancer can cause.

TABLE 46.15.
High Dose Rate (HDR) versus Low Dose Rate (LDR) Intracavitary Brachytherapy for Carcinoma of the Cervix, 1979 to 1981

Stage	Number of Patients (HDR/LDR)	5-Year Survival Rate (%) HDR	5-Year Survival Rate (%) LDR
I	160/422	76.9	71.6
II	358/796	58.1	54.4
III	386/588	38.1	38.4
IV	66/50	15.2	10.0

From: Annual report on the results of treatment in gynecological cancer. In: Pettersson F, ed. *Twentieth volume statements of results obtained in patients treated in 1979–81, including 5-year survival up to 1986.* Stockholm: International Federation of Gynecology and Obstetrics, 1987:52, with permission.

BIBLIOGRAPHY

Abu-Rustum NR, Hoskins WJ. Radical abdominal hysterectomy. *Surg Clin North Am* 2001;81(4):815.

Abu-Rustum NR, Lee S, Correa A, et al. Compliance with and acute hematologic toxic effects of chemoradiation in indigent women with cervical cancer. *Gynecol Oncol* 2001; 81(1):88.

Abu-Rustum NR, Lee S, Massad LS. Screening for HIV infection in indigent women with newly diagnosed cervical cancer. *J Acquir Immune Defic Syndr* 2001;27(1):95.

Abu-Rustum NR, Lee S, Massad LS. Topotecan for recurrent cervical cancer after platinum-based therapy. *Int J Gynecol Cancer* 2000;10(4):285.

Abu-Rustum NR, Rajbhandari D, Glusman S, et al. Acute lower extremity paralysis following radiation therapy for cervical cancer. *Gynecol Oncol* 1999;75(1):152.

Ahrens CA, Tschoke S. Lvmphknotenbefunde nach Wertheim Meigscher operation. *Geburtshilfe Frauenheilkd* 1961;21: 219.

Albores-Saavedra J, Gersell D, Gilks CB, et al. Terminology of endocrine tumors of the uterine cervix: results of a workshop sponsored by the College of American Pathologists and the National Cancer Institute. *Arch Pathol Lab Med* 1997;121:34.

Altgassen C, Possover M, Krause N, et al. Establishing a new technique of laparoscopic pelvic and paraaortic lymphadenectomy. *Obstet Gynecol* 2000;95(3):348.

Alvarez RD, Helm CW, Edwards RP, et al. Prospective randomized trial of LLETZ versus laser ablation in patients with cervical intraepithelial neoplasia. *Gynecol Oncol* 1994;52:175.

Alvarez RD, Potter ME, Soong S-J, et al. Rationale for using pathologic tumor dimensions and nodal status to sub-classify treated stage IB cervical cancer patients. *Gynecol Oncol* 1991;43:108.

Anderson B, LaPolla J, Turner D, et al. Ovarian transposition in cervical cancer. *Gynecol Oncol* 1993;40:206.

Angel C, DuBeshter B, Lin JY. Clinical presentation and management of stage 1 cervical adenocarcinoma: a 25-year experience. *Gynecol Oncol* 1992;44:71.

Arneson A, Kao MS. Long-term observations of cervical cancer. *Am J Obstet Gynecol* 1987;156:614.

Axelrod JH, Fruchter R, Boyce JG. Multiple primaries among gynecologic malignancies. *Gynecol Oncol* 1984;18:359.

Balega J, Michael H, Hurteau JA, et al. The risk of nodal metastasis in early adenocarcinoma of the uterine cervix. *Gynecol Oncol* 2000;76:235(abstr).

Bandy LC, Clarke-Pearson DL, Soper JT, et al. Long-term effects on bladder function of radical hysterectomy with and without postoperative radiation. *Gynecol Oncol* 1987; 26:160.

Barber HRK. Cervical cancer: pelvic and paraaortic lymph nodes sampling and its consequences. *Baillieres Clin Obstet Gynaecol* 1988;2:768.

Barnes W, Waggoner S, Delgado G, et al. Manometric characterization of rectal dysfunction following radical hysterectomy. *Gynecol Oncol* 1991;42:116.

Behbakht K, Abu-Rustum NR, Lee S, et al. Characteristics and survival of cervical cancer patients managed at adjacent urban public and university medical centers. *Gynecol Oncol* 2001;81(1):40.

Benedet JL, Anderson GH. Stage IA carcinoma of the cervix revisited. *Obstet Gynecol* 1996;87:1052.

Berman ML, Keys H, Creasman W, et al. Survival and patterns of recurrence in cervical cancer metastatic to periaortic lymph nodes: a Gynecologic Oncology Group study. *Gynecol Oncol* 1984;19:8.

Bleker OP, Ketting BW, van Wayjen-Eecen B, et al. The significance of microscopic involvement of the parametrium and or pelvic lymph nodes in cervical cancer stages IB and IIA. *Gynecol Oncol* 1983;6:56.

Blythe JG, Hodel KA, Wahl TP. A comparison between peritoneal sheathing of the ureters (Ohkawa technique) and retroperitoneal pelvic suction drainage in the prevention of ureteral damage during radical abdominal hysterectomy. *Gynecol Oncol* 1988;30:222.

Bonney V. The results of 500 cases of Wertheim's operation for carcinoma of the cervix. *J Obstet Gynaecol Br Emp* 1941;48:421.

Bosch FX, Castellsague X, Munoz N, et al. Male sexual behavior and human papillomavirus DNA: key risk factors for cervical cancer in Spain. *J Natl Cancer Inst* 1996;88:1060.

Bosch FX, Manos MM, Munoz N, et al. Prevalence of human papillomavirus in cervical cancer: a worldwide perspective. *J Natl Cancer Inst* 1995;87:796.

Brewer CA, Chan J, Kurosaki T, et al. Radical hysterectomy with the endoscopic stapler. *Gynecol Oncol* 1998;71:50.

Broders AC. The grading of carcinoma. *Mim Med* 1925;8:726.

Buchsbaum HJ. Extrapelvic lymph node metastases in cervical carcinoma. *Am J Obstet Gynecol* 1979;133:814.

Buller RE, Tamir IL, DiSaia PJ, et al. Early evaluation of the urinary tract following radical hysterectomy; structure and function relationships. *Obstet Gynecol* 1991;78:840.

Burghardt E, Baltzer J, Tulusan AH, et al. Results of surgical treatment of 1028 cervical cancers studied with volumetry. *Cancer* 1992;70:648.

Burghardt E, Pickel H. Local spread and lymph node involvement in cervical cancer. *Obstet Gynecol* 1978;52:138.

Burghardt E, Pickel H, Haas J, et al. Prognostic factors and operative treatment of stages IB to IIB cervical cancer. *Am J Obstet Gynecol* 1987;156:988.

Burghardt E, Girardi F, Lahousen M, et al. Microinvasive carcinoma of the uterine cervix (International Federation of Gynecology and Obstetrics stage IA). *Cancer* 1991; 67:1037.

Centers for Disease Control and Prevention. 1993 revised classification system for HIV infection and expanded surveillance case definition for AIDS among adolescents and adults. *MMWR* 1993;41:1.

Chamberlin DH, Hopkins MP, Roberts JA, et al. The effects of early removal of indwelling urinary catheter after radical hysterectomy. *Gynecol Oncol* 1991;43:98.

Chambers SK, Chambers JT, Holm C, et al. Sequelae of lateral ovarian transposition in unirradiated cervical cancer patients. *Gynecol Oncol* 1990;39:155.

Chapman JA, Mannel RS, DiSaia PJ, et al. Surgical treatment of unexpected invasive cervical cancer found at total hysterectomy. *Obstet Gynecol* 1992;80:931.

Chen MD, Lim PC, Spirtos NM. Laparoscopic radical hysterectomy. *CME J Gynecol Oncol* 2001.

Chen F, Trapido Ej, Davia K. Differences in stage at presentation of breast and gynecologic cancers among whites, blacks, and Hispanics. *Cancer* 1994;73:2838.

Chi DS. Laparoscopy in gynecologic malignancies. *Oncology (Huntington)* 1999;13(6):773.

Childers JM, Hatch K, Surwit EA. The role of laparoscopic lymphadenectomy in the management of cervical carcinoma. *Gynecol Oncol* 1992;47(1):38.

Chu KK, Chang SD, Chen FP, et al. Laparoscopic surgical staging in cervical cancer—preliminary experience among Chinese. *Gynecol Oncol* 1997;64(1):49.

Chung CK, Nahhas WA, Zaino R, et al. Histologic grade and lymph node metastasis in squamous cell carcinoma of the cervix. *Gynecol Oncol* 1981;12:348.

Clark JG. A more radical method of performing hysterectomy for cancer of the uterus. *Bull Johns Hopkins Hosp* 1895; 6:120.

Clarke-Pearson DL, DeLong E, Synan IS, et al. A controlled trial of two low-dose heparin regimens for the prevention of postoperative deep vein thrombosis. *Obstet Gynecol* 1990;75:684.

Clarke-Pearson DL, Jelovsek FR, Creasman WT. Thromboembolism complicating surgery for cervical and uterine malignancy: incidence, risk factors, and prophylaxis. *Obstet Gynecol* 1983;61:87.

Clarke-Pearson DL, Synan IS, Dodge R, et al. A randomized trial of low-dose heparin and intermittent pneumatic calf compression for the prevention of deep venous thrombosis after gynecologic oncology surgery. *Am J Obstet Gynecol* 1993;168:1146.

Cohn DE, Swisher EM, Herzog TJ, et al. Radical hysterectomy for cervical cancer in obese women. *Obstet Gynecol* 2000;96:727.

Corbett PJ, Crompton AC. Invasive carcinoma of one cervix in a uterus didelphys. Case report. *Br J Obstet Gynaecol* 1982;89:171–172.

Covens A, Shaw P, Murphy J, et al. Is radical trachelectomy a safe alternative to radical hysterectomy for patients with stage IA-B carcinoma of the cervix? *Cancer* 1999; 86(11):2273.

Creasman WT, Zaino RJ, Major FJ, et al. Early invasive carcinoma of the cervix (3 to 5 mm invasion): risk factors and prognosis. A Gynecologic Oncology Group study. *Am J Obstet Gynecol* 1998;178:62.

Creasman WT. New gynecologic cancer staging [editorial]. *Gynecol Oncol* 1995;58:157.

Currie JL. *A cosmetically-pleasing transverse incision for pelvic surgery.* ACOG Film Library, 1996.

Curtin JP, Hoskins WJ, Venkatraman ES, et al. Adjuvant chemotherapy versus chemotherapy plus pelvic irradiation for high-risk cervical cancer patients after radical hysterectomy and pelvic lymphadenectomy (RH-PLND): a randomized phase III trial. *Gynecol Oncol* 1996;61(1):3.

Dargent D, Ansquer Y, Mathevet P. Technical development and results of left extraperitoneal laparoscopic paraaortic lymphadenectomy for cervical cancer. *Gynecol Oncol* 2000;77(1):87.

Dargent D, Brun JL, Roy M, et al. Pregnancies following radical trachelectomy for invasive cervical cancer. *Gynecol Oncol* 1994;52:105 (abstr).

Dargent D, Martin X, Sacchetoni A, et al. Laparoscopic vaginal radical trachelectomy: a treatment to preserve the fertility of cervical carcinoma patients. *Cancer* 2000; 88(8):1877.

Dargent D, Mathevet P. Schauta's vaginal hysterectomy combined with laparoscopic lymphadenectomy. *Baillieres Clin Obstet Gynaecol* 1995;9(4):691.

Dargent D. A new future for Schauta's operation through presurgical retroperitoneal pelviscopy. *Eur J Gynaecol Oncol* 1987;8:292.

Dargent D. Using radical trachelectomy to preserve fertility in early invasive cervical cancer. *Contemp Ob/Gyn* 2000; 45:23.

deJesus M, Tang W, Sadjadi M, et al. Carcinoma of the cervix with extensive endometrial and myometrial involvement. *Gynecol Oncol* 1990;36:263.

Delgado G, Bundy BN, Zaino R, et al. Prospective surgical-pathological study of disease-free interval in patients with stage IB squamous cell carcinoma of the cervix: a Gynecologic Oncology Group study. *Gynecol Oncol* 1990;38:352.

Devesa SS, Grauman DJ, Blot WJ, et al. *Atlas of cancer mortality in the United States, 1950–1994.* Bethesda, MD: National Institutes of Health, National Cancer Institute, 1999 (NIH Publ No. 99-4564).

Downey GO, Potish RA, Adcock LL, et al. Pretreatment surgical staging in cervical carcinoma: therapeutic efficacy of pelvic lymph node resection. *Am J Obstet Gynecol* 1989;160:1055.

Drescher CW, Hopkins MP, Roberts JA. Comparison of the pattern of metastatic spread of squamous cell cancer and adenocarcinoma of the uterine cervix. *Gynecol Oncol* 1989;33:340.

Eifel PJ, Burke TW, Morris M, et al. Adenocarcinoma as an independent risk factor for disease recurrence in patients with stage IB cervical carcinoma. *Gynecol Oncol* 1995;59:38.

Ellerbrock TV, Chiasson MA, Bush TJ, et al. Incidence of cervical squamous intraepithelial lesions in HIV-infected women. *JAMA* 2000;283:1031.

Elliott P, Coppleseon M, Russell P, et al. Early invasive (FIGO stage IA) carcinoma of the uterine cervix: a clinico-pathologic study of 475 cases. *Int J Gynecol Cancer* 2000;10.42.

Ellsworth LR, Allen HH, Nisker JA. Ovarian function after radical hysterectomy for stage IB carcinoma of the cervix. *Am J Obstet Gynecol* 1983;145:185.

Estape R, Angioli R, Wagman F, et al. Significance of intraperitoneal cytology in patients undergoing radical hysterectomy. *Gynecol Oncol* 1998;68:169.

Fanning J, Kraus K. Surgical stapling technique for radical hysterectomy: survival, recurrence, and late complications. *Gynecol Oncol* 2000;79:281.

Fernando JN, Moskovic E, Fryatt I, et al. Is there a role for lymphography in the management of early-stage carcinoma of the cervix? *Br J Radiol* 1994;67:1052.

Ferrante JM, Gonzalez EC, Roetzheim RG, et al. Clinical and demographic predictors of late-stage cervical cancer. *Arch Fam Med* 2000;9:439.

Fletcher GH. Predominant parameters in the planning of radiation therapy of carcinoma of the cervix. *Bull Cancer* 1979;66:561.

Fowler JM, Carter JR, Carlson JW, et al. Lymph node yield from laparoscopic lymphadenectomy in cervical cancer: a comparative study. *Gynecol Oncol* 1993;51(2):187.

Franchi M, Ghezzi F, Zanaboni F, et al. Nonclosure of peritoneum at radical abdominal hysterectomy and pelvic node dissection: a randomized study. *Obstet Gynecol* 1997;90:622.

Freund WA. Eine neue methode der exstirpation des ganten uterus. *Zentralbl Gynakol* 1878;10:222.

Freund WA. Method of complete removal of the uterus. *Am J Obstet Gynecol* 1879;7:200.

Fuchtner C, Manetta A, Walker JL, et al. Radical hysterectomy in the elderly patient: analysis of morbidity. *Am J Obstet Gynecol* 1992;166:593.

Fuller AF Jr, Elliott N, Kosloff C, et al. Determinants of increased risk for recurrence in patients undergoing radical hysterectomy for stage IB and IIA carcinoma of the cervix. *Gynecol Oncol* 1989;33:34.

Gallion HH, van Nagell JR Jr, Donaldson ES, et al. Combined radiation therapy and extrafascial hysterectomy in the treatment of stage IB barrel-shaped cervical cancer. *Cancer* 1985;56:262.

Gallup DG, Jordan GH, Talledo OE. Extraperitoneal lymph node dissections with use of a midline incision on patients with female genital cancer. *Am J Obstet Gynecol* 1986; 155:559.

Garza-Leal J. Vaginally assisted laparoscopic radical hysterectomy in Mexico. *J Am Assoc Gynecol Laparosc* 1994;1(4):S12.

Geisler JP, Geisler HE. Radical hysterectomy in the elderly female: a comparison to patients age 50 or younger. *Gynecol Oncol* 2001;80:258.

Gilks CB, Young RH, Gersell D, et al. Large cell neuroendocrine carcinoma of the uterine cervix: a clinicopathologic study of 12 cases. *Am J Surg Pathol* 1997;21:905.

Gilliland JD, Spies JB, Brown SB, et al. Lymphoceles: percutaneous treatment with povidone-iodine sclerosis. *Radiology* 1989;171:227.

Girardi F, Lichtenegger W, Tamussino K, et al. The importance of parametrial lymph nodes in the treatment of cervical cancer. *Gynecol Oncol* 1989;34:206.

Goldberger SB, Rosen DJD, Fejgin MD, et al. An unusually aggressive verrucose carcinoma of the uterine cervix. *Acta Obstet Gynecol Scand* 1988;67:369.

Green TH Jr, Meigs JV, Ulfelder H, et al. Urologic complications of radical Wertheim hysterectomy: incidence, etiology, management and prevention. *Obstet Gynecol* 1962;20:293.

Greer BE, Easterling TR, McLennan DA, et al. Fetal and maternal considerations in the management of stage I-B cervical cancer during pregnancy. *Gynecol Oncol* 1989;34:61.

Greer BE, Figge DC, Tamimi HK, et al. Stage IB adenocarcinoma of the cervix treated by radical hysterectomy and pelvic lymph node dissection. *Am J Obstet Gynecol* 1989;160:1509.

Griffenberg L, Morris M, Atkinson N, et al. The effect of dietary fiber on bowel function following radical hysterectomy. *Gynecol Oncol* 1997;66:417.

Haas S. Recommendations for prophylaxis of venous thromboembolism: international consensus and the American College of chest physicians fifth consensus conference on antithrombotic therapy. *Curr Opin Pulm Med* 2000;6:314.

Hatch KD, Hallum AV 3rd, Nour M. New surgical approaches to treatment of cervical cancer. *J Natl Cancer Inst Monogr* 1996;21:71.

Herrero R. Epidemiology of cervical cancer. *Monogr Natl Cancer Inst* 1996;21:1.

Hoffman MS, Parsons M, Gunasekaran S, et al. Distal external iliac lymph nodes in early cervical cancer. *Obstet Gynecol* 1999;94:391.

Hoffman MS, Roberts WS, Cavanagh D. Neuropathies associated with radical pelvic surgery for gynecologic cancer. *Gynecol Oncol* 1988;31:462.

Hoffman MS, Roberts WS, Cavanagh D. Second pelvic malignancies following radiation therapy for cervical cancer. *Obstet Gynecol Surv* 1985;40:611.

Hopkins MP, Morley GW. The prognosis and management of cervical cancer associated with pregnancy. *Obstet Gynecol* 1992;80:9.

Hopkins MP, Schmidt RW, Roberts JA, et al. The prognosis and treatment of stage adenocarcinoma of the cervix. *Obstet Gynecol* 1988;72:915.

Horii T, Mitsumoto T, Noda K. Significance of paraaortic node irradiation in the treatment of cervical cancer. *Gynecol Oncol* 1988;31:371.

Hoskins WJ. Prognostic factors for risk of recurrence in stages IB and IIA cervical cancer. *Baillieres Clin Obstet Gynecol* 1988;2:817.

Howell EA, Chen YT, Concato J. Differences in cervical cancer mortality among black and white women. *Obstet Gynecol* 1999;94:509.

Hsieh YY, Lin WC, Chang CC, et al. Laparoscopic radical hysterectomy with low paraaortic, subaortic and pelvic lymphadenectomy. Results of short-term follow-up. *J Reprod Med* 1998;43(6):528.

Husseinzadeh N, Nahhas WA, Velkley DE, et al. The preservation of ovarian function in young women undergoing pelvic radiation therapy. *Gynecol Oncol* 1984;18:373.

IARC. Human papillomaviruses. *IARC Monogr Eval Carcinog Risk Chem Hum* 1995;64:407.

Inoue T, Morita K. 5-year results of postoperative extended-field irradiation of 76 patients with nodal metastases from cervical carcinoma stage Ib to IIIb. *Cancer* 1988;61:2009.

Janicek MF, Averette HE. Cervical cancer: prevention, diagnosis, and therapeutics. *CA Cancer J Clin* 2001;51:92.

Jemal A, Murray T, Samuels A, et al. Cancer statistics 2003. *CA Cancer J Clin* 2003;53:5–26.

Jensen JK, Lucci JA, DiSaia PH, et al. To drain or not to drain: a retrospective study of closed-suction drainage following radical hysterectomy with pelvic lymphadenectomy. *Gynecol Oncol* 1993;512:46.

Jobsen JJ, Leer JWH, Cleton FJ, et al. Treatment of locoregional recurrence of carcinoma of the cervix by radiotherapy after primary surgery. *Gynecol Oncol* 1989;33:368.

Jones HW, Jones GES. Panhysterectomy versus irradiation in early cancer of the cervix. *JAMA* 1943;122:930.

Jones WB. Surgical approaches for advanced or recurrent cancer of the cervix. *Cancer* 1987;60:2094.

Kadar N, Saliba N, Nelson JH. The frequency, causes, and prevention of severe urinary dysfunction after radical hysterectomy. *Br J Obstet Gynaecol* 1983;90:858.

Kadar N. Laparoscopic vaginal radical hysterectomy: an operative technique and its evolution. *Gynaecol Endosc* 1994;3:109–122.

Keys HM, Bundy BN, Stehman FB, et al. Cisplatin, radiation, and adjuvant hysterectomy compared with radiation and adjuvant hysterectomy for bulky stage IB cervical carcinoma. *N Engl J Med* 1999;340:1154–1161.

Kilgore LC, Soong S-J, Gore H, et al. Analysis of prognostic features in adenocarcinoma of the cervix. *Gynecol Oncol* 1988;31:137.

Kim DH, Moon JS. Laparoscopic radical hysterectomy with pelvic lymphadenectomy for early, invasive cervical carcinoma. *J Am Assoc Gynecol Laparosc* 1998;5(4):411.

Kim SH, Choi BI, Han JK, et al. Preoperative staging of uterine cervical carcinoma: comparison of CT and MR imaging in 99 patients. *J Comput Assist Tomogr* 1993;17:633.

Kinney WK, Egorshin EV, Podratz KC. Wertheim hysterectomy in the geriatric population. *Gynecol Oncol* 1988;31:227.

Kolstad P. Follow-up study of 232 patients with stage Ia1 and 411 patients with stage Ia2 squamous cell carcinoma of the cervix (microinvasive carcinoma). *Gynecol Oncol* 1989;33:265.

Kottmeier HL. Carcinoma of the uterine cervix: radiotherapy. *Curr Top Pathol* 1981;70:237.

Krebs HB, Helmkamp BF, Sevin B-U, et al. Recurrent cancer of the cervix following radical hysterectomy and pelvic node dissection. *Obstet Gynecol* 1982;59:422.

Kundrat R. Uber die ausbreitung des karzinoms in parametranen gewebe beim Krebs des collum uteri. *Arch Gynakol* 1903;69:355.

Kurman RJ, Norris HJ, Wilkinson F. *Atlas of tumor pathology, tumors of the cervix, vagina, and vulva*, third series, fascicle 4. Washington, DC: Armed Forces Institute of Pathology, 1992.

Kuwabara Y, Suzuki M, Hashimoto M, et al. New method to prevent bladder dysfunction after radical hysterectomy for uterine cervical cancer. *J Obstet Gynaecol Res* 2000;26:1.

Lagasse LD, Creasman WT, Shingleton HM, et al. Results and complications of operative staging in cervical cancer: experience of the Gynecologic Oncology Group. *Gynecol Oncol* 1980;9:90.

Landoni F, Maneo A, Cormio G, et al. Class II versus class III radical hysterectomy in stage IB–IIA cervical cancer: a prospective randomized study. *Gynecol Oncol* 2001;80:3.

Larson DM, Copeland LJ, Malone JM Jr, et al. Diagnosis of recurrent cervical carcinoma after radical hysterectomy. *Obstet Gynecol* 1988;71:6.

Larson Malone JM Jr, Copeland LJ, et al. Ureteral assessment after radical hysterectomy. *Obstet Gynecol* 1987;69:612.

Latzko W, Schiffmann J. Klinisches and anatomisches zur radikaloperation des gebarmutterkrebses. *Zentralbl Gynakol* 1919;43:715.

Lee RB, Neglia W, Park RD. Cervical carcinoma in pregnancy. *Obstet Gynecol* 1981;58:584.

Levrant SG, Fruchter RG, Maiman M. Radical hysterectomy for cervical cancer: morbidity and survival in relation to weight and age. *Gynecol Oncol* 1992;45:317.

Lin HH, Yu HJ, Sheu BC, et al. Importance of urodynamic study before radical hysterectomy for cervical cancer. *Gynecol Oncol* 2001;81:270.

Look KY, Brunetto VL, Clarke-Pearson DL, et al. An analysis of cell type in patients with surgically staged IB carcinoma of the cervix: a Gynecologic Oncology Group study. *Gynecol Oncol* 1996;63:304.

Lopes AD, Hall JR, Monaghan JM. Drainage following radical hysterectomy and pelvic lymphadenectomy: dogma or need? *Obstet Gynecol* 1995;86:960.

Lovecchio JL, Averette HE, Donato D, et al. 5-year survival of patients with periaortic nodal metastasis in clinical stage IB and IIA cervical cancer. *Gynecol Oncol* 1989;34:43.

Luesley DM, Cullimore J, Redman CWE, et al. Loop diathermy excision of the cervical transformation zone in patients with abnormal cervical smears. *Br Med J* 1990;300:1690.

Maiman M, Fruchter RG, Guy L, et al. Human immunodeficiency virus infection and invasive cervical carcinoma. *Cancer* 1993;71:402

Maiman M, Fruchter RG, Sedlis A, et al. Prevalence, risk factors, and accuracy of cytologic screening for cervical intraepithelial neoplasia in women with human immunodeficiency virus. *Gynecol Oncol* 1998;68:233.

Mann WJ, Vogel F, Patsner B, et al. Management of lymphocysts after radical gynecologic surgery. *Gynecol Oncol* 1989;33:248.

Martin XJ, Golfier F, Romestaing P, et al. First case of pregnancy after radical trachelectomy and pelvic irradiation. *Gynecol Oncol* 1999;74(2):286–287.

Martzloff KH. Carcinoma of the cervix uteri: a pathological and clinical study with particular reference to the relative malignancy of the neoplastic process as indicated by the predominant type of cancer cell. *Bull Johns Hopkins Hosp* 1923;34:141.

Massi G, Savino L, Susini T. Schauta-Amreich vaginal hysterectomy and Wertheim-Meigs abdominal hysterectomy in the treatment of cervical cancer: a retrospective analysis. *Am J Obstet Gynecol* 1993;168:928.

Matsuyama T, Inoue I, Tsukamoto N, et al. Stage Ib, IIa, and IIb cervical cancer postsurgical staging and prognosis. *Cancer* 1984;54:3072.

Matthews CM, Morris M, Burke TW, et al. Pelvic exenteration in the elderly patient. *Obstet Gynecol* 1992;79:773.

Maxwell GL, Synan I, Dodge R, et al. A prospective randomized comparison of pneumatic compression and low-molecular-weight heparin in the postoperative prophylaxis of gynecologic oncology patients. *Gynecol Oncol* 2001;80:284 (abstr).

McCall ML, Keaty EC, Thompson JD. Conservation of ovarian tissue in the treatment of carcinoma of the cervix with radical surgery. *Am J Obstet Gynecol* 1958;75:590.

McIntyre JF, Eifel PJ, Levenback C, et al. Ureteral stricture as a late complication of radiotherapy for stage IB carcinoma of the uterine cervix. *Cancer* 1995;75:836.

Meigs JV. Carcinoma of the cervix: the Wertheim operation. *Surg Gynecol Obstet* 1944;78:195.

Meigs JV. The Wertheim operation for carcinoma of the cervix. *Am J Obstet Gynecol* 1945;49:542.

Miller BA, Kolonel LN, Bernstein L, et al. *Racial/ethnic patterns of cancer in the United States 1988–1992.* Bethesda, MD: National Institutes of Health, National Cancer Institute, 1996 (DHHS Publ No. [NIH] 96-4104).

Mitra S. Radikale vaginale hysterektomie and extraperitoneale lymphadenektomie bei rvixkrebs. *Zentralbl Gynakol* 1951;73:574.

Montana GS, Fowler WC, Varia MA. Analysis of results of radiation therapy for stage IB carcinoma of the cervix. *Cancer* 1989;60:2195.

Montana GS, Hanlon AL, Brickner TJ, et al. Carcinoma of the cervix: patterns of care studies; review of 1978, 1983 and 1988–1989 surveys. *Int J Radiat Oncol Biol Phys* 1995;32:1481.

Moore DH, Fowler WC, Walton LA, et al. Morbidity of lymph node sampling in cancers of the uterine corpus and cervix. *Obstet Gynecol* 1989;74:180.

Morley GW, Hopkins MP, Lindenauer SM, et al. Pelvic exenteration, University of Michigan: 100 patients at 5 years. *Obstet Gynecol* 1989;74:934.

Morris M, Eifel PJ, Lu J, et al. Pelvic radiation with concurrent chemotherapy versus pelvic and paraaortic radiation for high-risk cervical cancer: a randomized radiation therapy oncology group clinical trial. *N Engl J Med* 1999;340:1137.

Morris PC, Haugen J, Anderson B, et al. The significance of peritoneal cytology in stage IB cervical cancer. *Obstet Gynecol* 1992;80:196.

Morrow CP, Curtin JP. Surgical anatomy. In: Morrow CP, Curtin JP, eds. *Gynecologic cancer surgery.* New York: Churchill Livingstone, 1996:67.

Morrow CP. Panel report: is pelvic radiation beneficial in the postoperative management of stage IB squamous-cell carcinoma of the cervix with pelvic node metastases treated by radical hysterectomy and pelvic lymphadenectomy? *Gynecol Oncol* 1980;10:105.

Mundy AR. An anatomical explanation of bladder dysfunction following rectal and uterine surgery. *Br J Urol* 1982;54:501.

Nagarsheth NP, Maxwell GL, Bentley RC, et al. Bilateral pelvic lymph node metastases in a case of FIGO stage IA1 adenocarcinoma of the cervix. *Gynecol Oncol* 2000;77:467.

Nahhas WA, Abt AB, Mortel R. Stage IB glassy cell carcinoma of the cervix with ovarian metastases. *Gynecol Oncol* 1977;5:87.

Navratil E. Indications and results of the vaginal and abdominal radical operation in the treatment of carcinoma of the cervix. *J Int Coll Surg* 1965;43:82.

Nelson JH, Boyce J, Macasaet M, et al. Incidence, significance and follow-up of paraaortic lymph node metastases in late invasive carcinoma of the cervix. *Am J Obstet Gynecol* 1977;128:336.

Nezhat CR, Burrell MO, Nezhat FR, et al. Laparoscopic radical hysterectomy with paraaortic and pelvic node dissection. *Am J Obstet Gynecol* 1992;166(3):864.

Nezhat CR, Nezhat FR, Burrell MO, et al. Laparoscopic radical hysterectomy and laparoscopically assisted vaginal radical hysterectomy with pelvic and paraaortic node dissection. *J Gynecol Surg* 1993;9(2):105.

Nori D, Valentine E, Hilaris BS. The role of paraaortic node irradiation in the treatment of cancer of the cervix. *Int J Radiat Oncol Biol Phys* 1985;11:1469.

Okabayashi H. Radical abdominal hysterectomy for cancer of the cervix uteri. *Surg Gynecol Obstet* 1921;33:335.

Orr JW Jr, Orr PJ, Bolen DD, et al. Radical hysterectomy: does the type of incision matter? *Am J Obstet Gynecol* 1995; 173:399.

Orr JW, Sisson PF, Patsner B, et al. Single-dose antibiotic prophylaxis for patients undergoing extended pelvic surgery for gynecologic malignancy. *Am J Obstet Gynecol* 1990;162:718.

Ostor AG, Rome R, Zuinn M. Microinvasive adenocarcinoma of the cervix: a clinicopathologic study of 77 women. *Obstet Gynecol* 1997;89:88.

Ostor AG. Pandora's box or Ariadne's thread? Definition and prognostic significance of microinvasion in the uterine cervix. Squamous lesions. *Pathol Ann* 1995;30:103.

Ostrzenski A. A new laparoscopic abdominal radical hysterectomy: a pilot phase trial. *Eur J Surg Oncol* 1996;22(6):602.

Owens S, Roberts WS, Fiorica JV, et al. Ovarian management at the time of radical hysterectomy for cancer of the cervix. *Gynecol Oncol* 1989;35:349.

Palella FJ, Delaney KM, Moorman AC, et al. Declining morbidity and mortality among patients with advanced human immunodeficiency virus infection. *N Engl J Med* 1998; 338:853.

Parkin DM, Pisani P, Ferlay J. Global cancer statistics. *CA Cancer J Clin* 1999;49:33.

Patsner B. Closed-suction drainage verus no drainage following radical abdominal hysterectomy with pelvic lymphadenectomy for stage IB cervical cancer. *Gynecol Oncol* 1995; 57:232.

Patsner B. Radical abdominal hysterectomy using the ENDO-GIA stapler: a report of 150 cases and literature review. *Eur J Gynaecol Oncol* 1998;19:215.

Patsner B, Hackett TE. Use of the omental J-flap for prevention of postoperative complications following radical abdominal hysterectomy: report of 140 cases and review of the literature. *Gynecol Oncol* 1997;65:405.

Patsner B, Sedlacek TV, Lovecchio JL. Paraaortic node sampling in small (3-cm or less) stage IB invasive cervical cancer. *Gynecol Oncol* 1992;44:53.

Peipert JF, Wells CK, Schwartz PE, et al. Prognostic value of clinical variables in invasive cervical cancer. *Obstet Gynecol* 1994;84:746.

Peters WA 3rd, Liu PY, Barrett RJ 2nd, et al. Concurrent chemotherapy and pelvic radiation therapy compared with pelvic radiation therapy alone as adjuvant therapy after radical surgery in high-risk early-stage cancer of the cervix. *J Clin Oncol* 2000;18(8):1606.

Piver MS, Chung WS. Prognostic significance of cervical lesion size and pelvic node metastases in cervical carcinoma. *Obstet Gynecol* 1975;46:507.

Piver MS, Rutledge F, Smith JP. Five classes of extended hysterectomy for women with cervical cancer. *Obstet Gynecol* 1974;44:265.

Plante M, Roy M. Radical trachelectomy. *Op Tech Gynecol Surg* 1997;3(3):187.

Podczaski ES, Palombo C, Manetta A, et al. Assessment of pretreatment laparotomy in patients with cervical carcinoma prior to radiotherapy. *Gynecol Oncol* 1980;33:71.

Porreco R, Penn I, Droegemueller W, et al. Gynecologic malignancies in immunosuppressed organ homograft recipients. *Obstet Gynecol* 1975;45:359.

Possover M, Krause N, Drahonovsky J, et al. Left-sided suprarenal retrocrural paraaortic lymphadenectomy in advanced cervical cancer by laparoscopy. *Gynecol Oncol* 1998;71(2):219.

Possover M, Krause N, Plaul K, et al. Laparoscopic paraaortic and pelvic lymphadenectomy: experience with 150 patients and review of the literature. *Gynecol Oncol* 1998;71(1):19.

Potish RA, Downey GO, Adcock LL, et al. The role of surgical debulking in cancer of the uterine cervix. *Int J Radiat Oncol Biol Phys* 1989;17:979.

Primicero M, Montanino-Oliva M, Casa A, et al. Laparoscopic lymphadenectomy and vaginal radical hysterectomy for the treatment of cervical cancer. *J Am Assoc Gynecol Laparosc* 1996;3(4):S40.

Querleu D, Dargent D, Ansquer Y, et al. Extraperitoneal endosurgical aortic and common iliac dissection in the staging of bulky or advanced cervical carcinomas. *Cancer* 2000; 88(8):1883.

Querleu D, Leblanc E, Castelain B. Laparoscopic pelvic lymphadenectomy in the staging of early carcinoma of the cervix. *Am J Obstet Gynecol* 1991;164(2):579.

Querleu D. Laparoscopically assisted radical vaginal hysterectomy. *Gynecol Oncol* 1993;51(2):248.

Ralph G, Tamussino K, Lichtenegger W. Urological complications after radical hysterectomy with or without radiotherapy for cervical cancer. *Arch Gynecol Obstet* 1990;248:61.

Recio FO, Piver MS, Hempling RE. Pretreatment transperitoneal laparoscopic staging pelvic and paraaortic lymphadenectomy in large (> or = 5 cm) stage IB2 cervical carcinoma: report of a pilot study. *Gynecol Oncol* 1996; 63(3):333.

Reiffenstuhl G. The clinical significance of the connective tissue planes and spaces. *Clin Obstet Gynecol* 1982;25:811.

Reiffenstuhl G. *The lymphatics of the female genital organs.* Philadelphia: JB Lippincott, 1964.

Reis E. Modern treatment of carcinoma of the uterus. *Chicago Med Res* 1895;9:284.

Renaud MC, Plante M, Roy M. Combined laparoscopic and vaginal radical surgery in cervical cancer. *Gynecol Oncol* 2000;79(1):59.

Roman LD, Felix JC, Muderspach LI, et al. Risk of residual invasive disease in women with microinvasive squamous cell cancer in a conization specimen. *Obstet Gynecol* 1997; 90:759.

Rose PG. Type II radical hysterectomy: evaluating its role in cervical cancer. *Gynecol Oncol* 2001;80:1 (editorial).

Rose PG, Bundy BN, Watkins EB, et al. Concurrent cisplatin-based radiotherapy and chemotherapy for locally advanced cervical cancer. *N Engl J Med* 1999;340:1144.

Rose PG, Lappas T. Analysis of cost effectiveness of concurrent cisplatin-based chemoradiation in cervical cancer: implications from five randomized trials. *Gynecol Oncol* 2000;78:3.

Rosenshein NB, Ruth JC, Villar J, et al. A prospective randomized study of doxycycline as a prophylactic antibiotic in patients undergoing radical hysterectomy. *Gynecol Oncol* 1983;15:201.

Rotmensch J, Rosenshein NB, Woodruff JD. Cervical sarcoma: a review. *Obstet Gynecol Surv* 1983;38:456.

Roy M, Plante M. Pregnancies after radical vaginal trachelectomy for early-stage cervical cancer. *Am J Obstet Gynecol* 1998;179(6):1491.

Roy M, Plante M, Renaud MC, et al. Vaginal radical hysterectomy versus abdominal radical hysterectomy in the treatment of early-stage cervical cancer. *Gynecol Oncol* 1996;62(3):336.

Russell AH, Anderson M, Walter J, et al. The integration of computed tomography and magnetic resonance imaging in treatment planning for gynecologic cancer. *Clin Obstet Gynecol* 1992;35:55.

Rutledge FN, Fletcher GH, MacDonald RJ. Pelvic lymphadenectomy as an adjunct to radiation therapy in treatment for cancer of the cervix. *Am J Roentgenol Radium Ther Nucl Med* 1965;93:607.

Rutledge FN, Mitchell MF, Munsell M, et al. Youth as a prognostic factor in carcinoma of the cervix: a matched analysis. *Gynecol Oncol* 1992;44:123.

Saigo PE, Cain JM, Kim WS, et al. Prognostic factors in adenocarcinoma of the uterine cervix. *Cancer* 1986;57:1584.

Sall S, Rini S, Pineda A. Surgical management of invasive carcinoma of the cervix in pregnancy. *Am J Obstet Gynecol* 1974;118:1.

Sampson JA. A careful study of the parametrium in twenty-seven cases of carcinoma cervices uteri and its clinical significance. *Am J Obstet* 1906;54:433.

Sardi J, Vidaurreta J, Bermudez A, et al. Laparoscopically assisted Schauta operation: learning experience at the Gynecologic Oncology Unit, Buenos Aires University Hospital. *Gynecol Oncol* 1999;75(3):361.

Schellhas HF. Extraperitoneal paraaortic node sampling in small stage IB invasive cervical cancer. *Gynecol Oncol* 1992;44:53.

Schiffman MII, Brinton LA. The epidemiology of cervical carcinogenesis. *Cancer* 1995;76:1888.

Schlaerth JB, Spirtos NM, Boike GM, et al. Laparoscopic retroperitoneal lymphadenectomy followed by laparotomy in women with cervical cancer. *Gynecol Oncol* 1999;72:443 (abstr).

Schneider A, Possover M, Kamprath S, et al. Laparoscopy-assisted radical vaginal hysterectomy modified according to Schauta-Stoeckel. *Obstet Gynecol* 1996;88(6):1057.

Schneidler J, Hricak H, Yu KK, et al. Radiologic evaluation of lymph nodes in patients with cervical cancer. Meta analysis. *JAMA* 1997;278:1096.

Scotti RJ, Bergman A, Bhatia NN, et al. Urodynamic changes in urethrovesical function after radical hysterectomy. *Obstet Gynecol* 1986;68:111.

Scribner DR, Kamelle SA, Gould N, et al. *Gynecol Oncol* 2001;81:481.

Sedlacek TV, Campion MJ, Hutchins RA, et al. Laparoscopic radical hysterectomy: a preliminary report. *J Am Assoc Gynecol Laparosc* 1994;1(4):S32.

Sedlacek TV, Campion MJ, Reich H, et al. Laparoscopic radical hysterectomy: a feasibility study. *Gynecol Oncol* 1995;56:126 (abstr).

Sedlis A, Bundy BN, Rotman MZ, et al. A randomized trial of pelvic radiation therapy versus no further therapy in selected patients with stage IB carcinoma of the cervix after radical hysterectomy and pelvic lymphadenectomy: a Gynecologic Oncology Group Study. *Gynecol Oncol* 1999;73(2):177.

Seibel MM, Freeman MG, Graves WL. The effect of surgical and radiation treatment for cervical carcinoma on sexual function. *South Med J* 1982;75:1195.

Sevin B-U, Ramos R, Lichtinger M, et al. Antibiotic prevention of infections complicating radical abdominal hysterectomy. *Obstet Gynecol* 1984;64:539.

Sheets EE, Berman ML, Hrountas CK, et al. Surgically treated, early stage neuroendocrine small-cell cervical carcinoma. *Obstet Gynecol* 1988;71:10.

Shepherd JH, Crawford RA, Oram DH. Radical trachelectomy: a way to preserve fertility in the treatment of early cervical cancer. *Br J Obstet Gynaecol* 1998;105(8):912.

Shepherd JH, Mould T, Oram DH. Radical trachelectomy in early stage carcinoma of the cervix: outcome as judged by recurrence and fertility rates. *Br J Obstet Gynaecol* 2001;108(8):882.

Shingleton HM, Bell MC, Fremgen A, et al. Is there really a difference in survival of women with early stage squamous cell carcinoma, adenocarcinoma and adenosquamous cell carcinoma of the cervix? *Cancer* 1995;76:1948.

Shingleton HM, Orr JW Jr. *Cancer of the cervix: diagnosis and treatment,* second ed. Edinburgh: Churchill Livingstone, 1987.

Shingleton HM, Orr JW, eds. *Cancer of the cervix.* Philadelphia: JB Lippincott, 1995.

Shingleton HM, Soong SJ, Gelder MS, et al. Clinical and histopathologic factors predicting recurrence and survival after pelvic exenteration for cancer of the cervix. *Obstet Gynecol* 1989;73:1027.

Shingleton HM, Thompson JD. Cancer of the cervix. In: Rock JA, Thompson JD, eds. *Te Linde's operative gynecology,* eighth ed. Philadelphia: Lippincott-Raven, 1997:1413–1499.

Smith HO, Tiffany MF, Qualls CR, et al. The rising incidence of adenocarcinoma relative to squamous cell carcinoma of the uterine cervix in the United States—a 24-year population-based study. *Gynecol Oncol* 2000;78:97.

Soisson AP, Geszler G, Soper JT, et al. A comparison of symptomatology, physical examination, and vaginal cytology in the detection of recurrent cervical carcinoma after radical hysterectomy. *Obstet Gynecol* 1990;76:106.

Soisson AP, Soper JT, Berchuck A, et al. Radical hysterectomy in obese women. *Obstet Gynecol* 1992;80:940.

Sood AK, Sorosky JI, Krogman S, et al. Surgical management of cervical cancer complicating pregnancy: a case-control study. *Gynecol Oncol* 1996;63:294.

Spirtos NM, Eisenkop SM, Schlaerth JB, et al. Laparoscopic radical hysterectomy (type III) with aortic and pelvic lymphadenectomy: surgical morbidity and intermediate-term follow-up. *Gynecol Oncol* 2000;76:232 (abstr).

Spirtos NM, Schlaerth JB, Ballon SC. Laparoscopic radical hysterectomy (type III) with aortic and pelvic lymphadenectomy. *Op Techn Gynecol Surg* 1997;2(3):200.

Spirtos NM, Schlaerth JB, Kimball RE, et al. Laparoscopic radical hysterectomy (type III) with aortic and pelvic lymphadenectomy. *Am J Obstet Gynecol* 1996;174(6):1763.

Spirtos NM, Schlaerth JB, Spirtos TW, et al. Laparoscopic bilateral pelvic and paraaortic lymph node sampling: an evolving technique. *Am J Obstet Gynecol* 1995;173(1):105.

Stallworthy J. Radical surgery following radiation treatment for cervical carcinoma. *Ann R Coll Surg Engl* 1964;34:161.

Stehman FB, Bundy BN, DiSaia PJ, et al. Carcinoma of the cervix treated with radiation therapy I: a multi-variate analysis of prognostic variables in the gynecologic oncology group. *Cancer* 1991;67:2776.

Stryker JA, Mortel R. Survival following extended field irradiation in carcinoma of cervix metastatic to paraaortic lymph nodes. *Gynecol Oncol* 2000;79:399.

Su TH, Wang KG, Yang YC, et al. Laparoscopic paraaortic lymph node sampling in the staging of invasive cervical carcinoma: including a comparative study of 21 laparotomy cases. *Int J Gynaecol Obstet* 1995;49(3):311.

Sun XW, Kuhn L, Ellerbrock TV, et al. Human papillomavirus infection in HIVB seropositive women; natural history and variability of detection. *N Engl J Med* 1997;337:1343.

Sutton G, Bundy B, Delgado G, et al. Ovarian metastases in stage IB carcinoma of the cervix. *Am J Obstet Gynecol* 1992;166:50.

Symmonds RE, Pratt JH. Prevention of fistulas and lymphocysts in radical hysterectomy: preliminary report of a new technique. *Obstet Gynecol* 1961;17:57.

Szarewski A, Cuzick J. Smoking and cervical neoplasia: a review of the evidence. *J Epidemiol Biostat* 1998;3:229.

Tabata M, Ichinoe K, Sakuragi N, et al. Incidence of ovarian metastases in patients with cancer of the uterine cervix. *Gynecol Oncol* 1987;28:255.

Tattersall MH, Ramirez C, Coppleson M. A randomized trial of adjuvant chemotherapy after radical hysterectomy in stage Ib-IIa cervical cancer patients with pelvic lymph node metastases. *Gynecol Oncol* 1992;46(2):176.

Thompson JD, Caputo TA, Franklin EW III, et al. The surgical management of invasive cancer of the cervix in pregnancy. *Obstet Gynecol* 1975;121:853.

Ting HC. Laparoscopic radical hysterectomy: a preliminary experience. *J Am Assoc Gynecol Laparosc* 1994;1(4):S36.

To ACW, Gore H, Shingleton HM, et al. Lymph node metastasis in cancer of the cervix: a preliminary report. *Am J Obstet Gynecol* 1986;155:388.

Underwood PB Jr, Lutz MH, Smoak DL. Ureteral injury following irradiation therapy for carcinoma of the cervix. *Obstet Gynecol* 1977;49:663.

van Nagell JR Jr, Donaldson ES, Parker JC, et al. The prognostic significance of pelvic lymph node morphology in carcinoma of the uterine cervix. *Cancer* 1977;39:2624.

Varia MA, Bundy BN, Deppe G, et al. Cervical carcinoma metastatic to paraaortic nodes: extended field radiation therapy with concomitant 5-fluorouracil and cisplatin chemotherapy: a Gynecologic Oncology Group study. *Int J Radiat Oncol Biol Phys* 1998;42(5):1015.

Vasilev SA. Obturator nerve injury: a review of management options. *Gynecol Oncol* 1994;53:152.

Vidaurreta J, Bermudez A, di Paola G, et al. Laparoscopic staging in locally advanced cervical carcinoma: a new possible philosophy? *Gynecol Oncol* 1999;75(3):366.

Walboomers JMM, Jacobs MV, Manos MM, et al. Human papillomavirus is a necessary cause of invasive cervical cancer worldwide. *J Pathol* 1999;189:12.

Webb JC, Key CR, Qualls CR, et al. Population-based study of microinvasive adenocarcinoma of the uterine cervix. *Obstet Gynecol* 2001;97:701.

Weber TM, Sostman HD, Spirtzer CE, et al. Cervical carcinoma: determination of current tumor extent versus radiation changes with MR imaging. *Radiology* 1995;194:135.

Weiser EB, Bundy BN, Hoskins WJ, et al. Extraperitoneal versus transperitoneal selective paraaortic lymphadenectomy in the pretreatment surgical staging of advanced cervical carcinoma (Gynecologic Oncology Group Study). *Gynecol Oncol* 1989;33:283.

Wentz WB, Reagan JW. Survival in cervical cancer with respect to cell type. *Cancer* 1959;12:384.

Wertheim E. *Die erweiterte abdominale operation bei carcinoma colli uteri (auf grund von 500 fallen)*. Berlin: Urban, 1911.

Wertheim E. Discussion on the diagnosis and treatment of carcinoma of the uterus. *Br Med J* 1905;2:689.

Wertheim E. The extended abdominal operation for carcinoma of the cervix. *Am J Obstet Gynecol* 1912;66:169.

Wertheim E. Zur frag der radikaloperation beim uteruskrebs. *Arch Gynakol* 1900;61:627.

Wertheim MS, Hakes TB, Daghestani AN, et al. A pilot study of adjuvant therapy in patients with cervical cancer at high risk of recurrence after radical hysterectomy and pelvic lymphadenectomy. *J Clin Oncol* 1985;3(7):912.

Whitney CW, Sause W, Bundy BN, et al. Randomized comparison of fluorouracil plus cisplatin versus hydroxyurea as an adjunct to radiation therapy in stage IIB-IVA carcinoma of the cervix with negative paraaortic lymph nodes: a Gynecologic Oncology Group and Southwest Oncology Group study. *J Clin Oncol* 1999;17:1339.

Wilkinson EJ, Hause L. Probability in lymph node sectioning. *Cancer* 1974;33:1269.

Wright TC. Pathogenesis and diagnosis of preinvasive lesions of the lower genital tract. In: Hoskins WJ, Perez CA, Young RC, eds. *Principles and practice of gynecologic oncology*, third ed. Philadelphia: Lippincott Williams & Wilkins, 2000:735.

Zaino RJ, Ward S, Delgado G, et al. Histopathologic predictors of the behavior of surgically treated stage IB squamous cell carcinoma of the cervix: a GOG study. *Cancer* 1990;69:1750.

Zweifel P. Zum Ancleken an die erste Totalexstirpation des Karzinomaatosen uterus. (Ausgefuhrt von Dr. John Neb Sauter in konstanz) *Much Med Wochem* 1922;69:19.

CHAPTER

47

Malignant Tumors
of the Uterine Corpus

WILLIAM T. CREASMAN

In the United States, cancer of the uterine corpus is the most common cancer of the female reproductive tract. The ACS (ACS) estimates that there will be 39,300 newly diagnosed corpus cancers in 2002, with 6,600 deaths. Most of these tumors are endometrial in origin, accounting for more than 95% of cases. Tumors of the uterine mesenchyme and mixed tumors (uterine sarcomas) account for a much smaller percentage. The incidence of uterine cancer is approximately one case per 1,000 postmenopausal women per year in the general population. It is the fourth most common cancer in women, exceeded only by carcinoma of the breast, bowel, and lung. Although the incidence of endometrial cancer increased appreciably during the first part of the 1970s, it has subsequently declined. The incidence rate for women age 50 and older declined from 116.1 per 100,000 in 1975 to 75.8 per 100,000 in 1986, and has remained stable since then. Among women 50 years of age and older, the mortality rate has declined from 17.4 per 100,000 in 1973 to approximately 13 per 100,000 in 1997.

EPIDEMIOLOGY

Endometrial adenocarcinoma occurs during both the reproductive and menopausal years. It is uncommon before the age of 40. The incidence increases with age,

peaking between 75 and 79 years. The median age at diagnosis is 66 years, but the largest number of patients is between the ages of 50 and 59 years. About one fourth of all endometrial cancers will occur before menopause.

The risk factors for endometrial cancer are united by the common theme of unopposed estrogen stimulation of the endometrium. This may be exposure to exogenous estrogens in the form of estrogen replacement therapy or tamoxifen. Or, it may be exposure to increased levels of endogenous estrogens because of morbid obesity or anovulatory states. This observation is consistent throughout epidemiologic studies of endometrial cancer risk factors, as well as in basic science studies of the biology of this disease.

The triad of obesity, nulliparity, and late menopause are factors that have been associated with endometrial cancer. In the case of obesity, this is related to the conversion of androgen to estrogen by the aromatase enzyme in adipocytes. The amount of body fat is also inversely associated with circulating levels of both progesterone and sex hormone binding globulin (SHBG). SHBG binds to circulating estrogen, making it unavailable to bind to the estrogen receptor and biologically inactive.

Studies have shown that women with a body weight over 200 lb or a body mass index (BMI) exceeding 27 have two- to four-fold increased relative risk of endometrial cancer compared with that of women of normal weight. Upper-body fat localization has also been suggested to be an important factor. Women with endometrial cancer have greater waist-to-hip circumference, abdominal-to-thigh skin fold thickness, and suprailiac-to-thigh skin fold thickness ratios than matched control women. As these ratios increase, the relative risk of endometrial cancer increases. The level of SHBG is progressively depressed with increasing upper-body fat localization.

Nulliparity appears to confer an approximately two-fold increased risk of developing endometrial cancer compared with a parity of one or more. Several studies have noted a marked decrease in the risk of endometrial cancer as the number of full term pregnancies increases. Menopause occurring after age 55 increases the risk of endometrial cancer two-fold. If a patient is nulliparous, is obese, and reaches menopause at age 52 or later, studies have suggested that she has a five-fold increase in the risk of endometrial cancer over the patient who does not satisfy these criteria.

Hypertension and diabetes have also been suggested as risk factors for endometrial cancer. Diabetes is an independent risk factor for endometrial cancer and confers about a two-fold increased relative risk, after adjusting for obesity. Hypertension has not been shown to be a risk factor independent of obesity.

Women with hereditary, nonpolyposis colon cancer (HNPCC) account for only 2% to 10% of all female cases of colon cancer; however, 5% of all endometrial cancers occur in women with this risk factor. These individuals have a 22% to 50% lifetime risk of developing endometrial cancer, according to several studies. The disease occurs at an earlier age (about 15 years younger) than in women without HNPCC. The greatest risk of developing endometrial cancer in women with HNPCC occurs between the ages of 40 and 60, during which time the absolute risk is greater than 1% per year.

Unopposed estrogen therapy in women with a uterus increases the risk of endometrial cancer two- to ten-fold, and the risk increases with the duration of use. The addition of either cyclic or continuous progestin to estrogen, reduces the risk of endometrial cancer to either equivalent to or, in some studies, less than, the expected risk of women not taking hormone replacement. Recent data would suggest that the length of cyclic progestin therapy is very important. If given cyclically, at least 10 days, and preferably 14 days, is necessary to decrease the risk of endometrial cancer. Withdrawal bleeding is expected for women taking cyclic progestin. With time, the amount and length of bleeding should decrease. Any other bleeding should be considered abnormal and investigated accordingly. In women who take continuous estrogen and progestin, amenorrhea is anticipated after a few months of use. Once this occurs, any spotting or bleeding should be investigated. It is important to remember that although progestin decreases the risk of endometrial hyperplasia and cancer, it does not confer absolute protection. Patients can still develop endometrial cancer on both adequate cyclic progestin and continuous progestin regimens.

Tamoxifen, the most common anticancer drug used today, has been suggested to increase the risk of endometrial cancer. Tamoxifen, the first selective estrogen receptor modifier (SERM), although labeled an antiestrogen, is truly a weak estrogen in some tissues. In contrast to steroidal estrogens, it appears to have inhibitory effects on the breast, yet stimulatory effects in the endometrium. It also appears to give some protection from osteoporosis and against heart disease. Its use is associated with decreased low-density lipoprotein (LDL) and total cholesterol.

There has been a considerable amount of publicity regarding the possible association between tamoxifen use and the development of endometrial cancer. The benefits of tamoxifen seem to be well documented. An early breast cancer cooperative study concluded that the drug is beneficial in preventing the recurrence of breast cancer or the development of contralateral disease in women who have a history of breast cancer. This includes both pre- and postmenopausal women with either positive or negative lymph nodes, as long as the tumor is estrogen-receptor positive. In the United States, more than 180,000 new invasive breast cancers are diagnosed each year, and the majority of these tumors are estrogen-receptor positive. Today the recommendation for such individuals is to take tamoxifen, 20 mg per day, for 5 years. Therefore, it appears that several hundred thousand women in the United States are on this drug at any given time. Recent data suggest tamoxifen is also of benefit to women with ductal cell carcinoma *in situ*. About 50,000 women in the United States have this diagnosis made each year.

A large study in the United States evaluated the role of tamoxifen prophylaxis in women at high risk for breast cancer, but without the disease. The investigators concluded that patients treated with tamoxifen had a significantly lower incidence of both invasive carcinoma and ductal cell carcinoma *in situ* than those who had been randomized to receive placebo. Two smaller European studies of the prophylactic use of tamoxifen in women at high-risk for breast cancer failed to show any benefit. Based on the results of the American study, it has been suggested that several million women each year in this country could potentially benefit from the prophylactic use of tamoxifen.

Although it is probably of considerable benefit, tamoxifen does have some potential adverse side effects. These include an increased incidence of thromboembolism, cataracts, endometrial pathology, and clinical hormonal effects. A large number of individuals on tamoxifen may have vasomotor symptoms and irregular bleeding. As noted previously, the most significant concern is the possibility of an increased risk of endometrial cancer among patients on tamoxifen.

The first report suggesting a link between tamoxifen and endometrial cancer was published in 1985. Three cases of endometrial cancer were reported in breast cancer patients taking the drug. Since then, this possible association was evaluated in many retrospective studies and several prospective, randomized studies of tamoxifen versus placebo in breast cancer patients. In essentially all of these studies, the development of endometrial cancer was not the primary end point of the study. Therefore, the status of the endometrium before initiating tamoxifen therapy was not evaluated. As already indicated, women on tamoxifen can have irregular bleeding. Because these are mainly postmenopausal individuals, this leads to histological evaluation of the endometrium. A detection bias could, therefore, influence a retrospective analysis. Of the 15 studies reported, 12 showed no relationship between tamoxifen use and the development of adenocarcinoma of the uterus. In one, the incidence of the disease was decreased, and in two, the researchers noted an increased incidence of endometrial cancer among women taking tamoxifen. It was the latter two studies that have received considerable publicity. When one considers that there is an increased incidence of endometrial cancer in breast cancer patients, latency, occult disease, and potential surveillance and ascertainment bias could explain the findings of these two studies. For example, in some patients, the diagnosis of endometrial cancer was made within a few months of beginning the tamoxifen. Most would agree that tamoxifen use and the development of endometrial cancer were purely coincidental, except that the tamoxifen use may have initiated the uterine bleeding earlier than it would have otherwise occurred.

In a recent case-controlled study using the SEER database, more than 300 breast cancer patients who took tamoxifen and subsequently developed endometrial cancer were compared with more than 600 breast cancer patients on tamoxifen who did not develop endometrial cancer. After controlling for confounding factors, no increased risk of endometrial cancer was associated with tamoxifen use. In a Japanese study, breast cancer patients were followed for an average of 9 years after the diagnosis of breast cancer. All patients underwent endometrial evaluation before either going on tamoxifen or not receiving the drug. Tamoxifen use was not randomized. A similar incidence of endometrial cancer was noted in both groups. It would appear that if there is an association between tamoxifen and endometrial cancer, it is very small.

In the asymptomatic patient on tamoxifen, the American College of Obstetricians and Gynecologists (ACOG) recommends only yearly pelvic exams and Papanicolaou (Pap) smears. Special studies to evaluate the endometrium in these women are not routinely recommended. Recent ACS guidelines on screening for endometrial cancer make the same recommendation. Obviously, if a woman on tamoxifen has uterine bleeding, her endometrium should be evaluated following the same protocol used for a postmenopausal patient.

The incidence and survival of endometrial cancer is higher in white women compared with blacks. The reason for this difference is unknown. In a study by the Gynecologic Oncology Group (GOG), it was noted that a larger number of black women were diagnosed after age 70. They also had a higher proportion of papillary serous and clear cell histologic types, more advanced disease, higher tumor grade, and greater depth of invasion and were more likely to have lymphvascular space involvement and lymph node metastases than were white women. Five-year survival for whites was 77%; for blacks, 60%. The survival difference remained even in subgroup analysis of high-risk groups, such as grade III (5-year survival 59% versus 37%, respectively). Although the adjusted risk ratio was only 1.2 (not a statistically significant difference), race did denote an increased risk for multiple poor prognostic factors. This may account for the observed decrease in survival among black women.

It is well accepted that combination oral contraceptives pills (OCPs) decrease the risk of developing endometrial cancer. There are now several case-controlled studies that have shown at least a 50% reduction in the risk of endometrial cancer in women who have ever used OCPs. Protection occurs in women who used OCPs for at least 12 months, and the protection continues for at least 10 years after OCP use is discontinued. This protection is most notable for nulliparous women. It has been estimated that about 2,000 cases of endometrial cancer are prevented each year in the United States by past or current OCP use.

Cigarette smoking apparently decreases the risk of endometrial cancer. A population-based case-control study noted a significant decline in the relative risk of endometrial cancer with increased smoking. The greatest reduction in the risk by smoking was in the heaviest women. Women who smoke usually go through a menopause 1 to 2 years earlier than do nonsmokers. Smoking also alters estrogen metabolism. Obviously, the advantage of smoking to reduce the risk of developing endometrial cancer is strongly outweighed by the increased risk of lung cancer and other major health hazards.

There are two phenotypic types of women with endometrial cancer. The classic findings are a woman who is white, nulliparous, and obese whose tumor tends to be well-differentiated, superficially invasive, and estrogen- and progesterone-receptor positive. These patients have a high cure rate when treated with standard therapy, including a hysterectomy and bilateral salpingo-oophorectomy. In contrast, the atypical patient is thin and parous, tends to be black, and has a tumor that is estrogen- and progesterone-receptor negative, poorly differentiated, deeply invasive, and tends to metastasize. These patients have a poor prognosis, regardless of the therapy used.

DIAGNOSIS OF ENDOMETRIAL CANCER

Screening

According to the 1989 ACOG bulletin on screening for gynecologic cancers, which was reaffirmed by the 1993 ACOG committee opinion, routine screening for endometrial cancer is neither cost-effective nor warranted. Should women who have any or all of the multiple risk factors for endometrial cancer undergo special screening tests? Certainly, all women approaching menopause or who are already menopausal should be aware of the risks and symptoms of endometrial cancer and should report any unexpected bleeding or spotting to their physicians. Based on a review of the available literature, the ACS has stated that there is no indication that screening for endometrial cancer should be recommended for women at increased risk owing to increasing age, history of unopposed estrogen therapy, late menopause, tamoxifen therapy, nulliparity, infertility, failure to ovulate, obesity, diabetes, or hypertension. The ACS did recommend annual screening for endometrial cancer with an endometrial biopsy for women with or at risk for HNPCC. It was suggested that this should be offered beginning at age 35. Women in this high-risk group should be informed about the risks and symptoms of endometrial cancer and should be informed about potential benefits, risks, and limitations of testing by either biopsy or pelvic ultrasound for early endometrial cancer detection.

Unfortunately, for corpus cancer there are no effective methods to satisfy the standard criteria for a good screening test; these criteria include patient acceptability and low cost. The often stenotic postmenopausal endocervical canal limits reliable screening for endometrial cancer. This stenosis impedes the flow of exfoliated cells from an early cancer, thus preventing a reliable cytologic screen. It also prevents an easy painless sampling of the endometrial lining. Attempts have been made to initiate screening programs for endometrial cancer. However, the routine Pap smear is notoriously unreliable in detecting endometrial cancer. Poor patient compliance with intrauterine sampling techniques has led clinicians to abandon this method of screening.

The Pap smear detects only 50% to 60% of endometrial carcinomas. Aspiration or scraping of the endocervical canal is normally 70% to 85% effective. Reagan and Ng reported 85% accuracy for all types of endometrial cancer by using a combination of endocervical aspiration and vaginal cytology. Vaginal cytology alone detected abnormal cells in only 50% of the patients with known endometrial carcinoma. Frost suggested sampling the cytologic material from the posterior fornix in combination with an endocervical scraping. The problem with this method is that the postmenopausal cervix does not always allow insertion of the tip of the spatula, so an endocervical specimen may not always be obtained. Even with the recent popularity of the endocervical brush, the Pap smear cannot be reliably used to detect endometrial cancer.

When certain Pap smear findings are present, they may be useful in identifying endometrial carcinoma. Zucker et al. evaluated 102 women with clinical pathologic correlation, by using six cytologic parameters: histiocytes, multinucleated histiocytes, nonspecific inflammation, blood, an elevated squamous maturation index, and the presence of glandular cell atypia. By using multivariate analysis, they determined that only cytologically atypical endometrial glandular cells were predictive of an endometrial lesion.

As discussed later, vaginal ultrasound has emerged as a useful technique to evaluate postmenopausal bleeding.

It has not been studied sufficiently as a widespread screening tool to recommend its use. Currie (1991) commented on the use of this modality to monitor estrogen replacement therapy. He warned that the best measurements for endometrial stripe thickness have yet to be finalized, and that even with minimal stripe measurements, endometrial pathology could be present. Therefore, this procedure is recommended only for evaluation in specific situations, not for routine screening.

Evaluation of Symptomatic Women

Abnormal uterine bleeding is the harbinger of endometrial cancer and should alert the clinician to rule out corpus cancer, regardless of the age of the patient. Five to ten percent of endometrial carcinomas occur in women younger than 40 years of age. Irregular, heavy bleeding in this age group should not be afforded the complacency of hormonal manipulation without appropriate endometrial evaluation. In the perimenopausal age group, it is even more important to sample the endometrium in situations of abnormal bleeding. Finally, any episode of postmenopausal bleeding represents endometrial cancer until proven otherwise.

Five basic categories of instruments are available to sample the endometrial cavity. They are listed in Table 47.1. Endometrial biopsy by various aspiration techniques or Novak curet, dilatation and curettage, hysteroscopy, and cytologic procedures provide the clinician

---

TABLE 47.1.
Techniques Used in the Diagnosis of Endometrial Cancer

DEFINITIVE TECHNIQUE

Dilatation and (fractional) curettage

CYTOLOGIC EVALUATION

Cervicovaginal Papanicolaou smear
Endometrial lavage
Endometrial brush

TRADITIONAL FOUR-QUADRANT BIOPSY

Novak curet

HISTOLOGIC SUCTION DEVICES

Vabra aspirator
Tis-U-Trap
Pipelle or equivalent

ENDOSCOPIC TECHNIQUES

Hysteroscopy
Operative hysteroscopy

IMAGING TECHNIQUES (OPTIONAL)

Ultrasound (vaginal or abdominal)
Computed tomography
Magnetic resonance imaging

with a suitable armamentarium to evaluate abnormal bleeding. Adjunctively, several imaging techniques may aid in the diagnosis, most notably vaginal ultrasound. Even with surgical staging, a separate endocervical curettage should be considered if there is a suspicion of primary endocervical cancer or if existing medical conditions might preclude hysterectomy.

Office endometrial biopsy is currently the most commonly used technique for histologic evaluation of endometrial pathology. Numerous devices are available for obtaining an endometrial sample in the office or clinic. The choice should be determined by the age of the patient, the experience of the clinician, anatomic considerations (e.g., stenosis), and the emotional milieu of the individual patient. Office endometrial biopsy is most commonly performed by using one of the various aspiration devices. The Vabra aspirator (Berkeley Medures, Berkeley, California) and the Tis-U-Trap (Milex Products, Chicago, Illinois) are two aspiration devices that use a pump as a vacuum source connected to a rigid metal or plastic cannula, usually 3 to 4 mm in diameter. The Pipelle (Unimar, Wilton, Connecticut), a softer, more flexible endometrial suction curet, has become a favorite of many clinicians. In our experience, this device is extremely well tolerated by patients and produces a satisfactory sample. With the use of a tenaculum on the cervix for traction, all but the most stenotic cervices can be traversed, usually without prior dilatation, leading to prompt sampling. Stoval et al. found that the Pipelle had a 97.5% sensitivity in patients with known endometrial cancer. Guido et al. noted the device was less sensitive in patients with disease confined to a polyp and in patients whose tumor occupied less than 5% of the endometrial surface. Many other devices have been introduced in recent years. The clinician should become completely familiar with the device he or she chooses and should monitor the results obtained. Complete reliance on any one device should be avoided. Clinical suspicion with continued monitoring and interval reevaluation should prevent failure of diagnosis when symptomatic bleeding persists despite a negative initial biopsy.

The traditional Novak curet, long the standard tool of endometrial dating, has been used in sampling the endometrium to detect endometrial carcinoma. Because of the discomfort associated with its use, as well as its limited sampling of the cavity, it is no longer used routinely as a first-line diagnostic technique.

A dilatation and fractional curettage (D&C) can provide definitive results, even though a thorough curettage may fail to sample the entire uterine cavity in 50% to 60% of patients. In a direct comparison of D&C with endometrial biopsy, Larson and associates (1995) showed that D&C was significantly more accurate in identifying cancer and predicting the final grade of disease. Even so, the false-negative rate of D&C for the diagnosis of endometrial cancer may be as high as 2% to 6%. This further reinforces the importance of maintaining a high index of suspicion and repeating the evaluation in women with persistent postmenopausal bleeding despite negative histology.

Some investigators advocate the use of hysteroscopy for the diagnosis of corpus cancer. Iossa et al. performed 2,007 consecutive outpatient hysteroscopies in self-referred women. They found 22 cases of malignancy but missed eight others. Several other studies have reported similar findings. Concerns have recently been raised regarding the possibility that hysteroscopy among patients with endometrial cancer may seed the peritoneal cavity with tumor cells via reflux of the distending medium through the fallopian tubes. Both Obermair and Zerbe in separate studies have reported an increased risk of positive peritoneal cytology among patients with endometrial cancer who underwent hysteroscopy as part of their evaluation, compared with women who did not undergo hysteroscopy. Positive peritoneal cytology when accompanied by other evidence of extrauterine disease is an adverse prognostic factor for patients with endometrial cancer. This observation, along with the known complications of hysteroscopy (some of which are serious), variations in expertise, anatomic malpositions and difficulties, and increased costs, indicate that hysteroscopy should not be routinely used in the initial evaluation of women with postmenopausal bleeding. It remains a useful adjunct to D&C in difficult cases. Many women can undergo D&C in the office. Premedication with ibuprofen followed by a paracervical block allows a comfortable dilatation and gentle curettage in all but the most apprehensive patients. Women with cervical stenosis, the very elderly, and those with high-risk cardiovascular or pulmonary disease may require the procedure to be performed in the operating room with concomitant monitoring. For circumstances in which cervical stenosis has occurred owing to prior radiation, sclerosing atrophy, advanced age, or multiple previous manipulations, real-time ultrasonography in the operating room can be used to guide the fine-wire probe into the cavity and help prevent false passages or perforation.

Many attempts have been made to brush, wash, or aspirate the endometrial cavity for intrauterine cytology. These require special instrumentation and special cytologic skills. They are no longer being advocated for the diagnosis of endometrial cancer.

Vaginal ultrasound has been suggested as a useful endometrial imaging technique. Indman examined 238 women with a combination of ultrasound, hysteroscopy, and suction curettage. He found a sensitivity of 96% in predicting abnormal uterine pathology. Karlsson et al., in a large Scandinavian multicenter study, used vaginal ultrasound before curettage to examine 1,168 women with postmenopausal bleeding. They found that when the thickness of the endometrial stripe was less than or equal to 4 mm, the chance of having abnormal pathology was 5.5%. A study by Brooks et al. evaluated 897 consecutive postmenopausal women with pelvic ultrasound. An endometrial thickness greater than or equal to 5 mm was considered abnormal among patients not on hormone replacement therapy. There were 184 patients with a normal endometrial stripe who underwent biopsy, and four atypical hyperplasias and four cases of endometrial cancer were detected. All eight of these patients were symptomatic. Only two cancers were diagnosed in the 129 patients with a thickened endometrial stripe, and both were asymptomatic. There is no general agreement as to the cut off for the definition of "thickened" endometrial stripe. This will vary depending on whether the patient is premenopausal or postmenopausal, length of time since menopause, and the use and type of hormone replacement therapy. Most experts recommend endometrial biopsy on all women with postmenopausal bleeding who have an endometrial stripe thickness greater than or equal to 5 mm and those women with persistent abnormal bleeding, no matter what the endometrial stripe thickness measured by transvaginal ultrasound.

Despite the apparent usefulness of the above-mentioned techniques, there is an important clinical caveat that must be observed when using these devices. Three basic facts must be remembered:

1. None of the devices provide results that are 100% sensitive. Failure to detect abnormal endometrium in persistently symptomatic patients should prompt a more thorough evaluation. Not only can endometrial cancers be missed but also the bleeding may be caused by a uterine sarcoma, fallopian tube cancer, or other pelvic pathology.
2. A close relationship must exist between the clinician and the pathologist who is interpreting the biopsy or D&C results. Concomitantly, it is the responsibility of the clinician to provide a complete and accurate clinical history on the requisition, so that the pathologist interpreting the results knows the patient's age, menstrual history, hormonal status, and symptoms.
3. Anatomic variation in the uterine cervix, such as stenosis or the presence of polyps, must warn the clinician against relying completely on office-based devices, which may not adequately sample the endometrial cavity.

Precursors of Endometrial Cancer

Over the years, a variety of different terms have been used to describe histologically distinct endometrial patterns. Various investigators have attempted to identify the malignant potential of these endometrial hyperplasias. Several years ago, Kurman and Norris introduced a terminology that has been widely accepted because of its simplicity and prognostic importance. They evaluated endometrial hyperplasia in 170 patients monitored for 1 to 26.7 years (mean, 13.4 years) by analyzing separately the cytologic and architectural alterations within the endometrial tissue specimens. When cytologic atypia alone was used to subdivide patients, 1.6% of those without cytologic atypia developed endometrial cancer, whereas 23% of those with cytologic atypia progressed to cancer, a highly significant ($p = 0.001$) difference. Further attempts to subdivide patients on the basis of glandular architectural features resulted in defining two categories: complex hyperplasias, which display marked glandular complexity and back-to-back glands, and simple hyperplasias, which are marked by prolifera-

tion in the number of glands but without architectural complexity. When these features were combined with cytologic characteristics to form four groups, they found that one of 93 patients with simple hyperplasia but no atypia developed cancer; however, cancer occurred in 29% of patients with complex atypical hyperplasias. Similarly, Ferenczy and Gelfand divided 85 patients with endometrial hyperplasia treated with oral medroxyprogesterone acetate therapy into two groups: those without and those with cytologic atypia. No patients without atypia developed cancer, although 20% had persistence or recurrence of hyperplasia. Seventy-five percent of those with atypia had persistence or recurrence, and 25% developed cancer, despite progesterone treatment. This occurred within 2 to 7 years of the initiation of hormonal therapy.

Data from these and other studies confirm that cytologic atypia is the prime factor to consider in estimating the malignant potential of endometrial hyperplasia. A woman with cytologic atypia is at high risk for endometrial cancer. Because a significant number of patients with atypical hyperplasia diagnosed by endometrial biopsy will actually have a coexistent adenocarcinoma, further histologic evaluation with a D&C is usually recommended. Even if cancer is not found, a hysterectomy is often recommended for women with complex atypical hyperplasia, unless fertility is a consideration. These patients have a very high risk of developing endometrial cancer within 5 years, if they do not already have it. Patients with architectural hyperplasia without cytologic atypia can be successfully treated with progestins.

Endometrial ablation is contraindicated in the management of hyperplasia. Horowitz and colleagues reported a case of endometrial carcinoma following endometrial ablation. Their case was diagnosed when metastatic.

STAGING OF ENDOMETRIAL CANCER

Preoperative Assessment Studies in Endometrial Cancer

Thorough pretreatment evaluation of the patient with endometrial cancer is essential. A detailed history and a complete general physical examination are the foundation of evaluation. Special attention should be paid to details of a family history of cancer. This may provide clues to the risk of concomitant cancers and may suggest that additional evaluation, such as colonoscopy, be performed. In addition to queries about the cardinal symptom of corpus cancer, abnormal uterine bleeding, the patient should be asked about the occurrence of symptoms such as pelvic pain or referred leg pain, leg edema or swelling, disturbances in bowel function, abdominal swelling, pelvic pressure, excessive flatulence, and early satiety. The presence of any of these symptoms may be indicative of advanced stage disease. During the general physical examination, attention should be paid to careful palpation of supraclavicular and inguinal lymph nodes.

Table 47.2 details staging and preoperative studies for patients with corpus cancer.

The pelvic examination is critical for patients with cancer of the uterus. After inspection of the vulva, palpation of Bartholin glands, and speculum evaluation of the vagina and cervix, careful bimanual and rectovaginal examination should discover any vaginal metastases, adnexal masses, or extension of the tumor into the parametrium or uterosacral ligaments. It is also used to establish a clinical estimate of the size of the uterus. Sounding of the uterus and endocervical curettage can be performed if the patient is deemed inoperable or if primary radiation therapy will be used.

Certain laboratory tests are useful in preoperative assessment. Complete blood count, liver and kidney function tests, serum electrolyte determinations, and a 12-lead electrocardiogram, although not useful for staging, form part of a thorough preoperative assessment of the patient with corpus cancer. Other tests should be performed as indicated by the patient's history and physical examination findings. For example, pulmonary function testing and arterial blood gas measurement should be considered in the preoperative assessment of the morbidly obese patient or the patient with a history of pulmonary disease.

There is no highly specific serum tumor marker for endometrial cancer, but the ovarian cancer antigen, CA-125, may be useful. In a retrospective study of 121 patients with endometrial cancer, Duk et al. in the Netherlands found that the incidence of elevated CA-125 increased with increasing stage of disease. Pretreatment CA-125 levels correlated with the finding at surgery of tumor outside the corpus, as well as with vascular invasion by malignant cells. After treatment, CA-125 levels paralleled the clinical course of the disease, with elevated CA-125 levels preceding clinical evidence of intraabdominal recurrence. Patsner et al. measured preoperative CA-125 levels in 89 patients before surgical staging. They found that 98% of patients with clinical or surgical stage I or II disease had normal preoperative CA-125 levels, whereas 28 of 31 patients (90.3%) with surgically proven extrauterine disease had elevated CA-125 levels. Kukura et al., in a study from Yugoslavia, reported a significantly higher CA-125 level when tumor had invaded more than one third of the myometrium. This suggests that CA-125 levels may have a predictive value in the preoperative assessment of patients with endometrial cancer. Elevated levels of CA-125 before surgery should alert the surgeon to search carefully for signs of extrauterine tumor. Postoperative levels may help to monitor disease status.

Ultrasonography is frequently used in the preoperative assessment of patients with endometrial cancer. Many women have already had a pelvic ultrasound as part of their evaluation for postmenopausal bleeding. But in addition to endometrial thickness, ultrasound can give the surgeon a good estimate of the depth of myometrial invasion and the presence of adnexal involvement. Because depth of invasion and tumor grade are predictors of lymph node metastases, preoperative knowledge of these tumor characteristics will help the surgeon to estimate the likelihood of nodal involvement and, perhaps, determine whether the patient should be referred to a gynecologic oncologist for primary surgery. Cacciatore et al. in Helsinki found that myometrial invasion was correctly predicted by ultrasonography in 80% of 93 patients, with polypoid growth being the most common reason for inaccuracy. Prompeler et al. studied myometrial invasion with vaginal ultrasound and reported a sensitivity of 93% when invasion was greater than 50%. The diagnostic accuracy was 81%; in 16% of the cases, the depth of invasion was overestimated, but in only 3% of the cases was it underestimated.

Radiographic assessment of the patient with endometrial cancer should certainly include a chest x-ray. This is used to look for metastatic disease and for preoperative assessment. Other imaging studies are not indicated, unless extrauterine metastases or other disease processes are suspected.

TABLE 47.2.
Staging and Preoperative Assessment Studies in Endometrial Cancer

---

History and complete physical examination
  Include careful evaluation of axillary, supraclavicular, and inguinal nodes.
Pelvic examination
  Careful inspection of vaginal vault
  Papanicolaou smear
  Endocervical curettage (for clinical staging)
  Sounding of endometrial cavity (for clinical staging)
  Palpation of fundal size, adnexa
  Rectovaginal examination to assess parametria, rectum, and cul-de-sac
Blood tests
  Complete hematology profile
  Chemistry screening panel, including liver and kidney function studies, electrolytes
  CA-125
  Optional: thyroid function tests, clotting profile
Urinalysis and urine culture
Imaging studies
  Chest radiograph (computed tomography of chest, if indicated)
  Computed tomography of pelvis and abdomen
  Magnetic resonance imaging (optional)
  Pelvic ultrasonography (optional; abdominal or vaginal technique)
  Barium enema (optional)
  Intravenous pyelography (optional)
Pulmonary function tests (for markedly obese patients or those with respiratory compromise) and arterial blood gas analysis
Proctosigmoidoscopy (colonoscopy if indicated)
Cystoscopy (if clinical stage II, III, or IV suspected)
Needle aspiration of suspicious nodes or masses
Indicated medical consultations

Some investigators obtain computed tomography (CT) scan of the pelvis and abdomen. The benefits of the CT scan are debatable, as lymph node metastases in endometrial cancer are mainly microscopic and therefore will not be detected on scan.

Hysterography has been used in the past to identify extent of endometrial disease. For the most part, this is not performed today because patients are surgically staged and the extent of disease is determined by surgical-pathologic evaluation.

Magnetic resonance imaging (MRI) shows some promise in the preoperative assessment of depth of myometrial invasion. Chen studied 50 consecutive patients with clinical stage I endometrial cancer and found that MRI accurately predicted deep myometrial invasion in 94% of cases and suggested an increase in clinical staging in 18%. Lien et al. reported that the overall accuracy of MRI in detecting deep invasion was 82%. They stated that the main limitation was false-positive results caused by large polypoid tumors that distended the uterus and distorted the thin rim of myometrium. We have found MRI to be useful in the management of young patients with low-grade cancers who wish conservative therapy to preserve their uterus. In such patients, myometrial invasion must be excluded before hormonal therapy can be considered.

The inclusion of cystoscopy in the preoperative work-up of patients with endometrial cancer depends on the index of suspicion that bladder invasion might be present or that there is a coexisting urologic problem which might affect pelvic surgery or radiation. Usually history and physical examination will give the clinician a good indication of the likelihood of bladder involvement. Cystoscopy is not routinely used.

Fine-needle aspiration of suspicious nodes or masses may provide documentation of distant metastases and greatly alter surgical plans. Appropriate timely use of this technique is important. Fine-needle aspiration of pelvic masses before definitive surgery is usually unnecessary.

Sound clinical judgment will dictate which of the extensive staging and preoperative evaluations in Table 47.2 is indicated for the individual patient. The wise surgeon is well prepared before surgery, and surgical staging of endometrial cancer is most proficiently accomplished after a thoughtful and thorough preoperative evaluation.

Surgical Staging of Endometrial Carcinoma

Thomas Cullen's textbook on uterine cancer published in 1900 states that the treatment of cancer of the endometrium is total abdominal hysterectomy and bilateral salpingo-oophorectomy. Hysterectomy remains the cornerstone of treatment of endometrial cancer to this day. In the mid-1930s, the use of preoperative radiation was popularized, and it remained the standard of care for many years. By the 1970s, the value of radiation therapy for early stage endometrial cancer was being questioned, and primary surgery for both treatment and staging was becoming more popular. GOG helped to firmly establish the importance of surgical staging by continued analysis of a prospective cohort of about 1,000 patients who underwent a standard staging operation. In 1988, the FIGO cancer committee changed the staging for endometrial cancer from a clinical to a surgical-pathologic staging system (Table 47.3). The FIGO staging systems have been used worldwide for all gynecologic cancers since they were first introduced for cervix cancer in 1937.

Surgical Staging Technique

After thoughtful preoperative evaluation, the plans for surgery are reviewed with the patient and her family and expected benefits of the operation, as well as the poten-

---

TABLE 47.3.
FIGO Clinical Staging of Endometrial Carcinoma

Classification	Description
Stage 0	Carcinoma *in situ*. Histologic findings suspicious of cancer. (Cases of stage 0 should not be included in statistics on invasive disease.)
Stage I	Carcinoma confined to the corpus, including the isthmus
IA	The length of the uterine cavity is 8 cm or less.
IB	The length of the uterine cavity is more than 8 cm.
	Stage I cases should be subgrouped with regard to the histologic type of adenocarcinoma as follows:
	Grade 1: Highly differentiated adenomatous carcinoma
	Grade 2: Differentiated adenomatous carcinoma with partly solid areas
	Grade 3: Predominantly solid or entirely undifferentiated carcinoma
Stage II	Carcinoma involving the corpus and cervix but not extending outside the uterus
Stage III	Carcinoma extending outside the uterus but not outside the true pelvis
Stage IV	Carcinoma extending outside the true pelvis or obviously involving the mucosa of the bladder or rectum. (Bullous edema alone does not permit a lesion to be considered stage IV.)
IVA	Spread to bladder or intestine
IVB	Spread to distant organs

tial risks and complications, are carefully discussed. An informed consent for surgery is signed.

We recommend mechanical bowel preparation before lymphadenectomy. Patients undergoing radical gynecologic surgery, including lymphadenectomy and staging of endometrial cancer, are at high risk for deep venous thrombosis and pulmonary embolus. Thus, all patients who are undergoing exploratory surgery for staging or therapy of endometrial cancer should receive prophylactic low-dose heparin or low-molecular-weight heparin, or should be fitted with intermittent pneumatic compression devices. The latter may be more comfortable and effective if used over TED stockings. Use of unfractionated heparin, but not low-molecular-weight heparin, is associated with a significantly increased transfusion requirement compared with use of intermittent pneumatic compression devices. A combination of both low-molecular-weight heparin and intermittent pneumatic compression devices should be used if the risk is extremely high. Preoperative antibiotics usually are recommended, and we prefer to use a broad-spectrum antibiotic with good anaerobic coverage. Positioning the patient for surgery in the operating room is done according to the surgeon's preference. Most surgeons prefer to have the patient in the supine position, but some gynecologic oncologists prefer to have the patient's legs elevated in a modified lithotomy position when performing radical surgery. This assists technically in performing the paraaortic lymph node dissection, if the operator stands between the patient's legs. Care should be taken in positioning to avoid neuropathy.

A lower midline incision should be used, except in extremely obese patients. For obese patients, a paramedian incision adjacent to the umbilicus works well, as does a transverse periumbilical incision. Both avoid the problems of the panniculus. Alternative incisions can be used; transverse incisions such as the Maylard or Cherney may be appropriate. We have used a panniculectomy before fascial incision in selected circumstances.

After entering the abdomen, peritoneal washings for cytologic examination are obtained by injecting 50 to 100 mL of saline or other physiologic solution into the pelvis and abdomen. By holding the intestines away and gently lifting the uterus forward, fluid can be collected after admixture with peritoneal fluid already present. It is important not to agitate or squeeze the uterus, because malignant cells may be dislodged and could cause a false-positive result. Also, it is important not to use overly warm irrigating saline, because this could cause coagulation and shrinkage of cytoplasm of mesothelial cells, rendering them difficult to interpret. After washings are aspirated, they are placed in a sterile container with dilute heparin and processed by standard cytologic techniques. The presence of malignant cells in the peritoneal washings is associated with a poor prognosis and a high risk of other extrauterine disease.

The peritoneal cavity is then thoroughly explored. The uterus, tubes, and ovaries are examined, and the retroperitoneal spaces are palpated for obviously suspicious lymph nodes. Care is taken to palpate the paraaortic area up to the level of the renal vessels. Thorough palpation and inspection of the hemidiaphragms, omentum, liver, kidneys, and the paracolic gutters is essential. After meticulous evaluation of the upper abdomen, the intestines are packed away and the pelvis is exposed, carefully dividing adhesions as necessary. Suspicious adhesions or suspected implants should be sampled and submitted for pathologic analysis. Some investigators recommend routinely obtaining a small biopsy of the omentum in patients who meet the criteria for surgical staging (see below).

Old techniques suggest suturing the ends of the fallopian tubes shut at this juncture to prevent reflux of tumor cells, but we prefer grasping each side of the fundus, tubes, and round ligaments with long Kelly clamps, which also serve as a handle to manipulate the uterus.

After ligation and division of the round ligaments, the retroperitoneal spaces are exposed. It is important to open the paravesical and pararectal spaces before initiating the hysterectomy. This not only allows discovery of obviously positive lymph nodes but also more clearly defines the anatomy and circumvents distortion that can accompany hysterectomy. Sometimes extension of uterine cancer to the lower segment can balloon out the isthmus. Opening the spaces will allow identification of the ureter down to its entry into the vesicouterine tunnel, where it may be necessary to ligate the uterine artery. The infundibulopelvic ligaments and ovarian vessels are divided and ligated with direct visualization of the ureter. The anterior peritoneum is incised, and the bladder is dissected off the lower uterine segment. The uterine vessels are skeletonized and cross-clamped at a level just below the internal os, cut, and sutured. One cardinal point needs to be continually emphasized: To accomplish an appropriate extrafascial hysterectomy, the technique of "bouncing off" the cervix when placing clamps on the uterine vessels and parametria should be avoided (Fig. 47.1). Likewise, after the clamps are appropriately placed, taking a wedge of the lower uterine segment or cervix to ensure a more voluminous pedicle is, in essence, leaving a portion of uterus in the patient. Many gynecologists make the mistake of attempting large bites of tissue (the "gyn hog" technique), creating a bulky pedicle; bites of no more than 1 cm will allow tying of the pedicles with appropriate approximation, and will also fulfill extrafascial total abdominal hysterectomy criteria. For circumstances in which the lower uterine segment is ballooned out, such as discussed in the section on uterine sarcoma, it is even more important that the "bouncing off" technique be avoided (Fig. 47.1). This can result in rupture of the cervix at the site of ballooning, allowing tumor to be extruded into the operative field and compromising traction on the cervix.

After the parametrium has been divided, dissection should continue to the upper vagina. The posterior peritoneum is dissected off the cervix, and the rectovaginal septum is developed. As the surgeon continues taking bites along the lower cervix and upper vagina, it is important not to incise the endopelvic fascia in an attempt to avoid injury to the bladder. Paravaginal bites should

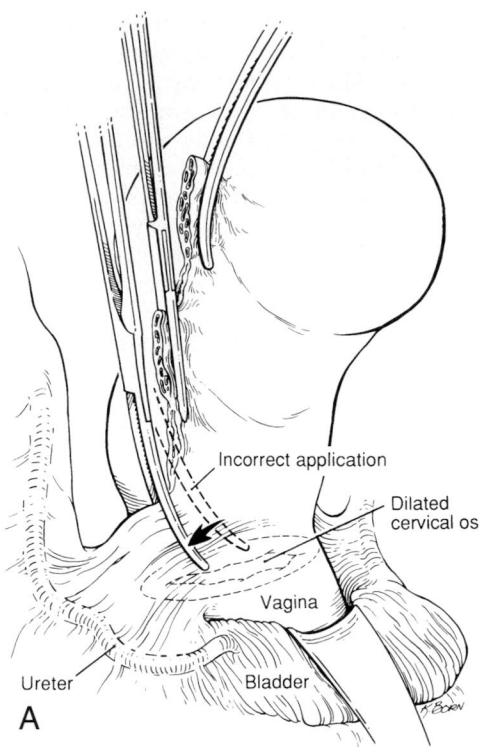

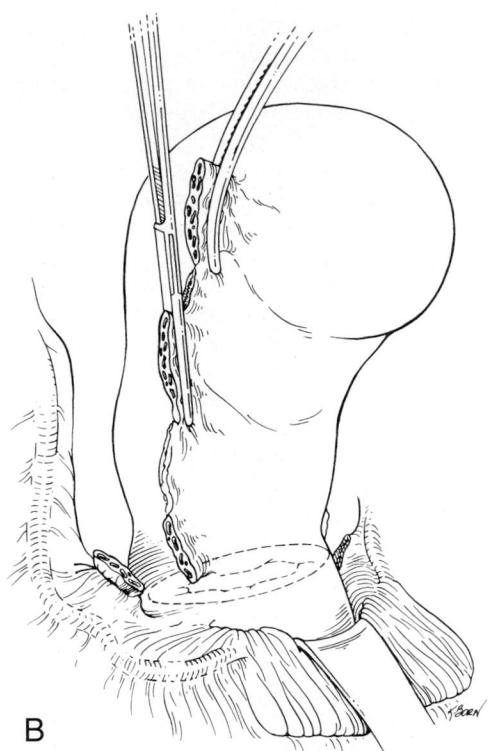

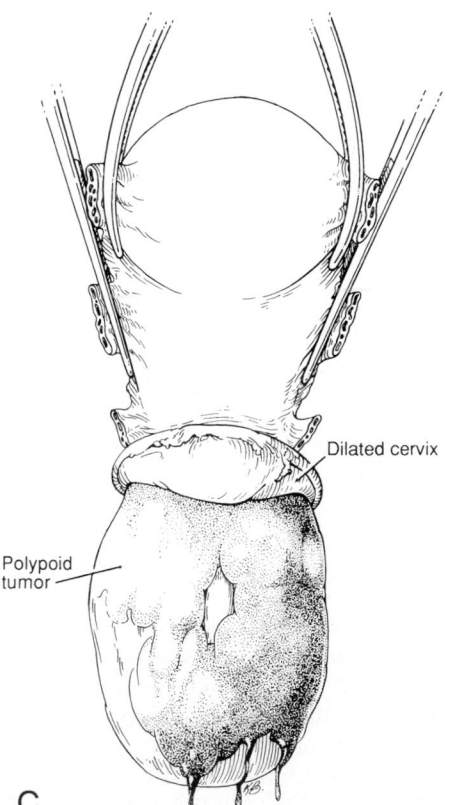

FIGURE 47.1. Correct technique for dissecting the lower broad ligament in parametria of patients with a ballooning out of the lower uterine segment and dilation of the cervix from polypoid sarcoma, or extended stage II endometrial cancer. **A:** The uteroovarian ligaments, round ligaments, and upper broad ligaments have been cross-clamped and divided. The uterine vesicles have been cross-clamped and divided at the level of the internal os, without extending into the endopelvic fascia and body of the lower uterine segment and cervix. The dotted line shows the incorrect application of the next series of clamps, which, in this schematic diagram, would have resulted in entering the cervix above the level of the external os and extruding tumor into the wound. Instead, the clamp is placed 2 to 3 mm lateral to the cervix so that a pedicle is obtained that is sufficient for hemostasis, and the cervix is not entered. To accomplish this maneuver safely, the ureter must be identified and dissected at a point just superior to its entry into the vesicouterine ligament (tunnel), and then retracted laterally. **B:** The outline of the ureter through the tunnel is seen, as is its entry into the bladder. Careful dissection of the bladder away from the lower ureter segment and vagina is essential to expose this area. The next application of clamps can begin in the paravaginal area before the necessary vaginal cuff is obtained. **C:** The removed specimen is shown with an appropriate vaginal cuff and a dilated cervix extending around the polypoid tumor. For a uterine sarcoma to be completely surgically excised, this technique must be used.

be taken at least 1 cm below the fornix to allow a full-cuff vaginal specimen. However, it is not necessary to remove the upper third of the vagina, as is done in a radical hysterectomy. The vaginal cuff should be closed with interrupted sutures. The pelvic peritoneum may or may not be closed.

In certain circumstances, a more radical hysterectomy may be necessary. When there is occult invasion outside the lower segment, when operative discovery of induration of the parametria occurs, or if gross disease is evident on the uterosacral ligaments, individualized wider margins must be taken according to the anatomic abnormality. Thus, the anterior vesicouterine ligament can be dissected away from the anterior surface of the ureter, the bladder can be dissected further down the vagina, or the uterosacral ligament can be excised more radically. The posterior vesicouterine ligament does not need extensive dissection; indeed, preservation of the posterior and inferior portions of the ureteral blood supply may prevent subsequent ureteral fistula or stenosis, if postoperative radiation is necessary.

When the tumor is moderately to poorly differentiated and surgical staging will most certainly be performed, the pathologist does not need to determine depth of invasion. In well-differentiated tumors, however, surgical staging may not always be necessary. In this situation, determination of depth of invasion is important. After hysterectomy, the uterus is opened and evaluated intraoperatively. This must be done according to the preference of the pathology department. Some pathologists prefer to open the uterus in the laboratory, and others come to the operating room and open the uterus with the surgeon. The latter method is preferred, as it facilitates direct communication between the surgeon and the pathologist. When this is not feasible, clear written instructions should accompany the specimen. In either circumstance, preoperative consultation with the pathologist can speed the process and improve the quality of the evaluation.

In some cases, it may be difficult to determine the depth of myometrial invasion or even to determine the location of the uterine tumor based on gross examination alone. Accordingly, frozen sections may be necessary. The method of determining the depth of myometrial invasion intraoperatively should be agreed upon preoperatively by the surgeon and pathologist. Docring et al. prospectively studied 148 patients with clinical stage I endometrial cancer. They found that gross visual examination of the cut surface of the tumor at the time of hysterectomy accurately determined the depth of myometrial invasion in 135 patients (91%), for a sensitivity of 72%, a specificity of 96%, and a positive predictive value of 80%. Malviya et al. in Detroit tested the reliability of intraoperative frozen section in 55 patients with clinical stage I corpus cancer. They assessed the depth of myometrial invasion by gross examination along with selected frozen section at the time of surgery, and compared it to the depth of myometrial invasion determined by extensive sampling and subsequent observation of permanent microscopic sections. They found that gross

examination with selective frozen section accurately predicted the depth of myometrial invasion in 96.5% of patients and accurately assessed the histologic grade of the tumor in 94.5% of patients. Furthermore, they found occult cervical invasion on frozen section in two thirds of patients who were later determined to have extension to the cervix. Combining gross inspection with frozen sections intraoperatively appears to offer reliable evaluation of the operative specimen.

After removal of the uterus with intraoperative evaluation of the depth of myometrial invasion and grade of tumor, the surgeon must decide whether or not to proceed with lymph node sampling to complete the surgical staging. If a well-differentiated tumor invades the outer one half of the myometrium, the tumor is moderately or poorly differentiated, the tumor is of a high-risk histologic subtype (i.e., papillary serous carcinoma, clear cell carcinoma, squamous cell carcinoma, or undifferentiated tumors), there is involvement of the cervix or adnexal structures, or there are palpably enlarged pelvic or paraaortic lymph nodes, complete surgical staging with pelvic and paraaortic lymphadenectomy is usually performed. Three issues are of paramount importance. First, is the safety of lymph node sampling sufficiently high to justify the additional operative time and possible complications? Second, is the operator sufficiently experienced to perform the lymph node sampling? Third, to what extent should lymphadenectomy be performed?

Moore et al. clearly demonstrated that the surgical morbidity of lymph node sampling is low. Their retrospective series included 292 patients with endometrial cancer and 262 patients with cervical cancer. All of the lymphadenectomies were performed by residents and fellows in training under the direct supervision of certified gynecologic oncologists. In this clinical setting, blood loss, transfusion requirements, operative time, and length of hospital stay were not significantly increased ($p < 0.05$) for these patients compared with similar patients who had surgical treatment without lymphadenectomy. Although vascular injuries, hematomas, and lymphocysts were more common after lymph node sampling, there was no significant increase in mortality or long-term sequelae. Chuang et al. at the M.D. Anderson Cancer Center in Houston reported a series of 295 patients with endometrial cancer, 193 (65%) of whom had lymph node sampling performed. They noted two intraoperative injuries (one ureteral transection and one major venous laceration) that apparently were repaired without sequelae. They believed that the information gained from the dissection greatly outweighed the operative risk. For patients who have a significant risk of lymph node metastases, lymphadenectomy is safe and provides valuable prognostic information that may help to determine the need for postoperative radiotherapy.

Certain medical problems may alter the safety of the procedure. In patients with severe arteriosclerosis (not an unlikely occurrence in the age group subject to the risk of endometrial cancer), lymph node dissection may be associated with difficulty in establishing hemostasis. Therefore, extensive sampling of nonsuspicious lymph nodes should probably be avoided. It is not uncommon to encounter medical problems intraoperatively that require termination of an operation. Additionally, in very obese patients, retraction may be compromised, and no attempt at lymph node removal (especially in the paraaortic area) should be undertaken if adequate exposure is not available.

In general, we believe that surgical therapy for endometrial cancer should not be undertaken by gynecologic surgeons who are not prepared to do a thorough staging procedure. For gynecologists not trained in lymph node removal, gynecologic oncologists are widely available to assist in these procedures.

The extent of the lymphadenectomy will determine its actual worth in establishing the presence or absence of lymph node metastases. Ideally, complete lymphadenectomy with evaluation of all the major lymph node areas should be performed. Obtaining one easy-to-dissect external iliac node and referring to this as lymph node removal is inadequate. When the GOG was conducting its endometrial surgical staging protocol, many such cases were encountered in the early years. Subsequent protocol revisions required at least 10 lymph nodes cumulatively from each patient to qualify for staging. The M.D. Anderson protocol, as reported by Chuang et al., divides the lymph-node bearing area at risk into 10 "lymphatic zones": right and left paraaortic, common iliac, external iliac, hypogastric, and obturator. Patients who had nodes removed from three zones, including one paraaortic site and at least one pelvic site on each side, had a mean of 6.2 sites biopsied, with an average yield of nine lymph nodes per patient. In this group, there were no tumor recurrences at retroperitoneal lymph node sites. Thus, for lymphadenectomy to be meaningful, lymph nodes from all the major node-bearing areas, as shown in Fig. 47.2, should be removed. Any palpable or enlarged lymph nodes should also be removed.

Kilgore et al. at the University of Alabama were the first to suggest that lymphadenectomy might actually have a therapeutic effect for patients with endometrial cancer. They evaluated the outcomes of 649 patients surgically managed for endometrial cancer. Of these patients, 212 patients had pelvic lymph nodes sampled from at least four separate sites (multiple-site lymph node sampling), 205 patients had pelvic lymph nodes sampled from fewer than four sites (limited-site lymph node sampling), and 208 patients had no pelvic lymph nodes sampled. Patients undergoing multiple-site lymph node sampling had a survival of approximately 85%, whereas patients in whom pelvic lymph nodes were not sampled had a survival of approximately 65%, a statistically significant difference ($p = 0.0027$). This survival advantage for patients with multiple-site lymph node sampling persisted even in a subgroup analysis of patients treated with postoperative whole pelvic radiotherapy.

Endometrial carcinoma spreads through three separate lymphatic pathways: Paracervical and parametrial lymphatics drain to the pelvic lymph nodes, ovarian lymphatics drain to the paraaortic lymph nodes, and round

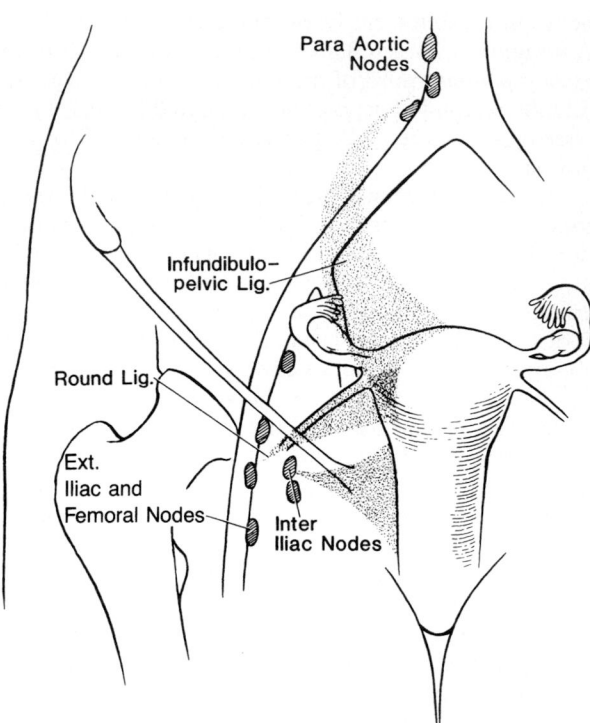

FIGURE 47.2. Lymphatic pathways of tumor spread of endometrial carcinoma to pelvic and extrapelvic nodes.

ligament lymphatics drain to the inguinal lymph nodes (Fig. 47.2). The lymphatic drainage of the uterine fundus and cervix directs most of the metastases to the pelvic lymph nodes. Although the paraaortic lymph nodes may be primary metastatic sites via spread through the infundibulopelvic ligament lymphatics, it is rare for an endometrial cancer patient to have isolated paraaortic lymph node metastases without concomitant pelvic lymph node metastases. In the GOG study, as reported by Boronow, only 1.5% of patients with negative pelvic lymph nodes had metastases to paraaortic lymph nodes.

Pelvic lymphadenectomy begins by extending the lateral peritoneal incision superiorly over the psoas muscle, from the round ligament to the pelvic brim. The ureter and its associated peritoneum are mobilized medially by using blunt dissection, exposing the common iliac, external iliac, and hypogastric vessels. The genitofemoral nerve is identified as it passes along the surface of the psoas muscle in order to avoid injury to it during the dissection. The fatty, node-bearing tissue overlying the anterior and medial surfaces of the common and external iliac arteries inferiorly to the level of the circumflex iliac vein, the medial surface of the external iliac vein, and the anterior surface of the hypogastric artery is carefully excised. Most surgeons use sharp dissection with Metzenbaum scissors and blunt forceps, such as Singley forceps. Small vessels are identified and secured with small hemoclips before being transected. As the dissection proceeds inferiorly along the hypogastric artery, the external iliac vein is elevated by using a vein retractor, and blunt dissection is used to identify the course of the obturator nerve through the obturator space. The lymph nodes in the obturator space, anterior to the obturator nerve, are excised by using sharp dissection. The superior vesical artery should be identified as it arises from the hypogastric artery and spared, in order to maintain the blood supply to the distal ureter. The lymph nodes can be sent to the pathologist in small groups, indicating their location in the pelvis. However, this does not have any prognostic significance and can increase pathology charges by increasing the number of specimens to be evaluated. It is important to communicate clearly the side and site (pelvic or paraaortic) of the lymph nodes being passed off to the circulating nurse, so that this can be accurately documented on the pathology sheet.

The paraaortic lymph node dissection can be performed from the surgeon's usual position at the side of the patient. However, many surgeons find that they can obtain better access to the paraaortic nodes by positioning the patient in low lithotomy at the beginning of the case and standing between the patient's legs to perform the dissection. The initial abdominal incision should be made to a level a short distance superior to the umbilicus in order to obtain adequate exposure for the paraaortic lymphadenectomy. Access to the paraaortic lymph nodes can be obtained either by extending the lateral peritoneal incisions superiorly along the paracolic gutters or by incising the peritoneum directly over the aorta. We prefer the prior approach. The colon on either side is mobilized medially by using blunt dissection in order to expose the aorta and vena cava on the right the lateral aspect of the aorta on the left. A Deaver or other large curved retractor is used to gently retract the peritoneum and associated ovarian vessels and ureter superiorly and medially. Care must be taken on the right side to avoid injury to the third portion of the duodenum from overvigorous retraction. The duodenum can be further protected by mobilizing the third portion superiorly by using blunt dissection. By using a similar technique to that used in the pelvis, the fatty, node-bearing tissues overlying the vessels are excised. On the right side, this is primarily the tissue overlying the inferior vena cava. On the left side, the lymph nodes lie somewhat more posteriorly. On this side, the surgeon should avoid taking the dissection too far posteriorly, where the lumbar arteries and veins can be injured. Also on the left side, the surgeon must identify and avoid injury to the inferior mesenteric artery, which arises from the anterior aorta approximately 8 to 10 cm superior to the aortic bifurcation. On either side, the dissection should be carried superiorly at least 4 to 5 cm, ideally to the level of the ovarian vessels. As a practical matter, many patients with endometrial cancer are obese, and adequate exposure cannot be obtained to extend the dissection that far superiorly.

The operative sites should be irrigated and adequate hemostasis ensured. Hemoclips can be used for this purpose. Small venous bleeders can often be controlled with direct pressure. Topical hemostatic agents can also be used. In the past, surgeons commonly placed retroperitoneal drains and closed the peritoneal incisions. Today, most surgeons do not routinely drain the pelvis after lymphadenectomy. Likewise, the peritoneal incisions are usually left open. The abdominal incision can be closed using a running far, far–near, near stitch, or continuous mass closure, using delayed absorbable or permanent suture material.

Uterine papillary serous carcinoma behaves in a manner similar to that of ovarian cancer, with a tendency toward intraperitoneal spread. Therefore, the staging of these patients should be performed as for an ovarian cancer. Initial washings should be obtained separately from the pelvis, the bilateral pericolic gutters, and the bilateral subdiaphragmatic spaces. In addition to total abdominal hysterectomy and bilateral salpingo-oophorectomy, all patients with uterine papillary serous carcinoma should have pelvic and paraaortic lymph node sampling, omentectomy, and systematic sampling of the peritoneum with biopsies being obtained from the bladder peritoneum, cul-de-sac peritoneum, bilateral pelvic side-wall peritoneum, and bilateral paracolic gutter peritoneum. Sampling of the bilateral diaphragm peritoneum can be performed either by biopsy or Pap smear.

In many circumstances, the need for lymphadenectomy can be determined preoperatively. In these situations, some gynecologic oncologists prefer to perform the lymphadenectomy first, when the surgeons are freshest, as this is the most tedious part of the procedure.

Postoperatively, early ambulation and attention to fluid and electrolyte balance in this patient group are important. Many patients are elderly and may be in precarious fluid balance preoperatively; thus, the use of a standing fluid order is contraindicated. Daily weights are helpful in monitoring patient fluid needs.

Surgical Debulking

Although the surgical staging procedure just described has gained wide acceptance, the role of surgical debulking in endometrial cancer is somewhat more controversial. Patients with bulky pelvic or paraaortic lymph node metastases may benefit from debulking, if all gross disease can be resected. There is a risk of significant vascular injury. However, external beam radiotherapy is unlikely to sterilize bulky nodal disease. Excision of these nodes may improve the patient's chances of responding to postoperative pelvic or extended field radiotherapy.

Several investigators have examined the role of surgical debulking, as is performed for patients with ovarian cancer, in the management of patients with stage IVB endometrial cancer. Goff et al. evaluated 47 patients with surgical stage IVB endometrial cancer who were treated at the Massachusetts General Hospital. The overall median survival was 12 months. The median survival of patients who underwent cytoreductive surgery was 18 months, compared with a median survival of 8 months among women who did not undergo cytoreductive surgery ($p = 0.0001$). Chi et al. at the Sloan-Kettering Cancer Center reported the outcomes of 55 patients who underwent cytoreductive surgery for stage IVB endometrial cancer. Optimal cytoreduction with the largest residual tumor measuring less than or equal to 2 cm was

TABLE 47.4.
Surgical Staging of Corpus Cancer

Stage	Grade	
IA	G123	Tumor limited to endometrium
IB	G123	Invasion to $<\frac{1}{2}$ myometrium
IC	G123	Invasion to $>\frac{1}{2}$ myometrium
IIA	G123	Endocervical glandular involvement only
IIB	G123	Cervical stromal invasion
IIIA	G123	Tumor invades serosa or adnexa, or positive peritoneal cytology
IIIB	G123	Vaginal metastases
IIIC	G123	Metastases to pelvic or paraaortic lymph nodes
IVA	G123	Tumor invasion of bladder or bowel mucosa
IVB	G123	Distant metastases, including intraabdominal or inguinal lymph nodes

HISTOPATHOLOGY: DEGREE OF DIFFERENTIATION

Cases of carcinoma of the corpus should be grouped with regard to the degree of differentiation of the adenocarcinoma as follows:

G1 = 5% or less of a nonsquamous or nonmorular solid growth pattern

G2 = 6%–50% of a nonsquamous or nonmorular solid growth pattern

G3 = more than 50% of a nonsquamous or nonmorular solid growth pattern

NOTES ON PATHOLOGIC GRADING

(1) Notable nuclear atypia, inappropriate for the architectural grade, raises the grade of a grade 1 or grade 2 tumor by 1.

(2) In serous adenocarcinomas, clear cell adenocarcinomas, and squamous cell carcinomas, nuclear grading takes precedent.

(3) Adenocarcinomas with squamous differentiation are graded according to the nuclear grade of the glandular component.

RULES RELATED TO STAGING

(1) Because corpus cancer is now surgically staged, procedures previously used for differentiation of stages are no longer applicable, such as the finding of dilatation and curettage to differentiate between stage I and stage II.

   (a) There may be a small number of patients with corpus cancer who will be treated primarily with radiation therapy. If that is the case, the clinical staging adopted by FIGO in 1971 would still apply, but designation of that staging system would be noted.

(2) Ideally, the width of the myometrium should be measured along with the width of tumor invasion.

FIGO, International Federation of Gynecology and Obstetrics.
From: International Federation of Gynecology and Obstetrics. Annual report on the results of treatment in gynecologic cancer. *Int J Gynaecol Obstet* 1989;28:189.

achieved in 24 patients. There were 21 patients who underwent suboptimal cytoreduction, with the largest residual tumor measuring greater than 2 cm. Ten patients had unresectable carcinomatosis. Those patients who were able to undergo optimal cytoreduction had a statistically significantly longer median survival of 31 months, compared with 12 months for patients who underwent suboptimal cytoreduction and 3 months for patients with unresectable disease ($p = 0.01$). Most recently, Bristow et al. have reported similar findings. They evaluated 65 patients with stage IVB endometrial cancer. They defined optimal cytoreduction as a maximal residual tumor less than or equal to 1 cm. In the 36 patients who had an optimal cytoreduction, the median survival was 34.3 months. This was a statistically significant advantage compared with the 29 patients who had a suboptimal cytoreduction, whose median survival was 11 months ($p = 0.0001$). Taken together, these data would argue for the performance of cytoreductive surgery in patients with stage IVB endometrial cancer, if a maximal residual disease of less than or equal to 1 to 2 cm can be achieved.

After the operative procedure and appropriate postoperative recovery, the pathologic findings should be reviewed and discussed, and the surgical staging system is outlined in Table 47.4. The indications for postoperative radiotherapy are reviewed later in this chapter.

Laparoscopic Surgical Staging

The advent of extensive laparoscopic surgery has included the management of endometrial carcinoma in investigational settings. Childers et al. from Arizona were the first to report a large series of patients who underwent complete surgical staging of endometrial cancer with laparoscopically assisted vaginal hysterectomy. Their successful completion rate was 93%; two obese patients were the only failures. Significant complications occurred in four patients, but there was minimal blood loss and the hospital stay averaged 2.9 days. The enthusiasm for this approach has extended to multiple institutions. It reached a crescendo that mandated study by the GOG to properly assess outcomes of minimally invasive surgery in the management of endometrial cancer. The first pilot study, Protocol 9206, was designed to determine if laparoscopic pelvic and paraaortic lymph node sampling would provide pathologic specimens and operative data comparable in detail to those obtained from a traditional staging laparotomy. In addition, the protocol was designed to evaluate whether the laparoscopic method fulfilled GOG safety and accuracy criteria. A second study, GOG Lap1, has much broader objectives, including evaluation of surgeon proficiency, outcome parameters, quality of life, and the therapeutic benefit of lymph node sampling in grade I, presumed stage I corpus cancers.

The proponents of minimally invasive surgery are universal in their claim that this approach will decrease complications and shorten hospital stay. In the early series reported by skilled laparoscopic surgeons, complication rates were at least comparable to, if not less than, those reported for staging laparotomy by Moore et al. (as noted earlier), Holmesly et al. (1992), and Larson et al. (1992). However, there is a steep learning curve associated with these techniques. The use of laparoscopic staging should be limited to the gynecologic oncologist with significant laparoscopic expertise. Further, equivalent survival of patients undergoing laparoscopic staging compared with staging laparotomy has yet to be demonstrated in a large, prospective trial. Until the GOG and other investigators have demonstrated efficacy, laparoscopic staging should be considered investigational. It is strongly recommended that patients undergoing laparoscopic staging be entered into institutional or, preferably, multi-institutional cooperative group protocols, such as those of the GOG.

The laparoscopic procedure begins with the standard preoperative preparation, including bowel preparation. General anesthesia and low dorsal lithotomy position on an operating table capable of steep Trendelenburg position are required. Instrumentation should consist of a high-flow electronic insufflator, a high-intensity light source, a high-resolution camera, two monitors, coagulation sources, (both bipolar and unipolar), state-of-the-art forceps, irrigators, and dissecting scissors. A 10- to 12-mm operating laparoscope is initially inserted at the umbilicus, with a similar port available above the symphysis. Accessory trocar sites in the right and left mid-abdomen are necessary, and additional trocar sites may be necessary for completion.

Laparoscopic exploration is performed by first estimating the volume of free fluid. If free fluid is present, one should determine if the quantity is sufficient for aspiration and submission for cytology. If free fluid is not present, peritoneal washings from the pelvis, paracolic gutters, and infradiaphragmatic areas are aspirated and sent for cytologic evaluation. Visualization of all peritoneal surfaces, the omentum, the diaphragm, and the mesenteric surfaces should be accomplished, and any suspicious areas should be biopsied.

The surgeon must choose the area in which the lymphadenectomy should begin. Paraaortic dissection requires the steep Trendelenburg position. Because this may cause anesthetic problems, especially in obese patients, it may be preferable to perform the pelvic dissection first. The retroperitoneal spaces in the pelvis are opened. The ureter, ovarian vessels, and superior vesical artery are retracted medially, and the lymph nodes are removed from the common iliac, hypogastric, obturator, and external iliac areas, primarily with use of the bipolar scissors. Some surgeons use hydrodissection and metallic clips. The high resolution and magnification afforded by quality equipment allow tiny vessels to be identified before coagulation and transection. This assists in minimizing blood loss. After the removal of pelvic nodes, which can be transported with ease through the large ports, a steeper Trendelenburg position is used and the posterior peritoneum medial to the right ureter is incised, providing access to the paraaortic region. After the anatomic landmarks are identified, the lymph nodes in the precaval, right paraaortic, aortic, and left paraaortic areas can be removed proximally to the level of the inferior mesenteric artery. Hemostasis can be aided with clips, pressure, or clotting matrix, if necessary. In performing this procedure, even an experienced laparoscopic surgeon must have adequate assistance, anesthesia, equipment, and operating room support. As seen in Fig. 47.3, an excellent harvest of pelvic and paraaortic lymph nodes can be accomplished.

Laparoscopic vaginal hysterectomy and bilateral salpingo-oophorectomy should be performed by standard

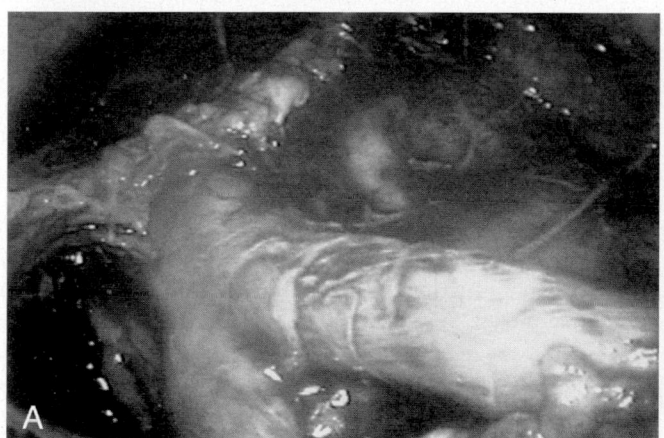
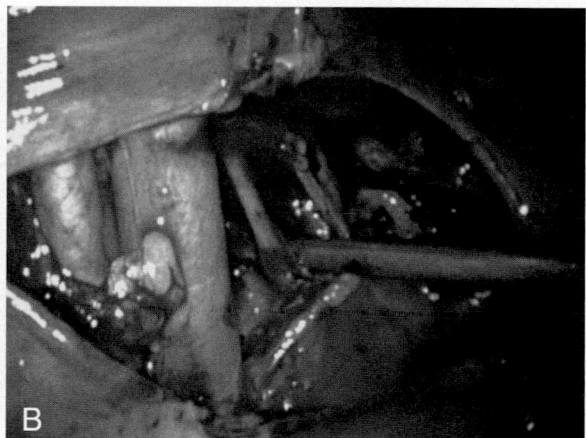

FIGURE 47.3. Laparoscopic node dissection. **A:** Paraaortic node dissection has been performed. All nodes from the aortic chains at the bifurcation have been removed, as have the precaval nodes. **B:** Pelvic node dissection in progress. The pelvic side-wall structures have been identified, and node dissection has been partially performed laparoscopically. (From: Dr. T.V. Sedlacek, with permission.) See color version of figure.

techniques. Irrigating the pelvis, reaffirming hemostasis, observing anatomic structures for signs of injury, and allowing escape of the pneumoperitoneum complete the procedure. Most surgeons close the 10- to 12-mm fascial defects to prevent the subsequent development of an incisional hernia, but this is usually unnecessary for 5-mm ports. As with laparoscopic surgery for other malignancies, port-site recurrences have been reported in patients who underwent laparoscopic surgery for endometrial cancer. The exact incidence and significance of this problem are unknown at this time.

PROGNOSTIC FACTORS

Multiple prognostic factors have been identified in endometrial cancer (Table 47.5). Although each one may have a significant impact in univariate analysis, determining which has independent prognostic significance has proven more difficult. The results of the GOG's surgical staging studies are a reliable source for analysis of prognostic factors, because each of the patients entered in the studies underwent the standard surgical staging procedure. Exact reporting and quality control were used throughout, so that the individual prognostic factors could be analyzed using both univariate and multivariate analysis. Many of the data have matured, and in general, the prognostic variables identified substantiate previous uncontrolled observations about the same characteristics. In the 2001 annual report, about 94% of all endometrial cancer patients had been surgically staged, indicating the acceptance of the surgical staging criteria by those institutions submitting data. The results of surgical staging allow the clinician to estimate prognosis and develop a plan for additional treatment or follow-up based on an accurate knowledge of the extent of disease.

Histologic Grade

Grade is a highly important prognostic variable in endometrial cancer. The current FIGO grading system includes three gradations of histopathologic differentiation

---

TABLE 47.5.

Prognostic and Staging Factors Determined by Surgical Staging in Endometrial Cancer

---

Histologic grade of tumor
Depth of myometrial invasion
Status of pelvic and paraaortic nodes
Presence of malignant cells in peritoneal washings
Histologic type
Lymphvascular invasion
Cervical invasion
Adnexal spread
Intraperitoneal disease
Estrogen and progesterone receptors
Oncogenes, ploidy, molecular markers

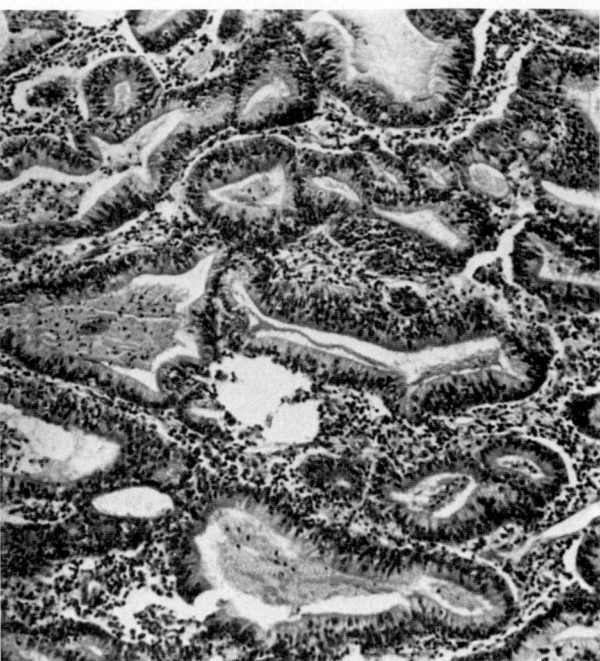

FIGURE 47.4. Well-differentiated adenocarcinoma (grade I). The distinct glandular pattern is preserved with minimal stroma. Nuclear atypia, palisading, and cribriforming usually are present.

of endometrial carcinoma, based on the percentage of solid component present in the tumor: well-differentiated, grade I, contains less that 5% solid tumor (Fig. 47.4); moderately differentiated, grade II, contains 5% to 50% solid tumor (Fig. 47.5); and poorly differentiated, grade III, contains greater than 50% solid tumor (Fig. 47.6). A grade I or II tumor can be upgraded by one grade if significant cytologic atypia is present. The significance of grade as a prognostic factor in endometrial cancer is demonstrated by evaluating the survival of patients with surgically staged, stage I tumors by grade. Patients with grade I tumors have a 5-year survival of 92% compared with a survival of only 74% for patients with grade III tumors. Histologic differentiation also is related to the risk of lymph node metastasis, as Lewis and associates found in a series of 107 patients who were treated by radical hysterectomy and lymph node dissection. Only 5% of the patients with well-differentiated tumors had positive pelvic lymph nodes, whereas 25% of the patients with poorly differentiated tumors had lymph node metastases.

Histologic Type

About 90% of epithelial tumors of the endometrium are of the endometrioid histologic type. Of these, more than 10% have mixed squamous elements. Unfortunately, the more virulent clear cell and papillary serous subtypes are seen more frequently today. Mucinous and pure squamous carcinomas of the endometrium are relatively rare (annual report, 2001). The uncommon types present

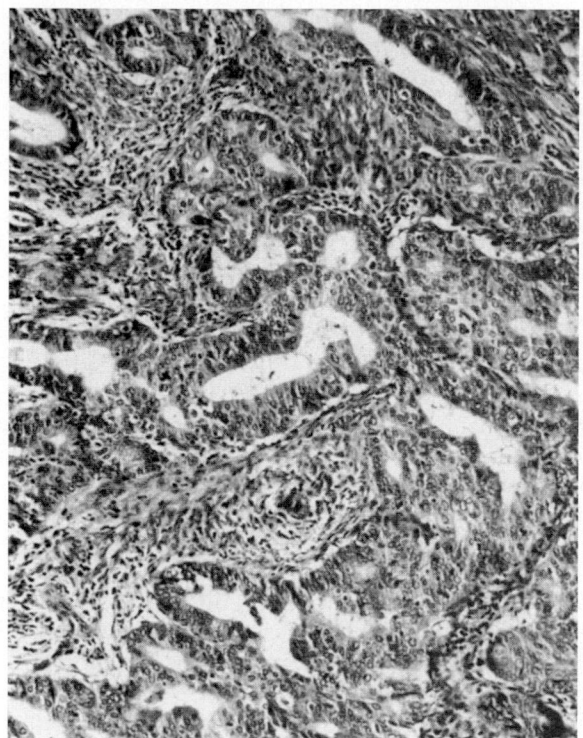

FIGURE 47.5. Moderately differentiated adenocarcinoma (grade II). Well-formed glands are mixed with solid sheets of malignant cells. Moderate pleomorphism and chromatin clumping are present.

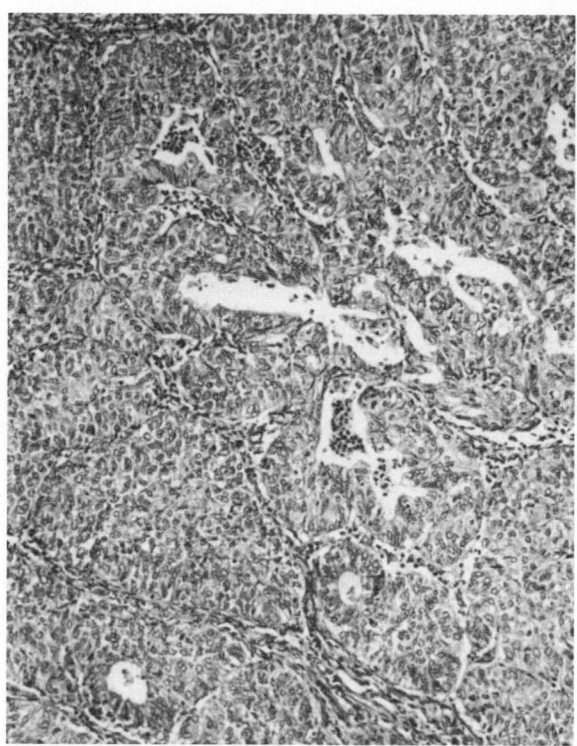

FIGURE 47.6. Poorly differentiated or undifferentiated adenocarcinoma (grade III). The tumor is virtually solid and has lost most glandular organization, with shells of atypical cells and prominent mitotic activity, pleomorphism, and chromatin clumping.

special problems in management, risk of recurrence, and overall prognosis.

Among the endometrioid tumors, the glandular grade is more important than the presence or absence of squamous elements in determining prognosis. The term *adenoacanthoma* is probably entrenched in the minds of generations of pathologists and clinicians. *Endometrioid carcinoma with benign squamous metaplasia* is the more current and more descriptive term. The prognosis for patients with endometrioid carcinoma with benign squamous metaplasia is probably slightly better than the prognosis for pure endometrioid carcinoma. Fanning et al. reported 418 cases of clinical stage I corpus cancer and found the absolute survival rate for endometrioid adenocarcinoma to be 88% and that for endometrioid adenocarcinoma with benign squamous metaplasia to be 91%. This supports the data of Connelly et al., which showed that grade for grade, endometrioid adenocarcinomas with benign squamous metaplasia have a somewhat better prognosis.

Although historically, women with adenosquamous carcinoma, in which both the squamous and the glandular elements are malignant, were felt to have a worse prognosis than pure adenocarcinoma, this is no longer thought to be the case. Salazar and coworkers (1991) compared the survival of 87 patients with adenosquamous carcinoma with that of 260 patients with pure adenocarcinomas and 29 patients with endometrioid adeno-

carcinoma with benign squamous metaplasia. The prognosis was similar, when corrected for stage.

Papillary serous adenocarcinoma is recognized as being an important histologic subtype with a poor prognosis. Christopherson et al. reported 46 patients with papillary serous carcinoma and described this lesion as a more aggressive type of papillary tumor. They found it to have a more anaplastic cellular pattern, to be associated with a more advanced stage of disease, and to have a 5-year cure rate of 51%. The pattern of spread of papillary serous adenocarcinoma is similar to that of ovarian carcinoma, and extrauterine disease is common even with clinical stage I disease and no myometrial invasion. The GOG finds this variant sufficiently virulent to include even early-stage cases in high-risk treatment protocols.

Similarly, *clear cell carcinoma* is associated with a more aggressive clinical course. Fanning and associates found clear cell tumors to have deep myometrial invasion in 36% of cases. Only 43% of their patients with stage I disease survived for 5 years.

Several other histologic types have been described, but cases are few and analysis is difficult. The secretory or *mucinous adenocarcinoma* has an appearance similar to that of other mucinous tumors of the genital tract. Its behavior appears to mimic adenocarcinoma of the endometrioid variety, when grade and myometrial invasion are considered. *Glassy cell carcinoma* of the endometrium has been reported, but most pathologists consider this a poorly differentiated adenosquamous carcinoma, as is the case for its counterpart in the cervix. Pure *squamous cell carcinoma* of the endometrium seldom occurs, but it appears to be moderately aggressive.

Depth of Myometrial Invasion

The use of depth of myometrial invasion for substaging stage I endometrial cancer emphasizes the importance of this finding. Although tumor grade is a reflection of aggressiveness, depth of invasion is the most reliable indicator of tumor volume.

The depth of tumor invasion into the myometrium correlates with the size of the uterine cavity, the frequency of pelvic lymph node metastases, and the 5-year survival rate. In an older study, Lewis and colleagues (1970) reported that no pelvic lymph node metastases were identified when the tumor involved only the endometrium or invaded the superficial one third of the myometrium. The 5-year survival rate was 93.7% in patients with no myometrial involvement and 88.1% in those with superficial myometrial involvement. Among patients who had tumors that extended to within 2 mm or less of the serosal surface, 36.2% were found to have positive pelvic lymph nodes and only 33% survived for 5 years, even though they received postoperative radiation therapy. These early data correlate well with the published pilot study of the GOG, as reported by Boronow et al. and discussed below in the section on lymph node metastases. Holmesly and coworkers observed 539 patients with carcinoma confined to the corpus (stage I), and found that only one of 93 patients with deep myometrial invasion had a grade I lesion. Of the other 92 pa-

tients with deep myometrial extension, 48 had grade II lesions, 32 had grade III lesions, and in 12 patients the tumor grade was not recorded. Deep myometrial invasion resulted in a 5-year survival rate of only 61%. In the 2001 FIGO report on endometrial cancer, data on depth of myometrial invasion were available in 6,260 operated cases. There were 3,996 patients with surgical stage I cancer. The 5-year survival rates were 88.9%, 90%, and 80.7% for stages IA, IB, and IC, respectively.

Lymph Node Metastasis

It was not until the early 1970s, when the pendulum of treatment began to swing away from preoperative radiotherapy, that pelvic lymph node involvement in endometrial carcinomas began to be more appreciated. This prompted collaborative attempts by the GOG and others to more accurately determine patterns of spread.

In the GOG collaborative pilot study, Boronow et al. made a clinicopathologic study of the uterus, fallopian tubes, ovaries, and pelvic lymph nodes of 222 patients who underwent surgery for clinical stage I endometrial carcinoma. They studied the paraaortic lymph nodes of 158 of these patients. In this study, 80% of stage I tumors were grade I or grade II (40% each) and 20% were grade III lesions. About 40% of the tumors were confined to the endometrium, and 20% showed deep myometrial invasion.

As shown in Table 47.6, both the tumor grade and the extent of myometrial invasion were important determinants of the frequency of pelvic lymph node metastases. Pelvic lymph nodes were involved in 10.3% of the patients, with a 2.2% incidence for grade I, 11.4% for

TABLE 47.6.

Node Metastasis in Patients with Clinical Stage I Endometrial Carcinoma by Invasion and Grade[a]

Invasion and Grade	Patients	Pelvic Node Metastasis		Aortic Node Metastasis in Sampled Patients		Aortic Node Metastasis Overall	
		Number	Percentage	Number	Percentage	Number	Percentage
Endometrium G1	58	1	1.7	1/47	2.1	1/58	1.7
Endometrium G2	27	1	3.7	0/15	0.0	0/27	0.0
Endometrium G3	7	0	0.0	0/06	0.0	0/07	0.0
Superficial G1	27	0	0.0	0/18	0.0	0/27	0.0
Superficial G2	40	1	2.5	0/26	0.0	0/40	0.0
Superficial G3	13	3	23.1	5/11	45.5	5/13	38.5
Intermediate G1	4	0	0.0	0/02	0.0	0/04	0.0
Intermediate G2	8	2	25.0	1/04	25.0	1/08	12.5
Intermediate G3	5	1	20.0	0/03	0.0	0/05	0.0
Deep G1	4	1	25.0	0/03	0.0	0/04	0.0
Deep G2	13	6	46.2	5/09	55.5	5/13	38.5
Deep G3	16	7	43.7	5/14	35.7	5/16	31.3
TOTALS	222	23	10.3	17/158	10.08	17/222	7.7

[a] It should be noted that patients were clinically staged and many would be up-staged on the new system. Also, depth of invasion is calculated by thirds of muscle thickness.

(From: Boronow RC, Morrow CP, Crasman WT, et al. Surgical staging in endometrial cancer: clinical pathologic findings of a prospective study. *Obstet Gynecol* 1984;63:825, with permission.)

grade II, and 26.8% for grade III tumors. The risk of pelvic lymph node metastases was negligible when the cancer was confined to the endometrium, regardless of the grade of the tumor. When superficial invasion to the inner one third of the myometrium occurred, only grade III lesions showed a significant incidence of pelvic lymph node metastases (23.1%). However, when the middle (intermediate) one third of the myometrium was invaded by tumor, the incidence of pelvic lymph node metastases for grade II and grade III tumors was 25% and 20%, respectively. When deep myometrial invasion occurred with extension of tumor to the outer one third of the uterine wall, all grades of tumor showed a high incidence of pelvic lymph node metastases: 25.0%, 46.2%, and 43.7%, respectively, for grade I, II, and III lesions.

Paraaortic lymph node metastases were detected in 10% of the 158 patients in the GOG study in whom these lymph nodes were sampled and in 7.7% of the entire 222 cases. The pelvic nodes provide a valid indicator of the risk of paraaortic lymph node metastases. In the study by Boronow et al., when pelvic lymph nodes were negative, only 1.5% of patient had involved paraaortic lymph nodes. When pelvic lymph node metastases were present, the paraaortic lymph nodes were positive in 60% of the cases. As noted in Table 47.6, when deep myometrial invasion occurs, between 25% and 46% of cases will have pelvic lymph node metastases, and more than 30% of the cases with grade II or grade III lesions will have paraaortic lymph node metastases.

The final update by Morrow and colleagues (1991) of the expanded group-wide GOG cohort of 895 patients that could be evaluated, emphasized the impact of myometrial invasion on paraaortic lymph node metastases: When there was no myometrial invasion, there were no paraaortic lymph node metastases. For invasion of one third and two thirds of the myometrium, paraaortic lymph node metastases were identified in 1.9% and 2.1% of patients, respectively. With invasion of the outer one third of the uterine wall, 38 of 224 (17%) patients were found to have tumor metastatic to the paraaortic lymph nodes.

The estimated overall risk for lymph node metastases for clinical stage I endometrial cancer ranges from 7.7% to 10.8%. The overall 5-year cure rate is reduced to 50% to 55% when pelvic lymph nodes are found to contain metastatic tumor.

Metastases to the pelvic lymph nodes are also related to tumor extension into the cervical canal (stage II). Because of the rich concentration of lymphatics in the paracervical tissues (cardinal ligaments), cervical involvement increases the potential for dissemination of tumor cells to pelvic lymph nodes. The frequency of extension of endometrial carcinoma to the isthmus and cervical canal increases with the extent of myometrial invasion. As reported by Lewis and Bundy, endocervical involvement (occult stage II) occurs in 7.3% of cases with tumor confined to the endometrium only and increases to 9.3% with superficial myometrial invasion, 10.8% with intermediate invasion, and 25% with deep myometrial invasion. About 15% of all cases of endometrial cancer will have either occult or clinical extension of tumor to the cervix. The incidence of pelvic node metastases in stage II disease is about 30% and increases to nearly 45% with grade III lesions.

Other Prognostic Variables

The prognostic factors most important in making treatment decisions are stage, tumor grade, histologic subtype, and depth of myometrial invasion. The following factors may alter the final surgical stage and also portend a statistically worse prognosis.

Increasing age of the patient continues to play an important role in predicting outcome. As stated earlier, the mean age at diagnosis continues to rise. The incidence of other adverse prognostic factors tends to increase with older age. The data from the twenty-fourth FIGO report demonstrate this. Among surgically staged patients with stage I disease, patients age 40 to 49 years had a 5-year survival of 97.7%, which decreased each decade thereafter. Patients age 60 to 69 years had a 5-year survival of only 88.4%. Age also affects grade and stage of disease. For the population as a whole, 70% to 75% of endometrial carcinomas present as stage I. However, Hoffman and associates (1995) found that 77% of women age 75 to 92 years presented with tumors that were deeply invasive or of advanced stage. In addition, the more virulent histologic types (undifferentiated, clear cell, papillary serous, and squamous cell) were disproportionately represented. The investigators suggested that such an increase in poor prognostic factors in the elderly might be related to a diminished immunologic defense rather than to hormonal factors, but this has not been substantiated. Age appears to be an independent variable of uncertain significance in treatment planning; the surgeon must not allow advanced age to compromise the patient's treatment, while at the same time considering all aspects of the patient's health and future quality of life.

Peritoneal cytology is considered by most investigators to be an important prognostic factor. In a comprehensive review of the existing literature, McLellan et al. combined 15 studies to establish an 11.4% incidence of positive peritoneal cytology among 3,091 patients with clinical stage I adenocarcinoma. Their review clearly indicated that patients with positive cytology are at higher risk for recurrent disease, and that the presence of malignant cells is predictive of other poor prognostic factors, including advanced histologic grade, depth of myometrial invasion, and lymph node metastases. Their cumulative data suggest that the importance of peritoneal cytology, a rather easy maneuver to accomplish, might rest in its predictive value for the presence of lymph node metastases. The incidence of positive lymph nodes among patients with positive cytology was 35% compared with only 8.7% in those with negative cytology ($p < 0.001$). Sutton confirmed the importance of peritoneal cytology in a series of 615 patients. In this series, survival for clinical stage I patients with negative cytology was superior to the survival of patients who had malignant cells in the washings.

Cervical invasion, lymph-vascular space invasion, adnexal spread, and *presence of intraperitoneal disease* are clear indicators of aggressive disease. All correlate well with other poor prognostic factors, and they are often found in combination. The report of the GOG pilot study by Boronow et al. confirmed that any of these factors portends a higher risk for lymph node metastases. This was confirmed by the 1987 report by Creasman and colleagues of the expanded series, as well as by a 1991 further analysis by Morrow and associates of the entire group of patients that could be evaluated. Three of these four factors increase the actual surgical stage, but the individual clinician must assign the prognostic weight of lymph–vascular invasion. In the GOG study, lymph–vascular invasion portended a much worse prognosis, so including this histologic observation in the pathology report is useful.

The expression of *steroid hormone receptors* is less well established as a prognostic indicator in women with endometrial cancer compared with women with breast cancer. Accumulated data have shown this information to be useful for predicting outcome, as well as for suggesting initial therapy of recurrent disease. Ehrlich et al. reported the relationship between of clinical outcome and estrogen- and progesterone-receptor content, as determined by the dextran-charcoal method, in 175 patients with endometrial adenocarcinoma. Progesterone-receptor content appeared to be more useful than estradiol-receptor content, correlating well with the risk of recurrence, grade, histology, adnexal spread, and age. Recurrence among patients with stage I disease was significantly more common if tumors were progesterone-receptor negative than if they were positive (37.2% versus 7%). Although a similar relationship to risk of recurrence was noted for estradiol receptor content (41.2% for receptor negative versus 12.7% for receptor positive patients), overall survival correlated only with progesterone receptor content ($p < 0.001$). The usefulness of receptor expression as a prognostic measure may be limited by available methods. Segreti et al. performed immunohistochemistry by using monoclonal antireceptor antibodies on paraffin-embedded tumor specimens and demonstrated significant expression of progesterone and estrogen receptors by adjacent benign tissue components, such as stroma, myometrium, and normal glandular epithelium. The expression of steroid hormone receptors by normal tissues cannot be differentiated from the expression of these receptors by tumor cells in biochemical assays.

The utility of steroid receptor expression analysis in endometrial cancer has yet to be established. It is not clear if the steroid hormone receptor data adds anything to the clinical picture, because a large number of excellent surgical–pathologic prognostic factors are already known for patients with endometrial cancer. The additional expense of obtaining steroid receptor studies has not yet been justified by the data.

Oncogenes, ploidy, and molecular markers are also being studied as prognostic factors. The virtual explosion in molecular biology, genetics, and biochemistry research has resulted in numerous efforts to translate such results into the clinical management of endometrial cancer patients. Berchuck et al. at Duke found high expression of the HER-2/neu oncogene in 27% of patients with metastatic disease, compared with 4% of patients with disease confined to the uterus. Investigation of this relationship is continuing at the GOG group-wide level. Ito et al. found a significant correlation between p53 tumor suppressor gene overexpression and poor prognosis in 221 cases of endometrioid endometrial adenocarcinoma. Podratz et al. published work that demonstrated that DNA ploidy and proliferative activity in pretreatment curettage specimens of patients with endometrial cancer were useful in identifying patients at high risk of extrauterine metastases and relapse. The clinical application of these parameters has yet to be established.

POSTOPERATIVE TREATMENT

After the comprehensive operation, the gynecologic surgeon can accurately assess the prognostic factors mentioned above (summarized in Table 47.7), assign the appropriate surgical stage, and plan postoperative treat-

TABLE 47.7.
Postoperative Treatment Plan for Endometrial Carcinoma

Stage	Grade	Treatment
IA	G1, G2, G3	Close follow-up
IB	G1	Close follow-up
IB	G2	Consider radiation
IB	G3	Postoperative radiation
IC	G1, G2, G3	Postoperative radiation
IIA	G1	Consider radiation
IIA	G2, G3	Radiation
IIB	G1, G2, G3	Radiation therapy
IIIA (positive washings only)	G1, G2, G3	Intraperitoneal ^{32}P
IIIA (adnexal spread)	G1, G2, G3	Radiation
IIIA (serosal spread)	G1, G2, G3	Radiation
IIIB	G1, G2, G3	Pelvic radiation Groin irradiation if lower $\frac{1}{3}$ of vagina involved
IIIC	G1, G2, G3	High-risk protocol treatment; if not available, pelvic radiation; consider whole-abdomen radiation
IVA	G1, G2, G3	Radiation
IVB	G1, G2, G3	Whole-abdomen radiation or chemotherapy

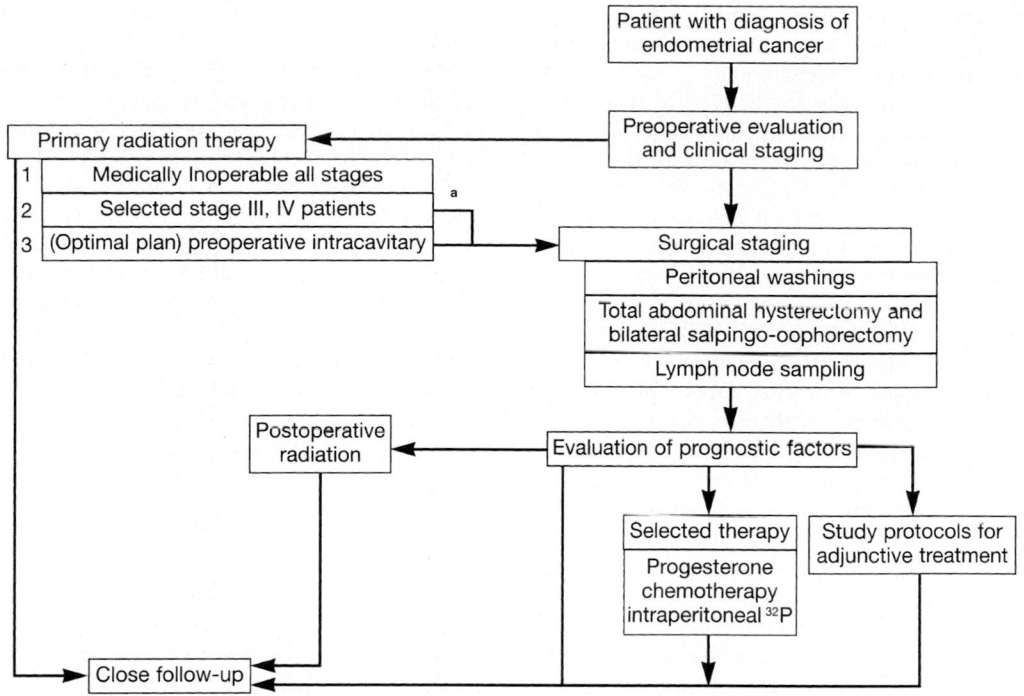

FIGURE 47.7. Algorithm for the overall treatment of endometrial cancer.

ment. Most patients will need no further therapy, but those with proven risk factors can have individualized treatment.

For patients who are thought to need additional therapy after definitive surgery, three basic modalities are available: radiation therapy, chemotherapy, and hormonal treatment (Table 47.7). Postoperative radiotherapy is commonly used for patients thought to be at increased risk of recurrence, although there are no prospective studies confirming its effectiveness. Chemotherapy and hormonal therapy are primarily used for patients with advanced stage disease or for palliative therapy. The overall treatment plan for endometrial cancer is schematically depicted in Fig. 47.7.

Irradiation Therapy

The options for the use of radiation therapy in endometrial carcinoma are summarized in Table 47.8. These should be used selectively after tumor board conference with close interaction and cooperation between the gynecologist and radiation therapist.

Radiation After Surgical Staging

Traditionally, patients with surgically staged endometrial cancer have been divided into three risk groups as an aid in making decisions about the need for postoperative radiotherapy. Low-risk patients have a high rate of cure without any postoperative therapy. This group includes individuals with grade I or II tumors confined to the en-

dometrium. Morrow's review of the GOG data has demonstrated that there is no benefit to these patients from receiving postoperative radiotherapy. Of 91 patients with stage IA, grade I or II tumors treated with hysterectomy, 19 received vaginal-cuff or whole-pelvic

---

TABLE 47.8.
Radiation Therapy in Endometrial Cancer

1. After surgical staging
   Vault radiation
   Whole-pelvis radiation
   Extended-field radiation (to paraaortic nodes)
   Whole-abdomen radiation with pelvic boost
2. Preoperatively
   Intracavitary and vault brachytherapy
   Whole-pelvis external therapy
3. As sole therapy
   Intracavitary
      Heyman packing
      Standard tandem with ovoids
   Whole pelvis with or without extended field
   Whole abdomen with pelvic boost
4. For recurrent disease
   Whole pelvis, with or without vault brachytherapy
   Spot irradiation for symptomatic metastasis
5. Special applications
   Intraperitoneal ^{32}P
   Template interstitial brachytherapy
   Intraoperative radiotherapy

radiation therapy postoperatively and 72 received no postoperative therapy. Treatment allocation was not randomized. No patient had a recurrence.

Intermediate risk patients are defined as those who demonstrate a reduced rate of surgical cure, but who may or may not benefit from additional therapy. This group includes patients with the following: myometrial invasion by tumor, cervical extension of tumor, lymph–vascular space invasion, positive peritoneal cytology, or grade III tumors with no myometrial invasion. Even today, many of these patients are treated with external beam whole pelvic radiotherapy. This is despite the fact that studies consistently show that whole-pelvic radiotherapy reduces local recurrence rates, but does not improve survival in patients with intermediate risk endometrial cancer. The GOG performed a prospective randomized study of surgical stage I and occult stage II endometrial cancer. Patients were randomized between 5,040 cGy whole-pelvic radiotherapy or no further treatment. There were 392 patients who could be evaluated. Those who received pelvic radiation had fewer local recurrences (6.8% in treated patients versus 15.3% in untreated patients), but there was no difference in survival (84.2% in treated patients versus 82.2% in untreated patients). A large randomized study was done by Dutch investigators of 715 patients with stage I endometrial cancer. Patients received either 46 Gy whole-pelvic radiotherapy or no postoperative radiotherapy. The 5-year local recurrence rate was 4% and 14%, respectively. The 5-year survival was 81% in patients who received radiotherapy and 85% in untreated patients.

As pointed out by Corn et al. in a study of 235 patients irradiated to a median dose of 45 Gy, pelvic radiotherapy after hysterectomy for endometrial cancer is not completely benign. Severe complications that required hospitalization or surgical intervention developed in 5% of patients. Age over 65 years, treatment of one portal per day, and previous lymph node dissection significantly predisposed patients to treatment-related morbidity. In the Dutch study, late complications occurred in 25% of the radiotherapy group compared with 6% of the control group. Most complications were grade I and involved mainly the gastrointestinal tract. There were seven grade III complications requiring surgery.

Evaluation of the GOG data revealed that most of the pelvic recurrences among patients with intermediate risk endometrial cancer occur at the vaginal cuff. This fact, along with the potential morbidity of external-beam whole-pelvic radiotherapy prompted the investigation of vaginal-cuff brachytherapy alone as adjuvant treatment for intermediate risk endometrial cancer. Chadha et al. treated 124 patients with stage IB, grade III or stage IC, any grade endometrial cancer with postoperative high-dose-rate vaginal-cuff brachytherapy. With a median follow-up of 30 months, there were no recurrences. Similarly, Anderson and colleagues treated 102 patients with stage IB and IC endometrial cancer who had undergone hysterectomy with high-dose-rate vaginal-cuff brachytherapy. The 5-year actuarial overall survival was 84%, and the 5-year disease-free survival was 93%. Pelvic control was excellent, with 97% of patients being free of pelvic disease at 5 years.

Most recently, Straughn et al. at the University of Alabama have suggested that patients with stage I endometrial cancer do not need any additional therapy after hysterectomy and surgical staging. They identified 613 patients with stage I endometrial cancer who had undergone comprehensive surgical staging, including pelvic and paraaortic lymphadenectomy. Of these patients, 239 were classified as intermediate-risk, and "most" were managed without radiotherapy. There were 16 (8%) recurrences among the intermediate-risk patients who were managed without postoperative pelvic radiotherapy. In comparison, there was one (4%) recurrence among the intermediate-risk patients who received adjuvant pelvic radiotherapy.

In this same study, there were 321 patients with stage IB endometrial cancer who did not receive any radiotherapy postoperatively. Of these patients, nine recurred in the pelvis or vagina, and all nine local recurrences were salvaged with whole-pelvic radiotherapy and vaginal-cuff brachytherapy. Fifty-three patients with stage IC disease received no postoperative radiotherapy. Two patients had vaginal recurrences and both were salvaged, one with surgery and radiotherapy and the other with radiotherapy alone. Although these numbers are small, they suggest that patients with stage I endometrial cancer may not benefit from adjunctive postoperative radiotherapy. The goal of this treatment is to prevent pelvic recurrences. Although pelvic (particularly vaginal) recurrences do occur in patients who do not receive postoperative pelvic radiotherapy, these patients are usually curable with radiotherapy given after the recurrence is diagnosed. A strategy of withholding pelvic radiotherapy postoperatively and treating only those patients who recur would decrease patient morbidity and significantly reduce the cost of treating endometrial cancer. Additional, preferably prospective, studies are needed to confirm these results. However, the role of postoperative radiotherapy in the treatment of patients with intermediate-risk endometrial cancer is clearly changing.

High-risk patients are unlikely to be cured without postoperative therapy. This group includes patients with pelvic or paraaortic lymph node metastases, patients with adnexal metastases, patients with intraperitoneal spread of disease, and those with high-risk histologic subtypes, such as papillary serous or clear cell carcinoma, but extrapelvic recurrences are common. Patients with pelvic lymph node or adnexal metastases are usually treated with pelvic radiotherapy. Patients with high pelvic or paraaortic lymph node metastases generally receive extended field radiotherapy. By using this approach, investigators have reported 5-year actuarial survival rates approaching 60%. It should be remembered that the efficacy of radiation therapy among patients with nodal metastases has not been proven in prospective studies, although it would be considered routine by many oncologists. There are reports of long-term survivors among patients with metastases to lymph nodes (even paraaortic) treated with surgery alone.

Whole-abdominal radiotherapy may be of benefit to high-risk group patients, particularly those with intraperitoneal disease. Greer and Hamberger from the M.D. Anderson Cancer Center reported on 31 patients who had intraperitoneal endometrial cancer treated by the whole-abdomen moving strip technique. Residual disease was equal to or less than 2 cm, and the corrected 5-year survival rate was 80%. Only one patient required operative intervention for a radiation complication. Although these results seem overly optimistic, they do suggest that aggressive irradiation therapy may be of benefit to patients with advanced disease. The GOG conducted a nonrandomized study of patients with ultra-high-risk disease by using whole-abdominal radiotherapy. Patients with all stages of papillary serous and clear cell carcinoma and surgical stage III and IV of all other cell types were included. The patients received radiotherapy to the whole abdomen along with a pelvic boost. Those patients with resected, positive paraaortic lymph nodes received a boost to the paraaortic chain. Three-year survival was 31% for patients with stage III/IV clear cell and papillary serous carcinoma and 33% for patients with stage III/IV endometrioid carcinoma.

Endometrioid adenocarcinomas are not particularly responsive to cytotoxic chemotherapy. However, for patients with papillary serous carcinoma, treatment with paclitaxel and carboplatin chemotherapy in combination with vaginal vault irradiation is sometimes used as an alternative to whole abdominal irradiation.

Preoperative or Radiation Therapy Alone

Although at one time preoperative radiation was standard therapy in many institutions, it is used rarely today. Surgical staging has essentially eliminated the need for this type of preoperative therapy.

When patients are medically inoperable, irradiation only may be used for definitive treatment. Despite general agreement that without surgery survival rates are lowered by 10% to 20%, good results have been provided with sophisticated radiotherapeutic techniques.

The M.D. Anderson Cancer Center and other expert radiotherapeutic centers have now achieved favorable results in the treatment of patients with serious medical complications or advanced disease. As reported by Landgren et al., a 5-year survival rate of 68% was achieved in the M.D. Anderson study, and a 10-year survival rate of 57% was achieved for patients with medical contraindications to surgery. Patients with an unresectable tumor treated with megavoltage irradiation had a 26% survival rate at both 5 and 10 years. The M.D. Anderson series stressed the use of intrauterine and intravaginal radiation sources combined with high-voltage external irradiation, when possible, to control the central tumor and any extension to the parametrium and pelvic wall. Autopsy reports from the medically inoperable patients showed that pelvic control of the disease was obtained in 89% of stage IA, 78% of stage IB, 82% of stage II, and 62% of stage III lesions.

Varia et al. from the University of North Carolina reported on 73 patients with clinical stage I and stage II disease who were poor operative risks and were treated with radiation only. Their data were broken down to show the impact of grade on survival. The 5-year survival rate for grade I was 72%; for grade II, 59%; and for grade III, only 31%, a profound and significant difference. In addition, they pointed out the limitations of radiation to even control disease in the treated field because 83% of the recurrences had a local or pelvic component. They suggested aggressive techniques, including chemoradiation, to improve local control.

Recurrent Disease

Radiation can be used for pelvic recurrent disease if the patient did not previously receive the maximum adjuvant radiation. Both intravaginal and external techniques can be used. Irradiation therapy is most effective for local recurrences confined to the central pelvis. The poor cure rates reported by Columbia–Presbyterian Hospital indicate the grave prognosis for recurrent endometrial carcinoma. Even when lesions recurred in the vagina, the survival rates were only 15% to 20%. Brown and coworkers from the Mayo Clinic reported a much more favorable survival rate of 50% for 30 patients with vaginal recurrences treated with irradiation.

When preoperative intracavitary irradiation is used before the initial surgical treatment, the secondary treatment should be limited to 5,000 cGy of betatron or linear accelerator megavoltage delivered to the mid-pelvis. If no irradiation was used during the initial treatment, 5,500 cGy of megavoltage irradiation can be given to the whole pelvis, followed by an additional 4,000 cGy given to the vaginal surface with vaginal ovoids. Normal tissue tolerance must be carefully observed. The total irradiation dose to the vesicovaginal wall should not exceed 8,000 cGy delivered to a depth of 0.5 cm. The rectovaginal wall should not be treated with doses higher than 7,000 cGy delivered to a depth of 0.5 cm. In many instances, small local recurrences can be treated with excision with or without subsequent radiation.

When endometrial cancer metastasizes to bone or peripheral nodal areas, spot irradiation can be used for pain control and to reduce unsightly and frightening lesions. The tolerance of adjacent tissues usually allows relatively high fractions, so that therapy can be completed quickly.

Special Applications

Customized radiation applications may be necessary in treating endometrial cancer. Interstitial therapy is often necessary in advanced disease when vaginal, parametrial, or pelvic disease needs higher doses than can be delivered by standard applicators. Similarly, intraoperative radiation, when available, may be useful for isolated unresectable metastasis. Although neither of these techniques can be relied on alone, they could be part of a comprehensive, customized therapy for advanced disease.

Intraperitoneal radioactive phosphorus (^{32}P) is a specialized intracavitary treatment used for patients with positive peritoneal cytology, but such treatment cannot yet be termed standard care for all centers. Soper et al. at

Duke University reported on 65 women with malignant cytology from endometrial cancer who were treated with intraperitoneal radioactive chromic phosphate suspension. The disease-free survival rate was 94% for surgical stage I (older staging system adaptation), and the incidence of intraperitoneal recurrences was low; only one of 11 patients who had recurrence had it solely in the peritoneal cavity. None of the 48 patients who received ^{32}P alone suffered chronic intestinal morbidity requiring surgery, but five of 17 patients who received adjuvant pelvic irradiation in addition to ^{32}P had complications necessitating surgical intervention. It was the investigators' conclusion that when peritoneal cytology was the only increased risk factor present, ^{32}P was the treatment of choice. We concur, but this is by no means a universal opinion. As previously pointed out, malignant cytology often is accompanied by other factors that indicate a poor prognosis. These patients might be better treated with whole-abdomen radiation, and they should be considered for advanced protocols in an oncology center.

TREATMENT OF ADVANCED DISEASE

Stage II

When the cervix is involved with endometrial cancer, the incidence of pelvic lymph node metastasis is 36.5%, as shown in a review by Morrow and coworkers (1991). Some may treat these patients with preoperative irradiation. A mid-pelvic dose of 5,400 cGy is given over 5 to 6 weeks by megavoltage external irradiation, which may be followed by a single intracavitary application of cesium with use of the Fletcher-Suit afterloading method and vaginal colpostats. The dose of irradiation to the vaginal surface should be adjusted appropriately. Four weeks after irradiation therapy, a total abdominal hysterectomy and a bilateral salpingo-oophorectomy are performed to remove the tumor in the uterus. Surgery should include an examination of the pelvic and paraaortic lymph nodes. All palpable nodes should be removed from the bifurcation of the aorta to the level of the inferior mesenteric artery because of the high incidence of extrapelvic node metastasis. Patients who are not able to undergo surgery should be treated with full external and intracavitary irradiation.

Other investigators have suggested a radical hysterectomy and pelvic lymphadenectomy should be done. In 1989, Boothby et al. reported on 42 patients with stage II disease treated at the Hospital of the University of Pennsylvania. In this retrospective, nonrandomized study, reported survival rate was in patients treated with radical hysterectomy and pelvic lymphadenectomy (68.5%), compared with combined surgery and radiation (46.1%) or radiation alone (36.5%), but the small numbers did not allow statistical significance. Andersen in Denmark reviewed 54 patients with clinical stage II corpus cancer and found a higher survival in patients treated with postoperative external and vaginal radiation after simple hysterectomy than in patients treated with radiation alone (70.6% versus 50%).

Today, many patients with presumed stage II disease undergo surgery first. Boente et al. retrospectively examined recurrence patterns and complications in 202 patients with cervical involvement. They divided the patients into five different groups according to treatment and found that the older conventional forms of treatment that used preoperative radiation therapy were not superior to primary surgical intervention and subjected patients to significant morbidity. Thus, they recommended consideration of the operative approach initially. We agree and do the primary surgical staging and plan postoperative therapy if needed, depending on surgical pathologic findings. Many investigators would give postoperative radiation therapy in patients with cervical involvement even though its effectiveness has not been evaluated in a prospective study. The last FIGO report (2001) would question the rational of postoperative radiation. In stage IIA, 5-year survival is 83% in the radiotherapy patients compared with 79.3% in nonradiated patients (not significant). In stage IIB, 74.9% compared with 73% survival is noted respectively, and again, this is not statistically significant.

Stage III

In the patient who is found to have stage III disease at the time of surgical staging, subsequent therapy depends on location of disease. If nodes are involved, many would treat with radiotherapy, the extent depending on site of metastasis. Patients with adnexal involvement or those in whom tumor penetrates to the uterine serosa are usually treated postoperatively with external pelvic radiation. Most recent studies have shown that peritoneal washings that contain malignant cells do not adversely affect prognosis unless there is other evidence of extrauterine disease. As noted previously, intraperitoneal ^{32}P has been used to treat these patients in the past. It is not clear if any additional treatment is necessary after surgery if positive washings are the only reason to assign a patient to stage III.

If the patient has disease in the vagina, (stage IIIB) some would treat with preoperative radiation. It is important to thoroughly evaluate the vagina. Disease can be limited to the upper vagina, although lower vaginal metastasis periurethrally is not uncommon. We prefer to surgically stage these patients so that if extra uterine disease is identified, radiation ports can be more exactly determined.

Stage IV

In the patient with intraabdominal or other stage IV disease, effective therapy currently is suboptimal. Certainly, all disease possible should be surgically removed. Fortunately, invasion into the bladder and rectum is unusual. Whether to do partial colectomy or cystectomy is a clinical decision made at the time of surgery. If all gross disease can be removed with excision of part of the bladder or rectum, this should lend itself to a more favorable prognosis. Intraperitoneal disease may be more difficult to remove if dissemination is present. Postoperative chemotherapy, much like ovarian cancer, is currently the treatment of choice, although most would add adriamycin to the regime. If inguinal nodes are involved, radiation after lymphadenectomy appears appropriate.

SPECIAL CONSIDERATIONS IN ENDOMETRIAL CANCER

The Role of Radical (Clark-Wertheim) Hysterectomy

Because radical hysterectomy and lymphadenectomy were used for cervical cancer, surgeons naturally extended the use of the procedure to the treatment of endometrial carcinoma. The followers of Bonney from London and then the Oxford school of pelvic surgeons, including Stallworthy and Hawksworth, practiced the radical method until statistical evaluations clearly showed that a radical procedure offered no improvement in patient survival. The best 5-year survival rate reported by Lewis and coworkers (1981) and by other investigators using radical hysterectomy and lymphadenectomy to treat stage I tumors was 71%. Better survival rates were achieved with less aggressive surgery with and without irradiation.

Even though Park et al. were able to report an excellent cure rate of 91% for stage I endometrial adenocarcinoma treated with the modified Wertheim procedure at the Walter Reed Hospital, patients had a high complication rate of 24%. Evaluation of the removed pelvic nodes showed that only 1.6% were positive for metastatic tumor. Rutledge reevaluated the role of radical hysterectomy for stage I disease and concluded that this procedure has a limited role, if any, in the treatment of endometrial carcinoma.

Many patients with endometrial carcinoma are elderly, obese, and fraught with multiple coexisting medical problems. Radical surgical procedures in these high-risk patients are all the more traumatic, and the complication rate naturally is increased; thus, the surgeon must exercise good judgment in treating such patients.

Vaginal Hysterectomy

Although vaginal hysterectomy occasionally has been used for treatment of endometrial tumors, use of the procedure should be limited. For instance, when a patient is so obese that abdominal surgery would be extremely difficult, performing vaginal surgery is better than not removing the tumor. The patient will tolerate vaginal surgery better, but the surgeon will have difficulty assessing the extent of the disease in the pelvis and abdomen. Examining the lateral pelvic walls and upper abdomen is virtually impossible from the vaginal route, but peritoneal washings can be obtained when entering the posterior cul-de-sac.

Butler and Pratt from the Mayo Clinic have reported more than 40 years experience with the use of vaginal hysterectomy for many selective cases, mainly those with well-differentiated endometrial carcinoma and a small uterus. These patients with stage IA tumors had an 84% survival rate, with only one vaginal recurrence. Peters and coworkers' (1983) report of 56 patients with stage I disease treated by vaginal hysterectomy, with or without adjunctive therapy, showed a 94% survival rate. The update of this series by Lelle et al. in 1994 added four additional patients. The crude survival rate at 5 and 10 years was 91.1% and 87.1%, respectively, with only one patient dying of cancer 6 years after primary treatment. Similar results were reported by Bloss et al., who used the vaginal approach on 31 patients; there was only one cancer-related death 4.5 years after surgery. Adjuvant radiotherapy was administered in 35% of patients who had either deep myometrial invasion or unfavorable histology. All of these studies should be viewed with extreme caution, because undoubtedly the candidates were carefully chosen.

Vaginal hysterectomy may be ideal for elderly, frail patients confined to nursing homes for multiple reasons. Surgically, these cases may be difficult, but with the use of Schuchardt incisions, proceeding slowly with small tissue bites, and with adequate retraction, the operation can proceed smoothly and can result in a paucity of postoperative care requirements. Removal of the ovaries is almost always possible. This is an important part of the treatment and should be performed if technically feasible during a vaginal procedure.

Unsuspected Endometrial Carcinoma

On rare occasions, an endometrial carcinoma is discovered during surgery for a supposedly benign disease. Although not originally planned, the ovaries and fallopian tubes must be removed, and if possible, the full staging procedure should be done if intraoperative evaluation of the uterus suggests poor prognostic factors. For cases in which the uterus has been removed for benign disease and the ovaries and tubes have been left in place, histologic study occasionally discloses unsuspected endometrial carcinoma. If there is no evidence of myometrial invasion and the lesion is a well-differentiated, grade I tumor, the adnexa need not be removed. If the uterine disease is grade III or shows deep myometrial invasion, the adnexa may be effectively treated with postoperative irradiation, or alternatively, the adnexa can be removed surgically. In postmenopausal patients, the small risk of ovarian metastasis alone should be compared with the stage of the disease and the grade of the tumor before an additional laparotomy is recommended for the specific purpose of removing the tubes and ovaries and completing the surgical staging.

In either case, the decision to reexplore the patient rests with the likelihood of the need for additional therapy. Even though a good estimate can be made on examination of the specimen, clear informed consent after patient appraisal of the facts is essential. For healthy women with moderate risk factors, we usually recommend the complete operation rather than blindly choosing either no further therapy or adjunctive radiation. Childers et al. in Arizona have demonstrated that the laparoscopic approach to restaging such patients can be accomplished not only with minimal morbidity and excellent information on which to base further therapy but also with the opportunity to remove the tubes and ovaries, perform lymph node sampling, and perform indicated biopsies. As mentioned earlier, restaging by this technique clearly requires laparoscopic and oncology expertise.

Concomitant Independent Ovarian Cancer

The coexistence of primary tumors in the ovary and uterus is not rare but causes considerable clinical discussion when it occurs. First, metastatic disease from either site or a remote primary tumor from a distant organ (e.g., breast) must be ruled out. In the former case, this can be quite difficult, because most synchronous tumors are endometrioid, and differentiation can be troublesome. Albright and Rath discussed 34 cases of simultaneous cancers of the uterus and ovary and found that 21 could be classified as endometrial primary tumors with ovarian metastasis. They established both major and minor criteria in reaching this decision: A multinodular ovarian pattern was a major criterion; minor criteria included small (less than 5 cm) ovaries, bilateral ovarian involvement, deep myometrial or vascular invasion, and tubal lumen involvement. Twelve of their patients had none of these criteria and were thought to have independent tumors. Interestingly, Gitsch and colleagues (1995b) found in a study of younger patients (less than 45 years old) that five of 17 cases (29.4%) had synchronous ovarian malignancies, and three others had secondary ovarian involvement. Thus, in the younger premenopausal patients, one should be especially cognizant of this possibility.

When this eventuality is encountered, the surgical staging procedure is virtually identical to the standard staging for endometrial cancer, except that evaluation of the diaphragm, omentum, and random peritoneal sites is indicated to properly assess the spread patterns of ovarian cancer. If full staging information is available, postoperative treatment usually is tailored to the disease with the worst prognosis or the most high-risk factors. Treatment can often be consolidated to cover both primary sites and their spread patterns. When exact staging has not been accomplished, the surgeon must surmise risk factors from available data and either plan treatment or reexplore surgically for definitive information.

Variable-Level Invasion Limited to Adenomyosis

Adenomyosis is a common occurrence in women at risk for endometrial cancer, and the presence of cancer deep in the uterine muscle may be solely owing to adenomyotic involvement. It is clear that myometrial invasion limited to foci of adenomyosis offers a better prognosis than true invasion to that depth. Jacques and Lawrence in Detroit provided more data supporting this concept in their clinicopathologic review of 23 cases. Their criteria included presence of stroma, adjacent benign glands, expansion patterns of the tumor, contour of myometrial lesions, and absence of peritumoral desmoplasia. When these criteria were properly identified, the data supported the earlier literature, and they also suggested that endometrial adenocarcinoma may arise *de novo* in adenomyosis. This may explain the occasional presentation of a patient with stage III or IV disease who never exhibits a classic bleeding pattern. Thus, patients who demonstrate this entity after careful review should be treated according to the grade of tumor and other surgical staging factors rather than according to myometrial invasion.

Simultaneous Cancers in Other Organs

A small percentage of patients with endometrial cancer may be found to have simultaneous cancers in other organs, discovered at the time of work-up for corpus disease or in the immediate post treatment period. In a review of 456 cases of endometrial cancer from the Johns Hopkins Tumor Registry, Abbas found 12 cases (2.5%) of nonovarian cancer that were diagnosed either at the time of work-up or within 6 months of treatment. In almost all patients who subsequently died, the other primary tumor was responsible for their demise. Therapy, therefore, should be complete for the corpus cancer, but treatment of the second primary tumor mandates vigorous regimens, and the corpus disease should not be considered a deterrent.

RESULTS OF TREATMENT AND PROGNOSIS

With the acceptance of FIGO's surgical staging by the gynecologic oncology community worldwide, for the first time comparison of like patients can now be accomplished. It was appreciated that clinical staging carried a large margin of error with studies noting clinical stage I cancers have extrauterine disease about a quarter of the time and clinical stage II with over 50% not having true stage II. In reviewing the FIGO annual reports since 1988 (date of surgical staging classification), volume 21, published in 1991, had 43% of reported patients surgically staged. This has increased with each subsequent volume so that with the current issue (volume 24), 94% of patients were surgically staged.

The current volume evaluated 5,694 patients surgically staged and only 391 clinically staged. The problem of inadequate staging and its impact on survival is apparent. The IB surgically staged patients experienced a 90% 5-year survival compared to 58% of those clinically staged. Certainly, one explanation for this disparity is in the clinically staged patients, a certain number had unrecognized extrauterine disease. This difference holds for stage I various grades of tumor differentiation. Surgical grade I has a 5-year survival of 92% compared with 52.5% clinical grade I.

Grade and depth of invasion in patients with disease limited to the uterus are prognostically important when evaluated separately. Again, data from FIGO's annual report (2001) notes surgical stage I has a 5-year survival of 92%, 86.9%, and 74% for grade I, II, and III, respectively. When depth of myometrial invasion is evaluated, IA and B cancers have similar survival (88.9% and 90%) but this decreased to 80.7% for stage IC disease.

In multivariant analysis of stage I and II, surgically staged patients, there was no difference in survival between grade I and II patients. The same was true for stage IA and IB patients. Grade III and less than 50% myometrial invasion had a statistically worse survival.

FOLLOW-UP AND RECURRENCE

After definitive treatment, patients should be carefully monitored according to the outline in Table 47.9. Emphasis should be placed not only on detection of recurrent disease but also on screening for other cancers or health problems. The follow-up outlined should allow detection of the most common sites of recurrence.

Whether or not to give estrogen replacement therapy during follow-up to patients with corpus cancer is an unsettled issue. Creasman (1991) audaciously addressed this previously taboo approach at a national presentation. His report was subsequently published. Many clinicians surveyed anonymously admitted giving low-risk patients estrogens. Several additional retrospective studies have been reported, as well as a cohort study, all suggestive of a low recurrence rate when estrogen is given to the postendometrial cancer patient. The GOG is currently conducting a prospective randomized study in these patients. The 1993 ACOG committee opinion on estrogen replacement therapy and endometrial cancer notes no contraindications to estrogen replacement therapy, obviously with informed consent.

The factors that influence the recurrence of endometrial carcinoma are the extent of disease at the time of initial treatment, the degree of differentiation of the tumor, the adequacy of the primary treatment, the individual host response, and the presence of other high-risk factors, including the patient's age. More than two thirds of all recurrent tumors develop within 2 years of initial therapy.

Flow cytometry of cell nuclei from endometrial cancers for DNA content and index has been shown to be a reliable prognosticator of treatment failure and recurrent disease. Iversen performed DNA indexing in a prospective study of 52 cases of cancer of the corpus and found 27% to be aneuploid, which was correlated with tumor grade but not with the other prognostic variables, such as stage, degree of invasion, or age. He found higher recurrence rates, shorter disease-free intervals, and higher death rates in the aneuploid group. Newbury et al. at Geisinger Medical Center reported 233 cases of endometrial cancer, with a median follow-up time of 8.7 years. In these cases, flow cytometry of archival paraffin blocks was used to determine DNA content. Aneuploidy was not detected in low-grade tumors and, similar to Iversen's work, was strongly predictive of death from disease when the DNA index was greater than 1.5. Thus, more sophisticated techniques in the future may assist standard staging methods to predict recurrence, including the ongoing oncogene studies.

The most frequent sites of recurrence of endometrial carcinoma are the upper vagina, uterus, pelvic lymph nodes, paraaortic nodes, and lungs. Dede et al. reported that in 75% of their patients with recurrent endometrial carcinoma, the secondary lesion developed outside the pelvis. This is in agreement with results from a multi-institutional report by DiSaia et al. in the GOG, in which 222 patients with clinical stage I carcinoma of the endometrium were studied. During the 36- to 72-month follow-up of this study, 79% of the recurrences were located outside the pelvis. When definable extrauterine disease was absent at the time of the original surgery, the recurrence rate was only 7%, but if disease was found anywhere outside the uterus, the recurrence rate was 43%. In this study, the undifferentiated grade III tumors, the tumors with deep myometrial invasion, and the tumors with either pelvic or aortic node involvement showed the highest incidence of recurrence. Curiously, of the 34 patients with recurrence among the 222 stud-

---

TABLE 47.9.
Follow-Up After Treatment for Endometrial Cancer

Examination or Test	Interval
History and physical examination, including pelvic examination, cuff Papanicolaou smear, and rectal examination	Every 3 months for 2 years, then every 6 months for 3 years, and then yearly for life
Chest radiography	Yearly
Mammography	Yearly
Computed tomography scan, magnetic resonance imaging, and ultrasonography	Only if clinically indicated

ied cases, local and distant recurrence was present in 3% of the patients treated by primary surgery and radium and in 5% of those treated by primary surgery alone.

Among 171 cases in studies by Malkasian et al., Salazar et al. (1977), and Aalders et al., the failure rate in the pelvis with surgery alone was 16.4%. In the abdomen or other sites, the rate was 11%. In contrast, among 198 patients with stage I, grade III tumors treated with radiotherapy and surgery, and reported by Aalders et al., Salazar et al., and Komaki et al. (1984), the rate of failure in the pelvis was only 5.6%, and in either the abdomen or distant sites, the rate was 15%. This large study gives clear evidence that the more advanced tumors that require surgery and external irradiation are more likely to recur. When such recurrences are found, they usually are in distant, extrapelvic sites.

Specific information about the original tumor and its treatment is needed to determine whether or not secondary treatment is possible. If secondary treatment is to be given, irradiation and chemotherapy are the primary methods used to attempt to arrest recurrent growth.

If the patient has an isolated vaginal vault recurrence, local excision with or without radiotherapy has been successful in a number of patients.

Exenteration for recurrent endometrial cancer is almost anecdotal. In a series of 100 patients at the University of Michigan who underwent pelvic exenteration, Morley et al. performed only four such procedures for adenocarcinoma of the endometrium, and only one patient survived for 5 years. Thus, before proceeding with radical surgery, a meticulous search for extant disease outside the pelvis must be accomplished.

SYSTEMIC TREATMENT OF RECURRENT DISEASE

Hormonal Therapy

Historically, progestins have been used both as an adjuvant and as definitive therapy for recurrence (Table 47.10). Objective remission has been reported in about one third of the patients treated with progestins. Response to the hormone is best when a long, tumor-free period existed before recurrence of a well-differentiated, slow-growing tumor with positive receptor activity.

TABLE 47.10.
Response to Hormonal Agents

Drug	Patients	Response (%)
Hydroxyprogesterone caproate	384	32
Medrogestone	56	49
Medroxyprogesterone acetate	195	41
Megestrol acetate	125	47
Tamoxifen	59	20

(Modified from: Deppe G. Chemotherapeutic treatment of endometrial cancer. *Clin Obstet Gynecol* 1982;25:93, with permission.)

Progestins appear to work at the cellular level by slowing both DNA and RNA replication. They also have a modulating effect on estrogen stimulation. The intracellular effects of hormonal therapy are mediated by the interaction of the steroid and its receptor. Estrogen and progesterone cytoplasmic receptors have been shown to be markedly involved in the tumor response to hormonal therapy. Tumors that lack receptors are presumably unresponsive to a specific hormone. Therefore, in the treatment of patients with recurrent endometrial carcinoma, one might expect a good response to progesterone therapy in patients who had a high concentration of progesterone receptors in the primary tumor. Also, progestins are known to effect a reduction in available estrogen receptors, thereby decreasing the response of tumors to circulating estrogens. Progesterone also stimulates the production of estradiol-17_β dehydrogenase, which converts the active form of estradiol to a weaker estrogen, estrone. Both of these physiologic events, decreasing the number of estrogen receptors and decreasing the concentration of intracellular estradiol, have an antiestrogenic effect on the tumor. Therefore, progesterone receptors commonly are measured at the time of initial treatment to determine the likely biologic effect of the hormone on a recurrent neoplasm. Ehrlich et al. have shown a strong correlation between the responsiveness of progestins in recurrent endometrial cancer and the presence of progesterone receptors. In their study, patients with high concentrations of progesterone receptors in the tumor responded more frequently to progesterone treatment. Many investigators have shown that levels of progesterone receptors are higher in well-differentiated than in poorly differentiated endometrial carcinoma. Limited experience to date suggests a greater than 90% correlation between receptor status and response to progestin therapy.

In 1961, Kelley and Baker reported the initial results of using Delalutin for the treatment of metastatic endometrial carcinoma. Objective remission occurred in six of 21 patients who had pulmonary metastasis and lasted from 9 months to 4.5 years. A more recent report listed a 32% remission rate. Kistner also reported a 30% remission rate. In a collaborative study reported by Reifenstein, the average duration of tumor regression was 30 months. The dosage of Delalutin used was 1 g or more each week for 12 or more weeks. Most patients showed a better response when treated for longer than 12 weeks. Of 314 women studied, 21 had complete arrest of the disease. Cure could not be considered the specific result of progestin therapy because the women in Reifenstein's study also received ancillary treatment. No correlations have been made between survival rates and the amount of drug given each week, the patient's age, or the type of concomitant anticancer therapy provided. About 15% of all poorly differentiated tumors that were treated by Reifenstein responded to progestin therapy. Progestins have been evaluated as adjunctive therapy. Lewis and associates treated endometrial cancer patients postoperatively in a randomized study with medroxyprogesterone (MPA) or placebo. The 4 year survival was similar in the two groups. Several other investigators have performed similar studies, and there was no difference in survival between those taking MPA or placebo.

A GOG study evaluated 420 patients with advanced or recurrent endometrial cancer treated with MPA, 50 mg t.i.d. Only 17 complete responses (8%) and 13 partial responses (6%) were seen in those with measurable disease. Median survival was 10.5 months. In another GOG study, almost 300 patients were treated with either MPA at 1,000 or 200 mg per day. No difference in response rate or survival was noted. Lentz reported another GOG trial of high-dose megestrol acetate (800 mg per day) in patients with advanced or recurrence endometrial carcinomas. Thirteen of 58 (24%) patients responded, six (11%) had a complete response. Four of the responses lasted greater than 18 months and were mainly in grade I or II lesions.

Other progestational agents have provided similar results. Deppe analyzed various reports of the treatment of advanced or recurrent endometrial carcinoma with various hormonal agents and found that response rates ranged from 30% to 49% (Table 47.10). Megace showed a 47% objective response rate in a combined series of studies when oral doses of 80 mg per day were given. Higher doses resulted in similar rates. Medroxyprogesterone (Depo-Provera) has been tried in doses of 400 to 800 mg three times a week for a month, then once a week for a second month, and then once a month for maintenance. The results currently available show a 42% response rate, but the drug appears to give results similar to those of the other progestins used.

The activity of tamoxifen, an antiestrogen nonsteroidal agent that blocks the estrogen receptor, was reported by Swenerton in 1980. Unfortunately, only three of 10 patients showed objective response when given an oral dose of 10 mg twice daily on a continuous basis for the treatment of recurrent endometrial carcinoma. Quinn and Campbell reported on 49 patients treated with tamoxifen, 20 mg twice daily, and noted 10 responses, six of which were complete. Significantly, the median survival of responders was 34 months, compared with only 6 months for those who did not respond. Again, grade I lesions were more responsive than other grades of tumor. In a recently completed study, the GOG found modest activity of tamoxifen against recurrent disease, similar to those studies reported above.

The toxicity of tamoxifen is minimal, and it is worth trying in patients who fail progestins. Quinn suggests concomitant tamoxifen therapy with progestins because in tumors that prove to be unresponsive to progestin, the antiestrogen tamoxifen can be used to block estrogen receptors in an effort to affect specific steroid receptor mechanisms. Studies of small groups of patients have not produced favorable results.

Cytotoxic Chemotherapy

Various chemotherapeutic agents have been used in limited trials. In an earlier collaborative study by the GOG, Cohen and associates (1984) observed the response of 358 patients with advanced (stage III and stage IV) or recurrent endometrial cancer when treated with one of two multiagent regimens: (a) melphalan and 5-fluorouracil daily for 4 days, repeated every 4 weeks with megestrol daily for 8 weeks, or (b) adriamycin, 5-fluorouracil, and cyclophosphamide, intravenous bolus every 21 days with Megace daily for 8 weeks. The objective response rate in patients with measurable disease was 36.8% in both groups; 36.8% of each group had stable disease, and 26.4% progressed with treatment. Response was not affected by age, site of recurrence, time to first recurrence, or presence or absence of previous treatment with progestational or irradiation therapy. However, grade of the tumor and performance status did affect response, although 44 of 57 objective responders had undifferentiated tumors. The median survival for complete responders of both groups was only 18.3 months, compared with 12.9 months for partial responders and 8.8 months for patients with stable disease. The overall objective response rate of 36.8% for the multidrug regimens is no higher than the objective response rate for adriamycin alone, which was reported by the GOG in 1979 (headed by Thigpen) as being 37%, with a median duration of response of 7.4 months for complete responders; survival for this group was a median of 14 months.

Thigpen et al. reported on cisplatin as first-line chemotherapy in a phase II GOG trial for advanced or recurrent disease in 49 patients who could be evaluated. There were only two complete responses and eight partial responses, but 45% of patients exhibited stable disease for at least 2 months. The investigators believed that this limited activity warranted further trials. Cisplatin chemotherapy has been used by Seski et al. at the M.D. Anderson Cancer Center for 26 women with advanced or recurrent endometrial carcinoma. Doses of 50, 70, and 100 mg/m^2 were used every 4 weeks. An objective response was obtained in 42% of the patients, but the median duration of the remission was only 5 months, with a range of 2 to 11 months. Although cisplatin was found to be active against endometrial cancer, the high rate of toxicity (31%) limited the use of this agent in high doses on an outpatient basis.

The newer platinum analog carboplatin was studied by the Southwest Oncology Group for activity in endometrial cancer, as reported by Green et al. They found two complete and five partial responses in 23 patients who could be evaluated, for an overall response rate of 30%. Four responders showed a significant (839 or more days) duration of response, which suggests that this newer drug may prove to be promising for corpus cancer. Similar results have been found with adriamycin, cyclophosphamide, and cisplatin, but the toxicity of this regimen has been significant and the durations of response disappointing. Although many ongoing studies appear promising, the preferential combination of therapeutic agents has not yet been defined.

In a more aggressive approach using four drugs in combination, Long and associates (1995), in a multiinstitutional study, found the combination of methotrexate, vinblastine, doxorubicin, and cisplatin to be effective for recurrent endometrial carcinoma, but with substantial toxicity. Although there was an overall response rate of 67%, with a complete response rate of 27%, the median survival of responders was 11 months (range, 2.6 to 34.2 months). There were two treatment-related deaths, and 93% of patients experienced grade III or greater neutropenia. Thus, although this regimen is effective, caution should be exercised with its use. Less hearty patients might have a better quality of life with less aggressive combinations.

In a GOG study, 336 patients with advanced or recurrent adenocarcinoma were treated with doxorubicin with or without cyclophosphamide. All of these patients had failed to respond when given MPA. Only seven (5.4%) of those treated with doxorubin had a complete response compared with 18 (12.5%) who received doxorubicin and cyclophosphamide. Total response rate was 22% and 30%, respectively. A randomized study of doxorubin and cisplatin versus doxorubin, paclitaxel, and filgrastim (GCSF, Neupogen) was done by the GOG. There were 317 patients with measurable stage III or IV or recurrent disease. There was no significant difference in response rate or survival between the two arms. Mean survival was a little over 1 year.

The results of these studies indicate that progestational agents alone should be used primarily in patients with well-differentiated tumors or high levels of progesterone receptors. Cytotoxic chemotherapy should be reserved for patients with less favorable prognoses, those with poor tumor differentiation, absent progesterone receptors, and reduced performance status, and then only after failed trials with progestins. If available, all patients with recurrent disease not amenable to radiation therapy should be considered for cooperative chemotherapy trials.

Unfortunately, chemical control of recurrent endometrial carcinoma is limited and temporary, but newer agents such as ifosfamide, etoposide (VP-16), and paclitaxel (Taxol), alone and in combination with other agents, are being studied in hopes of gaining control over recurrent disease. Although the newer drugs show activity and are encouraging, none appears to provide a major breakthrough in the treatment of metastatic corpus cancer.

The advent of standardized surgical staging along with detection of early disease may preclude or decrease the current need for advanced disease treatment in most patients.

UTERINE SARCOMAS

The uterine sarcomas constitute only about 3% of corpus cancers. Nevertheless, they are important neoplasms for multiple reasons. First, they are the most rapidly growing of the uterine tumors, reputedly having a tumor cell–doubling time as short as 4 weeks. Second, although a unifying theme is that all arise from mesoderm, their histologic diversity has made them interesting and intriguing. Third, because they appear most commonly in the older age group, the incidence appears to be increasing. Finally, because of the virulent nature of these aggressive tumors, the clinical management is challenging.

Unlike pure epithelial tumors, uterine sarcomas can occur in perplexing sarcoma-like states, presenting a spectrum of clinical behaviors for each individual category. This often confuses not only the clinician but also the pathologist. Distinguishing between the benign variants can be difficult, because overall treatment and prognosis vary markedly. Consultation, therefore, is advised when planning treatment.

There is no known cause for sarcomas of the uterus, but there has been a long association with prior pelvic irradiation. This relation appears to be more commonly linked to the mixed mesodermal tumors, but it has, on occasion, been remotely present in all histologic varieties. The incidence of this association varies, lending some doubt as to whether or not there is a causative factor. Podczaski et al., in a retrospective review of 42 patients with mixed mesodermal tumors seen at the Hershey Medical Center, found that six patients had a history of prior radiation, for an incidence of 14%. This figure is consistent with the median of several series relating a prior exposure. Thus, historical information about previous radiation in an older woman with a pelvic mass or bleeding should raise the suspicion of uterine sarcoma.

Staging and Classification

Although there is no official FIGO staging for uterine sarcoma, most clinicians tend to use the surgical staging for endometrial cancer. Most systems of classification that are purely pathologic can become overly verbose and clumsy; a much more practical system reflects the observed frequency of the different sarcomas. This system is detailed in Table 47.11. The system revolves around the three basic tissues in the uterus derived from mesoderm: myometrium, stroma, and mixed patterns. The mixed patterns include both epithelial and mesodermal elements. These are most often termed mixed mesodermal tumors, although the term mixed müllerian tumor and the more specific carcinosarcoma also have been used. Included in this classification are the sarcoma-like entities associated with each tissue of origin.

TABLE 47.11.
Classification of Uterine Sarcomas

Mixed mesodermal tumors
   Homologous
   Heterologous
   Adenosarcoma
Leiomyosarcoma
Stromal sarcoma
Other (hemangiopericytoma, angiosarcoma, and so forth)

The relative frequency of sarcoma type more often depends on referral patterns and practice type than on pure epidemiologic data, mainly because of the relatively rare occurrence of sarcomas. The GOG completed a comprehensive long-term staging study of uterine sarcomas that was presented by Major et al. Of 447 cases that could be evaluated, most were mixed mesodermal tumors (337, or 75%); but other studies in the literature would suggest that 50% of uterine sarcomas are mixed (mostly heterologous or homologous with a lesser number of adenosarcomas), with about one third of cases leiomyosarcomas, about one sixth arising from the stroma, and the rarer types occurring much less frequently.

OVERALL SURGICAL MANAGEMENT

Preoperative assessment of uterine sarcomas parallels that of the more common epithelial cell type. Indeed, as many as 15% to 25% of poorly differentiated endometrial cancers in elderly women prove to have sarcomatous changes on final pathology. Therefore, the surgical staging procedure should be virtually identical. Data from the recent GOG staging study suggest that lymph node metastasis may be less important prognostically than previously suspected in sarcomas, especially leiomyosarcoma. Therefore, during the initial surgical procedure, total extrafascial hysterectomy with bilateral salpingo-oophorectomy is the basis of treatment, accompanied by lymph node sampling of suspicious nodes. Pelvic washings are performed on entry to the abdomen. A total lymph node dissection is not recommended merely for staging purposes. Although previous staging studies recommended omentectomy, this procedure has proved not to be worthwhile unless there is gross evidence of intraperitoneal disease.

Some surgical aspects of uterine sarcomas are unique. A mass protruding through the cervix in a postmenopausal woman must be considered sarcoma until proven otherwise. Fig. 47.8 shows a surgical specimen from an older woman with a mixed mesodermal tumor of the uterus, which extended into the left broad ligament and adnexa. Because of cervical stenosis, there was no symptomatic bleeding until disease was advanced, and then curettage was thwarted by the false passage created (Fig. 47.8, inset). Thus, the gynecologist must take caution when attempting to sound the uterus in such patients; we have found ultrasonography useful intraoperatively to guide the surgeon to the uterine cavity.

More commonly, sarcomas tend to be polypoid masses that dilate and balloon out the cervix and lower uterine segment (Fig. 47.9). This is a surgical challenge, and dissection of the parametria must be performed in a more radical manner if complete removal of the uterus is to be accomplished; failure to do so may mean tumor extruded into the peritoneal cavity or a portion of tumor-laden cervix left behind, virtually assuring a vaginal recurrence. Fig. 47.1 shows the correct technique. Dissection of the ureter takes place more laterally, with the uterine vessels cross-clamped away from the cervix. This

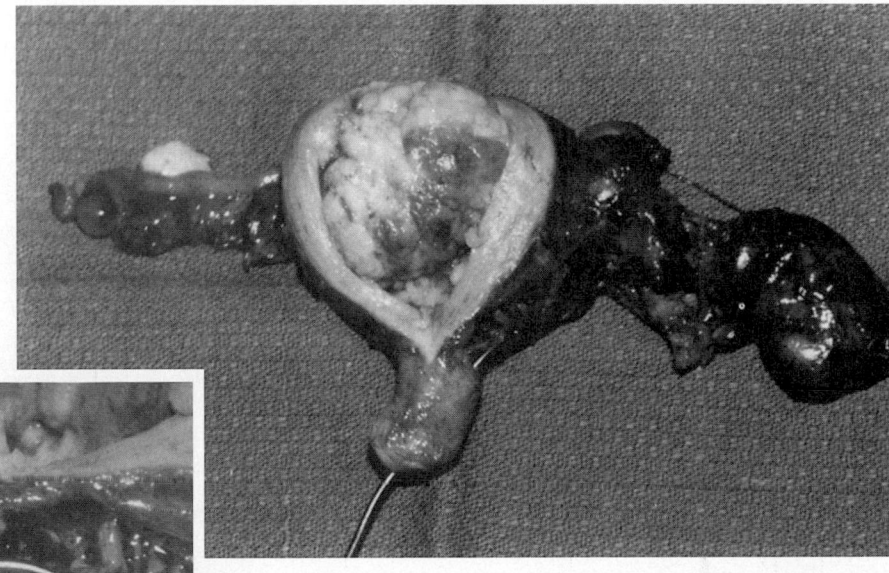

FIGURE 47.8. Typical appearance of mixed mesodermal tumor of the uterus, with extension into the left adnexa. **Inset:** How the preoperative dilatation and curettage created a false passage in the stenotic cervix.

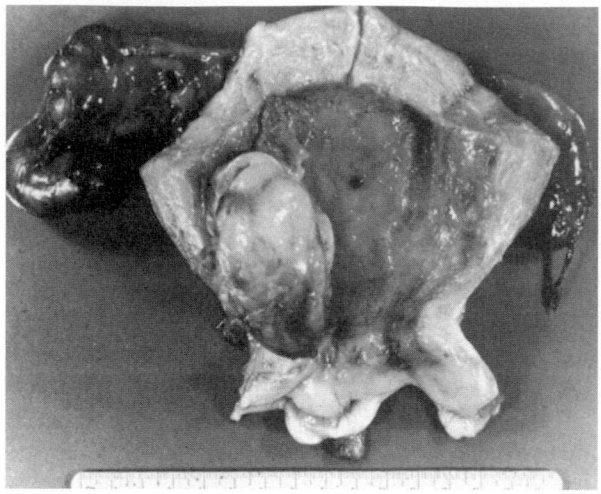

FIGURE 47.9. Characteristic polypoid pattern of a mixed mesodermal tumor of the uterus in an elderly woman. This tumor may appear grossly as a large endometrial polyp or as an aborting submucous leiomyoma.

avoids the "bounce off the cervix" maneuver when clamping the lower broad ligament and parametria. This also requires lower dissection of the bladder away from the upper vagina and allows a more complete vaginal cuff. If there is suspicion that the tumor actually invades the lower cervix, additional vaginal cuff can be removed, with frozen section guidance of free margins. The vaginal cuff should be closed with interrupted sutures. If closed-suction drainage is necessary, it should be accomplished transabdominally.

Postoperatively, there is no proven benefit to radiation therapy. Some investigators claim a reduction in the local failure rate if radiation therapy is given, but there is clearly no increase in overall survival. Salazar et al. (1978) suggested, in their review of radiation after surgery, a significant improvement in local control, but Spanos et al. found a local failure rate of 11% with combined treatment. Kohorn et al., by using both teletherapy and brachytherapy postoperatively, found an 18% failure rate in the pelvis, whereas Podczaski et al. reported a series with a 14% local persistence or recurrence with adjunctive radiation. Similarly, Echt et al. reported 66 patients treated with surgery alone, or surgery plus radiation. There was no difference in the incidence of failure, but there was a significant ($p = 0.0001$) decrease in pelvic failure.

We believe that postoperative treatment must be tailored to the surgical findings, but adjunctive treatment for advanced disease is mandatory. As recommended by Peters (1989) and others, we first administer vigorous chemotherapy systemically, by using agents that are protocol specified, if possible. The histologic type appears to have the most influence on the choice of drugs. Pelvic radiotherapy can then be given for local control, if indicated.

Ultraradical surgical therapy seldom is indicated for uterine sarcomas. In a series of nine patients with pelvic sarcomas treated with pelvic exenteration, as reported by Reid et al., four had primary uterine tumors. Two patients, one with stromal sarcoma and the other with leiomyosarcoma, were long-term survivors, but both patients with mixed mesodermal tumors succumbed to disease within a few months. As discussed below, we believe that extended surgical therapy plays an important role in the overall management of leiomyosarcomas, but in general, exenterative procedures and other ultraradical surgical maneuvers must be approached with caution in patients with uterine sarcomas.

Clinical Presentation and Management

Mixed Mesodermal Tumors

Mixed mesodermal tumors are the most common of the uterine sarcomas and constitute about 2% of all corpus cancers. This diverse group of tumors usually occurs in postmenopausal women age 55 to 65 years, and the incidence of the tumor appears to be increasing. These patients do not have the characteristics associated with endometrial carcinoma, such as prolonged estrogen stimulation or obesity, and they commonly present with uterine bleeding. Speculum examination often reveals polypoid masses extruding through the cervix. Diagnosis is rendered by histologic sampling of the endometrium, and the cellular patterns vary from one field to another. Further subdivision of these tumors depends on the cellular elements present (Figs. 47.10 and 47.11).

More benign-acting variants are *adenofibroma* and *adenosarcoma*, which can be defined histologically as showing a benign epithelial component intimately admixed with a benign or malignant mesenchymal component. Zaloudek and Norris presented a clinicopathologic

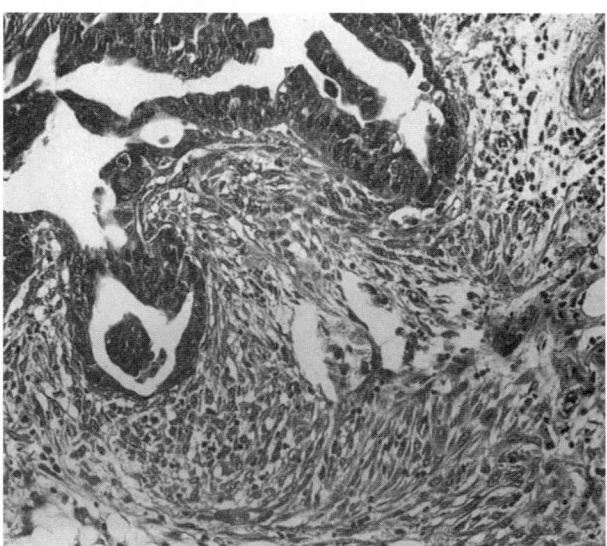

FIGURE 47.10. Homologous mixed mesodermal tumor. Malignant epithelial elements and malignant stromal sarcoma are admixed in this rather poorly differentiated tumor.

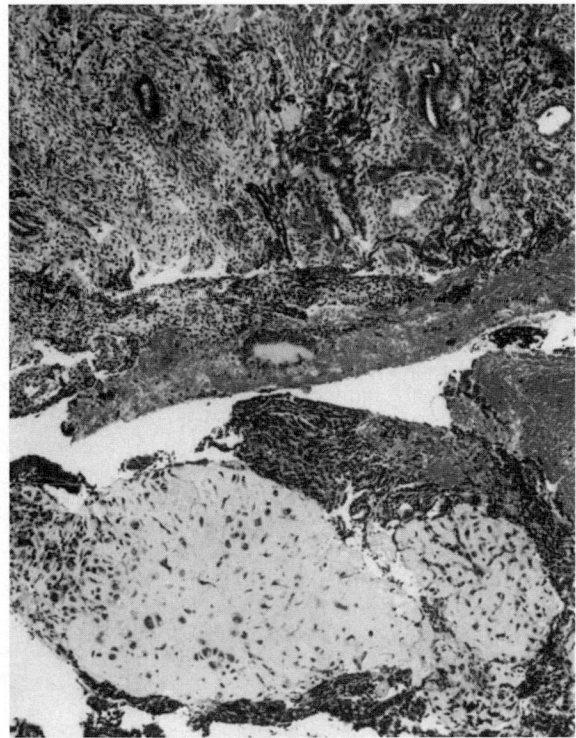

FIGURE 47.11. Heterologous mixed mesodermal tumor. The presence of sarcomatous elements ordinarily foreign to the uterus characterizes this variant of mixed mesodermal tumor.

study of 35 cases and found that adenofibromas had fewer than four mitotic figures per 10 high-power fields and behaved almost as benign tumors. On the other hand, the more malignant adenosarcoma, with more than four mitotic figures per 10 high-power fields histologically, behaved like other sarcomas, with a 40% recurrence rate and a median interval to recurrence of 5 years. These investigators found that the deeper the invasion of the myometrium, the worse the prognosis. About 11% of the mixed müllerian tumors in the GOG study were adenosarcomas, and their clinical behavior was less malignant when no heterologous elements were found. This supports our view that adenosarcoma as an entity must be closely examined with multiple pathologic samples to allow a prediction of a low incidence of recurrence.

Most mixed mesodermal sarcomas contain both malignant epithelial and mesenchymal components. The stromal component is basically a stromal sarcoma that contains rhabdomyoblasts, and the epithelial component demonstrates a wide variety of patterns from well-differentiated carcinoma to adenosquamous carcinoma. When the cell types are confined to these varieties only, the tumor is termed *homologous* mixed müllerian tumor, or the older term *carcinosarcoma*. In about half of the cases, these cancers contain tissues foreign to the endometrium, such as striated muscle, bone, cartilage, or adipose tissue; these are termed *heterologous* mixed mesodermal tumors. Heterologous tumors originally

were thought to have a worse prognosis than were the homologous variety, but all types have proved to have similar outcomes when extent of disease is the basis of comparison. This was borne out in the GOG study reported by Major et al. in which 42% of homologous tumors and 58% of heterologous tumors recurred. The group found that the presence of lymph node metastasis, adnexal spread, tumor size, lymph–vascular space involvement, and histologic grade were more predictive of recurrence than was cell type or mitotic index.

Postoperatively, patients with disease confined to the uterus should be closely followed, because there appears to be no proven benefit to adjunctive chemotherapy. In a randomized trial, Omura et al. (1985) from the GOG showed no benefit of adjuvant adriamycin in preventing recurrence, although adriamycin as a single agent and in combination with dacarbazine had shown activity in these sarcomas. Thigpen et al. from the GOG demonstrated activity of cisplatin in these tumors. It appears that ifosfamide is the most active single agent, and trials using ifosfamide in all uterine sarcomas, both as a single agent and in combination with cisplatin, are ongoing. Sutton et al. (1989), reporting for the GOG, found single-agent ifosfamide to effect a 32% response rate in patients who had not been exposed to prior chemotherapy, with five patients exhibiting complete response. In a subsequent study, Currie et al. from the GOG found modest activity with the regimen of hydroxyurea, dacarbazine, and VP-16 in similar untreated patients. Because none of these agents, alone or in combination, has been shown in a randomized study to prevent recurrence in early-stage patients, they should be used with caution in patients who have not demonstrated extrauterine disease.

In patients with advanced or recurrent MMT, the GOG performed a prospective randomized study comparing ifosfamide and mesna with or without cisplatin. In 194 patients, it was noted that the combined therapy results in higher response rate, greater toxicity, but no improvement in survival.

Leiomyosarcomas

Leiomyosarcomas arise from the myometrium and account for roughly one third of uterine sarcomas. Like their counterparts in the endometrium, these lesions demonstrate a spectrum of clinical diseases, from absolutely benign to highly malignant. Often there is great concern when a rapidly growing leiomyoma is excised and found to be a *cellular myoma*. These are characterized by dense cellularity but with rare mitotic activity and no pleomorphism. Thus, their behavior is benign, and surgical excision is the treatment of choice, either with myomectomy or hysterectomy. There are three variants of sarcoma-like conditions of the myometrium that can be mistaken for frank leiomyosarcoma: *intravenous leiomyomatosis, benign metastasizing leiomyoma,* and *leiomyomatosis peritonealis disseminata.* Although all have distinct clinical presentations, they are similar in their benign histologic appearance, and all appear to have sensitivity to progesterone treatment.

Intravenous leiomyomatosis involves vascular channels and often extends from the uterus into the veins of the broad ligament, and even into the major vasculature of the pelvis and upper abdomen. Grossly, it has a worm-like appearance, with swirls of tissue extruding from vessels that are cross-clamped and divided. The lesion may arise from adjacent myometrium and extend into the vessels, or it may develop *de novo* from the muscle of blood vessel walls. Surgically, care must be taken to remove all extension of disease into the pelvic vasculature, but otherwise, a simple hysterectomy is sufficient. The adnexa should be removed, and postoperative treatment with long-term progesterone is indicated.

Benign metastasizing leiomyoma is a rare condition in which apparently benign-appearing myomas can spread to the lungs and, occasionally, regional lymph nodes. In postmenopausal women, such nodules usually remain stable, but in premenopausal women, they can enlarge enough to cause pulmonary insufficiency. Treatment with progesterone can cause remission or stabilization, but surgical excision occasionally is required. Lesions that continue to grow despite hormonal therapy must be treated with systemic chemotherapy or excised; this growth is associated with a poor outcome.

Leiomyomatosis peritonealis disseminata is a diffuse, multifocal lesion in the peritoneal cavity that consists of benign-appearing leiomyomata that can reach several centimeters in size. Two thirds of the cases appear in black women, and most patients are diagnosed during the postpartum period or after taking oral contraceptives on a long-term basis. The origin of this entity is controversial, but Woodruff believes that it may be a consequence of fibrosis of the peritoneal decidua, or that it has some other multifocal cause. Treatment revolves around removing the estrogenic stimulus, either with delivery or discontinuation of oral contraceptives. When no apparent source of estrogen is evident, postoperative treatment with progesterone is indicated.

Frank *leiomyosarcoma* is a highly malignant tumor associated with a poor outcome, unless it develops in a pre-existing benign leiomyoma. Sarcomatous lesions of this kind are found in about 0.1% to 0.2% of all removed leiomyomata (Fig. 47.12). The accuracy of these figures was recently substantiated in an excellent review by Parker et al. Among 1,332 patients operated on for presumed leiomyoma, only one (0.075%) was found subsequently to have leiomyosarcoma; included in that series were 371 women who underwent surgery for "rapidly growing" myomas. Although this single patient was in that group, most patients with a uterus that enlarges in such a short interval have a very low chance of leiomyosarcoma being the culprit (one out of 371, or 0.27%, in this study). When the lesion is present in a pre-existing encapsulated tumor, the prognosis is excellent, even when there is a high mitotic count. Thus, simple surgical excision, preferably with total hysterectomy, is sufficient therapy.

The classic approach to determining cancer in a leiomyomatous lesion is to count the number of mitoses per 10 high-power fields. Unless the lesion in question is

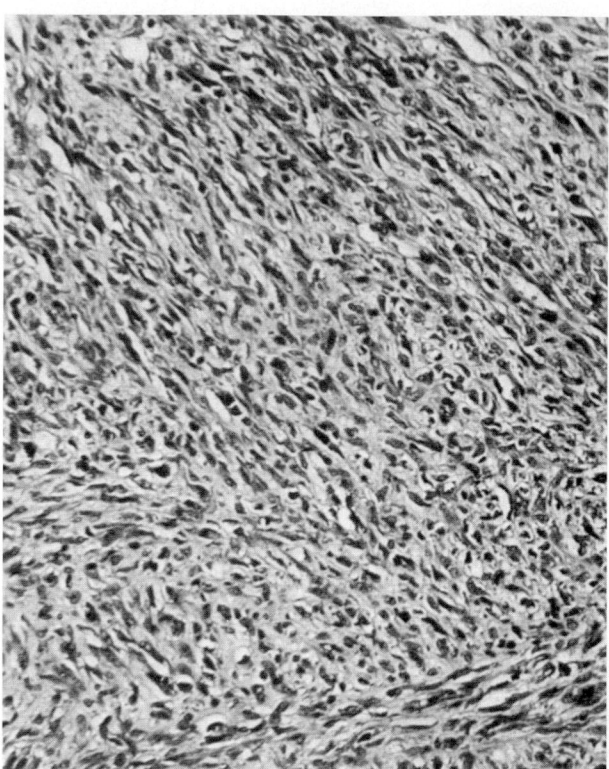

FIGURE 47.12. Sarcomatous change in leiomyoma showing frequent mitoses.

completely encapsulated in a benign leiomyoma, this approach appears to poorly predict clinical behavior until the mitotic count exceeds 20 mitoses per 10 high-power fields. Thus, the traditional approach of designating sarcomas with five to 10 mitoses per 10 high-power fields as low grade must be used with caution, because the extent of disease at the time of surgery offers a much better prediction of recurrence and, hence, survival. Interestingly, the propensity for these tumors to metastasize to regional nodes is surprisingly low—only 4% in the large GOG study.

Surgical treatment involves total hysterectomy with removal of the adnexa and any suspicious regional nodes or metastatic nodules. Adjunctive treatment with radiation appears to offer no benefit and may indeed impede future chemotherapy or surgical treatment.

In contrast to sarcoma arising in a leiomyoma, sarcoma developing *de novo* in the myometrium has an extremely poor prognosis. These lesions metastasize early and often to the lungs, and overall survival is rather dismal. In the GOG study, 36 of 56 patients with leiomyosarcomas had recurrence within 4 years of the original therapy, and similar results have been reported elsewhere. Size of tumor, vascular invasion, and extrauterine spread are poor prognostic factors.

Recurrent disease should be treated with chemotherapy. Currie et al. (1985) presented encouraging data using a combination of hydroxyurea, dacarbazine, and etoposide in recurrent leiomyosarcomas, and they noted several complete responses. When this regimen was tested in a group-wide phase II study in previously untreated patients, there were only two complete and five partial responses, for an objective response rate of 18.4%. However, 20 of 38 patients experienced stable disease while receiving a median of five courses of therapy. Using ifosfamide, Sutton and associates (1992) reported for the GOG a 17.2% partial response rate but no complete responses. In a subsequent GOG phase II study, Sutton and coworkers (1992) found an overall response rate of 33.3% with the addition of adriamycin, but only one complete response. Clearly, newer drugs and regimens are needed for a significant chemotherapy impact on metastatic leiomyosarcoma.

Currie and Rosenshein presented a group of seven patients with recurrent leiomyosarcoma who underwent surgical excision of abdominal disease followed by combination chemotherapy with subsequent long disease-free intervals. Thus, it appears that selected patients can benefit from aggressive surgical intervention, especially if chemotherapy is effective in controlling small-volume disease (see Chapter 43).

Primary Stromal Tumors

An isolated *stromal nodule* occasionally is encountered, and this raises the question of true sarcoma. These behave as a benign counterpart of malignant stromal disease and need no further therapy other than hysterectomy. If there is a possibility of extrauterine extension, postoperative progesterone is indicated. The most common stromal tumor usually is classified as *stromatosis,* or *endolymphatic stromal myosis* (Figs. 47.13 and 47.14). The typical patient is age 35 to 45 years. Although stromatosis normally is asymptomatic, some cases produce the same complaints as adenomyosis. Stromatosis is considered an adenomyosis without glandular involvement.

Because the lesions are primarily composed of proliferative stroma, mitoses occur frequently, and mitotic count is not a criterion of malignant potential. Although tumors with less than 10 mitoses per 10 high-power fields are considered low-grade stromal sarcomas, the 10-year survival rate is almost 100% when lesions are confined to the uterus.

As with all uterine tumors, the adnexa should be evaluated during surgery. If a diagnosis of stromatosis is made by frozen section of the uterine tumor, the tubes and ovaries should be removed, regardless of the patient's age. The lesions tend to spread without gross clinical evidence of the disease. Lesions extend through the myometrium, invade the adjacent tissues, and eventually metastasize.

Surgical evaluation of this entity is important because local recurrences are common and can lead to death by ureteral obstruction, intestinal obstruction, and massive

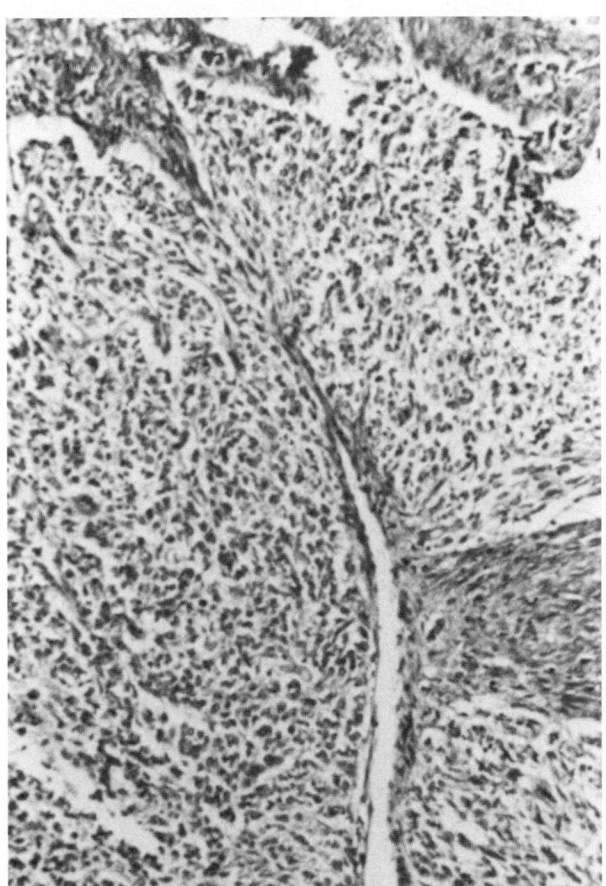

FIGURE 47.13. High-power microscopic view of stromatosis uteri or endolymphatic stromal myosis. The tumor is composed of proliferating endometrial stromal cells with many mitotic figures. Although relatively benign, it infiltrates the myometrium like adenomyosis without glands.

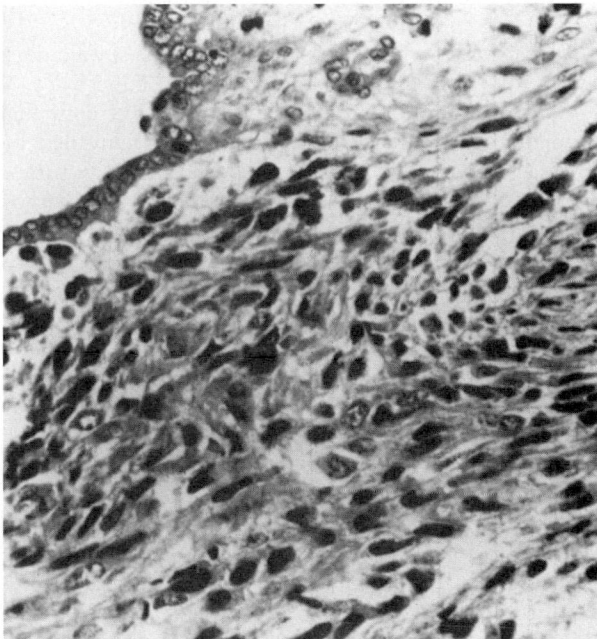

FIGURE 47.14. Endometrial stromal sarcoma. High-power microscopic view shows spindle cell pattern of stromal sarcoma cells. Bizarre nuclear changes of pleomorphism, hyperchromasia, and frequent mitoses are the features of this lesion (250×).

intravascular involvement. During removal of the uterus, the characteristic wormy extensions into the parametria may be obvious, and the cut surface of the freshly removed uterus virtually exudes low-grade sarcoma. Obtaining receptor data is vital to future therapy, because these lesions have high progesterone receptor content, as demonstrated by Baker et al. and others.

In a follow-up study of 33 patients reported by Thatcher and Woodruff, adjunctive progesterone treatment resulted in a high 10-year survival rate even when lesions had extended into adjacent tissue. Patients treated with irradiation had recurrences and eventually metastases. If more than 50% of the myometrium is involved, postoperative therapy with progestational agents (40 to 160 mg megestrol acetate daily) should be started. In a long-term follow-up of nine cases similarly treated, no recurrence was found in 10 years.

Montag and Manart reported on a patient with extensive venous recurrence treated with extirpation of intravascular disease extending up the inferior vena cava, as well as removal of the pelvic tumor. Postoperative treatment with progesterone resulted in good long-term follow-up. We encountered a similar case that presented with venous thrombosis and unilateral leg edema. Both of these recurrences probably could have been prevented by initial postoperative progesterone treatment. However, both demonstrate not only the ability of this disease to recur dramatically in vessels but also that aggressive surgical therapy is warranted.

The true stromal sarcoma is characterized by rapid mitotic activity, a loss of stromal cell differentiation, and frequent appearances of "strap cells" or rhabdomyoblasts (Fig. 47.12). The tumor is aggressive, and the adjacent myometrium often is destroyed by invasion and infiltration of inflammatory cells.

Treatment for the true stromal sarcoma should consist of total abdominal hysterectomy and adnectomy. A careful histologic search should be made for epithelial elements. One area of the uterus may be invaded by stromal sarcoma, whereas mixed mesodermal tumor may exist in another area. Adjunctive chemotherapy should be used in most cases, and preliminary data from the GOG suggest that ifosfamide-based regimens offer promise.

Other Uterine Sarcomas

Other pure heterologous sarcomas can arise from the uterus, but they, with other rare variants, constitute only a fraction of mesodermal tumors. Buscema et al. reported a series of patients with hemangiopericytoma, which is an extremely uncommon lesion that can occur at any site, in any age group, and in either sex. In female patients, the preoperative diagnosis usually is leiomyoma; the fundus is the most common site of origin. Although hemangiopericytomas are reported in many sizes, most are less than 10 cm in diameter. The surface of the tumor appears yellowish brown and greasy. When analyzed histologically, the lesion is characterized by a proliferation of the cells surrounding small blood vessels. The proliferating cells are known as pericytes of Zimmermann, which were identified more than 100 years ago by Rouget.

Although of vascular origin, the tumor is not as hemorrhagic as an angioma or an angiosarcoma. Because solitary tumors usually extend into the adjacent tissue, complete removal may be difficult. However, surgery reported to date, including a total abdominal hysterectomy and adnectomy, has resulted in a 5-year survival rate of almost 100% for patients with uterine hemangiopericytomas. Tumors in other parts of the body tend to recur, to extend into adjacent tissue, and to metastasize to the lungs. No adjunctive therapy is used for treatment of a hemangiopericytoma.

Sarcoma Prognostic Factors

In addition to the well-known indicators of sarcoma, such as grade, tumor size, depth of invasion, number of mitotic figures, extrauterine spread, lymph node metastasis, and clinical and surgical stage, numerous studies have indicated that there are additional prognostic factors. Wolfson and associates found that DNA content (ploidy level) had a clear prognostic value. Similarly, Malmstrom et al. from Sweden found that DNA ploidy and S-phase fraction showed significant value in predicting outcome, even when adjusted for stage, grade, and mitotic index.

Cytogenetic studies of uterine sarcomas are infrequent, but Laxman et al. from Johns Hopkins reported a series of 14 patients with sarcoma of the uterus who underwent chromosome analysis. They found abnormalities in 10 of 14 and suggested that chromosomes 1, 7, and 11 might play a role in tumor initiation or progression. Fresia et al. from the same institution reported an ongoing cell line of stromal sarcoma with an abnormal karyotype of 46,XX, del(5)(q31.1), der (7)t (6;7)(p21;p22), which remained unchanged in long-term culture. Finally, Liu et al. from Duke reported that mutation of the p53 tumor suppressor gene, with resultant overexpression of the p53 protein, frequently occurred in uterine sarcomas.

Clearly, continued investigation along these and other avenues is essential to improve the disappointing cure rate for uterine sarcomas that exists with the surgical and adjunctive tools currently available.

BIBLIOGRAPHY

Aalders J, Abeler V, Kolstad P, et al. Postoperative external irradiation and prognostic parameters in stage I endometrial carcinoma. *Obstet Gynecol* 1980;56:419.

American College of Obstetricians and Gynecologists. Report of Committee on Gynecologic Practice. *ACOG Committee Opin* 1993;126.

American College of Obstetricians and Gynecologists. Report of Task Force on Routine Cancer Screening. *ACOG Committee Opin* 1989;68.

Andersen ES. Stage II endometrial carcinoma: prognostic factors and the results of treatment. *Gynecol Oncol* 1990;38:220.

Anderson B, Marchant DJ, Munzenrider JE. Routine noninvasive hysterography in the evaluation and treatment of endometrial carcinoma. *Gynecol Oncol* 1976;4:354.

Annegers JF, Malkasian GD. Patterns of other neoplasia in patients with endometrial carcinoma. *Cancer* 1981;48:856.

Antunes CMF, Stolley PD, Rosenshein NB, et al. Endometrial cancer and estrogen use: report of a large cancer-control study. *N Engl J Med* 1979;30:9.

Barakat RB, Wong G, Curtin JPP, et al. Tamoxifen use in breast cancer patients who subsequently develop corpus cancer is not associated with a higher incidence of adverse histological features. *Gynecol Oncol* 1994;55:164.

Barbone F, Austin H, Partridge EE. Diet and endometrial cancer: a case-control study. *Am J Epidemiol* 1993;137:393.

Barnhill D, Heller P, Dames J, et al. Persistence of endometrial activity after radiation therapy for cervical carcinoma. *Obstet Gynecol* 1985;66:805.

Baum M, Odling-Smee W, Houghton J, et al. Endometrial cancer during tamoxifen treatment: Cancer Research Campaign Breast Cancer Trials Group. *Lancet* 1994;343:1291.

Bean HA, Bryant AJ, Carmichael JA, et al. Carcinoma of the endometrium in Saskatchewan: 1966 to 1971. *Gynecol Oncol* 1978;6:503.

Behbakht K, Yordan EL, Casey C, et al. Prognostic indicators of survival in advanced endometrial cancer. *Gynecol Oncol* 1994;55:363.

Berchuck A, Rodriguez G, Kinney RB, et al. Overexpression of HER-2/neu in endometrial cancer is associated with advanced stage disease. *Am J Obstet Gynecol* 1991;164:15.

Bloss JD, Berman ML, Bloss LP, et al. Use of vaginal hysterectomy for the management of stage 1 endometrial cancer in the medically compromised patient. *Gynecol Oncol* 1991;40:74.

Boente MP, Orandi YA, Yordan EL, et al. Recurrence patterns and complications in endometrial adenocarcinoma with cervical involvement. *Ann Surg Oncol* 1995;2:138.

Bonham DG, Donham RJC. Cancer of the endometrium, an improved epidemiological assessment. *Aust NZ J Obstet Gynecol* 1973;13:172.

Bonte J, Decoster JM, Ide P, et al. Hormonoprophylaxis and hormonotherapy in the treatment of endometrial adenocarcinoma by means of medroxyprogesterone acetate. *Gynecol Oncol* 1978;6:60.

Boothby RA, Carlson JA, Neiman W, et al. Treatment of stage II endometrial carcinoma. *Gynecol Oncol* 1989;33:204.

Boronow RC, Morrow CP, Creasman WT, et al. Surgical staging in endometrial cancer: clinical pathologic findings of a prospective study. *Obstet Gynecol* 1984;63:825.

Brinton LA, Barrett RJ, Berman ML, et al. Cigarette smoking and the risk of endometrial cancer. *Am J Epidemiol* 1993;137:281.

Brinton LA, Berman ML, Mortel R, et al. Reproductive, menstrual, and medical risk factors for endometrial cancer: results from a case-control study. *Am J Obstet Gynecol* 1992;167:1317.

Bristow RE, Zerbe MJ, Rosenshein NB, et al. Stage IV endometrial carcinoma. *Gynecol Oncol* 2000;78:85–91.

Broders AC. Microscopic grading of cancer. In: Pack GT, Livingston EM, eds. *Treatment of cancer and allied diseases,* vol. 1. New York: Hoeber & Harper, 1941.

Brooks SE, Yeatts-Peterson M, Boher SP, et al. Thickened endometrial stripe and/or endometrial fluid as a marker of pathology: fact or fancy? *Gynecol Oncol* 1996; 63:19.

Brown JM, Dockerty MD, Symmonds RE, et al. Vaginal recurrence of endometrial carcinoma. *Am J Obstet Gynecol* 1968;100:544.

Brown R. Clinical features associated with endometrial carcinoma. *J Obstet Gynaecol Br Commonw* 1974;81:933.

Brunschwig A. Surgical treatment of recurrent endometrial cancer. *Obstet Gynecol* 1961;18:272.

Burke TW, Heller PB, Woodward JE, et al. Treatment failure in endometrial carcinoma. *Obstet Gynecol* 1990;75:96.

Buscema J, Klein V, Rotmensch J, et al. Uterine hemangiopericytoma. *Obstet Gynecol* 1987;69:104.

Butler CF, Pratt JH. Vaginal hysterectomy for carcinoma of the endometrium: forty years' experience at the Mayo Clinic. In: Gray LA, ed. *Endometrial carcinoma and its treatment.* Springfield, IL: Charles C. Thomas, 1976.

Cacciatore B, Lehtovirta P, Wahlstrom T, et al. Preoperative sonographic evaluation of endometrial cancer. *Am J Obstet Gynecol* 1989;160:133.

Chadha M. Gynecologic brachytherapy-II: Intravaginal brachytherapy for carcinoma of the endometrium. *Semin Radiat Oncol* 2002;12:53–61.

Charpin C, Andrac L, Habib MC, et al. Immunocytochemical assays in human endometrial carcinoma: a multiparametric computerized analysis and comparison with nonmalignant changes. *Gynecol Oncol* 1989;33:9.

Chen SS. Propensity of retroperitoneal lymph node metastasis in patients with stage I sarcoma of the uterus. *Gynecol Oncol* 1989;32:215.

Chen SS, Rumancik WM, Spiegel G. Magnetic resonance imaging in stage I endometrial carcinoma. *Obstet Gynecol* 1990;75:274.

Chetkowski RJ, Meldrum DR, Steingold KA, et al. Biologic effects of transdermal estradiol. *N Engl J Med* 1986; 314:1615.

Chi DS, Welshinger M, Venkatraman ES, et al. The role of surgical cytoreduction in Stage IV endometrial carcinoma. *Gynecol Oncol* 1997;67:56–60.

Childers J, Brzechffa P, Hatch K, et al. Laparoscopically assisted surgical staging (LASS) of endometrial cancer. *Gynecol Oncol* 1993;51:33.

Christopherson WA, Alberhasky RC, Connelly PJ. Carcinoma of the endometrium, II: papillary adenocarcinoma: a clinical pathological study of 46 cases. *Am J Clin Pathol* 1982;77:534.

Chuang L, Burke TW, Tornos C, et al. Staging laparotomy for endometrial carcinoma: assessment of retroperitoneal lymph nodes. *Gynecol Oncol* 1995;58:189.

Clarke-Pearson D, DeLong E, Synan I, et al. Variables associated with postoperative deep venous thrombosis: a prospective study of 411 gynecology patients with creation of a prognostic model. *Obstet Gynecol* 1987;69:152.

Clement PB, Scully RE. Müllerian adenosarcoma of the uterus: a clinicopathologic analysis of ten cases of a distinctive type of müllerian mixed tumor. *Cancer* 1974;34:1138.

Cliby WA, Dodson MK, Podratz KC. Uterine prolapse complicated by endometrial cancer. *Am J Obstet Gynecol* 1995; 172:1675.

Cohen CJ, Brukner HW, Deppe G, et al. Multi-drug treatment of advanced and recurrent endometrial carcinoma: a gynecological oncology group study. *Obstet Gynecol* 1984; 63:719.

Cohen I, Rosen DJ, Shapira J, et al. Endometrial changes in postmenopausal women treated with tamoxifen for breast cancer. *Br J Obstet Gynaecol* 1993;100:567.

Cohen I, Rosen DJ, Shapira J, et al. Endometrial changes with tamoxifen: comparison between tamoxifen-treated and nontreated asymptomatic, postmenopausal breast cancer patients. *Gynecol Oncol* 1994;52:185.

Connelly PJ, Alberhasky RC, Christopherson WN. Carcinoma of the endometrium, III: analysis of 865 cases of adenocarcinoma and adenoacanthoma. *Obstet Gynecol* 1982;59:569.

Corn BW, Lanciano RM, Greven KM, et al. The impact of improved irradiation technique, age and lymph node sampling on the severe complication rate of surgically staged endometrial cancer patients: a multivariate analysis. *J Clin Oncol* 1994;12:510.

Coulam CB, Annegers JF, Kranz JS. Chronic anovulation syndrome and associated neoplasia. *Obstet Gynecol* 1983; 61:403.

Cramer DW, Cutler SJ, Christine D. Trends in the incidence of endometrial cancer in the U.S. *Gynecol Oncol* 1974;2:130.

Creasman WT. Estrogen replacement therapy: is previously treated cancer a contraindication? *Obstet Gynecol* 1991; 77:308.

Creasman WT. New gynecologic cancer staging. *Obstet Gynecol* 1990;75:287.

Creasman WT. Prognostic significance of hormone receptors in endometrial cancer. *Cancer Diagn Treat Res* 1993; 15:1467.

Creasman WT, DiSaia PF, Blessing J. Prognostic significance of peritoneal cytology in patients with endometrial cancer and preliminary data concerning therapy with intraperitoneal radiopharmaceuticals. *Am J Obstet Gynecol* 1981;141:921.

Creasman WT, Morrow CP, Bundy BN, et al. Surgical pathologic spread patterns of endometrial cancer. *Cancer* 1987;60:2035.

Creasman WT, Weed JC. Screening techniques in endometrial cancer. *Cancer* 1976;38:436.

Crentzberg CL, van Puttan WLJ, Kaper PCM et al. Surgery and postoperative radiotherapy versus surgery alone for patients with stage 1 endometrial carcinoma. *Lancet* 2000; 355:1404.

Cullen TS. *Cancer of the uterus*. Philadelphia: WB Saunders, 1900.

Currie JL. U.S. monitoring of endometrial thickness in estrogen replacement therapy. *Radiology* 1991;180:306.

Currie JL, Blessing JA, McGehee R, et al. Phase II trial of hydroxyurea, dacarbazine (DTIC), and etoposide (VP-16) in mixed mesodermal tumors of the uterus: a Gynecologic Oncology Group study. *Gynecol Oncol* 1996;61:94–96.

Currie JL, Blessing JA, Muss HB, et al. Combination chemotherapy with hydroxyurea, dacarbazine (DTIC), and etoposide in the treatment of uterine leiomyosarcoma: a Gynecologic Oncology Group study. *Gynecol Oncol* 1996;60.

Currie JL, Rosenshein NB. Surgical resection of recurrent leiomyosarcoma: aggressive intervention can result in long-term survival. *Gynecol Oncol* 1990;36:2.

Currie JL, Swiger T, Dudzinski M, et al. Combination chemotherapy for patients with recurrent or advanced uterine sarcomas. *Gynecol Oncol* 1985;20:254.

Dede JA, Plentl AA, Moore JG. Recurrent endometrial carcinoma. *Surg Gynecol Obstet* 1968;126:553.

Deppe G. Chemotherapeutic treatment of endometrial cancer. *Clin Obstet Gynecol* 1982;25:93.

Devore GR, Schwartz PE, Morris JM. Hysterography: a 5-year followup in patients with endometrial carcinoma. *Obstet Gynecol* 1982;60:369.

Dinh TV, Slavin RE, Bhagavan BS, et al. Mixed müllerian tumors of the uterus: a clinicopathologic study. *Obstet Gynecol* 1989;74:388.

DiSaia PJ, Creasman WT, Boronow RC, et al. Risk factors and recurrent patterns in stage I endometrial cancer. *Am J Obstet Gynecol* 1985;151:1009.

Doering DL, Barnhill DR, Weiser EB, et al. Intraoperative evaluation of depth of invasion in stage I endometrial adenocarcinoma. *Obstet Gynecol* 1989;74:930.

Duk JM, Aalders JG, Fleuren GJ, et al. CA-125: a useful marker in endometrial cancer. *Am J Obstet Gynecol* 1986; 155:1097.

Dunn LJ, Bradbury JT. Endocrine factors in endometrial carcinoma. *Am J Obstet Gynecol* 1967;97:465.

Dunn LJ, Merchant JA, Bradbury JT, et al. Glucose tolerance and endometrial carcinoma. *Arch Intern Med* 1968; 121:236.

Echt G, Jepson J, Steel J, et al. Treatment of uterine sarcomas. *Cancer Diagn Treat Res* 1990;66:35.

Ehrlich CE, Young PCM, Stechman FB, et al. Steroid receptors and clinical outcome in patients with adenocarcinoma of the endometrium. *Am J Obstet Gynecol* 1988;158:796.

Enriori CL, Vico CM, Calandra RS, et al. Cytoplasmic steroid receptors in tumoral and "normal" endometrial samples from symmetrical uterine zones. *Gynecol Oncol* 1989;33:40.

Fanning J, Evans MC, Peters AJ, et al. Endometrial adenocarcinoma histologic subtypes: clinical and pathologic profile. *Gynecol Oncol* 1989;32:288.

Ferenczy A, Gelfand M. The biologic significance of cytologic atypia in progestogen-treated endometrial hyperplasia. *Am J Obstet Gynecol* 1989;160:126.

FIGO. Annual report on the results of treatment in gynecological cancer. *Int J Gynecol Obstet* 1989;28:189.

FIGO. Annual report on the results of treatment in gynecological cancer. In: Pettersson F, ed. *Annual report on the results of treatment in gynecological cancer.* Stockholm: Panorama Press, 1994:65–82.

FIGO. Statements of results obtained in patients treated in 1979 to 1981. In: Pettersson F, ed. *Annual report on the results of treatment in gynecological cancer.* Stockholm: Panorama Press, 1988:75–109.

Fisher B, Costantino JP, Redmond CK, et al. Endometrial cancer in tamoxifen-treated breast cancer patients: findings from the National Surgical Adjuvant Breast and Bowel Project (NSABP) B-14. *J Natl Cancer Inst* 1994;86:527.

Fox H, Sen DK. A controlled study of the constitutional stigmata of endometrial adenocarcinoma. *Br J Cancer* 1970; 24:30.

Fresia AE, Currie JL, Farrington JE, et al. Uterine stromal sarcoma cell line: a cytogenetic and electron microscopic study. *Cancer Genet Cytogenet* 1992;60:60.

Friberg LG, Noren H. Prognostic value of steroid hormone receptors for 5-year survival in stage II endometrial cancer. *Cancer Diagn Treat Res* 1993;71:3570.

Friedl A, Gottardis JP, Buchler A, et al. Enhanced growth of an estrogen receptor–negative endometrial adenocarcinoma by estradiol in athymic mice. *Cancer Res* 1989; 49:4758.

Frost JF. Gynecologic clinical cytopathology. In: Noval ER, Jones GS, Jones HW, eds. *Novak's textbook of gynecology*, ninth edition. Baltimore: Williams & Wilkins, 1975:782.

Gal D, Weiselberg L, Runowicz CD. Re endometrial cancer in tamoxifen-treated breast cancer patients: findings from the National Surgical Adjuvant Breast and Bowel Project (NSABP) B-14. *J Natl Cancer Inst* 1994;86:1252.

Gambrell DR Jr. Role of hormones in the etiology and prevention of endometrial and breast cancer. *Acta Obstet Gynecol Scand* 1982;106:337.

Gapstur SM, Potter JD, Sellers TA, et al. Alcohol consumption and postmenopausal endometrial cancer: results from the Iowa Women's Health Study. *Cancer Causes Control* 1993;4:323.

Gelfand MM, Ferenczy A. A prospective 1-year study of estrogen and progestin in postmenopausal women: effects on the endometrium. *Obstet Gynecol* 1989;74:398.

Gitsch G, Friedlander ML, Wain GV, et al. Uterine papillary serous carcinoma: a clinical study. *Cancer Diagn Treat Res* 1995a;75,2239.

Gitsch G, Hanzal E, Jensen D, et al. Endometrial cancer in premenopausal women 45 years and younger. *Obstet Gynecol* 1995b;85:504.

Goff BA, Goodman A, Muntz HE, et al. Surgical stage IV endometrial carcinoma: a study of 47 cases. *Gynecol Oncol* 1994;52:237–240.

Gollard R, Kosty M, Bordin G, et al. Two unusual presentations of müllerian adenosarcoma: case reports, literature review, and treatment considerations. *Gynecol Oncol* 1995;59:412.

Gordon AN, Fleischer AC, Dudley BS, et al. Preoperative assessment of myometrial invasion of endometrial adenocarcinoma by sonography (US) and magnetic resonance imaging (MRI). *Gynecol Oncol* 1989;34:175.

Grady D, Gebretsadik T, Kerlikowske K, et al. Hormone replacement therapy and endometrial cancer risk: a meta-analysis. *Obstet Gynecol* 1995;85:304.

Green JB III, Green S, Alberts DS, et al. Carboplatin therapy in advanced endometrial cancer. *Obstet Gynecol* 1990;75:696.

Greer B, Hamberger AD. Treatment of intraperitoneal metastatic adenocarcinoma of the endometrium by whole abdomen moving strip technique and pelvic boost irradiation. *Gynecol Oncol* 1983;16:365.

Grimes D. Diagnostic dilatation and curettage: a reappraisal. *Am J Obstet Gynecol* 1982;142:1.

Gronroos M, Salmi TA, Vuento MH, et al. Mass screening for endometrial cancer directed in risk groups of patients with diabetes and patients with hypertension. *Cancer Diagn Treat Res* 1993;71:1279.

Guido RS, Kanbour-Shakir A, Rulin MC, et al. Pipelle endometrial sampling. *J Reprod Med* 1995;40:553.

Gusberg SB. Precursors of corpus carcinoma: estrogen in adenomatous hyperplasia. *Am J Obstet Gynecol* 1947;54:905.

Gusberg SB, Chen SY, Cohen CJ. Endometrial cancer: factors influencing the choice of therapy. *Gynecol Oncol* 1974;2:308.

Gusberg SB, Kaplan AL. Precursors of corpus cancer: adenomatous hyperplasia as stage 0 carcinoma of the endometrium. *Am J Obstet Gynecol* 1963;87:662.

Hachsug T, Sugimori H, Kaku T, et al. Case report: glassy cell carcinoma of the endometrium. *Gynecol Oncol* 1990;36:134.

Hammond CB, Jelovsek FR, Lee KL, et al. Effects of long-term estrogen replacement therapy. *Am J Obstet Gynecol* 1979;133:537.

Haqqani MT, Fox H. Adenosquamous carcinoma of the endometrium. *J Clin Pathol* 1976;29:959.

Herbst AL, Robboy SJ, Scully RE. Clear-cell adenocarcinoma of the vagina and cervix in girls: analysis of 170 registry cases. *Am J Obstet Gynecol* 1974;119:713.

Herbst AL, Scully RE. Adenocarcinoma of the vagina in adolescence: a report of seven cases including six clear cell carcinoma (so-called mesonephromas). *Cancer* 1970;25:745.

Herbst AL, Ulfelder H, Poskanzer EC. Adenocarcinoma: association of maternal stilbestrol therapy with tumor appearing in young women. *N Engl J Med* 1971;284:878.

Hoffman K, Nekhlyudov L, Deligdisch L. Endometrial carcinoma in elderly women. *Gynecol Oncol* 1995;58:198.

Hoffman MS, Roberts WS, Cavanagh D, et al. Treatment of recurrent and metastatic endometrial cancer with cisplatin, doxorubicin, cyclophosphamide, and megestrol acetate. *Gynecol Oncol* 1989;35:75.

Hofmeister EJ. Endometrial biopsy: another look. *Am J Obstet Gynecol* 1974;228:773.

Holmesley HD, Boronow RC, Lewis JL. Treatment of adenocarcinoma of the endometrium at Memorial-James Ewing Hospitals, 1949–1965. *Obstet Gynecol* 1984;47:200.

Holmesley HD, Kadar N, Barrett RJ, et al. Selective pelvic and periaortic lymphadenectomy does not increase morbidity in surgical staging of endometrial carcinoma. *Am J Obstet Gynecol* 1992;167:1225.

Hoogerland DL, Buchler DA, Crowley JJ, et al. Estrogen use: risk of endometrial carcinoma. *Gynecol Oncol* 1978;6:451.

Horowitz IR, Copas PR, Aaronoff M, et al. Endometrial adenocarcinoma following endometrial ablation for postmenopausal bleeding. *Gynecol Oncol* 1995;56:460.

Horowitz IR, Feinstein AR. Alternative analytic methods for case-control studies of estrogens and endometrial cancer. *N Engl J Med* 1978;299:1089.

Hulka CA, Hall DA. Endometrial abnormalities associated with tamoxifen therapy for breast cancer: sonographic and pathologic correlation. *AJR Am J Roentgenol* 1993;160:809.

Indman PD. Abnormal uterine bleeding: accuracy of vaginal probe ultrasound in predicting abnormal hysteroscopic findings. *J Reprod Med* 1995;40:545.

Iossa A, Cianferoni L, Ciatto S, et al. Hysteroscopy and endometrial cancer diagnosis: a review of 2007 consecutive examinations in self-referred patients. *Tumori* 1991;77:479.

Ito K, Watanabe K, Nasim S, et al. Prognostic significance of p53 overexpression in endometrial cancer. *Cancer Res* 1994;54:4667.

Iversen OE. Flow cytometric deoxyribonucleic acid index: a prognostic factor in endometrial carcinoma. *Am J Obstet Gynecol* 1986;155:770.

Iversen OE, Laerum OD. Ploidy disturbances in endometrial and ovarian carcinomas. *Anal Quant Cytol Histol* 1985;7:327.

Iwamori M, Sakayori M, Nozawa S, et al. Monoclonal antibody—defined antigen of human uterine endometrial carcinomas is Le^B. *J Biochem* 1989;105:718.

Jacques SM, Lawrence WD. Endometrial adenocarcinoma with variable-level myometrial involvement limited to adenomyosis: a clinicopathologic study of 23 cases. *Gynecol Oncol* 1990;37:401.

Jones HW. Treatment of adenocarcinoma of the endometrium. *Obstet Gynecol Surv* 1975;30:147.

Kaplan SD, Cole P. *Epidemiology of cancer of the endometrium,* 1980.

Karlan B. Where are we now and where are we going? *Gynecol Oncol* 1995;59:315.

Karlsson B, Granberg S, Wikland M, et al. Transvaginal ultrasonography of the endometrium in women with postmenopausal bleeding: a Nordic multicenter study. *Am J Obstet Gynecol* 1995;172:1488.

Kelley RM, Baker WH. Progestational agents in the treatment of carcinoma of the endometrium. *N Engl J Med* 1961;264:216.

Kennedy AW, Flagg JS, Webster KD. Gynecologic cancer in the very elderly. *Gynecol Oncol* 1989;32:49.

Kilgore LC, Partridge EE, Alvarez RD, et al. Adenocarcinoma of the endometrium: survival comparison in patients with and without pelvic node sampling. *Gynecol Oncol* 1995;56:29.

Kistner RW. Endometrial hyperplasia and carcinoma in situ. In: Stall BA, ed. *Endocrine therapy in malignant disease.* Philadelphia: WB Saunders, 1972.

Knab DR. Estrogen and endometrial carcinoma. *Obstet Gynecol Surv* 1977;32:267.

Kohorn EI, Schwartz PE, Chambers JT, et al. Adjuvant therapy in mixed müllerian tumors of the uterus. *Gynecol Oncol* 1986;23:212.

Komaki R, Cox JD, Hartz A, et al. Influence of preoperative irradiation on failures of endometrial carcinoma with high risk of lymph node metastases. *Am J Clin Oncol* 1984;7:661.

Komaki R, Mattingly RF, Hoffman RG, et al. Irradiation of paraaortic lymph node metastases from carcinoma of the cervix or endometrium. *Radiology* 1983;147:245.

Koonings PP, Moyer DL, Grimes DA. A randomized clinical trial comparing Pipelle and Tis-U-Trap for endometrial biopsy. *Obstet Gynecol* 1990;75:293.

Koss LG, Schreiber K, Oberlander SG, et al. Detection of endometrial carcinoma and hyperplasia in asymptomatic women. *Obstet Gynecol* 1984;64:1.

Kottmeier H. Individualization of therapy in carcinoma of the corpus. In: *Carcinoma of the uterus and ovary.* Chicago: Mosby–Year Book, 1969:102.

Kukura V, Zaninovic I, Hrdina B. Concentrations of CA-125 tumor marker in endometrial carcinoma. *Gynecol Oncol* 1990;37:388.

Kurjak A, Kupesic S, Shalan H, et al. Uterine sarcoma: a report of 10 cases studied by transvaginal color and pulsed Doppler sonography. *Gynecol Oncol* 1995;59:342.

Kurman RJ, Kaminski PF, Norris HJ. The behavior of endometrial hyperplasia. *Cancer* 1985;56:403.

Landgren RC, Fletcher GH, Delclos L, et al. Irradiation of endometrial cancer in patients with medical contraindication to surgery or with unresectable lesions. *AMJ Roentgenol Rad Ther Nucl Med* 1976;126:148.

LaPolla JP, Nicosia S, McCurdy C, et al. Experience with the EndoPap device for the cytologic detection of uterine cancer and its precursors: a comparison of the EndoPap with fractional curettage or hysterectomy. *Am J Obstet Gynecol* 1990;163:1055.

Larson DM, Johnson K, Olson KA. Pelvic and para-aortic lymphadenectomy for surgical staging of endometrial cancer: morbidity and mortality. *Obstet Gynecol* 1992;79:998.

Larson DM, Johnson KK, Broste SK, et al. Comparison of D&C and office endometrial biopsy in predicting final histopathologic grade in endometrial cancer. *Obstet Gynecol* 1995;86:38.

Lawrence C, Tessaro I, Durgerian S, et al. Advanced-stage endometrial cancer: contributions of estrogen use, smoking, and other risk factors. *Gynecol Oncol* 1989;32:41.

Laxman R, Currie JL, Kurman RJ, et al. Cytogenic profile of uterine sarcomas. *Cancer Diagn Treat Res* 1993;71:1283.

Lelle RJ, Morley GW, Peters WA. The role of vaginal hysterectomy in the treatment of endometrial carcinoma. *Int J Gynecol Cancer* 1994;4:342.

Lentz SS, Brady MF, Major FJ, et al. High-dose megestrol acetate in advanced or recurrent endometrial carcinoma: a Gynecologic Oncology Group study. *J Clin Oncol* 1996; 14:357.

Lesko SM, Rosenberg L, Kaufman DW, et al. Cigarette smoking and risk of endometrial cancer. *N Engl J Med* 1985;313:593.

Lesko SM, Rosenberg L, Kaufman DW, et al. Endometrial cancer and age at last delivery: evidence for an association. *Am J Epidemiol* 1991;133:554.

Levi F, Franceschi S, Negri E, et al. Dietary factors and the risk of endometrial cancer. *Cancer Diagn Treat Res* 1993a; 71:3575.

Levi F, LaVecchia C, Negri E, et al. Selected physical activities and the risk of endometrial cancer. *Br J Cancer* 1993b; 67:846.

Lewis B, Cowdell R, Stallworthy JA. Adenocarcinoma of the body of the uterus. *J Obstet Gynaecol Br Commonw* 1970; 77:343.

Lewis GC Jr, Bundy B. Surgery for endometrial cancer. *Cancer* 1981;48:568.

Lewis GC Jr, Slack NH, Mortel R, et al. Adjuvant progestogen therapy in the primary definitive therapy of endometrial cancer. *Gynecol Oncol* 1974;2:368.

Lien HH, Blomlie V, Trope C, et al. Cancer of the endometrium: value of MR imaging in determining depth of invasion into the myometrium. *AJR Am J Roentgenol* 1991;157:1221.

Liu FS, Kohler MF, Marks JR, et al. Mutation and over-expression of the p53 tumor suppressor gene frequently occurs in uterine and ovarian sarcomas. *Obstet Gynecol* 1994;83:118.

Long CA, O'Brien TJ, Sanders M, et al. *ras* Oncogene is expressed in adenocarcinoma of the endometrium. *Am J Obstet Gynecol* 1988;159:1512.

Long HJ III, Langdon RM Jr, Cha SS, et al. Phase II trial of methotrexate, vinblastine, doxorubicin, and cisplatin in advanced/recurrent endometrial carcinoma. *Gynecol Oncol* 1995;58:240.

Lurain JR, Runsey NK, Schink JC, et al. Prognostic significance of positive peritoneal cytology in clinical stage I adenocarcinoma of the endometrium. *Obstet Gynecol* 1989;74:175.

Lyon FA. The development of adenocarcinoma of the endometrium in young women receiving long-term sequential oral contraception. *Am J Obstet Gynecol* 1975;123:299.

Mach TM, Pike MC, Henderson BE, et al. Estrogens and endometrial cancer in a retirement community. *N Engl J Med* 1976;294:1262.

Magriples U, Naftolin F, Schwartz PE, et al. High-grade endometrial carcinoma in tamoxifen-treated breast cancer patients. *J Clin Oncol* 1993;11:485.

Mahle AE. The morphological history of adenocarcinoma of the body of the uterus in relation to longevity. *Surg Gynecol Obstet* 1923;36:385.

Major F, Silverberg S, Morrow P, et al. A preliminary analysis of prognostic factors in uterine sarcoma: a Gynecology Oncology Group study. *Gynecol Oncol* 1987;26:411(abst).

Malfetano JH, Hussain M. A uterine tumor that resembled ovarian sex-cord tumors: a low-grade sarcoma. *Obstet Gynecol* 1989;74:489.

Malkasian GD Jr, Annegers JS, Fountain KS. Carcinoma of the endometrium, stage I. *Am J Obstet Gynecol* 1980;136:872.

Malmstrom H, Schmidt H, Persson P, et al. Flow cytometric analysis of uterine sarcoma: ploidy and s-phase rate as prognostic indicators. *Gynecol Oncol* 1992;44:172.

Malviya VK, Deppe G, Malone J Jr, et al. Reliability of frozen section examination in identifying poor prognostic indicators in stage I endometrial adenocarcinoma. *Gynecol Oncol* 1989;34:299.

Marabini A, Gubbini G, DeJaco P, et al. A case of unsuspected endometrial stromal sarcoma removed by operative hysteroscopy. *Gynecol Oncol* 1995;59:409.

Marrett LD, Elwood JM, Epid SM, et al. Recent trends in the incidence and mortality of cancer of the uterine corpus in Connecticut. *Gynecol Oncol* 1978;6:193.

Martinex Monge R, Jurado M, Azinovic I, et al. Intraoperative radiotherapy in recurrent gynecological cancer. *Radiother Oncol* 1993;28:127.

Marziale P, Atlante G, Pozzi M, et al. Four hundred twenty-six cases of stage I endometrial carcinoma: a clinicopathologic analysis. *Gynecol Oncol* 1989;32:278.

Mazurka JL, Krepart GV, Lotocki RJ. Prognostic significance of positive peritoneal cytology in endometrial carcinoma. *Am J Obstet Gynecol* 1988;158:303.

McLellan R, Dillon MB, Currie JL, et al. Peritoneal cytology in endometrial cancer: a review. *Obstet Gynecol Surv* 1989; 44:711.

Meyer WR, Mayer AR, Diamond MP, et al. Unsuspected leiomyosarcoma: treatment with a gonadotropin-releasing hormone analogue. *Obstet Gynecol* 1990;75:529.

Montag TW, Manart FD. Endolymphatic stromal myosis: surgical and hormonal therapy for extensive venous recurrence. *Gynecol Oncol* 1989;33:255.

Moore DH, Fower WC Jr, Walton LA, et al. Morbidity of lymph node sampling in cancers of the uterine corpus and cervix. *Obstet Gynecol* 1989;74:180.

Morley GW, Hopkins MP, Lindenauer SM, et al. Pelvic exenteration, University of Michigan: 100 patients at 5 years. *Obstet Gynecol* 1989;74:934.

Morrow CP, Bundy BN, Kurman RJ, et al. Relationship between surgical-pathological risk factors and outcome in clinical stage I and II carcinoma of the endometrium: a Gynecologic Oncology Group study. *Gynecol Oncol* 1991;40:55.

Morrow CP, DiSaia PJ, Townsend DE. Current management of endometrial cancer. *Obstet Gynecol* 1973;42:399.

Nachtigall LE, Nachtigall RH, Nachtigall RD, et al. Estrogen replacement therapy, II: a prospective study in the relationship to carcinoma and cardiovascular metabolic problems. *Obstet Gynecol* 1979;54:74.

Nardone FD, Benedetto T, Rossiella F, et al. Hormone receptor status in human endometrial adenocarcinoma. *Cancer* 1989;64:2572.

Newbury R, Schuerch C, Goodspeed N, et al. DNA content as a prognostic factor in endometrial cancer. *Obstet Gynecol* 1990;76:251.

Niloff JM, Klug TL, Schaetzl E, et al. Elevation of serum CA-125 in carcinomas of the fallopian tube, endometrium, and endocervix. *Am J Obstet Gynecol* 1986;148:1057.

Nischan P, Ebeling K. Endometrial cancer incidence and oral contraception. *Int J Epidemiol* 1991;20:820.

Nisker JA, Kirk ME, Nunez-Troconis JT. Reduced incidence of rabbit endometrial neoplasia with levonorgestrel implant. *Am J Obstet Gynecol* 1988;158:300.

Novak E, Anderson DF. Sarcoma of uterus. *Am J Obstet Gynecol* 1937;34:740.

Novak E, Woodruff JD. *Gynecologic and obstetric pathology*, eighth edition. Philadelphia: WB Saunders, 1979.

Novak E, Yui E. Relation of endometrial hyperplasia to adenocarcinoma of the uterus. *Am J Obstet Gynecol* 1936; 32:674.

Nyholm HCJ, Christensen IJ, Nielsen AL. Progesterone receptor levels independently predict survival in endometrial adenocarcinoma. *Gynecol Oncol* 1995;59:347.

Omura GA, Blessing JA, Major FJ, et al. A randomized trial of adjuvant adriamycin in uterine sarcomas: a Gynecologic Oncology Group study. *J Clin Oncol* 1985;3:1240.

Omura GA, Major FJ, Blessing JA, et al. A randomized trial of adriamycin with and without dimethyl triazenoimidazole carboxamide in advanced uterine sarcomas. *Cancer* 1983;52:626.

Onsrud M, Kolstad P, Normann T. Postoperative external pelvic irradiation in carcinoma of the corpus stage I: a controlled clinical trial. *Gynecol Oncol* 1976;4:222.

Ortac F, Bahceci M, Salih M, et al. Myometrial invasion of endometrium cancer assessed by transrectal ultrasonography. *Gynecol Obstet Invest* 1991;32:115.

Ozasa H, Noda Y, Mori T. A dynamic test of hormonal sensitivity of gynecologic malignancy by use of an antiestrogen, tamoxifen. *Am J Obstet Gynecol* 1988;158:1120.

Padwick MB, Endacott J, Whitehead MB. Efficacy, acceptability, and metabolic effects of transdermal estradiol in the management of postmenopausal women. *Am J Obstet Gynecol* 1985;152:1085.

Parazzini F, LaVecchia C, Negri E, et al. Reproductive factors and risk of endometrial cancer. *Am J Obstet Gynecol* 1991;164:522.

Parazzini F, LaVecchia C, Negri E, et al. Smoking and risk of endometrial cancer: results from an Italian case-control study. *Gynecol Oncol* 1995;56:195.

Park RC, Patow WE, Petty WE, et al. Treatment of adenocarcinoma of the endometrium. *Gynecol Oncol* 1974;2:60.

Parker WH, Fu YS, Berek JS. Uterine sarcoma in patients operated on for presumed leiomyoma and rapidly growing leiomyoma. *Obstet Gynecol* 1994;83:414.

Patsner B, Mann WJ, Cohen H, et al. Predictive value of preoperative serum CA 125 levels in clinically localized

and advanced carcinoma. *Am J Obstet Gynecol* 1988; 158:399.

Pecorelli S, ed. Annual report of the results of treatment in gynecological cancer. *J Epidemiol Biostat* 2001;6:45.

Peters WA, Andersen WA, Tharton NJ, et al. The selective use of vaginal hysterectomy in the management of adenocarcinoma of the endometrium. *Am J Obstet Gynecol* 1983; 146:285.

Peters WA III, Riokis SE, Smith MR, et al. Cisplatin and adriamycin combination chemotherapy for uterine stromal sarcomas and mixed mesodermal tumors. *Gynecol Oncol* 1989;34:323.

Peterson EP. Endometrial carcinoma in young women: a clinical profile. *Obstet Gynecol* 1968;31:702.

Piver MS, Yazigi R, Blumenson L, Tsukada Y. A prospective trial comparing hysterectomy, hysterectomy plus vaginal radium, and uterine radium plus hysterectomy in stage I endometrial carcinoma. *Obstet Gynecol* 1985;54:85.

Podczaski ES, Woomert CA, Stevens CW, et al. Management of malignant, mixed mesodermal tumors of the uterus. *Gynecol Oncol* 1989;32:240.

Podratz KC, Wilson TO, Gaffey TA, et al. Deoxyribonucleic acid analysis facilitates the pretreatment identification of high-risk endometrial cancer patients. *Am J Obstet Gynecol* 1993;168:1206.

Pollow K, Lubbert H, Boquol E, et al. Characterization and comparison of receptors for 17_β-estradiol and progesterone in human proliferative endometrium and endometrial carcinoma. *Endocrinology* 1975;96:319.

Prompeler HJ, Madjar H, du Bois A, et al. Transvaginal sonography of myometrial invasion depth in endometrial cancer. *Acta Obstet Gynecol Scand* 1994;73:343.

Quinn MA, Campbell JJ. Tamoxifen therapy in advanced/recurrent endometrial carcinoma. *Gynecol Oncol* 1989; 32:1.

Reagan JW, Ng ABP. *The cells of uterine adenocarcinoma*. Baltimore: Williams & Wilkins, 1965.

Reddoch JM, Burke TW, Morris M, et al. Surveillance for recurrent endometrial carcinoma: development of a follow-up scheme. *Gynecol Oncol* 1995;59:221.

Reid GC, Morley GW, Schmidt RW, et al. The role of pelvic exenteration for sarcomatous malignancies. *Obstet Gynecol* 1989;74:80.

Reifenstein ECJ. The treatment of advanced endometrial cancer with hydroxyprogesterone caproate. *Gynecol Oncol* 1974;2:377.

Roberts JA, Brunetto VL, Keys HM, et al. A phase III randomized surgery vs. surgery plus adjunctive radiation therapy in intermediate risk endometrial adenocarcinoma. *Gynecol Oncol* 1998;68:135.

Rosenwaks Z, Weitz AC, Jones GS, et al. Endometrial pathology and estrogens. *Obstet Gynecol* 1979;53:403.

Rutledge F. Role of radical hysterectomy in adenocarcinoma of the endometrium. *Gynecol Oncol* 1974;2:331.

Salazar OM, Bonfiglio TA, Pattern SF, et al. Uterine sarcomas: natural history, treatment and prognosis. *Cancer* 1978;42:1152.

Salazar OM, DePapp EW, Bonfiglio TA, et al. Adenosquamous carcinoma of the endometrium. *Cancer* 1977;40:119.

Schapira DV, Kumar NB, Lyman GH, et al. Upper-body fat distribution and endometrial cancer risk. *JAMA* 1991; 266:1808.

Schink JC, Rademaker AW, Miller DS, et al. Tumor size in endometrial cancer. *Cancer Diagn Treat Res* 1991;67:2791.

Schroeder R. Nordwestdeutsche Gesellschaft fur Gynakolgie. *Zentralbl Gynakol* 1922;46:193.

Segreti EM, Novotny DB, Soper JT, et al. Endometrial cancer: histologic correlates of immunohistochemical localization of progesterone receptor and estrogen receptor. *Obstet Gynecol* 1989;73:780.

Seoud MA, Johnson J, Weed JC Jr. Gynecologic tumors in tamoxifen-treated women with breast cancer. *Obstet Gynecol* 1993;82:165.

Seski JC, Edwards CL, Herson J, et al. Cisplatin chemotherapy for disseminated endometrial cancer. *Obstet Gynecol* 1982;59:225.

Shimizu H, Inoue M, Tanizawa O. Adaptive cellular immunotherapy to the endometrial carcinoma cell line xenografts in nude mice. *Gynecol Oncol* 1989;34:195.

Shu XO, Hatch MC, Zheng W, et al. Physical activity and risk of endometrial cancer. *Epidemiology* 1993;4:342.

Siiteri PK, Schwarz BE, MacDonald PC. Estrogen receptors and the estrone hypothesis in relation to endometrial and breast cancer. *Gynecol Oncol* 1974;2:228.

Silverberg E, Boring CC, Squire TS. Cancer statistics, 1990. *CA Cancer J Clin* 1990;40:9.

Silverberg SG, Makowski EL. Endometrial carcinoma in young women taking oral contraceptives. *Obstet Gynecol* 1975;46:503.

Soper JT, Creasman WT, Clarke-Pearson DL, et al. Intraperitoneal chronic phosphate P-32 suspension therapy of malignant peritoneal cytology in endometrial carcinoma. *Am J Obstet Gynecol* 1985;153:191.

Sorbe B, Frankendal B, Risberg B. Intracavitary irradiation of endometrial carcinoma stage I by a high dose-rate afterloading technique. *Gynecol Oncol* 1989;33:135.

Spanos WJ Jr, Wharton JT, Gomez L, et al. Malignant mixed müllerian tumors of the uterus. *Cancer* 1984;53:311.

Stanford JL, Brinton LA, Berman ML, et al. Oral contraceptives and endometrial cancer: do other risk factors modify the association? *Int J Cancer* 1993;54:243.

Stovall TG, Photopulos GJ, Poston WM, et al. Pipelle endometrial sampling in patients with known endometrial carcinoma. *Obstet Gynecol* 1991;77:954.

Straughn JM, Huh WK, Kelly FJ, et al. Conservative management of stage I endometrial cancer after surgical staging. *Gynecol Oncol* 2002;84:194–200.

Stratton JA, Mannel RS, Rettenmaier MA, et al. Treatment of advanced and recurrent endometrial carcinoma: correlation of patient response to hormonal and cytotoxic chemotherapy and the response predicted by the subrenal capsule chemosensitivity assay. *Gynecol Oncol* 1989;32:55.

Sutton G. Hormonal aspects of endometrial cancer. *Curr Opin Obstet Gynecol* 1990;2:69.

Sutton GP, Blessing JA, Barrett RJ, et al. Phase II trial of ifosfamide and mesna in leiomyosarcoma of the uterus: a Gynecologic Oncology Group study. *Am J Obstet Gynecol* 1992;166:556.

Sutton GP, Blessing JA, Malfetano JH. A phase II trial of doxorubicin, ifosfamide and mesna in patients with advanced or recurrent uterine leiomyosarcoma. *Proc Am Soc Clin Oncol* 1993;12:291.

Sutton GP, Blessing JA, Rosenshein N, et al. Phase II trial of ifosfamide and mesna in mixed mesodermal tumors of the uterus: a Gynecologic Oncology Group study. *Am J Obstet Gynecol* 1989;161:309.

Swanson CA, Wilbanks GD, Twiggs LB, et al. Moderate alcohol consumption and the risk of endometrial cancer. *Epidemiology* 1993;4:530.

Swenerton KD. Treatment of advanced endometrial adenocarcinoma with tamoxifen. *Cancer Treat Rep* 1980;64:805.

Taina E, Maenpaa J, Erkkola R, et al. Endometrial stromal sarcoma: a report of nine cases. *Gynecol Oncol* 1989;32:156.

Tak WK, Marchant DJ, Munzenrider JE, et al. Preoperative irradiation for carcinoma of the endometrium: indications and results. *Gynecol Oncol* 1977;5:18.

Thatcher SS, Woodruff JD. Uterine stromatosis: a report of 33 cases. *Obstet Gynecol* 1982;59:428.

Thigpen JT, Blessing JA, Holmesley H, et al. Phase II trial of cisplatin as first-line chemotherapy in patients with advanced or recurrent endometrial carcinoma: a Gynecologic Oncology Group study. *Gynecol Oncol* 1989;33:68.

Thomas DB. Steroid hormones and medications that alter cancer risk. *Cancer* 1988;62:1755.

Tsukamoto N, Hirakawa T, Matsukuma K, et al. Carcinoma of the uterine cervix with variegated histological patterns and calcitonin production. *Gynecol Oncol* 1989;33:395.

Turner DA, Gershenson DM, Atkinson N, et al. The prognostic significance of peritoneal cytology for stage I endometrial cancer. *Obstet Gynecol* 1989;74:775.

Twiggs LB, DiSaia PJ, Morrow PC, et al. Gravlee jet irrigator: efficacy in diagnosis of endometrial neoplasia. *JAMA* 1976;235:2748.

Ulbright TM, Roth LM. Metastatic and independent cancers of the endometrium and ovary: a clinicopathologic study of 34 cases. *Hum Pathol* 1985;16:28.

Vardi J, Tadros GH, Simindokht Z, et al. Stage IV endometrial carcinoma in a 25-year-old woman: a case report and review of the literature. *Gynecol Oncol* 1989;34:244.

Varia V, Rosenman J, Halle J, et al. Primary radiation therapy for medically inoperable patients with endometrial carcinoma: stages I–II. *Int J Radiat Oncol Biol Phys* 1987;13:11.

Vasen HF, Watson P, Mecklin JP, et al. The epidemiology of endometrial cancer in hereditary nonpolyposis colorectal cancer. *Anticancer Res* 1994;14:1675.

Walker AM, Jick H. Declining rates of endometrial cancer. *Obstet Gynecol* 1980;56:733.

Wharam MD, Phillips TL. The role of radiation therapy in clinical stage I carcinoma of the endometrium. *Int J Radiat Oncol Biol Phys* 1976;1:1081.

Wolfson AH, Wolfson DJ, Sittler SY, et al. A multivariate analysis of clinicopathologic factors for predicting outcome in uterine sarcomas. *Gynecol Oncol* 1994;52:56.

Wynder EL, Escher GC, Mantel N. An epidemiological investigation of cancer of the endometrium. *Cancer* 1966;19:489.

Zaino RJ, Kurman R, Herbald D et al. The significance of squamous differentiation in endometrial carcinomas. *Cancer* 1991;68:2293-302

Zaino RJ, Kurman RJ, Diana KL, et al. The utility of the revised International Federation of Gynecology and Obstetrics histologic grading system: a Gynecologic Oncology Group study. *Cancer* 1995;75:81.

Zaino RJ, Silverberg SG, Norris JH, et al. The prognostic value of nuclear versus architectural grading in endometrial adenocarcinoma: a Gynecologic Oncology Group study. *Int J Gynecol Pathol* 1994;13:29.

Zaloudek CJ, Norris HJ. Adenofibroma and adenosarcoma of the uterus. *Cancer* 1981;48:354.

Ziel HK, Finkle WD. Increased risk of endometrial carcinoma among users of conjugated estrogens. *N Engl J Med* 1975;93:1167.

Zucker PK, Kasdon EJ, Feldstein ML. The validity of Pap smear parameters as predictors of endometrial pathology in menopausal women. *Cancer* 1985;56:2256.

Te Linde's Operative Gynecology, ninth edition, edited by John A. Rock and Howard W. Jones, III. Lippincott Williams & Wilkins, Philadelphia: © 2003.

CHAPTER

48

Ovarian Cancer: Etiology, Screening, and Surgery

JOHN R. VAN NAGELL, JR.   DAVID M. GERSHENSON

Ovarian cancer is the leading cause of death from gynecologic malignancies in the United States. This year, over 23,000 new cases of ovarian cancer will be detected and over 13,000 women will die of the disease. The lifetime risk for ovarian cancer in the US without a family history of the disease is 1 in 70 (1.4%). Because early ovarian cancer produces few specific symptoms, most women present with advanced-stage disease where the prognosis is poor. Approximately 90% of malignant ovarian tumors in adults are of epithelial origin, followed by sex cord stromal tumors (6%) and germ cell tumors (3%). Good surgery is a blend of good judgment and sound surgical technique. Much of this chapter is devoted to the natural history and results of various surgical and other treatment approaches for ovarian cancer. This background information provides the surgeon with the basis for clinical decision making concerning patient selections, choice of the right operation, and postoperative treatment recommendations. The operative techniques involved in surgery for ovarian cancer are illustrated in many of the other chapters in this text.

INCIDENCE AND RISK FACTORS

The incidence of ovarian cancer is highest in the Scandinavian countries (14.9/100,000) and the United States

(13.3/100,000), and lowest in Japan (2.7/100,000). In the United States, ovarian cancer incidence rates are highest in White women (15/100,000), intermediate in Black women (10.2/100,000), and lowest in Native American women.

Factors associated with an increase in ovarian cancer risk are age, nulliparity, and a family history of the disease. Ovarian cancer is rare before the age of 40, increases steadily thereafter, and peaks at age 65 to 75. Parity is the most important nongenetic factor affecting risk for ovarian cancer (Table 48.1). Whittimore and colleagues analyzed 12 case-controlled studies in the United States, and reported a significant risk reduction for ovarian cancer with each term pregnancy (odds ratio = 0.47). The risk of ovarian cancer decreased progressively with increasing numbers of pregnancies. Similarly, the use of oral contraceptives has been shown to reduce the risk of ovarian cancer. Ovarian cancer risk decreases approximately 11% per year of oral contraceptive use, to a maximum of 46% after 5 years of use. These observations have led to the theory of "incessant ovulation" in the etiology of ovarian cancer. According to this theory, the risk for epithelial ovarian cancer is related directly to the number of uninterrupted ovulatory cycles. With ovulation, the surface epithelium is ruptured and undergoes rapid proliferation and repair. At the time of ovulation, there is invagination of the surface epithelium

TABLE 48.1.
Risk Factors for Ovarian Cancer

Factor	Odds Ratio
Parity	
Nulliparous	1.0
Parous	0.47
OCP use	
Never	1.0
2–5 years	0.73
Estrogen use	
Never	1.0[a]
Ever	0.9
Clomid use	
No	1.0
Yes	2.3
Tubal ligation	
No	1.0
Yes	0.59
Hysterectomy	
No	1.0
Yes	0.66
Talc use	
No	1.0[a]
Yes	1.09
Breast feeding	
No	1.0
Yes	0.73
Family history	
1 FDR[b] with ovarian cancer	3.1
>2 FDRs with ovarian cancer	4.6

Whittemore et al., Gertig et al., Rossing et al., Kerlikowske et al.
[a] nonsignificant.
[b] FDR, first-degree relative.

into the underlying stroma forming inclusion cysts. The epithelium lining these inclusion cysts undergoes neoplastic transformation under the influence of oncogenic factors. The observation that early age of menarche and late menopause are associated with an increase in ovarian cancer risk is consistent with this theory because both increase the number of ovulatory cycles. The observed decrease in ovarian cancer risk in women who have undergone tubal ligation or hysterectomy also supports this hypothesis because these procedures prevent the ascent of potential oncogenic factors from the lower genital tract to the ovary.

A second hypothesis concerning the genesis of ovarian cancer is that exposure of ovarian epithelium to persistently high levels of pituitary gonadotropins results in neoplastic transformation. Follicle stimulating hormone (FSH) has been shown to promote the growth of epithelial ovarian cancer cells *in vitro,* and this effect can be blocked by luteinizing hormone (LH). A corollary to this hypothesis is that elevated circulating gonadotropin levels promote estrogen biosynthesis in the ovarian stroma, which in turn causes abnormal proliferation of the adjacent epithelium. Breast feeding, which has been associated with a lower risk of ovarian cancer, also is as-

sociated with reduced serum concentrations of LH and estradiol. Pregnancy and oral contraceptive use presumably lower the risk of ovarian cancer by inhibiting pituitary secretion of gonadotropins. This theory also is supported by the increased risk of ovarian cancer in women taking fertility drugs. These drugs stimulate ovulation by increasing levels of FSH, particularly in the follicular phase of the cycle.

Perhaps the most important risk factor for epithelial ovarian cancer is a family history of the disease. The estimated odds ratio for the development of ovarian cancer in a woman with one first-degree relative with ovarian cancer is 3.1 (95% CL = 2.1 to 4.5). This risk increases (odds ratio 4.6 CL = 1.1 to 18.4) in a woman with two or more primary or secondary relatives with ovarian cancer. These odds ratios translate to a lifetime risk for ovarian cancer of approximately 5% in a woman with one first-degree relative with the disease, and 7% in a woman with two or more relatives with the disease. It should be mentioned, however, that familial ovarian cancers comprise a relatively small proportion of total ovarian cancer cases. Only 5% to 10% of ovarian cancer patients report a positive family history of the disease.

Three familial ovarian cancer syndromes have been described. Hereditary breast-ovarian cancer syndrome (HBOC), hereditary site-specific ovarian cancer syndrome, and Lynch syndrome type II. Hereditary breast-ovarian cancer syndrome, the most common of the familial syndromes, is characterized by multiple cases of early-onset (<50 years of age) breast and ovarian cancers. This syndrome accounts for 75% to 90% of all hereditary ovarian cancer cases. Hereditary site-specific ovarian cancer syndrome is manifested only by an increase in cases of early-onset ovarian cancer, and accounts for about 5% of hereditary ovarian cancers. Women with hereditary site-specific ovarian cancer often are younger and more commonly have tumors with serous histology than women with sporadic ovarian cancer. Nonpolyposis colon cancer syndrome or Lynch syndrome type II is characterized by a predominance of early-onset proximal colon cancer in association with cancers of the endometrium and ovary. These three familial ovarian cancer syndromes are inherited by autosomal dominant transmission through either maternal or paternal lineage. Therefore, the children of an affected parent have a 50% risk of inheriting the genetic abnormality.

Germline mutations in BRCA1 or BRCA2 genes appear to account for most hereditary ovarian cancers. BRCA1, identified in 1994, is localized on the short arm chromosome 17. BRCA1 is thought to be a tumor suppressor because the normal copy of BRCA1 is always deleted in ovarian cancers that arise in women who inherit a mutant BRCA1 gene. It is estimated that germline mutations in BRCA1 are responsible for 80% to 90% of hereditary ovarian cancers. BRCA2, identified in 1995, is localized on the short arm of chromosome 13. In a recent report from the Breast Cancer Linkage Consortium, BRCA1 mutations were identified in 81% of ovarian cancer families, whereas BRCA2 mutations were detected in 14% of those families. Although penetrance is variable from one individual to another, it is estimated that the lifetime risk of ovarian cancer is approximately 30% in BRCA1 carriers, and slightly less in BRCA2 carriers.

SIGNS AND SYMPTOMS

Although most reports indicate that patients with early-stage ovarian cancer have few symptoms, a recent national survey of 1,725 ovarian cancer patients provides evidence that many of these patients actually had symptoms that they or their primary health providers ignored. The most common symptoms of patients with stage I or II ovarian cancer were abdominal bloating or pain, indigestion, urinary frequency, and constipation. Because many of these symptoms are nonspecific, patients were unaware that they could be associated with ovarian cancer. As a result, 22% of patients ignored their symptoms entirely, and 30% reported that the wrong diagnosis was made. A pelvic examination was performed in only two thirds of patients, and 45% had a delay in diagnosis of over 3 months. Patients with advanced disease commonly complained of abdominal swelling, fatigue, and weight loss. These observations emphasize the need for patient and physician education concerning the possible relationship of rather nonspecific abdominal symptoms to ovarian cancer.

Although vaginal bleeding is not commonly associated with ovarian cancer, it may be present in patients with metastatic involvement of the uterus. Likewise, endometrial hyperplasia and abnormal uterine bleeding can be caused by excess estrogen production from an ovarian stromal tumor. Ovarian cancer must be considered in a patient who presents with a pelvic mass and shortness of breath. A malignant pleural effusion from metastatic ovarian cancer is more common on the left side, and usually is associated with dullness to percussion and decreased breath sounds. Finally, any patient with a clinically detected pelvic tumor on pelvic examination should undergo careful palpation of both groins to rule out inguinal lymphadenopathy secondary to metastatic disease.

EARLY DETECTION

Although there have been advances in the evaluation and treatment of ovarian cancer, most patients continue to present with advanced disease when survival is limited. As a result, the past two decades have seen little improvement in the overall prognosis of patients with ovarian cancer. According to data from the Surveillance, Epidemiology, and End Results (SEER) program of the National Cancer Institute, the mortality rates of ovarian cancer patients have decreased from 7.7 per 100,000 in 1983 to 1987 to 7.5 per 100,000 in 1993 to 1997. Because early ovarian cancer produces few specific symptoms, recent efforts have focused on developing screening methods to detect ovarian cancer while it is still curable.

For screening to be effective, a disease should: (a) be a major cause of mortality; (b) have a reasonably high prevalence in the screened population; (c) have a preclinical phase detectable by the screening test; and (d) be amenable to therapy such that the survival rate of patients with early-stage disease is significantly higher than that of patients with advanced disease.

Unfortunately, knowledge concerning the duration of the preclinical phase of ovarian cancer is limited at best. Histologic transition from benign to borderline or malignant epithelium has been identified by light and electron microscopy in ovarian mucinous and serous cystadenocarcinomas. Likewise, transition from endometriosis to endometrioid ovarian carcinoma has been documented. These studies suggest that with time, certain benign or borderline epithelial ovarian tumors may undergo malignant transformation. However, the frequency with which neoplastic transformation occurs in these tumors is unknown and is probably rare. Theoretically, the identification and removal of premalignant ovarian tumors, particularly in postmenopausal women, should decrease the subsequent occurrence of ovarian cancer.

There is little doubt that early-stage ovarian cancer is significantly more curable than late-stage disease. The 5-year survival of patients with stage I epithelial ovarian cancer is approximately 90%. In contrast, the 5-year survival of patients with stage III or IV epithelial ovarian cancer is only 20% to 25%, despite optimal surgery and combination chemotherapy. It has been estimated that if the 25% of ovarian cancer patients currently diagnosed with stage I tumors could be increased to 75% through early detection, the number of women dying from this disease could be halved.

The statistical definitions used in ovarian cancer screening are illustrated in Table 48.2. Characteristics of

---

TABLE 48.2.
Statistical Definitions in Ovarian Cancer Screening

	Screen	Findings
True positive (TP)	Positive	Ovarian cancer
False positive (FP)	Positive	No ovarian cancer
True negative (TN)	Negative	Absence of ovarian cancer for 1 year, confirmed by annual screening examination
False negative (FN)	Negative	Ovarian cancer within 1 year of normal screen

Negative predictive value (NPV), TN/TN + FN; Positive predictive value (PPV), TP/TP + FP; Sensitivity, TP/TP + FN; Specificity, TN/TN + FP.

an optimal screening test include high sensitivity, high specificity, high positive predictive value (PPV) and high negative predictive value (NPV). In addition, the test should be easy to perform, time efficient, and well accepted by patients. An effective screening test should: (a) decrease stage at detection; (b) decrease case-specific mortality; and (c) cause a statistically significant reduction in site-specific cancer mortality in the screened population. Finally, the screening test should be cost effective such that its use would reduce the overall cost of health care in the screened population.

At present, the two most effective screening methods for ovarian cancer are transvaginal sonography (TVS) and serum Ca-125. TVS is usually performed using a standard ultrasound unit with a 5.0 mHz vaginal transducer. Each ovary is measured in three dimensions, and ovarian volume is calculated using the prolate ellipsoid formula (L × H × W × 0.523). An ovarian volume >20 cm^3 in premenopausal women or 10 cm^3 in postmenopausal women is defined as abnormal. In addition, any solid or papillary projection from the tumor wall is considered abnormal.

Transvaginal Sonography

Ovarian cancer screening in the United States using TVS as the initial screening method was initiated at the University of Kentucky Medical Center in 1987. The current screening algorithm used at this center is illustrated in

Fig. 48.1. A woman with an abnormal screen is scheduled to have a repeat sonogram in 4 to 6 weeks. A woman with a persisting ovarian tumor at the time of the second screen is scheduled to have a serum Ca-125 determination, tumor morphology indexing, and color Doppler sonography. Following these studies, laparoscopic tumor removal is recommended. At the time of laparoscopy, the ovarian tumor is placed in an endocatch bag intraabdominally and removed through a midline subumbilical incision. After removal, frozen section histologic examination is performed on all areas suspicious for malignancy. Patients with ovarian cancer on frozen section or those with obvious metastatic disease at laparoscopy undergo immediate exploratory laparotomy with tumor debulking and staging. Using this algorithm, 14,469 asymptomatic women were screened from 1987 to 1999. One hundred and eighty women (1.4%) with a persisting abnormality on TVS underwent surgical tumor removal. Seventeen of these patients were found to have primary ovarian cancer. Fourteen (82%) had stage I or II disease, and all were cured after conventional therapy. The 5-year survival of ovarian cancer patients detected by screening was 88% or approximately twice that of unscreened patients.

Annual TVS screening was found to decrease stage at detection and reduce case-specific ovarian cancer mortality. The sensitivity of TVS was 0.820, and the specificity was 0.989. However, the PPV of TVS screening in detecting ovarian cancer was only 9.4%. Therefore, approx-

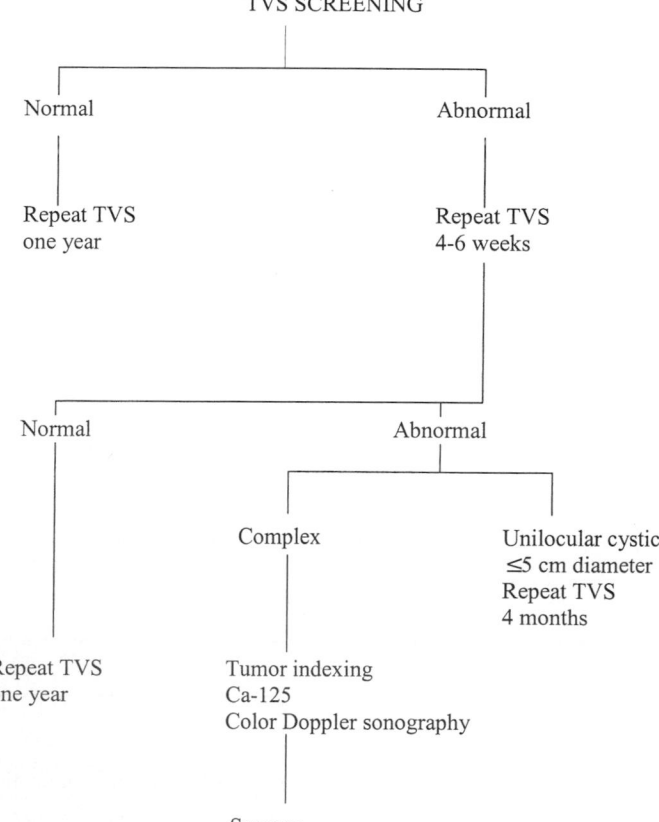

FIGURE 48.1. Ovarian cancer screening algorithm, University of Kentucky.

imately 10 benign ovarian tumors were removed for every ovarian cancer detected. Although these results are promising, a larger number of patients must be screened using this algorithm. Also, additional tests that can increase the PPV of TVS must be developed.

Morphology indexing is one of the adjuvant methods capable of increasing the PPV of TVS screening. Morphologic characteristics of ovarian tumors are related directly to the risk of malignancy. Unilocular cystic tumors usually are benign, whereas complex ovarian tumors with solid or papillary components are more often malignant. The addition of morphology indexing to TVS in postmenopausal women has been reported to increase the PPV of sonographic screening to 20%.

Serum CA-125

Ca-125 is an antigenic determinant on a high molecular weight glycoprotein recognized by a monoclonal antibody OC-125. Despite repeated attempts, the gene encoding this molecule has not yet been cloned. Ca-125 is expressed by epithelial ovarian cancers, and is present in highest concentrations on the tumor cell surface. Although serum levels of this marker are elevated (>35 μ/mL) in as many as 80% of patients with advanced ovarian cancer, they are elevated in only 25% to 50% of patients with clinically detected stage I ovarian cancers. Studies have indicated that a rising trend in serum Ca-125 levels over time is more predictive of ovarian cancer than a single elevated marker determination. Its value as a screening method is limited by its inability to detect ovarian cancer in earlier stages. Often, Ca-125 in serum levels is not sensitive enough to detect early stages of ovarian cancer. Furthermore, elevations in Ca-125 serum levels are present in a number of benign ovarian tumors, including endometriomas, inflammatory disease of the ovaries, and serous cystadenomas. This marker also has been reported to increase with a number of nongynecologic cancers, including cancers of the pancreas, breast, colon, and lung. Also decreasing the usefulness of Ca-125 screening for ovarian cancer is the presence of elevated levels of Ca-125 in many benign conditions, including endometriosis, pelvic inflammatory disease, and pregnancy.

The efficacy of serum Ca-125 as a screening method for ovarian cancer was evaluated in 22,000 asymptomatic postmenopausal women in England. Forty-one women (0.2%) had elevated (>30 μ/mL) serum Ca-125 levels and underwent surgery. Eleven of these patients had ovarian cancer, but seven had advanced disease (stage III or IV). Eight additional patients developed ovarian cancer despite having a normal serum Ca-125. A single serum Ca-125 determination in this trial had a sensitivity of 58%, a specificity of 98.5%, and a positive predictive value of 2%. When serum Ca-125 was used as the initial screening method, early stage cancers were missed, and stage at detection was not decreased appreciably. Subsequent studies have indicated that a rising trend in serum Ca-125 levels over time is more predictive of ovarian cancer than a single elevated marker determina-

tion. Nevertheless, the lack of sensitivity of serum Ca-125 in early-stage ovarian cancer and its inability to lower stage at detection has limited its value as a screening method.

The challenge of future ovarian cancer detection trials is to combine TVS with serum markers and morphology indexing in an algorithm which improves the sensitivity, specificity, and PPV of screening. Also, the optimal time interval between successive screens in various high-risk populations has yet to be determined.

ASSESSMENT OF RISK OF MALIGNANCY IN OVARIAN TUMORS

Once an ovarian tumor is identified, it is important to establish its risk of malignancy to properly inform the patient and plan the most appropriate surgical approach. Approximately 10% to 15% of ovarian tumors in premenopausal women and 40% of ovarian tumors in postmenopausal women are malignant. Tumor characteristics associated with malignancy include bilaterality, solid composition, fixation in the pelvis on bimanual examination, and increased size (>10 cm diameter). Interestingly, extremely large ovarian tumors often are benign mucinous or serous cystadenomas. Sonographically determined tumor morphology, serum markers, and color Doppler assessment of tumor vasculature also have been used to predict risk for malignancy. A number of studies have concluded that sonographically generated tumor morphology can be used to differentiate benign from malignant ovarian tumors, particularly in postmenopausal women. Unilocular cystic tumors <5 cm in diameter have been shown to have an extremely low risk of malignancy, whereas complex ovarian tumors with solid or papillary projections from the cyst wall have a higher risk of malignancy. Bailey and colleagues reported no cases of malignancy in 256 unilocular cystic ovarian tumors <10 cm in diameter, and recommended that these lesions could be followed with periodic transvaginal sonography rather than proceeding with operative intervention. Conversely, 7 of 135 complex ovarian tumors <10 cm in diameter were malignant. Using this reasoning, morphology indexes have been developed relating risk of malignancy to specific morphologic findings. DePriest and colleagues evaluated three variables: tumor volume, wall structure, and septal structure to risk of malignancy (Fig. 48.2). They found that tumor volume and wall structure were related directly to malignant potential, and developed a nomogram predicting risk of malignancy according to specific morphologic findings and volume calculations.

Once an adnexal mass has been identified, serum marker levels also have been used both independently and in conjunction with sonographic findings as a means to differentiate benign from malignant ovarian tumors. Alcazar and colleagues obtained serum Ca-125 values on 94 patients with suspicious adnexal masses confirmed sonographically. A serum CA-125 value <35 μ/mL was

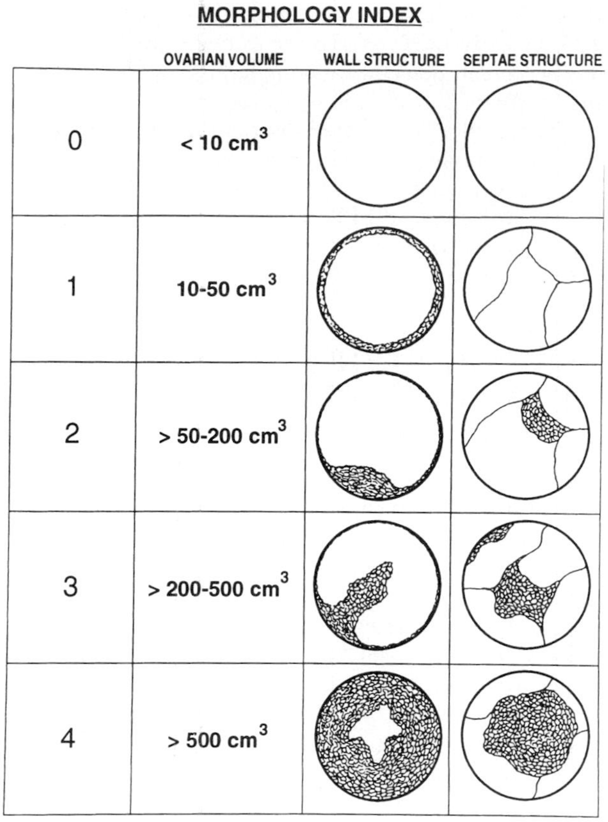

MORPHOLOGY INDEX

FIGURE 48.2. Morphology index used in evaluating sonographically confirmed ovarian tumors. (From: DePriest et al., with permission.)

designated as abnormal. Using this criterion, an elevated serum Ca-125 in a postmenopausal woman with a sonographically detected ovarian tumor had a PPV of 80%. The sensitivity and specificity of an elevated serum Ca-125 were highest in postmenopausal women. In addition, patients with an elevated serum Ca-125 of abnormal ovarian morphology had a significantly increased risk of ovarian malignancy.

The use of color flow Doppler as a method to assess risk of malignancy in ovarian tumors is based on observed differences in vascularity associated with neoplasia. Vessels supplying ovarian malignancies are characterized by central location, decreased medial thickness, and increased diastolic flow when compared to vessels within benign ovarian tumors. Transvaginal color flow Doppler can be used to measure blood flow patterns within ovarian vessels. A pulsatility index (PI) of <1.0 and a resistive index (RI) of <0.4 are indicative of low impedance to flow and a high risk of malignancy. Using these criteria, Weiner and colleagues reported that vessels supplying ovarian malignancies had an abnormally low pulsatility index in 16 of 17 cases. Conversely, the pulsatility index of vessels supplying benign ovarian tumors was normal (≥ 1.0) in 35 of 36 cases. Other studies have confirmed that the mean PI and RI are lower in malignant and borderline ovarian tumors than in benign ovarian tumors. However, the overlap in values is such that preoperative color Doppler cannot be used as a reliable preoperative indicator of malignancy.

More recently, contrast enhanced, three-dimensional power Doppler sonography has been shown to improve the visualization and diagnostic evaluation of tumor vascularity in complex adnexal masses.

Perhaps the most clinically valuable study concerning the differentiation of benign and malignant ovarian tumors was reported recently by Roman and colleagues. These investigators performed a prospective trial to evaluate the efficacy of pelvic examination, tumor markers, transvaginal gray scale sonography, and Doppler flow sonography in predicting ovarian malignancy. These tests were performed on 226 consecutive women prior to operative removal of an ovarian tumor. Positive findings included fixed or irregular consistency on pelvic examination, solid or papillary projections on transvaginal sonography, a serum Ca-125 >35 μ/mL, and a pulsatility index <1.0 or a resistive index <0.4 on color Doppler. If all four indicators were positive in a postmenopausal woman, the risk for malignancy was 83%. In contrast, if all indicators were negative, 100% of postmenopausal women had benign ovarian tumors. Logistic regression analysis revealed that sonographically determined ovarian morphology and serum Ca-125 were the most significant predictors of malignancy in the ovarian tumors of postmenopausal women. Spectral Doppler analysis of PI and RI did not improve diagnostic accuracy because of the overlap in values obtained between benign and malignant ovarian tumors.

Using sonographic technology and serum markers, it is now possible to assess risk of malignancy in an ovarian mass and to plan accordingly. A recent analysis of national data has indicated that the highest survival of women with ovarian cancer occurred when a gynecologic oncologist was involved in their care. Therefore, patients with a high risk of ovarian malignancy on preoperative evaluation should be referred directly to a gynecologic oncologist.

PREOPERATIVE EVALUATION

Prior to operative intervention, each patient should undergo a thorough evaluation designed to determine the anatomic location, size, and morphology of the ovarian tumor as well as possible sites of metastases. In addition, her general medical condition and ability to undergo a major surgical procedure should be established. All patients should undergo routine hematologic and biochemical testing. A chest x-ray provides valuable information concerning cardiac size, as well as the presence of pulmonary metastases or a pleural effusion. An EKG is indicated in all women over the age of 40 or in a patient with specific signs or symptoms of cardiac disease.

As mentioned, TVS is the most accurate test in assessing tumor size and morphology. In patients with large ovarian tumors, it may be necessary to perform abdominal sonography as well as vaginal sonography to determine the full extent of the tumor. TVS is also valuable in identifying an intrauterine tumor or occult ascites. A patient with an ovarian tumor and vaginal bleeding should undergo a dilatation and curettage to rule out coexisting endometrial cancer or a primary uterine cancer with spread to the ovaries. Likewise, a Pap smear should be performed in all patients who have not had a cervical cytology evaluation within 6 months. Any patient with abnormal cervical cytology should undergo colposcopy with directed biopsies and endocervical curettage.

Although intravenous urography is performed less frequently than it once was, this test provides useful information concerning urinary tract anomalies, ureteral obstruction, and retroperitoneal lymph nodal spread. In a patient with an ovarian tumor and no ascites, pelvic/abdominal computed tomography (CT) or magnetic resonance imaging (MRI) is rarely indicated. However, patients with ascites in the absence of an ovarian tumor should undergo CT or MRI scanning to identify liver or pancreatic malignancies, and to confirm omental disease and peritoneal nodularity consistent with primary peritoneal cancer. Likewise, liver function studies should be performed to exclude cirrhosis or liver disease as a cause of ascites. Rarely, the presence of right heart failure and hepatic congestion is be the cause of ascites. Although paracentesis is contraindicated in a patient with an ovarian tumor confirmed on sonography, it may be useful in a patient who presents with ascites and no evidence of an ovarian abnormality. The presence of malignant cells in ascitic fluid may help identify the primary site of intraabdominal malignancy.

Common sites of nongynecologic cancer that spreads to the ovary include gastric malignancy, colonic carcinoma, and breast carcinoma. Colonoscopy should be performed in patients >45 years of age, or in any woman with occult blood in the stool. Colonoscopy also is indicated in patients with suspicious findings on barium enema. Upper gastrointestinal endoscopy should be obtained in any patient with hematemesis, persisting epigastric pain, or symptoms of upper gastrointestinal obstruction. Mammography is indicated in any woman over the age of 40 years who has not had this test or in patients with a palpable breast mass.

Finally, serum markers should be obtained according to the age and clinical findings of each patient. Serum Ca-125 and CEA often are elevated in patients with epithelial ovarian cancer, whereas serum AFP, hCG, or LDH are more commonly increased in younger women with germ cell ovarian malignancies. Serum inhibin is the most reliable marker in patients with ovarian granulosa cell tumors. The specific marker associated with each type of ovarian cancer is illustrated in Table 48.3. It is important to obtain a baseline serum marker value prior to surgery so that it can be used to monitor response to therapy.

PATTERNS OF SPREAD

Ovarian cancer spreads by: (a) direct extension and exfoliation of tumor cells into the peritoneal cavity; (b) lymphatic metastases to regional and paraaortic lymph nodes; and (c) hematogenous dissemination (Fig. 48.3). The specific pattern of spread depends on the stage, cell type, and histologic differentiation of the tumor involved.

TABLE 48.3.
Serum Markers in Ovarian Cancer

Tumor Histology	Serum Marker
Epithelial ovarian cancer	Ca-125
Mucinous cystadenocarcinoma	CEA
Endodermal sinus tumor	AFP
Embryonal cell carcinoma	hCG, AFP
Choriocarcinoma	hCG
Dysgerminoma	LDH-1, LDH-2
Granulosa cell tumor	Inhibin

The earliest method of spread in epithelial ovarian cancer is by exfoliation of tumor cells from the ovarian surface. These cells migrate with the circulation of peritoneal fluid along the surfaces of the pelvic and mesenteric peritoneum. They also are carried cephalad in the paracolic spaces to the omentum and undersurface of the diaphragm. Spread to the right lung occurs through the transdiaphragmatic lymphatics in the right hemidiaphragm, often producing a right pleural effusion. Surface spread to the bowel and bladder is a common finding in advanced-stage ovarian cancer, but involvement of the bowel lumen or bladder mucosa is rare.

Lymphatic drainage from the ovary follows two pathways. The first involves lateral spread through the infundibula pelvic ligament to the external and common iliac lymph nodes. In patients with advanced-stage disease, there may be retrograde dissemination via this pathway to the external ilial and femoral lymph nodes. The second pathway of efferent lymphatic drainage follows the ovarian vein to the paracaval and paraaortic lymph nodes. Metastatic spread of ovarian cancer to lymph nodes is well documented even in early-stage disease (Table 48.4) and confirms that there may be separate pathways of dissemination to the pelvic and paraaortic lymph nodes. Li and coworkers, for example, reported that 14 of 91 patients (15%) with disease visibly confined to one ovary had positive lymph nodal metastases. Thirteen of the 14 patients with lymph nodal spread had poorly differentiated tumors. Isolated ipsilateral lymph nodal metastases occurred in five patients and isolated contralateral lymph nodal metastases in three patients. Pelvic lymph nodes were involved in 7% of patients, paraaortic lymph nodes in 5% of patients, and both in 3% of cases. As expected, the frequency of lymph node metastases is related to stage of disease, cell type, and histologic differentiation of the tumor. Chen and Lee reported that the frequency of pelvic lymph node metastases increased from 9% in patients with clinically apparent stage I ovarian cancer to 33% in patients with stage IV disease. Similarly, the frequency of paraaortic lymph node involvement increased from 18% in patients with clinically apparent stage I disease to 67% in patients with stage IV disease. These findings are similar to those of Burghardt and colleagues, who noted lymph node metastases in 74% of patients with stage III or IV ovarian cancer. The incidence of lymph nodal metastases in-

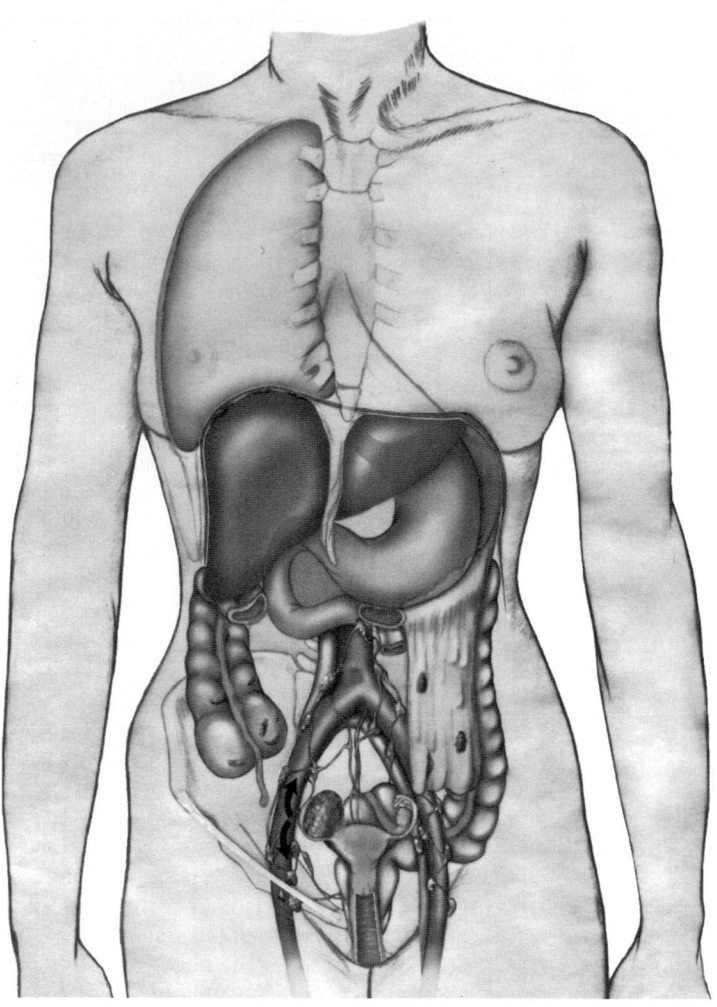

FIGURE 48.3. Patterns of spread of ovarian cancer.

creased from 20% in well-differentiated ovarian cancers to 65% in poorly differentiated tumors, and was higher in serous ovarian malignancies than in mucinous or endometrioid cancers.

Hematogenous spread of ovarian cancer to the parenchyma of the liver or lung fortunately is quite rare (<5%) at the time of initial diagnosis, but may occur, particularly in poorly differentiated tumors that become refractory to combination chemotherapy.

HISTOLOGIC CLASSIFICATION

Ovarian tumor specimens should be described, fixed, and sectioned according to the guidelines established by the College of American Pathologists (CAP). Tumor should be classified histologically according to the World Health Organization classification and nomenclature of ovarian tumors (Table 48.5). The three most common cell types are the epithelial, sex cord-stromal, and germ

TABLE 48.4.
Lymph Nodal Metastases in Patients with Clinically Apparent Stage I Epithelial Ovarian Cancer

Author	Patients	Pelivc Lymph Node Metastases	Paraaortic Lymph Node Metastases
Onda et al., (1996)	30	6 (18%)	5 (15%)
Carnino et al., (1997)	47	1 (4%)	0 (0%)
Burghardt et al., (1991)	20	3 (15%)	1 (5%)
Sakai et al., (1997)	46	1 (2%)	1 (2%)
Chen and Lee (1983)	11	1 (9%)	2 (18%)
Li et al., (2000)	91	9 (10%)	8 (9%)
TOTAL	245	21 (9%)	17 (7%)

TABLE 48.5.
World Health Organization Histological Classification of Ovarian Tumors

I. Surface epithelial-stromal tumors
  A. Serous tumors
    1. Benign
      a. Cystadenoma and papillary cystadenoma
      b. Surface papilloma
      c. Adenofibroma and cystadenofibroma
    2. Of borderline malignancy
      a. Cystic tumor and papillary cystic tumor
      b. Surface papillary tumor
      c. Adenofibroma and cystadenofibroma
    3. Malignant
      a. Adenocarcinoma, papillary adenocarcinoma, and papillary cystadenocarcinoma
      b. Surface papillary adenocarcinoma
      c. Adenocarcinofibroma and cystadenocarcinofibroma (malignant adenofibroma and cystadenofibroma)
  B. Mucinous tumors, endocervical-like and intestinal types
    1. Benign
      a. Cystadenoma
      b. Adenofibroma and cystadenofibroma
    2. Of borderline malignancy
      a. Cystic tumor
      b. Adenofibroma and cystadenofibroma
    3. Malignant
      a. Adenocarcinoma and cystadenocarcinoma
      b. Adenocarcinofibroma and cystadenocarcinofibroma (malignant adenofibroma and cystadenofibroma)
  C. Endometrioid tumors
    1. Benign
      a. Cystadenoma
      b. Cystadenoma with squamous differentiation
      c. Adenofibroma and cystadenofibroma
      d. Adenofibroma and cystadenofibroma with squamous differentiation
    2. Of borderline malignancy (of low malignant potiential)
      a. Cystic tumor
      b. Cytstic tumor with squamous differentiation
      c. Adenofibroma and cystadenofibroma
      d. Adenofibroma and cystadenofibroma with squamous differentiation
    3. Malignant
      a. Adenocarcinoma and cystadenocarcinoma
      b. Adenocarcinoma and cystadenocarcinoma with squamous differentiation
      c. Adenocarcinofibroma and cystadenocarcinofibroma (malignant adenofibroma and cystadenofibroma)
      d. Adenocarcinofibroma and cystadenocarcinofibroma with squamous differentiation (malignant adenofibroma and cystadenofibroma with squamous differentiation)
    4. Epithelial-stromal and stromal
      a. Adenosarcoma, homologous and heterologous
      b. Mesodermal (müllerian) mixed tumor (carcinosarcoma), homologous and heterologous
      c. Stromal sarcoma

  D. Clear cell tumors
    1. Benign
      a. Cystadenofibroma
      b. Adenofibroma and cystadenfibroma
    2. Of borderline malignancy (of low malignant potential)
      a. Cystic tumor
      b. Adenofibroma and cystadenofibroma
    3. Malignant
      a. Adenocarcinoma
      b. Adenocarcinofibroma and cystadenocarcinofibroma (malignant adenofibroma and cystadenofibroma)
  E. Transitional cell tumors
    1. Brenner tumor
    2. Brenner tumor of borderline malignancy (proliferating)
    3. Malignant Brenner tumor
    4. Transitional cell carcinoma (non-Brenner type)
  F. Squamous cell tumors
  G. Mixed epithelial tumors (specify types)
    1. Benign
    2. Of borderline malignancy (of low malignant potential)
    3. Malignant
  H. Undifferentiated carcinoma
II. Sex cord-stromal tumors
  A. Granulosa-stromal cell tumors
    1. Granulosa cell tumor
      a. Adult
      b. Juvenile
    2. Tumors in thecoma-fibroma group
      a. Thecoma
        Typical
        Luteinized
      b. Fibroma
      c. Cellular fibroma
      d. Fibrosarcoma
      e. Stromal tumor with minor sex cord elements
      f. Sclerosing stroma tumor
      g. Stromal luteoma
      h. Unclassified
      i. Others
  B. Sertoli-stromal cell tumors; androblastomas
    1. Well differentiated
      a. Sertoli cell tumor (tubular androblastoma)
      b. Sertoli-Leydig cell tumor
      c. Leydig cell tumor
    2. Sertoli-Leydig cell tumor of intermediate differentiation
      a. Variant—with heterologous elements (specify type)
    3. Sertoli-Leydig Cell Tumor, Poorly Differentiated (sarcomatoid)
      a. Variant—with heterologous elements (specify type)
    4. Retiform
      a. Variant—with heterologous elements (specify type)
  C. Sex cord tumor with annular tubules

TABLE 48.5. (continued)
World Health Organization Histological Classification of Ovarian Tumors

D. Gynandroblastoma	F. Teratomas
E. Unclassified	1. Immature
F. Steroid (lipid) cell tumors	2. Mature
1. Stromal luteoma	a. Solid
2. Leydig cell tumor	b. Cystic (dermoid cyst)
a. Hilus cell tumor	c. With secondary tumor (specify type)
b. Leydig cell tumor, nonhilar type	d. Fetiform (homunculus)
3. Unclassified (not otherwise specified)	3. Monodermal
III. Germ cell tumors	a. Struma ovarii
A. Dysgerminoma	1. Variant—with secondary tumor (specify type)
1. Variant—with synctiotrophoblast cells	b. Carcinoid tumor
B. Yolk sac tumor (endodermal sinus tumor)	1. Insular
1. Variants	2. Trabecular
Polyvesicular vitelline tumor	c. Strumal carcinoid tumor
Hepatoid	d. Mucinous carcinoid tumor
Glandular (Some glandular yolk sac tumors resemble endometrioid adenocarcinoma and have been called "endometrioid-like.")	e. Neuroectodermal tumors (specify type)
	f. Sebaceous tumors
	g. Others
C. Embryonal carcinoma	G. Mixed germ cell tumors (specify types)
D. Polyembryoma	IV. Gonadoblastoma
E. Choriocarcinoma	V. Mesothelial and other uncommon ovarian tumors
	VI. Secondary (metastatic) tumors

cell tumors. Although numerous grading systems for ovarian cancers use both architectural and nuclear features, it is recommended that four grades be used with grade 4 (undifferentiated) applied to tumors with minimal or no differentiation. Recommendations concerning the use of special staining techniques or flow cytometry in establishing the correct histologic diagnosis of ovarian tumors are made in the CAP report.

PRIMARY SURGERY

Ovarian cancer is one of the most challenging diseases facing gynecologic oncologists. Surgery remains the cornerstone in the management of ovarian cancer. For a patient suspected of having ovarian cancer, primary surgery accomplishes the following goals: (a) confirmation of the diagnosis of ovarian cancer; (b) precise determination of extent of disease, that is, surgical staging; and (c) maximum cytoreductive surgery in patients with advanced-stage disease.

Early-Stage Ovarian Cancer

Surgical Staging

Stage of disease is determined by the extent of tumor at initial diagnosis prior to any treatment. Ovarian cancer is surgically staged according to the staging system developed by the International Federation of Gynecology and Obstetrics (FIGO) (Table 48.6). Stage distribution varies depending on the type of ovarian malignancy. In addition, there is some variation from one study to another, especially with regard to sex cord-stromal tumors.

Invasive epithelial tumors are most often diagnosed after spread to the upper abdomen and beyond, whereas approximately 70% of borderline tumors are stage I at diagnosis. Sex cord-stromal tumors are rarely metastatic at diagnosis. Malignant germ cell tumors have intermediate metastatic potential, but the majority of these patients are still diagnosed with early-stage disease.

The gynecologic literature is replete with inadequate staging information. Several reports have documented occult metastases in patients with apparent stage I or II disease. The problem of incomplete staging in ovarian cancer is illustrated by the collaborative study of Young et al., in which 100 patients with apparent early disease (stages IA to IIB) underwent a variety of restaging procedures on referral to one of the member institutions. Thirty-one patients were found to have more advanced disease than originally thought, and 23 of the 31 patients (74%) actually had stage III disease. In 61% of patients found to have more advanced disease stage, procedures other than a second laparotomy, that is, laparoscopy or imaging study, confirmed the evidence.

McGowan et al. reported that only 54% of 291 patients with ovarian cancer received proper staging procedures. The completeness of staging varied depending on the type of specialist performing the procedure: gynecologic oncologists, 97%; obstetrician-gynecologists, 53%; and general surgeons, 35%. In a multicenter trial from the Netherlands, Trimbos et al. reported that surgical staging after one or two laparotomies was complete in only 53% of 86 patients. The most frequently omitted steps were biopsy of the paracolic gutter or pelvic peritoneum and sampling of the retroperitoneal lymph nodes.

TABLE 48.6.
FIGO Stage Grouping for Primary Carcinoma of the Ovary

Stage I	Growth limited to the ovaries.
Stage IA	Growth limited to one ovary; no ascites. No tumor on the external surface; capsule intact.
Stage IB	Growth limited to both ovaries; no ascites. No tumor on the external surface; capsules intact.
Stage IC[a]	Tumor either stage IA or IB but with tumor on the surface of one or both ovaries or with capsule ruptured or with ascites present containing malignant cells or with positive peritoneal washings.
Stage II	Growth involving one or both ovaries with pelvic extension.
Stage IIA	Extension and/or metastases to the uterus and/or tubes.
Stage IIB	Extension to other pelvic tissues.
Stage IIC[a]	Tumor either stage IIA or IIB but with tumor on the surface of one or both ovaries or with capsule(s) ruptured or with ascites present containing malignant cells or with positive peritoneal washings.
Stage III	Tumor involving one or both ovaries with peritoneal implants outside the pelvis and/or positive retroperitoneal or inguinal nodes. Superficial liver metastasis equals stage III. Tumor is limited to the true pelvis but with histologically verified malignant extension to small bowel or omentum.
Stage IIIA	Tumor grossly limited to the true pelvis with negative nodes but with histologically confirmed microscopic seeding of abdominal peritoneal surfaces.
Stage IIIB	Tumor of one or both ovaries with histologically confirmed implants of abdominal peritoneal surfaces, none exceeding 2 cm in diameter. Nodes negative.
Stage IIIC	Abdominal implants >2 cm in diameter and/or positive retroperitoneal or inguinal nodes.
Stage IV	Growth involving one or both ovaries with distant metastasis. If pleural effusion is present, there must be positive cytologic test results to allot a case to stage IV.

[a] To evaluate the impact on prognosis of the different criteria for allotting cases to stage IC or IIC, it would be of value to know whether rupture of the capsule was spontaneous or caused by the surgeon and whether the source of malignant cells detected was peritoneal washings or ascites.

In a survey of 785 ovarian cancer cases diagnosed in 1991, which were selected from the SEER program, Munoz et al. found that only approximately 10% of women with presumptive stage I and II ovarian cancer received recommended staging and treatment. The absence of lymphadenectomy and assignment of histologic grade were the primary reasons.

The emphasis on surgical staging has increased our awareness of retroperitoneal nodal involvement associated with epithelial ovarian cancer. In 1974, Knapp and Friedman reported finding aortic nodal metastases in 19% of 26 patients with apparent stage I ovarian cancer. Since then, other studies have shown nodal involvement in over 50% of patients with epithelial ovarian cancer. Recently, Li et al. reported on 91 patients with tumor visibly confined to one ovary at initial surgery. All patients underwent lymph node sampling. Fourteen patients (15%) had positive lymph nodes. Thirteen of these 13 patients had grade 3 tumors. Pelvic nodes were positive in six (7%), paraaortic nodes in five (5%), and both in three (3%). Forty-two patients had lymph node sampling only on the side ipsilateral to the involved ovary, of which four (10%) had lymph node metastases. Forty-nine patients had bilateral sampling, of which 10 (20%) had metastases; of these 10 patients, isolated ipsilateral lymph node metastases were found in five (50%) cases, isolated contralateral metastases were seen in three, and bilateral metastases were seen in two. The authors concluded that bilateral lymph node sampling significantly increased the identification of nodal metastases in patients with apparent stage IA invasive epithelial ovarian cancer.

A major dilemma facing gynecologic oncologists is the referral of a patient with apparent stage I ovarian cancer who has had an incomplete staging procedure. We are in the midst of an evolution in which we are attempting to strictly define a subset of patients with early ovarian cancer who require no adjuvant treatment; incomplete staging information obviously compounds the difficulty in decision making about the need for postoperative therapy in such patients. Reoperation with comprehensive surgical staging is one of the options to be considered in this subset.

Proper staging procedures should consist of the following (Table 48.7):

1. A vertical midline incision is usually preferable to a transverse incision in order to provide adequate expo-

TABLE 48.7.
Surgical Staging of Apparent Early Stage Ovarian Cancer

Vertical midline incision
Evacuation of ascites or multiple cytologic washings
Complete abdominal inspection and palpation
Resection of ovaries, fallopian tubes, and uterus[a]
Omentectomy
Random peritoneal biopsies
Retroperitoneal lymph node sampling

[a] Exceptions may be made in selected patients who wish to preserve fertility.

sure for appropriate staging biopsies or resection of metastatic disease in the upper abdomen.

2. Ascites, if present, should be evacuated and submitted for cytologic analysis. If no peritoneal fluid is noted, cytologic washings of the pelvis, bilateral paracolic gutters, and subdiaphragmatic areas should be performed prior to manipulation of the intraperitoneal contents. Cytologic washings are obtained by instilling approximately 50 to 100 mL of normal saline into each area.

3. The entire peritoneal cavity and its structures should be carefully inspected and palpated in a systematic manner. Generally, we prefer to begin with the subphrenic spaces and move caudad, toward the pelvis. In particular, the subdiaphragmatic areas, hepatic capsule, omentum, colon, all peritoneal surfaces, the entire retroperitoneum, and small intestinal serosa and mesentery should be checked. If any suspicious areas are noted, they should be excised or sampled. During this process, one should be vigilant for nongynecologic primary cancers.

4. The primary ovarian tumor and pelvis should be examined. Both ovaries should be carefully assessed for size, presence of obvious tumor involvement, capsular rupture, external excrescences, and adherence to surrounding structures. If the surgical findings are strongly suggestive of a benign ovarian mass in a young patient desirous of future child bearing, then ovarian cystectomy may be indicated. Otherwise, a unilateral salpingo-oophorectomy should be performed and the specimen submitted for frozen section examination. If bilateral ovarian masses are present, the more suspicious side should be dealt with initially. If frozen section analysis reveals a malignant epithelial tumor, standard surgical therapy consists of hysterectomy and bilateral salpingo-oophorectomy. Exceptions to this rule (e.g., conservative surgery) are discussed in the following.

5. If disease seems to be limited; that is, confined to the ovary or localized to the pelvis, then random staging biopsies of structures at risk for metastases should be performed. These sites include the omentum (either omentectomy or generous biopsies from multiple areas) and the peritoneal surfaces of the following sites: bilateral paracolic gutters, cul-de-sac, lateral pelvic walls, vesicouterine reflection, and subdiaphragmatic areas. Any adhesions should be generously sampled. Some surgeons, including the authors, prefer cytologic analysis by saline lavage rather than scraping or biopsy of clinically normal subdiaphragmatic surfaces. Others prefer scraping the subdiaphragmatic surfaces with a wooden spatula or tongue depressor and making a cytologic smear. Still others perform biopsies using laparoscopic equipment. The advantage of one technique over another, however, remains unclear and requires further study. In addition, no definitive studies demonstrate that total omentectomy or even infracolic omentectomy is more beneficial in terms of diagnostic accuracy or survival than generous sampling of the omentum in a patient without gross omental tumor.

6. If gross metastatic disease is present, it should be excised if feasible or at least sampled to document disease extent. The concept of cytoreductive surgery and supporting evidence is discussed in the following.

7. As noted, the retroperitoneum has historically been the area of greatest neglect. The paraaortic and bilateral pelvic lymph node-bearing areas should be carefully palpated. Any suspicious nodes should be excised or sampled. If no suspicious nodes are detected, then we generously sample these areas. There is no evidence at present that a complete paraaortic and/or pelvic lymphadenectomy are advantageous.

8. Appendectomy should be done in women with mucinous ovarian tumors because this can occasionally be the primary site.

Fertility-Sparing Surgery

Although the majority of ovarian malignancies occur in older women for whom bilateral salpingo-oophorectomy and hysterectomy are standard treatment, a significant subset of patients is young and can be managed more conservatively (Table 48.8). Conservative management is used here to denote surgery that preserves reproductive potential without compromising curability. With some exceptions, such a strategy may be applicable for women <40 years old who wish to bear children.

When contemplating surgery on a young patient with a suspected ovarian malignancy, it is important to discuss with her all possible operative findings and procedures and the long-term implications of the various options. If the patient is a child, the parents need to clearly understand this information.

In most instances, young patients have their initial surgery done outside major university hospitals or cancer centers. Common errors in surgical management include incomplete surgical staging and unnecessary bilateral salpingo-oophorectomy. In addition, some patients are mismanaged because of an error in the pathologic diagnosis of a rare ovarian neoplasm.

The optimal candidate for conservative surgical management is a young patient who has stage IA disease. If, on initial inspection, the suspected cancer is confined to one ovary, then unilateral salpingo-oophorectomy is appropriate. If the mass is thought to be benign, then ovar-

---

TABLE 48.8.

Criteria for Potential Fertility-Sparing Surgery in Ovarian Cancer Patients

---

Patient desirous of preserving fertility
Patient and family consent and agreement to close follow-up
No evidence of dysgenetic gonads
Specific situations
    Any unilateral malignant germ cell tumor
    Any unilateral sex cord-stromal tumor
    Any unilateral borderline tumor
    Stage IA invasive epithelial tumor

---

ian cystectomy may be preferable. The specimen should be sent for frozen section examination. If malignancy is diagnosed, then appropriate staging biopsies should be performed, as discussed. If the contralateral ovary appears normal, it is recommended that it be left undisturbed to avoid potential infertility caused by peritoneal adhesions or ovarian failure.

One should not rely too heavily on frozen section examination in making the decision to perform a hysterectomy and bilateral salpingo-oophorectomy. If the histologic diagnosis is in question, it is always preferable to wait for permanent section results for a young patient, even if this requires a repeat surgery.

The advent of *in vitro* fertilization technology should also have an impact on intraoperative management. Convention has dictated that if a bilateral salpingo-oophorectomy is necessary, a hysterectomy should also be performed. However, current technology for donor oocyte transfer and hormonal support allows a woman without ovaries to sustain a normal intrauterine pregnancy. Similarly, if the uterus and one ovary are resected because of tumor involvement, current techniques allow retrieval of oocytes from the patient's remaining ovary, *in vitro* fertilization with sperm from her male partner, and implantation of the embryo into a surrogate's uterus. Therefore, traditional guidelines concerning surgical management of ovarian cancer may no longer be applicable in selected young patients.

Approximately 50% to 70% of *malignant germ cell tumors* are stage I. Except for dysgerminoma, in which the incidence of bilaterality is 10% to 15%, bilateral ovarian tumors are exceedingly rare. Such a finding almost always signifies advanced disease with metastatic spread from one ovary to the other or a mixed germ cell tumor with a dysgerminoma component. Benign cystic teratoma is associated with malignant germ cell tumors in 5% to 10% of cases and may occur in one or both ovaries. Therefore, unilateral salpingo-oophorectomy, preserving the contralateral ovary and uterus, combined with surgical staging can be performed in most patients with these neoplasms, even many with advanced-stage disease. If the contralateral ovary is enlarged, most likely it represents a benign cystic teratoma that can be managed with an ovarian cystectomy only. With the exception of stage IA pure dysgerminoma or stage IA, grade 1 immature teratoma, these patients require postoperative chemotherapy. In the past few years, some investigators have advocated the practice of surgery alone for other categories of malignant germ cell tumors, including stage IA, grade 2 and 3 immature teratomas, and stage IA yolk sac tumors. Such an approach, however, should be taken with caution; many experts would still consider it experimental.

Most *sex cord-stromal tumors* are confined to the ovary. Stage I accounts for >50% (in some series as high as 100%) of granulosa cell tumors. More than 90% of Sertoli-Leydig cell tumors are stage IA. Bilaterality occurs in <5% of cases with either tumor type. Therefore, optimal surgical management of most patients with stromal tumors consists of unilateral adnexectomy combined with appropriate surgical staging. Endometrial curettage also should be performed in any young patient whose uterus is preserved because 5% to 15% of patients with granulosa cell tumors develop endometrial cancer or hyperplasia. Postoperative therapy may be indicated for patients with metastatic disease or for selected patients with stage I disease (e.g., poorly differentiated Sertoli-Leydig cell tumor or granulosa cell tumor with rupture).

Approximately 10% to 15% of all ovarian neoplasms are of the *borderline or low malignant potential* classification. Although they were first described over 70 years ago, only in the last few years have we begun to fully appreciate their biologic behavior. Approximately 33% to 60% of serous borderline tumors are limited to one ovary. Extraovarian spread is noted in approximately 20% to 30% of cases. Approximately 80% to 90% of mucinous borderline tumors are confined to one ovary. Both endometrioid and clear cell borderline tumors are almost always stage I, and the vast majority are unilateral. For patients with borderline tumors seemingly confined to one ovary, appropriate surgical management includes unilateral salpingo-oophorectomy with surgical staging. The use of ovarian cystectomy instead of unilateral adnexectomy also has been reported, although some patients treated in this manner require repeat surgery for a recurrence of tumor in the same or opposite ovary. If bilateral borderline tumors are present, portions of one or both ovaries may be preserved with ovarian cystectomy, if feasible. Whatever the surgical approach, reported 5-year survival rates for patients with stage I borderline tumors treated with surgery alone are 95% or better.

For patients with borderline tumors and peritoneal implants, the optimal management remains controversial. However, surgical excision is the mainstay of treatment. After frozen-section confirmation of borderline tumor, an effort should be made to resect all gross disease. In addition, staging biopsies of peritoneal surfaces and lymph nodes and cytologic washings are indicated. Even in the face of metastatic disease, a normal contralateral ovary may be preserved in young patients. In such cases, however, some recommend ovarian biopsy to eliminate the possibility of occult disease. In patients with advanced-stage serous disease, the incidence of bilateral tumors is approximately 75% in patients with advanced-stage serous tumors.

Invasive epithelial tumors account for approximately 70% of all ovarian malignancies. Despite the low overall survival rate associated with these tumors, selected young patients with stage I disease can be treated conservatively. The major factors that influence the selection process are histologic grade and bilaterality in addition to stage. Serous tumors are bilateral in about 50% of cases. The incidence of bilaterality for mucinous tumors varies widely in reported series from as low as 5% to as high as 50%, but probably is no greater than 10% to 20%. Approximately 30% to 50% of endometrioid and clear cell cancers are bilateral.

Brown et al. reported a retrospective review of 16 patients, all <40 years old at diagnosis, who had preservation of the uterus and contralateral ovary at the time of surgical staging. Adjuvant platinum-based chemotherapy was administered to 37% of these patients based on high-risk factors. With a median follow-up of 66 months, 14/16 (88%) patients were alive without disease. Two (12%) patients recurred in the retained ovary at 11 and 20 months; both died of tumor. Five patients had a total of eight successful pregnancies, two after adjuvant chemotherapy.

Risk Assessment

To begin making decisions about which patients might benefit from postoperative or adjuvant therapy, one must categorize them based on risk of relapse. The risk of relapse is approximately 1% for patients with stage I borderline ovarian tumors; thus, adjuvant therapy is not recommended.

For women with stage IA or IB *sex cord-stromal tumors*, no adjuvant therapy is recommended because of the low risk of relapse. For those with stage IC disease, however, the level of risk remains uncertain; some studies suggest that tumor rupture or the presence of ascites is prognostic, whereas others do not.

All patients with early-stage malignant ovarian *germ cell tumors* except those with stage IA dysgerminoma or stage IA, grade 1 immature teratoma require postoperative chemotherapy. As noted, there is some controversy about whether patients with stage IA yolk sac tumor or stage IA, grade 2 immature teratoma require adjuvant chemotherapy, but most experts in the United States favor treatment for such patients until such time as more information is available.

For patients with early-stage *epithelial ovarian cancer*, most experts currently accept a classification system of low and high risk (Table 48.9). Within the stage I category, histologic grade is the most powerful predictor of outcome. Patients with well-differentiated or grade 1 tumors have an excellent prognosis, with a 5-year survival rate of over 90%. On the other hand, the 5-year survival rates for patients with grade 2 or 3 tumors are approximately 75% to 80% and 50% to 60%, respectively. Other factors that have been found to have prognostic significance include large-volume ascites, dense adherence, and clear cell histology. Although older studies suggested that capsular rupture or excrescences may be associated with a worsened prognosis, more recent studies have found no independent influence of these features on prognosis. However, the issue about the influence of tumor rupture on prognosis remains controversial.

Therefore, low-risk early-stage epithelial ovarian cancer includes patients with the following factors: (a) stage IA or IB (intact capsule, no tumor excrescences, and no malignant ascites or negative peritoneal cytology); and (b) grade 1 or 2 disease. The standard treatment for this group of patients is surgery alone, and the 5-year survival is at least 95%. A controversy about whether grade 2 belongs in the low- or high-risk category remains unresolved; it is compounded by the lack of uniformity of grading systems.

High-risk early-stage epithelial ovarian cancer includes those patients with the following factors: (a) stages IC (ruptured capsule, tumor excrescences, positive peritoneal cytology, or malignant ascites)-II; (b) grade 3 disease; or (c) clear cell histology. In some classification systems, dense adherence is also included in the high-risk category; however, in the view of many experts, this designation is simply a surrogate for stage II disease. This high-risk subset is thought to have a relapse risk in the range of 40% to 50% and is the focus of adjuvant therapy trials.

Persistent problems with incomplete surgical staging and interobserver variability in assigning histologic grade leads one to the realization that more objective and reliable methods would be desirable for assessment of risk in early-stage ovarian cancer. Currently, there is no universally accepted prognostic molecular biomarker. There are, however, reports of several putative or potential biomarkers. Among these are DNA ploidy, computerized morphometry, Ki-67, p53, and HER-2/neu. Although none of the markers studied yet qualifies as prognostic, as technology advances, future studies will most certainly identify reliable biomarkers.

Adjuvant Treatment

For patients with *malignant ovarian germ cell tumors* who require adjuvant treatment, standard postoperative therapy consists of the combination of bleomycin, etoposide, and cis-platinum (BEP). For patients with high-risk *early-stage sex cord-stromal tumors* (stage IC or II), there is no standard postoperative treatment. The most commonly used regimens include the BEP combination or the combination of paclitaxel and carboplatin.

Platinum-based chemotherapy has emerged as the standard treatment for patients with *early-stage epithelial ovarian cancer*. The optimal regimen and duration of therapy remains elusive. In a prospective trial of 347 patients from the Norwegian Radium Hospital, patients with stage I, II, and III disease were randomized between intraperitoneal chromic phosphate or six cycles of cis-platinum. Patients who were randomized to 32p and were then found to have extensive peritoneal adhesions received whole abdominal radiotherapy instead. There was no difference in 5-year actuarial survival rates between the two arms; however, because of a 5% rate of in-

TABLE 48.9.
Early-Stage Epithelial Ovarian Cancer Risk Groups

Low-Risk	High-Risk
Stage IA or IB, $G_{1\&2}$	Stage IA or IB, G_3
	Stage IC
	Tumor on external surface
	Ruptured capsule
	Ascites or positive peritoneal washing
	All stage II

testinal injury requiring surgery in the 32p arm, it was not recommended for further study.

In nonrandomized studies, Piver et al. and Dottino et al. have reported excellent survival rates (>90%) in small series of patients treated with cis-platinum–based chemotherapy. Rubin et al. retrospectively reviewed 62 patients with stage I epithelial ovarian cancer, all of whom underwent comprehensive surgical staging followed by platinum-based chemotherapy. Fifteen patients (224%) relapsed. No patient was rendered disease-free after relapse. Patients with grade 3 tumors and clear cell histology had a higher risk of relapse.

Bolis et al. reported the results of two multicenter trials conducted by the Gruppo Italiano Collaborativo in Oncologia Ginecologica (GICOG). A total of 271 patients were included in these two trials. Trial 1 compared single-agent cis-platinum to observation in patients with stage IA and IB, grade 2 or 3. Trial 2 compared single-agent cis-platinum to intraperitoneal chromic phosphate in patients with stages IAii, IBii, and IC disease. In both trials, although the cis-platinum groups had a better disease-free survival, overall survival was not significantly different compared with the other arm. One possible explanation for these finding is that patients in the nonchemotherapy arm crossed over to cis-platinum at time of relapse.

The Gynecologic Oncology Group (GOG) has completed a randomized trial of cis-platinum plus cyclophosphamide for three cycles versus intraperitoneal chromic phosphate in patients with high-risk early-stage ovarian cancer. With 204 evaluable patients randomized, relapse-free rates were 77% for the chemotherapy arm and 66% for the 32p arm. After adjusting for stage and histologic grade, the group receiving chemotherapy had a 31% decrement in estimated relapse. Chemotherapy was recommended as standard adjuvant therapy for this subset of patients because of the superior progression-free survival and the late bowel toxicity associated with 32p.

There are several clinical trials of patients with early-stage epithelial ovarian cancer that either have been completed recently but results are not available or are ongoing. The GOG has recently completed a trial for patients with high-risk early-stage ovarian cancer in which patients were randomized between three versus six cycles of the combination of paclitaxel and carboplatin (GOG #157). No mature results are yet available from this study. In the current GOG trial for early-stage disease, all patients initially receive three cycles of paclitaxel/carboplatin and then are randomized between observation and 26 weekly doses of paclitaxel (GOG #175). This trial is obviously testing the potential benefit of so-called "maintenance therapy."

Other ongoing early-stage clinical trials include the International Collaborative Ovarian Neoplasms (ICON) trial and the Scandinavian trial. In both trials, high-risk early-stage patients are randomized between observation and single-agent carboplatin chemotherapy after primary surgery. There are some differences in these two trials, including minor differences in eligibility criteria and the lack of a requirement for comprehensive surgical staging in the ICON trial.

Advanced-stage Ovarian Cancer
Primary Cytoreductive Surgery

Cytoreductive or debulking surgery refers to a surgical procedure for which the goal is to reduce the amount of tumor as much as possible in a patient with metastatic ovarian cancer. Early studies suggested a relationship between the completeness of the surgery or the amount of residual tumor and survival. In a landmark paper, Griffiths demonstrated an inverse relationship between residual tumor diameter and survival; patients having residual disease <1.5 cm in diameter had a significantly improved survival compared with patients with bulky residual disease. Subsequent reports confirmed these findings. As our philosophy about cytoreductive surgery has evolved over the last two decades, "optimal debulking" has come to denote minimal residual disease ≤1.0 to 2.0 cm in greatest diameter; "suboptimal debulking" denotes bulky residual disease >1.0 to 2.0 cm in diameter. Defining the extent of residual disease when dealing with tumor plaques on the peritoneal surfaces remains problematic.

Cytoreductive surgery, of course, must be considered not in a vacuum but rather in the context of responsiveness of residual tumor to postoperative therapies. Both radiotherapy and chemotherapy trials have shown a higher response rate in patients with minimal residual disease. These observations are supported by basic studies that suggest that larger tumor masses have poorly perfused anoxic areas that are not accessible to cytotoxic agents. Furthermore, larger tumors may have a greater proportion of cells in the resting phase. These nonproliferating cells may be less sensitive to cytotoxic agents. Skipper espoused the "fractional cell kill hypothesis," stating that the ability of chemotherapeutic agents to eradicate cancer cells depends on both the dose of drug and the number of cells present. A given dose of drug kills a constant fraction of cells with each exposure. However, certain factors, such as cell repair mechanisms, tumor heterogeneity, the fraction of cells in Go phase, and the development of drug resistance serve to counteract this process. Goldie and Coldman have shown that tumor cells have an intrinsic spontaneous mutation rate; larger tumors that go untreated for an extended period theoretically have a greater probability of containing cell populations resistant to anticancer agents. Therefore, even though patients with advanced ovarian cancer may undergo optimal debulking, the small residual tumor masses may still contain drug-resistant cells that preclude ultimate cure.

Several reports have described the accomplishment of optimal cytoreductive surgery in a high percentage of patients. The morbidity and mortality associated with cytoreductive surgery also have been analyzed. These studies generally reflect an operative mortality rate of <2%, a mean operating time of 3 to 5 hours, and a mean blood loss of approximately 500 to 1,500 mL. There is a wide range of postoperative complications, the most common of which are infection, hemorrhage (at times requiring reexploration), prolonged ileus, and cardiopulmonary problems. The primary question concerning the efficacy of primary cytoreductive surgery is whether improved survival is related more to the biology of the tumor or the skill and aggressiveness of the surgeon. In other words, are those tumors that can be debulked optimally also tumors that are less invasive, less infiltrative, and more indolent? Earlier studies do not suggest that this is the case. All demonstrated that patients who required extensive surgery to achieve minimal residual disease and those who had minimal disease at the outset had similar survival rates. More recent studies, however, suggest that patients with *de novo* minimal disease have a superior prognosis to those who are debulked to minimal disease, supporting the prognostic influence of substage categories within the stage III classification. Unfortunately, there are no randomized studies to resolve important issues in this area. Moreover, prospects for such studies are not good because of several factors, including deeply established biases, the multiplicity of associated prognostic factors, and the highly individualized nature of each procedure. In the meantime, the efficacy of cytoreductive surgery remains controversial. Better information will be required ultimately to define its role.

Studies indicate that optimal cytoreductive surgery may confer a survival advantage, even for patients with stage IV ovarian cancer. Four large retrospective reports noted that patients with stage IV disease who were optimally cytoreduced had a statistically superior survival to patients who were suboptimally cytoreduced (Table 48.10).

EXPLORATION

The patient is placed in either the supine or semilithotomy or ski position, depending on the likelihood of a rectosigmoid resection. A vertical midline incision is employed and extended cephalad as much as necessary. On entering the abdomen, the initial steps outlined under surgical staging are followed. After evacuation of ascites, if present, and inspection and palpation, the size of the primary tumors(s) and size and extent of metastatic deposits should be noted.

During this initial phase of the operation, the surgeon must make an assessment of the feasibility of cytoreductive surgery. In a typical patient with advanced disease, the omentum may be totally replaced by tumor, and the pelvis may be filled with tumor, making it difficult or impossible for the surgeon to distinguish normal pelvic structures. Findings that may initially dissuade the surgeon from proceeding with aggressive tumor resection include extensive parenchymal hepatic involvement, massive diaphragmatic involvement, extensive infiltration of the small intestinal mesentery, or bulky nodal disease high in the paraaortic chain. On the other hand, even if minimal residual disease cannot be achieved, debulking of omental and pelvic masses may relieve production of ascites, reduce pressure on adjacent organs, and allow the patient increased comfort, at least temporarily. Moreover, intestinal resection still may be indicated for relief of impending or true obstruction.

OMENTECTOMY

It is our preference to perform an omentectomy prior to focusing on the pelvis if the omentum is largely or completely replaced by tumor. If the omental tumor is adherent to the parietal peritoneum of the anterior abdominal wall, the pelvic structures, or loops of small intestine, it should be dissected from these structures. Once the omentum is mobilized and lifted cephalad, a dissection plane is developed between it and the serosa of the transverse colon, extending the dissection laterally in both directions (Fig. 48.4A). If the supracolic omentum is heavily involved with tumor and densely adherent to the transverse colon, it also may be necessary to establish a plane between the greater curvature of the stomach and the omentum by ligating the right and left gastroepiploic arteries and the individual gastric branches (Fig. 48.4B). Entrance into the lesser sac allows traction on the greater curvature of the stomach and facilitates exposure and transection of the gastric branches of the gastroepiploic arch. Occasionally, omental tumor may

---

TABLE 48.10.
Effect of Debulking on Survival in Stage IV Ovarian Cancer

First Author	Year	Surgical Result	Patients	Optimal	Median Survival	p
Curtin	1997	Optimal ($<$2 cm)	41	45%	40	0.01
		Suboptimal	51		18	
Liu	1997	Optimal ($<$2 cm)	14	30%	37	0.02
		Suboptimal	33		17	
Munkarah	1997	Optimal ($<$2 cm)	31	34%	25	0.02
		Suboptimal	61		15	
Bristow	1999	Optimal ($\leq$1 cm)	25	30%	38	0.0004
		Suboptimal	59		10	

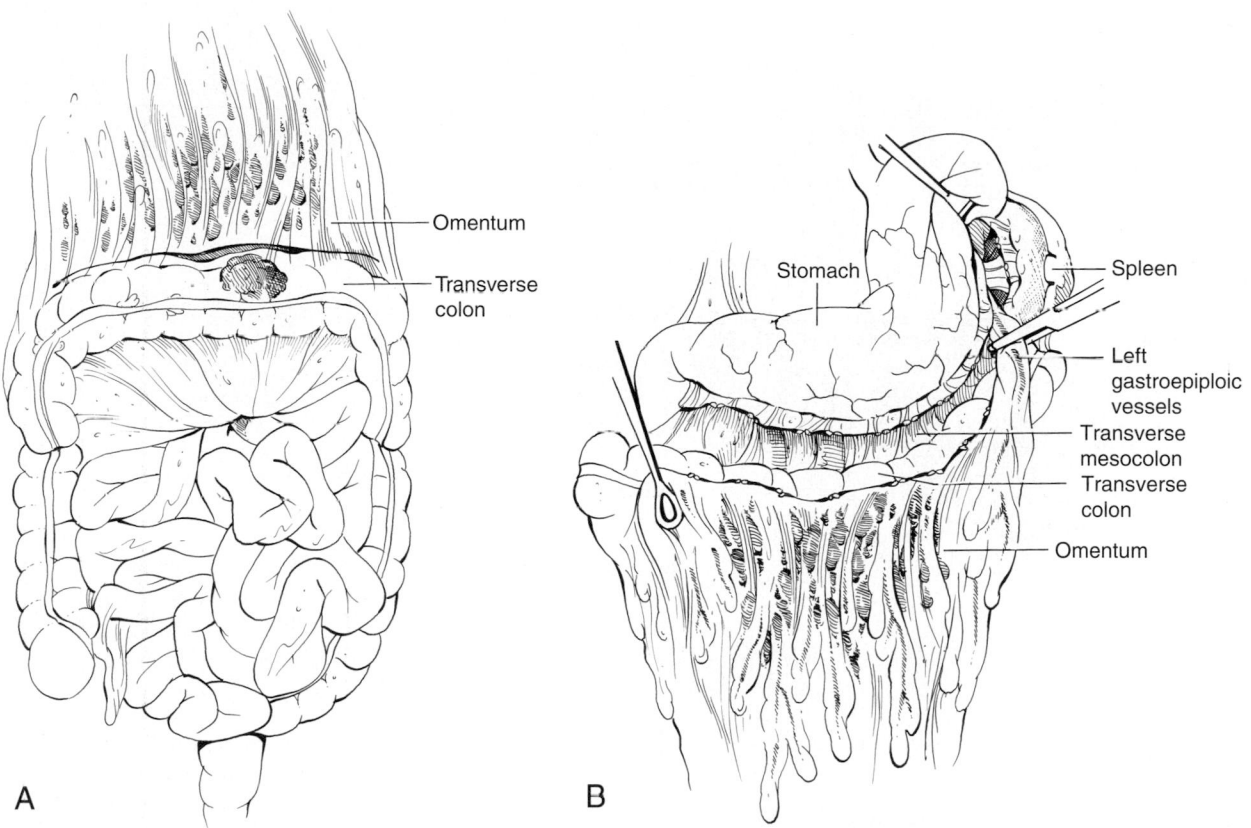

FIGURE 48.4. A. Omentectomy. Avascular dissection plane between omentum with metastatic ovarian tumor and transverse colon. **B:** Omentectomy. Dissection of omentum with tumor from stomach with ligation of gastric branches.

also involve the spleen or splenic hilum, necessitating splenectomy (see the following).

RESECTION OF PELVIC TUMOR

Any adhesions of small intestine or cecum to the pelvic structures should be lysed. A self-retaining retractor then may be inserted and the bowel packed for adequate exposure. If normal pelvic spaces and planes are obliterated by tumor, then the retroperitoneal approach is preferred (Fig. 48.5). The lateral pelvic peritoneum is incised, and the incision is carried cephalad and caudad. As part of this maneuver, the round ligament is identified and ligated as well. The retroperitoneal space is thus entered and the structures—ureter, iliac vessels, and ovarian vessels—identified by using both sharp and blunt dissection. A suction tip is a very nice instrument for dissecting areolar tissue planes if used properly. Next, the ovarian vessels are ligated. The identical procedure is performed on the opposite side of the pelvis, and the tumor mass(es) is mobilized medially.

If the ureters are densely adherent to the pelvic tumor, the surgeon may need to dissect them free, in some instances along the entire length of the pelvic portion of the ureter to the ureterovesical junction. In addition, the surgeon must establish a dissection plane between the sigmoid colon and the uterus and ovaries. This portion

of the procedure may take considerable effort if this plane is obliterated by tumor. On the other hand, if the surgeon determines that such dissection is not feasible or that the wall of the colon is heavily infiltrated with tumor, resection of the rectosigmoid colon may be indicated (Fig. 48.6) (see the following). Resection of the pelvic portion of the colon allows the surgeon access to the avascular retrorectal space. The uterus is dissected from the bladder as well. It is extremely rare for ovarian cancer to involve the bladder mucosa at the time of primary surgery, but the vesicouterine peritoneum may be heavily infiltrated. In such cases, resection of this area may be necessary, occasionally in conjunction with a partial cystectomy (see the following). Hysterectomy is then performed, the vagina is entered, and the mass is removed en bloc. In some instances, it may be necessary to ligate the uterine vessels at their origin rather than near the uterus if tumor is extensive in this area. Also, subtotal hysterectomy may be advisable if there is extensive unresectable tumor in the cul-de-sac.

RESECTION OF RECTOSIGMOID COLON

A rectosigmoid resection may be performed in approximately 10% of patients during primary debulking (Fig. 48.7). The decision to perform this procedure depends on several factors, including the presence or absence of

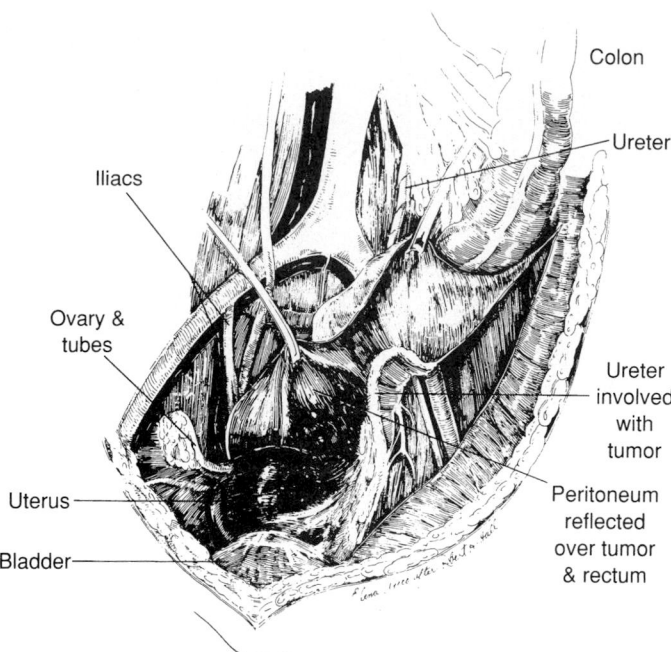

FIGURE 48.5. Retroperitoneal approach with lateral peritoneum incised, demonstrating the proximity of the left ovarian tumor to major pelvic vessels, the ureter, and the rectum.

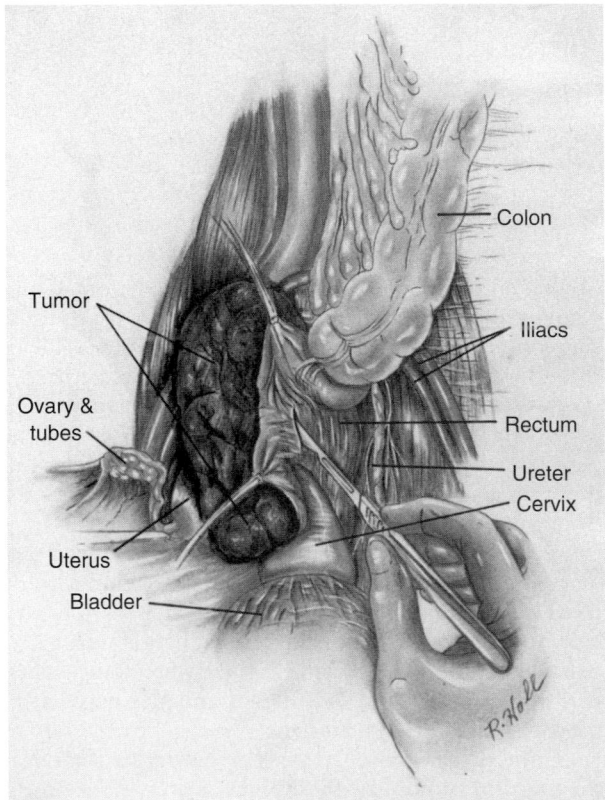

FIGURE 48.6. In the retroperitoneal approach, the proximity of the left ovarian tumor to the rectum is visualized before it is decided whether the tumor can be safely dissected from the rectum or resection of the rectosigmoid colon is required. (See Fig. 51.4 from Piver MS, Hempling RE. Ovarian cancer: etiology, screening, prophylactic oophorectomy, and surgery. In Rock JA, Thompson JD. *Te Linde's Operative Gynecology,* eighth edition. Philadelphia: Lippincott Williams & Wilkins, 1997:1557–1568.)

rectosigmoid obstruction, the amount of tumor infiltration of the lower colon and its contiguity with the ovarian tumor(s), and the probability that such a procedure will render the patient "optimally debulked." Occasionally, a patient will limit the surgeon's intraoperative decision-making ability by refusing to consent to possible colostomy. In our experience, resection of the rectosigmoid colon almost always can be accomplished with consequent minimal residual disease in the pelvis; the limiting factor in achieving optimal cytoreduction, however, may be unresectable bulky residual tumor in the upper abdomen or retroperitoneum. In such cases, palliative resection in the absence of obstruction is not recommended. If a rectosigmoid colon resection is performed, in most cases the colon can be reanastomosed using either a suture technique or the end-to-end anastomosis (EEA) stapler. For patients who undergo a reanastomosis, a protective hepatic flexure transverse loop colostomy or loop ileostomy protects the anastomosis for those who have received pelvic radiotherapy, those with unprepared colon, or those whose anastomosis is judged to be suboptimal. Occasionally, a colostomy with a Hartmann's pouch is necessary.

In 1984, Berek et al. reported their experience with 35 patients who underwent a rectosigmoid resection for ovarian cancer, 22 during primary debulking and 13 at secondary debulking. Twenty-four patients underwent a reanastomosis, and 11 had a colostomy without reanastomosis. Seventy-five percent of patients who underwent a reanastomosis did not require a protective colostomy. Optimal cytoreduction (residual tumor <1.5 cm in diameter) was accomplished in 94% of patients undergoing primary surgery and 57% undergoing secondary surgery. Although major morbidity occurred in seven patients (20%), it was temporary in all except one, who developed

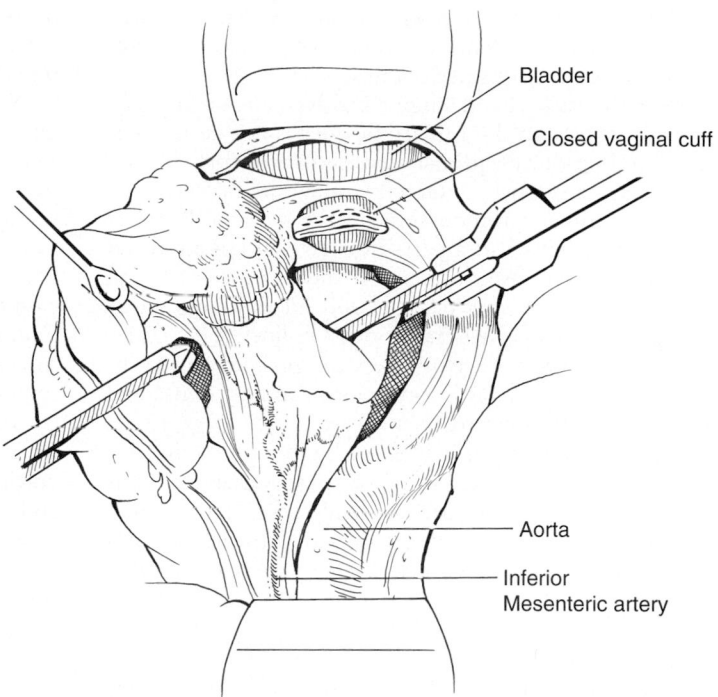

Bladder

Closed vaginal cuff

Aorta

Inferior
Mesenteric artery

FIGURE 48.7. Resection of rectosigmoid colon involved with ovarian cancer. The uterus and bilateral ovarian tumors have already been removed. After mobilization of the specimen and ligation of mesenteric vessels, transection is performed using GIA stapling devices (or reticulating stapler for distal transection) and remainder of mesentery is ligated. Usually, reanastomosis using EEA stapler can be accomplished.

an anastomotic stricture. There were no postoperative anastomotic leaks or pelvic abscesses.

Soper et al. described 40 women who underwent rectosigmoid colon resection during cytoreductive surgery, 21 (53%) as part of a primary procedure and 19 (47%) as part of a secondary procedure. Residual disease was <1 cm in 54% of patients. A permanent colostomy was avoided in 78% of patients. Twenty-five percent of patients experienced major morbidity, including one patient who developed an anastomotic dehiscence and pelvic abscess requiring a colostomy. One patient (3%) died in the immediate postoperative period. Despite aggressive surgical resection and postoperative therapy, the median survival for the entire group was only 14.5 months.

SMALL INTESTINAL RESECTION

Although the small intestine is a common site of metastasis, both to the serosa and the mesentery, extensive tumor involvement is an uncommon finding at primary surgery. If the small intestine is extensively involved with tumor, it is usually in the terminal ileum. Occasionally, small intestinal obstruction, either partial or complete, is present at diagnosis. As noted, complete surgical staging includes careful examination of the entire length of the small intestine from the ligament of Treitz to the cecum. If, on exploration, loops of small intestine are adherent to the pelvic tumor, omental tumor, or other loops of intestine, then these adhesions should be lysed. Indications for small intestinal resection include obstruction or impending obstruction by tumor infiltrating the serosa and muscularis of a segment or a nonobstructing extensive

lesion of the small intestine for which resection would result in minimal residual disease.

If the lesion involves the very terminal portion of the ileum, an ileocolectomy with resection of the cecum and portion of ascending colon adjacent to the small intestine may be necessary. Care should be taken to avoid the presence of tumor at the points of reanastomosis. The reanastomosis may be performed using either the suture or the stapling technique. In our experience and in the literature, small intestinal resection is indicated in approximately 5% to 10% of primary operations for ovarian cancer.

RESECTION OF THE URINARY TRACT

Indications for ureteral resection or partial cystectomy are uncommon during cytoreductive surgery. If ureteral obstruction is noted preoperatively, it is almost always a result of ureteral compression rather than tumor infiltration. Although adherence of the ureter(s) to masses of ovarian cancer is not an unusual finding, the surgeon can almost always separate the ureter from the tumor using sharp dissection. If the distal ureter is resected as part of cytoreductive surgery, it usually can be reimplanted into the bladder. More commonly, the ureter may be injured during the course of debulking surgery. Depending on the site of injury, a primary reanastomosis, transureteroureterostomy, or ureteroncocystostomy may be indicated. In a report by Berek and associates, 16 of 848 patients (2%) underwent partial ureteral resection. Five patients had transureteroureterostomy, two had reanastomosis, and four had urinary diversion. Twelve of the operations were part of primary cytoreductive surgery, and four were part of secondary surgery. Nine of these 16 patients had evidence of ureteral obstruction on preoperative intravenous pyelograms.

On the other hand, tumor involvement of the peritoneum overlying the urinary bladder is not an uncommon finding during primary cytoreductive surgery. Occasionally, a partial cystectomy may be necessary to achieve optimal cytoreduction. In the series of Berek et al., eight patients had a partial cystectomy for advanced ovarian cancer. Reconstruction necessitated ureteral reimplantation in two patients and an ileal conduit in one patient. If a partial cystotomy is indicated, we prefer a simple closure with two layers of chromic catgut suture, the inner layer as a continuous running suture and the outer layer as interrupted sutures.

In our experience, it is exceedingly rare to find involvement of the bladder mucosa with ovarian cancer at initial diagnosis. Such patients usually complain of hematuria in association with obvious massive disease. The definitive diagnosis can be made easily by preoperative cystoscopy.

SPLENECTOMY

Splenectomy is indicated occasionally during primary cytoreductive surgery (Fig. 48.8). Various series report the incidence of splenectomy during primary cytoreductive surgery in 5% to 11% of cases of advanced ovarian cancer. In addition, the indications for splenectomy and the procedure itself have been described in case re-

ports. Most commonly, the hilum of the spleen is involved with ovarian cancer in association with extensive omental involvement. Rarely, isolated splenic capsular involvement or even splenic parenchymal involvement may be found. In addition to tumor debulking, splenectomy also may be indicated during cytoreductive surgery because of a traction injury with avulsion of the splenic capsule during omentectomy or mobilization of the splenic flexure of the colon in association with descending colostomy or reanastomosis after rectosigmoid colon resection. If a splenic capsular avulsion injury does occur in the absence of tumor involvement, splenorrhaphy may be indicated before resorting to splenectomy.

In the series of Sonnendecker et al., five patients underwent splenectomy because of metastatic disease involving the spleen, one with parenchymal involvement, and one patient required splenectomy for capsular avulsion injury. In a report from M.D. Anderson Cancer Center, Morris et al. reported on 23 patients for whom the procedure was performed as part of cytoreductive surgery for advanced ovarian cancer. Splenectomy was planned preoperatively in only three of these patients. Seven patients had parenchymal involvement by tumor, 11 had capsular disease, and five have no pathologic involvement by tumor.

The methods of performing splenectomy during cytoreductive surgery may vary depending on the circumstances. Under controlled conditions (no uncontrolled

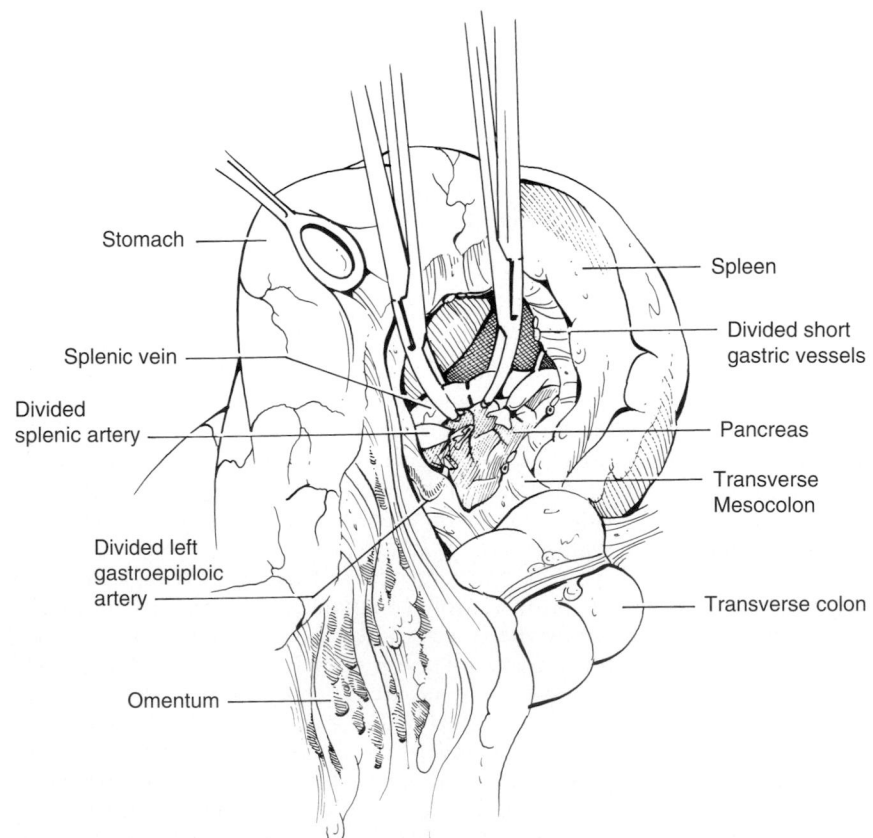

Stomach

Splenic vein

Divided splenic artery

Divided left gastroepiploic artery

Omentum

Spleen

Divided short gastric vessels

Pancreas

Transverse Mesocolon

Transverse colon

FIGURE 48.8. Splenectomy. Transection of splenic artery and vein along the superior border of the pancreas after access is gained to lesser sac with transection of gastrosplenic ligament.

hemorrhage), the surgeon may prefer to incise the gastrosplenic ligament, gain access to the lesser sac, and identify and ligate the splenic vessels as they run along the superior border of the pancreas. The spleen then can be mobilized by transecting its attachments to the colon, the left kidney, and the diaphragm. If hemorrhage is occurring or access to the lesser sac is limited by the distribution of tumor, the surgeon may prefer to first mobilize the spleen by dividing its peritoneal attachments while compressing the splenic vessels and then ligate the splenic vessels employing a posterior approach. The spleen is rotated anteriorly and medially in this technique.

Complications associated with splenectomy include hemorrhage, infection, thromboembolic phenomena, left-sided atelectasis or pneumonia, injury to the tail of the pancreas (with resultant pancreatic pseudocyst), or injury to the stomach (with resultant gastric fistula). Because of the risk of severe infection following splenectomy, the patient should receive perioperative antibiotic coverage and should be vaccinated with polyvalent pneumococcal vaccine. We also prefer to insert a drain in the splenic bed postoperatively to diagnose early postoperative hemorrhage and reduce the infection rate.

RESECTION OF DIAPHRAGMATIC TUMOR

Several recent reports have described experience with resection of diaphragmatic metastatic deposits in patients with advanced ovarian cancer (Fig. 48.9). To gain access to the diaphragmatic surfaces, the abdominal incision is extended to just below the xiphoid process, and the liver is mobilized by transecting the entire falciform ligament and the coronary and triangular ligaments. After it is adequately exposed, the diaphragmatic tumor may be resected by stripping the peritoneum from the diaphragmatic muscle using sharp dissection with either Metzenbaum scissors or electrocautery. Alternative techniques of debulking in this area are discussed in the following. The anesthesiologist should be notified if the pleural cavity is entered. Defects in the diaphragm may be closed with interrupted sutures. If a large defect cannot be closed primarily or can be closed only under tension, then the defect may be closed using synthetic mesh. If the pleural cavity is entered, then a thoracostomy tube should be placed.

Possible complications associated with resection of diaphragmatic tumor include pneumothorax, hemorrhage from the phrenic arteries, infection, injury to the pericardial sac, and injury to such structures as the lung, the vena cava, or the phrenic nerves.

Whether aggressive resection of diaphragmatic metastases with associated potential complications is justified is unclear. Montz et al. reported that 13 of 14 patients with diaphragmatic tumor could be optimally debulked. The size of resected specimens ranged from 12 × 7 cm to 17 × 11 cm. Kapnick et al. found that tumors that penetrated the entire thickness of the diaphragm to involve the pleura were ≥5.0 cm in diameter. Patients with tumors that penetrated the diaphragm had a median survival time of 8 months compared with a median survival time of 26 months for those patients without full-thickness diaphragmatic penetration by the tumor. Therefore, the assessment of the benefit of this procedure must await further studies.

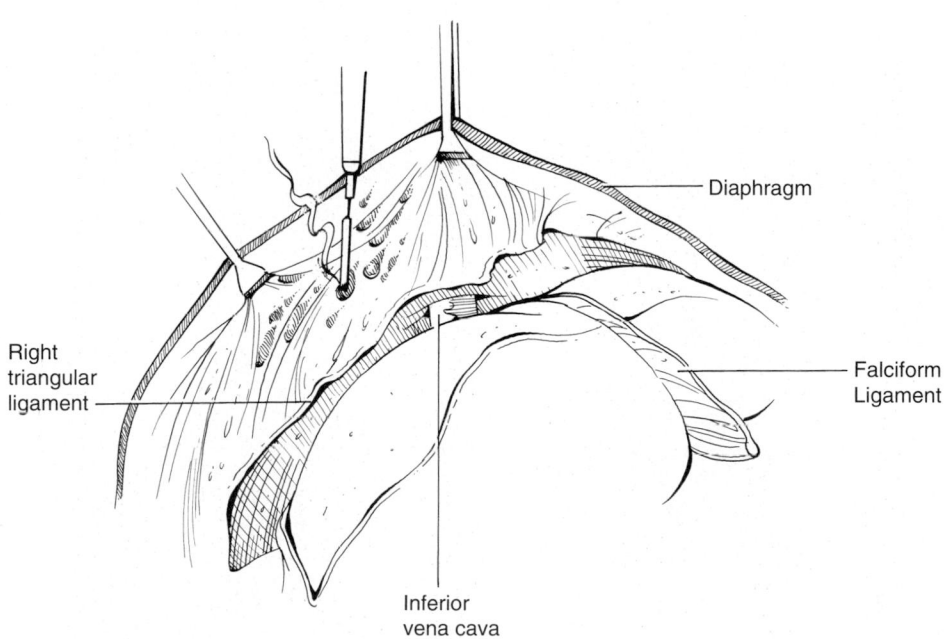

FIGURE 48.9. Ablation of subdiaphragmatic tumor implants with cautery after mobilization of liver. Sharp dissection, argon beam coagulator, of Cavitron ultrasonic surgical aspirator (CUSA) also may be used for the same purpose.

RESECTION OF RETROPERITONEAL LYMPH NODES
The initial retroperitoneal approach for cytoreductive surgery exposes the node-bearing areas. Lymph nodes are sampled as part of the staging technique, and every effort is extended to remove suspicious retroperitoneal nodes when the peritoneal cavity has been cleared of disease (Fig. 48.10). The benefit of radical resection of extensive retroperitoneal lymph node metastases also remains unclear. Burghardt et al. compared the survival of 70 patients with stage III ovarian cancer who had undergone radical pelvic lymphadenectomy with 40 patients with the same stage of disease treated without lymphadenectomy. The actuarial 5-year survival was superior for the former group—53% versus 13%, respectively. In the reports of Wu et al. and Burghardt et al., the role of pelvic and paraaortic lymphadenectomy at initial surgery for ovarian cancer is discussed, but there is no particular discussion of debulking of grossly enlarged retroperitoneal nodes. Benedetti Panici et al. reported the findings of a prospective study on the feasibility and morbidity of radical paraaortic and pelvic lymphadenectomy in patients with gynecologic malignancies. They observed acceptable morbidity—principally hemorrhage, lymphocyst formation, and deep venous thrombosis—and no operative mortality. Scarabelli et al. retrospectively evaluated the potential benefit on survival of systematic pelvic and paraaortic lymphadenectomy during both primary and secondary cytoreductive surgery in patients with stage IIIc or IV ovarian cancer. The previously untreated patients who underwent systematic lymphadenectomy had a significantly improved survival. The authors appropriately recommended a prospective randomized study to determine the efficacy of such an approach.

For patients with malignant germ cell tumors, especially dysgerminoma, the advantages of debulking metastatic retroperitoneal nodes are even less apparent, because these tumors are generally much more sensitive to chemotherapy than are other ovarian tumors.

Until further information becomes available, it is probably reasonable to consider debulking enlarged retroperitoneal nodes if peritoneal metastases can be cytoreduced optimally, if there is no fixation to blood vessels, and if the surgeon believes that the procedure can be successfully accomplished without undue risk.

ADDITIONAL TECHNIQUES FOR CYTOREDUCTIVE SURGERY
In the last few years, several reports described innovative techniques of debulking—the argon beam coagulator, the Cavitron ultrasonic surgical aspirator (CUSA), and various types of laser therapy.

The argon beam coagulator is a new electrosurgical device that conducts current to tissue in a beam of inert argon gas. Brand and Pearlman reported the use of the argon beam coagulator for debulking in seven patients with advanced ovarian cancer. Areas treated using the device included the diaphragm, stomach, duodenum, small intestine, colon, liver capsule, peritoneum, bladder and ureters, vaginal apex and parametrium, iliac vessels, and abdominal wall. Four of the patients had no gross residual tumor, and three had residual masses of ≤2 to 3 mm in diameter.

There have been several reports of the use of the CUSA for cytoreductive surgery. The CUSA combines

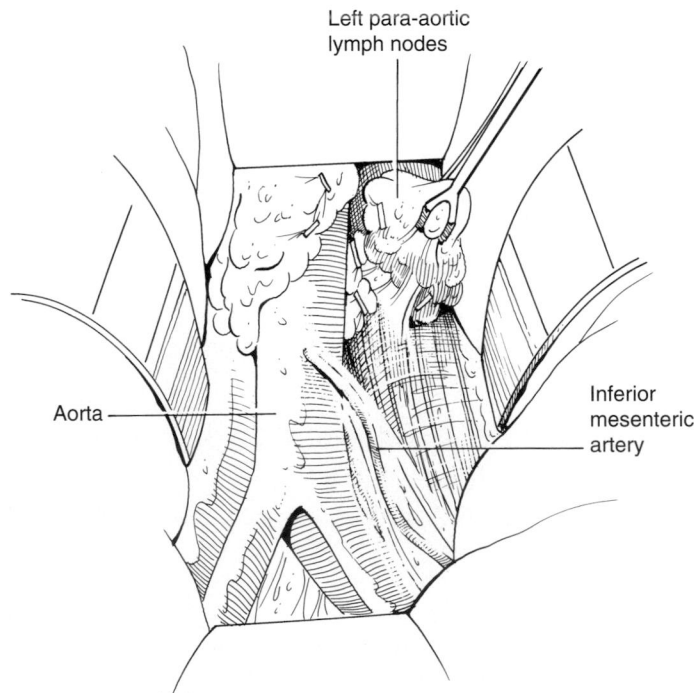

FIGURE 48.10. Retroperitoneal dissection of paraaortic lymph nodes involved with metastatic ovarian cancer.

tissue fragmentation, irrigation, and aspiration while dissecting tumor from blood vessels without injuring them. Adelson et al. described cytoreduction of tumors to <0.5 cm in nine of 10 patients. The authors particularly noted that intestinal resections were avoided because of the use of the CUSA. Deppe et al. reported on 11 patients who underwent optimal debulking using the CUSA. In other reports, the same authors described the utility of the CUSA in debulking diaphragmatic metastases and retroperitoneal lymph nodes. In the latter report, the authors were able to optimally resect extensive paraaortic and pelvic lymph node masses in five of six patients with advanced ovarian cancer. Two patients sustained lacerations of the inferior vena cava during the procedure.

Use of the neodymium-yttrium-aluminum-garnet (Nd-YAG) laser for the resection of intraabdominal tumors has been reported. Other reports of laser therapy for metastatic deposits of ovarian cancer undoubtedly will follow during the next few years.

The benefit of any of these new techniques for cytoreductive surgery remains unproved. Further studies will be necessary to elucidate their proper role.

Primary Chemotherapy for Advanced Ovarian Cancer

For patients with advanced-stage *malignant ovarian germ cell tumors*, the standard regimen is identical to that for patients with early-stage disease who require chemotherapy—the BEP regimen. The optimal number of cycles remains unknown, but for these patients with a potentially greater tumor burden than those with early-stage disease, four to six cycles may be required in some instances. Generally, administering two cycles following normalization of serum tumor markers may be a reasonable guide, although there are no definitive studies to support this practice.

For patients with advanced-stage *sex cord-stromal tumors*, platinum-based combination chemotherapy is generally recommended. As noted, the BEP combination regimen or the combination of paclitaxel/carboplatin are the most popular regimens in the United States.

For advanced-stage *epithelial ovarian cancer*, the combination of cis-platinum and cyclophosphamide was the standard postoperative regimen throughout most the 1980s and until the mid-1990s. Subsequently, based on encouraging results of phase II studies of paclitaxel in patients with refractory ovarian cancer, the GOG initiated a randomized trial comparing the standard regimen of cyclophosphamide/cis-platinum with the combination of paclitaxel/cis-platinum in patients with suboptimal advanced epithelial ovarian cancer. The findings of this study revealed a significant outcome advantage for the paclitaxel/cis-platinum regimen in terms of progression-free survival and overall survival. A subsequent similar study conducted by a European consortium confirmed the results of the GOG study.

Subsequently, based on the results of a GOG phase I trial, the GOG initiated a randomized study comparing paclitaxel/cis-platinum with paclitaxel/carboplatin. In the latter regimen, paclitaxel was administered over 3 rather than 24 hours, as in the previous GOG study. Recent data from that study suggest that the paclitaxel/carboplatin regimen is equally efficacious and has a superior toxicity profile compared with the paclitaxel/cis-platinum regimen. A subsequent study conducted by a German consortium (AGO) demonstrated similar results. Thus, because of its superior therapeutic index, the paclitaxel/carboplatin regimen has become the standard postoperative treatment for patients with advanced epithelial ovarian cancer.

Two other recent studies, however, have somewhat confused the issue. The GOG recently reported the results of a phase III randomized study in which the 24-hour infusion paclitaxel and cis-platinum regimen was compared with single-agent paclitaxel and single-agent cis-platinum. Response with single-agent paclitaxel was significantly inferior but overall survival was identical for all three arms of the study, probably because of significant crossover of patients on monotherapy to the other single agent. In another study conducted by the British Medical Research Council (MRC), the paclitaxel/carboplatin regimen was compared with a non–paclitaxel regimen (either single-agent carboplatin or a combination of cyclophosphamide/doxorubicin/cis-platinum). There is no difference in outcome between the two treatment arms with a relatively short follow-up time. However, approximately 20% of the patients in this trial had early-stage disease.

Intraperitoneal chemotherapy also has been studied as primary treatment for patients with optimally cytoreduced advanced epithelial ovarian cancer, but its precise role remains uncertain. In an Intergroup Study, 654 patients with <2 cm residual disease were randomized to receive intravenous cis-platinum/cyclophosphamide versus intraperitoneal cis-platinum plus intravenous cyclophosphamide. The median survival was significantly longer in the group receiving intraperitoneal cis-platinum (49 months) than in the group receiving intravenous cis-platinum (41 months). In addition, toxicity was worse in the intravenous group. The subsequent GOG study used intravenous versus intraperitoneal cis-platinum as part of initial therapy. Patients on the intraperitoneal arm received an initial two cycles of moderate-dose systemic carboplatin. The preliminary results of that study showed a significant improvement in recurrence-free survival for the intraperitoneal arm but no effect on overall survival. Because of significant design flaws associated with each of these GOG studies, the role of intraperitoneal chemotherapy in the management of advanced ovarian cancer remains unclear. The GOG is currently conducting an intraperitoneal chemotherapy trial that will provide more definitive results hopefully. This trial incorporates the use of intraperitoneal paclitaxel.

One of the most popular strategies in investigating the primary chemotherapeutic treatment of advanced ovarian cancer is either to add a third active agent to the paclitaxel/platinum foundation (doxil, gemcitabine, etc.) or to use sequential doublet regimens. A five-arm GOG trial using this type of design has been activated only recently.

Neoadjuvant Chemotherapy and Interval Cytoreductive Surgery

Over the past two decades, the concept of neoadjuvant chemotherapy followed by interval debulking (as a primary cytoreductive procedure after a few cycles of chemotherapy) emerged. This approach began to be reported in the late 1970s for certain subsets of patients: (a) patients who were referred to an oncologist after a surgical or nonsurgical biopsy; or (b) patients who initially were poor surgical candidates because of a debilitated state related to massive effusions or comorbid conditions. However, this approach has been proposed as a potential alternative for all patients with advanced epithelial ovarian cancer or for certain subsets, such as those predicted to be suboptimally resected. The potential advantage of such an approach is to operate on a patient with an improved nutritional status, a smaller tumor burden, and superior perioperative risk. A European cooperative group is currently studying this approach in a randomized clinical trial.

SECONDARY SURGERY

Second-Look Laparotomy

Second-look laparotomy for evaluation of disease status following treatment for cancer of the colon was proposed initially by Wangensteen and associates in 1948. Since the early 1960s, second-look laparotomy was employed extensively in the management of ovarian cancer. The procedure continued to gain popularity as more ovarian cancer patients were treated with chemotherapy and fewer received radiotherapy. Since the mid-1980s, however, there has been increasing skepticism about the benefits of this procedure.

Interpretation of reports of experience with second-look laparotomy has been complicated by the fact that no standard definition of the procedure exists. Most experts agree that the term second-look surgery should be restricted to an operation performed on a patient with no clinical evidence of persistent tumor for the purpose of determining disease status after a planned interval of treatment with chemotherapy. The term should not be applied to a surgical procedure performed in patients with clinical evidence of persistent or progressive disease for the primary purpose of debulking or treatment of complications. With current treatment regimens, at least 50% to 60% of patients with advanced ovarian cancer are clinically disease-free at the conclusion of chemotherapy.

Standard preoperative assessment of ovarian cancer patients at completion of the planned interval of chemotherapy includes physical examination, determination of serum tumor marker levels, and CT of the abdomen and pelvis. If these studies clearly document persistent ovarian cancer, then, with rare exceptions, second-look laparotomy is not performed. The operative technique of second-look laparotomy has been well described. It is essentially identical to a staging laparotomy, as discussed in the preceding. An adequate vertical midline abdominal incision is made. On entering the abdomen, cytologic washings from the pelvis, bilateral paracolic gutters, and subdiaphragmatic areas are obtained, and the entire contents of the peritoneal cavity are inspected and palpated. If obvious macroscopic tumor is present, then the procedure usually is limited. However, the extent of disease should be carefully determined, and a few biopsies should be taken for documentation of persistent disease (frozen as well as permanent section). If no obvious macroscopic disease is noted, then random biopsy specimens are taken routinely from the peritoneal surfaces, including the cul-de-sac, vesicouterine reflection, bilateral pelvic walls, bilateral paracolic gutters, and surfaces of the diaphragm. Omental biopsies and biopsies of the retroperitoneal lymph nodes also are performed. Lysis of adhesions is not uncommon in the process of performing these biopsies. Sites of previously documented tumor and adhesions should be carefully evaluated and generously sampled. An adequate procedure consists of a minimum of 20 to 30 biopsy specimens.

Second-look laparotomy is a major operative procedure, although it is a very safe one. The average duration of the operation is 2 hours, and the usual hospital stay is 4 to 5 days. Operative mortality is a rarity. Operative morbidity is low, and most complications are minor. The most common complications include wound infection and prolonged ileus. Other reported complications include urinary tract infection, small intestinal obstruction, pneumothorax, intestinal injury, hemorrhage, pneumonia, and thromboembolic phenomena.

Findings at second-look laparotomy are classified as negative (grossly and pathologically negative), microscopically positive (grossly negative, pathologically positive), and macroscopically positive (grossly and pathologically positive). The clinical variables most consistently associated with findings at second-look laparotomy and survival afterward are histologic grade, amount of residual disease, and FIGO stage. Patients with low-grade tumors, minimal residual disease, and early-stage disease have a greater probability of having negative findings at second-look laparotomy than do those with high-grade tumors, bulky residual disease, or advanced-stage disease. Other variables found to correlate with second-look findings and subsequent survival in some of these studies are histologic type, type of chemotherapy, amount of disease found at the initial surgery, age, performance status, and peritoneal cytology status.

Findings in approximately 50% of patients with advanced ovarian cancer (and a smaller percentage of those with early-stage disease) will be macroscopically positive at second-look laparotomy. Such patients, with the exception of those with low-grade tumors, have a very poor prognosis; most eventually develop progressive disease and die. With rare exceptions, they are candidates for experimental therapies. The issue of cytoreductive surgery in this setting is discussed in the following.

Approximately 20% of patients with advanced ovarian cancer who undergo second-look laparotomy have microscopically positive findings. In 1985, Copeland et al. reported 50 patients with advanced ovarian cancer who had microscopically positive findings. The 2- and 5-year actuarial survival rates of these patients were 81% and 70%, respectively—not statistically different from those achieved by patients with negative second-look findings. However, most of the patients with microscopic disease received chemotherapy after second-look surgery, whereas those with negative findings did not. Moreover, the microscopic disease group contained a higher percentage of patients with low-grade tumors. After these studies were reported, a detailed pathologic analysis of the microscopic disease group revealed that benign mullerian rests were misinterpreted as representing persistent tumor in several cases. Another updated analysis of these patients revealed that when grade 1 and borderline tumors were excluded, 58% of microscopic disease patients had recurrences. Treatment approaches currently under study for microscopically positive disease include abdominopelvic radiotherapy, intraperitoneal chemotherapy, high-dose chemotherapy with peripheral blood stem cell rescue, and radioisotope therapy.

Negative second-look laparotomy findings are noted in approximately 30% of patients with advanced ovarian cancer undergoing this procedure. Gershenson et al. initially found a recurrence rate of 24% in 85 patients with advanced ovarian cancer who had negative second-look results. An updated analysis revealed a recurrence rate of 44% in patients with grades 2 and 3 disease. Studies from other large centers have noted similar recurrence rates. The recurrence rates of 30% to 50% in patients with negative second-look findings after treatment for advanced ovarian cancer have prompted initiation of clinical trials evaluating a variety of therapies to follow negative second-look laparotomy. These treatments include external radiotherapy, intraperitoneal chemotherapy, high-dose chemotherapy, and radioisotope therapy.

There is limited information in the literature regarding second-look laparotomy in patients with *malignant germ cell tumors* and virtually no meaningful information about patients with *sex cord-stromal tumors*. In a review of the experience with second-look laparotomy in patients with malignant germ cell tumors at M.D. Anderson Cancer Center, findings were negative in 52 of 53 such patients. One patient with negative findings subsequently experienced a relapse and died. Thirteen patients had biopsy-proven evidence of mature teratoma—so-called chemotherapeutic retroconversion—at second-look laparotomy; treatment was discontinued in all patients and none developed a recurrence. Based on these observations, our group recommended limitation on the use of second-look laparotomy in this patient population as much as possible. Williams et al. reported the GOG experience, in which 117 patients with malignant germ cell tumors underwent second-look laparotomy after treatment with platinum-based chemotherapy. Based on their findings, the authors concluded that patients with either completely resected tumor or advanced-stage in-

completely resected tumor that does not contain elements of teratoma rarely, if ever, benefit from second-look laparotomy. They did recommend second-look surgery for patients with incompletely resected tumor that contains teratoma. However, a significant proportion of this latter subset of patients had clinically detectable tumor prior to second-look surgery. The procedure is not recommended for those patients with initially detectable levels of serum tumor markers, especially those with early-stage disease. Some patients with advanced disease, particularly those with initially undetectable serum tumor markers, continue to undergo second-look laparotomy. The issue of second-look surgery for patients with incompletely resected elements of teratoma remains unresolved. As better therapies are developed and refined, the procedure will inevitably become obsolete except in unusual situations.

A number of alternatives to second-look laparotomy have been investigated. Laparoscopy has been evaluated as a substitute. With the availability of improved equipment, we have witnessed a revitalization of interest in this procedure for cancer patients. Approximately 30% to 50% of patients with ovarian cancer undergoing laparoscopy after chemotherapy have positive findings, thus avoiding the need for laparotomy. However, second-look laparoscopy is associated with several potential problems: (a) several areas, including the bowel mesentery, the retroperitoneum, and areas obscured by adhesions, are not accessible with this procedure; (b) total operating time may be significantly longer if both laparoscopy and laparotomy are performed; and (c) 10% to 20% of patients develop complications, including hematomas and intestinal perforation.

The complication rate with the "open" laparoscopy technique is probably lower. With this technique, the surgeon makes a small incision through the abdominal wall layers into the peritoneal cavity and then inserts the scope. Such a maneuver is associated generally with a lower incidence of intestinal perforation. If second-look laparoscopy is employed, it should be recognized that the false-negative rate is approximately 35%. Therefore, a negative laparoscopy should be followed by laparotomy.

On the other hand, it should be mentioned that laparoscopy is superior to laparotomy for specific functions, such as visualization of the subdiaphragmatic surfaces and other upper abdominal peritoneal surfaces. As noted, there has been a recent resurgence in the use of laparoscopy for second-look surgery. To date, however, there have been no prospective randomized studies with sufficient power to resolve the issue of laparoscopy versus laparotomy.

Computed tomography has been evaluated as a substitute for second-look laparotomy also, but available information confirms the fact that tumor implants <2 cm in diameter are not reliably imaged. Therefore, a negative CT scan does not obviate the need for second-look laparotomy. However, a positive study may avoid second-look laparotomy in approximately 20% of patients. Positive CT studies should always be confirmed with fine needle aspiration. Whether MRI will prove superior to CT in defining persistent ovarian cancer remains unknown, although preliminary experience suggests that it will not.

The obvious substitute for second-look laparotomy is a reliable serum tumor marker. A negative CA-125 level at completion of chemotherapy, however, does not reliably predict lack of persistent disease. Second-look laparotomy has been negative in only 40% to 50% of patients with normal CA-125 levels. Therefore, a negative CA-125 level is not a substitute for second-look laparotomy. Patsner and associates reported that size of residual disease at second-look laparotomy did not correlate well with the serum level of CA-125. A positive CA-125 level, however, reliably predicts disease persistence and avoids a surgical procedure. Eventually, a battery of serum tumor markers or a more reliable single marker will probably replace second-look laparotomy.

Therefore, despite its shortcomings, second-look laparotomy remains the most reliable method for detection of persistent cancer. Theoretically, negative findings allow the clinician to stop potentially toxic therapy, and positive findings prevent premature cessation of therapy. On the other hand, for one of several reasons (most commonly patient refusal or physician preference), many patients do not undergo the procedure. Currently, the most widespread alternative to second-look laparotomy is simply discontinuation of chemotherapy after a fixed interval (usually six to nine cycles) for a patient with no clinical evidence of disease.

The benefits of second-look laparotomy have been seriously questioned in published articles and editorials. Few argue that the findings at second-look laparotomy are of prognostic value; patients with macroscopic tumor have a worse survival rate than do those with either microscopic tumor or negative findings. Critics state, however, that although second-look laparotomy is superior to other methods of detecting residual ovarian cancer, the procedure still does not accurately predict the presence or absence of disease. The high recurrence rate after negative second-look laparotomy has essentially eliminated our ability to identify a subgroup of patients for whom therapy can be discontinued safely.

A second major criticism of second-look laparotomy is the lack of evidence that the procedure or the therapeutic decisions made based on the findings enhance survival. No prospective randomized clinical trials have compared patients who undergo second-look laparotomy with those who do not. Although the results of GOG protocol #158 have not been published in manuscript form at the time of this writing, the author has presented data from this trial comparing patients who underwent second-look surgery with those who did not; these data reveal no difference in survival between the two groups. However, the presentation of these data has sparked a debate highlighting the fact that no randomization with regard to second-look surgery occurred in this study, and survival based on second-look surgery was not an end point of the study.

The greatest impediment to improvement in survival for patients undergoing the procedure is the lack of success of salvage therapies. Few patients with persistent disease found at second-look laparotomy (or diagnosed otherwise) are cured of their disease with second-line therapy. Although there has been a flurry of enthusiasm for such modalities as external radiotherapy and intraperitoneal chemotherapy for patients with minimal persistent tumor, results with the former have been generally quite disappointing, and the benefits of the latter are being questioned increasingly despite reports of responses and prolonged survival.

Proponents of second-look laparotomy claim that resection of residual tumor in this setting improves survival. The issue of debulking at second-look laparotomy is very controversial; it is discussed in the following. Until randomized clinical trials demonstrate a survival benefit of salvage therapies for patients with negative, microscopic, or macroscopic findings at second-look laparotomy, a cloud will remain over this procedure. Such trials are currently being conducted for patients with negative or microscopically positive findings. To our knowledge, no randomized trials are assigning patients with no clinical evidence of disease after completion of chemotherapy to undergo surgery or not. Such a study might be quite difficult to execute in the present environment. In the meantime, *it seems very reasonable to recommend that second-look laparotomy be performed only in a research setting until further information becomes available.* For patients with stage I epithelial ovarian cancer and those with malignant germ cell tumors, it is very difficult to justify second-look laparotomy because of the high probability of truly negative findings.

Secondary Cytoreductive Surgery

The term secondary cytoreductive surgery has no universal definition. It may denote cytoreductive surgery performed in one of several different settings: (a) in patients who are partial responders or nonresponders to primary chemotherapy; (2) in patients who have developed recurrent disease after receiving primary therapy and experience a prolonged disease-free interval off therapy (<6 months); (c) in patients who undergo a suboptimal debulking initially followed by three cycles of chemotherapy—so-called "interval debulking;" and (d) in patients who have persistent macroscopic tumor at second-look laparotomy.

Tumors in these subgroups of ovarian cancer patients may have very different natural histories, principally defined by whether they are "platinum-resistant" or "platinum-sensitive." For example, patients whose tumor progresses during first-line chemotherapy, whether progression is noted clinically or at second-look laparotomy, are by definition "platinum-resistant," whereas patients who have not yet received chemotherapy or are partial responders to chemotherapy, the response noted clinically or at second-look surgery, or who have developed recurrent disease after a prolonged interval off therapy may well be "platinum-sensitive." These subgroups thus may have very different survival rates based on their responsiveness to second-line chemotherapy after secondary cytoreductive surgery. Therefore, it is extremely important for studies designed to assess the impact of these various secondary procedures on survival rates to carefully define their study populations. Because of the lack of prospective randomized studies in this area, it is difficult if not impossible to draw any firm conclusions about the influence of secondary debulking in these settings.

Secondary Cytoreductive Surgery for Nonresponders or Partial Responders to Primary Chemotherapy

Very little information is available about the possible benefits of secondary surgery for patients who have no or partial response to primary chemotherapy. Morris and associates reported the experience at M.D. Anderson Cancer Center with 33 ovarian cancer patients who had progressive or stable disease and who subsequently underwent an attempt at secondary cytoreductive surgery. The tumors of 55% of the patients were cytoreduced to a residual diameter of ≤2 cm. Sixty-six percent of the patients required intestinal resection during the procedure. Operative morbidity occurred in 24% of patients, mostly in those who underwent bowel resection. The overall median survival after secondary surgery was 9.4 months. For patients with residual tumor <1 cm, median survival after secondary surgery was 19.5 months, compared with 8.3 months for patients with residual tumor of ≥1 cm ($p < 0.004$). Patients with an interval between primary cytoreductive effort and secondary surgery of <12 months survived a median of 7.3 months, compared with an 18.3-month median survival for patients with an interval of ≥12 months ($p < 0.004$). The authors concluded that there is no definite evidence that secondary cytoreductive surgery is of significant benefit in most patients with ovarian cancer that is progressive or stable during chemotherapy. This issue can be resolved only by a prospective randomized study, the outcome of which would be significantly influenced by the effectiveness of postoperative second-line therapy. It is quite unlikely, however, that such a randomized study will ever be conducted.

Secondary Cytoreductive Surgery for Recurrent Disease

Equally scant information is available about the impact of secondary cytoreductive surgery for recurrent disease. Morris et al. reported 30 patients who underwent secondary debulking for recurrent ovarian cancer. All had been treated initially with primary cytoreductive surgery and chemotherapy and had a period of clinical remission of at least 6 months thereafter. In 17 patients (57%), residual tumor was <2 cm. There were no postoperative deaths, but 40% of patients suffered postoperative morbidity, mostly prolonged ileus. The overall median survival after secondary surgery was 16.3 months. The authors concluded that, although secondary cytoreductive surgery for recurrent ovarian cancer is technically feasible, its value is limited in the absence of an effective second-line systemic therapy. In general, the longer the interval from completion of primary chemotherapy to

recurrence, the more favorable the survival. Subsequently, four retrospective studies did show an improved survival for patients secondarily cytoreduced to small residual disease compared with patients who were not optimally cytoreduced. Eisenkop et al. reported a prospective study of 36 patients with recurrent ovarian cancer who underwent secondary cytoreductive surgery. Thirty patients (83%) had complete resection of macroscopic tumor; their survival was significantly better than that for patients with macroscopic residual disease (43 versus 5 months, $p = 0.03$). Results of the five published studies on secondary cytoreduction for recurrent ovarian cancer are summarized in Table 48.11. Clearly, the true value of debulking surgery for recurrent ovarian cancer can be assessed only by a prospective randomized study. The GOG is in the process of planning such a study in the near future.

Secondary Attempt at Cytoreductive Surgery After Suboptimal Debulking

The term interval cytoreduction has been used to describe two distinct entities: (a) a true secondary cytoreduction performed after primary cytoreduction that is suboptimal (with bulky residual disease remaining) and three cycles of chemotherapy; or (b) cytoreduction after a biopsy (performed at surgery (by laparoscopy or laparotomy), fine needle aspiration, or paracentesis and a few (typically three) cycles of chemotherapy. The latter is really neoadjuvant chemotherapy followed by primary

TABLE 48.11.
Survival After Secondary Cytoreductive Surgery from Recurrent Epithelial Ovarian Cancer

Study	Patients	Median Survival (months)	Significance
Morris et al., 1988			
≤2 cm	17	18	$p < 0.2$
>2 cm	13	13	
Janicke et al., 1999			
Microscopic	14	29	$p = 0.004$
≤2 cm	12	9	
>2 cm	4	3	
Segna et al., 1993			
≤2 cm	61	27	$p = 0.0001$
>2 cm	39	9	
Vacarello et al., 1995			
<0.5 cm	14	41+	$p < 0.0001$
>0.5 cm	24	23	
No surgery	19	9	
Eisenkop et al., 1995			
Microscopic	30	43	$p < 0.01$
Macroscopic	6	5	
Gadducci et al., 2000			
Microscopic	17	37	$p = 0.04$
Macroscopic	13	19	

cytoreduction. These two entities have been confused and used interchangeably in the literature.

Several reports described secondary cytoreductive surgery as interval debulking after a suboptimal primary surgery and a few cycles of chemotherapy. Van der Burg et al. reported the findings of a large prospective randomized trial in which 278 patients with >1 cm residual tumor after primary cytoreductive surgery were enrolled. After three cycles of cis-platinum/cyclophosphamide chemotherapy, patients were randomized to receive either secondary cytoreductive surgery followed by three more cycles of chemotherapy or three more cycles of chemotherapy alone. Of the 140 patients randomized to the interval cytoreduction arm, 65% still had bulky tumor at the time of this secondary surgery; about 45% of them were able to be cytoreduced optimally. Both progression-free survival and overall survival were modestly improved in the interval cytoreduction group. The GOG currently is conducting a study with an identical study design in an effort to replicate the results of this European trial; the combination of paclitaxel/cis-platinum is being used rather than cyclophosphamide/cis-platinum.

Secondary Cytoreductive Surgery at Second-Look Laparotomy

The issue of cytoreductive surgery at second-look laparotomy is very controversial and its value unproved. No prospective randomized trials exist to resolve this controversy. Although some have questioned the value of secondary cytoreduction at second-look laparotomy, several authors have suggested a survival benefit associated with tumor resection at second-look surgery. In the study of Hoskins et al., the 5-year survival rate of patients found to have microscopic disease at second-look laparotomy was 62%, similar to that of patients whose disease was rendered microscopic by tumor resection— 51% ($p = 0.55$). Especially in these retrospective studies, it is extremely difficult to evaluate the influence of all prognostic factors. As with all studies on the subject of cytoreductive surgery, it is virtually impossible to distinguish the effects of secondary tumor resection from the influence of the inherent tumor characteristics. Noninfiltrating tumors may be easier to resect but may be inherently more indolent. In addition, survival after secondary debulking at second-look surgery is intimately linked to the skill of the surgeon and to the effectiveness of postoperative therapy.

MANAGEMENT OF INTESTINAL OBSTRUCTION

Approximately 25% of ovarian cancer patients develop intestinal obstruction in the terminal phase of their illness. One of the major dilemmas facing the gynecologic oncologist is whether to operate on a patient with refractory ovarian cancer and an intestinal obstruction. Although current information provides some guidelines, the decisions concerning the wisdom of surgical intervention and intraoperative management are based more on the art of the discipline and experience of the surgeon than on scientific criteria.

Signs and symptoms of intestinal obstruction resulting from ovarian cancer include nausea and vomiting, abdominal cramping, abdominal distention, and progressive constipation. In patients who have only partial obstruction, these complaints and findings may be episodic and more subtle. Plain films of the abdomen may support the diagnosis. Dilatation of the small intestine and air fluid levels suggest involvement of the small bowel. Dilatation of the colon may characterize large bowel obstruction. In patients with early partial obstruction, the radiographic findings may be nonspecific.

Although intestinal obstruction in patients with ovarian cancer may be caused by adhesions, progressive tumor usually is the inciting factor. Of course, if the patient has received abdominopelvic radiotherapy, this cause also should be considered. In our experience and that of others, however, most cases of intestinal obstruction in ovarian cancer patients who have received prior radiotherapy are related primarily to tumor progression.

The site(s) of the obstruction may be solitary or multiple. In 5% to 10% of patients, there is simultaneous obstruction of the small and large bowel. Colon obstruction in the area of the sigmoid portion usually occurs from growth of pelvic tumor and resultant extrinsic compression, although occasionally there may be obstruction of more proximal segments. Small bowel obstruction is usually the result of adherence of loops of bowel by mesenteric or serosal tumor implants.

The gynecologist must outline a plan of management once the appropriate evaluation is completed and the diagnosis of intestinal obstruction is made. Many factors influence this decision, including age, the nutritional status and general condition of the patient, the amount of tumor present, the presence or absence of ascites, the options for postoperative salvage therapy, the attitude of the physician, and the wishes of the patient and her family. The decision of whether to operate or manage the patient nonoperatively is colored by the fact that surgery for patients with refractory ovarian cancer is associated with significant morbidity and mortality, the obstruction cannot be relieved in almost 20% of those undergoing surgery, and postoperative survival is disappointingly brief. In reported series, the serious complication rate has ranged from 28% to 49%, and the operative mortality rate is in the range of 12% to 16%. The median survival rate for patients who have undergone surgery is in the range of 3 to 5 months.

Although some investigators have used projected survival (usually >2 months) as a parameter to decide on type of management, such an indicator is too unpredictable. Krebs and Goplerud devised a scoring system for selection of patients for surgery that included patient age, nutritional status, amount of palpable tumor, presence of ascites, previous chemotherapy, and previous radiotherapy. Outcome seemed to correlate with the prognostic score. Clarke-Pearson et al. later confirmed the influence of disease status, ascites, and nutritional status.

For initial management of a patient with small bowel obstruction, we prefer the insertion of a nasogastric tube rather than a long tube (Cantor, Miller-Abbott, or Dennis) for intestinal decompression. After extensive experience with both, we have found no advantage from the latter. Furthermore, long tubes are associated with considerably greater discomfort. Long intestinal tubes seem to have the greatest success rate in patients with postoperative adhesions but are fairly ineffective in relieving obstruction resulting from cancer. In the study of Krebs and Goplerud, only 10% of patients had their obstruction relieved by tube decompression. In patients for whom no surgery is planned, we have extensively used the technique of percutaneous gastrostomy since 1984. This procedure has resulted in excellent palliation for terminal-stage ovarian cancer patients, avoiding the discomfort of the nasogastric tube and allowing the patient to be easily cared for at home in most cases. With such a device, the patient may even continue to eat, although, the nutritional benefit is essentially nil of course.

Optimal preoperative preparation is desirable if a patient is judged to be a suitable candidate for surgical intervention. For patients with complete colonic obstruction or perforation of the small or large intestine, a surgical emergency exists unless the patient is in such poor condition that such an intervention is not feasible. In emergency cases, the patient should be stabilized with intravenous fluids and antibiotics prior to surgery. Emergency surgery is rarely indicated for patients with a small intestinal obstruction. It is preferable to optimize the patient's condition with nasogastric tube decompression and rehydration. In addition, a barium enema is indicated usually. If the patient is malnourished, then intravenous hyperalimentation may be indicated preoperatively. Ample information suggests that hyperalimentation places the patient in an anabolic state and reduces the incidence of postoperative morbidity; however, its effect on long-term survival is unclear.

Colonic obstruction usually is treated by performing a colostomy. The selection of the site of colostomy depends on the area of obstruction and the ability to find an adequate bowel segment free of cancer. Most commonly, a transverse loop colostomy is indicated in the presence of a descending colon or sigmoid colon obstruction. A number of options are available for small bowel obstruction, depending on the operative findings. Most commonly, there are multiple sites of obstruction in the terminal ileum, in which case an ileo-ascending colon bypass or ileo-transverse colon bypass is preferable. In such situations, it is usually both unwise and inappropriate to attempt resection and reanastomosis. If, on the other hand, there is an isolated area of obstruction, then a resection and reanastomosis may be indicated. The anastomosis may be either hand-sewn using a two-layer technique or approximated with surgical staplers. We generally prefer the latter because of the time-saving aspect. Frequently, there may be extensive tumor with multiple areas of obstruction, making both bypass and resection impossible. A tube gastrostomy is indicated in such a situation, if possible. Procedures such as these are among the most demanding because of the meticulous, often tedious dissection required. Enterotomies are not uncommon and should be repaired as soon as they are identified. Complications of small intestinal procedures include wound infection, intraperitoneal abscess, sepsis, pneumonia, "blind loop syndrome," and enterocutaneous fistula.

BIBLIOGRAPHY

Adelson MD. Cytoreduction of diaphragmatic metastases using the Cavitron ultrasonic surgical aspirator. *Gynecol Oncol* 1991;41:220–1222.

Adelson MD, Baggish MS, Seifer DB, et al. Cytoreduction of ovarian cancer with the Cavitron ultrasonic surgical aspirator. *Obstet Gynecol* 1988;72:140–143.

Alberts DS, Liu PY, Hannigan EV, et al. Intraperitoneal cisplatin plus intravenous cyclophosphamide versus intravenous cisplatin plus intravenous cyclophosphamide for stage III ovarian cancer. *N Engl J Med* 1996;335: 1950–1955.

Alcazar JL, Errasti T, Zornoza A, et al. Transvaginal color Doppler ultrasonography and Ca-125 in suspicious adnexal masses. *Int J Obstet Gynecol* 1999;66:255–261.

Allen DG, Baak J, Belpomme D, et al. Advanced epithelial ovarian cancer: 1993 consensus statement. *Ann Oncol* 1993;4(suppl 4):S83.

Aure JC, Hoeg K, Kalstad P. Clinical and histologic studies of ovarian carcinoma: long-term follow-up of 990 cases. *Obstet Gynecol* 1971;37:1–9.

Averette HE, Janicek MF, Menck HR. The national cancer data base report on ovarian cancer. *Cancer* 1995;76: 1096–1103.

Bailey CL, Ueland FR, Land GL, et al. Malignant potential of small cystic ovarian tumors in postmenopausal women. *Gynecol Oncol* 1998;69:3–7.

Barnhill D, Hoskins W, Heller P, et al. The second-look surgical reassessment for epithelial ovarian carcinoma. *Gynecol Oncol* 1984;19:148–154.

Barnhill DR, Kurman RJ, Brady MF, et al. Preliminary analysis of the behavior of stage I ovarian serous tumors of low malignant potential: a Gynecologic Oncology Group study. *J Clin Oncol* 1995;13:2752–2756.

Bast RC, Klug TL, St. John ER, et al. A radioimmunoassay using a monoclonal antibody to monitor the course of epithelial ovarian cancer. *N Engl J Med* 1983;308:883–887.

Bast RC, Xu FJK, Yu YH, et al. Ca-125: the past and the future. *Int J Biol Markers* 1998;13:179–187.

Benedetti-Panici GS, Baiocchi G, et al. Technique and feasibility of radical paraaortic and pelvic lymphadenectomy for gynecologic malignancies: a prospective study. *Int J Gynecol Cancer* 1991;1:133–140.

Berchuck A, Schildkraut JM, Marks JR, et al. Managing hereditary ovarian cancer risk. *Cancer* 1999;86(suppl): 1697–1704.

Berek S, Griffiths CT, Leventhal J. Laparoscopy for second-look evaluation in ovarian cancer. *Obstet Gynecol* 1981; 58:192–198.

Berek JS, Hacker NF, Lagasse LD. Rectosigmoid colectomy and reanastomosis to facilitate resection of primary and recurrent gynecologic cancer. *Obstet Gynecol* 1984;64: 715–720.

Berek JS, Hacker NF, Lagasse LD, et al. Lower urinary tract resection as part of cytoreductive surgery for ovarian cancer. *Gynecol Oncol* 1982;13:87–92.

Berek JS, Hacker NF, Lagasse LD, et al. Survival of patients following secondary cytoreductive surgery in ovarian cancer. *Obstet Gynecol* 1983;61:189–193.

Berek J, Knapp R, Malkasian G, et al. CA-125 serum levels correlated with second-look operations among ovarian cancer patients. *Obstet Gynecol* 1986;67:685–689.

Blythe JG, Wahl TP. Debulking surgery: does it increase the quality of survival? *Gynecol Oncol* 1982;14:396–408.

Bolis G, Colombo N, Pecorelli S, et al. Adjuvant treatment for early epithelial ovarian cancer: results of two randomised clinical trials comparing cisplatin to no further treatment or chromic phosphate (^{32}P). *Ann Oncol* 1995;6:887–893.

Bonazzi C, Peccatori F, Colombo N, et al. Pure ovarian immature teratoma, a unique and curable disease: 10 years' experience of 32 prospectively treated patients. *Obstet Gynecol* 1994;84:598–604.

Bostwick DG, Tazelaar HD, Ballon SC, et al. Ovarian epithelial tumors of borderline malignancy: a clinical and pathologic study of 109 cases. *Cancer* 1986;58:2052–2065.

Brand E, Pearlman N. Electrosurgical debulking of ovarian cancer: a new technique using the argon beam coagulator. *Gynecol Oncol* 1990;39:115–118.

Brand E, Wade ME, Lagasse LD. Resection of fixed pelvic tumors using the Nd:YAG laser. *J Surg Oncol* 1988;37:246–251.

Brenner D, Shaff M, Jones H, et al. Abdominopelvic computed tomography: evaluation in patients undergoing second-look laparotomy for ovarian carcinoma. *Obstet Gynecol* 1985;65:715–719.

Bristow RE, Montz FJ, Lagasse LD, et al. Survival impact of surgical cytoreduction in Stage IV epithelial ovarian cancer. *Gynecol Oncol* 1999;72:278–287.

Brown CL, Dharmendra B, Barakat RR. Preserving fertility in patients with epithelial ovarian cancer (EOC): the role of conservative surgery in treatment of early-stage disease. *Gynecol Oncol* 2000;76:240(abstr).

Burghardt E, Girardi F, Lahousen M, et al. Patterns of pelvic and paraaortic lymph node involvement in ovarian cancer. *Gynecol Oncol* 1991;40:103–106.

Burghardt E, Pickel H, Lahousen M, et al. Pelvic lymphadenectomy in operative treatment of ovarian cancer. *Am J Obstet Gynecol* 1986;155:15–19.

Carlson KJ, Skates SJ, Singer D. Screening for ovarian cancer. *Ann Intern Med* 1994;121:124–132.

Carnino F, Fuda G, Ciccone G, et al. Significance of lymph node sampling in epithelial carcinoma of the ovary. *Gynecol Oncol* 1997;65:467–472.

Casagrande JT, Louie EW, Pike MC. Incessant ovulation and ovarian cancer. *Lancet* 1979;2:170–173.

Castaldo TW, Petrilli ES, Ballon SC, et al. Intestinal operations in patients with ovarian carcinoma. *Am J Obstet Gynecol* 1981;139:80–84.

Chaitin BA, Gershsenson DM, Evans HL. Mucinous tumors of the ovary. A clinicopathologic study of 70 cases. *Cancer* 1985;55:1958–1062.

Chambers S, Chambers J, Kohorn E, et al. Evaluation of the role of second-look surgery in ovarian cancer. *Obstet Gynecol* 1988;72:404–408.

Chambers JT, Chambers SK, Voynick IM, et al. Neoadjuvant chemotherapy in stage × ovarian carcinoma. *Gynecol Oncol* 1990;37:327–331.

Chang J, Fryatt I, Ponder B, et al. A matched control study of familial epithelial ovarian cancer: patient characteristics, response to chemotherapy and outcome. *Ann Oncol* 1995;6:80–82.

Chen SS, Bochner R. Assessment of morbidity and mortality in primary cytoreductive surgery for advanced ovarian carcinoma. *Gynecol Oncol* 1985;20:190–195.

Chen SS, Lee L. Incidence of paraaortic and pelvic lymph node metastases in epithelial carcinoma of the ovary. *Gynecol Oncol* 1983;15:95–100.

Clarke-Pearson D, Bandy L, Dudzinski M, et al. Computed tomography in evaluation of patients with ovarian carcinoma in complete clinical remission. Correlation with surgical-pathologic findings. *JAMA* 1986;255:627–630.

Clarke-Pearson DL, Chin NO, DeLong ER, et al. Surgical management of intestinal obstruction in ovarian cancer. *Gynecol Oncol* 1987;26:11–18.

Clarke-Pearson DL, DeLong ER, Chin NE, et al. Surgical management of intestinal obstruction in ovarian cancer. II. Analysis of factors associated with complications and survival. *Arch Surg* 1988;123:42–45.

Colombo N. Randomized trial of paclitaxel and carboplatin versus a control arm of carboplatin or CAP: the Third International Collaborative Ovarian Neoplasm Study (ICON3). *Proc Am Soc Clin Oncol* 2000;19:A1500.

Copeland L, Gershenson DM. Ovarian cancer recurrences in patients with no macroscopic tumor at second-look laparotomy. *Obstet Gynecol* 1986;68:873–874.

Copeland L, Gershenson D, Wharton JT, et al. Microscopic disease at second-look laparotomy in advanced ovarian cancer. *Cancer* 1985;55:472–478.

Copeland L, Silva E, Gershenson D, et al. The significance of mullerian inclusions found at second-look laparotomy in patients with epithelial ovarian neoplasms. *Obstet Gynecol* 1988;71:763–770.

Cramer DW, Welch WR. Determinants of ovarian cancer. Risk II. Inferences regarding pathogenesis. *J Natl Cancer Inst* 1983;71:717–721.

Creasman WT, Rutledge F. The prognostic value of peritoneal cytology in gynecologic malignant disease. *Am J Obstet Gynecol* 1971;110:773–781

Curtin JP, Malik R, Venkatraman ES, et al. Stage IV ovarian cancer: Impact of surgical debulking. *Gynecol Oncol* 1997;64:9–12.

Dark GG, Bower M, Newlands ES, et al. Surveillance policy for stage I ovarian germ cell tumors. *J Clin Oncol* 1997;15:620–624.

Dauplat J, Ferriere JP, Monique G, et al. Second-look laparotomy in managing epithelial ovarian carcinoma. *Cancer* 1986;57:1627–1631.

Dembo AJ, Davy D, Stenwig AE, et al. Prognostic factors in patients with stage I epithelial ovarian cancer. *Obstet Gynecol* 1990;75:263–273.

Deppe G, Malviya VK, Boike G, et al. Use of Cavitron surgical aspirator for debulking of diaphragmatic metastases in patients with advanced carcinoma of the ovaries. *Surg Gynecol Obstet* 1989;168:455–456.

Deppe G, Malviya VK, Malone JM, et al. Debulking of pelvic and paraaortic lymph node metastases in ovarian cancer with the Cavitron ultrasonic surgical aspirator. *Obstet Gynecol* 1990;76:1140–1142.

Deppe G, Zbella EA, Skogerson K, et al. The rare indication for splenectomy as part of cytoreductive surgery in ovarian cancer. *Gynecol Oncol* 1983;16:282–287.

DePriest DP, Banks ER, Powell DE, et al. Endometrioid carcinoma of the ovary and endometriosis: The association in postmenopausal women. *Gynecol Oncol* 1992;47:71–75.

DePriest P, Shenson D, Fried A, et al.. Evaluation of Ca-125 levels in differentiating malignant from benign tumors in patients with pelvic masses. *Obstet Gynecol* 1988;72:23–27.

Dottino PR, Plaxe SC, Cohen CJ. A phase II trial of adjuvant cis-platinum and doxorubicin in stage I epithelial ovarian cancer. *Gynecol Oncol* 1991;43:203–205.

DuBois A, Lueck HJ, Meier W, et al. Cis-platinum/paclitaxel vs. carboplatin/paclitaxel in ovarian cancer: update of an Arbeitsgemeinschaft Gynaekolgische Onkologie study group trial. *Proc Am Soc Clin Oncol* 1999;18:A1374.

Easton DR, Bishop DT, Ford D. Genetic linkage analysis in familial breast and ovarian cancer: results in 214 families. The Breast Cancer Linkage Consortium. *Am J Hum Genet* 1993;52:678–701.

Einhorn N, Sjovak K, Knapp RC, et al. Prospective evaluations of serum Ca-125 levels for early detection of ovarian cancer. *Obstet Gynecol* 1992;8:14–18.

Eisenkop SM, Friedman RL, Wang H-J. Secondary cytoreductive surgery for recurrent ovarian cancer. *Cancer* 1995;76:1606–1614.

Fathalla MF. Incessant ovulation: a factor in ovarian neoplasia? (letter) *Lancet* 1971;2:163.

FIGO Staging for Carcinoma of the Ovary. In: Pecorelli S, ed. *Annual report on the results of treatment in gynecological cancer,* 24th ed. Milan, Italy: *J Epidemiol Biostat* 2001; 6(2).

Fiorica JV, Hoffman MS, LaPolla JP, et al. The management of diaphragmatic lesions in ovarian carcinoma. *Obstet Gynecol* 1989;74:927–929.

Fleischer AC, Cullinan JA, Kepple DM, et al. Conventional and color Doppler transvaginal sonography of pelvic masses: a comparison of relative histologic specificities. *J Ultrasound Med* 1993;12:705–712.

Ford D, Easton DF. The genetics of breast and ovarian cancer. *Br J Cancer* 1995;72:805–812.

Ford D, Easton DF, Stratton M, et al. Genetic heterogeneity and penetrance analysis of the BRCA1 and BRCA2 genes in breast cancer families. The Breast Cancer Linkage Consortium. *Am J Hum Genet* 1998;62:676–689.

Friedman J, Weiss N. Second thoughts about second-look laparotomy in advanced ovarian cancer. *N Engl J Med* 1990;322:1079–1082.

Gadducci A, Iacconi P, Cosio S, et al. Complete salvage surgical cytoreduction improves further survival of patients with late recurrent ovarian cancer. *Gynecol Oncol* 2000;79: 344–349.

Gershenson DM. Conservative management of ovarian cancer. *Curr Probl Obstet Gynecol Fertil* 1994;27:165–192.

Gershenson DM. Management of early ovarian cancer: germ cell and sex cord-stromal tumors. *Gynecol Oncol* 1994;55:S62–S72.

Gershenson DM. Update on malignant ovarian germ cell tumors. *Cancer* 1993;71:1581–1590.

Gershenson DM, Copeland L, Del Junco et al. Second-look laparotomy in the management of malignant germ cell tumors of the ovary. *Obstet Gynecol* 1986;67:789–793.

Gershenson D, Copeland L, Wharton JT, et al. Prognosis of surgically determined complete responders in advanced ovarian cancer. *Cancer* 1985;55:1129–1135.

Gershenson DM, Morris M, Burke TW, et al. Treatment of poor-prognosis sex cord-stromal tumors of the ovary with the combination of bleomycin, etoposide, and cis-platinum. *Obstet Gynecol* 1996;87:527–531.

Gershenson DM, Morris M, Cangir A, et al. Treatment of malignant germ cell tumors of the ovary with bleomycin, etoposide, and cisplatin. *J Clin Oncol* 1990;8:715.

Gershenson DM, Silva EG. Serous ovarian tumors of low malignant potential with peritoneal implants. *Cancer* 1990;65:578–585.

Gertig DM, Hunter DJ, Cramer DW, et al. Ovarian carcinoma diagnosis: results of a national ovarian cancer survey. *Cancer* 2000;89:2068–2075.

Goldhirsch A, Triller J, Greiner R, et al. Computed tomography prior to second-look operation in advanced ovarian cancer. *Obstet Gynecol* 1983;62:630–634.

Goldie JH, Coldman AJ. A mathematical model for relating the drug sensitivity of tumors to their spontaneous mutation rate. *Cancer Treat Rep* 1979;63:1727–1733.

Greenlee RT, Murray T, Bolden S, et al. Cancer statistics 2000. *Cancer* 2000;50:7–33.

Griffiths CT. Surgical resection of tumor bulk in the primary treatment of ovarian carcinoma: seminar on ovarian cancer. *NCI Monogr* 1975;42:101–104.

Rubin SC, Hoskins WJ, Saigo PE, et al. Prognostic factors for recurrence following negative second-look laparotomy in ovarian cancer patients treated with platinum-based chemotherapy. *Gynecol Oncol* 1991;42:137–141.

Griffiths CT, Parker LM, Fuller AF. Role of cytoreductive surgical treatment in the management of advanced ovarian cancer. *Cancer Treat Rep* 1979;63:235–240.

Hacker NF, Berek JS, Lagasse LD, et al. Primary cytoreductive surgery for epithelial ovarian cancer. *Obstet Gynecol* 1983;61:413–420.

Hankinson SE. Prospective study of talc use and ovarian cancer. *J Natl Cancer Inst* 2000;92:249–252.

Hankinson SE, Colditz GA, Hunter DJ, et al. A quantitative assessment of oral contraceptive use and risk of ovarian cancer. *Obstet Gynecol* 1992;180:708–714.

Hart WR, Norris HJ. Borderline and malignant mucinous tumors of the ovary: histologic criteria and clinical behavior. *Cancer* 1973;31:1031–1045.

Hartge P, Hoover R, McGowan L, et al. Menopause and ovarian cancer. *Am J Epidemiol* 1988;127:990–998.

Heintz APM, Hacker NF, Berek JS, et al. Cytoreductive surgery in ovarian carcinoma: feasibility and morbidity. *Obstet Gynecol* 1986;67:783–788.

Henriksen R, Runa K, Wilander E, et al. Expression and prognostic significance of platelet-derived growth factor and its receptors in epithelial ovarian neoplasms. *Cancer Res* 1993;53:4550.

Ho AG, Beller U, Speyer J, et al. A reassessment of the role of second-look laparotomy in advanced ovarian cancer. *J Clin Oncol* 1987;5:1316–1321.

Homesley HD, Bundy BN, Hurteau JA, et al. Bleomycin, etoposide, and cis-platinum combination therapy of ovarian granulosa cell tumors and other stromal malignancies: a Gynecologic Oncology Group study. *Gynecol Oncol* 1999; 72:131–137.

Hoskins W, Bundy B, Thigpen J, et al. The influence of initial surgery on progression-free interval (PFI) and survival (S) in optimal (<1 cm) stage III epithelial ovarian cancer (EOC). Society of Gynecologic Oncologist Abstract. *Gynecol Oncol* 1992;45:76.

Hoskins WJ, Rubin SC, Dulaney E, et al. Influence of secondary cytoreduction at the time of second-look laparotomy on the survival of patients with epithelial ovarian carcinoma. *Gynecol Oncol* 1989;34:365–371.

Hulka BS. Cancer screening: degrees of proof and practical application. *Cancer* 1987;62:1776–1789.

Hunter J, Andrews S, van Nagell, JR. Efficacy of a sonographic morphology index in identifying ovarian cancer: a multi-institutional investigation. *Gynecol Oncol* 1994;55:174–177.

Jacob J, Gershenson DM, Morris M, et al. Neoadjuvant chemotherapy and interval debulking for advanced epithelial ovarian cancer. *Gynecol Oncol* 1991;42:146–150.

Jacobs I, Bast RC. The Ca-125 tumour-associated antigen: a review of the literature. *Hum Reprod* 1989;4:1–12.

Jacobs I, Davies AP, Bridges J, et al. Prevalence screening for ovarian cancer in postmenopausal women by Ca-125 measurement and ultrasonography. *Br Med J* 1993;306: 1030–1034.

Janicke F, Holscher M, Kuhn W, et al. Radical surgical procedure improves survival time in patients with recurrent ovarian cancer. *Cancer* 1992;70:2129–2136.

Joyeux H, Szawlowski A, Saint-Aubert B, et al. Aggressive regional surgery for advanced ovarian carcinoma. *Cancer* 1986;57:142–147.

Kapnick SJ, Griffiths CG, Finkler NJ. Occult pleural involvement in stage III ovarian carcinoma: role of diaphragm resection. *Gynecol Oncol* 1990;39:135–138.

Kawai M, Kano K, Kikkawa F, et al. Transvaginal Doppler ultrasound with color flow imaging in the diagnosis of ovarian cancer. *Obstet Gynecol* 1992;79:163–167.

Keettel WX, Pixley EE, Buschbaum HJ. Experience with peritoneal cytology in the management of gynecologic malignancies. *Am J Obstet Gynecol* 1974;120:174–182.

Kerlikowske K, Brown JS, Grady DG. Should women with familial ovarian cancer undergo prophylactic oophorectomy. *Obstet Gynecol* 1992;80:700–707.

Knapp RC, Friedman EA. Aortic lymph node metastases in early ovarian cancer. *Am J Obstet Gynecol* 1974;119: 1013–1017.

Koch M, Gaedke H, Jenkins H. Family history of ovarian cancer patients: a case control study. *Int J Epidemiol* 1989;18:782–785.

Kohler MF, Kerns BM, Humphrey PA, et al. Mutation and overexpression of p53 in early-stage epithelial ovarian cancer. *Obstet Gynecol* 1993;81:643–650.

Krebs HB, Goplerud DR. Surgical management of bowel obstruction in advanced ovarian carcinoma. *Obstet Gynecol* 1983;61:327–330.

Krebs HB, Goplerud DR. The role of intestinal intubation in obstruction of the small intestine due to carcinoma of the ovary. *Surg Gynecol Obstet* 1984;158:467–471.

Kryscio RJ. The efficacy of transvaginal sonographic screening in asymptomatic women at risk for ovarian cancer. *Gynecol Oncol* 2000;77:350–356.

Kryscio RJ, van Nagell JR. A morphologic index based on sonographic findings in ovarian cancer. *Gynecol Oncol* 1993;51:7–11.

Kurjak A, Kupesic S, Anic T, et al. Three dimensional ultrasound and power Doppler improve the diagnosis of ovarian lesions. *Gynecol Oncol* 2000;76:28–32.

Kurjak A, Predanic M. New scoring system for prediction of ovarian malignancy based on transvaginal color Doppler sonography. *J Ultrasound Med* 1992;11:631–638.

Kurjak A, Schulman H, Zalud I, et al. Transvaginal ultrasound color flow and Doppler waveform of the postmenopausal adnexal mass. *Obstet Gynecol* 1992;80:917–921.

Larson JE, Podczaski ES, Manetta A, et al. Bowel obstruction in patients with ovarian carcinoma: analysis of prognostic factors. *Gynecol Oncol* 1989;35:61–65.

Lawton FG, Luesley D, Redman C, et al. Feasibility and outcome of complete secondary tumor resection for patients with advanced ovarian cancer. *J Surg Oncol* 1990; 45:14–19.

Lele S, Piver MS. Interval laparoscopy as predictor of response to chemotherapy in ovarian carcinoma. *Obstet Gynecol* 1986;68:345–347.

Levine D, Gossink B, Wolf SI, et al. Simple adnexal cysts: the natural history in postmenopausal women. *Radiology* 1992;184:653–659.

Li A, Otero F, Funowica CD, et al. Pattern of lymph node metastases in apparent Stage IA invasive epithelial ovarian carcinomas. *Gynecol Oncol* 2000;76:239.

Li AJ, Cass I, Otero F, et al. Pattern of lymph node metastases in apparent stage IA invasive epithelial ovarian carcinomas. *Gynecol Oncol* 2000;76:239(abstr).

Lim-Tan SK, Cajigas HE, Scully RE. Ovarian cystectomy for serous borderline tumors: a follow-up study of 35 cases. *Obstet Gynecol* 1981;72:775–780.

Liu PC, Benjamin I, Morgan MA, et al. Effect of surgical debulking on survival in stage IV ovarian cancer. *Gynecol Oncol* 1997;64:4–8.

Lu JL, Zheng Y, Yuan J, et al. Decreased luteinizing hormone receptor in RNA expression in human ovarian epithelial cancer. *Gynecol Oncol* 2000;79:158–168.

Luesley D, Chan K, Fielding J, et al. Second-look laparotomy in the management of epithelial ovarian carcinoma: an evaluation of fifty cases. *Obstet Gynecol* 1984;64:421–426.

Luesley D, Chan K, Lawton F, et al. Survival after negative second-look laparotomy. *Eur J Surg Oncol* 1989;15:205–210.

Lund B, Jaconsen K, Rasch L, et al. Correlation of abdominal ultrasound and computed tomography scans with second- or third-look laparotomy in patients with ovarian carcinoma. *Gynecol Oncol* 1990;37:279–283.

Lund B, Williamson P. Prognostic factors for outcome of and survival after second-look laparotomy in patients with advanced ovarian carcinoma. *Obstet Gynecol* 1990;76:617–622.

Lynch HT, Harris RE, Guirgis HA, et al. Familial association of breast/ovarian carcinoma. *Cancer* 1978;41:1543–1549.

Lynch HT, Lemon SJ, Karr B. Etiology natural history, management and molecular genetics of hereditary non-polyposis colorectal cancer (Lynch syndromes). *Cancer Epidemiol Biomarkers Prev* 1977;6:978–991.

Lynch HT, Watson P, Bewtra C. Hereditary ovarian cancer. Heterogeneity in age at diagnosis. *Cancer* 1991;67: 1460–1466.

Malfetano JH. Splenectomy for optimal cytoreduction in ovarian cancer. *Gynecol Oncol* 1986;24:392–394.

Malkasian GD, Knapp RC, Zurawaski VR, et al. Preoperative evaluation of serum Ca-125 levels in premenopausal and postmenopausal patients with pelvic masses. Discrimination from malignant disease. *Am J Obstet Gynecol* 1988;159: 341–346.

Malone JM, Koonce T, Larson DM, et al. Palliation of small bowel obstruction by percutaneous gastrostomy in patients with progressive ovarian carcinoma. *Obstet Gynecol* 1986;68:431–433.

Mann W, Patsner B, Cohen H, et al. Preoperative serum Ca-125 levels in patients with surgical Stage I invasive ovarian adenocarcinoma. *J Natl Cancer Inst* 1988;80:208–209.

Marina NM, Cushing B, Giller R, et al. Complete surgical excision is effective treatment for children with immature teratomas with or without malignant elements: a Pediatric Oncology Group/Children's Cancer Group intergroup study. *J Clin Oncol* 1999;17:2137–2143.

Markman M, Bundy B, Benda J, et al. Randomized phase III study of intravenous cis-platinum/paclitaxel versus moderately high dose carboplatin followed by intravenous paclitaxel and intraperitoneal cisplatin in optimal residual ovarian cancer: an intergroup trial (GOG, SWOG, ECOG). *Proc Am Soc Clin Oncol* 1998;17:A1392.

McGowan L, Lesher LP, Norris HJ, et al. Misstaging of ovarian cancer. *Obstet Gynecol* 1985;65:568–572.

McGuire WP, Hoskins WJ, Brady MF, et al. Cyclophosphamide and cis-platinum compared with paclitaxel and cisplatin in patients with stage III and stage IV ovarian cancer. *N Engl J Med* 1996;334:1–6.

McMahill HL, Calle EE, Koskinski AS, et al. Tubal ligation and fatal ovarian cancer in a large prospective cohort study. *Am J Epidemiol* 1997;145:349–357.

Miki Y, Swensen J, Shattuck-Eidens D, et al. A strong candidate for the breast ovarian cancer susceptibility gene BRCA1. *Science* 1994;266:66–71.

Miller D, Ballon S, Teng N, et al. A critical reassessment of second-look laparotomy in epithelial ovarian carcinoma. *Cancer* 1986;57:530–535.

Monga M, Carmichael JA, Shelley WE, et al. Surgery without adjuvant chemotherapy for early epithelial ovarian carcinoma after comprehensive surgical staging. *Gynecol Oncol* 1992;43:195–197.

Montz FJ, Schlaerth JB, Berek JS. Resection of diaphragmatic peritoneum and muscle: role in cytoreductive surgery for ovarian cancer. *Gynecol Oncol* 1989;35:338–340.

Morris M, Gershenson DM, Burke TW, et al. Splenectomy in gynecologic oncology: indications, complications, and technique. *Gynecol Oncol* 1991;43:118–122.

Morris M, Gershenson DM, Wharton JT. Secondary cytoreductive surgery in epithelial ovarian cancer: nonresponders to first-line therapy. *Gynecol Oncol* 1989;33:1–5.

Morris M, Gershenson DM, Wharton JT, et al. Secondary cytoreductive surgery for recurrent epithelial ovarian cancer. *Gynecol Oncol* 1989;34:334–338.

Morrow CP. An opinion in support of second-look surgery in ovarian cancer. (editorial) *Gynecol Oncol* 2000;79:341–343.

Muggia FM, Braly PS, Brady MF, et al. Phase III randomized study of cis-platinum versus paclitaxel versus cis-platinum and paclitaxel in patients with suboptimal stage III or IV ovarian cancer: a Gynecologic Oncology Group study. *J Clin Oncol* 2000;18:106–115.

Muir C, Waterhouse J, Mack T, et al. *Cancer incidence in five continents IARC.* Lyon, France: IARC Scientific Publication No. 88, 1987:892–893.

Munkarah AR, Hallum AV, Morris M, et al. Prognostic significance of residual disease in patients with stage IV epithelial ovarian cancer. *Gynecol Oncol* 1997;64:13–17.

Muñoz KA, Harlan LC, Trimble EL. Patterns of care for women with ovarian cancer in the United States. *J Clin Oncol* 1997;15:3408–3415.

Neijt JP, Huinink WW, van der Burg MEL, et al. Randomized trial comparing two combination chemotherapy regimens (CHAP-5 V CP) in advanced ovarian carcinoma. *J Clin Oncol* 1987;5:1157–1168.

Nelson BE, Rosenfeld AT, Schwartz PE. Preoperative abdominopelvic computed tomographic prediction of optimal cytoreduction in epithelial ovarian carcinoma. *J Clin Oncol* 1993;11:166–172.

Niloff JM, Bast RC, Schaetzl EM, et al. Predictive value of CA-125 antigen levels in second-look procedures for ovarian cancer. *Am J Obstet Gynecol* 1985;151:981–986.

Onda T, Yoshikawa H, Yokota II, et al. Assessment of metastases to aortic and pelvic lymph nodes in epithelial ovarian carcinoma. *Cancer* 1996;78:803–808.

Ozols R, Fisher R, Anderson T, et al. Peritoneoscopy in the management of ovarian cancer. *Am J Obstet Gynecol* 1981;140:611–618.

Ozols RF, Bundy BN, Fowler J, et al. Randomized phase III study of cis-platinum/paclitaxel versus carboplatin/paclitaxel in ovarian cancer: a Gynecologic Oncology Group trial. *Proc Am Soc Clin Oncol* 1999;18:A1373.

Parazzini F, Negri E, LaVecchia C, et al. Family history of reproductive cancers and ovarian cancer risk. An Italian case-control study. *Am J Epidemiol* 1992;135:35–40.

Partridge EE, Gunter B, Gelder M, et al. The validity and significance of substages in advanced ovarian carcinoma. *Gynecol Oncol* 1993;48:236–241.

Patsner B, Orr J, Mann W, et al. Does serum CA-125 level prior to second-look laparotomy for invasive ovarian adenocarcinoma predict size of residual disease? *Gynecol Oncol* 1990;37:319–322.

Pavlik EJ, DePriest PD, Gallion HH, et al. Ovarian volume related to age. *Gynecol Oncol* 2000;77:410–412.

Piccart MJ, Bertelsen K, James K, et al. Randomized intergroup trial of cis-platinum-paclitaxel versus cis-platinum-cyclophosphamide in women with advanced epithelial ovarian cancer: three-year results. *J Natl Cancer Inst* 2000;92:699–708.

Piver MS, Baker T. The potential for optimal (≤2 cm) cytoreductive surgery in advanced ovarian carcinoma at a tertiary medical center: a prospective study. *Gynecol Oncol* 1986;24:1–8.

Piver MS, Barlow JJ, Lele SB. Incidence of subclinical metastasis in stage I and II ovarian carcinoma. *Obstet Gynecol* 1978;52:100–104.

Piver MS, Malfetano J, Baker TR, et al. Adjuvant cis-platinum-based chemotherapy for stage I ovarian adenocarcinoma: a preliminary report. *Gynecol Oncol* 1989;35:69–72.

Plentl AA, Friedman EA. Lymphatics of the ovary. In: *Lymphatic system of the female genitalia.* Philadelphia, London, Toronto: Sanders, 1971:173–195.

Podczaski E, Stevens C, Manetta A, et al. Use of second-look laparotomy in the management of patients with ovarian epithelial malignancies. *Gynecol Oncol* 1987;28:205–214.

Podratz K, Malkasian G, Hilton J, et al. Second-look laparotomy in ovarian cancer: evaluation of pathologic variables. *Am J Obstet Gynecol* 1985;152:230–238.

Podratz K, Malkasian G, Wieand H, et al. Recurrent disease after negative second-look laparotomy in stages III and IV ovarian carcinoma. *Gynecol Oncol* 1988;29:274–282.

Podratz KC, Schwarz MF, Wieand HS, et al. Evaluation of treatment and survival after positive second-look laparotomy. *Gynecol Oncol* 1988;31:9–21.

Prorok PC. Evaluation of screening programs for the early detection of cancer. *Natl Cancer Inst Statistical Textbook Monogr* 1984;51:267–328.

Puls LE, Powell DE, DePriest PD, et al. Transition from benign to malignant epithelium in mucinous and serous ovarian cystadenocarcinoma. *Gynecol Oncol* 1992;47:53–57.

Raju KS, McKinna JA, Barker GH, et al. Second-look operations in the planned management of advanced ovarian carcinoma. *Am J Obstet Gynecol* 1982;144:650–654.

Reuter K, Griffin T, Hunter R. Comparison of abdominopelvic computed tomography results and findings at second-look laparotomy in ovarian carcinoma patients. *Cancer* 1989;63:1123–1128.

Risch HA, Marrett LD, Howe GR. Parity, contraception, infertility, and the risk of epithelial ovarian cancer. *Am J Epidemiol* 1994;146:585–597.

Risch HA. Hormonal etiology of epithelial ovarian cancer, with a hypothesis concerning the role of androgens and progesterone. *J Natl Cancer Inst* 1998;90:1774–1785.

Roberts W, Hodel K, Rich W, et al. Second-look laparotomy in the management of gynecologic malignancy. *Gynecol Oncol* 1982;13:345–355.

Roman LD, Muderspac LI, Stein SM, et al. Pelvic examination, tumor marker level and gray-scale and Doppler sonography in the prediction of pelvic cancer. *Obstet Gynecol* 1997;89:493–500.

Rossing MA, Daling JR, Weiss NS, et al. Ovarian tumors in a cohort of infertile women. *N Engl J Med* 1994;331:771–776.

Rubin S, Hoskins W, Hakes T, et al. Recurrence after negative second-look laparotomy for ovarian cancer: analysis of risk factors. *Am J Obstet Gynecol* 1988;159:1094–1098.

Rubin S, Hoskins W, Saigo P. Update on prognostic factors for recurrence following negative second-look laparotomy in ovarian cancer patients treated with platinum-based chemotherapy. *Gynecol Oncol* 1991;42:137–141.

Rubin SC, Hoskins WJ, Benjamin I, et al. Palliative surgery for intestinal obstruction in advanced ovarian cancer. *Gynecol Oncol* 1989;34:16–19.

Rubin SC, Wong GYC, Curtin JP, et al. Platinum-based chemotherapy of high-risk stage I epithelial ovarian cancer following comprehensive surgical staging. *Obstet Gynecol* 1993;82:143–147.

Russell P. The pathological assessment of ovarian neoplasms. I. Introduction to the common "epithelial" tumors and analysis of benign "epithelial" tumors. *Pathology* 1979;11:5–26.

Russell P, Merkur H. Proliferating ovarian "epithelial" tumours: a clinico-pathological analysis of 144 cases. *Aust NZ J Obstet Gynaecol* 1979;19:45–51.

Sakai K, Kamura T, Hirakawa T, et al. Relationship between pelvic lymph node involvement and other disease sites in patients with ovarian cancer. *Gynecol Oncol* 1997;65: 164–168.

Sassone M, Timor-Tritsch I, Artner A, et al. Transvaginal sonographic characterization of ovarian disease: evaluation of a new scoring system to predict ovarian malignancy. *Obstet Gynecol* 1991;78:70–76.

Scarabelli C, Campagnutta E, Perin A, et al. La splenectomia enl trattameno chirurgico radicale del carcinoma ovarico. *Minerva Ginecol* 1985;37:37–41.

Scarabelli C, Gallo A, Zarrelli A, et al. Systematic pelvic and paraaortic lymphadenectomy during cytoreductive surgery n advanced ovarian cancer: potential benefit on survival. *Gynecol Oncol* 1995;56:328–337.

Schildkraut JM, Thompson WD. Familial ovarian cancer: a population-based case control study. *Am J Epidemiol* 1988;128:456–466.

Schneider VL, Schneider A, Reed KL, et al. Comparison of Doppler with two dimensional sonography and Ca-125 for prediction of malignancy of pelvic masses. *Obstet Gynecol* 1993;81:983–988.

Schwartz PE, Chambers JT, Makuch R. Neoadjuvant chemotherapy for advanced ovarian cancer. *Gynecol Oncol* 1994;53:33–37.

Schwartz P, Smith J. Second-look operations in ovarian cancer. *Am J Obstet Gynecol* 1980;138:1124–1130.

Schwartz PE, Rutherford TJ, Chambers JT, et al. Neoadjuvant chemotherapy for advanced ovarian cancer: long-term survival. *Gynecol Oncol* 1999;72:93–99.

Scully RE, Henson DE, Nielsen ML, et al. Ovary. Reporting on cancer specimens: protocols and case summaries. In: *Cancer protocol manual*. CAP Cancer Committee, 1998:1–25.

SEER Cancer Statistics Review, 1973–1997. Bethesda, MD: National Cancer Institute, 1997.

Scully RE, Hensen DE, Nielson ML, et al. Practice protocol for the examination of specimens removed from patients with ovarian tumors. *Arch Pathol Lab Med* 1995;199: 1012–1022.

Segna RA, Dottino PR, Mandeli JP, et al. Secondary cytoreduction for ovarian cancer following cis-platinum therapy. *J Clin Oncol* 1993;11:434–439.

Sevelda P, Dittrich C, Salzer H. Prognostic value of the rupture of the capsule in stage I epithelial ovarian carcinoma. *Gynecol Oncol* 1989;35:321–322.

Skates SJ, Feng J, Yin-Hua Y, et al. Toward an optimal algorithm for ovarian cancer screening with longitudinal tumor markers. *Cancer* 1995;76:2004–2010.

Skipper HE. Stepwise progress in the treatment of disseminated cancer. *Cancer* 1983;5:1773–1776.

Slamon DJ, Godolphin W, Jones LA, et al. Studies of the HER-2/neu proto-oncogene in human breast and ovarian cancer. *Science* 1989;244:707–712.

Smirz L, Stehman F, Ulbright T, et al. Second-look laparotomy after chemotherapy in the management of ovarian malignancy. *Am J Obstet Gynecol* 1985;152:661–668.

Smith SA, Easton DF, Evans DG, et al. Allele losses in region 17 q12-21 in familial breast and ovarian cancer involving the wild-type chromosome. *Nat Genet* 1992;2: 128–131.

Smith W, Day T, Smith J. The use of laparoscopy to determine the results of chemotherapy for ovarian cancer. *J Reprod Med* 1977;18:257–260.

Sonnendecker EW. Is routine second-look laparotomy for ovarian cancer justified? *Gynecol Oncol* 1988;31:249–255.

Sonnendecker EW, Guidozzi F, Margolius KA. Splenectomy during primary maximal cytoreductive surgery for epithelial ovarian cancer. *Gynecol Oncol* 1989;35:301–306.

Soper JT, Couchman G, Berchuck A, et al. The role of partial sigmoid colectomy for debulking epithelial ovarian carcinoma. *Gynecol Oncol* 1991;41:239–244.

Stehman F, Calkins A, Wass J, et al. A comparison of findings at second-look laparotomy with preoperative computed tomography in patients with ovarian cancer. *Gynecol Oncol* 1988;29:37–42.

Stein S, Laifer-Narin S, Johnson MB, et al. Differentiation of benign and malignant adnexal masses: relative value of gray scale, color Doppler and spectral Doppler sonography. *Am J Radiol* 1995;164:381–386.

Stern J, Buscema J, Rosenshein N, et al. Can computed tomography substitute for second-look operation in ovarian carcinoma? *Gynecol Oncol* 1981;11:82–88.

Stuart GC, Jeffries M, Stuart JL, et al. The changing role of "second-look" laparotomy in the management of epithelial carcinoma of the ovary. *Am J Obstet Gynecol* 1982;142: 612–616.

Surwit E, Childers J, Atlas I, et al. Neoadjuvant chemotherapy for advanced ovarian cancer. *Int J Gynecol Cancer* 1996;6:356–361.

Taylor JWK, Ramas I, Carter D, et al. Correlation of Doppler US tumor signals with neovascular morphologic features. *Radiology* 1988;166:157–162.

Tazelaar HD, Bostwick DG, Ballon SC, et al. Conservative treatment of borderline ovarian tumors. *Obstet Gynecol* 1985;66:417–422.

Tortolero-Luna G, Mitchell MF. The epidemiology of ovarian cancer. *J Cell Biochem Suppl* 1995;13:200–207.

Trimbos JB, Schueler JA, van Lent M, et al. Reasons for incomplete surgical staging in early ovarian carcinoma. *Gynecol Oncol* 1990;37:374–377.

Vacarello L, Rubin SC, Vlamis V, et al. Cytoreductive surgery in ovarian carcinoma patients with a documented previously complete surgical response. *Gynecol Oncol* 1995; 57:61–65.

Valentin L, Sladkevicius P, Marsal, K. Limited contribution of Doppler velocimetry to the differential diagnosis of extrauterine pelvic tumors. *Obstet Gynecol* 1994;83:425–433.

Van der Burg MEL, van Lent M, Buyse M, et al. The effect of debulking surgery after induction chemotherapy. On the prognosis in advanced epithelial ovarian cancer. *N Engl J Med* 1995;332:629–634.

van Nagell, JR, Higgins RV, Donaldson ES, et al. Transvaginal sonography as a screening method for ovarian cancer: a report of the first 1000 cases screened. *Cancer* 1990;65:573–577.

van Nagell JR, DePriest PD, Reedy MB, et al. The efficacy of transvaginal sonographic screening in asymptomatic women at risk for ovarian cancer. *Gynecol Oncol* 2000;77: 350–356.

Vasilev SA, Schlaerth JB, Canpean J, et al. Serum Ca-125 levels in preoperative evaluation of ovarian masses. *Obstet Gynecol* 1988;71:751–756.

Vergote IB, Kaern J, Abeler VM, et al. Analysis of prognostic factors in stage I epithelial ovarian cancer: importance of degree of differentiation and deoxyribonucleic acid ploidy in predicting relapse. *Am J Obstet Gynecol* 1993;169: 40–52.

Vergote IB, Vergote-De Vos LN, Abeler VM, et al. Randomized trial comparing cis-platinum with radioactive phosphorus or whole-abdomen irradiation as adjuvant treatment of ovarian cancer. *Cancer* 1992;69:741–749.

Wangensteen OH, Lewis FJ, Tongen LA. The "second-look" in cancer surgery. *Lancet* 1951;71:303–307.

Webb M, Snyder J, Williams T, et al. Second-look laparotomy in ovarian cancer. *Gynecol Oncol* 1982;14:285–293.

Weiner Z, Thaler I, Beck D, et al. Differentiating malignant from benign ovarian tumors with transvaginal color flow imaging. *Obstet Gynecol* 1992;79:159–162.

Whittemore AS, Gong G, Itnyre J. Prevalence and contribution of BRCA1 mutations in breast cancer and ovarian cancer: results from three U.S. population-based case-control studies of ovarian cancer. *Am J Hum Genet* 1997;60: 496–504.

Whittemore AS, Harris R, Itnyre J. Collaborative Ovarian Cancer Group: characteristics relating to ovarian cancer risk, collaborative analysis of 12 U.S. case-control studies. II. Invasive epithelial ovarian cancers in white women. *Am J Epidemiol* 1992;136:1184–1203.

Williams S, Blessing JA, Liao S, et al. Adjuvant therapy of ovarian germ cell tumors with cisplatin, etoposide, and bleomycin: a trial of the Gynecologic Oncology Group. *J Clin Oncol* 1994;12:701–706.

Williams SD, Blessing JA, DiSaia PJ, et al. Second-look laparotomy in ovarian germ cell tumors: the Gyneoclogic Oncology Group experience. *Gynecol Oncol* 1994;52:287–291.

Wiltshaw E, Raju KS, Dawson I. The role of cytoreductive surgery in advanced carcinoma of the ovary: an analysis of primary and second surgery. *Br J Obstet Gynecol* 1985;92: 522–527.

Woods CII, Thompson EA. Transvaginal sonography as a screening method for ovarian cancer: a report of the first 1000 cases screened. *Cancer* 1990;65:573–577.

Wooster R, Bignell G, Lancaster J, et al. Identification of the breast cancer susceptibility gene BRCA2. *Nature* 1995;378:789–791.

World Health Organization histological classification of ovarian tumors. In: Scully RE, Young RH, Clement PB, eds. *Atlas of tumor pathology, tumors of the ovary, maldeveloped gonads, fallopian tube and broad ligament.* Bethesda, MD: AFIP, 199828–31.

Wu P-C, Qu J-Y, Lang J-H, et al. Lymph node metastasis of ovarian cancer: a preliminary survey of 74 cases of lymphadenectomy. *Am J Obstet Gynecol* 1986;155:1103–1108.

Young RC, Brady MF, Nieberg RM, et al. Randomized clinical trial of adjuvant treatment of women with early (FIGO I-IIA high risk) ovarian cancer. *Proc Am Soc Clin Oncol* 1999;18:357a(abstr).

Young RC, Decker DG, Wharton JT, et al. Staging laparotomy in early ovarian cancer. *JAMA* 1983;250:3072–3076.

Young RC, Walton LA, Ellenberg SS, et al. Adjuvant therapy in stage I and II epithelial ovarian cancer. Results of two prospective randomized trials. *N Engl J Med* 1990;322: 1021–1027.

Young RC. A second look at second-look laparotomy (editorial) *J Clin Oncol* 1987;5:1311–1313.

Te Linde's Operative Gynecology, ninth edition, edited by John A. Rock and Howard W. Jones, III. Lippincott Williams & Wilkins, Philadelphia: © 2003.

CHAPTER

49

▼

Pelvic Exenteration

THOMAS W. BURKE   GEORGE W. MORLEY

It has been more than 50 years since Brunschwig introduced surgical evisceration as an option to control cancers within the pelvic organs. Initially, significant morbidity and mortality rates ranging from 50% to 70% were encountered. These rates have decreased dramatically, allowing the survival rate for those treated to increase substantially. The results of ultraradical pelvic surgery have been enhanced by a number of advances.

Improved surgical techniques and training have decreased operative time and blood loss and limited the extent of disfigurement. Perioperative morbidity has been reduced through the control of infection and the use of blood component therapy, improved anesthetic techniques, parenteral nutrition, and intensive care facilities managed by expert medical teams. Although pelvic exenteration is a formidable procedure, the 5-year survival rate is greater than 50% for appropriately targeted women (Table 49.1). Exenteration has become the treatment of choice for certain types of advanced or recurrent tumors of the pelvis, and it provides another chance at survival for women in whom primary therapy has failed.

Careful patient selection using a thorough and detailed approach to preoperative assessment is essential. Strict guidelines regarding the indications and contraindications for operability must be met. The adaptive ability of patients who survive is dramatic given the magnitude of anatomic and physiologic change associated with exenteration. However, those who die of their disease despite this heroic surgical effort commonly experience intractable pain from intestinal obstruction or distant metastases.

Many modifications of the Brunschwig procedure have been instituted since its introduction in 1948. The most significant modification was introduced in 1950 when Bricker developed and reported his classic ileal conduit technique. This technique provided an isolated conduit for urinary diversion, which became a replacement option for the traditional "wet colostomies" or ureterosigmoidostomy. The separation of urinary and fecal streams represented a huge advance in terms of reducing complication rates from infection. Despite the requirement for two stomas, this technique also achieved greater patient acceptance. Other more recent advances, such as continent urinary diversion, the use of automatic stapling devices for the gastrointestinal portion of the procedure, pelvic floor coverage, vaginal reconstruction, and low rectal anastomosis, also have improved the overall results and rehabilitation of these patients.

Total pelvic exenteration encompasses removal of the genital organs (vagina, uterus, fallopian tubes, and ovaries) as well as the bladder and rectum. An isolated segment of bowel is used to construct a replacement urinary reservoir. A segment of small or large bowel or a combination of both may be considered. Modifications of the pelvic exenterative procedure include either an anterior or posterior exenteration or a total exenteration with a low rectal reanastomosis. Patients whose cancer is confined to the anterior pelvic structures are candidates for anterior exenteration, which removes the bladder and

TABLE 49.1.
Perioperative Mortality and 5-Year
Survival After Pelvic Exenteration

Report	No. Patients	Operative Mortality (%)	5-Year Survival (%)
Parsons and Friedell (1964)	112	14	21
Brunschwig (1965)	535	16	20
Rutledge and Burns (1965)	108	17	29
Kiselow et al. (1968)	207	8	35
Symmonds et al. (1968)	118	12	26
Ketcham et al. (1970)	162	7	38
Brunschwig (1970)	225	8	19
Symmonds et al. (1975)	198	8	33
Rutledge et al. (1977)	296	13	48
Averrette et al. (1984)	92	24	37
Morley et al. (1989)	100	2	61
Shingleton et al. (1989)	143	6	50

genital organs while leaving the gastrointestinal system intact. In this situation, a urinary conduit is developed from an isolated segment of bowel into which the ureters are anastomosed. For tumors limited to posterior structures, posterior exenteration can be used to remove the genital organs and rectum, allowing preservation of the urinary system. In selected patients who undergo a total pelvic exenteration, a low rectal anastomosis can be accomplished if the lower 6 to 10 cm of rectum is preserved. The end-to-end anastomosis (EEA) stapling device designed for this purpose is used to reconstruct the rectum low in the pelvis. Low anastomosis often requires a protective colostomy because the anastomosis has been constructed in an irradiated field. The colostomy can be reversed at a later date, eliminating one of the patient's stomas.

INDICATIONS AND CONTRAINDICATIONS

The decision-making process begins when the physician first sees the patient and takes her history. An initial diagnostic evaluation is obtained. If the patient appears to be a candidate for a pelvic exenterative procedure, she is referred to a gynecologic oncologist who is experienced in the evaluation and treatment of such patients. The best outcomes are achieved in patients who have recurrent squamous cell carcinoma of the cervix or vagina. Exenteration may be appropriate for some women with advanced vulvar cancer when more conventional therapy has failed. In rare cases, patients with large vulvar carcinomas may require pelvic exenteration as primary treatment because of geographic spread of the disease to involve adjacent organs. Infrequently, a recurrent adenocarcinoma of the cervix or endometrium or a sarcoma in

the pelvis may be isolated to the central pelvis and resectable by exenteration. Women with recurrent ovarian carcinomas are rarely candidates for exenterative resection because isolated pelvic recurrence is so unusual.

The primary indication for pelvic exenteration is recurrent or persistent squamous cell carcinoma of the cervix. This indication is most common because of the frequency of cervical cancer and because squamous cell lesions tend to spread by continuity and contiguity along tissue planes, often staying localized for long periods of time before metastasizing to more remote areas. The adjacent tissues, such as the bladder, urethra, and bowel, often are involved. Even when final pathologic examination shows no direct invasion of these adjacent organs, often it is not possible to obtain a satisfactory tumor-free margin in these previously irradiated, healing-impaired tissues without their removal. Control of the carcinoma cannot be achieved without their removal.

Total pelvic exenteration is the most common type of exenteration performed in most reported series. The more extensive resection ensures that an adequate margin beyond palpable disease is obtained. A philosophy of ensuring the widest margin of resection at the earliest possible moment must prevail if the disease is to be eradicated successfully. The less extensive forms of radical pelvic surgery, such as radical hysterectomy, produce a higher incidence of treatment failure and an unacceptably high incidence of urinary or bowel fistulization because the pelvic tissues in the operative field have already been compromised by radiotherapy. Although some patient's disease can be curatively resected by radical hysterectomy or anterior or posterior exenteration, these approaches should be limited to patients with very small and well-defined recurrences.

Prior to the introduction of current diagnostic techniques, clinical evaluation of the patient and intravenous pyelography were the only methods available to assess whether the disease could be resected by exenteration. The so-called "triad of trouble" used in this assessment consisted of: (a) an abnormal intravenous pyelogram demonstrating ureteral obstruction; (b) sciatic nerve distribution of pain suggesting neural sheath involvement at or near the lateral pelvic wall; and (c) lower-extremity edema, implying venous or lymphatic compromise of the iliac vessels. If none or one of these features were present, exploration to determine resectability was recommended. If two or more of these abnormalities were present, the patient's disease was considered unresectable. If there is any doubt whether the lesion can be resected, the patient should undergo exploratory surgery, since pelvic wall involvement is difficult to delineate clinically.

Several diagnostic techniques can aid in assessing resectability in a patient who is believed to have central pelvic disease on clinical grounds. Evaluation of resectability is important from both a technical and psychological standpoint. A preoperative study that demonstrates the presence of nonresectable disease helps to avoid not only the morbidity of exploratory laparotomy, but also its attendant false hope for cure. There is a tremendous negative psychological impact on the patient when she is prepared preoperatively for the exenterative procedure only to be told postoperatively that she had an inoperable lesion.

Computed tomography (CT) or magnetic resonance imaging (MRI) can be most beneficial in assessing the presence of lateral pelvic wall invasion and unsuspected liver metastases as well as in further evaluation of the retroperitoneal lymph nodes. MRI is especially useful in locating tumor invasion at the pelvic wall.

Transvaginal Tru-Cut needle biopsy can be used to evaluate a palpable pelvic mass at the lateral pelvic wall. These biopsies can differentiate between recurrent neoplasm and postirradiation fibrosis when thickened tissue is encountered throughout the pelvis. Fine-needle aspiration (FNA) of suggestive regional lymph nodes can be helpful in confirming unresectable metastases. McDonald and coworkers reported that FNA had an 85% accuracy rate in identifying positive nodes. Because the 5-year survival rate drops to 0% to 14% when the pelvic lymph nodes are positive, pelvic exenteration is unrewarding, and exploratory surgery is not recommended (Table 49.2). It must be remembered that a negative biopsy does not guarantee that cancer is not present, but merely that no cancer was identified at the focal point of the needle tip.

The final diagnostic decision concerning the operability of disease is made when the patient is examined under anesthesia and as the exploratory laparotomy is performed. Fixation of the tumor in the pelvis caused by recurrent disease extending to the pelvic side wall, penetration of the tumor into the peritoneal cavity with dissemination of cells intraabdominally, and extrapelvic involvement of regional lymph nodes, omentum, liver, and other structures are all contraindications to the performance of pelvic exenteration with curative intent. These areas must be completely assessed by thorough palpation, visualization, and multiple frozen section biopsies, when indicated. Transection of the ureters and bowel commit the surgeon and the patient to exenteration. The use of the avascular paravesical and pararectal spaces can be helpful in evaluating the extent of the disease under these circumstances. Incomplete resection with positive margins or metastatic disease is not curative and subjects the patient to an extended and difficult postoperative recovery without much hope of long-term survival.

Pelvic exenteration is an appropriate therapeutic option for relatively few women with recurrent cancer. About one third of recurrences appear to be central pelvic failure by clinical examination. Of these, one half are excluded from surgical therapy when diagnostic studies reveal unresectable disease. About one half of women who undergo exploration for exenteration are found to have inoperable disease and the procedure is aborted. Of those who undergo resection by exenteration, about one half obtain long-term survival and apparent cure.

Pelvic exenteration is not considered a treatment of choice for primary disease except in a limited number of patients with carcinoma of the vulva and in selected patients with nongynecologic lesions that involve the bladder, urethra, or colon. In the past, stage IVA carcinoma of the cervix involving the bladder or rectum was treated in this manner; however, the results were not considered superior to those achieved by full-course pelvic radiotherapy. Therefore, exenteration has been abandoned universally as primary therapy for this lesion since Rutledge and Burns treated stage IV lesions with radiation therapy and showed an acceptable 28% survival rate. The same concept exists in regard to primary carcinoma of the vagina, for which radiation therapy is the preferred initial treatment. Current chemoradiation protocols with or without conservative surgery appear to provide results equivalent or superior to those obtained with exenteration for advanced tumors of the cervix, vulva, and vagina. Consequently, primary exenteration has become a rare operation.

Disease-free interval—the time from primary diagnosis to recurrence—is highly predictive of survival following exenteration. In all series, there is a direct relation between time from primary treatment to time of recurrence and survival: 5-year survival rate of greater than 90% has been reported when the disease-free interval was greater than 10 years, compared with a survival rate less than 50% when this interval was 1 year or less.

Pelvic exenteration occasionally may be indicated to manage severely damaged irradiated tissue in the pelvis. Many patients with radiation necrosis experience in-

TABLE 49.2.
Effect of Pelvic Lymph Node Metastasis on Survival After Pelvic Exenteration

Report	Negative Nodes		Positive Nodes	
	No. Patients	5-Year Survival (%)	No. Patients	5-Year Survival (%)
Barber and Jones (1971)	166	17	97	5
Creasman and Rutledge (1974)	29	27	14	14
Symmonds et al. (1975)	139	39	59	13
Averette et al. (1984)	92	—	6	0
Morley et al. (1998)	87	70	13	0
Shingleton et al. (1989)	106	—	10	10

TABLE 49.3.
Pelvic Exenteration Outcomes in Women with Vulvar or Endometrial Cancer

	Site	No. of Patients	Morbidity (%)	5-Year Survival (%)
Hopkins and Morley (1992)	Vulva	19	53	60
Miller et al. (1995)	Vulva	21	57	52
Morris et al. (1996)	Endometrium	20	60	45
Barakat et al. (1999)	Endometrium	44	80	20

tractable pain, copious amounts of foul-smelling discharge, and both urinary and rectal fistulas from tissue necrosis. In many cases, symptoms can be relieved with urinary and/or bowel diversion procedures alone. Palliative exenteration should be considered only in extreme cases in which more conservative approaches have failed.

Similarly, pelvic exenteration should not be used as a palliative treatment for cancer. The morbidity, mortality, and complication rates are too high to justify this approach, especially when other palliative alternatives are available. The long-term hospitalization and protracted recovery after this procedure prevent the patient from spending more of her remaining time at home and usually exchange one set of troublesome symptoms for another.

Traditionally, the presence of recurrent or persistent adenocarcinoma of the female pelvic organs was a relative contraindication to pelvic exenterative therapy. These glandular lesions are more likely to disseminate through the hematologic or lymphatic routes and bypass the traditional, more orderly mode of spread seen with squamous tumors. However, small recent series suggest that exenteration can provide curative therapy for 30% to 50% of women with isolated central recurrence of adenocarcinoma of the endocervix and endometrium (see Table 49.3). A diligent search for unresectable metastases must be performed before and during the operation. High tumor grade and short disease-free interval are correlated with decreasing chance of survival. Locally advanced or recurrent pelvic sarcoma, although rare, occasionally may be managed by pelvic exenteration.

Age, religious orientation, obesity, and medical and psychological alterations must be evaluated as potential contraindications to exenteration. Although life expectancy beyond 70 years for women who undergo this procedure steadily diminishes, this factor alone is not an absolute deterrent to this procedure. A number of patients older than 70 years have been treated successfully with return to fully functional status. Religious orientation is seldom a contraindication; however, the high likelihood of blood replacement requires that the patient be willing to accept transfusion of blood and blood products.

Obesity is a relative contraindication to surgery. Most patients with recurrent cancer of the cervix have a protracted disease course and are rarely overweight. Obese patients present technical problems that further complicate an already difficult procedure, and they must be evaluated individually. Stomal construction can be difficult in these patients, operating time is prolonged,

infection rates are increased, and pulmonary function may be compromised during the postoperative period.

Medical condition and psychological state are important factors in deciding whether some patients should undergo operation. Surgical risks must be weighed against the benefit of the procedure. The patient's willingness to actively participate in her recovery and her ability to adapt psychologically are key components to the success of resection. In most settings where exenteration is offered, there is no favorable alternative therapy. The patient must clearly understand the implications of her decision to seek or refuse exenteration. Although small, the risk of perioperative mortality with this operation is definite. Complications of some type are seen in 30% to 50% of cases.

The preoperative medical and anesthetic assessments of the cardiopulmonary, renal, and nutritional status of the patient must be thorough. Consultants in these areas must be available during the perioperative period. All patients require close surveillance in a well-equipped and well-staffed intensive care unit postoperatively. Patients must also be psychologically prepared for the significant alterations in their excretory systems and their sexual function. These patients often benefit from counseling by an enterostomal therapist, psychologist, or psychiatrist prior to the operation. The consultant's aid in preparing the patient may be as important as the surgery itself. An informal discussion with another patient who has satisfactorily adjusted to the alterations of exenteration frequently is beneficial and should be considered.

The surgeon who undertakes pelvic exenterative therapy has responsibilities beyond the performance of surgery. The surgeon must consider the quality of life remaining for the patient after the operation, the long-term rehabilitation of the patient if the operation is successful, as well as the long-term terminal care of the patient if it is not.

EXENTERATION TECHNIQUE
Preoperative Preparation

The initial planning for pelvic exenteration begins in the outpatient office setting. A full discussion is undertaken with the patient before definitive surgery is planned. The complete operation, including the removal of the bladder, vagina, and rectum and the possible necessity of two ostomies is fully outlined. Occasional patients cannot psychologically adjust to the concept of the operation and elect to refuse further evaluation. Such decisions should be honored and ongoing supportive care of the patient should be offered. For the patient who can psychologically commit to the removal of her pelvic viscera, a further discussion is undertaken to assess her desire for vaginal reconstruction, creation of a continent urinary diversion, and, potentially, low rectal reanastomosis.

Patients are admitted the day before surgery for bowel preparation and intravenous hydration and to be marked by the stomal therapist for ostomy placement. Arterial blood gas analysis is obtained routinely. For patients whose oxygen saturation is adequate, pulmonary function testing is not routinely performed. A central venous catheter should be placed during anesthetic induction to provide appropriate vascular access. Preoperative total parenteral nutrition is not used routinely unless the patient has a nutritional deficit. Intravenous prophylactic antibiotics are given on call to the operating room, and the patient is shaved just before surgery. Either subcutaneous heparin or sequential compression devices (SCDs) may be used for prophylaxis against deep venous thrombosis.

The patient is positioned for surgery using Allen stirrups. This position allows simultaneous access to the abdominal and perineal areas for bimanual assessment of the lesion intraoperatively and to facilitate the "double team" approach to operating transabdominally and transvaginally simultaneously. A two-team approach should be considered in all cases to shorten anesthetic time, reduce blood loss, and minimize fatigue of the surgical team. Rotation of members of the operative team in and out of the operating room allows for rest and refreshment and minimizes the chance of fatigue-related operator errors during the critical reconstructive phase of the operation.

Intraoperative Exploration

The abdomen is opened using a vertical, midline incision. Although a transverse incision allows greater pelvic exposure and facilitates the lateral pelvic wall assessment, it limits the upper abdominal evaluation, aortic node dissection, and creation of continent urinary diversion (Fig. 49.1). On entry into the peritoneal cavity, the surgeon should carefully palpate all organs, surfaces, and lymph node areas. The liver is examined for evidence of metastatic disease. Cytologic washings and ascitic fluid, if present, can be recovered and sent for immediate cytologic analysis. Any areas that appear abnormal on the preoperative diagnostic studies are examined. Any questionable areas are biopsied and samples sent for frozen section analysis. Abnormal nodal findings are similarly analyzed, with a specific focus on the pelvic, high common iliac, and paraaortic lymph nodes.

Paraaortic lymph node dissection is performed by initially incising the peritoneum over the lower aorta (Fig. 49.2) or right common iliac vessels. The area is carefully

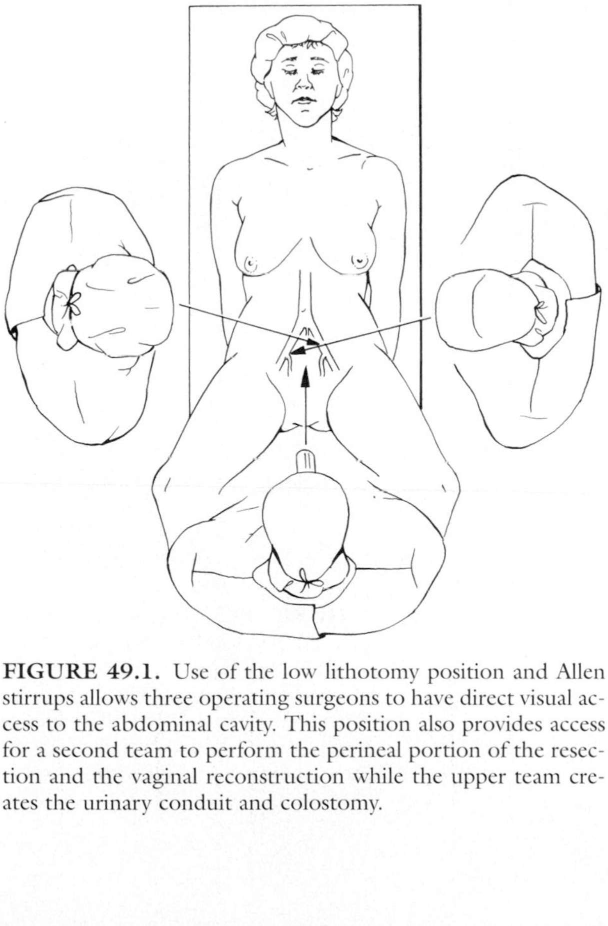

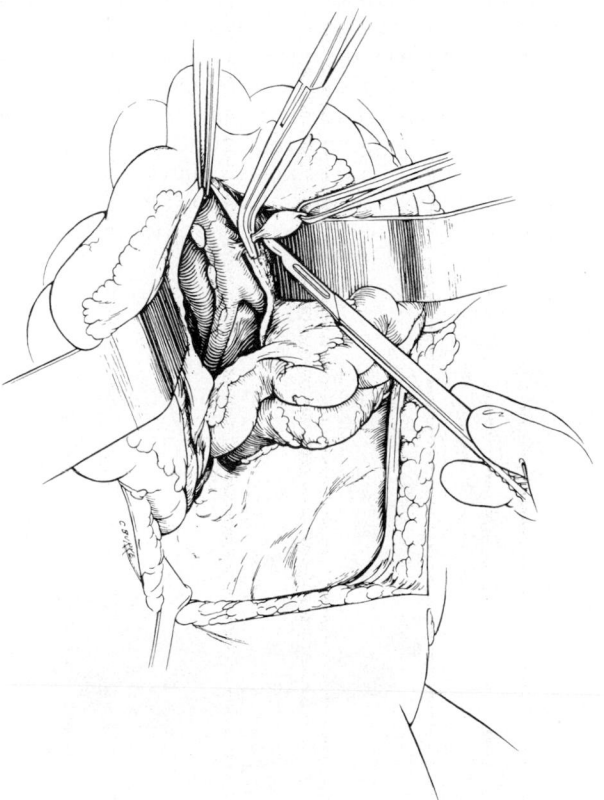

FIGURE 49.1. Use of the low lithotomy position and Allen stirrups allows three operating surgeons to have direct visual access to the abdominal cavity. This position also provides access for a second team to perform the perineal portion of the resection and the vaginal reconstruction while the upper team creates the urinary conduit and colostomy.

FIGURE 49.2. Lymph nodes are sampled by first incising the peritoneum overlying the aorta. Small vessels are ligated with hemoclips as the fat pad is elevated from the aorta fat pad over the inferior vena cava should then be isolated in a similar manner. Great care must be used over the inferior vena cava to avoid injury to this thin-walled great vessel. Complete mobilization of the aorta is not necessary.

evaluated by visual and tactile examination. The lymph node dissection is begun at or just below the bifurcation of the aorta and proceeds cephalad. The lymphatic tissue is carefully freed from the aorta; hemoclips are used to ligate the small perforating vessels. Using gentle upward traction and sharp dissection, the surgeon can isolate the nodes to about the level of the inferior mesenteric artery. The uppermost pedicle is tied or ligated with an appropriate hemoclip. A similar dissection is performed over the anterior wall of the inferior vena cava to obtain lymph nodes located on the right side of the aorta. Squamous cell carcinoma of the cervix spreads in a stepwise manner; thus, extensive paraaortic node dissection to the level of the renal artery is not necessary. If the lower paraaortic tissue is negative for metastatic disease, none is found at a higher level. The high common iliac and pelvic lymph nodes are dissected similarly and evaluated.

When this evaluation is completed and there are no contraindications to proceeding, the round ligaments are divided and the *pararectal and paravesical spaces* are opened. The paravesical space is developed by bluntly sweeping the bladder away from the pubic symphysis in the space of Retzius and continuing the dissection laterally, sweeping the bladder medially off the pelvic sidewall until the fibrovascular pedicles are encountered at the 4- and 8-o'clock positions. These fibrovascular pedicles, commonly referred to as "the web," contain the uterine artery and vein, the ureter, the base of the broad ligament extending from the upper vagina and cervix to the pelvic sidewall, and the superior hemorrhoidal vessels. One pelvic sidewall at a time should be evaluated. The round ligament is ligated and divided, and the peritoneum is incised over the iliopsoas muscle. This exposes the pararectal space, which is developed by bluntly freeing the medial leaf of the peritoneum with the attached

ureter from its areolar attachment to the pelvic sidewall structures. When the pararectal space is fully developed, the fibrovascular pedicle can be palpated between the operator's thumb and index finger, allowing for evaluation of the pelvic sidewall. Any nodular or suspicious area in this region is biopsied and frozen section is obtained (Fig. 49.3). At this early stage in the operation, the mass of neoplasm should be movable. Free spaces should be present between the neoplasm and the pelvic sidewalls in both the paravesical and pararectal spaces. If the tumor mass is not freely movable, lateral invasion is likely and a more extensive evaluation of resectability should be undertaken.

At this point in the operation, the patient has not been committed to an exenteration because neither the bowel nor the ureter has been transected. Once disease resectability has been confirmed and the decision to perform an exenteration is made, the specific type of procedure—total, posterior, or anterior—must be chosen. The extent of the disease, including its involvement of the bladder, bowel, or both, must be estimated. If preoperative studies have shown involvement of the bladder or rectum, these organs must be removed. The surgeon must consider the possibility of microscopic disease that cannot be palpated or seen without magnification. The selected procedure must encompass the entire neoplasm with a margin of uninvolved tissue. Contraindications to pelvic exenteration include intraabdominal metastases, malignant cells in ascitic fluid, metastatic disease to regional lymph nodes, breakthrough of the tumor through the peritoneal surfaces, and presence of malignant disease at or beyond a surgically resected margin. The decision is made to perform the exenteration when all frozen section reports are returned and are negative for metastatic disease.

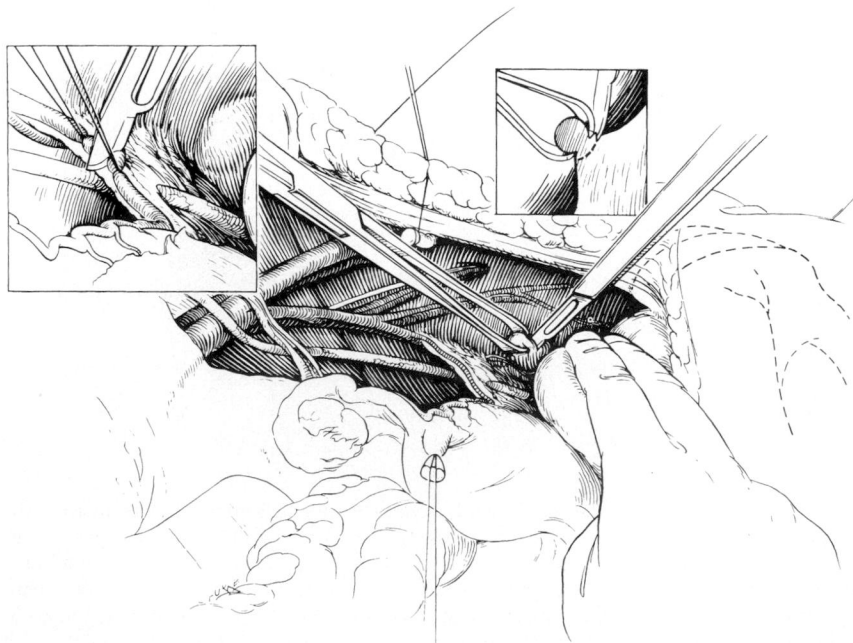

FIGURE 49.3. The pararectal and paravesical spaces have been developed. Thickened or suggestive areas of tumor extension to the sidewalls are sampled for frozen section analysis. The uterine artery is divided at its origin from the internal iliac and is tied with 2-0 silk.

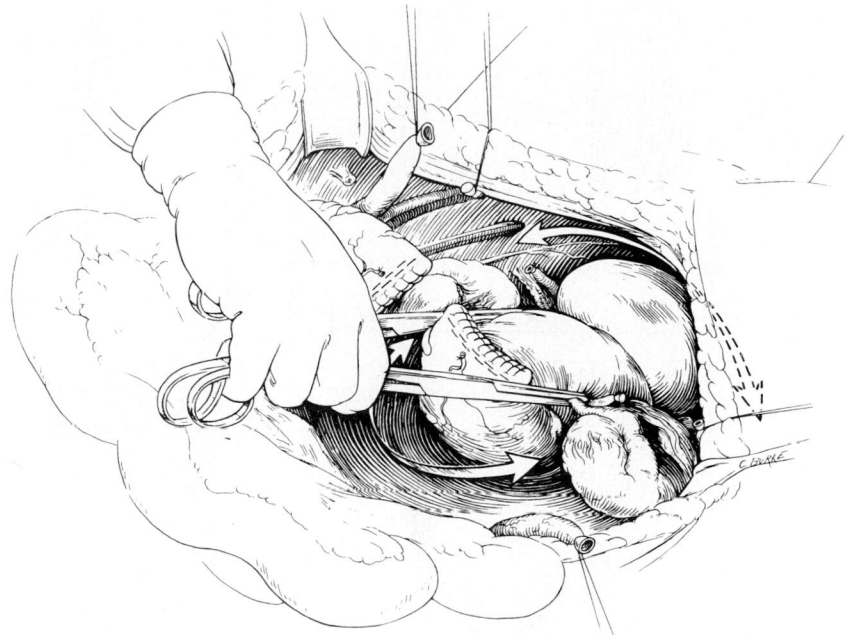

FIGURE 49.4. Ureters have been tied and divided. The colon has been isolated and divided with the gastrointestinal anastomotic stapler. The superior hemorrhoidal vessels have been clamped and divided previously. The colon is swept free by gentle blunt dissection from the sacrum. Similarly, the bladder is swept free from the symphysis pubis *(arrows)*.

Removal of Specimen

An en bloc dissection of the pelvic tissue is undertaken by clamping and dividing the web of tissue at the pelvic sidewalls. Large pedicle clamps are used to clamp the tissue and control the bleeding from this area. The tissue is divided and ligated with suture, using either suture ligatures or large hemostatic clips. We prefer to clamp, divide, and ligate the uterine artery at the top of the web lateral to the ureter separately, allowing the dissection to continue along the pelvic sidewall. The ureters are freed from the medial leaf of the peritoneum with sharp dissection, clipped with large hemoclips, and transected as distally as possible. The proximal ureters distend during the remainder of this part of the procedure, facilitating their later anastomosis into the urinary conduit.

The sigmoid colon is divided using the gastrointestinal anastomotic (GIA) stapler. Before this division, small epiploic vessels are divided and tied. A free space is developed in the bowel mesentery just beneath the bowel wall. This allows introduction of either a bowel clamp or the stapler. The peritoneum overlying the mesentery is incised, exposing the vessels to the sigmoid colon. These are cross-clamped and tied. Transillumination of the vascular arcade leading to the bowel allows for preservation of the major blood supply, which consists of the sigmoidal and superior hemorrhoidal arteries arising from the inferior mesenteric artery, the middle hemorrhoidal arteries coming bilaterally from the hypogastric vessels, and the inferior hemorrhoidal vessels from the pudendal arteries. The sigmoidal artery usually is preserved, whereas the superior hemorrhoidal vessel is ligated.

When the sigmoid colon is divided and the superior hemorrhoidal vessel is clamped and divided, the sigmoid is detached from the sacrum and a free space becomes apparent (Fig. 49.4). This is an avascular plane, and the dissection should be directed toward the colon and away from the sacrum. Using blunt dissection, the colon can be freed posteriorly to the levator ani muscles that compromise the lateral pelvic diaphragm. Care must be taken not to damage the sacral veins when dissecting the colon free in this area. If these sacral veins are torn, the resulting hemorrhage often is difficult to control. Attempts to clamp and ligate the sacral vessels are uniformly unsuccessful. Fine, absorbable figure-of-eight sutures or packing with the use of absorbable hemostatic substances may be more beneficial in these instances. Sterile thumbtacks placed directly into the sacrum also can be used to control this bleeding. The middle hemorrhoidal vessels are clamped, further freeing the pelvic specimen. These pedicles, entering from the 4- and 8-o'clock positions, are ligated with suture (Fig. 49.5).

As the pelvic diaphragm is approached abdominally, the second surgical team begins the perineal phase of the operation. The incision around the urethra, vagina, and rectum is outlined, and the dissection proceeds cephalad toward the pelvic diaphragm from below. These muscles are transected circumferentially, and the specimen is removed in toto through the pelvis. The pelvis is copiously irrigated and hemostasis is achieved. The perineum is supported by approximating the levator muscles with absorbable sutures. If a bilateral myocutaneous graft is to be used for vaginal reconstruction, the second team begins "harvesting" the grafts while the team operating in the abdomen begins construction of the urinary conduit.

Conduit Formation

We prefer either the continent urinary reservoir or the ileal conduit. About 15 cm of the terminal ileum is selected as the urinary conduit; it is divided with the GIA stapler. It

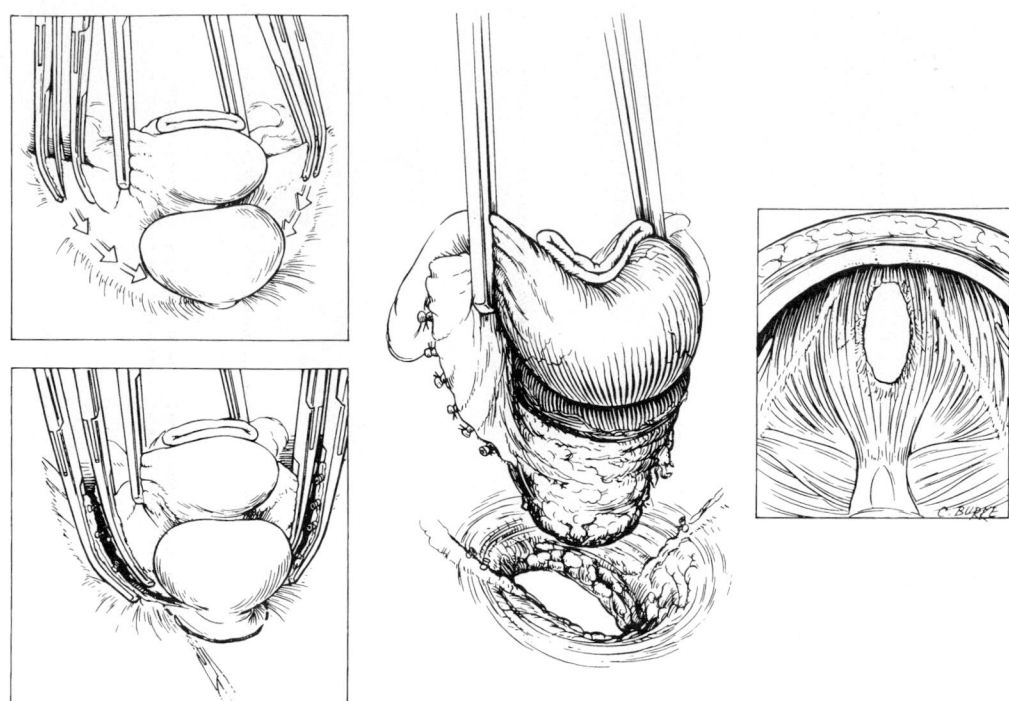

FIGURE 49.5. The fibrovascular pedicle (the "web") is progressively clamped and divided down to the pelvic floor. The perineal dissection is simultaneously performed with isolation and removal of the pelvic mass *in toto.*

is important to carefully estimate the length of the conduit segment. If the conduit is too short, stomal retraction and stenosis follows. An excessively long conduit can lead to stone formation or metabolic complications from fluid and electrolyte absorption across the bowel mucosa. In the obese patient, measurements for the conduit should be taken during the preoperative planning phase. In general, the conduit length should be 15 cm plus the thickness of the anterior abdominal wall when the patient is in the supine or standing position to account for the thickness of the patient's pannus. Alternatively, a segment of sigmoid colon may be used. If a colostomy is to be done, this saves a small bowel anastomosis because an isolated segment of ilium is not needed for the conduit. If there is significant radiation injury to the bowel in the pelvis, a transverse colon conduit can be constructed.

The ureters are further freed along their routes using blunt and sharp dissection. Care should be taken to select an area of the ureter for anastomosis that is relatively free of radiation damage. The left ureter should be freed superiorly and tunneled through an avascular window in the bowel mesentery to reach the isolated segment of ileum. After an appropriate site is selected to ensure a tension-free anastomosis, the ureters are sutured to the bowel segment (Fig. 49.6). This site usually is 2 to 3 cm from the proximal end of the conduit. The site is opened sharply for about 1 cm. Some surgeons choose not to use stents; however, we routinely place a silastic pediatric feeding tube through the lumen of the bowel and through the selected anastomotic site into the ureter.

The stent is sutured to the colon with fine absorbable suture passing through the bowel wall and the feeding tube. The ureter is then spatulated for a distance of about 4 to 5 mm. A full-thickness mucosa-to-mucosa anastomosis of the ureter to the antimesenteric border of the isolated segment of bowel is then performed using fine (3-0 or 4-0) absorbable suture. Six to ten interrupted sutures are used for the anastomosis. The ureter is anchored with long-acting absorbable suture to the underside of the conduit about 2 cm from the anastomosis to further reduce tension on the anastomosis. When the conduit is completed, the distal end is brought through the preselected site on the abdominal wall and, once positioned, is sutured to the peritoneum for stability. A "rosebud"-type stoma is fashioned to allow for ease of care and application of the urinary appliance. The proximal end of the conduit can be anchored to the sacral peritoneum to stabilize the unit.

Continent Reservoir

The continent urinary conduit has gained increasing acceptance and now provides a legitimate alternative to the ileal conduit. This modification of the urinary diversion procedure requires serial catheterization but eliminates the need for an external appliance. Construction of the continent conduit is more complex but is a preferred option for appropriate patients.

The continent conduit is formed from the right colon and the proximal portion of the transverse colon as well

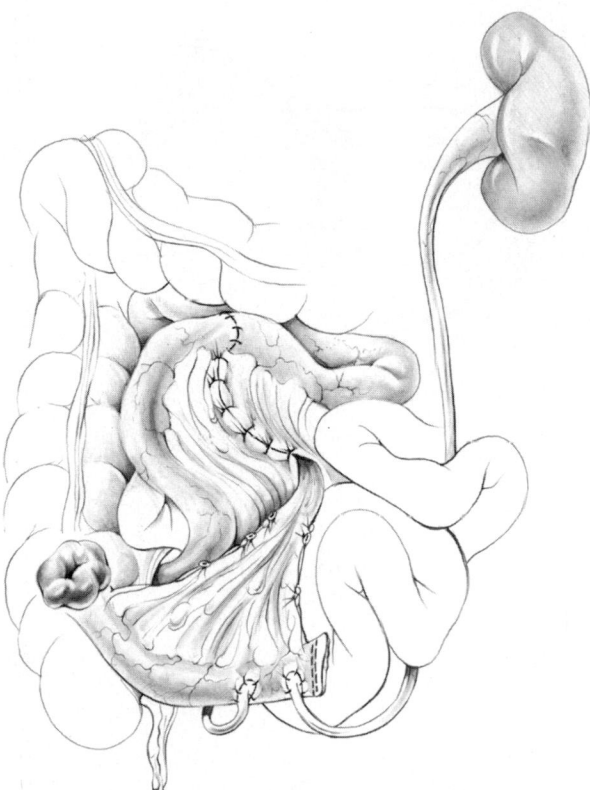

FIGURE 49.6. The ileal conduit is created by isolating a 15- to 20-cm segment of the distal ileum. The ureters are anastomosed near the closed end of the conduit. A "rosebud" stoma is constructed at the surface of the abdomen.

as a distal part of the terminal ileum. The details of this technique are provided in Chapter 50. Once the continent urinary conduit has been developed, the terminal ileum is brought through the abdominal wall. This site should be preselected, and care must be taken to bring the terminal ileum straight through the layers of the abdominal wall so that catheterization is not impeded postoperatively. A kink or turn in the ileum may cause the patient to have difficulty with catheterization. Ureteral stents are placed at the time of ureteral implantation; these are brought through separate stab incisions in both the cecum and the abdominal wall. A Foley or 14 F red Robinson catheter is placed through the stoma, and the conduit drains dependently for about 10 to 20 days.

For all urinary diversions, an intravenous pyelogram or loopogram is obtained about 10 to 14 days postoperatively. If there is no urinary leakage, the ureteral stents can be removed. The patient is instructed on methods of appliance application (ileal conduit) or self-catheterization and irrigation (continent conduit).

Stoma Construction

The sites for urinary and fecal stomas, which are selected preoperatively by the stomal therapist, are marked on the abdomen using scratch marks or sterile methylene blue

injections before the patient is draped. The urinary conduit is brought through the abdominal wall in the right lower quadrant, midway between the umbilicus and the anterior superior iliac spines, where a flat skin surface is available for attachment of the prosthesis. The sigmoid colostomy site is located in the left lower quadrant.

The abdominal wall aperture is prepared by removing a round segment, 2 to 3 cm in diameter, through its entire thickness to the level of the fascia. Skin, subcutaneous fat, and external oblique fascia must all be excised so that the flow of urine from the conduit is not obstructed. The urinary conduit is brought through the abdominal wall, and the serosa of the bowel is sutured to the peritoneum. The bowel mucosa is everted, creating a raised "rosebud" stoma, which projects over the abdominal wall. The stoma is fashioned with interrupted sutures of 3-0 delayed-absorbable suture, which passes initially through the dermis at the skin edge, then through the serosa and musculature of the adjacent bowel wall, and finally through the free margin of the bowel mucosa. When the sutures are tied, the mucosa is everted over the serosa of the bowel to produce a raised stoma that directs the urine away from the skin surface, thus reducing the chance for stricture and skin irritation. Application of the urinary stoma bag also is facilitated by the raised opening.

The fecal stream is diverted through the left abdominal wall in a similar manner. The free end of the sigmoid colon is brought through the abdominal wall to the skin through the previously marked site. If anatomically feasible, the colostomy bud should be placed below the waistline for cosmetic purposes (Fig. 49.7). Stoma construction is accomplished as described in the preceding.

Pelvic Floor Coverage

Attention is then directed to the pelvic floor. If vaginal reconstruction has been done using myocutaneous flaps, these effectively fill the pelvis and bring in new blood supply. Coverage of this raw surface enhances hemostasis and minimizes the risks of bowel adhesions and subsequent obstruction. If no vaginal reconstruction is done, an omental J-flap is used for this purpose with satisfactory results. The omental attachment to the greater curvature of the stomach is isolated, transected, and ligated (Fig. 49.8). Hemostasis must be meticulous. The operator must preserve the blood supply from the left gastroepiploic artery as the major blood supply to the omentum. The omental flap can be laid into the pelvic basin as a carpet and sutured in place with absorbable interrupted sutures. The omental coverage of the pelvic floor provides "new" blood supply to the surgical site and enhances healing. Some type of pelvic floor support should be provided to minimize the possibility of vaginal evisceration. Usually, this can be accomplished by suturing the remnants of the levator muscles together in the midline.

Anterior Exenteration

Anterior exenteration is a modification of total exenteration that leaves the rectosigmoid colon and posterior

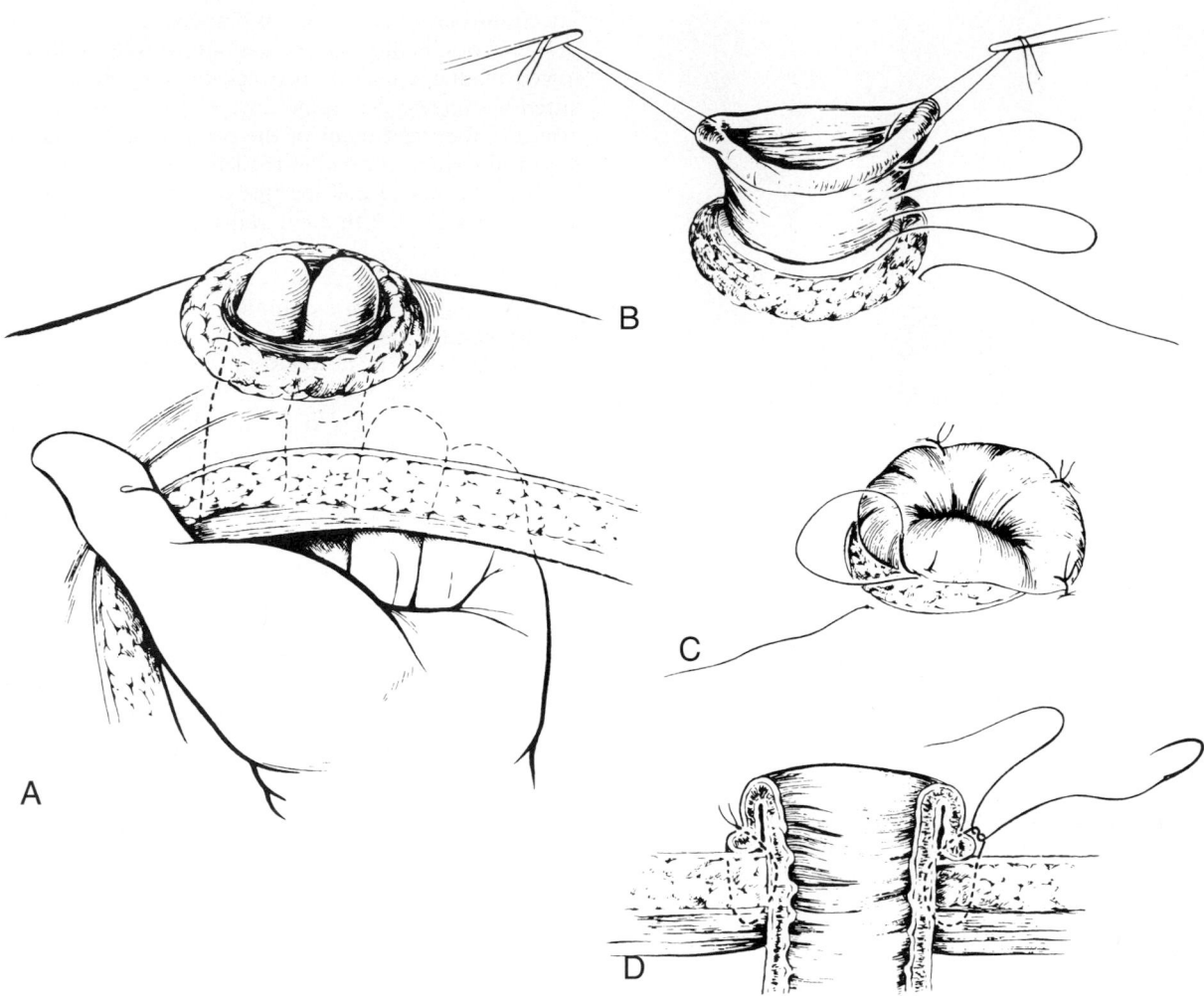

FIGURE 49.7. Technique for creating a bowel stoma that is elevated from the skin surface. This "rosebud" stoma is developed by excising a 3-cm circumferential segment of abdominal wall *(A)*, anchoring the skin margin with the adjacent wall of the exteriorized bowel *(B)*, and approximating the mucosal edge of the bowel to the skin *(C)*. The cross-sectional view demonstrates how the bowel wall is anchored to the skin margin to prevent retraction *(D)*.

vagina intact. After the ureters are isolated and divided, the rectum must be taken down from the posterior vagina. This is accomplished by incising the peritoneum along the rectovaginal peritoneal reflection. When this free space has been entered, the rectum can be bluntly dissected from the upper portion of the posterior vagina. It is freed laterally from the uterosacral ligament. The uterosacral ligaments are clamped, divided, and ligated with sutures as close to the sacrum as possible. The procedure is carried down the pelvic sidewalls, similar to the procedure for total exenteration. Great care is taken to ensure that the rectum and its blood supply are not damaged. When the perineal phase is performed, the vagina is entered in its midportion and dissection connected into the upper portion of the rectovaginal septum. An ileal conduit is constructed as described. Alternatively, a continent reservoir can be created. A single gracilis myocutaneous flap can be used to replace the anterior vaginal wall.

Posterior Exenteration

Posterior exenteration is most often used for vulvar cancer and is also a modification of total exenteration. In this procedure, the uterovesical peritoneum is incised and the bladder is freed, using sharp and blunt dissection, from the cervix and vagina. After the uterine artery is ligated, the ureter must be dissected free down to the bladder. This is performed in a manner similar to that used for a radical hysterectomy. This allows for visualization of the ureter and frees it from the vagina. The web can be divided in a manner similar to that used for total exenteration. The ureter and bladder are preserved under direct visualization of these structures. The perineal phase retains the anterior vagina adjacent to the base of the bladder in the lowermost portion of the pelvis. The upper and posterior vagina are resected along with the rectosigmoid colon. An end sigmoid colostomy is created. A single gracilis myocutaneous flap can be used to

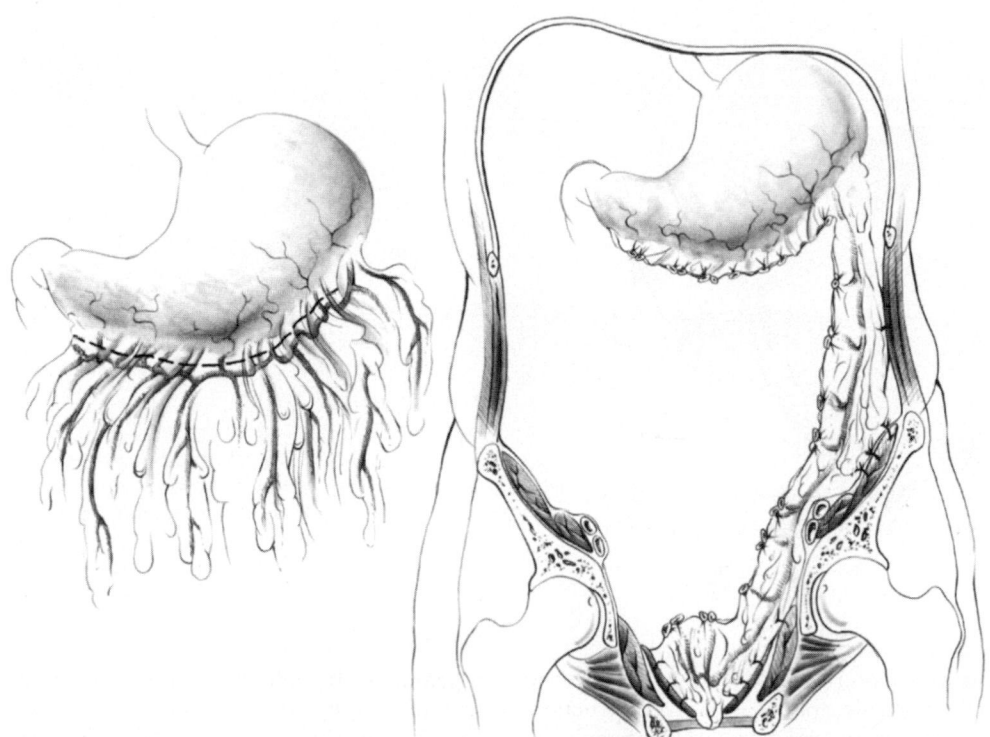

FIGURE 49.8. An omental "J-flap" can be developed by separating the right-sided portion of the omentum from the stomach and transverse colon. This pedicle then is positioned over the pelvic defect and loosely sutured in place.

replace the posterior vaginal wall and fill the surgical defect (Fig. 49.9). This is particularly useful because bladder prolapse is common following loss of the posterior support structures.

Total Exenteration with Low Rectal Reanastomosis

The lower 6 to 10 cm of rectum may be preserved in selected patients undergoing total pelvic exenteration. This depends on the location of the recurrent tumor. When this lower portion of the rectum is preserved, the sigmoid colon can be brought down and anastomosed to the rectal stump. This is greatly facilitated by use of the EEA stapler. In these patients, the colon has been previously divided using a GIA stapler proximally across the sigmoid and a TA-50 or reticulating stapler across the rectum. The staple line is cut off the sigmoid, and a running suture of 2-0 nylon or Prolene, starting on the outside, is placed on the open end of the sigmoid colon. The anvil of the EEA stapler is placed in the sigmoid and the pursestring is tied. The EEA stapler is introduced through the rectum and centered so that the spike can be advanced through or just above the staple line. The spike is removed, and the stem of the anvil is inserted. When the stapler is properly oriented, the two ends of the bowel are approximated and the stapler is fired. When the stapler is removed, a "doughnut" of tissue from each end of the bowel should be present in the re-

moved EEA stapler. The anastomosis is reinforced with interrupted sutures. A temporary diverting colostomy usually is necessary if the patient has been previously irradiated. Bowel continuity can be restored via colostomy closure in 3 to 6 months. This technique is illustrated in Chapter 42.

VAGINAL RECONSTRUCTION

Split-Thickness Skin Graft Vaginoplasty

The skin graft is taken from the buttocks or the posterior thigh as a split-thickness graft 10 to 15 cm in length at about 0.015 to 0.017 of an inch in thickness, using the air-powered dermatome. A vaginal stent is selected from commercially available supplies or fashioned from a foam obturator, the graft is sewn together over the obturator, and the visible end is sutured to the introitus. This technique is illustrated in Chapter 50. The patient is confined to bed for 3 days and ambulation allowed on the fourth or fifth day. The obturator is removed for the first time on about the fifth day, but may be left in place for up to 10 days. The patient leaves the obturator in place continuously for 4 to 6 months removing it for cleaning and vaginal irrigation every day or so. It is worn at night for another 4 to 6 months to minimize the risk of stricture of the skin graft. A new obturator can be fashioned inexpensively by shaping a piece of foam rubber and covering it with a condom. The patient can attempt inter-

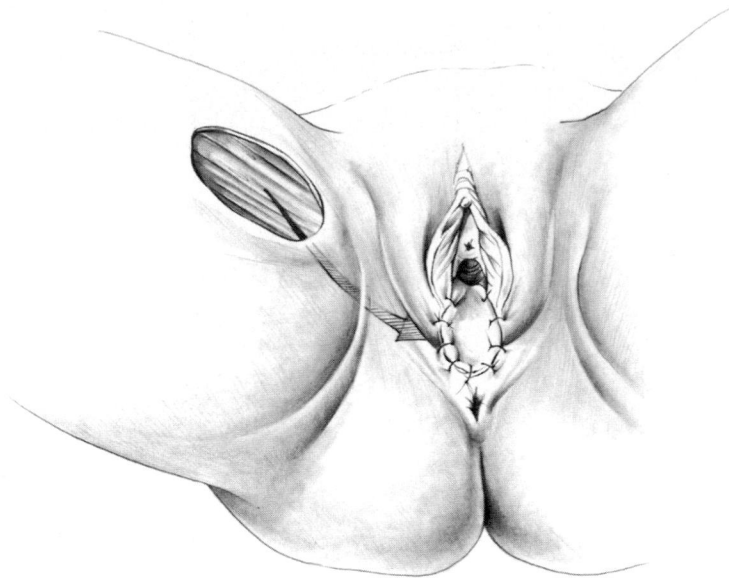

FIGURE 49.9. A single gracilis myocutaneous flap can be used for reconstruction when anterior or posterior exenteration is performed. The single flap can be harvested from either thigh, rotated into position and sutured to the remaining vagina.

course about 6 weeks after surgery. Skin grafts can provide an excellent result for vaginal reconstruction. Beemer and coworkers reported that 90% of their patients achieved satisfactory coitus.

Myocutaneous Gracilis Graft

The myocutaneous gracilis graft also can be used for creation of a neovagina. Construction at the time of initial exenteration surgery is required. The advantages include immediate reconstruction of the vagina, and the tissue mass itself helps to fill the pelvic defect as well as introduce a new blood supply to the area. An obturator is not required to maintain patency. When this approach is chosen, it is best to have a second operating team harvest the grafts and construct the neovagina while the primary surgical team completes the urinary diversion.

Myocutaneous grafts are constructed by obtaining bilateral full-thickness muscle, adipose, and skin flaps. The initial incision is made in an elliptical manner along an imaginary line extending from the superior aspect of the symphysis pubis to the medial condyle of the femur. The overlying skin to be taken should measure 10 to 12 cm in length by 6 to 8 cm in width. The underlying gracilis muscle is identified separate from the adductor group and is divided using the cautery about 2 cm distal to the skin paddle. This muscle is mobilized toward the symphysis. The perforating vessels on the underside of the muscle are about 10 cm from the symphysis and should be dissected with the myocutaneous unit. When the muscle and overlying skin are fully mobilized, they are brought through a subcutaneous tunnel to the perineal defect. The posterior edges of the grafts from both sides are sutured together with absorbable interrupted sutures, followed by a similar approximation of the anterior edges. This graft is introduced (or inserted) into the pelvic cavity and sutured to the sacral periosteum or levator remnants with long-acting absorbable sutures. The

opening to the new vaginal tube is sutured to the introitus with interrupted absorbable sutures (Fig. 49.10). The leg incisions are closed with skin staples. Jackson-Pratt drains are placed in the bed of each harvest site as well as in close proximity to the graft in the pelvis.

Postoperative Care

Patients are routinely admitted to the intensive care unit on completion of a pelvic exenteration. The continued oozing from the operative site with sequestration of fluids in the extravascular spaces causes significant fluid shifts; therefore, central venous pressure monitoring is essential. When left heart function and pulmonary function are adequate, a Swan-Ganz catheter is not routinely used. When ureteral stents are used, there is little chance of conduit obstruction from mucous plugging, and the urine output should accurately reflect kidney function. During the initial 24 hours after surgery, volume usually is replaced with crystalloid and blood products. Electrolytes and coagulation studies must be closely monitored, as well as calcium and magnesium levels. By the second to fourth postoperative day, the patient usually is ready to leave the intensive care unit. Hyperalimentation, which is started on the first postoperative day, is continued until the patient begins to have spontaneous bowel function. Intravenous antibiotics are continued for about 5 days. If vaginal reconstruction has not been performed or the perineum has not closed, the pelvic packing is changed daily after being left in place for the first 3 to 5 postoperative days.

Complications

The incidence of postoperative complications following pelvic exenteration is significant; complications occur in 30% to 50% of patients undergoing this procedure. The most common major complications after this operation

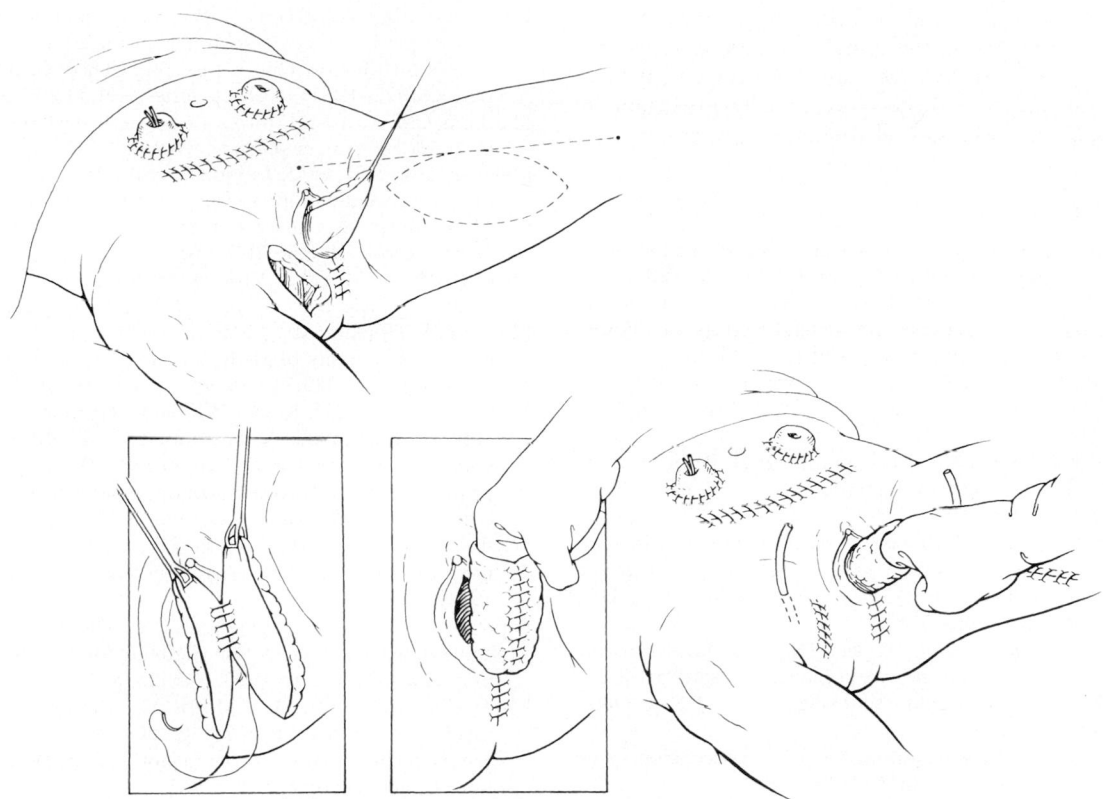

FIGURE 49.10. Full-thickness gracilis grafts, about 10 by 6 cm in dimension, are harvested from the medial thigh. They are tunneled through the thigh, sutured on themselves, and positioned in the pelvic cavity. The myocutaneous vaginoplasty is one of the alternative methods to a split-thickness skin graft vaginoplasty. Either one can be developed at the time of the pelvic exenteration.

primarily involve the urinary or gastrointestinal tracts and their reconstructions. Other complications include bleeding, infection, thromboembolism, and, some time later, stoma problems such as stenosis, prolapse, and hernia.

The occurrence of ureteral stricture and urinary leakage at the ureterointestinal anastomotic site has significantly decreased with current techniques. Ureteral stricture, especially if ureteral obstruction coexists, must be corrected surgically without delay or a percutaneous nephrostomy done to preserve renal function. Most anastomotic leaks heal spontaneously without requiring surgical repair. Renal calculus formation does occur but can be reduced by avoiding exposed staple lines and permanent sutures in the conduit.

Intestinal obstruction occurs both as an early and a late complication of exenteration and continues to be a serious problem in 10% to 15% of cases. The incidence of this complication has been reduced by use of the omental J-flap to cover the raw pelvic surface at the level of the pelvic diaphragm. Most paralytic ileus problems seen in the postoperative period can be treated conservatively with traditional nasogastric decompression. Enteral fistulas are seen uncommonly but are more common when omental flap or vaginal reconstruction is not employed. These fistulas may heal spontaneously with bowel rest and hyperalimentation.

Septicemia, which often originates as a urinary tract infection, usually responds to antibiotic therapy. Thromboembolic disease has become a less frequent postoperative complication since the use of low-dose heparin or SCDs began, even in the presence of a large denuded pelvic vault and exposed vessels. For wound and pelvic abscesses, CT-guided drainage, if feasible, is preferred to laparotomy.

The operative mortality rate related to pelvic exenterative surgery has improved dramatically since the 1970s. Earlier series reported a perioperative mortality rate ranging from 7% to 17%. In modern series, the reported mortality rate is less than 5% (see Table 49.1).

SUMMARY

During the past 50 years, there have been dramatic changes in our approach to patients with persistent or recurrent gynecologic cancer that is localized to the pelvis and that has been resistant to prior therapeutic measures. Advances in preoperative diagnostic aids, improved surgical techniques, and sophisticated postoperative intensive care facilities provide these patients a second chance at survival through exenterative pelvic therapy. This approach does require the expertise of a team well trained in ultraradical surgery and the constant vigilance of a tertiary care team during the immediate postoperative period. Long-term supportive care, encouragement, and motivation after the surgery are equally important in bringing about successful rehabilitation.

BIBLIOGRAPHY

Anderson BL, Hacker NF. Psychosexual adjustment following pelvic exenteration. *Obstet Gynecol* 1983;61:331–338.

Averette HE, Lichtinger M, Seven BU, et al. Pelvic exenteration: a 15-year experience in a general metropolitan hospital. *Am J Obstet Gynecol* 1984;150:179–184.

Beemer W, Hopkins MP, Morley GW. Vaginal reconstruction in gynecologic oncology. *Obstet Gynecol* 1988;72: 911–914.

Barakat RR, Goldman NA, Devendra AP, et al. Pelvic exenteration for recurrent endometrial cancer. *Gynecol Oncol* 1999;75:99–102.

Benson MC, Sawczuk IS, Hensle TW, et al. Modified Indiana University continent diversion. In: Olsson CA, ed. *Current surgical techniques in urology,* vol 1. Wilmington, DE: Medical Publications, 1988.

Bladou F, Houvnaeghel G, Delpero JR, et al. Incidence and management of major urinary complications after pelvic exenteration for gynecological malignancies. *J Surg Oncol* 1995;58:91–96.

Bricker EM. Bladder substitution for pelvic evisceration. *Surg Clin North Am* 1950;30:1511–1514.

Brunschwig A. Complete excision of the pelvic viscera for advanced carcinoma. *Cancer* 1948;177–183.

Brunschwig A. What are the indications and results of pelvic exenteration? *JAMA* 1965;194:274.

Buchsbaum HJ, White AJ. Omental sling for management of pelvis floor following exenteration. *Am J Obstet Gynecol* 1973;117:407–412.

Burke TW, Morris M, et al. Perineal reconstruction using single gracilis myocutaneous flaps. *Gynecol Oncol* 1995;57: 221–225.

Cavanagh D, Shepherd JH. The place of pelvic exenteration in the primary management of advanced carcinoma of the vulva. *Gynecol Oncol* 1982;13:318–328.

Copeland LJ, Hancock KC, et al. Gracilis myocutaneous vaginal reconstruction concurrent with total pelvic exenteration. *J Obstet Gynecol* 1989;150:1095–1101.

Creasman WT, Rutledge F. Is positive pelvic lymphadenectomy a contraindication to radical surgery in recurrent cervical cancer? *Gynecol Oncol* 1974;2:482–485.

Hatch KD, Gelder MS, Soong SJ, et al. Pelvic exenteration with low rectal anastomosis: survival, complications and prognostic factors. *Gynecol Oncol* 1990;38:462–467.

Hopkins MP, Morley GW. Pelvic exenteration for the treatment of vulvar cancer. *Cancer* 1992;70:2835–2838.

Ketcham AS, Deckers PJ, Sugarbaker EV, et al. Pelvic exenteration for carcinoma of the uterine cervix: a fifteen year experience. *Cancer* 1970;26:513–521.

Kiselow M, Butcher HR Jr, Bricker EM. Results of the radical surgical treatment of advanced pelvic cancer: a 15-year survey. *Ann Surg* 1967;166:428–436.

Lawhead RA Jr, Clark DG, et al. Pelvic exenteration for recurrent or persistent gynecologic malignancies: a 10-year review of the Memorial Sloan-Kettering Cancer Center experience (1972–1981). *Gynecol Oncol* 1989;33:279–282.

Matthews CM, Morris M, Burke TW, et al. Pelvic exenteration in the elderly patient. *Obstet Gynecol* 1992;79:773–777.

Miller B, Morris M, et al. Intestinal fistulae formation following pelvic exenteration: a review of the University of Texas M.D. Anderson Cancer Center experience, 1957–1990. *Gynecol Oncol* 1995;56:207–210.

Miller B, Morris M, et al. Pelvic exenteration for primary and recurrent vulvar cancer. *Gynecol Oncol* 1995;58:202–205.

Morley GW, Hopkins MP, Lindenauer SM, et al. Pelvic exenteration: University of Michigan 100 patients at five years. *Obstet Gynecol* 1989;74:934–942.

Morris M, Alvarez RD, Kinney WK, et al. Treatment of recurrent adenocarcinoma of the endometrium with pelvic exenteration. *Gynecol Oncol* 1996;60:288–291.

Parsons L, Friedell GH. Radical surgical treatment of cancer of cervix. *Proc Natl Cancer Conf* 1964;5:241–246.

Penalver MA, Bejany DE, Averette HE, et al. Continent urinary diversion in gynecology oncology. *Gynecol Oncol* 1989;34:274–288.

Popovich MJ, Hricak H, Sugimura K, et al. The role of MR imaging in determining surgical eligibility for pelvic exenteration. *Am J Roentgenol* 1993;160:525–531.

Ratliff CR, Gershenson DM, Morris M, et al. Sexual adjustment of patients undergoing gracilis myocutaneous flap vaginal reconstruction in conjunction with pelvic exenteration. *Cancer* 1996;78:2229–2235.

Reid GC, Morley GW, Schmidt RW, et al. The role of pelvic exenteration for sarcomatous malignancies. *Obstet Gynecol* 1989;74:80–84.

Roberts WS, Cavanagh D, et al. Major morbidity after pelvic exenteration: a seven-year experience. *Obstet Gynecol* 1987;69:617–621.

Rutledge FN, Burns BC Jr. Pelvic exenteration. *Am J Obstet Gynecol* 1965;91:692–708.

Rutledge FN, McGuffee VB. Pelvic exenteration: prognostic significance of regional lymph node metastasis. *Gynecol Oncol* 1987;26:374–380.

Rutledge FN, Smith JP, Wharton JT, et al. Pelvic exenteration: analysis of 296 patients. *Am J Obstet Gynecol* 1977;129: 881–892.

Shingleton HM, Soong SJ, Gelder MS, et al. Clinical and histopathologic factors predicting recurrence and survival after pelvic exenteration for cancer of the cervix. *Obstet Gynecol* 1989;73:1027–1034.

Soper JT, Berchuck A, et al. Pelvic exenteration: factors associated with major surgical morbidity. *Gynecol Oncol* 1989;35:93–98.

Symmonds RE, Pratt JH, Webb MJ. Exenterative operations: experience with 198 patients. *Am J Obstet Gynecol* 1975;121:907–918.

Symmonds RE, Pratt JH, Welch JS. Exenterative operations. *Am J Obstet Gynecol* 1968;101:66–77.

Vera MI. Quality of life following pelvic exenteration. *Gynecol Oncol* 1981;12:355–366.

Webb MJ, Symmonds RE. Management of the pelvic floor after pelvic exenteration. *Obstet Gynecol* 1977;50:166–171.

CHAPTER
50

▼

Pelvic Reconstruction After Gynecologic Cancer Surgery

LUIS E. MENDEZ   MANUEL PENALVER

The radical resection of pelvic malignancies to date remains an important procedure in the armamentarium of the gynecologic oncologist, despite significant advances in radiation therapy and chemotherapy. The trend toward minimization of surgical resective techniques has fared well for some patients in certain diseases such as vulvar cancer. However, en bloc resection can be the only hope for survival for some women with certain advanced or recurrent gynecologic cancers. Contemporary techniques in reconstructive surgery should be used to restore these women to an acceptable quality of life. Reconstruction is the surgical challenge of this and future generations of pelvic surgeons. This surgical challenge has been addressed by other subspecialties such as the oncologic surgical practices in head, neck, breast, and orthopedic surgery. It is imperative that pelvic surgeons begin to consider quality of life and the functional reintegration into society of the patients who undergo these radical surgical efforts.

This chapter reviews the techniques of reconstruction of a functional vagina, construction of an anatomically correct vulva, restoration of a functional rectum with elimination of colostomy, and construction of urostomy that allows for physiologic protection of the upper renal tracts and improves aesthetics as an alternative to the urine ostomy bag.

VAGINAL RECONSTRUCTION

Vaginal reconstruction has only been recently considered for patients undergoing radical pelvic procedures. Vaginectomy, whether simple or radical, can be a primary procedure or a part of a more extirpative procedure such as a pelvic exenteration. In addition, nonsurgical techniques such as radiation therapy can produce severe fibrosis or stenosis with the result of an essentially nonfunctional vagina.

With the advent of improved perioperative care and survival for radically resected patients, thoughts must extend to affording the patient acceptable sexual options. The loss of sexual gratification and function may be a devastating consequence to a woman even in the presence of a surgical cure. The oncologist has no way of knowing unless specific questions are presented to the patient as part of the routine preoperative history. The possibility of restoring a functional vagina may provide a woman with a tremendous source of psychological motivation in approaching her cancer therapy. It may alleviate some of the fears that she has toward her future psychosexual well-being as well as the domestic relationship with her partner. Physical sexual function, even though attempted, is not always successful. Depending on the procedure chosen and the commitment of the patient to maintain the neovagina, success rates of 80% are considered reasonable.

Besides its beneficial effects on psychosexual factors, reconstruction of the vagina after total pelvic exenteration has been shown to have a beneficial effect on wound healing, prevention of enteroperineal fistulae, and abscess or pelvic collection formation. The insertion of nonirradiated tissue in the previously radiated pelvis obliterates a great deal of dead space and provides a healthy vascular pedicle in an area with borderline blood supply resulting from extensive pelvic irradiation and radical resection.

Description of a neovagina using skin grafts attached to the colon posteriorly and bladder anteriorly supported by vaginal forms and stents was popularized by McIndoe as early as 1938. Techniques were also modified to use portions of the remaining viscera after less radical operations to fashion a neovagina. However, with the advent of ultraradical pelvic operations and the theory of en bloc resections to improve survival, it was evident that new efforts in reconstruction were needed. Classic reconstructive techniques that simply use skin grafts, as in the McIndoe procedure, are insufficient, because the supportive fasciae, rectum, bladder, and even pelvic floor have usually been extirpated.

Today there are various techniques to reconstruct the vagina. Some techniques, such as the pudendal thigh flap or the gluteal thigh flap, can be used for neovaginal construction. These are addressed in the section on vulvar reconstruction, where they are more commonly used. This section discusses the omental J-flap with skin graft, sigmoid neovagina, gracilis myocutaneous flap (GMF), and rectus abdominis flap.

Techniques for Vaginal Reconstruction

Gracilis Myocutaneous Flap

For the past 2 decades, the GMF has been the "workhorse" of neovaginal reconstruction in patients who have had radical resections. The GMF was introduced by McGraw in 1976 and had the immediate impact of decreasing perioperative morbidity and providing a potential for restoring coital function. The GMF is a versatile flap and has also been used for neovaginal and neovulvar reconstructions. However, it has not been without its problems. Initially, the GMF had rates of flap necrosis and prolapse as high as 65%. Techniques to anchor the neovagina and the trend to use smaller flaps have reduced this rate significantly to 13% to 37%. Infection is a problem and can complicate up to 37% of cases, but infection responds well to antibiotic therapy and local debridement if needed. Sexual adjustment has lagged and is reported to be significantly impaired in these women for various reasons, including the appearance of large inner thigh scars.

The GMF operation is begun with the patient in the dorsal supine position. The hips are abducted 45 degrees and flexed 30 degrees for exposure of the vulva, the knees are extended, and the feet are placed in gynecologic stirrups. This extended knee position provides maximum visualization of the gracilis muscle and the overlying cutaneous skin.

The approximate upper limit for flap viability is 8 × 20 cm (Fig. 50.1). After determining the length and width of flap needed, the gracilis muscle is palpated from its origin on the pubic ramus to its insertion on the medial aspect of the knee. The extension of the knee aids in the palpation of the gracilis muscle and reduces the possibility of mistaking the sartorius muscle for the gracilis muscle. A line is drawn along the length of the gracilis muscle and the skin island is marked carefully because only a 2- to 3-cm length of skin from the muscle edge will be supported (Fig. 50.2). The vascular supply is mainly based on the medial circumflex artery proximally. The distal muscle belly is supplied by minor vascular pedicles from the superficial femoral artery that can be sacrificed. Innervation is from the obturator nerve branches, resulting in a sensate flap.

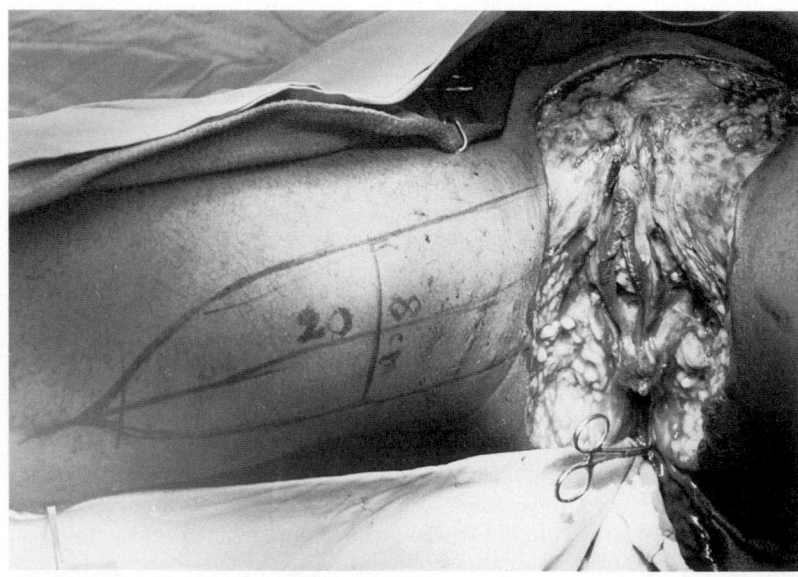

FIGURE 50.1. Vulva defect showing skin lines for gracilis myocutaneous flap.

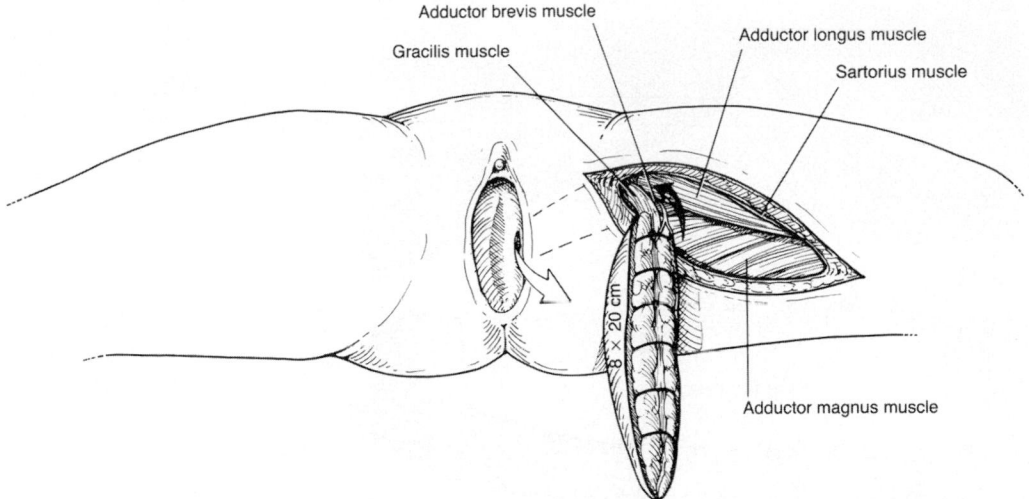

FIGURE 50.2. A mobilized gracilis myocutaneous flap. Note the 8- × 20-cm dimension and the critical muscle landmarks. (From: Gallup D, Talledo O. *Surgical atlas of gynecologic oncology.* Philadelphia: WB Saunders, 1994:235, with permission.)

An incision is made through the skin and subcutaneous tissue distally along the anterior border of the flap, down to the adductor longus fascia. It is extended along the line of the skin, outlining the paddle-shaped flap. Distally, at the edge of the flap, the gracilis is transected. We prefer to secure the muscle belly to the dermis with 3-0 synthetic absorbable suture to avoid shearing the flap. The vascular pedicle of the gracilis muscle is invested by the fascial layer that separates the adductor longus and adductor magnus muscles (Figs. 50.3 and 50.4). The surgical approach to the gracilis neurovascular bundle is made by reflecting the fascia to the adductor longus muscle. When the fascia is reflected, the adductor longus, adductor brevis, and the gracilis muscles are identified, exposing the vascular bundle of the gracilis muscle about 7 to 10 cm from the pubic ramus. The gra-

cilis muscle is isolated and divided at its origin on the pubic ramus. At this point, the gracilis vascular pedicle is located by sterile Doppler ultrasound. Repeated use of sterile Doppler ultrasonography confirms the location of the blood supply to the muscle and ensures its protection. When the flaps from both legs have been adequately dissected and are ready for rotation, 1 to 3 g of intravenous fluorescein is administered. The flaps are exposed to an ultraviolet Wood's light in a darkened room. Nonviable areas of the flaps are demonstrated by their failure to fluoresce, and these areas are excised (Fig. 50.4). Each flap is rotated into position (or tunneled under a skin bridge if no vulvar defect is present) and either secured to cover one half of a vulvar defect or sutured together, tubularized, and inserted into the pelvic cavity to form the neovagina (Figs. 50.2, 50.5, and 50.6).

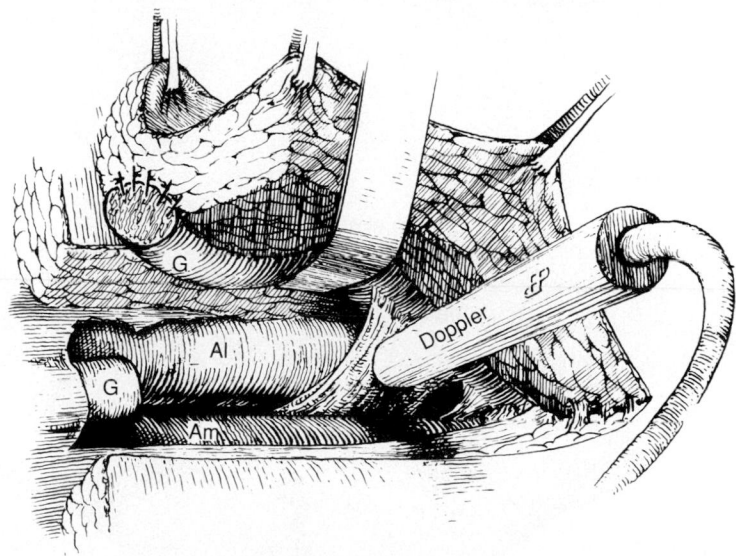

FIGURE 50.3. Gracilis myocutaneous flap. Doppler ultrasonography is used to confirm the neurovascular bundle emerging from the adductor longus (Al) and adductor magnus (Am) muscles. G, gracilis muscle.

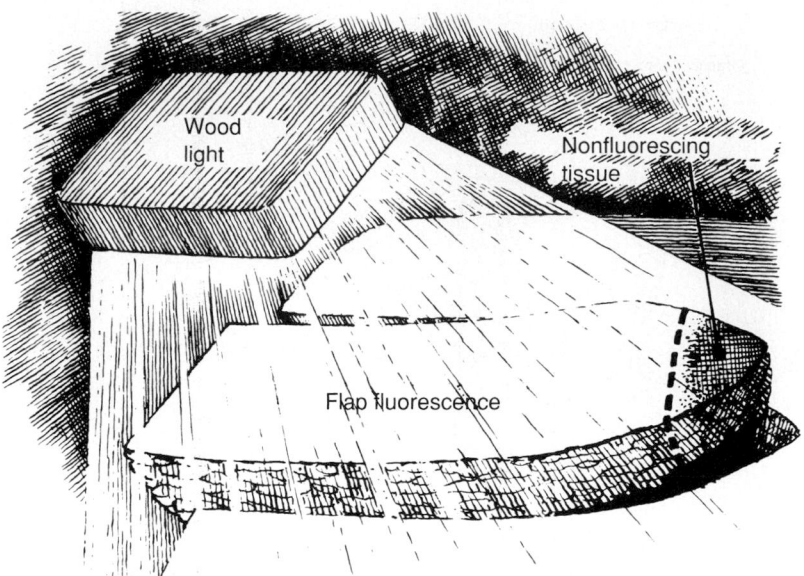

FIGURE 50.4. The Wood light focuses on a myocutaneous flap perfused with fluorescein dye. The avascular portion of the flap can be identified and excised.

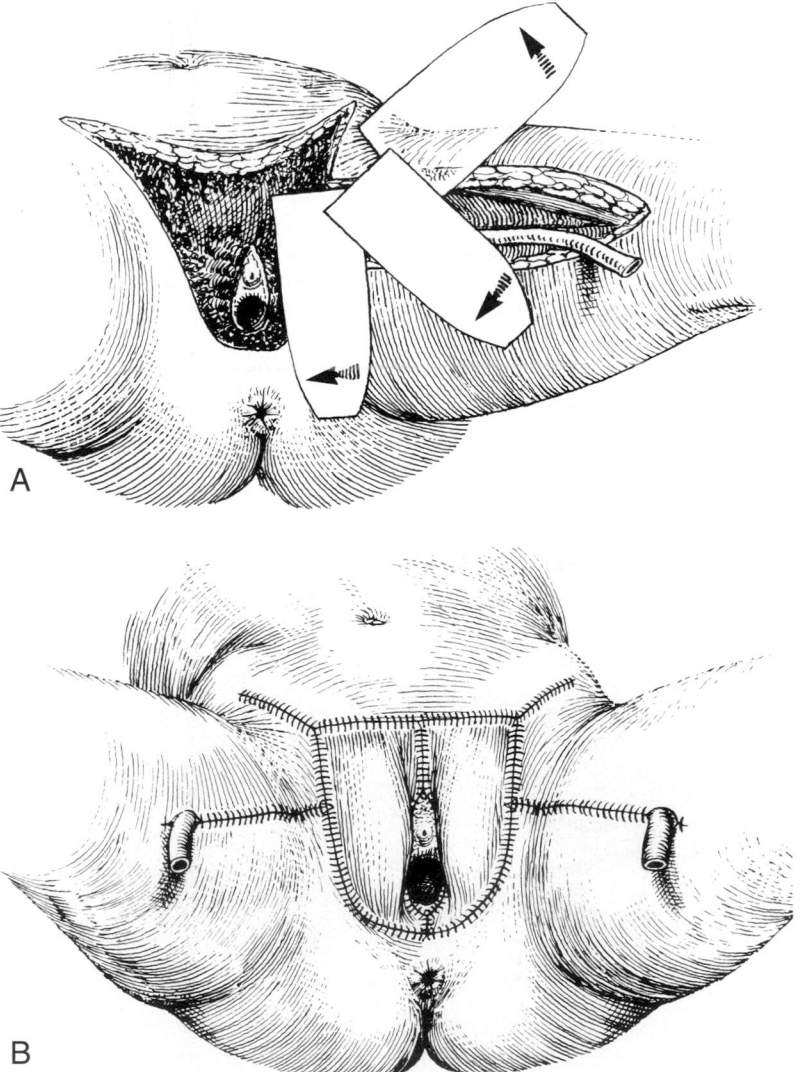

FIGURE 50.5. A: Bilateral myocutaneous flaps rotated into place. **B:** Completed neovulva.

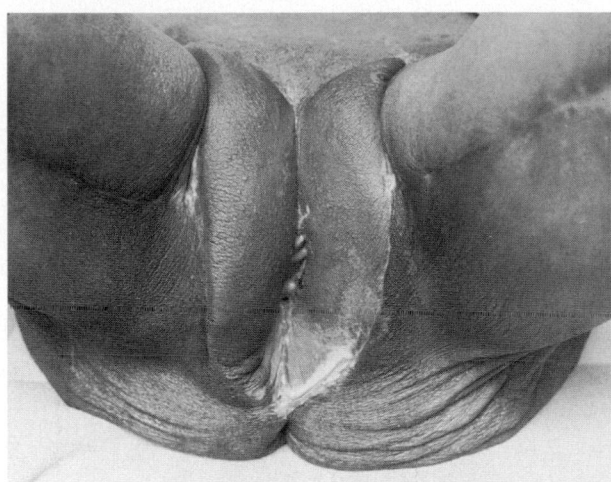

FIGURE 50.6. Completed myocutaneous flap, 8 weeks postoperatively.

The remaining subcutaneous tissue of the defect is sutured to the subcutaneous tissue of the flap with interrupted 3-0 synthetic absorbable sutures if a vulvar defect is present. Otherwise the flaps are tubularized and inserted into the empty pelvic cavity. Closed suction drains should be used at the harvest sites and the skin closed primarily. Sexual activity can commence after 6 to 8 weeks of recovery.

Omental J-Flap with Split-Thickness Skin Graft

By modifying the omental flap that is normally used to close off the pelvic inlet after exenteration (Fig. 50.7A), with or without low coloproctostomy, the surgeon can create an omental cylinder, providing anterior, posterior, and lateral walls for the neovagina. When the cylinder is sutured to the introitus and lined with a skin graft (split or preferably full thickness) and expanded in the postoperative period by a soft rubber vaginal form, a satisfactory functional neovagina can be created (Figs. 50.7B–D). The works of Morley as well as Wheeless have shown that a split-thickness skin graft for the neovagina may no longer be needed. Full-thickness skin grafts work well for all neovaginal reconstructions. The full-thickness skin graft survives equally well as the split-thickness graft but has reduced the tendency to contract postoperatively compared with the split-thickness skin graft.

In Figure 50.7C, the skin graft is laid out on a vaginal form. The form is fashioned from foam rubber and stuffed into a contraceptive latex condom. The split-thickness skin graft is folded over the vaginal form, and the edges of the graft are sutured with a running 4-0 synthetic absorbable suture. The completed operation is shown in Figure 50.7D.

In Figure 50.7D, a sagittal section shows a patient who has undergone a total pelvic exenteration. The rectal stump was retained, and the descending colon was mobilized and brought down into the pelvis for a very low (below 6 cm) coloproctostomy. The omentum has been detached from the greater curvature of the stomach and brought down as a flap based on the left gastroepi-

ploic artery. It is first sutured to the sacral promontory posteriorly, the pubic symphysis anteriorly, and pelvic walls laterally to form a pelvic lid. In patients who have insufficient omentum to form both the pelvic flap lid and walls of the neovagina, the omentum making the pelvic lid can be supplemented by the use of a sheet of synthetic, absorbable mesh.

The omentum, innervated by the vagus nerve, forms the wall of the neovagina. Normally, tugging or pulling on the omentum does not produce a sensation of pleasure that is associated with sexual intercourse; however, about 40% of the patients who have undergone this operation report that they experience sexual orgasm. Another possible physiologic change is the development of estrogen hormone receptors in the skin graft. The graft, taken from the skin on the buttocks or thigh, normally has no demonstrable hormone receptors. Once the skin is placed in the neovagina, the graft eventually becomes almost indistinguishable from normal vaginal mucosa on histologic examination. After the development of estrogen receptors, the maturation index from cells of the graft can be influenced by the administration of systemic estrogen similar to normal vaginal mucosa.

If construction of the neovagina is performed immediately following total pelvic exenteration, it is important to ensure that hemostasis in the pelvis is complete before applying the skin graft. If hemostasis is uncertain, the omental pocket for the neovagina should be packed with gauze. When hemostasis is secure and serous drainage has stopped, the packing can be removed and the graft can be taken and applied to a vaginal form and placed in the omental pocket.

After the skin graft is inserted, the neovagina must remain dilated with a vaginal form until healing is complete. For a period of 6 months thereafter, a soft Silastic vaginal form should be worn at all times except during intercourse and douching. After 6 months, the vaginal form is worn only at night if the patient is not sexually active.

Studies have demonstrated that this type of reconstruction works well and has minimal morbidity. Kusiak has reported a series of 20 patients in whom all grafts have taken, and there has been no postoperative morbidity as a result of the neovagina. Up to 80% of patients have reported satisfactory vaginal function.

Sigmoid Neovagina

A third procedure that can be used to fashion a neovagina uses the distal sigmoid colon. As early as 1955, Alexandrov reported on the use of a colon segment to create a new vagina. An impressive 89% success rate was reported. Kindermann subsequently published his experience with this technique for construction of neovaginas, also with good results.

The cardinal feature for use of an isolated segment of rectosigmoid colon is the integrity of the vascular supply of the colon via the superior hemorrhoidal artery (Fig. 50.8). Unlike secretions of the small bowel, the secretions of an isolated (10 to 12 cm) segment of sigmoid colon are not copious. Thus, the inconvenience to the patient of a copious vaginal discharge from the neo-

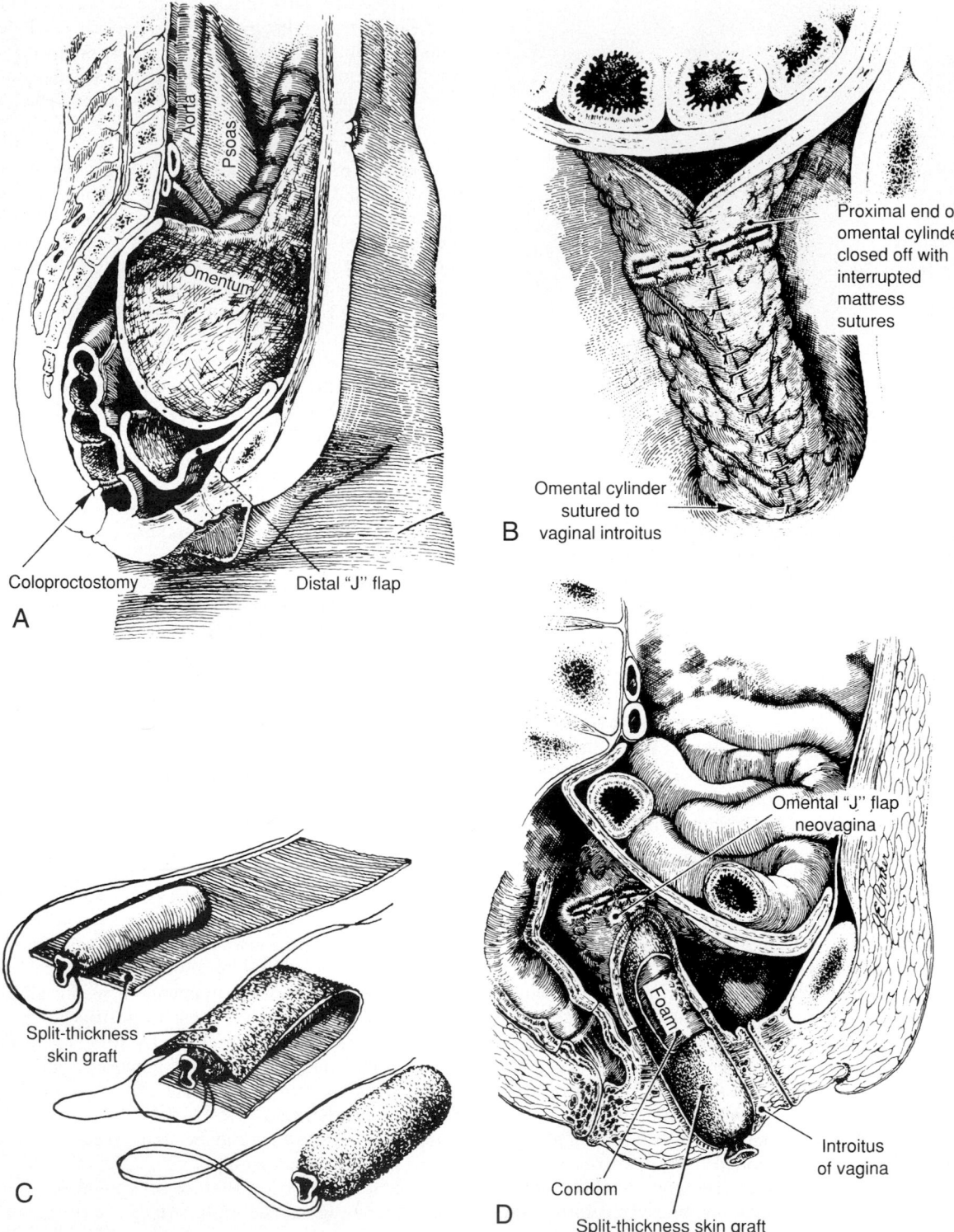

FIGURE 50.7. A: Drawing of the sagittal view of the pelvis after total exenteration. The colon has been reanastomosed to the rectum. The omentum has been taken off the stomach and brought into the pelvis as a J-flap for closing the pelvic inlet. The distal omentum of the J-flap is available for rolling into a cylinder, thus creating the walls of the neovagina. **B:** The distal omentum is rolled into a cylinder to be lined with a split-thickness skin graft. **C:** A foam rubber vaginal mold is covered with a condom. The split-thickness skin graft is sutured over the mold. **D:** Drawing of a sagittal view of the omental flap neovagina, lined with a split-thickness skin graft fashioned over a foam rubber vaginal mold covered with a condom.

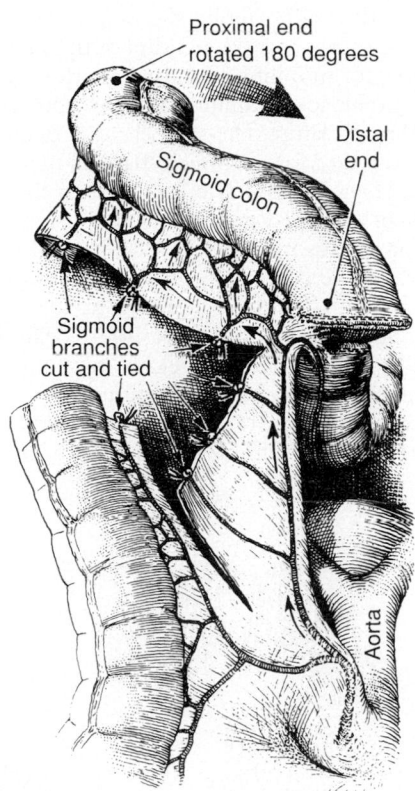

FIGURE 50.8. Colonic segment for a neovagina. The super-hemorrhoidal artery is the blood supply to the colonic segment. The sigmoid neovagina must prolapse through the introitus.

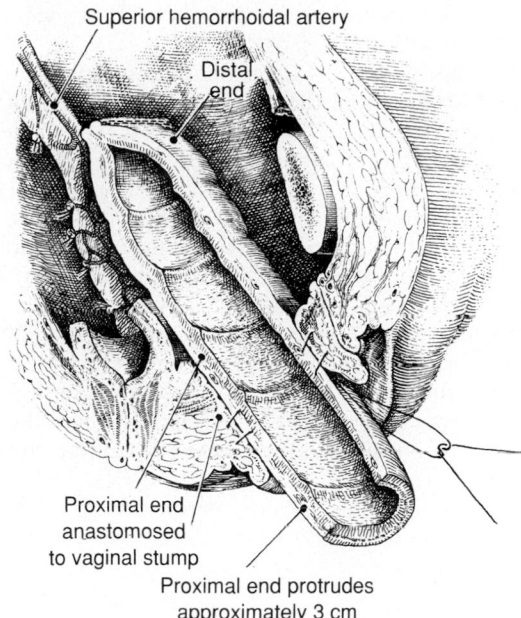

FIGURE 50.9. Prolapsed colon sutured to the vaginal introitus.

vagina is reduced. An additional anatomic advantage of the rectosigmoid colon over the use of isolated segments of small bowel is the unique anatomic feature of the marginal artery of the colon. This allows the surgeon to reverse the peristaltic direction of the colon to obtain greater mobility by transecting the mesentery medial to the marginal artery. The superior hemorrhoidal artery provides the appropriate vascular supply to the colonic segment via the marginal artery. Thus, by bringing down the proximal segment of the isolated colon, it reaches the desired vaginal introitus without tension. The wall of the colon is sutured to the introitus with interrupted 3-0 synthetic absorbable sutures (Fig. 50.9). The colonic neovagina tends to retract postoperatively. Often, the prolapsed segment extending through the vaginal introitus retracts enough that it may not need to be trimmed 2 to 3 weeks postoperatively. If trimming is needed, it is a minor procedure requiring local anesthesia.

Results in most studies reveal adequate patient satisfaction and few complications. There are cases reported with persistent malodorous discharge. In rare cases, the transplanted colon segment can develop an invasive adenocarcinoma or even ulcerative colitis.

Rectus Abdominis Myocutaneous Flap

More recently the rectus abdominis myocutaneous (RAM) flap has come into widespread use for vaginal re-construction. It is one of the most versatile myocuta-neous flaps to date. The flap provides for a wide array of procedures, including vulvar reconstruction. It has a long pedicle allowing for mobilization to most areas of groin, vagina, pelvis, and proximal thigh or even for contralateral procedures. Reports detailing the improved outcomes of these reconstructions when compared with other techniques are promising. The surgical procedure seems easier when compared with GMF, and there is a decreased incidence of flap necrosis and overall infection with the RAM flap. Both vertically oriented (VRAM) and transversely oriented (TRAM) flaps can be elevated to fit the specific needs of the surgeon.

The reported breakdown rate is 9% to 19%, better than with the GMF. Also, most studies report relatively few hernias or wound breakdowns with these flaps. The cosmetic benefits are obvious, in that the same midline vertical abdominal incision used for laparotomy can be continued to outline the flap. This usually allows for easy primary skin closure, with or without mesh reinforcement of the fascia. A unilateral RAM flap is usually sufficient to repair large vulvar defects or create an adequate-sized neovagina. The horizontal diameter of the skin should be at least 10 to 12 cm wide to make a vagina that is about 4 cm in diameter.

There are some perioperative factors that may play a role in flap viability such as obesity, diabetes, previous radiotherapy, smoking, and previous laparotomies. None of these factors seem to be absolute contraindications. However, a previous Maylard incision or one in which the inferior epigastric artery may be compromised is a contraindication because the flap is not viable without a reliable blood supply. Similar to the GMF, the RAM flap fills the pelvis with new blood supply and decreases dead space and postoperative pelvic infections. Prolapse is very uncommon with RAM flaps.

The flap itself is based on the inferior epigastric artery and is taken from the supraumbilical portion of the laparotomy incision (VRAM) (Fig. 50.10). Either a transverse or vertical skin island can be isolated depending on the anatomy of the individual patient (Fig. 50.11). Average skin diameters can range up to 8 × 12 cm. The flap is outlined and the cutaneous portion is mobilized to the edge of the palpable muscle belly. The anterior rectus fascia and muscle belly are transected with electrocautery at the superior portion of the flap. Blood supply from the superior epigastric is interrupted without consequence as the flap survives from the inferior epigastric supply (Fig. 50.12). We always secure the cutaneous portion to the muscle belly with all our flaps to prevent shearing. After mobilization inferiorly, the anterior rectus sheath is incised, mindful of the vascular pedicle, to allow for mobility. Vascular integrity is confirmed with the intravenous administration of fluorescein and use of a Wood's lamp. The skin island is folded over itself and sutured to form a pouch that will function as the neovagina (Fig. 50.13). The unit is then brought into the pelvis and secured to the introitus using 3-0 interrupted delayed absorbable suture. A vaginal form is inserted and can be coated with a sulfa cream or a topical estrogen cream. Care must be taken to adequately mobilize the muscle belly to its insertion to eliminate tension. The donor site is usually closed without tension as part of the primary incision with permanent suture (nylon or polypropylene). If need be, a synthetic mesh can be used to eliminate tension on the closures. Closed suc-

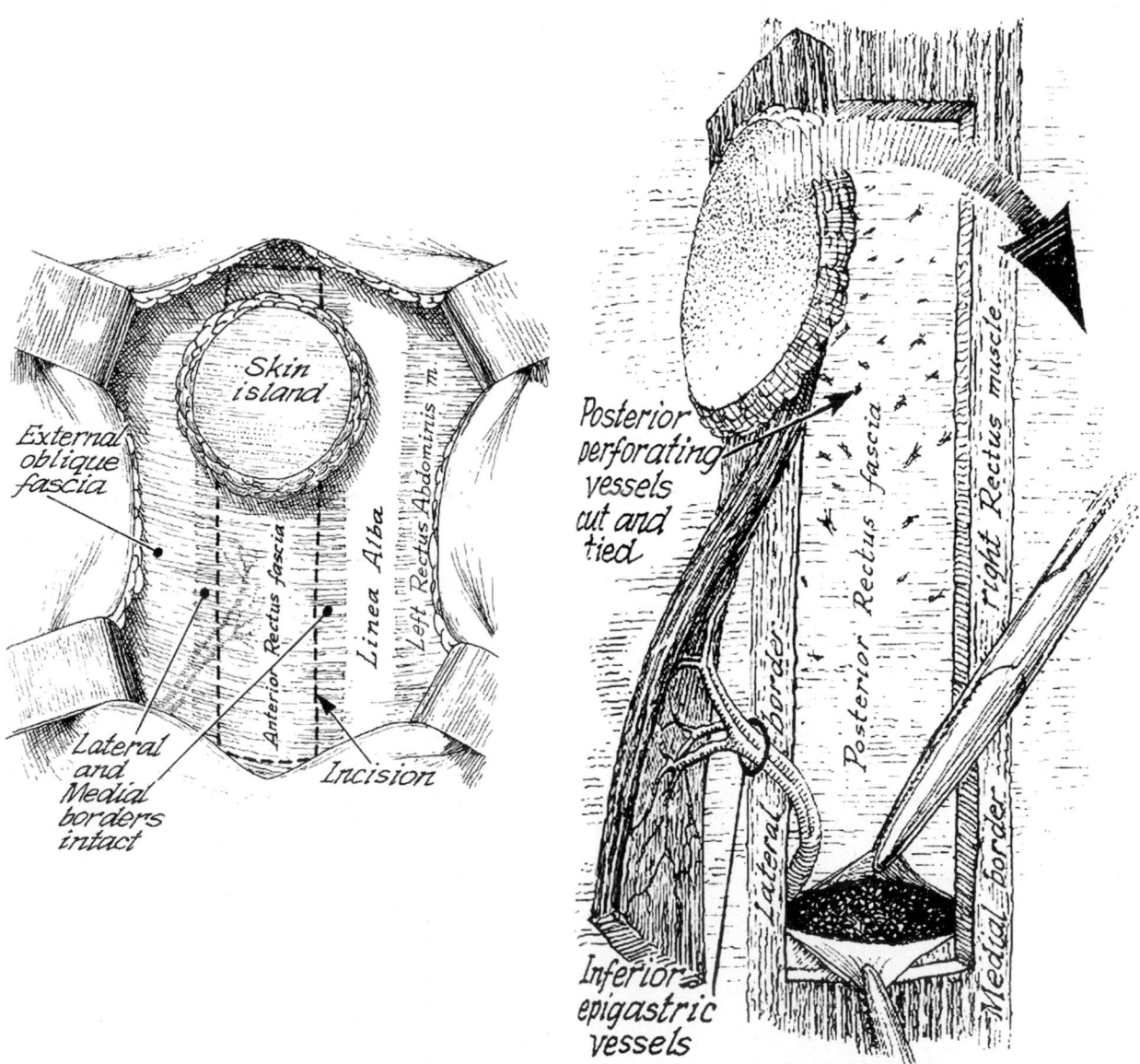

FIGURE 50.10. The vertical rectus abdominis flap. It is supplied inferiorly by the inferior epigastric artery and can be modified to fit the surgical defect and the patient's body habitus. (From: Wheeless C. *Atlas of pelvic surgery*, Baltimore: Williams and Wilkins, 1997:419, with permission.)

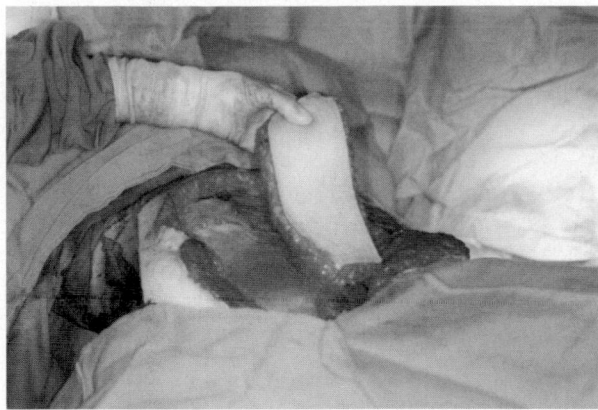

FIGURE 50.11. A vertical musculocutaneous segment isolated and elevated from the primary incision using rectus abdominis and overlying skin. See color version of figure.

tion drains can be used if indicated. The vaginal form is removed from 5 to 7 days postsurgically, and the patient can attempt intercourse after 6 weeks.

The RAM family of myocutaneous flaps is becoming the procedure of choice for vulvovaginal reconstructive procedures in gynecologic oncology. Long-term sequelae of RAM flaps are few and prolapse is greatly reduced. Carlson reported on a pilot series in 1993 with 100% flap viability. Subsequent studies are likewise very favorable. Nonetheless, reports exist of squamous carcinomas of RAM neovaginas and perioperative complications demanding that the utmost care be taken in developing this type of flap and in selecting the appropriate patient who will benefit from this extensive reconstructive procedure.

VULVAR RECONSTRUCTION

In the 1940s, the work of Taussig and Way demonstrated the efficacy of en bloc removal of the vulva, mons pubis, and inguinal lymph nodes from the anterior iliac spine to the adductor canal in patients with squa-

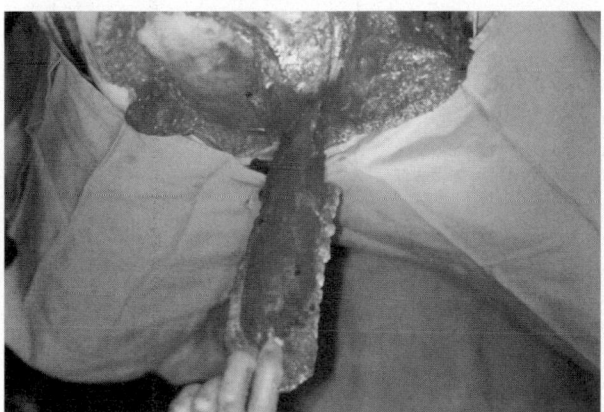

FIGURE 50.12. An elevated flap with the attached rectus abdominis muscle and supplying inferior epigastric pedicle. See color version of figure.

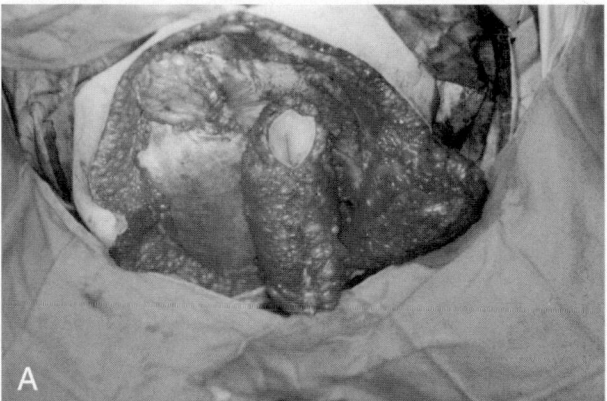

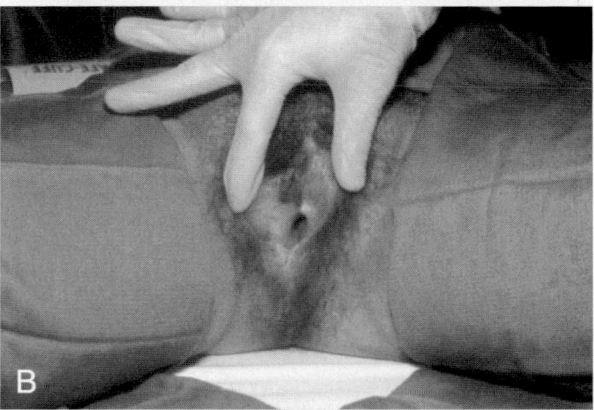

FIGURE 50.13. A: The vertically oriented rectus abdominis myocutaneous (VRAM) flap has been tubularized and is ready to be rotated into the pelvic cavity and secured to the introitus. **B:** A functional, well-healed VRAM neovagina. See color version of figure.

mous cell carcinoma of the vulva. By using a more extensive dissection, pelvic surgeons have removed more tissue and thereby enhanced the probability of increased survival. This type of radical excision, however, has been complicated by problems associated with closure of large wounds, that is, difficulties involving postoperative necrosis of the suture line over the mons pubis and the inguinal and lateral vulvar skin (Fig. 50.14). Attempts have been made to redesign the incisions for radical vulvectomy to allow for adequate surgical margins and, at the same time, provide better primary healing of the incision with reduced necrosis. This includes the use of "separate incisions" to approach the primary tumor and the inguinofemoral lymph nodes. Nonetheless, resection of the primary tumor can result in defects necessitating extensive plastic reconstruction. Although these modifications of the original Way incision have allowed some improvement in the incidence of necrosis and pelvic contracture, many patients have had significant wound breakdown, requiring a split-thickness skin graft to cover the area that has become necrotic during the postoperative period. The hospital stay of these patients has been prolonged, awaiting acceptable healing of the wound. In addition, patients have developed severe perineal contractions with significant distortion of the bladder neck and urethra, resulting in incontinence of urine,

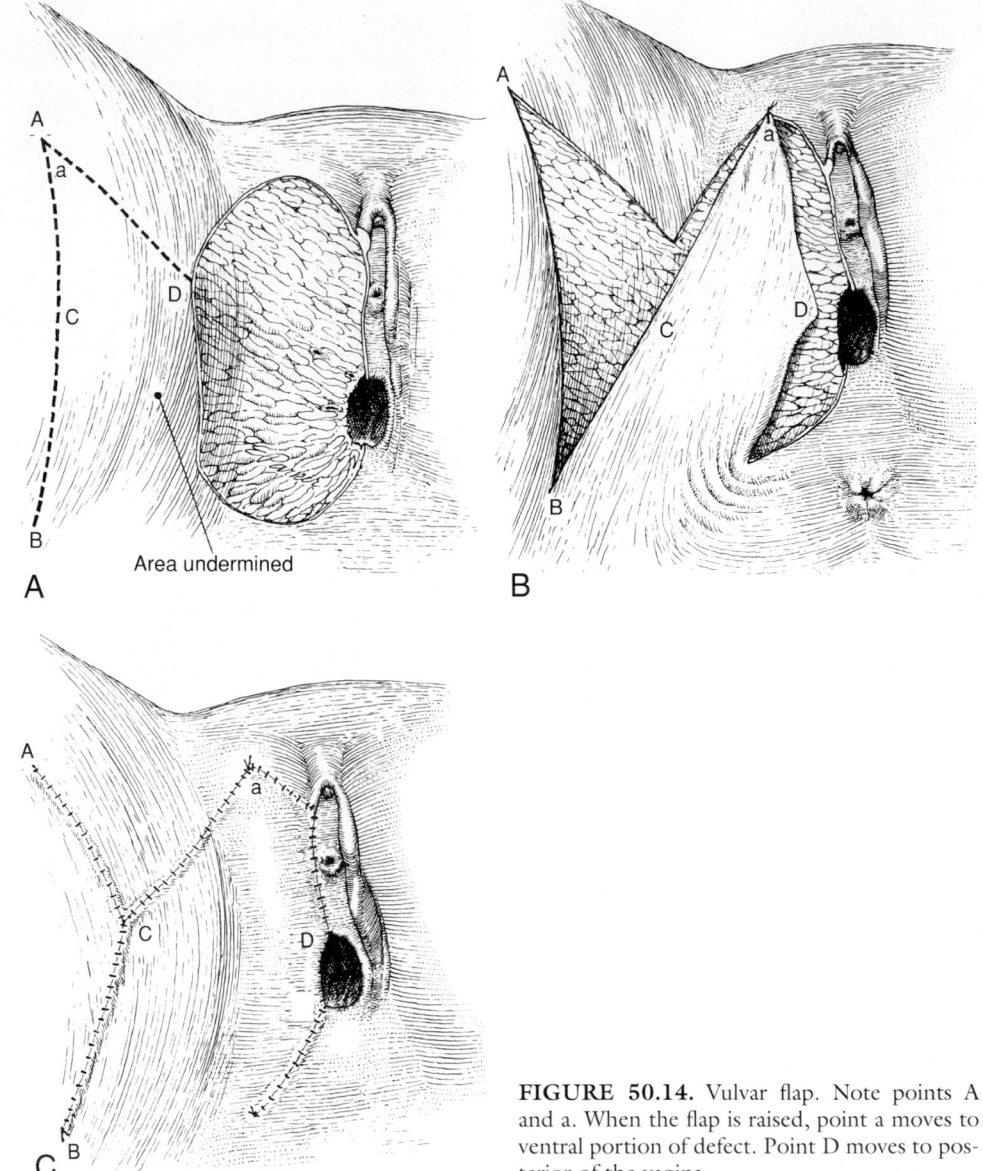

Area undermined

A

B

C

B

FIGURE 50.14. Vulvar flap. Note points A and a. When the flap is raised, point a moves to ventral portion of defect. Point D moves to posterior of the vagina.

perineal pain, pressure, and, in some cases, difficulty walking.

The ideal method of perineal reconstruction after a radical resection of the vulva should provide an immediate anatomic restoration and primary healing at the time of tumor resection. The neovulva should have as many of the anatomic characteristics of the original vulva as possible. The donor tissue ideally should be expendable from the donor site and transferable with minimal patient morbidity. Most radical vulvectomy operations can be closed primarily. Others can be closed with the assistance of the Z-plasty pedicle flaps advocated by Julian and colleagues (Fig. 50.14) and by the other techniques described below. There are occasional perineal resections, however, that are so extensive that none of the cited techniques is adequate for primary

closure. In these patients, myocutaneous flap is a means of primary closure. Efforts to reconstruct a radically resected vulva have been ongoing for decades. Many different techniques have been introduced and each has a particular risk:benefit profile. With the refinement of surgical therapies for vulvar carcinoma, emphasis has shifted to the use of fasciocutaneous and local flaps for reconstruction. Nonetheless, in certain cases the volume resected can only be reconstructed with a myocutaneous flap. This section describes split-thickness skin grafts, Z-plasty closures, the SURE Closure, V-Y advancement flaps, and the pudendal thigh flap. The gracilis and RAM flaps are discussed in the section on vaginal reconstruction. The myocutaneous flaps, however, continue to be the mainstay for vulvar reconstruction of very large defects.

Techniques for Vulvar Reconstruction

Split-Thickness Skin Graft

The use of the split-thickness skin graft for reconstruction of the vulva is not extensively described here. Most radical vulvar procedures resect deep to the perineal fascia requiring a reconstruction that needs to provide greater thickness than that of a simple graft. However, in the case of an extensive simple or "skinning" vulvectomy, this technique alone can be adequate. The procedure for harvesting a graft is available in standard surgical texts. In brief, it involves taking a 0.35-mm (12/1,000 inch) split-thickness skin graft from an acceptable donor site with a dermatome and applying the split-thickness graft to the denuded area of the vulva. The margin of the graft is sutured to the margin of the defect with fine sutures, and a moist stent pack is used to ensure that the split-thickness skin graft is adequately pressed against the wound. Small pockets of serum can be aspirated by needle to allow the graft to lie flat over the denuded area. We have found the use of meshed grafts to be of particular value in large wounds in which the potential for infection and subgraft seroma collection can be significant. The small defects in the mesh allow adequate drainage of the wound while epithelization takes place. The physiologic and logistic advantages of covering large, open wounds is well documented and is preferable to the long and costly process of granulation. Immobilization of the graft is an important key to success of the transplant.

Z-Plasty Full-Thickness Pedicle Flap

In cases in which primary closure of the vulvar wound cannot be performed without tension, the use of a pedicle flap, as advocated by Julian and Woodruff, has proven efficacious (Fig. 50.14). The flap is relatively easy to perform, but must be well designed before making the actual incision for the flap. Particular attention should be given to the width of the base of the flap to ensure an adequate blood supply to the distal points of the flap. A general rule to follow is that 2 cm of base should be present for each 1 cm of length of the flap. After measuring the defect and translating these measurements into the appropriate size of flap needed, the future flap is marked along the designated lines with a surgical marker before the incisions are made. The incision should be full thickness, including epidermis, dermis, and subcutaneous fat, down to the fascia. The flap is rotated into position and sutured to the midline of the perineum without tension. Generally, it is difficult to rotate the flap beyond the mid-perineal line. If additional tissue is needed to close the contralateral vulvar defect, a flap is elevated from the opposite side and similarly sutured in the midline. The flap is sutured to the underlying fascia, covering the pubic rami, and to the incision line on the opposite side. Preferably, 3-0 synthetic absorbable suture is used. The suture in the skin margin should be fine synthetic monofilament suture such as nylon or fine delayed absorbable suture. The medial margin of the flap is sutured to the margin of the vaginal mucosa with interrupted 2-0 synthetic absorbable

sutures. A soft Silastic closed suction drain is placed under the flap, sutured into place, and placed to low suction. The remaining skin adjacent to the flap is brought into position to close the donor site and is sutured with a subcutaneous row of interrupted 3-0 synthetic absorbable sutures and 4-0 nylon sutures in the skin. The cardinal feature of successful healing of these flaps is positioning without tension. If they are under tension, separation occurs.

Modification of full-thickness pedicled flaps includes the gluteal thigh flap, which can incorporate a much larger skin paddle, depending on the inferior gluteal artery, and can range up to 8 × 20 cm. It should not be performed in a patient with a previous bilateral hypogastric artery ligation because compromise may occur.

Mechanical Skin Stretcher (SURE Closure)

A contemporary technique for closure of skin defects or to obtain a full-thickness skin graft for neovagina construction from donor site on the body is the mechanical skin stretcher (SURE Closure, Life Medical Sciences, Inc.) (Fig. 50.15). The skin, because of its viscoelastic properties, can be stretched significantly. (For example, the abdominal skin of a woman who is 40 weeks pregnant is significantly stretched.) Through the extensive work of Hirshowitz and Lindenbaum and through the mechanical engineering of the Life Medical Sciences, Inc., it is possible to stretch skin in about 1 hour in the operating room to cover most defects (Fig. 50.16). This new device can have a significant role in pelvic surgery.

Large abdominal wall defects and certain vulvar defects may be closed without rotational flaps and split-thickness skin grafts. The application of the skin stretching device to each margin of the large open abdominal defect allows stretching of the skin gradually over a 1-hour period under general anesthesia in the operating room such that the skin can be sutured without tension. Large abdominal skin defects can be closed primarily without skin grafting. Full-thickness skin grafts can be harvested for neovagina reconstruction without leaving a donor site scar. This device is worthy of the attention of all who perform extensive gynecologic surgery.

V-Y Advancement Flap

A simple sliding design for a skin flap that is dependent on random perfusion of perforating musculocutaneous arteries can reconstruct even moderately large vulvar defects. The upper inner thigh is the usual donor site for vulvar defects. Circulation to that area has been reported distally via a rich suprafascial plexus from gracilis and adductor musculocutaneous perforators and proximally from the external pudendal. Bilateral triangles can be drawn while the patient is in the dorsal lithotomy position. The incision is carried down to include subcutaneous fat. After mobilization, the flap is "slid" toward the defect and secured to the remaining vaginal mucosa or to each other, if needed. The original "V" incision is then closed as a "Y" (Fig. 50.17). With a good blood supply and adequate mobilization, the incidence of wound dehiscence is small. Closed suction drains should

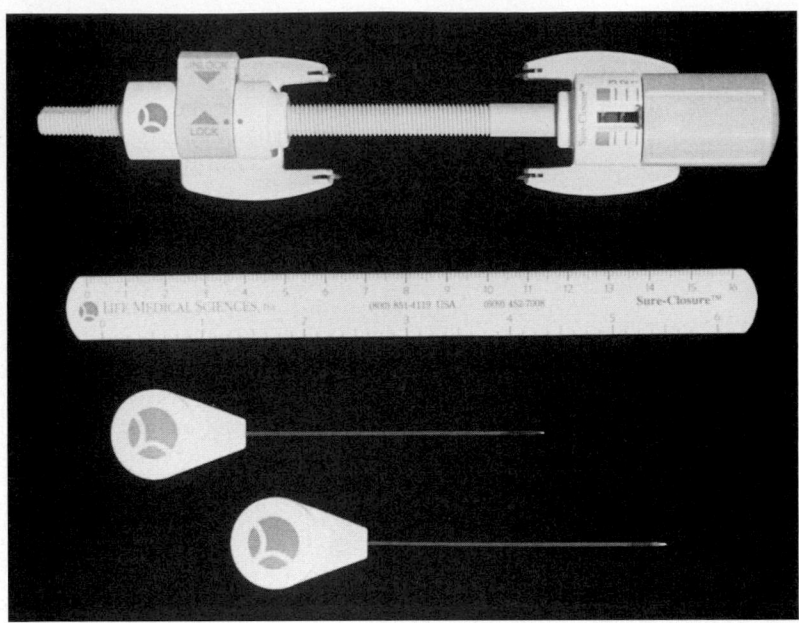

FIGURE 50.15. Mechanical skin stretcher instrument called the SURE Closure.

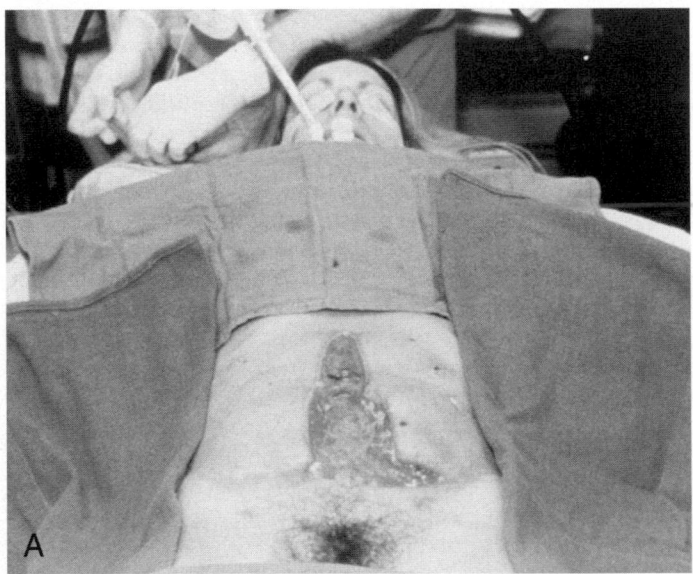

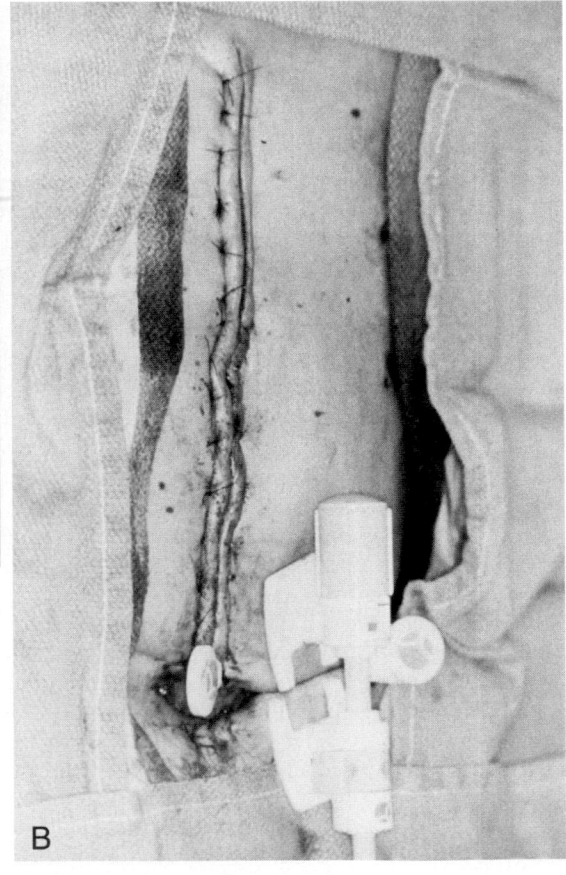

FIGURE 50.16. A: Photograph of an open abdominal wound to be closed with a skin stretcher instrument. **B:** Midline skin closed without tension. The transverse incision is stretched with the instrument before it is sutured.

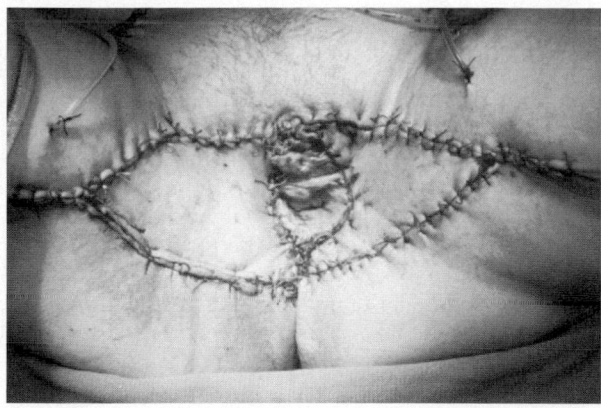

FIGURE 50.17. A completed V-Y flap used to reconstruct a patient who underwent radical vulvectomy. Notice the incision originally made as a "V" has been closed as a "Y." Closed suction drains are placed under the flaps to prevent fluid collections. See color version of figure.

be placed and left for 7 to 10 days. Ambulation may begin after 3 days. In the interim, prophylactic antibiotics and thromboprophylaxis should be administered, as with most moderately extensive vulvar flaps.

The V-Y flap can be used for even larger reconstructions, as described by Tateo, by transecting the gracilis toward the insertion and making it a type of sliding musculocutaneous flap after mobilization.

Gracilis and Rectus Abdominis Myocutaneous Flaps

The gracilis and RAM flaps are extremely versatile flaps, as described in the section on vaginal reconstruction. The same principles hold true for vulvar reconstruction in terms of elevating, rotating, and securing these flaps. The principal difference is that unilateral gracilis flaps can be used, depending on the vulvar defect, and no tubularization is necessary. Similar breakdown rates are seen with vulvar reconstruction as with vaginal reconstruction. We believe that the RAM flap continues to be a superior flap for all myocutaneous vulvovaginal reconstructions.

OPERATIONS TO PRESERVE URINARY CONTINENCE

Fecal and urinary diversion have been an essential part of total pelvic exenteration surgery. The early pioneer work of Brunschwig in total pelvic exenteration surgery used ureterosigmoidostomy for urinary diversion (a "wet colostomy"). Reflux of fecal contaminated urine resulted in unacceptable rates of pyelonephritis and secondary renal deterioration. In 1950, Bricker introduced the isolated ileal loop urinary diversion. Later, the colonic loop modification was preferred by some operators. These two techniques have been the preferred techniques for urinary diversion for more than 40 years. Long-term follow-up of patients with isolated intestinal loop urinary diversion, however, has revealed a high incidence of ureteral stenosis and upper renal tract deterioration, especially in those patients who have had pelvic irradiation for gynecologic malignancies. In addition, negative quality-of-life issues secondary to the required urostomy bag, including its odor, reduced self-image, and reduced sexuality, make an alternative technique without a bag desirable. This section discusses the Kock pouch, which introduced the idea of a continent reservoir, and the Miami pouch, which is a newer continent ileocolonic reservoir that has become popular in gynecologic oncology. Each patient should be evaluated individually as to the type of reservoir best suited for her needs. The surgeon should consider the various types but should always perform the procedure that he or she is most comfortable with and that is best suited for the patient.

Continent Urostomy Operations

There are unique pathologic and physiologic changes in pelvic organs after irradiation for gynecologic malignancies. The same levels of perioperative irradiation are not usually required for most urologic malignancies such as carcinoma of the prostate and bladder. The pathophysiologic changes of irradiation-induced endarteritis, resulting in ischemia and later fibrosis, are not present in urinary diversions required for congenital anomalies. In selecting a continent, nonrefluxing urostomy that meets the physiologic requirements, several features must be considered. The ureteral intestinal anastomosis must be as free as possible from potential stricture formation that would result in hydronephrosis and eventual upper renal unit deterioration. Techniques that require the irradiated ureter to be buried in the muscular layers of irradiated colon to achieve the nonrefluxing feature of continent urostomy may be associated with a risk of stenosis and secondary hydronephrosis that is higher than acceptable. The integrity of the upper renal tracts remains to be evaluated in prospective, randomized trials between the incontinent urostomies and the ileoascending colonic variety of these operations. All continent urostomy pouches should have similar physiologic characteristics including a low pouch pressure of less than 40 cmH_2O pressure, even at volumes greater than 500 mL. This reduces the chance of ureteral reflux and reduces the incidence of incontinence. Reflux and incontinence are reduced because, in the Kock pouch urostomy nipples, pressures are 90 cmH_2O. The use of small segments of irradiated large bowel in continent urostomies, that is, the Indiana pouch, may lead to unacceptable levels of pressure. This finding needs careful study with long-term follow-up.

The compliance of large bowel, especially after irradiation therapy, is less than that of small bowel. A larger segment of detubularized colon, that is, the entire ascending and proximal transverse colon (Miami pouch), may overcome this problem and allow pressures within the pouch to remain at acceptable low levels. Patients should catheterize their continent pouches at least four times per day.

The continent urostomy is favored in gynecologic oncology patients for two reasons. First, medically, the continent urostomy should help prevent contaminated urine from refluxing into the kidney. This contaminated urine reflux sets up a chronic pyelonephritis. After a prolonged period of time, there could be deterioration of the upper renal units commonly associated with ileal or colonic loops. Second, quality of life is improved by elimination of the urinary bag with its attendant problems of awkwardness, odor, reduced self-image, and reduced sexuality.

Continent Urostomy with Ileal Reservoir (Kock Pouch)

The Kock pouch, developed by Nils Kock in 1982, was devised as a continent nonrefluxing urostomy. Modifications by Skinner improved the surgical technique and reduced the postoperative complications of the original Kock technique. This alternative to ileal or colonic loop urinary diversion should be considered by gynecologic oncologists. Skinner and co-workers have shown that construction of an internal reservoir suitable for urinary bladder replacement must provide (1) retention of 500 to 1,000 mL of fluid, (2) maintenance of low pressure after filling, (3) elimination of intermittent pressure spikes that produce reflux, (4) true continence day and night, (5) ease of catheterization, and (6) prevention of reflux.

The mucosa of the ileum in the wall of the pouch appears to adapt well to urine. The height of the villi of the ileal mucosa gradually decreases, and, in time, the mucosa becomes nearly flat, thereby proportionally reducing the absorption of electrolytes from the urine.

Prerequisites for constructing a continent urostomy include reasonable renal function (creatinine level less than 3.0 mg/dL), an adequate length of small bowel so

that use of 80 cm of ileum taken out of the digestive tract does not result in significant short bowel syndrome, and a patient and her surgeon who are motivated for the procedure and who both understand the inherent risks (in irradiated bowel, an 8% to 16% incidence of malfunction of the continent valve mechanism, necessitating additional surgery). When the pouch procedure is performed in conjunction with total pelvic exenteration, resection of the pelvic organs is performed first. For the conversion of an existing ileal or colon conduit to a continent urostomy, all the intraabdominal adhesions of the intestine must be taken down and the bowel inspected for enterotomies before initiating the Kock pouch continent urostomy.

Technique for Kock Pouch Continent Urostomies: Skinner Modification

As seen in Figure 50.18, knowledge and understanding of the anatomy of the terminal ileum and ascending colon and of the blood supply to these structures is essential for the success of the operation. The terminal ileum is transected about 16 cm from the ileocecal junction in the area of the avascular plane of Treves. To ensure mobility of the pouch, an incision is carried up the avascular plane of Treves for 25 to 30 cm. The ileocolic artery must be lateral to this incision, with the branches of the superior mesenteric artery medial to the incision.

The pouch requires 17 cm of ileum for the efferent nipple valve and bowel limb, two 22-cm segments of ileum for the pouch itself, and one 17-cm segment of ileum for the afferent bowel limb and nipple valve. As seen in Figure 50.19, 5 cm of proximal ileum is sacrificed to allow greater mobility of the completed pouch. The anterior wall of the pouch is opened with electrocautery. The posterior wall is sutured with two layers of synthetic absorbable suture (Fig. 50.19A).

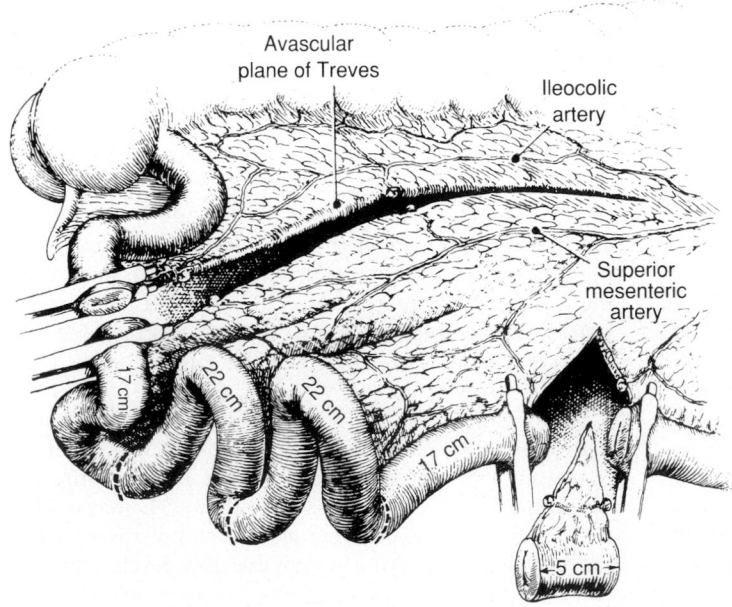

FIGURE 50.18. Anatomic drawing of the terminal ileum illustrating the avascular plane of Treves, the ileocolic artery, and the superior mesenteric artery. Note that the efferent system requires 17 cm of bowel, the Kock pouch requires two 22-cm segments of bowel, and the afferent system requires 17 cm of bowel. Five centimeters of intestine are resected to give additional mobility to the completed Kock pouch.

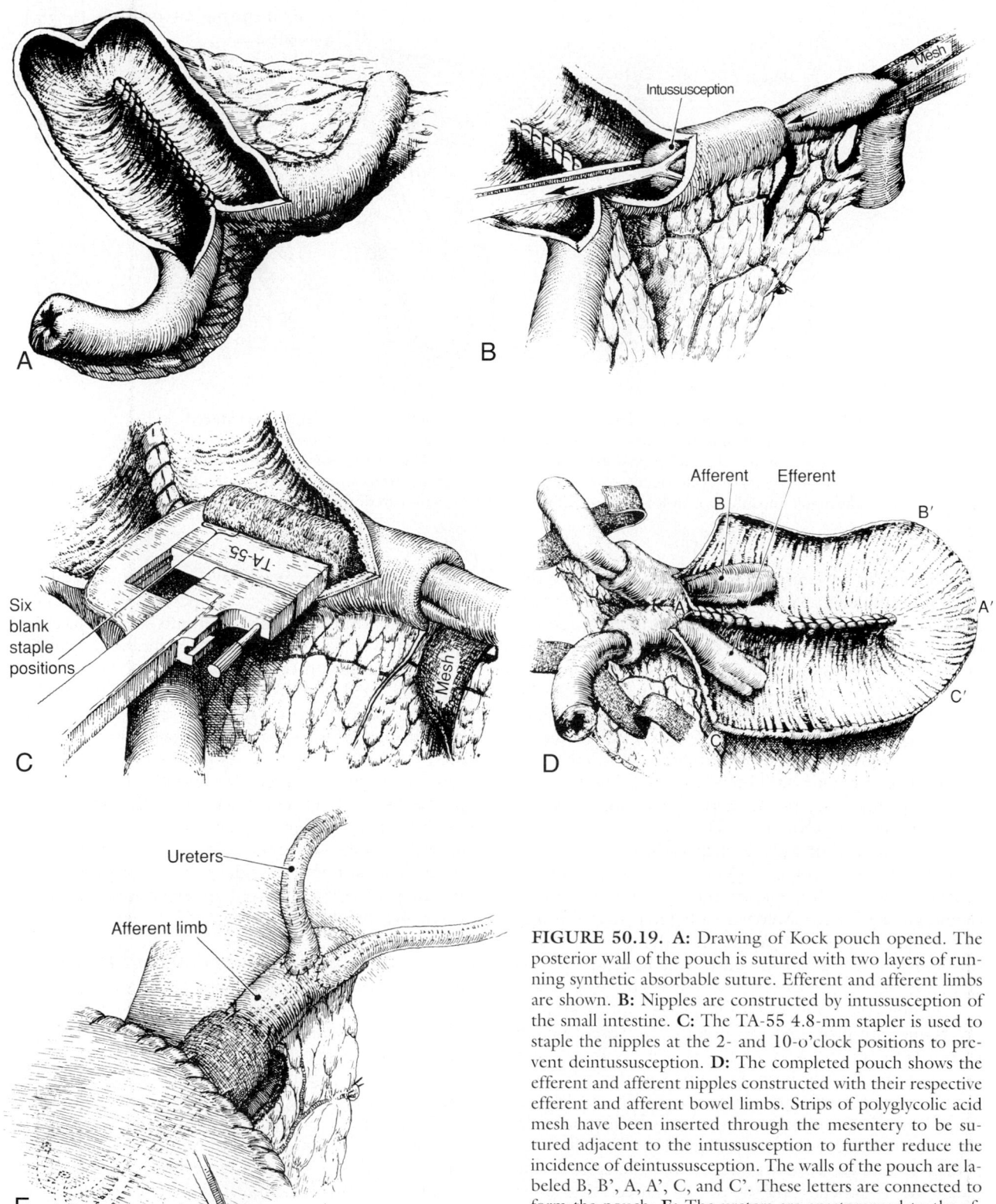

FIGURE 50.19. A: Drawing of Kock pouch opened. The posterior wall of the pouch is sutured with two layers of running synthetic absorbable suture. Efferent and afferent limbs are shown. **B:** Nipples are constructed by intussusception of the small intestine. **C:** The TA-55 4.8-mm stapler is used to staple the nipples at the 2- and 10-o'clock positions to prevent deintussusception. **D:** The completed pouch shows the efferent and afferent nipples constructed with their respective efferent and afferent bowel limbs. Strips of polyglycolic acid mesh have been inserted through the mesentery to be sutured adjacent to the intussusception to further reduce the incidence of deintussusception. The walls of the pouch are labeled B, B', A, A', C, and C'. These letters are connected to form the pouch. **E:** The ureters are anastomosed to the afferent bowel limb over the Silastic stents.

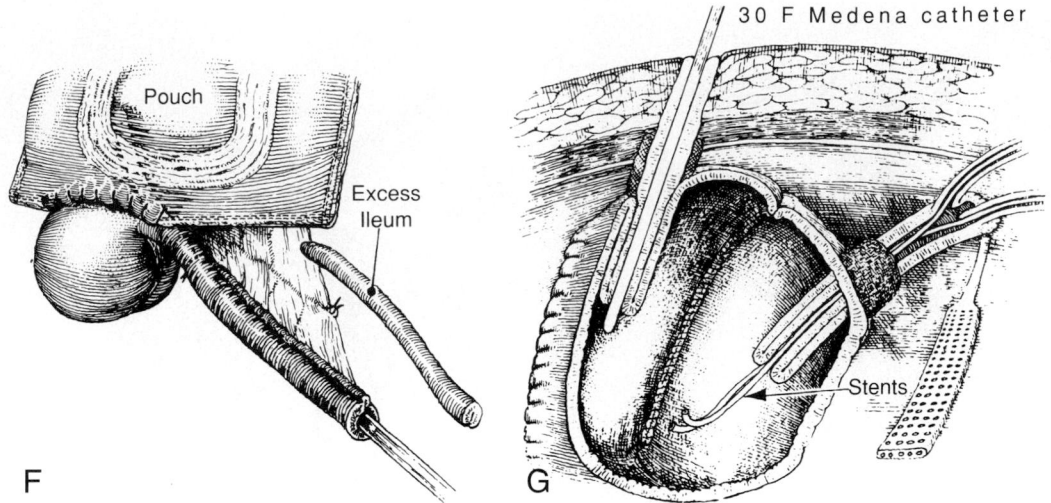

FIGURE 50.19. (*continued*): **F:** The diameter of the lumen of the terminal ileum was reduced by applying the gastrointestinal anastomotic stapler over a number 14-French catheter used as a sizer. **G:** The completed pouch is positioned in the pelvic inlet. The efferent system of the pouch requires a number 24-French Medena catheter placed through the stoma and passed through the efferent nipple into the pouch for drainage of urine. The stoma is exteriorized at the umbilicus.

The nipples are constructed by intussusception of the small intestine (Fig. 50.19B). Stapling the nipple intussusception with a TA-55 4.8-mm stapler to prevent deintussusception is a vital step in this procedure (Fig. 50.19C). The walls of the pouch are folded over and sutured in place to complete the pouch (see Fig. 50.19D). The ureters are anastomosed to the afferent bowel limb over Silastic stents (Fig. 50.19E). The efferent bowel limb is tapered and brought through a defect in the umbilicus. The afferent bowel limb is anchored with suture near the promontory of the sacrum. The pouch itself is positioned in the pelvic inlet. The efferent bowel is tapered to the size of a 20-French catheter with a gastrointestinal anastomotic (GIA) stapler before it is exteriorized (Fig. 50.19F). The efferent system of the pouch requires a 30-French Medena catheter placed through the stoma and passed through the efferent nipple into the pouch for drainage of urine and intestinal mucus (Fig. 50.19G).

During the postoperative phase, all continent urostomies are protected by an adjacent, closed-suction drain placed in the area of the pouch. Leakage from pouch suture lines has been frequent, and, if not drained, a urinoma with septic abscess may occur. The catheter in the efferent limb and nipple and the closed suction drain can be removed 3 weeks postoperatively. Thereafter, the patient is trained by the enterostomal therapist in the technique of catheterizing the pouch. Three weeks postoperatively, endoscopy is performed on the pouch, the Silastic stents are removed from the ureters, and the pouch is tested for ureteral reflux, as well as continence by filling the pouch with 200 mL of radiopaque contrast. An abdominal radiograph is obtained to observe reflux into the kidney. An intravenous pyelogram should be obtained after removal of the ureteral stents for baseline assessment of the kidney. Slight pyelocaliectasis (grade I) is not unusual in the postoperative period. For the first 3 weeks postoperatively, while the stents are in place, the patient is placed on a broad-spectrum antibiotic regimen.

Results of this procedure have been encouraging. In highly irradiated bowel, there is a higher percentage of nipple valve necrosis compared with the Kock and Skinner series that were predominately made up of nonirradiated patients. Long-term evaluation of upper renal tract deterioration in patients with ileal and colonic loops compared with upper renal tract deterioration in patients with continent urostomies awaits further study. Early results reported by Skinner indicate a protective effect on the upper renal tracts secondary to a reduction of contaminated urinary reflux and its associated subclinical chronic pyelonephritis.

Ileocolic Continent Urostomy (Miami Pouch)

Another procedure for continent urostomies following removal of the bladder is the use of a small portion (10 to 15 cm) of terminal ileum, the ascending colon, and proximal transverse colon.

Earlier series of patients having a modification of this procedure, that is, the Indiana pouch, using irradiated bowel were discouraging because the amount of colon used was small (ascending colon only). The smaller segment of irradiated colon may result in higher pouch pressures and, therefore, greater ureteral reflux and incontinence. In a technique described at the University of Miami, modifications used a larger segment of colon that included the entire ascending colon as well as the proximal portion of the transverse colon, resulted in reduced pouch pressure, less reflux, and reduced incontinence (Fig. 50.20). The Miami pouch was developed by Bejany and Politano and was reported in 1988. The intention of

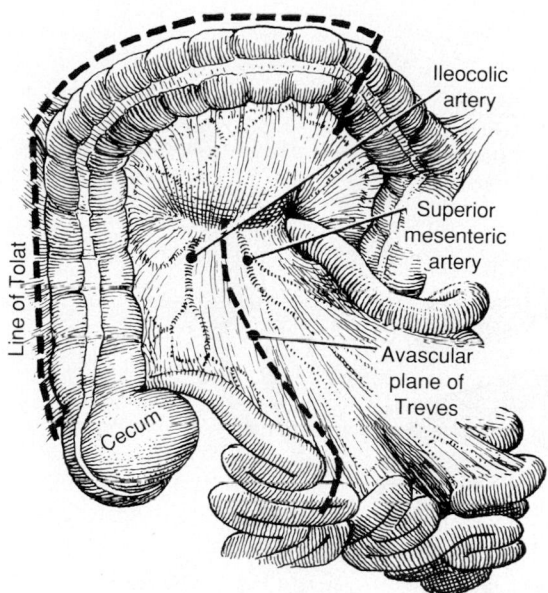

FIGURE 50.20. The ileocolic pouch requires a larger volume of colon. The small bowel is transected about 10 to 15 cm from the ileocecal valve. Incision is carried up the avascular plane of Treves. The transverse colon in transected to provide an equal segment of transverse colon to the right colon. Care is taken to preserve the middle colic artery.

the pouch was to improve the rate of urinary continence, allowing for both increased flexibility in reimplantation of the ureters and an adequate storage system. The alternative to the intussuscepted segment to prevent ureteral reflux was a nontunneled ureterocolonic anastomosis. Continence was achieved by reinforcing the ileocecal segment with three circumferential silk sutures, placed in a pursestring fashion, and tapering the distal segment of the ileum over a 14-French catheter. This technique created a low-pressure reservoir, high-pressure outlet to maximize continence.

The ileocolic continent urostomy (Miami pouch) does not require the intussusception of bowel to create the continent mechanism for the efferent system. A combination of the intact ileocecal valve, as well as reduction in the diameter of the lumen of the terminal ileum by tapering, elevates the pressure in the efferent system to about 80 to 90 cmH$_2$O. The pressure in the efferent system is higher than the pressure in the central pouch, which should be less than 40 cmH$_2$O. It is unclear whether patients who are continent after an ileocolic continent urostomy are continent secondary to an intact (competent) ileocecal valve or from the tapering of the terminal ileum. Furthermore, it is unclear which ureterocolic technique is the best for achieving a nonrefluxing anastomosis of the ureters to the colon. Further data are required to determine whether the traditional technique for achieving antireflux (i.e., embedding the ureter in the wall of the colon) prevents reflux because there is a naturally higher ureteral pressure compared with pouch pressure or because embedding the ureter in

the wall of the colon elevates ureteral pressure to a level greater than the pouch. Stenosis at the ureteral anastomotic site can result in hydroureter and hydronephrosis. A benefit of the ileocolic continent urostomy technique is the elimination of the need for intussusception of the small bowel, as in the Kock pouch, to produce the continent afferent and efferent systems. Construction of an ileocolic continent urostomy (Miami pouch) is technically simpler. It also lends itself to the use of a Polysorb (synthetic absorbable) surgical stapler for closure of the margins of the pouch walls, thereby reducing overall operative time. Finally, there is the potential decreased morbidity by sparing a large segment of small bowel absorptive function that can be seen with small bowel continent reservoirs.

Technique for Ileocolic Continent Urostomy (Miami Pouch)

The distal ileum is transected 10 to 15 cm proximal to the ileocecal valve. The cecum and the segment of ascending colon are mobilized up to the right colic flexure, and the transverse colon is transected just distal to the middle colic artery (Fig. 50.21). Continuity of the bowel is restored with an ileotransverse colon anastomosis. If an appendectomy has not been performed, it should be done during the procedure. The colon is opened with cautery along the tenia and folded onto itself to create a U-shaped intestinal plate (Fig. 50.22). The legs of the "U" are anastomosed in a side-to-side fashion with absorbable staples or interrupted absorbable sutures to form the posterior wall of the reservoir (Fig. 50.23).

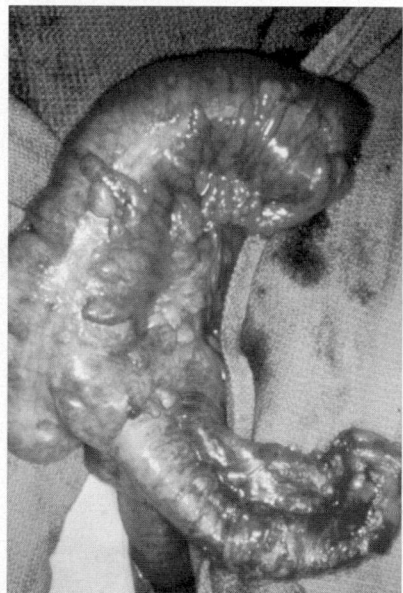

FIGURE 50.21. Pictured is the isolated segment of colon that will be used for construction of a Miami pouch. Approximately 10 to 15 cm of distal ileum are used as are the entire ascending and half of the transverse colon. (From: Estape R, Mendez L, et al. Urinary diversion in gynecologic oncology. *Surg Clin North Am* 2001;81:787, with permission.) See color version of figure.

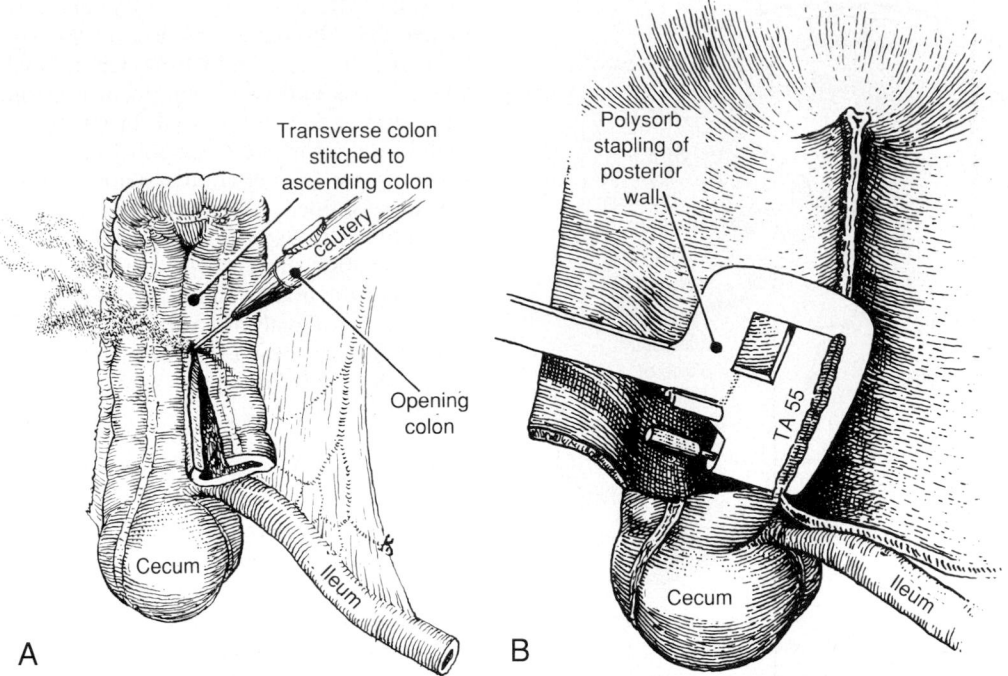

FIGURE 50.22. A: The transverse colon is brought along the side of the right colon. Interrupted sutures are placed in the adjacent segments of colon. A cautery is used to open the antimesenteric border of the transverse and right colon to the cecum. **B:** A TA-55 Polysorb stapler loaded with 0.6-mm staples is used to close the posterior wall of the opened pouch.

This detubularizes the segment of bowel and reduces the potential for high pressure in the colon segment.

The left ureter is passed through the sigmoid mesocolon before entering the reservoir, unless the sigmoid colon has been removed. A mucosal incision is made to create a sulcus in which the ureters will be anastomosed. The distal ends of the ureters are spatulated and, with 4-0 polyglycolic acid sutures, anastomosed to the submucosal layers of the colon. The muscular wall of the colon and the low-pressure reservoir provide the antireflux

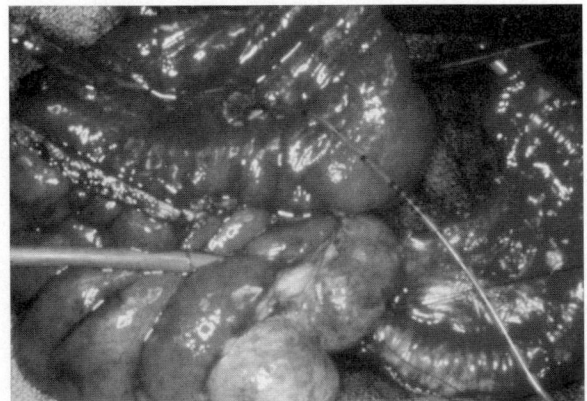

FIGURE 50.23. The opened segment of colon is brought together as a "U" and then the posterior wall is closed first. After this step, the ureters can be brought in to the pouch, secured to the mucosa, and catheterized, as seen here. See color version of figure.

mechanism. Extraluminally, the ureteral adventitia is fixed to the bowel serosa. The ureters are stented with 7-French single-J ureteral diversion stents that are secured distal to the ureterocolonic anastomosis with absorbable sutures or alternatively double-J indwelling catheters may be used. The nontunneled ureteral anastomosis has worked well for us in the colon. Incidence of reflux and obstruction has been similar to that recorded with other forms of intestinal anastomosis.

Tapering the segment of distal ileum and placing pursestring sutures at the level of the ileocecal valve helps create the continence mechanism. A 14-French rubber catheter is placed into the distal ileum. The ileum, with the rubber catheter in place, is clamped using four Babcock clamps on the mesenteric side. Allis clamps are placed on the antimesenteric border of the ileum and pulled to provide mild traction. A stapling instrument is applied to the ileum longitudinally between the Babcock and the Allis clamps to reduce the lumen diameter down to the underlying 14-French catheter (Fig. 50.24). This tapering is done to increase the pressure of this ileal segment and to provide continence by having a higher pressure than the colonic reservoir. Three pursestring sutures (0.5 cm apart) of 2-0 silk or polypropylene are placed in the seromuscular layer of the ileal segment at the level of the ileocecal valve to increase the final closure pressure and achieve urinary continence (Fig. 50.25). The tapered ileal segment is exteriorized as a stoma to the right lower quadrant of the abdomen for future self-catheterization by the patient.

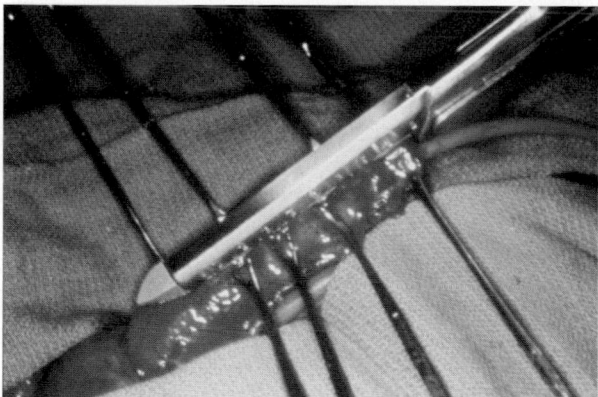

FIGURE 50.24. The second procedure to maintain continence when constructing a Miami pouch is tapering of the distal ileum. The ileal segment is tapered over a 14-French catheter. Care must be taken to taper the antimesenteric side so as not to disrupt blood supply. (From: Estape R, Mendez L, et al. Urinary diversion in gynecologic oncology. *Surg Clin North Am* 2001;81:788, with permission.) See color version of figure.

The anterior wall of the reservoir is then closed with absorbable staples or suture in an interrupted fashion. The reservoir is secured to the abdominal wall peritoneum and the 14-French catheter and single-J stents are secured to the skin after stoma formation low in the right lower quadrant (Fig. 50.26).

Reinforcing the ileocecal valve is considered essential for maintaining continence. The ileocecal junction normally acts as a valve, thus preventing reflux of colonic contents into the lumen. If a urinary reservoir becomes distended, the ileocecal valve alone may not be sufficient to prevent leakage. By tapering the segment of the distal ileum and placing pursestring sutures at the ileocecal valve, the pressure of this segment of bowel exceeds the reservoir pressure at all times, thereby resulting in full continence.

Approximately 2 weeks after surgery, a contrast study of the reservoir and an intravenous urogram are

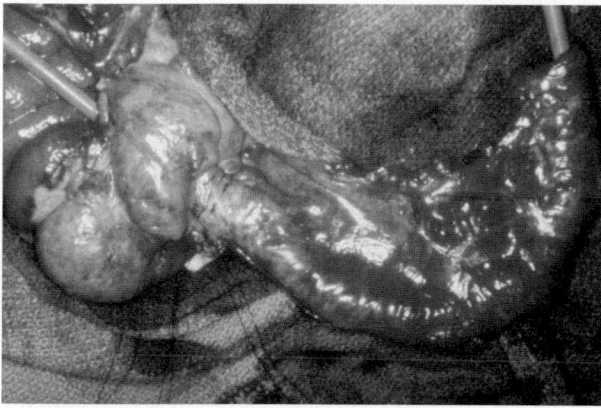

FIGURE 50.25. The continent feature of the efferent system is constructed by two separate surgical techniques. This drawing illustrates two pursestring sutures placed adjacent to the ileocecal junction. See color version of figure.

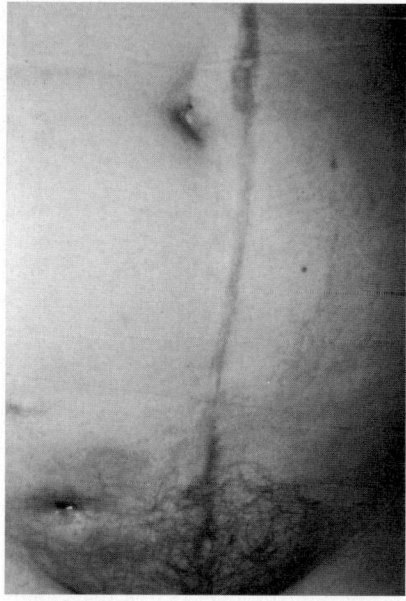

FIGURE 50.26. Shown is a patient who underwent pelvic exenteration with Miami pouch construction. Note the small catheterizable stoma in the right lower quadrant. (From: Estape R, Mendez L, et al. Urinary diversion in gynecologic oncology. *Surg Clin North Am* 2001;81:789, with permission.) See color version of figure.

performed to evaluate for leakage, reflux, or upper tract obstruction. If the radiographs show normal findings, the ureteral stents are removed and the patient is taught to irrigate and catheterize the pouch. Initially, the patient catheterizes the stoma every 2 to 4 hours and irrigates it four times a day. The patient gradually decreases the frequency of catheterization and irrigation if continence and/or obstruction of the catheter by mucus is not a problem. Patients describe a feeling of fullness or slight cramping in the right lower quadrant indicating the need to empty the reservoir. The average frequency of catheterization is five to six catheterizations in 24 hours. The time needed for emptying the reservoir is about 3½ minutes. The amount of urine for each catheterization averages 365 mL (range, 250 to 500 mL). Urodynamic evaluation of the reservoir reveals that the basal pressure fluctuates between 10 and 20 cm of water, whereas in the tapered ileum it varies between 50 and 60 cm of water.

We have recently reviewed the incidence and management of the urinary complications related to the creation of the Miami pouch at the Division of Gynecologic Oncology of the University of Miami. The majority of the patients who had urinary diversion, 68 of 90 (76%), underwent pelvic exenteration for recurrent cervical cancer and the majority of these (93.5%) were previously irradiated. The most common complications of the 90 patients evaluated were urinary tract infection/pyelonephritis (40%), ureteral stricture/obstruction (20%), difficult catheterization (18%), and pouch leakage (14%). It is now clear that most of the complications related to the urinary diversion can be safely treated conservatively. Conservative treatment was efficacious in most of the urinary complications related to the creation of the Miami pouch. In this study, ureteral strictures were encountered in 10 patients (13%). All strictures were noted at the level of the ureterocolonic anastomosis. Conservative management includes balloon dilation, stent placement, and nephrostomy placement. Conservative treatment was successful in 8 of the 10 patients. Ureteral obstruction due to stone formation was treated with lithotripsy in one patient, the other required surgical revision because of the dimension of the stones. Another five patients presented with ureteral obstruction, four of which cases were successfully managed conservatively. The total number of patients with stones was four (5.2%); only one, as previously mentioned, required surgical revision. Five patients developed a fistula with the Miami pouch; three of these cases were also managed conservatively.

In summary, although complications related to the creation of the Miami pouch are not infrequent, early detection and conservative management are now recommended to manage the majority of these patients safely. Conservative management should be attempted whenever possible, but surgical intervention should not be delayed when indicated. The optimal management of these complications consists of multidisciplinary approach with the active participation of endoscopists, urologists, and radiologists.

TECHNIQUES TO RESTORE RECTAL FUNCTION

In many gynecologic malignancies, resection of the rectosigmoid colon may be indicated to achieve optimal cure rates. In diseases ranging from primary ovarian cancer to recurrent cervical cancer, the rectosigmoid may need resection even with the anus for proper surgical management. In cases in which the anus is resected, the patient has few options except end colostomy. However, efforts have been made in patients who have rectal and anus-sparing procedures to improve the technical and functional results by reanastomosis. Metastasis of cervical cancer to the anus and lower rectum is rare. In 1954, Javert reported that the number of metastases of cervical carcinoma of the anus and rectum was less than 1%. Survival rates from sphincter-sparing supralevator pelvic exenteration procedures have not been statistically different from those in which the rectum is removed. Metastasis of ovarian cancer to the anus and lower rectum is also extremely rare. Therefore, in gynecologic oncology procedures, it seems reasonable to make every effort to retain the anus in order to preserve fecal continence and avoid permanent colostomy.

Rectosigmoid Colon Resection and "Straight" Colorectal Anastomosis

The first event that truly led to technically easier anastomosis operations was the widespread use of circular stapling devices in the 1980s . At first, fears existed that these stapled anastomoses would leak when compared with hand-sewing. Studies of the double staple line by Knight and Griffen confirmed the adequacy of the circular stapling device. The ability to resect tumors deep in the pelvis (>2 cm above the dentate line) with adequate margins (at least 2 cm) and perform a technically simple anastomosis procedure has spared many patients an undesirable end colostomy. This technique is described in Chapter 49.

The straight end-to-end colorectal anastomosis is not without its critics. Functional studies have revealed poor results with defecation disorders (leakage, urgency) in up to 30% of patients, usually related to residual rectal length. Wheeless reported in 1987 on incontinence and dysfunction in gynecologic patients undergoing very low straight colorectal anastomoses. An unacceptably high 70% of patients reported more than four bowel movements per day, even 2 years after surgery. Some physiologic studies seem to indicate that the incontinence is due to damage of the internal anal sphincter. Introduction of any instrument transanally should be done with the utmost caution.

Frequency disorders on the other hand are a result of loss of rectal storage function. Many patients tend to improve over time, probably from an increased reservoir function of the remaining rectal stump; however, this adaptive period may last up to 2 years. For this reason, surgical options to improve functionality in patients undergoing rectosigmoid colon resection and anastomosis have been introduced with good results.

Colonic J-Pouch Reservoir for Very Low Coloproctostomy

Patients in whom a very low anterior resection of the colon was performed were frequently left with an end sigmoid colostomy and low Hartmann pouch. Historical attempts to reestablish continuity of the fecal stream in patients requiring very low anastomosis (<5 cm from anus) of the colon to the rectum at or below the level of the levator sling met with discouraging results.

Tenesmus and fecal frequency are common side effects of very low end-to-end coloproctostomy after very low rectosigmoid resection. The creation of a rectal J-pouch reservoir, even in irradiated colon and rectum, appears to restore the rectal ampullae bulb reservoir and is an effective method of substantially decreasing these troublesome symptoms.

As shown in Figure 50.27, the sigmoid colon is folded on itself with 5 to 7 cm extending into the afferent and efferent segments. A defect is opened in the bottom of the J-pouch and the 10-cm in-line stapler with 4.8-mm staples is placed in both loops of the colon and fired. The end-to-end anastomosis (EEA) stapler is inserted through the rectum after two pursestring sutures are placed in the rectal stump and the bottom of the J-pouch. The EEA stapler is fired and the anastomosis is completed. The integrity of the anastomosis is tested by inserting a sigmoidoscope per anus, pumping air through the sigmoidoscope into the J-pouch, and ob-

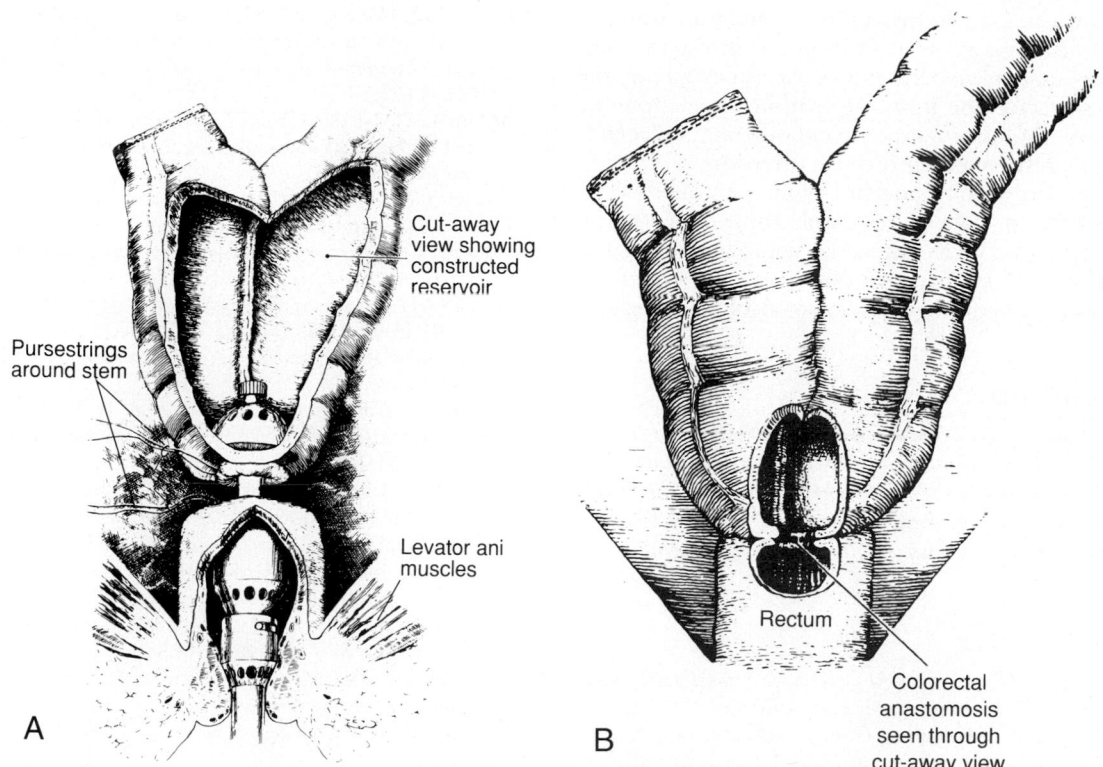

Cut-away
view showing
constructed
reservoir

Pursestrings
around stem

Levator ani
muscles

A

Rectum

Colorectal
anastomosis
seen through
cut-away view

B

FIGURE 50.27. A: A cutaway view of the completed rectal J-pouch is shown positioned over the anus and rectal stump with the end-to-end anastomosis stapler inserted through the anus up the rectum. The anvil of the stapler has been inserted into the pouch, and two adjacent pursestring sutures are applied and tied around the central rod. The stapler is closed and activated. **B:** Completed rectal J-pouch coloproctostomy.

serving all stapled sutured lines for air leaks under saline placed into the pelvis.

The problem of tenesmus and fecal frequency in very low anastomosis has been addressed by Lazorthes and co-workers in a study of 65 patients who underwent low anterior resection of the colon for rectal carcinoma. Forty of the 65 patients underwent end-to-end anastomosis at a mean distance of 2.3 cm from the anal verge, and 20 had construction of a rectal J-pouch reservoir with anastomosis to rectum at a mean distance of 1.4 cm from the anal verge. A statistically significant difference in the number of patients having fecal frequency was noted between the group with end-to-end anastomosis versus those having construction of a rectal J-pouch reservoir. A total of 60% of those with a J-pouch reservoir had one to two bowel movements per day versus 33% of those with an end-to-end anastomosis. Fecal frequency in these patients is due to the surgical removal of the rectal ampullae, which acts as a low pressure pouch that does not produce tenesmus until it is full. This improvement was ascribed to a manometrically confirmed and statistically significant higher maximum pressure and tolerable fecal volume in the neorectum of those patients with a neoreservoir (J-pouch) versus those having direct end-to-end anastomosis.

This is especially true in gynecologic oncology patients with irradiated rectosigmoid colons whose compliance is reduced. Therefore, the radius of the end-to-end anastomosis is small and, under Laplace's law, the pressure becomes high. In the J-pouch, the radius is larger; therefore, the pressure is lower. There is little tenesmus and fecal frequency is significantly reduced. A confirmatory study was published by Parc and colleagues who reported on 30 patients who underwent low anterior resection and rectal J-pouch coloproctostomy. After surgery, the mean number of bowel movements in this group was 1.1 per day, and no patients reported tenesmus.

The use of this technique in patients undergoing surgery for gynecologic malignancy, particularly those whose condition has been previously treated with total pelvic irradiation and brachytherapy, has not been extensive. Some suggestion has been made that with the J-pouch there is a better blood supply leading to a decreased incidence of anastomosis breakdown in patients with a history of pelvic radiotherapy.

The colonic J-pouch is not without complications itself. The principal shortcoming is incomplete emptying. Several studies have been directed at the limb length of the J-pouch. To minimize this problem, the consensus seems to be to construct a useful reservoir the limb length of 5 to 7 cm in length.

The issue of a protective colostomy or ileostomy when performing a colorectal anastomosis usually rears its ugly head at about this time. The literature at this time is unclear. Data in the colorectal literature suggests it is beneficial. However, data from our institution suggests, for patients undergoing pelvic exenteration, the major risk factor for fistula formation or anastomotic breakdown is a history of pelvic radiotherapy, independent of the presence of a protective diversion.

In summary, colon J-pouches significantly improve the quality of life for patients, especially those patients who have irradiated bowel and in whom significant portions of the small bowel have been removed. It should be considered by all who perform gynecologic oncology surgery.

ACKNOWLEDGMENT

We would like to acknowledge Clifford R. Wheeless, Jr., M. D., for his contributions to the current and prior editions of this chapter. Dr. Wheeless is a pioneer in the field of reconstructive gynecologic surgery and his work has continued the rich tradition of the true pelvic surgeon.

BIBLIOGRAPHY

Alexandrov MS. *Obrazovanie Iskustvennogo Vlagalishcha iz Sigmovidnoi Kishki.* Moskva: Medgiz, 1955:185.

Angioli R, Estape R, Cantuaria G, et al. Urinary complications of Miami pouch: trend of conservative management. *Am J Obstet Gynecol* 1998;179:343.

Bejany DE, Politano VA. Stapled and nonstapled tapered distal ileum for construction of a continent colonic urinary reservoir. *J Urol* 1988;140:491.

Berek JS, Hacker NF, Lagasse LD. Delayed vaginal reconstruction in the fibrotic pelvis following radiation or previous reconstruction. *Obstet Gynecol* 1983;61:331.

Berek JS, Hacker NF, Lagasse LD. Vaginal reconstruction performed simultaneous with pelvic exenteration. *Obstet Gynecol* 1984;63:318.

Bricker EM. Symposium on clinical surgery. Bladder substitution after pelvic evisceration. *Surg Clin North Am* 1950;30:1511.

Broderick GA, Stone AR. Neo-bladders: clinical management and considerations for patients receiving chemotherapy. *Semin Oncol* 1990;17:598.

Brown SR, Seow-Choen F. Preservation of rectal function after low anterior resection with formation of a neorectum. *Semin Surg Oncol* 2000;19:376.

Brunschwig A. Complete excision of the pelvic viscera for advanced carcinoma. *Cancer* 1948;1:177.

Burger RA, Riedmiller H, Friedberg V, et al. The ileocecal vagina. *Geburtshilfe Frauenheilkd* 1987;47:644.

Cain JM, Diamond A, Tamimi HK, et al. The morbidity and benefits of concurrent myocutaneous graft with pelvic exenteration. *Obstet Gynecol* 1989;74:185–188.

Carlson JW, Carter JR, Saltzman AK, et al. Gynecologic reconstruction with a rectus abdominis myocutaneous flap: an update. *Gynecol Oncol* 1996;61:364–368.

Carlson JW, Saltzman AK, Carter JR, et al. Recurrent squamous cell carcinoma in a rectus abdominis neovagina. *Gynecol Oncol* 1995;59:159–161.

Carlson JW, Soisson AP, Fowler JM, et al. Rectus abdominis myocutaneous flap for primary vaginal reconstruction. *Gynecol Oncol* 1993;51:323–329.

Coliger JC. Functional results from sphincter saving resection of the rectum. *Ann R Coll Surg Engl* 1951;8:42.

Copeland LJ, Hancock KC, Gershenson DM, et al. Gracilis myocutaneous vaginal reconstruction concurrent with total pelvic exenteration. *Am J Obstet Gynecol* 1989;160:1095–1101.

Cordonnier JJ, Nicolai CH. An evaluation of the use of an isolated segment of ileum as a means of urinary diversion. *J Urol* 1972;83:834.

Cormack GC, Lamberty BG. The blood supply of the thigh skin. *Plast Reconst Surg* 1985;75:342.

DiSaia PJ, Creasman WT. Invasive cervical cancer. In: *Clinical gynecologic oncology,* second ed. St. Louis: CV Mosby, 1984:61.

Froese DP, Haggitt RC, Friend WG. Ulcerative colitis in the autotransplanted neovagina. *Gastroenterology* 1991;100:1749–1752

Gleeson NC, Baile W, Roberts WS, et al. Pudendal thigh fasciocutaneous flaps for vaginal reconstruction. *Gynecol Oncol* 1994;54:269.

Gleeson NC, Baile W, Roberts WS, et al. Surgical and psychosexual outcome following vaginal reconstruction with total pelvic exenteration. *Eur J Gynecol Oncol* 1994;15:88.

Hallbook O, Johansson K Sjodahl R. Laser Doppler blood flow measurement in rectal resection for carcinoma—comparison between the straight and the colonic J pouch construction. *Br J Surg* 1996;83:389.

Harris WJ, Wheeless CR. Use of the end-to-end anastomosis stapling device in low colo-rectal anastomosis associated with radical gynecology surgery. *Gynecol Oncol* 1986;23:350.

Hartenbach EM, Saltzman AK, Carter JR, et al. Nonsurgical management strategies for the functional complications of ileocolonic continent urinary reservoirs. *Gynecol Oncol* 1995;56:127(abst).

Hida J, Yasutomi M, Maruyama T, et al. Functional outcome after low anterior resection with low anastomosis for rectal cancer using the colonic J pouch: prospective randomized study for determination of optimum pouch size. *Dis Colon Rectum* 1996;39:986.

Hida J, Yasutomi M, Maruyama T, et al. Indications for colonic J pouch reconstruction after anterior resection for rectal cancer. *Dis Colon Rectum* 1998;41:558.

Hirshowitz B, Lindenbaum E. A skin stretching device for harnessing of the visco-elastic properties of skin. *J Plast Reconstr Surg* 1993;92:260.

Ho YH, Tsang C, Tang CL, et al. Anal sphincter injuries from stapling instruments introduced transanally. Randomized, controlled study with endoanal ultrasound and anorectal manometry. *Dis Colon Rectum* 2000;43:169.

Javert CT. Lymph nodes and lymph channels of the pelvis. In: Meigs JV, ed. *Surgical treatment of cancer of the cervix.* New York: Grune & Stratton, 1954.

Julian CG, Woodruff JD. Surgery of the vulva: vulvectomy. In: Ridley JH, ed. *Gynecologic surgery errors, safeguards, salvage.* Baltimore: Williams & Wilkins, 1974:256.

Kindermann G. The sigmoid vagina: experiences in the treatment of congenital absence or later loss of vagina. *Geburtshilfe Frauenheilkd* 1987;47:650.

Knight CD, Griffen FD. An improved technique for low anterior resection of the rectum using the EEA stapler. *Surgery* 1980;88:710.

Kock NG, Nilson AE, Nilsson LO, et al. Urinary diversion via continent ileal reservoir: clinical results of 12 patients. *Urology* 1982;128:469.

Kusiak JF, Rosenblum NG. Neovaginal reconstruction after exenteration using an omental flap and split-thickness skin graft. *Plast Reconstr Surg* 1996;97(4):775–781.

Lahey FH. Disadvantages of sphincter preserving operations for cancer of the rectum. *JAMA* 1951;149:626.

Lazorthes F, Fages P, Chiotasso P, et al. Resection of the rectum with construction of a colonic reservoir and colo-anal anastomosis for carcinoma of the rectum. *Br J Surg* 1986;73:136.

Licklider D, Mauffray O. Conventional urostomy vs continent urostomy. *Ostomy Wound Management* 1991;34:26.

McCraw JB, Massey FM, Shanklin KD, et al. Vaginal reconstruction with gracilis myocutaneous flap. *Plast Reconstr Surg* 1976;58:176.

McIndoe A. Treatment of congenital absence and obliterative condition of vagina. *Br J Plast Surg* 1950;2:254.

McIndoe AH, Banister JB. An operation for the care of congenital absence of the vagina. *Obstet Gynaecol Br Emp* 1938;45:490.

Mirhashemi R, Averette H, Estape R, et al. Low colorectal anastomosis following radical pelvic surgery: a risk factor analysis. *Am J Obstet Gynecol* 2000;183(6):1375–1380.

Morley G, DeLancey JO. Full thickness skin graft vaginoplasty for treatment of the stenotic or foreshortened vagina. *Obstet Gynecol* 1991;77:485.

Orr JW, Shingleton HM, Hatch KD, et al. Urinary diversion in patients undergoing pelvic exenteration. *Am J Obstet Gynecol* 1982;142:883.

Pappalardo G, Toccaceli S, Dionisio P, et al. Preoperative and postoperative evaluation by manometric study of the anal sphincter after coloanal anastomosis for carcinoma. *Dis Colon Rectum* 1988;31:119.

Parc R, Tiret E, Frileaux P, et al. Resection and colo-anal anastomosis with colonic reservoir for rectal carcinoma. *Br J Surg* 1986;73:139.

Penalver MA, Angioli R, Mirhashemi R, et al. Management of early and late complications of ileocolonic continent urinary reservoir (Miami pouch). *Gynecol Oncol* 1998;69:185.

Pursell SH, Day TG, Tobin TG. Distally based rectus abdominis flap for reconstruction in radical gynecologic procedures. *Gynecol Oncol* 1990;37:234–238.

Ratliff CR, Gershenson DM, Morris M, et al. Sexual adjustment of patients undergoing gracilis myocutaneous flap vaginal reconstruction in conjunction with pelvic exenteration. *Cancer* 1996;78:2229-35.

Ravitch M, Steichen FM. A stapling instrument for end to end inverting anastomosis in the gastrointestinal tract. *Ann Surg* 1979;189:791.

Richie JP, Skinner DG, Waisman J. The effect of reflux on the development of pyelonephritis in urinary diversion. An experimental study. *J Surg Res* 1974;16:256.

Rowland RG, Mitchell ME, Bihrle, et al. Indiana continent urinary reservoir. *J Urol* 1987;137:1136.

Schmidt JD, Buchsbaum HJ, Jacoby EC. Transverse colon conduit for supra-vesical urinary tract diversion. *Urology* 1976;8:542.

Skinner DG, Boyd SD, Lieskovsky G. Ongoing experiences with the Kock continent ileal reservoir for urinary diversion. *World J Urol* 1985;3:155.

Skinner DG, Lieskovsky G, Boyd SD. Continuing experience in continent urinary diversion: the Kock pouch in 250 patients. Read before the American Urological Association. New York, 1986.

Skinner DG, Lieskovsky G, Boyd SD. Technique of creation of a continent internal ileal reservoir (Kock pouch) for urinary diversion. *Urol Clin North Am* 1984;11:741.

Smith HO, Genesen MC, Runowicz CD, et al. The rectus abdominis myocutaneous flap. Modifications, complications and sexual function. *Cancer* 1998;83:510–520.

Soper JT, Berchuck A, Creasman WT, et al. Pelvic exenteration: Factors associated with major surgical morbidity. *Gynecol Oncol* 1989;35:93–98.

Tateo A, Tateo S, Bernasconi C, et al. Use of the V-Y flap for vulvar reconstruction. *Gynecol Oncol* 1996;62:203.

Taussig F. Primary cancer of the vulva, vagina and female urethra. Five year results. *Surg Gynecol Obstet* 1935;60:477.

Thuroff JW, Alken P, Engelmann U, et al. Der Mainz-Pouch zur Blasenerweiterungsplastik und kontinenten Harnableitung. *Akt Urol* 1985;16:1.

Tobin GR, Day TG. Vaginal and pelvic reconstruction with a distally based rectus abdominis and myocutaneous flaps. *Plast Reconstr Surg* 1988;81:62–73.

Valle G, Ferraris G. Use of the omentum to contain the intestines in pelvic exenteration. *Obstet Gynecol* 1969;33:772.

Way S. The anatomy of the lymphatic drainage of the vulva and its influence on the radical operation for carcinoma. *Ann R Coll Surg Engl* 1948;3:187.

Wheeless CR. *Atlas of pelvic surgery.* Philadelphia: Lea & Febiger, 1988.

Wheeless CR. Estrogen/progesterone receptors in split-thickness skin graft used for neo-vagina in gynecologic oncology patients. *Trans South Surg Assoc* 1990;CII:215.

Wheeless CR. Gracilis myocutaneous flap in reconstruction of the vulva and female perineum. *Obstet Gynecol* 1979;54:97.

Wheeless CR. Incidence of fecal incontinence after coloproctostomy below 5 cm in the rectum. *Gynecol Oncol* 1987;27:373.

Wheeless CR. Neo-vagina constructed from an omental J flap and split thickness skin graft. *Gynecol Oncol* 1989;35:224.

Wheeless CR. Recent advances in surgical reconstruction of the gynecologic cancer patient. *Curr Opin Obstet Gynecol* 1992;4:91.

Wheeless CR, Hempling RE. Rectal J pouch reservoir to decrease the frequency of tenesmus and defecation in low coloproctostomy. *Gynecol Oncol* 1989;35:136.

Williams NS, Price R, Johnston D. The long term effect of sphincter preserving operations for rectal carcinoma on the function of the anal sphincter in man. *Br J Surg* 1980;67:208.

Te Linde's Operative Gynecology, ninth edition, edited by John A. Rock and Howard W. Jones, III. Lippincott Williams & Wilkins, Philadelphia © 2003.

CHAPTER

51

▼

Training the Gynecologic Surgeon

ROBERT M. ROGERS, JR.

A true crisis in the quantity and quality of gynecologic surgical training has been gradually evolving over the past 15 years. This crisis has acutely accelerated in the past several years with the various pressures to train many more laparoscopic and hysteroscopic surgeons. The traditional apprenticeship model of teaching surgery to gynecology residents has failed to keep up, especially in the training of the newer surgical modalities. Despairingly, there is now an exodus of many skilled surgeons and seasoned instructors out of academic and teaching centers because of the many reimbursement and financial pressures. Where are we now? Where are we going? What are we to do? What does the future hold for gynecologic surgery and the training of competent gynecologic surgeons?

WHERE ARE WE NOW?

Teachers of gynecologic surgery have noted a significant and generalized decrease in the number and types of major gynecologic cases from which they can teach the resident surgeon. These decreasing numbers of cases have resulted from the various financial pressures on many levels, a much better educated consumer, and the dramatic increase in medical management of previously surgically managed problems in gynecology. Financial constraints in the past decade have dramatically impacted the payment policies of the various payers of medical services—health maintenance organizations, fee-for-service payers,

and especially the government mandated health care programs, Medicare and Medicaid. There is less money available for medical and surgical care.

Previous requirements for second surgical opinions have rolled over into mandatory precertification protocols by the various payers. These protocols are administered by nonmedical personnel via fixed computer screen questions. These cascades of criteria do not allow for the unique and individual input that each caring physician and surgeon adds to the judgment mix in determining the final treatment course for the individual patient. This has significantly narrowed the surgical options for various gynecologic complaints. These financial constraints have resulted in a dramatic increase in the number of office and outpatient surgical procedures that are done, significantly decreasing the major surgical cases available for resident teaching.

In addition, the consumer herself has become much better educated via television reports and programs, radio talk shows, friends, women's organizations, various publications, and particularly the Internet. More and more, patients come to us as service providers with a full knowledge of the many options, both surgical and nonsurgical, that are available.

Surgical case loads have also decreased because of the increasing use of conservative medical management in dealing with previously defined surgical problems. Many cases of endometriosis and uterine fibroids are now managed by hormonal manipulation, such as with progesterones or gonadotropin agonists. In addition, more cases of ectopic pregnancy are managed with the administration of methotrexate and not necessarily through laparoscopic or laparotomy intervention.

Along with the decreasing gynecologic surgical case load, teachers of gynecologic surgery have also noticed a troublesome decrease in the quality of teaching within the more than 260 accredited residency programs in obstetrics and gynecology in the United States. These changes are the result of the changing curriculum in the residencies; the changing perceptions, attitudes, lifestyles, and goals of the residents themselves; the new financial pressures placed upon each individual academic teacher; and the overwhelming changes in the funding of individual departments of obstetrics and gynecology. In addition, with the maturation of operative hysteroscopy, operative laparoscopy, and more technically involved and challenging procedures, the traditional apprenticeship model of teaching residents in the operating room and in the procedure rooms has failed to keep up with the needed training.

Because of the decreasing reimbursements to all levels of hospital departments, including residency programs, the residents are taking on more and more clinical responsibilities with *less* dedicated time for educational activities. Yet with the advent of the primary care initiatives in gynecologic education and with the significantly increased knowledge base that the current Ob/Gyn resident must master within the same 4-year training period, there are real demands for *more* dedicated time blocks for resident teaching and learning. The present gynecology resident is physically and emotionally stressed with little time to concentrate on studying and learning. Little time is left for personal recreation and rejuvenation or family activities. A recent study concerning resident attitudes about work hours revealed that most residents would like to limit their work hours because of fatigue, the need for more personal and family time, and concerns of compromising the quality of their services. The most common reason for wanting more training time was for additional surgical experiences.

Although not formally documented, many gynecologic surgeons are concerned about medical-legal liability in teaching residents, particularly in the newer, more complex operative laparoscopic and operative hysteroscopic procedures. They are afraid of increasing the chances for medical and surgical errors.

Because of financial pressures, there has been an exodus of many skilled surgeons and seasoned instructors to private practice or into health-related industries, such as pharmaceutical companies or surgical products companies. Some have even chosen early retirement. Many medical doctors are now pursuing or have obtained their degrees in business administration. Some have found other nonacademic pursuits in which to supplement their incomes. All these pursuits take time away from effective and dedicated resident teaching in gynecologic surgery.

Those clinical instructors who remain to teach the residents no longer have dedicated time to teach. They have intense pressures upon them to generate within their departments the income to support themselves and their associated overheads, as well as the many departmental activities and financial obligations. These same pressures urge the attending surgeon to conduct operations himself or herself as much as possible to speed the case along, get the case done, and thus allow the next scheduled case to start sooner, so that more surgical cases can be performed in the same day of surgery. This is financially efficient. Obviously, the resident becomes a technical assistant with little opportunity for verbal and hands-on instruction. The teaching attending feels that he or she can perform the case faster and better with perceived significantly lessened medical-legal risk. This perception may not necessarily be true, however.

Just as importantly, gynecologic teachers have noted that there is significantly less time at the scrub sink to discuss surgical cases, including their presentations, findings, medical or surgical options, surgical techniques, and various approaches to performing that surgery. Fifteen years ago, there was a mandatory 5- to 10-minute scrub at the sink, at which time the teaching surgeon and resident could establish a personal rapport and initiate a friendly teaching environment. Now, to maximize the time efficiency of that particular room, the scrub time is only 1 to 2 minutes and the team is quickly in the operating room.

Furthermore, the vast majority of teaching in the apprenticeship model is teacher oriented rather than student oriented. Most times, this teaching is haphazard without structure, without goals, without purpose. Reznick from the Department of Surgery, The University of Toronto, wrote in 1993:

> An important aspect of teaching operative skills is a realization that residents are adult learners. As such, teaching principles developed from adult learning theory will apply.
> Adult learning is enhanced by an approach that is self-directed and centered on the learner rather than on the teacher. Adult learning is facilitated by focusing on a problem or task. Abstract, subject-centered learning is less effective as a motivator. Adults come to an education activity, such as a surgical rotation, with a vast amount of past experience that must be recognized and utilized.

Many times surgical knowledge is accumulated passively and is taught by "a trial by exhaustion and humiliation, as well as a journey of harassment and abuse" (Dunnington). As more and more clinical mentors leave the teaching of residents, the remaining instructors do not have the experience, maturity, time, interest, or expertise to do effective teaching. As a result of the unstructured, individual teacher-oriented model of surgical training and decreasing case loads, the surgical skills and surgical judgment of senior gynecologic residents remain highly variable, individual, and uniformly unmeasured.

The advent of laparoscopic procedures has also complicated the training of gynecologic surgeons in another way. A laparoscopic surgeon may be well trained in laparoscopic procedures and the use of laparoscopic instruments, but that surgeon is rendered most ineffective unless he or she has able, knowledgeable, and skilled assistance from a harmonious laparoscopic team. Laparoscopy is not an individual endeavor but is a team endeavor wherein the quality of the team determines the quality of laparoscopic surgery and not the individual skills of the laparoscopic surgeons.

A shift has occurred in the learning environment of many residencies. In the past, the older gynecologic surgeons spoke of a sense of community, a sense of purpose, a sense of pride in their individual residency training and gynecologic programs. Today, more residents appear to be overwhelmed by their patient responsibilities and lack real surgical training. There are presently no measurable standards by which to determine how well a gynecologic resident has been trained in various gynecologic surgical procedures. The surgical training method of apprenticeship with an individual mentor is no longer producing surgically qualified gynecologic surgeons. The role of "see one; do one; teach one" is wholly inadequate in this new era of laparoscopic surgery, operative hysteroscopy, and expansion of surgical and medical knowledge needed to treat previous surgical gynecologic problems. The operating room cases available for resident training vary widely. They cannot be standardized for resident training, they may or may not be of sufficient difficulty and complexity for training, and they may involve instructors who are not educated and experienced enough to do effective training in the operating room.

WHAT ARE WE TO DO?

> You will remember a little of what you hear, some of what you read, considerably more
> of what you see, but almost all of what you understand.—Roger C. Crafts

This statement not only applies to the learning of scientific knowledge and principles, but also applies to the learning of technical skills and medical/surgical judgments. Studies of highly successful individuals, particularly with athletic or musical talents, indicate that their success is dependent upon several factors (Gawande). The first is, of course, individual motivation and talent. In the surgical field, obviously, hand-eye coordination and other psychomotor technical skills are inherent within the individual, yet they must be developed. In addition, the successful resident has an inborn ability to face mistakes and failure with an eye to learning and improving rather than taking a guilty, defeatist attitude.

Second, the successful individual plans dedicated time for practice, practice, and more practice, yet in an effective and efficient positive way. Complex procedures must be broken down into individual, practiceable components with immediate feedback from a trained observer. As has been said, "Practice does not make perfect, perfect practice makes perfect." The repetitive performance of specific skills has been shown to be much more effective in surgical training than general training involving multitask procedures (Hamdorf).

Third, the highest performing successful individuals have clarity, purpose, and imagination in their chosen field. "The ability to improvise, to cope skillfully with novel situations, requires vision, which takes years to develop" (Gawande).

Equally important, the training of the skilled and talented gynecologic surgeon must involve a skilled, caring, and interested mentor. The teaching quality of surgery faculty does have an impact on positive student performance. This must also include a positive environment for immediate evaluation from both self and mentor. This environment many times is delicate and balances between confidence-building positive and self-defeating negative. Reznick from Toronto writes:

> Surgical preceptors serve as extremely potent and influential role models. We do so in all the aspects of an operation, from our approach to tissue handling to our interpersonal relationships in the operating room. The second aspect is coaching. This role as a coach reminds us of a need to provide encouragement and discipline to the resident. In this way, we help create a scaffold upon which the resident can build.

Levels of resident surgical training include the use of the individual senses: hearing, seeing, and tactile feeling. In addition, these individual surgical skills need to be practiced and then integrated into an operative framework. This framework enables the resident to perform a procedure step-by-step. However, fluidity of these skills, along with operative judgment, demands further refined practice and experience under close, critical supervision. This final maturation process, called *automization*, not only involves psychomotor skill development, clinical judgment, excellence, and knowledge of the literature, but also involves the development of interpersonal skills with emphasis on managing the operating room team.

Learning through hearing involves carefully crafted, presented, and coordinated lectures, case presentations, and discussions. Observational activities include seeing videos, watching various surgical exercises on inanimate trainers, watching cadaveric dissections, and, of course, observing live surgical procedures. The development of hand-eye coordination and hands-on surgical skills involves the use of inanimate trainers, computer simulators, animal models, human cadaveric dissections, and, of course, surgery on actual patients under the careful tutelage of a surgical instructor and mentor. Obviously, the teaching and evaluation of surgical skills and clinical judgment before entering the live operating room presents several distinct ethical, medical-legal, and financial advantages.

Lectures and case discussions must include patient presentations, appropriate history taking, focused physical examinations, discussion of findings, medical or surgical options including possible benefits, and possible risks and possible complications. The modern gynecologic surgeon must not have the mindset that "if you can cut it, you can cure it." Above all, the gynecologic surgeon must become an expert in the understanding, evaluation, and treatment options of gynecologic diseases and disorders. Auditory learning must include appropriate objectives, enthusiastic lecture presentations by the teacher, and appropriate postpresentation objective testing. Progress is only and truly achieved when it can be made accountable and measurable.

Likewise, observational learning when observing videos or surgery on animals, human cadavers, or alive patients needs to be focused and broken down into individual surgical skills and decision components. The observations by the residents again must involve individual accountability and appropriate testing and measurement. Hands-on training must focus on specific and individual tasks within each complex surgical procedure.

Beginning exercises involve minimal equipment to practice knot-tying and the ergonomic use of surgical instruments. *Knot-tying boards* and *simple plastic trainers* are available from various surgical instrument companies. In addition, *video laparoscopic trainers* are also available for practicing more involved laparoscopic skills. Anastakis from Toronto showed "that both bench and cadaver training were superior to text learning and that bench and cadaver training were equivalent." A formal surgical training program within a residency does objectively improve the resident's surgical skills.

Animal models, particularly anesthetized pigs, allow the emerging gynecologic surgeon to get the actual feel of tissue dissections, see physiologic response, and experience a physical realism of operating on a live patient, especially with the immediate feedback of hemorrhage. However, the drawback of animal models is that the anatomy is often much different and the dimensions within the pelvis are much smaller than those in the human patient. However, the cost is much more affordable than present human cadaver courses and computer-simulated models, and the student has a real, physiologic, hands-on operative experience. Other animal models may include various body parts of various animals to recreate the feel and texture of various human parts. However, to work on a live animal model, the technical support aspects can be complex, just as in the human model. The animal must be properly obtained, properly anesthetized in a properly prepared room with appropriate lighting, equipment, instrumentation, and technical and surgical support.

WHAT DOES THE FUTURE HOLD?

A more advanced model for surgical training is the performance of dissection techniques and procedures on *unembalmed human cadavers.* This excellent model has been successfully used in teaching vaginal surgery, open laparotomy, hysteroscopy, and, of course, operative laparoscopy. We are fortunate in the United States to have the opportunity to have resident and postgraduate education courses using unembalmed cadavers. The use of human cadavers for postgraduate surgical education is not allowed or feasible in most countries of the world today. The human cadaver model is an excellent model in which to learn human pelvic anatomy, including the dimensions and relations of the various structures and tissues within the human body, proper dissection techniques, and the performance of various surgical procedures.

Even though the overhead financial cost of these courses is high, the intense and concentrated nature of the learning is well worth the expense in the minds of many individuals who have taken such training. The overhead expenses include the cost of administering the willed body programs in the various states; the immediate testing of the bodies for human immunodeficiency virus, hepatitis B and C, and syphilis; the proper handling of the bodies for cold preservation; the appropriate shipping, preparation of the body at the course site, and cost of technical support personnel in setting up the body at each workstation; and setting up the appropriate audiovisual equipment, instrumentation, and appropriate universal safety precautions. Teaching institutions interested in organizing such human cadaver teaching opportunities must check and coordinate their programs with their local medical school and state board of anatomic gifts. They must conform to the prevailing rules, regulations, and laws that control the use of these voluntarily willed bodies. Students must be respectful, courteous, and appreciative of these individuals who allow their bodies to be used for learning.

The participants in such a learning exercise must realize the purpose of this teaching is to appreciate and understand structural and pelvic support anatomy, to allow for more confident dissections during surgical procedures. Further hands-on exercises allow each student to perform various gynecologic procedures. The purpose of cadaver learning is not to learn basic, individual surgical skills. The purpose of cadaver learning is to learn dissectional surgical anatomy and to integrate surgical skills, already mastered, into an entire operative procedure. The goal of cadaver training is to significantly improve the operative experience of each participating surgeon. Ideally, operative procedures on their own patients will become safer (fewer operative complications), more efficient (smoother dissections with less wasted motion and hesitation, and less blood loss to obscure the field), and more effective (better long-term results).

Teaching on human cadavers must have specific and directed objectives, because the gynecologic surgeon, when left to dissect a cadaver alone, may not have a clear understanding of the relevant anatomy that needs to be mastered. Dissectional techniques must be taught in a specific and directed manner likewise. The participant should already have the appropriate surgical skills to take full advantage of his or her learning on the cadaveric model. These skills can certainly be learned, as noted earlier, via training on the various inanimate trainers, animal models, and, eventually, the computer-simulated trainers.

All aspects of gynecologic surgery may be understood and practiced on the human cadaver. This includes the following: dissection of the anterior abdominal wall; correlation with surgical incisions and laparoscopic trocar placement; practicing of dissectional techniques, layer-by-layer within the pelvis itself, particularly in the retroperitoneal areas. The retroperitoneal areas include the presacral space, the pelvic brim area, the pelvic sidewall, the base of the broad ligament where the ureter passes underneath the uterine artery, the paravesical space anteriorly, the pararectal space posteriorly, the vesicocervical and vesicovaginal spaces, the rectovaginal space including the rectovaginal septum, and, of course, a thorough dissection and understanding of the anatomy of the retropubic space of Retzius. These dissections must be carried out carefully in a directed manner to find the structures contained within the dissection plane and to understand their relationships to other vital structures within the same and surrounding anatomic areas. Further dissections, whether open laparotomy or through the laparoscope, can also include appreciation of the various somatic nerves, such as the obturator nerve and even the femoral nerve in the iliopsoas groove. Other dissections can reveal the sacrospinous ligament; the sacral plexus of nerves including the pudendal nerve and the sciatic nerve; the visceral innervation of the presacral space; the many components of the pelvic sidewall, including the inferior hypogastric plexus and its many branches; the cardinal ligament and uterosacral ligament complexes, as well as the various support tissues, such as the pubocervical fascia and rectovaginal septum.

Unembalmed cadavers also allow the opportunity to understand and perform vaginal surgery. This enables the student to dissect and to understand the structural and relational anatomy, and to perform procedures through the vagina for understanding of anterior vaginal wall prolapse or cystocele repair, apical prolapse or enterocele repair, and posterior wall prolapse or rectocele repair. Within the pelvic cavity, the various tissue layers such as the peritoneum, visceral fascia, and anatomic structures have the feel of the live patient, but neither bleed much nor cause undue anxiety during the learning of dissectional techniques. The operating gynecologist has the opportunity to practice surgical skills in a specific, focused manner, step-by-step, integrating all the steps to perform an entire procedure without the pressures of medical-legal considerations.

A less effective but still viable method of learning anatomy is on the embalmed cadavers such as is found in medical schools. However, the opportunity to have the feel of live patient tissue is lost with the embalming process.

After these human cadaver specimens have been used for learning, these individual specimens are respectfully taken to a funeral home where they are cremated. Their remains are returned to their home states, and then to their families by the respective anatomic gifts registries. Again, we are appreciative for these individuals and their families who have voluntarily allowed their bodies to be used for anatomic and surgical training.

The program involving human cadavers must also have specific goals to allow the gynecologic resident and interested attending physician to develop a base of clinical and anatomic knowledge upon which to grow and develop as more experience is obtained in surgery. This core of knowledge and training in anatomy and surgical procedures is important so that the independent gynecologic surgeon can understand new techniques and surgical developments as the field of gynecology progresses in the future.

Several computer companies are well on their way in developing effective *computer-based simulators* to train gynecologic surgeons, particularly involving open surgery, laparoscopic surgery, and hysteroscopic surgery. These computer-based simulators not only give the perception of operating on a "normal" patient but also allow for anatomic and pathologic variations within the practice patient. The computer provides a "virtual attending mentor" that offers immediate objective and nonjudgmental feedback. These computers are being programmed to allow for realistic haptics, and the true feel of instrument motion and tissue pressure. The simulators provide skills maintenance, even with the decreasing case load of major surgical procedures found in gynecologic residencies today. They are accessible for on-demand training, 24 hours a day, every day of the week, 365 days of the year. The objective, unbiased, and nonjudgmental quantitative skills assessment motivates the individual because each resident is directly accountable for his or her own measured progress. Computer-based simulators allow for objective assessment of performance and outcome before the individual resident operates on a living patient.

The development of computer-based simulators by various research computer engineers is rapidly overcoming the challenges of computer costs, visual realism, anatomic realism, physical realism, haptic realism, and physiologic realism. Computer costs have decreased dramatically, thereby making this teaching modality much more affordable. Visual realism compares the look of the tissues on the computer screen compared with the real patient. Anatomic realism deals with the structural and relational anatomy within the field of operation. Physical realism deals with the size and feel of the instruments and tissues encountered. Haptic realism pertains to "how things feel," like the feel of live surgery. The feel of mass, elasticity, gravity, and moving instruments is important in psychomotor development. Physiologic realism deals with possible hemorrhage at the surgical site and various movements of the patient such as during respiration, and even pain perception by the poorly anesthetized patient. Visual realism and haptic realism allow the individual to practice hand-eye coordination. Issues of ethics, medical-legal concerns, and patient safety in teaching gynecologic surgery will be better solved as computer-based education becomes more affordable and more available.

As a result of the need to train surgeons in complex laparoscopic procedures, various training formats have evolved in recent years in various countries around the world. Many of these training models are based on individual laparoscopic procedures (see Bibliography). However, in August 1998, Brill and Rogers published "A Comprehensive Program for Resident Training in Operative Laparoscopy," using an outline form. The thesis of this outline is that the basic laparoscopic anatomy, pathology, and fundamental technical and ergonomic skills, even for the most advanced laparoscopic procedures, can be found and practiced on the most readily available and basic of laparoscopic cases. Using plentiful cases such as laparoscopic sterilizations and diagnostic laparoscopic procedures, the resident gynecologic surgeon can be shown and taught basic laparoscopic techniques and maneuvers in preparation for performing more complex and advanced laparoscopic cases. Each surgical procedure is reduced to its fundamental technical and ergonomic components. These components can then be practiced on laparoscopic trainers and then on the simplest laparoscopic cases. These earliest and most available cases then provide most of the technical components required for the more advanced laparoscopic cases. They further state:

> At each level, proctoring in relevant anatomy can be used to unite process with specific procedures. We believe that the quality and durability of the learning process is dependent on proper sequencing and specific behavioral milestones: hearing, observation, comprehension, integration, sensation, and simulation with inanimate models, animal models, fresh cadaver dissection, and live patient surgery with preceptorship. Ultimately, development of necessary skills represents a balance between an individual's capacity for visual-motor processing, while referencing two-dimensional imaging, and level of conditioned responses obtained by simulation and practice.

CONCLUSIONS

Millions of dollars are spent each year by commercial airlines and by the United States Military in training aviation pilots using computer modulated flight simulators, as well as actual training flights. Why has gynecologic surgical training lagged so far behind in the use of these modern modalities? Is a well-trained and seasoned surgeon not worth the expense to individuals in this society? Also, with the loss of many skilled and seasoned educators from academic and teaching centers, the problem of dedicated and available educators must be immediately and directly addressed. The teachers themselves need to be mentored and trained, and must have financial incentives to be the best possible teachers. This is a proven business method of developing quality.

The problem of dedicated and available surgical teachers must be addressed directly, not only by teaching institutions and the specialty, but most importantly, by the health care payers and the government policy makers. Postgraduate programs must be developed to increase the numbers of quality surgical instructors. These physicians should be getting PhDs in how to teach, not MBAs.

Testing of technical skills must be clearly addressed. The residents must be accountable for their own progress. Tests must be crafted so that they can measure their progress—both quantitatively and qualitatively. These tests must be feasible, reliable, and valid. Assessment and measurement leads to personal accountability, motivation to learn, and true measurable progress. Formal programs in surgical education are being developed.

Some have been shown to be effective in improving surgical skills.

In addition, training of the individual gynecologic surgeon must not only emphasize individual skill development but should also include training in creating effective and harmonious surgical teams, particularly involving the administration of and interpersonal relationships within these teams.

We need to train more effective and sensitive mentors. Mentors must provide each resident with a series of tasks and objectives to be achieved. The mentor must provide ongoing feedback in a positive and constructive manner. Without this continual feedback, deficiencies in an individual's training will not be corrected.

The caring and effective mentor will have a professional yet personal relationship with the learner. The effective mentor in surgical education must be skilled in questioning, must ensure a comfortable environment for learning, and must be willing to question present surgical practices. "Without effective mentoring, students feel alone, perplexed, overwhelmed" with a decreased enthusiasm for learning (Dunnington). Lastly, Resnick from Toronto concludes:

> What makes an excellent operative teacher is adherence to basic, almost simple principals: treat residents as adult learners; set specific objectives; realize that operative skills are multidimensional; and be there, observe, be patient, provide feed-back, be positive, take the job seriously and structure the assessment process.

BIBLIOGRAPHY

Anastakis DJ, Regehr G, Reznick RK, et al. Assessment of technical skills transfer from the bench training model to the human model. *Am J Surg* 1999;177:167–170.

Blue AV, Griffith CH, Wilson J, et al. Surgical teaching quality makes a difference. *Am J Surg* 1999;177:86–89.

Brill AI, Rogers RM. A comprehensive program for resident training in operative laparoscopy. *J Am Assoc Gynecol Laparosc* 1998;5(3):223–228.

Brill AI, Rogers RM. A new paradigm for resident training [Editorial]. *J Am Assoc Gynecol Laparosc* 1998;5(3):219–220.

Coates KW, Kuehl TJ, Bachofen CG, et al. Analysis of surgical complications and patient outcomes in a residency training program. *Am J Obstet Gynecol* 2001;184:1380–1385.

Crafts RC. *A textbook of human anatomy*, third ed. New York: Churchill Livingstone, 1985:Dedication page.

Cundiff GW. Analysis of the effectiveness of an endoscopy education program in improving residents' laparoscopic skills. *Obstet Gynecol* 1997;90:854–859.

Defoe DM, Power ML, Holzman GB, et al. Long hours and little sleep: work schedules of residents in obstetrics and gynecology. *Obstet Gynecol* 2001;97:1015–1018.

Dunnington GL. The art of mentoring. *Am J Surg* 1996;171:604–607.

Gawande AA. Creating the educated surgeon in the 21st century. *Am J Surg* 2001;181:551–556.

Goff BA, Lentz GM, Lee DM, et al. Formal teaching of surgical skills in an obstetric-gynecologic residency. *Obstet Gynecol* 1999;93:785–790.

Haluck RS, Krummel TM. Computers and virtual reality for surgical education in the 21st century. *Arch Surg* 2000;135:786–792.

Hamdorf JM, Hall AC. Acquiring surgical skills. *Br J Surg* 2000;87:28–37.

Hasser CJ, Merril G. *Design of an endoscopy simulator.* Presentation at the AAGL 30th Annual Meeting. San Francisco, Nov. 18, 2001.

Mandel LP, Lente GM, Goff BA. Teaching and evaluating surgical skills. *Obstet Gynecol* 2000;95:783–785.

Reznick RK. Teaching and testing technical skills. *Am J Surg* 1993;165:358–361.

Rosser JC, Rosser LE, Savalgi RS. Objective evaluation of a laparoscopic surgical skill program for residents and senior surgeons. *Arch Surg* 1998;133:657–661.

Royal Australian College of Obstetricians and Gynaecologists. *Guidelines for training in advanced operative laparoscopy.* East Melbourne:Royal Australian College, 1993.

Royal College of Obstetricians and Gynaecologists. *Working party report of the RCOG Working Party on Training in Gynaecological Endoscopic Surgery.* London: RCOG Press, 1994.

Royal College of Obstetricians and Gynaecologists Working Party. *Implementation of the recommendations of the Working Party in Gynaecological Endoscopy Surgery.* London: RCOG Press, 1994.

Society of Obstetricians and Gynaecologists of Canada. *Guidelines for training in operative endoscopy in the specialty of obstetrics and gynaecology.* Toronto: Society of Obstetricians and Gynaecologists of Canada, 1992.

Sorosky JI, Anderson B. Surgical experiences and training residents: perspective of experienced gynecologic oncologists. *Gynecol Oncol* 1999;75:222–223.

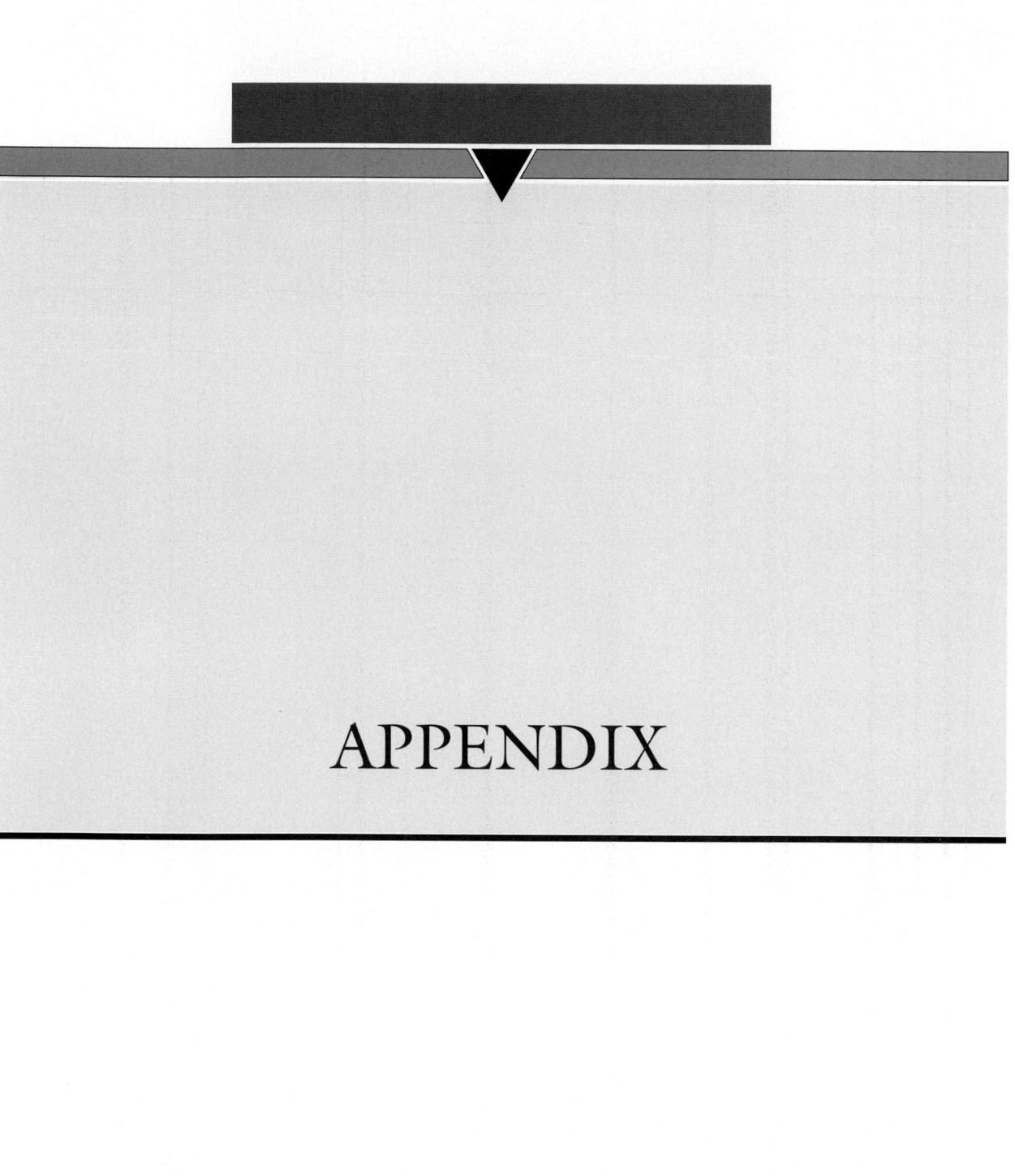

APPENDIX

Questions

CHAPTER 1

1. What factor was the most significant barrier to the development of surgery in ancient times?
   a) Lack of anesthesia
   b) Lack of real anatomic knowledge
   c) Lack of surgical instruments
   d) Lack of subjects

2. In what time period did the concept of hand washing and disinfection of instruments, sutures, and dressings become popularized?
   a) Hellenistic period
   b) Seventeenth century
   c) Eighteenth century
   d) Nineteenth century
   e) Twentieth century

3. In what year was the advent of effective and relatively safe anesthesia described?
   a) 1801
   b) 1846
   c) 1865
   d) 1901

4. One of the gynecologic procedures that was heralded as the beginning of the field of operative gynecology is
   a) Hysterectomy
   b) Salpingectomy
   c) Repair of vesicovaginal fistulas
   d) Episiotomy
   e) Tubal ligation

5. When was the term *oophorectomy* first formally defined?
   a) Late 1700s
   b) 1820s
   c) 1850s
   d) 1870s

6. When was the first journal devoted to the practice of obstetrics and gynecology published?
   a) 1878
   b) 1899
   c) 1905
   d) 1916

7. What physician described the first successful repair of vesicovaginal fistula?
   a) James Marion Sims
   b) Alexander Dunlap
   c) T.G. Thomas
   d) James McDowell
   e) Robert L. Dickinson

8. Which physician was considered the pioneer of surgical rubber gloves in the late nineteenth century?
   a) Howard Longyear
   b) William S. Halsted
   c) Robert L. Dickinson
   d) Emil Ries
   e) Ephraim McDowell

9. Which form of postoperative care described in the late nineteenth century has been most responsible for improved surgical recovery, shortened hospital stays, reduced costs, and reduced postoperative complications?
   a) Early ambulation after surgery
   b) Postoperative antibiotics
   c) Use of sterile dressings
   d) Use of compression stockings
   e) Early feeding after surgery

10. Which physician was responsible for formalizing gynecologic academic training at the turn of the twentieth century and publishing the first widely accepted textbook titled *Operative Gynecology*?
   a) George N. Papanicolaou
   b) Herbert Traut
   c) Richard Wesley Te Linde
   d) Howard Kelly

CHAPTER 2

1. Which one of the following is not one of the major goals of medicine?
   a) Provide relief from pain
   b) Provide relief from suffering
   c) Eradicate all disease
   d) Try to treat disease
   e) Minimize harm in the process of healing

2. When did medical ethics courses become formally offered during medical training?
   a) 1991
   b) 1981
   c) 1951
   d) 1901

3. In what year did the American Hospital Association issue the first "Patient Bill of Rights"?
   a) 1964
   b) 1971
   c) 1973
   d) 1981

4. In 1978, the National Commission for the Protection of Human Subjects of Biomedical and Behavioral Research issued a landmark paper governing the conduct of research and medical practice. This was called
   a) The Montgomery Doctrine
   b) The Hippocratic Oath
   c) The Human Manifesto
   d) The Belmont Report

5. Which of the following important concepts was not included in these advisory guidelines?
   a) Respect for persons
   b) Beneficence
   c) Justice
   d) Charity

6. In what year was the Nuremberg Code established?
   a) 1914
   b) 1918
   c) 1945
   d) 1949

7. Which governing body introduced the concept of the Institutional Review Board in 1966?
   a) World Health Organization
   b) American Medical Association
   c) U.S. Public Health Service
   d) Surgeon General

8. Which element is not included in the informed consent for operative procedures?
   a) Disclosure of information
   b) Competence of the patient to give consent
   c) Financial compensation of the physician
   d) Comprehension by the patient
   e) Voluntary transaction

9. In what year did the Supreme Court's decision on *Roe v. Wade* establish a national standard on abortion rights of women?
   a) 1965
   b) 1971
   c) 1973
   d) 1984

10. In what year did Congress pass the Patient Self Determination Act requiring hospitals to promote the use of advance directives by their patients to qualify for federal funds for Medicare and Medicaid?
   a) 1976
   b) 1981
   c) 1990
   d) 1995

CHAPTER 3

1. The most common cause of lower urinary tract trauma in women is
   a) Douching
   b) Vigorous intercourse
   c) Iatrogenic injury
   d) Chronic infection

2. The following are common themes in cross-cultural medicine that physicians should be aware of
   a) Fear of blood loss
   b) Poorly developed concept of preventive medicine
   c) Intolerance to side effects from medication
   d) All of the above

3. What is the most frequently performed major surgical procedure done on reproductive-aged women?
   a) Cesarean section
   b) Hysterectomy
   c) Laparoscopy
   d) Abdominoplasty

4. Which of the following factors is related to poor prognosis for excellent mental health after hysterectomy?
   a) Numerous hospitalizations or surgeries
   b) Fear of loss of libido
   c) Marital instability
   d) All of the above

5. The following are common emotional responses to surgery EXCEPT
   a) Suicidal ideation
   b) Insecurity
   c) Anxiety or fear
   d) Regression
   e) Grief

6. The stages of grief include
   a) Denial
   b) Guilt
   c) Depression
   d) Rage
   e) All of the above

7. Communication and counseling as part of psychologic preparation for surgery are effective determinants of all the following EXCEPT
   a) Potential of narcotic abuse
   b) Patient satisfaction
   c) Adherence to treatment
   d) Patient understanding of procedures

8. The four phases of crisis, as described by Kaplan, include all of the following EXCEPT
   a) Arousal occurs and attempts are made at problem solving
   b) Increased tension leads to distress and disorganization, as well as insomnia and fatigue
   c) Internal and external emergency resources are mobilized
   d) State of progressive deterioration, exhaustion, and decompensation
   e) None of the above

9. In the general population survey, what percentage range of women reported some form of sexual dysfunction?
   a) Less than 10%
   b) 16%–24%
   c) 23%–43%
   d) More than 50%

10. The following are all symptoms of rape trauma syndrome EXCEPT
    a) Inappropriate smiles or laughter
    b) Detachment toward others
    c) Demonstrations of fear, anger, or anxiety
    d) Matter-of-fact answering of questions
    e) Self-mutilation

CHAPTER 4

1. The standard of care requires that physicians must render the degree of care exercised by physicians under the same or similar circumstances in their
   a) Community
   b) State
   c) Region
   d) Nation

2. An indirect cause and effect relationship must exist between the breach in the standard of care and the adverse outcome for malpractice to legally occur.
   a) True
   b) False

3. It is the patient's responsibility to call for and obtain the results of studies or tests, such as mammograms, ordered by the physician.
   a) True
   b) False

4. The primary purpose of a well-documented medical record is to
   a) Protect the physician from a malpractice claim
   b) Provide adequate information to the patient's insurance company
   c) Communicate with members of the health care team
   d) Meet hospital requirements

5. The words _____ are legally correct words to be used in describing, in a progress note or an operative note, an adverse event that might have occurred during an operative procedure.
   I) Unintentionally
   II) Inadvertently
   III) Accidentally
   IV) Unfortunately
   a) I and IV
   b) I and III
   c) II and IV
   d) None of the above

6. Risk management's primary purpose is to keep physicians from being sued.
   a) True
   b) False

7. The physician is protected from being sued for malpractice for an adverse outcome when the physician's managed care plan has denied the physician's patient access to studies or treatments recommended by the physician.
   a) True
   b) False

8. In preparation for and during a deposition, it is generally prudent for a physician to
   I) Be unfamiliar with the office and hospital policies so that the plaintiff's attorney cannot question the physician about those areas
   II) Not attempt to educate your attorney about the medical facts of the case, because the insurance carrier would only use attorneys who are very knowledgeable about all the medical aspects of the case
   III) Always demand to be able to read and sign your deposition
   IV) Be unfamiliar with the alternative forms of therapy that you might have used, so that the plaintiff's attorney is unable to question you about them
   a) I and II
   b) I and IV
   c) III
   d) II and IV

9. During a trial, it is prudent for the physician to
   I) Attend only those sessions in which you have to give testimony, so that you convey to the jury your lack of concern about the matter
   II) Explain in complex medical terms the facts of your case so that the jury can be impressed with your medical knowledge
   III) Give your best educated guess to questions that you are not completely sure of the answer
   IV) Dress in a manner to convey to the jury that you are a rich and very successful physician
   a) I and III
   b) II and IV
   c) II and III
   d) None of the above

10. The emotional stress of a malpractice case has
    a) Been equated to the loss of a loved one
    b) Resulted in symptoms of major depression in 40% of sued physicians
    c) Resulted in 8% of sued physicians having the onset of physical ailments of which one fourth were life threatening
    d) All of the above

CHAPTER 5

1. Which of the following structures is not considered part of the vulva?
   a) Mons
   b) Labia
   c) Clitoris
   d) Vestibule
   e) Anus

2. Choose the *incorrect* statement pertaining to the pudendal artery and nerve.
   a) The pudendal nerve provides only sensory innervation to the perineum
   b) The pudendal nerve arises from the sacral plexus
   c) The pudendal artery originates from the anterior division of the internal iliac artery
   d) The nerve and vessels have three branches: clitoral, perineal, and inferior hemorrhoidal
   e) The perineal branch of the pudendal artery is the largest of the three branches

3. Choose the *incorrect* statement.
   a) Vulvar lymphatic channels lie medial to the labiocrural fold, establishing this as the lateral border of surgical resection
   b) The clitoris never drains directly into the deep pelvic nodes
   c) The superficial inguinal nodes lie in a T-shaped distribution 1 cm below the inguinal ligament
   d) The deep inguinal nodes are found beneath the fascia cribrosa
   e) Within the femoral triangle the most medial structure is the femoral vein

4. Choose the *incorrect* statement.
   a) The perineal membrane is a triangular sheet of fibromuscular tissue spanning the anterior half of the pelvic outlet
   b) The perineal membrane attaches medially with the urethra, walls of the vagina, and the perineal body
   c) The internal anal sphincter is indistinguishable from the external anal sphincter and it lies just outside the external anal sphincter
   d) The levator ani muscles and their fascia are called the pelvic diaphragm
   e) The urogenital hiatus allows passage of the urethra, vagina, and rectum through the pelvic diaphragm

5. Which of the following is a vaginal structure?
   a) Anterior and posterior columns
   b) Urethral carina
   c) Anterior and posterior fornices
   d) Lateral vaginal sulci
   e) All of the above

6. Choose the *incorrect* statement.
   a) In a woman of reproductive age, the uterine cervix is larger than the uterine corpus
   b) The muscle fibers of the uterine corpus are arranged in a complex diagonal crisscrossed pattern
   c) The cervix is divided into two portions: the portio vaginalis and the portio supravaginalis
   d) The external cervical os contains the transition from squamous to columnar epithelium
   e) The anterior portion of the uterine cervix is covered by the bladder

7. Choose the *correct* statement.
   a) The fallopian tubes are approximately 15 cm long
   b) The four portions of the fallopian tube from medial to lateral are the isthmus, interstitium, ampulla, and fimbriated end
   c) The outer layer of the tubal muscularis is composed of circular fibers, whereas the inner fibers are longitudinal
   d) The distal end of the fallopian tube is attached to the ovary by the fimbria ovarica

8. Choose the *incorrect* statement.
   a) The ovary attaches laterally to the pelvic sidewall with the infundibulopelvic ligament, which contains the ovarian vessels
   b) The ovary connects medially to the uterus with the uteroovarian ligament
   c) The normal ovary measures 7 cm long during reproductive life
   d) The ovary attaches to the broad ligament through the mesovarium
   e) Ovarian follicles, corpora lutea, and corpora albicantia are found within the ovarian cortex

9. Choose the *incorrect* statement.
   a) The blood supply of the upper adnexal structures comes from the ovarian arteries that arise from the aorta below the renal arteries
   b) The ovarian veins drain into the vena cava on the left and the renal vein on the right
   c) The uterine artery, which usually originates from the internal iliac artery, may have a common origin with the internal pudendal or vaginal arteries
   d) The uterine artery joins the uterus near the junction of the corpus and cervix
   e) The vagina receives blood supply from the uterine artery, vaginal artery, and the pudendal vessels

10. Choose the *incorrect* statement pertaining to the ureter.
    a) The ureter descends into the pelvis after passing over the bifurcation of the internal and external iliac arteries
    b) The ureter lies in a special connective tissue sheath within the medial leaf of the broad ligament
    c) The ureter crosses under the uterine artery in its course through the cardinal ligament
    d) The ureter lies approximately 3 cm from the anterolateral surface of the cervix
    e) The ureter receives blood supply from the common iliac, internal iliac, uterine, and vesical arteries

CHAPTER 6

1. Pelvic surgery should always be preceded by a recent cytologic study of the cervix because
   a) A negative Papanicolaou smear always excludes the possibility of cervical, endocervical, or endometrial neoplasm
   b) Most preclinical malignancies of the cervix demonstrate significant gross lesions indicating the need for cytologic evaluation
   c) Patients with abnormal Papanicolaou smears showing repeated dysplasia should be evaluated by colposcopy and suspicious lesions biopsied
   d) A sampling of cells taken from the portio of the cervix is simple, inexpensive, and is indicative of cervical and endocervical pathology
   e) A finding of abnormal glandular cell dysplasia requires only an endocervical curettage for a complete evaluation

2. Preoperative evaluation of a patient with an uncomplicated gynecologic pathology and an uncomplicated medical or surgical status should include all of the following laboratory tests EXCEPT
   a) Electrocardiogram if older than 40 years
   b) Pregnancy test if in the reproductive age, sexually active, not using contraception, or if using questionably effective contraception
   c) Blood type and screen if the potential exists for a more-than-minimal surgical blood loss
   d) Chemistry panel
   e) Hematocrit or hemoglobin if older than 6 months

3. In addition to good surgical skills and techniques, successful surgical outcomes of operative gynecologic procedures occur as the result of all of the following EXCEPT
   a) The ability to determine when surgical intervention is a necessary course of action
   b) The ability to convince the patient of a surgical approach even though she shows reluctance to undergo the procedure
   c) The ability to work with managed care organizations in obtaining preoperative approval and complying with individual health care plan guidelines
   d) The ability to accurately assess and diagnose gynecologic pathology, defects, and injury
   e) The ability to communicate to the patient both short- and long-term complications in a manner that can be understood

4. All of the following statements regarding preoperative patient preparation are true EXCEPT
   a) A full bowel prep should be carried out on all gynecologic surgeries
   b) Pelvic cleansing should be accomplished before all pelvic or abdominal surgeries
   c) Universal precautions should be used in all gynecologic surgeries
   d) Hepatitis B vaccination is recommended for all physicians accomplishing gynecologic surgery
   e) In those gynecologic surgeries in which hair removal is deemed necessary, hair clipping, rather than hair shaving, is recommended just before surgery

5. Studies on the use of "routine" preoperative laboratory testing before gynecologic surgery have revealed all of the following findings EXCEPT
   a) Between 30% and 60% of all unexpected abnormalities detected by preoperative laboratory tests were not actually noted or investigated before surgery
   b) "Routine" preoperative testing adds many millions of dollars to health care costs each year
   c) 60% to 70% of laboratory tests ordered preoperatively are not actually required based on a review of the patient's history and/or physical examination
   d) Only 1% or less of routinely ordered preoperative tests revealed abnormalities that might influence perioperative management
   e) Between 25% and 35% of routinely ordered preoperative tests revealed abnormalities that influenced perioperative management

6. Preoperative broad-spectrum antibiotic prophylaxis is suggested for which of the following uncomplicated gynecologic surgical procedures?
   a) Ovarian cystectomy
   b) Ectopic pregnancy
   c) Uterine myomectomy
   d) Tubal ligation
   e) Vaginal or abdominal hysterectomy

7. All of the following preoperative management actions are suggested in the preoperative care of gynecologic patients EXCEPT
   a) Discontinue the use of birth control pills 2 to 4 weeks before the planned gynecologic surgery
   b) Immediate preoperative examination by the gynecologic surgeon and anesthesia assessment by an individual anesthesiologist or in the anesthesia preoperative clinic
   c) Cleansing of the lower colon by a preoperative enema
   d) Use of vaginal estrogen cream in postmenopausal women undergoing vaginal surgery
   e) Use of a gonadotropin-releasing hormone agonist for 3 months before hysteroscopic resection of submucous uterine leiomyoma

8. The rectal examination, in combination with the abdominal-pelvic examination, offers all of the following benefits EXCEPT
   a) A more complete assessment of the broad and uterosacral ligaments
   b) A more effective assessment of the posterior bladder wall
   c) A more complete assessment of the cul-de-sac of Douglas
   d) A more effective assessment of the adnexa
   e) A more effective assessment of the anal sphincter, anal canal, and lower rectum

9. The purpose of the preoperative evaluation is to accomplish all of the following tasks EXCEPT
   a) Decrease surgical morbidity
   b) Evaluate and optimize patient health status
   c) Decrease the hospital length of stay
   d) Obtain informed consent
   e) Reduce patient anxiety through education

10. All of the following statements regarding preoperative evaluation are true EXCEPT
   a) Preoperative patient conditions are predictors of postoperative morbidity
   b) Routine batteries of preoperative tests have proven to decrease "less-than-desirable" surgical outcomes and to increase legal protection
   c) Preoperative evaluation should strive to determine if the patient is in optimal health, determine if the patient's physical or mental condition can be improved before surgery, and determine if the patient has any health problems or use of any medications that might adversely affect perioperative events
   d) During the preoperative evaluation process the patient must be given sufficient medical information relating to her gynecologic problem to allow her to make an educated decision regarding proceeding with the planned surgery
   e) Use of preprinted medical history and physical examination forms are felt to have merit in the preoperative management of gynecologic patients

CHAPTER 7

1. Low molecular weight heparin (LMWH) potentiates the inhibition of which factor?
   a) V
   b) VII
   c) Xa
   d) XI

2. With the perioperative use of thromboprophylaxis the percentage reduction of fatal pulmonary embolism is
   a) 10%
   b) 33%
   c) 75%
   d) 90%

3. All of the following are major risk factors for thromboembolic disease EXCEPT
   a) Age younger than 40
   b) Malignancy
   c) Trauma
   d) Prior history of DVT

4. All of the following have been implicated as risk factors for adult respiratory distress syndrome (ARDS) EXCEPT
   a) Sepsis
   b) Drug overdose
   c) Disseminated intravascular coagulation
   d) Renal failure

5. The last clinical stage of ARDS is characterized by which of the following?
   a) Intrapulmonary shunting leading to worsening hypoxia despite oxygen therapy
   b) Chest x-ray film changes showing air bronchograms and diffuse patchy infiltrates
   c) Rales on physical examination
   d) Acute lung injury causing respiratory alkalosis

6. Common manifestations of atelectasis include all of the following EXCEPT
   a) Hypoxia
   b) Rales
   c) Hypertension
   d) Decreased breath sounds

7. The cornerstone of therapy for ARDS is
   a) Inverse ration ventilation
   b) Mechanical ventilation with low tidal volume and positive end expiratory pressure
   c) Antiinflammatory agents
   d) Nitrous oxide

8. The least likely complication with insertion of a subclavian catheter placement is
   a) Injury to the subclavian artery
   b) Pneumothorax
   c) Brachial plexus injury
   d) Injury to the thoracic duct

9. All of the following are essential amino acids EXCEPT
   a) Histidine
   b) Glutamine
   c) Lysine
   d) Phenylalanine

10. All of the following have been associated with hormone replacement use EXCEPT
   a) Reduction in risk of colon cancer
   b) Improvement in cognitive function
   c) Inhibition of osteoclast action on the bony skeleton
   d) Glutamine

CHAPTER 8

1. Choose the *incorrect* statement.
   a) The human body is 60% water by weight
   b) Approximately 2 L of fluid are taken in orally each day
   c) 750–1500 mL of urine are produced per day
   d) 1 L of insensible fluid loss occurs per day

2. Choose the *incorrect* statement.
   a) The osmolality of extracellular fluid is determined almost entirely by potassium and its accompanying anions
   b) Glucose, mannitol, alcohol, and urea can contribute to plasma osmolality

   c) Serum sodium is lowered by 1.6 mEq/L for every increase in serum glucose of 100 mg/dL
   d) The osmolality of intracellular fluid and extracellular fluid is equal

3. Choose the *incorrect* statement.
   a) Ingestion or infusion of water results in expansion of all body fluid compartments
   b) Infusion of isotonic solution selectively expands the extracellular fluid compartment
   c) Infusion of hypertonic solution causes the extracellular fluid volume to contract
   d) Urea does not affect the steady state water distribution because it rapidly distributes throughout the body water space

4. Which of the following is the most effective means of assessing the effective intravenous volume?
   a) Body weight
   b) Tissue turgor
   c) Central venous pressure
   d) Pulmonary capillary wedge pressure

5. Normal pulmonary capillary wedge pressure is
   a) 5–12 cm water
   b) 8–12 mm Hg
   c) Less than 8 mm Hg
   d) More than 18 mm Hg

6. Which of the following is a symptom of serum sodium below 115 mEq/L?
   a) Convulsions
   b) Coma
   c) Possible death
   d) All of the above

7. Which of the following is associated with hyponatremia and renal sodium wasting?
   a) Diuretic therapy
   b) Gastrointestinal losses
   c) Severe burns
   d) All of the above

8. Choose the *incorrect* statement.
   a) A soaked laparotomy pad contains approximately 50 mL of blood
   b) Replacement of 3-mL crystalloid suspension per 1 mL of blood loss is recommended
   c) Replacement of 2-mL colloid suspension per 1 mL of blood loss is recommended
   d) Optimal intraoperative urine output is 0.5 mL/kg/hour

9. In which situation should colloid suspension be used instead of crystalloid?
   a) Large amounts of crystalloid are needed to maintain normal hemodynamics
   b) Assessment of circulatory status is difficult
   c) The patient has an elevated pulmonary capillary wedge pressure
   d) All of the above

10. Which of the following can be used to treat severe hyperkalemia?
    a) Infusion of 10 mL of 10% calcium gluconate
    b) Infusion of 50 g of glucose with 10 units of regular insulin
    c) Hemodialysis
    d) All of the above

CHAPTER 9

1. A 54-year-old woman underwent a total abdominal hysterectomy for uterine leiomyomata. The day after surgery, the patient's temperature is 38.4°C (101.2°F) and she complains of pelvic pain, chills, and rectal pressure. Your bedside examination of this patient reveals a vaginal cuff abscess. The most likely source of bacteria that caused this infection is
    a) Incompletely sterilized surgical instruments
    b) Vagina
    c) The surgeon's skin
    d) Residual peritoneal fluid

2. A 60-year-old woman is scheduled to undergo a vaginal hysterectomy for uterine prolapse. Which of the following is *not* a risk factor for postoperative infection?
    a) Bacterial vaginosis
    b) Diabetes mellitus
    c) Hypertension
    d) Obesity

3. A 45-year-old woman, gravida 4, para 4, has experienced chronic pelvic pain over the past 3 years. Her symptoms have continued despite conservative medical management, and the patient now elects to undergo a total abdominal hysterectomy. The scheduled surgery is performed 3 weeks later with no complications, and the patient is discharged from the hospital on the second postoperative day. Three days later, the patient presents to your office with fever, chills, and abdominal pain. A CT scan is ordered and a right-sided ovarian abscess is discovered. The microbe most likely to be implicated in this postoperative infection is
    a) *Bacteroides fragilis*
    b) *Staphylococcus aureus*
    c) *Escherichia coli*
    d) *Chlamydia trachomatis*

4. A 64-year-old woman undergoes a retropubic urethropexy for genuine stress urinary incontinence without complications. On the third postoperative day, the patient develops a fever and is treated empirically with intravenous ampicillin and gentamicin. Examination of the patient reveals no overt cause for febrile morbidity. The fever persists 48 hours after the first dose of these antibiotics, despite negative blood and urine cultures. Clindamycin and vancomycin are then added to the antibiotic regimen without defer-

vescence over the next 2 days. The appropriate next step in the management of this infection is
    a) Add metronidazole and order a chest radiograph
    b) Take the patient back to the operating room for exploratory laparotomy
    c) Start IV heparin
    d) Add doxycycline to the current antibiotic regimen

5. A 40-year-old woman is diagnosed by ultrasound with a left tubo-ovarian complex (6 × 6 cm). An open left salpingo-oophorectomy is performed without complications. On postoperative day number two, the patient complains of pain at the incision site, and her temperature is noted to be 38.1° C (100.6° F). Examination and gentle probing of the wound show purulent drainage with an intact fascia. Along with antibiotic therapy, the next appropriate step in the management of this postoperative infection is
    a) Return to the operating room for a thorough examination of the wound and fascial plane under general anesthesia
    b) Open the wound widely to allow drainage and debridement of necrotic tissue, then cleanse the wound thoroughly with povidone-iodine before reclosing the wound
    c) Open the wound widely and debride necrotic tissue, then insert a Penrose drain at the infected site before reclosing the wound
    d) Open the wound widely to allow drainage and debridement of necrotic tissue, then apply wet-to-dry packing until the wound closes by secondary intention

6. A 62-year-old woman undergoes a radical hysterectomy for pelvic organ prolapse. On the second postoperative day, the patient develops a low-grade fever and complains of dysuria. You suspect a urinary tract infection. The next step in management should be
    a) Obtain a urine culture and start a 7-day course of levofloxacin
    b) Obtain blood and urine cultures, beginning appropriate antibiotics when culture results are reported
    c) Obtain blood and urine cultures, then start ticarcillin-clavulanate
    d) Obtain urine cultures and start a 7-day course of amoxicillin

7. A 45-year-old woman who weighs 53 kg (120 lb) and is 163 cm (64 in.) tall undergoes total abdominal hysterectomy for multiple uterine leiomyomata without complications. Twelve hours after leaving the recovery area, the patient develops a fever of 100.1° F. The *least* likely cause of this elevated temperature is
    a) Pneumonia
    b) Atelectasis
    c) Hematoma formation
    d) Hypersensitivity to an anesthetic agent given in the recovery area

8. The hospital where you perform the majority of your gynecologic surgeries has recently implemented a policy to reduce postoperative infections and decrease the incidence of nosocomial morbidity. The most important step in preventing the spread of infection is
   a) Strict adherence to sterile technique during operative procedures
   b) Frequent handwashing
   c) Admitting patients to the hospital 12 to 24 hours before scheduled procedures
   d) Sterile placement of Foley catheters

9. A 44-year-old woman presents to your office with a 6-month history of menometrorrhagia. She reports having undergone an appendectomy and two Caesarian sections in the past 5 years. While performing a physical examination, you discover a suprapubic mass that is later verified by ultrasonography to be a uterine leiomyoma 5×5 cm in dimension. The patient elects total abdominal hysterectomy as definitive treatment. An appropriate precaution to take before this surgery is
   a) Instructing the patient to shave the anticipated incision site before surgery
   b) Having the bowel prepared with oral antibiotics and a cathartic agent
   c) Instructing the patient to refrain from sexual intercourse 2 weeks before the date of surgery
   d) Hospitalizing the patient preoperatively to control infection risk

10. A 23-year-old woman presents to the emergency department of the hospital with the sudden onset of left lower quadrant abdominal pain and tenderness. Laboratory evaluation of this patient reveals a positive pregnancy test and a hematocrit of 22%. She undergoes an emergent laparotomy, and a left salpingo-oophorectomy is performed to remove a 6-week ruptured ectopic pregnancy. The surgical technique *least* likely to prevent postoperative infection is
    a) Excise any necrotic tissue identified during surgery
    b) Place a closed-suction drain if the patient is obese
    c) Close the subcutaneous space
    d) Obtain adequate hemostasis to prevent hematoma formation

CHAPTER 10

1. Adult respiratory distress syndrome is characterized by
   a) Narrowing of the alveolar-arterial O_2 gradient
   b) Supplemental oxygen usually is able to maintain systemic oxygen saturation (arterial PaO_2 more than 65 mm Hg)
   c) Intrapulmonary shunting
   d) Increased pulmonary compliance
   e) Increased functional residual capacity

2. Initial manifestations of early, reversible shock include
   a) Reduced cardiac output
   b) An increase in the systemic vascular resistance
   c) Cold, clammy skin
   d) Disorientation
   e) Oliguria

3. Platelet transfusion is indicated
   a) For every four units of packed red cells transfused
   b) Whenever the platelet count falls below 50,000/mm³
   c) Persistent bleeding consistent with coagulopathy
   d) For platelet counts below 100,000/mm³ before surgery
   e) Persistent bleeding for coagulopathy following fresh frozen plasma replacement

4. At 5–12 µg/kg/min doses, dopamine has which of the following predominant effects?
   a) Maximizes cerebral, coronary artery, and renal blood flow
   b) α-Adrenergic effects predominate
   c) β_1-Adrenergic effects predominate
   d) β_2-Adrenergic effects predominate
   e) Inotropic and vasoconstrictive effects

5. Which of the following characterizes dobutamine?
   a) Indirect-acting inotropic agent
   b) Both β_1- and β_2-adrenergic effects
   c) Stimulation of β_1-adrenergic receptors reduces afterload
   d) Increases O_2 consumption
   e) Causes clinically significant tachycardia

6. Following an uneventful total abdominal hysterectomy for symptomatic uterine leiomyomata, a 47-year-old otherwise healthy patient is seen on morning rounds 24 hours after surgery. The estimated operative blood loss was approximately 1500 mL. Current vital signs reveal that she is afebrile, has a blood pressure of 110/80 mm Hg (consistent with her preoperative blood pressure), and does not appear to be in distress. Orthostatics reveal a positive tilt test. Her postoperative hemoglobin, checked 24 hours after surgery is 8 mg/dL. The best management initial treatment for this patient is
   a) Packed red blood cells (1 to 2 units)
   b) Crystalloid infusion (1 to 2 L)
   c) Colloid solution (50–100 mL 25% albumin)
   d) Central venous catheterization
   e) Observation

7. A 22-year-old G_0 woman presents to the emergency room with complaints of diffuse abdominal pain. She reports that she was treated last year for pelvic inflammatory disease. On admission, her temperature is 38.4° C, her blood pressure is 100/65 mm Hg, and her heart rate is 90 beats/min. Orthostatics reveal minimal change in blood pressure sitting and reclining. Abdominal examination reveals diffuse tenderness without rebound or guarding, and a bimanual examination reveals a left-sided mass. Laboratory in-

vestigation reveals a negative β-HCG titer; a white blood cell count is 21,000 /mm^{3}with 90% mature segmental neutrophils. There is a 5-cm complex adnexal mass on ultrasound and no cul-de-sac fluid. Of the following, which is the most appropriate next step?
   a) Immediate intravenous antibiotics
   b) Immediate exploratory laparotomy
   c) Hospitalization
   d) Plain x-ray films of the abdomen and pelvis
   e) Blood and cervical cultures

8. Oliguric prerenal azotemia characterized by
   a) Hyponatremic hyperchloremic metabolic alkalosis
   b) Urine-plasma creatinine less than 40 mEq/L/24 hr
   c) Urine sodium excretion less than 20 mEq/L/24 hr
   d) Fractional excretion of sodium greater than 1%
   e) Low urine osmolality less than 350 mOsm

9. A 46-year-old woman underwent a difficult abdominal hysterectomy and bilateral salpingo-oophorectomy for endometriosis, and the estimated blood loss was 950 mL. Twenty-four hours later, she is anxious. Vital signs reveal a heart rate of 110 beats/min, that increases to 125 beats/min on sitting, and her reclining blood pressure, 110/80 mm Hg, is 105/70 mm Hg in the sitting position. Over the past 8-hour shift, her urine output was 250 mL These findings are most consistent with which class of shock?
   a) Class I
   b) Class II
   c) Class III
   d) Class IV
   e) Class V

10. Classically, the order of organ system loss in patients with multiorgan failure syndrome is
   a) Lung, liver, GI, kidney
   b) Liver, lung, GI, kidney
   c) GI, kidney, liver, lung
   d) Kidney, GI, lung, liver
   e) Kidney, lung, liver, GI

11. Which of the following statements characterize the mechanism of action of an intact renin-angiotensinogen system?
   a) Angiotensin I is an active polypeptide
   b) Angiotensin II is a potent vasoconstrictor
   c) Aldosterone along with antidiuretic hormone promotes water and sodium excretion
   d) Angiotensin II decreases venous return, stroke volume, and cardiac output
   e) Increased sympathetic activation causes renin release

CHAPTER 11

1. From what material is catgut made?
   a) Bovine tendon
   b) Feline intestine
   c) Sheep intestine
   d) Feline tendon

2. Which of the following suture material has the largest tensile strength at 4 weeks?
   a) Dexon
   b) Maxon
   c) Vicryl
   d) Chromic gut

3. In the sequence of wound healing, which of the following biologic processes should come last?
   a) Wound contraction
   b) Scar maturation
   c) Fibroplasia
   d) Inflammation

4. Using third-intention wound closure (delayed primary closure), when is the ideal time for closure to occur to provide for decreased risk of infection?
   a) Before 2 days
   b) On or after the fourth day
   c) After 7–8 days
   d) On or after the sixth day

5. What is the most common cause of wound dehiscence?
   a) Incorrect choice of suture material
   b) Too few knots
   c) Patient noncompliance
   d) Intact sutures pulling through fascia

6. For a suture material to be classified as nonabsorbable, it must lose the majority of its tensile strength before _____ days when implanted in body tissues.
   a) 20 days
   b) 40 days
   c) 60 days
   d) 120 days

7. Which U.S. governing body sets standards for sutures marketed in the United States?
   a) The Bureau of Weights and Measures
   b) The United States Pharmacopeia
   c) The U.S. Department of Health
   d) The Office of the Surgeon General
   e) Johnson & Johnson

8. By postoperative week four, how much of its original strength is restored to a fascial incision?
   a) 10%
   b) 25%
   c) 40%
   d) 50%

9. Which of the following retractors is considered the most versatile?
   a) Balfour retractor
   b) O'Conner-O'Sullivan retractor
   c) Bookwalter retractor
   d) Heaney retractor

10. What percentage of tensile strength is lost in the first 7 days after implantation when using Vicryl or Dexon suture?
    a) 0%
    b) 10%
    c) 20%–30%
    d) 50%

CHAPTER 12

1. The lymphatic drainage of the abdominal wall passes DIRECTLY to all of the following EXCEPT
   a) Axillary lymph nodes
   b) Para-aortic lymph nodes
   c) Liver
   d) Inguinal nodes

2. The blood supply of the muscles of the anterior abdominal wall include all of the following EXCEPT
   a) Deep circumflex iliac artery
   b) Superficial epigastric artery
   c) Musculophrenic artery
   d) Inferior epigastric artery

3. Which of the following statements regarding the nervous supply to the abdominal wall is true?
   a) The ilioinguinal and iliohypogastric nerves are motor nerves
   b) The ilioinguinal and iliohypogastric nerves are frequently injured during midline incisions
   c) Injury to the iliohypogastric nerve results in sensory deficits in the area of the mons
   d) Injury to the iliohypogastric nerve results in sensory deficits to the labia majora

4. The four phases of wound healing include all of the following EXCEPT
   a) Migration
   b) Reconstruction
   c) Inflammation
   d) Maturation

5. A simple total hysterectomy is associated with which of the following wound classifications?
   a) Clean
   b) Clean-contaminated
   c) Contaminated
   d) Dirty

6. Which of the following statements regarding drains is incorrect?
   a) Drains should be brought out through the incision
   b) Passive drains may be associated with increased wound infection rates
   c) Drains in the subcutaneous space should be advanced when their output is less than 50 mL/day
   d) Drain catheters should never be "stripped"

7. All of the following are characteristics of transverse abdominal incisions EXCEPT
   a) Better cosmetic result
   b) Less painful than midline incisions
   c) Weaker than midline incisions
   d) Less interference with postoperative respirations when placed in the lower abdomen

8. The most appropriate incision for a patient with impaired circulation to the lower extremities secondary to obstruction of the terminal aorta is
   a) Maylard
   b) Cherney
   c) Midline
   d) Pfannensticl

9. All of the following are true regarding evisceration EXCEPT
   a) Occurs in 0.3%–0.7% of gynecologic patients
   b) Carries a 10%–35% mortality rate
   c) Is associated with paroxysmal coughing or retching
   d) Wound infection is an associated factor in less than 10% of cases

10. Reasonable candidates for delayed primary closure include all of the following EXCEPT
    a) Ruptured TOA
    b) Suppurative appendicitis
    c) Bowel injury to an unprepared bowel
    d) Uncomplicated radical hysterectomy

CHAPTER 13

1. In what year did Arsenne d'Arsonoval receive credit for being the first to use high-frequency currents for medical therapy?
   a) 1790
   b) 1851
   c) 1893
   d) 1911

2. For what type of surgery did Harvey Cushing and William T. Bovie describe their use of electrosurgery to control hemorrhage in 1928?
   a) Hand surgery
   b) Neurosurgery
   c) Vascular reanastomosis
   d) Laparoscopic oophorectomy

3. Cutting/desiccation (CUT) is generally produced by what type of energy frequency?
   a) Interrupted (damped or modulated waveform)
   b) Continuous (undamped or nonmodulated waveform)
   c) Harmonic
   d) Sonic

4. Coagulation (COAG) is generally produced by what type of energy frequency?
   a) Interrupted (damped or modulated waveform)
   b) Continuous (undamped or nonmodulated waveform)
   c) Harmonic
   d) Sonic

5. For general surgical use, most electrosurgical generators can produce a maximum of _____ volts in the COAG mode.
   a) 8000
   b) 10,000
   c) 15,000
   d) 20,000

6. The stages of grief include
   a) Denial
   b) Guilt
   c) Depression
   d) Rage
   e) All of the above

7. A grounding pad is essential for the use of both monopolar and bipolar electrosurgery.
   a) True
   b) False

8. Which of the following media would be the worst choice when performing operative hysteroscopy using electrosurgical techniques?
   a) Hyskon
   b) Sorbitol
   c) Glycine
   d) Lactated Ringer's

9. Direct coupling is a source of unintended electrical injury that
   a) Occurs as a result of miswiring of the electrosurgical generator
   b) Occurs when two conductors in close proximity, each insulated from one another, induce an electrical current from one to the other
   c) Occurs when the active electrode touches other metal instruments within the abdomen
   d) Occurs when a power surge causes a temporary spike in voltage

10. When performing a LEEP or LLETZ procedure, which of the following parameters are important to ensure good surgical outcome?
    a) Electrode size
    b) Waveform
    c) Power density
    d) Speed of incision
    e) All of the above

CHAPTER 14

1. The frequency of diagnostic ultrasound differs from that of the Cavitron ultrasonic surgical aspirator (CUSA). The average diagnostic ultrasound frequency is greater than 1 million Hertz (cycles/sec). The average frequency of the CUSA is
   a) 2 million Hz
   b) 100,000 Hz
   c) 50,000 Hz
   d) 25,000 Hz
   e) 1000 Hz

2. What is the maximum power recommended for the CUSA's use?
   a) 1000 watts
   b) 100 watts
   c) 10 watts
   d) 1 watt

3. There are three mechanisms of action *in vitro* of the CUSA. One of these is through viscous stress. This involves acoustic microstreaming of small-scale fluid motion. The gas bubbles give rise to motion creating circular flow. What is the best scenario to achieve this action?
   a) High irradiation intensity
   b) Medium irradiation intensity
   c) Low irradiation intensity
   d) Irradiation intensity is irrelevant

4. The harmonic scalpel produces hemostasis as it cuts by
   a) The piezoelectric effect
   b) Thermal effects that produce a denatured protein clot
   c) High-frequency microwave energy
   d) Electrical energy

5. *In vivo* use of the Cavitron ultrasonic surgical aspirator includes all of the following techniques EXCEPT
   a) Stroking motion
   b) Plunging motion
   c) Dragging motion
   d) Direct tissue application

6. Use of the CO_2 laser compared with the CUSA resulted in no significant difference in each of the following areas EXCEPT
   a) Depth of tissue damage
   b) Width of tissue damage
   c) Rates of wound healing
   d) Time to peak inflammation

7. The CUSA selectively removes tissues with a
   a) High collagen content
   b) High nuclear density
   c) High water content
   d) Low density of intracellular bridges

8. The potential risks of the CUSA include
   a) High-frequency hearing loss
   b) Increased tissue thrombin activation
   c) Viable cancer cells in the spray
   d) Transient nerve injury in the operative field

9. The most common use of the CUSA in gynecologic surgery has been
   a) Excision/ablation of vulvar intraepithelial neoplasia
   b) Skeletonizing the uterine vessels during hysterectomy
   c) Debriding infected wounds
   d) Cytoreduction in ovarian cancer

10. All of the following are advantages of the CUSA EXCEPT
    a) Rapid tissue destruction/dissection
    b) Decreased blood loss
    c) Improved visibility because of lack of plume
    d) Lack of tissue adherence to instruments
    e) Kidneys

CHAPTER 15

1. Which of the following types of laser energy is *not* able to be conducted along a quartz fiber?
   a) Carbon dioxide
   b) KTP
   c) YAG
   d) Argon

2. Choose the *incorrect* answer pertaining to laser effects on tissue.
   a) The primary tissue effect is one of heat damage and vaporization
   b) Carbon dioxide laser energy causes minimal deep penetration, allowing for destruction of cells layer by layer
   c) YAG laser energy is able to penetrate tissue to depths of 4 mm or more
   d) Argon and KTP laser energy penetrates tissues to a greater depth than both carbon dioxide and YAG

3. Choose the *incorrect* statement about laser use for cervical intraepithelial neoplasia (CIN).
   a) CIN typically involves the endocervical crypts that have a depth of 4 mm
   b) Atypical epithelial changes almost always start in the transformation zone
   c) Multifocal CIN or skip lesions are common
   d) It is necessary to destroy the entire transformation zone, including the visible cervical lesion, to a measured depth of 5 mm

4. Choose the *incorrect* statement.
   a) When performing vaporization conization of the cervix, tissue should be vaporized to a depth of 7 mm with an additional 2–3 mm up into the endocervical canal
   b) For excisional conization of the cervix, low power with a large spot size is used for cutting purposes
   c) Combination vaporization and excisional procedures may be used for certain cases that involve the cervix along with the vagina or vulva
   d) CIN treatment by laser shows an overall success rate of 96%–97%

5. Choose the correct statement about laser use for vulvar intraepithelial neoplasia.
   a) General anesthesia must be used
   b) 0.4% acetic acid is applied to the vulva to demonstrate areas of neoplastic change
   c) The laser should first be used to mark the limits of the disease before landmarks are lost
   d) A spot size of 10 mm should be used

6. Which of the following are advantages of using the carbon dioxide laser instead of skinning vulvectomy for vulvar intraepithelial neoplasia?
   a) The ability to ablate large areas of disease
   b) More controlled depth of tissue removal
   c) Rapid healing with little residual thermal damage
   d) Maintenance of normal vulvar anatomy
   e) All of the above

7. Which of the following is not used as an adjuvant therapy to laser surgery for HPV?
   a) Trichloroacetic acid
   b) Methotrexate
   c) 5-fluorouracil
   d) Interferon

8. Choose the *incorrect* statement pertaining to use of laser in laparotomy.
   a) Flame-resistant surgical drapes should be used
   b) An appropriate backstop should be selected to prevent damage to surrounding tissues
   c) Dental mirrors may be used to facilitate operating in inaccessible areas
   d) Removal of the laser plume is important

9. Choose the *incorrect* statement about laparoscopic ovarian cystectomy.
   a) Most young women with cystic adnexal masses will be found to have a malignancy so laparoscopy is rarely indicated
   b) Cystic adnexal masses should be evaluated by ultrasound or MRI before surgery
   c) Ovarian endometriomas larger than 2 cm should be excised rather than vaporized
   d) Tumor markers may be obtained before surgery to aid in differentiating malignant adnexal masses

10. Which of the following statements are *incorrect* pertaining to laser safety?
    a) Flammable liquids and paper drapes may be ignited by the laser
    b) The laser smoke should be collected by a suction device no farther than 5 cm from the target site
    c) Carbon dioxide laser energy can produce eye injury by damaging the cornea
    d) The fiberoptic lasers can produce eye injury by damaging the retina

CHAPTER 16

1. Which of the following is not a contraindication for laparoscopy?
   a) Bowel obstruction
   b) Intraperitoneal hemorrhage
   c) Inguinal hernia
   d) Severe cardiorespiratory disease

2. Relative contraindications for laparoscopy include
   a) Extremes of body weight
   b) Inflammatory bowel disease
   c) Presence of a large abdominal mass
   d) Advanced pregnancy
   e) All of the above

3. Choose the *incorrect* statement.
   a) Modem electrosurgical generators are safer due to their low-voltage, high-frequency, insulated circuitry
   b) Cutting current provides a constant high-energy waveform
   c) Coagulating current creates an initial high-voltage peak, which quickly dissipates
   d) Unipolar cautery may cause tissue damage 4–5 cm from the point of coagulation
   e) Bipolar cautery may cause tissue damage 1–2 cm from the point of coagulation

4. Choose the *incorrect* statement.
   a) The major types of lasers used in surgery are the carbon dioxide, argon, KTP-532, and Nd:YAG
   b) The power density of a laser is expressed in W/mm^2
   c) The carbon dioxide laser is the most commonly used laser for laparoscopy
   d) The carbon dioxide laser is able to seal off blood vessels up to 2.0 mm in diameter

5. All of the following are essential before beginning a laparoscopic procedure EXCEPT
   a) Reviewing the indications for the procedure
   b) Ruling out contraindications to endoscopic surgery
   c) Obtaining appropriate informed consent
   d) Providing the patient with adequate regional anesthesia

6. Choose the *correct* answer pertaining to patient positioning for gynecologic laparoscopic procedures.
   a) The patient's arms should both be placed on extended arm supports
   b) The patient should be in dorsal supine position
   c) The video monitor should be placed at the patient's head
   d) Stirrups that support the foot and knee are necessary

7. Choose the *incorrect* statement.
   a) The patient's stomach and bladder should be emptied before initial trocar insertion
   b) Carbon dioxide gas is used to insufflate the abdomen because there is less risk for embolism compared with nitrous oxide
   c) Alternate entry sites including the left upper quadrant may be chosen for patients who have had multiple previous surgeries
   d) Intraabdominal pressure should never exceed 10 mm Hg

8. Choose the *incorrect* statement.
   a) Results with laparoscopic lysis of adhesions are comparable to those obtained at laparotomy
   b) Blunt dissection should never be used for adhesiolysis
   c) Other methods of adhesiolysis include sharp dissection, aquadissection, and electrodissection
   d) Adhesions involving the tube and ovary should be incised at both ends and removed from the peritoneal cavity

9. Laparoscopic myomectomy
   a) Is usually easier to perform and has less blood loss than hysterectomy
   b) Still requires that the uterine incisions are closed in multiple layers
   c) Results in lower pregnancy rates than abdominal myomectomy
   d) Is more difficult in patients who have received GnRH agonists before surgery

10. Choose the *incorrect* statement dealing with complications of laparoscopy.
    a) Thin, smaller patients are at increased risk for vascular injury with trocar placement
    b) Most bowel injuries caused by the Veress needle require laparotomy for repair
    c) Bladder lacerations less than 5 mm will heal spontaneously with 4–5 days of bladder drainage
    d) Trocars larger than 7 mm increase the risk of bowel herniation

CHAPTER 17

1. Choose the *incorrect* statement.
   a) Hysteroscopes are available with 0-degree straight on or 30-degree fore-oblique views
   b) The telescope is composed of the eyepiece, the barrel, and the objective lens
   c) Three types of light generators are available: tungsten, metal halide, and xenon
   d) The tungsten light source is superior to other sources

2. Choose the *incorrect* statement.
   a) The diagnostic hysteroscope is 4–5 mm in diameter
   b) The operative hysteroscope is 15 mm in diameter
   c) The operating electrodes include a ball, barrel, and cutting loop
   d) Most resectoscopes are equipped with a 30-degree telescope

3. Which of the following are available as accessory instruments for hysteroscopy?
   a) Grasping forceps
   b) Scissors
   c) Biopsy forceps
   d) Monopolar electrode
   e) All of the above

4. Which of the following is the distending medium of choice for office hysteroscopy?
   a) Carbon dioxide
   b) Hyskon
   c) Normal saline
   d) Glycine 1.5%

5. Which of the following should not be used with monopolar cautery?
   a) Carbon dioxide
   b) Hyskon
   c) Normal saline
   d) Glycine 1.5%

6. Which of the following should not be instilled in an amount greater than 500 mL because of its hyperosmotic activity?
   a) Carbon dioxide
   b) Hyskon
   c) Normal saline
   d) Glycine 1.5%

7. Because of its hypoosmolarity, while using which of the following should caution be taken when a fluid deficit of greater than or equal to 500 mL occurs?
   a) Carbon dioxide
   b) Hyskon
   c) Normal saline
   d) Glycine 1.5%

8. Choose the *incorrect* statement.
   a) Hysteroscopy should be performed during the luteal phase for best visualization of the endometrial cavity
   b) Routine cervical dilatation should be avoided at time of hysteroscopy
   c) Uterine position should be determined by pelvic examination before beginning hysteroscopy
   d) The hysteroscope should be advanced into the uterine cavity under direct visualization

9. Simultaneous laparoscopy should be performed with all of the following hysteroscopic procedures EXCEPT
   a) Metroplasty
   b) Resection of uterine synechiae
   c) Cannulation of the fallopian tube
   d) Endometrial ablation

10. Which is the most common complication of operative hysteroscopy?
    a) Infection
    b) Uterine perforation
    c) Carbon dioxide embolism
    d) Bleeding

CHAPTER 18

1. All of the following techniques have been shown to decrease the risk of postoperative deep venous thrombosis and pulmonary embolism EXCEPT
   a) Lower extremity pneumatic sequential compression devices
   b) TED stockings
   c) Low-dose unfractionated heparin
   d) Low molecular weight heparin

2. A 38-year-old woman presents to the gynecology clinic desiring permanent sterilization in the form of bilateral tubal ligation. As you review the patient's history, you discover that the patient's father and grandmother "bled very easily" from cuts and formed bruises easily. On further questioning of this patient, she reports having frequent bouts of epistaxis since childhood and easy bruising. Before scheduling the desired operation, you decide to send blood for testing to assess the presence of a hereditary bleeding disorder. The most common hereditary bleeding disorder is
   a) Hemophilia A
   b) von Willebrand disease
   c) Platelet-activating factor (PAF) deficiency
   d) Hereditary thrombocytopenia

3. A 38 year-old-woman who is scheduled to undergo abdominal hysterectomy for extensive endometriosis asks about the risk of blood transfusion. Which of the following risks is incorrect?
   a) HIV 1:1.9 million
   b) Hepatitis B 1:180,000
   c) Hepatitis C 1:500,000
   d) Anaphylactic reaction 1:150,000

4. During a difficult operation for ovarian cancer, acute blood loss has required transfusion of 15 units of packed red blood cells to maintain sufficient blood volume. The anesthesiologist recommends fresh frozen plasma to ensure adequate hemostasis. Based on the amount of estimated blood loss, this patient should receive how many units of fresh frozen plasma?
   a) 1–2 units (250 mL per unit)
   b) 4–5 units
   c) 7–8 units
   d) 10–12 units
   e) 14–16 units

5. A 62-year-old woman is undergoing pelvic exenteration for recurrent cervical carcinoma. The surgical team estimates operating time from start to finish to be approximately 6 hours and that estimated blood loss in this case could exceed 2 L. Which of the following methods of maintaining intravascular volume in contraindicated in this surgery?
   a) Haemonetics Cell Saver
   b) Predeposit autologous blood transfusion
   c) Intraoperative allogenic blood transfusion
   d) Intravenous crystalloid infusion

6. On the morning following a fairly routine hysterectomy for endometrial cancer, a 72-year-old, 240-lb patient has a hematocrit of 20% (down from 40% preop) and decreased urine output. CT scan shows free blood in the abdomen and pelvis. Her hematocrit continues to fall slowly despite transfusion. What would be the best way to achieve hemostasis in this patient?
   a) Reoperation with ligation of the bleeder
   b) Transfuse 6 units of platelets
   c) Transvaginal placement of an umbrella pack
   d) Arterial embolization of the bleeding vessel

7. A 30-year-old woman presents to you complaining of infertility. She reports that she and her husband have engaged in nonprotected sexual intercourse (with no contraceptive use of any kind) for over a year with no success. She asks you to initiate an infertility workup. After physical examination and ultrasound of the pelvis, an intramural uterine leiomyoma (5 × 5 cm) is identified. The patient elects to undergo transabdominal myomectomy. In addition to myomectomy, in which other procedure can a tourniquet be used to control bleeding?
   a) Uterine unification operation
   b) Cesarean hysterectomy
   c) Resection of a parasitic leiomyoma
   d) Transabdominal sacrocolpopexy

8. Which of the following statements about hypogastric artery ligation is true?
   a) It decreases pulse pressure by 75%–85%
   b) High ligation prevents collateral blood flow to the pelvis
   c) Bilateral ligation is required to be effective
   d) Pregnancy is contraindicated after bilateral ligation

9. Autologous blood donation before surgery is generally not recommended for women undergoing hysterectomy because
   a) The risk of transfusion-related hepatitis C is increased
   b) The patient must donate the blood more than 6 weeks before surgery
   c) Transfusion during hysterectomy is too uncommon to make autologous donation cost-effective
   d) Blood which is unused by the donor cannot be used for other patients

10. During pelvic surgery on a 45-year-old-woman with a large broad ligament leiomyoma, bleeding is encountered from a small vein in the obturator space. Which method should be used first to control the bleeding?
    a) Pressure with a gauze pack
    b) Small hemoclips
    c) 2-0 synthetic absorbable suture
    d) Ligation of the obturator artery

CHAPTER 19

1. In what decade did the use of microsurgical technology and *in vitro* fertilization begin to signal a new therapeutic approach to impairments of reproduction?
   a) 1960s
   b) 1970s
   c) 1980s
   d) 1990s

2. According to U.S. guidelines issued by the American Society for Reproductive Medicine, the maximum number of preembryos that may be transferred per IVF cycle is
   a) 3
   b) 4
   c) 5
   d) No limit

3. GnRH agonists are used in the IVF ovarian stimulation cycle for all the following reason EXCEPT
   a) Improved synchrony of nuclear oocyte maturation
   b) Decreased release of toxic mediators from endometriosis implants
   c) Blocking of the LH surge
   d) Suppressing pituitary gonadotropin output

4. During what stage of cell replication is insemination of harvested oocytes performed?
   a) Interphase
   b) Meiosis I
   c) Meiosis II
   d) Blastocyst stage

5. The following techniques are all acceptable options in the treatment of distal tubal obstruction EXCEPT
   a) Macrosurgical salpingostomy
   b) Microsurgical salpingostomy
   c) Operative laparoscopy

d) IVF
e) Ovarian hyperstimulation with intrauterine insemination

6. Which of the following is an absolute contraindication to tubal reanastomosis following surgical interruption?
   a) Isthmic portion of the tube less than 3 cm in length
   b) Patient age older than 35 years old
   c) Ampullary portion of the tube less than 4 cm in length
   d) Interruption for more than 5 years

7. Which form of tubal sterilization leads to the worst success rate for a tubal reanastomosis procedure?
   a) Cautery
   b) Clips
   c) Bands
   d) Partial salpingectomy

8. How long following the LH surge should mature oocytes be collected during an IVF cycle?
   a) 12–24 hours
   b) 24–36 hours
   c) 34–36 hours
   d) 36–48 hours

9. During an IVF cycle, how long after insemination of the oocytes with washed sperm should transfer by transcervical route occur?
   a) 16–24 hours
   b) 24 hours
   c) 24–36 hours
   d) 48–72 hours

10. Which testing parameter is the most valuable predictor of response to gonadotropin stimulation for the potential IVF patient?
    a) Initial ovarian size
    b) Thickness of endometrial stripe
    c) FSH level
    d) Estradiol level

CHAPTER 20

1. Choose the *incorrect* statement.
   a) Polymenorrhea is a menstrual cycle interval of less then 21 days
   b) Oligomenorrhea is a menstrual cycle interval of more than 37 days
   c) Amenorrhea is the absence of menstrual bleeding for more than 12 months
   d) Postmenopausal bleeding is uterine bleeding occurring more than 12 months after the last menstrual period in a postmenopausal woman

2. Choose the *incorrect* statement.
   a) There are two estrogen receptors, alpha and beta
   b) Estrogen receptors reach a maximum concentration in the early proliferative phase

   c) Progesterone receptors reach maximum concentration in the late proliferative phase
   d) The net effect of estrogenic stimulation is to induce DNA synthesis and mitotic activity with proliferation of endometrial glands and stroma

3. Choose the *incorrect* statement.
   a) The postmenstrual endometrium consists of a thin layer of basalis cells and the stratum spongiosum
   b) In the early proliferative phase the endometrium grows to a thickness of 1–2 mm
   c) Abnormal VEGF mRNA expression may play a role in the pathogenesis of menorrhagia
   d) In the luteal phase the endometrium reaches its maximum thickness of 5–6 mm
   e) The luteal phase functional endometrium consists of a superficial compactum and a deeper spongiosum

4. All of the following limit menstrual blood loss EXCEPT
   a) Recovery of myometrial tone
   b) Cessation of cellular autolysis
   c) Coagulation factors in menstrual blood
   d) Clotting over the endometrial surface
   e) Active regeneration of glands, stroma, and vessels in the basalis layer

5. Choose the *incorrect* answer.
   a) Menstrual flow of 7 days or less is normal
   b) Total blood loss of 20–80 mL is normal
   c) Mean menstrual blood loss is 40 mL
   d) 50 mg of iron is lost in a normal menstrual cycle

6. Which of the following can produce DUB?
   a) Hypothyroidism
   b) Hyperthyroidism
   c) Hyperprolactinemia
   d) Cushing's disease
   e) All of the above

7. Which of the following is the procedure of choice for imaging the endometrial cavity?
   a) Saline infusion sonography
   b) Transvaginal ultrasound
   c) MRI
   d) CT scan

8. The differential diagnosis of DUB in the perimenarchal girl includes
   a) Anovulation
   b) Pregnancy
   c) Coagulopathies
   d) Functional ovarian neoplasm
   e) All of the above

9. Which of the following can be used to treat DUB?
   a) Progestin-impregnated IUD
   b) Step-down regimen of combination oral contraceptive pills
   c) Nonsteroidal antiinflammatory medications
   d) GnRH agonists
   e) All of the above

10. Choose the *incorrect* statement.
    a) In cases of postmenopausal bleeding, endometrial thickness less than 4 mm on transvaginal ultrasound may be used to exclude endometrial cancer
    b) Sampling of the endometrium may be performed with either a silastic curette or dilation and curettage
    c) When unopposed estrogen is used in postmenopausal patients with an intact uterus, endometrial hyperplasia develops in 50% of patients
    d) Endometrial sampling in postmenopausal patients may be complicated by cervical stenosis

CHAPTER 21

1. The most frequent outcome of human fertilization is which one of the following?
    a) Early embryonic mortality
    b) Induced abortion
    c) Premature birth
    d) Term birth
    e) Ectopic pregnancy

2. According the Medical Research Council/Royal College of Obstetricians and Gynaecologists/MRC randomized controlled trial of cervical cerclage, about how many women will have to undergo this operation in order for one to benefit (i.e., the "number needed to treat")?
    a) 4
    b) 10
    c) 15
    d) 25
    e) 40

3. According to World Health Organization estimates, a minimum of how many women die worldwide each year from complications of unsafe abortion?
    a) 4,000
    b) 10,000
    c) 20,000
    d) 30,000
    e) 50,000

4. According to a randomized controlled trial of cervical priming by Singh and others, the optimal dose of misoprostol to be given vaginally 3–4 hours before suction curettage is
    a) 25 μg
    b) 50 μg
    c) 200 μg
    d) 400 μg
    e) 800 μg

5. Which one of the following uterotonic drugs is not marketed in the United States?
    a) 15-Methyl-prostaglandin $F_{2\alpha}$
    b) Prostaglandin E_2 suppository
    c) Misoprostol
    d) Gemeprost
    e) Methylergonovine maleate

6. When added to the local anesthetic, which one of the following has been shown to reduce significantly blood loss during D&E abortion?
    a) Epinephrine
    b) Oxytocin
    c) Vasopressin
    d) Ergot
    e) Misoprostol

7. The risk of death from induced abortion in the United States per 100,000 procedures is about
    a) Less than 1
    b) 5
    c) 10
    d) 20
    e) 40

8. When followed by a prostaglandin for early medical abortion, the lowest single dose of oral mifepristone that provides comparable efficacy as 600 mg is
    a) 50 mg
    b) 100 mg
    c) 200 mg
    d) 400 mg
    e) 500 mg

9. Which of the following is medically essential as part of suction curettage abortion?
    a) Vaginal ultrasonography to confirm gestational age
    b) Follow-up examination in approximately 2 weeks to exclude failed attempted abortion
    c) Formal pathology examination of the products of conception
    d) Examination of the products of conception before the patient is discharged
    e) Oxytocin administration during the operation

10. For suction curettage abortion, randomized controlled trials have established the superiority of which of the following?
    a) Prophylactic antibiotics versus placebo
    b) Oral ergot for 3 days after operation versus no treatment
    c) Preoperative ergot versus intraoperative oxytocin
    d) Preoperative washing the vagina with chlorhexidine versus povidone-iodine
    e) Single-tooth versus atraumatic tenaculum

CHAPTER 22

1. Choose the *correct* answer.
    a) Ectopic pregnancy is the leading cause of maternal death in the first trimester
    b) The total number of pregnancies has declined over the past 30 years, causing the rate of ectopic pregnancy to decline
    c) Increased physician awareness and improved diagnostic and therapeutic alternatives have not affected the risk of death from ectopic pregnancy
    d) A rising incidence of sexually transmitted diseases has not influenced the rate of ectopic pregnancy

2. Which of the following increases the rate of ectopic pregnancy?
   a) Improved antibiotics used to treat pelvic inflammatory disease
   b) Intrauterine device
   c) *In vitro* fertilization
   d) Cigarette smoking
   e) All of the above

3. In a patient with prior tubal surgery
   a) The ectopic risk is higher following neosalpingostomy than reversal of a sterilization procedure
   b) Following tubal sterilization, a patient with a positive pregnancy test has an 80% risk that the pregnancy is ectopic
   c) Following tubal sterilization, the 10-year cumulative probability of ectopic pregnancy for all methods of sterilization is 18.5 per 1000 procedures
   d) Patients undergoing postpartum partial salpingectomy have a higher risk of ectopic pregnancy than those undergoing sterilization by bipolar tubal coagulation

4. Choose the *incorrect* answer.
   a) 95% of ectopic pregnancies occur in the fallopian tube
   b) The most common site of tubal pregnancy is the isthmic portion
   c) Cornual pregnancy accounts for 2%–4% of all tubal pregnancies
   d) Abdominal pregnancy is the rarest site of ectopic implantation

5. In terms of diagnosis of ectopic pregnancy, choose the *incorrect* answer.
   a) 15% of all tubal pregnancies rupture before the first missed menstrual period
   b) An adnexal mass is palpable in only ½ of the cases of ectopic pregnancy
   c) Most patients with pain, uterine bleeding, and an adnexal mass will be diagnosed with ectopic pregnancy
   d) Diagnostic accuracy is improved in repeat ectopic pregnancies, leading to less tubal rupture in these patients

6. Which of the following have improved early diagnosis of ectopic pregnancy?
   a) Highly sensitive beta-hCG assays
   b) Transvaginal sonography
   c) Increased use of laparoscopy
   d) Serum progesterone level less than 5 ng/mL
   e) All of the above

7. Using transvaginal ultrasound in the diagnosis of ectopic pregnancy
   a) An extrauterine pregnancy must be visualized to confirm the diagnosis of ectopic pregnancy
   b) The "double-line" image indicated a pseudogestational sac within the uterus
   c) The discriminatory zone at which an intrauterine pregnancy is expected to be seen is 6500 IU/L (Third IS)
   d) Intrauterine gestations are detectable as early as 1 week after missed menses

8. Choose the *incorrect* answer as it pertains to treatment of ectopic pregnancy.
   a) Expectant management is reasonable in a patient with decreasing beta-hCG levels, absent intrauterine pregnancy by transvaginal ultrasound, and an adnexal mass less than 4 cm without embryonic cardiac activity
   b) Methotrexate is a folic acid antagonist that eradicates trophoblastic tissue
   c) Long-term follow-up of patients given methotrexate for gestational trophoblastic disease has demonstrated an increase in congenital malformations and spontaneous abortions in subsequent pregnancies
   d) Methotrexate can be administered by single-dose, multiple-dose, and local injection regimens

9. Choose the *incorrect* answer concerning single-dose methotrexate therapy.
   a) This regimen is administered as a single intramuscular dose of 50 mg/m²
   b) An increase in serum beta-hCG between day 1 and day 4 indicates probable failure of therapy
   c) A decline in serum beta-hCG of less than 15% from day 4 to day 7 indicates failure of therapy
   d) Analysis has demonstrated that serum beta-hCG level before treatment is the only factor that contributes to treatment outcome

10. Choose the *correct* answer in regard to surgical treatment of ectopic pregnancy.
    a) Linear salpingotomy is considered the gold standard for distal tubal pregnancy in patients who desire future fertility
    b) Subsequent intrauterine pregnancy rates are higher in patients undergoing conservative surgical treatment by laparoscopy than in those undergoing laparotomy
    c) It is not necessary to follow beta-hCG measurements after linear salpingostomy
    d) It is always appropriate to remove the ipsilateral ovary at time of salpingectomy for ectopic pregnancy

CHAPTER 23

1. In what year did James Blundell first propose the concept of tubal sterilization?
   a) 1789
   b) 1824
   c) 1842
   d) 1903

2. In what year was the first successful tubal sterilization performed?
   a) 1795
   b) 1840
   c) 1880
   d) 1903

3. By 1987, what percentage of tubal sterilizations were performed via the laparoscope?
   a) 30%–40%
   b) 40%–50%
   c) 60%–70%
   d) 70%–80%

4. What country accounts for the highest percentage of total tubal sterilizations performed in the world?
   a) India
   b) United States
   c) Brazil
   d) China

5. Worldwide, most tubal sterilization procedures are performed using what kind of anesthesia?
   a) General
   b) Spinal
   c) Local
   d) Epidural

6. What figure is most commonly cited as the failure rate for tubal sterilization?
   a) 4 pregnancies per 1000 sterilization procedures
   b) 7.5 pregnancies per 1000 sterilization procedures
   c) 24 pregnancies per 1000 sterilization procedures
   d) 36.5 pregnancies per 1000 sterilization procedures

7. Which method of sterilization is reported to result in the highest proportion of ectopic pregnancies among all pregnancies after sterilization?
   a) Bipolar coagulation
   b) Interval partial salpingectomy
   c) Unipolar coagulation
   d) Silicone rubber band application

8. The strongest predictor of poststerilization regret is
   a) Parity
   b) Marital status
   c) Timing of procedure in relation to pregnancy
   d) Age

9. The generally reported postvasectomy pregnancy rate is
   a) Less than 1%
   b) 1%
   c) 1.5%
   d) 2%

10. In the United States, the most commonly used method of contraception among married couples is
    a) Intrauterine device
    b) Oral contraceptive pills
    c) Tubal sterilization
    d) Withdrawal

CHAPTER 24

1. The physiologic functions of the fallopian tube include all of the following EXCEPT
   a) Pro-ovarian sperm transport to the site of fertilization
   b) Ovum pickup and pro-uterine transport of the ovum
   c) Ampullary retention of the ovum for approximately 7 days
   d) Transport of the zygote from the ampulla to the uterine cavity

2. Which of the following is a common organism responsible for sexually transmitted pelvic infections?
   a) *Chlamydia trachomatis*
   b) *Neisseria gonorrhoeae*
   c) *Mycoplasma hominis*
   d) Mixed aerobic and anaerobic flora
   e) All of the above

3. Which of these statements is *incorrect*?
   a) The classic clinical picture of PID consisting of pain, fever, and lower genital tract infection occurs in less than 50% of patients
   b) Nearly all patients investigated for infertility and found to have a hydrosalpinx give a history of acute PID
   c) PID occurs at a rate of 10 cases per 1000 women per year age 15–39
   d) A single episode of PID will leave residual tubal damage sufficient to cause infertility in nearly 20% of women

4. Which technique is not recommended for evaluation of tubal patency?
   a) Tubal insufflation
   b) Hysterosalpingogram
   c) Chromopertubation at time of laparoscopy
   d) Selective salpingography

5. According to data collected by SART for the whole year of 1997
   a) 33,032 IVF cycles were initiated
   b) 21.7% of cycles were canceled
   c) The rate of delivery per initiated cycle was 22.3%
   d) The rate of delivery per initiated cycle with ICSI was 27.0%
   e) All of the above are correct

6–10. Match the type of tubal disease with the best treatment.

6. Periadnexal adhesive disease

7. Fimbrial phimosis

8. Distal tubal occlusion with mild tubal damage

9. Proximal tubal occlusion

10. Combined proximal and distal tubal occlusion
    a) Laparoscopic adhesiolysis
    b) Open, microsurgical adhesiolysis
    c) Laparoscopic fimbrioplasty

d) Open, microsurgical fimbrioplasty
e) Laparoscopic salpingostomy
f) Open, microsurgical salpingostomy
g) Selective tubal cannulation
h) Open, microsurgical tubo-cornual anastomosis
i) *In vitro* fertilization

CHAPTER 25

1. Choose the *incorrect* statement.
   a) The prevalence of endometriosis in reproductive age women is 3%–10%
   b) The incidence of endometriosis in women with dysmenorrhea is 40%–60%
   c) 60%–70% of women with infertility are diagnosed with endometriosis
   d) The possibility of familial tendency to develop endometriosis has been reported

2. Which of the following have been proposed as possible mechanisms for development of endometriosis?
   a) Retrograde menstruation and direct implantation
   b) Coelomic metaplasia
   c) Vascular dissemination
   d) Alterations in cellular immunity
   e) All of the above

3. Choose the *correct* statement.
   a) Endometriosis appears to be progressive in most untreated patients
   b) Pregnancy always results in regression of endometriosis
   c) Postmenopausal women do not experience symptoms of endometriosis
   d) Progression of endometriosis occurs in 25% of patients who receive treatment with Danazol or GnRH agonists

4. Choose the *incorrect* statement.
   a) 0.7%–1.0% of patients with endometriosis have lesions that undergo malignant transformation
   b) Atypical glandular changes have been found in 20% of cases of ovarian endometriosis
   c) Endometrioid adenocarcinomas account for nearly 70% of lesions
   d) Rapidly enlarging endometriomas or those measuring more than 10 cm should be sectioned carefully to search for malignant foci

5. By which of the following mechanisms can endometriosis affect fertility?
   a) Local inflammatory response within the pelvis
   b) Anatomic distortion of the pelvic organs
   c) Diminished oocyte pickup
   d) Altered folliculogenesis
   e) All of the above

6. Choose the *correct* statement.
   a) The classic triad associated with endometriosis includes dysmenorrhea, dyschezia, and infertility
   b) Pain associated with endometriosis is strongly linked to deep infiltration of the pelvis
   c) Pain typically does not correlate to steroid hormone fluctuations
   d) Surgical castration does not decrease pain in most patients

7. Choose the *incorrect* statement pertaining to diagnosis of endometriosis.
   a) Bimanual examination may reveal uterosacral ligament tenderness and nodularity, induration of the rectovaginal septum, and fixed retroversion of the uterus
   b) CA-125 levels are not adequately sensitive to screen for endometriosis
   c) Ultrasonography can provide specific information to classify extent and severity of disease
   d) A painful swelling of suspected implants before or during the time of menstruation is a classic sign of endometriosis

8. Choose the *correct* statement pertaining to the classification of endometriosis.
   a) The AFS classification system was revised in 1995 to better categorize disease states
   b) Evaluation of disease is limited by a lack of recognition of atypical implants
   c) Parameters have been determined to indicate the present activity and state of evolution of the disease
   d) The classification system does address disease involving the intestines and urinary tract

9. Choose the *incorrect* statement regarding treatment of endometriosis.
   a) Progestins inhibit pituitary LH release and suppress ovarian production of estrogen to promote secretory changes in the glandular epithelium
   b) Danazol has direct androgenic action on endometrial implants antagonistic to endometriosis
   c) Oral contraceptive pills can induce a "pseudopregnancy" state that improves symptoms of endometriosis
   d) GnRH agonists function to upregulate the pituitary-ovarian axis over time, which decreases symptoms of endometriosis

10. Choose the *incorrect* statement.
    a) Surgery is successful in relieving pain symptoms in a high percentage of women and offers a better prognosis for pregnancy in cases of advanced disease
    b) Preoperative sigmoidoscopy and IVP are recommended in patients with symptoms suggestive of deeply invasive endometriosis
    c) Laparoscopy provides inferior visualization of the posterior cul-de-sac than laparotomy
    d) Conservative resection of endometriosis by laparotomy is most valuable in cases of extensive pelvic adhesions or endometriomas more than 5 cm

CHAPTER 26

1. Choose the *incorrect* statement.
   a) At 4 to 5 weeks' gestation, two gonadal ridges develop on the medial aspect of the coelomic cavity
   b) The epithelial and mesenchymal cells of the gonadal primordia are of mesodermal origin
   c) The gonads of the two sexes remain morphologically indistinguishable until the sixteenth week of gestation
   d) The ovarian stroma is made up of fibroblasts, smooth muscle, and interstitial cells

2. Choose the *correct* statement.
   a) Sexual differentiation requires initiation by a gene determinant on the X chromosome
   b) Maternal ovarian hormone production is required for differentiation of the fetal reproductive tract
   c) Thecal cells play an essential role in development of the fetal ovary
   d) There is a lack of evidence that fetal gonadotropins influence development of the fetal ovary

3. Choose the *incorrect* statement.
   a) The onset of meiosis in the fetal ovary occurs at 11 to 12 weeks' gestation
   b) Cells passing through the various stages of the first meiotic prophase are designated oocytes
   c) Follicular formation begins at 18 to 20 weeks' gestation
   d) The newborn ovary contains 100 million oocytes

4. Choose the *incorrect* answer.
   a) The ligamentous attachments of the ovary include the utero-ovarian, mesovarian, and the infundibulopelvic ligaments
   b) The ovarian arteries originate from the aorta inferior to the renal arteries
   c) The ovarian vein terminates in the inferior vena cava on the left and the renal vein on the right
   d) The main lymphatic vessels of the ovary drain into the periaortic nodes

5. Indications for visualization of an adnexal mass with laparoscopy or laparotomy include which of the following?
   a) Ovarian mass greater than 6 cm
   b) Adnexal mass greater than 10 cm
   c) Any mass developing after menopause
   d) Failure to discover the nature of the mass with radiologic techniques
   e) All of the above

6. In adnexal masses discovered during pregnancy
   a) The rate of adnexal masses was found to be 12.3%
   b) The rate of torsion was 1%
   c) The rate of malignancy was 10%
   d) Laparoscopic surgery was found to be safest in the third trimester

7. Choose the *incorrect* statement pertaining to ultrasound.
   a) Ultrasound has a positive predictive value of 74% and a sensitivity of 88% in predicting malignancy in ovarian neoplasms
   b) A pulsatility index above 1:16 suggests malignancy in an adnexal mass
   c) Cysts containing papillations, septa, or solid components suggest malignancy
   d) None of the above

8. Which of the following are nongynecologic causes of an adnexal mass?
   a) Appendiceal abscess
   b) Diverticulosis
   c) Pelvic kidney
   d) a and c
   e) All of the above

9. Choose the *incorrect* statement.
   a) Adnexal torsion is a common gynecologic surgical emergency with a prevalence of 5%
   b) The classic presentation for adnexal torsion includes acute onset of abdominal pain with clinical evidence of peritonitis and an adnexal mass
   c) Torsion is more likely to occur during ovulation
   d) Unwinding the involved adnexa to observe for tissue reperfusion and viability is safe

10. Choose the *incorrect* statement.
    a) Multiple small adhesions on the ovarian surface should be coagulated then removed
    b) Gentle tissue handling need not be observed during ovarian reconstruction because adhesion formation is uncommon
    c) Resection of an ovarian cyst through the laparoscope decreases incidence of de novo adhesion formation
    d) Interceed, Ringer's lactate solution, and Seprafilm may be used to prevent adhesion formation

CHAPTER 27

1. Choose the *correct* answer.
   a) Chronic pelvic pain must be constant for 6 months or longer
   b) The Cartesian theory states that pain should be proportional to the extent of tissue damage
   c) The gate control theory does not differentiate between acute and chronic pain
   d) Patients with a history of physical or sexual abuse never have concomitant organic pathology

2. Choose the *incorrect* answer.
   a) Not every woman with endometriosis will necessarily have pain
   b) Of patients undergoing laparoscopy for chronic pelvic pain, 41% will have endometriosis
   c) Severity of pain correlates poorly with amount of peritoneal endometriosis
   d) Severity of pain correlates poorly with presence of deep, infiltrative endometriosis

3. Choose the *correct* answer.
   a) Hysterectomy with bilateral salpingo-oophorectomy is an ineffective treatment for endometriosis-related pain
   b) Hysterectomy with ovarian preservation does not affect the recurrence rate of endometriosis
   c) Most patients undergoing laparoscopy for recurrent pain following TAH-BSO for endometriosis will have evidence of recurrent disease
   d) Most pain following TAH-BSO will be due to pelvic adhesions, levator spasm, or irritable bowel syndrome

4. Choose the *incorrect* answer.
   a) Pelvic adhesions are a common cause of chronic pelvic pain
   b) Site of pelvic adhesions does not correlate with site of pelvic pain
   c) Intensity of pelvic pain was unrelated to the extent of adhesions present
   d) Adhesions are anatomically stable a few months after surgery or infection

5. Which of the following are possible etiologies for chronic pelvic pain?
   a) Pelvic organ prolapse
   b) Ovarian remnant
   c) Pelvic floor myalgia
   d) Nerve entrapment
   e) All of the above

6. Choose the *correct* answer.
   a) Urologic problems are the most common cause of nongynecologic pelvic pain
   b) Constipation and irritable bowel syndrome are the most frequent GI causes of chronic pelvic pain
   c) GnRH agonists are ineffective as treatment for irritable bowel syndrome
   d) Women with irritable bowel syndrome have decreased relaxin levels compared with controls

7. Patients with chronic pelvic pain
   a) More frequently score in the depressed range on the Center for Epidemiologic Studies Depression Scale at the time of their initial visit
   b) More frequently meet criteria for major depression, substance abuse, sexual dysfunction, and somatization than controls
   c) Have a higher prevalence of sexual abuse in their histories
   d) Report a high incidence of marital distress
   e) All of the above

8. In patients with true chronic pelvic pain syndrome
   a) Duration of pain is 12 months or longer
   b) The patient has experienced relief from most previous treatments
   c) Physical function is significantly impaired at home or work
   d) Symptoms of depression are rarely exhibited

9. In management of chronic pelvic pain
   a) It is preferable to administer pain medication continuously rather than in a pain-contingent fashion
   b) Antidepressants are ineffective
   c) Anxiolytics do not have potential for addiction and should be used liberally
   d) Pain relief after administration of GnRH agonists is proof that the cause of pain is endometriosis

10. Choose the *incorrect* answer.
    a) In the United States, 12% of hysterectomies are performed for pelvic pain
    b) In one third of hysterectomies performed for pelvic pain, no pathology is found
    c) Laparotomy is superior to laparoscopy in treatment of pelvic adhesive disease
    d) Patients with preoperative depression or sexual dysfunction are more likely to continue to experience pain after surgery

CHAPTER 28

1. Choose the *incorrect* statement pertaining to acute pelvic inflammatory disease (PID).
   a) Generates 2.5 million visits to physicians per year
   b) Requires 150,000 surgical procedures per year
   c) Occurs in 10% of young, sexually active women each year
   d) Is the most common serious infection in women aged 16–25

2. Choose the *incorrect* statement.
   a) 85% of cases of acute PID are sexually transmitted, whereas 15% occur after procedures that break the cervical mucus barrier
   b) Anaerobic bacteria are frequently cultured in the first 48 hours of infection, whereas *Neisseria gonorrhoeae* is cultured late in the disease
   c) Because of a slow growth cycle and lack of clinical symptoms *Chlamydia trachomatis* can produce extended tissue damage
   d) Most cases of acute PID are polymicrobial in etiology

3. Which of the following is a risk factor for acute PID?
   a) Early age of first intercourse
   b) Increased frequency of intercourse
   c) Increased number of sexual partners
   d) Unmarried status
   e) All of the above

4. Choose the *incorrect* statement.
   a) The incidence of PID decreases with advancing age
   b) IUD users have an increased risk of PID
   c) Use of oral contraceptive pills increases the risk of PID
   d) A previous episode of acute PID is a risk factor for future episodes

5. Which is *not* included in the differential diagnosis of acute PID?
   a) Appendicitis
   b) Adnexal torsion
   c) Ectopic pregnancy
   d) Ruptured ovarian cyst
   e) All of the above should be considered in the differential diagnosis

6. Choose the *incorrect* statement.
   a) The classic triad in diagnosis of acute PID includes pelvic mass, fever, leukocytosis
   b) The classic triad of symptoms is seen in only 15–30% of patients with acute PID
   c) The most common symptom of acute PID is pelvic pain
   d) Fitz-Hugh-Curtis adhesions develop in 1%–10% of patients with acute PID

7. Choose the *incorrect* statement.
   a) 20% of patients who have had acute PID will have subsequent infertility
   b) Ectopic pregnancy is 6–10 times more frequent in patients with previous acute PID
   c) 50% of ectopic pregnancies occur in tubes damaged by previous salpingitis
   d) The chance that a woman will develop chronic pelvic pain after acute PID is 5%

8. Choose the *incorrect* statement.
   a) In the United States one out of every four women with acute PID are treated as outpatients
   b) 10%–20% of women treated as outpatients will experience treatment failure
   c) Patients should be reevaluated within 48–72 hours of initiating therapy to determine response to treatment
   d) Patients who fail to respond to oral antibiotics should be hospitalized for parenteral antibiotic therapy

9. Which of the following is *not* an indication for inpatient treatment for acute PID?
   a) Adolescent
   b) Pelvic pain
   c) Pelvic abscess
   d) Questionable diagnosis of PID
   e) Nausea and vomiting

10. Choose the *incorrect* statement.
    a) Laparoscopy is an underused tool in the diagnosis of acute PID
    b) Cultures taken from the peritoneal cavity at the time of surgery can guide antibiotic therapy
    c) Tubo-ovarian abscesses should never be drained laparoscopically
    d) Posterior colpotomy is an option for drainage of midline pelvic abscesses
    e) Ruptured tubo-ovarian abscesses should be treated with immediate exploratory laparotomy

CHAPTER 29

1. The müllerian anomalies associated with ipsilateral renal agenesis include all of the following EXCEPT
   a) Unilateral vaginal obstruction
   b) Septate uterus
   c) Unilateral obstruction of a cavity of a double uterus
   d) Unicornuate uterus with a non communicating horn

2. Which of the following is true regarding vaginal development?
   a) The vagina develops from both the müllerian ducts and the urogenital sinus
   b) A transverse septum is more common in the lower or distal vagina
   c) Partial vaginal agenesis has a high incidence of associated renal anomalies
   d) Abnormal development of the vagina never accompanies other anomalies

3. All of the following are characteristics of women with müllerian agenesis EXCEPT
   a) Genetic sex is female (XX)
   b) Congenital absence of a normal uterus and vagina
   c) Impaired ovarian function
   d) Frequent association of other anomalies, including skeletal, urologic, and renal

4. Evaluation of patients with müllerian agenesis should include all of the following EXCEPT
   a) Psychologic support
   b) Genetic evaluation
   c) Ultrasonography or MRI
   d) Complete physical examination
   e) Laparoscopy

5. Which of these important issues in successful nonsurgical creation of a neovagina is true?
   a) Nonsurgical creation of a neovagina is not appropriate as a first line approach
   b) Greater than 90% patients have been shown to achieve anatomic and functional success by vaginal dilation
   c) A "buddy" support system is not helpful in achieving success with vaginal dilation
   d) Vaginal dilation should be initiated in any age patient, even in prepubertal girls

6. According to Sir Archibald McIndoe, the important principles in successful surgical creation of a neovagina include all EXCEPT
   a) Dissection of an adequate space between the rectum and bladder
   b) Inlay split-thickness skin grafting
   c) Continued and prolonged dilatation during the contractile phase of healing
   d) Adequate preoperative dilatation

7. Which of the following is true regarding cervical dysgenesis?
    a) Cervical agenesis is the most common müllerian anomaly
    b) There is only one type of cervical dysgenesis
    c) Creation of a passage between the uterus and vagina is a simple, highly successful procedure
    d) Conservative management, with hormonal suppression of endometrial stimulation, is appropriate for young patients

8. Lateral fusion disorders of the müllerian ducts include all of the following EXCEPT
    a) Bicornuate uterus
    b) Septate uterus
    c) Didelphic uterus
    d) Rokitansky syndrome

9. The müllerian anomaly associated with the most reproductive success is
    a) Septate uterus
    b) Bicornuate uterus
    c) Didelphic uterus
    d) Unicornuate uterus

10. Benefits of hysteroscopic resection of a uterine septum include all of the following EXCEPT
    a) The potential for a vaginal delivery with future pregnancies
    b) A prolonged postoperative recovery period
    c) Similar success as an abdominal metroplasty
    d) Transcervical lysis may also be used to repair a complete septate uterus

CHAPTER 30

1. Typical characteristics of uterine leiomyomata include all of the following EXCEPT
    a) Typical locations are subserosal, submucosal, and intramural in nature
    b) The most common change is hyaline degeneration
    c) Red or carneous degeneration is never seen during pregnancy
    d) A subserosal, pedunculated myoma may outgrow its blood supply

2. Which degenerative changes are the least common?
    a) Hyaline degeneration
    b) Red or carneous degeneration
    c) Necrosis
    d) Sarcomatous degeneration

3. Which of the following is true regarding intravenous leiomyomatosis?
    a) The condition is quite common and may be found in up to 50% patients with leiomyoma
    b) The tumor behaves clinically as a benign entity
    c) Wormlike extensions of tumor involve only the ovarian veins
    d) The most common site of metastases is the brain

4. In describing the clinical features of leiomyomata, it is important to remember that
    a) Most leiomyomata are asymptomatic and may not require any treatment
    b) If the uterine size is believed to be greater than 12 weeks size, a hysterectomy is recommended
    c) Most women will have an increase in symptomatology after menopause

5. Hormonal management options for patients with a myomatous uterus may include all of the following EXCEPT
    a) Mifepristone (RU486)
    b) Danazol
    c) GnRH analogues
    d) Oral contraceptives (30 to 35 μg ethinyl estradiol)

6. Which of the following is a true statement regarding hysteroscopic resection of submucous myomata?
    a) By combining the procedure with endometrial ablation, pregnancy rates are increased
    b) Menorrhagia is only rarely controlled
    c) It is recommended to combine laparoscopic guidance with the hysteroscopic procedure
    d) Success rates are not dependent on the experience or skill of the surgeon

7. Appropriate candidates for a laparoscopic myomectomy include which of the following?
    a) A postmenopausal patient with incidentally detected myomata on an annual examination
    b) A 34-year-old woman, desiring future fertility, with two intramural myomas each measuring 3 cm in diameter
    c) A 34-year-old woman, desiring future fertility, with two submucosal myomas each measuring 3 cm in diameter
    d) A 40-year-old woman, completed childbearing, with a 20-week size uterus with multiple myomas

8. Methods to control intraoperative blood loss during an abdominal myomectomy may include all of the following EXCEPT
    a) Preoperative treatment with oral contraceptive pills
    b) Local injection with vasoconstrictive agents
    c) Controlled induced hypotension
    d) Use of a uterine tourniquet

9. Postoperative morbidity commonly associated with an abdominal myomectomy includes all of the following EXCEPT
    a) Significant blood loss
    b) Intraabdominal adhesion formation
    c) Febrile morbidity
    d) Pulmonary embolus

10. Which of the following statements is true regarding uterine artery embolization?
    a) Most patients report an improvement in menorrhagia and bulk related symptoms
    b) The overall success rate with an experienced team of providers is only about 25%
    c) Less than 1% of patients develop postembolization syndrome with fever and malaise.
    d) The major complication rate approaches 50%

CHAPTER 31

1. The mortality rate from hysterectomy is approximately
    a) 1–2 per 100 patients
    b) 1–2 per 1000 patients
    c) 1–2 per 10,000 patients
    d) 1–2 per 100,000 patients

2. Which of the following statements regarding the treatment of dysfunctional uterine bleeding is true?
    a) Approximately 10% of hysterectomies are performed with dysfunctional uterine bleeding as the primary indication
    b) The quality of life scores of women treated with endometrial ablation for dysfunctional uterine bleeding are equivalent to those of women treated with hysterectomy
    c) In women older than 40 years, endometrial sampling should be performed before the initiation of hormonal therapy, but it is not necessary before surgical therapy
    d) After endometrial ablation for the treatment of dysfunctional uterine bleeding, approximately 12%–15% of patients will require a hysterectomy for persistent bleeding and/or pain

3. The most common indication for the performance of hysterectomy is
    a) Uterine leiomyomata
    b) Dysfunctional uterine bleeding
    c) Uterine prolapse
    d) Adenomyosis

4. Which of the following statements regarding uterine leiomyomata is true?
    a) The incidence of leiomyosarcoma in patients undergoing hysterectomy for presumed uterine leiomyomata is 1%–2%
    b) The risk of complications from abdominal hysterectomy increases when the uterine weight exceeds 500 g
    c) The best treatment for a prolapsing uterine myoma is immediate abdominal hysterectomy
    d) Uterine leiomyomas frequently continue to enlarge and cause new symptoms after menopause

5. A 40-year-old, otherwise healthy woman who has completed her family undergoes a cervical conization for evaluation of an abnormal Pap smear. Pathology reveals a cervical cancer with a depth of invasion of 2.5 mm, lateral extent of 5 mm, and no evidence of lymphovascular space invasion. All cone margins are free of dysplasia or cancer. The next best step in the treatment of this patient would be
    a) Chemoradiation
    b) Observation
    c) Radical hysterectomy
    d) Vaginal hysterectomy

6. Which of the following factors is *not* associated with an increased risk of postoperative complications following hysterectomy?
    a) Use of the vaginal approach
    b) Increasing age
    c) Diagnosis of malignancy
    d) Presence of concurrent medical illnesses

7. Which of the following is the correct order in which to perform an abdominal hysterectomy?
    a) 1) Incise vagina; 2) clamp, transect, and ligate the uterine arteries; 3) dissect the bladder off of the anterior cervix; 4) isolate, clamp, transect, and ligate the utero-ovarian ligaments
    b) 1) Clamp, transect, and ligate the uterine arteries; 2) incise vagina; 3) isolate, clamp, transect, and ligate the utero-ovarian ligaments; 4) dissect the bladder off of the anterior cervix
    c) 1) Isolate, clamp, transect, and ligate the utero-ovarian ligaments; 2) dissect the bladder off of the anterior cervix; 3) clamp, transect, and ligate the uterine arteries; 4) incise vagina
    d) 1) Dissect the bladder off of the anterior cervix; 2) incise vagina; 3) clamp, transect, and ligate the uterine arteries; 4) isolate, clamp, transect, and ligate the utero-ovarian ligaments

8. A 35-year-old woman, G3P3003, is considering a hysterectomy for the treatment of uterine leiomyomata with resultant menorrhagia. She has failed a trial of medical management. She is otherwise healthy and has no family history of cancer. On examination, her uterus is 12-week size and mobile. There is good uterine descensus. During your preoperative counseling of this patient, you should tell her that
    a) Hysterectomy often results in a loss of sexual function
    b) Performance of vaginal hysterectomy in this clinical situation is associated with a shorter operative time and fewer complications than abdominal hysterectomy
    c) Concurrent bilateral salpingo-oophorectomy should be performed to decrease her risk of ovarian and breast cancer
    d) Supracervical hysterectomy has been demonstrated to decrease the risk of subsequent bladder dysfunction

9. Which of the following is *not* a part of the routine preoperative preparation of a healthy 40-year-old women before the performance of an abdominal hysterectomy for benign disease?
    a) Hemoglobin or hematocrit
    b) Pregnancy test
    c) Recent Pap smear
    d) Computerized tomographic (CT) scan of the pelvis

10. Which of the following is the MOST important factor in decreasing the risk of postoperative infection following hysterectomy?
    a) Diagnosis and treatment of bacterial vaginosis preoperatively
    b) Leaving the vaginal cuff open
    c) Povidone-iodine douche preoperatively
    d) Administration of intravenous second-generation cephalosporin preoperatively

CHAPTER 32

1. A 28-year-old woman, gravida 3, para 2, with a single intrauterine pregnancy, has failed induction of labor at 42 weeks' gestation. As you explain the risks and benefits of cesarean delivery, you mention the possibility of emergency hysterectomy. The patient desires future fertility and is concerned about this potential complication. The most common condition leading to an emergent cesarean hysterectomy is
    a) Uterine rupture
    b) Placental abruption
    c) Placenta accreta
    d) Uterine atony

2. A 28-year-old woman, gravida 2, has a routine obstetrical ultrasound at 18 weeks gestation and a 3.5-cm smooth walled cyst is noted in the right ovary. The best plan of management would be
    a) Ultrasound guided needle aspiration of the cyst with cytologic examination of the fluid
    b) Repeat ultrasound in 6 weeks
    c) Exploratory laparotomy with right oophorectomy
    d) Plan for cesarean delivery with right ovarian cystectomy at that time

3. A 40-year-old woman, gravida 3, para 2, presents in active labor at 39 weeks' gestation. A brief ultrasound performed in the office 2 days previously showed a single intrauterine pregnancy with amniotic fluid index (AFI) of 15. The duration of active labor is 2 hours; the second stage of labor lasts 90 minutes. The patient undergoes a spontaneous vaginal delivery of a 4026 g (8 lb 14 oz) infant complicated by postpartum hemorrhage. The most likely cause of postpartum hemorrhage in this patient is
    a) Infant birthweight
    b) Length of the active phase of labor
    c) Amniotic fluid volume
    d) Duration of the second stage of labor

4. A 19-year-old woman, gravida 1, with suboptimally controlled asthma during her pregnancy presents in active labor at 40 weeks' gestation. She undergoes a spontaneous vaginal delivery of a 3005 g (6 lb 10 oz) infant. As you perform uterine massage, you note a boggy uterus and continued vaginal bleeding. Which of the following measures would *not* be appropriate

in the management of this patient's postpartum hemorrhage?
    a) Intravenous infusion of crystalloid
    b) Intravenous oxytocin
    c) Intramuscular methylergonovine (Methergine)
    d) Intramuscular carboprost (Hemabate)

5. A 22-year-old woman, gravida 1, presents in active labor at 39 weeks' gestation. The patient has an uneventful first stage of labor; as the patient begins to push after complete cervical dilation has occurred, you note her blood pressure is 145/90 mm Hg. After 2 hours of pushing, you perform both an episiotomy and a forceps-assisted vaginal delivery. Which of the following is an acceptable indication for an episiotomy in this scenario?
    a) Maternal blood pressure
    b) Prevention of trauma to the fetus
    c) Prevention of future pelvic muscle relaxation
    d) Forceps-assisted vaginal delivery

6. A 30-year-old woman undergoes a midline episiotomy to assist in the vaginal delivery of a 3175 gram (7 lb 0 oz) infant. The episiotomy repair is performed without complication. On the first postpartum day, you examine the perineum and note that dehiscence of the episiotomy has taken place. The patient asks to be discharged from the hospital, despite your advice that she remain in the hospital for repair of this dehiscence. You explain that a potential disadvantage of delayed repair of an episiotomy dehiscence is
    a) Loss of sexual function
    b) Decreased incidence of primary healing
    c) Need to use permanent suture material
    d) Increased risk of fourth-degree laceration with future deliveries

7. A 35-year-old woman undergoes a midline episiotomy to assist in the vaginal delivery of a 4111 gram (9 lb 1 oz) infant. Her medical history is significant for class C gestational diabetes during this pregnancy. On postpartum day number two, the patient develops a fever of 39.1° C (102.4° F). You examine the patient at the bedside and are concerned for possible necrotizing fasciitis. A common etiologic agent of necrotizing fasciitis is
    a) *Chlamydia trachomatis*
    b) *Clostridium perfringens*
    c) *Escherichia coli*
    d) *Proteus mirabilis*

8. The most common complications of emergency peripartum hysterectomy is
    a) Blood transfusion
    b) Urinary tract injury
    c) Infection
    d) Pelvic thrombophlebitis

9. A 34-year-old woman, gravida 3, para 2, with a twin intrauterine pregnancy presents to your office at 34 weeks' gestation complaining of mild, intermittent left lower quadrant abdominal pain. She also notes the recent development of sparse, dark facial hair on her mandible. You perform an ultrasound and note a solid 2-cm mass on the left ovary. Subsequent biopsy of this lesion shows a luteoma of pregnancy. The next appropriate step in the management of this condition is
   a) Induction of labor
   b) Laparoscopic left salpingo-oophorectomy
   c) Laparoscopic bilateral salpingo-oophorectomy and pelvic lymph node sampling
   d) Observation

10. Fetal endoscopy has proved to be most useful in which of the following conditions?
   a) Obstructed fetal bladder
   b) Spina bifida
   c) Twin-twin transfusion syndrome
   d) Myelomeningocele repair

CHAPTER 33

1. An ulcerating perianal lesion is found on examination that clinically is very concerning for a malignancy. The lesion is biopsied and is negative for malignancy. Because of the clinical appearance, the lesion is again biopsied and again the biopsy is negative. Cytology and biopsy with which of the following tests is most likely to establish the true diagnosis?
   a) Schiff's stain
   b) Tzanck smear
   c) Warthin-Starry stain
   d) Fontana-Masson stain

2. A patient is diagnosed with early hidradenitis suppurativa, characterized by chronic pruritus and the occasional development of superficial pustules, especially at the time of menses. The lesions are mildly tender and nonfluctuant. In this early stage of the disease, which of the following would be the best initial choice of treatment?
   a) A course of clindamycin at the first sign of each outbreak
   b) A daily topical steroid cream
   c) Incision and drainage of each pustule
   d) Hormonal therapy
   e) Accutane

3. Each of the following characteristics, except which, would cause an increased consideration of excision rather than marsupialization of a Bartholin duct cyst?
   a) Greater than 3 cm in diameter
   b) Patient age older than 40 years
   c) Induration at the base
   d) Patient with coexisting Paget's disease

4. All patients with vulvar vestibulitis should have which of the following as at least part of their medical regimen to treat this condition?
   a) Antifungals (oral or topical)
   b) Alfa-interferon
   c) Amitriptyline
   d) Topical steroids

5. You have a patient with condyloma acuminatum, which you decide to treat with trichloroacetic acid (TCA). Which of the following statements is false, regarding TCA treatment of condyloma acuminatum?
   a) Lesions treated with TCA should rapidly turn white
   b) TCA should not be used intravaginally during pregnancy
   c) Sodium bicarbonate can be used to rapidly neutralize TCA
   d) A suitable concentration is 90% TCA

6. While examining the external genitalia of a patient a lesion is noticed in the interlabial fold that is 0.5 cm in diameter, is of medium firmness, and has a reddish-brown pulpy material on the surface. Which of the following is the most likely diagnosis?
   a) Hidradenoma
   b) Hemangioma
   c) Granular cell tumor
   d) Basal cell carcinoma

7. Which of the following is the predominant symptom of vulvar cancer?
   a) Bleeding
   b) Pain
   c) Itching
   d) A palpable lump

8. For the treatment of *in situ* vulvar neoplasia, which of the following best describes the recurrence risk for local excision verses total vulvectomy?
   a) Local—70% recurrence; total vulvectomy—20% recurrence
   b) Local—25% recurrence; total vulvectomy—75% recurrence
   c) Local—35% recurrence; total vulvectomy—35% recurrence
   d) Local—80% recurrence; total vulvectomy—80% recurrence

9. Which of the following patients have an indication for simple vulvectomy?
   I) 45 year old with granulomatous disease unresponsive to medical therapy and wide local excision
   II) 67 year old with marked atypical hyperplasia
   III) 39 year old with vulvar intraepithelial neoplasia (VIN)
   IV) 55 year old with Paget's disease of the vulva
   a) I and III only
   b) I, II, and IV only
   c) I, II, III, and IV
   d) II and IV only

10. Which of the following nerves would not have branches broken by the Mering procedure for vulvar pruritus?
    a) Ilioinguinal nerve
    b) Genitofemoral nerve
    c) Pudendal nerve
    d) Inferior gluteal nerve

CHAPTER 34

1. The hymen
    a) Is usually imperforate during embryonic life
    b) Becomes patent when canalization of the most caudal portion of the vaginal plate at the urogenital sinus occurs
    c) Most frequently has a folded shape with an eccentric orifice in the newborn
    d) Is found to be imperforate in 1% of newborns

2. Choose the *incorrect* answer.
    a) Ambiguous external genitalia are remarkably constant in appearance regardless of etiology
    b) Most patients have a high (suprasphincteric) urethral-vaginal connection
    c) Reconstruction must be timed properly to allow easy identification of all structures while preventing psychologic stress to the patient
    d) Most hermaphrodites reared as girls do have a vagina or vaginal pouch

3. Choose the *incorrect* answer.
    a) In the group of patients undergoing reconstruction of the external genitalia, 87% required further vaginal reconstructive surgery to allow intercourse
    b) The most common long-term problem following reconstruction procedures is intravaginal stenosis
    c) Vaginoplasty should be performed in infancy to prevent vaginal stenosis
    d) In patients who underwent clitoridectomy, 29% reported no orgasms

4. Classic bladder exstrophy is characterized by all of the following EXCEPT
    a) Male to female ratio of 2:1
    b) Absence of anterior abdominal wall
    c) Absence of the posterior wall of the bladder exposing the ureteral orifices
    d) Poorly defined bladder neck and urethra
    e) Wide separation of the pubic symphysis

5. Other possible anomalies associated with bladder exstrophy include
    a) Bifid clitoris
    b) Rectal prolapse
    c) Imperforate anus
    d) Renal agenesis
    e) All of the above

6. Choose the *incorrect* statement about vaginal carcinoma.
    a) The average age at presentation is 35 years
    b) Vaginal carcinoma must meet specific FIGO criteria to be considered a primary vaginal carcinoma
    c) Vaginal carcinoma comprises less than 2% of gynecologic malignancies
    d) Clinicians must find the urethra, cervix, and vulva to be histologically negative to diagnose primary vaginal carcinoma

7. Choose the *incorrect* statement about diethylstilbestrol (DES).
    a) DES is a nonsteroidal estrogenic hormone that was used in patients with a history of recurrent pregnancy loss until 1970
    b) The incidence of vaginal adenocarcinoma in young women exposed to DES *in utero* is 0.14–1.4 per 1000
    c) 75% of women exposed to DES *in utero* have anatomic abnormalities
    d) Vaginal adenosis has been found in 34%–90% of women exposed to DES *in utero*

8. Choose the *incorrect* answer pertaining to vaginal carcinoma.
    a) Stage 0 disease can be treated with surgery, carbon dioxide laser, or 5-fluorouracil cream
    b) Stage 1 disease lesions can be treated with radiation therapy or total abdominal hysterectomy
    c) Stage 2 or 3 lesions are treated with radiotherapy
    d) Stage 4 lesions are treated with pelvic exenteration or radiotherapy

9. Which of the following is not a possible cause of urethral diverticulum?
    a) *Neisseria gonorrhoeae* infection
    b) Trauma associated with childbirth
    c) Urethral stone
    d) Surgical trauma
    e) Infection of the Bartholin's gland

10. Choose the *incorrect* answer.
    a) Dysuria, frequency, urgency, and hematuria occur in 85%–90% of patients with urethral diverticula
    b) Urethral diverticula frequently cause a palpable lump in the vagina
    c) Most urethral diverticula are located in the proximal urethra
    d) Urethral diverticula can be diagnosed with cystourethroscopy, positive-pressure urethrography, or voiding cystourethrography

CHAPTER 35A

1. The pelvic diaphragm is composed of all of the following muscles EXCEPT
    a) Ileococcygeus
    b) Puborectalis
    c) Transversus perinei
    d) Pubococcygeus

2. The goal of defect-specific pelvic reconstructive surgery is to identify and reattach the endopelvic connective tissue to which central pelvic structure?
   a) Arcus tendineus fascia pelvis
   b) Sacrospinous ligament
   c) Levator plate
   d) Pericervical ring

3. It is now believed that the most important cause of pelvic organ prolapse is
   a) Low estrogen levels
   b) Vaginal delivery
   c) Straining with constipation
   d) Coughing resulting from chronic lung disease

4. With the Baden-Walker halfway system for grading pelvic prolapse, the fixed anatomic reference point to which measurements are referred is the
   a) Ischial spine
   b) Vaginal introitus
   c) Cervix or vaginal vault
   d) Halfway between the cervix and vaginal introitus

5. In most patients, pelvic organ prolapse can be best managed via which approach?
   a) Vaginal
   b) Abdominal
   c) Laparoscopic
   d) Combined approach

CHAPTER 35B

1. A 39-year-old gravida 4 para 4 presents complaining of a "bulge" in her vagina. When ring forceps are placed against the anterior vaginal wall and directed laterally and posteriorly toward the ischial spines, the defect is corrected. Which of the following is the most likely defect(s)?
   a) Transverse defect alone
   b) Midline defect alone
   c) Paravaginal defect alone
   d) Paravaginal and midline defect
   e) Midline and transverse defect

2. A 24-year-old nulliparous woman presents for her annual examination and for birth control with no complaints. On examination she is noted to have bilateral sulci in the anterior vagina. Which of the following best describes the anatomic structure(s) responsible for these sulci?
   a) This is where the pubocervical fascia blends into the pericervical ring of fibromuscular tissue
   b) This is where the cardinal ligament inserts
   c) The sulci are a result of a midline defect prolapsing between them
   d) This is where the pubocervical fascia attaches to the arcus tendineus fascia pelvis

3. The pubocervical fascia is attached to all of the following structures EXCEPT
   a) The pericervical ring of biromuscular tissue
   b) The arcus tendinous fascia pelvis
   c) The pubic ramus
   d) The endopelvic fascia

4. During an open retropubic pelvic support defect repair, palpation of the pelvis reveals an "button-hole" like opening along the inferior border of the superior pubic ramus about 7–10 cm lateral to the midline. This is the obturator canal. From this landmark where would one expect to locate the ischial spine?
   a) 7–8 cm dorsally
   b) 3–4 cm superiorly
   c) 5–6 cm medially
   d) 1–2 cm ventrally

5. Generally, where is easiest point of identification of the arcus tendineus fascia pelvis?
   a) The ischial spine
   b) At the attachment to the pubocervical fascia near the pelvic sidewall
   c) The posterior aspect of the pubic bone
   d) Medial to the obturator canal

6. Which of the following structures contribute to the "white line"? (Select all that apply)
   a) The levator ani fascia
   b) The coccygeus fascia
   c) The obturator externus fascia
   d) The piriformis fascia

7. The bladder should never be dissected off of the anterior vaginal surface during an open retropubic paravaginal defect repair because doing so is likely to result in which of the following? (Select one)
   a) Excessive bleeding
   b) Denervation of part of the bladder
   c) Creation of midline support defect
   d) Weakness of the paravaginal repair

8. A 73-year-old para 3 woman presents complaining of "a fallen bladder." She describes urinary incontinence for several years. She is also a smoker who was recently diagnosed with emphysema, but she does not require supplemental oxygen. She is found on examination to have a right paravaginal defect. Furthermore, on examination her suprapubic arch is two fingerbreadths wide. Which of the following pieces of information make an open approach more likely to be the best approach for this patient instead of the vaginal approach? (Select all that apply)
   a) Her age
   b) The fact that her defect is paravaginal
   c) The width of her pubic arch
   d) Her medical history (emphysema)

9. On a vaginal reconstruction of an anterior defect, where is the first suture usually placed?
   a) Close to the posterior surface of the pubic bone
   b) About halfway between the urethrovesical junction and the urethral meatus

c) Just through the vaginal epithelium near the lateral edge of the pubocervical fascia

d) Into the tendinous arch and obturator fascia anterior to the ischial spine

10. Transvaginally, the sutures that are used to close the paravaginal defect are
   a) Placed individually from the ischial spine anteriorly toward the symphysis
   b) 0 chromic sutures
   c) Tied one at a time starting with the suture nearest the vaginal apex
   d) Placed carefully to avoid penetration of the vaginal mucosa

CHAPTER 35C

1. Name the four major anatomic constituents that determine vaginal axis configuration.

2. What is the specific type of lesion in the rectovaginal septum that leads to rectocele and what is the principal cause of it?

3. If a perineal body defect is present, even though asymptomatic, why is anatomic restitution important in conjunction with any form of urethropexy or cystourethropexy?

4. What are the principal reasons for doing a rectal examination during posterior pelvic compartment repair surgery?

5. Are imaging studies of any value in diagnosing rectocele and what are the reasons for your answer?

6. Can estrogen play a role in pelvic reconstructive surgery and, if it does, how does this work?

7. What is considered appropriate conduct in the event the anorectal lumen is entered inadvertently during dissection?

8. In what situations should one consider combining a McCall procedure or a sacrospinous ligament fixation with a rectocele repair?

9. Under what circumstances, and why, should an asymptomatic but distinct rectocele and perineal body defects scenario demand repair?

10. When should one consider using a graft in posterior reparative surgery and should it ever be invoked in a primary operation?

CHAPTER 35D

1. To prevent vaginal vault prolapse after the performance of a vaginal hysterectomy for uterine prolapse, the surgeon should
   a) Secure the vaginal angle to the ipsilateral cardinal ligament
   b) Perform a Kelly plication

c) Obliterate the cul-de-sac of Douglas
   d) Perform a posterior colpoperineorrhaphy

2. At the completion of a total vaginal hysterectomy with repair of enterocele, cystocele, and rectocele for uterine prolapse, the MOST desired anatomic outcome is
   a) The vagina is shortened and narrowed to one finger in depth and diameter
   b) The upper one third of the vagina is parallel to the floor when the patient is standing
   c) The apex of the posterior suture line points toward the sacral promontory
   d) The perineal body is shortened as much as possible

3. During the performance of a vaginal hysterectomy for total procidentia, the ureter can BEST be identified
   a) On the medial leaf of the broad ligament
   b) At the bladder base, where it enters the trigone
   c) Outside the vagina, just cephalad to the uterosacral ligament tie
   d) By seeing a gush of clear fluid when it is cut

4. Which of the following statements regarding a McCall culdoplasty is TRUE?
   a) Enterocele repair is rarely necessary at the time of surgery for total procidentia
   b) The procedure results in narrowing of the levator hiatus
   c) The internal McCall suture should include the pararectal fascia on both sides and the posterior vaginal wall
   d) The McCall sutures should be tied after the performance of the anterior colporrhaphy

5. Which of the following statements regarding the goals of surgical correction of uterine prolapse is FALSE?
   a) The length of the uterosacral and cardinal ligaments should be maintained
   b) The cul-de-sac of Douglas should be obliterated
   c) The upper vagina should be restored over the levator plate
   d) The endopelvic fascial attachments of the vagina should be reconstructed

CHAPTER 35E

1. After performing a hysterectomy, to what ligament complex should one attach the vaginal apex to prevent vaginal vault prolapse?
   a) Pubourethral ligament
   b) Sacrospinous ligament
   c) Round ligament
   d) Uterosacral cardinal ligament

2. According to DeLancey, where does a Level III defect occur?
   a) Lateral attachment of the midvagina
   b) Perineal body
   c) Uterosacral ligament
   d) Paracolpium and parametrium

3. Abdominal support procedures should be performed in patients who meet all of the following criteria EXCEPT
   a) Previous vaginal support procedure
   b) Multiple previous abdominal procedures
   c) Have a foreshortened vagina
   d) Would benefit from long duration of mesh grafts

4. Which one of the following structures is at risk for injury during a McCall's culdoplasty?
   a) Sciatic nerve
   b) Rectum
   c) Internal iliac vein
   d) Pudendal nerve

5. Operative complications of the McCall's culdoplasty include all of the following EXCEPT
   a) Bowel or rectum lacerations
   b) Hematomas
   c) Cuff abscess or infection
   d) Cervical lacerations

6. Which of the following structures lies posterior to the ischial spine?
   a) Pudendal nerve/vessels
   b) Sciatic nerve
   c) Hypogastric venous plexus
   d) Inferior gluteal vessels

7. What type of stitch can be used for a sacrospinous ligament fixation?
   a) Vertical mattress stitch
   b) Horizontal mattress stitch
   c) Pulley stitch
   d) Interrupted stitch

8. One of the late complications following sacrospinous ligament fixation is
   a) Uterine prolapse
   b) Anterior wall prolapse
   c) Rectal prolapse
   d) Dyspareunia

9. Uterosacral ligament suspension is a relatively new technique in the management of enterocele and vaginal vault prolapse. Permanent sutures are used in each of the following steps EXCEPT
   a) Tagging the uterosacral ligaments
   b) Securing the proximal uterosacral ligament
   c) Securing the posterior peritoneum to the uterosacral ligaments
   d) Suspending the anterior and posterior walls to the ridge of the uterosacral ligament

10. Steps involved in performing an abdominal sacral colpopexy include all of the following EXCEPT
    a) Suturing the sacrospinous ligaments to each other
    b) Dissecting the peritoneum away from the vagina
    c) Placing nonabsorbable sutures through the posterior vagina
    d) Suturing the mesh halfway down the posterior vagina
    e) Suturing the mesh to the longitudinal ligament over the sacral promontory

CHAPTER 35F

1. Which of the following is not a use for a vaginal pessary?
   a) Genital prolapse
   b) Fecal incontinence
   c) Urinary incontinence
   d) Cervical incompetence
   e) Administration of local estrogen

2. What is the most common reason a woman stops using her pessary?
   a) Inability to hold it in place
   b) Difficulty of removal
   c) Inadequate relief of symptoms
   d) Discomfort
   e) Inability to urinate

3. Which of the following factors is associated with successful use of a pessary?
   a) Young age
   b) History of pelvic surgery
   c) Stress urinary incontinence
   d) Lower parity

4. When types of pessaries are divided by mechanism of action, space-filling pessaries include all of the following EXCEPT
   a) Cube
   b) Donut
   c) Gehrung
   d) Schaatz
   e) Gellhorn

5. Which of the following pessaries can be worn during intercourse?
   a) Cube
   b) Gellhorn
   c) Donut
   d) Ring

6. The ring pessary is the most commonly used pessary according to the AUGS. Which of the following statements does not describe the ring?
   a) It contains a spring mechanism providing support
   b) It is made from silicone
   c) It can be worn during coitus
   d) It provides support to anterior vaginal wall defects
   e) It is supported by the levator muscles

7. Which of the following pessaries would not be suitable for an obese, disabled patient whose mobility is restricted, yet she has severe prolapse?
   a) Ring
   b) Cube
   c) Gellhorn
   d) Donut

8. A 32-year-old G4P0 woman already had a prophylactic cerclage placed for cervical incompetence at 12 weeks' gestation. She is now 18 weeks' gestation and complains of pelvic pressure. A colleague recommends a pessary to alleviate pressure on the cervix. Which pessary should you choose?
   a) Ring
   b) Smith-Hodge
   c) Cube
   d) Gellhorn

9 A patient complains of severe pruritus, burning, and erythema with her last pessary. She was subsequently diagnosed with a latex allergy. However, she wants to continue using her pessary. Which pessary was she previously using?
   a) Cube
   b) Schaatz
   c) Inflatoball
   d) Donut

10 Three months after being fitted for a pessary, a patient returns for evaluation. You notice bleeding, ulcers, and mucosal abrasions. You recommend withholding its use for 2–3 weeks, topical estrogen cream, and trying a smaller pessary to prevent which of the following complications?
   a) HSV outbreak
   b) Atrophy
   c) Fistula formation
   d) Other sexually transmitted infection

CHAPTER 36

1. What are the therapeutic mainstays for treatment of detrusor instability?
   a) Anticholinergic drug therapy
   b) Behavioral modification
   c) Surgery
   d) a and b
   e) b and c

2. Sacral reflexes that should be elicited in the physical examination of all patients with complaints of urinary incontinence include all of the following EXCEPT
   a) Anal "wink" reflex
   b) Babinski reflex
   c) Cough reflex
   d) Bulbocavernous reflex

3. Common side effects of anticholinergic medications used to treat urinary incontinence include all the following EXCEPT
   a) Dry mouth
   b) Blurred vision
   c) Decreased heart rate
   d) Constipation

4. The maximal normal straining angle by convention on Q-tip test is
   a) 30 degrees
   b) 45 degrees
   c) 20 degrees
   d) 35 degrees

5. The muscle strengthen by routine Kegel exercises is
   a) Obturator internus
   b) Piriformis
   c) Ileococcygeus
   d) Pubococcygeus

6. There has been a decreasing therapeutic role for phenylpropanolamine in treating stress urinary incontinence. This is due to studies showing that taking medications containing this was an independent risk factor for
   a) Hemorrhagic stroke
   b) Myocardial Infarction
   c) Pulmonary embolism
   d) Pneumonia

7. What is the most common mistake made by surgeons performing sling operations?
   a) Choice of incision site
   b) Choice of sling material
   c) Postoperative management
   d) Making the sling too tight

8. Injection therapy works by
   a) Decreasing inflammation
   b) Bulking up tissue at the bladder neck
   c) Decreasing scar tissue
   d) Treating infection

9. The most important component of postoperative bladder care is
   a) Making sure that the bladder is well drained
   b) Checking frequently for infection
   c) Kegel exercises
   d) Prophylactic antibiotics

10. Potential points of reattachment of the endopelvic fascia during retropubic bladder neck suspension operations include all of the following EXCEPT
   a) Arcus tendineus fascia pelvis
   b) Periosteum of pubic symphysis
   c) Rectus fascia
   d) Cooper's ligament

CHAPTER 37

1. The most important factor in preventing operative injuries to the ureter is
   a) Obtaining preoperative intravenous pyelogram
   b) Insertion of prophylactic ureteral stints
   c) Surgeon's knowledge of where the ureters are located
   d) Obtaining preoperative CT scan to locate the ureters

2. In gynecologic surgery, the most common procedure and the site of injury are
   a) Vaginal hysterectomy, tunnel of Wertheim
   b) Bladder neck suspension, tunnel of Wertheim
   c) Laparoscopic oophorectomy, pelvic brim near the IP ligament
   d) Simple abdominal hysterectomy, pelvic brim near the IP ligament

3. All of the following statements are correct regarding a repair of the ureteral transection EXCEPT
   a) Ureteral stint should be placed through the ureterotomy
   b) Closed suction drain is placed at the base of the repair to aid in detecting the leakage of urine after the repair
   c) At least three individual sutures are needed to repair the ureter to achieve a watertight closure
   d) The surgeon should be assured that the repair is tension free

4. Management of ureteral transection within 6 cm of the ureterovesical junction or at the time of any resection of the lower third of the ureter should be
   a) Uretero-neocystotomy with psoas hitch over ureteral stint
   b) Primary repair over the ureteral stint
   c) Uretero-ileal interposition
   d) Resection of transected margins, then primary repair over the ureteral stint

5. In gynecologic surgery, the most common type of ureteral injury and "activity" leading to the injury are
   a) Crushing, at the time of ligation of the uterine artery
   b) Obstruction, attempting to obtain hemostasis
   c) Transection, at the time of ligation and transection of the IP ligament
   d) Ligation, at the time of ligation of the uterine artery

6. The following statements regarding the advantages of renal/proximal ureter ultrasound over CT scan or intravenous pyelogram (IVP) in identifying ureteral injuries are true EXCEPT
   a) It prevents renal damage that may result from intravenous contrast medium
   b) It is noninvasive and relatively easily obtained
   c) There is no risk of radiation exposure
   d) It has a low false-negative rate in detecting ureteral obstruction

7. A surgeon should *not* defer surgical attempt to repair an ureteral injury when
   a) Patient is too unstable to undergo reoperation
   b) The obstruction is caused by a metal clip
   c) The diagnosis of ureteral injury is not certain
   d) Leakage of urine is stopped with ureteral stint placement

8. Compared with ureteral injuries caused by laparotomy, laparoscopy-associated ureteral injuries are
   a) More likely to have increased long-term or even fatal complications
   b) More likely to be diagnosed sooner after surgery
   c) More likely to be mechanical, rather than thermal injuries
   d) Likely to be repaired just as easily by laparoscopy

9. Which statement correctly describes one of the recommended steps to enter the retroperitoneum to identify the ureters?
   a) Transect the round ligament as close to the sidewall as possible to maximize the exposure of the retroperitoneum
   b) Incision into the lateral leaf of the broad ligament should be carried in a caudolateral to cephalomedial fashion
   c) You can assure yourself of the location of the ureter by "plucking" it
   d) The ureter will be visible on the medial leaf of the broad ligament

10. During radical hysterectomy, which is not the recommended step universally taken by the author to minimize injury to the ureter?
    a) Ureters are always freed from the medial leaf of the broad ligament, while leaving them inside of their adventitial sheath
    b) Space of Morrow is developed to facilitate entrance into the tunnel of Wertheim
    c) Prophylactic ureteral stints are placed to facilitate identification of the ureters
    d) Making sure that ureteral dissection is always staying outside of the ureteral sheath

CHAPTER 38

1. A 41-year-old patient undergoes a total abdominal hysterectomy for a fundal uterine fibroid. After about 10 minutes have been spent dissecting the bladder off of the uterus, the anesthetist notes that the urine appears bloody and was clear before surgery. Cystoscopy is performed. Where is the most likely location, in this situation, to find an injury to the urinary system?
   a) Superior to the interureteric ridge
   b) The trigone
   c) The bladder neck
   d) The dome of the bladder

2. A 38-year-old patient who had a total abdominal hysterectomy presents 2 months postoperatively complaining of leaking urine form the vagina. On examination, no fistula can be identified. Dilute methylene blue (100 mL) is injected into the bladder through a Foley catheter and a tampon is placed in the vagina. The patient is asked to walk for about 15 minutes, after which time the tampon is removed. The tampon

is found to be wet, but there is no blue dye anywhere on the tampon. Which of the following is true?
a) 100 mL was probably not enough methylene blue, and the test should be repeated with a higher volume
b) The patient probably has stress incontinence not a fistula
c) The patient probably has a ureterovaginal fistula
d) The patient most likely has a small apical vesicovaginal fistula that was too small to leak the dye in 15 minutes

3. The postoperative course of patients who have had an abdominal hysterectomy complicated by an unrecognized vesicovaginal fistula often have
a) Prolonged postoperative fever
b) Costovertebral angle tenderness
c) Hyperactive bowel sounds
d) No abnormal signs or symptoms

4. After evaluating a patient with a vesicovaginal fistula several things can be done preoperatively that may be beneficial for the patient. Which of the following strategies has *not* been shown to help?
a) A short course of oral steroids
b) Preoperative estrogen to estrogen-deficient patients
c) Zinc oxide ointment for the perineum and vulva
d) Diversion of the urinary stream by catheterization

5. Which of the following statements regarding the "flap-splitting technique" of vesicovaginal fistula repair is false?
a) The bladder should be closed in two layers
b) Trigonal defect repairs should be made in the vertical direction.
c) Adequate vaginal length is preserved with this procedure
d) Cure rates approach those achieved with the Latzko procedure

6. What is the occurrence of stress incontinence after the successful repair of a vesicovaginal fistula?
a) Less than 5%
b) 10%–20%
c) About 50%
d) More than 70%

7. During a difficult dissection of the bladder at the time of hysterectomy in a woman with two previous cesarean sections, which of the following has *not* been recommended as a way to decrease the risk of bladder injury?
a) Careful blunt dissection to isolate the bladder
b) Use of a two-way indwelling catheter
c) An extraperitoneal cystotomy
d) Retrograde filling of the bladder

8. In the United States the most common reason for vesicovaginal fistulas is
a) Trauma such as motor vehicle accidents
b) Obstetrical delivery
c) Gynecologic surgery
d) Pelvic radiation for cancer

9. Advantages of the Latzko technique for vesicovaginal fistula repair include all of the following EXCEPT
a) There is early catheter removal
b) The vagina is not shortened
c) There are no sutures in the bladder mucous
d) Operating time is short

10. After a prolonged labor and difficult forceps delivery you are asked to consult on a 26-year-old woman who is otherwise in good health. On examination, she has a 1-cm vesicovaginal fistula in the anterior, upper one third of the vaginal wall with associated edema. The best chance of a successful repair is with
a) Immediate vesicovaginal fistula repair
b) High-dose oral steroids for 2 days and then fistula repair
c) Wait 4 weeks, then repair
d) Wait 3 to 6 months, then repair

CHAPTER 39

1. Which of the following is not a risk factor for anal incontinence?
a) Neurologic disease
b) Age older than 60 years
c) Concomitant urinary incontinence
d) Cognitive decline

2. The mechanism of anal continence is multifactorial. Which of the following is necessary for maintaining continence?
a) Soft or liquid stools
b) Perineal sensation
c) An intact puborectalis muscle sling
d) Urinary continence

3. The anal canal and lower rectum are under both voluntary and involuntary mechanisms. Which of the following structures is under voluntary control?
a) Internal anal sphincter
b) Inner rectal mucosa
c) Mucosal glands in the distal rectum
d) Medial portion of the puborectalis muscle

4. Which of the following is *not* a cause of anal incontinence?
a) Obstetrical injury
b) Infectious diarrhea
c) Previous radiation
d) Anal intercourse

5. Which of the following increases one's risk of an obstetric-related injury leading to anal incontinence?
a) Fundal pressure
b) Prematurity
c) Suprapubic pressure
d) Preeclampsia

6. In addition to direct anatomic disruption of the anal sphincter, denervation injuries can occur during vaginal birth. By what mechanism can this occur?
   a) Dissection of the nerves
   b) Ischemic injury
   c) Massage of the perineum during the second stage of labor
   d) Idiopathic

7. Many nonobstetrical conditions can lead to anal incontinence. Which of the following is the most common?
   a) Fecal impaction with overflow
   b) Trauma
   c) Inflammatory bowel disease
   d) Radiation fibrosis and related conditions

8. In addition to the history and physical examination, what tools should be used in aiding the diagnosis of anal incontinence?
   a) Abdominal x-ray film (KUB)
   b) CT scan
   c) Ultrasound
   d) Stool cultures

9. Anal manometry provides information regarding function, sensation, compliance, and the presence of intact reflexes within the anal canal and distal rectum. Measurements of resting and contraction pressures are obtained. What is a "normal" maximum squeeze pressure?
   a) 0–60 cm H_2O
   b) 60–120 cm H_2O
   c) 200–300 cm H_2O
   d) 100–200 cm H_2O

10. Which of the following is not a complication of anal incontinence surgery?
    a) Wound infection
    b) Wound hematoma
    c) New onset urinary incontinence
    d) Incomplete continence

CHAPTER 40

1. Choose the *incorrect* statement.
   a) Embryologic differentiation of the paired mammary glands begins in the fifth or sixth week of development
   b) Transient breast enlargement and nipple secretion in the newborn typically resolves in the sixth week postpartum
   c) At the time of menarche, breast transformation begins with ductal branching and proliferation of interductal stroma
   d) During pregnancy, prolactin function is inhibited at the alveolar level by progesterone until the time of delivery

2. Which of the following is *not* a congenital breast abnormality?
   a) Amastia
   b) Nipple inversion
   c) Polymastia
   d) Polythelia
   e) All of the above are congenital breast abnormalities

3. Choose the *incorrect* statement.
   a) The organisms most commonly responsible for acute mastitis are *Staphylococcus aureus* and *Streptococcus*
   b) Nonpuerperal mastitis is associated with a bloody nipple discharge and is found in individuals who are immunocompromised
   c) Duct ectasia is most commonly seen in women in the fifth or sixth decade of life
   d) Galactocele presents as a firm, nontender mass in the outer quadrants of the breast

4. Fibrocystic change of the breast
   a) Occurs mainly in menopausal women
   b) Presents with breast discomfort in 85%–90% of cases
   c) Increases the risk of developing breast cancer
   d) Occurs in 25% of women younger than 21 years

5. Choose the *incorrect* statement.
   a) Women find most breast masses themselves, either by chance or during self-breast examination
   b) Two thirds of masses found during the reproductive years are benign
   c) Fibroadenomas are the most common benign breast tumors and are typically seen in women younger than 30 years
   d) Multiple fibroadenomas are found in the same patient in approximately 50% of cases

6. Which of the following is *not* a treatment for cyclic breast pain?
   a) Danazol
   b) Bromocriptine
   c) Oral contraceptive pills
   d) Tamoxifen
   e) All of the above may be used to treat cyclic breast pain

7. Which category of medications does *not* result in galactorrhea?
   a) Diuretics
   b) Antidepressants
   c) Opiates
   d) Oral contraceptive pills
   e) Tranquilizers

8. Choose the *incorrect* statement.
   a) Breast cancer accounts for 15% of cancer deaths in women
   b) Mammography is the gold standard for early detection of breast cancer
   c) Self-breast examination should be performed monthly beginning at age 30
   d) Clinical breast examination has been shown to have a sensitivity of 57%–70% in detecting breast cancer

9. Choose the *incorrect* statement.
   a) 30% of breast cancers are inherited in an autosomal dominant pattern
   b) *BRCA1* and *BRCA2* are the only known breast cancer genes
   c) Approximately 600 mutations have been found in the *BRCA1* gene and 500 in the *BRCA2* gene
   d) *BRCA1* accounts for 50% of all inherited breast cancers and 90% of hereditary ovarian cancers, whereas *BRCA2* accounts for 40% of familial breast cancers and 5%–10% of familial ovarian cancer

10. The Gail Model Risk Assessment Tool uses which of the following to estimate the risk of developing breast cancer?
    a) Number of previous breast biopsies and pathology results
    b) Age at menarche
    c) Age at first live birth
    d) Number of first-degree relatives with breast cancer
    e) All of the above

CHAPTER 41

1. Which of the following statements regarding antibiotic therapy in the setting of appendicitis is false?
   a) Preoperative antibiotic therapy significantly reduces the morbidity of appendicitis
   b) The incidence of appendiceal perforation is significantly less with preoperative antibiotics
   c) Second-generation cephalosporins, such as cefotetan, are an acceptable antibiotic choice for most cases of appendicitis
   d) Perioperative antibiotics alone are usually adequate for nonruptured, nongangrenous cases of appendicitis

2. Which of the following statements regarding imaging studies in the diagnosis of appendicitis is true?
   a) CT scan has a much higher rate of providing a specific diagnosis of appendicitis than ultrasound
   b) The loss of the right psoas shadow on plain abdominal x-ray films is an early sign of appendicitis
   c) An appendiceal wall thickness on ultrasound of 12 mm would be consistent with likely appendicitis
   d) Because it is a superior test, CT scan should always be the first choice for imaging, even in pregnant patients

3. A 23-year-old G0 woman presents to the emergency department complaining of right lower quadrant abdominal pain. All of her symptoms as well as her physical examination are consistent with the diagnosis of appendicitis. If all patients such as this were taken to the OR for surgery without the benefit of laboratory tests and imaging, about what percentage would actually have appendicitis?
   a) Less than 10%
   b) 25%
   c) 50%
   d) 75%
   e) More than 90%

4. If all commonly available laboratory tests and imaging are used to confirm the diagnosis, what percentage of patients would actually have appendicitis?
   a) Less than 10%
   b) 25%
   c) 50%
   d) 75%
   e) More than 90%

5. A 21-year-old G1P0 at 33 weeks' gestation with a history of a previous cesarean section presents with right-sided abdominal and flank pain for the past 8 hours. The pain has gotten progressively worse and she has also developed anorexia and nausea. She has a fever of 100.9°F. Fetal heart monitoring shows a fetal heart rate of 160 beats/min with moderate variability and two accelerations during the first 15 minutes of monitoring. The tocometer shows one discreet contraction and some irritability but is mostly flat. Ultrasound shows a normal placenta, AFI of 11.5, with the fetus in vertex presentation. Point tenderness is noted while performing the ultrasound on the right side of the uterus. An ultrasound obtained in the radiology department shows a displaced appendix with a wall thickness of 14 mm, luminal distention, and a lack of compressibility. Which of the following would be an appropriate course of action?
   a) Begin a course of steroids for fetal lung maturity and perform a cesarean section and appendectomy when the course is complete
   b) Immediately go to surgery and perform an appendectomy and cesarean hysterectomy
   c) Immediately go to surgery and perform an appendectomy without cesarean section or hysterectomy
   d) Begin IV antibiotics, monitor patient for signs of sepsis, and perform appendectomy if her condition worsens
   e) Begin IV antibiotics, induce labor, and perform appendectomy after delivery

6. A 48-year-old perimenopausal woman with chronic pelvic pain and irregular menses decides to have a total abdominal hysterectomy and bilateral salpingo-oophorectomy. Her gynecologist routinely performs incidental appendectomies at the time of TAH-BSO. This patient's appendix looks completely normal but is removed and sent to pathology. Which of the following statements is true?
   a) There is an approximately 10% chance that her appendix will be found to have significant pathology
   b) Her risk of morbidity is significantly higher than if the appendectomy were not performed
   c) Informed consent does not need to specifically include "appendectomy" because it is a routine part of the surgeon's TAH-BSO
   d) If not removed, her chance of developing appendicitis at some point in the future is approximately 80%
   e) If carcinoid tumor is found in her appendix, it is most like malignant

7. Acceptable techniques for managing the appendiceal stump include all of the following EXCEPT

a) Inverting the stump into the cecum with a purse-string suture
b) Ligating the stump with permanent suture
c) Covering the stump with periappendiceal fat
d) Cauterizing the stump and leaving it exposed

8. Which of the following maneuvers is not used to elicit the obturator sign?
a) Flexion of the right hip
b) Flexion of the right knee
c) Straight by elevation of the right leg
d) External rotation of the right leg

9. Which of the following is not an advantage of laparoscopic appendectomy versus open appendectomy?
a) Lower morbidity
b) Lower operative cost
c) Shorter hospitalization
d) Lower rate of abdominal wall infection
e) Less postoperative pain

10. In which of the following patient or patients would an incidental appendectomy be indicated even if informed consent for appendectomy was not specifically obtained before surgery? (Select all that apply)
a) A 63-year-old woman with an ovarian mass that is sent for pathology after removal and found to be a mucinous tumor
b) A 35-year-old woman with a history of chronic pelvic pain who is undergoing a TAH-BSO and is found to have several implants of endometriosis on the uterosacral ligaments
c) A 41-year-old woman who is undergoing a radical hysterectomy for Stage IIA cervical cancer whose appendix appears normal on gross examination
d) A 21-year-old woman undergoing a left salpingo-oophorectomy for a dermoid cyst whose appendix is found to have a small granuloma on it
e) The appendix should never be removed without specific informed consent for "appendectomy"

CHAPTER 42

1. An 18-year-old nulliparous woman presents to your clinic for her annual examination. On examination there is a right adnexal mass which is about 5×5 cm. Ultrasonographically it is consistent with a dermoid cyst. Although without pain for the past several weeks, she has a history of right lower quadrant pain that has occurred intermittently over several years, and she has had guaiac-positive stool in the past but none currently. She is taken to the operating room where she is found to have a dermoid, as expected, but is also found to have a diverticulum 9 cm in length arising from the antimesenteric border of the ileum 13 inches from the ileocecal valve. There is a slight thickening of the tip of the diverticulum but the tissue otherwise appears totally healthy. Which of the following statements about the management of this case of Meckel's diverticulum is true?

a) The patient's symptoms have now resolved and the dermoid has been removed so there is no need to remove the diverticulum, which likely will remain asymptomatic the patient's entire life
b) The diverticulum should be removed because the patient has a history of symptoms that it may have caused and it has slightly atypical features
c) The diverticulum should be removed because any time a Meckel's diverticulum is discovered incidentally is should be removed to prevent future complications
d) The diverticulum should not be removed at this time, but if the patient has recurrent symptoms she should be referred to general surgery for removal

2. In which of the following patient(s) would sodium phosphate probably not be a good choice for a bowel prep?
a) A 26 year old with SLE who has end-stage renal disease
b) A 54-year-old alcoholic with cirrhosis
c) A 64 year old with stage IIB ovarian cancer
d) A 48 year old with Class II heart failure
e) A 35-year-old diabetic with a hemoglobin A_{1c} of 6.7

3. A patient is undergoing a laparoscopic tubal ligation and on insertion of the laparoscope intraluminal bowel mucosa is seen, as well as reflux of enteric contents. Which of the following would be the best course of action?
a) Remove the trocar, convert to an open laparotomy, and repair the injury
b) Leave the trocar in place, convert to an open laparotomy, and repair the injury
c) Insert another trocar to confirm that bowel injury has occurred, then attempt to repair the injury laparoscopically
d) Withdraw and reposition the trocar so that the injury is visible with the laparoscope and then decide if laparoscopic repair is feasible

4. A 37-year-old patient undergoes a laparoscopy for fulguration of endometriosis and is discharged the same day. Which of the following presentations would be most consistent with an electrosurgical injury that was unrecognized during surgery?
a) The patient presents to the ER 3 days postoperatively complaining of nausea, vomiting, and fever
b) The patient becomes hypotensive and tachycardic in the recovery room but responds to fluid boluses
c) The patient presents to the ER on postoperative day one complaining of worsening abdominal pain, fever, and constipation
d) The patient calls the clinic 1 week postoperatively complaining of nausea, vomiting, diarrhea but denies fever
e) The patient presents to clinic 1 month postoperatively complaining of irregular bowel movements since surgery and continued abdominal pain

5. Which of the following statements regarding early feeding in patients who have undergone a bowel anastomosis is true?
   a) The rate of ileus is significantly higher in patients who are fed before passing flatus
   b) The rate of anastomotic complications is significantly decreased by delaying feeding
   c) Return of bowel function generally occurs at the same rate regardless of early or delayed feeding
   d) Early feeding decreases the probable length of hospital stay
   e) None of the above

6. Which of the following are the three most common reasons for bowel obstruction? (Select all that apply)
   a) Adhesions
   b) Intestinal polyps
   c) Volvulus
   d) Hernias
   e) Malignancy

7. A 62-year-old patient undergoes a bowel resection and because there is only 5 cm of rectum conserved, the decision is made to create a sigmoid J-pouch. Which of the following regarding the J-pouch is true?
   a) The patient is less likely to suffer from frequency, urgency, and incontinence of stool
   b) The patient is less likely to have a sense of incomplete evacuation after bowel movements
   c) Slight tension on the J-pouch will resolve over time and need not be a source of concern
   d) Enemas should be avoided in patients who have had a J-pouch created

8. A 34-year-old patient undergoes a TAH-BSO for leiomyomata. During the surgery the small bowel sustains a thermal injury requiring resection of 4 cm of small bowel. The remaining bowel appears healthy. Which of the following types of anastomosis should probably not be used because of the higher potential for excessive luminal narrowing?
   a) End-to-end hand-sewn anastomosis
   b) Side-to-side hand-sewn anastomosis
   c) End-to-end staple anastomosis
   d) Side-to-side staple anastomosis (functional end-to-end anastomosis)

9. A 38-year-old patient with a history severe endometriosis who is known to have extensive adhesive disease presents to the ER with abdominal pain. Physical examination and radiologic imaging lead to the diagnosis of small bowel obstruction. During surgery, which of the following characteristics of her injured bowel indicate viability most reliably? (Choose two)
   a) Tissue color
   b) Bleeding from a cut edge
   c) Extent of edema
   d) Peristalsis
   e) Fluorescence of bowel wall under Wood's lamp 10 minutes after IV fluorescein

10. Designate whether each of the following statements is true or false.
    a) Intraluminal fluid collection in a complete obstruction is unlikely to exceed 2 L
    b) Less than 20% of bowel injuries during gynecologic surgery occur during lysis of adhesions
    c) Absent bowel sounds are usually indicative of ileus
    d) Peristaltic waves causing pain every 12 minutes indicate a relatively high obstruction
    e) Sodium phosphate generally provides better bowel prep for colonoscopy than polyethylene glycol
    f) Stair-step air fluid levels from RLQ to LUQ is most consistent with adynamic ileus
    g) The tissue edges on a bowel anastomosis should be everted
    h) Colonic dysfunction following surgery usually resolves within 6–8 hours

CHAPTER 43

1. A 62-year-old gravida 4, para 4 woman presents to your office complaining of occasional "streaks of blood" in her stool. Although she has been seen at your gynecology clinic on a yearly basis for routine well-woman care for over 10 years, she admits that she has not seen her internist in 7 years. After performing a thorough review of her past medical and surgical history, you perform a physical examination that is significant only for a heme-positive digital rectal examination. The next step you should take to provide appropriate care to this patient is
   a) Order a magnetic resonance imaging (MRI) study of the abdomen and pelvis
   b) Refer the patient to a gastroenterologist for a colonoscopy
   c) Ask the patient to return to your clinic in 6 weeks to repeat the digital rectal examination
   d) Encourage the patient to see her internist for a flexible sigmoidoscopy
   e) Perform a pelvic ultrasound in your clinic

2. A 25-year-old nulligravid woman presents to your office complaining of fevers and chills over the past 3 months. Without any conscious attempt to lose weight, she reports a 40 lb (17.8 kg) weight loss, vague abdominal discomfort, and joint pain in her hands and feet. Physical examination reveals diffuse abdominal discomfort to palpation that is greatest in the left lower quadrant, erythematous skin nodules on the back and chest, and supraclavicular and axillary lymphadenopathy. Appropriate steps in the workup of this patient would include
   a) Biopsy of an enlarged peripheral lymph node
   b) Mammography
   c) Diagnostic laparoscopy to evaluate the abdomen and pelvis
   d) Technetium-99 bone scan
   e) Intravenous antibiotics

3. A 50-year-old gravida 2, para 2 woman presents to your office complaining of pelvic pain. She reports feeling a "dull, ache-like sensation" after intercourse and occasional bouts of this pain occur two or three times per week. Review of systems is positive for urinary frequency and constipation. After reviewing her medical, social, and family history, you perform a physical examination. This examination reveals moderate-to-severe pain on deep palpation of the right adnexal tissues with no identifiable mass. Subsequent laboratory studies are obtained with notable hypercalcemia. MRI reveals a bony tumor of the pelvis arising from the anterior sacrum. The most likely diagnosis in this case is
   a) Chordoma
   b) Gardner's syndrome
   c) Chondrosarcoma
   d) Breast cancer with bony metastases
   e) Giant cell tumor

4. A 32-year-old gravida 1, para 1 woman presents to your clinic with abdominal pain that began 2 weeks before this visit. She did not take her temperature at home but reports feeling feverish. She has been working her normal schedule as an accountant during this time, but her ability to exercise regularly has been somewhat curtailed because of this pain. Her vital signs reveal tachycardia (pulse = 102 beats/min) and a low-grade fever. Physical examination reveals left lower quadrant abdominal pain without guarding or rebound. Rectal examination is negative for masses or blood. Laboratory studies show leukocytosis. Likely diagnoses to consider in this case would *not* include
   a) Pyelonephritis
   b) Cancer of the ovary
   c) Acute viral gastroenteritis
   d) Pelvic inflammatory disease
   e) Chronic appendicitis

5. A general surgeon consults you about possible intraoperative consultation in a 36-year-old gravida 3, para 3 woman with early colon cancer. His is planning a curative sigmoid resection and asks you to counsel the patient about possible oophorectomy. You discuss the options and recommend
   a) Left oophorectomy
   b) Bilateral oophorectomy
   c) Bilateral oophorectomy and hysterectomy
   d) No gynecologic surgery if the uterus and ovaries are normal

6. A 28-year-old woman with chronic pelvic pain is operated on for chronic pelvic inflammatory disease and bilateral adnexal masses. In addition to bilateral tubo-ovarian abscesses, she is found to have chronic disease with extensive small bowel involvement and perforation. You call a general surgeon to assist you and you proceed with
   a) Total abdominal hysterectomy, bilateral salpingo-oophorectomy, and ileostomy
   b) TAH-BSO, ileal resection, and protective ileostomy

   c) BSO only
   d) Ileal resection and reanastomosis only

7. A 72-year-old woman undergoes total abdominal hysterectomy and bilateral salpingo-oophorectomy for a mass in the left adnexa. The pathology report shows metastatic carcinoma of the colon involving the left ovary. The uterus, fallopian tubes, and right ovary contain no evidence of disease. The most appropriate serum tumor marker to obtain is
   a) Human chorionic gonadotropin
   b) CC-17 (colon cancer) antigen
   c) Carcinoembryonic antigen (CEA)
   d) CA-125 (cancer antigen)
   e) Alpha-fetoprotein

8. A 42-year-old woman undergoes exploratory laparotomy for acute left-sided pelvic pain. Although ovarian torsion was suspected, a diverticular abscess is noted on the left side with no evidence of ovarian torsion. The best treatment option, assuming appropriate consent is given by the patient, would be
   a) Drainage of the abscess, resection of the diseased segment of bowel, and a diverting colostomy
   b) Closure of the abdomen and inpatient intravenous antibiotics until the patient is afebrile for 24–48 hours
   c) Drainage of the abscess with inpatient intravenous antibiotics until the patient is afebrile for 24–48 hours
   d) Drainage of the abscess, resection of the disease segment of bowel with primary anastomosis

9. A 19-year-old nulligravid woman presents to your clinic complaining of a 3-month history of right lower quadrant pain ("it just aches intermittently"), diarrhea between five and ten times per day, fatigue, and a 15 lb (7 kg) weight loss. After a complete history and physical examination, you refer her to a gastroenterologist. The gastroenterologist informs you (after performing laboratory studies and a colonoscopic biopsy) that Crohn's disease is present involving a focal segment of the ileum. There is no evidence of fistula formation, abscess, or bowel obstruction. The best treatment of Crohn's disease in this patient's case is
   a) Resection of the diseased portion of the ileum with primary anastomosis
   b) Resection of the ileum, cecum, and distal jejunum to prevent local spreading of the disease
   c) Endoscopic or colonoscopic thermal ablation of the diseased portion of the intestinal mucosa
   d) Nonsurgical management with salicylates and other medications

10. Your are consulted intraoperatively by another surgeon who is operating on a 34-year-old gravida 2, para 2 with left-sided pelvic pain and low back pain. He has found a retroperitoneal mass that may represent a pelvic kidney. The following are appropriate methods to determine whether or not the mass is a pelvic kidney EXCEPT

a) Aspiration with a 22-guage needle to see if urine can be withdrawn from the mass
b) Palpation of the ipsilateral and contralateral side to ascertain that a kidney is present on both sides
c) Excretory urography during surgery (intravenous injection of contrast material followed by a supine film after 15 minutes)
d) Injection of 5 to 10 mL of indigo carmine intravenously and aspirate the suspected renal pelvis 5 to 10 minutes later

CHAPTER 44

1. Which of the following is a recognized risk factor for vulvar malignancy?
   a) Diabetes
   b) Cigarette smoking
   c) Obesity
   d) Immunosuppression

2. You may consider omitting lymphadenectomy as part of the staging procedure for squamous cell vulvar carcinoma when
   a) Lesion 1.5 cm diameter, less than 5 mm invasion
   b) Unilateral lesion, less than 5 mm invasion
   c) Any location, less than 1 mm invasion
   d) Unilateral lesion 1.3 cm diameter, 3 mm invasion

3. What factors predispose patients to develop local recurrence with squamous cell vulvar carcinoma?
   a) Midline location
   b) Enlarged inguinal nodes
   c) Close resection with margin less than 1 cm
   d) Poorly differentiated histology

4. The use of preoperative adjuvant therapy in patients with squamous cell vulvar carcinoma is generally recommended for
   a) Patients with suspicious groin nodes
   b) Locally advanced disease or lesions encroaching on midline structures where surgical removal is accompanied by significant morbidity
   c) Poorly differentiated histologic type in stage 1 disease
   d) Multifocal lesions in stage 1 disease

5. What is the single most effective method of reducing groin wound breakdown?
   a) Prophylactic antibiotics
   b) Ligation of draining lymphatics
   c) Prophylactic suction drainage
   d) Separate groin incisions

6. When a woman has a Bartholin mass, what features would prompt you to consider biopsy or excision?
   a) Age younger than 40
   b) History of previous Bartholin's abscess
   c) Failure to improve promptly with conservative therapy
   d) Negative culture
   e) Bilateral masses

7. The recurrence-free survival of patients with invasive squamous cell carcinoma of the vulva correlates most closely with
   a) Tumor differentiation
   b) Tumor location
   c) Radiation tumor dose
   d) Pathologic status of the inguinal lymph nodes
   e) Age of the patient

8. A vulvar cancer with the lowest risk for inguinal lymph node metastases would be a tumor that
   a) Is well differentiated
   b) Only involves the labia major
   c) Is infiltrative
   d) Invades 0.9 mm
   e) Had not incited an inflammatory response

9. The second most common histologic type of vulvar cancer is
   a) Squamous cell carcinoma
   b) Melanoma
   c) Bartholin gland carcinoma
   d) Basal cell carcinoma
   e) Invasive Paget's disease

10. Characteristics of Paget's disease of the vulva include all of the following EXCEPT
    a) Presentation as a patchy, eczematous lesion
    b) The presence of underlying invasive disease in more than 90% of patients
    c) The development of another malignancy in about 25% of patients
    d) Histologic extension beyond that which is clinically apparent
    e) Tends to occur in white postmenopausal women

CHAPTER 45

1. In the 2002 Bethesda System terminology, "low grade squamous intraepithelial lesion" combines which older designation into the LSIL category?
   a) Mild and moderate dysplasia
   b) CIN 1 and HPV changes
   c) ASCUS and CIN 1
   d) Koilocytosis and atypia

2. In the United States, the most common abnormal Pap test diagnosis is
   a) ASC
   b) AGC
   c) LSIL
   d) HSIL

3. Human papillomavirus DNA has been detected in what percent of women with carcinoma in situ of the cervix?
   a) Less than 10%
   b) 50%–60%
   c) 75%
   d) Greater than 90%

4. Current practice guidelines recommend HPV testing as an adjunctive test to help direct management in women with which Pap test diagnosis?
   a) Inflammation, atypia
   b) ASC
   c) ASC-H
   d) LSIL

5. The transformation zone is defined as
   a) The area of white epithelium on the cervix
   b) The area around the squamocolumnar junction
   c) The area of abnormal epithelium on the cervix
   d) The area between the original and current squamocolumnar junction

6. Cellular transformation of cervical epithelial cells is thought to be caused by which of the following HPV DNA mechanisms?
   a) E_6 and E_7 proteins inactivate *p53* and *RB* antioncogenes
   b) L_1 protein blocks DNA repair genes
   c) E_2 causes deregulation of cellular apoptosis mechanisms
   d) HPV DNA incorporation into cellular DNA causes mitotic deregulation

7. According to large, careful meta-analyses, a single Pap test has a sensitivity to diagnose cervical dysplasia or cancer of about
   a) 50%–60%
   b) 75%–85%
   c) 90%
   d) Greater than 95%

8. Referral for colposcopy is recommended for patients with all of the following diagnoses EXCEPT
   a) LSIL
   b) ASC-US on two consecutive Paps 6 months apart
   c) ASC-US, low-risk HPV positive
   d) AGC

9. Experts generally recommend traditional cold knife cone biopsy for management of which of the following patients?
   a) Cervical biopsy = CIN 3 with endocervical glandular involvement
   b) Cervical biopsy = CIN 3, SCJ cannot be seen on colposcopy
   c) Cervical biopsy = CIN 3, patient is 24 weeks pregnant
   d) ECC = adenocarcinoma in situ, SCJ is visible on colposcopy

10. Initial workup of a 40-year-old woman with a Pap showing atypical glandular cells should include all of the following EXCEPT
    a) Colposcopy
    b) Endocervical curettage
    c) Pelvic ultrasound
    d) Endometrial biopsy

CHAPTER 46

1. The etiology of cancer of the cervix is most likely related to
   a) Sexual promiscuity
   b) Genital herpes zoster
   c) Cigarette smoking
   d) HPV infection

2. A 3-cm cancer on the cervix with no signs of spread is probably
   a) Stage IA2
   b) Microinvasive disease
   c) Stage IB
   d) Stage IIA

3. The most important determinant of prognosis of cervical cancer is
   a) Depth of invasion into the cervix
   b) FIGO clinical stage
   c) Presence of lymph node metastasis
   d) Histologic differentiation

4. The best rationale for choosing radical surgery over radiation for treatment of early stage carcinoma of the cervix is
   a) Better survival with surgery
   b) Fewer complications
   c) Preservation of ovarian function
   d) Decreased short-term recurrence

5. The middle segment of the ureter derives it blood supply from
   a) Collateral circulation from the superior portion of the ureter
   b) A nutrient branch from the common iliac or hypogastric artery
   c) Longitudinal collateral branches of pelvic vessels
   d) All of the above

6. Which of the following tests is used for FIGO staging of cervical cancer?
   a) Intravenous pyelogram
   b) CT scans of abdomen and pelvis
   c) Lymphangiogram
   d) PET scan

7. Which of the avascular pelvic spaces lies immediately inferior to the cardinal ligament?
   a) Space of Trezius
   b) Pararectal space
   c) Paravesical space
   d) Rectovaginal space

8. In a classic type III radical hysterectomy, the uterine artery is ligated at which point?
   a) Its origin from the hypogastric artery
   b) Where it crosses over the ureter
   c) 1 cm lateral to the uterus
   d) As it enters the parametrial "web"

9. The most common late sequela of radical hysterectomy and pelvic lymphadenectomy is
   a) Vesicovaginal fistula
   b) Numbness of the medial thigh
   c) Leg edema
   d) Bladder dysfunction

10. If postoperative pelvic radiation is expected, how can ovarian function be saved?
    a) The ovaries are transplanted to the splenic bed
    b) The ovaries are suspended high in the lateral paracolic gutters
    c) The ovaries are covered with the omentum
    d) The patient is given intravenous amifostine (Ethyol) 30 minutes before radiation

CHAPTER 47

1. Endometrial cancer is the fourth most common cancer in women in the United States. The incidence of newly diagnosed cases in 2001 was estimated to be 38,300. Known risk factors for endometrial cancer include all of the following EXCEPT
   a) Age
   b) Obesity
   c) Oral contraceptive use
   d) Nulliparity
   e) Diabetes

2. Tamoxifen is a selective estrogen receptor modulator (SERM) commonly used as adjuvant therapy in treatment of breast cancer, as well as prophylaxis against breast cancer in high-risk women. According to the SEER database (2001), when controlled for confounding factors, no increased risk of endometrial cancer could be attributed to tamoxifen use. Which of the following has been associated with tamoxifen use?
   a) Ovarian cancer
   b) Osteoporosis
   c) Benign breast disease
   d) Thromboembolism
   e) Infertility

3. For which group of women should annual screening for endometrial cancer be performed?
   a) Positive family history of endometrial cancer
   b) History of anovulation/anovulatory disease
   c) History of unopposed estrogen
   d) Family history of hereditary nonpolyposis colon cancer (HNPCC)
   e) Tamoxifen use

4. There are no effective methods currently available in use for adequate screening for endometrial cancer. However, certain findings on Pap smears are suggestive of endometrial cancer. Which of the following is most predictive of an endometrial lesion?
   a) Cytologically atypical endometrial glandular cells
   b) Elevated squamous maturation index
   c) Atypical histiocytes
   d) Bleeding (RBCs)
   e) Nonspecific inflammation

5. A 39-year-old obese, diabetic para 1 patient presents with a history of 8 months of menorrhagia. She states she is not interested in preserving her fertility (she is status post BTL) and NSAIDs have not helped her menstrual bleeding. What should be the next step in management of this patient?
   a) Trial of oral contraceptives
   b) Endometrial biopsy
   c) Endometrial ablation
   d) Hysterectomy
   e) GnRH agonist therapy (i.e., Lupron)

6. An endometrial biopsy performed on the patient described above returns positive for simple hyperplasia. What is her risk of developing endometrial cancer?
   a) 1%
   b) 3%
   c) 8%
   d) 29%

7. According to FIGO, endometrial cancer should be surgically staged. Which of the following radiographic studies should be part of the preoperative staging evaluation?
   a) CT abdomen and pelvis
   b) MRI Abdomen and pelvis
   c) IVP
   d) CXR
   e) HSG

8. A patient with a Grade I endometrial adenocarcinoma undergoes an exploratory laparotomy, TAH-BSO, and pelvic washings. Which of the following prognostic factors would mandate pelvic and paraaortic lymphadenectomy?
   a) Lymph-vascular space invasion
   b) Invasion of the myometrium to the outer $\frac{1}{3}$
   c) History of tamoxifen use
   d) Patient age

9. On performing lymphadenectomy for surgical staging, at least 10 lymph nodes are required to qualify for adequate staging. Which of the following groups of lymph nodes is most important prognostically?
   a) External iliac
   b) Hypogastric
   c) Obturator
   d) Paraaortic
   e) Common iliac

10. Of the histologic subtypes of endometrial adenocarcinoma, which has the poorest prognosis?
    a) Endometrioid
    b) Mucinous
    c) Adenoacanthoma
    d) Clear cell

11. Prognosis depends on all of the following factors EXCEPT
    a) Depth of invasion
    b) Stage of disease
    c) Grade of tumor
    d) Histologic subtype
    e) Hysteroscopy during diagnostic evaluation

CHAPTER 48

1. A 23-year-old patient is diagnosed with a stage IA malignant ovarian germ cell tumor. Which of the following would be the standard treatment?
   a) Unilateral oophorectomy
   b) Bilateral oophorectomy and hysterectomy
   c) Unilateral oophorectomy followed by chemotherapy
   d) Ovarian biopsy followed by chemotherapy

2. A 63-year-old patient is diagnosed with stage IB serous ovarian cancer, grade. Which of the following treatment regimens would generally be recommended, with a 5-year survival of at least 95%?
   a) Surgery followed with chemotherapy
   b) Surgery alone
   c) Surgery followed by pelvic radiation
   d) Chemotherapy followed by surgery

3. Which of the following factors has not been shown to have prognostic significance in epithelial ovarian cancer?
   a) Large volume ascites
   b) Clear cell histology
   c) Capsular rupture
   d) Histologic grade

4. You are consulted intraoperatively by a colleague who has a 33-year-old G2P0A2 patient diagnosed with endometrioid borderline tumor of the right ovary. The tumor appears to be confined to that ovary that was 20 cm in diameter and was removed intact. The patient strongly desires to maintain her fertility. Which of the following treatments would you recommend?
   a) Unilateral salpingo-oophorectomy with surgical staging
   b) Unilateral salpingo-oophorectomy of the opposite ovary
   c) Bilateral salpingo-oophorectomy without hysterectomy, with the possibility of donor oocyte pregnancy remaining
   d) TAH-BSO with surgical staging

5. Several large studies have found that early ovarian cancer can be detected successfully using which of the following screening techniques?
   a) Serum Ca-125
   b) Cul-de-sac aspiration cytology
   c) *BRCA1* genetic testing
   d) Transvaginal pelvic ultrasound

6. Which of the following tumor markers is most often elevated in patients with ovarian granulosa cell tumors?
   a) Serum inhibin
   b) Ca-125
   c) AFP
   d) Beta hCG

7. Which of the following findings on color flow Doppler are consistent with a benign mass (as opposed to a possible malignant mass)?
   a) Peripheral vasculature
   b) Increased diastolic blood flow
   c) Pulsatility index of greater than 1
   d) Resistive index of 0.2

8. A 56-year-old G3P3 patient presents for her annual examination with no complaints. She experienced menopause at the age of 51 and has no complaints. She has been on combination hormone replacement therapy. Her mother died of metastatic cancer (unknown primary) at the age of 68. She is found on examination to have a mobile, firm, nontender right adnexal mass. Her bimanual and rectal examination have no other abnormal findings. An ultrasound shows a simple, unilocular cyst of the right ovary measuring $4 \times 3 \times 5$ cm. Which of the following would be the best course of action?
   a) Check a CA-125 level, and if normal, repeat the ultrasound in 3 months to determine if any change has occurred
   b) Assure the patient that everything looks all right and that she should return for her next annual examination in 1 year
   c) Recommend laparoscopy with laparoscopic RSO if the ovarian cyst looks benign
   d) Order a CT scan to reevaluate the findings seen on ultrasound

9. What percentage of ovarian tumors in premenopausal women of malignant?
   a) Less than 10%
   b) 10%–15%
   c) 25%–50%
   d) More than 75%

10. A 65-year-old G1P1A1 of Native American descent presents complaining of bloating and weight loss for 6 months. Her mother is alive and well in her 80s. Her maternal aunt died of breast cancer at the age of 43. Her single pregnancy ended in spontaneous abortion at 10 weeks gestation, and she was on birth control pills for 8 years over her life. Menarche had been at the age of 15 and menopause at the age of 56. Which of the following place the patient at increased risk of having ovarian cancer?
    a) History of oral contraceptive use
    b) Age of menarche (15)
    c) Native American ethnicity
    d) Nulliparity

CHAPTER 49

1. Survival rates for surgical evisceration have decreased substantially because of all of the following EXCEPT
   a) Control of infection
   b) Use of blood products
   c) Use of synthetic mesh to reclose the incision
   d) Improvements in intensive care therapy

2. Pelvic exenteration should usually be considered only after primary therapy has failed.
   a) True
   b) False

3. For which of the following neoplasias does exenteration typically achieve its best outcome?
   a) Recurrent adenocarcinoma of the cervix or vagina
   b) Recurrent squamous cell carcinoma of the cervix or vagina
   c) Primary uterine sarcoma
   d) Recurrent endometrial adenocarcinoma

4. All of the following are poor prognostic indicators for survival after pelvic exenteration EXCEPT
   a) Unilateral ureteral obstruction
   b) Sciatic leg pain
   c) Tumor causing a vesicovaginal fistula
   d) Unilateral leg edema

5. Intraoperative findings that should lead to cancellation of a planned exenteration include all of the following EXCEPT
   a) Metastases to the right ovary
   b) Metastases to an external iliac lymph node
   c) Direct extension of tumor surrounding the obturator nerve
   d) A 2 cm, resectable, omental metastasis

6. Important surgical spaces that are used in total pelvic exenteration include all of the following EXCEPT
   a) Pararectal space
   b) Pouch of Douglas
   c) Paravesical space
   d) Space of Retzius
   e) Presacral space

7. At the time of pelvic exenteration for central recurrence of squamous cell carcinoma of the cervix after radiation, which of the following node groups do not need dissection?
   a) High para-aortics (ovarian vessels)
   b) External iliacs
   c) Obturator
   d) Internal iliac

8. Advantages of a myocutaneous flap for vaginal reconstruction do *not* include
   a) It brings new blood supply to the pelvic
   b) It is a rapid, technically easy procedure
   c) It fills the pelvic deflect
   d) It does not require an obturator to maintain patency

9. Which is not a contraindication to pelvic exenteration?
   a) Obesity
   b) Significant psychiatric illness
   c) Distant metastases
   d) Lack of supportive care during the postoperative period

10. Which of the following complications requires immediate surgical intervention?
    a) Stricture of the ureteral stent to an ileal conduit
    b) Postoperative ileus
    c) Enterocutaneous fistula formation
    d) Pelvic abscess

CHAPTER 50

1. One technique for vaginal reconstruction after vaginectomy includes the omental J-flap with split thickness skin graft (STSG). Which of the following is *not* considered a benefit of this technique?
   a) Psychosexual factors/satisfactory intercourse
   b) Prevention of enteroperineal fistulas
   c) Abscess collection
   d) Urinary continence

2. Incorporating which vessel is crucial to ensuring success of the sigmoid neovagina procedure?
   a) Inferior hemorrhoidal artery
   b) Superior hemorrhoidal artery
   c) Pudendal artery
   d) Dorsal clitoral artery

3. When identifying the structure for the gracilis myocutaneous flap, which muscle can be confused for the gracilis?
   a) Adductor longus
   b) Adductor brevis
   c) Adductor magnus
   d) Sartorius

4. When performing a rectus abdominus myocutaneous (RAM) flap, what is an absolute contraindication to the procedure?
   a) Previous Maylard incision
   b) Diabetes
   c) Obesity
   d) Previous radiotherapy

5. All of the following are considered disadvantages of the traditional vulvectomy EXCEPT
   a) Perineal contractions
   b) Distortion of the bladder neck/urethra leading to incontinence
   c) Increased risk of recurrence
   d) Wound breakdown

6. To ensure adequate closure with a Z-plasty pedicle flap, each of the following should be included EXCEPT
   a) Adequate blood supply
   b) A flap length 2 cm long and a base of 1 cm
   c) Full-thickness skin graft
   d) Rotation of the flap to the midperineal line

7. Physiologic characteristics of a continent urinary pouch are designed to prevent reflux, infection, and incontinence. Which describes the ideal situation for a continent urinary pouch?
   a) 40 cm H_2O pressure, 500 mL volume
   b) 80 cm H_2O pressure, 500 mL volume
   c) 80 cm H_2O pressure, 1000 mL volume
   d) 40 cm H_2O, 1000 mL volume

8. The Kock pouch is suitable for urinary bladder replacement because it possesses features necessary for maintaining continence. These include all of the following EXCEPT
   a) Maintenance of low pressure after filling
   b) Prevention of reflux
   c) Retention of 1000–1500 mL of fluid
   d) Elimination of intermittent pressure spikes (promoting reflux)

9. Variations of the original Kock procedure have been designed that do not require intussusception of the bowel. One of these is the Miami pouch. In what way is it different from the Kock procedure?
   a) The distal terminal ileum is transected proximal to the ileocecal valve
   b) Appendectomy is performed
   c) The ureters are anastomosed directly into the muscular wall of the colon
   d) Reinforcing the ileocecal valve by tapering the distal segment is essential for maintaining continence

10. Rectosigmoid colon resection (RSc) can lead to several defecation disorders, including all of the following EXCEPT
    a) Fecal incontinence
    b) Constipation
    c) Fecal urgency
    d) Tenesmus

CHAPTER 51

1. Choose the *incorrect* statement.
   a) There has been a significant decrease in the number and types of major gynecologic cases
   b) Financial constraints have dramatically affected the payment policies of the various payers of medical services
   c) The surgical options available for various gynecologic complaints have significantly narrowed because of mandatory precertification protocols
   d) A decrease in the number of surgical cases has resulted from a better educated consumer
   e) Decreased use of conservative medical management has increased the number of major surgical cases

2. A decrease in the quality of gynecologic surgical training is due to
   a) Changing residency curriculum
   b) Changing attitude and goals of residents
   c) Financial pressures on academicians
   d) Decreased funding in Ob/Gyn departments
   e) All of the above

3. Decreased time for resident educational activities results from which of the following?
   a) Increased departmental funding
   b) Decreased resident clinical responsibility
   c) Significantly increased Ob/Gyn knowledge base
   d) Decreased physical and emotional stress for residents
   e) Decreased medical-legal liability for surgeons who teach residents

4. Which of the following is required for the learning of surgical skills?
   a) Individual motivation and talent
   b) Dedicated time for practice
   c) Clarity, purpose, and imagination
   d) A skilled, caring, interested mentor
   e) All of the above

5. Which of the following is not an effective component of teaching surgical skills?
   a) Lectures, case presentations, and discussions
   b) Observing surgical videos
   c) Use of inanimate trainers and computer simulators
   d) Surgery on actual patients without supervision
   e) Human cadaveric dissections

Te Linde's Operative Gynecology, ninth edition, edited by John A. Rock and Howard W. Jones, III. Lippincott Williams & Wilkins, Philadelphia, © 2003.

Answers

CHAPTER 1

1. b) Lack of real anatomic knowledge
2. d) Nineteenth century
3. b) 1846
4. c) Repair of vesicovaginal fistulas
5. d) 1870s
6. c) 1905
7. a) James Marion Sims
8. b) William S. Halsted
9. a) Early ambulation after surgery
10. d) Howard Kelly

CHAPTER 2

1. c) Eradicate all disease
2. b) 1981
3. c) 1973
4. d) The Belmont Report
5. d) Charity
6. d) 1949
7. c) U.S. Public Health Service
8. c) Financial compensation of the physician
9. c) 1973
10. c) 1990

CHAPTER 3

1. c) Iatrogenic injury
2. d) All of the above
3. b) Hysterectomy

4. d) All of the above
5. a) Suicidal ideation
6. e) All of the above
7. a) Potential of narcotic abuse
8. e) None of the above
9. c) 23%–43%
10. e) Self-mutilation

CHAPTER 4

1. d) Nation
2. b) False
3. b) False
4. c) Communicate with members of the health care team
5. d) None of the above
6. b) False
7. b) False
8. c) 3
9. d) None of the above
10. d) All of the above

CHAPTER 5

1. e) Anus
2. a) The pudendal nerve provides only sensory innervation to the perineum
3. b) The clitoris never drains directly into the deep pelvic nodes

4. c) The internal anal sphincter is indistinguishable from the external anal sphincter and it lies just outside the external anal sphincter
5. e) All of the above
6. a) In a woman of reproductive age, the uterine cervix is larger than the uterine corpus
7. d) The distal end of the fallopian tube is attached to the ovary by the fimbria ovarica
8. c) The normal ovary measures 7 cm long during reproductive life
9. b) The ovarian veins drain into the vena cava on the left and the renal vein on the right
10. d) The ureter lies approximately 3 cm from the anterolateral surface of the cervix

CHAPTER 6

1. c) Patients with abnormal Papanicolaou smears showing repeated dysplasia should be evaluated by colposcopy and suspicious lesions biopsied
2. d) Chemistry panel
3. b) The ability to convince the patient of a surgical approach even though she shows reluctance to undergo the procedure
4. a) A full bowel prep should be carried out on all gynecologic surgeries
5. e) Between 25% and 35% of routinely ordered preoperative tests revealed abnormalities that influenced perioperative management
6. e) Vaginal or abdominal hysterectomy
7. a) Discontinue the use of birth control pills 2 to 4 weeks before the planned gynecologic surgery
8. b) A more effective assessment of the posterior bladder wall
9. c) Decrease the hospital length of stay
10. b) Routine batteries of preoperative tests have proven to decrease ``less-than-desirable'' surgical outcomes and to increase legal protection

CHAPTER 7

1. c) Xa
2. c) 75%
3. a) Age younger than 40
4. d) Renal failure
5. a) Intrapulmonary shunting leading to worsening hypoxia despite oxygen therapy
6. c) Hypertension
7. b) Mechanical ventilation with low tidal volume and positive end expiratory pressure
8. d) Injury to the thoracic duct
9. b) Glutamine
10. d) Glutamine

CHAPTER 8

1. d) One liter of insensible fluid loss occurs per day
2. a) The osmolality of extracellular fluid is determined almost entirely by potassium and its accompanying anions
3. c) Infusion of hypertonic solution causes the extracellular fluid volume to contract
4. d) Pulmonary capillary wedge pressure
5. b) 8–12 mm Hg
6. d) All of the above
7. a) Diuretic therapy
8. c) Replacement of 2-mL colloid suspension per 1 mL of blood loss is recommended
9. d) All of the above
10. d) All of the above

CHAPTER 9

1. b) Vagina
2. c) Hypertension
3. a) *Bacteroides fragilis*
4. c) Start IV heparin
5. d) Open the wound widely to allow drainage and debridement of necrotic tissue, then apply wet-to-dry packing until the wound closes by secondary intention
6. a) Obtain a urine culture and start a 7-day course of levofloxacin
7. a) Pneumonia
8. b) Frequent hand washing
9. b) Having the bowel prepared with oral antibiotics and a cathartic agent
10. c) Close the subcutaneous space

CHAPTER 10

1. c) Intrapulmonary shunting. Clinically, adult respiratory distress syndrome is characterized by intrapulmonary shunting, widening of alveolar-arterial O_2 gradient, and reduced pulmonary compliance and functional residual capacity. Although supplemental oxygen is used, arterial PaO_2 typically remains less than 65 mm Hg. In patients with significant pulmonary injury, hypoxemia is progressive despite adequate oxygen supplementation, and assisted mechanical ventilation is required.
2. e) Oliguria. For both hypovolemic and septic shock, oliguria is a manifestation of early, early reversible shock and is also a clinical finding for patients with irreversible shock. Characteristics of late, irreversible shock include a reduction in cardiac output, systemic vascular resistance, and cardiac index. Cold, clammy skin is present because of poor peripheral circulation, and disorientation or obtundation from decreased cerebral perfusion is present. In contrast, early reversible septic shock is characterized by an increase in cardiac output re-

sulting from compensatory cardiac dilatation and sympathetic response; tachycardia is also present. Systemic vascular resistance is decreased but may be normal in the absence of hypotension. The skin is usually warm, secondary to an increase in cardiac output and peripheral vasodilatation and to the febrile response.

3. c) Persistent bleeding consistent with coagulopathy. Platelet transfusion is indicated intraoperatively whenever there is persistent bleeding consistent with coagulopathy. In general, one unit of platelets will increase the platelet count by 5000–10,000/mm^3. It is recommended that when blood loss exceeds 25% of the total intravascular volume and is ongoing or when there is bleeding consistent with coagulopathy, packed red blood cells are indicated in a 4:1 ratio with fresh frozen plasma. There are isolated reports of satisfactory outcome in asymptomatic patients with solid tumors, who did not receive platelet transfusions in the absence of bleeding unless the counts were below 10,000/mm^3. Depending on the bleeding risks, currently accepted indications for preoperative and intraoperative platelet transfusion include platelet counts of less than 50,000/mm^3.

4. e) Inotropic and vasoconstrictive effects. Dopamine stimulates dopaminergic, α-adrenergic and β-adrenergic receptors. Dopamine is unique in that it stimulates these receptors in a dose-dependent fashion. At low doses (1–3 μg/kg/min) dopaminergic receptors are mainly affected. This results in preferential cerebral, renal, and mesenteric arterial vasodilatation. The net effect is an increase in urine output and blood flow to the brain and gastrointestinal tract without increasing the heart rate or significantly affecting blood pressure. In moderate doses (5–12 μg/kg/min), both α- and β- adrenergic receptors are affected. The effects are inotropic; that is, the effect is an increase in myocardial contractility, sinoatrial rate impulse conduction, and cardiac output. With increased myocardial contractility, myocardial oxygen consumption is increased with no compensatory increase in coronary blood flow. In a patient with a history of coronary artery disease, this effect could lead to myocardial ischemia. At high doses (20 μg/kg/min) α-adrenergic effects predominate, resulting in severe generalized vasoconstriction, and the severity of vasoconstriction is similar to the effects of epinephrine or norepinephrine. Dopamine has little β$_2$-adrenergic activity.

5. b) Both β$_1$- and β$_2$-adrenergic effects. Dobutamine is a direct-acting inotropic agent that stimulates β$_1$- and β$_2$-adrenergic receptors. Its β$_2$ effects reduce afterload and pulmonary congestion without increasing O$_2$ consumption or causing significant tachycardia. Because of these effects, dobutamine is the drug of choice for the treatment of cardiogenic shock.

6. b) Crystalloid infusion (1 to 2 L). The most common types of shock in obstetrics and gynecology are hypovolemic and septic. A healthy, young patient who is otherwise asymptomatic and is tolerating a hemoglobin of 8 mg/dL may be managed adequately with crystalloid infusion and oral iron, as soon as she is able to begin oral feeding. Blood transfusion is not indicated in this patient at this time. Although colloids such as 5% and 25% albumin, and synthetic colloid preparations have been used in the past for volume replacement, most studies have found no advantage of colloids over crystalloids in this clinical setting.

When hemorrhagic shock is identified, the initial management consists of placement of a large-bore peripheral intravenous catheter, and infusion of 1 to 2 L of an isotonic electrolyte solution. The rate of fluid administration is proportionate to the caliber and length of the catheter; thus, placement of a central venous catheter will not improve the rate of fluid administration. Furthermore, central venous catheterization carries a risk of pneumothorax and other life-threatening complications and is unnecessary in an otherwise healthy patient.

7. e) Obtain blood and cervical cultures. In all probability, this patient has a tubo-ovarian abscess. In this young, nulliparous patient, to preserve fertility, aggressive intravenous antibiotic therapy specific for genital tract pathogens (chlamydia and anaerobes) is recommended. When the diagnosis of tubo-ovarian abscess is suspect, antibiotic therapy in the hospitalized setting is warranted, regardless of concerns for future fertility. Before initiation of intravenous antibiotics, a pelvic examination with appropriate cultures for gonorrhea and chlamydia and blood cultures should be obtained in a patient who is febrile and has a significant leukocytosis. Because this patient has no evidence of a perforated viscus, plain x-ray films for free air are not indicated at this time. If the patient does not respond to antibiotic therapy, exploratory laparotomy may be indicated, but the initial management should be intravenous antibiotics, after obtaining appropriate cultures.

8. c) Urine sodium excretion less than 20 mEq/L/24 hr. Oliguric prerenal azotemia is an early reversible injury. It is characterized by urine-to-plasma creatinine ratio greater than 40 mEq/L/24 hr, a urine sodium excretion of less than 20 mEq/L/24 hr, a fractional excretion of sodium less than 1% and a high urine osmolality (greater than 500 mOsm). Patients can have normal, increased, or reduced serum sodium, depending on volume replacement and intake. Contraction alkalosis is characteristic of prolonged diuretic use. Acute tubular necrosis, which results from prolonged hypoperfusion and cellular damage, is typically characterized by the loss of ability to concentrate urine. Osmolality of the urine is usually less than 350 mOsm.

9. b) Class II. Based on presenting signs and symptoms, hypovolemic shock is subdivided into four classes. Class I is generally characterized by blood loss of less than 750 mL, Class II with volume losses of 750–1500 mL, and Class III, with uncompensated blood or volume loss of more than 1500 mL. Any volume loss may be associated with tachycardia, which can be a sympathomimetic response to pain or anxiety. In patients with less than 1500 mL of volume loss, renal perfusion and urine output is typically maintained. The major clinical distinction between Class I and Class II hypovolemic shock is the presence of postural hypotension.

10. a) Lung, liver, GI, kidney. Multiorgan system dysfunction is a syndrome characterized by progressive manifestations of the systemic inflammatory response, even when there is no evidence of ongoing sepsis or insult. Mortality is high and depends on the number and severity of organ systems affected and patient reserve. This syndrome remains the predominant cause of death from shock in patients who appear to have received adequate resuscitation and who have no culture evidence of ongoing bacteremia. Classically, multiorgan failure affects the lungs first, followed by the liver, the gastrointestinal tract, and finally the kidneys, although clinical presentation is variable.

11. b) Angiotensin II is a potent vasoconstrictor. In response to hypovolemia, which results in decreased wall tension, decreased sodium, or increased sympathetic activation, renin is released from the juxtaglomerular cells. Renin converts angiotensinogen into angiotensin I, which is an inactive polypeptide. In the liver, angiotensin I is converted to angiotensin II. Angiotensin II is a potent vasoconstrictor that stimulates aldosterone release from the renal cortex. Aldosterone along with ADH promotes sodium and water retention. The net effect is an increase in venous return, stroke volume, cardiac output, and blood pressure.

CHAPTER 11

1. c) Sheep intestine
2. b) Maxon
3. b) Scar maturation
4. b) On or after the fourth day
5. d) Intact sutures pulling through fascia
6. c) 60 days
7. b) The United States Pharmacopeia
8. c) 40%
9. c) Bookwalter retractor
10. a) 0%

CHAPTER 12

1. B) Para-aortic lymph nodes
2. b) Superficial epigastric artery
3. d) Injury to the iliohypogastric nerve results in sensory deficits to the labia majora
4. b) Reconstruction
5. b) Clean-contaminated
6. b) Passive drains may be associated with increased wound infection rates
7. c) Weaker than midline incisions
8. c) Midline
9. d) Wound infection is an associated factor in less than 10% of cases
10. d) Uncomplicated radical hysterectomy

CHAPTER 13

1. c) 1893
2. b) Neurosurgery
3. b) Continuous (undamped or nonmodulated waveform)
4. a) Interrupted (damped or modulated waveform)
5. a) 8000
6. e) All of the above
7. b) False
8. d) Lactated Ringer's
9. c) Occurs when the active electrode touches other metal instruments within the abdomen
10. e) All of the above

CHAPTER 14

1. d) 25,000 Hz
2. b) 100 watts
3. c) Low irradiation intensity
4. b) Thermal effects that produce a denatured protein clot
5. d) Direct tissue application
6. b) Width of tissue damage
7. c) High water content
8. c) Viable cancer cells in the spray
9. d) Cytoreduction in ovarian cancer
10. a) Rapid tissue destruction/dissection

CHAPTER 15

1. a) Carbon dioxide
2. d) Argon and KTP laser energy penetrates tissues to a greater depth than both carbon dioxide and YAG
3. c) Multifocal CIN or skip lesions are common
4. b) For excisional conization of the cervix, low power with a large spot size is used for cutting purposes
5. c) The laser should first be used to mark the limits of the disease before landmarks are lost
6. e) All of the above

7. b) Methotrexate
8. c) Dental mirrors may be used to facilitate operating in inaccessible areas
9. a) Most young women with cystic adnexal masses will be found to have a malignancy so laparoscopy is rarely indicated
10. b) The laser smoke should be collected by a suction device no farther than 5 cm from the target site

CHAPTER 16

1. c) Inguinal hernia
2. e) All of the above
3. d) Unipolar cautery may cause tissue damage 4–5 cm from the point of coagulation
4. b) The power density of a laser is expressed in W/mm^2
5. d) Providing the patient with adequate regional anesthesia
6. d) Stirrups that support the foot and knee are necessary
7. d) Intraabdominal pressure should never exceed 10 mm Hg
8. b) Blunt dissection should never be used for adhesiolysis
9. b) Still requires that the uterine incisions are closed in multiple layers
10. b) Most bowel injuries caused by the Veress needle require laparotomy for repair

CHAPTER 17

1. d) The tungsten light source is superior to other sources
2. b) The operative hysteroscope is 15 mm in diameter
3. e) All of the above
4. a) Carbon dioxide
5. c) Normal saline
6. b) Hyskon
7. d) Glycine 1.5%
8. a) Hysteroscopy should be performed during the luteal phase for best visualization of the endometrial cavity
9. d) Endometrial ablation
10. d) Bleeding

CHAPTER 18

1. b) TED stockings
2. b) von Willebrand disease
3. c) Hepatitis C, 1:500,000
4. c) 4–5 units
5. a) Haemonetics Cell Saver
6. d) Arterial embolization of the bleeding vessel
7. a) Uterine unification operation
8. a) It decreases pulse pressure by 75%–85%

9. c) Transfusion during hysterectomy is too uncommon to make autologous donation cost-effective
10. b) Small hemoclips

CHAPTER 19

1. c) 1980s
2. c) 5
3. b) Decreased release of toxic mediators from endometriosis implants
4. c) Meiosis II
5. e) Ovarian hyperstimulation with intrauterine insemination
6. c) Ampullary portion of the tube less than 4 cm in length
7. a) Cautery
8. c) 34–36 hours
9. d) 48–72 hours
10. c) FSH level

CHAPTER 20

1. a) Amenorrhea is the absence of menstrual bleeding for more than 12 months
2. b) Estrogen receptors reach a maximum concentration in the early proliferative phase
3. b) In the early proliferative phase the endometrium grows to a thickness of 1–2 mm
4. c) Coagulation factors in menstrual blood
5. d) 50 mg of iron is lost in a normal menstrual cycle
6. e) All of the above
7. a) Saline infusion sonography
8. e) All of the above
9. e) All of the above
10. c) When unopposed estrogen is used in postmenopausal patients with an intact uterus, endometrial hyperplasia develops in 50% of patients

CHAPTER 21

1. b) Induced abortion
2. d) 25
3. e) 50,000
4. d) 400 µg
5. d) Gemeprost
6. b) oxytocin
7. a) Less than 1
8. d) 400 mg
9. b) Follow-up examination in approximately 2 weeks to exclude failed attempted abortion
10. a) Prophylactic antibiotics versus placebo

CHAPTER 22

1. A) Ectopic pregnancy is the leading cause of maternal death in the first trimester
2. e) All of the above
3. a) The ectopic risk is higher following neosalpingostomy than reversal of a sterilization procedure
4. b) The most common site of tubal pregnancy is the isthmic portion
5. c) Most patients with pain, uterine bleeding, and an adnexal mass will be diagnosed with ectopic pregnancy
6. e) All of the above
7. d) Intrauterine gestations are detectable as early as 1 week after missed menses
8. c) Long-term follow-up of patients given methotrexate for gestational trophoblastic disease has demonstrated an increase in congenital malformations and spontaneous abortions in subsequent pregnancies
9. b) An increase in serum beta-hCG between day 1 and day 4 indicates probable failure of therapy
10. a) Linear salpingotomy is considered the gold standard for distal tubal pregnancy in patients who desire future fertility

CHAPTER 23

1. c) 1842
2. c) 1880
3. d) 70%–80%
4. d) China
5. c) Local
6. a) 4 pregnancies per 1000 sterilization procedures
7. a) Bipolar coagulation
8. d) Age
9. b) 1%
10. c) Tubal sterilization

CHAPTER 24

1. c) Ampullary retention of the ovum for approximately 7 days
2. e) All of the above
3. b) Nearly all patients investigated for infertility and found to have a hydrosalpinx give a history of acute PID
4. a) Tubal insufflation
5. e) All of the above are correct
6. a) Laparoscopic adhesiolysis
7. c) Laparoscopic fimbrioplasty
8. f) Open, microsurgical salpingostomy
9. g) Selective tubal cannulation
10. i) *In vitro* fertilization

CHAPTER 25

1. c) 60%–70% of women with infertility are diagnosed with endometriosis
2. e) All of the above
3. a) Endometriosis appears to be progressive in most untreated patients
4. b) Atypical glandular changes have been found in 20% of cases of ovarian endometriosis
5. e) All of the above
6. b) Pain associated with endometriosis is strongly linked to deep infiltration of the pelvis
7. c) Ultrasonography can provide specific information to classify extent and severity of disease
8. b) Evaluation of disease is limited by a lack of recognition of atypical implants
9. d) GnRH agonists function to upregulate the pituitary-ovarian axis over time, which decreases symptoms of endometriosis
10. c) Laparoscopy provides inferior visualization of the posterior cul-de-sac than laparotomy

CHAPTER 26

1. c) The gonads of the two sexes remain morphologically indistinguishable until the sixteenth week of gestation
2. d) There is a lack of evidence that fetal gonadotropins influence development of the fetal ovary
3. d) The newborn ovary contains 100 million oocytes
4. c) The ovarian vein terminates in the inferior vena cava on the left and the renal vein on the right
5. e) All of the above
6. b) The rate of torsion was 1%
7. b) A pulsatility index above 1:16 suggests malignancy in an adnexal mass
8. e) All of the above
9. a) Adnexal torsion is a common gynecologic surgical emergency with a prevalence of 5%
10. b) Gentle tissue handling need not be observed during ovarian reconstruction because adhesion formation is uncommon

CHAPTER 27

1. b) The Cartesian theory states that pain should be proportional to the extent of tissue damage
2. d) Severity of pain correlates poorly with presence of deep, infiltrative endometriosis
3. d) Most pain following TAH-BSO will be due to pelvic adhesions, levator spasm, or irritable bowel syndrome
4. b) Site of pelvic adhesions does not correlate with site of pelvic pain
5. e) All of the above
6. b) Constipation and irritable bowel syndrome are the most frequent GI causes of chronic pelvic pain
7. e) All of the above

8. c) Physical function is significantly impaired at home or work
9. a) It is preferable to administer pain medication continuously rather than in a pain-contingent fashion
10. c) Laparotomy is superior to laparoscopy in treatment of pelvic adhesive disease

CHAPTER 28

1. c) Occurs in 10% of young, sexually active women each year
2. b) Anaerobic bacteria are frequently cultured in the first 48 hours of infection, whereas *Neisseria gonorrhoeae* is cultured late in the disease
3. e) All of the above
4. c) Use of oral contraceptive pills increases the risk of PID
5. e) All of the above should be considered in the differential diagnosis
6. a) The classic triad in diagnosis of acute PID includes pelvic mass, fever, and leukocytosis
7. d) The chance that a woman will develop chronic pelvic pain after acute PID is 5%
8. a) In the United States one out of every four women with acute PID are treated as outpatients
9. b) In the United States one out of every four women with acute PID are treated as outpatients
10. c) Tubo-ovarian abscesses should never be drained laparoscopically

CHAPTER 29

1. b) Septate uterus
2. a) The vagina develops from both the müllerian ducts and the urogenital sinus
3. c) Impaired ovarian function
4. e) Laparoscopy
5. b) Greater than 90% of patients have been shown to achieve anatomic and functional success by vaginal dilation
6. d) Adequate preoperative dilatation
7. d) Conservative management, with hormonal suppression of endometrial stimulation, is appropriate for young patients
8. d) Rokitansky syndrome
9. c) Didelphic uterus
10. b) A prolonged postoperative recovery period

CHAPTER 30

1. c) Red or carneous degeneration is never seen during pregnancy
2. d) Sarcomatous degeneration
3. b) The tumor behaves clinically as a benign entity
4. a) Most leiomyomata are asymptomatic and may not require any treatment

5. b) Danazol
6. c) It is recommended to combine laparoscopic guidance with the hysteroscopic procedure
7. b) A 34-year-old woman, desiring future fertility, with two intramural myomas each measuring 3 cm in diameter
8. a) Preoperative treatment with oral contraceptive pills
9. d) Pulmonary embolus
10. a) Most patients report an improvement in menorrhagia and bulk-related symptoms

CHAPTER 31

1. b) 1–2 per 1000 patients
2. d) After endometrial ablation for the treatment of dysfunctional uterine bleeding, approximately 12%–15% of patients will require a hysterectomy for persistent bleeding and/or pain
3. a) Uterine leiomyomata
4. b) The risk of complications from abdominal hysterectomy increases when the uterine weight exceeds 500 g
5. d) Vaginal hysterectomy
6. a) Use of the vaginal approach
7. c) 1) Isolate, clamp, transect, and ligate the utero-ovarian ligaments; 2) dissect the bladder off of the anterior cervix; 3) clamp, transect, and ligate the uterine arteries; 4) incise vagina
8. b) Performance of vaginal hysterectomy in this clinical situation is associated with a shorter operative time and fewer complications than abdominal hysterectomy
9. d) Computerized tomographic (CT) scan of the pelvis
10. d) Administration of intravenous second generation cephalosporin preoperatively

CHAPTER 32

1. c) Placenta accreta
2. b) Repeat ultrasound in 6 weeks
3. a) Infant birthweight
4. d) Intramuscular carboprost (Hemabate)
5. d) Forceps-assisted vaginal delivery
6. a) Loss of sexual function
7. b) *Clostridium perfringens*
8. a) Blood transfusion
9. d) Observation
10. c) Twin-twin transfusion syndrome

CHAPTER 33

1. c) Warthin-Starry stain
2. d) Hormonal therapy
3. a) Greater than 3 cm in diameter
4. d) Topical steroids

5. b) TCA should not be used intra-vaginally during pregnancy
6. a) Hidradenoma
7. c) Itching
8. c) 35%, 35%
9. b) I, II, and IV only
10. d) Inferior gluteal nerve

CHAPTER 34

1. b) Becomes patent when canalization of the most caudal portion of the vaginal plate at the urogenital sinus occurs
2. b) Most patients have a high (suprasphincteric) urethral-vaginal connection
3. c) Vaginoplasty should be performed in infancy to prevent vaginal stenosis
4. c) Absence of the posterior wall of the bladder exposing the ureteral orifices
5. e) All of the above
6. a) The average age at presentation is 35 years
7. c) 75% of women exposed to DES *in utero* have anatomic abnormalities
8. b) Stage 1 disease lesions can be treated with radiation therapy or total abdominal hysterectomy
9. e) Infection of the Bartholin's gland
10. c) Most urethral diverticula are located in the proximal urethra

CHAPTER 35

1. c) Transversus perinei
2. d) Pericervical ring
3. b) Vaginal delivery
4. b) Vaginal introitus
5. a) Vaginal

CHAPTER 35B

1. c) Paravaginal defect alone
2. d) This is where the pubocervical fascia attaches to the arcus tendineus fascia pelvis
3. d) The endopelvic fascia
4. a) 7–8 cm dorsally
5. c) The posterior aspect of the pubic bone
6. a) The levator ani fascia
7. a) Excessive bleeding
8. c) The width of her pubic arch
9. d) Into the tendinous arch and obturator fascia anterior to the ischial spine
10. a) Placed individually from the ischial spine anteriorly toward the symphysis

CHAPTER 35C

1. Cardinal-uterosacral ligaments, rectovaginal septum, perineal body, and levator plate

2. Tears or detachments of the RVS from adjacent structures in a variety of locations or tears in the RVS itself
3. Anterior compartment repairs pull the anterior vaginal wall forward, further widening the already enlarged introitus. This interferes even more with the already compromised intrinsic valve-flap mechanism of the pelvic floor and thus markedly potentiates the development of enterocele
4. A. Aids in identifying sites of RVS tears
   B. Tests the integrity of the reunified RVS
   C. Assists in locating a posterior enterocele that is difficult to isolate secondary to scarring
   D. Crucial in identifying cardinal-uterosacral ligament stumps in posthysterectomy cases requiring a McCall procedure
   E. Helps to evaluate extent of perineal body defects
5. They are of no value at all because there are essentially no difficulties in delineating a rectocele from the patient's history and an appropriate bidigital bimanual examination conducted in the erect posture in association with a Valsalva maneuver
6. Because of conclusively demonstrated estrogen receptors throughout the pelvis, estrogen-primed tissues preoperatively and continued ERT postoperatively contribute unquestionably both to more reliable surgery and significantly greater durability than when estrogen influence is absent
7. Thorough and frequent jet-propelled lavage of the entire operative field, continued dissection taking advantage of the opening with a helping index finger in the rectum, then standard simple closure of the luminal entry with rapidly absorbable synthetic suture. If one closes the inadvertently created defect immediately, the surgeon is back to "square one" and faces the same dissecting problems that were present before the miscue
8. A. When the rectocele is accompanied by an enterocele
   B. When the rectocele is associated with a prolapsed uterus removed initially in the same operation
   C. When two or more previous colporrhaphies have failed
   D. When there is a clear indication of congenital collagen deficiency syndrome
   E. When there is a history of medical conditions involving intermittent episodes of increased intraabdominal pressure
9. Whenever any other pelvic surgery is being conducted to correct symptomatic defects, the "silent" posterior lesions should simultaneously be repaired to prevent an almost certain return to the OR in the future
10. The answer is the same as that for Question 8.

CHAPTER 35D

1. a) Secure the vaginal angle to the ipsilateral cardinal ligament

2. b) The upper one third of the vagina is parallel to the floor when the patient is standing
3. c) Outside the vagina, just cephalad to the uterosacral ligament tie
4. d) The McCall sutures should be tied after the performance of the anterior colporrhaphy
5. a) The length of the uterosacral and cardinal ligaments should be maintained

CHAPTER 35E

1. d) Uterosacral cardinal ligament
2. c) Uterosacral ligament
3. b) Multiple previous abdominal procedures
4. b) Rectum
5. d) Cervical lacerations
6. a) Pudendal nerve/vessels
7. c) Pulley stitch
8. b) Anterior wall prolapse
9. d) Suspending the anterior and posterior walls to the ridge of the uterosacral ligament
10. a) Suturing the sacrospinous ligaments to each other

CHAPTER 35F

1. b) Fecal incontinence
2. c) Inadequate relief of symptoms
3. d) Lower parity
4. c) Gehrung
5. d) Ring
6. e) It is supported by the levator muscles
7. b) Cube
8. b) Smith-Hodge
9. c) Inflatoball
10. c) Fistula formation

CHAPTER 36

1. d) Anticholinergic drug therapy; behavioral modification
2. b) Babinski reflex
3. c) Decreased heart rate
4. a) 30 degrees
5. d) Pubococcygeus
6. a) Hemorrhagic stroke
7. d) Making the sling too tight
8. b) Bulking up tissue at the bladder neck
9. a) Making sure that the bladder is well drained
10. c) Rectus fascia

CHAPTER 37

1. c) Surgeon's knowledge of where the ureters are located

2. d) Simple abdominal hysterectomy, pelvic brim near the IP ligament
3. c) At least three individual sutures are needed to repair the ureter to achieve a water-tight closure
4. a) Uretero-neocystotomy with psoas hitch over ureteral stint
5. b) Obstruction, attempting to obtain hemostasis
6. d) It has a low false-negative rate in detecting ureteral obstruction
7. b) The obstruction is caused by a metal clip
8. a) More likely to have increased long-term or even fatal complications
9. d) The ureter will be visible on the medial leaf of the broad ligament
10. c) Prophylactic ureteral stints are placed to facilitate identification of the ureters

CHAPTER 38

1. a) Superior to the interureteric ridge
2. c) The patient probably has a ureterovaginal fistula
3. a) Prolonged postoperative fever
4. a) A short course of oral steroids
5. b) Trigonal defect repairs should be made in the vertical direction
6. b) 10%–20%
7. a) Careful blunt dissection to isolate the bladder
8. c) Gynecologic surgery
9. b) The vagina is not shortened
10. d) Wait 3 to 6 months, then repair

CHAPTER 39

1. b) Age greater than 60 years
2. c) An intact puborectalis muscle sling
3. d) Medial portion of the puborectalis muscle
4. d) Anal intercourse
5. a) Fundal pressure
6. b) Ischemic injury
7. a) Fecal impaction with overflow
8. c) Ultrasound
9. d) 100–200 cm H_2O
10. c) New onset urinary incontinence

CHAPTER 40

1. b) Transient breast enlargement and nipple secretion in the newborn typically resolves in the sixth week postpartum
2. e) All of the above are congenital breast abnormalities
3. b) Nonpuerperal mastitis is associated with a bloody nipple discharge and is found in individuals who are immunocompromised
4. b) Presents with breast discomfort in 85%–90% of cases

5. d) Multiple fibroadenomas are found in the same patient in approximately 50% of cases
6. e) All of the above may be used to treat cyclic breast pain
7. a) Diuretics
8. c) Self-breast examination should be performed monthly beginning at age 30
9. a) 30% of breast cancers are inherited in an autosomal dominant pattern
10. e) All of the above

CHAPTER 41

1. b) The incidence of appendiceal perforation is significantly less with preoperative antibiotics
2. c) An appendiceal wall thickness on ultrasound of 12 mm would be consistent with likely appendicitis
3. c) 50%
4. e) More than 90%
5. c) Immediately go to surgery and perform an appendectomy without cesarean section or hysterectomy
6. a) There is an approximately 10% chance that her appendix will be found to have significant pathology
7. b) Ligating the stump with permanent suture
8. d) External rotation of the right leg
9. b) Lower operative cost
10. a) A 63-year-old woman with an ovarian mass that is sent for pathology after removal and found to be a mucinous tumor; b) A 35-year-old woman with a history of chronic pelvic pain who is undergoing a TAH-BSO and is found to have several implants of endometriosis on the uterosacral ligaments; and d) A 21-year-old woman undergoing a left salpingo-oophorectomy for a dermoid cyst whose appendix is found to have a small granuloma on it

CHAPTER 42

1. b) The diverticulum should be removed because the patient has a history of symptoms that it may have caused and because it has slightly atypical features
2. a) A 26 year old with SLE who has end-stage renal disease; b) A 54-year-old alcoholic with cirrhosis; and d) A 48 year old with Class II heart failure
3. b) Leave the trocar in place, convert to an open laparotomy, and repair the injury
4. a) The patient presents to the ER 3 days postoperatively complaining of nausea, vomiting, and fever
5. c) Return of bowel function generally occurs at the same rate regardless of early or delayed feeding
6. a) Adhesions; d) Hernias; and e) Malignancy
7. b) The patient is less likely to have a sense of incomplete evacuation after bowel movements
8. c) End-to-end staple anastomosis

9. b) Bleeding from a cut edge and e) Fluorescence of bowel wall under Wood's lamp 10 minutes after IV fluorescein
10. a) False; b) False; c) True; d) False; e) True; f) False; g) False; h) False

CHAPTER 43

1. b) Refer the patient to a gastroenterologist for a colonoscopy
2. a) Biopsy of an enlarged peripheral lymph node
3. a) Chordoma
4. b) Cancer of the ovary
5. d) No gynecologic surgery if the uterus and ovaries are normal
6. b) TAH-BSO, ileal resection, and protective ileostomy
7. c) Carcinoembryonic antigen (CEA)
8. a) Drainage of the abscess, resection of the diseased segment of bowel, and a diverting colostomy
9. d) Nonsurgical management with salicylates and other medications
10. b) Palpation of the ipsilateral and contralateral side to ascertain that a kidney is present on both sides

CHAPTER 44

1. d) Immunosuppression
2. c) Any location, less than 1 mm invasion
3. c) Close resection with margin less than 1 cm
4. b) Locally advanced disease or lesions encroaching on midline structures where surgical removal is accompanied by significant morbidity
5. d) Separate groin incisions
6. c) Failure to improve promptly with conservative therapy
7. d) Pathologic status of the inguinal lymph nodes
8. d) Invades 0.9 mm
9. d) Basal cell carcinoma
10. b) The presence of underlying invasive disease in more than 90% of patients

CHAPTER 45

1. b) CIN 1 and HPV changes
2. a) ASC
3. d) Greater than 90%
4. b) ASC
5. d) The area between the original and current squamocolumnar junction
6. a) E_6 and E_7 proteins, which inactivate *p53* and *RB* antioncogenes
7. a) 50%–60%
8. c) ASC-US, low-risk HPV positive
9. d) ECC = adenocarcinoma in situ, SCJ is visible on colposcopy
10. c) Pelvic ultrasound

CHAPTER 46

1. d) HPV infection
2. c) Stage IB
3. b) FIGO clinical stage
4. c) Preservation of ovarian function
5. d) All of the above
6. a) Intravenous pyelogram
7. c) Paravesical space
8. a) Its origin from the hypogastric artery
9. d) Bladder dysfunction
10. b) The ovaries are suspended high in the lateral paracolic gutters

CHAPTER 47

1. c) Oral contraceptive use
2. d) Thromboembolism
3. d) Family history of hereditary nonpolyposis colon cancer (HNPCC)
4. a) Cytologically atypical endometrial glandular cells
5. b) Endometrial biopsy
6. a) 1%
7. d) CXR
8. b) Invasion of the myometrium to the outer one third
9. d) Paraaortic
10. d) Clear cell
11. e) Hysteroscopy during diagnostic evaluation

CHAPTER 48

1. c) Unilateral oophorectomy followed by chemotherapy
2. b) Surgery alone
3. c) Capsular rupture
4. a) Unilateral salpingo-oophorectomy with surgical staging
5. d) Transvaginal pelvic ultrasound
6. a) Serum inhibin
7. a) Peripheral vasculature
8. a) Check a CA-125 level, and if normal, repeat the ultrasound in 3 months to determine if any change has occurred

9. b) 10%–15%
10. d) Nulliparity

CHAPTER 49

1. c) Use of synthetic mesh to reclose the incision
2. a) True
3. b) Recurrent squamous cell carcinoma of the cervix or vagina
4. c) Tumor causing a vesicovaginal fistula
5. a) Metastases to the right ovary
6. b) Pouch of Douglas
7. a) High para-aortics (ovarian vessels)
8. b) It is a rapid, technically easy procedure
9. a) Obesity
10. a) Stricture of the ureteral stent to an ileal conduit

CHAPTER 50

1. d) Urinary continence
2. b) Superior hemorrhoidal artery
3. d) Sartorius
4. a) Previous Maylard incision
5. c) Increased risk of recurrence
6. b) A flap length 2 cm long and a base of 1 cm
7. b) 80 cm H_2O pressure, 500 mL volume
8. c) Retention of 1000–1500 mL of fluid
9. d) Reinforcing the ileocecal valve by tapering the distal segment is essential for maintaining continence
10. b) Constipation

CHAPTER 51

1. e) Decreased use of conservative medical management has increased the number of major surgical cases
2. e) All of the above
3. c) Significantly increased Ob/Gyn knowledge base
4. e) All of the above
5. d) Surgery on actual patients without supervision

SUBJECT INDEX

Page numbers followed by f *indicate figures;* t *following a page number indicates tabular material.*